D1444731

CURRENT DIAGNOSIS 9

Edited by

REX B. CONN, M.D.
Professor and Vice Chairman
Department of Pathology, Cell Biology and Anatomy
Jefferson Medical College of Thomas Jefferson University
Director, Clinical Laboratories
Thomas Jefferson University Hospital
Philadelphia, Pennsylvania

WILLIAM Z. BORER, M.D.
Associate Professor
Department of Pathology, Cell Biology and Anatomy
Jefferson Medical College of Thomas Jefferson University
Director, Clinical Chemistry
Thomas Jefferson University Hospital
Philadelphia, Pennsylvania

JACK W. SNYDER, M.D., Ph.D.
Associate Professor
Departments of Emergency Medicine and Pathology
Thomas Jefferson University
Philadelphia, Pennsylvania

CURRENT DIAGNOSIS

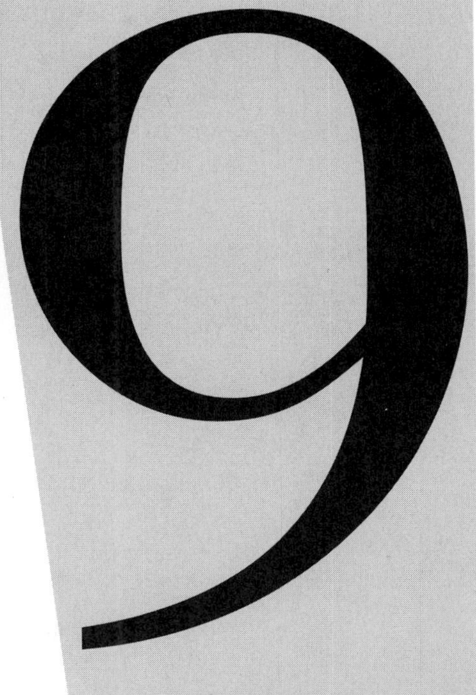

W. B. SAUNDERS COMPANY
A Division of Harcourt Brace & Company
Philadelphia • London • Toronto • Montreal • Sydney • Tokyo

W.B. SAUNDERS COMPANY
A Division of Harcourt Brace & Company

The Curtis Center
Independence Square West
Philadelphia, Pennsylvania 19106

Library of Congress Cataloging-in-Publication Data

Current diagnosis, 1966–

Philadelphia, W.B. Saunders Co.

v. ill. 28 cm.

Biennial.

Editors: 1966— H. F. Conn, R. J. Clohecy, and R. B. Conn.

1. Diagnosis. I. Conn, Howard Franklin, 1908–1982, ed. II. Clohecy, Robert J., ed. III. Conn, Rex B., ed.

RC71.A13 616.075

[DNLM: W1 CU788CX] 66-15617 MARC-S

CURRENT DIAGNOSIS 9 ISBN 0–7216–5843–1

Printed in the United States of America.

Last digit is the print number: 9 8 7 6 5 4 3 2 1

Contributors

Adil A. Abbasi, M.D. Assistant Professor, Medical College of Wisconsin Affiliated Hospitals, Milwaukee, WI
Nutritional Assessment

Frank J. Aberger, M.D. Gundersen Clinic/Lutheran Hospital Teaching Staff, University of Wisconsin, Madison; Chief of Gastroenterology, Gundersen Clinic/Lutheran Hospital, La Crosse, WI
Chronic Diarrhea and Malabsorption

Walid Abou-Jaoude, M.D. Surgery Resident, University of Louisville, School of Medicine Louisville, KY
Peritonitis and Intra-abdominal Abscesses

Aitezaz Ahmed, M.D. Staff Physician, Charter Oak Clinic, Hartford, CT
Bursitis and Tendinitis

Ziauddin Ahmed, M.D. Assistant Professor of Medicine, Medical College of Pennsylvania, and Director of Dialysis, Allegheny University Hospital, Philadelphia, PA
Nephrotic Syndrome

Giuseppe Aliperti, M.D. Associate Professor of Medicine, and Head, Section of Pancreaticobiliary Endoscopy, Washington University School of Medicine; Director, Interventional Endoscopy, Barnes-Jewish Hospital, St. Louis, MO
Acute and Chronic Pancreatitis

Jo Ann Allen, M.D. Assistant Professor of Medicine, West Virginia University School of Medicine, Morgantown, WV
Polymyalgia Rheumatica and Giant Cell Arteritis

Nancy B. Allen, M.D. Associate Professor of Medicine, Division of Rheumatology, Allergy and Immunology, Duke University Medical Center, Durham, NC
Wegener's Granulomatosis

Elaine J. Alpert, M.D., M.P.H. Assistant Professor of Medicine and Public Health, Boston University Medical Center; Assistant Dean for Student Affairs, Boston University School of Medicine, Boston, MA
Domestic Violence

Martin A. Alpert, M.D. Professor of Medicine and Director, Division of Cardiology, University of South Alabama Medical Center, Mobile, AL
Chest Pain

William A. Alto, M.D., M.P.H. Associate Professor, Department of Family and Community Medicine, Dartmouth University; Maine-Dartmouth Family Practice Residency, Fairfield, ME
Acute Rheumatic Fever

Sujata H. Ambardar, M.D. Suburban Hospital, Bethesda, MD
Sepsis and Septic Shock

Bhupinderjit S. Anand, M.D. Associate Professor, Department of Internal Medicine, Baylor College of Medicine; Staff Physician, Veterans Administration Medical Center, Houston, TX
Gastritis

E. Everett Anderson, M.D. Professor of Urology, Duke University Medical Center, Durham, NC
Dysuria, Pyuria, and Hematuria

Gregory A. Anderson, M.D. Urologist, Marshfield Clinic, Marshfield, WI
Cystic Disorders of the Kidney

Mary-Margaret Andrews, M.D. Clinical Fellow in Infectious Disease, Dartmouth-Hitchcock Medical Center, Lebanon, NH
Nonpolio Enterovirus Infections

Joseph H. Antin, M.D. Associate Professor of Medicine, Harvard Medical School; Director, Bone Marrow Transplant Program, Brigham and Women's Hospital, Boston, MA
Chronic Myelogenous Leukemia

Barbara S. Apgar, M.D., M.S. Clinical Associate Professor, Department of Family Practice, University of Michigan Medical School, Ann Arbor, MI
Hyperplasia and Carcinoma of the Endometrium

Joanne Armstrong, M.D., M.P.H. Clinical Assistant Professor, Jefferson Medical College of Thomas Jefferson University, Philadelphia, PA
Diagnosis and Selected Medical Problems in Pregnancy

Lee I. Ascherman, M.D., M.P.H. Associate Professor, Director of Training, Child and Adolescent Psychiatry, Department of Psychiatry, University of Alabama at Birmingham, Birmingham, AL
Attention-Deficit/Hyperactivity Disorder

Douglas Ashinsky, M.D. Clinical Instructor, Department of Medicine, University of Medicine and Dentistry of New Jersey, Robert Wood Johnson Medical School, New Brunswick; Attending Physician, Department of Internal Medicine, Overlook Hospital, Summit, and Muhlenberg Regional Medical Center, Plainfield, NJ
Pulmonary Hypertension

Nicolaos Athienites, M.D. Instructor in Medicine, Tufts University School of Medicine; Staff Physician, Division of Nephrology, New England Medical Center Hospitals, Boston, MA
Chronic Renal Failure

Louis N. Aurisicchio, M.D. Our Lady of Mercy Medical Center, Bronx; New York Medical College, Valhalla; Attending Physician, Department of Gastroenterology, Putnam Hospital Center, Carmel; Hudson Valley Hospital Center, Peekskill, NY
Intestinal Disaccharidase Deficiency

Boaz Avitall, M.D., Ph.D. Associate Professor of Medicine, University of Illinois at Chicago, Chicago, IL
Cardiac Arrhythmias

Gloria A. Bachmann, M.D. Professor, Department of Obstetrics and Gynecology (Reproductive Sciences), University of Medicine and Dentistry of New Jersey, Robert Wood Johnson Medical School; Chief of Obstetrics and Gynecology Service, Robert Wood Johnson University Hospital, New Brunswick, NJ
The Menopause

Bruce R. Bacon, M.D. Professor of Internal Medicine, and Director, Division of Gastroenterology and Hepatology, Saint Louis University School of Medicine, St. Louis, MO
Viral Hepatitis

R. Eugene Bailey, M.D. Residency Faculty, St. Joseph's Hospital Family Practice Residency Program; Assistant Professor, State University of New York Health Science Center at Syracuse, Syracuse, NY
Infectious Mononucleosis

Roy A. E. Bakay, M.D. Professor, Neurosurgery, Emory University/Emory Clinic, Atlanta, GA
Trauma of the Central Nervous System

Daniel G. Baker, M.D. Associate Professor of Medicine, Medical College of Pennsylvania–Allegheny University; Director of Clinical Services, Rheumatology, Philadelphia Veterans Administration Medical Center, Philadelphia, PA
Septic Arthritis

George L. Bakris, M.D. Associate Professor, Preventive and Internal Medicine, Rush Medical College; Director, Rush University Hypertension Program, Rush-Presbyterian/St. Luke's Medical Center, Chicago, IL
Pheochromocytoma

Alan F. Barker, M.D. Professor of Medicine, Pulmonary and Critical Care Division, Oregon Health Sciences University, Portland, OR
Bronchiectasis

Walter G. Barr, M.D. Associate Professor of Medicine, Loyola University Stritch School of Medicine, and Director, Division of Rheumatology, Loyola University Medical Center, Maywood, IL
Scleroderma

Diane Barton, M.D. Assistant Professor of Clinical Medicine, University of Medicine and Dentistry of New Jersey, Robert Wood Johnson Medical School; Attending, Cooper Hospital/University Medical Center, Camden, NJ
Back and Extremity Pain

James C. Barton, M.D. Medical Director, Southern Iron Disorders Center, Birmingham, AL
Iron Storage Disorders

Thaddeus Bartter, M.D. Associate Professor of Medicine, Division of Pulmonary and Critical Care Medicine, University of Medicine and Dentistry of New Jersey, Robert Wood Johnson Medical School; Director, Pulmonary Function Laboratory, Cooper Hospital/University Medical Center, Camden, NJ
Chronic Cough

Thomas M. Bashore, M.D. Director, Fellowship Training Program, Duke Medical Center, Durham, NC
Valvular Heart Disease

Marc D. Basson, M.D., Ph.D. Assistant Professor of Surgery, Yale University School of Medicine; Attending Physician, Yale-New Haven Hospital, New Haven; Chief, Surgical Endoscopy, West Haven-VA Medical Center, West Haven, CT
Carcinoid Tumor and Carcinoid Syndrome

John Baum, M.D. Professor Emeritus of Medicine, Allergy, Immunology, Rheumatology Unit; Co-Director, Pediatric Rheumatology, Department of Pediatrics, University of Rochester School of Medicine and Dentistry, Rochester, NY
Rheumatoid Arthritis

Kathleen G. Beavis, M.D. Clinical Assistant Professor, Thomas Jefferson Medical College; Assistant Director, Clinical Microbiology, Thomas Jefferson University Hospital, Philadelphia, PA
Systemic Mycoses

Philip M. Becker, M.D. Clinical Associate Professor, Department of Psychiatry, University of Texas Southwestern Medical Center at Dallas; Director and Medical Director, Presbyterian Hospital of Dallas, Dallas, TX
Sleep Disorders

Norman H. Bell, M.D. Professor of Medicine, Medical University of South Carolina; Senior Investigator, Ralph H. Johnson Veterans Affairs Medical Center, Charleston, SC
Rickets and Osteomalacia

H. Michael Belmont, M.D. Assistant Professor of Medicine, New York University School of Medicine; Assistant Director of Rheumatology, Hospital for Joint Diseases, New York, NY
Systemic Lupus Erythematosus

Robert Benjamin, M.D. Assistant Clinical Professor, Department of Psychiatry, Temple University School of Medicine, Philadelphia; Regional Medical Director, Progressions Health Systems, Inc., and Northwestern Institute of Psychiatry, Fort Washington, PA
Personality Disorders

Robert M. Bennett, M.D., F.R.C.P. Professor of Medicine, and Chairman, Division of Arthritis and Rheumatic Diseases, Oregon Health Sciences University, Portland, OR
Ankylosing Spondylitis and Related Arthropathies

Michael L. Bennish, M.D. Associate Professor, Division of Geographic Medicine and Infectious Disease, Departments of Medicine and Pediatrics, Tufts University School of Medicine; Pediatrician, Floating Hospital for Children, New England Medical Center, Boston, MA
Bacterial Diarrheas

David I. Bernstein, M.D. Associate Director and Professor, Infectious Diseases, Children's Hospital Medical Center, Cincinnati, OH
Viral Gastroenteritis

Laura L. Bilodeau, M.D. Assistant Professor of Pathology and Laboratory Medicine, University of Colorado Health Sciences Center; Medical Director, Clinical Chemistry, University Hospital, Denver, CO
Acute Myocardial Infarction

Louis S. Binder, M.D. Professor of Emergency Medicine and Associate Dean for Academic Affairs, University of Illinois at Chicago College of Medicine, Chicago, IL
Periodic Paralyses

C. Laird Birmingham, M.D., M.H.Sc., F.R.C.P.C., F.A.C.P. Professor and Head, Division of Internal Medicine, University of British Columbia; Director, Division of Internal Medicine, Co-Director, Eating Disorder Clinic, St. Paul's Hospital, Vancouver, British Columbia, Canada
Obesity

Michelle Biros, M.D., M.S. Assistant Professor, Departments of Neurosurgery and of Emergency Medicine, University of Minnesota, Minneapolis, School of Medicine; Senior Associate Physician, Department of Emergency Medicine, Hennepin County Medical Center, Minneapolis, MN
Psychiatric Emergencies

Fred E. Boehmke, M.D. Clinical Instructor in Surgery (Colon and Rectal), State University of New York at Buffalo; Attending Surgeon, Millard Fillmore Hospital, Buffalo General Hospital, Sisters of Charity Hospital, St. Joseph's Hospital, Buffalo, NY
Anorectal and Perianal Disorders

Scott J. Boley, M.D., F.A.C.S. Professor of Surgery and Pediatrics and Chief of Pediatric Surgical Services, Albert Einstein College of Medicine and Montefiore Medical Center, Bronx, NY
Mesenteric Vascular Diseases

John H. Bond, M.D. Professor, University of Minnesota; Chief, Gastroenterology Section, Minneapolis Veterans Administration Medical Center, Minneapolis, MN
Polyps and Tumors of the Colon

Henry G. Bone, M.D. Senior Staff Physician, Bone and Mineral Division, Henry Ford Hospital, Detroit, MI
Paget's Disease of Bone

William Z. Borer, M.D. Associate Professor of Pathology and Cell Biology, Thomas Jefferson University, Philadelphia, PA
Nausea, Vomiting, and Dyspepsia; Peripheral Venous Disease; Reference Intervals for the Interpretation of Laboratory Tests

Kevin L. Boyer, M.D. Chief Resident, Neurosurgery, Emory University Hospital, Atlanta, GA
Trauma of the Central Nervous System

George C. Brainard, Ph.D. Professor of Neurology, Thomas Jefferson University, Jefferson Medical College, Philadelphia, PA
Seasonal Affective Disorder

George J. Brewer, M.D. Professor, Department of Human Genetics and Internal Medicine, University of Michigan, Ann Arbor, MI
Hepatolenticular Degeneration (Wilson's Disease)

James E. Brick, M.D. Professor of Medicine, West Virginia University School of Medicine, Morgantown, WV
Polymyalgia Rheumatica and Giant Cell Arteritis

Malcolm L. Brigden, M.D. Clinical Instructor, Department of Medicine, University of British Columbia; Associate Head of Hematology, Metro-McNair Clinical Laboratories, Victoria, British Columbia, Canada
Iron Deficiency Anemia

Michael H. Bross, M.D. Associate Professor, Department of Family Medicine, University of Mississippi Medical Center, Jackson, MS
Delirium and Dementia

Gregory Brotzman, M.D. Associate Professor, Department of Family and Community Medicine, Columbia Family Care Center, Medical College of Wisconsin, Milwaukee, WI
Hyperplasia and Carcinoma of the Endometrium

Robert D. Brown, Jr., M.D. Assistant Professor of Neurology, Mayo Medical School; Consultant, Division of Cerebrovascular Diseases and Department of Neurology, Mayo Clinic, Rochester, MN
Cerebrovascular Disease

Glenn J. Bubley, M.D. Assistant Professor of Medicine, Harvard Medical School; Hematology/Oncology Division, Beth Israel Hospital, Boston, MA
Hypereosinophilic Syndrome

R. Michael Buckley, M.D. Director of Clinical Services, Clinical Professor of Medicine, and Director of Fellowship Program, Division of Infectious Diseases, Thomas Jefferson University Hospital, Philadelphia, PA
Acquired Immunodeficiency Syndrome (AIDS)

Ronald M. Bukowski, M.D. Professor of Medicine, Ohio State University Medical School, Columbus; Staff, Department of Hematology/Oncology, Cleveland Clinic Foundation, Cleveland, OH
Multiple Myeloma and Other Plasma Cell Disorders

Pongamorn Bunnag, M.D. Assistant Professor of Medicine, Mahidol University; Department of Endocrinology, Ramathibodi Hospital, Bangkok, Thailand
Primary Aldosteronism

Gerard N. Burrow, M.D. Dean and Professor, Yale University School of Medicine; Attending Physician, Yale-New Haven Hospital, New Haven, CT
Thyroid Nodules and Goiter

Marla M. Buth, R.D. Section of Dietetics, VA Medical Center, Milwaukee, WI
Nutritional Assessment

Brenda Byrne, Ph.D. Psychologist, Margolis and Shrier Health Psychology Associates, Philadelphia, PA
Seasonal Affective Disorder

Jason H. Calhoun, M.D., M.Eng. Professor and Chairman, Department of Orthopaedic Surgery and Rehabilitation, University of Texas Medical Branch at Galveston, Galveston, TX
Osteomyelitis

José F. Caro, M.D. Magee Professor of Medicine and Chairman of the Department, Thomas Jefferson Medical College, Philadelphia, PA
Diabetes Mellitus

Angelina Carvalho, M.D. Associate Professor of Medicine, Brown University; Chief, Hematology, Veterans Administration Medical Center, Providence, RI
The Purpuras: Vascular and Platelet Disorders as Causes of Bleeding

Joseph T. Chambers, M.D., Ph.D. Associate Professor, Yale University School of Medicine, New Haven, CT
Dysfunctional Uterine Bleeding

James P. Chandler, M.D. Chief Resident, Division of Neurological Surgery, Northwestern University Medical School, Chicago, IL
Brain Abscess

Lisa Chen, M.D. Resident (General Surgery), Department of Surgery, Yale University School of Medicine, New Haven, CT
Hernias of the Abdominal Wall

Jen-Tse Cheng, M.D. Assistant Professor of Clinical Medicine, College of Physicians and Surgeons of Columbia University; Assistant Attending Physician; Attending Nephrologist; Chief, Biochemistry Consultation Laboratory of the Department of Medicine, Harlem Hospital Center, New York, NY
Rhabdomyolysis and Myoglobinuria

Lawrence J. Cheskin, M.D. Associate Professor of Medicine (Gastroenterology) and International Health (Human Nutrition), Johns Hopkins University School of Medicine, and School of Public Health; Active Staff, Johns Hopkins Bayview Medical Center, Baltimore, MD
Diverticular Disease of the Colon

Asha N. Chesnutt, M.D. Fellow, Pulmonary and Critical Care Medicine, University of California, San Francisco, CA
Acute Respiratory Distress Syndrome

Robert Chin, Jr., M.D. Associate Professor of Internal Medicine, Section of Pulmonary and Critical Care Medicine, Bowman Gray School of Medicine of Wake Forest University, Winston-Salem, NC
Acute Adrenal Insufficiency

Michael E. Clark, M.D. Assistant Professor, Department of Family and Community Medicine, Dartmouth University, Maine-Dartmouth Family Practice Residency, Fairfield, ME
Acute Rheumatic Fever

Iain G. M. Cleator, M.B., Ch.B., F.R.C.S.(C), F.R.C.S.(E), F.R.C.S., F.A.C.S. Professor of Surgery, University of British Columbia; Head of Gastrointestinal Clinic, St. Paul's Hospital, Vancouver, British Columbia, Canada
Obesity

Thomas H. Cogbill, M.D. Program Director of Surgical Residency and Vice-President, Gundersen Lutheran Medical Center, La Crosse, WI
Acute Abdominal Pain

Stanley L. Cohan, M.D., Ph.D. Professor and Chairman, Department of Neurology, Georgetown University; Chief of Service, Neurology, Georgetown University Hospital, Washington, DC
Coma

Philip R. Cohen, M.D. Assistant Professor, Departments of Dermatology and Pathology, University of Texas-Houston Medical School; and Section of Dermatology, Department of Medical Specialties, University of Texas M.D. Anderson Cancer Center, Houston, TX
Paraneoplastic Syndromes of the Skin

Lawrence H. Cohn, M.D. Professor of Surgery, Harvard Medical School; Chief Cardiac Surgery, Brigham and Women's Hospital, Boston, MA
Aneurysms of the Aorta

Kathryn Colby, M.D., Ph.D. Clinical Instructor in Ophthalmology, Harvard Medical School; Resident in Ophthalmology, Massachusetts Eye and Ear Infirmary, Boston, MA
Common Ocular Disorders

Richard J. Comi, M.D. Associate Professor, Dartmouth Medical School, Hanover; Program Director for Internal Medicine, Dartmouth Hitchcock Medical Center, Lebanon, NH
Hypoglycemia

Gregory S. Cooper, M.D. Assistant Professor of Medicine, Case Western Reserve University; Attending Physician, Division of Gastroenterology, University Hospitals of Cleveland, Cleveland, OH
Dysphagia, Esophageal Obstruction, and Esophagitis

Gene R. Corbman, M.D. Clinical Instructor, Temple University School of Medicine; Attending, Albert Einstein Medical Center, Philadelphia, PA
Anxiety Disorders

Jorge E. Cortes, M.D. Head, Department of Hematology-Oncology, Instituto Nacional de la Nutricion Salvador Zubirán, Tlalpan, Mexico
Adult Acute Leukemia

Albert C. Cuetter, M.D. Professor of Neurology, Texas Tech University Health Sciences Center, El Paso, TX
Periodic Paralyses

Burke A. Cunha, M.D. Professor of Medicine, State University of New York School of Medicine, Stony Brook; Chief, Infectious Disease Division, Winthrop-University Hospital, Mineola, NY
Lyme Disease; Acute Pharyngitis; Atypical Pneumonias

James R. Curtiss, M.D. Clinical Instructor and Fellow, Division of Gastroenterology, University of South Alabama, Mobile, AL
Functional Disorders of the Gastrointestinal Tract

Gary W. Cushing, M.D. Clinical Instructor in Medicine, Harvard Medical School, Boston; Section Head, Endocrinology, and Endocrinology Fellowship Program Director, Lahey Hitchcock Clinic, Burlington, MA
Hypothyroidism

Michael B. Dabrow, D.O. Clinical Associate Professor of Medicine, Jefferson Medical College, Thomas Jefferson University, Philadelphia; Member, Department of Medicine, Division of Hematology/Oncology, The Lankenau Hospital and Medical Research Center, Wynnewood, PA
Acquired Hemolytic Anemia

Chi Van Dang, M.D., Ph.D. Associate Professor of Medicine, Oncology, Pathology, and Molecular Biology & Genetics, Johns Hopkins University School of Medicine; Chief, Division of Hematology, Department of Medicine, Johns Hopkins Medical Institutions, Baltimore, MD
Myelodysplastic Syndromes and Sideroblastic Anemias

William C. Daniel, M.D. Cardiology Fellow, University of Texas Southwestern Medical Center, Dallas, TX
Cardiomyopathy

Holly Dastghaib, M.D. Resident in Pathology and Laboratory Medicine, LAC/USC Medical Center, Los Angeles, CA
Transfusion Reactions

Andrew M. Davidoff, M.D. Chief Surgical Resident, The Children's Hospital of Philadelphia, Philadelphia, PA
Intestinal Obstruction

James M. Davison, D.O. Assistant Professor, Obstetrics and Gynecology, University of Missouri–Kansas City, Kansas City, MO
Intraepithelial and Invasive Cervical Cancer

Tom R. DeMeester, M.D. Professor and Chairman, Department of Surgery, University of Southern California School of Medicine, Los Angeles, CA
Diaphragmatic Hernias

Richard Depp, M.D. Professor and Chairman, Department of Obstetrics and Gynecology, Jefferson Medical College of Thomas Jefferson University, Philadelphia, PA
Diagnosis and Selected Medical Problems in Pregnancy

Howard S. Derman, M.D. Associate Professor of Neurology, Baylor College of Medicine; Attending Physician, Methodist Hospital, Ben Taub Hospital, Houston, TX
Migraine Headaches

Kathleen De Wolf, M.D. Assistant Professor of Dermatology, Free University of Brussels; Staff Dermatologist, Hôpitaux Universitaires Saint-Pierre et Brugmann, Brussels, Belgium
Granuloma Inguinale

Jack A. DiPalma, M.D. Associate Professor of Medicine and Director, Division of Gastroenterology, University of South Alabama, Mobile, AL
Functional Disorders of the Gastrointestinal Tract

Richard M. Dubinsky, M.D. Associate Professor, Department of Neurology, University of Kansas Medical Center, Kansas City, KS
Extrapyramidal Disorders

George F. Duna, M.D. Staff, Department of Rheumatic and Immunologic Diseases, Cleveland Clinic Foundation, Cleveland, OH
Fibromyalgia

Barry Egener, M.D. Assistant Clinical Professor, Oregon Health Sciences University; Faculty, Portland Program in Internal Medicine; Faculty, Northwest Center for Physician-Patient Communication, Portland, OR
Working With a Difficult Patient

Burton L. Eisenberg, M.D. Professor of Surgery, Temple University School of Medicine; Chairman, Department of Surgical Oncology, Fox Chase Cancer Center, Philadelphia, PA
Neck Masses

William J. Ellis, M.D. Assistant Professor, Department of Urology, University of Washington, Seattle, WA
Benign Prostatic Hyperplasia

D. Michael Elnicki, M.D. Associate Professor, Section of General Internal Medicine, West Virginia University School of Medicine, Morgantown, WV
Hereditary Angioedema

Paul Enright, M.D. Assistant Professor of Medicine, University of Arizona, Tucson, AZ
Tests of Respiratory Function

W. James Evans, M.D. Clinical Assistant Professor, Department of Neurology, Medical University of South Carolina, Charleston; Medical Director, Electroneurodiagnostic Laboratory, Carolinas Hospital System; Florence Neurological Clinic, Florence, SC
Disorders of Taste and Smell

E. Dale Everett, M.D. Professor of Medicine, University of Missouri, Columbia, MO
Rickettsial Diseases

Rose Mary Fair-Covely, D.O. Endocrine Fellow, Thomas Jefferson University Hospital, Philadelphia, PA
Diabetes Mellitus

Crayton A. Fargason, Jr., M.D., M.M. Assistant Professor of Pediatrics, The University of Alabama at Birmingham, Birmingham, AL
Attention-Deficit/Hyperactivity Disorder

Rachel E. Fargason, M.D. Assistant Professor of Psychiatry, The University of Alabama at Birmingham, Birmingham, AL
Attention-Deficit/Hyperactivity Disorder

Donald F. Farrell, M.D. Professor of Neurology, and Associate Director, Center for Human Development and Developmental Disabilities, University of Washington School of Medicine; Director, EEG and Clinical Neurophysiology, University of Washington Medical Center, Seattle, WA
The Sphingolipidoses

Kellie L. Faulk, M.D., M.P.H. Fellow, Endocrinology and Metabolism, Bowman Gray School of Medicine of Wake Forest University, Winston-Salem, NC
Diabetes Insipidus

Donald A. Feinfeld, M.D. Professor of Clinical Medicine, State University of New York Health Sciences Center at Stony Brook, Stony Brook; Co-Director of Nephrology, Nassau County Medical Center, East Meadow, NY
Rhabdomyolysis and Myoglobinuria

Steven H. Feinsilver, M.D. Associate Professor of Medicine, State University of New York at Stony Brook, Stony Brook; Director, Pulmonary and Critical Care Training Program, Winthrop-University Hospital, Mineola, NY
Diseases of the Pleura

David T. Felson, M.D. Professor of Medicine and Public Health, Boston University School of Medicine, Boston, MA
Osteoarthritis

M. Brian Fennerty, M.D. Associate Professor of Medicine, Division of Gastroenterology, Oregon Health Sciences University, Portland, OR
Small Bowel Tumors

Gregory A. Filice, M.D. Associate Professor of Medicine, University of Minnesota; Chief, Infectious Disease Section, Veterans Affairs Medical Center, Minneapolis, MN
Toxoplasmosis

James W. Findling, M.D. Clinical Professor of Medicine, Medical College of Wisconsin; Director, Endocrine-Diabetes Center, St. Luke's Medical Center, Milwaukee, WI
Cushing's Syndrome

Christina Finlayson, M.D. Instructor, Temple University; Fellow, Fox Chase Cancer Center, Philadelphia, PA
Tumors of the Pharynx and Larynx

Anthony E. Fiore, M.D. Fellow, Center for Vaccine Development, University of Maryland School of Medicine, Baltimore, MD
Cholera

James E. Fish, M.D. Professor of Medicine, Director, Pulmonary Medicine and Critical Care, Jefferson Medical College, Philadelphia, PA
Asthma

Andrew J. Fishleder, M.D. Chairman, Division of Education, Staff, Department of Clinical Pathology, Cleveland Clinic Foundation, Cleveland, OH
Hemoglobinopathies

James F. Flaherty, M.D. Clinical Instructor/Senior Registrar, St. James's Hospital, Trinity College, Dublin, Ireland; Chief Resident, University of Connecticut School of Medicine, Farmington, CT
Appendicitis

Timothy P. Flanigan, M.D. Associate Professor of Medicine, Brown University School of Medicine; Chief, Division of Clinical Immunology and Infectious Diseases, Miriam Hospital, Providence, RI
Cryptosporidiosis

Lucio Fortunato, M.D. Attending, Rome American Hospital, Rome, Italy
Pulmonary Tumors

Scott W. Fosko, M.D. Assistant Professor, Department of Dermatology, St. Louis University School of Medicine, St. Louis, MO
Skin Tumors

David C. Foster, M.D., M.P.H. Associate Professor, Obstetrics and Gynecology, Strong Memorial Hospital, University of Rochester, Rochester, NY
Vulvar and Vaginal Disease

Mary H. Foster, M.D. Assistant Professor of Medicine, Renal-Electrolyte and Hypertension Division, University of Pennsylvania; Attending, Hospital of the University of Pennsylvania, Philadelphia, PA
Glomerulonephritis

Robert I. Fox, M.D., Ph.D. The Scripps Research Institute Department of Immunology; Member, Division of Rheumatology, Scripps Clinic and Research Foundation, La Jolla, CA
Sjögren's Syndrome

Ian Frank, M.D. Assistant Professor, Division of Infectious Diseases, University of Pennsylvania; Director, Antiretroviral Clinical Research, Hospital of the University of Pennsylvania, Philadelphia, PA
Pneumocystis *Infection*

David Frankfurter, M.D. Clinical Instructor, Tufts University School of Medicine, Boston, MA
Dysfunctional Uterine Bleeding

Herbert L. Fred, M.D. Professor of Internal Medicine, University of Texas Health Science Center at Houston; Clinical Chief of Medicine, Lyndon B. Johnson General Hospital, Houston, TX
Hypoparathyroidism

Nancy J. Freeman, M.D. Clinical Assistant Professor of Medicine, Brown University; Assistant Chief of Hematology, Providence Veterans Administration Medical Center, Providence, RI
The Purpuras: Vascular and Platelet Disorders as Causes of Bleeding

Thomas G. Gabuzda, M.D. Professor of Medicine, Jefferson Medical College, Philadelphia; Chief, Division of Hematology-Oncology, Lankenau Hospital, Wynnewood, PA
Acquired Hemolytic Anemia

Patrick G. Gallagher, M.D. Assistant Professor, Department of Pediatrics, Yale University School of Medicine; Attending Physician, Yale-New Haven Hospital, New Haven, CT
Hereditary Spherocytosis, Hereditary Elliptocytosis, and Related Disorders

Tracy F. Gannon, M.D. Clinical Assistant Professor, University of Minnesota; Staff Dermatologist, Hennepin County Medical Center, Minneapolis, MN
Approach to Skin Disorders

Morie A. Gertz, M.D. Consultant, Division of Hematology and Internal Medicine, Mayo Clinic and Mayo Foundation; Associate Professor of Medicine, Mayo Medical School, Rochester, MN
The Amyloidoses

Fathia Gibril, M.D. National Institutes of Health, Bethesda, MD
Endocrine Disorders of the Gastrointestinal Tract

D. J. Gillespie, M.D., Ph.D. Consultant in Pulmonary and Critical Care Medicine, Mayo Clinic, Rochester, MN
Dyspnea

Jean L. Goens, M.D. Assistant Professor of Dermatology, Free University of Brussels; Staff Dermatologist, Hôpitaux Universitaires Saint-Pierre et Brugmann, Brussels, Belgium
Granuloma Inguinale

John W. Goethe, M.D. Associate Clinical Professor of Psychiatry, University of Connecticut School of Medicine, Farmington, and Yale University School of Medicine, New Haven; Director of Clinical Research, Institute of Living, Hartford, CT
Schizophrenia

Melvyn Goldberg, M.D., F.R.C.S.C. Professor, Department of Surgery, Temple University School of Medicine; Chief, Thoracic Surgical Oncology, Fox Chase Cancer Center, Philadelphia, PA
Pulmonary Tumors

Lewis R. Goldfrank, M.D. Associate Professor of Clinical Medicine, New York University School of Medicine; Medical Director, New York City Poison Center, Director, Department of Emergency Medicine, Bellevue Hospital Center, New York, NY
Food-Borne Neurotoxins

Elliot M. Goldner, M.D. Assistant Professor, University of British Columbia; Psychiatric Director, Eating Disorders Program, St. Paul's Hospital, Vancouver, British Columbia, Canada
Obesity

Marvin E. Gozum, M.D. Thomas Jefferson University, Jefferson Medical College; Consultant, Wills Eye Hospital, Philadelphia, PA
Computer-Assisted Diagnosis

Linda K. Green, M.D. Associate Professor of Pathology, Baylor College of Medicine; Director of Cytology and Flow Cytometry, Veterans Administration Medical Center, Houston, TX
Gastritis

Georgina Groleau, M.D., F.A.C.E.P., F.A.C.P. Assistant Professor of Surgery and Medicine, University of Maryland Medical School; Attending Physician, University of Maryland Medical System and Baltimore Veterans Hospital, Baltimore, MD
Rabies

Gene L. Gulati, Ph.D., S.H.(A.S.C.P.)D.L.M. Clinical Associate Professor of Pathology, Jefferson Medical College, Thomas Jefferson University; Associate Director, Hematology Laboratory, Thomas Jefferson University Hospital, Philadelphia, PA
Agnogenic Myeloid Metaplasia and Essential Thrombocythemia

Jeffrey P. Gumprecht, M.D. Clinical Instructor, Mt. Sinai School of Medicine of the City University of New York; Assistant Attending, Mt. Sinai Medical Center, New York, NY
Other Intestinal Parasites

José A. Gutrecht, M.D., M.Sc. Lecturer, Harvard University, Cambridge; Senior Staff, Department of Neurology, Lahey Hitchcock Clinic, Burlington, MA
Paraneoplastic Central Neural Syndromes

Steven M. Hacker, M.D. Assistant Clinical Professor of Dermatology, University of Florida, Gainesville, FL
Common Bacterial and Fungal Infections of the Integument

Stephanos J. Hadziyannis, M.D. Professor of Internal Medicine, University of Athens School of Medicine; Head of the Second Department of Medicine and of the Liver Research Unit, Hippouration General Hospital, Athens, Greece
Echinococcosis

Romaine Hain, M.D. Psychiatrist, Private Practice, Alabama Psychotherapy and Wellness Center, P.C., Brookwood Medical Center, Birmingham, AL
Somatoform Disorders

Roxanne Halencak, P.A.-C. Physician's Assistant-Certified, University of Texas Medical Branch at Galveston, Galveston, TX
Osteomyelitis

Katherine A. Halmi, M.D. Professor of Psychiatry, Cornell University Medical College, New York; Attending Psychiatrist and Director, Eating Disorder Program, New York Hospital-Westchester, White Plains, NY
Anorexia and Bulimia

John G. Halvorsen, M.D., M.S. Associate Professor and Chairman, Department of Family and Community Medicine, University of Illinois College of Medicine at Peoria, Peoria, IL
Sexual and Gender Identity Disorders

Richard J. Ham, M.D. State University of New York Health Science Center at Syracuse, College of Medicine, Program in Geriatrics, Syracuse, NY
Nutrient Deficiency Disorders

Richard J. Hamilton, M.D. Instructor in Clinical Surgery/Emergency Medicine, New York University School of Medicine; Fellow, Medical Toxicology, New York City Poison Center, New York, NY
Food-Borne Neurotoxins

J. Kevin Harrison, M.D. Assistant Director, Cardiac Catheterization Laboratories, Duke University Medical Center, Durham, NC
Valvular Heart Disease

Christine J. Hashem, M.D. Resident in Dermatology, Bowman Gray School of Medicine of Wake Forest University, Winston-Salem, NC
Dermatitis

Houria I. Hassouna, M.D., Ph.D. Associate Professor and Medicine Director, Special Coagulation Laboratory, College of Human Medicine, Michigan State University, East Lansing, MI
Hypercoagulable States

H. Bradford Hawley, M.D. Professor of Medicine, Chief, Division of Infectious Diseases, Wright State University School of Medicine; Director, Sexually Transmitted Diseases Clinic, Montgomery County Health Department, Dayton, OH
Gonorrhea

Ian D. Hay, M.B., Ph.D., F.A.C.P., F.R.C.P. Professor of Medicine, Mayo Medical School; Consultant in Endocrinology and Internal Medicine, Mayo Clinic and Foundation, Rochester, MN
Hyperthyroidism

Steven E. Hearne, M.D. Cardiology Fellow, Duke University Medical Center, Durham, NC
Valvular Heart Disease

Vivien Herman, M.B., Ch.B. Assistant Professor, University of California, Los Angeles; Staff Endocrinologist, Cedars-Sinai Medical Center, Los Angeles, CA
Acromegaly

L. David Hillis, M.D. James M. Wooten Chair in Cardiology, University of Texas Southwestern Medical Center, Dallas, TX
Cardiomyopathy

Seok-Chan Hong, M.D. Assistant Professor, Department of Otolaryngology, Kon-Kuk University College of Medicine; Chairman of Otolaryngology, Kon-Kuk University Hospital, Chungju-Si, Chungbuk-Do, South Korea
Disorders of the Nose and Paranasal Sinuses

Mary Hooks, M.D. Clinical Instructor of Surgery, Temple University School of Medicine; Surgical Fellow, Department of Surgical Oncology, Fox Chase Cancer Center, Philadelphia, PA
Neck Masses

Stan Houston, M.D. Associate Professor, Department of Medicine, University of Alberta; Admitting Staff, Divisions of Infectious Disease and General Internal Medicine, University of Alberta Hospitals, Edmonton, Alberta, Canada
Other Trematodes

Jane Chen Huang, M.D. Fellow in Hematopathology, Northwestern University Medical School, Chicago, IL
Thalassemia

Jean P. Hubble, M.D. Assistant Professor, Department of Neurology, Parkinson's Disease Center of Excellence and Movement Disorders Clinic, Columbus, OH
Extrapyramidal Disorders

Richard W. Hudgens, M.D. Professor of Psychiatry and Vice Chairman for Clinical Affairs, Washington University School of Medicine, St. Louis, MO
Mood Disorders

Anne E. Hull, M.D. Assistant Professor of Medicine, Section of Infectious Diseases, Louisiana State University School of Medicine, New Orleans, LA
Salmonellae

Verda Hunter, M.D. Clinical Associate Professor, University of Missouri–Kansas City, Kansas City, MO
Intraepithelial and Invasive Cervical Cancer

Howard Hurtig, M.D. Clinical Professor of Neurology, University of Pennsylvania; Chairman, Department of Neurology, and President, Neurologic Center, Graduate Hospital, Philadelphia, PA
Spinocerebellar Degenerative Disorders

Mohamad A. Hussein, M.D. Staff, Hematology/Medical Oncology; Staff, Cleveland Clinic Cancer Center, Cleveland Clinic Foundation, Cleveland, OH
Multiple Myeloma and Other Plasma Cell Disorders

David P. Huston, M.D. Cullen Professor of Immunology, Departments of Medicine and Microbiology & Immunology; Chief, Immunology Section, Baylor College of Medicine; Director, Immunology Service, Baylor College of Medicine Affiliated Hospitals, Houston, TX
Urticaria

Joel C. Hutcheson, M.D. Chief Resident in Urological Surgery, Harvard Program in Urology (Longwood Area), Harvard Medical School, Boston, MA
Intrascrotal Masses and Tumors

Florence N. Hutchison, M.D. Associate Professor of Medicine, Medical University of South Carolina; Chief, Dialysis Service, Ralph H. Johnson Veterans Affairs Medical Center, Charleston, SC
Rickets and Osteomalacia

Bong H. Hyun, M.D., D.Sc. Professor of Pathology and Director of Hematology, Thomas Jefferson University Hospital, Philadelphia, PA; Honorary Professor, Yanbian Medical College, Yanji, China
Agnogenic Myeloid Metaplasia and Essential Thrombocythemia

Steven Idell, M.D., Ph.D. Professor of Medicine, Associate Chairman for Subspecialty Care, and Chief, Pulmonary Division, The University of Texas Health Center at Tyler, Tyler, TX
Hemoptysis

Silvio E. Inzucchi, M.D. Assistant Professor of Medicine, Yale School of Medicine; Attending Physician, Yale-New Haven Hospital, New Haven, CT
Thyroid Nodules and Goiter

Richard F. Jacobs, M.D., F.A.A.P. Horace C. Cabe Professor of Pediatrics and Chief, Pediatric Infectious Diseases, University of Arkansas for Medical Sciences and Arkansas Children's Hospital, Little Rock, AR
Acute Viral Encephalitis and Meningitis

William G. Jamieson, M.D., F.R.C.S.(C.), F.R.C.S.(Eng.) Professor of Surgery, University of Western Ontario; Chief of Vascular Surgery, Victoria Hospital, London, Ontario, Canada
Peripheral Venous Disease

Camila K. Janniger, M.D. Clinical Associate Professor, Dermatology and Pediatrics, Chief, Pediatric Dermatology, University of Medicine and Dentistry of New Jersey–New Jersey Medical School, Newark, NJ
Chancroid; Lymphogranuloma Venereum

Robert T. Jensen, M.D. National Institutes of Health, Bethesda, MD
Endocrine Disorders of the Gastrointestinal Tract

H. Royden Jones, Jr., M.D. Associate Clinical Professor of Neurology, Harvard Medical School, Boston; Chairman, Department of Neurology, Lahey Hitchcock Medical Center, Burlington, MA
Paraneoplastic Syndromes: Disorders of the Peripheral Motor Sensory Unit

Lawrence J. Kagen, M.D. Professor of Medicine, Cornell University Medical College; Attending Physician, Hospital for Special Surgery, New York Hospital, New York, NY
Myopathies

Ronald N. Kaleya, M.D., F.A.C.S. Associate Professor of Surgery, Albert Einstein College of Medicine, Bronx, NY
Mesenteric Vascular Diseases

Stephan L. Kamholz, M.D. Professor and Chairman, Department of Internal Medicine, State University of New York Health Science Center at Brooklyn; Chief of the Medical Service, and President of the Medical Board, Kings County Hospital Center, Brooklyn, NY
Anaerobic Lung Infections

Gregory C. Kane, M.D. Assistant Professor of Medicine, Director, Medical-Respiratory Intensive Care Unit, Thomas Jefferson University Hospital, Philadelphia, PA
Chronic Obstructive Pulmonary Disease; Asthma; Pulmonary Embolism and Infarction

Hagop Kantarjian, M.D. Head, Leukemia Section, Department of Hematology, M.D. Anderson Cancer Center, Houston, TX
Adult Acute Leukemia

Gary R. Kantor, M.D. Associate Professor, Departments of Dermatology and Pathology and Laboratory Medicine, Medical College of Pennsylvania and Allegheny University, Philadelphia, PA
Pruritus

Andre A. Kaplan, M.D. Professor of Medicine, University of Connecticut School of Medicine; Director, Dialysis Program, John Dempsey Hospital, Farmington, CT
Interstitial Nephritis

Wishwa N. Kapoor, M.D., M.P.H. Professor of Medicine, University of Pittsburgh, School of Medicine; Chief, Division of General Internal Medicine, and Department of Medicine, University of Pittsburgh Medical Center, Pittsburgh, PA
Syncope

Elton Katagihara, M.D. Fellow, Pulmonary and Critical Care Medicine, University of Southern California School of Medicine, Los Angeles, CA
Interstitial Lung Disease

Athanasios Katsarkas, M.D. Royal Victoria Hospital, Montreal, Quebec, Canada
Dizziness and Vertigo

Richard T. Katz, M.D. Associate Professor of Clinical Internal Medicine (Physical Medicine and Rehabilitation), St. Louis University School of Medicine; Medical Director, SSM Rehabilitation Institute, St. Louis, MO
Carpal Tunnel Syndrome

Lee D. Kaufman, M.D., F.A.C.P. Associate Professor of Medicine and Chief, Division of Rheumatology, State University of New York at Stony Brook, Stony Brook, NY
Polyarteritis Nodosa

Arthur Kavanaugh, M.D. Associate Professor of Internal Medicine, University of Texas Southwestern Medical Center at Dallas; Chief of Rheumatology, Dallas Department of Veterans Affairs Medical Center, Dallas, TX
Immunodeficiency

Rosemary A. Kearney, M.D. Clinical Instructor, Thomas Jefferson University Hospital; Internist, Department of Medicine, Pennsylvania Hospital, Philadelphia, PA
Infective Endocarditis

Herbert J. Keating, III, M.D. Professor of Clinical Medicine, University of Medicine and Dentistry of New Jersey, Robert Wood Johnson Medical School, Piscataway; Head, Division of General Internal Medicine and Primary Care, Cooper Hospital/University Medical Center, Camden, NJ
Back and Extremity Pain

Michael J. Keating, M.B.B.S. Associate Head for Clinical Research, University of Texas M.D. Anderson Cancer Center, Houston, TX
Chronic Lymphocytic Leukemia

Ellen C. Keeley, M.D. Cardiology Fellow, University of Texas Southwestern Medical Center, Dallas, TX
Cardiomyopathy

David A. Keith, B.D.S., D.M.D. Associate Professor, Oral and Maxillofacial Surgery, Harvard School of Dental Medicine; Visiting Professor and Director, Harvard Community Health Plan, Massachusetts General Hospital, Boston, MA
Cephalic Neuralgias

Rick Kellerman, M.D. Associate Professor, University of Kansas School of Medicine–Wichita, Wichita; Program Director, Smoky Hill Family Practice Residency, Salina, KS
Tetanus

Gary J. Kennedy, M.D. Associate Professor, and Director of Fellowship Training Program in Geriatric Psychiatry, Albert Einstein College of Medicine; Director, Division of Geriatric Psychiatry, Montefiore Medical Center, Bronx, NY
Geriatric Psychiatry

Ali S. Khan, M.D. Medical Epidemiologist, Centers for Disease Control and Prevention, Atlanta, GA
Viral Hemorrhagic Fevers and Hantavirus Pulmonary Syndrome

Robert J. Kiltz, M.D. Private Practice, Women's Health Specialists, Auburn, NY
Leiomyoma Uteri

Hueston C. King, M.D., F.A.C.S., F.A.C.A.A.I., F.A.O.O.A. Clinical Professor, Department of Otolaryngology, University of Texas Southwestern Medical Center at Dallas, Dallas, TX; Emeritus Staff, Venice Hospital; Bon Secours–Venice Hospital, Venice, FL
Rhinitis

Louis V. Kirchhoff, M.D., M.P.H. Associate Professor, Department of Internal Medicine, University of Iowa; Staff Physician, Department of Veterans Affairs Medical Center, Iowa City, IA
American Trypanosomiasis (Chagas' Disease)

Jeffrey T. Kirchner, D.O., F.A.A.F.P. Clinical Instructor, Department of Family and Community Medicine, Family Practice Residency Program, Lancaster General Hospital, Lancaster, PA
Primary Hyperparathyroidism

Lloyd W. Klein, M.D. Associate Professor of Medicine, Rush Medical College; Co-Director, Cardiac Catheterization Laboratories and Director, Interventional Cardiology, Rush-Presbyterian/St. Luke's Medical Center and The Rush Heart Institute, Chicago, IL
Ischemic Heart Disease

Robert L. Knobler, M.D., Ph.D. Professor, Neurology, Thomas Jefferson University; Attending Neurologist, Thomas Jefferson University Hospital, Philadelphia, PA
Multiple Sclerosis and Other Demyelinating Diseases

Michael K. Koehler, M.D. Assistant Clinical Professor, Case Western Reserve School of Medicine, University Hospitals of Cleveland, Cleveland, OH
Dysphagia, Esophageal Obstruction, and Esophagitis

Orly F. Kohn, M.D. Assistant Professor of Medicine, University of Connecticut School of Medicine, Farmington, CT
Interstitial Nephritis

William C. Koller, M.D., Ph.D. Professor and Chairman, Department of Neurology, University of Kansas Medical Center, Kansas City, KS
Extrapyramidal Disorders

Kinga Kowalewska-Grochowska, M.D. Associate Professor, University of Alberta; Medical Microbiologist, Microbiology and Public Health, Provincial Laboratory, Edmonton, Alberta, Canada
Other Trematodes

Kris V. Kowdley, M.D. Assistant Professor of Medicine, University of Washington; Attending Physician, University of Washington Medical Center, Seattle, WA
Cirrhosis of the Liver

Jesse C. Krakauer, M.D., F.A.C.P. Staff Physician, William Beaumont Hospital, Nutritional Medicine Center, Birmingham, MI
Chronic Adrenal Insufficiency

Kurt Kroenke, M.D. Associate Professor of Medicine, and Director, Fellowship Program in General Internal Medicine, Uniformed Services University of the Health Sciences, Bethesda, MD
Fatigue

Razelle Kurzrock, M.D. Professor of Medicine and Chief, Section of Cytokines, Department of Bioimmunotherapy, University of Texas M.D. Anderson Cancer Center, Houston, TX
Paraneoplastic Syndromes of the Skin

James N. Kvale, M.D. Clinical Associate Professor, Department of Family Medicine, Case Western Reserve University, Cleveland, OH; Program Director, Family Practice Residency, Central Texas Medical Foundation, Austin, TX
Urethritis and Stress Incontinence

Janice K. Kvale, Ph.D., C.N.M. Assistant Professor, Frances Payne Bolton School of Nursing, Case Western Reserve University, Cleveland, OH
Urethritis and Stress Incontinence

Robert A. Kyle, M.D. Consultant, Division of Hematology and Internal Medicine, Mayo Clinic and Mayo Foundation; Professor of Medicine and of Laboratory Medicine, Mayo Medical School, Rochester, MN
The Amyloidoses

Richard D. Lackman, M.D. Professor and Co-Director, Musculoskeletal Tumor Center, Department of Orthopaedic Surgery, Medical College of Pennsylvania and Allegheny University, Philadelphia, PA
Skeletal Neoplasms

Robert Lamport, M.D. Senior Fellow, Johns Hopkins University School of Medicine; Staff Physician, Johns Hopkins Bayview Medical Center, Baltimore, MD
Diverticular Disease of the Colon

Jeffrey Landercasper, M.D. Chairman, Department of Surgery, and Attending Surgeon, Gundersen Lutheran Medical Center, La Crosse, WI
Acute Abdominal Pain

Richard A. Lange, M.D. Jonsson-Rogers Chair in Cardiology, Associate Professor of Internal Medicine, and Director, Cardiac Catheterization Laboratory, University of Texas Southwestern Medical Center, Dallas, TX
Cardiomyopathy

Victor R. Lavis, M.D. Associate Professor, Internal Medicine (Endocrinology), University of Texas Medical School; Attending Physician, Hermann Hospital and Lyndon B. Johnson General Hospital, Houston, TX
Hypoparathyroidism

Jeffry B. Lawrence, M.D. Clinical Associate Professor of Pathology, Indiana University School of Medicine, Indianapolis, IN; Adjunct Associate Professor of Pathology, Case Western Reserve University School of Medicine, Cleveland, OH; Clinical Research Pathologist, Lilly Research Laboratories, Indianapolis, IN
Hemorrhagic Diseases Due to Circulating Anticoagulants

William Lawson, M.D., D.D.S. Professor of Otolaryngology, Mount Sinai School of Medicine, New York; Chief of Otolaryngology, Veterans Affairs Medical Center, Bronx; Attending Physician, Mt. Sinai Hospital and Elmhurst Hospital Center, New York, NY
Neoplastic and Non-neoplastic Lesions of the Oral Mucosa

Billy R. Ledbetter, M.D. Fellow, Marine Medicine Facility, University of Texas Medical Branch at Galveston, Galveston, TX
Osteomyelitis

Jean Lee, M.D. Assistant Professor of Medicine, Medical College of Pennsylvania; Director of CAPD, Dialysis Clinics, Inc., Philadelphia, PA
Nephrotic Syndrome

K. Philip Lee, M.D. Instructor in Neurology, Washington University School of Medicine, St. Louis, MO
Myasthenia Gravis

Jack L. LeFrock, M.D. Columbia Doctors Hospital of Sarasota, Sarasota, FL
Acute Bacterial Meningitis

Barbara M. Leighton, M.D. Fellow, Division of Pulmonary Medicine and Critical Care, Thomas Jefferson University Hospital, Philadelphia, PA
Chronic Obstructive Pulmonary Disease

Frank T. Leone, M.D. Fellow, Pulmonary and Critical Care Medicine, Thomas Jefferson University Hospital, Philadelphia, PA
Pulmonary Embolism and Infarction

Donald A. Leopold, M.D. Associate Professor, Johns Hopkins Medical Institutions, Baltimore, MD
Disorders of the Nose and Paranasal Sinuses

Murray L. Levin, M.D. Professor of Medicine, Northwestern University Medical School; Chief, Patterson Teaching Firm, Northwestern Memorial Hospital, Chicago, IL
Acute Renal Failure

Myron M. Levine, M.D., D.T.P.H. Professor and Director, Center for Vaccine Development, University of Maryland School of Medicine, Baltimore, MD
Cholera

Michael J. Levinson, M.D., F.A.C.P., F.A.C.G. Associate Professor of Medicine, University of Tennessee College of Health Sciences, Memphis, TN
Jaundice

Wendy Levinson, M.D. Professor of Medicine, Oregon Health Sciences University; Assistant Chief of Medicine, Good Samaritan Hospital, Portland, OR
Working With a Difficult Patient

Robert M. Levy, M.D., Ph.D. Associate Professor of Neurosurgery and Physiology, Northwestern University Medical School; Director, Northwestern Multidisciplinary Pain Clinic, Chicago, IL
Brain Abscess

J. Brad Lichtenhan, M.D. Private Practice, Family Medicine, Travis Physician Associates, Austin, TX
Tetanus

Philip R. Liebson, M.D. Professor of Internal Medicine and Preventive Medicine, Rush Medical College; Attending Physician, Senior Echocardiographer and Consultant in Preventive Cardiology, Section of Cardiology, Rush-Presbyterian/St. Luke's Medical Center, Chicago, IL
Ischemic Heart Disease

Barry Lifson, M.D. Chief Resident, New York Medical College, Valhalla, NY
Obstructive Nephropathy

Evan Loh, M.D. Assistant Professor of Medicine, University of Pennsylvania Medical School; Medical Director, Congestive Heart Failure and Cardiac Transplantation Program, Hospital of the University of Pennsylvania, Philadelphia, PA
Congestive Heart Failure

Larry I. Lutwick, M.D. Professor of Clinical Medicine, State University of New York, Health Science Center; Director, Division of Infectious Diseases, Department of Medicine, Maimonides Medical Center, Brooklyn, NY
Herpesviruses

Richard L. Mabry, M.D. Professor of Otorhinolaryngology, University of Texas Southwestern Medical Center, Dallas, TX
Rhinitis

Philip A. Mackowiak, M.D. Professor and Vice Chairman, Department of Medicine, University of Maryland School of Medicine; Chief, Medical Service, Department of Veterans Affairs Medical Center, Baltimore, MD
Fever

Jon T. Mader, M.D. Professor, Department of Internal Medicine, Division of Infectious Disease, and Chief, Marine Medicine Facility-Marine Biomedical Institute, University of Texas Medical Branch at Galveston, Texas, Galveston, TX
Osteomyelitis

Barbara A. Majeroni, M.D. Assistant Professor, Director of Continuing Medical Education, Department of Family Medicine, State University of New York at Buffalo, School of Medicine and Biomedical Sciences; Attending Physician, Erie County Medical Center, Buffalo, NY
Chlamydial Infections

Paris T. Mansmann, M.D. Associate Professor, West Virginia University School of Medicine; Staff Physician, West Virginia University Hospitals, Morgantown, WV
Hereditary Angioedema

Thomas J. Marrie, M.D. Professor of Medicine and Associate Professor of Microbiology, Dalhousie University; Attending Staff Physician, Victoria General Hospital, Halifax, Nova Scotia, Canada
Bacterial Pneumonia

John B. Marshall, M.D. Associate Professor of Medicine, University of Missouri-Columbia School of Medicine; Director of Gastroenterology, University of Missouri Hospital and Clinics, Columbia, MO
Gastrointestinal Hemorrhage

Mary C. Massa, M.D. Associate Professor of Medicine and Director, Division of Dermatology, Loyola University Stritch School of Medicine, Maywood, IL
Scleroderma

Michael A. Matthay, M.D. Professor, Medicine and Anesthesia, University of California, San Francisco; Senior Member, Cardiovascular Research Institute, University of California, San Francisco, CA
Acute Respiratory Distress Syndrome

Suzanne Maxson, M.D., F.A.A.P. Pediatric Infectious Diseases, Cook-Ft. Worth Children's Medical Center, Ft. Worth, TX
Acute Viral Encephalitis and Meningitis

Rex M. McCallum, M.D. Associate Professor and Vice Chair for Clinical Services, Department of Medicine, Duke University School of Medicine, Durham, NC
Wegener's Granulomatosis

Geraldine M. McCarthy, M.D., F.R.C.P.I. Associate Professor of Medicine, Department of Medicine, Division of Rheumatology, Medical College of Wisconsin; Attending Physician, Froedtert Memorial Lutheran Hospital, Milwaukee, WI
Hyperuricemia and Gout

James S. McCarthy, M.B.B.S., M.D., D.T.M.H., F.R.A.C.P. Visiting Associate, Laboratory of Parasitic Diseases, National Institutes of Health, Bethesda, MD
Filarial Infection

Daniel J. McCarty, M.D. Will and Cava Ross Professor of Medicine, and Director, Arthritis Institute, Medical College of Wisconsin; Attending Physician, Froedtert Memorial Lutheran Hospital, Department of Rheumatology, Milwaukee, WI
Hyperuricemia and Gout

Joseph R. McClellan, M.D. Assistant Professor of Medicine, University of Pennsylvania School of Medicine; Director of Cardiac Care Unit, Co-Director, Nuclear Cardiology, Hospital of the University of Pennsylvania, Philadelphia, PA
Congestive Heart Failure

Peter McLaughlin, M.D. Associate Internist and Associate Professor of Medicine, University of Texas M.D. Anderson Cancer Center, Houston, TX
The Lymphomas

Shlomo Melmed, M.B., Ch.B. Professor of Medicine, University of California, Los Angeles, School of Medicine; Director, Research Institute, Cedars-Sinai Medical Center, Los Angeles, CA
Acromegaly

Geno J. Merli, M.D. Clinical Professor of Medicine, Jefferson Medical College of Thomas Jefferson University; Deputy Chairman, Department of Medicine, and Director, Division of Internal Medicine, Thomas Jefferson University Hospital, Philadelphia, PA
Perioperative Medical Consultation

Donald B. Middleton, M.D. Director, St. Margaret Memorial Hospital Family Practice Residency; Clinical Associate Professor, University of Pittsburgh School of Medicine, Pittsburgh, PA
Other Arthropod-Borne Infections

David K. Miller, M.D. Staff Physician, Department of Internal Medicine, Gundersen Clinic, La Crosse, WI
Chronic Abdominal Pain

Debra Q. Miller, M.D. Assistant Professor of Medicine, Pennsylvania State University College of Medicine, Hershey, PA
Iatrogenesis

G. Klaud Miller, M.D. Assistant Clinical Professor of Orthopedics, Northwestern University Medical School, Chicago; St. Francis Hospital, Evanston, IL
Sports Medicine

Geoffrey Miller, M.D., M.B., Ch.B., M.R.C.P., F.R.A.C.P. Professor of Pediatrics and Neurology, Baylor College of Medicine; Child Neurologist, Texas Children's Hospital, Houston, TX
Muscular Dystrophies

Larry K. Miller, M.D. Head, Infectious Diseases Division, Naval Medical Center, San Diego, CA
Malaria

Larry E. Millikan, M.D. Professor and Chairman, Department of Dermatology, Tulane University Medical Center, New Orleans, LA
Flies, Lice, Mites, and Bites

John F. Modlin, M.D. Professor of Pediatrics and Medicine, Dartmouth Medical School, Hanover; Attending Physician, Infectious Diseases, Dartmouth-Hitchcock Medical Center, Lebanon, NH
Nonpolio Enterovirus Infections

Mark E. Molitch, M.D. Professor of Medicine, Center for Endocrinology, Metabolism and Molecular Medicine, Northwestern University Medical School; Attending Physician, Northwestern Memorial Hospital, Chicago, IL
Hyperprolactinemia

Basanti Mukerji, M.D. Associate Professor of Medicine (Rheumatology), University of South Alabama Medical Center, Mobile, AL
Chest Pain

Vaskar Mukerji, M.D. Professor of Medicine and Director, Cardiovascular Training Program, University of South Alabama Medical Center, Mobile, AL
Chest Pain

David L. Nahrwold, M.D. Loyal and Edith Davis Professor and Chairman, Department of Surgery, Northwestern University Medical School; Surgeon-in-Chief, Northwestern Memorial Hospital, Chicago, IL
Disorders of the Gallbladder and Bile Ducts

Ratanavadec Nanagara, M.D. Associate Professor of Medicine, Khonkaen University; Director of Allergy-Immunology, Rheumatology Unit, Department of Medicine and Srinagarind Hospital, Khonkaen, Thailand
Septic Arthritis

Neena Natt, M.B., B.Chir., M.R.C.P. (U.K.) Senior Clinical Fellow, Division of Endocrinology, Mayo Graduate School of Medicine, Rochester, MN
Hyperthyroidism

Kevin R. Nelson, M.D. Associate Professor of Neurology, University of Kentucky, Lexington, KY
Poliomyelitis

Brent A. Neuschwander-Tetri, M.D. Assistant Professor of Internal Medicine, Division of Gastroenterology and Hepatology, St. Louis University School of Medicine, St. Louis, MO
Viral Hepatitis

Maria I. New, M.D. Professor, Department of Pediatrics, Harold and Percy Uris Professor of Pediatric Endocrinology and Metabolism, Cornell University Medical College; Chairman, Department of Pediatrics, and Chief, Division of Pediatric Endocrinology, New York Hospital, Cornell Medical Center, New York, NY
Congenital Adrenal Hyperplasia

Herbert B. Newton, M.D. Assistant Professor of Neurology, and Director, Division of Neuro-Oncology, The Ohio State University Hospitals and Arthur James Cancer Hospital and Research Institute, Columbus, OH
Intracranial Neoplasms

Albert H. Niden, M.D. Professor of Medicine, Interim Chief, Division of Pulmonary Disease and Critical Care Medicine; Associate Chair, Department of Medicine, University of Southern California School of Medicine, Los Angeles, CA
Diagnostic Procedures in Respiratory Disease

Kathryn North, M.B.B.S., B.Sc.(Med.), M.D., F.R.A.C.P. Senior Lecturer, University of Sydney, Sydney; Pediatric Neurologist, Clinical Geneticist, Director, Neurogenetics Unit, Royal Alexandra Hospital for Children, Sydney, New South Wales, Australia
Muscular Dystrophies

Jeffrey A. Norton, M.D. Professor of Surgery, Washington University School of Medicine, St. Louis, MO
Multiple Endocrine Neoplasia

Thomas B. Nutman, M.D. Head, Helminth Immunology Section, Laboratory of Parasitic Diseases, National Institutes of Health, Bethesda, MD
Filarial Infection

K. Patrick Ober, M.D. Professor of Internal Medicine (Endocrinology and Metabolism), Bowman Gray School of Medicine of Wake Forest University, Winston-Salem, NC
Diabetes Insipidus

Susan O'Brien, M.D. Associate Professor of Medicine, University of Texas M.D. Anderson Cancer Center, Houston, TX
Chronic Lymphocytic Leukemia

Jeanne O'Connell, M.D. Chief Resident, Emergency Medicine, University of Maryland Medical System, Baltimore, MD
Rabies

Stephen T. Olin, M.D. Clinical Assistant Professor of Family and Community Medicine, College of Medicine of the Pennsylvania State University, Hershey; Temple University School of Medicine, Philadelphia; Associate Director, Department of Family and Community Medicine, Lancaster General Hospital, Lancaster, PA
Superficial Mycoses

David L. Olive, M.D. Associate Professor and Chief, Reproductive Endocrinology and Infertility, Department of Obstetrics and Gynecology, Yale University School of Medicine, New Haven, CT
Endometriosis

E. J. Olson, M.D. Fellow in Pulmonary and Critical Care Medicine, Mayo Clinic, Rochester, MN
Dyspnea

Anthony M. Ortega, M.D. Clinical Assistant Instructor in Medicine, State University of New York School of Medicine, Stony Brook; Fellow, Infectious Disease Division, Winthrop-University Hospital, Mineola, NY
Atypical Pneumonias

Constance T. Pachucki, M.D. Assistant Professor of Medicine, Stritch School of Medicine, Loyola University, Maywood; Assistant Chief, Section of Infectious Diseases, Department of Veterans Affairs, Hines VA Hospital, Hines, IL
Influenza

Rajesh Pahwa, M.D. Assistant Professor, Department of Neurology, University of Kansas Medical Center, Kansas City, KS
Extrapyramidal Disorders

Robert M. Pascuzzi, M.D. Professor and Vice Chairman of Education, and Chief of Wishard Section, Department of Neurology, Indiana University School of Medicine, Indianapolis, IN
Conversion Disorders, Malingering, and Dissociative Disorders

David A. Paslin, M.D. Assistant Clinical Professor, Department of Dermatology, University of California, San Francisco, School of Medicine, San Francisco, CA
The Porphyrias

Susan Pauker, M.D. Assistant Professor of Pediatrics, Harvard Medical School; Chief, Department of Medical Genetics, Harvard Community Health Plan; Director, Genetics Clinic, Massachusetts General Hospital, Boston, MA
Genetic Disease

Henry Paulson, M.D., Ph.D. Fellow in Movement Disorders and Neurogenetics, Research Associate, Department of Pharmacology, University of Pennsylvania Medical Center and Graduate Hospital, Philadelphia, PA
Spinocerebellar Degenerative Disorders

Deborah Pavan-Langston, M.D. Associate Professor of Ophthalmology, Harvard Medical School; Surgeon and Director, Clinical Virology, Massachusetts Eye and Ear Infirmary, Boston, MA
Common Ocular Disorders

Zbigniew S. Pawlowski, M.D., D.T.M.&H. Professor and Head, Clinic of Parasitic and Tropical Diseases, University of Medical Sciences, Poznań, Poland
Trichinosis (Trichinellosis)

S. Kirk Payne, M.D. Fellow in Hematology and Oncology, University of Virginia School of Medicine, Charlottesville, VA
Anemias Caused by Decreased Erythrocyte Production

Richard Pazdur, M.D. Professor of Medicine and Assistant Vice President for Academic Affairs, University of Texas M.D. Anderson Cancer Center, Houston, TX
Pancreatic Cysts and Neoplasms

Starr P. Pearson, M.D. Assistant Professor of Medicine, Temple University School of Medicine, Philadelphia, PA
Quantitative Disorders of Granulocytes

Neal S. Penneys, M.D. Department of Dermatology, St. Louis University School of Medicine, St. Louis, MO
Skin Tumors

Mark A. Peppercorn, M.D. Associate Professor of Medicine, Harvard Medical School; Director, Center for Inflammatory Bowel Disease, Beth Israel Hospital, Boston, MA
Ulcerative Colitis and Crohn's Disease

Bruce Perlman, M.D. Assistant Professor of Clinical Medicine, University of Illinois at Chicago; Director of Electrophysiology, West Side Veterans Administration Hospital, Chicago, IL
Cardiac Arrhythmias

Ronald D. Perrone, M.D. Associate Professor of Medicine, Tufts University School of Medicine; Physician, Nephrology Division, New England Medical Center, Boston, MA
Chronic Renal Failure

Alan Pestronk, M.D. Professor of Neurology, Washington University School of Medicine, St. Louis, MO
Myasthenia Gravis

Jeffrey H. Peters, M.D. Assistant Professor of Surgery, University of Southern California School of Medicine; Chief, Section of General Surgery, USC University Hospital, Los Angeles, CA
Diaphragmatic Hernias

LoAnn Peterson, M.D. Professor, Northwestern University; Director of Hematopathology, Northwestern Memorial Hospital, Chicago, IL
Thalassemia

Martin D. Phillips, M.D. Assistant Professor in Internal Medicine (Hematology), University of Texas Medical School, Houston, TX
Bleeding Due to Intravascular Coagulation and Fibrinolysis

C. S. Pitchumoni, M.D., F.A.C.P., F.A.C.G. Professor of Medicine and Chairman, Department of Gastroenterology, Our Lady of Mercy Medical Center, Bronx; New York Medical College, Valhalla, NY
Intestinal Disaccharidase Deficiency

Hiram C. Polk, Jr., M.D. Ben A. Reid, Sr., Professor and Chairman, Department of Surgery, University of Louisville School of Medicine, Louisville, KY
Peritonitis and Intra-abdominal Abscesses

Claire Pomeroy, M.D. Associate Professor, Infectious Disease, University of Minnesota Medical School; Staff Physician, Infectious Disease, Veterans Affairs Medical Center, Minneapolis, MN
Mumps

David L. Porter, M.D. Assistant Professor of Medicine, University of Pennsylvania; Director, Allogeneic Bone Marrow Transplantation, Hospital of the University of Pennsylvania, Philadelphia, PA
Chronic Myelogenous Leukemia

Bertram A. Portin, M.D. Clinical Professor of Surgery, School of Medicine and Biomedical Sciences, State University of New York at Buffalo; Chief, Colon and Rectal Surgery, Sisters of Charity Hospital, Buffalo, NY
Anorectal and Perianal Disorders

Melvin R. Pratter, M.D. Professor, Division of Pulmonary and Critical Care Medicine, University of Medicine and Dentistry of New Jersey/Robert Wood Johnson Medical School at Camden; Head, Division of Pulmonary and Critical Care Medicine, Cooper Hospital/University Medical Center, Camden, NJ
Chronic Cough

L. Michael Prisant, M.D. Professor of Medicine, Medical College of Georgia School of Medicine, Augusta, GA
Hypertension

Rajiv K. Pruthi, M.D. Fellow in Hematology, Mayo Graduate School of Medicine, Rochester, MN
Pernicious Anemia and Other Megaloblastic Anemias

Martin A. Quan, M.D. Professor of Clinical Family Medicine, Director of Residency Training, UCLA Division of Family Medicine, and Director, Office of Continuing Medical Education, University of California, Los Angeles, School of Medicine, Los Angeles, CA
Pelvic Inflammatory Disease

Robert J. Quinet, M.D. Clinical Associate Professor of Medicine, Louisiana State University School of Medicine, and Clinical Assistant Professor of Medicine, Tulane University Medical School; Chief, Section on Rheumatology, Department of Medicine, Ochsner Clinic, New Orleans, LA
Whipple's Disease (Intestinal Lipodystrophy)

Jeffrey Rapp, M.D. Clinical Assistant Professor of Medicine, Thomas Jefferson University Hospital, Philadelphia, PA
Acquired Immunodeficiency Syndrome (AIDS)

G. Daniel Rath, M.D. Clinical Instructor, Department of Family Medicine, University of South Dakota School of Medicine, Sioux Falls; Staff Physician, Canton-Inwood Memorial Hospital, Canton, SD
Bladder and Ureteral Cancers

Jeffrey H. Reese, M.D. Clinical Associate Professor of Urology, Stanford University School of Medicine, Stanford; Associate Chief, Division of Urology, Santa Clara Valley Medical Center, San Jose, CA
Carcinoma of the Kidney

Robert V. Rege, M.D. Associate Professor, Surgery, Northwestern University School of Medicine; Acting Chief of Surgery, Veterans Administration Lakeside Medical Center, Chicago, IL
Disorders of the Gallbladder and Bile Ducts

James H. Reichheld, M.D. Fellow in Gastroenterology, University of Massachusetts Medical School; Physician, University of Massachusetts Medical Center, Worcester, MA
Ulcerative Colitis and Crohn's Disease

Anthony J. Reino, M.D., M.Sc. Assistant Professor of Clinical Otolaryngology, Mount Sinai School of Medicine, New York; Staff Physician, Veterans Affairs Medical Center, Bronx, NY
Neoplastic and Non-neoplastic Lesions of the Oral Mucosa

Virginia Rhodes, M.D. Oncologist and Hematologist, Grant/Riverside Hospitals, Columbus, OH
Pancreatic Cysts and Neoplasms

Jerome P. Richie, M.D. Elliott C. Cutler Professor of Surgery, and Chairman, Harvard Program in Urology (Longwood Area), Harvard Medical School; Chief of Urology, Brigham and Women's Hospital, Boston, MA
Intrascrotal Masses and Tumors

John A. Ridge, M.D., Ph.D. Assistant Professor, Temple University School of Medicine; Chief, Head and Neck Surgery Section, Fox Chase Cancer Center, Philadelphia, PA
Tumors of the Pharynx and Larynx

Robert J. Rizzo, M.D. Assistant Professor of Surgery, Harvard Medical School; Cardiac Surgeon, Brigham and Women's Hospital, Boston, MA
Aneurysms of the Aorta

Thomas N. Roberts, M.D. Assistant Clinical Professor, Pediatrics, University of Wisconsin, Madison; Attending, La Crosse Lutheran Hospital, La Crosse, WI
Otitis (Media and Externa)

Stephen H. Robinson, M.D. Professor of Medicine, Harvard Medical School; Chief, Division of Hematology, and Associate Chairman, Department of Medicine, Beth Israel Hospital, Boston, MA
Diseases of the Spleen

Sarah M. Roddy, M.D. Associate Professor of Pediatrics and Neurology, Loma Linda University School of Medicine, Loma Linda, CA
Tics

William E. Roland, M.D. Assistant Professor of Medicine, University of Missouri; Staff Physician, Harry S. Truman Memorial Veterans Hospital, Columbia, MO
Rickettsial Diseases

Steven J. Romano, M.D. Clinical Assistant Professor, Cornell University Medical College, New York, NY; Clinical Research Physician, Eli Lilly & Company, Indianapolis, IN
Anorexia and Bulimia

Clifford J. Rosen, M.D. Research Professor, University of Maine, Orono; Chief of Medicine, St. Joseph Hospital, Bangor, ME
Osteoporosis

Howard G. Rosenthal, M.D. Clinical Associate Professor, University of Missouri—Kansas City School of Medicine; Medical Director, Limb Preservation Institute, University of Missouri–Kansas City, Kansas City, MO
Tumors of Muscle and Soft Tissue

Ronnie Ann Rosenthal, M.D. Associate Professor of Surgery, Yale University School of Medicine, New Haven; Chief, General Surgery, Veterans Administration Medical Center, West Haven, CT
Hernias of the Abdominal Wall

Susan Rosenthal, M.D. Professor of Oncology in Medicine, University of Rochester School of Medicine and Dentistry; Chief of Medical Oncology, Rochester General Hospital, Rochester, NY
Breast Cancer

Leonard J. Rossoff, M.D. Assistant Professor of Medicine, Albert Einstein School of Medicine; Section Head, Pulmonary Medicine, Long Island Jewish Medical Center, New York, NY
Occupational Lung Disease

Ranjan Roy, M.D. Staff Physician, Department of Veterans Affairs Medical Center, Northport, NY
Polyarteritis Nodosa

Deborah Rubens, M.D. Associate Professor of Radiology, University of Rochester School of Medicine and Dentistry; Director of Ultrasound, Department of Radiology, University of Rochester Medical Center, Rochester, NY
Breast Cancer

Rebecca E. Rudolph, M.D. Research Fellow in Gastroenterology, University of Washington; Research Fellow in Cancer Prevention, Fred Hutchinson Cancer Research Center, Seattle, WA
Cirrhosis of the Liver

Stanley J. Russin, M.D. Associate Professor of Medicine, Deputy Chairman for Clinical Affairs, Chief of Section of General Internal Medicine, Department of Medicine, Temple University School of Medicine, Philadelphia, PA
Qualitative Disorders of Granulocytes

Gregory W. Rutecki, M.D. Associate Professor of Medicine and Associate Program Director, Northeastern Ohio Universities College of Medicine, Affiliated Hospitals at Canton, Canton, OH
Syndrome of Inappropriate Antidiuretic Hormone Secretion

Thomas J. Rutherford, M.D., Ph.D. Assistant Professor, Gynecologic Oncology, Yale University School of Medicine, New Haven, CT
Benign and Malignant Ovarian Tumors

Stephen J. Ryan, M.D. Assistant Professor, Department of Neurology, University of Kentucky, Lexington, KY
Poliomyelitis

Geronimo Sahagun, M.D. Fellow, Division of Gastroenterology, Oregon Health Sciences University, Portland, OR
Small Bowel Tumors

Roland Sakiyama, M.D., F.A.C.P. Professor of Family Medicine, University of California, Los Angeles, School of Medicine, Los Angeles, CA
Thyroiditis

William L. Salzer, M.D. Associate Professor of Medicine, University of Missouri-Columbia, Columbia, MO
Rickettsial Diseases

Mark H. Sanders, M.D. Associate Professor of Medicine and Anesthesiology, Division of Pulmonary, Allergy and Critical Care Medicine, University of Pittsburgh School of Medicine; Chief, Pulmonary Sleep Disorders Program, University of Pittsburgh Medical Center; Assistant Chief, Pulmonary Service, Veterans Affairs Medical Center, Pittsburgh, PA
Sleep-Related Upper Airway Obstruction

Jay P. Sanford, M.D. Clinical Professor of Medicine, University of Texas Southwestern Medical Center, Dallas, TX; Dean Emeritus and Professor of Military Medicine, Uniformed Services University of the Health Sciences, Bethesda, MD
Bacterial Zoonoses

Arif R. Sarwari, M.D. Fellow in Infectious Diseases, Department of Medicine, University of Maryland School of Medicine, Baltimore, MD
Fever

Joseph D. Schmidt, M.D. Professor of Surgery/Urology, University of California, San Diego, School of Medicine, San Diego; Head, Division of Urology, UCSD Medical Center, San Diego; Staff Physician, Veterans Affairs Medical Center, San Diego; Thornton Hospital, La Jolla, CA
Carcinoma of the Prostate

Paul Schoenfeld, M.D. Staff Cardiologist, Gundersen-Lutheran Heart Institute, La Crosse, WI
Pericardial Disease

Patricia Schram, M.D. Attending Physician, Lenox Hill Hospital, New York, NY
Congenital Adrenal Hyperplasia

David E. Schteingart, M.D. Professor of Internal Medicine, University of Michigan Medical School; Associate Division Chief for Clinical Affairs, Division of Endocrinology and Metabolism, University of Michigan Hospitals, Ann Arbor, MI
Endocrine Paraneoplastic Syndromes

H. Ralph Schumacher, Jr., M.D. Professor of Medicine, University of Pennsylvania School of Medicine; Director, Arthritis-Immunology Center, Veterans Affairs Medical Center, Philadelphia, PA
Septic Arthritis

M. David Schwalb, M.D. Clinical Assistant Professor, Urology, New York Medical College, Valhalla; Lincoln Hospital Attending, Bronx, NY
Obstructive Nephropathy

Peter E. Schwartz, M.D. Professor, Obstetrics and Gynecology, Division Director, Gynecologic Oncology, Vice Chairman, Department of Obstetrics and Gynecology, Yale University School of Medicine; Chief, Gynecologic Oncology, Yale-New Haven Medical Center, New Haven, CT
Benign and Malignant Ovarian Tumors

Robert A. Schwartz, M.D., M.P.H. Professor and Head, Dermatology, and Professor of Medicine, Pediatrics, Pathology, and Preventive Medicine, New Jersey Medical School; Chief, Dermatology Service, University of Medicine and Dentistry of New Jersey University Hospital, Newark, NJ
Chancroid; Granuloma Inguinale; Lymphogranuloma Venereum

Steven J. Scrivani, D.D.S. Professor, Harvard University; Fellow, Oral and Maxillofacial Surgery, and Assistant Surgeon, Massachusetts General Hospital, Boston, MA
Cephalic Neuralgias

Carlos Seas, M.D. Associate Professor, Universidad Peruana Cayetano Heredia, Instituto de Medicina Tropical "Alexander von Humboldt"; Attending Physician, Hospital Cayetano Heredia, Lima, Peru
Bacterial Diarrheas

E. James Seidmon, M.D. Professor of Urology, Temple University School of Medicine; Attending, Temple University Hospital, St. Christopher's Hospital for Children, Philadelphia, PA
Urethritis and Prostatitis

Joel L. Sereboff, Ph.D. Clinical Director, IMPACT, and CEO, Associated Assessment and Consulting Service, Owings Mills, MD
Substance Use Disorders

Om P. Sharma, M.D. Professor of Medicine, University of Southern California School of Medicine; Senior Physician, LAC-USC Medical Center, Los Angeles, CA
Interstitial Lung Disease

Kevin W. Shea, M.D. Assistant Clinical Instructor of Medicine, State University of New York at Stony Brook School of Medicine, Stony Brook; Fellow, Infectious Disease Division, Winthrop-University Hospital, Mineola, NY
Lyme Disease

Jeremy M. Shefner, M.D., Ph.D. Associate Professor of Neurology, Harvard Medical School; Director, Neurology Clinical Research Unit, Co-Director, Muscular Dystrophy Association Clinic, Brigham and Women's Hospital, Boston, MA
Motor Neuron Diseases

Elizabeth F. Sherertz, M.D. Professor of Dermatology, Bowman Gray School of Medicine of Wake Forest University, Winston-Salem, NC
Dermatitis

Ira A. Shulman, M.D. Professor, Pathology, University of Southern California, School of Medicine; Chief, Transfusion Medicine and Microbiology, LAC-USC Medical Center, Los Angeles, CA
Transfusion Reactions

Michael E. Shy, M.D. Associate Professor of Neurology and Molecular Medicine and Genetics, Wayne State University School of Medicine; Co-Director of Division of Neuromuscular Disease, Harper Hospital and Detroit Receiving Hospital, Detroit, MI
Peripheral Neuropathies

Richard T. Silver, M.D. Clinical Professor of Medicine, Cornell University Medical College; Attending Physician, The New York Hospital, New York, NY
Polycythemia Vera and Other Polycythemia Syndromes

Pamela Silverman, M.D. Assistant Professor of Psychiatry, Albert Einstein College of Medicine; Assistant Director, Division of Geriatric Psychiatry, Montefiore Medical Center, Bronx, NY
Geriatric Psychiatry

Gary L. Simon, M.D., Ph.D. Professor of Medicine, Biochemistry and Molecular Biology, Director, Division of Infectious Diseases, and Associate Chairman, Department of Medicine, George Washington University School of Medicine, Washington, DC
Sepsis and Septic Shock

Richard J. Simons, Jr., M.D. Associate Professor of Medicine, Associate Chairman for Education, Pennsylvania State University College of Medicine, Hershey, PA
Iatrogenesis

Donald A. Smith, M.D., M.P.H. Assistant Professor of Medicine and Community Medicine, Mount Sinai School of Medicine of the City University of New York; Assistant Attending, Mount Sinai Medical Center, New York, NY
Cardiovascular Risk Factors

Jack W. Snyder, M.D., J.D., Ph.D. Associate Professor of Emergency Medicine and Laboratory Medicine, Thomas Jefferson University, Philadelphia, PA
Disorders of Vitamin and Supplement Excess

Rosemary Soave, M.D. Associate Professor of Medicine and Public Health, Cornell University Medical College; Associate Attending Physician, The New York Hospital-Cornell Medical Center, New York, NY
Cryptosporidiosis

Perry W. Stafford, M.D. Assistant Professor of Pediatric Surgery, University of Pennsylvania School of Medicine; Director of Trauma and Surgical Critical Care, Children's Hospital of Philadelphia, Philadelphia, PA
Intestinal Obstruction

Samuel L. Stanley, Jr., M.D. Associate Professor, Departments of Medicine and Molecular Microbiology, Division of Infectious Diseases, Washington University School of Medicine; Attending, Jewish Hospital, and Chief Medical Consultant, Barnes Care Traveler's Health Center, Barnes Hospital, St. Louis, MO
Amebiasis

John R. Steinberg, M.D. Assistant Professor of Family Medicine and Psychiatry, University of Maryland School of Medicine, Baltimore, MD
Substance Use Disorders

David P. Stevens, M.D. Vice Dean and Professor of Medicine, Case Western Reserve School of Medicine, Cleveland, OH
Giardiasis

Michael B. Stevens, M.D. Associate Professor, Division of Family and Community Medicine, Stanford University School of Medicine, Stanford; Associate Director, San Jose Medical Center, Family Practice Residency Program, San Jose, CA
Headache and Facial Pain

Susan K. Stevens, M.D. Clinical Assistant Professor of Radiology, University of California, San Francisco School of Medicine, San Francisco; Staff Radiologist, Open MRI, Hayward, CA
Carcinoma of the Kidney

Ronald A. Stiller, M.D., Ph.D. Assistant Professor of Medicine, Division of Pulmonary, Allergy and Critical Care Medicine, University of Pittsburgh School of Medicine; Associate Director, Pulmonary Sleep Evaluation Center, Pittsburgh, PA
Sleep-Related Upper Airway Obstruction

Sheldon S. Stoffer, M.D., F.A.C.P., F.A.C.E. Endocrine Consultant, Oakland Internists-Sinai Hospital, Southfield, MI
Chronic Adrenal Insufficiency

Timothy E. Stone, M.D. Staff Physician, Bradford Health Services, Carraway Methodist Medical Center, Birmingham, AL
Somatoform Disorders

Dale W. Stovall, M.D. Assistant Professor, Department of Obstetrics and Gynecology, Division of Reproductive Endocrinology, University of Iowa College of Medicine, Iowa City, IA
Infertility

Larry J. Strausbaugh, M.D. Professor of Medicine, Oregon Health Sciences University, School of Medicine; Hospital Epidemiologist and Staff Physician, Veterans Affairs Medical Center, Portland, OR
Toxic Shock Syndrome

Michael B. Streiff, M.D. Senior Clinical Fellow, Division of Hematology, Johns Hopkins University School of Medicine, Baltimore, MD
Myelodysplastic Syndromes and Sideroblastic Anemias

Judy A. Streit, M.D. Fellow-Associate, Division of Infectious Diseases, University of Iowa Hospitals and Clinics, Iowa City, IA
Leishmaniasis

G. Thomas Strickland, M.D., Ph.D. Professor of International Health; Epidemiology and Preventive Medicine; Microbiology and Immunology; and Medicine; and Director, International Health Program, University of Maryland School of Medicine, Baltimore, MD
Schistosomiasis

Patrick J. Strollo, Jr., M.D. Assistant Professor of Medicine, Division of Pulmonary, Allergy, and Critical Care Medicine, University of Pittsburgh School of Medicine; Associate Director, Pulmonary Sleep Evaluation Center, and Director, Pulmonary Sleep Disorders Training Program, Pittsburgh, PA
Sleep-Related Upper Airway Obstruction

José S. Subauste, M.D. Assistant Professor of Medicine, University of Mississippi; Staff Physician, Veterans Administration Hospital, Jackson, MS
Endocrine Paraneoplastic Syndromes

Byungse Suh, M.D., Ph.D. Professor of Medicine, Microbiology and Immunology, Section of Infectious Diseases, Temple University School of Medicine; Attending Physician, Temple University Hospital, Philadelphia, PA
Infections of the Urinary Tract

John L. Sullivan, M.D. Professor of Pediatrics, University of Massachusetts Medical Center; Division Director, Immunology and Rheumatology, University of Massachusetts Medical Center, Worcester, MA
Benign and Malignant Histiocytic and Dendritic Cell Disorders

Faisal Sultan, M.B.B.S. Fellow in Infectious Diseases, Department of Medicine, Washington University School of Medicine, St. Louis, MO
Amebiasis

Imad A. Tabbara, M.D., F.A.C.P. Associate Professor of Medicine, George Washington University School of Medicine; Attending Physician and Director, Bone Marrow Transplant Program, George Washington University Medical Center, Washington, DC
Hemolytic Anemia Caused by Erythrocyte Enzyme Deficiency

Duane W. Taebel, M.D., F.A.C.P., F.A.C.G. Attending Physician, Gundersen Lutheran Medical Center, La Crosse, WI
Nausea, Vomiting, and Dyspepsia

Ira N. Targoff, M.D. Associate Professor, Department of Medicine, University of Oklahoma Health Sciences Center, Oklahoma City, OK
Polymyositis and Dermatomyositis

Nancy O. Tatum, M.D. Assistant Professor, Department of Family Medicine, University of Mississippi Medical Center, Jackson, MS
Delirium and Dementia

Ayalew Tefferi, M.D. Consultant, Division of Hematology and Internal Medicine, Mayo Clinic and Mayo Foundation; Assistant Professor of Medicine, Mayo Medical School, Rochester, MN
Pernicious Anemia and Other Megaloblastic Anemias

Ronald F. Teitler, M.D. Clinical Instructor in Surgery, State University of New York at Buffalo, School of Medicine and Biomedical Sciences, Buffalo, NY
Anorectal and Perianal Disorders

Edward E. Telzak, M.D. Associate Professor, Departments of Medicine and Epidemiology and Social Medicine, Albert Einstein College of Medicine; Chief, Division of Infectious Diseases, Bronx-Lebanon Hospital Center, Bronx, NY
Tuberculosis

Bradley C. Thaemert, M.D. Resident, General Surgery, Gundersen Lutheran Medical Center, La Crosse, WI
Acute Abdominal Pain

Isabelle Thomas, M.D. Assistant Professor, Department of Dermatology, New Jersey Medical School, University of Medicine and Dentistry of New Jersey, Newark; Chief, Dermatology Service, East Orange Veterans Affairs Medical Center, East Orange, NJ
Lymphogranuloma Venereum

Jerry S. Trier, M.D. Professor of Medicine, Harvard Medical School; Senior Physician, Brigham and Women's Hospital, Boston, MA
Celiac Sprue

Theodore F. Tsai, M.D., M.P.H. Medical Officer, Centers for Disease Control and Prevention, Ft. Collins, CO
Viral Hemorrhagic Fevers and Hantavirus Pulmonary Syndrome

Michael L. Tuck, M.D. Professor of Medicine, University of California, Los Angeles, School of Medicine, Los Angeles; Chief, Endocrinology and Metabolism, UCLA San Fernando Valley Medical Program, Veterans Administration Hospital, Sepulveda, CA
Primary Aldosteronism

Nadine M. Tung, M.D. Instructor in Medicine, Harvard Medical School; Associate in Medicine, Beth Israel Hospital, Boston, MA
Diseases of the Spleen

Glenn Turett, M.D. Assistant Professor, Albert Einstein College of Medicine; Attending Physician, Division of Infectious Diseases, Bronx-Lebanon Hospital Center, Bronx, NY
Tuberculosis

George Tweddel, M.D. Clinical Instructor, Obstetrics and Gynecology/Reproductive Sciences, University of Medicine and Dentistry of New Jersey, Robert Wood Johnson Medical School; Staff, Robert Wood Johnson University Hospital, New Brunswick, NJ
The Menopause

Mary Lee Vance, M.D. Professor of Medicine and Neurosurgery, University of Virginia School of Medicine, Charlottesville, VA
Hypopituitarism

Chitra Venkatraman, M.D. Fellow, Hematology/Oncology, George Washington University Medical Center, Washington, DC
Hemolytic Anemia Caused by Erythrocyte Enzyme Deficiency

Joseph Venzor, M.D. Senior Fellow, Immunology Section, Department of Medicine, Baylor College of Medicine; Senior Fellow, Baylor College of Medicine Affiliated Hospitals, Houston, TX
Urticaria

Thomas R. Viggiano, M.D. Associate Professor of Medicine, Mayo Medical School; Consultant, Internal Medicine, Gastroenterology, and Geriatric Medicine, Mayo Clinic, Rochester, MN
Peptic Ulcer Disease

Miriam T. Vincent, M.D. Associate Professor, Interim Chair, Department of Family Practice, State University of New York Health Science Center at Brooklyn; Chief of Service, Family Practice, Kings County Hospital Center, Brooklyn, NY
Anaerobic Lung Infections

Evan Vosburgh, M.D. Assistant Professor of Medicine, Boston University School of Medicine; Associate Chief, Section of Hematology and Oncology, Boston University Medical Center Hospital, Boston, MA
Hemophilia and Other Inherited Hemostatic Disorders

David G. Vossler, M.D. Clinical Assistant Professor of Neurology, University of Washington; Director, Neurodiagnostic Laboratory, Swedish Medical Center, Seattle, WA
Epilepsy and Seizure Disorders

Mark R. Wallace, M.D. Director, Infectious Disease Fellowship, Naval Medical Center, San Diego, CA
Malaria

Richard J. Wallace, Jr., M.D. Professor of Medicine, John Chapman Professorship in Microbiology, and Chairman, Department of Microbiology, University of Texas Health Center at Tyler, Tyler, TX
Nontuberculous Mycobacterial Infections

Richard L. Ward, Ph.D. Research Professor, University of Cincinnati; Staff, Division of Infectious Diseases, Children's Hospital Medical Center, Cincinnati, OH
Viral Gastroenteritis

John R. Waterman, M.D. Assistant Professor of Medicine, University of Connecticut School of Medicine; Staff, University of Connecticut Health Center, Farmington, CT
Bursitis and Tendinitis

Mary E. Watson, M.D. Clinical Instructor, University of South Dakota School of Medicine, Sioux Falls; Staff, Canton-Inwood Memorial Hospital, Canton; Sioux Valley Hospital, Sioux Falls, SD
Bladder and Ureteral Cancers

Gayle J. Weaver, M.D. Infectious Disease Physician, St. Joseph's Hospital, Syracuse, NY
Infections of the Urinary Tract

Mary C. Weber, M.D. Clinical Assistant Professor of Psychiatry, Indiana University School of Medicine; Staff, Indiana University Hospitals, Indianapolis, IN
Conversion Disorders, Malingering, and Dissociative Disorders

Benjamin Wedro, M.D. Clinical Assistant Professor, Department of Medicine, University of Wisconsin, Madison; Staff, Department of Emergency Medicine, Gundersen Clinic, La Crosse, WI
Approach to the Patient in the Emergency Department

Louis M. Weiss, M.D., M.P.H. Associate Professor of Medicine and Pathology, Albert Einstein College of Medicine; Attending Physician, The Jack D. Weiler Hospital/Montefiore Medical Center, Bronx Municipal Hospital, Bronx, NY
Other Cestodes

Howard H. Weitz, M.D. Clinical Associate Professor of Medicine, Jefferson Medical College of Thomas Jefferson University; Director, Division of Cardiology, Thomas Jefferson University Hospital, Philadelphia, PA
Perioperative Medical Consultation

Jeanna L. Welborn, M.D. Associate Professor, Internal Medicine and Pathology, University of California at Davis Medical Center, Sacramento, CA
Anemia

Peter F. Weller, M.D. Professor of Medicine, Harvard Medical School; Chief, Infectious Diseases Division, Beth Israel Hospital, Boston, MA
Hypereosinophilic Syndrome

Sandra S. Hsu Werbel, M.D. Assistant Professor of Internal Medicine, Section on Endocrinology and Metabolism, Bowman Gray School of Medicine of Wake Forest University, Winston-Salem, NC
Acute Adrenal Insufficiency

Giles F. Whalen, M.D. Associate Professor of Surgery, University of Connecticut School of Medicine; Attending Surgeon, University of Connecticut Health Sciences Center, Farmington, CT
Appendicitis

Munsey S. Wheby, M.D., F.A.C.P. Professor and Interim Chair, Department of Internal Medicine, University of Virginia School of Medicine, Charlottesville, VA
Anemias Caused by Decreased Erythrocyte Production

Jane V. White, Ph.D., R.D. Professor, Department of Family Medicine, Graduate School of Medicine, University of Tennessee, Knoxville, TN
Nutrient Deficiency Disorders

Frederick C. Whittier, M.D. Professor and Program Director, Internal Medicine, Northeastern Ohio Universities College of Medicine, Affiliated Hospitals at Canton, Canton, OH
Syndrome of Inappropriate Antidiuretic Hormone Secretion

Mary E. Wilson, M.D. Associate Professor, Department of Internal Medicine and Department of Microbiology, University of Iowa; Staff Physician, Iowa City Veterans Affairs Medical Center, Iowa City, IA
Leishmaniasis

Murray Wittner, M.D., Ph.D. Professor of Pathology and Parasitology, Albert Einstein College of Medicine; Attending Physician, Director, Parasitology and Tropical Medicine Clinic, Director, Parasitology and Tropical Medicine Laboratory, Jacobi Medical Center, Bronx, NY
Other Cestodes; Other Intestinal Parasites

Bruce A. Woda, M.D. Professor of Pathology, University of Massachusetts Medical Center, Worcester, MA
Benign and Malignant Histiocytic and Dendritic Cell Disorders

Judith E. Wolf, M.D. Clinical Associate Professor of Medicine, University of Pennsylvania School of Medicine; Attending Physician, Infectious Diseases Unit, The Graduate Hospital, Philadelphia, PA
Syphilis; Infective Endocarditis

Bartholomew O'Beirne Woods, M.D. Assistant Clinical Professor, Department of Medicine, Tufts University School of Medicine, Boston; Senior Staff Physician, Consultant in Vascular Medicine and Hypertension, Lahey Hitchcock Clinic, Burlington, MA
Chronic Arterial Occlusive Disease of the Lower Extremity

Timothy A. Woodward, M.D. Assistant Professor of Medicine, Mayo Clinic, Rochester, MN; Staff Physician, St. Luke's Hospital, Jacksonville, FL
Neoplasms of the Stomach

Hilary Worthen, M.D. Instructor in Medicine, Harvard Medical School, Boston; Attending Physician, Cambridge Hospital, Cambridge, MA
Genetic Disease

Paul W. Wright, M.D. Professor of Family Practice, University of Texas Health Center at Tyler, Tyler, TX
Nontuberculous Mycobacterial Infections

Allen R. Wyler, M.D. Medical Director, Neurosciences, Swedish Medical Center, Seattle, WA
Epilepsy and Seizure Disorders

Woon-Chee Yee, M.D. Assistant Professor in Neurology, Washington University School of Medicine, St. Louis, MO
Myasthenia Gravis

Jong-Yoon Yi, M.D. Fellow in Hypertension, Rush Medical College; Instructor in Preventive Medicine, Rush-Presbyterian/St. Luke's Medical Center, Chicago, IL
Pheochromocytoma

Leo J. Yoder, M.D. Chief of Medicine, Gillis W. Long Hansen's Disease Center, U.S. Public Health Service, Carville, LA
Leprosy (Hansen's Disease)

John A. Zaia, M.D. Professor of Pediatrics and Director, Virology and Infectious Diseases, City of Hope National Medical Center, Duarte, CA
Cytomegalovirus Infections

Susan M. Zurowski, M.D. Staff, Boone Hospital Center, Columbia, MO
Mycosis Fungoides and Sézary Syndrome

Preface

It has been a challenging and gratifying experience to prepare a new edition of *Current Diagnosis,* a text that has been used by the medical community, both here and abroad, for more than 30 years. The task has been challenging because the rapid developments in medicine have required nine new editions during this time, and each new edition has involved a search for more than 400 expert physicians who could accept our invitation to write on well over 200 topics. Publication of another completely revised and rewritten edition of *Current Diagnosis* indicates that a single-volume source of the best currently available information on medical diagnosis has been useful to a large group of practicing physicians, and this usefulness is the source of the gratifying experience.

The utility and, inevitably, the viability of a medical book are not determined by publishers, editors, or authors; this judgment is made by the readers who use the book in their practices or in their medical studies. The success of *Current Diagnosis* can be attributed to the editorial objectives adopted for the first edition in 1966 and followed in all subsequent editions. *Current Diagnosis* was never intended to be a comprehensive textbook of medicine, which must include information on etiology, pathogenesis, epidemiology, and treatment, as well as diagnosis. The editorial objectives remain unchanged in this edition: to bring together in concise, definitive articles the best available current information on medical diagnosis to assist the physician in arriving at the correct diagnosis as efficiently as possible. While the accumulation of new medical information mandates the periodic revision of most medical books, one of our objectives is to provide a fresh, critical look at all of the available information, both new and old. Authors were asked not only to describe the diagnostic procedures that will assist in leading to the correct diagnosis but also to mention previously used procedures that have become obsolete. Common diagnostic errors, identified as "pitfalls," are discussed in most of the articles. Significant changes, made independently by many authors, include data on diagnostic sensitivity and specificity as well as suggestions for cost-effective approaches to diagnosis. The former suggests development of a more critical attitude toward the usefulness of diagnostic procedures, while the latter reflects the current medical environment, which requires more intense scrutiny of the cost of medical care.

This edition retains the format used in previous editions. The first section covers the differential diagnosis of frequently encountered clinical problems, while the following sections discuss specific disease entities or clinical conditions grouped according to etiology or organ system. Many articles refer the reader to other articles on related topics, and a comprehensive index will lead the reader to all locations in the book that mention a specific sign, symptom, syndrome, or condition. This edition contains articles on 293 topics selected because they are of interest to many practicing physicians. We have attempted to respond to suggestions from readers of previous editions, and new articles reflect more widespread interest in areas such as domestic violence, sports medicine, iatrogenic diseases, disorders due to excessive vitamin and dietary supplement intake, and computer-assisted diagnosis. Although it was not possible to include comprehensive coverage in some areas, this edition contains articles on suggested approaches to skin disorders and diseases of the eye. Other new topics, such as the difficult patient and the emergency patient, were included because physicians in all types of practice encounter them. To restrain growth in the size of the book, some topics were combined, such as articles on abdominal pain in children and in adults.

Contributors were selected not only because they are familiar with recent advances in their fields but also because they are physicians who apply this information in daily patient care. To ensure that the information in *Current Diagnosis* is truly current, new contributors have been selected to write the vast majority of articles appearing in this edition. Progressive improvement in the articles is a result of this policy because virtually all physician-authors will accept the challenge of attempting to enhance a previously published article.

For this edition, the number of editors has grown from one to three. This increase permitted review of each manuscript by at least two, and sometimes three, editors and greatly reduced editorial stress. The three editors would like to thank many colleagues at Thomas Jefferson University for suggestions on topics and potential authors, and especially to thank those who are among the authors. The W.B. Saunders Company has been a most understanding and helpful publisher, and special thanks go to Raymond Kersey, Senior Acquisitions Editor; David Kilmer, Developmental Editor; Gina Scala, Copy Editing Supervisor; Shelley Hampton, Production Manager; Ellen Zanolle, Senior Book Designer; and Christine Cantera, Cover Designer. The editors also express their thanks to the Editorial Assistant for this edition, Ms. Loretta Jacobs, who kept track of all manuscripts, galley proofs, and page proofs, and saw that the authors and editors adhered to the publication schedule. Above all, of course, the editors express their thanks to the more than 400 authors who took time from their professional and personal activities to write for *Current Diagnosis*. To them we are truly grateful.

REX B. CONN, M.D.
WILLIAM Z. BORER, M.D.
JACK W. SNYDER, M.D.
Philadelphia, Pennsylvania

NOTICE

Medicine is an ever-changing field. Standard safety precautions must be followed, but as new research and clinical experience broaden our knowledge, changes in treatment and drug therapy become necessary or appropriate. The editors of this work have carefully checked the generic and trade drug names and verified drug dosages to ensure that the dosage information in this work is accurate and in accord with the standards accepted at the time of publication. Readers are advised, however, to check the product information currently provided by the manufacturer of each drug to be administered to be certain that changes have not been made in the recommended dose or in the contraindications for administration. This is of particular importance in regard to new or infrequently used drugs. It is the responsibility of the treating physicians, relying on experience and knowledge of the patient, to determine dosages and the best treatment for the patient. The editors cannot be responsible for misuse or misapplication of the material in this work.

THE PUBLISHER

Contents

Helminthic and Other Parasitic Diseases

Section Three
EAR, NOSE, AND THROAT

Section Four
RESPIRATORY SYSTEM

Section Five
CARDIOVASCULAR SYSTEM

Section Six
BLOOD AND BLOOD-FORMING ORGANS

Section Seven
GASTROINTESTINAL TRACT

Section Eight
METABOLIC DISEASE

Section Nine
ENDOCRINE SYSTEM

Section Ten
NERVOUS SYSTEM

Section Eleven
PSYCHIATRY

Section Twelve
MUSCLE, BONE, AND JOINT DISORDERS

Section Thirteen
CONNECTIVE TISSUE AND AUTOIMMUNE DISORDERS

Section Fourteen
GENITOURINARY SYSTEM

Section Fifteen
GYNECOLOGIC MEDICINE

Section One

DIAGNOSTIC PROBLEMS

FEVER

By Arif R. Sarwari, M.D.,
and Philip A. Mackowiak, M.D.
Baltimore, Maryland

Fever is a complex physiologic response to disease in which body temperature is increased above the normal range as a result of the action of pyrogenic cytokines on the hypothalamic thermoregulatory center. In adult humans, body temperature (as reflected by oral readings) is usually tightly controlled between 35.6 and 37.7°C (96.0 and 99.9°F) and exhibits a circadian rhythm characterized by an evening peak and an early morning trough. Such circadian rhythmicity is maintained during fever, even during conditions such as bacterial endocarditis, in which circulating concentrations of exogenous pyrogens (i.e., bacteria) are constant throughout the day.

THERMOMETRY

In defining the febrile state, the quantitative effects of anatomic site and oral stimulation on estimates of body temperature must be considered. In adults, mean rectal temperatures exceed concurrent oral temperatures by 0.4 ± 0.4°C (0.8 ± 0.7°F), which in turn exceed concurrent tympanic membrane temperatures by 0.4 ± 1.1°C (0.7 ± 2.0°F). Tympanic membrane readings show significantly more intrasubject and intersubject variability than rectal or oral temperatures, especially when cerumen is present in the external canal. Mastication, smoking, and exercise cause significant increases in oral temperature that may persist for periods of approximately 20 minutes.

UTILITY OF FEVER

Considerable data indicate that fever and its mediators have the capacity both to potentiate and to impair resistance to infection. Phylogenetic studies, for example, have shown the febrile response to be widespread within the animal kingdom. Such data constitute some of the most persuasive evidence that fever is an adaptive response, based on the argument that this metabolically expensive rise in body temperature would not have evolved and been so faithfully preserved within the animal kingdom unless fever had some net benefit to the host. Nevertheless, there are equally convincing data to suggest that the mediators of the febrile response (i.e., pyrogenic cytokines such as tumor necrosis factor [TNF] and interleukin-1 [IL-1]) also contribute to the morbidity and mortality of gram-negative sepsis. It is difficult to reconcile these apparently contradictory observations if they are viewed solely from the standpoint of the individual. However, when viewed from the perspective of the species, both fever's salutary effects on mild to moderately severe infections and its pernicious influence on fulminating infections become plausible. If one accepts preservation of the species, rather than survival of the individual, as the essence of evolution, fever and its mediators may have evolved as mechanisms both for accelerating recovery of individuals from localized or mild to moderately severe systemic infections in the interest of continued propagation of the species and for hastening the elimination of fulminantly infected individuals who pose a threat of epidemic disease to the species.

THERMOREGULATION

The preoptic area of the anterior hypothalamus is the thermal control center responsible for establishing the body's thermal set-point. This area is the site of integration of thermal stimuli, and through its input into the autonomic nervous system, it initiates thermal homeostatic mechanisms. These mechanisms include both physiologic and behavioral responses. An increase in blood flow to the skin, sweating, and moving to a cooler environment increase heat loss, whereas a decrease in blood flow to the skin, shivering, and the use of heavy clothing decrease heat loss and increase heat production.

The postulated physiologic pathway for the febrile response suggests an indirect effect of exogenous pyrogens (e.g., bacteria and viruses) on the hypothalamic thermoregulatory center, which is mediated by endogenous pyrogens produced by activated leukocytes. The principal endogenous pyrogens currently recognized are IL-1, IL-2, IL-6, TNF, interferon (IF) and prostaglandin E_2 (PGE_2), all of which are capable of raising the thermal set-point of the thermoregulatory center (Fig. 1).

FEVER OF UNKNOWN ORIGIN

In clinical practice, most febrile illnesses are caused by readily apparent infections of the respiratory, genitourinary, or gastrointestinal systems. A few, however, are persistent and go undiagnosed despite intensive investigation. These disorders belong to a class known as "fever of unknown origin," or FUO. In general, a febrile illness is designated a FUO only if:

1. Fever has persisted for at least 2 to 3 weeks.
2. Oral temperatures of at least 38.3°C (101°F) have been documented on several occasions.
3. There has been a failure to establish a diagnosis after at least 1 week of intensive study.

Etiology

Although the list of possible causes of FUO is long and complex, most cases are ultimately proved to be caused by common diseases presenting in an atypical fashion. The three most common causes of FUO are infections, which account for more than one third of patients reported in most series; malignant neoplasms, which account for about a fifth of such patients; and connective tissue disorders,

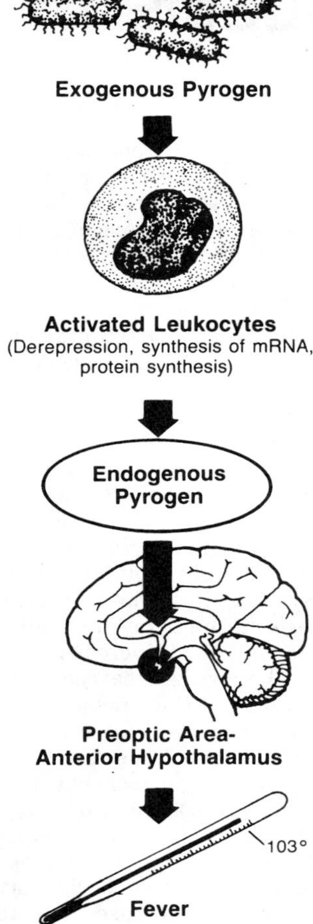

Figure 1. Postulated physiologic pathway for fever. (From Mackowiak, P.A.: *In* Kelley, W.N. [ed.]: Textbook of Internal Medicine, 2nd ed. Philadelphia, J.B. Lippincott, 1992, p. 1616, with permission.)

which account for approximately 10 per cent. The remainder of patients suffer from a variety of less common conditions (Table 1).

Infections

Infections responsible for FUO can be divided into two general categories: systemic and localized infections. Tuberculosis and endocarditis are two of the most important systemic infections. Most of the cases of tuberculosis presenting as FUO are disseminated infections, occurring among frail, elderly persons and those with acquired immunodeficiency syndrome (AIDS) or chronic alcoholism. Subacute bacterial endocarditis, another important cause of FUO, has changed in presentation in recent years, in that patients with this disorder tend to be diagnosed earlier in the course of their illness than in the past. As a result, clubbing, splenomegaly, splinter hemorrhages, and other classic stigmata of endocarditis are now uncommon findings when such patients first seek medical attention. In addition, prior antibiotic therapy may cause difficulty in isolating the causative bacterium from initial blood cultures. In other instances, positive cultures of the fastidious or slowly growing bacteria responsible for the infections (e.g., *Haemophilus aphrophilus* or *Cardiobacterium hominis*) require special culture media or prolonged periods of incubation. Similar difficulties are encountered in diagnosing endocarditis caused by organisms such as *Aspergillus* species, other fungi, and *Coxiella burnetii*. Each are potential etiologic agents in cases of culture-negative endocarditis. Marantic endocarditis—a thrombotic, nonmicrobial form of endocarditis—is clinically indistinguishable from bacterial endocarditis and should be considered in the cancer patient with signs or symptoms of endocarditis and sterile blood cultures.

Occasionally, localized infections are causes of FUO. Liver abscess, due to either bacteria or amebae, and cholangitis may produce fever without obvious hepatomegaly or jaundice. Other sites of occult abscesses that cause FUO are the subphrenic area, the pelvis, the pericholecystic area, the perinephric space, and the prostate.

Neoplasms

In patients with FUO, lymphomas deserve special attention, because they are responsible for as many as 40 per cent of patients in some series. Although both Hodgkin's and non-Hodgkin's lymphomas usually present with readily identifiable lymphadenopathy and/or hepatosplenomegaly, such presentation is not always the case. Diagnostic difficulty arises when disease is confined to the abdomen or retroperitoneal area. In such cases fever, FUO, may be the only manifestation of the underlying lymphoma.

Rarely, leukemias present as protracted febrile illnesses. Patients with such leukemias usually are pancytopenic and do not exhibit leukemic cells in the peripheral blood. The correct diagnosis is established by demonstrating malignant cells in a bone marrow aspirate or biopsy.

Renal cell carcinoma (hypernephroma) and hepatoma are two of the most important solid tumors that cause FUO. Both malignant neoplasms also occasionally produce paraneoplastic abnormalities, such as polycythemia and hypoglycemia. Malignant neoplasms of virtually any organ may be associated with fever. Among the metastatic neoplasms, those involving the liver are especially likely to be associated with prolonged febrile courses.

Collagen Vascular Diseases

In adults, the collagen vascular diseases most likely to cause FUO are the vasculitides and adult Still's disease. The latter disorder usually affects young adults and presents with high fever, rash, and intense arthralgias and myalgias. Since there is no specific test for adult Still's disease, the diagnosis is based purely on clinical grounds. Today, diseases such as rheumatoid arthritis and systemic lupus erythematosus seldom elude diagnosis for long, even when they present as febrile disorders. Giant cell arteritis and polymyalgia rheumatica, however, may be occult causes of FUO and should be considered in elderly patients with prolonged fever, anemia, and markedly increased erythrocyte sedimentation rates (ESR).

Granulomatous Diseases

Sarcoidosis occasionally presents as FUO and may be particularly difficult to diagnose when localized to organs other than the lung. Idiopathic granulomatous hepatitis may also present with fever as its only manifestation, as may granulomatous colitis and regional enteritis on rare occasions.

Table 1. Diseases Responsible for Fever of Unknown Origin (FUO)

Infections

Pyrogenic Infections

Abdominal, upper
- Subphrenic abscess
- Hepatic abscess
- Subhepatic abscess
- Splenic abscess
- Cholecystitis
- Cholangitis
- Lesser sac abscess

Abdominal, lower
- Diverticular abscess
- Appendiceal abscess
- Pelvic abscess

Renal infections
Osteomyelitis
Sinusitis
Mycotic aneurysm
Wound infection
Catheter infection
Whipple's disease

Mycobacterial and Granulomatous Infections

Mycobacterium tuberculosis
Atypical mycobacterial infections
Fungal and higher bacterial infections (candidiasis, histoplasmosis, nocardiosis, actinomycosis)

Bacteremias

Subacute bacterial endocarditis
Brucellosis
Listeriosis
Typhoid fever
Gonococcemia
Meningococcemia (chronic)

Viral, Rickettsial, and Chlamydial Infections

Human immunodeficiency virus (HIV)
Cytomegalovirus
Epstein-Barr virus
Coxsackievirus group B
Q fever
Psittacosis

Parasitic Infections

Amebiasis
Trichinosis
Malaria
Babesiosis

Spirochetal Infections

Borrelia recurrentis
Syphilis
Lyme disease
Leptospirosis

Neoplasms

Tumors of the Reticuloendothelial System

Lymphoma
Leukemia
Malignant histiocytosis
Lymphomatoid granulomatosis

Solid Tumors

Hypernephroma
Hepatoma
Pancreatic carcinoma
Atrial myxoma
Other intra-abdominal tumors

Metastatic Tumors

From gastrointestinal tract
From lungs, kidneys, and bone
Melanoma

Connective Tissue and Immune Disorders

Systemic lupus erythematosus
Rheumatic fever
Still's disease
Giant cell arteritis
Polymyalgia rheumatica
Polyarteritis nodosa
Hypersensitivity vasculitis

Granulomatous Diseases

Sarcoidosis
Granulomatous colitis
Granulomatous hepatitis

Miscellaneous Causes

Drug fever
Factitious fever
Hematomas
Multiple pulmonary emboli
Subacute thyroiditis
Familial Mediterranean fever
Nonspecific pericarditis

Undiagnosed FUO

Drugs

Drugs must always be considered as a cause of persistent fever. Many and possibly all drugs have the capacity to induce fever as an adverse reaction. Fever induced by drugs may result from a pharmacologic effect of the drug, an idiosyncratic reaction, or a complication related to administration of the drug (e.g., phlebitis). Most cases of drug-induced fever appear to be immune-mediated reactions to the offending agent. Certain drugs, such as alphamethyldopa, quinidine, and penicillin, appear to be particularly prone to causing such reactions. The time between initiation of administration of a drug and the onset of fever induced by the drug varies, with antineoplastic agents having some of the shortest lag times and cardiac drugs some of the longest. The interval between initiation of drug therapy and the onset of drug-induced fever is occasionally extremely long and, in rare cases, may exceed a year. The average lag time has been reported to be 6 days for antineoplastic agents, 8 days for antimicrobial agents, and 45 days for cardiac drugs. In patients with suspected drug fever, a history of prior drug allergy is elicited in only 10 per cent of patients.

Generally, drug fever is a diagnosis of exclusion made in a febrile patient whose fever abates within 24 to 72 hours of discontinuing the suspected pyrogenic medication.

Miscellaneous Causes

A variety of uncommon disorders are responsible for as many as 25 per cent of episodes of FUO. Occult hematomas and multiple pulmonary emboli are two such disorders. Factitious fever is another and should be considered in the chronically febrile young woman with a history of psychiatric illness and/or a background of having worked in the medical field. Familial Mediterranean fever, another rare cause of FUO, is a hereditary disorder characterized by recurrent episodes of unexplained fever, frequently accompanied by peritonitis, pleuritis, and arthritis and seen primarily among males of Armenian, Sephardic Jewish, and Arab descent.

DIAGNOSTIC WORK-UP

Probably nowhere else in clinical medicine is a systematic approach to diagnosis as important as it is in the work-up of FUO. The history and physical examination are the cornerstones of this evaluation. In cases that elude diagnosis for protracted periods, it may be necessary to repeat a complete history and physical examination at regular intervals. Meticulous attention to every aspect of the review of systems, travel and occupational history, and information about food and animal exposures may provide vital clues to diagnosis. In the physical examination, particular attention should be given to the funduscopic evaluation, palpation of less prominent lymph node chains (e.g., epitrochlear and occipital), and examination of the prostate, testis, and epididymis. An epididymal nodule, for example, may be the sole manifestation of extrapulmonary tuberculosis.

Given the wide range of possible diagnoses, blood tests ordered reflexively generally fail to provide useful new information. Laboratory testing in FUO must be tailored to specific ongoing diagnostic hypotheses. The initial studies should include a complete blood count, urinalysis, biochemical tests (including hepatic enzyme determinations), chest radiograph, and tuberculin skin test. The ESR, although nonspecific, may be helpful if it is found to be markedly elevated. Blood should be drawn for culture at least two or three times (two sets each time), and the microbiology laboratory alerted to the need to process such cultures with particular attention to fastidious microorganisms. Other tests that may be useful in the preliminary evaluation include thyroid function tests, creatine kinase (CK) activity, lumbar puncture, and serologic tests for connective tissue disorders.

In the patient with FUO, the chest radiograph may reveal evidence of tuberculosis, lymphoma, carcinoma, or an abnormal diaphragm contour suggestive of a subphrenic abscess. In the past, gastrointestinal radiographic studies were used to evaluate the upper and lower gastrointestinal tract. Today, however, endoscopic procedures are more commonly used for this purpose. An abdominal ultrasound examination is useful in detecting subphrenic, subhepatic, splenic and hepatic abscesses as well as lymphadenopathy and other masses in the abdomen and retroperitoneal area. The computed tomography (CT) scan is similarly useful and can also detect intracranial pathology, sinus disease, and pulmonary disorders not evident on the standard chest radiograph. Angiography may be required to establish a diagnosis of cranial vasculitis or polyarteritis nodosa. Echocardiography is useful in identifying valvular vegetations in the patient with suspected endocarditis.

Radioisotope scans only occasionally provide clinically useful information in the evaluation of the patient with FUO. The liver-spleen scan has for the most part been replaced by the ultrasound and CT scan. However, the ventilation-perfusion scan is useful in evaluating pulmonary emboli as a potential cause of FUO. Gallium and indium scans are occasionally useful as crude screening tests for areas of localized inflammation that can be evaluated with more sensitive examinations such as CT and magnetic resonance imaging (MRI).

In some cases, tissue biopsies for microbiologic and histologic examination are required to establish a definitive diagnosis. Bone marrow biopsies should be considered in patients with abnormal complete blood cell counts. Such biopsies are useful in diagnosing not only leukemia and lymphoma but also disseminated tuberculosis and histoplasmosis. Similarly, biopsies of clinically abnormal skin, muscle, or lung may prove diagnostic in appropriate cases.

THERAPEUTIC TRIALS

A clinical diagnosis may be strongly suspected but may remain histologically or microbiologically unconfirmed. In such circumstances, a therapeutic trial may be considered. Antituberculosis therapy, for example, may be instituted as a therapeutic trial in suspected cases of extrapulmonary tuberculosis. Similarly, corticosteroids may be administered empirically in patients with persistent fever and a suspected autoimmune disorder. Such empirical treatments, when effective in relieving fever and other manifestations of FUO, constitute both effective therapy and indirect support for the suspected diagnosis.

DIAGNOSTIC FAILURE

In 5 to 20 per cent of patients with FUO, no diagnosis is obtained despite the most intensive evaluation. In most of these patients, fever usually subsides spontaneously after several weeks. Such cases are generally thought to be hypersensitivity reactions or undiagnosed viral infections. If fever persists, a complete re-evaluation in 6 to 8 weeks should be considered.

HYPERTHERMIA

Hyperthermia—as distinguished from fever—is an unregulated increase in body temperature in which endogenous pyrogens do not appear to play a role and standard antipyretics are ineffective in lowering body temperature. This condition results from a failure of thermoregulatory

Table 2. Causes of Hyperthermia

Causes
Increased Heat Production
Exercise-induced hyperthermia
Thyrotoxicosis
Pheochromocytoma
Malignant hyperthermia
Neuroleptic malignant syndrome
Decreased Heat Loss
Heat stroke
Drugs (e.g., atropine)
Autonomic dysfunction
Dehydration
Occlusive dressings
Severe anemia
Congestive heart failure
Absence of sweat glands
Hypothalamic Disorders
Infection (e.g., granulomas)
Tumors
Trauma
Vascular accident
Drugs (e.g., phenothiazines)

homeostasis in which there is uncontrolled heat production, inadequate heat dissipation, or failure of hypothalamic thermoregulation. Some causes of hyperthermia are listed in Table 2.

Malignant hyperthermia is a rare hereditary disease transmitted by autosomal dominant inheritance, with variable penetrance. This disease is characterized by rapidly evolving hyperthermia, muscular rigidity, and acidosis in patients undergoing general anesthesia. Although various inhalational anesthetic agents have been incriminated in the disorder, halothane (alone or in conjunction with succinylcholine) has been the most common offender. The condition is often presaged by sudden ventricular ectopic activity, tachypnea, circulatory instability, and a sharp rise in body temperature. Metabolic acidosis and rhabdomyolysis are common and frequently severe. The mortality in acute cases varies between 28 and 70 per cent.

Neuroleptic malignant syndrome, another form of hyperthermia, is characterized by an increased body temperature, diffuse muscular rigidity, autonomic instability, and altered consciousness. This syndrome most often occurs as a side effect of haloperidol, but it has also been reported in association with other antipsychotic drugs, such as the phenothiazines and thioxanthenes.

CHEST PAIN

By Basanti Mukerji, M.D.,
Martin A. Alpert, M.D.,
and Vaskar Mukerji, M.D.
Mobile, Alabama

The causes of chest pain are diverse. Some causes, such as acute myocardial infarction and aortic dissection, may be life-threatening, whereas others, such as the various forms of chest wall pain, may be aggravating but pose no threat to life. An assessment of the probable cause of chest pain can usually be made from data obtained from the medical history and physical examination. The chest radiograph and resting electrocardiogram, the two most frequently ordered studies in patients with chest pain, are perhaps the most useful. More sophisticated laboratory studies are usually employed to confirm clinical suspicions, to delineate the extent of disease, or to investigate more complex cases.

HISTORY

The history, the first step in evaluating a patient with chest pain, should be carefully elicited. Did the patient experience a single episode of chest pain, or has this been a recurring symptom? Many patients report chest discomfort rather than pain. What factors precipitate the symptom, and what relieves it? The patient should be questioned about the location and radiation of the chest pain as well as the quality, intensity, frequency, and duration. Questions should be asked regarding associated symptoms, such as dyspnea, diaphoresis, palpitations, fatigue, and nausea or vomiting. The patient should also be asked about any medication that is being used and about the response to that medication.

EXAMINATION

The physical examination may be normal in many patients with chest pain resulting from coronary artery disease, esophageal dysfunction, or psychiatric disorders. The diagnosis of hypertrophic cardiomyopathy or aortic stenosis is suggested by the presence of the characteristic systolic murmur. A diastolic murmur with severe chest pain may signal involvement of the aortic valve in a patient with aortic dissection. Pericarditis frequently causes a friction rub. With mitral valve prolapse, a systolic click may be heard, with or without a systolic murmur. Patients with coronary artery disease may have a fourth heart sound, but this may also be heard in some healthy individuals and in those with ventricular hypertrophy. Abnormal breath sounds or crackles on auscultation of the lungs suggest pulmonary disease. Fever generally indicates an infectious disease. Musculoskeletal tenderness and pain with movement of the shoulders, arms, or spine suggest that the patient's symptoms are of arthritic origin. The presence of multiple, paired tender points, referred to as "trigger points," may be diagnostic of fibromyalgia. Tenderness of the costal cartilages is found in costochondritis. In selected cases, examination of the breasts may be useful. Palpation of the abdomen may reveal a subdiaphragmatic source of the patient's symptoms.

LABORATORY STUDIES

The chest radiograph is the most useful study in the diagnosis of pulmonary conditions and should be carefully reviewed. The cardiac shadow can also be assessed. On the electrocardiogram, ST-segment depression suggests myocardial ischemia, whereas acute ST-segment elevation may be diagnostic of acute myocardial infarction. Transient ST-segment elevation that occurs during episodes of chest pain and that later reverts to normal occurs with Prinzmetal's angina or coronary artery spasm. Cardiac enzyme assays should be ordered whenever recent myocardial injury is suspected. A technetium pyrophosphate scan of the heart or a troponin T assay can also be helpful in the diagnosis of acute myocardial infarction. Exercise testing is indicated for stable patients with occasional chest pain. A standard treadmill protocol is generally employed, although a stationary bicycle or an arm ergometer can also be used. Thallium (or sestamibi) scintigraphy or echocardiography with exercise testing improves the reliability of the study. For patients who cannot exercise, the dipyridamole thallium test may be a useful alternative. Coronary angiography provides the most accurate definition of the coronary arteries. Valvular disorders and cardiomyopathy can be evaluated with echocardiography or cardiac catheterization. For pulmonary embolism, a lung scan is commonly ordered along with tests to assess the leg veins. Bronchoscopy, thoracentesis, and pleural biopsy should be considered in the appropriate setting. X-ray studies of the vertebral spine and rib cage are helpful when musculoskeletal causes are suspected. Esophageal conditions can be evaluated with a barium esophagogram, endoscopy, a motility study, or even pH monitoring. The history and physical examination provide clues for the selection of appropriate tests.

DIFFERENTIAL DIAGNOSIS

Cardiovascular System

Angina pectoris is chest pain due to myocardial ischemia. It results from an imbalance between myocardial oxygen supply and demand and is usually caused by atherosclerosis. The discomfort is usually located substernally but may occasionally be localized in the left anterior chest or in the epigastrium. Angina pectoris may radiate to the left (the most common site) or right shoulder or arm (usually the medial aspect), the neck or jaw, the upper abdomen, or the back. Occasionally, pain in one of these sites of radiation occurs in the absence of chest pain. The intensity of angina pectoris pain is highly variable, ranging from mild to severe. Most episodes are characterized as moderate to severe but are less intense than chest pain associated with acute myocardial infarction. Various descriptive terms have been used to characterize angina pectoris, including "tightness," "pressurelike," "viselike," "crushing," "choking," "suffocating," "oppressive," "bursting," and "burning." Angina pectoris is characterized by a crescendo-decrescendo pattern. It is frequently but not invariably associated with dyspnea, diaphoresis, weakness or lassitude, nausea, and a sense of impending doom. Occasionally, dyspnea or intense lassitude may occur with myocardial ischemia in the absence of chest pain and may serve as angina pectoris equivalents. Stable angina pectoris is angina pectoris that predictably recurs in response to exertion and sometimes with exposure to emotional stress or cold or following ingestion of a large meal. Removal of the exacerbating factor or use of sublingual nitroglycerin typically produces relief of pain within 5 minutes. Unstable angina pectoris is characterized by an increase in the frequency, intensity, or duration of anginal symptoms. Variant angina pectoris, or Prinzmetal's angina, refers to angina pectoris caused by coronary artery spasm, which itself may occur in the presence or absence of coronary atherosclerosis. Variant angina pectoris typically occurs at rest without discernible exacerbating factors. It tends to occur at similar times of day and not infrequently exceeds 5 minutes in duration.

Acute myocardial infarction occurs with total occlusion of a coronary artery, usually in association with coronary atherosclerosis. The chest pain of acute myocardial infarction shares several characteristics with that of angina pectoris. The quality, location, and sites of radiation are identical to those of angina pectoris. There is a gradual increase in intensity. The peak intensity of chest pain associated with acute myocardial infarction is generally greater than that of angina pectoris. Most patients who experience acute myocardial infarction have chest pain that exceeds 1 hour in duration. Acute myocardial infarction may be provoked (e.g., by exertion) but more often occurs without apparent precipitating factors. Unlike angina pectoris, the chest pain of acute myocardial infarction typically is not relieved by removal of exacerbating factors or sublingual nitroglycerin. Associated symptoms, including diaphoresis, nausea, and lassitude, are more protracted and often more intense in patients with acute myocardial infarction than in patients with angina pectoris.

Chest pain may occur in association with a variety of forms of valvular heart disease. It is encountered frequently in severe aortic stenosis, less commonly in severe aortic insufficiency, and often with mitral valve prolapse. In approximately 10 per cent of individuals with chest pain and mitral valve prolapse, angina pectoris–like pain occurs. In the remainder, chest discomfort is characterized chiefly by its lack of resemblance to other known causes of chest pain. The pain is usually located in the left anterior chest, often over the cardiac apex. It is frequently characterized as sharp or stabbing but occasionally is described as achy or dull. The duration of chest pain in mitral valve prolapse is highly variable, ranging from seconds to hours. The actual intensity ranges from mild to moderate but is sometimes exaggerated by worry. The pain may be associated with other symptoms of mitral valve prolapse, such as palpitations, effort intolerance, and presyncope. There are no consistent exacerbating or relieving factors. Chest pain can occur at any time but tends to occur more frequently during periods of emotional stress.

Chest pain is commonly encountered in patients with hypertrophic cardiomyopathy (idiopathic hypertrophic subaortic stenosis), is infrequently observed in patients with dilated cardiomyopathy, and is rare in acute myocarditis. In each case, the chest pain is angina pectoris–like in character.

The most common symptom of acute pericarditis is chest pain. Three types have been described. The most common form is sharp and stabbing. It is typically located in the left precordium and occasionally radiates into the neck, back, or flank. The pain may be exacerbated by inspiration, swallowing, sudden movements of the thorax, or reclining. The pain is sometimes relieved by sitting up and leaning forward. The intensity of the pain is variable but is generally rated as moderate to severe. Most episodes of pain are momentary, occurring in association with exacerbating factors. Episodes may recur for several days, weeks, or months. Sharp, stabbing interscapular pain is less commonly encountered. Rarely, sharp pains located at the cardiac apex and associated with each heartbeat are described by patients with acute pericarditis. Associated symptoms reflect the underlying causes of acute pericarditis or the presence of pericardial effusion.

Chest pain occurs in 90 per cent of patients with acute aortic dissection and is typically characterized as ripping or tearing. It is extremely intense and is often described as the most severe pain the patient has ever experienced. The location of the pain depends on the site of dissection. Involvement of the aortic root produces substernal pain in the neck or jaw. Involvement of the descending aorta produces interscapular, lumbar, or abdominal pain. The pain is most intense at the onset of the episode and dissipates with time. Associated symptoms reflect compromise of vital organs by the dissecting hematoma. Aortic dissection may involve the right coronary artery, producing myocardial ischemia or infarction. The aortic valve may be involved, resulting in aortic insufficiency, and it may extend into the pericardium, producing pericarditis and pericardial effusion. Each of these complications may produce distinctive forms of chest pain.

Pulmonary System

A persistent cough for any reason can result in chest soreness. Thus, tracheobronchitis represents one of the most common causes of chest pain, although it is prognostically less important than other causes and is easily treatable.

Pleuritic chest pain is a sharp, stabbing pain that is exacerbated by chest wall movements, breathing, or coughing. It is usually characterized as being of moderate to severe intensity. Individual episodes are typically of short duration. This type of pain is caused by diseases that produce pleural irritation, including pneumonia, empyema, pulmonary embolism and infarction, pneumothorax, and neoplasm. The location of pleuritic chest pain depends on the site of pleural irritation.

Acute pulmonary embolism causes dyspnea with accompanying chest pain in fewer than 25 per cent of patients. Angina pectoris–like substernal pain has been described and is thought to result from right ventricular subendocardial ischemia caused by acute right ventricular pressure overload. Pleuritic chest pain may also occur with pulmonary embolism and is probably attributable to pleural ischemia. Both forms of chest pain are short-lived, lasting several minutes to several hours.

Tumors of the lung may produce a chronic, sustained, deep, aching chest pain. Apical tumors may also produce pain in the shoulder of the involved side.

Controversy exists as to whether chronic pulmonary hypertension actually produces chest pain. Patients with pulmonary hypertension have variously described chest pain as angina pectoris–like, sharp, dull, central, and peripheral.

The Esophagus

Esophageal disorders are a fairly common cause of chest pain, which may occur from esophageal reflux or various types of motility disorders.

Reflux esophagitis is caused by irritation of the lower esophageal mucosa from reflux of gastric acid. It is typically characterized by a burning epigastric pain (heartburn, or pyrosis) that may also be perceived in the substernal region. The pain commonly starts during a meal or shortly thereafter and lasts for a variable period. Esophageal reflux is commonly exacerbated on assuming the supine position (thus precipitating episodes of pain at night) or on bending over at the waist. The pain is mild to moderate in intensity and is readily relieved with antacids. Associated symptoms include water brash, nocturnal wheezing from aspiration of refluxed gastric acid, and angina pectoris–like pain usually from concurrent esophageal spasm.

There are essentially five forms of esophageal motility disorder diagnosed by manometric study: nutcracker esophagus, diffuse esophageal spasm, nonspecific esophageal motility disorder, hypertensive lower esophageal sphincter, and achalasia. The last is esophageal aperistalsis accompanied by incomplete relaxation of the lower esophageal sphincter, but this condition infrequently causes chest pain. Nutcracker esophagus is characterized by high-amplitude peristaltic contractions of pressures of 180 mm Hg or more. Diffuse esophageal spasm is characterized by intermittent, simultaneous, prolonged contractions in the esophagus. Nonspecific esophageal motility disorder is a mixed type of condition. Nutcracker esophagus and nonspecific esophageal motility disorder are the two types most commonly identified in patients with chest pain. The chest pain of esophageal spasm may mimic angina pectoris in quality, intensity, location, and radiation. The duration of chest pain is variable, ranging from seconds to minutes to hours. Episodes of esophageal spasm may occur spontaneously or may be exacerbated by swallowing a food bolus or ingesting hot or cold liquids or by gastric acid reflux. The pain is typically nonexertional, which helps differentiate it from stable angina pectoris. Sublingual nitroglycerin may be effective in aborting episodes. Dysphagia may be encountered in patients with esophageal spasm. Angina pectoris and esophageal spasm may occur together in the same patient, making it difficult to ascertain the precise cause of chest pain.

Rheumatic Disorders

A musculoskeletal cause can be identified in 13 to 20 per cent of patients with chest pain. The causes include fibromyalgia, costochondritis (and Tietze's syndrome), arthritis (rheumatoid or osteoarthritis), injury to the chest wall, and vertebrospinal disease.

Fibromyalgia is characterized by diffuse musculoskeletal pain and the inability to get a restful night's sleep. The disease commonly affects women in the third or fourth decade of life. Patients with fibromyalgia often awaken aching, fatigued, and stiff, with burning pain in the muscles around joints. The intensity of pain varies from day to day and is accentuated by cold, damp weather, fatigue, inactivity or excessive exertion, mental stress, and poor posture. Palpation over the musculotendinous junctions elicits multiple, paired tender points, or "trigger" points.

Costochondritis is a benign condition characterized by pain and tenderness of the cartilaginous articulations of the anterior chest wall. This condition commonly affects young individuals of either sex. Although typically localized to the involved joints, this pain may radiate widely over the chest wall. Its intensity varies and is increased when the patient coughs, breathes deeply, or lies prone. The principal diagnostic feature is tenderness over the affected costal cartilage or cartilages, commonly the second to fifth. The disorder is self-limited, but there may be remissions and exacerbations; the pain usually resolves in weeks to months. Patients with Tietze's syndrome experience nonsuppurative, painful swelling of the cartilaginous ends of the ribs.

Ankylosing spondylitis and seronegative spondyloarthropathies may affect the thoracic vertebrae, causing pain to radiate to the anterior chest. Rheumatoid arthritis and osteoarthritis can also cause chest pain by involving the facet joints of the vertebrae, the costovertebral and costotransverse joints, the sternoclavicular joints, and the manubriosternal joint. Xiphoidalgia refers to pain and tenderness of the xiphoid cartilage that radiates to the precordium, epigastrium, shoulders, and back.

Trauma to the rib cage, with or without fracture, may cause chest wall pain. In patients with osteoporosis, ribs may fracture from apparently trivial injury. Metastatic bone disease from carcinoma of the breast, kidney, lung, thyroid, or prostate can cause rib tumors that may produce painful rib swelling or pathologic fracture. Pain in the intercostal and accessory thoracic muscles can occur after unaccustomed exertion, for example, from painting, chopping wood, excessive coughing, or lifting heavy weights. Pain originating around the shoulders from either subacromial bursitis or arthritis of the shoulder or the acromioclavicular joint can be referred to the upper anterior chest wall. The thoracic outlet syndrome involves compression of the structures lying in the space bounded inferiorly by the first rib, superiorly by the clavicle, anteriorly by the scalenus anticus muscle, and posteriorly by the scalenus medius muscle. Nerve impingement in this area causes pain that is referred to the upper chest wall.

Psychiatric Disorders

The psychiatric causes of chest pain include panic disorder, generalized anxiety disorder, agoraphobia and other phobias, depression, somatization, conversion, malingering, and Munchausen syndrome. Before assigning a psychiatric origin to the patient's chest pain, it is important to exclude organic (particularly cardiac) causes. Proper diagnosis of the patient's psychiatric condition may be expected to reduce morbidity and in some cases preclude the need for costly and potentially dangerous diagnostic tests.

Among the psychiatric causes of chest pain, panic disorder deserves special attention. It is a subtype of anxiety that is estimated to affect 2 to 5 per cent of the general population, but the prevalence may be as high as 10 to 14 per cent in cardiac patients. Some studies indicate that 30 to 40 per cent of patients with chest pain and angiographically confirmed normal coronary arteries have panic disorder. Conversely, 60 per cent of patients with panic disorder report chest pain as a prominent symptom. Eighty per cent of panic disorder patients are women. A familial trend has been demonstrated by genetic studies. The illness runs a chronic, fluctuating course. Some patients with panic disorder may progress to the development of anticipatory anxiety and agoraphobia. Although agoraphobia is uncommon among cardiac patients, major depression can be found in about 50 per cent of patients with chest pain and panic disorder. Somatic symptoms that accompany the chest pain in patients with panic disorder include dyspnea, palpitations, sweating, dizziness, paresthesias, and hot and cold flashes.

Other Causes

Disorders that affect the abdominal viscera can cause chest pain. Peptic ulcer disease typically produces a gnawing pain in the epigastrium 1 to 2 hours after a meal, or sooner with a gastric ulcer. Occasionally, such pain is felt in the substernal region. The pain is usually relieved promptly with antacids, which helps differentiate it from pain of cardiac origin. Acute pancreatitis usually occurs in patients with biliary disease or alcoholism. The pain of acute pancreatitis is usually epigastric in location. It is a severe, boring pain that commonly radiates through to the back. It is usually constant and can sometimes be relieved by sitting. It is frequently accompanied by nausea and vomiting, fever, abdominal tenderness, guarding, and loss of bowel sounds. Acute cholecystitis is typically characterized by severe right upper quadrant and epigastric pain. Radiation to the right shoulder is common, and pain involving the right or left anterior chest may occur. These pains usually have an achy quality. Fever, jaundice, and a palpable, painful gallbladder may help localize the source of pain. Cholelithiasis and choledocholithiasis typically produce episodes of steady, achy, or colicky right upper quadrant pain. Distention of the splenic flexure of the colon by trapped gas may produce sharp or colicky pain in the left upper quadrant of the abdomen. Referral of pain to the left shoulder or upper anterior chest occurs frequently and may be the dominant presentation.

Chest pain in drug abusers is a problem of particular concern today. Cocaine and its nonionic complex form called "crack" are potent vasoconstrictive agents. According to estimates, more than 5 million individuals in the United States are occasional or regular users of cocaine. About 15 per cent of cocaine users experience acute chest pain. Myocardial infarction, presumably the result of coronary artery spasm in susceptible individuals, can result in sudden death.

Herpes zoster can affect the thoracic nerves, causing severe burning and pain for 2 to 5 days, followed by the appearance of a vesicular rash along the affected dermatome. Epidemic pleurodynia is an acute viral illness characterized by pain in the chest wall and epigastrium, usually caused by infection with group B coxsackievirus affecting the intercostal and upper abdominal muscles and, rarely, the pleura. Various conditions that affect the breast can also cause chest pain.

Patients with chest pain frequently present a diagnostic challenge that requires careful investigation and follow-up. A definitive diagnosis is important before specific therapy can be instituted.

CHRONIC COUGH

By Thaddeus Bartter, M.D.,
and Melvin R. Pratter, M.D.
Camden, New Jersey

Chronic cough is most often defined as cough of more than 3 weeks' duration. Cough is different from many conditions in clinical medicine because it is defined by the patient, not by an objective study performed by the physician. Although severity is not part of the definition, most patients who come to a physician with a chronic cough declare that it has caused some interruption of daily function, and many have been coughing for years. Studies of chronic cough have traditionally excluded active smokers because smoking is a common cause of chronic cough. A "new" chronic cough in a long-term smoker is nevertheless usually due to one of the common causes listed in the following paragraph and can be worked up with the use of the algorithm presented in this article with certain caveats.

Despite the large number of possible causes of chronic cough, repeated studies have demonstrated that three causes—postnasal drip (PND) syndrome, asthma, and gastroesophageal reflux (GER)—cause chronic cough in the vast majority (more than 95 per cent) of cases. The complexity of most difficult cases derives not from an expanded differential but from the fact that any two or all three of the preceding causes may be contributing to chronic cough in an individual patient. This knowledge has simplified the approach to chronic cough (Table 1); it has also led to the understanding that cancer is *not* a common cause of chronic cough (Table 2). Most patients with chronic cough do not need a chest roentgenogram. Bronchoscopy is rarely indicated or useful in the work-up of chronic cough.

A sequential approach is most useful in the evaluation of patients with chronic cough. It begins with consideration of PND, the most common cause, followed by consideration of less likely causes. The algorithm stops when the cough has resolved. A patient may have bronchial hyperresponsiveness (BHR) with methacholine challenge or GER by 24-hour pH-probe monitoring, but if cough has resolved with treatment of PND, there is no reason for the physician to evaluate for another condition unless other symptoms prompt a work-up. The sequential approach avoids both the expense of unnecessary testing and the awkwardness of abnormal findings with no known clinical significance. It also proceeds from initial approaches available to any internist to more specialized testing. The primary care physician can initiate the work-up and effect resolution of

Table 1. Chronic Cough: Diagnostic Studies

Etiology	Diagnostic Studies
PND	Trial of A/D therapy
	Nasal steroids
	Sinus roentgenograms
Asthma	Pulmonary function studies with methacholine challenge
GER	24-hour pH-probe monitoring
Other	Chest roentgenogram
	Bronchoscopy
	Cardiac ultrasound

PND = postnasal drip; GER = gastroesophageal reflux; A/D = antihistamine and decongestant.

Table 2. Chronic Cough in Nonsmokers

Common Causes
Postnasal drip syndrome
Asthma
Gastroesophageal reflux
Uncommon Causes
Lung tumor
Endobronchial lesion
benign
malignant
foreign body
Drug-induced: angiotensin converting enzyme inhibitors
Bronchiectasis
Pleural disease
Upper airway problems
tonsillar hypertrophy
laryngeal inflammation, polyps, or cancer
Cardiac disorder
pericardial disease
heart failure
Ear canal disease
Psychogenic causes (diagnosis of exclusion)

cough in most patients. Referral to diagnostic laboratories or specialist physicians, if needed, may be made at a later stage of the work-up. The timing of the referral depends on the physician's level of comfort with the diagnosis.

HISTORY AND PHYSICAL EXAMINATION

The history and physical examination rarely provide the cause of chronic cough. In many individuals, PND is present, and observation of discharge in the nares or phlegm in the posterior pharynx is evidence of PND but not proof of a linkage between PND and cough. Neither a history of dyspnea nor wheezing on physical examination confirms a diagnosis of asthma or a causative relationship to cough. Gastroesophageal reflux may be suspected from the history, but physical examination cannot confirm its presence; even if GER is present, linkage with cough cannot be established. The history and physical examination can help one to focus suspicion but should not alter the approach except when a blatant condition or evidence of a serious underlying cause other than PND, asthma, or GER is present. For example, a patient who is taking an angiotensin converting enzyme inhibitor should have the medication stopped for at least 2 weeks prior to evaluation. A smoker with a chronic cough and scant hemoptysis should have a chest roentgenogram and bronchoscopy immediately after the initial evaluation. For the vast majority of patients, however, the history and physical examination are nondirective, and the most rapid and efficient resolution of cough will be achieved with the stepped algorithm.

THE ALGORITHM

Step 1: Postnasal Drip Syndrome

Postnasal drip syndrome is the most common cause of chronic cough. The term "postnasal drip syndrome" is used because there are several causes of PND. They include allergic rhinitis, vasomotor rhinitis, and sinusitis, and all can present as chronic cough. Some patients are aware of the PND, whereas others who have been shown to have had PND by their response to therapy were unaware of it. Added to the difficulty in diagnosing PND is the fact that there is no specific diagnostic test that can quantify PND or any causative role it may play in a cough.

Patients with chronic cough are treated with an initial diagnostic and therapeutic trial of a 2-week course of a long-acting antihistamine and decongestant (A/D). The authors have had therapeutic success with an A/D preparation containing 1 mg of azatadine maleate plus 120 mg of sustained-release pseudoephedrine sulfate (Trinalin).

Re-evaluation begins on day 7. If the cough shows no improvement, the authors immediately move on to evaluation for asthma (step 2). If the cough has diminished, A/D therapy is continued until either the cough has resolved or a new plateau short of resolution is reached. At this time, symptoms become a branch point in the decision tree. Those patients with no PND symptoms are moved on to step 2. Those with PND symptoms unresponsive to A/D therapy are treated with a nasal steroid spray in addition to the A/D. If the PND still does not resolve, the patient is evaluated for sinusitis. Whether to obtain plain films first or to go directly to a computed tomography (CT) scan of the sinuses is not clear. The authors often use plain films, as they are widely available and relatively inexpensive and have a good record of diagnosing chronic sinusitis as a cause of cough, but coronal CT scanning is clearly the definitive study. Patients with sinusitis are treated with antibiotics in addition to nasal therapy, with referral to an ear-nose-throat (ENT) specialist for those who have refractory sinusitis.

Some patients (about 16 per cent) do not tolerate even a short course of A/D therapy. If the side effect is drowsiness, a nonsedating antihistamine plus pseudoephedrine, 60 mg twice daily, can be substituted. If the side effects are insomnia, agitation, and/or urinary obstruction, a nonsedating antihistamine plus nasal corticosteroids twice daily can be substituted.

Step 2: Asthma

Patients who are still coughing after receiving treatment for PND are evaluated for asthma. Asthma is the second most common cause of chronic cough. Cough can occur along with a history of dyspnea and wheezing that had been unrecognized, or asthma may present solely as "cough-variant asthma," in which cough is the only symptom of asthma. Bronchoprovocation challenge (BPC) testing is the cornerstone of the diagnosis of BHR in this population: some patients who show airflow obstruction on pulmonary function testing will respond to beta-agonists, but the majority will need provocation testing to demonstrate BHR. Asthma should not be eliminated from the differential diagnosis of chronic cough in a patient with normal spirometry results unless either the cough has resolved with other therapy or bronchoprovocation testing has demonstrated that BHR is not present.

Step 2 consists of pulmonary function testing and spirometry with provocation testing. (Patients with airflow obstruction should be given a bronchodilator during pulmonary function testing.) Those without BHR can proceed immediately to step 3. Those with BHR or with airflow obstruction should be treated for asthma. A 7-day trial of regular (not "as necessary" [PRN]) beta-agonist therapy should be given first. If cough persists, a therapeutic trial of prednisone, 1 mg/kg per day for 7 days orally, with a maximum of 60 mg per day should be initiated. Asthma-associated cough usually is not relieved until the course of steroids is given.

Patients who respond to treatment for asthma may proceed to maintenance therapy, usually inhaled steroids. Patients whose cough responds partially or not at all to asthma therapy should go on to the next step, with asthma therapy continued for those with a partial response.

Step 3: Radiologic Imaging

Radiologic evaluation should consist of sinus films (if not obtained as part of step 1) and a chest roentgenogram (unless a recent one is available). The sinus films constitute a search for an occult sinusitis that may present only with chronic cough. The chest roentgenogram may reveal a tumor or other abnormality that could explain the cough. The chest films only occasionally yield an answer (about 5 per cent of patients), but they are indicated here because (1) the next step is invasive and expensive and (2) patient fears of a serious underlying process, such as a malignancy.

Patients who have an abnormality should be treated or evaluated accordingly. Patients with persistent cough after completing step 3 should be evaluated according to step 4.

Step 4: Evaluation for GER

The third most common cause of chronic cough, gastroesophageal reflux is also the most difficult cause to prove. The gold standard of diagnosis is 24-hour pH-probe monitoring, which is relatively invasive. Barium swallow is not recommended for the diagnosis of GER because it documents only one point in time and is insensitive compared with the 24-hour study. Twenty-four hour pH-probe monitoring is also more sensitive than endoscopy, which is useful primarily in the search for a structural lesion. Even if GER is diagnosed, appropriate therapy may take weeks to affect the cough.

For patients with persistent cough and a history strongly consistent with GER (acid taste in mouth, heartburn, frequent use of antacids), a 2-week trial with an H_2 antagonist is reasonable. Many patients do not respond. The patients who do not respond and those who do not have classic reflux symptoms should undergo 24-hour pH-probe monitoring. Patients with pathologic GER established by monitoring should be treated with omeprazole, 20 mg per day orally for up to 8 weeks, before the therapy is considered ineffective. In selected patients, adding a prokinetic agent—cisapride, 20 mg 4 times a day orally—may be helpful.

Step 5: Special Studies

Approximately 95 per cent of patients should experience resolution of cough during the sequential evaluation. Occasionally, patients with a known causative diagnosis, such as chronic sinusitis, continue to cough because the condition is refractory to treatment. For the rare patient who is still coughing and whose condition is undiagnosed, bronchoscopy should be considered. Patients who do not have an endobronchial lesion or other cause evident on bronchoscopy should be approached with the differential diagnosis of less common causes, as listed in Table 2. The diagnostic work-up must be tailored to the patient according to the causes listed and the results of the physical examination.

DYSPNEA

By D.J. Gillespie, M.D., Ph.D.,
and E.J. Olson, M.D.
Rochester, Minnesota

Dyspnea, although a common complaint, is not specifically defined and can result from a wide variety of disorders. The terms used to describe dyspnea include "difficult," "labored," "heavy," "uncomfortable," or "unpleasant" breathing. Most commonly, the symptoms reflect pulmonary or cardiac disease and, occasionally, a neuromuscular disorder. However, a hyperventilation syndrome of organic or psychogenic origin must also be considered. Additional conditions are less common and may require an extensive evaluation with the use of specialized testing.

The sensation of dyspnea or breathlessness involves reaction to subjective or perceptual stimuli as well as objective or neuromuscular stimuli. Receptor signals and central interpretations are involved in a complex interaction that contributes to the sensation of dyspnea. Important receptors include mechanoreceptors from lung, airway (vagal afferent); and respiratory muscles; chemoreceptors in carotid and aortic bodies plus the central medullary area; afferent signals from the central nervous system; and possibly vascular receptors.

The factors leading to dyspnea are not well understood, but there is some correlation between the degree of dyspnea and the extent of the disease or condition. The pulmonary disorders that lead to dyspnea include airway disease, parenchymal disease, pleural or chest wall conditions, and pulmonary vascular disease. The cardiac disorders that result in dyspnea most commonly include ventricular dysfunction, valvular disease, pericardial disease, and arrhythmias. Neuromuscular conditions, such as systemic neuromuscular disorders, central nervous system disease, and phrenic nerve or diaphragmatic dysfunction, can also result in dyspnea. Age-related conditions may also present with progressive dyspnea in the elderly population, reflecting a decline in pulmonary and/or cardiac function in addition to less common causes of dyspnea, including anemia, metabolic (thyroid) disorders, poor nutrition, and generalized deconditioning.

A large number of conditions can produce dyspnea, and they can be generally divided into disorders that result in symptoms of acute dyspnea or those with more long-standing symptoms that cause chronic dyspnea. Some of the conditions that can result in acute or chronic dyspnea are outlined in Table 1.

ACUTE DYSPNEA

The sudden onset of dyspnea can result in severe symptoms and frequently leads to an emergency room evaluation. Clinical evaluation and radiographic findings commonly establish the cause of dyspnea, with asthma, congestive heart failure, and exacerbation of chronic obstructive pulmonary disease (COPD) being most common.

Pulmonary Disease

Airway Disease

Upper airway obstruction from laryngospasm, foreign-body aspiration, trauma, anaphylaxis, and infection (epiglottitis, compressing abscess) commonly produces inspiratory stridor. Acute bronchospasm, however, produces diffuse wheezing and evidence of hyperinflation on the chest roentgenogram. Hyperventilation is usually associated with other symptoms, such as dizziness, lightheadedness, and paresthesias of the hands and perioral region.

Pulmonary Parenchymal Disease

Pneumonia can result in acute dyspnea of varying degrees and is associated with cough (productive or nonproductive), fever (possibly low grade), and infiltrate on the

Table 1. Some Causes of Dyspnea

Acute Dyspnea	Chronic Dyspnea	Other Causes
Pulmonary	***Pulmonary***	***Neuromuscular***
Airways	Airways	Amyotrophic lateral sclerosis
Upper airway obstruction	Asthma	Muscular dystrophy
Acute bronchospasm	Chronic obstructive pulmonary disease	Myasthenia gravis
Parenchymal	Major airway obstruction	Diaphragm dysfunction
Pneumonia	Parenchymal	***Cardiac***
Pulmonary edema	Interstitial fibrosis	Valvular disease
Pneumothorax	Hypersensitivity pneumonitis	Mycocardial ischemia
Cardiovascular	Drug-induced	Intracardiac shunting
Arrhythmias	Malignancy	Pericardial disease
Acute left ventricular failure	Vascular	Atrial myxoma
Acute mitral valve dysfunction	Primary pulmonary hypertension	***Miscellaneous***
Pulmonary emboli	Chronic pulmonary emboli	Anemia
Thoracic Trauma	Arteriovenous malformation	Deconditioning
Pneumothorax	Veno-occlusive disease	Psychogenic causes
Pulmonary contusion	Vasculitis	Hypo- and hyperthyroidism
Rib fractures	Chest wall and pleural	Gastrointestinal reflux
	Kyphoscoliosis	
	Ankylosing spondylitis	
	Trauma	
	Obesity	
	Pleural fibrosis	
	Pleural effusion	

chest radiograph. Pulmonary edema from a noncardiac cause and pulmonary hemorrhage are less common but may be life-threatening and result in respiratory failure. Spontaneous pneumothorax, usually from rupture of a subpleural bleb, presents with chest pain and dyspnea.

Cardiovascular Disease

Arrhythmias can result in sudden dyspnea, in addition to acute left ventricular failure with pulmonary edema or acute mitral valve dysfunction from papillary muscle rupture, and are usually evident on physical examination. An acute pulmonary embolus may present with no specific clinical findings, although chest pain and dyspnea are the most common complaints. A high index of suspicion is needed when the initial findings are nondiagnostic.

Thoracic Trauma

Pneumothorax and pulmonary contusion can result from both penetrating and nonpenetrating injuries caused by severe trauma. In some patients, these conditions may be delayed if the injury is less serious. Fractured ribs, however, are most common, and in uncomplicated fractures, pain during respiration can result in difficult breathing.

CHRONIC DYSPNEA

Unexplained or slowly progressive dyspnea lasting weeks or months can result from a variety of causes. These symptoms result from increased work of breathing, increased respiratory drive, or decreased power from neuromuscular dysfunction.

Pulmonary Disease

Airway Disease

Asthma can result in chronic dyspnea with prolonged episodes of bronchospasm of variable degrees and poor response to therapy. Some airway responsiveness to bronchodilators may also be seen in COPD with chronic bronchitis and/or emphysema, but these conditions also exhibit hyperinflation with chest wall changes and diaphragmatic dysfunction. Airway obstruction from tumor or tracheal stenosis and vocal cord dysfunction must be considered also.

Pulmonary Parenchymal Disease

Interstitial fibrosis from idiopathic causes, hypersensitivity pneumonitis, and drug-induced interstitial disease are diagnostic considerations when interstitial changes are seen on chest roentgenograms. Malignancy is also a consideration with advanced disease and lymphangitic spread. Other forms of interstitial pulmonary disease are less common.

Pulmonary Vascular Disease

Pulmonary hypertension results in progressive dyspnea, which may not be evident on initial examination. Chronic pulmonary emboli may present with similar symptoms. Less common vascular causes of chronic dyspnea include arteriovenous malformation, veno-occlusive disease, and vasculitis.

Chest Wall and Pleural Disease

Severe chest wall deformity from kyphoscoliosis, ankylosing spondylitis, or severe trauma can result in restrictive pulmonary disease with impaired gas exchange. Obesity restricts chest wall and diaphragm movement, resulting in increased work of breathing. Extensive pleural fibrosis restricts chest wall function and lung expansion, whereas pleural effusions reduce lung volumes, causing dyspnea.

Neuromuscular Disease

Respiratory muscle weakness can be the result of neuromuscular disease or diaphragm dysfunction or weakness. The progression of amyotrophic lateral sclerosis and muscular dystrophy initially leads to dyspnea, followed by hypercapnia and respiratory failure. Myasthenia gravis may present with dyspnea of varying degree or episodes of acute respiratory failure, especially with a superimposed respiratory infection. When unilateral, diaphragm dysfunction may result in only mild dyspnea with activity. However, bilateral diaphragm dysfunction causes more symptomatic dyspnea, particularly when the patient is supine.

Cardiac Disease

Left-sided cardiac disease involving the aortic or mitral valve and myocardial dysfunction or ischemia can lead to increased pulmonary capillary pressure and dyspnea. These effects occur initially via stimulation of intrapulmonary receptors and later as the result of pulmonary edema. Less frequent causes include intracardiac shunting, pericardial disease, and, rarely, atrial myxoma.

Miscellaneous Conditions

Severe anemia occasionally results in dyspnea, especially during activity. Hyperthyroidism and hypothyroidism occasionally are causes of dyspnea, and gastroesophageal reflux can produce a sensation of breathlessness. In the deconditioned state, submaximal exercise can produce a sensation of excessive respiratory effort and a disproportionate sensation of dyspnea. Psychological factors may influence breathing pattern, and anxiety can result in hyperventilation or an inappropriate sensation of breathlessness that leads to a frequent need to take a deep breath.

OTHER FORMS OF DYSPNEA

Body position can result in dyspnea from a variety of causes. Unilateral pulmonary disease can lead to dyspnea when the patient is in the lateral decubitus position, which is referred to as trepopnea. Dyspnea occurs when the diseased side is dependent in conditions of unilateral pulmonary disease or pleural effusion. Rarely, severe COPD with asymptomatic bullous disease or a variably (intermittently) obstructing major airway mass can produce similar effects. Dyspnea is sometimes seen in liver disease when the individual is in the upright position (platypnea), with arterial desaturation (orthodeoxia) resulting from intrapulmonary shunting that occurs at the lung bases. Orthopnea, dyspnea that occurs when the individual is in a recumbent position, is a well-known symptom of cardiac dysfunction, but it can also be caused by bilateral diaphragmatic paralysis.

The cause of dyspnea may not be evident on initial clinical examination, and the diagnosis may depend on specialized testing. Although unexplained dyspnea may not always be specifically diagnosed, the majority of such cases result from pulmonary disease, cardiac disorders, and psychogenic hyperventilation. In fact, for patients younger than 40 years of age with a normal clinical evaluation, mild asthma and hyperventilation are the main causes of dyspnea. In cases of chronic dyspnea, pulmonary diseases are the most common causes, followed by cardiovascular diseases and deconditioning.

Assessment of the degree of dyspnea is usually subjective, and, in general, the degree of dyspnea correlates with cardiopulmonary function. The use of clinically derived grading scales, or psychophysical testing, has been useful, as has cardiopulmonary exercise testing or therapeutic intervention programs to assess the degree of dyspnea.

INITIAL ASSESSMENT

The initial assessment of dyspnea (Table 2) is based on the clinical evaluation. It is important to define the degree and course of dyspnea as it relates to daily activities. The history should include potential exposures (e.g., work environment, hobbies), trauma, past diseases, medication for drug-induced disease, and past surgery. The findings on physical examination, with emphasis on heart, lungs, and chest wall, may define a pulmonary or cardiac disorder that explains the dyspnea in addition to a chest wall condition or neuromuscular disease. Basic laboratory testing may also explain the underlying cause of dyspnea. A chest roentgenogram may provide clues to pulmonary or cardiac disease in addition to diaphragm position and chest wall abnormalities, and an electrocardiogram may show arrhythmias or possible cardiac ischemia. Spirometry, including maximal voluntary ventilation and bronchodilator administration, is a useful screening test for airway disease. Blood studies should include hemoglobin analysis for anemia and thyroid function (hypothyroidism and hyperthyroidism). The cause of dyspnea may not be evident after initial assessment, and specialized testing (Table 3) may be needed, based on selected cases.

SPECIALIZED TESTING

Pulmonary Disorders

Airway Disease

In patients with normal spirometry results and suspected obstructive airway disease, a bronchoprovocation test can be performed. Most commonly, spirometry is performed before and after a challenge with methacholine. Depending on the pattern of symptoms, however, cold air or exercise may be a more appropriate challenge. With upper or large airway lesions that are causing stridor, a flow-volume loop will define a significant, variable intrathoracic obstruction noted by a flattened peak expiratory curve, whereas a variable extrathoracic obstruction will show a flattened peak inspiratory curve. Fixed airway obstruction results in a flattening of both the peak inspiratory and the peak expiratory flow-volume curves. Computed tomography (CT) that uses high-resolution techniques can be useful in the diagnosis of unexplained dyspnea with airway obstruction and a normal chest roentgenogram in rare cases, such as early lymphangioleiomyomatosis and mild emphysema.

Parenchymal Disease

Pulmonary function testing is helpful in defining restrictive disorders. The carbon monoxide diffusing capacity of the lungs is a useful indicator of a pulmonary vascular or parenchymal abnormality. Also, the measurement of total

Table 2. Initial Assessment of Dyspnea

Comprehensive history
Physical examination
Basic laboratory testing
Electrocardiography
Chest roentgenography
Hemoglobin
Thyroid function
Spirometry including bronchodilator administration and maximal voluntary ventilation

Table 3. Specialized Testing for Dyspnea

Pulmonary Disorders
Airway Diseases
Bronchoprovocation
Flow-volume curves
High-resolution chest CT scanning
Parenchymal-Vascular Disease
Carbon monoxide diffusing capacity
Total lung capacity
Pulse oximetry or arterial blood gases
Rest and exercise
High-resolution chest CT scanning
Lung biopsy
Ventilation-perfusion scanning
Venous leg studies
Pulmonary angiography
Cardiac Disorders
Echocardiography
Radionuclide cardiac studies
Cardiac catheterization, coronary angiography
Ambulatory cardiac rhythm monitoring
Neuromuscular Disease
Maximal inspiratory and expiratory respiratory pressures
Electromyography
Unexplained
Cardiopulmonary exercise studies

CT = computed tomography.

lung capacity with body plethysmography will determine whether a restrictive process exists, but the test will not differentiate among chest wall, parenchymal, and diaphragmatic disorders. Pulse oximetry or arterial blood gas analysis (the latter being more accurate) during both rest and exercise will help determine whether gas exchange abnormalities exist. More specifically, a good indicator of pulmonary disease is a widening of the alveolar-arterial Po_2 gradient. High-resolution computed tomography scanning may also be helpful in detecting subtle interstitial or fibrotic changes that may characterize an early disease process. Tissue diagnosis may be performed with bronchoscopic biopsy. Rarely, an open lung biopsy is needed, but thoracoscopy has made this a less extensive procedure.

Pulmonary Vascular Disease

The evaluation of a pulmonary embolism requires ventilation-perfusion scanning and venous leg studies (ultrasonography, impedance plethysmography, or venography). Pulmonary angiography should be performed if pulmonary embolism is strongly suspected in an acute situation. Abnormal gas exchange or pulmonary hypertension may occur with chronic pulmonary embolism, and a more extensive evaluation may include ventilation-perfusion scanning, echocardiography, and/or right-sided cardiac catheterization, and ultimately pulmonary angiography. Echocardiography may be helpful in primary pulmonary hypertension, but in many patients right-sided cardiac catheterization is required.

Cardiac Disease

The most useful study in the initial evaluation of a patient suspected of having dyspnea of cardiac origin is echocardiography, which can define left-sided valvular disease, pericardial disease, ventricular dysfunction, and "restrictive" physiology. In some patients, transesophageal echocardiography may also be helpful. In addition, radionuclide studies may further characterize left ventricular function, and in some patients cardiac catheterization and coronary angiography may be indicated. Intermittent arrhythmic disorders may require ambulatory cardiac monitoring.

Occasionally, esophageal reflux can produce a sensation of dyspnea with accompanying chest pain. In these patients, 24-hour monitoring of esophageal pH is helpful.

Neuromuscular Disorders

Pulmonary function studies may help define neuromuscular conditions that produce muscle weakness involving respiratory muscles, including the diaphragm. A severely reduced maximal voluntary ventilation in the absence of major airway obstruction suggests respiratory muscle weakness. This can be confirmed with measurement of maximal inspiratory and expiratory pressures; however, abnormally low pressures can also be the result of submaximal effort. Another useful study is electromyography (EMG), which can be used to document phrenic nerve dysfunction and other neuromuscular disorders.

CARDIOPULMONARY EXERCISE TESTING

The cause of dyspnea may not be evident even after extensive testing, or it may not correlate with findings, and exercise testing is needed to define cardiac and pulmonary status. In addition, deconditioning and psychogenic factors, such as hyperventilation, can be defined. The results of exercise testing, when abnormal, may determine which organ system is responsible for dyspnea and will help assess the level of physical fitness. Exercise testing will include the electrocardiogram, blood pressure, heart rate, oxygen saturation, oxygen uptake, and carbon dioxide output. In specific patients, arterial blood gas determinations are needed to evaluate gas exchange abnormalities, and cardiac output should be calculated in patients with cardiac dysfunction.

In general, patients with pulmonary disease have decreased maximal oxygen consumption and increased ventilation. Specifically, patients with COPD show a decreased maximal oxygen uptake and an increased maximal ventilation in relation to maximal voluntary ventilation. Patients with interstitial pulmonary disease show abnormal gas exchange leading to hypoxemia, increased ventilation, and abnormal pulmonary mechanics. Patients with cardiac disease have a decreased maximal heart rate with decreased cardiac output and decreased maximal oxygen uptake. In these patients, arrhythmias may develop or angina may occur. Deconditioning results in a reduced maximal oxygen uptake in an otherwise normal study.

HEMOPTYSIS

By Steven Idell, M.D., Ph.D.
Tyler, Texas

Hemoptysis is defined as expectoration or coughing up of blood from the respiratory tract. As such, the source of bleeding can be in the trachea, the major airways, or the lung parenchyma. Hemoptysis encompasses coughing up of either large or small amounts of blood and includes expectoration of blood-streaked sputum. Massive hemoptysis is an alarming problem that demands rapid assessment and treatment. Although massive hemoptysis has been variably defined in the literature, it has included a range of 100 to 600 mL in a 24-hour period. The amount of expectorated blood is, however, often difficult to quantitate accurately in an emergency situation, and the physiologic consequences depend, in large part, on the underlying pulmonary function and effectiveness of cough in the individual patient. For these reasons, some have chosen to define massive hemoptysis as expectorated blood in an amount that is life-threatening.

The course of hemoptysis depends on the underlying problem and can be self-limited or recurrent. In cases of massive hemoptysis, there can be an initial cessation of bleeding followed by life-threatening recurrences. Mortality rates of up to 70 per cent were initially reported in patients with massive hemoptysis. Follow-up series report more encouraging mortality rates of about 15 per cent. Unfortunately, the rate of bleeding is not a reliable predictor of fatal outcome. For this reason, patients presenting with massive hemoptysis require rapid evaluation and careful intensive care unit (ICU) monitoring and management. The diagnostic approach to patients with hemoptysis is therefore guided by the specific clinical setting. The history, physical examination, and laboratory and radiographic findings allow the selection of the most appropriate tests.

HISTORY

The initial diagnostic concern is whether the patient is experiencing hemoptysis rather than hematemesis or bleeding from the oropharynx. Occasionally, it may be difficult to distinguish between hemoptysis and hematemesis because blood from the gastrointestinal tract can be aspirated and induce coughing and respiratory distress. Conversely, gross hemoptysis can induce nausea or vomiting. Blood originating in the lungs can be swallowed, causing stomach secretions to be bloody or produce positive results on Hematest evaluation. Hemoptysis is likely if there is known underlying pulmonary disease, and hematemesis is favored in the presence of a known predisposing gastrointestinal condition. A history of alcoholism, liver disease, or peptic ulcer disease should be sought. Conversely, a history of tuberculosis, pulmonary neoplasm, bronchiectasis, mitral valve disease, or long-term smoking should increase suspicion for hemoptysis. Patients may have underlying problems that could predispose to either hemoptysis or hematemesis, including several of the preceding conditions. A known bleeding diathesis or anticoagulation therapy may also contribute to the development of hemoptysis in the presence of such underlying pulmonary diseases.

An additional historical feature favoring hemoptysis is the occurrence of the problem over several days. Blood expectorated during hemoptysis may be described as frothy or associated with cough and purulent sputum, whereas hematemesis is most often described in association with vomiting. Based on these historical considerations, it may be worthwhile to examine the bloody material further. The presence of macrophages points toward hemoptysis, whereas the presence of food particles and an acid pH suggests hematemesis. Several historical points help narrow the differential diagnosis of hemoptysis (Tables 1 and 2).

Table 1. Historical Information for Narrowing the Differential Diagnosis of Hemoptysis

History of cigarette smoking
Cough and sputum production
Chest pain
Cardiopulmonary disease
Illicit drug use
Hematuria

A history of cough and associated sputum production over several years suggests either chronic bronchitis or bronchiectasis. Acute bronchitis, particularly in patients with chronic obstructive pulmonary disease (COPD), can be associated with hemoptysis, usually presenting as blood-streaked sputum. Close follow-up of these patients is mandatory, and radiographic screening and sputum cytologic studies should be strongly considered. The possibility of underlying neoplasm is further raised by recurrence of hemoptysis after completion of antibiotic therapy for acute bronchitis. A history of heavy smoking for several years should also increase suspicion for bronchogenic carcinoma. Although smokers older than 40 years of age are at increased risk of lung cancer, the diagnosis should be considered even in patients younger than 40 years if there is a history of heavy smoking beginning in the teenage years. In patients with cancer of the lung, hemoptysis is often a relatively late finding and there are often associated symptoms that may include a change in chronic cough, weight loss, chest pain, and fatigue.

Other infectious pulmonary diseases, including necrotizing pneumonias, pulmonary abscess, and bronchiectasis of any cause can all be associated with hemoptysis, cough, and purulent sputum. Patients with necrotizing pneumonia or pulmonary abscess often have foul-smelling sputum caused by anaerobic pathogens. In some cases, patients with pulmonary abscess or bronchiectasis may present with hemoptysis and little or no sputum production. Bronchiectasis can occur in patients with a history of severe or recurrent lower respiratory tract injuries or in patients with immotile cilia syndrome or cystic fibrosis. Mycetomas may develop in persistent lung cavities, such as those associated with inactive tuberculosis or sarcoidosis, and can produce brisk, recurrent hemoptysis. Patients with pneumococcal pneumonia may present with rusty sputum production, which may be confused with hemoptysis. Tuberculosis can also lead to hemoptysis, with the development of bleeding from cavitary pneumonitis or secondary bronchiectasis. Patients with tuberculosis or other granulomatous diseases may experience hemoptysis related to broncholithiasis when a calcified lymph node erodes through the wall of a proximate bronchus.

Chest discomfort in patients with hemoptysis can sometimes enable a patient to localize the bleeding site, but

Table 2. Commonly Encountered Causes of Hemoptysis

Infections, including bronchitis, bronchiectasis, pneumonia, and tuberculosis
Neoplasms: benign and malignant
Cardiovascular causes
Arteriovenous malformations and other structural causes
Trauma and inhalational injuries
Vasculitides

further characterization may be necessary to narrow the differential diagnosis. Chest pain in patients with hemoptysis commonly occurs in infectious or cardiovascular diseases. A history of trauma should also be sought in patients presenting with chest pain. Pleuritic-quality chest pain can occur in patients with pneumonia, and similar chest discomfort can develop in patients with pleural extension of a pulmonary abscess. In immunocompromised patients, hemoptysis and pleuritic chest pain suggest the diagnosis of underlying invasive pulmonary aspergillosis. Pleuritic chest pain and occasional nonproductive cough occur in patients with pulmonary embolism. This diagnosis is further supported by a history of shortness of breath and immobility. In patients with anginal pain, hemoptysis may be associated with pulmonary edema and myocardial ischemia. A history of valvular heart disease raises the possibility of underlying mitral stenosis.

Hemoptysis can also be a presenting feature of illicit drug abuse, particularly in patients who use cocaine. This possibility should be considered in young patients without a history of prior pulmonary or cardiac disease. Massive hemoptysis can occur in these patients.

A history of hematuria suggests the presence of a pulmonary-renal syndrome such as Wegener's granulomatosis, Goodpasture's syndrome, or rapidly progressive glomerulonephritis. Gross or microscopic hematuria can be associated with these disorders. A history of sinusitis also suggests the possibility of Wegener's granulomatosis.

A history of easy bleeding or anticoagulant use should also be sought. Patients with a systemic bleeding diathesis can present with hemoptysis. Alternatively, the development of hemoptysis in a patient receiving anticoagulant therapy in proper therapeutic dosage suggests the presence of an underlying structural cause.

Lastly, hemoptysis can be iatrogenic in origin. Patients undergoing endobronchial or transbronchial biopsy or right-sided heart catheterization can experience hemoptysis as a complication of these procedures. Occasionally, the cause of hemoptysis defies diagnosis and is termed "cryptogenic."

PHYSICAL EXAMINATION

The cause of hemoptysis may be suggested by examination of the upper airway. Sinusitis, sinus tenderness, or ulceration of the nasal septum can occur in Wegener's granulomatosis. A bleeding site may actually be identified on the gums or in the nasopharynx rather than the lungs. Laryngoscopy may be needed to identify a laryngeal source of bleeding. Telangiectases on the oral mucosa suggest the presence of hereditary hemorrhagic telangiectasia, a condition associated with arteriovenous malformations of the lungs or extensive telangiectases in the gastrointestinal tract. Poor dentition raises the possibility of anaerobic pulmonary abscess or necrotizing pneumonia.

Examination of the neck and chest can likewise be helpful. Ecchymoses suggest chest trauma. Physical findings including cachexia and supraclavicular adenopathy suggest the diagnosis of an underlying neoplasm. A tracheal shift in the supraclavicular notch can occur if there is significant volume loss associated with endobronchial obstruction. Obstructing lesions in the upper airway, including the trachea, can be associated with wheezing or hemoptysis. The symptoms and findings of tracheal neoplasms can be virtually indistinguishable from those of asthma, and a high index of suspicion is necessary to arrive at the correct diagnosis. Localized wheezing on auscultation of the chest may be associated with more distal lesions of the bronchial tree. Clubbing of the phalanges may be seen in bronchogenic carcinoma but also occurs in pulmonary abscess, bronchiectasis, or pulmonary arteriovenous malformations.

The cardiovascular examination is also important. The findings of bilateral basilar rales, neck vein distention, and peripheral edema strongly suggest that congestive heart failure could be the cause of apparent hemoptysis. A diastolic rumble and opening snap on auscultation of the heart indicates mitral stenosis. The physical findings in cases of pulmonary embolism may include a pleural friction rub associated with pulmonary infarction or peripheral edema associated with deep venous thrombosis. Arteriovenous malformations may be associated with an auscultatable bruit, which can be increased by inspiration. These patients may also complain of dyspnea, which worsens with sitting or standing (platypnea).

LABORATORY EVALUATION

Coagulation studies should be performed, particularly in patients with massive hemoptysis. A complete blood count, prothrombin time, partial thromboplastin time, and platelet count should be considered, although coagulopathies and thrombocytopenia do not usually cause spontaneous hemoptysis by themselves. A urinalysis along with serum urea nitrogen and serum creatinine determinations should be obtained to assess renal function. Abnormalities of renal function or hematuria may suggest underlying vasculitis. A sputum sample should be sent for Gram staining and culture. Sputum should also be sent for acid-fast stains and mycobacterial cultures, fungal cultures, and cytologic studies. Arterial blood gas determinations should be obtained in patients with massive hemoptysis to assess the adequacy of oxygenation and ventilation.

Other laboratory examinations depend on the clinical situation. A tuberculin skin test and anergy panel should be considered to evaluate the possibility of tuberculosis. Fungal serologic studies may be used to screen for underlying fungal disease. Circulating precipitins and sputum cultures that are positive for *Aspergillus* species are associated with mycetoma. The finding of *Pseudomonas* species in the sputum may suggest the presence of underlying bronchiectasis. Sputum studies can also help in the diagnosis of parasitic diseases. If paragonimiasis is being considered, ova can be identified in sputum by the Papanicolaou smear or in stool specimens sent for ova and parasite analysis. Ascariasis can likewise be diagnosed by finding larvae in sputum specimens. Amebiasis can be diagnosed by finding amebic cysts in the sputum, and a hemagglutination test usually produces positive results in extraintestinal infections. Echinococcal cysts found in the sputum confirm this diagnosis. Additional testing can be helpful in identifying the cause of bronchiectasis. The most reliable test for cystic fibrosis is the quantitative pilocarpine iontophoresis sweat test. Diagnosis of the immotile cilia syndrome can be made by electron microscopic analysis of nasal mucosa biopsy specimens.

Serologic studies can help in the diagnosis of the underlying causes of diffuse alveolar hemorrhage. A circulating antineutrophil cytoplasmic antibody (ANCA) determination may be helpful if Wegener's granulomatosis or related renal diseases are suspected. Goodpasture's syndrome is confirmed by the presence of antiglomerular basement membrane antibodies in the serum. In diffuse alveolar hemorrhage associated with systemic lupus erythematosus, antinuclear and antinative DNA antibodies may be detected, and cryoglobulins may be found in association with vasculitis. These studies can take considerable time to process and are therefore of limited value in acute disease.

CHEST RADIOGRAPHY FINDINGS

A chest radiograph is invariably indicated. Localized lesions may suggest a source of hemoptysis, but endoscopic confirmation is required. Diffuse infiltrates occur in pulmonary edema, extensive pneumonitis, or parenchymal hemorrhage. Cavitary lesions occur with pulmonary abscess, bronchogenic carcinoma, and mycobacterial or other infectious pulmonary diseases. Fibrocavitary disease of the upper lobes and/or superior segments of the lower lobes suggests reactivated tuberculosis. Cavitating infiltrates also occur with necrotizing pneumonia. Localized cystic lesions or increased bronchial markings are associated with bronchiectasis. Mycetomas or fungus balls occur in pre-existing cavities and present as intracavitary opacities, often associated with localized pleural thickening. Pleural effusion or blunting of a costophrenic sulcus can be seen with pulmonary emboli, and peripheral infiltrates can occur with pulmonary infarction. In patients with a normal chest roentgenogram, the possibility of bleeding from the oropharynx, gastrointestinal tract, or nose should also be considered as should pulmonary embolus. The lateral chest film should be carefully examined to exclude a mass in the tracheal air column.

BRONCHOSCOPY

Bronchoscopy is usually the most important initial diagnostic study in the evaluation of hemoptysis and is indicated in most patients. Exceptions include patients in whom a cause has been established previously and possibly patients with chronic bronchitis who have recurrent blood-streaked sputum and respond rapidly to medical therapy. In smokers with bronchitis and refractory hemoptysis, bronchoscopy should be strongly considered to exclude the possibility of an underlying neoplasm. Flexible fiberoptic bronchoscopy is usually performed initially, but rigid bronchoscopy may be required in cases of massive hemoptysis. There is good evidence that the early performance of bronchoscopy, particularly during active bleeding, is more effective in identifying the bleeding source. Bronchoscopy is useful in identifying the type and endobronchial extent of neoplasms and their staging and can document infectious causes of hemoptysis. Despite early bronchoscopy (performed within 48 hours of the acute episode of hemoptysis), a bleeding site is often not identified. In such patients, repeat bronchoscopy is indicated if hemoptysis recurs. Long-term smokers older than 40 years of age with a normal or nonlocalizing chest roentgenogram often have an underlying neoplasm that is causing hemoptysis. In these patients, especially males, and in those who bleed more than 30 mL daily, bronchoscopy should be strongly considered. In up to 20 per cent of patients, the cause of hemoptysis remains unknown despite evaluation including bronchoscopy. Careful follow-up of these patients is necessary.

OTHER DIAGNOSTIC STUDIES

An echocardiogram may confirm the presence of suspected mitral stenosis and can be helpful in documenting left ventricular dysfunction as a cause of hemoptysis. High-resolution computed tomography (CT) scanning of the chest is now the preferred procedure to diagnose bronchiectasis, although bronchography is still advocated by some when surgical resection is being considered. Computed tomography scanning is also useful in identifying vascular abnormalities such as aneurysms or broncholithiasis. Ventilation-perfusion lung scanning is indicated in patients with suspected pulmonary embolism. A normal perfusion scan excludes the diagnosis. A low-probability scan in the setting of low clinical suspicion can also be used to exclude the diagnosis, particularly if noninvasive studies of the lower extremities are also normal. A high-probability scan strongly suggests that pulmonary embolism has occurred, except if the patient is known to have had a prior episode of pulmonary embolism. In cases in which the ventilation-perfusion scan is equivocal and the clinical index of suspicion for pulmonary embolism is high, pulmonary arteriography can be used to exclude the diagnosis. Pulmonary angiography is also useful in documenting the presence of pulmonary arteriovenous malformations, particularly since multiple lesions may be present. Bronchial arteriography is occasionally needed to identify a bleeding site but is often nondiagnostic in patients in whom bronchoscopy has failed. Other tests that have limited clinical applicability include serial measurement of the diffusion capacity to document ongoing alveolar hemorrhage or the use of radiolabeled erythrocytes to localize the bleeding site.

SPECIAL CONSIDERATIONS

The role of lung biopsy in the diagnosis of hemoptysis is generally limited, but it can be used in selected patients to confirm the presence of underlying infection or vasculitis. The choice of transbronchial or open biopsy depends on the clinical presentation. Massive hemoptysis is a true medical emergency, and referral to a thoracic surgeon in consultation with a pulmonologist should be arranged. Mild to moderate hemoptysis can cause respiratory distress in patients with limited pulmonary reserve or serious associated illnesses. In such patients, invasive options may be limited, and the diagnostic strategy should be individualized to the clinical circumstances.

NECK MASSES

By Mary Hooks, M.D.,
and Burton L. Eisenberg, M.D.
Philadelphia, Pennsylvania

Although the differential diagnosis of a mass in the neck is complex, most neck masses can be diagnosed accurately prior to surgical intervention. In adults, 85 per cent of neck masses are neoplastic, and 85 per cent of these neoplastic lesions are malignant. The majority of these are metastatic from a source above the clavicles and can be identified with a complete physical examination. All neck masses in those older than 40 years of age should be considered malignant and should be diagnosed and treated expeditiously. The clinical assessment of a neck mass includes pertinent history, physical findings, useful laboratory tests, and radiographic studies. A brief review of the most common clinical entities that may present with a neck mass is also provided (Table 1).

Age is an important guideline in the differential diagnosis. After age 40, a neck mass should be considered malignant until proved otherwise. A rapidly enlarging mass is more likely to be malignant, whereas congenital and infectious or inflammatory lesions are more commonly associated with an indolent course and are more commonly seen in pediatric patients. The location of a mass is extremely helpful in the differential diagnosis. A mass in the midline of the upper neck is likely to be a thyroglossal duct cyst, whereas a lesion in the lower neck is more likely to be of thyroid origin. A mass at the anterior border of the sternocleidomastoid is likely to be a branchial cleft cyst or an enlarged lymph node. Because head and neck cancers metastasize in an orderly and predictable progression, the location of an enlarged cervical lymph node may direct the physician to the primary tumor site (Fig. 1 and Table 2).

Table 1. Differential Diagnosis of a Neck Mass

Differential Diagnosis: First Think Malignancy

Neoplasms

- Malignant
  - Primary
    - Thyroid carcinoma
    - Salivary gland carcinoma, including parotid
    - Sarcoma
    - Neuroblastoma
    - Lymphoma, skin, including melanoma
  - Metastatic
    - Sources above the clavicles (85%): tumors of the head and neck, skin, sinuses, oropharynx, larynx, thyroid, and salivary gland
    - Sources below the clavicles: tumors of the lung, breast, kidney, and gonads
- Benign
  - Thyroid mass
  - Salivary gland mass, including parotid
  - Lipoma
  - Epidermoid cyst
  - Hemangioma
  - Paraganglioma
  - Neurofibroma
  - Schwannoma

Congenital

- Thyroglossal duct cyst
- Branchial cleft cyst
- Cystic hygroma
- Teratoma
- Dermoid
- Vascular malformation

Inflammatory

- Bacterial and viral infections
  - Cervical adenitis
  - Abscesses
  - Mononucleosis
  - Brucellosis
  - Toxoplasmosis
  - Cat-scratch disease
  - Histoplasmosis
  - Actinomycosis
- Granulomatous disorders
  - *Mycobacterium tuberculosis*
  - Atypical mycobacteria
  - Sarcoidosis

Others

- Zenker's diverticulum
- Laryngocele
- Normal structures
  - Hyoid bone, submandibular gland, transverse processes of the cervical vertebrae

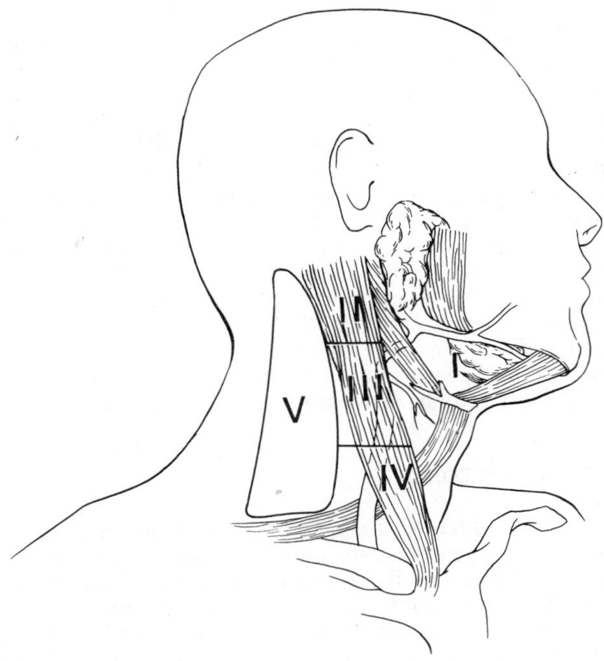

Figure 1. Lymph node levels within the neck.

ASSOCIATED SYMPTOMS

The patient's sense of well-being can reflect the chronicity of the disease process. Constitutional symptoms, including fever, weight loss, and night sweats, may indicate an inflammatory or infectious process or a lymphoma. Pain around the orbits or skull base may be associated with a

Table 2. Primary Tumor Site of Lymph Node Metastasis

Lymphatic Drainage	Possible Primary Sites
Level I	
Submental	Lower lip; chin; anterior oral cavity, including anterior third of tongue and floor of mouth
Submandibular	Upper and lower lip, anterior floor of the mouth, facial skin
Level II	Oral cavity; oropharynx, hypopharynx, including soft palate, base of tongue, piriform sinus
Level III	Hypopharynx, thyroid, lung, gastrointestinal tract
Level IV	Thyroid, cervical esophagus, trachea
Level V	Nasopharynx, oropharynx, hypopharynx, thyroid, paranasal sinuses, scalp
Supraclavicular	Infraclavicular, including lung, esophagus, breast, pancreas, gastrointestinal tract, genitourinary and gynecologic sources

carcinoma of the nasopharynx, tongue base, or hypopharynx. Otalgia may be caused indirectly by inflammation of tissues innervated by the facial nerve (including nose, paranasal sinuses, nasopharynx, mandible, and salivary glands) or by direct impingement by a mass in the ear canal. Odynophagia may be secondary to a mass in the tongue base or hypopharynx. Impingement of the recurrent laryngeal nerve or facial nerve may cause hoarseness or hypoesthesia, respectively. A change in the sense of smell or the development of epistaxis and nasal obstruction suggests a maxillary or nasopharyngeal mass. A complete dental history is of paramount importance. It may reveal an inflammatory or infectious process or a malignancy if healing is incomplete. Productive cough, hemoptysis, or shortness of breath may indicate pulmonary involvement by a primary tumor or metastatic disease.

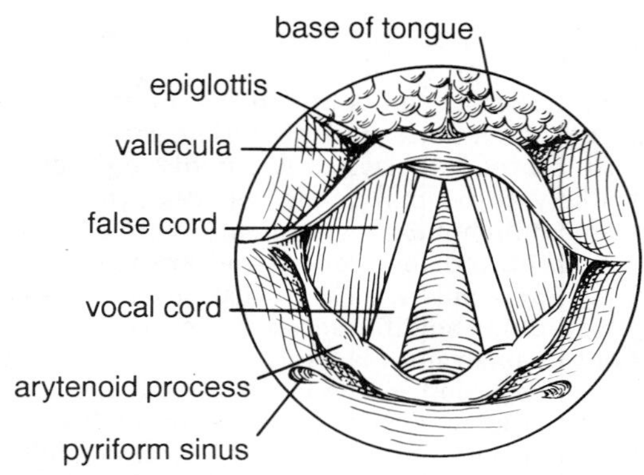

Figure 2. Anatomic structures in the supraglottic and glottic larynx.

MEDICAL HISTORY

A previous history of cancer of the skin or scalp, head or neck, or lung is obviously important but frequently overlooked. Squamous cell carcinomas arising in the same area more than 3 years later are usually new primaries, rather than recurrent disease. Family history is particularly important in thyroid carcinoma. A history of cigarette and alcohol use is very important in adults. Exposures to radiation, asbestos, and pets are also helpful in the differential diagnosis.

PHYSICAL EXAMINATION

The physical examination is the most important part of the diagnostic evaluation. Fifty to sixty-five per cent of adults will have an obvious primary tumor of the head or neck. The examination must be thorough and consistent and proceed in an orderly progression. To avoid distraction, the physician should examine the mass at the end of a thorough head and neck examination. Cachexia, if present, provides a measure of the severity and chronicity of the disease. Abnormal vital signs, including tachycardia and fever, may indicate infection or dehydration. Ulcerations, nodules, and pigmented or other suspicious lesions should be carefully sought during the evaluation. A complete cranial nerve evaluation is essential in any patient with a neck mass of unclear etiology. The ears, nose, and eyes should be examined for any sign of mass effect, abnormal drainage, discharge, or bleeding.

Dentures *must be removed* for the examination of the mouth. Halitosis may be the first indication of a lesion in the upper aerodigestive tract. The entire mucosal surface must be visualized. The physician should palpate the floor of the mouth using a bimanual technique (the finger of one hand inside the mouth and the second hand submandibular). *Any suspicious lesion should be biopsied.* A systematic examination of the neck should provide detailed documentation of mass location (see Fig. 1). Bimanual palpation contributes the most information. This maneuver is performed by grasping the sternocleidomastoid muscle and feeling nodes between the thumb and the first two fingers. The relationship of the mass to the thyroid should be noted, and the thyroid should be palpated for the presence, number, and location of nodules. Important qualities of the mass include location, firmness, tenderness, size, mobility, and associated thrill or bruit. The nasopharynx, hypopharynx, and larynx all should be thoroughly examined with indirect laryngoscopy (Fig. 2). The flexible nasopharyngoscope facilitates a thorough inspection of the upper aerodigestive tract, painlessly, in the clinical setting.

If the history and physical examination do not reveal a diagnosis, a unilateral, enlarged lymph node in an adult patient must be considered a metastasis. Proceed with further investigation, including triple endoscopy as outlined below, computed tomography (CT) evaluation, and more complete physical examination. Primary tumors below the clavicles most frequently metastasize to the neck. Primaries include the lung, breast, genitourinary, and gynecologic malignancies, and the physical examination should focus on these organ systems.

Triple endoscopy, which includes direct laryngoscopy, esophagoscopy, and bronchoscopy with "guided" biopsy, should be performed in all patients with an unidentified primary or a *known* head and neck primary. The most common areas of silent primary tumor are the tonsils, base of the tongue, and piriform sinus. The nasopharynx has become a less common site, with increased use of flexible nasopharyngoscopy. Aggressive biopsies should be performed in these common areas of silent primary and in the anatomic areas associated with lymphatic drainage of these primary sites. Triple endoscopy can provide information regarding the extent of tumor and the possibility of a second primary.

LABORATORY EVALUATION

A complete blood count may reveal lymphocytosis or atypical lymphocytes. Thyroid function studies are essential in any patient with an anterior neck mass. Monospot and purified protein derivative (PPD) may demonstrate infectious mononucleosis or tuberculosis, respectively. Epstein-Barr virus, anticapsid antibodies, and serum IgG correlate with nasopharyngeal carcinoma. A positive Kveim test may indicate sarcoidosis. Urinalysis and liver function studies may further define the disease process. Any wound drainage should be cultured. Any patient with productive cough should have sputum submitted for culture, cytology, and acid-fast bacillus testing.

DIAGNOSTIC IMAGING

Plain films provide limited information; they usually cannot rule out an abnormality. A Panorex film may demonstrate bone erosion or other lesions of the oral cavity. Posteroanterior and lateral chest radiographs should be obtained in all adults. Ultrasound may distinguish solid from cystic lesions of the thyroid but otherwise has limited utility.

The CT scan can be the single most informative test in the diagnosis of a cervical mass. It may delineate the extent of tissue or lymphatic involvement, and it may distinguish cystic from solid lesions. Offering high spatial resolution with discrimination between fat, muscle, bone, and other soft tissues, CT surpasses magnetic resonance imaging (MRI) in the ability to detect bony erosion. Dynamic CT helps distinguish vessels from enlarged lymph nodes or masses and maintains image quality with the use of less contrast agent. Spiral CT provides a faster approach using multiplanar reconstruction while maintaining the quality of the image. Computed tomography scans of the chest, abdomen, and pelvis may be helpful in identifying the site of an occult primary.

Magnetic resonance imaging may provide more accurate information regarding the size, location, and extent of a tumor. The advantages of MRI over CT include high spatial resolution, multiplanar imaging without patient repositioning, and the ability to clearly depict vessels without the use of intravenous contrast media. Gadolinium may be used as a contrast agent to enhance the border between neoplastic and normal tissues and to detect perineural invasion. Gadolinium accumulates primarily on mucosal surfaces. Its uptake in tumors is variable. Gadolinium does not bind to fibrous tissue, muscle, or fat. The main disadvantage of MRI is movement artifact, especially in laryngeal or hypopharyngeal images. However, MRI is superior to CT in the diagnosis of tumors of the nasopharynx, oral cavity, and oropharynx.

Two indications for arteriography are a pulsatile neck mass and clinical evidence of a paraganglioma. High-resolution angiography is preferred over digital subtraction angiography because it provides more information and embolization may be performed.

BIOPSY

Punch biopsy aids in the diagnosis of mucosal lesions. The biopsy should be obtained at the border, avoiding areas of obvious necrosis. Fine-needle aspiration (FNA) is rapid, inexpensive, and increasingly useful. At least six passes are made through the lesion with a fine-gauge (22G) needle while suction is applied. Once the needle is outside the lesion, suction should be released before withdrawing the needle from the neck. Fine-needle aspiration has an associated false-negative rate as low as 7 per cent. The diagnostic accuracy depends on the physician's skill and the cytopathologist's experience. However, a negative result *cannot* be interpreted as the absence of malignancy. Cytology may be particularly useful in distinguishing metastatic carcinoma from lymphoma. *Core biopsy should not be performed on a neck mass!*

Open biopsy should be performed only when clinical evaluation, laboratory tests, and FNA have not provided a diagnosis. The operation should be performed only by a surgeon who can undertake an immediate complete neck dissection. Thorough, informed consent for a complete neck dissection should be obtained prior to open biopsy. It deserves emphasis that patients who have undergone pretreatment biopsies have a higher incidence of late regional and distant metastases as well as an increased rate of local wound complications.

MALIGNANT PRIMARY NEOPLASMS

Thyroid enlargement accounts for 50 per cent of all neck masses and is usually apparent by its location in the lower neck. The most important issue in the diagnosis of a thyroid mass is distinguishing benign from malignant lesions. The patient's age, sex, family history, and previous radiation exposure all are important. A thyroid lesion is more likely to be cancer in men than in women and in younger patients than in older ones. Thyroid carcinoma is matched with lymphoma as the most common neoplasm of the pediatric and young adult age groups. A family history of thyroid cancer suggests medullary carcinoma. The signs and symptoms that suggest malignancy include a change in the size of the mass, hoarseness, dysphagia, and dyspnea. The physical examination should focus on whether the mass is solitary (more likely to be malignant) or multiple, and whether there is associated lymphadenopathy (greater suspicion of malignancy). Lymph node metastases are the initial finding in 15 per cent of thyroid carcinoma patients. Fine-needle aspiration is the gold standard in diagnosis. Its accuracy may approach 97 per cent, depending on tumor type; FNA is extremely accurate in the diagnosis of papillary and medullary carcinomas. It is less useful for follicular lesions, because the criteria for malignancy (capsular or vascular invasion) cannot be determined with FNA. Indeterminate cytology requires repeat FNA or thyroid lobectomy when the diagnosis remains unclear.

Fewer than 3 per cent of all head and neck tumors are salivary gland neoplasms. Seventy per cent of these tumors occur in the parotid, and three quarters of these are benign. The diagnosis of parotid tumor should be considered whenever a patient presents with a mass anterior to or below the ear, at the angle of the mandible, or in the submandibular triangle. Seventy per cent of parotid tumors are pleomorphic adenomas, which are more common in women than in men and have a peak incidence in the fifth decade. These benign adenomas usually present as painless, slowly growing, freely moveable masses of variable size with no associated paralysis or ulceration. Facial nerve paralysis is usually associated with malignancy. Submandibular gland tumors are more commonly malignant. Computed tomography or MRI is helpful in delineating the extent of disease, particularly in lesions that involve the deep lobe, but CT and MRI do not generally distinguish benign from malignant disease. The gold-standard diagnostic maneuver and safest approach to biopsy is a superficial parotidectomy. When the deep lobe is involved, it can be excised after removal of the superficial lobe and identification of the facial nerve and its branches.

Hodgkin's disease has a bimodal age distribution, with early incidence between ages 10 and 13 years, and late incidence in patients older than 55 years. Hodgkin's disease in the neck usually consists of nontender, matted, rubbery nodes found primarily in the posterior triangle. Lymphadenopathy may be present in other areas, including the axilla and groin. Constitutional symptoms including fever, night sweats, and weight loss may also be present. The incidence of non-Hodgkin's lymphoma increases steadily from childhood to late adulthood. It is otherwise similar to Hodgkin's disease in its presentation. Important diagnostic studies include FNA, bone marrow biopsy, and CT scan.

METASTATIC NEOPLASMS

Twelve per cent of head and neck tumors present as an asymmetric neck mass. Ninety-five per cent of all head and neck tumors are squamous cell carcinomas. The ratio of male-to-female patients is 9:1, but the incidence is increasing in women. Tobacco is the principal carcinogen associated with these tumors, and alcohol may be a co-carcinogen. Oral cavity lesions tend to present early, while oropharyngeal lesions tend to present at a more advanced and more poorly differentiated stage. Fifty per cent of nasopharyngeal carcinomas initially present with a neck mass. Mucosal punch biopsy may provide the diagnosis in oral cavity lesions. Fine-needle aspiration of a neck mass positive for squamous cell carcinoma suggests a primary tumor of the head and neck. Both CT scans and triple endoscopy are important in assessing the extent of disease. Triple endoscopy can also provide biopsy information important in assessing the possibility of a second primary tumor.

Carcinoma of the lung is the most common origin of an isolated cervical metastasis, emphasizing the importance of an initial chest x-ray study. Other possible primaries include pancreas, esophagus, stomach, breast, ovary, and prostate. Primary tumors in these locations usually metastasize to supraclavicular lymph nodes. Fine-needle aspiration of a neck mass that shows adenocarcinoma is more suspicious for a primary tumor outside the head and neck.

A thorough history and physical examination will identify the site of the primary tumor in 95 per cent of patients with a neck mass. Computed tomography is also helpful. Occult tumors usually originate in the nasopharynx, hypopharynx (piriform sinus), or oropharynx (tonsillar fossa and base of the tongue). At the time of endoscopy, these areas should be aggressively biopsied.

BENIGN NEOPLASMS

Paragangliomas originate from neural crest cells and are found mainly in the carotid body and jugular bulb. They are generally benign neoplasms that present as painless masses in the upper neck along the anterior border of the sternocleidomastoid. These lesions occasionally transmit a carotid pulsation and may have an associated thrill or bruit. They are pulsatile, compressible masses that rapidly refill on release of pressure and can be moved laterally but not vertically. Arteriography is diagnostic and demonstrates a vascular blush. Schwannomas are usually solitary and may be painful. Radicular pain or unpleasant paresthesias may be present on light palpation.

Thyroglossal duct cyst presents as a mass anywhere in the midline of the upper neck during late childhood or early adulthood. Eighty per cent are at or just above the hyoid bone. Unless associated with infection, these cysts are firm and painless and typically rise with swallowing or tongue protrusion. They often appear following an upper respiratory infection. Acute inflammation may be controlled with antibiotic therapy. After resolution of the acute inflammation, ultrasonography may be used to differentiate them from a lymph node or dermoid cyst. Unlike branchial cleft cysts, thyroglossal duct cysts usually do not have a sinus tract. The diagnosis is made on clinical course and ultrasonographic findings. Although 5 per cent of thyroglossal duct cysts contain functioning thyroid tissue, radionuclide scanning is usually not necessary.

Branchial cleft cyst is the most common congenital abnormality seen in the lateral neck. Most of these congenital abnormalities appear before age 10 years. They can be found anywhere from the preauricular area to the upper neck along the anterior border of the sternocleidomastoid. These lesions are soft, nontender, and mobile. The presence of a sinus tract confirms the diagnosis. The most common branchial cleft cyst arises from the second cleft and presents at the inferior to middle third of the sternocleidomastoid. The cyst includes a fistulous tract that courses superiorly along the carotid sheath between the internal and the external carotid arteries and ends at the pharynx. The less common first cleft cyst presents above the level of the hyoid bone, just below the angle of the mandible, extends through the parotid gland, and ends in the external auditory canal. The diagnosis is based on clinical findings.

Cystic hygromas are benign lymphatic tumors. Fifty per cent of them are present at birth, and more than 90 per cent present prior to age 1 year. These characteristically fluctuant, diffuse, spongy masses with indiscrete margins are usually found in the posterior triangle or supraclavicular area and may extend to the face or mediastinum. Transillumination may be diagnostic. The CT scan or MRI assists in delineating the extent of disease.

Inflammatory lesions usually occur in children in association with viral upper respiratory infections. Associated symptoms include fever, chills, and leukocytosis. Bacterial infections usually respond well to appropriate antibiotic therapy, with significant improvement within days. Wound drainage or abscess aspiration fluid should be submitted for culture and sensitivity to direct antibiotic therapy. Computed tomography is useful in defining the extent of disease.

Many disease entities can present as a neck mass. A complete history and systematic physical examination will reveal the diagnosis in most cases. Close observation and antibiotics provide a reasonable approach in the pediatric and young adult population. In adults, however, these lesions are usually malignant and a vigorous diagnostic approach is indicated. Any neck mass in an adult patient should be considered malignant until proved otherwise.

ACUTE ABDOMINAL PAIN

By Jeffrey Landercasper, M.D.,
Thomas H. Cogbill, M.D.,
and Bradley C. Thaemert, M.D.
La Crosse, Wisconsin

The approach to patients presenting with acute abdominal pain requires a rapid initial assessment to judge the severity of illness. Attempts to arrive at an accurate diagnosis should not delay resuscitation and treatment of patients who present with shock and obvious peritonitis. These patients may have a fatal outcome if vigorous hemodynamic resuscitation is not instituted immediately. Selected patients may require laparotomy, with minimal time spent on diagnostic work-up.

Most patients presenting with acute abdominal pain are not gravely ill. The crucial question facing the clinician caring for these patients is whether an urgent abdominal operation is necessary. A systematic evaluation of the patient's pain should be undertaken to answer this question. This methodical evaluation includes an accurate history, a complete physical examination (which includes a rectal and pelvic examination), blood studies, and a judicious radiographic work-up. A search for extra-abdominal (Table 1) and nonsurgical (Table 2) causes of acute pain is essential. Intra-abdominal causes of acute abdominal pain stratified by organ system are listed in Table 3. The

Table 1. Extra-abdominal Causes of Abdominal Pain

Thoracic Cage
Lower rib fractures
Empyema
Pleuritis (any cause)

Heart
Myocardial infarction
Pericarditis
Congestive heart failure with congestive hepatomegaly

Thoracic Aorta
Dissection of thoracic aorta
Ruptured thoracic aorta

Thoracic Esophagus
Rupture
Diffuse esophageal spasm
Reflux esophagitis

Lung
Infarction
Pneumonia

Spine
Fracture
Spinal cord compression
Herpes zoster
Osteomyelitis

Genital
Testicular torsion
Epididymitis
Prostatitis

Other
Septic hip

medical history must be complete to maximize the chance that a clinician will reach a timely, accurate diagnosis. A history of medication administration and disease states that may predispose the patient to specific conditions should be sought. For example, patients with atrial fibrillation may have embolic events. Alcoholism and oral steroids and nonsteroidal anti-inflammatory medications predispose to gastroduodenal ulcer disease. Female gender, obesity, and multiple pregnancies are associated with gallstones. Multiple prior laparotomies predispose a patient to the risk of small bowel obstruction. Intravenous drug abuse and alcoholism are associated with hepatitis and pancreatitis. Many other associations exist and justify the need for an interview that includes a prior social history, family history, and medication and surgical history in addition to the complete medical history and characterization of pain. The characteristics of abdominal pain to be elucidated include location, timing of onset, severity, and character as well as associated symptoms and modifying factors that precipitate or alleviate the pain.

LOCATION

The location of abdominal pain provides the first clue to its origin. Most visceral disease causes the patient to perceive pain near the organ's position in the body cavity. For example, biliary colic usually presents with right upper quadrant pain, sigmoid diverticulitis presents with left lower quadrant pain, and appendicitis presents with right lower quadrant pain. An initial and nearly complete list of conditions causing a patient's pain can therefore be generated simply by discerning the location of the pain (especially if the pain is focal) and listing all the organs and structures in the area of pain. Exceptions to this rule may occur when the diseased organ is located in an unusual location (e.g., appendix and cecum located in the right upper quadrant) or when the pain is "referred" to a distant location. A gastroduodenal origin of pain is usually perceived by the patient as being upper abdominal, a small intestinal origin is perceived as central or periumbilical, and a colonic origin is perceived as lower abdominal. Referred pain is a phenomenon whereby the patient perceives a noxious sensation in the somatic nervous system distribution at the same spinal cord level as the afferent nerve fibers that supply the diseased organ or structure. Patterns of referred pain in certain conditions are common enough to provide valuable clues to the cause of pain. For example, pain at the tip of the left shoulder in a patient with left upper quadrant discomfort after trauma suggests diaphragmatic irritation by blood from a ruptured spleen. Pain is sensed by the patient in the cutaneous somatic distribution of the phrenic nerve (C4). Other common patterns of referred pain are listed in Table 4. In addition to recognition of referred pain patterns, a history of a changing location of pain over time may be helpful in the diagnosis. In the classic presentation of appendicitis, for example, pain begins centrally in the abdomen and later moves to the right lower quadrant.

Table 2. Nonsurgical Causes of Acute Abdominal Pain

Metabolic and Endocrine
Acute intermittent porphyria
Diabetic ketoacidosis
Uremia
Acute adrenal insufficiency
Hereditary Mediterranean fever
Pleuritis (any cause)

Toxic
Cocaine
Drugs
Heavy metals (especially lead)
Black widow spider envenomation
Narcotic withdrawal

Hematologic
Sickle cell crisis
Leukemic crisis
Vasculitis (SLE, PAN)
Porphyria

Infectious
Spontaneous (primary) bacterial peritonitis
Tuberculous peritonitis
Gastroenteritis

Hepatobiliary and Pancreatic
Hepatitis
Hepatomegaly
Acute pancreatitis (uncomplicated)

Neurogenic
Herpes zoster
Nerve root compression
Tabes dorsalis

Miscellaneous
Rectus sheath hematoma

SLE = systemic lupus erythematosus; PAN = periarteritis nodosa.

Table 3. Intra-abdominal Causes of Acute Abdominal Pain by Organ System

Gastrointestinal
Perforated viscus (any cause)
Gastric or duodenal ulcer
Regional enteritis
Gastritis
Gastroenteritis
Bowel infarction
Appendicitis
Diverticulitis (any site)
Colitis (any cause)
Obstruction (any site, any cause), pseudo-obstruction
Volvulus (any site)
Trauma

Biliary and Pancreatic
Cholecystitis or colic
Cholangitis
Liver abscess
Hepatic hemorrhage (any cause)
Pancreatitis (or pseudocyst)
Trauma

Gynecologic
Endometritis
Ectopic pregnancy
PID, tubo-ovarian abscess
Ovarian torsion
Ruptured ovarian cyst
Endometriosis
Fibroid infarction

Liver and Spleen
Hepatitis
Infarction (segmental or organ)

Liver and Spleen *(Continued)*
Congestive hepatomegaly
Rupture or hemorrhage
Abscess

Genitourinary
Stones
Pyelonephritis
Obstruction (any cause)
Perinephric abscess
Renal infarction (any cause)
Acute retention
Acute cystitis

Peritoneal
Abscess
Primary peritonitis
Spontaneous primary bacterial peritonitis

Retroperitoneal
Abscess
Hemorrhage

Vascular
Aortic, iliac, or visceral artery aneurysm
Mesenteric venous thrombosis
Mesenteric arterial ischemia (any cause)
Spontaneous arterial rupture

Miscellaneous
Omental infarction
Infarcted appendices epiploicae
Mesenteric adenitis

PID = pelvic inflammatory disease.

TIMING OF ONSET

The mode of onset and progression of pain varies with the inciting process causing the pain. A ruptured abdominal aortic aneurysm or a perforated duodenal ulcer often has an explosive, rapid onset. These patients may have felt entirely well until the rupture or perforation occurred and may be able to inform the examiner about the exact hour of onset of their symptoms. The majority of patients with other causes of abdominal pain do not have an instantaneous onset of pain. Common conditions having progressive symptoms over hours include acute cholecystitis, pancreatitis, mesenteric infarction, appendicitis, and ureteral colic. Many other processes initially lead to vague and mild abdominal symptoms for 1 to 2 days and then progress to sufficient severity to cause the patient to seek medical advice. Small and large bowel obstruction, walled-off enteric perforations, appendicitis, diverticulitis, penetrating peptic ulcer, pyelonephritis, spontaneous bacterial peritonitis, and pelvic inflammatory disease may present in this manner. The timing of the onset of pain depends on many factors, including the patient's ability to tolerate pain, underlying medical conditions, the effectiveness of host defenses, medications being taken (especially antibiotics, narcotics, and steroids), and the severity of the condition (e.g., partial mechanical small bowel obstruction versus complete small bowel obstruction with strangulation and infarction).

CHARACTER AND SEVERITY

The character and severity of pain provide additional clues to the diagnosis. Patients may experience a "visceral" type of pain, which they often describe as dull, deep, aching, poorly localized, vague, of slow onset, and sometimes crampy. Visceral pain may be accompanied by anorexia, nausea, vomiting, sweating, and salivation. Visceral pain usually results from distention of a hollow viscus or organ capsule or from ischemic, inflammatory, or malignant stimulation of autonomic nervous system afferent fibers in an organ. In contrast, "parietal" or "somatic" pain is perceived as superficial, sharp, stabbing, pricking, localized, more abrupt in onset, and more intense and constant. Somatic pain is often exacerbated by patient movement, coughing, or sneezing. Blood, pus, feces, and infected bile or urine may be the inciting caustic stimulators of pain from the parietal peritoneum, a condition termed "peritonitis." The parietal pain of peritonitis is often more severe than visceral pain. Instantaneous onset of severe and unbearable pain often indicates gastroduodenal perforation or massive hemorrhage. In contrast, the pain of peritonitis from a perforated appendix, small intestine, or colon is usually a crescendo, building from a tolerable to intolerable level as bacterial contamination increases. The pain of bowel obstruction is usually visceral in character, increases in severity over hours to days, and is crampy. Obstruction of the gallbladder and ureter is often visceral too, but the onset and severity is more rapid. "Colicky" pain implies pain-free periods. Colicky pain may occur with bowel and ureteral obstruction when smooth muscle contraction alternates with relaxation. Biliary "colic" is rare because pain from cystic duct obstruction is usually constant and persists for 30 minutes to 6 hours. Pain of biliary origin lasting more than 6 to 12 hours suggests that an acute inflammatory response (acute cholecystitis) is contributing

Table 4. Causes of Referred Pain by Location

Shoulder
Gallbladder
Liver capsule
Spleen
Diaphragm
Pneumoperitoneum
Right Scapula
Biliary
Left Scapula
Spleen
Back
Aorta
Pancreas
Kidney
Ureter
Groin and Scrotum
Kidney
Ureter, bladder
Iliac artery
Prostate gland
Chest and Substernal Area
Biliary tract
Esophagus
Stomach
Pancreas
Lower Back and Sacral Area
Rectum
Uterus

to the pain. Severe, agonizing pain that is resistant to narcotics suggests advanced disease, hemorrhagic pancreatitis, or mesenteric infarction.

ASSOCIATED SYMPTOMS

Symptoms associated with abdominal pain include anorexia, nausea, vomiting, constipation, diarrhea, and melena or hematochezia. These symptoms are nonspecific but do help diagnostically and therefore should be elicited in the medical history. Nausea and vomiting may occur with most abdominal disorders but are of paramount importance in bowel obstruction. In general, the more proximal the obstruction in the alimentary tract, the greater the severity of vomiting and the less the patient is distended. In contrast, distal colonic obstruction may lead to profound distention but not necessarily severe vomiting. Feculent vomiting heralds well-established, nearly complete or complete obstruction of the small intestine. Vomiting may also be severe as a response to regional inflammatory changes, such as with pancreatitis. Vomiting may cause the Mallory-Weiss syndrome and Boerhaave's syndrome.

A history of constipation, especially in the elderly, does not usually correlate with bowel obstruction. However, a recent change in bowel habits, with progressive constipation and then obstipation (no stool or flatus) accompanied by crampy pain, bloating, and distention is significant. Paradoxically, intermittent diarrhea associated with the preceding symptoms may indicate distal colonic obstruction because only liquid stool is able to pass through a narrowed channel. Diarrhea and bloody stools are clues to a host of potential causes of abdominal pain, such as colitis (any cause), gastroenteritis, and Crohn's disease.

Other symptoms, such as jaundice, hematemesis, and hematuria, provide putative evidence that the hepatobiliary, esophagogastroduodenal, or genitourinary system is involved, respectively. Pneumaturia and fecaluria suggest an enterovesical fistula, and passage of feces via the vagina suggests a colovaginal fistula.

MODIFYING FACTORS

After the onset of pain, patients may notice factors that exacerbate or ameliorate it. Pain relieved by eating or antacids suggests a peptic origin. Pain markedly worsened by movement, coughing, or the "bumps in the road on an automobile ride" is usually imputable to peritoneal irritation. Pain worsened by deep breathing and coughing may be attributable to diaphragmatic irritation. Patients with inflammatory changes adjacent to the bladder may have urinary frequency or pain with micturition (e.g., in sigmoid diverticulitis).

PHYSICAL EXAMINATION

The physical examination must be complete. Abdominal, rectal, and pelvic examinations are essential, but so too is the remainder of the examination because abdominal disease may have extra-abdominal manifestations. Furthermore, the primary pathologic condition may be outside the abdomen (see Table 1). Examination begins with simple observation of the patient and assessment of vital signs. Witnessing the patient ambulate and observing the willingness to move are helpful in assessing the severity of pain. An effort should be made to exclude extra-abdominal sources of pain (e.g., basilar pneumonia with pleural friction rub) and to identify extra-abdominal markers of potential gastrointestinal disease (e.g., jaundice, scleral icterus, stigmata of multiple polyposis syndromes). Evidence of trauma and physical signs of alcoholism and intravenous drug abuse should be identified. Signs of peripheral and cerebrovascular disease and atrial fibrillation are pertinent if present. Periumbilical and flank ecchymoses may be apparent.

The evaluation of the abdomen includes inspection, auscultation, percussion, and palpation. Inspection involves a search for scars, masses, hernias, ecchymoses, and distention. Auscultation is important but lacks sensitivity and specificity. Characteristic intermittent, high-pitched bowel sounds alternating with splashes, rushes, and tinkles of gas are associated with bowel obstruction. The complete absence of bowel sounds over 1 to 2 minutes is associated with diffuse peritonitis, but the presence of active bowel sounds does not exclude a significant, even life-threatening, pathologic condition. Bruits should be noted during auscultation.

Gentleness and patience are the key to percussion and palpation if these maneuvers are to be of value. Preferably, percussion and palpation begin at sites distant from where the patient localizes pain. Percussion aids in distinguishing whether gas or fluid is the cause of abdominal distention. Percussion is also used to establish whether involuntary guarding is present. Involuntary guarding connotes reflex contraction of the abdominal wall muscles overlying intra-abdominal pathology. It is present when the minimal stimulation of light percussion or palpation elicits contraction. "Heavy-handed" guarding and "deep" rebound tenderness may be found in nonsurgical causes of abdominal pain. A single rough touch to the abdomen hinders all subsequent examinations. In addition to palpation for masses, the main focus of physical examination is to try to discern whether the patient has evidence of peritoneal irritation, which, if present, suggests that laparotomy may be indicated. The factors that suggest peritoneal irritation include the patient's reluctance to move or allow hip extension, a preference for the fetal position or hip flexion, involuntary guarding to light palpation or percussion, and exacerbation of pain with shaking the bed or the pelvis. In advanced peritonitis, a patient may have a "boardlike," rigid abdomen. The back and flanks should also be examined, with attempts to elicit tenderness. Inguinal and femoral hernias, masses, and points of tenderness should be noted. Pelvic and rectal examinations complete the abdominal examination. Stool should be checked for occult blood. Cervical cultures may be appropriate.

LABORATORY EVALUATION

The patient history and examination should suggest a list of diagnostic possibilities and direct a laboratory and imaging evaluation. Laboratory tests are essential for excluding medical causes of pain (e.g., an electrocardiogram to exclude heart disease) and for assisting in preoperative resuscitation. Recommended tests for almost all patients include a complete blood count with differential and urinalysis. Further studies may be indicated in more complicated cases or in critically ill patients. Serum electrolyte, creatinine, and amylase determinations; liver function tests; and clotting studies are appropriate in selected patients but need not be ordered routinely. Arterial blood gas monitoring is appropriate in patients who appear severely ill or who have hypotension. Metabolic acidosis may be present in conditions causing major intravascular volume depletion (hemorrhage or dehydration) or in conditions causing sepsis or ischemia. Serum pregnancy tests are performed in women of reproductive age, especially if their pain is pelvic or lower abdominal in location.

IMAGING STUDIES

The menu of imaging studies available to investigate origins of abdominal pain varies from institution to institution. No single algorithm has gained widespread acceptance. Improvements in technology and cost are factors that mandate constant reassessment. No imaging study should be obtained without consideration of whether the results will affect patient management. Two groups of patients need no imaging studies. Those with overt, diffuse peritonitis and those with a classic presentation for appendicitis do not require even a plain film of the abdomen prior to operation. The remainder of patients with abdominal pain but equivocal abdominal findings benefit from upright chest and two-view abdominal roentgenograms. These films may reveal air-fluid levels, distended bowel, gallstones, ureteral stones, aneurysms, fecaliths, obliterated psoas shadows, ascites, elevated diaphragm, pneumoperitoneum, foreign bodies, or other findings that suggest the origin of pain. Abdominal ultrasonography is beneficial in patients with a suspected biliary or pancreatic pathologic condition or aortic aneurysms. Transvaginal ultrasonography is useful in detecting gynecologic sources of pain. Computed tomography (CT) is valuable in identifying inflammatory, obstructive, hemorrhagic, and malignant disease throughout the abdomen. In selected patients, CT offers not only diagnosis but also therapy, such as CT-guided drainage of intra-abdominal and retroperitoneal abscesses. Computed tomography scans are especially beneficial in patients who are difficult to examine or who have been found historically to have unreliable examinations. Such patients include those with mental retardation, obtundation, or ventilator dependence; those receiving steroid treatment; patients of advanced age; those who have suffered trauma; and individuals who have had a recent laparotomy. Computed tomography scans provide the most sensitive test for pneumoperitoneum and small collections of extraluminal gas. They also identify retroperitoneal and abdominal wall pathology. With advances in CT scanning, fewer alimentary tract contrast studies are necessary. Contrast evaluation of the esophagus may still be appropriate in searching for esophageal leaks; small bowel follow-through examinations may be useful for detecting small bowel obstruction; and barium or meglumine diatrizoate (Gastrografin) enemas may be worthwhile for ruling out colon obstruction and perforation. In patients with suspected sigmoid diverticulitis and focal abscess formation, however, CT scans are now often preferred over contrast enemas because therapeutic drainage may be possible.

Other imaging modalities that are occasionally useful include angiography, endoscopy, cholescintigraphy, intravenous pyelography, and laparoscopy. The latter is the most invasive of all diagnostic maneuvers but may be of benefit to distinguish pelvic inflammatory disease and other gynecologic sources of pain from acute appendicitis. Similar to CT, laparoscopy is a diagnostic tool with therapeutic potential. Diagnostic peritoneal lavage is an alternative technique to consider in patients who are felt to be too unstable or ill to transport to a radiology suite. Lavage findings of hemoperitoneum or a ruptured viscus may obviate the need for any further radiologic work-up.

PERIOD OF OBSERVATION

The source of abdominal pain remains a mystery in some patients despite a comprehensive examination and thorough laboratory and imaging evaluations. For these patients, hospital admission is warranted. Subsequent observation and serial examinations serve as the final diagnostic tool to determine if laparotomy is required.

ABDOMINAL PAIN IN THE PREGNANT PATIENT

Abdominal pain during pregnancy is common; however, this should not evoke complacency. Pregnant patients have an incidence of abdominal pain from nonobstetric causes similar to that of the age-matched general population. Appendicitis is the most frequent nonobstetric cause of acute abdominal pain during pregnancy. Biliary colic and acute cholecystitis also occur commonly.

A history of presenting symptoms is useful but must be differentiated from normal variants of pregnancy, such as morning sickness, gastric reflux symptoms, back pain, and constipation. Findings on physical examination may be atypical, as visceral anatomy changes in the gravid abdomen. During pregnancy, particularly in the third trimester, there is a separation of visceral from parietal peritoneum with a subsequent change in normal localization of pain. For example, the appendix usually ascends toward the right upper quadrant. Typical findings such as McBurney's point tenderness, psoas, and obturator signs may be absent. In the face of vaginal bleeding, a speculum and digital examination is performed only after a diagnosis of placenta previa has been excluded by ultrasound.

Diagnostic evaluation of the pregnant patient is difficult. Normal physiologic changes include a progressive leukocytosis (up to 15,000 white blood cells/mm^3) but should not include a left shift, anemia, elevated alkaline phosphatase levels, or bacteriuria. Mild tachycardia and orthostasis may also be normal variants of pregnancy. Ultrasonography is a useful study for both nonobstetric and obstetric causes of abdominal pain during pregnancy. Laparoscopy, particularly during the second trimester, is another helpful diagnostic aid. Patients who present with upper abdominal pain and shock during the third trimester of pregnancy require special consideration to identify ruptured hepatic adenomas or visceral artery aneurysms. Eclampsia of pregnancy may also be associated with abdominal pain.

Early diagnosis of atypical obstetric abdominal pain is essential. Physicians are justified in using all diagnostic approaches necessary (including roentgenograms) to attain a definitive diagnosis and avoid the high incidence of perinatal loss associated with peritonitis or hemorrhage.

ACUTE ABDOMINAL PAIN IN THE IMMUNOCOMPROMISED PATIENT

To differentiate between surgical and nonsurgical causes of pain, physicians must be aware of special presentations of abdominal pain in immunocompromised patients. Human immunodeficiency virus (HIV)-infected patients are susceptible to opportunistic pathogens, lymphomas, and Kaposi's sarcoma, which may lead to acute abdominal pain. The clinical presentations of appendicitis and cholecystitis are similar to the presentation in the non–HIV-infected population, and standard evaluation as outlined earlier should follow. Immunosuppression may blunt the normal inflammatory response to infection, however, occasionally leading to diffuse, poorly contained abdominal infections. Usual signs and symptoms of infection, such as fever, erythema, and leukocytosis, may be diminished. Expected symptoms in the HIV-infected patient, such as chronic diarrhea, fatigue, low-grade fevers, and night sweats, may also obscure a new onset of abdominal pain. Certain medications used in HIV-infected patients, such as pentamidine, are associated with pancreatitis, a possible cause of abdominal pain.

The diagnostic approach includes flat and upright abdominal and chest roentgenograms. Pneumoperitoneum and pneumatosis cystoides intestinalis are general indications for surgical exploration. Blood and stool cultures should be obtained to search for infectious causes of abdominal pain, specifically cytomegalovirus and mycobacterial pathogens. In stable patients without pneumoperitoneum, limited upper and lower gastrointestinal studies using water-soluble contrast agents are useful to demonstrate ulcerations, colitis, and/or lesions causing mass effect. Abdominal CT is useful in patients with nonspecific findings to distinguish mycobacterial infections from neoplastic lesions on the basis of anatomic site and densitometric features. The majority of HIV-infected patients with abdominal pain do not require surgical intervention, but a heightened index of suspicion is necessary. Perioperative mortality rates are low in HIV-infected patients with simple appendicitis or cholecystitis but are high in patients with acquired immunodeficiency syndrome (AIDS) with enteric perforation.

Abdominal pain in solid organ transplant patients presents a unique problem for the clinician. The immunocompromised state resulting from antirejection therapy increases the risk of infectious complications and post-transplantation malignancies. Acute colonic ileus, usually related to corticosteroid administration, is common. As with all immunocompromised patients, transplant patients are at increased risk for gastrointestinal hemorrhage and perforation.

Rejection of a transplanted kidney, liver, or pancreas may cause abdominal pain over the site of the transplant. Definitive diagnosis is made with ultrasound-guided core needle biopsy of the transplanted organ. Liver function and creatinine levels may be elevated with liver and kidney transplants, respectively. Graft-versus-host disease is another entity specific to the transplant patient—typically bone marrow transplant patients. Presenting signs and symptoms include skin rash and diarrhea followed by abdominal pain and ileus. Diagnosis is based primarily on clinical suspicion with occasional elevation of bilirubin, aspartate aminotransferase, and alkaline phosphatase levels.

Patients receiving chemotherapy also present the clinician with unique problems because of altered immunity. Abdominal pain and tenderness may be more significant because of the blunted inflammatory response, neutropenia, or administration of corticosteroids. Certain chemotherapeutic agents can cause nausea, vomiting, abdominal pain, adynamic ileus, and constipation. A disorder unique to the cancer patient undergoing intensive induction chemotherapy has been termed "neutropenic enterocolitis." This cecal or ascending colitis may cause abdominal pain and tenderness, gastrointestinal bleeding, and occasionally a mass in the right lower quadrant of the abdomen. The diagnosis may be suggested by peritoneal signs, pneumatosis cystoides intestinalis, or free air on abdominal roentgenograms, but it is often made at surgical exploration. Enteric perforations may occur after induction chemotherapy, especially in patients with full-thickness intestinal infiltration by lymphoma. Abdominal CT is indicated in many oncology patients presenting with new complaints of abdominal pain because progression of malignancy, new metastases, inflammation, and obstructive causes of pain may be found.

Conditions compromising host defenses typically lead to late diagnosis with a disease process at a more advanced stage. A high index of suspicion with liberal use of imaging techniques is crucial in this patient population.

VASCULAR CAUSES OF ABDOMINAL PAIN

Abdominal pain from a vascular cause is usually the result of hemorrhage or ischemia. Significant arterial hemorrhage is most frequently due to a ruptured abdominal aortic or iliac artery aneurysm and less often to ruptured visceral aneurysms, spontaneous retroperitoneal or mesenteric hemorrhage in association with anticoagulation, or arterial rupture in patients with collagen abnormalities. A history of an acute onset of severe back, abdominal, flank, or groin pain in a patient older than 50 years of age must raise the suspicion of a ruptured abdominal aortic or iliac artery aneurysm. Severe pain of this nature associated with a syncopal episode or significant hypotension mandates immediate resuscitation and surgical treatment without the need for any further diagnostic studies. Although a large aneurysm may be palpable as a pulsatile mass on abdominal examination, absence of this finding does not exclude the diagnosis. A large internal iliac artery aneurysm may be palpable on rectal examination. In a hemodynamically stable patient with back or abdominal pain, expeditious diagnostic evaluation may include a lateral abdominal x-ray film, abdominal ultrasound, or abdominal CT scan to visualize an aortic or iliac artery aneurysm. Abdominal CT scanning may also be useful to visualize retroperitoneal hemorrhage from contained rupture of a known aortic or iliac artery aneurysm. Other sites of hemorrhage (e.g., adrenal glands, visceral aneurysms) may also be seen on an abdominal CT scan. Arteriography is occasionally indicated to diagnose and treat visceral artery aneurysms.

Intestinal ischemia may result from mesenteric arterial embolism, thrombosis, or dissection. A history of atrial fibrillation, hypertension, or arteriosclerosis obliterans may facilitate the diagnosis. The degree of abdominal pain is classically out of proportion to any physical findings. An abdominal bruit may be a diagnostic clue. Peritoneal irritation and metabolic abnormalities are late signs and are apparent only with advanced ischemia or intestinal perforation. Diagnostic aids include color flow duplex ultrasound scanning of the main mesenteric arteries and selective celiac or mesenteric arteriography.

Abdominal pain from mesenteric venous thrombosis is poorly localized and often described as abdominal distention and a "gut ache." No specific physical signs may be apparent. Color flow duplex ultrasound scanning can visualize thrombosis of the large mesenteric veins, but venous-phase views of mesenteric arteriograms are often necessary to establish the diagnosis. Patients with mesenteric venous thrombosis should be screened for hypercoagulable disorders.

ABDOMINAL PAIN DUE TO BLUNT TRAUMA

Abdominal pain after blunt trauma is the result of hemorrhage from solid organs, disruption of hollow viscera, injury to retroperitoneal structures, or abdominal wall injury. A history of the injury mechanism may be essential to discovering significant injury. Free intraperitoneal blood, bile, pancreatic juices, and intestinal contents may not cause peritoneal irritation early after trauma. Therefore, physical signs may be poorly localized or absent despite serious abdominal injury. This is especially true in patients with an altered sensorium caused by head injury or alcohol and drug use. Adjunctive diagnostic tests are critical in the evaluation of blunt trauma patients. The goal of diagnostic tests in this situation is not necessarily to identify the specific organ or organs injured but rather to help the clinician decide whether or not an urgent operation is necessary. Useful diagnostic tests include abdominal CT scanning, peritoneal lavage, abdominal ultrasound, and laparoscopic examination. Single determinations of serum amylase levels are notoriously inaccurate; however, serial determinations may be useful in identifying pancreatic injury. Finally, it must be emphasized that no diagnostic evaluation is necessary in a patient with clinical evidence of abdominal injury who presents with profound shock or persistent hypotension. The most appropriate diagnostic test in this subset of patients is exploratory laparotomy.

CHRONIC ABDOMINAL PAIN

By David K. Miller, M.D.
La Crosse, Wisconsin

Chronic abdominal pain is a common problem. Although there seems to be no precise definition, chronic abdominal pain may be considered pain that is continuously or nearly continuously present for weeks, months, or years. Chronic abdominal pain also includes pain that recurs in discrete episodes lasting hours, days, or weeks. The interval between episodes may be variable and the patient may be entirely normal between attacks.

Disorders of the abdominal or pelvic viscera are frequent causes of chronic abdominal pain. Pain may be referred to the abdomen by diseases of thoracic viscera. Abdominal pain can also result from neuropathic mechanisms caused by disease of the spinal cord or the lower six thoracic nerves. Injury or disease of muscles, fascia, and other somatic structures that are part of the abdominal wall can also cause abdominal pain. Certain systemic diseases cause abdominal pain through various mechanisms, some of which are not well understood. Finally, functional disorders cause abdominal pain without associated specific structural or biochemical disorders, probably through a mechanism of visceral hyperalgesia.

TYPES OF ABDOMINAL PAIN

Classically, abdominal pain is subdivided into three categories: visceral, parietal (somatic), and referred pain. The clinical recognition of these pain patterns has some diagnostic value.

Visceral Pain

When noxious stimuli affect an abdominal organ, visceral pain results. Pain-receptive afferent fibers lie within the walls of hollow organs and in the capsule of solid organs. Visceral pain is poorly localized and tends to be felt in the midline at approximately the level of the diseased organ's innervation. Visceral pain is dull, aching, or colicky and at times may have a deep burning or gnawing quality. Secondary autonomic events such as sweating, restlessness, nausea, vomiting, and pallor may accompany visceral pain. The patient with visceral pain tends to move around restlessly and may writhe in agony when pain is severe.

Parietal (Somatic) Pain

Parietal pain is produced when the parietal peritoneum is irritated by noxious stimuli such as pH changes, chemical substances, temperature changes, and pressure. Parietal pain is mediated by spinal nerves that supply the abdominal wall. Fibers reach the spinal cord in the peripheral nerves corresponding to dermatomes T6–L1. The quality of parietal pain is sharp, severe, pricking, and relatively constant. Parietal pain is more localized than is visceral pain and is perceived as arising from one of the four quadrants of the abdomen. Lateralization is possible because only one side of the nervous system innervates a given part of the parietal peritoneum. The pain is aggravated by cough, jarring movement, and palpation. The patient with parietal pain tends to remain motionless. Muscle guarding and rebound tenderness are features of parietal pain. The pain appears when an inflamed organ contacts the overlying peritoneum, as in cholecystitis or diverticulitis. Parietal pain is unreferred, or local, when the inflammation of the parietal peritoneum produces pain localized in the body wall directly over the site of inflammation, such as the localized pain in acute appendicitis produced by inflammation of the parietal peritoneum at McBurney's point. Referred parietal pain is felt in an area remote from the site of nociceptive stimulation. A typical example is pain felt in the shoulder when the parietal peritoneum of the middle portion of the diaphragm is inflamed and stimulated.

Referred Pain

Pain that is referred to a site distant from the affected organ is a typical feature of abdominal pain. Generally, referred pain appears as the noxious visceral stimulus becomes more intense. Pain referred from an abdominal source is usually a deep aching sensation perceived to be near the surface of the body. Skin hyperesthesia and increased abdominal wall muscle tone are features associated with referred pain. Knowledge of characteristic patterns of pain referral can be helpful in making a diagnosis.

HISTORY AND PHYSICAL EXAMINATION

In the evaluation of chronic abdominal pain, the history is the single most important diagnostic tool available to the clinician. The history alone may allow a functionally accurate diagnosis in a majority of patients, as high as 80 per cent by some estimates. The history should be orderly, systematic, and detailed. It should be obtained from all available sources, including the patient, relatives, previous medical records, and referring physician. The family history and the social and occupational histories may provide clues to the diagnosis and should be included. The history should attempt to characterize the abdominal pain according to its location, quality, type of onset, temporal features, intensity, circumstances that produce or modify the pain, and associated symptoms.

The physical examination should be thorough and complete, recognizing that abdominal pain occurs during many different diseases often associated with physical signs distant from the abdomen. The examination of the abdomen should be systematic. Inspection may reveal contour changes suggestive of intestinal distention, a mass, or ascites. Downward displacement of the umbilicus may occur in long-standing hepatomegaly or ascites. Upward displacement may occur with pelvic tumors. Auscultation of the abdomen may reveal a spectrum of bowel sounds, from hyperactive (suggesting obstruction) to complete absence (suggesting ileus). No particular feature of bowel sounds, or their absence, is diagnostic, and they must be interpreted in the setting of associated clinical findings. A bruit may indicate a vascular lesion. Bruits over the liver suggest cirrhosis or hepatoma. A friction rub can occasionally be heard over the liver in hepatoma or metastatic carcinoma. Percussion of the abdomen may detect ascites, estimate liver size, detect gaseous distention, or suggest peritonitis when light percussion elicits pain. Palpation identifies local tenderness, guarding, organ enlargement, and abdominal masses. The rectal and pelvic examinations are important as they may reveal a pelvic mass or tenderness or other important clues to a diagnosis.

LABORATORY EXAMINATION

The laboratory, radiographic, and endoscopic evaluation of the patient with chronic abdominal pain is based on the working diagnosis derived from the history and physical examination. A complete blood count, determination of the sedimentation rate, urinalysis, electrolyte determination, and a general blood chemistry panel give valuable information concerning the general nutritional state, hydration, presence of inflammation, and hepatobiliary, renal, hematologic, and endocrine function.

Plain x-ray films of the abdomen may be helpful in conditions causing chronic abdominal pain. Pancreatic calcifications may be noted in chronic pancreatitis. Dilated loops of bowel may be seen in recurrent intestinal obstruction, internal hernias, and chronic intestinal pseudo-obstruction. Renal calculi, calcified gallstones, and vascular calcifications may also be noted.

Upper gastrointestinal endoscopy permits evaluation of the esophagus, stomach, and duodenum. Endoscopy is generally the procedure of choice when the clinical history suggests a mucosal or structural lesion in these areas. Air-contrast barium examination of the upper gastrointestinal tract is an alternative if endoscopy is not readily available or if the precise definition of mucosal disease is not critical. More specialized forms of upper gastrointestinal endoscopy, such as endoscopic retrograde cholangiopancreatography (ERCP) and fiberoptic enteroscopy, are available for evaluation of the biliary tree, pancreatic duct, and small intestine.

The small intestine can be evaluated with small bowel series using barium by mouth or peroral intubation and enteroclysis using a mixture of barium and methylcellulose. The latter technique is more invasive and costly but may provide better identification of strictures and small bowel mucosal lesions. A normal small bowel enteroclysis has been reported to have a specificity of 92 per cent in excluding small bowel disease.

Flexible sigmoidoscopy or colonoscopy is useful when abdominal pain is associated with diarrhea. The colonoscope enables visualization of the entire colon and often the terminal ileum, allowing more accurate diagnosis of mucosal inflammation and mass lesions. However, it is probably rare for the colonoscopist to identify a colonic source of abdominal pain that was not apparent from a barium enema and flexible sigmoidoscopy. An exception might be the occasional patient with Crohn's disease not diagnosed radiographically.

Both ultrasonography (US) and computed tomography (CT) are valuable imaging techniques in the diagnosis of abdominal and pelvic disease. Ultrasonography is noninvasive, generally readily available, and portable and does not expose the patient to ionizing radiation. It is more operator-dependent than CT because the reliability and reproducibility of sonography are functions of the skill and experience of the sonographer. A skilled ultrasonographer is able to detect gallbladder stones; dilated intrahepatic bile ducts; a thickened gallbladder wall; pericholecystic fluid; a dilated common bile duct; intrahepatic, intra-abdominal, and pelvic abscesses; liver and kidney cysts; periappendiceal fluid; ascites; hydronephrosis; and pelvic cysts and neoplasms. Computed tomography exposes the patient to radiation and is more expensive than US but gives excellent high-resolution views readily understood with a knowledge of cross-sectional anatomy. The CT scan is usually superior to US for lesions of the pancreas and kidneys and for assessment of intra-abdominal and pelvic abscesses and lymphadenopathy. Sonography is more sensitive in detecting gallstones in the gallbladder. Abdominal angiography is useful in the evaluation of suspected mesenteric vascular insufficiency and abdominal pain caused by conditions associated with large- and medium-vessel vasculitis, such as polyarteritis nodosa.

Except in the case of chronic pelvic pain in the female and in suspected tuberculous peritonitis, laparoscopy is rarely used in the evaluation of chronic abdominal pain. There is also a rather limited role for exploratory surgery in the diagnosis of chronic abdominal pain.

The optimal use of the laboratory and endoscopic and radiographic imaging techniques depends on a knowledge of the inherent advantages and limitations of each modality. Only the clinician can determine whether the information provided is sufficient to confirm or exclude a diagnosis suggested by the history and physical findings. Likewise, only the clinician can determine whether abnormal findings are the cause of the patient's symptoms or are simply incidental.

DISEASES ASSOCIATED WITH CHRONIC OR RECURRENT ABDOMINAL PAIN

Diseases of the Esophagus, Stomach, and Duodenum

The recurrent pain of reflux esophagitis or esophageal motility disorders is usually retrosternal but often radiates to the epigastrium. The pain of reflux esophagitis is temporarily relieved with antacids, whereas anginalike pain from mucosal irritation responds less readily. Upper gastrointestinal endoscopy usually confirms the diagnosis, but 24-hour ambulatory pH monitoring and esophageal motility studies may be helpful if endoscopy does not confirm esophagitis or if a motility disorder is suspected. Although dysphagia is the most common symptom of esophageal cancer, this lesion can also cause epigastric pain.

Chronic peptic ulcer is associated with the classic symptoms of burning epigastric pain occurring 1 to 3 hours after meals and at night. Symptomatic periods lasting a few weeks are followed by symptom-free intervals lasting weeks to months. Heartburn occurs in 20 to 60 per cent of patients, reflecting the frequent occurrence of gastroesophageal reflux rather than referral of pain from gastroduodenal lesions. A change in the character of the pain, especially the new onset of pain referred to the back, suggests penetration of the ulcer. In the case of nonsteroidal anti-inflammatory drug (NSAID)-induced ulcers, the presence of symptoms does not reliably predict the presence of an ulcer nor does the absence of symptoms decrease the likelihood of finding an ulcer. Despite the "classic" ulcer pain pattern, gastric ulcer, duodenal ulcer, NSAID-induced ulcers, nonulcer dyspepsia, gastroesophageal reflux, gastric malignancy, and biliary tract disease cannot be reliably differentiated by history and physical examination alone. Upper gastrointestinal endoscopy establishes the diagnosis most precisely, but the double-contrast upper gastrointestinal series may be an acceptable alternative.

Chronic gastritis is an ill-defined entity that can be diagnosed only by performing a biopsy of the gastric mucosa. There is a long history of epigastric pain or discomfort that is unrelated to meals. Gastroscopy shows no ulceration, but chronic inflammation is often observed in the gastric mucosa.

The postgastrectomy syndromes can cause recurrent abdominal pain. The dumping syndrome is relatively common and results from rapid gastric emptying and distention of the proximal intestine. Crampy, periumbilical pain develops 20 to 60 minutes after eating and is associated with vasomotor phenomena, including flushing, palpitation, diaphoresis, tachycardia, lightheadedness, and postural hypotension. Affective symptoms, such as lassitude and a decreased attention span, may also be described. Diarrhea or vomiting may or may not be present. The afferent loop syndrome is relatively rare and consists of epigastric and right upper quadrant pain following meals, which is relieved by bilious vomiting. The syndrome is caused by obstruction of the afferent loop of a Billroth II anastomosis. The upper gastrointestinal series occasionally demonstrates the obstructing loop. The alkaline reflux syndrome also consists of upper abdominal pain and bilious vomiting. It is associated with intense gastritis due to excessive reflux of bile into the gastric remnant. Recurrent ulcer is also associated with epigastric pain and sometimes vomiting. The pain tends to be less clearly related to meals than in the syndromes mentioned previously. Endoscopy is the best method of diagnosis. The Roux-en-Y syndrome is a postgastrectomy syndrome characterized by chronic abdominal pain as well as persistent nausea and vomiting that is exacerbated by eating. It is postulated that the Roux-en-Y limb acts as a functional obstruction that causes the symptoms.

Gastric neoplasms are asymptomatic early; these lesions may reach considerable size before the patient feels unwell. Symptoms consist of vague epigastric pain similar to that of peptic ulcer disease, early satiety, and decreasing appetite. Later, local invasion may cause severe and continuous abdominal and back pain, as well as symptoms related to complications such as pancreatitis and gastrocolic fistula. At first there are no physical findings. As the disease progresses, the patient loses weight and there may be epigastric tenderness and a palpable mass. Metastases may cause hepatic enlargement and pelvic masses. Endoscopy is the best method of diagnosis; CT scanning may detect metastatic disease.

The most frequent symptom of a gastric bezoar is epigastric pain, occurring in 70 per cent of cases. Associated symptoms include intermittent attacks of nausea, vomiting, early satiety, and epigastric fullness.

Chronic gastric volvulus is rare but is probably underdiagnosed. In contrast to acute gastric volvulus, the chronic form is associated with mild, nonspecific symptoms such as epigastric discomfort, heartburn, abdominal fullness, bloating, and borborygmus after meals. The primary or subdiaphragmatic form accounts for one third of cases and results from laxity of the stabilizing ligaments of the stomach. The secondary or supradiaphragmatic form of gastric volvulus accounts for two thirds of cases and is associated with a paraesophageal hiatal hernia or a congenital or acquired defect of the diaphragm. A sliding hiatal hernia is not usually associated with gastric volvulus.

Gastric outlet obstruction secondary to peptic ulcer disease, neoplasm, or adult hypertrophic pyloric stenosis causes symptoms of recurrent vomiting, epigastric pain, early satiety, and nausea. Weight loss is an associated finding. The duration of symptoms before diagnosis is estimated to be less than 3 months in a third of patients, 1 to 3 months in a third of patients, and greater than 3 months in the remaining third. Only 10 per cent of patients have symptoms for more than 1 year prior to diagnosis.

Intestinal Diseases

Isolated nonspecific ulcers of the small intestine tend to be located in the ileum and are associated with the use of potassium chloride tablets and prolonged NSAID use. The clinical picture is most commonly one of intermittent small bowel obstruction with chronic periumbilical colic, nausea, or vomiting. Bleeding and acute abdominal crisis associated with perforation are the other modes of presentation.

In lactose intolerance, frequent bouts of colicky midabdominal pain are accompanied by bloating and diarrhea following lactose consumption. A history, lactose tolerance test, or breath hydrogen analysis suggests the diagnosis.

The late symptoms of radiation enteritis may develop after a variable and often prolonged latent period of 3 months to 30 years. The most common late symptom is recurrent colicky abdominal pain due to partial small bowel obstruction. Symptoms often begin in a subacute manner and may progress to complete obstruction. There may be associated malabsorption due to mucosal damage, bile salt malabsorption, and bacterial overgrowth.

Jejunal diverticulosis is an uncommon acquired condition that may be asymptomatic, but some patients may complain of chronic abdominal pain. Acute complications include diverticulitis, bleeding, perforation, and intestinal obstruction. Chronic complications consist of intractable abdominal pain, malabsorption, and intestinal pseudo-obstruction.

Nonrotation of the midgut usually presents in the neonatal period with duodenal obstruction or midgut volvulus. Rarely this condition can present in adolescents and adults as chronic abdominal pain or as an abdominal emergency.

Periodic abdominal pain, consistent with intermittent bowel obstruction, is the most common clinical presentation for small bowel carcinoid tumors. An abdominal mass is palpable on initial presentation in one in five patients. The median duration of symptoms before diagnosis is 2 years.

Abdominal pain is the most common presenting complaint in lymphoma of the small intestine. In proximal lesions, the pain may resemble that of peptic ulcer disease, whereas in more distal disease, the pain may be more variable and is often colicky. Nausea and vomiting may occur with proximal lesions. Abdominal distention is more common with distal lesions. Weight loss, anorexia, and malaise are common.

Other primary malignant tumors of the small intestine cause symptoms of abdominal pain, nausea, vomiting, and usually low-volume gastrointestinal bleeding.

In patients with acquired immunodeficiency syndrome (AIDS), symptoms of chronic or subacute abdominal pain, nausea, vomiting, early satiety, and weight loss suggest an obstructing lesion caused by lymphoma or Kaposi's sarcoma.

The classic symptoms of Crohn's disease are recurrent right lower quadrant abdominal pain and diarrhea resulting from transmural inflammation of the distal ileum and colon. Other common patterns of involvement include small bowel alone and colon alone. Fever is commonly present and is usually low grade. Gross bleeding is not common but may occur with deep colonic ulceration. Perianal disease and extraintestinal manifestations are frequent and are often important clues to the diagnosis.

The major symptoms of chronic ulcerative colitis include diarrhea, rectal bleeding, the passage of mucus, and abdominal pain. In contrast to Crohn's disease, diarrhea and bleeding rather than pain are the more prominent symptoms. The diagnosis is made by the clinical history, sigmoidoscopic or colonoscopic findings, and abnormal mucosal histologic features. Biopsy results can also help distinguish acute colitis from chronic ulcerative colitis.

The most common symptom of colonic diverticulosis is lower abdominal pain, more often on the left than on the right side. It may persist for several hours to several days with variable intensity. It is often worse after eating, and relief may follow the passage of gas or stool. Associated symptoms include diarrhea, constipation, flatulence, and dyspepsia. Physical signs include a tender, firm sigmoid colon. In contrast to diverticulitis, signs of inflammation (such as fever, leukocytosis, an elevated sedimentation rate, and signs of peritoneal irritation) are absent. The clinical features of symptomatic diverticulosis may be difficult to distinguish from diverticulitis; CT scanning can be helpful in the differential diagnosis.

Abdominal pain is a relatively late symptom in colorectal cancer. Cecal and ascending colon lesions rarely obstruct and may cause only vague abdominal discomfort. Symptoms referable to iron deficiency anemia are far more common. Because of the narrower lumen of the left side of the colon, obstructive symptoms occur. Intermittent colicky pain, particularly after meals, is associated with a change in bowel habit. Hematochezia is more common with distal lesions. Rectal cancers may cause tenesmus associated with obstructive symptoms, changes in bowel habit, and bleeding. Diagnosis is made by colonoscopy or flexible sigmoidoscopy and air-contrast barium enema.

In the elderly or those with chronic debility, lack of mobility, or depressed mental status, fecal impaction may be chronic or recurrent and associated with abdominal pain and incontinence resulting from "overflow" of small amounts of liquid stool around the impaction.

Diversion colitis is an inflammation in segments of colon excluded from the fecal stream by surgical bypass procedures (typically colostomy with Hartmann's pouch). Although not always symptomatic, diversion colitis can cause crampy lower abdominal pain, tenesmus, anorectal pain, and a purulent or bloody rectal discharge.

Collagenous and lymphocytic colitis most commonly occurs in women in the fifth and sixth decades of life. The cardinal symptom is chronic watery diarrhea, up to 2 L daily. Colicky abdominal pain is also common. Barium examinations of the small intestine and colon are normal. At colonoscopy, the appearance of the mucosa is usually normal but may show patchy edema and mild erythema. The diagnosis is made by biopsy of the colonic mucosa at the time of endoscopy. Ideally the biopsy specimens should be taken from the right side of the colon, where the changes are more frequent.

Diseases of the Gallbladder and Biliary Tree

Biliary colic is the most common complaint in the majority of symptomatic patients with gallstones. It is a visceral pain, the result of transient obstruction of the gallbladder neck or of the cystic duct by a gallstone. Except when complicated by acute cholecystitis, biliary colic is not associated with inflammation. The pain is located in the epigastrium or right upper quadrant and may radiate to the region of the right scapula. The pain is steady, not intermittent as the term "colic" might suggest. It gradually increases over 15 to 60 minutes, remaining at a plateau for an hour or more, and then diminishes slowly. The attack may be associated with vomiting and diaphoresis. Pain lasting more than 6 hours should suggest the development of acute cholecystitis. The attacks are recurrent and occur at unpredictable intervals of weeks, months, or years. Dyspeptic symptoms such as fatty food intolerance; excessive belching or flatus; postprandial abdominal bloating, fullness, and discomfort; early satiety; epigastric burning; and nausea and vomiting occur with equal frequency in patients with and without gallstones and therefore are not specific for biliary tract disease.

Attacks of biliary pain associated with intermittent mild jaundice and fever suggest choledocholithiasis. The peak bilirubin level is typically in the range of 2 to 10 mg/dL. The alkaline phosphatase level is usually mildly elevated. Marked elevations of the transaminases suggest associated cholangitis. The diagnosis is supported by the finding of gallbladder stones, but the common bile duct is not necessarily dilated. Confirmation is obtained by ERCP.

Cholangitis occurs with bacterial infection of an obstructed bile duct. The cardinal features are pain, jaundice, and fever (Charcot's triad). Only 70 per cent of patients with cholangitis display all three features, and diagnosis is more difficult in the incompletely expressed syndrome. With more severe cholangitis, hypotension and confusion may occur; these signs, along with pain, jaundice, and fever, are sometimes called Reynold's pentad. Attacks of cholangitis can be recurrent if the underlying obstruction is not identified and relieved.

The "postcholecystectomy syndrome" is a term used to describe abdominal symptoms that occur in 10 to 40 per cent of patients following cholecystectomy. Most will have dyspepsia, but severe pain and more serious symptoms occur in 25 per cent of those patients experiencing postcholecystectomy distress. The symptoms characteristically occur within a few weeks of surgery in half of patients and months to years later in the remainder. The causes of this syndrome are numerous and include biliary disorders such as choledocholithiasis, stricture, a cystic duct remnant, papillary stenosis, sphincter of Oddi dyskinesia, malignancy, and choledochocele; pancreatic disorders such as pseudocyst, malignancy, and pancreatitis, and pancreas divisum; and other gastrointestinal disorders such as gastroesophageal reflux, esophageal motor disorders, peptic ulcer disease, and irritable bowel syndrome.

Sclerosing cholangitis, a syndrome of many causes, results in progressive fibrosis and the ultimate disappearance of intra- or extrahepatic bile ducts, or both. The usual symptoms at presentation are jaundice, pruritus, and pain. The pain is rarely severe and is localized to the right upper quadrant. The onset and progress are insidious. There are associated features of weight loss and chronic fatigue. Acute cholangitis is unusual unless the patient has had biliary surgery or instrumentation. Jaundice and hepatomegaly are the most common physical signs. The diagnosis is confirmed by liver biopsy and cholangiography.

Caroli's disease, or congenital intrahepatic biliary dilatation, is associated with hepatomegaly and episodes of abdominal pain and fever with gram-negative sepsis. Jaundice is mild or absent but may increase during attacks of cholangitis. Choledochal cyst (congenital biliary dilatation) in the adult form is marked by intermittent jaundice, pain, and abdominal tumor. Occasionally, an intraduodenal choledochal diverticulum will cause chronic upper abdominal pain and high gastrointestinal obstruction without either cholangitis or pancreatitis.

Abnormalities of the biliary tract can occur in AIDS as a result of infection with *Cryptosporidium*, cytomegalovirus, or Microsporidia. The syndromes include intrahepatic and extrahepatic sclerosing cholangitis, papillary stenosis, and acalculous cholecystitis. The presenting symptoms may include intermittent upper abdominal pain, tenderness, and diarrhea; painless cholestasis; or acute cholangitis. Computed tomography and US show biliary dilatation. ERCP shows an irregularly dilated common bile duct with papillary stenosis.

Carcinoma of the gallbladder most commonly presents with jaundice. Abdominal pain, when present, may mimic biliary colic or it may be dull and unrelenting. A right upper quadrant mass is commonly palpable.

Malignant tumors of the extrahepatic bile ducts most commonly present with jaundice as the initial manifestation. Abdominal pain is relatively common and is a chronic dull ache in the right upper quadrant. It is uncommon for a mass to be palpated, but hepatomegaly may be present in as many as 25 per cent of patients. In carcinoma of the ampulla of Vater, jaundice is also the most common presenting symptom, with pain occurring in 50 per cent of patients. There may be intermittent obstruction, causing episodes of cholangitis and pancreatitis.

Diseases of the Liver

Pyogenic liver abscess may present insidiously, with symptoms lasting several weeks before diagnosis occurs. Malaise, low-grade fever, and dull aching abdominal pain that is increased by movement are the usual features. If there is subdiaphragmatic or pleuropulmonary spread of infection, there may be right shoulder pain and cough. The liver is enlarged and tender, and the spleen may be palpable in chronic cases. Jaundice is mild or absent unless there is suppurative cholangitis. The alkaline phosphatase level, sedimentation rate, and white blood cell count are increased. Computed tomography is the imaging method of choice in most patients. Needle aspiration provides confirmation and drainage.

Amebic liver abscess is associated with the insidious onset of dull aching pain and hepatic tenderness. Amebic liver abscess may occur as long as 30 years after the primary bowel infection. Active dysentery is present in only 10 per cent of patients with hepatic amebiasis. Fever is usually intermittent or remittent. Unless the abscess becomes secondarily infected, the fever is usually less than 40°C (104°F). Right upper quadrant pain begins as a dull ache that later becomes sharp and stabbing. Leaning to the left tends to ease the pain. The liver is enlarged and tender. The spleen is not enlarged. Serologic test results for amebiasis are positive. Ultrasonography is useful in the diagnosis and for following progress. Computed tomography is more sensitive for smaller abscesses and for extrahepatic involvement. The diagnosis is supported by a history of residence in an endemic area; positive serologic test results; an enlarged, tender liver; and a positive response to metronidazole challenge.

Nonparasitic cysts of the liver, if large enough to be symptomatic, present with symptoms of chronic abdominal pain and right upper quadrant tenderness.

In hepatocellular carcinoma, pain is frequent but rarely severe and is experienced as a continuous dull ache in the epigastrium, right upper quadrant, or back. Associated symptoms include malaise, abdominal fullness, and weight loss. The liver is enlarged and jaundice, if present, is rarely severe. Ascites is present in half of cases. Systemic effects, such as hypercalcemia, hypoglycemia, hypercholesterolemia, hyperthyroidism, pseudoporphyria, and painful gynecomastia, may occur. Hepatic metastases may cause similar pain, weight loss, malaise, lassitude, and fever.

Budd-Chiari syndrome consists of hepatomegaly, abdominal pain, ascites, and hepatic histologic features showing zone 3 venous dilatation, congestion with hemorrhage, and central necrosis. In the more common chronic form, the patient presents with an enlarged, painful liver and ascites that develops over 1 to 6 months. Some patients run a more fulminant course, presenting with encephalopathy and dying within 2 to 3 weeks. Budd-Chiari syndrome is caused by obstruction of the hepatic venous outflow at any level. The syndrome is usually associated with diseases having an increased risk of thrombotic complications such as polycythemia rubra vera, systemic lupus erythematosus, paroxysmal nocturnal hemoglobinuria, renal carcinoma, and primary carcinoma of the liver. A syndrome similar to Budd-Chiari may be seen in constrictive pericarditis and right-sided heart failure.

In AIDS, liver involvement with non-Hodgkin's lymphoma is usually metastatic but may also be primary. It presents with right upper quadrant pain associated with fever, weight loss, and night sweats. The transaminases and alkaline phosphatase levels are elevated. There may be jaundice with a large lesion. Ultrasonography and CT show large, multifocal, space-occupying lesions.

Diseases of the Pancreas

Pain is a prominent feature of chronic pancreatitis. In about half of patients, the pain is constant and unrelenting. It may vary in intensity but never completely subsides. The pain frequently radiates to the back. Eating and alcohol exacerbate the symptoms. Weight loss is frequent. In the other half of patients, the pain is episodic, lasting for days to weeks with pain-free intervals in between. The pain may eventually disappear in some patients after years of symptoms. Insulin dependency may develop in 15 per cent of patients and pancreatic exocrine insufficiency in 50 per cent of patients with chronic pancreatitis.

Pancreatic pseudocyst may develop as a complication of acute pancreatitis but more commonly appears during chronic pancreatitis. Regardless of the way in which the cyst develops, the most frequent symptom is pain, usually located in the epigastrium and radiating to the back. A tender, palpable mass is present in half the patients. Abdominal US may facilitate the diagnosis of pancreatic pseudocyst.

Pain is not an early symptom of carcinoma of the pancreas, and for most patients there are few characteristic symptoms or signs early in the course of the disease. Vague, dull midepigastric pain occasionally going to the back usually implies direct invasion of adjacent retroperitoneal organs or splanchnic nerves. Jaundice, insidious weight loss, anorexia, vomiting, diarrhea, and weakness are commonly associated symptoms. When carcinoma of the pancreas is suspected, CT should be considered as the initial diagnostic procedure because it is accurate, noninvasive, and generally available.

Diseases of the Spleen

Massive splenomegaly from any cause may result in constant dull aching pain in the left hypochondrium. Splenic abscess is an uncommon occult deep-seated infection that follows a bacteremic episode. The clinical manifestations include the subacute onset of fever and left-sided abdominal pain. The pain is often located in the flank, upper abdomen, or lower chest and can radiate to the left shoulder. The symptoms may be present for 3 weeks or more before diagnosis. Left upper abdominal tenderness, splenomegaly, and dullness to percussion in the left lung base are common physical findings. Diagnosis is facilitated by US or CT.

Urologic Disease

Autosomal dominant polycystic kidney disease (PKD) causes chronic intermittent dull flank pain that may increase with hyperextension of the spine. Intermittent gross hematuria, abdominal mass, urinary tract infection, and hypertension also occur. Renal failure may develop later. In adults, more than five distinct cysts per kidney suggest the diagnosis of autosomal dominant PKD. Computed tomography scanning with contrast enhancement aids the diagnosis of autosomal dominant PKD in any age group.

The onset of perinephric abscess is insidious. Patients are often ill for 1 to 3 weeks before they seek medical care. The most frequent symptoms are unilateral flank pain in 80 per cent of patients and chills and fever in almost all patients. On examination, abdominal tenderness may be present, but flank and costovertebral angle tenderness is more common. Computed tomography provides the most precise diagnostic information and is helpful in planning surgical drainage.

The subacute form of papillary necrosis can run a protracted course with recurrent attacks of lumbar pain and hematuria simulating ureteral colic. Chills, fever, evidence of urinary tract infection, and the passage of papillary fragments differentiate this disease from other causes of ureteral colic.

Xanthogranulomatous pyelonephritis (XGP) is an atypical form of renal infection. The inflammatory response is characterized by a hard, lobulated, dull yellow renal mass. Patients with XGP are usually women in the fourth to seventh decades of life. They have chronic symptoms of flank pain, fever, chills, malaise, and urosepsis. Flank tenderness and a palpable mass are present in about half of patients. Computed tomography is useful for differentiating XPG from renal carcinoma. XPG is characterized by a low-attenuating nonfunctional kidney and negative attenuation due to fat; renal cell carcinoma shows enhancement with contrast material.

Renal malacoplakia is a chronic granulomatous disorder associated with gram-negative urinary tract infection. An association with debilitating disease, such as diabetes mellitus, transplant immunosuppression, and tuberculosis, suggests that an immunologic defect is instrumental in the development of malacoplakia. Patients present with fever, flank pain, hematuria, and pyuria. A urinary tract infection is present 90 per cent of the time. A flank mass may be palpable.

Approximately 4 to 9 per cent of patients with pulmonary tuberculosis experience destructive genitourinary tuberculosis. Renal tuberculosis may cause flank pain, gross hematuria, and ureteral colic secondary to calculi, clots, and debris. Systemic complaints such as fever, chills, sweats, and malaise are uncommon.

The classic triad of renal cell carcinoma consists of flank pain, hematuria, and a flank mass. Hypertension, weight loss, and a variety of paraneoplastic syndromes may be associated with renal cell carcinoma.

In Fraley's syndrome (infundibular stenosis), there is obstruction of the superior infundibulum and its calyces by intrarenal vessels impinging on the infundibular channel. The patient complains of dull, steady pain in the costovertebral angle and flank for months or years. Pain relief on lying down is the key to the diagnosis. The pyelogram shows a linear filling defect caused by vascular compression crossing the infundibulum to the superior calyx. A delayed drainage film shows contrast retained in the superior calyx.

Idiopathic nephralgia is a rare condition consisting of renal-like pain and other urologic symptoms such as frequency, nocturia, and dysuria, without demonstrable pathology.

Intra-abdominal Vascular Disease

As many as two thirds of patients with a ruptured abdominal aortic aneurysm may have abdominal pain or backache over the weeks before rupture. If the patient reports the symptoms and an examination is made, diagnosis is possible. Diagnosis may be difficult because some patients complain more of backache or "lumbago" than abdominal pain, and in obese individuals palpation of a pulsatile mass may be difficult. If a symptomatic aneurysm is suspected, its presence may be confirmed by US. The triad of chronic abdominal pain, weight loss, and an elevated erythrocyte sedimentation rate in a patient with an abdominal aortic aneurysm suggests an inflammatory aneurysm.

Chronic mesenteric insufficiency (abdominal angina) is suggested by abdominal pain that begins 15 to 30 minutes after eating. The pain follows a crescendo-decrescendo pattern, slowly abating over 1 to 3 hours. It is dull, gnawing, or cramping and is located in the epigastrium or periumbilical area. The patient reduces meal size and eventually becomes reluctant to eat in attempts to avoid the pain. Weight loss is common. The diagnosis is based on the history, the angiographic demonstration of significant splanchnic arterial stenoses or occlusions, and the exclusion of other diseases that might account for abdominal pain and weight loss. Atypical gastric antral ulcers associated with chronic abdominal pain and healing only after revascularization have been reported in association with chronic mesenteric vascular insufficiency.

The gastrointestinal tract may be involved in virtually all disorders associated with systemic vasculitis, including polyarteritis nodosa, Churg-Strauss syndrome, systemic lupus erythematosus, and Henoch-Schönlein purpura. With such vasculitis, chronic relapsing manifestations of abdominal pain, fever, gastrointestinal bleeding, diarrhea, and intestinal obstruction are common. In scleroderma, small bowel involvement causes intermittent bloating, abdominal cramps, intermittent or chronic diarrhea, and intestinal obstruction.

Diseases of the Peritoneum, Mesentery, and Diaphragm

Retractile mesenteritis and mesenteric panniculitis are rare idiopathic chronic inflammatory diseases manifested by fever, weight loss, abdominal pain, intestinal obstructive symptoms, and a mass. Usually, laparotomy is necessary to make the diagnosis.

Primary mesothelioma presents with the gradual onset of abdominal pain and distention associated with anorexia, nausea, vomiting, weight loss, and ascites. There is a history of asbestos exposure. Ultrasonography and CT often demonstrate ascites and sheetlike masses that may suggest the diagnosis.

Metastatic cancer is the most common peritoneal tumor. Most metastases are adenocarcinomas from the ovary, pancreas, or colon. Symptoms consist of diffuse abdominal pain, ascites, weight loss, and weakness.

Connective tissue disorders may lead to painful peritonitis as a manifestation of serositis in systemic lupus erythematosus, polyarteritis, and scleroderma. Fever and migratory abdominal pain caused by starch peritonitis formerly occurred in 1 of 1000 patients undergoing laparotomy. The incidence has decreased with changes in glove lubricants.

Familial Mediterranean fever, more common in Europe and the Middle East, causes recurrent bouts of peritonitis associated with moderate to severe abdominal pain, arthritis, fever, and leukocytosis. Attacks occur suddenly, subside after 6 to 12 hours, and the patient is well in 24 to 48 hours. Recurrences occur at irregular and unpredictable intervals.

Tuberculous peritonitis should be considered in any patient with ascites and chronic abdominal pain. The illness develops insidiously over a period of months. Typical symptoms include lassitude, weight loss, intermittent fever, and night sweats. Laparoscopy may allow visualization and biopsy of the peritoneal tubercles.

A foramen of Bochdalek hernia may cause vague intermittent abdominal pain in 50 per cent and chest pain in 25 per cent of patients.

Systemic Disease

Various systemic, toxic, allergic, hematologic, and endocrine disturbances can cause episodes of severe deep abdominal pain that can simulate visceral disease. The pain of porphyria or colic resulting from lead poisoning is usually difficult to distinguish from that of intestinal obstruction because severe hyperperistalsis is a feature of both. The pain of uremia or diabetes is nonspecific and the pain and tenderness frequently shift in location and intensity.

Lead poisoning is associated with recurrent abdominal colic when the blood lead level is approximately 80 μg/dL or greater. At times, severe colic may suggest the need for emergent surgery. In more chronic cases, the symptoms are milder, and intermittent colic, constipation, and lethargy occur. Coarse basophilic stippling of the erythrocytes and a blue-black lead line on the gingival margin may provide clues to the diagnosis.

Extreme hypertriglyceridemia, associated with either primary or secondary hyperlipoproteinemia, may cause recurrent episodes of acute pancreatitis. Recurrent, severe abdominal pain may occur in association with diabetic ketoacidosis. Diabetic gastroparesis may be associated with abdominal pain as well as anorexia, weight loss, bloating, nausea, and vomiting. Diabetic radiculopathy involving the thoracic nerve roots causes chronic severe abdominal pain that is often associated with anorexia and weight loss.

Hypercalcemia of primary hyperparathyroidism may cause abdominal pain by inducing peptic ulcers and acute and chronic pancreatitis. Other gastrointestinal symptoms include constipation, anorexia, nausea, vomiting, weight loss, and diarrhea.

Apathetic thyrotoxicosis may simulate intra-abdominal malignant disease with colicky abdominal pain, marked weight loss, and altered bowel habits. Myxedema may lead to abdominal pain through ileus, pseudo-obstruction and constipation, obstipation, and sigmoid volvulus.

In Addison's disease, anorexia and weight loss are present in almost all patients and vomiting and abdominal pains are common.

Gastrinoma (multiple endocrine neoplasia, type 1 [MEN 1]) is associated with abdominal pain due to severe peptic ulcer disease. Mucosal neuromas (multiple endocrine neoplasia, type 2B [MEN 2B]) affect the colon, causing abdominal pain associated with colonic dilatation, diverticulosis, and diverticulitis.

Myelodysplastic syndromes such as agnogenic myelofibrosis and agnogenic myeloid metaplasia (AMM), polycythemia vera, and essential thrombocythemia may cause abdominal pain because of hepatic vein thrombosis and the Budd-Chiari syndrome. Agnogenic myeloid metaplasia can also cause pain through massive splenomegaly. Multiple myeloma may directly involve the gastrointestinal tract with amyloidosis or local infiltration by plasmacytomas leading to dysmotility and abdominal pain. Blood coagulation disorders may involve the intestinal tract by intramural, submucosal, or intramesenteric bleeding, causing obstruction, intussusception, or pain. Paroxysmal nocturnal hemoglobinuria, sickle cell anemia, and chronic hemolytic anemias may be associated with episodes of abdominal pain.

Systemic mastocytosis is commonly associated with dyspeptic as well as nondyspeptic abdominal pain, accompanied by nausea, vomiting, and diarrhea.

In sickle cell anemia, episodes of severe abdominal pain may occur during hemolytic crises. Clumping of red blood cells leads to thrombosis and rupture of capillaries in the gut. The usual features of a hemolytic anemia will be found in the blood, and a raised leukocyte count is common during an attack.

Fabry's disease causes impaired intestinal motility and recurrent episodes of crampy abdominal pain with frequent liquid stools.

Acute intermittent porphyria causes recurrent attacks of abdominal pain ranging in severity from mild abdominal discomfort to agonizing colic. The pain may be associated with low-grade fever, mild leukocytosis, tachycardia, hypertension, postural hypotension, and sweating. Neurologic symptoms and peripheral neuropathy may be noted. Attacks are triggered by drugs and environmental factors. In variegate porphyria, attacks of abdominal pain and neurologic symptoms accompany light-sensitive skin rashes on exposed parts of the body. Elevated urinary levels of porphyrin metabolites help establish the diagnosis.

Gynecologic Disease

Mittelschmerz occurs at the middle of the cycle around the time of ovulation. It recurs at the same relative time each month. The pain is caused by rupture of the ovarian follicle, leading to leakage of blood and irritation of the peritoneum. Follicular fluids rich in prostaglandin E and F_1 are released into the peritoneal cavity and may stimulate painful uterine contractions.

Dysmenorrhea is cyclic pain associated with the menses. It can begin a few hours or days before bleeding and usually lasts through the initial flow and sometimes throughout the period. The pain is cramping in nature and located in the midportion of the lower abdomen. Dysmenorrhea is considered to be primary if no pelvic or structural abnormalities are found as causes and secondary if it is the result of organic pathology. The pain of primary dysmenorrhea is caused by relative uterine ischemia from hypercontractility of the myometrium. Secondary dysmenorrhea occurs as the result of an organic pelvic pathologic condition, such as endometriosis, adenomyosis, submucosal fibroids, or endometrial polyps, or from the use of an intrauterine device.

Chronic pelvic inflammatory disease causes damage to the pelvic nerves and adhesions so that painful stretching is produced by activities such as exercise, sexual intercourse, or alimentary tract function. Adhesions occurring after extensive pelvic surgery can also be a cause of chronic pelvic pain.

Ovarian neoplasms are asymptomatic in the early stages, but with advanced growth they become symptomatic, presenting with lower abdominal pain or discomfort in 60 per cent of patients, distention or mass in 50 per cent of patients, abnormal uterine bleeding in 34 per cent of patients, urinary tract symptoms in 17 per cent of patients, and gastrointestinal symptoms in 16 per cent of patients. Ovarian carcinoma spreads primarily by implantation on peritoneal surfaces. Tumor growth causes progressive interference with the function of abdominal organs, leading to disturbed bowel motility, obstruction, serous effusions, and often a protracted terminal course.

Neurologic Disease

Lesions of the lower thoracic spinal cord from trauma, tumors, syringomyelia, multiple sclerosis, hemorrhage, and so on can cause pain in the trunk, including the abdominal wall. The pain is burning, diffuse, and poorly localized. In some cases, the pain has a radicular (segmental) distribution associated with hyperalgesia, hyperpathia, and paresthesia. Epidural cord compression produces localized low back pain at the site of the lesion in 95 per cent and bilateral radicular pain involving the abdominal wall in 55 per cent of patients. The pain is aggravated by neck flexion, straight leg raising, coughing, sneezing, and the Valsalva maneuver. Percussion and firm palpation produce back tenderness. Compression radiculopathy resulting from tumors, disk protrusion, vertebral fractures, osteophytes, and adhesive arachnoiditis may cause abdominal pain. Herniation of lower thoracic disks produces radicular pain in the lower abdomen. Initially the pain is vague and poorly localized and it may be referred laterally or bilaterally in the abdomen. Typically pain is aggravated by neck flexion and by an increase in intraspinal pressure resulting from coughing, sneezing, or straining. The pain is usually relieved by lying down.

Arachnoiditis characterized by inflammation and fibrosis of the arachnoid membrane is a well-recognized cause of chronic pain. Arachnoiditis can occur at any spinal level and it can be focal, involving only one root, causing a segmental pain syndrome associated with variable sensory and motor functional loss. Arachnoiditis can also affect multiple segments and lead to a more diffuse pain syndrome involving the lower trunk and abdomen. The pain of arachnoiditis is constant but is increased by physical activity. There is often a dysesthetic component and paresthesias are common.

Herpes zoster produces a continuous aching, itching, or burning pain with superimposed bouts of severe lancinating pain. Some patients experience postherpetic neuralgia, which is a chronic condition that causes severe, intractable, continous, unrelenting, and burning pain. A typical rash usually develops and may involve the skin of the abdominal wall; pain may precede the rash by several days.

Tabes dorsalis, a now rare form of tertiary syphilis, may cause brief shocklike or girdlelike pains in the thorax or abdomen. Most patients with this condition also have pain in the limbs. More severe is the tabetic pain syndrome known as "gastric crisis," occurring in 10 per cent of tabetic patients. The patient has a sudden onset of agonizing epigastric pain associated with nausea and vomiting. Attacks may last for days, but spontaneous remission occurs. A similar pain syndrome may involve the lower abdomen and pelvis. Associated signs include altered position sense, absent deep tendon reflexes, hypotonia, ataxia, and Argyll Robertson pupils.

Intercostal neuropathy involving the lower intercostal nerves may cause unilateral pain of a superficial burning nature in the lower part of the posterior and lateral chest and abdominal wall.

Entrapment of the anterior cutaneous branches of the thoracoabdominal intercostal nerves in the rectus sheath causes intermittent dull aching pain that can be associated with sharp piercing pain in the distribution of the dermatome, along with paresthesia, hyperesthesia, and local tenderness. The distribution of pain depends on the site of entrapment and the number of nerves involved. In most cases, one anterior cutaneous nerve is involved, causing pain in the medial part of the anterior abdominal wall over the rectus muscle. Pain can be reproduced by increasing tension in the rectus abdominis muscle. Ilioinguinal-iliohypogastric nerve entrapment may also cause chronic lower abdominal pain.

Musculoskeletal Disease

Neuromuscular mechanisms involving the back and the abdominal wall produce chronic abdominal pain that may be impossible to distinguish from visceral pain by the clinical history. This is sometimes called the "back-gut syndrome." A spinal reflex mechanism characterized by a vicious cycle of reflex pain and spasm initiated by an often transient, painful trigger stimulus has been proposed. Spasm of abdominal, rectus, intercostal, or paraspinous muscles amplifies the pain, especially if nerve entrapment occurs. Similar mechanisms may underlie chronic abdominal pain after surgery. The presence of the syndrome is suggested by pain of segmental distribution, abdominal wall or paraspinal muscle tenderness, altered cutaneous sensation, and an increase in pain with tensing of abdominal muscles or twisting of the spine. Psychological factors amplify the pain, presumably by enhancing muscle spasm, facilitating spinal reflexes, altering afferent sensory thresholds, or causing preoccupation with pain. Although parietal pain can mimic visceral symptoms, visceral disease can also precipitate referred pain; thus, underlying visceral disease may need to be excluded despite an obvious neuromuscular element to the pain.

The back-gut syndrome, the gastroenterologist's version of fibromyalgia, is important because it may contribute to the symptoms of patients with functional bowel disorders. If the musculoskeletal contribution to the pain syndrome is not sought and recognized, it will continue to obscure or mimic other disease processes.

Periostitis pubis is characterized by lower abdominal pain that is present for weeks to years. Physical findings consist of tenderness in one of the lower abdominal quadrants and over the os pubis on the affected side. The diagnosis can be confirmed by injecting lidocaine into the area of point tenderness over the os pubis, which should relieve tenderness in both sites.

The slipping rib syndrome (rib tip syndrome or slipped rib cartilage syndrome) is characterized by sharp stabbing pain localized to the upper quadrant or to the epigastrium. The pain is present at rest and is aggravated by movement, especially twisting, hyperextension, or raising the arm. Occasionally the pain is dull, aching, or burning and radiates to the back. The symptoms are easily confused with pain originating from abdominal viscera, especially in patients with nausea and vomiting. The pathognomonic test involves hooking the curled fingers under the inferior rib margin and pulling anteriorly. This maneuver produces a clicking noise as the detached cartilage slides over the rib cartilage above and aggravates the pain. Because the condition is usually unilateral, performing the hooking maneuver on the contralateral side should not produce a similar pain.

Xiphoidalgia is characterized by spontaneous deep aching or sharp pain that varies in intensity from slight to agonizing, simulating myocardial infarction. The pain is felt around the xiphoid process and radiates to the epigastrium and occasionally to the lower chest. The pain increases with movements that act on the xiphoid process, such as bending, stooping, or turning, or by an increase in intragastric pressure caused by a large meal. The pain can be constant or recur several times a day, lasting for several minutes to several hours. The condition can persist for weeks or months. Pressure over the xiphoid process produces pain.

Functional Abdominal Pain

A functional gastrointestinal disorder is a variable combination of chronic or recurrent gastrointestinal symptoms not explained by structural or biochemical abnormalities. The functional causes of abdominal pain include irritable bowel syndrome (IBS), nonulcer dyspepsia, (NUD), biliary dyskinesia, and chronic intractable abdominal pain (CIAP). In these disorders, the pathogenesis is thought to involve disordered motility or altered visceral sensation, although no consistent abnormality has been identified.

Irritable bowel syndrome is the most common gastrointestinal disorder seen in clinical practice and is also among the most common causes of chronic abdominal pain. It is estimated to affect 10 to 15 per cent or more of the adult population. There is a slight predominance in women. Symptoms typically begin in young adult life, but the prevalence is similar in younger and older adults. The majority of patients with IBS do not consult a physician for this disorder. Currently IBS is defined as 3 months or more of continuous or intermittent symptoms of abdominal pain or discomfort associated with a change in the frequency or consistency of stool. In addition, there is an irregular pattern of defecation at least 25 per cent of the time, including three or more of the following: (1) altered stool frequency, (2) altered stool form (hard, loose, or watery stool), (3) altered stool passage (straining or urgency, feeling of incomplete evacuation), (4) passage of mucus, and (5) bloating or feeling of abdominal distention. Patients with IBS may have associated symptoms of gastroesophageal reflux with heartburn, dysphagia, and a globus sensation, as well as noncardiac chest pain, although these symptoms are not a part of the diagnostic criteria. There may also be nongastrointestinal symptoms such as fatigue, gynecologic problems, and urologic dysfunction. Patients with IBS who see a physician tend to have a higher frequency of psychological problems than do those with irritable bowel symptoms who do not seek medical attention. Those IBS patients not seeking medical attention have psychological profiles similar to healthy subjects, suggesting that psychological factors influence how the illness is perceived and handled by the patient.

To make a diagnosis of CIAP, certain diagnostic criteria must be met. The abdominal pain must be present much or all the time for longer than 6 months. No pathophysiologic process is identifiable to explain the symptoms despite investigations appropriate to the findings on repeated histories and physical examinations. For patients initially diagnosed as having chronic, unexplained pain who are followed prospectively, fewer than 10 per cent are ever given a specific medical diagnosis. Highly characteristic features in the history include childhood physical or sexual abuse; multiple procedures and/or surgeries, usually with negative results; and multiple somatic complaints, including pain outside the abdomen. The abdominal pain has certain characteristic features: (1) it does not vary in intensity, character, or location in response to physiologic states such as defecation, meals, and so forth or does so in a nonpredictable way; (2) the description of the pain is dramatic and idiosyncratic; (3) the pain may be triggered or exacerbated by psychological factors; (4) the pain is often associated with major interference with work, family, and social functioning; and (5) the pain tends to be unresponsive to usual treatments. Patients with CIAP tend to display certain psychological features, including depression, anxiety, preoccupation with the pain, illness behavior, pain-prone personality, and a high prevalence of somatoform disorders.

Symptoms that tend to suggest organic disease rather

than functional abdominal pain include fever, weight loss, visible or occult blood in the stool, diarrhea that awakens the patient from sleep, pain on awakening from sleep, and pain that interferes with normal sleep patterns.

The physical examination in functional abdominal pain is usually normal with the exception of mild abdominal tenderness. Physical findings such as marked abdominal tenderness, rebound tenderness, a palpable mass, hepatosplenomegaly, jaundice, ascites, evidence of weight loss, fever, lymphadenopathy, or fecal occult blood are not consistent with functional abdominal pain and demand further investigation.

The differential diagnosis of IBS includes neoplasia, inflammatory bowel disease, giardiasis, drugs, celiac disease, constipation, intermittent volvulus, mesenteric vascular insufficiency, bacterial overgrowth, and lactase deficiency. A feature distinguishing CIAP from IBS or NUD is that the pain of CIAP tends to be present most of the time, whereas the pain of IBS or NUD is generally cyclical or associated with abnormal bowel function and eating, respectively.

Laboratory studies are usually normal but are indicated to help exclude other diseases. The tests should include a complete blood count, sedimentation rate, thyroid function tests, chemistry panel, and urinalysis. Flexible sigmoidoscopy is performed to exclude neoplasm, especially in patients older than 40 years of age, and inflammatory bowel disease. With persistent diarrhea, the stool should be examined for occult blood; fecal leukocytes, ova, and parasites; and excess fat. A sigmoidoscopic mucosal biopsy may be performed to exclude collagenous or lymphocytic colitis. In selected cases, a barium enema or colonoscopy may be needed. When symptoms suggestive of upper gastrointestinal or biliary tract disease are present, additional diagnostic studies appropriate to these areas must be considered.

In conclusion, chronic abdominal pain is a common problem of multiple and diverse causation. A diagnosis should be possible in most cases by obtaining a complete history, careful physical examination, and selected laboratory, radiographic, and endoscopic evaluations.

GASTROINTESTINAL HEMORRHAGE

By John B. Marshall, M.D.
Columbia, Missouri

Gastrointestinal (GI) hemorrhage is a common clinical problem with variable presentation, depending on the rapidity of blood loss and its source. At one end of the spectrum is acute massive GI bleeding, a life-threatening emergency that presents with the obvious passage of large amounts of blood and hemodynamic compromise. At the other end of the spectrum is chronic occult GI bleeding, which presents insidiously as iron deficiency anemia or a positive result on fecal occult blood testing.

Acute GI bleeding presents as hematemesis, melena, and/or hematochezia. Hematemesis, the vomiting of blood, always arises from an upper GI tract bleeding site (i.e., proximal to the ligament of Treitz, located at the duodenojejunal junction). The color of vomited blood can vary from bright red to a black coffee-ground appearance (the black color results from the action of hydrochloric acid on blood).

Melena, the passage of black tarry stools, usually has an upper GI tract origin (about 95 per cent of cases) but is occasionally caused by bleeding from a lesion in the jejunum, ileum, or right colon. It takes at least 50 to 60 mL of blood passed acutely to produce a single melenic stool. The tarry (sticky) consistency of melena is a useful characteristic that helps distinguish it from black stools caused by ingestion of iron or bismuth-containing products.

Hematochezia is the passage of red blood through the rectum. The anorectum or colon is likely to be the source when the blood is bright red. When bright red blood is passed in small amounts, this helps localize the bleeding source even further, usually implying bleeding from the anorectum or distal colon. Conversely, the passage of large-volume maroon stools constitutes a more difficult problem, as it can originate from any point in the upper GI tract, small bowel, or colon.

Occult GI bleeding occurs when the degree of blood loss is low grade and does not cause visible changes in the color of the stool. It presents as iron deficiency anemia or as a positive chemical test result for occult blood.

Other clinical manifestations of GI hemorrhage depend on the magnitude and rate of blood loss as well as on the patient's age and the presence of concomitant medical illnesses (e.g., cardiovascular disease, pulmonary disease, or pre-existing anemia). Manifestations include fatigue, dyspnea on exertion, orthostatic hypotension or lightheadedness, worsening of angina pectoris, and shock.

ACUTE UPPER GASTROINTESTINAL TRACT HEMORRHAGE

Acute bleeding from the upper GI tract (esophagus, stomach, or duodenum) is characterized by hematemesis and/or melena, but if bleeding is massive and associated with rapid transit, it can present with hematochezia (large-volume maroon stools). Most episodes are self-limited, but they can be recurrent if the causative lesion persists. However, occasional cases are manifested as exsanguinating hemorrhage (most common with aortoenteric fistula and varices but can occur with ulcer bleeding as well). The mortality rate with severe acute upper GI bleeding is 8 to 10 per cent and is highest in the elderly and in patients with serious underlying illnesses.

Etiology

Specific causes of acute upper GI tract hemorrhage and their approximate frequency are listed in Table 1. Duode-

Table 1. Sources of Acute Upper Gastrointestinal Bleeding

Source	% of Cases
Duodenal and gastric ulcers	45
Gastroduodenal erosions	25
Varices	10
Mallory-Weiss tear	7
Esophagitis	6
Neoplasm	3
Dieulafoy lesion	1
Angiodysplasia	1
Aortoenteric fistula	<0.5
Hemobilia	<0.5
Other	2

nal and gastric ulcers are the most common cause (some 45 per cent of cases), followed by gastroduodenal erosions, varices, and Mallory-Weiss tears. Although most patients with a bleeding peptic ulcer will give a history of pain, about a quarter will present without pain or dyspepsia. The regular use of aspirin or nonsteroidal anti-inflammatory drugs (NSAIDs) suggests the possibility of gastric or duodenal ulcer disease or erosions. Likewise, ulcer disease is also suspected in a patient with prior peptic ulcer disease or bleeding ulcer. Critically ill patients in the intensive care unit commonly bleed from gastroduodenal mucosal stress ulcers or erosions. Although this is most commonly low-grade bleeding, serious hemorrhage can sometimes occur.

After gastroduodenal ulcers and erosions, varices are the next most frequent cause of upper GI bleeding. The presence of varices should be considered in patients with longstanding alcohol abuse or liver disease. Bleeding is usually from varices in the esophagus, although it can also arise from gastric varices. Also, patients with cirrhosis and portal hypertension can sometimes bleed from gastric mucosal lesions termed "congestive, or portal hypertensive, gastropathy." Most patients with congestive gastropathy have concomitant esophagogastric varices.

The next most common cause of bleeding is mucosal tears of the esophagogastric junction, so-called Mallory-Weiss tears. Patients with these lesions give a history of retching or vomiting. Acute upper GI bleeding is also an occasional complication of reflux esophagitis. Most patients give a history of frequent heartburn. Tumors are a relatively infrequent cause of acute GI bleeding (examples of such tumors include esophageal and gastric carcinomas, lymphomas, leiomyomas). Depending on the type and location of the tumor, associated symptoms may include anorexia, weight loss, dysphagia, and abdominal or chest pain.

The clinician should also be aware of several other relatively rare causes of upper GI bleeding. Dieulafoy's lesion is an unusually large submucosal artery protruding through a tiny mucosal defect of uncertain pathogenesis. It is most frequent in the proximal stomach but can also occur in other areas of the GI tract. It is important to be aware of this lesion because it is sometimes difficult to visualize endoscopically, and multiple examinations are sometimes required. Although it is a rare cause of upper GI bleeding, angiodysplasia of the upper GI tract (small vascular ectasias) should be considered in patients with hereditary hemorrhagic telangiectasia (Osler-Weber-Rendu syndrome) and chronic renal failure. An aortoenteric fistula should be considered in patients who have undergone previous aortic reconstructive surgery. Early diagnosis of such lesions is essential because they are usually associated with catastrophic hemorrhage. The distal duodenum is the most common site of graft rupture into the bowel (about 80 per cent of the time).

History and Physical Examination

The physician should ask if the patient has epigastric or upper abdominal pain, heartburn, retching, dysphagia, loss of appetite, or weight loss. Other pertinent points include a past history of peptic ulcer disease, previous GI bleeding, liver disease, alcohol abuse, abdominal surgery, and other significant medical problems. The patient should also be asked specifically about the use of aspirin and NSAIDs.

Physical examination may also provide diagnostic clues. Cirrhosis is suggested by the presence of spider angiomas, jaundice, hepatosplenomegaly, and ascites. Epigastric tenderness is commonly seen in peptic ulcer disease. Non–GI tract telangiectasias may be seen in patients with Osler-Weber-Rendu syndrome (e.g., involving the mucous membranes of the mouth or nose, the face, or the distal extremities, including under the nails). Examination of the stool (e.g., that obtained on rectal examination) is important and may provide clues to the magnitude and location of bleeding; the presence of melena or maroon stools should be noted.

Diagnostic Approach

All patients with hematemesis and most with melena (about 95 per cent) have an upper GI tract bleeding source. As noted earlier, patients with large-volume maroon stools present a more difficult situation, since bleeding may be from either the upper or the lower GI tract. Gastric aspiration for gross blood is an easy and rapid technique for localizing the source of bleeding to the upper GI tract in patients with melena or maroon stools. Blood loss is localized to the upper GI tract if significant amounts of red blood or "coffee grounds" are aspirated. The finding of a few specks of bright red blood in the aspirate is of little import, however, since it may have arisen from trauma related to passage of the nasogastric tube or to the overzealous use of suction. It is not helpful (and is potentially misleading) to check for the presence of occult blood if the gastric aspirate does not contain gross blood. A normal gastric aspirate is much less helpful than an abnormal aspirate and does not exclude an upper GI bleeding source since (1) bleeding may have stopped and blood may have been cleared from the stomach and (2) blood from an actively bleeding duodenal ulcer does not always reflux back through the pylorus into the stomach.

Because of its greater diagnostic accuracy and therapeutic potential, endoscopy has largely replaced barium x-ray studies in the evaluation of patients with presumed acute upper GI tract bleeding. It is important that patients be resuscitated and hemodynamics restored before endoscopy is attempted. Upper GI bleeding usually stops spontaneously and most patients can undergo endoscopy electively. Indications for emergent (including nighttime) endoscopy include severe persistent or recurrent bleeding (since an attempt at hemostatic control with endoscopy or surgery is required in such patients) and a history of previous aortic reconstructive surgery (which would raise the possibility of an aortoenteric fistula). Patients with suspected variceal hemorrhage should also be considered for early endoscopy, since it has a considerably worse prognosis than do most other causes of bleeding and is treated differently. In addition, early endoscopy can also be helpful in making decisions about the necessity of admission to the intensive care unit (ICU) and early discharge from the hospital.

A high-quality double-contrast barium x-ray study is a reasonable alternative to endoscopy in nonactively bleeding patients who refuse endoscopy or who are considered at high risk from the procedure.

Angiography is used in the diagnosis and treatment of upper GI tract bleeding when massive bleeding obscures endoscopic visualization. To detect active extravasation of contrast requires a rate of bleeding of at least 0.5 mL per minute.

LOWER GASTROINTESTINAL TRACT BLEEDING

Lower GI tract bleeding is defined as bleeding arising from below the ligament of Treitz (including the jejunum, ileum, colorectum, and anal canal). The passage of bright red blood through the rectum implies that the bleeding site is in the anal canal, rectum, or colon. The passage of small amounts of bright red blood tends to localize the bleeding source distally to the anal canal, rectum, or sigmoid colon. In contrast, large-volume maroon stools may originate in either the lower or upper GI tract. Only about 5 per cent of cases of melena arise from the lower GI tract. As with upper GI tract bleeding, most lower GI tract bleeding will stop spontaneously.

Etiology

Hemorrhoids are a common cause of mild, intermittent passage of bright red blood through the rectum, with blood typically seen on the toilet tissue or around the feces but not mixed in with it. Hemorrhoidal bleeding is rarely severe. Anal fissures, another common cause of similar anal canal bleeding, are usually associated with local pain. Bleeding from hemorrhoids and anal fissures is often associated with straining or passage of hard stools.

The causes of major hematochezia are listed in Table 2. Most cases of severe or hemodynamically significant hematochezia will arise from the colorectum; however, some 15 per cent of cases will be related to lesions in the small bowel or the upper GI tract.

Bleeding from a colonic diverticulum is the most common cause of severe hematochezia. Although diverticulosis is more common in the distal colon than in the proximal colon, hemorrhage is more likely to arise from diverticula in the proximal colon. Diverticular bleeding is characteristically painless. Only rarely is it associated with acute diverticulitis.

Angiodysplasia with focal vascular ectasia is another common cause of acute major lower GI tract bleeding. Although such lesions, which are often multiple, may occur anywhere in the gut, they are most common in the cecum and ascending colon (the small bowel is the next most common site). Approximately two thirds of patients with colonic angiodysplasia are older than 70 years of age. Bleeding from angiodysplasia is also painless. Angiodysplasia can be difficult to detect; the lesions are not identified on barium contrast x-ray studies. Endoscopy may be more sensitive than angiography but neither represents a "gold standard."

Colorectal cancer and large polyps represent another important cause of acute lower GI bleeding, particularly in persons older than 40 to 50 years of age. However, chronic occult GI blood loss and mild intermittent hematochezia are much more common presentations than is major hemorrhage. Some patients with colorectal neoplasms will give a history of a recent change in bowel habits or a family history of colorectal cancer.

Patients with acute hematochezia resulting from ischemic colitis or infectious colitis usually have associated acute abdominal cramping and diarrhea as significant symptoms. Risk factors for ischemic colitis include advanced age, known arteriosclerotic vascular disease, history of major abdominal surgery, and use of certain drugs (e.g., estrogens, cocaine). Severe hemorrhage is a rare complication of chronic inflammatory bowel disease (ulcerative colitis or Crohn's disease); such patients are much more likely to present with mild chronic hematochezia. Other symptoms, such as chronic diarrhea, cramping, and rectal urgency, are common. Patients with radiation proctocolitis may have acute or chronic rectal bleeding that is rarely massive.

Although small bowel lesions are a relatively infrequent source of hematochezia, they present a particular diagnostic challenge because the small bowel is less accessible for evaluation than either the upper GI tract or the colon. Sources of GI bleeding in the small intestine are summarized in Table 3. Angiodysplasias followed by neoplasms are the two most common causes in adults. Other causes of bleeding in the small intestine include Crohn's disease, Meckel's diverticulum (the most common cause in young persons), NSAID-ulcers, and aortoenteric fistula.

The most common upper GI tract causes of hematochezia are bleeding ulcers of the stomach or duodenum and esophagogastric varices.

Table 2. Sources of Moderate to Severe Rectal Bleeding

Source	% of Cases
Upper GI Tract	10
Small Bowel	5
Angiodysplasia	
Neoplasm	
Crohn's disease	
Meckel's diverticulum	
Aortoenteric fistula	
Colon	85
Diverticulosis	
Angiodysplasia	
Neoplasm	
Inflammatory bowel disease	
Ischemic colitis	
Radiation-induced colitis	
Other	

GI = gastrointestinal.

Table 3. Small Bowel Sources of Obscure Gastrointestinal Bleeding

Angiodysplasia
Neoplasm
NSAID- or drug-induced erosions or ulcers
Crohn's disease
Meckel's diverticulum
Jejunal diverticula
Ulcerative jejunitis
Aortoenteric fistula
Other

NSAID = nonsteroidal anti-inflammatory drug.

History and Physical Examination

The physician should ask the patient about the duration and magnitude of blood loss, as well as the color of the blood passed. Not infrequently, however, patients overestimate the amount of blood they have passed. The presence of other symptoms, such as abdominal pain, diarrhea, constipation, straining with bowel movements, change in bowel habits, rectal urgency, and weight loss, is also significant. A past history of pelvic irradiation or a history of chronic inflammatory bowel disease has obvious importance. Other pertinent findings include a past history of serious vascular disease, other medical illness, medication history, and a family history of colorectal cancer.

The rectal examination (including perianal inspection and inspection of the stool) is the most important aspect of the physical examination of suspected lower GI tract bleeding. Abdominal tenderness may be present with infectious colitis, ischemic colitis, and chronic inflammatory bowel disease. An abdominal mass is occasionally palpable in patients with carcinoma of the colon and Crohn's disease.

Diagnostic Approach

The diagnostic approach to hematochezia depends on its nature and severity and the clinical setting. In patients with suspected minor bleeding from the anal canal or rectum, rigid proctoscopy or flexible proctosigmoidoscopy with anoscopy may be all that is needed.

For most patients in whom a colonic source is suspected, colonoscopy is the preferred diagnostic approach. This can usually be performed electively. In patients with persistent acute bleeding, however, the procedure can be performed urgently after rapid lavage preparation. Advantages of colonoscopy over air-contrast barium enema include an increased diagnostic yield, the ability to obtain biopsy specimens, and therapeutic applications (e.g., removal of polyps and bipolar coagulation of angiodysplasia). In addition, an abnormal barium enema study often necessitates colonoscopy anyway. An air-contrast barium enema study can be helpful in patients who are not actively bleeding and in whom total colonoscopy is not technically possible or is nondiagnostic.

Angiography is indicated in patients with ongoing lower GI bleeding who have undergone nondiagnostic colonoscopy or in whom the rate of bleeding is so great as to preclude an attempt at colonoscopy. Many angiographers will request that a radionuclide-tagged red blood cell (RBC) GI blood loss localization study be performed prior to angiography to document that the patient is actively bleeding and to help direct their study. An abnormal radionuclide scan will detect active blood loss down to about 0.1 mL per minute, which can hopefully be localized to the small bowel or some segment of the colon.

The passage of large-volume maroon stools with a normal nasogastric aspirate (hematochezia of uncertain origin) presents a more difficult diagnostic challenge. I will usually perform upper GI endoscopy as the initial diagnostic study in this situation. My rationale for initially performing upper GI endoscopy rather than colonoscopy includes the following reasons. Upper endoscopy can usually be performed in just a few minutes and is generally well tolerated. If the examination is normal, an upper GI tract site can virtually be excluded. Conversely, if an upper GI bleeding site is identified, an attempt to pass a colonoscope through a bloody colon can be avoided.

If the bleeding site is not identified on upper GI endoscopy, colonoscopy is performed after rapid lavage preparation. Patients with nondiagnostic colonoscopy results and active bleeding warrant radionuclide scanning and angiography. Examination with an enteroscope can also be useful, as discussed in the next section.

OBSCURE GASTROINTESTINAL BLEEDING

Chronic GI bleeding or recurrent acute bleeding can occur without careful evaluation of the upper GI tract and colon identifying a bleeding source. A lesion in the small bowel will be the site of bleeding in the majority of such cases, although it is possible to miss some lesions in the upper GI tract and colon even with repeated endoscopic examinations (e.g., angiodysplasias, Dieulafoy's lesion).

Enteroclysis is recommended to evaluate the small bowel provided that the patient is not actively bleeding and an aortoenteric fistula is not considered likely. This special type of infusion small bowel x-ray study requires that the radiologist pass a tube (via the mouth or nose) to the duodenojejunal junction. Barium is instilled through the tube, followed by a methylcellulose solution. The study has a much greater sensitivity for detecting small bowel bleeding lesions than does a conventional small bowel x-ray series (which is performed by having the patient drink an oral barium suspension and intermittently taking x-rays) because (1) the double-contrast effect of enteroclysis permits greater mucosal detail and also allows overlying loops of small bowel to be better examined and (2) the infusion is carried out under fluoroscopic visualization, theoretically allowing the entire small bowel to be specifically visualized.

Tagged red blood cell–radionuclide studies can be performed during episodes of apparent active bleeding. The yield of angiography is highest in patients with an abnormal radionuclide study, but angiography results are occasionally abnormal even when the radionuclide study is normal, allowing detection of some angiodysplasias and small bowel tumors. Radionuclide scanning using technetium-99m pertechnetate for Meckel's diverticulum ("Meckel's scan") is another consideration. Bleeding from a Meckel's diverticulum is the most common cause of small bowel bleeding in individuals younger than 30 years of age, but it can also occur in older adults. The rationale for a Meckel scan is that most, although not all, bleeding Meckel's diverticula contain gastric mucosa capable of secreting acid and taking up radiolabeled technetium. Ulceration is thought to arise from acid production by the ectopic gastric mucosa.

Patients whose bleeding remains obscure are considered for enteroscopy. "Push enteroscopy" is a technique in which a pediatric colonoscope or dedicated push enteroscope is advanced as far into the small bowel as possible. The jejunum is accessible with this procedure. Enteroscopy can also be performed using a very long, thin enteroscope (referred to as a "Sonde-type" enteroscope). Although the ileum can be reached with this technique, the procedure is tedious, uncomfortable, and not widely available. Furthermore, Sonde-type enteroscopes lack fine tip control (meaning the small bowel mucosa cannot be completely visualized) and therapeutic capability. Intraoperative enteroscopy is another way of visualizing the small bowel endoscopically. It can be helpful in selected patients with recurrent obscure GI bleeding and permits visualization of the entire small bowel. Angiodysplasias of the small bowel are visible with this technique through a combination of direct intraluminal visualization and transluminal endoscopic illumination. Other small bowel lesions can also be identified by this procedure. Lesions identified during intraoperative endoscopy can be treated definitively by endoscopic or surgical means.

OCCULT GASTROINTESTINAL BLEEDING

The approach to occult GI bleeding depends on which of three settings is encountered: (1) a positive fecal occult blood test in an asymptomatic, nonanemic individual undergoing routine colorectal cancer screening, (2) unexplained iron deficiency anemia, or (3) a positive result on fecal occult blood testing carried out to evaluate a patient presenting with GI symptoms. In the first setting, the major goal is to exclude colorectal malignancy and large polyps. Colonoscopy is usually recommended, although the combination of flexible proctosigmoidoscopy and air-contrast barium enema represents an alternative approach.

Study of the upper GI tract is usually not necessary in patients whose colons have been cleared provided that they are not anemic or symptomatic.

In asymptomatic adults with iron deficiency anemia resulting from suspected occult GI blood loss, colonoscopy is performed first. If no abnormality is found, endoscopy of the upper GI tract is performed, usually at the same sitting. If both studies are normal, enteroclysis is recommended. If all three studies are normal, I usually treat the patient with an iron supplement and observe for further bleeding. Patients who fail to respond to iron therapy and who have continued documented GI blood loss are considered for additional evaluation (outlined in the section on obscure GI bleeding).

Patients with a positive fecal occult blood test result and GI symptoms are evaluated with either upper GI endoscopy or colonoscopy, depending on the level of symptoms.

NAUSEA, VOMITING, AND DYSPEPSIA

By William Z. Borer, M.D.
Philadelphia, Pennsylvania
and Duane W. Taebel, M.D.
La Crosse, Wisconsin

NAUSEA AND VOMITING

Nausea is an unpleasant subjective sensation of illness characterized by the imminent need to vomit. Nausea may precede vomiting or it may occur in varying degrees of severity without subsequent vomiting. Severe nausea is often accompanied by increased parasympathetic activity that results in skin pallor, diaphoresis, hypersalivation, and bradycardia with hypotension (vasovagal response). Anorexia usually accompanies nausea, and both may be symptoms of a wide range of gastrointestinal or nongastrointestinal diseases (Table 1).

Vomiting, or emesis, is the forceful oral ejection of gastric contents. Retching, or the "dry heaves," refers to the labored effort of vomiting without significant loss of gastric contents. It may precede or follow the act of vomiting. With both, the expulsive force is generated by strong rhythmic contractions of the respiratory and abdominal muscles. The gastric fundus is rendered hypotonic and hence plays only a passive role in the process. Concomitant contraction of the pylorus and relaxation of the gastroesophageal sphincter direct the gastric contents into the esophagus, where increased intrathoracic pressure further propels them through the mouth after reflex closure of the glottis, which prevents aspiration.

Nausea, vomiting, and retching are probably primordial responses that serve to eliminate toxins or potentially injurious substances. They are initiated and coordinated by a complex set of neurologic controls in specialized areas of the brain. The vomiting center in the lateral reticular formation of the medulla coordinates the patterned response to many noxious stimuli and receives visceral afferent impulses directly from the gastrointestinal tract. The chemoreceptor trigger zone (CTZ) in the area postrema of the fourth ventricle, where the "blood-brain barrier" is virtually nonexistent, functions as an emetic chemoreceptor that responds to chemical stimuli in the circulation.

Vomiting should be distinguished from regurgitation, which is an overflow phenomenon related to a weak or an incompetent lower esophageal sphincter. Regurgitation does not require complex neuronal mediation, and little or no physical effort is needed. Regurgitated gastric contents are often returned to the stomach by voluntary swallowing or tertiary esophageal contractions (see the article on esophageal diseases).

Clinical Correlations

The timing, duration, frequency, and intensity of vomiting may offer clues to the underlying clinical disorder. Early morning nausea and vomiting (morning sickness) occurs in more than one half of pregnant women during the first trimester. Sudden and forceful (projectile) vomiting is often associated with increased intracranial pressure. If the vomitus consists of food eaten more than 12 hours earlier, gastric outlet obstruction or gastric atony should be strongly considered. Obstruction or a motility disorder, such as diabetic or postvagotomy gastroparesis, is suggested by recurrent vomiting that is delayed for an hour or more after eating (see the article on functional disorders of the gastrointestinal tract). Psychogenic vomiting typically occurs during or soon after a meal. Pain caused by peptic ulcer disease is frequently relieved by vomiting, but pain due to pancreatitis or biliary tract disease is not.

The character of the vomitus also has clinical significance. Blood (hematemesis) or "coffee grounds" (partially digested blood) emesis is the clinical hallmark of upper gastrointestinal bleeding (see the article on gastrointestinal hemorrhage). Bile in the vomitus attests to an open communication between the duodenal ampulla and the stomach virtually excluding obstruction between these two points. Undigested food may not have reached the stomach and is typically seen in the vomitus associated with esophageal disease (achalasia or diverticulum) or with pharyngeal (Zenker's) diverticulum. Old or partially digested food with no bile suggests obstruction at the pylorus or in the proximal duodenum. Small bowel obstruction distal to the duodenum is usually associated with severe colicky periumbilical pain that may be temporarily relieved by vomiting, and the vomitus is typically bile stained with the appearance of small bowel contents. Lower quadrant or epigastric pain with vomitus that looks and smells like feces is virtually diagnostic of colonic obstruction (see the articles on abdominal pain and intestinal obstruction). Feculent vomitus may also occur in patients with ischemic bowel injury, gastrocolic fistula, ileus due to peritonitis, or bacterial overgrowth syndrome in either the stomach or the duodenum.

Infections

Acute gastroenteritis ranks as one of the most common infections worldwide and is second in frequency only to acute upper respiratory illnesses. The viral syndrome includes nausea, vomiting, abdominal cramps, diarrhea, headache, and myalgias. Various viral agents (see the article on viral gastroenteritis) have been implicated in this illness, which is usually mild and self-limited except in patients who are immunocompromised, very old, or very young. Bacterial enterotoxins associated with "food poisoning" cause nausea of sudden onset, vomiting, abdominal cramping, and diarrhea within 2 to 24 hours of ingestion of contaminated food. Nausea, vomiting, and diarrhea accompanied by fever suggest an invasive or inflammatory bacterial enteritis (see the article on bacterial diarrheas).

Table 1. Causes of Anorexia, Nausea, and Vomiting

Gastrointestinal
- Inflammatory or neoplastic diseases of the oropharynx
- Esophagus
  - Esophagitis and/or esophageal stricture
  - Malignancy
  - Motility disorders
- Stomach and duodenum
  - Gastritis
  - Peptic ulcer disease
  - Malignancy
  - After gastric surgery
  - Motility disorders
- Small bowel and colon
  - Appendicitis
  - Obstruction
  - Inflammatory bowel disease
  - Malignancy
  - Vascular insufficiency
  - Diverticulitis
  - Food poisoning
  - Parasitic infestation

Pancreas
- Pancreatitis, acute and chronic
- Malignancy

Liver and Gallbladder
- Hepatitis
- Alcoholic liver disease
- Malignancy, primary or secondary
- Congestive hepatomegaly
- Hepatic abscess
- Cholecystitis, cholelithiasis, cholangitis
- Biliary obstruction, intrahepatic or extrahepatic

Peritoneum and Mesentery
- Peritonitis
- Mesenteritis
- Neoplasm, primary or metastatic
- Retroperitoneal malignancies

Cardiovascular
- Congestive heart failure
- Pericarditis
- Myocardial infarction

Pulmonary
- Pulmonary insufficiency
- Malignancy
- Pulmonary infections

Renal
- Renal colic
- Urinary tract infections
- Renal malignancy

Metabolic and Endocrine
- Pituitary or adrenal insufficiency
- Hypothyroidism
- Hyperparathyroidism
- Diabetic ketoacidosis
- Electrolyte abnormalities
  - Hyponatremia
  - Alkalosis

Hematologic
- Lymphoma
- Pernicious anemia

Infectious
- Most febrile infectious illnesses
- Tuberculosis
- Gastroenteritis, viral and bacterial

Neurologic
- Intracranial malignancy
- Meningitis
- Brain abscess
- Degenerative and vascular diseases
- Migraine
- Labyrinthine disturbances
- Tabes

Psychiatric and Psychogenic
- Psychogenic vomiting
- Depression
- Schizophrenia
- Anorexia nervosa
- Acute psychoses
- Neuroses

Miscellaneous
- Alcoholism
- Drugs
  - Digitalis
  - Antibiotics
  - Narcotic drugs (including withdrawal)
  - Chemotherapeutic drugs
  - Theophylline
- Pregnancy
- Collagen vascular disease
- Erotic vomiting

Modified from Mitchell, R.D.: Anorexia, nausea, and vomiting. *In* Conn, R.B. (ed.): *Current Diagnosis,* 8th ed. Philadelphia, W.B. Saunders Company, 1991, p. 46.

Nausea and anorexia with or without vomiting may precede the icteric phase of viral hepatitis by several days.

Drugs

Many different classes of drugs are associated with nausea and vomiting, including antibiotics such as erythromycin, opiates, cardiac glycosides, and several cancer chemotheraputic agents. Many drugs act directly on the CTZ, whereas others (aspirin, alcohol, and nonsteroidal anti-inflammatory agents) cause gastritis and may activate the vomiting center via afferent pathways from the stomach. Commonly used drugs such as codeine, hydromorphone, digitalis, and theophylline are easily overlooked by both patient and physician as potential causes of nausea and vomiting. Several cytotoxic agents (cisplatin, vinblastine, and etoposide) are notorious for their emetic effect, which typically occurs a few hours after administration. This delay suggests that the drugs act peripherally or via an intermediate factor to produce nausea and vomiting. Some cancer patients develop anticipatory nausea and vomiting in response to multiple chemotherapy treatments.

Visceral Pain

The association between nausea and vomiting and visceral pain is common and is presumed to be mediated via visceral afferent pathways. Examples include the obstruction and subsequent distention of a hollow viscus, such as the intestine, ureter, and cystic or common bile duct. Physical trauma or inflammation involving the kidney, testis, ovary, gallbladder, pancreas, or myocardium is often accompanied by nausea as well as pain (see the articles on abdominal pain).

Central Nervous System

Sudden and forceful (projectile) vomiting is the clinical hallmark of increased intracranial pressure. Associated anorexia and nausea are typically minimal or absent. The physical findings, such as papilledema and neurologic changes, are variable, and imaging studies (e.g., computed tomography [CT] and magnetic resonance imaging [MRI] scans) of the head can be very useful if an intracranial space-occupying lesion is suspected. Vascular headache (migraine) is often associated with nausea and vomiting and must be differentiated from an intracranial lesion. Vestibular stimulation (labyrinthitis, motion sickness, Ménière's disease) results in activation of the vomiting center, but it can be distinguished from other intracranial causes of nausea and vomiting by the presence of vertigo and nystagmus (see the articles on intracranial neoplasms, migraine, and vertigo).

Pregnancy

Early-morning nausea (morning sickness) is reported by as many as 90 per cent of pregnant women during the first trimester. Vomiting, however, is reported by fewer than half. The onset occurs around the time of the first missed menstrual period, and symptoms typically resolve by the end of the first trimester. The nausea and vomiting of pregnancy are not associated with adverse outcomes of pregnancy, but the pathogenesis remains obscure. If vomiting persists (hyperemesis gravidarum), fluid and electrolyte abnormalities and nutritional deficiencies can develop. Severe, untreated hyperemesis gravidarum carries a high mortality rate, but appropriate fluid and electrolyte replacement and supportive psychotherapy can prevent maternal and fetal compromise.

Complications of Vomiting

Damage to the esophagus and the gastroesophageal junction can occur as the result of the substantial pressure and shear forces generated during acute vomiting or retching. Laceration of the mucosa into the submucosa at the gastroesophageal junction (Mallory-Weiss tear) can cause severe hemorrhage with hematemesis that is typically preceded by an episode of blood-free emesis. Rarely, with violent vomiting, the laceration may extend transmurally through the serosa (Boerhaave's syndrome), causing perforation with intense pain, pneumothorax (usually left-sided), pneumomediastinum, and pleural effusion. Patients with impaired consciousness, neurologic deficits, or acute intoxication (alcohol or drugs) are at risk for aspiration of vomitus, with resultant pneumonitis and anaerobic lung abcess (see the article on anaerobic lung infections).

The metabolic consequences of protracted vomiting are the result of water loss and electrolyte imbalances. When severe, these disturbances carry a high mortality rate, especially in young and old patients. The loss of acid (hydrochloric acid) from the stomach and potassium from the proximal small intestine cause a syndrome of hypochloremic, hypokalemic alkalosis with varying degrees of dehydration. Sodium and water depletion lead to volume contraction and activation of the renin-angiotensin-aldosterone pathway, which exacerbates renal potassium loss. If the alkalosis is severe, the renal tubular maximum (T_m) for bicarbonate reabsorption may be exceeded, a situation that results in further renal sodium (or potassium) and bicarbonate loss (Fig. 1).

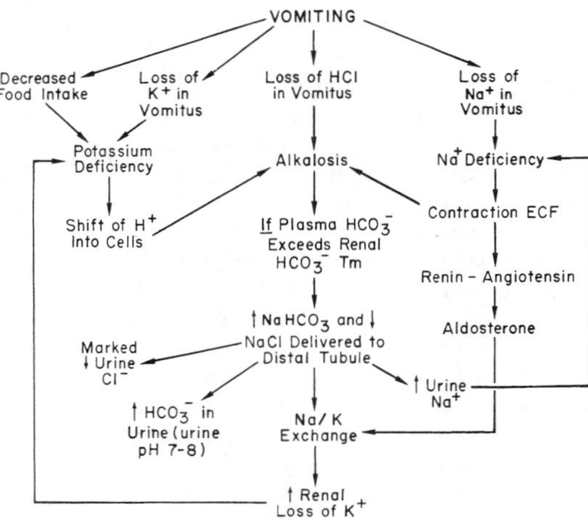

Figure 1. Metabolic consequences of vomiting. (From Feldman, M.: Nausea and vomiting. *In* Sleisenger, M., and Fordtran, J. [eds.]: *Gastrointestinal Disease: Pathophysiology, Diagnosis, Management,* 4th ed. Philadelphia, W.B. Saunders, 1989, p. 233, with permission.)

Dyspepsia

Nonulcer dyspepsia (NUD) is a poorly defined and heterogeneous constellation of symptoms that usually involves epigastric pain or discomfort. About one third of patients with dyspepsia describe pain that is typical of duodenal ulcer ("ulcerlike dyspepsia") with epigastric "burning" or "gnawing" 1 to 3 hours after meals. The pain is often nocturnal, is relieved by antacids or food, and is characterized by periods of remission and relapse. Other dyspeptic patients describe symptoms of fullness, bloating, gas (belching and flatulence), distention, early satiety, and nausea that are typically precipitated by eating. Terms such as "functional indigestion" and "dysmotilitylike dyspepsia" have been used to characterize this group. "Refluxlike dyspepsia" refers to a small group of patients who report symptoms of heartburn and regurgitation. About half the patients with NUD describe a complex that is a combination of symptoms from the three categories.

The key to the diagnosis of this disorder is the exclusion of organic disease. For example, myocardial ischemia must be considered when epigastric pain or discomfort is precipitated by exercise or is not relieved by 5 minutes of rest. The clinical evaluation should be directed toward the identification of any structural abnormality that would cause the symptoms reported by the patient (see the section on gastrointestinal diseases). Panendoscopy of the upper gastrointestinal tract should reveal no evidence of peptic ulcer disease, esophageal disease, or malignancy. Gallstones should be excluded by radiography or ultrasound, and irritable bowel syndrome and gastroesophageal reflux should be excluded by objective clinical criteria. Patients with persistent symptoms may require re-evaluation, including a search for stress factors and psychological precipitants as well as occult organic disease.

JAUNDICE

By Michael J. Levinson, M.D.
Memphis, Tennessee

Jaundice is yellowing of the skin, sclera, and mucous membranes that results from hyperbilirubinemia. The diagnosis should become apparent to the careful observer when the concentration of bilirubin in serum begins to exceed 2.5 mg/dL. Once bilirubin has reached levels greater than 7 mg/dL, jaundice is striking and should be noticeable to everyone. Jaundice is more difficult to detect in black or Asian patients, unless there is marked yellowing of the sclera. On the other hand, a patient may look jaundiced in artificial light and need to be examined by sunlight, if possible.

The conventional approach to the differential diagnosis always brings up a "prehepatic" or hemolytic process. Yes, such a condition has to be considered, but most important in the differential diagnosis is deciding between a "medical" hepatic cause and a "surgical" extrahepatic cause of jaundice. To operate on a patient with alcoholic hepatitis, which may mimic a surgical cause, leads to significant morbidity and mortality. On the other hand, to miss severe gallstone disease and the development of bile peritonitis also leads to prolonged morbidity and an increase in mortality. A brief review of normal bilirubin metabolism will facilitate a better understanding of the differential diagnosis of jaundice.

BILIRUBIN METABOLISM

Heme is the exclusive source of bilirubin. Eighty per cent of bilirubin derives from the hemoglobin of senescent erythrocytes (Fig. 1), and the remaining 20 per cent from ineffective erythropoiesis and other hemoproteins, including cytochromes and myoglobin. A small fraction of daily bilirubin production is the result of premature destruction of newly formed erythrocytes, a process termed "ineffective erythropoiesis."

Bilirubin is formed as the result of a multistep process in which the porphyrin ring of heme is first opened by selective enzymatic oxidation of the alpha-bridge carbon by a microsomal enzyme designated heme oxygenase, leading to the formation of a green tetrapyrrolic pigment, biliverdin. The oxidized alpha-bridge carbon is liberated as carbon monoxide, with one molecule of biliverdin and one molecule of carbon monoxide being produced for each molecule of heme degraded. Biliverdin is rapidly and quantitatively converted to the orange-yellow pigment bilirubin by a second enzyme, biliverdin reductase. Heme oxygenase is present not only in Kupffer cells and in a population of macrophages throughout the reticuloendothelial system but also in certain epithelial cells, including hepatocytes and renal tubules. Biliverdin reductase is widely distributed in many cell types throughout the body, including macrophages. As a consequence of the presence of both enzymes in macrophages, the sequential steps in the degradation of heme to bilirubin are readily visualized at the site of any bruise, where the color changes from purple to green to yellow reflect the conversion of extravasated and deoxygenated hemoglobin first to biliverdin, and then to bilirubin. Hence, large resolving hematomas may add to the bilirubin load.

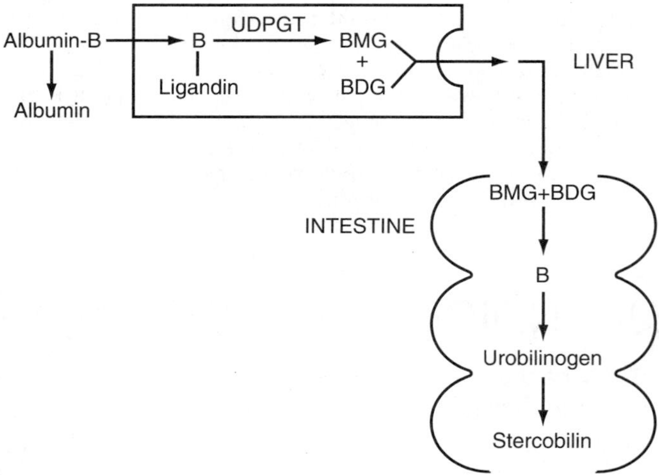

Figure 1. The metabolism of bilirubin. B = unconjugated bilirubin; UDPGT = uridine diphosphoglucuronyl transferase; BMG = bilirubin monoglucuronide; BDG = bilirubin diglucuronide.

The newly synthesized, unconjugated bilirubin is insoluble in water because intramolecular hydrogen bonding prevents ionization of the carboxylic acid groups. The unconjugated bilirubin is transported in the blood tightly bound to albumin. The adult human albumin molecule has one high-affinity binding site for bilirubin and at least one class of lower affinity sites. As a result, until the molar ratio of bilirubin to albumin in the circulation exceeds 1:1, which normally occurs only at bilirubin concentrations in excess of 35 mg/dL, the concentration of unbound bilirubin in the circulation is very small. This small concentration of unbound bilirubin is nevertheless a major driving force for bilirubin uptake by the hepatocytes. It is also a critical pathogenic factor in the development of bilirubin encephalopathy and kernicterus, both in the newborn period and, occasionally, in the setting of the rare hereditary hyperbilirubinemia designated Crigler-Najjar syndrome type I. The endothelial cells that line the hepatic sinusoids are unique in possessing fenestrae whose size can be physiologically and pharmacologically regulated, and that permit the exchange of albumin molecules and even larger proteins between the flowing plasma stream and the extracellular fluid within the space of Disse. This anatomic arrangement permits the delivery of albumin-bilirubin complexes virtually to the surface of the hepatocyte.

The hepatocyte has also evolved specialized mechanisms for facilitating the transport of bilirubin across the sinusoidal plasma membrane by means of a carrier, for keeping it in solution by binding to cytosolic proteins, for converting it to more polar metabolites by conjugating its propionic acid side chains with glucuronic acid, and for excreting the resulting water-soluble bilirubin glucuronidase across the canalicular plasma membrane into bile. Bilirubin binds mainly to the ligandin glutathione acetyltransferase B in the hepatocyte cytoplasm. The enzyme uridine diphosphoglucuronyl transferase conjugates bilirubin to glucuronic acid in the endoplasmic reticulum of the hepatocyte, forming water-soluble bilirubin monoglucuronides and diglucuronides. Normal human bile typically contains 70 to 90 per cent bilirubin diglucuronide, 5 to 25 per cent bilirubin monoglucuronide, and traces of other glycosidic conjugates.

When the ratio of unconjugated bilirubin to available enzyme is increased, as the result of either an increased bilirubin load (e.g., hemolysis) or reduced enzyme activity (Gilbert syndrome), the proportion of monoglucuronide increases, whereas that of the diglucuronide decreases. This situation is attributed to an increased intracellular concentration of unconjugated bilirubin, which successfully competes with bilirubin monoglucuronide for binding to the enzyme, favoring the formation of bilirubin monoglucuronide over that of bilirubin diglucuronide. These products are excreted in the bile canaliculus by a carrier-mediated process.

In the intestine, the conjugated bilirubin first undergoes deconjugation by the bacterial enzyme β-glucuronidase.

This step is followed by reduction to urobilinogens, which are mostly reabsorbed in the colon and circulated enterohepatically, although a small fraction reaches the systemic circulation and is excreted by the kidneys. Most of the urobilinogen undergoes spontaneous oxidation to stercobilin, the orange-brown pigment that gives stool its color.

MEASUREMENT OF BILIRUBIN

The "normal" serum bilirubin level in adults is 1.0 mg/dL. In clinical laboratories, bilirubin in plasma is typically measured by modifications of the diazo reaction first described in 1916. In this procedure, unconjugated bilirubin reacts slowly with the diazo reagent. In the presence of ethanol, caffeine, or the accelerators that disrupt the internal hydrogen bonding, the reaction can be accelerated. Accordingly, the concentration of prompt or *direct-reacting bilirubin* in serum or plasma, considered a measure of the amount of conjugated bilirubin present, is determined a short time interval (typically 30 to 60 seconds) after addition of the diazo reagent to the sample in the absence of an accelerator. The *total bilirubin concentration,* a measure of both unconjugated and conjugated bilirubin, is typically measured at some more prolonged interval (e.g., 30 to 60 minutes) after addition of an accelerator substance. The *indirect-reacting bilirubin*, calculated as the total minus the direct-reacting bilirubin, is a proxy for the amount of unconjugated bilirubin. (The tests for direct and indirect bilirubin are least sensitive at close to normal concentrations.) Hence, with nearly normal concentrations of bilirubin, the ability to identify purely unconjugated hyperbilirubinemia depends heavily on the index of suspicion of the clinician. At the same time, the ability to use the presence of small amounts of direct-reacting bilirubin in excess of 0.3 mg/dL as a subtle and sensitive indicator of hepatic dysfunction has largely become a casualty of automation in the clinical laboratory.

Three bilirubin levels are very important: A bilirubin level above 5 mg/dL in a chronic steady-state hemolysis means liver disease. On the other hand, a bilirubin level above 30 mg/dL, "hyper-hyperbilirubinemia," means something plus liver disease; that is, renal disease and/or hemolysis. A bilirubin level above 15 mg/dL in hepatic jaundice means severe liver disease and may be one of the reasons to admit the patient to the hospital.

DIFFERENTIAL DIAGNOSIS OF JAUNDICE

The differential diagnosis of jaundice (Table 1) can be divided into two major pathophysiologic categories, bilirubin overproduction and decreased bilirubin clearance. The diagnostic key remains to separate surgical conditions from medical ones as rapidly, safely, and cost-effectively as possible.

Table 1. Differential Diagnosis of Jaundice

- I. Increased Bilirubin Production
  - A. Hemolysis
  - B. Resorption of hematomas
- II. Decreased Bilirubin Clearance
  - A. Selective defects in hepatic bilirubin clearance
    - 1. Unconjugated bilirubin
      - a. Gilbert syndrome
      - b. Crigler-Najjar syndrome types 1 and 2
    - 2. Conjugated bilirubin
      - a. Dubin-Johnson syndrome
      - b. Rotor syndrome
- III. Cholestasis
  - A. Hepatocellular
    - 1. Drug-induced
    - 2. Cholestatic hepatitis
  - B. Biliary tract obstruction
    - 1. Stone
    - 2. Cancer

Bilirubin Overproduction

Bilirubin overproduction is most commonly caused by hemolysis. The liver has enormous reserve function, but, at times, with massive hemolysis or crush injuries, the bilirubin level may exceed 5 mg/dL. On the other hand, hemolysis, by itself, cannot account for a sustained bilirubin concentration above 5 mg/dL. Concentrations higher than this usually indicate the additional presence of hepatic dysfunction, even if it is not clinically significant.

The remainder of the bilirubin reflected in the "early labeled peak" has multiple sources, which include ineffective erythropoiesis in the bone marrow and turnover of short-lived nonhemoglobin heme proteins, including cytochrome P-450 and b_5, catalase and peroxidase. Ineffective erythropoiesis is seen in folic acid or vitamin B_{12} deficiency, the thalassemias, and the congenital and acquired dyserythropoietic anemias.

Defects in Bilirubin Metabolism or Transport

Hyperbilirubinemia and jaundice may also result from decreased hepatic bilirubin clearance owing to a hereditary defect in either hepatic metabolism or transport of bilirubin (Table 2). The tables outline the key features in these rare syndromes. Of note, Gilbert syndrome is seen in as many as 7 per cent of the white population in the United States and Western Europe.

Gilbert syndrome is one of the most common sources of patient referral to practicing gastroenterologists and hepatologists. In Gilbert syndrome, serum bilirubin concentrations for indirect bilirubin are most often less than 3 mg/dL. Bilirubin concentrations tend to fluctuate substantially in a given individual with higher concentrations associated with stress, fatigue, alcohol ingestion, and intercurrent illness, which is perhaps mediated by reduced caloric intake. In the earlier series, most patients were

Table 2. The Familial Hyperbilirubinemias

- I. Unconjugated Hyperbilirubinemias
  - A. Due to increased bilirubin production
    - 1. Hemolytic anemias
      - a. Hemoglobinopathies
      - b. Thalassemia syndromes
      - c. Enzyme defects
      - d. Membrane defects, etc.
    - 2. Shunt hyperbilirubinemias
      - a. Congenital dyserythropoietic jaundice syndromes
      - b. Miscellaneous
  - B. Due to defective hepatic bilirubin clearance
    - 1. Gilbert syndrome
    - 2. Crigler-Najjar syndrome
      - a. Type 1: Phenobarbital-resistant
      - b. Type 2: Phenobarbital-responsive
- II. Conjugated Hyperbilirubinemias
  - A. Dubin-Johnson syndrome
  - B. Rotor syndrome
  - C. Hepatic storage syndrome

diagnosed just after puberty, age 18 years. Now, many adults do not know they have Gilbert syndrome. In this disease, males have predominated by at least 1.5:1. This gender discrepancy may be due to sex steroids (Gilbert syndrome is rarely detected before puberty). Of note, an interesting variant of Gilbert syndrome in women is characterized by marked premenstrual accentuation of the hyperbilirubinemia.

Many patients with Gilbert syndrome have nonspecific complaints, fatigue, weakness, abdominal pain, and various gastrointestinal complaints that may be mistaken for liver disease.

Unconjugated hyperbilirubinemia is the *only abnormality present* on conventional hepatic biochemical tests in Gilbert syndrome. Recent studies have shown that some patients with Gilbert syndrome have reduced protoporphyrinogen oxidase in peripheral blood leukocytes, while levels of δ-aminolevulinic acid synthase may be increased fivefold.

Gilbert syndrome results from hepatic clearance of unconjugated bilirubin that is decreased by one third of normal. The exact cause is still under investigation. There may also be an abnormality in acetaminophen metabolism. Thus, patients with Gilbert syndrome should be warned not to exceed routine doses of acetaminophen.

In Gilbert syndrome, the liver biopsy is generally unremarkable. However, many patients and their families want further proof that there is no liver disease. The simplest provocative test is a 36- to 72-hour dietary restriction to 1680 calories a day, which produces a twofold to threefold increase in total bilirubin, but mostly indirect bilirubin. In normal subjects, the serum bilirubin level should increase by 0.4 mg/dL. The major reason to establish the diagnosis of Gilbert syndrome is to reassure the patient and to avoid unnecessary surgical procedures.

Cholestasis

It remains crucial to identify the patient with cholestasis, that is, impairment of bile formation, or bile flow, or both, resulting from extrahepatic biliary tract obstruction or hepatic parenchymal disease. Cholestasis can also occur without jaundice.

APPROACH TO THE PATIENT WITH JAUNDICE

Most conditions *should* be diagnosed by history and physical examination complemented by routine complete blood count (CBC) and liver function studies. A practical approach is outlined in Figure 2, but nothing is more important than individualizing the approach to the specific patient.

History and Physical Examination

It is very important that the first physician who sees the patient obtain a good history. The key point on the history is the presence or absence of pain. True painful jaundice, with pain as an unsolicited presenting feature, makes the diagnosis of extrahepatic or obstructive jaundice 95 per cent accurate. On the other hand, painless jaundice is only 90 per cent accurate in making the diagnosis of medical jaundice. An in-depth history of predisposing factors for viral hepatitis must be elicited. An equally careful drug history, especially regarding the use of over-the-counter

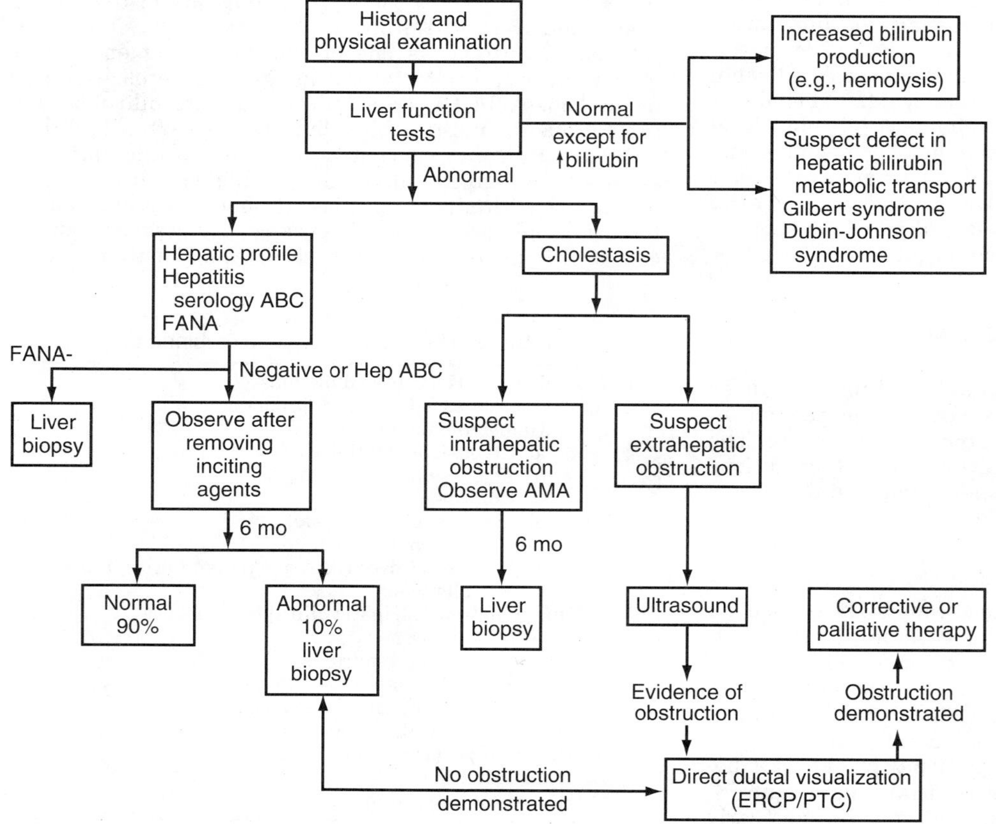

Figure 2. Approach to the patient with jaundice. AMA = antimitochondrial antibody; ERCP/PTC = endoscopic retrograde cholangiopancreatography/percutaneous transhepatic cholangiography; FANA = fluorescent antinuclear antibody; Hepatitis serology ABC = serologic tests for hepatitis A, B, and C.

medications, and products containing acetaminophen, must be obtained.

The diagnostic key during the physical examination is the size of the liver. It is rare to have extrahepatic obstruction present for any length of time with a normal-sized liver. Also, do not forget to search for the stigmata of liver disease. At this point, a tentative diagnosis should be made, and a differential diagnosis constructed if appropriate.

Laboratory Tests

Cost-consciousness tends to generate "short-cut," cheaper profiles, but in the case of liver disease, the physician should obtain a CBC with differential and reticulocyte count, total and direct bilirubin, alanine aminotransferase (ALT), aspartate aminotransferase (AST), alkaline phosphatase (ALP), gamma-glutamyl transferase (GGT), prothrombin time, protein electrophoresis, and, at times, a lactate dehydrogenase (LD) if hemolysis is a concern. The CBC helps in many ways. A polymorphonuclear response with pain suggests surgical jaundice. Lymphocytosis points to viral hepatitis, and eosinophilia to drug or parasitic disease.

The presence of anemia with a high reticulocyte count and LD level suggests hemolytic anemia. If the patient is anemic and the reticulocyte count is inappropriately low, the diagnosis of ineffective erythropoiesis is suggested. When the CBC and liver function studies are normal in the presence of indirect hyperbilirubinemia think Gilbert syndrome. With direct hyperbilirubinemia think Dubin-Johnson syndrome; with evidence of hemolysis think increased bilirubin production.

When the liver function studies are abnormal and the transaminases are more than three times the upper limit of the reference range, think hepatic process, that is, viral hepatitis. If the ALP and GGT levels are greater than three times the upper limit of the reference range with unremarkable ALT and AST levels, think cholestasis (Table 3).

When the patient has a history of pain and abnormal cholestatic liver function studies, there is a 97 per cent likelihood of a surgically treatable cause of jaundice. However, the patient may be a poor historian or have multiple risk factors for jaundice, or the liver function studies may show a mixed picture (hepatic-cholestatic). Hepatic imaging may then be helpful.

Hepatic Imaging

In challenging cases, an important question is: Are the bile ducts dilated? The cheapest and safest (no radiation, no intravenous contrast), albeit operator-dependent, method of imaging is ultrasound. In skillful hands, intrahepatic and extrahepatic bile duct dilation should be found in more than 85 per cent of patients in whom dilatation is eventually confirmed at surgery.

Table 3. Patterns of Biochemical Abnormalities in Liver Disease

Enzyme	Pattern *Cholestatic*	*Hepatocellular*
AST and ALT	N to ↑	↑↑ to ↑↑↑
Alkaline phosphatase	↑↑ to ↑↑↑	N to ↑
GGT	↑↑ to ↑↑↑	↑ to ↑↑

ALT = alanine aminotransferase; AST = aspartate aminotransferase; GGT = gamma-glutamyl transferase; N, normal; ↑ to ↑↑↑, degree of elevation.

If the bile ducts are dilated, endoscopic retrograde cholangiopancreatography (ERCP) can facilitate definitive diagnosis and/or treatment (see the article on biliary diseases). In some institutions, if the clotting studies are normal, a percutaneous transhepatic cholangiogram can also be performed.

If the clinical impression, liver function studies, and ultrasound findings are consistent with hepatocellular injury, a reliable patient can be watched for 6 months or until liver function test results return to baseline. At the end of 6 months, the patient may fulfill the criteria of chronic hepatitis, but in 90 per cent of patients, the liver function studies will return to baseline. If they do not, a liver biopsy should be performed.

When there is substantial evidence of extrahepatic biliary obstruction with normal ultrasound findings, ERCP or transhepatic cholangiography should be performed. If either test is nondiagnostic, then follow the liver function studies until baseline is reached or until 6 months have passed. ERCP should be performed on the patient with previous cholecystectomy (especially laparoscopic cholecystectomy) who has not undergone preoperative ERCP. Biliary scintigraphy may be best used in patients with known gallstones when the clinician wants to determine whether pain and/or jaundice is secondary to the gallstones.

EXCEPTIONS TO THE RULES

Three exceptions to the rules can cause trouble with the diagnosis. Two are common, one is relatively rare. The first is cholestatic hepatitis A, especially the relapsing variety. In the presence of pain, fever, and hepatomegaly, the IgM Hep A antibody test will be positive. Second, alcoholic hepatitis can cause pain, fever, and a tender, enlarged liver. This condition is accompanied by a 25 per cent chance of gallstones, and operative morbidity and mortality are rather significant. The third exception, which is rare, is the reverse situation, in which an extrahepatic surgical condition mimics acute hepatitis. Specifically, Klatskin's tumor, which may have normal bile ducts early, can present with a hepatitic or, at least, a mixed liver function panel and with a liver biopsy that looks like cholestatic (non-extrahepatic) hepatitis.

The evaluation of jaundice is a classic evaluation in medicine and surgery. In the majority of patients, a history and physical examination produce the answer, especially when the liver function studies are compatible. Ultrasonography helps confirm the diagnosis in as many as 90 per cent of cases. Direct visualization of the biliary tree is required for diagnosis and possible therapy in cases of extrahepatic obstruction and that rare case in which the physician's impression leans toward extrahepatic obstruction.

COMA

By Stanley L. Cohan, M.D., Ph.D.
Washington, D.C.

Coma is a pathologic state of brain function in which the baseline level of consciousness is severely impaired and in which responses to stimulation are reflexive, stereotyped, and noncognate. Comatose patients cannot be elevated by any stimulus to a level of consciousness in which they are aware of their surroundings. Coma superficially resembles sleep, but sleep is a physiologic process that is actively generated and from which patients can be aroused to a normal level of consciousness. On the other hand, coma is a pathologic state due to impaired brain function at one or more levels that precludes arousal, by any means, to a normal level of consciousness. Coma must also be distinguished from brain death, the latter being a state of irreversible, total brain destruction in which no brain response, reflex or otherwise, can be elicited, irrespective of the type or intensity of stimulus employed.

In the analysis of the comatose patient, it is important to determine the anatomic sites of dysfunction responsible for the coma, since location of dysfunction within the brain may provide important clues to the cause of coma and may be valuable in determining whether the patient is improving or deteriorating clinically. For example, a patient in coma with dysfunction at the level of the cerebral hemispheres on initial assessment and who has evidence of dysfunction to the level of the lower brain stem several days later is a patient who has obviously worsened. It is also important to have multiple clinical clues in patient assessment, since contemporary patient management so frequently employs intubation, mechanical ventilation, sedation, pharmacologic paralysis, and mechanical immobilization, all of which can significantly interfere with diagnostic testing in comatose individuals.

LEVEL OF CONSCIOUSNESS

When describing a patient's level of consciousness, avoid the use of single-word descriptions such as stupor, obtundation, and lethargy because these terms may have different meanings to different physicians and nurses. Instead, describe the patient's baseline appearance, the stimuli used to arouse the patient (noise, shaking, rotating the head from side to side, or supraorbital or nail bed pressure), and the patient's responses to these stimuli (see later). Normal consciousness requires both normal cerebral hemispheric and normal brain stem function. The latter contains the reticular activating system, which, from the diencephalon to the distal pons, contains neuronal nuclei that provide the cortical arousal required for maintaining consciousness. Disease at either level of the neuraxis may result in coma. In the brain stem reticular formation, discrete anatomic lesions, such as stroke, intraparenchymal hemorrhage, and tumor, can produce coma. By contrast, coma due to cerebral hemispheric disorders most often results from processes that produce diffuse bilateral changes, such as metabolic impairment or intoxication (Table 1). Strictly speaking, unilateral hemispheric disease will not result in coma unless there is extension of disease by herniation that secondarily involves the contralateral hemisphere or brain stem, or extension of dysfunction due to increased intracranial pressure. Thus, by locating the cause of coma in either the brain stem or the cerebrum, the clinician begins to distinguish anatomic insults (brain stem) from metabolic or toxicologic causes of coma (cerebrum). Unfortunately, the appearance of the coma and the level of consciousness, by themselves, cannot be used to determine the primary site of disease or often to distinguish improvement from deterioration.

Table 1. Coma Due to Diffuse Cortical Suppression

Metabolic and Toxic Causes
Postanoxic insult
Hypoxia
Diffuse cerebral ischemia
Hypoglycemia
Hyperglycemia and hyperosmolar state with or without ketosis
Renal failure
Hepatic failure
Sepsis and systemic acidosis
Hypothyroidism
Hypothermia
Hyponatremia
Hypercalcemia
Hypoadrenocortical state (Addison's disease or withdrawal from steroids)
Pharmacologic Causes
Barbiturates
Benzodiazepines
Alcohol
Glutethimide
Phenothiazines and butyrophenones
Meprobamate
Opiates (small pupils)
Cocaine, amphetamines, and other sympathomimetics (dilated pupils, flushed skin, hypertension, tachycardia, and arrhythmias)
Anticonvulsants, particularly carbamazepine and phenytoin (ophthalmoplegia with sparing of pupils)

RESPIRATION

Assessment of the level of consciousness and arousability should be supplemented by analysis of the patient's respiration (Table 2). Although the rate and pattern of respiration are the net result of the interaction of numerous regulatory mechanisms functioning at multiple levels of the neuraxis, including blood gas and pH receptors, respiratory muscle stretch receptors, and respiratory pacemakers within the brain stem and upper cervical spinal cord, these varying inputs into the control of respiratory function appear to be integrated and regulated by neurons deep within the frontal lobes to produce the regular respiratory rate of the normal conscious individual. Bilateral frontal lobe impairment may diminish this regulatory integration action and unmask the respiratory input of primary subcortical driving mechanisms, particularly variations in blood gas concentrations. With regulation by the frontal lobes absent, as may occur in coma due to diffuse hemispheric dysfunction, increased but still regular respirations produce a respiratory alkalosis, which will be metabolically compensated if renal function is normal. Thus, a comatose patient with a regular, rapid respiratory rate and respiratory alkalosis is most likely in coma secondary to diffuse hemispheric dysfunction. Of course, other causes of sustained hyperventilation, such as airway obstruction, pneumonia, pulmonary infarction, congestive heart failure, and systemic acidosis, should be ruled out with chest film and measurement of arterial blood gases, blood glucose, and serum salicylate concentrations. The patient may evolve into a pure blood gas breather, with the oscillating, waxing and waning pattern known as Cheyne-Stokes respiration (CSR). Patients in coma with CSR have severe bilateral cerebral hemispheric suppression, and most are functioning at a diencephalic level. It deserves emphasis that the *appearance of CSR may be the earliest indication of brain herniation.* Since other types of periodic breathing,

Table 2. Clinical Presentation of Comatose Patients

Disease Level	Respiratory Pattern	Pupillary Reaction	Reflex Oculomotor Responses (Oculocephalic Reflexes)	Motor Responses of Extremities
Diffuse cerebral cortical depression	Normal sustained or hyperventilation with respiratory alkalosis	Midposition and normally reactive to light	Full extraocular response	Diffusely hypotonic or diffusely hypertonic
Diffuse deep cerebral hemispheric depression	Sustained hyperventilation with respiratory alkalosis, or Cheyne-Stokes respiration	Midposition and normally reactive to light	Full extraocular response	Diffusely hypertonic, with decorticate responses to noxious stimulation
Thalamic impairment	Cheyne-Stokes respiration, possible periods of sustained hyperventilation	*Small* pupils that are *reactive* to light	Third nerve paresis, i.e., medial and superior rectus muscle weakness with eyes in abducted position	Decerebrate response to noxious stimulation
Pontine impairment	Apnea or irregular pattern and depth of respiration ("ataxic" breathing)	Midposition unreactive, or pinpoint and unreactive	Sixth nerve paresis, i.e., lateral rectus muscle, or complete ophthalmoplegia	Flaccid quadriplegia No decerebrate or decorticate responses
Medullary impairment	Apnea or ataxic breathing	Midposition unreactive pupils or pinpoint pupils	Complete ophthalmoplegia	Flaccid quadriplegia No decerebrate or decorticate responses

which are poorly characterized anatomically and pathophysiologically, may be confused with CSR, it is important to remember that CSR results from loss of frontal lobe control of respiration driven by the concentrations of blood gases. Thus, patients with CSR have respiratory alkalosis and develop sustained hyperventilation if their P_{CO_2} is increased, as may be produced by rebreathing of expired carbon dioxide. These latter two characteristics should distinguish CSR from other types of periodic breathing.

Patients with rapidly progressive deterioration due to devastating acute insults may present with coma and sustained hyperventilation with rates of 30 to 50 breaths per minute. This respiratory drive is unresponsive to changes in arterial pH or in blood gas concentrations. The only known way of controlling the breathing of such patients is mechanical ventilation with simultaneous neuromuscular paralysis induced with curarelike agents. If this breathing is not controlled by paralysis, these patients will literally breathe themselves to death, with the development of severe alkalosis, hypocalcemia, and an increased risk of cardiac electromechanical dissociation. The neurologic insults that produce coma and sustained hyperventilation unresponsive to P_{CO_2}, P_{O_2}, and pH are so severe that it is highly unlikely that these patients will ever regain consciousness. The common insults associated with central neurogenic hyperventilation include the following:

1. Deep intracerebral hypertensive hemorrhage that produces herniation beneath the falx cerebri, compression of the contralateral hemisphere, extension of blood into the ventricles, acute obstructive hydrocephalus, and herniation through the tentorium cerebelli
2. Cerebral abscess that ruptures through the wall of the lateral ventricle and produces acute ventriculitis, obstruction of the sylvian aqueduct, hydrocephalus, and herniation
3. Massive subarachnoid hemorrhage with diffuse, multifocal arterial vasospasm that produces secondary multifocal infarction, as well as edema and decreased reabsorption of cerebrospinal fluid due to the excess blood in the subarachnoid space, producing acute, nonobstructive communicating hydrocephalus.
4. A depressed skull fracture that produces laceration of the brain and overlying dura mater with secondary acute intracerebral and subdural-epidural hemorrhage, rapid increased intracranial pressure, and herniation beneath the falx and through the tentorium

In general, acute insults of this magnitude have a grim prognosis. Computed tomography (CT) of the brain early in the course speeds recognition of the cause. However, CT of the brain may not be immediately available, and the presence of coma and sustained hyperventilation in the absence of congestive heart failure, airway obstruction, or other causes of hypoxemia, hypercapnia, or acidosis should clearly point to rapidly evolving, devastating brain injury with herniation and extremely poor prognosis.

Comatose patients may have irregular breathing in which brief, gaspinglike respiratory efforts are intermixed with periods of apnea and occasional seemingly normal breaths. These breathing efforts do not seem to be influenced by the presence of hypoxemia, hypercapnia, acidosis, or alkalosis. Such patients appear to be functioning at the level of the medulla, their breathing patterns resulting from disinhibition of respiratory pacemaker mechanisms arising within the deep tegmental nuclei of the medulla and upper cervical spinal cord. Although seemingly unresponsive to blood gas concentrations and arterial pH, these mechanisms are *selectively vulnerable to suppression by opiates, barbiturates, and benzodiazepines. Avoid the use of these agents unless the patient is intubated and under ventilatory control.* Although this level of respiratory drive alone cannot provide sufficient brain oxygenation, loss of these mechanisms (in bilateral brain stem stroke or in skull base and upper cervical spine trauma) may produce apnea, particularly during sleep or when the patient is under sedation or under opiate analgesia. *Thus, patients with medullary–upper cervical spinal cord lesions, who appear to ventilate adequately when awake, must be observed closely for periodic apnea during sleep and may require intubation and ventilatory assist during sleep or when analgesics are administered.* Patients with bilateral medullary and upper cervical cord lesions may be alert despite impairment of the central tegmentum, because cerebral cortical stimulation by the reticular activating systems depends on neurons extending from the diencephalon to the middle-to-distal pons. Thus, significant deep parenchymal lesions at the level of the medulla and spinal cord may not suppress consciousness.

PUPILLARY FUNCTION

Proper characterization of the breathing patterns described above helps establish prognosis and determine improvement or deterioration. However, the aforementioned patterns may not be seen because patients with severely depressed consciousness are commonly intubated (to prevent aspiration) and mechanically ventilated (frequently with the aid of sedation and/or neuromuscular paralysis to keep them from fighting the ventilator). Thus, other clues must be sought to determine the location of disease, clinical improvement, or clinical deterioration. Pupillary examination may provide such clues. Pupillary size and reactivity to light and dark depend on the relative inputs of the sympathetic nervous system, which when stimulated causes pupillary dilatation, and the parasympathetic nervous system, which when stimulated causes pupillary constriction. Since both of these systems arise in the brain stem and are in close anatomic proximity to the central tegmentum, brain stem lesions that produce coma are commonly associated with pupillary functional abnormalities (Fig. 1). *The observation that a comatose patient has normal pupillary function provides strong presumptive evidence that coma is due to diffuse cerebral hemispheric dysfunction* caused by disorders such as hypoglycemia, diffuse ischemia, renal or hepatic failure, and postanoxic encephalopathy. By contrast, primary insults of the brain stem that result in coma are also likely to produce pupillary dysfunction. The sympathetic nervous system originates in the hypothalamus as a poorly localized polysynaptic neuronal system (see Fig. 1) that descends the lateral brain stem and does not exit the central nervous system until it reaches the T1 segment of the spinal cord. At each spinal level from T1 to L2 or L3, the sympathetic system gives off fibers that synapse in the corresponding sympathetic ganglion, with postsynaptic fibers providing sympathetic autonomic innervation to viscera, blood vessels, and the integument. Some of the fibers that exit at T1, however, do not synapse at the T1 level. Instead, they ascend in the neck and synapse in the superior cervical ganglion, with postsynaptic fibers reaching the pupil in association with the common carotid, internal carotid, and ophthalmic arteries. Stimulation of the sympathetic nervous system anywhere along this pathway, from the hypothalamus to the orbit, results in pupillary dilatation. The parasympathetic innervation of the pupil arises in the pretectal and tectal regions of the mesencephalon (see Fig. 1). These parasympathetic fibers leave the mesencephalon with the oculomotor fibers of the third cranial nerve, covering the surface of the third nerve. This anatomic arrangement may disassociate pupillomotor and oculomotor function when *extrinsic or compressive lesions of the third nerve produce pupillary dilatation* (due to parasympathetic impairment) *while sparing oculomotor function* (i.e., eye movement). *By contrast, intrinsic lesions of the third nerve or its nucleus* caused by diabetes or ischemia *produce oculomotor impairment while sparing pupillary function.* The parasympathetic fibers that exit the mesencephalon with the third nerve enter the orbit, leave the third nerve, and synapse in the ciliary ganglion. Postsynaptic fibers then innervate the pupil. Stimulation of this parasympathetic arc anywhere along its length produces pupillary constriction.

Evaluation of the sympathetic-parasympathetic pupillomotor system can help distinguish diencephalic, mesencephalic, pontine, and medullary causes or contributions to coma (see Table 2). As mentioned previously, coma due to hemispheric disease per se does not produce pupillary abnormalities. However, in *diencephalic* disorders, such as thalamic hemorrhage, tumors of the third ventricle, and tumors of the sella turcica that compress the hypothalamus, coma is associated with sympathetic impairment, resulting in small pupils. Because the pupillary parasympathetic system arises in the mesencephalon and is caudal to the lesion, pupillary reactivity to light is spared. *Thus, coma due to diencephalic impairment is associated with small pupils that react to light with constriction* ("small but reactive pupils"). By contrast, coma produced by mesencephalic lesions arising from basilar artery aneurysm or thrombosis or from thalamic masses compressing the dorsal mesencephalon manifests as impairment of both sympathetic and parasympathetic innervation of the pupil. Thus, mesencephalic lesions cause midposition pupils that are unreactive to light. Lesions of the pons, most commonly due to hypertensive pontine hemorrhage or infarction, may completely inhibit sympathetic outflow, producing maximal pupil constriction due to parasympathetic disinhibition ("pinpoint pupils"). The clinician should recall, however, that opiate overdose—and not anatomic lesions of the pons—is the most common cause of coma with pinpoint pupils. Thus, every patient who presents with altered mental status and small or pinpoint pupils should immediately receive an opiate antagonist, such as naloxone. The absence of enhanced responsiveness and increased pupillary size following administration of naloxone strongly suggest that the coma is the result of pontine disease. At death, the uncontrolled sympathetic release of norepinephrine causes

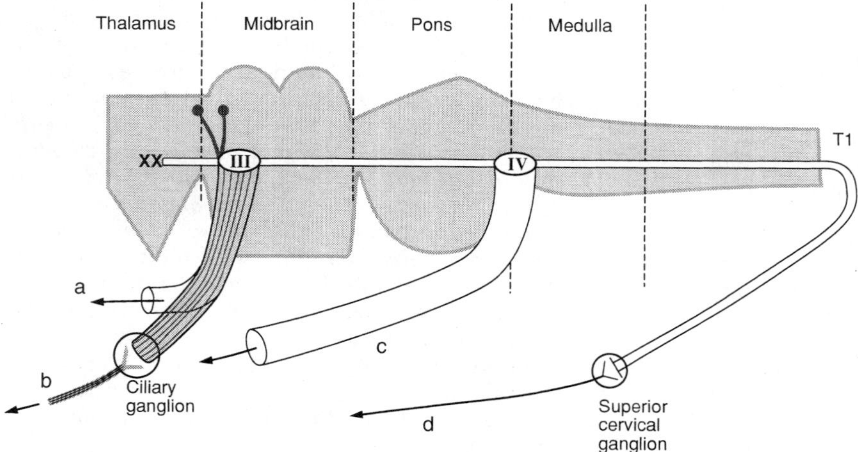

Figure 1. Diagram of the brain stem in sagittal view. *a,* The oculomotor portion of cranial nerve III. *b,* The parasympathetic portion of cranial nerve III, which innervates the pupil, stimulation of which produces pupillary constriction. *c,* Cranial nerve IV. *d,* The postsynaptic sympathetic innervation of the pupil, stimulation of which produces pupillary dilatation.

widely dilated pupils that do not constrict in response to light ("fixed and dilated" pupils). However, with death of the pupillomotor fibers, the pupil may return to midposition. Importantly, the presence of fixed and dilated pupils, by itself, should not serve as the basis for refusals to resuscitate the patient.

EXTRAOCULAR MUSCLES

As with pupillomotor function, abnormalities in extraocular muscle motility in comatose patients are usually the result of structural lesions in the brain stem (see Table 2). If extraocular movements are completely intact, it is highly unlikely that the cause of coma is anatomic disease of the brain stem. In the conscious patient who does not have significant cerebral hemispheric disease, reflex eye movements generated by brain stem and vestibular-cerebellar mechanisms are not observed because of cerebral suppression of these reflexes. Patients with coma from bihemispheric disease, however, have disinhibition of those reflex eye movements. To assess integrity of the oculomotor system in coma, examine reflex eye movements with the oculocephalic maneuver. Place the head of the supine patient 15 to 30 degrees above the horizontal, and then turn the head repeatedly from side to side. If the brain stem is intact, the clinician will observe tonic, conjugate deviation of the eyes in the opposite direction of the head rotation. By contrast, comatose patients with mesencephalic disease have impairment of cranial nerve III (see Fig. 1); therefore, the oculocephalic maneuver just described will demonstrate medial rectus muscle impairment with reduction or loss of adduction. When coma accompanies pontomedullary lesions, impairment of cranial nerve VI causes reduction or loss of abduction on oculocephalic testing owing to lateral rectus muscle weakness. Although lateral rectus muscle palsy may occur with parenchymal disease of the lower brain stem, patients may also have "false localizing" or "nonspecific" lateral rectus muscle weakness due to increased intracranial pressure that causes downward displacement of the brain stem and compression or stretching of the sixth cranial nerve as it passes beneath the pons in the subarachnoid space.

Complete loss of extraocular movements on oculocephalic testing suggests impairment of the brain stem from the mesencephalon to the medulla. However, loss of oculocephalic reflexes can result from causes other than brain stem impairment or destruction. In the hysterical or malingering patient, the cerebral hemispheres suppress the oculocephalic reflexes. Alternatively, the oculocephalic maneuver may not provide sufficient stimulus in patients whose reflexes have been suppressed by phenytoin, carbamazepine, or benzodiazepines. Therefore, when oculocephalic reflexes are not elicited, a second maneuver, cold caloric stimulation, should be employed. With the patient supine, the head 30 degrees above the horizontal, and the tympanic membranes unobstructed by cerumen or clotted blood, 40 to 50 mL of ice water is infused over 15 to 30 seconds into the external auditory canal through a small catheter, such as butterfly needle tubing. Within 30 to 60 seconds, a slow conjugate deviation of the eyes *toward* the irrigated side should be seen. In patients with mesencephalic lesions, adduction by the contralateral eye will be reduced or absent, and in patients with pontomedullary disease, abduction of the ipsilateral eye will be impaired. Complete ophthalmoplegia is consistent with brain stem impairment from the mesencephalon to the medulla. In the malingering or hysterical patient, slow tonic conjugate deviation of the eyes will alternate with rapid corrective eye movement in the opposite direction (i.e., nystagmus). Nystagmus in response to caloric testing is not seen in comatose patients.

MOTOR SYSTEM

Examination of the motor system may also provide clues to the etiology of coma and the extent of improvement or deterioration. Perhaps more important, however, is the value of the motor examination in determining whether potentially serious organic disease of the central nervous system is present in the alert patient. Frequently, patients who have sustained significant physical trauma present with an apparent psychiatric disorder. Likewise, the state of some intoxicated patients in the aggressive or belligerent stages of delirium may be mistaken for a psychologically based behavioral disorder. The pyramidal motor system, which has substantial metabolic requirements, appears selectively vulnerable to various physical, metabolic, and pharmacologic insults. Thus, the earliest objective clinical evidence of serious organic impairment may reflect pyramidal motor dysfunction, as demonstrated by the inability to button clothing, to place a key in a keyhole, or to open and close a safety-pin with one hand. Repetitive hand or finger movements may be slowed, and motor overflow may cause simultaneous dyskinesia of the ipsilateral foot or side of the face. Palmar grasps and snout reflexes may also be elicited. Such signs of cerebral cortical pyramidal impairment may be the earliest, or the only, signs consistent with significant cerebral hemispheric dysfunction. They should raise the index of suspicion of potentially serious cerebral impairment. As cortical suppression progresses, worsening motor coordination and pathologic motor reflexes such as snout, grasp, and Babinski's sign emerge. In patients with partially suppressed consciousness due to diffuse hemispheric impairment, cortical motor arousal may still be elicited by a noxious stimulus such as firm, sustained supraorbital pressure, which may elicit arm movement toward the stimulus, a facial grimace, or no discernible motor response appropriate to the stimulus. With complete cortical motor suppression in deep coma, stereotyped motor responses emerge. Patients functioning at a subcortical to an upper thalamic level may respond to a stimulus with *decorticate* posturing in which fingers are clenched in a fist with flexion at the elbows. In comatose patients functioning at a low thalamic to mesencephalic level, *decerebrate* responses to stimuli are characterized by hyperextension and inward rotation of the arms and hyperextension of the neck. In the patient with coma due to pontomedullary impairment, flaccid quadriplegia is seen. Finally, motor system changes are not as useful as pupillary or extraocular muscle abnormalities in pinpointing the anatomic location of disease. However, changes in motor responses may be the only valid clinical indication of further improvement or deterioration in a deeply comatose patient.

INTERPRETING THE FINDINGS

Ideally, the clinician should be able to elicit and utilize all potential findings to locate and define the cause of the lesion and to monitor the clinical progress of the comatose patient. On occasion, the available information may be severely limited. Scanning facilities may not be available, or the patient may be too unstable or too immunocompromised to move from the intensive care or isolation care environment. The use of sedatives, paralytic agents, and ventilators may preclude elicitation of helpful clinical signs, pharmacologic agents may alter pupillary function, and physical injuries to the patient may preclude oculocephalic and/or caloric testing. Thus, the physician may have to glean much meaning from few data.

COMA SYNDROMES

Diffuse Cerebral Hemispheric Dysfunction

Anoxia-hypoxia, severe global ischemia, hypoglycemia, hyperglycemia–hyperosmolar state with or without ketosis, hepatic or renal failure, meningitis, subarachnoid hemorrhage, and toxicity of environmental agents may produce diffuse bilateral cerebral hemisphere suppression that results in coma. Pupillary and extraocular muscle function are preserved. Motor tone may be reduced and, if not mechanically ventilated, patients may spontaneously hyperventilate, unless there has been drug-induced respiratory depression as in opiate, barbiturate, or benzodiazepine intoxication. Some patients may not worsen neurologically but nevertheless fail to regain consciousness because of diffuse cerebral cortical damage ("chronic vegetative state"). Others may worsen neurologically and undergo "rostrocaudal" deterioration as dysfunction moves down the neuraxis to a *subcortical hemispheric level,* with persisting coma, normal pupillary and extraocular reflexes, and decorticate motor responses of the extremities to stimulation. Over time, these patients may deteriorate to a *thalamic level,* remaining in coma, possibly with CSR, small but reactive pupils, normal extraocular reflexes, and decorticate or decerebrate motor responses. Deterioration to a mesencephalic level produces coma, Cheyne-Stokes or central neurogenic hyperventilation, *midposition fixed* pupils, third nerve paresis (medial and superior rectus muscle weakness are most obvious), and decerebrate motor responses. Extension of dysfunction to the *pontomedullary* level results in irregular, "ataxic" ventilation, complete ophthalmoplegia, and flaccid extremities without motor response to noxious stimulation. Extension to the *medulla* adds apnea to the picture of the comatose patient with fixed pupils, ophthalmoplegia, and flaccid quadriplegia of the extremities.

Unilateral Hemisphere Syndrome With Secondary Spread

Unilateral mass lesions, including intracerebral or subdural hemorrhage, cerebral infarction, brain abscess with associated cerebral edema, and brain tumor with a focal increase in intracranial pressure, can present with contralateral hemiparesis. Secondary herniation beneath the falx cerebri may compress the contralateral hemisphere with bihemispheric impairment and reduction in consciousness. If further deterioration occurs, subsequent progressive thalamic and brain stem impairment resembles that seen in rostrocaudal deterioration following severe diffuse hemispheric insults. Motor impairment may be more pronounced on the side of the initial lesion (i.e., decerebrate on one side and decorticate on the other). In some cases, mass effect from a unilateral hemispheric lesion causes the uncus of the temporal lobe to herniate over the free edge of the tentorium. This herniation compresses the mesencephalon and the third cranial nerve, causing unilateral pupillary dilatation followed by oculomotor paralysis and ipsilateral eye abduction. Further compression of the mesencephalon and destruction of the reticular activating system produce coma followed by continued rostrocaudal deterioration.

Coma Due To Direct Brain Stem Insult

Common causes of direct impairment of brain stem function include intraparenchymal hemorrhage, basilar artery ischemia, and brain stem–cerebellar tumors. Although coma due to brain stem ischemia or hemorrhage is of sudden onset, this history is frequently not available. One of the cardinal features of direct brain stem insult is the association of coma with asymmetric cranial nerve dysfunction. Recall, however, that third nerve paresis or unilateral pupillary dilatation can result from uncal herniation, and sixth nerve paresis can be produced solely by increased intracranial pressure.

Primary thalamic lesions produce coma with small reactive pupils, preserved extraocular reflexes, and decorticate-decerebrate posturing. Mesencephalic insults produce coma with midposition fixed pupils, medial and superior rectus muscle palsy, and decerebration. Finally, pontine insults result in coma with small to midposition pupils, lateral rectus muscle palsy, and flaccid quadriplegia. *Remember to rule out opiate overdose!*

Brain Death

Deeply comatose patients may be mistaken for patients with brain death. In coma, however, loss of consciousness occurs in the presence of residual brain function. Therefore, for some patients, there is a possibility of partial or complete recovery. In contrast, brain death occurs as the result of irreversible destruction. There is no evidence of any central nervous system function above the level of the cervical spinal cord, and there is no possibility of recovery of any brain function regardless of the therapeutic strategy. Unresponsiveness of the patient to any stimulus (except for possible preservation of tendon reflexes), apnea, flaccid quadriplegia, and unelicitable pupillary, extraoculomotor, gag, snout, and tracheal reflexes are essential for the diagnosis of brain death. These observations must be made in the absence of pharmacologic agents that block these responses. In some situations, such as before organ removal for transplantation or on request of the patient's family prior to discontinuing supportive care, confirmatory laboratory studies may be utilized. These tests include a "flat" (isoelectric) electroencephalogram (EEG) in the absence of hypothermia or drugs that may suppress the EEG; absent somatosensory evoked responses; and absent cerebral circulation as determined by radionuclide blood flow, transcranial Doppler, brain scan, or cerebral angiogram.

HEADACHE AND FACIAL PAIN

By Michael B. Stevens, M.D.
San Jose, California

HEADACHE

Headaches are common. They represent one of the top ten reasons for patients to seek medical care. The estimated lifetime prevalence rate for all types of headache is

Table 1. Thirteen Basic Types of Headaches Proposed by the International Headache Society (1988)

Primary Code	Primary Headache Type
1	Migraine
2	Tension-type headache
3	Cluster headache and chronic paroxysmal hemicrania
4	Miscellaneous headaches unassociated with structural lesion
5	Headache associated with head trauma
6	Headache associated with vascular disorders
7	Headache associated with nonvascular intracranial disorders
8	Headache associated with substances or their withdrawal
9	Headache associated with noncephalic infections
10	Headache associated with metabolic disorders
11	Headache or facial pain associated with disorders of the cranium, neck, eyes, ears, nose, sinuses, teeth, mouth, or other facial or cranial structures
12	Cranial neuralgias, nerve trunk pain, and deafferentation pain
13	Headache not classifiable elsewhere

93 per cent for males and 99 per cent for females, with 6.1 per cent of males and 14 per cent of females reporting four or more headaches per month. Headaches account for 18 million outpatient visits and 2.5 per cent of all emergency room visits each year. The cost of lost work hours is exceedingly high. The cost of unnecessary diagnostic testing is also extremely high. Social bias toward headache patients is found in both lay and medical populations.

Early scientific study of headaches was hampered by the lack of demonstrable physical findings and the lack of consistent, exacting nomenclature. To address the latter, the Headache Classification Committee of the International Headache Society outlined a new system in 1988 for the diagnosis, classification, and study of various headache and facial pain disorders.* Although extremely complex, detailed, and rigid, the scheme classifies headaches using a 1- to 4-digit number. The first digit represents the major headache type (e.g., migraine) and the second digit represents the major subtypes (e.g., migraine with aura, migraine without aura). The third and fourth digits represent further delineation into subclasses. The first-digit classifications are summarized in Table 1. Note that the primary code numbers represent both primary headaches and secondary headaches. Primary headaches are idiopathic disorders without identifiable structural or physiologic cause. Examples of primary headaches are tension-type headaches and migraine headaches. Secondary headaches are disorders caused by identifiable structural or physiologic changes, such as meningitis and cerebrovascular accidents. Although the 1988 Headache Classification Committee of the International Headache Society system is the most commonly used classification system, other systems have been proposed.

An adage in medicine states that some 80 per cent of diagnoses are made by history alone. This is particularly true in the diagnosis of headache disorders. A complete and thorough history is crucial for accurate diagnosis and treatment. Table 2 lists critical historical data that should be obtained by the physician. Importantly, the physician must appreciate the typical patterns of the patient's headaches because many of these patients have more than one type of headache. For example, many patients have frequent tension-type headaches and occasional migraine headaches, whereas others may have "mixed headaches," with symptoms that do not accurately fit into any of the "classic" primary headache disorders. Some patients have migraine headaches with clusteroid features; others have "crossover headaches" that start as one type of headache and progress to another type. The most common crossover headache is a tension-type headache that develops into a migraine headache. Often, a patient's headache in early life "transforms" to a different type of headache in later life (e.g., migraine to chronic daily headache). Physicians should consider headaches a continuum of conditions rather than a set of multiple, discrete primary headache disorders.

Primary Headache Disorders

Migraine

Migraine headaches occur in about 4 to 15 per cent of the general population yet account for 20 to 25 per cent of all headaches treated by physicians. Females are three times more likely to experience migraines than are males. The peak incidence of migraine headaches occurs at 20 to

Table 2. Critical Historical Data for Headache Patients

Age of onset
Typical pattern of headache
- Frequency
- Usual time of onset
- Location
- Radiation
- Progression
- Perceived intensity, usually on a scale of 1 to 10
- Duration
- Triggers or precipitating events
- Current treatment modalities, conservative or medicinal

Absence or presence of neurologic symptoms before, during, or after headache
Recent changes in pattern of headaches
Prior medical encounters
- "Diagnoses" given by physicians
- Diagnostic tests performed
- Past treatment modalities, conservative or medicinal

Other concurrent medical problems and medications
Social history
- Occupation, family, and social stressors
- Alcohol, tobacco, and recreational drug use

Family history of headache disorders
General review of system, including a specific focus on possible symptoms of depression
- Sleep patterns
  - Trouble falling asleep
  - Difficulty staying asleep
  - Early morning awakening
  - Feel rested on arising
- Fatigue
- Anhedonia
  - Appetite and weight changes
  - Sexual drive
- Sad or depressed mood or affect, crying spells
- Constipation

*Headache Classification Committee of the International Headache Society: Classification and diagnostic criteria for headache disorders, cranial neuralgias and facial pain. Cephalalgia, 8(Suppl. 7):1–96, 1988.

35 years of age. Thereafter, these headaches decrease in both frequency and severity. Migraines typically decrease during pregnancy but often rebound post partum. Migraine headaches can be triggered by various agents, situations, and environmental changes. Some common precipitants are listed in Table 3.

According to the International Headache Society, the diagnosis of migraine encompasses 14 separate diagnoses, including the broad category "migrainous disorder not fulfilling above criteria." For simplicity, migraine headaches can be divided into three major subcategories: migraine with aura, migraine without aura, and complicated migraine.

Migraine with aura (formerly classic migraine, classical migraine, ophthalmic migraine, and others) is the "typical" migraine. This headache has three distinct phases: the aura, the headache, and the sequelae following the headache. The aura is a premonitory stage lasting 5 to 60 minutes in which patients describe various symptoms that precede the headache. A common aura is scintillating scotoma, which is a triphasic event manifested by a sparkling or twinkling leading edge (the scintillation), followed by visual loss (the scotoma) and then restoration of vision. Other auras include other visual distortions, paresthesias, sensory and motor dysfunctions, and affective symptoms (e.g., depression, food cravings). With sensory and motor dysfunctions, the symptoms and physical manifestations are noted contralateral to the resulting headache. The aura typically resolves before the onset of headache pain, which is generally deep, throbbing, and unilateral. The headache is often associated with anorexia, irritability, photophobia, phonophobia, nausea, and occasionally vomiting. The latter may lead to resolution of the headache, and some patients may try vomiting in an attempt to end the migraine. Without intervention, migraine headaches with aura will generally resolve within 4 to 6 hours. The final stage of the migraine headache with aura includes lassitude and fatigue following the headache.

Migraine without aura (formerly common migraine, hemicrania simplex) is the most common class of migraine headache, accounting for 75 to 80 per cent of all migrainous attacks. In this type of headache, the pain is not preceded by an aura. The headache often begins on awakening and gradually intensifies. The pain can last from 4 to 72 hours. The protracted nature of migraine without aura can be more debilitating than migraine with aura. Migraine without aura can be unilateral or bilateral. Associated symptoms and sequelae following the headache are similar to those found in patients whose migraine is preceded by aura.

Complicated migraine is the last major category of migraine headache. Of the three major types of migraine, it is the least common and most worrisome to patients and physicians. Complicated migraines are associated with intense, atypical, and often prolonged neurologic deficits. The migraine begins with an aura that persists during the headache or after it resolves. Complicated migraines can sometimes lead to permanent neurologic deficits. Complicated migraine includes hemiplegic, basilar, and ophthalmoplegic migraines.

Hemiplegic migraine follows the course of a migraine with aura, except that neurologic deficits during the aura are severe and may persist during the headache and after its resolution. Persisting hemiparesis or hemiplegia can mimic a stroke. These headaches may follow a strikingly similar pattern among family members (*familial hemiplegic migraine*).

Basilar migraine (formerly basilar artery migraine, vertebrobasilar migraine, syncopal migraine) is a migraine with aura whose neurologic symptoms clearly originate from the brain stem or both occipital lobes. The neurologic symptoms include temporal and nasal visual field changes, diplopia, dysarthria, vertigo, tinnitus, ataxia, decreased hearing, bilateral paresthesias, bilateral paresis, and a decreased level of consciousness. This form of migraine is seen mostly in young adults. Basilar migraine is important because it can resemble symptoms of a carotid aneurysm.

Ophthalmoplegic migraine is a rare form of headache that begins as focal periorbital head pain associated with nausea, vomiting, and photophobia. After 1 to 4 days, the headache usually subsides, and ipsilateral extraocular muscle paralysis develops. Diplopia, ptosis, ocular muscle weakness, and unilateral pupillary changes can occur. These eye changes may be protracted but are rarely permanent.

Many other types of migraine headaches exist. *Status migrainosus* is a migrainous attack that lasts more than 72 hours despite adequate medical treatment. *Migraine aura without headache* (formerly acephalic migraine, migraine equivalents) is a migraine variant in which the aura of a migraine headache is experienced, but headache does not ensue. Migraine equivalents are characterized by recurrent attacks of abdominal pain, nausea, vomiting, vertigo, and other symptoms. A patient may have headache with or without aura interspersed with migraine aura without headache. Some investigators believe that carsickness in children may represent a migraine aura without headache and thus be a harbinger of more typical migraines later in life.

Benign exertional headache is a severe, bilateral, throbbing headache caused by physical exercise. This headache, which can last 5 minutes to 24 hours, has many variations, depending on the inciting cause. For example, benign exertional headaches caused by the strain of weightlifting have been labeled "weightlifter's headache." Benign exertional headaches can also develop migrainous features.

Headache associated with sexual activity (formerly be-

Table 3. Common Precipitants of Migraines

- Infection (especially with a fever)
- Vasoactive substances
  - Nitrites, e.g., reddened hot dogs, sausages, and luncheon meats
  - Phenylethylamines: e.g., tyramine found in aged or ripened cheeses, red and blush wines, champagne, sour cream, yogurt, and certain nuts
  - Monosodium glutamate: a common food preservative-enhancer, used especially in Asian cooking and prepared foods
  - Drugs: medicinal nitrites or nitrates (e.g., nitroglycerin, nitrate paste), amyl or butyl nitrite, histamine, alcohol, and estrogens
- Withdrawal from caffeine, chocolate, ergot compounds, or analgesics
- Allergens, food sensitivities, and foreign protein reactions: e.g., dairy products, citrus fruits, and shellfish
- Hypoglycemia, to include headache from erratic eating patterns or "skipping" a meal (probably secondary to norepinephrine release)
- Menses
- Nasal sinus disease
- Bright lights, loud or noxious noises
- Environmental factors: e.g., changes in weather, cigarette smoke, strong odors (perfumes, incense)
- Lifestyle changes, such as sleep, exercise, and sexual activity patterns

nign sex headache, coital cephalalgia) is a headache precipitated by masturbation or coitus, usually beginning as a dull bilateral headache that progresses and suddenly intensifies at orgasm. These headaches are often more frequent during particularly intense sexual activity. Headache associated with sexual activity may be prevented by easing or temporarily ceasing sexual activity. This headache can mimic a headache associated with impending rupture of a vascular malformation.

Tension-Type Headaches

Tension-type headache (formerly tension, muscle contraction, stress, ordinary, and psychogenic headache) is the most common primary headache disorder. The estimated lifetime prevalence for tension-type headaches is 69 per cent for males and 88 per cent for females, with a 63 and 68 per cent prevalence, respectively, within the previous year. Traditionally, tension-type headaches were attributed to maladaptive responses to life stressors. Today, some investigators view tension-type headaches as perhaps on the same continuum as migraine headaches.

Of the primary headache disorders, tension-type headaches are the most variable in onset, character, location, severity, and duration. If a typical tension-type headache were to exist, it might consist of bilateral, steady, nonpulsatile, "bandlike" or nuchal "tightness" in the frontal, temporal, parietal, and/or occipital regions. These headaches are often associated with photophobia and phonophobia, but nausea and vomiting are rare. No true prodrome or aura exists; however, patients often perceive muscle tightness in the "hat-band" distribution of the head or in the occipital and nuchal regions of the neck before the onset of the headache pain. Whether this perceived muscle tightness is actually true muscle contraction is controversial. This is the reason that the previous term "muscle contraction headache" was discarded. Tension-type headaches often increase during periods of emotional conflict, hence the older term "stress headache." Tension-type headaches may be acute and self-limited or chronic and persistent. A patient's headache is termed an "episodic tension-type headache" if it occurs less than 15 times per month and a "chronic tension-type headache" if it occurs more than 15 times per month. Chronic tension-type headaches can last for days, weeks, months, or years and are often associated with depression. These headaches that occur daily are generally referred to as "chronic daily headaches." The distinction between episodic and chronic tension-type headaches influences treatment. Analgesics are recommended for episodic tension-type headaches, and antidepressants are recommended for chronic tension-type headaches.

Physical examination of patients with tension-type headaches is generally unrevealing. Subjective tenderness in the temporalis and trapezius muscles and palpable myofascial "trigger points" in the trapezius muscle may be noted.

Cluster Headaches

Cluster headache (formerly ciliary neuralgia, migrainous neuralgia, Horton's headache, histaminic cephalalgia, petrosal neuralgia, and many others) is an excruciating unilateral, periorbital, and/or temporal lancinating pain lasting 15 minutes to 3 hours. Cluster headache is given its name because this headache "clusters" in both time and location. Thus, a patient with cluster headaches may have a series of sudden-onset headaches every other day to eight times a day, each in exactly the same location. These "cluster periods" can last up to 6 to 8 weeks. Cluster periods are more frequent in the spring and fall seasons and may vary in duration and frequency. Cluster headaches often become more protracted and severe with age. Some 10 to 15 per cent of patients with cluster headaches will develop daily headaches with cluster-type pain. Cluster headaches are rare, occurring in an estimated 0.05 to 1 per cent of headache patients. Unlike migraine headaches, cluster headaches are five to six times more common in males, especially in the third and fourth decades of life. There is no hereditary component. Cluster headaches are often caused by rapid eye movement (REM) sleep, so the patient often awakens with severe pain. This is different from migraine headaches, which are generally relieved by sleep. Cluster headaches may be accompanied by *unilateral* conjunctival injection, lacrimation, nasal congestion or rhinorrhea, forehead or facial sweating, miosis, ptosis, and blepharitis. Many of these findings can be noted on clinical examination during the cluster headache. These headaches are refractory to most interventions, including large doses of narcotics. Even with appropriate treatment, the pain of cluster headaches is so intense and unrelenting that depression and suicide are common.

Secondary Headache Disorders

A complete description of all secondary headache disorders is not included here, but detailed articles may be found elsewhere.* Some common secondary headaches are discussed in the following sections.

Rebound Headache

Rebound headache (formerly toxic headache) follows the withdrawal of an acutely or chronically used substance. The latter may be an important factor in patients with chronic headaches because the chronic use of analgesics may perpetuate the headaches. Rebound headaches can occur after the use of caffeine, vasoconstrictors (e.g., ergot medications), or any analgesic from over-the-counter acetaminophen to prescribed narcotics. Cephalalgia phobia, the fear of getting a headache, may also play a role in analgesic abuse and rebound headache because a patient may self-medicate to prevent the onset of headache pain. Any patient with chronic daily headache should be considered a candidate for rebound headaches. Treatment includes the slow withdrawal of the offending agent and may require hospitalization.

Post-traumatic Headache

Post-traumatic headache commonly follows head trauma—from minor concussions to more severe insults to the skull or brain. Head trauma can lead to headache pain in two ways: (1) aggravation and perpetuation of a pre-existing headache disorder or (2) creation of a new type of headache in a patient with or without prior headaches. A common presentation of the latter is headache associated with nuchal limitations, occipital and cervical tenderness, and trapezius muscle tenderness.

In patients with moderate to severe post-traumatic headache, complete resolution of symptoms occurs within 12 to 36 months in about 75 per cent of patients. In the remaining 25 per cent, a slower resolution may occur, or a chronic headache disorder may develop.

Patients with post-traumatic headache are among the small subset of headache patients that routinely warrant

---

*Dalessio, D.J., and Silberstein, S.D. (eds.): Wolff's Headache and Other Head Pain, 6th ed. New York, Oxford University Press, 1993, pp. 59–95.

further diagnostic work-up, including computed tomography (CT) or magnetic resonance imaging (MRI).

Headache Resulting From Infection

Headaches resulting from infection may be of cephalic or noncephalic origin. Headaches caused by *intracranial* infection arise with meningitis, encephalitis, brain abscess, and subdural empyema and are detailed in textbooks of infectious disease. Usually, the presence of other clinical symptoms and signs (e.g., nuchal rigidity, fever, and increased leukocyte count) is sufficient to suggest a more detailed work-up, starting with lumbar puncture. A higher index of suspicion is warranted in the very young and the very old because the symptoms and signs of infection are often attenuated or absent. Headaches caused by *extracranial* infection accompany viral, bacterial, or other infections. Headaches associated with viral infections (e.g., upper respiratory infections) can be severe and may represent a form of nonrecurrent migraine headache. Lyme disease should be considered in patients with new-onset constant headache if other data are consistent with this diagnosis.

Headache Resulting From Blood Vessel Inflammation

Giant cell arteritis (formerly temporal arteritis, Horton's disease) is an inflammatory disorder of the elderly. It is rare in individuals younger than 50 years of age. The headache of giant cell arteritis generally involves one or both temporal regions, and it may accompany a swollen, tender scalp artery, usually the superficial temporal artery. Jaw claudication is pathognomonic but uncommon. Diagnosis is supported when the erythrocyte sedimentation rate (ESR) exceeds 50 mm per hour (Westergren method), and the headache relents within 48 hours after starting steroid therapy. Diagnosis can be confirmed with biopsy of the affected vessel, but careful histologic examination is required because the abnormality is segmental and nonuniform. Systemic findings include fever, weight loss, and other symptoms. Polymyalgia rheumatica (PMR) is often associated.

Headache From Other Causes

Perhaps the most worrisome headache is the premonitory *"sentinel bleed" headache associated with impending rupture of a vascular malformation*. The vascular malformation can be either an arteriovenous malformation or a saccular aneurysm. Patients often describe this headache as the "worst headache ever." Sentinel bleed headaches can be associated with nausea, vomiting, nuchal rigidity, and loss of consciousness. Computed tomography, MRI, or angiography may facilitate the diagnosis of an impending rupture of a vascular malformation. Blood in the cerebrospinal fluid suggests a subarachnoid hemorrhage. Normal scans and normal lumbar puncture results within 48 hours of the onset of headache usually rule out impending rupture of a vascular malformation.

Headache resulting from arterial hypertension can be caused by an external pressor agent, pheochromocytoma, malignant hypertension, pre-eclampsia, and eclampsia. The nature and characteristics of these headaches are unremarkable, except for their association with increased blood pressure and resolution when blood pressure normalizes.

Headache resulting from intracranial neoplasm can be caused by benign or malignant tumors because both are space-occupying, can compress brain matter, and may increase intracranial pressure.

Headache resulting from benign intracranial hypertension (also known as idiopathic intracranial hypertension [IIH]; formerly pseudotumor cerebri, otitic hydrocephalus) is characterized by chronic elevation of cerebrospinal fluid pressure without evidence of hydrocephalus or deformation of the ventricular system. The annual incidence of this disorder is 1 per 100,000 persons; however, its incidence is 19.3 per 100,000 persons in obese women between the ages of 20 and 44 years. Several medical disorders (e.g., hypothyroidism) and several medications (e.g., oral contraceptives) have been implicated but not verified as causes of this disorder. The only verifiable risk factor is obesity, which is found in 90 per cent of patients with benign intracranial hypertension. The symptoms of this disorder reflect the increase in intracranial pressure. Patients complain of headache, transient visual disturbances, and diplopia. Permanent visual loss can occur in 5 to 15 per cent of patients. Many of these symptoms are relieved with a reduction in cerebrospinal fluid pressure, either by frequent (daily or twice weekly) lumbar puncture to remove fluid or by lumboperitoneal shunting.

Physical Examination in Headache Disorders

In general, the examination of patients with primary and secondary headache disorders reveals few abnormalities. Blood pressure should be assessed to eliminate the rare headache caused by malignant hypertension. The pericranial muscles of the frontal, temporal, parietal, occipital, and nuchal regions should be palpated for muscle spasm. Although muscle tightness may be present with tension-type headaches, true nuchal rigidity (positive Brudzinski's or Kernig's sign) is present only in headaches caused by meningeal inflammation. Funduscopy may reveal papilledema, a finding consistent with increased intracranial pressure and the presence of a secondary headache disorder requiring urgent treatment. A brief and superficial mental status examination may reveal the patient to be normal, anxious, or depressed.

Adjunctive Diagnostic Tests for Headache Disorders

With a detailed headache history and appropriate physical examination, adjunctive diagnostic tests are seldom required. These tests should be ordered only when the history or physical examination reveals any of the markers for potential serious disease listed in Table 4. Common adjunctive tests include lumbar puncture and CT or MRI of the brain. Less common are laboratory (ESR, rapid plasma reagin [RPR] test, and nasal drainage culture), radio-

Table 4. Markers for Potential Serious Disease Requiring Further Evaluation

Acute onset of headaches after age 25 years without an appreciable prior history of headaches
Frequent headaches with localization to the same side (except cluster headaches)
Headaches associated with neurologic deficits
Seizure activity
Paralysis of extraocular muscles
Persistent visual field defects
Speech disorders
Persistent paresthesias or motor dysfunction
Meningismus
Changes in mental status
Other persistent neurologic deficits
Headaches caused by coughing, sneezing, or bending over
Headaches refractory to standard, usual treatment regimens

graphic (cranial, sinus, or cervical spine radiographs), and electroencephalographic tests.

Differential Diagnosis of Headache Disorders

The first goal in the assessment of headache is to eliminate the possibility of serious structural or systemic disorders whose principal manifestation is headache. If the patient's symptoms fit the classic description of a primary headache disorder, lack alarming physical findings, and lack any markers for potentially serious disease, the physician can safely make a presumptive diagnosis of that primary headache disorder. If the patient's headache has atypical features, worrisome physical findings, or any marker for potentially serious disease, additional diagnostic testing is warranted to exclude the possibility of a secondary headache disorder.

As noted earlier, most patients with headaches have more than one type of headache. Thus, more than one diagnosis may be necessary. For example, patients may present with frequent tension-type headaches and less frequent migraine headaches. Also common are patients whose headaches have features of more than one type of headache disorder. For example, a patient may have migraine headaches with cluster features or sinus headaches that lead to migraine. In such cases, the physician should diagnose and treat the more frequent or severe headache.

FACIAL PAIN SYNDROMES

Facial pain is subdivided into three main categories: (1) facial pain associated with disorders of cranial and facial structures; (2) cranial neuralgias, nerve trunk pain, and deafferentation pain; and (3) facial pain not associated with either of the preceding categories.

Facial pain or headache associated with a disorder of the cranium, neck, eyes, ears, nose, sinuses, teeth, mouth, or other facial or cranial structures is a vast category. Headache may or may not accompany these disorders. Common examples of facial pain and/or headaches associated with disorders of these structures are listed in Table 5. Among these examples are two disorders that commonly cause headache and facial pain.

Sinus headache (also known as facial or headache pain associated with a disorder of the nose and sinuses) is a dull, pressurelike pain affecting patients with either sinus congestion or infection. The pain is generally felt in the area overlying the affected frontal, maxillary, and sphenoethmoidal regions. The pain may also radiate. Frontal sinus involvement may radiate pain to the vertex or retro-orbitally. Maxillary sinus involvement may radiate pain to the upper teeth or forehead. Sphenoethmoidal sinus involvement may radiate pain to the retro-orbital or temporal area. Transillumination may demonstrate opacification of the frontal or maxillary sinuses. Because acute sinusitis is a clinical diagnosis, sinus x-ray films and CT are best reserved for evaluation of chronic sinusitis. Facial pain and headache from sinus involvement resolve completely after appropriate treatment.

Table 5. Common Examples of Disorders of Head and Facial Structures Resulting in Facial Pain or Headache

Structure	Disorder
Cranial bone	Fractures of cranium
	Primary and metastatic lesions
	Osteomyelitis
	Paget's disease
Neck	Fractures of cervical spine
	Rheumatoid arthritis or osteoarthritis
	Myofascial disorders of the trapezius muscle
Eyes	Acute glaucoma
	Uncorrected refractive errors
	Heterophoria, heterotropia ("squint")
Ears	Otitis externa
	Otitis media
Nose and sinuses	Nasal congestion from allergic or viral causes
	Acute sinusitis (mucopurulent)
Teeth, jaw, and related structures	Periodontal disease
	Temporomandibular joint disease

Facial or headache pain resulting from temporomandibular joint disease is common, but it is only rarely related to definable organic disease. Patients with this disorder experience mild to moderate jaw pain triggered by movement of the jaw and clenching of the teeth. Temporomandibular joint disease is three times more common in women than in men and is usually found in persons older than 40 years of age. Examination of the jaw demonstrates a decreased range of motion, and crepitus can be heard during movement. Disease can be confirmed by radiographic and isotope scintigraphic studies.

Cranial neuralgias, nerve trunk pain, and deafferentation pain is also a vast category whose predominant symptom is facial pain. Examples of cranial neuralgias include trigeminal, glossopharyngeal, and occipital neuralgia. *Trigeminal neuralgia* (formerly tic douloureux) presents with a rapid onset of lancinating pain that lasts for seconds to minutes. The pain is localized in the distribution of the branches of the trigeminal nerve, especially the second and third divisions. Pain may be spontaneous or triggered by seemingly trivial stimuli such as talking, brushing the teeth, or light touch. Spasm ("tic") of the facial muscle may occur. Trigeminal neuralgia is paroxysmal, with the patient being free of pain between episodes. *Anesthesia dolorosa* involves painful anesthesia or dysesthesia in the distribution of the trigeminal nerve following surgical trauma of the trigeminal ganglion. This disorder often follows surgical rhizotomy or thermocoagulation for the treatment of trigeminal neuralgia.

Glossopharyngeal neuralgia presents with severe, stabbing, episodic pain in the distribution of the auricular and pharyngeal branches of the vagus nerve and the glossopharyngeal nerve. Pain may be experienced in the ear, at the base of the tongue, in the tonsillar fossa, or beneath the angle of the jaw. The characteristics and paroxysmal nature of the pain are similar to trigeminal neuralgia.

Occipital neuralgia involves paroxysmal lancinating pain with hypesthesia or dysesthesia in the distribution of the greater or lesser occipital nerve. *Optic neuritis* (also known as retrobulbar neuritis) involves impairment of central or paracentral visual acuity with unilateral retro-orbital pain most likely related to demyelination of the optic nerve. Some 13 to 85 per cent of patients with optic neuritis will later acquire multiple sclerosis. *Diabetic neuritis* manifests as periorbital and facial pain associated with oculomotor nerve palsy of diabetic origin. The pupil is usually spared.

Although *acute herpes zoster* can involve any of the cranial nerves, it affects the trigeminal nerve in 10 to 15 per cent of patients. Facial pain occurs first and is followed by vesicular eruptions in the distribution of the nerve. Pain begins to subside after eruption of the rash, usually within a few days to weeks. The pain can, however, take up to 6 months to completely resolve. *Chronic postherpetic neural-*

gia occurs when the pain from herpes zoster lasts beyond 6 months. This protracted neuralgia increases in frequency as the age of the patient increases; more than half of the patients are older than 60 years of age.

Thalamic pain manifests as unilateral facial pain or dysesthesia attributed to a lesion of the quintothalamic pathway or thalamus. Symptoms may also involve the trunk and limbs of the affected side. A lesion in the region of the thalamus may be observed on CT or MRI.

Atypical facial pain (formerly atypical odontalgia) is a vague diagnosis that encompasses other facial pain disorders with characteristics of cranial neuralgias yet does not fulfill specific criteria for the diagnosis. Atypical facial pain occurs most commonly in women between the ages of 30 and 50 years. The pain is usually unilateral and constant and does not seem to involve the triggers found with other cranial neuralgias. Some of these patients may have structural disorders (e.g., tumors, abscesses) that cause the pain.

Like the diagnosis of headache disorders, the diagnosis of facial pain disorders requires a thorough history. Physical examination should include careful examination of the head and neck and a methodical neurologic examination. The examining physician should attempt to "map out" the location of the pain, hypesthesia, or dysesthesia. When the pain is focused on a specific anatomic location such as the eye or mouth, referral of the patient to the appropriate specialist to exclude other pathologic conditions causing facial pain is medically prudent. Because facial pain is more likely to be caused by structural and therefore potentially life-threatening disorders, a CT scan or MRI study is usually warranted.

SYNCOPE

By Wishwa N. Kapoor, M.D., MPH
Pittsburgh, Pennsylvania

Syncope is defined as a sudden transient loss of consciousness associated with loss of postural tone with spontaneous recovery that does not require electrical or chemical cardioversion. The episode may be abrupt without prodromal symptoms or it may be preceded by sweating, pallor, warmth, nausea, and vomiting. Patients often have symptoms after the episode that include recurrence of syncope or presyncope on standing immediately after the episode as well as fatigue, diaphoresis, and headaches.

CAUSES OF SYNCOPE

Table 1 lists most of the causes of syncope. They can be categorized broadly as neurally mediated syncope syndromes, orthostatic hypotension, neurologic diseases, and cardiac syncope. Prior studies of syncope, primarily from referral centers, show wide variation in the proportion of patients with various causes. This variation is largely due to patient selection (differences ranging from emergency department to intensive care unit [ICU] patients) and use of diagnostic criteria for assigning causes of syncope. The most common causes are vasovagal syncope (1 to 29 per cent), situational syncope (1 to 8 per cent), orthostatic hypotension (4 to 12 per cent), and drug-induced syncope (2 to 9 per cent). Organic heart disease resulting in syncope is found in 3 to 11 per cent of patients and arrhythmias are found in 5 to 30 per cent of individuals. Other causes are present in less than 5 per cent of patients. In many patients (up to 45 per cent), a cause could not be determined. Recent studies employing upright tilt testing, electrophysiologic studies, and psychiatric evaluations show that three different areas need to be considered in patients with syncope of unknown origin.

Table 1. Causes of Syncope

Neurally mediated syndromes	*Cardiac disease*
Vasovagal	*Obstruction to flow*
Situational	Obstruction to left ventricular outflow
Micturition	Aortic stenosis, idiopathic hypertrophic subaortic stenosis
Cough	Mitral stenosis, myxoma
Swallow	Obstruction to right ventricular outflow
Defecation	Pulmonic stenosis
Carotid sinus syncope	Pulmonary embolism, pulmonary hypertension
Neuralgias	Myxoma
High altitude	*Other heart disease*
Psychiatric disorders	Pump failure
Others (exercise, selected drugs)	Myocardial infarction, coronary artery disease, coronary spasm
Orthostatic hypotension	Tamponade, dissection
Neurologic diseases	Arrhythmias
Migraines	
Transient ischemic attacks (TIAs)	
Seizures	

Vasovagal Syncope

Vasovagal syncope is often diagnosed clinically. In many patients, however, precipitating factors and associated autonomic symptoms are not present. In such patients, upright tilt testing may provoke vasovagal syncope in the laboratory in approximately 50 to 70 per cent of patients. Thus, vasovagal syncope appears to be the most common cause of syncope in patients in whom cause is not determined by other means.

Psychiatric Disorders

Psychiatric disorders, including generalized anxiety disorder, panic disorder, major depression, and somatization disorder, can cause syncope. It is estimated that as many as 15 to 20 per cent of patients presenting with syncope may have psychiatric disorders that are potential causes of syncope. These patients are generally young, do not have underlying heart disease, and often have multiple episodes of syncope prior to presentation.

Miscellaneous Disorders

In a small group of patients (<5 per cent), the cause becomes apparent following the evaluation of the recurrence of syncope. Such entities include supraventricular tachycardias, seizures and, occasionally, bradycardias.

DIAGNOSTIC EVALUATION

Is This Syncope?

Syncope must be separated clinically from other disorders causing loss or alteration of consciousness, including dizziness, vertigo, coma, narcolepsy, and seizures. A particularly difficult distinction is that between seizures and syncope. Seizures are often associated with a blue face (patients are not pale), aching muscles, frothing at the mouth, tongue biting, disorientation, and sleepiness after the event. The duration of loss of consciousness is often more than 5 minutes. In contrast, independent symptoms associated with syncope are sweatiness or nausea before the event and no disorientation after the event. Disorientation after the episode appears to be the best distinguishing symptom between seizure and syncope.

History and Physical Examination

The work-up of syncope begins with a careful history and physical examination, which establishes most of the diagnoses. The characteristics of the events leading to the episode and symptoms associated with loss of consciousness help determine the potential causes of syncope. Table 2 provides historical findings that are particularly useful.

The history and physical examination may suggest specific entities that require further diagnostic testing. For example, syncope with arm exercise and differences in blood pressure between the two arms (>10 to 20 mm Hg) suggest subclavian steal syndrome. Syncope associated with effort and cardiovascular findings consistent with aortic stenosis suggest aortic valvular disease as the cause of syncope.

Useful findings on physical examination include the presence of orthostatic hypotension, cardiovascular abnormalities, and neurologic signs. Orthostatic hypotension is generally defined as a systolic blood pressure decline of 20 mm Hg or greater on standing. In determining the cause of syncope, the presence of symptoms on standing in association with an orthostatic blood pressure decline is required. To accurately document orthostatic hypotension, baseline blood pressure measurements should be obtained after the patient remains supine for 5 to 10 minutes. Blood pressures must be measured immediately on standing and several times during a 2-minute period. Blood pressure measurements on sitting are inaccurate and generally do not reflect orthostatic hypotension found on standing. Since orthostatic hypotension may be worse at certain times during the day (e.g., in the morning or in the middle of the night), repeated blood pressure measurements may be needed to diagnose orthostatic hypotension. This condition may also be a problem 45 minutes to an hour after meals. Thus, blood pressure measurements after meals should be obtained in patients with symptoms after eating.

Cardiovascular examination is important in determining the cause of syncope. Causes include aortic dissection and subclavian steal syndrome, in which differences in pulse intensity and blood pressure (generally >20 mm Hg) in the two arms are important. Other cardiovascular findings include signs of aortic stenosis, idiopathic hypertrophic subaortic stenosis, pulmonary hypertension, myxomas, and pulmonary embolism.

In patients in whom a specific cause is not determined by history and physical examination, further assessment should focus on the following areas: (1) arrhythmias, (2) tilt testing, and (3) psychiatric assessment.

Table 2. Clinical Features Suggestive of Specific Causes

Symptom or Finding	Diagnostic Consideration
After sudden unexpected pain, unpleasant sight, sound, or smell	Vasovagal syncope
During or immediately after micturition, cough, swallow, or defecation	Situational syncope
With neuralgia (glossopharyngeal or trigeminal)	Bradycardia or vasodepressor reaction
On standing	Orthostatic hypotension
Prolonged standing at attention	Vasovagal
Well-trained athlete after exertion	Neurally mediated
Changing position (from sitting to lying, bending, turning over in bed)	Atrial myxoma, thrombus
Syncope with exertion	Aortic stenosis, pulmonary hypertension, pulmonary embolus, mitral stenosis, idiopathic hypertrophic subaortic stenosis, coronary artery disease, neurally mediated
With head rotation, pressure on carotid sinus (as in tumors, shaving, tight collars)	Carotid sinus syncope
Associated with vertigo, dysarthria, diplopia, and other motor and sensory symptoms of brain stem ischemia	Transient ischemic attack, subclavian steal syndrome, basilar artery migraine
With arm exercise	Subclavian steal syndrome
Confusion after episode	Seizure

Arrhythmias

Arrhythmias are primarily of concern in patients who have underlying organic heart disease or an abnormal electrocardiogram (ECG) with symptoms suggestive of arrhythmic syncope. Clinically, cardiac syncope is associated with a sudden brief loss of consciousness without a prodrome, with rapid and full recovery. Electrocardiographic findings that are particularly important include bundle branch block, first-degree atrioventricular (AV) block, ventricular arrhythmias, Wolff-Parkinson-White syndrome, and significant bradycardia. The following tests are available for detection of arrhythmias:

ELECTROCARDIOGRAM–RHYTHM STRIP. Electrocardiography leads to a diagnosis rarely (2 to 11 per cent of patients with syncope). It is useful, however, since diagnoses can be established rapidly and therapy can be instituted based on the findings. Additionally, a normal ECG identifies a low-risk subgroup of patients who have a low likelihood of arrhythmias or sudden death.

PROLONGED ELECTROCARDIOGRAPHIC MONITORING. The results of monitoring are most helpful if symptoms are concurrent with arrhythmias. Symptom correlation occurs in about 4 per cent of patients monitored. In 15 per cent of patients undergoing monitoring, symptoms occur but no arrhythmias are found, thereby excluding arrhythmias as a cause of syncope. In most patients (approximately 80 per cent), there are no symptoms. In these patients, arrhythmias are not excluded as a cause of syncope because significant rhythm disturbances with symptoms can be episodic and may not be captured by 24 hours of Holter monitoring. In patients with underlying heart disease or an abnormal ECG, further testing is often required for detection of arrhythmias.

Prolonged monitoring for weeks to months is possible through the use of patient-activated, intermittent event recorders (loop monitors). These monitors capture arrhythmias during an episode if the patient activates it after regaining consciousness. They are helpful in patients who have frequent recurrences of syncope, since the likelihood of capturing an episode during the period of monitoring is increased.

ELECTROPHYSIOLOGIC STUDIES. In patients with structural heart disease or an abnormal ECG, electrophysiologic studies should be considered if arrhythmias are suggested clinically but are not diagnosed by electrocardiography, Holter monitoring, or event recorders. These tests are generally not useful in patients without heart disease or an abnormal ECG because the yield is low. In patients undergoing electrophysiologic studies, approximately 60 per cent of these studies are abnormal. The abnormalities consist of inducible ventricular tachycardia in approximately 45 per cent of patients, supraventricular tachycardia in 22 per cent of patients, conduction system disorders (abnormal sinus node, atrioventricular node, or His-Purkinje function) in 28 per cent of patients, and other abnormalities (e.g., hypervagotomia and carotid sinus hypersensitivity) in 5 per cent of patients. The interpretation of electrophysiologic studies can often be difficult; experienced cardiologists and laboratories may be required for accurate diagnosis and treatment of the arrhythmias.

Upright Tilt Testing

Vasovagal syncope (also termed "neurally mediated" or "neurocardiogenic syncope") can be provoked by standing upright on a tilt table with or without concurrent administration of an adrenergic agent such as isoproterenol. Upright tilt testing leads to pooling of blood in the lower extremities with decreased venous return. In individuals susceptible to vasovagal syncope, this decrease in venous return leads to more forceful ventricular contractions, which may activate cardiac mechanoreceptors triggering neural discharges to the vasomotor center in the central nervous system (CNS), leading to hypotension and bradycardia. Catecholamine release or administration of catecholamines may increase the force of ventricular contraction, activating these nerve endings responsible for triggering this reflex.

Two major types of tilt testing protocols include (1) passive testing (without the use of chemical agents) and (2) tilt testing in conjunction with intravenous isoproterenol. During this test, blood pressure and heart rates are measured. After baseline measurements, patients are brought to an upright posture. If isoproterenol is used, patients are brought to a supine position after a brief period of passive tilt testing. The isoproterenol infusion is begun slowly and gradually increased as long as the patient does not reach an endpoint of positive response such as syncope or presyncope in association with hypotension and/or bradycardia.

Passive tilt studies show that positive responses are found in approximately 50 per cent of patients tested. With isoproterenol, approximately 66 per cent of patients have positive responses. The specificity of the test is approximately 90 per cent with passive upright tilt testing and 75 per cent with testing using isoproterenol. Reproduction of symptoms that occur during spontaneous episodes can be considered a positive response. When the syncopal event is different from the spontaneous episode, it should be considered a false-positive response.

Psychiatric Assessment

Young patients with syncope of unknown cause may have psychiatric disorders, including generalized anxiety, panic attack, depression, and somatization disorder. Additionally, alcohol and substance abuse can rarely cause syncope. These disorders should be assessed clinically and with the use of psychiatric screening instruments.

Low-Yield Tests

Many tests used in the evaluation of syncope often do not establish a cause of syncope. These studies include radionuclide brain scans, skull radiographs, lumbar puncture, routine blood tests, and glucose tolerance tests. However, electroencephalography (EEG) and computed tomography (CT) scans may be useful in patients whose history and physical examination suggest seizures or other neurologic problems.

OVERALL APPROACH TO DIAGNOSTIC EVALUATION

A detailed clinical assessment (by history and physical examination) leads to a determination of most causes of syncope. In a smaller proportion of patients, clinical assessment may suggest specific entities (e.g., aortic stenosis or neurologic signs and symptoms suggestive of a seizure disorder). These findings then guide further testing to aid diagnosis. An ECG is appropriate in most patients with syncope, except when the cause, as determined by the history and physical examination, is clearly not cardiac.

When a cause of syncope is not established by the history, physical examination, and an ECG, the approach detailed in the following sections can be used.

Patients With Heart Disease

The initial step in evaluating patients with structural heart disease or an abnormal ECG is prolonged electrocardiographic monitoring. Event recorders are recommended in patients with recurrent syncope and normal or unclear findings on electrocardiographic monitoring (e.g., asymptomatic brief nonsustained ventricular tachycardia). If ambulatory and event recorders are nondiagnostic, electrophysiologic studies are recommended. Finally, to diagnose vasovagal syncope, upright tilt testing is recommended in patients with normal results on electrophysiologic testing who report recurrent or disabling symptoms.

Patients Without Heart Disease

Since the likelihood of arrhythmias is low in young patients without heart disease who have a normal ECG, prolonged electrocardiographic monitoring or electrophysiologic studies are generally normal and are not required. Vasovagal syncope and psychiatric disorders should be pursued as the initial step in the evaluation. A similar diagnostic approach can be taken with older patients without heart disease who have normal ECGs, but further studies are needed to define the role of prolonged electrocardiographic monitoring in these patients. In this group, multiple pathologic and physiologic abnormalities should be considered and treated.

Recurrent Syncope

The initial approach to diagnostic testing should be based on the presence or absence of heart disease (as noted previously). If a cause of syncope is not established in this group of patients, event recorders may be useful for the evaluation of brief episodic arrhythmias.

FATIGUE

By Kurt Kroenke, M.D.
Bethesda, Maryland

Fatigue is one of the most common nonpainful physical complaints in adult outpatients, accounting for an estimated 10 million clinic visits in the United States each year; yet what the health care provider sees is only the tip of the iceberg. Fatigue is often a self-limited symptom accompanying acute viral illnesses, recuperation from medical diseases or surgery, overwork, stress, sleep deprivation, jet lag, and other temporary conditions. Since such precipitants are well recognized by the general public, most individuals who experience temporary or episodic tiredness never present for medical care. Persistent fatigue is what usually brings a patient to medical attention, especially when it is accompanied by occupational or social impairment or by patient concerns that the fatigue may signify a serious underlying illness.

MEDICAL CAUSES OF FATIGUE

Fatigue as an isolated symptom is seldom an occult manifestation of a serious organic illness. Use of medication by the patient is one of the most important considerations, particularly when there is a temporal correlation between the initiation of a new medication and the onset of fatigue. Although certain classes of medications (central-acting antihypertensive agents, psychotropic drugs, antihistamines, anticholinergic medications) are associated with a higher incidence of fatigue, a clinical rule of thumb is to "believe the patient," that is, if a new symptom occurs after the patient begins a new medication, consider it a potential suspect. In addition, the clinician should ask about exposure to alcohol, illicit drugs, and other environmental agents.

Organic diseases are usually evident from the history, physical examination, or simple laboratory testing. Thyroid dysfunction, especially hypothyroidism, is frequently considered, although it accounts for relatively few cases of unexplained fatigue. Diabetes mellitus is a second endocrine cause to consider, although changes in appetite or weight, increased thirst, urinary frequency, visual blurring, or other symptoms typically accompany hyperglycemia severe enough to cause persistent fatigue. Adrenal dysfunction is uncommon and need not be pursued unless the patient manifests other signs and symptoms of excessive or deficient cortisol production.

Anemia severe enough to produce fatigue—typically a hemoglobin value less than 8 to 10 g/dL—can be excluded by a simple hemoglobin determination. Cardiopulmonary causes of fatigue, such as congestive heart failure or chronic pulmonary disease, should be evident from clinical signs or symptoms. Exhaustive searches for a "hidden cancer" can generally be avoided unless something else in the review of systems prompts a concern about malignancy, such as blood in the stool or urine, a new lump, a nagging cough, involuntary weight loss, or unexplained pain.

Autoimmune diseases, such as systemic lupus erythematosus or rheumatoid arthritis, are systemic diseases in which joint or skin findings will be found in addition to specific serologic abnormalities. Patients with multiple sclerosis will manifest other neurologic signs or symptoms. Tuberculosis, human immunodeficiency virus (HIV) disease, and other chronic infections should be considered in the setting of fever, night sweats, pulmonary symptoms, weight change, adenopathy, or other systemic clues. Recent studies suggest that sleep disorders are more prevalent than once thought. Marked snoring or apneic spells noted by a partner or excessive daytime somnolence, particularly daytime naps and inadvertently falling asleep, should prompt further evaluation for sleep apnea, narcolepsy, or other sleep disorders.

PSYCHOSOCIAL CAUSES

At least two thirds of patients with unexplained fatigue have a diagnosable psychiatric disorder, most commonly depression, anxiety, or somatization. Clues to a potential psychiatric cause include the following:

1. Isolated fatigue, that is, no other abnormal clinical symptoms or signs
2. Depression or anxiety symptoms other than fatigue, such as depressed mood, anhedonia, insomnia, nervousness or irritability, and feelings of guilt or worthlessness
3. Prior episodes of depression or anxiety, particularly if severe, disabling, prolonged, or requiring treatment
4. Chronic history of multiple, unexplained symptoms, suggestive of a somatoform disorder

In fact, these mental disorders are such common causes of fatigue that they should be considered early in the evaluation and not simply reserved as diagnoses of exclusion after an exhaustive pursuit of organic causes.

CHRONIC FATIGUE SYNDROME

About one fourth of patients with persistent fatigue have neither a clear-cut physical nor a psychiatric cause of their symptoms. In the past decade, the entity of chronic fatigue syndrome (CFS) has received a lot of attention. A research definition was developed in 1988 and recently revised and simplified.* In the new proposal, the duration for *prolonged* and *chronic* fatigue is 1 and 6 months, respectively. For a patient to be diagnosed with CFS, the following severity (A) and symptom (B) criteria must be met: (1) clinically evaluated, unexplained, persistent or relapsing chronic fatigue that is not the result of ongoing exertion, is not substantially alleviated by rest, and results in substantial reduction in previous levels of occupational, educational, social, or personal activities; and (2) concurrent occurrence of four or more of the following symptoms, all of which must have persisted or recurred during 6 or more consecutive months of illness and must not have predated the fatigue:

a. Impairment of memory or concentration severe enough to cause a substantial reduction in the patient's usual activities
b. Sore throat
c. Tender cervical or axillary lymph nodes
d. Muscle pain
e. Multijoint pain without joint swelling or redness
f. Headaches of a new type, pattern, or severity
g. Unrefreshing sleep

*Fukuda, K., Straus, S.E., Hickie, I., et al.: The chronic fatigue syndrome: A comprehensive approach to its definition and study. Ann. Intern. Med., 121:953–959, 1994.

h. Malaise following exertion and lasting more than 24 hours

Even as revised, CFS remains an operational, consensus-defined illness, the "reality" of which remains controversial. Many of its symptoms overlap with primary psychiatric disturbances, fibromyalgia, and viral syndromes, as well as neurasthenia, a diagnosis that has been around for more than a century and is still widely used by clinicians around the world. Also, it is not clear that CFS usefully describes a unique subset of patients with chronic fatigue. One characteristic feature of a typical CFS patient, however, is the abrupt onset of disabling fatigue in someone who was previously in excellent medical and psychological health.

EVALUATION

Fatigue—a pervasive sense of tiredness or lack of energy not strictly related to exertion—should be distinguished from symptoms such as weakness and fatigability—a temporary, exertion-related tiredness that resolves with rest. The latter are not usually the symptoms patients describe when they complain of fatigue, but when these symptoms are present, the clinician should consider organic causes more carefully, for example, cardiopulmonary disorders, neuromuscular disease, and deconditioning. The *duration* of the fatigue can arbitrarily be divided into less than 1 month, 1 to 6 months, and greater than 6 months. In the absence of other obvious signs or symptoms, patients with fatigue for less than a month often do not require an extensive evaluation. The clinician can inquire about recent viral illnesses; new medications; sleep disturbances or deprivation; changes or stress at home, school, or the workplace; and symptoms of depression or anxiety, particularly depressed mood, loss of interest or pleasure, and/or feelings of nervousness or irritability.

As a nonspecific symptom, fatigue that persists beyond a month should prompt a thorough review of systems to identify constitutional complaints (fevers, night sweats, changes in appetite or weight) or symptoms pointing to a particular body organ or region, such as localized pain, bleeding, new lumps or masses, cough, bowel or urinary complaints, arthralgias, or skin lesions. Likewise, the physical examination must be complete, including a careful evaluation of the cardiopulmonary, abdominal, musculoskeletal, neurologic, and lymphoreticular systems.

Routine laboratory testing can be simple: a complete blood count; serum electrolytes; glucose, calcium, creatinine, alanine aminotransferase, and alkaline phosphatase determinations; erythrocyte sedimentation rate (ESR); thyroid-stimulating hormone (TSH) levels; and a urinalysis. Although thyroid-stimulating hormone elevations greater than 15 mU/L may be diagnostic of hypothyroidism, borderline range elevations of 5 to 15 mU should be interpreted cautiously, since clinical trials of replacement therapy in patients with this degree of "subclinical hypothyroidism" and vague symptoms have been inconclusive in terms of symptomatic improvement. In the absence of other worrisome or localizing signs, fatigue is seldom a warning sign of an occult malignancy, and it is usually sufficient to make sure that screening recommendations for cervical, colorectal, breast, and possibly prostate cancer have been followed. Abdominal computed tomography (CT) scanning, endoscopy, and other costly or invasive procedures are seldom warranted in evaluating isolated fatigue.

Several types of testing described in studies of CFS are expensive, do not affect patient management at present, and should not be performed outside the setting of a research protocol. The first is immunologic testing. A variety of markers of mild immunologic activation have been reported in some patients with CFS, including decreased immunoglobulin levels (particularly IgG subsets), low levels of circulating immune complexes, anergy, increased cytokines, and a decrease in natural killer cell numbers and activity. Such tests are problematic, however, because (1) they are unremarkable in more than half of patients with classic CFS, (2) they are nonspecific in that subtle immunologic abnormalities have also been reported in reaction to depression or stress, (3) they are costly, and (4) there is no specific therapy available. Second, testing for Epstein-Barr virus, human herpesvirus type 6, Lyme disease, and other infectious agents is not clinically useful. Viral causes for chronic fatigue still remain speculative and lack specific therapy, and patients with positive *Borrelia* titers and isolated fatigue do not respond to standard therapy for Lyme disease. Third, neuroimaging studies such as magnetic resonance imaging (MRI) and single photon emission computed tomography (SPECT) scanning, which have been reported to show nonspecific abnormalities in selected CFS patients, are not clinically indicated at present.

Sleep studies may be indicated in the occasional patient with chronic fatigue who has marked snoring or apneic episodes observed by a sleep partner; excessive daytime sleepiness, particularly if accompanied by narcolepsy; or multiple potential markers of sleep apnea, such as male gender, obesity, hypertension, and hypersomnolence. Because of the cost, as well as the nonspecific abnormalities that can be difficult to interpret, more research is needed before sleep studies become an important part of the evaluation of chronic fatigue. Finally, neuropsychological testing is occasionally performed in certain CFS patients who complain of impaired concentration and memory problems, particularly when disability determinations are an issue. However, such testing can be substantially influenced by patient effort and cooperation, and its role in evaluating CFS remains to be determined.

Inquiring about potential psychosocial causes or aggravating factors remains the single most important task in the evaluation of chronic fatigue. Depression is the most frequent treatable condition, but anxiety disorders, somatization, family dysfunction, and stress are also common. Simple questionnaires for detecting mental disorders in primary care, such as PRIME-MD,* have recently been developed. Antidepressants or psychotherapy are clearly indicated in the fatigued patient with a definite depressive disorder, but preliminary evidence indicates that low doses of antidepressants may also be useful in selected patients with CFS.

PROGNOSIS

As many as 70 per cent of patients presenting with fatigue in the primary care setting have improved by 6 months. Since studies of CFS contain highly selected groups of chronically ill individuals, the outcome in chronic fatigue is not well established. There is some evidence, however, that even many CFS patients gradually show some improvement 2 to 3 years after diagnosis. Patients who are convinced of a viral or organic basis for their symptoms as well as those who fail to return to work or

---

*Spitzer, R.L., Williams, J.B.W., Kroenke, K., et al.: Utility of a new procedure for diagnosing mental disorders in primary care: The PRIME-MD 1000 study. JAMA, 272:1749–1756, 1994.

other productive activities seem to experience less improvement. Although there does not appear to be an increased risk of mortality or the emergence of serious medical disorders, significant occupational and social impairment is common. Disability payments are often denied, however, and many CFS experts believe the optimal approach is one of gradual rehabilitation rather than permanent disability.

BACK AND EXTREMITY PAIN

By Herbert J. Keating, III, M.D.,
and Diane Barton, M.D.
Camden, New Jersey

Back and extremity pain are common presenting complaints and can tax the diagnostic acumen of the most skilled clinician. Because of the importance of practicing cost-effective medicine, the utility of a pertinent, directed history and physical examination cannot be overestimated. Selective use of laboratory and radiographic examinations may follow but often is not required. Once initial examination has excluded life-threatening or limb-threatening processes, observation over time can often be a useful diagnostic approach. Continued vigilance for cancer and infectious causes of pain is essential, however, especially in aged or immunocompromised patients.

Back and extremity pain may arise independently or occur together, either from the same traumatic or inflammatory process (e.g., herniated disk or ankylosing spondylitis) or as a result of a systemic disease, which may potentially cause problems at other sites (e.g., multiple myeloma).

In the initial approach to back or extremity pain, the diagnostician must first determine whether there is an emergency aspect. Are there signs of hemodynamic compromise? Are there signs of limb-threatening ischemia, such as cyanosis or livedo reticularis? Is there evidence of neurologic deficit suggesting myelopathy from cord compression (particularly at the sensory or motor "level") or sphincter dysfunction? The next step is to determine whether there is a systemic process underlying the back or extremity pain. Symptoms such as fever, chills, night sweats, anorexia, and weight loss, especially in the patient with a history of neoplastic or immunosuppressive disease, suggest a systemic process that will likely progress if not recognized and treated (Table 1).

Most back and extremity pain arises as a result of local pathology, which can cause pain at the site of local involvement (e.g., a ruptured Baker cyst) or referred pain (e.g., shoulder pain from inferior wall myocardial infarction), or both (e.g., sciatica).

Table 1. Factors That Increase the Possibility of Serious Causes of Back and Extremity Pain

History of malignancy
Severe trauma
Unexplained weight loss
Steroid or anticoagulant use
Severe pain, especially if not related to trauma and not relieved by rest
Fever
Neurologic deficits, especially saddle anesthesia, urinary retention

BACK PAIN

Back pain is usually acute or chronic in nature. In most patients, the history and physical examination enable etiologic diagnosis. Back pain is usually "mechanical" in nature, characterized by a musculoskeletal cause and benign course. Pain unrelated to mechanical use of the back should suggest an unusual cause, which may be life-threatening.

Obtaining a complete history is essential in the evaluation of the patient with back pain. This must include a detailed chief complaint; a past medical history, including neuropsychiatric, family, social, and occupational histories; and a review of systems. Important questions in obtaining the history follow:

1. Where is the pain located and does it radiate?
2. Is the pain acute or chronic?
3. Is the pain mechanical?

Most back pain originates from the spine or paraspinal structures, including the intervertebral disks, facet joints, spinal ligaments, and paraspinal muscles. Such pain usually occurs after movement or trauma and is exacerbated by movement and relieved by rest. Back pain can also be referred from intra-abdominal, pelvic, or retroperitoneal sites. Many of the causes of referred back pain are serious, even life-threatening, diseases. It must be noted, however, that occasionally a "nonmechanical" cause of back pain may result in pain precipitated by movement.

Acute onset of back pain following an injury suggests a mechanical cause of back pain. Pain that is more insidious suggests a nonmechanical, medical cause. The duration of pain is important. Mechanical back pain may last weeks to months, whereas spondyloarthropathies and tumors cause chronic, unremitting pain.

Pain originating in the back and radiating down the leg is suggestive of nerve root irritation. Bilateral sacroiliac joint pain suggests spondyloarthropathy. Pain from musculoskeletal causes may be localized to an area of "point tenderness." Pain from gallbladder disease may originate in the right upper quadrant and radiate to the right paraspinal area. Pain with a sudden onset may suggest serious conditions such as aortic dissection, ruptured ectopic pregnancy, or renal colic.

Clues to the cause of back pain may arise from the medical history, including the occupational, social, and psychiatric history. For instance, a patient with psoriasis and low back pain may have spondyloarthropathy associated with psoriasis.

Factors that exacerbate or alleviate back pain should be elicited. Pain worsened by prolonged standing or extension of the body suggests spinal stenosis. Cough, sneeze, and the Valsalva maneuver tend to worsen the pain of disk herniation. Patients with spondyloarthropathies feel worse after bed rest. Pain associated with acute infection or fracture may improve only with complete immobility. Referred visceral pain usually does not change with position; patients with colicky pain, for example, constantly shift position, unable to find a comfortable one. Psychogenic pain does not fit into any specific pattern.

Table 2. Important Causes of Back Pain

Name of Condition	History and Physical	Studies	Comments
Metabolic and Endocrine			
Osteomalacia	↑ Pain with activity; bone pain on percussion	Calcium, vitamin D, PO_4, alk phos, PTH bx: Inadequate mineralization; x-ray findings: codfish vertebrae; bone scan: hot spots–Looser's zones	Treat cause; prognosis depends on cause, reversibility
Infectious			
Osteomyelitis	+/− Fever, tenderness	Cultures, x-ray films	Early diagnosis → good prognosis; can progress → epidural abscess or meningitis if untreated
Pyogenic sacroiliitis	SI joint pain, fever, soft tissue abscess	Cultures +, MRI, bone scan; x-rays lag	Early treatment → good results
Sciatic diskitis	Local pain, limited motion	+ synovial fluid culture, x-ray, MRI	Usually good prognosis
Epidural abscess	Radicular pain, fever; risk factors: IVDA, DM, ETOH	CSF culture, bone scan, CT, MRI	IV antibiotics or drainage; can progress to paraplegia if untreated
Herpes zoster	Fever, vesicular dermatomal rash	H + P, culture, Tzanck preparation	Postherpetic neuralgia may occur; may have occult malignancy
Hematologic			
Hemoglobinopathy, i.e., sickle cell disease	Bone tenderness, repeated episodes	Anemia, Hgb electrophoresis, "Fishmouth vertebrae"	Variable
Tumors			
Metastatic	May have malignancy history	Anemia, ↑ alk phos; bone bx if no "primary" found	Can cause cord compression
Multiple myeloma	Fatigue, bone pain	Anemia, ↑ calcium; light-chain proteinuria, M protein, abnormal plasma cells in marrow	
Neurologic and Psychological			
Neuropathy	Sharp pain ↑ at night, +/− weakness	H + P, EMG	Depends on cause
Psychogenic rheumatism	Sleepiness, anorexia	H + P	
Malingering	Does not fit anatomic pattern; inconsistency	H + P	

Physical Examination

The general physical examination of the patient with possible referred back pain should include abdominal, rectal, and gynecologic examinations, percussion of the costovertebral angles, and assessment of the limbs for evidence of vascular insufficiency. If spondyloarthropathy is suspected, measurement of chest wall excursion is also indicated. With the patient's arms over the head, a tape measure placed below the breasts in women or at the fourth intercostal space in men should demonstrate an excursion of at least 2.5 cm with inspiration.

The components of the musculoskeletal examination in the patient with back pain include (1) *observation,* (2) testing the back's *range of motion,* (3) *palpation* of the spine and paraspinal structures, (4) *traction maneuvers,* and (5) *neurologic examination.*

First, the patient is observed, noting gait, position, and demeanor. The shape of the back is then examined, looking for curvature and posture. The patient who sits comfortably is unlikely to have a mechanical disorder, since this is usually the least comfortable position. Patients with muscle spasm or radicular pain often move slowly and experience discomfort while sitting. Those with radicular pain caused by disk herniation are least comfortable sitting, bending, straining, or lifting and are more comfortable in a supine position or standing or walking. Patients with spondylosis or spinal stenosis may be more comfortable in positions of spinal flexion. Evidence of weight loss or obesity should be noted. Skin lesions may be important. Psoriasis or hidradenitis suppurativa is associated with spondyloarthropathy. Dermatomal vesicles suggest a diagnosis of herpes zoster, and track marks on the skin may suggest drug abuse. Lymphadenopathy may suggest malignant, infectious, or idiopathic processes (e.g., sarcoidosis).

Pain unaffected by maneuvers that test the patient's range of motion suggests a nonmechanical disorder. Spinal flexion and extension may be assessed by orthopedic maneuvers such as the Schober test and the Flech test. Patients with spondyloarthropathies exhibit decreased lumbar flexion. Back extension may exacerbate referred pain from the retroperitoneum (hemorrhage, abscess, appendicitis) and may also worsen pain from spinal stenosis, facet joint disease or, rarely, a high lumbar disk. Lateral flexion and torsion testing may help localize the level of the herniated disk.

Severe point tenderness to palpation suggests an inflammatory, infectious, or malignant process but is not specific for these conditions. Unilateral or bilateral paravertebral muscle spasm suggests a mechanical back condition. "Trigger points" are local points of tenderness in the

Table 2. Important Causes of Back Pain *(Continued)*

Name of Condition	History and Physical	Studies	Comments
Mechanical			
Muscle strain	Low back pain → thigh-buttock; point tenderness, spasm	—	Treat with NSAIDs, controlled activity, resolves days → 2 wk
Spondylolisthesis	Pain low back → legs, point tenderness	X-ray films	Controlled activity—grade I, II; surgery—grade III, VI
Cauda equina	Loss of bladder-bowel control, saddle anesthesia, ↓ rectal tone	Myelogram, MRI	Causes disk herniation; surgical emergency
Herniated nucleus pulposus	Radicular pain +/− neurodeficits	CT, MRI, myelogram; MRI most sensitive	80% improve without surgery
Spinal stenosis	Pain in legs ↑ with extension; pseudoclaudication	X-ray films, CT; myelogram confirmatory	Multiple causes (osteoarthritis, metabolic bone disk, trauma); Most respond to conservative tx
Scoliosis	Deformity	X-ray films	Curve <40 degrees tends to remain stable; severe cases can result in premature death
Rheumatologic			
Ankylosing spondylitis	Male predominance, bilateral SI joint pain, ↓ with exercise, AM stiffness, ↓ chest expansion, ↓ lumbar motion	↑ ESR; 90% HLA-B27 +; x-ray findings: bamboo spine sacroiliitis, syndesmophytes	Remissions and exacerbations; destructive vertebral lesions can develop Cardiac involvement
Reiter syndrome	Male predominance, unilateral or bilateral SI joint pain, ↓ LS motion, urethritis, conjunctivitis, skin lesions, GI or GU infection	80% HLA-B27 +; x-ray findings: syndesmophytes, heel periostitis	Variable course, may have severe peripheral arthritis
Diffuse idiopathic skeletal hyperostosis	Dysphagia with cervical involvement	X-ray findings: T/L spine—flowing calcification; anterolateral aspect four contiguous vertebral bodies	Benign course
Vertebral osteochondritis (Scheuermann's)	Hip, paravertebral muscle pain, thoracic kyphosis	Irregular endplates, wedge vertebral body	Usually benign, can have severe kyphosis
Fibromyalgia	Female predominance, tender points, sleep disturbance, fatigue	Diagnosis of exclusion	Exacerbations and remissions can cause ↓ productivity

PO_4 = phosphate; alk phos = alkaline phosphatase; PTH = parathormone; bx = biopsy; SI = sacroiliac; IVDA = intravenous drug abuse; DM = diabetes mellitus; ETOH = ethanol; MRI = magnetic resonance imaging; CSF = cerebrospinal fluid; CT = computed tomography; H+P = history and physical; IV = intravenous; Hgb = hemoglobin; EMG = electromyography; NSAIDs = nonsteroidal anti-inflammatory drugs; tx = treatment; LS = lumbosacral; GI = gastrointestinal; GU = genitourinary; ESR = erythrocyte sedimentation rate; TL = thoracolumbar.

subcutaneous or muscular tissue that trigger a patient's pain. They occur in patients with chronic pain, for example, those with myofascial pain syndromes. The coccyx, ischial tuberosity, greater trochanter, sciatic notch, and rectum should be examined.

Traction or "tension" maneuvers (e.g., straight leg raising) identify disorders that produce lumbosacral nerve root compression. With the patient supine and the contralateral leg flat, each leg is passively flexed at the hip with the knee extended. This maneuver elicits traction on the lower lumbosacral nerve roots, primarily L5–S1. When these nerve roots are compressed or inflamed, straight leg raising elicits pain along the distribution of these nerve roots, especially down the back of the leg. If this maneuver worsens pain, no conclusion can be drawn. A positive test result should occur between 30 and 60 degrees of hip flexion and should have a sharp, shooting, or tingling quality. Also, pain down the asymptomatic leg when the painful leg is raised ("crossed straight leg raising") is highly suggestive of nerve root involvement.

The "flip sign" is performed with the patient in the sitting position and unaware of the examiner's intent. The patient's knee is passively extended. If the patient shows no discomfort while the knee is fully extended, doubt is cast on a positive straight leg raising test result.

Several other traction tests that may be performed include Yeoman's test for lumbosacral mechanical pain, Patrick's test for hip or sacroiliac disease, Laguerre's test for hip disease, and Gaenslen's test for sacroiliac disease.

If the history and tension maneuvers suggest neurologic disease, a full neurologic examination should be performed, otherwise a brief screening examination is carried out, including a motor assessment as well as examination of reflexes and sensation (including perineum, sacrum, and rectal tone). The sensory nerve supply in the saddle area comes from S3–S5. Every evaluation of back pain should include pinprick testing between the upper buttocks. Although rare, massive midline posterior lumbar disk protrusion causing saddle anesthesia and diminished rectal tone (cauda equina syndrome) can result in permanent bowel and bladder incontinence.

Laboratory and Imaging Studies

In cases of simple mechanical back pain, laboratory or radiologic studies are usually unnecessary. Erythrocyte sedimentation rate (ESR), serum protein electrophoresis, calcium, phosphate, alkaline phosphatase, and prostate specific antigen (PSA) or prostatic acid phosphatase determinations are appropriate in certain clinical settings, when back pain pattern is atypical, or in the elderly with new-onset back pain. Plain radiographs should be ordered for recurrent back pain, trauma, failure to improve with therapy, or when there are other clues to serious disease. Bone scans may be useful in suspected malignancy, fracture, or osteomyelitis, especially if radiographs are normal. Computed tomography (CT), magnetic resonance imaging (MRI), and myelography may be appropriate when there are neurologic findings or there is suspected spinal stenosis, disk disease, neoplasm, or infection. Generally myelography, which is an invasive study, is used only to confirm or extend CT or MRI findings. Electromyography assesses nerve and muscle damage but does not usually provide a specific diagnosis.

Table 2 summarizes important and relatively common causes of back pain and clues to diagnosis. Table 3 lists causes of referred back pain, and Table 4 lists infrequent causes of back pain.

Table 4. Infrequent Causes of Back Pain

Rheumatoid arthritis
Enteropathic arthritis
Whipple's disease
Postintestinal bypass arthritis
Behçet's syndrome
Familial Mediterranean fever
Hidradenitis suppurativa
Gout and calcium pyrophosphate disease
Vertebral sarcoidosis
Retroperitoneal fibrosis
Lyme disease
Paget's disease
Psoriatic arthritis
Ochronosis
Fluorosis
Myelofibrosis
Gaucher disease
Endocarditis
Tumors: osteoid osteoma, osteoblastoma, osteochondroma, bone cyst, hemangioma, giant cell tumor, eosinophilic granuloma, sacral lipoma, chordoma
Marfan's syndrome
Hyper- or hypoparathyroidism
Acromegaly

SHOULDER PAIN

Although shoulder pain usually arises from the supporting structures of the rotator cuff, it is critical to consider whether intrathoracic, diaphragmatic, or cervical lesions may be causing the pain. Important intrathoracic causes include myocardial infarction and dissection of the thoracic aorta. These conditions usually exhibit other features in addition to the shoulder pain, such as acute hemodynamic changes (hypotension or a disparity between upper extremity blood pressures and lower extremity blood pressures), nausea, and diaphoresis. A cause of more indolent shoulder pain is the Pancoast tumor, named for the involvement of the superior sulcus (apex) of the lung by bronchogenic carcinoma. Shoulder pain, when it seems to be "local" but escapes definitive diagnosis on the basis of physical examination (see further on), should be evaluated by chest radiography in addition to the shoulder film. If normal, the chest film excludes the Pancoast tumor. Important causes of pain referred to the shoulder from intra-abdominal sources include irritation of the diaphragm from gallbladder and liver disease, gastric disease, hemoperitoneum, and a ruptured abdominal viscus. Historical symptoms of gastrointestinal disease (pain, nausea, vomiting), icterus, tenderness on abdominal examination (particularly with excursion of the diaphragm), and increased serum amylase or liver enzyme activity may suggest these diagnoses.

Table 3. Causes of Referred Back Pain

Gastrointestinal
Gastric carcinoma
Peptic ulcer
Pancreatitis or pancreatic carcinoma
Cholecystitis
Irritable bowel
Diverticulosis
Colon carcinoma
Retrocecal or pelvic appendix
Vascular Disease
Aortic aneurysm or occlusion
Genitourinary
Kidney stones, infection, malignancy, infarction
Prostate carcinoma, prostatitis
Cystitis
Testicular carcinoma
Gynecologic
Leiomyoma
Endometriosis
Gynecologic carcinoma
Uterine or ectopic pregnancy
Ovarian cyst or torsion
Pelvic inflammatory disease
Retroperitoneal Disorders
Abscess, tumor
Retroperitoneal bleed
Aortic dissection

Cervical spine disease of several different origins (e.g., cervical disk disease, osteoarthritis, tumor) can also cause shoulder pain. If muscle strength is lost, if pain of a shock-like nature with numbness and tingling in a dermatomal distribution occurs, or if asymmetric reflexes are found, cervical spine disease should be suspected. Occasionally, the Valsalva maneuver may make the pain worse. Extension of the neck may cause the pain to radiate into the upper extremities. Cervical radiographs, electromyography, and CT or MRI may be necessary to confirm the diagnosis and will help define the pathology.

Very infrequently, shoulder pain may arise from vascular disease, including arterial insufficiency and thrombophlebitis. Most pain in the shoulder arises from its periarticular structures (bursae, tendons, muscles) and joints (the glenohumeral, acromioclavicular, and sternoclavicular). When pain originates from any of these sources, inflammation may result in more pain and muscle spasm, followed by dystrophic changes that then interfere with joint function.

Calcific tendinitis is a frequent cause of both acute and chronic shoulder pain. This often follows excessive use of the shoulder (as in house painting) and is associated with pain that may radiate into the upper arm and neck. There is usually local tenderness over the inflamed site and pain on motion. Radiographs may show calcium deposition that appears as linear densities in the perihumeral tendons. Bursitis of the subacromial and subdeltoid bursae may also occur from continuation of the calcium into the bursal space. Overuse, gout, and rheumatoid arthritis may also cause bursitis, which characteristically causes severe pain that is exaggerated by shoulder motion. Calcification of the bursae may be seen on x-ray film.

Bicipital tendinitis is associated with inflammation, subluxation, or rupture of the biceps tendon over the bicipital groove. Usually there is tenderness on palpation that is worsened with pronation of the arm (internal rotation and abduction). If the biceps tendon ruptures, the patient may recall a "snap," followed by immediate pain and a lump in the upper arm. In biceps tendinitis, local injection of a corticosteroid into the bicipital groove may cause immediate relief of pain, which is diagnostic.

Rotator cuff tears with tendon or ligament injury usually follow sports or work-related trauma and demonstrate pain on abduction. There may be radiographic changes (cysts or sclerosis) of the greater tuberosity of the humerus or osteophytes at the anterior margin of the acromion, with narrowing of the distance between the humeral head and the acromion. *Adhesive capsulitis* ("*frozen shoulder*"), which may follow shoulder injury from any cause or arise on its own, is a syndrome of progressively worsening pain and decreased range of motion of the glenohumeral joint. Radiographs may show humeral head osteoporosis but are often not useful.

Brachial plexus injury or inflammation ("plexitis") may cause neuropathic pain with muscle dysfunction.

Reflex sympathetic dystrophy (RSD), also called the "shoulder-hand syndrome," combines shoulder and upper extremity pain with evidence of vasomotor changes, including swelling and thickening of the skin. The pain is unilateral, intense, and prolonged and is often described as burning in nature. Classically, three stages occur. Stage I ("acute") presents with pain, edema, and decreased range of motion. This may last up to 3 months. Stage II ("dystrophy") may develop over 6 months and demonstrates dystrophic changes in the shoulder and arm such as shiny skin, hair loss, and brittle nails. Stage III ("atrophy") culminates with skin atrophy and osteopenia seen on radiographs. A bone scan may demonstrate periarticular uptake before osteoporosis. Reflex sympathetic dystrophy can follow prolonged immobilization from myocardial infarction, stroke, or trauma to the upper extremity.

Like RSD, the thoracic outlet syndrome (TOS) can cause shoulder pain that radiates into the arm. This is a controversial disorder, potentially arising from any condition in which the neurovascular supply to the arm is impinged on by other anatomic structures. Most easily understood, perhaps, is a cervical rib compressing the subclavian artery or the lower trunk of the brachial plexus (C8–T1)(occurring in about 1 per cent of the population). The anterior scalene syndrome refers to a thoracic outlet syndrome in which compression of the neurovascular bundle occurs between the scalene muscles and the first rib. The "Adson maneuver" is said to be diagnostic when the radial artery pulse disappears with the patient holding the breath, extending the neck, looking at the affected side, and abducting and externally rotating the arm.

Common causes of bilateral shoulder pain include the myofascial pain syndromes (e.g., fibromyalgia and polymyalgia rheumatica [PMR]). Myofascial pain syndromes are more common in women and are often associated with fatigue, multiple somatic complaints, nonrestorative sleep, and depression. The hallmark of fibromyalgia is the presence of characteristic "tender points" or trigger points—locally tender areas that may radiate pain; about 50 per cent of fibromyalgia patients have shoulder musculature trigger points. Polymyalgia rheumatica tends to involve the upper arms in addition to the painful shoulders (often with loss of abduction capabilities) but does not cause the vasomotor changes seen in RSD. Usually it affects elderly individuals, classically with an abrupt onset, and is associated with a high ESR, anemia, and, in some cases, the symptoms and signs of temporal arteritis (e.g., visual disturbances, jaw claudication, temporal artery tenderness or nodularity). Polymyalgia rheumatica may also affect the proximal musculature of the lower extremities.

Dislocation of the shoulder joint or fracture as a result of trauma causes shoulder pain, the reason for which is usually obvious. Other important but unusual causes of localized shoulder pain include rheumatoid arthritis and septic arthritis, gout, ankylosing spondylitis, steroid arthropathy, and osteomyelitis. Just like the femoral head, the humeral head may undergo aseptic necrosis. Because amyloid arthropathy can infiltrate the periarticular structures, it may cause thickening of the shoulder, the so-called shoulder pad sign.

EXTREMITY PAIN

Extremity pain is common and usually arises in isolation from other discomforts or diseases. When first presented with extremity pain, however, the clinician must be alert to processes that may, if not rapidly identified and treated, threaten serious consequences. The probability of one of these processes increases with (1) advancing age; (2) known medical problems, especially cancer; and (3) the presence of systemic symptoms (e.g., fever, weight loss, anorexia), suggesting underlying cancer or infectious disease.

Most extremity pain will arise from the musculoskeletal system, and most of this pain, in turn, will arise from some sort of trauma, either a one-time event or repetitive trauma. Therefore, the history is critical in the evaluation of extremity pain. Acute trauma is usually obvious as an explanation for pain involving the extremities and is usually perceptible at the site of injury. Importantly, however, pain originating in the proximal skeleton can be felt further down the axial skeleton. For example, hip pain may be perceived in the knee; therefore, during the evaluation of knee pain, attention should be paid to the hip as well. Puzzling extremity pain is often occupational or recreational in origin, and careful detective work may help uncover these causes.

Several "site-specific" musculoskeletal pains should be emphasized. In the elbow, epicondylitis is an important cause of pain. It has an insidious onset and is seen in individuals whose jobs or hobbies require repetitive wrist and forearm movements. Lateral epicondylitis ("tennis elbow") is seen when extension or supination is involved, and medial epicondylitis ("golfer's elbow") is seen when flexion and pronation are involved. Usually this pain is traumatic in nature, following repetitive injury. Rarely an autoimmune enthesopathy (an inflammation of the site where the tendon is inserted at the bone) from disorders such as Reiter syndrome can cause epicondylitis. The diagnosis is made on clinical examination when there is local tenderness in either the lateral or medial region. Relief of symptoms with injection of a local anesthetic can confirm the diagnosis.

Olecranon bursitis is usually traumatic in origin (from elbows leaning on the table), but it can also be caused by rheumatoid arthritis, gout, pseudogout, and, occasionally, microorganisms (e.g., staphylococci). Like bursae in other areas (housemaid's knee in the prepatellar area or trochanteric bursitis), the bursa may fill with fluid, and the synovial lining may become inflamed and thickened. This causes a tender bulge in the elbow, which can be aspirated. Gram stain and examination under the microscope should be performed to identify microorganisms and crystals. Occasionally, peripheral blood leukocyte counts may be deceptively low despite infection.

Nerve entrapment syndromes may present with elbow or more distal pain, usually accompanied by paresthesias, numbness, and/or weakness of various muscle groups. Ulnar entrapment presents with elbow or forearm pain, paresthesias, and numbness of the fourth and fifth digits. Often, there will be hand weakness. Median nerve entrapment near the medial epicondyle may occur with sensory loss and weakness in the median distribution, as occurs in the carpal tunnel syndrome, and may also arise from the pronator syndrome, in which the medial nerve is compressed by the two heads of the pronator teres muscle. This injury may arise from jobs requiring repetitive supination and pronation of the arm. Pain and tenderness in the area of the supinator, with weakness of the finger extensors and the ulnar wrist extensors, may suggest the posterior interosseous syndrome. The anterior interosseous syndrome will demonstrate vague forearm or elbow pain without sensory loss but with weakness of the flexors of the distal interphalangeal (DIP) joints. DeQuervain's disease, a tenosynovitis of the extensor tendons of the thumb, produces pain and tenderness over the radial styloid, which is worsened by traction on the thumb. Ganglion cysts, frequently arising over the tendon sheaths of the dorsal wrist, may be painful but usually are not.

Apophysitis of the tibial tubercle (Osgood-Schlatter disease) causes bilateral pain in adolescents at the site of tendon insertion at the tibial tubercles. This pain is insidious and increases with activity; fortunately, it tends to be self-limited, ceasing when skeletal growth stops. Knee pain is common. In general, if fluid is evident, it should be tapped and examined for cells, microorganisms, and crystals. Sizable knee effusions that occur after trauma should be aspirated to identify hemarthrosis, which should prompt draining and further diagnostic testing. Common orthopedic causes of knee pain include patellofemoral joint pain, chondromalacia patellae, osteoarthritis of the patella, plica syndromes, meniscus and ligamentous injuries, patellar tendinitis, and bursitis, particularly in the prepatellar and anserine area. Baker cyst, a synovial cyst of the popliteal space, may by itself cause local discomfort. With trauma or strenuous exertion, the cyst may rupture and cause acute swelling and tenderness, often traveling distally and resembling symptomatic thrombophlebitis.

Common foot and ankle disorders arising from trauma include ankle sprains, which have been classified according to location and degree of injury to the supporting ligaments of the ankle. The most common ankle sprain is the inversion type, with tearing of the anterior talofibular ligament. History will suggest ankle inversion combined with plantar flexion. A first-degree sprain is one in which there is partial tearing of the fibers. Mild to moderate tenderness and lack of joint instability confirm this diagnosis. Higher degrees of ankle sprain suggest the possibility of fracture. If the patient has severe pain, moderate diffuse swelling or ecchymosis, tenderness over the lateral aspect of the foot and ankle, and joint laxity, a radiograph should be obtained. The peroneal tendons pass beneath and behind the lateral malleolus and may tear with eversion and dorsiflexion of the ankle.

Rupture of the Achilles tendon can occur, particularly in "weekend warriors." Examination of the calf reveals a palpable interruption in the Achilles tendon. The belly of the gastrocnemius may be retracted into the upper portion of the calf. There may be ecchymosis around the heel and an inability to raise up on one's toes. Other common trauma-related musculoskeletal disorders in the foot and ankle include "stone bruises," a painful contusion of the plantar surface of the heel with swelling and tenderness of the calcaneal fat pad, plantar calcaneal spurs (heel spurs) and fasciitis. Plantar fasciitis is an inflammation of the plantar fascia of the foot, whereas heel spurring refers to a bony prominence that develops on the anterior plantar aspect of the calcaneus just anterior to the tuberosity where the plantar fascia inserts. Pain may present on the medial undersurface of the heel with standing, walking, and running. Metatarsalgia refers to pain over the metatarsal heads and/or the metatarsophalangeal (MTP) joints. Overweight and wearing high-heeled shoes are probably risk factors for development of this condition, but middle-aged individuals with a tendency to pronate their feet can also have this pain. Direct pressure over the metatarsal heads will elicit pain. Patients may report pain only on weight bearing. Night pain is uncommon.

Other causes of distal lower extremity traumatic pain include *stress fractures*, most commonly in the metatarsal bones (march fracture), occasionally in the tibia and fibula. A sharp pain without a history of acute injury is typical; however, there usually is a history of a particularly repetitive or stressful activity in the recent past. Palpable tenderness at the involved site is common. X-ray findings commonly may be normal initially. Two or three weeks later, an increased density appears at the area of callus formation, indicating that a stress fracture occurred.

"Shin splints" is an overuse syndrome, presenting with a dull ache that is often seen in runners. The pain progresses during and after the run and may be more common in individuals who are just beginning a training program. The origin of this anterior tibial inflammation may be multifactorial and may in rare instances progress to an anterior compartment syndrome with vascular compromise.

The tarsal tunnel syndrome is an entrapment neuropathy of the posterior tibial nerve under the medial malleolus (tarsal tunnel). Tenderness and local swelling with paresthesias into the plantar surface or heel occur. Pain is worsened with eversion of the foot and dorsiflexion. Night "burning" or tingling of the toes that interferes with sleep may be reported. By tapping over the posteroinferior region of the medial malleolus, a Tinel-like tingling may be elicited.

Middle-aged females wearing tight, high-heeled shoes may experience Morton's neuroma, with pain between the third and fourth or second and third metatarsal heads at the bottom of the feet. Local pain and paresthesias, which are improved by removing the shoe and massaging the ball of the foot, are the presenting symptoms. Pain may be present on walking or may awaken the patient at night. There is local tenderness. Other causes of mechanical traumatic pain in the ankle region include Achilles tendinitis, posterior calcaneal bursitis, pain from the deformity of hallux valgus (bunion), pain arising from pressure over the medial bony prominence, and bursitis. Pes planus (flat foot) may contribute to gradual development of degenerative arthritis changes, even extending up to the knees, hip, and lower back. Pes cavus is characterized by an extremely high medial arch in the forefoot and may also cause discomfort. Hammertoes (fixed flexion contractures of the proximal interphalangeal [PIP] joints with dorsiflexion of the MTP joints) may develop a painful corn on the dorsum of the foot, but this is usually an obvious source of pain, as are calluses and plantar warts. Hallux rigidus, referring to a painfully restricted motion of the first MTP joint in the foot, causes increasing stiffness, with pain at the base of the first toe when walking.

Vascular disease commonly causes extremity pain on the basis of inadequate arterial perfusion, capillary leak, or inadequate venous return. Ischemic injury to the vasonervorum may also cause painful mononeuropathy. This can arise from arteritis (classically, polyarteritis nodosa), atherosclerosis, or emboli. Clues to the diagnosis of important vascular causes are listed in Table 5. *Claudication* is exertional pain in the extremities (usually the leg) that is relieved by rest. It is most commonly caused by atherosclerosis; however, similar pain (pseudoclaudication) may be seen in patients with spinal stenosis, type V glycogen storage disease (McArdle's syndrome), hypokalemia, and amyloid myopathy. Conditions resembling deep vein thrombophlebitis (pseudothrombophlebitis) can also cause calf swelling and pain. These conditions include cellulitis, Baker cyst, muscle tears, hemarthrosis of the knee, gout, and postphlebitic syndrome.

Chilblain (pernio) is an uncommon angiitis related to cold exposure. The patient, often a woman or child, notes burning pain and bluish or red edematous discoloration in the lower extremities. Erythromelalgia, an episodic burning pain that occurs most often in the feet, may be associated with abnormal platelets.

Neuropathic pain in the extremities is common. Pain from radiculopathy refers to pain originating between the point where the dorsal (sensory) and ventral (motor) nerve roots join the spinal cord and the more distal point where the two roots fuse to form the peripheral nerve. Impingement on the dorsal nerve root is classically the cause of radicular pain. Peripheral neuropathies, both polyneuropathy and mononeuropathy, may cause pain. Both radicular pain and mononeuropathy pain tend to be more localized than polyneuropathy, which usually arises from a generalized, symmetric process and causes pain in a more widespread distribution.

Ruptured intervertebral disks in either the cervical spine or the lumbar spine will cause pain that may radiate toward the extremities. Prodromal symptoms include pain and stiffness in the neck or back. Although the pain may be dull, deep, or vague in character, classically it is sharp, superficial, and stabbing, as the disk hits the nerve root. Pain radiating to the shoulders suggests disk pathology between C3 and C4 (see earlier discussion). Sciatica, which is pain along the distribution of the sciatic nerve, radiating down the back of the leg to the lateral aspect of the distal lower extremity, may arise from impingement on the dorsal root.

Sciatica may also arise from processes causing mononeuropathy (e.g., diabetes), including that resulting from impingement by mass lesions anywhere along the sciatic nerve. Lesions such as soft tissue sarcomas, hematomas, or cysts, or even a wallet in the back pocket, have been reported culprits. Although controversial, spasm or trauma to the piriformis muscle is said to cause sciatica.

Neurologic pain may arise from lumbar stenosis, syringomyelia, hematomyelia, and central cord tumors, which are rare. It may also arise from the cauda equina syndrome, vertebral osteomyelitis, or epidural abscess.

Lesions anywhere along the sensory tracts may cause pain, often with "dysesthesia," a commonly used but poorly defined term describing an unpleasant sensation produced by a stimulus that ordinarily is painless. Tabes dorsalis from tertiary syphilis causes lancinating pain in the legs. Early loss of vibration and position sense, pupillary abnormalities, lower extremity areflexia, and the Romberg sign may also be seen. Transverse myelitis and amyotrophic

Table 5. Important Vascular Causes of Extremity Pain

Name of Condition	History and Physical	Studies	Comments
Atherosclerosis	Older individuals, especially males, may present with lower extremity pain with exercise (claudication)	Noninvasive vascular studies; angiography if therapeutic procedure considered	Exclude pseudoclaudication
Thromboangiitis obliterans	Young male smokers		Buerger's disease
Leriche syndrome	Pain in legs, hips, buttocks; impotence	Angiography shows arteriosclerotic disease in iliac vessels	
Acute ischemia	From emboli or thrombosis; acute pain, often severe, throbbing; livedo or pallor in limb	Angiography if therapeutic procedure considered	Underlying reason for emboli or thrombosis (e.g., atrial fibrillation, vasculitis, hypercoagulable state) usually apparent
Raynaud's phenomenon	Cold or stress-induced; three-color change; upper extremities more common		Idiopathic or associated with underlying reason (e.g., rheumatologic disease, drugs, or trauma)
Thrombophlebitis	Risk factors for deep vein thrombosis; pain at site, better with leg elevation	*IPG* or ultrasound examination shows clot	Pain is not usually severe and may be minimal
Postphlebitic syndrome	Aching pain after episode of deep vein thrombosis	Clinical diagnosis: *IPG*; ultrasound normal	Pain worse with dependency
Superficial thrombophlebitis	Local pain; tenderness at superficial vein site		May have symptoms or signs of underlying malignancy

IPG = impedance plethysmography.

lateral sclerosis may also be accompanied by pain corresponding to the level of involvement.

Peripheral neuropathies of either the polyneuropathy or mononeuropathy type may also cause extremity pain. Polyneuropathy is most commonly a distal axonopathy and can be seen with a variety of metabolic disorders (particularly diabetes), toxic exposures (e.g., alcohol, lead), and deficiency syndromes. Clinical features include a gradual onset, a stocking-glove combined sensory-motor loss, and slow recovery. Other painful polyneuropathies may be caused by a myelinopathy or neuronopathy (e.g., motor neuron disease, herpes zoster, paraneoplastic carcinomatous sensory neuropathy). In general, peripheral neuropathies cause bilateral discomfort in a stocking-glove distribution. The discomfort often moves proximally. Numbness, tingling, or burning pain is characteristic.

Mononeuropathy from ischemia, trauma, or infiltrative processes may cause pain. Pain usually coexists with motor and other sensory symptoms. Trauma is the most common cause; however, infiltration by tumor, amyloid, or ischemia is frequently responsible. Nerve conduction studies determine the presence of a neuropathy and may also indicate whether a symmetric polyneuropathy is of an axonal or demyelinating type, which may help in the diagnosis. Occasionally, biopsy of the sural nerve (at the ankle) or radial nerve may be necessary to identify the cause of mononeuritis multiplex, particularly in the presence of vasculitis (e.g., polyarteritis nodosa).

Well-localized pain in the extremity can originate from bone and this bone pain originates from the periosteum. Any process with periosteal involvement will produce pain. Pain is often associated with tenderness over the area of involvement and can be described as throbbing and worse at night. Periosteal processes such as hemorrhage (from coagulopathy, scurvy, trauma) or periostitis from cancer (either primary bone cancer or metastatic disease) may cause pain. An unusual cause of severe bone pain is hypertrophic pulmonary osteoarthropathy, manifested by periostitis and polyarthritis. It is seen in chronic pulmonary disease, including non–small cell lung cancer and mesothelioma. In the latter the pain may improve with successful treatment of the primary tumor. Osteomyelitis can cause local bone pain. Paget's disease causes pain, usually in the lower extremities, and initially with weight bearing. Metabolic bone disease, osteitis fibrosa or osteomalacia, may cause bone pain, generally in the lower parts of the body—the hips, knees, and legs. The pain is generally vague. When sharp pain appears in the setting of known bone disease (e.g., osteogenesis imperfecta), spontaneous fracture should be considered. Evidence of renal failure, hyperparathyroidism, and calcium, vitamin D, and phosphate abnormalities may be found. Osteomalacia associated with aluminum toxicity may cause severe bone pain, characteristically with low levels of parathyroid hormone. The sources of aluminum-associated osteomalacia may include the ingestion of phosphate binders containing aluminum in patients with chronic renal failure, but occasionally the osteomalacia results from environmental sources. Radiographs may show the typical changes of osteomalacia and/or osteitis. Subperiosteal erosion (particularly in the terminal phalanx or the second or third digit), bony erosions in the long bones and the skull, and brown tumors may be found on radiographs in osteitis fibrosa. The x-ray finding of osteomalacia in the adult is the pseudofracture (Looser's or Milkman's zones).

The muscles may be sources of pain in the extremities. Myalgia, the painful cramping caused by metabolic or electrolyte imbalance (e.g., hypokalemia, hypocalcemia) may cause significant extremity pain and tetany. Polymyositis and dermatomyositis, sometimes appearing as part of an overlap syndrome with other autoimmune diseases such as

Table 6. Selected Cutaneous Signs of Systemic Causes of Extremity Pain

Finding	Dermatologic Term	Systemic Disorder
Painless nodules on extensor surface	Rheumatoid nodule	Rheumatoid arthritis
Malar erythema	Butterfly rash	Systemic lupus erythematosus
Hyperkeratotic lesions on palms and soles	Keratoderma	Reiter syndrome
Subcutaneous nodules, painless, over bony surfaces or tendons		Rheumatic fever, juvenile rheumatoid arthritis
Erythema, advancing edge, central clearing	Erythema marginatum or erythema chronicum migrans	Rheumatic fever or Lyme arthritis
Superficial erythema, scaling of glans penis	Balanitis	Reiter syndrome
Painful anterior tibial nodules	Erythema nodosum	Coccidia, sarcoid, others
Salmon pink macular rash, transient		Still's disease (juvenile rheumatoid arthritis)
Purplish upper eyelids, edema	Heliotrope eruption	Dermatomyositis
Papular rash over fingers	Gottron's papules	Dermatomyositis
Nodules on helix of ear or extremities	Tophi	Gout
Subcutaneous calcifications of fingers		Scleroderma, polymyositis
Splinter hemorrhages		Infective endocarditis, vasculitis
Lipid deposits in skin or over tendons, around eyes	Xanthelasma or xanthoma	Hyperlipoproteinemia, higher risk of vascular disease
Hidebound acral skin, fingertip ulcers, telangectasias		Scleroderma, cheiroarthropathy in diabetes mellitus

scleroderma, rheumatoid arthritis, or lupus, may cause extremity pain. The pain is described as an aching associated with weakness. Usually the proximal muscles of the extremities are involved and are tender. Increased muscle enzyme activity is characteristic, and electromyography will show the changes of a myopathy.

Muscle stiffness or cramps with or without fasciculations can be seen in diseases such as systemic amyloidosis with a myopathy, the stiff man syndrome (a progressive disease of adult life, sometimes associated with diabetes and characterized by intermittent spasm of axial muscles followed by immobilizing stiffness), neuromyotonia, myotonia congenita and paramyotonia congenita, and "rippling muscle" syndrome. Myophosphorylase deficiency (type V glycogen storage disease, McArdle's disease) may cause a pseudoclaudication pain. Most patients with this disease are not diagnosed until the second or third decade of life when they present with postexertional muscle pain, myoglobinuria, and increased serum creatine kinase (CK) muscle isoenzyme activity. The diagnosis is established by the failure of the muscle to produce increased serum lactate with exercise as well as the demonstration on muscle biopsy of elevated glycogen and reduced phosphorylase activity. Muscle injury from rhabdomyolysis and paroxysmal myoglobinuria will often be associated with muscle pain and tenderness.

Systemic diseases often cause extremity pain and should be suspected when the pain is symmetric. The presence of cutaneous abnormalities, if not tender and clearly responsible for extremity discomfort, may suggest a systemic cause of extremity pain (Table 6). When more than one joint is involved and trauma has been excluded, an inflammatory arthritis is generally the cause of extremity pain. Systemic lupus erythematosus may cause myalgia as well as produce joint involvement that is characterized by an arthritis causing severe transient pain. The arthritis usually is not destructive. Rheumatoid arthritis, ankylosing spondylitis, Reiter syndrome, reactive enteropathies, amyloidosis, Lyme disease, gout, pseudogout, familial Mediterranean fever, serum sickness, and Behçet's and Whipple's disease all cause extremity pain from arthritis.

Many of these arthritic disorders are infectious or postinfectious in origin. Disorders such as acute rheumatic fever, dengue fever ("break bone fever"), and acute coccidioidomycosis ("Valley fever") are commonly associated with extreme musculoskeletal pain. Typhoid fever may cause painful subperiosteal nodular abscesses. Myalgia commonly accompanies infectious disease. Trichinosis causes muscle pain and tenderness.

Endocrine and metabolic diseases, particularly as they affect bone (e.g., hyperparathyroidism, osteomalacia), may cause extremity pain. Acromegaly may cause pain in muscles, bones, and joints. It accelerates osteoarthritis and is associated with crystal arthropathy. Endocrine insufficiency states (hypothyroidism, adrenal insufficiency, steroid withdrawal syndrome) cause muscle aches and stiffness. Diabetes may cause an aching pain in the hands, accompanied by sclerodactyly and joint contractures (diabetic cheiroarthropathy). The hands often cannot be brought together flat, resulting in the "prayer sign." Storage diseases (Hurler and Morquio syndromes) cause muscle stiffness. Vitamin A excess and vitamin C deficiency cause extremity pain.

Miscellaneous causes of extremity pain include psychogenic pain and nocturnal leg cramps. After extremity amputation, pain may arise from neuromas at the amputation site or from the phantom limb syndrome.

DYSURIA, PYURIA, AND HEMATURIA

By E. Everett Anderson, M.D.
Durham, North Carolina

DYSURIA

Dysuria is defined as painful or difficult urination but is universally used to describe only painful urination. Dysuria that is often associated with urgency and frequency is usually a symptom of lower urinary tract infection, prostatitis, or urethritis in the male and cystitis in the female. Urethritis and cystitis are associated with pyuria (more than 5 leukocytes/high-power field [HPF]) and positive urine culture results. Acute prostatitis is also usually associated with pyuria and positive urine culture results. In chronic prostatitis, urinalysis and urine culture results are often negative because the infection is focal and distant from the urethra. The diagnosis of chronic prostatitis is made by examination of prostatic secretions after prostatic massage (more than 10 leukocytes/HPF), the first 30 mL of voided urine after prostatic massage, or seminal fluid after ejaculation. If the diagnosis of lower urinary tract infection can be made by urinalysis without urine culture, it is not cost-effective to obtain a urine culture specimen. Urine cultures are indicated in recurrent or refractory lower urinary tract infections. Dysuria urgency and frequency when not associated with urinary tract infection may be caused by "prostatalgia" or "prostatosis," "urethral syndrome," "pelvic pain syndrome," interstitial cystitis, hypersensitive bladder, or unstable bladder. The entities surrounded by quotation marks are poorly understood and in fact may not exist. Interstitial cystitis can be identified by symptom complex: suprapubic or pelvic pain relieved by micturition and cystoscopic findings of small vesical capacity and stellate ulcers. Hypersensitive and unstable bladders are identified by urodynamic study. A calculus within the intravesical ureter produces vesical irritation manifested by burning, urgency, and frequency (and microscopic hematuria).

PYURIA

Pyuria (more than 5 leukocytes/HPF) most often is a sign of upper or lower urinary tract infection. Upper urinary tract (kidney) infections (pyelonephritis) are manifested by flank pain, chills, and fever. Lower urinary tract (bladder, prostate, urethra) infections have already been discussed. Approximately 95 per cent of urinary tract infections involve the lower urinary tract. Upper urinary tract infections are often associated with congenital or acquired ureteral obstruction or primary diseases of the kidney (e.g., renal calculi) and therefore require imaging of the urinary tract by intravenous pyelography or renal ultrasonography. A specimen for urine culture should be obtained in every patient with an upper urinary tract infection because immediate, appropriate antimicrobial therapy is indicated.

Pyuria without evidence of urinary tract infection by urine culture (abacterial pyuria) is a common occurrence after lower urinary tract operations (transurethral prostatectomy, transurethral resection of vesical tumors, and so on). It also can be a manifestation of renal calculi, urinary tract tuberculosis, cystitis glandularis, and enterovesical fistula. Virtually all diseases of the urinary tract that produce an inflammatory response can produce abacterial pyuria. Unexplained abacterial pyuria warrants investigation of the lower urinary tract by cystoscopy and the upper urinary tract by intravenous pyelography.

Pyuria in children is always significant because uncomplicated urinary tract infections in this age group are rare. Congenital anomalies of the urinary tract are often responsible for urinary tract infections in children. Specimens for urine culture should always be obtained, and the urinary tract should be examined by cystourethrography and renal ultrasonography. Vesicoureteral reflux is a common cause of urinary tract infections in girls and prostatic urethral valves in newborn boys.

HEMATURIA

Hematuria is the most common presenting sign of cancer of the urinary tract and renal parenchymal disease. Usually cancer of the urinary tract is associated with gross or macroscopic hematuria, but microscopic hematuria is occasionally the only clinical finding. All malignancies of the urinary tract bleed intermittently, and this accounts for the unfortunate delay in their diagnosis and treatment. When not associated with urinary tract infection, one episode of gross hematuria and persistent microscopic hematuria warrant investigation by cystoscopy and intravenous pyelography.

Red blood cells identified in urine can originate from the glomeruli or the urothelium. Glomerular red blood cells have uneven hemoglobin distribution and irregular shapes and cellular membranes with varied configurations because of osmotic and physical changes encountered during passage through nephrons. Epithelial red blood cells have even hemoglobin distribution and smooth, rounded, or crenated cellular membranes. This differentiation can be made with a phase-contrast microscope or by lowering of the condensor on any microscope. An abnormal number of glomerular red blood cells (more than 2 erythrocytes/HPF) suggests parenchymal renal bleeding, and an abnormal number of epithelial red blood cells (more than 1 erythrocyte/HPF) suggests urothelial bleeding and possible malignancy. Most laboratories do not distinguish between glomerular and epithelial red blood cells. In microscopic hematuria, large numbers of white blood cells that are out of proportion to the numbers of red blood cells and bacteriuria suggest an infectious origin. Significant proteinuria that is out of proportion to the degree of hematuria (more than 2+ proteinuria by dipstick technique with microscopic hematuria) and the presence of red blood cell and cellular-granular casts suggest renal parenchymal disease. Many patients with glomerulonephritis present with microscopic hematuria without proteinuria, red blood cell casts, cellular-granular casts, or other stigmata of renal parenchymal disease. Berger's disease (IgA nephropathy) is the most common glomerulopathy. It is found in up to 30 per cent of all renal biopsies, and one third of patients present with microscopic hematuria as the only clinical finding. Berger's disease is thought by some to be the most common cause of microscopic hematuria in patients with no other demonstrable cause.

Gross hematuria associated with lower urinary tract irritative symptoms—burning, urgency, and frequency of urination ("painful hematuria")—is usually the result of acute prostatitis in the male and acute hemorrhagic cystitis in the female. Occasionally, however, infiltrative vesical carcinoma with secondary infection will present as "painful" hematuria. "Painless" gross hematuria suggests a noninfectious origin and is the most common presenting symptom in patients with malignancy of the urinary tract. Males have the opportunity to examine their urinary stream and can often distinguish between bleeding from the anterior urethra (initial gross hematuria that clears during voiding), bleeding from the prostate gland (initial clear urine followed by terminal gross hematuria), and bleeding from the bladder or above (equal quantities of gross hematuria throughout the stream). Blood from the lower urinary tract is often bright red, whereas blood from the upper urinary tract may be smoky or reddish brown. Hematuria associated with flank pain suggests upper urinary tract calculi or ureteral colic from passage of blood clots or sloughed renal papillae (papillary necrosis). In the presence of atrial fibrillation, sudden onset of flank pain and a nonfunctioning kidney seen on intravenous pyelography suggest renal artery embolism. Cyclic hematuria associated with menses suggests endometriosis involving the urinary tract.

Fever associated with hematuria suggests an infectious origin and may be present with acute prostatitis, acute cystitis, or acute pyelonephritis. The latter condition does not produce hematuria per se but may be the result of ureteral obstruction from calculi or urothelial tumors. Blood pressure should be measured and may be elevated in parenchymal renal disease. A palpable kidney suggests renal tumor, but usually renal tumors are not palpable even when they are large. Flank tenderness suggests ureteral calculi or pyelonephritis. A palpable bladder after voiding indicates incomplete vesical emptying from outflow obstruction (benign hyperplasia of the prostate gland, urethral stricture, carcinoma of the prostate gland, acute prostatitis). A pelvic examination should be performed on women to exclude carcinoma of the vagina or uterus invading the bladder, and a rectal examination should be performed on men to exclude acute prostatitis, carcinoma of the prostate gland, and rectal carcinoma invading the bladder. Hematuria from carcinoma of the prostate gland does not occur until there is advanced disease because prostatic cancer develops on the periphery of the gland and does not encroach on the urethral lumen until late in the disease. Benign hyperplasia of the prostate gland is a much more common cause of hematuria.

There are innumerable causes of hematuria (Table 1), but in the majority of patients the differential diagnosis will include malignancy, infection, benign prostate gland hyperplasia, and urinary tract calculi. Malignancies usually present with intermittent, gross, "painless" hematuria. Carcinoma of the bladder is the most common malignancy producing hematuria. Renal cell carcinoma and transitional cell carcinoma of the renal pelvis and ureter account for the majority of other neoplasms producing hematuria. Cystitis in the female and acute prostatitis in the male are the most common infections and may present with gross, "painful" hematuria or microscopic hematuria. Benign hyperplasia of the prostate gland may present with either gross, "painless" hematuria or microscopic hematuria. Urethral stricture disease may be associated with hematuria. Renal and ureteral calculi usually present with microscopic hematuria. Urinary tract calculi obstructing the renal pelvis or ureter produce renal colic and flank pain, nausea, and vomiting.

The age, race, and sex of the patient are important factors and will often suggest the origin of hematuria. In children, the most common causes of hematuria, in order of frequency, are urinary tract infections, hypercalciuria, glomerulonephritis, and idiopathic hematuria. Wilms' tu-

Table 1. Common Causes of Hematuria

Glomerular
- Berger's disease (IgA nephropathy)
- Glomerulonephritis
- Lupus nephritis
- Familial nephritis (Alport's syndrome)
- Benign familial hematuria
- Sports (following exercise) hematuria

Renal
- Polycystic renal disease
- Papillary necrosis
- Renal artery embolism
- Lymphoma
- Multiple myeloma
- Amyloidosis
- Vascular malformations

Urologic
- Neoplasms
- Infections
- Calculi
- Benign prostate gland hyperplasia
- Urethral stricture
- Endometriosis
- Abdominal aortic aneurysm
- Trauma

Hematologic
- Therapeutic anticoagulation
- Coagulopathies
- Sickle cell hemoglobinopathies

Factitious
- Vaginal bleeding

False Hematuria (Red Urine)
- Hemoglobinuria
- Myoglobinuria
- Natural food pigments (beets, berries)
- Artificial food coloring
- Drugs—phenothiazines, phenazopyridine, phenolphthalein
- Porphyrins

mor, in contradistinction to renal cell carcinoma, usually grows away from the collecting system, and less than a third of cases are associated with hematuria. Young women experience hemorrhagic cystitis and young men have prostatitis. Older (>40 years) women usually have either hemorrhagic cystitis or urinary tract neoplasia. In older (>40 years) men, one should entertain the possibility of urinary tract neoplasia. In men older than 60 years, the most common causes of hematuria are bladder cancer and benign hyperplasia of the prostate gland. Eight per cent of African Americans have sickle cell trait (hemoglobin SA), and hematuria is the most common presenting symptom of this disease. This hematologic disorder is the cause of hematuria in one third of African American patients. However, all African American patients should be evaluated for other causes of hematuria. The diagnosis of sickle cell trait can be made by sickle cell preparation, but the result of this test may be negative and the test should be replaced by hemoglobin electrophoresis, which is the gold standard for identifying sickle cell hemoglobinopathy.

A familial history of hematuria and/or renal disease should be obtained and may suggest sickle cell hemoglobinopathy, familial nephritis (Alport's syndrome), benign familial hematuria, or polycystic renal disease.

A previous drug history is important—particularly anticoagulant, aspirin, nonsteroidal analgesic, and cyclophosphamide (Cytoxan) use. Anticoagulation with heparin or warfarin sodium (Coumadin) results in hematuria in 5 to 10 per cent of patients even when coagulation test results are in the therapeutic range. Anticoagulants can enhance bleeding from urinary tract neoplasms, and therefore significant hematuria during anticoagulation requires investigation. Aspirin and nonsteroidal analgesics may produce a coagulopathy that can be identified by obtaining a prothrombin time, partial thromboplastin time, thrombin time, platelet count, and bleeding time. Patients with known bleeding tendencies should also undergo a coagulopathy evaluation. Hemorrhagic cystitis occurs frequently after long-term cyclophosphamide therapy, and patients with a history of cyclophosphamide treatment are also at risk for the development of carcinoma of the bladder and rarely carcinoma of the upper urinary tract.

Pelvic irradiation can produce hemorrhagic cystitis that may develop years after the cessation of treatment.

Strenuous sports activity commonly results in microscopic hematuria and on occasion gross "painless" hematuria. This phenomenon can occur after both contact (football, boxing) and noncontact (running, swimming) sports. It is most commonly identified in runners. The pathophysiologic cause in runners may be traumatic (repetitive impact of posterior bladder wall against the bladder base) or nontraumatic (increased glomerular permeability and/or increased filtration) pressure at the nephron level. In the latter situation, proteinuria and red blood cell casts may also be present. Sports hematuria can be differentiated from other causes of red urine occurring after exercise—hemoglobinuria and myoglobinuria—by identification of erythrocyturia. Sports hematuria has a benign course, but the possibility of a coexisting pathologic lesion of the urinary tract should be excluded.

Patients who have no known explanation for hematuria are categorized as having benign idiopathic hematuria.

Urinary tract malignancy is the chief concern and can usually be identified or excluded by intravenous pyelography and cystoscopy. One must remember that cancer of the bladder is at least three times as common as cancer of the kidney, and cancer of the urinary tract (kidneys, ureters, bladder, and urethra) is three times as common in men as in women, except for cancer of the urethra, which is rare and found more often in women. Cancer of the bladder can be excluded only by cystoscopy. Therefore, all patients with unexplained hematuria should undergo intravenous pyelography and cystoscopy. In patients with an allergy to contrast material or with renal insufficiency, renal ultrasonography is the study of choice. The indeterminate intravenous pyelogram is supplemented by a renal ultrasonogram. Suggestion of a solid renal mass requires an enhanced abdominal computed tomography (CT) scan, which is the gold standard imaging study for renal cell carcinoma. Cystoscopy ideally should be performed while the patient is experiencing gross hematuria because cystoscopic visualization of an effluence of urine from the ureteral orifices can document or exclude bleeding from the upper urinary tracts. Further, if there is bleeding from the upper urinary tracts, the involved kidney or ureter producing the hematuria can be identified. Intravenous pyelography should be performed prior to cystoscopy because urothelial tumors of the renal pelvis and ureter are best delineated by retrograde pyelography.

Cytologic studies of urine should be reserved for patients who have persistent, unexplained hematuria. An abnormal cytologic study of urine in a patient with a normal intravenous pyelogram and cystoscopy findings suggests flat transitional cell carcinoma in situ of the bladder or transitional cell carcinoma of the prostate gland. These patients should receive random transurethral vesical and prostatic biopsies and bilateral ureteral catheterization with lavage of renal pelves for cytologic studies of the urine.

Unexplained, recurrent gross hematuria demands more careful surveillance than does microscopic hematuria because it is more commonly a manifestation of urinary tract malignancy. Enhanced abdominal computed tomography should be performed to rule out renal cell carcinoma in these patients, even if all other urographic studies (intravenous pyelogram, renal ultrasonogram) are normal. Cytologic studies of the urine and random transurethral vesical and prostatic biopsies are also indicated. When feasible, cystoscopy should be performed while gross hematuria is present to detect the bleeding site. Unexplained microscopic hematuria should also be followed; in general, however, if a patient has one normal intravenous pyelogram, as well as normal cystoscopic and urine cytologic findings, further diagnostic studies for malignancy are unrewarding. Many of these patients have Berger's disease, for which there is no immediate treatment. Patients with Berger's disease are at risk for the development of hypertension and renal failure, and therefore serial blood pressure, serum creatinine, and urinary protein determinations are appropriate.

A positive Hematest result on dip tape in the absence of microscopic hematuria on urinalysis can be the result of myoglobinuria, hemoglobinuria, or other conditions that do not warrant investigation.

PRURITUS

By Gary R. Kantor, M.D.
Philadelphia, Pennsylvania

Pruritus, the most common symptom related to dermatologic disease, may or may not occur with apparent clinical skin rash. Itching can be localized or generalized and may be troublesome enough to interfere with daytime activities or sleep.

When patients present with a complaint of pruritus, the physician must decide whether the patient's itching is related to primary dermatologic disease, systemic disease, or other causes. A thorough history and physical examination with or without laboratory studies are needed to identify the underlying cause.

HISTORY

The clinical history is the single most important source of information for determining the cause of a patient's itching. This information can often be obtained from the patient, but occasionally a family member, a caregiver, a health provider, or the patient's medical record may provide valuable insight.

Table 1 lists the most important points in the medical history that may provide clues to the cause of pruritus. Pruritus of acute onset that lasts several days is less likely to be associated with an underlying systemic disease than is chronic, progressive, generalized pruritus that lasts weeks to months. Localized itching is seldom a consequence of systemic disease. The severity of pruritus may vary during the course of the day, with itching becoming especially troublesome in the evening or at bedtime. This history is often elicited from patients with scabies infestation. Itching that causes the patient to awaken from sleep may be a symptom of underlying systemic disease. Itching that is described by the patient as "burning" may occur in senile pruritus and dermatitis herpetiformis. The itching associated with polycythemia vera and aquagenic pruritus is often described as "pricking."

Table 1. Important Points in the History

Description of Pruritus
Onset—abrupt or gradual
Nature—continuous, intermittent, pricking, or burning
Duration—days, weeks, or months
Severity—e.g., interference with normal activities
Time—nighttime, cyclical
Location—generalized or localized, unilateral or bilateral
Relationship to activities—occupation, hobbies
Provoking factors—e.g., water, skin-cooling, exercise
Medical History Related to Pruritus
Medications—prescribed, over-the-counter, illicit
Allergies—systemic, topical
Atopic history—asthma, hay fever, eczema
Family history—atopy or skin disease
Social history—household and other personal contacts
Bathing habits
Pets and their care
Sexual history
Travel history
Other diseases

One of the most common causes of generalized itching without an observable rash is a reaction to a systemic medication. When patients are taking several medications, drug interactions must be considered. Itching can precede the development of a rash in a patient who has a drug hypersensitivity, and absence of a rash does not exclude a drug cause. A history of contact with animals may also be important in determining the cause of pruritus. Treatment of pets infested with fleas or mites is likely to improve the symptoms of pruritus in their owners. Lymphoma (e.g., Hodgkin's disease) should be considered in the patient who complains of itching and also gives a history of fever and night sweats.

PHYSICAL EXAMINATION

The involuntary response to a perceived itch is to scratch, which produces excoriations that often assume a linear configuration. Rubbing the skin produces a reactive thickening with accentuation of the skin lines (lichenification). Localized rubbing of the skin may produce papules, plaques, or nodules. These lesions are often seen on the extremities, scalp, and posterior neck. It is important to differentiate a pruritic rash associated with a primary dermatologic disease from the secondary changes that occur in the skin as the result of scratching associated with itching from other causes.

The middle of the upper back should be examined in the patient with itching. Because it is relatively inaccessible to the hands, this site is spared in most patients with systemic diseases associated with itching. It may, however, be involved when primary dermatologic disease is the cause of the patient's itching. Patients with primary biliary cirrhosis associated with chronic severe itching rub and scratch their skin so severely that they may develop a secondary hyperpigmentation of the skin. Often the skin on the middle upper back appears normal (butterfly sign) in these patients. Vesicles are the primary lesions of dermatitis herpetiformis. They may group together on the extensor surfaces of the skin, including the upper back. The upper back is one of the best areas for biopsy, because lesions in this area are spared from the secondary changes that may occur from scratching.

Scabies infestation often presents subtly with itching that is out of proportion to the physical findings. A careful cutaneous examination may reveal burrows. Scrapings of skin from affected sites may demonstrate mites, ova, or feces on microscopic examination.

The skin, hair, and nails should be examined for skin signs of systemic disease. For example, the finding of "half-and-half" nails in which the nailplate shows a proximal white band and a distal red-brown band of equal size in the patient with generalized itching suggests chronic renal disease. Lymphadenopathy and palpable abnormalities of the liver or spleen suggest systemic disease, such as malignancy.

DIFFERENTIAL DIAGNOSIS (Table 2)

Xerosis, or dry skin, is a frequent cause of itching in cooler climates during the fall and winter seasons ("winter itch"). It has a predictable seasonal onset and is associated with bathing in hot water and the use of harsh soaps. Xerosis is exacerbated by the effects of cold air, low humidity, and central heating, especially forced hot air heating. The physical examination may reveal fine platelike scaling, especially on the legs, with or without an associated dermatitis. A simple 2-week trial consisting of less frequent bathing, the use of a mild soap, and the application of baby oil or moisturizing cream right after bathing greatly improves or cures the itching associated with xerosis.

Scabies infestation is an important cause of severe itching. The mite, *Sarcoptes scabiei*, burrows in the skin, mates, and lays eggs. The characteristic sites of involvement include the interdigital finger webs, volar wrists, elbows, axillae, nipples, genitals, buttocks, and upper thighs. If the skin scraping reveals mites or their products, treatment with topical lindane lotion or permethrin cream is curative.

Fiberglass dermatitis is an irritant dermatitis that occurs after contact with fiberglass insulation or fabrics. The glass particles mechanically pierce the skin and produce severe itching with the later development of a rash. The history, including the patient's occupation, is crucial for making the diagnosis. Fiberglass particles can be demonstrated in skin scrapings microscopically.

Table 2. Skin Diseases Associated With Pruritus

Xerosis*	Pediculosis
Scabies*	Urticaria
Dermatitis herpetiformis	Folliculitis
Atopic dermatitis	Sunburn
Lichen simplex chronicus	Polymorphous light eruption
Psoriasis	Bullous pemphigoid
Lichen planus	Pemphigus foliaceus
Contact dermatitis	Pityriasis rosea
Miliaria	Fiberglass dermatitis*
Drug reactions	Fungal infections
Insect bites	Mycosis fungoides
Pruritic urticarial papules and plaques of pregnancy	

*Specific skin findings may be subtle.

Table 3. Systemic Diseases Associated With Generalized Pruritus

Group 1. Diseases Known to be Associated With Pruritus
- Uremia
- Obstructive hepatobiliary disease
- Polycythemia vera
- Hyperthyroidism
- Hodgkin's disease and other lymphomas

Group 2. Diseases Possibly Associated With Pruritus
- Diabetes mellitus
- Hypothyrodism
- Iron deficiency anemia
- Systemic carcinoma

Group 3. Diseases Associated With Pruritus in Case Reports
- Acquired immunodeficiency syndrome
- Benign gammopathy
- Bullous pemphigoid
- Carcinoid syndrome
- Dumping syndrome
- Mastocytosis
- Multiple myeloma
- Neurologic disorders
- Sjögren's syndrome

Table 3 lists the systemic diseases that are associated with pruritus.

The most common systemic disease associated with severe itching is uremia. Itching occurs in as many as 90 per cent of patients receiving hemodialysis. It is paroxysmal in nature, localized or generalized, and more severe in the summertime. These patients may develop nodules on the skin from chronic rubbing and scratching (prurigo nodularis). Patients who do not respond to moisturizers and antihistamines may be treated with ultraviolet light (UVB) therapy.

Obstructive hepatobiliary disease may produce intense generalized itching, and in contrast with uremia, itching may be the first sign of this disease. Both intrahepatic and extrahepatic causes of biliary obstruction may produce pruritus. Of the diseases that produce hepatobiliary obstruction, primary biliary cirrhosis is the one most closely associated with severe generalized itching.

Hyperthyroidism—not hypothyroidism—is associated with generalized itching. Pruritus may occur after the disease has been diagnosed, although some patients may present with a complaint of generalized itching. The return to a euthyroid state is associated with improvement of the itching.

The most common cancer by far that produces generalized itching is Hodgkin's disease. Pruritus occurs in as many as 50 per cent of patients with polycythemia vera. Itching is often associated with bathing ("bath pruritus"). This history is not diagnostic because patients with aquagenic pruritus or xerosis may have the same complaint.

Internal malignancy (with the exception of Hodgkin's disease) is rarely associated with itching unless there is alteration in liver or renal function. An exhaustive search for internal cancer is not indicated unless the history and physical examination direct otherwise. One possible exception may be carcinoma of the colon associated with a low serum ferritin in elderly men.

DIAGNOSTIC APPROACH

A decision algorithm (Fig. 1) is often useful in the evaluation of a patient with a complaint of pruritus. If there is

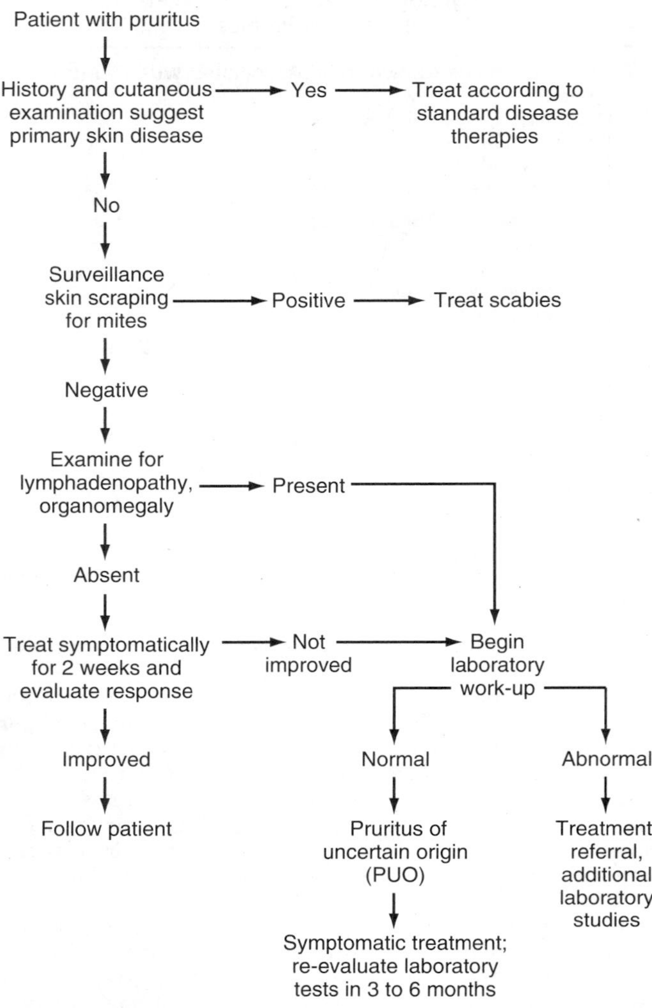

Figure 1. Decision algorithm for evaluating patients with pruritus.

no evidence of a primary dermatologic disorder, evidence for infestation should be sought based on physical findings and examination of skin scrapings. The signs, symptoms, or physical findings of systemic illness and the absence of primary dermatologic disease should direct the investigator to the laboratory evaluation. If the index of suspicion for internal disease is low, a 2-week trial course of conservative treatment is indicated. This therapy includes an oral antihistamine and a soothing topical nonsteroidal emollient lotion or cream. Approximately one half to two thirds of patients who undergo this therapeutic treatment experience partial or complete abatement of their itching.

Table 4. Suggested Screening Laboratory Evaluation for Pruritus

Complete blood count with differential white blood cell count
Serum urea nitrogen, creatinine
Alkaline phosphatase, bilirubin
Thyroxine (T_4), thyroid-stimulating hormone (TSH)
Glucose
Stool for occult blood (if patient older than age 40 years)
Chest x-ray film

Table 5. Further Laboratory Evaluation of Pruritus in Selected Cases

Serum iron, ferritin
Serum protein electrophoresis, serum immunoelectrophoresis
Skin biopsy for special stains (to exclude mastocytosis)
Skin biopsy for direct immunofluorescence (to exclude dermatitis herpetiformis, bullous pemphigoid)
Stool for ova and parasites
Urine for 5-hydroxyindoleacetic acid (5-HIAA) and mast cell metabolites
Additional radiologic studies
Human immunodeficiency virus (HIV) testing

When no improvement occurs, screening laboratory tests are indicated.

LABORATORY EVALUATION

The screening studies shown in Table 4 may detect undisclosed systemic disease that is causing the itching. Screening radiologic studies (except for a chest radiograph) are not particularly helpful in detecting underlying systemic disease unless the history and physical examination direct otherwise.

One test that may be helpful in some instances is the skin biopsy, which ideally should be performed on a nontraumatized primary lesion. The middle upper back area is often a good biopsy location. Histopathology may not always yield a specific diagnosis, but it may help narrow the differential diagnosis and yield specific information in selected cases. In some elderly patients, a perilesional biopsy of normal skin adjacent to a traumatized or nonspecific lesion may show dermatitis herpetiformis or bullous pemphigoid when tested by direct immunofluorescence studies. Other laboratory tests (Table 5) may be helpful in some patients with pruritus.

If no internal cause of the itching is found on initial evaluation, the diagnosis of pruritus of uncertain origin (PUO) should be considered. The absence of findings during the first evaluation does not necessarily preclude an associated systemic disease. Approximately 10 per cent of patients with PUO may be shown to have a systemic disease on clinical follow-up. The patient with chronic PUO should be re-evaluated with a history, a physical examination, and appropriate laboratory tests after about 6 months. Most patients with pruritus need support, empathy, and reassurance. Some patients are only concerned that they may have a serious underlying disease, such as cancer, and reassurance that the disease is not present can alleviate the itch. Many other patients, such as those with xerosis, will respond to simple empirical therapy.

PERIOPERATIVE MEDICAL CONSULTATION

By Geno J. Merli, M.D.,
and Howard H. Weitz, M.D.
Philadelphia, Pennsylvania

Over the past 25 years, the role of the medical consultant in perioperative consultation has undergone significant change. This transformation has resulted from a rapidly expanding information base and the impact of the insurance industry on the responsibilities of the primary care physician as medical consultant. Also contributing to the consultant's changing role are the new demographics of the surgical patient. Procedures are being performed on patients with multiple medical problems that, collectively, would have eliminated their candidacy for surgery in the recent past. In addition, more surgery is being performed on an outpatient basis than ever before. The often-used phrase "cleared for surgery" at the completion of a consultation is an archaic term without meaning or substance, in the present arena of preoperative assessment. The job of the perioperative consultant is to estimate the patient's perioperative risk, to reverse risk factors if possible, to advise the surgical-anesthesia team in the care of medical problems that are irreversible, and to aid in the care of postoperative medical problems. To fulfill this role in the 1990s, the medical consultant must possess the expertise and skill to appropriately orchestrate the role of consultant.

ASSESSING OPERATIVE RISK

The risk from inpatient noncardiac surgery for patients with cardiac disease has been estimated by computing multifactorial indices (Tables 1 and 2). This computation provided a method not only for risk determination but also for identification of several reversible risk factors that, if eliminated, could result in fewer complications. Earlier studies suggested that the only clinical parameter that was indicative of postoperative cardiac complications was postoperative myocardial ischemia. However, increased risk for deep vein thrombophlebitis and pulmonary embolism is related to venous stasis, vascular intimal injury, and hypercoaguability resulting from the surgical procedure. After the physician has completed the history and physical examination, the patient may be placed in the category of high, moderate, or low risk for the development of thrombosis based on patient age, length and type of procedure, and secondary risk factors (Table 3). After assessing the risk to the surgical patient, the consultant has the responsibility of recommending or prescribing the most effective prophylaxis to prevent or reduce the likelihood of the complication.

Table 1. Computation of Cardiac Risk Index

Criteria	Points
1. History	
Age over 70 years	5
Myocardial infarction within previous 6 months	10
2. Physical examination	
Protodiastolic third heart sound (S_3 gallop) or jugular vein distention	11
Important valvular aortic stenosis	3
3. Electrocardiogram (ECG)	
Rhythm other than sinus or premature atrial contractions	7
More than five premature ventricular contractions per minute	7
4. General status	
$Po_2 < 60$ mm Hg; $Pco_2 > 50$ mm Hg; potassium < 3.0 mEq/L; bicarbonate < 20 mEq/L; serum urea nitrogen > 50 mg/dL or creatinine > 3.0 mg/dL; abnormal aspartate aminotransferase (AST); signs of chronic liver disease; or patient bedridden from noncardiac causes	3
5. Operation to be done	
Intraperitoneal, intrathoracic, or aortic operation	3
Emergency operation	4
TOTAL POSSIBLE	53

Adapted from Goldman, L., Caldera, D.L., Nussbaum, S.R., et al.: Multifactorial index of cardiac risk in noncardiac surgical procedures. N. Engl. J. Med., 297:845–850, 1977, with permission.

Table 2. Cardiac Risk Index

Class	Point Total	Life-Threatening Complication*	Cardiac Deaths
I	0–5	4 (0.7%)	1 (0.2%)
II	6–12	16 (5 %)	5 (2%)
III	13–25	15 (11%)	3 (2%)
IV	≥26	4 (22%)	10 (56%)

*Documented intraoperative or postoperative myocardial infarction, pulmonary edema, or ventricular tachycardia without progression to death.

Adapted from Goldman, L., Caldera, D.L., Nussbaum, S.R., et al.: Multifactorial index of cardiac risk in noncardiac surgical procedures. N. Engl. J. Med. 297:845–850, 1977, with permission.

Risk stratification for patients undergoing peripheral revascularization procedures is evolving. The approach employs consideration of pre-existing risk factors, physical signs and symptoms, laboratory testing, and both invasive and noninvasive studies to evaluate underlying cardiovascular disease in the high-risk population (Fig. 1). Classic risk stratification indices underestimate the risk of perioperative cardiac complications in the patient undergoing major vascular surgery. To assess whether a patient is at low, intermediate, or high cardiac risk during and after vascular surgery, five cardiac risk factors have been used: myocardial infarction with Q wave on electrocardiogram (ECG), age greater than 70 years, diabetes mellitus that requires medical treatment, ventricular premature contractions that require medical treatment, and angina. The intermediate-risk patients are further evaluated with the use of dipyridamole thallium scanning. This procedure has become a mainstay of preoperative evaluation in vascular surgery, but it has a low positive predictive value. Dobutamine echocardiography, dipyridamole echocardiography, and dobutamine thallium scanning show promise but require more study.

ISSUES FOR THE PERIOPERATIVE CONSULTATION

Diabetes Mellitus

In nondiabetic patients, the stress of surgery postoperatively produces hyperglycemia secondary to catecholamines, which inhibit pancreatic insulin release and increase insulin resistance in the periphery. Fatty acids and amino acids become the substrate for gluconeogenesis. In addition, increased concentrations of anti-insulin hormones, such as cortisol, glucagon, and growth hormone, enhance gluconeogenesis and glycogenolysis, which further exacerbate hyperglycemia. Patients with diabetes mellitus are likely to have exaggerated responses to these changes during the postoperative period. The goal of the medical consultant is to maintain metabolic homeostasis, to monitor for complications arising from diabetic target organ disease, and to treat these problems as they arise.

The initial evaluation focuses on the assessment of tar-

Table 3. Risk Classification for Postoperative Deep Vein Thrombophlebitis (DVT) and Pulmonary Embolism (PE)

Risk Categories	Calf DVT (%)	Prox DVT (%)	Fatal PE (%)
1. High Risk	40 to 80	10 to 20	1 to 5
a. Age >40 yr			
b. Surgery >30 min			
(1) Orthopedic surgery			
(2) Pelvic or abdominal cancer surgery			
c. Previous DVT or PE			
d. Secondary risk factors*			
e. Hereditary or acquired coagulopathies†			
2. Moderate Risk	20 to 40	4 to 8	0.4 to 1.0
a. Age >40 yr			
b. Surgery >30 min			
c. Secondary risk factors*			
3. Low Risk	2	0.4	.002
a. Age <40 yr			
b. Surgery minor <30 min			
c. No secondary risk factors			

PROX = proximal.
*Secondary risk factors: obesity, immobilization, malignancy, varicose veins, estrogen use, paralysis.
†Hereditary or acquired coagulopathies: protein C, S, antithrombin III, anticardiolipin antibodies.
Modified from Clagett, P.G., Anderson, F., Heit, J., et al: Prevention of venous thromboembolism. Chest, 4:312S–334S, 1995, with permission.

get organ damage and on stability and control of blood glucose (Table 4). One third to one half of the usual total daily dose of neutral protamine Hagedorn (NPH) insulin is typically given on the morning of surgery along with 5 per cent dextrose intravenous fluid infusion. Blood glucose is monitored every 6 hours after surgery with the use of sliding-scale regular insulin coverage. Diet-controlled diabetic patients or those taking oral hypoglycemic agents do not receive insulin unless the blood glucose rises above 250 mg/dL. Hypoglycemic agents should be discontinued the day before surgery or 36 to 48 hours prior to surgery for long-acting chlorpropamide. Blood glucose monitoring should be implemented postoperatively. Normal or half-normal saline is typically used for fluid replacement during the perioperative period.

Hypertension

More than 30 per cent of patients undergoing surgery have hypertension. The primary concern of the consultant is the impact of hypertension on operative risk and its management during the perioperative period. The two hemodynamically unstable periods during anesthesia are the induction and the recovery phases. During laryngoscopy and endotracheal intubation, activation of the sympathetic nervous system occurs, with a concomitant rise in blood pressure and heart rate. After initial intubation and with further deepening of anesthesia, mean arterial pressure declines below the preoperative baseline. During the recovery period, blood pressure increases with the waning effects of anesthesia and sympathetic nervous system activity. Patients with a preoperative diastolic blood pressure above 110 mm Hg have an increased risk of perioperative blood pressure lability, dysrhythmias, myocardial ischemia, myocardial infarction, and transient or permanent neurologic complications. Those patients with systolic pressures above 200 mm Hg have an increased incidence of postoperative hypertension and neurologic complications. The consultant must assess the duration and degree of preoperative blood pressure changes in the context of maintenance antihypertensive medications.

Hypertensive patients who are undergoing surgery require control of both systolic and diastolic pressures. With

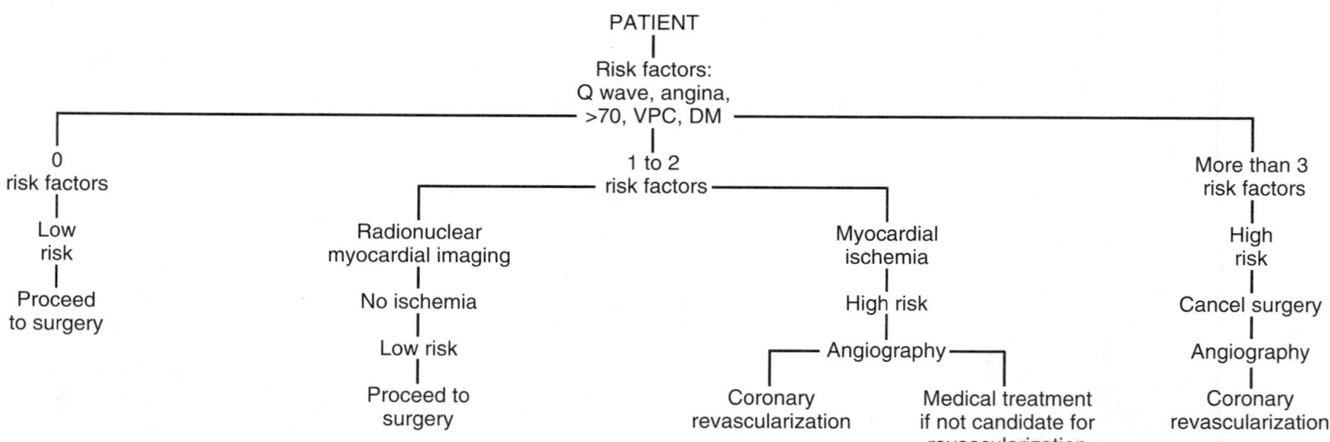

Figure 1. Assessing patient risk for peripheral revascularization surgery.

Table 4. Perioperative Management of the Diabetic Patient

STEP I.	Serum glucose range below 250 mg/dL
STEP II.	Assess target organ involvement Creatinine Urinalysis Electrolytes Electrocardiogram (ECG)
STEP III.	Perioperative management Intravenous fluid, based on glucose, electrolytes, and cardiovascular and renal status Give one third to one half of the total daily dose of insulin as NPH on the morning of surgery Oral hypoglycemic agents are discontinued the day before surgery Follow blood glucose levels every 6 hours and give regular insulin according to sliding scale Obtain laboratory testing, such as electrolytes, creatinine, or ECG, as clinically indicated Re-establish patient's usual diabetic regimen when the patient has resumed oral intake

NPH = neutral protamine Hagedorn.

the exception of guanethidine and monoamine oxidase (MAO) inhibitors, which should be discontinued 2 weeks before surgery, all medications may be continued up to and including the morning of surgery. Diuretics are usually not prescribed during the preoperative period unless diuresis is required. The risk of volume depletion and electrolyte disturbance secondary to these agents should be avoided. Patients who are unable to resume oral medications postoperatively should receive the parenteral form. When the surgery is not urgent and the blood pressure is either greater than 200 mm Hg systolic or greater than 110 mm Hg diastolic, the procedure should be postponed, and the blood pressure brought under control. Urgent or emergent surgery should proceed with perioperative blood pressure controlled with appropriate antihypertensive medication. Caution is warranted when patients are taking more than 1 mg per day of clonidine for hypertension or beta-blockers for ischemic heart disease. Discontinuing the former medication can cause rebound hypertension and ischemia, while withdrawal of the latter can cause worsening of ischemia.

Pulmonary Disease

The focus of the consultant is the assessment of pulmonary function and extrinsic nonpulmonary risk factors, such as surgical site, duration of the procedure, patient age, and obesity. Cigarette smoking is the single most important factor in the genesis of airflow obstruction. This, coupled with bronchial epithelial abnormalities and eventually chronic cough with phlegm production, results in an increased incidence of postoperative pulmonary complications. Patients with chronic obstructive pulmonary disease have reduced forced vital capacity (FVC) and forced expiratory volume in 1 second (FEV_1). These two changes in lung function have also been associated with increased postoperative pulmonary complications. Patients with poorly controlled asthma have a greater risk of postoperative problems related to bronchospasm and atelectasis. A complete history and physical examination combined with pulmonary function and arterial blood gas studies provide the information necessary for the consultant to formulate a management strategy. An FVC lower than 70 per cent of predicted and a partial pressure of carbon dioxide (Pco_2) greater than 45 mm Hg are important predictors of significant postoperative pulmonary complications.

Cessation of cigarette smoking should begin as soon as possible prior to surgery. Six to eight weeks is the minimal time for a significant physiologic improvement in pulmonary function to occur following the cessation of smoking. Patients with chronic bronchitis, cough, or phlegm production related to infection should receive a course of antibiotics 10 to 14 days prior to the procedure. Patients with chronic obstructive pulmonary disease (COPD) and decreased FVC and FEV_1, in addition to any of the problems described earlier, should have aggressive chest physical therapy and incentive spirometry following surgery. Patients with asthma or COPD who are taking bronchodilators, steroids, or beta-adrenergic agonists should be maintained on these medications until the day of surgery. During the immediate postoperative period, these drugs should be given via the parenteral and/or aerosol route.

Seizure Disorder

All surgical candidates who have a seizure disorder should be evaluated and classified with respect to control of their seizures. The major issues for the medical consultant are the history of seizure activity and the types of medications currently being used for control. Contributing factors are sought for the patient with a poorly controlled seizure disorder, such as noncompliance with drug therapy, alcohol use, and/or intercurrent illness. The critical periods for seizure activity during anesthesia are stage I (excitation) and stage II (delirium). Patients with a poorly controlled seizure disorder are at greatest risk at these times.

The assessment of the effects of anticonvulsant medication should include a complete blood count, creatinine, liver function tests, and an anticonvulsant drug concentration in the serum. There are about six frequently used anticonvulsant medications, but only phenytoin and phenobarbital are available in parenteral forms for perioperative administration. Phenytoin is given in a loading dose of 15 to 18 mg/kg intravenously and 4 to 8 mg/kg per day in divided doses for maintenance. It must be administered in saline solution, at a rate no faster than 50 mg per minute. This dosage avoids the risk of hypotension and asystole. Phenobarbital is given in a loading dose of 2 to 6 mg/kg and 1 to 5 mg/kg per day in divided doses for maintenance. This drug can be given intramuscularly or intravenously. Patients with head trauma (penetrating or contusion), brain tumors, and brain abscesses should receive seizure prophylaxis with phenytoin perioperatively and for at least 3 months postoperatively.

Prophylaxis for Deep Vein Thrombosis (DVT) and Pulmonary Embolism (PE)

After assessing the postoperative risks for deep vein thrombosis (DVT) and/or pulmonary embolism (PE) (see Table 3), the consultant may elect to institute prophylaxis to reduce the probability of occurrence of this potentially lethal complication. Fortunately, many options for prophylaxis are available, depending on the surgical procedure (Table 5).

TEN COMMANDMENTS OF PERIOPERATIVE CONSULTATION

I. Respond Promptly

When a request for a consultation is received by the medical consultant, it is the consultant's responsibility to complete this request in a timely fashion. If circumstances should arise that preclude completion of the consultation,

Table 5. Prophylaxis for Deep Vein Thrombosis and Pulmonary Embolism

Surgical Procedure	Prophylaxis
General surgery	LDH, EPCS
Orthopedic surgery	
Total hip replacement	Enoxaparin, warfarin, EPCS, ALDH
Fractured hip	Warfarin, enoxaparin, ALDH
Total knee replacement	Enoxaparin, warfarin, EPCS
Spinal cord injury	LDH, EPCS
Gynecologic surgery	LDH, EPCS, combination
Urologic surgery	LDH, EPCS, combination
Neurosurgery	EPCS, LDH

LDH = low-dose heparin 5000 U subcutaneously every 8–12 hr.
EPCS = external pneumatic compression sleeves.
ALDH = adjusted low-dose heparin.
Enoxaparin = low-molecular-weight heparin 30 mg subcutaneously every 12 hr.

the consultant must notify the requesting surgeon in ample time for another consultant to complete the task.

II. Focus the Consultation

The consultant should focus initially on those issues that the requesting physician has indicated. Sometimes the request for consultation is not clear. Communication with the surgeon or house officer is important for defining the reason for the consultation.

III. Assess the Case Completely

A complete history, physical examination, assessment of pertinent laboratory tests, and review of appropriate medical records must be provided. The consultant is responsible for acquiring, reviewing, and documenting all data relevant to the consultation.

IV. Summarize the Problems

All the pertinent medical problems must be identified with respect to their current status and perioperative management.

V. Identify New Problems

New problems or diagnoses discovered by the consultant must be brought to the attention of the requesting physician.

VI. Provide a Management Plan

The management plan should be concise, with the therapeutic approach clearly defined. Unnecessarily lengthy plans will not be read or followed by the requesting physician. Options and alternatives for management should be offered so that the requesting physician does not feel bound to follow one single management plan.

VII. Document Clearly

The consultant must provide clear documentation of the plan in the record for the requesting physician. Verbal communication with the surgeon and/or house officer improves the likelihood that the therapeutic plan will be followed.

VIII. Provide Follow-Up Consultation

Follow-up care focuses on the medical problems identified in the preoperative evaluation. This follow-up may include investigation of abnormal laboratory results, medication adjustment, or assessment of new problems. When the care of the patient is completed during the postoperative period, the consultant should document this fact in the medical record.

IX. Communicate Frequently

The consultant must develop a rapport with the requesting surgeon in order to define the patient care responsibilities during the perioperative period. This relationship will define the role as pure consultant or co-manager, with its associated order-writing, test-ordering, and day-to-day care.

X. Teach

The requesting physician will appreciate a consultant who provides insightful information concerning the management of the patient. This communication should be done tactfully and without condescension.

ANEMIA

By Jeanna L. Welborn, M.D.
Sacramento, California

Anemia is a manifestation of an underlying disorder, and the selection of appropriate treatment requires identification of this underlying cause. The procedures necessary for defining the precise etiology can be determined by reviewing three parameters that are available from a routine hemogram: the size of the red blood cells, the reticulocyte count, and the presence or absence of pancytopenia. Classifying the anemia as microcytic, normocytic, or macrocytic obviates the memorization of a long list of possible etiologies and, rather, focuses the clinical evaluation in a direct and cost-effective manner. An appropriately elevated reticulocyte count assesses the marrow response to the anemia and distinguishes a hemolytic, or blood loss, mechanism from bone marrow dysfunction. The presence of pancytopenia suggests disorders distinctly different from those that result in a simple deficiency of hemoglobin. Based on these three parameters, a protocol for the evaluation of anemia can accurately and easily determine the cause of the anemia with few additional tests.

HISTORY

Symptoms may be absent if the anemia has developed over a length of time sufficient to permit physiologic adaptation to a low hemoglobin concentration. A precipitious decrease in hemoglobin concentration may be manifested by pallor, weakness, and circulatory collapse. Older patients may complain of angina or symptoms of congestive heart failure, and these may be the presenting symptoms. The medical history should include questions about bleeding from the gastrointestinal tract or other sites. The family history should include questions regarding relatives with anemia or jaundice. Jaundice suggests hereditary hemolytic disease. The early development of gallstones in family members may also be due to a hemolytic disorder.

PHYSICAL EXAMINATION

The physical examination should specifically note pallor of the conjunctivae, mucous membranes, and nail beds; jaundice; lymphadenopathy; splenomegaly; glossitis; and evidence of peripheral neuropathy or loss of vibration and position sense (posterior column disease). These findings may point the way to hemolytic disease, neoplastic processes, or vitamin B_{12} or folate deficiencies.

MICROCYTIC ANEMIAS

Microcytic anemia is defined as the presence of anemia with a mean corpuscular volume (MCV) of less than 80 fL (Fig. 1). If pancytopenia is present, a bone marrow aspirate and biopsy are required to diagnose leukemia, marrow fibrosis or infiltration, marrow aplasia due to drug-induced marrow suppression, or aplastic anemia. If the platelet count and white blood cell count (WBC) with differential are in the normal range, the reticulocyte count will determine whether the marrow is responding appropriately. An increased reticulocyte count is seen in anemias due to shortened red blood cell survival, whereas an inappropriately normal to low reticulocyte count occurs in anemias due to impaired marrow erythropoiesis. The physician can find distinctive morphologic features by reviewing the peripheral blood smear. Hemoglobinopathies are associated with microcytosis with polychromasia, target cells, and minor anisopoikilocytosis. The degree of anisopoikilocytosis, indicated by the red blood cell distribution width (RDW) on the hemogram, is increased in iron deficiency and normal in thalassemia. The diagnosis of a hemoglobinopathy is confirmed by hemoglobin electrophoresis, which shows elevated fetal and A_2 hemoglobins in beta-thalassemia. Alpha-thalassemia has a normal hemoglobin electrophoretic pattern and is a diagnosis of exclusion supported by a family history of Asian extraction in the presence of normal iron body stores (see the article on the thalassemias).

A normal or low reticulocyte count in a patient with microcytosis, hypochromia, marked anisopoikilocytosis, and mild thrombocytosis suggests iron deficiency anemia (see the article on iron deficiency anemia). If the patient does not have liver disease, a chronic infection, inflammatory condition, or malignancy, then a serum ferritin level lower than 10 μg/L is compatible with iron deficiency. The serum ferritin is an acute phase reactant that is synthesized in the liver and is increased in a variety of chronic diseases. In the presence of chronic disease, a serum ferritin level lower than 50 μg/L is suggestive of iron deficiency. Normal or increased serum ferritin concentrations are seen in anemia of chronic disease and sideroblastic anemia, which can be associated with microcytic red blood cells. Sideroblastic anemia is an acquired disorder that shows a dimorphic population of microcytic and normocytic red blood cells, and the marrow iron stain shows characteristic ringed sideroblasts (see the article on myelodysplastic syndrome and sideroblastic anemia). A bone marrow aspirate stained for iron remains the gold standard for confirming the absence of iron in iron deficiency. The presence of iron in the reticuloendothelial system (RES) and its absence in red blood cell precursors is diagnostic of anemia of chronic disease.

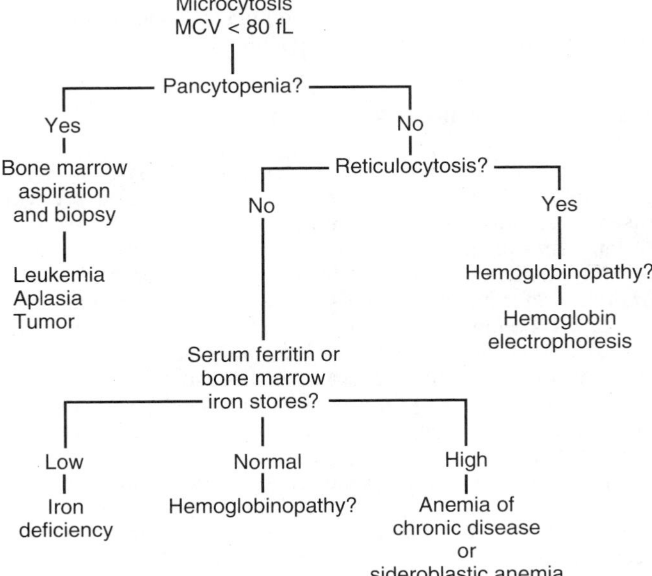

Figure 1. Algorithm for the evaluation of a microcytic anemia.

NORMOCYTIC ANEMIA

Normocytic anemia with an MCV of 80 to 100 fL is the most common type of anemia encountered and encompasses diverse etiologies (Fig. 2). When pancytopenia is present, a careful evaluation for splenomegaly, which results in the sequestration of normally circulating blood cells, and a bone marrow aspirate and biopsy are required to detect primary marrow disease, such as fibrosis, or infiltrative disease, leukemia, or aplasia. In patients with a normal platelet count and WBC with differential, a reticulocyte count differentiates a hypoproliferative marrow with a low reticulocyte count from an appropriate marrow response with an increased reticulocyte count.

An absolute reticulocyte count greater than 100,000 cells/μL or a corrected reticulocyte index greater than 1.0 is the appropriate marrow response to acute blood loss, hemolysis, or hypersplenism and may be present within 1 day of onset. Hemolytic anemias are commonly due to Coombs' test–positive or other immune-mediated mechanisms, fragmentation, acute infections, drugs, or hereditary red blood cell enzyme deficiencies (see the articles on acquired hemolytic anemia and hemolytic anemias due to erythrocyte enzyme deficiency). The peripheral blood smear shows polychromasia and spherocytes in the immune hemolytic anemias. Schistocytes and helmet cells are seen in the fragmentation syndromes, such as disseminated intravascular coagulation, and intracellular organisms or Döhle's bodies are present in white blood cells in acute infections (see the article on bleeding due to intravascular coagulation and fibrinolysis).

A normal or low reticulocyte count is inappropriate in any patient with anemia and indicates marrow dysfunction or impairment. Renal insufficiency with a creatinine clearance of less than 30 mL per minute is the most common cause of a mild normocytic anemia with a hemoglobin in the range of 8 to 10 gm/dL (see the article on chronic renal failure). There is a linear relationship between decreasing renal function and lack of the hormone erythropoietin, which is synthesized in the kidney and directly stimulates red blood cell production by the marrow. A low serum erythropoietin concentration is diagnostic, and patients will respond to therapeutic erythropoietin administration

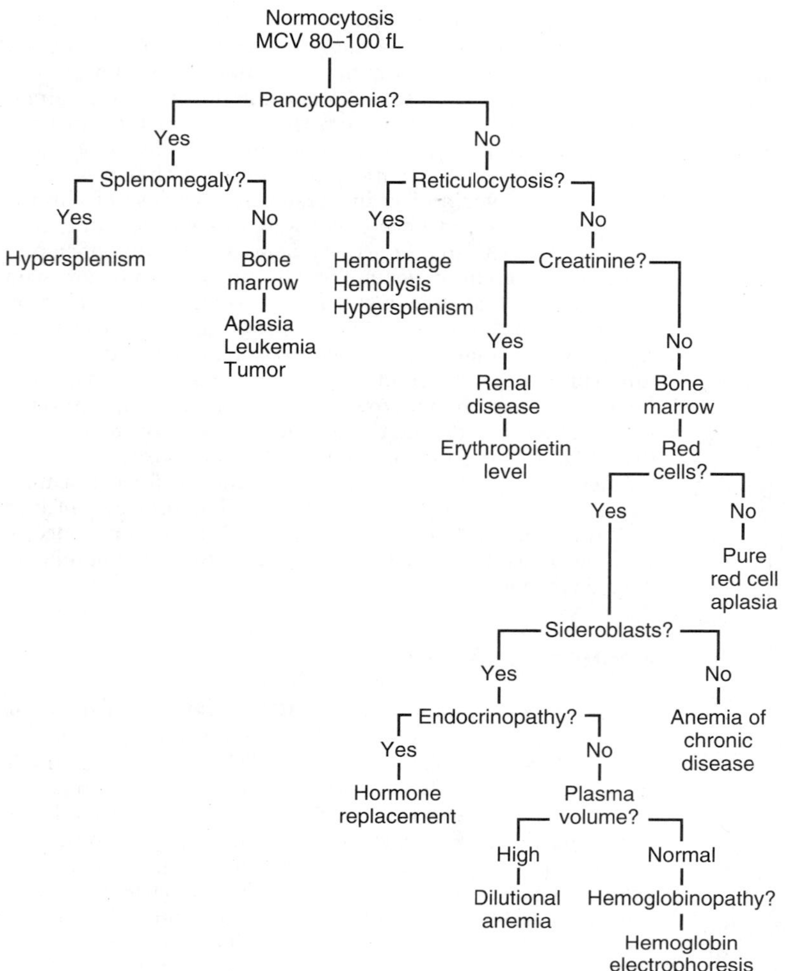

Figure 2. Algorithm for the evaluation of a normocytic anemia.

within 1 to 2 weeks. Other endocrinopathies, such as thyroid, adrenal, and pituitary hypofunction, result in hypoproliferative marrow and a mild normocytic anemia until adequate hormone replacement is achieved. In the presence of normal renal and endocrine function, a bone marrow aspirate is required to evaluate the patient for a primary hematopoietic disease. Occasionally, red blood cell precursors are singularly absent from the marrow aspirate. This condition is diagnostic of pure red blood cell aplasia, which may be primary or may be associated with autoimmune disorders, drugs, and infectious agents such as parvovirus. The marrow aspirate should always be stained with Prussian blue to assess iron stores. The anemia of chronic disease is characterized by adequate iron stores in the marrow reticuloendothelial cells but an absence of iron in the developing red blood cell precursors. Iron utilization by the red blood cells is blocked by the action of cytokines that are increased in states of chronic infection, inflammation, or malignancy. A bone marrow aspirate is usually not necessary in a patient with mild anemia and an obvious reason for anemia of chronic disease. The hemoglobin is in the range of 10 gm/dL, unless complicated by another condition, and does not generally require intervention. Rarely, an increased plasma volume results in a spurious anemia because of dilution and typically is seen in Waldenström's macroglobulinemia, myeloma, pregnancy, or conditions of fluid overload.

When a patient with a normocytic anemia has a normal reticulocyte count and a normal marrow aspirate with adequate iron stores and sideroblasts and without pancytopenia, the physician should investigate for the presence of a hemoglobinopathy by reviewing the family history and ethnic origin and by performing hemoglobin electrophoresis (see the article on hemoglobinopathies).

MACROCYTIC ANEMIAS

Macrocytic anemias are characterized by an MCV greater than 100 fL and almost always are due to liver disease, alcoholism, or drugs and less commonly are due to leukemia or megaloblastosis secondary to folate or vitamin B_{12} deficiency (Fig. 3) (see the article on pernicious anemia and other megaloblastic anemias). The reticulocyte count will be low or normal, and the peripheral smear will show distinctive morphologic abnormalities. Round macrocytes and target cells suggest liver disease and alcoholism, whereas oval macrocytes, marked anisopoikilocytosis, hypersegmented neutrophils, and pancytopenia are the hallmarks of a megaloblastic anemia. The platelet count may be mildly depressed in patients with alcoholism or liver disease but is generally greater than 50,000 cells/mm^3.

Reticulocytes are larger than mature erythrocytes, and occasionally a significant reticulocytosis will increase the MCV, which is easily detected on the peripheral blood smear by marked polychromasia and is confirmed by a

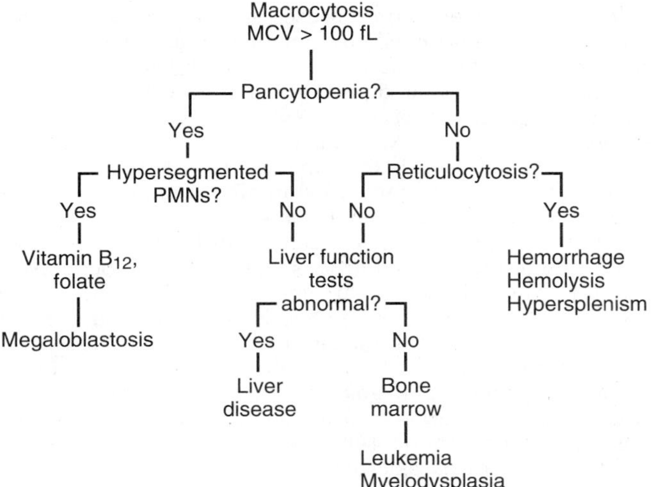

Figure 3. Algorithm for the evaluation of a macrocytic anemia.

reticulocyte count. The peripheral smear in leukemia or myelodysplastic syndromes may reveal anisopoikilocytosis, atypical neutrophils, and generally decreased WBC and platelet counts. A bone marrow aspirate shows impaired maturation involving all three cell lines, and more than half of the patients will have abnormal cytogenetic studies, which is diagnostic of a malignancy (see the articles on the leukemias).

Hospitalized patients or patients with several disease processes may have an anemia that is multifactorial in etiology. Repeated phlebotomy for laboratory tests, shortened red blood cell survival due to infections, and suppression of normal erythropoiesis by drugs, liver and renal impairment, or nutritional deficiencies all may contribute to the development of a complex anemia. A review of the peripheral blood smear generally shows nonspecific morphology and an inappropriately low reticulocyte count. Serum iron studies and serum ferritin concentrations may be uninterpretable because they are acute phase reactants and may be artifactually altered. When the etiology of the anemia is important to the overall medical care during the acute illness, a bone marrow aspirate with a Prussian blue iron stain is necessary to differentiate iron deficiency, chronic disease, or marrow suppression as the primary cause of the anemic state.

GENETIC DISEASE

By Hilary Worthen, M.D.
Cambridge, Massachusetts
and Susan Pauker, M.D.
Boston, Massachusetts

Although the famous comment by Victor McKusick that all of medicine is genetics may be an overstatement, it seems more credible with each issue of the major medical journals. Basic research, spurred on by the Human Genome Project, is uncovering the genetic mechanisms of disease at an accelerating pace, and physicians unfamiliar with genetics are finding themselves incorporating more genetic responsibilities into their practices. Most of these are variations on the traditional activities of primary care, ranging from *patient education* (e.g., the use of folate for the prevention of neural tube defects) through *screening* (e.g., carrier detection for Tay-Sachs or cystic fibrosis, or evaluation of relatives of patients with familial hypercholesterolemia), *diagnosis* (e.g., a patient with seizures due to neurofibromatosis), *surveillance for complications* (e.g., monitoring aortic root expansion in a patient with Marfan's syndrome or renal cyst size in a patient with von Hippel–Lindau disease), *treatment* (e.g., excision of suspicious dysplastic nevi), and *counseling* (e.g., a couple concerned about the risk of recurrence of cleft palate in a second child). As primary care physicians, under managed care, increasingly play the role of gatekeeper and coordinator for all medical services, patients and families with genetic problems will rely more frequently on them for diagnosis, treatment, and referral.

In January 1995, the American Society of Human Genetics recommended a Core Curriculum in genetics, listing 51 objectives in the areas of knowledge, skills, and attitudes. However, as recently as 1988, nearly half of all medical schools had inadequate or nonexistent teaching in genetics, and few continuing education courses have filled the gap. Thus, physicians who finished medical school before 1985 have had few opportunities to master these areas, yet they provide most of the clinical care for patients. Because approximately 1000 board-certified clinical medical geneticists and more than 800 board-certified genetic counselors remain unevenly distributed throughout the United States, primary care physicians will most likely play a continuing and expanding role in the care of genetic disorders. Unfortunately, however, the incorporation of genetic information into clinical practice poses formidable challenges (Table 1).

The fatalism that often accompanies the diagnosis of genetic disorders continues to influence clinical practice: Why diagnose an untreatable disorder? The history of medicine suggests that our understanding of genetic disorders is at the point where diagnosis is possible, but treatment is not highly developed. This situation creates ethical dilemmas that will eventually be resolved as treatment improves. Gene therapy offers promise, but advances in more traditional methods of treatment have contributed the most to the care of patients with genetic diseases.

GENETIC DISEASE AND GENETIC DIAGNOSIS

How is genetic disease defined? Strictly speaking, genetic disorders are disorders caused partly or entirely by

Table 1. Deterrents to Incorporating Genetic Concepts Into Practice

Arcane terminology drawn from diverse disciplines, multiple naming conventions
Enormous scale of the genome, myriad of types of mutations
Vast number of individually rare disorders
Skepticism about genetic determinism and legacy of eugenics movement
Genetic disorders' aura of immutability
"Syndromology" approach requiring knowledge of a plethora of anomalies
Lack of adequate teaching programs in medical schools and thereafter
Unfamiliarity with computerized and print resources
Rapid explosion of information in genetics

alterations of DNA. This definition, however, encompasses nearly every condition except trauma, since most disorders have at least some genetic contribution to susceptibility. Diseases are traditionally classified by organ system, as are the subspecialties of medicine, and genetic diseases, with the exception of inborn errors of metabolism, are generally categorized under the organ system most affected. What all genetic disorders share is their etiology in DNA, with its implications for heritability, permanence, and, up to now, imperviousness to intervention. As an etiologic category, then, genetic disease includes disorders customarily considered under almost every other grouping of diseases.

Of what benefit is recognizing and identifying the genetic basis of a disease? The most obvious benefit is the identification of other people at risk, such as siblings and unborn children. Second, the degree to which a diagnosis can support a prognosis and the choice of therapy or further workup depends on comparison of the case with a group of others who have the same disease, in whom the natural history, response to treatment, and results of testing have been observed. The more homogeneous that group, and the more the case resembles it, the stronger the predictive power of the diagnosis. Diagnosis at the genetic level can be much more specific than organ system, histopathologic, or pathophysiologic diagnosis. For example, in familial hypertrophic cardiomyopathy, different mutations in the cardiac beta-myosin heavy chain gene produce identical echocardiographic findings but widely different predispositions to sudden death.

What, then, is a complete genetic diagnosis? Theoretically, it would specify the disorder, its mode of occurrence or inheritance, the affected gene or genes, the exact mutation involved, key modifying genes, and any important environmental factors. In practice, this is currently possible for very few disorders and is probably not required in most situations. It is important, however, for the clinician to be aware of the limitations of working with a less than fully specific diagnosis and of the situations in which a more specific diagnosis is possible.

SCOPE AND VARIABILITY OF THE GENOME

The vast number of known genetic disorders present an astonishing degree of clinical variation. This diversity is not surprising, since the 60,000 to 100,000 genes in the human genome all are subject to numerous types of mutations. McKusick's *Mendelian Inheritance in Man* lists more than 6500 loci known to be inherited in mendelian fashion. Most of these loci are associated with at least one disorder. Patterns of inheritance as well as clinical, pathologic, biochemical, and cytogenetic features permit genetic diseases to be organized into major categories (see later), yet within these categories, many diseases still exhibit substantial variation in inheritance, features, and clinical course. This variation has been described with terms such as pleiotropy, heterogeneity, penetrance, and expression. As advances in cytogenetics and molecular genetics have illuminated the molecular basis of genetic disorders, the mechanisms of this variation have become clearer. An appreciation of the scope and nature of this variation is important for the clinician whose patient may have one of a vast array of disorders that even the most experienced geneticist may never have seen.

FREQUENCY OF GENETIC DISEASE

It is difficult to imagine a disease, with the possible exception of trauma, in which genetics does not play some role. At one extreme are diseases such as achondroplasia, which is caused primarily by genetic alterations with minimal environmental contribution. At the other extreme are diseases such as polio, diphtheria, and scurvy, to which all humans are "genetically susceptible." With these latter disorders, however, environmental factors strongly influence which individuals are affected. In between are most other disorders, determined by an often complex interplay of genetic variation and environmental factors.

The incidence of genetic disease can be estimated from surveys that differ in definitions, approach, and population studied. There is some agreement that the incidence of significant congenital anomalies is between 3 and 4 per cent of live births, the incidence of single gene disorders (including late-onset disorders) about 1 per cent, and that of major chromosomal abnormalities about 0.6 per cent. Multifactorial disorders, or those with a combination of genetic and environmental causes, constitute some of the most common diseases (Table 2).

Prior to birth, the toll of genetic errors is even greater. About 15 to 20 per cent of recognized pregnancies (and 50 per cent of all conceptions) end in miscarriage; in early spontaneous abortion, the rate of chromosomal abnormalities exceeds 60 per cent. Many chromosomal disorders associated with occasional survival lead much more frequently to spontaneous abortion. Turner's syndrome (45,X), for example, is 150 times more frequent among miscarried fetuses than among liveborns. Between 6 and 7 per cent of stillbirths and neonatal deaths have a chromosome abnormality. Thus, only a small fraction of zygotes with chromosome abnormalities survive to be born.

The prevalence of genetic disease in medical patients is considerably higher than in the general population. As a percentage of those who visit physicians or those admitted to a hospital, the incidence of genetic disease is even higher. Between 30 and 50 per cent of pediatric admissions are due wholly or in part to genetically determined disorders, and about 10 per cent of adult admissions are due to genetic disease. These statistics have not escaped the attention of the insurance industry, which frequently denies coverage to patients suspected of having a genetic disorder.

Most chromosomal disorders and single gene disorders are diagnosed during the first year of life, but some are diagnosed in childhood and adolescence as developmental abnormalities manifest themselves. Disorders with a delayed age at onset, including many neurodegenerative disorders, may first come to the attention of the primary care physician. The adult with a previously diagnosed genetic disorder may also present with a new manifestation, and new information may require a revision of a previous diagnosis. Genetic disease, then, must be a diagnostic concern for physicians who deal with any age group.

MOLECULAR BASIS OF GENETIC DISEASE

Knowledge of the normal and morbid anatomy of the genome is required for understanding how aberrations in

Table 2. Genetic Contribution to Common Disorders

Example	Affected in U.S.	Genetic Component (%)
Obesity	20 million	60–90
Type II diabetes	13 million	70–95
Asthma	10 million	50–75
Rheumatoid arthritis	4 million	30–50
Coronary artery disease	400,000 (per yr)	30–50

DNA sequence occur, produce disease, and are passed on to progeny. The human genome consists of about 3.5×10^9 base pairs of DNA organized into 23 chromosomes (22 autosomes and the sex chromosome). Only about 3 to 5 per cent of this DNA serves a coding function, the rest being intergenic "junk" DNA or intragenic noncoding segments *(introns)*. Each *diploid cell* has two copies of each autosomal chromosome and two sex chromosomes.

During cell division, this entire complement of DNA is replicated so that each daughter cell receives a copy. In *mitosis*, the resulting cells have two copies of each chromosome, like the parent cell. In the special case of *meiosis*, two cell divisions reduce the chromosome complement to a single copy of each, creating a *haploid germ cell,* or gamete. *Crossing over*, or the exchange of *homologous* (corresponding) *parts* between chromosomes during cell division, is responsible for the mixing of genes that otherwise would travel through cell divisions together because of their location on the same chromosome. It is thought that most mutations occur during these processes of replication (Fig. 1).

The effects of mutations, however, are the result of alterations in *gene expression*. A gene, which is the segment of DNA needed for *transcription* of a messenger RNA (mRNA) molecule and which, with some exceptions, leads to *translation* into a protein, has a complex structure (Fig. 2).

The segments of DNA that actually code for polypeptide sequences, *exons*, are separated by intervening sequences called *introns*. Outside the exons and introns lie *regulatory regions,* where sequences such as *promoters* and *enhancers* control the transcription process. The initial mRNA copy, or *primary transcript*, which includes all the exons and introns, undergoes further processing: It is capped at one end, gets a tail at the other, and has the RNA representing the introns spliced out. The *splice sites* are marked with particular sequences, and the same gene product may be spliced differently in different tissues or phases of development *(alternative splicing)*. On completion of this process, the *mature transcript* leaves the nucleus, to be translated into protein in the cytoplasm.

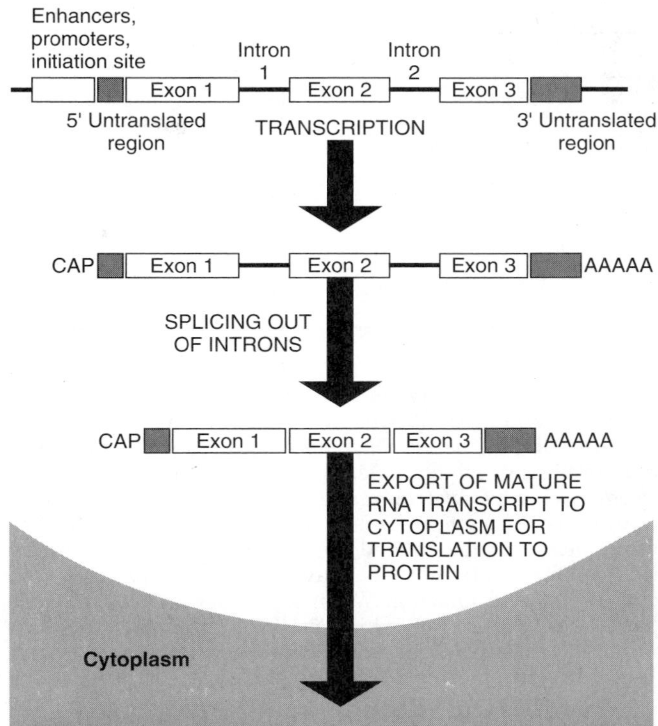

Figure 2. Gene structure and expression. A schematic diagram of a gene, showing enhancers and promoter regions before the transcription initiation site at the 5′ end of the gene, three exons and two introns, and the untranslated regions at both ends. For gene expression, the genetic code is transcribed from DNA to RNA, which is then processed by the addition of a cap and tail and splicing out of introns before it is ready to move to the cytoplasm, where it will be translated into protein in the ribosomes.

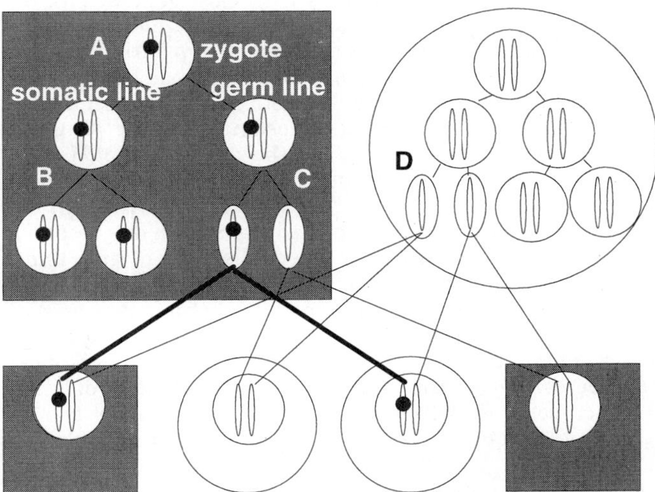

Figure 1. Occurrence and inheritance of mutations. The black dot and the shaded pedigree figures indicate the inheritance of an autosomal dominant single gene disorder. For clarity, only one chromosome pair is shown. In this case, the mutation was present in the father as a zygote (A) and is passed to two of his four offspring, as well as all of his own somatic cells. If a new mutation were to occur at B during mitosis of somatic cells, a clonal somatic cell disorder could result. In cases of autosomal dominant disease in which no parent is affected, a new mutation is likely to have occurred at C (spermatogenesis). Most chromosomal mutations seem to happen through nondisjunction events, at D (oogenesis).

Types of Mutation

Mutations, or changes in DNA sequence, can occur at many points in replication and affect any aspect of gene expression or protein sequence.

Mutations comprise three broad categories, depending on the scale: genomic, chromosomal, and gene (Table 3). *Genomic mutations* result in a loss or gain of an entire set of chromosomes. Since these mutations are not compatible with life, they are not discussed further here. *Chromosomal mutations* include *numerical* aberrations (*aneuploidy*) and *structural rearrangements,* such as *translocation* of segments between chromosomes or changes within a chromosome such as deletions, duplications, and inversions. With the exception of *balanced translocations*, in which the total amount of DNA is preserved but in the wrong location, chromosomal mutations involve the loss or gain of large numbers of genes and are generally associated with fetal loss or severe and multiple congenital anomalies. Chromosomal mutations are discussed in detail elsewhere in this volume. Most of the following discussion focuses on *gene mutations* that involve a single gene and are the molecular basis of disorders inherited in a mendelian pattern (see later).

The function of a gene can be altered in various ways. An entire gene can be *deleted,* as in most cases of alpha-

Table 3. Categories of Mutations

Category	Definition	Examples
Genomic	Gain or loss of entire set of chromosomes	Triploidy, tetraploidy
Chromosomal	Aberrations in number or structure of chromosomes, on a scale detectable with cytogenetic techniques	Number: (aneuploidy) Monosomy, trisomy Structure: Deletions Duplications Rearrangements
Gene	Aberrations on the scale of a gene or part of a gene	Deletions, duplications, insertions, point mutations, fusion genes

thalassemia, probably because of misalignment and *unequal crossing over* during replication. A part of a gene can be deleted, as in Duchenne and Becker's muscular dystrophies, in which at least two preferential "hot spots" in the enormous dystrophin gene seem predisposed to such mutations. A *codon,* or set of three bases that code for one amino acid, can be deleted, as in the most common mutation causing cystic fibrosis, leaving a protein product with one amino acid missing. When a deletion affects multiple bases, the number of which is not a multiple of 3 (the number of "letters" in each "word" of the genetic code specifying an amino acid), the result is a disruption of the *reading frame*, which can change the meaning of all the codons further along the gene. Such *frameshift mutations* often cause severe effects because the radically altered protein product is truncated or unstable and rapidly degraded.

The same process that leads to deletions can result in duplication and insertion of all or part of a gene. When this disrupts the reading frame, the consequences may be severe. At least one disease (Charcot-Marie-Tooth disease type I) is due to the complete duplication of a gene, resulting in a triple dose of the gene product.

Point mutations, the simple substitution of one base for another, may change the meaning of a codon to specify another amino acid (a *missense* mutation) or a "stop" signal (a *nonsense mutation*). When the substituted amino acid is similar in charge and size to the original, or is not in a critical functional area *(domain)* of the gene, the effect can be minimal. When the new amino acid brings about a significant alteration in characteristics of the protein, however, as in sickle cell anemia, or leads to a truncated or unstable product, as in common forms of beta-thalassemia and hemophilia A, the clinical effects can be severe.

The rate of mutation in humans has been estimated at 10^{-6} per gene per cell division. Where mutations occur is clearly significant. Most involve "junk" DNA. These mutations are phenotypically silent but may serve as gene-tracking markers. Other mutations have neutral or minimal phenotypic effect. A rare mutation may offer some survival advantage, but most mutations that have any significant phenotypic effect disrupt the complex balance of the organism. The location of a mutation can determine what aspect of gene function it disrupts. Mutations in the regulatory regions cause an abnormal amount (usually less) of a normal gene product. Mutations in a stop codon can result in an elongated gene product. Mutations in sites that specify the boundaries of introns and exons can disrupt splicing and lead to a radically altered product. In general, mutations that affect the amino acid sequence of a protein account for 50 to 60 per cent of single gene disorders, while 40 to 50 per cent result from mutations that affect the quantity or timing of gene expression.

There is no sharp dividing line between chromosomal mutations that can be detected through cytogenetic techniques and gene mutations that are detected with the tools of molecular biology. The intermediate zone is occupied by the *contiguous gene syndromes,* in which a number of adjacent genes are affected. Because these genes may have little in common besides location, the resulting clinical syndromes can defy pathophysiologic analysis, as in the WAGR syndrome (Wilms' tumor, aniridia, genitourinary malformations, and mental retardation), caused by a deletion of multiple genes on the short arm of chromosome 11. In this regard, the development of *FISH* (fluorescent in situ hybridization) is rapidly closing the gap between cytogenetics and molecular genetics.

The expansion of *unstable trinucleotide repeat sequences* is a newly described mutation that has been implicated in at least 11 neurologic disorders, including Huntington's disease, myotonic dystrophy, and fragile X mental retardation. Because these segments of DNA made up of three bases repeated over and over become unstable in replication after a certain size, they can expand from one cell division to the next, leading to previously unexplainable clinical phenomena, such as *anticipation* (increasing severity and earlier onset of disease with each generation). *Imprinting* is a mutation thought to involve methylation of certain DNA sequences. The impact of imprinting on male gametogenesis may differ from that on female gametogenesis. Various mishaps of replication cause inappropriately imprinted genes or entire chromosomes, leading to underexpression or overexpression of the gene product. *Uniparental disomy,* a condition in which an individual has two copies of a chromosome but both copies derive from one parent, can lead to the unexpected expression of a recessive disorder in a child with only one carrier parent and, under some circumstances, can reveal the effects of imprinting. For example, although the clinically distinct Prader-Willi and Angelman syndromes are generally due to identical deletions in the same section of chromosome 15, they can also be caused by uniparental disomy without a deletion. In each case, Prader-Willi syndrome is caused by the absence of a paternal copy of the region, and Angelman's syndrome by the absence of a maternal copy. Finally, nondisjunction during mitosis can result in replacement of one allele by the other, leading to homozygosity at that location. When this *loss of heterozygosity* (LOH) produces a cell with two nonfunctional copies of a tumor suppressor gene, malignancy may ensue (see later).

Timing of Mutations

The timing of a mutation may influence its effect on a person and that person's progeny (see Fig. 1). Mutations may be *inherited* (carried by a parent and passed on to the offspring, as in most single gene disorders) or may occur *de novo*, that is, arising in a parental germ-line cell or in the developing embryo, as in most chromosomal mutations. Of course, all inherited mutations were once de novo. If a de novo mutation occurs during parental gamete formation, all the cells of the embryo will be affected. If it occurs *postzygotically* but very early, before the determination of the primordial *germ cells* (which are apparent during the fourth week), it may affect some of the cells of the individual, including germ cells, but not others. If a de novo mutation occurs in a *somatic cell* after the germ line has separated, it will affect the cells of the individual that are descendants of that somatic cell—but not the other cells—and will not be passed on to offspring. In this vein, many authorities believe that most—if not all—human cancers are caused by such somatic cell mutations in genes that regulate cell growth.

Mutations that occur in some intervals can thus give rise to an individual with two lines of cells: one with the mutation and one without. The condition of having multiple lines of cells that differ in their genetic constitution, called *mosaicism*, is emerging as an important phenomenon in genetic disease. Since female cells undergo random inactivation of one X chromosome (lyonization), all females are mosaics for those genes. This fact may explain, for example, the variable degree of impairment in female carriers of the fragile X gene. In de novo mutations, postzygotic occurrence usually leads to mosaicism, which may produce a milder or an unusual phenotype. For example, in McCune-Albright polyostotic fibrous dysplasia, only mosaics are viable, since the mutation is lethal even in heterozygous form when all cells are affected.

Causes of Mutation

Most mutations seem to occur during cell division. Chromosomal mutations are the result of *nondisjunction*, the failure of appropriate separation of paired chromosomes or chromatids. This failure can occur during meiosis, leading to a germ line disorder, or during mitosis, resulting in mosaicism or a somatic cell disorder. Smaller deletions and duplications may result from *unequal crossing over* due to misalignment of homologous regions during meiosis. The smallest mutations are probably copy errors that have escaped the mismatch repair mechanism. Although exposure to radiation and toxic chemicals can certainly cause mutation, and there is a background level of each to which humans are exposed, the contribution of environmental agents to the baseline rate of mutation in humans is difficult to assess. It is likely that other factors contribute to most of the mutations that lead to disease. Chromosomal mutations are more frequent with advancing maternal age; autoimmune processes and a tendency for inappropriate association of repeating sequences in the acrocentric chromosomes may contribute as well. New gene mutations seem to occur more frequently during spermatogenesis and are more frequent with advancing paternal age. This frequency may result from a fundamental difference in paternal and maternal gamete formation: By age 25 years, some 310 cell divisions have taken place in spermatogenesis, compared with 23 in oogenesis. Certain base sequences are inherently susceptible to copy errors (so-called mutational hot spots). Some environmental agents preferentially cause mutations in a particular location. For example, aflatoxin and hepatitis B cause different characteristic mutations of the p53 tumor suppressor gene, leading to hepatoma; ultraviolet light causes a unique mutation that results in squamous cell skin cancer; and tobacco smoke causes another set of typical mutations that lead to lung cancer. In addition, *transposons*, also known as *jumping genes*, are increasingly recognized as important causes of mutations. These mutations are segments of DNA that are capable of using the intracellular enzymatic machinery to excise themselves and reinsert themselves in other locations of the genome, resulting in various mutational effects.

MAJOR CATEGORIES OF GENETIC DISEASE

What sort of picture emerges clinically from this jigsaw puzzle of mutational possibilities? Genetic diseases are customarily divided into four major categories: *chromosomal disorders*, *single gene (mendelian) disorders*, *multifactorial disorders,* and *somatic cell disorders* (Table 4). Recently, the recognition of mitochondrial DNA and its maternal inheritance has added another category, *mitochondrial disorders,* and some would include *contiguous gene syndromes* as a sixth category. These disease categories have just enough correspondence to the categories of mutation to create confusion. While it is intuitive that chromosomal disorders are due to chromosomal mutations, and single gene disorders to gene mutations, the other categories are not as simple. Multifactorial disorders are due to the combined effects of multiple genes or to the effects of one or more genes plus environmental factors. Somatic cell disorders are defined by their timing: They are due to mutations that occur in a somatic cell after the differentiation of the germ line. Mitochondrial disorders are classified by their location in the extranuclear mitochondrial DNA and are characterized by the unique inheritance pattern that results. Contiguous gene syndromes are due to mutations large enough to affect several genes but not large enough to be detected by traditional cytogenetic methods. Although this classification may seem illogical, it is clinically very useful because it distinguishes groups that share many characteristics.

Chromosomal Disorders

Most chromosomal disorders represent new mutations that occur during the formation of the parental germ cells, generally through *nondisjunction* events, in which homologous pairs fail to separate in meiosis I or II. Although heritable in theory, most such mutations are not passed on because their severe effects preclude reproduction (i.e., they are *genetic lethals*). The exception to this, as mentioned earlier, is the balanced translocation.

Single Gene (Mendelian) Disorders

Mutations in a single gene may have effects that are incompatible with life, compatible with life but with phenotypic changes, neutral in clinical effect (a *polymorphism*), or even beneficial to adaptation. Although probably rare, these latter mutations form the basis of evolutionary change. Mutations that do not eliminate reproductive success may be passed on and inherited according to the patterns first described by Mendel in 1866. The classic patterns of mendelian inheritance in families should be familiar to every clinician and provide a framework for diagnosis as well as prognosis and prevention. The *family pedigree* is the format in which this pattern is elicited and recorded with the use of conventional symbols (Figs. 3 and 4).

Certain characteristics and pedigree patterns typify each of the major categories of disease inherited in mendelian fashion and are briefly described in Tables 5, 6, and 7 and

Table 4. Major Categories of Genetic Disease

Type	Explanation	Example
Chromsome	Caused by chromosome mutations	Down syndrome
Single gene (mendelian)	Caused by a mutation in a single gene, and inherited in mendelian patterns:	
	Autosomal dominant	Neurofibromatosis 1
	Autosomal recessive	Cystic fibrosis
	X-linked recessive	Fragile X retardation
	X-linked dominant	Hypophosphatemic rickets
	Y-linked	XY female with gonadal dysgenesis
Multifactorial	Caused by the interaction of more than one gene or the interaction of a gene or genes with environmental factors	Diabetes Hypertension Asthma
Somatic cell	Caused by a mutation occurring in a somatic cell and resulting in a clone of altered somatic cells	Neoplastic diseases Some localized congenital malformations
Contiguous gene	Caused by mutations large enough to affect more than one gene but too small to be visualized cytogenetically	WAGR syndrome Prader-Willi syndrome
Mitochondrial	Caused by mutations in the DNA of mitochondrial chromosomes	MELAS syndrome Leber's optic atrophy

MELAS syndrome = mitochondrial encephalopathy, lactic acidosis, and strokelike episodes; WAGR = Wilms' tumor, aniridia, genitourinary malformations, and mental retardation.

Figures 5, 6, and 7. Note that if the status of an adequate number of family members cannot be ascertained, it can be quite difficult to establish an inheritance pattern.

Although the basic mechanism of inheritance is the same for mutations that cause mendelian disorders, clinically these mutations are conveniently divided into *dominant* and *recessive categories,* according to whether one or two mutant copies of the gene are required to produce disease. Importantly, the terms "dominant" and "recessive" refer to the *effect* of an allele on the observable phenotype. Closer scrutiny of the genes that contribute to phenotype, however, reveals that most diseases involve *codominant mutations.* For example, partial enzyme deficiencies can be detected in clinically unaffected carriers of a single allele for a recessive disorder, such as Tay-Sachs disease. Conversely, many dominant disorders, such as achondroplasia and familial hypercholesterolemia, produce a more severe phenotype in the homozygous form. This condition is called *incomplete dominance*, suggesting that the normal allele substantially influences the phenotype of the heterozygote. Although the distinction between dominant and recessive blurs at the gene level, at the clinical level it remains an important distinction, since the patterns formed by affected individuals in a pedigree are quite different.

Autosomal dominant disorders (Table 5; Fig. 5) constitute 50 per cent of mendelian disorders and include many of the serious genetic diseases of adult life. Mutations that cause dominant disorders are frequently lost from the gene pool because even a single copy of the mutant allele often decreases the reproductive success of the affected individual. Since the overall frequency of these disorders is stable, new presentations of severe dominant disorders most likely represent new mutations, for example, in osteogenesis imperfecta. The high frequency of new mutations in dominant disorders means that in many, such as Marfan's syndrome or hypertrophic cardiomyopathy, different families have different mutations, a fact that complicates the development of a generally applicable direct DNA test for a mutation. Exceptions to this include late-onset disorders such as Huntington's disease, and "mutational hot spot" disorders, such as achondroplasia, in which specific base sequences seem especially prone to mutation. Autosomal dominant disorders may also frequently display *variable expressivity* (see later).

Recessive disorders (Table 6; Fig. 6) account for 40 per cent of mendelian disorders. They frequently result from mutations that affect the genes for enzymes. In more than one third of recessive disorders, a specific enzyme deficiency has been identified. In a particular population, most of the alleles for a recessive disorder will be found in clinically unaffected heterozygotes, with only a small pro-

Table 5. Characteristics of Autosomal Dominant Disorders

Vertical pedigree pattern (except for new mutations, every affected child has an affected parent)
Males and females equally affected
50% chance of transmitting disorder to each offspring
Male-to-male transmission may be present
High frequency of new mutations in diseases that reduce reproduction
Frequently involve structural proteins
Incomplete penetrance can make cases look sporadic
New mutations show some association with advanced paternal age

Table 6. Characteristics of Autosomal Recessive Disorders

Horizontal pedigree pattern (siblings affected but not parents)
Males and females equally affected
Each offspring of two heterozygous carriers has
25% chance of being homozygous affected
50% chance of being heterozygous carrier
25% chance of being homozygous unaffected
Increased frequency with consanguinity
Clustering of specific disorders within ethnic groups
Enzymes and peptide hormones frequently affected
Small family size can make many cases look sporadic
Offspring of affected (homozygous) parent are heterozygous, unless other parent carries affected allele

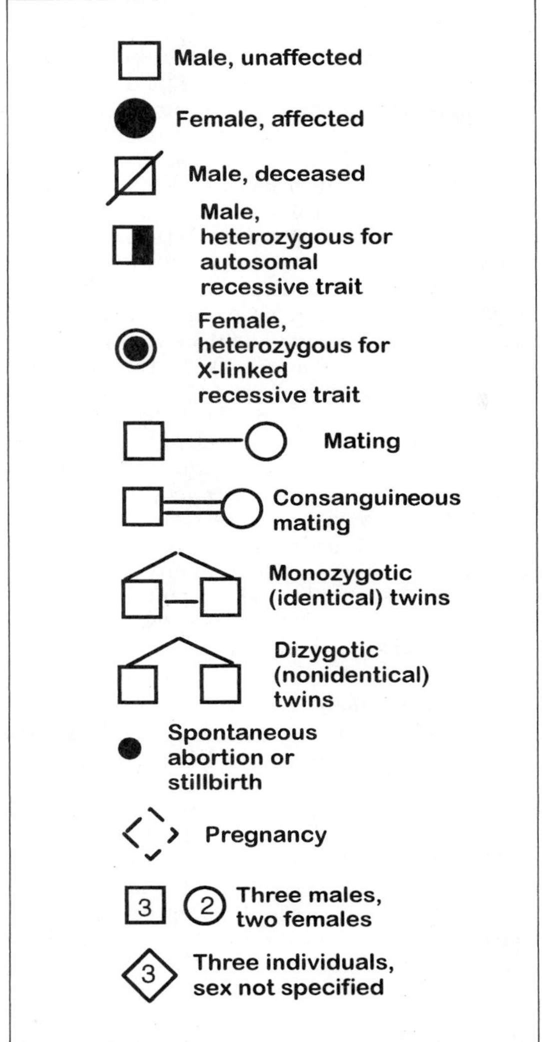

Figure 3. Standard symbols for recording pedigrees.

portion found in homozygotes (the *Hardy-Weinberg equation* is used to describe the specific ratio). Therefore, a mutation can easily be passed on and may even increase in frequency when the population is expanding, or when the mutation offers some advantage to heterozygotes. Consistent with this is the fact that most recessive disorders result from inherited rather than new mutations, cluster in certain ethnic groups, and are more likely to emerge in the setting of *consanguinity.*

A distinctive pedigree pattern occurs when mutations affect genes on the X or Y chromosome (Table 7; Fig. 7). Because the small Y chromosome renders males essentially *hemizygous* for large parts of the X chromosome, mutations in the areas that act recessively in females will be dominant in males (although lyonization may modify this pattern, as noted earlier). Also, since males pass their X chromosome to their daughters and their Y chromosome to their sons, there is no male-to-male transmission of X-linked traits. These two concepts explain the pedigree patterns of X-linked recessive and the rarer X-linked dominant disorders, which together make up 10 per cent of mendelian disorders. Y-linked disorders, due to mutations

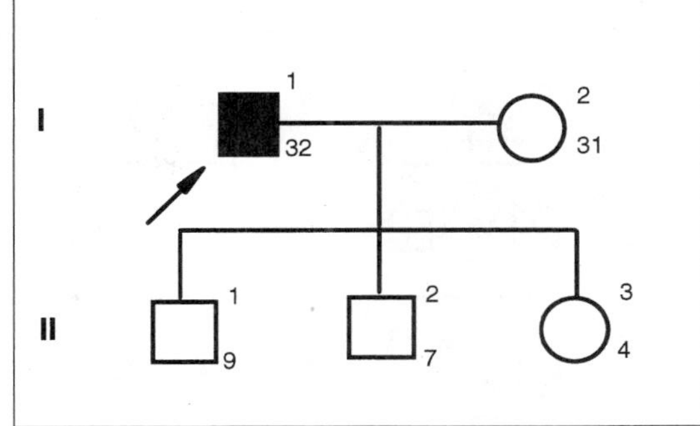

Figure 4. Explanation of pedigree diagram. The generations are designated with Roman numerals, the individuals within generations with Arabic numerals. In this pedigree, the father, 32 years old, is the affected proband *(arrow).* His wife, age 31 years, and his two sons and one daughter, ages 9, 7, and 4 years, are unaffected.

in the small, sex-determining section of the Y chromosome, are extremely rare.

The manifestations of genetic disease are often extremely variable, particularly for autosomal dominant disorders. Some of this variability is the result of *genetic heterogeneity,* or multiple genetic causes: What appears clinically to be a single but variable disease is really a reflection of mutations in different genes *(locus heterogeneity)* or different mutations in one gene *(allelic* heterogeneity, forming an *allelic series).* Heterogeneity is particularly probable if the variability is between unrelated families.

When the variability is also intrafamilial, in which case it may be presumed that the underlying mutation is the same for all members, the complexity of the relationship of the genotype to the phenotype, and the influence of other factors on the ultimate clinical expression of a change in DNA, become readily apparent. These factors are thought to include the presence of major modifier genes, minor variations in the corresponding normal allele, minor variations in the disease allele that normally would have no effect, the polygenic background, and environmental factors. This variability in the degree of severity of manifestations of a disorder is called *variable expressivity.* In some disorders, the expression is so variable that a portion of individuals who inherit the mutation show no clinical man-

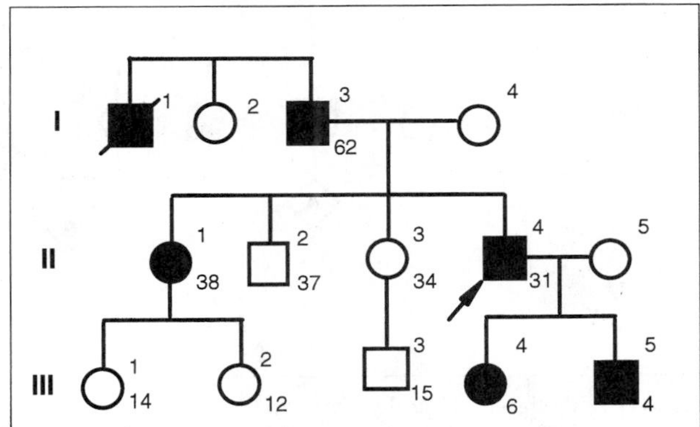

Figure 5. Pedigree of family with autosomal dominant disorder. This family has members with familial hypercholesterolemia. Note the "vertical" inheritance pattern. Both genders are affected, male-to-male transmission is present. Roughly half of the offspring of affected parents are affected.

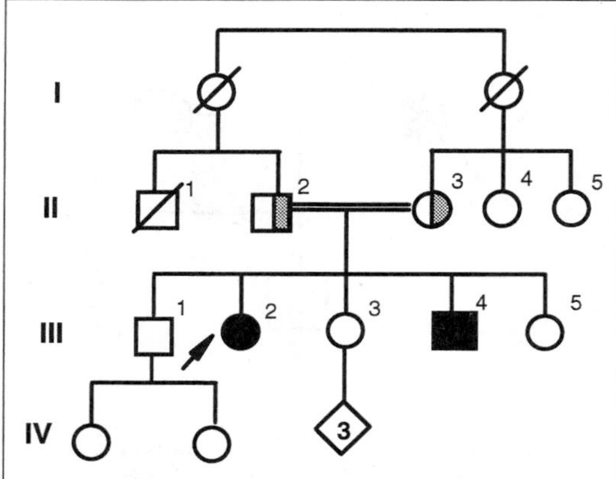

Figure 6. Pedigree of family with autosomal recessive disorder. This family has members with Gaucher disease type 1, an autosomal recessive disorder generally presenting in adolescence. Note the "horizontal" pattern of clustering: Siblings but not parents are affected. The parents (II-2 and II-3) are first cousins (consanguinity). Each parent must be a carrier of the disease allele (*obligate heterozygotes*, indicated by half-tone shading). The status of other at-risk members of the family (III-1, III-3, III-5, and all of generation IV) is unknown. It is likely that some are heterozygotes. Note that occasionally the noninformative member of a mating is omitted from the pedigree. Note also the effect of small family size: If the parents had had only 3 children, individual III-2 would have appeared to be a sporadic case.

ifestations at all. This situation is termed *incomplete penetrance*. Penetrance and expressivity may depend on age or gender, as in polycystic kidney disease, in which cysts do not develop before adolescence, or in *BRCA1* mutations, in which women have an 85 per cent lifetime risk of breast cancer but men have minimal risk. Thus, at the biochemical (gene) level, all disorders are probably 100 per cent penetrant, whereas at the clinical level, incomplete penetrance may complicate the recognition of a mendelian pattern of inheritance. Awareness of variable expression should prevent the clinician from declaring minimally or unaffected family members as free from risk of transmitting or developing complications of a disorder unless genetic testing has confirmed that they have not inherited the mutation.

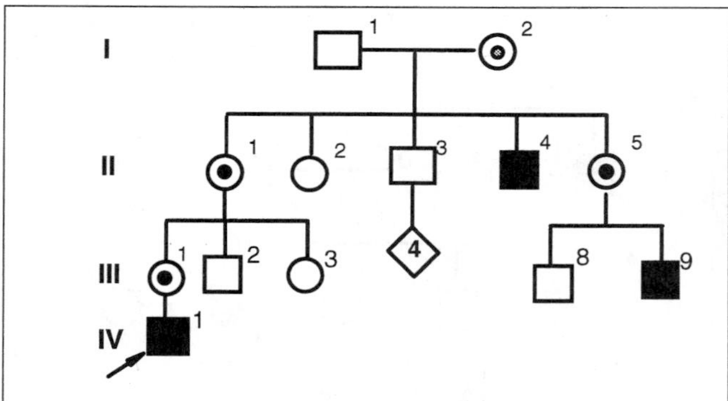

Figure 7. Pedigree of family with an X-linked disorder. This family has members with fragile X mental retardation. Note the "oblique" pattern of inheritance. No male-to-male transmission is present, and all affected males have a carrier mother. Individual IV-1 is severely affected. His great-uncle, II-4, was less severely affected. His mother, III-1, has very mild evidence of the disorder, suggestive of a mosaic effect.

Many genetic disorders manifest diverse clinical effects through a wide range of systems, a phenomenon called *pleiotropy*. This phenomenon is not surprising when one considers that many genes are active in different tissues and are turned on and off at different phases of development. The physician's awareness of pleiotropy facilitates recognition of a disorder through one or more of its minor, unusual, or hidden manifestations. For example, the skeletal features of Marfan's syndrome may trigger a search for a dilated aortic root. Within a pedigree, pleiotropy can cause a pattern of different problems that are really due to the inheritance of a single allele, as in myotonic dystrophy, in which early cataracts may be the clue linking a minimally affected grandparent to a hypotonic neonate with the severe congenital form of the disease.

In summary, a carefully researched pedigree provides a foundation for understanding mendelian disorders. The pattern of inheritance may be clear, or it may be obscured by small family size, variable expression, or pleiotropy. The features of a disorder within a family often have predictive significance for members of that family, but multifamily comparisons can be complicated by genetic heterogeneity. The more specific the genetic diagnosis, the greater the confidence in predictions based on multiple families.

Multifactorial Inheritance

Through comparisons of monozygotic and dizygotic twins, many common diseases have been clearly shown to have a significant genetic component, even though they do not follow an inheritance pattern that indicates that a single gene is at fault (see Table 2). Rather, the picture is one of inheritance of an increased susceptibility to a disorder. In these disorders, the risk of developing the disease decreases more sharply from first-degree to second- and third-degree relatives than it does in mendelian disorders. The risk is higher when the *proband*, or first identified patient, is affected severely or earlier than usual or is not of the more commonly affected gender. Several possible explanations for these phenomena have been advanced (Table 8), and it is likely that all of them occur.

Susceptibility to insulin-dependent diabetes mellitus (IDDM) is inherited: The risk for an identical twin of an affected proband is 82 times that of the general population. Yet there is also strong evidence of an *environmental component*, probably a virus. Because identification of individuals at high risk has allowed trials of early intervention that seems to prevent the onset of IDDM, there is great interest in clarifying the genetic basis. There is one *major susceptibility gene,* the major histocompatibility (MHC) locus on chromosome 6. There are, however, 19 other independent chromosomal associations, suggesting *genetic heterogeneity.* Of interest, the *IDDM2* locus near (but not in) the gene encoding insulin on chromosome 11 has multiple

Table 7. Characteristics of X-Linked Recessive Disorders

Behave as dominant in males and recessive in females
Only males and, rarely, homozygous females affected
No male-to-male transmission: Sons of affected males are unaffected
Daughters of affected males have 50% risk of being heterozygous carrier
Sons of carrier females have 50% chance of being affected
Lyonization can produce variably affected female heterozygotes (mosaics)

Table 8. Possible Genetic Mechanisms of Common Nonmendelian Disorders

Mechanism	Explanation
Genetic heterogeneity	Clinical disorder is actually several different disorders at genetic level
Genetic susceptibility	One major gene plus environmental factors
Multilocus	Two or more major genes acting together
Multifactorial	Several genes plus environmental factors
Polygenic	Additive effects of many genes

alleles that contain different numbers of a repeating sequence of 14 bases (a *variable number of tandem repeats,* or *VNTR*). The length of this repeat has major effects on the transcription of insulin.

Somatic Cell Disorders

When a mutation occurs during mitosis anytime after the differentiation of the germ line cells in early embryogenesis, only somatic cells that are descendants of the cell in which the mutation occurred are affected. Disorders that result from this phenomenon, called somatic cell disorders, include neoplasia, mosaic states, some localized congenital malformations, and, possibly, autoimmune diseases. This brief discussion focuses on cancer and, in particular, the aspects of that disease that make a genetic paradigm useful in approaching the patient or family with cancer.

Cancer arises as a clone of a single cell. A genetic basis of this clonal proliferation was suspected from characteristic chromosomal aberrations seen in tumor tissue and from the 5 per cent of cancers that show a mendelian inheritance pattern. One model of carcinogenesis holds that various mutations cause hyperactivation of normal cell growth–promoting genes (*proto-oncogenes*) and inactivation of normal cell growth–constraining genes (*tumor suppressor* genes). Cell growth is normally stimulated or controlled by signals from surrounding tissues, and loss of control of that process leads to oncogenesis. The cell growth control system is complex and has many components, such as growth factor receptors at the cell surface (e.g., the *RET* proto-oncogene involved in multiple endocrine neoplasia 2), cytoplasmic signal transducers (e.g., the *RAS* proto-oncogene involved in bladder cancers), and nuclear transcription factors that help control gene expression (e.g., the *RB* tumor suppressor gene of retinoblastoma). Mutations in any of the genes that code for these components can start a clone of cells with accelerated growth. A further mutation in one of the cells of that clone can start a subclone with even less control of growth. Through this process of *clonal evolution,* a cell eventually develops that has all the characteristics of cancer.

Oncogenes act in a dominant fashion, so it is not surprising that the transformation from proto-oncogene to oncogene is almost always the result of a new mutation. By contrast, tumor suppressor genes are, at least at the cellular level, recessive: A cell with one working copy obeys the rules of growth. This situtation allows mutations in such genes to be passed on through the germ line. Unfortunately, the risk that the normal allele will become mutated in some cell at some point in life (usually by *loss of heterozygosity*) is statistically high. The frequency of "second hits" may be sufficient to create the pedigree pattern of a dominant disorder, as in retinoblastoma.

The loss of both normal alleles for the *RB* gene in a retinal cell is sufficient to cause the development of retinoblastoma, but many other tumors conform to a model known as the "multistep theory," in which a series of mutations in critical genes leads to the stepwise development of a clone of cells with malignant characteristics, as has been shown for familial adenomatous polyposis, astrocytoma, and other tumors. In some cancers, familial forms appear to have the same cause as the more common sporadic forms. The difference is that the individual who has inherited the first mutation in a series begins with an unfortunate head start in the process.

Other genes that participate in the neoplastic process are being discovered rapidly. In particular, mutations in the genes that control the stability of the replication process can lead to numerous other mutations. Examples include the DNA mismatch repair genes mutated in hereditary nonpolyposis colon cancer (HNPCC) and the genes mutated in Bloom syndrome or xeroderma pigmentosum. Recent work suggests a role for telomerase, an enzyme that keeps germ cells from undergoing the progressive chromosomal shortening that normally limits replication of somatic cells to a certain number of generations.

This emerging model of carcinogenesis suggests several diagnostic approaches to the problems of inherited susceptibilities to cancer. To date, there are well over 100 mendelian disorders that have malignant tumors as a feature. In some, such as neurofibromatosis 1 (NF1), the frequency of malignant tumors is increased but not drastically. In others, such as Li-Fraumeni, von Hippel–Lindau, or *BRCA1* mutations, tumors constitute the major or only feature. It is important to distinguish familial from sporadic cases of cancer because the high risk of occurrence in family members and of recurrence in the patient warrants increased surveillance. The clinician concerned about this risk should scrutinize four areas: the pedigree, the clinical examination for other features of a syndrome, the presentation of the tumor in the affected people, and the possibility of genetic testing. These strategies are discussed further below.

Contiguous Gene Syndromes

A number of syndromes that had been clinically described but whose molecular basis had been unknown have now been shown, with the use of methods such as FISH (see later), to be due to deletions or duplications of chromosomal regions too small to be cytogenetically detectable but large enough to encompass several genes. Because of the altered function of several genes that may have little connection other than location, these syndromes resist embryologic or pathophysiologic analysis. These diseases are often very pleiotropic and may exist in partial forms, depending on the size of the mutation. Examples include the WAGR syndrome, the Prader-Willi syndrome, and the DiGeorge malformation complex.

Mitochondrial Inheritance

Mitochondria, cytoplasmic organelles in which oxidative energy metabolism takes place, are unusual in that they have their own extranuclear chromosomes. This small, circular chromosome, of which about 10 copies exist in each mitochondrion, has a slightly different version of the genetic code, and its 37 genes make its own transfer RNAs (tRNAs) as well as some enzymes for oxidative phosphorylation. Although most mitochondrial enzymes are coded for by nuclear DNA in the usual fashion, those made from the mitochondrial DNA are important enough that a number of diseases have been recognized as being due to mutations in mitochondrial DNA. These disorders generally affect the brain, muscles, heart, and eye, organs which depend on oxidative glucose metabolism for energy. Since mitochondria are exclusively maternally inherited (sperm contribute no cytoplasm to the zygote), and each cell has hundreds or thousands of copies of mitochondrial chromosomes, the resulting inheritance pattern is *matrilineal* with significant variability.

GENETIC TESTING

A few points may clarify the process of genetic diagnosis. For some disorders, standard radiologic or electrodiagnostic testing may be adequate. For others, a biochemical test is sufficient for diagnosis (e.g., a lipid profile in familial hypercholesterolemia or a hexosaminidase A level in Tay-Sachs disease). Because all genes are present, but not necessarily active, in all tissues, and many gene products remain intracellular, tests based on a gene product, even if it is known, have limitations. Therefore, in some settings, more direct evaluation of DNA is required for understanding the problem at the most specific level possible. Recognizing these settings, making the proper choice of tests, understanding the constraints and limitations of the test, interpreting the results, and providing appropriate pretesting and post-testing counseling to the patient and family is a complex process generally best undertaken in consultation with a geneticist.

Chromosome Studies

For conditions in which a chromosome disorder is suspected, a chromosome study, or *karyotype,* is appropriate. A widely available test that costs about $500 in most areas, a karyotype is performed on peripheral blood lymphocytes that have been cultured, stimulated, and then arrested in metaphase. The lymphocytes are spread out on a slide and the chromosomes stained with Giemsa, bringing out a banding pattern that allows identification of individual chromosomes, which are then photographed and placed in order for analysis. With high-resolution techniques, as many as 850 individual bands can be distinguished per haploid set of chromosomes. The smallest stretch of DNA that can be distinguished with these methods is on the order of 2000 kilobases, which is nearly 10 times the size of the largest known gene and could contain as many as 100 smaller genes.

When a DNA sequence from the area in question is known, it can be labeled with fluorescent stain and used as a *probe* to match *(hybridize)* with the homologous areas of a chromosome spread. The fluorescent marker then reveals the number of copies of that region and whether they are in the proper location or translocated to another chromosome. Panels of probes tagged with different color dyes can be used to examine several areas at once. This technique, called *fluorescence in situ hybridization,* or FISH, can reveal deletions, duplications, and translocations that are too small to be seen with standard Giemsa staining. This technique is particularly useful in evaluating suspected contiguous gene syndromes.

Molecular Testing for Mendelian Disorders

When a pedigree or clinical diagnosis implicates a mendelian disorder, and the location of the responsible gene has been narrowed down to a particular chromosomal region but has not yet been identified, it is still possible to predict whether an individual has inherited the disorder. The goal is to determine whether the person inherited the copy of the region that, in affected relatives, is associated with the disease. This technique is a clinical application of the *positional cloning approach* (identifying a gene by its location rather than its product), which has been the most effective strategy in the effort to map the human genome. For distinguishing one copy (or *haplotype*) of a region from its homologous copy, positional cloning relies on *DNA markers*, which are being identified in ever-increasing numbers. These markers are usually *polymorphisms:* segments of DNA in which two or more versions exist in significant numbers in the population but no phenotypic effect is evident. These innocent variations include VNTRs, restriction fragment length polymorphisms (*RFLPs;* places where a sequence difference causes a change in susceptibility to being cut by a restriction enzyme), and *microsatellites*, which are repeating pairs of bases, so named for their behavior in the ultracentrifuge. The more closely a marker is linked (i.e., the closer it sits on the chromosome) to the actual gene, the better proxy it makes for tracking the inheritance of the disease allele through a pedigree. This form of testing requires the existence and participation of a number of family members, as well as accurate clinical diagnosis of those who are already affected. If these conditions are met, this approach, called *linkage analysis,* can be a powerful tool for predicting whether an individual at risk has actually inherited a disease.

In some situations involving mendelian disorders, the gene has been cloned and studied, and one or more specific mutations associated with the disease identified. One can then ask whether a particular individual who is at risk for the disease has one of these mutations. This situation arises in three settings: where the mutation in a family has been characterized and a relative is being tested, where a particular ethnic group has a high frequency of a certain mutation (as in cystic fibrosis), and where there is only one or a few mutations known to cause the disorder (as in Huntington's disease or achondroplasia). In such cases, a direct test for the mutation may be appropriate. Such testing is usually performed either with the use of the *polymerase chain reaction* (PCR) to amplify the small segment of DNA in question into a quantity that can be sequenced, or with the use of *restriction endonucleases* (bacterial enzymes that cut DNA only at particular sequences) to reveal a change in a *restriction site* caused by the mutation. This approach becomes difficult when, as is the case in many autosomal dominant disorders, there is a large allelic series of different mutations that can cause the disorder, and either a new mutation is suspected or a family's particular mutation is unknown. In such circumstances, the only option may be to look for the new mutation, a laborious process usually done only in research settings. Even if the mutation is found in this way, a causal connection to the disease can be made only by testing others with the disorder in the family to see whether the mutation travels with the disease.

Restriction enzyme cleavage, the *polymerase chain reaction, Southern blotting, probes,* and *DNA sequencing* are the tools used to obtain sufficient copies of a discrete segment of DNA for analysis, and to compare that segment to known normal and abnormal versions.

DIAGNOSTIC STRATEGIES FOR GENETIC DISORDERS

Clinical Reasoning

The diagnostic process begins with the generation of candidate hypotheses to explain findings, followed by refinement and verification phases until a hypothesis has become a working diagnosis sufficient to guide further testing or support prognosis or treatment. The clinician generates these hypotheses by comparing the findings to his or her knowledge of disease, stored in the memory essentially as case stories, which includes some information about prevalence and clinical spectrum. Certain "heuristic devices" or shortcuts have been identified that help the clinician come up with a candidate hypothesis, including the familiarity of the disease (or freshness in the clinician's mind), the degree of resemblance of the hypothesized disorder to the condition of the patient at hand, and the seriousness or urgency it implies. Once the hypotheses are generated, the clinician refines or rejects them using probabilistic, causal, and deterministic reasoning.

The application of this model to genetics reveals some of the sources of the difficulty clinicians can experience in diagnosing genetic disorders. First, the existence of so many individually rare genetic disorders means that no single clinician can have detailed familiarity with more than a few specific disorders, making the "familiarity" heuristic much less useful. Second, the great clinical variation typical of many genetic disorders, described as pleiotropy, variable expression, variable penetrance, and genetic heterogeneity, makes it less likely that a case story stored in the clinician's memory will so closely resemble the patient in question that the former patient's disease will pop up as a hypothesis. Furthermore, the new patient may represent only a partial picture of the disorder—the full picture may be spread out over the extended family. Third, although there occasionally are genetic emergencies, the seriousness of most genetic disorders stems more from the long-term prognosis than from the urgency of an immediate crisis. This situation may delay the generation of genetic hypotheses in settings focused on urgent and episodic care, such as hospitals, emergency rooms, and busy office practices.

Finally, the causal pathophysiologic mechanisms in genetic disorders are often obscure, because of gaps in our knowledge of the relevant biochemistry, chromosomal anatomy, or embryology. This lack makes causal reasoning more difficult and complicates the process of hypothesis verification and refinement. Some of these very features, which make genetic diseases resistant to the usual heuristics, can be overcome or even turned to advantage with the use of the following principles:

1. Although genetic disorders may be individually rare, their vast number and total burden of serious long-term effects mean that encounters with patients with genetic disorders are common in medical practice. This knowledge, plus awareness of the scope of the genome, the complexity of its workings, and the number of ways gene function can be altered, will lower the threshold for the perception of variation and the generation of a genetic hypothesis.
2. An appropriate family history and pedigree may suggest inheritance patterns that aid in hypothesis generation and refinement.
3. An attempt to attribute diverse findings to a single cause, especially in patients with traces of an embryologic or a developmental process and findings not obviously related to nongenetic pathophysiology, will often produce a genetic hypothesis.
4. Awareness of pleiotropy, and the fact that in many syndromes no single feature is invariably part of the constellation of findings, can heighten the physician's sensitivity to minor findings as clues to genetic disease. Numbers 3 and 4 reflect the approach developed by dysmorphologists who deal with malformation syndromes, often called "syndromology."
5. Quick access to, and a low threshold for using, computerized, print, and consultative resources are more important than memorizing lists.
6. Unhurried examination and careful construction of a detailed pedigree may also create a less hectic atmosphere, facilitating the generation of genetic hypotheses that may not emerge under the normal pressures in a busy office.
7. Verification of a hypothesis with genetic testing provides the opportunity to consult with a geneticist, who may enrich and add to the hypotheses already generated.

Clinical Suspicion of Genetic Disease

When should a clinician include genetic disorders among his or her diagnostic hypotheses? Clearly, a comprehensive list is impossible. There are certain clues, however, that can be grouped in four categories: setting, syndrome, pedigree, and presentation.

The factors that make the combination of two identical alleles for a recessive disorder more likely include consanguinity and the patient's belonging to certain ethnic populations that historically have been reproductively isolated (Table 9). With advanced maternal age, the physician should think of chromosome disorders. With advanced paternal age, think of new dominant mutations. When a single unusual finding is noted, consider a genetic etiology. Also with two or more unusual features in the same person and no obvious common cause, seriously consider a genetic contribution. Any pedigree containing two members with the same disorder should suggest an inherited form of or susceptibility to that disorder. A pedigree with many members chronically ill or deceased at a young age should trigger thoughts of a single pleiotropic disorder even when the illnesses are described as different. Numerous spontaneous abortions should raise the question of a balanced translocation in one of the parents. A pedigree with significantly more healthy females than males may suggest an X-linked recessive disorder. Table 10 lists some specific presentations that are likely to have a genetic basis.

In addition, think genetics in any patient with a rare or puzzling finding, or an undiagnosable degenerative disorder. Where recent information may shed new light, unusual past diagnoses should be reconsidered. Finally, an unusual presentation of a common disorder should raise the question of an inherited form. Examples include very early age at onset, occurrence in the less common gender, multiple or bilateral findings that are usually few or solitary, unusual clinical course, and appearance in a patient

Table 9. Examples of Increased Frequency of Mendelian Disorders in Ethnic Groups

Ethnic Group	Disorder
Africans	Sickle cell anemia G-6-PD deficiency
Ashkenazi Jews	Tay-Sachs disease Gaucher disease
French Canadians	Morquio syndrome Myotonic dystrophy
Italians and Greeks	Beta-thalassemia Mediterranean fever
Northern Europeans	Cystic fibrosis Phenylketonuria

G-6-PD = glucose-6-phosphate dehydrogenase.

Table 10. Examples of Presentations Suggestive of Genetic Disorders

Timing	Presentation
Prenatal	Multiple miscarriages Abnormal ultrasound or triple screen
Neonatal	Multiple congenital malformations Single birth defects Three or more minor anomalies Skeletal dysplasias Abnormal sex differentiation Hypotonia or hypertonia Seizures Overwhelming illness or coma Metabolic acidosis Hyperammonemia Bleeding Hyperbilirubinemia Meconium ileus Abnormal screen for metabolic errors Anemia
Infancy and childhood	Mental retardation Hypotonia or hypertonia Unexplained recurrent severe vomiting Visual or hearing impairment Any loss of previously learned skills Growth failure Disproportionate growth Visceromegaly Coarse facial features Abnormal odor Recurrent infections Anemia Chronic renal disease Liver dysfunction Bleeding or hemarthrosis Malignancy
Adolescence	Failure of sexual maturation
Adulthood	Malignancies characteristic of syndromes Infertility Neurologic deterioration Anemia Increased iron stores

already known to have or suspected of having a genetic disorder.

Clinical Evaluation

The clinical evaluation of the patient suspected of having a genetic disorder should include the same history, physical examination, and testing that would be done for nongenetic causes of the same problem. However, a more extensive family history, a careful search for minor as well as major anomalies, a search of computer or print resources, and, in some circumstances, genetic testing may be helpful. Consultation should be available, and efforts should be made to mitigate the effects of the evaluation process on the patient and family.

History

The history should focus not only on acute or recent events but also on long-term trends. In children, this includes questions about gestation, development, and education. In adults, who often restrict activities unconsciously in response to degenerative changes, questions about specific activities during specific periods of life are helpful. The examination of old photographs can reveal slow changes in appearance.

Family History and Pedigree

The family history may provide clues to the effects of the patient's genes in other people. A complete family history is not appropriate for most visits; it must be tailored to the setting (Table 11). Is there anything about this family's background that puts them at risk? What genetic disorders occur in this family? Is a particular problem acquired or inherited? What is the spectrum of the disorder in this family? Who is at risk? Early-onset preventable disorders deserve special attention because diagnosis may indeed lead to prevention. Disorders with marked pleiotropy and variable expression require attention because these factors can obscure syndromes and inheritance patterns.

The family history should be recorded with the use of standard pedigree symbols. The drawing can be used to educate the patient. Begin with the patient and work outward, asking about first-degree relatives, then second-degree, on both sides of the family. Record the age or date of birth and name of family members. If a comprehensive family history is obtained, ask permission to contact family members. Get the most specific information possible, including medical records. Finally, review and update the pedigree periodically, especially for patients and families followed for many years.

Confounding factors can make the interpretation of the

Table 11. Types of Family History Appropriate to Different Contexts

Purpose and Setting	Contents of Family History
Screening family history, appropriate, for initial encounter, preventive health maintenance review or preconceptual counseling visit	A pedigree, to include first-degree relatives (sibs, parents, children), with current age, any illnesses, age, cause of death; ethnic background. *Specific questions about extended family:* Does anyone else have a problem similar to yours? Is there any problem affecting two or more people? Does anyone have a problem with the kidneys or blood? Is there anyone with early heart disease, cancer, or death? Is there anyone with a progressive disability? Are there any cases of infertility, miscarriages, or infant death? Does anyone have birth defects or mental retardation? Is there any consanguinity? (Are your mother's and father's families related to each other in any way?)
Detailed family history, appropriate when there is suspicion of a genetic disease	*All of the above plus:* For first- and second-degree relatives: specific questions about signs and symptoms of the suspected disorder
Comprehensive family history, appropriate for the genetics consultation	*All of the above plus:* Complete pedigree, including all known family members All relevant medical information on informative members, including medical records, pathology, and autopsy reports

pedigree unreliable. Patients' memories may not be accurate, or the information they were given may be erroneous. Nonpaternity can introduce paradoxes. In many families, there are blocks to communication. Adoption, immigration, and wars can truncate the obtainable pedigree. Despite this, the pedigree is the single most useful tool for genetic diagnosis.

Physical Examination

Depending on the disorder, the physical examination may be expanded to include complete neurologic and developmental components. When there are major anomalies, they should be quantified with the use of tables of norms for anthropometric data (see later). Minor anomalies, such as hair patterns and dermatoglyphics, are important clues: 90 per cent of infants with three or more minor anomalies also have major malformations. Available family members should be examined as well, since a person cannot be declared free from a disorder unless they have been examined by a clinician who is looking for the specific disorder. Special attention should be paid to findings that suggest disorders with serious preventable complications, such as multiple dysplastic nevi (melanoma) or lens dislocation (aortic dissection in Marfan's syndrome).

Routine Testing

When ordering biochemical, histologic, electrodiagnostic, or radiologic tests for a suspected rare disorder, the physician should consult with the pathologist, surgeon, neurologist, or radiologist beforehand. In many cases, special handling of specimens, special stimuli, or special views are crucial for the acquisition of reliable data.

Genetic Testing

Most genetic testing, including chromosome analysis, family linkage studies, and direct mutation analysis, is performed at centers staffed with clinical geneticists, genetic counselors, cytogeneticists, and molecular biologists. Although commercial testing is widespread, there are advantages to consulting a geneticist during the planning of genetic testing. Because printed lists are quickly outdated, computer databases, described later, provide better information about the existence and availability of specific tests.

Data Repositories

In broadening a differential diagnosis to include unfamiliar disorders, it is essential to have the support of comprehensive, searchable databases and access to specialists familiar with the disorders in question. In this regard, several resources are helpful to the clinician and should be used regularly.

The single most useful resource for clinicians in the diagnosis of genetic disorders is the on-line computerized version of Victor McKusick's catalog of mendelian traits, *On-Line Mendelian Inheritance in Man* (OMIM), which is updated daily. Access is available without charge over the Internet, and a search algorithm facilitates immediate generation of a ranked list of disorders that feature the findings in question. Monographs on these disorders are detailed and include copious references. Within minutes the clinician who uses OMIM can find out whether a particular finding or constellation of findings may be caused by a known single gene disorder, what disorders may be involved, what groups have done recent work on these disorders, and what diagnostic approaches are sensible. Similar databases are maintained for birth defects, inherited bone disorders, teratogens, and so forth (see below for details).

Smith's Recognizable Patterns of Human Malformation provides descriptions and illustrations of malformation syndromes, anthropometric tables, and an index of hundreds of major and minor malformations and their frequencies in genetic disorders.

The Alliance of Genetic Support Groups publishes the *Directory of National Genetic Voluntary Organizations and Related Resources*. This organization and others can be enormously helpful to the clinician through their identification of regional, national, or international experts in the particular disorder and through the supplying of recent literature.

Genetics Consultation

Given the complexity of genetic diagnosis and the implications of such a diagnosis for the patient and family, clinicians must have access to and feel comfortable using the consultative services of geneticists and other professionals. These services are generally available through genetics units.

There are now about 500 clinical genetics centers or units throughout the country that can provide comprehensive consultative services. These units, staffed by clinical geneticists and genetic counselors, usually offer primary diagnosis, diagnosis of complications, prenatal diagnosis, laboratory services, management and treatment, and genetic counseling. It is estimated that only about 2 per cent of patients and families who could benefit from referral are actually referred to such units. Although there is currently no national directory of such units, state health departments generally have regional listings.

The genetics consultation often begins with a phone call to discuss the patient. The primary care physician can greatly facilitate the referral by organizing and providing as much relevant history as possible, gathering results of radiologic and other studies, and helping the patient enlist the participation of family members.

The genetics consultation is often a prolonged process, involving multiple telephone contacts with the family; a detailed family history; examination (with permission) of medical records, radiographs, pathology reports, and even slides from all relevant family members; examination of the patient and relevant family members; further clinical, biochemical, radiologic, electrodiagnostic, and other testing; genetic testing, such as chromosome analysis, linkage analysis, and mutation analysis; diagnosis of the disorder; development of a treatment plan; identification of other family members at risk; and genetic counseling. During this process, the primary care physician plays an important role in supporting the patient and family and facilitating the evaluation. Frequent telephone contact helps all parties stay current. At the end, the clinician can expect a detailed report and a discussion of further screening and management recommendations.

Concerns of Patients and Families

Surveys of patients and families have revealed several common concerns. First, many report misdiagnosis or substantial delays in diagnosis. Second, a cooperative working relationship between the primary care physician and the genetic specialists is extremely helpful to patients. Third, learning that one has a genetic disorder can have powerful emotional effects, including relief at finding an explanation, fear of the implications, guilt over passing on a disorder, and anger that the disorder is not better understood.

An attitude of respectful engagement and empathy on the part of the physician is valued by these patients. Voluntary genetic support groups can assist many patients and families at the time of diagnosis, and the clinician should know how to locate the appropriate organizations for them.

Genetic information has lifelong implications not only for the patient but also for relatives. Many parties other than patients, their families, and care providers seek information about genetic diagnoses. These range from researchers to insurance companies, employers, and even political organizations. Therefore, confidentiality is paramount; the patient must be fully aware of and in control of the release of any information.

Genetic knowledge and skills are important in primary care practice. Specific diagnosis is becoming increasingly possible and has important implications for prognosis, surveillance, treatment, and prevention. An understanding of the scope of the genome and its mechanisms of variation can help the clinician appreciate the patterns of genetic disease and develop an effective diagnostic approach. Cognitive strategies for genetic diagnosis must consider the enormous variety and syndromic nature of genetic disorders. The family history as recorded in the pedigree and the syndromology approach are powerful tools. Computer, print, and consultative resources are readily available but probably underutilized. Genetic testing can lead to a more specific diagnosis, but such testing is complex and should generally be done in consultation with a specialist. Since patients and families often find the process of genetic diagnosis extremely harrowing, clinicians should be prepared to offer support and access to voluntary genetic support organizations.

COMMON OCULAR DISORDERS

By Kathryn Colby, M.D., Ph.D.,
and Deborah Pavan-Langston, M.D.
Boston, Massachusetts

EYE EXAMINATION EQUIPMENT

Relatively little equipment is needed to perform the basic ophthalmologic examination. A standardized vision chart is useful, although the lack of a chart does not preclude an assessment of vision. Readily available reading material, such as newspapers and magazines, can be used to test near vision. Patients older than 45 years of age should be tested with their reading correction in place. Inexpensive +2.00 glasses from a local store may be used when the patient has no reading glasses. Each eye should be tested individually, with the other eye covered.

Proparacaine anesthetic eye drops greatly facilitate the examination. Stains such as fluorescein and rose bengal are helpful in diagnosing corneal pathology. The authors recommend the use of paper strips impregnated with these stains, rather than pre-made solutions that may become contaminated with bacteria if used improperly or allowed to grow old. The strips are dipped in proparacaine or sterile saline and touched to the eye inside the lower lid.

Some type of magnifying device is needed as well. While a slit lamp is ideal, several ocular disorders can be detected with loupes or hand-held magnifiers. Ocular pressure is measured with a tonometer after proparacaine instillation. Hand-held "pen-type" tonometers are convenient and easy to use with minimal training, an advantage in circumstances in which intraocular pressure measurements are made infrequently.

To view the retina, one needs an ophthalmoscope. The direct (hand-held) ophthalmoscope will probably best serve most nonophthalmologists, as it is relatively inexpensive and provides a magnified view. With practice, one can easily evaluate the posterior pole (optic nerve head, macula, and retinal blood vessels), especially through a dilated pupil.

BASIC EYE ANATOMY

Figure 1 shows a schematic diagram of the internal structures of the eye. The cornea is the transparent anterior surface that acts as the main refracting surface of the eye. It is continuous with the sclera at the limbus. The sclera forms the tough, fibrous outer coat of the eye, into which the extraocular muscles insert. The anterior sclera is covered by a thin, translucent mucous membrane, the bulbar conjunctiva. The conjunctiva also lines both the superior and the inferior fornices, and covers the inner surfaces of the eyelids (the palpebral conjunctiva). The bulbar and palpebral conjunctiva form a continuous layer. This arrangement prevents a contact lens or surface foreign body from getting lost "behind the eye."

The anterior chamber is located between the iris and the cornea. It contains aqueous fluid that is produced by the ciliary processes. Aqueous fluid drains from the eye via the trabecular meshwork and Schlemm's canal, structures located in the angle of the eye. Angle structures can be visualized only with the use of special gonioscopic lenses.

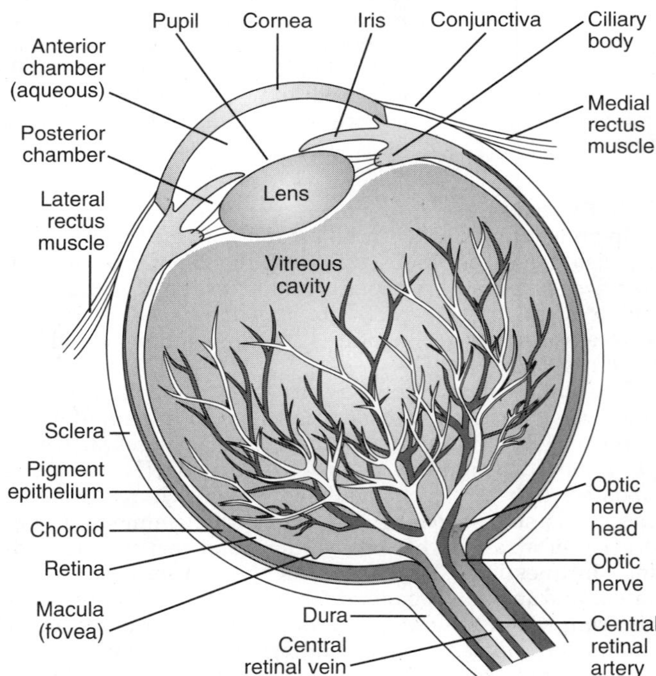

Figure 1. The internal structures of the human eye.

The iris is part of the uveal tract, the pigmented vascular layer of the eye. The crystalline lens is located immediately posterior to the iris. Zonular fibers attach the lens to the ciliary body, which contains the smooth muscle fibers responsible for accommodation, the process by which the lens changes shape to allow focusing for near work.

The vitreous cavity, posterior to the lens, is filled with vitreous humor, a gelatinous material. With age, the vitreous may liquefy and detach from the retina, leading to the common complaint of "floaters," small black flecks that move when the eye moves.

The retina lines the back of the eye and can be divided into the neurosensory retina (the photoreceptors and supporting cells) and the underlying retinal pigment epithelium, which supports and nourishes the neurosensory retina. The choroid is the vascular layer that lies between the retina and the posterior sclera. It supplies blood to the retinal pigment epithelium and the outer portion of the neurosensory retina.

The optic nerve contains the axons of the retinal ganglion cells and serves as a pathway to higher visual centers. The central retinal artery and vein travel within the optic nerve and then arborize at the optic disc to supply the inner part of the retina. The macula, the area of the retina located between the temporal vascular arcades, is responsible for fine central and color vision. The fovea lies at the center of the macula.

REFRACTIVE ERRORS OF THE EYE

Several common refractive errors may initially present to the nonophthalmologist. Myopia, or "nearsightedness," occurs when the eye is too long. Light rays from distant objects are focused in front of the retina, and the image on the retina is blurred. Patients with myopia have decreased distance vision, but good near acuity. Myopia is corrected by concave, diverging ("minus") lenses that move the focused image back to the retina.

When the eye is too short, hyperopia ("farsightedness") results as light rays are focused behind the retina. Good distance acuity is present, but near images are blurred. Children and young adults may be able to accommodate sufficiently to clear up the blurred near image. As patients age and their accommodation naturally decreases, symptoms of asthenopia (uncomfortable vision) or frontal headache may occur with prolonged near work. Hyperopia is corrected by convex, convergent ("plus") lenses.

Astigmatism results when the curvature of the eye is not uniform; that is, when the power of the eye differs in different meridians. Light rays from the different meridians of the eye are refracted in a nonuniform manner, leading to distortion of the retinal image. Astigmatism can be corrected with toric lenses, in which the power of the lens differs in different meridians.

Presbyopia ("old eyes") results from the physiologic decrease in accommodation that occurs with aging and hardening of the eye's lens. As patients approach age 40 years, many notice difficulty with near work, requiring reading material to be held a longer distance from the eyes. This symptom may worsen as the day goes on. Uncorrected hyperopes will notice presbyopic symptoms at a younger age than those without refractive error or with myopia. Low-strength-plus lenses compensate for presbyopia. The strength of the reading glasses will gradually need to be increased as the patient ages, until about age 60 years, when there is essentially no accommodation left.

COMMON ANTERIOR SEGMENT PROBLEMS

Corneal Abrasions

The cornea has a dense sensory innervation and is thus exquisitely sensitive. Corneal abrasions, disruption of the epithelium or front surface of the cornea, are very painful. Corneal abrasions are often caused by trauma. The diagnosis is made by instillation of fluorescein with topical anesthetic and examination under cobalt blue light. Areas that have been denuded of their epithelium will stain with fluorescein, appearing fluorescent green under blue light. A 2- to 3-mm abrasion may be visible without magnification, but a slit lamp is needed to detect small or subtle defects.

After diagnosing a corneal abrasion, the physician should check for the presence of foreign bodies. A foreign body embedded in the cornea may be visible. The physician can lift it off the cornea with a sterile needle on a syringe. Clues that a foreign body may be lodged beneath the upper lid include fluorescein-staining vertical linear epithelial defects on the cornea, from the continuous friction of the trapped particle. To check for a trapped foreign body, evert the upper lid. While the patient looks down, place the stick end of a cotton swab on the upper lid just posterior to the lid crease. With the other hand, grasp the upper eyelashes and gently pull the lid down, out, and up over the stick. The foreign body will often be found on the palpebral conjunctiva of the everted lid and may be removed with the cotton swab. With topical anesthetic in place, this procedure is not painful, and the patient is more cooperative.

Chemical Burns of the Cornea

Alkali burns of the cornea are a true ocular emergency. Chemicals such as lye, fresh lime, plaster of Paris, ammonia, and sodium or potassium hydroxide cause severe damage to anterior segment structures related to both the degree of alkalinity and the time of exposure. Alkali compounds combine with components of cell membranes to cause cellular disruption and rapid tissue penetration. Immediate copious irrigation is essential, and often should be continued for an hour or more.

Acid burns are often less serious than alkali burns because the acid precipitates tissue proteins, which then act as a barrier to further penetration. Nonetheless, acid burns can also be quite serious. Prompt irrigation is needed.

The extent of injury from a chemical burn can be assessed with the use of the following criteria. In a mild chemical injury, corneal epithelial defects may be present, as discussed earlier. The eye is red, and there is no blanching or whitening of the limbal blood vessels, indicating ischemia of the conjunctiva or underlying sclera. In moderate injuries, the physician may discern corneal haze, obscuring iris details. Blanching of part of the limbus may be present, and there may be a mild inflammatory reaction within the anterior chamber. Following severe injuries, there may be complete denudation of the corneal epithelium, marked corneal haze, and blanching of more than two thirds of the limbal blood vessels. This type of injury may be associated with severe intraocular inflammation and elevation of intraocular pressure. There is a risk of corneal perforation and loss of the eye following very severe chemical injuries.

Ocular Radiation Burns

Excessive exposure to ultraviolet radiation can lead to corneal damage. Common sources include sunlamps and welding arcs. Ordinary sunlight can also cause ultraviolet keratopathy under conditions where there is a great deal of light reflection, such as snow skiing on a bright, sunny day. The symptoms of ultraviolet keratopathy usually begin 6 to 10 hours after exposure and vary, depending on the severity of the exposure. Mild symptoms such as irritation and foreign body sensation occur after short exposures, while longer exposures can cause severe photophobia and pain.

On clinical examination, the lids may appear edematous and reddened. The conjunctiva may be injected. Staining of the cornea with fluorescein and topical anesthetic reveals multiple punctate defects in the corneal epithelium, so-called "superficial punctate keratopathy." Most ultraviolet corneal burns can be avoided with the use of appropriate protective eyewear, such as welding shields and sunglasses.

Dry Eyes

Insufficient tear production is a very common, and often overlooked, cause of ocular complaints, especially in older patients. Keratoconjunctivitis sicca, or dry eye syndrome, may be associated with menopause and with systemic collagen vascular diseases, including rheumatoid arthritis and systemic lupus erythematosus. Many patients with dry eyes, however, have no associated systemic disease. A natural decline in tear production occurs with aging. In addition, medications such as oral contraceptives or antispasmodics can produce tear hyposecretion as a side effect.

Clinically, patients complain of a low-grade ocular irritation and a gritty or sandy foreign-body sensation. Dryness of the ocular surface often triggers an increase in reflex tearing, and patients may complain of epiphora or excess tearing when there is actually an underlying tear hyposecretion.

On examination, patients may have a decreased tear meniscus. Rose bengal, which stains devitalized cells, demonstrates punctate staining of the cornea and conjunctiva, most concentrated in the interpalpebral fissures. Measurements of actual tear production can be made with the use of the Schirmer test, in which small pieces of filter paper are placed in the inferior fornix to collect the tears produced during a 5-minute period.

In addition to producing discomfort, chronically inadequate tear production predisposes to contact lens intolerance and to bacterial infections that may lead to serious corneal damage. Borderline tear production can be "tipped over the edge" by other factors, such as a dry environment during the heating season, meibomian gland dysfunction (see the section on blepharitis, below), or medications with anticholinergic side effects.

OCULAR TRAUMA

Hyphema

Direct blunt trauma to the eye, such as that from a squash ball, champagne cork, or fist, can lead to a number of potentially serious injuries. Hyphema, blood in the anterior chamber of the eye, is a common sequela of blunt trauma and results from the tearing of small blood vessels within the iris. The symptoms and clinical findings depend on the size of the hyphema. A microscopic hyphema, in which suspended red blood cells can be detected only with a slit lamp, may cause few symptoms and would not be apparent to the nonophthalmologist. At the other extreme, a complete or "eight-ball" hyphema, in which the anterior chamber is completely filled with blood, causes a marked decrease in vision and is visible on penlight examination. Partial hyphemas, in which the anterior chamber contains layered blood but is not completely filled, cause decreased vision that may improve spontaneously within hours as the blood cells settle. On examination, the physician will see a layer of blood within the anterior chamber. The suspended erythrocytes that have yet to settle may cause a hazy view of the iris and posterior segment structures.

The complications of hyphema include rebleeding and increased intraocular pressure. As the red blood cells are cleared, they may clog the outflow pathways of the eye and cause glaucoma. In addition, there is always the possibility of other associated ocular trauma. For these reasons, it is always prudent to refer patients who have sustained ocular trauma to an ophthalmologist for a comprehensive, dilated-eye examination.

Ocular Perforation

Several types of injuries can disrupt the integrity of the globe. Blunt injuries of sufficient force can cause rupture of the sclera at its relatively weak points (the insertions of the extraocular muscles and the optic nerve), leading to a "ruptured globe." Penetrating injuries, on the other hand, are caused by sharp objects, such as pencils, glass fragments, and tools. A laceration of the cornea and/or sclera often is seen clinically after a penetrating injury.

The signs and symptoms of these two types of injuries can be similar. In evaluating the patient with ocular trauma, a careful history to determine the exact mechanism of injury is crucial in helping the physician decide which type of perforation is present. Sometimes, it is not possible to obtain a complete history following accidents involving unsupervised children or unconscious adults.

Decreased visual acuity typically occurs after a perforating injury to the globe. In addition, the anterior chamber may be markedly shallowed or even flat. The pupil may be abnormal in size, shape, or location. Intraocular pressure is usually extremely low (hypotony). If an ocular perforation is suspected, manipulations that press on the globe should be deferred until an ophthalmologist can examine the patient. When a corneal-scleral laceration is present, there may be extrusion of intraocular structures, such as the iris. Any patient who presents with a history or examination suggestive of ocular perforation should be referred to an ophthalmologist. In this situation, minimal interventions such as covering the eye with a metal shield, giving antiemetics as needed, and instructing the patient not to ingest anything (NPO) can be useful prior to arrival of the ophthalmologist.

Orbital Fractures

Orbital wall or floor fractures ("blowout fractures") can occur as the consequence of facial trauma. On examination, there is often periocular ecchymosis and edema. There may be a palpable "step-off" or discontinuity of the orbital rim. If air from the adjacent sinuses has been trapped in the subcutaneous tissue, crepitus of the periocular skin may be present. Decreased sensation in the V1 or V2 dermatome may occur.

When the floor fracture is small, entrapment of extraocular muscles, most commonly the inferior rectus, can occasionally occur, leading to complaints of diplopia and restriction of motility on examination. Orbital computed tomography is useful for the definitive diagnosis of orbital floor fractures, although one can often make the diagnosis clinically. Additional ocular injuries are often found in association with floor and wall fractures. Any patient who sustains significant periocular trauma should be evaluated by an ophthalmologist.

OCULAR INFECTIONS

Blepharitis

Blepharitis, chronic inflammation of the eyelids often associated with staphylococcal infection, is an extremely common condition. Patients present with complaints of ocular irritation and foreign-body sensation. Crusting of the eyelid margins may occur, most commonly in the morning.

Clinically, the margins of the eyelids are thickened and erythematous. Crusted debris at the bases of the lashes can be seen with magnification. There may be plugging of the orifices of the meibomian glands, the small sebaceous glands of the eyelids ("meibomitis"). Left untreated, these blocked glands may become infected, leading to a hordeolum (colloquially known as a "stye"). Inflammation from an acute hordeolum usually resolves. Occasionally, however, a chronic inflammatory focus forms, and the patient is left with a hard lump—a chalazion—at the site of the previous hordeolum. Treatment of the chalazion includes local steroid injection or incision and curettage for elimination.

Conjunctival injection often accompanies active blepharitis. In addition, corneal changes such as superficial punctate keratopathy can result from blepharitis. Patients with significant blepharitis often have associated skin findings of acne rosacea.

Conjunctivitis

Conjunctivitis is an inflammation of the conjunctiva, the thin, transparent mucous membrane that lines the inner surface of the eyelids (palpebral conjunctiva) and the anterior sclera (bulbar conjunctiva). Conjunctival injection is present. Swelling of the conjunctiva (chemosis) can also be seen. A discharge may be present as well. There are multiple possible causes of conjunctivitis, including bacterial or viral infection and allergic or toxic reactions. There are a number of differentiating clinical signs. A careful history is also important in the attempt to define an etiology for conjunctivitis.

Viral infection is a very common cause of conjunctivitis. Usually caused by an adenovirus or the common cold virus, viral conjunctivitis presents with moderate injection and a scant watery discharge. There is usually a history of concurrent or recent upper respiratory infection. Often, other members of the patient's family or some of the patient's co-workers have similar complaints. A preauricular lymph node is usually present with adenovirus infection. Follicles, accumulations of inflammatory cells surrounded by blood vessels, are seen in the inferior palpebral conjunctiva. Follicles are especially prominent after fluorescein instillation, which highlights the areas between the follicles. Adenoviral subepithelial deposits in the cornea may be seen in about 30 per cent of patients. Adenoviral conjunctivitis is extremely contagious. A case can last up to 3 weeks, with remissions and exacerbations before final resolution occurs. The common cold conjunctivitis resolves in a few days.

On the other hand, bacterial conjunctivitis is often associated with a mucopurulent discharge and marked conjunctival injection. Chemosis is often seen. The common causative agents include *Staphylococcus aureus* or *epidermidis*. Children can be infected with *Streptococcus pneumoniae* or *Haemophilus influenzae*. A preauricular node may or may not be present in cases of bacterial conjunctivitis. If definitive identification of the causative agent is necessary, a conjunctival culture can be taken. Ideally, cultures should be done before instillation of anesthetic drops, which may lessen the yield. Special culture kits are commonly available and consist of a sterile cotton-tipped swab and a culture medium. Cultures are taken by moistening the swab with sterile saline and wiping the lid margin or inferior fornix. The swab is used to inoculate the culture medium. If a Gram stain is to be done, a new swab can be used to place a specimen on a glass slide. Alternatively, a conjunctival scraping for a Gram stain can be performed with a sterile spatula after topical anesthetic has been applied.

Serious hyperacute conjunctivitis can be caused by *Neisseria* species, *Corynebacterium diphtheriae*, and some species of *Haemophilus* and *Streptococcus*. These infections can start as a routine mucopurulent conjunctivitis but can rapidly progress to a severe infection with marked chemosis, copious discharge, and lid edema. An expedient Gram stain is important for diagnosis and institution of appropriate systemic antibiotics. A hyperacute form of neonatal conjunctivitis (ophthalmia neonatorum) can be caused by *Neisseria* species as well. This infection typically presents 2 to 4 days following vaginal delivery. The signs are the same as those for adult hyperacute conjunctivitis. Rapid and accurate diagnosis is essential for preventing vision loss.

Inflammation of the conjunctiva can also be caused by allergy or toxic agents. Patients with seasonal allergic conjunctivitis report intermittent ocular itching, watering, and redness. These symptoms are usually present in association with seasonal rhinitis or sinusitis. The symptoms, particularly itching, usually far outweigh the clinical signs in this disorder. In fact, there may be no findings on clinical examination, despite dramatic symptomatology, and the diagnosis is made on history alone. The signs, if present, include mild conjunctival injection and chemosis. A watery discharge may be noted.

Allergic or toxic reactions from medications can occur. One should inquire about ocular medications in patients with conjunctival injection. Neomycin-containing solutions and the glaucoma medication apraclonidine are notorious for causing allergic conjunctivitis.

It is important to mention that conjunctival injection occurs in ophthalmic disorders other than conjunctivitis. Acute elevations in intraocular pressure, such as that in angle-closure glaucoma (see the section on glaucoma, below), also present with a red eye. In addition, inflammation of the pigmented layers of the eye (uveitis, iritis) can cause conjunctival inflammation in association with the intraocular inflammation. Subconjunctival hemorrhage, which presents as a localized, flat, deep-red hemorrhage under the conjunctiva, is often associated with minor trauma but is occasionally idiopathic. Injection of the sclera, the layer beneath the conjunctiva, is a potentially serious condition often associated with systemic disorders, such as rheumatoid arthritis and Wegener's granulomatosis. In scleritis, the injected vessels lie deeper than those in conjunctivitis, and they are not freely movable with a cotton-tipped swab. The injected vessels in scleritis do not blanch after instillation of dilating drops such as phenylephrine, whereas those in conjunctivitis do. When one is in doubt about the etiology of a red eye that seems atypical for routine viral or bacterial conjunctivitis, it is advisable to seek an opinion from an ophthalmologist.

Bacterial Keratitis

Bacterial keratitis can be categorized according to location on the cornea, either central or peripheral (limbal).

Central corneal ulcers can lead to severe vision loss and must be taken seriously. These ulcers are often associated with contact lens use, especially overnight use of extended-wear lenses. Because of the dramatically increased risk of corneal ulcer, the authors do not recommend overnight use of lenses. The causative organisms for central corneal ulcers include *Staphylococcus* and *Streptococcus* species. *Pseudomonas* is common in contact lens–associated ulcers. *Moraxella* may be found in alcoholic or debilitated hosts.

On clinical examination, the eye appears red. A white infiltrate is seen in the central cornea with an overlying epithelial defect that is visible with fluorescein staining. A hypopyon, layered white cells within the anterior chamber, may be seen with a severe ulcer. A cellular reaction within the anterior chamber can be visualized with a slit lamp.

Central corneal ulcers require definitive identification of the causative agent to ensure appropriate antibiotic coverage. Scraping of the ulcer for Gram stain and cultures should be performed before institution of antibiotic therapy. This procedure is best performed by an ophthalmologist, and immediate referral should be made when a corneal ulcer is suspected.

Multiple small infiltrates located at the limbus may be seen in association with staphylococcal blepharitis. These so-called marginal ulcers are immune in nature, rather than infectious, and are believed to represent hypersensitivity reactions to bacterial antigens. Cultures of these ulcers are sterile.

Viral Keratitis

Herpes simplex virus (HSV) keratitis is the most common infectious cause of blindness in the United States. Nearly half a million cases of herpes simplex virus keratitis occur yearly. Primary ocular herpes usually presents as an acute follicular keratoconjunctivitis with regional lymphadenopathy. Vesicular ulcerative blepharitis or lesions of the surrounding skin may occur as well. Like other herpesvirus infections, the initial course is self-limited, but the virus establishes a latent infection in the trigeminal ganglion. Reactivation of the virus due to physical or emotional stress leads to recurrent disease, which can often be challenging to treat.

Recurrent disease can take a number of different forms. Most common is the epithelial infection that is manifested by a corneal dendrite. Dendrites are branching forms with terminal bulbs on the corneal surface, visible after instillation of fluorescein or rose bengal dye. Dendrites represent live virus particles within the basal layers of the corneal epithelium and are typically associated with conjunctival injection. Iritis may be present as well.

Herpes simplex keratitis can also trigger various immune reactions throughout all layers of the cornea. These reactions are not due to the presence of active virus, but rather to immune reaction to viral antigens. Focal corneal haze may be seen with immune keratitis. Both primary and recurrent herpetic keratitis should be managed by an ophthalmologist.

Varicella-Zoster Virus Ocular Infection

Reactivation of the herpes zoster (chickenpox) virus within the trigeminal ganglion can lead to ocular involvement. Reactivation is associated with defective cell-mediated immunity that may occur with advancing age, immunosuppression, or acquired immunodeficiency. Cases of herpes zoster have increased dramatically since the onset of the acquired immunodeficiency syndrome (AIDS) epidemic. AIDS should be considered in any zoster patient younger than 45 years of age.

Clinically, patients present with the typical vesicular skin lesions located in the V1 dermatome. Ocular involvement occurs in about half of these patients. Milder presentations may show conjunctival injection only. Keratitis, ranging from fine superficial punctate keratopathy to frank dendritic ulceration, is common. Iritis can occur. Inflammation of the trabecular meshwork can lead to acute glaucoma. Retinitis, optic neuritis, and cranial nerve palsies have been reported in association with herpes zoster infection.

Although the acute phase of herpes zoster ophthalmicus is usually short-lived, the disease can have severe long-term sequelae. Dense corneal anesthesia often occurs after ocular zoster, predisposing to corneal ulceration. In addition, postherpetic neuralgia can be difficult to treat and frustrating for the patient.

Ocular Infection With Human Immunodeficiency Virus (HIV)

Ocular manifestations of HIV are protean. Almost 60 per cent of HIV patients have ocular involvement at some point in the disease. Patients with HIV are prone to multiple opportunistic infections with viral, bacterial, fungal, and parasitic agents.

Anterior segment lesions include follicular conjunctivitis, Kaposi's sarcoma of the conjunctiva, a punctate ulcerative keratitis that may mimic herpes infection, and anterior uveitis. Herpes zoster and simplex infections are more common, and often more complicated, in AIDS patients. There is an increased incidence of fungal and bacterial corneal ulcers as well.

The majority of ocular conditions in HIV patients involve the retina and choroid. Cytomegalovirus (CMV) retinitis is estimated to occur in 30 to 40 per cent of AIDS patients, especially when CD4 counts fall below 50 cells/μl. Symptoms of CMV retinitis include decreased visual acuity. Patients may note an increase in the number of "floaters" as well. On examination, cells may be noted within the vitreous. The fundus shows exudates and hemorrhages, especially along the vascular arcades (so-called "pizza pie" fundus). Vascular sheathing may be seen. Treatment of CMV retinitis is lifelong and fraught with serious side effects. Retinal atrophy from regressed CMV can lead to retinal detachments. Routine dilated-eye examinations should be performed every 6 months on patients with CD4 counts less than 200 cells/μl, and sooner should symptoms develop.

Retinitis from *Toxoplasma gondii* also occurs in HIV patients, although it is less common than CMV retinitis. Distinguishing between these entities may be difficult for the nonophthalmologist. Acute retinal necrosis can also occur in AIDS patients, occasionally in association with infection with herpes zoster or simplex.

Periorbital and Orbital Cellulitis

Bacterial infections of the periorbital tissues can be categorized according to location. Preseptal cellulitis denotes infection anterior to the orbital septum. The eye itself is *uninvolved* in preseptal cellulitis. Vision, pupillary reactions, and extraocular motility are normal. The clinical signs include dramatic edema and erythema of the eyelids and periorbital skin. The eyes may be swollen shut. As with cellulitis elsewhere, *Staphylococcus* and *Streptococcus* species are common causative agents. *Haemophilus* may be found in children with preseptal cellulitis.

Orbital cellulitis, on the other hand, involves structures posterior to the orbital septum. In addition to eyelid swelling and redness, chemosis and conjunctival injection are present. The eye may be proptotic. There is often limitation of extraocular motility. Visual acuity or color vision may be impaired. Pupillary reactions may be abnormal. Orbital cellulitis often results from contiguous spread from infected sinuses, especially in children. This is a life-threatening condition that requires emergency treatment. Rapid referral to an ophthalmologist and to an otolaryngologist is mandatory.

CATARACTS

Changes with age occur within the lens in most patients, although not all of these changes are visually significant. Patients with visually significant cataracts report decreased visual acuity. Whether distance or near vision is more severely affected depends on the type of cataract. Cataracts in which nuclear sclerosis predominates often cause decreased distance vision with relatively preserved near vision. Surgery may often be deferred with refraction and new glasses. Cortical cataracts, on the other hand, cause greater reduction of near vision. Posterior subcapsular cataracts, common in diabetics and patients receiving steroids, often cause tremendous difficulty with glare, even in relatively low-light situations.

The diagnosis of cataract can be made with a penlight when the cataract is advanced. In the case of a hypermature cataract, the white lens is visible through the pupil. In less advanced cases, the color of the lens has changed to shades of yellow or brown. Cortical cataracts may be visible as white, spokelike projections into the visual axis. Posterior subcapsular cataracts can be visualized with the use of the high-plus (green) lenses on the direct ophthalmoscope. While looking through the ophthalmoscope at approximately 1 foot from the patient, the physician can occasionally see a plaquelike opacification in the posterior portion of the lens. Significant cataracts of all types decrease the examiner's view into the posterior pole, a finding that can be used to confirm the diagnosis.

GLAUCOMA

Glaucoma is a general term used for various disorders that have in common damage to the optic nerve in association with increased intraocular pressure. The at least 40 different types of glaucoma differ in their epidemiology and presumed mechanism of increased intraocular pressure.

Most common is primary or chronic open-angle glaucoma in which there is increased eye pressure without a clinically detectable structural alteration in the eye. This is an insidious disease, causing peripheral vision loss that is unrecognized by the patient until very late in the disorder. The diagnosis of open-angle glaucoma is made with detection of increased intraocular pressure in association with visual field and/or optic nerve changes. In advanced glaucoma, there is "cupping" of the optic nerve, in which the central physiologic depression in the nerve head expands to fill the entire nerve. There may be optic nerve pallor and displacement of the retinal blood vessels to the nasal side of the disc. The two optic nerves may be affected asymmetrically. These changes correlate with the death of the ganglion cells that serve as the conduit from the retina to the higher portions of the visual system. Optic nerve changes such as these may be detected on direct ophthalmoscopy. By the time changes are this advanced, however, significant visual field loss has occurred, although the patient may be unaware of the defect. Thus, a yearly check of intraocular pressure by an eye care provider is an important piece of preventive medicine.

Acute forms of glaucoma are also seen, and these are more likely to present to the nonophthalmologist. In angle-closure glaucoma, an acute, symptomatic increase of intraocular pressure is caused by blockage of the trabecular meshwork, the drainage pathway of the eye, usually by peripheral iris tissue. Patients with particularly "short" eyes (e.g., those with high hyperopia) and those with anatomically narrow "angles" or outflow paths are more prone to this disorder. These patients present with acute onset of a unilateral, painful red eye. There may be headache or nausea and vomiting. The pupil is fixed in mid-dilation. The cornea may be hazy. Patients may give a history of similar, short-lived episodes in the past. When a penlight is shown from the temporal side of the eye, the nasal part of the iris is in shadow (Fig. 2). Intraocular pressures can be as high as 70 mm Hg. Immediate referral to an ophthalmologist is essential.

RETINAL DISEASES

Age-Related Macular Degeneration

Age-related macular degeneration (ARMD) is a very common and, as yet, poorly understood degeneration of the macula, the part of the retina responsible for our fine, central vision. In ARMD, there is deposition of drusen, thought to represent discharged material from the phagosomes of the retinal pigment epithelial cells, beneath the retinal pigment epithelium. Continued accumulation of drusen causes disruption of Bruch's membrane, the layer between the retinal pigment epithelium and the vascular choroid.

The presence of drusen, which are seen clinically as small, bright, yellow-white circular points deep in the retina, constitutes the "dry" form of ARMD. The exudative, or "wet," type of ARMD occurs when new blood vessels grow from the choroid through the breaks in Bruch's membrane to lie beneath the retinal pigment epithelium. These subretinal neovascular membranes are fragile and bleed easily, leading to a loss of central vision. Clinically, the exudative form of ARMD is suggested by the presence of subretinal hemorrhage, which appears greenish gray, and elevation of the macula. Drusen often are seen in the other eye. The diagnosis is confirmed by fluorescein angiography,

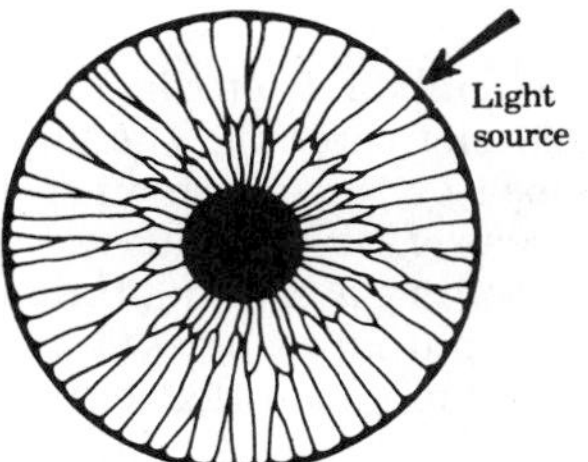

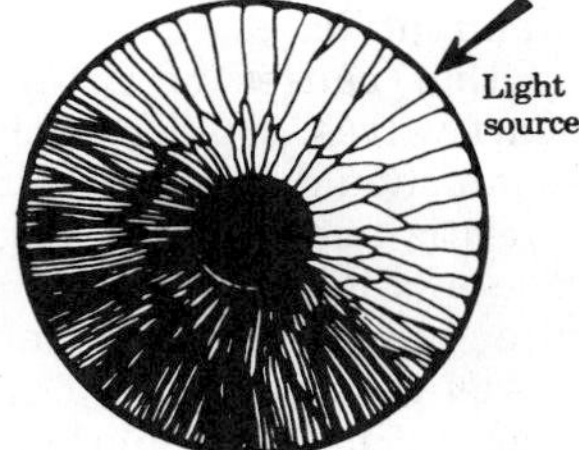

A Deep **B** Shallow

Figure 2. Estimation of anterior chamber depth by oblique illumination. *A,* Safe for dilation. *B,* Risk of acute-angle closure, spontaneous or on dilation. (Adapted from D. Paton and J. Craig, *Glaucomas: Diagnosis and Management.* Clinical Symposia. Summit, N.J.: Ciba Pharmaceutical Co., 1976, and *Manual of Ocular Diagnosis and Therapy,* 4th ed. [D. Pavan-Langston], Little, Brown and Co. [Inc.], Boston, 1995. With permission.)

which demonstrates the leaking blood vessels. In the end stage of exudative ARMD, an area of atrophy, often extensive, can be seen in the macula, corresponding to the site of the involuted neovascular membrane.

Diabetic Retinopathy

Diabetic retinopathy is a common cause of visual loss. The major risk factor for retinopathy is duration of diabetes. All patients with diabetes need routine ophthalmologic evaluation at regular intervals.

Diabetic retinopathy can be broadly divided into nonproliferative and proliferative forms. Nonproliferative retinopathy is characterized by microaneurysms and intraretinal, "dot-and-blot" hemorrhages. Changes in the caliber of the veins, so-called venous beading, and cotton-wool spots, representing infarction of the nerve fiber layer, may be seen. In proliferative retinopathy, there is growth of new blood vessels, thought to be stimulated by an as yet unidentified angiogenic factor produced by the ischemic retina. These new blood vessels are fragile and thus may bleed, leading to preretinal or vitreous hemorrhage. Another consequence of diabetes is swelling of the macula (macular edema), a common cause of visual loss in patients with adult-onset diabetes.

The direct ophthalmoscope can be used to detect microaneurysms and hemorrhages. One may also see new vessels on the optic disc. When vitreous hemorrhage has occurred, the patient's vision is diminished, and the examiner's view of the posterior pole may be obscured by blood. Dulling or loss of the foveal light reflex may be a sign of macular edema.

Central Retinal Artery Occlusion

Central retinal artery occlusion (CRAO), most commonly caused by emboli from carotid artery atherosclerotic plaques, is an ocular emergency. Ischemia of the inner retina results in irreversible damage within 1 hour. Patients typically present with sudden, dramatic painless loss of vision in one eye, often to bare light perception. On examination, the infarcted retina is milky white and edematous. There may be a "cherry-red spot" within the fovea, reflecting the underlying choroidal blood flow. An embolus may be seen within the central retinal artery, often lodged at a vessel bifurcation. The retinal arterioles are markedly constricted. Slowing of blood flow so that the passage of individual red blood cells can be seen, so-called "boxcarring," may be noted. When the embolus lodges within a branch artery, only part of the patient's vision is lost and part of the retina appears milky white on clinical examination.

Other causes of CRAO include emboli from diseased heart valves, septic emboli, and platelet thrombi. The physician should rule out systemic diseases, such as temporal arteritis and collagen vascular diseases, as the cause of a case of CRAO by immediately obtaining a sedimentation rate. Immediate treatment by an ophthalmologist is required to prevent the permanent loss of vision that occurs when retinal ischemia continues for more than 1 hour.

Central Retinal Vein Occlusion

Occlusion of the central retinal vein (CRVO) causes an obstruction of venous outflow from the eye and resulting stagnation of blood flow. The elevation of intravascular pressure causes vessel leakage, hemorrhage, and retinal edema.

Clinically, CRVO presents with a wide spectrum of appearances, depending on the severity of the outflow obstruction. Early in the course of disease, the veins may appear minimally dilated. Rare hemorrhages and limited macular edema are noted. The patient may notice only a mild decrease in vision. Later, optic disc edema develops. The retinal veins are markedly dilated and tortuous. Extensive retinal hemorrhages and cotton-wool spots extending to the retinal periphery are present (so-called "blood and thunder" fundus). Severe macular edema may be noted. Vision may be decreased to hand motions.

The causes of CRVO are varied. Possible mechanisms include retro-ocular tumors, external compression of the retinal veins, thrombus formation, and primary vasculitis. There is no acute treatment for CRVO. However, patients with CRVO should be evaluated by an ophthalmologist to prevent potentially devastating long-term sequelae such as neovascular glaucoma.

Retinal Detachment

In retinal detachment, fluid collects in the potential space between the sensory retina (containing photoreceptors, ganglion, and intervening cells) and the underlying retinal pigment epithelium, the layer that supports and nourishes the photoreceptors. Rhegmatogenous retinal detachments, in which subretinal fluid accumulates through a tear or hole in the retina, are the most common type.

The symptoms of a retinal detachment include a large number of new "floaters" with associated flashes of light. Patients also report a visual field cut, usually described as a gray or black curtain over part of the visual field.

Visual acuity is typically reduced; the extent depends on whether the detachment involves the macula. The detached retina may be visible with the direct ophthalmoscope as a billowing translucent membrane. A retinal hole may be noted. Detachments and holes outside the posterior pole usually are not visible with the direct ophthalmoscope. For this reason, patients with the aforementioned symptoms should be referred to an ophthalmologist for a dilated-eye retinal examination.

NEURO-OPHTHALMIC DISORDERS

Optic Neuritis

Optic neuritis is often secondary to demyelination and may be a harbinger of multiple sclerosis. There are also idiopathic cases of optic nerve inflammation. The symptoms include decreased visual acuity and pain on eye movements. The acuity may worsen over several days before it reaches its nadir. On examination, there is decreased visual acuity, ranging from relatively mild (20/30) to dramatic (counting fingers). Dyschromatopsia (color vision alteration) can be detected with the use of Ishihara pseudoisochromic plates. Subjective red desaturation may be noted as well. To test this, simply show a brightly colored red object to each eye separately. The red will often appear "washed out" to the involved eye. A relative afferent pupillary defect will also be seen, although this may be subtle. The swinging flashlight test is used to detect an afferent pupillary defect. To test pupillary responses, the patient should be instructed to look in the distance. The examiner shines a bright light in one eye, then quickly alternates to the other eye. The normal response to light is a brief constriction and then a slight release to a slightly larger, constant diameter. When a relative afferent defect is present, both pupils become larger as the light is shone into the affected eye and smaller as the light is directed toward the uninvolved eye. Dimming the room lights may help detect a subtle afferent defect.

If the intraocular portion of the optic nerve is affected, disc swelling and hyperemia may be present, ranging from mild to florid. Splinter hemorrhages may be seen. In retrobulbar optic neuritis, the fundus is normal at the time of active inflammation. Optic atrophy typically occurs as a late sequela of optic neuritis.

Temporal Arteritis

Temporal, or giant cell, arteritis is a systemic vasculitis of the elderly. Although usually idiopathic, it may be associated with systemic conditions, such as polymyalgia rheumatica. Patients present with complaints of headache, jaw claudication, neck ache, fever, chills, weight loss, and general malaise. Amaurosis fugax, transient monocular vision loss, may be described as momentary blurred vision or obscuring of vision by a gray cloud. This symptom represents retinal ischemia and may be a harbinger of severe vision loss. Episodes of transient monocular vision loss that alternate between eyes must be considered to be giant cell arteritis until proved otherwise. A delay in instituting systemic therapy for this disorder can result in severe vision loss in both eyes.

The signs on examination include decreased vision, dyschromatopsia, and an afferent pupillary defect. Funduscopic examination may reveal pallid swelling of the optic disc, which may be seen in association with segmental disc infarction. Small peripapillary hemorrhages may be noted. Cotton-wool spots, representing focal infarction of the nerve-fiber layer of the retina, may be seen. Temporal arteritis can also cause a CRAO, in which signs would be as described earlier.

The sedimentation rate is elevated in temporal arteritis, although this is not a specific sign, as the sedimentation rate may be high in other disorders as well. If temporal arteritis is suspected, treatment should be started. Confirmation of the diagnosis can then be made with temporal artery biopsy, which reveals the characteristic inflammation within the arterial wall. One must maintain a high index of suspicion for temporal arteritis in any patient older than 55 years of age with visual complaints and other systemic symptoms. This treatable disorder can have devastating visual consequences if it is missed.

Papilledema

Papilledema has a very specific definition, namely, optic disc swelling secondary to increased intracranial pressure. Papilledema is a bilateral process, although the discs may be affected asymmetrically. Unilateral disc swelling accompanies a number of other ophthalmic disorders, some of which were mentioned earlier. These are not papilledema.

The signs of papilledema include blurring of the margins of the optic disc, disc hyperemia, and obscuration of the retinal vessels as they cross the disc. Disc elevation, sometimes dramatic, may occur with papilledema. Although best demonstrated with stereoscopic viewing techniques such as indirect ophthalmoscopy, disc elevation can be detected with the use of the direct ophthalmoscope. The physician notes what power lens is required for a clear view of the retina and then focuses on the disc. Every 1 mm of disc elevation requires a compensatory 3 diopters of plus power (green or black numbers on the direct ophthalmoscope) for clear focus.

The symptoms of papilledema include transient visual obscurations and visual field defects from enlargement of the blind spot. Headache, especially on awakening or with straining or coughing, is common. True papilledema requires referral to a neurologist.

PEDIATRIC EYE DISORDERS

The diagnosis of pediatric eye disorders can be challenging. A history must be obtained from the parents, the physician is often unable to obtain an accurate assessment of visual acuity, and the examination itself may be difficult because of a lack of patient cooperation. Nonetheless, it is important to be experienced with the basics of a pediatric eye examination and a few of the more common pediatric ophthalmic conditions.

Routine physical examinations in children should include measurement of visual acuity as soon as the child is able to cooperate with testing. Most children older than 2 years of age are able to perform some rudimentary distance acuity test, either naming or matching pictures (Allen's cards). It is important to test each eye separately. This is best done with an adhesive patch over the eye not being tested. Children are remarkably adept at peeking around occluders. Many pediatric eye disorders affect only one eye, leaving the other eye with normal acuity. Thus, a serious problem may be missed if acuity is measured in both eyes simultaneously.

The direct ophthalmoscope should be used to evaluate the red reflex in children of all ages. While looking through the ophthalmoscope at about a foot from the patient, the examiner shines the light through the pupil. A sharp red reflex should be noted. This maneuver screens for media opacities such as cataracts, as well as for gross lesions of the posterior pole. A more detailed view of the optic disc should be obtained as soon as the child is old enough to cooperate.

A common eye problem that may be detected by the nonophthalmologist is misalignment of the eyes, or strabismus. Horizontal misalignment can be divided into esotropia (in-turning of the eyes) and exotropia (out-turning of the eyes). There are a number of different causes of strabismus, which vary in age at onset, treatment, and prognosis. Often a family history of strabismus is present. Transient misalignment of the eyes is not uncommon during the first 6 months of life. However, constant deviations at any age are abnormal, and such patients should be promptly referred to an ophthalmologist.

The diagnosis of strabismus can be made by examining the location of the pupillary light reflexes. When one eye is turned in, the pupillary light reflex is displaced temporally. Conversely, when the eye is turned outward, the light reflex moves nasally. The magnitude of the misalignment is proportional to the degree of decentration of the pupillary light reflex. Additional tests, including cycloplegic retinoscopic refraction, are needed to determine the exact type of strabismus present. Detection and treatment of strabismus in young children is critical for avoiding the development of amblyopia. If both eyes are not used equally during childhood, for whatever reason—strabismus, anisometropia (unequal refractive error), or media opacity such as cataract—the pathways in the brain are not "wired up" properly. Vision will be permanently diminished even if the eye appears normal on examination. In addition, stereovision will not develop properly if significant amblyopia is present.

WORKING WITH A DIFFICULT PATIENT

By Barry Egener, M.D.,
and Wendy Levinson, M.D.
Portland, Oregon

In the era of managed care, the nature of the doctor-patient relationship is changing from a paternalistic to a more collaborative one. The patient of a generation ago commonly expected to "follow doctor's orders," whereas the patient of the 1990s expects to be educated about health care options and to have an equal voice in decision-making. The impact of this change on the physician has been equally significant. The physician's power to effect healthy change depends less on professional image and more on technical and interpersonal skills. The more empowered patient may openly challenge the physician, viewing the professional as having to balance medical needs against the economic needs of the health plan.

Particular types of patients may present challenges, for example, the patient with a list, the patient who is angry because of having to wait, the patient with a 5-day headache who needs proof of the nonexistence of a tumor, or the injured worker who is tired of suffering and feels entitled to "real pain medications." Of course these patients existed before managed care, but patients' newly recognized power makes them more likely to express disagreement or distrust. Physicians are more likely to feel threatened by such challenges to their authority.

Some patients are challenging for all or most physicians. Such patients include those who elicit feelings of hopelessness, patients who have poor treatment outcomes, and patients who do not conform to expectations. In addition, patients with psychosocial and psychiatric problems, especially somatization disorder, are often considered "difficult." The common theme may be that these patients challenge the physician's ability to bring about a favorable medical outcome. Similarly, patients who are unable to change poor health habits are frustrating because physicians cannot change their behavior.

In workshops conducted on this topic, a curious phenomenon has emerged—that the most challenging patients for some doctors are not at all challenging for others. This suggests that in some instances, differences among physicians may explain the different perceptions of what constitutes a difficult patient. Differences in physician personality traits may create potential "mismatches" with certain kinds of patients. When physicians encounter particular types of patients uniquely challenging to them, discussions with colleagues may provide useful insights about working with and caring for these patients. A general approach to the medical interview may set the stage for a successful encounter. However, specific approaches may be required for certain types of patients that doctors commonly describe as "difficult."

INTERACTION BETWEEN DOCTOR AND PATIENT

The medical interview establishes the set of problems to be addressed and begins the process of compiling the data to be used in clinical reasoning. It also begins to define the nature of the doctor-patient relationship, the degree of compliance that may be achieved in the care process, and the level of satisfaction of both patient and physician with the process (Table 1). Information obtained in the interview is crucial for the physician's understanding the context of the illness and the patient's views and attitudes about it. Time constraints require that the medical interview be made as effective and efficient as possible. Specific communication skills can help achieve this goal. These skills facilitate data gathering during routine visits and also help prevent breakdowns in communication between physicians and difficult patients.

Physicians gather data from both the verbal and nonverbal communications of patients. From the moment of introduction, patients send clues about their lifestyle and self-image as well as their illnesses. Sometimes these initial clues can help the physician make patients more comfortable. Comments that convey compassion; for example, "*You look anxious,*" and the use of open questions; for example, "*Can I help you feel comfortable so that we can begin?*" can greatly help put the patient at ease.

Most interviews begin by eliciting the reason for the patient's visit. Again the use of open-ended questions; for example, "*What is the problem that brings you here today?*" or "*What concerns have led to your visit today?*" allow patients to begin telling their story. Studies support the importance of letting patients complete their opening statement about their concerns in an uninterrupted fashion. Interrupting patients before they have completed their initial statement may be interpreted as a lack of interest or a lack of time. Furthermore, interrupting early in the interview may lead patients to delay expressing their real concerns until late in the visit or not at all. Physicians often worry that patients will take too long, but most patients complete their opening statements within 90 seconds and provide important historical details.

After the patient has explained the initial concern, another open-ended question, for example, "*What else concerns you?*" may elicit descriptions of other medical problems. On average, patients have three problems at a first visit, and often the concern mentioned initially is not the most important to the patient. Allowing patients to express all their concerns at the beginning of the interview can make the interview more efficient, often avoiding last minute worries being brought up in the closing moments of the interview. Problems expressed by the patient as the physician is leaving the room, for example, "*Oh, by the way. . .*" can be particularly frustrating. Sometimes it is not possible to cover all the patient's concerns in one visit; in this situation, the physician and patient must negotiate the highest priorities for the time available (see discussion of patients with lists).

Data gathering is often most efficient when physicians use open-ended questions; for example, "*Tell me about your chest pain*" to begin each line of inquiry. These questions invite patients to convey their experience in an unrestricted fashion. Once patients have presented the story, physicians can focus on details, using more closed-ended questions about details not covered. This technique, often called "open to closed cone" of questions, has been documented as an efficient interviewing style associated with high patient satisfaction.

Table 1. Functions of the Medical Interview

Gathering data
Building the doctor-patient relationship
Educating the patient about diagnosis and treatment

As the story of the illness unfolds, the physician can learn about the patient as a person. Understanding the contexts of patients' lives, how illnesses affect them, and their beliefs about their problems is vital to patient satisfaction and good health outcomes. Often patients complain that physicians treat them like a disease, for example, *"the diabetic in room 101"* or *"the patient with gallstones,"* rather than showing compassion for the person. An efficient strategy for the physician is to follow up on clues mentioned by the patient. For example, the patient may state, *"I have these headaches whenever I'm at work,"* to which the physician may respond *"work?"* By simply repeating the patient's word, the physician opens the opportunity for the patient to provide important details about his or her life.

It is also important for physicians to discover what patients believe about their disease and its possible treatments. Most patients come to physicians with information about what their symptoms might represent. They have read such information or have heard it from friends. They have often heard of treatments that have been successful for others and hope that the physician will prescribe these treatments for them. It is efficient to discover these beliefs early so that they can be incorporated into plans for diagnostic investigations or therapeutic management. For example, a postmenopausal woman may believe that hormones lead to cancer, and she may be resistant to the physician's suggestion for estrogen replacement therapy. Understanding the patient's fears and beliefs may allow discussion about the risks and benefits. Patients will not always state their beliefs in the discussion because they fear criticism or derision. Again, this information may be elicited by a concerned, tactful line of questioning; for example, *"Most patients have ideas about what might be causing their problem. Do you have any ideas about what is causing your problem?"*

Patients visiting physicians are often worried about their health problems or feel emotional distress about issues in their personal life. They may come to the appointment feeling sadness, anger, frustration, or anxiety. To build trust and make the interview effective, the physician must recognize and address patients' feelings. This can be challenging for the physician and is often neglected. When patients are experiencing strong emotions, physicians may fear that discussing these emotions will slow the interview by "opening a can of worms." In fact, talking to patients about their feelings and understanding their emotional experience is therapeutic and actually builds the doctor-patient relationship. Physicians should address these feelings when they first appear in the interview by commenting on them directly; for example, *"You seem pretty sad about the things that have happened."* After the patient confirms the feelings, the physician may make a statement that shows compassion for the patient's situation; for example, *"I can understand feeling like that. It must be so disappointing to you to have it turn out this way."* Such brief comments indicate recognition of the patient's pain and understanding of the patient's life experience. If appropriate, a further statement of empathy may be made; for example, *"Many people would feel the same way in this situation."* Even if the physician disagrees with the patient's point of view, a statement of understanding may comfort the patient; for example, *"I can understand feeling angry with the delay in getting an appointment when you were worried something was seriously wrong."* The physician shows acceptance of the patient's feelings even though the patient's response seems unreasonable.

Physicians can also use nonverbal communication to indicate their concern for patients' feelings. Touching a patient who is feeling sad or tearful is a strong statement of caring. Similarly, maintaining a relaxed and nondefensive body posture when a patient is expressing anger can communicate acceptance rather than defensiveness.

Patients often complain that they do not receive enough information from physicians or that physicians use jargon to explain medical concepts. Explaining a patient's diagnoses in a simple fashion allows time for questions. Spending additional time to discuss the treatment plan and the next steps in the patient's care can be timesaving. Misunderstandings can be minimized by asking the patient to write notes about the treatment plan. Compliance can be improved by exploring potential barriers to therapy; for example, *"It's often hard to remember to take pills three times a day. What will the hard part of this be for you?"* This allows the patient to anticipate difficulties and plan a strategy to deal with them.

DIFFICULT ENCOUNTERS

Some visits will be difficult even with the skillful use of interviewing techniques. Specific communiation strategies are often helpful in these situations. The physician may not recognize that a breakdown in communication has occurred until the patient has actually left the room. Awareness of the problem while it is happening is crucial to improving the situation. A negative attitude toward the patient may be the physician's first clue to a communication barrier. Physicians' recognition of their own feelings at a conscious level can be useful in establishing effective lines of communication with patients. The physician, like the patient, may feel frustrated and hopeless about the therapeutic effectiveness of the treatment. Often the physician's feelings of helplessness really mirror the patient's experience. Physicians who recognize their own feelings may be able to improve a negative encounter.

Patients may express anger or blame the physician for problems beyond the physician's control. For example, patients may be frustrated by rules and regulations of the managed care plan that limit access to subspecialists, or they may express frustration and anger that the diagnosis of their illness is not immediately apparent or that tests have been unrevealing. These feelings may then be diverted toward the physician, who must avoid defensiveness, remain calm, and convey understanding and compassion to the patient. This can be accomplished by naming the feeling that the patient is expressing, (e.g., sadness, anger, and so on). The exact emotions the patient is experiencing may be unknown, but a comment on a specific observation; for example, *"I notice a tear in your eye"* may allow the patient to openly express feelings. The physician can then indicate empathy by accepting the patient's feelings as legitimate even when patient and physician disagree. For example, a patient may be angry that a physician is unwilling to write a referral to a specialist. From the physician's perspective, the patient may be making an unreasonable request, but these relationships can be strengthed by conveying empathy and understanding.

The physician and patient should become partners in solving a problem. The use of language such as "we" and "together" demonstrates that physician and patient are on the same team. It is useful to recognize differences and underscore areas of agreement. The physician can state the common goal, cite the differences of opinion, and propose a solution. Seeking the patient's opinion communicates respect and an effort to collaborate with the patient.

Occasionally the patient requests something that is not acceptable to the physician, such as narcotics for treatment of chronic pain. Under these circumstances, personal limits must be stated clearly. Although the physician may not be willing to prescribe narcotics, the statement should clearly define the issue as a professional guideline. Most patients respect the physician's professional (or sometimes personal) boundaries when they are stated clearly.

Despite the physician's helpful intent and clear communication, the patient may still have a strong negative reaction. The patient may appear to be purposely attempting to anger the physician. Feelings such as frustration, rejection, and anger directed toward the physician provide important insights into the patient's personality. An emotional response by the physician is inappropriate and can precipitate an unfavorable outcome.

DIFFICULT PATIENTS

Patients With Lists

Some patients visit the physician with a list of complaints or questions. They may not reveal their most serious concern first, but instead wait until they have established a relationship and a sense of trust. This is especially true when the problem is confidential or embarrassing (e.g., sexual dysfunction).

The most effective approach is to ask the patient to mention everything he or she wants to discuss early in the visit and then to ask "What else is on your list?" Scanning the list to look for patterns of symptoms may be useful. Dealing with all the problems on the list during the first visit may be impossible. The physician can also ask the patient which problems are most important, while understanding that priorities may differ between physician and patient (Table 2).

Angry Patients

Anger is common in illness and physicians must deal with it appropriately. A patient's anger can be directed at the physician, and it is often a manifestation of other feelings such as frustration, fear, and humiliation. Anger may be the outward expression of a deeper emotion that is more difficult to express. Physicians must avoid reacting to the anger in kind and instead convey understanding for the patient's condition. Expression of anger may be therapeutic, especially when it fails to trigger an emotional response from the physician (Table 3).

Substance Abusers

Patients who abuse medications may be suffering from physical illnesses, such as chronic back pain, or psychiatric illnesses, such as depression or anxiety. The physician should help the patient clearly express the goal for the visit. The patient's objective may be to obtain a drug or relief from a symptom. If the goal is relief, the physician and patient can collaborate on finding ways to help the patient. The medical history should include the success (if any) of treatment modalities other than drugs and the impact of the illness on family and friends. Any history of disability claims or treatment for substance abuse should be noted. Alcohol use should also be documented.

If the patient's goal is to obtain drugs, a limit-setting strategy becomes important. The physician's initial verbal response to the patient should show an understanding of the patient's request. Restating the patient's goal does not necessarily imply agreement. The empathy conveyed by the physician's response is as important as its content. Most physicians agree that scheduled drugs should not be used on a chronic basis, whether or not the patient's symptoms have an organic basis. This is best stated clearly early in the relationship so that the patient understands the "terms of the contract."

If the patient is a long-term user of a scheduled drug, it may be appropriate at the first meeting to set the ultimate goal of discontinuing the medication. The contract for the tapering schedule may be set at a later date. It should be clear and adhered to firmly but empathetically. Negotiation should concentrate on areas of agreement rather than disagreement. The common goal may be discontinuation of scheduled drugs, relief of suffering, or simply improved functioning. Complete elimination of symptoms may not be possible. If the patient continues to demand what the physician is unwilling to give, the refusal may be framed in terms of the physician's comfort, rather than the patient's limitation. A nondefensive, calm statement of the physician's professional position is less likely to escalate negative feelings than focusing on issues surrounding the patient's pain (e.g., whether the pain is "real" or whether too much medication is being used for too long).

Patients under the influence of drugs or alcohol may be particularly difficult because their behavior is unpredictable and often disturbing to other patients and staff. Many doctors refuse to see patients who are intoxicated, but at times this cannot be avoided. When interviewing intoxicated individuals, one's speech should be calm, simple, and clear. Specific patient instructions should be written. If violence is a possibility, the physician should sit between the patient and the door, with the door open. A security officer should be visible but not close enough to be perceived as a threat by the patient.

Psychotic patients often resemble intoxicated patients in their misinterpretation of their surroundings. Physicians

Table 2. Strategies for Patients With Lists

Strategy	Suggested Phrases
Invite the "list"	What else?
Look at the list, if written	
Ask patient's priorities	What is most important for us to cover today?
Negotiate the agenda for the visit	In the time we have together let's make sure we cover the headache (patient priority) and the chest pain (physician priority)
Plan strategy to deal with remaining problems	What do you think may be causing your problem?

Table 3. Strategies for the Angry Patient

Strategy	Suggested Phrases
Avoid becoming defensive	
Listen to the patient without interrupting	
Name patient's emotion and check underlying feelings	You seem very angry about this and maybe frustrated too.
Validate feelings (the physician does not need to argue to do this)	I can understand feeling angry in your situation, since you feel that the health plan has not met your needs
Build a common goal	I'd like to help solve your health problem if I can. I'd like to work together on this.

disagree about whether they should adopt the reality of the patient in order to communicate. A sense of how threatened the patient feels by his delusions can be gained from some discussion of their content. Clearly it is pointless to attempt to convince a delusional patient of the unreality in his universe.

Patients With Limited Capacity

Preverbal children, the severely retarded, and very demented patients are often unable to understand spoken language and are much more likely to respond to body language. Fearing the atmosphere of a physician's office or hospital, these patients may soften in response to smiles, a calm voice, and gentle touch. A simulated examination on a parent, who suffers no apparent ill effects, may gain the trust of an infant. Similarly, allowing an infant to handle medical equipment may provide a sense of control and comfort.

DOMESTIC VIOLENCE

By Elaine J. Alpert, M.D., M.P.H.
Boston, Massachusetts

Domestic violence is a public health problem of near-crisis proportions (Table 1). During the course of routine practice, nearly every physician encounters patients suffering from the short-term and long-term effects of domestic violence. Physicians can provide a supportive and confidential environment in which patients can safely disclose a history of domestic violence. The prerequisites for effective routine and emergency care of victims of domestic violence include the acquisition of a core body of knowledge, utilization of basic information-gathering skills, and employment of nonjudgmental attitudes.

The impact of domestic violence on the health of patients and on the health care system is substantial. Victims of violence not only suffer the acute effects of trauma but also are at risk for the long-term physical and psychological sequelae of victimization. Victims of domestic violence often perceive their health to be poor and present frequently for treatment of injuries as well as for evaluation and treatment of a variety of chronic medical conditions, including headaches, atypical chest pain, abdominal pain, pelvic pain, anxiety, depression, insomnia, and alcohol and other substance abuse.

Because physicians are often the first—and sometimes the only—health care professionals to whom victims of domestic violence may turn for care, they can play a crucial role in diagnosis, treatment, referral, and breaking the often intergenerational cycle of violence. Physicians who incorporate inquiry about domestic violence into the routine medical history can screen, assess, and intervene effectively, taking no more than a few minutes of the patient's visit. Effective intervention, however, also requires awareness of and collaboration with community resources, such as battered women's shelters, community-based advocates, support groups, and hospital social service departments, among others. Treatment begins at the time of diagnosis by ensuring safety and confidentiality in the doctor-patient relationship, addressing and reducing the nearly universal feelings of self-blame and humiliation experienced by the patient, and developing with the patient a safety plan, individualized according to her needs and the resources that she is able to access.

Table 1. Synonyms for Domestic Violence

Partner violence
Relationship violence
Dating violence
Teen dating violence
Intimate partner abuse
Spouse abuse
Domestic abuse
Wife abuse
Wife beating
Battering

Domestic violence can be defined as intentional violent or controlling behavior exhibited by a person who is currently, or was previously, in an intimate relationship with the victim. The battering syndrome encompasses a spectrum of intentional coercive behaviors that include not only actual or threatened physical injury but also sexual assault; social isolation; repetitive belittling verbal abuse; threats and intimidation; economic control; restriction of access to transportation, telephone, and other forms of communication; and denial of the woman's ability to receive education, health care, and other customary rights, privileges, and benefits generally available to individuals in a free society. These behaviors can occur in any combination, in sporadic episodes or chronically, for a short period of time or for many years.

Domestic violence may occur in the context of a married or unmarried heterosexual or homosexual relationship that may be, but is not necessarily, cohabitating; a traditional or a nontraditional family; or an extended kinship network. Most domestic abuse is perpetrated by men against women, although violence is also known to occur in both male and female homosexual relationships and, in a small proportion of cases, is perpetrated by women against men. Because violence against women represents the predominant expression of this syndrome, the victim is referred to as "she" and the perpetrator as "he" in the paragraphs that follow.

Any person who is disempowered is at risk for abuse. In domestic violence, the strongest risk factor is being female. Domestic violence occurs in all segments of society, independent of racial, ethnic, religious, educational, or socioeconomic factors. However, the prevalence of domestic violence does appear to be increased in certain groups (Table 2).

BEHAVIORAL DYNAMICS

The goal of the perpetrator in cases of domestic violence is to assert power and maintain control of the victim. The abuse can be physical, sexual, psychological, and/or economic. There is a strong association between abuse of women and child abuse and/or neglect. The abuse is generally one-way, although victims have been known to strike back in self-defense. In general, the victims of domestic violence are not constantly being beaten. Batterers may act in a caring and apologetic manner at times when no

Portions of this chapter have been adapted with permission from *Partner Violence: How to Recognize and Treat Victims of Abuse: A Guide for Physicians.* Copyright 1992, 1993, 1994, Massachusetts Medical Society.

Table 2. Risk Factors for Domestic Violence

Risk Factors
Women who are single or who have recently separated or divorced
Women who have recently sought an order of protection
Women younger than 28 years of age
Women who abuse alcohol or other drugs
Women who are pregnant
Women whose partners are excessively jealous or possessive
Women who have witnessed or experienced physical or sexual abuse as children
Women whose partners have witnessed or experienced physical or sexual abuse as children

overt abuse is taking place. Therefore, there may be no physical evidence of abuse at the time the physician sees the patient.

In general, abusive relationships do not begin with violence, but violence increases with time, as the perpetrator acts to exert progressive control over the victim. Abusive acts, whether physical, sexual, emotional, or of another nature, are rarely isolated events. Violent behavior is usually recurrent, and, in fact, violent acts tend to increase in both frequency and severity over time. There are many reasons why it is very difficult for battered women to leave their abusers. Any or all of these may be used by the perpetrator to exert control over the victim.

Fear

The batterer may threaten to hurt or even kill his victim, or to take away or hurt the children if she attempts to leave. Indeed, more battered women are murdered after obtaining a restraining order or while in the process of leaving their abusers than at any other time.

Economic and Other Constraints

The batterer often controls the financial resources of his victim as well as her access to telephones, transportation, and other sources of independence, making it impossible for the woman to leave because she would be unable to support herself and her children.

Social Isolation

The batterer often prevents his victim from communicating with friends and family. Isolation leaves the victim psychologically dependent on the batterer as her sole social support.

Feelings of Failure

Many battered women have been made to feel that they are failures and are responsible for having brought on the abuse. The woman may also adhere to personal, societal, or religious beliefs that her children deserve a two-parent family. She may thus believe that she is the one who must adapt or change to halt the abuse.

Promises of Change

Many women believe the batterer's apparent contrition for his abusive acts, and his promise that it will never happen again. While some women want the relationship to continue, most clearly want the violence to stop.

Prior Lack of Intervention

Historically, the desperate situations of many victims of abuse have not been acknowledged or taken seriously by family members, clergy, health care providers, educators, and law enforcement authorities; therefore, such women feel even more helpless and vulnerable.

CLINICAL EVALUATION

In addition to physical injuries, battered women experience serious but less readily visible sequelae. In addition to physical trauma, battered women may present with various health problems, including atypical chest pain, chronic abdominal pain, chronic musculoskeletal pain, chronic headaches, chronic pelvic pain, post-traumatic stress disorder, anxiety, depression, alcoholism, and other forms of substance abuse.

History

As part of routine patient care, all patients should be asked periodically about domestic violence. The patient should be interviewed in private, without her partner or children present. A history of previous trauma, chronic pain complaints, or psychological distress should be sought from direct history or from the medical record. A single question, asked routinely and nonjudgmentally during the course of the history, can significantly increase the detection rate of domestic violence in office practice and can allow the patient to feel safer in disclosing a history of abuse (Table 3). An example of such a question follows:

> "Because domestic violence is unfortunately so common and so devastating, I am now asking all my patients whether their lives have ever been touched by violence. At any time (or, in the case of an annual visit, in the last year), have you been hit, hurt, threatened, or frightened by a current or former partner or by anyone who took care of you as a child?"

If the patient discloses a history of domestic violence, it is important to determine who (first and last names) the batterer is, and the nature of his relationship with the patient. Ask the patient whether the batterer is living with her or whether he lives outside her home. Ask her whether anyone who is close to her or whom she trusts knows about the violence and has been supportive to the patient. It is important to determine whether the violence is escalating, because escalating violence commonly precedes homicide attempts.

If battering is diagnosed or suspected, even in the absence of disclosure, a few specific questions (Table 4), asked in the setting of a safe and confidential environment, may help determine the extent of abuse and the possible risk to the patient.

Table 3. Questions for Eliciting a History of Violence

Questions
Have you ever (or, "Since your last visit to my office, have you. . .") been hit, hurt, or threatened by your husband (or boyfriend or partner)?
What happens when you and your husband (or boyfriend or partner) have a disagreement at home?
Have you ever been threatened, intimidated, or frightened by your husband (or boyfriend or partner)?
Do you feel safe in your home?
Have you ever needed to see a doctor or go to an emergency room because someone did something to hurt or frighten you?
Are you afraid for your safety or for that of your children because of anyone you live with or are close to?
Would you leave your husband (or boyfriend or partner) if you could?

Table 4. Questions for the Victim of Domestic Violence

How were you hurt?
Has this happened before?
Could you tell me about the first episode?
How badly have you been hurt in the past?
Have you needed to go to an emergency room for treatment?
Have you ever been threatened with a weapon, or has a weapon ever been used on you?
Are you afraid for your children?
Have your children ever seen you threatened or hurt?
Have your children ever been threatened or hurt by your husband (or boyfriend or partner)?

Physical Examination

When domestic violence is suspected or confirmed by history-taking, the physician should conduct a thorough medical examination and document the findings carefully in the medical record (Table 5). Visible marks or deformities should be noted, and appropriate documentation is imperative. A picture may be drawn freehand, or findings may be noted on a preprinted line drawing (Fig. 1). Alternatively, a labeled photograph may be included as a supplement to a written description. It is important to accurately describe the patient's symptoms and signs and to identify the problem as "intentional injury," "domestic violence," or "partner violence."

Accurate documentation in the medical record can be a source of invaluable information should the patient ever seek legal redress from the batterer. Clear documentation in the medical record not only decreases the physician's risk of being required to personally appear in a legal proceeding (e.g., assault trial, custody hearing) but also helps ensure that the patient's allegations are viewed as legitimate in a court of law.

RISK ASSESSMENT, SAFETY PLANNING, AND INTERVENTION

Once a woman has disclosed that she is currently in a threatening or violent relationship, the physician should assess her level of risk, and initiate discussion of a safety plan with her. An important determinant in assessing risk is the woman's sense of her own fear and her own safety. However, since patients may minimize or deny the danger of their situation, indicators of escalating risk (Table 6) should be explored with the patient.

Table 5. Physical Findings That Often Occur With Domestic Violence

Any evidence of injury, especially to central areas of the body (face, torso, breasts, or genitals)
Bilateral or multiple injuries
Injuries in different stages of healing
Delay between the time of injury and the arrival of the patient to the health care facility
Explanation by the patient that is inconsistent with the type of injury
Prior, repetitive use of emergency services for trauma
Chronic pain symptoms when no etiology is apparent
Psychological distress: dissociation, suicidal ideation, depression, anxiety, or substance abuse
Evidence of rape or sexual assault
Pregnant woman with any injury, particularly to the abdomen or breasts

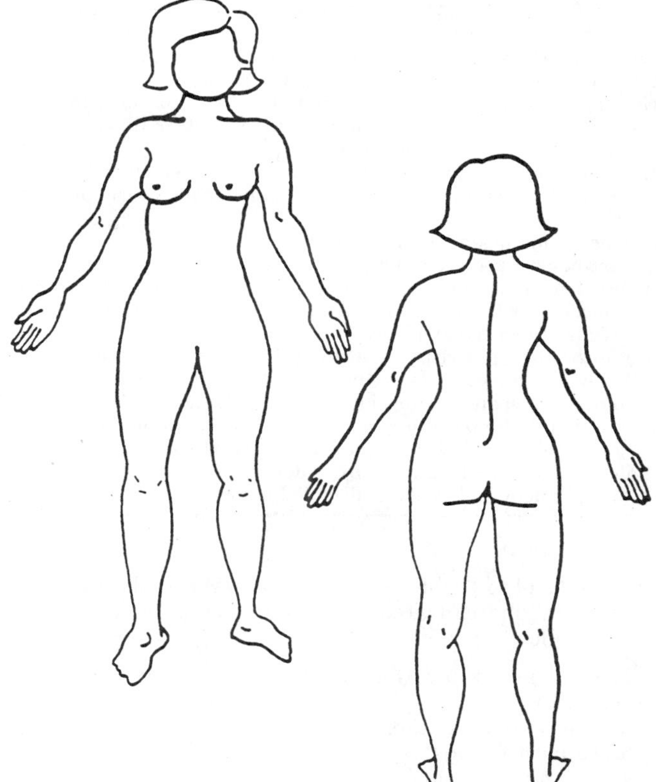

Figure 1. Body injury map.

The role of the physician is to convey to the patient his or her concern for her safety and to provide her with a framework for finding support to ensure her own safety and that of her children (Table 7). A simple statement such as "I am prepared to stand by you and help you when you feel you are ready to take action" can have a strongly positive effect on the patient.

Physicians are mandated reporters for domestic violence in a small number of states; however, most experts in domestic violence believe that it is *absolutely contraindicated* to report cases of domestic violence to any agency or authority without the woman's direct request and consent. Mandatory reporting of domestic violence often increases the woman's sense of powerlessness related to her own situation and may increase the risk of further harm, including the risk of homicide.

The physician must ensure that a safety plan is discussed once domestic violence has been identified. The physician may formulate a safety plan directly with the patient or may refer the patient to an appropriate resource, based on the patient's individual needs and the urgency of the situation. An individualized safety plan should be designed for each patient. Recall that each woman's needs and resources are unique, and that when children are involved, the woman should include the children's needs in

Table 6. Indicators of Escalating Risk

An increase in the frequency or severity of assaults
Increasing or new threats of homicide or suicide by the partner
The abuser's known criminal record of violent crime
The presence or availability of a firearm

Table 7. Specific Interventions by the Physician

Reframing the violent behavior as unacceptable and criminal
Conveying to the patient concern for her safety
Helping the patient understand that she did not deserve to be hit, hurt, or threatened by anyone under any circumstances, particularly by someone she loves
"Leaving the door open" for future discussion if she is not prepared to disclose the abuse or to take action at the present time
Diagnosis, management, and referral as appropriate for treatment of specific injuries and medical sequelae
Referral of the patient, as appropriate, for psychological counseling with providers who have expertise in caring for victims of domestic violence
Minimizing the prescription of tranquilizers or other sedating psychoactive medications (these could impair the victim's ability to respond appropriately should she need to flee)
Evaluation of the need to report the violence to an outside agency (physicians in all states must report suspected child abuse and/or neglect; in many states, they must report elder mistreatment and abuse of disabled persons)

her safety plan (Table 8). The patient should be informed about how she can access available community agencies for the following:

1. legal assistance (for orders of protection and victim assistance)
2. emergency shelters
3. support groups
4. emergency funds

It is the woman's role to decide when it is safe for her to leave, and when she has the economic and emotional resources and support to do so. It is the physician's role to provide the woman with options, support, and information about pertinent resources. The woman who does not leave a potentially dangerous relationship does not constitute a treatment failure or a noncompliant patient; the failure of such a woman to leave an abusive situation usually reflects the complex nature of the situation and the limited resources available to battered women.

DIAGNOSTIC PROBLEMS AND PITFALLS

It is clearly important to ask patients the right questions and to maintain privacy and confidentiality. It is equally important, however, to refrain from asking certain other questions, to avoid placing the patient in a situation that increases her danger or her sense of shame and humiliation about the violence. Most battered women do not identify themselves as "battered" per se because of the perception of utter shame and worthlessness associated with such a value-laden term. Therefore, the physician should avoid the use of terms such as "domestic violence," "abused," or "battered" when speaking initially with the patient. Do not inquire about the cause of the violence in the presence of the partner, because the victim may feel forced to lie to the physician to protect her immediate and future safety. Avoid disruption of patient confidentiality by disclosing any information to, or discussing your concerns with, the victim's partner. Never ask the patient why she has not left her partner. Quite commonly, a woman may leave her batterer, only to return later for financial, emotional, religious, or even safety reasons. Do not risk humiliating her by asking her why she keeps returning to her batterer. Never ask the victim what she did to bring on the violence.

For various reasons, the patient may be reluctant to disclose information about current or past abuse, even if specifically asked. She may not fully recognize the nature or extent of her distress and may not even recognize her condition as being attributable to domestic violence. She may not have access to regular medical care, and thus will not have had an opportunity to develop a trusting relationship with a physician or other health care provider. She may be troubled by comorbid conditions, such as alcoholism or other substance abuse, that impair her ability to offer a detailed and accurate history. She may believe that physicians and other health care providers have not been educated about this problem and thus may not know how to help her. She may feel that her physician may not have the time or interest to address the abuse. She may fear that her situation will not be taken seriously, and thus she may refuse to risk further humiliation by disclosing the abuse. She may also perceive that revealing her situation may mean further victimization as well as increased danger to herself or her children.

For various reasons, physicians may find it difficult to address domestic violence in the context of patient care. They may not be aware of the prevalence of domestic violence in their practice or in society at large. They may deny or minimize the seriousness of this problem, or may blame the victim by attributing responsibility for the abuse to her behavior. Physicians, like other members of society, often adhere to an idealized vision of the family and have difficulty in admitting that such a problem could even exist. Many members of society have taken the position that conflict in families is a private matter, that such strife should be kept "behind closed doors," and that it is not the business or responsibility of physicians, other health care providers, or anyone else to intervene. Because violence in all its manifestations is so prevalent, physicians may feel powerless to intervene and thus may avoid raising the subject entirely. Some physicians fear that asking patients about domestic violence may open a "Pandora's box," unleashing an overwhelming and unmanageable burden of responsibility for ongoing care. Furthermore, some physicians have been personally touched by victimization, either as child witnesses to family violence or as adult victims or perpetrators. Busy practices are constrained by the restric-

Table 8. Topics for Safety Planning

List of emergency phone numbers: shelter, hotline, police, legal advocacy, medical
A place to go (friends, family, or shelter)
A way of getting to a place of safety
Financial resources (cash, checkbook, credit card)
Personal information for the woman and her children: social security numbers, health insurance plan information, Medicaid, or other public assistance numbers
Miscellaneous items: keys to the car and house, changes of clothing, diapers, formula, medications, toothbrush, etc.

Table 9. Use Your "Radar"

1. *R*emember to be concerned about domestic violence in your own practice.
2. *A*sk about domestic violence as part of the routine of patient care.
3. *D*ocument your findings in the medical record.
4. *A*ssess your patient's immediate and future safety.
5. *R*eview options with your patient, and refer her, as appropriate, to community and legal agencies.

tive requirements of managed care with respect to time, resources, paperwork, and confidentiality and by concerns about workplace safety and security. These constraints may result in the perception that seeking out and intervening in domestic violence is beyond the scope of modern clinical practice.

The effects of domestic violence account for substantial morbidity and mortality in this and other countries, while underdiagnosis and misdiagnosis of this serious problem are common in medical practice. Violence identification, intervention, and prevention skills can be incorporated into the routine care of patients and can be an integral part of the diagnostic and therapeutic repertoire of every physician (Table 9).

IATROGENESIS

By Debra Q. Miller, M.D.,
and Richard J. Simons, Jr., M.D.
Hershey, Pennsylvania

Iatrogenesis refers to an unintended, adverse condition resulting from a diagnostic, therapeutic, or prophylactic intervention or an accidental injury occurring in a medical setting. Iatrogenic events may also occur from an error or delay in diagnosis, failure to perform an intervention when indicated, or failure to take necessary preventive measures. Thus, iatrogenesis may result from errors of omission as well as errors of commission. An iatrogenic event is independent of the natural progression of a patient's underlying disease. It may be the result of the patient's interaction with a physician, nurse, or other ancillary medical personnel (e.g., a respiratory technician or transport attendant) or may be secondary to a medication or equipment malfunction. Equally important, a physician's words and behavior may also cause immeasurable harm.

Every diagnostic and therapeutic action has the potential to cause injury. Depending on their nature and degree, some iatrogenic events may be minor, whereas others may result in substantial morbidity or even mortality. Iatrogenic events should not be equated with negligence. The latter is the failure to meet a standard of care that is expected of a reasonably prudent physician in the relevant specialty. Negligence does not occur every time there is an error, and most medical errors do not result in injury or harm to the patient. Adverse events that result from negligence, however, are more often associated with serious disability.

MAGNITUDE OF THE PROBLEM

Iatrogenic events may occur in the outpatient setting, in the hospital, or in extended medical care facilities. Most adverse events that occur in the outpatient setting are the result of interventions in the physician's office. Approximately 5 per cent of all hospital admissions are precipitated by some type of iatrogenic occurrence. The degree of morbidity and mortality is significantly lower for events occurring outside the hospital than for those occurring in hospitalized patients. Twenty to thirty per cent of hospitalized patients experience some type of iatrogenic event; 20 per cent of these events are life-threatening.

The risk of iatrogenic complications increases with patient age, the number of medications being taken, and the severity of the acute illness. The elderly are more susceptible to iatrogenic complications, but it is not clear whether age is an independent risk factor or just a correlate of disease severity. Complications that are well tolerated by young, healthy individuals can be fatal in older patients. Elderly patients are more likely to have complications such as myocardial infarction, pulmonary embolus, or pneumonia. Patients who have a history of alcohol or tobacco abuse also are more likely to experience a poor outcome.

The frequency of hospital admissions due to iatrogenesis has not changed significantly over the past 15 years, but the most common causes for admission have continued to change. A list of the most common causes of iatrogenesis can be found in Table 1. Medication-related complications are the most common cause of iatrogenic disease. Complications related to procedures may be surgical in nature, medical subspecialty–related, or secondary to bedside procedures such as arterial catheterization or thoracentesis. Impairment may also result from treatment modalities such as blood transfusions or radiotherapy or from injuries endemic to the hospital setting, such as nosocomial infections, complications associated with prolonged bed rest, falls, and other accidental injuries. Harm may also result from improper or delayed diagnosis. Underdiagnosis and failure to recognize illness occurs most commonly in the elderly because symptoms of disease tend to be less characteristic with advancing age and because the elderly may have inadequate access to appropriate care.

MEDICATIONS

As already stated, drugs are the most important cause of iatrogenic illness. As many as 10 to 20 per cent of patients admitted to a hospital will experience an iatrogenic complication secondary to medication. Many of these complications are serious and sometimes life-threatening. For example, the inappropriate use of drugs has been reported to be the major cause of preventable cardiac arrest in hospitals. The number of potent drugs available for the treatment of a wide array of clinical disorders has risen dramatically over the past two decades, and there appears to be no end in sight as new drugs are added to the market almost weekly. Thus, the practicing clinician must be familiar with the adverse effects of drugs prescribed and be alert for drug-induced illness.

Although any drug can cause iatrogenic disease, certain agents deserve special mention because they cause most drug-related disorders (Table 2). Antibiotics are commonly administered medications that may cause hypersensitivity reactions (penicillins, cephalosporins), acute renal failure (aminoglycosides), bone marrow suppression (chloramphenicol, penicillins), and *Clostridium difficile* infection. Diarrhea from *C. difficile* is a well-recognized complication

Table 1. Causes of Iatrogenic Illness

Medication-related
Procedures
Blood transfusions
Nosocomial infections
Radiotherapy
Falls
Bed rest
Diagnostic errors

Table 2. Drugs Most Frequently Implicated in Iatrogenic Illness

Antibiotics
Cardiovascular agents
Antihypertensives
Antiarrhythmics
Digoxin
Antineoplastic agents
Anticoagulants
Sedative hypnotic-psychoactive agents

of the use of broad-spectrum antibiotics. Although the infection usually responds to discontinuation of the antibiotic and oral administration of metronidazole or vancomycin, some patients experience severe illness with high fever, volume depletion, and even toxic megacolon requiring total colectomy.

Cardiovascular drugs are taken by many patients, especially the elderly, and have the potential for causing serious complications. Hypertension affects nearly one of three adults in the United States. Antihypertensive medications clearly reduce complications such as stroke or congestive heart failure, and these drugs may also help prevent myocardial infarction. Antihypertensive agents frequently cause adverse affects, however, and may interfere with the quality of life. For example, diuretics may cause hyponatremia and volume depletion, especially in the elderly. Beta-blockers have been associated with numerous side effects, including depression, fatigue, impotence, exacerbation of asthma, and heart block. Calcium channel blockers may cause dizziness, edema, constipation, and bradycardia. Angiotensin converting enzyme inhibitors commonly cause cough but also may cause life-threatening angioedema.

All antiarrhythmic agents have the potential to induce cardiac dysrhythmias. They should be used only for specific indications. Quinidine has well-known side effects, including gastrointestinal upset and cinchonism. Both quinidine and procainamide have been associated with the drug-induced lupus syndrome. Lidocaine and mexiletine frequently cause neurologic symptoms. Amiodarone, which is used in patients with refractory arrhythmias, may produce serious side effects, including pulmonary fibrosis, hepatotoxicity, skin rash, and thyroid dysfunction.

Digoxin has been instrumental in the management of patients with atrial fibrillation and congestive heart failure. The toxic effects of this drug have been recognized for centuries and include anorexia, nausea and vomiting, visual disturbance, and provocation of ventricular arrhythmias. Digoxin has a narrow therapeutic index and must be used with caution, especially in patients with underlying renal disease in whom lower doses are required. Serum digoxin levels are useful in monitoring patients for toxicity, although toxic symptoms may occur even in patients with therapeutic digoxin levels.

Antineoplastic agents have been used increasingly in the treatment of many cancers and hematologic malignancies. Side effects occur frequently and include bone marrow suppression, nausea and vomiting, and mucositis, among others. Although advances have been made in preventing and reducing the severity of these complications (e.g., more effective antiemetic agents, granulocyte-stimulating factors for neutropenia), the morbidity and sometimes mortality from these drugs continues to be a major problem for patients with cancer.

Anticoagulants carry a major risk of bleeding and should be prescribed only after the relative benefits and risks have been appropriately considered and discussed with the patient. The elderly are particularly susceptible to gastrointestinal hemorrhage when taking warfarin. Patients must be warned about the potential for drug-drug interactions that may either augment or diminish the anticoagulant effect of warfarin. The combination of nonsteroidal anti-inflammatory agents and warfarin is particularly hazardous. The dosage of warfarin should be adjusted to maintain the prothrombin time in the therapeutic range. The literature supports using lower therapeutic ranges (prothrombin time ratio of 1.2 to 1.5 or a target International Normalized Ratio [INR] of 2 to 3) for most groups of patients.

Drug-induced delirium is common in the elderly and is frequently underrecognized and overlooked by medical caregivers. Delirium has been associated with increased morbidity and mortality, longer hospital stays, and increased risk of nursing home placement. Delirium tends to occur in the older hospitalized patient who often has several medical problems and is receiving multiple medications. Although many factors contribute to delirium, drugs are the most common single cause. The drugs that have been most closely associated with delirium include sedative hypnotics, antidepressants, narcotics, antihistamines, and benzodiazepines. (Many of these agents have anticholinergic properties.) These drugs should be used with caution in the elderly, starting with the lowest dose possible. Other drugs associated with drug-induced delirium include digoxin, nonsteroidal anti-inflammatory agents, amantadine, and antiparkinsonian agents. Physicians should suspect delirium in any elderly patient with a change in mental status and discontinue any drugs capable of inducing the delirium syndrome.

Although some adverse effects of drugs are neither preventable nor predictable (e.g., idiosyncratic drug reactions), many, if not most, adverse events can be prevented if basic principles of pharmacotherapy are kept in mind. First, drugs should be used for specific indications related to an established disease or clinical syndrome. Physicians should resist the temptation to prescribe medications to treat vague or nonspecific symptoms. Second, patient characteristics and pharmacokinetic factors must be considered when prescribing any medication. Drugs should be given in dosages based on the patient's age and body weight. For example, the metabolism and elimination of many drugs are prolonged in the neonate and the elderly; thus, lower doses are indicated. The general rule, "start low and go slow," should be followed when prescribing drugs for the elderly.

Adverse drug reactions occur more often in patients taking multiple medications. In fact, the risk of a drug reaction increases exponentially when the number of concomitant drugs is four or more. There are several well-documented drug-drug interactions of clinical importance. Erythromycin and other macrolide antibiotics increase the serum concentration of the "nonsedating" antihistamines terfenadine and astemizole, which can result in fatal ventricular arrhythmias. Erythromycin also inhibits the metabolism of theophylline, predisposing the patient to theophylline toxicity. Quinidine increases the serum concentration of digoxin. Cimetidine increases serum theophylline concentrations. Bile acid resins interfere with the absorption of many drugs, leading to a decreased drug effect. Phenobarbital accelerates the metabolism of many drugs. Finally, numerous drugs interact with warfarin, either potentiating or inhibiting the anticoagulant effect. Although it is impossible for anyone to remember every specific drug-drug interaction, physicians should refer to drug inserts or other literature when prescribing new medications to patients who are already receiving other drugs.

Medication *errors* may also result in iatrogenic injury. Sloppy or illegible prescriptions or medication orders can translate into an incorrect dosage or the wrong medication. For example, a patient hospitalized for evaluation of recurrent episodes of hypoglycemia may have ingested acetohexamide (a hypoglycemic agent) instead of the intended acetazolamide prescribed for the treatment of glaucoma. In another example, patients may die of colchicine poisoning when they inadvertently receive a toxic amount of the drug. If a physician intends to give a patient only two doses of intravenous colchicine, the order should not read "colchicine, 1 mg intravenously every 12 hours," which may lead to treatment for several days, with accumulation of the drug and multisystem organ failure.

Medication errors may also result from lack of standardized procedures for drug administration. For example, the pharmacy of one hospital documented more than 70 different methods associated with orders for parenteral aminophylline. The same issue arises with insulin, heparin, and potassium, which may be administered intravenously in various concentrations and solutions. The lack of standardization makes recognition of potentially toxic infusion orders difficult. Standardization of drug doses and times of administration could, therefore, enhance efficiency and reduce errors.

In summary, the majority of adverse reactions to drugs are preventable if physicians carefully select and prescribe drugs, keeping in mind the pharmacokinetic principles discussed. Advances in knowledge, improved information access (e.g., computerization of the medical record), and standardization should prove beneficial in the future.

IATROGENIC ILLNESS IN HOSPITALS

Many adverse events that occur in hospitals are related to procedures, especially those carried out in operating rooms. Adverse events are most frequently associated with thoracic surgery, neurosurgery, and obstetrics. The increased frequency of occurrences most likely arises from the technical nature of the procedures. There is, as yet, no evidence that negligence or deficient standards of care are more prevalent in operating rooms. In general, surgical complications are more common in the elderly, who account for 30 per cent of surgical procedures but up to 75 per cent of operative mortality. Older patients often have a greater severity of illness that renders them more vulnerable to complications.

Medical subspecialty procedures account for fewer injuries than do surgical procedures, but some of the complications may be equally severe. Cardiac catheterization may be complicated by dissection of a coronary artery; colonoscopy or paracentesis may lead to colonic perforation with a subsequent need for surgical bowel resection.

The potential for iatrogenesis in the intensive care unit is great. The most common complications are those associated with vascular catheters such as arterial lines, central venous catheters, and pulmonary artery catheters. Inflammation at the insertion site, sepsis, thrombosis, and pulmonary artery catheter–associated arrhythmias are well documented. Mechanical ventilation may also cause problems, such as barotrauma, pneumothorax, and equipment failure. Adverse events commonly arising during intubation and extubation include trauma, aspiration, and unrecognized esophageal or selective bronchial intubation. The average length of stay in the intensive care unit and in-hospital mortality tend to be greater in patients who experience iatrogenic events.

Physicians must determine whether the benefit from a specific diagnostic test or therapeutic intervention outweighs the risk of complications (risk-to-benefit ratio). Importantly, surgical patients, especially the elderly, require an individualized preoperative evaluation to determine the need for further preoperative assessment, intraoperative monitoring, or correction of acute or chronic conditions. Moreover, postoperative management must include early ambulation, adequate skin care, and close attention to cardiac, fluid, and renal status to decrease prolonged hospitalization.

The second most prevalent site in the hospital for injury to occur is the patient's own room, where accidents occur most commonly in the bathroom and at the bedside. Falls are the most frequent type of accident in these settings. Such falls occur mainly in older patients during their first few days in a new environment, when they are unfamiliar with the surroundings. Factors that contribute to falls include generalized deconditioning, confusion or delirium, impaired vision, and environmental hazards. Mechanical restraints are often used to prevent falls, but ironically many of these restraining devices actually increase the risk of injury. The elderly often are placed in Posey devices, which may lead to strangulation. Patients often try to climb over bed rails, which may increase the severity of injury if falls occur. Many other devices, such as intravenous lines, urinary catheters, and oxygen supply lines, also effectively function as patient restraints, creating the potential for harm.

Falls can be reduced by familiarizing the patient with the environment, eliminating unnecessary medications that may cause orthostatic hypotension or confusion, and providing assistance with transfers to and from the bed, wheelchair, and toilet. Furthermore, hospital and nursing home rooms should be equipped with appropriate safety features, including sufficient lighting, bathroom handrails, nonslip surfaces, and accessible call buttons and telephones.

Prolonged bed rest and immobilization may lead to the physiologic decline of many organ systems. These changes begin within the first 24 hours of bed rest, and their degree of severity increases with time. Bed rest causes orthostasis, vasomotor instability, and decreased exercise tolerance, with subsequent development of atelectasis and an increased risk of pneumonia. Immobilization can cause demineralization of bones, with resultant hypercalcemia, constipation, and renal stones. Another common consequence of extended bed rest is decubitus ulcers, which may become infected, especially when functional urinary incontinence exists, and may lead to osteomyelitis. Prolonged bed rest also leads to muscle atrophy, contractures, and compression neuropathies. The isolation and sensory deprivation caused by prolonged bed rest may have psychological consequences, such as chronic depression or anxiety. Hospitalization often leads to irreversible functional decline that is independent of the acute illness or its treatment for which the patient was admitted. The elderly are particularly susceptible to this deterioration, and many older patients who were independently functional at the time of admission to the hospital are ultimately placed in nursing homes at the time of discharge.

Many of the conditions that predispose the patient to functional decline in hospitals can be modified. Physicians who are aware of the deleterious effects of prolonged bed rest can encourage physical therapy for immobile patients and early ambulation when possible. Pressure ulcers can be prevented by frequent repositioning to avoid prolonged pressure at any one site.

Nosocomial infections also complicate the lives of hospitalized patients and patients in extended care facilities. The overall risk of infection acquired during a hospital stay is about 5 per cent. This risk increases with the length of hospital stay and with previous exposure to antibiotics. Approximately 1.5 million infections occur annually in nursing home residents, and infections are the leading cause of transfer to acute care facilities. The most common nosocomial infections include urinary tract infections (UTIs), pneumonia, wound infections, and bacteremia. Although UTI is the most frequently occurring nosocomial infection, pneumonia causes the greatest mortality. Among the risk factors for the development of these infections are the use of urinary and venous catheters, malnutrition, continuous ventilator support, and nasogastric feeding. Sedatives can lead to aspiration and subsequent pulmonary infections. External condom and indwelling urinary catheters cause bacteriuria and subsequent symptomatic UTIs. Highly prevalent *Pseudomonas aeruginosa* infection in hospitals and nursing homes is extremely difficult to eradicate. Other infections can be transmitted from one patient to another or from a health care worker to a patient. Tuberculosis, *C. difficile*, human immunodeficiency virus (HIV), and methicillin-resistant *Staphylococcus aureus* (MRSA) are several examples.

Physicians must emphasize the importance of removing urinary catheters expeditiously, limiting mechanical ventilation time, and encouraging incentive spirometry to treat atelectasis. Strict hand-washing procedures must be enforced to decrease the spread of infections such as methicillin-resistant *S. aureus* and *C. difficile*. An infection control program for both patients and employees should include tuberculosis screening, maintenance of immunizations (influenza and pneumonia vaccine [Pneumovax]), an annual health assessment, and general education regarding infectious disease policies.

Some iatrogenic complications are apparent immediately, whereas others may not become manifest for several years. Iatrogenesis from blood transfusions may range from acute intravascular hemolysis resulting from ABO incompatibility to hepatitis C or human immunodeficiency virus infection, which may not become apparent until years later. Acute side effects of radiation may include gastrointestinal distress and bone marrow suppression. With time, radiation enteritis or pneumonitis may develop. The most important late effect of ionizing radiation is the increased risk of malignancy, especially leukemia or thyroid cancer.

DIAGNOSIS AND PREVENTION

In order to recognize iatrogenic disease, the health care team must be aware of the potential for harm caused by diagnostic and therapeutic measures. The risk factors and susceptibility of each patient must be identified. When an adverse reaction to a prescribed drug occurs, or a patient's symptoms or course are not as anticipated, the physician must consider the possibility of iatrogenic disease.

Many, if not most, iatrogenic events are preventable. Health care workers are trained to be careful and efficient in providing health care. Physicians, nurses, and other health care workers are human, however, and will make mistakes. Given the complex and increasingly sophisticated nature of medical practice and the many interventions that occur every day in the care of a patient, it is not surprising that iatrogenic events are frequent both in and out of the hospital. What, then, can be done to reduce iatrogenic injuries?

First, the education and training of physicians, nurses, pharmacists, and other health care personnel should emphasize prevention of errors and testing performance. For example, residents should be more closely supervised as they learn to perform new procedures. Second, improved information access through development of the computerized medical record will reduce the reliance on memory by health care workers. Automatic "fail-safe" systems—such as computers that make it impossible to order or dispense a drug to a patient with a known sensitivity—are likely to have an increasing role. Third, standardized patient care processes should be developed and advocated whenever possible. Fourth, the adoption of total quality management principles in hospitals and offices may help reduce errors through a concentrated, organized, and systematic approach, in which errors and deviations are not regarded as human failures, but rather as opportunities to improve the medical care system. Finally, the development and use of practice guidelines and clinical pathways should result in more efficient, higher quality care with a reduced rate of iatrogenesis.

COMPUTER-ASSISTED DIAGNOSIS

By Marvin E. Gozum, M.D.
Philadelphia, Pennsylvania

Computer-assisted, or -aided, diagnosis may be defined as the use of computer-based operations to aid the diagnosis of disease. It was created to manage large medical knowledge databases quickly and economically. Early work flourished in the 1970s amid an environment of high expectation surrounding artificial intelligence (software attempting to duplicate human cognition) in which researchers found many problems but managed to create tools for analyzing medical data within computers. A significant development was the creation of expert systems (see later discussion). Continued growth of computer applications in health care developed into the multidisciplinary specialty of medical informatics. Informatics tools have revolutionary implications for health care delivery and education: a diminished need for memorization in medical education; an emphasis on general principles of disease, using computers to provide details; a diminished need for "keeping up with the literature"; a renewed emphasis on problem-based learning; and cost control through the efficiency of computer-based processes. The time saved through computer processes provides incentive to enhance the humanities in medical education, a move that encourages an understanding of patients as humans rather than organisms.

Reflecting on the scientific method, the art of diagnosis may be categorized into four processes: observe, hypothesize, test the hypothesis, and conclude. Informatics attempts to augment hypothesis generation and test selection. Informatics treats the diagnostic process as a classification scheme in which diseases are labels for unique, but complex, patterns of findings. These findings consist of physical, electronic, laboratory, imaging, and tissue data. Findings are modified by additional characteristics such as time, specificity for disease, frequency of occurrence, or probability of occurrence. Physicians must properly identify and interpret data for software at appropriate moments in time; that is, they must observe an event. Once identified, findings must be entered into software using a specialized computer vocabulary. With data, software presents users with labels for patterns of findings and thus a differential diagnosis list, which is a list of hypotheses for the cause of an event. With a differential diagnosis list, physicians must not only rank diseases for consideration but also contemplate what may not be listed. A diagnostic hypothesis may be confirmed by a demonstration of software-recommended findings. This represents a potentially useful test of hypothesis and derivation of a conclusion. In methodology, treatments are assigned to diseases and thus are a consequence of the classification scheme. Using computers, physicians need not ponder what treatment to consider but may choose among treatment options, with subsequent monitoring of the effects of the treatment selected. In practice, the use of new treatments is justified only as research or when existing therapies are ineffective.

With studies supporting the deterioration of human memory with time, the flow of new knowledge provides a dilemma for physicians. However, the expertise of older physicians is well known. Equally well known is the high reliability of computer memory over time. These observations suggest that the imperative of clinical expertise is experience, a proficiency that may be enhanced by computer methods conscripted to manage the flow of new medical knowledge. With medical informatics, memorization may be limited to emergency, surgical, and general principles of medicine, that is, situations in which time constraints limit the use of electronic consultations. Thus, expert systems in medicine support medical management by modeling differential diagnosis as a classification scheme. However, these same systems rely heavily on skilled physicians to provide good data, narrow a differential diagnosis list, and effect treatment.

Computer-assisted diagnosis may exist in several forms: expert system software, automated literature searching (e.g., Medline), e-mail, clinical calculators, and electronic textbooks.

Expert Systems

Expert systems are computer programs that serve as specialized consultants in a narrow field of expertise, such as differential diagnosis or electrocardiographic interpretation, providing users with expert knowledge previously obtained only by consultation with human specialists. Expert system expertise, however, does not extend beyond its field. Thus, although an expert system may be able to cross-reference thousands of possible diseases, it will be inept in recommending intravenous fluids. Two popular techniques used by medical expert systems are heuristics and bayesian analysis. Developments using other techniques, such as genetic programming or neural networks, offer future benefits.

The quality of expert system judgment depends on the quality of information used, making the development of data for expert systems crucial. Informaticians surmise that 1500 diseases cover most ailments in human beings, recognizing that disease, its diagnostic approach, and its treatment may evolve over time. Findings, therefore, need to be updated periodically. Expert system developers evaluate the medical literature for appropriateness, review case studies for relevant rare manifestations, or simply update probability tables. Considering the size and variation in the quality of medical studies, literature review is a large task made larger by the number of diseases represented in an expert system. However, the rigor used by informaticians in reviewing medical literature for expert systems frees users from repeating this task for diagnostic education. Thus, physicians versed in expert system use need only maintain a general knowledge of disease obtained through journal review articles or review texts. In sum, expert systems simplify the task of maintaining current medical knowledge for diagnosis.

Bayesian analysis essentially calculates the probability of diagnosis given a probability of each mutually exclusive finding associated with a diagnosis. When accurate probabilities are available for a large number of findings, bayesian analysis offers a theoretical model for calculating risk based on statistical fact. In practice, however, bayesian analysis is encumbered by many limitations—many medical findings are not mutually exclusive and there is wide regional variation in disease prevalence and incidence as well as wide variation in the probabilities of findings associated with disease (expected because of variations of prevalence). With these limitations, bayesian systems must incorporate elements of expert judgment in defining probabilities for findings. Thus, Bayes' theorem constitutes only one part of a methodology incorporated into expert systems. A principal advantage of expert systems using Bayes' theorem is the potential to consider findings as a probability: What is the probability of a hypertensive male having angina if he has only a 50% chance of having chest pain?

Heuristics are rules developed by human experts. This approach is rooted in the tradition of experts adjudicating conditions in which definite conclusions remain vague. For example, experts ruled that diabetes mellitus will be defined as fasting serum glucose levels of 140 mg/dL or greater on two separate occasions, coalescing the various findings of the American Diabetes Association's study. Experts define categories in studies and may clarify whether smokers of 15 cigarettes a day are valid members of groups defining smokers in packs per day. Since heuristics are based on the opinions of experts, they may be subject to a contrary opinion by another expert. Thus, heuristics have been criticized as being built on opinion rather than fact. However, the concept of "standard practice" is rooted in a consensus of experts in clinical medicine. Expert judgment often forms *a priori*, and obtains validation prospectively via pragmatic results. Studies have demonstrated nearly humanlike responses of heuristic systems in providing judgment and argue for an evaluation of expert systems as *full* systems rather than merely databases.

Historically, two programs serve as models for expert systems in medicine: Quick Medical Reference, from the University of Pittsburgh (employing heuristics), and Iliad, from the University of Utah (employing Bayes' theorem). Both programs are extensively documented in the literature. They both provide a meaningful differential diagnosis list. Both programs have two limitations: use of a specialized vocabulary that must be mastered by users and an incomplete collection of findings and diseases seen in practice, based on the idealized total of 1500 diseases.

Automated Literature Searches

Medline is the National Library of Medicine's electronic version of the *Index Medicus.* It serves as an index, including abstracts, to the most frequently used journals in medical literature. Medline provides a rapid and cost-effective method for obtaining citations using three computer-based modes: software that accesses the National Library of Medicine's computers directly via telephone lines (e.g., Grateful Med); subsets of Medline on CD-ROM for use at a local site; and indirect access to Medline via commercial providers of Medline data (e.g., PaperChase on CompuServe). A choice of search strategy is controlled by how frequently a physician consults the literature, access costs, search time, and the user's proficiency with relevant software. Effective methods for individuals include Grateful Med and direct access via the Internet. Institutions, by contrast, are best served by access to Medline subsets in CD-ROM. Occasional users may find services provided by commercial vendors cost-effective, where charges are based on fees for service.

Electronic Mail

E-mail stands for electronic mail and is widely available in two forms: access to the Internet and private networks such as CompuServe. Unlike conventional mail, e-mail provides rapid-access delivery and distribution to large audiences for costs equal to those of conventional mail. Distribution to thousands of network subscribers can be performed with the effort needed for addressing a conventional letter, with delivery time measured in minutes or seconds. With more than 20 million Internet users and a growth rate in excess of 20 per cent monthly, Internet access is important to e-mail. Local networks provide gateways to the Internet and, thus, to other networks connected to the Internet. Limited networks support users who append voice, computer files, and images to mail, a function being developed for general e-mail. One cost-effective method for individual e-mail is via commercial vendors such as CompuServe, which provide indirect access to Medline, the Internet, and many other resources. There are many commercial computer networks to consider. Choice of network should be dictated by costs and services provided.

Clinical Calculators

Clinical calculators are programs that help clinicians to calculate. Programs can be rapidly created by users of spreadsheets or purchased from vendors. For example, clinicians may find programs to calculate dopamine dosing, fluid replacement, or creatinine clearance. Clinical calculators are best used in two modes: as programs distributed via networks or as stand-alone programs in palmtop computers carried by clinicians. The flexibility of palmtop computers offers many advantages to busy clinicians by freeing them from network dependence and its politics.

Electronic Textbooks

Paper-based medical textbooks and journals are being converted into electronic form to make use of computer capacities for quick text searches and the "cutting and pasting" of relevant citations. Electronic publications are best used as reference sources by allowing readers to collate required citations in a single source document. These publications are available in two modes: distributed via a computer network or as stand-alone items in CD-ROM or other media used in portable computers. Physicians may have access to either modality but may find palmtop computers best suited to busy schedules in which immediate access to information is required.

USING COMPUTER-ASSISTED DIAGNOSIS IN A CLINICAL SETTING

A practicing physician may encounter fewer than 50 diseases on a regular basis, a case mix that is less diverse than the several hundred diseases taught in medical school. However, recurrent encounters with particular disorders enhance the ability to manage typical and atypical disease manifestations within the scope of that physician's specialty training. Limited case mix experience not only nurtures a physician's talents but also provides a community with an expert physician skilled in the management of diseases that principally affect a community. However, this same phenomenon limits a physician's exposure to rare diseases that may afflict patients. The busy nature of practice limits the effectiveness of mandatory continuing medical education (CME). Even with effective CME, theoretical knowledge is less applicable than real world experience. Even if real world experience is obtained, sporadic encounters with a disease may not provide physicians with the level of expertise provided by recurrent encounters with disease. A rare disease that attracts numerous medical students is paradoxical: if the disease is rare, chances are it will never be seen again, and if a rare disease were to be seen in the future, it probably would not be recognized quickly. Thus, a physician's limited case mix experience increases the likelihood of overlooking a number of diseases during a diagnostic work-up, making assistance via computer beneficial.

An inconclusive result obtained by an unaided diagnostic evaluation may indicate a need for consultation. A physician has several options: consult a standard textbook, consult an electronic textbook, consult journals using Medline as an index, consult a human expert, or consult an expert system. The physician should realize that textbooks and journals offer a limited capacity for cross-referencing, whereas a human consultation may be delayed by hours to weeks. Between electronic textbooks and human consultations lies the domain of expert systems, software providing immediate access with outstanding cross-referencing capacity. In a cost-conscious health care environment, the use of software provides an option to further a work-up without traditional human consultation. Since data entry into software is time-consuming, consulting software is justified by expected returns.

A first encounter with a diagnostic dilemma may be solved by a textbook reference. If available, electronic textbooks facilitate an information search by cross-indexing multiple search terms. If texts provide no answers, a physician should consider a run through a familiar expert system.

In expert systems, a physician or designate enters findings deemed important in a case analysis. These findings are abstracted from a case just as summaries are prepared for presentation to human consultants on rounds. All expert systems have limited vocabularies, and it is important to match appropriate software terms to findings presented for analysis. For example if a patient "coughs blood," a judgment must be made to map this finding to the program's statements of either "blood-streaked sputum" or "hemoptysis." Once a differential diagnosis list is created, a physician must draw on principles of disease acquired from medical training to rank or differentiate useful diagnostic hypotheses obtained from a differential diagnosis list. A physician may query diseases on a list to determine what additional findings may be helpful to support a potential diagnosis.

Two common mistakes made by users of medical expert

systems are mismapping vocabulary terms and presuming that diseases not listed on a differential list are excluded from consideration. Since software-based diagnosis is a classification scheme, using fewer findings for analysis produces a greater chance for error. Omitting a critical finding produces a critical error. Generally, it advisable to use as many relevant findings as are available, since using multiple findings for a disease strengthens its classification by software and blurs any omission of critical findings. For example, an omission of an antinuclear antibody titer may be compensated for by an entry for malar rash, arthralgia, and leukopenia. Further, users should begin with the most specific representation for a finding and use as many of the synonyms listed by the software as possible. When faced with a potential absence of a finding within a computer's vocabulary, select the most likely match from the listed vocabulary to minimize any omissions of actual case findings. For example, for a finding of "chest pain near the breasts," the computer may present a user with "chest pain lateral wall," and if not, the term "chest pain" remains a less specific but valid entry. If presented with the option of using two or more terms, do so. Users should understand that entering many findings, including synonyms, may produce a larger differential diagnosis list or point to a narrow set of syndromes! However, it remains more useful to scan and omit a diagnosis from a list rather than not have a disease within a list. Difficulty in entering data into expert systems is a major stimulus for informaticians to pursue work in computer-based interpretation of human speech, *or natural language*. Until natural language issues are resolved, users of expert systems must serve as translators between their needs and expert system software. As a computer cliché goes, "garbage in, garbage out."

Most users assume that a differential diagnosis list presented by expert systems contains all diagnostic possibilities provided by the software's approach. This is not true. Additional findings can be added or eliminated and the list re-evaluated. Technology and time constraints may limit knowledge bases, so databases may be incomplete. Diseases listed may be only manifestations of a syndrome. It is important to look at patterns presented by diseases in a differential diagnosis list and consider broader concepts, such as disease categories. Are listed diseases all infectious? What organ is principally affected? Are diseases all collagen vascular diseases? Are there common tests to confirm or exclude diagnoses, such as biopsies or imaging tests? What diseases are not included in the database? Reviewing patterns provides users with additional insight into an unlisted potential diagnosis by exploiting the similarity of diseases within categories, such as causes or affected organs.

When an expert system or textbook fails to deliver useful information, a Medline search offers another alternative before a human consultation. Medline allows a quick search of current journals via electronic indexing. Medline searches are expanded by search topics using synonyms. However, the cognitive approach to Medline is close to the paper-based *Index Medicus.* Once relevant articles are located, the user must proceed through them as with paper-based processes. Medline-based diagnosis confirms preconceived associations of findings with diseases, made by physicians with or without expert system help, by relying on its indexing engine to map findings to "diseases" represented by the title of a journal article. Medline's principal advantage lies in an up-to-date database. Unlike expert system knowledge bases, however, Medline search strategies are not optimized for diagnosis; accuracy of the search depends on terms used to index articles or on the contents of abstracts. Furthermore, except for reviews undertaken by journal editors in screening articles indexed by Medline, its information is not evaluated for appropriateness.

When expert systems and textbooks provide inconclusive results, physicians may consult specialists or colleagues locally. Alternatively, a human consultation may be performed by e-mail, if the required specialists are involved in an e-mail culture. E-mail cultures have three essential characteristics: users log on frequently; users are willing to provide information; and e-mail connections are reliable. Only when these characteristics are met should the user consider e-mail for medical consultations. Generally, physicians participating in larger networks, such as the Medical Special Interest Group, MedSig on CompuServe, or the Internet, meet these characteristics. Extant for more than a decade, large networks have thousands of users, and a less than 1 per cent response rate provides a large return. A majority of e-mail responses are without charge, a phenomenon of the medium. Since e-mail is time-consuming in complex cases with lengthy documents, it is most effective when cases are abstracted succinctly or discussed in generalities. However, e-mail suffers from lack of depth provided by a face-to-face consultation or by an expert system evaluation. E-mail's speed is most useful for the transmission of records and data between physicians. E-mail security measures continue to evolve, so care must be exercised to avoid a breach of patient confidentiality. The legal issues surrounding e-mail remain unresolved.

USING COMPUTER-ASSISTED TREATMENT IN A CLINICAL SETTING

Treatment recommendations by computer are less sophisticated than the process of diagnosis. The primary goal is to clearly and completely outline the current therapeutic options for a diagnosis. Electronic sources are rapidly cross-indexed and are as current as paper-based sources. Electronic textbooks that succinctly present treatment options for disease provide the best sources for computer-assisted treatment. Essentially, treatment programs outline protocols to institute treatment. Since treatment actions require simple decision trees, the application of an expert system for treatment is limited and, beyond electronic publishing, few projects have been undertaken that justify the cost of software development. Rapid development in treatment options compounds the problem of creating software for treatment.

In summary, computer-assisted diagnosis and treatment open doors to a new model of medical education and practice that involves resource management. Human resources may be considered the effective interaction and management of consultants, surgeons, nurses, residents, students, and other health care workers. Laboratory and imaging resource management considers the judicious use of tests and procedures. Cognitive resource management considers the informed use of electronic databases and expert systems. Finally, financial resource management considers cost as a limiting factor in *all* resource management strategies developed for patient care.

APPROACH TO THE PATIENT IN THE EMERGENCY DEPARTMENT

By Benjamin Wedro, M.D.
La Crosse, Wisconsin

The physician in the emergency department must efficiently manage patients whose presentations tend to be more dramatic and stressful than those seen in usual office practice. The approach to care is significantly different, and the patient-physician interaction is often brief. In emergencies, the physician who uses an office-style approach may not offer the best care and advice to the patient.

The time span from introduction to treatment and disposition in the emergency department is compressed and complicated by the likelihood of numerous concurrent patient interactions. The physician in this circumstance must use time efficiently and allocate the resources of the department wisely.

Time-honored thought processes in the practice of medicine are also suspended in the emergency department. Although the office physician will dutifully progress through a history, physical examination, and testing protocol to render a diagnosis and specific treatment, the emergency physician's approach to the emergency patient may not be so ordered. In many patients, treatment precedes the history and physical examination. In others, evaluation and therapy occur concurrently while a differential diagnosis is entertained. In general, emergency medicine is disposition-driven rather than diagnosis-driven—that is, the desirability of diagnostic precision often yields to the need to decide on appropriate therapy and on the best place for that therapy to occur. In a busy emergency department, the limiting (least available) resources are nursing care and treatment space. With expectations of future patient arrival so great, there is constant pressure to move patients along, thereby freeing nurses and space for the next wave of arrivals.

The condition of most patients who come to an emergency department is nonemergent. Only 5 per cent of patients present with true emergencies that are life- or limb-threatening, including patients with chest pain, dyspnea, or major trauma. Another 15 per cent have urgencies that require intervention but not immediately (within minutes). These patients may include those with lacerations, fractures, or abdominal pain. The rest of the patients tend not to have urgent conditions and can safely undergo triage to receive care when time allows. The initial requirement in emergency medicine is to differentiate the emergent from the nonemergent patient, and this triage skill must be applied at every stage of assessment in the department, from the personnel at the front entrance to the physician ultimately providing care.

The physician must first decide if a particular patient needs emergency intervention. If not, the astute physician should consider whether the patient needs admission or can be treated as an outpatient. The role of the emergency physician changes according to these decisions. In the true emergency, the physician is responsible for stabilization as well as coordination of hospital resources and consulting specialist care so that timely and specific treatments can be undertaken. Remember that resources held for one patient cannot be used for another. Holding an operating theater empty "just in case" may not be in the best interest of another patient in the hospital. If, however, the patient requires more leisurely evaluation and admission, the emergency physician becomes a facilitator, and if the decision for outpatient care is made, the role becomes that of therapist. Throughout, the emergency physician remains diagnostician, therapist and, of course, patient advocate.

INITIAL EVALUATION

Although the usual routes for obtaining information are undertaken for many patients in the emergency department, those with life- or limb-threatening illness or injury may require initial stabilization prior to diagnostic evaluation.

Screening Examination

In an active emergency department, time for the individual patient encounter is limited. The physician must assess patient stability, general quality and severity of illness, and probable disposition in an abbreviated time frame. The luxury of leisurely evaluations does not commonly exist in emergency medicine, yet the physician must facilitate precise diagnosis and treatment. Often, an initial screening examination is performed, followed by general treatment that can be undertaken while the physician moves to the care of another patient.

Observation is the key to optimal screening of emergency patients. All senses must be used. General visual inspection should focus on a patient's demeanor, habitus, hydration status, and level of consciousness. Much of the screening examination can be performed at the foot of the bed in a few seconds.

1. Are the patient's vital signs stable?
2. Is the respiratory status strained?
3. Are cardiac dysrhythmias present?
4. Is the patient alert?
5. Is there symmetry to observed movement, including observed cranial nerves?
6. What is the hydration status of the patient?

The initial history may already be documented by nursing staff but must be obtained again by the physician. Significant information can be acquired by a second history, since the time interval between questions may enable the patient or family to recall pertinent information. History taking should be directed to the specific problems that the physician recognizes as active in the encounter. Extraneous complaints or tangential requests may be handled at a later time if warranted, but the emergency department patient-physician encounter is not an office visit, and the physician is not obliged to address and solve all patient concerns.

The physical examination should be specific to the problem in question. A full examination may be warranted at a later time, but the initial encounter is meant to begin diagnostics and treatments that may need to run concurrently. The diagnoses that are most commonly missed in the emergency department and lead to patient mortality and morbidity include myocardial infarction, meningitis, fracture, and appendicitis. Some examples of basic evaluation are presented in the following sections.

Airway

All patients, including those with complaints that may seem benign, must be continually reassessed regarding the ABCs (airway, breathing, and circulation) of resuscitation. To comply with Advanced Cardiac and Trauma Life Support guidelines, airway, breathing, and circulation must be stabilized regardless of cause. All too often, patients are left unattended, and they deteriorate because of lack of airway support. Patients who are intoxicated, those who are septic, or those who present with cardiac or pulmonary problems require appropriate monitoring and repeated assessment to assure the basics of tissue oxygenation and perfusion.

Vital Signs

All too often, the patient's vital signs are discarded as trivial information by the emergency physician. However, vital signs can cause the physician to approach the patient more aggressively. Monitoring of vital signs must be accurate and should include, at a minimum, temperature, blood pressure, pulse rate, and respiratory rate. The blood pressure measurement may be omitted in the pediatric patient if clinically appropriate.

The physician has an opportunity to evaluate the patient visually and determine the stability or instability of the patient, using the vital signs as well. Patients who are hemodynamically unstable should be easy to identify. They include the victims of hemorrhagic shock or cardiac decompensation from myocardial infarction or heart failure. Of equal or greater concern, however, are those patients whose occult instability is not readily apparent because of their age or underlying pathologic condition. The physician must retain a healthy respect for the ability of the body to maintain vital signs at reasonably normal levels until precipitous decompensation occurs. Representative examples are presented in the following sections.

Blood Pressure

Following trauma, the body augments tissue perfusion and sympathetic stimulation and maintains peripheral resistance in the face of intravascular fluid and blood loss. A prime example of this phenomenon occurs daily with people who volunteer to donate blood. A 500-mL blood loss is adequately compensated for by various protective mechanisms. Imagine the same mechanisms at work in the trauma patient with an encapsulated splenic rupture.

The body can also adapt to slow losses of blood volume caused by malaria, occult gastrointestinal blood loss, or dietary insufficiency. A "normal" blood pressure may not equate with a normal hematocrit.

Pulse Rate

The youth with hemorrhagic shock may maintain adequate blood pressure and exhibit *paradoxical bradycardia* while losing significant volumes of blood. Reliance on a "normal" set of vital signs may give the physician a false sense of security.

A patient with spinal cord trauma can experience bradycardia and mild hypotension resulting from sympathetic denervation and dilatation of the distal vascular bed. Appreciating constellations or patterns of vital signs can also help define disease processes. For example, the Cushing response is characterized by raised intracranial pressure, increased blood pressure, and persistent bradycardia.

Temperature

In the septic patient, fever should develop in response to the underlying infection. This may not occur in extremely young or extremely old patients or in patients with underlying medical conditions that suppress the immune response.

Postural Vital Signs

In a busy emergency department, *postural vital signs* may be neglected. Some patients never seem to be evaluated in an upright position. They arrive by wheelchair or stretcher and are assisted onto an examination table, with no opportunity to ambulate independently. Taking vital signs in both supine and upright positions allows staff to observe not only the numbers but also the patient's response to position change. Does the patient have symptomatic postural hypotension? Is there difficulty in ambulating because of pain? or loss of balance? or weakness?

This information is sometimes obtained after the patient is evaluated and discharged, at which point observers note that the patient cannot sit or stand independently. If the patient cannot stand, sitting vital signs may be compared with those obtained with the patient in a supine position.

Respiratory Rate

Finally, a word of caution regarding assessment of the respiratory rate. There is a tendency for this vital sign to be estimated rather than accurately measured. The number of breaths per minute varies; it is seldom 20 breaths per minute. Thus, along with the rate, the physician may also obtain significant information from respiratory patterns that can distinguish underlying illness. Central neurogenic hyperventilation, Kussmaul breathing, and Cheyne-Stokes respirations are examples.

Recent advances in technology permit continual monitoring of patient oxygenation and ventilation via pulse oximetry. This has enhanced the safety of anesthesia in the emergency department, especially in the area of conscious sedation. However, in the initial evaluation of the emergency patient, there is a tendency to misuse this information. Pulse oximetry cannot measure the adequacy of oxygen content or ventilation. Only an arterial blood gas (ABG) determination can give that specific information. Thus, reliance solely on oximetry is not advised. Rather, pulse oximetry should be correlated with ABG measure-

Table 1. Pulse Oximetry*

Potential Confounder	Rationale
Motion artifact	
Abnormal hemoglobin	Anemia, carboxyhemoglobin, methemoglobin
Intravascular dyes	Methylene blue and green dyes
Exposure of probe to ambient light	Caused by inappropriate application to site
Low perfusion states	Central sites may be more accurate
Skin pigmentation; nail polish or coverings	
Low oxygen saturation	Oxygen saturation less than 83% unreliable
Hyperoxemia	Oximetry cannot quantify hyperoxygenation

*Factors that may limit precision, performance, and application of the pulse oximeter.

Table 2. Glasgow Coma Scale

Eye opening	Spontaneous	4
	To verbal command	3
	To pain	2
	No response	1
Best verbal response	Oriented and converses	5
	Disoriented and converses	4
	Inappropriate words	3
	Incomprehensible sounds	2
	No response	1
Best motor response	Obeys commands	6
	Localizes pain	5
	Withdraws from pain	4
	Abnormal flexion—decorticate	3
	Abnormal extension—decerebrate	2
	No response	1
Total		3–15

ments. Once acid-base balance is established and the disease process defined, oximetry may be used to adjust and monitor oxygen therapy (Table 1).

Glasgow Coma Scale

The Glasgow Coma Scale (GCS) is not a diagnostic tool and should not be used as a one-time score. The GCS is designed for health workers who need a common, easily understood scale to measure the condition of a patient with head trauma or altered mental status. Important information regarding improvement, deterioration, or stability of the patient can be ascertained if the GCS is applied at the time of presentation and at reasonable intervals thereafter.

A patient may interact with several members of the medical staff before entering an emergency department. On-scene first responders, paramedics, hospital nurses and physicians seen initially, transferring paramedics, and accepting hospital nurses and physicians may all evaluate a patient. Ideally, each will apply the GCS, thereby producing an important piece of time-defined clinical history. Recall that the patient who is dead has a GCS score of 3 (Table 2).

Laboratory and Radiologic Testing

Just as the history and physical examination must be problem-focused, so must the use of testing services. Because they are expensive and time-consuming, laboratory and radiologic tests should be requested only when it is clear that the results will more likely than not influence diagnosis, therapy, or disposition. Also, recall that the transport to a radiology suite may reduce the intensity and quality of monitoring of a critically ill patient.

THE PATIENT WITH ALTERED MENTAL STATUS

This section focuses on patients who present with altered mental status who are *not* victims of trauma. At the outset, the lack of a firm diagnosis should not delay rapid intervention in these patients. Assessment and maintenance of airway, breathing, and circulation are paramount, closely followed by empirical administration of intravenous dextrose, 50 per cent, plus thiamine and naloxone. Dextrose can be withheld if glucose testing rules out hypoglycemia. Intravenous access and cardiac monitoring should be maintained throughout the emergency department evaluation.

Concurrent history taking, physical examination, and laboratory testing are required to define the cause of the altered mental state. The history is often obtained from family or personnel who have examined the patient before the hospital was reached, but it may not be readily available or helpful. Nevertheless, the physician should communicate with someone who knows the patient's past medical history, current medications, and current living and social situation. Although almost any organ failure or compromise can lead to central nervous system dysfunction, the physical examination performed at the time of presentation should focus on the cardiopulmonary and nervous systems.

When stability of cardiopulmonary function is assured, the neurologic examination should begin with determination of the GCS score. Movements should then be assessed for symmetry consistent with global cerebral dysfunction or asymmetry, which favors focal neurologic deficit. In addition, pupillary response; cranial nerve function, including gag reflex; the presence or absence of meningismus (to evaluate meningeal irritation from infection or subarachnoid hemorrhage); abdominal mass or tenderness; deep tendon reflexes; and plantar responses should all be documented.

Pertinent laboratory testing should not be delayed. A complete blood count (CBC); electrolyte, glucose, serum urea nitrogen, and creatinine determinations; and ABG studies aid the detection of most metabolic abnormalities associated with coma. ABG studies should include measurement of carboxyhemoglobin and methemoglobin by co-oximetry. Specific drug blood levels are useful only when directed by the history, but in suspected intentional overdose, salicylate and acetaminophen levels may be diagnostic.

Imaging of the brain by computed tomography should be undertaken primarily when an intracerebral event is strongly suspected. Otherwise, repeated clinical evaluation of the patient is of greatest use. As noted earlier, specialized radiology suites are geographically removed from the emergency department, thereby requiring maximal patient stability prior to testing.

Unless the patient awakens or the neurologic status improves in the emergency department, admission to a monitored hospital unit is appropriate. For patients who improve enough to warrant discharge, the physician should be convinced that adequate observation of the patient can be undertaken by family or friends who will assume responsibility for the patient's welfare. Finally, some patients who are physically stable following intentional ingestion may require psychiatric evaluation prior to consideration for discharge from the emergency department.

Section Two

INFECTIOUS DISEASES

Sexually Transmitted Diseases

CHLAMYDIAL INFECTIONS

By Barbara A. Majeroni, M.D.
Buffalo, New York

Chlamydial diseases include any condition caused by the genus of parasites that includes *Chlamydia trachomatis, C. psittaci, and C. pneumoniae.* These organisms are similar to gram-negative bacteria but are obligate intracellular parasites.

Chlamydia trachomatis is a common, sexually transmitted organism that can cause cervicitis, endometritis, salpingitis, and urethritis in women; urethritis, epididymitis, and proctitis in men; and vaginitis in prepubertal girls. Twenty to forty per cent of sexually active women in the United States show serologic evidence of exposure. Pregnant women with genital infections are at higher risk for preterm rupture of membranes, premature birth, low-birth-weight infants, spontaneous abortion, and intrauterine death. Untreated, 60 to 70 per cent of women will transmit the organism to their infants during vaginal delivery. Neonatal conjunctivitis will develop in up to 50 per cent of exposed babies; chlamydial pneumonia will develop in 10 to 16 per cent of such newborns; and 15 to 20 per cent of these infants will carry the organism in the nasopharynx for up to 18 months.

Chlamydia trachomatis has also been associated with prolonged tonsillitis, Reiter syndrome, and seronegative arthritis. In both sexes, the same organism can infect pelvic lymph nodes, causing the swelling, ulceration, and scarring of lymphogranuloma venereum or granuloma inguinale, which are discussed elsewhere in this book. Infection of the eye with *C. trachomatis* causes conjunctivitis. In rural areas of nonindustrialized countries, trachoma is very common and is caused by serovars A, B, Ba, and C. Serovars D through K cause the sexually transmitted forms of *C. trachomatis* that are common in the United States, and serovars L1 through L3 are associated with lymphogranuloma venereum. Serovars D, G, L1, and L2 are associated with rectal infections in homosexual men.

Chlamydia psittaci is a respiratory pathogen usually transmitted by birds. Atypical pneumonia is frequently complicated by infection of the liver, spleen, and heart. *Chlamydia pneumoniae*, also known as the Taiwan acute respiratory (TWAR) agent, causes pharyngitis, bronchitis, and atypical pneumonia. These agents are covered elsewhere in this book.

PRESENTING SIGNS AND SYMPTOMS

Infection in Women

Genital chlamydial infection in women is frequently asymptomatic but should be treated to decrease the risk of salpingitis with scarring, which leads to infertility and ectopic pregnancy. Some women note a vaginal discharge resulting from the purulent cervicitis. On examination, a yellow or green cervical discharge, cervical friability (easy bleeding), and the presence of 20 or more leukocytes/high-power field on endocervical Gram staining all suggest cervicitis, but no physical findings are reliable predictors of chlamydial infection. Historical factors such as a new or multiple sexual partners, age less than 25 years, the presence of another sexually transmitted disease, and failure to use barrier contraception may further define the population that should be screened.

In salpingitis, dyspareunia, lower abdominal tenderness, pain with cervical motion, and adnexal tenderness are common. Fever and leukocytosis are variable. Symptoms may be milder than those seen in salpingitis caused by *Neisseria gonorrhoeae*. Since many women are infected with both organisms, the presence of *N. gonorrhoeae* suggests that *C. trachomatis* may also be present.

Infection in Men

Symptoms in men vary from acute urethritis with dysuria and urethral discharge to no symptoms at all. *Chlamydia trachomatis* can be recovered from 30 to 50 per cent of men with nongonococcal urethritis, whereas *Ureaplasma urealyticum* is associated with another 10 to 20 per cent. The presence of leukocytes in the first 10 mL of voided urine suggests urethritis. Onset frequently occurs 7 to 10 days after a new sexual contact. The persistence of symptoms of urethritis after adequate treatment of gonococcal infection suggests concurrent chlamydial infection. Epididymitis may present with scrotal swelling and pain, which must be distinguished from torsion of the testicle. Chlamydial proctitis and proctocolitis are more common in homosexual men. Symptoms include rectal pain, discharge, tenesmus, and constipation. The rectal mucosa is erythematous and friable.

Ocular Disease

Neonatal inclusion conjunctivitis appears 3 to 25 days after birth. A mucoid discharge that progressively becomes more purulent accompanies conjunctival erythema. Infants are typically alert but have swollen eyelids, and pseudomembranes may develop. Adult inclusion conjunctivitis presents with a similar discharge accompanied by a foreign body sensation.

Infant Pneumonia

A fourth of all infants younger than 6 months of age who are admitted to the hospital with lower respiratory disease and three fourths of all infants with afebrile pneumonia are infected with *Chlamydia*. Patients typically present at 3 to 16 weeks of age but may have been ill for several weeks prior to evaluation. These infants are usually afebrile and alert, with increasing cough and tachypnea developing. Physical examination may reveal rales and, at times, wheezing. Chest radiographs show hyperinflation with diffuse interstitial or patchy infiltrates.

CLINICAL COURSE

Untreated chlamydial cervicitis in women may resolve, but the infection may ascend to the endometrium and fallopian tubes, where chronic inflammation causes scarring that can lead to infertility and ectopic pregnancies. Similarly, in men the acute symptoms may resolve, resulting in an asymptomatic carrier state. Men with untreated chlamydial urethritis have a 1 to 2 per cent risk of epididymitis and are also at increased risk for the development of Reiter syndrome. In pregnancy, treatment with appropriate antibiotics returns the risk factors to baseline and eliminates transmission to the infant. Inclusion conjunctivitis will clear with or without treatment, but it tends to recur. Pneumonitis lasts several weeks without treatment, but roentgenographic abnormalities may persist for months. Pulmonary function abnormalities may persist for years.

PHYSICAL EXAMINATION

Women

No physical findings reliably predict chlamydial infection. Signs of cervicitis include a purulent discharge, ectopy, friability, and tenderness, but many women with chlamydial disease have none of these signs. Cervical motion pain and adnexal tenderness suggest salpingitis, but other causes, such as ectopic pregnancy and appendicitis, must be ruled out.

Men

In chlamydial urethritis, stripping of the penis typically produces a urethral discharge, which may range from thin and watery to yellow-green and purulent. Some men with chlamydial urethritis have no expressible discharge, so a urethral specimen should be obtained if the diagnosis is suspected. Inguinal adenopathy is not generally present with chlamydial urethritis. Prominent adenopathy suggests another diagnosis, such as lymphogranuloma venereum. With epididymitis, the patient will have a red, swollen, and tender scrotum. In chlamydial proctitis, there is a mucoid discharge and the rectum is red, tender, and friable.

Ocular Disease

Purulent discharge from one or both eyes, erythema of the conjunctiva, and eyelid swelling in an otherwise alert infant suggest inclusion conjunctivitis.

Infant Pneumonitis

Tachypnea and cough in an afebrile infant suggest chlamydial infection. Rales and wheezing may be present.

LABORATORY PROCEDURES

Bacterial Culture

Chlamydia can be cultured in specially treated McCoy, hamster kidney, or HeLa cell lines. Sensitivity ranges from 70 to 90 per cent for a single cervical specimen. Storing and freezing specimens may lower sensitivity. The use of enzyme immunoassays with cultures increases the sensitivity to 95 per cent. Because *C. trachomatis* is an obligate intracellular organism, an adequate cervical specimen should include endocervical columnar epithelial cells, so it is essential to remove cervical mucus before the sample is taken. Polyester (Dacron) swabs on metal or plastic handles should be used because chemicals released into the transport medium by wooden-handled swabs can interfere with the growth of this fastidious organism. Other specimens appropriate for culture include those collected by swabbing the male urethra as well as scrapings from the conjunctiva. In lymphogranuloma venereum, aspirates or biopsy specimens from infected nodes are cultured to confirm the clinical diagnosis. In children, only culture is considered reliable, especially if there is a question of sexual abuse.

Nonculture Tests

Nonculture methods include enzyme assays, such as Clearview Chlamydia (Unipath Ltd., Bedford, U.K.), Chlamydiazyme (Abbott Laboratories, North Chicago, IL), the Kodak SureCell Chlamydia assay (Eastman Kodak Co., Rochester, NY), AntigEnz Chlamydia enzyme immunoassay (Baxter-Bartels, Bellevue, WA), and Syva MicroTrak EIA test (Syva, Palo Alto, CA). These tests are acceptable alternatives when culture is not possible, but they lack the sensitivity of culture. A DNA probe assay (PACE 2 [Gen-Probe, San Diego, CA]) is reported to be equivalent to tissue culture. In women, enzyme assays should be used only on cervical specimens because of an unacceptably high rate of false-positive results in vaginal specimens.

In sexually active men 25 years of age and younger, screening a first-voided urine specimen for leukocytes followed by testing of positive samples with an enzyme immunoassay has been shown to be an effective method of screening asymptomatic men for chlamydial urethritis. The Amplicor *C. trachomatis* test (Roche Diagnostics Systems, Branchburg, NJ) combines polymerase chain reaction and colorimetric DNA hybridization for detection of *Chlamydia* in first-voided urine specimens in males. In the high-prevalence population seen in a sexually transmitted disease clinic, this test has been shown to be highly sensitive and specific. With cervical specimens, Amplicor *C. trachomatis* is more sensitive and specific than enzyme assay or culture alone. No urine screen has been approved for use in women.

Serologic Tests

Because 40 to 80 per cent of sexually active adults have serum antichlamydial antibodies, serologic testing generally is not useful in the diagnosis of urogenital chlamydial infection. Elevated *Chlamydia*-specific IgA levels may persist up to 5 years after eradication of infection. In infants, the presence of antichlamydial IgM is diagnostic for an acute chlamydial infection.

Ocular Infections

Conjunctival specimens from infants or adults with inclusion conjunctivitis usually reveal the organism by culture, antigen testing, or direct fluorescent antibody testing.

Infant Pneumonia

In infants with pneumonia, nasopharyngeal specimens can be cultured for *Chlamydia*. Eosinophilia is common.

DIAGNOSTIC PROCEDURES

Salpingitis

The sonographic finding of an abscess suggests anaerobic infection but does not rule out *Chlamydia* because salpingitis is usually polymicrobial. If the diagnosis is in doubt or a trial of antibiotics has failed to produce improvement, laparoscopy to obtain specimens for tubal cultures may aid the diagnosis.

Proctitis

Sigmoidoscopy provides the opportunity to visualize the mucosa, biopsy lesions if indicated, and collect specimens to culture for *C. trachomatis* and *N. gonorrhoeae*.

DIAGNOSTIC PROCEDURES THAT MAY NOT BE HELPFUL

The Frei test, an intradermal skin test for *C. trachomatis,* is no longer used because it is unreliable. Findings from Papanicolaou smears are also unreliable in the diagnosis of *Chlamydia*.

DIAGNOSTIC ERRORS AND PITFALLS

Screening

Because of the insidious nature of chlamydial infections, the clinician must maintain a high index of suspicion. The Centers for Disease Control and Prevention recommends screening all pregnant women. In addition, asymptomatic sexually active women with historical risk factors, such as age less than 25 years, a new sexual partner or a partner with other sexual partners, and the presence of any sexually transmitted disease should be screened.

Specimens

In women, specimens must be taken from the cervix, since the organism does not infect squamous epithelium, which lines the vagina. In prepubertal girls, the transitional epithelial cells that line the vagina can be infected with *C. trachomatis*, leading to vaginitis. In this setting, vaginal cultures are appropriate.

Differential Diagnosis

Any woman of childbearing age with abdominal pain should have a serum human chorionic gonadotropin (HCG) determination to rule out ectopic pregnancy before a diagnosis of salpingitis is made. Treatment of any salpingitis must include a drug that covers *C. trachomatis,* even if cultures are negative.

False-Negative and False-Positive Results

Because of the relatively poor sensitivity of available tests, a negative test result does not exclude infection. When infection is likely, such as with concurrent gonorrhea, nongonococcal urethritis, or a partner with either of these conditions, empirical therapy to treat *Chlamydia* should be initiated. False-positive test results occur, particularly with enzyme assays. Because *C. trachomatis* can remain asymptomatic for years, the new diagnosis of disease does not necessarily mean that it was recently acquired.

GONORRHEA

By H. Bradford Hawley, M.D.
Dayton, Ohio

Gonorrhea is a bacterial infection of noncornified epithelium, including that of the urethra, rectum, conjunctiva, pharynx, and endocervix. It is caused by *Neisseria gonorrhoeae*. Transmission is nearly always by sexual contact or perinatally. Gonorrhea is the most common reportable communicable disease in the United States, with 690,169 cases reported in 1990. The annual incidence decreased by 30 per cent from a decade earlier, but the incidence increased in adolescents. The Youth Risk Behavior Survey conducted by the Centers for Disease Control and Prevention, which was a telephone survey of 11,631 representative high school students, revealed that 54 per cent of students reported having sexual intercourse, and 40 per cent of students had had intercourse within the 3 months prior to the survey. A history of a sexually transmitted disease was reported by 4 per cent of all students surveyed. Other studies have shown an association between crack cocaine usage and gonorrhea, particularly in young women who exchange sex for drugs or money. In the United States, the incidence of gonorrhea is about 10 times higher for nonwhites than for whites. This higher incidence is only partially explained by greater attendance and reporting at public clinics and seems to correlate with the increased sexual activity of nonwhite, compared with white, high school students. Other risk factors for gonorrhea are low socioeconomic status, urban dwelling, early sexual intercourse, unmarried status, and past gonococcal infection.

An uninfected woman exposed to a man with gonorrhea will acquire the infection approximately 50 per cent of the time, which increases to more than 90 per cent with several exposures. Transmission from female to male is about 20 per cent per episode of vaginal intercourse. In both cases, the infecting partner is usually asymptomatic, and recent studies suggest that the asymptomatic male (20 to 40 per cent of patients) may contribute significantly to the spread of disease. The rates of transmission for other forms of sexual intercourse have not been accurately determined. Exposed infants will have an incidence of gonococcal ophthalmia ranging from 2 to 30 per cent. Ocular silver nitrate prophylaxis reduces this incidence to 0 to 5 per cent.

Human immunodeficiency virus (HIV) infection does not appear to influence the clinical presentation, diagnostic tests, or efficacy of treatment of gonorrhea. However, HIV-infected women may be more susceptible to endocervical gonococcal infection and local complications such as tubo-ovarian abscesses.

PRESENTING SYMPTOMS AND SIGNS

Acute urethritis is the most common clinical gonococcal infection in men. After an incubation period of 1 to 14 days (usually 2 to 5 days), a urethral discharge develops, which is associated with or followed closely by dysuria. The discharge may be scant or mucoid initially but usually becomes more purulent and profuse by the second day.

The endocervix is the most common site of infection in women and is associated with urethral colonization in 70 to 90 per cent of infected women. The most common symptoms include increased vaginal discharge, dysuria, abnormal uterine bleeding, and menorrhagia occurring within

10 days of exposure. Lower abdominal pain usually heralds spread of the infection to the fallopian tubes, resulting in acute salpingitis. Up to 80 per cent of infected women may be asymptomatic or have symptoms mild enough that they do not seek medical attention. The physical examination typically reveals a purulent or mucopurulent cervical discharge, with areas of cervical erythema and mucosal bleeding. Occasionally the examination will reveal no abnormalities. Cervical or adnexal tenderness usually indicates ascending spread of the infection.

Rectal gonococcal infection occurs in homosexual men as a result of direct inoculation through rectal intercourse and is the only site of infection in 40 per cent of these men. Most homosexual men with gonococcal infection have rectal symptoms, but it is difficult to attribute them to this infection because up to 40 per cent of such individuals from whom no gonococci can be cultured have rectal symptoms. Symptoms range from mild pruritus and painless mucopurulent discharge to severe pain, tenesmus, and constipation. The external anus is usually unremarkable, but anoscopy will often reveal mucosal erythema and mucoid or purulent discharge. Rectal infection in women is most often asymptomatic and occurs as a result of local spread via cervical secretions rather than rectal intercourse. Rectal cultures will be positive in 35 to 50 per cent of women with gonococcal cervicitis. Occasionally, the rectum will be the only site that yields a positive culture.

Gonococcal pharyngitis occurs as a result of oropharyngeal sexual contact with an infected individual. More than 90 per cent of patients with gonococcal pharyngitis are asymptomatic. The occasional symptomatic patient may have pharyngeal erythema and exudate sometimes associated with fever and cervical lymphadenopathy. Pharyngeal gonorrhea seems to be more common in pregnancy.

Gonococcal conjunctival infection in the newborn produces an acute purulent conjunctivitis 2 to 5 days after birth. Occasionally a more indolent or chronic conjunctivitis results after a delayed incubation period. Because of this variable clinical presentation, gonococcal infection must be investigated in all cases of newborn conjunctivitis. Conjunctivitis can rarely be seen in the adult patient as a result of direct contact with infected secretions and is usually less severe.

CLINICAL COURSE

The symptoms of gonococcal urethritis will gradually resolve over several weeks, and nearly all untreated patients will be free of symptoms by 6 months. The natural history of endocervical gonorrhea is less well understood because of mild and nonspecific symptoms and frequent coinfection with other pathogens. Since most patients with rectal and pharyngeal gonococcal infection are asymptomatic, little is known about the course of untreated infection. Without prompt treatment of neonatal gonococcal ophthalmia, the infection will extend into deeper layers of the conjunctiva and cornea, resulting in severe ocular damage. Further spread of the infection into the bloodstream may result in the death of the infant.

COMPLICATIONS

Local complications of gonococcal urethritis include epididymitis, acute or chronic prostatitis, inguinal lymphadenitis, urethral stricture, and periurethral abscesses. Repeated infections and the lack of effective antibiotic therapy contributed greatly to these complications in the past; however, they are uncommon today. Extension of infection from the endocervix to the fallopian tubes resulting in salpingitis or pelvic inflammatory disease still occurs in 10 to 20 per cent of women with acute gonococcal infection. The infection may spread to the pelvic peritoneum and may cause tubo-ovarian abscess. The late complications of healing include peritubal damage and tubal occlusion with infertility. Abscess of Bartholin's gland is another urogenital complication in women. When salpingitis spreads to the upper abdomen, it can be associated with perihepatitis (Fitz-Hugh-Curtis syndrome). This syndrome may be caused by gonococci or *Chlamydia*. The disorder is characterized by the sudden onset of upper abdominal pain, which is usually on the right side and may radiate to the shoulder. The pain is made worse by breathing or coughing.

Dissemination of gonococcal infection via the bloodstream occurs in 0.5 to 3 per cent of patients and is usually manifested by fever, rash, and joint pain—the acute arthritis-dermatitis syndrome. The skin rash varies in appearance and may be petechial, papular, pustular, hemorrhagic or necrotic. The joint discomfort is migratory and is most commonly a result of tenosynovitis or polyarthralgias rather than true arthritis. However, true septic arthritis may occur as part of this syndrome or as a separate process. The arthritis is monarthric and usually affects large joints. Tenosynovitis and migratory polyarthralgias may precede the arthritis.

Other systemic complications due to bacteremia include endocarditis, meningitis, and acute respiratory distress syndrome. Endocarditis occurs in 1 to 3 per cent of patients with disseminated infection and can lead to rapid valvular destruction with catastrophic consequences.

LABORATORY DIAGNOSIS

Gram-stained smears of urethral, endocervical, anorectal, pharyngeal, or conjunctival exudate may provide immediate diagnostic information. The sensitivity and specificity of these smears is clinically adequate if the collection technique is proper and the experience of the microscopist is substantial. Vaginal speculums and anoscopes should be lubricated with warm water only, as other lubricants may be toxic to gonococci. Polyester (Dacron) or rayon swabs on a metal or plastic shaft are preferred because some cotton or calcium alginate swabs and wooden shafts are toxic to the organisms. Urethral specimens may be obtained by swabbing the discharge or inserting and rotating the swab about 2 cm into the urethra. The swab is rolled across a microscopic slide and then across a plate for culture. Alternatively, separate swabs may be used to obtain specimens for slide and culture preparation. If urethral swabbing is not possible, the sediment from 10 to 15 mL of centrifuged urine may be cultured. Endocervical specimens are obtained by first wiping away cervical mucus and then inserting the swab into the external os with rotation. One must avoid touching the walls of the vagina with the swab. Rectal specimens are best obtained by swabbing exudate visualized during anoscopy. Alternatively, a swab may be inserted 4 to 5 cm into the rectum with rotation; swabs with heavy fecal contamination should be discarded and the procedure repeated. Pharyngeal or conjunctival exudate is simply swabbed. Slide and culture inoculation for all specimens is as previously described for urethral specimens. Gram-stained smears should be interpreted as positive only when gram-negative diplococci with typical morphologic features are observed in association with neutrophils.

Material for culture is best inoculated immediately onto a selective media, such as modified Thayer-Martin or New York City agars, and placed into a candle jar. Agar plates should be at room temperature or 35°C at the time of inoculation, since inoculation of plates taken directly from the refrigerator can result in microbial death. The plates can be transported to the laboratory in the candle jar. If plates are not directly inoculated and a bacterial transport medium is used, transit time should not exceed 4 to 6 hours. Blood for culture is best obtained and inoculated immediately into appropriate media. Blood collection tubes containing sodium polyanetholesulfonate (SPS) may be used but should be inoculated into broth within 1 hour of collection to avoid the toxic effects of sodium polyanetholesulfonate. Joint fluid can be transported in a capped syringe or sterile container and slides prepared and plates inoculated as soon as possible. Skin lesions are best examined by punch biopsy, with the specimen transported on a chocolate agar plate to prevent drying.

Nucleic acid probes (Gen-Probe) can detect gonococci directly in urogenital specimens within 2 to 3 hours. The sensitivity and specificity of nucleic acid procedures compare favorably with traditional culture techniques. Furthermore, specimens may be frozen up to a week prior to nucleic acid testing.

Susceptibility testing is not routinely performed on gonococcal isolates. All isolates, however, should be tested for beta-lactamase production. With disseminated or serious systemic disease or treatment failure, minimal inhibitory concentrations of appropriate antibiotics may be determined using an agar dilution method.

PITFALLS IN DIAGNOSIS

Inadequate sexual history and lack of suspicion are probably the most common factors leading to misdiagnosis. Inadequate culturing can also reduce diagnostic yield. Women should undergo endocervical and rectal swabbing to obtain material for cultures. If there is a history of orogenital contact, specimens for pharyngeal cultures should also be obtained. Only urethral specimens are required for culture in heterosexual men. Homosexual men should have urethral, rectal, and pharyngeal cultures performed. All patients with suspected disseminated infection should have blood cultures in addition to the previous categorical cultures. If appropriate, skin lesions and joint fluid may also be sampled in these patients.

In patients who are suspected of having or who have been proved to have gonococcal infection, other sexually transmitted diseases (including HIV) may coexist, and evidence for them should be sought by both clinical and laboratory methods. *Chlamydia* may coexist with gonococci in up to 45 per cent of patients, and dual treatment is generally recommended.

SYPHILIS

By Judith E. Wolf, M.D.
Philadelphia, Pennsylvania

Know syphilis in all its manifestations and relations, and all other things clinical will be added unto you.

SIR WILLIAM OSLER, 1897

Syphilis is a systemic disease with protean manifestations caused by the spirochete *Treponema pallidum*. Most often transmitted sexually or transplacentally (congenital syphilis), it has also been called "the French disease," "bad blood," and lues (from the Latin *lues venereum*).

The risk of acquiring syphilis from an infected individual is highest early in the course of disease when contact with lesions containing high concentrations of treponemes (e.g., chancre, mucous patch, condyloma latum) is more likely to lead to spirochete penetration through skin and mucous membranes. Transmission occurs in approximately 30 to 50 per cent of individuals exposed to a sexual partner with early syphilis. Acquisition is followed by rapid dissemination throughout the body—including the central nervous system (CNS)—via the bloodstream and lymphatics.

PRESENTING SIGNS AND SYMPTOMS

Because of its varied clinical manifestations that often mimic other medical conditions, syphilis has earned the nickname "the great imitator." In the adult, syphilis can be divided into several clinical stages that are useful in estimating the duration of infection and degree of infectivity and in determining therapeutic interventions. These stages include incubating, primary, secondary, latent, and tertiary syphilis. Congenital syphilis is discussed separately.

Incubating Syphilis

After inoculation there is a period of incubation that averages 3 weeks. Despite the absence of visible lesions during this time, spirochetes have already begun to disseminate, rendering the patient's blood potentially infectious.

Primary Syphilis

The primary skin lesion or *chancre* develops at the site of inoculation about 3 weeks after exposure, with a range of 10 to 90 days depending on inoculum size. The chancre is classically described as a round or oval solitary painless ulcer arising from a papule, measuring a few millimeters to 2 cm in diameter, and exhibiting well-defined raised borders, an indurated dull red base, and scant serous exudate. Although these features are often helpful in distinguishing syphilitic chancres from other ulcerative genital lesions, such as chancroid, herpes genitalis, donovanosis, lymphogranuloma venereum, aphthous ulcers, traumatic lesions, furuncles, or carcinomas, considerable overlap in clinical characteristics exists. For example, chancres can be multiple, especially in human immunodeficiency virus (HIV)–infected patients and can also be painful if they are extragenital (especially on the fingers) or become secondarily infected. Since most primary lesions are asymptomatic, however, they may go unnoticed. Because untreated

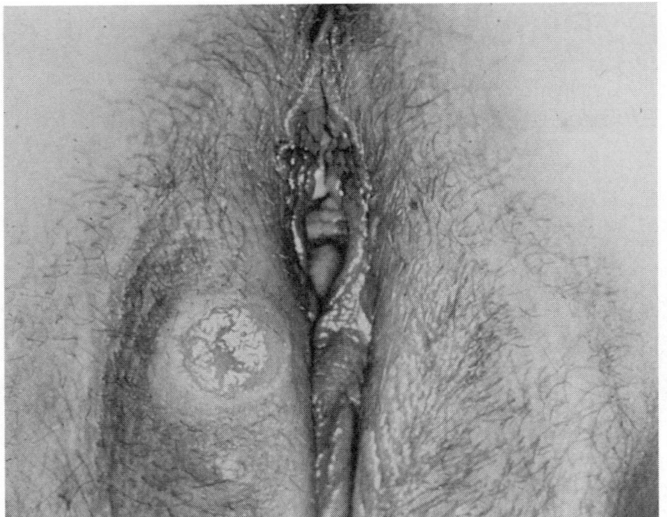

Figure 1. Primary syphilis: chancre of labium majoris. (Courtesy of the M. Harris Sametz, M.D., Dermatology Slide Collection, The Graduate Hospital, Philadelphia.)

chancres heal spontaneously in 3 to 6 weeks, patients may fail to seek medical attention.

Chancres in men most often arise on the inner prepuce, coronal sulcus of the glans, and the shaft and base of the penis. In women, lesions may be observed less frequently because they arise in the vagina or cervix as well as on the vulva and clitoris (Fig. 1). The distribution of extragenital chancres (anus or rectum, breast, lips, tongue, and fingers) may relate to sexual practices. Homosexual men, for example, may present with oral lesions or anorectal chancres accompanied by pruritus or painful discharge.

Regional lymphadenopathy develops within a week of the appearance of the chancre. Lymph nodes are characteristically firm, rubbery, nontender, nonsuppurative, and either unilateral or bilateral, the latter most often associated with genital and anal chancres. In approximately 30 per cent of patients, there is no obvious lymph node enlargement.

Secondary Syphilis

The most florid stage of infection, secondary syphilis, begins 2 to 6 months after primary infection and 2 to 12 weeks after the the appearance of the chancre. The second stage may even develop while the chancre is still visible. During this systemic phase, widespread dissemination of *T. pallidum* causes lesions at sites distant from the original site of inoculation. Because most of these lesions involve the skin and mucous membranes and are teeming with spirochetes, they should be considered highly contagious. Constitutional signs and symptoms such as fever, chills, malaise, sore throat, headache, myalgias, weight loss, and generalized lymphadenopathy may be prominent.

A generalized nonpruritic maculopapular skin rash involving the palms and soles is the hallmark of secondary syphilis (Fig. 2). However, lesions may be macular, papular, pustular, acneform, papulosquamous, annular, or follicular, thus mimicking dermatologic conditions such as fixed drug eruptions, pityriasis rosea, viral exanthems, impetigo, acne, dermatophyte infections, scabies, and guttate psoriasis (Fig. 3). Rarely, lesions may ulcerate with necrosis ("lues maligna"). Vesiculobullous lesions are seen only in congenital syphilis. Papules located at the angles of the mouth, nasolabial fold, and behind the ears may become fissured ("split papules") (Fig. 4). In intertriginous zones, papules may enlarge and flatten into moist plaques or condylomata lata. The lesions of secondary syphilis heal, with or without treatment, in 2 to 10 weeks. This usually occurs without scarring, but sometimes residual areas of hypo- or hyperpigmentation may be found, especially on the neck.

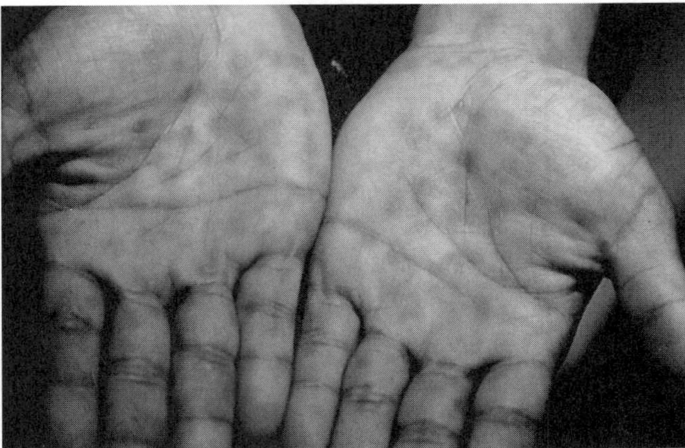

Figure 2. Secondary syphilis: maculopapular skin lesions involving the palms. (Courtesy of the M. Harris Sametz, M.D., Dermatology Slide Collection, The Graduate Hospital, Philadelphia.)

Asymptomatic superficial erosions of the oral or genital mucosa known as "mucous patches" are usually covered by a hyperkeratotic gray-white membrane and surrounded by an erythematous margin. Diffuse or patchy ("moth-eaten") alopecia may occur on the scalp and beard, along with loss of eyelashes and the lateral third of the eyebrows. Other manifestations of secondary syphilis include immune complex glomerulonephritis, transient carditis, gastritis, hepatitis, splenomegaly, myositis, arthritis, osteitis, iritis, anterior uveitis, aseptic meningitis, and cranial nerve palsies.

Latent Syphilis

By definition, latent syphilis is the quiescent phase in which there are no overt clinical manifestations of disease. Subdivided, although somewhat arbitrarily, into early (in-

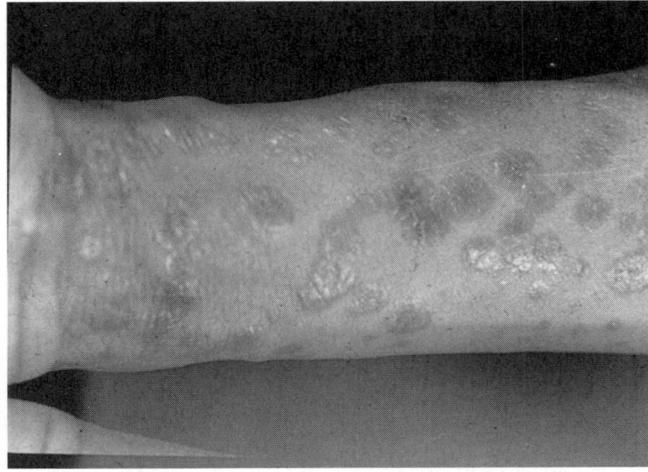

Figure 3. Secondary syphilis: papulosquamous or "psoriasiform" lesions. (Courtesy of the M. Harris Sametz, M.D., Dermatology Slide Collection, The Graduate Hospital, Philadelphia.)

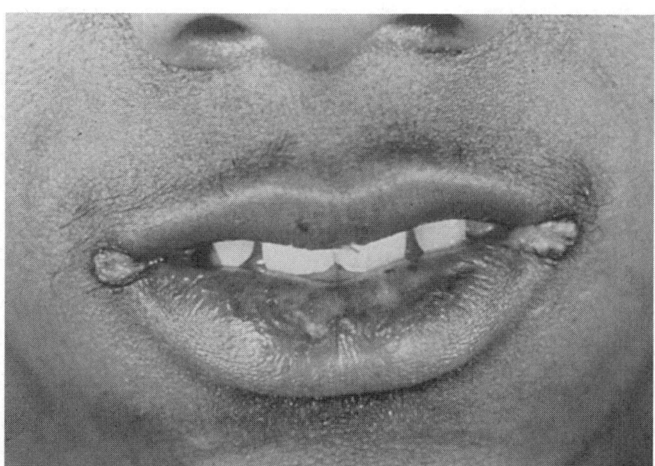

Figure 4. Secondary syphilis: "split papules." (Courtesy of the M. Harris Sametz, M.D., Dermatology Slide Collection, The Graduate Hospital, Philadelphia.)

fectious or relapsing) and late (noninfectious) latent disease on the basis of the estimated duration of illness, latency per se should not imply lack of infectivity or lack of disease progression. For example, a pregnant woman with latent syphilis can infect her unborn child. Although the exact definition of early latent syphilis varies—the Centers for Disease Control and Prevention (CDC) defines it as infection for less than 1 year, whereas the World Health Organization (WHO) defines it as infection for 2 years—these differences are less important than the clinical implications of early latency and their impact on treatment decisions. Specifically, since 85 to 90 per cent of spontaneous mucocutaneous relapses occur in early latency, patients in this stage of disease should be considered infectious to their sexual partners. Overall, latency may last from several months to many years. In general, as the duration of latency increases, infectivity decreases.

Tertiary Syphilis

After a variable period of latency, usually 5 to 20 years, late or tertiary syphilis develops in about 30 per cent of untreated patients. Although almost any tissue or organ may be involved, the most common manifestations include infiltrative lesions of skin, bone, and liver (gummas) as well as cardiovascular and CNS syphilis. Previously termed "late benign syphilis" because of the brisk clinical response to antibiotic therapy, gummas are rarely seen in clinical practice today. As chronic inflammatory lesions, they are believed to represent a hypersensitivity response to *T. pallidum* antigen. Complications are most often due to local mass effects such as tissue destruction, perforation, or obstruction. In addition, gummas must be distinguished from granulomas and malignancy.

Cardiovascular syphilis, also uncommon today, had previously been documented in 10 to 35 per cent of autopsy specimens from patients with syphilis. Its pathogenesis involves an arteritis of the supracardiac region of the aorta, which ultimately leads to the development of saccular aortic aneurysms, aortic insufficiency, and narrowing of the coronary ostia. Luetic aneuryms almost always involve the thoracic aorta and have fusiform or saccular morphologic features. Because the degree of chronic inflammation leads to wall thickening and medial scarring, dissection is a rare event. Pure aortic insufficiency without stenosis is a classic presentation of cardiovascular syphilis and is due to aortic root dilatation.

NEUROSYPHILIS

Syphilis can involve the CNS at any time after primary infection and is not limited to tertiary disease. Laboratory manifestations of CNS involvement, often referred to as "asymptomatic neurosyphilis," are relatively common even in early syphilis and must be distinguished from "symptomatic clinical disease," which historically developed in 4 to 9 per cent of patients with untreated infection. This latter category can be subdivided into several neurologic syndromes, each of which can develop at different stages in the natural history of the infection. Early forms of neurosyphilis, including meningeal, meningovascular, and ocular disease, presumably develop in patients who are inadequately treated for early syphilis. Theoretically, although partial therapy clears peripheral infection, thus attenuating the normal immune response, it fails to eradicate organisms in the eye and CNS. Supporting this hypothesis is the increased frequency with which uveitis, optic neuritis, and seizures have been observed in the penicillin era despite the overall decline in the incidence of neurosyphilis in non–HIV infected individuals.

Syphilitic meningitis presents as an aseptic meningitis in the first 2 years following infection, often in patients with secondary syphilis. Involvement of the cranial nerves secondary to basilar meningitis can lead to hearing loss, facial nerve palsies, and oculomotor problems (e.g., irregular pupils with abnormal light and accomodation reflexes), accompanied by headache and irritability. Rarely, syphilitic meningitis presents as meningomyelitis or pachymeningitis, with radicular pains and paresthesias, loss of tendon reflexes, muscle wasting, segmental sensory loss, and spastic paraparesis. Fever is generally low grade or absent.

Meningovascular syphilis is typically manifested as focal ischemia or stroke secondary to syphilitic endarteritis 5 to 10 years after infection. The spectrum of clinical signs and symptoms varies with the degree of arteritis in the cerebrum, brain stem, and spinal cord and includes headaches, seizures, confusion, hemiparesis, aphasia, cranial nerve palsies, optic neuritis, optic atrophy, altered deep tendon reflexes, and Argyll Robertson pupils that react normally to convergence-accomodation but not to light. The differential diagnosis includes other causes of stroke syndromes such as hypertension, cerebral embolic disease, or vasculitis (e.g., systemic lupus erythematosus).

Parenchymal neurosyphilis, or true tertiary disease, tends to develop later in the course of untreated syphilis, usually more than 10 years after the initial infection. Presenting as general paresis or tabes dorsalis, or a combination of the two, this form of neurosyphilis is generally considered irreversible. Tabes dorsalis is a chronic progressive degenerative process of the posterior columns of the spinal cord, sensory ganglia, and nerve roots. Among the sensory abnormalities observed with this disorder are severe lower extremity shooting pains ("lightning pains"), abdominal pain secondary to visceral crises, paresthesias, and areas of analgesia that can lead to the development of painless ulcers ("mal perforant") and joint damage ("Charcot's joints") of the lower extremities. The ataxic or high stepping-slapping gait classically associated with syphilis results from impaired proprioception and is worse in the dark. Altered vibration sense, hyporeflexia and Argyll Robertson pupils are also commonly seen.

General paresis is an insidiously progressive dementia

that results from diffuse involvement of the cerebral cortex. It is of interest that in the prepenicillin era patients with neuropsychiatric illness secondary to general paresis (also known as dementia paralytica and general paresis of the insane) accounted for a significant number of admissions to psychiatric hospitals. Symptoms include gradual memory loss, dysarthria, tremor, irritability, emotional lability, loss of concentration, personality changes, delusions, depression, confusion, and frank psychosis. The most common neurologic findings observed are pupillary abnormalities, lack of facial expression (paralytic facies), tremors, and dysarthria. Other organic brain syndromes found with tumors, subdural hematoma, multi-infarct dementia, chronic alcoholism, and Alzheimer's disease may have certain features in common.

CONGENITAL SYPHILIS

Syphilis can be transmitted transplacentally from untreated or inadequately treated mothers to their fetuses. The risk of transmission is highest in the first year after acquisition of infection and declines thereafter. Although it had been previously held that infection of the fetus prior to the fourth month of gestation was rare (passage of *T. pallidum* through the placenta being prevented by the Langhans' cell layer), more recent data suggest that first-trimester infection may, in fact, not always be recognized because of the paucity of organisms and the absence of inflammation. Conversely, the inflammatory changes in the placenta may at times be striking.

Traditionally, congenital syphilis has been classified into two clinical syndromes, early and late, depending on whether the features appear within or after the first 2 years of life. Either stage can result in permanent abnormalities or stigmata. Physical findings can be variable. Most often abnormalities are minimal or absent at birth or may be delayed until 6 to 8 weeks of age. Examination of the skin and mucous membranes may reveal serous nasal discharge ("snuffles"), mucous membrane patches, a diffuse maculopapular desquamative rash that is most pronounced on the palms and soles and around the mouth (rhagades) and anus, and condylomata lata in intertriginous zones. In contrast to the rash of acquired secondary syphilis in adults, lesions of congenital syphilis may be vesicular or even bullous ("syphilitic pemphigus"). Regardless of the morphologic features, all these lesions should be considered highly infectious.

Generalized osteochondritis and perichondritis may be present throughout the skeletal system but are most prominent in the nose and the metaphyses of the lower extremities. Left untreated, permanent sequelae may develop, for example, "saddle nose" deformity (Fig. 5), frontal bossing, protruding mandible, high palatal arch or palatal perforation, clavicular deformity (Higouménakis' sign), scaphoid scapulae, symmetric recurrent arthropathy and knee effusions (Clutton's joints), or anterior bowing of the legs (saber shins). Acutely, pseudoparalysis may result from pain on motion of the limbs. Joint dislocation and pathologic fractures can also be seen. Dental manifestations include mulberry (Moon's) molars, enamel dystrophy, and notched (Hutchinson's) incisors (Fig. 6).

Liver involvement, which can be severe, may be associated with splenomegaly and jaundice. Other findings include generalized lymphadenopathy, an immune complex glomerulonephritis with nephrotic syndrome and ascites, iritis, interstitial keratitis, uveitis, and chorioretinitis. Cardiovascular involvement in congenital infection is rare, but CNS infection may result in eighth nerve deafness, mental retardation, hydrocephalus, seizure disorders, paresis, and paralysis. These findings must be distinguished from other congenital infections such as rubella, cytomegalovirus, and toxoplasmosis.

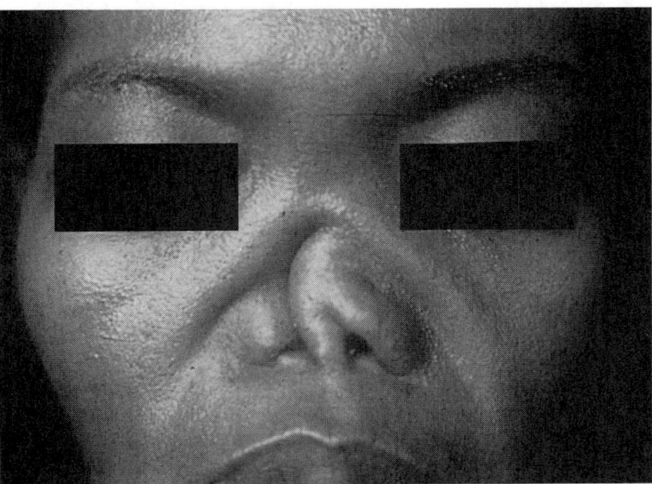

Figure 5. Congenital syphilis: destruction of vomer and nasal septum. (Courtesy of the M. Harris Sametz, M.D., Dermatology Slide Collection, The Graduate Hospital, Philadelphia.)

LABORATORY DIAGNOSIS OF SYPHILIS

Depending on the stage of disease, syphilis may be diagnosed either by direct microscopic identification of *T. pallidum* in specimens (exudate or tissue) taken from lesions of primary, secondary, or congenital syphilis or indirectly through the use of serologic tests, since the spirochete cannot be readily cultured. Although not yet widely available, new monoclonal antibody techniques, antigen detection tests, and the polymerase chain reaction may soon expand our diagnostic capabilities.

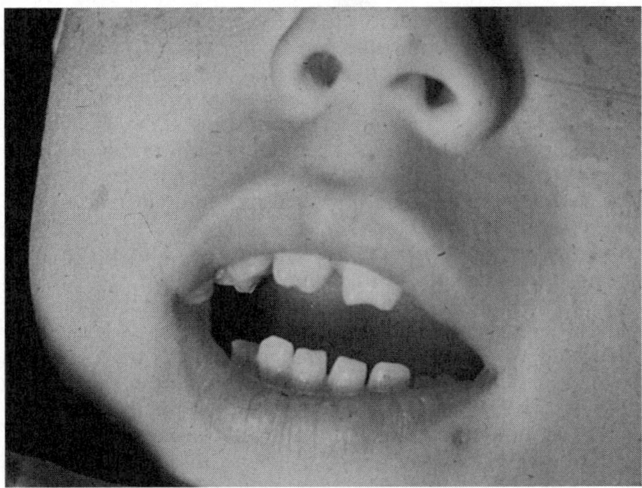

Figure 6. Congenital syphilis: Hutchinson's teeth (incisors). (Courtesy of the M. Harris Sametz, M.D., Dermatology Slide Collection, The Graduate Hospital, Philadelphia.)

Direct Examination of Specimens

T. pallidum is a thin, elongated bacterium that cannot be seen readily by light microscopy. Visualization can be achieved with dark-field microscopy, however, which uses oblique light to illuminate the organism. The technique is performed by collecting serous fluid expressed from the base of a lesion onto a glass slide after cleaning the lesion with sterile saline. A coverslip is then applied to the transudate and the slide is examined immediately with a compound microscope equipped with a dark-field condenser. The organisms can be identified by their characteristic corkscrew morphologic features and "hairpin" motility. Moist lesions such as chancres, condylomas, and mucous patches usually have large numbers of treponemes. Dark-field microscopy should not be used to evaluate oral or rectal specimens because other nonpathogenic treponemes are part of the normal oral and gastrointestinal flora.

An alternative technique for the identification of *T. pallidum* in clinical specimens is fluorescent antibody microscopy. One of its advantages over dark-field examination is that live organisms are not required. Therefore, specimens can be collected on a glass slide and fixed with acetone or transported in a capillary tube. Specimens are incubated with fluorescein isothiocyanate (FITC)–conjugated antibodies to *T. pallidum* (direct fluorescence) or *T. pallidum*-specific antibodies and fluorescein isothiocyanate–conjugated anti-immunoglobulin antibodies (indirect fluorescence) and examined.

Biopsy specimens of suspicious skin lesions can also be examined histopathologically. Lymphocytic and plasmacytic infiltration, proliferation of capillaries, and lymphatics with endarteritis are often seen. Although not definitive, in the appropriate clinical setting, a positive Dieterle or Warthin-Starry stain demonstrating spirochetes makes the diagnosis likely.

Serologic Tests

The diagnosis of syphilis is most often made serologically. Two kinds of antibody tests are commonly used to provide complementary information regarding the presence and activity of the disease. Measurements of nontreponemal antibodies with the Venereal Disease Research Laboratory (VDRL) test or the rapid plasma reagin (RPR) test are used to screen for syphilis as well as monitor disease activity. Nonspecific IgG and IgM antibodies are directed against a lipoidal antigen produced by the interaction of host tissues with *T. pallidum.* Because they cross-react with reagin (a purified cholesterol-lecithin-cardiolipin antigen used as a substrate in performing both the VDRL and RPR tests), they are sometimes called reaginic antibodies. However, they should not be confused with atopic reagin, an IgE class of antibody.

In the VDRL test, heated serum or unheated cerebrospinal fluid (CSF) is mixed with reagin on a glass slide, and flocculation is read microscopically as "reactive" or "nonreactive." The test may be quantitated by serial dilution of serum and, in this way, used to follow disease activity. A fourfold change in titer (which corresponds to a difference of two dilutions) is required to demonstrate a significant difference between two tests. Since reaginic activity may also be present transiently after immunizations, various febrile illnesses, and chronic conditions ("biologic false-positive results"), VDRL test reactivity is not specific for syphilis (Table 1). The VDRL test may also be relatively insensitive in early primary and late disease.

The VDRL test usually becomes reactive some time during the primary syphilis stage, about 4 to 7 days following the appearance of a lesion, although it can remain nonreactive in 13 to 41 per cent of patients. The VDRL test is virtually always reactive during secondary syphilis. Occasionally, false-negative results can occur in patients with very high antibody titers. This "prozone reaction" can be overcome with appropriate serum dilution. The VDRL test reactivity peaks during the first year of infection (secondary or early latent stage) and then slowly declines so that low titers are seen in late syphilis. In about 25 per cent of untreated patients, the VDRL test result ultimately reverts to nonreactive. In treated patients, the VDRL test reactivity declines or becomes nonreactive more rapidly, depending on the stage and severity of disease. For example, in primary syphilis, the test result should revert to nonreactive within 1 year of successful therapy. In secondary syphilis, this should occur within 2 years. However, a small percentage of patients may remain serum-fast at a low titer ($\leq$1:4). Therefore, the presence of a positive test result after 1 year in primary syphilis, or 2 years in secondary syphilis, must be interpreted with caution, as it may represent persistent infection, reinfection, or a biologic false-positive result.

Table 1. Causes of False-Positive Nontreponemal Serologic Test Results for Syphilis

Bacterial Infections	
Pneumococcal pneumonia	Lymphogranuloma venereum
Scarlet fever	Chancroid
Bacterial endocarditis	Rickettsial disease
Tuberculosis	Leptospirosis
Leprosy	Relapsing fever
Mycoplasmal pneumonia	Malaria
Psittacosis	Trypanosomiasis
Viral Infections	
Vaccinia vaccination	Infectious mononucleosis
Chickenpox	Viral hepatitis
Measles	HIV
Mumps	
Noninfectious Causes	
Connective tissue disease	Pregnancy
Chronic liver disease	Multiple myeloma
Intravenous drug use	Advanced malignancy
Multiple blood transfusions	Advancing age

HIV = human immunodeficiency virus.

The RPR card test is a simplified version of the VDRL test and uses unheated serum reagin and carbon particles in the antigenic suspension, enabling flocculation to be interpreted with the naked eye. The RPR test can be quantitated and usually correlates with VDRL titers to within one dilution. Since there can be some divergence of results, however, the same test should be used to follow the course of infection in a particular patient.

Specific treponemal antibody tests are used as confirmation to distinguish patients with syphilis from those with a false-positive screening test result. They establish a high likelihood of treponemal infection either currently or at sometime in the past but cannot be used to monitor disease activity because they remain reactive for an indefinite period. The first treponemal test in use was the *T. pallidum* immobilization (TPI) test, a complement fixation test employing live treponemes. Despite its specificity, however, it was less sensitive and convenient than two other methods that replaced it, the FTA-ABS (fluorescent treponemal antibody absorption) test and the MHA-TP (microhemagglutination *Treponema pallidum*) test. In these tests, the patient's serum is first heated and mixed with nonpathogenic treponemes to remove cross-reacting antibodies. In the FTA-ABS test, the serum is then incubated on slides containing fixed *T. pallidum*. Fluorescein-labeled antihuman globulin is applied to the slides, which are examined by fluorescence microscopy. The intensity of fluorescence is quantified using a 0 to 4+ scale. The MHA-TP test uses agglutination of sheep erythrocytes coated with *T. pallidum* antigen.

Because treponemal tests are more expensive and technically more difficult to perform than nontreponemal tests, they are more appropriate for confirmation than for screening. They are very specific and very sensitive. False-positive results do occur, but this happens much less commonly than with nonspecific antibody tests. False-positive FTA-ABS results have been associated with autoimmune or connective tissue disorders, genital herpes, narcotic addiction, and technical factors.

Cerebrospinal Fluid Studies in the Diagnosis of Neurosyphilis

The diagnosis of neurosyphilis is based on various parameters, including seropositivity, abnormalities of CSF (cell count and protein), and a reactive CSF VDRL test result. Unfortunately, there is no "gold standard" with which to make a definitive diagnosis. CSF leukocytosis and elevated protein concentrations are nonspecific findings, and serologic test results may be negative in 25 per cent of patients with late-stage syphilis. Although classically there should be a mild mononuclear pleocytosis (10 to 400 cells/μL), an elevated protein concentration (46 to 200 mg/dL), and a positive CSF VDRL test result, the CSF may be completely normal, especially in patients with HIV coinfection (see further on). The CSF VDRL test is so highly specific that false-positive results occur only with significant blood contamination of spinal fluid. Its sensitivity, however, ranges between 30 and 70 per cent. Thus, although a reactive CSF VDRL test can be used to diagnose neurosyphilis, a nonreactive result does not exclude the diagnosis.

The yield from screening all asymptomatic patients with positive serologic test results is low. However, patients with syphilis who have not responded to treatment adequately, those who have neurologic abnormalities, or those who are coinfected with HIV are at increased risk for the development of neurosyphilis. For these individuals, as well as those with confirmed penicillin allergy and all infants suspected of having congenital syphilis, CSF examination is indicated.

Laboratory Tests in Congenital Syphilis

The serologic status of an infant's mother should be determined at least once during pregnancy. The goal is to prevent congenital syphilis through detection and treatment of infection in the mother. Infants born to seropositive women who have untreated syphilis as well as those who were treated with a nonpenicillin regimen, those who were treated with an appropriate penicillin regimen but whose antibody titer either did not decrease sufficiently after treatment or is unknown, or those who were treated less than 1 month before delivery should be evaluated for congenital syphilis.

Evaluation of infants should include a quantitative nontreponemal serologic test for syphilis performed on the infant's serum (not on cord blood), CSF analysis for cells and protein, a VDRL test performed on CSF, and dark-field examination of material from lesions of the skin and mucous membranes. Pathologic examination of the placenta or umbilical cord using specific fluorescent antitreponemal antibody staining can also be performed. Infants should be treated for presumed congenital syphilis if they have a reactive CSF VDRL test, an abnormal CSF white blood cell count or protein level (provided that the mother is seroreactive), a quantitative nontreponemal serologic titer that is at least fourfold greater than the mother's titer (both drawn at birth), or specific FTA-ABS-10S IgM antibody.

Infection acquired near the time of delivery may result in negative serologic test results at birth because there has been insufficient time for an antibody response to develop. These infants should receive careful follow-up examinations at 1, 2, 3, 6, and 12 months. Conversely, in noninfected, seroreactive infants whose positive titers are the result of passive transplacental transfer of IgG from the mother, nontreponemal antibody titers should decline by 3 months of age and should be nonreactive by 6 months of age. Passively transferred treponemal antibodies may be present for as long as 1 year.

SYPHILIS IN HUMAN IMMUNODEFICIENCY VIRUS–INFECTED INDIVIDUALS

Syphilis is disproportionately common among patients with HIV infection (and vice versa). As such, complex interactions between the two diseases have had significant impact on diagnostic and therapeutic decision-making. Like other genital ulcer diseases, syphilis may increase the risk of acquisition and transmission of HIV. As a result, the Centers for Disease Control and Prevention recommends serologic testing for HIV infection in all patients with newly diagnosed syphilis and serologic testing for syphilis in patients with newly diagnosed HIV.

Concurrent infection with HIV alters the natural history of syphilis. HIV-infected individuals may have an atypical clinical presentation, an altered serologic response, and an increased incidence of complications, including more rapid progression to CNS disease. Although unusual or florid presentations of syphilis have been described in patients with HIV, they have generally occurred in individuals with advanced disease and significantly compromised cell-mediated immunity. Similarly, although serologic testing appears to be reliable in most patients with HIV, unusually high, unusually low, delayed, and fluctuating nontreponemal titers have been observed. Therefore, if there is a high index of suspicion for syphilis, but serologic test results are negative, the diagnosis should be pursued using alternate methods such as dark-field microscopy, direct fluorescent antibody tests for *T. pallidum,* or silver staining of lesion exudate or biopsy material. Patients with HIV infection are also more likely to have false-positive serologic test results, presumably because of polyclonal B-cell activation that is present early in the course of the disease.

In HIV-seropositive individuals, the incubation period for the development of neurosyphilis appears to be unusually short (months) and the course of infection more aggressive than in patients without HIV infection. Neurosyphilis has developed in many patients despite previous treatment for early or latent infection. This raises the question of whether the CSF should be examined routinely in all coinfected patients regardless of the clinical stage of syphilis. The interpretation of CSF test results, however, may be difficult or misleading. For example, although the spinal fluid may appear completely normal in HIV-seropositive individuals, it may still contain viable *T. pallidum*. In addition, HIV infection of the CNS can cause CSF abnormalities and clinical signs and symptoms (strokes, myelopathy, dementia) that mimic those of neurosyphilis. Given these uncertainties, the most prudent approach appears to be careful assessment and monitoring of each patient, including serial serologic tests and CSF examinations, on an individual basis.

CHANCROID

By Camila K. Janniger, M.D.,
and Robert A. Schwartz, M.D., M.P.H.
Newark, New Jersey

Chancroid is an infrequently reported disease caused by *Haemophilus ducreyi,* a gram-negative coccobacillus that is difficult to culture. This bacterium is endemic in some tropical and semitropical regions. The global incidence of chancroid may actually exceed that of syphilis; *H. ducreyi* is probably the most common cause of genital ulcers in Kenya, Gambia, and Zimbabwe.

By contrast, chancroid is not common in the United States; it typically occurs in small epidemics. The incidence of chancroid in North America peaked in 1947, when 9515 infections were reported. The number of cases gradually declined until 1981, when only 93 infections were reported. The decrease has been attributed to the effectiveness of sulfonamide therapy. With increased antibiotic resistance, however, outbreaks of chancroid resurfaced in the early 1980s. By 1989, 4697 infections were reported. Contact with infected, often asymptomatic prostitutes is the most likely method of disease spread. More then 80 per cent of patients are men. Asymptomatic women provide the main reservoir of *H. ducreyi.*

CLINICAL PRESENTATION

The incubation period for chancroid is typically 4 to 5 days, ranging from 1 to 14 days. The first lesion is a small, tender papule or pustule surrounded by erythema. It rapidly erodes into an ulcer. One to several ulcers may appear; each ulcer is shallow and exquisitely painful. Unlike the indurated ulcers of syphilis and granuloma inguinale, chancroid lesions have a soft consistency resembling putty. The ulcer has a ragged, indistinct, undermined border that may spread to adjacent normal skin.

The chancroid ulcer is shaped like an Erlenmeyer flask, with its opening at the skin surface. The ulcer base is yellowish and may produce purulent drainage. In men, the sites of predilection are the prepuce, coronal sulcus, glans, and frenulum of the penis. In women, labial chancres are common, but lesions may also be found on the anogenital skin, within the vagina, or on the cervix. Several patients have been described with conditions that mimic herpes, syphilis, or granuloma inguinale. Ulcers resulting from autoinoculation are frequent and are characteristic of classic chancroid. Dwarf chancroid presents with a small ulcer. Giant chancroid enlarges rapidly and may first present as a ruptured inguinal lymph node. Phagedenic chancroid is highlighted by severe destruction of the external genitals. Concomitant infection with fusobacteria may substantially contribute to the necrosis. With effective therapy, ulcers tend to resolve within 1 or 2 weeks; left untreated, they may persist for 1 to 3 months.

Thirty to sixty per cent of patients have enlarged regional lymph nodes, which may also ulcerate. The lymphadenopathy is likely to be unilateral. Nodes may be firm initially but often become fluctuant, sometimes rupturing through the overlying skin, forming single-track sinuses. Untreated chancroid gradually progresses by direct extension, increasing the likelihood of inguinal ulceration. The primary ulcer may extend to the inguinal ulcer created by the ruptured, fluctuant lymph node. Lymphatic swelling may result, with genital edema caused by lymphatic blockage. Extensive lymphedema produces lower extremity elephantiasis.

DIAGNOSIS

Laboratory diagnosis of chancroid is aided by a substantially improved culture technique for *H. ducreyi.* Selective media should be inoculated directly from exudates. On occasion, these media may produce the pure culture required for confirmatory biochemical tests. Unfortunately, culture remains difficult without considerable laboratory support and an optimal growth environment.

DNA probes and use of the polymerase chain reaction may facilitate the diagnosis of chancroid in the future. Cytologic examination of exudate from the ulcer base, using a Giemsa or Gram stain, may show the classic "school of fish" or "railroad tracking" parallel chains of pleomorphic gram-negative rods. This method is suboptimal, however, because it lacks both sensitivity and specificity.

Skin biopsy is an important part of the patient evaluation. Microscopically, the ulcer consists of a superficial necrotic layer of neutrophils, red blood cells, and fibrin overlying a relatively large area of blood vessel formation, with endothelial cell proliferation and vascular thromboses. The deepest zone contains a dense infiltrate of plasma cells and lymphocytes.

PITFALLS IN DIAGNOSIS

Herpes simplex presents with multiple painful ulcers resembling the classic form of chancroid. Herpetic lymph nodes are symmetrically involved, however, and are not suppurative. The ulcer of granuloma inguinale is not tender, rapidly enlarges, and is often indurated. It may be confused with the phagodenic type of chancroid. In lymphogranuloma venereum, enlarged suppurative lymph nodes may be seen, but they are usually bilateral and appear after the primary ulcer has healed. The syphilitic ulcer is painless and indurated; lymphadenopathy is not suppurative. The clinician should remember that a patient with chancroid may have coexistent sexually transmitted diseases within the ulcer. Concurrent syphilis is most commonly seen.

GRANULOMA INGUINALE

By Jean L. Goens, M.D.
Brussels, Belgium
Robert A. Schwartz, M.D., M.P.H.
Newark, New Jersey
and Kathleen De Wolf, M.D.
Brussels, Belgium

Granuloma inguinale, also called donovanosis, is a chronic, painless ulcerogranulomatous infection caused by an encapsulated gram-negative pleomorphic rod-shaped bacterium, *Calymmatobacterium granulomatis,* formerly known as *Donovania granulomatis*. The distribution of the disease is worldwide, but it is endemic in the tropics and subtropics. Donovanosis may account for 20 per cent of sexually transmitted disease in male patients in certain tropical regions. The incidence has fallen dramatically in developed countries. There are fewer than 100 cases per year reported in the United States. Donovanosis is generally associated with low socioeconomic status and poor hygiene. Although the frequency and contagiousness of granuloma inguinale are generally considered to be low, persons with defective cellular immunity may be at increased risk for the development of clinically significant infection with *C. granulomatis*.

Infection occurs most frequently between the ages of 20 and 40 years; the incidence is two times greater in men than in women. Sexual activity is the most common route of transmission, but infections among children and sexually inactive persons suggest that other modes of transmission are possible, especially in highly endemic areas. Contaminated feces could provide one source of transmission; indeed, the gastrointestinal tract may be the natural habitat of *C. granulomatis*.

PRESENTING SIGNS AND SYMPTOMS

The incubation period of granuloma inguinale varies from 1 week to 3 months, with an average of 2 to 4 weeks. The initial lesion is an evanescent, infrequently detected solitary papule or nodule that rapidly evolves to a firm, painless, irregular, clean-based, sharply bordered, granulomatous ulcer that bleeds on contact and produces a serosanguineous exudate.

Primary lesions arise on the genitals in more than 90 per cent of patients. In men, the sites of predilection are the prepuce, the coronal sulcus, and the frenulum. In women, lesions are more common on the labia than on the vagina or cervix. Women may initially present with genital bleeding. Extragenital primary lesions are uncommon but may arise in the buccal (orogenital contact) and perianal (anogenital contact) regions.

The course of granuloma inguinale can be divided into three clinical stages: exuberant, ulcerovegatative, and cicatricial. In the exuberant stage, nodules of pink to dull red hypertrophic granulation tissue are noted in the perianal region. In the more commonly observed ulcerovegetative stage, coalescence of lesions and foul-smelling, shallow ulcers are described. The cicatricial stage is characterized by fibrosis, keloid, and scar formation. Lymph nodes are not typically involved, except in the presence of superinfection, often with fusospirochetal organisms.

CLINICAL COURSE

The clinical course is usually chronic. The granulomatous lesion spreads slowly, especially in the warm, moist, intertriginous areas of the inguinal and perineal regions. Extragenital lesions may arise through autoinoculation. In some patients, granuloma inguinale undergoes spontaneous resolution; in others, untreated or inadequately treated lesions progress to marked atrophic and depigmented scarring. By contrast, extension by contiguity or via satellite ulcers coalescing with the primary lesion can produce extensive serpiginous lesions that spread slowly for many years, with formation of deep scars. Deep granulomas, especially in the inguinal area, can mimic fluctuant lymph nodes ("pseudobuboes"), with subsequent erosion and genital ulceration. Hematogenous dissemination is rare.

COMMON COMPLICATIONS

Extensive granuloma inguinale can cause destruction and deformities of the external genitals. With superinfection by fusospirochetal organisms, rapidly spreading destructive ulceration leads to necrosis, foul-smelling exudate, and impressive lymphadenopathy. Deep scarring can cause cicatricial stenosis or narrowing of the urethra, vagina, and anus; genitoinguinal scarring may also interfere with lymphatic drainage and result in elephantiasis of the genitals and the lower extremities. Rarely, squamous cell carcinoma of the penis, vulva, or cervix arises after prolonged infection. Carcinoma must be distinguished from pseudoepitheliomatous epidermal hyperplasia, which occurs frequently in granuloma inguinale. Also rarely, *C. granulomatis* infection may become life-threatening as a result of bone, liver, and spleen involvement.

Like all genital ulcers, those due to granuloma inguinale can predispose the patient to human immunodeficiency virus (HIV) infection. Mucosal discontinuity, chronicity, and the presence of target cells in the granulomatous tissue may facilitate human immunodeficiency virus transmission. Coinfection with other sexually transmitted organisms may also occur.

LABORATORY FINDINGS

Diagnosis of granuloma inguinale requires identification of the infectious agent by direct cytologic or histologic examination. Skin specimens should contain a fragment of tissue from the ulcer border obtained by either punch biopsy or scalpel incisional biopsy. Superficial smears and scrapings usually are not adequate for proper interpretation but may be examined nevertheless. Punch biopsies are preferred, and the undersurface of the specimen can be used to make a smear. For direct examination, the tissue is placed between two slides, air dried, and stained with Wright's or Giemsa stain.

Microscopy reveals an ulcer bordered by hyperkeratosis and acanthosis. Pseudoepitheliomatous hyperplasia must be distinguished from the rare squamous cell carcinoma. A dense dermal infiltrate contains many plasma cells and histiocytes, small clusters of neutrophils, and a few lymphocytes. The rod-shaped, oval microorganisms can usually be seen as intracytoplasmic inclusions within the histiocytes found in the granulation tissue. These inclusions, called Donovan bodies, typically have a bipolar appearance, often characterized as "safety pin–like." Donovan bodies stain red with Giemsa stain and purple with Wright's stain and are surrounded by a lighter staining capsule. In some patients, the inclusions are better seen on semithin sections or by electron microscopy, which may be required for definitive diagnosis.

Other laboratory methods may be considered. Electron microscopy may reveal cytoplasmic inclusions at the periphery of the bacteria. Culture generally is neither practical nor useful because it is difficult to perform and requires special media prepared and inoculated under strict conditions. Serologic tests are not used routinely, but a promising indirect immunofluorescence technique has been evaluated in South Africa.

PITFALLS IN DIAGNOSIS

Granuloma inguinale must be distinguished from other genital ulcers, especially syphilis, chancroid, necrotic genital herpes simplex, and lymphogranuloma venereum. The ulcer of donovanosis is typically larger—it is also painless, irregular in shape, and granulomatous; bleeds on contact; and is not accompanied by lymphadenopathy. The differential diagnosis includes ulcerative tuberculosis, bacterial phagodenic ulcers, squamous cell carcinoma (including cervix carcinoma), leishmaniasis, amebiasis, filariasis, histoplasmosis, and other deep mycoses. The clinical impression of granuloma inguinale must be confirmed by microscopic identification of Donovan bodies, which are usually smaller than the histiocytic inclusions seen in leishmaniasis, rhinoscleroma, and histoplasmosis.

LYMPHOGRANULOMA VENEREUM

By Isabelle Thomas, M.D.,
Camila K. Janniger, M.D.,
and Robert A. Schwartz, M.D.
Newark, New Jersey

Lymphogranuloma venereum (LGV) is a sexually transmitted infection caused by *Chlamydia trachomatis*, serotype L1, L2, or L3. *C. trachomatis* is also responsible for several other venereal infections, as well as trachoma, neonatal conjunctivitis, and pneumonia. *Chlamydia* is the most common cause of venereal disease in the United States, but fewer than 1000 cases are caused by serotypes L1, L2, and L3—the agents responsible for LGV. This disease occurs worldwide but is endemic to the tropics and subtropics. Classically, LGV has been described in sailors, soldiers, or travelers to endemic areas and their sexual contacts, particularly in large urban areas. An outbreak in Florida in 1986 and 1987 revealed the major role of asymptomatic prostitutes in the transmission of LGV. The course of LGV may be divided into primary, secondary, and tertiary stages, reflecting the progression from inoculation to lymphatic spread to late manifestations. The primary lesion often goes undetected, particularly in women. The most common presentation in men is lymphadenitis. The diagnosis relies on clinical examination supported by serologic tests and culture results.

PRESENTING SIGNS AND SYMPTOMS

Stage I

The primary stage of lymphogranuloma often goes undetected but is more likely to be seen in men. Incubation ranges from a few days to a month, and the initial lesion typically appears after 7 days, most often in the genital area. The lesion is usually small and asymptomatic, is often hidden in women, and heals rapidly without scarring. It is located on the glans penis, prepuce, or frenulum in men and in the vagina or on the labia minora, cervix, or urethra in women, where it can easily be missed. Rarely, LGV presents as diffuse ulcerative glossitis resulting from orogenital contact. LGV presents as a solitary papule or vesicle, a small group of herpetiform vesicles, one or several small ulcers, or a nonspecific urethritis. In a study of 27 men, only 5 individuals recalled having a genital sore within weeks of the onset of inguinal lymphadenopathy or proctitis.

Stage II

The second stage is characterized by regional lymphadenopathy, which is often the presenting sign of LGV in men. Lymphatic spread of the organism involves the inguinal nodes in about two thirds of patients. Adenopathy is typically unilateral, or bilateral, involving both the inguinal and femoral chains in about 20 per cent of patients. A depression created by Poupart's ligament between the inguinal and femoral nodes is referred to as the "groove sign." At first, the nodes are enlarged, tender, and mobile. They may coalesce into a matted mass, or bubo, which becomes fixed to the overlying skin. The bubo may heal spontaneously or become fluctuant and rupture into multiple fistulas and sinus tracts that drain a chronic seropurulent discharge.

In women, lymphatics from the external genitals and the lower third of the vagina drain into the inguinal nodes. The rest of the vagina and the cervix drain into deep rectal and iliac nodes. The spread of LGV from primary lesions to somewhat deeper nodes can further delay diagnosis.

Second-stage systemic manifestations include fever, nausea, headache, meningismus, arthralgia, polyarthritis, hepatosplenomegaly, and pneumonitis. Cutaneous signs may include erythema multiforme, erythema nodosum, urticaria, or maculopapular eruptions.

Atypical presentations such as follicular conjunctivitis and maxillary lymphadenitis (due to autoinoculation) have also been described. Oropharyngeal disease and submaxillary or cervical lymphadenopathy may follow orogenital activity.

Stage III

The third stage is known as the anogenitorectal syndrome and is seen in about 25 per cent of patients with LGV. Women may present in the third stage because the disease remains latent for prolonged periods. In men, the third stage is usually described in homosexuals.

Complaints of rectal pain, tenesmus, and a chronic mucopurulent, sometimes bloody, discharge may be the first signs of acute proctocolitis. Rectosigmoidoscopy reveals a friable, hemorrhagic, and hypertrophic mucosa with necrotic ulcerations.

COMPLICATIONS

If left untreated, LGV proctocolitis may cause strictures and fibrosis of the bowel wall. Partial or complete obstruction, bowel perforation, and peritonitis may ensue. Chronic rectal lymphadenitis may rupture, creating rectovaginal or anal fistulas and perirectal abscesses. Chronic lymphatic obstruction may lead to chronic edema and elephantiasis of the penis and scrotum in men or the vulva in women. Elephantiasis is more frequent in women, in whom cobblestoning and gross distortions of the vulva are observed. Elephantiasis associated with painful ulcerations is known as esthiomene. Finally, squamous cell carcinoma may arise at the site of fistulas, strictures, or ulcers following many years of chronic or recurrent inflammation.

CLINICAL COURSE

LGV is a systemic disease characterized by lymphatic spread resulting in chronic obstruction and occasional systemic involvement. Thus, LGV differs from other chlamydial infections, which are typically restricted to the mucosa.

In general, the primary lesion appears at the site of inoculation within 1 to 4 weeks of contact with the organism. It is often ignored, and men commonly present with inguinal adenopathy (male-to-female ratio of 20:1) 2 to 8 weeks after contact. Two thirds of the nodes rupture, and the rest resolve spontaneously within 8 to 12 weeks. Women may present at this stage but are more often seen with proctocolitis or late complications.

Latent LGV may be reactivated in patients infected with the human immunodeficiency virus, leading to multiple ulcers in the groin and a poor response to therapy. Response to tetracyclines or sulfonamides is better in acute cases and requires at least 2 to 3 weeks of therapy.

DIAGNOSIS

The diagnosis relies on clinical findings, supported by serologic or histologic examination or isolation and immunotyping of the organism. The Frei skin test is no longer available or used.

Serologic tests include a complement fixation test and a microimmunofluorescence test. The latter is more sensitive but less available. Both lack specificity, as they cross-react with other *Chlamydia* serotypes. Patients with LGV, however, tend to have higher serologic titers. Complement fixation titers of 1:64 or greater are considered positive for LGV. Histologic examination of lymph nodes reveals nonspecific necrotic abscesses with a stellate or triangular shape. Biopsy of lymph nodes or buboes should be avoided, as this may cause them to rupture. The most specific test is culture and immunotyping of the organism from an ulcer, a lymph node aspirate, or pus from a ruptured bubo or an anorectal biopsy specimen. Unfortunately, this technique is expensive and is not always available, with a recovery rate of about 50 per cent.

PITFALLS IN DIAGNOSIS

Patients with LGV are at increased risk for other sexually transmitted diseases, including human immunodeficiency virus infection.

In patients presenting with genital ulcers, the possibility of coexistent venereal disease means that primary syphilis, herpes simplex, chancroid, and granuloma inguinale must be excluded. Lymphadenopathy can be seen in all of these diseases and in other infections such as cat-scratch disease, tularemia, plague, and tuberculosis. The anogenitorectal stage of LGV may resemble Crohn's disease, hidradenitis suppurativa, and anal or rectal carcinoma. Finally, the late elephantiasis of LGV can be confused with filariasis.

Bacterial Diseases

SEPSIS AND SEPTIC SHOCK

By Sujata H. Ambardar, M.D.,
and Gary L. Simon, M.D., Ph.D.
Washington, D.C.

Bacteremia, which is the presence of microorganisms in the bloodstream, may be symptomatic or asymptomatic (Table 1). The terms "bacteremia" and "septicemia" have often been used interchangeably to describe symptomatic bacteremia, although the latter term actually refers to the presence of either microbes or microbial products in the blood. Many clinicians have reserved the term "septicemia" to imply a more severe illness, which has led to confusion. In general, the term "septicemia" should be avoided. The term "sepsis" defines the degree of systemic response as characterized by fever, tachycardia, and tachypnea. "Sepsis syndrome" is the term used when there is evidence of altered organ perfusion in addition to systemic signs, and "septic shock" occurs when altered organ perfusion is accompanied by hypotension.

The systemic inflammatory response syndrome (SIRS) is a broader term that includes not only infectious causes of sepsis but also noninfectious entities such as burns or pancreatitis in which the clinical findings may mimic those of sepsis.

The incidence of microbial sepsis and septic shock has been increasing. The Centers for Disease Control and Prevention estimated the incidence at 425,000 cases of sepsis in 1987 and identified this condition as the 13th leading cause of death. Among certain high-risk patients, such as oncology and transplant patients, newborns, and intensive care unit patients, sepsis is a major cause of morbidity and mortality. In patients in whom septic shock develops, the mortality rate may approach 70 to 90 per cent.

Sepsis and septic shock can occur with infections involving a wide variety of microorganisms, including gram-positive and gram-negative bacteria, viruses, rickettsia, fungi, and protozoa. Of these, gram-negative bacteria are the most commonly identified etiologic agents, although several recent studies have indicated that the incidence of septic shock due to gram-positive bacteria is increasing.

CLINICAL MANIFESTATIONS OF SEPSIS

The clinical features of sepsis include signs and symptoms that represent the systemic host response to microbial challenge—fever, chills or rigors, tachycardia, and tachypnea.

Fever is an essential feature of sepsis, although there are many noninfectious conditions associated with fever. Temperature regulation in most individuals is remarkably consistent, so increases in temperature greater than or equal to 38°C (100.4°F) indicate abnormal host physiology. In some septic patients, especially the elderly or debili-

Table 1. Definitions of Infection

Disorder	Definition
Bacteremia	Bacteria present in blood, confirmed by culture
Sepsis	Clinical evidence of infection plus evidence of a systemic response as manifested by two or more of the following: Temperature >38°C (>100.4°F) or <36°C (<96.8°F); Heart rate >90 beats per minute; Respiratory rate >20 breaths per minute or $Pa{CO_2}$ <32 mm Hg
Sepsis syndrome	Sepsis plus evidence of altered organ perfusion with at least one of the following: hypoxemia, elevated serum lactate, oliguria, or altered mentation
Early septic shock	Sepsis syndrome with hypotension that lasts for less than 1 hr and responds to fluid resuscitation
Refractory (late) septic shock	Sepsis syndrome with hypotension that lasts for more than 1 hour and requires intervention with vasopressors to restore blood pressure
Systemic inflammatory response syndrome	Response to a wide variety of clinical insults, which can be infectious or noninfectious in origin

Adapted from Bone, R.C.: The pathogenesis of sepsis. Ann Intern Med 115:457–469, 1991 *and* American College of Chest Physicians/Society of Critical Care Medicine Consensus Conference Committee: Definitions for sepsis and organ failure and guidelines for use of innovative therapies in sepsis. Crit Care Med 20:864–874, 1992.

tated, fever may be absent. Hypothermia may occasionally be a manifestation of sepsis and is associated with a poor prognosis. Increases in temperature may be masked by antipyretics such as aspirin, acetaminophen, and nonsteroidal anti-inflammatory drugs. In general, the use of such agents should be avoided until a diagnosis is established and the effectiveness of therapy determined.

Neither the magnitude of a temperature increase nor the pattern of fever is particularly useful. The well-synchronized malarial fevers are seldom seen in nonendemic areas. Prolonged fevers are consistent with many conditions, including infectious entities such as bacterial endocarditis, intra-abdominal abscess, and occult tuberculosis. Herpesvirus infections, such as cytomegalovirus and Epstein-Barr virus, may also be associated with prolonged fever. In addition, there are a number of noninfectious causes of prolonged fever, including drugs, tumors, and collagen vascular diseases.

Chills are often associated with fever; sometimes patients describe the sensation of feeling cold rather than an elevation in temperature. Occasionally, a patient will describe a rigor or shaking chill, which should be distinguished from the sensation of feeling chilled. Rigors are relatively violent chills with uncontrolled shaking and teeth chattering that usually last about 30 minutes, after which there is a rapid rise in temperature. The presence of a rigor often indicates bacteremia, but it may also be seen in other infections such as influenza, candidemia, and malaria.

Tachypnea is frequently associated with sepsis and may be recognized even before an increase in temperature or chills. Monitoring of intensive care unit patients has indicated that the earliest clinical findings in sepsis are apprehension and hyperventilation with resultant respiratory alkalosis. Hyperventilation may also be secondary to clumping and entrapment of white cells in the lungs as a result of early cytokine activity. Tachypnea and hyperventilation also occur late in sepsis to compensate for metabolic acidosis.

Tachycardia is often associated with sepsis; it may be due to fever but may also reflect relative hypovolemia resulting from cytokine-induced vasodilatation. Occasionally, patients present with fever and a heart rate that is relatively slow for the degree of temperature increase. This pulse-temperature dissociation is seen in a number of conditions such as typhoid fever, brucellosis, mycoplasmal infection, Legionnaires' disease, and psittacosis.

There are a number of other clinical manifestations of sepsis that may be present, and they can often provide clues to the site of infection and the infecting organism. For example, cough, dyspnea, and chest pain suggest a respiratory focus, whereas back pain and urinary frequency point to pyelonephritis as the primary disease process. Identification of the specific site of infection helps direct the diagnostic evaluation as well as the selection of an antibiotic.

Cutaneous manifestations of sepsis may be seen with bacterial, viral, or fungal diseases and, in many patients, may help guide the diagnostic and therapeutic approach. Diffuse erythroderma may be seen with a number of viral infections, such as measles, rubella, and roseola. An erythematous, blanching eruption is also seen in some patients with enteroviral infections and with parvovirus B-19 infection. Approximately 30 per cent of patients with typhoid fever will develop rose spots, which are faint salmon-colored maculopapular lesions on the trunk. Erythematous eruptions may also be seen with infections caused by *Staphylococcus aureus, Streptococcus* species, *Corynebacterium haemolyticum* (a cause of pharyngitis in young adults), and mycoplasma. In patients with toxic shock syndrome, which may be caused by either *S. aureus* or *Streptococcus pyogenes,* intense cutaneous erythema is followed by desquamation, most notably at the tips of the extremities.

Ecthyma gangrenosum is typically associated with *Pseudomonas aeruginosa* bacteremia but also occurs with other bacterial species such as *Serratia marcescens* and *Aeromonas hydrophila*. Similar lesions are seen in some patients with fungal infections caused by *Aspergillus, Mucor,* and *Candida* species. The lesions are round or oval and have a raised halo or rim of erythema and induration that surrounds a necrotic central area. These "bull's-eye" type lesions have been seen in 2 to 3 per cent of patients with *Pseudomonas* bacteremia.

The presence of petechiae in the conjunctiva or on other mucus membranes, splinter hemorrhages, tender nodular swellings under the tips of the fingers or toes (Osler nodes), or macular lesions on the palms and soles (Janeway lesions) are, in the appropriate clinical setting, suggestive of bacterial endocarditis. Diffuse petechiae and hemorrhagic purpuric lesions are seen in Rocky Mountain spotted fever, meningococcemia, and overwhelming staphylococcal sepsis. Patients who acquire disseminated intravascular coagulation may have peripheral gangrene. Such gangrene can also occur as a result of high-dose vasopressor therapy.

Maculonodular skin lesions may be seen in patients with disseminated candidiasis. Gram staining and culture of material obtained by needle aspiration of these lesions may reveal the hyphal forms of this organism. Pustular lesions on a small erythematous base are characteristic of gonococcemia, but such lesions may be seen in staphylococcal infections as well.

Funduscopic examination may also be quite useful in selected patients. Roth spots are rarely seen in patients with endocarditis, but their presence may help establish the diagnosis in patients in whom such findings are noted. Both *Candida* and cytomegalovirus are associated with specific findings in the retina of patients with these infections. *Candida* endophthalmitis is characterized by fluffy white chorioretinal infiltrates, whereas cytomegalovirus retinitis presents as a discrete area of white or yellow retinal opacification associated with hemorrhage.

SEPSIS SYNDROME

The sepsis syndrome includes the clinical findings of sepsis combined with evidence of organ dysfunction. This can include laboratory evidence of organ dysfunction, such as hypoxemia, increased serum lactate levels, coagulopathy, or increased levels of serum urea nitrogen or creatinine. Clinical manifestations of the sepsis syndrome include dyspnea, oliguria (defined as hourly urine outputs of less than 20 mL), and alterations in mental status.

Dyspnea and hypoxemia may be due to respiratory insufficiency caused by the adult respiratory distress syndrome. This syndrome is characterized by diffuse pulmonary infiltrates, evidence of a right-to-left shunt, normal pulmonary wedge pressures, and high pulmonary arterial pressures.

Changes in mentation can be an important clue to the diagnosis of sepsis syndrome. The most frequently encountered alteration in mental status is lethargy or obtundation; however, some patients may become excited or agitated or display bizarre behavior. There are a number of potential etiologic considerations in the septic patient who has significant alterations in mental status. They include primary central nervous system infections such as meningitis, encephalitis, or brain abscesses; the toxic and metabolic effects of sepsis; and, in the patient with septic shock, hypoperfusion of the central nervous system resulting from systemic hypotension.

SEPTIC SHOCK

Septic shock is defined as the clinical manifestations of sepsis and the sepsis syndrome accompanied by hypotension. Early in the course of septic shock, patients may not be hypotensive, but with decreasing systemic vascular resistance as a result of progressive vasodilatation, cardiac demand exceeds cardiac output, and blood pressure falls.

An accepted definition of hypotension is a systolic blood pressure less than 90 mm Hg or a reduction of greater than 40 mm Hg from baseline in the absence of other causes. Early septic shock is characterized by hypotension that lasts less than 1 hour and is correctable with a fluid challenge, whereas late or refractory septic shock lasts longer than 1 hour, does not respond to fluid challenge, requires treatment with vasopressors, and usually has a worse outcome. Management of patients with septic shock requires hemodynamic monitoring of pulmonary capillary wedge and ventricular filling pressures.

In some patients, septic shock progresses from an initial phase of hypotension, tachycardia, and peripheral vasodilatation (warm shock) to a phase of deep pallor, intense vasoconstriction, and anuria (cold shock). Hemodynamically, the initial phase is characterized by increased cardiac output and diminished vascular resistance. In the latter phase, cardiac output is diminished and systemic vascular resistance is increased.

The impact of prolonged hypotension and organ hypoperfusion results in widespread derangements in host physiology. Impairment of renal function and oliguria may progress to anuria because of acute tubular necrosis. Hepatic failure with the development of "shock liver" may occur in patients who have severe and prolonged hypotension. In this condition, there is marked elevation of the serum aminotransferases as a result of widespread hepatocellular damage and necrosis. Less frequently, patients may have ischemic damage to the gastrointestinal tract as a consequence of redistribution of blood flow away from the splanchnic circulation. Mortality is substantially increased in patients with septic shock that is subsequently complicated by multiorgan system failure.

LABORATORY FINDINGS

Laboratory abnormalities in sepsis and septic shock reflect the ongoing systemic response to infection. The diagnosis is often based solely on clinical findings because culture results may not be available for several days. Proper techniques should be used in obtaining blood culture specimens to minimize contamination. Two or three sets of specimens should be obtained using separate venipuncture sites. It is rarely necessary to wait more than a few minutes between each venipuncture. Recovery of infecting organisms is dependent on the volume of blood cultured, so at least 10 mL and preferably 20 mL should be obtained with each venipuncture. The effectiveness of adding ion exchange resins to blood culture media to remove antimicrobial agents is still being evaluated. Lysis centrifugation is a new, more sensitive method that is being used for the detection of mycobacteria and fungi in blood cultures.

Leukocytosis with neutrophil predominance is a common finding in septic patients. In patients with bacterial infections, increases in the neutrophil population may occur as a result of demargination of mature neutrophils as well as the release of both mature and early granulocytic forms from marrow reserves. Leukopenia and neutropenia may be seen in viral infections and occasionally in bacterial infection with intracellular pathogens such as *Brucella*, *Salmonella*, and *Listeria*. Leukopenia can also be seen in patients with overwhelming bacteremia, especially in alcoholics and elderly patients who may have limited marrow reserves. It is generally associated with a poor prognosis.

Acid-base disturbances are characterized by a primary respiratory alkalosis early in the course of sepsis, followed by lactic acidosis. This metabolic acidosis may be partially compensated for by a secondary respiratory alkalosis, but as septic shock progresses, perfusion to tissue decreases and energy requirements are met increasingly by anaerobic metabolism, resulting in increased production of lactic acid.

Coagulation defects may present with prolongation of the prothrombin time (PT) and partial thromboplastin time (PTT), along with thrombocytopenia, hypofibrinogenemia, increases in fibrin degradation products, and prolongation of the thrombin time. This is characteristic of disseminated intravascular coagulation (DIC), which is most commonly associated with gram-negative organisms such as *Pseudomonas* or meningococcus, but it may also occur with gram-positive organisms, plasmodia, and viruses. Isolated mild thrombocytopenia may also occur in septic patients without evidence of disseminated intravascular coagulation.

Renal dysfunction may present initially as azotemia but may later progress to acute renal failure caused by acute tubular necrosis or cortical necrosis with oliguria or anuria and a rising serum creatinine level. Urinalysis may be helpful in following this progression; the unremarkable urine sediment of prerenal azotemia may later be replaced by an active sediment with hyaline casts and tubular epithelial cells.

Abnormalities in liver function may present as cholestatic jaundice in both gram-positive and gram-negative bacterial infections. Severe red cell lysis resulting from hemolytic processes, such as in malaria, may result in an increase in the serum bilirubin level. Hepatocellular damage may be reflected by precipitous increases in the serum aminotransferases, which may be indicative of shock liver from a hypotensive episode. Hypoglycemia may complicate sepsis and may occur more commonly in patients with underlying liver disease.

ANATOMIC SITES AND PATHOGENS

In most patients, bacteremia is not a primary process but is secondary to infection at some specific site. The most commonly identified site from which bacteremic illness occurs is the genitourinary tract. Other sources of bacteremic infection include the gastrointestinal and biliary tracts, the respiratory system, and the skin and soft tissues. However, nearly one third of patients have no identifiable site of infection. Some of these patients have bacterial endocarditis, although in many patients it is likely that the source is a subclinical focus of infection in the gastrointestinal tract or infection related to indwelling catheters.

Identifying the anatomic site of origin and the epidemiology of a particular bacterial infection may have important therapeutic implications. The frequency and types of organisms involved depend on whether the infection was acquired in the community or in the hospital as well as on the particular site of infection. Although a community-acquired bacteremic urinary tract infection (UTI) might result from a strain of *Escherichia coli* that is susceptible to most antibiotics, a patient with a nosocomial urinary tract infection might have a multidrug-resistant *P. aeruginosa* or *Serratia marcescans* infection.

Streptococcus pneumoniae is the most common cause of community-acquired pneumonia, but hospitalized patients who often require intubation and mechanical ventilation tend to acquire pneumonias with enteric gram-negative rods, including *Klebsiella*, *Enterobacter*, *Serratia*, and *Pseudomonas* species.

Intravascular catheters are frequently associated with bacteremia caused by coagulase-negative staphylococci or *S. aureus*. Methicillin-resistant strains of *Staphylococcus* are often present, especially in patients with hospital-acquired infections. Enterococci are also becoming more commonly recognized nosocomial pathogens and are associated with increasing antimicrobial resistance, which has complicated the therapeutic approach for patients with these infections.

DIAGNOSTIC APPROACH

The diagnostic approach to a patient with possible sepsis must begin with an assessment of any predisposing factors such as surgery, transplantation, chemotherapy, or trauma. A history of previous infections and antimicrobial treatment should be obtained, along with any microbiologic data that may be available. The physical examination should include a neurologic assessment and evaluation of skin and fundi for clues to the microbial cause. Clinical findings that suggest a localized site of infection should be evaluated promptly. It is important to obtain potentially infected secretions or body fluids for a microbiologic evaluation that includes appropriate stains and cultures. In the patient with diarrhea, stool samples should be obtained for a leukocyte determination, *Clostridium difficile* toxin assay, cultures, and microscopic examination for ova and parasites. A patient with an altered mental status should have a lumbar puncture performed provided that there is no evidence of increased intracranial pressure or a supratentorial mass.

Laboratory studies should include a urinalysis, a urine Gram stain, and culture. An arterial blood gas determination may be helpful in evaluating the degree of hypoxemia and acid-base status. Radiographic studies may include chest roentgenograms or an abdominal series, depending on the clinical scenario. Further diagnostic studies or procedures should be guided by the clinical situation and the patient's progress. Surgical or mechanical intervention may be necessary in some patients who do not respond rapidly to antibiotic therapy. Such procedures include removal of foreign bodies such as intravascular catheters or urinary catheters, drainage of abscesses, and relief of an obstructed viscus.

PROGNOSTIC FACTORS

The outcome in patients with sepsis is dependent on a number of factors. The ability to maintain the function of vital organs in patients with sepsis is related to both the adequacy of host defense mechanisms and the appropriate use of antimicrobial agents. Mortality is increased when there are underlying conditions that compromise host defense mechanisms, such as neutropenia, diabetes mellitus, cirrhosis, renal failure, hypogammaglobulinemia, and acquired immunodeficiency syndrome (AIDS). Complications such as shock or anuria worsen the prognosis. Similarly, absence of an identifiable focus, delay in instituting therapy, and inappropriate antibiotic selection are associated with an adverse outcome. Age is also a prognostic indicator; decreased survival is seen in both the very young and the elderly.

PITFALLS IN DIAGNOSIS

The major pitfalls in the diagnosis of sepsis often result from an atypical presentation. Signs and symptoms of sepsis may be subtle in elderly and immunocompromised patients, leading to a delay in diagnosis. In addition, many noninfectious processes can mimic sepsis or septic shock. In patients with multisystem disease, such as trauma patients, hemodynamic monitoring may help to distinguish between hypotension secondary to hypovolemia and septic shock. An increased cardiac output with a low systemic vascular resistance is suggestive of septic shock, whereas a high vascular resistance is more indicative of hypovolemia.

The interpretation of the results of blood cultures often presents a dilemma. Infections involving fastidious bacteria, fungi, or mycobacteria may be difficult to detect by blood culture, leading to a delay in diagnosis. In some patients, prior antibiotic administration can also lead to falsely negative blood culture results. False-positive blood cultures are usually caused by contamination from commensal skin flora such as diptheroids or coagulase-negative staphylococci, although these organisms have been implicated as pathogens in patients with endocarditis, infected intravascular catheters, and infected prosthetic devices. Distinguishing contaminants from true pathogens is often a difficult process. A second blood culture is useful in distinguishing true bacteremia from contamination.

Bacteremia and its progression to sepsis and septic shock poses a challenging problem for the clinician. In some patients, the diagnosis may not be readily apparent. At the same time, a delay in initiating appropriate therapy is associated with increased mortality. Nevertheless, it is not necessary to initiate antibiotic therapy in every patient with a fever without an evident source. However, for patients who are at high risk for the development of sepsis and septic shock (e.g., neutropenic patients or those in the intensive care unit), empirical antibiotic therapy will help reduce the morbidity and mortality associated with this condition.

TOXIC SHOCK SYNDROME

By Larry J. Strausbaugh, M.D.
Portland, Oregon

Toxic shock syndrome (TSS) is an acute illness characterized by fever, hypotension, and multisystem involvement. Two forms are recognized: staphylococcal TSS caused by *Staphylococcus aureus* and streptococcal TSS caused by *Streptococcus pyogenes*. Both forms arise when persons lacking immunity to staphylococcal or streptococcal toxins become colonized or infected by toxin-producing strains, and growth conditions promote toxin elaboration.

Both forms of TSS occur in all age groups, but individuals between the ages of 20 and 50 years are affected most frequently. The male-to-female ratio is 1:1 for streptococcal TSS and 2:1 for staphylococcal TSS. Most patients with streptococcal TSS do not have significant predisposing conditions, whereas most patients with staphylococcal TSS report recent tampon use during menstruation (about 50 per cent of patients), trauma, surgery, parturition, barrier contraceptive use, or recent infection. Other distinguishing features of the two syndromes are highlighted in Table 1.

CLINICAL FEATURES

Staphylococcal TSS begins abruptly with the rapid development of malaise, fever, myalgias, vomiting, and watery diarrhea. Other common symptoms include headache, sore throat, listlessness, arthralgias and, less commonly, confusion. Hypotension, heralded by dizziness on standing, and a generalized, erythematous, sunburnlike rash appear within hours. Patients generally seek medical attention within a day or two of the onset of symptoms. Symptoms referrable to localized staphylococcal infection—such as sinusitis, skin or soft tissue infection, and osteomyelitis—often stand out in nonmenstrual cases. In menstruating tampon users, symptoms referrable to localized infection are distinctly unusual.

Physical examination of patients with staphylococcal TSS discloses fever, tachycardia, hypotension or marked orthostatic blood pressure changes, diffuse erythroderma, hyperemia of conjunctivae and other mucosal surfaces, muscle tenderness, generalized abdominal tenderness, and marked prostration. In menstrual cases, vaginal hyperemia is frequently observed. In nonmenstrual cases associated with wound or skin infections, gross purulence of the wound is infrequent. Lastly, confusion, agitation, disorientation, and other signs of encephalopathy are common, especially on the second or third day of illness. The diagnosis of staphylococcal TSS is established on clinical grounds using the Centers for Disease Control and Prevention case definition (Table 2).

In streptococcal TSS, pain is the most common initial symptom, often beginning at the site of minor local trauma. It usually begins abruptly, involves an extremity, and rapidly becomes severe. Occasionally, abdominal pain or chest pain initiates the illness. Some patients describe a flulike syndrome, with fever, chills, myalgias, and diarrhea that antedates the pain. Once symptoms appear, disease progression is rapid, with development of fever, chills, vomiting, diarrhea, and agitation or confusion.

Physical examination of patients with streptococcal TSS usually reveals fever (although 10 per cent of patients may be hypothermic), tachycardia, hypotension, and confusion. Maculopapular or petechial rashes occur in less than 20 per cent of patients, and hyperemia of mucosal surfaces is variable. Approximately 80 per cent of patients exhibit evidence of localized soft tissue infection, with swelling and erythema initially and often progressing to vesicles and bullae with a violaceous or bluish discoloration. These soft tissue infections commonly evolve to necrotizing fasciitis or myositis. Recently, a case definition has been proposed to facilitate the diagnosis of streptococcal TSS (Table 3).

ATYPICAL PRESENTATIONS

Patients with staphylococcal TSS who are seen early in the course of disease may present with clinical findings that are suggestive of a diagnosis of acute gastroenteritis, food poisoning, acute abdomen, pneumonia, or pyelonephritis. Patients with prominent neurologic findings or cervical myalgias and tenderness may appear to have encephalitis or meningitis.

Patients with streptococcal TSS without soft tissue infection have presented with symptoms and signs of endophthalmitis, salpingitis, postpartum myometritis, pharyngitis, pneumonia, perihepatitis, peritonitis, myocarditis, and overwhelming sepsis.

COURSE AND COMPLICATIONS

Both forms of TSS tend to be rapidly progressive, with clinical deterioration often ensuing within a few hours of presentation. Toxin-induced damage to capillaries throughout the body leads to hypotension, shock, and organ dysfunction. Acute renal failure and acute respiratory distress syndrome are encountered frequently, especially in streptococcal TSS. Necrotizing fasciitis and myositis, the most common complications of streptococcal TSS, necessitate debridement, fasciotomy, amputation, or other surgical interventions with their attendant morbidity. Uncommon complications of staphylococcal TSS include arrhythmias, congestive heart failure, centrilobular hepatic necrosis, dis-

Table 1. Differences Between Staphylococcal and Streptococcal Toxic Shock Syndrome

Feature	Staphylococcal Toxic Shock Syndrome	Streptococcal Toxic Shock Syndrome
Localization of colonization or infection	Focus generally not obvious, especially in menstrual cases	Focus of soft tissue infection in 80 per cent of patients; usually affecting extremities
Dermatologic features	Diffuse erythroderma in virtually all patients; occasionally diffuse maculopapular or petechial rash; desquamation in 1 to 2 wk in most patients	Maculopapular or petechial rash in <20 per cent of patients; erythema, swelling, vesicles, and bullae at site of soft tissue focus; desquamation in 25 per cent
Bacteremia	Rare	60 per cent of patients
Outcome	Mortality rate <5 per cent; morbidity variable but usually not severe if diagnosis timely	Mortality rate 30 per cent; debridement, fasciotomy, or amputation in 65 per cent; ARDS in 55 per cent; irreversible renal failure in 10 per cent
Recurrence	In up to 30 per cent of patients	Not reported

ARDS = adult respiratory distress syndrome.

seminated intravascular coagulation, and tetany. Desquamation, especially of palms and soles, usually occurs 1 to 2 weeks after the onset of staphylococcal TSS in virtually all patients. Hair and nail loss have also been reported. Only 25 per cent of patients with streptococcal TSS undergo some degree of desquamation.

Table 2. Case Definition for Staphylococcal Toxic Shock Syndrome

Major criteria (all four must be met)
- Fever: temperature ≥38.9°C (102°F)
- Rash: diffuse macular erythroderma
- Hypotension: systolic blood pressure ≤90 mm Hg for adults or below the fifth percentile by age for children less than 16 yr, orthostatic drop in diastolic blood pressure ≥15 mm Hg from lying to sitting position, orthostatic syncope, or orthostatic dizziness
- Desquamation: 1 to 2 wk after onset of illness, particularly affecting palms and soles

Multisystem involvement (three or more must be met)
- Gastrointestinal: vomiting or diarrhea at onset of illness
- Muscular: severe myalgia or creatine kinase activity at least twice upper limit of normal
- Mucous membrane: vaginal, oropharyngeal, or conjuctival hyperemia
- Renal: urea nitrogen or creatinine concentration at least twice upper limit of normal or urinary sediment with pyuria (≥5 leukocytes/high-power field) in absence of urinary tract infection
- Hepatic: total bilirubin, AST, ALT levels at least twice upper limit of normal
- Hematologic: platelets ≤100,000/mm^3
- Central nervous system: disorientation or alterations in consciousness without focal neurologic signs when fever and hypotension are absent

Negative results on the following tests (if performed)
- Blood, throat, or CSF cultures (blood culture may be positive for *Staphylococcus aureus*)
- Rise in titer in antibody tests for Rocky Mountain spotted fever, leptospirosis, or rubeola

AST = aspartate aminotransferase; ALT = alanine aminotransferase; CSF = cerebrospinal fluid.

Adapted from Shands, K.N., Schmid, G.P., Dan, B.B., et al: Toxic-shock syndrome in menstruating women. Association with tampon use and *Staphylococcus aureus* and clinical features in 52 cases. N. Engl. J. Med. 303:1436–1442, 1980.

LABORATORY FINDINGS

Laboratory findings vary considerably in both forms of TSS, depending on the duration and severity of disease. Characteristic hematologic findings include an increased hematocrit, leukocytosis with a high percentage of imma-

Table 3. Proposed Case Definiton for the Streptococcal Toxic Shock Syndrome*

I. Isolation of group A streptococcus *(Streptococcus pyogenes)*
  A. From a normally sterile site (e.g., blood, cerebrospinal, pleural, or peritoneal fluid, tissue biopsy, surgical wound)
  B. From a nonsterile site (e.g., throat, sputum, vagina, superficial skin lesion)

II. Clinical signs of severity
  A. Hypotension: systolic blood pressure ≤90 mm Hg in adults or < fifth percentile for age in children
     and
  B. Two or more of the following signs
    1. Renal impairment: creatinine level ≥2 mg/dL for adults or ≥ twice the upper limit of normal for age. In patients with pre-existing renal disease, a ≥ twofold increase over the baseline concentration.
    2. Coagulopathy: platelets ≤100,000/mm^3 or disseminated intravascular coagulation defined by prolonged clotting time, low fibrinogen level, and the presence of fibrin degradation products
    3. Liver involvement: alanine aminotransferase (ALT), aspartate aminotransferase (AST), or total bilirubin concentration twice the upper limit of normal for age. In patients with pre-existing liver disease, a ≥ twofold increase over the baseline concentration.
    4. Adult respiratory distress syndrome defined by acute onset of diffuse pulmonary infiltrates and hypoxemia in the absence of cardiac failure, or evidence of diffuse capillary leak manifested by acute onset of generalized edema, or pleural or peritoneal effusions with hypoalbuminemia
    5. A generalized erythematous macular rash that may desquamate
    6. Soft tissue necrosis, including necrotizing fasciitis or myositis, or gangrene

*An illness fulfilling criteria IA and II (A and B) is defined as toxic shock syndrome (TSS). An illness fulfilling criteria IB and II (A and B) is defined as *probable* TSS if no other cause for the illness is identified.

Adapted from The Working Group on Severe Streptococcal Infections: Defining the group A streptococcal toxic shock syndrome. JAMA 269:390–391, 1993.

ture forms, and thrombocytopenia. Serum chemistry panels typically demonstrate some decrease in sodium, potassium, calcium, magnesium, albumin, phosphate, and bicarbonate concentrations and some increase in lactate, creatine kinase, bilirubin, hepatic enzymes, urea nitrogen, and creatinine concentrations. Urinalysis frequently discloses pyuria, hematuria, and proteinuria.

OTHER DIAGNOSTIC PROCEDURES

In severe cases of TSS, chest roentgenograms may reveal diffuse interstitial infiltrates, especially after vigorous volume replacement. In patients with streptococcal TSS, surgical biopsies of the involved extremity provide pathologic evidence of necrotizing fasciitis and myositis (if present).

In both forms of TSS, Gram-stained smears of wound exudates may identify gram-positive cocci in clumps or chains, depending on the site of infection and cause. Depending on the site of colonization or infection, bacterial cultures of vaginal secretions, respiratory secretions, or wound exudates generally yield *S. aureus* from patients with staphylococcal TSS, but blood cultures are rarely positive. Cultures of blood and localized soft tissue infection yield *Streptococcus pyogenes* from the majority of patients with streptococcal TSS. Culture results are supportive but not definitive because tests for toxin production and serum antitoxin antibodies are not commercially available.

DIFFERENTIAL DIAGNOSIS

The differential diagnosis for staphylococcal and streptococcal TSS varies across a wide spectrum. On one extreme, patients presenting with prominent systemic symptomatology, especially rashes, suggest a variety of diagnoses, such as septic shock, systemic lupus erythematosus, Kawasaki disease, leptospirosis, or Rocky Mountain spotted fever. On the other extreme, patients presenting with localized findings may raise the possibility of gastroenteritis, pyelonephritis, thrombophlebitis, or dermatologic disorders.

AVOIDANCE OF ERRORS AND PITFALLS IN DIAGNOSIS

Appreciation of the expanding spectrum of TSS is essential for diagnosis in the 1990s, especially the recognition that TSS occurs in men and children and not just in menstruating women. Knowing that TSS can ensue within hours after surgery or trauma is also important. TSS is a serious consideration in any severely ill patient with the three cardinal manifestations—fever, hypotension, and multisystem involvement—when staphylococcal or streptococcal colonization or infection is a possibility, whether rash is present or not. When these three features are present, a reluctance to accept more limited diagnoses—for example, acute gastroenteritis to explain diarrhea or pyelonephritis to explain pyuria—may be critical in the diagnostic process. Attention to other details will also keep diagnostic reasoning on track, especially the notation of systemic toxicity or pain that is disproportionate to local findings, rapid clinical deterioration, rapidly evolving soft tissue lesions, unexplained mental status changes, and unanticipated laboratory findings such as pronounced leukocytosis with many immature forms, increased serum creatinine levels, acidosis, or increased creatine kinase levels. Recognizing the presence of multisystem involvement in a hypotensive patient with an acute febrile illness is often the key to a timely diagnosis.

BACTERIAL DIARRHEAS

By Michael L. Bennish, M.D.
Boston, Massachusetts
and Carlos Seas, M.D.
Lima, Peru

Diarrhea is a common problem in clinical practice. Community surveys in the United States document an incidence of 1.5 episodes per person per year, with higher rates in young children, especially those in day care centers. The incidence in persons living in developing countries, persons traveling to developing countries, and persons living in custodial facilities, including nursing homes, is also high. Although diarrhea is an uncommon cause of death in healthy adults, it can be lethal in infants, the debilitated of any age (but especially the elderly), and patients with immune deficiencies. In developing countries, diarrhea and respiratory infections are the two leading causes of death among children.

DEFINITION

The most common definition of diarrhea used in surveys is three or more unformed stools in 24 hours. Diarrhea remains primarily a subjective determination, however, based on the patient's perception of changes in the pattern of defecation. Bowel habits differ markedly among individuals and among cultural groups. What is normal for an Andean highlander who eats a high-fiber diet and defecates at will is not normal for a city dweller who consumes highly refined foods and defecates only as time permits. Therefore, a single definition of diarrhea probably does not suffice. A functional definition of an increase in stool frequency or a decrease in stool consistency that is of concern to either the patient or the physician is probably the most pragmatic approach to defining diarrhea.

Although this article is entitled Bacterial Diarrheas, the clinical findings of diarrhea caused by bacteria, viruses, and protozoa overlap. Thus, this article describes an approach to diarrhea caused by any infection, since there is no way to know a priori that a patient's diarrhea is caused by a bacterium.

CLINICAL FEATURES AND NATURAL HISTORY

If, for diagnostic purposes, the definition of diarrhea is pragmatic, so also is its further subdivision into type. A categorization of diarrhea as watery or dysenteric is a useful starting point for the evaluation of a patient with diarrhea, with watery diarrhea defined as stool that is watery in character (with or without fecal matter) and dysentery defined as passage of unformed stool that contains blood and mucus. Such a categorization generally correlates with the site of infection (small bowel for watery diarrhea, colon for dysentery), pathogenesis (often toxin-mediated for watery diarrhea and cytolytic for dysentery), inflammatory response (absent in watery diarrhea and

Table 1. Bacterial Enteric Pathogens Categorized by the Type of Diarrhea They Cause

Watery Diarrhea	Dysentery or Bloody Diarrhea
Clostridium difficile	*Campylobacter jejuni*
Enteropathogenic *Escherichia coli*	*Clostridium difficile*
Enterotoxigenic *E. coli*	Enterohemorrhagic *E. coli*
Salmonella species	Enteroinvasive *E. coli*
Shigella sonnei	*Salmonella* species
Vibrio cholerae O1 or O139	*Shigella boydii, S. flexneri, S. dysenteriae*
	Yersinia enterocolitica

present in dysentery), and the need for antimicrobial therapy (typically not needed in watery diarrhea but often required for dysentery). Although different bacterial species prototypically cause either watery diarrhea or dysentery, infection with many of the common enteric bacterial pathogens (*Campylobacter jejuni*, *Salmonella*, *Shigella*) can result in either of the two types of diarrhea (Table 1). The precise factors influencing the clinical expression of infection are uncertain but include species or serotype (*Shigella sonnei* is more likely to cause watery diarrhea and *S. dysenteriae* type 1 almost always causes severe dysentery) and possibly pre-existing host immunity.

Most episodes of infectious diarrhea abate without specific intervention. Therefore, efforts to establish a cause are not required in most patients who present with diarrhea. Such efforts should focus on patients who have dysentery that may require treatment with antibiotics, patients who have severe watery diarrhea causing dehydration, patients who have prolonged watery diarrhea (lasting >3 days, or at least not substantially decreasing in intensity by that time), and debilitated or immunocompromised patients at risk of potentially lethal complications. A comprehensive diagnostic evaluation of all patients with diarrhea is not required and may even be discouraged by managed care organizations and insurance companies attempting to reduce patient care expenditures. The futility of evaluating all patients with diarrhea is reflected in the experience at the New England Medical Center, where from April 1994 to March 1995, 1370 stool samples from inpatients and outpatients were submitted to the hospital laboratory; a bacterial pathogen was found in only 67 (4.9 per cent) of these samples. These 67 isolates included the following organisms: 32 *Salmonella*, 18 *Campylobacter jejuni*, 12 *Shigella*, 2 enterohemorrhagic *Escherichia coli*, 2 *Yersinia enterocolitica*, and 1 *Aeromonas hydrophila*. Fifteen of the 18 *Campylobacter* isolates and 9 of the 12 *Shigella* isolates were obtained in the warmer months of April to September.

DIAGNOSTIC EVALUATION

A thoughtful and directed history is critical in the evaluation of diarrhea. The clinician should obtain the patient's description of stool character, stool frequency, the presence of nausea or vomiting (suggesting a small intestine locus of infection), and the presence of fever and tenesmus (suggesting an inflammatory diarrhea). Important epidemiologic clues include the simultaneous presence of diarrhea in friends, colleagues, or members of the patient's household. Outbreaks from a common source are more frequent with some bacterial pathogens, such as *Salmonella,* than with others, such as *Shigella*. Recent ingestion of an antimicrobial agent suggests diarrhea caused by *Clostridium difficile*. Ingestion of undercooked or uncooked shellfish increases the risk of infection with *Vibrio* and pathogenic viruses, whereas ingestion of undercooked hamburger increases the risk of infection with *E. coli* strains causing hemorrhagic colitis. Travel to a developing country suggests infection with toxigenic *E. coli,* which is a pathogen not commonly encountered in industrialized countries. The physical examination of the patient with diarrhea includes assessment of hydration and of the abdomen. Dryness of oral mucous membranes, increased skin elasticity (determined by pinching the skin), and changes in level of consciousness suggest severe dehydration, whereas abdominal tenderness suggests dysentery. Systemic findings other than those related to hydration are uncommon. Patients with typhoid fever and diarrhea (an inconsistent finding in this disease) may have splenomegaly and a characteristic rash (rose spots on the abdomen). Characteristic rashes do not occur with any of the other bacterial enteric pathogens.

Examination of the stool is the next step in the evaluation of the patient with diarrhea. Watery and dysenteric stools can usually be distinguished by visual examination of a specimen. The clinician should not rely entirely on history for categorization of stool type. Many persons are reluctant to examine the stool, and stool passed into the toilet is often difficult to characterize. Also, many persons are "hemophobic," and the quantity of blood in the stool can be greatly exaggerated. The only costs for the physician who visually examines a stool are the container required to collect the sample and the minute required to view the specimen.

LABORATORY DIAGNOSIS

Microscopic examination and culture of stools are useful primary laboratory tests for identification of bacterial causes of diarrhea (Table 2). Microscopy may reveal leukocytes and erythrocytes in stool, thereby confirming (or rejecting) the initial categorization of the diarrhea as watery or dysenteric. Parasites and protozoa can also be detected. Infections with more than one type of organism may rarely occur.

Most bacteria that can cause diarrhea are identified from a culture of stool. These pathogens include *Aeromonas hydrophila*, *Campylobacter jejuni*, *Plesiomonas shigelloides*, *Salmonella* species, *Shigella* species, *Vibrio* species, and *Yersinia enterocolitica.* Not all these pathogens will be routinely identified when a stool or rectal swab sample is submitted for culture. Most clinical microbiology laboratories will routinely identify *Salmonella* and *Shigella*. Identification of the other pathogens, however, requires the use of special selective culture media or special conditions for incubation. Thus, many microbiologic laboratories will attempt to identify these pathogens only if a specific request is made. Infection with *Vibrio* species is usually associated with ingestion of raw or undercooked seafood and rarely with travel to areas where *V. cholerae* is epidemic or endemic. Travelers from industrialized countries are at extremely low risk of infection with the serotypes of *V. cholerae* (O1 and O139) that cause clinical cholera. Although *Vibrio* causing enteric infection may grow on media routinely used for processing stool samples, optimal identification of *Vibrio* requires the use of a selective differential medium. A rapid presumptive diagnosis of *V. cholerae* infection can be made by identifying characteristic motile vibrios on dark-field or phase-contrast microscopy

Table 2. Diagnosis of Bacterial Pathogens Commonly Associated with Diarrheal Illness

Pathogen	Epidemiologic Features	Clinical Features	Diagnosis	Antimicrobial Therapy
Campylobacter jejuni	Currently the most common cause of bacterial diarrhea in most industrialized countries; commercial poultry products major source of infection; person-to-person transmission can also occur	Fever, malaise, abdominal cramps, watery or dysenteric stools; extraintestinal complications rarely include bacteremia, cholecystitis, postinfectious arthritis, and Guillain-Barré syndrome; prolonged infection can occur in patients with immunoglobulin deficiencies	Isolation of organism from culture of stool; isolation methods include incubation on selective media at 42°C under microaerobic conditions	Treatment with erythromycin early in the course of illness has a modest effect on clinical manifestations of this usually self-limited infection
Clostridium difficile colitis	Commonly associated with antibiotic use or seen in ill persons who have not received antibiotics; can occur with use of any antibiotic	Range from watery diarrhea to severe pseudomembranous colitis with high fever, leukocytosis, and mucoid, bloody stool	Detection of *C. difficile* toxin either A or B in stool by bioassay or antigen detection	Treatment with oral vancomycin or metronidazole
Escherichia coli				
Enterohemorrhagic *E. coli* (EHEC)	Increasing incidence in the United States; associated with ingestion of undercooked hamburgers and other beef products	Bloody diarrhea, often without fever or mucus in the stool; hemolytic-uremic syndrome is the major complication; disease associated with strains that produce Shiga toxin	Majority of EHEC infections in the United States caused by a single serotype, O157:H7, that does not ferment sorbitol; the latter feature is used by clinical laboratories to screen *E. coli* isolates from patients with suspected infection; methods now available to detect toxin in stool or culture supernatants	Role of antimicrobial therapy uncertain
Enteroinvasive *E. coli* (EIEC)	Rare in all settings	Dysentery similar to that caused by *Shigella* infection	Detection of invasive capability by gene probe or Sereny (rabbit keratoconjunctivitis) test; methods not routinely available in clinical laboratories	Role of antimicrobial therapy uncertain
Enteropathogenic *E. coli* (EPEC)	Infants, including those in nurseries; identification now relatively uncommon	Watery diarrhea	Caused by multiple different serotypes; no method of routinely identifying EPEC strains in clinical laboratories	Role of antimicrobial therapy uncertain
Enterotoxigenic *E. coli* (ETEC)	Common in developing countries, especially in young children; most common cause of travelers' diarrhea	Watery diarrhea that is mediated by toxin similar to cholera toxin; organism is noninvasive and, other than dehydration, extraintestinal manifestations do not occur	Detection of toxin by gene probe, antigenically, or by bioassay; these methods are not routinely available	Antibiotics can shorten duration of illness, although they are not routinely used in endemic settings; choice of antibiotic for travelers' diarrhea depends on local resistance pattern of *E. coli*

Salmonella species	Common in both developing and developed countries; large outbreaks in the United States associated with contaminated food, including milk products, meat, and eggs	Watery diarrhea or mild dysentery; bacteremia relatively common, especially in children and immunocompromised persons; septic complications most common in persons with hemolytic anemia (sickle cell disease)	Isolation from stool using methods routinely available in clinical laboratories	Treatment reserved for infants and patients at risk for septic complications; routine therapy does not affect clinical course and prolongs carriage
Salmonella typhi	Common in developing countries	Prolonged fever with or without diarrhea	Isolation from stools or blood using standard methods; culture of bone marrow aspirates useful in suspect cases in which preceding cultures are negative	Antimicrobial therapy indicated and determined by susceptibility of isolate
Shigella species	Common anywhere hygiene is poor—developing countries, custodial institutions, day care centers, Native American reservations	Clinical features vary with the four different species of *Shigella;* watery diarrhea is common with *S. sonnei,* the most common serotype in the United States, and severe dysentery is common with *S. dysenteriae,* which is rarely identified in the United States; systemic complications include seizures with *S. sonnei* infections in young children and hemolytic-uremic syndrome with *S. dysenteriae* type 1 infection	Isolation of *Shigella* from stool using standard methods available in clinical laboratories	Antimicrobial therapy determined by susceptibility of isolate
Vibrio cholerae O1 and O139	Endemic and epidemic throughout much of the world where potable water is not routinely available; travelers rarely affected	Profuse watery diarrhea mediated by a toxin	Rapid identification of organism from stool by darkfield microscopy or antigen detection or culture of the organism from stool; in epidemic situations, diagnosis is clinical	Treatment with doxycycline, furazolidone, or a quinolone, depending on susceptibility pattern
Yersinia enterocolitica	Uncommon everywhere, but most commonly identified in children in northern climates; both food-borne and person-to-person transmission occurs	Febrile enterocolitis, mesenteric adenitis (mimicking appendicitis), reactive polyarthritis, septicemia in compromised host	Isolation of organism from stool, mesenteric lymph node obtained at surgery, or blood in septicemic patients; isolation rate from stool enhanced by use of selective media and incubation at reduced temperature	Role of antimicrobial therapy uncertain

and by neutralizing them with specific antisera to the O1 or O139 serogroup. Such methods are typically available only in areas where cholera is endemic, but they can be rapidly established during epidemics if basic facilities are available. Like *Vibrio*, *Aeromonas* species and *P. shigelloides* infections are associated with tropical or semitropical climates and ingestion of shellfish. As with *Vibrio*, isolation of these organisms is enhanced by the use of selective media. By contrast, *Y. enterocolitica* infections are more common in Canada and in countries such as Belgium, where undercooked pork is consumed. Isolation of *Y. enterocolitica* is enhanced by incubation of culture plates at temperatures below the 37°C routinely used for processing stool specimens. *Campylobacter jejuni* is now epizootic and most commonly associated with processed poultry. In many laboratories, it is the most commonly identified bacterial enteric pathogen. Infection with *Campylobacter jejuni* is often associated with mild dysenteric symptoms.

Several well-recognized bacterial pathogens cannot be identified with conventional culture techniques alone. One such pathogen is *C. difficile*, the cause of antibiotic-associated pseudomembranous colitis as well as milder forms of antibiotic-associated diarrhea. *C. difficile* causes diarrhea by producing a cytolytic toxin. Because *C. difficile* can colonize the gut without causing disease, diagnosis of clinically significant infection requires detection of toxin in the stool rather than isolation of the organism. Therefore, stool specimens should be submitted to the laboratory for detection of toxin, using a cytotoxicity or latex agglutination assay.

There are at least four well-defined groups of diarrheogenic *E. coli*. They include *E. coli* that elaborates a choleralike toxin causing watery diarrhea (known as *e*ntero*t*oxigenic *E.* *c*oli, or ETEC), *E. coli* that adheres to small intestinal epithelium and produces a watery diarrhea (*e*ntero*p*athogenic *E.* *c*oli, or EPEC), *E. coli* that causes dysentery by invading and destroying colonic epithelial cells (*e*ntero*i*nvasive *E.* *c*oli, or EIEC), and *E. coli* that secretes a *Shigella*-like toxin that causes hemorrhagic colitis and hemolytic-uremic syndrome (*e*ntero*h*emorrhagic *E.* *c*oli, or EHEC). Routine culture does not distinguish these four types of *E. coli* from other nonpathogenic *E. coli*. The first three of the pathogenic types of *E. coli* (ETEC, EPEC, and EIEC) are uncommon in the United States; identification of these strains is primarily performed in research laboratories. The fourth type (EHEC) is increasingly common in the United States, and well-publicized outbreaks associated with ingestion of hamburgers from fast-food chain restaurants, as well as from other foodstuffs, have been reported. On request, many laboratories screen for EHEC with a sorbitol-containing medium, because most EHEC strains can be distinguished from other *E. coli* by their inability to ferment sorbitol. Confirmation of EHEC requires serotyping or detection of *Shiga* toxin production; most EHEC strains in the United States and Europe belong to the O157:H7 serotype. Screening for EHEC should be undertaken in any patient with painless bloody diarrhea (patients with EHEC usually do not have the tenesmus that accompanies the bloody diarrhea of *Shigella* infection) or who develops hemolytic-uremic syndrome in association with diarrhea.

Samples for microscopy and culture are best processed and examined while they are fresh. A delay in plating samples allows the less hardy organisms, such as *Shigella*, to be lysed or to be overgrown by nonpathogens. Delays also decrease the likelihood of a correct identification of protozoa and helminths. Ostensibly, the rapid processing of stool samples should be easier to accomplish in the hospital than in the clinic or private office, but this may not happen without specific efforts to assure rapid processing of the specimen. If a patient is not able to provide a stool sample, whether in the office or in the hospital, cultures can be obtained from a rectal swab sample. The yield of bacterial pathogens from rectal swab samples is equivalent to that obtained from samples of stool, but microscopic features will not be identified. Most bacterial pathogens are identified from the initial stool sample, whereas the additional yield from repetitive cultures of stool or rectal swab samples is relatively low.

Blood cultures may aid the diagnosis of *Salmonella* infections, in which an appreciable number of patients (especially children) may be bacteremic. By contrast, bacteremia is exceedingly rare with other types of bacterial diarrhea. Endoscopy is generally contraindicated in acute infectious diarrhea. Cultures of small intestine or colonic fluid obtained at endoscopy add little to the information obtained by the culturing and microscopic examination of stool. Endoscopy is most useful in prolonged diarrhea when a possible noninfectious cause of diarrhea (such as inflammatory bowel disease) is being sought.

Imaging procedures generally do not help establish the diagnosis. Abdominal films typically show nonspecific findings, including air-fluid levels in the small bowel. In severe colitis, thumbprinting and edema of the bowel wall may be detected.

THERAPEUTIC TRIALS

Because identification of a bacterial pathogen by culture requires a minimum of 36 to 48 hours, empirical antimicrobial treatment of moderately to severely ill patients is sometimes indicated. Patients with dysentery who are at risk of shigellosis because of travel or residence in an area endemic for *Shigella* infection or because an outbreak is occurring are often treated with an antimicrobial agent effective against *Shigella*. Similarly, patients with choleralike illness in a cholera endemic area may receive antimicrobial therapy. Response to such empirical treatment suggests, but does not prove, a specific diagnosis, as most infectious diarrhea is self-limiting. Another bacterial condition for which a therapeutic trial of empirical antimicrobial therapy is occasionally indicated is the small bowel overgrowth syndrome, which is caused when increased numbers of normal colonic flora can be found in the small bowel. This condition occurs occasionally in persons who are residents in tropical countries and in persons with altered gut motility. Methods to diagnose this condition are limited by the difficulty of reliably sampling small bowel contents for culture.

In general, because many (if not the majority) of the acute diarrheal episodes in the United States are caused by nonbacterial pathogens, or by bacterial pathogens such as *Campylobacter* or *Salmonella* for which antimicrobial therapy does not affect the course of illness, the use of therapeutic trials of empirical therapy is discouraged.

CHOLERA

By Anthony E. Fiore, M.D.,
and Myron M. Levine, M.D.
Baltimore, Maryland

Cholera is caused by *Vibrio cholerae* strains that produce cholera toxin. In its most severe forms, the disease causes copious diarrheal purging, severe dehydration, and death within 24 hours of onset. Not surprisingly, cholera inspires fear unmatched among the diarrheal pathogens. The epidemiologic hallmark of cholera is the occurrence of explosive outbreaks of disease, often with multiple, seemingly distinct foci. True pandemic spread through susceptible populations is possible—an event that has been documented at least seven times in the last two centuries. Until the advent of rehydration therapy, case fatality rates during epidemics often exceeded 50 per cent. Synonymous terms in the literature include Asiatic cholera, which refers to the geographic origin of many outbreaks, and cholera gravis, the most severe form of the disease. For many years, epidemic cholera was thought to be caused only by strains from the O1 serogroup. In 1992, however, a large scale epidemic of cholera in southern Asia was linked to a newly recognized serogroup designated O139. Molecular characterization of the epidemic strains suggests that they are *Vibrio cholerae* O1 biotype El Tor that have acquired genetic material from a non-O1 strain, including the genes responsible for capsule formation.

EPIDEMIOLOGY

V. cholerae is acquired by ingestion of contaminated water or food. In endemic areas, contaminated water is the most important vehicle of spread; epidemics may erupt across a large area, overwhelming the local health care resources. A seasonal pattern is seen in endemic areas, with rates of illness increasing in late summer and fall and usually coinciding with the highest mean temperature, peaking several months later, and then diminishing in colder, drier weather. Introduction of the organism into developed countries by imported foods, international travelers, or even ship ballast discharged into coastal waters, is well documented and is responsible for sporadic cases in the United States and Europe. Over the last 22 years, a strain of *V. cholerae* unique to the Gulf of Mexico has caused more than 50 cases of cholera in the United States, most associated with consumption of raw or undercooked shellfish.

ETIOLOGY AND MICROBIOLOGY

V. cholerae is a motile, gram-negative, facultative anaerobe. The organism is 1.4 to 2.6 μm in length and may be curved or straight. The pH range for optimal growth is 6 to 10, and it is oxidase-positive. Microbiologic diagnosis can be achieved by culturing a stool or rectal swab specimen. The numbers of excreted organisms are greatest early in the course of diarrhea and diminish soon after, especially if antibiotics are given. Transport media, preferably Cary-Blair, should be used if a delay of more than 2 hours is anticipated prior to plating for culture, and the specimen must be kept at room temperature during transport. *V. cholerae* grows poorly on most standard selective media, and thiosulfate citrate bile salts sucrose (TCBS, commercially available) agar should be used if *Vibrio* infection is suspected. Most laboratories in endemic areas enrich the culture in alkaline peptone water for 6 hours prior to plating.

Two biotypes of the O1 group are recognized, classic and El Tor. Although either biotype may cause the entire range of clinical manifestations, the ratio of asymptomatic infections to clinical infections is considerably higher for the El Tor biotype. The El Tor strain is distinguished by its resistance to polymyxin B, its ability to agglutinate chicken erythrocytes, and a susceptibility to certain vibriophages. For many years, most disease outside of Bangladesh was caused by the El Tor strain (the seventh pandemic). In 1992, a new toxigenic strain appeared in India and quickly spread through much of Asia. This is the O139 or Bengal strain, and imported cases of cholera due to this strain have been recognized in travelers returning to the United States and the United Kingdom.

IMMUNOLOGY

Volunteer studies and epidemiologic observations indicate that long-lasting immunity can be conferred by infection with O1 serotypes. However, field studies in Bangladesh indicate that although infection with the classic biotype confers complete protection against subsequent episodes of cholera caused by either the classic or El Tor biotype, infection with the El Tor biotype provides protection against subsequent El Tor infection in a minority of patients and no protection against subsequent classic biotype infection. Volunteer studies demonstrate that infection with either biotype confers 90 per cent (El Tor) to 100 per cent (classic) protection against subsequent infection with the same biotype. In the epidemic caused by the O139 (Bengal) strain, many individuals with a history of infection with O1 strains acquired clinical cholera, suggesting that cross-protective immunity does not extend to other serogroups. Immunity to O1 strains correlates best with the production of serum vibriocidal antibodies.

CVD 103-HgR, an attenuated, live oral vaccine derived from a classic O1 strain, confers complete protection against severe and moderate diarrhea on challenge with O1 strains of either biotype or serogroup in volunteer studies. An oral vaccine consisting of killed whole cell *V. cholerae* combined with purified cholera enterotoxin B subunit has demonstrated 50 per cent overall protection at 3 years of follow-up in a field trial. A parenteral killed whole cell vaccine currently available in the United States has limited efficacy, is frequently reactogenic, and is not recommended.

PRESENTATION

As with many diarrheal pathogens, *V. cholerae* produces a range of clinical manifestations, from mild diarrhea to massive, life-threatening purging. Volunteer studies indicate that as few as 10^3 organisms can cause diarrhea and that larger numbers of organisms correlate with the severity of purging. Decreased gastric acidity lowers the required inoculum. The inoculum size required in naturally occurring infection is unknown but may be on the order of 10^3 organisms based on the numbers present in contaminated household water samples. The incubation period is typically 1 to 3 days but may be as long as 7 days. This range is influenced by inoculum size. Many of the persons infected are asymptomatic or experience undiagnosed mild diarrheal illness; these patients may serve as a reservoir for the spread of disease. Long-term carriage of the organism in stool is distinctly unusual.

Certain hosts are at particularly high risk for severe disease. Pregnant women with severe dehydration have a higher fatality rate, and when infection occurs in the third trimester, fetal loss is common. Hypochlorhydria, whether due to surgical or medical intervention, or perhaps even to concurrent infection with *Helicobacter pylori,* increases the risk of severe disease, presumably by allowing more vibrios to reach their site of colonization in the small intestine. Individuals with blood type O have a more severe form of disease, perhaps because of increased accessibility of the cholera enterotoxin receptor in the small intestine. Marijuana use, common in many parts of the world, may also predispose to more severe infection.

Only 2 to 5 per cent of persons infected present with severe disease, characterized by an acute onset of voluminous diarrhea. Some patients may have a prodrome of malaise, nausea, vomiting, and abdominal discomfort or simple diarrhea. Stools initially consist of fecal material but rapidly clear and increase in volume to resemble the opalescent liquid created by the washing or soaking of rice in water. Flecks of mucus and a mild, slightly fishy odor are often reported. The patient may experience only mild abdominal discomfort, and emesis is common early in the disease, sometimes hampering efforts at oral rehydration. As dehydration progresses, the signs of intravascular volume loss appear, with a rapid, weak pulse; falling blood pressure and urine output; diminished skin turgor with characteristic wrinkling of the hands and feet; and dry mucous membranes. Mentation may be surprisingly clear but apathetic, or a marked restlessness or irritability may be present. Elecrolyte and glucose losses may lead to muscle cramping, tetany, or seizures. The respiratory rate is increased, and Kussmaul's respirations may be seen, presumably as a compensatory mechanism provoked by bicarbonate loss. Low-grade fever may be seen in up to 20 per cent of patients. Stool losses may reach extraordinary levels, up to 1.25 L per hour and usually peak at 12 to 14 hours. Very rarely, circulatory collapse may precede significant passage of stool. This has been termed "cholera sicca" and is thought to result from massive pooling of secretions in the gastrointestinal tract.

Laboratory studies reveal signs of hemoconcentration and diminished renal function, with an increased hematocrit, plasma protein levels, urine specific gravity, and serum urea nitrogen and serum creatinine levels. Serum bicarbonate levels and pH may be decreased from stool bicarbonate losses and lactic acidosis. Symptomatic hypoglycemia is common, especially in children. The leukocyte count is often increased, with an average of 21,000 cells/mm^3 in one series. The stool is isotonic, and no leukocytes are seen with methylene blue staining. Bacteremia with toxigenic *V. cholerae* is extremely rare.

DIAGNOSIS

Confirmation of *V. cholerae* O1 or O139 infection is achieved by isolation of the organism in stool culture, followed by agglutination with polyvalent antisera against O1 or O139 strains. Although other serogroups are capable of producing cholera enterotoxin and/or diarrheal disease, only these two serogroups are known to produce epidemic disease. DNA probes for detecting cholera enterotoxin genes may be used to confirm the isolation of a toxigenic strain.

Dark-field microscopy provides rapid, presumptive diagnosis in the field with visualization of motile vibrios and immobilization with specific antisera. More sensitive methods for rapid diagnosis have recently become available. The polymerase chain reaction technique detects the presence of toxigenic *V. cholerae* in both stool and food samples. A coagglutination test using monoclonal antibodies against the cholera O1 antigen (CholeraScreen [New Horizons Diagnostics Corp.]) rapidly detects organisms in stool specimens and is almost as sensitive as a stool culture. A recently developed colorimetric immunoassay directed against the O1 antigen (Cholera SMART [New Horizons Diagnostics Corp.]) may make rapid diagnosis even easier. Immunoassays to detect the O139 antigen are being developed.

Diagnosis may also be made serologically. Serum vibriocidal antibodies appear 3 to 5 days after the onset of illness on O1 serogroup infection and peak after 10 days. A fourfold rise in titer, or a single titer greater than 1:1280, is diagnostic of new *V. cholerae* O1 infection. Measurement of serum antibodies to the cholera enterotoxin may also be used for diagnosis, although the presence of cross-reacting antibodies to the heat-labile toxin in persons previously infected with heat-labile toxin–producing *Escherichia coli* makes this test less specific.

DIFFERENTIAL DIAGNOSIS

No other diarrheal pathogen causes such widespread, rapid, life-threatening diarrhea in a population. Sporadic cases, such as those associated with imported foods or uncooked shellfish, may be more difficult to recognize rapidly. Point-source outbreaks in the United States have recently been associated with airline food prepared in an endemic country and with imported frozen coconut milk. Early diagnosis, even in severe cholera, substantially reduces mortality when appropriate oral and intravenous hydration are administered prior to circulatory collapse. Many infections will present as nonspecific diarrheal illness that is clinically similar to that seen with numerous other pathogens. This underscores the point that early management of any severe diarrheal illness should focus on replacement of fluid losses. If a patient with diarrhea has traveled to an endemic region or has a food risk factor for infection with *V. cholerae,* special microbiologic or serologic testing is warranted, as outlined earlier. The public health implications of *V. cholerae* infection are substantial, and it is an internationally reportable disease.

SALMONELLAE

By Anne E. Hull, M.D.
New Orleans, Louisiana

Salmonellae are among the most prevalent human pathogens in nature. Found throughout the world, these adaptable microbes colonize the gastrointestinal tract of humans, domestic and wild animals, reptiles, and birds. Some serotypes, such as *Salmonella typhi* and *S. paratyphi,* are exclusively human pathogens and cause the prolonged bacteremic illnesses of typhoid and paratyphoid fevers. They are endemic only in developing countries, where poor sanitation and impure drinking water allow their wide dissemination. Nontyphoidal salmonellae, such as *S. typhimurium* and *S. enteritidis,* infect a broad range of hosts and can infect humans through contaminated food and water as well as person-to-person contact. This group of salmonella is increasingly important in developed countries because of the mass production and distribution of poultry and eggs, the primary vehicles of salmonellae transmission.

EPIDEMIOLOGY

Salmonellae are transmitted to humans by ingestion of food or water contaminated by a strain capable of causing disease. The major transmitters of *S. typhi* are food handlers with acute disease or, more commonly, asymptomatic carriers. In the case of nontyphoidal salmonellae, nearly 50 per cent of commercially available chickens harbor the organism. It is estimated that 0.01 per cent of eggs are infected with *S. enteritidis*. Contaminated milk and hamburger also have been implicated in outbreaks. Infections caused by unusual strains such as *S. arizonae* have been associated with pet reptiles. Ninety per cent of these creatures are colonized with salmonellae.

INCREASED HOST SUSCEPTIBILITY

A number of clinical conditions predispose patients to disease when they are exposed to salmonellae in the environment. Since gastric acidity is the first line of defense against these organisms, patients with decreased stomach acid are at increased risk of infection. Patients with achlorhydria and those taking agents that reduce gastric pH require a challenge with fewer organisms to acquire disease. The presence of normal intestinal flora may be protective. Administration of antibiotics disrupts this flora and predisposes the person to *Salmonella* infection.

Various immune disorders may increase the risk of serious disease after *Salmonella* infection. Transplant recipients and patients with lymphoproliferative disease are more likely to experience severe or disseminated disease. Patients with acquired immunodeficiency syndrome more commonly experience recurrent *Salmonella* bacteremia.

Macrophage function is important in the host defense against salmonellae. Patients with histoplasmosis or schistosomiasis have defective macrophage function and are at increased risk for disseminated disease. Macrophage overload syndromes, as seen in chronic hemolysis resulting from sickle cell disease or malaria, also place patients at increased risk for metastatic infection. In fact, salmonellae are the most common organisms isolated from patients with sickle cell disease and osteomyelitis. Neonates and elderly patients are prone to systemic manifestations of nontyphoidal salmonellosis, such as bacteremia, osteomyelitis, and meningitis.

CLINICAL SYNDROMES

Infection with salmonellae produces four major clinical syndromes: gastroenteritis, enteric fever, bacteremia (with or without extraintestinal foci), and the chronic carrier state. Despite considerable overlap among these categories, they remain useful in the differential diagnosis. All strains of *Salmonella* have been reported to cause each of the four syndromes, but specific strains have a strong association with particular clinical presentations. For instance, *S. typhi and S. paratyphi* usually present as enteric fever, whereas *S. enteritidis* typically produces gastroenteritis. *S. choleraesuis* often causes metastatic infection, whereas *S. typhimurium* is the strain most frequently linked to the entire spectrum of clinical syndromes.

Gastroenteritis

Gastroenteritis is the most common manifestation of *Salmonella* infection, accounting for more than 10 per cent of cases of food poisoning in the United States. The symptoms of gastroenteritis caused by *Salmonella* do not distinguish it from other causes of acute diarrhea. Nausea and vomiting typically occur within 48 hours of ingesting contaminated food or water. Diarrhea and periumbilical abdominal pain rapidly follow. The diarrhea varies from a few loose stools to an explosive, choleralike, watery product to dysentery with bloody stools and tenesmus. The choleralike syndrome occurs more often in patients with achlorhydria, whereas persons with inflammatory bowel disease experience dysentery that is easily confused with exacerbations of the underlying disease. The severity of abdominal pain also varies and can mimic acute appendicitis, cholecystitis, or perforated bowel. *Salmonella*, as well as *Yersinia enterocolitica* and *Campylobacter*, may cause the pseudoappendicitis syndrome.

Fever is present in more than 90 per cent of patients and reaches 39°C (102.2°F) in almost half of those with gastroenteritis resulting from *Salmonella* infection. Direct microscopic examination of the stool usually reveals neutrophils, underscoring the invasive nature of the pathogen. Although grossly bloody stools are rare in gastroenteritis caused by salmonellae, the presence of occult blood in the stool is relatively common. Leukocyte counts may be increased but are most often within the reference range.

Fever characteristically resolves within 2 to 3 days, and diarrhea resolves without specific therapy. Transient bacteremia occurs in 1 to 4 per cent of patients. If fever persists, however, the possibility of persistent bacteremia or metastatic infection should be considered. If diarrhea persists beyond a week in the noncompromised patient, an alternative diagnosis should be sought. Patients with *Salmonella* infection rarely require hospitalization for treatment of dehydration, and the mortality rate is less that 1 per cent. Stool cultures remain positive for a mean of 4 to 5 weeks after an episode of gastroenteritis; most patients have cleared the organism after 2 to 3 months.

Enteric Fever

Enteric fever, also known as typhoid or paratyphoid fever, is a severe, acute systemic infection that may lack abdominal symptoms. The most common strain causing this syndrome worldwide is *S. typhi*, which also causes the most severe disease. In the last 10 years, the incidence of typhoid fever in the United States has steadily dropped to approximately 500 patients per year. An increasing number of these patients (now >60 per cent) acquire the infection abroad, especially in Mexico, India, and South America.

The incubation period is typically 1 to 2 weeks, but ranges from 3 to 60 days, varying with inoculum size and the state of host defenses. During this stage of intestinal proliferation, diarrhea is uncommon, occurring in roughly 25 per cent of patients. Symptoms of enteritis usually resolve before the onset of fever. One to two weeks after ingestion of salmonellae, a classically stepwise increase in fever occurs. Influenzalike symptoms predominate and include malaise, myalgias, headache, anorexia, cough, and sore throat. The sustained, high, spiking fever that is the hallmark of typhoid fever is well established by the second week after inoculation. At this stage, confusion may be present, and cough, coryza, abdominal pain, and constipation are the most prominent manifestations. Psychosis is noted in 5 to 10 per cent of patients with typhoid fever. Patients with neurologic involvement characteristically pick at the bedclothes, wave at imaginary objects, and experience muscle twitching.

Physical examination of the patient with typhoid fever reveals an acutely ill person whose pulse is classically slow, given the height of the fever. Unfortunately, this helpful diagnostic clue is not often observed. The abdomen is tender to deep palpation, and increased peristalsis may be detected. Hepatosplenomegaly can be demonstrated in half the patients. Rose spots, which are small, slightly raised, blanching red macules, are seen most often on the anterior chest in about 30 per cent of patients. Rose spots occur in the first week of illness and evolve to small hemorrhages that may be difficult to see in dark-skinned persons. Cervical nodes may be enlarged; pulmonary findings are rare.

The leukocyte count is usually normal, but leukopenia is found in 25 per cent of patients. High, spiking fevers in the absence of corresponding leukocytosis are characteristic of typhoid fever. Mild anemia is common. If untreated, most symptoms of typhoid fever resolve by the fourth week of illness. With appropriate antibiotic therapy, symptoms resolve within a few days.

Complications of typhoid fever usually occur during the third to fourth weeks of disease in patients with unrecognized infection. Intestinal perforation, which occurs in less than 3 per cent of patients in the United States, is more common in the developing world. Intestinal hemorrhage has been reported in as many as 10 per cent of patients worldwide. Less frequent complications include acute cholecystitis, myocarditis, and orchitis. Spontaneous abortion and premature labor are more frequent in patients with typhoid fever.

A diagnosis of enteric fever should be considered in any patient with prolonged unexplained fever, especially those who have traveled to tropical regions where typhoid is endemic. In a returning traveler who presents with prolonged high fever, rose spots, and abdominal pain, the diagnosis is evident. However, most patients lack these classic manifestations. The differential diagnosis should include other illnesses that feature prominent and prolonged fever such as malaria, tularemia, rickettsial illnesses, leptospirosis, viral hepatitis, dengue, miliary tuberculosis, and other viral syndromes.

Bacteremia and Metastatic Infection

Once salmonellae have invaded the bloodstream, they tend to seed areas of underlying abnormalities, such as atherosclerotic lesions, mural thrombi, and bone infarctions. High-grade sustained bacteremia suggests intravascular infection. Endocarditis is rare after infection with salmonellae; when it does occur, it can involve unusual sites, leading to ventricular aneurysms or mural thrombi. Endocarditis caused by salmonellae can be aggressive, with the mortality rate approaching 70 per cent. Intravascular infection without endocarditis occurs most frequently in men older than 50 years and typically involves the abdominal aorta in areas of aneurysmal dilatation or atherosclerotic plaques. This complication should be suspected in elderly patients with sustained fever, back or chest pain after an episode of gastroenteritis, recurrent bacteremia after treatment, or a paravertebral abscess. A rare complication is massive gastrointestinal bleeding from erosion of an infected aneurysm into the small bowel.

Osteomyelitis from infection with *Salmonella* is most common in children. It can involve any bone but has a predilection for the long bones and vertebral bodies; it rapidly crosses intervertebral junctions. Multiple bones are infected in 15 per cent of patients. Seeding of *Salmonella* typically occurs at sites of underlying abnormality. Thus, patients with sickle cell disease and joint prostheses are at increased risk for osteomyelitis. Blood cultures are frequently positive in patients with osteomyelitis resulting from salmonellae, and 60 per cent of these patients present with diarrhea.

Septic arthritis occurs most often in children, patients with sickle cell disease, and immunosuppressed persons. It commonly results from contiguous spread from bone, especially around the knees and shoulders. Septic arthritis should not be confused with postdiarrheal reactive arthritis, which is characterized by a culture-negative inflammation of multiple joints. More than half the patients with reactive arthritis are HLA-B27–positive. Nearly 25 per cent have a triad of signs associated with Reiter syndrome: arthritis, urethritis, and conjunctivitis. Patients with Reiter syndrome are typically young adults with a mean age of 22 years.

Meningitis is a serious complication seen primarily in neonates (75 per cent of cases) or young children. Infection may be acquired at birth from mothers with diarrhea and may be transmitted nosocomially to other neonates in a nursery. Infants with meningitis caused by salmonellae tend to have a fulminant course, with the mortality rate approaching 40 per cent. Neurologic sequelae—including seizures, intellectual impairment, hydrocephalus, visual disturbances, and paresis—are frequent. Gram stains of cerebrospinal fluid are usually positive for *Salmonella*.

The most common intra-abdominal infection associated with salmonellae is cholangitis in patients with pre-existing gallstones and biliary cirrhosis. Splenic abscesses are seen less often. Salmonellae account for 15 per cent of splenic abscesses, which are most common in patients with sickle cell disorders. Urinary tract infection with *Salmonella* accompanies urinary stones or immunosuppression. Other rare examples of metastatic infection include pneumonia, empyema, brain abscess (in acquired immunodeficiency syndrome [AIDS] patients), orchitis, and subdural empyema.

Chronic Carrier State

The chronic carrier state is defined as the persistence of salmonellae in the stool for at least 1 year. Less than 0.5 per cent of patients with nontyphoidal *Salmonella* infection become chronic carriers. In patients with *S. typhi*, the percentage increases to 1 to 4 per cent. A major predisposing factor to chronic carriage is biliary tract disease, particularly gallstones. Chronic urinary carriage may also arise with urolithiasis or urinary tract fibrosis following infection with *Schistosoma haematobium*.

DIAGNOSIS

Definitive diagnosis of gastroenteritis caused by *Salmonella* requires isolation of the organism from stool cultures. Culture of fresh stool is preferred; cultures of rectal swab specimens have lower recovery rates. The presence of leukocytes in the stool aids diagnosis but does not distinguish *Salmonella* gastroenteritis from other invasive diarrheal disorders.

Isolation of *Salmonella* is also required to make the diagnosis of typhoid fever. Stool cultures usually are not positive until the third week of illness, however, and then only in 80 per cent of patients. Blood cultures are positive in up to 90 per cent of patients in the first to third weeks of illness, but the sensitivity throughout the illness is only about 70 per cent. Cultures of bone marrow and rose spots are positive in 90 per cent and 60 per cent of patients with established disease (weeks 2 to 4), respectively. The Enterotest (HEDECO, Palo Alto, CA) or string test is useful for culture of intestinal secretions and increases the diagnostic yield of culture, especially in children. The combination of blood cultures and the string test may be as sensitive as culture of bone marrow aspirates.

Although various serologic tests have been developed for *S. typhi*, none is more sensitive than cultures. The most widely used is the Widal test, which measures titers of agglutinins to the O and H antigens of *Salmonella*. Carriers and patients with gastroenteritis do not have an antibody response to these antigens. In patients with suspected typhoid fever, a rise in antibody titer (>1:640) to the O antigen in the absence of prior immunization is sensitive but not specific for disease. The H antigen has an even higher rate of cross-reactivity. Effective antibiotic therapy may blunt the response to these antigens. The use of the Widal test adds little to culture in the diagnosis of disease caused by salmonellae.

In conclusion, salmonellae are ubiquitous organisms that have successfully adapted to colonization of mass-produced poultry and other food products. The protean clinical manifestations of *Salmonella* require a high index of suspicion on the part of the physician and the inclusion of *Salmonella* infection in the differential diagnosis of various clinical syndomes. Culture of the organism remains the mainstay of diagnosis.

BACTERIAL ZOONOSES

By Jay P. Sanford, M.D.
Dallas, Texas

Zoonoses are diseases that are communicable from animals to humans under natural conditions. Transmission may result from direct contact with animal tissues or from the ingestion of contaminated body fluids or secretions (e.g., milk). Transmission may also occur by means of insect vectors and by the inhalation of aerosols containing infectious materials. For most zoonoses, a confirmed diagnosis depends on laboratory tests that are specific for the organism. A detailed epidemiologic history covering the 4 to 6 weeks prior to the illness is essential because the symptoms and signs of various bacterial zoonotic infections often overlap. When a history is taken, it is best to use a calendar and to review specifically, day by day, the patient's location, activities, and contacts with animals, insects, and other individuals who were ill.

I am reminded of a patient in whom brucellosis was strongly suspected and who, when asked repeatedly whether he drank raw milk, denied it. When asked when he stopped drinking raw milk, he replied, "a month or so ago because my cow had Bang's disease" (brucellosis).

ANTHRAX

Anthrax is an acute infection of animals and humans that is caused by the gram-positive spore-forming bacillus *Bacillus anthracis*. Animals (primarily herbivores) acquire the disease following inoculation or ingestion of spores present in the soil. Viable spores persist in the soil for years. On germination, *B. anthracis* may produce two toxins—edema toxin and lethal toxin—as well as capsular material that is antiphagocytic. Production of the toxins and capsular material is regulated by plasmids. Anthrax occurs throughout the world, predominantly in developing countries. In the United States, rare human cases arise in occupational or agricultural settings. Work-related infections usually involve contact with contaminated animal materials, such as goat hair. *Bacillus anthracis* is endemic in the soils of Texas, Louisiana, Oklahoma, and the lower Mississippi Valley.

Epidemiology and Clinical History

Anthrax in humans occurs in three clinical syndromes: cutaneous (95 per cent), respiratory (5 per cent), and gastrointestinal (<1 per cent). A history of occupational exposure to goats, cattle, sheep, horses, or imported animal products, including the hair or skins of herbivores, can be obtained from almost all patients. The time from exposure to onset of disease is typically 3 to 7 days. The incubation period of inhalational anthrax is shorter than that of the cutaneous form, which may be up to 10 days.

Presenting Symptoms and Signs

Cutaneous Anthrax

Three to ten days after inoculation, a painless, pruritic papule develops. Lesions typically occur on the arms, neck, or face. After several days, the papule evolves into a vesicle about 4 to 6 cm in diameter. The vesicular fluid, initially serous, typically becomes hemorrhagic. Within 1 to 2 days, the lesion ulcerates, forming a central dark eschar, which is usually round, with surrounding vesicles and edema. Painful regional adenopathy develops during the eschar stage, which persists for 1 to 3 weeks, leaving a scar on healing. Multiple lesions are uncommon. Systemic manifestations, including fever, malaise, and headache, occur in only half of patients.

Respiratory (Inhalational) Anthrax

The clinical course of respiratory anthrax is often biphasic. Initial symptoms are those of an undifferentiated benign respiratory infection, with malaise, myalgia, low-grade fever, nonproductive cough, and occasionally substernal discomfort. Physical examination is usually unremarkable, but rales may be noted. After 2 to 4 days, the patient experiences the sudden onset of severe, rapidly progressive respiratory distress, with severe dyspnea and hypoxia. Examination typically reveals cyanosis, tachycardia, tachypnea, and fever. Bilateral rales and edema of the neck and chest may occur. On chest film, widening of the mediastinum may be seen. Inhaled spores move from the alveoli to mediastinal lymph nodes, where they germinate to produce edema and lethal toxins, which, in turn, produce a hemorrhagic mediastinitis. Pleural effusions are common. Patients rapidly become hypotensive and meningitis can occur.

Gastrointestinal Anthrax

The syndrome of gastrointestinal anthrax has never been reported in the United States. In developing countries, both abdominal and oropharyngeal syndromes are reported. With abdominal anthrax, symptoms include nausea, vomiting, anorexia, abdominal pain, and fever. Primary lesions typically arise in the cecum. Over 2 to 5 days, patients experience increasing abdominal pain and bloody diarrhea. The oropharyngeal syndrome is cutaneous anthrax of the oropharynx, characterized by sore throat, dysphagia, ulceromembranous lesions on the hard or soft palate or pharynx, regional adenopathy, and nonpitting edema in the cervical region.

Laboratory Findings

Systemic Findings

Leukocytosis with neutrophilia occurs in half of patients with cutaneous anthrax and in almost all patients with respiratory or gastrointestinal syndromes. *B. anthracis* is not fastidious and grows readily in the usual blood culture media. Blood cultures are positive in only 10 per cent of patients with cutaneous anthrax, whereas they usually are positive with respiratory or gastrointestinal anthrax. Chest films are abnormal with respiratory anthrax (see earlier discussion).

Specific Findings

The diagnosis requires a high index of suspicion. A cutaneous lesion at the vesicular stage should be aspirated, examined with Gram stain, and cultured on usual laboratory media such as blood agar and trypticase soy agar plates. *B. anthracis* is a large encapsulated gram-positive bacillus; the capsule can best be demonstrated using a polychrome methylene blue stain. *B. anthracis* usually grows overnight, producing gray-white, nonhemolytic, catalase-positive colonies. Identification of isolates is based on fluorescent antibody staining or the API 50 CH test strip used in conjunction with the API 20 E test strip (bioMérieux, St. Louis, MO). *B. anthracis* is not found in the sputum of patients with respiratory anthrax.

Pitfalls in Diagnosis

Cutaneous Anthrax

Depending on the stage at which the patient is seen, early papular lesions in cutaneous anthrax may resemble those of orf, especially if there has been contact with sheep or goats. Although the time courses differ, papular lesions also resemble those of cutaneous leishmaniasis. At the vesicular stage, the lesions can mimic those of bullous impetigo (readily distinguished on Gram stain), the sting of the wooly caterpillar (wooly caterpillar stings are extremely painful), and the brown recluse spider bite (also painful). With the development of an eschar and regional adenopathy, the differential diagnosis includes tularemia, cat-scratch disease, plague, cutaneous diphtheria, and thermal burns.

Respiratory Anthrax

Initially, most patients with respiratory anthrax present with an undifferentiated upper respiratory infection. With the onset of tachypnea and hypoxemia, the differential diagnosis includes Hantavirus pulmonary syndrome, primary influenza virus pneumonia, pneumonic plague, legionellosis, Q fever, and pulmonary tularemia. In the immunocompromised patient, *Pneumocystis carinii* pneumonia must be considered. The presence or absence of mediastinal widening is the key to the diagnosis.

Gastrointestinal Anthrax

The major mimic of gastrointestinal anthrax is *Yersinia enterocolitis* gastroenteritis. In areas where gastrointestinal anthrax occurs, enteritis necroticans caused by the ingestion of spores of *Clostridium perfringens* clinically resembles gastrointestinal anthrax.

BRUCELLOSIS

Brucellosis in humans is evenly divided between an acute and insidious onset. Infection in animals and humans can be caused by one of four species of *Brucella: Brucella abortus, Brucella melitensis, Brucella suis,* and *Brucella canis*. Brucellae are small, nonmotile aerobic gram-negative coccobacilli. Most human disease can be traced to domesticated food animals: cattle, sheep, goats, buffalo, yak, and camels. Transmission to humans is by one of three routes: direct contact of conjunctivae or broken skin with excretions, secretions, or tissues of infected animals; inhalation of aerosols; or ingestion of tissues or foodstuffs containing the organisms. Brucellosis occurs throughout the world but is most prevalent in the Mediterranean basin, the Arabian peninsula, the Indian subcontinent, Mexico, and Central and South America. In the United States, the majority of cases are reported in Texas, California, Virginia, and Florida. The incubation period between exposure and the onset of symptoms is usually 2 to 8 weeks.

Epidemiology

In animals, brucellae localize in the female and male reproductive organs and persist for life. Organisms are shed in large numbers in milk, urine, and products of pregnancy. Brucellae are transmitted to humans by direct contact with infected animals or their carcasses or by ingestion of unpasteurized milk or milk products. Occupations associated with an increased risk include animal husbandry, slaughterhouse work, and veterinary medicine. Ingestion of unpasteurized dairy products (especially goat cheese) carries the greatest risk for the general population. Meat products are rarely a source of *Brucella*. Inadvertent self-inoculation of the live attenuated calf vaccine, *Brucella abortus* strain 19, can produce disease in humans (typically veterinarians).

Presenting Symptoms and Signs

Brucellosis is characterized by symptoms typically associated with an unremarkable physical examination. Classic symptoms include weakness (92 per cent), chills (79 per cent), sweats (77 per cent), anorexia (73 per cent), generalized aching (68 per cent), headache (64 per cent), and fever (57 per cent). The fever "undulates" in one third of patients with *B. melitensis* and in 10 per cent of those with *B. suis*. Hepatomegaly and splenomegaly occur in two thirds and lymphadenopathy is reported in 40 per cent of patients. Other symptoms may also raise the index of suspicion for brucellosis. Spondylitis, typically of the lumbar spine, occurs in 3 to 15 per cent of patients. *Brucella* spondylitis may present without fever. Peripheral arthritis is usually monarticular and may relapse in children or young adults. Prepatellar bursitis may be a classic hallmark in patients with brucellosis. Unilateral epididymo-orchitis occurs in 10 per cent of adult males.

Laboratory Findings

Systemic Findings

Routine hematologic studies are of little help. About one third of patients show evidence of iron deficiency anemia. Leukocyte counts are slightly increased (10,000 to 20,000 cells/mm^3) in one third of patients, normal in one third of patients, and slightly decreased (2000 to 5000 cells/mm^3) in one third of patients. Brucellosis is one of the infectious diseases that may be associated with a normal erythrocyte sedimentation rate (ESR). Early in the course of disease in one third of patients, the erythrocyte sedimentation rate is less than 10 mm per hour; however, during the course of illness, increases are usually seen. Tests of hepatocellular function show mild abnormalities in about half of patients.

Specific Findings

A confirmed diagnosis of brucellosis is based on the isolation and identification of brucellae from blood, bone marrow, or other tissues. *Brucella abortus* requires an atmosphere of 5 to 10 per cent carbon dioxide for primary isolation. In the past, prolonged incubation (up to 4 weeks) was often required. Today most laboratories employ rapid isolation methods to identify organisms within a few days; however, when brucellosis is suspected clinically, the clinician should request retention of cultures for 4 weeks. The frequency of positive blood cultures in brucellosis is 15 to 70 per cent. Once isolated, species can be identified using API 20 NE test strips, although misidentification as *Moraxella phenylpyruvica* has been reported. When blood cultures are negative, serologic tests may be used to make a presumptive diagnosis. The most widely used is the serum agglutination test (SAT). The lipopolysaccharide (LPS) of brucellae contains A and M antigens that cross-react with *B. abortus, B. melitensis,* and *B. suis* but not *B. canis*. In most laboratories, the SAT employs killed whole cells of *B. abortus* strain 1119. Because cross-reactivity occurs with other smooth brucellae, specific tests for *B. melitensis* and *B. abortus* are not required. An SAT titer of greater than or equal to 1:160 is presumptively diagnostic. Unfortunately, false-negative titers caused by prozoning may occur. This can be overcome by diluting the serum to greater than 1:320. False-positive reactions can also occur, especially with sera containing antibodies to *Y. enterocolitica* 0:9, cholera, and tularemia. The antigen used in "febrile agglutinins" screening tests is insensitive and unreliable. Therefore "febrile agglutinins" should not be used to diagnose or exclude brucellosis. Several enzyme-linked immunosorbent assays (ELISAs) have been developed, but standardized reagents are not available.

Pitfalls in Diagnosis

The major pitfall involves ordering an inappropriate serologic test such as "febrile agglutinins" and then overinterpreting a low-dilution positive titer (e.g., 1:40) in a patient with numerous chronic symptoms, no signs, vague history of exposure, and failure of response to one or more courses of appropriate antibiotics. These patients may have persisting foci of infection, including abscesses in bone, spleen, or liver. Imaging procedures are helpful in detecting such foci. Other individuals with "chronic brucellosis" overlap with patients with the chronic fatigue syndrome. The second major pitfall is the failure to associate brucellosis with specific focal syndromes such as arthritis, spondylitis, and orchitis, resulting in failure to obtain appropriate materials for culture and failure to perform serologic tests. Other pitfalls include false-negative titers due to the prozone phenomenon and false-positive cross-reactions.

TULAREMIA

Tularemia is an acute disease caused by *Francisella tularensis,* a small pleomorphic gram-negative coccobacillus. *F. tularensis* is a strict aerobe, grows optimally at 37°C (98.6°F), and requires cysteine for growth. The organism is readily killed by heat; 56°C (132.8°F) for 10 minutes is typically sufficient. Therefore, cooking renders the meat of animals and game birds safe. *F. tularensis* is not killed by freezing; organisms remain viable in frozen animal carcasses for as long as 3 weeks.

Epidemiology

Tularemia occurs in the Northern Hemisphere between 30 and 71 degrees north latitude except in the United Kingdom. It has not been reported in South America or Africa. In the United States, most cases are reported in Missouri, Arkansas, Tennessee, Oklahoma, Kansas, and Utah. *F. tularensis* has been isolated from more than 100 species of wild mammals (rabbits, hares, squirrels, moles, muskrats, and beavers), at least 9 species of domestic animals, and 25 species of birds, amphibians, and fish. In addition, it has been isolated from more than 50 species of arthropods and from mud and water. In the United States, the most common sources of infection are bites by ticks or deer flies and contact with infected animals or their carcasses. In Scandinavia, mosquitoes are the most important vector. Outbreaks associated with exposure to water contaminated by beavers or muskrats have been reported. In the United States, tick exposure now accounts for three fourths of human infections, and wild rabbits and hares are the most common reservoirs. Domestic rabbits have not been implicated in natural disease.

Presenting Symptoms and Signs

Tularemia has been classified into six clinical syndromes: ulceroglandular, glandular, oculoglandular, oropharyngeal, typhoidal, and pneumonic. This classification is a matter of convenience and may be misleading. The preconception that tularemia is an ulceroglandular disease may preclude consideration of its other presentations, which represent a quarter to half of all cases. The usual incubation period is 3 to 5 days (range 1 to 21 days). The onset of symptoms is abrupt. Initial symptoms consist of fever, chills, headache, cough, pharyngitis, and myalgia. The initial fever and constitutional symptoms usually subside after 1 to 4 days, and a remission of 1 to 3 days is followed by recurrence of fever and symptoms.

Ulceroglandular Tularemia

Ulceroglandular tularemia occurs in 45 to 85 per cent of patients. Twenty-four to forty-eight hours after the onset of initial fever, lymph nodes draining the site of inoculation become enlarged, firm, and tender. The overlying skin is usually inflamed. Concurrently or within a day, a local lesion or lesions (about 10 per cent are multiple) develop. They begin as painful, small, red papules that progress to pustules and then to ulcers with sharp undermined borders. Occasionally, dry, cracked lesions resembling chapped skin are associated with regional nodes. Over the course of 1 to 2 weeks, the ulcers become covered with a dark crust. Lymphangitis is rare. Enlarged nodes may persist for a mean period of 3 months.

Other Forms of Tularemia

The glandular form of tularemia is similar to the ulceroglandular type except that a local lesion is not found. Oculoglandular tularemia refers to the site of inoculation in the conjunctiva. A syndrome similar to that of ulceroglandular tularemia is complicated by striking edema of the eyelids and conjunctivitis. Oropharyngeal disease is analogous to ulceroglandular tularemia, but the oropharyngeal ynx is the portal of entry. Typical features include exudative pharyngitis and/or tonsillitis with cervical adenopathy. Clinically, the typhoidal form presents as sepsis without localizing features or as a subacute fever of unknown origin. The typhoidal form is usually not associated with lymphadenopathy. Secondary pneumonitis is common with each of the clinical syndromes. Chest films are abnormal in about half of the patients, typically showing infiltrates in one of the lower lobes. One third of the patients have associated pleural effusions. Symptoms are similar with primary pneumonic tularemia following aerosol transmission.

Laboratory Findings

General Findings

The hemogram is usually normal. Leukocyte counts vary from 5000 to 20,000 cells/mm^3. Urinalysis reveals sterile pyuria in 20 to 30 per cent of patients. The basis and significance of this finding are unclear, but recognition of its occurrence may preclude unnecessary diagnostic studies. Alanine aminotransferase (ALT), aspartate aminotransferase (AST), and lactate dehydrogenase (LD) levels are abnormal in 5 to 15 per cent of patients, but results do not correlate with clinical abdominal findings.

Specific Findings

The diagnosis of tularemia is usually based on serologic tests rather than culture. *F. tularensis* requires cysteine for growth, and successful cultivation poses a laboratory hazard. Thus, confirmation of tuleremia requires a fourfold or greater increase in SAT titer. An acute-phase titer of 1:160 or greater is presumptive, but this increase seldom develops before the 11th day of illness and sometimes not until the third week. Positive SAT titers of 1:10 to 1:50 occur in about 1 per cent of the general American population.

Pitfalls in Diagnosis

Misdiagnosis of ulceroglandular tularemia most often results from failure to obtain a history of contact with wild animal carcasses or a history of tick or deer fly bites or failure to consider acute ulceroglandular syndromes caused by organisms other than *F. tularensis*. Such syndromes include impetigo with lymphadenitis, cat-scratch disease, plague, rat-bite fever, brown recluse spider bites, and wooly caterpillar stings. The diagnosis of typhoidal tularemia requires a high index of suspicion and is now most often made serendipitously when *F. tularensis* is isolated from blood cultures.

PLAGUE

Plague is a flea-borne disease of rodents, caused by *Yersinia pestis*, an aerobic gram-negative coccobacillus or bacillus. *Y. pestis* is enzootic in various native rodent species in Asia, Africa, and North and South America. In the United States, enzootic or sylvatic plague exists in the rodent and flea populations ranging from the Pacific coast to western Texas, western Oklahoma, and Colorado. In the United States, the most important reservoirs are the ground squirrel, rock squirrel, and prairie dog.

Epidemiology

Plague is most often transmitted to humans by the bite of vector fleas, less often by direct contact and inoculation from infected animals, and rarely by aerosols. In the United States, most patients are infected by direct contact with tissues from plague-infected animals, not from the bites of vector fleas. In endemic areas such as the southwestern United States, domestic cats pose a risk to pet owners and veterinarians. *Y. pestis* may be carried on the teeth or claws of cats and transmitted through bites or scratches.

Presenting Symptoms and Signs

Bubonic Plague

Following exposure, the incubation period is usually 4 to 6 days (range 2 to 8 days). The onset of symptoms is abrupt, with fever, rigors, headache, and myalgia. Concomitantly or within 24 hours, the patient notices intense pain in regional lymph nodes. The pain is often so intense that the patient avoids motion or pressure on the nodes. Inguinal and femoral node involvement causes the patient to limp. The skin over the affected nodes may be erythematous. Edema usually surrounds the nodes. Lymphangitis is not a feature of bubonic plague. One quarter or fewer patients have skin lesions at the site of the bite or inoculation.

Septicemic Plague

Septicemic plague is plague with bacteremia but without lymphadenitis. In New Mexico, approximately one fourth of patients present with the septicemic syndrome. Transmissible pneumonic infection occurs in only about 5 per cent of septicemic patients.

Pneumonic Plague

Pneumonia in the patient with plague is usually secondary to hematogenous dissemination from lymph nodes. The patient experiences chest pain, cough, and occasional "raspberry"-streaked hemoptysis. Chest film shows patchy bronchopneumonia. Primary pneumonic plague has a shorter incubation period (2 to 3 days) than does bubonic plague. Progression to death occurs within 24 to 48 hours. Fortunately, primary pneumonic plague is now rare in the United States.

Laboratory Findings

Leukocytosis is common, and liver function test results are frequently abnormal. A bacteriologic diagnosis is readily made in most patients by smear and culture of the aspirate from a bubo. Because the bubo may not contain pus, saline injection (about 1 mL) with immediate reaspiration may be required to produce a specimen. Drops of pus or aspirate are placed on slides for staining with both Gram and Wayson methylene blue stains. *Y. pestis* organisms are gram-negative bacilli or coccobacilli. With Wayson stain, the organisms appear as bipolar rods resembling safety pins. Aspirates should be plated directly on blood or nutrient agar plates. *Y. pestis* grows slowly, requiring 48 hours to develop small colonies. Optimal temperature for growth is 28°C, not the 35°C used in most laboratories. Blood cultures should also be obtained.

Serologic tests are of less value in the diagnosis of plague. A passive hemagglutination test using fraction I of *Y. pestis* can be performed at the Centers for Disease Control and Prevention, Plague Branch, Ft. Collins, CO. A fourfold or greater rise in titer or a single titer of greater than or equal to 1:16 is presumptive evidence for plague infection.

Pitfalls in Diagnosis

The major pitfall in diagnosis is the failure of a physician in a nonendemic area to include plague in the differential diagnosis of acute lymphadenitis, acute sepsis, or rapidly developing and progressive pneumonia in a person who has visited endemic areas of the southwestern or western United States and has had contact with wild animals such as prairie dogs or domestic animals such as cats. Other diagnostic considerations in the patient with bubonic plague include tularemia and cat-scratch disease. The differential diagnosis for patients with pneumonic plague includes hantavirus pulmonary syndrome, primary influenzal pneumonia, acute fungal pneumonia (especially coccidioidomycosis), pneumonic tularemia, and acute eosinophilic pneumonia. If the diagnosis of plague, especially septicemic or pneumonic plague, is suspected on epidemiologic grounds, empirical treatment with streptomycin, gentamicin, or tetracycline should be initiated immediately after specimens are obtained for culture. Plague pneumonia is invariably fatal if appropriate antibiotic treatment is delayed 18 to 24 hours.

RAT-BITE FEVER

Rat-bite fever represents two clinically similar but etiologically distinct diseases that may follow a rodent bite. Streptobacillary rat-bite fever, caused by the pleomorphic gram-negative bacillus *Streptobacillus moniliformis*, is more common in the United States. Spirillary rat-bite fever, caused by *Spirillum minus*, is more common in Asia. Rat-bite fever occurs following a bite in up to 10 per cent of bite victims.

Epidemiology

Fifty to one hundred per cent of both wild and laboratory rats harbor *S. moniliformis* in the nasopharynx. Rat-bite fever is mainly a disease of individuals (especially children) living in crowded urban dwellings or in rural areas infested with rats. Also at risk are biomedical laboratory personnel. Carnivores that prey on rodents may also mechanically transmit *S. moniliformis* through scratches or bites. The epidemiology of *Spirillum minus* infections is similar, but the frequency of colonization of the rat oropharynx with *Spirillum minus* is lower (25 per cent) than with *S. moniliformis*.

Presenting Symptoms and Signs

Streptobacillary Rat-Bite Fever

Following an incubation period of 1 to 22 days, the patient experiences the abrupt onset of fever, rigors, headache, vomiting, myalgia, and severe migratory arthralgia. At the onset of symptoms, the bite has usually healed. Two to four days after the onset of fever, a nonpruritic maculopapular morbilliform or petechial rash occurs on the palms, soles, and extremities. Regional lymphadenopathy is minimal or absent. One half of these patients experience an asymmetric polyarthritis, most commonly involving knees, ankles, elbows, wrists, shoulders, and hips.

Spirillary Rat-Bite Fever

The incubation period of *Spirillum minus* infection is 4 to 28 days (usually >10 days). During this time, the initial bite wound heals. With the onset of disease, the initial lesion becomes painful, swollen, and violaceous and is accompanied by lymphangitis and lymphadenitis. The lesion progresses to an eschar. Concurrent systemic symptoms of fever, rigors, headache, and malaise occur. Myalgia and arthralgia are uncommon. During the first week of fever, a blotchy macular rash develops over the extremities, face, and trunk.

Laboratory Findings

The leukocyte count with both forms of rat-bite fever is in the range of 5000 to 30,000 cells/mm^3. With *Spirillum minus* infection, VDRL (Veneral Disease Research Laboratories) test results are false-positive in one half of patients.

Streptobacillus moniliformis is a highly pleomorphic gram-negative bacillus. It requires 8 to 10 per cent carbon dioxide and 10 to 20 per cent horse or rabbit serum for primary isolation, but it can be grown on most solid or liquid media. Serum agglutinins develop within 10 days of onset of illness. A fourfold rise in titer or an initial titer of greater than or equal to 1:80 is considered diagnostic. *Spirillum minus* is a short spiral bacillus (spirochete) with two to six regular helical turns. *Spirillum minus* cannot be cultured on artificial media. Diagnosis requires demonstration of characteristic spirochetes in blood or lymph node aspirate using Giemsa or Wright stain or dark-field microscopy. There are no serologic tests available for *Spirillum minus*.

Pitfalls in Diagnosis

In the patient with fever, rash, and recent rat exposure, the differential diagnosis is limited. Leptospirosis is a consideration. Often there is no history of a rat bite, especially in children who may be bitten at night. Without a history of rat exposure, the differential diagnosis includes viral exanthems, Rocky Mountain spotted fever, meningococcemia, disseminated gonococcal infection, secondary syphilis, and Lyme disease as well as collagen vascular disease, acute rheumatic fever, and infective endocarditis. With *Spirillum minus* disease, the differential diagnosis includes the ulceroglandular syndromes of tularemia and plague.

LEPTOSPIROSIS

Leptospirosis is a spirochete infection acquired by humans through contact of skin or mucous membranes with contaminated urine from infected wild or domestic mammals. Leptospires are motile, flexible rods that must be identified using silver stains or dark-field microscopy. More than 200 serovars of *Leptospira* may infect more than 180 species of animals. Mammals appear to be the only epidemiologically important reservoirs. In the United States, the most important transmitters are dogs, cattle, rats, swine, racoons, goats, and mice. Leptospirosis occurs throughout the world except in Antarctica. In the United States, leptospirosis has been reported from all states but is most common in Hawaii and the southern states.

Epidemiology

Animals who survive acute leptospirosis can harbor the spirochete in renal tubules and shed leptospires in urine for years. Humans then contact urine directly or more commonly contact soil or surface water contaminated with animal urine. Leptospires can survive in clean water for several weeks at an alkaline pH and a temperature above 22°C (71.6°F). They do not survive in salt water. Viable leptospires may be isolated from fresh urine spots for 6 to

48 hours. Portals of entry include abraded skin and the mucous membranes. In the United States, 20 per cent of patients have swimming or immersion exposure. Occupational groups at risk include persons in agriculture, sewer workers, miners, slaughterhouse workers, veterinarians, and laboratory personnel.

Presenting Symptoms and Signs

The incubation period is typically 7 to 13 days, with extremes of 2 to 26 days. Leptospirosis may present as one of three major syndromes: mild anicteric leptospirosis, severe hepatorenal syndrome (Weil's disease), or aseptic meningitis. Leptospirosis is classically a biphasic illness, with a leptospiremic phase followed by an immune phase. The leptospiremic phase is typically abrupt in onset and characterized by severe myalgia, cutaneous hyperesthesia, fever, and rigors. Anorexia, nausea, and vomiting occur in one half of patients. Cough occurs in 25 to 85 per cent of patients and is associated with blood streaking or hemoptysis in one half of patients. During the initial phase, most patients show conjunctival suffusion (dilatation of conjunctival vessels without signs of inflammation). Pharyngeal injection, cutaneous hemorrhage, and skin rashes are less common, whereas splenomegaly, hepatomegaly, and lymphadenopathy are uncommon. After 4 to 9 days, symptoms improve as leptospires disappear from the blood and cerebrospinal fluid. The second phase is characterized by recurrence of fever and signs of "aseptic" meningitis or, less commonly, iridocyclitis.

Weil's disease accounts for 1 to 6 per cent of cases of leptospirosis and is characterized by continued fever, jaundice, azotemia, hemorrhagic manifestations, anemia, and disturbances in consciousness. The onset is similar to mild anicteric disease, with the features of Weil's syndrome appearing on the third to sixth day of illness. Either renal or hepatic dysfunction may predominate.

Laboratory Findings

General Findings

In anicteric patients, leukocyte counts vary around the reference range. In patients with jaundice, leukocytosis as high as 70,000 cells/mm^3 may occur. Neutrophilia of greater than 70 per cent is typical. Urinalysis during the first phase reveals mild proteinuria, casts, and an increase in cellular elements. Azotemia has been reported in one fourth of patients and is usually associated with jaundice. During the first phase, one half of patients have increased creatine kinase activity in their serum (mean value five times normal), with minimal increases in aminotransferase activity.

Specific Findings

Leptospires can be cultured from blood or cerebrospinal fluid during the first week or from urine after the first week. One to three drops of fluid to be cultured are added to 3 to 5 mL of Tween 80-albumin medium (EMJH). Cultures are then incubated at 28 to 30°C in the dark for 5 to 6 weeks. Leptospires remain viable in anticoagulated blood (not citrated) for up to 11 days, so specimens can be shipped to a reference laboratory for culture. Leptospires can be seen on darkfield microscopy, but this examination should not be performed on urine because there is a high frequency of false-positive results.

The diagnosis is usually based on serologic tests. The macroscopic slide agglutination test uses antigen from killed leptospires and is widely used for screening. Unfortunately, its specificity and sensitivity are marginal. The microscopic agglutination test, using live leptospires as the antigen, is most specific but is used primarily in reference or research laboratories. More recently, highly specific and sensitive enzyme-linked immunosorbent assay techniques have been developed. Such tests are available in reference laboratories.

Pitfalls in Diagnosis

As with the other zoonotic infections, the likelihood of a correct and definite diagnosis is greatly enhanced if a careful epidemiologic history is correlated with clinical observations. For the initial 48 hours, it is extremely difficult to differentiate leptospirosis from diseases such as hemorrhagic fever with renal syndrome resulting from hantaviruses, scrub typhus, or viral diseases such as dengue and influenza. When leptospirosis and scrub typhus cannot be excluded based on the epidemiologic history, doxycycline should be given because it is effective against both agents.

Mycobacterial Diseases

TUBERCULOSIS

By Edward E. Telzak, M.D.,
and Glenn Turett, M.D.
Bronx, New York

Mycobacterium tuberculosis infects one third of the world's population, and tuberculosis (TB) remains one of the most common infectious diseases of humans. Each year, 8 million new patients and 3 million deaths are reported worldwide. In the United States, for decades, there had been a steady decline in the incidence and prevalence of TB until 1985, when the number of infected persons leveled off. Although the annual incidence decreased by approximately 5 per cent in 1993, compared with 1992, from 1985 to 1992 the annual incidence increased by more than 20 per cent, from 22,201 to 26,673. The factors that contribute to the resurgence of TB in the United States include homelessness, increased immigration from TB-endemic areas outside the United States, and inadequate support of both the public health infrastructure and TB control programs. However, the most important factor responsible for the increasing rates of TB is the epidemic of human immunodeficiency virus (HIV) infection. All these factors have also contributed to the dramatic rise in resistant TB, especially multidrug-resistant TB (MDRTB). In addition to HIV-infected populations, the elderly, especially in nursing homes, and foreign-born Americans are at increased risk for TB.

The HIV epidemic has influenced the rates of TB in

numerous ways. Regions with the highest prevalence of patients with acquired immunodeficiency syndrome (AIDS) have also had the greatest increases in the number of patients with TB. The demographic groups in whom HIV infection is increasing at the highest rates (African American and Latino men, aged 25 to 44 years) have also had the greatest increases in TB rates. HIV seroprevalence studies in TB clinics have documented HIV-seropositivity rates between 0 and 61 per cent, with the highest rates reported in New York City. There is also a growing incidence of both reactivation TB and primary, progressive TB after initial infection. Institutional and community transmission of both drug-susceptible and drug-resistant strains has been well documented. These dual epidemics are characterized by a greater prevalence of multidrug-resistant strains and atypical clinical presentations.

TUBERCULOSIS AND TUBERCULOSIS INFECTION

The clinician should distinguish between TB infection and TB. Tuberculosis infection in immunocompetent persons is most often silent and typically detectable only with the development of skin test reactivity to tuberculin purified protein (PPD) derivative. During the course of a lifetime, it is estimated that 10 per cent of persons with a reactive skin test to PPD will develop TB, which has protean signs and symptoms that may involve any organ system. Furthermore, in severely immunosuppressed persons, especially those co-infected with HIV, atypical manifestations may predominate, and TB can produce an extraordinary range of clinical signs and symptoms.

PULMONARY TUBERCULOSIS

Tuberculosis typically involves the lungs and produces a febrile, wasting syndrome. In immunocompetent persons, more than three fourths of patients with TB have disease confined to the lungs. Cough, usually productive, is the most common symptom of TB and is frequently accompanied by fever, night sweats, weight loss, and malaise. Hemoptysis, not usually life-threatening, may occur, and pleuritic chest pain is not unusual. Dyspnea is distinctly uncommon in the absence of substantial pulmonary parenchymal disease.

Because the incidence of extrapulmonary disease remains low in immunocompetent persons, symptoms related to organs other than the lung remain relatively uncommon. Nevertheless, extrapulmonary involvement can produce both symptoms related to that organ and systemic features such as fever, night sweats, weight loss, and malaise.

EXTRAPULMONARY TUBERCULOSIS

In the past, extrapulmonary TB was unusual, affecting primarily the very young and the elderly. In the 1990s, however, extrapulmonary TB has become a prominent feature of the presentation of TB. Prior to the HIV epidemic, 20 per cent of patients with TB in the United States developed extrapulmonary disease. By contrast, among patients co-infected with HIV, extrapulmonary involvement occurs in as many as 70 per cent. Extrapulmonary involvement is also far more likely to occur in HIV-infected patients when they have advanced HIV disease. In fact, among patients with early HIV disease and TB, as in HIV-uninfected immunocompetent patients with TB, approximately 80 per cent have pulmonary disease with typical radiographic findings, such as upper lobe alveolar infiltrates, with or without cavitation. With greater degrees of immunosuppression, the likelihood of extrapulmonary disease increases. In addition to advanced HIV infection, other immunosuppressive processes are associated with extrapulmonary TB, including end-stage renal disease, jejunoileal bypass, and bone marrow transplantation.

Any organ system may be involved in TB, either singly or as part of a disseminated process. Brief discussions of genitourinary, central nervous system, bone and joint, disseminated, and lymphadenopathic TB are provided below as examples of the myriad presentations of extrapulmonary TB.

GENITOURINARY TUBERCULOSIS

Genitourinary TB accounts for nearly 10 per cent of cases of extrapulmonary TB in the United States. Genitourinary TB may involve the urologic system and/or the male or female genital organs. Renal TB originates from a primary lung focus with subsequent lymphohematogenous seeding of the cortical areas of the kidneys. Renal cortical tubercles usually remain silent for many years. Granulomas may eventually rupture into the collecting system, and the infection spreads via the ureter into the bladder, contralateral kidney, or genitalia. Cavitation, abscess formation, fibrosis, and calcification are typical local features of genitourinary TB. Untreated TB may eventually lead to end-stage renal disease through ureteral strictures, hydronephrosis, and progressive destruction of one or both kidneys. There is no typical clinical presentation of urologic TB, but many patients develop dysuria, hematuria, pyuria, flank pain, and, occasionally, recurrent urinary tract infections or a flank mass.

The male genitalia become infected by contiguous, urinary, or hematogenous spread. In men, the prostate is the most common site of infection, followed by the seminal vesicles, epididymis, and testes. Painful inflammation of the testes, prostate, vas deferens, and seminal vesicles may occur. The most common clinical presentation of male genital TB is epididymitis, with a palpable mass and chronic draining sinus due to abscess formation.

Tuberculosis of the female genital tract most often follows lymphohematogenous spread from a pulmonary or an abdominal focus. The distal end of the salpinx is the most common site of infection in the female genital tract, followed by the endometrium and ovary. Systemic symptoms are generally absent in female genital TB, but pelvic-abdominal pain, menstrual disorders, leukorrhea, and dyspareunia may occur.

TUBERCULOSIS OF BONES AND JOINTS

Half of all cases of skeletal TB occur in the spine. The process, known as Pott's disease, typically begins in the anterior vertebral body and destroys the disc space between two adjacent vertebrae. This produces the characteristic spine film showing anterior wedging of two adjacent vertebrae and loss of the intervening disc space, the so-called gibbus deformity. Pus from the vertebrae typically ruptures anteriorly, may dissect along tissue planes, and presents as a paraspinal, supraclavicular, groin, or buttock mass.

Tuberculosis of peripheral bones and joints is typically a monoarticular combination of osteomyelitis and arthritis.

In general, localized pain is the first clinical manifestation with or without associated inflammation.

CENTRAL NERVOUS SYSTEM TUBERCULOSIS

Central nervous system TB presents in various ways. Tuberculous meningitis most often develops when a subependymal tubercle ruptures into the subarachnoid space. Although the meninges are most severely infected at the base of the brain, the clinical spectrum of TB meningitis is very broad, ranging from subtle changes in mentation and mild headache to severe, fulminant meningitis. The typical clinical features include fever, nausea, vomiting, anorexia, headache, apathy, and altered mental status. The physical findings may be minimal but are more likely to include one or more of the following: nuchal rigidity, basilar cranial nerve deficits, papilledema, and focal neurologic deficits. Concomitant extraneurologic TB is present in one third to three quarters of patients with TB meningitis.

Importantly, tuberculomas in the central nervous system are also reported. These may be asymptomatic or may present with the symptoms and signs of a focal brain or spinal cord mass.

MILIARY OR DISSEMINATED TUBERCULOSIS

Historically, miliary TB was defined as disseminated TB with diffuse 1- to 2-mm densities on chest film that often resembled "millet seeds." However, the term "miliary TB" now refers to all forms of extensive hematogenous spread. Miliary TB may result from newly acquired infection or from reactivation disease, and it may present in an acute form or a more chronic form. The acute form is rapidly progressive and fatal if not treated promptly. The signs and symptoms are generally nonspecific, may not localize, and frequently include fever, weight loss, fatigue, and malaise. The physical findings include hepatomegaly, splenomegaly, and lymphadenopathy. The more chronic form of miliary TB lacks the typical radiographic and clinical features of miliary TB. The disease is insidious and usually presents as a fever of unknown origin. The diagnosis of TB is often delayed, and overall mortality exceeds 80 per cent.

Among HIV-infected persons, bacteremia and disseminated disease are not unusual. As previously mentioned, extrapulmonary TB may occur in as many as three quarters of severely immunosuppressed HIV-infected persons, and as many as one third of these patients may have a miliary pattern.

LYMPHATIC TUBERCULOSIS

Tuberculous lymphadenitis is the most common form of extrapulmonary TB in both normal and immunocompromised hosts. Scrofula is tuberculous adenitis of the cervical or supraclavicular nodes. The anterior triangle of the neck, just below the mandible, is the most frequent site of adenopathic disease, although any lymph node can be involved. In the normal host, these nodes frequently enlarge without systemic manifestations. Evidence of active TB outside the nodes is found in approximately 20 per cent of patients, and the PPD is positive in approximately 75 per cent of patients. In general, tuberculous nodes are not tender and are rubbery rather than hard. By contrast, HIV-infected patients with tuberculous adenitis often have fever, weight loss, and multiple tender nodes. Sampling the involved nodes with needle aspiration, needle biopsy, or excisional biopsy is crucial for making a microbiologic diagnosis.

OTHER SITES OF EXTRAPULMONARY TUBERCULOSIS

Any organ system may be involved in TB, either singly or as part of a disseminated process. Tuberculosis of the abdomen includes disease of the peritoneum, gastrointestinal tract, liver and biliary tract, pancreas, tonsils, tongue, and mouth. Cardiac TB typically presents as pericarditis, with fever, chest pain, friction rub, and occasional tamponade. If cardiac TB goes untreated, constrictive pericarditis often occurs. Pleural disease, one of the more common forms of extrapulmonary TB, may occur with primary or reactivation disease. Pleural TB most often follows rupture of a subpleural focus into the pleural space, causing an aggressive immune response and subsequent serofibrinous pleurisy. Chest pain, cough, and fever occur in most patients. Less common sites of tuberculous involvement include the adrenal glands, the skin, and the eye.

DIAGNOSTIC EVALUATION

Skin Testing

In the United States, screening for TB attempts to identify infected persons at high risk for developing disease who would benefit from preventive therapy. In immunocompetent patients, the intracutaneous tuberculin test, with PPD as the antigen, is a reliable method for the detection of prior mycobacterial infection. The tuberculin test is typically performed with intradermal injection of 0.1 mL of PPD (5 tuberculin units) into the volar aspect of the forearm. The injection should be made just beneath the surface of the skin, with the needle bevel facing upward to produce a discrete wheal 6 mm to 10 mm in diameter. Reactions are determined by measuring the transverse diameter of induration. In turn, induration is assessed with palpation between 48 and 72 hours after intradermal inoculation. A positive reaction to PPD is presumptive evidence of current or prior *M. tuberculosis* infection.

Patients with TB and those who are infected but who have not yet developed the disease have a broad range of reaction sizes. In addition, a positive skin test may result from contact with relatively nonpathogenic mycobacteria in the environment, making interpretation of skin tests occasionally problematic. Consequently, guidelines exist to aid clinicians in the interpretation of the tuberculin reaction. A tuberculin reaction of 5 mm or more is classified as positive in the following three groups: persons with known or suspected HIV infection; persons who have chest radiographs with fibrotic lesions likely to represent old healed TB; and persons who have had close recent contact with a patient with infectious TB. A tuberculin reaction of 10 mm or more is classified as positive in persons who do not meet the above criteria but who are from population groups that have an increased risk of TB, such as the medically underserved, low-income groups, foreign-born persons from high prevalence countries, and those with medical conditions known to substantially increase the risk of TB once infection has occurred (e.g., diabetics and people with silicosis). A tuberculin reaction of 15 mm or more is classified as positive in persons from the low-risk general population, especially in locales known to have a high prevalence of nonspecific tuberculin reactivity. Absence of a reaction to the tuberculin test does not exclude a diagnosis of TB or tuberculous infection. Reactions may decrease or disappear during any severe febrile illness, including TB, Hodgkin's disease, and other immunosuppressive malignancies, during HIV infection, and during the administration of immunosuppressive drugs such as corticosteroids. In addition, it requires 4 to 6 weeks after initial infection to develop a reaction to the tuberculin skin test; thus, persons who have been very recently infected may not have developed a reaction. False-negative tuberculin tests may result from technical errors, including subcutaneous or deeper injection and the use of PPD that is outdated or has remained in syringes for too long prior to injection.

A significant problem in identifying newly infected persons is the so-called "booster" phenomenon. In general, repeated skin testing with PPD does not lead to a positive reaction in uninfected persons. However, gradually waning immunity to PPD is well documented in those with bacille Calmette-Guérin (BCG) vaccination or with established infection by any species of mycobacteria. Thus, infected patients, when skin-tested, may have a false-negative reaction. However, the injection of tuberculin in these patients may recall hypersensitivity such that subsequent tests elicit a "boosted" response. Caution is therefore required when the physician attributes an increase in reactivity to a new infection. Although the booster reaction may occur at any age, its frequency increases with age and it is most often encountered in persons older than 55 years of age. The "booster" phenomenon can be seen on a second test done as little as a week after the initial stimulating test. Moreover, the boosted response can persist for a year or longer.

Bacteriology

The definitive diagnosis of TB requires isolation of *M. tuberculosis* via culture from human specimens. Given the high rate of pulmonary disease, sputum (not saliva) is the most appropriate sample to send for culture. However, because TB can occur in almost any anatomic site, various clinical specimens other than sputum should be submitted for examination when nonpulmonary mycobacterial disease is suspected (e.g., urine, cerebrospinal fluid, pleural fluid, pus, biopsy specimens). Proper technique is critical for the diagnosis of pulmonary TB in the laboratory. The patient must produce a "deep-cough" specimen for collection in an appropriate container. Collect at least three fresh specimens on three successive days, preferably on the patient's awakening and prior to meals. If the patient cannot produce a deep-cough specimen, sputum should be induced with hypertonic saline. If a specimen cannot be delivered to the laboratory as soon after it is produced, it should be refrigerated because sputum contains rapidly dividing bacteria that may overgrow any mycobacteria present. The detection of mycobacteria on acid-fast smears varies widely, with sensitivities ranging from 22 to 78 per cent. Although not accurately quantified, the sensitivity depends on factors such as specimen type, number of specimens examined, observer experience, clinical conditions, and the number of acid-fast bacilli (AFB) present. The fluorochrome stain is generally more sensitive than the more traditional Kinyoun or Ziehl-Neelsen stains, but any of these methods are acceptable. However, stained smears are not useful for species identification. Moreover, even nonviable bacilli will stain; therefore, a positive smear does not necessarily indicate the presence of live organisms.

Sputum culture increases the diagnostic yield, facilitates species identification of AFB, and allows the determination of drug susceptibilities. Mycobacteria may be isolated with conventional media or radiometric techniques. Conventional media include egg-based media (i.e., Löwenstein-Jensen culture) and agar-based media (i.e., Middlebrook 7H10 agar). With conventional media, visual analysis of colonies facilitates preliminary identification of AFB. However, mycobacteria grow very slowly; thus, identification with the use of conventional biochemical profiles may require 6 to 8 weeks. The preferred method for culturing mycobacteria employs a radiometric system, which offers greater sensitivity and more rapid growth of mycobacteria, facilitating earlier detection. Radiometric media allow cultivation in 1 or 2 weeks, but confirmation of the identity of an isolated organism may require more time. Once growth in the radiometric system occurs, DNA probes can identify *M. tuberculosis* on the same day.

With the advent of HIV and MDRTB, susceptibility testing is critical. All patients with TB should have at least one isolate of *M. tuberculosis* tested for susceptibility to therapeutic agents. The radiometric method usually provides results within 7 days, whereas the conventional proportional method may take several weeks. The results of susceptibility testing are critical for decisions on therapy.

When sputum cannot be obtained through spontaneous expectoration or induction with irritating normal saline, other diagnostic maneuvers may be employed. Samples may be obtained through nasotracheal aspiration or through early-morning gastric aspiration. The latter technique provides excellent material for AFB smear and culture despite the occasional appearance of nonpathogenic mycobacteria in smears of gastric aspirates. When the above simpler methods fail to produce adequate specimens for culture or a diagnosis remains in doubt, fiberoptic bronchoscopy may yield diagnostic material from lavage, brushings, or biopsies. All tissue specimens should be submitted for both histopathologic analysis and mycobacteriologic smears and cultures. Sputum collected after bronchoscopy may also prove diagnostically useful. It should be emphasized, however, that this diagnostic procedure is to be employed only when less invasive techniques do not produce adequate specimens or a diagnosis. In addition to potentially exposing the patient to additional risk, the staff performing the procedure is at relatively high risk for exposure to and acquisition of infection.

The diagnostic yield of sputum smear and culture is directly related to the extent of pulmonary disease. When a patient with cavitary disease has repeatedly negative AFB smears, diagnoses other than TB should be sought. Conversely, those with a normal chest radiograph often do not have a positive smear.

Newer Diagnostic Tests

Newer diagnostic tests such as the polymerase chain reaction (PCR) and restriction fragment length polymorphism (RFLP) analysis are now available as research tools. Until these methods are better standardized and more readily available, acid-fast staining and culture of sputum, body fluids, or tissue remain the primary methods for diagnosis. In reference laboratories, high-performance chromatographic techniques can rapidly identify mycobacteria by their characteristic lipids.

Chest Radiography

The chest roentgenogram is central to the diagnosis, the determination of the extent of disease, and the evaluation of the response to therapy. No radiographic abnormality is specific for TB; however, certain patterns remain highly suggestive of the diagnosis. Primary TB typically produces noncavitary infiltrates in the middle or lower lung fields and is often associated with hilar adenopathy. This is most often seen in children. Recent studies of epidemic TB in nursing homes, however, indicate that infection contracted in the elderly often causes nondescript lower lobe pneumonitis, implying that local progression of the inhaled organism may be as typical in this age group as it is in children. Scars that result from primary TB are called Ghon complexes. Primary TB most often resolves spontaneously, but, on occasion, the primary focus may become an area of advancing pneumonia, so-called progressive primary infection. Also, typically in children, massive hilar or mediastinal node enlargement may cause bronchial collapse with distal atelectasis. Pleural effusions may also result from primary infection.

Classically, reactivation TB produces disease in the apical and posterior segments of the upper lobe. The superior segment of the lower lobe is also commonly involved. Consolidation with or without cavitation is the typical radiographic pattern seen. Cavities are typically thick-walled and do not contain air-fluid levels. In fact, the presence of an air-fluid level in a patient with TB implies a secondary bacterial superinfection or intracavitary hemorrhage. It deserves emphasis that recognition of the typical features of pulmonary TB, by itself, cannot serve as the basis for a diagnosis in the absence of careful bacteriologic evaluation.

There is also a role for radiography in the diagnosis and evaluation of extrapulmonary TB. Intravenous pyelograms for the evaluation of genitourinary TB and computed tomography scanning and magnetic resonance imaging for the evaluation of central nervous system and spinal and/or paraspinal TB are just some examples.

Useful Laboratory Procedures

In most laboratories, a definitive diagnosis of TB depends on the isolation of the organism. However, numerous other laboratory examinations are commonly abnormal, and these may provide sufficient basis for starting empirical therapy in the absence of confirmatory microbiology test results.

Anemia of chronic disease and an elevated white blood cell count are commonly observed, especially in long-standing disease. On occasion, and especially with miliary TB, a leukemoid reaction may occur, with white blood cell counts exceeding 40,000. Isolated cytopenias, monocytosis or lymphocytosis, and disseminated intravascular coagulation all have been attributed to, and associated with, TB. Although not accurately quantified, hyponatremia and hypercalcemia are thought to be common metabolic complications of TB. Hyponatremia may result from the syndrome of inappropriate secretion of antidiuretic hormone (SIADH) or, less commonly, from tuberculous involvement of the adrenal gland with adrenal insufficiency.

Evaluation of pleural, peritoneal, joint, and cerebrospinal fluid is critical in patients with appropriate clinical presentations. These fluids, when abnormal as a result of TB, share several characteristics. The protein level is usually increased, and the glucose level is reduced, although normal protein and glucose levels can be observed. An increased number of white blood cells in the fluid is common. Generally, polymorphonuclear cells predominate early, with a gradual shift to lymphocyte predominance over days to weeks. Eosinophilia, though described, is unusual.

Sterile pyuria and microscopic hematuria should lead to consideration of genitourinary TB. Given the high rates of positive urine cultures in patients with HIV infection, urine should be cultured even when the sediment is unremarkable.

Therapeutic Tests

Since AFB smears and cultures are not 100 per cent sensitive, there is a role for empirical treatment when clinical suspicion of TB is high. Smear-negative, culture-positive TB occurs with varying frequency and seems to be more common in patients with advanced HIV infection. Also, from a specimen that is smear-negative, it may take several weeks or longer for mycobacteria to grow. In addition, as culture is not absolutely sensitive, there may be no growth of mycobacteria from clinical specimens. When the decision is made to start empirical antituberculous therapy, every effort should be made to obtain appropriate specimens prior to initiating treatment. A response to empirical therapy in this setting can be diagnostic, but without an organism growing in culture, drug susceptibilities cannot be determined and tailoring of the drug regimen is problematic.

A definitive diagnosis of TB can be made only by identifying *M. tuberculosis* in culture from a clinical specimen. Without this, a response to anti-TB therapy, in the proper clinical setting, provides strong suggestive evidence of TB. In patients without a diagnostic culture or response to empirical therapy, another disease process is present, the patient is not taking medication as prescribed, or the organism is resistant to the therapeutic regimen.

Diagnostic Errors and Pitfalls

Diagnostic errors include failure to recognize TB when the infection is present and diagnosing TB when it is not present. By maintaining a high index of suspicion, especially in areas where the disease is prevalent and in HIV-infected patients in whom extrapulmonary involvement and atypical presentations are common, the clinician can readily diagnose TB. Finally, patients may be wrongly considered to have TB because other diseases may have similar presentations (malignancies; sarcoidosis; other bacterial, fungal, viral, or parasitic infections); AFB identified on smear or culture may be nontuberculous mycobacteria or, more rarely, other acid-fast staining organisms (*Nocardia, Rhodococcus, Cryptosporidium,* and *Isospora*); and *M. tuberculosis* may be a laboratory contaminant.

NONTUBERCULOUS MYCOBACTERIAL INFECTIONS

By Paul W. Wright, M.D.,
and Richard J. Wallace, Jr., M.D.
Tyler, Texas

The genus *Mycobacterium* contains more than 50 species, of which approximately half are associated with human disease. Nontuberculous mycobacterial infections include all mycobacterial infections not caused by *M. tuberculosis, M. bovis, M. africanum,* and *M. microti* (the tuberculosis group) and *M. leprae* (the causative agent of

Table 1. Diseases Due to Commonly Encountered NTM Pathogens

Species	Disease
M. avium complex	Disseminated, lymph node, pulmonary
M. kansasii	Pulmonary
M. marinum	Cutaneous
M. fortuitum	Cutaneous, pulmonary
M. chelonae	Cutaneous, disseminated
M. abscessus	Cutaneous, pulmonary
M. scrofulaceum	Lymph node
*M. gordonae**	Pulmonary

**M. gordonae* occurs commonly in the environment but is rarely associated with human illness.
NTM = nontuberculous mycobacteria.

leprosy). Commonly encountered nontuberculous mycobacteria (NTM) include *Mycobacterium avium* complex (MAC), *M. kansasii, M. marinum, M. scrofulaceum, M. gordonae,* and the rapidly growing mycobacteria (RGM) *M. fortuitum, M. abscessus,* and *M. chelonae* (Table 1). The synonyms for NTM include atypical mycobacteria, mycobacteria other than tuberculosis, atypical acid-fast organisms, and enviromental mycobacteria.

These organisms behave as opportunistic pathogens, originating from the environment, mostly water and soil. Human-to-human transmission is rare, but nosocomial infection with case clustering occasionally occurs, usually from contaminated tap water or contaminated water in hospital equipment and supplies (Table 2).

NONTUBERCULOUS MYCOBACTERIAL INFECTION IN HIV-NEGATIVE PATIENTS

Pulmonary Infections

Pulmonary disease accounts for almost 90 per cent of NTM infections in persons who do not have the acquired immunodeficiency syndrome (AIDS). The most commonly isolated pathogens include MAC, *M. kansasii,* and *M. abscessus.* Two groups of patients are infected with MAC. The best known are typically white males 50 to 60 years of age who have a history of smoking and chronic obstructive pulmonary disease (COPD). The second group consists primarily of women 60 to 70 years of age who have bronchiectasis documented with computed tomography. Both groups tend to come from rural settings. Pulmonary infection due to MAC presents a variable picture similar to tuberculosis, but usually with less intensity. The symptoms include productive cough, weakness, fatigue, mild fever, and hemoptysis. Chest films in the first group of patients (underlying COPD) typically show upper lobe cavitation that mimics tuberculosis. The second group of patients have reticulonodular interstitial disease that involves the middle lung fields and upper lobes, but usually without cavitation. On computed tomography scan, clusters of small nodules as well as bronchiectasis are most often seen. Infection with MAC results in a chronic and indolent illness that is slowly progressive when it goes untreated. A few severely ill patients may experience massive hemoptysis, respiratory failure, and death.

Table 2. Common Clinical Syndromes Due to Nontuberculous Mycobacteria

Cervical lymphadenitis
Chronic pulmonary disease
Disseminated disease
Post-traumatic wound infections
Postsurgical wound infections

Patients who develop pulmonary infection due to *M. kansasii* tend to be white, middle-aged, urban males whose presentation is typically indistinguishable from pulmonary tuberculosis but is typically milder. Approximately half of these patients have underlying COPD; many have thin-walled cavitation on chest film. Most patients respond to antibiotics, whereas untreated illness is progressive and can result in massive hemoptysis, respiratory failure, and death.

Pulmonary infection due to RGM (*M. abscessus,* 82 per cent; *M. fortuitum,* 13 per cent) occurs most commonly in nonsmoking middle-aged, white females. Two thirds of these women have pre-existing conditions such as previous mycobacterial lung infections, cystic fibrosis, and lipoid pneumonia. Like the second group of patients with MAC, most patients with no apparent underlying disease have (undiagnosed) bronchiectasis. RGM infection produces an indolent lung disease: patients present initially with only cough. Because the radiographic features are not typical of tuberculosis, sputum cultures are often not obtained and found positive until 2 years after the first symptoms appear. Compared with tuberculosis, the fever, weight loss, sputum production, hemoptysis, and dyspnea of RGM infection are less severe and present much later in the course of disease. Chest films typically show bilateral, reticulonodular upper lobe infiltrates; cavitation is noted in 16 per cent of patients with RGM infection. These features are quite similar to the second group of patients with MAC, and approximately 15 per cent of patients known to have either *M. abscessus* or MAC infection subsequently manifest coinfection with the other microbe (Table 3).

Laboratory diagnosis of NTM lung disease is most often accomplished by isolating the organism from multiple sputum specimens. Acid-fast stains of NTM compare favorably with those of *M. tuberculosis. Mycobacterium kansasii* and *M. marinum* may be suspected by their larger and more beaded microscopic appearance. However, definitive diagnosis of species cannot be made solely by acid-fast microscopy, which has a sensitivity of 60 per cent and depends on the quality of sputum collection, slide preparation, laboratory experience, and the amount of time dedicated for slide examination. Fluorescence acid-fast microscopy, which uses the fluorescent dyes auramine and/or rhodamine, offers higher sensitivities than those of carbolfuchsin (e.g., Kinyoun stain) in detecting mycobacteria. Cytocentrifugation (Cyto-Tek, Ames Division, Miles Laboratories, Inc., Elkhart, IN), a new technique for identifying acid-fast organisms on smear, concentrates the liquefied and decontaminated sputum specimen. Early reports suggest that this technique is rapid and efficient, with a sensitivity approaching 100 per cent.

Table 3. Common Clinical Signs and Symptoms of NTM Wound Infections

Serous, watery drainage
Sinus tract formation
Delay of 3 to 6 weeks from injury to clinical disease
Absent systemic signs or symptoms
Normal host
History of penetrating trauma

NTM = nontuberculous mycobacteria.

Nontuberculous mycobacteria can be isolated by culture on standard tuberculosis media. For each sample, laboratories should employ at least one liquid (or broth) medium (e.g., Middlebrook 7H9) and one solid medium (either Löwenstein-Jensen egg-potato or Middlebrook 7H10/7H11 with soluble nutrients). Positive cultures can be observed in 2 to 3 weeks for slow-growing NTM and 2 to 5 days for rapid-growing NTM. By contrast, the BACTEC broth system (Becton-Dickinson, Sparks, MD) facilitates recovery of slow-growing NTM in 5 to 10 days, and RGM in 2 to 5 days. BACTEC detects radiolabeled carbon dioxide produced by mycobacterial metabolism of a labeled broth substrate. The disadvantages of BACTEC include the carbon dioxide, the use of radioactive materials, the cost of the substrate, and the need for a carbon dioxide instrument. Another culture system, BBL MGIT (Mycobacteria Growth Indicator Tube, Becton Dickinson Microbiology Systems, Cockeysville, MD), may also offer rapid diagnosis (comparable to the BACTEC System) with high accuracy. This system has not been fully evaluated, but it may offer a more "user-friendly" technique. The loss of oxygen from broth due to mycobacterial growth is detected by a substrate that fluoresces. This method could allow more laboratories to utilize a rapid broth culture system for the mycobacteria.

While the NTM as a group have culture and staining properties similar to those of *M. tuberculosis*, certain NTM exhibit different growth requirements. *Mycobacterium marinum, M. chelonae,* and *M. haemophilum* (all cutaneous pathogens) grow at lower temperatures (28°C to 32°C), and *M. haemophilum* requires iron or hemin in its culture medium for growth. *Mycobacterium xenopi* grows optimally at 42°C. *Mycobacterium genavense*, a newly described NTM that causes disseminated disease in AIDS, is reliably recovered only in broth media, such as BACTEC 13A medium, and then only after incubation for 4 to 12 weeks.

Even more rapid techniques for the identification of NTM are undergoing evaluation. Commercially available DNA probes for *M. tuberculosis,* MAC, *M. kansasii,* and *M. gordonae* allow species identification within 2 hours. These probes are used by numerous laboratories. Other new technologies include the polymerase chain reaction (PCR) of sputum samples for mycobacterial specific gene sequences, and PCR of selected gene sequences followed by restriction endonuclease digestion of grown cultures that allows species identification by restriction fragment length polymorphism (RFLP) patterns within 24 hours (neither are yet commercial). By contrast, skin tests are not helpful in diagnosing NTM infection because many people who do not have disease test positive because of environmental exposure.

Because certain NTM are commonly encountered as contaminants or colonizers, isolation of the NTM is not necessarily diagnostic of NTM infection. This fact is especially true for pulmonary disease, in which NTM such as *M. terrae* complex, *M. fortuitum, M. scrofulaceum,* and *M. gordonae* are commonly isolated from sputum specimens but may not represent the etiologic agents of disease. When NTM are recovered from normally sterile tissue or body fluid such as liver, spleen, blood, bone marrow, and spinal fluid, the likelihood of colonization is much less, but contamination is still possible. Factors that increase the likelihood that the isolated NTM represents real infection include the following: a clinical illness compatible with that reported for the species of NTM isolated; an abnormal chest film not otherwise explained; the presence of an acid-fast organism on smear, especially in high numbers (2+ to 4+); and the isolation of the NTM from multiple samples. Most physicians require two positive cultures to make a diagnosis of disease caused by NTM. However, when *M. kansasii* is isolated from a single sputum, the presence of true infection is strongly suggested because this organism rarely occurs as a contaminant. However, even with *M. kansasii,* two or more positive sputum specimens are preferred for definitive diagnosis.

Cutaneous Infections

Cutaneous disease due to NTM often occurs in the normal host who sustains a penetrating injury to an extremity. Signs and symptoms of NTM infection may arise at the site of trauma as early as 1 month or as late as 6 months following the incident. Skin and soft tissue infection from NTM most commonly involves *M. fortuitum, M. abscessus, M. chelonae, M. marinum, M. haemophilum,* and *M. ulcerans* (in geographic areas where this organism occurs). These local infections present as abscesses, granulomas, diffuse inflammations, cellulitis with draining fistulas, and rheumatoidlike nodules.

The diagnosis of skin and soft tissue NTM infection is made by isolating the organism from the lesion by vigorous swabbing; tissue biopsy is usually not necessary. A single positive culture is acceptable for diagnosis. Skin infections with RGM are often nosocomial and may be associated with long-term intravenous catheters, cardiac bypass, and other surgery. RGM may cause either single or clustered outbreaks, especially in the southern coastal United States. Of note, 80 per cent of RGM infections of the breast and sternum are due to *M. fortuitum*.

Skin disease due to *M. marinum* most commonly arises from trauma that occurs in swimming pools, fishtanks, and freshwater or saltwater aquariums. Infection with *M. marinum* may also follow exposure to fish or other aquatic animals. The fingers, hands, elbows, and knees are commonly involved. Patients typically present with granulomatous-type lesions, reddish nodules, papules, pustules, or ulcerative lesions resembling sporotrichosis. Symptoms usually occur about 3 to 8 weeks after trauma and/or exposure, with a range of 10 days to 2 years. The prognosis for recovery is excellent; 80 per cent of *M. marinum* infections resolve spontaneously within 36 months. Almost all cases remain localized, but deep tissue involvement, especially involving the synovia, does occur.

Localized bone and joint infection due to NTM arises independently, usually following trauma, and is not the result of disseminated disease. The most commonly isolated organisms are *M. kansasii,* MAC, *M. marinum,* and RGM. These infections tend to produce chronic, indolent, and localized (not systemic) lesions. When draining, the fluid may appear more serous than purulent. The sites involved in NTM bone and joint infection include the knees, wrists, fingers, elbows, feet or ankles, spine, and long bones. The diagnosis of NTM infection often requires biopsy with histology and culture, but sometimes the NTM may be recovered from the culture of joint fluid alone.

Systemic Infection

Disseminated NTM infection occurs mostly in AIDS patients and is relatively rare in other clinical settings. Among patients who do not have AIDS, disseminated disease is seen usually in the immunocompromised and rarely in normal hosts. The diagnosis is made when the NTM are isolated from cultures of blood, bone marrow, and other body fluids. The most common isolates in disseminated NTM disease (in the absence of AIDS) are *M. kansasii, M. chelonae, M. haemophilum,* and *M. genavense.* Disseminated diseases due to *M. kansasii, M. chelonae,* and *M. haemophilum* tend to present with multiple skin nodules or abscesses. *M. chelonae,* the most commonly encountered disseminated RGM, is seen almost exclusively in patients receiving immunosuppressive drugs, especially low-dose corticosteroids.

Disseminated disease due to RGM has been described in three clinical forms. Patients in group 1 receive low-dose corticosteroids for collagen-vascular disease or chronic renal disease. Ninety per cent develop *M. chelonae* infection, and none have been known to have immunodeficiency. These patients have disseminated skin disease with few systemic symptoms.

Group 2 patients are immunodeficient or have leukemia or lymphoma. These patients develop severe multiorgan disease that often requires intensive therapy. The severity of the signs and symptoms in the third group falls in between these first two groups of patients.

Lymph node infection with NTM is most common in children 1 to 10 years of age, who typically present with unilateral and often painless cervical, submandibular, submaxillary, and/or preauricular lymphadenopathy. MAC and *M. scrofulaceum* are the most commonly recovered NTM that infect lymph nodes. Adult mycobacterial lymph node disease is most often (90 per cent) due to *M. tuberculosis* infection rather than NTM.

In NTM lymphadenitis, the causative organism can be isolated in only 50 to 75 per cent of patients. A presumptive diagnosis may occasionally be made when biopsy material shows granulomas despite a failure to isolate either *M. tuberculosis* or NTM. The use of newer diagnostic techniques such as PCR with DNA sequencing or restriction endonuclease analysis may improve the frequency of identification of causative NTM in the future. Complete excisional biopsies are preferred to partial biopsies because complete removal of nodes can be curative and may prevent the development of chronic fistulas and drainage. Although some infections resolve spontaneously, most lymph nodes undergo necrosis and chronically drain. The diseases to be distinguished from NTM lymphadenitis include infectious mononucleosis, brucellosis, tularemia, fungal infections, tuberculosis, sarcoidosis, cat-scratch disease, and malignancy.

DISSEMINATED INFECTION IN AIDS PATIENTS

Disseminated disease due to MAC (DMAC) and, much less frequently, to *M. kansasii, M. xenopi, M. haemophilum, M. celatum,* and *M. genavense* is a common occurrence in patients with AIDS. More than 50 per cent of AIDS patients develop DMAC 30 months after their diagnosis; DMAC occurs late in the course of the AIDS illness. In these patients, a major risk of DMAC infection exists when their CD4 cell counts fall below 60 cells per cm^3. Infection due to MAC is now the most common bacterial infection in AIDS and the most common mycobacterial infection in the United States.

Since DMAC occurs late in the course of AIDS, patients with DMAC present with symptoms and signs that overlap other AIDS-related illnesses. Fever, weight loss, malaise, anemia, and neutropenia are commonly reported with DMAC. Other overlapping problems include chronic diarrhea, abdominal pain, and jaundice due to extrabiliary obstruction (periportal lymphadenopathy). Occasionally, patients with DMAC (positive blood cultures for MAC) are initially asymptomatic.

The occurrence of DMAC parallels the distribution of AIDS in the United States and does not distribute according to the geographic-environmental pattern seen with MAC infection in the non-AIDS population. Furthermore, the prevalence of DMAC infection is not influenced by race, sex, ethnicity, or risk behavior. These patterns of disease distribution are the same for Europe and Australia. However, for reasons that are unclear, MAC infection is rarely encountered in African nations, despite the great prevalence of AIDS seen in these countries.

The current diagnosis of DMAC is most often made through a positive blood culture. The diagnosis can also be made with more invasive procedures that result in recovery of MAC from other normally sterile body tissues and fluids, such as bone marrow, liver, spleen, lymph node, and cerebrospinal fluid. The significance of stool and sputum cultures that grow MAC when blood cultures are negative is controversial because only two thirds of patients with such findings subsequently develop DMAC. Stool and sputum cultures frequently become positive at the same time as do blood cultures. Blood cultures are commonly positive for MAC when MAC is isolated from biopsy specimens as well. Rapid diagnosis of DMAC can be expected when acid-fast organisms are identified on Kinyoun carbolfuchsin–stained or auramine-stained buffy-coat blood smears.

Infection with *M. kansasii* is the second most commonly occurring NTM infection in AIDS patients but is far less common than MAC. Patients present with pulmonary infections, extrapulmonary infections, and mycobacteremia or disseminated disease. Chest films typically show focal or diffuse interstitial upper lobe infiltrates with thin-walled cavities in fewer than one third of cases. Extrapulmonary disease involves the bone or gastrointestinal tract. Isolation of *M. kansasii* in blood or even sputum is usually diagnostic of infection because the organism is rarely recovered as a contaminant. Most patients with localized pulmonary disease respond to antibiotic therapy, but patients with widespread disseminated disease often do not, and this illness can be the cause of death in patients with AIDS.

Mycobacterium xenopi is the next most commonly recovered pathogenic NTM in AIDS patients. It is prevalent in southeast England, Canada, and Brooklyn, New York, and is associated with hospital hot water systems. While some isolates represent nonpathogens, others cause pulmonary disease and rarely bacteremia in AIDS patients, with mortality in some cases.

Disseminated infection due to *M. haemophilum* has been reported in patients infected with the human immunodeficiency virus (HIV), especially in New York City. As with DMAC, the CD4 cell counts are markedly depressed. *Mycobacterium genavense* and *M. celatum* are two newly recognized NTM that also cause illness in patients with AIDS.

Disease due to RGM is rarely associated with HIV infection. Almost all of the few (less than 15) cases reported involve *M. fortuitum* complex organisms isolated from lymph nodes, blood, or pleural fluid.

LEPROSY (HANSEN'S DISEASE)

By Leo J. Yoder, M.D.
Carville, Louisiana

Leprosy (Hansen's disease) is a chronic mycobacterial infection of humans that involves primarily the skin and peripheral nerves. In some patients, organs such as the eyes, nose, testicles, and bone may be involved. The causative agent, *Mycobacterium leprae,* was first described by Armauer Hansen in 1873, but even today a number of significant unanswered questions remain. *Mycobacterium leprae* still has not been cultured in vitro. The mode of transmission, the sources of infection, and the nature of the immune defect in susceptible individuals are still not well defined. The stigma associated with the disease persists in most nations of the world, including the United States. Despite these problems, research has now rendered leprosy a treatable and curable disease. In the last decade, the prevalence of the disease has decreased dramatically. The incidence may also be decreasing, albeit more slowly. Worldwide, approximately 600,000 new cases are reported annually, while in the United States, about 200 new cases are reported each year.

Leprosy is an immunologic disorder as well as a bacterial infection. More than 95 per cent of individuals possess natural immunity to this disease, whereas 3 to 5 per cent of any population have a defect in the cell-mediated immune response that is specific for *M. leprae,* thereby increasing the risk of onset of disease following exposure of these persons to the bacteria. The immune defect is variable and thus results in a spectrum of clinical disease. At one end is localized disease, with one or two skin lesions and relatively few bacteria (tuberculoid [TT]). At the other end is diffuse disease, with many lesions and a large number of bacteria (lepromatous [LL]). Tuberculoid patients have a high degree of cell-mediated immunity to *M. leprae,* whereas lepromatous patients have no cell-mediated response to the bacteria. Between the polar tuberculoid and lepromatous forms is a broad range of disease known as borderline leprosy. The widely recognized Ridley-Jopling classification divides the borderline group into three additional classifications and an indeterminate (I) group. The complete classification of leprosy then has six categories, indeterminate (I), tuberculoid (TT), borderline tuberculoid (BT), midborderline (BB), borderline lepromatous (BL), and lepromatous (LL). Most patients fall somewhere in the borderline range. The Ridley-Jopling classification is useful for research and clinical studies but is generally too complex for routine patient management. For treatment purposes, patients are classified into two groups: paucibacillary (PB), which includes I, TT, and BT, and multibacillary (MB), which includes BB, BL, and LL.

CLINICAL PRESENTATION

Early leprosy most often presents with a slowly evolving skin lesion. Usually no itching, pain, or burning is present, and the patient may be unaware of the lesion. Lepromatous changes often cannot be distinguished from other disorders by mere visual examination of the skin. Thus, the clinician should look for sensory loss, anhidrosis, or hair loss in a lesion that does not respond to the usual treatments for common skin disorders. The presence of skin lesions plus a sensory or motor deficit in a hand or foot strongly suggests leprosy. Rarely, however, the disease presents as a peripheral neuropathy with no skin lesions.

The earliest skin lesion is indeterminate (I)—most often a single hypopigmented macule with minimal sensory loss. Detection of indeterminate lesions is rare in the United States because the diagnosis is usually not made until the disease has progressed to a more definitive stage. Even a biopsy may be inconclusive at the indeterminate stage.

Tuberculoid (TT) leprosy presents as one or two macules or plaques that may be hypopigmented or erythematous. The lesions are well defined, and there is diminished sensation or even complete anesthesia within the lesion. These early changes can appear almost anywhere, including the face, extremities, and buttocks. Peripheral nerves in the area of the skin lesions may also be involved. Borderline tuberculoid (BT) lesions are similar to tuberculoid lesions but are more numerous and may be larger. BT lesions have diminished sensation; peripheral nerves in the area of the skin lesions may be enlarged or tender. Often, BT lesions have a healing center with the most active process at the edge. Larger BT lesions often have smaller satellite lesions. More numerous are midborderline (BB) lesions, which are raised, well-defined, and inflamed erythematous plaques with punched-out centers and donut-shaped morphology. BB disease is considered a rare, unstable immunologic state; most patients eventually shift toward either BT or BL disease.

Borderline lepromatous (BL) patients have numerous and varied skin changes ranging from large, well-defined lesions to vague, ill-defined macules. Some lesions have sensory loss, whereas others do not, and there is often a wide range of sizes of lesions in the same patient. Multiple peripheral nerves may be involved, often asymmetrically. The presentation in lepromatous (LL) leprosy is also quite variable and usually generalized. The skin lesions may be disseminated, faint, hypopigmented, hyperpigmented, or erythematous macules. In other patients, there may be a generalized papular or nodular eruption or a diffuse skin infiltration with no distinct lesions. Early in LL disease, there may be no sensory changes in the skin. Later, sensation may decrease in the distal extremities and may progress to near-total body anesthesia, sparing only the warmer regions, such as the axillae and groin. The peripheral neuropathy that develops late in LL disease may also lead to motor loss, with clawhands, clawtoes, or footdrop. In advanced LL, there may be loss of eyebrows, lagophthalmos with insensitive cornea, nasal stuffiness with septal perforation, collapse of the bridge of the nose, epistaxis, hoarseness, and the classic "leonine" facies.

The most serious aspect of all types of leprosy is the peripheral neuropathy. Neuritis may not be clinically evident in all new patients, but aggressive attempts to detect it should nevertheless be made. The commonly involved mixed nerves are the ulnar nerve at the elbow, the median nerve at the wrist, the peroneal nerve just below the knee, the posterior tibial nerve just behind the medial malleolus, and the upper portion of the facial nerve. Rarely, the radial nerve can be affected in the upper arm and produce a wristdrop. Although not of major functional significance, the radial cutaneous nerve at the wrist is the most commonly enlarged nerve in leprosy. This finding can be important in confirming the diagnosis. The earliest sign of peripheral nerve damage is the loss of sweating in the palms of the hands or the soles of the feet. This sign is followed by decreased sensation and mild intrinsic muscle weakness in the hands. Later, intrinsic muscle atrophy and paralysis of the hands, or footdrop and clawtoes in the lower extremities, may develop. Mild to severe lagophthalmos indicates damage to the facial nerve. (Paralysis of the orbicularis oculi muscle suggests damage to the zygomatic branch of the facial nerve.)

As many as 50 per cent of patients develop acute reactions at some time during the course of the illness. These reactions are most common after treatment has begun, but they may also be a presenting symptom. Acute reactions are immunologic disorders with acute skin eruptions and occasionally serious nerve and eye problems. These reactions are sometimes confused with acute or chronic febrile illnesses, such as sepsis and rheumatoid arthritis. The reactions are of two main types. Type 1, or reversal reaction, can occur in all borderline patients. A cell-mediated immune response to *M. leprae,* reversal reaction presents as erythema, edema, and tenderness of previously existing skin lesions accompanied by edema of the extremities, enlarged and painful nerves, and evidence of nerve damage in the extremities. Type 2 reaction, or erythema nodosum leprosum (ENL), is a humoral immune disorder that occurs only in BL and LL patients. ENL presents with fever and crops of erythematous painful nodules in previously normal skin. If the disease goes untreated, new crops of nodules will appear as the older ones fade away. The severity ranges from a few nodules to an extensive eruption with an acute toxic illness. Edema of the extremities is common; some lesions are plaquelike and may ulcerate. Associated findings include neuritis, iridocyclitis, lymphadenitis, orchitis, and arthritis. Leukocytosis is common. The most serious complication of both types of reactions is nerve damage. Therefore, the evaluation of nerves is very important in managing patients with such reactions.

DIAGNOSIS

The diagnosis of leprosy relies primarily on the history and physical examination. Rarely is the diagnosis made with laboratory studies in the absence of physical findings. The cardinal signs include anesthetic skin lesions, enlarged peripheral nerves, and acid-fast bacilli (AFB) in skin smears and biopsies. The examination for leprosy should focus on five major areas: the skin, nerves, hands, feet, and eyes. Examine the skin of the entire body in good light. Document the size, number, and character of the lesions. Use nylon monofilaments, wisps of cotton, and pinprick to test for loss of light touch or pain sensation. The loss of light touch in the skin lesion may be the earliest sign of leprosy. The examination of peripheral nerves should focus on nerve enlargement and tenderness. Palpate the great auricular nerve in the neck, the ulnar nerve at the elbow, the radial cutaneous nerve at the wrist, the peroneal nerve at the lateral aspect of the knee, and the posterior tibial nerve behind the medial malleolus.

Examine the hands and feet for loss of sweating and for loss of sensation to light touch or pain. Look for weakness of the intrinsic muscles of the hand. In advanced cases, the clinician may observe intrinsic muscle atrophy with claw deformity. In the lower extremities, look for footdrop and clawtoes. Again, remember that the major nerve damage occurs in the distal extremities. In general, the large muscles of the arms and legs are not involved except for rare wristdrop due to radial nerve damage. Finally, examine the eyes for lagophthalmos and signs of scleritis or iritis.

LABORATORY STUDIES

The two laboratory procedures most useful for routine diagnosis of leprosy are skin smears and skin biopsies. Skin smears are obtained by pinching a fold of skin to diminish blood flow, wiping the area with an alcohol sponge, and making a small slit about 5 mm long and 3 mm deep into the dermis with a sterile scalpel (e.g., size 15 Bard-Parker blade). The slit is gently scraped, and the tissue fluid expressed is smeared on a microscopic slide. Bacilli are most abundant on the cool areas of the skin, such as the earlobes. In the United States, the routine skin smear sites are the ears, elbows, and knees. However, in new patients, additional smears can be obtained from active or suspected skin lesions regardless of location. Smears are usually negative in I and BT patients, mildly positive in BB patients, and strongly positive in BL and LL patients. Skin smears should be analyzed in all patients who may have leprosy. Negative smears, however, do not exclude the diagnosis. Those patients with positive sites should have smears repeated at least annually to monitor the clearance of bacilli.

Skin smears are stained for AFB with the Fite modification of the Ziehl-Neelsen stain. AFB are quantified in each smear with the use of a semilogarithmic scale called the bacterial index (BI), which ranges from 0 to 6+ (as shown in Table 1). The percentage of intact, solid-staining bacilli is also documented as the morphologic index (MI), which typically ranges from 1 to 5 per cent in the newly diagnosed multibacillary patient. The MI reasonably correlates with viability and should become 0 within 3 to 6 months after the start of therapy. The BI decreases from 0.5+ to 1+ per year.

Biopsies are not always required in the diagnosis of leprosy. In areas of the world where leprosy is common, most patients are not biopsied. However, in the United States, where the disease is rare, all patients should have at least an initial biopsy taken within the margin of the chosen lesion and fixed in 10 per cent formalin. Some sections are stained with hematoxylin-eosin, and others with a modified Fite-Ferraco stain for AFB. Biopsies should be evaluated by workers familiar with the histopathology of leprosy. A positive diagnosis requires the presence of AFB or evidence of nerve involvement.

Mycobacterium leprae cannot be cultured in the laboratory. In specialized centers, the bacteria are injected into mouse footpads for drug sensitivity studies. However, this is not required for routine case management. Several serologic tests have been studied as possible aids to diagnosis. The most important is antibody to phenolic glycolipid 1 (PGL-1), the immunologically specific outer surface component of the leprosy bacillus. Although PGL-1 antibody tests are invariably positive in new multibacillary patients, they are negative in about 50 per cent of paucibacillary persons. Moreover, antibody levels vary widely among patients and are not generally useful in diagnosis and management. The polymerase chain reaction is very specific, but its sensitivity is unacceptably low in cases with relatively few bacteria. At present, these tests remain research tools.

The lepromin test (intradermal injection of autoclaved bacilli from human lepromas) is not a diagnostic test, and the skin test material is not commercially available. A positive lepromin reaction indicates that an individual is able to mount a cell-mediated immune response to *M. leprae*. The test is generally positive in TT and BT patients and negative or weakly positive in LL and BL patients. The lepromin reaction is also positive in nearly all normal

Table 1. The Bacterial Index (BI)

0	No bacilli in 100 OIF
1+	1–10 bacilli per 100 OIF
2+	1–10 bacilli per 10 OIF
3+	1–10 bacilli per OIF
4+	10–100 bacilli per OIF
5+	100–1000 bacilli per OIF
6+	More than 1000 bacilli per OIF

OIF = oil immersion fields.

adults. The test may help classify the occasional patient who may be difficult to classify with the usual methods.

DIFFERENTIAL DIAGNOSIS

The list of possibilities in the differential diagnoses of leprosy includes fungal infections, allergies, and various other hypopigmented, hyperpigmented, and erythematous lesions of the skin. Many of these can be excluded by the history and physical examination and the evidence of nerve involvement. When uncertainty remains, skin smears and biopsies often provide the answer. Other diagnoses in patients who have, or are suspected of having, leprosy include sarcoidosis, rheumatoid arthritis, allergies of undetermined etiology, lymphomatoid granulomatosis, cutaneous leishmaniasis, carpal tunnel syndrome, and nasal obstruction. Among the most difficult patients are those with a single or a few hypopigmented macules but no other confirmatory findings and an inconclusive biopsy. Here it is best to simply recheck the patient periodically for 3 to 6 months for signs of progression. When there is strong suspicion of leprosy neuropathy in the absence of skin lesions, a nerve biopsy can occasionally be helpful. The nerves most often biopsied are the radial cutaneous nerve at the wrist and the sural nerve at the ankle. It deserves emphasis that the clinician should not make a diagnosis of leprosy unless objective evidence of the disease is documented. Therapeutic trials are not recommended.

When a case of leprosy is confirmed, the members of the patient's immediate household should be evaluated. Is there a history of visible skin lesions or symptoms of sensory changes in the hands or feet? Because early skin lesions may be very subtle, a careful and complete skin examination is required. A brief examination of nerves, hands, feet, and eyes, as outlined earlier, should also be undertaken. If there are any suspicious skin lesions, skin smears and biopsies should be obtained. These evaluations should be done every year for 5 years after the index case is detected. Early detection means early treatment that may prevent the onset of permanent disability.

Information and consultation regarding the diagnosis and management of leprosy, including evaluation of biopsies and/or skin smears, can be obtained by contacting the Clinical Branch at Gillis W. Long Hansen's Disease Center, U.S. Public Health Service, Carville, Louisiana 70721 (1-800-642-2477).

Viral Diseases

ACQUIRED IMMUNODEFICIENCY SYNDROME (AIDS)

By Jeffrey Rapp, M.D.,
and R. Michael Buckley, M.D.
Philadelphia, Pennsylvania

The acquired immunodeficiency syndrome (AIDS) is the most advanced stage of an infectious disease process caused by the human immunodeficiency virus (HIV). The spectrum of disease caused by HIV ranges from an asymptomatic state to total destruction of the immune system and may take more than 10 years to manifest itself clinically. As the progression of immunosuppression accelerates, patients infected with HIV become more susceptible to infections, malignancies, and other life-threatening illnesses. HIV has a predilection for cells that have a CD4 molecule on their membrane. The most vulnerable of these cells includes the CD4 T lymphocyte ("CD4 cells," or "T cells"), but other cells include monocytes-macrophages, megakaryocytes, cells found in lymph nodes, cells within the central nervous system, cervical cells, renal epithelial cells, cardiac myocytes, and retinal cells. The Centers for Disease Control and Prevention (CDC) case definition of AIDS includes the following signs, symptoms, infections, malignancies, and other disease entities (Table 1).

Human immunodeficiency virus has been transmitted most commonly through sexual contact, but other modes of transmission have included mother-to-fetus or mother-to-child transmission (in utero, peripartum, breast-feeding), intravenous drug use, transfusion of contaminated blood products, and occasionally nosocomial spread via needlestick or other routes. Because there is currently no cure for HIV infection, emphasis has been placed on prevention of transmission. Condom use and other "safer sex" practices have unequivocally decreased the spread of other sexually transmitted diseases within the gay community, and the rate of new HIV infections among white gay men may have plateaued. Antenatal and perinatal use of the antiretroviral, zidovudine (AZT), reduces vertical transmission of HIV by over 70 per cent. Communities in which clean needles are provided for intravenous drug users seem to show a decrease in HIV transmission in select populations. Finally, routine screening of all blood products since the mid-1980s has dramatically decreased the incidence of transfusion-related HIV transmission.

CLINICAL MANIFESTATIONS OF HIV INFECTION

Many cases of acute HIV infection go undetected. However, 50 to 65 per cent of patients develop an acute retroviral syndrome within 1 to 6 weeks following exposure to HIV. This syndrome is nonspecific and variable and resembles acute mononucleosis, with fever, night sweats, malaise, anorexia, sore throat, and gastrointestinal symptoms (Table 2). Cervical, occipital, and axillary lymphadenopathy may be noted, along with rashes ranging from morbilliform exanthem to frank urticaria. Hepatosplenomegaly, oropharyngeal ulcers, or candidiasis may be accompanied by lymphopenia, an increased erythrocyte sedimentation rate, a negative Monospot (horse cell) test, and abnormal liver function tests. Because the acute retroviral syndrome develops soon after exposure to HIV, antibodies may not be detected at that point (see later). Rather, an HIV core protein, p24, can be detected in the blood as early as 2 weeks after exposure. The differential diagnosis of the acute retroviral syndrome includes infectious mononucleosis, influenza, measles, rubella, and secondary syphilis.

Following the acute retroviral syndrome, a decade may pass before the patient progresses clinically to AIDS. In the interim, relatively nondescript signs and symptoms often do not point directly to HIV infection. Thus, a high index of suspicion must be maintained to make the diagnosis (Table 3). However, nearly every organ system may be involved at any point during the disease process, especially as the patient becomes more immunocompromised. What follows is an overview by organ system of various clinical manifestations of HIV infection.

Persistent Generalized Lymphadenopathy

Persistent generalized lymphadenopathy (PGL) occurs in more than 50 per cent of HIV-positive patients. It often follows the acute retroviral syndrome and may persist throughout the patient's life, although involution of the nodes may signal progression to the later stages of infection. Cervical, submandibular, occipital, and axillary nodes may be involved. Epitrochlear and femoral lymphadenopathies have been reported. The lymphadenopathy is usually bilateral, painless, and symmetric, with each node measuring 0.5 to 2.0 cm. Biopsy generally reveals benign follicular hyperplasia.

Table 1. Conditions Included in the 1993 AIDS Surveillance Case Definition

Condition
Bacterial infections, multiple or recurrent[1]
Bacillary angiomatosis[3]
CD4+ T-lymphocyte counts of <200, or $<14\%$[2]
Candidiasis of bronchi, trachea, or lungs
Candidiasis, esophageal
Candidiasis, oropharyngeal (thrush)[3]
Candidiasis, vulvovaginal; persistent, frequent, or poorly responsive to therapy[3]
Cervical cancer, invasive[2]
Cervical dysplasia (moderate or severe)[3]
Coccidioidomycosis, disseminated or extrapulmonary
Constitutional symptoms, such as fever (38.5°C) or diarrhea lasting >1 month[3]
Cryptococcosis, extrapulmonary
Cryptosporidiosis, chronic intestinal (>1 month's duration)
Cytomegalovirus disease (other than liver, spleen, or nodes)
Cytomegalovirus retinitis (with loss of vision)
Encephalopathy, HIV-related
Hairy leukoplakia, oral[3]
Herpes simplex viral infection: chronic ulcer or ulcers (>1 month's duration); or bronchitis, pneumonitis, or esophagitis
Herpes zoster infection (shingles), involving at least two distinct episodes or more than one dermatome[3]
Histoplasmosis, disseminated or extrapulmonary
Idiopathic thrombocytopenic purpura[3]
Isosporiasis, chronic intestinal (>1 month's duration)
Kaposi's sarcoma
Listeriosis[3]
Lymphoid interstitial pneumonia and/or pulmonary lymphoid hyperplasia[1]
Lymphoma, Burkitt's (or equivalent term)
Lymphoma, immunoblastic (or equivalent term)
Lymphoma, primary, of brain
Mycobacterium avium-intracellulare complex or *M. kansasii* infection, disseminated or extrapulmonary
Mycobacterium tuberculosis infection, any site (pulmonary[2] or extrapulmonary)
Mycobacterium infection, other species or unidentified species, disseminated or extrapulmonary
Pelvic inflammatory disease, particularly if complicated by tubo-ovarian abscess[3]
Peripheral neuropathy[3]
Pneumocystis carinii pneumonia
Pneumonia, recurrent[2]
Progressive multifocal leukoencephalopathy
Salmonella septicemia, recurrent
Toxoplasmosis of brain
Wasting syndrome due to HIV

[1]Children younger than 13 years of age.
[2]Added in the 1993 expansion of the AIDS Surveillance Case Definition for Adolescents and Adults (MMWR 1992; vol. 41, RR-17).
[3]Must occur with CD4+ T-lymphocyte counts <200 cells/μL.

Table 2. Frequency (%) of Signs and Symptoms Associated with the Acute Retroviral Syndrome

Sign/Symptom	%
Fever	96
Adenopathy	74
Pharyngitis	70
Rash	70
Myalgia or arthralgia	54
Thrombocytopenia	45
Leukopenia	38
Diarrhea	32
Headache	32
Nausea, vomiting	27
Elevated aminotransferases	21
Hepatosplenomegaly	14
Thrush	12
Neuropathy	6
Encephalopathy	6

Constitutional Symptoms

The constitutional symptoms that accompany HIV infection become increasingly common as the degree of immunosuppression increases. Intermittent periods of malaise, fatigue, anorexia, weight loss, and low-grade fevers are described by many patients throughout the course of their infection, with escalation as CD4 counts drop below 200 cells/μL. However, attributing all constitutional symptoms solely to HIV can be misleading. More than half of HIV-infected patients who present with fever have definable causes, such as sinusitis, pneumonia, cytomegaloviral infection, and *Mycobacterium avium-intracellulare* (MAI).

Hematologic Complications

The hematologic complications of HIV infection include idiopathic thrombocytopenic purpura (ITP) due to peripheral destruction of platelets. Of note, HIV replication may occur in megakaryocytes. Thrombocytopenia may occur anytime after initial infection and may respond to antiretrovirals alone. Other nonspecific hematologic complications include anemia (most commonly normocytic, normochromic) and lymphopenia.

Oral Disease

Oral disease is common during all stages of HIV infection. The acute retroviral syndrome may be accompanied

Table 3. Symptoms That May Alert the Clinician to Occult HIV Infection

Symptom
Candidiasis, oropharyngeal
Candidiasis, vulvovaginal; persistent, frequent, or poorly responsive to therapy
Diarrhea, persistent, lasting >1 month
Mycobacterium tuberculosis infection
Pelvic inflammatory disease, particularly if complicated by tubo-ovarian abscess
Wasting syndrome

by aphthous stomatitis and mucocutaneous candidiasis. These manifestations are usually short-lived, and many patients remain asymptomatic while CD4 counts remain greater than 300 cells/μL. However, with the decline of immune function, the incidence of oral disease increases. Oral candidiasis, or "thrush," may be the first indication that immunosuppression has progressed to the point where other opportunistic infections may now occur. For this reason, many clinicians begin prophylaxis against *Pneumocystis carinii* pneumonia (PCP) at the first sign of thrush, except during the acute retroviral syndrome. Other common oral manifestations of advancing HIV infection include aphthous stomatitis (ulcers of unknown etiology), increasing frequency and severity of herpes simplex stomatitis, oral hairy leukoplakia (secondary to Epstein-Barr viral infection), and gingivitis-periodontitis.

Gastrointestinal Syndromes

Gastrointestinal syndromes, related to both routine gut pathophysiology and opportunistic infection, present significant challenges. In particular, chronic gastroenteritis with persistent prolonged diarrhea not only may severely compromise the quality of life but also may cause profound malnutrition and weight loss. Infections of the lower gastrointestinal tract with *Salmonella, Cryptosporidium, Isospora,* cytomegalovirus, and microsporidia occur more frequently in HIV-infected patients, and the role of *Clostridium difficile, Giardia,* and *Entamoeba* cannot be overstated. Despite aggressive work-ups, however, the etiology of some lower gastrointestinal disorders in AIDS remains elusive. An AIDS-associated enteropathy may account for some cases, but the pathophysiology of this entity is poorly understood.

Candida esophagitis is the most common infection in the upper gastrointestinal tract among HIV-infected individuals, followed closely by cytomegalovirus and herpes simplex virus. Odynophagia and dysphagia are the most common symptoms, and these infections may occur together. Endoscopy with biopsy is often required for diagnosis. Cytomegalovirus ulceration, peptic ulcer disease, gastroesophageal reflux, or malignancy may present with epigastric pain late in the course of HIV infection. Again, endoscopy with biopsy is required for diagnosis. Finally, both cytomegalovirus and *Cryptosporidium* may cause acalculous cholecystitis, with the former also causing a hepatitis.

HIV Nephropathy

HIV nephropathy with proteinuria and increased serum creatinine was initially observed among intravenous drug users. This entity is now also recognized among nonusers, and the histopathology includes focal glomerulosclerosis, mesangial proliferation, and glomerulonephritis. HIV nephropathy is usually, but not always, discovered incidentally in patients with CD4 counts below 200 cells/μL. The prognosis when the condition is discovered late in the course of AIDS is poor. Many centers, however, have had substantial success in dialyzing selected patients with HIV nephropathy.

Pulmonary Disease

Pulmonary disease in HIV-positive patients is very common. The physician confronts a wide spectrum of clinical disease and a long list of possibilities in the differential diagnosis when evaluating the patient with pulmonary symptoms. Knowledge of the degree of immunosuppression is essential for rapid and correct diagnosis. Although exceptions to the rule exist, most opportunistic infections are unlikely to occur with CD4 counts in excess of 200 cells/μL. Pulmonary processes likely to occur more frequently in patients with relatively intact immune systems include routine bacterial infections (notably encapsulated organisms), tuberculosis, and Kaposi's sarcoma. As the CD4 count approaches 200 cells/μL and below, the list of possible pathogens in the differential diagnosis broadens exponentially. In addition to routine pulmonary pathogens, bacteria such as *Pseudomonas, Nocardia, Legionella, Rhodococcus,* and Enterobacteriaceae assume greater prominence. Infections, including *Pneumocystis carinii, Cryptococcus,* and *Histoplasma,* must be considered. *Pneumocystis carinii* pneumonia remains the most common opportunistic pulmonary infection to occur in severely immunocompromised patients. Cytomegalovirus, by itself an infrequent cause of pneumonitis, is often a coinfecting pathogen with other organisms, especially *Pneumocystis;* respiratory syncytial virus (RSV) and adenovirus can be lethal in the severely immunocompromised HIV patient. *Toxoplasma* pneumonitis is increasingly recognized as a complication that cannot be overlooked.

Because the list of possibilities in the differential diagnosis is so lengthy in the severely immunocompromised HIV-infected patient, definitive diagnostic procedures are usually required. An induced sputum for PCP may be helpful, but brochoscopy with lavage and biopsy is often required to make the diagnosis. Remember that multiple pathogens may coinfect, a possibility that makes bronchoscopy even more attractive.

Neurologic Complications

Neurologic complications may occur at any stage of HIV infection. The acute retroviral syndrome may be complicated by meningismus, and cerebrospinal fluid analysis is often consistent with aseptic meningitis. Demyelinating processes resembling Guillain-Barré syndrome are uncommon but may occur early in the course of infection. As the CD4 count approaches 200 cells/μL and below, opportunistic infections increasingly contribute to neurologic complications. In patients presenting with focal abnormalities, magnetic resonance imaging may be appropriate. The lesions of toxoplasmosis and primary central nervous system lymphoma often appear ring-enhancing, with the former being more common. Statistically, multiple lesions most often mean toxoplasmosis, while single, ring-enhancing lesions are more likely to be lymphoma. Definitive diagnosis generally rests on biopsy or on the patient's response to therapy. Focal lesions that may be confused with the two disease entities mentioned above include tuberculomas, aspergillomas, progressive multifocal leukoencephalopathy, and bacterial abscess. Most clinicians now start empirical antitoxoplasmosis medication for 2 to 3 weeks. If repeat imaging shows that one or more lesions have not decreased in size during therapy, biopsy is undertaken for definitive diagnosis.

Meningeal signs and symptoms, such as severe headache, should be further defined with lumbar puncture. The most likely cause of meningitis in patients with CD4 counts below 200 cells/μL is *Cryptococcus neoformans*. Cerebrospinal fluid data, like clinical presentation, can vary considerably. Early meningitis may reveal no cells and normal glucose and/or protein concentration, despite a significant cryptococcal antigen titer, which may provide the only objective basis for diagnosis. Other frequent causes of meningitis in the AIDS patient include encapsulated organisms and an aseptic "HIV" meningitis.

AIDS dementia complex, seen in the late stages of the disease, is manifested by a constellation of symptoms including memory loss, decreased cognitive skills, behavioral change, and motor symptoms. Imaging studies of the brain show atrophy out of proportion to the age of the patient.

Infections of the Genital Tract

Infections of the genital tract influence the efficiency of HIV transmission and are more severe in those already infected with HIV. Sexually transmitted diseases that produce genital ulcers (e.g., syphilis, chancroid, and herpes) create an environment that enhances infection with HIV. The role of nonulcerating diseases (e.g., gonorrhea and veneral warts) is less certain, but they probably increase the efficiency of HIV transmission as well.

Infections of the female genital tract can be more severe in HIV-infected women. Candidal vaginal infections in HIV-positive women may be more frequent, more symptomatic, and more difficult to treat than those in uninfected women. More frequent hospitalization due to pelvic inflammatory disease has been documented, although the mechanism and microbiology of this disease in HIV-positive women are poorly understood. Cervical dysplasia occurs more frequently in HIV-infected women, and the risk of developing invasive carcinoma is thought to be higher. Thus, all HIV-infected women should have regular gynecologic examinations throughout the course of the disease.

Managing syphilis in AIDS patients presents a challenge. Following penicillin therapy, the immunologic response may be impaired at any stage of syphilis, and the rapid plasma reagin test (RPR) or VDRL (Veneral Disease Research Laboratories) may decline more slowly. The incidence of neurosyphilis may be higher than originally appreciated because of an accelerated clinical course. Many authorities recommend lumbar puncture for all HIV-positive patients found to be RPR-positive; if any abnormalities are noted, treatment for neurosyphilis should be instituted parenterally. However, such therapy may be logistically difficult, especially where the incidence of syphilis is high and resources may be severely limited. In addition, the common finding of an increased cerebrospinal fluid protein level and mild leukocytosis in uninfected HIV-positive patients may confound the interpretation of cerebrospinal fluid results.

Musculoskeletal Complications

The musculoskeletal complications include myositis and arthralgias. A diffuse myositis may primarily involve proximal muscles. Patients may notice difficulty with hip flexion and may report pain. Serum aspartate aminotransferase (AST) and creatine kinase (CK) levels may be increased. Confounding factors include a myositis associated with antiretrovirals, most notably AZT, with identical clinical and laboratory findings. Distinguishing between these two entities may be difficult, and may require biopsy. Diffuse and debilitating arthralgias associated with HIV infection have been described, but the mechanism is poorly understood and treatment is restricted to symptomatic relief.

Cutaneous Manifestations

The cutaneous manifestations of HIV infection are increasingly recognized as a barometer of disease progression. The onset of Kaposi's sarcoma (see below), cutaneous viral infections, bacillary angiomatosis, or other skin conditions suggests that the patient is prone to further opportunistic infections.

The papular lesions of molluscum contagiosum (MC), caused by a poxvirus, are more common in the HIV patient and are transmitted by sexual and/or close contact. Occasionally, MC may be confused with cryptococcal papules, but the latter most often arise in conjunction with clinically evident cryptococcosis. MC lesions are found primarily on the face, trunk, and/or genital regions and are generally smooth, nonerythematous, and painless.

Mucocutaneous herpes simplex virus (HSV) infection is more frequent in patients infected with HIV. Perirectal involvement tends to recur in gay men as the degree of immunosuppression increases. Other areas of mucocutaneous involvement include the lips, buccal mucosa, gingiva, and soft palate.

HIV-infected patients are at greater risk for both complicated primary varicella-zoster infection (chickenpox) and reactivation (shingles). Because the complications of primary infection may be severe in the immunocompromised host, all HIV-positive patients who do not have a history of varicella infection who have been exposed to an individual with chickenpox within the preceding 96 hours should receive varicella-zoster immune globulin (VZIG). The role of VZIG in immunosuppressed individuals (both immune and nonimmune to varicella) exposed to persons with shingles is more controversial. All HIV-infected patients with chickenpox or shingles should receive acyclovir.

The raised, violaceous papules associated with bacillary angiomatosis may sometimes be confused with Kaposi's sarcoma. Although the incidence of this bacterial process is low, the clinician should maintain a high index of suspicion when encountering nodules or plaques that are erythematous and friable. Biopsy specimens require special stains (Warthin-Starry), and the bacterial process may respond to antibiotics. The most likely cause of bacillary angiomatosis is a species of *Bartonella (Rochalimaea)*.

Other common cutaneous manifestations of HIV infection include seborrheic dermatitis, psoriasis, tinea infections, onychomycosis, eosinophilic folliculitis, xerosis, and ichthyosis.

Detection of HIV Infection

The most widely used test for confirmation of the diagnosis of HIV infection involves detection of antibodies to proteins unique to the human immunodeficiency virus. The most widely used screening test is the enzyme immunoassay (EIA). Several variations of EIA are available commercially. A positive result requires that the serum be retested to confirm the reaction. Sensitivities and specificities in excess of 99 per cent are reported for EIA.

All positive EIA results are confirmed by Western blot analysis. After lysis of HIV-infected cells, the proteins are separated by electrophoresis. The separated proteins bind antibodies in the patient's serum. Opinions differ as to which protein or proteins should be used to characterize a positive result. Tests may sometimes be called indeterminate if some, but not all, antibodies to HIV proteins are detected. Both false-positive and false-negative Western blots occur, but they are rare.

Both EIA and Western blot detect antibodies in the patient's serum. Because antibodies may not appear in the serum for at least 6 weeks, other techniques are required to diagnose acute HIV infection. Perhaps the most sensitive method for detecting acute HIV infection is the viral culture. This technique, however, is cumbersome, costly, and currently confined to research laboratories. The most widely used test for diagnosing acute HIV infection is the detection of one of the viral proteins, the p24 antigen, in the patient's serum. The p24 antigen is the first marker to be detected in the serum and can be detected within several days of infection. Unfortunately, despite its high specificity, the test is not considered particularly sensitive.

Finally, the role of the polymerase chain reaction (PCR) in the diagnosis of HIV infection has yet to be defined. Since only the smallest amount of viral material is required to produce a positive result, it is unclear whether a transient and minute exposure to HIV translates necessarily to a latent (and, consequently, active) infection. Given the superb sensitivity of PCR, however, the use of newly available quantitative PCR kits will undoubtedly supplement the clinician's ability to diagnose HIV infection even in the unusual setting.

INFLUENZA

By Constance T. Pachucki, M.D.
Hines, Illinois

Influenza, or the flu, is an epidemic illness seen in temperate zones in the northern hemisphere between October and March, and in the southern hemisphere between May and September. It is caused by influenza virus types A and B. Typically, influenza is characterized by the overwhelming presence in the community of a febrile, upper respiratory illness among adults and children that may be debilitating for several days.

Because influenza is an epidemic disease, recognizing the signs of an outbreak in the community is crucial to its diagnosis in an individual patient. The most sensitive indicators that the influenza virus is circulating and causing infection in the community are the occurrence of febrile respiratory illness in increased numbers of children and increased numbers of visits by patients of all ages to the emergency room and primary care clinics. School absenteeism peaks around the time that influenza is epidemic. State health departments document the local occurrence of influenza infection by isolating influenza from specimens obtained from patients with febrile upper respiratory illness. The Centers for Disease Control and Prevention document the incidence of influenza A infections by city, state, and patient age. The clinician can acquire information on influenza incidence and prevalence by calling state or local health departments or by reviewing the *Morbidity and Mortality Weekly Report*. Primary care physicians may also recognize outbreaks of influenza when patients have similar symptoms and physical findings and influenza A is isolated from at least one of these patients

PRESENTING SIGNS AND SYMPTOMS

The most common symptoms of influenza in adults are fever, prostration, cough, and myalgia. Additional symptoms include headache, malaise, backache, rhinorrhea, nasal obstruction, pharyngitis, and otalgia. In specific patients, the constellation of signs and symptoms varies with the interval between the onset of infection and the clinical evaluation. Early in the illness, the systemic symptoms of myalgias, chills, and fever are more prominent. As the illness progresses, upper respiratory symptoms become more frequent. Toward the end of the infection, approximately 5 days after the onset, fever resolves, but dry cough and weakness may persist. Gastrointestinal symptoms are uncommon in adults; the "stomach flu" is a misnomer. Note that the symptoms of influenza also vary with the age and immune status of the patient. For example, in children younger than 5 years of age, fever and rhinitis predominate and vomiting and diarrhea may become a significant part of the presentation. By contrast, patients with pre-existing low titers of antibody to the virus may become infected and shed virus but may have no or very minimal symptoms.

The physical findings are few. Oral temperatures of 100 to 102°F (38 to 39°C) are recorded. The patients appear uncomfortable, acutely ill, and toxic. They may have watery eyes and erythematous nasal and pharyngeal mucosa with a clear discharge. Auscultation of the lungs is generally unremarkable.

Influenza that occurs in institutions may be more difficult to identify than influenza in ambulatory settings. Nosocomial influenza does occur in hospitalized patients who present with fever and no obvious source of infection. However, influenza is not usually part of the differential diagnosis of nosocomial infection in hospitalized patients with fever. Upper respiratory symptoms are frequently overlooked, and patients are treated empirically with antibiotics despite sterile cultures. Fever often resolves, and the diagnosis of nosocomial influenza is missed. Viral isolation can be useful for the diagnosis of influenza in hospitalized patients. Appropriate infection control measures can then be initiated. Hospitalized patients with exacerbations of chronic obstructive pulmonary disease (COPD) may have coexisting influenza that has contributed to an episode of bronchospasm. These patients have signs of upper respiratory viral infection and bronchitis. Without a high index of suspicion for viral respiratory infection, and without confirmatory viral isolation, the diagnosis will be missed. In immunocompromised or hospitalized patients, influenza may present as viral pneumonia with progressive hypoxemia, few lung findings, and interstitial infiltrates or changes of adult respiratory distress syndrome on chest roentgenogram.

CLINICAL COURSE

Influenza infection generally resolves in 5 to 7 days. Patients with cardiovascular disease, pulmonary disease, and diabetes mellitus are at higher risk for the complications of influenza, including bronchitis, sinusitis, otitis media, and pneumonia. Two types of pneumonia complicate influenza: primary influenza viral pneumonia and secondary bacterial pneumonia. Croup and exacerbation of COPD are other respiratory complications of influenza infections. Other nonpulmonary complications include myositis, myocarditis and pericarditis, toxic shock syndrome, Guillain-Barré syndrome, and Reye's syndrome.

Primary influenza viral pneumonia occurs after a typical case of influenza. It is more frequent in high-risk patients but may occur in healthy adults. The signs and symptoms of influenza do not remit. Rather, they progress to dyspnea and cyanosis. The physical examination reveals respiratory distress with few rales and no signs of consolidation. Patients are severely hypoxemic, and the chest film shows bilateral interstitial infiltrates and/or adult respiratory distress syndrome. Sputum cultures grow normal respiratory flora, and influenza A is isolated. Mortality is very high.

Secondary bacterial pneumonia may occur on the heels of an influenza infection. Approximately 4 to 14 days following resolution of an influenza infection, patients may have recrudescence of fever with productive cough, dyspnea, and physical signs of consolidation of the lungs.

DIAGNOSIS

The diagnosis of influenza is generally based on clinical evidence of similar widespread illness, accompanied by isolation of influenza virus type A or B or by detection of a fourfold increase or decrease in antibody titers to influenza A or B virus. On occasion, however, serologic and/or virologic confirmation of influenza may be used retrospectively to identify the presence of circulating influenza virus, which then defines the clinical syndrome

In individual patients, confirmation of the diagnosis of influenza requires viral isolation or the use of rapid serologic tests to identify influenza virus type A or B. Importantly, other respiratory viruses, including respiratory syncytial virus, adenovirus, and parainfluenza, may circulate simultaneously with influenza virus. Because influenza A infections may be treated with amantadine or rimantadine, it is useful to distinguish influenza from other respiratory viral infections. Routine laboratory tests are unremarkable, but rapid diagnostic tests for influenza A and B are commercially available. These tests employ direct immunofluorescence or enzyme immunoassay to identify influenza virus types A and B in nasal swab specimens, throat gargles, nasal aspirate specimens, and throat swabs. The sensitivity and specificity of these assays depend on the type of specimen and range from 80 to 95 per cent. Rapid diagnostic tests should be supplemented with isolation of virus in tissue culture. Accurate identification may require as little as 1 day or as much as 1 week. If laboratory confirmation of influenza infection is accomplished within 24 hours of contact with the patient, treatment with antiviral agents may be possible. Using the algorithm in Figure 1, laboratories can increase the likelihood of detecting influenza virus, especially from nasal washes, nasal and throat aspirates, throat gargles, and nasal swabs. Peak shedding of influenza virus occurs on days 1 to 3 of the illness, so recognition of the virus by rapid test or viral isolation is more likely during this period.

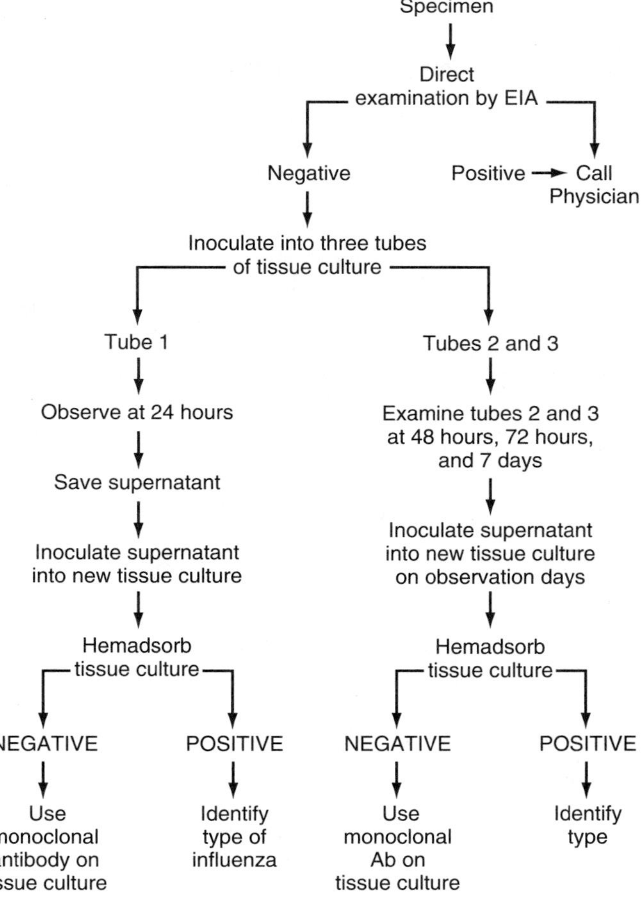

Figure 1. Algorithm for identification of influenza virus.

Because most influenza infections are diagnosed clinically and may not be confirmed for up to 7 days, several diagnostic pitfalls and errors must be kept in mind. The most important infection to be distinguished from influenza is the common cold, which does not have the systemic findings of influenza. That is, despite nasal discharge and sneezing, myalgias, malaise, and high fevers are uncommon. The differential diagnosis of influenza also includes streptococcal pharyngitis, bronchitis, sinusitis, and other viral upper respiratory infections. Some patients with influenza may appear very toxic because of high fever. In patients with chronic disease, the list of possibilities in the differential diagnosis of high fever includes serious bacterial infections such as sepsis, pneumonia, and meningitis. In the hospitalized patient, even during outbreaks in the community, nosocomial influenza is uncommon; whereas intravenous catheter line sepsis, urosepsis, and pneumonia are frequent and should be considered before influenza. The recognition of the influenza virus as the cause of an infection discourages the inappropriate use of antibacterial agents, suggests the use of rimantadine (a specific antiviral agent for influenza type A), and may prevent unnecessary hospitalizations.

VIRAL GASTROENTERITIS

By David I. Bernstein, M.D.,
and Richard L. Ward, Ph.D.
Cincinnati, Ohio

Viral infections of the gastrointestinal tract are a leading cause of morbidity in developed countries and mortality in developing countries. Each year in the United States, more than 200,000 infants and children are hospitalized and more than 500 people die as a result of such infections, at a cost of 1 billion dollars. For clinicians confronted with cases of diarrhea, the most important tasks are to assess the degree of dehydration and to distinguish viral infections from other treatable causes of diarrhea. Diagnosis begins with a complete physical examination and history, emphasizing key epidemiologic concerns. Information should be sought on travel, exposure to others with gastrointestinal symptoms, common-source exposures, exposure to young infants or day care settings, history of antimicrobial therapy, and whether the patient is immunocompromised. The answers to these questions, along with knowledge of the season at presentation, the age of the patient, and the description of the diarrhea, provide the cornerstone of the diagnostic approach to patients who may have viral gastroenteritis.

Many pathogens can cause gastroenteritis. Establishing the exact cause is often difficult, and the sophisticated tests required for diagnosis are sometimes available only in research laboratories. Over the past decade, there have been significant advances in characterizing the viral agents responsible for causing gastroenteritis and in developing new diagnostic tests.

Viral etiologies of gastroenteritis include rotavirus, both typical (group A) and atypical (groups B to G, but only groups B and C identified in humans); enteric adenovirus; caliciviruses and calici-type viruses, including Norwalk agent; astrovirus; coronavirus; enterovirus; and picobirnavirus. The heterogeneous group of viruses that includes many of the caliciviruses, calicilike viruses, and astroviruses has also been called small round structure viruses (SRSV). Many of these viruses are also named for the location where they were first identified, such as Norwalk agent, Snow Mountain virus, Hawaii virus, and Sapporo virus. By contrast, diarrheal diseases associated with such colorful names as Tourista, Montezuma's revenge, Delhi belly, Greek gallop, Aztec two-step, Turkey trots, Rome ruins, and backdoor sprint are not generally caused by viruses. The major viral agents and their distinguishing characteristics are summarized in Table 1.

Diarrhea is also common among patients with the acquired immunodeficiency syndrome (AIDS). Although the etiology often remains unknown, viruses can often be detected in stool specimens from these subjects at a higher frequency than from asymptomatic HIV-infected subjects. Astroviruses, picobirnaviruses, caliciviruses, and adenoviruses have now been implicated as causes of diarrhea in AIDS, along with cytomegalovirus, rotavirus, enterovirus, and HIV itself.

PRESENTING SIGNS AND SYMPTOMS

Viruses that cause gastroenteritis can produce asymptomatic infection or rapidly dehydrating illness with profuse watery diarrhea and vomiting. All the viral agents that cause gastroenteritis produce a nonbloody, watery diarrhea with or without vomiting as a major manifestation. These agents are also characterized by differences in the season at onset, the severity of symptoms, the incidence of dehydration, and the age range of patients with gastroenteritis. The incubation period is generally short, and the illness self-limited, except in the immunocompromised or when substantial dehydration goes untreated. The signs of dehydration in infants and children include lethargy, tachycardia, dry skin with decreased turgor, dry sunken eyes, sunken fontanelles, and dry mucous membranes.

CLINICAL DIAGNOSIS

The nature and extent of the work-up for viral gastroenteritis depend on the age of the patient, the severity and duration of the illness, the availability of tests, and the history, as mentioned earlier. If the history and physical examination indicate more than a mild, short-term illness or the presence of bloody diarrhea, fresh stool should be examined for the presence of fecal leukocytes, mucus, and/or blood. If fever and fecal leukocytes are present, then culture for *Campylobacter jejuni, C. coli, Salmonella,* and *Shigella* is indicated. Other inflammatory etiologies such as ulcerative colitis are, however, also possible.

Gastroenteritis that presents with vomiting, watery diarrhea, little or no fever, and varying levels of dehydration without fecal leukocytes or blood is more likely of viral origin. The differential diagnostic clues for each of the major viral pathogens are detailed below. In general, cases of gastroenteritis occurring during the cooler months in temperate climates, especially in young children, are most likely due to rotavirus, while cases of diarrhea in the warmer months are more likely caused by enteric adenovirus. Common-source outbreaks of diarrhea in adults are more likely due to calicilike viruses.

Table 1. Common Causes of Viral Gastroenteritis

Agent	Season	Age	Distinguishing Characteristics	Detection
Rotavirus	Drier, winter months in temperate zones	Usually 6–24 mo Can affect adults	Most common cause of dehydrating gastroenteritis in 6–24 month olds Seasonal	EIA Latex
Calicivirus (Norwalk virus–like)	More in winter and spring, but throughout the year	All ages, especially adults	Source outbreak from contaminated food or water All ages affected Vomiting prominent	Research only EIA PCR
Enteric adenovirus	None	All ages	Occurs year-round Milder than rotavirus, but second leading cause of hospitalization	EIA Latex Types 40, 41
Astrovirus	Similar to rotavirus	Usually less than 3 yr	Vomiting less common Milder than rotavirus	Research only EM EIA PCR
Coronavirus	Like rotavirus	Young infants	May be more mucoid and less watery stool than rotavirus	Research only EIA

EIA = enzyme immunoassay; EM = electron microscopy; PCR = polymerase chain reaction.

ROTAVIRUS

Rotavirus infection is the primary cause of severe gastroenteritis in infants worldwide, resulting in nearly 1 million deaths annually. Rotaviruses also account for 35 to 45 per cent of hospitalizations due to diarrhea in infants between 6 and 24 months of age in developed countries. Rotavirus illness can also occur in elderly or immunosuppressed adults, and in neonates who are often asymptomatic and develop little immune response to the infection. Although infected neonates are not protected against subsequent rotavirus illness, the severity of these episodes may decrease.

Human rotaviruses were first identified by electron microscopy in 1973 in the stool and vomitus of symptomatic infants. As members of the Reoviridae family, rotaviruses are nonenveloped, icosahedral-shaped viruses 70 nm in size, with 11 segments of double-stranded RNA. Their name derives from the Latin word *rota,* meaning "wheel," which describes the characteristic appearance of the virus with a hub, spokes, and a rim. Multiple groups of rotavirus are found in mammals and birds, and three of these groups (A to C) have been identified in humans, but relatively little is known about the clinical importance of any except group A. Within this group, four serotypes have been associated with most human infections (serotypes G1 to G4), and strains belonging to all four appear to be equally pathogenic. Animal strains of rotavirus have been associated with some episodes of human disease. As with influenza viruses, reassortants (recombinants) have been found among human and animal strains, thus greatly expanding the possibility of significant antigenic changes in circulating rotavirus strains.

Rotavirus is transmitted by the fecal-oral route, and symptoms can begin within 2 days of exposure, even in previously infected adults challenged with a virulent human rotavirus. The most characteristic signs of rotavirus disease in hospitalized children are extensive vomiting for 2 to 3 days followed by watery diarrhea for 3 to 9 days, accompanied by fever, nausea, and abdominal cramping. Severe illness results in dehydration and electrolyte imbalance. Oral rehydration therapy with solutions containing glucose and electrolytes is the usual recommended treatment, but cases of severe dehydration can require hospitalization for intravenous replacement of fluids. There are no antivirals and no licensed vaccines yet available to combat or prevent rotavirus disease.

Most infants are naturally protected against rotavirus disease during the first 6 months of life, possibly by maternal antibodies whose disappearance coincides with susceptibility to the disease. The most severe illnesses typically occur between 6 and 24 months of age worldwide, although this age span is probably more extended in developed countries. Few hospitalizations due to rotavirus infection occur after age 4 years; by that time, almost every child has experienced at least one rotavirus infection. Rotavirus disease occurs almost exclusively during the colder months in temperate climates, but its occurrence is less restricted in tropical and developing areas. A yearly pattern of rotavirus disease has been reported in the United States, where illnesses begin in the west in early fall and spread like a wave across the country, reaching the eastern seaboard in late winter. This pattern occurs regardless of latitude or climatic conditions.

Although the mechanism of protection against rotavirus disease is not understood, evidence suggests that immunity is associated primarily with intestinal responses. Because infants may be protected during the first months of life by circulating maternal antibodies, and animals can be protected by parenteral immunization, humoral immunity may also play a role in protection. Factors other than neutralizing antibody have also been implicated in protection against rotavirus disease. In general, natural rotavirus infection seems to provide protection against subsequent rotavirus disease. Therefore, live-virus vaccines delivered orally have been developed and are being tested. Most provide partial protection against all rotavirus disease and better protection against severe diarrhea in developed countries.

In many patients, rotavirus is shed in quantities of more than 10^{10} particles per gram of stool, so infection is generally not difficult to detect. Commercially available enzyme-linked immunosorbent assay (ELISA) and latex agglutination kits routinely detect rotavirus antigen in stool specimens collected from symptomatic patients. Their sensitivity and specificity seem adequate, but almost all kits for rotavirus detection lack reagents for detecting false-positive reactions. Such reactions have been a particular problem with stools collected from neonates, and rotaviruses have been wrongly associated with a variety of ailments in these patients. Thus, kits that are prone to this problem should not be used for neonatal specimens.

CALICIVIRUS (NORWALK AGENT)

Recognized as animal pathogens since 1932, caliciviruses were first identified as human pathogens in 1976. These agents are small, round RNA viruses 26 to 34 nm in size. There are at least five antigenic types of human calicivirus (HCV). Minireoviruses that cause gastroenteritis are also included in the Caliciviridae family. Numerous outbreaks of gastroenteritis have been attributed to caliciviruses, and many are named for the geographic location of the outbreak, such as Norwalk, Snow Mountain, Sapporo, and Hawaii. Norwalk virus, the prototype of this group, was isolated from an outbreak in Norwalk, Ohio.

Human caliciviruses have been identified worldwide and have been detected in 0.5 to 6.6 per cent of sporadic cases of pediatric gastroenteritis. A smaller percentage are implicated in diarrhea that requires hospitalization. Outbreaks can occur in all age groups and are associated with seafood and water contamination and, less commonly, with epizootic disease from domestic pets. Caliciviruses should be considered in outbreaks in closed settings for all age groups. Serosurveys suggest that infection with some strains occurs by 4 to 6 years of age, while infection with others is delayed. Norwalk virus is the most carefully studied; it is acquired throughout adulthood in developed countries, but earlier in those developing countries where it causes infantile diarrhea.

Calicivirus gastroenteritis is a short-lived (2 to 3 days) illness manifested by nausea, vomiting, and abdominal cramps. Low-grade fever is observed in 50 per cent of cases. Human calicivirus has an incubation period of 1 to 2 days and a high secondary attack rate. Forty per cent of outbreaks with these characteristics are caused by Norwalk virus, whereas other HCV types are not as well characterized. Outbreaks occur year-round but are more common in the winter and spring. Infection with Norwalk virus causes sudden-onset diarrhea and vomiting that is more pronounced than that associated with other viral agents. In the original outbreak, 44 per cent of patients had diarrhea, and 84 per cent had vomiting. In children, vomiting is observed more often than diarrhea, whereas in adults diarrhea is more frequent than vomiting.

Immune electron microscopy is the most widely used method for detection because the HCV viruses do not grow in culture. Antibody is required for detection because of the small number of particles present in the stool. Particles of similar size found in the stool may be enteroviruses or other unidentified matter. Radioimmunoassay (RIA) and enzyme immunoassay (EIA) are also available in research laboratories for the detection of Norwalk, Snow Mountain, or Hawaii virus or the Japanese variety of HCV. In these laboratories, recently cloned Norwalk virus capsid antigens can be used to make high-titered serum for use in various immunoassays. In addition, a polymerase chain reaction (PCR)–based assay has been described that recognizes consensus nucleotide sequences. The amplified region can be used to identify particular HCV strains. Confirmation of Norwalk virus infection, however, is more efficient by serology than by antigen detection, with an increase in antibody seen in 10 to 14 days.

ENTERIC ADENOVIRUSES

Adenoviruses are large (65 to 80 nm), nonenveloped, double-stranded, DNA-containing viruses that are icosahedral-shaped and have the appearance of a satellite with antennae (fibers) extending from their 12 vertices. These viruses are second only to rotaviruses as leading causes of hospitalizations due to viral gastroenteritis in infants. Forty-one serotypes have been designated within six subgenera (A to F); enteric adenoviruses (types 40 and 41) in subgenera F are most frequently associated with gastrointestinal illnesses, particularly those requiring hospitalization. The importance of adenoviruses as enteric pathogens has been established in both developed and developing nations. In developed countries, enteric adenoviruses account for 7 to 17 per cent of acute gastroenteritis in infants and young children. The median age for hospitalization due to enteric adenovirus disease is 7 months. Twenty per cent of children between 1 and 6 months of age demonstrate antibody to these viruses; 50 per cent are seropositive by 4 years of age. There appears to be no seasonality associated with enteric adenovirus infection.

Enteric adenoviruses appear to replicate only in the gastrointestinal tract. Thus, they are probably transmitted by the fecal-oral route. The incubation period is approximately 1 week; the duration of diarrhea is typically 10 days but commonly extends beyond 14 days. Other symptoms include mild fever, nausea, and vomiting, with a median duration of 2 days. These symptoms are analogous to those found with rotavirus but are generally less severe. Although vaccines have long been used in military recruits against respiratory adenovirus types 4 and 7, no vaccine has been developed against enteric adenoviruses.

Serotype-specific EIA kits for enteric adenoviruses are commercially available and used routinely. The high reactivity and specificity of these assays compare favorably to electron microscopy. Latex agglutination can also detect enteric adenoviruses in stool specimens.

ASTROVIRUSES (SMALL ROUND STRUCTURE VIRUSES, MARIN COUNTY VIRUS)

First identified in 1975, astroviruses are small RNA viruses with a characteristic star-shaped appearance by electron microscopy. There are at least five serotypes of astrovirus, with type 1 the most common. They have been detected in 2 to 9 per cent of children who seek medical attention because of diarrhea. Like rotavirus, they are more prevalent during the winter in temperate zones but occur year-round in tropical climates. Astroviruses have been associated with outbreaks of disease in a newborn nursery, day care centers, schools, and a home for the elderly and have been implicated in nosocomial infection on pediatric wards. By the age of 5 years, more than 70 per cent of children have serologic evidence of infection with astroviruses, suggesting that most infections occur in young children. Astrovirus secretion has been detected for 2 to 30 days, with excretion 1 to 8 days prior to the manifestation of symptoms. Thus, the incubation period appears to be longer than that of Norwalk virus. Children younger than 1 year of age may be at greatest risk. Diarrhea and, less often, vomiting are the most common symptoms and are usually mild, lasting less than 5 days. Astrovirus infections appear to be less common in adults, occur only in a minority of volunteers challenged with astrovirus, and, unlike Norwalk agent, do not cause illness in antibody-positive volunteers.

Astroviruses are shed in large amounts and thus are readily detected with electron microscopy. An ELISA directed at a group antigen is used most often in epidemiologic studies, although a PCR assay has been described and the virus can be cultured under select conditions. No commercial assay is available.

CORONAVIRUSES AND TOROVIRUSES

In 1965, a virus obtained from an adult with common cold–like symptoms was propagated in organ culture and later identified as a coronavirus. Coronaviruses are enveloped RNA viruses 60 to 120 nm in size. In 1992, the prototype torovirus, Berne-like or Breda-like virus, was also placed in the coronavirus family. Thus, an unofficial designation for this family is coronaviruslike superfamily.

Coronaviruses are more commonly implicated in respiratory diseases. However, enteric coronaviruses have been identified both in animal diarrheal diseases (e.g., transmissible gastroenteritis virus of swine) and in human gastroenteritis.

The clinical manifestations of enteric coronavirus infection are not clear. Gastroenteritis in infants, children, and young adults has been associated with the detection of coronaviruslike particles (CVLPs) in the stool. Similarly, CVLPs have been associated with several outbreaks of bloody stools or necrotizing enterocolitis in neonates. One study of diarrhea in infants and children attempted to characterize and compare CVLP-associated diarrhea with rotavirus-associated diarrhea. Both occurred during the fall and winter in children younger than 2 years of age. Shedding of CVLPs was detected for 5 to 25 days and was associated with diarrhea (94 per cent), fever (63 per cent), and vomiting (51 per cent). Compared with rotavirus stools, coronavirus stools were more often positive for occult blood (18 per cent versus 0 per cent), less often watery (66 per cent versus 92 per cent), and more often mucoid (32 per cent versus 8 per cent).

Coronaviruses are difficult to grow, but they can be propagated in organ cultures. A recent ELISA assay has been described, but there are no commercially available tests.

PICOBIRNAVIRUSES

These viruses have only recently been identified as a possible cause of gastroenteritis in humans. They are RNA viruses 32 to 34 nm in size. They have also been suggested as a cause of diarrhea in HIV-infected individuals, where they can be excreted for prolonged periods.

These viruses appear to be detected best with acrylamide gel electrophoresis.

INFECTIOUS MONONUCLEOSIS

By R. Eugene Bailey, M.D.
Syracuse, New York

Infectious mononucleosis (IM), or "mono," is caused by the Epstein-Barr virus (EBV), one of the herpesviruses, and most commonly affects young adults from 15 to 35 years of age. The diagnosis is made by accurate assessment of clinical, hematologic, and serologic manifestations of the illness. The manifestations include the classic triad of fever, pharyngitis, and cervical lymphadenopathy; lymphocytosis with a predominance of atypical lymphocytes; a positive heterophil (Monospot) antibody test and other serologic markers, the most important being the presence of IgM antibody to the EBV viral capsid antigen. Other agents included in this classification include cytomegalovirus (CMV), varicella-zoster virus, herpesvirus types 1 and 2, and human herpesvirus type 6.

EPIDEMIOLOGY

The incidence of mononucleosis is surprisingly low when one considers the regular shedding of the virus in oropharyngeal secretions among infected persons. Early childhood infection is especially common in persons among low socioeconomic levels; it is estimated that 50 to 85 per cent of children will acquire EBV antibodies by age 4 years. In affluent populations, however, EBV infection tends to occur in adolescence. Infectious mononucleosis is uncommon in persons older than 40 years of age.

The mode of transmission of EBV is mainly exchange of oropharyngeal secretions, usually by kissing. There is a preinfectious phase of approximately 2 to 4 weeks, when the virus invades local tissues in the oropharynx (the primary infection), and then over the next few weeks it invades the bloodstream (secondary infection). The virus most often replicates in B lymphocytes during this time, and after an additional incubation period of 4 to 6 weeks the patient develops the classic clinical manifestations of IM.

CLINICAL MANIFESTATIONS

In very young children, the most frequent manifestations of IM are upper respiratory tract symptoms and prolonged febrile illness with or without lymphadenopathy. These manifestations are in marked contrast with the classic signs and symptoms in older children, adolescents, and adults younger than 35 years of age. In this population, prodromal symptoms may occur for several days and include malaise, fatigue, headache, arthralgia, fever and chills, dysphagia, and anorexia. The classic triad of symptoms and signs at presentation is fever, pharyngitis, and lymphadenopathy, accompanied by an enlarged spleen and/or liver. In older patients, IM is often associated with more atypical features and may be difficult to diagnose. The physician should suspect EBV infection in a patient older than 40 years of age who presents with unexplained fever for more than a week, especially when liver function tests are abnormal or hepatomegaly, jaundice, unexplained peripheral neuropathy, or Guillain-Barré syndrome is present. In addition, consider IM in a patient with the diagnosis of lymphoma, lymphocytic leukemia, cholestatic jaundice, or fever of unknown origin.

Other organ systems can also manifest EBV infection. For example, the neurologic symptoms may include Guillian-Barré syndrome, Bell's palsy, encephalitis, optic neuritis, mental impairment, transverse myelitis, cerebellar ataxia, and demyelinating disease. Reye's syndrome has also been observed in association with EBV. Eye manifestations include eyelid and periorbital edema, dry eyes, keratitis, uveitis, conjunctivitis, retinitis, oculoglandular syndrome, chondritis, papillitis, and ophthalmoplegia. The pulmonary manifestations, although rare, include hilar and mediastinal lymphadenopathy, interstitial pneumonitis, and pleural effusions. A characteristic skin rash is observed when amoxicillin is used during IM that does not appear to be an allergic reaction.

Infectious mononucleosis is usually a self-limited disease. Although previous reports postulated a link between EBV infection and chronic fatigue syndrome, this association does not appear to be causal. Based on numerous studies, the Centers for Disease Control and Prevention do not support EBV as a cause of chronic fatigue syndrome.

DIAGNOSTIC EVALUATION

Accurate diagnosis of IM depends on a combination of clinical, hematologic, and serologic evidence of the disease.

Clinical

The incubation period for IM is approximately 4 to 6 weeks after initial EBV infection. Most patients present with the triad of fever, pharyngitis, and lymphadenopathy. Other helpful signs and symptoms include splenomegaly with or without hepatomegaly, jaundice, eyelid edema, and maculopapular exanthem. Table 1 lists common signs and symptoms of IM by age group.

Table 1. Signs and Symptoms of Infectious Mononucleosis by Age Group

	Patients <35 Years of Age		Patients >40 Years of Age	
Sign or Symptom*	***No.***	**%**	***No.***	**%**
Fever	229/256	89	70/74	95
Sore throat, pharyngitis	338/432	78	34/79	43
Lymphadenopathy	407/432	94	36/77	47
Splenomegaly	184/376	49	17/51	33
Hepatomegaly	6/100	6	22/52	42
Jaundice	10/256	4	14/51	27
Rash	29/432	7	6/50	12

*Information about signs and symptoms was not available for all patients.
Adapted from Bailey, R. E.: Diagnosis and treatment of infectious mononucleosis. Am. Fam. Physician, 49:879–888, 1994, with permission.

Table 2. EBV-Specific Antigens/Antibodies in Infectious Mononucleosis

Antigen	Method of Detection	Antibody Titers: Acute	Antibody Titers: Long-Term Postprimary Infection
Viral capsid antigen (VCA)	Indirect immunofluorescence	IgM >160 IgG >160	Nondetectable >40
Early antigens			
Diffuse (D-EA)	Indirect immunofluorescence	>40	<40
Restricted (R-EA)		<10	<10
Nuclear antigen (EBNA or NA)	Anticomplement immunofluorescence (ACIF)	<2	>40
Heterophile antigen (not coded by EBV)	Agglutination Paul-Bunnell test (PBT)	IgM (+) up to 1 year	Negative after 1 year

Adapted from Bailey, R. E.: Diagnosis and treatment of infectious mononucleosis. Am. Fam. Physician, 49:879–888, 1994, with permission.

Hematologic

An increased leukocyte count of 10,000 to 15,000 cells/mm^3 usually occurs 2 to 3 weeks after infection, and there is a relative lymphocytosis. Both B and T cells contribute to the characteristic increase in atypical lymphocytes seen in 30 to 50 per cent of patients. Atypical lymphocytes may also be associated with CMV infections, viral hepatitis, measles, rubella, and serum sickness. Mild thrombocytopenia is seen in about 50 per cent of patients with IM; severe thrombocytopenia may occur infrequently.

Serologic

The first serologic test for IM, the Paul-Bunnell test, assayed the production of heterophil antibody by detecting the highest antibody titer that would agglutinate sheep erythrocytes. This test was further developed into the popular rapid latex agglutination test (Monospot test). Despite its ease and rapidity of performance, this test is limited by its false-negative results (failure to produce or detect heterophil antibody) of approximately 10 to 20 per cent and false-positive rates of 5 to 15 per cent because of cross-reactivity with antibodies produced by other infections, such as CMV infection, adenovirus infection, and toxoplasmosis.

There are three key groups of antigens that are directly produced by EBV. Techniques have been developed to measure antibodies to these antigens. Table 2 summarizes important points about the antigens directly produced by the virus: EBV viral capsid antigens, diffuse (D) and restricted (R) antigens of the EBV-induced early antigen complex, and EBV-associated nuclear antigen (EBNA). These tests allow identification of current, recent, and past infection.

Current Infection

Acute EBV infection is marked by increased IgM and IgG antibodies to viral capsid antigen (VCA-IgM and VCA-

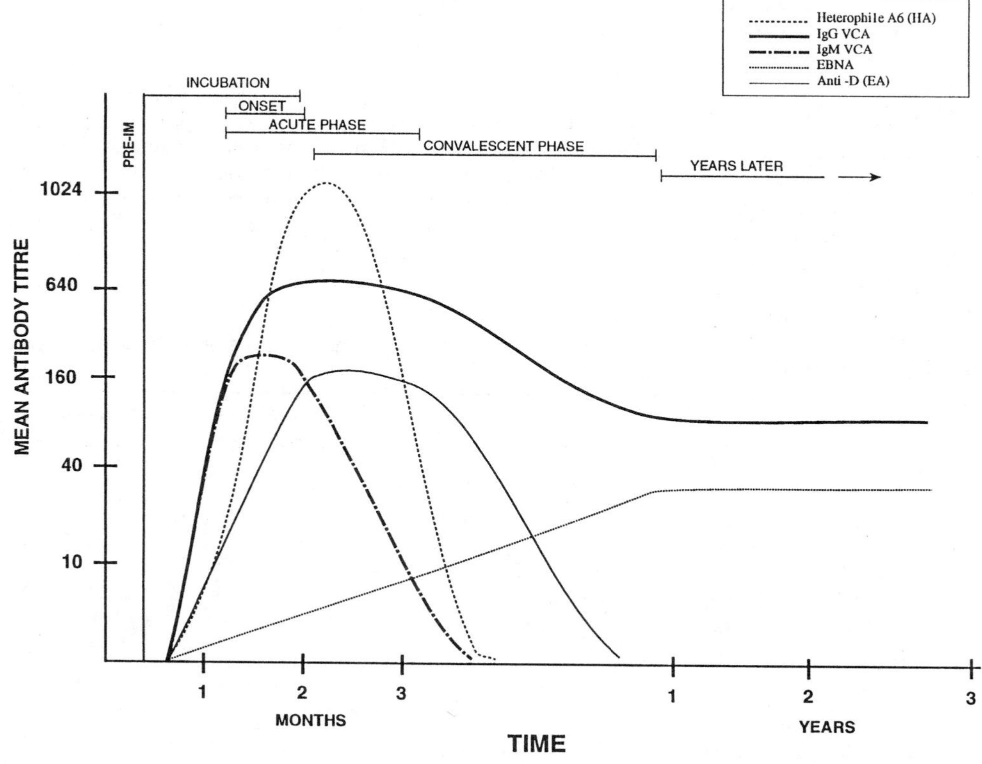

Figure 1. Antibody responses during the course of infectious mononucleosis. (From Bailey, R. E.: Diagnosis and treatment of infectious mononucleosis. Am. Fam. Physician, 49:879–888, 1994, with permission.)

IgG, respectively), transient antibodies to diffuse antigen (anti-D), and no antibodies to EBV-associated nuclear antigen (anti-EBNA). Since most persons seek medical attention after VCA-IgG titers have reached peak concentration, the VCA-IgM titer is the most accurate and useful marker for early diagnosis of acute primary infection.

Recent Infection

Recent EBV infection is identified by low (or no longer detectable) levels of VCA-IgM, high titers of VCA-IgG, and no (or very low) titers of anti-EBNA. Detectable anti-D may also be observed or may be replaced by low, transient titers of anti-R.

Past Infection

In persons already exposed to IM, only moderate titers of VCA-IgG and anti-EBNA are found, and these antibodies probably persist for life. Rarely, anti-D and anti-R may be detected if VCA-IgG is sufficiently high (Fig. 1).

Immunosuppressed states may cause a variation in the typical antibody patterns by reactivating VCA-IgG production to anti-D or anti-R, but VCA-IgM antibodies do not re-emerge. In addition, the absence of anti-EBNA is observed in certain immunodeficiencies and therefore does not always reflect EBV infection. For EBV-associated Burkitt's lymphoma, high antibody titers to VCA and R antigen are characteristic; for undifferentiated nasopharyngeal carcinoma, both IgG and IgA antibody titers to VCA and D antigen are characteristic.

DIFFERENTIAL DIAGNOSIS

Infectious mononucleosis can be diagnosed in most patients by carefully considering the clinical and laboratory findings and demonstrating a positive Monospot test. Detection of VCA-IgM antibody is the most accurate and important assay for confirming acute infection during IM. However, IM must be differentiated from other illnesses associated with the signs and symptoms of pharyngitis, fever, and lymphadenopathy. These illnesses may be caused by agents such as bacteria (*Streptococcus* or *Corynebacterium diphtheriae*), other viruses (CMV, rubella, adenovirus, hepatitis A and B viruses, or human immunodeficiency virus [HIV]), and *Toxoplasma gondii*.

Cytomegalovirus infection may be associated with signs and symptoms similar to those of IM, including splenomegaly, hepatomegaly, and atypical lymphocytosis. However, CMV is more likely to occur in adults, is typically not accompanied by sore throat and lymphadenopathy, and is not associated with the production of heterophil antibodies. Lymphoproliferative disorders, such as leukemia, Hodgkin's disease, and lymphomas, should be considered in patients who present with central nervous system involvement. Differentiation between IM and a lymphoproliferative disorder can often be difficult, since these conditions or their treatments can cause immunosuppression and reactivation of EBV antibody responses. Human immunodeficiency virus infection may produce signs and symptoms similar to those of IM.

MUMPS

By Claire Pomeroy, M.D.
Minneapolis, Minnesota

Mumps is a contagious, acute viral infection caused by a paramyxovirus and characterized by parotitis. Systemic involvement may result in serious manifestations, including meningoencephalitis, pancreatitis, and orchitis. The availability of an effective vaccine has dramatically reduced the incidence of mumps in the United States, but outbreaks still occur and may involve groups outside the usual childhood age range, including college students and adults in the workplace. Because of this changing epidemiology, the diagnosis of mumps may be delayed or missed, especially when parotitis is absent.

PRESENTING SIGNS AND SYMPTOMS

Infection with mumps is asymptomatic in up to one third of patients. When symptomatic, mumps may present with varying severity, ranging from a mild upper respiratory illness to viremia with generalized organ involvement.

After an average incubation period of 16 to 18 days (range, 14 to 25 days), the patient often notes 1 or 2 days of nonspecific prodromal symptoms, including low-grade fever, anorexia, malaise, and headache. Then, most patients develop painful swelling of one or both parotid glands. Enlargement of the parotid glands progresses for several days, with bilateral involvement in 75 per cent of patients. In 10 per cent, additional salivary glands are involved. Glandular swelling diminishes over the next week, occasionally lasting as long as 2 weeks.

Parotitis is usually obvious to both the patient and the examining physician. The symptom severity varies from mild discomfort to dramatic enlargement and tenderness of the face and jaw. Patients may complain of earache and pain with chewing or drinking sour or bitter liquids. On physical examination, parotitis may be obvious, with glandular enlargement resulting in the classic "chipmunk appearance." Swelling of the parotid gland may result in disappearance of the angle of the mandible and asymmetry of the neck, with the earlobe pushed upward and outward. On palpation, the involved parotid gland may be boggy and tender, but in severe infections the gland can become firm and tense. Erythema over the glands speaks against the diagnosis of mumps. Parotitis is usually obvious for 2 to 5 days and rarely lasts longer than 10 days. The orifices of Stenson's or Wharton's duct may be red and edematous with petechial hemorrhages. Patients with submandibular gland involvement can develop lymphatic obstruction, manifested as presternal pitting edema and laryngeal swelling. In unusual presentations with sublingual gland involvement, swelling of the tongue and dysphagia may occur.

It is critical to remember that mumps is a generalized illness with potential involvement of many glandular and neural tissues (Table 1). Although parotitis is usually the predominant manifestation, symptoms can result from any of a number of involved organs. Extra–salivary gland involvement can occur before, during, after, and even in the absence of parotitis and appears to be more common in older children and adults. The physician must be careful not to overlook the diagnosis of central nervous system (CNS), gonadal, pancreatic, or myocardial involvement by mumps in patients without parotitis.

Meningoencephalitis

The CNS is the most common extraglandular site of mumps, and involvement is more common in males than females. Mumps must be considered in the differential diagnosis of aseptic meningitis. Mumps caused 10 per cent of aseptic meningitis cases in the United States prior to

Table 1. Organ Involvement in Mumps

Organ Involvement	Incidence
Parotitis	60–70% (other salivary glands, 10%)
Meningitis	Asymptomatic, 50%; symptomatic, 10%
Encephalitis	~1 in 6000
Cranial nerve VIII	Transient deafness, 4%; permanent deafness, 1 in 15,000–20,000; usually unilateral
Orchitis and epididymitis	20% of postpubertal men
Mastitis	7–30% of postpubertal women; also in men
Oophoritis	5% of postpubertal women
Pancreatitis	~5%
Myocarditis	Electrocardiographic abnormalities, 5–15%; symptomatic, rare
Nephritis	Mild laboratory abnormalities, 60%; symptomatic, rare
Arthritis	~0.4%

Other: Thyroiditis, conjunctivitis, keratitis, iritis, uveitis, hepatitis, prostatitis, and infection of other glandular and neural tissues

the availability of the vaccine and still accounts for about 1 per cent of cases. More than half of patients with mumps have a cerebrospinal fluid (CSF) pleocytosis, but only about 10 per cent of patients have symptomatic meningitis. Interestingly, nearly half of patients with mumps meningitis lack clinical evidence of parotitis. The clinical features of mumps meningitis are not distinguishable from those of many other viral meningitides. Fever, headache, mild nuchal rigidity, and lethargy are common and generally last 3 to 10 days. The CSF laboratory abnormalities (see later) may last longer, for as long as 1 month. The prognosis is excellent, with complete recovery as the norm.

Mumps encephalitis is, fortunately, less common than meningitis, occurring in about 1 in 6000 cases. Although the prognosis for mumps encephalitis is better than that for many other types of viral encephalitis, long-term sequelae and fatalities occur in 1 to 2 per cent of patients. As with other forms of encephalitis, seizures, focal neurologic abnormalities, and depressed level of consciousness provide nonspecific clues to the diagnosis. Both primary encephalomyelitis with direct neuronal invasion manifesting at the time of parotitis and postinfectious demyelinating encephalomyelitis occurring later in the disease course have been described. Like mumps meningitis, mumps encephalitis can occur in the absence of salivary gland involvement. Other manifestations of neuronal mumps include transverse myelitis, cranial nerve neuritis, polyneuritis, Guillain-Barré syndrome, cortical blindness, and cerebellar ataxia.

Hearing Loss

Damage to the eighth cranial nerve by mumps infection can result in sensorineural deafness. Transient deafness occurs in as many as 4 per cent of patients with mumps. Rarely, permanent deafness may occur; hearing loss is usually unilateral but may be bilateral. The risk of deafness is not related to the severity of the systemic illness, and deafness usually occurs coincidentally with or shortly after parotitis.

Epididymo-orchitis

Epididymo-orchitis occurs in about 20 per cent of adult men with mumps but is quite uncommon in prepubescent boys. Involvement is usually unilateral, but bilateral orchitis occurs in 15 to 25 per cent of patients. Orchitis may develop in the absence of parotitis but is most commonly observed shortly after parotitis has peaked. Patients with mumps orchitis present with the abrupt onset of testicular pain. On physical examination, the involved testicle may be swollen to several times the normal size and is tender and warm to palpation. Scrotal edema and erythema may be noted. Epididymitis accompanies orchitis in about 85 per cent of patients and may precede or coincide with the onset of orchitis. The signs and symptoms of epididymo-orchitis generally wane over about 1 week.

Mastitis

Mumps may involve the breast in both men and women, occurring in 7 to 30 per cent of postpubertal women with mumps. Mastitis is characterized by the painful, nonerythematous swelling of one or both breasts.

Oophoritis

The signs and symptoms of oophoritis are noted in about 5 per cent of postpubertal women with mumps and include fever and abdominal or pelvic pain. An enlarged, tender ovary may be palpable during pelvic examination.

Pancreatitis

Pancreatitis probably occurs in about 5 per cent of mumps patients, but the diagnosis is often missed when increased serum amylase values are attributed to parotid gland involvement. Patients report signs and symptoms of fever, nausea, vomiting, and epigastric pain. Tenderness to palpation over the abdomen can be elicited on physical examination. Like the other extra–salivary gland manifestations of mumps, pancreatitis may occur without parotitis and should be considered in the differential diagnosis of otherwise unexplained pancreatitis. Pancreatitis may be particularly severe in patients with cystic fibrosis. However, in most patients, recovery occurs in about 1 week.

Myocarditis

Although symptomatic cases of mumps myocarditis or pericarditis have been reported, the vast majority of infections are asymptomatic and are noted only because of electrocardiographic changes. ST-T wave abnormalities and atrioventricular conduction delays may be seen in as many as 15 per cent of patients with mumps but are, of course, not specific and usually not clinically significant. Deaths from mumps myocarditis have been rarely reported.

Nephritis

Asymptomatic viruria and mild laboratory abnormalities of renal function are common in mumps. Microscopic hematuria and proteinuria are also reported. Although symptomatic impairment is quite unusual, rare deaths have been reported.

Arthritis and Arthralgias

Joint involvement is noted in about 0.4 per cent of mumps patients and may occur before, after, or in the absence of parotitis. Most commonly, signs and symptoms begin about 2 weeks after the onset of parotitis and persist for an average of 2 weeks but occasionally last for up to 5 weeks. The manifestations include migratory polyarthritis or monoarticular arthritis, usually of large joints. Complete recovery is generally anticipated.

Other

A variety of other organs may be involved in mumps. Thyroiditis, conjunctivitis, keratitis, iritis, uveitis, hepatitis, and prostatitis all have been reported.

DISEASE COURSE AND PROGNOSIS

Mumps is usually a benign, self-limited illness, with recovery expected after supportive treatment only. Long-term sequelae and/or fatalities occur in about 1.3 per cent of patients with mumps encephalitis. A few reports suggest that aqueductal stenosis and hydrocephalus may rarely follow mumps encephalitis. Optic atrophy may result from mumps infection of the optic nerve. Infections characterized by involvement of the eighth cranial nerve can cause permanent deafness in 1 in 15,000 to 20,000 patients, usually with unilateral involvement. With mumps epididymo-orchitis, testicular atrophy may occur in up to one third of patients but is usually unilateral. Although fertility may be impaired in 10 per cent of patients after mumps orchitis, sterility is very unusual. Anxiety after mumps orchitis and psychogenic impotence are more frequent problems. Rare fatalities have been reported in mumps pancreatitis, myopericarditis, and nephritis. However, chronic pancreatic, cardiac, or renal impairment has not been reported.

DIAGNOSIS

The diagnosis of mumps is usually made on clinical grounds, based on the symptoms and signs described earlier, especially when there is a history of exposure in the past 2 to 3 weeks. Obviously, the diagnosis is more likely in unvaccinated individuals. However, since both inadequate immune responses to vaccination and waning immunity over time are possible, a history of being immunized does not preclude the diagnosis. Clinicians should consider the diagnosis not only in the patient with classic parotitis but also in patients with aseptic meningitis, orchitis, or pancreatitis of uncertain etiology.

Laboratory confirmation of typical mumps is not necessary. However, in atypical presentations, laboratory evaluation may be necessary to make the diagnosis. The diagnosis of mumps is generally confirmed by virus isolation or by serologic studies. The mumps skin test is unreliable and is no longer commercially available.

Routine Laboratory Assessment

Most routine laboratory values do not provide specific clues to the diagnosis of mumps. The peripheral leukocyte count is most often normal or nearly normal. As with many other viral infections, a predominance of lymphocytes and atypical lymphocytes may be observed. Extraparotid involvement may be associated with a higher percentage of neutrophils.

Increased serum amylase activities can be due to parotitis, pancreatitis, or both. Differentiation between the two sources can be made by determination of amylase isoenzymes, but this is rarely necessary. An increased serum lipase value is suggestive of pancreatic involvement.

Mild abnormalities of renal function are not uncommon in mumps. Microscopic hematuria and proteinuria can be observed. An active urinary sediment with red blood cell casts is suggestive of the rare case of mumps nephritis.

In mumps meningitis, the CSF shows a lymphocytic pleocytosis, usually with leukocyte counts of less than 500 cells/mm^3, although counts as high as 2500 cells/mm^3 have been reported. In up to one fourth of patients, a predominance of neutrophils may occur. The CSF protein level is usually mildly increased, and the glucose level is most often normal. However, mumps meningitis is unusual for a viral meningitis in that CSF glucose concentrations are low in nearly one third of patients.

Virus Culture

Mumps virus has been isolated from saliva, blood, urine, CSF, and infected tissues. Cultures of urine or saliva and swab specimens from the area around Stensen's duct are of most value. Mumps virus has been recovered from the saliva in patients without clinically obvious salivary gland involvement. Virus has been isolated from saliva as long as 1 week after the onset of symptoms, and urine cultures may detect virus for up to 2 weeks after the onset of parotitis. However, specimens should be obtained as early as possible in the course of the illness, when virus titers are higher. Cerebrospinal fluid cultures are useful in cases of possible mumps meningitis; CSF cultures may be positive for as long as 6 days after the onset of meningeal symptoms. Since viremia is rarely detected and then only in the first 2 days of illness, viral blood cultures for mumps should not be pursued.

The receiving laboratory should be contacted regarding the specifics of specimen collection and transport. Urine, swab specimens, and CSF will be inoculated into cell cultures, usually monkey kidney cells or Vero cell lines. The presence of mumps virus is suggested by formation of multinucleated giant cells, but a cytopathic effect is often absent. The method of choice for confirming the presence of mumps virus in cell culture is the hemadsorption test. With this test, guinea pig or chicken erythrocytes added to cell culture adhere to mumps-infected cells because of the virus-specific hemagglutinins expressed on the cell surface. The presence of mumps virus is confirmed when mumps-specific antisera block the hemadsorption. It is critical that the laboratory include appropriate controls to eliminate the possibility of cross-reactivity with other paramyxoviruses, including parainfluenza viruses and simian viruses present in the cells used for culture.

Serology

Serology is the most common approach used to confirm the diagnosis of mumps (Table 2). For serologic diagnosis, acute and convalescent specimens should be collected. The acute sample should be drawn as soon as the diagnosis is suspected, and the convalescent titer should be obtained 14 or more days later. Mumps-specific IgM can be assessed on a single serum specimen. Antibody titers can also be determined on CSF, but a serum sample should be run in parallel.

A variety of serologic tests for mumps have been developed, although most clinical laboratories appropriately offer only one test. Traditionally, the complement fixation (CF) test has been used for the diagnosis of mumps. This test requires acute and convalescent serum samples. The CF test detects antibody against the soluble (S) antigen (corresponding to the NP, one of three nucleocapsid-associated proteins) and the virion (V) antigen (corresponding to the hemagglutinin-neuraminidase antigen). S antibody usually rises within the first week of illness, whereas V antibody appears 1 to 2 weeks later. Therefore, detection of S antibody in the absence of V antibody has been interpreted as representative of acute mumps. However, some

Table 2. Serologic Tests for Mumps

Test	Comment
Complement fixation	Traditionally used for diagnosis Requires acute and convalescent specimens
Enzyme-linked immunosorbent assay (ELISA)*	Commercially available assays for IgG and IgM +IgM suggests acute disease 4-fold rise in IgG generally confirms diagnosis of recent mumps +IgG alone suggests immunity
Immunofluorescence assay (IFA)	Commercially available Interpreted as for ELISA above Solid-phase IFA for IgG also available
Virus neutralization	Most sensitive but technically difficult and not widely available
Radioimmunoassay (RIA)	Less commonly available
Hemagglutination inhibition (HI)	No longer used frequently Nonspecific inhibitors in serum may preclude detection of low antibody titers

*Antibody capture techniques appear to result in increased sensitivity.

have questioned the reliability of these antibody patterns and suggest that documentation of seroconversion is required for definitive diagnosis. A fourfold rise in either antibody between the acute and the convalescent specimens confirms the diagnosis of mumps. Generally, S antibody disappears after several months, but V antibody can be detected for years. Therefore, an increase of V antibody without S antibody suggests prior, resolved infection.

Currently, in many laboratories, the use of CF has been supplanted by enzyme-linked immunosorbent assay (ELISA) tests, which are considered to have improved sensitivity. A variety of ELISA assays to measure IgG and IgM antibodies to mumps virus have been developed and are now commercially available. The diagnosis of mumps is made on the basis of a significant rise in IgG antibody between acute and convalescent specimens or, if available, a positive test for IgM. Mumps-specific IgM is detectable during the first week of clinical symptoms in 80 per cent of patients and may persist for several months. In addition, mumps-susceptible individuals can be identified by a negative ELISA test for IgG on a single serum sample.

Immunofluorescence (IF) assays are also currently used by many laboratories to detect antibodies to mumps. Both IgG and IgM mumps antibodies can be detected with commercially available kits. As with the ELISA assays, mumps infection is suggested by a positive IgM assay or by a fourfold rise of IgG between acute and convalescent specimens. A solid-phase IF assay is available for measurement of IgG to mumps and is useful for determining immune status and susceptibility to mumps.

To reduce the potential for false-positive and false-negative results in ELISA assays, a variation of the ELISA test called "antibody capture" has been developed recently. For example, in one report, IgM antibody capture ELISA was more reliable than the routine ELISA and detected IgM antibody by the third or fourth day of mumps illness and at least 6 weeks after recovery. Human IgM antibody in the sample is selectively attached to a surface coated with antihuman IgM antibody. Mumps-specific IgM is then detected by addition of mumps antigen followed by labeled antimumps antibody.

Antibody to mumps can also be detected with the neutralization test. However, this assay is technically challenging and is not routinely available. The hemagglutinin inhibition (HI) test is no longer widely available. Nonspecific serum inhibitors may prevent detection of low levels of antibody by HI, and the assay is less sensitive than ELISA or IF assay. Radioimmunoassays have also been developed to detect mumps antibodies but are used less frequently because of the requirement for radioactive labels.

Regardless of the specific serologic test used, caution must be exercised in the interpretation of serologic results. Problems can arise because of cross-reactions between IgG antibody against mumps and other paramyxoviruses. If paired sera suggest a fourfold rise in antibody against mumps, the samples should also be tested for antibodies against the parainfluenza viruses. False-positive IgM assays can arise for a number of other reasons, including the presence of rheumatoid factor, and false-negative results may occur when high levels of IgG inhibit binding of IgM antibodies. IgM capture assays appear to be the most reliable.

For detection of mumps-specific antibody in CSF, the ELISA is generally more sensitive than the CF test. CSF IgG is usually present within a few days of the onset of clinical CNS symptoms and peaks about 7 days later.

DIFFERENTIAL DIAGNOSIS

A variety of other conditions can cause parotid enlargement and inflammation that may be confused with the parotitis of mumps (Table 3). Importantly, parainfluenza viruses can cause parotitis and cross-react with mumps on serologic testing. Other viruses such as coxsackievirus A and B, echoviruses, lymphocytic choriomeningitis virus, and influenza A all can cause parotitis. Other infectious etiologies of parotitis include staphylococci and streptococci. Acute suppurative parotitis usually occurs in elderly, debilitated or dehydrated patients, and pus in Stensen's duct may be expressed on examination. In addition, drugs, tumors, and a number of metabolic conditions can cause parotid enlargement. Parotid gland enlargement should

Table 3. Differential Diagnosis of Parotitis

Infectious	Noninfectious
Acute Viral Parotitis Mumps, parainfluenza types 1 and 3, coxsackievirus A and B, echovirus, lymphocytic choriomeningitis virus, influenza A ***Suppurative Parotitis*** Staphylococci, pneumococci, other streptococci, gram-negative bacilli, anaerobes ***Other*** *Mycobacterium tuberculosis*, actinomycosis, fungi, cat-scratch disease	***Drugs*** Iodides, thiouracil, sulfa drugs, phenothiazines, phenylbutazone, heavy metals, alpha-methyldopa, bretylium, bromides, others ***Other Medical Conditions*** Diabetes mellitus, bulimia nervosa, obesity, alcoholism, vitamin deficiency, pregnancy, thyrotoxicosis, uremia, cystic fibrosis Sialolithiasis, benign or malignant tumors, cysts, pneumatocele in buglers and glassblowers Lupus erythematosus, amyloidosis, sarcoidosis, Sjögren's syndrome, Mikulicz syndrome

be distinguished from other conditions such as cervical lymphadenitis, dental abscess, otitis externa, cervicofacial actinomycosis, and extraparotid tumors.

COMPLICATIONS

An increased frequency of spontaneous abortions has been reported in women with mumps during the first trimester. However, no significant increase in congenital malformations has been established. The observation that mumps virus can infect islet cells has prompted hypotheses that mumps virus may play an etiologic role in diabetes mellitus. However, careful epidemiologic studies have found no evidence for this association. The proposed association between endocardial fibroblastosis and congenital mumps has also not been confirmed.

ERRORS AND PITFALLS IN DIAGNOSIS

The major error in diagnosing mumps is the failure to consider mumps as a potential etiologic agent in the patient who presents without classic parotitis. Mumps is an important consideration in the differential diagnosis of meningoencephalitis, epididymo-orchitis, and pancreatitis. With the decreased incidence of this disease in the United States since the availability of an effective vaccine, many young physicians have never seen a patient with mumps and may fail to recognize the wide variety of manifestations of this generalized viral illness. In addition, the use of the vaccine has shifted the epidemiology of the disease. Patients are not routinely exposed as children and thus may be at risk for developing mumps later in life, especially as young adults, owing to missed vaccination, ineffective immune response to the vaccine, or waning immunity. Thus, physicians must now consider the diagnosis of mumps in patients outside of the traditional childhood age range.

NONPOLIO ENTEROVIRUS INFECTIONS

By Mary-Margaret Andrews, M.D.,
and John F. Modlin, M.D.
Lebanon, New Hampshire

Coxsackieviruses and echoviruses are enteroviruses commonly transmitted via the fecal-oral route. These viruses replicate in the upper respiratory and gastrointestinal tracts, and hematogenous spread causes a wide spectrum of disease. The human enteroviruses include the polioviruses, group A coxsackieviruses, group B coxsackieviruses, and echoviruses. Because naturally occurring polioviruses have been eradicated in the Western Hemisphere, and only rare cases of poliomyelitis occur with the use of live, attenuated polio vaccine viruses, they are not considered further in this article. Historically, the nonpolio enteroviruses have been separated into 23 group A coxsackievirus serotypes, 6 group B coxsackievirus serotypes, 32 echovirus serotypes, and 4 newer serotypes designated enteroviruses 68 to 71.

Although enterovirus infections occur throughout the calendar year, there is a distinct seasonal peak during summer and early fall in temperate climates. Typically, several serotypes circulate during a season, but a single serotype may predominate during periodic epidemics. Attack rates are generally higher in children. Spread of infection is common within households, with 50 to 80 per cent of susceptible persons experiencing secondary infection.

While most enterovirus infections cause either no symptoms or nonspecific upper respiratory complaints, there are several distinctive clinical syndromes attributed to enterovirus infection.

CLINICAL SYNDROMES

Nonfocal Febrile Illness

Many enteroviruses cause acute febrile illness without apparent source, especially in infants and young children. These infections may lead to evaluation for sepsis in infants younger than 3 to 4 months of age; half of these infants also have aseptic meningitis. Similar illnesses among older children and adults are typically self-limited and are often termed "summer grippe." The same symptoms, however, may herald aseptic meningitis, myopericarditis, or other serious disease.

Exanthems and Enanthems

Many echoviruses cause nonspecific maculopapular and morbilliform eruptions. A characteristic but relatively uncommon syndrome known as "Boston exanthem" has been linked to echovirus 16, which may produce centimeter-sized maculopapular lesions on the head and upper trunk following defervescence of the preceding fever.

Group A coxsackieviruses, especially serotype A16, are the principal agents of *hand-foot-and-mouth disease,* a.k.a. vesicular stomatitis with exanthem. Children younger than 10 years of age are the most common victims. Fever and shallow, painful vesicles of the buccal mucosa and tongue are commonly noted. Seventy-five per cent of patients also have small cutaneous vesicles of the distal extremities, which may be confused with those of varicella or rickettsialpox. *Herpangina* is a vesicular enanthem of the tonsillar fauces and soft palate in preschool and grade-school children. Fever, sore throat, and dysphagia are often present. Many group A coxsackievirus serotypes have been implicated. The disease must be distinguished from other causes of pharyngitis.

Aseptic Meningitis and Encephalitis

Group B coxsackieviruses and echoviruses are the most common causes of acute *aseptic meningitis.* Attack rates are highest among infants younger than 3 months of age. Common manifestations include fever, nausea, vomiting, and signs of meningeal irritation. Young infants typically present with only fever, irritability, and poor feeding.

Leukocyte counts in the cerebrospinal fluid (CSF) generally range from 10 to 500 cells/mm^3, but lower and higher cell counts are sometimes noted. Neutrophils predominate during the first 2 days, but thereafter more than 50 per cent are lymphocytes. The CSF glucose level is usually normal or slightly depressed, and the protein level may be mildly increased.

The diagnosis of viral meningitis is confirmed by isolation of virus in cell culture or by demonstration of viral RNA in the CSF with the use of the polymerase chain reaction. Many echovirus and group B coxsackievirus serotypes have been isolated from patients with aseptic meningitis, especially coxsackievirus serotypes B2 and B5 and echovirus serotypes 4, 6, 9, 11, 16, and 30. Group A coxsackieviruses are rarely identified. The differential diagnosis of viral meningitis includes partially treated bacterial meningitis, and meningitis caused by mumps virus, lymphocytic choriomeningitis virus, herpes simplex virus, human immunodeficiency virus, and arboviruses, leptospirosis, and Lyme disease. Patients with persistent symptoms should also be evaluated for tuberculosis, cryptococcal infection, and coccidioidomycosis.

Encephalitis is a less common manifestation of enteroviral infection. The presenting symptoms and neurologic signs may suggest either focal or generalized involvement of the central nervous system. Many serotypes of enterovirus have been implicated in all age groups. The CSF abnormalities are similar to those observed in aseptic meningitis.

The muscle weakness and paralysis seen in poliomyelitis may rarely be caused by some nonpolio enteroviruses. The prognosis for recovery of strength following infection with nonpolio enteroviruses is better than that following infection with polioviruses.

Pleurodynia

Pleurodynia (epidemic myalgia, Bornholm disease) is a distinctive illness caused primarily by group B coxsackieviruses and characterized by the acute onset of fever, malaise, and sharp thoracic pain. Enteroviral pleurodynia affects adults more often than children, causing both community outbreaks and major epidemics.

The term "pleurodynia" is misleading, since infection is confined to the skeletal muscles of the chest wall and abdomen rather than the pleura. The hallmark of pleurodynia is intermittent, painful muscle spasm. Fifty per cent of patients with pleurodynia also complain of concurrent abdominal pain. Physical examination reveals fever and localized tenderness in the chest or abdominal wall; the heart and lungs are typically unremarkable. The differential diagnosis includes pneumonia, pulmonary embolus, pericarditis, myocardial ischemia, and prodromal herpes zoster. The electrocardiogram and chest radiograph are usually normal; rare pleural effusions have been reported. The diagnosis is confirmed by isolation of group B coxsackievirus from throat and stool specimens.

Myopericarditis

The term "myopericarditis" refers to a spectrum of disorders with overlapping etiologic, clinical, and pathologic features of pericarditis and myocarditis. Among the viruses associated with myopericarditis, group B coxsackieviruses are most prominent, followed by other enteroviruses, adenoviruses, influenza viruses, and mumps virus. Myopericarditis affects all ages, but adolescents and young adults are at particular risk, perhaps because of the well-established association with exercise. In two thirds of patients, upper respiratory illness precedes the onset of fever, dyspnea, and chest pain. The quality of chest pain varies from sharp to dull; the pain may be worse when the patient is supine. The physical examination may reveal a pericardial friction rub, cardiac gallop, aberrant cardiac rhythm, or signs of congestive heart failure. The chest radiograph shows enlargement of the cardiac silhouette in half of the patients. Electrocardiograms may reveal ST-segment elevation and ST- and T-wave abnormalities. Severe myocarditis can lead to heart block, arrhythmias, and Q waves. Assessment of ventricular function with echocardiography is now routine.

Etiologic diagnosis is made by isolation of virus from the oropharynx or stool. Enterovirus RNA has been amplified from myocardial biopsies by the polymerase chain reaction. The differential diagnosis includes myocarditis due to other viruses and myocardial ischemia.

Neonatal Enteroviral Disease

Neonates younger than 10 days of age may develop systemic, life-threatening infections with enteroviruses acquired vertically from the mother or nosocomially. Two syndromes of severe infection are seen in neonates. *Neonatal myocarditis* is associated with the group B coxsackieviruses. Concurrent encephalitis is common; some infants also develop hepatitis, pancreatitis, or pneumonia. Fifty per cent of cases are complicated by heart failure and circulatory collapse, resulting in death. Several echovirus serotypes, particularly echovirus 11, cause fulminant *neonatal hepatitis.* Jaundice, hypertension, profuse, uncontrollable bleeding, and multiple organ system dysfunction develop within 2 to 4 days. Mortality exceeds 80 per cent, with most deaths occurring within 1 week.

The diagnosis of neonatal enteroviral infection requires isolation of virus from the upper respiratory tract, stool, urine, CSF, serum, or feces. Typically, high concentrations of virus are present.

Conjunctivitis

Global epidemics of *acute hemorrhagic conjunctivitis* caused by enterovirus 70 and coxsackievirus A24 affect millions of people in tropical climates. These highly contagious illnesses are characterized by the abrupt onset of eye pain, photophobia, and lid swelling. Prominent subconjunctival hemorrhages that develop within several hours and resolve spontaneously within a week are typical of enterovirus 70 infections. Virus can be recovered from conjunctival swabs during the first 3 days of the illness. The differential diagnosis includes acute foreign body injury and epidemic keratoconjunctivitis caused by adenovirus. Rare complications include keratitis, secondary bacterial infection, and motor paralysis. Treatment is symptomatic.

Other Enteroviral Infections

Pancreatitis has been associated with infections with coxsackievirus B. The role of the group B coxsackieviruses in the onset of insulin-dependent diabetes mellitus is currently a subject of intense investigation.

Coxsackievirus and echovirus infections in immunocompromised hosts may follow an unusual course. For example, children with X-linked agammaglobulinemia may have persistent central nervous system infections, skeletal muscle inflammation, and chronic hepatitis.

LABORATORY DIAGNOSIS OF ENTEROVIRAL INFECTIONS

Virus Isolation

Viral culture remains the "gold standard" for diagnosis of enteroviral infection. Enteroviruses replicate only in primate cells. Three or four primate cell lines are used by most laboratories to increase the chance for recovery. The most popular are primary monkey kidney cells and human fibroblasts. The addition of human heteroploid cells such as RD or Hep-2 increases recovery of some group A coxsackieviruses, which characteristically grow poorly in cell culture. Optimal isolation of group A coxsackieviruses requires inoculation of newborn mice, an impracticality for most clinical virology laboratories.

Virus replication is detected by recognition of characteristic cytopathic changes in the morphology of the cultured cells. The demonstration of a cytopathic effect (CPE) typically requires 3 to 7 days for most clinical specimens. Serotypic identification is limited to reference or research laboratories where antibody neutralization with the Lim Benyesh-Melnick equine antiserum pools is employed to "type" an enterovirus isolate.

Cerebrospinal fluid, pericardial fluid, urine, blood, stool, upper respiratory tract specimens, and tissue all may be submitted for viral culture. Because the concentration of infectious viruses tends to be low in most specimens, the culturing of multiple sites increases the diagnostic yield. Enteroviruses are shed in low titers for short periods (i.e., days) from the upper respiratory tract. By contrast, virus may be shed in the stool for weeks after resolution of the primary clinical syndrome, for example, meningitis. Therefore, the recovery of viruses from stool samples or rectal swabs is considered less specific than the recovery of viruses from other sites.

Polymerase Chain Reaction

The use of the polymerase chain reaction (PCR) technique may enhance the speed and sensitivity of enterovirus detection. For the enteroviruses, genomic RNA must be transcribed to the complementary DNA. The PCR then amplifies a portion of the 5′ noncoding region of the genome, which is highly conserved among most enteroviruses and which can be positively identified with Southern blot hybridization or other methods.

Enteroviral PCR can be useful in the diagnosis of aseptic meningitis, myopericarditis, and recurrent enteroviral meningitis in children with hypogammaglobulinemia. During outbreaks of enteroviral aseptic meningitis, the PCR has been used to detect enteroviral RNA in CSF in as many as 40 per cent of culture-negative patients. In those undergoing endomyocardial biopsy for suspected myocarditis, 10 to 20 per cent reveal evidence of enterovirus infection on PCR testing. Recurrent bouts of culture-negative meningoencephalitis in agammaglobulinemic patients thought to have chronic enteroviral infections had previously defied diagnosis. Enterovirus has now been detected by PCR in the CSF of these patients during periods of clinical exacerbation, suggesting a persistent inability to eradicate the virus.

The PCR technique is more sensitive than culture, and false-positive results are uncommon when the PCR is performed in an experienced laboratory. Currently, the assay is limited to CSF and endomyocardial biopsy specimens. Serotype-specific diagnosis still depends on isolation of a virus in cell culture. Echovirus types 22 and 23 are not detected with the PCR, because their RNA sequences differ sufficiently from other enteroviruses at the amplified site.

Serology

Human antibodies generated against enteroviruses are serotype-specific. Thus, serologic diagnosis is practical only when a specific enteroviral serotype is suspected. The microneutralization assay is labor-intensive, poorly standardized, and not widely available. Several immunoassays for more common enteroviral infections are available commercially but lack specificity.

HERPESVIRUSES

By Larry I. Lutwick, M.D.
Brooklyn, New York

The term "herpes" is derived from the Greek word for reptile and is used because of the serpiginous pattern of lesions that may occur in recurrent cutaneous herpesvirus infection. Herpesviruses can cause characteristic primary infections, with development of a latent state in neural ganglia or leukocytes. Reactivation from latency can be clinically overt, usually is less severe than the primary component, and can occur multiply, only once in a lifetime, or not at all. Reactivation is often manifested only by asymptomatic viral shedding but may be particularly overt and prolonged in cellular immunoincompetent hosts.

In recent years, the number of known human herpesviruses has grown to eight with the description of human herpesviruses 6, 7, and 8 (Table 1). This article does not discuss Epstein-Barr virus (EBV), human cytomegalovirus (HCMV), or a simian herpesvirus, herpes B, which can cause a severe encephalitis in humans.

HERPES SIMPLEX VIRUS

Presenting Signs and Symptoms and Course of Disease

Orolabial Infection

Primary oral herpes simplex virus (HSV) infection is usually acquired in childhood but may present in an adult. Although this infection is generally due to HSV-1, it can be associated with HSV-2 as the result of orogenital contact in adults or abused children. The spectrum of severity ranges from asymptomatic seroconversion to significant disease that requires hospitalization of the patient for rehydration. Overt infection is associated with small vesicles that progress to ulcers on the buccal mucosa, palate, gingivae, and tongue with a sore throat and mouth and dysphagia. Vesiculoulcerative lesions also occur on the lips and periorally. This systemic process is associated with fever, malaise, myalgias, and regional lymphadenopathy and, if untreated, can last for 1 to 3 weeks. Autoinoculation via fingers to other body surfaces, especially in young children, is not uncommon. In teenagers and young adults, the process may be localized to the posterior pharynx and can be indistinguishable from bacterial pharyngitis or mononucleosis. Among the conditions that need to be considered in the differential diagnosis of herpetic gingivostomatitis are Vincent's disease (acute necrotizing ulcerative gingivostomatitis, or trench mouth), hand-foot-and-mouth disease (coxsackievirus), malnutrition, chemotherapy effect, and drug reaction.

Recurrent oral HSV infection (cold sores, fever blisters) can be triggered by fever, sunburn, trauma (including dental extraction), or stress. Typically, the process is heralded by burning or tingling and presents as a painful group of vesicles at the lip vermilion border or on perioral areas of the face (Fig. 1). Episodes can be frequent or uncommon in any individual and often decrease in frequency over time. In both oral and genital infections, symptomatic recurrences may be associated with a subclinical primary infection. The lesions usually heal in 5 to 7 days, and the period during which virus is shed is short. Asymptomatic recurrences are common, so isolation of HSV from saliva cannot be definitely identified as the cause of respiratory

Table 1. Human Herpesviruses

Virus	Designation	Primary Infection	Usual Reactivation Infection*
Herpes simplex virus type 1	HSV-1	Herpetic gingivostomatitis	Cold sores (fever blisters)
Herpes simplex virus type 2	HSV-2	Primary genital herpes simplex	Recurrent disease
Varicella-zoster virus	VZV	Varicella (chickenpox)	Herpes zoster (shingles)
Epstein-Barr virus	EBV	Heterophil-positive mononucleosis	Asymptomatic shedding
Human cytomegalovirus	HCMV	Heterophil-negative mononucleosis	Asymptomatic shedding
Human herpesvirus 6	HHV-6	Roseola (exanthema subitum)	Asymptomatic shedding
Human herpesvirus 7	HHV-7	Roseola	Asymptomatic shedding
Human herpesvirus 8	HHV-8	Unknown	?Kaposi's sarcoma

*Herpesviruses are associated with severe infection, with reactivation in cellular immunoincompetent hosts.

tract pathology, but the asymptomatic state can be a source of transmission of the virus to others. Recurrent aphthous ulcers (canker sores) can be confused with recurrent HSV infection, but the former are usually intraoral.

Genital Infection

Primary genital infection—asymptomatic or overt—may be caused by HSV-2 or HSV-1, depending on the mode of transmission. The clinical course of the first episode of genital infection is similar for either type of HSV. In males, painful vesicles progress to ulcers that may involve the penis, perineum, and urethra. Females can have cervical, vaginal, urethral, and vulvar lesions, with proctitis occurring in females and homosexual males. Autoinoculation via the fingers may cause spread to other sites. Associated systemic symptoms include fever, fatigue, and myalgias, and, if untreated, the infection may last 1 to 3 weeks. The severity of genital HSV-2 infection is modified, in part, by previous oral HSV-1 infection, which results in a shorter, milder course with fewer systemic signs and symptoms.

Even though first-episode genital herpes infection can be due to either type of virus, most recurrences are due to HSV-2. The frequency of recurrence is higher, and the time to recurrence shorter, after primary genital HSV-2 compared with HSV-1. This difference appears to reflect a difficulty for HSV-1 in establishing and maintaining latency in this area. Recurrence rates vary drastically between individuals and can diminish over time. The recurrences present as painful vesicular lesions on the penis or adjacent areas in males and vulvar lesions in females without systemic signs and symptoms, often associated with a painful or dysesthetic prodrome. The only manifestation in females may be mucosal lesions involving the cervix or urethra and presenting with minimal or no symptoms, mucoid discharge, or dysuria. Asymptomatic shedding occurs in both sexes and can be the cause of transmission of the disease. Recurrences also may involve the sacral area, be zosteriform in character, and be associated with aseptic meningitis.

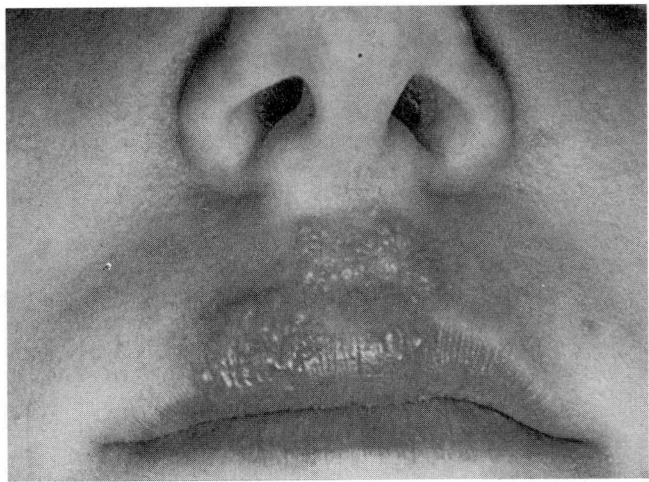

Figure 1. Recurrent labial HSV-1 infection. (From Shafer, W. G., Hine, M. K., and Levy, B. M.: *A Textbook of Oral Pathology.* Philadelphia, W. B. Saunders, 1983, p. 368, with permission.)

The physician must make the distinction between genital herpes and other ulcerative venereal diseases. Syphilitic lesions are generally painless, but it may be difficult to distinguish between chancroid and HSV infection, especially without a history of recurrences. Pyoderma and scabies can also be confused with late, crusted HSV infection. The presence of either a prodrome or recurrences is highly suggestive of HSV rather than other infectious or noninfectious causes.

Cutaneous Infection

Any site can be infected by either HSV type, and infection is facilitated by focal trauma. One classic form is the herpetic whitlow. The whitlow presents as acute redness, swelling, and pain of the distal finger, with vesicular lesions. Fever, lymphadenitis, and lymphangitis can occur with these signs and symptoms, making it difficult for the physician to differentiate HSV from the bacterial felon. HSV-1 whitlows are found in children and health care workers, and HSV-2 disease is related to genital exposure. Recurrent whitlows may be more common with HSV-2. Other syndromes include herpes gladiatorum in contact sports, such as wrestling, and more serious infections with widespread disease may be associated with HSV in burns or eczema.

Ocular Involvement

A recurring form of infection of the cornea and conjunctiva is usually due to HSV-1. It is the leading infectious cause of corneal blindness in the United States. Primary infection is associated with a unilateral follicular conjunctivitis and blepharitis with vesicles on the lid margin. Pain, tearing, chemosis, photophobia, and blurry vision may occur. The cornea shows dendritic ulcers (Fig. 2) or epithelial opacities. Herpes simplex virus eye disease can be confused with bacterial, chlamydial, adenoviral, or allergic conjunctivitis. Topical corticosteroids may aggravate the infection.

Reactivation disease often involves only the cornea, with irritation and photophobia. The recurrent superficial kera-

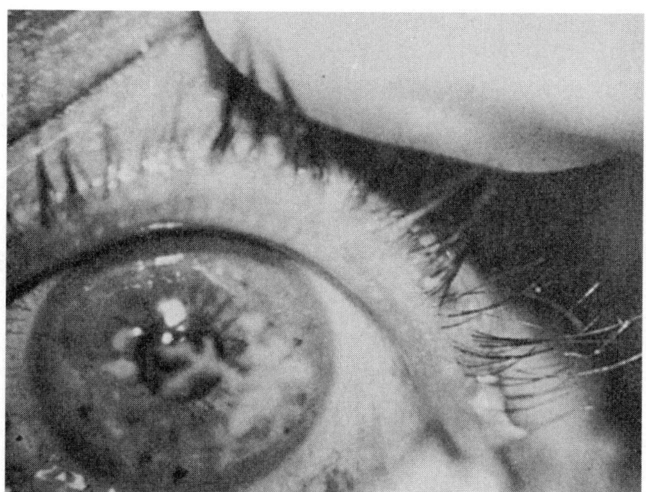

Figure 2. Herpetic corneal dendritic ulcer seen under a Wood's light after fluorescein staining. (From Biswell. *In* Vaughan, D., and Asbury, T.: *General Ophthalmology,* 13th ed. East Norwalk, CT, Appleton & Lange, 1992, p. 133, with permission.)

titis heals, but deeper corneal involvement and uveitis develop—these may be immunologically mediated. If the infection goes untreated, corneal scars, thinning, and neovascularization can eventually result in visual loss.

Complications of HSV Infection

Herpes Encephalitis

In the United States, HSV encephalitis remains the most commonly reported viral encephalitis, with a rate of 1 to 2 cases per 1 million persons per year. Most non-neonatal cases are due to HSV-1. The disease may be related to primary infection or reactivation, or it may be the consequence of reinfection with an exogenous HSV strain. Herpes simplex encephalitis presents with fever, altered mental status, and focal findings that may be related to the temporal lobe. The signs and symptoms include abnormal behavior, speech difficulties, focal seizures, and olfactory hallucinations.

As herpes encephalitis is one of the few treatable forms of viral encephalitis, its differentiation from other viral causes, such as enteroviruses and arthropod-borne viruses, is important. Since infections with these latter groups are more frequent in the summer and fall, winter-onset encephalitis is more commonly due to HSV. The presence of active orolabial HSV or HSV isolation from saliva in an encephalitic patient is of little diagnostic help. The cerebrospinal fluid (CSF) reflects a necrotizing process with erythrocytes, a lymphocytic pleocytosis, mildly elevated protein level, and normal glucose concentration. Electroencephalography and computed tomography or magnetic resonance imaging of the brain should reveal focal encephalitis, which can assist the physician in locating the lesion if a brain biopsy is needed. Brain pathology demonstrates a necrotizing inflammatory process with intranuclear inclusion bodies. The tissue should be positive on culture for HSV. Importantly, the biopsy may identify as many as 10 to 15 per cent of patients with nonviral and potentially treatable conditions, including tubercular and fungal infections and vasculitic diseases.

The course of this HSV complication usually involves rapid deterioration over several days, progressing to coma and death. If the disease goes untreated, mortality is roughly 70 per cent, and many survivors have significant neurologic residua.

Neonatal Infection

The newborn may acquire HSV-2 at the time of parturition by passage through an infected birth canal or from ascending infection. Transmission is more likely to occur with primary maternal infection but is due to symptomatic or asymptomatic reactivation in two thirds of patients. Perinatal HSV-1 can be acquired from nursery workers or family members. Transplacental congenital infection with HSV also occurs.

The manifestations may range from a mild, localized, nonprogressive cutaneous focus to one that disseminates fatally. Disseminated HSV infection in the neonate often presents with a cutaneous focus on the birth presentation part of the body (usually the scalp) and, over a few days, can progress to multiorgan involvement, including the liver, adrenals, lung, kidneys, and brain. The absence of a cutaneous focus is not uncommon, and in this circumstance, it may be difficult to distinguish the viral infection from a bacterial one. Untreated, the entity has a mortality rate of 85 per cent or higher in the disseminated form. It may be difficult to distinguish congenital HSV from other congenital infections due to HCMV, toxoplasmosis, or rubella.

Infection in the Immune-Compromised Host

The immune-compromised host commonly sheds HSV-1 in oral secretions, and its presence in culture does not necessarily connote a pathogenic role. Individuals with cellular immunosuppression (human immunodeficiency virus [HIV] disease, organ or marrow transplant, chemotherapy) may develop chronic progressive mucocutaneous disease involving the orolabial or genital areas. The virus may spread to adjacent areas, such as the esophagus (infection of which may be difficult to differentiate from candidal disease) and trachea. Rarely, HSV infection may involve visceral organs in this population. This process may infect the liver, lungs, adrenals, and kidneys in a manner similar to that of neonatal infection. Encephalitis is no more common in immune-compromised hosts than in normal ones.

VARICELLA-ZOSTER VIRUS

Presenting Signs and Symptoms and Course of Disease

Varicella

Primary varicella-zoster virus (VZV) infection is also called chickenpox, a misnomer because it has nothing to do with fowl and is not due to a poxvirus. The term probably came from the Old English word for itch, "gican." "Gican pox" eventually became chickenpox.

Primary VZV infection occurs with an incubation period of 11 to 21 days (average 14 to 15 days). Transmission is by air and highly efficient in the household setting where more than 90 per cent of susceptible individuals develop disease. Infection can also spread in reactivation infection (herpes zoster) from direct lesion contact, but this mode is much less efficient. Adequate exposure to herpes zoster in a susceptible individual causes varicella—not zoster.

Varicella usually presents with a rash that begins on the neck hairline or scalp. Erythematous macules and papules rapidly progress to vesicles within 24 hours. Central vesiculation of a red macule can appear as a "dewdrop on a rose petal." Usually significantly pruritic, the rash progresses through vesicles, umbilicated vesicles, ulcers, and crusted lesions over several days. High fever may be present early, but recurrence or persistence after 48 hours of rash is suggestive of bacterial superinfection or varicella pneumonia.

The rash is usually concentrated on the head and torso, with fewer lesions on the extremities. Areas of increased skin blood flow, such as from a sunburn, can develop more concentrated disease. Importantly, affected areas contain lesions in all developmental stages. The vesicles are not loculated and they completely collapse when aspirated. Varicella may also mildly involve mucosal surfaces, such as the mouth and conjunctivae. Other nonherpetic vesiculoulcerative cutaneous diseases that may be confused with varicella include *Pseudomonas* folliculitis, atypical measles, Stevens-Johnson syndrome, coxsackievirus infections, drug reactions, pemphigus, pemphigoid, rickettsialpox, disseminated vaccinia, and, when it existed, smallpox. In its classic form following an exposure, varicella is easily diagnosed.

Varicella develops in successive crops over 3 to 4 days, or slightly longer in adults. The evolution to complete crusting is usually complete in 1 week in children and after a few more days in adults. The total number of lesions varies from fewer than 50 to more than 1000. Subclinical infections are uncommon. Secondary household infections in siblings of a primary patient are often more severe. This severity may be due to a larger inoculum from the closeness of exposure but also to viral passage through a genetically similar host. Varicella is usually considered infectious from 1 day prior to the onset of rash until all of the lesions are crusted.

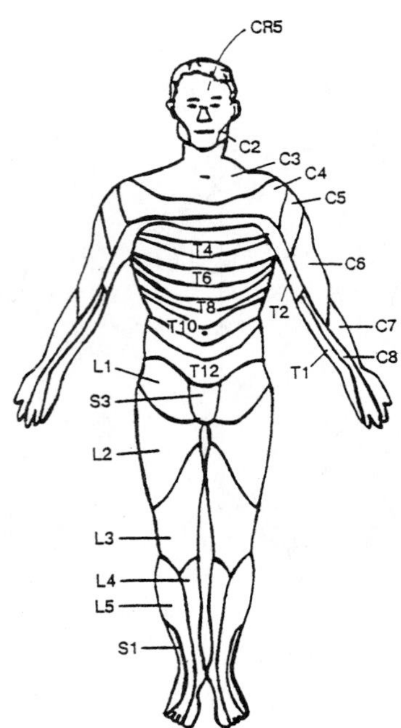

Figure 3. Anterior view of cutaneous dermatomal distributions. (CR5 = trigeminal nerve.)

Herpes Zoster

This process, also called shingles, is reactivation VZV infection. The term "zoster" is derived from a Greek word for belt and refers to the segmental distribution of the infection. It occurs at a rate of 2 to 4 in 1000 persons per year and is 15 times more frequent in the eighth decade than in the first. About 20 per cent of people develop zoster at some time, rarely more than once. The rate is quite high in those who are cellularly immunocompromised by HIV, other diseases, or chemotherapy. Uncomplicated zoster in an otherwise well individual with no other physical findings should not arouse concern about a covert malignancy.

The disease manifests as vesicular lesions in a dermatomal distribution (Fig. 3). Unlike those with varicella, many patients manifest pain and/or paresthesias in the area for several days prior to the rash. Prelesional pain may be severe enough to be confused with a myocardial infarction or abdominal catastrophe. The most common dermatomes involved are those on the torso (usually thoracic) or in the trigeminal nerve distribution, representing the usual predilection of the varicella eruption. Zoster on the extremities is less common. The lesions often do not occupy the entire dermatome but occur in patches. Lesion progression over the 7- to 10-day "attack" is similar to that with varicella but can be associated with significant pain and paresthesias. Because of the appearance and pain, Norwegians have called zoster a "belt of roses from hell." In most cases, only one dermatome is affected, but adjacent dermatomes may be involved (duplex zoster). A few extradermatomal lesions can be present (10 to 20) without a diagnosis of disseminated zoster.

Fever is generally minimal in dermatomal zoster, but regional lymphadenopathy is common. The pain and dysesthesias associated with acute zoster may persist for several weeks after the rash has healed. In its characteristic form, the clinical diagnosis of zoster is rarely difficult. Sacral zosteriform lesions, if recurrent, can be due to HSV-2.

Complications of Varicella

Secondary Bacterial Infection

The skin lesions of varicella and zoster may become superinfected. Staphylococci and group A streptococci are the most common causes of impetigo and cellulitis in these patients, and residual scarring is more likely with superinfection. Bacterial dissemination causing bacteremia, meningitis, or endocarditis is well described, and the VZV lesion can be an entry site for toxin-producing strains that cause toxic shock syndrome.

Varicella Pneumonia

Pneumonia is the most frequent viral complication of varicella. It is more commonly recognized in the adult, even if immunocompetent, and increases morbidity and mortality significantly. Although the pneumonia may be mild, with x-ray changes and no symptoms, it can present with cough, dyspnea, pleuritic chest pain, and hemoptysis beginning up to several days to a week after the onset of varicella. The severity of the diffuse nodular infiltrates on the chest film correlates well with the degree of the skin rash—but not with the pulmonary physical findings. On resolution, multiple small calcifications can be seen, similar to those with histoplasmosis. The pneumonia is more significant in immune-compromised hosts and pregnant women, especially in the third trimester. The older literature reported more than 40 per cent maternal and fetal mortality with this complication, but it is now significantly lower, even before the availability of antiviral interventions.

Varicella Embryopathy

A syndrome associated with maternal varicella in the first trimester of pregnancy has been described. In the fetus, it consists of a hypoplastic limb, scarred lesions on the affected limb, ocular involvement (cataracts, microphthalmia), and nervous system features (microcephaly, autonomic dysfunction). The risk of this syndrome is low, probably less than 5 per cent.

Varicella in the Neonate

Perinatal chickenpox is associated with substantial morbidity and mortality when varicella in the mother begins less than 5 days before delivery or up to 2 days after. The severity of the process reflects the immaturity of the neonatal immune response and the absence of maternal VZV antibodies, which are passively transferred to neonates delivered more than 5 days after the onset of maternal varicella. Visceral involvement is common, especially of the lung, and overall mortality may be 30 per cent.

Disease in Immune-Compromised Hosts

These patients, especially those with leukemia, are prone to severe varicella with more lesions that are often hemorrhagic and that heal more slowly. Bacterial superinfection is common in those who are neutropenic. Visceral spread to the lungs and other organs is common, and the mortality can be as high as 15 per cent. The appropriate use of varicella vaccine can decrease the impact of this illness. Chronic varicella has been described in children with HIV infection.

Neurologic Complications

The central nervous system manifestations of varicella include meningoencephalitis and Reye's syndrome. The former most often presents as cerebellar ataxia, usually within 1 week of the onset of rash, and occurs in 1 in 4000 children. A more progressive encephalitis can occur less commonly with seizures, altered mental status, and a significant risk of sequelae or death. Reye's syndrome has been linked to a number of viral infections, including varicella. Reye's syndrome is associated with liver disease (coagulopathy, elevated ammonia levels), hypoglycemia, and cerebral edema. Aspirin used as an antipyretic in varicella may be a risk factor.

Complications of Zoster

Postherpetic Neuralgia

This entity is the most dreaded complication of zoster, defined as persistence of pain after the acute dermal process has healed. The pain, which can be quite severe and can adversely affect the individual's lifestyle, usually diminishes over time. The pain can be constant or intermittent and may increase at night or on exposure to temperature changes. Overall, as many as 5 to 15 per cent of patients may still be symptomatic after 1 year. This statistic approaches 50 per cent in those older than 70 years of age. It is not entirely clear whether antiviral therapy during the acute process modifies the incidence or severity of postherpetic neuralgia. Likewise, since zoster is associated with a waning immune response, attenuated varicella vaccine given to adults could modify the likelihood or severity of subsequent zoster.

Neurologic Sequelae of Zoster

A variety of neurologic events may occur. Isolated muscle weakness in the involved dermatome (segmental zoster paresis) is more likely noted when an extremity is involved. Herpes zoster ophthalmicus may be complicated by a delayed contralateral hemiplegia that is due to cerebral angiitis. A palsy of cranial nerve VII can occur in association with zoster of the eighth cranial nerve (Ramsay Hunt syndrome), with loss of taste over the anterior two thirds of the tongue and altered lacrimal function. Additionally, seventh nerve palsy or intercurrent dermatomal pain without a rash can be diagnosed as related to VZV by an increase in antibody titer (zoster sine zoster).

Aseptic meningitis (based on a lymphocytic CSF pleocytosis) occurs in 40 to 50 per cent of uncomplicated zoster infections and may cause headache and mild meningismus. Rarely, encephalitis or myelitis occurs at the time of acute zoster or afterward.

Ocular Complications

Ocular complications occur commonly in zoster involving the ophthalmic branch of the trigeminal nerve. Zoster lesions near the tip of the nose indicate involvement of the external nasal nerve, a branch of the nasociliary nerve, and a higher probability of ocular involvement. When the supraorbital and supratrochlear branches of the ophthalmic nerve are the only nerves involved, vesicles develop on the upper eyelid, forehead, and scalp, but the eye itself is spared (Fig. 4). The cornea is involved in about 50 to 55 per cent of infections with ophthalmic zoster. Uveal tract infection is common as well and can predispose to glaucoma or cataracts. Rarely, there is retinal involvement, usually related to ischemia. The delicate skin of the eyelid is susceptible to permanent changes with pitting, scarring, and altered pigmentation. Ocular motor palsies occur but usually are noted only in positions of extreme gaze.

Disseminated Zoster

The appearance of more than 20 lesions in extradermatomal locations defines this complication. It is generally associated with immunosuppression but occurs rarely in normal hosts. Visceral dissemination can complicate cutaneous spread involving the lung, central nervous system, or liver. Even before the availability of antiviral therapy, the process was usually self-limiting. Dissemination is common in HIV-infected people, may be prolonged, and often occurs without primary dermatome involvement.

Zoster in Pregnancy

The occurrence of zoster in pregnancy is not considered a risk to the gestation.

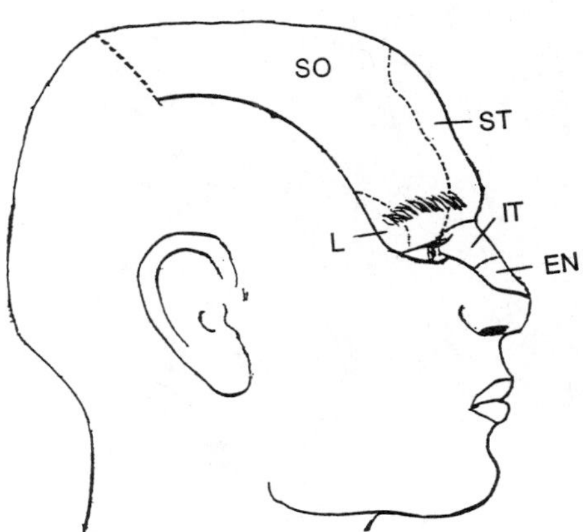

Figure 4. Branches of the ophthalmic division of the trigeminal nerve. (SO = supraorbital nerve; ST = supratrochlear nerve; IT = infratrochlear nerve; L = lacrimal nerve; EN = external nasal branch of nasociliary nerve.)

LABORATORY DIAGNOSTIC TECHNIQUES

Confirmatory testing is useful in atypical or complicated infections with HSV and VZV or those in immune-compromised hosts. The usual patient with varicella or recurrent oral HSV infection does not need virologic confirmation. Because of the potential psychosocial impact of recurrent genital HSV infection, however, virologic confirmation of the agent is indicated. It may be accepted practice soon that more routine viral isolation will be done to determine antiviral susceptibility patterns. With the increased use of antiherpes prophylaxis and treatment, more drug-resistant HSV and VZV will result.

Evaluation of the Vesicle

The simplest diagnostic procedure is the Tzanck test, in which stained scrapings of the base of an unroofed vesicle are examined. A positive test reveals multinucleated giant cells (Fig. 5). The Papanicolaou stain is preferred, since it can better reveal intranuclear inclusion bodies. A positive Tzanck test is specific for a herpesvirus infection but cannot distinguish HSV-1, HSV-2, or VZV. It has a sensitivity of 40 to 80 per cent. Material from the scraping can also be stained with fluorescein-labeled reagents to identify specific agents.

Electron Microscopy

Election microscopic studies of vesicular fluid or tissue may reveal the presence of a herpesvirus but, by themselves, cannot distinguish the specific pathogen. Herpesviruses are enveloped, about 200 nm in size, and contain a 90-nm nucleocapsid with icosahedral symmetry.

Viral Culture

Culture remains the diagnostic "gold standard." To optimize yields, culture is best performed early in the illness. HSV yield is highest in the vesicular (95 per cent) and pustular (90 per cent) stages and lowest in crusted lesions (20 per cent). Herpes simplex virus can be easily recovered from the crusted lesions of chronic mucocutaneous HSV infection in immune-compromised hosts. Varicella-zoster virus is optimally isolated during the first 3 days of the rash. Again, in disseminated VZV of impaired hosts, cultures may be positive even with atypical or crusted lesions. Body fluids or tissue biopsies can be cultured as indicated, and the latter should be combined with histopathologic studies.

Once obtained, the specimen should be quickly transferred to viral transport media. Transient storage can be done at 4°C, but specimens should be frozen at −70°C if there is to be prolonged storage before culture. A standard kitchen-type freezer is not optimal for maintaining virus viability, and inappropriate handling markedly decreases culture yields.

HSV replicates and produces cytopathic effect in a variety of tissue culture cell lines within 4 days, while it takes VZV up to 2 weeks or more. Immunostaining with the use of fluorescein or horseradish peroxidase can identify the isolate and type the HSV. Typing first-episode HSV isolates can aid in predicting clinical outcome. Immunostaining also reduces the time for identification, since virus-specific proteins are detected prior to cytopathic changes. Viral isolation should be successful if performed in a timely and appropriate manner, but the CSF in HSV encephalitis is usually culture negative. HSV-2 may be isolated from the CSF in meningitis associated with a sacral recurrence.

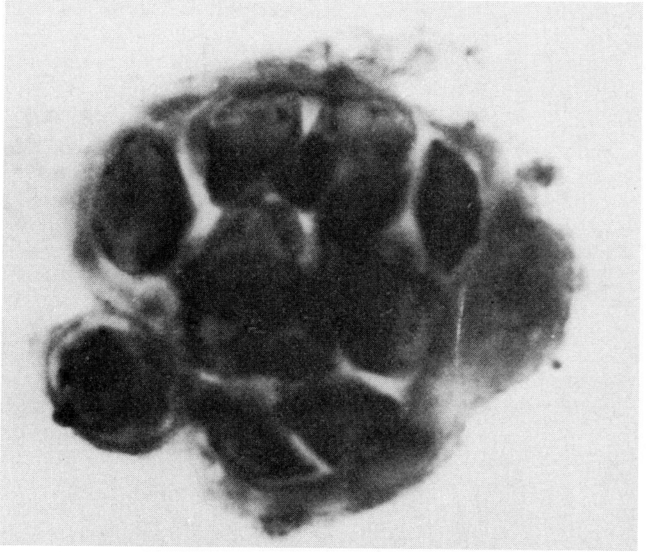

Figure 5. Tzanck test showing multinucleated giant cell. (From Stewart, W. D., Danto, J. L., and Maddin, S.: *Synopsis of Dermatology,* 2nd ed. St. Louis, Mosby–Year Book, 1970, p. 21, with permission.)

Virus Protein and Genome Detection

This methodology offers rapid herpesvirus detection. Vesicle fluid cells or tissue specimens, after cellular disruption, can be used to detect viral proteins by methods including enzyme-linked immunosorbent assay (ELISA). Testing may not be sensitive enough to detect subclinical viral excretion as may occur late in pregnancy. These antigen assays should be done together with culture to optimize results.

The viral genome can be measured directly from clinical specimens or extracts of cultured virus with the use of DNA hybridization techniques to detect the specific agent. Polymerase chain reaction (PCR) methods can be used to amplify herpesvirus DNA in clinical specimens, facilitating identification. PCR can detect the genome in specimens after cultures are no longer positive. Because the sensitivity of PCR assays is so great, care must be taken in interpretation, as the test is prone to producing false-positive results owing to contamination. Cerebrospinal fluid PCR can be useful in the diagnosis of HSV encephalitis and, if positive, obviates the need for brain biopsy.

Epidemiologic Methodology

Restriction endonucleases are bacterial enzymes that break apart DNA at highly specific short nucleotide sequences. The use of endonucleases on viral DNA creates a specific, reproducible DNA fragment pattern in epidemiologically linked isolates. Antigenically identical, nonepidemiologically linked viruses can be shown to differ with the use of these endonuclease "maps." It is therefore possible to show whether isolates of HSV or VZV are linked in nosocomial or medicolegal situations. Studies of VZV with the use of this technique have shown that varicella and subsequent zoster in the same individual are due to the same virus and that "clusters" of zoster are not.

Serologic Methods

HSV antibodies can be detected with the use of different methods, including ELISA, radioimmunoassay, and indirect immunofluorescence. The finding of antibody serves only to demonstrate that HSV infection occurred at some time in the past. Commercial HSV antibody assays do not distinguish HSV-1 from HSV-2. Since HSV-1 is very commonly acquired in childhood with a demonstrable seroconversion, an infected individual who develops primary genital HSV-2 later in life will not seroconvert, as the person is already positive. Tests for IgM HSV antibodies are not useful for identifying primary infection, since reactivation may be associated with a transient IgM response and false-positive results may be due to technical factors. The distinction between HSV-1 and HSV-2 antibody can be made with the use of HSV glycoprotein G antibody assays, since this antigen is type-specific. This test may show seroconversion to HSV-2 even in the presence of HSV-1 antibody. A Western blot technique is currently the gold standard for type-specific testing and is available in some research laboratories. Cerebrospinal antibodies are increased in HSV encephalitis, but this response occurs late and is not useful initially.

Antibodies to VZV can be detected with the use of a variety of techniques and can indicate seroconversion during varicella. Detection of antibodies to VZV is useful in atypical infections. Results obtained with some antibody assays, such as complement fixation, wane with time and are not useful for assessing subsequent susceptibility. ELISA or fluorescent antibody assays for membrane antigen (FAMA) may be used in evaluating health care workers or immunosuppressed patients at high risk for varicella morbidity with no history of previous infection. Many adults without a clear history of chickenpox may still be seropositive, but those from rural areas or who are foreign born are more likely to be susceptible. In reactivation VZV infection, a four-fold rise in antibody titer can be seen, which is in contradistinction to reactivation HSV infection.

HUMAN HERPESVIRUSES 6 AND 7

Human herpesvirus 6 (HHV-6) was called human B lymphotropic virus (HBLV) based on its initial isolation, but it can infect a variety of cells and cell lines. HHV-6 seems most closely related to HCMV, and cross-reactivity of antibody may occur. It is grouped into two variants, A and B, based on restriction endonuclease patterns and growth characteristics. Human herpervirus 7 (HHV-7) has been described more recently and has been less well studied. Both viruses are quite prevalent in the population, with as many as 70 to 80 per cent of infants acquiring HHV-6 during the first year of life; nearly all individuals are seropositive for HHV-7 by age 5 years.

Clinical Illness

Roseola infantum (exanthema subitum) is the classic illness related to primary infection with these agents. Most infections can be shown to be caused by HHV-6, with a smaller number due to HHV-7. A relatively benign disease of children, usually younger than 2 years of age, it manifests as a few days of fever and a maculopapular rash on the torso following defervescence. Roseola may be associated with febrile seizures and/or a meningoencephalitis in children. HHV-6 is a major cause of febrile episodes warranting hospital visits in infants. The B variant is more common in symptomatic disease in infants, while HHV-6 A is more frequent in adults.

Seroconversions may be asymptomatic or related to nonspecific illnesses without rash. In adults, primary HHV-6 infection can cause a mononucleosislike illness or hepatitis. Reactivation HHV-6 infection in immunosuppressed hosts has been associated with fever and rash with hepatic, neurologic, or bone marrow involvement.

Diagnosis

Primary HHV-6 infection can be confirmed by seroconversion. An IgM response occurs but also may be seen transiently with reactivation. In the United States, the seroprevalence of HHV-6 decreases with age: close to 100 per cent are seropositive at age 3 years, with this figure dropping to as low as 35 per cent after age 60 years. This waning of demonstrable antibodies in older adults makes serologic diagnosis in adults more difficult. Likewise, HHV-6 isolation from saliva is commonly noted in both healthy and immunosuppressed people without increases in serologic titers. The physician must take care in using either HHV-6 serology or culture alone in assessing disease causation. Because of the possibility of cross-reactivity, antibody to CMV should be done in parallel.

HUMAN HERPESVIRUS 8

With the use of nucleic acid detection technology, evidence of a unique herpesvirus (HHV-8) has been found in tissues of AIDS-related and AIDS-unrelated Kaposi's sarcoma. Whether this virus, also called Kaposi's sarcoma–associated herpesvirus (KSHV), causes this malignancy has yet to be determined.

VIRAL HEMORRHAGIC FEVERS AND HANTAVIRUS PULMONARY SYNDROME

By Theodore F. Tsai, M.D.
Ft. Collins, Colorado
and Ali S. Khan, M.D.
Atlanta, Georgia

The viral hemorrhagic fevers are exotic, principally rodent- or vector-borne infections caused by more than 20 RNA viruses in four viral families (Table 1). The illnesses are associated with high mortality and infectiousness and share a common feature of sometimes prominent alterations in hemostasis and hemorrhage as a clinical hallmark. Hantavirus pulmonary syndrome (HPS), although not typically associated with a hemorrhagic diathesis, is considered here because of its etiologic relationship to other hantavirus-associated hemorrhagic fevers.

With the exception of Seoul virus, a rat-associated hantavirus that causes hemorrhagic fever with renal syndrome (HFRS), these viruses are exotic to the United States. Only rare cases of viral hemorrhagic fever have been imported to the United States, Europe, and Japan. As international tourism and air travel increase, however, additional imported cases are likely to occur. Although these diseases have specific geographic, ecologic, and vector associations, their clinical presentations may be indistinguishable, and

Table 1. Salient Epidemiologic Features of Viral Hemorrhagic Fevers and Hantavirus Pulmonary Syndrome

Disease, Virus	Geographic Distribution	Ecology and Transmission	Incubation Period (d)
Argentine hemorrhagic fever* (AHF), Juniń	Argentina—Buenos Aires, Cordoba and Santa Fe provinces	Rural campestral; occupational disease of agricultural workers Transmitted by rodents	7–14
Bolivian hemorrhagic fever* (BHF), Machupo	Bolivia—Beni province	Rural peridomestic Transmitted by rodents	7–14
Venezuelan hemorrhagic fever (VHF), Guanarito	Venezuela—Portuguesa and Baraquenas states	Rural peridomestic Transmitted by rodents	7–14
Unnamed Sabiá viral infection, Sabiá	Brazil	Unknown	8
Lassa fever,* Lassa	West and Central Africa	Rural peridomestic Transmitted by rodents	5–16
Hantavirus pulmonary syndrome (HPS), Sin Nombre, Black Creek Canal, Bayou, unnamed Brazilian virus, probably others	United States, Canada, Brazil, Argentina, Americas?	Rural peridomestic; recreational and occupational infections Transmitted by rodents	7–21
Hemorrhagic fever with renal syndrome (HFRS), Hantaan, Seoul, Dobrava, Puumula	Asia (Hantaan, Seoul); Europe (Puumula, Dobrava); rare Seoul virus infections worldwide	Rural campestral and sylvatic; urban peridomestic Transmitted by rodents	4–42
Rift Valley fever (RVF), Rift Valley fever	Africa	Rural Transmitted by mosquitoes; mechanically transmitted by other insects and directly from blood and tissues of infected livestock	3–5
Crimean-Congo hemorrhagic fever* (CCHF), Crimean-Congo	Asia, Africa, Southern Europe	Rural-sylvatic; occupational disease of herders and butchers Transmitted by ticks; directly from blood, tissues of infected livestock	2–7
Marburg hemorrhagic fever,* Marburg	Africa (imported to Europe in monkeys)	Rural Natural reservoir and primary transmission unknown	3–16
Ebola hemorrhagic fever,* Ebola Sudan, Zaire, Côte d'Ivoire	Africa	Rural Natural reservoir and primary transmission unknown	3–16
Dengue hemorrhagic fever (DHF), dengue types 1–4	Tropics, wordwide	Urban, peridomestic Transmitted by mosquitoes	2–7
Yellow fever, yellow fever	South America; Africa	Forests; urban peridomestic and savanna Transmitted by mosquitoes	3–6
Omsk hemorrhagic fever (OHF), OHF	Western Siberia	Sylvan Transmitted by ticks; direct contact, waterborne	3–8
Kyasanur forest disease (KFD), KFD	India, Karnataka state	Human modified forests Transmitted by ticks	3–8

*Documented nosocomial transmission.

their initial differentiation from other tropical infections may be difficult. Therefore, a detailed history of a patient's travel itinerary and activities within the incubation period is essential to suggest a specific cause (see Table 1).

Clinicians should be alert to the possibility of viral hemorrhagic fever in travelers who have returned for three reasons: (1) Untreated infections are associated with a high mortality rate (5 to 50 per cent), (2) for Lassa fever, HFRS, and other fevers, specific antiviral therapy and immunotherapy are available and may be life-saving if initiated early, and (3) the many of the hemorrhagic fevers are easily spread to medical personnel and others who have close contact with infected body fluids. Hospital and community outbreaks, with frightening rates of secondary transmission and mortality, have occurred. An imported case constitutes a medical and public health emergency. Rapid recognition of this possibility and institution of appropriate barrier nursing precautions and disinfection of clinical specimens have thus far prevented nosocomial transmission and community spread from cases imported to the United States and Europe.

PRESENTING SIGNS AND SYMPTOMS

Early symptoms are nonspecific, and differentiation from other common febrile illnesses can be difficult. Initial symptoms may have an abrupt onset and include fever, myalgia, headache, and gastrointestinal symptoms. The subsequent development of hypotension, a flushed appearance, and hemorrhages such as epistaxis, gum bleeding, and petechiae should stimulate consideration of these illnesses in returned travelers with the appropriate history of exposure. Rash is uncommon except in Ebola hemorrhagic fever (EHF) and Marburg hemorrhagic fever (MHF) and in some patients with dengue hemorrhagic fever (DHF), and Lassa fever.

Although a hemorrhagic diathesis is common to this

group of diseases, the pathogenesis of this alteration is variable, and bleeding is seldom of an extent to be of clinical significance. The often critical course of illness is more directly attributable to vascular endothelial injury leading to fluid transudation, edema, and shock. Infection is pantropic. Parenchymal infection, especially of the liver, as well as microscopic hemorrhages and infarction may lead to dysfunction of multiple organ systems.

POTENTIAL ERRORS AND PITFALLS IN DIAGNOSIS

Imported cases have been extremely rare; however, the potential public health consequences of a single case are such that clinicians should retain the possibility in the differential diagnosis of severe febrile illnesses in travelers who have returned from areas where these diseases occur. Conversely, a potential pitfall is to entertain the diagnosis at the expense of a thorough evaluation of more common and treatable conditions such as malaria, leptospirosis, or typhoid fever. The final challenge is the inherent difficulty of making the correct etiologic diagnosis, especially in a traveler who has returned from Africa, where many of these diseases are endemic in overlapping regions.

LABORATORY FINDINGS

Transient leukopenia or leukocytosis with a left shift is frequently found. The peripheral smear may disclose atypical lymphocytes or the Pelger-Huët nuclear anomaly. Thrombocytopenia is a nearly universal feature but is most marked in DHF, HFRS, Crimean-Congo hemorrhagic fever (CCHF), MHF, and severe cases of yellow fever. Transient bone marrow depression may produce a heterotypic appearance of platelets. Liver damage in yellow fever, RVF, CCHF, and filoviral infections may be extensive and may lead to reduced levels of coagulation factors and a prolonged prothrombin time (PT); some patients exhibit features of consumptive coagulopathy. Alterations in other laboratory measures of hemostasis are variable. Elevated hepatic aminotransferases and bilirubin levels are common, and in yellow fever, RVF, and CCHF, they may be markedly raised. Azotemia from prerenal and renal insufficiency is common. The absence of proteinuria and/or hematuria is helpful in excluding the diagnosis of yellow fever, arenaviral hemorrhagic fevers, and HFRS.

DIAGNOSTIC PROCEDURES

Except for the hantaviruses, these viruses are readily recoverable from samples retrieved in the acute phase of illness. Infection may be transmitted percutaneously or potentially by aerosol from clinical samples. Therefore, acute samples should be collected, handled, and shipped with due caution to an appropriate high-containment laboratory for diagnostic evaluation (see addresses further on).

The enzyme-linked immunosorbent assay (ELISA) and the indirect immunofluorescent antibody (IFA) test have proved to be the most convenient approaches to serologic diagnosis, especially for detection of IgM. Hemagglutination inhibition (HI), complement fixation (CF), and neutralization tests still have specific diagnostic utility in some instances. Antibodies are detected very late in the arenaviral and filoviral diseases (usually not at all in fatal cases) and may be detected falsely in patients given passive immunotherapy. For some of these infections, assays have been developed to detect viral antigen or genomic sequences directly in acute specimens by ELISA or polymerase chain reaction (PCR), respectively.

NOSOCOMIAL TRANSMISSION

CCHF, the filoviral and arenaviral hemorrhagic fevers, and others as noted in Table 1, are associated with nosocomial transmission; therefore, appropriate precautions should be taken while evaluating these patients to limit patient and specimen contact to essential personnel. Communication among physicians, nursing, housekeeping, and laboratory staff is essential. However, fear of nosocomial transmission must not delay diagnostic evaluation and institution of appropriate therapy for more common treatable diseases. Specific guidelines on patient management, precautions, and diagnostic testing can be obtained at any time from Special Pathogens Branch, Division of Viral and Rickettsial Diseases, Centers for Disease Control and Prevention (CDC), 1600 Clifton Road (MS G-14), Atlanta GA, 30333, telephone (404)639-1511 (days) and (404)639-2888 (evenings).

ARENAVIRAL HEMORRHAGIC FEVERS

Definition

The arenaviral hemorrhagic fevers are acquired by contact with or inhalation of aerosolized infected rodent excreta. The diseases are generally divided into those caused by Old World viruses (Lassa fever) and those resulting from New World viruses (Juniń, Machupo, Guanarito, and Sabiá-associated hemorrhagic fevers). Lymphocytic choriomeningitis virus (an Old World arenavirus) has rarely been associated with generalized hemorrhages. Lassa fever may be the cause of as many as 300,000 human infections and 5000 deaths annually in rural villages of West and Central Africa. Outbreaks of the New World arenaviral hemorrhagic fevers have been highly localized in rural populations who also have peridomestic contact with specific rodent species that function as viral reservoirs. The exception is Argentine hemorrhagic fever (AHF), which is principally an occupational disease of adult male agricultural workers infected in rodent-infested fields (Fig. 1).

Presenting Signs and Symptoms

An insidious onset of several days to a week is typical; early symptoms include fever, weakness and generalized malaise, lower backache, substernal chest or epigastric pain, dizziness, cough, and gastrointestinal symptoms. There may be few physical findings other than fever, hypotension, conjunctivitis, a flushed appearance, and abdominal tenderness. An exudative pharyngitis may be seen in some Lassa fever patients. Arthralgia, lymphadenopathy, petechial enanthem, neurologic signs (e.g., confusion and gait disturbances), and epistaxis may be part of the initial presentation of South American arenaviral fevers.

Course of the Process

Lassa Fever

Illness and fever are protracted and may extend for up to several weeks with various degrees of hemorrhage and edema, hepatic damage, and pulmonary symptoms. Some patients have a fulminant course of illness marked by acute shock, hemorrhage, generalized and pulmonary edema, and encephalitis. A rash may be visible in white

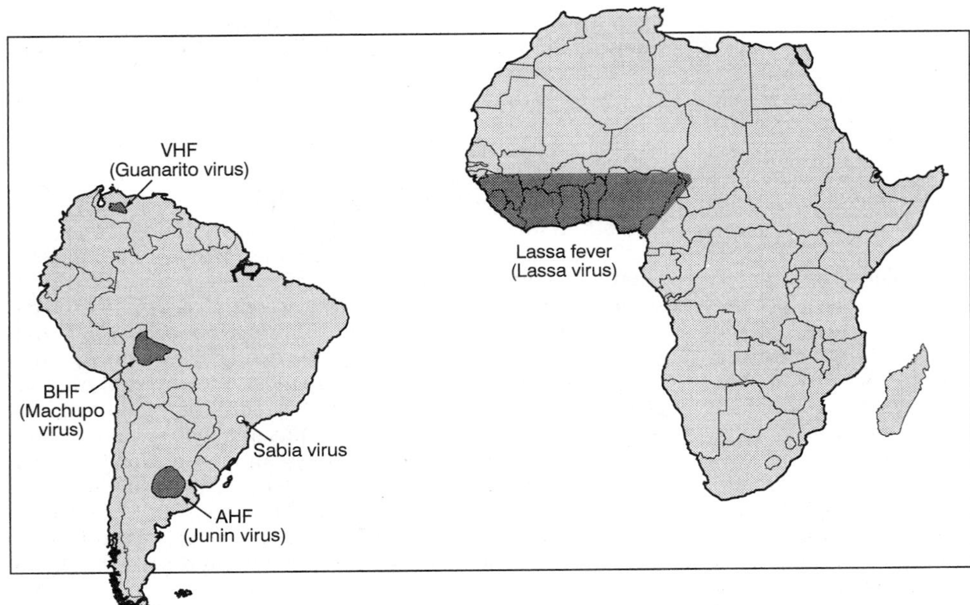

Figure 1. Geographic distribution of arenaviral hemorrhagic fevers.

patients. Recovery usually is gradual. About 20 per cent of all hospitalized cases are fatal.

New World Arenaviral Hemorrhagic Fevers

During the second week of illness, some patients deteriorate, with hemorrhagic manifestations including gastrointestinal bleeding, metrorrhagia, purpura and oral mucosal bleeding, oliguria, and shock resulting from capillary leakage. Others may have prominent neurologic symptoms, including tremor, bulbar signs, convulsions, and coma. The case fatality rate in untreated patients is about 15 per cent.

Complications

Secondary bacterial infections should be anticipated and treated. Complications of Lassa fever include abortion, pleural and pericardial effusions and, in recovered patients, permanent sensorineural hearing loss. Hearing loss and transient hair loss have also been reported following Bolivian hemorrhagic fever. A late neurologic syndrome may develop in 10 per cent of AHF patients 3 to 6 weeks after treatment with immune plasma.

Expected and Unusual Findings on Physical Examination

Lassa Fever

Patients hospitalized with Lassa fever appear toxic with profuse sweating, tachypnea, and tachycardia commensurate with the degree of fever. Pharyngitis is a common feature and may appear purulent. Conjunctivitis, with occasional conjunctival hemorrhage, occurs in about a third of patients. Edema of the neck and face is noted in severe cases. Some patients have a maculopapular rash. Fine, dry, diffuse rales; pleural rubs; and basilar effusions may be found on auscultation of the chest. Pericardial rubs can be heard late in the disease.

New World Arenaviral Hemorrhagic Fevers

Patients with New World arenaviral hemorrhagic fevers are acutely ill and irritable. Nonexudative bulbar and palpebral conjunctival injection associated with edematous and flushed facies are common. There may be confusion and global neurologic signs such as fine intention tremors.

Useful Laboratory Procedures

Lassa Fever

The complete blood count (CBC) is generally unremarkable in Lassa fever; leukocytosis may occur in severe infections, and the platelet count may be moderately reduced. Proteinuria is common; pyuria and hematuria are variable. Hepatic aminotransferase levels are slightly elevated; an aspartate aminotransferase (AST) greater than 150 U/L is associated with a fatal outcome. Increased activity of amylase and creatine kinase (CK) (>2000 U/L) is also noted. Minimal cerebrospinal fluid (CSF) pleocytosis and elevated levels of CSF protein are seen in symptomatic patients.

New World Arenaviral Hemorrhagic Fevers

Leukopenia (1000 to 2000 cells/mm^3) and thrombocytopenia (50 to 100,000 cells/mm^3) are usually noted. Atypical lymphocytes and giant platelets may be seen. Proteinuria is a common feature. Moderately elevated CK, lactate dehydrogenase (LD), and alanine aminotransferase levels may be seen. Typically the CSF is normal.

Other Useful Diagnostic Procedures

Electrocardiographic changes of myocarditis (low-voltage ST-segment elevation and T-wave inversion) may be seen in AHF. Nonspecific ST-T wave changes may occur in Lassa fever. Chest radiographs may show pleural effusions, interstitial infiltrates, and pericardial effusion in Lassa fever patients.

Diagnostic Procedures

Lassa viral antigen is often detected early, followed by IgM antibodies in the first 3 to 6 days of illness. IgG antibodies are detected late in the illness and may be absent in fatal cases. Antigen detection tests have been successful in the early diagnosis of Bolivian hemorrhagic fever.

Errors and Pitfalls in Diagnosis

Malaria and typhoid fever can mimic Lassa fever, although gingival petechiae and purulent pharyngitis, if present, are unusual for the former two diseases. Other conditions to exclude are the other locally endemic viral hemorrhagic fevers, streptococcal pharyngitis, typhoid fever, and bacterial pneumonia. Common viral hepatitis, yellow fever, DHF, and leptospirosis are important in the differential diagnosis of the New World arenaviral hemorrhagic fevers. AHF infections with a neurologic presentation may be difficult to distinguish from other causes of encephalitis or encephalopathy.

HANTAVIRUS PULMONARY SYNDROME (HANTAVIRUS DISEASE, HANTAVIRUS-ASSOCIATED ADULT RESPIRATORY DISEASE, FOUR CORNERS MYSTERY ILLNESS)

Definition

HPS, first recognized following the investigation of a cluster of unexplained respiratory deaths in the southwestern United States in the spring of 1993, is characterized by a febrile prodrome and acute noncardiogenic pulmonary edema presenting as adult respiratory distress syndrome (ARDS). In the United States, HPS is caused by at least three newly identified hantaviruses: Sin Nombre, Black Creek Canal, and Bayou viruses. The identified rodent reservoir hosts for these viruses—*Peromyscus maniculatus* (deer mouse) and *P. leucopus* (white-footed mouse) for Sin Nombre virus, *Sigmodon hispidus* (cotton rat) for Black Creek Canal virus, and *Oryzomys palustris* (rice rat) for Bayou virus—exist across the continental United States. Infection follows direct contact or inhalation of aerosolized rodent excreta. The majority of infected individuals are young adults (median age of 35 years), although the age of patients has ranged from 11 to 69 years. As of November 1995, national surveillance identified 124 confirmed cases of HPS in 24 states (52 per cent of cases were fatal); 31 of these cases occurred in 1994.

Presenting Signs and Symptoms

Patients usually present after a brief 3- to 5-day febrile prodrome of myalgia, headache, cough, nausea or vomiting, and chills. Malaise, diarrhea, shortness of breath, and dizziness or lightheadedness are also reported in approximately half of these patients and, less frequently, there are complaints of arthralgia, back pain, and abdominal pain.

Course of the Process

Within 24 hours of the initial evaluation, most patients experience some degree of hypotension and progressive evidence of pulmonary edema and hypoxia, usually requiring mechanical ventilation. Approximately 50 per cent of cases are fatal and decline inexorably over several days (median 5 days), with severe hypotension and terminal sinus bradycardia, electromechanical dissociation, or ventricular tachycardia or fibrillation. A multiorgan dysfunction syndrome is rarely seen. Survivors, who frequently have a positive fluid balance, undergo diuresis early in recovery and show improvement almost as rapidly as they underwent decompensation.

Expected and Unusual Physical Findings

The initial physical examination is usually unremarkable except for fever, tachypnea, and tachycardia. Rashes, conjunctival or other hemorrhages, throat or conjunctival erythema, petechiae, and peripheral or periorbital edema are absent. Rapidly progressive respiratory and hemodynamic compromise are reflected by increasing tachypnea, hypotension, and physical findings of pulmonary edema and pleural effusions. In contrast to HFRS, overt hemorrhage is rare in HPS except in severe cases with associated disseminated intravascular coagulation (DIC).

Useful Laboratory Procedures

Notable hematologic findings on presentation or shortly thereafter include neutrophilic leukocytosis with increased myeloid precursors, circulating immunoblasts, thrombocytopenia, and hemoconcentration that is most pronounced in patients with florid pulmonary edema. The presence of the complete tetrad may help in early diagnosis. Hypoalbuminemia, proteinuria, and mild increases of aminotransferase, CK, amylase, and creatinine levels have also been reported. Other abnormalities mirror the extent of hemodynamic and pulmonary involvement, including signs of metabolic acidosis and rising serum lactate levels. Marked renal insufficiency has been noted in patients from the southeastern United States. The PT and partial thromboplastin time (PTT) time are prolonged in some patients, but increased fibrin split products and decreased fibrinogen levels suggestive of DIC are uncommon.

Diagnostic Procedures

Diagnosis can be rapidly confirmed by ELISA detection of Sin Nombre virus–specific IgM and IgG antibodies (available at all state health departments and the CDC). Specific antibodies are almost always present on admission, and patients should have measurable antibodies by the seventh day of illness. With prior consultation, the CDC can provide postmortem diagnosis on frozen or fixed tissues using immunohistochemical techniques or the PCR technique.

Useful Imaging Procedures

In almost all patients, initial chest radiographs have been abnormal with findings indicative of interstitial edema, specifically Kerley's B lines, indistinct hilar shadows, or peribronchial cuffing with normal cardiothoracic ratios. A third of patients also have had evidence of airspace disease on the initial radiograph. By 48 hours after admission, all patients have had evidence of interstitial edema and two thirds have extensive consolidations with an initial bibasilar or perihilar distribution and some degree of pleural effusion. The absence of peripheral airspace disease initially, the prominence of interstitial edema, and the presence of pleural effusions early in the disease process contrast with the typical radiographic findings in adult respiratory distress syndrome.

Other Useful Diagnostic Procedures

Flow-directed pulmonary artery catheterization is helpful for managing the patient and anticipating the normal to low pulmonary wedge pressure, decreased cardiac index, and increased systemic vascular resistance in patients who progress to shock.

Errors and Pitfalls in Diagnosis

It is important to consider treatable conditions such as sepsis and pneumonia caused by *Streptococcus pneumoniae, Chlamydia pneumoniae, Mycoplasma pneumoniae*, and

Legionella pneumophilia. Other considerations include influenza A, adenoviral pneumonia, diffuse pulmonary hemorrhage as in Goodpasture's syndrome and, depending on history of exposure, septicemic plague, tularemia, leptospirosis, Q fever, coccidioidomycosis, and histoplasmosis.

HEMORRHAGIC FEVER WITH RENAL SYNDROME (NEPHROPATHIA EPIDEMICA, KOREAN HEMORRHAGIC FEVER, EPIDEMIC HEMORRHAGIC FEVER, AND HEMORRHAGIC NEPHROSONEPHRITIS)

Definition

Since early in this century, outbreaks of hemorrhagic fever with acute renal insufficiency, appearing in Asia and Europe, have been given assorted regional names. These diseases, caused by at least four rodent-borne hantaviruses, are now known collectively as HFRS. Clinically, they exhibit a broad spectrum of severity, with mortality rates ranging from 5 to 15 per cent for Hantaan virus infection (Korean or epidemic hemorrhagic fever) to rates of less than 0.2 per cent for Puumala virus infection (nephropathia epidemica).

HFRS has been reported principally from countries on the Eurasian landmass. The disease is a major public health problem in China, where 40,000 to 100,000 cases are reported each year. HFRS resulting from the Hantaan and Seoul viruses is endemic in Korea, China, Japan, and the former USSR; Puumala virus–associated nephropathia epidemica is endemic in Scandinavia and western Europe; in eastern Europe, Puumala, Hantaan, and Dobrova viruses overlap. *Rattus*-associated Seoul viral infections have a virtual cosmopolitan distribution. In the United States, Seoul virus–infected rats can be found in virtually every city; sporadic cases have been reported only from Baltimore, MD.

Presenting Signs and Symptoms and Course

The most severe form of HFRS is caused by Hantaan virus and classically follows five clinical phases, which are described in the following sections.

There is considerable variation in the clinical severity of these infections. This is most apparent in Puumala virus infection, the mildest form of HFRS, in which hypotension rarely leads to shock, renal insufficiency generally is mild, and overt hemorrhagic manifestations may be completely absent or include only epistaxis and scattered petechiae. HFRS caused by Seoul and Dobrova viruses is similar in severity to Hantaan virus infection or somewhat milder.

Febrile Phase

The onset of HFRS is usually abrupt with high fever (often >39°C [102.2°F]), chills, lethargy, and weakness. Other associated symptoms include frontal or retro-orbital headache exacerbated by eye movement, myalgia, lumbar back pain, diffuse abdominal pain, blurred vision and, later, nausea and vomiting. The face and trunk appear flushed, and there may be a generalized petechial rash that is most prominent in the axilla and intertriginous areas. Oropharyngeal and conjunctival membranes may be injected and exhibit minor hemorrhages.

Hypotensive Phase

Shock or hypotension, often of sudden onset, develops during the last 24 to 48 hours of the febrile phase or on about the fifth day of illness. Hypotension, narrowed pulse pressure, and tachycardia reflect decreased circulating volume and interstitial fluid loss resulting from increased capillary permeability. Hemodynamic changes may be brief, lasting several hours, or may be protracted over several days; shock accounts for one third of all deaths.

Oliguric Phase

By the ninth day of illness, when blood pressure tends to normalize albeit with occasional episodes of brief hypertension, oliguria ensues. The degree of renal insufficiency ranges from modest oliguria to anuria with associated azotemia, hyperkalemia, and metabolic acidosis. Fluid resuscitation during the hypotensive phase may lead to hypervolemia and pulmonary edema. Hemorrhagic manifestations caused by increased capillary fragility become more prominent, with bleeding from venipuncture sites, petechiae, hematuria, hemoptysis, and gastrointestinal and internal bleeding, including the central nervous system (CNS).

Diuretic Phase

Progressive improvement is heralded by the onset of diuresis, sometimes of a volume exceeding several liters per day. The simultaneous problems of massive diuresis, previous interstitial fluid accumulation, and rapid changes in electrolyte levels are a clinical challenge.

Convalescent Phase

Full recovery, although gradual, is the rule. Some patients may have minor residual renal tubular dysfunction, including loss of urine concentrating ability, renal tubular acidosis, and proteinuria. A connection between hantaviral infection and chronic hypertension has been proposed.

Complications

Infection is pantropic and all organs including the liver, lungs, spleen, pancreas, heart, thymus, brain, and spinal cord may be affected by direct infection, edema, and infarction. Myocarditis and right atrial hemorrhage are common; some degree of hepatitis and pulmonary abnormalities are expected. Delirium is common in the acute hypotensive and oliguric phases and may have multiple causes, with the possibilities of CNS and pituitary hemorrhage, metabolic derangements secondary to renal failure and shock, and primary meningoencephalitis. Adrenal infarction may occur as a catastrophic event.

Expected and Unusual Physical Findings

Initial findings include flushed facies, upper torso petechiae, and conjunctival injection or suffusion. There may be a petechial enanthem and mild generalized lymphadenopathy. Vision may be blurred from ciliary body edema. Modest hepatosplenomegaly and jaundice may develop. Tachycardia and hypotension and narrowed pulse pressure are the hallmarks of the hypotensive phase. Pleural and peritoneal fluid accumulations may be significant.

Useful Laboratory Procedures

Laboratory findings in the initial febrile phase include leukocytosis with a left shift, atypical lymphocytes, and moderate thrombocytopenia. The hematocrit increases with hemoconcentration and fluid loss. Proteinuria and variable numbers of red and white blood cells and granular casts are seen in the urine sediment on about the fifth day of illness. Renal failure is due to interstitial nephritis, and red cell casts are rarely seen. Azotemia, hyperkalemia, hypocalcemia, and chemical signs of metabolic acidosis parallel impaired renal function.

Diagnostic Procedures

Measurement of IgM-specific antihantaviral antibodies (by ELISA) is the method of choice for the early diagnosis of HFRS. Specific antibodies are usually present on admission, and most patients have measurable antibodies by the seventh day of disease. HI and neutralization tests also may be used on paired serum samples.

Errors and Pitfalls in Diagnosis

Disseminated meningococcal septicemia is the most important alternative diagnosis. HFRS potentially could be confused with hemolytic-uremic syndrome, leptospirosis, scrub typhus, dengue hemorrhagic fever, idiopathic thrombocytopenic purpura, drug-related interstitial nephritis, renal vein thrombosis, acute glomerulonephritis, pyelonephritis, and other conditions with tubulointerstitial nephritis and fever. Differentiation of this interstitial nephritis from acute tubular necrosis may be a clinical challenge.

MARBURG AND EBOLA HEMORRHAGIC FEVERS (GREEN MONKEY DISEASE [MARBURG])

Definition

Marburg and Ebola hemorrhagic fevers are caused by unusually large RNA viruses with a tubular morphologic appearance (>700 μm in length) called filoviruses. All cases caused by Marburg virus and the three Ebola viruses that are pathogenic for humans (Zaire, Sudan and Côte d'Ivoire strains) have been acquired in Africa or were connected to monkeys or tissues from that continent. Ebola Reston virus, evidently enzootic in Asian monkeys, produces infection but no known disease in humans.

Most cases of filoviral hemorrhagic fever have resulted from secondary human-to-human transmission after the unexplained occurrence of single or multiple primary cases. The several sporadic cases that have occurred have provided little insight into the viruses' reservoirs in nature or their mode of transmission to humans. Outbreaks have been associated with frightening mortality: 23 per cent in the Marburg outbreak in 1967 among European laboratory personnel handling tissues from African green monkeys; 53 per cent and 91 per cent in nearly simultaneous outbreaks in Sudan and Zaire, respectively, in 1976, and 17 per cent in the recent 1995 outbreak in Kikwit, Zaire.

Presenting Signs and Symptoms

The usual onset is abrupt, with development of sudden fever, headache, arthralgia, myalgia, and malaise followed by diarrhea, vomiting, chest pain, and dry painful throat or sore throat. The conjunctivae may be injected, and the pulse may be disproportionately slow. Patients appear prostrate.

Course of the Process

Patients frequently become disoriented and delirious and may have other encephalopathic signs. A nonpruritic morbilliform rash appears 5 to 7 days after the onset of illness, starting on the trunk and spreading to the face and limbs. A bleeding diathesis, evident within several days of onset, may be dramatic and may progress inexorably with oral and nasal mucosal bleeding, oozing from venipuncture sites, petechiae and purpuric lesions, and severe gastrointestinal hemorrhage. There may be profuse vomiting, diarrhea, and abdominal pain. Hepatitis, pancreatitis, and renal failure may develop. Worsening neurologic signs, convulsions, and coma signal a poor prognosis. Progressive hypotension, hemorrhage, and organ failure lead to death. Survivors recover within a week to 10 days, during which time the rash desquamates. Convalescence is prolonged.

Expected and Unusual Physical Findings

A morbilliform rash appearing on the fifth to seventh day of illness and fading with desquamation in 48 hours is a helpful diagnostic feature that occurs in about half of white EHF patients. Signs of dehydration are present, with drawn facies, sunken eyes, and poor skin turgor. The oral cavity is usually dry with small aphthouslike ulcers and posterior pharygeal injection. The conjunctivae appear slightly injected and rarely are icteric. Examination of the chest commonly reveals bibasilar rales; abdominal pain is often intense and may suggest a surgical abdomen; hepatomegaly and right subcostal tenderness may be present.

Useful Laboratory Procedures

Typical findings include thrombocytopenia, normal to depressed leukocyte counts (<2000 cells/mm^3), and the presence of atypical lymphocytes, immature mononuclear cells, and Pelger-Huët–like anomalies of neutrophils. Proteinuria and microscopic hematuria are also present in some patients. Mild to severe elevations in liver aminotransferase and serum amylase levels are noted. A prolonged PT and PTT, increased fibrin degradation products, and DIC have been reported in several patients with MHF.

Diagnostic Procedures

In survivors, antibody can be detected by ELISA and IFA techniques in the second week of illness. Fatal infections are best diagnosed by ELISA detection of antigen in serum samples or by IFA or immunohistochemical examination of liver, other tissue, or skin sections. Diagnosis can also be made by electron microscopic examination of negatively stained preparations of centrifuged serum or fixed tissues (liver, kidney).

Errors and Pitfalls in Diagnosis

The filoviral hemorrhagic fevers cannot be easily differentiated from Lassa fever and CCHF. Other diseases to consider include bacterial sepsis, yellow fever, and RVF.

YELLOW FEVER

Definition

Yellow fever (Spanish, fiebre amarilla; French, fievre jaune) is a mosquito-borne flaviviral infection occurring only in Africa and South America. Sporadic cases occur in savanna and forested areas where the sylvatic cycle of mosquito-monkey viral transmission is maintained (Fig. 2). Periodically, extensive epidemics develop when viremic persons bring the virus from these enzootic areas to towns, and human-to-human spread occurs by *Aedes aegypti* mosquitoes (urban yellow fever).

Presenting Signs and Symptoms

Illness begins suddenly with headache, fever, muscle aches, and low back pain. Prostration, conjunctival

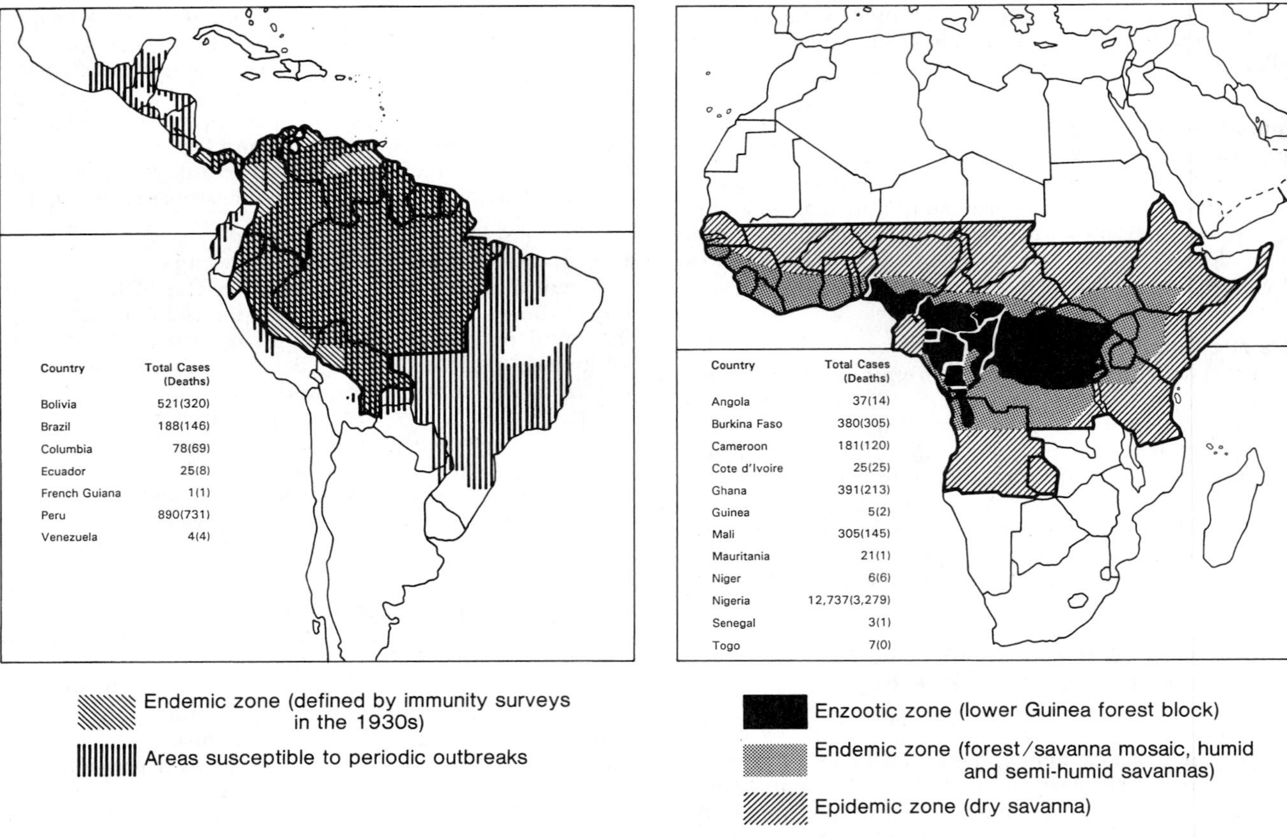

Figure 2. Geoecologic distribution of yellow fever and reported cases, 1980 to 1990.

injection, epistaxis, dehydration from vomiting, abdominal tenderness, and relative bradycardia (Faget's sign) are the initial findings. Scleral icterus is evident in some patients.

Course of the Process

Most infections resolve without further complication; however, after a period of remission as brief as several hours, about 10 to 20 per cent of patients have a sudden reversal with increased prostration, generalized hemorrhages, progressive hepatitis, renal insufficiency, and encephalopathy (the so-called toxic stage of yellow fever). Gastrointestinal bleeding, especially hematemesis, melena, and oral and nasal mucosal bleeding, is prominent. About 25 per cent of such patients die of shock, multiorgan failure, and/or secondary bacterial infections. In other patients, hepatitis and renal insufficiency resolve after a prolonged convalescence.

Common Complications

Combined hepatorenal failure, myocarditis and arrhythmias, and secondary bacterial infections may occur. Fulminant hepatic failure is common in pregnant women. Encephalopathy, possibly caused by petecchial CNS hemorrhages, may be present.

Expected and Unusual Physical Findings

Jaundice, petechiae, oral and nasal mucosal bleeding, dehydration, and a thready pulse are typical findings in severe cases.

Useful Laboratory Procedures

Examination of the peripheral blood discloses lymphopenia followed by lymphocytosis. Thrombocytopenia, a prolonged PT and PTT, and the presence of fibrin degradation products may be noted. Hepatic enzyme levels (>1000 U/L aspartate aminotransferase) and direct and indirect bilirubin levels (>10 to 20 mg/dL) are increased. Hypoalbuminemia, increased serum urea nitrogen, and proteinuria appear in varying degrees.

Diagnostic Procedures

Viral isolation from acute-phase blood is diagnostic. Detection of specific IgM by capture ELISA is the recommended serologic procedure. Serodiagnosis also is possible by measuring HI, CF, or neutralizing antibodies. Liver biopsy should not be performed in acutely ill patients. Immunohistochemical staining of liver specimens obtained at autopsy can provide a specific diagnosis.

Pitfalls in Diagnosis

Other African and South American viral hemorrhagic fevers, ordinary viral hepatitis, leptospirosis, and fatty liver of pregnancy can mimic yellow fever. Toxins, possibly including those in native herbal remedies, can cause similar hepatic damage. A history of immunization is an important clue in ruling out the diagnosis. Previous flaviviral infections may obscure the serologic diagnosis.

DENGUE HEMORRHAGIC FEVER AND SHOCK SYNDROME

Definition

A complication of mosquito-borne dengue, dengue hemorrhagic fever (DHF) and shock syndrome occurs mainly in children in Asia and adults and children in the Caribbean region and Latin America. DHF is transmitted from human to human by *A. aegypti* mosquitoes in urban areas throughout the tropics. Four distinct serotypes of dengue virus cause an identical flulike illness without cross-protection among the types. Ordinary dengue infections may be complicated by self-limited mucosal and gastrointestinal bleeding and petechiae (hemorrhagic dengue). The definition of DHF and shock syndrome requires further evidence of increased capillary permeability and altered hemostasis: thrombocytopenia less than 100,000 cells/mm^3, hemoconcentration with a hematocrit greater than 20 per cent higher than that of recovery value, and hypotension or a pulse pressure of less than 20 mm Hg.

Presenting Signs and Symptoms

Two to five days after the onset of fever and grippelike symptoms of ordinary dengue, there is a rapid clinical deterioration, with pallor, lethargy, acute abdominal pain, and sudden collapse from hypovolemic shock resulting from capillary leakage. Infants may be in shock, with dehydration, hypotension, tachycardia, peripheral edema, and pleural and peritoneal effusions. Examination discloses petechiae, nasal and oral mucosal bleeding, and bleeding from venipuncture sites. The liver is usually enlarged.

Course of the Process

Shock from capillary leakage and third space fluid accumulation is fatal in 5 to 40 per cent of patients if it is not quickly and carefully treated. Return of capillary integrity and recovery usually occurs within 36 hours.

Common Complications

Complications include hepatitis, gastrointestinal hemorrhage, and secondary bacterial infection. Fatty liver with encephalopathy resembling Reye's syndrome has been reported in a few patients; other encephalopathic patients may have CNS hemorrhages or edema. Congestive heart failure and pulmonary edema follow overvigorous fluid resuscitation.

Expected and Unusual Physical Findings

Examination discloses depressed consciousness, petechiae, and mucosal hemorrhages. Peripheral edema, cool and clammy skin, hypotension, and tachycardia reflect shock and capillary leakage. The liver may be enlarged.

Laboratory Procedures

Examination of the peripheral blood discloses thrombocytopenia, giant platelets, leukopenia, and an elevated hematocrit (>50 per cent). DIC occurs in some patients. There may be mild prolongation of the PT, PTT, and thrombin time. Elevated hepatic enzyme levels and proteinuria are common.

Diagnostic Procedures

Virus isolation from blood is diagnostic. Viral-specific IgM is found in more than 95 per cent of patients by 1 week after the onset of illness. Other serologic procedures such as HI, CF, and neutralization require paired serum samples. PCR detection of viral genomic sequences appears as sensitive as IgM ELISA.

Pitfalls in Diagnosis

Meningococcemia should be ruled out. Early detection and hospitalization of patients with DHF before the onset of vascular collapse may be life-saving. Outpatients should be followed with serial hematocrit and platelet determinations and tourniquet tests.

KYASANUR FOREST DISEASE AND OMSK HEMORRHAGIC FEVER

Definition

Kyansanur forest disease (KFD) is a tick-borne flaviviral infection that is seasonally transmitted in geographically delimited regions of Karnataka state, India. Omsk hemorrhagic fever (OHF) is endemic to the Omsk, Novosibirsk, Kurgan, and Tjunem regions of western Siberia. KFD occurs mainly among villagers and lumbermen with forest contact. OHF is transmitted directly from infected muskrats as well as by ticks and may also be waterborne.

Presenting Signs and Symptoms

In half of these patients illness consists of a self-limited acute fever with chills, myalgia, headache, vomiting, and diarrhea lasting 4 to 10 days. Examination discloses relative bradycardia, hyperemia, conjunctival injection, gingivitis, epistaxis, and petechiae. Lymphadenopathy, papulovesicular enanthem, and hepatomegaly are common in KFD.

Course of the Process

Both illnesses progress with hemorrhagic phenomena, hypotension, neurologic signs, and pneumonia or bronchitis. Hemorrhages tend to be minor in OHF and are present from the onset of illness; gastrointestinal bleeding may be prominent in KFD. Hypotension persists for several days. Neurologic signs, including depressed consciousness, neck stiffness, tremor, rigidity, pyramidal signs, and convulsions, appear in one half of KFD patients but are less prominent in OHF. Bronchitis, pneumonia, and hemorrhagic pulmonary edema develop in 40 per cent of patients. Hepatitis and acute renal failure are components of both illnesses. The case fatality rate is less than 3 per cent for OHF and 5 to 10 per cent for KFD. About 1 to 3 weeks after the acute phase of illness, 15 to 50 per cent of recovered patients experience a recurrence of fever and symptoms, although of a milder degree. In some KFD patients, neurologic symptoms predominate. A prolonged convalescence is typical.

Common Complications

Secondary pulmonary infections, keratitis, and iritis may occur in KFD.

Expected and Unusual Physical Findings

Petecchial and other hemorrhages, hepatomegaly, neurologic signs, and pulmonary abnormalities are usually present.

Laboratory Procedures

Hematologic examination discloses leukopenia and a left shift, thrombocytopenia, and an increased hematocrit reflecting hemoconcentration. In KFD, hepatic enzymes, bilirubin, and serum urea nitrogen are increased; the CSF is normal in most cases.

Diagnostic Procedures

KFD virus can be readily isolated from acute-phase blood specimens, HI, CF, and neutralization tests can be used for serologic diagnosis.

Pitfalls in Diagnosis

Mild infections resemble influenza. Rickettsial infections, meningococcemia, leptospirosis, typhoid, and malaria should be considered in the differential diagnosis of severe infections.

RIFT VALLEY FEVER

Definition

RVF is a mosquito-borne bunyaviral infection causing livestock epizootic disease and sporadic human cases principally in sub-Saharan Africa. Outbreaks in Egypt since 1977 signal the emerging importance of this zoonotic disease over a broader geographic area. Although the virus is transmitted by and can be maintained exclusively in mosquitoes, during outbreaks spread may also occur by mechanical transmission from other flying insects and by direct contact with blood and tissues of infected animals.

Presenting Signs and Symptoms

Illness begins with a sudden onset of fever, chills, malaise, myalgia, headache, and photophobia.

Course of the Process

In the majority of patients, symptoms are self-limited, lasting 2 to 10 days and sometimes interrupted by a brief remission of 1 to 2 days. Nausea and signs of mild hepatitis are common. Most patients make an uneventful recovery.

Common Complications

Three syndromes are recognized, each constituting about 1 per cent of all cases.

1. The most common of the complications are disturbances in vision principally resulting from retinitis and less commonly from optic atrophy, retinal detachment, and uveitis. Central vision may be lost. The onset is usually delayed until late into the illness or several weeks into convalescence.
2. Hemorrhagic manifestations, including epistaxis, profuse gastrointestinal hemorrhage, and bleeding from venipuncture sites, typically develop toward the end of the febrile period, around 1 week after the onset of illness. Fulminant hepatitis and renal failure may develop, and 50 per cent of such cases are fatal.
3. The onset of encephalitis, a relatively rare complication, also may be delayed to several days or weeks after the beginning of fever. Neurologic manifestations include headache, meningismus, confusion, and coma; after recovery, some patients have residual neurologic deficits.

Expected and Unusual Findings on Physical Examination

The face appears flushed, conjunctivae are injected, and there may be a faint petechial rash on the trunk and extremities. The liver may be tender and enlarged. In patients with visual disturbances, the most common findings are retinal hemorrhages and exudates.

Useful Laboratory Procedures

Findings include leukopenia and, in patients with hemorrhagic disease, mild thrombocytopenia and prolonged coagulation and bleeding and prothrombin times. Serum hepatic enzyme and bilirubin levels are increased and may reflect hepatic necrosis. In encephalitic patients, the CSF exhibits a moderate lymphocytic pleocytosis and slightly increased protein levels.

Diagnostic Procedures

Virus, viral antigen, and viral RNA can be detected in acute-phase blood samples. Most infections are diagnosed serologically by the increases in ELISA or other IgG antibody titers or by detection of IgM antibodies in serum or CSF.

Pitfalls in Diagnosis

Most RFV infections are mild and cannot be distinguished from other common infections. RVF associated with hemorrhagic complications and hepatitis cannot be clinically differentiated from yellow fever and other African viral hemorrhagic fevers. Visual deficits have been the presenting feature of RVF in travelers returning from enzootic locations. The late onset of visual disturbances and retinitis after a severe flulike illness in a traveler returning from Africa or the Middle East should stimulate consideration of RVF in the differential diagnosis.

CONGO-CRIMEAN HEMORRHAGIC FEVER

Definition

CCHF is a tick-borne bunyaviral hemorrhagic fever with a widespread distribution in Africa, eastern Europe, and central Asia. Most infections occur sporadically among herders and woodsmen bitten by infected *Hyalomma* ticks or in persons who have had contact with livestock animals or their blood or tissues. Some patients have no specific recollection of tick or animal exposure but give a history of travel to a known enzootic area. There are numerous instances of secondary transmission to family members and hospital staff who had contact with infected patient blood or tissues.

Presenting Signs and Symptoms

Onset is typically sudden, with intense headache, eye pain, and neck stiffness, fever and chills, and severe muscle, joint, and back pain. A sore throat, abdominal pain, nausea, vomiting, and diarrhea are common. The face and upper trunk may be flushed, and conjunctivae and oropharyngeal membranes may appear injected and congested.

Course of the Process

Alterations in mood and mentation develop, with progressive lassitude, stupor, or agitation. The patient may complain of tender hepatomegaly. Hypotension and tachycardia develop, and hemorrhagic manifestations appear 3 to 6 days after onset. Epistaxis and a generalized petechial rash are the first signs of hemorrhage, followed rapidly by hematemesis, melena, metrorrhagia, bleeding from venipuncture sites, and dramatic extensive purpuric bruising.

Hemorrhagic bullae may appear in the mouth. Some patients recover spontaneously after 1 to 2 weeks; however, in others a progressive deterioration, with hepatic necrosis, renal failure, and internal hemorrhage, leads to death in 30 per cent of patients. A prolonged period of asthenia and convalescence is typical. Mild or even asymptomatic infections must occur, given the prevalence of seropositive individuals in some enzootic locations.

Common Complications

Various degrees of consumptive coagulopathy contribute to the hemorrhagic state. CNS hemorrhages probably account for many of the neurologic disturbances. Fulminant hepatic necrosis and hepatorenal syndrome may develop. Secondary bacterial infections are a treatable cause of mortality.

Expected and Unusual Physical Findings

Purpuric hemorrhages in CCHF often are more extensive than in other African viral hemorrhagic fevers. Jaundice may be pronounced in patients with extensive hepatic involvement.

Useful Laboratory Procedures

There may be an initial brief leukocytosis followed by leukopenia. In patients with hemorrhagic disease, there may be a dramatic drop in the platelet count to less than 20,000 cells/mm^3. A prolonged PT, PTT, and thrombin time; the presence of fibrin degradation products; and decreased fibrinogen and hemoglobin concentrations are found in various degrees. Serum hepatic enzymes, bilirubin, and urea nitrogen levels are increased.

Diagnostic Procedures

Virus and viral antigen can be detected in blood early in the illness. Detection of specific IgM antibodies or a rise in IgG antibodies by immunofluorescence provides a serologic diagnosis. Viral antigen can be demonstrated in liver tissue.

Pitfalls in Diagnosis

Tick-borne typhus, infection with *Rickettsia conorii*, may be acquired under similar circumstances but is less fulminant and usually is associated with a characteristic cutaneous lesion. Bacterial septicemia with purpura fulminans can have a similar presentation. Hemorrhagic CCHF cannot be easily differentiated from the other African viral hemorrhagic fevers.

CYTOMEGALOVIRUS INFECTIONS

By John A. Zaia, M.D.
Duarte, California

Human cytomegalovirus (CMV) is a herpesvirus that infects humans worldwide but rarely produces disease. The virus is usually transmitted by close contact with infectious saliva, seminal fluid, breast milk, blood, and body organs. Thus, infection occurs following perinatal and neonatal exposure to maternal or nosocomial sources, during early childhood in association with day care and preschool centers, and in early adulthood during periods of increasing sexual activity.

Most infection with CMV is asymptomatic. CMV is one of the most prominent opportunistic pathogens, however, causing life-threatening disorders during states of immunodeficiency. Disorders associated with CMV include congenital cytomegalic inclusion disease, CMV mononucleosis (heterophil-negative mononucleosis), post-transfusion CMV mononucleosis, and organ-specific or systems-specific syndromes associated with CMV infection in the immunosuppressed person. In acquired immunodeficiency syndrome (AIDS) patients and in organ and marrow transplant recipients, CMV causes retinitis, hepatitis, interstitial pneumonitis, and other syndromes.

CMV infection is defined as (1) the isolation of CMV in tissue culture inoculated with a body fluid or tissue specimen, (2) the identification of CMV in tissue specimens by histologic and histochemical means, (3) the identification of CMV DNA by direct detection in tissue using in situ hybridization or in amplified tissue-derived DNA using the polymerase chain reaction (PCR) assay, or (4) a fourfold or greater increase in CMV antibody titer. CMV pneumonia is defined as a progressive interstitial pulmonary process seen radiographically with concomitant evidence of CMV infection in the lung and without evidence of other causes of pneumonitis. CMV enteritis is defined as an enteropathic syndrome with pain, nausea, vomiting or diarrhea, and evidence of CMV infection at the site of an erythematous or ulcerative mucosal lesion. In general, other CMV-associated organ-related syndromes (e.g., hepatitis and encephalitis) are defined as syndromes with specific organ dysfunction and the concomitant presence of active CMV infection. In the absence of histologic evidence of CMV infection in the involved organ, the diagnosis of CMV disease cannot be made with confidence, except for retinitis, which is recognized by characteristic perivascular exudative inflammation.

In immunosuppressed persons, identification of asymptomatic CMV infection improves patient management because it predicts the risk of eventual overt disease, especially in solid organ and marrow transplant recipients and possibly in persons with AIDS. Antiviral agents such as ganciclovir and foscarnet provide effective treatment for CMV retinitis and pneumonitis, but their toxicity requires that assays of virus infection be used to decide when to begin treatment in the absence of symptoms. In solid organ and marrow transplant recipients, the use of ganciclovir based on asymptomatic blood or pulmonary infection can prevent evolution of overt disease, a treatment strategy termed "pre-emptive" therapy.

INFECTIONS IN THE NORMAL SUBJECT: HETEROPHIL-NEGATIVE MONONUCLEOSIS

When symptomatic CMV infection occurs in normal children and adults, it most often presents as a mononucleosis syndrome that is clinically indistinguishable from Epstein-Barr virus (EBV) or heterophil-positive mononucleosis. The differential diagnosis of heterophil-negative mononucleosis includes not only CMV infection but also EBV infection, toxoplasmosis, and hepatitis A, B, or C infection. EBV mononucleosis usually occurs in the teenage and college years, whereas CMV mononucleosis typically occurs between 25 and 35 years of age. The clinical hallmarks are prolonged fever, lymphocytosis or lymphopenia with atypical lymphocytes, and hepatitis without severe pharyngitis or lymphadenopathy. Jaundice and marked hepatomegaly usually are not observed. Less common manifestations include skin rashes (which may be associated with ampicillin administration), pneumonitis, conjunctivitis, myocarditis, thrombocytopenia, hemolytic anemia, and aseptic meningitis (including Guillain-Barré syndrome). In normal persons, the course of most CMV infections is benign and recovery is usually complete.

CMV mononucleosis should be suspected in young adults who have children in day care or have been exposed to CMV in the workplace. Multiple transfusions of blood or platelets are also an important source of infection, especially after major surgery, at which time CMV mononucleosis is an important source of postoperative fever of unknown origin.

INFECTIONS IN THE IMMUNOSUPPRESSED PATIENT

CMV-associated syndromes are a major cause of morbidity and mortality in AIDS patients and in organ transplant recipients, especially in marrow, lung, and liver transplantation. More than 95 per cent of AIDS patients have CMV infection, and the prevalence of symptomatic disease, especially retinitis, is increasing as survival of AIDS patients improves with antiretroviral chemotherapy. As noted previously, the hallmark of serious CMV infection is the detection of virus in peripheral blood by culture, antigenemia assay, or plasma PCR assay. The risk of disease after organ transplantation or marrow transplantation and in AIDS patients correlates with these positive markers for CMV infection in blood.

The course of CMV infection in the immunocompromised person is determined by the degree of immunocompetence and by the duration of the immunodeficiency. In patients with transient immunodeficiency, as observed during chemotherapy for leukemia, CMV infection rarely causes severe symptoms. By contrast, in transplant recipients, CMV disease typically arises 30 to 60 days after transplantation. In this period, infection can be asymptomatic, or patients can present with fever and malaise, thrombocytopenia, neutropenia, gastroenteritis including gastrointestinal bleeding, and interstitial pneumonitis. These syndromes are often associated with intensified immunosuppressive regimens designed to suppress host-versus-graft disease after solid organ transplantation or graft-versus-host disease after marrow transplantation. By contrast, retinitis is rarely seen during acute immunosuppression and is unusual even in patients requiring chronic immunosuppression for maintenance of the graft.

In AIDS patients, CMV infection of blood can be asymptomatic for many months prior to the onset of retinitis. When retinitis occurs, the course is determined by the initial and continued responses to anti-CMV chemotherapy. CMV retinitis may be asymptomatic, discovered only on routine funduscopy. Many patients, however, complain of blurred vision, decreased visual acuity, and blind spots in one or both eyes. The retinal examination will disclose a vascular pattern of white necrotic patches that may be superimposed on flame-shaped intraretinal hemorrhages. These lesions typically begin in the periphery of the retina but may progress to involve the central retina. The diagnosis of retinitis requires oculoretinal signs and symptoms as well as evidence of systemic CMV infection. Presenting symptoms of CMV gastroenteritis include abdominal pain, nausea, poor appetite, and/or diarrhea. The diagnosis most often requires endoscopy, biopsy, and microscopic evidence of CMV infection in ulcerated or inflamed tissue.

CMV infection is not eradicated by treatment. If the anti-CMV agent is withdrawn, progression of CMV infection typically occurs. Even with continued antiviral therapy, the inexorable course of CMV retinitis, enteritis, or encephalitis in persons with AIDS is not significantly altered. The lung, pancreas, and adrenal gland become infected, and death occurs within days to weeks.

LABORATORY DIAGNOSIS

Conventional Methods of Cytomegalovirus Detection

The conventional method for detection of CMV involves observation of the cytopathogenic effects of the agent in tissue culture or in tissue specimens. Virus can be isolated easily from urine, blood, and other body fluids and tissues by tissue culture methods, and all diagnostic evaluations in which CMV infection is part of the differential diagnosis should include this simple and relatively inexpensive assay. A common method of virus culture is conventionally referred to as the "shell vial" method because the original tissue culture vials used for centrifugal inoculation of the specimen onto the monolayer of tissue culture cells consisted of thin-walled glass. Current assays are performed in plastic microtiter plates that permit efficient processing of multiple specimens and detection of infection with appropriate stains at 24 to 48 hours. However, the newer, rapid method does not permit retrieval of the virus isolate for later testing. Thus, to isolate CMV, negative specimens, or specimens from which the actual virus is needed, conventional techniques can still be used. The rapid method is as good as or better than such conventional culture methods in terms of sensitivity, but if the specimen itself is likely to be toxic to the cell monolayer, such as occurs with some urine or leukocyte specimens, the rapid method is less sensitive than conventional tissue culture. Thus, both methods should be used for diagnostic evaluation.

Detection of Cytomegalovirus Antigens or DNA

Newer assays permit direct detection of CMV antigens or CMV DNA in blood and other tissues. The antigen that has been most useful for indicating CMV infection, particularly of granulocytes in peripheral blood, is the 65-kd internal tegument protein of the virion, termed "CMVpp65," which is present in nuclei of infected cells shortly after infection. By staining peripheral blood leukocytes with a monoclonal antibody to CMVpp65, CMV "antigenemia" can be detected. The presence of this antigen in leukocytes means that either the phagocytes ingested virus particles or were actually infected by the virus. By counting the number of infected leukocytes, one can predict the risk of subsequent disease. This is particularly useful in organ and marrow transplant recipients because it permits pre-emptive treatment of infection before the occurrence of disease. CMV antigenemia occurs in organ transplant recipients before virus can be detected in tissue culture. In addition, when culture is used to identify CMV infection, the onset of disease can occur simultaneously with the first documented infection in approximately 12 per cent of patients. Use of the antigenemia assay permits earlier detection of serious CMV infection, typically prior to the onset of symptoms. Thus, as a good marker for CMV blood infection, the antigen assay helps the clinician define persons who may require pre-emptive antiviral treatment.

Similarly, the PCR technique facilitates detection of

CMV DNA either in peripheral blood leukocytes or in plasma, and in situ cytohybridization reveals the presence of CMV DNA in tissue and biopsy specimens. However, the ubiquity of CMV infection, even in asymptomatic persons, makes the clinical relevance of PCR-based assays unclear. In high-risk populations, such as AIDS patients and organ transplant recipients, it is likely that the DNA detection systems will become useful in determining indications for pre-emptive antiviral therapy. At this time, however, these assays remain experimental, and recommendations cannot be made for clinical use of such DNA-based methods.

The author gratefully acknowledges the technical assistance of Ms. Joan LeBlanc with the preparation of this manuscript.

Arthropod-Borne Infections

RICKETTSIAL DISEASES

By E. Dale Everett, M.D.,
William L. Salzer, M.D.,
and William E. Roland, M.D.
Columbia, Missouri

Rickettsiae are tiny gram-negative obligate intracellular bacteria that produce disease in both humans and animals. Rickettsiae are found worldwide, but specific species are limited to certain regions. In general, rickettsiae are maintained in nature by various vertebrate hosts and/or transovarial passage in their vectors. The known pathogenic species are transmitted by invertebrate vectors such as ticks, mites, fleas, and lice. One exception is *Coxiella burnetii,* which is primarily spread through aerosolization.

Illnesses produced by rickettsiae tend to be nonspecific febrile syndromes. Therefore, many types of presentations warrant inclusion of rickettsial infections in the differential diagnosis. The geographic distribution of agents, the season of the year, a history of exposure to vectors, and careful physical examination are key factors in the clinician's effort to diagnose rickettsial disease. In most patients, therapy is based on clinical suspicion, since confirmation by laboratory studies often requires several days to a few weeks.

ROCKY MOUNTAIN SPOTTED FEVER

Rocky Mountain spotted fever (RMSF) is the predominant rickettsial spotted fever in the Western Hemisphere and the most commonly reported rickettsial disease in the United States. It is caused by *Rickettsia rickettsii*, an obligate intracellular parasite. Recognition of the disease in the mountainous areas of Idaho and western Montana in the late 19th century resulted in its name. Today, most patients in the United States are reported in the southeastern and south central United States, but occasional patients are found in all parts of the country. RMSF occurs in Canada, Mexico, Central America, and South America. The organism is most often transmitted to humans through the bite of an infected tick. In the United States, the predominant vectors are *Dermacentor variabilis* and *D. andersoni*. These ticks provide not only the vector but also the reservoir for the organism. *R. rickettsii* persists in ticks through their developmental stages and is passed transovarially. Most human infections occur during the warmer months, but in temperate climates, RMSF has been reported in every month of the year. RMSF has also been acquired via aerosol and percutaneous exposure in research laboratories and by persons who remove and crush ticks.

Clinical Illness

One half to two thirds of patients report a recent tick bite. Symptoms usually develop abruptly 5 to 7 days (range 2 to 14 days) after exposure. Fever, headache, malaise, and myalgia are almost always present early in the illness. Gastrointestinal complaints are reported by 50 per cent of patients; the abdominal examination occasionally suggests an acute abdomen. Ultimately, a rash develops in 90 per cent of patients, typically 3 to 5 days after the onset of symptoms. The characteristic rash, which begins as fine macules on the wrists and ankles, spreads centripetally and becomes petechial. The rash frequently involves the palms and soles. An eschar or tache noire does not occur at the site of the tick bite.

Prompt diagnosis and treatment minimizes complications. When RMSF goes untreated, the mortality rate is 25 per cent. Mortality is increased in patients older than 40 years and in those who start therapy more than 7 days after the onset of symptoms. Patients with severe, often untreated RMSF resemble those with overwhelming sepsis and multiorgan failure. Disseminated intravascular coagulation, purpura fulminans, and skin necrosis are often seen in patients who die.

Laboratory Findings

Routine laboratory testing may suggest the diagnosis of RMSF, but the abnormalities are not specific. Peripheral leukocyte counts are typically normal or low, often with a striking left shift toward immature granulocytic cells. Careful examination of peripheral blood smears may reveal toxic granules or Döhle's bodies in the neutrophils. Thrombocytopenia is common, occurring in more than 50 per cent of cases. Roughly half of the patients with RMSF have hyponatremia or increased serum aminotransferase or lactate dehydrogenase levels. Headache is often a prominent complaint, but cerebrospinal fluid examination is usually unremarkable. Occasionally, however, mild pleocytosis (often neutrophilic) and/or increased protein levels are found in the cerebrospinal fluid.

Diagnosis

The key to making an early diagnosis in RMSF is clinical suspicion based on a constellation of nonspecific signs and symptoms, history suggesting tick exposure, and residence in or travel to an area where the disease is prevalent. Prior to treatment, *R. rickettsii* can be isolated from blood or tissues of patients with RMSF using tissue culture techniques, embryonated eggs, or animal inoculation. However, these techniques require specialized laboratory facilities that are not available to most clinicians, the organism is hazardous to laboratory personnel, and it takes 5 to 14 days for the organism to grow. A polymerase chain reaction (PCR) assay has been developed for rapid diagnosis of RMSF prior to therapy. However, the PCR technique has limited availability, and its sensitivity has been inconsistent in the testing of whole blood.

Rickettsial infections may occasionally be detected by histologic examination. *R. rickettsii* invades and multiplies in endothelial cells and occasionally smooth muscle cells of the walls of blood vessels. The organism is not seen with routine stains but can be visualized with Wolbach's Giemsa, Pinkerton's, Macchiavello's, or modified Brown-Hopps stains in tissue specimens. These stains may confirm the diagnosis of rickettsial infection early in the disease, but they do not define the species.

One of the most rapid and specific methods for the early diagnosis of RMSF is direct immunofluorescent staining of a biopsy specimen from a rickettsial skin lesion. This procedure requires a fluorescein-conjugated anti–*R. rickettsii* antibody, which can be obtained from the Centers for Disease Control and Prevention. This antibody cross-reacts with other members of the spotted fever group of rickettsiae. With a biopsy specimen taken from the center of an active skin lesion, this technique approaches 70 per cent sensitivity and 100 per cent specificity for the diagnosis of RMSF. The sensitivity of immunofluorescence markedly decreases after 48 hours of effective antimicrobial therapy. The clinical value of this test is highly dependent on the availability of appropriate reagents and technical expertise in direct immunofluorescent staining. A similar technique using the specific antibody with immunoperoxidase staining has also been developed.

The best way to confirm the diagnosis of RMSF is to detect an antibody response to RMSF-specific antigens in convalescent serum. Unfortunately, RMSF-specific antibodies are seldom detected in the first week of illness, rendering them of little practical value for early diagnosis. A serum specimen should be obtained as soon as possible after the onset of symptoms, and another should be acquired 3 to 4 weeks later. The diagnosis is confirmed by demonstrating either a fourfold or greater rise in titer or a single increased titer on a late specimen. Importantly, early effective antimicrobial therapy may delay the serologic response and reduce the peak titer. Furthermore, cross-reacting antibodies occur with other members of the spotted fever group of rickettsiae.

The most widely used tests are the indirect hemagglutination assay (IHA), the indirect immunofluorescence antibody (IFA) method, latex agglutination (LA) test, and enzyme-linked immunoassay (EIA). A fourfold or greater rise or fall or a single increased titer (1:128 for LA or 1:64 for IHA) is diagnostic. IHA is the most sensitive (94 to 100 per cent) and specific (approximately 100 per cent) serologic test; titers usually persist for a year or longer. LA is less sensitive (71 to 94 per cent) but is easier to perform, and titers decline after 2 months.

The Weil-Felix test measures the agglutination of *Proteus vulgaris* strains OX-2 and OX-19. Patients with RMSF and other rickettsial infections often have antibodies against cross-reacting antigens on the surface of OX-2 and OX-19. Although this test is available in many hospital laboratories as part of the "febrile agglutinins" panel, results should be interpreted with caution. A titer of 1:320 or greater or a fourfold or greater rise is considered positive. For RMSF, *Proteus* OX-19 has a sensitivity of 70 per cent and a specificity of 78 per cent, whereas *Proteus* OX-2 has values of 47 per cent and 96 per cent, respectively. Measuring Weil-Felix titers in patients with a low likelihood of having RMSF will significantly reduce the specificity of a positive titer for diagnosing RMSF. In a patient with a clinical illness consistent with RMSF, positive Weil-Felix test results are suggestive. In all such patients, however, the diagnosis should be confirmed with an RMSF-specific serologic test.

Making a specific diagnosis of RMSF early in its course remains problematic. The most rapid test is direct immunofluorescent staining of a skin biopsy specimen. This test is not readily available in smaller hospitals or in facilities outside highly endemic areas. It also requires that the patient have a rash, which may occur late or not at all. Antimicrobial therapy must be started early in the course of illness to decrease the morbidity and mortality of this serious illness significantly. Therefore, in a patient with epidemiologic and clinical features that suggest RMSF, an empirical trial of tetracycline or chloramphenicol is prudent. Except in patients with overwhelming infection and shock, there is significant clinical improvement after 2 to 3 days of therapy. The diagnosis can be confirmed with specific serologic tests for RMSF on acute-phase and convalescent-phase serum.

EPIDEMIC TYPHUS

Epidemic typhus is caused by infection with *R. prowazekii*. It occurs most commonly in the colder months among people living in crowded, unhygienic conditions. It is classically associated with times of war or natural disaster. Humans are the reservoir for the organism, which is transmitted by the bite of an infected body louse. The disease is locally endemic in mountainous regions of Mexico, Central and South America, Africa, and parts of Asia. In the United States, epidemics have not occurred since the early part of this century. In the last two decades, however, sporadic human cases have occurred in the United States, mostly along the East Coast. Flying squirrels have been implicated as the reservoir, and infection is thought to be transmitted to humans by squirrel lice or fleas. Most of these infections have occurred in the winter in persons residing in rural areas.

Clinical Illness

Symptoms begin abruptly with severe headache, myalgia, chills, and fever, typically 1 to 2 weeks after exposure. These symptoms persist, and a macular rash that blanches with pressure typically appears in the axillary folds and upper trunk on the fifth day. The rash spreads centrifugally, sparing the face, palms, and soles, and it may become confluent or petechial. There is no eschar at the site of inoculation. Untreated, the fever and rash usually resolve spontaneously after 2 weeks. In the preantibiotic era, mortality rates of 10 to 40 per cent were reported and were highest in the elderly. Illness linked to flying squirrel reservoirs may be less severe than classic epidemic typhus.

Complications involving the central nervous system, skin, kidneys, and heart may result from infectious vasculitis. Meningismus, deafness, delirium, and coma can occur. Cutaneous necrosis and gangrene, renal failure requiring dialysis, myocarditis, and pulmonary infiltration have been reported.

Laboratory Findings

Routine laboratory studies reveal nonspecific abnormalities. The total leukocyte count is usually normal or low. Thrombocytopenia or hyponatremia occurs in some patients; serum urea nitrogen and creatinine levels may be increased. Electrocardiograms may reveal nonspecific ST-segment and T-wave changes and chest films may show infiltrates. Examination of cerebrospinal fluid may disclose a lymphocytic pleocytosis.

Diagnosis

As with other rickettsial diseases, establishing a rapid and specific diagnosis of epidemic typhus in the acute phase is difficult using currently available tests. The disorder should be suspected in any patient with a compatible illness who has recently traveled to or lived in an endemic area. In the United States, a history of exposure to flying squirrels should be sought in any patient with suggestive signs and symptoms.

R. prowazekii can be isolated from blood or tissues, but this requires animal inoculation or tissue culture, which can be hazardous to laboratory personnel. Organisms may be detected with immunohistologic techniques, but the required specific reagents are not widely available. At least one patient with epidemic typhus has been diagnosed by PCR using primers derived from the genome of *R. rickettsii*. Unfortunately, these techniques are available only in research facilities.

The diagnosis of epidemic typhus is usually confirmed by measuring antibodies against typhus-group antigens in convalescent serum. The most commonly used serologic tests are IFA, LA, and solid-phase EIA. Given the low incidence of disease in the United States, these tests are performed only in reference laboratories. Most patients with epidemic typhus have a diagnostic serologic titer within 2 weeks after the onset of symptoms (fourfold or greater rise or a titer of 1:128 or greater by IFA).

R. prowazekii, *R. canada*, and the agent of endemic or murine typhus, *R. typhi,* are antigenically similar and cannot be distinguished by currently available serologic tests. If speciation is required, toxin neutralization or antibody absorption studies must be performed. These tests are available only in reference laboratories and are used mainly for epidemiologic studies.

The Weil-Felix agglutination test should not be used to confirm epidemic typhus. Compared with the specific typhus-group serologic tests, Weil-Felix titers are much less sensitive and specific. Conversely, the test is widely available. A patient with a consistent clinical illness and an increased OX-2 or OX-19 titer should have the diagnosis of typhus or other rickettsial diseases confirmed or excluded with specific serologic tests.

Definitive diagnosis of epidemic typhus during its acute stage is currently impossible for most clinicians. The diagnosis is usually based on the serologic response to typhus-group antigens several weeks later. Therapy must be started early in the illness to reduce complications and mortality. Therefore, a trial of therapy is warranted in the patient with possible exposure and a rash that begins in the axillary fold or upper body with blanching macules.

BRILL-ZINSSER DISEASE

Brill-Zinsser disease (BZD) is the recrudescent form of epidemic typhus caused by reactivation of infection with *R. prowazekii*. Most patients seen in the United States were infected in Europe during World War II, but the disease can occur in anyone with previously untreated epidemic typhus. Why such patients develop recurrent infection is poorly understood. The person with BZD may serve as a reservoir for the reintroduction of epidemic (louse-borne) typhus under conditions conducive to the spread of disease, especially poor sanitation, crowding, and human louse infestation.

Clinical Illness

The signs and symptoms of BZD are similar to but generally milder than those of epidemic typhus. The illness begins with nonspecific symptoms including malaise, anorexia, myalgia, and headache. These are followed by fever, worsening headache, and a rash that begins on the trunk and spreads to the extremities. Even without treatment, mortality and complications are rare, and the symptoms generally remit within 2 weeks.

Diagnosis

The methods used to diagnose BZD are similar to those used for epidemic typhus. *R. prowazekii* can be isolated from the blood of patients with BZD, but few facilities are capable of this. The serologic tests are the same as those for epidemic typhus. The serologic distinction between BZD and epidemic typhus rests in the demonstration of both an IgG and IgM antibody response to typhus antigen in epidemic typhus, whereas patients with BZD have a response to IgG without IgM. Unlike most other typhus- and spotted fever–group infections, patients with BZD usually have negative Weil-Felix test results.

BZD should be suspected in a patient with a remote history of epidemic typhus. There are no readily available tests to make the diagnosis during the clinical illness. Diagnosis is confirmed by rising IgG antibody titers against typhus antigen.

ENDEMIC TYPHUS

Endemic typhus is caused by infection with *R. typhi*, previously referred to as *R. mooseri*. *R. typhi* is a member of the typhus group and is antigenically similar to *R. prowazekii*, the agent of epidemic typhus. The infection is transmitted to humans through the bite of infected rat fleas and possibly cat fleas. Infected rats are the predominant reservoir, but mice and opossums may also harbor the organism. Endemic typhus occurs worldwide, particularly in areas where large numbers of rats live in close proximity to humans. In the United States, most patients are reported in southern Texas, especially during the warmer months.

Clinical Illness

Symptoms usually begin abruptly 1 to 2 weeks after the bite of an infected flea. Fewer than half of patients with endemic typhus report contact with fleas. Compared with epidemic typhus, symptoms are generally less severe and more variable. Almost all patients have fever, but only three fourths report headache, and one half report myalgia. An obvious rash, typically macular and concentrated on the trunk, is found in 50 per cent of patients. Petechial lesions are seen in about 5 per cent of patients with endemic typhus. Rash involves the face in about 10 per cent of patients but rarely the palms and soles.

Complications involving the central nervous system,

lungs, kidney, and liver occur infrequently. The mortality rate is less than 5 per cent. Severe disease with organ complications and death is more common in the elderly.

Routine laboratory testing may reveal nonspecific abnormalities. Leukopenia occurs in the first 7 days in 50 per cent of patients, whereas moderate leukocytosis may be found in the later stages. Thrombocytopenia is common. Increased serum aspartate aminotransferase and lactate dehydrogenase levels and decreased serum albumin levels are noted in 90 per cent of patients with endemic typhus. Hyponatremia occurs in 50 per cent, and patients with more severe illness tend to have leukocytosis; low serum sodium, potassium, calcium, and albumin levels; and increased serum urea nitrogen and creatinine levels.

Diagnosis

The challenges in diagnosing endemic typhus are similar to those in epidemic typhus and are described in more detail in that section. *R. typhi* can be isolated from blood samples in specialized laboratories. PCR assays have also been described. *R. typhi* can be detected in tissues using specific immunohistologic techniques. These three techniques are not readily available to most clinicians. As with epidemic typhus, the specific diagnosis of endemic typhus is typically based on the detection of antibodies against typhus-group antigens. IFA and EIA are the most widely used serologic tests. Virtually all patients with endemic typhus have a diagnostic titer (1:128 or greater by IFA) after 2 weeks of symptoms. Elevated Weil-Felix titers may suggest the diagnosis, but they are significantly less sensitive and specific and should not be relied on to confirm the diagnosis of endemic typhus.

As with most other rickettsial diseases, a firm diagnosis of endemic typhus is difficult to establish in the acute phase. Serologic confirmation after the fact is the rule. A patient with the appropriate history, signs, and symptoms should be given a trial of tetracycline or chloramphenicol. Patients with endemic typhus usually respond promptly.

RICKETTSIALPOX

Most of the documented cases of rickettsialpox have occurred in urban areas of the eastern United States, notably New York City, and in the former Soviet Union. Rodents, especially the house mouse, provide the reservoir, and transmission to humans occurs from the bite of the mite *Liponyssoides sanguineus*. The incubation period typically lasts 9 to 14 days. The causative agent of rickettsialpox is *R. akari*.

Clinical Illness

Rickettsialpox is usually abrupt in onset with fevers of 38 to 40°C (101 to 104°F) accompanied by headache, malaise, and myalgias. Chills and drenching sweats occur in half of the patients. Less frequent symptoms include photophobia, rhinorrhea, sore throat, cough, and nausea or vomiting. Skin lesions usually appear within 3 days of systemic symptoms and not later than 7 days. The number of lesions typically ranges from 5 to 30, but as many as 100 lesions have been described, including red macules, papules, and papulovesicular lesions. An eschar at the site of the primary inoculation is characteristic. Patients rarely recognize the presence of the eschar, so the clinician must search for it in patients with papulovesicular eruptions. Conjunctival injection, regional lymphadenopathy in the area draining the eschar, an enanthem, and rarely generalized lymphadenopathy may accompany the skin lesions. Untreated, the illness typically resolves over a period of 6 to 10 days. The eschar heals in 3 to 4 weeks. The major consideration in the differential diagnosis is chickenpox. Routine laboratory studies are rarely helpful, but as many as 75 per cent of patients may have leukopenia.

Diagnosis

Although the diagnosis of rickettsialpox can be confirmed by animal inoculation, complement fixation or IFA testing of acute and convalescent sera is preferred. The latter should be performed 3 to 4 weeks after the onset of illness. Direct immunofluorescence of biopsy specimens of eschar tissue using fluorescein-tagged antibody to *R. rickettsii* antigen may provide a more rapid test in some laboratories.

EHRLICHIOSIS

The vector for *Ehrlichia* is thought to be the tick. Most patients seen in the United States have an acute, nonspecific febrile illness with the sudden onset of fever, chills, and headache, often accompanied by nausea, myalgia, arthralgia, and malaise. Indolent cases with prolonged fever have also been observed, and occasional fatalities have occurred. The etiologic agents, *E. chaffeensis* and another, yet to be named *Ehrlichia* species resembling *E. phagocytophila* and *E. equi*, infect monocytes and granulocytes, respectively, where they grow within cytoplasmic membrane–bound vacuoles called morulae.

Epidemiology

Outdoor activity in tick-infested areas is a risk factor for disease. The Lone Star tick, *Amblyomma americanum*, and possibly the common dog tick, *D. variabilis*, are the likely vectors. The majority of patients are male. The onset of illness usually occurs between March and October, with most infections occurring in May, June, and July. With two possible exceptions, disease due to *E. chaffeensis* has been diagnosed only in the United States. Ehrlichiosis caused by *E. sennetsu* has been described in Japan, where the clinical presentation resembles that of infectious mononucleosis.

Clinical Illness

After an incubation period of about 10 days, infected patients experience the sudden onset of high fever and headache, often accompanied by nausea, myalgia, and malaise. Physical examination is typically unrevealing, with a rash of varying morphologic appearance found in about 20 per cent of patients. Pharyngitis, respiratory symptoms, and lymphadenopathy are usually absent. With proper therapy, symptoms usually decrease within 48 hours. Rare complications include pulmonary edema, hemorrhage, mental confusion, renal failure, and/or death. Some patients have a more indolent, prolonged infection with fever, thrombocytopenia, and abnormal liver function test results.

Laboratory Findings

Thrombocytopenia, leukopenia, and abnormal liver profiles are common. Other findings include lymphopenia during the acute phase, prolongation of the activated partial thromboplastin time, and increased fibrin split products. Observation of the membrane-bound vacuoles or morulae of *Ehrlichia* within leukocytes is diagnostic. A marked lymphocytosis has been observed during convalescence, typically on the second to third day of antimicrobial therapy.

Diagnosis

Because isolation of blood-borne *E. chaffeensis* in tissue culture is laborious and insensitive, the diagnosis of ehrlichiosis must be confirmed serologically. An IFA method using *E. chaffeensis* antigen for human ehrlichiosis and *E. phagocytophila* and/or *E. equi* antigen for human granulocytic ehrlichiosis demonstrates a rise or fall in antibody titers between acute and convalescent sera. PCR techniques using *E. chaffeensis*–specific primers for amplification and detection of *E. chaffeensis* DNA from peripheral blood provides a timely diagnosis of human ehrlichiosis. PCR techniques using *E. phagocytophila*– and *E. equi*–specific primers provide a rapid diagnosis for human granulocytic ehrlichiosis. Immunohistologic demonstration of *Ehrlichia* morulae can also provide a rapid specific diagnosis, but tissue samples that reliably contain demonstrable organisms have not been identified. The differential diagnosis includes RMSF, tularemia, Lyme disease, babesiosis, meningococcemia, hepatitis, enteroviral infection, influenza, murine typhus, Q fever, collagen vascular diseases, and leukemia.

Q FEVER

Q fever is a rickettsial disease caused by *Coxiella burnetii*. Acute illness is characterized by the abrupt onset of high fever, chills with rigors, and severe headaches, often resembling an atypical pneumonia syndrome. A few patients have chronic infection with endocarditis. Hepatitis may occur with or without accompanying pneumonia.

Epidemiology

Q fever is a worldwide zoonosis infecting a wide variety of animals. The most common reservoirs are cattle, sheep, and goats. Parturient cats have recently been implicated as a source of human infection. *C. burnetii* is found in urine, feces, milk, and birth products of infected animals. Human infections arise from inhalation of contaminated aerosols or ingestion of raw milk or fresh goat cheese. The disease has a high male-to-female ratio, probably resulting from the occupational exposure of farmers and slaughterhouse workers.

Clinical Illness

After an incubation period of 2 to 6 weeks, infected patients experience the acute onset of high fever, chills, headache and/or retro-orbital pain, malaise, and myalgia. Additional symptoms may include chest pain, cough, nausea, vomiting, and diarrhea. Physical signs often include hepatomegaly and splenomegaly. Rash is unusual. The most common acute syndromes are self-limited febrile illness, granulomatous hepatitis, pneumonia, and meningoencephalitis, whereas the predominant chronic syndrome is endocarditis, in which symptoms are often present for several months before medical care is sought. Q fever endocarditis typically occurs on a previously damaged heart valve.

Laboratory Findings

The radiographic picture of Q fever pneumonia is variable. Subsegmental and segmental pleural-based opacities are common. Multiple rounded opacities have been seen in patients exposed to infected cat placentas. One third of patients have an increased leukocyte count. Two- to threefold increases in serum aminotransferase levels are noted in almost all patients. Q fever is one of several causes of "culture-negative" endocarditis.

Diagnosis

Confirmation of the diagnosis of Q fever usually requires serologic testing. *C. burnetii* displays a phase-variation phenomenon in which the smooth-type phase I lipopolysaccharide (LPS) is found in wild-type strains, whereas the rough-type phase II lipopolysaccharide is detected only after in vitro cultivation or other laboratory manipulation. Antibodies to both phase I and phase II antigens can be detected by complement fixation, IFA tests, and the EIA technique. The ratio of phase II to phase I antibodies is 1 in acute disease, greater than or equal to 1 in subacute disease, and less than 1 in chronic disease. High phase I antibody titers are diagnostic of chronic active infection. On occasion, PCR techniques aimed at unique genetic sequences of *C. burnetii* have been used for rapid diagnosis.

The organism can be detected in blood and tissue using shell vial culture followed by immunofluorescent antibody staining to detect the presence of *C. burnetii* antigen within cells. The differential diagnosis includes influenza, viral hepatitis, atypical pneumonias, brucellosis, infectious mononucleosis, leptospirosis, toxoplasmosis, cytomegalovirus infection, ehrlichiosis, and typhoid fever.

SCRUB TYPHUS

The geographic distribution of scrub typhus includes East and Southeast Asia, India, Pakistan, the islands of the eastern Pacific, and northern Australia. Although many mammals may be infected with the agent of scrub typhus, the principal reservoirs and vectors are several mite species of the genus *Leptotrombidium*. The incubation period lasts from 6 to 21 days. The causative agent of scrub typhus is *R. tsutsugamushi,* which has several distinct serotypes.

Clinical Illness

The intensity of disease varies from very mild to severe. Scrub typhus most often has an insidious onset, with fever, headache, chills, cough, and myalgia. Alternatively, approximately one third of patients may have an abrupt onset. Less frequent symptoms include nausea, sore throat, vomiting, diarrhea, back pain, abdominal pain, and arthralgia. The most consistent physical finding is diffuse lymph node enlargement. An important clue to the diagnosis, detected in about 50 per cent of patients, is the presence of an eschar at the site of the mite bite. Other physical findings include splenomegaly in 40 per cent of patients and the appearance of a nonpruritic maculopapular rash beginning on the trunk and spreading to the extremities in one third of patients. Conjunctivitis, pharyngitis, and hepatomegaly may also be found. Hearing loss and tinnitus are relatively common in scrub typhus.

Complications generally appear during the second week of untreated illness and include pneumonitis, cerebritis with coma and seizures, myocarditis with heart failure, and disseminated intravascular coagulation. The mortality rate may be as high as 30 per cent in unrecognized and untreated cases.

Laboratory Findings

Routine laboratory findings are nonspecific. Leukocyte counts are often normal but range between 3000 and 22,000 cells/μL. Lymphocytosis develops during the second week of illness in up to 70 per cent of patients. Abnormalities of liver enzymes, hyperbilirubinemia, and increased serum urea nitrogen and serum creatinine levels may be noted in severe illness. In patients with altered levels of consciousness or seizures, the cerebrospinal fluid reveals mild to moderate pleocytosis, mononuclear cell predominance, and increased protein and normal to borderline-low glucose concentrations.

Chest films show prominent hilar markings, interstitial infiltrates, frank consolidation, or patchy bronchopneumonic infiltrates.

Diagnosis

The diagnosis of scrub typhus can be confirmed by intraperitoneal inoculation of mice with anticoagulated blood from appropriate patients. However, methods to detect a fourfold or greater rise or fall in antibodies in acute- and convalescent-phase sera are more readily available, including complement fixation, microimmunofluorescence, and immunoperoxidase procedures. The Weil-Felix test for agglutination of the OX-K strain of *Proteus* can be used, but it is neither sensitive nor specific. A method for rapid diagnosis using a PCR technique on whole blood samples shows promise.

OTHER RICKETTSIAL DISEASES

Five other spotted fever group rickettsial species are known pathogens for humans (Table 1). These agents produce disease similar to RMSF, only milder. All five of these rickettsiae are maintained in nature in both Ixodidae (hard shell) ticks and animals. Humans enter the natural cycle of infection only by accident. Infections occur in designated areas (as their names imply) primarily in the warmer months. Many imported infections occur in travelers returning to the United States and northern Europe from Africa and southern Europe.

Clinical Features

Diseases caused by these rickettsiae are characterized by a local eschar at the site of tick attachment. After a mean incubation period of 7 days, the illness is manifested as fever, headache, myalgia, malaise, and maculopapular eruptions that may become petechial. The maculopapular erythematous rash typically appears on the fifth day of illness and often involves the palms and soles. Physical examination may reveal a tache noire (eschar) at the site of the tick bite and enlarged regional lymph nodes. These disorders usually resolve within 2 weeks. Complications are rare. Severe disease can occur in persons with glucose-6-phosphate dehydrogenase (G-6-PD) deficiency, diabetes mellitus, cardiac insufficiency, or alcoholism and in old age.

Laboratory Findings

The leukocyte count shows no consistent changes. Abnormal liver function, transient proteinuria and hematuria, and an increased erythrocyte sedimentation rate have been reported.

Diagnosis

Clinical diagnosis is based on the primary lesion (tache noire), the geographic location, fever, rash, and regional lymphadenopathy in patients exposed to ticks in endemic areas. The diagnosis can be confirmed serologically by demonstrating antibody production to the spotted fever group of rickettsiae during the convalescent phase using microimmunofluorescence, LA, EIA, Western blot, or complement fixation techniques. Boutonneuse fever can be diagnosed before the onset of rash by immunofluorescence detection of *R. conorii* in circulating endothelial cells collected by immunomagnetic beads coated with a monoclonal antibody to the human endothelial cell surface. *R. conorii* can also be isolated with shell vial cell culture. The differential diagnosis of these spotted fever rickettsioses includes typhus fevers, meningococcal infections, leptospirosis, and measles.

Table 1. Other Spotted Fever Group Rickettsioses

Disease	Synonyms	Agent
Boutonneuse fever	South African tick bite fever Kenya tick typhus Indian tick typhus Marseilles fever Mediterranean spotted fever Israel tick typhus	*Rickettsia conorii*
North Asian tick typhus	Siberian tick typhus	*R. sibirica*
Queensland tick typhus		*R. australis*
Spotted fever rickettsiosis of Japan		*R. japonica*
Spotted fever rickettsiosis of Africa		*R. africae*

BARTONELLA *(ROCHALIMAEA)* INFECTIONS

Understanding of the diseases and syndromes caused by *Bartonella (Rochalimaea)* species and the taxonomy of these organisms continue to evolve. The organisms are small, slow-growing, aerobic, gram-negative rods that are presumed to be worldwide in distribution. Within the past few years, molecular biologic techniques, improved culture methods, development of serologic tests, and the acquired immunodeficiency syndrome (AIDS) epidemic have influenced the incidence and provided the means for diagnosis of diseases caused by these infectious agents. At least three species other than *B. bacilliformis* (not addressed in this article) have been linked to human disease. They include *B. quintana*, *B. henselae,* and *B. elizabethae*. The last-named has been isolated only from an immunocompromised patient with endocarditis and will not be addressed further.

Bartonella Henselae

Several clinical syndromes have been attributed to *B. henselae* infections. These include cutaneous bacillary angiomatosis, extracutaneous infections, bacillary peliosis of the liver and spleen, fever and bacteremia, and cat-scratch disease.

The syndrome of cutaneous bacillary angiomatosis has been identified most frequently but not exclusively in immunocompromised patients, namely, those with AIDS. Most patients present with cutaneous or subcutaneous lesions that appear vascular. Lesions are occasionally solitary but are usually multiple. Patients frequently have accompanying fever, chills, and malaise. Some patients have visceral lesions in addition to the cutaneous lesions. The differential diagnosis is rather extensive, but the lesion most likely to be confused with bacillary angiomatosis is Kaposi's sarcoma. Biopsy is often necessary to distinguish between the two processes.

Extracutaneous *B. henselae* infections also occur more often in the AIDS population. Typically insidious and nonspecific signs and symptoms include anorexia, fever, vomiting, and weight loss. Occasionally, the presentation is acute with a rapid course. Pulmonary, gastrointestinal mucosa, myocardial, endocardial, liver, spleen, bone, lymph node, and central nervous system infection have all been described. Most but not all are accompanied by skin lesions.

Bacillary peliosis of the liver and/or spleen may also occur with or without concomitant skin lesions. Symptoms may include nausea, vomiting, diarrhea, fever, chills, and bloating; hepatosplenomegaly may be present.

A chronic syndrome of fever with bacteremia has been described in both immunocompetent and immunocompromised hosts. Recurring fever, malaise, fatigue, anorexia, and weight loss can last for weeks to months.

B. henselae is the primary causative agent of cat-scratch disease. Typically, the disease begins with a scratch, bite, or lick (often by a young kitten), followed by the formation of a red papule or a pustule at the site and then enlargement of regional lymph nodes within 2 weeks of inoculation. A minority of patients report no contact with a cat or other animal. Most patients do not have systemic symptoms, but up to 30 per cent will report low-grade fever, malaise, and fatigue. Rarely, fever may be quite high. In most patients, disease is confined to lymph nodes. Extranodal disease such as encephalopathy, radiculopathy, bone lesions, thrombocytopenic purpura, oculoglandular disease, and severe systemic disease has been reported. Most patients recover in 1 to 6 months.

Bartonella Quintana

B. quintana, the causative agent of trench fever, has again become a clinically significant organism. After the epidemics of trench fever transmitted by the body louse during World War I and World War II, *B. quintana* infection had been largely forgotten. However, it is now clear that all of the syndromes caused by *B. henselae* can also be caused by *B. quintana* (except cat-scratch disease). The true incidence of *B. quintana* infection has yet to be fully defined.

Routine laboratory studies rarely facilitate the diagnosis of *Bartonella* species infection. In patients with bacillary peliosis hepatitis, serum alkaline phosphatase and gamma glutamyl transferase levels may be increased. Computed tomography may highlight lesions in the liver and spleen, and routine radiographs may show lytic bone lesions.

Blood cultures should be performed in patients with suspected *Bartonella* infection. Lysis-centrifugation methods are preferred. Because these organisms are fastidious and slow growing, cultures should be observed for 15 to 30 days. Cultures of skin lesions or biopsy specimens from cat-scratch lymph nodes can be set up with various media, but rabbit or human blood agar appears to support growth best.

Tissue biopsy specimens stained with Warthin-Starry silver may reveal organisms, but speciation is not possible with this technique. PCR techniques using specific primers for the various *Bartonella* species are not yet widely available.

By contrast, serologic tests are available for *B. henselae* and *B. quintana*. To confirm cat-scratch disease, the clinician should request an IFA test for *B. henselae,* which has a reported sensitivity of 84 per cent and specificity of 96 per cent. A skin test using crude "homemade" antigen has been used in the past, but it is not commercially available and has been replaced by serologic studies.

LYME DISEASE

By Kevin W. Shea, M.D.,
and Burke A. Cunha, M.D.
Mineola, New York

Lyme disease, or Lyme borreliosis, is a multisystem infection caused by the spirochete *Borrelia burgdorferi.* Transmission occurs via the tick vector *Ixodes scapularis* (formerly *I. dammini*) during the late spring and early summer months. Although the causative organism was discovered in 1982, the criteria for the diagnosis of Lyme disease are still primarily clinical. Laboratory confirmation relies on serologic tests; culture of *B. burgdorferi* remains difficult, impractical, and rather insensitive.

Lyme disease has increasingly entered the consciousness of both physicians and the public; therefore, many persons advocate earlier diagnosis and treatment of the disease. Unfortunately, increased awareness has led to overdiagnosis of Lyme disease in patients with nonspecific signs and symptoms. This, in turn, has led to inappropriate treatment of many uninfected patients.

Only by understanding the clinical and laboratory manifestations of Lyme disease can physicians make an accurate diagnosis. Careful history taking and physical examination combined with the proper interpretation of a well-timed test performed in a reliable laboratory will almost always yield diagnostically useful information. The most common problem is overdiagnosis in patients with nonspecific symptoms and a positive IgG Lyme titer. An isolated positive IgG titer is not diagnostic of disease but most often represents past exposure or a false-positive test result.

CLINICAL FEATURES

Lyme disease is a systemic disorder in which organ-specific clinical manifestations can be divided into three categories or stages: early localized infection, early disseminated infection, and late or chronic disease (Table 1). Manifestations overlap among groups (stages), and progression of disease can be variable.

Early Localized Infection (Stage I)

Erythema chronicum migrans (ECM) is the classic early sign of Lyme disease and has been used to define the

Table 1. Clinical Manifestations of Lyme Disease

	Localized (Stage I)	Early Disseminated (Stage II)	Chronic Disease (Stage III)
Dermatologic	Erythema chronicum migrans (ECM)	Secondary annular lesions, diffuse erythema, lymphocytoma	Acrodermatitis chronica atrophicans (ACA), sclerotic "sclerodermalike" lesions
Rheumatologic	None	Migratory myalgia, arthralgia	Prolonged acute arthritis, chronic arthritis
Cardiac	None	Atrioventricular nodal block, myopericarditis	Cardiomyopathy (rare)
Neurologic	Headache (if any)	Meningitis, encephalitis, cranial neuritis, mononeuritis multiplex, motor or sensory radiculoneuritis	Chronic meningoencephalitis, ataxia, chronic axonal polyradiculopathy, dementia, multiple sclerosis–like syndrome

syndrome clinically. ECM usually develops a few days to a few weeks after a tick bite but may occur as soon as several hours following exposure. The lesion begins as an erythematous macule or papule at the site of the tick bite. It gradually expands centrifugally, over days to weeks, to form an erythematous annular lesion with partial central clearing. Variants of ECM do occur and include vesicular, necrotic, scaling, and homogeneous erythema with a well-defined border. Lesions are typically warm, nonpruritic, and painless, and the color is intensified by heat, as from a warm bath or shower.

The lesion of ECM arises at the site of the tick bite, which is most commonly found in intertriginous areas, along the waistline of clothing, or on the lower extremities. To be considered diagnostic, the ECM lesions of Lyme disease are typically greater than 5 cm in diameter and usually few in number. Smaller lesions are not specific and may be confused with a normal host response to the tick bite. Many patients with ECM are unable to recall a preceding tick bite. Constitutional signs and symptoms are frequently associated with ECM or may be the only manifestation of early infection. They include headache, neck pain, arthralgia, myalgia, fever, chills, sore throat, anorexia, nausea, vomiting, and lymphadenopathy. Untreated, ECM lesions typically fade within 1 to 2 months. With appropriate antibiotic therapy, however, lesions usually resolve within a few days. Persistent or recurrent lesions suggest that therapy has been inadequate and retreatment is indicated.

Unfortunately, only two thirds of patients acquire the characteristic ECM lesion. The remaining one third of patients are diagnosed later in the course of infection after demonstration of an immune response to *B. burgdorferi* in a clinical setting that suggests early disseminated or late Lyme disease.

Early Disseminated Infection (Stage II)

Within days to weeks after inoculation, *B. burgdorferi* disseminates hematogenously. Systemic signs and symptoms are more prominent at this stage, with fever, headache, stiff neck, arthralgia, and malaise occurring in most patients. Secondary ECM lesions occur in up to one half of patients but are generally smaller than the primary lesion and rarely number more than 10. In Europe, *Borrelia* lymphocytoma, a form of B-cell pseudolymphoma, occurs in approximately 1 per cent of Lyme disease patients. Lymphocytoma presents as a bluish or purplish lesion, most often found on the earlobes of children or the nipple and areola area of adults. The lesion may be tender and is usually accompanied by regional adenopathy. Biopsy is required for accurate diagnosis.

Cardiac involvement occurs in approximately 8 per cent of patients within several weeks after the onset of illness. Typically, patients experience low-grade myocarditis and varying degrees of atrioventricular (AV) node block; progression to complete heart block occurs in approximately 50 per cent of patients. The duration of cardiac abnormalities is brief, lasting days to weeks, and heart block is almost always reversible. Mild left ventricular dysfunction occurs in half of these patients, but congestive heart failure is rare, and Lyme disease is only rarely implicated as a cause of chronic cardiomyopathy.

The musculoskeletal symptoms during early disseminated disease are nonspecific and often consist of migratory and intermittent arthralgia lasting only hours to days. Both articular and periarticular structures may be involved, and up to 60 per cent of patients in the United States may subsequently acquire an asymmetrical oligoarthritis, preferentially affecting large joints, especially the knee. The onset of oligoarthritis usually follows a longer latent period than that for cardiac or neurologic abnormalities, occurring an average of 6 months after the onset of disease. The involved joints are painful and may have large effusions, but these episodes are brief, lasting days to weeks.

Early neurologic involvement occurs in 15 to 20 per cent of patients with Lyme disease within 4 to 6 weeks of exposure. Early manifestations include cranial nerve palsies, meningitis, meningoencephalitis, or peripheral radiculoneuropathy. The most frequent cranial neuropathy involves the facial nerve (Bell's palsy). It may be unilateral or bilateral and is frequently associated with cerebrospinal fluid (CSF) pleocytosis. For most patients, recovery is complete within 1 to 2 months and is not hastened by antibiotic therapy. Other cranial nerves may also be involved. Transient deafness and vertigo have been recognized in association with auditory nerve involvement. Peripheral neuritis is usually asymmetrical and may involve motor or sensory fibers or both. Neurophysiologic studies reveal primarily axonal nerve involvement with mild demyelination of both proximal and distal nerve segments. Histologically, epineural vasculitis is evident at sites of axonal injury.

Headache, photophobia, and mild neck stiffness may occur in patients with meningitis, but Kernig's and Brudzinski's signs are notably absent. Fatigue and malaise are common, and a concomitant mild encephalitis is often present, predominantly manifested by loss of short-term memory, lack of concentration, and emotional lability. Examination of the CSF typically shows a mild to moderate lymphocytic pleocytosis with normal glucose and elevated protein levels.

In Europe, the most common neurologic presentation of Lyme disease is the Garin-Bujadoux-Bannworth syndrome, characterized by painful radiculitis in association with CFS pleocytosis and occasionally concomitant cranial nerve palsy. Headache and other signs of meningeal irritation are absent. As in cranial nerve involvement, these other neurologic manifestations usually resolve within 2 to 3 months regardless of treatment. In the absence of antibiotic therapy, however, they may recur or become chronic.

Late or Chronic Disease (Stage III)

The episodes of arthritis tend to become more frequent and last longer, often months, during the second and third years of illness in patients who had earlier joint manifestations. Although typically a mono- or oligoarthritis affecting predominantly large joints, a symmetrical pattern affecting smaller joints and resembling rheumatoid arthritis occurs rarely. In approximately 10 per cent of patients per year, the arthritis will resolve completely, whereas 10 per cent of patients overall will go on to acquire chronic arthritis, defined as an episode of joint inflammation lasting longer than 1 year. This chronic arthritis has been associated with an increased frequency of the class II major histocompatibility complex (MHC) alleles HLA-DR4 and, somewhat less frequently, HLA-DR2. Arthritis associated with the combination of HLA-DR4 and specific antibodies to the OspA and OspB proteins of the spirochete often fails to respond to antibiotic therapy.

Late neurologic involvement may develop months to years after the onset of *B. burgdorferi* infection, with several distinct clinical syndromes being well described, including peripheral neuropathy, subacute encephalopathy, and, rarely, progressive encephalomyelitis. The peripheral neuropathy is most often manifested by intermittent distal paresthesias and/or radicular pain in the absence of motor findings. Physical examination may be completely normal, but electromyography reveals evidence of axonal neuropathy. Subacute Lyme encephalopathy may present quite subtly with symptoms of headache, fatigue, short-term memory impairment, sleep or mood disturbance, and difficulty with verbal expression. Cognitive abnormalities, especially memory impairment, are evident on formal neuropsychological testing. The CSF at this stage often shows increased protein, whereas intrathecal production of antibody to the spirochete is an inconsistent finding. Progressive encephalomyelitis, a particularly severe disorder described primarily in Europe, is characterized by spastic paraparesis, ataxia, bladder dysfunction, cognitive impairment, and cranial neuropathies. Intrathecal antibody production is uniformly found in this condition.

A unique late manifestation of Lyme disease is acrodermatitis chronica atrophicans (ACA), a skin lesion found in Europe in 10 per cent of patients with untreated Lyme disease but rarely reported in the United States. Initial ACA lesions are erythematous or violaceous and appear as doughy plaques or nodules. They are typically found on the extremities in an acral distribution and are often bilateral. ACA lesions commonly occur 5 to 10 years after the initial exposure and last for weeks to years. The skin gradually becomes atrophic, resembling cigarette paper. Sclerotic lesions resembling localized scleroderma (morphea) or lichen planus atrophicus also occur. This latter stage is irreversible.

Congenital Infection

Although transplacental transmission of *B. burgdorferi* has been reported, prospective studies have not identified an association between maternal seropositivity and subsequent congenital malformations. Case reports and a retrospective review suggest that adverse fetal outcome may be associated with congenital Lyme infection, but it seems to be an unusual event. Appropriately treated, Lyme disease during pregnancy apparently portends little risk for the developing fetus.

IMMUNOLOGIC RESPONSE

Understanding the immune response to *B. burgdorferi* is essential for the clinician, as it is the characteristic humoral antibody response that forms the basis of the serologic diagnosis of Lyme disease. An initial specific IgM antibody response develops 2 to 4 weeks after exposure to the spirochete. At the same time, mononuclear cells in peripheral blood begin to show increased responsiveness to *B. burgdorferi* antigens. Initially, the IgM antibodies are specific for the 41-kd flagella-associated antigen. Antibodies develop to higher molecular weight proteins and are followed by antibodies to lower molecular weight proteins as infection continues. The specific IgM antibody response is often associated with nonspecific B-cell activation, resulting in increased total serum IgM, cryoglobulins, and immune complexes. The initial IgG antibody response begins at weeks 4 to 8 and evolves over months, following the same specific pattern for *B. burgdorferi* proteins and nonprotein antigens as with the preceding IgM response. The IgM titer peaks at 6 to 8 weeks and then declines gradually over several months. In some patients, however, the IgM response may persist for many months. IgG titers increase later in the course of active infection, but in successfully treated or spontaneously resolving disease, they slowly decline over years, often remaining positive at low titers for a lifetime.

Standing alone, the results of serologic tests cannot be considered diagnostic of active Lyme disease. Rather, serologic studies must be interpreted in the appropriate clinical context. During the first days to weeks of illness, an antibody response is notably absent. Therefore, serologic testing should not be requested in the early stages of clinically apparent Lyme disease (presence of typical ECM) or immediately following evidence of a tick bite. In general, an IgM titer should be obtained 4 weeks after exposure. IgG antibodies may remain increased for the patient's lifetime; thus, their presence does not prove current infection or treatment failure. The diagnosis and treatment of Lyme disease should be based primarily on clinical presentation, with appropriate laboratory testing used for confirmation.

LABORATORY DIAGNOSIS: SEROLOGIC ASSAYS

Serologic tests that are currently available for the diagnosis of Lyme disease include the indirect immunofluorescence assay (IFA), the indirect enzyme-linked immunosorbent assay (ELISA), the antibody-capture immunoassay (enzyme immunoassay [EIA]), and the Western blot (immunoblotting). Although their sensitivity and specificity are acceptable, these methods have not been standardized and interlaboratory variation is problematic. In general, the ELISA is more sensitive, more reproducible, and less subjective than the IFA.

Most of the serologic tests use sonicated whole cell lysates of *B. burgdorferi*. Some of the less commonly available tests use partially purified or recombinant antigens. The initial IgM antibody response is directed against the 41-kd flagellar protein and the 21-kd outer surface protein (OspC). Subsequent antibodies (IgM followed by IgG) target the 31-kd (OspA) and 34-kd (OspB) outer surface proteins. Finally the 60-kd common antigen response is expressed. Unfortunately, the high degree of cross-reactivity between *B. burgdorferi* antigens and those found on other organisms decreases the specificity of serologic testing. The 41-kd flagellar protein is found on other spirochetes and may cross-react with other bacterial flagellins; the 60-kd antigen is also common to most bacteria. Importantly, low titers of these cross-reactive antibodies are found in uninfected persons, and it is the amount of reactivity in the serum of normal controls that defines the reference range for ELISA testing.

Western blot, or immunoblotting, can help distinguish true-positive from false-positive ELISA results. Proteins are extracted from the spirochete and subjected to polyacrylamide gel electrophoresis (PAGE). The separated proteins are transferred to nitrocellulose paper and incubated overnight with the patient's serum. The blots are detected with an enzyme- or radioisotope-labeled secondary antibody. The interpretation of specific band patterns is limited by subjectivity and, as with the ELISA, there is poor standardization among laboratories. The Western blot lacks the specificity required for a screening test. Many uninfected persons have detectable bands that correspond to nonspecific antigens. For clinical practice, at least two IgM or five IgG bands should be present to consider a blot positive. Those found to be most specific for *B. burgdorferi* infection include the 31-kd (OspA), the 34-kd (OspB) and, in late-stage infection, the 94-kd protein. Newer adsorption techniques to remove cross-reactive antibodies and the addition of highly specific recombinant antigens such as P39 have substantially improved the specificity of serologic testing. These newer tests allow confirmation and should be used when available.

The clinical diagnosis of neuroborreliosis can be corroborated by demonstrating the intrathecal production of antibody to the spirochete. Using antibody-capture immunoassay, a ratio of CSF to serum-specific antibody greater than a factor of 1 strongly suggests the diagnosis. The timing of such testing is critical because intrathecal production of antibody may persist after treatment, which should not be interpreted as treatment failure. In addition, intrathecal antibody may not be present in all patients, especially those with primarily peripheral nervous system involvement.

Some investigators use the polymerase chain reaction (PCR) assay to diagnose Lyme disease. Although the PCR can detect *B. burgdorferi* DNA in synovial fluid of patients with chronic arthritis, it has not proved useful in the evaluation of blood, urine, or CSF. Since the PCR detects fragments of DNA or mRNA, a positive result should not be interpreted as indicating active infection. The detection of *Borrelia* in ticks by the PCR has no clinical significance. The risk of acquiring Lyme disease from a known infected tick is on the order of 5 to 10 per cent.

The laboratory diagnosis of Lyme disease remains problematic. The burden of an appropriate diagnosis lies with the clinician; serologic tests should be used only to confirm the diagnosis in patients without ECM. False-positive results may occur in association with other spirochetal infections, Rocky Mountain spotted fever, and echovirus, varicella, human immunodeficiency virus (HIV), and Epstein-Barr viral infections; in various autoimmune disorders, such as rheumatoid arthritis and lupus erythematosus; and in conditions resulting in hypergammaglobulinemia. Recall that a positive IgG titer to *B. burgdorferi* may only indicate past exposure and is not, by itself, indicative of disease. Conversely, when clinical evidence of Lyme disease is substantial, a negative serologic test result should not refute the diagnosis. Early in the course of illness, a detectable antibody response may not have developed, and early treatment may blunt the evolution of the normal humoral response.

The clinician should also remember that although Lyme disease is easily treated, the absence of therapy seldom leads to permanent sequelae. Finally, Lyme disease remains a clinical diagnosis in patients with ECM. In the absence of objective findings, however, a serologic diagnosis should be made with caution.

OTHER ARTHROPOD-BORNE INFECTIONS

By Donald B. Middleton, M.D.
Pittsburgh, Pennsylvania

RELAPSING FEVER

Relapsing fever is synonymous with famine fever, recurrent fever, spirillum fever, African tick fever, bilious typhoid, febris recurrens, and various other titles. Several species of *Borrelia*, a vector-borne, gram-negative, loosely wound spirochete, can produce an acute systemic infection known as relapsing fever that is characterized by recurrent 3- to 6-day-long febrile episodes. Louse-borne illness is "epidemic," whereas tick-borne episodes are "endemic."

Epidemiology

Epidemic or body louse–borne relapsing fever develops when populations infested with *Pediculus humanus* crowd together, especially during seasonal rains or in times of poor hygiene such as war or famine. Humans are the only hosts and *B. recurrentis* is the only infective agent. Transmission occurs when infected lice are crushed against bites or scratches in the skin or rents in the mucous membranes or when contaminated materials, usually under fingernails, are rubbed into the conjunctivae or scratches.

Epidemic relapsing fever is most prevalent in Ethiopia, the Sudan, and other parts of Central and East Africa. Cases also have been reported from Peru and China, but such cases in the United States are imported.

Endemic or tick-borne relapsing fever is caused by many species of *Borrelia*, especially *B. duttonii* in Africa and *B. hermsii* in the United States. *Borrelia* species are named after specific ticks belonging to the genus *Ornithodoros*, a soft-shelled rodent tick that feeds at night. At least 15 *Borrelia* species have been described. Tick bites are painless and often brief and hence often go unnoticed. In the United States, most cases are reported in spring and summer when overnight camping in tick-infested cabins is common. Major outbreaks have developed in the Grand Canyon, Arizona and parts of California and Washington. Although transovarial passage of *Borrelia* occurs in ticks, the rodent population of chipmunks, mice, rats, and squirrels serves as the major reservoir. Rodent urine is also a vector of transmission.

Clinical Course

After infection, *Borrelia* multiplies in the bloodstream and invades virtually every body organ. Endothelial damage may be extensive. An incubation period of 3 to 18 days (mode 7 days) is followed by a fever of 39°C (102.2°F) to 41°C (105.8°F), with chills, headaches, myalgia, and arthralgia. Various organ systems are affected: the gastrointestinal tract (abdominal pain, nausea, vomiting, diarrhea), the respiratory tract (sore throat, cough, shortness of breath), the eyes (photophobia), and the central nervous system (dizziness, delirium). Signs and symptoms include conjunctival erythema, petechiae, diffuse abdominal tenderness, nuchal rigidity, pulmonary and peripheral edema, lymphadenopathy, hematuria, hemoptysis, hematemesis, iritis, otitis media, pneumonia, coma, cranial nerve palsies, hemiplegia, meningitis, and seizures. A truncal rash often develops during the last few days of the primary episode; the rash may be macular, papular, or petechial. Additional features are listed in Table 1. The duration of fever is usually 3 days in tick-borne disease and 6 days in louse-borne illness.

The first attack ends by crisis, with rigors, marked fever, elevated blood pressure, tachycardia, and tachypnea. Abrupt profuse sweating, hypotension, and falling temperature follow 10 to 20 minutes later. Intractable myocarditis, hepatic failure, or disseminated intravascular coagulation may cause death. Patients either die or recover during the crisis, appearing well for 5 to 10 days until a recurrent febrile episode erupts. The relapse is generally milder and shorter than the first attack. Each progressive relapse (up to 10) is likely to be less intensive. Louse-borne disease has a much higher fatality rate (4 to 40 per cent) than does tick-borne disease (0 to 5 per cent).

Diagnosis

Definitive diagnosis requires demonstration of spirochetes in peripheral blood smears, preferably prepared during a febrile episode, when spirochetemia is most intense. Repeat smears may be necessary. Buffy coat smears stained with Giemsa or acridine orange are most likely to reveal spirochetes, but Wright's stains are often positive as well. *Borrelia* can be found in urine, sputum, cerebrospinal fluid, and effusions. Blood can be injected into mice and their blood later smeared for culture of *Borrelia*.

Serum antibody tests typically are not helpful. Reasonably sensitive indirect fluorescent antibody tests may be falsely positive in Lyme disease or syphilis. *Proteus* OXK agglutinins may be present.

The leukocyte count is usually normal, but thrombocytopenia and anemia are common. Increases in serum creatinine and serum urea nitrogen levels, prothrombin time, partial thromboplastin time, serum bilirubin concentration, sedimentation rate, aminotransferase levels, and cerebrospinal fluid protein concentrations are common. Chest films can show pulmonary edema, cardiomegaly, or pneumonia, whereas the electrocardiogram can show prolonged Q-T intervals and various arrhythmias. A trial of antibiotic therapy (penicillin, tetracycline, or erythromycin) followed by a Jarisch-Herxheimer reaction occasionally confirms the diagnosis of relapsing fever.

Table 1. Clinical Features of Relapsing Fever

Condition	Tick-Borne (Endemic)	Louse-Borne (Epidemic)
Splenomegaly	40%	75%
Truncal rash	30%	10%
Hepatomegaly	20%	65%
Pulmonary symptoms	15%	35%
Central nervous system abnormality	10%	30%
Jaundice	5%	35%
Epistaxis	3%	30%
Relapses	3 (up to 10)	1 (rarely 2)
Fatality rate	Up to 5%	Up to 40%
Jarisch-Herxheimer reaction	33%	100%

Differential Diagnosis

The differential diagnosis of relapsing fever includes other infections that target endothelium such as leptospirosis and Rocky Mountain spotted fever (RMSF). Occasionally, the clinician must also consider tick typhus, malaria, dengue fever, or meningococcemia. Of greatest importance, epidemiologic evidence of exposure, a relapsing clinical course, and a positive blood smear remain the keys to correct diagnosis of relapsing fever.

COLORADO TICK FEVER

Colorado tick fever, also known as tick fever, was formerly called mountain fever. It is an acute, febrile, often biphasic disease caused by a double-stranded RNA orbivirus, one of only two tick-borne viruses found in the United States (the other is Powassan virus).

Epidemiology

Colorado tick fever is transmitted by the large, adult, hard-bodied wood tick, *Dermacentor andersoni*. In the Rocky Mountains, up to 25 per cent of these ticks may be infected with the orbivirus. The natural reservoir is the small rodent population, but tick transovarial viral transmission has been established. Nearly all patients have traveled in endemic regions (Colorado, Utah, Wyoming, and Montana), 90 per cent report tick contact, and half report tick bites. Cases peak in April to June but can occur from March through September. Persons who camp frequently often have neutralizing antibodies that confirm prior infection. In endemic regions, Colorado tick fever is roughly 20 times as common as RMSF. Of the 140 infections reported annually, most arise in young men, but both sexes and all ages can be infected. Transfusion-related transmission has been reported.

Clinical Course

Mild, inapparent infection probably occurs frequently. In some patients, an incubation period of 3 to 6 days (range 1 to 14 days) is followed by the sudden onset of myalgia (especially in the legs and back), chills, fever to 40°C (104°F), headache, photophobia, and eye pain. These patients often are severely stricken or bedridden, and up to 20 per cent are admitted to a health care facility. Nausea, vomiting, abdominal pain, stiff neck, sensitive skin, and mild sore throat are common, but diarrhea is rare.

Patients with tick fever are lethargic and have facial flushing, fever, and tachycardia, with occasional splenomegaly or conjunctival injection. Rarely, an ulcer may be found at the site of the tick bite. Up to 12 per cent of patients acquire a rash, with petechiae on the arms and legs, maculopapular lesions over the trunk and extremities, or localized purpura. From 3 to 8 per cent of patients have aseptic meningitis, with vomiting, neck stiffness, or encephalitis with delirium or coma. A few patients experience gastrointestinal bleeding, epistaxis, epididymo-orchitis, pneumonitis, hepatitis, or pericarditis. Most of these patients are less than 10 years of age. Three reported deaths have followed bleeding, all in children.

Although fever typically and abruptly abates within 2 days, the patient remains lethargic. In 50 per cent of patients, fever recurs within 2 to 3 days, lasting up to 3 days. A third recurrence of fever is rare. Young patients recover in 1 week, but many older individuals require 4 weeks or more to convalesce despite clearing of viremia.

Diagnosis

Virus infects erythrocytes for up to 120 days, the life span of the red blood cell. Blood cultures are positive in up to 90 per cent of patients with tick fever in the first 2 weeks and in 50 per cent of patients in the first month. Serum cultures are positive up to 5 days after the onset of illness, but virus can be obtained from washed erythrocytes for as long as 4 months.

Cerebrospinal fluid culture may also be positive. Although the complete blood count (CBC) is initially unremarkable, by the fifth day of illness, a marked leukopenia to less than 3000 cells/μL is typical. Toxic granulations, thrombocytopenia, and maturation arrest of the bone marrow are common. Serial CBCs may be required to demonstrate the leukocyte nadir. Slight increases in serum creatine kinase (CK) and aspartate aminotransferase (AST) have been noted.

Usually, a combination of fluorescent antibody stains of erythrocytes plus mouse inoculation or Vero cell culture provides the highest diagnostic accuracy. Within 30 days of infection, about 90 per cent of patients have fourfold increases in neutralizing antibody. Complement fixation or enzyme immunoassay antibodies also can be assessed, but these methods are less sensitive.

Differential Diagnosis

Persons from endemic areas with typical biphasic disease are likely to have Colorado tick fever. Confusion arises when fever, rash, and a history of tick bite suggest RMSF. Thus, tick fever victims may require antibiotic (tetracycline) treatment until the diagnosis is established. In persons without rash, the diagnosis of relapsing fever should be considered, but it has a more abrupt onset, more dramatic conclusion, and longer period of remission than Colorado tick fever. Antibiotic treatment often produces a Jarisch-Herxheimer reaction in patients with relapsing fever. Q fever, tularemia, and Powassan encephalitis may rarely enter the differential picture.

When ticks are carried to nonendemic areas via cars or clothes, persons who have not traveled may acquire infection if bitten. For campers, the use of tick repellent is prudent.

BABESIOSIS

Babesiosis, also called babesiasis or piroplasmosis, is a malarialike infection caused by *Babesia*, a protozoan with worldwide distribution.

Epidemiology

In the United States the highest incidence is found in the Northeast (especially Massachusetts), but cases have been reported from the northern Midwest, West Coast, and South. Nantucket Island, Martha's Vineyard, Cape Cod, eastern Long Island, Block Island (Rhode Island), and Fire Island and Shelter Island (New York) are well-known sites of disease.

The rodent strain *Babesia microti* is the major infecting agent in the United States, where babesiosis is transmitted by *Ixodes scapularis*, which is also the tick vector of Lyme disease. Victims may experience both illnesses simultaneously. Re-emergence of the white-tailed deer, which is not infected by *Babesia*, has nevertheless increased the *I. scapularis* population. Meanwhile, white-footed mice, which serve as hosts for both *B. burgdorferi* and *Babesia*, are the major food source for *I. scapularis* larvae and nymphs. The nymphs most frequently transmit the agents of Lyme disease and babesiosis to humans.

Babesia microti infects human erythrocytes, which are the site of trophozoite maturation to merozoites. The latter forms damage the red cell membrane and are released to reinfect other erythrocytes. Because the maturation process is asynchronous, malarialike hemolytic crisis rarely, if ever, occurs. More than 120 patients with babesiosis have been reported. A few of these infections have been associated with transfusion of red cells or platelets. The peak incidence is from May through September. Most infections are probably subclinical, with delayed detection via antibody titers. Four to seven per cent of the inhabitants of Shelter Island and Nantucket have positive serologic tests.

Clinical Manifestations

The incubation period for babesiosis is usually 1 to 3 weeks but may be up to 9 weeks, especially in transfusion-related cases. Most patients do not remember the small (2 mm) nymphal tick or a bite. Healthy persons more than 60 years of age, persons older than age 45 years with preexisiting medical conditions, and those without spleens are more likely to demonstrate clinical illness.

Onset is gradual. Nonspecific symptoms such as fatigue, headache, myalgia, sore throat, cough, fever, chills, sweats, arthralgia, nausea, emesis, and abdominal pain often do not allow the clinician to distinguish babesiosis from viral syndromes. By contrast, photophobia, petechiae, splinter hemorrhages, ecchymoses, darkened urine, conjunctival erythema, and emotional upset, especially depression, should raise the specter of babesiosis. The temperature may rise to 40°C (104°F). Hepatosplenomegaly without lymphadenopathy can be observed. Although spontaneous recovery is typical, parasitemia may continue for up to 10 months. Those who do poorly acquire adult respiratory distress syndrome, myocardial infarction, or renal failure. Although the disease is only rarely fatal, hospitalization for up to 20 days is common. Splenectomized patients may have a greater risk of dying.

Laboratory Findings

Hemolytic anemia is the hallmark of babesiosis. Five to ten per cent of red blood cells typically harbor the parasite. Occasionally, severe anemia may be complicated by thrombocytopenia, leukopenia, reticulocytosis, decreased serum haptoglobin levels, an increased erythrocyte sedimentation rate, and sometimes a positive direct Coombs' test. Proteinuria, hemoglobinuria, and increased serum urea nitrogen, serum bilirubin, aminotransferase, and lactate dehydrogenase (LD) levels are also commonly noted.

Diagnosis

Infection with *Babesia* should be suspected in any person traveling or living in an endemic area who experiences fever and hemolytic anemia with or without a history of tick bite. Diagnosis is confirmed with a Giemsa- or

Wright's-stained blood smear that demonstrates intraerythrocytic parasites. A single ring form lacking pigment is typical, but tetrads or Maltese crosses are sometimes found. Multiple smears may be required because many patients have low levels of parasitemia. Black pigmentation or multiple rings suggest *Plasmodium falciparum*. The rings of *Babesia* have white centers and are about one fifth the size of the red cell.

Other laboratory tests for babesiosis have surfaced, but their exact role is unclear. Polymerase chain reaction, Western blot, and DNA probe assays may prove useful. Currently, the indirect immunofluorescence antibody titer for *Babesia microti* is favored. A titer of 1:256 or greater is considered diagnostic. Titers of greater than or equal to 1:1024 are common during acute infection, whereas unchanging titers of greater than or equal to 1:32 indicate past infection. Indirect immunofluorescence has a 92 per cent sensitivity, a 95 per cent specificity, and a 98 per cent negative predictive value. Inoculation of the golden hamster to demonstrate late parasitemia is only rarely required.

Differential Diagnosis

Confusion with Lyme disease is common, but the blood smear is diagnostic. Other tick-borne illnesses like RMSF and Colorado tick fever are usually found in different regions of the United States and have a typical rash (RMSF) or a biphasic course (Colorado tick fever).

Mycotic Diseases

SYSTEMIC MYCOSES

By Kathleen G. Beavis, M.D.
Philadelphia, Pennsylvania

The term "systemic mycoses" traditionally describes systemic infections in healthy hosts caused by fungi such as *Histoplasma capsulatum, Blastomyces dermatitidis, Coccidioides immitis, Paracoccidioides brasiliensis*, and *Cryptococcus neoformans*. Of these fungi, four are dimorphic; that is, they are mycelial at 30°C (mould phase) and unicellular at 37°C (yeast phase). *C. neoformans* is monomorphic and grows as a yeast; it usually has a prominent mucopolysaccharide capsule. *Candida* species, Zygomycetes, and *Aspergillus* species are opportunistic pathogens that typically cause systemic disease only in immunosuppressed hosts. *Nocardia* species and *Actinomyces israelii* cause diseases that have traditionally been included with the mycoses, even though these organisms are bacteria. Fungi should be cultured and the species identified, rather than presumptively identifying the organism in histopathologic or cytologic preparations. For example, textbook descriptions of *Aspergillus* species seem clear-cut; however, this mould can be mistaken for Zygomycetes or even *Fusarium* species.

HISTOPLASMOSIS

Histoplasmosis is caused by *H. capsulatum* var. *capsulatum*, a dimorphic fungus whose conidia are inhaled most frequently in the midwestern valleys of the United States and in Central America. Although chickens, starlings, and blackbirds do not carry the organism, the mycelial form thrives in the acidic, superficial soil enriched by their guano. Bats carry the organism and excrete it in their feces. Outbreaks of histoplasmosis have followed not only caving expeditions but also many recreational and excavating activities.

Clinical Presentation

More than 80 per cent of long-term residents of the Ohio and Mississippi River valleys show skin test reactivity to histoplasmin, yet most infections are asymptomatic. The inoculum size and the immune status of the individual correlate with the severity of symptoms. Infants, young children, and immune-compromised adults are vulnerable; serious illness can also develop in healthy adults inhaling a heavy inoculum. Skin test reactivity probably gives some immunity to subsequent infection, but exposure to a large inoculum can trigger especially severe pulmonary disease. When the conidia and hyphal fragments reach the alveoli, they convert to the yeast form, probably after phagocytosis by neutrophils and macrophages. The yeasts can multiply rapidly within macrophages, causing the host cell to burst, with infection of neighboring macrophages. *H. capsulatum* spreads through lymphatics to regional lymph nodes and hematogenously to the liver, spleen, bone marrow, and other organs.

Approximately 10 per cent of infected individuals have symptoms, most commonly an acute flulike illness with fever, nonproductive cough, headache, and lethargy that resolve without therapy. In immunocompetent patients, disease is usually confined to the lungs, draining lymph nodes, and adjacent structures and can present as acute or chronic pulmonary histoplasmosis with or without mediastinitis or pericarditis. Patients with defective cell-mediated immunity, especially those with decreased CD4+ cells, can present with disseminated histoplasmosis. The very young and the immunosuppressed patient are most likely to have symptoms. A positive skin test suggests some immunity against reinfection, but a heavy re-exposure can trigger severe pulmonary disease in these individuals, probably because of an anamnestic cellular immune response.

Clinical Manifestations

Acute Pulmonary Histoplasmosis

Most persons are asymptomatic following the initial pulmonary infection. Symptoms can begin from 3 days to 3 weeks after exposure and often include fever, headache, lethargy, anorexia, and chest pain. Fever typically lasts several days and can persist for more than a week. About 5 per cent of patients, mostly women, exhibit joint abnormalities such as arthralgia and arthritis and dermatologic findings such as erythema multiforme and erythema nodosum.

About 5 per cent of patients experience pericarditis. The

pericardial fluid is typically bloody or xanthochromic and the cell count shows primarily lymphocytes, but neutrophils can sometimes predominate. Organisms infrequently are seen in tissue section or grown in cultures. Occasionally, acute tamponade will require drainage, but pericarditis usually resolves without antifungal therapy. Severely ill patients can experience dyspnea and hypoxia, requiring intensive care. The normal outcome is full recovery, but this can take several weeks.

Physical examination and laboratory findings are nonspecific. The chest film in acute pulmonary histoplasmosis typically shows patchy infiltrates and hilar adenopathy; sicker patients have confluent, nodular infiltrates and pleural effusions. Rarely a cavitary lesion will form a few weeks into the illness, but these typically resolve spontaneously.

Because physical, laboratory, and radiologic findings are nonspecific, a high index of suspicion for histoplasmosis must be derived from the occupational, recreational, and travel histories. The differential diagnosis includes influenza, community-acquired pneumonia, tuberculosis, and infection with other fungal pathogens. Both sarcoid and histoplasmosis can share the granulomatous histopathologic features and increased angiotensin converting enzyme (ACE) activity of histoplasmosis.

Sequelae can include mediastinal fibrosis and histoplasmomas. As the pneumonia spreads to the regional lymph nodes, an initial caseating granulomatous response is followed by fibrosis entrapping the necrotic nodes. Although they usually heal without complications, cystic lesions resembling tumor or tuberculosis can follow. Calcified debris can erode into the bronchi, causing broncholithiasis. The small broncholiths are asymptomatic; larger "stones" can cause coughing, hemorrhage, and bronchiectasis. The fibrotic process can encase the mediastinal structures and cause the superior vena cava syndrome. The pulmonary veins and artery can also be constricted by reactive fibrosis. Some of the larger pulmonary lesions become nodular, forming the "coin lesion" seen on chest films. These histoplasmomas are typically asymptomatic, subpleural, and less than 4 cm in diameter. The nodules can enlarge and calcify in reaction to antigens persisting in the central caseation. Central calcifications or laminar calcification, when seen on chest film, can help differentiate a histoplasmoma from tumor.

Chronic Pulmonary Histoplasmosis

In contrast to the lower lobe parenchymal damage in acute pulmonary histoplasmosis, chronic pulmonary histoplasmosis typically involves the upper lobes. Cavity formation is common, and men older than 50 years who have chronic obstructive pulmonary disease make up the greatest portion of patients. Radiologic findings usually include calcification in the hilar nodes or pulmonary parenchyma; hilar adenopathy is uncommon. The source of chronic disease may be exogenous reinfection or the reactivation of prior disease. Symptoms are nonspecific and include low-grade fever, weight loss, and cough. The pneumonitis that often develops in emphysematous bullae can be confused radiologically with cancer. Infiltrates that do not cavitate may take up to 6 months to form a scar. The disease can recur.

Progressive Disseminated Histoplasmosis

Only 0.05 per cent of patients with histoplasmosis will experience disseminated disease, but the very young and he immune-compromised—especially acquired immunodeficiency syndrome (AIDS) patients—are at risk. The course can be acute or chronic following a primary pulmonary infection, an exogenous reinfection, or a reactivation of a quiescent focus.

Before the advent of AIDS, the very young and patients with Hodgkin's disease or lymphocytic leukemia accounted for most of the patients with acute progressive disseminated histoplasmosis. This disease is now seen most frequently in AIDS patients; it is an AIDS-defining illness and in endemic areas is as prevalent as cryptococcosis. Most signs and symptoms are nonspecific, and they include fever, weight loss, and malaise. Erythematous maculopapular skin eruptions can be a clue; they are seen in 10 per cent of patients. Biopsy of these cutaneous lesions shows dermal necrosis without granulomatous inflammation; intracellular and extracellular yeasts are typically present. Most of the patients are anergic and have a negative skin test result, consistent with their inability to mount a granulomatous response to contain the organisms. Without therapy, patients with acute progressive disseminated histoplasmosis die within 6 weeks of complications, which include adult respiratory distress syndrome, encephalopathy, multiorgan failure, disseminated intravascular coagulation, and leukopenia.

Chronic progressive disseminated disease is seen in adults who complain of fatigue and weight loss. Oropharyngeal ulcers are seen in approximately 50 per cent of patients; they are not seen in acute progressive disseminated histoplasmosis. The ulcers can involve the tongue, buccal mucosa, gums, and larynx. With their heaped edges, these painful ulcers resemble cancer. Microscopic sections show acute and chronic inflammation with many yeast cells. Oral ulcers differ from the typical lesions seen in chronic progressive disseminated histoplasmosis, which are well-organized granulomas with yeast rarely seen. The course is chronic, and disease in the adrenal glands, meninges, heart, and gastrointestinal tract can punctuate periods of inactivity.

Diagnosis

Culture

Definitive diagnosis requires culture and identification of the organism. Cultures should be held for 4 to 6 weeks at 30°C for the mycelial form to appear. Confirmation is made after the mycelial form converts to the yeast form at 37°C, or when exoantigen testing or probes are carried out. The culture yield depends on the clinical presentation and the laboratory's expertise. Sputum from patients with acute pulmonary histoplasmosis has a 10 per cent yield; a 60 per cent yield is obtained from patients with chronic pulmonary histoplasmosis. The yield in AIDS patients with acute progressive disseminated disease is 85 per cent from bronchoscopic aspirates and 50 to 90 per cent from bone marrow.

The yeast forms can be seen on hematoxylin and eosin, but silver stains highlight the organism. Wright-Giemsa stain is useful on peripheral smears on which yeasts can be seen in the circulating neutrophils and monocytes. *H. capsulatum* yeast forms are intracellular but can be differentiated from the amastigotes of *Leishmania* species and the trophozoites of *Toxoplasma gondii* because these parasites do not stain with silver stains. In contrast to the cysts of larger extracellular *Pneumocystis carinii, H. capsulatum* is intracellular and smaller.

Serologic Findings

Detection of complement-fixing antibodies and immune precipitins can be useful in diagnosing histoplasmosis. Because 10 per cent of the population in an endemic area can have low titers of complement-fixing antibodies, the lowest dilution for a positive result is 1:8. A titer of 1:32 strongly suggests active disease, yet titers of 1:8 and 1:16 should also give pause, especially in immunosuppressed patients. These antibodies are detectable after 6 weeks in most symptomatic patients with a primary pulmonary infection. Paired sera should be tested; at least a fourfold increase in titer is seen between acute and convalescent specimens. Cross-reactivity is seen with *C. immitis* and *B. dermatitidis,* but the titers are lower. Consistent with their inability to mount an immune response, up to 50 per cent of immunosuppressed patients will not produce diagnostic titers.

Immunodiffusion can detect precipitating antibodies to the H and M antigens from mycelial filtrates. Anti-H antibodies are seen in only 10 to 20 per cent of patients and, when present, appear 2 to 3 weeks after infection and disappear within 6 months. Anti-M antibodies are seen in three fourths of patients 2 to 3 weeks after complement fixation antibodies appear; these antibodies can persist for years, confusing the diagnosis of recurring disease. Therefore, even though the anti-H antibodies appear in fewer individuals, they are more specific for active disease.

Skin Testing

Most individuals have a positive delayed-type hypersensitivity skin test response to histoplasmin. As useful as the test is for documenting infection in endemic areas, it is useless for diagnosis because of the high prevalence of positive skin test results in endemic areas. A further danger that exists with the use of skin tests for diagnosis is that the skin test can cause production of complement-fixing and precipitin antibodies to titers consistent with acute disease.

BLASTOMYCOSIS

Blastomycosis (Chicago disease, Gilchrist's disease, North American blastomycosis) is a systemic pyogranulomatous disease caused by inhaling the conidia of *B. dermatitidis*. The epidemiology and incidence of blastomycosis are not as well defined as those of many of the other systemic mycoses because a sensitive and specific skin test has not been developed and the niche of the organism in the environment has not been described. Based on sporadic and epidemic disease in humans and dogs, the endemic area is the North American Midwest, the Southeast and South Central United States, and the states and provinces bordering the St. Laurence River. Isolation of the organism from its environment is difficult.

Blastomycosis was initially thought to be a cutaneous disease caused by a protozoan until it was shown that inhalation usually causes the primary, often subclinical, pulmonary infection. Hematogenous dissemination follows, and the lungs, skin, bones, and genitourinary system are the most frequent sites of symptomatic disease. Primary cutaneous blastomycosis can also occur, usually following dog bites or accidental inoculation during autopsies or laboratory work.

Clinical Manifestations

Inhalation of the *B. dermatitidis* conidia produces the primary pulmonary infection. About one half of those infected experience acute, nonspecific symptoms, including fever, chills, arthralgia, and myalgia. Transient pleuritic pain can occur, and an initially nonproductive cough can later produce purulent sputum. Chest films are nonspecific. Lobar or segmental consolidation can be seen, but pleural effusions and hilar adenopathy are uncommon. Spontaneous resolution of acute pulmonary symptoms can occur, but chronic pulmonary or disseminated disease is more common.

The symptoms of chronic pulmonary blastomycosis are those of chronic pneumonia, including hemoptysis, productive cough, pleuritic pain, and low-grade fever. Findings on chest film are variable, but lobar or segmental infiltrates or lesions resembling bronchogenic cancer are seen most commonly. Unlike the radiologic findings of histoplasmosis, calcification of hilar nodes or parenchymal nodules is uncommon. Hematogenous spread within the lungs can cause miliary disease; respiratory failure and death occur in more than half of these patients.

The skin is the most frequent site of extrapulmonary blastomycosis. The lesions can be either ulcerative or verrucous with an appearance similar to that of squamous cell carcinoma. Although cutaneous blastomycosis typically occurs with symptomatic or asymptomatic pulmonary blastomycosis, it can occur alone. Nevertheless, skin involvement is a useful indicator of disseminated disease.

After the skin, bones and joints are the most frequent sites of extrapulmonary blastomycosis. Osteolytic lesions are typically seen in the long bones, vertebrae, and ribs, but most bones can become infected. The bony lesions typically present with adjacent soft-tissue abscesses or draining sinuses.

Other sites of blastomycosis include the subcutaneous tissue and infrequently the central nervous system (CNS). Subcutaneous nodules are usually seen in acutely ill patients with disseminated disease; drainage from the nodules teems with organisms. The CNS is infrequently involved in immunocompetent patients, but up to 40 per cent of AIDS patients have intracranial or spinal abscesses and meningitis.

Diagnosis

Culture

Because the clinical symptoms are nonspecific, definitive diagnosis can be made only with culture. Initial growth of the culture will produce the mycelial phase at 30°C; this phase should then be converted to the yeast phase at 37°C or tested with exoantigens for confirmation. By contrast, only a presumptive identification can be made when the organism is seen on direct examination of sputum or bronchial washings or in tissue sections. The 8- to 15-μm organism has a thick refractile cell wall with a single, broad-based bud. The endospores of *C. immitis* can be mistaken for *B. dermatitidis,* but *C. immitis* lacks budding. *B. dermatitidis* can also be confused with *C. neoformans,* but the buds of *C. neoformans* have a broader base. In tissue, pyogranulomas should suggest *B. dermatitidis*, but the budding yeast forms can be difficult to see in hematoxylin-and-eosin–stained sections. Organisms are better seen with the Gomori methenamine silver or periodic acid–Schiff (PAS) stain. Mayer's mucicarmine stain can help distinguish *B. dermatitidis* from *C. neoformans* by highlighting the capsule of *C. neoformans* but not that of *B. dermatitidis.*

Serologic Findings

Complement fixation is neither sensitive nor specific for blastomycosis. A sensitive commercial enzyme immunoassay (enzyme-linked immunosorbent assay [ELISA]) that uses A antigen has been developed. An immunodiffusion test that detects antibody to A antigen is specific, exhibiting almost no cross-reactivity with other fungi. Initial screening with the sensitive enzyme-linked immunosorbent assay, followed by testing of positive patients with the more specific immunodiffusion test, may be useful.

COCCIDIOIDOMYCOSIS

Coccidioidomycosis is caused by *Coccidioides immitis* and is endemic in the American Southwest, especially in the Sonoran desert. The organism is closely associated with the creosote bush and rodent burrows. Soil disturbances can precipitate outbreaks; recent cases have occurred among archeologists digging for Native American artifacts and in California following earthquakes. Human-to-human transmission has not been documented.

Coccidiodes immitis appears as septate hyphae in the soil; alternate cells become barrel-shaped and break off. When these fragmented arthroconidia land in soil and germinate, the saprophytic phase continues and more hyphae and arthroconidia are produced. When the airborne arthroconidia are inhaled, they become spherical and develop a thick capsule. Within the spherule, small endospores develop to be released when the spherule opens. Each of the released endospores repeats this parasitic cycle, developing into a spherule and releasing more endospores. When infected tissue is cultured in the laboratory, the endospores revert to hyphal form and gray colonies appear within 3 to 4 days. The smooth gray colonies become tufted and cottony white-gray material fills the plate.

Clinical Manifestations

In the healthy human, symptoms develop within 2 weeks (range 7 to 28 days) in approximately 40 per cent of those infected. Rashes, especially erythema nodosum, may precede acute pulmonary disease. Symptoms include productive cough, fever, chills, night sweats, and lethargy. Some chest films show no change; others demonstrate infiltrates, pleural effusions, and prominent hilar nodes suggesting sarcoid. Most episodes of acute pulmonary coccidioidomycosis resolve spontaneously, but recovery can take longer than a month.

Approximately 1 in 200 persons infected experience disseminated disease. Such disease is associated with Filipino, Asian, or African-American background; a primary infection late in pregnancy; or immunosuppression. In endemic areas, coccidioidomycosis is a significant cause of maternal mortality. Only 15 per cent of pregnant patients survive disseminated disease, and premature birth and neonatal mortality are high. When fever occurs in pregnant residents of or travelers to endemic areas, a high index of suspicion, followed by diagnosis and therapy, increases the survival of mother and infant.

Disseminated disease can closely follow acute pulmonary disease or can develop months or years later. Except for endocardium and intestinal mucosa, all organs can be infected. Disseminated disease can be seen as pustular skin lesions or as diffuse involvement of many organs. Meningeal coccidioidomycosis carries a poor prognosis; untreated patients die and therapy is not always effective. The most common symptom is headache, whereas meningeal irritation commonly seen in bacterial meningitis is uncommon. Cerebrospinal fluid (CSF) examination typically shows a mononuclear pleocytosis, decreased glucose levels, and increased protein concentrations. A pulmonary nodule or cavity develops in about 5 per cent of those infected; coccidioidomycosis is often diagnosed when the nodules are biopsied to rule out cancer.

Diagnosis

The diagnosis of coccidioidomycosis can be made from histologic examination of infected tissue or cytologic examination of sputum or by culture of pus, sputum, joint fluid, or tissues. Cultures of blood, urine, CSF, and pleural and peritoneal fluid are typically negative. It is important to look for the large (up to 100 μm in diameter) spherules; the 2- to 5-μm endospores can resemble pollen and small yeasts. Because the cultured arthroconidia are potentially infectious in the laboratory, all gray-white cottony moulds should be manipulated in a biologic safety cabinet by experienced technologists. Arthroconidia can be present in many saprobic fungi; media with cycloheximide will inhibit many of the saprobes. Definitive identification is based on conversion of the spherule to the hyphal phase, exoantigen testing, or probes.

Skin Testing

Skin testing with mycelial coccidioidal antigens can document previous exposure in a patient with a lung nodule. Serial testing of patients with negative results on skin testing can give a false-positive result. Coccidioidin is a mycelial-phase antigen that remains the standard antigen used in skin testing. Spherulin is a parasitic-phase antigen that may be as specific as coccidioidin and more sensitive in detecting dermal delayed hypersensitivity.

Most symptomatic patients with a prior infection will have a positive skin test result (>5 mm induration) within 3 weeks of the onset of symptoms. Because skin tests frequently produce positive results before serologic tests do, skin testing can also be useful in patients with suspected disease whose serologic findings are still negative. Because patients with erythema nodosum can have severe reactions to coccidioidin, they should be tested only with 1:100 dilutions of the regular strength. Some cross-reactivity occurs with antigens from *H. capsulatum* and *B. dermatitidis*. Anergy is common in disseminated disease, and a negative skin test result in primary disease suggests latent or future dissemination.

Serologic Findings

The mycelial-phase antigen, coccidioidin, is most frequently used to detect antibody production. IgM precipitin antibodies develop 1 to 4 weeks after the onset of symptoms in three fourths of patients and are detectable for up to 4 months or more in disseminated or reactivated disease. IgG complement-fixing antibodies appear later and are more prevalent in sicker patients. They can persist up to 8 months. Higher or rising titers of IgG complement-fixing antibodies typify disseminated disease, and paired sera should be tested simultaneously. Ninety-five to 99 per cent of patients without disseminated disease have titers less than 1:32, and 61 per cent of patients with disseminated disease have titers greater than or equal to 1:32. An important exception is coccidioidomycosis disseminated only to the meninges; the serologic findings of patients with spread only to the meninges resemble the serologic findings of patients without disseminated disease. Only when *C. immitis* spreads to sites other than the meninges are the serologic findings useful in predicting disseminated disease.

Because the tube precipitin and complement fixation

tests can be difficult to perform, latex particle agglutination and immunodiffusion are often used. The latex agglutination kit is available commercially, is easily performed, and is the most sensitive method of detecting precipitin antibodies. Specificity is approximately 90 to 95 per cent. Immunodiffusion methods detect both precipitin antibodies and complement-fixing antibodies.

Disseminated coccidioidomycosis is an AIDS-defining event in patients who are positive for human immunodeficiency virus (HIV). Approximately 10 per cent of HIV-positive patients in endemic areas acquire disseminated primary or reactive disease each year. Disseminated disease in HIV infection correlates strongly with a CD4 cell count of less than 250 cells/mm^3 and a diagnosis of AIDS. Length of residence in the area, positive skin test results, and prior disease are not risk factors. Biopsy is often required for diagnosis because the organism is not easily cultured from sputum and bronchial alveolar lavage fluid. Because most of the immunocompromised patients can mount some type of serologic response, routine serologic testing is often performed.

CRYPTOCOCCOSIS

Cryptococcosis (torulosis, European blastomycosis) is caused by *Cryptococcus neoformans*, a fungus with worldwide distribution. Although serotypes A and D (*C. neoformans* var. *neoformans*) do not infect pigeons, *C. neoformans* grows well in pigeon droppings, and the organism is often found in soil contaminated with the droppings, on window ledges, and in barns. Serotypes B and C (*C. neoformans* var. *gatti*) are usually found in tropical and subtropical areas, especially in the air under flowering Eucalyptus trees. Disease follows inhalation of aerosolized organisms. Although the lungs are the major site of infection, the organism typically spreads to the brain and meninges.

Person-to-person spread via the pulmonary route has not been documented, but spread has resulted from infected transplanted kidneys and corneas. Persons with heavy exposure to pigeon droppings and laboratory workers exposed to aerosols from cultures have an increased likelihood of a positive skin test result but no increased rate of disease. Skin tests show that exposure to *C. neoformans* is widespread, but disease is uncommon in individuals with intact immune systems. Persons with AIDS account for approximately 85 per cent of cases, and approximately 10 per cent of AIDS patients in the United States have cryptococcosis. HIV-infected individuals are most susceptible when their CD4+ counts drop to less than 200 cells/mm^3. Transplant recipients also have an increased risk for cryptococcosis, largely because of steroids and other immunosuppressive therapy. Other risk factors include idiopathic CD4 lymphopenia, lymphoreticular malignancies, and sarcoid.

Clinical Manifestations

Pulmonary cryptococcosis is often asymptomatic and frequently diagnosed when a solitary pulmonary nodule seen on a chest film is biopsied to exclude cancer. Symptomatic cryptococcal pneumonia accompanied by minimal, sometimes blood-streaked sputum can present with coughing and shortness of breath. Pleural effusions are uncommon. In otherwise healthy persons who have infection confined to the lungs, the infection resolves, often spontaneously. In HIV-positive patients, cryptococcal pneumonia can be rapidly progressive and fatal.

Meningitis is the most common form of cryptococcosis. The organisms are spread hematogenously from the lungs to the meninges. Neither history nor symptoms are specific, but history can include changes in behavior or memory. The symptoms include headache and fever of several weeks' duration. The signs include papilledema in approximately 30 per cent of patients and cranial nerve deficits in 20 per cent. Onset can be acute or insidious. The onset is more often acute in immunosuppressed patients. The predilection toward CNS localization is explained by the lack of normal host defense mechanisms. Cerebrospinal fluid is an excellent culture medium for the organisms; it lacks soluble anticryptococcal factors present in serum. In addition, the alternate complement pathway is activated in serum by *C. neoformans,* but no complement activity accompanies *C. neoformans* in the CSF. Finally, the vigorous inflammatory response by macrophages, neutrophils, and lymphocytes seen in the rest of the body does not occur at all in the brain and occurs only slightly in the meninges.

Other organs in addition to the lungs and CNS can be involved. Painless skin lesions, especially on the face and scalp, are seen in 10 per cent of patients, and 5 to 10 per cent of these patients have osteolytic bony lesions that resemble tuberculosis or malignancy.

Localized pulmonary infections are frequently self-limited or cured by surgical resection, but untreated disseminated disease is usually fatal. Complete cures are unusual in immunosuppressed patients. Relapses and neurologic deficits are common in these patients after initial therapy. Hydrocephalus, high titers of antigen, and widespread infection are associated with a poor prognosis.

Diagnosis

Immunocompromised patients with CNS cryptococcosis typically have an increased opening pressure, decreased glucose and increased protein levels, and leukocyte counts greater than 20 cells/mm^3 with a lymphocytosis. These findings are often lacking in AIDS patients, but the organisms are easily cultured from CSF and are often visible with an India ink preparation.

The India ink test is rapid and simple to perform, but strict criteria must be used to prevent false-positive results. A drop of sediment from CSF is dropped onto a slide and mixed with an equal amount of India ink. A coverslip is added and the slide is examined under a light microscope. The mucopolysaccharide capsule repels the ink and forms a halo around the organism. Because artifacts, including red blood cells, can be mistaken for the organism, one should search for budding yeast forms. When no budding is seen, other characteristics of the organism should be sought, including a refractile double cell wall, a distinct capsule, and cytoplasmic inclusions. The appearance of the organism varies with the stain used. With a Wright-Giemsa stain, one sees a reddish purple sunburst, but with Gram staining, the organism has variable morphologic and staining characteristics. Nonpathogenic *Cryptococcus* species can be present in staining reagents; positive results on staining should be confirmed with culture.

Another rapid procedure for the detection of cryptococcal antigen in serum and CSF is a latex agglutination test. Unlike other systemic mycoses, the serologic test for *C. neoformans* detects antigen, not antibody. This commercial test is routinely available in clinical laboratories and is sensitive and specific. Latex particles coated with rabbit anticryptococcal antibody are mixed with the patient's serum or CSF, and capsular polysaccharides in the patient's specimen bind to and agglutinate the latex particles. Because rheumatoid factor can cause false-positive results, it is important to use appropriate controls. Serum (not CSF) can be treated with pronase, which reduces noncryptococcal agglutination as well as the occurrence of the prozone effect in which a positive specimen does not test positive until the specimen has been diluted. Titers can be useful; a favorable prognosis is associated with low titers.

Cultures remain the gold standard for documenting infection. Because organisms in the CSF may be sparse, repeated cultures may be required. Urine and sputum cultures should be taken, even in the absence of suspected pulmonary or genitourinary involvement. Blood cultures are positive in widespread infection, which is most frequent in patients with AIDS, neutropenia, or steroid-related immunosuppression. Cycloheximide added to the culture media will inhibit *C. neoformans* as well as many saprobes. The organism grows at 37°C but grows more rapidly at 30°C.

C. neoformans can also be presumptively identified from histologic examination of tissue specimens. *C. neoformans* is difficult to discern with hematoxylin and eosin, but silver and PAS stains highlight the organism and its characteristic narrow-based budding. Mayer's mucicarmine stains the capsule red; this differentiates the organism from artifacts and other encapsulated yeasts.

CANDIDIASIS

Candidiasis, which ranges from superficial cutaneous infection to severe systemic disease, can be caused by many species of *Candida*. Although *Candida* does not routinely colonize skin except sporadically in the intertriginous areas, about 80 per cent of healthy individuals will have some colonization of mucosal areas in the oral cavity, vagina, gastrointestinal tract, and rectum (see article on superficial mycosis). Species found as part of the normal flora include *Candida albicans, Candida tropicalis, Candida kefyr (pseudotropicalis), Candida glabrata (Torulopsis glabrata)*, and *Candida parapsilosis*. When the normal defenses of the skin or mucosa are breached, the organisms can enter and spread hematogenously to many organs, especially the lungs, liver, spleen, kidneys, heart, brain, and eyes. Most healthy persons can resist systemic infections by *Candida*. Immune defenses include humoral and, more importantly, cell-mediated processes. Many normal individuals have antibodies against the cell wall glycoprotein antigens of *Candida*; therefore, serologic findings are not very useful in diagnosis.

Clinical Manifestations

Disseminated Candidiasis

Both diagnosis and management of disseminated candidiasis are difficult. Blood cultures from patients with disseminated disease can be negative, and isolation of *Candida* from sputum, urine, feces, and skin is difficult to interpret because of colonization at these sites. The patients most at risk for disseminated disease are those with burns, cancer (especially acute leukemia), and recent complicated surgery (especially transplantation and cardiac and gastrointestinal surgery). In addition to larger abscesses, diffuse microabscesses with suppurative and granulomatous reactions can be seen, especially in the liver and spleen.

Candidal Endocarditis

Fungal endocarditis was once uncommon, but with the increased incidence of candidal infections, candidal endocarditis is seen more frequently. Risk factors include damaged cardiac valves, prosthetic cardiac valves, intravenous drug use, antineoplastic agents, long-term intravenous catheter use, and concurrent bacterial endocarditis. *Candida albicans* is responsible for more than half of all cases; *Candida parapsilosis* is the most frequent organism seen in heroin addicts. The aortic and mitral valves are most commonly involved, and the signs, symptoms, and complications are those of bacterial endocarditis except that the vegetations can be larger. As with disseminated candidiasis (and in contrast to bacterial endocarditis), blood cultures can be negative.

Central Nervous System Candidiasis

Infection of the parenchyma and meninges can be seen in disseminated candidiasis. Multiple small abscesses are typical. Symptoms of parenchymal disease are variable and depend on the size and distribution of the lesions. Meningitis can present with headache, stiff neck, and irritability. A lymphocytic pleocytosis is seen in 50 per cent of cases, and organisms can often be visualized by Gram stain. Candidal meningitis can also follow trauma, lumbar puncture, neurosurgery, and an infected ventricular shunt. *Candida albicans* is responsible for 90 per cent of infections.

Respiratory Tract Candidiasis

Pneumonia caused by *Candida* can be a focal or diffuse bronchopneumonia originating from an endobronchial location, or it can be a hematogenously seeded, nodular, diffuse infiltrate that resembles congestive heart failure or *Pneumocystis* pneumonia. Necrotizing pneumonias are rare. Definitive diagnosis depends on biopsy-proven tissue invasion, because yeast recovered from sputum is often colonizing and chest films are nonspecific.

Urinary Tract Candidiasis

Urethral candidiasis often follows antibiotic use. It can occur in women (typically spread from vaginal candidiasis) and in men (usually as a result of sexual contact). *Candida* is commonly found in urine, especially in patients with Foley catheters or those receiving antibiotics, and its presence does not necessarily indicate infection. Colony counts usually do not help to separate colonization from true infection; casts in the urine suggest invasion of the renal tissue. Kidney or upper urinary tract infection more commonly results from hematogenous dissemination, and microabscesses can be seen in the renal cortex. Less commonly, the kidney or upper urinary tract is the target of an ascending infection, particularly in patients with diabetes mellitus, renal stones, or other urinary tract obstruction. Papillary necrosis, caliceal invasion, and perinephric abscess can follow an ascending infection.

Diagnosis

In sputum and tissue section, budding yeasts, pseudohyphae, and blastospores can be seen. Although the pseudohyphae of *Candida* are generally constricted at the septations and have septations at branch points, they can be confused with the septate hyphae of *Aspergillus* species.

Hyphal outgrowths from blastospores in serum (germ tube formation) are presumptive evidence of *Candida albicans*, but the tubes must be read within 2 to 3 hours because other species of *Candida* can form germ tubes if the specimen is evaluated later. Definitive identification relies on chlamydospore formation on corn meal agar or sugar assimilation tests.

ZYGOMYCOSIS

Zygomycosis (mucormycosis, phycomycosis) refers to various diseases caused by fungi in the class Zygomycetes. These fungi include *Mucor, Rhizopus, Rhizomucor*, and *Absidia*. Like aspergillosis and candidiasis, zygomycosis is often regarded as an opportunistic infection; predisposing conditions include metabolic acidosis in poorly controlled diabetes and leukopenia.

Clinical Syndromes

Rhinocerebral Zygomycosis

Rhinocerebral zygomycosis is the most common disease caused by the Zygomycetes. The paranasal sinuses are the starting point of the infection, which can spread rapidly through the hard palate and into the ocular orbit and brain. The symptoms include facial pain and headache, and fever or cellulitis can be present. Orbital invasion is followed by a decline of extraocular muscle function and proptosis. Continued involvement leads to ptosis, dilated pupils, cerebral abscesses, and thromboses of the cavernous sinus and internal carotid artery.

Plain films of the sinuses and orbit often show mucosal thickening, with or without air-fluid levels. Because of their rapid growth, these organisms are referred to as "lid lifters" in the laboratory, and this characteristic is reflected in the dramatic changes (sometimes seen on a daily basis) as the organisms fill the sinus. Computed tomography scans show the bone and soft-tissue destruction caused by these angioinvasive organisms. Those who survive the infection should be examined periodically because patients who have apparently been cured can harbor residual organisms.

Pulmonary Zygomycosis

Most patients with pulmonary zygomycosis are leukemics with markedly decreased circulating neutrophils following chemotherapy. These patients, who are often receiving broad-spectrum antibiotics, present with fever and dyspnea. As the infection progresses, hemoptysis can occur, and when these angioinvasive organisms erode a major pulmonary vessel, pulmonary hemorrhage ensues. Chest films typically show infiltrates or cavity formation initially in one segment, but the unchecked infection can spread contiguously.

Diabetic patients can acquire a subacute form of pulmonary zygomycosis. Other patients at risk include those in intensive care units who are hyperglycemic or immunosuppressed following steroid administration or malnutrition.

Diagnosis

Invasion of the hard palate can sometimes be seen on physical examination. The tissue necrosis following angioinvasion can cause a black nasal discharge that should not be mistaken for and dismissed as dried blood. Black necrotic lesions of the hard palate or nasal mucosa also suggest zygomycosis. A presumptive diagnosis can be made quickly with the use of a PAS stain read with a light microscope or a Calcofluor stain read with a fluorescent microscope. Potassium hydroxide (KOH) applied to touch preparations is also helpful. Gomori methenamine silver stains the organism but the procedure takes longer to perform.

Tissue specimens sent to a surgical pathology laboratory may show both the organisms and the extent of invasion with routine stains. Although the organisms can be presumptively identified from the stains performed in the microbiology, cytology, or histology laboratory, definitive species identification requires culture. Like the Zygomycetes, *Aspergillus* species are angioinvasive. The broad ribbonlike aseptate hyphae of the Zygomycetes can usually be distinguished from the more rigidly parallel, septate, dichotomously branching hyphae of *Aspergillus* species. However, the hyphae of the Zygomycetes can twist and turn on themselves, giving the appearance of septations.

Definitive identification is usually based on the gross and microscopic morphologic features of cultures. Growth at higher temperatures and carbohydrate assimilation are sometimes useful. These organisms grow rapidly (2 to 5 days) on most media, except for media containing cycloheximide.

ASPERGILLOSIS

Aspergillosis refers to allergy, colonization, or tissue invasion by *Aspergillus* species. These organisms are ubiquitous, and disease can be caused by many species. Humans usually inhale the airborne conidia, which can then invade the nose, paranasal sinuses, and lungs. The skin can also be a portal of entry, especially around burns, catheter insertion sites, and incisions. The most important determinant of subsequent infection is not the exposure but rather the immune status of the patient. Acute leukemia, bone marrow and other organ transplantation, high-dose steroids, and chronic granulomatous disease are important risk factors. *Aspergillus fumigatus* is the most frequent cause of invasive and noninvasive disease. *Aspergillus flavus* is especially common in immunosuppressed patients and in nasal or sinus infections. *Aspergillus niger* and *Aspergillus fumigatus* are the most common causes of "fungus balls."

Clinical Manifestations

Allergic Bronchopulmonary Aspergillosis

Allergic bronchopulmonary aspergillosis occurs in asthmatics who present with eosinophilia, bronchial plugging that causes pulmonary infiltrates, and an immediate cutaneous reaction to *Aspergillus* antigen. Symptoms typically increase with age and the bronchial plugs can lead to bronchiectasis. These plugs are sometimes coughed up, and tangled masses of hyphae can be seen in them.

Fungus Ball (Aspergilloma)

A fungus ball can develop in patients with structural abnormalities due to prior lung disease, such as sarcoid, tuberculosis, or histoplasmosis, as colonizing organisms grow to fill parenchymal defects. Diagnosis can sometimes be suspected radiologically when air is seen surrounding a cavitary mass. Symptoms are not increased beyond those due to the underlying disease except for hemoptysis, which can sometimes be severe or fatal. Fungus balls can also occur in the maxillary and other paranasal sinuses when anatomic abnormalities or poor drainage is present. Immunosuppressed patients are at risk for acute invasive disease into the hard palate or nasal turbinates, as is seen in rhinocerebral zygomycosis.

Invasive Aspergillosis

Invasive aspergillosis is often rapidly fatal unless treated aggressively. Granulocytopenic patients are at greatest risk. High fever is followed by pulmonary consolidation; the lesion spreads hematogenously as well as directly through the lungs and contiguous tissues without regard to tissue planes. The blood vessels within the lesions often contain tangles of matted hyphae, causing both hemorrhage and infection. A "halo sign" around the lesion can sometimes be seen on computed tomography scans.

Other Sites

Normal, damaged, or replacement heart valves can be infected with *Aspergillus* species. Clinically, *Aspergillus* endocarditis resembles routine bacterial endocarditis except that it is difficult to isolate the fungus from blood cultures. Immunosuppressed patients are at risk for hematogenous dissemination, causing lesions in the bones, skin, kidney, and prostate.

Diagnosis

The hyphae have nearly parallel walls and are 2 to 4 μm wide, septate, and dichotomously branched at 45-degree angles. The spores and distinctive fruiting head are rarely seen in tissue (except occasionally in fungus balls in cavities containing air). Cross-sections through hyphal tangles can be mistaken for spores. Although *Aspergillus* species may be suspected after direct examination of smears or histologic examination of tissue, definitive species identification can be made only from culture.

The organism is easy to grow and identify in the standard clinical laboratory. When organisms are seen, the site, clinical state of the patient, and histologic evidence of invasion all help determine whether the organism is a contaminant or pathogen. As with other fungi, potassium hydroxide preparations, the PAS stain, and the Calcofluor stain can rapidly outline the organism in direct specimens. The PAS and Gomori methenamine silver stain highlight the organism in tissue. Stains for elastin can dramatically illustrate invasion of the arteries and the splaying of elastin fibers by the hyphae.

NOCARDIOSIS

Nocardiosis refers to diseases caused by *Nocardia* species, which are classified as bacteria. *Nocardia asteroides* complex is responsible for most systemic infections. *Nocardia* can cause subcutaneous disease and form mycetomas; *N. brasiliensis* and *N. otitidiscaviarum* (*N. caviae*) are other human pathogens that usually cause cutaneous disease. The organisms are found worldwide in soil and are not part of normal human flora. Although cutaneous disease and mycetomas can be seen in persons with intact immune systems, the bronchopulmonary disease and systemic hematogenous dissemination are usually seen in immune-compromised individuals with decreased T-cell function, especially that resulting from AIDS, leukemia, and immunosuppressive therapy following organ transplantation.

Clinical Manifestations

Bronchopulmonary infections due to *Nocardia* are similar to infections caused by other pyogenic bacteria. Fever, cough, and shortness of breath as well as cavitation and pleural spread are typical but not specific for *Nocardia*. Chest films often show multiple and confluent abscesses, but coin lesions and a miliary pattern can also be seen. Extension to the chest wall can cause sinus tract formation and bony involvement resembling actinomycosis. The disease can be acute, subacute, or chronic, punctuated by remission and exacerbation. Bronchopulmonary infections, even minor ones, often spread hematogenously, and the CNS is an affected target in one third of cases. Multilocular abscesses with "daughter" abscesses are common; meningitis is usually associated with a contiguous abscess.

Diagnosis

Multiple early morning sputum specimens should be collected from the patient. The laboratory should be alerted that *Nocardia* is part of the differential diagnosis because the organism can require a week to grow and most routine bacterial sputum cultures are held less than 5 days. The *Nocardia* bacilli are strict aerobic actinomycetes. They initially form gram-positive, beaded, branching filamentous rods, but these filamentous rods can fragment into shorter rods and cocci. Sometimes these organisms retain the Gram stain poorly and appear to be gram-negative rods studded with gram-positive beads. Some of the other actinomycetes such as *Rhodococcus* species, *Actinomadura, Streptomyces*, and *Actinomyces* stain similarly with the Gram stain. Like the mycobacteria, however, *Nocardia* has mycolic acid in its cell wall, and it can partially retain a modified acid-fast stain. *Rhodococcus* can also be partially acid-fast.

Nocardia grows well on most routine media over a wide temperature range. Added carbon dioxide enhances growth. Another reason to alert the laboratory to the possibility of *Nocardia* is that specimens can be plated on selective media to prevent some of the rapidly growing respiratory flora from obscuring the slower growing *Nocardia. Nocardia* will grow on routine acid-fast bacilli media, but it may not survive the decontamination procedure for mycobacteria.

A preliminary identification of *Nocardia* can be made based on the stains. Definitive species identification typically requires 3 weeks because *N. asteroides*, the species most frequently isolated, is inert in most biochemical tests.

Serologic findings are not helpful in diagnosis because there is a high degree of cross-reactivity among *Nocardia* species, *Mycobacteria* species, and *Streptomyces* species. Skin tests showing delayed cutaneous hypersensitivity are not available.

ACTINOMYCOSIS

Actinomycosis is most commonly caused by *Actinomyces israelii*, an anaerobic gram-positive bacillus. Like nocardiosis, actinomycosis is caused by bacteria, yet it is traditionally discussed in the context of fungal diseases. Because they have branching morphologic features and hyphal-like appearance in sulfur granules, *Actinomyces* species were once thought to be fungi. They lack the nuclear membrane, mitochondria, and chitin that are found in fungi; as bacteria, they reproduce by fission and are inhibited by penicillin, not antifungal agents.

Despite early reports that actinomycosis was acquired by chewing grass or straw, it is clear that it is an endogenous infection. In humans older than 3 years, it is always found in the oral cavity and often in the respiratory, gastrointestinal, and female genital tracts when appropriate anaerobic methods are used. The disease is not rare, but with improved dental care the frequency has decreased.

Almost any site can be affected; the organism enters through a break in the mucosal barrier. Oral lesions follow trauma or dental procedures; pulmonary disease follows aspiration; and gastrointestinal disease can be precipitated by diverticulitis, appendicitis, surgery, or foreign objects. Pelvic actinomycosis is associated with intrauterine devices (IUDs). Once a nidus for disease is established, it spreads slowly but progressively to adjacent structures, ignoring tissue planes, as do many fungal infections. Although associations with steroid use and HIV infection have been described, a causal relationship with specific humoral or cellular immune defects has not emerged.

Clinical Manifestations

Oral Cervicofacial Disease

The face and neck area is the most common site for actinomycosis; it presents as a soft-tissue swelling or mass lesion and spreads through tissue planes to contiguous structures. Pain, fever, and leukocytosis are typical; enlarged lymph nodes are uncommon. When the mass seems solid, cancer needs to be excluded. The most common location is at the submandibular angle of the jaw, but other sites can be affected. The skin over the lesion is often discolored, appearing blue or red, and sinus tracts can open and close spontaneously.

Thoracic Actinomycosis

Thoracic disease usually follows aspiration; spread from oral lesions is now uncommon because antibiotic treatment is effective. Disease presents slowly with fever, chest pain, and sometimes a productive cough. Radiographic findings are nonspecific. Infection should be suspected when a sinus tract draining an empyema forms in the chest wall or when pulmonary disease spreads through fissures and pleura to involve the chest wall and bony structures. Without the classic presentation of chest wall extension or a draining sinus, thoracic actinomycosis may elude rapid diagnosis.

Pelvic Actinomycosis

Although it can follow lower gastrointestinal tract disease, pelvic actinomycosis occurs most frequently in association with the use of an IUD for more than 2 years. A history of IUD use is also important because disease can occur months after its removal. Patients can present with fever, abdominal pain, or unusual discharge, but recognition of the entity is often delayed until an initial endometritis has spread through the genital tract and pelvis. The use of cervical screening for detection of *Actinomyces*-like organisms in women with IUDs is controversial, because *Actinomyces* species can also be part of the normal vaginal flora.

Diagnosis

Actinomycotic sulfur granules in the proper clinical setting are presumptive evidence of actinomycosis. Confirmation depends on identifying the organisms from the sulfur granules or in normally sterile tissue.

Sulfur granules are lumps of organisms that can be difficult to identify in purulent material or sinus tracts. Despite their name, they can be white, pink, gray, or brown, in addition to yellow. In tissue sections, the granules are eosinophilic at least on the periphery. It is difficult to see the filamentous bacteria with a hematoxylin and eosin stain, but Giemsa stains and tissue Gram and silver stains highlight the organisms. Proteinaceous, eosinophilic material can surround the granule (Splendore-Hoeppli phenomenon), but this also can be seen in nonactinomycotic granules.

The differential diagnosis often includes nocardiosis. Only the cutaneous, not the visceral, nocardial lesions can contain sulfur granules. The granules seen in cutaneous nocardiosis stain with a modified acid-fast stain; the granules of actinomycosis do not. Another bacterial infection that can produce granules is botryomycosis. Causative organisms include *Staphylococcus, Streptococcus, Escherichia, Pseudomonas*, and *Proteus*, all of which can be easily distinguished from the filamentous gram-positive actinomycetes with Gram stains and cultures.

Laboratory diagnosis can be difficult unless the clinician carefully avoids contaminating the specimen with normal flora that can contain *Actinomyces* species. Swabs provide misleading information. To obtain material from a sinus tract, the surface should be well cleansed and the specimen collected by curettage or needle and syringe. When actinomycosis is suspected, the laboratory should be alerted so that the specimens are incubated for at least 2 weeks under anaerobic conditions. Colonies are white with an irregularly domed surface resembling a molar tooth. Definitive identification follows biochemical tests.

SUPERFICIAL MYCOSES

By Stephen T. Olin, M.D.
Lancaster, Pennsylvania

Superficial fungal skin infections are the most common skin diseases affecting humans and are frequently seen by primary care physicians and dermatologists. Because the incidence of superficial mycoses is increasing, and highly effective treatment is available, it is important that accurate diagnosis be feasible with the use of relatively simple and inexpensive procedures. The superficial mycoses include the dermatophytoses, cutaneous candidiasis, and the yeast *Pityrosporum ovale* (also called *P. orbiculare* and, previously, *Malassezia furfur*).

DIAGNOSTIC PROCEDURES

Three simple and readily available diagnostic procedures can confirm the presence of a superficial mycotic skin infection. These procedures are the potassium hydroxide (KOH) preparation, fungal culture on dermatophyte test medium (DTM; the most commonly used culture medium in office practice), and the Wood's light examination.

Potassium Hydroxide Preparation

The KOH examination is the most valuable, simple, and inexpensive diagnostic technique for identifying superficial mycoses, specifically dermatophytes and yeasts (*Candida* and *Pityrosporum* species). By separation and destruction of the cells of the stratum corneum, the alkaline KOH solution allows easy identification of spores and hyphae, which are less readily altered. Proper site selection and specimen collection, together with specimen preparation and examination, will greatly facilitate positive identification of disease-producing organisms.

Creams, powder, ointment, and make-up should be removed with acetone-containing swabs, such as those available for removing fingernail polish. Use a No. 15 scalpel, dermal curette, plastic serrated knife, or edge of a micro-

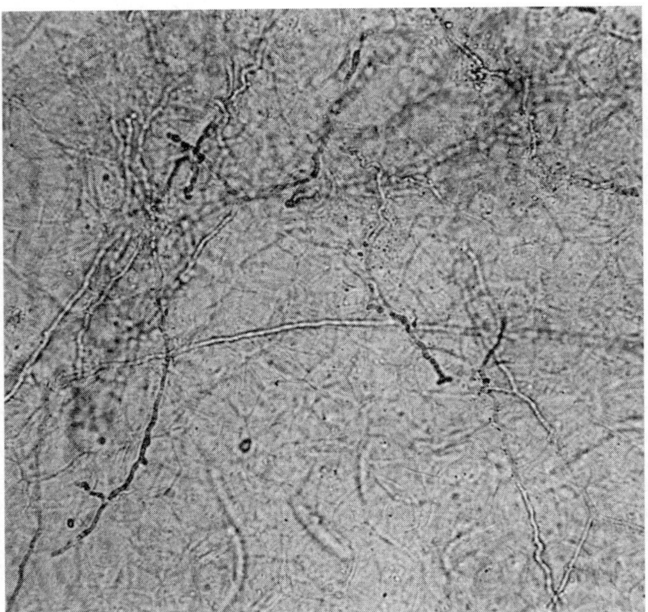

Figure 1. Dermatophyte hyphae. (Courtesy of Robert J. Pariser, M.D.)

scope slide to scrape scales onto a microscope slide. A soft-bristle children's toothbrush is particularly useful in obtaining scalp scale. Collect scales from the border next to the normal skin. When vesicles or pustules are present, remove their roofs for examination. Collect subungual nail debris or scales from white patches on nail surfaces. Remove remnants of broken hairs or scalp scales for examination, depending on the site affected.

Push the collected material to the center of the microscope slide using a coverslip or scalpel blade. Place the coverslip on the specimen before adding a drop or two of KOH (usually 15 to 20 per cent) on either side of the

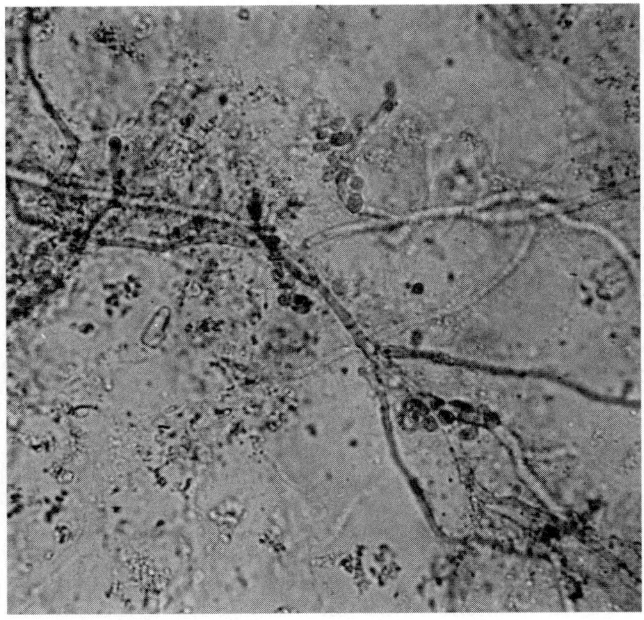

Figure 2. Hyphae and spores of *Candida*. (Courtesy of Robert J. Pariser, M.D.)

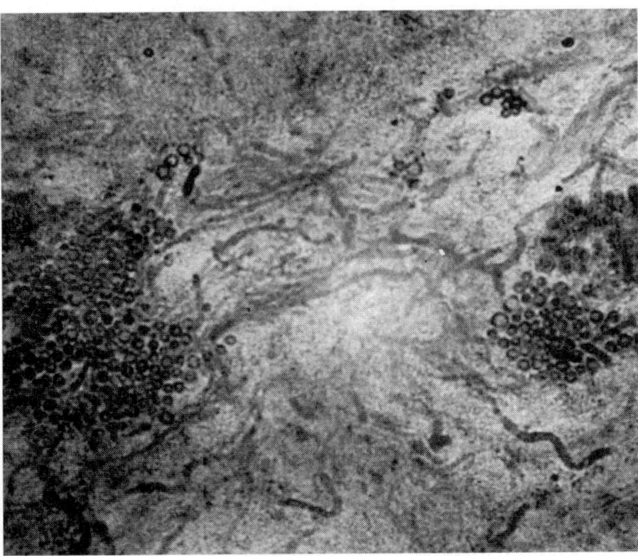

Figure 3. Hyphae and spores of tinea versicolor. (Courtesy of Robert J. Pariser, M.D.)

coverslip. Capillary action draws the KOH into the specimen without disturbing it. Gently warm the slide but only to the point at which it can still be touched without burning. This prevents boiling of the solution, which disrupts the specimen and produces KOH crystallization, creating artifact sometimes mistaken for hyphae. Place the heated microscope slide under the edge of a C-fold paper towel and gently compress coverslip and specimen to remove excess KOH (which can ruin expensive microscope objectives).

Examine the specimen with low-intensity light under the 10× objective with the substage condenser lowered. Constantly rotate the fine focus knob while scanning the specimen; this allows the entire depth of the specimen to be examined. Typical "positive" KOH findings are illustrated in Figures 1 through 3. Dermatophyte hyphae (see Fig. 1) are long structures, usually straight or wavy, that branch and have a fairly uniform diameter. Hyphae and spores of *Candida* are sometimes difficult to distinguish from dermatophytes; however, *Candida* hyphae are usually shorter, and budding spores are often seen (see Fig. 2). The typical "spaghetti and meatball" hyphae and spores of tinea versicolor are illustrated in Figure 3. Spores are clustered around short and stubby hyphae, which are best seen under 40× power. Scanning under 10× power will quickly identify the preferred location for high-power viewing. A "negative" KOH examination does not exclude the diagnosis of a superficial fungal infection. Errors in technique that can result in false-negative results include the following:

- A KOH solution that was improperly made or stored
- A specimen that was insufficiently "cleared," resulting in diagnostic features being missed
- Insufficient material collected or obtained from a site lacking diagnostic structures
- A specimen that was incompletely examined and/or examined with improper lighting and focusing

Dermatophyte Test Medium

DTM is supplied in wide-mouthed bottles with screw tops. DTM contains gentamicin sulfate and chlortetracycline to inhibit bacterial growth, cycloheximide to inhibit moulds, and phenol red to indicate pH. Growth of a dermatophyte changes the culture medium from yellow to red.

The appropriate specimen can be scraped, brushed, or plucked directly onto the culture medium or transferred from a microscope slide or paper. Some or all of the specimen should be pressed into the medium with a scalpel. The top of the bottle containing DTM should not be tightened but should be partially screwed on to provide oxygen to the growing organism. DTM should be incubated at room temperature; dermatophytes will turn the media red within 14 days. Dermatophyte colonies are typically white or off-white, with a fluffy, powdery, or crystalline texture. *Candida*, moulds, or other fungi and bacteria rarely turn the medium red. Dark-colored, black, or green colonies (especially when isolated, large, and few in number) are never dermatophytes.

Although specifically developed for isolating dermatophytes, DTM will also grow *Candida*. Although the medium will usually remain yellow, *Candida* may cause it to turn red. However, the colonies are distinct from those of dermatophytes (or mould contaminants); *Candida* appears lemon-yellow or cream-colored and consists of smooth, translucent, dome-shaped, pasty colonies.

Wood's Light Examination

The Wood's lamp produces invisible long-wave ultraviolet (UV) radiation (365 nm). This lamp induces visible fluorescence, thereby facilitating diagnosis of some superficial mycoses. Wood's light is produced by filtering a UV light source with barium silicate glass containing approximately 9 per cent nickel oxide. Wood's lamps produce some visible blue-white light, which is reflected, as well as UV light, which induces fluorescence. The long-wave UV energy from a Wood's lamp is converted to visible light after interacting with pteridine, a substance that produces fluorescence, mainly in ectothrix tinea capitis infections (Table 1).

DERMATOPHYTOSES

Dermatophytosis translates into "skin plant." Dermatophytes are a group of fungi responsible for most superficial infections of the skin, nails, and hair. They infect and survive only within superficial keratin layers of the epidermis; they rarely invade living epidermis and its appendages. A breakdown of the cutaneous barrier by heat, maceration, fissures, or immunocompromise increases the risk of cutaneous fungal infection. The dermatophyte or "ringworm" fungi are acquired by humans from three sources: (1) soil (geophilic), (2) animals (zoophilic), or (3) most commonly pathogens that infect only humans (anthropophilic) and cannot survive elsewhere. Geophilic and zoophilic fungi tend to produce more highly inflammatory skin infections than do the anthropophilic fungi. The dermatophytes belong to one of three genera: *Trichophyton*, *Microsporum*, and *Epidermophyton*. The individual clinical entities caused by these fungi are called "tinea" infections. Specific infections are commonly named for the site of involvement (e.g., tinea capitis, referring to a dermatophyte infection of the scalp, or tinea cruris, referring to an infection of the groin).

Table 1. Wood's Light Examination

Condition	Fluorescent Color
Tinea capitis	
Microsporum audouinii	Bright yellow-green
Microsporum canis	Bright yellow-green
Trichophyton schoenleinii	Pale green
Tinea versicolor	Golden yellow
Erythrasma	Coral red

TINEA CAPITIS

Clinical Features

Also known as ringworm of the scalp, tinea capitis occurs chiefly in school-aged children, although it is occasionally found in adults and infants. In the 1950s, most tinea capitis was caused by *Microsporum audouinii*, whereas today the most common pathogen is *Trichophyton tonsurans*, followed by *Microsporum canis*. Most patients are asymptomatic, although significant pruritus may occur. Presentations vary widely and include diffuse or localized alopecia, with or without scaling; "black dot" ringworm, in which hairs break off close to the scalp; thick scaling or crusting resembling seborrheic dermatitis or psoriasis; and kerion formation, which mimics a bacterial infection and presents as a large, painful, boggy, inflammatory lesion (typically caused by *M. canis* and, less commonly, *T. tonsurans*). Kerion is associated with delayed hypersensitivity and a local inflammatory response to fungal antigen. Regional lymphadenopathy, especially posterior cervical lymphadenopathy, is often prominent.

Tinea barbae is a fungal infection of the beard, predominantly seen in men infected by animals, especially in rural areas. Also known as "cattle ringworm," tinea barbae has clinical features similar to those of tinea capitis.

Complications are uncommon, but kerion formation may cause permanent scarring and alopecia. Some patients may also have a diffuse papular eruption on the face and trunk, a form of hypersensitivity reaction known as an "id reaction."

Diagnostic Procedures

Culture with DTM represents the most reliable means of diagnosing tinea capitis. Scalp scale can be obtained most easily with a small children's toothbrush; plucked hair, including the bulb end and 2 to 4 mm of hair shaft, should also be placed on DTM, along with the scale.

KOH examination of scale and plucked hair may also be useful but is less reliable. Tinea capitis results from invasion of the hair shaft. When the spores remain within the shaft, it is referred to as an endothrix infection; this condition usually results in a noninflammatory tinea capitis (alopecia without scale, erythema, or pustules) and is often caused by *T. tonsurans*. When the spores spread beyond the hair shaft, it is referred to as an ectothrix infection, and a sheath of the spores forms on the outside of the hair. This often leads to inflammatory tinea capitis and is often caused by *M. audouinii* or *M. canis*.

Wood's light examination previously was extremely helpful when *M. audouinii* (which causes an ectothrix infection with spores on the hair surface resulting in characteristic fluorescence) was the most common cause of tinea capitis. However, today *T. tonsurans* is the most common causative organism (at least 90 per cent of cases). *T. tonsurans* produces an endothrix infection with spores contained within the hair shaft and thus does not produce fluorescence.

Pitfalls in Diagnosis

Because dandruff does not develop in prepubertal school-aged children, their scaling scalps almost always represent dermatophytoses. Scaling scalps are often mistakenly diagnosed as seborrheic dermatitis. Other causes of scaling include psoriasis, atopic dermatitis and, occasionally, pediculosis. Other causes of hair loss include alopecia areata, trichotillomania, and secondary syphilis. Inflammatory tinea capitis may resemble bacterial pyodermas such as impetigo or folliculitis. Kerion formation may be confused with a carbuncle, and scarring tinea must be differentiated from discoid lupus erythematosus, radiodermatitis, the cicatricial alopecias, and folliculitis decalvans.

TINEA CORPORIS

Clinical Features

Also known as ringworm of the skin, tinea corporis is a dermatophyte infection of the glabrous, or nonhairy, skin; it occurs in all ages, but children are most susceptible. Tinea corporis occurs worldwide but is more common in hot, humid climates and rural areas. Similar eruptions on the face, aside from the beard area, are referred to as tinea faciei. The most common pathogens are *T. rubrum*, *T. mentagrophytes*, *T. tonsurans*, and *M. canis*. The latter is commonly acquired from infected dogs and kittens.

The typical presentation is that of annular, erythematous, papulosquamous plaques. The borders are well defined, with raised margins that are occasionally studded with vesicles or pustules. The infection may be asymptomatic or mildly pruritic. The annular lesions frequently demonstrate central clearing. Rarely, the lesions become granulomatous and produce ulceration of the skin. Nodular perifolliculitis may be associated with infections by *T. rubrum* or *T. verrucosum*, the only organisms that can invade hair follicles. Majocchi's granuloma is a granulomatous folliculitis caused by *T. rubrum*, usually affecting the lower legs of women who shave.

Diagnostic Procedures

KOH preparation and examination of scale obtained from the active edge of a lesion provides the most useful diagnostic procedure. Long, straight or wavy, filamentous, thin, branching hyphae are diagnostic. When the KOH examination is equivocal or negative, culture on DTM of scale obtained from an active border is useful. Wood's light examination is useful only in rare cases of tinea corporis caused by *M. canis*, which produces moist, crusted annular plaques.

Pitfalls in Diagnosis

Partially treated lesions may produce negative KOH examinations or cultures. A useful statement to remember is "not all that rings is ringworm." Other diagnostic possibilities include nummular eczema, contact dermatitis, psoriasis, the "herald patch" of pityriasis rosea, granuloma annulare, subacute cutaneous lupus erythematosus, secondary syphilis, erythema annulare centrifugum, seborrheic dermatitis, bullous impetigo, tinea versicolor, candidiasis, and erythrasma.

TINEA CRURIS

Clinical Features

Also known as "jock itch," tinea cruris is an extremely pruritic infection of the groin and surrounding areas and represents the second most common dermatophytosis. Heat, humidity, excessive sweating, obesity, and occlusive undergarments can predispose to this condition, which most commonly occurs in men. The most frequent pathogens are *Epidermophyton floccosum*, *T. rubrum*, and *T. mentagrophytes*. Tinea cruris may be unilateral or bilateral and typically presents as an erythematous plaque with a slightly raised, scaly, advancing edge, which is well demarcated and symmetric.

Diagnostic Procedures

KOH examination is the most useful diagnostic procedure. Again, when the KOH examination is negative, DTM culture should be obtained. Wood's light examination is useful only in differentiating tinea cruris from erythrasma (caused by *Corynebacterium minutissimum*), which produces a characteristic coral red fluorescence under Wood's light.

Pitfalls in Diagnosis

Several conditions mimic tinea cruris, including psoriasis, candidiasis, contact dermatitis, erythrasma, seborrheic dermatitis, and nonspecific intertrigo. Tinea cruris seldom involves the scrotum, and the penis is never involved because of the sparse amount of keratin present in these locations. Erythrasma has a uniform, fine, bran-colored scale and lacks a raised border. Psoriasis is usually a deeper red and usually contains more scale. Candidiasis has a wet, weeping appearance. Intertrigo is also moist and often red and tender. Contact dermatitis usually does not have a raised border.

TINEA PEDIS AND TINEA MANUUM

Clinical Features

Also known as athlete's foot, tinea pedis is the most common superficial mycotic skin infection, affecting 50 per cent of individuals at some time in life. The disease is more prevalent in males than in females and is spread indirectly from person to person by exposure to infective fungal elements in public facilities such as locker room floors or showers or carpeted flooring. Occlusive footwear and socks predispose to disease because of promotion of heat and sweating that encourage fungal growth. *T. rubrum*, *T. mentagrophytes*, and *E. floccosum* are the dermatophytes most often responsible for causing tinea pedis.

Four clinical varieties of tinea pedis have been described: interdigital, moccasin-type, vesicular, and ulcerative. *Interdigital* infection is the most common and is characterized by mild scaling to marked maceration with fissures; the web spaces between the third and fourth and/or fourth and fifth toes are most frequently affected. A foul odor is often present as a result of a breakdown of the epidermal barrier, thus allowing invasion of gram-negative, staphylococcal, and streptococcal organisms. Painful, deep, erosive lesions may occur, as may intense pruritus. Cellulitis may also develop and may spread to the lower extremity, especially in diabetics.

The *moccasin type* of tinea pedis is also common, with one or both plantar surfaces affected with diffuse scale and hyperkeratosis. Itching is usually mild and the distribution may be patchy; however, diffuse erythema may be present and the process often extends to the medial and lateral aspect of the foot, thus resembling a moccasin. Although symptoms are mild, the condition is extremely persistent.

The *vesicular* form of tinea pedis is uncommon, but it

can be severe enough to cause great disability with acute eruption of highly inflammatory, pruritic vesicles, generally occurring on the instep of one or both feet. This form is caused by *T. mentagrophytes,* which also causes the *ulcerative* form, and similarly is uncommon. This fulminating form of the disease results in epidermal ulceration, purulent vesicular fluid, and rapid spread. The ulcerative form usually affects the web spaces and most often occurs in immunocompromised persons and those with diabetes mellitus. Secondary bacterial infection is common.

Tinea pedis occasionally involves one or both hands, with two-foot and one-hand or two-hand and one-foot presentations. Hand infection is almost never found in the absence of foot involvement.

Diagnostic Procedures

The diagnosis is readily confirmed by examination of a KOH preparation of the macerated scale within the web spaces or the fine, silvery white scale present in the moccasin type of tinea pedis. When vesicles or pustules are present, they should be gently unroofed with a No. 15 scalpel and the roof examined with a KOH preparation. Blister fluid alone may not contain diagnostic hyphal elements. Again, when the KOH examination is negative, DTM culture of scale or blister roofs serves to confirm one's clinical diagnosis. Wood's light examination is not useful.

Pitfalls in Diagnosis

The many varieties of tinea pedis must be distinguished from dyshidrotic eczema, allergic and primary irritant dermatitis, psoriasis, bacterial and candidal infections, atopic dermatitis, secondary syphilis, drug eruptions, the various keratodermas, and acrodermatitis continua.

ONYCHOMYCOSIS

Clinical Features

Onychomycosis, also known as tinea unguium, occurs more frequently in toenails than in fingernails. As with tinea pedis, this condition typically affects persons wearing occlusive shoes. The most common causative organisms are those responsible for tinea pedis: *T. rubrum* (most common), *T. mentagrophytes*, and *E. floccosum*, which invade the nail unit via the nail bed or nail plate. *Candida albicans* and nondermatophyte moulds may also cause onychomycosis.

There are four presentations of onychomycosis:

- *Distal subungual* onychomycosis is the most common variety, affecting both fingernails and toenails, in which the distal nail plate develops yellow to brown discoloration, hyperkeratotic debris accumulates beneath the nail, and onycholysis develops. Affected individuals usually have tinea pedis or, to a lesser extent, tinea manuum.
- *White superficial* onychomycosis is seen primarily in toenails and is characterized by surface invasion of the nail plate, which becomes soft, dry, and powdery. *T. mentagrophytes*, as well as several nondermatophyte moulds, are responsible for this variant.
- *Proximal subungual* onychomycosis is the least common type, in which the fungus invades under the cuticle into the proximal nail bed. The nail plate remains intact, and the proximal region of the nail bed turns white. This variety is common in human immunodeficiency virus (HIV)–infected individuals or those with other immunodeficiencies and is caused by *T. rubrum*. Both fingernails and toenails may be involved.
- *Candidal onychomycosis* is rare and is limited to individuals who have chronic mucocutaneous candidiasis or whose hands are frequently in water. The entire nail plate becomes thick and opaque with a yellowish discoloration. Fingernails are affected more often than are toenails.

In all four types of onychomycosis, infected nails may coexist with normal-appearing nails.

Diagnostic Procedures

KOH examination of subungual debris will usually reveal hyphae; nail clippings usually require overnight soaking in 40 per cent KOH to obtain the best results. Culture of subungual debris or nail clippings on DTM will often yield positive results. However, when both KOH examination and DTM culture fail to yield a diagnosis, nail plate clippings can be sent for histologic analysis. Wood's light examination is not useful.

Pitfalls in Diagnosis

Not all dystrophic nails are due to fungal pathogens. Other diseases of the nails that may mimic onychomycosis are psoriasis, lichen planus, allergic contact or atopic dermatitis involving the proximal nail fold, *Pseudomonas* infections, traumatic onycholysis or onychodystrophy, acrodermatitis continua, and pachyonychia congenita.

TINEA VERSICOLOR

Clinical Features

Also known as pityriasis versicolor, tinea versicolor is a mycotic invasion of the stratum corneum by the lipophytic, dimorphic yeast *Pityrosporum ovale* (also known as *P. orbiculare*, and previously *Malassezia furfur,* as stated earlier). *P. ovale* is considered a skin saprophyte that normally colonizes the hair follicle in areas of the body with high sebum production. Although in the yeast phase *P. ovale* normally produces no rash, under certain environmental or host conditions, the organism converts to its mycelial or filamentous form spreading into the superficial dermal layers and producing a rash. Tinea versicolor occurs most commonly during the years of greatest sebum production, beginning during puberty and decreasing during the fifth and sixth decades of life. Tinea versicolor occurs more commonly during the summer months because heat, humidity, and perspiration facilitate growth of the filamentous forms. Greasy skin, hereditary predisposition, systemic corticosteroid use, malnutrition, chronic illnesses, pregnancy, and immunosuppression are other predisposing factors.

P. ovale produces macular lesions or patches ranging in size from several millimeters to several centimeters in diameter. Lesions appear in the "turtle-neck" distribution (back, chest, shoulders, and neck), although the face and entire trunk may be affected. Tinea versicolor causes pigmentary alterations in skin color from salmon pink to red to brown or white, thus the name "versicolor." The color is usually light brown on untanned skin and white on tanned skin. In dark-skinned individuals, tinea versicolor often produces dark brown macules. Gentle scraping of the involved skin produces a characteristic fine, powdery scale. Patients usually present during the summer months, when hypopigmentation is more likely to be observed. The lesions usually produce no symptoms but can be pruritic in some persons.

A recent hypothesis suggests that *P. ovale* contributes to the cause of dandruff and seborrheic dermatitis because of a markedly increased prevalence of this organism in affected patients. In addition, *P. ovale* may cause *Pityrosporum* folliculitis, which is characterized by pruritic follicular papules and pustules on the upper back.

Diagnostic Procedures

KOH examination is the most reliable diagnostic test. Scale from a suspected lesion will reveal characteristic short, blunt hyphae and clusters of round spores, commonly known as "spaghetti and meatballs." Partially treated infections may result in negative findings on KOH examination of skin scrapings.

Wood's light examination produces characteristic golden yellow fluorescence, although it may not be present in those who have recently showered because the fluorescent substance is water-soluble. Culture is difficult to perform and typically not required.

Pitfalls in Diagnosis

Tinea versicolor must be distinguished from seborrheic dermatitis, tinea corporis, pityriasis alba, pityriasis rosea, guttate psoriasis, nummular eczema, vitiligo and melasma, tuberculoid leprosy, and secondary syphilis. *Pityrosporum* folliculitis must be differentiated from acne vulgaris, drug-induced or steroid acne, hot tub folliculitis, and eosinophilic folliculitis in human immunodeficiency virus–infected individuals.

CANDIDIASIS

Clinical Features

Also known as moniliasis or thrush, candidiasis is caused by the dimorphous yeast *Candida albicans*, which is part of the normal flora of the pharynx, gastrointestinal tract, and vagina. Although there are many species of *Candida*, most human disease is due to *C. albicans*. Conditions that disrupt the corneum increase the risk of cutaneous candidiasis. Factors that predispose to infection include obesity; maceration; hot, humid environments; prolonged systemic antibiotic or corticosteroid use; diabetes mellitus; pregnancy; immunodeficiencies; oral contraceptive use; Cushing's disease; and debilitating states.

There are many clinical presentations of candidiasis, which depend on the site of involvement. The following represent the more common candidal infections.

Thrush represents oral candidiasis and is characterized by white plaques loosely attached to bright red oral mucous membranes. Infections are common in infants; passage of the yeast through the gastrointestinal tract can result in seeding of the perineum, causing diaper dermatitis. Immunocompromised individuals and those taking antibiotics are also frequently infected.

Perlèche is also known as candidal angular cheilitis and presents as erythematous, painful, macerated fissures at the corners of the mouth. Predisposing factors include dental malocclusions, braces, or dentures; diabetes; prolonged antibiotic use; and frequent lip-licking.

Intertriginous infections most often occur in the axillary, inframammary, groin, intergluteal, or perianal regions, which are warm and moist. Affected skin folds become red, macerated, and occasionally scaly, with well-defined borders and satellite papules or pustules. Obesity, diabetes, and immunodeficiency are common predisposing conditions.

Vulvovaginitis is characterized by vulvar erythema, edema, and pruritus, with an associated white, curdlike vaginal discharge. Diabetes, pregnancy, oral contraceptive use, and antibiotic use frequently trigger this disorder.

Paronychia caused by *C. albicans* is usually found in persons who have frequent contact with water. Invasion of the proximal and lateral nail folds results in erythema and edema of the folds, with resultant green or brown discoloration of the nail and dystrophic ridging.

Diaper dermatitis usually appears as bright red confluent patches or plaques with well-demarcated serpiginous borders. Satellite papules and pustules are often present. The warm, moist perineum and friction from the diaper create an environment conducive to this condition.

Erosio interdigitalis blastomycetica specifically denotes web space infection of the fingers caused by *Candida*, most commonly occurring between the third and fourth fingers. The web space becomes macerated, red, and fissured; sloughing of the epidermis leaves the area painful, raw, and denuded. Individuals constantly exposed to water or strong alkalis are more prone to the development of this disorder.

Chronic mucocutaneous candidiasis is a condition associated with an underlying defect in T-cell–mediated immunity, usually occurring in childhood and characterized by thickened, dystrophic nails; paronychia; and hyperkeratotic, hornlike, or granulomatous lesions affecting the scalp and fingers. The disorder may be inherited, may occur with associated endocrinopathies, or may appear sporadically.

Diagnostic Procedures

KOH preparation and examination of skin scrapings, mucosal discharge or plaques, or unroofed pustules will usually reveal the typical pseudohyphae and budding spores. *C. albicans* grows readily on DTM, and although usually will not turn the media red, it will demonstrate the characteristic lemon-yellow or cream-colored, smooth, translucent dome-shaped, pasty colonies. Wood's light examination is not useful, except in differentiating intertriginous infections caused by *C. albicans* from erythrasma, which produces a characteristic coral red fluorescence.

Pitfalls in Diagnosis

Candidal dermatitis can be mistaken for many other conditions because of its wide distribution and clinical appearance. Diaper dermatitis is a complex syndrome with multiple potential causes. The following should be considered in the differential diagnosis: contact or primary irritant dermatitis, psoriasis, seborrheic dermatitis, atopic dermatitis, bacterial infection, acrodermatitis enteropathica, and histiocytosis.

Pseudomonal paronychia also causes nail discoloration and dystrophy, as does *C. albicans*; however, pseudomonal infections are often foul-smelling and may have a blue-green discoloration resulting from pyocyanin, a pigment elaborated by *Pseudomonas aeruginosa*. In addition, *Pseudomonas* produces another pigment, pyoverdin, which fluoresces a bright aqua-green to white-green under Wood's light.

Thrush must be distinguished from lichen planus and leukoplakia. Intertriginous candidiasis may closely resemble tinea cruris, erythrasma, seborrheic dermatitis, and psoriasis. Perineal itching, although commonly resulting from candidiasis, has multiple causes, including contact or primary irritant dermatitis, psoriasis, atrophic vaginitis, and lichen sclerosus et atrophicus.

SPOROTRICHOSIS

Clinical Features

Sporotrichosis is a chronic infection caused by the dimorphic fungus *Sporothrix schenckii* following accidental implantation of the organism into the skin. *S. schenckii* lives as a saprophyte on certain grasses, shrubs, and other plants. Sources of inoculation include rose bushes, barberry shrubs, carnations, sphagnum moss, and contaminated soil or mine timbers. Primary invasion is usually seen as an occupational disease in farmers, florists, gardeners, laborers, or nursery workers. Transmission to humans has been documented from cat scratches.

The earliest manifestation is a small nodule or chancriform ulceration that may heal and disappear. Within a few weeks, the infection spreads along the lymphatics, producing multiple subcutaneous painless nodules. Unusual clinical patterns include a solitary ulcer without regional lymphangitis, a systemic visceral pattern via hematogenous dissemination, and a pulmonary pattern.

Diagnostic Procedures

Even with special stains, *S. schenckii* is rarely found in histologic tissue samples; however, the organism is readily cultured or identified via fluorescent antibody staining. KOH and Wood's light examinations are not helpful.

Pitfalls in Diagnosis

Several infectious diseases produce nodular lesions that spread along lymphatics and resemble sporotrichosis: atypical mycobacterial infection, cutaneous tuberculosis, syphilis, furunculosis, cat-scratch disease, anthrax, tularemia, and the primary inoculation of other deep fungal organisms. Therefore, specific culture techniques and staining are required to establish the correct diagnosis.

Protozoal Diseases

MALARIA

By Mark R. Wallace, M.D.,
and Larry K. Miller, M.D.
San Diego, California

Malaria, one of the world's most common infectious diseases, is prevalent throughout the tropics and subtropics. Each year an estimated 30,000 American and European travelers to endemic areas acquire the disease. Transmitted by the bite of an infected female anopheline mosquito, human malaria is caused by four species of the protozoan genus *Plasmodium. Plasmodium falciparum*, which causes 40 to 60 per cent of infections worldwide, is also the organism most likely to cause death. *P. vivax* causes 30 to 40 per cent of infections and is most likely to produce relapsing infection. Resistance to chloroquine is common with *P. falciparum* and also occurs in *P. vivax* from Irian Jaya and Papua New Guinea. *P. ovale* and *P. malariae* occur much less frequently and have remained uniformly sensitive to chloroquine.

PRESENTING SIGNS AND SYMPTOMS

The classic presentation of nonimmuine patients with malaria remains the "febrile paroxysm" of diaphoresis, high fever, chills, headache, myalgia, and malaise. Although patterns of fever may help to distinguish malaria from other febrile illnesses (*P. ovale* and *P. vivax* produce fever every other day, whereas *P. malariae* causes fever every third day), the pattern of fever must not be relied on for diagnosis. *P. falciparum*, the most dangerous species, typically produces hectic, irregular spiking fevers in nonimmune hosts. The nonspecific "flulike" symptoms may be mistaken for upper respiratory infection. Gastrointestinal symptoms (nausea, vomiting, and diarrhea), which are present in 30 to 50 per cent of patients (especially children), may be mistaken for gastroenteritis. All nonspecific febrile conditions in patients who have visited endemic zones in the past 3 years *must* be evaluated for possible malaria.

CLINICAL COURSE

Acute Malaria

All four species of malaria cause similar acute symptoms. *P. falciparum*, however, most commonly causes life-threatening illness because it has the greatest capacity to parasitize red blood cells of all ages. Acute falciparum malaria is a true medical emergency. Although residents of endemic regions acquire partial immunity that modifies the course of illness, nonimmune hosts with falciparum malaria often have a fulminant, fatal course. Infections with nonfalciparum species produce less severe illness and are rarely fatal, regardless of treatment.

Recurrent Malaria

P. vivax and *P. ovale* can form dormant hepatic hypnozoites that may cause latent infection. Patients may relapse after a primary attack or present with an apparent first attack up to 3 years later. Patients with *P. malariae* may have clinical recurrences up to 50 years after leaving an endemic area, but these are usually mild symptomatic recrudescences of chronic, persistent parasitemia rather than relapses.

The Chief, Navy Bureau of Medicine and Surgery, Washington, D.C., Clinical Investigation Program sponsored this report, No. 84-16-1968-519, as required by HSETCINST 6000.41A. The views expressed in this article are those of the authors and do not reflect the official policy or position of the Department of the Navy, Department of Defense, or the U. S. Government.

COMPLICATIONS

The clinician not only must diagnose malaria but also must recognize severe or complicated illness, which is defined as altered mental status (cerebral malaria); hematocrit less than 20 per cent; hypoglycemia; significant pulmonary, cardiac, or renal dysfunction; disseminated intravascular coagulation; prolonged pyrexia; severe gastrointestinal symptoms; or the presence of a coexisting bacterial sepsis (algid malaria). Severe or complicated malaria most often follows infection with *P. falciparum* and usually occurs with parasitemias in which more than 3 per cent of red blood cells are infected. Cerebral malaria (delirium or decreased mental status with *P. falciparum* infection) is the most feared complication, with a mortality rate of 50 per cent. Whenever possible, patients with complicated falciparum malaria should be treated in a critical care unit. The other malarial species rarely cause serious sequelae, but *P. vivax* can produce splenic rupture and *P. malariae* can produce an immune complex glomerulonephritis.

PHYSICAL EXAMINATION

The physical examination is not helpful in the diagnosis of malaria. Most patients have nonspecific fever, chills, diaphoresis, and tachycardia, but no focal findings. In endemic areas, chronic *P. falciparum* infection can lead to massive splenomegaly (tropical splenomegaly syndrome), but less than 10 per cent of nonimmune hosts presenting with acute malaria have a palpable spleen.

DIAGNOSTIC STUDIES

The diagnosis of malaria still requires the careful evaluation of Giemsa- or Wright's-stained blood films. Thin smears are easier to prepare and read, but thick smears are more sensitive for diagnosis of malaria because the blood volume examined is 10 to 40 times that of individual thin smears. The latter are required for species identification. Optimal smears are obtained with 3 per cent Giemsa stain (pH 7 to 7.2); lower pH impairs identification and species identification of malarial parasites. Many laboratories without extensive thick smear experience prefer to make multiple thin smears instead.

The primary goal of species identification on blood smears is to distinguish *P. falciparum* from *P. vivax* or *P. ovale*. The distinction is crucial, as falciparum malaria is typically a life-threatening infection that is refractory to chloroquine, whereas *P. vivax* and *P. ovale* are less dangerous and usually chloroquine-sensitive. The most useful morphologic clues to falciparum malaria are (1) small ring forms and banana-shaped gametocytes (gametocytes occur later in infection and may not be seen early in the course), (2) infected red cells of all sizes, and (3) multiple parasites per cell. *P. vivax* and *P. ovale* can be distinguished, as they (1) occur primarily in larger (younger) red cells, (2) may have Schüffner's dots, (3) may have multiple parasite life stages on the same slide, and (4) rarely have more than one parasite per cell. The degree of malarial parasitemia is reflected in the percentage of red blood cells infected. When more than 2 per cent of all red blood cells are infected, *P. falciparum* is the presumed infecting agent. When species identification is uncertain, the clinician should institute treatment for *P. falciparum*. Despite occasional "overtreatment" of *P. vivax* and *P. ovale,* this approach will avoid the much greater risk of undertreated falciparum malaria.

Quantitative Buffy Coat Tube

The quantitative buffy coat (QBC) method uses acridine orange fluorescent staining of malarial parasites following centrifugation of microhematocrit tubes. Although simpler and faster than thick smears, the QBC evaluation does require experience and training in fluorescence microscopy. QBC can detect very low-grade parasitemias, and in experienced hands it may be more sensitive than thick films. The QBC is not, however, reliable for species identification or quantitation of parasite burden, so it must be used in conjunction with thin films. For clinicians who have access to laboratories with the specialized tubes (Becton-Dickinson, Sparks, MD), centifuges, microscopes, and experience, QBC is an excellent rapid diagnostic technique.

Dipstick Antigen Capture Assay

The dipstick method is an antigen capture assay based on the qualitative detection of *P. falciparum* histidine-rich protein (HRP). This assay is simple to perform and specific for *P. falciparum*. Sensitivity ranges from 70 to 99 per cent (depending on parasite load), and specificity approaches 90 per cent. Thus, antigen capture is not as sensitive or specific as blood smears or QBC and does not quantitate parasitemia. Antigen capture (ParaSight F, Becton-Dickinson Tropical Disease Diagnostics, Sparks, MD) is not yet licensed in the United States but is available in Europe and the developing world. A similiar test for detection of *P. vivax* is under development.

DNA Probes and Polymerase Chain Reaction

DNA-based methods for the detection of malaria are being tested in various research centers. Although these techniques are sensitive (at least equal to thick smears), they are unlikely to reach widespread use in the near future because of economic and technical problems associated with performing individual tests in less specialized laboratories.

THERAPEUTIC TRIALS

In the developing world, empirical antimalarial treatment is common for the patient with some immunity with no obvious localizing cause of fever. This frequently results in overdiagnosis of malaria and underdiagnosis of other conditions. However, empirical treatment of the acutely febrile nonimmune patient whose exposure history is compatible with malaria should not be withheld when proper diagnostic facilities are not available. Blood samples should be obtained for later analysis, and the patient should also receive a broad-spectrum antimicrobial agent (such as ceftriaxone) to cover rapidly fatal conditions such as meningococcal or pneumococcal sepsis.

DIAGNOSTIC PITFALLS

Most cases of malaria are "missed" because the clinician fails to obtain a travel history with complete itineraries. All febrile patients who have visited endemic regions in the past 2 to 3 years must be evaluated for malaria promptly. Even patients who have made a brief airport stop in endemic areas without deplaning have been infected.

Nonimmune hosts can be severely ill before parasites are detectable on smears or QBC. Negative smears should be repeated every 8 to 12 hours until another diagnosis is established or the patient's febrile illness resolves.

False-positive diagnoses of malaria are common, and they usually occur when inexperienced observers mistake platelets on smears for malarial parasites.

Although antibody assays for the malarial species are available, they are of limited clinical value and should not be used for the evaluation of acute malaria. The development of positive antibody titers requires weeks, whereas decisions on malaria treatment must be made in hours. Antibody assays may, on occasion, aid the evaluation of chronic or recurrent fevers that defy diagnosis by standard methods. There is no specifically useful diagnostic imaging technique for malaria, but a baseline chest film helps to exclude other causes of fever.

AMEBIASIS

By Faisal Sultan, M.B., B.S.,
and Samuel L. Stanley, Jr., M.D.
St. Louis, Missouri

Amebiasis, caused by the protozoan parasite *Entamoeba histolytica*, remains a global health concern and is probably responsible for more than 50 million cases of diarrhea and 40,000 to 100,000 deaths annually. *Entamoeba histolytica* exists in one of two stages—trophozoite or cyst. Trophozoites are motile and can invade colonic mucosa. By contrast, cysts are nonmotile, can survive outside the human host, and are resistant to gastric acid. Cysts are the infectious form of the parasite. In the past, as many as 90 per cent of the individuals thought to be infected with *E. histolytica* (estimated at 500 million individuals worldwide) were asymptomatic. Today, the organism previously called *E. histolytica* has been divided into two morphologically identical but genetically distinct species—*E. histolytica* and *E. dispar*. *Entamoeba histolytica* is the causative agent of amebic dysentery and amebic liver abscess (ALA), whereas *E. dispar* appears to be commensal, colonizing the large intestine without causing disease. *Entamoeba dispar* is probably responsible for the vast majority of asymptomatic infections. Unfortunately, the most widely used technique to diagnose intestinal disease, microscopic examination of the stool for the presence of *E. histolytica* trophozoites or cysts, cannot distinguish *E. histolytica* from *E. dispar*.

CLINICAL PRESENTATION

Intestinal Amebiasis

Asymptomatic Infection (Cyst Passers)

As noted, most asymptomatic patients are probably colonized with *E. dispar*, but a few may have *E. histolytica* infection. By definition, these patients are asymptomatic, and cysts may be observed in their stools during the evaluation of another condition. Most of these individuals clear the cysts from their stools in 3 to 6 months. When trophozoites are seen, they do not exhibit erythrophagocytosis.

Amebic Colitis (Amebic Dysentery)

Colitis is the most common form of symptomatic amebiasis. The illness is subacute, typically lasting less than a month. Patients classically present with multiple small volume bloody stools; some patients have abdominal pain, and nearly one third have fever. Even when the stool is not visibly bloody, it is invariably positive for occult blood, reflecting the invasion of the colonic mucosa by *E. histolytica* trophozoites. The differential diagnosis includes dysentery caused by shigellae or other invasive bacteria, pseudomembranous colitis, and inflammatory bowel disease.

Nondysenteric Amebic Colitis

In the relatively unusual syndrome of nondysenteric amebic colitis, patients typically have a chronic diarrheal illness complicated by abdominal pain and weight loss. This condition should not be confused with inflammatory bowel disease.

Fulminant Amebic Colitis

In fulminant amebic colitis, a more severe and rapidly progressive form of dysenteric amebic colitis, individuals present with bloody diarrhea, diffuse abdominal pain, and fever. As many as 75 per cent of patients may progress to perforation of the colon, with resultant peritonitis and high mortality. Liver abscess can be present concurrently. The risk of fulminant amebic colitis is higher in children, pregnant women, and patients receiving corticosteroids.

Toxic Megacolon

Toxic megacolon is a rare complication that is associated with corticosteroid administration and has a high mortality rate despite treatment.

Ameboma

Localized infection in the cecum or ascending colon may produce a concentric granulomatous lesion that is palpable as a firm mass. Ameboma may cause intestinal obstruction and must be distinguished from cancer of the colon.

Extraintestinal Amebiasis

Amebic Liver Abscess

In 10 per cent of patients with intestinal disease, amebae travel through the portal circulation to the liver, producing the most common extraintestinal manifestation of amebiasis—ALA. Individuals with ALA generally present with fever and dull or pleuritic right upper quadrant pain, which may be referred to the right shoulder. In half of the patients, hepatomegaly and point tenderness of the liver are prominent on physical examination. Individuals may present with fever alone. Thus, the diagnosis of ALA should be entertained in any patient with fever of unknown origin who resides in, or has traveled to, an area endemic for amebiasis. Concurrent diarrhea occurs in only one third of the patients.

Complications of ALA include rupture into the pleural space or lung parenchyma. This occurs in as many as 10 to 20 per cent of individuals with ALA. In some cases, this causes a bronchopleural fistula leading to the expectoration of profuse amounts of the odorless, brown, "anchovy paste" contents of the ALA. Rupture into the peritoneal space (2 to 7 per cent of cases) and pericardial sac (rare, often from left lobe abscesses) are also known to occur.

Other Extraintestinal Sites of Amebiasis

Amebic brain abscess occurs rarely but has a high mortality rate. Patients with genitourinary amebiasis, including perinephric abscesses, infected renal cysts, rectovaginal fistulas, cervical ulcers, uterine involvement, and vaginal lesions, have also been described but have not been present in large series of amebic disease. Skin lesions, especially in the perianal region, have also been reported.

DIAGNOSTIC STUDIES

Leukocytosis greater than 10,000 cells/mm^3 is present in three fourths of patients with ALA. Eosinophilia is unusual, but almost all patients have an increased erythrocyte sedimentation rate. About 50 per cent of patients with ALA have slight increases in aminotransferase levels, which usually resolve within weeks of therapy. Alkaline phosphatase is increased in 75 per cent of individuals with ALA and may remain abnormal for months after successful treatment. In some patients with ALA, abnormal chest films invariably involve the right lung field, with elevation of the right hemidiaphragm, subsegmental and lobar atelectasis, and pleural effusion.

Microscopic Examination of Specimens

The diagnosis of intestinal amebiasis still requires demonstration of organisms in the stool or in colonic samples obtained by sigmoidoscopy or colonoscopy. Examination of three separate stool samples will detect 75 to 90 per cent of cases of intestinal amebiasis. Direct examination of fresh stool requires rapid transport (<30 minutes) to the laboratory. Prior use of radiographic contrast material, laxatives, antibiotics, or antidiarrheal compounds can interfere with the visualizaton of the organism and should be avoided. The stool sample should be resuspended in a drop of saline and examined under low light. Trophozoites range in size from 12 to 60 μm, display linear motility, and have a clear ectoplasm. The presence of ingested red blood cells in trophozoites indicates invasive disease. Cysts are 10 to 20 μm in diameter, have one to four nuclei, and are nonmotile. Chromatid bodies appear as elongated, blunt-ended structures. Addition of iodine to the sample enhances morphologic detail in trophozoites and cysts and can facilitate diagnosis. The concentration of specimens by formalin–ethyl acetate sedimentation or zinc sulfate flotation probably increases the diagnostic yield.

The use of preservatives allows a second examination of the same sample and examination of the sample after long intervals. Commonly used fixatives include polyvinyl alcohol and Schaudinn's fixative. Merthiolate iodine formalin and formalin (5 or 10 per cent) may also be used. Sodium acetate–acetic acid–formalin (SAF) combines fixation and staining of specimens in a single step. Staining is commonly used; it allows discrimination of *E. histolytica* from other intestinal protozoa by demonstrating finer details of the trophozoite or cyst structure. The laboratory can stain both fresh and fixed specimens, but the latter provide higher diagnostic yield. The two most widely used stains are trichrome (showing pink nuclei) and iron-hematoxylin (showing dark blue organisms). Biopsy specimens may be stained with periodic acid–Schiff (PAS).

Unfortunately, microscopy cannot distinguish *E. histolytica* from the morphologically identical, but apparently nonpathogenic, *E. dispar*. Thus, in asymptomatic individuals, or in patients whose symptoms are not consistent with invasive amebiasis, caution is required when stool microscopy reveals *E. histolytica* cysts or trophozoites. Serologic findings can be helpful in this situation.

Serologic Findings

Amebic serologic findings are crucial in the diagnosis of ALA and can be used to confirm amebic intestinal disease. The widely used indirect hemagglutination assay (IHA) is positive in almost all patients with ALA (the rare false-negative results are found almost exclusively in patients tested within the first week of infection) and in up to 80 per cent of patients with invasive colonic disease. IHA results are typically negative in asymptomatic cyst passers (presumably infected with *E. dispar*) and may be valuable in interpreting microscopic results. The IHA remains positive for years and thus may be difficult to interpret when there is a history of prior amebic infection. Other serologic methods employed include gel precipitins, counterimmunoelectrophoresis (CIE), and indirect immunofluorescence (IFA). Following resolution of acute illness, the counterimmunoelectrophoresis and indirect immunofluorescence assays may return to normal sooner than the IHA and thus may have marginally greater utility in patients with a history of prior amebiasis. Enzyme-linked immunosorbent assays (ELISAs) to detect antiamebic antibodies have also been designed, and most have reasonably good specificity and sensitivity.

Several enzyme-linked immunosorbent assays that detect amebic antigen are being developed to replace stool microscopy for the diagnosis of intestinal amebiasis. Some of these tests use monoclonal antibodies that can distinguish between antigens of *E. histolytica* and *E. dispar*. If these tests are confirmed to be sensitive and specific in widespread trials, they could replace microscopy as the standard technique for the diagnosis of intestinal amebiasis and would resolve the problem of distinguishing between *E. histolytica* and *E. dispar* infection.

DNA-Based Diagnostic Methods

Although several protocols that use DNA hybridization and polymerase chain reaction (PCR) to detect amebic DNA sequences in stool have been reported, these are research tools that may one day be clinically useful in distinguishing *E. histolytica* from *E. dispar*.

Imaging

Imaging should be performed in all suspected cases of ALA. Sonography is a reasonable and inexpensive first step. Classically, ALA appears as a single, large, round or oval-shaped, hypoechoic lesion in the right lobe of the liver; however, multiple abscesses are not unusual, and 5 to 10 per cent of patients will have abscesses in the left lobe of the liver. Abdominal computed tomography (CT) and magnetic resonance imaging (MRI) are sensitive but more expensive alternatives for visualizing ALA. When space-occupying lesions consistent with ALA are seen, the usual differential diagnosis includes bacterial (pyogenic) liver abscess, hydatid cyst, or tumor. Amebic serologic findings are required to establish or exclude the diagnosis of ALA.

Other Diagnostic Procedures

Sigmoidoscopy and/or colonoscopy may be useful in patients with suspected amebic colitis when stool examinations are initially negative. Gross examination may show punctate hemorrhage and/or discrete shallow ulcers covered with a yellowish white exudate. Amebae are most often detected at the border of the ulcers; therefore, the leading edge of the ulcer should be included in any biopsy specimen or scrapings. The intervening colon may be normal, or in severe cases a diffuse colitis may be present.

Pseudomembranes have been reported occasionally. A saline wet mount of fresh colonic material should be prepared and immediately examined microscopically for motile trophozoites. Additional material should be fixed and stained. Suspicious areas should be biopsied.

Aspiration of an ALA is usually not required for cure. As a diagnostic procedure, aspiration should be carried out only when rapid amebic serologic testing is not available, pyogenic abscess is a major concern, and the condition of the patient warrants an immediate diagnosis. Other indications for aspiration of suspected or proven ALA include failure of medical therapy and possibly left-sided ALAs (because of risk of rupture into the pericardium). The aspirate is typically sterile, odorless, and brown, and amebae are rarely seen. Open drainage of ALA is almost never needed because computed tomography and ultrasound are now available to guide needle aspiration.

PITFALLS IN DIAGNOSIS

E. histolytica may be confused with other intestinal protozoa on microscopic examination and, in some cases, false-positive microscopic results can occur when white blood cells in the stool are mistakenly identified as *E. histolytica* trophozoites. Referral of samples to an experienced reference laboratory may be warranted.

Barium enema is generally not useful, as there is no specific finding consistent with amebic colitis, and the preparative regimen, as well as the barium, will interfere with the examination of the stool for parasites.

PNEUMOCYSTIS INFECTION

By Ian Frank, M.D.
Philadelphia, Pennsylvania

The report of an outbreak of pneumonia in homosexual men in 1981 established *Pneumocystis carinii* as the first opportunistic infection reported in association with what is now known as acquired immunodeficiency syndrome (AIDS). Today, *Pneumocystis* infection ranks among the most common causes of community-acquired pneumonia. However, individuals with other causes of defects in cellular immunity are also at increased risk for acquiring *Pneumocystis* pneumonia. Such individuals include premature or debilitated infants; children with primary immunodeficiency diseases, particularly severe combined immunodeficiency; individuals with protein malnutrition; patients with lymphoreticular malignancies; and those receiving corticosteriods and other immunosuppressive medications for cancer chemotherapy or organ transplantation.

AIDS has replaced all other conditions as the most common predisposing cause of *Pneumocystis* infection. In the absence of chemoprophylaxis, more than 80 per cent of AIDS patients will experience *Pneumocystis* infection during their lifetimes. The degree of immunologic impairment is important in estimating the likelihood of a human immunodeficiency virus (HIV)–infected individual acquiring *Pneumocystis* pneumonia. In adults, initial episodes of *Pneumocystis* pneumonia are most commonly seen in persons with CD4+ lymphocyte counts between 50 and 75 cells/mm^3, and it is uncommon in individuals with CD4+ lymphocyte counts greater than 200 cells/mm^3 or a CD4+ lymphocyte percentage greater than 20 per cent of the absolute lymphocyte count. However, HIV-infected infants with normal CD4+ lymphocyte counts may experience *Pneumocystis* infection. Therefore, an expeditious diagnosis of *Pneumocystis* pneumonia requires obtaining a careful history to elicit risks for HIV infection, as well as a strong index of suspicion in other individuals with impaired cellular immunity.

CLINICAL MANIFESTATIONS

In AIDS patients, *Pneumocystis* pneumonia frequently has an insidious onset, and patients may have symptoms for weeks prior to the establishment of the diagnosis. The most commonly reported symptoms include fever, nonproductive cough, shortness of breath, and retrosternal chest tightness that is worse with inspiration or cough. On occasion, the cough produces mucoid sputum or, rarely, hemoptysis. Other immunocompromised patients may be symptomatic for 1 to 2 weeks before they seek medical attention. Individuals receiving chronic corticosteroid treatment are more likely to become symptomatic after the steroids are tapered. Children may present with poor feeding, and they progress to have fever, cough, respiratory distress, and cyanosis. Physical findings are not helpful in establishing the diagnosis. Symptomatic patients may have tachypnea or tachycardia. Rales are present in one third of patients. Findings of consolidation are unusual.

The natural history of untreated *Pneumocystis* pneumonia in immunocompromised patients is progressive respiratory insufficiency and death. Early diagnosis is associated with more favorable outcomes. Prognosis is related to the alveolar-arterial (A-a) oxygen gradient at presentation, the extent of infiltrates on the chest radiograph, neutrophilia in a bronchoalveolar lavage (BAL) specimen, increased serum lactate dehydrogenase (LD), and an increase in general markers of disease severity, such as the Acute Physiology and Chronic Health Evaluation (APACHE) II score. Spontaneous pneumothorax related to thin-walled cavitary lung disease occurs in as many as 10 per cent of patients and is the most common complication of *Pneumocystis* pneumonia. Bronchopleural fistulas may be refractory to closure short of chemical pleurodesis. Spontaneous pneumothorax may be the presenting manifestation in some patients; therefore, all HIV patients with spontaneous pneumothorax should be evaluated for *Pneumocystis* infection. In addition, the use of aerosolized pentamidine for prophylaxis is a major risk factor for pneumothorax.

In AIDS patients, extrapulmonary pneumocystosis has become recognized more frequently. Reports initially described isolated patients with visceral infection. Now as many as one half of patients with extrapulmonary pneumocystosis have concurrent pneumonia, and extrapulmonary disease can be a complication of pneumonia in 0.5 to 3 per cent of these patients. Infection of lymph nodes, spleen, liver, bone marrow, gastrointestinal tract, eyes, thyroid gland, adrenal gland, and kidneys is described most often, but mastoiditis, cutaneous lesions, vasculitis, brain abscess, and myopericarditis have also been reported. The clinical presentation of extrapulmonary pneumocystosis includes fever and signs and symptoms referable to the organ involved. Pancytopenia is the most common manifestation of bone marrow involvement. Disease in the liver, spleen, or adrenal gland appears as multiple hypodense lesions on computed tomography (CT) or magnetic resonance imaging

(MRI). Thyroid disease may present as hyperthyroidism or hypothyroidism. Ocular disease typically is manifested as choroiditis with characteristic elevated plaques limited to the choroid without vascular involvement or intraocular inflammation. Extrapulmonary pneumocystosis is more commonly seen in individuals receiving prophylaxis with aerosolized pentamidine, compared with agents taken orally, because aerosolized pentamidine is not absorbed systemically to any significant extent. The prognosis following treatment of isolated extrapulmonary disease is good. However, the few individuals who have presented with widely disseminated pneumocystosis have followed rapidly fatal courses.

USEFUL LABORATORY TESTS

Although nonspecific, hypoxemia is the most common laboratory abnormality that indirectly supports the diagnosis of *Pneumocystis* pneumonia. All patients suspected of having *Pneumocystis* infection should be evaluated for hypoxemia. More than 80 per cent of persons with *Pneumocystis* pneumonia have a room air Pa_{O_2} concentration less than 80 mm Hg or an A-a oxygen gradient greater than 15 mm Hg. These determinations serve as prognostic indicators, with higher mortality expected in individuals who present with a room air Pa_{O_2} concentration less than 70 mm Hg or an A-a oxygen gradient greater than 35 mm Hg. In 5 to 20 per cent of patients, however, room air arterial blood gas concentrations may be normal. In this situation, clinicians can use pulse oximetry before and after exercise to detect widening of the A-a oxygen gradient. This maneuver demonstrates oxygen desaturation in almost all *Pneumocystis* pneumonia patients with normal blood gas determinations; pulse oximetry is also rapid and inexpensive and can be performed in the office. Another pulmonary function test that is abnormal in nearly all patients with *Pneumocystis* pneumonia is the carbon monoxide diffusing capacity, which is typically less than 70 per cent of the predicted value. This test is helpful in AIDS patients with asthma because it can distinguish hypoxemia secondary to bronchospasm.

Hematologic and chemical analyses provide supportive evidence of *Pneumocystis* infection. As stated earlier, *Pneumocystis* pneumonia is rare in AIDS patients with absolute CD4+ lymphocyte counts greater than 200 cells/mm^3 or percentages greater than 20 per cent. LD is increased in 90 per cent of hospitalized patients with *Pneumocystis* pneumonia; patients whose LD values exceed 500 IU/L are more likely to die.

USEFUL RADIOLOGIC TESTS

The chest radiograph of patients with *Pneumocystis* infection classically exhibits diffuse, bilateral interstitial infiltrates that extend from the perihilar region and spare the apices (Fig. 1). More extensive disease can have an alveolar pattern. In 5 to 20 per cent of patients, chest films are normal, whereas in 10 to 30 per cent of patients, atypical patterns can be seen. These patterns include unilateral or asymmetric disease, single or multiple nodules, cysts or cavities, pneumatoceles, pneumothorax, hilar adenopathy, postobstructive infiltrates secondary to endobronchial nodules, and effusion. Patients receiving prophylaxis with aerosolized pentamidine may present with apical infiltrates due to preferential deposition of the aerosol in the lower lung fields.

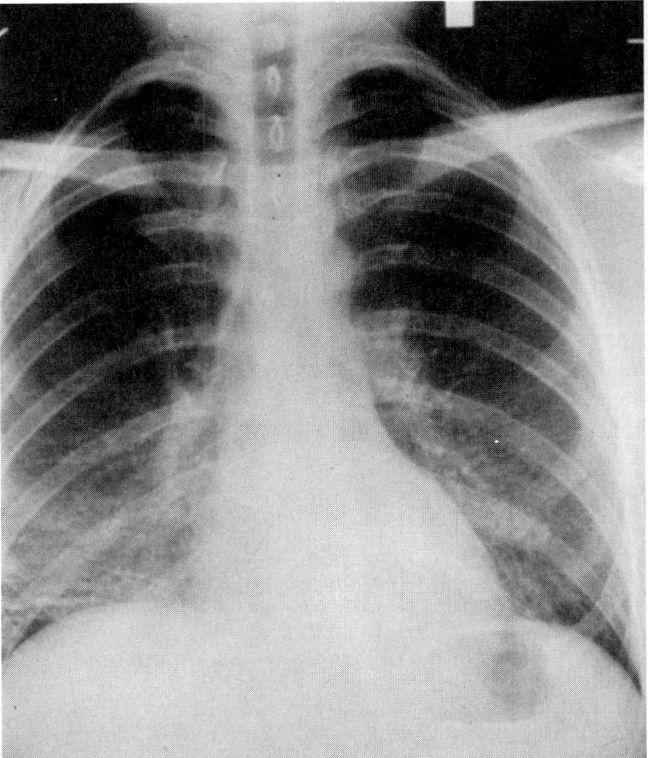

Figure 1. Chest radiograph of a patient with *Pneumocystis* pneumonia demonstrating diffuse bilateral interstitial infiltrates.

In patients with normal chest radiographs, CT of the chest can detect fine diffuse alveolar consolidation. CT can also detect low-density lesions or calcifications due to *Pneumocystis* infection in lymph nodes, liver, spleen, or kidney when extrapulmonary disease is suspected. Nuclear imaging techniques can also enhance the detection of *Pneumocystis* infection in the lungs in the setting of an unremarkable chest film. Increased uptake of gallium-67 citrate or indium-111 human IgG or clearance of technetium-99m diethylenetriaminepentaacetate are consistent with *Pneumocystis* infection. However, these tests are expensive, and they lack specificity. Moreover, they do not enhance the sensitivity of testing for oxygen desaturation following exercise in patients with normal chest films. Their use should therefore be restricted to the rare patient with chronic lung disease who may have baseline abnormalities in blood gas concentrations and chest films and whose worsening respiratory symptoms make *Pneumocystis* pneumonia a concern.

DIAGNOSTIC PROCEDURES

A definitive diagnosis should be attempted in anyone with hypoxemia or an abnormal chest film and a clinical presentation consistent with *Pneumocystis* pneumonia. Definitive diagnosis of *Pneumocystis* pneumonia requires visualization of the organism in pulmonary secretions or biopsy material. As many as 20 per cent of persons with clinical, laboratory, and radiographic evidence of *Pneumocystis* infection will have another diagnosis. In addition, patients treated empirically may have a worse outcome than those in whom a definitive diagnosis is made. Therefore, empirical treatment for *Pneumocystis* pneumonia is not recommended, except in persons whose confirmed diagnosis was followed by incomplete treatment of their acute illness or persons who fail to comply with prophylaxis after completion of a course of treatment.

Pneumocystis is rarely found in expectorated sputum without induction. A sputum sample induced with nebulized hypertonic saline is adequate to diagnose *Pneumocystis* pneumonia in 15 to 90 per cent of patients. The procedure requires the cooperation of the patient and an experienced staff to increase the diagnostic yield. Patients should brush their teeth and gargle with 3 per cent saline to decrease contamination with oral organisms and debris. Breathing normally with occasional deep breaths, patients then inhale 3 per cent saline from an ultrasonic nebulizer. Forty-five minutes may be required to obtain an adequate sample.

When induced sputum cannot be produced, or when sputum yields a negative result, fiberoptic bronchoscopy should be performed. Specimens obtained by BAL have a diagnostic yield of 86 to 97 per cent. BAL is more sensitive than bronchial washing and brushing, and sensitivity can be enhanced if lavage of both lungs is performed. Transbronchial biopsy, which has a sensitivity similar to BAL, may detect some infections that are missed by BAL. When BAL and biopsy are combined, sensitivity approaches 100 per cent in some centers. Others, however, have not been able to demonstrate an increased diagnostic yield when transbronchial biopsy is performed. Citing the increased risk of hemoptysis or pneumothorax, these groups prefer to perform BAL alone. When a diagnosis is not made, a second bronchoscopy with BAL and biopsy is then performed. Used alone, BAL is probably not sufficient to diagnose *Pneumocystis* pneumonia in patients receiving aerosolized pentamidine for prophylaxis. In this setting, BAL should always be combined with transbronchial biopsy. Thoracoscopic or open lung biopsy is rarely needed to make the diagnosis of *Pneumocystis* pneumonia in AIDS patients but should be reserved for patients in whom bronchoscopy has been unrevealing. Lung biopsy can be helpful if pulmonary Kaposi's sarcoma is suspected in addition to *Pneumocystis* pneumonia.

BAL following a course of treatment often reveals persistent *Pneumocystis* organisms in the collected specimen. Semiquantitative estimates of microbe burden can be made; failure to reduce the number of *Pneumocystis* organisms by 50 per cent following a completed course of therapy suggests persistent disease or increased risk of recurrence. However, patients who have a clinical response to anti-*Pneumocystis* therapy should not undergo BAL to assess their response cytologically.

Various stains are used to identify *Pneumocystis* in sputum, bronchoalveolar secretions, or biopsy material. To enhance detection, stains that label the cyst wall should be combined with those that identify trophozoites. In 30 minutes, the Wright-Giemsa or Diff-Quik stain can detect nuclei of cysts and intermediate forms of *Pneumocystis* (Fig. 2). The sensitivity of these stains is 85 to 90 per cent. The Papanicolau stain highlights nonspecific, foamy, eosinophilic material that surrounds clumps of organisms. Gomori's methenamine silver and toluidine blue O stain cyst walls with a sensitivity exceeding 95 per cent. Calcofluor white, a chemifluorescent brightening agent that binds to beta-linked polysaccharides of fungi and *Pneumocystis*, has a reported sensitivity approaching 100 per cent. Immunofluorescent staining with monoclonal antibodies (now commercially available) can also enhance detection of organisms in induced sputum as well as BAL fluid.

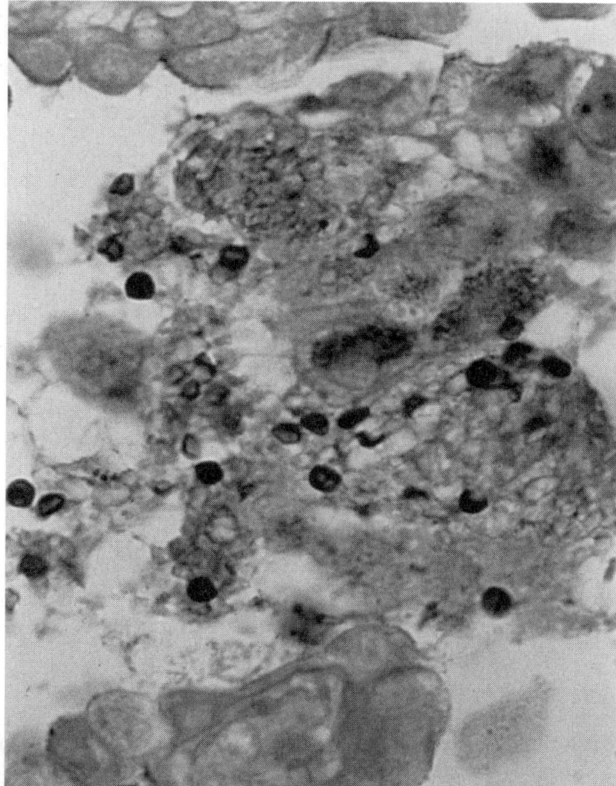

Figure 2. Lung biopsy specimen demonstrating trophozoites of *Pneumocystis carinii* together with the characteristic frothy exudate filling the alveolar space. (H & E stain, ×1000.)

Immunohistochemical methods may detect *Pneumocystis* in tissue specimens.

DNA amplification by the polymerase chain reaction (PCR) may also aid the diagnosis of *Pneumocystis* pneumonia. However, PCR may generate too many false-positive results. Thus, clinical correlates remain to be established so that positive results do not detect subclinical infection that may not require treatment. PCR may also identify *Pneumocystis* DNA in blood, suggesting disseminated disease.

THERAPY AS A CLUE TO DIAGNOSIS

Early diagnosis of *Pneumocystis* pneumonia is correlated with improved survival. Furthermore, survival is higher in centers that have more experience in caring for patients with HIV. As stated earlier, empirical therapy of *Pneumocystis* pneumonia should be avoided. However, when diagnostic studies such as induced sputum analysis and bronchoscopy are not readily available, there may be few options other than empirical treatment. By contrast, empirical treatment can and often should be started while diagnostic evaluation is under way. The ability to make a definitive diagnosis from induced sputum or bronchoscopy is not altered during the first days of therapy.

Pneumocystis pneumonia can be classified by severity of illness based on the patient's A-a oxygen gradient at presentation. Gradients less than 35 mm Hg are associated with mild disease; gradients between 35 and 45 mm Hg are associated with moderate disease, and gradients exceeding 45 mm Hg indicate severe disease. Patients may deteriorate clinically with decreased oxygenation and increased markings on chest film during the first 7 days of treatment. Therefore, when no improvement is observed after 1 week of therapy, patients lacking a definitive diagnosis of *Pneumocystis* pneumonia should undergo bronchoscopy. In patients with an established diagnosis of *Pneumocystis* pneumonia, a second copathogen should be sought.

Patients who have had *Pneumocystis* pneumonia as well as those with CD4+ lymphocyte counts less than 200 cells/mm^3 or a CD4+ lymphocyte percentage less than 20 per cent should receive lifelong chemoprophylaxis. *Pneumocystis* is uncommon in patients who are taking trimethoprim-sulfamethoxazole (TMP-SMX) appropriately, and alternative diagnoses should be preferentially considered in these patients who present with an illness consistent with *Pneumocystis* pneumonia. *Pneumocystis* pneumonia frequently presents atypically in persons receiving prophylaxis. In these patients, the time course of illness is often protracted, and fever rather than cough may be the predominant symptom. Atypical presentations on the chest radiograph are more frequent in patients receiving prophylaxis; apical disease is often seen in patients receiving aerosolized pentamidine. Extrapulmonary pneumocystosis is rare in patients receiving systemic prophylaxis.

AVOIDING ERRORS IN DIAGNOSIS

The most important factor in establishing the diagnosis of *Pneumocystis* pneumonia is to consider it in the differential diagnosis. As the HIV epidemic widens, more patients will present without a known or admitted risk of infection. *Pneumocystis* pneumonia should always be considered in the differential diagnosis of bilateral interstitial pneumonia. *Pneumocystis* pneumonia should be considered in the differential diagnosis of fever of unknown origin in the AIDS patient with a normal chest radiograph and no hypoxemia. This disease is not restricted to patients with HIV infection; all patients with cellular immune defects are at risk for infection with *Pneumocystis*. Importantly, patients with immune defects may have more than one disorder causing their symptoms. Therefore, *Pneumocystis* infection should be sought in patients with a compatible illness who are not responding to treatment for another established diagnosis. Finally, because increased mortality and toxicity are associated with empirical therapy, definitive diagnosis of *Pneumocystis* pneumonia should always be the goal.

TOXOPLASMOSIS

By Gregory A. Filice, M.D.
Minneapolis, Minnesota

The term toxoplasmosis refers to infection with the apicomplexan protozoan parasite *Toxoplasma gondii*. Although *T. gondii* infects mammals, birds, reptiles, and nearly one third of humans worldwide, most infections are of little consequence. During an initial proliferative phase, tachyzoites enter various cells, replicate, burst the cells, and then enter other cells. In most animals, this phase is followed by encystation, especially within muscle and nervous tissue. Cysts containing thousands of bradyzoites remain viable in tissues for years, probably for the life of the animal. In felines, *T. gondii* has a sexual, enteroepithelial cycle in the gastrointestinal tract that results in excretion of persistent, highly infectious oocysts.

Humans become infected by ingesting oocysts or tissue cysts. Oocysts are ingested from hands or fomites or in food that has come into contact with cat feces. Tissue cysts in meat are infectious for humans when the meat has not been adequately cooked. The four major clinical presentations of toxoplasmosis in humans are new infection in immunocompetent persons, progressive infection in immunocompromised persons, congenital infection, and isolated chorioretinitis.

CLINCAL SIGNS AND SYMPTOMS

New Infection in Immunocompetent Persons

Ninety per cent of people infected with *T. gondii* have no signs or symptoms. Most of the rest have symptomatic lymph node enlargement at a single site, most commonly in the cervical, suboccipital, supraclavicular, axillary, or inguinal regions. Some patients have fever, headache, or fatigue. Node enlargement may wax and wane over a period of weeks to months. *Toxoplasma gondii* causes approximately 5 per cent of cases of lymphadenopathy in the United States.

A few immunocompetent people with newly acquired infection have fever, fatigue, malaise, myalgias, sweats, rash, sore throat, hepatomegaly, or splenomegaly. Rarely, myocarditis, pericarditis, pneumonitis, or encephalitis occurs. The signs and symptoms usually resolve within weeks to months, rarely more than 12 months. Death is exceedingly rare in postnatal immunocompetent persons. Chorioretinitis occurs rarely after infection of immunocompetent persons, usually in only one eye.

The differential diagnosis of toxoplasmosis includes lymphoma, infectious mononucleosis with Epstein-Barr virus or cytomegalovirus (CMV), cat-scratch disease, sarcoidosis, tuberculosis, tularemia, or metastatic cancer. Fewer than 1 per cent of patients with infectious mononucleosis–like syndrome in the United States have *Toxoplasma* infection. Most episodes of toxoplasmosis in nonpregnant immunocompetent people are not severe enough to warrant treatment with currently available drugs.

Toxoplasmosis in Immunocompromised Persons

Toxoplasmosis in immunocompromised persons occurs primarily in people with acquired immunodeficiency syndrome (AIDS). Toxoplasmosis in adults with AIDS is typically due to reactivation of dormant infection. The incidence varies with the prevalence of latent infection in the population, which in turn varies regionally and reflects culinary habits, climate, and human contact with felines. The incidence of disease also varies with the prevalence of prophylaxis for *Pneumocystis* infection with co-trimoxazole or other compounds that may also provide prophylaxis against toxoplasmosis. Toxoplasmic encephalitis (TE) is the most common cause of focal central nervous system (CNS) lesions in persons with AIDS.

The brain is the most commonly involved organ during active toxoplasmosis in AIDS patients. Lesions are most common in the cortex but may be present anywhere in the CNS. Disease usually begins with the subacute onset of focal neurologic signs, but onset may be abrupt, with focal changes or diffuse cerebral dysfunction. Delirium, obtundation, coma, seizures, cranial nerve abnormalities, focal sensory abnormalities, movement disorders, psychiatric disturbances, and ataxia have been reported. The most common focal motor findings are dysphasia and unilateral weakness. Spinal lesions present with bowel or bladder dysfunction, or motor or sensory dysfunction of the limbs. Uncommon CNS manifestations include panhypopituitarism, diabetes insipidus, and the syndrome of inappropriate antidiuretic hormone secretion.

Pneumonia is the second most common manifestation of toxoplasmosis in persons with AIDS. It usually begins insidiously with dyspnea, cough, and fever, and the most common initial impression is that the patient has *Pneumocystis* pneumonia. One half of patients with pulmonary toxoplasmosis develop extrapulmonary disease either concurrently or later.

Chorioretinitis occurs uncommonly in persons with AIDS and is usually associated with active toxoplasmosis elsewhere in the CNS. The symptoms typically include eye pain and loss of visual acuity. Other uncommon manifestations of toxoplasmosis in persons with AIDS include orchitis, peritonitis, hepatitis, gastritis, pancreatitis, colitis, acute respiratory distress syndrome, and shock.

Toxoplasmosis also occurs in persons with depressed cell-mediated immunity from conditions other than AIDS. Three quarters of these patients have CNS disease, but it presents as a diffuse encephalitis more commonly than in persons with AIDS. Forty per cent of patients have myocardial disease, and 25 per cent have pneumonia.

In bone marrow transplant patients, toxoplasmosis usually follows reactivation of dormant infection in the recipient after transplantation of marrow from an uninfected and thus immunologically naive donor. In heart transplant patients, disease usually occurs after transplantation of a heart from an infected donor into a naive recipient. Asymptomatic increases in IgG and IgM antibody titers frequently occur in dormantly infected heart transplant recipients regardless of the infection status of the donor, presumably as the result of subclinical reactivation from immunosuppressive therapy. Toxoplasma can be transmitted in a transplanted organ or in blood products from an infected individual.

Ocular Toxoplasmosis

In immunocompetent people, almost all chorioretinitis is due to congenital infection. Ocular toxoplasmosis is most commonly diagnosed in the second or third decade of life, but patients typically have old, healed lesions when they first present. Lesions are usually found in both eyes. Congenitally acquired chorioretinitis is rarely detected after the 40th year. Acquired toxoplasmosis rarely results in chorioretinitis and is then usually confined to one eye.

The typical lesion is a focal area of retinitis. Occasionally, panuveitis is present. Involvement of the optic nerve usually reflects CNS disease. The symptoms may include blurred vision, scotomata, pain, photophobia, or epiphora. As the lesion heals, vision that has been lost may be partially or completely restored. Damage to the macula typically causes permanent impairment of central vision.

The differential diagnosis includes posterior uveitis of tuberculosis, syphilis, leprosy, or presumed ocular histoplasmosis syndrome. Cytomegalovirus retinitis occurs commonly in immunosuppressed persons and may even coexist with toxoplasmic chorioretinitis.

Congenital Toxoplasmosis

Congenital infection is nearly always the result of primary infection of a woman during pregnancy. The risk of congenital infection is minimal when a woman is infected during the 8 weeks prior to conception. The major obstacle to diagnosis is the absence, or minimal and nonspecific nature, of symptoms. Congenital transmission can also occur when immunocompromised women with dormant *T. gondii* infection become pregnant. Babies born to women with AIDS and *T. gondii* infection are at substantial risk for congenital toxoplasmosis.

In immunocompetent women, the risk of transmission increases by trimester (about 15 per cent in the first trimester, about 30 per cent in the second, and about 60 per cent in the third). The incidence of congenital transmission is reduced 60 per cent when primary infection in the mother is promptly treated with antiparasitic therapy.

In contrast, the severity of damage due to congenital infection decreases by trimester. When women are infected in the first trimester, most pregnancies end with spontaneous abortion, stillbirth, or severe disease in the newborn. When maternal infection occurs during the second or third trimester, only 15 and 5 per cent of newborns, respectively, have signs of disease at birth. However, many asymptomatic congenitally infected neonates will develop complications later in life, including chorioretinitis, hearing abnormalities, decreased intelligence, and seizures. Treatment during the first year of life seems to prevent most of these sequelae.

The signs of infection present at birth include chorioretinitis, strabismus, blindness, seizures, retardation, anemia, jaundice, rash, petechiae, encephalitis, pneumonia, microcephaly, hydrocephalus, diarrhea, and hypothermia. In babies infected later in pregnancy, the signs may be detected only by detailed, focused examination. Infants with congenital toxoplasmosis born to mothers infected with the human immunodeficiency virus (HIV) are likely to be infected with HIV, and their congenital toxoplasmosis tends to run a more severe and rapid course. These infants typically have fever, hepatomegaly, splenomegaly, myocardial involvement, pneumonia, chorioretinitis, seizures, and failure to gain weight. The differential diagnosis includes rubella, CMV, herpes simplex, syphilis, listeriosis, other bacterial infections, other encephalopathies, and erythroblastosis fetalis.

PHYSICAL EXAMINATION

In patients with lymphadenopathy, the most commonly recognized nodes are cervical, but any or all lymph node groups may be affected. Nodes vary in size up to 3 cm in diameter. Palpable nodes are smooth to firm or rubbery—not hard or fibrotic—and usually are not fixed to other nodes or tissues. Immunocompetent patients with primary infection may have hepatomegaly, splenomegaly, or maculopapular rash. Rales may be present in persons with pneumonia, but consolidation is unlikely.

The typical signs of toxoplasmosis in immunocompromised patients include focal neurologic deficits corresponding to necrotic lesions in the CNS. Meningismus may be present. If pneumonia is present, rales are heard over affected areas.

In the acute stage of chorioretinitis, focal necrotizing retinitis appears as a pale yellow, elevated cotton patch with indistinct margins. Focal or diffuse vitreal inflammation often overlies the retinal lesion, and this inflammation makes underlying structures indistinct. The acute lesion may resemble "headlights in the fog." After weeks to months, the lesions appear more distinct. The sclera is revealed and appears pale yellow or white, and there are focal regions of black pigmentation. The margins are sharp, and retinal tissue surrounding the lesions is normal. Retinal examination may reveal multiple lesions in one or both eyes. In immunocompetent patients with congenitally acquired *Toxoplasma* infection, lesions are often in different stages of development, the stages reflecting episodic activity over several years. Optic nerve involvement is detected in 10 per cent of patients with AIDS. Chorioretinitis in persons with AIDS tends to be more diffuse and atypical than in other persons; thus, the diagnosis in this group is more difficult.

In congenitally infected infants who are ill at birth, the signs include chorioretinitis, strabismus, blindness, jaundice, petechial rash, rales, bulging fontanelles or frank hydrocephalus, diarrhea, and hypothermia. Congenitally infected infants who appear normal at birth may have signs of chorioretinitis, hearing loss, or seizures later in life. Infants born with AIDS and toxoplasmosis typically have fever, hepatomegaly, splenomegaly, signs of myocardial failure, rales, chorioretinitis, seizures, and weight loss or failure to gain weight.

USEFUL LABORATORY PROCEDURES

The peripheral blood smear from immunocompetent patients with primary infection may show up to 10 per cent atypical lymphocytes. Liver enzymes may be mildly abnormal. Other routine laboratory tests are usually normal. In immunosuppressed persons with toxoplasmosis, nonspecific laboratory values are of little help. Congenitally infected infants often have thrombocytopenia and markedly increased cerebrospinal fluid protein levels.

In general, IgG antibodies appear 1 to 2 weeks after infection, peak within 1 to 2 months following infection, and fall to low concentrations over months to years. IgG antibodies usually persist for life. IgM, IgA, and IgE antibodies usually appear 1 week after infection and persist for weeks to months. They occasionally are detectable after reactivation of dormant infection. Many tests have been described to measure IgG, IgM, IgA, and IgE antibodies. Few of them are readily available to most clinicians, and the reliability of commercially available tests varies substantially. In difficult cases, samples should be sent to reference laboratories.

IgG Serologic Tests

In the Sabin-Feldman dye test, IgG antibodies in patient samples kill tachyzoites in the presence of added complement. Killing is detected with phase-contrast microscopy, and Sabin-Feldman remains the "gold standard" test performed in reference laboratories. The titer, however, does not correlate with clinical severity. The IgG enzyme-linked immunosorbent assay (IgG-ELISA) measures antibodies similar to those measured with the dye test. Antibodies measured with the indirect fluorescent antibody test (IFA) are similar to those measured with the dye test, but IFA is less sensitive and more difficult to quantify. Also, antinuclear antibodies may react with *Toxoplasma* nuclei in the IFA test, yielding false-positive results. The agglutination test for IgG antibodies employs 2-mercaptoethanol to inactivate IgM and measures antibodies similar to those measured with the dye test.

The indirect hemagglutination (IHA) and complement fixation (CF) tests measure antibodies that appear later than those detected with the IgG tests mentioned previously. IHA antibody titers remain elevated longer than dye test titers, whereas CF antibodies disappear more quickly. These are older tests that are rarely available and seldom used.

Early during infection, IgG antibodies have a broad spectrum of avidity to *T. gondii*. By the sixth month of infection, plasma cell clones that make more specific antibodies have been selected. The degree of avidity can be measured with the IgG avidity test to determine how long infection has been present.

The differential agglutination test (AC/HS test) compares titers with formalin-fixed tachyzoites (HS antigen) and acetone- or methanol-fixed tachyzoites (AC antigen). IgG antibodies to AC antigen appear earlier during infection, and the AC to HS antibody ratio can be used to help determine the time of infection.

IgM, IgA, and IgE Serologic Tests

The IgM immunofluorescent antibody (IgM-IFA) test was the first to detect IgM antibody to *T. gondii*. Titers rise rapidly starting 1 week after infection, peak within a week or two, fall rapidly to low levels, and usually disappear by 6 months. Antinuclear antibodies and rheumatoid factor can produce false-positive results, and high titers of IgG antibody can interfere, yielding false-negative results. The double-sandwich IgM enzyme-linked immunosorbent assay (DS-IgM-ELISA) is more sensitive and specific than the IgM-IFA test. Results are frequently positive for up to a year or more after infection. Rheumatoid factor and antinuclear antibodies do not produce false-positive results. The IgM immunosorbent assay (IgM-ISAGA) test gives results similar to those of the DS-IgM-ELISA.

The IgA enzyme-linked immunosorbent assay (IgA-ELISA) is positive soon after infection, and this test is positive more often than the DS-IgM-ELISA with sera from congenitally infected infants. IgA-ELISA may also be more sensitive in patients with flares of chorioretinitis. The IgE enzyme-linked immunosorbent assay (IgE-ELISA) gives results similar to the DS-IgM-ELISA and the IgA-ELISA in most groups, and it may be positive in 40 per cent of patients with AIDS and toxoplasmic encephalitis.

Cytology

Tachyzoites can be demonstrated in body fluids with common stains such as Giemsa, Papanicolaou, silver impregnation, and Wright's. Tachyzoites are often missed because observers are not experienced or do not expect to see them. Bronchoalveolar lavage fluid from patients with pneumonia and cytocentrifuge smears of cerebrospinal fluid from patients with CNS disease commonly reveal tachyzoites.

Biopsy

The observation of tachyzoites in tissues documents that an infection is active. The presence of tissue cysts near a site of inflammatory necrosis implies active infection without proving it. Tissue cysts alone are compatible with acute or dormant infection. Immunofluorescent antibody staining of tissue improves sensitivity but is prone to artifact. Peroxidase-antiperoxidase immunostaining is even more sensitive and specific. Endomyocardial biopsy has facilitated diagnosis of myocardial toxoplasmosis in cardiac transplant recipients and other immunosuppressed patients.

Most cases of lymphadenopathy should be diagnosed with serology, but toxoplasmosis is frequently not considered before the lymph node is removed and examined. Lymph node histopathology in immunocompetent adults and older children is characteristic and easily recognized by experienced observers. To confirm the histopathology, serologic tests should be performed.

Antigenemia

ELISA techniques can also detect antigen in the blood of recently infected immunocompetent adults, but these tests are not widely available.

DNA Detection Methods

DNA from as little as one tachyzoite can be detected in tissue, blood, or other body fluids after amplification with the polymerase chain reaction (PCR). DNA in tissues may reflect tissue cysts or active infection. By contrast, DNA in blood or other body fluids probably represents tachyzoites and, thus, active infection. Contamination is a widely recognized problem that must be prevented. DNA testing has the potential to substantially improve the diagnosis of congenital infection.

Mouse Inoculation

Tissues or body fluids may be inoculated into mice, which are then observed for illness and tested serologically for antibodies to *T. gondii.* Mouse inoculation is sensitive and specific, but it is slow, cumbersome, and expensive and is offered only in specialized reference laboratories. As with DNA testing, a positive result with a tissue sample indicates the presence of active or dormant infection, while a positive result with a body fluid specimen indicates active disease.

USEFUL IMAGING PROCEDURES

In persons with AIDS and toxoplasmic encephalitis, the typical computed tomography (CT) scan shows multiple low-density ring-enhancing lesions in both cerebral hemispheres. Single lesions occur in approximately 20 per cent of patients, and CT scans are negative in fewer than 5 per cent. Lesions tend to occur at the corticomedullary junction and are frequent in the basal ganglia. Contrast-enhanced magnetic resonance imaging (MRI) is more sensitive and often shows more lesions, but it is also more expensive. In a patient with a typical computed tomogram, a magnetic resonance scan is unlikely to show additional clinically useful information. Lymphoma is the most common disorder that produces similar images. Lymphoma usually presents with a single mass. Imaging produces similar results in persons without AIDS, but diffuse encephalitis is more common in these patients than in people with AIDS. Chest films in people with *Toxoplasma* pneumonia typically reveal diffuse, bilateral interstitial infiltrates.

DIAGNOSTIC APPROACHES IN SPECIFIC CLINICAL SETTINGS

New Infection in Immunocompetent Persons

The diagnosis is usually made with serologic tests that show a high titer of IgG antibodies and the presence of IgM or IgA antibodies. With a compatible clinical picture, it is appropriate to observe the patient for recovery. In patients with lymphadenopathy, the diagnosis can usually be made with serology alone. Often, the diagnosis is made with lymph node biopsy because toxoplasmosis was not considered and serology was not performed. The potential toxicities of antimicrobial therapy usually outweigh its benefits.

Active Toxoplasmosis in Immunocompromised Persons

The diagnosis of toxoplasmic encephalitis is most often made presumptively, based on typical symptoms and signs and a characteristic CT or magnetic resonance image in a person with IgG antibodies to *T. gondii.* IgG antibody status should be determined; IgG antibodies are usually positive in low or moderate titer. By contrast, IgG antibodies may not be present in rare cases where infection is newly acquired or where IgG antibodies have been lost because of immunosuppression. In general, however, IgG antibodies are so commonly present that their absence should prompt the clinician to reconsider a diagnosis of toxoplasmosis. IgM, IgE, or IgA antibody tests should be performed when the diagnosis is not clear, because the presence of these antibodies confirms the diagnosis in some patients.

Most patients with characteristic presentations are treated with antimicrobials against *T. gondii* and observed for a response. Signs and symptoms should improve in 50 per cent of responders by 3 days and in the remainder within 7 to 14 days. Improvement on CT scan should occur by 3 weeks. When improvement in symptoms or scans is not observed, the lesion should be biopsied to confirm the diagnosis. Since empirical therapy is often used for people with AIDS who are also known to have underlying infection with *T. gondii,* providers should test for IgG antibodies to *T. gondii* in persons with HIV infection before CD4 counts drop below about 250 cells/mm^3.

Chorioretinitis can usually be diagnosed by the characteristic appearance and response to therapy. Disease outside the CNS is usually diagnosed by observing tachyzoites in tissue or cytology specimens. When myocarditis is suspected, endomyocardial biopsy may reveal the organisms, especially when peroxidase-antiperoxidase immunostaining is performed. Detection of DNA in blood or other body fluids may soon prove to be clinically useful.

Infection During Pregnancy

The clinician should seek to determine whether the mother became newly infected during or just before gestation. If so, IgG antibodies will be present in high or rising titers, and IgM, IgA, or IgE antibodies to *T. gondii* will often be present. Since IgM antibodies may be detected for more than a year after infection, their presence does not prove that infection occurred during pregnancy.

If infection was acquired during pregnancy, the parents must decide whether to continue the pregnancy. Fetal infection is not certain, it is often possible to diagnose infection in the fetus, and treatment of the mother will prevent many congenital infections and ensuing fetal damage. If the parents decide to continue the pregnancy, fetal blood and amniotic fluid are obtained 20 to 24 weeks after conception for detection of the organism, for serologic tests, and for certain nonspecific tests. In decreasing order of sensitivity, the tests for detection of the organism include mouse inoculation, detection of DNA in amniotic fluid with the use of PCR, and tissue culture. Sensitive serologic tests for IgM and IgA antibodies to *T. gondii* should be performed on fetal blood. For proper interpretation, the fetal blood sample should be tested for contamination by maternal blood. Eosinophilia, thrombocytopenia, increased γ-glutamyltransferase, and increased lactate dehydrogenase suggest that congenital transmission has occurred in suspect cases. From the time of fetal blood sampling until the end of pregnancy, ultrasonography should be performed every 2 to 4 weeks to detect cerebral ventricular enlargement, intracranial calcification, hepatomegaly, ascites, or an increase in the width of the placenta. Fetal diagnosis can be made in about 80 per cent of cases of congenital transmission. When fetal transmission has been documented, the mother should be treated with sulfadiazine and pyrimethamine if the pregnancy is to be continued.

Congenital Toxoplasmosis

The diagnosis should be sought in any infant born to a mother who had primary infection during or within 8 weeks before pregnancy and in any infant with signs of congenital infection. Maternal IgG antibody crosses the placenta, and titers will decrease by half every 28 days. Maternal IgM, IgA, and IgE antibodies cross the placenta only rarely when there is leakage of maternal blood, and then these antibodies disappear rapidly. The presence of IgM, IgA, or IgE antibodies in the fetus strongly suggests congenital infection, especially when titers are stable or increase. Western blotting has shown that maternal and infant sera often recognize different antigens. Thus, Western blotting has been proposed as a test for distinguishing between maternal and fetal infection.

CRYPTOSPORIDIOSIS

By Timothy P. Flanigan, M.D.
Cleveland, Ohio

and Rosemary Soave, M.D.
New York, New York

Human cryptosporidiosis is a cause of severe diarrhea in patients with the acquired immunodeficiency syndrome (AIDS) and a common cause of sporadic and epidemic gastroenteritis in immunocompetent persons. The protozoan parasite *Cryptosporidium* has been recognized for decades as a cause of disease in animals, including livestock, but its role as a human pathogen has been brought to light only in the last decade during the AIDS epidemic.

Infection in humans results from ingestion of oocysts. They release sporozoites that in turn infect epithelial cells, primarily in the small intestine. Although the developing parasite appears to be loosely attached to the surface of the cell, it actually maintains an intracellular, although extracytoplasmic, position. The sporozoite subsequently undergoes asexual reproduction (schizogony). Schizogony can go through multiple cycles with release of merozoites that can reinfect the epithelial cells, or, alternatively, the parasite may undergo sexual reproduction (gametogony). Gametogony results in an oocyst that is capable of reinfecting the same host or may be excreted in the stool and thus can infect another host.

EPIDEMIOLOGY

Cryptosporidium is thought to be the etiologic agent in 1 to 4 per cent of patients with diarrhea worldwide and in up to 16 per cent of patients with enteritis in less developed countries. Infection occurs more commonly in children and during the wet summer months. *Cryptosporidium* is spread from person to person, from animal to human, and through fecal contamination of the environment, particularly water. Person-to-person spread accounts for sequential infections among families and outbreaks in day care centers that occasionally have infected more than 50 per cent of children and staff. Outbreaks among animal handlers and veterinary students have been reported in association with illness in sheep, pigs, cows, and horses. Cryptosporidiosis, much like giardiasis, is an occasional cause of diarrhea in travelers returning from abroad. There have been outbreaks in this country when public water supplies become contaminated with feces. Among homosexual men, the protozoa are possibly spread through sexual contact, much like other protozoa that can cause "the gay bowel syndrome."

CLINICAL PRESENTATION

Typically, acute infection with *Cryptosporidium* is characterized by watery diarrhea, crampy epigastric abdominal pain, weight loss, anorexia, malaise, and flatulence. Nausea and vomiting may be present. Diarrhea and abdominal pain are usually exacerbated by eating. Recently, a broader spectrum of symptoms from cryptosporidial infection has been appreciated. There are reports of asymptomatic carriage of *Cryptosporidium*. Also, patients with vague epigastric abdominal pain or dyspepsia and mild or no diarrhea have had *Cryptosporidium* oocysts in their duodenal aspirates.

The initial physical examination is often unrevealing. The patient may have orthostatic hypotension due to dehydration. Temperature above 38°C (100.4°F) is not uncommon. Borborygmi are often present on abdominal examination. Examination of the liver and spleen is normal. Laboratory examination often reveals electrolyte disturbances consistent with diarrhea and dehydration. Leukocytosis is not uncommon. Fecal examination may reveal mucus, but blood and leukocytes are rarely seen. Charcot-Leyden crystals are characteristic of *Isospora belli* infection and amebiasis but not cryptosporidiosis. Lactose intolerance and fat malabsorption have been well documented, and the D-xylose test is uniformly abnormal. The incubation period may vary from a day to 2 weeks. In immunocompetent individuals, the illness is always self-limited, but the diarrhea may be so severe that intravenous rehydration is sometimes necessary. The duration of illness in immunocompetent hosts ranges from 2 days to a month, but most individuals become asymptomatic within 2 weeks.

CRYPTOSPORIDIOSIS IN AIDS

In patients with AIDS, symptoms often begin insidiously with only mild diarrhea, but they increase in severity over time. The majority of these patients experience profound voluminous watery diarrhea ranging from 1 to 25 L per day, loss of more than 10 per cent of total body weight, and severe abdominal pain. Without adequate rehydration (either oral or intravenous), the disease may be quickly fatal. Severe malabsorption is the rule, and many patients avoid eating because it worsens the diarrhea and abdominal pain. Occasionally symptoms may remit, but these respites are usually brief. The majority of patients with AIDS never clear the infection and die of cryptosporidial diarrhea.

A subset of patients with AIDS and cryptosporidiosis have biliary tract involvement (Table 1). This complication

Table 1. Clinical Manifestations: Human Cryptosporidiosis, The New York Hospital, 6/82 to 4/88

	AIDS	Non-AIDS
Total number of patients	79	22
Watery diarrhea (bowel movements/d)	5–20	3–8
Weight loss (kg)	6–23	2–10
Nausea, vomiting	+ +	+
Abdominal pain	+ + +	+ +
Duration of diarrhea (d)	4–720	10–38
Fecal parasite shedding (d)	4–720	10–50
	Number of Patients	
Biliary tract involvement	15	0
Pulmonary involvement	2	0
Other intestinal parasites	21	2

Presented at the First International Conference on Cryptosporidiosis, Moredun Research Institute, Edinburgh, Scotland, 1988.
\+ = mild, + + = moderate, + + + = severe.

is invariably associated with severe right upper quadrant pain, nausea, and vomiting. Physical examination reveals right upper quadrant tenderness. Laboratory examination indicates elevated levels of serum alkaline phosphatase and γ-glutamyltransferase. Serum aminotransferase levels may be mildly elevated. Serum bilirubin levels are usually normal. Endoscopic retrograde cholangiopancreatography reveals dilation of bile ducts with multiple luminal irregularities and distal duct strictures consistent with either partial obstruction or sclerosing cholangitis. Thickening of the gallbladder wall occurs commonly. Biliary tract disease in patients with AIDS may have many causes, including cytomegalovirus and possibly even human immunodeficiency virus itself. Initial reports described concurrent infection with *Cryptosporidium* and cytomegalovirus in the biliary epithelium of patients with sclerosing cholangitis and biliary tract obstruction.

There is still no effective therapy for cryptosporidiosis, and thus management of infected patients should focus on appropriate hydration and nutrition. Antidiarrheal agents such as loperamide may produce some relief, although they may also make the symptoms worse.

Fulminant cryptosporidiosis is rare among immunodeficient patients without human immunodeficiency virus infection, but it does occur. The initial reports of human cryptosporidiosis in immunodeficient patients involved two 6-year-old children with congenital hypogammaglobulinemia and two patients with impaired humoral and cellular immunity due to chemotherapy. Cryptosporidiosis has also been reported in renal transplant and bone marrow transplant patients. Patients with reversible immune deficiencies usually recover when the cause of the immunosuppression is removed.

DIAGNOSIS

Diagnosis of cryptosporidiosis is based on identification of the oocyst in stool specimens. More than 15 different staining techniques have been tried, and the modified acid-fast stain is optimal because it is both easy to perform and inexpensive. The acid-fast oocyst stains red with varying intensity and may appear round or crescentic. It is 4 to 6 μm in diameter. Yeast, which are morphologically similar to cryptosporidial oocysts, are not acid fast and hence do not stain red. A fluorescein-labeled immunoglobulin G monoclonal antibody (Meridien) is commercially available and appears to be more sensitive but not necessarily more specific than the acid-fast stain. It is presently being evaluated clinically.

It is not yet clear how many stool specimens are needed to confirm that a patient does not have cryptosporidial enteritis. In acute cryptosporidiosis, oocysts are easily detected without concentration techniques. Concentration of oocysts from stool is carried out by centrifugation, flotation in Sheather's sugar solution, hypertonic sodium chloride, or zinc sulfate. Concentration techniques are most helpful when one is examining stool with low numbers of organisms, such as that from asymptomatic individuals with formed stool. When cryptosporidiosis is a diagnostic consideration, special studies should be specifically requested because many laboratories do not routinely look for the organism in ova and parasite examinations. Care should be taken in the handling of infected specimens to prevent leakage or aerosolization because infection of laboratory workers has been reported.

Biopsy of the small intestine is not usually necessary to make the diagnosis of cryptosporidiosis. In fact, biopsy results may be false-negative owing to the sampling of uninfected areas that result from patchy parasite distribution. Biopsy specimens from AIDS patients with cryptosporidiosis typically show villous atrophy, a mononuclear cell infiltrate of the lamina propria, and an absence of inflammatory changes.

Anticryptosporidial IgM, IgG, and IgA can be detected in infected persons by enzyme-linked immunosorbent assay (ELISA) or the immunofluorescent antibody test. Although useful in epidemiologic evaluation, serologic studies have no role in the diagnosis of acute illness.

DIFFERENTIAL DIAGNOSIS OF DIARRHEA IN AIDS

Diarrhea is a prominent feature of AIDS and is present in 50 per cent of patients in this country and in more than 70 per cent of patients from Haiti and Africa. Diarrhea may be acute, intermittent, or chronic, and both infectious (bacterial, fungal, viral, and protozoan) and noninfectious causes (neoplasm and autoimmune) have been implicated. Multiple concurrent enteric infections are not uncommon; therefore, even if *Cryptosporidium* is found, other treatable pathogens must be looked for as well. Acute enteritis may be caused by protozoa or bacteria, such as *Giardia lamblia, Entamoeba histolytica, Salmonella, Shigella,* and *Campylobacter.* Despite appropriate therapeutic intervention, relapses may occur. Pseudomembranous colitis caused by *Clostridium difficile* toxin may cause acute diarrhea even in the patient without a history of recent antibiotic use. *I. belli* commonly causes malabsorptive diarrhea that is indistinguishable from cryptosporidiosis in patients from Africa and Haiti. The work-up of AIDS patients with diarrhea should include bacterial stool culture, ova and parasite examination (including acid-fast examination for *Cryptosporidium*), and a test for *C. difficile* toxin. Patients with persistent diarrhea and no obvious etiologic agent on stool examination should undergo endoscopy with biopsies. Other causes of chronic diarrhea include *Mycobacterium avium-intracellulare,* cytomegalovirus, perhaps microsporidia, and visceral infiltration with neoplasms such as Kaposi's sarcoma or lymphoma. Histopathologic examination of tissue is required to make these diagnoses. Finally, even in patients with persistent diarrhea due to cryptosporidiosis, repeated periodic stool examination for pathogenic bacteria, other parasites, and *C. difficile* toxin should be done to exclude the development of dual infections.

GIARDIASIS

By David P. Stevens, M.D.
Cleveland, Ohio

Giardiasis is an infection of the small intestine caused by the protozoan *Giardia lamblia*. This organism exists either as a motile flagellated trophozoite that is usually found in the small intestine or as a tough-walled cyst that is excreted in stool and is resistant to environmental stresses outside the host. The clinical presentation of giardiasis ranges from a totally asymptomatic infection to severe malabsorption, diarrhea, and weight loss. On histologic examination, the infected small intestine appears atrophic and is characterized by shortened villi and elongated crypts. The pathogenesis of the malabsorption is not well explained.

COURSE

A careful history is the most important step to a correct, swift, and efficient diagnosis. Infection starts by oral inoculation via contaminated water, food, or fomites. After an incubation period of 6 to 21 days, the symptomatic patient has frequent, loose, foul-smelling stools accompanied by malaise, cramping abdominal pain, and, eventually, weight loss (Table 1). The symptoms progress until treated; infrequently, they may recede spontaneously. Selected manifestations of malabsorption may dominate the clinical picture, for example, temporary lactase deficiency that results in a dominant picture of milk intolerance and overshadows other symptoms.

Giardiasis occurs most frequently in (1) travelers returning from endemic areas, (2) residents of areas where breakdown of purification systems results in contaminated water supplies, and (3) situations that facilitate person-to-person spread.

Giardiasis in Travelers

The disease should be suspected in travelers who return from endemic areas where the organism is prevalent in drinking water. Typical locations are Central America, Southeast Asia, India, and Russia, particularly St. Petersburg. In the United States, campers and hikers in the Rocky Mountains frequently become infected by contaminated streams and rivers. The source of this contamination is probably beaver, canine, or human feces.

Table 1. Frequency of Symptoms in Giardiasis

Symptom	Frequency (%)
Diarrhea	96
Weakness	72
Weight loss	62
Abdominal cramps	61
Nausea	60
Greasy stools	57
Abdominal distention	42
Flatuence	39
Vomiting	29
Belching	26
Fever	17

Adapted from Brodsky, R. E., Spencer, H. C., and Schultz, M. G.: Giardiasis in American travelers to the Soviet Union. J. Infect. Dis., 130:319–323, 1974, with permission.

Table 2. Differentiating Factors in Traveler's Diarrhea Caused by *Giardia* and Bacteria

	Giardiasis	Toxicogenic *E. coli*
Incubation period	5–21 days	2–3 days
Typical onset	After arrival home	While traveling
Course	Indolent	Acute
Diarrhea	Soft, loose	Watery, explosive

Giardiasis can be distinguished from other frequent causes of traveler's diarrhea, such as toxicogenic *Escherichia coli,* by the longer incubation period of giardiasis (Table 2). The diarrhea often occurs after the traveler returns home and is more gradual in its onset. The stool is soft and voluminous—typical of malabsorption. The symptoms may wax and wane. Indeed, *G. lamblia* is the most common cause of chronic diarrhea in travelers. The shorter incubation period of toxicogenic diarrheas, on the other hand, usually results in illness while the traveler is still away from home. Its onset is more explosive and the watery diarrhea more urgent.

Breakdown of Community Water Supplies

Community outbreaks of giardiasis are usually associated with failure of filtration systems in water treatment plants, cross-contamination of water supplies with sewage, or contamination of wells and other local water sources. More than two thirds of community outbreaks documented by the Centers for Disease Control and Prevention have resulted from failed filtration systems. The concentration of chlorine usually found in treated water supplies is inadequate to kill *Giardia* cysts.

Person-to-Person Spread

Infection can be spread by the fecal-oral route. This assumption is based on the frequent observation of epidemics in day care centers and among sexually active gay men. Spread of infection can occur among people living closely together in institutional residences and even among family members. The detection of infection in any residential setting should prompt the evaluation of symptomatic contacts.

PHYSICAL EXAMINATION

The pertinent physical findings in giardiasis are confined to the abdomen. There may be modest nonlocalized tenderness, tympany, and increased intensity of bowel sounds. The rectal examination is normal and notable for the absence of occult blood or fecal leukocytes in the stool.

RADIOGRAPHIC EVALUATION

Radiographic findings are nonspecific, and radiographic evaluation cannot be justified except to exclude other suspected diagnoses. The plain film of the abdomen may show increased small and large bowel gas. The barium meal examination generally shows the nonspecific picture of small intestinal edema and thickened folds. The barium enema study is unrewarding except for the exclusion of other processes.

LABORATORY PROCEDURES

Studies of the blood are not helpful in making the diagnosis. Chemistry examinations may show reduced albumin after prolonged infection. The complete blood count is generally normal. Eosinophilia is not seen in giardiasis but is a finding in helminth infections.

The diagnosis is confirmed by detection of *Giardia* organisms in stool or duodenal contents. Stool specimens must be examined in either the fresh state or in a specially preserved form because of the rapid loss of viability of trophozoites. The complex interpretation of stool specimens is best left to trained laboratory personnel. Unless a laboratory technician is at hand for a proper examination of a "warm" specimen, a stool preservative system should be used. Polyvinyl alcohol–formalin preservatives, such as Para-Pak LV-PVA Systems (Meridian Diagnostics, 3471 River Hills Drive, Cincinnati, OH 45244), are used for preservation, transportation, and storage of stool specimens.

Even under the best circumstances, *Giardia* organisms are inconsistently found in the stool because their excretion may be intermittent. Three separate specimens should be examined before a negative conclusion is reached. Direct examination of wet-mount preparations of stool specimens with iodine or Wheatley's trichrome may be successfully done by the clinician, but trained laboratory assistance is preferable. Several hazards can complicate detection of the organism. Laxatives and antibiotics as well as barium contrast material should be avoided for 3 days before stool examination. Along with other substances such as antacids and antidiarrheal preparations, they may result in false-negative test results by causing the disappearance of organisms from the stool or by altering the morphologic features of the organism.

An enzyme-linked immunosorbent assay for *Giardia* antigen will soon be available for use in the diagnostic laboratory. This technique may circumvent many complexities of direct microscopic examination of stool specimens.

If the stool does not reveal *Giardia,* examination of duodenal specimens may be warranted. Small bowel biopsy provides specimens to use in touch preparations for fresh wet-mount examination and in histologic sections for examination after hematoxylin-eosin staining. Intubation and aspiration of duodenal contents provide material for wet-mount examination. A more economical technique for obtaining small bowel fluid employs the Entero-test (HDC Corp., 2551 Casey Avenue, Mountain View, CA 94043). This device is a nylon string contained in a gelatin capsule. One end of the string is held while the capsule is swallowed by the patient; the string is withdrawn after 1 to 3 hours. The material from the bile-stained end of the string is expressed onto a microscope slide for direct examination. Motile organisms are seen on a positive wet-mount specimen.

THERAPEUTIC TRIAL

A clinical trial of therapy for giardiasis is considered reasonable in situations where the typical clinical picture cannot be substantiated by laboratory confirmation of *Giardia* infection in small bowel contents or stool. The use of quinacrine hydrochloride, 100 mg three times daily for 10 days, or metronidazole, 250 mg three times daily for 7 days, is effective in 85 to 90 per cent of cases. Manufacturers' precautions regarding the use of these drugs in children and pregnant women must be observed.

AMERICAN TRYPANOSOMIASIS (CHAGAS' DISEASE)

By Louis V. Kirchhoff, M.D., M.P.H.
Iowa City, Iowa

American trypanosomiasis, or Chagas' disease, is caused by the protozoan parasite *Trypanosoma cruzi*. This organism is found only in the Americas, where it is distributed unevenly from southern Mexico to Argentina and Chile in many species of wild and domestic mammals, humans, and insect vectors called reduviid bugs. An estimated 16 to 18 million persons are infected with *T. cruzi*, and it is thought that 50,000 deaths result from Chagas' disease annually. Transmission of *T. cruzi* to humans usually occurs through contact with feces of infected vectors, but transfusion-associated and congenital transmission are also important. Infections associated with laboratory accidents have occasionally been reported. The clinical syndromes of acute *T. cruzi* infection and chronic Chagas' disease are quite different and are described separately.

ACUTE CHAGAS' DISEASE

Clinical Manifestations

Acute Chagas' disease is usually an illness of children, but it can occur at any age. The frequency and intensity of the manifestations of acute Chagas' disease are highly variable. Only a small percentage of acute *T. cruzi* infections are diagnosed, because the signs and symptoms are mild and nonspecific in most patients. The first signs of illness occur 7 days or more after invasion by the parasites, and with transfusion-associated disease, signs may not appear for 20 to 40 days. When the parasite has entered through a break in the skin, a chagoma may be formed, consisting of an indurated area of erythema and swelling accompanied by local lymph node enlargement. Romaña's sign, the classic finding in acute Chagas' disease, consists of unilateral painless edema of the palpebrae and periocular tissues and may appear when the conjunctiva is the portal of entry. These initial local signs may be followed by fever, tachycardia, malaise, anorexia, and edema of the face and lower extremities. Generalized lymphadenopathy and mild hepatosplenomegaly also may appear.

Severe myocarditis develops in a small proportion of patients with acute Chagas' disease, and it is frequently accompanied by pericardial effusion. The clinical findings are those of congestive heart failure, and most deaths due to acute *T. cruzi* infection result from this cause. Overt central nervous system signs are also uncommon, but meningoencephalitis develops in a small percentage of patients and is associated with a poor prognosis. In most untreated patients, the clinical manifestations of acute Chagas' disease resolve gradually over a period of weeks to months. Areas of local reaction around the eye or other sites of parasite entry can persist for several weeks, as can the lymphadenopathy and splenomegaly.

Acute Chagas' disease that results from congenital transmission of *T. cruzi* is generally more severe than the vector-borne or transfusion-acquired forms and merits special mention here. The incidence of *T. cruzi* infection in infants born to infected mothers is less than 5 per cent and varies considerably from one region to another. Stillbirths occur occasionally, and surviving infants with congenital Chagas' disease are often severely affected. Prematurity and hepatosplenomegaly are nearly constant features. Edema is also frequent, and many congenitally infected infants have hemorrhagic chagomas in the skin and mucosal surfaces. The heart also is often involved, resulting in conduction abnormalities, but frank cardiac insufficiency is uncommon. Central nervous system involvement is common, resulting in seizures, hypotonia, motor retardation, and tremors. The prognosis in severely affected infants is poor.

A second special case of acute Chagas' disease is the reactivation of the parasitosis that can occur when persons with chronic *T. cruzi* infections become immunosuppressed. This reactivation often occurs with a severity greater than that of the initial *T. cruzi* infections in immunocompetent patients. The frequency of central nervous system involvement in immunosuppressed patients is greater than that in patients with acute Chagas' disease who are immunocompetent. This increased frequency is especially true of patients with chronic *T. cruzi* infections who become immunosuppressed by human immunodeficiency virus (HIV). These patients generally present with neurologic findings resulting from *T. cruzi* brain abscesses.

Diagnostic Procedures

The first consideration in the diagnosis of acute Chagas' disease is a history consistent with exposure to *T. cruzi.* This exposure can include residence in an area in which transmission of the parasite occurs, a recent blood transfusion in an endemic area, being born to a mother known to be or suspected of being infected with *T. cruzi,* or a laboratory accident. No infections among tourists returning to the United States from endemic areas have been reported, and only a handful of autochthonous *T. cruzi* infections have been described here.

The diagnosis of acute Chagas' disease is made by detecting parasites. Serologic tests for anti–*T. cruzi* IgM, which are not standardized and are not widely available, play a limited role. Circulating parasites are motile and can often be seen in wet preparations of anticoagulated blood or buffy coat. The parasites can also be seen in Giemsa-stained smears. In acutely infected immunocompetent patients, examination of blood preparations is the cornerstone of detecting *T. cruzi*. In immunosuppressed patients suspected of having acute Chagas' disease, however, other specimens such as lymph node and bone marrow aspirates, pericardial fluid, and cerebrospinal fluid should be examined microscopically. When these methods fail to detect *T. cruzi* in a patient whose clinical and epidemiologic histories suggest that the organism is present, culturing the parasite from blood or other body fluids in specialized liquid media may be attempted. One major problem with this method is that it takes at least a month to complete, and this is far beyond the time by which decisions regarding drug treatment must be made. Moreover, although it is thought that blood culture is more sensitive than microscopic examination of blood and other specimens, its sensitivity may be no greater than 80 per cent. Polymerase chain reaction (PCR)–based assays for detecting *T. cruzi* are being developed and have shown promise under research laboratory conditions, but none is available commercially.

Patients with acute Chagas' disease may have a variety of conduction abnormalities on electrocardiogram, radiographic signs of cardiomegaly, or indications of pericardial effusion on echocardiography. Cerebrospinal fluid parameters also may be abnormal. None of these findings is specific, however, and the diagnosis of acute *T. cruzi* infection must rest on demonstration of the parasite.

CHRONIC CHAGAS' DISEASE

After the spontaneous resolution of the acute illness, the patient enters what is called the *indeterminate phase* of Chagas' disease, which is characterized by asymptomatic parasitemia and IgG antibodies to a variety of *T. cruzi* antigens. Only 10 to 30 per cent of persons with chronic *T. cruzi* infections develop symptoms related to the infection, and the percentage is lower in Central America, for example, than it is in central Brazil, Argentina, and Chile.

Clinical Manifestations

Symptomatic chronic Chagas' disease becomes apparent years or even decades after the initial infection. The heart is the organ most commonly involved, and signs and symptoms reflect underlying rhythm disturbances, cardiomyopathy, congestive failure, and thromboembolism. Palpitations, dizziness, syncope, seizures, and sudden death can result from a wide variety of dysrhythmias. The cardiomyopathy that develops can affect primarily the right ventricle, leading to the classic signs of right heart failure, but biventricular failure is also common. Typical symptoms and signs include dyspnea on exertion, orthopnea, paroxysmal nocturnal dyspnea, cough, and lower extremity edema. Although some patients have both cardiomyopathy and arrhythmias, most do not. As is the case in patients with cardiomyopathies caused by other diseases, thrombus formation is common and the clinical course is frequently complicated by embolization to the lungs, brain, and other organs. The physical findings in patients with chronic cardiac Chagas' disease are similar to those found in persons with dysrhythmias and cardiomyopathies due to other causes.

The second system frequently affected in patients with chronic *T. cruzi* infection is the gastrointestinal tract. Megaesophagus and megacolon (mega syndrome) resulting from denervation of these organs are the most common anatomic changes. In patients with megaesophagus, symptoms are similar to those of idiopathic achalasia and may include cough, dysphagia, odynophagia, heartburn, retrosternal pain, and regurgitation. Hypersalivation and salivary gland hypertrophy have been observed. Aspiration can be a recurrent problem, especially during sleep, and repeated episodes of aspiration pneumonitis are common. Weight loss and even cachexia in patients with megaesophagus can combine with pulmonary infection to cause death. As in idiopathic achalasia, an increased incidence of cancer of the esophagus has been reported in patients with esophageal Chagas' disease.

Patients with megacolon associated with chronic *T. cruzi* infection are plagued by abdominal pain and chronic constipation. Persons with advanced disease can go for several weeks without having bowel movements, and acute obstruction, occasionally with volvulus, can lead to perforation, septicemia, and death.

Diagnostic Procedures

Chronic Chagas' disease is usually diagnosed by detection of IgG that binds specifically to *T. cruzi* antigens. Unlike acute Chagas' disease, it is not necessary to demonstrate the presence of the parasite to make the diagnosis of chronic Chagas' disease. Several highly sensitive serologic tests are used widely in Latin America, such as complement fixation (CF), indirect immunofluorescence (IIF), hemagglutination, and enzyme-linked immunosorbent assay (ELISA). A persistent problem with these conventional serodiagnostic assays, however, has been the occurrence of false-positive reactions. These reactions often occur with serum specimens from patients who have diseases such as leishmaniasis, malaria, syphilis, autoimmune diseases, and other parasitic and nonparasitic illnesses. Therefore, most experts recommend that sera be tested in two or three conventional assays before being accepted as positive. This latter approach obviously carries with it an enormous logistical and economic burden, especially for blood banks. For example, in the largest blood bank in São Paulo, Brazil, three serologic tests for antibodies to *T. cruzi* are used, and 3.4 per cent of donated units are discarded because they test positive with these assays. As many as two thirds of these may be false positives, but the blood must be discarded because of inconsistent test results. Therefore, it is important to keep in mind the possibility of false-positive reactions when evaluating the results of testing for antibodies to *T. cruzi.*

In Latin America, a number of test kits for detecting antibodies to *T. cruzi* are available commercially, but these are not used in the United States. There are several options here, however, for testing for chronic *T. cruzi* infection. Specimens can be sent to the Centers for Disease Control and Prevention (404-488-4414) for testing by IIF and CF. In addition, an assay based on an ELISA format, manufactured by Gull Laboratories (Salt Lake City, UT), has been approved by the FDA for clinical, but not blood bank, testing. This product has undergone only limited evaluation, and its sensitivity and specificity need to be defined further. In addition, Abbott Laboratories (Abbott Park, IL) recently has received similar FDA approval for marketing an ELISA-based test kit. Diagnostic assays in which recombinant *T. cruzi* proteins are used as the target antigens are being developed, as are PCR-based *T. cruzi* detection assays. These tests are not available commercially, and none has been approved for use in the United States.

In patients with chronic cardiac Chagas' disease, the most frequent electrocardiographic changes include premature ventricular contractions (PVCs), first- and third-degree atrioventricular (AV) block, left anterior fascicular block, and right bundle branch block (RBBB). The latter is perhaps the most representative conduction abnormality of Chagas' cardiopathy. Nonetheless, it is a nonspecific finding, and in nonendemic areas the vast majority of persons with RBBB do not have Chagas' disease. The radiographic and echocardiographic signs of chronic cardiac Chagas' disease are similar to those found in patients with cardiomyopathies and heart failure caused by other diseases. Megaesophagus and megacolon are best diagnosed with barium contrast studies. The clinician must recall, however, that the diagnosis of chronic Chagas' disease rests on demonstrating IgG antibodies to *T. cruzi.*

LEISHMANIASIS

By Judy A. Streit, M.D.,
and Mary E. Wilson, M.D.
Iowa City, Iowa

Leishmaniasis is a term that includes a spectrum of clinical syndromes caused by species of the dimorphic protozoan *Leishmania.* At one extreme is localized cutaneous leishmaniasis, a relatively benign and self-limited ulceronodular disease. At the other extreme is visceral leishmaniasis, a potentially fulminant disease that is fatal if left untreated. Manifestation of the syndrome depends on a complex interplay among the parasite's tropism for different organs, its invasiveness, and the host's immune status. The sandfly vector is necessary for transmission of infection, and often rodent or canine populations serve as reservoirs. The disease is widely distributed in the tropics and subtropics, with an estimated 12 million people infected and 350 million people at risk for infection. These figures are probably inaccurate because many infected individuals live in regions where epidemiologic surveillance is poor, and because the disease is often subclinical. Only by active immunologic testing of asymptomatic populations can total numbers of infected individuals be estimated.

Each clinical syndrome is usually caused by one or a group of *Leishmania* species endemic to a geographic region. Table 1 lists the species, the characteristic clinical syndromes resulting from infection, and the usual geographic locations where the organisms are found. Additionally, there are also unusual presentations or syndromes caused by many of the species. Knowledge of the distribution of *Leishmania* species is useful for clinical decisions, such as antibiotic selection and decision-to-treat. For example, drug resistance to first-line antimonial agents found in *L. aethiopica* of Africa may lead the clinician to consider an alternative regimen. Also, untreated localized cutaneous disease caused by *L. braziliensis* is often severe and slow to heal, and it carries a risk of subsequent mutilating mucocutaneous leishmaniasis. Hence, even mild cases are treated when this species is considered as the probable agent.

CUTANEOUS LEISHMANIASIS

Clinical Features

Cutaneous leishmaniasis (CL) is the most common form of disease caused by *Leishmania* spp. A papule develops at the site of parasite inoculation by the sandfly, usually in exposed areas, such as the legs, arms, and face. Over several weeks to months, the lesion slowly enlarges and eventually forms a shallow, nontender ulcer with indurated margins and a base of granulation tissue that may reach several centimeters in diameter. Serous drainage, satellite lesions, and regional lymphadenopathy may develop, along with occasional cutaneous horns at the site of the ulcer. The major morbidity is cosmetic, especially when the ulcer involves the face. Patients with CL are also at risk for secondary bacterial infection with *Staphylococcus* or *Streptococcus.* Spontaneous resolution may take months, often leaving an atrophic, hypopigmented scar.

Old World CL, referred to as "oriental sore," "bouton d'orient," or Baghdad boil, has classically been divided into the "wet," rurally acquired disease caused by *L. major* and the "dry," urban-acquired disease associated with *L. tropica.* New World CL, often caused by *L. amazonensis* or *L. mexicana,* has alternatively been called chiclero ulcer, pian bois, and uta. The number and size of lesions vary in CL. With infection by *L. braziliensis,* marked adenopathy occasionally precedes the development of the ulcer by several weeks. Infection with *L. guyanensis* can produce a sporotrichoid pattern of skin nodules or ulcers. Other complications of infection with *L. braziliensis* are discussed later, under the section on mucocutaneous leishmaniasis.

Several unusual forms of cutaneous disease can occur.

Table 1. Species of *Leishmania* That Commonly Cause Clinical Syndromes

Clinical Syndrome	Species of *Leishmania*	Distribution
Cutaneous Leishmaniasis—New World		
Localized	*L. (Leishmania) amazonensis**	Brazil, especially Amazon basin
	L. (L.) mexicana	Central America, Mexico
	L. (L.) pifanoi	Venezuela
	L. (L.) venezuelensis	Venezuela
	L. (Viannia) braziliensis	Latin America
	L. (V.) guyanensis	Guyana, Surinam, Amazon basin
	L. (V.) peruviana	Peru, Argentina
	L. (V.) panamensis	Costa Rica, Panama, Colombia
Diffuse cutaneous	*L. (L.) amazonensis*	Brazil, especially Amazon basin
	L. (L.) pifanoi	Venezuela
	L. (L.) mexicana	Central America, Mexico
Cutaneous Leishmaniasis—Old World		
Localized	*L. (L.) major*	Middle East, northwestern China, northwestern India, Pakistan, Africa
	L. (L.) aethiopica	Ethiopia, Kenya
	L. (L.) tropica	Middle East, western Asia, India, Mediterranean littoral
Diffuse cutaneous	*L. (L.) aethiopica*	Ethiopia, Kenya
Visceral Leishmaniasis—New World		
	L. (L.) chagasi	Latin America
Visceral Leishmaniasis—Old World		
	L. (L.) donovani	India, northern and eastern China, Nepal, Pakistan
	L. (L.) infantum	Africa, Middle East, Mediterranean littoral, Balkans, southwestern and central Asia, northwestern China
	L. (L.) archibaldi	Africa
Viscerotropic Leishmaniasis		
	L. (L.) tropica	Israel, India, Saudi Arabia (Desert Storm troops)
Mucocutaneous Leishmaniasis		
	L. (V.) braziliensis	Latin America

*The subgenus *Leishmania* or *Viannia* is indicated in parentheses. Often the subgenus name is not specified when referring to the organism (e.g., *L. amazonensis*).

In the Old World variety, a chronic, relapsing tuberculoid form is known as leishmaniasis recidivans. Disfiguring nodules on the face exhibit central healing as the lesions spread outward; biopsies show few organisms. By contrast, biopsies of the lesions of diffuse cutaneous leishmanisis (DCL) show many intracellular parasites in broad areas of the skin with little immune response. Nodules of DCL often disseminate to the face and upper extremities. These two clinical syndromes have been likened to the tuberculoid (paucibacillary) and the lepromatous (multibacillary) forms of leprosy, respectively.

Differential Diagnosis

The differential diagnosis of lesions consistent with CL includes sporotrichosis, chromoblastomycosis, lobomycosis, mycobacterial infection (*M. tuberculosis, M. leprae,* and atypical mycobacterial infections), treponemal infection, malignancy, and sarcoidosis.

Parasite Detection

A diagnosis of CL is firmly made by identification of the organism in tissue or in cultures obtained from appropriate lesions. After careful cleansing of a lesion, a 4- or 6-mm punch biopsy is obtained from intact, involved skin at the periphery of the ulcer. Alternatively, dermal scrapings can be obtained from a small incision or aspiration. Touch preparations from biopsy specimens should be air-dried, fixed in methanol, and stained with Wright's or Giemsa stain. Touch preparations from lesions of less than 6 months' duration typically contain more parasites than do older lesions. Histopathologic features include a histiocytic infiltrate with intracellular amastigotes present in macrophages. Identified by their characteristic kinetoplast and nucleus, amastigotes can be seen on the Giemsa stain, hematoxylin and eosin stain, or both. The use of fluoresceinated monoclonal antibodies directed against parasite antigens can markedly increase the ability to detect parasites in tissues, but these antibodies are not yet commercially available. Detection rates for *Leishmania* infection can also be improved by culture. Disrupted tissue, aspirate, or scraped materials are inoculated into parasite growth media, such as Novy, McNeal, and Nicolle (NNN) medium, maintained at 22 to 26°C, and checked for growth over the course of 2 to 5 weeks. Species such as *L. braziliensis* are traditionally difficult to grow in culture. Thus, lesion material may also be inoculated into the skin of a hamster or mouse to observe for characteristic changes at the injection site.

Leishmanin Skin Test

A positive leishmanin skin test, or Montenegro skin test, with the use of standard preparations of either killed promastigotes or promastigote extract, indicates the presence of cell-mediated delayed-type cutaneous hypersensitivity to parasite antigens. A positive test result correlates well with active or healed CL. Standard antigen (0.1 mL) is injected intradermally and evaluated at 48 to 72 hours for induration. Induration of 5 mm or more indicates a positive test result. During the first month of cutaneous disease, the Montenegro test is negative. Over the ensuing months, nearly 85 per cent of patients infected with diverse species of *Leishmania* will develop a positive test result, and patients who have tested positive may continue to test positive for years.

Serology

When antibodies are detected during the course of localized CL, they are usually present at low titer. For populations in whom leishmaniasis is endemic, positive serologic test results do not provide useful information about acute infection. In expatriates, a positive serologic test result may be more useful for supporting a diagnosis of leishmaniasis. Unfortunately, cross-reactivity with *Trypanosoma cruzi* and other parasites decreases specificity. Thus, serology is often not requested in patients with CL. In contrast with localized disease, patients with DCL may have significant antileishmanial titers (see the discussion of visceral leishmaniasis for serologic techniques).

MUCOCUTANEOUS LEISHMANIASIS

Clinical Features

Months to many years after the healing of the cutaneous ulcer caused by *L. braziliensis,* a destructive process of nasal and upper airway mucosa can develop, referred to as mucocutaneous leishmaniasis (MCL) or espundia. The initial signs and symptoms include central facial fullness and discomfort, epistaxis, and lip edema. These findings are followed by exophytic growths of the palate and destruction of nasal cartilage, lips, and, occasionally, the larynx. Destruction of the nasal septum results in the tapir-nose appearance. Three to twenty per cent of patients with CL caused by *L. braziliensis* eventually develop MCL. These numbers vary with the geographic area and with the racial origin of the host. Often, the atrophic scar of CL can be found in MCL patients, indicating the original site of parasite entry.

Differential Diagnosis

The lesion of MCL can resemble those seen in paracoccidioidomycosis, histoplasmosis, oropharyngeal carcinoma, tertiary treponemal infections (*T. pallidum* and *T. pertenue*), midline granuloma, and sarcoidosis.

Parasite Detection

In MCL, few organisms are present, especially early in the course of the disease. Therefore, biopsy material often does not contain detectable amastigotes on microscopy. Unfortunately, *L. braziliensis* is notoriously difficult to culture, and animal models often do not develop lesions. Multiple specimens for histologic examination can enhance detection of organisms. As the disease progresses, the number of organisms increases, so a repeat biopsy may be useful.

Leishmanin Skin Test

More than 85 per cent of patients with MCL have a positive Montenegro skin test. In an endemic region, with a scar consistent with previous localized CL and with a positive Montenegro skin test and typical mucocutaneous lesions, a presumptive diagnosis of MCL may be made.

Serology

Patients with MCL typically have higher antileishmanial titers than patients with CL. Thus, indirect fluorescent antibody tests that use amastigote antigen yield positive results in more than 85 per cent of patients. During the first 2 years of MCL infection, similar sensitivities are obtained with the use of the enzyme-linked immunosorbent assay (ELISA).

VISCERAL LEISHMANIASIS

Clinical Features

Visceral leishmaniasis (VL), or kala-azar, results from widespread reticuloendothelial involvement by species in the *L. donovani* complex. The onset of disease usually occurs several months after initial infection and can be insidious or fulminant. The signs and symptoms include fever, night sweats, abdominal distention, weight loss, anorexia, and epistaxis. Physical examination can reveal a markedly enlarged, soft, nontender spleen, hepatomegaly, emaciation, and thin skin with hair loss on the extremities. Lymphadenopathy may be notable, particularly in Sudan. Peripheral edema and petechiae may be seen, and generalized hyperpigmentation has been attributed to adrenal insufficiency. Laboratory studies reveal pancytopenia, mildly elevated aminotransferases, hyperglobulinemia with circulating immune complexes, and proteinuria. Secondary bacterial infections of the skin and lower and upper respiratory tract are common and account for much of the mortality directly related to the disease.

A number of cases of VL have been reported in patients with compromised cellular immunity, including those infected with human immunodeficiency virus (HIV) or patients who have received transplanted organs. The presentation can be similar to that in noncompromised persons, although a number of cases document unusual presentations without splenomegaly in HIV disease.

Following the deployment of United States troops to areas in the vicinity of the Persian Gulf endemic for *L. tropica,* systemic illness was seen. The presentation was highly variable and included headache, prolonged fever, abdominal pain with diarrhea, lymphadenopathy, mild anemia, and minor elevations in serum aminotransferases. A diagnosis of leishmaniasis was made by isolation of *L. tropica* from the bone marrow of patients and a few asymptomatic but epidemiologically linked individuals. *Leishmania tropica* had not previously been known to involve organs other than the skin. This relatively novel form of leishmaniasis was termed viscerotropic leishmaniasis.

A complication of VL seen in Africa and India is post–kala-azar dermal leishmaniasis (PKDL). Months to years after treatment of VL, hyperpigmented macules or nodules can appear on multiple areas of the body, including the mucous membranes. Associated peripheral neuropathy has been reported. PKDL develops more readily after incomplete treatment of VL and can persist chronically. Thus, the syndrome may contribute to the existence of a human reservoir of disease.

Differential Diagnosis

Visceral leishmaniasis must be distinguished from hematologic malignancies, malaria (especially tropical splenomegaly syndrome), schistosomiasis, typhoid fever, typhus, infectious mononucleosis, miliary tuberculosis, and brucellosis.

Parasite Detection

A definitive diagnosis of VL relies on the demonstration of the parasite in a tissue or fluid sample. A bone marrow aspirate is typically acquired for stain with Wright's or Giemsa stain. Splenic puncture often yields diagnostic information but may be complicated by hemorrhage and therefore is avoided if possible. When lymphadenitis is present, aspiration of the node may be performed. In immunocompromised patients, buffy coat of the blood may demonstrate amastigotes in peripheral monocytes. In addition, culture of bone marrow aspirate specimens notably increases the rates of diagnosis. Similarly, cultures of blood, buffy coat, lymph node, and spleen have also yielded isolates of *Leishmania*.

Serology

Most patients with active VL have antileishmanial antibodies, which can persist at low levels for years even after effective therapy. Titers are often quite high, except in patients with HIV infection. The percentage of patients with positive serology varies with the detection method used, and, overall, the sensitivity of serology is said to be roughly equal to that of the combination of the definitive microscopic and culture methods. The diagnostic techniques employed have included ELISA, complement fixation, direct and indirect hemagglutination, indirect immunofluorescence, and Western blot. Some reports indicate improved sensitivity when combinations of tests are used. Currently, the Centers for Disease Control and Prevention (CDC) use indirect immunofluorescence and employ a panel of three *Leishmania* species as antigen. Cross-reactivity with other parasitic diseases, especially *T. cruzi* and *M. leprae* infection, creates difficulties in interpretation of the test in endemic populations. Some recombinant *Leishmania* antigens are being tested for their ability to circumvent the problem of cross-reactivity, and several look quite promising. The direct agglutination test (DAT) is an assay of the ability of dilutions of serum to agglutinate fixed, stained promastigotes. Reports from Sudan indicate good sensitivity and specificity when specific parameters are used for interpretation of a positive test. Titers achieved with this technique vary with disease activity and therefore can be used as a marker for recrudescence of active VL. The ease with which this test can be performed in the field makes it useful where fluoresceinated or radioactive materials cannot be used.

Leishmanin Skin Test

Patients with active VL do not have delayed cutaneous hypersensitivity to parasite antigen, and this test is not useful in the diagnosis of the illness. After successful therapy, the test usually becomes positive and remains so for years. It is a marker for protection against reinfection. Thus, leishmanin skin test reactivity is useful in epidemiologic studies that assess the prevalence of immunity to *Leishmania*. This test does not distinguish among the different *Leishmania* species, however.

Future Molecular Techniques

Recombinant techniques have allowed the development of probes that can detect *Leishmania* DNA in tissue or aspirated material with greater sensitivity than microscopic techniques. Parasite detection by in situ hybridization with the use of probes specific for *Leishmania* species DNA requires at least a moderate parasite burden in tissues. However, the use of the polymerase chain reaction (PCR) to amplify *Leishmania* sequences allows for the detection of one organism. Neither of these tests is commercially available. Obviously, nonradioactive variations of these techniques will be needed before they can be useful in many locations where leishmaniasis is epidemic. Also being developed are tests for species identification, including Southern blot, dot blot, and restriction fragment analysis. Such rapid techniques for determination of the etiologic agent could be a significant improvement over the isoenzyme analysis currently being used.

Helminthic and Other Parasitic Diseases

SCHISTOSOMIASIS

By G. Thomas Strickland, M.D., Ph.D.
Baltimore, Maryland

Schistosomiasis is a parasitic disease with a wide distribution in the tropics and subtropics (Figs. 1 and 2). The worldwide prevalence of infection is estimated at 200 million; three times that number are potentially exposed.

Infection with schistosomes occurs after skin exposure in fresh water contaminated by cercariae. In endemic areas, the most common exposures are from swimming, bathing, playing, and washing utensils or clothes in streams, rivers, or canals, and water contact during irrigation of fields. Expatriates or travelers are usually exposed during recreational activities in streams, lakes, ponds, canals, or rivers. The patient with schistosomiasis must have an exposure history in an endemic area (see Figs. 1 and 2). Depending on the stage of illness, exposure could have been as recent as 2 weeks or in the distant past.

Infection in humans is caused by three species of this digenetic trematode (i.e., *Schistosoma mansoni, S. haematobium,* and *S. japonicum*) and other less common, less widely distributed species (e.g., *S. mekongi, S. intercalatum*). Infection occurs after exposure of intact skin to fresh water containing a motile larval stage, the cercaria. Cercariae are shed into the water from the specific snail host and penetrate the skin of the definitive human host. After skin penetration, cercariae shed their tails to become schistosomules, which migrate through the body to specific sites (i.e., the mesenteric venules for *S. mansoni* and *S. japonicum* and the bladder venules for *S. haematobium*)

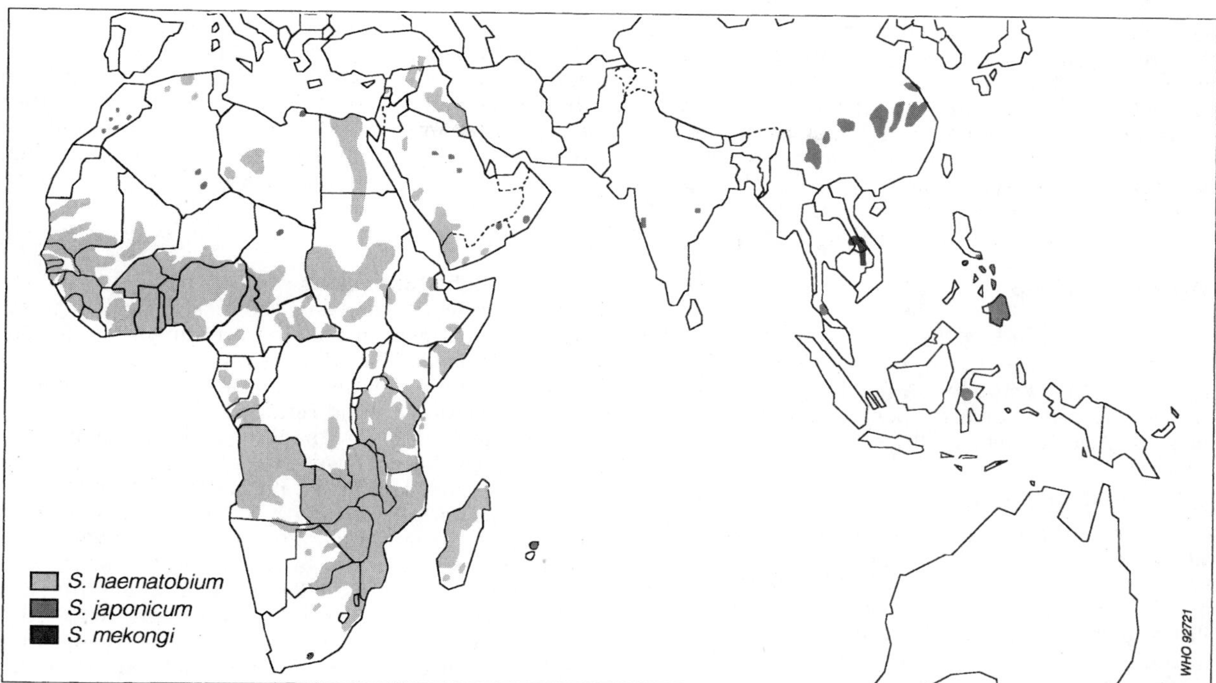

Figure 1. Global distribution of schistosomiasis due to *Schistosoma haematobium, S. japonicum,* and *S. mekongi.* (From The Control of Schistosomiasis: Second Report of The WHO Expert Committee. Geneva, World Health Organization, 1993. WHO Technical Report Series, No. 830, with permission.)

where the adult flukes reside. These migrations are not absolute; some clinical syndromes are caused by adult worms and/or ova in ectopic sites. After maturation and fertilization, the adult female blood flukes begin to lay eggs. Some 50 per cent of eggs exit the body in feces and urine, reach fresh water, and hatch to release a motile larval stage, the miracidium, which can infect the snail intermediate host. About 50 per cent of the ova are retained in the liver, intestines, urinary bladder, and elsewhere, triggering granulomatous reactions and disease.

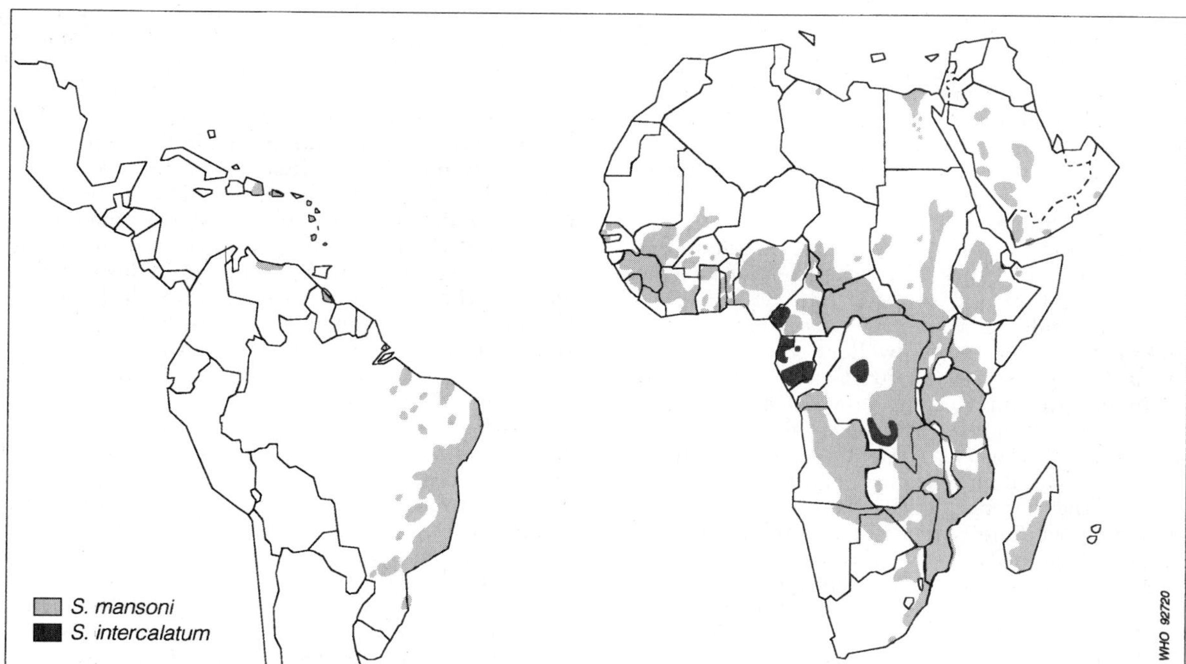

Figure 2. Global distribution of schistosomiasis due to *Schistosoma mansoni* and *S. intercalatum.* (From The Control of Schistosomiasis: Second Report of The WHO Expert Committee. Geneva, World Health Organization, 1993. WHO Technical Report Series, No. 830, with permission.)

Although recognizable disease caused by *Schistosoma* dates to antiquity in China and Egypt, the parasite was not identified until 1851 when Theodor Bilharz, working in the Kasr El Aini Hospital in Cairo, detected the etiologic worm of Egyptian endemic hematuria and named it *Distoma haematobium* (later changed to *Schistosoma haematobium*). Bilharziasis is synonymous with the clinical human disease caused by schistosomes.

SIGNS AND SYMPTOMS

The majority of patients with schistosomiasis have repeated infections resulting in chronic manifestations, often without recognizable symptoms. A few have skin manifestations associated with cercarial penetration or an acute, immunologically caused febrile illness.

Schistosome Cercarial Dermatitis

Cercarial dermatitis is a pruritic papular eruption that occurs at the site of cercarial skin penetration. It is often called swimmers' or clam diggers' itch. The pathologic lesion typically consists of edema and heavy dermoepidermal eosinophil and mononuclear infiltrates around the dying schistosomules. The lesions are commonly caused by nonhuman avian and small mammal schistosomes that penetrate the skin but are unable to develop further. A milder form of cercarial dermatitis occurs in individuals who have been sensitized to the cercariae of human parasites. Symptoms vary from a mild, brief pruritic rash at the site of exposure to more severe lesions in those who have marked hypersensitivity.

Acute Schistosomiasis (Katayama Fever)

Nineteenth century reports from the Katayama River Valley in Japan (an area formerly hyperendemic for schistosomiasis japonica) detailed a clinical syndrome of abrupt onset of fever, chills, abdominal pain, diarrhea, nausea, vomiting, cough, headache, urticaria, hepatosplenomegaly, and lymphadenopathy. This syndrome was later shown to be associated with marked eosinophilia and increased concentrations of immunoglobulins G and E in the serum. This illness, now thought to be a serum sickness–like reaction, occurs 4 to 6 weeks after heavy infection when the first schistosome egg production and release takes place. The acute disease lasts up to several weeks and may be associated with a significant mortality.

Acute schistosomiasis is exceedingly rare in endemic areas where children are exposed to schistosomal antigens and antibodies in utero and to infection early in life. It occurs focally in endemic countries where transmission spreads to new sites and in city dwellers who are exposed while visiting the countryside. Tourists and other nonimmune individuals who enter cercariae-infested waters may also have acute schistosomiasis. Because the illness occurs 4 to 6 weeks after exposure, patients often seek initial medical care from local practitioners, when diagnosis is complicated by the absence of the characteristic ova in the excreta. In descending frequency, acute schistosomiasis occurs from infections with *S. japonicum, S. mansoni,* and *S. haematobium.* Acute infections from one species may also occur in patients with chronic schistosomiasis caused by another species.

Another form of acute illness is spinal schistosomiasis. This syndrome, most often seen in *S. mansoni* infections, usually presents as a transverse myelitis with variable neurologic signs such as paraplegia, loss of bladder control, and loss of anal sphincter function. Spinal disease is caused by ova or migrating worms in the anterior spinal arteries and/or the spinal cord. This relatively rare syndrome has typically been reported in tourists or other expatriates after initial exposure to cercaria-contaminated water. Spinal schistosomiasis is even rarer in individuals who have been chronically and repeatedly exposed to infection since birth.

Chronic Schistosomiasis

Chronic schistosomiasis, the most prevalent form of the disease, is the condition most frequently referred to as schistosomiasis. The pathophysiologic process is basically the same in all patients: a chronic granulomatous and fibrous reaction around retained ova in the tissues.

Most individuals with chronic schistosomiasis do not seek medical care. However, they may have symptoms and signs that are considered normal in the endemic population: blood in the stool (with *S. mansoni* and *S. japonicum* infections), terminal hematuria (in *S. haematobium* infections), and malaise and fatigue (from anemia in infections caused by any species). These patients may have hepatosplenomegaly. However, in most endemic areas, there are other infections that can cause enlarged spleens and livers, and many with schistosomiasis do not have these manifestations. The most frequent finding in those with ova-associated inflammatory lesions of the gut (with *S. mansoni* or *S. japonicum* infections) is repeated episodes of blood in the stool. These patients may also be anemic. A relatively rare complication, intestinal polyposis, can lead to malabsorption and cause considerable loss of blood and protein.

Hepatosplenic schistosomiasis is the most important complication associated with *S. mansoni* and *S. japonicum* infections. It occurs most frequently in patients with longstanding heavy infections. The periportal fibrosis resulting from presinusoidal trapping of ova in the liver leads to portal hypertension with relatively normal liver function (except in those with concomitant hepatitis B or C). The enlarged liver gradually involutes, and splenomegaly is almost universal. These patients bleed from ruptured esophageal varices and may have repeated bouts of hematemesis if they survive the bleeding episodes.

The inflammatory response around *S. haematobium* ova in the bladder wall causes terminal hematuria, dysuria, frequency, and urgency. Red blood cells and protein may be detected on urinalysis. More chronic complications include bladder wall polyposis, calcification, squamous cell carcinoma, and obstructive uropathy. Granulomatous lesions of *S. haematobium* in the bladder and lower ureters may obstruct the outflow of urine, leading to hydroureter and hydronephrosis. Pyelonephritis is a complication of obstruction, and renal failure may ensue if both the schistosomiasis and the bacterial infections are not treated and cured.

Less frequent clinical syndromes occurring with chronic schistosomiasis include bladder carcinoma; intestinal polyposis; cor pulmonale (from trapping of ova in the pulmonary arterioles due to shunting of ova around the liver in some patients with portal hypertension); epilepsy (from cerebral granulomas usually caused by ectopic ova and worms of *S. japonicum*); glomerulonephritis in patients with chronic *S. mansoni* infections; and eosinophilic pneumonitis (after heavy larval migration through the lungs in initial infections). Chronic persistent low-grade enteric fever that is unresponsive to antibacterial therapy has been reported in patients with chronic schistosomiasis. An association of schistosomiasis (particularly schistosomiasis mansoni and schistosomiasis japonica) with chronic hepatitis B and C infections has also been documented.

Schistosomiasis in Expatriates and/or Travelers

Nonimmune travelers may seek medical care for either the febrile immune complex or the transverse myelitis form of acute schistosomiasis. These acute syndromes typically occur 4 to 8 weeks after exposure to cercaria-contaminated fresh water. The first manifestations of chronic schistosomiasis are usually terminal hematuria in those infected with *S. haematobium* and mucohemorrhagic loose stools in those with *S. mansoni* or *S. japonicum* infections. Hepatomegaly and a palpable spleen may be present.

PARASITOLOGIC EXAMINATIONS

If schistosomiasis is suspected, the stool (for *S. mansoni* and *S. japonicum*) and urine (for *S. haematobium*) should be microscopically examined to detect the parasite ova (Fig. 3). Serologic tests, biopsies, endoscopy, and imaging can supplement the parasitologic examinations, but parasitologic studies of stool and urine are the linchpins of diagnosis.

Stool Parasitology

Direct wet-film examination is performed by placing a small portion of a fresh stool mixed with a drop of normal saline on a microscope slide, applying a coverslip, and scanning the entire slide under the microscope. Because *Schistosoma* ova are relatively large, the slide is best reviewed at low power (×100). *S. mansoni* ova are oval, 115 to 175 μm in length and 45 to 70 μm in width; they have a prominent lateral spine (see Fig. 3*B*). *S. japonicum* ova are more rounded, 70 to 100 μm in length and 50 to 65 μm in width; they have a small lateral hook (see Fig. 3*C*). Iodine and other stains may be used if desired. The sensitivity of a direct wet film is low, especially in patients with mild infections, because the amount of stool examined is exceedingly small.

Methods that concentrate the stool increase the sensitivity of the microscopic examination. Some methods separate the eggs from the bulk of fecal material on the basis of specific gravity. In sedimentation methods such as formalin-ether and zinc sulfate, eggs more dense than the suspending liquid concentrate at the bottom of the tube. In the formalin-ether method, an ether layer at the top is separated from the larger formalin layer by debris and fat. The eggs are found in the sediment at the bottom of the tube. After the supernatant is poured off, the sediment is placed on a microscope slide and scanned at low power (×100). Although the sensitivity of the sedimentation methods is better than that of the direct wet film, several examinations must be performed on different specimens before it is concluded that schistosomiasis is unlikely.

The Kato thick smear is used to screen stool for schistosomal ova and provides an estimate of relative intensity of infection. A sample of feces that has been pressed through a 105-mesh steel sieve is packed into a steel template that holds 50 mg of stool (about the size of a pea) and then placed on a glass slide. This sample is covered with a cellophane coverslip impregnated with glycerin and then inverted and pressed onto a bed of filter paper. The slide is left for 24 to 48 hours to allow the fecal material to clear. All eggs on the slide are counted under low power (×100). Multiplying this number by 20 gives the number of ova per gram of stool.

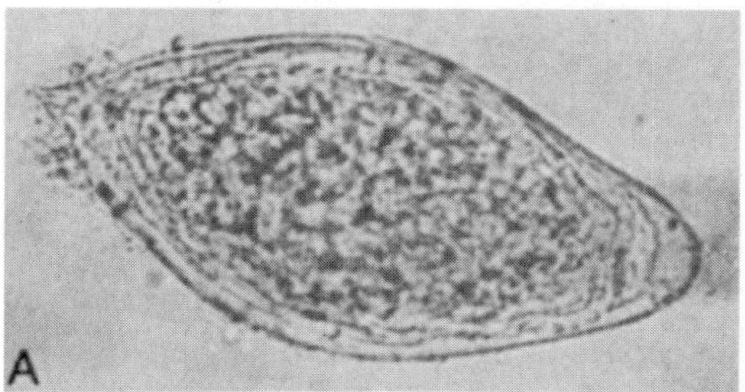

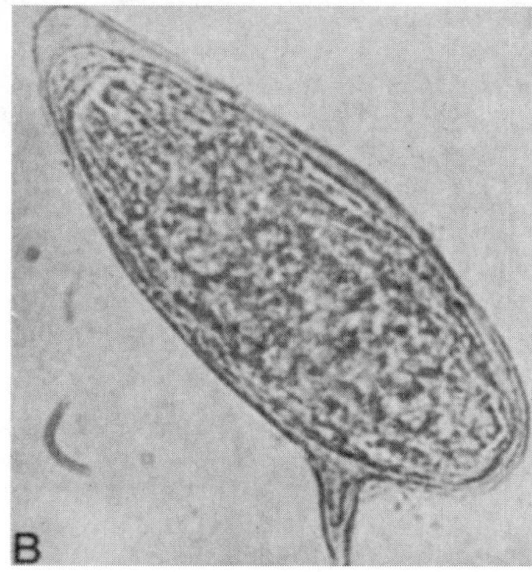

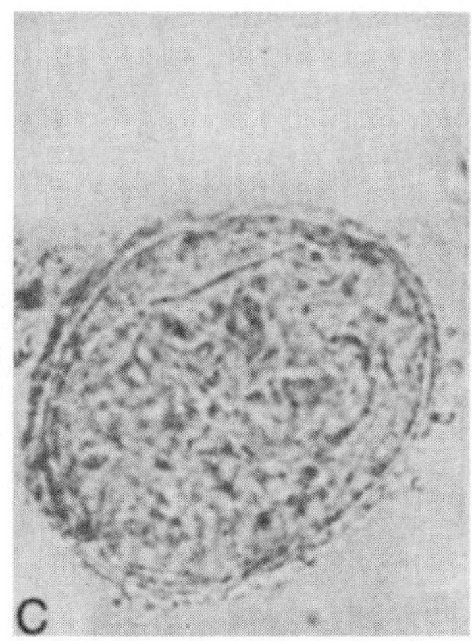

Figure 3. Ova of schistosomes commonly infecting humans. *A, S. haematobium* with terminal spine, taken from urine (×500). *B, S. mansoni* with prominent lateral spine, taken from feces (×500). *C, S. japonicum* taken from feces (×500). (Courtesy of Dr. R. L. Roudabush. Ward's Natural Science Establishment, Rochester, NY.)

The Kato smear has the same limitations as the direct smear and concentration methods do. Sensitivity can be improved by performing duplicate examinations on three separate stool samples.

Urine Parasitology

Eggs in the urine can be detected either by simple sedimentation or by membrane filtration (see Fig. 3*A*). A specimen obtained between 10 AM and 2 PM provides the best opportunity to detect parasites. A 10-mL aliquot of urine is allowed to deposit sediment, or it can be spun briefly in

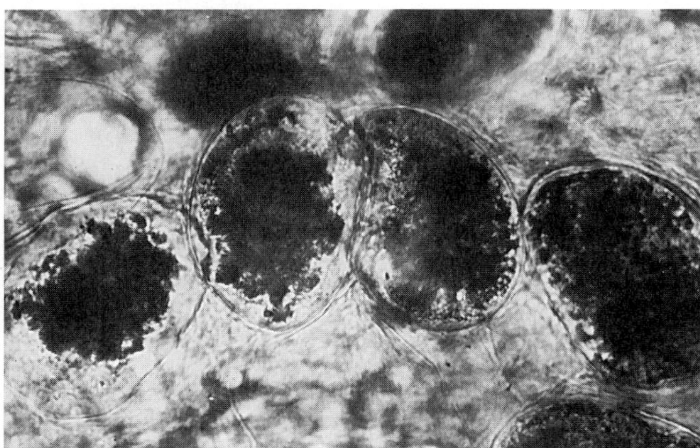

Figure 4. Calcified *S. japonicum* ova in a rectal snip biopsy from a patient with a chronic infection (×500).

a centrifuge. The supernatant is removed and the sediment poured onto a microscope slide. After a coverslip is applied, all eggs on the slide are counted under low power (×100). This provides the number of ova in 10 mL of urine and permits the detection and measurement of red and white blood cells in the specimen. Membrane filtration using a Nucleopore or similar filter to trap the eggs provides a similar quantitative count.

Other Tests for Parasites

Rectal snip biopsy is the least invasive means of establishing the diagnosis in patients who do not have detectable eggs in stool and urine. A snip of the rectal mucosa is taken during sigmoidoscopy, placed between two slides, and observed microscopically under low power (×100). The ova are easily visualized, particularly under reduced light. Active infections can be confirmed by movement of the miracidium within the egg (flame cell activity). Older inactive infections are characterized by calcified black eggs (Fig. 4). Biopsy specimens taken from small inflamed or granulomatous mucosal lesions (sandy patches) are more likely to reveal ova; but in the absence of lesions, biopsy samples of normal mucosa should be taken. Some rectal snips can be fixed in formalin for histopathologic examination, but direct microscopy provides the quickest and least expensive approach to establishing the diagnosis.

In patients who might have schistosomiasis haematobia, mucosal biopsy of the bladder during cystoscopy often confirms the diagnosis. These specimens are handled in the same manner as rectal biopsy specimens.

SEROLOGIC DIAGNOSIS

Serology can be helpful in light and in prepatent infections in which eggs are difficult to detect microscopically. Antibodies to *Schistosoma* signify current or past infection. Circulating schistosomal antigen detection remains a research tool, not yet clinically available. At best, it has a sensitivity of 80 per cent and a specificity of 95 per cent compared with carefully performed multiple examinations of the stool or urine. A positive result generally means the subject has, or recently had, an active schistosomal infection.

Antibody Tests

The Parasitic Disease Division of the National Center for Infectious Diseases in Atlanta, Georgia (telephone: 404–488–4050), routinely screens sera for schistosomal antibody with a Falcon assay screening test enzyme-linked immunosorbent assay (FAST-ELISA). Positive samples are confirmed and speciated with the enzyme-linked immunoelectro-transfer blot (EITB). The FAST-ELISA and EITB use microsomal antigens of adult schistosomes to detect serum antibodies.

OTHER BLOOD TESTS

Patients from endemic areas with chronic schistosomiasis often have characteristic abnormalities in blood tests. They may have anemia, and if there is an associated splenomegaly with hypersplenism, they may have leukopenia and thrombocytopenia. A mild eosinophilia (3 to 8 per cent) is the rule. Liver function tests, with the exception of alkaline phosphatase, are usually unremarkable in the absence of concomitant infection with hepatitis B or C virus. Tests of renal function are usually normal unless obstructive uropathy is present in patients with *S. haematobium* infections. These patients may have increased serum urea nitrogen and serum creatinine concentrations. Hypergammaglobulinemia with marked increases in IgG isotypes is frequent in chronic schistosomiasis, and hypoalbuminemia may be detected in hepatosplenic schistosomiasis. Patients with acute schistosomiasis have a marked eosinophilia (10 to 30 per cent) as well as increased IgG and IgE concentrations in their serum. They often do not have ova in their stool or urine during initial examination. Expatriates, or other nonimmune adults, may also demonstrate eosinophilia and increased immunoglobulin G and E concentrations. However, these patients often have no, or no other, serum or blood cell abnormalities.

DIAGNOSTIC PROCEDURES

Some diagnostically useful tests demonstrate lesions of schistosomiasis that are reversible after specific chemotherapy with praziquantel. These include endoscopy, radiography, ultrasonography, and, rarely, computed tomography or magnetic resonance imaging.

Endoscopy

Esophagoscopy demonstrates esophageal varices in patients with portal hypertension. Sigmoidoscopy and colonoscopy permit detection and biopsy of large bowel lesions, including polyps. Cystoscopy allows visualization and biopsy of bladder wall lesions in those with urinary schistosomiasis. Rarely, retrograde pyelography performed during cystoscopy provides useful anatomic information about the ureters and kidneys.

Radiography

Esophageal varices can be detected with barium swallow examination. A barium enema study may reveal colonic lesions, including polyps and rarer strictures. Evidence of pulmonary hypertension may be seen on the chest film of patients with schistosomal cor pulmonale. A plain film of the abdomen may show calcified bladder wall in a patient with long-standing heavy infection with *S. haematobium.* Intravenous pyelography could show hydronephrosis and/or hydroureters in patients with obstructive uropathy and may show renal, ureteral, or urinary bladder stones. Angiography occasionally reveals ectopic lesions in the brain and elsewhere.

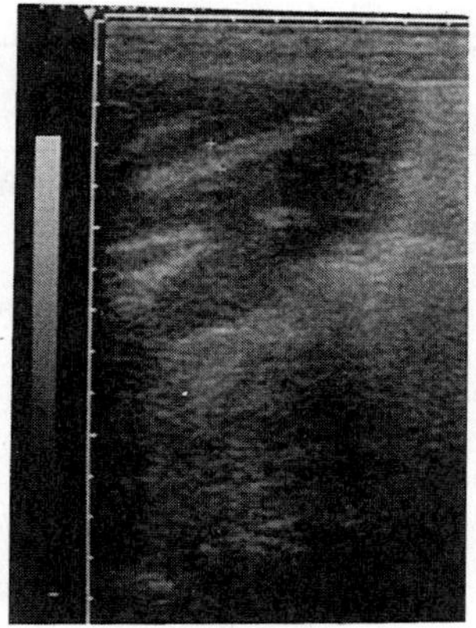
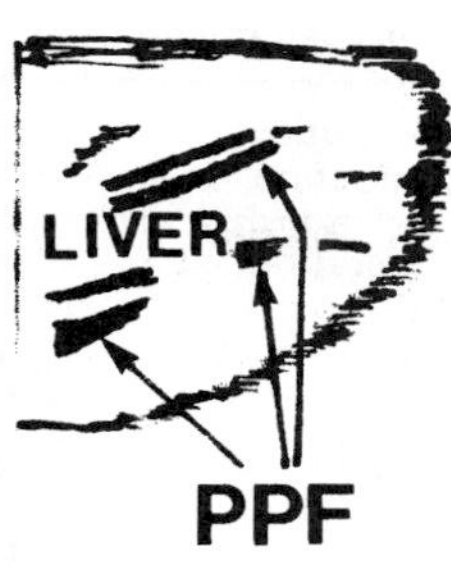

Figure 5. Grade II periportal fibrosis (PPF) detected by ultrasonography in the liver of an Egyptian patient with schistosomiasis due to *Schistosoma mansoni.*

Ultrasonography

Abdominal ultrasonography has revolutionized the evaluation of schistosomal morbidity. Its numerous advantages include production of low-cost real-time images in multiple planes without revision of format. Biologic hazard is negligible, and portability permits ease of use in rural or urban communities. The speed of the technique makes it ideal for screening populations and directing interventions (e.g., biopsies or aspirations).

Abdominal ultrasonography can accurately measure liver and spleen size and configuration. It can detect and grade periportal fibrosis (Fig. 5), with good sensitivity and specificity for schistosomal hepatic fibrosis. Ultrasonography can detect thickening of the gallbladder wall and the presence of gallstones. It can also detect and grade portal hypertension and predict the presence and severity of esophageal varices. It can detect bladder wall thickening, irregularities, polyps, and tumors (Fig. 6) and can often demonstrate bladder wall calcifications. Hydronephrosis and renal and bladder stones are easily visualized.

Computed Tomography and Magnetic Resonance Imaging

These procedures add little to other procedures except to better delineate lesions in the brain, abdomen, and pelvis. They are expensive and do not provide as much information as ultrasonography does.

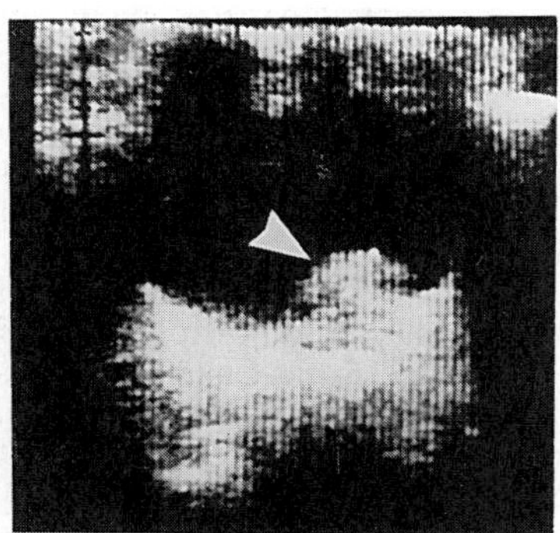
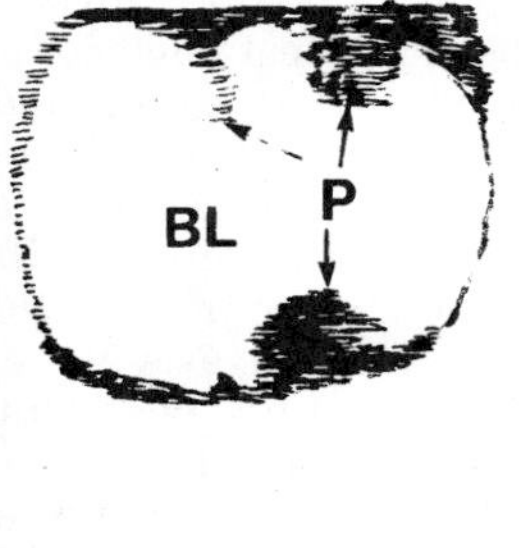

Figure 6. Large polyps (P) in the bladder (BL) in an Egyptian patient infected with *S. haematobium.*

OTHER TREMATODES

By Stan Houston, M.D.,
and Kinga Kowalewska-Grochowska, M.D.
Edmonton, Alberta, Canada

The nonschistosomal trematodes that infect humans are flat and symmetrical, resemble a fleshy leaf in appearance, and vary widely in size. All are capable of zoonotic infection, although in some settings humans may serve as the major reservoir host. Unlike the case with schistosomes, human infections with other trematodes are acquired by ingestion of the infective stage, usually in association with aquatic vegetation, aquatic animals, or fish. The life cycle of trematodes involves a snail and, in some species, a second intermediate host (Table 1). Most species are hermaphroditic and capable of self-fertilization. Trematode eggs in clinical specimens are oval and equipped with a lid (operculum), which raises to release a ciliated larva.

The three factors listed below are crucial in the diagnosis of trematode infections in humans.

EPIDEMIOLOGIC HISTORY. Most species of trematodes have limited and specific geographic distributions, and infections are associated with ingestion of specific foods.

CLINICAL FINDINGS. Human infection with each trematode species is associated with characteristic sites of involvement and symptom complexes. However, symptoms are usually nonspecific and fail to differentiate trematode infection from other possible causes of illness. In addition, trematode infections are often asymptomatic.

IDENTIFICATION OF OVA. Identification of ova usually involves stool examination, but ova of some trematode species may be found in biliary aspirates, sputum, or pleural fluid.

Trematode infections are encountered infrequently in many clinical laboratories, and subtle distinctions in microscopic findings may be clinically important. Therefore, specimens should be examined by a reference laboratory when the microscopic diagnosis is difficult or unusual. In the diagnosis of trematode infections, formalin-ether concentration techniques are preferred to the zinc sulfate flotation techniques because the latter technique may rupture operculated eggs. Occasionally, adult flukes are detected in vomitus, duodenal or biliary aspirate, or stool, especially following antihelmintic treatment. In some circumstances, examination of an adult form is the only means of identifying species.

The value of serology is limited in trematode infections because cross-reactions between species commonly occur and seropositivity may persist for many years after seroconversion. Serology, however, may be useful in some well-defined clinical situations. A range of assays for detection of parasite antigens and products in serum or feces is available in research laboratories; new methods, including DNA hybridization and enzyme immunoassay (EIA), are under development. Imaging procedures may also be useful in a few specific situations.

INTESTINAL TREMATODES

Fasciolopsiasis

Fasciolopsis buski is the largest human trematode; adult flukes reach 75 mm in length. The geographic distribution of this trematode is patchy; the disease has been reported

Table 1. Features of Nonschistosomal Trematode Infections in Humans

Fluke	Geographic Distribution	Usual Source of Infection	Usual Site and Symptoms
Fasciolopsis buski	S.E. Asia, S. China, India	Aquatic vegetation, e.g., water caltrop	*Small Bowel:* diarrhea and abdominal pain
Heterophyes and *Metagonimus*	Nile, Middle East, Far East, S.E. Asia	Uncooked fish	*Small Bowel:* abdominal pain, diarrhea, rare metastatic lesions
Opisthorchis viverrini	Thailand, Laos, Cambodia	Uncooked fish	*Biliary Tract:* biliary symptoms, cholangiocarcinoma
O. felineus	Central and eastern Europe, Asia	Uncooked fish	*Biliary Tract:* biliary symptoms, cholangiocarcinoma
Clonorchis sinensis	China, Taiwan	Uncooked fish	*Biliary Tract:* biliary symptoms, cholangiocarcinoma
Fasciola	Wide, patchy temperate and tropical distribution	Aquatic plants (watercress)	*Liver to Biliary Tract:* RUQ pain, fever, eosinophilia, biliary symptoms
Paragonimus	Mainly Far East, also W. Africa, Latin America	Uncooked crabs, crayfish	*Lung* *Other: subcutaneous, CNS, abdomen.* Symptoms include chronic cough, chest pain, hemoptysis, migratory subcutaneous swelling, CNS symptoms
Other *Echinostoma, Gastrodiscoides*	S.E. Asia, India	Varies with species	*Small Bowel, Colon:* diarrhea

RUQ = right upper quadrant; CNS = central nervous system.

from central and south China, India, Bangladesh, and Southeast Asia. The prevalence of *F. buski* infection appears to be greatest where pig raising accompanies the cultivation of water caltrop. The reservoir hosts are humans and pigs. The intermediate host, a freshwater snail, releases cercariae that encyst on the water caltrop, water chestnut, or other aquatic vegetation. Human infection occurs when these are ingested. The eggs then hatch in the gastrointestinal tract and mature in about 3 months to adult worms, which attach to the duodenal or jejunal mucosa and cause inflammation and ulceration.

The majority of infections are asymptomatic. Upper abdominal "hunger pains" suggestive of peptic ulcer disease may occur. Diarrhea is probably the most common symptom and is related to worm burden. In heavy infestations, gastrointestinal hemorrhage, obstruction, protein-losing enteropathy, or systemic allergic manifestations can occur. Death is rare, and this parasite is not known to cause metastatic or extraintestinal disease.

The diagnosis is typically made by identification of the characteristic eggs in stool. The ova of *Echinostoma* species, *Fasciola hepatica,* and *Fasciolopsis buski* overlap in size and shape, and, therefore, exact species identification cannot be made from examination of the eggs alone. The distinction between *Fasciola* and *Fasciolopsis* is clinically important and must be made by considering geographic source of infection, clinical findings, anatomic source of specimen, and, possibly, *Fasciola* serology. If an adult fluke can be obtained, the distinction is easily made. A peripheral eosinophilia may be found.

Heterophyiasis and Metagonimiasis

These diseases are caused by the closely related intestinal flukes *Heterophyes heterophyes* and *Metagonimus yokogawai*. Human infection with these tiny flukes (1 to 2 mm × 0.4 mm) has a patchy distribution in the Nile delta, the Middle East, and parts of Southeast Asia. The life cycle involves two intermediate hosts: a freshwater snail and a fish. Humans are infected by ingestion of inadequately cooked freshwater fish. Several animal species can serve as reservoir hosts. The tiny flukes live deep in the wall of the small intestine, where they can cause colicky abdominal pain and diarrhea, particularly with heavy infections. Rarely, either ova or adult flukes may penetrate the intestinal wall and metastasize hematogenously to other sites, such as the heart and brain.

The diagnosis is usually based on identification of ova in feces or duodenal aspirates. Experience is required to distinguish these ova from those of *Clonorchis* or *Opisthorchis.* Antigen detection methods may facilitate diagnosis in the near future. Peripheral eosinophilia may be present.

Less Well-Known Fluke Infections

Echinostomiasis refers to infection with one of at least 12 species of *Echinostoma*. Their geographic distribution includes Thailand, the Philippines, and Indonesia. Infection occurs following ingestion of raw freshwater snails or other second intermediate hosts. The flukes attach to the small intestine. Although the clinical features have not been well established, heavy infections appear to be associated with diarrhea and abdominal pain. Eggs of *Echinostoma* species can be demonstrated in the stool, but they overlap in size and shape with *Fasciola* and *Fasciolopsis* species. Certain identification may not be possible without examination of the adult fluke.

Gastrodisciasis is reported to be common in parts of India and has been found in Vietnam, the Philippines, and Kazakhstan. The 5- to 14-mm-long fluke *Gastrodiscoides* attaches to the cecum and ascending colon in humans and pigs. The infection is believed to be asymptomatic in most patients but may be associated with diarrhea.

A number of other flukes have been reported to cause human disease, either rarely or within specific geographic locations. Recently, for example, *Metorchis conjunctus*, a parasite of fish-eating mammals in northern Canada, has been found to cause clinical illness in humans.

LIVER FLUKES

Fascioliasis

Fascioliasis is most commonly caused by *Fasciola hepatica* and rarely by *F. gigantica*. This fluke is unusual in its widespread geographic distribution, including temperate zones, and it is the only important human trematode that does not respond to praziquantel treatment. Human infections occur in Latin America, across Europe and Asia, and in parts of Africa. Outbreaks resulting from local transmission have been described in England. However, fascioliasis is not recognized as either a common infection or a major health problem in any of these areas. *Fasciola gigantica* is primarily a bovine parasite. Human disease occurs occasionally, often with ectopic lesions.

Adult flukes of *F. hepatica* may be up to 30 mm in length. Sheep are the main reservoir host in most of the world, but cattle and other ungulates may also host the parasite, which is sometimes called the sheep liver fluke, causing "liver rot" in its natural host. Eggs shed in feces infect the intermediate host, a snail, which subsequently produces cercariae that, in turn, encyst on aquatic vegetation. Eating raw watercress containing the cysts is the most common route of transmission for fascioliasis in humans.

Once ingested, the parasite excysts and migrates, usually asymptomatically, through the small intestinal wall and into the peritoneal cavity. It then penetrates the liver capsule and migrates through the liver parenchymal tissue. The larvae develop into adults after reaching the bile ducts, where they attach and produce eggs, which subsequently reach the small intestine and are excreted in feces.

The signs and symptoms may be associated with the initial liver invasion, usually 1 to 3 months after ingestion of metacercariae. Local hepatic parenchymal damage has been demonstrated in animals and is thought to occur along the path of the parasite's migration through the hepatic parenchyma. The signs and symptoms associated with this stage may persist for several weeks or months and include nausea and vomiting, dyspepsia, right upper quadrant pain, and fever. Hepatomegaly and liver tenderness may occur, but jaundice is uncommon. A marked peripheral eosinophilia is typical. The severity of the illness is related to the parasite burden. Most human disease is mild, but in animals heavy infestations can be fatal. After the parasites reach the bile ducts, most patients are asymptomatic, but some may have persistent biliary symptoms related to irritation and obstruction of the biliary tract. Eosinophilia is more variable at this stage. Ectopic sites of parasite migration in the abdomen, chest, and even brain have been described.

The diagnosis in the acute stage of the disease should be suspected in an individual who may have been exposed through consumption of raw freshwater plants in an endemic area and who presents with fever, right upper quadrant pain or hepatomegaly, and eosinophilia. At this stage of the parasite's development, ova are usually not detectable in a stool or bile specimen, but serologic diagnosis may be helpful.

Ultrasound or computed tomography (CT) scans of the liver may show lucent areas in the early hepatic migration stage. Percutaneous needle liver biopsy is rarely helpful. Ultrasound and endoscopic retrograde cholangiopancreatography (ERCP) or percutaneous cholangiography may be useful in the biliary stage of the disease. Motile flukes have occasionally been seen on ultrasound. In addition, ERCP permits direct sampling of bile for parasitologic examination, and flukes can sometimes be visualized directly by cholangiography (Fig. 1).

Definitive diagnosis is based on demonstration of ova (or, rarely, flukes) in stool or bile. Spurious infection has been described, with ova seen in the stool for a few days after ingestion of *Fasciola*-infected animal liver. The ova are not reliably distinguishable from those of *Echinostoma ilocanum* or *Fasciolopsis buski*. Because treatment is different for fascioliasis, the distinction must be made by epidemiologic history, clinical syndrome, anatomic source of specimen, serology, or—best of all—microscopic examination of the adult fluke.

Numerous serologic tests for *Fasciola hepatica* have been developed. They can be very useful, particularly in early acute disease or in patients with ectopic infection. The results should be interpreted with caution, because *Fasciola hepatica* shares antigens with other trematodes (e.g., *Schistosoma mansoni, F. gigantica*) as well as with other parasites, and cross-reactions in immunologic assays are not unusual. Patients with infections remain seropositive for years; therefore, these tests usually fail to distinguish between acute infection and past exposure. New tests are being developed to detect parasite antigen in serum or stool, but these are not yet widely available.

Opisthorchiasis and Clonorchiasis

Opisthorchiasis and clonorchiasis are similar clinical conditions caused by the closely related species, *Opis-*

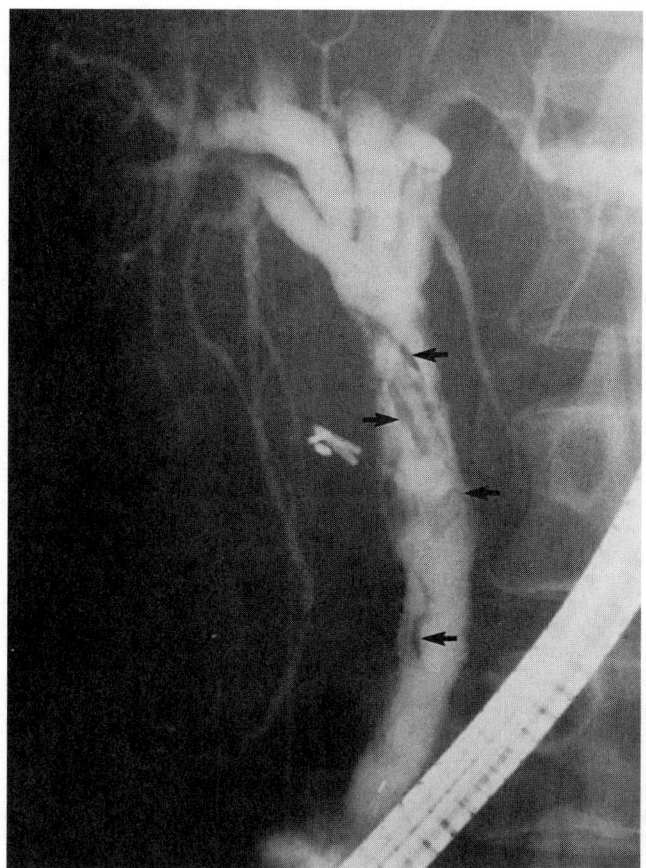

Figure 1. ERCP showing adult *Fasciola hepatica (arrows)* in a Canadian woman with biliary symptoms after travel to Indonesia. (Courtesy of Dr. Terry Talbot.)

thorchis viverrini, O. felineus, and *Clonorchis sinensis*. The geographic distribution of *O. viverrini* is primarily in north and northeast Thailand, Laos, and Cambodia, where some communities may have prevalence rates of 90 per cent. As many as 7 million people may be infected globally. *Opisthorchis felineus* has a patchy distribution across central and eastern Europe and western Siberia. It is estimated that *C. sinensis* affects some 25 million people, mainly in China and Taiwan, and immigrants from these areas.

The life cycle involves excretion of ova in the feces of humans or other reservoir hosts, such as dogs, cats, and fish-eating mammals. Several species of freshwater snails act as first intermediate hosts, and freshwater fish (usually carp) provide the second intermediate host. Human infection occurs from ingestion of inadequately cooked or raw pickled fish. Transmission of the disease is facilitated by the production of fish in ponds fertilized with human or animal feces. In humans, adult flukes can survive for at least 2 decades. After ingestion, the parasites excyst in the gut and migrate through the ampulla of Vater into the biliary tract, where they mature into 10- to 20-mm flukes, attach, and produce eggs. Pathologic changes and signs and symptoms are thought to be due to the irritation caused by worm attachment, inflammatory reaction, and secondary bacterial infection in the bile ducts. Disease generally correlates with worm burden; as many as 20,000 worms have been found in a single individual.

Most infected individuals have light infections, are asymptomatic, and suffer no demonstrable ill effects. Individuals with higher parasite burdens may experience a poorly defined spectrum of biliary and right upper quadrant symptoms. A syndrome of recurrent bacterial cholangitis, "Oriental cholangitis," has been attributed to *Clonorchis.* There is strong and consistent epidemiologic evidence of an association between infection with *Opisthorchis* or *Clonorchis* and the development of cholangiocarcinoma. Cholangiocarcinoma can be produced in an animal model by the combination of *Clonorchis* infection and carcinogen administration.

The diagnosis is usually made by finding ova in the stool or ova or adult flukes in bile aspirates. Experience is necessary to distinguish these ova from those of *Heterophyes* or *Metagonimus*. Several serologic tests have been developed, but they are unreliable and unavailable. Antigen detection tests for stool are under development. Ultrasound scans may show a number of abnormalities, including enlarged gallbladder, gallbladder sludge, hepatomegaly, and occasionally changes in or dilation of the common bile duct. Ultrasound or CT scans may also provide evidence of the presence of cholangiocarcinoma. ERCP may show irregularly dilated bile ducts, and flukes can sometimes be visualized as filling defects (Fig. 2).

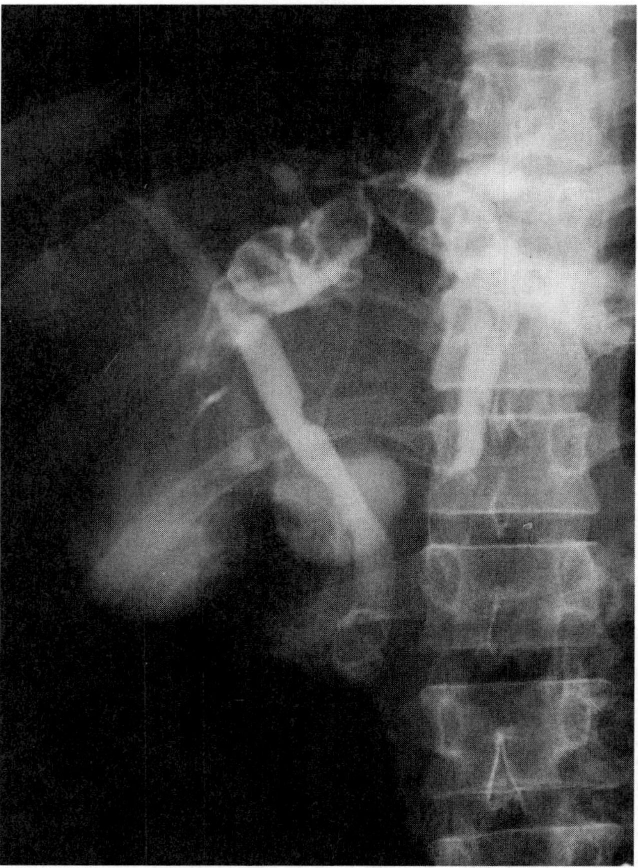

Figure 2. ERCP showing adult *Opisthorchis* in an immigrant from Vietnam. Note dilated bile ducts and multiple filling defects. (Courtesy of Drs. T. Alexander and R. Henning.)

LUNG FLUKES (PARAGONIMIASIS)

Infections with members of the genus *Paragonimus* may occur in many body sites, but they typically involve the lung. Several million people in Korea, China, Japan, and Taiwan are infested with *Paragonimus westermani.* Less commonly, paragonimiasis is found in other areas of Southeast Asia, as far east as Papua New Guinea. The disease has also been reported, associated with different species of *Paragonimus,* in West Africa and in Central and South America.

The life cycle involves freshwater snails as the first intermediate host and freshwater crabs or crayfish as the second intermediate host. Humans are usually infected by ingesting crabs that have been inadequately cooked or prepared by pickling without cooking, or from preparations made with juice from raw crabs. Reservoir hosts include a variety of carnivorous animals. After ingestion, the metacercariae excyst in the duodenum and penetrate the intestinal wall into the peritoneal cavity. From there they eventually migrate through the diaphragm into the pulmonary parenchyma, where the adults may reach 12 mm in length. The clinical signs and symptoms are often subacute or chronic and include cough, sputum production, hemoptysis, and chest pain, depending on the location of the lesion. Radiologic abnormalities may be the first indication of the presence and nature of the disease. Other important metastatic sites include the central nervous system, infection of which results in meningitis or focal lesions of the brain or spinal cord, and the abdomen. Migratory subcutaneous nodules, reminiscent of gnathostomiasis, appear to be more common with certain regional strains of *Paragonimus*.

The diagnosis is made by detection of characteristic ova in sputum, or in stool where they may be found after having been swallowed, or less commonly in pleural fluid or other sites. *Paragonimus* ova can be confused with those of *Diphyllobothrium latum*, the fish tapeworm, because of similarity of size, but essential morphologic details should allow experienced microscopists to make the diagnosis. Serology can be very helpful in distinguishing paragonimiasis from the many other diseases that may cause similar clinical syndromes or radiographic findings and is of particular

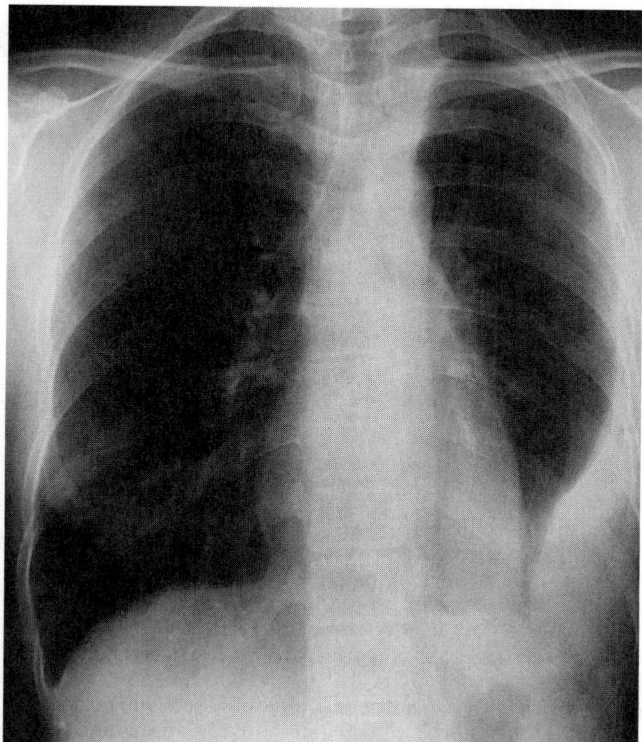

Figure 3. Chest film of a woman who had emigrated from Korea 20 years previously showing left pleural effusion. Pleural aspirate showed ova of *Paragonimus*. (Courtesy of Dr. Eric Wong.)

value in extrapulmonary disease. Unfortunately, serologic testing is available only in specialized centers or major endemic areas, and it is not well standardized. Radiologic findings can include ill-defined infiltrates, cavitary lesions, calcifications, and pleural fluid or thickening (Fig. 3). In endemic areas, tuberculosis must be distinguished from paragonimiasis, and the differential diagnosis may also include other pulmonary infections or carcinoma of the lung. Infiltrates in paragonimiasis are likely to change more quickly than those in tuberculosis, and they are less likely to produce fibrosis. Eosinophilia may occur, but it is uncommon in patients with chronic paragonimiasis. Radiologic evidence of coexisting pulmonary disease is seen in most patients with central nervous system paragonimiasis. Plain films of the skull may show a "soap bubble" appearance, and cysts similar to those of cysticercosis may be seen on CT scan.

FILARIAL INFECTION

By James S. McCarthy, M.B.B.S., M.D., D.T.M.H.,
and Thomas B. Nutman, M.D.
Bethesda, Maryland

Eight different filarial parasite species are known to infect humans; however, disease manifestations are classified into only three general groups: lymphatic filariasis, onchocerciasis, and loiasis (Table 1). The infective larvae are transmitted by an insect vector (fly or mosquito), and a minimum of 3 to 6 months elapses before adult worms develop to produce the microfilarial stage of the disease.

LYMPHATIC FILARIASIS

Lymphatic filariasis is caused primarily by the filarial species *Wuchereria bancrofti* and *Brugia malayi*. It is prevalent throughout the tropics, with *W. bancrofti* found worldwide and *B. malayi* confined to tropical Asia. Infection may rarely be caused by a second *Brugia* species, *B. timori* (found only on islands of the Indonesian archipelago). Adult worms reside in the lymphatics, primarily in the limbs, the scrotum (in the male), and the pelvis. Through the direct effect of the worms and the host inflammatory response, lymphatic dysfunction develops and results in lymphedema, which can progress to elephantiasis. Microfilariae of *W. bancrofti* and *B. malayi* circulate in the bloodstream, generally with nocturnal periodicity.

Asymptomatic Disease

Infected individuals may be identified by an unexpected discovery of eosinophilia or microfilariae on a blood film. Other patients may harbor cryptic infection and require indirect diagnostic methods, such as antifilarial serology or antigen tests. While asymptomatic subjects may have completely normal clinical and laboratory evaluations, the natural history of infection in this group is not clearly defined, and such subjects may be at risk for developing more pronounced manifestations of the disease.

Lymphatic Disease

Lymphatic disease, the best recognized manifestation of filariasis, most commonly involves the lower limbs, the upper limbs, or the female breast. The early stages of pitting edema may progress to significant nonpitting edema and, eventually, to elephantiasis. Patients may report a history of recurrent episodes of fever and lymphangitis, with retrograde lymphangitis a characteristic feature of lymphangitis of filarial origin. Acute bacterial lymphangitis generally proceeds in an antegrade pattern. Acute lymphadenitis may lead to the development of sterile abscesses (particularly in *B. malayi* infection). Lymphatic dysfunction induced by the filarial infection predisposes to secondary bacterial and fungal infections, infections that are probably important cofactors in the progression to the deforming complications of lymphatic filariasis (elephantiasis).

Hydrocele and Scrotal Disease

Infected males frequently develop disease in the scrotum owing to the presence of adult worms in the lymphatics of the spermatic cord (more than 25 per cent of infected subjects in some studies). Scrotal disease may present acutely as funiculitis or epididymitis. Nodules due to the presence of dead or dying adult worms may be palpable. The testis and epididymis may become enlarged, and a hydrocele may develop, which in advanced stages may evolve into scrotal elephantiasis. The clinician must distinguish scrotal disease of filarial origin from bacterial epididymo-orchitis, testicular torsion, and testicular tumors.

Tropical Pulmonary Eosinophilia (TPE)

This condition, the least common manifestation of lymphatic filariasis, typically manifests in young adult men as paroxysmal nocturnal cough, dyspnea, and wheezing

Table 1. Principal Clinical Syndromes in the Major Filarial Infections

Clinical Syndrome	Principal Clinical Manifestations	Causative Organism	Distribution	Location of Adult Worm	Location of Microfilariae	Periodicity of Microfilariae
Lymphatic filariasis	Lymphedema Hydrocele Elephantiasis Tropical pulmonary eosinophilia	*Wuchereria bancrofti*	Tropics worldwide	Lymphatic vessels	Bloodstream	Nocturnal or subperiodic
		Brugia malayi	India, Sri Lanka, China, Southeast Asia	Lymphatic vessels	Bloodstream	Nocturnal or subperiodic
		Brugia timori	Southeast Asia			
Onchocerciasis (river blindness)	Dermatitis Eye disease	*Onchocerca volvulus*	Central and west Africa Central and South America	Subcutaneous nodules	Skin	None
Loiasis (eyeworm)	Migratory angioedema (Calabar swellings) Eyeworm	*Loa loa*	Central and west Africa	Migratory in subcutaneous tissues	Bloodstream	Diurnal

accompanied by fatigue, weight loss, and fever. While the clinical and laboratory features of TPE resemble those seen in other interstitial lung diseases (e.g., Löffler's syndrome, systemic vasculitis, eosinophilic pneumonia, hypersensitivity pneumonitis, allergic bronchopulmonary aspergillosis [ABPA]), the markedly increased eosinophil count (>3000/μL), IgE concentration, and antifilarial antibody concentration, along with the rapid response to antifilarial chemotherapy, distinguish this infection from these other conditions. Without antifilarial chemotherapy, this syndrome can lead to irreversible fibrotic lung disease.

ONCHOCERCIASIS

Onchocerciasis (river blindness) is caused by infection with the filarial species *Onchocerca volvulus.* Infection is prevalent in central and western Africa, and in certain areas of Central and South America. Adult worms typically reside in subcutaneous nodules but may occasionally be found in deeper structures, including internal organs. Microfilariae in the skin and ocular tissues account for the primary clinical manifestations.

Asymptomatic Disease

Infection may occasionally be found in asymptomatic subjects with a history of exposure. Patients may seek attention for evaluation of subcutaneous nodules, which vary in size from 5 mm to more than 3 cm and are often palpable over bony structures such as the iliac crest and scapula.

Onchodermatitis

Pruritus and rash are the most frequent manifestations of onchocerciasis. They may be localized to particular regions of the body or may be more generalized. The intensity of pruritus varies, and it is usually only partially relieved by oral antihistamine or topical corticosteroid therapy. The appearance of the rash ranges from a faint erythematous papular eruption frequently seen in mild or early infection to more severe changes that include lichenification and dermal atrophy with hyperpigmentation or hypopigmentation seen in long-standing, severe infection. Localized onchodermatitis, or sowda, is an uncommon but more florid manifestation of skin disease. It is typically confined to one area, where a severe inflammatory response to microfilariae causes the affected skin to become intensely pruritic, markedly swollen, and hyperpigmented.

Eye Disease

While less common than skin disease, blinding eye disease gives onchocerciasis its eponymous name. The inflammatory response to invasion of the cornea and anterior segment of the eye by microfilariae results in a punctate keratitis that may eventually progress to sclerosing keratitis. These changes may be accompanied by anterior uveitis. Blinding eye disease may also involve the posterior segment of the eye, with the development of chorioretinitis, optic neuritis, and optic atrophy independent of anterior segment disease.

Lymphatic Disease

Lymphadenopathy is frequently present in onchocerciasis. In advanced disease, the subcutaneous tissue surrounding the inguinal nodes may lose its elasticity, and the appearance of "hanging groin" may result.

LOIASIS

Infection with the filarial parasite *Loa loa,* the cause of "eyeworm," is confined to central and west Africa. Adult worms reside in subcutaneous tissue, where they move about freely, while microfilariae are found in the blood where they exhibit diurnal periodicity (parasite counts in the blood peak in the early afternoon).

Asymptomatic Disease

Despite severe microfilaremia, in which counts may occasionally reach thousands of parasites per milliliter of blood, patients in endemic areas may be completely asymptomatic. However, these individuals may develop immune complex–induced glomerulonephritis. Treatment with antifilarial medication in patients with microfilaremia has resulted in life-threatening encephalopathy.

Systemic Effects

Despite the absence of demonstrable parasites, patients from nonendemic areas may suffer significant systemic effects, principally malaise, urticaria, and arthralgia. Eosinophil counts may be extremely high, and untreated patients may develop exaggerated immune responses, leading to endomyocardial fibrosis and glomerulonephritis.

Calabar Swellings

These painless angioedematous swellings, which may be a reaction to antigens released by the adult worm, can be found on any part of the body but occur most frequently on the limbs, especially around the joints. The frequency of occurrence and the location of the swellings are extremely variable. Calabar swellings may last up to 3 days and generally resolve without lasting effect. If the swelling occurs in a location susceptible to nerve compression, entrapment neuropathy may result.

Eyeworm

The most dramatic presentation of loiasis is the passage of an adult worm beneath the conjunctiva. Such episodes cause minor irritation and pose no threat to vision. The worm will continue to migrate freely if not surgically removed.

LESS COMMON FILARIAL INFECTIONS

Three filarial species of the *Mansonella* genus may occasionally cause disease in humans. *Mansonella streptocerca,* the cause of streptocerciasis, is endemic in west Africa. Both adult worms and microfilariae inhabit the dermis, and infected subjects may have skin findings similar to those found in onchocerciasis. *Mansonella perstans* is widely distributed throughout central Africa, and is also found in Latin America. Adult worms reside in serosal cavities (pleural, pericardial, peritoneal, and retroperitoneal spaces), while the microfilariae circulate in the blood without periodicity. In addition, they may be found in cerebrospinal fluid. Apart from a clinical picture of hypersensitivity resembling that seen in loiasis, clinical illness with *M. perstans* is poorly defined. *Mansonella ozzardi* is endemic in Latin America. Like the case with *M. perstans* infection, *M. ozzardi* microfilariae circulate in the blood without periodicity; similarly, the clinical features are ill defined.

Dirofilaria immitis, the cause of dog heartworm, cannot fully develop in the human but lodges in the lung, where the resulting granuloma occasionally causes cough and hemoptysis. Alternatively, such granulomas may lead to the appearance of a "coin lesion" on chest film that is indistinguishable from malignancy.

LABORATORY DIAGNOSIS

Demonstration of microfilariae is the most definitive means of diagnosis of filarial infection. In lymphatic filariasis and loiasis, in which microfilariae circulate in the blood, the specimen should be collected at the time of peak parasitemia. Infection is generally nocturnally periodic in lymphatic filariasis; thus, it is necessary to collect blood late at night (with peak parasitemia between 10 PM and 2 AM). In parts of Southeast Asia and the Pacific, where infection is subperiodic, specimens should be collected in the morning or early evening. For *Loa loa*, which exhibits diurnal periodicity, blood specimens are best collected in the early afternoon. Microfilariae survive in anticoagulated blood at room temperature for several days, which allows storage of specimens for later processing. While microfilariae may be visualized on Giemsa- or Wright-stained thin blood smears in heavily infected subjects, sensitivity of the test is increased by sampling larger volumes of blood. This can be accomplished by filtration of 1 mL of blood through a polycarbonate filter (3 μM pore size), followed by staining of the filter membrane. The Knott concentration method uses 1 mL of blood added to 9 mL of 2 per cent formalin. The centrifuged sediment is then microscopically examined. Microfilariae may be distinguished by the identification and characterization of a sheath, tail, and terminal nuclei.

In onchocerciasis, detection of microfilariae in the skin is accomplished by taking a bloodless 1-mm skin biopsy, the "skin snip." This is typically performed with the use of a corneoscleral punch, but it may also be obtained by lifting the skin with the tip of a needle and excising a small piece (1 to 3 mm in diameter) with a sterile blade. The skin biopsy is placed in physiologic saline and incubated to permit the emergence of motile microfilariae, which are visualized with low-power microscopy. Sensitivity of the procedure is increased by obtaining three pairs of snips bilaterally (generally from the shoulders, hips, and thighs) and by incubating the biopsies for 24 hours.

The diagnosis of onchocerciasis is occasionally made by pathologic examination of a surgically removed nodule. Similarly, the removal of a subconjunctival worm or the discovery of a nematode within lymphatic tissue may lead to a definitive diagnosis of loiasis or lymphatic filariasis, respectively.

Serology

Antifilarial antibody estimation with enzyme-linked immunosorbent assay (ELISA) that utilizes crude parasite extract is available for serologic diagnosis of filariasis. The test result is uniformly positive in active filarial infection but lacks specificity for the filarial species responsible, and may reflect exposure to filarial antigen without active infection. Further, low-positive values may represent infection with other nonfilarial nematode parasites. Antifilarial antibody concentrations are extremely increased in tropical pulmonary eosinophilia and may also be greatly increased in nonendemic subjects with loiasis. Specific serologic tests that use recombinant antigens have been developed for *O. volvulus*. They offer high specificity and are in use in large-scale control programs for diagnosing prepatent infection before microfilariae can be detected in the skin.

Other Diagnostic Tests

The total eosinophil count may be increased in filarial infection, particularly in nonendemic subjects, and is universally increased in tropical pulmonary eosinophilia. However, a high eosinophil count is a relatively nonspecific finding. Further, a normal eosinophil count does not exclude infection, especially in subjects with long-standing infection.

Increased IgE concentrations are frequently seen in filarial infection; these may be extremely high in tropical pulmonary eosinophilia. Assays for circulating filarial antigen have been developed for *W. bancrofti* infection and permit diagnosis of microfilaremic and cryptic (amicrofilaremic) infection from daytime blood samples. A polymerase chain reaction (PCR)–based assay for *O. volvulus* DNA present in the skin snip is available in some research laboratories. It is more sensitive than microscopy for detection of microfilariae in the skin. Similarly, PCR-based assays for *W. bancrofti* and *B. malayi* DNA in blood are under development.

Imaging Procedures

Evaluation of lymphatic function with lymphoscintigraphy can provide useful information in lymphatic filariasis. The procedure involves injection of ^{99}Tc-radiolabeled albumin or dextran (the latter not FDA-approved) into the dermis, followed by sequential imaging with a gamma camera. In patients with suspected lymphatic filariasis, examination of the scrotum by ultrasound may reveal nodules or lymphatic dilatation. The use of high-frequency transducers and Doppler techniques may reveal motile worms within the scrotal lymphatics. Ultrasound or magnetic resonance imaging modalities may identify nodules in onchocerciasis and distinguish them from other subcutaneous masses. However, such studies are not generally clinically useful.

Patients with tropical pulmonary eosinophilia should have pulmonary function tests and a chest radiograph performed. Bronchoscopy with bronchoalveolar lavage is useful for following the response to therapy.

Ophthalmologic Evaluation

Slit-lamp examination and indirect ophthalmoscopy are necessary for evaluation of eye disease in onchocerciasis. Motile microfilariae may be seen in the anterior chamber after the subject rests with the head down for at least 10 minutes.

Mazzotti Test

This provocative test for diagnosis of cryptic infection with *O. volvulus* involves administration of 50 mg of the antifilarial drug diethylcarbamazine to induce pronounced pruritus and rash caused by death of microfilariae. The reaction generally begins within 2 to 24 hours after administration of the drug. The absence of microfilariae in the skin *must* be confirmed before the physician gives the drug because severe reactions and permanent eye damage may occur in heavily infected patients.

PITFALLS IN DIAGNOSIS

The species likely to be responsible for infection can generally be defined by the exposure history (see Table 1) because each of the filarial parasites has restricted regions in which it is endemic. The prolonged interval between exposure and development of patency frequently leads to a delay in presentation and hinders consideration of filarial infection as a cause of the symptom. The manifestations of infection in patients with long-term residence in an endemic area and long-standing infection may differ from those seen in individuals from nonendemic areas (tourists or temporary residents) who may have become infected after a relatively brief period of exposure. Individuals of the latter group, when compared with endemic populations, typically have relatively more prominent clinical and laboratory findings with a lower parasite burden.

ECHINOCOCCOSIS

By Stephanos J. Hadziyannis, M.D.
Athens, Greece

Echinococcosis is a parasitic disease caused by infection with the larval form of tapeworms (cestodes) of the genus *Echinococcus,* phylum Platyhelminthes, order Cyclophyllidea, family Taeniidae. It is characterized by the development of cysts in various organs, predominantly the liver and lung. It is one of the most important zoonoses, has a worldwide distribution, and is a serious human health problem in some areas of the world, particularly in sheep-rearing countries.

Echinococcus means sea urchin (*echinus*) plus grain (*coccus*). It is a composite term used to designate both the thorny appearance and the small size of the tapeworm, particularly of its scolices (heads), which are contained in the cysts.

Echinococcosis is also referred to as *hydatid disease* or *hydatidosis* from the Greek word meaning watery, a term emphasizing the clear, watery appearance of the fluid content of the cysts (hydatid cysts or simply hydatids) that form in humans and other intermediate hosts.

There are several species and subspecies of the genus *Echinococcus.* The most common and worldwide species causing human disease is *Echinococcus granulosus* or *cysticus.* Another relatively rarer species, *E. multilocularis* or *alveolaris,* can also affect humans, causing a malignantlike disease, mainly of the liver. This is usually described under the terms alveolar echinococcosis, alveolar hydatid disease, alveolar hydatidosis, alveolosis, and alveococcosis.

Recently, molecular biologic techniques have been applied successfully to the study of genetic variability of the genus *Echinococcus,* with implications for taxonomy, diagnosis, and epidemiology. Echinococcal species, subspecies, and strains can be rapidly discriminated by polymerase chain reaction (PCR) based on the restriction fragment length polymorphism (RFLP) method and by other molecular biologic techniques.

This article deals primarily with echinococcosis caused by the common species *E. granulosus.* When necessary, echinococcosis due to *E. multilocularis* is also briefly discussed, being specifically designated with the adjective *alveolar.* Two other species, *E. oligarthrus* and *E. vogeli,* have also been reported to affect humans. However, the number of described cases is small, and further information is needed to define the diagnostic features of these diseases.

LIFE CYCLE OF THE PARASITE AND PATHOLOGY

All species of *Echinococcus* are maintained in nature by a cycle of transmission between an intermediate and a definitive host. The cycles of the various species differ only in the species of the hosts involved. The modes of transmission to humans are identical. The usual epidemiologic cycle of *E. granulosus* is a rural one, but it can become sylvatic and, even, urban.

Definitive hosts are several carnivorous and omnivorous animals, the usual one for *E. granulosus* being the dog and for *E. multilocularis* the red fox. The mature worms live in the small intestine of the definitive host. In dogs, the life span of *E. granulosus* is 3 to 6 months.

Echinococci are the smallest of all tapeworms (1.5 to 9 mm) and consist of a head (scolex), a neck, and usually three segments (proglottids), the last one being gravid and containing many eggs. The various species and subspecies of *Echinococcus* can be differentiated morphologically.

Eggs pass in the feces of the definitive host. They contaminate grass and farmland and are ingested by intermediate host animals. Humans can be infected easily by handling dogs or by eating contaminated vegetables.

The most frequent intermediate hosts for *E. granulosus* are sheep, cattle, pigs, and occasionally a human; for *E. multilocularis,* they are various rodents, especially field mice, and occasionally a human. With a related species of *E. oligarthrus,* the cat is the definitive host and the small rodent is an intermediate one.

The eggs of *Echinococcus* have an outer chitinous shell and an inner spherical larva (oncosphere) with six hooklets. They are resistant to temperature and to various physical and chemical agents and may remain viable for as long as 2 or 3 months at −16 to −18°C (−0.4 to 3.2°F). Eggs are swallowed by the intermediate host, and the chitinous shell is digested in the duodenum. Embryos are liberated, penetrate the intestinal wall, and are carried by the portal bloodstream until trapped in a small capillary. The first capillary filter is the liver, where about 65 to 70 per cent of the larvae are arrested, and the next most common is the lung (20 per cent). About 10 per cent of the larvae gain access to the systemic circulation, so that almost any organ and tissue of the body can be affected (e.g., the spleen, brain, bone, kidneys).

The parasite develops in the intermediate host into a bladderlike cyst, which grows at a rate of approximately 1 cm per year. The growing hydatid cyst becomes isolated from adjacent tissues by a connective tissue membrane that represents a host defense mechanism. Calcification of this membrane is not exceptional. Inside this outer wall develops a semipermeable laminated cuticle and an inner germinal layer consisting of nucleated epithelium, which gives rise to brood capsules. In these capsules, scolices develop that are released into the fluid of the cysts and fall to the bottom by gravity. This is referred to as hydatid sand, and it may contain as many as 400,000 scolices per milliliter. Daughter and granddaughter cysts may develop in the germinal layer, and some cysts may thus become huge (50 cm or more). The largest cyst ever found was recorded in a patient in Australia and contained 57 L of fluid.

Alveolar cysts are minute cysts containing a jellylike substance. They have a thin, laminated membrane and are not surrounded by connective tissue; they grow by exogenous budding, forming conglomerates of small vesicles (alveolosis), which penetrate the surrounding tissues. They can metastasize via the circulation, and their growth is considered to be malignant.

Carnivorous and omnivorous definitive hosts eat infected carcasses and offal of intermediate hosts; scolices contained in the cysts are liberated in the duodenum and adhere to the small intestine, where they develop into adult worms. The eggs are excreted in the feces and are ingested by intermediate hosts, and the whole cycle starts again.

GEOGRAPHIC DISTRIBUTION

Echinococcosis caused by *E. granulosus* occurs worldwide. It is common in livestock-raising countries in both developed and developing parts of the world. Sheep- and goat-herding populations that keep dogs as pets or work animals are at highest risk for hydatid disease. Until recently, echinococcosis was endemic in the entire Mediterranean littoral; the Middle East; many areas of Africa, particularly in the north, east, and south; southeast Australia; New Zealand; and some South American countries (Argentina, Uruguay, and Chile). Currently, the area with the highest prevalence in the world is the Turkana and Somburu region of northwestern Kenya. Significant disease transmission is also found in central Asia, particularly China. Echinococcosis is rare in the United States, where it is encountered mainly in immigrants.

On the other hand, human disease due to *E. multilocularis* is encountered only in the Northern Hemisphere. Alaska, Canada, some areas of Switzerland, Austria, some parts of Germany, and Russia, including Siberia, are the main regions where it remains endemic.

PRESENTING SYMPTOMS AND SIGNS

Clinical symptoms of echinococcosis do not usually develop until the hydatid cyst has attained a considerable size. Symptoms may be delayed for a period of 20 years or more after the initial infection. Thus, although most infections occur in childhood, the average age of a patient at presentation is about 35 years. As many as 20 per cent of *E. granulosus* cysts of the liver and about 50 per cent of cysts of the lung may never cause symptoms. Silent cysts are not an uncommon autopsy finding in endemic areas.

Symptoms and signs are not characteristic. They depend entirely on the organs involved, on the size of the cysts, on the mechanical effects on affected organs and adjacent tissues, and on the development of complications.

LIVER. About 70 per cent of the cysts are located in the liver, and 90 per cent of these are in the right lobe. Liver hydatidosis is usually manifested after the cyst has attained a size of 10 or even 20 cm. About 50 per cent of liver cysts are discovered incidentally in patients hospitalized for other reasons. The most frequent presentation is an enlarged liver or a slowly growing liver mass, either painless or accompanied by right upper quadrant abdominal pain (50 per cent) and discomfort. Patients with liver cysts may occasionally present with symptoms and signs caused by pressure on the biliary tract (obstructive jaundice), on the portal vein (portal hypertension), or on the hepatic veins (Budd-Chiari syndrome). Not rarely, liver echinococcosis may first present with symptoms and signs of the complications discussed later, particularly rupture in the biliary tract (15 to 25 per cent), or with allergic manifestations.

LUNG. Patients usually present with cough and chest pain that is not severe and is frequently reported as discomfort or a feeling of weight in the chest. Hemoptysis is not rare and may be induced by coughing. Many patients (50 per cent) are completely asymptomatic, whereas others first present with clinical features of some complication, such as cyst rupture and infection.

BRAIN. Hydatidosis may present with symptoms and signs of increased intracranial pressure, convulsions, and sometimes focal neurologic signs. The patients are younger than those with cysts of other organs.

CARDIAC. Cysts may be silent or may present with arrhythmias or with pericardial symptoms caused by rupture into the pericardium.

KIDNEY. Echinococcosis may cause pain, hematuria, or altered renal function.

BONE. Echinococcosis often presents as a relatively painless cystic mass or as a pathologic fracture. Soft-tissue cysts also present as painless masses.

ALVEOLAR. In alveolar echinococcosis, 90 per cent of the cysts are located in the liver. Hepatic manifestations are therefore predominant. Usual initial symptoms include vague right upper abdominal pain, epigastric discomfort, anorexia, and weight loss. Jaundice is frequently included among the initial manifestations, in contrast to infection due to *E. granulosus,* in which jaundice is usually related to rupture of a cyst in the biliary tract. The liver is enlarged and sensitive, and its surface is often nodular. Clinical features of pulmonary and brain metastases may also be present.

COURSE

Hydatid cysts increase in size progressively. The rate of their growth is generally slow (1 cm per year) although extremely variable, depending on the resistance of the involved tissue. With increasing size, complications develop and may cause the death of the patient. However, rupture of a cyst with evacuation of its content (e.g., into intestine or bronchi) may also lead to spontaneous healing. In the natural course of untreated cysts, calcification and death of the parasite are also included; however, calcification should not necessarily be regarded as synonymous with eradication of *Echinococcus*.

The course of alveolar echinococcosis is characterized by progressive deterioration, and untreated disease frequently (75 per cent) runs a fatal course in a mean period of 5 years from presentation. The initial manifestations become progressively more severe, and massive hepatomegaly, shortness of breath, ascites, and even neurologic signs due to brain metastases are frequently encountered.

COMMON COMPLICATIONS

Complications of echinococcosis due to *E. granulosus* are rupture, infection, and allergic reactions (Table 1).

RUPTURE. This is the most frequent complication and is either spontaneous, after high intracystic pressure and pressure necrosis, or induced by manipulations and trauma. Rupture is a dangerous complication and is usually associated with dissemination, infection, and allergic reactions that have a potentially fatal outcome; however, it may occasionally lead to spontaneous healing of the disease.

Liver cysts are usually located in the right lobe (90 per cent) either superficially or deeply. According to their location, rupture can occur:

1. Into the biliary tract (15 per cent), producing pain, obstructive jaundice, and cholangitis with chills and fever
2. Into the peritoneal cavity, causing generalized infestation and a usually catastrophic syndrome with anaphylaxis and peritonitis
3. Through the diaphragm (3.5 per cent) into the pleural space, causing pleurisy and empyema containing bile followed by bronchopleural fistula and expectoration of hydatid sand; into the lung and bronchi, causing hepatobronchial fistula; or, rarely, into the pericardium
4. With perforation; cysts projecting from the liver surface may be in contact with other abdominal organs and can perforate them (e.g., duodenum, colon, right renal pelvis, vena cava, or even the abdominal wall)

Table 1. Major Complications of Echinococcosis

Rupture of Liver Cyst
Peritoneal cavity
Biliary tract (obstructive jaundice, cholangitis)
Pleural space, lung, bronchi, pericardium (through diaphragm)
Stomach, duodenum, colon, and other sites
Infection
Liver or lung abscess
Subphrenic abscess
Pleural effusion and empyema
Peritonitis
Cholangitis
Septicemia
Allergic Reactions
Urticaria and other rashes with pruritus
Fever and eosinophilia
Wheezing
Anaphylactic shock

Rupture of lung cysts may cause pneumonia, anaphylactic shock, pleural invasion, or simply evacuation of the cyst contents through the bronchus by coughing up a salty-tasting clear fluid and pieces of membranes. A coexisting biliary communication may produce biliptysis.

INFECTION. This complication usually occurs in ruptured cysts, especially of the liver, with invading organisms being introduced through the biliary system. Active infection of the cyst results in death of the scolices, and the condition then presents as liver abscess. A suppurative process in the liver may extend to the subphrenic space, causing a subphrenic abscess, or to the peritoneal cavity, causing peritonitis.

ALLERGIC REACTIONS. These are relatively common (10 to 25 per cent). With slow leakage of cyst fluid, urticaria and other allergic manifestations may occur; whereas with cyst rupture or needle puncture, severe anaphylactic shock may develop. Urticaria, fever, wheezing, abdominal pain, and delirium may accompany such a reaction, which can be fatal.

PHYSICAL EXAMINATION

In the absence of complications and with small cysts, physical findings are usually completely negative. Most patients remain in good health, even those with cysts that are large. Liver cysts of large size deeply located in the organ are accompanied only by hepatomegaly; inferior and high anterior cysts are palpable as rounded, smooth, sometimes tender masses. Cysts in other organs and in soft tissues are also felt as slowly growing, smooth, cystic tumors, but they may become hard if calcified.

A characteristic physical sign over a cyst is a vibration or tremor produced by ballottement, known as the hydatid thrill. This sign is rarely elicited and should not be depended on for diagnosis.

Physical examination findings may be negative for cysts but positive for signs indicative of some of the described complications; such findings, particularly in areas in which echinococcosis is endemic, are of considerable diagnostic value.

LABORATORY PROCEDURES

Several laboratory tests aid in diagnosis:

EOSINOPHIL COUNT. A count above 5 per cent is present in half the cases and above 7 per cent in about one quarter. Eosinophil counts are even higher (up to 20 and 25 per cent) in the presence of ruptured cysts. *Leukocytosis* accompanies an infected cyst.

LIVER FUNCTION TESTS. These are of little value in the diagnosis of uncomplicated hepatic disease, but increased serum bilirubin, alkaline phosphatase, and γ-glutamyltransferase are found if cysts rupture into the biliary tract or on the rare occasions when pressure is produced on large ducts. Abnormal liver test results are found mostly in patients with alveolar echinococcosis.

CASONI'S TEST. The standardized intradermal Casoni test has been widely used for years, being considered a sensitive diagnostic procedure. Its use is now limited, and it may soon be abandoned completely partly because of a shortage of suitable antigenic material and partly because of the availability of superior tests. The test should be performed with 0.2 mL of sterile hydatid fluid. Characteristic is the development of a wheal within 15 minutes. Casoni's test results should always be compared with those from a control injection. Results are positive in about 75 per cent of cases, but false-positive reactions may occur in as many as 18 per cent of normal control subjects.

IMMUNOSEROLOGIC TESTS. Several tests are used, aiming at the demonstration of serum antibodies against specific echinococcal antigens. These are complement fixation (Weinberg test), indirect hemagglutination, latex agglutination, bentonite flocculation, immunofluorescence, radioimmunoassay, enzyme-linked immunosorbent assay, immunodiffusion, counterelectrophoresis in agarose or cellulose acetate, and immunoelectrophoresis tests. The results are influenced not only by the sensitivity of each technique but also by the composition of the antigenic material used; by cross-reactivities between other serum antibodies and the antigens in the tests; and, of course, by various other factors influencing the titer, class, and specificity of antibodies produced by the host. As a result, none of these tests is 100 per cent sensitive and entirely specific. In practice, it is advisable to use a highly sensitive, easy-to-perform test like indirect hemagglutination, enzyme immunoassay, or latex hemagglutination and to subject the positive reactions to specificity control by immunoelectrophoresis or counterelectrophoresis in cellulose acetate, looking for the diagnostic antibodies against the echinococcus-specific arc 5 antigen. Detection of circulating hydatid antigen in serum is also possible by ELISA.

MICROSCOPIC EXAMINATION. The finding of suspicious material in sputum, gastric juice, bile, or urine in cases of ruptured cysts may be helpful in detecting scolices and parts of membranes. In the case of suspected liver echinococcosis, needle liver biopsy and needle aspiration are contraindicated, because of the risk of anaphylaxis and of implantation of germinal membranes. However, recent reports suggest that percutaneous ultrasonography or computed tomography–guided thin-needle aspiration may be safe and applied in diagnosis and treatment with drainage of fluid and instillation of a scolicidal solution, such as ethanol.

RADIOLOGIC EVALUATION

A plain film of the abdomen may give important information, showing calcified cysts, a calcified rim, or irregular calcifications. Diaphragmatic distortion, an opaque line around the cyst, intrahepatic gas bubbles, and the "water lily" sign (caused by membranes and vesicles floating on the surface of fluid in a cyst) may be detected by radiologic examination in liver echinococcosis.

Cholangiograms are also of value, mainly to check the patency of the biliary system.

Lung hydatids typically appear radiologically as oval opacities or as a cavity with a fluid level. The water lily sign may be present. In complicated cases, pleural effusion or hydropneumothorax may be detected.

Angiography, once useful for the differential diagnosis of cysts from tumors and for demonstrating their location, number, and size, has been replaced by computed tomography and by ultrasonography.

OTHER DIAGNOSTIC PROCEDURES

RADIOISOTOPE SCANNING. Liver scans are of great value in demonstrating hepatic cysts more than 3 cm in size. The cysts appear as cold areas and cannot be differentiated with confidence from tumors.

ULTRASONOGRAPHY. This technique has been found to be extremely helpful in detecting cysts in various organs and is the method of choice for differentiating cystic from solid lesions. It may also help in differentiating between unilocular and multilocular cysts. However, it is not applicable in the diagnosis of lung and other cysts and may also give some false-positive results in neoplastic lesions with central necrosis and cavitation, particularly in hepatocellular carcinoma. Distinguishing hydatid from simple cysts may also be difficult.

COMPUTED TOMOGRAPHY. This is the imaging technique of choice in the diagnosis of echinococcosis. It shows clearly and precisely the presence, number, and size of hepatic, pulmonary, kidney, brain, and other cysts. Computed tomography can easily differentiate echinococcosis from solid tumors and even from abscesses. However, differentiation from simple cysts is not always possible. Magnetic resonance scanning is also a useful technique for visualizing and characterizing hydatid cysts.

POTENTIAL ERRORS AND PITFALLS IN DIAGNOSIS

The diagnosis of echinococcosis is seldom mistaken in an endemic area, particularly when a cystic swelling is detected and radiography shows compatible findings. Immunologic and other laboratory procedures usually confirm the diagnosis. However, the clinical picture may be extremely puzzling and misleading, particularly in complicated disease, with uncommon localizations of the cysts, and mostly in alveolar echinococcosis, which resembles malignant disease. In such cases, the appropriate confirmatory immunologic tests, which are also positive in *E. alveolaris* infections, are not ordered, and diagnostic errors by internists and surgeons are common. The high degree of suspicion required for diagnosis is practically achieved only in endemic areas. Even so, laboratory procedures may be misleading, giving rise to diagnostic errors. Thus, in patients with calcified or dead cysts, serologic test results may be falsely negative because of low or negative titers of serum antibodies. Confusing serologic test results due to nonspecific reactions may also be obtained in patients with other hepatic disorders.

Lung cysts frequently give negative results on immunologic tests, and radiologic appearances may be confused with those of solid tumors.

Intrahepatic calcifications may be due to other causes such as hemangiomas or old bacterial abscesses. They can also be confused with calcifications of adjacent structures such as the adrenals, kidney, diaphragm, and costal cartilages, leading to unnecessary or wrong operations.

Errors and pitfalls in diagnosis have been significantly reduced with the use of computed tomography and ultrasonography; but even so, multilocular cysts and alveolar disease may still be confused with some neoplastic and other lesions. Moreover, a clear-cut distinction between hydatid and simple cysts is not always possible.

OTHER CESTODES

By Murray Wittner, M.D., Ph.D.,
and Louis M. Weiss, M.D., M.P.H.
Bronx, New York

Tapeworm infection is probably one of the oldest recognized afflictions of mankind. The tapeworm's huge size and, at times, the untimely egress of the parasite from the body could hardly go unnoticed. Tapeworms (i.e., Cestoda), a subclass of the phylum Platyhelminthes, are exclusively parasitic. (The other important human parasitic platyhelminths belong to the class Trematoda, or flukes.) Tapeworms are flattened and do not possess a body cavity. They infect members of all vertebrate classes, whereas their larvae may infect both vertebrates and invertebrates. Adult tapeworms typically possess a scolex, or head, which may be modified or adorned with structures or organelles that serve as holdfast organs for attachment to the small intestinal mucosa. The scolex is clinically important because therapy is aimed at its destruction or elimination. Failure to destroy the scolex results in regrowth of the entire tapeworm.

Two of the four main groups of cestodes are important parasites of humans and domestic animals. Members of the order Pseudophyllidea are characterized by the presence of a scolex, or attachment organ, containing sucking grooves; this group includes members of the genus *Diphyllobothrium* such as *D. latum* (the broad, or fish, tapeworm) and worms that infect humans only at the larval stage, such as the sparganum. The life cycles of pseudophyllidean organisms involve a minimum of three hosts. Members of Cyclophyllidea, the order that includes all other tapeworms that parasitize humans, are characterized by a scolex with four suckers and include the beef and pork tapeworms, that is, *Taenia* (see previous articles *Echinococcus* and *Taeniae*). The life cycle of the Cyclophyllidea typically involves two hosts, but occasionally the definitive host can also serve as the intermediate host. Adult tapeworms that are medically important range in size from the minute *Echinococcus*, which has a scolex and three segments and is 2 cm in size, to *D. latum*, which can reach 25 to 30 m in length.

With the exception of *Hymenolepis nana*, tapeworms that infect humans require one or more intermediate hosts to complete their life cycles. The life cycle of diphyllobothriid cestodes involves two or more intermediate hosts. Coracidia, ingested by water fleas or copepods, develop in the body cavity of these hosts into procercoid larvae that retain the embryonic six hooklets and show evidence of developing bothria. When infected copepods are ingested by the appropriate piscine hosts, the procercoid larva enters the musculature of the fish, where it becomes a plerocercoid, or sparganum, larva. These larvae may have a number of transfer, or paratenic, hosts. For example, a plerocercoid that has developed in a minnow may next parasitize a larger fish, and so on until its final piscine host is ingested by a suitable mammal, in which the sparganum will develop to the adult stage.

Some cestodes infect only humans in the larval stage (e.g., the plerocercus [sparganum] of *Spirometra mansonoides)*, while others infect humans in both the adult and the larval stages (e.g., *Taenia solium)*. In the genera *Multiceps* and *Echinococcus,* larval development produces considerable multiplication. Thus, when these larvae are ingested by a suitable host, there may be large numbers of adult worms produced. The clinical manifestations of tapeworm infection may be due to infection with either the adult or the larval stage. Adult tapeworm infections may persist for many years or even for the life of the host and may be either asymptomatic or persistently symptomatic, with the parasite depriving the host of essential nutrients. In general, however, these infections are well tolerated. In contrast to infection with the adult stage, infection with the larval stage of a tapeworm often causes serious or fatal disease and can be of great economic consequence.

DIPHYLLOBOTHRIASIS

The fish, or broad, tapeworm *D. latum* is a frequent human intestinal parasite in many areas where uncooked freshwater fish are consumed. Raw fish, lightly cooked fish, pickled fish, and fresh roe are considered delicacies by many people. Carefully cooking freshwater fish, freezing at −10°C (14°F) for 24 hours, or brining fish before smoking prevent transmission of this parasite. Infection is most prevalent in those northern temperate and subarctic zones where freshwater fish are commonly consumed. In the past decade, the prevalence of diphyllobothriasis has decreased and is now estimated at 9 to 10 million people worldwide. In North America, endemic foci have been found among Eskimos in Alaska and Canada, particularly in the smaller lakes of the Great Lakes region. In the endemic regions of Finnish and Soviet Karelia, prevalence ranges from 25 to 100 per cent of the local population.

The characteristic light yellow eggs are 40 to 50 μm by 60 to 75 μm. They possess an operculum, or lid, at one end; at the abopercular end, there is often a characteristic tiny knob. In fresh water, the eggs mature in 2 weeks, and ciliated coracidia emerge to be ingested by one of several crustacean species of copepods. The larvae penetrate the midgut and enter the hemocoelom of the copepod, where in 2 to 3 weeks, they transform into elongated procercoid larvae, each about 0.5 mm in length, which are soon ingested by various species of freshwater plankton-eating fish. The procercoid larvae then migrate through the tissues of the fish until they reach muscle fibers, where they transform within a month to plerocercoid or sparganum larvae. The latter has the characteristic rudiments of a scolex but is unsegmented. When these fish are eaten by larger carnivorous fish, such as rainbow trout, wall-eyed pike, and burbot (paratenic, or transport, hosts), the plerocercoid larvae migrate again to the muscle of the new host. When fish are consumed raw or inadequately cooked by a suitable host (i.e., humans), the larvae attach to the wall of the small intestine and become mature tapeworms in 5 to 6 weeks.

A large tapeworm comprising 3000 to 4000 segments or proglottids, *D. latum* inhabits the ileum and jejunum and reaches a length of 3 to 12 m. These tapeworms possess a scolex that is characteristically elongated or spoon-shaped, with ventral and dorsal sucking grooves, or bothria. Egg production usually occurs in many proglottids simultaneously over days to weeks. The mature proglottid is broader than it is long and contains both male and female reproductive organs. In the center of the mature proglottid is a characteristic dark, "rosette," that is, the egg-filled uterus that aids in identification of the organism. The uterus leads to a uterine pore on the ventral surface of the segment through which the eggs pass into the feces. Typically, proglottids do not break off and migrate out of the body, as occurs in taeniasis. Occasionally, however, a long chain of proglottids may pass with the stool. More than a million eggs per day are extruded into the small intestinal lumen by contractions of the muscular uterine pore. Humans are the primary definitive host and the most important reservoir of infection. Other definitive and reservoir hosts include fish-eating mammals, such as the fox, mink, bear, domestic and wild cats, dog, pig, walrus, and seal.

Other adult diphyllobothriid species that are normally

parasites of fish-eating mammals have occasionally been found in humans, dogs, and cats. *Diphyllobothrium pacificum* is found in seals (its natural host) and marine fish (its intermediate host) in Peru and Chile. Unlike *D. latum* infection, human infection with *D. pacificum* is acquired by eating marine fish that have been prepared in lime juice, that is, ceviche, or consuming raw fish.

Clinical Manifestations

Infection with this large tapeworm is often associated with surprisingly few symptoms or pathologic changes in the intestinal mucosa. It is often first recognized in an asymptomatic patient when a stool examination is performed for other reasons. Some individuals, however, complain of vague abdominal pain and some patients describe the sensation that "something is moving inside." Others describe bloating, sore tongue, sore gums, allergic symptoms, headache, hunger pains, and decreased or increased appetite. Mechanical intestinal obstruction may rarely occur when several worms become entangled. Diarrhea has also been described. Almost all patients become aware of the infection when they spontaneously pass a large section of the spent proglottids; typically this startling event brings the patient to the office or clinic. Unlike the proglottids of *Taenia saginata,* those of *D. latum* do not spontaneously crawl through the anus.

In a few patients, megaloblastic and pernicious anemia are caused by infection with *D. latum* ("bothriocephalus anemia"). Approximately 40 per cent of persons harboring the worm have decreased vitamin B_{12} concentrations, but fewer than 2 per cent develop anemia. When fully manifest, this anemia is hyperchromic, macrocytic, and megaloblastic, with thrombocytopenia and mild leukopenia. Importantly, weakness, numbness, paresthesiasis, disturbances of motility and coordination, and impaired sensation can occur in the absence of hematologic abnormalities. Worms in the ileum or jejunum successfully compete with the host for vitamin B_{12}. Folate absorption by the host may also be impaired, and decreased concentrations of ascorbic acid, thiamine, and riboflavin have been described. For unknown reasons, anemia associated with diphyllobothriasis is found primarily in Scandinavia. The anemia and neurologic manifestations respond to vitamin B_{12} and do not recur after the worm has been eliminated.

Diagnosis

Fish tapeworm infection can be diagnosed readily by finding characteristic ova in the feces. Concentration methods are usually unnecessary because the number of eggs present is typically so great that direct examination of a small amount of feces in a drop of saline is sufficient. Uncommonly, a strobila may be expelled in the feces, or portions of worm may be vomited. Tapeworm-induced anemia is usually associated with hydrochloric acid in the gastric juice, whereas pernicious anemia is accompanied by achlorhydria. No reliable serologic test is available. Eosinophilia of 5 to 10 per cent is common in patients with *D. latum* infection and is accompanied by a minimal leukocytosis.

HYMENOLEPIASIS

Two species of small tapeworms of the genus *Hymenolepis* infect humans. Infection with the dwarf tapeworm, *Hymenolepis nana*, is common in children and can be passed from human to human. In moderate to heavy infections, it may cause various abdominal and neurologic signs and symptoms. *Hymenolepis diminuta* is a parasite primarily of rodents and infrequently infects humans.

Hymenolepis Nana

The smallest adult tapeworm to regularly infect humans, *H. nana* measures about 25 to 30 mm in length and consists of 175 to 220 segments. Infection with this parasite is worldwide in distribution, with millions of people infected. Commonly regarded as a hand-to-mouth infection, hymenolepiasis is encountered most frequently in children, inhabitants of institutions for the mentally retarded, and chronic care psychiatric hospitals. The minute, rounded scolex (3 mm in diameter) possesses four sucking discs and a short, armed, retractable rostellum. The eggs are characteristic, measuring 35 to 50 μm in diameter and containing a hexacanth embryo or oncosphere residing within an inner membrane, with two polar thickenings from which arise four to eight polar filaments. The eggs are released by the gradual disintegration of the terminal gravid proglottids and are immediately infective when passed in the feces. Unlike most other tapeworms that infect humans, no intermediate host is required. When the eggs are ingested by another or the same host, they hatch and cysticercoid larvae develop in the villi. In 4 days the larvae re-enter the lumen and attach to the small intestine via the scolex. The larvae mature within 2 to 3 weeks. Hyperinfection or autoinfection occurs when ova liberated in the small intestine spontaneously hatch and immediately penetrate a villus to undergo a new cycle. Individual worms live about a year. However, as a result of hyperinfection, individuals may have a large worm burden for many years.

Humans are the natural reservoir for the parasite, and transmission is generally direct from human to human by ingestion of eggs from feces of infected individuals. Transmission may occur via fomites, water, and food, but is uncommon because the eggs quickly die outside the host. Larvae of fleas and grain beetles can become infected after ingesting *H. nana* eggs and develop cysticercoids in the hemocoelom. However, these insects are of little importance as intermediate hosts in human infection. Some murine strains have been shown to be infectious to humans, with pet mice, rats, and hamsters occasionally sources of infection.

Clinical Manifestations

Light infections generally cause no significant mucosal damage and either are asymptomatic or cause vague abdominal complaints. Even heavy burdens of parasites are usually well tolerated. Young children, however, are particularly prone to symptoms, especially when they are infected with many worms. Diffuse, persistent abdominal pain is the commonest complaint. Commonly these children have loose bowel movements or occasionally frank diarrhea with mucus; however, bloody diarrhea is unusual. Pruritus ani and nasi and urticaria are occasionally encountered. Many children have headaches, dizziness, and sleep and behavioral disturbances, which improve with treatment. Rarely, more severe neurologic complications, such as seizures, have been reported. A moderate eosinophilia of 5 to 10 per cent is often seen.

Diagnosis

The diagnosis is made by identifying the characteristic ova in a fecal specimen. Proglottids are usually not found because they degenerate before passage.

Hymenolepis Diminuta

This tapeworm is closely related to *H. nana* and infrequently infects humans. More than 200 human cases have been reported, with most frequent occurrence in children younger than 3 years of age. The adult worm is 10 to 60 cm in length and has 800 to 1000 proglottids. The scolex is club shaped, with a rudimentary apical unarmed rostellum and four small suckers. The eggs are spherical and 60 to 86 μm in diameter; their thin, yellowish outer membrane is separated from the inner embryonic envelope by a clear area that, in contrast to the eggs of *H. nana*, contains no polar filaments. Development of this tapeworm requires an intermediate host. Presumably, rat fleas (*Nosopsyllus*, *Xenopsylla*) and mealworms infected with larvae are accidentally ingested, and mature adults develop in about 3 weeks. Cockroaches may also serve as intermediate hosts. These insects become infected by ingesting eggs passed in rodent feces. The eggs develop into cysticercoids in the hemocoelom of the insect; when ingested, the cysticercoids are infectious to rodents or humans. Human infection probably occurs by accidental ingestion of mealworms, or grain beetles found in dry grains, cereals, flour, and dried fruits. Human infections are light, and the life span in humans is short. The diagnosis is made by finding ova in the stool.

DIPYLIDIASIS

Dipylidium caninum is a cestode of dogs, cats, and wild carnivores that occasionally infects humans. Most of the infections have occurred in children younger than 8 years of age, with one third occurring in infants younger than 6 months. Transmission is thought to be due to accidental swallowing of infected adult fleas, most likely because of the close association between children and dogs and cats. Transmission may also occur as the result of hand-to-mouth contamination.

Adult tapeworms are 15 to 20 cm in length, with 60 to 175 proglottids. *Dipylidium caninum* has a characteristic rhomboidal scolex with four oval suckers and an armed, retractable, conical rostellum containing 30 to 150 thorn-shaped hooks arranged in transverse rows. The vase-shaped proglottids possess a double set of reproductive organs with genital pores at the midpoint of each lateral margin. Gravid proglottids contain 25 to 30 eggs. Each egg is 35 to 60 μm in diameter and contains an oncosphere with six hooklets. Strobila are capable of moving several inches per hour passing out of the anus or in the feces. Eggs are expelled by contraction of the proglottids or disintegration of the proglottid outside of the intestine on the perianal region. The intermediate hosts of *Dipylidium* are larval fleas that infect dogs, cats, or humans. Those cysticercoid larvae that survive the metamorphosis of the larval flea are ingested by the definitive host, where the larvae are liberated in the small intestine to become adults in about 20 days.

Most patients are asymptomatic, but clinical findings attributed to *D. caninum* infection include abdominal pain, diarrhea, urticaria, and pruritus ani. Multiple infections are not uncommon. Definitive diagnosis is made by finding typical eggs or proglottids in stool. However, examination for eggs may be unreliable, since proglottids usually do not release eggs within the intestines. There may be moderate eosinophilia.

TRICHINOSIS (TRICHINELLOSIS)

By Zbigniew S. Pawlowski, M.D.
Poznań, Poland

Synonyms for trichinosis are trichinellosis and trichiniasis. The term trichinosis implies both the infection with *Trichinella spiralis* and the disease caused by *T. spiralis,* a nematode that parasitizes the intestinal tract and muscle tissue of humans and many domesticated and wild mammals. In its acute stage, trichinosis is characterized by hypersensitivity reactions, acute myositis, and metabolic disorders. Circulatory, neurologic, and pulmonary complications are not uncommon and may be fatal.

Trichinosis tends to occur in epidemic form, with each epidemic caused by the same infected meat; however, isolated cases in which the diagnosis may be more difficult are occasionally reported. The disease is not as common in the United States as it was 30 to 50 years ago; 32 cases were reported in 1994.

BIOLOGIC BACKGROUND

Trichinosis is acquired by ingestion of *T. spiralis* larvae encysted in meat. Pork, horse, wild boar, bear, and walrus are the most common sources of infection. Adult worms develop in the small intestine and start to produce newborn *T. spiralis* larvae as early as the fifth day after consumption of infected meat. The larvae are carried in the bloodstream to different tissues and organs but develop further only in the muscle tissue. Adult worms may survive in the human intestine for about 2 months, but most of the larvae are produced in the first few weeks. The muscle larvae may live for many years, but usually they die off gradually and become calcified or absorbed.

Five separate species of *Trichinella* have been identified recently by isoenzyme electrophoresis and genotype (DNA, r-DNA) characterization. The various species differ in epidemiology and clinical expression. *Trichinella nelsoni* in Africa and *T. britovi* in Palearctic cause a relatively mild trichinellosis in humans; *T. nativa* in the Arctic is more likely to cause more serious disease than widely spread *T. spiralis* sensu stricto. It is only recently that *T. pseudospiralis* has been identified in a human case. In the text, the term *T. spiralis* is used because it is the most common in human infections and the best known species.

SIGNS AND SYMPTOMS

Trichinosis is characterized by a remarkable variety of signs and symptoms that occur in a sequence reflecting the successive pathologic processes.

The abdominal syndrome, consisting of abdominal pain and diarrhea, may be the first to appear as a result of trichinous enteritis. It may also occur or recur between the third and fifth weeks of disease, probably because of a delayed hypersensitivity reaction.

The general trichinous syndrome involves fever, followed by myalgia and malaise. The pathomechanism of the fever remains unclear; some toxins or immunologic phenomena are suspected of activating endogenous pyrogens. Myalgia is related to acute myositis; there is some spontaneous muscle pain, but intensity normally increases greatly with movement. Immobilization of untreated patients may lead to fixed contractures in the later stage of disease.

The allergic vasculitis, present early in moderate and severe trichinosis, manifests itself in the leakage of fluid from the vascular to the interstitial compartment, best visible as periorbital edema, and in hemorrhages. The hemorrhages may occur in many organs but can be seen most easily in the conjunctiva and as splinter hemorrhages in fingernail beds.

Metabolic disorders, such as hypoalbuminemia, hypokalemia, and hypoglycemia, are usually related to the intensity of infection and do not occur before the third week of trichinosis. Hypoalbuminemia is clinically expressed by hydrostatic edema and effusions in the peritoneal and pleural cavities. Signs of hypokalemia may best be seen in electrocardiographic tracings in the later stages of disease.

COURSE

The clinical course of trichinosis usually varies considerably among individuals, even in the same epidemic outbreak. The incubation period of acute trichinosis (fever, myalgia, periorbital edema, eosinophilia) is between 5 and 51 days, but it is usually shorter in severe cases.

Trichinosis may be asymptomatic, or it may follow one of five clinical courses:

1. In *asymptomatic* cases, history of exposure and positive results of serologic tests (if performed 4 to 8 weeks after ingestion of infected meat) may be the only positive findings; eosinophilia may be transient.
2. In *abortive* cases, eosinophilia is usually present in addition to a few transient signs (some fever and/or myalgia for 1 to 2 days).
3. *Mild* cases usually show a complex of signs (fever, myalgia, periorbital edema) mildly expressed. Temperature in patients not treated with steroids is below 38°C (100.4°F), and fever lasts for less than a week.
4. In *moderate* cases, the full complex of signs is well expressed, with body temperatures above 38°C (100.4°F) for up to 2 weeks and hypoalbuminemia with serum albumin levels below 3 g/dL, in untreated cases. Complications are still rare and/or transient, and recovery occurs within 5 to 7 weeks.
5. In *severe* cases, the full complex of signs is intensively expressed. High fever, with temperatures above 39°C (102.2°F), may be present for more than 2 weeks; hypoalbuminemia may be significant, with serum albumin levels below 2.5 g/dL; and eosinophilia may be absent. Circulatory, neurologic, and/or pulmonary complications are common and may be fatal. Recovery is slow and takes at least 7 weeks.

COMMON COMPLICATIONS

The diagnosis may be difficult in the later stages of trichinosis, when complications may dominate the clinical picture. The complications are mainly due to the ectopic migration of *T. spiralis* larvae and/or inflammatory or hypersensitive reactions of the host. Sometimes the complications are secondary, for example, to metabolic disorders.

Orbital manifestations, such as periorbital edema and conjunctival hemorrhages, are sometimes the first signs to suggest trichinosis. Later, pain in the eyeball, disturbed vision, photophobia, and blurring may occur.

Neurologic manifestations can appear early or late; they may be of a diffuse or focal character. Signs and symptoms of meningitis and encephalitis, such as strong headache, insomnia, delirium, and apathy, are usually early and diffuse. Focal manifestations, such as hemianopia, aphasia, anisocoria, tinnitus, ataxia, seizures, and various types of paralysis and paresis, usually develop during or after the third week of disease.

Cardiovascular complications of trichinosis are the most frequent and the most serious. Focal necrosis and/or cellular infiltration of myocardial fibers can later become more diffuse and cause an eosinophilic myocarditis that may eventually evolve into an interstitial myocarditis. The myocardial changes are only one cause of circulatory complications; others are arrhythmias, adrenal gland insufficiency, and functional changes of blood vessels. Extreme hypotension, thrombosis, emboli, and pulmonary complications are not uncommon.

The major causes of death in trichinosis are myocarditis, encephalitis, and pneumonitis. Sudden death without premonitory cardiac symptoms may occur in the first week of the disease but is more likely to occur later as a result of pulmonary embolism or paroxysmal tachycardia.

PHYSICAL EXAMINATION

In trichinosis, physical examination has a somewhat limited diagnostic importance. The clinician may suspect trichinosis only by finding signs and symptoms that are not pathognomonic, a history of exposure to infected meat, and high eosinophilia. Trichinosis may be confirmed by the observation of a characteristic clinical course, by a positive reaction to corticosteroid and/or mebendazole or albendazole treatment, and by positive serologic test results. However, the definitive diagnosis of trichinosis can be based only on finding the parasite.

Fever, myalgia, and malaise are common in many other diseases (e.g., viral infections). However, muscle signs and symptoms have some characteristic features:

1. Myalgia follows fever and does not precede it.
2. Pain is referred to the muscles most frequently used (masseters, tongue, extraocular and respiratory muscles, neck, and flexor muscles of the extremities).
3. Because pain increases greatly with movement, patients usually keep their elbows, hips, and knee joints flexed and do not like to change position.
4. The muscles of the extremities are tender to palpation and painful with induced movement or deeper pressure.
5. Flexor contractions may induce tetanic rigidity.

Characteristic but by no means universal symptoms of trichinosis include periorbital edema and conjunctival or fingernail hemorrhages.

LABORATORY PROCEDURES

Eosinophilia, leukocytosis, increased activity of some enzymes, and positive specific serologic test results are of much help in the diagnosis of trichinosis.

Eosinophilia is an early, common, and characteristic finding in human trichinosis. It occurs during the second week after ingestion of infected meat, remains high for several weeks, and gradually declines; it can be diminished by corticosteroid therapy. Eosinophilia is usually well pronounced (1000 to 3000/mm^3) and protracted for many weeks; only in aborted infections may it be slight (500/mm^3) and transient. In severe trichinosis, eosinophilia may be as high as 89 per cent or may fall sharply; either finding is a poor prognostic sign.

Leukocytosis is usually less consistent, less evident, and less persistent than eosinophilia. The count is usually around 15,000/mm^3, but it may be as high as 50,000/mm^3.

Leakage of some enzymes from muscle fibers into the serum results in an increase in serum levels of creatine kinase, aldolase, and lactate dehydrogenase in the second week of disease. Less common and less pronounced is the increase of aspartate and alanine aminotransferases.

A high serum creatine level and creatinuria are usually present in intensive trichinosis.

Serologic tests, such as the IgG enzyme-linked immunosorbent assay (ELISA) and double-sandwich IgM, identify most of the diseased patients 3 to 4 weeks after exposure, and results become negative after 2 to 8 months. The indirect immunofluorescence test is less sensitive. IgE antibodies occur only in about 20 per cent of patients and show inconsistent patterns during the disease. Circulatory antigens occur late and usually disappear when acute symptoms fade away. Flocculation or agglutination techniques with bentonite, latex, or cholesterol are highly specific but have low sensitivity; the same is true for counterelectrophoresis and double-diffusion tests. In practice, it is good to use two different tests at the same time and to repeat the serologic examination after 10 to 14 days to observe a positive conversion or an increase in their titers, which would suggest a recent infection.

PARASITOLOGIC DIAGNOSIS

A definite diagnosis of trichinosis by finding the parasite is important in a sporadic case or in an index case in an epidemic outbreak. Attempts to find adult *T. spiralis* worms in the duodenal content or in the feces are impractical. Finding adult worms in small intestinal mucosa scrapings during postmortem examination has been reported. A few newborn *T. spiralis* larvae can be isolated by filtration of several milliliters of blood through filters with 3-μm pores.

Finding the older larval stages of *T. spiralis* requires biopsy of muscle tissue. Muscle biopsy not only confirms the presence (or absence) of *T. spiralis* but also gives an idea of the intensity of infection and enables taxonomic identification. The character and intensity of some pathologic changes found in the muscle tissue on biopsy may also be helpful for a better understanding of the clinical picture and for decisions concerning specific therapy.

The preferred superficial skeletal muscles for biopsy are the deltoid of the shoulder and the gastrocnemius of the leg. The muscle sample (0.5 to 1.0 g) is usually divided into a smaller part (one fourth) for fixation and subsequent histopathologic examination and a larger part (three fourths) for parasitologic examination. This consists of trichinoscopy (microscopic examination of tiny cuts of muscle compressed between two glass slides) and digestion of the muscle tissue. The muscle tissue samples used for trichinoscopy can be digested in 1 per cent pepsin and 1 per cent hydrochloric acid solution at 38°C (100.4°F). After a few hours, the excysted larvae can be collected from the washed sediment. The digestion technique is not practicable for nonencysted *T. spiralis* larvae (i.e., younger than 16 days). After trichinoscopy, a small sample with *T. spiralis* encysted larvae may be fed to mice to keep the isolate for further investigations.

POTENTIAL DIAGNOSTIC ERRORS AND PITFALLS

Human trichinosis frequently remains undiagnosed or is incorrectly diagnosed, especially in sporadic or index cases, because of the diversity and wide variation in signs and symptoms during different periods of the disease.

During the incubation period of trichinosis, food intoxication and nonspecific gastroenterocolitis are common misdiagnoses. The acute general trichinosis syndrome (fever, myalgia, and malaise) is similar to the clinical picture in several viral infections, typhoid fever, leptospirosis, rheumatic fever, and septicemia.

The syndrome of allergic vasculitis may be confused with dermatomyositis, periarteritis nodosa, angioneurotic edema, serum sickness, and drug allergy. Neurologic, pulmonary, or cardiac complications may sometimes overshadow other signs and symptoms of trichinosis.

In some severe cases, the lack of eosinophilia or a false-positive serologic test response for typhoid may be misleading.

Trichinosis is most likely to occur in people who live in the well-known endemic areas, but it should also be considered in tourists and hunters who visit exotic states or countries (e.g., Alaska, Hawaii, Egypt, Kenya, Tanzania, and Thailand).

OTHER INTESTINAL PARASITES

By Jeffrey P. Gumprecht, M.D.
New York, New York

and Murray Wittner, M.D., Ph.D.
Bronx, New York

Parasites are recognized as increasingly important causes of illness in the United States as a result of (1) more immigrants from Third World countries, (2) more travel by Americans to Third World countries, and (3) an increase in the population of immunocompromised individuals including those with human immunodeficiency virus infection.

MEDICAL HISTORY

Unless parasitic illness is specifically considered and diagnostic clues are actively sought, the diagnosis is likely to remain obscure. Diagnosis begins with a careful history, including the central question, Where have you been? Important clues from the travel history include any exposure to environments in which the level of sanitation is poor, thus resulting in possible fecal-oral transmission or fecal contamination of food or water. Such environments are not limited to the Third World; institutions for the retarded or disturbed, day care centers, and Indian reservations in developed countries are also areas of high risk. Another risk is drinking untreated water, whether from private wells or directly from streams or lakes in North America, or even drinking tap water in St. Petersburg, Russia (a high risk for giardiasis).

In some parasitic infections, the organisms excreted by a human are directly infectious to other persons, and the history should include information about exposure to an ill child, traveler, or immigrant. Consumption of unusual foods should be indicated, especially raw meat or seafood and uncooked items that were preserved by pickling, smoking, or drying. Employment may also be a significant risk factor, if it involves exposure to an unsanitary environment (as described before). A sexual history may be appropriate to elicit the possibility of oral-anal contact, particularly among homosexual men. The physician should inquire about prior history of parasitism and its treatment.

A search for gastrointestinal symptoms should include (1) development of intolerance to particular foods, especially milk; (2) diarrhea with or without the passage of obvious worms, blood, or mucus; (3) presence of significant weight loss; and (4) abdominal pain and its characteristics, as well as provoking and alleviating factors or evidence of malabsorption. Extraintestinal symptoms of fever, pruritus, jaundice, myalgias, and respiratory disorders may also be important clues to parasitosis.

It is important to determine through the patient's history and laboratory report whether the patient has or has had a dysenteric syndrome marked by the presence of red blood cells in the stool and noted by the patient as abdominal pain, tenesmus, frequent stools, and visible pus, blood, and mucus. Alternatively, the patient may be experiencing a watery diarrheal syndrome defined as a change in stool habit and consistency but without tenesmus or the passage of red or white blood cells in the stool. Differentiating these two syndromes is necessary because they suggest different groups of infectious agents.

LABORATORY INVESTIGATION

Microscopic examination of the stool remains the primary method of identifying intestinal parasitism. Diligent examination by skilled technicians of properly collected and processed specimens is an expensive, but irreplaceable, diagnostic tool. The laboratory has available a variety of special stains and concentration techniques that often permit vastly increased diagnostic sensitivity for specific organisms. These procedures, however, may substantially increase the time and expense of the stool examination; to use them appropriately, the clinician must inform the laboratory of the organism being sought and the patient's travel history.

Specimens for examination should be collected in clean containers free of urine, water, soap, and disinfectants. Stools are unsuitable for parasitologic examination for about a week after a patient has been given barium, antidiarrheal agents (especially those containing antibiotic or amebicidal agents), antacids, bismuth, or certain enema preparations. Identification of protozoa is much more sensitive to interference from these substances than is identification of helminth larvae or eggs. Appropriate handling of the stool specimens before examination is of paramount importance. Formed stool specimens may be kept under refrigeration for up to 16 hours; unformed and liquid stools must be examined within 1 hour of being passed or protozoal trophozoites may have lysed. If examination within these time limits is impractical, specimens should be preserved by a technique of the laboratory's choice.

In the choice of a parasitology laboratory, an important criterion is its participation in proficiency testing programs administered by the College of American Pathologists or another recognized agency. Parasitologic examinations performed outside of North America, particularly in Third World countries, are of uncertain validity and should not be accepted as diagnostic, especially if results are negative. New techniques using fluorescein-labeled antibodies for stool examination are commercially available, but their appropriate roles are still being explored. The patient should be given instructions, in the event that a macroscopic worm is passed, to preserve the specimen for examination by an expert. This can be done by placing it in ethanol (70 per cent), vodka, or other clear grain spirits.

Serologic diagnosis of parasitic infections is rapidly evolving, and analysis of coproantibodies may be useful in the future, especially when nursing or transportation problems prevent the collection of adequate stool samples or when substances that interfere with analysis are present in the stool. Serology is also useful when repeated examination of the stool fails to demonstrate parasites in a setting of high clinical suspicion.

As a rule of thumb, three stools obtained on alternate days should be examined to ensure that adequate diagnostic sensitivity and specificity are achieved. The presence of one parasite is often a marker of exposure to an environment with poor sanitation; multiple parasitosis is frequent, and an important organism may be present in small numbers. Three stool examinations should then be repeated some weeks after treatment is completed to detect the occasional treatment failures expected with all drug regimens.

It is important to understand the mechanisms and requirements for transmission of the various parasites described in the following. Appropriate isolation practices must be instituted to protect others from the patient, and the source of the patient's infection must be determined and its public health implications analyzed.

TRANSMISSION, SYMPTOMS, AND DIAGNOSIS

Protozoa

Enterocytozoon bienusi

This protozoan parasite and *Encephalitozoon intestinalis* are in the phylum Microspora, whose members are best known for causing illnesses of economic significance in fish and insects. It is an obligate intracellular parasite that has been discovered in some patients with acquired immunodeficiency syndrome (AIDS) who are afflicted with chronic diarrhea and weight loss. Diagnosis is made by examining Giemsa-stained biopsy specimens of intestinal mucosa with the use of light or electron microscopy. Stool examination can be useful if staining with calcifluor white, Giemsa, or modified trichrome is employed. Information on the prevalence of this infection and an effective treatment awaits further studies.

Isospora belli

Most frequently found in tropical climates in areas of poor sanitation, this protozoan has also caused clusters of infection in developed countries where sanitation is inadequate. Humans are the only known host. Ingested oocysts liberate sporozoites on reaching the small intestine; these enter epithelial cells and initiate both asexual and sexual reproductive cycles. Infection spreads to adjacent epithelial cells, and infective oocysts are produced and passed in the stool. In immunocompetent hosts, the illness is self-limited and typically consists of colicky abdominal pain, watery diarrhea, and flatulence lasting 2 to 3 weeks. However, the syndrome can persist for months in otherwise normal patients and may be accompanied by eosinophilia, malabsorption, and weight loss. In patients with AIDS, the infection is often chronic or relapsing and causes a progressive and severe wasting syndrome. Diagnosis is usually made by examination of the stool. However, the organism may be shed intermittently and in small numbers; stool concentration techniques or duodenal sampling by string or intubation may be required to demonstrate the organism. Diagnosis may also be accomplished by examination of biopsy material. Even in the presence of symptomatically effective treatment, normal hosts may continue to shed the organism for several months.

Blastocystis hominis

The taxonomic position of this organism, as well as its validity as a human pathogen, remains uncertain. Distribution of the organism is ubiquitous, and it was found in up to 18 per cent of asymptomatic individuals in some population surveys. However, in some individuals, the organism appears to be associated with a mild to severe diarrheal syndrome with nonspecific abdominal discomfort. Some patients respond to treatment with resolution of symptoms and disappearance of the organism from the stool. The diagnosis is made by identifying characteristic cysts or trophozoites in the stool.

Balantidium coli

This is the only ciliated protozoan known to be pathogenic to humans and also the largest protozoan that infects humans. It is found in both temperate and tropical climates, usually in areas where humans have close contact with pigs, sheep, and a variety of other animals and also in settings of poor hygiene. The infection is acquired by fecal-oral contact or from contaminated water. After the cysts are ingested, trophozoites are liberated in the small intestine and passed to the colon. There they may live in the lumen or invade the bowel wall and cause ulceration of the mucosa. Cysts are shed in the stool and are immediately infective.

Most patients are asymptomatic, but either a diarrheal or a dysenteric syndrome of variable severity may occur. The dysentery is clinically and pathologically similar to that of amebiasis; however, extraintestinal disease is rare. Diagnosis is made by examination of the stool or material scraped from the base of an ulcer during sigmoidoscopic examination. Serology is being developed.

Dientamoeba fragilis

This protozoan is found in both temperate and tropical settings, independent of the level of sanitation. The details of its life cycle remain unknown, but an association has been noted between infection with *Enterobius vermicularis* (pinworm) and infection with *D. fragilis*; it has been suggested that it is transmitted with *E. vermicularis* ova. Infection produces symptoms that include abdominal discomfort, nausea, vomiting, diarrhea, and sometimes low-grade fever. Diagnosis is accomplished by careful examination of trichrome-stained preparations of either fresh stool or stool preserved in polyvinyl alcohol.

Nematodes

Anisakid Nematodes

These parasites infect various saltwater fish and squid. Humans, as accidental hosts, represent a dead end for the larvae, which are then unable to mature. Human infection is acquired by eating raw or improperly prepared fish, often as sashimi, sushi, or ceviche. Implicated fish include salmon, Pacific red snapper, cod, mackerel, herring, and occasionally tuna. After ingestion, the larvae are exceedingly active; they may travel up the esophagus into the mouth or pharynx, they may be passed into the stool, or they may burrow into or through the wall of the gastrointestinal tract. With time, the worms become lodged, most often in the wall of the stomach or intestine but occasionally elsewhere in the peritoneal cavity, and a host response leads to abscess or granuloma formation.

Patients may present several hours after ingestion of raw fish and appear to have appendicitis or other causes of an acute abdomen with severe pain, nausea, vomiting, and diarrhea. The symptoms may wane after several days, but the patient may present later with symptoms of inflammatory bowel disease or other causes of chronic abdominal pain. Variable degrees of eosinophilia may be seen. The definitive diagnosis is often made during acute disease by retrieving a worm at laparotomy or endoscopy. In a patient with a compatible history, the diagnosis of chronic disease is suggested by finding a granuloma or small mass in the wall of the stomach or intestine that is infiltrated with eosinophils. Careful pathologic examination of this tissue for the remains of the worm is indicated. Serologic techniques for the diagnosis of anisakiasis are currently under evaluation.

Trichuris trichiura

This organism causes trichuriasis or whipworm infection. It has a worldwide distribution but is seen most frequently in warm, moist regions, including the southern United States. Infection is acquired by ingestion of mature eggs. Larvae emerge from the eggs in the small intestine and mature there before passing to the cecum, where the adult worms attach to the mucosa. The adults produce large numbers of eggs, which are passed in the stool. These eggs are noninfectious until they have matured in appropriate soil.

Most patients with moderate or light infections are asymptomatic. Heavy infections may cause a chronic dysenteric syndrome with marked rectal tenesmus, rectal prolapse, abdominal cramping, and weight loss similar to amebic dysentery. Eosinophilia is unusual and rarely, if ever, is greater than 15 per cent. Coinfection with *Entamoeba histolytica, Ascaris lumbricoides,* or hookworms occurs frequently. The diagnosis is usually made by identification of the characteristic eggs in the stool; Charcot-Leyden crystals may be present. If stool samples are difficult to obtain, the diagnosis in heavy infections is made by proctoscopic examination, which can reveal the adult worms embedded in the rectal mucosa.

Enterobius vermicularis

Also known as the seatworm or pinworm, this parasite causes enterobiasis and has a worldwide distribution. It is usually acquired by the fecal-oral route, but transmission by ingestion of recently passed eggs and by objects contaminated with these eggs has been demonstrated. The eggs hatch in the small intestine and attach to the mucosa in the area of the cecum. After 1 month the worms are mature, and gravid females migrate out of the colon onto the perianal skin, where they lay their eggs; these become infective within hours of deposit. Diagnosis is rarely made by stool examination, but rather the perianal skin is touched with clear plastic tape. The tape is then applied to a glass slide and examined for characteristic eggs or adult worms. This examination is most useful if performed in the morning before the patient bathes or has a bowel movement.

Ascaris lumbricoides

The human roundworm that causes ascariasis, this organism has worldwide distribution. Infection is acquired by ingestion of eggs that have matured in appropriate soil. The eggs hatch in the stomach and intestine and release larvae, which penetrate the mucosa and enter capillaries. The larvae are carried to the lungs, where they pass into the airspaces and travel up the bronchial tree. They are then swallowed in the pharynx. When they reach the small intestine, the larvae attach to the walls and mature into adults.

Symptoms due to adult worms in the intestine are unusual unless large numbers are present; in such cases, abdominal pain, nausea, and vomiting may occur. Rarely, intestinal obstruction may result from intussusception or a mass of worms. Because adult worms tend to probe small channels, they may ascend the biliary tree and cause cholangitis, pancreatitis, and hepatic abscesses. During their passage through the lungs, larvae may produce a syndrome of bronchospasm, fever, marked eosinophilia, and fleeting infiltrates (seen on chest radiograph) known as Löffler's syndrome, or *Ascaris* pneumonia. In the absence of larval migration, eosinophilia is usually mild (10 to 15 per cent). Eggs are usually found in the feces in large numbers and make the diagnosis straightforward; occasionally, adult worms are also found. Immunodiagnosis, currently limited by cross-reactivity among different species of helminths, is of little value. The presence of *A. lumbricoides* suggests exposure to an environment with poor sanitation, and a multiple parasitosis should be carefully excluded.

Ancylostoma duodenale *and* Necator americanus

These parasites cause human hookworm infection. They are found throughout tropical and subtropical areas of the world. Infection is acquired by contact of bare skin with soil contaminated by infective filariform larval worms. After penetration of the skin, the larvae travel to the lungs via the bloodstream and pass into the airspaces. They then ascend the bronchial tree and are swallowed. Subsequently, they mate, attach to the mucosa of the small intestine, and on maturation lay eggs, which are passed in the feces. In soil, the larvae hatch, feed, and molt to infective filariform larvae.

Symptoms of pruritus and an erythematous rash may occur when the larvae pass through the skin. Löffler's syndrome (described before) occurs rarely but may produce symptoms. The intestinal worms cause only mild abdominal discomfort; but in the presence of a heavy worm burden, they may cause significant losses of iron and protein that lead to a microcytic hypochromic anemia and weight loss. Diagnosis is made by discovering characteristic eggs in the stool. Eosinophilia is usually present but is mild except during the period of larval migration or in instances of heavy infection.

Strongyloides stercoralis

The threadworm that causes strongyloidiasis, this parasite is found in areas of poor sanitation throughout tropical and temperate climates. Infective filariform larvae produced by free-living worms in the soil penetrate the human skin. The larvae travel through the venous system into the lungs, where they enter the airspace and then migrate up to the pharynx and are swallowed. On arriving in the small intestine, the female burrows into the mucosa, matures, and deposits eggs. These hatch immediately and release rhabditiform larvae, which may be excreted in the feces. If deposited in appropriate soil, the larvae either develop into filariform larvae or initiate the free-living sexual cycle of the worm. However, during passage through the lumen of the colon, some rhabditiform larvae may molt into infective filariform larvae. These may penetrate the bowel wall and cause internal autoinfection, or they may penetrate the perineal skin and cause a rash (larva currens) and external autoinfection. Filariform larvae that have penetrated the bowel wall or perineal skin then enter the venous system, repeat the migration through the lung, and return to the intestine.

When small numbers of larvae produce autoinfection, they cause few, if any, symptoms and appear to maintain a persistent infection for decades after the host has left the endemic zone. At the onset of infection, a pruritic rash at the site of larval penetration may occur. Löffler's syndrome can follow in exceptionally heavy infections. During replication in the intestines, midepigastric pain often mimics peptic ulcer disease. A dysenteric syndrome with colicky abdominal pain may occur, but this is uncommon except in heavy infections. A few patients have malabsorption and weight loss.

In patients who harbor even a small number of worms, immunosuppression due to malnutrition, steroids, or antineoplastic agents may lead to the hyperinfection syndrome. This occurs when autoinfection intensifies, with massive larval migration through the gut wall into the peritoneum, lungs, and other distant sites. Perforation of the bowel, gram-negative sepsis, shock, and death often follow. The hyperinfection syndrome should be avoided by careful screening for *S. stercoralis* before therapeutic immunosuppression if the patient has an appropriate exposure history.

Typical infection is diagnosed by finding characteristic larvae in the stools; concentration techniques are useful if small numbers are present. Sampling of duodenal fluid may also demonstrate the larvae in some occult infections. Serology is available. In cases of hyperinfection syndrome, larvae are easily found in stool and sputum and occasionally in pleural fluid and cerebrospinal fluid. Eosinophilia may be absent or markedly increased; the former may have a poor prognosis.

Cestodes

Taeniasis

The pork tapeworm, *Taenia solium,* and the beef tapeworm, *Taenia saginata,* are the common tapeworm parasites of humans. These infections have been known since ancient times and occur whenever infected, insufficiently cooked beef or pork is consumed. Adult worms vary in size from 4 to 12 m and may be composed of 1000 to 2000 proglottids. In multiple infections, however, a "crowding effect" is noted so that each worm is usually smaller.

The adult is found only in humans and is generally attached in the jejunum. Their eggs are 30 to 40 μm in diameter and are similar in morphologic appearance among all members of the genus. Cattle or hogs become infected by ingesting mature eggs. The action of gastric juice, intestinal enzymes, and bile is required to stimulate hatching. Embryos then penetrate the intestinal mucosa, enter the circulation, and migrate throughout the body. Encystment usually occurs in striated muscle, and within 10 to 11 weeks the larvae, termed *Cysticercus cellulosae* in hogs or *Cysticercus bovis* in cattle, are infectious. On ingestion, the cysticercus is activated by digestive juices in the gut. The scolex then evaginates and attaches to the jejunal wall, becoming a mature tapeworm in 10 to 12 weeks for *T. saginata* and in 5 to 12 weeks for *T. solium.*

Humans are the definitive host for both *T. saginata* and *T. solium.* Human infection with the pork tapeworm has become uncommon in the United States, although cysticercosis in hogs still occurs. Human infection with *C. cellulosae,* or cysticercosis, is found wherever adult *T. solium* infection is common. *T. saginata* infection occurs among those who prefer to eat raw or insufficiently cooked beef. In the United States, raw beef is often found on menus as steak tartare at "chic" metropolitan restaurants, indicating the extent of the popularity of this food.

The scolex generally lodges in the upper jejunum. Most individuals who harbor *T. solium* or *T. saginata* infection either are asymptomatic or have mild to moderate complaints. The infection can occasionally cause serious, life-threatening disease by intestinal, appendiceal, biliary, or pancreatic obstruction resulting in an acute surgical abdomen. Among the most frequently reported signs or symptoms of adult *Taenia* infection are spontaneous discharge of proglottids per rectum, abdominal pain, nausea, weakness, loss of appetite, increased appetite, headache, constipation, dizziness, diarrhea, pruritus ani, and hyperexcitability. Abdominal pain and nausea are more common in the morning and characteristically relieved by food. Children are symptomatic more frequently than adults. Eosinophilia can rarely rise to more than 50 per cent, but it usually ranges from 5 to 15 per cent. Serum immunoglobulin E concentrations may be increased.

Because detection of *Taenia* eggs in the stool is not sufficient to make a specific diagnosis, a gravid proglottid must be obtained. Proglottids are passed in the stool or emerge on the perianal or perineal region frequently and spontaneously, but at irregular intervals. Identification of proglottids is done by pressing the segment between two glass microscope slides and counting the main lateral branches of the uterus. *T. solium* has 10 to 13 primary branches on each side, and *T. saginata* has 15 to 20 lateral primary branches per side. Fecal examination, especially for *T. saginata,* is often unrewarding because gravid proglottids tend to migrate or "crawl" out on the perianal area before ovipositing. Anal swabs, such as the cellophane tape method usually done for the diagnosis of pinworm, are recommended to detect the ova. In addition, the embryophore of *T. saginata* can be stained with the Ziehl-Neelsen stain, but that of *T. solium* does not stain.

The prevention of beef and pork tapeworm infection can be accomplished by adequate cooking or freezing of these meats. *Cysticercus cellulosae* is killed by moderate temperatures of 65°C (149°F) or if the pork is frozen at −20°C (−4°F) for at least 12 hours. Pickling in brine and salted pork are not always adequate methods. *Cysticercus bovis* is killed by thorough cooking at 55°C (131°F) or freezing at −10°C (14°F) for 5 days. Pickling of beef in 25 per cent brine for 5 to 6 days may render the beef safe. Treatment of all infected individuals would eliminate the source of soil and sewage pollution with *Taenia* eggs. However, meat inspection would help reduce transmission to humans who fail to properly prepare meat.

Cysticercosis

Cysticercus cellulosae is a well-known cause of central nervous system disease in endemic areas. When humans (or hogs) ingest mature eggs of *T. solium*, the embryos hatch (when stimulated by gastric juice, intestinal enzymes, and bile), enter the circulation, and disseminate throughout the body. They often encyst in striated muscle and other tissues, where in 10 to 11 weeks they become infectious larvae termed *C. cellulosae.* Cysticerci are bladderlike cysts in which an inverted scolex has developed. Symptomatic disease results when these larvae become encysted in the central nervous system, eye, or heart.

The clinical manifestations depend on the number and anatomic localization of the cysts and the inflammatory response of the host. Cysticerci have been found in almost every tissue and organ of the body. Cerebral cysticercosis may remain asymptomatic for years, until symptoms arise from inflammation that accompanies the death of the cysts. If a cysticercus is located in the cerebral ventricles, noncommunicating hydrocephalus can occur; rarely, a ball-valve mechanism causes sudden blockage and syncope. In the basilar cisterns, cysts may cause communicating hydrocephalus and cranial nerve palsy. Racemose forms may occur in this location and are associated with a poor prognosis. Heavy cyst burdens may cause dementia and personality changes. Ocular cysticercosis can present as disturbances of vision, scotoma, free-floating parasites in the vitreous, or retinal detachment.

Computed tomographic scanning may demonstrate active cysts with edema and/or calcifications. Magnetic resonance imaging is more likely to detect active lesions with edema and less likely to detect old calcified lesions. Calcified cysticerci can often be seen on skull films as multiple comma-shaped or arclike calcifications in the brain or soft tissues. Careful physical examination may reveal subcutaneous cysticerci, of which biopsy can be done for diagnosis. In some patients with hydrocephalus or aseptic meningitis, myelography may demonstrate extraventricular cysts.

Lumbar puncture is useful to obtain cerebrospinal fluid for diagnostic studies. Active meningitis is an indication for treatment. Cerebrospinal fluid eosinophilia may be observed. Glucose concentration in the cerebrospinal fluid may be as low as 2 mg/dL.

Serologic studies are useful in the diagnosis of *Cysticercus* infection. Both cerebrospinal fluid and serum should be examined. Western blot has replaced indirect hemagglutination as the diagnostic test of choice. Western blot (from the Centers for Disease Control and Prevention) has also eliminated the previous problems of cross-reactivity with *Echinococcus.* With isolated cysts, however, the sensitivity of Western blot may be lower.

Although the yield is low, patients with cysticercosis should have stool examinations for *T. solium.* Family members may also require screening.

Section Three

EAR, NOSE, AND THROAT

OTITIS (MEDIA AND EXTERNA)

By Thomas N. Roberts, M.D.
La Crosse, Wisconsin

OTITIS EXTERNA

Otitis externa refers to inflammation of the external ear canal and pinna. For practical purposes, otitis externa can be classified as acute otitis externa, chronic otitis externa, dermatoses of the external ear, and necrotizing malignant otitis externa.

Acute Otitis Externa

The normal external ear is protected by sebaceous gland secretions and exfoliated cells that provide a waxy, water-repellent coating. If this coating is compromised, acute infections may occur. For example, excess moisture in the external canal due to swimming or increased humidity often causes maceration of the canal, promoting secondary bacterial infection. The protective barrier can also be breached by trauma during cleaning or scratching of the canal. The most common infecting agents are *Pseudomonas*, *Proteus*, *Escherichia coli*, and *Klebsiella pneumoniae*; less commonly involved microbes include *Staphylococcus epidermidis* and streptococci. Most patients present with pain that may be accompanied by fever and swelling. Physical examination reveals marked discomfort during traction of the pinna or direct palpation of the tragus. The external canal often appears circumferentially hyperemic. Extensive edema of the canal may prevent adequate examination of the tympanic membrane. Conductive hearing loss is not uncommon when edema is extensive.

Staphylococcal furunculosis typically presents with pain, hyperemia, and localized swelling in the outer third of the hair-containing portion of the external canal. Acute cellulitis of the external canal and pinna, commonly caused by staphylococci or streptococci, is characterized by generalized swelling, edema, and systemic manifestations of illness. By contrast, herpetic infection of the canal and pinna presents with pain, fever, and groups of crusted vesicles. The differential diagnosis of acute otitis externa includes otitis media and mastoiditis. In both of these conditions, however, tenderness on traction of the pinna or pressure on the tragus is not typically noted. Systemic manifestations of illness are more prevalent in both otitis media and mastoiditis. The swelling of mastoiditis tends to be localized over the mastoid process and may elevate the pinna anteriorly and inferiorly.

Chronic Otitis Externa

Chronic otitis externa, which is relatively uncommon, occurs when inflammation lasts for more than 1 month. Itching is more prominent than severe pain or discomfort. The most common cause of chronic otitis externa is *Pseudomonas* infection, but tuberculosis, syphilis, and sarcoidosis have also been implicated.

Acute Dermatoses

Acute dermatoses of the external canal are common in children. Examples include acute seborrheic dermatitis, eczema, and contact dermatitis. Dermatoses of the external canal and pinna are characterized by extensive pruritus and crusting. Pain is relatively minimal compared with that of acute otitis externa. Nickel dermatosis, which is characterized by a localized crusting of the earlobe, is common and is most frequently associated with the use of pierced earrings.

Necrotizing Malignant Otitis Externa

Necrotizing malignant otitis externa typically arises in diabetics, the elderly, and the debilitated. In this condition, *Pseudomonas* infection causes fever, prostration, vasculitis, thrombosis, and necrosis that may extend to the mastoid, parotid gland, and facial nerve and regional lymph nodes.

OTITIS MEDIA

Otitis media is defined as inflammation of the middle ear that may extend to contiguous structures, such as the mastoid. A practical classification of otitis media includes acute otitis media, otitis media with effusion, atelectasis of the tympanic membrane and middle ear, chronic otitis media with perforation (COMP), and chronic serous otitis media.

Epidemiology

Otitis media is the most common treatable condition for which children seek medical care. It is second only to viral upper respiratory infection as a reason for pediatric office visits. Seventy per cent of children have at least one episode of acute otitis media by age 3 years (30 per cent have one to three infections, and 40 per cent have four or more). Otitis media occurs with equal frequency in males and females. The condition is more frequent during the winter and spring, when viral infections tend to cluster. Other factors positively associated with otitis media include cleft palate, allergic rhinitis, exposure to passive smoke, and day care participation. Infants who are breast-fed have fewer ear infections than do children who are formula-fed.

Pathogenesis

Eustachian tube dysfunction is the cardinal event in the development of otitis media. Normally, the eustachian tube blocks passage of nasopharyngeal secretions to the middle ear, equalizes pressure between the middle ear and the external ear, and permits drainage of fluids from the middle ear. Mechanical or functional obstruction of the eustachian tube leads to persistent negative pressure in the middle ear, which stimulates the mucus-secreting epithelial cells to produce fluid. Obstruction of the eustachian tube also prevents the normal egress of fluid into the nasopharynx. Infants are more susceptible to eustachian tube dysfunction than are older people. The eustachian tube in infants is shorter and more horizontal than it is in older children. The cartilaginous support of the eustachian tube in infants is less rigid than that in older children. The most common cause of eustachian tube dysfunction is viral infection. Other causes include allergic rhinitis, mechanical obstruction due to nasopharyngeal tumors, and functional obstruction that occurs in children with cleft palate.

The fluid that forms in the middle ear provides an excellent medium for infection with the normal flora of the nasopharynx. These bacteria access the middle ear through reflux into the eustachian tube or by aspiration from high negative middle ear pressure. The bacteria most commonly responsible for otitis media are *Streptococcus pneumoniae*, *Haemophilus influenzae*, and *Moraxella catarrhalis*. Viruses have been implicated in middle ear infection in fewer than 10 per cent of patients. The most commonly recovered viruses are respiratory syncytial virus and influenza A virus.

Acute Otitis Media

Acute otitis media, also known as suppurative or purulent otitis media, is defined as fluid in the middle ear accompanied by signs or symptoms of infection. Typically, acute otitis media follows a viral upper respiratory infection. Accumulation of fluid in the middle ear is often rapidly followed by acute infection. The child with acute otitis media may have hearing loss, otalgia, and fever, although fever does not occur in all patients. The younger child with acute otitis media may present with irritability, poor feeding, and nocturnal awakening. Pulling or batting at the ear is also seen in the young child with acute otitis media. Other symptoms include cough, vomiting, diarrhea, malaise, headache, and occasional ataxia.

Physical examination often reveals a bulging, hyperemic tympanic membrane, conductive hearing loss, and distortion of the light reflex. By contrast, isolated hyperemia of the tympanic membrane, which may occur in any crying child, can be difficult to interpret. Differential hyperemia of the two tympanic membranes, however, may differentiate infection from mere crying. Bulging of the tympanic membrane is the most reliable physical indicator of acute otitis media. Pneumatic otoscopy in acute otitis media reveals a poorly mobile tympanic membrane. Tympanometry reveals a flat pattern or an effusion pattern. The positive predictive value of this pattern varies from 50 to 90 per cent. In general, a normal tympanometric pattern excludes the diagnosis of otitis media.

Two variations on the presentation of acute otitis media are perforation and bullous myringitis. In acute otitis media with perforation, middle ear pressure increases to the point at which the tympanic membrane ruptures. The process leading up to and including perforation is often quite painful. After perforation, otalgia may decrease markedly. The external canal may contain a foul-smelling, watery, purulent drainage that is occasionally quite bloody. Bullous myringitis represents acute inflammation within the various layers of the tympanic membrane. The signs and symptoms are typically the same as those in acute otitis media. A large, fluid-filled vesicle arises on the surface of a bulging tympanic membrane. The bacteriology of bullous myringitis is similar to that of acute otitis media.

The child with multiple episodes of otitis media must be evaluated for the presence of tumors and submucous cleft palate. The latter diagnosis is strongly suggested by palpation of a deep V-shaped defect of the palate and by detection of a bifid uvula.

The differential diagnosis of acute otitis media includes otitis media with effusion, atelectasis of the tympanic membrane, otitis externa, and severe pharyngitis with pain referred to the ear. Children with otitis media typically do not have pain on traction of the pinna, whereas this maneuver is quite painful in patients with otitis externa.

Acute otitis media usually resolves in 10 to 14 days. With appropriate treatment, the otalgia resolves even sooner.

Otitis Media With Effusion

Otitis media with effusion is also known as secretory, serous, or nonsuppurative otitis media. This condition is defined as fluid in the middle ear in the absence of signs or symptoms of infection. Otitis media with effusion may develop spontaneously, or it may be a resolution phase of acute otitis media.

Otitis media with effusion may be asymptomatic or may present with only mild loss of conductive hearing. Children may have otalgia that is typically less severe than that seen in acute otitis media; they also complain of a plugged feeling or a sense of popping in the ears, especially while swallowing. Although symptoms may be annoying, they rarely interfere with sleep or other daily activities.

In otitis media with effusion, the tympanic membrane may bulge, but more commonly it is retracted. When the tympanic membrane is retracted, the long process of the malleus prominently resembles a finger protruding from behind the tympanic membrane. The eardrum often appears thickened and dull. The light reflex may be normal or distorted. If fluid and air are present in the middle ear, bubbles may be seen behind the tympanic membrane. Pneumatic otoscopy reveals a sluggish, poorly mobile tympanic membrane. Tympanometry reveals a flat or an effusion pattern. A conductive hearing loss is often present. Otitis media with effusion usually resolves within a few weeks, although the condition may be chronic. Also, recurrent episodes of acute otitis media may develop from otitis media with effusion.

Atelectasis of the Tympanic Membrane and Middle Ear

Atelectasis of the tympanic membrane and middle ear is defined as eustachian tube dysfunction without subsequent inflammation of the middle ear. This condition, like otitis media with effusion, may be asymptomatic, or it may present with otalgia, hearing loss, and a feeling of fullness in the ear. Physical examination demonstrates a translucent, retracted tympanic membrane and a normal light reflex. Pneumatic otoscopy reveals immobility to positive pressure and either decreased or absent motility to negative pressure. Tympanometry reveals a high negative middle ear pressure tracing. Conductive hearing loss may be present. Occasionally, a retraction pocket or localized atelectasis at the pars flaccida or the posterosuperior portion of the pars tensa of the tympanic membrane can be observed. Atelectasis of the tympanic membrane and middle ear is often transient but may become chronic.

Chronic Otitis Media With Perforation

COMP is an infection of the middle ear that does not resolve within 2 months. It may result from inappropriate treatment of acute otitis media (either failure to complete the course of antibiotics or incorrect choice of antibiotics), persistent eustachian tube dysfunction, or an immunodeficient state. The signs and symptoms of COMP include hearing loss, otalgia, and foul-smelling, purulent otorrhea. The external canal contains a serous to purulent discharge and may be hyperemic. The tympanic membrane typically has a large central perforation, through which an inflamed middle ear mucosa may be seen. The tympanic membrane is generally thickened and may be retracted. Pneumatic otoscopy reveals impaired mobility of the tympanic membrane.

Because COMP typically begins as acute otitis media, the initial bacteriology of the middle ear fluid is the same as that for acute otitis media. Over time, the fluid in the middle ear becomes secondarily infected. The most common organisms in COMP are *Staphylococcus*, *Pseudomonas*, and anaerobic bacteria.

Chronic Otitis Media With Effusion

Chronic otitis media with effusion, or persistent otitis media with effusion, occurs when middle ear fluid has been present for 3 months. The natural evolution of middle ear fluid is to spontaneously resolve. More than 50 per cent of effusions resolve within 3 months, and effusion persisting for more than 1 year is uncommon. Hearing loss is the most common symptom in children with chronic otitis media with effusion. In general, patients with this condition do not have otalgia. They may experience a sensation of fullness or popping in their ears. The tympanic membrane appears thickened and is usually retracted. Air-fluid levels in the middle ear may be detected. Pneumatic otoscopy reveals either an immobile tympanic membrane or sluggish motility. A flat or an effusion pattern is noted with tympanometry. Any child or adult with chronic otitis media with effusion should have a careful examination of the nasopharynx to rule out an inapparent cleft palate or nasopharyngeal tumor.

Complications of Otitis Media

Hearing Loss

Virtually all children and adults with otitis media have conductive hearing loss. This hearing loss occurs because the middle ear fluid is quite viscous and dampens the vibrations through the ossicular chain. Usually, this hearing loss resolves spontaneously after the middle ear effusion is absorbed. Any child with an effusion that lasts 3 months or longer should undergo audiometric testing. A child with a loss greater than 20 dB may require more aggressive therapy. Children with speech and language delay, learning disability, or any pre-existing sensorineural hearing loss should also be evaluated for more aggressive therapy.

Ossicular chain disruption can cause conductive hearing loss. This disruption may complicate atelectasis of the tympanic membrane and middle ear or result from tympanosclerosis or a cholesteatoma. Chronic or recurrent otitis media may produce tympanosclerosis. Tympanosclerosis is the deposition of whitish plaques in the tympanic membrane and nodular deposits in the submucosal layers of the middle ear. In tympanosclerosis, the ossicles in the middle ear may become embedded. Finally, acute and chronic perforation of the tympanic membrane leads to hearing loss owing to inappropriate mobility of the tympanic membrane.

Mastoiditis

The mastoid air cells directly communicate with the middle ear. In most cases of acute otitis media, an acute mastoiditis may coexist. This condition usually resolves as the otitis media clears. If the disease within the mastoid process progresses, causing disruption and coalescence of the bony trabeculae, an empyema may form. The clinical manifestations of acute mastoiditis include fever, lethargy, and a tender, hyperemic mastoid process. The pinna is displaced downward and outward. Swelling of the superior posterior portion of the external auditory canal may be noted. COMP may lead to chronic mastoiditis. In this condition, the mastoid becomes sclerotic and poorly pneumatized.

Cholesteatoma

A cholesteatoma is a saclike structure that contains desquamated keratinized epithelial cells, usually derived from the squamous epithelial cells of the tympanic membrane. Cholesteatoma is usually a complication of an atelectatic tympanic membrane and middle ear, chronic otitis media with effusion, or COMP. Secondary bacterial infections may occur, usually with the same organisms as those seen in COMP. As the cholesteatoma grows, it may destroy middle ear and contiguous structures. Ossicular disruption may occur. The facial nerve may become compressed, producing a facial nerve palsy. Progression into the labyrinth can produce labyrinthitis and subsequent labyrinth destruction. Extension into the cranial cavity can produce meningitis and dural sinus thrombosis. The signs and symptoms of cholesteatoma develop very insidiously. Adults may notice hearing loss, but this is uncommon in children. A sense of fullness in the ears and mild vertigo may also be described. If the cholesteatoma is associated with persistent perforation of the tympanic membrane, foul otorrhea may occur. A retraction pocket, particularly in the posterosuperior region of the tympanic membrane or in the attic, is often present. Bright, shiny, greasy flakes of debris may be seen in defects of the tympanic membrane. When cholesteatoma is suspected, computed tympanography helps delineate the extent of the lesion.

DISORDERS OF TASTE AND SMELL

By W. James Evans, M.D.
Florence, South Carolina

Intact senses of taste and smell underlie many of the daily pleasures that enhance the quality of human life. These senses also enable humans to avoid unpleasant, noxious, or even hazardous chemicals. There is even some evidence that humans communicate by smell, subconsciously altering hormone production in response to the secretion of pheromones by others. Odors also influence mood, a phenomenon that has been successfully exploited by the perfume industry for centuries. The chemical senses, however, are often ignored by physicians. The National Institutes of Health estimate that in the United States 2 million people with chemosensory disorders account for at least 200,000 patient visits annually. More effective treatment is needed for these disorders, and the first step is to make an accurate diagnosis. This article outlines a practical clinical approach to the differential diagnosis of olfactory and gustatory disorders. Clinically relevant anatomy and physiology are reviewed, and classification schema for chemosensory disorders and testing methods are offered. For further information on these topics, the reader is referred to *Smell and Taste in Health and Disease* (Getchell, T.V. et al. [eds.], Raven Press, 1991).

ANATOMY AND PHYSIOLOGY OF CHEMOSENSATION

Within the past 10 years, the basic mechanisms of taste and smell have been elucidated, advances that have prompted revisions of many theories and concepts of chemosensation. Given the fundamental nature of the discoveries, a re-examination of chemosensory anatomy and physiology may cast new light on these disorders and help clinicians rethink their approach to diagnosis. This article provides a brief but up-to-date overview that necessarily excludes many interesting details and controversies.

Gustation

The word "taste" is often linked to the flavor of foods, but gustation is classically described as the sensations of salty, sweet, sour, and bitter.* Each one of the 10,000 taste buds distributed over the surface of the tongue and oropharynx is composed of clusters of 50 to 150 neuroepithelial cells known as taste cells. These taste cells and taste buds mature, die, and regenerate new cells every 10 to 14 days. Each taste cell projects a microvillar process through the taste pore at the apex of the taste bud, where sensory transduction occurs by one of four stimulus-dependent mechanisms. First, monovalent salts pass directly through ion channels. Second, hydrogen ions block potassium channels. Third, some amino acids bind directly to cationic channels that gate the passage of ions. Finally, sugars and some bitter compounds bind to taste receptors coupled to second messenger systems via G proteins linked to adenylate cyclase or phospholipase C. All four mechanisms ultimately produce an increased intracellular ionized calcium concentration that triggers depolarization, local action potentials, and neurotransmitter release at synapses between the taste cells and the primary gustatory neurons within the taste bud. Putative primary gustatory neurotransmitters include acetylcholine, serotonin, norepinephrine, and vasoactive intestinal peptide.

The taste buds are embedded in and around three types of papillae on the tongue. The fungiform papillae, each containing as many as a dozen taste buds, are located anteriorly and dorsally. A dozen circumvallate papillae, each holding possibly hundreds of taste buds, are arranged in a V shape posteriorly. The foliate papillae, which contain hundreds of taste buds, appear as vertical folds on the lateral aspects of the tongue. The conical and filiform papillae do not exhibit chemosensory activity. Most taste cells and taste buds respond to most tastants. Furthermore, sensitivity for the four taste qualities does not differ significantly among receptors in different parts of the tongue.

The cell bodies of the primary gustatory neurons that innervate the fungiform and foliate papillae on the anterior two thirds of the tongue are located in the geniculate ganglion and reach the taste cells via the facial, chorda tympani, and lingual nerves. The primary neurons that innervate the circumvallate papillae, posterior foliate papillae, and taste buds on the oropharynx originate in the petrosal ganglion and form connections to the receptor cells through the glossopharyngeal nerve. The third and final group of primary sensory neurons resides in the nodose ganglion and projects via the superior laryngeal branch of the vagus nerve to taste buds in the posterior tongue, esophagus, and epiglottis. All primary gustatory neurons project centrally to the rostral part of the nucleus tractus solitarius in the medulla, where they synapse with secondary gustatory neurons. The secondary neurons project to tertiary neurons in ipsilateral pontine parabrachial nuclei. Secondary medullary and tertiary pontine neurons project bilaterally to the thalamus and amygdala. Tertiary and quaternary gustatory neurons in the ventral posteromedial nucleus of the thalamus send fibers to the lateral postcentral gyrus and the anterior insular cortex, mostly contralateral to the originating taste buds. Gustatory cortex does not appear to be distinct from oral somatosensory cortex, since neurons that subserve gustation and somatesthesia are intermixed in cortical areas. Cells in the anterior insula project to an associative secondary gustatory area in the orbitofrontal cortex.

Olfaction

Most of what humans regard as the flavor of food derives from the sense of smell. Variations in olfactory experience are due primarily to 150 different types of olfactory receptors that are located throughout the mucus layer on the cilia of 5 million primary olfactory neurons. These neurons, as well as taste cells, die and regenerate every 4 to 6 weeks throughout life. Each primary olfactory neuron typically expresses only one receptor type. This means that new axons not only must grow from nasal mucosa through the cribriform plate to synapse in the olfactory bulb every 6 weeks, but also must synapse in the same glomerular structures as their predecessors! Olfactory sensory transduction occurs via cyclic adenosine monophosphate (cAMP)–dependent mechanisms that open ion channels in the ciliary membrane. Odorants must also be removed rapidly and continuously from the nose via uptake into the circulation, desorption into the air compartment, mucociliary transport, or cellular uptake and enzymatic degradation. In addition, olfactory epithelial cells contain cytochrome P-450 and other enzymes that perform the following functions: (1) detoxification and protection of the nasal mucosa, lungs, and brain; (2) activation of inhaled nonodorants into odorants; (3) modification of odorants for clearance from olfactory receptors, permitting reactivation of the receptors; and (4) generation of potentially toxic or carcinogenic metabolites.

Primary olfactory nerve axons project to glomerular structures in the paired, radially-symmetrical olfactory bulbs. The main output cells of the olfactory bulb are the mitral and tufted cells, which send axons to the primary olfactory cortex, amygdala, and supraoptic region of the hypothalamus. Primary olfactory cortex is composed of the anterior olfactory nucleus, piriform cortex, entorhinal cortex, and olfactory tubercle. Pyramidal cells in piriform and/or entorhinal cortex project back to the olfactory bulb, synapsing on inhibitory granule cells that form reciprocal dendrodendritic synapses with mitral and tufted cells. Periglomerular cells function as inhibitory interneurons between glomeruli in the olfactory bulb. The putative neurotransmitters include glutamate for primary olfactory neurons and mitral or tufted cells, dopamine for periglomerular cells, and gamma-aminobutyric acid for glomerular cells. Odors may be encoded by local feedback loops within the olfactory bulb, with a distinct spatial distribution of activation for different odors. Odor learning proba-

*The Japanese add to this list the taste of monosodium salts of glutamic and aspartic acid known as "umami."

bly involves feedback loops from the olfactory cortex to the olfactory bulb, mediated by the development of long-term potentiation in pyramidal cells of the piriform cortex. The piriform cortex also sends axons to the following structures: (1) the hippocampus, a structure implicated in memory functions; (2) the nucleus accumbens in the ventral striatum, an area that integrates visceral and somatic inputs with motor functions; (3) the insular cortex, a structure that regulates visceral autonomic responses; and (4) the orbitofrontal cortex via the mediodorsal nucleus of the thalamus. These pathways mediate odor discrimination and integration of multiple sensory modalities.

Trigeminal Chemesthesis

The sense of irritation that follows inhalation or ingestion of noxious chemicals (e.g., ammonia capsules) is mediated primarily by trigeminal afferents interspersed among olfactory receptor neurons in nasal epithelium and taste cells in the tongue and oropharynx. This chemesthetic property of the trigeminal nerve is probably mediated by nociceptors and enables the detection of chemosensory stimulants in the absence of olfactory and gustatory functions. The trigeminal nerve may exhibit greater or lesser chemosensitivity than the olfactory and gustatory nerves, depending on the stimulant. The trigeminal nerve also responds to mechanical, thermal, and proprioceptive stimuli in the nose and anterior portions of the mouth. In the posterior mouth, the glossopharyngeal nerve subserves these trigeminal functions as well as the gustatory functions described earlier. Stimulation of chemesthetic neurons causes release of neuropeptides, such as substance P and calcitonin gene–related peptide either locally or from peripheral, collateral, and central terminals. Thus, trigeminal neurons may directly influence olfactory and gustatory neuronal activity at multiple levels from receptor to brain stem and cortex. Trigeminal neurons also indirectly influence chemosensation via reflexes that regulate intranasal vasomotor tone, nasal patency, mucociliary activity, nasal secretions, turnover and differentiation of olfactory epithelial basal cells, bronchial motor tone, cardiac and respiratory rate, and the immunologic function of respiratory mucosa.

Saliva and Mucus Secretion

Saliva is critical for the delivery of stimuli to taste buds. The parotid, submandibular, and sublingual glands contribute 90 per cent of the total saliva volume, with labial, palatine, and buccal glands producing the remaining 10 per cent. Saliva is 99 per cent water and 1 per cent organic and inorganic components. The inorganic components include sodium, potassium, chloride, bicarbonate, calcium phosphate, fluoride, thiocyanate, magnesium sulfate, and iodide. The organic components of saliva include digestive enzymes (e.g., amylase, lipase), tissue- and tooth-coating agents (e.g., mucus and proline-rich glycoproteins, lysozyme), and other substances (e.g., secretory IgA, growth factors, and regulatory peptides).

Salivary secretion is under sympathetic and parasympathetic control. Parasympathetic secretomotor neurons in the salivatory nucleus of the medulla send cholinergic preganglionic fibers via the glossopharyngeal, tympanic, and lesser petrosal nerves to the otic ganglion, which innervates the parotid gland, and via the lingual-tonsillar branch of the glossopharyngeal nerve to Remak's ganglion in the tongue, which innervates the lingual salivary glands. Parasympathetic neuronal innervation of the submandibular and sublingual glands is mediated by fibers traveling in the facial, chorda tympani, and lingual nerves to reach the submandibular ganglion. Cholinergic preganglionic sympathetic neurons in the intermediolateral nucleus of the upper thoracic spinal cord ascend in the paravertebral sympathetic trunk to synapse in the superior cervical ganglion. The noradrenergic postganglionic fibers travel along blood vessels to the different salivary glands. Stimulation of oral mechanoreceptors or taste buds increases autonomic outflow to the salivary glands via brain stem reflexes that are modulated by descending fibers from the hypothalamus.

Olfactory mucus plays a critical role in the sense of smell. Mucus not only protects the mucosa but also promotes the adsorption and diffusion of odorant molecules. The primary mucus-secreting cells of the olfactory mucosa are the acinar cells of subepithelial Bowman's glands, whose mucus secretions differ from those in respiratory mucosa. Bowman's glands secrete the water, electrolyte, and protein constituents of mucus that include the following: secretory IgA, which immobilizes pathogens in mucus and opsonizes them for destruction by cytotoxic cells; sialylated glycoproteins, which increase the viscosity of mucus and may bind specific pathogens; lysozyme and lactoferrin (bacteriostatic enzymes); uric acid, an antioxidant; odorant-binding protein, a transport protein for some odorant molecules; and xenobiotic-transforming enzymes. Both sympathetic and parasympathetic fibers innervate Bowman's glands via the pterygopalatine ganglion. Cholinergic agonists stimulate mucus secretion directly, whereas adrenergic agonists tend to reduce secretions via vasoconstriction. Other agents that activate Bowman's glands include prostaglandins, calcium channel blockers, cAMP, and theophylline. Substance P and vasoactive intestinal peptide selectively increase the water content of mucus secretions. Age-related changes in Bowman's glands include alterations in mucus glycoprotein composition and diminished sensitivity of glandular neurotransmitter receptors. Inflammation and glandular destruction in Sjögren's syndrome and in sarcoidosis lead to decreased mucus secretion. Cystic fibrosis is associated with a defect in chloride channels that decreases the water content of epithelial mucus.

CLASSIFICATION OF CHEMOSENSORY DISORDERS

Disorders of olfaction can be classified by type of dysfunction and underlying cause. Olfactory loss can be classified as *anosmia* (complete loss of smell) or *hyposmia* (partial loss of smell) and qualified as to the number of odors affected, that is, *general* (all odors), *partial* (some odors), and *specific* (one odor). Specific anosmia is akin to color blindness and is usually hereditary. *Hyperosmia,* or hypersensitivity to odors, should be distinguished from *dysosmia,* which is distortion of smell in the presence of chemosensory stimulants, and *phantosmia* or *olfactory hallucinations,* which are sensations of odor in the absence of chemosensory stimulants. Dysosmia (also known as parosmia or cacosmia) and phantosmia often occur in association with anosmia or hyposmia. *Osmagnosia* (olfactory agnosia) is the inability to recognize the qualities of an odorant despite a normal ability to detect the presence or absence of odors.

Olfactory disorders can be categorized according to cause. *Conduction disorders* result from impaired transport of odor molecules to the receptors in the olfactory epithelium. *Sensory disorders* result from impaired sensory transduction at the receptor or in the second messenger

Table 1. Disorders of Smell

Conduction Disorders
Adenoid hypertrophy
Allergic rhinitis
Nasal polyposis
Vasomotor rhinitis
Atrophic rhinitis
Chronic sinusitis
Septal deviation
Intranasal tumors
Laryngectomy
Cholinergic drugs
Alpha-adrenergic drugs
Sensory Disorders
Viral infections
Intranasal surgery
Radiation therapy
Toxic inhalation
Cigarette smoke
Hepatic and renal disease
Specific anosmia
G-protein deficiency
Drugs
Neural Disorders
Head trauma
Stroke
Intracranial tumors
Meningitis
Encephalitis
Temporal lobe epilepsy
Alzheimer's disease
Parkinson's disease
Progressive supranuclear palsy
Guam parkinsonian dementia
Huntington's chorea
Korsakoff's psychosis
Down's syndrome
Kallman's syndrome
Depression
Schizophrenia
Drugs

cascade that produces cAMP. *Neural disorders* are attributed to impaired function of neurons in various parts of the olfactory pathway. The major disorders in each category are summarized in Table 1.

A similar classification of gustatory dysfunction can be made. *Ageusia* is defined as the total loss of taste sensitivity, *hypogeusia* is a partial loss, and *hypergeusia* refers to increased sensitivity to tastants. These disorders may be general, partial, or specific, depending on the number of altered taste qualities. *Dysgeusia* is defined as a distorted sense of taste in the presence of a taste stimulus, whereas *phantogeusia* and *gustatory hallucinations* are defined as the perception of taste in the absence of taste stimuli. *Gustatory agnosia* is the inability to recognize qualities of taste despite normal abilities to identify the presence or absence of tastants.

Gustatory dysfunction may also be classified according to cause. *Conduction disorders* relate to impaired transport of tastants to the taste buds. *Sensory problems* are caused by functional impairment or destruction of taste cells, and *neural disorders* are most likely related to impaired function or destruction of either central or peripheral neurons in the gustatory pathways. The main gustatory disorders in each of these categories are summarized in Table 2.

TESTS OF CHEMOSENSORY FUNCTION

Objective testing of chemosensory dysfunction with the use of quantitative measures increases the accuracy of diagnosis and establishes a baseline against which treatment responses can be compared.

Odor Identification

The Smell Identification Test (S.I.T.) is a forced-choice, 40-item "scratch-and-sniff" test commercially available from Sensonics, Inc. (telephone: 609-547-7702, $24.95 each). This clinically useful test has been extensively validated across all ages, and it offers corrections for age and gender. Scores on the S.I.T. correlate highly with odor detection threshold test scores, and an S.I.T. can be self-administered by most patients in 10 to 20 minutes. For each item, the patient identifies the odor by selecting one of four descriptors. Thus, chance performance yields a score of 10, allowing detection of malingering in those who score significantly below 10. Answering in various patterns (e.g., selecting all "A's") may still subvert the test, but such patterns do not necessarily imply malingering. The 3-item Pocket Smell Test is also available from Sensonics, Inc., at a cost of $80 for a package of 50 tests.

Odor Detection Thresholds

Detection thresholds should be determined for as many odorants as practical to avoid pitfalls related to specific anosmias. Thresholds for three to five odorants can be tested with the use of commercially available kits from Olfacto-Labs (telephone: 510-235-0203). Each "Utility Kit" sells for $400 and includes 18 squeeze bottles containing nine different concentrations of one odorant paired with nine control bottles. The patient is handed one pair of bottles at a time and asked to select or guess which bottle contains the odorant. For this test, threshold is defined as the lowest concentration at which the patient correctly identifies three in a row. These tests have been validated in a population of normal young adults; corrections for age and gender are not available. Concentrations are given in decismels (abbreviated dS), a semilog scale similar to the decibel scale used in audiometry. The average threshold is defined as 0 dS, with each standard deviation from the mean equal to 10 dS. For clinical purposes, the normal range for detection threshold for every odor is 0 ± 25 dS.

Table 2. Disorders of Taste

Conduction Disorders
Periodontal disease
Xerostomia
Prosthodontic devices
Cholinergic drugs
Alpha-adrenergic drugs
Blood-borne chemicals
Sensory Disorders
Viral infections
Smoking
Drugs
Neural Disorders
Viral infections
Bell's palsy
Diabetes
Head trauma
Stroke
Intracranial tumors
Aneurysms
Meningoencephalocele
Meningitis
Encephalitis
Burning mouth syndrome
Drugs

A Bedside Olfactory Test

Olfactory tests can often be improvised with materials available in the office or nurses' station. For olfactory testing, choose four aromatic spices, e.g., vanilla, coffee, oregano, and cloves. Do not use pungent or cooling chemicals, such as menthol, vinegar, and ammonia, unless you intend to test trigeminal function. Test the patient with the eyes closed. First, ask the patient to identify each odorant. If the patient identifies at least three of the four odorants, olfactory function may be intact. If the patient identifies fewer than three, perform an odor discrimination test with the same odorants. Using a forced-choice paradigm, present pairs of the four odorant stimuli, including pairs in which the same odorant is used both times. For each pair of stimuli, ask the patient whether the two odors are the "same" or "different." In this design, chance performance is 50 per cent correct. To pass the test, the patient should get at least six of eight pairs correct. If the patient gets fewer than six correct on this test, perform a suprathreshold detection test for each of the four odorants. Again, using a forced-choice paradigm, present stimulus pairs in which one of the stimuli is always a blank. For each pair of stimuli, ask the patient to determine which stimulus has an odor. Chance performance is 50 per cent, so the patient must correctly detect each odorant three of four times, for a total of 12 of 16 pairs correct. Although such testing is not quantitative, simple bedside tests at least give some objective indication of olfactory dysfunction. Bedside olfaction may also be used to detect malingering because a cumulative score of fewer than 6 correct out of 24 on the combined odor discrimination and detection tests indicates a level of performance that is significantly less than chance.

Psychophysical olfactory tests can provide limited information regarding the anatomic site of a lesion. For example, chance performance on both the odor discrimination and detection tests is often noted when severe general anosmia accompanies nasal disease, upper respiratory tract infection, or complete transection of the olfactory nerves. Good performance on the odor detection test with impaired odor discrimination is seen in thalamic disorders, such as Korsakoff's amnestic confabulatory syndrome. Good performance on odor detection and odor discrimination with poor odor identification is seen in olfactory agnosia and suggests a central disorder. However, the finding of impaired olfactory thresholds does not exclude a central etiology because patients with Parkinson's disease suffer a loss of sensitivity early in the course of that disorder. Patients with Alzheimer's disease progress from odor memory and odor identification deficits in the earlier stages to increased odor thresholds in the later stages of the disease.

Taste Detection Thresholds

The detection threshold is the lowest concentration of a tastant that can be detected. A forced-choice, up-down paradigm is preferred, with the use of log-step dilutions of sucrose, sodium chloride, and citrate. Two cups are presented to the patient, one containing water and the other containing a tastant solution. The patient is instructed to taste the solution in both cups and select or guess which cup contains the stimulus. When the patient guesses incorrectly, the next higher concentration is given. When the patient correctly identifies the cup, the same concentration is repeated. When the patient correctly identifies the stimulus two times in a row, the next lower concentration is given. A reversal is defined as the concentration at which the patient's responses change from correct to incorrect and vice versa. Threshold is defined as the mean of the concentrations at six reversals. This method is repeated for each of the tastants. Since saliva contains sodium chloride and may act as an adapting agent, it is important for the patient to rinse the mouth with water before each tasting to remove saliva from the tongue. Another problem to consider in threshold determinations is that sodium chloride, citric acid, and quinine may produce stinging sensations that confound test interpretation by enabling ageusic patients to detect these solutions.

Spatial Taste Test

A modification of the Spatial Taste Test developed at the Connecticut Chemosensory Clinical Research Center may help define the specific nerves involved in gustatory dysfunction. Solutions of sodium chloride (1 M), sucrose (0.5 M), and citrate (0.032 M) are painted on specific areas of the tongue with a cotton-tipped applicator. Paired presentations of a tastant and water are made to different areas in the front and the back of the tongue. The tastant is applied first to one side of the tongue, and the water control is applied to the other. After each paired presentation, the patient is asked to identify the side of the tongue where the tastant was perceived, to describe the taste, and to give an estimate of the intensity on a six-point scale. Normally, patients should be able to identify each taste quality correctly over the four areas of the tongue.

OLFACTORY DISORDERS

Evaluation

Initially, olfactory dysfunction should be characterized in terms of severity, nature of onset, and any relationship to allergies, viral infections, head trauma, surgery, radiation, or exposure to other environmental agents. Determine whether there are fluctuations in symptomatology and whether there are any provocative or palliative factors, such as changes in humidity, temperature, or medications. Ask about nonolfactory symptoms involving the nose and head and whether they fluctuate in association with the olfactory symptoms. For example, in allergic rhinitis, hyposmia typically fluctuates with the severity of nasal congestion and tends to be seasonal. However, when the hyposmia persists after the allergies have resolved, other causes must be considered. Inquire about previous nasal and sinus surgery and response to antibiotics or steroid treatment. Is there a history of smoking or other toxic inhalation? Was the exposure sufficient to cause the observed deficit or, if the exposure persists, could it impede the regeneration of olfactory neurons? Determine the degree to which the olfactory symptoms have changed the patient's activities and whether they interfere with job performance or home safety.

Examine the head and neck, including the remainder of the cranial nerves. In the nose, look for airway obstruction due to septal deviation, inflammation, or masses. Examine the mucosa for abnormal color, atrophy, exudates, erosions, and ulcerations. Determine the origin of any purulent rhinorrhea. Palpate over the sinuses and look for allergic stigmata. Inspect the optic discs for atrophy or for signs of retinitis. Examine the tympanic membranes for signs of fluid collection or inflammation. Check pupillary reflexes, visual fields, and extraocular movements. Test sensitivity over the face, cornea, and tongue and buccal mucosa. Observe face and tongue movements to ascertain symmetry and bulk. Smell the patient's breath for fetid odor. Listen to the speaking voice and breathing pattern to assess lower cranial motor nerve function and patency of upper airways. In younger patients, examine the genitalia for anomalies and the skin for neurocutaneous stigmata. In older patients, look for parkinsonian signs, including resting tremor, cogwheeling rigidity, shuffling gait, or bradykinesia. In the elderly, do a brief mental status examination, including tests of short-term memory, confrontational naming, and praxis to screen for dementia.

Initial laboratory testing is confined to screening blood tests. Additional testing should be tailored to the major categories of disease. Screening tests include a complete blood count, glucose, electrolytes, renal and liver function tests, sedimentation rate, thyroid function, and serum IgA and IgE concentrations. More specific tests include (1) skin testing in allergic rhinitis to identify specific allergens, (2) selective mucosal biopsy, (3) computed tomography scan for suspected nasal and paranasal sinus disease, and (4) magnetic resonance imaging for suspected neural disorders.

Conduction Disorders

Conductive olfactory disorders are usually characterized by variable and incomplete olfactory loss that is associated with nasal congestion and a sensation of pressure in the face and sinuses. The severity of olfactory loss corresponds with the severity of the nasal disease. For example, when obstruction is complete and the patient cannot breathe through the nose, he or she will probably be anosmic. In chronic sinusitis, hyposmia may be associated with dysosmia due to anaerobic bacterial growth. In these patients, a trial of antibiotic therapy may be diagnostically useful. When symptoms progress despite treatment, or clear abnormalities are seen on direct and endoscopic examination, then computed tomography scanning of the nose and paranasal sinuses is indicated.

Rhinorrhea is characteristic of both allergic and nonallergic vasomotor rhinitis. In allergic rhinitis, the rhinorrhea is due to the release of histamine, prostaglandins, tryptase, and other mediators during mast cell degranulation. By contrast, in vasomotor rhinitis, normal autonomic tone in the nose gives way to predominant parasympathetic influences. Vasomotor rhinitis is a nonspecific phenomenon, and a number of causes must be considered, including pregnancy, hypothyroidism, inhaled toxins, nasal trauma, infections, and chronic inflammatory conditions. In addition, medications that may contribute to vasomotor rhinitis include beta-blockers, hydralazine, neuroleptics, and tricyclic antidepressants. Also, rebound rhinitis may result from the chronic use of nasal decongestants. Nasal obstruction without prominent symptoms of rhinorrhea can be seen with septal deviation but may also be the presenting feature of a variety of benign, intermediate, and malignant intranasal neoplasms. Tumors can cause rhinorrhea via vasomotor mechanisms or secondary infections due to sinus obstruction or mucosal ulceration.

Sensory Disorders

Upper respiratory viral infections cause acute conductive olfactory deficits due to swelling of the mucosa. In many patients, olfactory function returns to normal as the nasal congestion resolves. However, some patients experience persistent olfactory loss and distortions after the infection, presumably because of alterations in the olfactory receptor neurons. Although the degree of deficit usually correlates with histopathologic changes in the mucosa, it does not seem to correlate with the clinical severity of the acute infection. These deficits can persist for years, if not permanently, although a number of patients show spontaneous recovery. Radiation therapy to the head and neck decreases the turnover and regeneration of olfactory and respiratory epithelium, including olfactory receptor neurons and mucus-secreting glands. Inhalation of cigarette smoke and other toxic agents also destroys olfactory epithelium in a dose-related manner that is usually reversible.

Neural Disorders

The mechanism of olfactory loss in head trauma is most often attributed to transection of the olfactory nerves at the cribriform plate. However, mesiotemporal and orbitofrontal contusion and/or concussion also may have contributed to olfactory deficit in closed head trauma, especially when psychophysical testing indicates that is odor identification and discrimination are more impaired than is odor detection. Post-traumatic chemosensory losses may not be noticed immediately, espcially when more life-threatening or disabling conditions may prevail. During hospitalization, patients may expect food to be bland. Only with resumption of regular diet and home activity do they begin to recognize their deficit. Patients with post-traumatic olfactory loss have reported a return to normal sensitivity after periods ranging from 6 weeks to 20 years. In general, the more severe the olfactory deficit at 6 weeks after trauma, the worse the prognosis for recovery.

Neurologic and psychiatric disorders associated with olfactory loss are listed in Table 1. Most patients with olfactory dysfunction due to central neurologic disease are not aware of their olfactory deficits unless they experience phantosmia or olfactory hallucinations. Thus, olfactory testing should be performed on all patients presenting with neurologic or psychiatric symptoms related to the limbic system, even if there is no complaint of olfactory loss or distortions. Olfactory dysfunction is known to occur early in the course of schizophrenia and neurodegenerative disorders such as Alzheimer's disease and Parkinson's disease, but the clinical utility of olfactory testing in the early diagnosis of these disorders has not yet been established. In Korsakoff's amnestic confabulatory syndrome, odor discrimination deficits are well documented.

Odor phantoms and hallucinations can be characterized in the same manner as hallucinations involving the other senses. "Simple" or "unformed" hallucinations involve perceptions of an odor in the absence of chemical stimuli. The perceived odor may be pleasant or unpleasant, and may be familiar or unfamiliar, but will otherwise have no significant meaning. "Formed" olfactory hallucinations implicate the limbic system and are associated with feelings of disgust, pleasure, or sexuality. "Complex" olfactory hallucinations are characterized by illusions or delusions regarding the source of the odor or its purpose. Simple phantoms are often associated with severe olfactory deficits; these events are analogous to simple visual hallucinations in the blind, or perceptions of touch and pain in an amputated limb. Formed and complex olfactory hallucinations have been associated with temporal lobe epilepsy and schizophrenia. In temporal lobe epilepsy, hallucinations may be accompanied by a sense of déja vû, changes in sexuality and religiosity, rage, epigastric sensations, nausea, and intense emotions that are "indescribable." Seizures may generalize to produce loss of consciousness, tonic-clonic movements, and incontinence. Olfactory hallucinations in schizophrenia may be associated with auditory hallucinations and paranoid delusions. Patients with temporal lobe epilepsy or schizophrenia often show deficits in olfactory function, primarily related to odor identification. In both conditions, the hallucinations typically involve external odors (outside the body). The opposite is noted in patients with olfactory reference syndrome, a fixed delusion or obsession that the patient's body emits a foul odor.

GUSTATORY DISORDERS

Evaluation

Examine the mouth in detail. Check the mucosa for signs of inflammation, atrophy, leukoplakia, exudate, erosion, or ulceration. Inspect the gums for signs of periodontal disease. Are prosthodontic devices present? Evaluate salivary production by observing the moistness of the mucosa. Palpate for masses in the tongue, the gums, and the lips inside the mouth, as well as the parotid and sublingual glands externally. Smell the patient's breath. Assess somatesthesia on the buccal mucosa, tongue, palate, and oropharynx using a cotton-tipped applicator. Examine eye movements, look for nystagmus, and test hearing. Observe movements of the soft palate during phonation. Test the gag reflex on both sides. Inspect the tongue again for bulk, symmetry, and strength. Look closely at the appearance of the papillae.

Conduction Disorders

Dysgeusia and phantogeusia typically originate in the mouth and are often produced by stimuli that are not recognized, including medications in saliva, free blood, reflux, postnasal drip, halitosis, tooth and gum disease, and oral prostheses. Chemotherapeutic and contrast agents circulating in the blood can also act as tastant stimuli after diffusing into the taste buds. In the evaluation of dysgeusia, topical anesthesia of the mouth may help distinguish neurologic abnormalities from the direct effects of chemicals in the mouth. If the dysgeusia is abolished by anesthesia, it is probably due to the presence of a tastant stimulus. If the dysgeusia intensifies with anesthesia, a neural origin is implicated. Incomplete anesthesia of the mouth confounds the results of testing because the unaffected taste buds become more sensitive. This phenomenon may be related to disinhibition of intact gustatory neural fields via central mechanisms that have yet to be defined.

Sensory Disorders

Viral infections of the upper respiratory tract may cause dysgeusia and ageusia as late sequelae. Head and neck irradiation decreases the turnover and renewal of mucosal epithelium, taste cells, and salivary glands, with subsequent profound and lasting effects on taste. Chemotherapy with vinblastine causes ageusia, whereas cisplatin, bleomycin, and methotrexate are associated with dysgeusia.

Neural Disorders

Unilateral gustatory deficits are typically caused by neural disorders. However, unilateral gustatory deficits usually do not cause subjective change in the sense of taste despite demonstrable impairments on psychophysical testing. In addition, testing often reveals increased sensitivity on the contralateral side that may be related to the disinhibition mechanisms discussed earlier. Thus, progressive loss of gustatory function may occur without symptoms until that critical point when the patient perceives a sudden and total loss of taste. Mononeuropathies involving the gustatory neurons of the facial nerve include the following: (1) Bell's palsy, an acute inflammatory reaction of the nerve; (2) diabetes mellitus, which causes nerve infarction; and (3) the Ramsay-Hunt syndrome, due to herpes zoster oticus. Mononeuropathies of the glossopharyngeal and vagus nerves are rare. Polyneuropathies that may involve gustatory nerves are seen in Wegener's granulomatosis, a necrotizing vasculitis of the upper respiratory tract and kidneys; basilar meningitis, due to fungi, mycobacteria, or sarcoidosis; acoustic neuromas, schwannomas, and meningiomas of the pontocerebellar angle; basilar and vertebral artery aneurysms; tumors of the jugular foramen; and trauma.

Brain stem infarction in the lateral medulla may cause ipsilateral loss of taste and tactile sensation in addition to Horner's syndrome, ataxia, vertigo, nausea, hiccups, dysphagia, and hoarseness. Pontine hemorrhage in the parabrachial nucleus may produce ipsilateral ageusia. Thalamic lesions produce contralateral gustatory and tactile deficits. Thalamic hemorrhage, which is the most common lesion of the midline thalamus, often produces coma and death before these patients can be evaluated for chemosensory deficits.

Burning mouth syndrome is an intraoral disorder characterized by pain and dysgeusia, primarily in postmenopausal females. The oral examination is usually normal except for gustatory deficits and reduced heat pain tolerance on the tongue. The most effective therapy consists of treatment with antidepressants. These factors have suggested that the disorder may be a variant of the thalamic pain syndrome of Déjerine-Roussy.

DISORDERS OF THE NOSE AND PARANASAL SINUSES

By Seok-Chan Hong, M.D.,
and Donald A. Leopold, M.D.
Baltimore, Maryland

HISTORY

The mainstay of any clinical assessment of the nose and paranasal sinuses remains the history. The clinician must accurately understand the patient's reported symptoms and the degree to which they affect his or her life. For instance, "nasal congestion" may refer to a feeling of generalized pressure in the face area, or it may relate to nasal airflow. Because the nose and paranasal sinuses are intimately connected, disease usually involves both regions, and signs and symptoms are typically referred to the nose. The clinician must document the presence or absence of nasal symptoms, such as anterior rhinorrhea, nasal airway obstruction, postnasal drip, pressure symptoms, sneezing, hyposmia or anosmia, and headache or facial pain. The times of the day, week, month, or year when symptoms are most frequent should also be noted. General health, other neurologic symptoms, and other medical conditions may warrant consideration, especially respiratory tract disease (e.g., asthma, bronchiectasis, recurrent pneumonia, sarcoidosis, Wegener's granulomatosis); diabetes mellitus; cardiovascular problems; facial palsy; thyroid disease; and immune deficiency, such as acquired immunodeficiency syndrome (AIDS). Drugs may also contribute to disorders of the nose and paranasal sinuses. For example, some antihypertensive agents produce a sensation of nasal obstruction. Abuse of decongestants may lead to the rebound congestion of rhinitis medicamentosa. In women, hormonal changes during pregnancy and menopause may contribute to the problem. The patient's occupation, pets, and consumption of tobacco, alcohol, and coffee may also be relevant. The physician's clinical decision-making ability is also enhanced by the knowledge of what treatment the patient has already received and how successful it was.

PHYSICAL EXAMINATION

In the context of a full ear, nose, and throat examination, the clinician must concentrate on a systematic evaluation of the nasal cavity, paranasal sinuses, and nasopharynx.

Anterior Rhinoscopy

Anterior rhinoscopy, with the use of a head mirror or fiberoptic headlight, provides an excellent view of the nostrils and anterior nasal cavity but limits views of areas posterior to the nasal valves. Nostril patency and lateral nasal wall strength can be assessed, and gentle palpation of the inferior turbinates and septum may reveal thickened or engorged mucosa or bony enlargement that contributes to nasal symptoms. Septal deflection, the presence and character of secretions, and the color and turgor of the mucosa all must be noted. The clinician should also inspect the space between the middle turbinate and the lateral nasal wall. This maneuver may require the application of decongestants.

Nasal Endoscopy

Since 1960, the availability of cold-light flexible fiberoptic and rigid-rod lens systems has significantly enhanced our understanding of the physiology and pathology of the nose and sinuses. Flexible nasoendoscopy and nasopharyngoscopy can be performed with instruments 1 to 4 mm in diameter, with the use of 90-degree bidirectional tip deflection. The optics are less desirable for photography, but these versatile instruments facilitate examination of the entire upper respiratory tract in most patients. Rigid telescopes vary in length, diameter, and tip angle; the 0-degree and 30-degree scopes at diameters of 2.7 and 4 mm are the most useful.

The telescope is initially inserted posteriorly as far as is possible without causing the patient discomfort. The undisturbed nasal cavity can then be assessed. Careful attention to anterior nasal structures is important, because most nasal resistance is in the valve area. If the telescope cannot be passed beyond the anterior attachment of the middle turbinate, a local anesthetic such as 4 per cent lidocaine and a decongestant such as 1 per cent phenylephrine hydrochloride should be applied. The first pass of a thorough nasal endoscopic examination is made along the floor of the nose, into the inferior meatus. If an inferior meatal antrostomy is present, this is visualized and the antrum can sometimes be entered through the opening. The scope can be passed back into the nasopharynx, and the orifices of the eustachian tube can then be observed. The second pass is made between the inferior and the middle turbinates. If an ostium is seen, it is usually an accessory maxillary ostium. The scope is passed back as far as the sphenoethmoidal recess, with the physician noting mucus drainage from the lateral middle meatus or the sphenoethmoid region. The third pass enters the middle meatus, which is best viewed with a 30-degree scope. In 30 per cent of normal people, the 4-mm scope cannot enter and a 2.7-mm scope must be passed and rotated up into the middle meatus. The angled scope provides a better view into the infundibulum and nasofrontal recess. Various abnormalities may now be apparent, especially those that cause obstruction of the ostiomeatal region.

IMAGING STUDIES

Plain Sinus Films

Plain sinus films are rarely used, because they are only slightly less expensive than are computed tomography (CT) scans and give much less information, especially in the important ethmoid region. Moreover, a normal sinus x-ray result does not preclude disease. The Caldwell and Waters views best demonstrate the frontal and maxillary sinuses. The lateral view best displays the sphenoid sinus. The fine bony anatomy of the ethmoid sinuses is poorly displayed on all views owing to structural superimposition. Despite their limited value in the evaluation of chronic inflammation, plain sinus films occasionally help identify acute inflammation or aggressive lesions.

Computed Tomography

Computed tomography is currently the preferred method of imaging of the nose and paranasal sinuses. Computed tomography can help distinguish bone, soft tissue, and air, thereby enhancing the detection of abnormalities and providing an accurate map for subsequent surgery. Scans should be undertaken when the patient is as well as possible, preferably after treatment such as antibiotics, topical steroids, and possibly oral steroids. The coronal cross-sectional plane most closely correlates with the surgical approach and best shows both the ostiomeatal complex and the relationships of the brain and orbit to the ethmoid sinus. Slice thickness is 3 to 4 mm, extent of examination is from the anterior frontal sinus through the sphenoid sinus, and windowing is set for soft tissue, air passages, and bone structures. Reformatting can produce sagittal views. Axial imaging is important in the evaluation of trauma, sphenoid disease, and sinus neoplasms.

Magnetic Resonance Imaging

Magnetic resonance imaging (MRI) provides better visualization of paranasal soft tissue but does not detail the anatomy of the region as well as CT. Because bone and air produce no signal intensities on MRI, precise definition of the ostiomeatal air passages and their bony perimeter is difficult. Furthermore, in the patient with extensive inflammation, the signal intensity of the pathologic process is indistinguishable from that of the normal mucosa in the edematous phase of the nasal cycle. Thus, MRI has little or no role in routine evaluation of paranasal sinuses, but it is indicated when tumor is suspected. Ninety per cent of paranasal neoplasms are squamous cell carcinomas. Most of these lesions assume an intermediate bright signal on T2-weighted images, whereas bacterial and viral inflammation produce high signal intensity on T2-weighted images. Fungal concretions have a very low signal intensity on T2-weighted images. On occasion, MRI may aid evaluation and surgical treatment of regional and intracranial complications of inflammatory sinus disease. In addition, MRI can improve the display of anatomic relationships between intraorbital and extraorbital compartments and may enhance the evaluation of the sphenoid sinus after pituitary surgery.

LABORATORY TESTS

Rhinomanometry

Rhinomanometry attempts to characterize nasal airway resistance (R) by measuring nasal flow rate (V) and pressure (P). To resolve the complex mathematics, in 1984 the European Committee for Standardization of Rhinomanometry selected $R = \Delta P/V$ at a fixed pressure of 150 Pa, a formula that has been widely accepted. This standardization has allowed comparison of results not hitherto possible and the production of normal ranges, taking into account such factors as size, height, and age. Rhinomanometry can be performed with active or passive techniques and by anterior or posterior approaches. Active techniques are the most physiologic and the most widely used. The anterior active technique can be performed with commercially available, standardized equipment. Pressure is recorded in one nostril while the patient breathes through the other. The pressure-sensing catheter is secured and made airtight with adhesive tape, and flow is measured though the other (open) nasal cavity. The results are presented in an xy format so that the curve for flow or pressure in each breath cycle can be observed for errors. The consistency of the curve over four to six breaths is checked, and a small computer calculates averages for five respirations. The resistance at a fixed pressure of 150 Pa is expressed in SI units (Sytème International d'Unités).

Acoustic Rhinometry

In this technique, an audible sound pulse (150 to 10,000 Hz) generated by a spark is propagated in a sound tube and reflected by local variances in acoustic impedance attributed to changing cross-sectional area with distance. The clinician can determine the magnitude of the change in cross-sectional area as a function of distance from the nostril, and from this a total volume can be derived. Several measurements are taken to ensure the accuracy of the result, and the test can be performed both before and after decongestion. The data provide accurate sequential measurements of the abnormalities and the patient's response to medical or surgical treatment. Correlation between the nasal examination and these measurements of nasal airflow and cross-sectional shape is necessary.

Immunodeficiency Tests

As many as 10 per cent of patients with chronic or recurrent acute sinusitis have defects of immune functions, especially defects of humoral immunity. The most common problems are deficiencies of immunoglobulin A (IgA), IgG_3 subclass, and antipolysaccharide antibody. Secondary immunodeficiencies caused by infection with human immunodeficiency virus (HIV), lymphoreticular neoplasm, and neutropenia also influence the course of sinusitis. The most cost-effective screening tests for immunodeficiency in these patients include quantitative determination of immunoglobulin levels (IgG, IgA, IgM), response to immunization with a polysaccharide vaccine (Pneumovax), complete blood count with differential, and HIV serology in high-risk patients.

Mucociliary Tests

Mucociliary flow in the nose is directed toward the nasopharynx, but in the sinuses flow is directed toward the natural ostia. Humidity, cold, age, and the nasal cycle may dynamically vary the mucociliary flow. In the maxillary sinus, the flow is roughly circular; studies suggest that even inferior meatal punctures do not disrupt this pattern. Early investigations of the frontal sinus showed clockwise flow on the right side and counterclockwise flow on the left, with areas of high turbulence near the ducts.

Saccharin Test

Place a drop of saccharin in front of the inferior turbinate in the anterior nasal vestibule and record the time required for the patient to identify a sweet taste in the throat. Objectivity can be enhanced by staining the saccharin drops with methylene blue and viewing color in the throat.

Measurement of Ciliary Beat Frequency

Ciliated epithelium from the inferior turbinate is obtained with brushing that does not require local anesthesia. Strips of ciliated epithelium are placed in a vial of nutrient medium for transfer to a sealed microscope apparatus. Beating cilia are visualized and positioned to obstruct intermittently the passage of light through a small diaphragm into a photometer. The transduction of light energy into an electrical signal is recorded, and the rate of beating is calculated. Ten consecutive measurements of vigorously beating cilia are taken from each sample, and the result is expressed as the mean and standard deviation (SD).

Olfactory Tests

Patients with an abnormal sense of smell typically experience problems with the intensity and quality of olfaction. A change in intensity is reflected in either a total loss (anosmia) or a partial loss (hyposmia) of olfaction. A change in quality may involve distortion of regular olfactory stimulation (parosmia or troposmia) or perception of olfactory stimulation when none is present (phantosmia, or hallucination). The most common causes of loss of olfaction, in order of decreasing frequency, are nasal disease, upper respiratory infection, trauma, and aging. There are very few life-threatening causes of olfactory loss, but a thorough work-up, including imaging of the brain and nasal cavities, should disclose any space-occupying lesions that may alter olfaction.

Odor Identification Tests

The most popular clinical assessment of olfaction employs the University of Pennsylvania Smell Identification Test (Sensonics, Haddonfield, NJ). The patient is asked to "scratch and sniff" a patch containing microencapsulated particles. For each of 40 patches, the patient must choose one of four possible odors, even if the choice would be a guess. The patient's score is then compared with that of normal subjects of similar age and gender. A quantitative percentile value is derived from standardized norms.

Odor Detection Threshold Tests

Widely used odor detection threshold tests are variants of the so-called method-of-limits procedure, in which the concentration of a stimulus is increased (or decreased) incrementally until the stimulus is just barely perceived. The increasingly popular staircase procedures, in which odorant concentrations are increased or decreased as a function of the correctness of the subject's responses, provide a reliable measure of threshold with a minimum number of trials.

Allergy Testing

If the history suggests that allergy contributes to the patient's sinus problem, the following investigations are available: (1) skin prick test, (2) measurement of IgE antibodies (radioallergosorbent assay), (3) measurement of serum IgE, (4) blood eosinophil count, (5) nasal smears cytology, and (6) nasal provocation test. Often a therapeutic trial of topical nasal steroids and/or antibiotics can control a patient's symptoms, making allergy testing unnecessary.

NEOPLASTIC AND NON-NEOPLASTIC LESIONS OF THE ORAL MUCOSA

By William Lawson, M.D., D.D.S.,
and Anthony J. Reino, M.D.
New York, New York

Infectious agents, metabolic disorders, endocrinopathies, traumatic injuries, neoplasms, developmental abnormalities, genetic syndromes, and immunologic disturbances may contribute to disease of the oral cavity. However, expression of disease in the mouth is typically limited to various mucosal abnormalities, destructive changes, and proliferative lesions.

Authors of textbooks and atlases of oral medicine have classified lesions either by appearance or by origin. This chapter classifies oral mucosal abnormalities according to appearance to enhance the clinician's ability to construct an appropriately finite differential diagnosis.

WHITE LESIONS

Thickening of one or more layers of the oral epithelium may lead to one or more white mucosal lesions of varying size and depth, usually with an irregular outline. White lesions most commonly arise from the buccal mucosa, lateral border of the tongue, floor of the mouth, and hard palate, with the remainder arising in the tongue, soft palate, lips, and gingiva (Table 1). Various causal factors may contribute to white lesions, including chronic inflammation, genetic disorders, microbes, and chemicals. Accordingly, a complete physical examination and personal, social, and family histories are required, including data on all past and present use of prescription and proprietary medications. Few lesions are visually diagnostic; biopsy is usually required.

The most common cofactor contributing to white lesions is chronic irritation from all forms of smoking. Less commonly, the direct application of tobacco to the oral mucosa by snuff dipping or chewing can lead to white lesions, including verrucous carcinoma, an uncommon, low-grade oral malignancy characterized by extensive hyperkeratosis and rugose surface proliferations. Other irritant factors include ill-fitting dentures, rough teeth, and dental restorations.

Leukokeratosis, Hyperkeratosis, and Leukoplakia

In general, the terms leukokeratosis and leukoplakia interchangeably refer to any white, plaquelike lesion of the oral cavity. A few authors, however, reserve the term leukoplakia for white lesions that show dyskeratosis under the microscope. Nondyskeratotic lesions are then classified as pachyderma oris.

Microscopically, white lesions may reveal hyperkeratosis (thickening of the outer keratin layer), parakeratosis (persistence of pyknotic nuclei in the outer epithelial layer), acanthosis (enlargement or edema of the stratum spinosum), and dyskeratosis. The latter term identifies disordered maturation of epithelial layers, loss of polarity of basal cells, and cytologic features, such as hyperchromatism, pleomorphism, enlarged nucleoli, increased mitoses, and increased nuclear-cytoplasmic ratios. In white lesions of the oral cavity, the incidence of dyskeratosis varies from 2 to 24 per cent, and the incidence of invasive carcinoma varies from 2 to 11 per cent.

Because it is often clinically impossible to differentiate benign from malignant white lesions, biopsy is essential. Lesions that demonstrate high-grade dyskeratosis are considered premalignant, with significant propensity to transform into carcinoma in situ or invasive squamous cell carcinoma. Accordingly, these leukoplakic growths must be excised completely, and the region followed closely for recurrence.

As noted, white lesions can arise anywhere in the oral cavity, with the most frequent occurrence on the buccal mucosa and the least frequent on the soft palate and gingiva. The peak incidence is in middle life, with a male preponderance. Most lesions are discovered on routine physical examination of asymptomatic patients, although a few patients report an area of roughness or burning.

In patients with white lesions, the clinician must identify and eliminate irritative causal agents. This strategy may lead to involution of many but not all lesions. New ones may even appear. Periodic follow-up examination and repeat biopsy are essential in such patients. With widespread oral disease, multiple areas should be sampled.

White, Hairy Leukoplakia

This lesion typically arises on the lateral border of the tongue but can also involve the buccal and labial mucosa. White, hairy leukoplakia is an excellent example of virally induced epithelial hyperplasia arising primarily in patients infected with human immunodeficiency virus (HIV). The name derives from the filamentous nature of the plaques. Under the microscope, hyperkeratosis, parakeratosis, and koilocytosis are prominent. The inclusion body of the koilocyte may represent opportunistic infection with the Epstein-Barr virus.

White, hairy leukoplakia appears as unilateral or bilateral whitening of the borders of the tongue. This white surface is irregular and usually contains prominent folds or projections that resemble hairs. The lesions are painless and may extend to the buccal mucosa, floor of the mouth, palate, and dorsal and ventral surfaces of the tongue. The lesions cannot be removed by scraping and are refractory to antifungal treatment.

Squamous Cell Carcinoma

Squamous cell carcinoma accounts for more than 90 per cent of the malignant tumors of the oral cavity and 5 per cent of all cancers. Carcinoma of the oral cavity causes painful ulcers as it grows insidiously. Otalgia is often present with advanced tumors of the posterior oral cavity and

Table 1. White Lesions

Disease	Location	Lesion Characteristics	Diagnosis	Treatment
Leukoplakia	Buccal mucosa most common, but may occur anywhere in oral cavity	Histology—hyperkeratosis, parakeratosis, dyskeratosis, acanthosis. 2–11% SCCA	Biopsy	Remove irritant, laser ablation, wide local excision
White, hairy leukoplakia	Lateral border of tongue more often than buccal or labial mucosa	Occurs exclusively in HIV-positive patients	HIV testing Biopsy	None
Squamous cell carcinoma	Tongue more often than floor of mouth	Hyperkeratotic, erythroplakic, granular, ulcerative with zone of central necrosis	Biopsy	Wide excision
Lichen planus	Skin and/or oral cavity, especially buccal mucosa	Reticular, ulcerative, erythematous, atrophic, bullous, plaque, and nummular forms	Biopsy Direct immunofluorescence	None
Stomatitis nicotina	Hard and soft palates	Microkeratotic papules with elevated red centers	Biopsy	None
Benign intraepithelial dyskeratosis	Buccal mucosa, oral commissure, conjunctiva	Pathology—hyperkeratosis	Biopsy	None
White, spongy nevus of Cannon	Buccal mucosa, anogenital region	Onset—infancy Pathology—parakeratosis/acanthosis	Biopsy	None
Leukoedema	Bilateral buccal mucosa	Dark-skinned patients	Stretch mucosa with tongue blades	None
Darier-White disease	Predilection—buccal mucosa; also skin and genitalia	Broad areas of yellow-white papular keratotic lesions	Biopsy	Topical vitamin A
Pachyonychia congenita	Bilateral buccal lesions	Pathology—parakeratosis, acanthosis, dystrophic changes in nails, palmar/plantar hyperkeratosis	Biopsy	None
Candidiasis	Nonspecific oral cavity	Thick, white plaques that can be rubbed off to show bleeding base	Culture	Antifungals
Allergy	Mucosal area apposed to dental restoration	Lichenoid-type keratotic reaction	History	Remove offending agent
SLE	Buccal mucosa	Central atrophy or ulceration with peripheral radial hyperkeratotic striae	Biopsy ANA	Systemic steroids

> = greater than; SCCA = squamous cell carcinoma; HIV = human immunodeficiency virus; SLE = systemic lupus erythematosus; ANA = antinuclear antibody test.

oropharynx. The peak incidence is in the sixth and seventh decades, with a strong male preponderance. A history of smoking and alcohol use is usually, but not invariably, elicited. Syphilitic glossitis and poor oral hygiene are strong predisposing factors. Common sites of involvement, in descending order of frequency, are the lateral border of the tongue, floor of mouth, gingiva, buccal mucosa, and palate.

Routine examination of the oral cavity seeks to detect malignant lesions early, because the prognosis for patients with oral cancer is directly related to its extent. Although the region is easily examined and early diagnosis should be standard, one third of oral carcinoma patients are dead within 5 years of tumor detection. There is also a 20 to 25 per cent rate of synchronous or metachronous second primary carcinoma in the same region owing to field cancerization. Consequently, panendoscopy should be performed in these patients to identify another primary aerodigestive cancer. The lesions primarily are squamous cell carcinomas, and most are invasive. Microscopically, hyperchromatic and pleomorphic tumor cells with various degrees of mitotic activity have clearly penetrated the basement membrane of the epidermis. Keratin pearls are seen in more differentiated lesions.

On physical examination, squamous cell tumors are typically hyperkeratotic but may be erythroplakic, granular, or ulcerative with a zone of central necrosis. To assess the true extent of the lesion, the clinician should palpate for induration beyond the apparent mucosal portion of the tumor. Induration suggests infiltrative spread of carcinoma into deeper tissues, especially in the tongue, where the tumor can spread along muscle bundles. Squamous cell cancer can be exophytic, with mainly surface spread, or endophytic, with substantial submucosal infiltration. Rarely, the lesion is totally submucosal, as in the tonsil and base of the tongue; however, this presentation is more typical of lymphoma or minor salivary gland tumors. The clinician should biopsy nonulcerated parts of the lesion with scalpel or biting forceps under local or topical anesthesia. However, with larger lesions and with painful ulcerated tumors, general anesthesia may be required for proper assessment of true size. The neck should be carefully palpated for the presence of lymph node metastases. Computed tomography scanning may detect not only small, necrotic lymph nodes not clinically apparent but also bone erosion of the mandible and maxilla. The treatment depends on the site and stage of the tumor and may involve surgery, radiotherapy, chemotherapy, or some combination of these modalities.

Lip

Squamous cell carcinomas arise primarily on the lower lip and appear to be related to actinic changes or pipe smoking. The lesions can be exophytic, verrucous, or ulcerative. The ulcerative type has the poorest prognosis owing to early invasion and spread to regional lymph nodes. Metastases are also related to the degree of differentiation of the tumor. The overall 5-year survival rate is 80 to 90 per cent.

Buccal Mucosa

Tumors here typically develop in tobacco chewers and are most often associated with antecedent leukoplakia. Buccal carcinomas are most commonly exophytic, but verrucous or ulcerative types also occur. The anterior lesions have a better prognosis than the posterior lesions, which may invade the pterygomaxillary space. The prognosis also correlates with the degree of tumor differentiation.

Gingiva

These tumors constitute 10 per cent of all oral malignancies. The lesions may be confused with inflammation of the gingiva, which may obscure and delay the correct diagnosis. Most of the tumors arise on the posterior mandibular gingiva. They may present as nodular, plaquelike lesions or as exophytic, papillary, or ulcerative growths. Because they may occur in the edentulous patient, whose only complaint may be an ill-fitting denture, the clinician must examine the edentulous patient with the dentures removed. Bone invasion is found in 50 per cent of patients with gingival tumors. Some patients may present with loose teeth at the site of the lesion. Metastatic spread is to the regional lymph nodes.

Tongue

This is a common tumor, most prevalent in patients with poor oral hygiene who smoke or chew tobacco, drink alcohol, or have a history of syphilis. Most of the lesions are found on the lateral border of the middle third of the tongue, but they may also arise on the ventral surface, dorsum, and tip. Consequently, all areas of the tongue must be carefully examined. Most lesions infiltrate and ulcerate, and they commonly present with local pain or a sore throat. Tumors of the posterior third are often asymptomatic until they enlarge, when they produce dysphagia and otalgia. These posterior tumors are not easily seen, and palpation of the base of tongue is essential for making the diagnosis. Metastases from tongue lesions are more common than from other oral carcinomas, and they are often bilateral owing to extensive lymphatic drainage. The prognosis varies with the anteroposterior location, the degree of differentiation and size of the primary tumor, and the presence and extent of lymph node involvement.

Floor of the Mouth

This is the second most common site for oral cancer after the tongue. The lesions usually arise anteriorly and tend to infiltrate. They spread along the periosteum of the mandible and into the tongue. Twenty per cent of these lesions are multifocal.

Palate

These tumors are usually well differentiated; they commonly appear as ulcerated masses. The size of the lesion is the most important factor in the prognosis. Cervical lymph node metastases usually occur late. Death is related to uncontrolled local disease; therefore, wide local resection should always be performed.

Lichen Planus

Lichen planus is a common skin disorder of unknown cause that typically presents as dermal and oral lesions. The oral lesions, however, may occur without skin involvement. Lichen planus is typically reticular in appearance, but it can also show atrophic, erythematous, plaquelike, papular, bullous, ulcerative, and nummular patterns. With the reticular form, the clinician often detects a network of interlacing white bands (striae of Wickham) on the buccal mucosa bilaterally. However, lesions may also appear on the tongue, palate, gingiva, and lip. On the lip, lichen planus may resemble a thumbprint (nummular type) and may be misdiagnosed as a fungal infection. Keratotic lesions may also assume papular and plaquelike forms. The erosive form is considered separately.

Typically, there are multiple admixed lesions scattered throughout the oral cavity. The clinician must detect the reticular pattern to establish the correct diagnosis, because random biopsy may reveal only acute and chronic inflammation. The cause of lichen planus is unknown, but it seems to involve immune degeneration of the basal epithelium. Grinspan's syndrome describes an association among oral lichen planus, diabetes, and hypertension.

Under the microscope, parakeratosis, elongation of the rete pegs of the surface epithelium, and submucosal lymphocytic infiltrates are prominent. The lesion usually occurs in middle life, more often in females. The patient is usually asymptomatic, and no treatment is necessary. Biopsy is performed to establish the diagnosis.

Direct immunofluorescence is positive in the superficial dermis and deep epidermis in 14 to 27 per cent of patients.

The differential diagnosis of oral lichen planus includes leukoplakia, carcinoma, candidiasis, pemphigus, benign mucous membrane pemphigoid, and systemic lupus erythematosus (SLE). Patients with lichen planus should be periodically re-examined, because malignant transformation to a squamous cell carcinoma can occur.

In the erosive form, erythema and ulceration develop secondary to vesicle formation within the keratotic lesion. Occasionally, the condition may present as desquamative gingivitis with oral pain and burning.

Stomatitis Nicotina

This condition occurs on the palate of pipe and cigar smokers. The hard and soft palate are covered with keratotic papules with elevated red centers corresponding to inflamed mucous gland orifices. Biopsy may be performed to rule out malignancy. Histologically, the epithelium reveals hyperkeratosis, parakeratosis, squamous metaplasia, obstruction of minor salivary gland ducts, and chronic inflammation of stroma. The disease is self-limited, and carcinomatous transformation does not occur. Treatment requires cessation of smoking.

Genetic Lesions

At least five autosomal dominant hereditary syndromes manifest with white lesions in the oral cavity. They typically affect the buccal mucosa bilaterally.

Benign Intraepithelial Dyskeratosis

Superficial, soft, white plaques arise on the buccal mucosa, oral commissures, and conjunctiva during childhood in a limited group of triracial families living in Halifax County, North Carolina. Histologically, as the name of the disorder implies, hyperkeratosis with disordered maturation is prominent. No treatment is required because the lesions are not considered precancerous.

White, Spongy Nevus of Cannon

Diffuse, soft, folded, white lesions typically appear on the buccal mucosa, but they may also arise elsewhere in the oral cavity and in the anogenital region. Nevi appear in infancy, with maximal severity during adolescence. The microscopic features include parakeratosis, acanthosis, and bands of parakeratin in the surface layers of the epithelium. No treatment is indicated.

Leukoedema

This condition presents primarily in dark-skinned persons as a diffuse, pearly sheen of the buccal mucosa bilaterally. Edema of the stratum spinosum is the most prominent microscopic feature. The clinical diagnosis is made by stretching the buccal mucosa with two tongue blades, which may cause the lesion to disappear, thereby obviating the need for biopsy. No treatment is indicated.

Darier-White Disease (Keratosis Follicularis)

Keratosis follicularis is often, but not exclusively, a combined cutaneous and mucosal disorder characterized by yellow to white papular and keratotic lesions as well as cobblestonelike plaques of the skin, oral cavity, and genital tract. Like other genetic conditions, Darier-White disease has a predilection for the buccal mucosa but can also occur in the palate, tongue, and lips. The prominent microscopic features include intraepithelial lacunae, hyperkeratosis, acanthosis, and "cell-within-a-cell" dyskeratosis. Biopsy is diagnostic. Treatment with topical vitamin A to decrease keratinization has had limited success.

Pachyonychia Congenita

This condition presents as bilateral buccal lesions that resemble those seen in the white, spongy nevus of Cannon. Histologically, the two lesions are similar, but pachyonychia is accompanied by dystrophic changes in the nails and palmar-plantar hyperkeratosis. The disease is self-limited, and no treatment is required.

Pseudolesions

Candidiasis

Various forms of candidiasis can appear anywhere in the mouth. Usually, candidiasis presents as a thick, white plaque produced by a matted collection of mycelia and desquamated epithelium. The plaque is actually a pseudomembrane and can be rubbed off readily with a tongue blade, producing a punctate, bleeding base. In contrast, hyperplastic candidiasis is a variant in which chronic, low-grade fungal infection stimulates keratin formation and leukoplakic lesions that cannot be scraped away. Microscopically, pseudohyphae found within the keratin suggest the diagnosis.

Occasionally, oral candidiasis presents as an erythroplakic lesion. *Candida* infections of the oral commissure (angular cheilosis) appear as multiple fissures. The diagnosis can be confirmed by culture demonstrating the budding yeast cells of *Candida albicans* and staining of the pellicle to show hyphae. The predisposing factors to this focal fungal overgrowth are chronic antibiotic therapy, diabetes, and immunodeficiency, especially acquired immunodeficiency syndrome. The common occurrence of oral candidiasis in HIV-positive patients, in either the pseudomembranous or the angular cheilosis form, should be kept in mind during clinical evaluation.

Aspirin Burn of the Oral Mucosa

Aspirin tablets may be placed inside the cheek to reduce regional pain. Aspirin is caustic and causes coagulation necrosis, forming a region of white slough. The diagnosis is primarily based on the history.

Other White Lesions

Occasionally, SLE presents as a white plaque of the buccal mucosa. Both discoid lupus erythematosus and SLE can produce lesions with central atrophy or ulceration and peripheral radial hyperkeratotic striae. Biopsy reveals hyperkeratosis, thickening of the basement membrane, and lymphocytic infiltrates in the submucosa resembling lichen planus.

ERYTHEMATOUS LESIONS

Erythematous lesions, or red lesions, reflect the vascularity of the underlying tissues (Table 2). Red lesions often result from thinning or ulceration of the epithelium accompanied by increased local blood supply secondary to chronic inflammation. This section highlights true mucosal lesions rather than focal hemorrhage due to trauma, hematologic disorders, or vascular abnormalities.

Erythroplasia and Erythroplakia

Erythroplasia simply describes any red patch; this term does not have a pathologic connotation. Some workers in-

Table 2. Erythematous Lesions

Disease	Location	Lesion Characteristics	Diagnosis	Treatment
Erythroplakia	Floor of mouth and retromolar trigone	Loss of surface keratin, painless, 50% invasive carcinoma	Biopsy	Wide local excision
Geographic tongue	Dorsum and lateral tongue	Loss of filiform papillae, appear as smooth erythematous patches with gray-white rims Prominent fungiform papillae Changing patterns	History—increased in patients with psoriasis and juvenile diabetes	Bland diet and antihistamine mouthrinses if symptomatic, treatment does not eliminate condition
Stomatitis areata migrans	Buccal mucosa>labial and oral vestibules>floor of mouth>ventral tongue>soft palate>gingiva	Nonlingual form of geographic tongue; multiple flat, painless, irregularly shaped red patches; raised keratotic rims; heal and reappear	History—geographic tongue and fissured tongue associated with this condition	Antihistamine mouthrinses, antibiotics
Candidiasis	Dorsum of tongue and palate Areas under dental prostheses	Erythematous or atrophic form—loss of epithelium and papillae	History Culture	Clotrimazole, nystatin
Allergy	Nonspecific oral cavity	Erythema multiforme Lichenoid	Clinical	Remove offending agent
Plasma cell gingivitis (atypical allergic gingivostomatitis)	Gingiva>lips>buccal mucosa>tongue	Intense gingival erythema Plasma cell infiltration	History—allergic reaction to ingredients in gum and toothpaste; biopsy	Remove offending agent
Pemphigus vulgaris	Nonspecific oral cavity or tongue Skin	Intense erythema of oral cavity, geographic tongue, or small scattered white plaques	Clinical	Symptomatic

> = greater than.

terchangeably employ the term erythroplakia. Others, however, designate erythroplakia as the red analogue to leukoplakia. That is, erythroplakia is a specific histologic entity with a distinct premalignant potential. In fact, the diagnosis of erythroplakia is more ominous because about 50 per cent of these lesions reveal invasive carcinoma under the microscope.

Erythroplakia typically occurs as a painless, solitary, flat or slightly raised red patch of varied size. Its color derives from loss of surface keratin. The lesion may be homogeneous or admixed with small foci of leukoplakia (speckled form). The most common sites are the floor of the mouth and the retromolar triangle. The gingiva is rarely involved. The incidence peaks after the sixth decade, with a male preponderance. The preferred treatment is wide local excision.

Stomatitis Migrans

Geographic Tongue

Migratory glossitis occurs primarily in 1 to 2 per cent of young adults, especially females. Its cause is unknown, but some authors suggest either allergic or autoimmune phenomena. The incidence may increase in psoriasis and juvenile diabetes. The lesions develop on the lateral borders and dorsum of the tongue, where depapillated areas appear as smooth, erythematous patches with gray-white rims. The fungiform papillae become prominent owing to selective loss of filiform papillae. The patterns formed by the lesions change at intervals ranging from days to weeks or months, and recurrences are the rule. Histologically, localized inflammation, inflammatory cell infiltrates, and spongiotic epithelium (spongiform pustules) are prominent. Geographic tongue is usually asymptomatic, but a few patients report the symptom of burning. Bland diet and antihistamine mouthrinses are occasionally prescribed in symptomatic patients.

Erythema Migrans (Stomatitis Areata Migrans)

Although geographic tongue is commonly recognized as a migratory stomatitis, the nonlingual form, stomatitis areata or erythema migrans, is not. The latter appears as multiple, flat, irregularly shaped (circinate) red patches with raised keratotic rims, which spontaneously heal and reappear with constantly changing patterns. Common sites of occurrence include the buccal mucosa and the labial and oral vestibula, but the floor of the mouth, ventral tongue, soft palate, and gingiva may also be involved. Geographic tongue and fissured tongue are commonly associated with erythema migrans. The lesions are usually painless despite the presence of acute and chronic inflammation on biopsy. Those affected are usually young adults. The migratory character of the lesions points to the diagnosis. Management in symptomatic cases includes antihistamine mouthwash and oral antibiotics for secondary bacterial infection.

Candidiasis

Oral candidiasis characteristically presents as a pseudomembranous lesion mimicking keratosis, but it also appears in several other forms. The erythematous type, also known as atrophic candidiasis, is caused by the loss of the surface epithelium, including the filiform and fungiform papillae. Lesions arise most commonly as bright red patches without ulceration, especially on the dorsum of the tongue and palate. One variant is denture stomatitis, in which *Candida* colonizes desquamated mucosa beneath a dental prosthesis.

Allergy

Red lesions caused by hypersensitivity reactions to drugs administered systemically or topically can arise anywhere in the oral cavity. Sulfa drugs, barbiturates, and iodine preparations are traditionally, albeit rarely, associated with allergic stomatitis. More common is contact allergy associated with denture adhesives, toothpastes, mouthrinses, and dental materials. The patient describes local pain, burning, or itching. On clinical examination, lesions appear nonspecific. A thorough drug history, including use of oral and dental preparations, must be elicited.

Allergic red lesions have been broadly subdivided into those resembling erythema multiforme and those resembling lichen planus. The former have been reported after use of various antibiotics (penicillin, clindamycin, sulfa, rifampin, tetracycline), and anti-inflammatory agents (salicylates, nonsteroidal compounds). Lichenoid drug reactions can be produced by methyldopa, beta-blockers, thiazides, systemic gold, penicillamine, nonsteroidal anti-inflammatory agents, and lithium.

Plasma Cell Gingivitis

Described in 1968 and also known as atypical gingivostomatitis, this entity is characterized by intense and diffuse gingival erythema. Biopsy reveals plasma cell infiltration. Lesions may also arise on the lips, buccal mucosa, and tongue (with loss of filiform papillae). Plasma cell gingivitis may be an allergic reaction to various components of chewing gums and toothpastes. Treatment means avoidance of the offending substance.

Other Erythematous Lesions

Many of the vesiculobullous oral disorders may resemble erythematous lesions because of loss of surface epithelium that leaves an irregular, inflamed base. This is especially true of lupus erythematosus and erythema multiforme. The clinician must therefore search for residual mucosal fragments that suggest the true nature of the disease. Moreover, the bullous disorders tend to have widespread oral involvement, often with cutaneous lesions. Finally, pemphigus vulgaris may also present as oral lesions, including scattered small, white plaques, intense erythema, and geographic tongue.

PIGMENTED LESIONS

Pigmentation in the mouth (Table 3) has been linked to racial traits, genetic syndromes, hormone imbalance, extrinsic metals, drugs, foreign bodies, chronic irritation, developmental lesions (nevi), and tumors (melanoma). Pigment may result from endogenous production and deposition of melanin or of hemosiderin, the former being more common. Exogenous agents most often associated with pigment include lead, mercury, bismuth, and silver. The color of the lesion may suggest its nature, but biopsy is usually required for definitive diagnosis. Occupational and medication histories are essential. Vascular lesions can be distinguished from pigmented ones by pressing a glass slide against the lesion, which tends to blanch if blood vessels are prominent.

Physiologic Pigmentation

Racial Pigmentation

Melanocytes reside in the basal layer of the oral epithelium of all individuals except albinos. Melanin pigmentation of the oral cavity is sufficiently common in dark-skinned races of all nationalities to be considered physiologic. Common sites of deposition include the gingiva and buccal mucosa, but pigment may be detected anywhere in the mouth. Lesions may be punctate (macular) or diffuse, even forming broad sheets of stained tissue called melanoplakia. Color may vary from blue-black to brown, and these deposits have no pathologic implications.

Oral Melanotic Macule

Arising in light-skinned persons, these solitary, dark lesions are typically less than 1 cm in diameter. Twenty-nine per cent of these macules appear on the lower lip; 23 per cent on the gingiva; 16 per cent on the buccal mucosa; and 7 per cent on the hard palate. A variant of this lesion is the ephelis, or freckle, which is generally seen as a small (2 to 3 mm) brown spot on the lip. Melanotic macules are benign and biopsy usually differentiates them from melanoma.

Genetic Syndromes

Peutz-Jeghers Syndrome

Peutz-Jeghers syndrome is an autosomal dominant disorder consisting of oral melanosis and intestinal polyposis. Macular deposits of melanin most often involve the lips, buccal mucosa, and fingers, and, less often, the gingiva, palate, and tongue. The polyps of the small intestine are benign and do not undergo malignant transformation, but may be a cause of intussusception in childhood. No treatment is required.

Von Recklinghausen Disease

Some patients with neurofibromatosis develop lightly pigmented café au lait spots, and others develop macular melanotic pigmentation of the lips. No treatment is necessary.

Albright's Syndrome

Albright's syndrome produces the triad of polyostotic fibrous dysplasia, precocious puberty, and café au lait skin pigmentation, which may extend to the lips and mouth. The nature of the genetic defect in Albright's syndrome remains unclear.

Hormonal Imbalance

Addison's Disease

The classic endocrine syndrome characterized by oral melanosis is adrenal insufficiency, or Addison's disease, in which the loss of feedback inhibition of pituitary release of adrenocorticotropic hormone (ACTH) causes increased pigmentation. Causes of adrenal insufficiency include tuberculosis and fungal infections, idiopathic adrenal atrophy, tumor metastases, and amyloidosis. The oral lesions are usually diffuse and multifocal (but may be macular) and are accompanied by darkening of the skin, hypotension, hyponatremia, hyperkalemia, hypoglycemia, and lym-

Table 3. Pigmented Lesions

Disease	Location	Lesion Characteristics	Diagnosis	Treatment
Racial pigmentation	Gingiva Buccal mucosa	Dark-skinned individuals; diffuse blue, black, brown color	Clinical	None, phenol peel for cosmesis
Oral melanotic macule	Lower lip>gingiva>buccal mucosa	Solitary dark lesion, <1 cm in diameter, light-skinned patients	Biopsy	None
Peutz-Jeghers syndrome	Lips, buccal mucosa, fingers, gingiva, palate, tongue	Autosomal dominant Oral melanosis, benign intestinal polyposis, macular deposits	Clinical	None
Neurofibromatosis	Lips and skin	Café au lait	Clinical	None
Albright's syndrome	Lips and skin—café au lait	Polyostotic fibrous dysplasia, precocious puberty, and cutaneous pigmentation	Clinical	None
Addison's disease	Diffuse/multifocal	Macular darkening of skin and mucosa	Clinical	None
Chloasma	Gingiva and skin	Macular darkening of skin and mucosa	Clinical	None
Drug reactions—quinacrine	Hard palate	Diffuse pigmentation	History	None
Drug reactions—Minocin, chlorpromazine, Myleran	Nonspecific oral pigmentation	Diffuse	History	None
Amalgam tattoo	Adjacent to dental silver restoration; buccal mucosa or gingiva	Solitary gray-black	Clinical	None
Lead line Argyria Graphite	Free gingival margin Skin/mucous membrane Submucosa	Lead—precipitation of metal by sulfide-producing bacteria Silver—blue-gray Graphite—black	Clinical	Remove offending agents/treat systemic disease
Smoker's melanosis	Anterior mandible and attached gingiva	Brown-black macules	Biopsy	None
Nevi	Hard palate>buccal mucosa>lip>gingiva>labial mucosa>soft palate>retromolar trigon>tongue	Flat or slightly raised gray, brown, or black macular lesions with irregular borders	Biopsy	Excision if lentigo maligna
Melanoma	Palate>maxillary gingiva>buccal mucosa>lip>mandibular gingival>tongue>floor of mouth	Pigmented macule or nodule, exophytic mass, 25% amelanotic, ulceration with irregular borders	Biopsy	Complete excision

> = greater than; < = less than.

phocytosis. The diagnosis of adrenal insufficiency is aided by the 24-hour ACTH stimulation test.

Chloasma

Physiologic changes in late pregnancy produce the characteristic pigmentation of the facial skin termed chloasma gravidarum, or mask of pregnancy. Chloasma is attributed to melanocyte stimulation by maternal ACTH, placental corticotropin-releasing hormone, and beta-endorphin release. Uncommonly, there is an intraoral variant of this condition wherein women experience melanin pigmentation, especially of the gingiva, during or after pregnancy. No treatment is required.

Drug Reactions

A number of chemical agents can produce oral melanin pigmentation. Quinacrine, originally used as an antimalarial and presently used to treat rheumatoid disorders, occasionally causes oral melanosis, especially of the hard palate. Chlorpromazine, minocycline (Minocin), and busulfan (Myleran) also can produce pigmentation. The diagnosis is established by taking a careful history.

Foreign Bodies

Amalgam Tattoo

Amalgam tattoos are relatively common pigmented lesions of the oral cavity, produced by scuffing of the oral mucosa adjacent to the site of a dental restoration. Fragments of the silver or mercury in the amalgam used as a cavity filler become embedded in the soft tissue, causing precipitation of proteins in immature collagen fibers. These lesions are usually solitary, localized, gray-black, and adjacent to a restored tooth on the buccal mucosa or gingiva. Biopsy helps differentiate the typical lesion from a melanoma. Under the microscope, fragments of foreign material are seen within the connective tissue matrix.

Graphite

Graphite is typically embedded when a child playing with a pencil accidentally falls and breaks the tip off in the palate. The carbon remains inert and presents as a dark submucosal mass.

Other Foreign Bodies

Embedded foreign bodies or perforating injuries to the oral mucosa may ultimately become pigmented. The foreign substance itself may have been extruded or phagocytized, but hemosiderin deposited at the injury site remains as a marker. Biopsy may be required to differentiate the lesion from a nevus or melanoma.

Heavy Metals

The ingestion of heavy metals, principally lead but also mercury and bismuth, may cause distinctive oral pigmentation known as "lead line." A scalloped band of dark (brown-black) discoloration along the free gingival margin of the teeth results from precipitation of the metal by sulfide-producing bacteria in the gingival crevice. Lead line is rare, but it has been observed in persons drinking moonshine whiskey distilled in automobile radiators containing high lead concentrations. It is also seen in children with pica who eat lead-containing paints; however, by the time the lead line appears, these children usually have other signs of lead poisoning, including anemia, basophilic stippling of erythrocytes, and neurologic manifestations. Bismuth and mercury ingestion can also produce gingival border discoloration, but chronic use of these agents is of only historical interest because these agents are no longer used to treat syphilis.

Chronic inhalation of silver fumes by photography workers in the past has caused argyria, with blue-gray discoloration of the skin and mucous membranes. Early in the 20th century, the popularity and overuse of silver-containing nose drops caused tissue staining of a lesser degree.

Smoker's Melanosis

This term denotes pigmentation of the gingiva associated with tobacco smoking. Unlike heavy metal pigmentation, which involves the free gingival margin, smoker's melanosis develops on the attached gingiva, especially the mandibular anterior gingiva. The degree of melanin deposition is related to the amount of tobacco use.

Nevi

Every type of nevus that develops on the skin can also arise, albeit rarely, in the oral cavity. One study of 130 intraoral nevi reported that 63 per cent were intramucosal, 19 per cent blue, 9 per cent compound, 5 per cent junctional, and 4 per cent combined nevi. The mean age was 32 years, and most patients were female. Forty per cent of the intraoral nevi were found on the hard palate. Other sites included the buccal mucosa (19 per cent), lip (11 per cent), gingiva (9 per cent), labial mucosa (7 per cent), soft palate (7 per cent), retromolar pad (6 per cent), and tongue (1 per cent).

Nevi appear as flat (28 per cent) or slightly elevated (72 per cent) gray, brown, blue, or black macular lesions with irregular borders. Microscopically, clusters of epithelioid nevus cells are noted along with melanin granules.

It is virtually impossible to clinically distinguish between nevi, melanotic macules, and early spreading melanoma; biopsy is essential.

Lentigo maligna, or Hutchinson's melanotic freckle, is a slow-growing, pigmented lesion that typically arises on the face and is considered precancerous. A few lesions have been reported in the oral cavity; 50 per cent of these became malignant. Accordingly, complete excision should be performed. Lentigo maligna should not be confused with the nevus of Ota (oculodermal melanocytosis), which involves the eye, facial skin, and oral cavity. Although the nevus of Ota clinically resembles lentigo maligna, it rarely becomes malignant. The diagnosis is clinical and is most often made in Japanese infants and children.

Melanoma

Melanoma of the oral cavity represents about 1 per cent of all melanomas. Oral melanoma is slightly more common in men than in women, and most of these tumors arise after age 40. In the mouth, melanoma most frequently occurs in the palate, followed by the maxillary gingiva, buccal mucosa, lip, mandibular gingiva, unspecified gingiva, tongue, and floor of the mouth. Concomitant or preexisting melanosis is detected in one third of patients with oral melanoma.

These tumors may take the form of a pigmented macule, a pigmented nodule, an exophytic mass, or an amelanotic lesion. Melanoma often begins as a localized, blue-black patch with diffuse borders. With continued growth, mucosal streaking is observed. Melanoma often ulcerates in the oral cavity. One quarter of oral melanomas are amelanotic, and these lesions may be mistaken for pyogenic granuloma. Accordingly, all amelanotic lesions require biopsy.

Oral melanoma is highly malignant and carries a poor prognosis (5-year survival rate, 3 to 20 per cent). Treatment involves radical surgery. Local, regional, and distant recurrences are common.

EROSIVE LESIONS

Erosions of the oral mucosa may be grossly subdivided into punctate and bullous lesions. Erosive lesions, which are relatively superficial and involve primarily loss of surface epithelium, should be differentiated from destructive lesions that produce deep ulcers and significant submucosal damage.

Punctate Lesions

Punctate lesions (Table 4) are erosions that are typically 1 to 5 mm in diameter, single or multiple, sporadic or

Table 4. Punctate Erosive Lesions

Disease	Location	Lesion Characteristics	Diagnosis	Treatment
Herpes simplex virus	Lips and gingiva, may occur throughout the oral cavity	Vesicular phase, then ulcerative with erythematous halo; clustered on fixed mucosa	Tzanck preparation	Supportive and/or acyclovir for recurrent infection or immunosuppressed host
Coxsackievirus A and B	Predilection for posterior pharyngeal structures: tonsils, tonsillar pillars, soft palate	Multiple vesicles	Coxsackievirus B1-B5—throat swab with plating on PMK medium/serology; coxsackievirus A1-A10 and A27—exclusionary diagnosis	Supportive
Coxsackievirus A16	Lips, buccal mucosa, extremities (hands and feet)	Multiple vesicles	Clinical	Supportive
Herpes zoster	Extremities Palate	Exanthem, multiple vesicles	Tzanck preparation, serology, direct immunofluorescence	Supportive, acyclovir
Aphthous stomatitis	Affinity for lateral tongue, buccal mucosa, lips, floor of mouth	Solitary/multifocal shallow ulcers 2–5 mm, necrotic center with erythematous borders	Biopsy if lesions are large and persistent	Supportive, 1% triamcinolone in Orabase
Sutton's disease (giant aphthae)	As for aphthous stomatitis	Lesions may be 10–15 mm and can be associated with ulcerative colitis, Crohn's disease, gluten-sensitive enteropathy	As for aphthous stomatitis	As for aphthous stomatitis
Behçet's syndrome	Oral cavity, genitalia, eyes, and skin	Painful oral ulcerative lesions, yellow necrotic base, erythema	Clinical, HLA-B5	Supportive, prednisone, triamcinolone in Orabase, diphenhydramine syrup, colchicine
Reiter's syndrome	Soft palate, buccal mucosa, dorsum of tongue	Painless ulcers, arthritis, ocular and genital lesions	Culture to exclude gonorrhea, HLA-B27	NSAIDs, steroids
Neutropenia	Favors gingiva, but there may be diffuse oral cavity involvement	Ulcers with central necrosis	Medical and drug histories, CBC	Treat underlying condition
ANUG	Gingiva	Loss of interdental papillae, gray pseudomembrane with bleeding base	Clinical	Penicillin, oral rinses, gingival sealing, periodontal treatment
Drug reaction	Buccal mucosa, gingiva	Ulcerations of variable depth	Medical and drug histories	Remove offending agent
Crohn's disease and ulcerative colitis	Lips, gingiva, vestibular sulci	Small ulcers, fissures, angular cheilitis, hyperplastic lesions, glossitis	Medical history, biopsy, direct immuno-fluorescence	Steroids
Contact allergy	Adjacent to gold dental restoration	Erythematous, ulcerations	Clinical skin tests not reliable	Remove restoration

NSAIDs = nonsteroidal anti-inflammatory drugs; CBC = complete blood count; ANUG = acute necrotizing ulcerative gingivostomatitis.

recurrent. Before erosion or ulceration occurs, a vesicle or fluid-filled bleb may be present. Most vesicles are caused by viruses. What begins as a blister or vesicle rapidly becomes abraded, creating an ulcer. Detection of early mucosal vesicles may significantly aid diagnosis.

Herpes Simplex

Infection with the human herpes simplex virus type 1 (HSV-1) appears in several clinical forms. Most people acquire HSV-1 infection silently in early life, with activation developing in adulthood. In some children and young adults, however, primary infection causes an explosive febrile disorder. In primary herpetic gingivostomatitis, ulcers appear diffusely throughout the oral cavity, especially on the lips and gingiva. The lesions have an erythematous halo, and intense gingivitis is common. Treatment is supportive and includes maintenance of hydration and alimentation. Oral herpes is self-limiting, and most lesions disappear in 10 to 14 days. Rarely, disseminated herpes (Pospischill-Feyrter syndrome) develops in debilitated infants.

Recurrent HSV-1 infection within the oral cavity was believed to be rare, presenting typically as a crop of vesicles limited to the palate. However, in the immunocompromised host, ulcers of varying diameters that culture positive for HSV-1 may be found anywhere in the oral cavity. Serologic tests are usually not performed. Although treatment with systemic acyclovir has met with limited success in many viral infections, it is of proven benefit in preventing or delaying recurrence of herpetic lesions in immunocompromised hosts.

Recurrent HSV-1 infection is most commonly seen as herpes labialis. This represents a reactivation of the latent herpes virus on the lips following trauma, sunlight exposure, stress, or another viral or febrile illness (cold sore). In the affected host, the condition tends to recur and usually appears on the vermilion border of either lip as a cluster of vesicles soon covered by a fibrin crust. The lesions may extend onto the adjacent skin. There may be a prodrome of burning and itching several hours to 24 hours before the eruption appears. Viral shedding is highest with ulcerative lesions and least with crusted ones. The lesions are distinguished by their focal nature, lack of involvement of the oral mucosa, and spontaneous healing. Topical application of acyclovir ointment decreases the duration of viral shedding but does not shorten the duration of the condition and does not promote healing. Similarly, oral administration of the drug has not been shown to be of consistent benefit. However, acyclovir may reduce relapses in normal and immunocompromised patients with severe recurrent disease.

Oral herpes must be differentiated from aphthous ulcers, which have no preliminary vesicular phase but do have a more intense erythematous halo. Recurrent herpetic ulcers tend to be smaller (<5 mm), occur in clusters, and arise on fixed mucosa (palate, gingiva, alveolus).

Coxsackieviruses

Both the A and B groups of the coxsackieviruses (as well as some echoviruses) produce oral lesions, primarily in children and young adults. Multiple vesicles typically arise in the soft palate, tonsillar fauces, and tonsils, producing a condition called herpangina. Constitutional signs (fever, malaise, lymphadenopathy) accompany an extremely sore throat that produces marked difficulty in swallowing. This condition is self-limiting, with ulcers spontaneously healing in 7 to 10 days.

Hand-foot-and-mouth disease similarly afflicts children and young adults and is produced by the coxsackievirus A16. Vesicles, which rapidly ulcerate, simultaneously appear in the oral cavity, particularly on the lips and buccal mucosa, and on the extremities. The cutaneous lesions involve both surfaces of the hands and feet. As with other coxsackievirus infections, constitutional signs are present. The clinical picture is virtually diagnostic. The disease is contagious and may achieve epidemic proportions in school children.

Herpes Zoster

Primary infection with the varicella-zoster virus presents as an explosive, diffuse, intensely painful vesicular eruption of the face, trunk, and hands. Constitutional signs are usually present, including fever and lymphadenopathy. In addition to the exanthem, oral vesicles often appear, especially on the palate. The illness is self-limiting, and crusting of the lesions occurs within 7 to 10 days. Treatment is supportive.

After initial infection with varicella-zoster, the virus remains latent in the dorsal root ganglia of sensory nerves until it becomes activated. Secondary varicella-zoster infections (shingles) characteristically appear as a unilateral vesicular eruption on the skin in a dermatome distribution. However, if the gasserian ganglion is infected, clusters of skin and oral mucosal lesions may appear in the distribution of the maxillary and mandibular nerves, accompanied by fever and regional lymphadenopathy.

Meningitis is a well-documented complication of varicella-zoster infection. Herpes zoster infections have also been linked to occult lymphoma, leukemia, and carcinoma. Therefore, in varicella-zoster patients, an underlying malignancy must be ruled out.

Rarely, herpes zoster infects the ninth and tenth cranial nerves. Vesicles appear along the posterior pharyngeal wall, tonsils, and base of the tongue. Patients complain of severe pain in the throat and difficulty swallowing. This condition is distinguished from herpangina by its unilateral nature. Again, a search for occult malignancy must be made.

Management includes supportive care and acyclovir, which may reduce pain in the acute phase and promote healing in normal and immunocompromised hosts.

Aphthous Stomatitis

Aphthous stomatitis is the most common ulcerative condition of the oral cavity. It occurs at all ages and equally in both sexes. Initially, aphthous stomatitis was confused with herpes simplex infection; however, there is no evidence that Sutton's disease has a viral origin. Autoimmunity may play a role. The lesions may be precipitated by emotional stress.

The aphthous ulcer (canker sore) is typically a solitary or multifocal, shallow, round or oval ulcer, 2 to 5 mm in diameter, with an erythematous border and a necrotic center. Existence of a preliminary vesicle has never been demonstrated. Canker sores can occur anywhere in the mouth but are most common on the lateral border of the tongue, buccal mucosa, lips, and floor of the mouth. Gingival lesions are uncommon. Occasionally, a few large ulcers develop. In some patients, crops of lesions reappear at varying intervals.

Recurrent oral ulcers may be subdivided into minor aphthous ulcers (several ulcers smaller than 10 mm that heal without scarring); major aphthous ulcers (one or several ulcers larger than 10 mm that heal with scarring); and herpetiform ulcers (numerous 1- to 2-mm ulcers that become confluent and may heal with scarring). Despite the name of the third type, there is no evidence for a viral cause of this variant.

There is a well-recognized association between recurrent aphthous stomatitis and ulcerative colitis, Crohn's disease, and gluten-sensitive enteropathy, but the significance is unknown.

The clinical course is usually 7 to 10 days, with spontaneous healing and little or no scarring. Pain is the predominant symptom. Various agents such as antibiotics, basic dyes, ether, and vaccination have been employed with limited success. Cautery of single lesions with silver nitrate eliminates the pain but results in scarring. Topical antihistamines (diphenhydramine syrup) promote healing and serve as topical anesthetics. Topical steroids provide effective treatment; intralesional injection and systemic administration of steroids have also been tried.

The large aphthous ulcers (10 to 15 mm in diameter) that heal with scarring are termed Sutton's disease, or periadenitis mucosa necrotica recurrens. They last longer than their smaller counterparts and recur more rapidly. Very large lesions (2 to 3 cm) may persist for several weeks or months, mimicking carcinoma. Biopsy is indicated in these patients. Oral corticosteroids may reduce the severity of the attack.

Behçet's Syndrome

This syndrome is characterized by oral, genital, ocular, and skin lesions as well as visceral involvement. The term complex aphthosis has been used to describe patients with recurrent oral and genital lesions without systemic involvement. The mean age at onset is in the twenties, with a male preponderance. The prevalence of Behçet's syndrome is highest in Japan and the Middle East and is low in Europe and the United States.

The ulcers of Behçet's syndrome, indistinguishable from those of aphthous stomatitis, appear in the oral cavity, eyes, and genitourinary tract. The oral ulcers may be single or multiple, shallow or deep, and many have a yellow, necrotic base. Ocular problems include conjunctivitis, uveitis, and hypopyon. Genital lesions may be cutaneous or mucosal. The cause of Behçet's syndrome may be autoimmune. The tissue antigen HLA-B5 has been found mainly in Turkish patients; its significance is unclear. Microscopically, a nonspecific epithelial ulcer filled with necrotic debris and chronic inflammation is typically observed.

Reiter's Syndrome

This condition principally affects young males, who present with arthritis as well as oral, ocular, genital, and skin lesions. The classic triad described by Reiter was arthritis, conjunctivitis, and urethritis. The arthritis is seronegative and involves the peripheral joints. The skin lesions typically are yellowish macules that arise on the soles of the feet (keratoderma blennorrhagicum), and pustular and psoriatic lesions also occur. The oral lesions consist of multiple small ulcers indistinguishable from those of aphthous stomatitis and Behçet's syndrome. They usually appear on the buccal mucosa, palate, and tongue. Occasionally, large erosions and a migratory stomatitis develop. The histologic findings are also nonspecific (epithelial ulceration with acute and chronic inflammation in the dermis).

The cause of Reiter's syndrome is unknown, but the tissue antigen HLA-B27 may play a permissive role. An attack may be precipitated by bacillary dysentery or *Mycoplasma* infection. Reiter's syndrome is associated with psoriasis and ankylosing spondylitis.

Neutropenia

Decreased numbers of circulating neutrophils may be associated with multifocal oral ulcers of varied size, containing necrotic debris in their craters. Neutropenia may result from primary hematologic disorders, sepsis, or cytotoxic suppression of the bone marrow with chemotherapeutic agents. Oral lesions are especially prominent after use of methotrexate. Other drugs associated with agranulocytosis include aminopyrine and chloramphenicol, which are seldom used today because of their established toxicity. Occasionally, neutropenia also follows administration of penicillin, barbiturates, sulfonamides, or cimetidine. The ulcers of neutropenia are not clinically distinguishable from other forms of punctate erosive stomatitis. Lesions usually appear when the leukocyte count falls below 2000 cells/mm^3.

Cyclic neutropenia is an uncommon childhood condition of unknown cause in which arthralgias, lymphadenitis, and periodic eruptions of gingival ulcers accompany a decrease in the number of granulocytes. Healing occurs when the leukocyte count returns to normal. However, the pattern is one of multiple exacerbations. Another oral manifestation of the impaired host defense is premature development of advanced periodontal disease.

Acute Necrotizing Ulcerative Gingivostomatitis

Acute necrotizing ulcerative gingivostomatitis (ANUG), also called trench mouth, Vincent's disease, and acute ulceromembranous gingivitis, is a severe form of gingivitis characterized by loss of the interdental papillae and free gingiva, leaving a gray pseudomembrane over a bleeding base. The papillae are characteristically blunted or "punched out." Uncommonly, the ulcers involve the palate and gingivobuccal fold. The clinical picture is virtually diagnostic; the cause is related to decreased host resistance and poor oral hygiene, which promote invasion of normally nonpathogenic, oral anaerobic fusiform bacteria and spirochetes (especially *Borrelia vincentii*). These factors were most likely present in the combat trenches of World War I, where the common term "trench mouth" originated. Microbiologic studies are not usually performed, but tissue smears may reveal fusiform and mobile spirochetes. The symptoms consist of fever, pain, foul breath, and metallic taste in the mouth.

Drug Reactions

Drugs can induce multiple small ulcers or large, irregular areas of mucosal destruction of varied depth. Drug-induced lesions may appear anywhere in the mouth, but they have a predilection for the buccal mucosa and gingiva. Ulcerative stomatitis produced by chemotherapeutic agents results from myelosuppression or from direct cytotoxic injury to the oral mucosa. Virtually any chemotherapeutic drug (e.g., antimetabolites, alkaloids, alkylating agents, antibiotics) can cause oral ulcers. Both herpes simplex and *Candida* have been isolated from such ulcers.

Other drugs associated with ulcerative stomatitis include salicylates, nonsteroidal anti-inflammatory agents, gold, and immunosuppressive agents. Among the latter, penicillamine, azathioprine, and cyclosporine are especially well known to produce erosive stomatitis.

Finally, captopril can cause tongue ulcers, and procainamide, penicillamine, and gold can produce the clinical picture of SLE.

Inflammatory Bowel Disease

Ulcerative colitis and Crohn's disease (regional enteritis) are inflammatory bowel conditions that may produce lesions anywhere along the alimentary tract from the mouth to the rectum. In Crohn's disease, inflammation is more severe and granulomas arise in the submucosal regions.

Oral manifestations precede intestinal symptoms in 60 per cent of patients with Crohn's disease. The lips, gingiva, and vestibular sulci are commonly the sites of small ulcers, ulcerated fissures, angular cheilitis, and hyperplasia. The latter lesions are termed pyostomatitis vegetans and are considered pathognomonic for inflammatory bowel disease. Remission of the oral lesions is induced by systemic and topical steroids. The most common sites of pyostomatitis vegetans are the gingiva, lips, and buccal mucosa. Typically, multiple pustules cover an area of hyperplastic mucosa.

The authors believe that oral lesions are more severe in Crohn's disease. By contrast, aphthouslike ulcers are the principal manifestation of ulcerative colitis. In both forms of inflammatory bowel disease, depapillated and erythematous areas of glossitis arise secondary to folic acid deficiency.

Contact Allergy

Dental restorations containing gold can induce mucosal changes ranging from erythema to ulceration. The slow release of gold salts may induce contact allergy. Lesions present adjacent to the restoration and this aids diagnosis; skin patch testing is not completely reliable. Healing occurs with removal of the restoration.

BULLOUS LESIONS

By definition, bullous lesions start with a preliminary bulla. In the moist oral environment, the bullae are transient. They rupture, leaving an irregular erythematous patch that forms a pseudomembrane centrally and fragments of sloughed epithelium at the margins. Bullous lesions tend to be multiple and may involve the lips. Bullous lesions are typically associated with dermatologic disorders (Table 5).

Erythema Multiforme

This common disorder is characterized by widespread irregular erythematous lesions of the skin and mouth. In some patients, oral lesions accompany skin manifestations. In others, oral lesions may be the only clue to the diagnosis. Multiple large areas of erosion with reddened margins and sloughing can be detected throughout the oral cavity. The erosions often coalesce to give the appearance that a caustic substance has been ingested. The lips may be covered by a fibrinous exudate.

Erythema multiforme is most common in young males but can appear at any age. The cause is unknown, but speculative links have been made to bacterial, viral, or fungal infection, malignancy, irradiation, autoimmune disease, allergy, and/or drug sensitivity. Prominent among the last group of causes is the use of sulfa drugs, which has been associated with a particularly severe, potentially fatal form of erythema multiforme, especially in combination with methotrexate.

Diagnosis typically requires the presence of diffuse oral and labial lesions and target lesions on the skin. Microscopically, degeneration of the entire epithelium, subepithelial clefting, and intense acute and chronic inflammation are prominent.

Stevens-Johnson syndrome (erythema multiforme pluriorificialis hemorrhagicum) is a disseminated disorder found in children, in young adults, and in persons with sensitivity to sulfa drugs. Bullous lesions cover the entire body, including the mucosa of the eye, mouth and genitourinary tract.

Pemphigus Vulgaris

Pemphigus vulgaris is an autoimmune disorder of skin and mucous membranes characterized by the formation of bullae of varied size. The mouth is almost invariably involved, with oral lesions often the first manifestation of

Table 5. Clinical Features of Bullous Stomatitis

Disease	Age/Sex	Bulla	Skin	Oral	Other Mucous Membranes	Gingiva	Lip	Immuno-fluorescence
Erythema multiforme	30/Male	Subepithelial	Occasional (target lesions)	100%	Rare (except Stevens-Johnson syndrome)	Absent	+ + + +	Cytoid bodies in dermis 40–50%
Pemphigus vulgaris	50/Equal	Intraepithelial	100%	80–90%	Pharynx, larynx, GU, anus, eye (+)	Desquamation + +	+ + +	IgG, IgA, IgM intraepithelial
Bullous pemphigoid	60/Equal	Subepithelial	100%	30–40%	Rare	Desquamation, erythema + +	+ +	IgG, C3 in basement membrane
Mucous membrane pemphigoid	60/Female	Subepithelial	10–30%	100%	Pharynx, larynx, GU, anus, nose, eye (+ + +)	Desquamation, erythema + + + +	+	IgG, C3 in basement membrane
Erosive lichen planus	30/Female	Subepithelial, ulcers	Variable	100%	Rare	Desquamation + +	+	Cytoid bodies in dermis 100%
Lupus erythematosus	30/Female	Subepithelial	Variable	25–40%	Rare	+	+	IgG in basement membrane, cytoid, bodies 40–50%

GU = genitourinary; C3 = complement; + = occasional involvement; + + = infrequent involvement; + + + = common involvement; + + + + = frequent involvement.

the disorder. However, the presence of a bulla in the oral cavity is transient; the most frequently observed lesion is a nonspecific erosion with fragments of surface epithelium present at its borders. Usually, multiple lesions are present, most commonly on the soft palate and buccal mucosa.

On occasion, pemphigus vulgaris may present as a desquamative gingivitis. It may also involve the oropharynx, hypopharynx, and larynx. The predominant symptom is pain. The disease is potentially fatal, with widespread skin ulcers progressing to sepsis. Even with high-dose steroid therapy, pemphigus is associated with significant morbidity and mortality (as high as 32 per cent). Pemphigus vulgaris has also been linked to the development of thymic neoplasms.

Under the microscope, clefting of the epithelium is noted above the stratum germinativum. The fluid-filled cleft contains acantholytic Tzanck cells, and the submucosa is variably inflamed. Biopsy diagnosis requires tissue removal from the margin of the lesion. However, epithelial loss and inflammatory infiltration alone may not yield a definitive diagnosis. Direct immunofluorescence demonstration of IgG, IgA, and IgM immune complexes in the intraepithelial layer confirms the diagnosis and differentiates pemphigus vulgaris from the other bullous disorders. In the active stage, tests for serum antibodies (indirect immunofluorescence) are positive in 95 per cent of patients; however, with remission, the titer is lower, or even normal. Consequently, indirect immunofluorescence may be used to monitor the effectiveness of drug therapy.

Bullous Pemphigoid

This condition resembles pemphigus vulgaris but has different features. Among these are (1) a decreased incidence of oral lesions; (2) the development of oral lesions after, rather than before, the appearance of skin lesions; (3) the nature of the oral lesions; and (4) the histologic picture. The mean age at onset is one decade later than for pemphigus vulgaris.

Most of the lesions are bullae, but vesicles may also occur. The distribution of lesions is similar to that in pemphigus vulgaris. The most common sites of pemphigoid in the mouth are the buccal mucosa (52 per cent), soft palate (40 per cent), tongue (24 per cent), lower lip (20 per cent), gingiva (16 per cent), upper lip (8 per cent), and floor of the mouth (8 per cent). However, of greater diagnostic importance is the more intense and widespread desquamative gingivitis in bullous pemphigoid.

Histologically, the bullae are subepithelial, and cleavage occurs at the epithelial–connective tissue junction. The epithelium is unremarkable, acantholysis is absent, and the submucosa is inflamed. Direct immunofluorescence confirms the diagnosis by revealing immune complexes binding IgG and the third component of complement (C3) in the epidermal basement membrane.

Mucous Membrane Pemphigoid

In this disorder, most lesions occur in the conjunctiva and oral cavity, but they can also arise in the nose, pharynx, esophagus, larynx, urogenital tract, rectum, and skin. Ocular involvement occurs in 10 to 62 per cent of patients. The lesions are vesiculobullous and often heal with scarring (hence the term cicatricial pemphigoid), except in the oral cavity. Adhesions commonly occur in the eye (symblepharon). The mean age at onset is 60 years, and the disease occurs two to three times more often in females. Mucous membrane pemphigoid typically is chronic, but it may undergo protracted intervals of remission.

Regional involvement occurs as follows: oral cavity (100 per cent), conjunctiva (50.8 per cent), genitalia (19.6 per cent), skin (8.9 per cent), nose (8 per cent), rectum (5.4 per cent), urethra (5.4 per cent), and esophagus (2.6 per cent). The most common sites of oral involvement, in descending order, are the gingiva (94 per cent), palate (32 per cent), buccal mucosa (29 per cent), floor of the mouth (5 per cent), and tongue (5 per cent). However, the authors have also seen lesions arising in the oropharynx and larynx, usually in conjunction with oral cavity involvement.

In mucous membrane pemphigoid, oral lesions are usually smaller and develop more slowly than in pemphigus vulgaris or bullous pemphigoid. Intense erythematous and desquamative gingivitis may also develop. Microscopy reveals subepithelial clefting of the mucosa, no acantholysis, and intense inflammatory infiltrate. Direct immunofluorescence shows deposition of immune complexes (IgG and C3) in the basement membrane. Although tissue studies may not differentiate mucous membrane pemphigoid from bullous pemphigoid, the clinical picture is helpful. The intense oral and ocular involvement and scarcity of skin lesions in mucous membrane pemphigoid differ from the extensive skin involvement and infrequent oral lesions seen with bullous pemphigoid.

Epidermolysis Bullosa

In this genetic dermatosis, cutaneous and oral mucosal subepidermal bullae appear in young individuals. The degree of severity of the disease is related to genetic penetrance. There are numerous variants of epidermolysis bullosa; however, they can be broadly subdivided into three categories, based on the level of tissue cleavage after trauma: the simplex form (epidermolytic); the junctional form (lamina lucidolytic); and the dystrophic form (dermolytic). The extent of oral involvement varies with type, ranging from small vesicles to large bullae. Numerous milia are also present in all three types. The entire oral cavity is at risk, with no preferential site of lesion formation. The recessive dystrophic type produces the most severe scarring, with vestibular stenosis, ankyloglossia, and microstoma often present.

Diagnosis is based on the distribution of the skin lesions (involvement of the skin over the joints of the extremities in the dystrophic form), presence of oral and cutaneous scarring, family history, and onset in childhood.

Erosive Lichen Planus

The erosive form of lichen planus has already been mentioned in the section on white lesions. The mean age at onset is 50 years, with a female and Caucasian preponderance. The sites of involvement include the buccal mucosa, tongue, gingiva, palate, lips, and floor of the mouth. Most patients complain of pain. Erosions typically arise from areas of atrophy in the keratotic plaques, which undergo desquamation. Rarely, actual bullae form. Microscopically, the epithelium is absent and the underlying connective tissue has mixed acute and chronic inflammation. Immunofluorescence reveals cytoid bodies, which are globular deposits of immunoglobulins in the papillary dermis, in more than 90 per cent of patients with lichen planus. Unfortunately, these bodies also occur in 40 to 50 per cent of patients with discoid lupus erythematosus, SLE, erythema multiform pemphigus, pemphigoid, and normal persons. Periodic re-examination of patients with lichen planus is required because a few patients develop squamous cell carcinoma.

Lupus Erythematosus

SLE is an autoimmune disorder with visceral involvement occurring primarily in young females. The term discoid lupus erythematosus denotes disease primarily of the skin, which has a better prognosis. Oral lesions occur in both forms, and in the absence of skin changes. The principal sites of occurrence are the buccal mucosa, labial mucosa, gingiva, and lips. The classic lesion is an erythematous patch having white striae radiating from the center. Microscopically, the picture is nonspecific and may be confused with lichen planus.

With SLE, the lesions can appear white, red, or bullous. The sites of occurrence, in descending order of frequency, are the hard palate, buccal mucosa, lips, and alveolar ridges. In half the patients, the lesions are multicentric. The bullae are fleeting; the typically observed lesions are erythematous patches with whitish fragments of sloughed epithelium either centrally or at the margins. SLE may also cause erythematous gingivitis and desquamative cheilitis.

Microscopically, hyperkeratosis, acanthosis, degeneration of the basal lamina, and subepithelial lymphocytic infiltrates are prominent. IgG is present in the basement membrane in 100 per cent of patients with SLE and in 73 per cent of those with the discoid form. IgM is likewise commonly found in this region. Because the clinical profile and histologic appearance of the lesions are nonspecific, diagnosis often requires a positive antinuclear antibody test and laboratory data that suggest multisystem disease.

Other Erosive Lesions

Mucous Patch

Secondary syphilis is usually accompanied by lymphadenopathy, a skin eruption, fever, malaise, and oral lesions. The latter may take the form of condylomata or mucous patches. The mucous patch typically appears on the buccal mucosa, tongue, and lips as a slightly elevated lesion with a grayish center, surrounded by a erythematous halo. Its appearance is nonspecific, and the diagnosis is confirmed by serology and by detecting spirochetes with darkfield microscopic examination of smears.

Drug-Induced Lesions

Various drugs may cause large, irregular ulcers of variable depth as a result of liquefaction necrosis of the oral mucosa. Drug-induced lesions can arise anywhere in the oral cavity but are most common on the buccal mucosa and gingiva.

Drugs can also induce acantholysis, producing a pemphiguslike clinical picture, by immunologic and nonimmunologic mechanisms. Culprits include anti-inflammatory agents used for rheumatoid disorders (penicillamine, pyritinol, tiopronin, gold), antihypertensives (captopril, beta-blockers), antibiotics (rifampin, penicillin, cephalexin), barbiturates, and hormones (progesterone). A common chemical feature shared by many of these drugs is the presence of sulfhydryl groups. The lesions are usually cutaneous, with the oral cavity rarely involved.

ACUTE PHARYNGITIS

By Burke A. Cunha, M.D.
Mineola, New York

The major task for the clinician faced with acute pharyngitis is to differentiate viral from group A streptococcal pharyngitis. This task is complicated by the fact that many patients with viral pharyngitis are colonized by group A streptococci. Thus, the clinician must distinguish among viral pharyngitis, group A streptococcal colonization, and group A streptococcal pharyngitis. Acute pharyngitis may also be caused by microbes other than viruses and group A streptococci. Non–group A streptococci uncommonly cause acute pharyngitis and are not reported from throat cultures unless specifically requested. Pharyngitis caused by these non–group A streptococci is observed most commonly in patients with recurring pharyngitis or in health care workers. Gonococcal pharyngitis may occur in young adults with appropriate sexual histories. To make this diagnosis, the clinician must specifically request that the laboratory attempt to culture *Neisseria gonorrhoeae*.

An important and frequently overlooked cause of acute pharyngitis is *Mycoplasma pneumoniae.* This organism often causes systemic illness associated with pharyngitis, with or without pneumonia. The clinician must consider *M. pneumoniae* pharyngitis in patients who are negative for group A streptococci. The acute pharyngitides caused by *Candida*, herpes simplex, or coxsackievirus A are characteristic, and the diagnosis is made clinically or by culture. The important viruses that cause acute pharyngitis include adenovirus, enterovirus, cytomegalovirus, and Epstein-Barr virus (EBV). Microbes cultured from the throat that colonize the oropharynx but do not cause pharyngitis include anaerobes, *Staphylococcus aureus, Streptococcus pneumoniae, Haemophilus influenzae,* and *Haemophilus parainfluenzae.* Recovery of these organisms from a patient with acute pharyngitis should not lead the clinician to ascribe the illness to them. To avoid unnecessary antibiotic therapy, it must be understood that colonization frequently accompanies viral pharyngitis. Finally, some microbes, such as *Neisseria meningitidis, Arcanobacterium haemolyticus* (formerly *Corynebacterium haemolyticum*), *Francisella tularensis,* measles, rubella, *C. pneumoniae, Toxoplasma gondii,* and *Coxiella burnetii,* typically cause pharyngitis as part of a systemic illness (Table 1).

STREPTOCOCCAL PHARYNGITIS VERSUS COLONIZATION

Group A streptococcal pharyngitis usually occurs in children between 5 and 15 years of age but may occur uncommonly in adults until age 30. Streptococcal pharyngitis is most prevalent between February and April but may occur at any time of the year. Pharyngitis due to group A streptococci is typically associated with peripheral leukocytosis, headache, cough, fever, sore throat, and anterior cervical adenopathy.

Unfortunately, the same signs and symptoms may occur with pharyngitis caused by other microbes. Up to 20 per cent of children and young adults may be colonized by group A beta-hemolytic streptococci. The rate of colonization is even higher during the winter and in patients with viral pharyngitis. Thirty per cent of patients with EBV infectious mononucleosis may have pharyngeal carriage of group A streptococci. If these normal throat commensals are not recognized as colonizers, clinicians may treat the patient unnecessarily with beta-lactam antibiotics, which not infrequently cause an erythematous rash.

Thus, it is clinically important to differentiate viral pharyngitis colonized with group A streptococci from bacterial pharyngitis caused by group A streptococci. In both situations, rapid streptococcal antigen agglutination assays and throat cultures are positive. The best way of distinguishing

Table 1. Oropharyngeal Microorganisms

Colonizing Organisms	Pharyngitis as Part of Systemic Infectious Disease	Pathogens in Acute Pharyngitis
Group A, B, C, and G streptococci	Epstein-Barr virus	Group A, B, C, and G streptococci
Oral anaerobes	Cytomegalovirus	Adenovirus
Streptococcus pneumoniae	*Mycoplasma pneumoniae*	Respiratory viruses
Haemophilus influenzae	*Chlamydia pneumoniae*	*Candida albicans*
Haemophilus parainfluenzae	*Franciscella tularensis*	Herpes simplex
Staphylococcus aureus	Enteroviruses	*Neisseria gonorrhoeae*
	Influenza A and B	*Corynebacterium diphtheriae*
	Rubella	*Corynebacterium haemolyticum*
	Measles	
	Toxoplasma gondii	
	Coxiella burnetii	
	Bordetella pertussis	

streptococcal colonization from infection is to perform a Gram stain of pharyngeal exudate. This is not done to detect bacteria or to identify their type by morphology. Rather, the Gram stain facilitates proper interpretation of the results of throat culture. If the group A streptococci that grow on the culture show few organisms and few neutrophils with Gram staining, then colonization is more likely than infection. In contrast, in a patient with group A streptococcal pharyngeal infection and positive throat culture for group A streptococci, the Gram stain reveals cellular debris and abundant neutrophils, suggesting active mucosal invasion (Table 2).

PERTUSSIS

Pertussis should be considered in adults with chronic, nonproductive cough and lymphocytosis. No other infection produces such intense lymphocytosis, which may exceed 60 per cent of the differential count.

Bordetella is transmitted by airborne droplets, and pertussis is extremely contagious. Signs and symptoms of the first ("catarrhal") phase appear after an incubation period of 1 to 3 weeks; the patient may feel listless and have tearing eyes, sneezing, and a hacking cough at night. Except for lymphocytosis, the syndrome may resemble mycoplasmal pneumonia and other common respiratory infections. Signs that may distinguish pertussis from upper respiratory infection include conjunctival injection, which rarely accompanies mild viral illness, and periorbital or eyelid edema. Children may have lacerations of the lingual frenulum and epistaxis from violent paroxysms of coughing. Both adult and pediatric patients with pertussis tend to appear relatively healthy throughout the illness and usually have little pharyngitis or fever.

The cough typically worsens gradually over 1 to 2 weeks during the catarrhal phase until it becomes diurnal and paroxysmal. The characteristic staccato cough is quite distinct from the dry cough of mycoplasmal pneumonia and most viral illnesses. Coughing paroxysms are precipitated by drinking, eating, exercising, sneezing, or yawning. During the paroxysmal stage of pertussis, the patient neither feels nor looks sick between coughing attacks.

A clinical diagnosis may be made with confidence during epidemics and in patients with full-blown manifestations of pertussis (Table 3). If necessary, culture confirms the

Table 2. Streptococcal Colonization Versus Infection

Clinical Parameters	Clinical Situation: *Colonization*	Clinical Situation: *Infection*
Laboratory		
Throat culture positive for group A streptococcus	+	+
Rapid streptococcal tests	±	+
↑ ASO titer	−	+
↑ WBC	−	±
Gram stain of throat		
PMNs	−	+
mononuclear cells	+	−
cellular debris	−	+
Physical Examination		
Exudative pharyngitis	−	+
EBV pharyngitis	−	+
Anterior cervical adenopathy	−	−
Postcervical adenopathy (if + consider EBV, CMV, etc.)	−	−
Therapy		
Clinical response to beta-lactam antibiotics	−	+

ASO = antistreptolysin; WBC = leukocyte count; PMNs = polymorphonuclear neutrophils; EBV = Epstein-Barr virus; CMV = cytomegalovirus; + = present; ± may be present or absent; − = absent.

Adapted from Cunha, B.A.: Group A streptococcal pharyngitis versus colonization. Intern. Med., 15:18–19, 1994.

Table 3. Clinical Features of Pertussis

Clinical Stages	Length	Indications/Symptoms
Incubation	6–21 days (usually 7)	Exposure by epidemic or household contact
Catarrhal	7–14 days	Runny nose and lacrimation Nocturnal cough Malaise and lassitude Sneezing Conjunctival injection Periorbital/eyelid edema Frenulum laceration (in children) Epistaxis (in children)
Paroxysmal	About 14 days	Diurnal spasms of hacking whooping cough followed by vomiting Persistence of symptoms "Shaggy heart sign" (in children)
Convalescent	After 14 days	Gradual decrease in frequency and intensity of cough and other symptoms

Adapted from Cunha, B.A.: Pertussis. Emerg. Med., 26:123–124, 1994.

diagnosis. Dacron-tipped calcium alginate swabs rather than cotton swabs should be used to obtain culture material. Rapid plating on Bordet-Gengou or Regan-Lowe agar increases accuracy of results. Early identification of pertussis can also be made with direct fluorescent antibody testing of oral pharyngeal secretions.

DIPHTHERIA

Corynebacterium diphtheriae causes the various upper respiratory tract manifestations of diphtheria, including acute pharyngeal or faucial inflammation. The posterior oropharynx is frequently involved, and the temperature is typically low grade (<39°C [102°F]) in this toxin-mediated disease. Membrane formation is characteristic of diphtheria, usually involves both tonsillar pillars, and may extend to the uvula or soft palate. The dark gray to black membrane is adherent and may bleed when scraped. Early in the disease process, the membrane is shiny and lighter in color. As the disease progresses, so does the extent of the membrane. In full-blown diphtheria, neck swelling (bull neck) may be accompanied by stridor and respiratory difficulty. The diagnosis of diphtheria is suggested by membranous pharyngitis, especially in the presence of a serosanguineous nasal discharge (i.e., nasal diphtheria). The leukocyte count is increased, but the differential count is nondiagnostic. Swabs of the membrane should be plated on Loeffler or tellurite medium, because *C. diphtheriae* does not grow on conventional blood agar plates. Methylene blue–stained smears of the exudate may reveal the typical club-shaped, pleomorphic gram-positive bacilli.

Arcanobacterium haemolyticus (formerly *C. haemolyticum*), in contrast to *C. diphtheriae,* presents as a scarlatiniform rash and is more likely to be confused with scarlet fever than with pharyngeal diphtheria. *Arcanobacterium haemolyticus is* easily cultured on human blood but not on sheep blood agar and grows best at 35 to 38°C (95 to 100°F).

OTHER COMMON CAUSES OF PHARYNGITIS

Candidal pharyngitis is characterized by white patches on the tongue and pharynx that adhere to the mucosa and may bleed when scraped. A Gram stain of the lesion reveals typical gram-positive, large candidal organisms. A KOH preparation is not required because there is no cellular debris to be dissolved by the KOH in patients with pharyngitis. Candidal esophagitis is common in alcoholics, children, diabetics, patients with acquired immunodeficiency syndrome, and patients receiving antibiotics or steroids.

Herpetic gingivostomatitis is frequently accompanied by a sore throat. The herpetic lesions are extremely painful, are characteristically located in the anterior oropharynx, and may involve the tongue and lips. The gums are hemorrhagic and there is no halitosis, in contrast to patients with Vincent's angina (trench mouth).

In contrast to herpetic gingivostomatitis, the ulcers of herpangina are located primarily in the posterior oropharynx. Herpangina is not associated with gingival involvement and is caused by coxsackievirus A.

DIAGNOSTIC CONSIDERATIONS

Because group A streptococcal pharyngitis is treatable but viral pharyngitis is not, the clinician must distinguish between group A streptococcal colonization superimposed on a viral process and group A streptococcal pharyngitis. This is most easily achieved by throat culture plus Gram stain of the pharyngeal exudate plus acute and convalescent anti–streptolysin O titers. Viruses are the most common cause of acute pharyngitis, but other treatable causes such as *Mycoplasma* should be considered. Pharyngitis occurring as part of systemic infection is typically not the predominant problem on clinical presentation. Pertussis and diphtheria are uncommon but important causes of pharyngitis that can be treated with antibiotics. Accurate diagnosis of the cause of acute pharyngitis is essential for providing effective therapy to patients with treatable disorders and for avoiding needless and potentially harmful antibiotic therapy in those who are only colonized or who have viral pharyngitis.

TUMORS OF THE PHARYNX AND LARYNX

By Christina Finlayson, M.D.,
and John A. Ridge, M.D., Ph.D.
Philadelphia, Pennsylvania

Tumors of the pharynx and larynx are uncommon and may go unrecognized on initial presentation. Frequently, progression of disease is documented while the patient is under medical care. Such delay in diagnosis contributes to the poor prognosis of patients with these tumors. A high index of suspicion plus skill in physical examination enhances the likelihood of timely identification of these potentially curable cancers.

Pharyngeal and laryngeal tumors arise from the epithelial lining of the head and neck, and 90 per cent are squamous cell cancers. Their incidence correlates strongly with environmental exposure, primarily to tobacco and alcohol. Consequently, a patient who presents with cancer of the pharynx or larynx must be evaluated for synchronous lesions and undergo lifetime surveillance for the detection of metachronous tumors. Physical examination is the mainstay of this diagnostic approach.

ANATOMY

The anatomy of the pharynx is shown in Figure 1.

Nasopharynx

The nasopharynx can be entered anteriorly from the nasal cavity or inferiorly from the oropharynx. The superior border is the base of the skull. The lateral and posterior pharyngeal walls are composed of pharyngeal constrictors. Posteriorly, the pharyngeal wall overlies the first and second cervical vertebrae. The eustachian tubes open into the lateral walls. The soft palate divides the inferior nasopharynx from the superior oropharynx.

Oropharynx

The opening to the oropharynx is a ring bounded by the anterior tonsillar pillar (faucial arch) that extends upward to blend with the uvula and medially across the base of the tongue behind the circumvallate papillae. The walls of the oropharynx are formed by the pharyngeal constrictor muscles, which overlie the cervical spine posteriorly. The superior boundary is the soft palate, which separates the oropharynx from the nasopharynx. Inferiorly, the oropharynx is separated conceptually from the hypopharynx (laryngopharynx) at the level of the epiglottis.

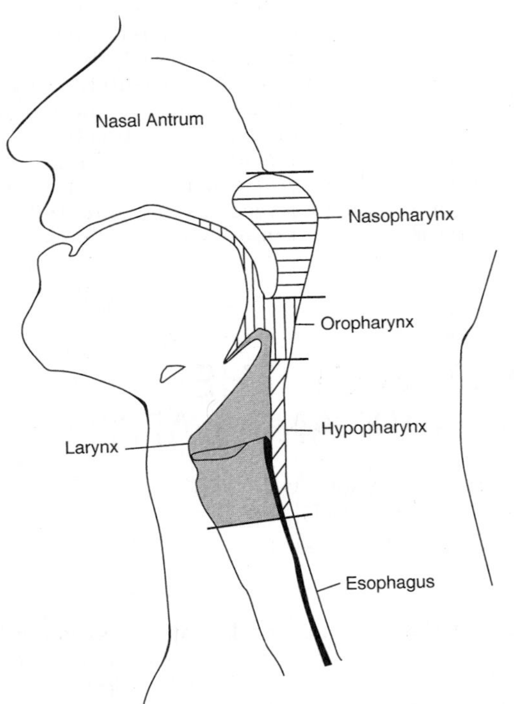

Figure 1. Anatomy of the pharynx and larynx indicating the boundaries of each site.

Hypopharynx

The hypopharynx (or laryngopharynx) is the entrance to the esophagus. The superior border is in the plane of the hyoid bone, and the inferior border is in the plane of the lowest part of the cricoid cartilage. The anterior surface (postcricoid area) is contiguous with the posterior surface of the larynx. The pharyngeal musculature forms the lateral and posterior walls. Included within its confines are the pyriform sinuses.

Larynx

The larynx is divided into three areas: supraglottis, glottis, and subglottis. The supraglottic larynx includes both the lingual and the laryngeal sides of the epiglottis, the arytenoids and the aryepiglottic folds, and the ventricular bands (false cords). The glottic larynx begins at the laryngeal side of the ventricles and extends 1 cm inferiorly to encompass the true vocal cords. The subglottis is the region below the glottis and behind the cricoid.

PHYSICAL DIAGNOSIS

Visual inspection and manual palpation are the basis of the head and neck examination. Seat the patient in a relaxed and comfortable position in front of the examiner. Assess external symmetry and color. Evaluate the cranial nerves. Inspect the anterior nasal antrum and the oral cavity after dentures and bridges have been removed. Palpate bimanually the oral cavity and pharynx for masses of the cheek, floor of the mouth, hard and soft palate, and base of the tongue. Examine the larynx by mirror or pharyngolaryngoscope; the mirror, which affords a wider field of view, is preferred. Examine the piriform sinuses, tongue base, pharyngeal walls, epiglottis, and arytenoids as well as the true and false vocal cords, assessing movement and contour. Finally, because the lymphatic drainage patterns are predictable with head and neck cancer, palpate the cervical and supraclavicular lymph nodes.

This comprehensive and systematic approach to examination of the head and neck will identify most tumors in this region and should be employed in its entirety when evaluating symptomatic patients and screening asymptomatic individuals.

NASOPHARYNX

The open cavity of the nasopharynx is difficult to see, and a tumor can grow to large size with very few symptoms. Although squamous cell carcinoma is still the predominant tumor of the nasopharynx, lymphoma comprises 10 per cent of the presenting tumors. In children, the most common tumor is rhabdomyosarcoma.

Presenting Signs and Symptoms

The local effects of a nasopharyngeal tumor include a "stuffy" nose, bleeding, or a "sinus" headache. A tumor that arises on the lateral wall may occlude the opening of the eustachian tube and cause unilateral serous otitis media. Most patients present with symptoms related to the local spread or regional metastasis of these tumors. Invasion of the base of the skull can extend into the middle cranial fossa and involve cranial nerves III, IV, V, and VI. Extension into the parapharyngeal space may affect cranial nerves IX, X, XI, and XII, the structures of the carotid sheath, and the sympathetic chain. Anteriorly, a tumor can penetrate the cribriform plate and involve the olfactory and optic nerves. It may also involve the maxillary antrum or posterior orbit. Submucosal infiltration may extend into the oropharynx or posteriorly into the cervical vertebrae.

The rich lymphatic network of the nasopharyngeal mucosa explains the predilection of tumors in this location to lymphatic spread. It is not uncommon for the first presentation to be a mass in the neck. Particularly suspicious for a nasopharyngeal tumor is an enlarged lymph node in the posterior triangle. Because the nasopharynx is a midline structure, lymph node metastases often occur bilaterally.

Diagnostic Procedures

Among the historical clues that suggest nasopharyngeal tumor is the ethnic background of the patient. The highest incidence of nasopharyngeal cancers occurs in southeast Asia. First-generation immigrants from this area remain at high risk, but future generations have a risk similar to that of others in their new environment. Such nasopharyngeal carcinoma is associated with Epstein-Barr virus infection.

Physical examination of the head and neck must include a detailed examination of the cranial nerves and all mucosal surfaces. The nasopharynx is difficult to examine with a mirror; a flexible or rigid nasopharyngoscope facilitates inspection and biopsy. If an occult primary is suspected on the basis of an involved cervical lymph node, directed biopsies of what may appear to be normal tissue are indicated.

The most useful radiographic evaluation is a computed tomography (CT) scan. An appropriately performed scan extends from the middle cranial fossa to the thoracic inlet, and an intravenous contrast agent should be used if there are no absolute contraindications. Computed tomography with contrast helps characterize local extension into the surrounding bone, soft tissues, or the airway. Plain films or conventional tomograms are not required, because positive findings prompt further evaluation with CT scanning.

Serologic tests are available to detect the antibody to Epstein-Barr virus as a tumor marker, but specificity is low.

OROPHARYNX

Because the area bounded by the oropharynx is relatively insensitive to pain and mass effect, a tumor may grow to a relatively large size before it interferes with swallowing or speech. Hence, cancers in this region often present or are detected at an advanced stage.

Presenting Signs and Symptoms

Tumors of the oropharynx often present with a mass in the neck, representing metastatic disease to the cervical lymph nodes. Careful questioning may reveal a history of earlier, more subtle, warning signs indicative of malignancy. Unilateral otalgia with visibly unremarkable tympanic membranes should alert the clinician to look for malignancy of the oropharynx. A persistent sore throat, often unilateral, is also a frequent complaint. Difficulty with phonation, or "hot potato" voice, suggests a more advanced tumor with deep infiltration into the base of the tongue. Other symptoms include dysphagia, pain with acid foods, malodorous breath, bleeding, and weight loss from difficulty in eating. An asymmetric enlargement of one tonsil, particularly in a young person, should be considered suspicious for lymphoma.

Tumors of the lateral and posterior walls often present as multiple ulcerations with areas of unremarkable mucosa intervening. These cancers are actually infiltrating in the submucosa and the entire field should be considered one tumor. Aphthous and herpetic ulcers rarely persist longer than 10 days in an immunocompetent individual. Therefore, any ulcerated lesion present longer than 2 weeks must be evaluated with biopsy.

Natural History

Tumors beginning in the tonsillar space infiltrate inferiorly to involve the tongue and its base and superiorly across the soft palate toward the uvula. If left to grow unchecked, they can extend across the midline to involve the opposite tonsillar pillar.

There are no barriers to growth within the tongue; therefore, tumors arising from the base of the tongue infiltrate anteriorly throughout the tongue musculature and deeply into the root of the tongue or posteriorly toward the epiglottis.

Tumors arising from the lateral or posterior pharyngeal wall tend to spread superiorly and inferiorly and can infiltrate deeply. Deep infiltration of the posterior wall abuts the cervical spine, and potential fixation of tumor mass in this area must be assessed.

Initial lymph node drainage is predictably to levels II and III in the cervical chain and is often bilateral.

Diagnostic Procedures

The value of physical examination with direct inspection cannot be overemphasized. Most of the oropharynx can be seen directly or with a mirror and headlamp. Endoscopy should be used to better examine the base of the tongue and the vallecula. In addition, the base of the tongue and tonsils should be palpated for masses or areas of tenderness. The patient should be warned that she or he may gag and asked not to bite. If the patient is uncooperative or it is impossible to obtain a good view in the office, an examination with anesthesia is required.

Tumors of the oropharynx, particularly at the base of the tongue, have the highest incidence of associated second primary malignancies. Panendoscopy should be employed to search for these lesions at the time of diagnosis and during follow-up. If there are no pulmonary symptoms and chest films are unremarkable, the yield from bronchoscopy is quite low and it need not be performed.

Radiographic evaluation of the oropharynx rarely reveals a lesion not seen on physical examination; it more often discloses the extent of infiltration and provides staging information for the primary tumor. CT with contrast or magnetic resonance imaging (MRI) aids evaluation of deep structures not accessible by observation or palpation. The technique of choice depends on local expertise. Other imaging modalities are not helpful but posteroanterior and lateral chest films should be obtained for staging.

There are no laboratory tests specific for the screening, diagnosis, or follow-up of tumors of the oropharynx.

HYPOPHARYNX

The hypopharynx lies at the inlet to the esophagus. Tumors here can enlarge with minimal symptoms; they are rarely detected at an early stage.

Presenting Signs and Symptoms

Although at least half of patients with hypopharyngeal cancer present with a cervical mass, a few have symptoms specific to the site of the primary tumor. Piriform sinus tumors are characterized by unilateral otalgia. Any patient with persistent pain in the ear and a normal otic examination requires thorough evaluation of the upper aerodigestive tract. Dysphagia, odynophagia, hemoptysis, cough, hoarseness, a globus sensation, or weight loss may be reported, depending on the size of the lesion. Tumors of the hypopharynx are associated with heavy smoking and drinking. Consequently, early symptoms are often ignored by the patient or attributed to environmental irritants. Any symptom that persists for longer than 2 weeks needs evaluation.

Natural History

The hypopharynx has a rich lymphatic network, and early metastasis to the cervical lymph nodes is the rule rather than the exception. All lymph node levels of the neck are at risk, especially levels II and III. Adjoining structures such as the larynx are at risk for local invasion. Lesions of the posterior pharyngeal wall can spread inferiorly in the submucosa to form "skip" lesions in the esophagus. The true extent of hypopharyngeal tumors is often underestimated during initial evaluation.

Diagnostic Procedures

Again, the mainstay of diagnosis is the visual examination afforded by either indirect or fiberoptic laryngoscopy. However, examination under anesthesia may be required. Obviously inadequate is the "flashlight and tongue blade" examination, which illuminates only the oral cavity. All folds and depressions must be examined and appropriate biopsies obtained.

No radiographic or laboratory tests are available to aid the diagnosis of a hypopharyngeal tumor. Contrast swallows or esophagrams are often performed, but they provide less information than do "cross-sectional" images. After a tumor has been identified, CT or MRI can delineate the degree of local extension and the possibility of metastases to cervical lymph nodes.

LARYNX

Interference with the intricate functional anatomy of the larynx usually produces symptoms that herald a tumor in this region. Tumors involving different parts of the larynx may have distinct presentations.

Presenting Signs and Symptoms

Tumors of the supraglottic larynx may become rather large before they cause significant problems. As with pharyngeal tumors, a mass in the neck is often the presenting sign. However, earlier signs include pain at the tumor site, unilateral otalgia, dysphagia, odynophagia, bleeding, or repetitive aspiration of liquids. Hoarseness is usually a late sign of supraglottic tumors.

In contrast to tumors at other sites that have been discussed, a tumor of the glottis is often diagnosed at an early stage. Even small lesions on the true vocal cords can cause significant changes in the voice and present as hoarseness. However, hoarseness is often ignored because many of the affected patients are smokers. Any voice change that persists longer than 2 weeks warrants examination and consideration for biopsy. Neglected tumors produce local invasion and destruction of the laryngeal cartilage. Because of the relative lack of lymphatics in the vocal cords themselves, cervical metastases are a late sign of advanced disease.

Tumors arising in the subglottis cause few early symptoms. Advanced cancer may present with airway obstruction. Fortunately, these tumors are very uncommon.

Diagnostic Procedures

Again, the best tool for diagnosis is a careful physical examination. Direct inspection with early biopsy is imperative. Computed tomography or MRI aids further staging, but these techniques may not detect small primary tumors.

There is no laboratory evaluation specific to tumors of the larynx.

Section Four

RESPIRATORY SYSTEM

CHRONIC OBSTRUCTIVE PULMONARY DISEASE

By Barbara M. Leighton, M.D.,
and Gregory C. Kane, M.D.
Philadelphia, Pennsylvania

Chronic obstructive pulmonary disease (COPD) is a broad term used to describe a group of respiratory diseases characterized by chronic airflow obstruction. These diseases include chronic bronchitis, emphysema, and asthmatic bronchitis. Asthma (see article on asthma) is a distinct disorder characterized by episodic reversible airflow obstruction, typically in patients who have not had significant exposure to tobacco products. Affecting an estimated 15 million people, COPD is the fifth leading cause of death in the United States. The mortality rate 10 years after the diagnosis is greater than 50 per cent.

Other terms used to describe COPD include chronic obstructive lung disease, obstructive lung disease, obstructive airway disease, chronic bronchitis, and emphysema. The last two terms really represent distinct disorders that make up COPD. Only a minority of patients have pure chronic bronchitis or emphysema. Most patients have a disorder that includes features of both diseases. Therefore, the term COPD is used most widely. The terms "blue bloater" and "pink puffer" were used in the past to describe chronic bronchitis and emphysema, respectively. Their use is now discouraged, but the concepts can be helpful in understanding these disorders.

Chronic bronchitis is defined as the presence of cough productive of mucopurulent sputum during 3 months of the year for 2 consecutive years, after other causes of chronic sputum production have been excluded. Emphysema, on the other hand, is a pathologic entity, although its clinical and laboratory characteristics are easily recognized, making biopsy unnecessary for diagnosis. Emphysema is defined by abnormal permanent enlargement of air spaces distal to the terminal bronchioles, accompanied by destruction of alveolar walls, without obvious fibrosis. Most patients with COPD have features of both chronic bronchitis and emphysema.

Asthmatic bronchitis is an overlapping condition between asthma and COPD. Patients with asthmatic bronchitis may be heavy smokers with chronic productive cough who have a history of childhood asthma. They may have an illness with features of chronic bronchitis combined with reversible airflow obstruction. Other patients may be lifelong nonsmokers with chronic asthma that leads to irreversible airflow obstruction over many years. It is important to recognize these patients because their treatment differs from the treatment of those with COPD.

PRESENTING SIGNS AND SYMPTOMS

The earliest symptom of chronic bronchitis is usually a productive cough, which may begin insidiously in the chronic smoker or may be first recognized after a viral upper respiratory tract infection. Sputum is usually mucopurulent and either yellow, green, tan, or brown. In some patients with advanced disease, sputum may be quite thick, leading to difficulty with expectoration and occasional violent paroxysms of cough. Other associated symptoms include exertional breathlessness, chest tightness or discomfort, and wheezing. Symptoms are usually worse after a cold or exposure to respiratory irritants, and scant hemoptysis may occur under these circumstances. Nocturnal worsening of symptoms is rare in COPD unless the patient has a history of allergies or asthmatic features, making asthmatic bronchitis a better descriptive term for such patients. The insidious onset of exertional dyspnea is the most common symptom of emphysema, although some patients can report a specific time for the onset of breathlessness. These patients tend to adjust their activity level rather than to take note of symptoms. Sedentary individuals are usually not aware of any limitation until they are unable to do simple daily tasks. Patients may date the onset of symptoms to a "cold that never cleared," because viral upper respiratory tract infections can initiate early symptoms. Patients with emphysema may have varying degrees of sputum, chest tightness, or wheezing. Because most patients with COPD have features of both chronic bronchitis and emphysema, combinations of the above symptoms are frequently observed.

HISTORY

A thorough history can give clues to the cause of COPD and can help the physician assess the patient's functional limitations. Of course, presenting symptoms should be carefully described as above. A thorough history of the use of tobacco products is essential and should include the type of tobacco (pipe, cigar, or cigarette), total duration of use, and information regarding current use or the time interval since quitting. Pack years (packs of cigarettes per day times total years smoked) serves as the best means of recording this information for cigarette smokers. For current smokers, this history can serve as a platform for launching a discussion of smoking cessation. Other factors may contribute to the development of COPD; therefore, questions of exposure to pollutants, drug use, early childhood infections, and family history are also important. Moreover, because tobacco smoke is also a risk factor for cardiac disease, detailed questions about heart disease, including chest pain, palpitations, claudication, and orthopnea, help in differential diagnosis.

PHYSICAL EXAMINATION

Physical examination may yield several clues helpful in the diagnosis of COPD. General appearance may be particularly striking. Chronic bronchitis patients may be overweight and cyanotic with lower extremity edema when disease is advanced. Emphysema patients tend to be thin, especially those with more severe disease, but this may be obscured by the presence of a barrel chest. Patients with advanced illness may have callus formation over their elbows, sometimes referred to as "thinker's sign," as a result of supporting the thorax and aiding the mechanical function of the respiratory muscles. Patients may breathe through pursed lips, a technique that can improve airflow obstruction by preventing airway collapse. Auscultation of the chest demonstrates decreased breath sounds with occasional wheezing and a prolonged expiratory phase. A right ventricular heave, an increased pulmonic component of the second heart sound, and dependent edema suggest cor pulmonale, a late complication resulting from hypoxemia. Digits may be cyanotic, but clubbing is usually absent.

During exacerbations, use of accessory muscles is often prominent. Wheezing may be increased but can disappear if airway obstruction markedly decreases airflow. Sinus tachycardia or atrial tachyarrhythmias are invariably present, especially during severe exacerbations. Pulsus paradoxus, cyanosis, or paradoxical abdominal muscle excursion may signify a severe exacerbation and alert the physician to impending respiratory failure.

PULMONARY FUNCTION TESTS

Pulmonary function tests are an essential component of the evaluation of patients with suspected COPD (Table 1). Usually, only spirometry is needed, but measurements of lung volumes and diffusion capacity can be helpful in more complicated cases. The most important variables determined by spirometry are the 1-second forced expired volume (FEV_1), the forced vital capacity (FVC), and the FEV_1/FVC ratio. By definition, obstructive lung disease reduces the FEV_1/FVC ratio below 70 per cent of predicted normal. After obstruction is present, the FEV_1 alone is a better index of severity. An absolute FEV_1 of less than 0.8 to 1.0 L (or 40 per cent of the predicted normal value) indicates advanced illness. A flow volume loop is helpful if an upper airway obstruction is suspected. Administration of a bronchodilator usually produces no significant change in spirometry results, although some patients with COPD show a reversible component, demonstrated by a 10 to 15 per cent improvement in absolute FEV_1. The lack of response to bronchodilators in the laboratory does not mean that a clinical benefit will not occur with these medications.

Lung volumes show hyperinflation and air trapping, with an elevated total lung capacity, functional residual capacity, and residual volume. Measurement of lung volumes is important if spirometry shows a low FVC in order to rule out a coexisting restrictive process. The single-breath carbon monoxide diffusion capacity (DLCO) is decreased in emphysema, a sign attributable to the loss of alveolar surface area for gas exchange. This measurement may help differentiate asthma from COPD, because the DLCO is usually preserved in asthma.

Table 1. Typical Pulmonary Function Changes in COPD

Baseline	After Bronchodilation
FEV_1 reduced	Unchanged or improved†
FVC normal or reduced	Unchanged or improved†
FEV_1/FVC reduced (less than 70%)	
TLC normal or increased*	
DLCO reduced	

*May be reduced in patients with large, poorly communicating bullae.

†Some patients with COPD have improvement of greater than 10–15 per cent.

FEV_1 = one-second forced expiratory volume; FVC = forced vital capacity; FEV_1/FVC = ratio between these measurements; TLC = total lung capacity; DLCO = carbon monoxide diffusing capacity.

EXERCISE TESTING

Exercise testing is required in selected patients to evaluate the degree to which a patient's poor lung function contributes to functional impairment. It can also help determine the effect of therapy. In the cardiopulmonary exercise test, a patient exercises on either a bicycle or a treadmill while having cardiac and ventilatory parameters continuously monitored. This sophisticated test can help determine whether the patient's dyspnea is caused by underlying heart disease, pulmonary disease, or another condition. In patients unable to exercise, a 12-minute walk test may be just as helpful in determining the degree of limitation or the response to therapy.

RADIOLOGIC STUDIES

Routine posteroanterior and lateral chest films should be obtained on all new patients undergoing evaluation for dyspnea. Several findings can suggest the presence of obstructive lung disease. Emphysema typically shows a low, flat diaphragm, increased retrosternal air space, a paucity of vascular markings, and perhaps the presence of bullae. Chronic bronchitis may show a diffuse increase in lung markings with thickened bronchial walls—so-called "dirty lungs." An increase in pulmonary artery size or an enlarged right heart suggests cor pulmonale. None of these findings is diagnostic. The greatest benefit of obtaining the chest film is for ruling out other conditions that may also cause symptoms of cough and dyspnea, such as neoplasm, pneumonia, tuberculosis, and heart disease.

Computed tomography (CT) scans have been used to help determine the severity of emphysema, especially now that high-resolution images are readily available. Patchy attenuation of lung parenchyma due to air space enlargement and bullae can be seen. Despite the remarkable resolution of these scans, they add little to the evaluation in uncomplicated cases. Such studies are useful if a coexistent interstitial process, such as usual interstitial pneumonitis or asbestosis, is suspected.

Magnetic resonance imaging (MRI) has not been helpful in the diagnosis of COPD. Although radioisotope ventilation-perfusion scanning is not indicated in COPD, certain findings are typical. The ventilation scan usually shows prolonged washout of radiolabeled gas consistent with air trapping, and bullae show an absence of uptake on the perfusion portion of the scan. An echocardiogram is useful if pulmonary hypertension or left ventricular dysfunction is suspected. On occasion, the transthoracic echocardiogram may not yield satisfactory images in patients with hyperinflated lungs. In these patients, a transesophageal echocardiogram may be performed.

LABORATORY EVALUATION

A complete blood count and electrolyte determination should be done on every patient. Anemia must be ruled out as a cause or contributing factor to explain breathlessness. Conversely, polycythemia secondary to severe COPD and hypoxemia may suggest the need for supplemental oxygen or phlebotomy. Electrolytes may show hypokalemia due to treatment with diuretics or beta-adrenergic agonists. An increased bicarbonate concentration may indicate compensation for hypercapnia in patients with chronic respiratory acidosis. Sputum evaluation is not helpful unless the patient is suffering from an upper respiratory infection.

ARTERIAL BLOOD GASES

It is helpful in more severe pulmonary disease to examine arterial blood gases. The results help determine whether the patient needs oxygen therapy and serve as a baseline for comparison when the patient experiences an acute exacerbation. Patients typically require oxygen if their PaO_2 is less than 55 mm Hg or if there is evidence of pulmonary hypertension or polycythemia. Some, but not all, patients with COPD have a chronic respiratory acidosis with increased $PaCO_2$ but a normal pH due to bicarbonate buffering. During an acute exacerbation, an uncompensated respiratory acidosis may be present. Such acute increases in $PaCO_2$ cannot rapidly be compensated (more than 24 to 48 hours is required). Marked increases in $PaCO_2$ with a pH less than 7.25 can indicate impending respiratory failure that requires rapid medical intervention.

ELECTROCARDIOGRAPHY (ECG)

There are five characteristic findings on the electrocardiogram in patients with COPD: prominent P waves in leads II, III, and aVF (P pulmonale); exaggerated T waves producing more than 1 mm depression of the ST segment in leads II, III, and aVF; rightward shift of both QRS and P axis (the P wave axis is usually shifted +70 to +90 degrees); marked clockwise rotation in the precordial leads; and low voltage of the QRS complexes, especially over the left precordium. Many of these changes are caused by chest hyperinflation and clockwise repositioning of the heart. Patients who have pulmonary hypertension may have all of the changes noted plus evidence of right ventricular hypertrophy or an rS pattern across the precordium. In early COPD, the ECG is usually normal, although sinus tachycardia may be present. During exacerbations, sinus tachycardia or atrial tachydysrhythmias (atrial fibrillation, atrial flutter, or multifocal atrial tachycardia) usually occur.

DEFICIENCY OF ALPHA$_1$-ANTITRYPSIN

The inhalation of cigarette smoke in susceptible individuals is the most important risk factor that has been demonstrated to lead to the development of COPD. Emphysema may develop in nonsmokers who have a genetic predisposition because of a lack of circulating alpha$_1$-antitrypsin (AAT). AAT is a serum protein that inhibits several types of proteolytic enzymes, the most important being elastase. The normal phenotype is PiMM, which corresponds to a normal ATT serum concentration of 150 to 350 mg/dL. Most patients who have a deficiency of the protein have the phenotype PiZZ and are of northern European descent. The serum concentration of AAT below which there is an increased risk of developing emphysema is 80 mg/dL. Patients heterozygous for the disease (phenotype PiMZ) do not progress like homozygous individuals but may have a higher incidence of COPD than normal smokers.

The severity of the disease varies among individuals and cannot be predicted by their serum AAT concentration. Some patients with marked AAT deficiency never develop symptoms. Smoking significantly increases the risk of developing emphysema in AAT deficiency. Affected patients may develop disease in adulthood (fourth decade) but typically do not experience symptoms before the age of 25. They usually present with dyspnea, but they can also have problems with wheezing and recurrent respiratory infections. On chest film, emphysematous changes are pronounced at the bases of the lungs, a pattern characteristic of this disorder. The diagnosis of AAT deficiency is made by measuring a serum AAT concentration and by determining the phenotype of selected patients. The test should be performed in patients with early-onset emphysema, especially if emphysema is predominantly at the lung bases. Patients who have a family member with the disease should also be tested.

COURSE AND PROGNOSIS

The long-term prognosis is best determined by the patient's age and baseline FEV_1. Patients who are older and have more respiratory impairment (lower FEV_1) do worse. In general, the 3- to 5-year survival rate varies from 50 to 70 per cent when the FEV_1 is 1 L or less. Predictors of poor prognosis are a resting tachycardia, hypercapnia, cor pulmonale, and poor nutritional status. One factor that has been found to improve survival is smoking cessation. Figure 1 shows that when patients stop smoking, the rate of decline in FEV_1 slows to a normal rate of loss related to aging. Lung function, however, never returns to normal. Oxygen therapy in patients with hypoxemia and cor pulmonale has also been shown to improve survival.

DIFFERENTIAL DIAGNOSIS

In patients with suspected COPD based on history and physical examination, the approach to diagnosis is uncomplicated. The usual evaluation should include those studies shown in Table 2. More detailed testing is often unnecessary and expensive. However, unexpected or atypical findings should prompt further diagnostic testing to substantiate the diagnosis. Other disorders to be considered when

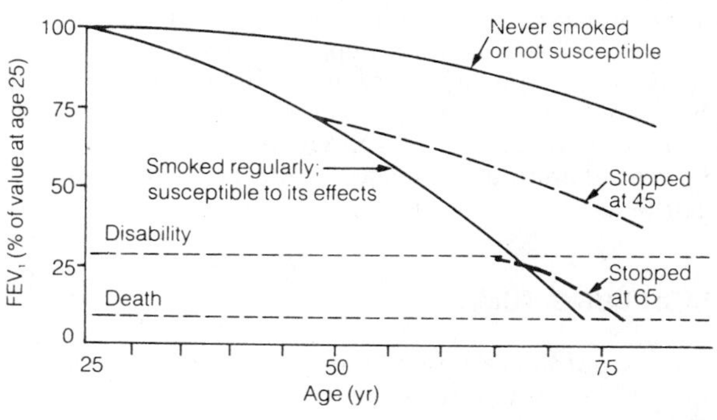

Figure 1. Rate of decline of FEV_1 in patients with COPD. By ceasing smoking, patients can slow the deterioration caused by the disease. (From Petty, T.L.: COPD and asthma: Practical steps for early detection and treatment. J. Resp. Dis 6[Suppl.]:35–39, 1985.)

Table 2. Evaluation for Suspected Chronic Obstructive Pulmonary Disease

History and physical examination
Chest radiograph
Electrocardiogram
Complete blood count, electrolytes, arterial blood gases
Spirogram with measurements made before and after bronchodilator use

evaluating the complaint of dyspnea include cardiovascular conditions (coronary artery disease, left ventricular failure, cardiomyopathy, valvular disease, and arrhythmia), other pulmonary disorders (infections, malignancy, pulmonary vascular disease or embolism, restrictive disorders, or other obstructive disorders), and anemia. Careful evaluation with attention toward these disorders is essential. In patients with known COPD, these disorders must also be considered if a sudden change in symptoms occurs.

COMPLICATIONS

The most common complication is infection, either viral or bacterial, which can lead to worsening of respiratory function. Other complications include pneumothorax, cor pulmonale, lung carcinoma, mycobacterial infections, and arrhythmia. Pulmonary hypertension with right-sided heart failure (cor pulmonale) usually occurs with advanced disease, especially if FEV_1 is less than 800 mL. Death may occur after progressive respiratory failure or as a result of complicating pneumonia.

PULMONARY TUMORS

By Lucio Fortunato, M.D.,
and Melvyn Goldberg, M.D.
Philadelphia, Pennsylvania

Primary bronchogenic carcinoma is the leading cause of cancer mortality in the United States and is caused largely by tobacco smoking. Most often, a solitary pulmonary nodule on a chest film is the initial finding. This finding may represent a primary lung cancer, a metastatic tumor, a bronchial adenoma, or a benign tumor of the lung, including pulmonary hamartoma or one of various mesenchymal tumors. Because treatment depends on histology, biopsy is crucial in the diagnosis of any new abnormality that arises in the lung. In patients undergoing surgical resection for a new solitary nodule, malignancy is identified in 40 per cent, granulomatous disease in 40 per cent, and other benign lesions in 20 per cent.

BENIGN LUNG TUMORS

Solitary pulmonary nodule, isolated granuloma, and coin lesion are descriptive terms defining solitary abnormalities seen on chest films in lung parenchyma. These tumors usually present as round or oval radiographic shadows up to 5 cm in diameter; they are surrounded by normal lung tissue and have well-defined margins. Because they are found in the periphery, they cannot be seen with the flexible bronchoscope. Benign tumors typically grow slowly and may contain central calcium deposits, although these criteria are not absolute. Review of previous chest films is essential in differentiating between new and old disease.

Mesenchymal Tumors

Pulmonary hamartoma presents as a slow-growing, isolated lung nodule, usually identified on a previous chest film, if available. It is composed primarily of cartilage and represents normal cellular constituents of lung that are abnormally organized. It has an appearance of "popped corn" on both chest film and computed tomography (CT) scan. Needle aspiration biopsy is usually diagnostic. Patients with pulmonary hamartomas do not require resection unless growth is rapid or the diagnosis is in doubt. Other rare mesenchymal tumors include lipoma, papilloma, fibroma, hemangioma, chondroma, neuroma, and leiomyoma. They are clinically significant only as diagnostic challenges.

Granulomatous Tumors

An isolated lung nodule can represent the late appearance of granulomatous disease. Tuberculosis is the most common cause, but rare fungal infections, particularly in endemic geographic locations, may be responsible. Other noninfectious inflammatory processes that are granulomatous in nature include sarcoidosis, silicosis, pneumoconiosis, Wegener's granulomatosis, and rheumatoid nodular disease (see the articles on interstitial lung disease and occupational lung disease).

LUNG CANCER

The most common lung cancer is adenocarcinoma (Table 1). It usually has a glandular pattern on histologic examination. Occasionally, it may show a multifocal or diffuse bronchioloalveolar pattern. Epidermoid carcinoma and large cell carcinoma are less common. Approximately 15 to 20 per cent of all lung cancers are small cell carcinomas. Frequently, mixed cell types are noted on pathologic examination. Neuroendocrine tumors encompass a spectrum from high-grade malignant small cell carcinoma to low-grade carcinoid. Despite their name, bronchial adenomas are not benign tumors, and they behave as low-grade malignancies. Most bronchial adenomas (85 to 95 per cent) are carcinoid tumors. The remaining tumors are represented by salivary gland tumors, which include adenoid cystic carcinoma (cylindroma), mucoepidermoid carcinoma, and pleomorphic mucous gland adenoma. Atypical carcinoids behave more like malignant tumors and commonly metastasize to regional lymph nodes and, rarely, to distant organs.

Natural History

The median survival of patients with *untreated lung cancer* from the onset of symptoms is 8 to 10 months, with

Table 1. Prevalence of Histologic Cell Types in Lung Cancer

	%
Adenocarcinoma	55
Epidermoid carcinoma	25
Small cell undifferentiated	15
Large cell undifferentiated	5

an overall 5-year survival rate of less than 2 per cent. Treatment increases this figure to 10 per cent, but usually only if patients undergo resection. Non–small cell cancer may take 3 to 5 years to reach 2 to 3 cm in diameter. Small cell carcinoma grows more rapidly and disseminates earlier. Forty-five per cent of small cell cancers have metastasized to bone marrow at the time of diagnosis, and survival rates are uniformly low.

Like other cancers, lung cancer spreads by direct invasion of adjacent tissues and by lymphatic and blood metastases. Adenocarcinoma and large cell undifferentiated carcinoma metastasize relatively early in their course, whereas squamous cell carcinoma metastasizes later. Bronchioloalveolar carcinoma may display a multicentric origin, diffusely covering the alveolar surface. It may rarely present with severe bronchorrhea (profuse expectoration).

At postmortem examination of patients with lung cancer, 26 per cent are found to have brain metastases, 15 per cent bone metastases, 39 per cent liver metastases, and 33 per cent adrenal gland metastases.

Clinical Manifestations

No Symptoms

Frequently, patients are asymptomatic, and the malignancy is detected on routine chest film, on a CT scan of the chest performed for another reason, or by routine sputum cytology in high-risk patients.

Symptoms of Endobronchial Tumor

Persistent cough is the most common presenting symptom and finding in patients with lung cancer (Tables 2 and 3). However, because most patients are smokers, this symptom is nonspecific and is often disregarded. It is caused by stimulation of nerve endings in a bronchus secondary to direct tumor involvement or to retained secretions distal to a bronchial obstruction. Involvement of the parietal pleura by tumor, inflammation, or effusion can also stimulate nerve endings and produce cough.

Dyspnea may occur secondary to airways obstruction and hypoventilation, resulting in a ventilation-perfusion mismatch. Atelectasis and recurrent or persistent pneumonias may be caused by partial or complete airway obstruction. Major airway involvement may produce an expiratory stridor. Hemoptysis develops in fewer than 10 per cent of patients. Usually, only a small amount of bright red blood is produced, which can be frightening to the patient. The tumor undergoes central necrosis and ulceration with involvement of the arterial blood supply of the involved bronchus.

Table 2. Presenting Symptoms in 1000 Patients With Lung Cancer

	%
Cough	55
Pain	15
Pneumonitis	6
Dyspnea	6
Hemoptysis	6
Weakness	5
None	5
Hoarseness	3
Weight loss	3
Wheezing	2

Table 3. Incidence of Symptoms in 1000 Patients With Lung Cancer

	%
Cough	92
Weight loss	
>15%	30
<15%	30
Excess sputum production	58
Pain	55
Dyspnea	50
Hemoptysis	50
Discomfort	38
Weakness	35
Pneumonia	35
Wheezing	30
Hoarseness	12
None	5

Symptoms of Intrathoracic Spread

Pleural pain with dyspnea suggests pleural invasion and a pleural effusion. The effusion is usually bloody. Persistent local somatic pain over one or two ribs suggests intercostal nerve involvement or invasion of the rib.

Tumors of the apex of the lung (superior sulcus tumors, or Pancoast tumors) cause pain in the ipsilateral shoulder and may involve the ulnar distribution of the arm and hand. Horner's syndrome (ptosis, miosis, unilateral loss of facial sweating, and, more rarely, enophthalmos) may develop. The tumor is often difficult to see on chest film. It frequently invades the brachial plexus, cervical sympathetic nerves, and first or second ribs.

Superior vena cava (SVC) obstruction leads to venous distention and engorgement of the face, neck, chest, and upper arms and suggests malignant invasion of the right superior mediastinum. Lung cancer is the most common cause of SVC obstruction.

Hoarseness suggests involvement of the left recurrent laryngeal nerve as it travels under the aortic arch just beyond its vagal origin. Involvement of the phrenic nerve can produce hiccups or paralysis of the hemidiaphragm with elevation. A paradoxical movement of the diaphragm is sometimes seen on fluoroscopy.

Pericardial involvement is usually manifested by increasing dyspnea, symptoms of heart failure, tamponade, or sudden onset of arrhythmia. Dysphagia suggests malignant invasion or compression of the esophagus by the primary tumor or by secondary lymph node involvement. Tracheoesophageal fistula can present with cough and aspiration while eating. Subsequent complications include pneumonia and lung abscess.

Symptoms of Distant Metastases

Brain metastases are most common with small cell tumors. At the time of diagnosis, approximately 10 per cent of patients with squamous cell carcinoma have symptoms of brain metastasis, and another 5 per cent have asymptomatic involvement. Tumors of the lung usually metastasize to the frontal lobes. Brain metastases may cause seizures, gradual hemiparesis, a change in mental status, or cerebellar ataxia.

Bone metastases are common. Ten per cent of patients with squamous cell carcinoma and normal biochemical and hematologic profiles have demonstrable bone metastases. The most common sites of bone metastasis are the spine (70 per cent), pelvic bones (40 per cent), and femur (25 per cent). Metastasis can present with pain due to compression or pathologic fracture.

Adrenal metastases are noted on CT scan in up to 15 per cent of patients with lung cancer. These are usually located in the adrenal medulla and therefore spare cortical function. Liver metastases are most frequent in patients with small cell lung cancer and can present with abdominal discomfort or distention, jaundice, or hepatomegaly.

Lung cancer infrequently metastasizes to the gastrointestinal tract and the pancreas. Skin metastases are rare. Lymph node metastases to the supraclavicular and axillary regions may occur. Small cell lung cancer also has a propensity to metastasize to endocrine organs, including the thyroid gland. Choroidal metastases may cause blurred vision and are almost always associated with widespread disease. Metastases to the kidney, uterus, ovaries, and testis may also occur.

Although metastases from lung cancer are common, extensive routine radiologic investigation is unnecessary unless patients are symptomatic, present at an advanced stage, have small cell lung cancer, or need to be entered in an investigational protocol.

Extrathoracic Nonmetastatic Symptoms (Paraneoplastic Syndromes)

Several neurologic symptoms have been described in association with lung cancer in the absence of metastatic disease. They may appear several months or even years before the tumor becomes apparent (in 83 per cent of patients), and they occur in 16 per cent of patients with small cell carcinomas. They include encephalopathies, myelopathies, neuropathies (sensory with dorsal column degeneration, peripheral motor-sensory), and muscular disorders such as dermatomyositis, carcinomatous myopathy, myasthenialike state (Eaton-Lambert syndrome), and metabolic myopathies caused by excessive production of corticotropin, parathyroid hormone–like substance, and thyroid-stimulating hormone. Various endocrine paraneoplastic syndromes may be caused by hormonelike substances produced and secreted by lung cancer (Table 4). Hematologic disorders include microcytic anemia, erythrocythemia, and a leukemoid reaction to tumor or tumor necrosis. Coagulation disorders include recurrent migratory thrombophlebitis, thrombocytopenic purpura, fibrinolytic purpura, cryofibrinogenemia, and nonbacterial thrombotic endocarditis.

Physical Examination

A complete physical examination should be carried out for all patients, but it is often unremarkable. There may be signs of pleural effusion, atelectasis, consolidation, stridor due to severe obstruction of the trachea or main stem bronchus, a persistent localized rhonchus suggesting a bronchus narrowed by endobronchial tumor, or a chest wall mass. Painful, swollen joints, particularly the wrists, ankles, and knees, may occur in patients with hypertrophic pulmonary osteoarthropathy.

In addition, clinical findings that are highly suggestive of incurability should be recognized. An SVC obstruction is associated with a suffused face and upper extremities with collateralized circulation on the anterior chest. Supraclavicular or axillary lymph node enlargement, subcutaneous metastases, liver metastases with hepatomegaly or abdominal distention, and central or peripheral nervous system abnormalities are present in approximately 25 per cent of patients with lung cancer.

Synchronous cancers of the upper aerodigestive tract are not rare, and a systematic examination of the head and neck should be carried out. Additionally, patients with lung cancer often have cardiopulmonary diseases, including chronic obstructive pulmonary disease and myocardial ischemia.

Table 4. Endocrine Paraneoplastic Syndromes Associated With Lung Cancer

Associated Hormone	Syndrome
Corticotropin (ACTH)	Hypercortisolism
Serotonin	Carcinoid syndrome
Parathyroid hormone	Hypercalcemia
Thyroid-stimulating hormone	Hyperthyroidism
Melanocyte-stimulating hormone	Hyperpigmentation
Antidiuretic hormone	SIADH,* hyponatremia
Erythropoietin	Erythrocythemia
Gonadotropin	Gynecomastia
Insulin	Hypoglycemia
Glucagon	Diabetes

*Syndrome of inappropriate antidiuretic hormone

Diagnosis

Early diagnosis in lung cancer is difficult. Several studies have failed to identify a survival advantage from yearly chest films and sputum cytology, even in the high-risk group. Therefore, most patients with lung cancer have regional or metastatic disease by the time the disease is diagnosed.

Imaging

The chest film is the touchstone for diagnosis of lung tumors. Posteroanterior and left lateral views should routinely be obtained. Features of malignancy include the size of the tumor (>3 cm in diameter), the presence of irregular or spiculated borders, and the absence of calcifications. However, the absence of these signs does not exclude a diagnosis of cancer. Approximately 30 to 40 per cent of nodular lesions are overlooked. The radiographs must be compared with old films whenever possible. The presence of an unchanged lung nodule over a 2-year period justifies the diagnosis of a benign lesion, but this criterion should not be used prospectively to follow new lung nodules.

A CT scan, enhanced with intravenous injection of contrast medium, defines the primary lesion and the presence or absence of mediastinal lymphadenopathy. This study is essential for staging lung cancer and for planning appropriate therapy. One-centimeter cuts should be performed throughout the thorax, and 5-mm cuts at the level of the hila are needed to define the bronchi and their relation to the hilar vessels and lymph nodes. The CT scan should include the upper abdomen to evaluate the liver and adrenal glands. If no lymph nodes are identified, the negative predictive value is approximately 95 per cent. If paratracheal, carinal, or hilar lymph nodes are identified on CT scan, the location, size, and number of involved nodes must be noted. In general, lymph nodes less than 1 cm in diameter should be considered negative, those between 1 and 1.5 cm are indeterminate, and those larger than 1.5 cm are suspicious and require histologic confirmation.

Nuclear bone scans are usually obtained if the patient is symptomatic or has an increased alkaline phosphatase activity or serum calcium concentration. The suspicious area should be further investigated with other x-ray studies, and confirmatory studies are often needed, including magnetic resonance imaging (MRI) and fine-needle aspiration biopsy (FNA).

Magnetic resonance imaging of the brain should be performed in patients with small cell lung cancer and in patients with symptoms of central nervous involvement. This procedure may also be valuable in assessing the bone and spinal cord in patients with a posterior mediastinal tumor and the brachial plexus in patients with superior sulcus tumor. Angiography and venography are now used less frequently for defining vessel invasion, because enhanced CT scans or MRI usually can define the adjacent structures or involvement by tumor masses. Echocardiography is useful in diagnosing pericardial effusion.

Diagnostic Procedures and Examinations

Sputum cytology is diagnostic in approximately 90 per cent of lung cancers but in only 20 per cent of peripheral tumors. Bronchoscopy is the mainstay for the diagnosis of lung cancer and is an important examination for planning of the operative resection. If a tumor is identified, a histologic diagnosis can be obtained in the vast majority of patients by direct biopsies or brushing. In rare patients, the lesion is peripheral and not readily accessible. Selective washings can be used in these situations. Transbronchial biopsies under fluoroscopic guidance can be obtained for diagnosis of more peripheral lesions or in patients in whom a bronchoalveolar carcinoma is suspected. Transcarinal biopsies can also be obtained to evaluate mediastinal adenopathy.

Percutaneous FNA has reduced the need for diagnostic thoracotomy. Most procedures can be performed with fluoroscopy, reserving CT-guided aspirations for patients with difficult lesions or previous unsuccessful attempts. A pneumothorax develops in approximately 20 to 30 per cent of patients with transthoracic FNA, but a thoracostomy tube is necessary in only 5 per cent.

Cervical mediastinoscopy is used to sample the paratracheal and subcarinal lymph nodes. In most patients, the status of these mediastinal lymph nodes determines the form of therapy for lung cancer. Evidence of regional disease in these stations is an indication of incurability in most circumstances. Mediastinoscopy is often used in the preoperative evaluation of patients with large and central tumors, or if CT identifies mediastinal nodes larger than 1.5 cm. Small, peripheral tumors with no evidence of mediastinal involvement by CT scan do not need staging mediastinoscopy.

Anterior mediastinotomy (Chamberlain's procedure) allows direct observation and biopsy of lymph nodes situated on or under the aortic arch. These stations are inaccessible by conventional cervical mediastinoscopy. Hilar fixation, which may preclude an operation, can be also assessed.

Thoracoscopy (video assisted thoracoscopic surgery) may be used to assess the pleura, a pleural effusion, mediastinal lymph nodes, and chest wall involvement. It requires general anesthesia and a double-lumen endotracheal tube, so that the pleural space can be viewed completely with a collapsed ipsilateral lung. After a small intercostal incision is performed, a thoracoscope is inserted into the chest cavity. Biopsies can be obtained under direct vision if indicated.

Esophagoscopy should be obtained at the time of bronchoscopy in patients with symptoms of dysphagia, or if an involvement of the esophagus is questioned. Diagnostic thoracotomy is still necessary in the rare patient in whom a definitive tissue diagnosis cannot be obtained from less invasive techniques.

Laboratory Procedures

Increased liver enzyme activity, particularly alkaline phosphatase, reflects either liver or bone metastasis. In the majority of patients with bone metastases, both the serum calcium and the serum alkaline phosphatase are increased.

An increased leukocyte count may reflect a leukemoid reaction to the tumor, central necrosis of the tumor and subsequent infection, or airways obstruction, pneumonia, and lung abscess. The hemoglobin concentration may be decreased secondary to chronic infection or bone marrow suppression.

The syndrome of inappropriate antidiuretic hormone (SIADH) can be diagnosed by simultaneous serum and urine osmolality analysis. Usually, an abnormally high urine osmolality is present despite low serum osmolality.

Pulmonary Function Studies

Pulmonary function studies are performed routinely in all patients undergoing pulmonary resection. Patients with a history of cardiac disease must have a cardiac functional assessment performed by a cardiologist. Standard guidelines require a preoperative 1-second forced expiratory volume (FEV_1) of at least 1 L, a diffusion capacity of 50 per cent, and an acceptable blood gas analysis with no carbon dioxide retention.

The functional residual lung capacity after resection of any portion of lung should not be less than 1 L to ensure the patient's survival postoperatively. Therefore, a patient evaluated for pneumonectomy must have a preoperative FEV_1 of 1.8 to 2 L, unless a ventilation-perfusion scan demonstrates that the majority of the functioning lung is present on the unresected side.

Complications

Most complications are secondary to an endobronchial tumor. Partial or complete airway obstruction may lead to recurrent or persistent pneumonia and sepsis requiring antibiotic therapy. Bronchoscopy should be performed to confirm the diagnosis. Laser or radiation therapy has been used in these circumstances to relieve the airway obstruction.

Hemoptysis is also related to an endobronchial lesion and is usually mild to moderate. Bronchoscopy should be performed in high-risk patients who have a single episode of hemoptysis and in patients with recurrent hemoptysis. Dyspnea usually complicates airways obstruction by producing regional hypoventilation and a ventilation-perfusion mismatch.

Pleural effusion may also produce dyspnea and occurs in approximately 10 per cent of patients. Diagnostic thoracentesis should be performed, and if cytology is positive for malignancy, a pleurodesis should be carried out by one of the many accepted methods to preclude recurrence. Tumor extension or nodal involvement in the mediastinum may produce a tracheoesophageal or bronchoesophageal fistula with aspiration pneumonitis and recurrent sepsis. A diagnosis of this abnormality must be made rapidly, and treatment must be aggressive to avoid further soiling of the tracheobronchial tree.

Common Errors in Diagnosis

Failure to review old chest films

Failure to obtain an absolute cytologic or histologic diagnosis before treatment

Failure to follow up patients with a presumed benign coin

lesion and patients with persisting or recurring pneumonias
Failure to exclude metastatic disease in high-risk patients with small cell carcinoma, large central lesions, or highly anaplastic lesions, or in the presence of signs and symptoms of distant disease
Failure to assess adequately the pulmonary and cardiac reserve in patients undergoing treatment by resection
Failure to differentiate between a primary and a secondary lung cancer
Failure to diagnose a second primary tumor of the upper aerodigestive tract

ASTHMA

By Gregory C. Kane, M.D.,
and James E. Fish, M.D.
Philadelphia, Pennsylvania

The definition of asthma incorporates both physiologic and pathologic criteria and includes three main elements: (1) reversible air flow obstruction that varies spontaneously or with therapy, (2) bronchial hyperresponsiveness to multiple stimuli, and (3) airway inflammation. Asthma is a heterogeneous disorder, not only with respect to etiologic factors but also in terms of pathologic features and clinical manifestations. The typical clinical manifestations are chronic but episodic symptoms of chest tightness, wheezing, cough, and dyspnea. Some patients experience rare symptomatic episodes that are mild, whereas others experience frequent severe symptoms superimposed on a level of chronic disability. Yet other patients experience extreme lability with near-fatal episodes interspersed with symptom-free intervals.

CLINICAL DIAGNOSIS

The diagnosis of asthma is usually clinical, based on a history of typical symptoms with confirmatory physiologic evidence of variable airflow obstruction. In the young patient, a diagnosis of asthma is facilitated by the relative scarcity of other disorders that either mimic asthma or complicate its clinical presentation. In older adults, however, the diagnosis of asthma is more problematic because cardiovascular diseases and other forms of chronic lung disease become more prevalent. In elderly asthmatic patients, allergic factors appear to play a diminishing role, and a component of fixed airway obstruction appears more common. These factors complicate the task of distinguishing between asthma and other forms of chronic airway obstruction such as chronic obstructive pulmonary disease (COPD), especially in current and former smokers. As a rule, the predictive values of clinical and laboratory findings in the diagnosis of asthma decline with age.

Signs and Symptoms

Episodes of wheezing with chest tightness, cough, and shortness of breath usually suggest a diagnosis of asthma in a young individual. Symptomatic episodes interspersed with long, symptom-free intervals often occur in mild asthmatics. If the disease is poorly controlled, symptoms can occur on a daily basis. Some patients state that the greatest difficulty is in getting air out, or that their lungs are "full." Nocturnal symptoms of wheezing, chest tightness, and cough are typical of asthma, and their absence should prompt a search for alternative diagnoses. These symptoms typically occur in the early morning hours, between 3:00 and 6:00 AM. This is in contrast to gastroesophageal reflux (GER), which causes similar symptoms soon after reclining at night, or cardiac decompensation and orthopnea, which can occur within a few hours of elevating edematous lower extremities.

Although COPD and cardiovascular disease are characterized by chronic dyspnea and disability, the same chronic symptoms may be experienced by older asthmatic patients, who tend to demonstrate a significant degree of persistent airway obstruction. Asthma can occur in conjunction with chronic bronchitis, cardiac disease, and other illnesses, which further confounds attempts to ascribe symptoms to a single diagnosis. In general, the diagnosis of asthma should be strongly suspected if episodic wheezing occurs in a nonsmoker. However, because many elderly asthmatic patients are either current smokers or former smokers, a smoking history does not exclude asthma.

No single symptom is specific for asthma. Wheezing is perhaps the most useful finding, because most asthmatics report more than just rare episodes of wheezing and nonasthmatics rarely report wheezing. Chronic cough with sputum production is usually associated with chronic bronchitis rather than asthma, although in elderly asthmatics productive cough is not uncommon. In older patients who have smoked for many years, asthma and chronic bronchitis can occur together. This overlap condition is usually referred to as asthmatic bronchitis.

Symptom patterns are often useful in the diagnosis of asthma, because asthma is usually associated with defined triggers. For example, symptoms that occur in association with seasonal pollen exposure, after viral respiratory infections, after heavy exercise, or in association with strong odors or fumes are typical of asthma. Likewise, symptoms that occur after ingestion of drugs such as aspirin and beta-blocking agents are also suggestive of asthma.

A history of other disorders known to be associated with asthma, such as rhinitis, sinusitis, and nasal polyposis, is important in the diagnosis. The presence of these conditions increases the likelihood that pulmonary symptoms are attributable to asthma.

The clinical history should include details about the patient's environment and how symptoms are influenced by the environment. Establishment of an association between asthma symptoms and aeroallergens helps confirm the diagnosis and suggests appropriate avoidance measures for facilitating treatment. Relevant questions include whether symptoms appear when the patient is visiting a house where there are indoor pets, or when there is exposure to pollen. Alternatively, if there are pets in the home, do symptoms improve when away from home (on vacation), and do they reappear within 24 hours after returning to home? If animals are involved, the clinician should inquire whether itching of the eyes or skin occurs after contact with the animal. Other questions include whether symptoms occur when carpets are being vacuumed or when the patient is breathing the air in a damp basement.

Physical Examination

Physical signs during a typical acute episode of asthma can be helpful in establishing the diagnosis. These signs include wheezing, which is most prominent on expiration, tachypnea, tachycardia, and a prolonged expiratory phase of respiration. Most often, however, patients seek medical advice when they are symptom-free, and physical findings may be absent. In such patients, certain nonspecific findings may give a clue to the diagnosis. For example, rhinitis, sinusitis, and nasal polyps are seen more commonly in patients with asthma than in those with other chronic lower respiratory tract diseases. Chronic sinus disease is difficult to diagnose on clinical grounds alone, and specialized imaging procedures may be required for confirmation. The presence of wheezing on forced expiration is nonspecific for the presence of airway obstruction. This finding can be reproduced in normal adults because increased intrathoracic pressure during forced expiration can lead to airway constriction.

Physical findings are quite dramatic during severe episodes of asthma. They include marked tachypnea, tachycardia, a paradoxical pulse, and use of accessory muscles of respiration. Diaphoresis, cyanosis, inability to lie flat, and the absence of breath sounds are signs of life-threatening disease. Marked weight loss or severe wasting in association with pursed-lip breathing, hyperinflation, and a quiet chest on auscultation with diminished breath sounds suggest severe emphysema rather than asthma. Patients with asthma may also show signs of hyperinflation with diminished breath sounds and heart sounds, but only during an acute exacerbation. Lower-extremity edema, neck vein distention, and other signs of cardiac decompensation should be evaluated to exclude heart failure as a cause of wheezing. Another finding of importance is clubbing, which is frequently associated with interstitial lung disease and bronchiectasis but not asthma. Audible inspiratory and expiratory wheezing that is heard best over the upper airways should prompt a search for causes of upper airway obstruction rather than asthma.

LABORATORY TESTS

A diagnosis of asthma is usually suggested by the medical history. Confirmation usually requires physiologic tests showing the presence of reversible or variable airflow obstruction. Other laboratory tests may be helpful in either supporting the diagnosis of asthma or eliminating other diagnoses from consideration.

Pulmonary Function Testing

Pulmonary function tests (see the article on tests of respiratory function) are important not only in confirming a diagnosis of asthma but also in monitoring the course of the patient's disease. The diagnosis of asthma is usually confirmed by objective demonstration of airway obstruction by spirometry showing significant variation (>15 per cent and >200 mL) in the 1-second forced expired volume (FEV_1), either after bronchodilator administration or with repeated measurements over time. The lack of an acute bronchodilator response in the laboratory or office does not exclude asthma. Longer-term therapy, often with corticosteroids, may be necessary for achieving appreciable improvement and documentation supportive of the diagnosis. The peak expiratory flow can also be used to confirm the presence of variable airflow obstruction. A variation of more than a 15 per cent in peak expiratory flow from day to day (measured at the same time each day) confirms variable obstruction.

Complete pulmonary function tests, including lung volume and flow-volume curves, are often useful in excluding a diagnosis of restrictive lung disease (e.g., pulmonary fibrosis) or upper airway problems that mimic asthma (which are characterized by abnormal inspiratory flow patterns or a plateau on the expiratory portion of the flow-volume curve, or both). The carbon monoxide diffusing capacity (DLCO) may be useful in distinguishing between asthma and emphysema. In emphysema, air space enlargement and alveolar destruction with loss of effective alveolar surface area leads to a reduction in DLCO. By contrast, the DLCO is usually normal in patients with asthma.

The typical pulmonary function findings in asthma are listed in Table 1 and compared with typical findings in COPD. Although spirometric testing is usually adequate for the diagnosis of asthma, complete pulmonary function studies with measurement of the DLCO should be considered if the chest film shows interstitial abnormalities or "small lung volumes" or if the spirogram reveals a low forced vital capacity (FVC) and FEV_1, but a normal FEV_1/FVC per cent ratio.

Arterial blood gas analysis is not useful in the stable asthmatic, but it may be helpful in assessing the status of patients with severe exacerbations. Arterial blood gas measurements are necessary if cyanosis is present or if the FEV_1 or peak expiratory flow is less than 25 per cent of the predicted normal value. The typical blood gas abnormality in acute asthma is hypoxemia due to ventilation-perfusion mismatching. Increased Pa_{CO_2} indicates potentially life-threatening asthma and respiratory failure. Because the initial Pa_{CO_2} is often low during mild to moderate exacerbations of asthma, a normal Pa_{CO_2} could indicate early respiratory failure and the need for careful monitoring until the patient responds to appropriate therapy.

RADIOGRAPHIC STUDIES

Because the chest film is usually unremarkable in patients with uncomplicated asthma, it is most useful for excluding other causes of respiratory symptoms. Radiographic evidence of hyperinflation has been reported in asthmatic patients with severe disease, in those with chronic versus intermittent symptoms, and during acute exacerbations. Hyperinflation with flattened diaphragms and evidence of decreased markings are prominent features in emphysema. The chest film is an integral part of both the initial diagnostic evaluation and the assessment of acute exacerbations that require hospitalization or unscheduled visits to the emergency room. Routine chest films in the uncomplicated asthmatic are not recommended.

Table 1. Comparison of Pulmonary Function in Asthma and Chronic Obstructive Pulmonary Disease

Test	Asthma	Chronic Obstructive Pulmonary Disease
FEV_1	Decreased	Decreased
FVC	Decreased	Decreased
FEV_1/FVC	Decreased	Decreased
Bronchodilator response	Usually	Sometimes
Total lung capacity	Normal	Normal or increased
Residual volume	Increased	Increased
DLCO	Normal	Decreased
Methacholine challenge	Almost always positive	Occasionally positive

FEV_1 = 1-second forced expiratory volume; FVC = forced vital capacity; FEV_1/FVC = ratio between these measurements; DLCO = carbon monoxide diffusing capacity.

ELECTROCARDIOGRAPHY

Electrocardiographic abnormalities are usually not observed in stable asthma. During an exacerbation, however, several abnormalities may occur, including sinus tachycardia, right axis deviation, right bundle branch block, repolarization abnormalities, right ventricular strain, and a variety of atrial tachyarrhythmias. The electrocardiogram is usually recommended in the initial evaluation of elderly asthmatic patients, not only to evaluate cardiac status but also to assess risk-benefit aspects of certain types of therapy.

BLOOD TESTS

Peripheral eosinophilia (>4 per cent or an absolute count of 300 to 400 cells/mm^3) or increased serum concentration of immunoglobulin IgE, or both, are often seen in asthmatic patients, but they are not specific for asthma and normal values do not exclude the diagnosis. Eosinophilia may be absent if the patient is being treated with corticosteroids. Marked increases in IgE (>1000 IU/mL), peripheral eosinophilia, and infiltrates on the chest film in a patient with a history of asthma and allergies strongly suggest a diagnosis of allergic bronchopulmonary aspergillosis (ABPA). This disorder is caused by an immune reaction to *Aspergillus* fungal species that colonize the airways. In general, ABPA is considered a distinct phenomenon, although it has been reported primarily in patients with a history of asthma.

ALLERGY TESTING

An allergy evaluation is appropriate if the history suggests that specific aeroallergens are important triggers of symptoms or if asthma is accompanied by other symptoms typical of allergic disease, such as rhinitis and conjunctivitis. The components of an allergy evaluation include a detailed environmental history to detect triggers, followed by tests for allergic sensitivity. Sensitivity can be verified by skin tests or by in vitro antibody studies. The presence of IgE antibodies, as determined by skin tests or serologic tests, does not necessarily mean that the patient has clinically significant allergic disease. Positive skin tests are demonstrable in many individuals with no allergic symptoms; therefore, the clinical history must be linked to the results of the allergy testing to evaluate the importance of allergic triggers.

BRONCHIAL CHALLENGE TESTING

Exercise and pharmacologic challenge have been used widely as diagnostic tests for asthma. Demonstration of a decrease of 15 per cent or more in FEV_1 after strenuous exercise is considered specific for asthma, although the sensitivity of such a test is limited. Pharmacologic challenges with histamine or methacholine are more sensitive, but the positive predictive value of tests using methacholine or histamine increases only if asthma is suspected from the history (i.e., with increased prevalence of disease).

Pharmacologic challenge tests also provide a measure of nonspecific airway responsiveness. Hyperresponsiveness has been shown in asthma and other conditions, including cystic fibrosis, COPD, congestive heart failure, viral respiratory infections, and exposure to allergens or oxidant pollutants. Changes in responsiveness that occur with acute inflammatory conditions such as viral respiratory infections or after exposure to allergens or pollutants are usually transient. Abnormal responsiveness associated with COPD tends to be fixed, and it correlates with the severity of pulmonary function decrement. For this reason, pharmacologic challenge tests cannot be used to discriminate between asthma and COPD in patients who have abnormal spirograms. In the presence of airway obstruction, the spirometric response to an inhaled bronchodilator provides the best assessment of reversibility of the process. In patients with asthma, abnormal responsiveness is usually demonstrable even if the baseline spirogram is normal. Therefore, pharmacologic challenge tests are most appropriately used in the evaluation of patients with normal spirograms who have unexplained respiratory tract symptoms suggesting asthma.

Abnormal response to methacholine or histamine is a sensitive test with a high negative predictive value (i.e., low rate of false-negative results). False-negative results usually occur in patients who experience symptoms only at times of relevant exposure and who are asymptomatic at the time of testing, such as patients with seasonal asthma who are tested out of season. Abnormal responses to methacholine or histamine may occur in up to 8 to 10 per cent of "normal" individuals with no respiratory symptoms and in a similar number of allergic patients without asthma. Thus, in a randomly selected population, the predictive value of a positive pharmacologic challenge for a diagnosis of asthma would be low because the prevalence rate of asthma is low (4 to 6 per cent). The predictive value of a positive test is increased if the pretest probability of asthma, based on the clinical history, is increased. Pharmacologic challenge tests are rarely required to confirm a diagnosis of asthma. Even in patients with normal spirograms and suggestive symptoms, such as patients with cough as the sole presenting manifestation, challenge tests can give equivocal results. Demonstration of symptomatic improvement after administration of bronchodilator medication often provides superior diagnostic information.

DIFFERENTIAL DIAGNOSIS

The differential diagnosis of asthma depends on the age of the symptomatic patient. In young adults, only a few conditions can mimic asthma (Table 2). Some of these conditions are quite rare, such as cystic fibrosis, bronchiectasis, and ABPA. Cystic fibrosis, suggested by recurrent pulmonary infections and chest symptoms, can be excluded by sweat chloride measurements. Bronchiectasis may occur after severe childhood pneumonia or tuberculosis and leads to chronic cough with mucus production. This mucus is often purulent and tenacious, but in some patients it may be scant. Thickening of the bronchi may be seen on routine chest film, but computed tomography scans are usually needed. ABPA is suggested if a patient with a clinical

Table 2. Differential Diagnosis of Asthma in Young Adults

Cystic fibrosis
Bronchiectasis
Allergic bronchopulmonary aspergillosis
Gastroesophageal reflux
Rhinosinusitis with cough
Acute viral respiratory infection

history of asthma is found to have markedly increased IgE, peripheral blood eosinophilia, and changing infiltrates on chest film.

Gastroesophageal reflux may produce cough, dyspnea, and chest tightness that can be confused with or complicate asthma. GER is not invariably associated with symptomatic heartburn, so symptoms that occur when assuming recumbency or after ingesting a large meal should be sought. GER is suggested by a barium swallow showing reflux into the esophagus, but more detailed pH probe testing may be necessary in some patients. Rhinosinusitis with posterior nasal drainage can produce cough and chest tightness. Although some of these patients may also have asthma, others may improve with therapy directed at rhinosinusitis alone. Conversely, known asthmatic patients may have poorly controlled chest symptoms when sinus disease is active. Viral respiratory tract infections can also mimic asthma by causing cough and wheezing that persist for many weeks after resolution of the acute infection. These infections can be associated with increased methacholine reactivity as well. Asthma should not be diagnosed on the basis of symptoms that occur only after an isolated viral respiratory infection, but if symptoms become chronic, the diagnosis of asthma should be further investigated.

In older adults, asthma must be differentiated from chronic pulmonary disorders and from cardiac and other diseases (Table 3). COPD can usually be differentiated from asthma by a history including tobacco exposure and a lack of nocturnal symptoms. Still, some patients may have features of asthma, but also have a significant smoking history. Here, the term asthmatic bronchitis may be a useful designation when chronic bronchitis and asthma are coexistent. Pulmonary function tests can help substantiate the diagnosis of COPD based on lack of reversibility of obstruction and a decreased DLCO. Ischemic heart disease is common in older smokers, and electrocardiography with or without cardiac stress testing should be considered for patients with episodic symptoms or dyspnea associated with chest pressure. Because congestive heart failure may present with wheezing and dyspnea, careful attention to signs and symptoms of left ventricular failure is also important. Pulmonary thromboembolism (see separate article) can produce sudden dyspnea, occasionally associated with wheezing. This diagnosis should be considered in older adults without pre-existing history of asthma. Lesions obstructing the major airways can generate dyspnea and wheezing that mimics asthma. If they are too small to be seen radiographically, the obstructing lesion may be diagnosed bronchoscopically. This procedure is indicated if the physical examination shows markedly asymmetric wheezing, or if symptoms are persistent and fail to respond to bronchodilator therapy. GER is common in all age groups, especially in the elderly because of changes in the lower esophageal sphincter with age. In younger patients, GER may be the only cause of wheezing and chest tightness, or it may exacerbate established asthma. Finally, airway hyperreactivity can be a normal finding after viral tracheobronchitis in older adults, just as in children or young adults.

Table 3. Differential Diagnosis of Asthma in Older Adults

Chronic obstructive pulmonary disease
Ischemic heart failure
Congestive heart failure
Mitral stenosis
Pulmonary thromboembolism
Lesions obstructing the major airways
Gastroesophageal reflux
Acute viral respiratory infection

COMPLICATIONS

Complications of mild asthma are rare. Patients with severe asthma may experience treatment-related side effects secondary to administration of systemic corticosteroids, including hyperglycemia, cataracts, glaucoma, osteoporosis, changes in body habitus, and edema. Intubation for life-threatening asthma can lead to barotrauma (pneumothorax, pneumomediastinum). Therapy in an intensive care unit can also have untoward effects, including vascular catheter-associated infections or prolonged neuromuscular weakness, especially if the use of neuromuscular blocking agents is required. Although the goal of outpatient treatment is to avoid hospitalization, hospital admission and appropriate care is life-saving for severe acute asthma.

COURSE AND PROGNOSIS

The course of asthma is highly variable, but for most patients the outlook is quite good. Asthma seems to be most severe at the extremes of life (i.e., in young children or older adults), and many patients with childhood asthma experience prolonged symptom-free periods during middle life. Symptoms recur in some of these patients; other patients may develop asthma de novo in late adulthood without predating childhood illness. For most patients, asthmatic symptoms are mild and intermittent with long, symptom-free intervals. Still, some patients experience severe symptoms that limit performance of daily activities and participation in school or work and may even require frequent hospitalization. Deaths from asthma have been uncommon, but the mortality rate has been increasing, possibly because of increasing populations at high risk. These populations include urban minority groups, persons exposed to high levels of airborne pollutants, and patients without access to appropriate medical care. With appropriate medical care and treatment, most patients should have normal lifestyles and participate fully in work and recreational activities.

BACTERIAL PNEUMONIA

By Thomas J. Marrie, M.D.
Halifax, Nova Scotia, Canada

Pneumonia is defined as inflammation and consolidation of lung tissue in response to an infectious agent. It is the sixth leading cause of death in the United States (12.7 deaths per 100,000 population), and the estimated cost of treating this illness is 23 billion dollars per year (14 billion in direct patient care costs and 9 billion in lost wages). Changes in the microorganisms that cause pneumonia and in the population at risk have resulted in major changes in the epidemiology of the disease. In the 1930s, *Streptococcus pneumoniae* accounted for most cases of pneumonia; in the 1990s, *Legionella pneumophila*, *Legionella micdadei*, other

Legionella species, and *Chlamydia pneumoniae* have emerged as new causes of community-acquired pneumonia. Penicillin-resistant *S. pneumoniae* is now a significant problem in North America.

The population at risk has changed; elderly individuals now represent the fastest-growing segment of the population. The incidence of pneumonia requiring hospitalization in this age group is much higher than that for younger adults. The nursing home population has increased, and pneumonia in this group resembles hospital-acquired, rather than community-acquired, disease. The success of organ transplantation and aggressive therapy for cancer and collagen vascular diseases has resulted in an increased number of immunosuppressed patients. The acquired immunodeficiency syndrome has produced a subset of patients with community-acquired pneumonia who may present with severe or atypical manifestations of pneumonia caused by conventional pathogens as well as opportunistic agents.

HISTORY AND PHYSICAL EXAMINATION

The diagnosis of pneumonia is based on the history, physical examination, and chest film. Fever, chills, pleuritic chest pain, and cough productive of purulent sputum are signs and symptoms that suggest bacterial pneumonia. However, these findings are not specific for pneumonia.

The history should include an assessment of the patient's risk factors for pneumonia. Table 1 lists items in the history that should suggest a particular etiology for the pneumonia. For example, rapidly progressive pneumonia in a young person who has returned from a trip to Spain suggests *L. pneumophila* infection. Pneumonia that occurs 10 to 14 days after exposure to a parturient cat, particularly if it involved cleaning up the products of conception, suggests *Coxiella burnetii* pneumonia. An occupational history should be taken because certain occupations predispose to different types of infection. Pneumonia occurring in a patient with diabetic ketoacidosis is more likely to be due to *S. pneumoniae* or *Staphylococcus aureus* than to other pathogens. Patients with alcoholism or chronic obstructive pulmonary disease are predisposed to certain pathogens, as are recipients of solid organ transplants (see Table 1). Patients with sickle cell disease or multiple myeloma are most likely to develop pneumococcal pneumonia. Those with human immunodeficiency virus (HIV) infection and a CD4 count of less than 200 cells/mm^3 may become infected with *Pneumocystis carinii*, *S. pneumoniae*, *Haemophilus influenzae*, *Cryptococcus neoformans*, *Rhodococcus equi*, or *Mycobacterium tuberculosis*.

A history of cigarette smoking is important not only because lung defenses against infection are impaired but also because smoking predisposes to carcinoma of the lung. Pneumonia distal to an obstructed bronchus (postobstructive pneumonia) can be a manifestation of cancer of the lung. An assessment should be made of risk factors for aspiration, such as recent stroke or neuromuscular diseases that interfere with swallowing.

The physical findings vary with the length of time since onset of symptoms, the state of the lungs before the onset of pneumonia (normal or chronic obstructive lung disease), and the size of the inoculum of the infecting microorganism. About 80 per cent of patients with pneumonia are febrile, and a few are hypothermic (core temperature less than 35°C [95°F]). Hypothermia is more likely to occur in elderly or alcoholic patients. Crackles are found on auscultation of the chest in about 80 per cent of patients, and 30 per cent have the physical findings of consolidation. Occasionally, a pleural friction rub is audible, and some patients have a pleural effusion. The physical examination should assess the severity of the pneumonia. Is the patient in respiratory distress? Is there a suggestion of hypoxemia as manifested by cyanosis or confusion? Does the patient have evidence of sepsis syndrome as manifested by hypotension? Table 2 gives physical findings that may suggest a specific etiology for the pneumonia.

CHEST FILM

The chest film is the "gold" standard for the diagnosis of pneumonia. It must be interpreted in the context of the history and physical examination. An opacity on the chest film may be caused by infection, blood, edema fluid, malignancy, inflammation, or a wide variety of processes such as vasculitis or the pulmonary manifestations of an adverse drug reaction. Pulmonary embolism can mimic pneumonia in its presentation. The opacification seen in bacterial pneumonia may be segmental, subsegmental, or lobar. Cavitation can complicate the mixed aerobic-anaerobic infection that follows aspiration. However, cavitation may also be seen in pneumonia caused by aerobic gram-negative bacilli such as *Escherichia coli*, *Klebsiella* spp., *Proteus* spp., or *Serratia* spp. *Mycobacterium tuberculosis* and *L. pneumophila* are other bacterial causes of cavitation. Pneumatoceles may complicate *S. aureus*, *Streptococcus pyogenes*, or *P. carinii* pneumonia. Small pleural effusions are seen in 20 per cent of patients with pneumonia. If the patient remains febrile and the pleural effusion increases, empyema should be considered. This finding can be confirmed by a computed tomography scan of the chest followed by needle aspiration.

Segmental or lobar pneumonia with lymphadenopathy suggests primary infection with *M. tuberculosis*. If the pneumonia is interstitial and there is lymphadenopathy, *Francisella tularensis* or *Chlamydia psittaci* should be considered. Other causes include *M. pneumoniae* and Epstein-Barr virus. The bulging fissure sign has been associated with *Klebsiella pneumoniae* but may also occur with *L. pneumophila* infection.

SPUTUM EXAMINATION

Critical evaluation of sputum is important in determining the cause of pneumonia. A considerable number of patients with pneumonia do not produce any sputum, but a determined effort should be made to obtain a sputum sample. Inhalation of an aerosol of hypertonic saline may help induce sputum production. The hypertonic saline causes bronchial irritation, leading to coughing and bronchorrhea. Visual inspection of the sputum is a time-honored technique. Rusty-colored sputum is associated with pneumococcal pneumonia, whereas "red currant jelly sputum" is characteristic of *K. pneumoniae.* Foul-smelling sputum suggests anaerobic infection.

The sputum Gram stain must be properly performed if it is to be interpreted correctly. When there are fewer than 10 epithelial cells and more than 25 leukocytes per low-power field, the specimen is indeed sputum—and not saliva. Samples that do not meet this criterion should not be processed for culture. When more than 10 gram-positive diplococci per high-power field are seen, the specificity for diagnosing pneumococcal pneumonia is 85 per cent, and the sensitivity 62 per cent. Clusters of gram-positive cocci

Table 1. Clues to the Source of Pneumonia From the History

Feature	Organism
Environmental Exposure	
Exposure to contaminated air conditioning cooling towers; recent travel associated with a stay in a hotel; exposure to a grocery store mist machine; visit or recent stay in a hospital (with potable water contaminated by *L. pneumophila)*	*Legionella pneumophila*
Exposure to infected parturient cats, cattle, sheep, or goats	*Coxiella burnetii*
Pneumonia following windstorm in an endemic area	*Coccidioides immitis*
Outbreak of pneumonia in shelters for homeless men; jails	*Streptococcus pneumoniae* *Mycobacterium tuberculosis*
Military training camps	*Streptococcus pneumoniae* *Chlamydia pneumoniae*
Animal Contact	
Exposure to contaminated bat caves, excavation of soil in endemic areas	*Histoplasma capsulatum*
Exposure to turkeys, chickens, ducks, or psittacine birds	*Chlamydia psittaci*
Travel History	
Travel to Thailand or other countries in Southeast Asia	*Pseudomonas pseudomallei* (melioidosis)
Immigrants from Asia or India	*Mycobacterium tuberculosis*
Occupational History	
Pneumonia in a health care worker who works with patients infected with human immunodeficiency virus in a large city	*Mycobacterium tuberculosis*
Host Factor	
Diabetic ketoacidosis	*Streptococcus pneumoniae* *Staphylococcus aureus*
Alcoholism	*Streptococcus pneumoniae* *Klebsiella pneumoniae* *Staphylococcus aureus*
Chronic obstructive lung disease	*Streptococcus pneumoniae* *Haemophilus influenzae* *Moraxella catarrhalis*
Solid organ transplant recipient (> 3 mo after transplant)	*Streptococcus pneumoniae* *Haemophilus influenzae* *Legionella* spp. *Pneumocystis carinii* Cytomegalovirus *Strongyloides stercoralis*
Sickle cell disease	*Streptococcus pneumoniae*
Human immunodeficiency virus infection with CD4 count <200 cells/μL	*Pneumocystis carinii* *Streptococcus pneumoniae* *Haemophilus influenzae* *Cryptococcus neoformans* *Mycobacterium tuberculosis* *Rhodococcus equi*
Multiple myeloma	*Streptococcus pneumoniae*

Table 2. Physical Findings Suggestive of a Specific Cause of Pneumonia

Periodontal disease with foul-smelling sputum	Anaerobes; may be mixed aerobic, anaerobic infection
Bullous myringitis	*Mycoplasma pneumoniae*
Absent gag reflex, altered level of consciousness, or a recent seizure	Polymicrobial (oral aerobic and anaerobic bacteria), macro- or microaspiration
Encephalitis	*Mycoplasma pneumoniae* *Coxiella burnetii* *Legionella pneumophila*
Cerebellar ataxia	*Mycoplasma pneumoniae* *Legionella pneumophila*
Erythema multiforme	*Mycoplasma pneumoniae*
Erythema nodosum	*Chlamydia pneumoniae* *Mycobacterium tuberculosis*
Ecthyma gangrenosum	*Pseudomonas aeruginosa* *Serratia marcescens*
Cutaneous nodules (abscesses) and central nervous system findings	*Nocardia* species

Table 3. Guidelines for Determining the Etiology of Community-Acquired Pneumonia

Definite
Blood culture positive for a pathogen
Pleural fluid positive for a pathogen
Presence of *Pneumocystis carinii* in induced sputum or in bronchoalveolar lavage fluid
A ≥4 fold rise in antibody titer to *Mycoplasma pneumoniae*
Isolation of *Legionella pneumophila* or a fourfold rise in antibody titer or positive urinary antigen test for *Legionella*
Positive direct fluorescence antibody test for *Legionella* plus an antibody titer of ≥1:256 for *Legionella*
Serum or urine positive for *Streptococcus pneumoniae* antigen
Probable
Heavy or moderate growth of a predominant bacterial pathogen on sputum culture and a compatible Gram stain
Light growth of a pathogen in which sputum Gram stain reveals a bacterium compatible with the culture results
Aspiration pneumonia diagnosed on clinical grounds

suggest *S. aureus*. *Haemophilus influenzae* is easily missed on Gram stain, because these small, gram-negative coccobacilli may be lost among the background proteinaceous material.

Sputum may be examined for the presence of *Legionella* with the use of a direct immunofluorescent antibody staining technique. If *M. tuberculosis* is suspected, Ziehl-Neelsen, Kinyoun, or auramine-rhodamine staining can be performed. *Pneumocystis carinii* can be detected with a monoclonal antibody in a direct immunofluorescence procedure. Sputum may also be examined for malignant cells when postobstructive pneumonia is suspected.

SPUTUM CULTURE

The sputum specimen should be delivered to the laboratory as soon as possible, and if it cannot be processed immediately it should be kept at 4°C, because pneumococci die very quickly. When anaerobic infection is suspected, the specimen should be obtained by either transtracheal aspiration or protected bronchial brush. Sputum is not acceptable for a culture for anaerobes because of the rich endogenous anaerobic flora in the mouth, through which the sputum has passed. Sputum culture results are usually available within 36 to 48 hours. Isolation of a microorganism from a sputum specimen does not mean that it is the causative organism. From Table 3 it is evident that, at best, an organism isolated from sputum can be interpreted as only a probable cause of the pneumonia. Sputum cultures should be interpreted with knowledge of the sputum Gram stain results.

All patients who are sick enough to be admitted to a hospital for treatment of pneumonia should have blood cultures done. Two sets should be done 15 minutes apart. About 10 per cent of the blood cultures will be positive. The leukocyte count is usually increased in pneumonia, accompanied by an increase in the polymorphonuclear leukocytes and immature forms. Leukopenia, if present, is a poor prognostic sign. Liver function tests are often mildly abnormal.

SEROLOGY

Acute and convalescent serology is important in the diagnosis of *Mycoplasma* and *C. pneumoniae,* but these tests are usually not used for bacterial pneumonias. Legionella infection can also be diagnosed serologically; here, however, the convalescent serum sample should be collected 6 weeks after the onset of signs and symptoms. Serology will be positive in only 75 per cent of patients with legionnaires' disease.

If legionnaires' disease is suspected, the urine should be tested for the presence of *L. pneumophila* antigen. A radioimmunoassay is available to detect the antigen of *L. pneumophila* serogroup 1. This test is 99 per cent sensitive and 99 per cent specific. *Legionella pneumophila* serogroup 1 causes about 90 per cent of all community-acquired legionnaires' disease. Recently, an enzyme-linked immunosorbent assay for the detection of *Legionella* antigen in urine has become available.

SPECIAL PROCEDURES

Transtracheal aspiration (puncture of the cricothyroid membrane by needle and passage of a catheter into the trachea followed by instillation of saline and aspiration of respiratory secretions) is now rarely carried out because the potential for bleeding is high. The procedure is contraindicated in patients who cannot cooperate, in those who are hypoxic, and in those who have ischemic heart disease. Fiberoptic bronchoscopy with a protected bronchial brush can be used to collect samples of respiratory secretions for culture. Quantitative bacterial cultures can be carried out on the specimen obtained with bronchial brush. In addition, bronchoalveolar lavage can be done. This technique samples a wider area of lung tissue and is useful for the diagnosis of *P. carinii* pneumonia and for cytomegalovirus. If necessary, tissue can be obtained by transbronchial biopsy. Bronchoscopy is mandatory in cases in which postobstructive pneumonia is suspected.

Thoracentesis should be performed when empyema is present. Not all patients with pleural effusion require thoracentesis. Aspirated pleural fluid should have cell counts, protein, glucose, pH, and lactate dehydrogenase (LD) determinations. Pleural effusion that is free-flowing with a pH greater than 7.3, glucose concentration greater than 60 mg/dL, and and LD less than 1000 U/L should resolve as the pneumonia is treated with antibiotics. If pus is found at the time of thoracentesis, chest tube drainage is necessary. The pleural fluid should also be cultured for *M. tuberculosis* and should be submitted for cytologic analysis.

Table 4. Noninfectious Causes of Cough, Fever, and Pulmonary Opacities

Pulmonary infarction
Atelectasis
Collagen vascular disease, especially Wegener's granulomatosis
Congestive heart failure
Sarcoidosis
Hypersensitivity pneumonitis
Lymphangitic carcinomatosis
Lymphoma
Eosinophilic pneumonia
Drug-induced pulmonary disease (a considerable number of drugs can do this: busulfan, bleomycin, cyclophosphamide, methotrexate, nitrofurantoin, sulfasalazine, amiodarone, gold salts)
Noncardiogenic edema due to salicylates, narcotics, chlordiazepoxide
Septic pulmonary emboli (in such instances, remember right-sided endocarditis)

Table 5. Stratification of Patients With Pneumonia

Place of acquisition	Community, nursing home, hospital
Comorbidities	Ischemic heart disease, chronic obstructive pulmonary disease, etc.
Immunosuppression	Corticosteroids, cytotoxic agents, human immunodeficiency virus
Severity of illness	Mild, moderate, severe
Place of treatment	Home, hospital ward, intensive care unit, nursing home

Pleural biopsy is often necessary for diagnosing tuberculosis pleuritis.

Percutaneous aspiration of consolidated lung tissue may also be used to obtain a specimen for culture. This procedure is probably best done by a radiologist under fluoroscopic guidance unless there is massive consolidation of the lung extending all the way out to the pleura. This test is rarely performed on immunocompetent adults. Diagnostic yield ranges from 33 to 85 per cent.

Open lung biopsy is rarely necessary in the investigation of patients with community-acquired pneumonia; fewer than 2 per cent of patients require this procedure. The diagnostic yield is about 25 per cent. However, the information is invariably helpful because it can exclude malignancy and because it allows modification or discontinuation of antibiotic therapy.

PITFALLS IN DIAGNOSIS

Failure to consider noninfectious causes of cough, fever, and pulmonary opacities (Table 4).

Failure to consider tuberculosis. Reactivated tuberculosis is occasionally seen in nursing home residents. Primary infection is again rising and can occur in HIV-infected patients and health care workers who provide care to HIV patients with tuberculosis (see the articles on tuberculosis and mycobacteria).

Table 6. Risk Factors for a Complicated Course or Mortality in Patients With Community-Acquired Pneumonia

Age >65 years
Comorbid illnesses, such as chronic renal failure, ischemic heart disease, congestive heart failure, or severe chronic obstructive lung disease
Concurrent malignancy
Postsplenectomy state
Altered mental status
Alcoholism
Immunosuppression
Respiratory rate >30 breaths per minute
Diastolic blood pressure <60 mm Hg; systolic blood pressure <90 mm Hg
Hypothermia
Creatinine >1.7 mg/dL or urea nitrogen >20 mg/dL
Leukopenia <3000 cells/mm^3 or leukocytosis >30,000 cells/mm^3
Pa_{O_2} <60 mm Hg or Pa_{CO_2} >48 mm Hg while breathing room air
Albumin <3.0 mg/dL
Hemoglobin <9.0 gm/dL
Pseudomonas aeruginosa or *Staphylococcus aureus* as the cause of the pneumonia
Bacteremic pneumonia
Multilobe involvement on chest film
Rapid progression of the pneumonia, defined as increase in the size of the pulmonary opacity on chest radiograph of ≥50% within 36 hours

Failure to appreciate the systemic complications of bacterial pneumonia. In the elderly, confusion caused by meningitis may be erroneously attributed to dementia or Alzheimer's disease. Endocarditis can also complicate bacteremic pneumonia, especially in the elderly.

Failure to consider that the infectious agent may be resistant to antibiotic therapy. *Streptococcus pneumoniae* resistant to penicillin, erythromycin, and tetracycline is common in several European countries and is now beginning to emerge as a significant problem in North America.

The physician can avoid many diagnostic errors and pitfalls by employing a disciplined stratification of patients with pneumonia, according to place of acquisition, comorbidity, immune status, severity of illness, and place of treatment (Table 5). If, on admission, the patient's respiratory rate is 30 per minute or faster, diastolic blood pressure is 60 mm Hg or lower, pulse is 140 beats per minute or faster, Pa_{O_2} is lower than 60 mm Hg, or mental status is acutely altered, the risk of death is increased. Factors that can help predict mortality or a complicated course in patients with community-acquired pneumonia are outlined in Table 6. Almost all the factors required for stratification and risk assessment can be obtained from the history, physical examination, and readily available laboratory tests.

ATYPICAL PNEUMONIAS

By Burke A. Cunha, M.D.,
and Anthony M. Ortega, M.D.
Mineola, New York

DIAGNOSTIC APPROACH

Atypical pneumonias are caused by unusual bacteria such as *Mycoplasma pneumoniae, Legionella* species, *Chlamydia pneumoniae* (formerly TWAR agent), *Francisella tularensis* (tularemia), *Coxiella burnetii* (Q fever), and *Chlamydia psittaci* (psittacosis). These disorders are best viewed as systemic infections with a pulmonary component. Extrapulmonary manifestations, however, often provide clues to the presumptive diagnosis of the atypical pneumonias. The clinician should subdivide patients with pneumonias into zoonotic atypical pneumonias, such as tularemia, Q fever, and psittacosis, and nonzoonotic atypical pneumonias, such as *Mycoplasma, Legionella,* and *C. pneumoniae*. A history of animal or animal product contact suggests a zoonotic atypical pneumonia. Otherwise, the differential diagnosis is most often narrowed to the common atypical pneumonias, namely, *Mycoplasma, Legionella,* and *C. pneumoniae*. Each of the atypical pneumonias has a characteristic pattern of organ involvement. To distinguish among the atypical pneumonias, the clinician should look for relative bradycardia, upper respiratory tract involvement, diarrhea, abnormal liver function tests, cold agglutinin titers, and hypophosphatemia (Table 1).

LEGIONNAIRES' DISEASE

Legionnaires' disease, which may be caused by any of the *Legionella* species, is transmitted by aerosolized droplets. The disease is reported most often in late summer or early fall, but cases may occur at any time of the year.

Table 1. Diagnostic Features of the Atypical Pneumonias

Key Characteristics	Zoonotic Atypical Pneumonias			Nonzoonotic Atypical Pneumonias		
	Psittacosis	*Q Fever*	*Tularemia*	Mycoplasma *Pneumonia*	*Legionnaires' Disease*	Chlamydia *Pneumonia*
Symptoms						
Mental confusion	−	−	−	±	±	−
Prominent headache	+	+	−	−	−	−
Meningismus	+	−	−	−	−	−
Myalgias	+	+	−	+	+	±
Ear pain	−	−	−	±	−	−
Pleuritic pain	−	−	−	±	+	−
Abdominal pain	−	−	−	−	+	−
Diarrhea	−	−	−	±	+	−
Signs						
Rash	± (Horder's spots)	−	−	± (erythema multiforme)	−	−
Nonexudative pharyngitis	±	−	±	+	−	+
Hemoptysis	+	−	−	−	+	−
Lobar consolidation	±	±	±	±	±	−
Cardiac involvement	± (myocarditis)	± (myocarditis)	−	± (myocarditis, heart block, or pericarditis)	−	−
Splenomegaly	+	+	−	−	−	−
Relative bradycardia	+	±	−	−	+	−
Chest Film						
Infiltrate	Patchy, consolidation	Patchy, consolidation	Ovoid bodies	Patchy	Patchy, consolidation	"Circumscribed" lesions
Bilateral hilar adenopathy	−	−	±	−	−	−
Pleural effusion	−	−	+ (bloody)	± (small)	±	±
Laboratory Abnormalities						
WBC count	↓	↑/N	↑/N	↑/N	↑	N
Hyponatremia, or hypophosphatemia	−	−	−	−	+	−
Increase in AST/ALT	+	+	−	−	+	−
Cold agglutinins	−	−	−	+	−	−
Microscopic hematuria	−	−	−	−	±	−
Diagnostic Tests						
Direct isolation (culture)	±	−	−	±	±	+
Serology (specific)	CF	CF	TA	CF	IFA	CF
Psittacosis CF titers	↑↑↑	−	−	−	↑	↑
Legionella IFA titers	−	−	↑	−	↑↑↑	−

↑ = increased; ↓ = decreased; ↑↑↑ = markedly increased; ALT = alanine aminotransferase; AST = aspartate aminotransferase; CF = complement fixation; IFA = indirect fluorescent antibody test; N = normal; TA = tularemia agglutinins; WBC = white blood cell.

Outbreaks in hospitals have been associated with contaminated water sources or nearby excavation or construction. The onset of legionnaires' disease is usually subacute but may be fulminant. Pulmonary manifestations of legionnaires' disease do not permit a specific diagnosis. Therefore, the most important clinical clues must be sought beyond the respiratory system.

Legionnaires' disease typically presents as a pneumonia that does not respond to beta-lactam antibiotics. Relative bradycardia, changes in mental status, abdominal discomfort, and diarrhea are features of legionnaires' disease.

Slightly increased serum aminotransferases in a patient who does not have a history of liver disease who presents with atypical pneumonia immediately limits the diagnostic possibilities to psittacosis, Q fever, or legionnaires' disease. Hyponatremia is more common in legionnaires' diseases than in other atypical pneumonias but is not specific for *Legionella*. Hypophosphatemia in a patient with atypical pneumonia strongly suggests *Legionella* infection. By contrast, cold agglutinin titers that exceed 1:64 strongly suggest the diagnosis of *Mycoplasma* pneumonia.

When a patient with *Legionella* pneumonia has a productive cough and has not received antibiotics, a diagnosis of legionnaires' disease can be rapidly confirmed with a direct fluorescent antibody (DFA) stain of sputum for *Legionella*. Unfortunately, *Legionella* DFA positivity decreases rapidly after effective antibiotic therapy has begun. Because most patients with legionnaires' disease do not have detectable serum antibody to *Legionella* early in the illness, a negative initial titer does not exclude the diagnosis. Furthermore, some patients never mount an effective antibody response, and antimicrobial therapy itself may blunt, delay, or eliminate subsequent antibody responses. Nevertheless, convalescent *Legionella* titers should be obtained 6 to 8 weeks after the onset of illness; a diagnostic rise in titer is typically present at that time.

In the absence of a positive sputum DFA for *Legionella*, a syndromic approach to diagnosis may be warranted. The syndromic approach combines history, physical, and laboratory findings, which of themselves are nonspecific but, when taken together, increase diagnostic specificity. For example, when a patient presents with a community-acquired pneumonia and extrapulmonary findings, the patient has an atypical pneumonia. When a patient with an atypical pneumonia also has diarrhea, the differential diagnosis is clearly limited to *Mycoplasma* or *Legionella* pneumonia. Hyponatremia is a common, though nonspecific, finding, whereas hypophosphatemia in a patient with atypical pneumonia often limits the diagnostic possibilities to legionnaire's disease.

With atypical pneumonia, a specific etiologic diagnosis cannot be made from the chest film alone. Legionnaires' disease does not have a characteristic appearance by chest film, but rapidly progressive asymmetrical infiltrates strongly suggest *Legionella* infection.

MYCOPLASMA PNEUMONIA

Mycoplasma pneumoniae is a common cause of atypical pneumonia. Although *Mycoplasma* pneumonia occurs at any time of year, small epidemics repeatedly occur during late fall or winter. The onset of the disease is usually insidious, following an incubation period of 2 to 3 weeks. The most common symptom is nonproductive cough. Other symptoms include fever up to 102°F (39°C), headache, and general malaise. Frank chills are uncommon. Diarrhea and other gastrointestinal complaints are reported by patients with *Mycoplasma* pneumonia as well as by those with *Legionella* pneumonia or adenoviral pneumonia.

Physical examination of the chest seldom reveals evidence of consolidation. Although extrapulmonary manifestations may be less evident than in legionnaires' disease, any organ system may be involved, since *Mycoplasma* pneumonia is a systemic infectious disease. Skin manifestations are common and range from maculopapular eruptions to Stevens-Johnson syndrome, which occurs in 5 to 10 per cent of patients. Cardiac involvement is the next most common extrapulmonary manifestation; abnormalities include arrhythmias, conduction defects, and congestive heart failure. Neurologic complications, including meningoencephalitis and reversible transverse myelitis, are uncommon. Asplenic or otherwise compromised hosts may be particularly susceptible to severe and overwhelming infections with *Mycoplasma pneumoniae*.

Routine laboratory tests other than cold agglutinins are not typically useful in the diagnosis of *Mycoplasma* pneumonia. Cold agglutinins are not specific for *Mycoplasma*; they can be detected in viral infections. Fewer than 75 per cent of patients with *Mycoplasma* pneumonia develop significant cold agglutinin titers; however, when titers exceed 1:64, the diagnosis of *Mycoplasma* is more likely. The "agglutinin-dissociation test" is a quick bedside test performed by collecting blood from the patient in an oxalated tube and immersing it in wet ice for 1 to 2 minutes, along with a control specimen. Observation of clumped or agglutinated erythrocytes on the sides of the glass tube and their disappearance on rewarming to 37°C correlates with the presence of cold agglutinins in a titer of 1:64 or more. (As noted earlier, a cold agglutinin titer of 1:64 or higher is presumptive evidence of *Mycoplasma* pneumonia.) By contrast, viral cold agglutinins typically do not exhibit the agglutination-dissociation phenomenon.

CHLAMYDIA PNEUMONIAE PNEUMONIA

Chlamydia pneumoniae (TWAR agent) is an organism that commonly causes disease of the respiratory tract. Pneumonia due to *C. pneumoniae* occurs sporadically but may also arise from outbreaks among college students and military recruits. The agent is spread from person to person via respiratory droplets.

Pneumonia due to *C. pneumoniae* may present in a manner similar to that of *Mycoplasma* pneumonia, but sinusitis, laryngitis, and pharyngitis sometimes precede the onset of pneumonia by a few days to a week. Otitis and pharyngitis often occur with *Mycoplasma* infection, but sinusitis is not a typical feature of *Mycoplasma* pneumonia. Laryngitis and hoarseness, when present, point to *C. pneumoniae*. Laryngitis is not seen with the other atypical pneumonias. The laboratory findings are not specific in *C. pneumoniae* infections, and chest films usually reveal patchy consolidation or interstitial infiltrates. *Chlamydia pneumoniae* infiltrates are sometimes described as funnel shaped. Pleural effusions are uncommon. Serologic studies may confirm the diagnosis, but *C. pneumoniae* grows poorly in cell culture. Primary infection is accompanied by a rise in the serum IgM titer within 2 to 4 weeks of illness, and a rise in the serum IgG titer within 6 to 8 weeks. Reinfection may not cause an IgM response, but the increase in the IgG titer will occur earlier than that in primary infection. Complement fixation (CF) testing is sensitive, but not specific. *Chlamydia pneumoniae* titers—not "chalamydia titers"—should be requested.

When empirical therapy is considered, tetracycline is the drug of choice. By contrast, erythromycin has often proved ineffective. That is, *Chlamydia* infections have sometimes presented as "mycoplasmalike" illnesses that have not responded to erythromycin.

ANAEROBIC LUNG INFECTIONS

By Miriam T. Vincent, M.D.,
and Stephan L. Kamholz, M.D.
Brooklyn, New York

Anaerobic lung infections involve the pulmonary parenchyma or pleural space as a locus for the proliferation of anaerobic bacteria, which in turn promote a necrotizing inflammatory response. These infections include aspiration pneumonitis, necrotizing pneumonias (hematogenous spread of anaerobic organisms from other foci), lung abscess, and pleural empyema. Pulmonary gangrene refers to rapidly progressive necrotizing parenchymal lung infection with interruption of local blood supply due to septic thrombosis.

Aspiration of oropharyngeal contents is the most frequent initiating event for anaerobic lung infections. Conditions in which consciousness is compromised are most likely to set the stage for aspiration. These conditions include seizures, alcohol or depressant drug abuse, central nervous system disease (e.g., stroke, encephalitis, metabolic coma), and general anesthesia. Other predispositions for aspiration include impaired swallowing; esophageal disorders, such as obstruction, dysmotility, and reflux; and protracted vomiting. Contributory factors that impair subglottic bronchopulmonary defense mechanisms include tobacco smoking, alcohol use, and ciliary dysmotility syndromes. Postobstructive pneumonia may be associated with airway lesions, such as neoplastic masses, saccular bronchiectasis, foreign bodies, and bronchostenosis, with anaerobic organisms as a component of the flora. The ability to contain and control small volumes of aspirated material (termed "microaspiration") is a crucial component of the pulmonary defense mechanism and is impaired in the face of alveolar macrophage functional defects and systemic immunodeficiency states. Poor oral hygiene is associated with gingival disease and intraoral proliferation of anaerobic bacteria, increasing the volume and pathogenic potential of the aspirate. Other routes for pulmonary anaerobic infection include hematogenous spread from various sources (e.g., abdominal infections, septic thrombophlebitis), transdiaphragmatic spread, and direct inoculation during penetrating thoracic trauma.

PRESENTING SIGNS AND SYMPTOMS

The anatomic location of the infectious process defines the symptomatic presentation. Parenchymal infections (aspiration pneumonia, necrotizing pneumonitis, lung abscess) are associated with cough, sputum production (mucopurulent or purulent early in the course, usually putrid in later stages), dyspnea, night sweats, anorexia, fevers, chills, including true rigors, and pleuritic chest pain of varying severity. Streaky, moderate, or massive hemoptysis can complicate any of these parenchymal processes, and hemoptysis is occasionally the dramatic initial presenting symptom. Patients or their family members may complain of profound halitosis. In more chronic presentations, weight loss, asthenia, fatigue, or intermittent fevers (with or without cough) may bring the patient to medical attention. Anaerobic pleural infection may cause severe pleuritic chest pain. Depending on the extent of adjacent parenchymal involvement, any or all of the characteristic symptoms may be present.

The physical examination in parenchymal pulmonary anaerobic infection typically reveals fever, tachycardia, and tachypnea. Localized thoracic findings may include rales, coarse rhonchi, wheezes, egophony, diminished breath sounds, percussion dullness, increased tactile fremitus (in the absence of a bronchial obstruction), and amphoric breathing. Other findings may include poor dentition and oral hygiene, halitosis, muscle wasting, weight loss, and digital clubbing. With empyema, percussion dullness is more profound and is accompanied by absent tactile fremitus and profoundly decreased or absent breath sounds. A focal area with signs of consolidation may be detected above the superior margin of the pleural fluid. Signs of coexisting parenchymal involvement may also be present (already discussed). Clubbing may accompany pleural empyema in the absence of abscess or other detectable parenchymal involvement.

COURSE AND COMPLICATIONS

Anaerobic lung infections evolve through a common series of stages after the arrival of the infecting organisms at the parenchymal destination. The aspirated inoculum consists of particulate material composed of food and oral secretions contaminated by a polymicrobial flora that includes both aerobes and anaerobes. The local evolution of the anaerobic lung infection is essentially independent of the route of infection. The bacteria are engulfed by resident phagocytic cells, which in turn release cytokines and other chemotactic factors leading to an influx of inflammatory cells, predominantly neutrophils. As a component of the exuberant inflammatory response, proteolytic enzymes and other inflammatory mediators such as toxic oxygen radicals are released to participate in the necrotizing process. Pulmonary consolidation, microabscess formation, and coalescence into frank abscesses may then ensue. Inocula localized to the periphery of the lung in immediate subpleural locations are probably responsible for isolated empyema in which parenchymal involvement is inapparent. More frequently, anaerobic empyema accompanies adjacent pneumonia or lung abscess.

Patients typically develop progressive signs and symptoms of an untreated infectious process, with fevers, localizing thoracic symptoms, and generalized weakness and malaise. Cough with sputum production is usually present, and foul-smelling, viscous, greenish-brown expectorate is common. Chest pain varies in severity and is a prominent complaint in those with frank empyema. The presentation may be indolent or modified by intercurrent administration of oral antibiotics. Delayed diagnosis due to patient inattention can lead to the development of a large, thick-walled, chronic abscess that is less likely to respond to medical therapy and may require surgical intervention. This finding is the most common complication of acute lung abscess.

Catastrophic complications of anaerobic parenchymal lung infection may supervene. These complications include massive hemoptysis and acute rupture of lung abscess into the pleural space with tension pyopneumothorax or bronchopleural fistula. Massive discharge of abscess contents into the airway can cause diffuse pneumonitis or the adult respiratory distress syndrome. Pulmonary gangrene is a rare complication of necrotizing parenchymal infection in which the involved lung parenchyma is infarcted, a complication that frequently requires surgical intervention. Although secondary hematogenous dissemination of lung abscess is rare, one complication is brain abscess. The complications of empyema include the development of fibrothorax and, occasionally, pleurocutaneous fistulae. The severity and extent of the anaerobic lung infection depends on host response to the pathogens. The virulence and volume of the inoculum are critical factors, as are the effectiveness of airway defense mechanisms and the strength of the immune system.

USEFUL LABORATORY AND IMAGING PROCEDURES

The hemogram often reveals chronic hypoproliferative anemia and leukocytosis with immature forms. The erythrocyte sedimentation rate is typically increased. Serum chemistries may show hyponatremia due to inappropriate secretion of antidiuretic hormone (SIADH). In chronic lung abscess, hypoalbuminemia and polyclonal hyperglobulinemia are typical. Dyspneic patients and those with concurrent or pre-existing cardiopulmonary disease should have arterial blood gases measured. Although the value of routine expectorated sputum cultures is debated, appropriately collected specimens submitted for both aerobic and anaerobic culture may be very helpful. These should be obtained with a plugged, sheathed microbiology catheter during fiberoptic bronchoscopy, or by sterile percutaneous fine-needle aspiration. Blood cultures should be drawn before antibiotic therapy is instituted.

All patients require chest films, both initially and during the course of management to define the nature, locale, and extent of involvement. The typical findings in aspiration pneumonitis include infiltration or consolidation in a dependent lung segment, usually the apical segments of lower lobes, posterobasal segments of lower lobes, or posterior segments of upper lobes. When a necrotizing pneumonitis is present, small rounded or cystic lesions may be seen within the infiltrate. Lung abscess is characterized by a cavity with walls of varying thickness. Often, an air-fluid level and surrounding parenchymal infiltrate are seen. In the presence of pleural fluid, bilateral decubitus views of the chest are useful. A horizontal air-fluid level extending to the chest wall on the upright chest film suggests bronchopleural fistula. In empyema, the decubitus views may reveal free-flowing pleural effusion, although loculation may occur in patients with long-standing effusion. Computed tomographic scans are often helpful in delineating and localizing abnormalities detected on chest film.

OTHER DIAGNOSTIC PROCEDURES

If pleural effusion is detected, thoracentesis is mandatory. Simple needle thoracentesis usually suffices, but when fluid is difficult to obtain, ultrasonographic guidance may facilitate aspiration of the diagnostic specimen. Aliquots should be submitted for aerobic, anaerobic, mycobacterial, and fungal cultures, as well as for cell count, chemistries, and pH analysis. The characteristic fluid in anaerobic empyema is thick, viscous, turbid or cloudy, foul-smelling, and often brownish or green. Microscopic examination reveals polymorphonuclear leukocytes, and the total leukocyte count usually exceeds 10,000 cells/mm^3. Gram stain of the pus demonstrates polymicrobial flora. Marked decrease in glucose concentration (often to <20 mg/dL) and increased total protein and lactate dehydrogenase are typical. The pleural fluid pH (with specimen collected and submitted anaerobically in a heparinized syringe) is usually less than 7.0. Nonempyematous parapneumonic effusions accompanying anaerobic pneumonitis or lung abscess may evolve to empyema during the clinical course. A second thoracentesis may be necessary when parapneumonic effusion increases in the setting of anaerobic lung infection.

Bronchoscopic examination is usually not required in anaerobic lung infection. The indications for bronchoscopy include hemoptysis, bronchial obstruction, and worsening disease. Similarly, fluoroscope-guided percutaneous lung aspiration biopsy is not often needed, but it may be helpful in establishing a bacteriologic diagnosis when initial therapy is not effective. Magnetic resonance imaging (MRI) is costly and rarely adds to the diagnostic assessment of these patients. Respiratory motion artifact degrades the MRI images and further limits diagnostic utility.

PITFALLS IN DIAGNOSIS

If signs of bronchopulmonary infection accompany a history of significant respiratory symptoms (productive cough, fever, auscultatory findings) lasting more than 7 to 10 days, a thorough evaluation, with chest films, is mandatory. This approach may decrease the frequency with which such patients are "presumptively" treated with oral antibiotics and may diminish the incidence of "missed" pneumonia, abscess, and empyema. When roentgenographic abnormalities are detected, appropriate diagnostic tests and follow-up are essential.

BRONCHIECTASIS

By Alan F. Barker, M.D.
Portland, Oregon

Bronchiectasis is a chronic respiratory disease with high morbidity and mortality. Bronchiectasis patients who have daily viscous sputum production and recurrent lower respiratory infections require frequent office visits and hospitalization. Bronchiectasis has been defined as an abnormal permanent dilation of subsegmental airways. These features were identified by bronchographic imaging at autopsy or in surgical specimens. Bronchography is rarely performed, and surgical resection for bronchiectasis has only a limited role in management.

CLINICAL FINDINGS

The hallmark, or key symptom, is cough with daily mucopurulent and tenacious sputum production lasting months to years. The older literature has described "dry bronchiectasis" with episodic hemoptysis but no sputum production; however, most patients produce phlegm daily. Dyspnea, wheezing, and pleuritic chest pain may accompany frequent bouts of "bronchitis" treated with antibiotics. Rhinosinusitis is almost always present. The remote history may identify a specific virulent pneumonia (e.g., pertussis, tuberculosis, *Mycoplasma*, or viral) or repeated respiratory tract infections over several years.

Foreign-body aspiration contributing to airway obstruction and bronchiectasis is important to recognize because surgical resection often produces a cure. Bronchiectasis as a sequela of foreign-body aspiration typically occurs in the lower lobes or posterior segments of the upper lobes. Although witnessed or recognized aspiration is uncommon, an episode of choking and coughing or unexplained wheezing or hemoptysis should raise the suspicion of foreign-body aspiration. In adults, an altered state of consciousness is associated with particulate aspiration. A history of seizures, stroke, inebriation, or emergent general anesthesia is typical. The foreign body is often unchewed food or part of a tooth or crown. An obstructive pneumonia with poor resolution or subsequent lung abscess may follow the aspiration. Delays in therapy or ineffective therapy and poor nutrition may contribute to prolonged pneumonitis with resultant focal bronchiectasis.

Several specific host defense defects have been associated with bronchiectasis. Humoral immunodeficiency is associated with low concentrations of immunoglobulins (IgG, IgA, and IgM). These patients are usually diagnosed during childhood with repeated sinopulmonary infections, but middle-aged adults may present with few or unrecognized previous respiratory infections. IgG subclass deficiency may also play a role in a few patients. IgG subclass concentrations may be decreased in the presence of a normal IgG concentration. Humoral immunodeficiency should not be overlooked, because gamma globulin replacement slows down or halts the respiratory tract infections and subsequent damage.

The major respiratory manifestations in cystic fibrosis are sinusitis and bronchiectasis. In adults, bronchiectasis may be the sole feature of cystic fibrosis. The clues to cystic fibrosis include upper lobe lesions on chest film and sputum cultures showing mucoid *Pseudomonas aeruginosa*. The sweat chloride determination is typically increased above 55 to 60 mEq/L. Some patients with suspected cystic fibrosis have a normal sweat chloride level. Cystic fibrosis is an autosomal recessive genetic disorder reflecting mutations in the transmembrane conductance regulator gene. Variations of the most common mutation (ΔF508) are being identified with normal sweat chloride concentration (see the article on cystic fibrosis).

Two rheumatologic diseases, rheumatoid arthritis and Sjögren's syndrome, may be accompanied by bronchiectasis. The arthropathy and sicca features are usually present and advanced. Some patients with bronchiectasis subsequently develop rheumatoid arthritis, but other causes of the bronchiectasis (e.g., tuberculosis) can sometimes be identified.

Although immotile cilia were originally described in the respiratory tract and sperm of patients with Kartagener's syndrome (dextrocardia, situs inversus, bronchiectasis), many other patients have been identified with dyskinetic cilia leading to poor mucociliary clearance and repeated respiratory infections. An epithelial (nasal or bronchial) brush or biopsy confirms the diagnosis.

Mycobacterium avium-intracellulare (MAI) has traditionally been viewed as a secondary pathogen in an abnormal host (e.g., in acquired immunodeficiency syndrome) or already-damaged lung (e.g., in bullous emphysema). More recently, several reports have described persons who appear to be normal hosts who have developed bronchiectasis with primary MAI infection. In addition to sputum smear showing acid-fast bacilli and a culture confirming MAI, the computed tomography (CT) scan of the chest is relatively specific, showing small, irregular nodules. It is important that the physician recognize primary MAI infection because antituberculous therapy may be effective.

Another association involves the fungus *Aspergillus*. Patients with a long history of asthma (often resistant to bronchodilator therapy) may also have a cough productive of sputum plugs or mucopurulence, suggesting respiratory infection. Sputum cultures in these patients may be positive for *Aspergillus* species. Laboratory results may show peripheral eosinophilia and high serum IgE as well as precipitating and specific antibodies to *Aspergillus*. This syndrome, allergic bronchopulmonary aspergillosis (ABPA), probably represents a hyperimmune reaction to the presence of the *Aspergillus* organism rather than a true infection. Chest CT scans show central airway bronchiectasis, unlike bronchiectasis from most other causes.

Cigarette smoking is responsible for chronic bronchitis and emphysema. Cigarette smoking and repeated infections may worsen pulmonary function and accelerate the progression of bronchiectasis, but cigarette smoking has not been shown to cause bronchiectasis.

PHYSICAL EXAMINATION

Pertinent physical signs are confined to the respiratory system. Nasopharyngeal examination reveals erythematous mucosa with pooling of secretions in the nose or throat. Nasal polyps are frequently found and may obstruct sinus drainage. Adventitial breath sounds are universal but not specific, with rhonchi reflecting airway secretions and collapse, crackles suggesting parenchymal damage or small airway collapse, and wheezing consistent with narrow and collapsible airways. Observation of expectorated sputum in a tissue or container confirms mucoid (clear) and purulent (yellow-green) components as well as bloody admixture. Digital clubbing has been described in earlier texts but is an uncommon finding.

Table 1. Laboratory Tests in Bronchiectasis

Blood Tests
Complete blood count
Immunoglobulins IgG, IgM, IgA
Aspergillus precipitins, antibodies*
Rheumatoid factor*
Imaging
Chest posteroanterior and lateral x-rays
High-resolution computed tomography
Sinus computed tomography
Sputum
Culture and sensitivity–smear for leukocytes
Mycobacterium culture
Fungal culture
Other Tests
Respiratory tract biopsy for ciliary ultrastructure*
Fiberoptic bronchoscopy (focal obstructing lesion suspected)*
Pulmonary function tests

*Not part of routine evaluation.

LABORATORY STUDIES

An underlying cause is found in fewer than 50 per cent of patients with suspected bronchiectasis. The tests in Table 1 include some that may suggest a disease or condition that is treatable. Imaging studies are always necessary to substantiate the diagnosis. In most patients, spirometry with a bronchodilator provides satisfactory assessment of pulmonary function. Obstructive impairment (reduced or normal forced vital capacity [FVC], low 1-second forced expiratory volume [FEV_1], and low FEV_1/FVC ratio) are the most frequent findings, but a very low FVC is seen in advanced disease.

IMAGING STUDIES

An imaging revolution has occurred in the assessment of bronchiectasis. Until the mid-1980s, contrast bronchography was the defining tool of bronchiectasis. Although bronchography is seldom performed anymore, the radiographic changes seen on chest films and bronchography reflect the terminology applied to modern CT.

All patients suspected of having bronchiectasis should have frontal (PA) and lateral chest films. The chest film is abnormal in 93 per cent of patients with bronchiectasis. Suspicious but not diagnostic findings include linear atelectasis, dilated and thickened airways (tram or parallel lines, ring shadows on cross-section), and irregular peripheral opacities that may represent mucopurulent plugs. A central (perihilar) distribution of this abnormal shadowing suggests ABPA. A predominant upper lobe distribution is typical of cystic fibrosis or one of its variants. In many patients, the combination of clinical signs and plain chest film findings may be enough to confirm the diagnosis. Further imaging with chest CT is indicated if (1) suspicious clinical findings are seen in the setting of a relatively normal chest film; (2) the chest film shows other abnormal findings (pneumonic infiltrate) and bronchiectasis is strongly suspected; (3) management depends on extent of bronchiectasis; or (4) the presence or absence of other confounding disorders (e.g., chronic obstructive pulmonary disease (COPD), interstitial lung disease) must be defined. If surgical resection is contemplated, mapping of the chest is required to define suspected abnormal areas and demonstrate the degree of involvement of the rest of the lungs.

The major features of the CT diagnosis include bronchial wall dilatation and thickening and the effects of airway obstruction. Airway dilation can be assessed when parallel (tram) lines or end-on ring shadows are seen. A luminal airway diameter 1.0 to 1.5 times that of the adjacent vessel is normal. A diameter greater than 1.5 times that of the adjacent vessel is typical of cylindrical bronchiectasis. Bronchial wall thickening is a more subjective feature, but it can also be observed in dilated airways. Obstructed airways in bronchiectasis may contain mucopurulent plugs or debris accompanied by postobstructive air trapping. Cysts off the bronchial wall are a feature of more destructive bronchiectasis. Blebs seen in emphysema are thinner walled and not accompanied by proximal airway changes. Consolidation of a segment or lobe (from pneumonia) may be seen, but this feature is not diagnostic of bronchiectasis by itself. CT may show enlarged lymph nodes, suggesting reaction to infection. Another confounding finding is "traction bronchiectasis," which is seen in pulmonary fibrosis. With distortion of lung parenchyma by fibrosis, airways can be dilated or stretched to simulate bronchiectasis. With this condition, other features of bronchiectasis are absent.

PITFALLS IN DIAGNOSIS

Asthma and chronic bronchitis are chronic respiratory conditions often manifested by cough and variable sputum production. Patients with asthma often have cough, but sputum production is scant and the chest film is usually normal. A complication of asthma is ABPA, as has been noted. Chronic bronchitis is almost always associated with a long history of cigarette smoking. The sputum production is usually foamy or mucoid, rather than viscous and purulent as in bronchiectasis. Coughing and shortness of breath may be disabling features of the interstitial lung diseases (pulmonary fibrosis), but sputum production is not apparent unless a respiratory infection intervenes. An acute pneumonia may linger for weeks or months, manifesting cough and sputum production. Other chronic conditions, such as diabetes mellitus, congestive heart failure, or COPD, may have contributed to the delayed resolution. If findings do not resolve after 6 to 12 weeks, an evaluation for bronchiectasis should be undertaken.

ACUTE RESPIRATORY DISTRESS SYNDROME

By Asha N. Chesnutt, M.D.,
and Michael A. Matthay, M.D.
San Francisco, California

The acute respiratory distress syndrome (ARDS) is a clinical syndrome of acute respiratory failure that is characterized by severe arterial hypoxemia, diffuse infiltrates on the chest film, and reduced lung compliance. Unfortunately, the term ARDS has not been uniformly applied or well defined. A recent North American–European Consensus Conference on ARDS has recommended more specific guidelines for the diagnosis of ARDS. The conference concluded that the clinical spectrum of acute respiratory failure represents a continuum of pulmonary physiologic and radiographic abnormalities. "ARDS" is now reserved for the more severe end of the spectrum, whereas the term acute lung injury (ALI) applies to the other pulmonary diseases seen in this syndrome. Thus, all patients with ARDS have ALI, but not all patients with ALI have ARDS. Other terms that have been used synonymously with ALI and ARDS in the past include noncardiogenic pulmonary edema, shock lung, and increased permeability pulmonary edema. ALI is now the preferred term.

DEFINITION

The specific criteria for ALI and ARDS include (1) acute onset, (2) bilateral infiltrates on the chest film, (3) arterial hypoxemia, and (4) lack of evidence of left atrial hypertension (Table 1). The degree of impairment of oxygenation is estimated by the ratio of the partial pressure of oxygen in arterial blood to the fraction of inspired oxygen (PaO_2:FIO_2 ratio), which must be less than 300 mm Hg for ALI and less than 200 mm Hg for ARDS. For example, oxygenation impairment criteria for ALI are met when the PaO_2 is less than 120 mm Hg despite supplemental oxygen therapy with an FIO_2 of 0.40. Part of the rationale for recommending a higher PaO_2:FIO_2 ratio for ALI is to identify patients earlier in the clinical course. The early identification of patients with impaired oxygenation may allow earlier application of appropriate treatment strategies to patients with ALI. This is an important objective because the mortality rate for ALI and ARDS remains high at 45 to 60 per cent.

The need for mechanical ventilation and/or positive end-expiratory pressure (PEEP) is not a prerequisite for making the diagnosis of either ALI or ARDS. Some patients with ALI never require mechanical ventilation, but in those who do, PEEP is nearly always used to improve oxygenation. The optimal level of PEEP remains controversial and should not be used as a prerequisite for the diagnosis. It may, however, be a useful parameter in the Lung Injury Score (LIS), which was developed to help quantitate the extent of ALI (Table 2). The Lung Injury Score shows little prognostic value early in the course of ALI and ARDS, but it does help clinicians assess changes in the severity of ALI over time. This scoring system is also useful in clinical studies of ALI and ARDS.

Histologically, ALI appears as diffuse alveolar damage. Although the injury can result from direct effects on lung cells as a complication of either a local or systemic inflammatory response, the pathologic features show little variation and include interstitial and alveolar edema fluid accumulation, hyaline membrane formation, and alveolar wall scarring. These pathologic changes result from injury to the pulmonary endothelium and occasionally to the alveolar epithelium. The acute exudative stage is characterized by protein-rich edema fluid in the interstitial and alveolar spaces of the lung, usually accompanied by neutrophils and red blood cells. The exuded protein may precipitate, forming hyaline membranes in the alveoli. Increased quantities of fluid cross the microvascular barrier, exceeding the capacity of the pulmonary lymphatics to remove the excess interstitial fluid. When the capacity of the interstitial space is exceeded, the edema fluid leaks into the alveolar spaces. The mechanisms for the arterial hypoxemia in ALI probably include shunting and a ventilation-perfusion mismatch.

CLINICAL DIAGNOSIS

Lung injury can develop within minutes to days following the inciting event, with the onset usually occurring within

Table 1. Recommended Criteria for Acute Lung Injury and Acute Respiratory Distress Syndrome

Criteria	Timing	Oxygenation Impairment	Chest Film	Pulmonary Artery Wedge Pressure
ALI	Acute onset	PaO_2:FIO_2 ≤300 mm Hg	Bilateral infiltrates on chest film	≤18 mm Hg when measured, or clinical absence of left atrial hypertension
ARDS	Acute onset	PaO_2:FIO_2 ≤200 mm Hg	Bilateral infiltrates on chest film	≤18 mm Hg when measured, or clinical absence of left atrial hypertension

ALI = acute lung injury; ARDS = acute respiratory distress syndrome.

48 hours. Clinically, the patient may present with nonspecific signs and symptoms such as dyspnea, tachypnea, and tachycardia. Rapid, shallow breathing is typical. Labored breathing with intercostal and suprasternal muscle retraction may presage impending respiratory failure. Auscultation of the chest can be unremarkable or can reveal rales and rhonchi. Signs of congestive heart failure or CHF (jugular venous distention, S_3 gallop, hepatojugular reflux, pedal edema, and weight gain) may complicate the diagnosis.

Hypoxemia

The earliest clinical sign may be tachypnea with an increasing oxygen requirement. Refractory arterial hypoxemia is the clinical hallmark of the disease (see Table 1). The degree of hypoxemia is estimated by the PaO_2:FIO_2 ratio (see earlier discussion). However, the severity of hypoxemia alone defines more of a continuum than a distinction between ALI and ARDS. Other defining variables for the severity of lung injury include the need for mechanical ventilation, the level of PEEP required, and the compliance of the lung.

Table 2. Components of the Lung Injury Score

Component	Point Values
Chest radiograph score, extent of alveolar consolidation	
No consolidation	0
1 quadrant	1
2 quadrants	2
3 quadrants	3
All 4 quadrants	4
Hypoxemia score (PaO_2:FIO_2 ratio)	
300 or more	0
225–299	1
175–224	2
100–174	3
100 or less	4
Total respiratory system compliance, mL/cm H_2O (if ventilated)	
80 or higher	0
60–79	1
40–59	2
20–39	3
<20	4
Positive end-expiratory pressure (PEEP) score cm H_2O (if ventilated)	
5 or less	0
6–8	1
9–11	2
12–14	3
15 or higher	4
The score is calculated by dividing the aggregate sum by the number of components included	
SCORE: No injury	0
Mild to moderate injury	0.1–2.5
Severe injury (ARDS)	≥2.5

ARDS = acute respiratory distress syndrome.

Radiologic Findings

The chest film in ALI reveals diffuse bilateral pulmonary infiltrates. The progression of the disease on chest film parallels the evolution of edema, with the initial interstitial edema typically progressing to a pattern of alveolar edema. Correlation between the chest film and clinical signs and symptoms is inconsistent, but a peripheral distribution of patchy infiltrates is the single most reliable radiologic criterion and is relatively specific for increased permeability edema. Although edema may not be seen initially, even with severe hypoxemia, infiltrates usually develop within the first 12 to 24 hours. Some patients with extensive pulmonary infiltrates may have only mild ALI with the use of the criterion of the PaO_2:FIO_2 ratio. Conversely, other patients may experience blood gas abnormalities only after alveolar edema has developed. Further studies are needed to correlate oxygenation abnormalities and the extent of pulmonary infiltrates on the chest film.

Absence of Left Atrial Hypertension

The exclusion of hydrostatic pulmonary edema in critically ill patients can be difficult, and physical findings of CHF do not necessarily exclude ALI. When hydrostatic pulmonary edema due to heart failure or volume overload is suspected, a therapeutic trial of diuretics and venodilators may improve oxygenation. Unfortunately, renal function may be impaired in many critically ill patients, and diuretics may be ineffective. When physical findings are equivocal, pulmonary artery catheterization should be considered (Table 3). The risks of central venous puncture and insertion of the pulmonary arterial catheter (arrhythmias, pulmonary infarction, infection) must be weighed against the potential value of the hemodynamic data. No arterial hemodynamic profile is diagnostic of ALI, but a high pulmonary arterial wedge pressure (PAWP) suggests that pulmonary edema is related to hydrostatic causes such as volume overload or CHF. A normal or high cardiac output and a pulmonary arterial wedge pressure less than 18 mm Hg are consistent with ALI. In some patients, echocardiography can be used as a noninvasive method of obtaining similar information. Surface echocardiography can assess left ventricular size and function and estimate the size of the inferior vena cava.

Pulmonary Edema Fluid–to–Plasma Total Protein Ratio

The integrity of the alveolar epithelial-endothelial barrier can be evaluated by measuring the protein content of the alveolar fluid. A sample of edema fluid (1 to 2 mL) is

Table 3. Indications for Pulmonary Artery Catheterization

Assessment of left atrial pressure
Definition of cause of shock (septic, hypovolemic, cardiogenic)
Management of fluid status, especially in oliguric renal failure
Management of fluids and vasopressors in refractory shock

collected in a specimen trap by aspiration through the endotracheal tube with the use of a standard 14-gauge suction catheter. Total protein concentration is then measured in the edema fluid and in a serum or plasma specimen drawn the same day. The ratio of pulmonary edema fluid–to–plasma (or serum) total protein is calculated. A ratio less than 0.65 is typically seen in hydrostatic edema associated with fluid overload or CHF, and a ratio greater than 0.75 suggests increased permeability edema seen with ALI. Ratios between 0.65 and 0.75 are indeterminate. Edema fluid must be collected early (within one-half hour of intubation) in the course of the disease, because reabsorption of edema water can artifactually increase the protein concentration.

Associated Clinical Disorders

The two most common predisposing factors for the development of ALI are aspiration of gastric contents and sepsis (Table 4). These two events are associated with a 30 to 40 per cent probability of ALI developing. Aspiration of gastric contents injures the lung when the pH is less than 2.5, even when the volume of aspirated fluid is small (50 mL). The acidic fluid causes an increase in pulmonary endothelial and epithelial permeability, with the subsequent development of pulmonary edema. Atelectasis also occurs as a result of alteration of surfactant activity and subsequent collapse of alveoli. Aspiration pneumonia is likely to develop in patients who aspirate oropharyngeal organisms and should be considered early in the disease course.

Table 4. Acute Lung Injury: Causes and Associated Diseases

Direct Injury
Aspiration
Gastric contents
Fresh and salt water (drowning)
Primary pulmonary infection
Bacterial
Viral
Fungal
Mycobacterial
Pneumocystis carinii
Toxic inhalation
Smoke
Corrosive chemicals (NO_2, Cl_2, NH_3)
Thoracic trauma
Lung contusion
Drugs
Heroin
Aspirin
Indirect Injury
Sepsis syndrome
Nonthoracic trauma
Fat embolism
Multiple fractures
Massive blood transfusions
Cardiopulmonary bypass
Acute pancreatitis
Neurogenic pulmonary edema

ALI develops in about 60 per cent of patients with sepsis syndrome. When sepsis is suspected or diagnosed, an exhaustive and complete search for potential sources of infection is required. Blood cultures and Gram staining of the sputum are necessary steps in the evaluation. Early bronchoalveolar lavage may be indicated when opportunistic infection is suspected in immunosuppressed patients. Judicious use of empirical antibiotic therapy may be indicated.

CLINICAL COURSE AND COMPLICATIONS

The only intervention consists of treatment of the underlying disorder and prompt institution of supportive measures. The major complications of ALI are (1) multiple organ dysfunction syndrome (MODS), (2) nosocomial infection, and (3) barotrauma. MODS occurs in up to 50 per cent of patients with ALI. Sepsis syndrome is the most common clinical problem associated with the development of MODS. Other patients at high risk for the development of MODS include those with severe trauma and hypotension requiring emergency surgery and multiple transfusions. Also at risk are patients with advanced chronic liver and kidney disease and immunosuppressed patients with underlying malignancy. Management remains supportive with an emphasis on early, aggressive treatment of infection and shock. The mortality rate increases with the number of failing organ systems and approaches 100 per cent when MODS persists beyond 4 hospital days.

The most common causes of nosocomial infection are ventilator-associated pneumonia, catheter-associated sepsis, and sinusitis (especially with nasotracheal intubation). When sepsis precedes ALI, the source is often extrapulmonary; when sepsis follows ALI, the source is likely to be pneumonia. Gram-negative organisms are the most common pathogens in ventilator-associated pneumonia. They colonize oropharyngeal secretions and gastric secretions in patients receiving H_2 antagonists or antacids and enter the lower respiratory tract by aspiration around the endotracheal tube.

Barotrauma is a complication of mechanical ventilation resulting in pneumothorax, pneumomediastinum, or subcutaneous emphysema. The incidence of barotrauma in ALI patients is about 10 to 15 per cent. It occurs most frequently with high levels of PEEP and tidal volumes greater than 12 mL/kg. On physical examination, subcutaneous emphysema is often present. The chest film reveals pneumothorax or air in the mediastinum, soft tissues, and neck. Barotrauma in the presence of nonpulmonary organ dysfunction is associated with a high mortality rate.

When the patient survives to be discharged from the hospital, the long-term survival is good. Restrictive ventilatory defects are common during the first 6 months after recovery, but they usually resolve. A few patients experience treatable airway hyperreactivity. Decreased diffusing capacity, especially with exercise, is the most common late abnormality. Nonetheless, the majority of survivors of ALI lose relatively little pulmonary function.

OCCUPATIONAL LUNG DISEASE

By Leonard J. Rossoff, M.D.
New Hyde Park, New York

The link of pulmonary disease to occupation dates back to antiquity. The recent interest in this problem is evi-

Table 1. Classification of Occupational Lung Disease by Major Site of Injury

Site	Disease
Nose	Allergic rhinitis
	Vasomotor rhinitis
	Nasal septal perforation
	Nasal cancer
Tracheobronchial tree	Allergic asthma
	Reactive airway dysfunction
	Tracheobronchitis
	Industrial bronchitis
	Byssinosis
	Bronchiolitis obliterans
	Lung cancer
Parenchyma	Hypersensitivity pneumonitis
	Pneumoconiosis
	Fibrogenic
	Nonfibrogenic
	Noncardiac pulmonary edema
	Emphysema
	Pulmonary alveolar proteinosis

Table 2. Common Materials Linked to Occupational Asthma

Animal / Vegetable	Chemical / Drugs / Metals
Animal	**Chemical**
Dander (rodent, birds)	Diisocyanates
Excreta (chicken, pigs)	Acid anhydrides
Fish feed	Acrylates
Enzymes	Epoxy resins
Larvae (locust, silkworm, screw worm)	**Drugs**
Shellfish	Cephalosporins
Vegetable	Tetracycline
Western red cedar	Penicillins
Mahogany	Isoniazid
Colophony (rosin)	Piperazine
Cotton	Methyldopa
Grain	Cimetidine
Green coffee beans	**Metals**
Tea	Platinum
Flour (wheat, rye)	Vanadium
Tobacco	Nickel
Gum acacia	Cobalt
Hops	Tungsten carbide
Hemp	

Adapted from Cullen, M.R., Cherniack, M.G., and Rosenstalk, L.: Occupational Medicine. N. Engl. J. Med. 322:594, 1990, with permission.

denced by a growing list of identified toxic environmental exposures and government agencies mandated to protect us from them. The respiratory system is constantly sampling the environment in large volume, with the risk that the inhalation of gases, mists, or particles may result in injury at various sites (Table 1). The impact of an injurious agent is determined by its physical and chemical properties, the length of exposure, and genetic and acquired host factors. The occupational exposure may be compounded by the effects of cigarette smoking, aging, and pre-existing lung disease. In addition, it may be difficult to distinguish these states from occupational exposure. This article focuses on the non-neoplastic impact of environmental agents on the airways and parenchyma.

AIRWAYS DISEASE

Occupational Asthma

Occupational asthma may be the most prevalent occupational pulmonary disorder and may account for up to 15 per cent of all patients with asthma in the industrialized world. It can be loosely defined as limitation of reversible airflow produced by an exposure in the workplace. Two types have been widely recognized: allergic asthma and reactive airways dysfunction syndrome (RADS). They are basically characterized by the latency of onset and mechanism of injury. A longer latency usually suggests an allergic or immunologic response (especially to high-molecular-weight substances). This type of asthma represents more than 80 per cent of occupational cases. A short latency and possibly single exposure suggest an as yet poorly defined irritant-induced asthmalike condition frequently referred to as RADS. In RADS, the exposure is short and the agent is usually a gas (e.g., chlorine) or vapor in high concentration. The onset is acute (<24 hours), but symptoms persist without a previous history of airways disease. Regardless of the mechanism, nearly 250 agents have been reported to induce asthma, and no simple classification is satisfactory (Table 2).

The diagnosis of occupational asthma requires (1) the recognition and confirmation of asthma (response to an inhaled bronchodilator or hyperreactivity to a nonspecific bronchial challenge), (2) suspicion of a workplace association, and (3) an attempt to isolate a single, specific cause. The initial reported symptoms are similar to those of idiopathic asthma and include cough, easy fatigability, and wheezing. Symptoms may first occur after departure from the job site and may initially be nocturnal. Physical examination may reveal bilateral rhonchi and evidence of hyperinflation. The timing of symptoms and signs in relation to the job and measurements of reduced airflow are essential to the diagnosis. Unfortunately, symptoms may subside outside the workplace and may not be detected in the physician's office.

Byssinosis

Byssinosis is an occupational airways disorder caused by exposure to textile dusts, including cotton, flax, and hemp. Signs and symptoms occur several hours after exposure and include chest tightness, cough, and dyspnea, which diminish on subsequent exposure but return after a hiatus from the job. It is distinguished from occupational asthma because it is unlikely to be immunologic in origin and does not demonstrate nonspecific bronchial hyperresponsiveness. It affects most exposed workers and progresses toward nonreversible airways obstruction.

Industrial Bronchitis

Industrial bronchitis refers to occupational disorders of the airways that usually present with cough and sputum production. They are not classified as asthma because they do not induce airways hyperreactivity, and progression to irreversible airways obstruction is uncommon. They appear to be associated with the inhalation of larger dust particles (3 to 10 μm) than those that cause pneumoconiosis. Coal and gold miners and foundry, textile, steel, and cement workers are at highest risk. As inducers of bronchitis, the dusts associated with these occupations are not nearly as potent as cigarette smoking, and they do not result in significant emphysema.

Bronchiolitis Obliterans

Bronchiolitis obliterans has been reported following exposure to various irritant gases, such as the nitrogen oxides, sulfur dioxide, and ammonia. Initial dyspnea and hypoxemia worsened by exertion may progress to respiratory failure characterized by the adult respiratory distress syndrome (ARDS). In 2 to 6 weeks, initial improvement may progress to extensive obliterative fibrosis of the bronchioles. The use of systemic corticosteroids may improve the usually dismal prognosis. Pulmonary function studies may reveal airflow limitation without hyperreactivity and impaired diffusion, but definitive diagnosis requires a lung biopsy.

PARENCHYMAL DISEASE

Hypersensitivity Pneumonitis

Allergic alveolar diseases (hypersensitivity pneumonitis, extrinsic allergic alveolitis) are colorfully described according to the etiologic nature of the organic dust exposure, for example, farmer's lung, pigeon-breeder's lung, and bagassosis (Table 3). The antigenic materials, which may also include organic compounds, have been identified in most cases, and they are small enough (1 to 5 μm) to penetrate deeply, resulting in granulomatous disease. Patients usually present with fever, cough, and dyspnea about 4 to 6 hours after exposure, with physical findings that are often mistaken for a respiratory infection. A more insidious form that is associated with chronic low-dose antigen exposure may present with only progressive dyspnea and eventual respiratory failure. Radiographic findings are nonspecific, with bilateral acute alveolar, nodular, or interstitial infiltrates in the middle and lower lung fields progressing to diffuse fibrosis in the later stages. Pulmonary function abnormalities typically show a restrictive pattern with decreased diffusing capacity, but in the acute stage airways obstruction may also be detected.

The best treatment is elimination of exposure to the sensitizing agent. Systemic corticosteroids may hasten recovery in the acute phase, but steroids have little or no long-term benefit. Inhaled bronchodilators may also be helpful when bronchospasm is detected.

Pneumoconioses

The word "pneumoconiosis" links the Greek words *pneumo,* the word for lung, and *konis,* the word for dust.

Table 3. Some Causes of Hypersensitivity Pneumonitis

Name	Source of Antigen
Vegetable	
Farmer's lung	Moldy hay
Mushroom worker's disease	Compost
Bagassosis	Sugar cane
Humidifier lung	Contaminated water
Coffee worker's lung	Green coffee beans
Tea grower's disease	Tea plant
Cheese washer's disease	Cheese casings
Maple bark disease	Contaminated logs
Sequoiosis	Wood dust
Wood pulp worker's disease	Wood pulp
Animal	
Pigeon breeder's lung	Droppings
Duck fever	Feathers
Turkey handler's disease	Turkey products
Laboratory worker's disease	Rat dander
Chemical	
TDI pneumonitis	Toluene diisocyanate
TMA pneumonitis	Trimellitic anhydride
Epoxy resin lung	Epoxy resin

TDI = toluene diisocyanate; TMA = trimellitic anhydride.

Table 4. Occupations at Risk for Silicosis

Occupation	Exposure
Miner	Gold
Driller	Copper
Excavator	Iron
Stoneworker	Tin
	Uranium
	Coal
	Iron
	Granite
	Sandstone
	Slate
	Clay
Foundry worker	Ferrous and nonferrous metals
Abrasives handler	Metal or glass polish
	Sandpaper
	Paint, rubber, and plastic fillers
	Sandblasting
	Tombstone engraving
Ceramics worker	Pottery
	Stoneware
	Bricks
Miscellaneous	Glass making
	Dental laboratory
	Gemstones

The modern connotation of pneumoconiosis is limited to permanent alteration of the structure and function of the lung (excluding emphysema and bronchitis) attributable to the inhalation of mineral dust. Some dusts produce more extensive fibrosis (e.g., silica, asbestos) than others (e.g., iron, barium). Some induce a granulomatous reaction (e.g., beryllium) that is difficult to distinguish from sarcoidosis. Immunologic mechanisms are most likely responsible for the injury. These diseases can produce significant morbidity and premature death, and they should always be suspected in the setting of chronic pulmonary disease, especially when typical findings are present on the chest film.

Silicosis

Silicosis results from the inhalation of silica (usually as quartz) during mining or quarrying of rock. Silicosis has declined in prevalence with the use of engineering controls and substitute materials, but it is still a potential problem in several occupations (Table 4). The disease often presents with nodules that are detected on chest film and is rarely associated with peripheral "eggshell" calcified hilar lymph nodes. The nodules are small (1 to 3 mm), are found mainly in the upper lobes, and may coalesce into larger aggregates. Large masses found in association with rheumatoid arthritis are reported as Caplan's syndrome. Clinical findings are typically few until late in the disease, when cor pulmonale may develop. Pulmonary function abnormalities, when present, typically include reduced diffusion capacity and lung volumes. Silicosis predisposes to tuberculosis, which must be excluded if corticosteroid treatment is considered. There is no specific treatment, and prevention requires elimination of exposure or the use of efficient face masks or other respiratory protective gear.

Coal Worker's Pneumoconiosis

Coal worker's pneumoconiosis (CWP), also known as anthracosis and black lung disease, results from exposure to coal, graphite, or synthetic carbon dust. The quartz contained in the coal is the likely pathogenic agent. Workers at the face of a mine are at highest risk, and the extent of fibrosis correlates with the total dust burden. A chest film may reveal nodules or diffuse interstitial markings often similar to, but less dramatic than, silicosis. There are no specific clinical findings or treatments.

Asbestos-Related Disease

The adverse effects of asbestos, a group of magnesium and calcium-containing fibrous silicates, were first observed and reported at the beginning of this century. There are two basic types of asbestos fibers: serpentine chrysolite, which is long and silky, and the more penetrating amphiboles. There are three types of amphiboles; crocidolite is probably the most significant carcinogen and inducer of fibrosis. Inhalation of asbestos has been associated with pulmonary fibrosis (asbestosis), pleural effusion, pleural plaques, mesothelioma, and carcinoma of the lung.

Asbestos predominantly affects the lower lobes and usually presents with dyspnea, dry cough, and fine bibasilar crackles. Progression of disease may lead to cor pulmonale. Interpretation of the chest films is difficult; significant inter-reader variability persists even with the use of the standardized International Labor Organization (ILO) system. Computed tomography (CT) is useful but is too expensive for ordinary screening. Pulmonary function testing typically reveals a restrictive defect and decreased diffusing capacity.

Chest pain, weight loss, and a large pleural effusion suggest mesothelioma, a diagnosis that requires percutaneous core needle biopsy or thorascopic or open biopsy for confirmation. There is no cure for mesothelioma, and the value of surgery, radiation, and chemotherapy is unproved. Relief of dyspnea and pain is the major goal. Pleural plaques, rounded atelectasis, and small benign pleural effusions (BAPEs), when seen on chest film or CT, are virtually pathognomonic of asbestos exposure but have little or no impact on functional status.

The risk of carcinoma of the lung in patients with asbestosis is nearly five times greater than that of nonexposed individuals. Cigarette smoking multiplies the risk by five again. Some studies have also associated asbestos exposure with an increased risk of colorectal and laryngeal carcinomas.

Talcosis

Clinically and radiographically, talc pneumoconiosis is similar to silicosis, coal worker's pneumoconiosis, and sarcoidosis. Inhalation of pure talc may cause acute or chronic bronchitis, and continued exposure results in chronic interstitial disease with multiple nodules. Crystalline talc contaminated by silica causes disease that is indistinguishable from silicosis. Talc that is contaminated by asbestos fibers causes all the asbestos-related diseases, including pleural plaques and malignancy.

Berylliosis

Exposure to beryllium results in a disease that is indistinguishable from sarcoidosis. Exposure to beryllium in the manufacture of fluorescent lights has been replaced by exposure in nuclear plants, weapons facilities, and plants that produce beryllium-metal alloys. The acute disease presents as inflammation of the upper airways along with bronchitis and pneumonitis. The chest film may show diffuse infiltrates with hilar adenopathy, and pulmonary function tests show reduced lung volumes and diffusion capacity. Treatment requires avoidance of exposure and supportive care with oxygen and possibly systemic steroids if significant hypoxemia is detected. Less than 20 per cent of exposures lead to chronic disease.

Hard Metal Disease

The drilling, grinding, or cutting of metals and other hard materials requiring high-speed metal tools with cemented tungsten carbide tips has resulted in occupational asthma and pulmonary fibrosis. The cause of the pulmonary disorder may not be the tungsten carbide—but the cobalt catalyst that promotes its binding. Pulmonary fibrosis is typically preceded by desquamative pneumonitis and a virtually pathognomonic infiltration of multinucleated giant cells.

Miscellaneous Conditions

Exposure to the fumes of zinc oxide and other metals may cause the flulike illness known as metal fume fever. The respiratory complaints are typically mild, and there may be no significant radiographic or pulmonary function abnormality. Repeated exposure may result in tolerance. The inhalation of iron compounds by miners or welders may cause siderosis, and rare pneumoconioses associated with exposure to tin, aluminum, barium, antimony, and zirconium has been reported.

GENERAL APPROACH TO OCCUPATIONAL LUNG DISEASE

History

The possibility of occupational and other environmental exposure should always be considered. A diagnosis of asthma should always be accompanied by a detailed occupational and avocational history, including a chronologic list of all jobs and chemical or biologic exposures. The clinician may need to seek information from the employer. When a specific substance is identified, the proximity, duration of exposure, adequacy of ventilation, and use of respiratory or other protective devices should be documented. Important clues include coworkers with similar symptoms or previous monitoring by the employer or health agencies. A variation of symptoms, especially improvement on weekends and vacations, may be useful. The widening array of allergens and irritants requires diligence and inquiry to arrive at the correct diagnosis.

Specialized Testing

Imaging Studies

The routine chest film is usually helpful in both asbestosis and pneumoconiosis. The extent and pattern of involvement may also be further elucidated with high-resolution CT studies. In asthma, the chest film will probably be interpreted as either normal or showing hyperinflation.

Pulmonary Function

Pneumoconiosis typically shows a restrictive pattern and reduced diffusing capacity. Hypoxemia is usually seen later. Exercise testing may also be useful in the detection of early disease. Serial testing is essential to follow the course of disease and response to treatment. Occupational asthma should show airflow limitation with reversibility after use of a bronchodilator. A history of worsening symptoms at work with improvement away from the job is typical. Objective evidence of these variations may be obtained with the use of an inexpensive portable peak flowmeter. Confirming the presence of bronchial hyperactivity with bronchoprovocation by nonspecific bronchoconstrictors (e.g., methacholine) may occasionally be useful. Specific bronchial challenge with a suspected offending agent is rarely performed outside specialized centers.

Biopsy

Fiberoptic, bronchoscopically guided biopsies may occasionally be helpful in the diagnosis of non–asbestos-related pneumoconiosis. The major role of bronchoscopy and biopsy is to exclude other disease processes. Bronchoalveolar lavage may prove increasingly valuable in the evaluation of hypersensitivity pneumonitis. Open lung or pleural biopsy is usually required to confirm mesothelioma or asbestosis. Thoracoscopy with guided biopsy of lung and pleura is a promising and less invasive approach.

INTERSTITIAL LUNG DISEASE

By Om P. Sharma, M.D.,
and Elton Katagihara, M.D.
Los Angeles, California

Pulmonary interstitium is the collagen framework that supports the airways, the pulmonary vasculature, and the lymphatics. As the airways reach the periphery of the lung, the connective tissue supporting the terminal airways blends with the alveolar basement membrane. The capillary connective tissue tends to fuse with alveolar capillary basement membrane. In many areas, the basement membrane remains separated by the interstitial space, which contains interstitial cells, reticulin threads, and elastic fibers. The interstitial cells can proliferate and differentiate into fibroblasts.

The clinical syndrome of *interstitial lung disease* encompasses a number of disorders that affect the alveolar walls, pulmonary interstitium, and small airways. The syndrome has more than 200 causes, including bacterial, fungal, viral, protozoal, and parasitic infections; collagen-vascular diseases (systemic lupus erythematosus, rheumatoid arthritis, progressive systemic sclerosis, ankylosing spondylitis, and mixed connective tissue disease); hypersensitivity lung disease or extrinsic allergic alveolitis; inorganic pneumoconioses (silicosis, asbestos, and berylliosis); drug-induced and iatrogenic entities; and disorders of unknown origin (sarcoidosis, idiopathic pulmonary fibrosis, eosinophilic granuloma, alveolar proteinosis, lymphangioleiomyomatosis, and bronchiolitis obliterans organizing pneumonitis [BOOP]). The sheer diversity and number of disorders make the task of arriving at a single diagnosis extremely arduous. Many of these diseases are benign and self-limited; others are chronic, progressive, and irreversible. All interstitial lung diseases, however, have common clinical, radiologic, and physiologic features (Table 1).

DIAGNOSTIC APPROACH

History

A thorough occupational history is of paramount importance in evaluating interstitial lung disease. Every occupation or job that the patient ever had should be recorded, including summer and part-time activities. Also list the occupations of spouses or live-in partners, because many disorders, particularly asbestosis, may be transmitted by dust brought home with clothing. History of recent or past exposures to inorganic or mineral particles, to organic dust, and to animal antigens (pets) should be identified. Drugs and chemicals that are known to cause interstitial lung disease, pulmonary infections (particularly human immunodeficiency virus [HIV] infection), immune disorders, and collagen-vascular diseases should be investigated. A smoking history may influence the evaluation: Many interstitial lung diseases, including histiocytosis X, alveolar proteinosis, amiodarone toxicity, idiopathic pulmonary fibrosis, and asbestosis, are common in smokers, whereas nonsmokers tend to be susceptible to sarcoidosis and hypersensitivity pneumonitis. The country of origin and recent travel history are often critical: A diffuse nodular interstitial roentgenographic pattern suggests tropical eosinophilia in a patient from India, but a similar roentgenographic abnormality may be related to pulmonary schistosomiasis in an Egyptian patient.

Clinical Features

Symptoms

Dyspnea is the most frequent symptom of interstitial lung disease. At first, dyspnea is evident only on exercise. Later, it progresses to breathlessness at rest. The duration of progressive dyspnea usually ranges from months to years. Dyspnea is commonly associated with fatigue. Dry cough, particularly on exertion, is frequently present. Fever, chills, and weight loss are the main symptoms in interstitial pulmonary infections but may also occur in collagen-vascular diseases. The combination of fever, cough, and dyspnea in an immunosuppressed patient is often due to *Pneumocystis carinii* pneumonitis, cytomegalovirus infection, miliary tuberculosis, or fungal infection. On the other hand, the constellation of fever, cough, chest tightness, and dyspnea that occurs 4 to 6 hours after exposure to an organic dust strongly suggests hypersensitivity pneumonitis. Severe dyspnea and weight loss without fever occurs in lymphangitic carcinomatosis, collagen-vascular diseases, and, rarely, disseminated tuberculosis.

Signs

Tachypnea is present in 10 to 15 per cent of patients with interstitial lung disease. Auscultation of the lungs reveals diffuse end-inspiratory crackles or rales in 60 to 95 per cent of the patients with idiopathic pulmonary fibrosis, acute hypersensitivity pneumonitis, or asbestosis. On the other hand, rales are heard in only about 20 per cent of patients with sarcoidosis. Rhonchi or wheezing, present in 10 to 20 per cent of patients with hypersensitivity pneumonitis, is not a feature of interstitial lung disease. Clubbing of the fingers is common in idiopathic pulmonary fibrosis and asbestosis. Erythema nodosum, uveitis, and parotid enlargement are important features of sarcoidosis. Multiorgan involvement is present in sarcoidosis, collagen-vascular diseases, histiocytosis X, and neurofibromatosis. The pulmonary valve second sound is usually loud, and a right-sided third heart sound is often heard in patients with severe hypoxemia, pulmonary hypertension, and right-sided heart failure secondary to interstitial lung disease.

Chest Radiographic Findings

The chest radiograph is abnormal in more than 90 per cent of patients with interstitial lung disease. Often the

Table 1. Interstitial Lung Disease at a Glance*

Group	Disease	Key Features: Clinical	Key Features: Chest X-ray	Key Features: Laboratory	Biopsy: Needed	Biopsy: Tissue
I. Infection	PCP, tuberculosis, viral, fungal	Fever, weight loss	Hilar and/or mediastinal adenopathy (unilateral)	HIV positive, tuberculin test ⊕, increased LD; cocci and histo-complement test ⊕	Yes	Lung
II. Inhalational						
Inorganic	Silicosis, asbestos	History of exposure	Eggshell calcification pleural plaques, lower lobe distribution	None	No	—
Organic	Farmer's lung	History of exposure	Upper lobe distribution	Precipitating (IgG) antibodies	Yes	Lung
III. Immunologic						
Collage-vascular	Systemic lupus erythematosus	Multisystem disease	Bilateral linear atelectasis, small pleural effusions	ANA positive, >15% DNA binding, positive smooth muscle antibody	No	—
	Rheumatoid arthritis	Polyarticular arthritis	Fibrosis, nodules, pleural effusion	Rheumatoid factor >1:80	No	—
	Scleroderma	Skin changes, dysphagia	Fibrosis	None	No	—
	Ankylosing spondylitis	Low back pain (men)	Upper lobe fibrotic changes	HLA B-27	No	—
	Polymyositis/ Dermatomyositis	Muscle weakness, heliotrope rash	Fibrosis, patchy pneumonitis	Increased serum muscle enzyme	Yes	Muscle
Granulomatous vasculitis	Wegener's granulomatosis	Triad of upper airway, lower respiratory, and kidney involvement	Nodular solid or cavitary lesions	ANCA positive	Yes	Lung
	Churg-Strauss syndrome	Asthma	Patchy infiltrate	Eosinophilia	Yes	Lung
Granulomas without vasculitis	Sarcoidosis	Multisystem involvement: uveitis, erythema nodosum, arthritis, heart block	Bilateral hilar adenopathy with or without lung involvement	ACE positive (60%)	Yes	Lung, skin, lymph nodes
Others	Goodpasture's syndrome	Hemoptysis, anemia	Diffuse ground-glass alveolar infiltrate	AGBM antibodies present	Yes	Lung, kidney
	Lymphomatoid granulomatosis	Skin, CNS lesions	Nodular, solid or cavitary lesions	None	Yes	Lung
IV. Iatrogenic						
Drugs	Pneumonitis	History of exposure	None	Lymphocytes in BAL	Yes	Lung
Radiation	Fibrosis	History of exposure	None	Lymphocytes in BAL	No	—
Oxygen	Fibrosis	History of exposure	None	Lymphocytes in BAL	No	—
V. Idiopathic	Idiopathic pulmonary fibrosis	Clubbing, end-inspiratory rales	Honeycombing	Increased LD	Yes	Lung
	Histocytosis X or Langhans' cell granulomatosis	Usually men, smokers	Upper lobe, honeycombing (fine lacework pattern), pneumothorax, HRCT diagnostic	Langhans' cells in BAL	Yes	Lung
	Lymphangioleiomyomatosis	Usually women, hemoptysis	Pneumothorax, HRCT diagnostic	—	Yes	Lung
	BOOP	Fever	Patchy, alveolar infiltrate	—	Yes	Lung
VI. Inherited	Alveolar microlithiasis	None	Micronodular infiltrate	None	Yes	Lung
	Gaucher's disease	Multisystem involvement	None	Gaucher's cells in BAL	No	—
	Neurofibromatosis	Café au lait spots, skin nodules	Nodules, fibrosis	None	No	—
VII. Inexorable	Lymphangitic carcinomatosis	Weight loss, dyspnea	Linear reticular infiltrate, Kerley's B lines, HRCT helpful		Yes	Lung

*Authors' note: There are seven groups, each beginning with the letter I; remember the seven I's.

PCP = *Pneumocystis carinii* pneumonia; BOOP = bronchiolitis obliterans organizing pneumonitis; CNS = central nervous system; HIV = human immunodeficiency virus; LD = lactate dehydrogenase; ANA = antinuclear antibody; DNA = deoxyribonucleic acid; ANCA = antineutrophil cytoplasmic antibody; ACE = angiotensin-converting enzyme; AGBM = antiglomerular basement membrane; HRCT = high-resolution computed tomography; BAL = bronchoalveolar lavage.

Table 2. Suggestions for Interpretation of Chest Radiographs

If Diffuse Interstitial Lung Infiltrate is Associated With the Following	Think of the Following	
	First	***Followed By***
Bilateral hilar adenopathy	Sarcoidosis, lymphoma	Tuberculosis, coccidioidomycosis, drug-induced lung disease, lymphangitic carcinomatosis
Unilateral hilar adenopathy		
Young (<40 years)	Lymphoma, tuberculosis, coccidioidomycosis	Sarcoidosis
Old (>40 years)	Carcinoma	
Mediastinal adenopathy	Lymphoma	Histoplasmosis, sarcoidosis
Eggshell calcification	Silicosis, histoplasmosis	Tuberculosis, sarcoidosis, lymphoma after radiotherapy
Pleural thickening/calcification	Asbestosis	Histoplasmosis
Pneumothorax		
Men	Eosinophilic granuloma	Idiopathic pulmonary fibrosis, sarcoidosis
Women	Lymphangioleiomyomatosis	
Parenchymal calcification	Alveolar microlithiasis, histoplasmosis, chickenpox pneumonia	Miliary tuberculosis, silicosis
Kerley's B (septal) lines	Left ventricular failure, lymphangitic carcinomatosis	Idiopathic pulmonary fibrosis, pulmonary hemosiderosis, sarcoidosis

first abnormalities to be recognized, the radiographic changes, are of paramount importance in elucidating the diagnosis. Although the chest film may not provide the definitive diagnosis, certain patterns are highly suggestive (Table 2). In general, parenchymal shadows may be classified into four categories: (1) normal; (2) ground-glass haziness; (3) linear, nodular, or reticulonodular infiltrate; and (4) honeycombing, representing end-stage fibrosis (Table 3).

Laboratory Tests

Laboratory tests are of limited value in establishing the cause and nature of interstitial lung disease. Only tests that are directly relevant to a clinical situation should be requested (Table 4). Complete blood count, sedimentation rate, total eosinophil count, screening for HIV, collagen-vascular panel, and serum angiotensin converting enzyme are some of the useful tests.

Table 3. Interpretation of Lung Involvement

Solely or Predominantly	Think of the Following
Upper zones	Eosinophilic granuloma or histiocytosis X
	Progressive massive fibrosis
	Ankylosing spondylitis lung
	Sarcoidosis
	Bronchopulmonary aspergillosis
	Cystic fibrosis
	Tuberculosis
Middle zones	Left ventricular failure
	Alveolar proteinosis
	Pneumocystis carinii pneumonia
	Sarcoidosis
Lower zones	Progressive massive fibrosis
	Idiopathic pulmonary fibrosis
	Alveolar microlithiasis
	Pulmonary hemosiderosis (chronic)
	Dermatomyositis
	Tropical eosinophilia
Uniformly diffuse	Miliary tuberculosis
	Lymphangitic carcinomatosis
	Disseminated fungal infection
	Alveolar microlithiasis
	Acute pulmonary hemosiderosis
	Bleomycin lung
	Pneumoconiosis
	Sarcoidosis

Pulmonary Function Tests

As a result of inflammation and fibrosis of the alveolar walls and the supporting structures, the lungs become stiff and have decreased compliance. Lung volumes are reduced, the diffusing capacity is impaired, and the alveolar-arterial oxygen difference is widened either at rest or on exercise. Although large airway function usually remains normal, small airway dysfunction is often present. Airway obstruction is prominent in hypersensitivity pneumonitis, Langhans' cell granulomatosis, lymphangioleiomyomatosis, and sarcoidosis. As a rule, pulmonary function tests correlate poorly with the degree of histopathologic changes, but the tests provide a baseline that can be used to monitor the course of the disease.

Histologic Diagnosis

When and why should a lung biopsy be performed in diffuse interstitial lung disease? An attempt to obtain a lung biopsy early in the disease should be made, particularly in young and middle-aged patients. This approach provides lung tissue before end-stage fibrosis obliterates any identifying disease hallmarks. Transbronchial biopsy is useful in the diagnosis of sarcoidosis, alveolar proteinosis, *Pneumocystis* pneumonia, and miliary tuberculosis, but the procedure has limitations because the amount of tissue obtained is often insufficient for extensive diagnostic studies. Open lung biopsy, the gold standard for diagnosis of interstitial lung disease, is now being replaced by thoracoscopic lung biopsy. Usually, diagnosis of idiopathic interstitial fibrosis, Langhans' cell granulomatosis, collagen-vascular disease, or BOOP requires an open lung biopsy (Fig. 1).

Assessment of Disease Activity

Chest radiographs and pulmonary function tests may indicate the extent and severity of functional abnormality. However, it is difficult to assess the activity of inflammation except by repeated lung biopsies. The following three

Table 4. Laboratory Tests Commonly Used in Interstitial Lung Disease

Complete blood count, sedimentation rate
Sputum (smears and culture): acid-fast bacilli, fungi
Skin tests: tuberculin, Kveim, coccidioidin, histoplasmin
Rheumatoid factor, ANA, LE cells in pleural fluid, immunoglobulins
Liver function tests
Angiotensin converting enzyme
Hypersensitivity pneumonitis panel
Inhalational challenge tests for occupational and hypersensitivity diseases
Bronchoscopy: bronchoalveolar lavage, transbronchial biopsy
Bone marrow and liver biopsies
Lung biopsy: thoracotomy, thoracoscopy
Lymphocyte transformation test (berylliosis, gold pneumonitis)
Gallium lung scan (to assess activity)
Spirometry, diffusing capacity for carbon monoxide, and arterial blood gases

ANA = antinuclear antibody; LE = lupus erythematosus.

methods have been proposed to evaluate the intensity of inflammation.

Bronchoalveolar Lavage

Bronchoalveolar lavage (BAL) has enhanced our knowledge of the pathogenesis of several interstitial lung diseases, including sarcoidosis, hypersensitivity pneumonitis, and idiopathic pulmonary fibrosis, but the utility of the test is far from established. In patients with idiopathic pulmonary fibrosis, the BAL fluid contains more neutrophils and eosinophils than are found in normal control subjects. BAL lymphocytosis often is a feature of sarcoidosis and hypersensitivity pneumonitis. Immunoglobulin G (IgG) concentrations are increased in interstitial pulmonary fibrosis, whereas IgM is increased in hypersensitivity

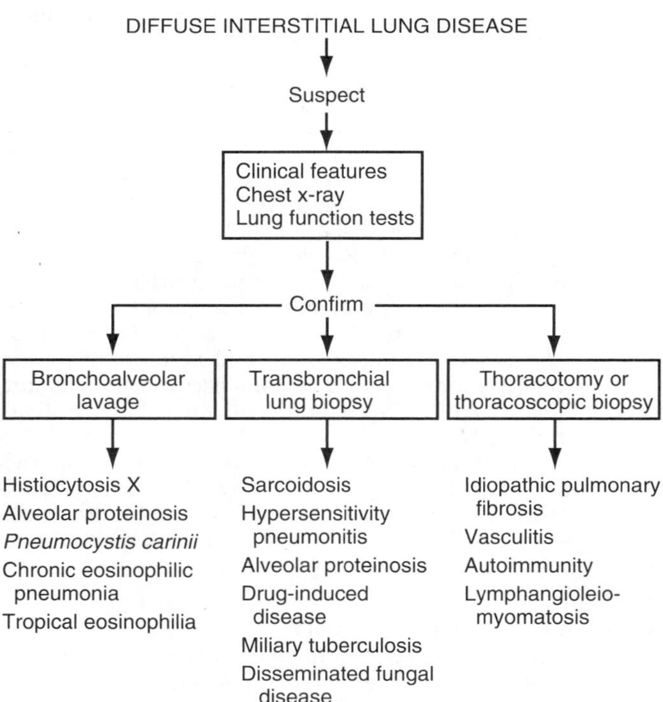

Figure 1. Diagnosis of interstitial lung disease: An algorithm.

pneumonitis. Both the percentage of inflammatory cells and the immunoglobulin concentrations decrease during treatment with corticosteroids.

Gallium Scanning

The ^{67}Ga isotope tends to localize in areas of inflammation. This increased concentration of the isotope occurs in about two thirds of patients with interstitial fibrosis. After the disease becomes chronic, the ^{67}Ga uptake diminishes, indicating low or absent inflammation. Although ^{67}Ga reflects the intensity of alveolar inflammation, it does not clearly reflect the functional capacity of the lung.

High-Resolution Computed Tomography

Both high-resolution computed tomography (HRCT) and the traditional (CT) examination are superior to conventional radiography and magnetic resonance imaging (MRI) in delineating the presence and extent of parenchymal abnormalities in interstitial lung disease. HRCT can help distinguish reversible, mostly inflammatory, changes from irreversible, presumably fibrotic, changes. Reversible changes include nodules, irregular nodules, and alveolar or pseudoalveolar consolidation. Irreversible changes include ground-glass opacity in patients with chronic disease, septal or nonseptal lines, cysts, bronchiectasis, and honeycombing. HRCT may be particularly helpful in distinguishing sarcoidosis from idiopathic pulmonary fibrosis (Table 5).

Indications for use of BAL, gallium scan, and HRCT in assessing activity, extent, and severity of the interstitial process are not clearly defined, and their value in day-to-day management is uncertain.

IMPORTANT INTERSTITIAL DISEASES

Two thirds of all patients with interstitial pulmonary disorders have sarcoidosis, collagen-vascular disease, idiopathic pulmonary fibrosis, or BOOP. Less common entities include drug-induced pulmonary disease, pulmonary infiltration with eosinophilia (PIE) syndrome, hypersensitivity pneumonitis, histiocytosis X, pulmonary alveolar proteinosis, pulmonary vasculitis, and granulomatous and nongranulomatous infections.

Sarcoidosis

Sarcoidosis is a multisystem granulomatous disorder of unknown cause that most frequently affects young adults. Although the disease is associated with other conditions (Table 6), the lungs are the most commonly affected organs. About 20 to 50 per cent of patients have symptoms of dyspnea, cough, and chest discomfort. Irritation, photophobia, and loss of visual acuity result from acute uveitis. A form of sarcoidosis with ocular involvement, parotid enlargement, and cranial nerve palsy is called Heerfordt's syndrome. Occasionally, chronic skin lesions, polyuria, polydipsia, facial palsy, arthritis, heart block, and neurologic lesions are the presenting features.

There are four types of pulmonary changes: (1) bilateral hilar adenopathy; (2) bilateral hilar adenopathy accompanied by diffuse pulmonary infiltration; (3) pulmonary infiltration or fibrosis without hilar adenopathy; and (4) bullae, cysts, and emphysematous changes. If indicated, a lung biopsy should be performed for histologic confirmation. The histologic lesion in sarcoidosis is a discrete, round granuloma made up of densely packed epithelioid cells, a few

Table 5. High-Resolution Computed Tomography Findings in Sarcoidosis and Idiopathic Interstitial Fibrosis

	Sarcoidosis	Diffuse Interstitial Fibrosis
Abnormalities	Nodular or beaded bronchovascular bundles, interlobular septa, and subpleural interstitium	Irregular
Distribution	Central, parahilar, medullary	Peripheral, patchy, subpleural, cortical
Predominance	Upper lobes	Lower lobes
Nodule	Frequent	Rare
Adenopathy	Present	Absent

multinucleated giant cells, and a scanty layer of lymphocytes. A granulomatous response similar to that of sarcoidosis is found in many other conditions, and the histologic findings should be correlated with the clinical and laboratory information to arrive at the most probable diagnosis (see the article on sarcoidosis).

Idiopathic Pulmonary Fibrosis

Idiopathic fibrosis, or cryptogenic fibrosing alveolitis, is second in frequency to sarcoidosis as a cause of chronic interstitial lung disease. Patients are usually in the fourth to seventh decades of life; men and women are equally affected. There is no clear racial or familial predisposition for the disease. The patient typically complains of shortness of breath and dry cough. Hemoptysis is rare. About one third of patients give a history of viral pneumonitis. Characteristic fine end-inspiratory crackles are present in about 90 per cent of patients. Another curious and unexplained but very helpful clinical sign is clubbing of the fingers, present in about 65 to 70 per cent of these patients (hypertrophic pulmonary osteoarthropathy). Although transbronchial biopsy may be helpful in excluding granulomatous and infectious processes, either a thoracoscopic or an open lung biopsy should be performed to obtain lung tissue. In early stages of idiopathic pulmonary fibrosis, the alveolar spaces are filled with alveolar macrophages, and the walls are infiltrated with inflammatory cells including plasma cells, lymphocytes, eosinophils, and neutrophils.

Corticosteroids are often effective in early stages of idiopathic pulmonary fibrosis. The chronic stage shows fibrosis, honeycombing, and loss of lung architecture. At this stage, medical therapy is futile. Single-lung transplantation in such patients is an encouraging option.

Several histologic descriptions are related to the clinical syndromes.

Usual Interstitial Pneumonitis

Usual interstitial pneumonitis (UIP) is characterized by a patchy distribution of the lesions in various developmental stages. Parts of the lung may appear normal, while other areas may reveal dense fibrosis, honeycombing, and cystic spaces. UIP is clinically and histologically distinct from *acute* interstitial pneumonitis.

Desquamative Interstitial Pneumonitis

Desquamative interstitial pneumonitis (DIP) is characterized by the uniform filling of air spaces by macrophages, mononuclear cells, lymphocytes, and plasma cells. Thickening and fibrosis of the alveolar septa are minimal. DIP most likely represents an early stage of UIP.

Lymphocytic Interstitial Pneumonitis

In lymphocytic interstitial pneumonitis (LIP), the diffuse interstitial infiltrate consists primarily of lymphocytes that crowd alveolar walls and lymphatic pathways. Small, noncleaved lymphocytes may form small nodules. The wide spectrum of lymphocytic interstitial pneumonitis includes idiopathic LIP and LIP associated with connective tissue disorders, Sjögren's syndrome, hypogammaglobulinemia,

Table 6. Collagen Vascular Disease Associated With Diffuse Interstitial Lung Disease

Entity	Clinical Features	Chest X-ray Features	Diagnostic Tests	Lung Biopsy
Rheumatoid arthritis	Polyarticular arthritis, rheumatoid nodules	Interstitial fibrosis, nodules, pleural effusion	Rheumatoid factor >180	No
Systemic lupus erythematosus	Arthritis, skin rash, renal disease, anemia, leukopenia	Bilateral linear atelectasis, pleural effusion	Positive ANA; antibody to dsDNA; anti-Sm Ab; anticardiolipin	No
Polymyositis, dermatomyositis	Muscle weakness, skin rash	Interstitial infiltrate	Increased serum muscle enzymes, anti-Jo antibody	Muscle biopsy diagnostic; lung biopsy not needed
Progressive systemic sclerosis	Dyspnea, dysphagia, skin changes	Interstitial infiltrate	Anti-Scl-70 Ab	No
Mixed connective tissue disease	Polyarthritis, pleuritis, Raynaud's phenomenon, dysphagia	Diffuse interstitial infiltrate	Anti-RNP Ab	No
Ankylosing spondylitis	Low back pain, hemoptysis, anterior uveitis, aortic valve incompetence	Upper lobe disease	HLA-B27	No

ANA = antinuclear antibody; dsDNA = double-stranded DNA; anti-Sm Ab = antibodies to the Smith antigen; Anti-Scl-70 Ab = antibody to DNA topoisomerase (Scl-70); Anti-RNP Ab = antibody to nuclear ribonucleoprotein.

and acquired immunodeficiency syndrome. Although the outcome of LIP varies with the primary cause, an excellent therapeutic response to corticosteroids occurs in some patients. On the other hand, some patients with LIP subsequently develop lymphomas.

Plasma Cell Interstitial Pneumonitis

The pathologic picture of plasma cell interstitial pneumonitis (PIP) suggests it is a variant of LIP. PIP is uncommon, and response to corticosteroids or immunosuppressive drugs has been documented.

Giant Cell Interstitial Pneumonitis

Giant cell interstitial pneumonitis (GIP) is caused by tungsten and cobalt used in the hard metal and diamond polishing industries. Measles pneumonitis is also characterized microscopically by the presence of giant cells.

Eosinophilic Interstitial Pneumonitis

Drugs, environmental agents, parasites, and various vasculitides may induce alveolar and eosinophilic interstitial pneumonitis (EIP). Tropical pulmonary eosinophilia and hypereosinophilic syndrome are important causes of eosinophilic lung disease.

Collagen-Vascular Diseases

The connective tissue disorders are a heterogenous group characterized by acute and chronic inflammation of synovial and serosal membranes and small blood vessels. There is a high frequency of visceral involvement that includes the lungs, heart, and kidneys. The lungs are frequently affected in all connective tissue disorders, including rheumatoid arthritis, systemic lupus erythematosus, scleroderma, polymyositis-dermatomyositis complex, ankylosing spondylitis, and mixed connective tissue disease (see Table 6). Rarely, lung involvement appears long before the other systemic manifestations of the disease and may lead to restrictive pulmonary impairment. Except for chest pain associated with pleural inflammation, the most common symptom of lung affliction is dyspnea, which occasionally may occur even when the chest film and pulmonary function tests are normal.

Bronchiolitis Obliterans Organizing Pneumonitis

BOOP is characterized by fever, cough, dyspnea, malaise, and muscle aches. Both sexes are affected equally, but the patients tend to be younger than those with idiopathic pulmonary fibrosis (Table 7). Physical examination may demonstrate rales and rhonchi. The chest film shows typical patchy alveolar densities occupying predominantly the peripheral areas of the lung. Hilar adenopathy, pleural effusions, honeycombing cavities, and bullous areas are absent. Fiberoptic bronchoscopy or thoracoscopy should be done in all patients. The diagnostic feature of the illness is the presence of connective tissue plugs in small airways. The granulation tissue, alveoli, and alveolar walls are infiltrated with lymphocytes, plasma cells, and occasional eosinophils. Prednisone is the treatment of choice. Response to prednisone is a diagnostic feature of the disease; 65 to 70 per cent of patients show complete clinical, radiologic, and physiologic recovery within a period of 2 to 3 months.

Iatrogenic Pulmonary Disease

A high index of suspicion and a meticulous clinical history are required to recognize iatrogenic pulmonary disease because the clinical, physiologic, and radiographic features are nonspecific. The patients receiving the offending drugs, radiation, or oxygen often have other complex illnesses. Furthermore, the pathologic changes are not always sufficient to exclude opportunistic infections and other interstitial disorders.

Histiocytosis X

Histiocytosis X (Langhans' cell granuloma; pulmonary eosinophilic granuloma) is characterized by an abnormal collection of histiocytes or Langhans' cells in the lung. The disease primarily affects young and middle-aged smokers. Cough, dyspnea, and chest discomfort are common symptoms. Spontaneous pneumothorax occurs in about 25 to 30 per cent of patients. A few patients develop bone lesions and diabetes insipidus. The chest radiograph shows interstitial disease, with or without honeycombing, involving the upper lung fields.

Pulmonary Vasculitis and Alveolar Hemorrhage Syndrome

Pulmonary vasculitis is defined as necrotizing inflammation of vessel walls in the lungs. Patients usually have complex multisystemic disease, and the diagnosis is often based on characteristic histopathologic features. Wegener's granulomatosis, Churg-Strauss disease, polyarteritis nodosa, bronchocentric granulomatosis, and lymphomatoid granulomatosis are the important entities. Many of these vasculitides produce hemoptysis as the initial clinical manifestation. In patients with diffuse interstitial disease and hemoptysis, Goodpasture's syndrome and idiopathic pulmonary hemosiderosis should be considered. Alveolar hemorrhage is rare in other collagen-vascular diseases.

Pulmonary Infiltration With Eosinophilia Syndrome

PIE syndrome is the association of pulmonary infiltrates and systemic eosinophilia. The patient usually has fever,

Table 7. Distinguishing Features of Idiopathic Pulmonary Fibrosis (IPF) and Bronchiolitis Obliterans Organizing Pneumonia (BOOP)

Feature	IPF	BOOP
Age (years)	40–70	40–60
Course	Chronic	Subacute
Symptoms	Dyspnea, fever, cough	Dyspnea, fever, cough
Signs	Rales, clubbing of fingers	Rales, rhonchi
Chest radiographs	Honeycombing	Patchy peripheral densities
Pathologic features	Interstitial neutrophils, eosinophils, plasma cells	Intraluminal plugs
Corticosteroids	1 mg/kg daily, orally	1 mg/kg daily, orally
Response to treatment	Moderate (20%)	Favorable (75%)

Table 8. Causes of Pulmonary Infiltration With Eosinophilia (PIE) Syndrome

Extrinsic (Known Causes)
- Allergic bronchopulmonary aspergillosis
- Tropical eosinophilia
- Infections (tuberculosis, fungi)
- Parasites
- Drugs (methotrexate)

Intrinsic (Causes Not Known)

Associated With Multisystem Involvement
- Sarcoidosis
- Vasculitides
- Eosinophilic granuloma

Not Associated With Multisystem Involvement
- Loeffler's syndrome
- Chronic eosinophilic pneumonia
- Hypereosinophilic syndrome

cough, and an abnormal chest film. There are many causes of PIE syndrome (Table 8). Many of these disorders are benign and do not require treatment.

Pulmonary Alveolar Proteinosis

Although pulmonary alveolar proteinosis is an alveolar-filling disease with little interstitial involvement, it often is included in the differential diagnosis of interstitial lung disease. Adults in the third to sixth decades of life are most likely to be affected. Chest films show bilateral alveolar space densities. Two characteristic features of alveolar proteinosis are a very high serum lactate dehydrogenase (LD) activity that reflects impaired function of alveolar macrophages and type II pneumocytes, and a large alveolar-arterial oxygen difference indicating severe ventilation-perfusion abnormality.

In summary, the term interstitial lung disease encompasses a wide spectrum of clinical entities that share certain common radiologic and physiologic features. Some of these illnesses run a benign course, whereas others progress to severe cor pulmonale resulting in death. A logical approach to diagnosis of interstitial lung disease is essential in order to treat and prevent the consequent severe morbidity and considerable mortality.

TESTS OF RESPIRATORY FUNCTION

By Paul Enright, M.D.
Tucson, Arizona

Pulmonary function (PF) tests are performed most commonly when a patient has symptoms suggesting pulmonary disease or a history of pulmonary disease, but they are also performed when risk factors such as cigarette smoking are known (Table 1). Spirometry is the most readily available and most useful PF test. It takes 10 to 15 minutes to perform in an outpatient clinic and carries no risk. Spirometry should be performed in all smokers past the age of 40 years who see a physician, since more than one fourth of these persons will have abnormal results. Other indications for PF tests include symptoms such as chronic, persistent cough; dyspnea, cough, or chest pain during exertion; the need for objective assessment of bronchodilator therapy; exposure to dusts or chemicals at work; and the evaluation of patients prior to thoracic or upper abdominal surgery.

Many pulmonary diseases begin slowly and insidiously and finally manifest themselves with the nonspecific symptom of dyspnea on exertion. PF tests are an essential part of the evaluation of patients with such conditions. In the outpatient clinic, where plenty of time is available to make the diagnosis, a cost-efficient approach to PF testing is to start with spirometry and then to refine the diagnosis with further testing as necessary (Fig. 1). When a patient is hospitalized and the diagnosis must be made within a day or two, a battery of PF tests may be ordered, which often includes spirometry before and after bronchodilator therapy, absolute lung volumes, and diffusing capacity (DLCO).

SPIROMETRY INTERPRETATION

Before interpreting spirometry results, examine the flow-volume graphs for maximal effort (sharp peak flows) and reproducibility of the three or more maneuvers (should be within 5 per cent). Poorly performed maneuvers give numeric results that mimic those of pulmonary disease (Fig. 2). When the quality of the effort is good, look for the pattern of airway obstruction or restriction (Fig. 3). Finally, analyze the numeric results. Because diseases causing airway obstruction are common, the forced expiratory volume in 1 second (FEV_1) is the most important spirometry variable. The FEV_1 measures the average flow rate during the first second of the forced vital capacity (FVC) maneuver. The FEV_1 declines in direct and linear proportion to clinical worsening of airway obstruction. Likewise, the FEV_1 increases with successful treatment of airway obstruction. The FEV_1 is used for determining the degree of obstruction (mild, moderate, or severe) and for serial comparisons

Table 1. Indications for Specific Pulmonary Function Tests

Test	Indications
Spirometry	Smokers past age 40 years to detect COPD; check recovery from exacerbation of asthma, COPD, CHF
Spirometry with BD	Chronic cough or chest tightness; suspected asthma or COPD
	Determine response to specific BD therapy
DLCO	Differential diagnosis of abnormal spirometry
	Obstruction: asthma versus COPD
	Restriction: interstitial versus chest wall
	Infiltrates on chest film
	Suspected pulmonary vascular disease
TLC	Low FVC on spirometry: restriction versus hyperinflation or mixed
Oximetry with exercise	Dyspnea on exertion, disability evaluation; check adequacy of supplemental oxygen
	During sleep: screen for sleep apnea syndrome
Methacholine challenge	Suspected asthma but normal spirometry results
Respiratory pressures	Muscle weakness, diaphragm paralysis, myasthenia, ALS, polio follow-up
FV loop (FIVC)	Inspiratory stridor
	Suspected *upper* airway obstruction: vocal cord paralysis, tracheal stenosis

COPD = chronic obstructive pulmonary disease; CHF = congestive heart failure; BD = bronchodilator; DLCO = diffusing capacity of the lung for carbon monoxide; TLC = total lung capacity; FVC = forced vital capacity; ALS = amyotrophic lateral sclerosis; FIVC = forced inspiratory vital capacity.

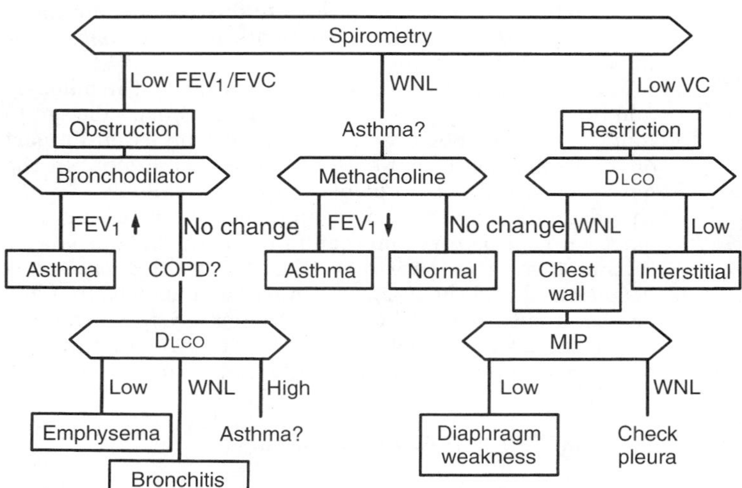

Figure 1. An efficient stepwise method of determining the cause of chronic dyspnea using pulmonary function tests. WNL = within normal limits; VC = vital capacity; TLC = total lung capacity; DLCO = diffusing capacity; MIP = maximal inspiratory pressure; FEV_1 = forced expiratory volume in 1 second.

when following patients with asthma or chronic obstructive pulmonary disease (COPD).

To determine whether a patient's measured FEV_1 falls below the normal range, it is usually expressed as a per cent of the predicted value (per cent pred). Values less than 80 per cent of the predicted FEV_1 are considered abnormal. As a rule of thumb, when predicted values have not been calculated, patients with severe COPD have an FEV_1 of 0.5 to 1 L, and those with moderate COPD have an FEV_1 of 1 to 1.5 L. It is unusual for patients with an FEV_1 of more than 2 L to have dyspnea from airway obstruction. The predicted FEV_1 for a healthy 50-year-old man of average height is about 4 L, and it is about 3 L for a healthy 50-year-old woman.

Typically, a gradual transition occurs between normal function of the airways and mild airway obstruction. The index obtained by dividing the FEV_1 by the FVC is the most sensitive PF test for early detection of borderline to mild COPD. The FEV_1/FVC ratio is the percentage of the vital capacity that can be exhaled in 1 second. As a rough rule of thumb for middle-aged patients, 70 per cent is the lower limit of the normal range (LLN) for the FEV_1/FVC ratio. This ratio is used to detect borderline to mild obstruction, but once it has been determined that a patient

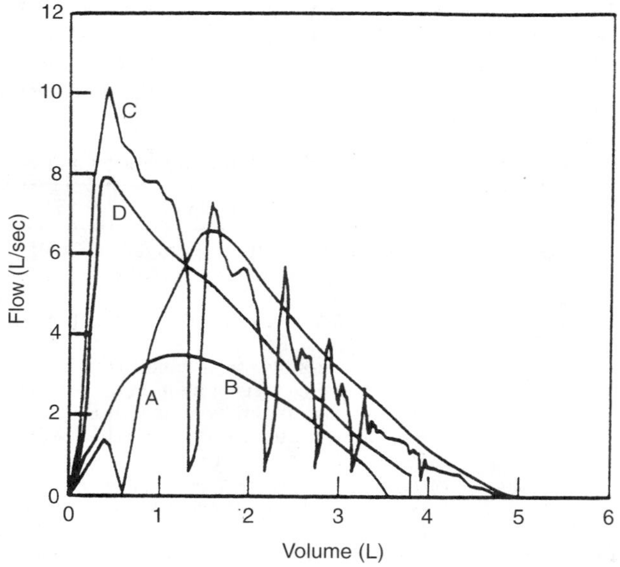

Figure 2. Flow-volume curve patterns from unacceptable maneuvers. *Curve A* has a small "tent" at the beginning (lower left corner) of the exhalation. The patient exhaled a little air (500 mL), stopped, and then blew out the remainder of the air forcefully. The FEV_1 was underestimated because of this hesitating start. *Curve B* is common, showing a Sugarloaf Mountain–shaped curve, without a sharp peak flow at the onset of the maneuver. The FEV_1 was falsely reduced by this poor expiratory effort. *Curve C* has an excellent initial blast (a sharp peak flow to 10 L per second), but the maneuver triggered coughing, shown by multiple valleys (due to the glottic closure, which initiates each cough). *Curve D* is good until the end, when it suddenly stops. This premature termination of effort caused the reported vital capacity to be underestimated by more than 1 L.

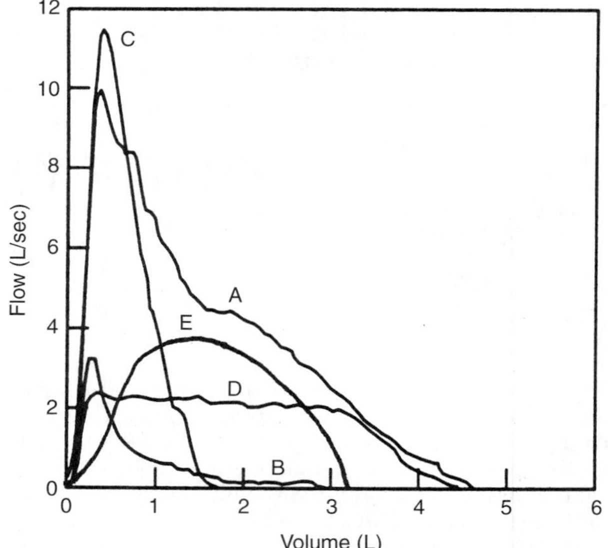

Figure 3. Flow-volume curves from a healthy person *(A)*, a patient with severe obstruction (emphysema) *(B)*, a patient with severe interstitial restriction (radiation fibrosis) *(C)*, a person with upper airway obstruction (tracheal stenosis) *(D)*, and an individual showing poor effort *(E)*, but no lung disease.

has airway obstruction, the FEV_1/FVC ratio is no longer useful.

"Restriction" refers to a decrease in lung volume. Spirometry measures the FVC—the volume of air that can be exhaled rapidly after the patient takes as deep a breath as possible. At the end of a maximal exhalation, there is still air left in the lungs—the residual volume (RV). The total lung capacity (TLC) is the sum of the FVC and the residual volume. In the absence of obstruction, a reduction in the FVC measured by spirometry is consistent with restriction because all restrictive disorders cause a decrease in *both* the TLC and FVC.

The many disorders that cause reduction of lung volumes (restriction) may be divided into three groups: (1) intrinsic pulmonary diseases that cause inflammation or scarring of the lung tissue or fill the airspaces with exudate or debris, (2) extrinsic disorders (chest wall) that mechanically compress the lungs or limit their expansion, and (3) neuromuscular disorders that decrease the ability of the respiratory muscles to inflate and deflate the lungs. Spirometry is useful in detecting restriction (reduction) of lung volumes, but it rarely helps in differentiating among the preceding causes. Some are obvious from the history, physical examination, or chest film.

POST–BRONCHODILATOR TESTING

Administration of an inhaled bronchodilator such as isoproterenol or albuterol is indicated when baseline spirometry demonstrates airway obstruction or when asthma is suspected. An increase in the FEV_1 of more than 12 per cent (and more than 200 mL) suggests a significant response. The lack of an acute bronchodilator response should not dissuade the clinician from a trial of bronchodilators and/or prednisone with follow-up assessment of FEV_1 and clinical status.

DIFFUSING CAPACITY

Measurement of the DLCO (single-breath uptake of carbon monoxide) is quick, safe, and useful in distinguishing between emphysema and other causes of chronic airway obstruction (see Fig. 1). Emphysema decreases the DLCO, obstructive chronic bronchitis does not affect the DLCO, and asthma frequently increases the DLCO. In patients with reduced lung volumes (restriction), a low DLCO suggests a pulmonary interstitial process or pneumonitis, whereas a normal DLCO suggests a "chest wall" cause such as pleural effusion or diaphragm weakness. The DLCO may be reduced because of pulmonary embolism, collagen vascular disease, drug toxicity, and *Pneumocystis carinii* pneumonia before the FVC falls to less than predicted values. When the patient is anemic, the DLCO must be corrected for the decreased hemoglobin concentration.

FORCED INSPIRATORY MANEUVERS

Flow-volume loops, which include forced *inspiratory* maneuvers (forced inspiratory vital capacity [FIVC]), should be performed whenever stridor is heard over the neck during forced breathing. Airway obstruction located in the pharynx, larynx, or trachea (upper airway) is usually impossible to detect from standard FVC maneuvers. Reproducible FIVC maneuvers detect variable upper airway obstruction (UAO) due to conditions such as vocal cord paralysis, which causes a characteristic limitation of flow (plateau) during forced inhalation but little if any obstruction during exhalation. A less common fixed UAO, for example, from tracheal stenosis, causes flow limitation during both forced inhalation (FIVC) and forced exhalation (FVC) maneuvers (Fig. 4). Poor effort mimics the flow-volume loop shapes of UAO but can be reasonably excluded when three or more maneuvers are seen to be reproducible.

METHACHOLINE CHALLENGE

Airway hyperreactivity may not be detected by pre– and post–bronchodilator therapy spirometry when the patient is asymptomatic at the time of testing. Cough or chest tightness with exercise or exposure to cold air, dusts, ani-

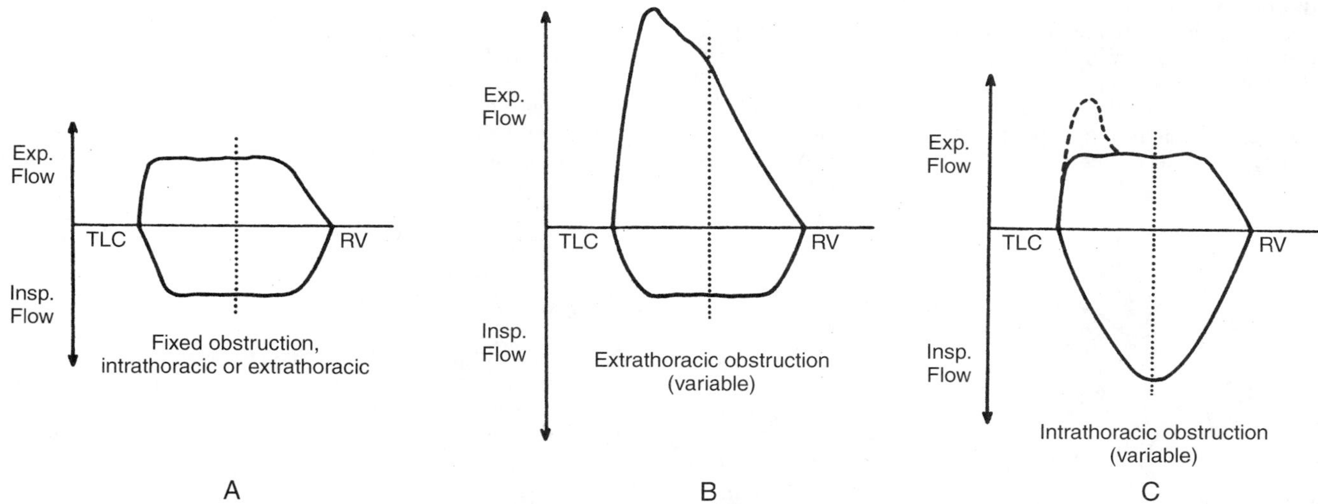

Figure 4. Flow-volume curve patterns in upper airway obstruction. *A,* The size of the upper airway is fixed in diseases such as tracheal stenosis and tumors invading the area of the carina, causing a plateau of flow limitation during both forced exhalation and forced inhalation. *B,* The obstruction of the trachea outside the thoracic cage is variable in cases of vocal cord paralysis. The negative pressure in the trachea during forced inspiration pulls the cords together, limiting the inspiratory flow, but during exhalation the cords are pushed apart, resulting in normal expiratory flow. *C,* Variable intrathoracic obstruction is rarely observed. Exp Flow = expiratory flow; Insp Flow = inspiratory flow.

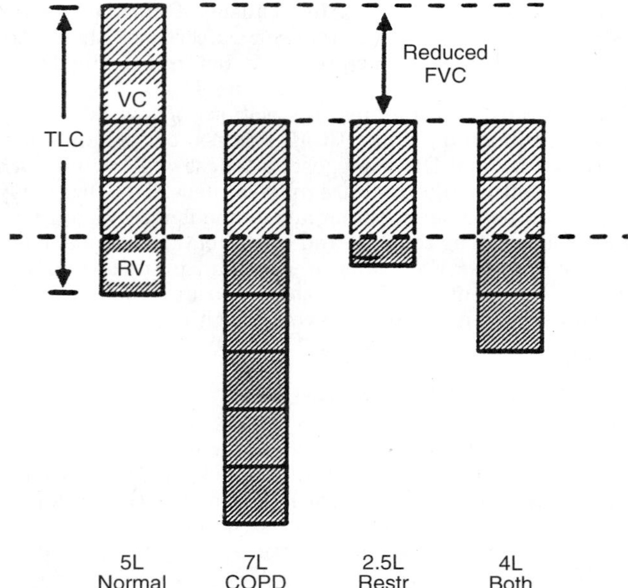

Figure 5. The absolute lung volumes of four patients are graphed, with each block representing 1 L of volume. Spirometry measures only the vital capacity above the dashed line. The first patient demonstrates normal predicted volumes. The latter three all have a vital capacity (*VC* or *FVC*) of only 50 per cent of predicted (2 L). Note the widely varying total lung capacities (*TLC*) caused by differences in the residual volume (*RV*), which is not measured by spirometry. COPD = chronic obstructive pulmonary disease—emphysema with hyperinflation and air-trapping that increase the residual volume; Restr = restriction of lung volumes by interstitial lung fibrosis; Both = restriction (e.g., a large pleural effusion) superimposed on COPD.

mals, or fumes suggest airway hyperreactivity. Baseline spirometry may be near normal in these patients, with only a small increase in the FEV_1 following bronchodilator therapy. Outpatients may be asked to return for retesting when symptoms occur; however, this delays the diagnosis and may be impractical. A methacholine challenge test (MCT) is safe when baseline spirometry is near normal, and it usually confirms the diagnosis in less than an hour. A 20 per cent or greater decrease in the FEV_1 following five or fewer inhalations of methacholine at a concentration of 10 mg/mL or less suggests an abnormal degree of airway reactivity that is typically seen in asthmatics. A negative methacholine challenge test virtually rules out asthma, but a positive test is sometimes seen with hay fever.

PULSE OXIMETRY

Instruments that estimate arterial oxygen saturation continuously and noninvasively are now ubiquitous. Indications for oximetry tests performed in the PF laboratory include screening for oxygen desaturation in patients with exercise limitation and determining the adequacy of supplemental oxygen therapy. Oximetry is also useful during sleep in patients with symptoms such as daytime somnolence, which suggests sleep apnea. (See the article on sleep-related respiratory dysfunction.) A fall of more than 4 per cent (ending at $<$93 per cent) suggests significant desaturation, and confirmation with arterial blood gas (ABG) measurements may be indicated.

MAXIMAL RESPIRATORY PRESSURES

Measurement of maximal respiratory pressure is indicated whenever there is an unexplained decrease in the vital capacity or maximal voluntary ventilation (MVV) and whenever respiratory muscle weakness is suspected clinically. MIP is the maximal inspiratory pressure that can be produced by the patient trying to inhale from a blocked mouthpiece (like sucking a thick milkshake through a straw). MEP is the maximal expiratory pressure measured (with cheeks bulging) after a full inhalation. Repeated measurements of MIP and MEP are useful in following the course of patients with neuromuscular disorders. The slow vital capacity may also be followed, but it is less specific.

MIP is easily measured with the use of a simple mechanical pressure gauge connected to a mouthpiece. MIP measures the ability of the diaphragm and other respiratory muscles to generate inspiratory force, reflected by a negative airway pressure. The average MIP for adult men is −100 cm H_2O, and for adult women it is about −70 cm H_2O. The lower limit of the normal range is about two thirds of these values.

SLOW VITAL CAPACITY

The slow vital capacity may be useful when the FVC is reduced and airway obstruction is also present. The FVC is often reduced in obstructive disease, but with a slow

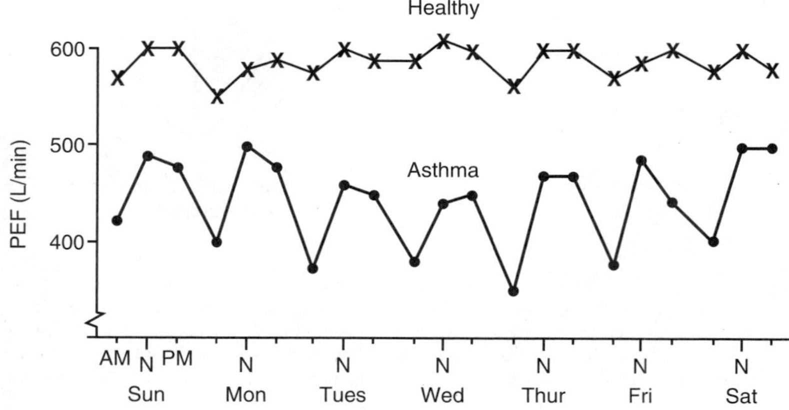

Figure 6. When a patient has symptoms suggesting asthma, but spirometry in the office is normal, giving the patient a peak flowmeter and diary may confirm the diagnosis without resorting to a methacholine challenge test. Persons with asthma have an exaggerated diurnal variation in peak flow (*PEF*) and FEV_1, as in this example. Their morning values are often more than 20 per cent lower than their values later in the day. N = noon.

exhalation there is less airway narrowing, and frequently the patient can exhale a larger volume, even normal, vital capacity. In contrast, in restrictive disease the vital capacity is reduced during both slow and fast maneuvers. Thus, when the slow vital capacity is within normal limits, a significant restrictive disorder is ruled out and the measurement of absolute lung volumes is unnecessary.

ABSOLUTE LUNG VOLUMES

The measurement of the TLC may be helpful whenever there is a decrease in vital capacity. When a patient has COPD and a decrease in vital capacity, measurement of the TLC can help determine whether there is a superimposed restrictive disorder (Fig. 5). The TLC may be reasonably assessed simply by viewing the chest film. Hyperinflation (large TLC) that results from severe COPD is associated with flattened diaphragms. The restriction (small TLC) that results from parenchymal diseases is often associated with pulmonary infiltrates and an elevated diaphragm. However, small changes in TLC are not easily detected by inspection.

PEAK FLOWMETERS

A rough measure of the degree of airway obstruction can be made inexpensively by the patient at home with the use of a peak flowmeter. Such a device is no substitute for spirometry when making a diagnosis, but it is useful in the management of many patients with asthma. The normal decrease in airway diameter (and forced airflow) seen in the early morning hours (the *morning dip*) is exaggerated in patients with asthma (Fig. 6). A decrease of more than 30 per cent in the patient's usual morning peak flowmeter reading presages an impending asthma attack and the need for treatment.

PULMONARY EMBOLISM AND INFARCTION

By Frank T. Leone, M.D.,
and Gregory C. Kane, M.D.
Philadelphia, Pennsylvania

Pulmonary embolism (PE), or more precisely pulmonary thromboembolism, is a common disorder, particularly among hospitalized patients, with an annual incidence in excess of 250,000 cases and a mortality rate of approximately 10 per cent. It is an important diagnostic entity not only because of its incidence but also because it is frequently unsuspected and often difficult to diagnose. Although the timely diagnosis and treatment of PE is gravely important, the spectrum of presenting signs and symptoms is so vast and nonspecific that the diagnosis of PE is often overlooked. It remains one of the most common unsuspected premorbid diagnoses made at autopsy in the United States. More than with any other pathologic entity, the accurate diagnosis of PE relies heavily on the clinician's ability to formulate a "pretest probability of disease," the degree of suspicion that the disease exists. The clinician must be vigilant and should suspect PE in any patient who presents with an acute change in cardiopulmonary status.

DEFINITION AND SYNONYMS

The term "PE" is often used, but it is somewhat imprecise. PE is not a specific disease per se but rather a specific complication of many diseases; it has become synonymous with pulmonary thromboembolism. The term "pulmonary thromboembolism" is preferred because it indicates more accurately the nature of the problem; thrombi form in the venous system, dislodge, and travel to the pulmonary vascular bed. Although most thromboemboli are from the deep venous system of the lower extremities, they can also form in the pelvic veins, renal veins, chambers in the right side of the heart, and veins of the upper extremities when venous catheters are in place. Other forms of embolism to the pulmonary vasculature can also occur, including amniotic fluid and fat emboli as well as air and septic emboli. These disorders may share some of the clinical manifestations of pulmonary thromboembolism, but their specific presentations can have unique characteristics.

HISTORY

It is important to recall that the presenting symptoms of pulmonary thromboembolism may be so varied and nonspecific as to make the diagnosis difficult. Thus, PE should be considered in *any patient who experiences a sudden change in respiratory or cardiovascular status.* Some patients may be nearly asymptomatic; others may present with cardiopulmonary collapse and sudden death. Although there is no "typical" presentation, many patients with PE will present with the sudden onset of dyspnea and chest discomfort, at times accompanied by a slightly increased temperature. Apprehension commonly accompanies the onset of dyspnea. It is unusual for patients to have concurrent complaints referable to venous thrombosis. The clinician must remember that the risk of a pulmonary complication from thrombotic disease is linked to the risk of thrombosis itself. Thus, the initial assessment of each patient suspected of having a pulmonary thromboembolism should include an assessment of the risk of thrombotic disease. In assessing the probability of thrombosis, the risk factors are best remembered as Virchow's triad, namely: (1) venous stasis, (2) intimal injury, and (3) a "hypercoagulable state." Table 1 represents a partial list of conditions associated with an increased risk for thrombosis. The risk factors are cumulative and not independent. For example, the patient who is obese and bed-bound after lower extremity vascular surgery is at an elevated risk for venous thrombosis and consequently PE. A thorough history obtained from the patient with suspected PE should attempt to identify these pre-existing conditions.

PHYSICAL EXAMINATION

Physical examination is rarely confirmatory but may be helpful in the diagnosis of PE. Tachypnea and tachycardia are generally present. Hypotension suggests that a large embolus has occluded 50 per cent or more of the pulmonary vascular tree. Typically, cardiac examination will not show signs of right ventricular (RV) overload when emboli are small, but RV lift and a new tricuspid regurgitation murmur may accompany large, life-threatening events. Auscul-

Table 1. Risk Factors for Hypercoagulability and Pulmonary Thromboembolism

Historical and Physical	Laboratory
Surgical and nonsurgical trauma, including burns—particularly those involving the pelvis or lower extremities—or requiring prolonged anesthesia	Lupus anticoagulant
Congestive heart failure (specifically right ventricular failure of any cause)	Antithrombin III deficiency
Immobilization from any cause, including bed rest, stroke, casting, and so on	Protein C deficiency
Occupations of an unusually sedentary nature or those requiring prolonged travel	Protein S deficiency
Malignancy	Disorders of the fibrinolytic system, including plasminogen activator deficiency and elevated plasminogen activator inhibitor
Previous deep venous thrombosis, especially with residual venous obstruction	Resistance to activated protein C
Pregnancy, especially immediately postpartum and following cesarean section	
Use of estrogen-containing compounds	
Age greater than 70 years	
Inflammatory bowel disease	
Nephrotic syndrome	
Polycythemia vera	
Homocysteinuria	
Obesity (as it relates to degree of immobility)	

tation of the lungs may reveal crackles and a pleural friction rub. Breath sounds may be decreased because of splinting or pleural effusion. In the lower extremities, tenderness, asymmetrical edema, or the presence of Homan's sign (slight pain at the back of the knee or calf when the ankle is slowly dorsiflexed) may suggest that a lower extremity clot is present. If a central venous line is in place, the upper extremities should be carefully compared for asymmetrical edema.

LABORATORY DATA

The most important initial laboratory test in the evaluation of the patient with acute shortness of breath is the arterial blood gas (ABG). In PE, the ABG usually reveals a respiratory alkalosis with mild hypoxemia. Blood gas disturbances are commonly linked to hyperventilation and a ventilation-perfusion (V/Q) mismatch. The extent of change in the ABG depends not only on the degree of vascular occlusion but also on pre-existing heart or lung conditions. The alveolar-arterial (A-a) oxygen gradient can be normal in up to 5 per cent of patients with PE.

THE CHEST RADIOGRAPH

In the absence of pre-existing lung disease, patients with pulmonary thromboembolism most often have normal chest films. When the chest radiograph is abnormal, the findings are generally subtle and never pathognomonic. The principal radiographic changes associated with pulmonary thromboembolism include (1) local oligemia or decreased vascular perfusion (Westermark's sign), (2) a change in hilar vessel size, (3) a change in the cardiac shadow, (4) loss of lung volume, and (5) a small pleural effusion. When changes are visible on the plain film, they are typically associated with a significant embolic event.

Peripheral pulmonary oligemia should increase clinical suspicion of pulmonary thromboembolism. Westermark's sign is most useful when comparison with a previous chest film can be made. Local oligemia is usually associated with occlusion of a segmental or larger artery. Enlargement of a major hilar artery may be a useful sign, especially when comparison with previous chest films can be made; progressive enlargement of a specific great vessel strongly suggests PE. Massive central embolization may cause acute cor pulmonale with rapid enlargement of the azygous vein and superior vena cava, enlargement of the main pulmonary artery (PA), and occasional abrupt tapering of the pulmonary vasculature. Loss of lung volume is a nonspecific radiologic sign typically seen as atelectasis or displacement of the hemidiaphragm upward.

THE ELECTROCARDIOGRAM

The electrocardiogram (ECG) typically aids diagnosis of PE when acute RV overload has occurred. A normal ECG does not rule out pulmonary thromboembolism, however, since as many as 25 per cent of patients with submassive emboli can have a normal ECG. The ECG is most helpful in excluding other causes of acute symptoms, including myocardial infarction (MI) and pericarditis. In otherwise healthy persons, the ECG typically reveals sinus tachycardia or even normal sinus rhythm. In patients with underlying heart disease, atrial tachyarrhythmias are more frequent. The classic changes of rightward axis deviation and right bundle branch block, associated with a prominent S wave in lead I, a Q wave in lead II, and new T-wave inversion in lead III (S_1, Q_3, T_3 pattern), typically accompany acute cor pulmonale following a massive embolic event.

PULMONARY ARTERY CATHETERIZATION

Massive pulmonary thromboembolism can lead to cardiogenic shock or hemodynamic collapse and sudden death. The major differential diagnoses in such patients include embolism, acute MI, and cardiac tamponade. In the critical care setting, the PA catheter can help distinguish among these causes and can also guide management. In massive embolism, the right atrial (RA) and RV diastolic pressures are increased, typically to greater than 10 mm Hg, with a normal pulmonary capillary wedge pressure (PCWP). RV and PA systolic pressures are only moderately increased to about 35 to 40 mm Hg. Acute increases in the PA systolic pressure are due to an abrupt increase in pulmonary vascular resistance to about 2.5 times normal. Acute increases in resistance to greater than three times normal place an enormous workload on the right ventricle, which is ill-equipped to handle a high afterload. RV failure, acute cor pulmonale, and death are associated with sudden PA systolic pressures greater than 40 mm Hg. Again, pre-existing heart and lung disease is important in determining outcome. In contrast, shock from RV infarction reveals right-sided diastolic pressures that are also increased, but the RV and PA systolic pressures are decreased (a narrow PA pulse pressure). In tamponade, increased and relatively equalized filling pressures (including RA and RV diastolic, PA diastolic, and pulmonary capillary wedge pressure) are observed.

VENTILATION-PERFUSION (V/Q) RADIONUCLIDE SCANNING

The radionuclide perfusion scan has proved only modestly useful in detecting PE because other conditions such as pneumonia or chronic obstructive pulmonary disease (COPD) can significantly alter distribution of blood flow through the lung. The addition of ventilation scanning enhances the utility of the perfusion scan because parenchymal lung disease not only affects perfusion but also causes a corresponding ventilation defect, whereas PE typically produces a discrete perfusion defect with intact ventilation; an "unmatched defect." Early investigators attempted to make the study even more useful by not only classifying results as abnormal but also adding the qualifiers "high probability," "low probability," and "moderate (indeterminate) probability" of thromboembolic disease.

In 1990, the Prospective Investigation of Pulmonary Embolism Diagnosis (PIOPED) investigators successfully evaluated the post-test probability of PE in relation to the clinical pretest probability of disease using V/Q scanning. Of all patients evaluated, 87 per cent of those with high-probability scans, 30 per cent of those with moderate-probability scans, and 14 per cent of those with low-probability scans had PE. Of note, 4 per cent of patients with normal V/Q scans had emboli. Further stratification by clinical index of suspicion (low, moderate, or high) yielded clinically relevant results (Table 2). Of particular interest are the patients in whom a high index of suspicion was combined with a high-probability scan; 96 per cent of these patients had PE. Also, a high index of suspicion coupled with a low-probability scan still resulted in a 40 per cent chance of PE. Even an indeterminate result (moderate probability), in a patient for whom there is a low clinical suspicion of PE, indicates a 16 per cent chance of pulmonary thromboembolism and may require further investigation.

Table 2. Probability of Pulmonary Embolism Based on Clinical Suspicion Versus Ventilation-Perfusion Scan Results

	High Suspicion (%)	Moderate Suspicion (%)	Low Suspicion (%)
High-probability scan	96	88	56
Moderate-probability or "indeterminate" scan	66	28	16
Low-probability scan	40	16	4
Normal scan	0	6	2

Data from the PIOPED Investigators: Value of the ventilation/perfusion scan in acute pulmonary embolism. Results of the Prospective Investigation of Pulmonary Embolism Diagnosis (PIOPED). JAMA 263:2753–2759, 1990.

Thus, the PIOPED study illustrates the absolute importance of formulating an estimate of clinical suspicion of disease before performing the V/Q scan. The correct interpretation of the diagnostic study and the need for further testing are intimately dependent on the physician's assessment of the pretest probability of disease.

PULMONARY ARTERIOGRAPHY

Although unnecessary when the index of suspicion and V/Q results are concordant, pulmonary arteriography remains the "gold standard" of diagnostic procedures in the evaluation of pulmonary thromboembolism. Arteriography is most valuable when significant doubt about the diagnosis persists (Table 3). Although the test has inherent risks, they are far outweighed by the need for an accurate, timely diagnosis in symptomatic patients. With appropriate evaluation before the procedure and in the hands of experienced personnel, pulmonary angiography should be considered safe. Safety is sometimes enhanced by "selective" angiography in which only those sections of the lung that are abnormal on the V/Q scan are studied. This limits the dye load and time requirements for the procedure.

Although interpretation can be influenced by the quality of the images, two angiographic findings are considered diagnostic of acute embolism. The "filling defect" is an intra-arterial, nonopacifying shadow that is felt to represent an intraluminal space-occupying clot. In addition, precipitous obstruction to flow of contrast material indicates the presence of a large, occlusive thrombus preventing downstream opacification.

CAVEATS

In the patient with mild symptoms of PE, one could argue that confirmation of a pulmonary thromboembolic event is not necessary if the presence of clot in the lower

Table 3. Recommended Diagnostic-Therapeutic Approach Based on Clinical Suspicion and Ventilation-Perfusion Scan Results

	High Suspicion	Moderate Suspicion	Low Suspicion
High-probability scan	Treat PE	Treat PE	Pulmonary arteriogram
Moderate-probability or "indeterminate" scan	Pulmonary arteriogram	Pulmonary arteriogram	Pulmonary arteriogram*
Low-probability scan	Pulmonary arteriogram	Pulmonary arteriogram	No PE
Normal scan	No PE	No PE	No PE

*Some clinicians may consider pulmonary arteriography optional here; diagnostic interventions must be individualized.
PE = pulmonary embolism.

extremities can be documented. In such a patient, the diagnosis of deep venous thrombosis (DVT) would be sufficient to begin anticoagulant therapy. Documenting a PE will do little to alter therapy, and further investigation may be unnecessary. The diagnostic plan must be individualized.

The diagnosis of DVT is accomplished in much the same way as is the diagnosis of PE. The history and physical examination serve to qualify the risk of thrombosis, and diagnostic testing is used to confirm the clinical suspicion. Although diagnostic studies that are useful in confirming the presence of DVT can also be used to influence assessment of the probability of pulmonary thromboembolism, they are not of themselves *diagnostic* of embolic complications. Useful studies include duplex Doppler scanning, impedance plethysmography, contrast venography, and radionuclide-tagged fibrinogen scanning. Doppler imaging of the lower extremities is often the easiest procedure to perform quickly and imparts no risk to the patient. Reliability, however, depends on the skill and experience of the operator.

OTHER FORMS OF PULMONARY EMBOLISM

Although much less common, other forms of PE are no less important or devastating. Fat embolism is unique and dramatic in its presentation. Typically occurring 24 to 48 hours after traumatic fracture of a long bone, fat embolism causes severe dyspnea, confusion, and diffuse petechiae. The systemic complications are attributed more to intrapulmonary lipolysis and production of toxic fatty acids than to vascular occlusion by fat. Embolism of fat may also induce intravascular coagulation. Diagnosis requires clinical suspicion and examination of urine for fat droplets. Therapy is supportive.

Similarly, amniotic fluid embolism occurs primarily during or shortly after spontaneous or cesarean delivery, often associated with premature placental separation. Manifestations include sudden severe dyspnea, disseminated intravascular coagulation, cardiovascular compromise, and occasionally death. Emboli consisting of squamous cells, amorphous debris, and mucin can be identified on direct examination of maternal lung tissue. Attempts to recover fetal squamous cells and trophoblast cells from the maternal pulmonary arterial circulation have met with only limited success. Amniotic fluid embolism is often a clinical diagnosis; definitive diagnosis usually occurs only at autopsy.

Both septic and air emboli are typically iatrogenic; however, septic emboli can also occur as a result of intravenous drug use. These emboli are frequently a complication of indwelling venous catheters and should be suspected when the patient experiences a sudden "spiking" fever, cough, and dyspnea, with or without pleuritic pain. The diagnosis is further supported by the characteristic presence of multiple, diffuse peripheral infiltrates that can undergo cavitation. Isolating the responsible pathogen in the blood or on the catheter tip is helpful in guiding therapy. Once the source of infection is identified and treated (including removal of the catheter when possible), resolution of clinical signs and symptoms confirms the diagnosis. Involvement of the tricuspid valve is not infrequent and can be evaluated using echocardiography.

The most common causes of air embolism are thoracic, abdominal, and craniofacial trauma. Air embolism can also be iatrogenic, often related to improper insertion technique during central venous cannulation. Other iatrogenic causes include craniotomy, total hip arthroplasty, liver transplantation, and cardiovascular procedures necessitating cardiopulmonary bypass as well as hemodialysis and forced injection of radiocontrast media. Sequelae depend on the amount of air entrained but range from no symptoms to sudden cardiac death. Significant air embolism may cause agitation, confusion, tachypnea, dyspnea, pleuritic pain, tachycardia, or hypotension. The diagnosis is primarily dependent on clinical suspicion. Rarely, a chest radiograph will reveal the presence of air within the chambers of the right side of the heart and the pulmonary trunk. An abdominal film may show air in the hepatic veins. Other potential radiographic abnormalities that are less specific for air embolism include pulmonary edema, focal oligemia, and enlarged central pulmonary arteries. Most commonly, the chest film is normal.

PULMONARY INFARCTION

Although logic may suggest that infarction is a common sequela of PE, in fact it is not. The lungs remain highly resistant to tissue hypoxia and cell death primarily because of an abundant supply of oxygen from three sources—the pulmonary arteries, bronchial arteries, and airways. Infarction is therefore rare in patients without previous heart or lung disease but may occur in up to 20 per cent of patients with pre-existing conditions. The cardinal manifestations include pleuritic pain, dyspnea, and hemoptysis. Pulmonary infarction may display characteristic wedge-shaped consolidations on chest film. Typically these opacifications are peripherally located in the lower lobes, with the apex of the wedge pointing toward the hilum. The size, number, and distribution of the infarcts depend on the caliber and frequency of embolization. Radiographic changes may resolve but often result in linear scarring and volume loss.

COMPLICATIONS AND PROGNOSIS

Chronic dyspnea may follow PE when emboli fail to lyse spontaneously and pulmonary vessels remain occluded by organized thrombi. These patients may display signs of pulmonary hypertension or cor pulmonale. The diagnosis of chronic pulmonary thromboembolism is suggested when repeated V/Q scans or arteriography show persistent perfusion abnormalities.

Most pulmonary emboli are submassive and well tolerated hemodynamically. Patients who die either have large initial emboli or suffer recurrent PE before the diagnosis is suspected. With prompt, appropriate anticoagulant therapy, recurrent embolism is infrequent. In patients with underlying malignancy or a hypercoagulable state, emboli often recur after anticoagulants are discontinued, and placement of an inferior vena cava filter or long-term anticoagulant therapy may be required.

DISEASES OF THE PLEURA

By Steven H. Feinsilver, M.D.
Mineola, New York

Clinical disorders of the pleural space are exceedingly common because they can be produced by a wide variety of both local and systemic illnesses. Examples include disruption of the pleural surface, which allows the lung to collapse (pneumothorax); inflammation in the pleural space, which causes pain (pleurisy); and the formation of pleural fluid (effusion). Although the pleura can be accessed relatively easily, the diagnosis of pleural diseases is more often empirical, based on other clinical information, rather than exact.

NORMAL PLEURA

Knowledge of the normal physiology of the pleural space is required for an understanding of pleural disease. The visceral and parietal pleural surfaces are lined with mesothelial cells that have abundant microvilli capable of fluid transport. Systemic capillaries provide the blood supply of the parietal pleura. Systemic capillaries also supply the visceral pleura, with a small contribution from the pulmonary circulation, which has a lower pressure. Accordingly, the hydrostatic pressure in parietal pleural capillaries is slightly higher than in the visceral pleura, favoring the net transport of fluid from the parietal to visceral surfaces. This fluid transport is currently thought to be rather small in the normal human. Fluid can also be removed by lymphatics. These lymphatics are present in both parietal and visceral pleural surfaces, but only the parietal pleura has stomas of 2- to 12-μm diameter to remove cells, protein, and particulate matter. Lymphatic drainage is thought to account for the lack of significant fluid accumulation in the normal individual despite hydrostatic forces favoring its formation.

Only the parietal pleura is innervated with pain fibers. Clinically, this means that any disease causing pleuritic pain implies involvement of the parietal pleura. The normal pleural space is under negative pressure because of opposing forces of elastic recoil of the lung and chest wall. In the normal upright human, this pressure varies from approximately -8 cm H_2O in the apex to -2 cm H_2O at the base, with a mean pleural pressure of -5 cm H_2O. The normal pleural space contains a 10- to 15-μm layer of pleural fluid, for a total of 5 to 10 mL of fluid in each hemithorax. Approximately 17 mL of fluid is formed each day in the normal pleural space. The pleura can remove up to 25 times this baseline amount of fluid without the development of clinically apparent pleural effusion.

PNEUMOTHORAX

Because the pleural pressure is normally negative and lower than the alveolar pressure, if the visceral pleura is disrupted and a connection is established between the alveoli and the pleural space, air will accumulate in the pleural space. Similarly, a communication between the pleural space and the atmosphere will cause air to enter the pleural space until the pleural pressure becomes atmospheric or the communication is sealed.

Pneumothoraces may be divided into those resulting from physical trauma (often iatrogenic) and those occurring spontaneously. Spontaneous pneumothoraces are further divided into primary pneumothoraces (no antecedent lung disease) and those secondary to underlying lung disease. Patients generally present with both chest pain localized to the affected side and dyspnea. The latter is more common in secondary pneumothorax because of already compromised pulmonary function.

Primary spontaneous pneumothorax is thought to be caused by rupture of small subpleural blebs near the apices. The condition occurs more often in taller, thinner individuals. Although these patients have no clinical antecedent lung disease, cigarette smoking is a strong risk factor. Secondary pneumothorax has been reported in a wide variety of diseases but is most common in chronic obstructive pulmonary disease.

Examination of the patient with a pneumothorax typically reveals decreased breath sounds, tympanitic percussion, and decreased vocal resonance on the affected side. Severe distress with cyanosis and hypotension suggests a tension pneumothorax, in which the disease process causes a one-way valve phenomenon to develop, leading to greater than atmospheric pressure in the pleural space. The catastrophic effects of a tension pneumothorax appear to relate more to sudden profound hypoxemia than to decreased venous return to the heart, as previously postulated. The finding on examination of shift of the heart and trachea away from the affected hemithorax is further evidence suggesting tension pneumothorax.

The diagnosis of pneumothorax is generally confirmed on chest radiography by the finding of a radiolucent area at the periphery without lung markings, separated from the partially collapsed lung by a radiopaque pleural stripe. In doubtful cases, repeat radiography in expiration may make the pneumothorax more evident. The size of the pneumothorax is often underestimated on the radiograph. It must be remembered that the volume of air is estimated by subtracting the diameter of the lung cubed from the diameter of the hemithorax cubed.

PLEURITIC PAIN WITHOUT EFFUSION (DRY PLEURISY, PLEURODYNIA)

Pleuritic chest pain without effusion usually denotes either underlying pulmonary parenchymal disease or early pleural disease that has not yet produced fluid. When pleuritic pain persists with a normal radiograph, the possibilities include collagen vascular disease such as rheumatoid disease or systemic lupus erythematosus, trauma, and cytotoxic agents including radiation and medications (e.g., methotrexate).

PLEURAL EFFUSION

Examination of the physiology of the normal pleural space reveals a relatively limited number of ways that fluid formation can occur. The most common mechanism for pleural effusion is increased capillary pressure, as in congestive heart failure. A second mechanism for fluid formation is increased protein or cells in the pleural space, which raises the oncotic pressure, as seen in infection or tumor invasion of the pleural space. A third mechanism is decreased lymphatic drainage, as seen in malignancy or following trauma. A fourth potential mechanism is decreased oncotic pressure; pleural effusions are not seen spontaneously until oncotic pressure is extremely low, probably requiring a serum albumin concentration of less than 1.5 g/dL.

SIGNS AND SYMPTOMS

As fluid accumulates in the pleural space, patients experience various symptoms and signs. Pleuritic chest pain—a sharp pain that worsens on deep inspiration—implies involvement of the parietal pleura. With increasing fluid, pain may diminish. Similarly, a pleural friction rub, which is characterized by a harsh loud sound over the chest in the latter part of inspiration and early expiration, is caused by the rubbing together of roughened or inflamed pleural surfaces; it may decrease as pleural effusions become larger. More reliable signs of pleural effusion are decreased chest wall movement on respiration, a dullness to percussion, decreased vocal fremitus, and decreased breath sounds. A larger effusion, causing collapse of adjacent lung tissue, can lead to egophony or bronchial breath sounds just above the effusion. A very large effusion may also cause the trachea to deviate to the contralateral side.

RADIOLOGY FOR PLEURAL EFFUSIONS

Fluid in the pleural space generally appears as a homogeneous radiodensity, the position of which is dependent on gravity. Blunting of the costophrenic angle on an upright posteroanterior (PA) radiograph is seen with 200 to 500 mL of fluid. On occasion, up to 1000 mL of fluid can remain in an infrapulmonary location without filling the costophrenic angle or extending up the chest wall. Such "subpulmonic" effusions can be difficult to recognize without a lateral decubitus film. One clue is the appearance of the highest part of the apparent diaphragm in a more lateral location than usual.

Fluid that does not appear to obey the laws of gravity is referred to as loculated. This may occur when the fluid is extremely inflammatory, as in empyema, or if the pleural space is abnormal because of previous disease. When fluid becomes loculated in a fissure, it may simulate a mass ("pseudotumor").

Decubitus radiographs are extremely helpful in assessing effusions. Generally, bilateral decubitus views should be obtained. In the view with the affected side dependent, the amount of fluid can be roughly quantitated by the measurement of the distance between the outer border of the lung and the inner border of the chest wall. If this distance exceeds 1 cm, thoracentesis will generally be successful. The view with the nonaffected side dependent is often useful for assessing the portion of lung otherwise obscured by fluid and for looking for small contralateral effusions often missed on the posteroanterior film.

The cross-sectional view afforded by computed tomography (CT) of the chest can be useful for distinguishing pleural from parenchymal disease and for assessing the underlying lung. The important and sometimes difficult distinction between pulmonary abscess and empyema can often be aided by computed tomography.

THORACENTESIS AND FLUID ANALYSIS

In most patients, the finding of significant pleural effusion should prompt thoracentesis unless there is a strong clinical suspicion of a transudate. A rule of thumb for significant fluid accumulation is the finding of at least 1 cm of fluid layering out on a decubitus radiograph. Thoracentesis is generally performed safely, given a cooperative patient without coagulopathy. It is usually safe even in the presence of anticoagulant therapy or mild thrombocytopenia.

Thoracentesis is performed most comfortably with the patient sitting forward on the edge of a bed, resting the head on a pillow on a tray table or similar stand. The upper extent of the effusion is determined by percussion and marked. The interspace just below this is palpated, and a small weal is raised with a 25-gauge needle and 1 or 2 per cent lidocaine in the skin overlying the top of the rib below this interspace. Next, a 20-gauge needle is inserted into the interspace immediately above the superior aspect of the rib to avoid injury to intercostal vessels and nerves running just below each rib. Additional lidocaine is injected, with care taken to aspirate before each injection, until the pleural space is entered and fluid is obtained. Removal of 20 to 50 mL is often adequate for diagnosis. If larger amounts are to be drained therapeutically, a catheter-over-needle system is generally employed so that the needle can be removed during drainage, minimizing trauma to the underlying lung. It is important to maintain a closed system during drainage, as an air leak is likely the most common cause of thoracentesis-induced pneumothorax.

Table 1. Diagnostic Criteria for Exudative Effusion*

Protein: pleural fluid-to-serum ratio >0.5
Lactate dehydrogenase (LD): pleural fluid-to-serum ratio >0.6
LD: absolute value in pleural fluid greater than two thirds of upper limit of reference range for serum

*The diagnostic criteria can include any of these.

The appearance of the pleural fluid immediately offers some information. Grossly purulent fluid is diagnostic of empyema and generally indicates a need for urgent drainage. A true hemothorax (hematocrit of pleural fluid greater than 50 per cent of peripheral blood hematocrit) is most common following trauma. Fluid with a hematocrit between 1 and 50 per cent of peripheral blood suggests trauma, tumor, or thromboembolism. A hematocrit less than 1 per cent of peripheral blood has no diagnostic significance. Milky-appearing fluid suggests chylothorax, but a true chylothorax is defined by a triglyceride concentration greater than 110 mg/dL. Other conditions can produce a milky appearance (pseudochylothorax).

Following gross examination of the fluid, a few laboratory tests are used to distinguish between transudates, which are caused by abnormal hydrostatic or osmotic forces, and exudates, which are caused by inflammation in the pleural space. Protein and lactate dehydrogenase (LD) in pleural fluid and serum are most commonly used to make this distinction; if any criteria are positive for exudate, the effusion is so considered (Table 1).

Transudates have a relatively limited differential diagnosis (Table 2). Generally the cause will be found outside the pleural space, and further investigation of the pleura will not be rewarding. The differential diagnosis of exudative effusions, by contrast, is very large and involves most diseases found in pulmonary medicine (Table 3). More than 90 per cent of exudates, however, are caused by pneumonia, malignancy, pulmonary embolism, or gastrointestinal disease. A few additional laboratory studies are useful for diagnosing some of the more common causes of effusions (Table 4). Pleural fluid cytologic studies are extremely accurate for diagnosing malignancy, and the sensitivity of

Table 2. Differential Diagnosis of Transudative Effusion*

Congestive heart failure	Nephrotic syndrome
Cirrhosis with ascites	Myxedema
Pericardial disease	Pulmonary embolism (usually exudate)

*The preceding are in approximate order of incidence.

Table 3. Differential Diagnosis of Exudative Effusion*

Malignancy	Tuberculosis
Parapneumonic	Asbestos exposure
Pulmonary embolism	Mesothelioma
Viral pleurisy	Following cardiotomy or myocardial infarction
Pancreatitis	Drug-induced
Collagen vascular disease (rheumatoid arthritis, systemic lupus erythematosus)	Yellow nail syndrome
	Miscellaneous

*The preceding are in approximate order of incidence.

these tests approaches 70 per cent. In most patients, however, thoracentesis information is used to make a presumptive diagnosis; the cause of an effusion is determined only after additional clinical information is considered.

After initial analysis, about 20 per cent of exudative effusions will remain undiagnosed. Options at this time include closed pleural biopsy or a more invasive procedure. Closed pleural biopsy with a Cope's or Abrams' needle significantly increases the yield only for malignancy and tuberculosis. For malignant effusions, cytologic evaluation of the fluid alone is nearly as sensitive as needle biopsy. The prognosis for malignant effusions is so poor that invasive work-up is often not warranted. The therapeutic implications of the diagnosis of tuberculosis are much greater, and this is the most important indication for closed pleural biopsy. The best single test for tuberculous pleurisy is culture of biopsy material, but obtaining results requires several weeks. Finding granulomas on biopsy is highly suggestive of tuberculosis, but they are found in only 60 to 80 per cent of patients. Thus, many patients should be treated empirically for tuberculosis if clinical suspicion is high.

Other possible approaches to unexplained pleural effusions include bronchoscopy and thoracoscopy. The most common final diagnosis for patients with unexplained pleural effusions is malignancy, most commonly bronchogenic carcinoma. However, the yield for bronchoscopy in the absence of a radiographic abnormality or hemoptysis is too small to recommend its routine use. Thoracoscopy allows direct examination and biopsy of the pleura after creating a controlled pneumothorax. Its sensitivity significantly exceeds that of pleural fluid cytologic studies or closed biopsy, particularly for malignancy. This relatively invasive procedure is not warranted in all patients.

Table 4. Pleural Fluid Analysis

Test	Abnormal Finding	Possible Diagnosis
Red blood cells	>100,000 cells/mm³	Malignancy, trauma, pulmonary embolism
White blood cells	>10,000 cells/mm³	Infection
Neutrophils	>50%	Acute pleuritis
Lymphocytes	>90%	Tuberculosis, malignancy
Eosinophils	>10%	Asbestosis, pneumothorax, resolving infection
Mesothelial cells	>5%	Tuberculosis
Glucose	<60 mg/dL	Empyema, tuberculosis, malignancy, rheumatoid disease
pH	<7.3	Parapneumonic (complicated), malignancy, tuberculosis, rheumatoid arthritis
	<7.1	Empyema, esophageal rupture
Amylase	Greater than serum value	Pancreatitis, esophageal rupture

DIAGNOSTIC PROCEDURES IN RESPIRATORY DISEASE

By Albert H. Niden, M.D.
Los Angeles, California

The appropriate use of diagnostic studies to evaluate and manage patients with pulmonary disease begins with a careful, detailed history and physical examination as well as a review of the chest film. This initial evaluation naturally leads to the judicious, cost-efficient use of selective diagnostic tests. This article briefly outlines various diagnostic modalities, such as examination of the sputum; chest imaging techniques; bronchoscopy and associated procedures; biopsy of the lung, pleura, and mediastinum; skin tests; and serologic studies. Pulmonary function testing, use of arterial blood gas determinations, exercise testing, and sleep studies are discussed in the articles on tests of respiratory function and sleep-related respiratory dysfunction.

SPUTUM EXAMINATION

A fresh, deep-cough sputum specimen is obtained for examination. Collection of sputum specimens should be observed. The quantity and character of the sputum should be noted to determine the adequacy of the specimen (i.e., sputum and not saliva). Objective criteria for an adequate sputum specimen are established cytologically by the presence of less than 10 epithelial cells and greater than 25 leukocytes per low-power field. Examination of expectorated sputum has been the key procedure for the diagnosis of bacterial pneumonia. However, because of oropharyngeal contamination, difficulties in culturing fastidious pathogens from mixed flora, previous antibiotic therapy, inadequate specimen processing, and uneven distribution of pathogens in the sputum, it is necessary to use care in interpreting the results. When compared with uncontaminated specimens (culture of blood, transthoracic aspirate, or surgical specimen), Gram staining and culture of expectorated sputum are diagnostically accurate only 50 per cent of the time. Therefore, the clinician should use such data as a guide to antibiotic therapy and not necessarily as an absolute bacteriologic diagnosis of the pneumonia (see article on bacterial pneumonia).

For smear and culture of *Mycobacterium tuberculosis,* three consecutive early-morning specimens have replaced the traditional 24-hour sputum collection. For fungal disease, a fresh, preferably early-morning sputum specimen is needed. The finding of *M. tuberculosis* or pathogenic fungi (*Histoplasma*, *Coccidioides*, *Blastomyces,* or *Cryptococcus*) in a sputum smear or culture is diagnostic of infection with that organism. In contrast, finding a saprophytic fungus (*Candida* or *Aspergillus*) in the sputum does not distinguish colonization of the tracheobronchial tree by the organism from invasive involvement of the lung. Demonstration of a saprophytic fungus involving the lung parenchyma by transbronchial biopsy (TBB) or open lung biopsy (OLB) is necessary for establishing the diagnosis of invasive pulmonary disease. Alternatively, isolating the organism from a protective sheath brushing of the involved area is highly suggestive of infection. The protective sheath greatly reduces, but does not eliminate, the problem of oropharyngeal and upper airway contamination (see section on fiberoptic bronchoscopy and related procedures). A direct immunofluorescent antibody (DFA) assay of fresh sputum (or bronchial washings) for *Legionella* can be used to identify the organism and establish the diagnosis of *Legionella* pneumonia within a few hours.

Induced sputum with the inhalation of an aerosolized solution of hypertonic saline or distilled water may stimulate a productive cough in those patients who cannot produce an adequate sputum specimen. This method of obtaining diagnostic specimens is useful in patients with tuberculosis, those with acquired imunodeficiency syndrome (AIDS) with *Pneumocystis carinii* pneumonia (PCP), and bronchogenic carcinoma.

SPUTUM CYTOLOGIC STUDIES

When properly performed, cytologic study of sputum is positive for malignant cells in 10 per cent of peripheral lesions and in 50 per cent of central endobronchial lesions. A fresh, early-morning, deep-cough sputum specimen is stained for neoplastic cells. If no sputum is produced spontaneously, an induced sputum specimen is obtained. There is a significant improvement in the detection rate of malignant cells (24-fold increase) if sputum is collected over several days in a jar containing fixative (50 per cent ethyl or isopropyl alcohol). The specimen is emulsified in a blender and centrifuged; the sediment is examined on glass slides (Saccomanno method).

CHEST IMAGING

The routine screening chest film is of little clinical value in patients without respiratory symptoms for the early diagnosis of either lung cancer or tuberculosis. Routine hospital admission chest films for patients without respiratory symptoms or relevant physical findings are also unwarranted except at hospitals caring for patients with an increased incidence of tuberculosis or AIDS.

In contrast, posteroanterior (PA) and lateral chest radiographs are an essential part of the initial evaluation of patients with respiratory symptoms or physical findings related to the lungs. These films should be considered part of the physical examination. If a radiographic abnormality is observed, the clinician should obtain old films for comparison to determine the activity or inactivity of localized or diffuse pulmonary disease. Time-consuming and expensive investigative studies may be avoided for lesions that have been present and stable for several years. Serial radiographs may be helpful in determining the significance of a lesion. For example, infiltrates that clear over a 2- to 3-day period may indicate localized atelectasis or edema fluid.

Oblique views may show pleural changes, whereas lateral decubitus views may distinguish among free effusions, loculated effusions, and pleural thickening. Lateral decubitus views are overused and are not required in the presence of a large pleural effusion. Portable chest radiographs should be reserved for critically ill, unstable patients. Because of their lesser quality—poor inspiration, geometric distortion, and apical lordotic tilt—overinterpretation of such studies should be avoided.

Fluoroscopy of the chest helps guide special invasive procedures. It is of diagnostic value only in demonstrating hemidiaphragmatic paralysis. The "sniff test" produces sudden negative intrathoracic and positive intra-abdominal pressure, resulting in the paradoxical upward movement of the paralyzed diaphragm, whereas the functioning diaphragm moves downward.

Conventional tomography and bronchography have been replaced by computed tomography (CT). With the use of consecutive 10-mm-thick horizontal radiographic slices of the chest, CT is a reliable means of studying abnormalities of the hilum, mediastinum, trachea, major bronchi, lung, and pleural space. The procedure is used to detect enlarged lymph nodes for the staging of lung cancer. It is also useful for detecting metastases to the lung not visualized on standard chest radiographs, for detecting calcification within a granuloma, and for distinguishing a pulmonary abscess from empyema. However, CT cannot distinguish lymph nodes enlarged by inflammation from those enlarged by tumor.

High-resolution CT (HRCT) of the chest uses 1.5- to 2-mm horizontal slices of the lung to better visualize normal anatomy and characterize pulmonary pathologic conditions in diffuse pulmonary disease. It has been proposed that the pattern and distribution of changes may be diagnostic of specific diffuse pulmonary diseases, but a recent double-blind study failed to demonstrate such specificity. Further studies are needed to define the role of HRCT in the diagnosis of diffuse pulmonary infiltrates. Ground-glass patterns may correlate with active inflammation and linear densities with fibrosis, but the capacity of HRCT to distinguish "active" from "inactive" disease remains to be determined.

Magnetic resonance imaging (MRI) of the thorax can provide horizontal or coronal sections with greater soft tissue specificity than can CT, but with less resolution. Because MRI can distinguish functioning blood vessels from soft tissue structures, it is particularly useful for assessing the hilum. MRI can distinguish flowing blood from clot; in the future this may facilitate the noninvasive diagnosis of pulmonary thromboembolic disease involving the major pulmonary arteries.

Selective bronchial arteriography can be used to demonstrate the source of pulmonary hemorrhage in patients with chronic infection. Embolization of the bronchial artery at the time of the study may achieve hemostasis when surgical resection is contraindicated.

The ventilation-perfusion lung scan (V/Q scan) is used in the examination of patients with suspected pulmonary embolism. The ventilation scan is performed first with inhalation of radioactive xenon-133 (^{133}Xe) gas. The equilibrium images reveal a deficit in radioactivity in areas of poorly ventilated or nonventilated lung, whereas washout images demonstrate retained ^{133}Xe activity in areas of air-trapping. Perfusion scans are performed following the intravenous injection of radioactive technetium-99m (^{99m}Tc) macroaggregated albumin. The perfusion scan reveals the pattern of pulmonary capillary blood flow and not anatomic obstruction per se. The pulmonary circulation is a low-pressure system that is sensitive to pressure changes caused by lung parenchymal and/or airway disease. Thus, perfusion defects are seen not only in pulmonary embolism but also in areas of parenchymal and/or airway disease. A normal perfusion scan virtually excludes the diagnosis of pulmonary embolism. In patients suspected of having pulmonary embolism, a single large perfusion defect or multiple segmental perfusion defects with normal ventilation (V/Q mismatch) is highly predictive of pulmonary embolism (high-probability scan means more than 90 per cent probability), whereas matching V/Q defects are unlikely to be due to embolism (low-probability scan means less than 10 per cent probability). In patients with radiographic abnormalities—for example, lung parenchymal changes—the V/Q scan results in unacceptably high false-positive and false-negative findings of approximately 33 per cent each. In this situation, the clinician should bypass the V/Q scan and proceed directly to pulmonary angiography. Patients who have an intermediate- or indeterminant-probability V/Q scan should have pulmonary angiography to establish the diagnosis.

The V/Q scan can also be used preoperatively to assess the ability of patients with marginal pulmonary reserve to withstand resectional surgery. The percentage of perfusion to the tissue to be resected compared with total perfusion accurately predicts the percentage of pulmonary function lost following resection.

Gallium-67 (^{67}Ga) lung scanning is of limited value in pulmonary disease. Following intravenous injection, gallium is bound to transferrin in the blood. The tracer accumulates in areas of the lung involved in bacterial and nonbacterial inflammatory and neoplastic processes. The CT scan has replaced gallium scans in detecting mediastinal involvement in bronchogenic carcinoma. In diffuse infiltrative pulmonary disease, such as sarcoidosis, idiopathic pulmonary fibrosis (usual interstitial pneumonitis), and collagen vascular pulmonary disease, lack of specificity and sensitivity limits the value of the gallium scan in staging disease or monitoring response to therapy. The gallium scan should not be used by itself to decide which patients to treat. It still may be used on occasion—for example, to evaluate diffuse pulmonary infiltrates in the elderly clinically stable patient in whom it is not clear whether lesions are active or inactive. In this situation, an abnormal scan may indicate the need for an immediate, more aggressive diagnostic evaluation, whereas a normal scan may suggest careful observation with a follow-up chest radiograph and pulmonary function tests.

Positron emission tomography (PET) provides both physiologic and metabolic information regarding normal and abnormal pulmonary function. Radioactive substrates can be either injected or inhaled as a gas. PET has been employed to stage lung cancer: with the use of radioactive glucose (fluorine-18 deoxyglucose) as a substrate, PET can detect the increased metabolism from a metastatic neoplasm in normal-sized hilar and mediastinal lymph nodes. PET is more sensitive than CT in this regard; however, PET cannot distinguish the increased metabolic activity of neoplasm from that of an inflammatory reaction such as sarcoidosis or tuberculosis.

Ultrasound in diagnostic imaging of the chest is used primarily to guide thoracentesis in the presence of loculated fluid, a small amount of fluid, or after failed attempts at thoracentesis.

FIBEROPTIC BRONCHOSCOPY AND RELATED PROCEDURES

The advent of flexible fiberoptic bronchoscopy (FOB) in 1965 revolutionized the practice of pulmonary medicine. The procedure is extremely well tolerated by patients, can be performed in outpatients by qualified physicians using conscious sedation, and has a very low rate of morbidity and mortality. Diagnostic indications for FOB include, but are not limited to, an abnormal chest film, hemoptysis, a new onset of unexplained cough or a change in cough, unresolved pneumonia or pulmonary abscess, or an unexplained loss of lung volume (atelectasis). It can also be used for the diagnosis of diffuse pulmonary lesions due to granulomatous disease (sarcoidosis, tuberculosis, fungal disease), carcinomatosis, or PCP.

Although FOB can be performed on critically ill unstable patients, the decision to proceed in such a patient requires good clinical judgment based on a careful risk-to-benefit evaluation. Absolute contraindications for FOB include an uncooperative patient and hypoxemia uncorrected with supplemental oxygen. Insertion of the bronchoscope results in a 20 mm Hg reduction in Pa_{O_2}. Thus, the Pa_{O_2} must be corrected to 80 mm Hg or greater. All patients undergoing bronchoscopy must have access to supplemental oxygen with electrocardiographic and Sa_{O_2} monitoring.

The tracheobronchial tree can be visualized to the fifth- or sixth-order subsegmental bronchi. The central channel of the scope permits aspiration of secretions, lavage of fluid (bronchial washing, bronchoalveolar lavage), brushing (bronchial brushing), forceps biopsies (endobronchial, transbronchial biopsy, TBB), and fine-needle aspiration (FNA; transbronchial needle aspiration). Specimens are sent for cytologic examination, smear and culture for acid-fast bacilli (AFB), fungi, silver staining for PCP, and histologic examination. Lavage of the lung with the scope wedged peripherally (bronchoalveolar lavage [BAL]) allows the clinician to obtain samples from the peripheral airways and alveoli.

Bronchial washing is used to obtain material for AFB and fungal smears and cultures as well as for cytologic examination for malignant cells. Bronchial brushings for cytologic and AFB and fungal examinations are made of endobronchial lesions and areas of extrinsic bronchial compression. Under fluoroscopic guidance, parenchymal lesions can also be explored. Protected sheath brushings from such regions can provide specimens that are relatively uncontaminated by organisms from the upper airways. A quantitative bacterial colony count of more than 10^3 colonies/mL correlates with pneumonia caused by the identified organism in difficult undiagnosed patients with pulmonary bacterial infections, particularly those receiving mechanical ventilation. A quantitative bacterial colony count of more than 10^5 colony-forming units (CFU)/mL from BAL of the area provides similar information. BAL is particularly useful for the diagnosis of PCP in patients with AIDS and is now the initial procedure of choice in such patients with clinical evidence of pulmonary disease. BAL has also facilitated cellular and molecular studies of the function of the lungs in health and disease.

Prior to a biopsy or brushing of an endobronchial lesion, 5 mL of 1:10,000 epinephrine can be injected into the airway at the site of the procedure. The resulting vasoconstriction reduces the amount of bleeding from such procedures. For neoplastic lesions visible by FOB, the diagnostic yield is greater than 95 per cent with the use of a combination of biopsy, brushings, and washings. With the use of fluoroscopic guidance for peripheral lesions not visualized by FOB, the diagnostic yield is 10 to 20 per cent. The skill of the operator may increase that yield.

TBB aids the diagnosis of focal and diffuse pulmonary lesions. During FOB, the biopsy forceps is wedged peripherally with the use of fluoroscopic guidance to avoid pleural penetration and pneumothorax. Five or six biopsy specimens containing lung parenchyma are obtained. TBB is useful for the diagnosis of lung cancer, but its greatest value is in patients with diffuse infiltrative pulmonary disease. The diagnostic yield is greater than 90 per cent in patients with pulmonary carcinomatosis, diffuse granulomatous disease (sarcoidosis, disseminated tuberculosis), and AIDS-associated PCP. However, the small size of specimens (1.5 to 3 mm) makes TBB relatively insensitive (40 per cent accuracy) for diagnosis of other causes of diffuse infiltrative pulmonary disease. TBB is contraindicated in patients with uncorrected coagulopathy.

Transbronchial needle aspiration (TBNA) can also be performed by FOB, primarily for the staging of lung cancer. Mediastinal, hilar, paratracheal, and subcarinal lymphadenopathy identified on CT scan, areas of extrinsic compression of trachea or bronchus, and widening of primary or secondary carinae can be aspirated with an 18-gauge needle, which provides material for histologic eximination. By contrast, a 21-gauge needle for cytologic specimens is used to aspirate more peripheral lesions under fluoroscopic guidance. The sensitivity of the procedure depends on the skill of the operator. An 80 per cent positive diagnostic yield has been reported for central metastatic lymphadenopathy.

THORACENTESIS AND NEEDLE PLEURAL BIOPSY

A diagnostic thoracentesis is indicated for *any* undiagnosed pleural effusion. In addition, any parapneumonic effusion greater than 300 mL should be aspirated to exclude empyema. The clinician should recall that a ground-glass radiographic appearance through which lung markings can be seen, with the upper margin forming a concave-upward meniscus, represents more than simple blunting of the costophrenic angle. Aerobic and anaerobic cultures of the fluid may prove to be the only means for identifying the organism responsible for the pneumonia. Relative contraindications for thoracentesis include an uncorrected coagulopathy, a limited cardiorespiratory reserve such that a small pneumothorax would not be tolerated, and an uncooperative patient. If, after assessing risk and benefit, the physician believes that thoracentesis is still indicated, the procedure should be performed by skilled personnel.

In general, patients with uncomplicated pleural effusions (absence of fever, chest pain) secondary to congestive heart failure, hepatic failure, or renal failure should not undergo thoracentesis. When inserting a needle into the pleural space, the rib should be located with the point of the needle, and the needle should then be inserted over the top of the rib. This maneuver avoids contact with the neurovascular bundle located along the inferior border of the rib and greatly reduces the risk of a hemothorax.

Pneumothorax occurs in 15 per cent of patients undergoing thoracentesis, and 20 per cent of those with pneumothorax require chest tube placement. The incidence of pneumothorax can be reduced in patients with small or loculated effusion by performing ultrasound-guided thoracentesis. An equally effective approach is to meticulously avoid entering the pleural space with a sharp needle. Significant pneumothoraces almost always result from lacerating the lung with a sharp needle—and not from air entering through the chest wall. The intercostal space is anesthetized with 2 per cent lidocaine, avoiding penetration of the pleural space with the anesthesia needle. After a Cope (pleural biopsy) needle with trocar in place is inserted into the intercostal space, the trocar is removed and the flat end of the Cope needle is pushed bluntly into the pleural space. Fluid can be withdrawn safely through the biopsy needle. This method can also be used to remove fluid safely from patients receiving mechanical ventilation. Alternatively, to drain a large pleural effusion, a 16-gauge intracatheter can be inserted. As fluid is withdrawn, the re-expanding lung will not be lacerated by a sharp needle.

One can safely remove up to 1500 mL of fluid slowly over 20 minutes. More rapid withdrawal of fluid may result in acute pulmonary edema secondary to a high negative intrathoracic pressure. Also, the volume of fluid removed may be limited if there is evidence that the underlying lung may not be re-expandable. This should be suspected if the trachea is deviated toward the side of the effusion or the ipsilateral diaphragm is elevated. With the development of any cardiorespiratory symptoms, the thoracentesis should be discontinued.

To improve the diagnostic yield from a thoracentesis, the fluid is anticoagulated with heparin to minimize the loss of cells and organisms in fibrin clots, and up to 1000 mL of fluid is submitted for centrifugation. The sediment is used for cytologic and/or microbiologic examination. Aliquots of noncentrifuged fluid can be submitted as indicated for a differential cell count; glucose, protein, and lactate dehydrogenase (LD) determinations; amylase (pancreatitis, ruptured esophagus) determinations; and/or triglyceride-cholesterol determinations (chylous-pseudochylous effusion). A pleural effusion protein-to-serum protein ratio greater than 0.5 or an effusion LD–to–serum LD ratio greater than 0.6 defines an exudative effusion rather than a transudate (see article on diseases of the pleura).

A pH of the pleural fluid less than or equal to 7 has been used to define the need for immediate chest tube drainage in the presence of parapneumonic effusions. This measurement, however, may not accurately predict which patients require chest tube drainage. Moreover, pleural fluid glucose levels ($\leq$40 mg/dL) often correlate with pleural fluid pH. Thus, a pH measurement on parapneumonic effusions may not be clinically indicated.

Transthoracic needle biopsy of the pleura is indicated in the presence of an undiagnosed pleural effusion in which granulomatous (tuberculous or fungal) or malignant disease is a suspected cause of the effusion. The biopsy is performed with either a Cope or an Abrams needle. Diagnostic yield is comparable with either needle so that the choice of needle is subjective. Pleural biopsy is contraindicated in the presence of an uncorrected coagulopathy or empyema (pus) or in an uncooperative patient. Five or six biopsies are taken from the 4 to 8 o'clock positions at one site over the top of the rib. One specimen is sent for culture; the others are sent for histologic examination. The diagnostic yield from thoracentesis of tuberculous and malignant effusions is only 25 per cent and 50 per cent, respectively, whereas that from needle biopsy of the pleura is 70 per cent for both tuberculous and neoplastic effusions. Thoracentesis plus pleural biopsy increases the diagnostic yield to 85 per cent. Transthoracic needle biopsy of the pleura is a remarkably safe procedure. Pneumothorax occurs 3 to 8 per cent of the time, chest tube placement is rarely required (0.1 per cent incidence), and hemothorax is rare. There are fewer complications reported following thoracentesis plus needle biopsy of the pleura than with thoracentesis alone. This apparent paradox occurs because the former is performed by physicians experienced in the field of pleural disease.

Some authorities recommend that a thoracentesis be performed initially, and if the fluid is an exudate and nondiagnostic, the thoracentesis be repeated with a pleural biopsy. If a malignant or tuberculous effusion is suspected, the author prefers to perform a pleural biopsy at the time of the initial thoracentesis. The reasoning is that (1) with appropriate selection of patients for thoracentesis and in the absence of pneumonia, almost all fluid specimens are exudates; (2) the diagnostic yield from thoracentesis alone is relatively low; and (3) there is a significant improvement in diagnostic yield with little, if any, additional risk, leading to earlier diagnosis, shorter hospital stays, and avoidance of repeated thoracentesis and pleural biopsy.

With clinical evidence of active tuberculous or malignant pleuritis, needle biopsy of the pleura can be safely performed in the absence of fluid. Using the flat end of the Cope pleural biopsy needle, the operator bluntly enters the pleural space and obtains tissue biopsy specimens. The diagnostic yield and complications are similar to those following pleural biopsy in the presence of an effusion. This technique has also been safely employed, when indicated, to obtain a pleural biopsy specimen from patients receiving mechanical ventilation. If hospitalization is not otherwise indicated, thoracentesis and pleural biopsy may be performed in outpatient facilities.

Transthoracic FNA of the lung is used primarily to determine the cause of solitary or multiple lung masses or nodules. In immunocompromised patients, FNA may help establish the cause of a localized pulmonary infection. Complications are minimal in experienced hands and with meticulous attention to detail (aspiration biopsy performed under fluoroscopic guidance, anesthesia needle not entering the pleural space, respirations suspended when FNA needle is inserted into the lung and whenever needle is held or immobilized by the operator, respirations allowed when the needle is not immobilized, and five or six thrusts made throughout the lesion while maintaining constant suction). Complications have included a small pneumothorax in 16 per cent of patients, minimal hemoptysis in 11 per cent of patients, and chest tube insertion in 3 per cent of patients. There were no deaths in the series reported by the author and colleagues. The diagnostic yield in the presence of malignancy is 96 per cent, with a false-positive rate less than 1 per cent. Although several effective needles are available, the author uses the 18-gauge EZEM needle. This needle obtains small cores of tissue for histologic examination, whereas thinner needles (21 to 25 gauge) provide cytologic specimens only. Larger needles improve the diagnostic yield, not only for cell-specific diagnosis of malignancy but also for nonmalignant lesions, without a significant increase in complications. A specific diagnosis can be made in 60 per cent of nonmalignant lesions. The diagnostic yield is also improved if a cytopathologist evaluates a Papanicolaou stain at the time of the biopsy; if the specimen is inadequate, an additional aspiration can be performed. The cytopathologist also expedites the proper processing of the specimen. FNA may be performed under fluoroscopic or CT guidance if possible. The diagnostic yield is comparable with either approach. Since the former is simpler, faster, and less costly to perform, I prefer it. CT-guided needle aspiration can be reserved for small lesions not visualized fluoroscopically and for hilar-mediastinal lesions in close proximity to large vessels.

Contraindications to percutaneous needle aspiration biopsy include patients in whom biopsy results would not alter management, uncooperative patients, and patients receiving mechanical ventilation. Other contraindications include uncontrollable cough, noncorrectable bleeding diathesis, a suspected vascular lesion, a suspected echinococcal cyst, severe pulmonary hypertension, hypoxemia not corrected with oxygen, and blebs or bullae in the biopsy path.

OTHER BIOPSY TECHNIQUES

Mediastinoscopy is useful for staging bronchogenic carcinoma as well as for evaluating mediastinal adenopathy caused by lymphoma, tuberculosis, sarcoidosis, or fungi. A rigid scope is introduced just above the suprasternal notch and passed down through the pretracheal fascia. The right and left paratracheal, the left peribronchial, and the subcarinal nodes are accessible through the scope. The hilar, aorticopulmonary, and anterior mediastinal nodes are not accessible. Complications are infrequent (3 per cent incidence) and most commonly involve pneumothorax.

Anterior mediastinotomy (Chamberlain's procedure) is used to access the hilar and anterior mediastinal nodes.

Thoracoscopy—the insertion of a rigid scope into the pleural space—is increasingly employed in patients with undiagnosed exudative pleural effusions. The parietal and visceral pleura, ipsilateral mediastinum and hilum, and lung parenchyma can be visualized and suspicious lesions biopsied. The role of thoracoscopy in the diagnosis of diffuse infiltrative pulmonary disease appears promising, and the size of the lung biopsy approaches that of an OLB.

OPEN LUNG BIOPSY

OLB through a limited thoracotomy is a safe, highly accurate procedure (92 per cent diagnostic yield) in a select group of patients. OLB is indicated in two types of patients: (1) those (often immunocompromised) with acute life-threatening pulmonary disease that does not respond to therapy and (2) those with chronic progressive pulmonary disease (often diffuse) in which a TBB has not been diagnostic. OLB can be performed in the presence of pulmonary hypertension and in patients receiving mechanical ventilation with high positive airway pressure. Selection of the biopsy site is important. The tip of the lingula or middle lobe should be avoided because passive congestion, inflammatory changes, and scarring unrelated to the diffuse disease are often present in these areas. At least two specimens from different locations are recommended. Tissue from an area of greatest involvement may represent end-stage nondiagnostic pulmonary fibrosis, whereas tissue from more normal-appearing lung may be diagnostic of early active disease. OLB tissue should be cultured and preserved for light and electron microscopy and immunofluorescence studies. Another portion of tissue should be frozen for unanticipated additional studies as indicated by the initial histopathologic examination. OLB should be undertaken only if the results of the biopsy are likely to influence the management of the patient.

SKIN TESTS

Skin tests can be placed in two categories: (1) those that produce delayed reactions and are used to diagnose bacterial, fungal, and parasitic disease and (2) those that produce immediate reactions and are used to detect hypersensitivity to specific allergens.

The delayed-type skin test helps identify tuberculosis (purified protein derivative [PPD]) or fungal disease (histoplasmin for histoplasmosis, coccidioidin or spherulin for coccidioidomycosis). A positive reaction 72 hours after intradermal injection indicates the patient has or has had the disease. False-positive results are rare. False-negative results are not uncommon because of anergy, lack of reagent potency, faulty interpretation of the reaction, and faulty application technique. Anergy panels are often used to screen for a diminished immunologic response in patients with suspected active pulmonary disease. A recent conversion of the skin test results to positive indicates a recent or active infection.

The tuberculin skin test should be performed with intermediate-strength PPD. Polysorbate (Tween)-stabilized PPD prevents absorption or adhesion of the protein to glass or plastic and is used to maintain the antigen's potency. The tine or Heath skin tests should not be used because they produce an unacceptable incidence of false-positive results. Less frequently, false-negative results may occur. The tuberculin skin test result may wane with time and become negative (less than 5-mm induration), but it may have a booster effect and a subsequent test administered as early as 1 week after the initial test may produce positive results (more than 10-mm induration) and falsely lead to the conclusion of a conversion. For tuberculosis control programs, a second skin test should be performed 1 week after the first test if any induration is noted so that true conversion can be distinguished from the booster effect in serial testing.

A positive allergic hypersensitivity skin test (immediate reaction) is not in itself diagnostic of the cause of asthma, but it may confirm a history of or direct the clinician's attention to an association of asthmatic attacks with a specific allergen. For patients with a history suggesting asthma but whose physical examination and pulmonary function tests are always normal, a bronchial provocation test or inhalation challenge with the inhalation of methacholine or histamine can be performed. A positive test of airway hyperreactivity may confirm the clinical diagnosis. When a specific allergen is suspected, an inhalation challenge with the aerosolized antigen can be used to confirm or exclude the allergen as a cause of the asthma.

SEROLOGIC TESTS

Serologic tests measure serum antibodies to specific antigens by agglutination, precipitation, or complement fixation. Serologic tests can be used to identify the pathogen in acute or chronic infections and in immunologic disorders involving the lung.

In acute bacterial (including *Mycoplasma, Legionella,* and *Chlamydia*) and viral pneumonias, a rising antibody titer may help establish the diagnosis (see article on atypical pneumonia). Serologic testing is most useful in chronic fungal and parasitic infections (e.g., histoplasmosis, coccidioidomycosis, cryptococcosis, aspergillosis, amebiasis, toxoplasmosis, and hydatid disease). The clinician must closely correlate serologic tests with all other clinical information to ensure appropriate interpretation of the data (see article on systemic mycoses).

Radioallergosorbent test (RAST) measures specific serum IgE antibodies to specific allergens. RAST provides an alternative to allergy skin testing for determining the cause of allergic pulmonary diseases. Properly performed and interpreted, allergy skin tests provide the same information as RAST. However, RAST provides a more convenient and semiquantitative form of testing.

Antineutrophil cytoplasmic antibody (ANCA) is present in the serum of patients with certain forms of vasculitis. There are two types of ANCA: (1) a diffuse cytoplasmic staining pattern (c-ANCA) and (2) a perinuclear staining pattern (p-ANCA). c-ANCA is specific for and is found in more than 90 per cent of patients with generalized active Wegener's granulomatosis. It is present in 75 per cent of patients with the limited form of Wegener's granulomatosis. Elevations in c-ANCA titers precede relapses, and the titers can be used to monitor the course of disease and the response to therapy. p-ANCA is nonspecific and occurs in a wide variety of vasculitides, including polyarteritis nodosa, the Churg-Strauss syndrome, and vasculitis overlap syndromes. Therefore, p-ANCA is of limited diagnostic value.

Anti–glomerular basement membrane antibody (anti-GBM) is found in the serum of patients with Goodpasture's syndrome. In these patients, the pulmonary alveolar basement membrane will stain positively with immunofluorescent anti-IgG antibodies that react with anti–glomerular basement membrane antibodies.

MISCELLANEOUS PROCEDURES

Catheterization of the right side of the heart with a flow-directed, balloon-tipped Swan-Ganz catheter is a relatively safe bedside procedure for obtaining essential hemodynamic data in patients with acute and chronic pulmonary disease. The catheter enables the clinician to monitor fluid status, ventricular function, and inotropic therapy for patients receiving mechanical ventilation who are in respiratory failure; to detect the presence and degree of primary or secondary pulmonary hypertension; and to determine the presence or absence of left ventricular failure in patients with chronic pulmonary disease. Right heart catheterization also provides data that help distinguish cardiogenic pulmonary edema (left heart failure) from noncardiogenic pulmonary edema (adult respiratory distress syndrome).

SLEEP-RELATED UPPER AIRWAY OBSTRUCTION

By Patrick J. Strollo, Jr., M.D.,
Ronald A. Stiller, M.D., Ph.D.,
and Mark H. Sanders, M.D.
Pittsburgh, Pennsylvania

Sleep-related upper airway obstruction is a common clinical problem. The prevalence of sleep apnea approaches that of asthma and diabetes mellitus, and its occurrence may be associated with significant pathophysiologic consequences (Table 1). This condition and its variants have been referred to as the pickwickian syndrome, the obesity-hypoventilation syndrome, sleep-disordered breathing, the obstructive sleep apnea syndrome, and the obstructive sleep hypopnea syndrome. Recently, the upper airway resistance syndrome has also been included in the category of sleep-related upper airway obstruction.

The obstructive sleep apnea syndrome is best defined as "repetitive obstructive apneas and hypopneas occurring during sleep resulting in excessive daytime sleepiness and/or altered cardiopulmonary function." Obstructive apnea is characterized by the cessation of airflow for 10 seconds or more in association with persistent ventilatory effort (Fig. 1*A*). Obstructive hypopnea is defined as a reduction in

Supported in part by VA Medical Research Service and NIH Training Grant No. 5T32HLO7563.

Table 1. Pathophysiologic Consequences of Obstructive Sleep Apnea

Vascular Morbidity-Mortality	Neurobehavioral Morbidity-Mortality
Systemic hypertension	Excessive daytime sleepiness
Nocturnal dysrhythmias	Impaired quality of life
Pulmonary hypertension	Adverse personality change
Right or left ventricular failure	Motor vehicle accidents
Myocardial infarction	
Stroke	

airflow by 30 to 50 per cent in response to increased upper airway resistance (see Fig. 1*B*). Both are typically terminated by a brief arousal from sleep and are associated with a 4 per cent or greater oxyhemoglobin desaturation. Although frequently considered to be synonymous with obstructive sleep apnea, the pickwickian and obesity-hypoventilation syndromes are distinguished by daytime hypercapnia as well as obesity. The upper airway resistance syndrome differs from obstructive sleep apnea in that transient arousals occur because of augmented ventilatory effort in the absence of discrete obstructive apnea or hypopnea (see Fig. 1*C*). Central sleep apnea (repeated apneic episodes in the absence of airflow or ventilatory effort for 10 seconds or more) is uncommon. Some patients may experience mixed apneas; that is, apneic events containing both central and obstructive components (see Fig. 1*D*). From a clinical perspective, distinguishing patients with mixed apnea from patients who have only obstructive apnea and/or hypopnea is irrelevant because the clinical presentation and approach to treatment is the same.

The diagnosis of sleep-related upper airway obstruction is established on the basis of data obtained from the patient's history and physical examination in conjunction with an assessment of cardiopulmonary function during sleep. Failure to establish a diagnosis may result in a missed opportunity to significantly improve a patient's quality of life and to decrease the risk of death.

CLINICAL PRESENTATION (Table 2)

Patients with obstructive sleep apnea frequently present during middle age, and men are affected three times as often as women. The sentinel symptom is loud snoring, which may be confusing because snoring is reported to occur in up to 40 per cent of adults in some populations. It is essential to differentiate benign snoring (snoring without pathophysiologic sequelae) from obstructive sleep apnea. The report of habitual snoring in conjunction with observed apnea and/or resuscitative snorting during sleep significantly increases the odds that obstructive sleep apnea is present.

If the patient reports excessive daytime sleepiness, habitual snoring, and observed apnea, a diagnosis of obstructive sleep apnea is further substantiated. The easily administered Epworth Sleepiness Scale (Table 3) is useful for identifying daytime sleepiness. This scoring system quantitates daytime sleepiness in a variety of soporific conditions and has been validated against objective monitoring of the propensity to fall asleep in a quiet darkened room (Multiple Sleep Latency Test). A score of greater than or equal to 9 out of a possible 24 correlates with the presence of daytime sleepiness when measured by the Multiple Sleep Latency Test. Unfortunately, a significant number of patients may underestimate their degree of daytime sleepiness. This may be partially related to gradual onset of the sleepiness over time or denial that significant sleepiness is present.

Table 2. Clinical Predictors of Obstructive Sleep Apnea

History	Physical Examination
Middle-aged male	Upper body obesity
Habitual snoring	Tonsillar hypertrophy
Observed apnea	Retrognathia
Excessive daytime sleepiness	Systemic hypertension

The complaint of daytime sleepiness is not unique to obstructive sleep apnea and may occur in patients with nonpulmonary sleep disorders. However, all patients who report habitual snoring and complain of difficulty maintaining alertness while driving or report an accident related to falling asleep while driving require evaluation for obstructive sleep apnea.

The physical examination often reveals evidence of upper body obesity in patients with obstructive sleep apnea. This can be identified by measuring the neck circumference at the cricothyroid membrane while the patient is sitting. A neck circumference of greater than or equal to 42 cm in men and greater than or equal to 40 cm in women correlates with the presence of upper body obesity. Discrete anatomic abnormalities such as tonsillar hypertrophy or retrognathia place the airway at increased risk for narrowing and/or closure during sleep and should not be overlooked. Tonsillar hypertrophy, although common in children with sleep apnea, is decidedly uncommon in adults.

The finding of hypertension on physical examination should also alert the clinician to the possibility of obstructive sleep apnea. Sleep apnea is an independent risk factor for systemic hypertension after controlling for age, sex, and obesity. The prevalence of significant sleep apnea is about 30 to 40 per cent in hypertensive populations.

NOCTURNAL SYMPTOMS (Table 4)

Nocturnal gastroesophageal reflux may be precipitated or exacerbated by the large negative intrathoracic pressures that are generated during the attempts to inhale against an obstructed upper airway. The large pressure gradient violates the integrity of the lower esophageal sphincter, promoting reflux. Patients who experience this symptom are frequently obese, which may place the stomach at an anatomic disadvantage, contributing further to nocturnal reflux.

Nocturia in patients with severe obstructive sleep apnea may be related to increased release of atrial natriuretic peptide in response to right ventricular overload. Treatment with positive pressure frequently decreases atrial natriuretic peptide release and improves nocturia. Patients may also experience nocturnal diaphoresis similar to that seen with occult malignancy. The increased work of breathing associated with sleep-disordered breathing events during non–rapid eye movement sleep is most likely responsible for the sweating. Some patients may complain of restless sleep or excessive nocturnal motor activity. This perception is linked to the movements that accompany the arousal from sleep at the termination of a sleep-disordered breathing event.

Nocturnal choking can be a particularly frightening symptom. If the patient awakens at the termination of the apnea, the inability to breathe may be experienced briefly.

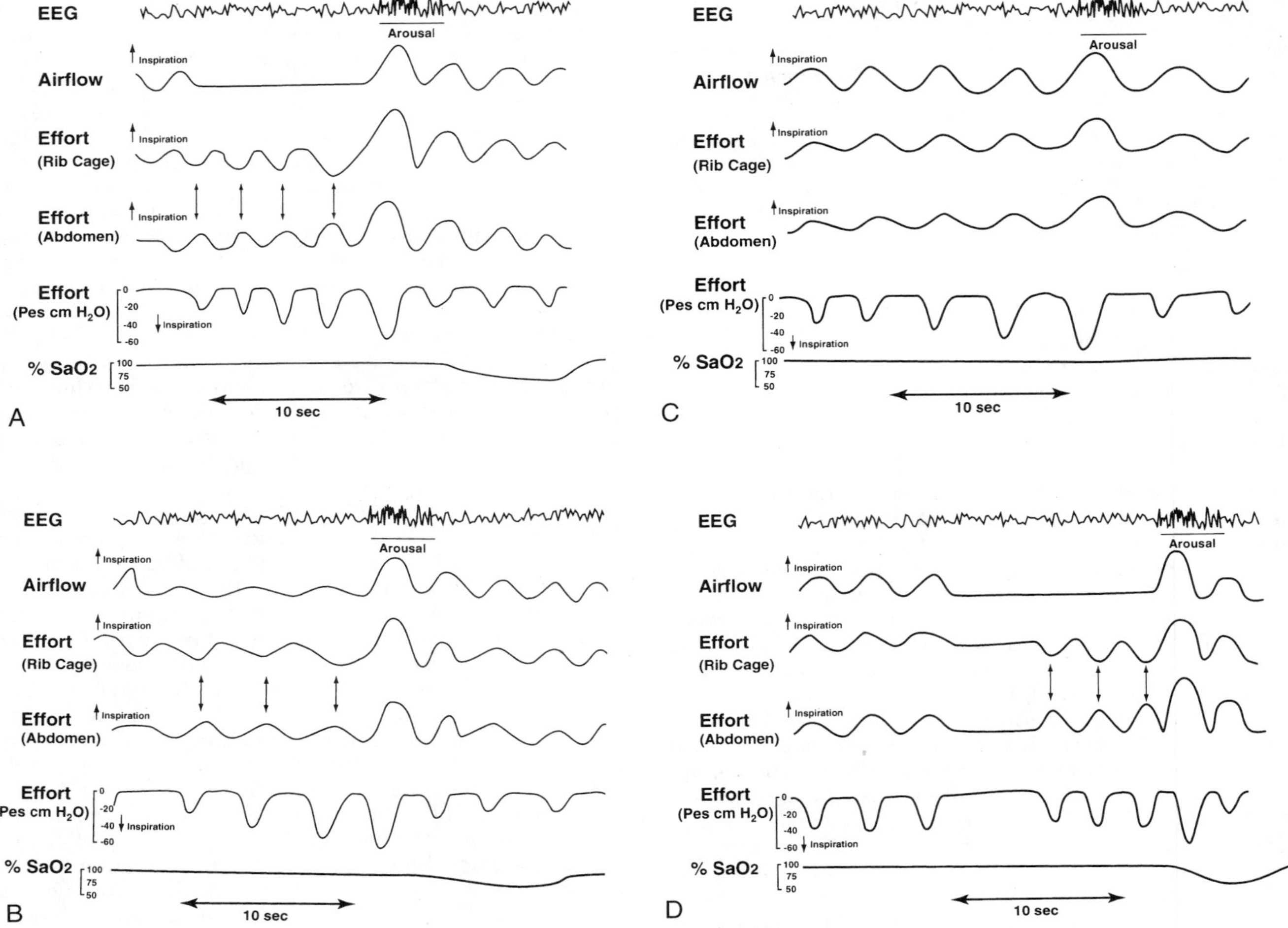

Figure 1. *A, Obstructive apnea.* Increasing ventilatory effort seen in the rib cage, abdomen, and Pes channels despite lack of airflow. The arousal seen on the EEG is associated with increasing ventilatory effort seen in the Pes channel. An oxyhemoglobin desaturation follows the termination of the apnea because of increased transit time to the finger oximeter. Note that during the apneic episode, the movements of the rib cage and the abdomen are in opposite directions *(arrows)* as a result of attempting to breathe against a closed airway. Once airway opening occurs in response to the arousal, rib cage and abdominal movements become synchronous. *B, Obstructive hypopnea.* Decreased airflow associated with increasing ventilatory effort (Pes channel) and subsequent arousal seen on the EEG. Rib cage and abdomen movements are in opposite directions during the hypopnea *(arrows),* reflecting breathing effort against a partially closed airway. Rib cage and abdominal movements become synchronous after the arousal with airway opening. The oxyhemoglobin desaturation follows the termination of the hypopnea because of increased transit time to the finger oximeter. *C, Upper airway resistance.* No significant decrease in airflow or out-of-phase movements of the rib cage and abdomen. Arousal seen on the EEG is associated with increasing ventilatory effort due to increased airway resistance as seen in the Pes channel. There is no significant oxyhemoglobin desaturation. *D, Mixed apnea.* Lack of ventilatory effort in the rib cage, abdomen, and Pes channel during the initial portion of the apnea followed increasing effort despite lack of airflow. The arousal seen on the EEG is associated with increasing ventilatory effort seen in the Pes channel. An oxyhemoglobin desaturation follows the termination of the apnea resulting from increased transit time to the finger oximeter. Note that during the obstructive portion of the apnea, the rib cage and abdomen movements are in opposite directions *(arrows)* but become synchronous after the arousal. EEG = electroencephalogram; Airflow = oronasal airflow; Effort (Rib Cage) = motion of rib cage; Effort (Abdomen) = motion of abdomen; Effort (Pes cm H_2O) = esophageal pressure as measured by an esophageal balloon in centimeters of water; $\%SaO_2$ = percent oxygen saturation.

This may be related to the uvula and/or the tongue blocking the airway. Assuming an upright position in association with awakening usually relieves this symptom. Rarely, patients with obstructive sleep apnea may present with the primary complaint of insomnia, which is usually related to difficulty maintaining rather than initiating sleep.

DIURNAL SYMPTOMS (see Table 4)

Irritability and/or other adverse personality changes are commonly found in patients with obstructive sleep apnea. They appear to be related to sleep deprivation and are usually reversed with treatment. Headache may be associated with the presence of obstructive sleep apnea. The headache is typically of the muscle tension type that is present on awakening and improves as the day progresses. It is not directly related to nocturnal hypoxia but may be related to nocturnal hypercapnia. Sexual dysfunction in patients with obstructive sleep apnea may be manifested as a decrease in sexual drive or complaints of impotence. The exact pathophysiologic mechanism of the sexual dysfunction is unclear. Treatment can result in improved libido in select patients. The effect of treatment on impotence is less certain.

Table 3. The Epworth Sleepiness Scale

Name: ____________________

Today's date: ____________ Your age (years): ________

Your sex (male = M; female = F): ____________

How likely are you to doze off or fall asleep in the following situations, in contrast to feeling just tired? This refers to your usual way of life in recent times. Even if you have not experienced some of these things recently, try to work out how they would have affected you.

Use the following scale to choose the *most appropriate number* for each situation:

0 = would *never* doze
1 = *slight* chance of dozing
2 = *moderate* chance of dozing
3 = *high* chance of dozing

Situation	Chance of dozing
Sitting and reading	________
Watching television	________
Sitting, inactive in a public place (e.g., theater or a meeting)	________
As a passenger in a car for an hour without a break	________
Lying down to rest in the afternoon when circumstances permit	________
Sitting and talking to someone	________
Sitting quietly after lunch without alcohol	________
In a car, while stopped for a few minutes in traffic	________

Thank you for your cooperation

Adapted from Johns, M.W.: A new method for measuring daytime sleepiness: The Epworth Sleepiness Scale. Sleep 14:541, 1991.

SPECIAL CONSIDERATIONS

Women may not report habitual snoring or apnea, but instead complain of fatigue. Recent studies have shown that these patients have a higher rate of divorce than men with obstructive sleep apnea. They often sleep alone and may not have a spouse or significant other accompany them to the appointment to corroborate their history.

Some patients at or close to ideal body weight may have abnormal upper airway anatomy that places them at risk for obstructive sleep apnea. Large tonsils (uncommon in adults) or facial skeletal abnormalities (i.e., high arched hard palate; midfacial deficiency; retrognathia; or micrognathia) may be found in these patients. Subtle but clinically important retrognathia may not be appreciated by the clinician.

The finding of tachy- or bradydysrhythmias that are encountered only during sleep should prompt the clinician to consider the possibility of concomitant obstructive sleep apnea. Upper airway obstruction with increased vagal tone can be associated with bradycardia and/or heart block. The termination of an apneic event is accompanied by increased sympathetic traffic that may augment tachydysrhythmias, particularly in the presence of hypoxia. Pulmonary hypertension and/or right ventricular failure is uncommonly encountered in obstructive sleep apnea unless concomitant obstructive pulmonary disease or morbid obesity is present. However, a diagnosis of obstructive sleep apnea should be considered if pulmonary hypertension is out of proportion to the degree of pulmonary disease or intrinsic heart disease does not explain the presence of right ventricular failure.

Table 4. Obstructive Sleep Apnea: Associated Symptoms

Nocturnal	Diurnal
Reflux	Irritability or adverse personality change
Nocturia	Headache
Diaphoresis	Sexual dysfunction
Increased motor activity	
Choking	
Insomnia	

Patients with primary neurologic problems occasionally experience upper airway obstruction during sleep. This may occur in the absence of concomitant obesity. Diseases that diffusely affect skeletal muscle function, such as the muscular dystrophies and amyotrophic lateral sclerosis, as well as stroke syndromes affecting bulbar muscle function can be complicated by sleep apnea or hypopnea. Syndromes resulting in ventilatory muscle discoordination such as the Shy-Drager or Arnold-Chiari syndrome may also be associated with upper airway obstruction during sleep.

Patients with endocrine disorders such as acromegaly or hypothyroidism are at risk for sleep-disordered breathing. Both conditions can increase tongue size, escalating the risk for upper airway obstruction during sleep. Acromegaly and hypothyroidism may also affect central ventilatory drive. Even with adequate endocrine treatment of these disorders, obstructive sleep apnea may persist and require treatment.

Patients with Marfan's syndrome are at increased risk for obstructive sleep apnea. This is presumably related to an increase in the compliance of the upper airways of these individuals. Substantial increases in negative pleural pressure are found in patients with sleep apnea or hypopnea. This increases aortic transmural pressure and may increase the risk for aortic dissection.

The cardiopulmonary consequences of obstructive sleep apnea can be amplified by the presence of concomitant pulmonary or cardiac disease. Patients with these underlying conditions may experience more profound oxygen desaturation and/or cardiac complications. Oxygen stores may be lower prior to the onset of the sleep-disordered breathing event, the ventricle may be more irritable, or the ventricular function may be impaired.

Patients usually do not present with a sudden onset of obstructive sleep apnea symptoms. These circumstances should suggest a new abnormality of the upper airway or of central control of ventilation. Tonsillar hypertrophy that is asymmetric or associated with bleeding should raise the suspicion of a malignancy. New-onset tonsillar hypertrophy can also be associated with lymphadenopathy due to human immunodeficiency virus (HIV) infection.

LABORATORY TESTS

There is currently no laboratory test, other than a sleep study, that can be used to confirm a diagnosis of obstructive sleep apnea. Hypothyroid patients may have concomitant sleep apnea, although the incidence of hypothyroidism in obstructive sleep apnea patients is low. Routine screening for hypothyroidism in all patients with suspected obstructive sleep apnea is not recommended. Screening spirometry and arterial blood gas determinations in nonsmokers without signs or symptoms of pulmonary disease are usually not indicated. "Saw-toothing" on the flow-volume loop is specific but not sensitive for obstructive sleep apnea. However, an incidental finding of saw-toothing or a ratio of

FEF_{50} to FIF_{50} greater than 1 should prompt the clinician to consider obstructive sleep apnea as a possible diagnosis (FEF_{50} = forced expiratory flow at 50 per cent of vital capacity; FIF_{50} = forced inspiratory flow at 50 per cent of vital capacity). A variety of imaging studies have been performed on patients with obstructive sleep apnea, but no single test can confirm a diagnosis. Assessment of skeletal anatomy with lateral cephalometric radiographs may be helpful for patients in whom maxillofacial surgery is contemplated.

SLEEP STUDIES

Sleep studies are performed not only to confirm a suspected diagnosis of obstructive sleep apnea but also to stratify the risk for pathophysiologic complications and to assess the level of urgency for initiation of treatment. Holter monitoring and overnight oximetry lack sufficient sensitivity and specificity to make them adequate screening tests for obstructive sleep apnea. Sleep studies performed in the home or the hospital without a trained technician in attendance have been used to diagnose obstructive sleep apnea. A variety of diagnostic systems are now commercially available. Unfortunately, little validation data are available to provide unqualified support for their use. Many of these systems do not monitor the electroencephalogram; therefore, a sleeping or waking state cannot be documented, and arousals that are not associated with nocturnal oxygen desaturation (typical of the upper airway resistance syndrome) cannot be identified. A negative study does not rule out a breathing disorder during sleep.

Laboratory-based nocturnal polysomnography with a trained technician in attendance is regarded as the "gold standard" for the diagnosis of sleep-related breathing disorders. The ability to monitor sleep and breathing allows the clinician to carefully examine patients with obstructive sleep apnea as well as patients with the upper airway resistance syndrome. Objective testing of daytime sleepiness with the Multiple Sleep Latency Test may assist the clinician in identifying patients who are significantly sleepy. Unfortunately, these tests do not identify those patients who are unable to drive safely.

THERAPEUTIC STUDIES

Occasionally, a therapeutic trial of positive airway pressure via a mask can assist the clinician in establishing the diagnosis of sleep-related upper airway obstruction. Patients who snore heavily and complain of daytime sleepiness or fatigue, despite a negative diagnostic polysomnogram, may have the upper airway resistance syndrome. If the application of positive pressure abolishes the snoring, decreases the degree of sleep fragmentation, and improves sleep architecture, treatment with positive pressure may be warranted.

Section Five

CARDIOVASCULAR SYSTEM

HYPERTENSION

By L. Michael Prisant, M.D.
Augusta, Georgia

Blood pressure is a continuous physiologic variable like temperature and heart rate. The blood pressure normally rises in the early morning hours before or at the time of awakening and declines in the evening hours, reaching its nadir between 12 midnight and 4 AM. The mean level of blood pressure rises with increasing age from birth to adulthood. With continued aging, there is progressive fragmentation of elastin in the aorta and other large blood vessels, resulting in a rise in the systolic blood pressure with little change in the diastolic blood pressure.

For adults aged 18 years and older, a systolic blood pressure less than or equal to 130 mm Hg and a diastolic blood pressure less than or equal to 85 mm Hg are considered optimal. The systolic blood pressure normally increases with pain, stress, or dynamic exercise (e.g., jogging). The diastolic blood pressure stays the same or falls with dynamic exercise but rises with isometric exercise (e.g., weight lifting) and myocardial ischemia.

Approximately 25 per cent of American adults have elevated blood pressure, which increases their risk of cardiovascular morbidity and mortality. The relative risk of systolic versus diastolic blood pressure on mortality from coronary heart disease is demonstrated in Figure 1. Although both systolic and diastolic blood pressure contribute to overall mortality, systolic blood pressure has a greater impact. The reason that diastolic blood pressure heretofore has received more attention is that most of the morbidity and mortality trials have used diastolic blood pressure as the goal of treatment. The recently published Systolic Hypertension in the Elderly Population (SHEP) trial supports intervention in isolated systolic hypertension.

DEFINITIONS

Hypertension is defined as systolic and/or diastolic blood pressure greater than or equal to 140/90 mm Hg. Table 1 categorizes hypertension according to the criteria of the Fifth Joint National Committee on Detection, Evaluation, and Treatment of High Blood Pressure. Labile hypertension refers to episodically normal and abnormal blood pressure. The term "borderline hypertension" should be used instead, however, because blood pressure is no more (or no less) variable in normotensive persons than in individuals with fixed hypertension. Secondary hypertension refers to hypertension for which there is a known cause (e.g., renovascular hypertension, hyperthyroidism, pheochromocytoma, primary renal disease). If there is no known secondary cause, the diagnosis of essential hypertension (also referred to as idiopathic or primary hypertension) is established by default. Isolated systolic hypertension indicates an elevated systolic blood pressure with a normal diastolic blood pressure. Pseudohypertension denotes a falsely elevated blood pressure that is an artifact of measurement. "White coat hypertension" (also called "office hypertension") refers to blood pressure elevation that occurs only in the medical environment. White coat hypertension does not appear to be free of cardiovascular risk.

The presence of resistant, accelerated, or malignant hypertension should increase the suspicion of secondary hypertension. Accelerated or malignant hypertension describes hypertension associated with ongoing vascular damage, including flame-shaped hemorrhages and/or retinal infarcts ("cotton wool" spots); however, with malignant hypertension, papilledema is also present (Fig. 2). Resistant hypertension refers to uncontrolled blood pressure (160/100 mm Hg) despite rational, maximal three-drug therapy in a compliant patient. If the initial blood pressure is less than 180/115 mm Hg, resistance is defined as failure to achieve pressures less than 140/90 mm Hg. Although resistant (or refractory) hypertension is more likely to result from suboptimal drug therapy (43 per cent) and medication intolerance (14 per cent) than secondary hypertension (11 per cent), the presence of the advanced retinopathy in accelerated and malignant hypertension is associated with a higher yield of secondary hypertension on further evaluation.

GOAL OF EVALUATION

Forty-three million Americans older than 17 years of age have hypertension. Essential hypertension accounts for 90 per cent of diagnoses (Table 2). It is not a homogeneous disease state; it is viewed as a polygenic trait. First-degree relatives of hypertensive persons are more likely to have hypertension than are the first-degree relatives of normotensive individuals. The risk increases with age, and the risk in men is greater than in women prior to 55 years of

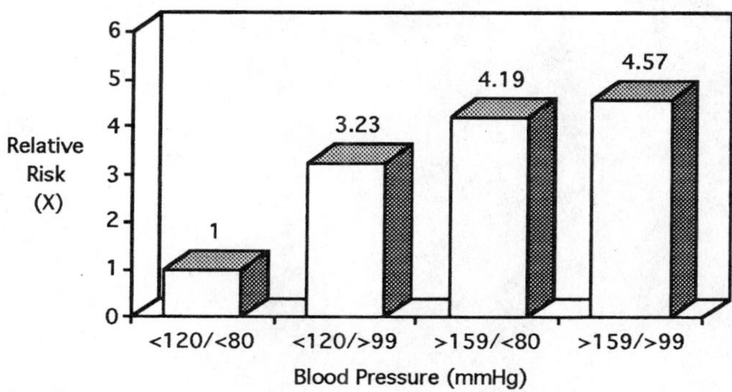

Figure 1. Comparison of the effect of systolic versus diastolic blood pressure on the adjusted relative risk of coronary heart disease for men. Relative risk adjusted for age, race, serum cholesterol level, cigarettes smoked per day, diabetes, and income. (Data from Stamler, R., and Neaton, J.D.: Arch. Intern. Med. 153:598–615, 1993, with permission.)

Table 1. Classification and Follow-Up of Blood Pressure for Adults 18 Years and Older*

Category	Systolic (mm Hg)	Diastolic (mm Hg)	Recommended Follow-Up
Normal	<130	<85	Recheck in 2 years
High normal	130–139	85–89	Recheck in 1 year
Hypertension			
Stage 1 (mild)	140–159	90–99	Confirm within 2 months
Stage 2 (moderate)	160–179	100–109	Evaluate or refer within 1 month
Stage 3 (severe)	180–209	110–119	Evaluate or refer within 1 week
Stage 4 (very severe)	≥210	≥120	Evaluate or refer immediately

*Based on the average of two or more readings taken at each of two or more visits following an initial screening with the patient not receiving antihypertensive agents. The classification should be based on the higher stage when the systolic and diastolic blood pressures fall into different categories. Follow-up recommendations are based on initial screening measurements.

age (Fig. 3). African Americans are more likely to have earlier onset, more severe hypertension, and higher mortality rates. Excess body weight, psychosocial stress, sodium ingestion, alcohol consumption, decreased physical activity, and potassium ingestion may modify the level of blood pressure for an individual patient.

Most patients have no symptoms from hypertension, which is called "the silent killer." With severe hypertension, morning headache is more common. When symptoms are present, they usually are caused by hypertensive or atherosclerotic target organ damage (Table 3), secondary hypertension, or side effects of drug therapy.

Hypertension is the most common cardiovascular reason for an office visit. The goals for the initial evaluation of the suspected hypertensive patient are to (1) prove that the patient has a sustained elevation in blood pressure, (2) identify the presence of hypertensive and atherosclerotic target organ damage, (3) screen for other cardiovascular risk factors, (4) identify factors that may modify treatment, and (5) identify correctable causes of secondary hypertension.

Medical History

The medical history should assess the apparent duration of hypertension and the degree of elevation. Previous drug therapy and adverse reactions to drugs—such as nightmares or wheezes in patients receving beta-blockers and angioneurotic edema (Fig. 4) or cough in patients receiving an angiotensin-converting enzyme inhibitor—are obviously important. The clinician should seek symptoms suggesting target organ damage (see Table 3) as well as a history of prior hospitalizations for unstable angina, myocardial infarction, congestive heart failure, transient ischemic attacks, cerebrovascular accidents, or aortic dissection. A history directed specifically at common causes of secondary hypertension (see Table 2) can detect correctable causes of hypertension. For example, intermittent claudication suggests coarctation of the aorta in young patients and atherosclerotic peripheral vascular disease in older patients.

An often neglected aspect of the history is a careful and complete accounting of all prescribed and over-the-counter medications and illicit drugs (Table 4). A daily alcohol intake of greater than 24 ounces of beer, 8 ounces of wine, or 2 ounces of 100-proof whiskey raises blood pressure and interferes with blood pressure control. Concomitant diseases (e.g., asthma, diabetes) that may alter the choice of drug must be considered. Evaluation of other cardiovascular risk factors and family history (Table 5) permits clinical assessment of overall risks for morbid events. Dietary habits and social history provide important information that may have an impact on blood pressure regulation.

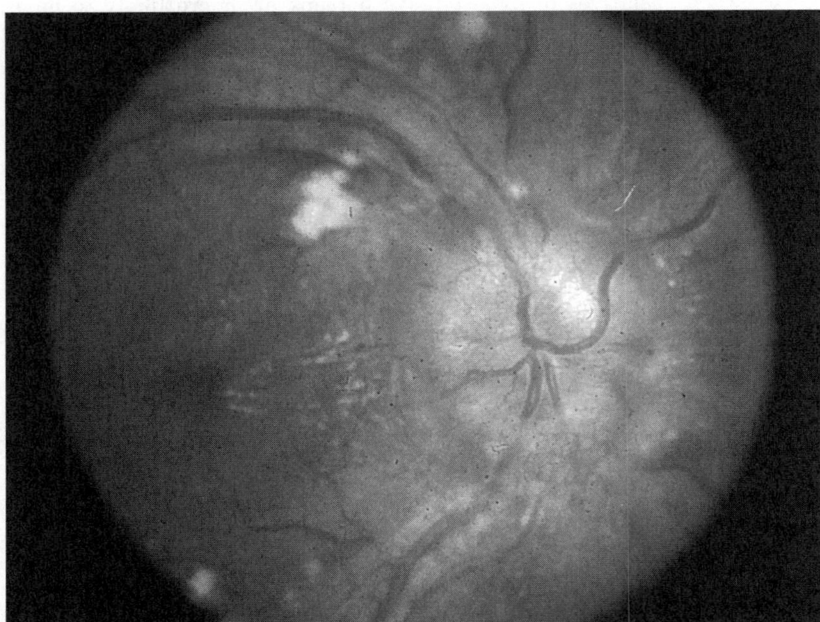

Figure 2. Retinopathy associated with malignant hypertension.

Table 2. Estimated Prevalence of Causes of Adult Hypertension

Cause	Percentage
Essential hypertension	89.0–92.1
Chronic renal disease	2.4–5.6
Renovascular hypertension	0.7–4
Aortic coarctation	0.1–1
Primary aldosteronism	0.1–0.3
Cushing's syndrome	0.1–0.2
Pheochromocytoma	0.1–0.2
Oral contraceptive use	0.2–1

Physical Examination

Blood pressure should initially be measured in both arms and the higher value used for all subsequent follow-up visits. Waist and hip circumference, height, and weight should also be recorded at the initial examination. Follow-up weight determinations are necessary. The general evaluation should include a funduscopic examination; a neck assessment for jugular venous distention, carotid bruits, and thyromegaly; and a pulmonary examination for wheezes and rales. Careful cardiovascular assessment of the heart rate and rhythm, the apical impulse, gallops, and murmurs should be routine. Palpation of the abdomen for masses, enlarged kidneys, and a dilated, expansile aorta as well as auscultation for bruits is required. In addition to examining the peripheral vascular system for reduced pulses and bruits, a neurologic assessment of hand dominance, communicative abilities, gait, paresis, or paralysis, Babinski's and Romberg's signs should be performed. Table 6 includes additional physical findings that may affect clinical management and treatment.

Laboratory Examination

Prior to initiating therapy, the routine laboratory tests recommended for the initial evaluation include (1) a fasting chemistry profile (including potassium, creatinine, calcium, glucose, uric acid, total and high-density lipoprotein cholesterol, triglyceride levels), (2) a complete blood count, (3) urinalysis, and (4) an electrocardiogram. Clinical information that can be derived from the chemistry data are shown in Table 7. Testing for plasma renin activity, plasma norepinephrine, sensitive thyroid-stimulating hormone (TSH), and urinary microalbumin levels is not routinely performed but may be useful in selected patients. In contrast to previous policy statements, the chest film is no longer routinely ordered. However, if the patient smokes, it is reasonable to obtain this study.

Echocardiography is useful for assessing cardiac anatomy and function. Wall thickness can be directly measured, and left ventricular mass, indexed for height or body sur-

Table 3. Symptoms of Target Organ Disease in Hypertension

Cardiac Damage
- Exertional dyspnea
- Orthopnea
- Paroxysmal nocturnal dyspnea
- Edema
- Angina
- Palpitations
- Syncope

Cerebrovascular Symptoms
- Morning headache
- Transient ischemic attacks
- Stroke
- Dementia
- Altered mental status
- Coma
- Seizures

Retinal Symptoms
- Visual blurring
- Blindness

Renal Symptoms
- Polyuria
- Nocturia
- Lethargy
- Nausea

Aorta and Peripheral Vascular Disease
- Pain of aortic dissection
- Pain of abdominal aneurysm rupture
- Intermittent claudication

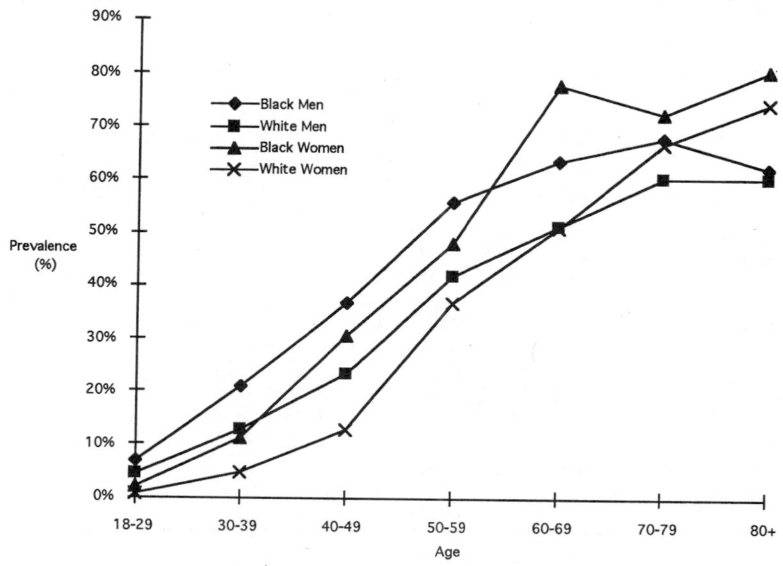

Figure 3. Prevalence of hypertension (≥140/90 mm Hg) by age, race, and gender of United States adult population from Third National Health and Nutrition Examination Survey, 1988–1991. (Data from Burt, V.L., Whelton, P., Roccella, E.J., et al.: Hypertension 25:305–313, 1995.)

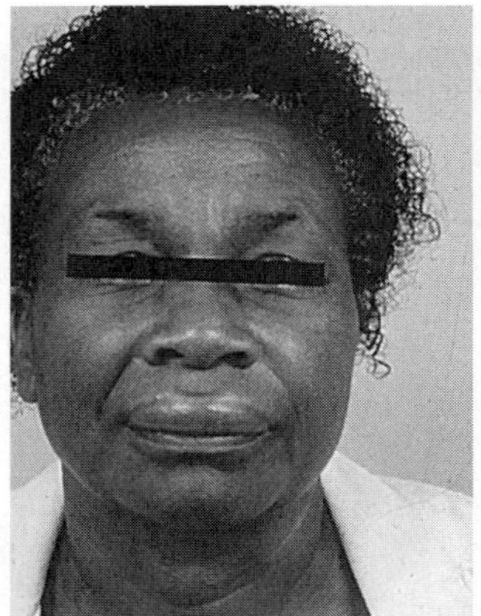
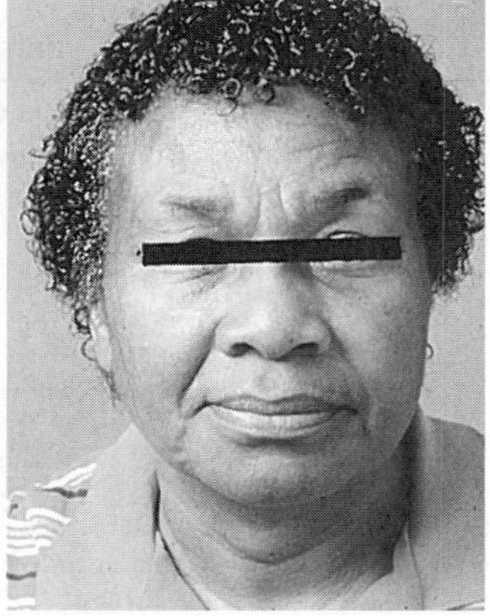

Figure 4. Angioneurotic edema following treatment with converting enzyme inhibitor and with resolution.

face area, can be computed (Fig. 5). The prognostic value of an increased left ventricular mass is greater than electrocardiographic left ventricular hypertrophy. Cost considerations preclude the use of routine echocardiography; however, if nonanginal cardiac symptoms are present, it is reasonable to perform the test.

Ambulatory blood pressure monitoring refers to portable blood pressure recording devices that measure blood pressure every 7.5 to 30 minutes over a period of 24 hours. The equipment does not measure blood pressure accurately during ambulation. Day-to-day repeatability of 24-hour blood pressure is not remarkable, but office measurements are also highly variable. Few prognostic data are available, but group measurements correlate better with hypertensive target organ damage than do office measurements. Although it is not recommended for the routine diagnosis of hypertension, reasonable uses of ambulatory blood pressure monitoring include (1) absence of target organ damage and suspected white coat hypertension, (2) resistant hypertension, (3) documentation of autonomic dysfunction or transient hypotension secondary to antihypertensive medications, and (4) episodic hypertension (associated with panic attacks or pheochromocytoma).

Table 4. Drugs or Substances That Cause or Aggravate Hypertension

9-α-Fluorocortisol
9-α-Fluoroprednisolone
Alcohol*
Aminophylline
Amphetamines
Anabolic steroids
Beta-blocker withdrawal
Central alpha-stimulant (e.g., clonidine) withdrawal
Cocaine*
Corticosteroids*
Cyclosporine
Ephedrine*
Epinephrine*
Ergot preparations
Erythropoietin
Levodopa
Licorice and licorice-containing chewing tobaccos*
Monoamine oxidase inhibitors with tyramine-containing foods
Nonsteroidal anti-inflammatory drugs (e.g., ibuprofen, indomethacin, naproxen)*
Oral contraceptives (high doses in premenopausal patients)
Racepinephrine*
Phenylephrine*
Phenylpropanolamine*
Pseudoephedrine*
Theophylline*
Tricyclic antidepressants
Yohimbine

*Available without a prescription.

Table 5. Assessment of Other Cardiovascular Risk Factors

Risk Factor	Assessment
Diabetes mellitus	Fasting plasma glucose ≥140 mg/dL twice *or* Random plasma glucose ≥200 mg/dL with symptoms
Family history	Risk of premature cardiovascular disease in parent or other first-degree relative before age 55 years in males and 65 years in females; also assess history of hypertension, diabetes mellitus, and dyslipidemia
Left ventricular hypertrophy (LVH)	Electrocardiographic diagnosis of LVH: Cornell criteria: voltage = R_{aVL} + S_{V3} >2.8 mV in men; >2.0 mV in women Framingham: The presence of voltage with "strain" (ST-T segment vector opposite QRS) identifies patients with a dismal prognosis Echocardiographic diagnosis of abnormal mass: Framingham: men ≥143 g/m; women ≥102 g/m [mass (g) corrected for height (m)] Cornell criteria: ≥125 g/m² [mass corrected for body surface area]; risk higher if relative wall thickness ≥0.45
Lipid disorder	Nonfasting total and HDL cholesterol: If HDL <35 mg/dL or total cholesterol ≥240 mg/dL, perform a lipoprotein analysis The risk of an LDL cholesterol level depends on other risk factors and manifested atherosclerosis
Obesity	Weight >10% more than ideal weight Waist-to-hip ratio: male: >0.95; female: >0.85 Body mass index = weight (kg)/height (m²) Male: ≥27.8 kg/m² (severe ≥31.1 kg/m²) Female: ≥27.3 kg/m² (severe ≥32.3 kg/m²)
Physical inactivity	Aerobic activity <20 to 30 min three times per wk
Premature menopause: no estrogen therapy	History
Smoking	History

HDL = high-density lipoprotein; LDL = low-density lipoprotein.

Table 6. Physical Examination

Test	Implication
Blood Pressure Measurement	
Isolated increased systolic blood pressure	Anemia Aortic regurgitation Arteriovenous fistula Atherosclerosis Beri-beri Hyperthyroidism
Inequality of pressures in arms	Cervical rib Dissection of the aorta Scalenus anticus syndrome Subclavian atherosclerosis Subclavian steal syndrome Supravalvular aortic stenosis Variability of measurements
Orthostatic changes	Autonomic failure Diabetes mellitus Hypovolemia Pheochromocytoma
General Appearance	
Angioneurotic edema	ACE inhibitor therapy
Café au lait spots, neurofibromatosis	Pheochromocytoma Renal artery stenosis
Central obesity, acne, moon face, hirsutism, thin skin striae, bruises, wasted limbs, "buffalo hump"	Cushing's syndrome
Coarse hair, thick lips and tongue, puffy eyelids, myxedema	Hypothyroidism
Exogenous obesity	Possibility of pseudohypertension
Exophthalmos, lid retraction, tremulousness, wasting, goiter	Hyperthyroidism
Marfanoid features, mucosal neuromas	Pheochromocytoma
Periorbital edema, pallor	Renal disease
Plethora, conjunctival suffusion	Polycythemia
Prognathism; enlarged tongue, nose, hands, and feet	Acromegaly
Webbing of the neck, broad chest, wide-spaced nipples, low posterior hairline, short stature	Turner's syndrome (coarctation of aorta)
Fundus	
Cotton wool spots	Anemia Diabetic retinopathy Accelerated hypertension Hyperviscosity Vasculitis
Linear retinal hemorrhages	Accelerated hypertension
Papilledema	Malignant hypertension
Neck	
Carotid bruits	Atherosclerosis of carotid artery
Jugular venous distention	Right-sided heart failure
Thyroid enlargement	Hyperthyroidism Hypothyroidism
Lungs	
Rales	Heart failure
Wheezes	Asthma Beta-blocker therapy Chronic lung disease Heart failure
Heart	
Tachycardia	Heart failure Hyperthyroidism Pheochromocytoma Anemia
Atrial fibrillation	Hyperthyroidism Ischemic heart disease Left atrial enlargement
Palpable pulses of intercostal arteries of posterior thorax	Coarctation of the aorta
Sustained and enlarged (>3 cm) apical impulse	Left ventricular hypertrophy
Apical impulse outside midclavicular line	Left ventricular hypertrophy Left ventricular dilatation

Table continued on following page

Table 6. Physical Examination *(Continued)*

Test	Implication
Heart *(Continued)*	
Tambour S_2	Aortic root dilatation
S_3 gallop	Heart failure Regurgitant lesions Anemia AV fistula Hyperthyroidism Cardiomyopathy
S_4 gallop	Left ventricular hypertrophy Coronary artery disease Anemia AV fistula Hyperthyroidism Cardiomyopathy
Basal systolic murmur	Hypertension Coarctation of aorta Aortic stenosis Benign murmur
Basal diastolic murmur	Aortic insufficiency Dissecting aorta
Pericardial rub	Uremic pericarditis
Abdomen	
Bilateral palpable kidneys	Polycystic kidney disease
Mass with expansile pulsation	Abdominal aneurysm
Systolic or systolic-diastolic bruit	Renal artery stenosis Mesenteric artery stenosis Arteriovenous malformation
Small testes or clitoromegaly	Anabolic steroid use
Priapism	Alpha-blocker therapy
Bilateral decreased femoral pulses	Coarctation of the aorta Aortoileofemoral atherosclerosis
Femoral bruits	Aortoileofemoral atherosclerosis
Radial-femoral delay	Aortoileofemoral atherosclerosis Coarctation of the aorta
Peripheral Edema	Right-sided heart failure Nephrotic syndrome Chronic renal failure Calcium antagonist therapy Direct vasodilator therapy

ACE = angiotensin-converting enzyme; AV = arteriovenous.

DIAGNOSIS OF HYPERTENSION

It is the physician's responsibility to be certain that the technique of blood pressure monitoring is implemented correctly by support personnel. Meticulous measurement of blood pressure is important because inaccurate labeling results in adverse insurance ratings, psychological trauma, and unnecessary medication. The short-term effect on medication adjustment must also be considered.

A single blood pressure measurement should not be used for the diagnosis of hypertension in stable patients. Instead, the average of the last two of three measurements, each obtained on different days, is used (see Table 1). The first of these three blood pressure measurements is used to determine the systolic and diastolic blood pressure. A mercury manometer should be used to measure blood pressure. If an aneroid or electronic sphygmomanometer is used, it should be calibrated against a mercury manometer every 3 months. Nonphysicians should measure blood pressure to avoid the "physician pressor effect" (white coat or office hypertension).

Baseline evaluation of blood pressure requires that the patient not smoke or ingest caffeine within 30 minutes of the measurement. The procedure should be performed after a 5- to 15-minute period of rest. An uncovered and supported arm at heart level is necessary *prior* to cuff application. The length and width of the cuff are critical: The *length* of the cuff bladder should surround 80 per cent of the arm circumference and the *width* of the cuff bladder should be 40 per cent of the arm circumference. The use of a small cuff in obese patients is a common cause of pseudohypertension.

Once the cuff is applied snugly and evenly over the brachial artery, palpation of the radial artery to estimate the systolic blood pressure is vital to avoid the underestimation of systolic blood pressure or the overestimation of diastolic blood pressure that is associated with the silent period (the auscultatory gap) that is sometimes present

Table 7. Laboratory Assessment of Hypertension

Test	Implication
Hypokalemia	Diuretic use Primary hyperaldosteronism Cushing's syndrome
Hypercalcemia	Thiazide diuretic use Hyperparathyroidism
Hyperglycemia	Diuretic use Diabetes mellitus Cushing's syndrome Acromegaly Pheochromocytoma
Hypercholesterolemia	Primary lipid disorder Hypothyroidism Nephrotic syndrome Hyperparathyroidism Hypercortisolism Progestational agents Anabolic steroids
Increased serum creatinine	Primary renal disease Acromegaly ACE inhibitor use Renovascular hypertension Avoid renally excreted drugs
Hyperkalemia	Chronic renal failure ACE inhibitor therapy Potassium-sparing diuretics Type IV renal tubular acidosis Salt substitutes Potassium chloride supplement
Hyperuricemia	Early sign of renal disease Gout Diuretics Chronic renal failure Polycythemia Hyperparathyroidism Hypothyroidism Polycystic kidney disease Toxemia of pregnancy
Hypertriglyceridemia	Obesity Diabetes mellitus Chronic renal failure Liver disease Ethanol abuse Estrogen use Beta-blocker use Diuretic use
Abnormal liver function	Ethanol abuse Avoid hepatically metabolized drugs

ACE = angiotensin-converting enzyme.

between the systolic and diastolic blood pressure. In addition, estimating the systolic blood pressure potentially avoids the pain of excess inflation pressure. The presence of a palpable, pulseless radial artery after inflation of the cuff to greater than the systolic blood pressure is called the Osler sign. This sign was thought to be a symptom of pseudohypertension resulting from atherosclerosis in older patients; however, it has been observed in normotensive patients and is probably not discriminatory.

The cuff should be distended about 20 mm Hg above the palpable systolic blood pressure. The *bell* of the stethoscope should be used to auscultate low-intensity Korotkoff sounds over the brachial artery while slowly deflating the cuff with each heart beat, or 2 to 3 mm Hg per second. The systolic blood pressure is the first faint tapping sound of two successive beats (Korotkoff phase I) after cuff deflation, and the diastolic blood pressure is the point at which Korotkoff sounds completely disappear (Korotkoff phase V). In adults whose Korotkoff sounds approach zero (and in infants and children aged 3 to 12 years), the diastolic blood pressure is specified as the period marked by an abrupt muffling of sound quality (Korotkoff phase IV). All values are reported to the nearest 2 mm Hg. The technique of blood pressure measurement should be used for follow-up measurements to decrease the variability in technique. Blood pressure may fall over time even without active drug therapy; this has been referred to as the placebo effect.

Home blood pressure monitoring may be a useful adjunct in defining white coat hypertension. The patient needs appropriate instruction to measure the blood pressure correctly. Furthermore, the equipment must be calibrated by means of a Y connection to a mercury manometer and correlated over a wide range of blood pressures to be certain that the equipment is accurate. This is recommended as the initial screening procedure for white coat hypertension in the absence of target organ damage.

HYPERTENSIVE AND ATHEROSCLEROTIC TARGET ORGAN DAMAGE

Myocardial infarctions and strokes are the first and third leading causes of death in the United States. Age, male gender, smoking, diabetes, hyperlipidemia, systolic blood pressure, and left ventricular hypertrophy are the cardiovascular risk factors associated with the development of angina, unstable angina, myocardial infarction, sudden death, stroke, congestive heart failure, and peripheral vascular disease (see article on cardiovascular risk factors). Reduction of blood pressure decreases the rate of stroke, myocardial infarction, congestive heart failure, and accelerated hypertension. Aortic aneurysm and dissection, retinal damage, renovascular hypertension, and renal insufficiency are other consequences of elevated blood pressure.

Target organ damage may be due to the alteration or rupture of arteries or arterioles in the brain, eyes, heart, and kidneys (hypertensive events) or to progressive atherosclerosis involving the aorta or the carotid, coronary, or renal arteries, and iliofemoral (atherosclerotic) events. The target organ damage from accelerated or malignant hypertension is different from the damage caused by chronic hypertension.

Accelerated or Malignant Hypertension

Active damage to the small arteries and arterioles, causing tissue ischemia, is the hallmark of accelerated or malignant hypertension. Involvement of the renal interlobular, preglomerular, cerebral, retinal, myocardial, gastrointestinal, and peripheral arterioles results in red blood cell casts, hematuria, heavy proteinuria, azotemia, oliguria, mental alteration, retinal hemorrhages and infarcts (cotton wool spots), papilledema, myocardial scarring, gastrointestinal hemorrhages and pancreatitis (rarely), and microangiopathic hemolytic anemia. Severe headaches, visual changes, and heart failure are common. Plasma volume may be reduced and the renin-angiotensin-aldosterone system is usually activated, resulting in hypokalemia. Untreated accelerated or malignant hypertension causes death in 6 to 12 months, usually because of uremia. Other

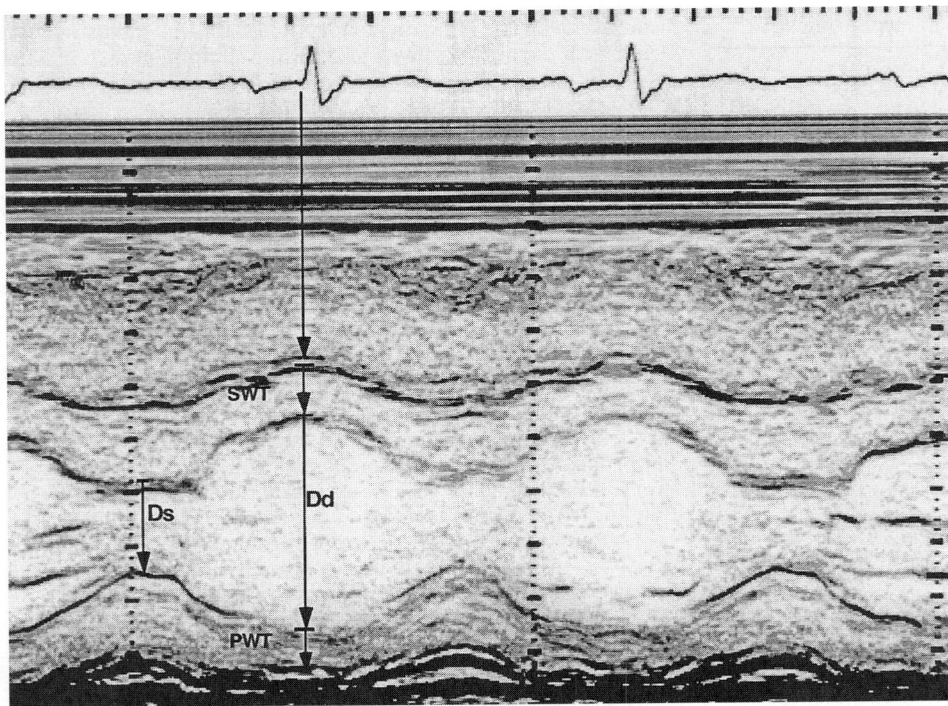

Figure 5. M-mode echocardiogram. The measurements of chamber dimension and thickness are made in diastole at the onset of the QRS complex from the leading edge to leading edge. Dd = diastolic diameter; SWT = septal wall thickness; PWT = posterior wall thickness; Ds = systolic diameter; left ventricular mass = $0.8 \times [((SWT + Dd + PWT)^3 - Dd^3) - 13.6] + 0.6$; relative wall thickness = $(2 \times PWT)/Dd$.

risks include hypertensive encephalopathy, acute intracerebral hemorrhage, subarachnoid hemorrhage due to rupture of a berry aneurysm, acute myocardial infarction, and acute aortic dissection.

Hypertensive encephalopathy refers to cerebral edema, microinfarcts, and petechial hemorrhages that occur when the blood pressure exceeds the upper limits of cerebral autoregulation. Headache, nausea, vomiting, visual disturbances, seizures, impaired consciousness, and reversible focal neurologic signs may be present with retinal hemorrhages, cotton wool spots, and papilledema. Symptoms and signs typically resolve with antihypertensive therapy after 48 to 72 hours. Computed tomography is useful to rule out other neurologic events that may produce similar findings.

The clinical picture of accelerated or malignant hypertension is less common today than it was in the past. When it appears, it is more likely to occur in young, urban, indigent minority men. Drug withdrawal (e.g., clonidine), cocaine use, noncompliance, and secondary hypertension (especially renovascular hypertension and pheochromocytoma) should be considered as precipitating factors.

Chronic Hypertension

Heart Damage

Hypertensive cardiomyopathy (left ventricular hypertrophy) not only is the target organ response of pressure overload on the left ventricle but also is the most potent of all the cardiovascular risk factors. In the absence of epicardial coronary artery disease, left ventricular hypertrophy is associated with angina, myocardial infarction, congestive heart failure, atrial and ventricular arrhythmias, and sudden death. Congestive heart failure may occur early in the natural history of the disease because of diastolic filling abnormalities with normal systolic function without a dilated ventricle or late because of reduced systolic function with a dilated ventricle. In addition to ventricular arrhythmias, atrial fibrillation may appear and increase the risk for embolic strokes.

A diagnosis of left ventricular hypertrophy suggests the need for pharmacologic therapy. Diagnosis may be obtained by physical examination, chest radiography, electrocardiography, or echocardiography. The usual physical finding is a sustained and forceful apical impulse within or outside the

Table 8. Test Performance for Diagnosis of Epicardial Coronary Artery Disease

	Bruce Treadmill* (%)	Exercise Nuclear Ventriculography (%)†	Thallium (± Dipyridamole) Scintigraphy (%)‡
Sensitivity	46.7	76.5	94.4
Specificity	37.5	25.0	63.5
Positive predictive value	41.2	46.4	38.6
Negative predictive value	42.9	55.6	97.9
False-positive rate	62.5	75.0	36.5
False-negative rate	53.3	23.5	5.6
Overall accuracy	41.9	48.6	69.6

*Horizontal or downsloping ST-segment depression ≥1 mm 0.08 seconds after J point.
†Failure of ejection fraction to increase by 5 per cent and development of a wall motion abnormality.
‡Development of a reversible perfusion defect.

midclavicular line. On chest film, an increased cardiothoracic ratio greater than 0.5 is neither sensitive nor specific for left ventricular enlargement (LVE). The prognosis is worse with an increased cardiothoracic ratio, however, and reversion of radiographic LVE is associated with decreased coronary mortality. A chest film is no longer routinely recommended. The identification of left ventricular hypertrophy on the electrocardiogram usually ensures its presence; it is a late finding associated with a worsened prognosis. The absence of electrocardiographic criteria for left ventricular hypertrophy does not exclude the anatomic diagnosis. LVE, according to the Cornell criteria, is present if the sum of the voltage in R_{aVL} and S_{V3} exceeds 2.8 mV in men and 2 mV in women. The Cornell voltage criteria are simpler than those of Romhilt-Estes, with improved sensitivity and overall test accuracy. The presence of repolarization changes or "strain" in the lateral precordial leads was associated with death within 5 years in 33 per cent of men and 21 per cent of women in the Framingham cohort. If echocardiographic measurements are meticulously performed, they not only provide accurate measurements of wall and chamber dimensions but also add a measure of left ventricular performance (which may influence the choice of antihypertensive agents and determine the cause of congestive heart failure). Finally, the use of echocardiography does not obviate the need for electrocardiography in assessing rhythm disturbances, myocardial infarction, and advanced heart block that may preclude the use of certain antihypertensive agents (e.g., verapamil).

Hypertensive patients may experience myocardial ischemia on the basis of atherosclerotic narrowing of epicardial coronary arteries, impaired coronary flow reserve, or small vessel disease. Atherosclerosis in the large coronary arteries may require a revascularization procedure, whereas small vessel disease requires rigorous antihypertensive therapy. Unfortunately, no tests are helpful in making the distinction. Table 8 shows the performance characteristics of various methods of detecting large vessel coronary disease. Routine exercise stress testing is associated with a high rate of both false-positive and false-negative results. Exercise radionuclide ventriculography is also inadequate for screening purposes. Thallium stress testing (with dipyridamole if the patient cannot achieve a heart rate systolic pressure product $\geq$20,000) is a test of exclusion that can be used when investigating the possibility of large vessel coronary disease. A positive test result necessitates coronary arteriography to determine the presence or absence of large vessel disease.

Kidney Damage

Hypertension may result in or be secondary to chronic renal insufficiency. Hypertensive nephropathy is suggested by the absence of other causes of renal disease. African Americans are more likely than whites to experience hypertensive nephrosclerosis. This condition reduces renal blood flow, resulting in early increases of uric acid and progressive excretory failure, characterized by rising serum urea nitrogen and creatinine levels. A fasting serum creatinine level greater than 1.4 mg/dL (or 1.3 mg/dL in patients older than 60 years) is defined as early renal insufficiency. Persistent and progressive changes in creatinine levels greater than 0.3 mg/dL from baseline are the best indicators of renal involvement. Microalbuminuria (excretion of 30 to 300 mg albumin per 24 hours) does not confirm the presence of hypertensive renal disease. In chronic hypertension, proteinuria is not greater than 2 g per 24 hours, and there are no cells or casts on microscopic examination of the urine.

Cerebrovascular Disease

Strokes may be embolic, thrombotic, or hemorrhagic. Transient ischemic attacks sometimes precede strokes. These transient attacks begin abruptly, manifest focal neurologic dysfunction of the carotid or vertebrobasilar artery, and resolve within 24 hours. Common symptoms include hemiparesis or hemiplegia, focal sensory deficits, amaurosis fugax, ataxia, vertigo, diplopia, dysphagia, and aphasia. Doppler ultrasound can help select the patients who may benefit from carotid endarterectomy. Computed tomography is used to localize strokes precisely and to differentiate infarction from hemorrhage.

Large Vessel Disease

Aortic dissection should be considered in any patient presenting with chest or back pain, congestive heart failure, or cerebrovascular accident. The onset of pain is sudden and usually is described as "tearing" or "ripping." The pain is maximal from the onset. When the chest pain is anterior, it may radiate to the back. When the pain occurs in the back, it may radiate to the flanks or abdomen. Most patients are elderly hypertensive individuals; however, aortic coarctation, Marfan's syndrome, Turner's syndrome, and pregnancy are common predisposing factors. After initiating drug therapy, diagnostic transesophageal echocardiography or computed tomography with contrast medium should be performed in consultation with a thoracic surgeon.

Hypertension and atherosclerosis cause abdominal aortic aneurysms. The normal width of the aorta is 1.5 to 2 cm. An aneurysm is said to be present when the aortic width is 3 to 4 cm. In thin patients, aneurysms may be detected by abdominal palpation, but in other patients ultrasound or computed tomography is necessary to detect an abdominal aneurysm. Patients with an aneurysm larger than 4 to 5 cm should be evaluated for resection.

Cramping or tightness in the hip, buttocks, thigh, or calf, precipitated by exercise and relieved by rest, is the primary symptom of aortoiliac or lower extremity peripheral vascular disease. Pain at rest suggests advanced peripheral vessel disease. All pulses should be checked and compared for symmetry. Segmental Doppler pressures before and after exercise confirm the clinical picture. Arteriography helps select which patients may benefit from balloon angioplasty or surgical reconstruction.

CAUSES OF SECONDARY HYPERTENSION

Renal Parenchymal Disease

The cause of renal parenchymal disease often can be determined by history and physical examination; urinalysis with microscopic examination; renal sonography; serum urea nitrogen, creatinine, and albumin determinations; and 24-hour urine collection for protein and creatinine clearance determination. The presence of diabetes mellitus, systemic lupus erythematosus, scleroderma, polyarteritis nodosa, recurrent urinary tract infections, prostatic hypertrophy, nephrolithiasis, analgesic use (including nonsteroidal anti-inflammatory drugs), and moonshine liquor use are pertinent historical items. Renal sonography can be used to determine the presence of cystic kidney disease, ureteral obstruction, renal masses, and kidney size. Hematuria often requires a urologic evaluation. Red cell casts indicate glomerular disease and may require a renal biopsy. Proteinuria greater than 3.5 g per 24 hours is associated with the nephrotic syndrome.

Primary Aldosteronism

Adrenocortical aldosterone secretion causes salt and water retention, renin suppression, and potassium excretion by the kidney. Primary aldosteronism is rare, occurring in only 0.1 to 0.3 per cent of hypertensive patients. The cause is usually a solitary, surgically treatable adrenocortical adenoma in about 60 per cent of patients and nonsurgical bilateral adrenal hyperplasia in the remaining patients. Black licorice, chewing tobacco, carbenoxolone, high-dose ketoconazole, topical 9-α-fluoroprednisolone, and intranasal 9-α-fluorocortisol may induce a reversible aldosteronelike state.

There is no unique clinical presentation for primary aldosteronism. Common symptoms include proximal muscle weakness, polyuria, nocturia, headaches, and tachycardia. A serum potassium level less than 3.5 mEq/L when the patient is not receiving diuretics, a serum potassium level less than 3 mEq/L when the patient is receiving diuretics, and refractory hypertension provide additional clues. A normal serum potassium level does not exclude the diagnosis of primary aldosteronism.

Several screening tests may be useful; however, isolated elevated plasma aldosterone levels or suppressed plasma renin activity is not usually helpful. Computed tomography should not be used as an initial screening test because it does not detect small (<1 cm) adenomas and may identify nonfunctioning adenomas or other causes of adrenal enlargement. Diuretics (including potassium-sparing agents), beta-blockers, calcium antagonists, and angiotensin-converting enzyme inhibitors should be discontinued for at least 2 weeks prior to evaluation because they affect renin and aldosterone levels. A 24-hour urinary potassium excretion or RBC greater than 40 mEq supports a nongastrointestinal tract cause of hypokalemia. After a diet to which 10 to 12 g of sodium chloride is added for 3 days, a urinary aldosterone greater than 14 μg per 24 hours with urinary sodium greater than or equal to 250 mEq per 24 hours provides optimal sensitivity for the outpatient diagnosis of primary aldosteronism. The unexpected postural decrease in plasma aldosterone levels with increased plasma 18-hydroxycorticosterone levels greater than 100 ng/dL is corroborative evidence of an adrenal adenoma. Computed tomography using 0.5-cm slices will aid in the localization. A biochemical picture of aldosteronism without radiographic localization may necessitate the performance of adrenal vein aldosterone sampling to differentiate an adrenal adenoma from hyperplasia.

Renovascular Hypertension

Renal artery stenosis is not equivalent to renovascular hypertension. Normotensive patients can have significant renal artery stenosis without hypertension. Renovascular hypertension refers to hypertension caused by renal ischemia from renal artery stenosis; the hypertension remits with relief of the obstruction. The actual prevalence is low in the general population, but the probability increases with resistant or severe hypertension, generalized atherosclerosis, retinal hemorrhages and/or infarcts with or without papilledema, an epigastric systolic-diastolic or flank bruit, renal insufficiency, a history of smoking, or new onset of hypertension before age 30 years or after age 55 years. An often-stated indication is a rise in serum creatinine levels when drug therapy is initiated with an angiotensin-converting enzyme inhibitor; however, a rise in serum creatinine is more likely to occur with pre-existing renal insufficiency, especially if renal function is dependent on the presence of angiotensin II to maintain adequate glomerular filtration. The cause of renovascular hypertension is more likely to be medial fibromuscular hyperplasia in young female patients and atherosclerosis in older patients. Peripheral renin activity is increased with unilateral renovascular hypertension. Renin is quantitated by measuring the rate of generation of angiotensin I, as determined by radioimmunoassay. It is exquisitely sensitive to variations in sodium balance and posture. About 12 per cent of patients with essential hypertension have increased renin concentrations. Results of peripheral measurements are highly variable in many laboratories. Diuretics, direct vasodilators, and angiotensin-converting enzyme inhibitors increase renin activity, and beta-blockers, alpha$_2$-stimulants, and nonsteroidal anti-inflammatory agents decrease renin activity. Furthermore, renin must be indexed to 24-hour urine sodium excretion (sodium excretion is inversely related to renin activity). Ideally, patients should not receive antihypertensive medication for 21 days prior to measurement of peripheral renin levels, but the reality is that many patients cannot safely have their medications withdrawn. As a result, the sensitivity and specificity are much lower.

Both the oral captopril test (measurement of renin activity after administration of oral captopril) and captopril renography using technetium-99m-diethylenetriamine penta-acetic acid (DTPA) as a measure of the glomerular filtration rate and/or iodine-133-orthoiodohippurate (IOH) as a measure of effective renal blood flow are associated with false-positive and false-negative results. Captopril renography detects asymmetry of uptake or excretion by comparing both kidneys before and after administration of 25 to 50 mg of oral captopril with or without furosemide stimulation. This test also predicts the blood pressure response to renal revascularization. Renal artery duplex sonography attempts to detect an increased renal artery velocity compared with the velocity of the aorta. This test is operator-dependent and is associated with difficulties in extremely obese patients. Simultaneous renal vein renin levels invasively demonstrate the physiology of lateralization: the renin activity of stenotic kidney is at least 1.5 times greater than that of the uninvolved kidney, and the renin activity of the uninvolved kidney is suppressed. The rapid-sequence intravenous pyelogram is no longer used because of the dye load, radiation exposure, and 12 per cent false-positive rate with essential hypertension.

A renal arteriogram, with or without intra-arterial digital subtraction angiography, will define the anatomy of the renal arteries but will not determine whether a 50 per cent (or greater) anatomic obstruction is causing renovascular hypertension. Intravenous digital subtraction arteriography is less useful. Magnetic resonance imaging can be useful for identifying proximal, but not distal, renal artery stenosis.

The clinical utility of all tests is determined by the test sensitivity and specificity as well as the disease prevalence. The tests shown in Figure 6 are adequate to exclude renovascular hypertension when the prevalence is 5 per cent or less; positive test results are not as useful. A reasonable alternative approach is to perform selective renal arteriography in patients who have a high likelihood of disease if they are willing to undergo surgical revascularization. If there is significant renal artery stenosis, it is important to prove that the hypertension is renin-dependent and normalizes with a converting enzyme inhibitor.

Pheochromocytoma

A pheochromocytoma usually presents as a norepinephrine-producing tumor of the adrenal medulla. About 10 per

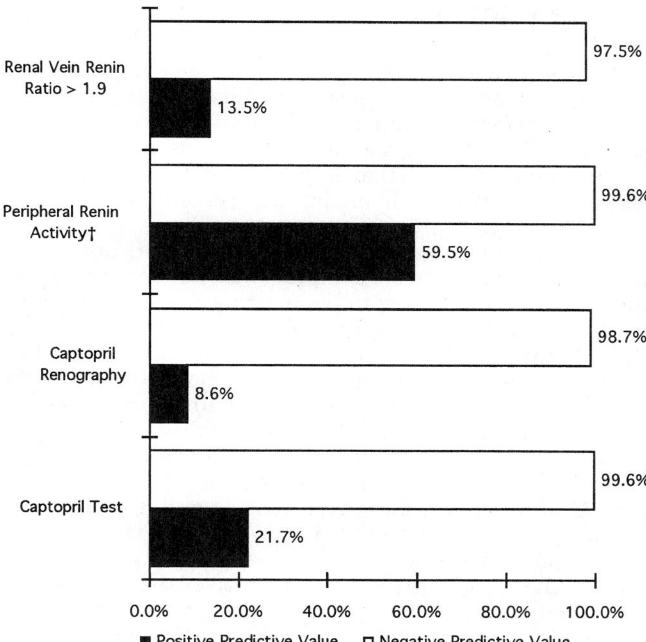

Figure 6. Positive and negative predictive values of tests for renovascular hypertension according to a disease prevalence of 5 per cent. Dagger indicates cessation of all medication for 21 days. (Data from Carr, A.A., Prisant, L.M., and Bottini, P.B.: Evaluation and management of hypertensives for renovascular hypertension. *In* Mandal, A.K., and Jennette, J.C. [eds.]: *Diagnosis and Management of Renal Disease and Hypertension.* Durham, N.C., Carolina Academic, 1994, pp. 389–409.)

cent occur bilaterally, 10 per cent are malignant, and 10 per cent are extra-adrenal. Pheochromocytoma is most likely to occur in young adults. About 10 per cent are associated with familial multiple endocrine neoplasia syndromes (hyperparathyroidism and medullary thyroid carcinoma in type II and mucosal neuromas, thickened corneal nerves, gastrointestinal ganglioneuromatosis, marfanoid habitus, and medullary thyroid carcinoma in type III).

Headaches, excessive sweating, palpitations (with or without tachycardia), anxiety, and tremulousness are common symptoms of pheochromocytoma. Flushing is unlikely to be associated with a pheochromocytoma. Hypertension does not have to be paroxysmal. Orthostatic hypotension may occur simultaneously because of volume depletion. Neurofibromatosis and café au lait spots are visual clues of disorders associated with pheochromocytomas (as well as renal artery stenosis). A catecholamine cardiomyopathy is seen in some patients. Glucose intolerance is frequently present. The occurrence of hypertension during the induction of anesthesia or initiation of tricyclic antidepressant therapy is an important clue to pheochromocytoma.

Plasma catecholamine levels determined by high-performance liquid chromatography and 24-hour urinary catecholamine and/or metanephrine excretion are usually increased with pheochromocytoma. When the secretion is paroxysmal, these biochemical tests may produce normal results. Congestive heart failure, renal failure, and administration of tricyclic antidepressants, levodopa, labetalol, appetite suppressants, nose drops, chlorpromazine, monoamine oxidase inhibitors, isoproterenol, erythromycin, and tetracycline may be associated with apparent increased catecholamine levels. Methylglucamine contained in radiocontrast agents may result in a false-negative test result with urinary metanephrines.

In the absence of drugs or conditions that increase catecholamine levels, plasma norepinephrine concentrations greater than 2000 pg/mL support the diagnosis. If the concentrations are 500 to 2000 pg/mL, clonidine (0.3 mg) may be given and plasma catecholamine determinations repeated 3 hours later (the clonidine suppression test). The absence of a 50 per cent decline in catecholamine levels are supportive of the diagnosis. The clonidine suppression test should be conducted in the fasting patient, and an indwelling catheter for blood collection should be inserted 30 minutes prior to the procedure to avoid pain, which might increase plasma catecholamine levels. The patient should remain supine during the 3 hours required for the test, and blood pressure and heart rate should be monitored every 30 minutes. Beta-blockers should be discontinued 48 hours prior to testing to avoid bradycardia. Testing should not be performed in volume-depleted patients.

If there is biochemical evidence of pheochromocytoma, computed tomographic scanning or magnetic resonance imaging of the abdomen and pelvis should be performed for tumor localization, along with an oblique chest film. If the tumor is not localized, ^{131}I-metaiodobenzylguanidine scintigraphy of the entire body is employed for localization. Uptake of ^{131}I-metaiodobenzylguanidine may be inhibited by beta-blockers, calcium antagonists, reserpine, tranquilizers, tricyclic antidepressants, and sympathomimetic agents.

PULMONARY HYPERTENSION

By Douglas Ashinsky, M.D.
Warren, New Jersey

Pulmonary hypertension develops when the resistance to flow across the pulmonary circulation increases. The natural history of pulmonary hypertension and its response to treatment depend on the mechanism of its initiation. When the cause is reversible, pulmonary hypertension may be prevented or treated by appropriate therapies. However, if the cause is not reversible or is unknown, sustained pulmonary hypertension typically follows an inexorably progressive course, and management is limited to supportive measures to keep the patient as comfortable as possible.

The pulmonary circulation is normally a high-flow, low-resistance, highly distensible circuit that is capable of accommodating the entire right ventricular outflow volume at a pressure that is only one fifth that of the systemic circulation. The resistance to blood flow in the pulmonary circulation is one twelfth the resistance across the systemic bed in normal individuals. The mean pulmonary artery pressure is 12 ± 2 mm Hg, and the mean left atrial pressure is 6 ± 2 mm Hg. A normal cardiac output of 5 to 6 L per minute flows from the right ventricle to the left atrium with a pressure drop of only 6 mm Hg, as opposed to a pressure drop of about 90 mm Hg in the systemic circulation between the left ventricle and the right atrium.

The pulmonary vascular bed has the capacity to regulate vascular tone and to recruit unused vessels to accommodate physiologic changes. This is done through the large aggregate cross-sectional area of the pulmonary circulation where its arterioles are thinner and lack the more muscular media found in systemic arterioles. Thus, a large runoff of blood from the pulmonary arterial tree occurs during each systole, and a large number of minute vessels that are held in reserve can be opened when cardiac output increases during exercise.

In the normal pulmonary circulation, blood flow is generally passive, and there are no baroreceptors similar to those found in the systemic circulation. Stimulation of pulmonary vasomotor nerves exerts a minimal effect on the pulmonary blood flow and on its resistance. Vasoactive mediators including histamine, serotonin, angiotensin II, and eicosanoids have not been shown to cause changes in the pulmonary blood flow that would lead to pulmonary hypertension.

CLASSIFICATION OF PULMONARY HYPERTENSION

Pulmonary hypertension exists when the mean pulmonary artery pressure exceeds 20 mm Hg and occurs in the majority of patients secondary to cardiac or pulmonary disease. Pulmonary hypertension can be subdivided into two groups on the basis of its pathophysiologic mechanism: precapillary (due to primary pulmonary vascular disease) and postcapillary (secondary to various cardiac or pulmonary diseases). In precapillary pulmonary hypertension, constriction, obstruction, or obliteration of a substantial component of the pulmonary bed occurs, but in postcapillary pulmonary hypertension, an obstruction to pulmonary venous return increases pulmonary vascular pressure (Table 1).

Table 1. Causes of Pulmonary Hypertension

Precapillary Pulmonary Hypertension
Pulmonary vascular obliteration/obstruction
Parenchymal lung disease
Interstitial lung disease
Emphysema
Pulmonary embolism
Vasculitis
Progressive systemic sclerosis
Pulmonary schistosomiasis
Miscellaneous
Intravenous drug use
Hepatic cirrhosis
L-Tryptophan
Reactive hypoxic vasoconstriction
Altitude
Hypoxia due to pulmonary, neuromuscular, or chest wall disease
Sleep apnea syndrome
Mechanical compression
Positive-pressure ventilation
Chest wall abnormalities (kyphoscoliosis)
Overperfusion (left-to-right shunt)
Postcapillary Pulmonary Hypertension
Cardiac causes
Left ventricular failure
Mitral valve disease
Left atrial obstruction
Pulmonary venous causes
Pulmonary veno-occlusive disease
Mediastinal fibrosis or neoplasm
Anomalous pulmonary venous return

CLINICAL FEATURES

The symptoms associated with pulmonary hypertension are usually nonspecific. Because pulmonary hypertension rarely occurs as an independent entity, symptoms and signs usually relate to the primary disease process, especially in mild cases. Patients with chronic respiratory disease who have cor pulmonale may present merely with worsening of their previous symptoms.

Exertional dyspnea, tachypnea, chest pain, and lightheadedness are common symptoms in pulmonary hypertension. They are related to the increased right ventricular work and the pulmonary vascular limitations to the increasing cardiac output. Syncope, pedal edema, and ascites are indicative of more critical impairments in the right ventricular function and more severe pulmonary hypertension. Hemoptysis, due to rupture of small vessels, is seen in precapillary pulmonary hypertension and more commonly in pulmonary venous hypertension. Hoarseness may occur in severe pulmonary hypertension and is due to compression of the left laryngeal nerve by the enlarged proximal pulmonary arteries. Raynaud's syndrome may be present in those patients with connective tissue diseases associated with pulmonary hypertension.

PHYSICAL EXAMINATION

Most patients with pulmonary hypertension have physical signs that are due to the underlying disease process. Often no detectable abnormalities are found on examination of the lungs. Crackles, a pleural friction rub, or signs of pleural effusion may be heard in the patient with pulmonary hypertension due to pulmonary embolism. Examination of the neck may show jugular venous distention and prominent cv waves, which result from tricuspid insufficiency. Pulmonary hypertension eventually leads to right ventricular hypertrophy with a palpable right ventricular heave. This causes an increasingly prominent right atrial a wave transmitted to the neck veins owing to the increased force of the right atrial systolic contraction that is in turn needed to overcome the increased end-diastolic right ventricular pressure of the compromised right ventricle. Atrial fibrillation may then develop as a late manifestation of this right ventricular compromise.

Auscultation of the heart often reveals a right ventricular third heart sound, frequently with an atrial fourth sound superimposed, producing a summation gallop. The pulmonary valve may become incompetent, causing a basal diastolic murmur (Graham Steell's murmur) that becomes louder on inspiration. An early pulmonary systolic ejection sound or even a short murmur may be heard when sufficient dilation of the main pulmonary trunk occurs. This may be confused with the presence of a soft systolic murmur, which increases during inspiration, due to the development of tricuspid valve incompetence. This can be verified by the presence of a right ventricular v wave visible in the jugular venous pulse.

Examination of the abdomen may disclose tender hepatomegaly from venous congestion or a "pulsatile liver" due to tricuspid insufficiency. Ascites and edema may indicate overt right-sided heart failure in the absence of other potential causes.

Clubbing is a common finding in patients with pulmonary hypertension due to chronic obstructive lung disease, pulmonary fibrosis, cystic fibrosis, and congenital heart disease. Clubbing is not a common physical finding in other conditions that cause pulmonary hypertension or in primary pulmonary hypertension itself.

Central cyanosis is an uncommon feature of pulmonary hypertension unless there is an associated reversal of a left-to-right intracardiac shunt. Occult recurrent pulmonary embolism with pulmonary hypertension is the likely diagnosis if the patient has dyspnea at rest, central cyanosis, and clinical signs of pulmonary hypertension *without* evidence of an intracardiac shunt.

IMAGING STUDIES AND LABORATORY DIAGNOSIS

Chest Film

The chest film in pulmonary hypertension commonly shows little overall cardiac enlargement until heart failure occurs, unless the causative condition leading to pulmonary hypertension is responsible for specific chamber enlargement. Broadening of the main pulmonary trunk is usually seen on chest films. This causes a prominent convexity of the upper left mediastinum between the aortic knuckle and the upper left border of the heart (left ventricle and left atrial appendage). The left and right main pulmonary arteries and their proximal branches are also typically widened. When pulmonary hypertension becomes severe, the peripheral pulmonary arteries appear to have been "pruned." They appear much narrower than normal, which causes increased radiologic translucency in the peripheral lung fields.

The size of the peripheral pulmonary arteries correlates with pulmonary blood flow. Patients with large septal defects and hyperdynamic pulmonary hypertension show plethoric lung fields with engorged peripheral vessels. Patients with pulmonary hypertension and low pulmonary blood flow (secondary to congenital septal defects, Eisenmenger's syndrome, or primary pulmonary hypertension) have severe vascular changes that show conspicuous peripheral vascular pruning. The appearance of the lung fields provides clues to the association of pulmonary hypertension with primary lung disease, such as emphysema. Areas of increased density on chest film are typical of fibrosis, whereas areas of translucency suggest pulmonary embolism.

Electrocardiogram

The electrocardiogram of patients with pulmonary hypertension usually shows evidence of right ventricular hypertrophy with a right axis deviation of more than +120 degrees. Dominant R and T inversion in the right precordial leads and a dominant S wave in the left precordial leads are typical. Right atrial enlargement associated with pulmonary hypertension is seen as tall, peaked P waves in the right precordial and inferior leads.

If pulmonary hypertension is due to mitral stenosis, the electrocardiogram may show bifid P waves and negative terminal deflection in the V_1 lead associated with dilation and hypertrophy of the left atrium. Biventricular hypertrophy (secondary to ventricular septal defects) produces tall R waves in the left precordial leads with large biphasic RS complexes in the mid-precordial leads. Right bundle branch block is seen in some patients with pulmonary hypertension and is present from birth in patients with congenital atrial septal defects.

Echocardiogram

The echocardiogram can assist the clinician in assessing the severity of the pulmonary hypertension. The pulmonary valve echo typically shows a reduced a wave excursion, an increased b to c slope, a prolonged right ventricular pre-ejection period, and a midsystolic notch. The echocardiogram is also useful for determining the underlying cause of the pulmonary hypertension. Chamber size and wall motion can be assessed, and if present, the severity of tricuspid and pulmonic insufficiency can be evaluated, especially if the clinician adds Doppler flow studies. The echocardiogram can provide information about the presence of mitral valve disease or left ventricular dysfunction. The presence of a right-to-left shunt can be determined through the use of contrast-enhanced echocardiography. This method can determine the size of an intracardiac septal defect.

Ventilation-Perfusion Scans and Arteriography

A ventilation-perfusion scan is an absolute necessity in the diagnosis of pulmonary hypertension. Patients with primary pulmonary hypertension have normal ventilation-perfusion scans. Pulmonary hypertension due to veno-occlusive disease shows a mottled or patchy distribution on perfusion scanning. Patients with recurrent or unresolved pulmonary embolism show multiple perfusion defects.

Pulmonary arteriography should be performed in patients with suspected pulmonary embolism and abnormal lung scans. This will help to clarify the diagnosis and to determine the extent and site of the embolus. Arteriography in this setting carries increased risk and should be performed with newer contrast materials that have lower osmotic properties.

Laboratory Tests

The arterial blood gas measurement is useful in the diagnosis of pulmonary hypertension secondary to intracardiac shunts. It is also helpful in the detection of thromboembolism and ventilation-perfusion abnormalities. Routine blood studies may be useful in determining the cause of pulmonary hypertension. A positive antinuclear antibody test response occurs in about 25 per cent of patients with primary pulmonary hypertension. An increased hematocrit suggests hypoxemia due to chronic parenchymal lung disease, sleep apnea, or a right-to-left shunt. Coagulation studies on patients with pulmonary hypertension due to thromboembolism can exclude deficiencies in antithrombin III, protein C, and protein S or confirm the presence of a circulating anticoagulant.

Open Lung Biopsy

Open lung biopsy may be helpful but should be used only in selected patients to establish the presence of interstitial lung disease, pulmonary vasculitis, small vessel thromboembolism, sarcoidosis, or polyarteritis nodosa. However, in the patient who is fragile hemodynamically, this procedure carries a substantial risk. A therapeutic trial with steroids or immunosuppressive agents with oral anticoagulants is a less hazardous course to follow.

Cardiac Catheterization

Cardiac catheterization enables the clinician to quantitate the severity of the pulmonary hypertension, to relate this to the pulmonary blood flow, to calculate the pulmonary vascular resistance, and to obtain direct evidence of pulmonary venous and arterial pressures. The measurements obtained on cardiac catheterization can be correlated with the results of pulmonary angiography to determine the cause of unexplained severe pulmonary hypertension.

PROGNOSIS AND NATURAL HISTORY

The presence of coexisting pulmonary hypertension in the setting of chronic respiratory disease is a poor prognostic sign. Death resulting from respiratory failure or cardiopulmonary decompensation usually occurs within 3 to 5 years. Most patients whose mean pulmonary artery pressure at rest is greater than 50 mm Hg typically die within 5 years. Deterioration is often rapid and treatment palliative. At best, treatment only postpones progressive right-sided heart failure. Death due to lethal cardiac arrhythmias or from pulmonary embolism may be sudden.

The mean survival time after the initial diagnosis of primary pulmonary hypertension is 2 to 3 years. Primary pulmonary hypertension is usually far advanced before it is recognized. Survival depends on right-sided heart function. Symptoms related to reduced cardiac output, such as syncope, are an ominous sign. Spontaneous remissions have been reported but are unusual. Improved survival with vasodilator therapy or transplantation has yet to be evaluated by a prospective multicenter study.

ISCHEMIC HEART DISEASE

By Philip R. Liebson, M.D.,
and Lloyd W. Klein, M.D.
Chicago, Illinois

The principal cause of mortality in the United States and in other western countries is ischemic heart disease. In the United States, more than 500,000 deaths per year can be attributed to coronary artery disease.

Ischemic heart disease and its clinical expressions are the result of coronary blood flow (CBF) that is inadequate to meet myocardial oxygen demand; consequently, an insufficient amount of oxygen is provided to the myocardium in a segment of the distribution of the coronary circulation (Fig. 1). Any reduction in CBF (supply) relative to myocardial oxygen consumption ($M\dot{V}O_2$; demand) causes ischemia. The degree of myocardial ischemia is influenced by both the presence of fixed atherosclerotic obstruction limiting flow and dynamic alterations in smooth muscle tone, either at the site of stenosis or distally in the arterioles. In addition, changes in the characteristics of the formed and fluid elements of the blood may transiently or permanently alter flow. It is the complex relationship involving (1) the severity, distribution, and progression of organic coronary atherosclerosis; (2) alterations in the tone of coronary vascular smooth muscle; and (3) alterations in the blood elements, which underlies the heterogeneity of presentations and outcomes of the syndromes characterizing myocardial ischemia. These consequences include reversible myocardial dysfunction (ischemia), myocardial necrosis (infarction—see article on myocardial infarction), and sudden cardiac death. The characteristic clinical presentation for ischemia or infarction is chest discomfort; angina pectoris refers to reversible ischemia. The approach to the diagnosis of ischemic heart disease must include consideration of the

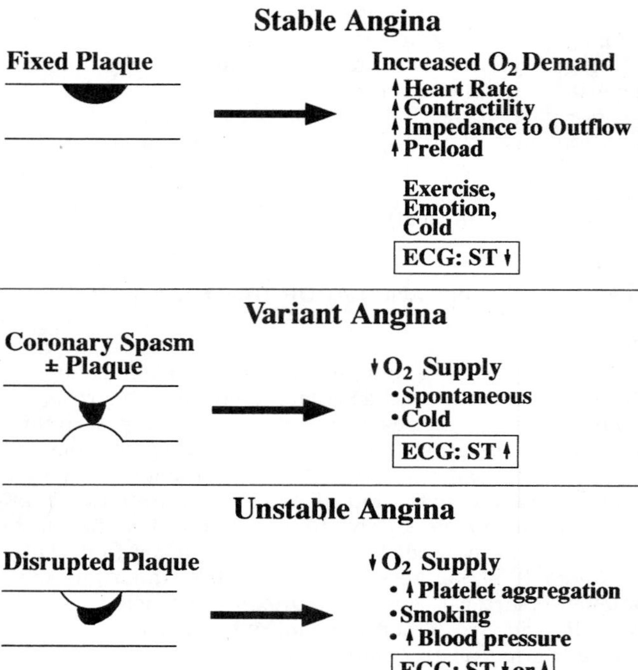

Figure 1. Myocardial ischemia and angina. The relationships among coronary anatomy, symptomatology, and pathophysiologic mechanisms. *Top,* Fixed plaque is associated with stable angina. Increased oxygen demand usually produces the anginal symptoms. The electrocardiogram (ECG) demonstrates ST-segment depression in leads from affected myocardium. *Middle,* Coronary spasm with or without plaque is associated with variant angina. Spasm is associated with decreased oxygen supply, spontaneously or with cold weather, or with other non-exercise stimuli. ECG shows ST-segment elevation in affected leads. *Bottom,* Plaque disruption leads to thrombus causing abrupt decrease in oxygen supply, usually associated with unstable angina. ST-segment depression or elevation may develop. An early infarction may produce findings similar to those seen in unstable angina.

presence and degree of both coronary artery disease and reversible myocardial dysfunction during ischemia.

Coronary artery disease is a general term that usually implies atheromatous disease resulting from the interaction of cholesterol-laden macrophages, fibroblasts, and smooth muscle cells. Thrombus formation is frequently superimposed on an atheromatous plaque, especially in unstable angina and acute myocardial infarction. Coronary artery disease also often causes fibrotic and calcified walls, medial smooth muscle proliferation and hypertrophy, and inflammatory cell infiltration, which compromises blood flow by impinging on the coronary lumen. Transient coronary artery occlusion, usually in the smaller vessels, may result from microembolization from valvular vegetations or left-sided heart thrombi. The larger epicardial vessels may transiently become occluded from spasm, either with or without underlying mild atheromatous changes.

Myocardial ischemia as a consequence of decreased CBF leads to reversible dysfunction of left ventricular myocardium resulting from an imbalance of the ratio of CBF to myocardial oxygen requirement ($CBF:M\dot{V}O_2$). Prolonged akinesis or hypokinesis may occur after an episode of myocardial ischemia even when arterial flow has been restored (stunned myocardium). When blood flow to viable myocardium is persistently low, a prolonged decrease in metabolism with myocardial akinesis (hibernating myocardium) may occur. Improved blood flow typically results in rapid restoration of function.

The terminology for the clinical presentation of ischemia includes stable and unstable angina (classic angina). Variant angina refers to a presentation that does not relate to effort and produces electrocardiographic changes that are not usually characteristic of classic angina. Combined characteristics of classic and variant angina may be called "mixed angina" (see further on). Angina pectoris may be atypical in location, may present as a symptom other than chest discomfort, or may be completely absent (silent ischemia). In describing the discomfort itself, patients may note angina at characteristic locations other than the chest, with or without evidence of physical exertion or psychological stress (atypical angina). Symptoms such as breathlessness or diaphoresis with exertion or stress may be anginal equivalents. Any chest discomfort that does not meet the criteria of typical or atypical angina, such as sharp stabbing pains anywhere in the chest, is called nonanginal chest pain. Finally, a syndrome of angina with abnormal stress test results and normal coronary arteriograms with evidence of lactate production in the coronary sinus with tachycardia has been called syndrome X. This condition is presumably due to microvascular coronary artery disease.

PATHOPHYSIOLOGY

CBF occurs primarily during diastole because increased intramyocardial tension occurs during systole, preventing blood from reaching the innermost myocardial layer—the subendocardium, which normally has a higher wall stress per unit area than does the subepicardium. Therefore, this region has a greater oxygen requirement and needs higher blood flow. Consequently, the subendocardium is more vulnerable to ischemia than is the subepicardium.

Atheromatous disease is by far the most frequent cause of diminished coronary artery flow. Fixed lesions due to atheromatous disease usually limit coronary flow and cause ischemia involving the subendocardium, especially during exercise. When a thrombus develops in association with an ulcerated atheroma, complete or partial occlusion of the vessel may occur with transmural ischemia at rest and/or myocardial infarction. Coronary artery spasm is also a cause of ischemia and may be superimposed on an atheromatous lesion or develop in an angiographically normal segment of coronary artery (see Fig. 1).

Rarely, ischemic heart disease may develop from calcification of the coronary ostia, coronary artery anomalies such as arteriovenous fistulas, or inadequate perfusion pressure in normal coronary arteries. The latter may result from aortic stenosis or regurgitation. Ischemia may be associated with severe anemia and conditions in which oxygen saturation is severely diminished. Severe myocardial hypertrophy (e.g., hypertrophic cardiomyopathy) may lead to subendocardial ischemia even without coronary artery anatomic lesions.

Fixed obstructions of the coronary arteries exhibit great variability. The individual lesion may be concentric or eccentric with respect to the lumen; it may be short or long, single or multiple, and affect dominant or nondominant coronary arteries. The hemodynamic effects of a coronary obstruction are determined by the severity of the luminal narrowing it produces. A cross-sectional area reduction of 50 per cent or less appears to have little or no effect on coronary artery blood flow in most circumstances. Significant limitations in the ability of an epicardial artery to conduct increased flow on demand occur when the cross-sectional area of the vessel is reduced by approximately 70 per cent. Significant reductions in resting flow appear at reductions in cross-sectional area of 90 per cent and greater. Further decreases in effective cross-sectional area can cause a profound reduction of flow, resulting in myocardial hypoperfusion and, if not corrected, myocardial infarction.

Myocardial oxygen demand ($M\dot{V}O_2$) is increased by increasing heart rate, contractility, and systolic myocardial wall tension. Systolic wall tension is, in turn, increased by increasing left ventricular end-diastolic volume (preload), increasing peripheral vascular resistance, and increasing stiffness of the aorta. In ventricular diastole, decreased myocardial compliance hinders left ventricular diastolic filling and increases $M\dot{V}O_2$ (see Fig. 1). Altered compliance can be due to anatomic or functional changes in the interstitial elements of the myocardium. Systolic contraction in the presence of increased myocardial stiffness also increases the demand for energy substrate. Hence, both systolic and diastolic factors determine myocardial blood supply; both are important in the development of myocardial ischemia; and both interact in a complex manner. The duration of diastole and mean diastolic coronary perfusion pressure are the prime determinants of myocardial blood flow.

Myocardial performance during acute ischemia adjusts proportionately to CBF changes. Thus, a graded decrease in myocardial function develops with decrements in CBF until function ceases, beginning when flow is less than 80 per cent of normal baseline value. Decreases in myocardial flow develop first in the subendocardium and then in the subepicardium. Subendocardial blood flow somewhat less than 50 per cent of normal can be associated with subendocardial hypokinesis or akinesis. Greater reduction in flow is needed to produce similar effects on the epicardium. Normally perfused myocardium may become hypercontractile during ischemia of another segment in order to maintain normal global systolic performance. Stunned and hibernating myocardium are colloquial terms given to two conditions of ischemia with differing pathogenesis and metabolic substrates (Table 1).

Either an acute decrease in CBF or an increase in the oxygen requirement of the myocardium that is supplied by a persistently compromised coronary artery produces a decreased contraction velocity and decreased diastolic compliance almost immediately (Fig. 2). Electrophysiologic changes can develop simultaneously and are typically manifested by ST-segment depression on the electrocardiogram (ECG). Occasionally ST-segment elevation is seen instead. The former is usually associated with subendocardial ischemia produced by exertion and a fixed coronary athero-

Table 1. Stunned and Hibernating Myocardium

	Stunned	Hibernating
Coronary flow	Reperfusion after profound ischemic episode	Persistently low
Contraction	Decreased or absent	Decreased or absent
Necrosis	Absent	Absent
Adenosine triphosphate levels	Low	Normal
Reversibility	Slow with adequate perfusion	Rapid with adequate perfusion

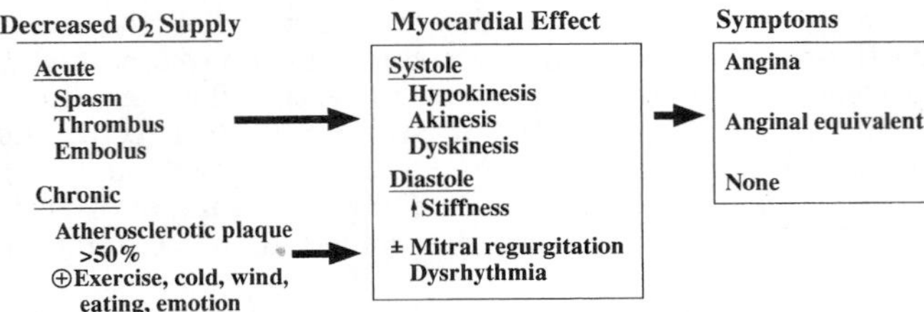

Sequence of Ischemic Events
(usually < 1 minute)

1. Decreased contraction, increased diastolic stiffness.
2. ST↑ or ↓.
3. Dyskinesis or Akinesis.
4. Angina or equivalent.

Figure 2. The pathogenesis of ischemia is associated with decreased coronary arterial perfusion as the underlying cause *(left)*, whether due to the acute effects of spasm or thrombus or a chronic fixed atheromatous plaque. *Middle,* The resulting myocardial effects on left ventricular systole and diastole are listed, producing either no symptoms (silent ischemia) or angina and/or anginal equivalent *(right).*

matous plaque obstructing 50 to 60 per cent of the lumen. If a clot or spasm develops, complete or nearly complete occlusion can ensue, leading to transmural ischemia (subepicardial and subendocardial) and ST elevation. Anginal symptoms can occur seconds to minutes after the preceding events. Sometimes angina does not develop, and evidence of ischemia can be found only by ambulatory electrocardiographic monitoring showing transient ST-segment abnormalities (silent ischemia). Ischemia associated with acute superimposed clot may lead to myocardial infarction if flow is not quickly restored to preocclusion levels.

CLINICAL PRESENTATIONS OF ISCHEMIA

The history leads to diagnosis of significant coronary artery disease in more than 80 per cent of individuals seen in the general internal medicine clinic. An additional 10 per cent are diagnosed on physical examination. Diagnostic criteria for anginal presentations are listed in Table 2 and those for the diagnosis of myocardial ischemia are seen in Table 3.

The symptoms of myocardial ischemia can include classic angina with exertion, vague discomfort, or no symptoms. The term "angina pectoris" means "chest choking," and classic angina is characterized by a sense of pressure, heaviness, or burning that is seldom described as pain. Angina is the initial presentation of coronary artery disease in 50 to 60 per cent of women and 40 to 50 per cent of men. However, many women referred for coronary arteriography on the basis of chest discomfort have minimal or no more coronary artery disease than men. An anginal attack that lasts for less than 20 seconds, with sharp, lancinating, or tearing pains that can be localized in the chest by pointing with one finger, are rarely if ever considered angina.

The temporal characteristics of angina can be used to differentiate stable from unstable angina. Stable angina usually occurs less than three or four times daily. An episode typically lasts 5 to 10 minutes; is produced by exertion, emotion, cold air, or eating a heavy meal; and stops within 2 to 3 minutes after these conditions cease. Unstable angina describes all other anginal attacks, such as increasing frequency or duration of attacks, including new-onset angina, angina at rest (with some exceptions), angina

Table 2. Clinical Classifications of Angina Pectoris Severity

Diagnosis of Angina Pectoris Presence and Severity*

Presence of pain or discomfort in chest (Y/N)
Location of pain or discomfort in chest (Indicate)
Characteristics of pain and discomfort:
  When walking uphill or hurrying (Y/N)
  When walking on level or ordinary pace (Y/N)
Response in activity to pain or discomfort:
  Stopping, slowing down, continued activity
Does pain/discomfort go away when standing still? (Y/N)
How soon? (<10 min, >10 min)

Functional Classifications of Activity Leading to Angina Pectoris

Class	*New York Heart Association*	*Canadian†*
I	Greater than ordinary activity	Strenuous or prolonged exertion
II	Ordinary activity	Walking or climbing stairs rapidly Walking uphill Regular or climbing after meals, in cold, wind, with emotional stress Walking more than 2 blocks on level Climbing more than 1 flight
III	Less than ordinary activity	Walking 1 to 2 blocks on level Climbing 1 flight normally
IV	Any activity or at rest	

*Modified from Rose, G.A., et al.: Self-administration of a questionnaire on chest pain and intermittent claudication. Br. J. Prev. Soc. Med. 31:42, 1977.

†Data from Cox, J., and Naylor, C.D.: The Canadian Cardiovascular Society rating scale for angina pectoris: Is it time for refinements? Ann. Intern. Med. 117:677–683, 1992.

Table 3. Diagnosis of Myocardial Ischemia

Clinical Presentation (Symptoms)

Typical: Usually retrosternal with or without radiation to inner arms, jaw, neck, upper back, epigastrium; lasts 30 sec to 15 min
Atypical: (1) only in areas of radiation; (2) sharp, fleeting pains, or other uncharacteristic presentations of chest discomfort but in appropriate location
Anginal equivalent: diaphoresis, breathlessness, anxiety, nausea, vomiting, occurring in response to ischemia that may develop without pressure or pain
Nonanginal chest pain: uncharacteristic pain in relation to location, character of pain, and cause

Physical Findings During Angina Attack

Transient S_4 gallop, mitral regurgitation murmur, paradoxically split S_2, abnormal precordial systolic impulse

Electrocardiographic Findings (Rest or Exercise)

Transient ST depression or elevation 0.08 sec after J-point, associated with J-point depression or elevation of 1 mm or more from baseline (TP interval at rest, PR segment with exercise)

Radionuclide Scan Findings (Exercise)

Filling defect with exercise that fills at rest (perfusion imbalance during exercise with viable myocardium at rest)

Echocardiographic Findings

Segmental decrease in systolic endocardial wall motion and thickening with exercise compared with rest lasting more than 10 minutes (especially if inciting conditions have ceased), and anginal episodes that are more frequent than four times daily.

The development of angina during exposure to cold has been attributed to an increase in blood pressure (because of peripheral vasconstriction) without a compensatory decrease in heart rate. Postprandial angina appears to be more common in men, is associated with angina at rest, and frequently occurs with left main or three-vessel disease. The association of coronary artery vasospasm and thrombosis with cocaine use must be considered in drug abusers. Intranasal administration of cocaine produces heart rate and blood pressure increases and CBF decreases, suggesting significant coronary artery vasoconstriction.

Evidence exists for circadian variation in the frequency of expression of myocardial ischemia and its anginal presentation. Ischemia is more likely to occur in the 6 hours after awakening than in any other 6-hour period during the day. This is also true for myocardial infarction and sudden cardiac death. This phenomenon is related to the increased catecholamine concentrations and the ability of platelets to aggregate and to decreased intrinsic tissue plasminogen activator (t-PA) coupled with increased heart rate and blood pressure during the morning hours. The result is an increased myocardial oxygen requirement and an increased propensity for thrombus formation in disrupted coronary plaques.

The differentiation of stable and unstable angina is important because more adverse prognostic implications are associated with unstable angina. Other terms have been used for unstable angina, including intermediate coronary syndrome, preinfarction angina, crescendo angina, rest angina, and acute coronary syndrome. The term "unstable angina" should be used to avoid confusion and because there is no difference in prognostic implications when any of these other terms are used.

The location of anginal pain is usually over the lower retrosternal area of the chest, but it may extend to the inner left arm, the inner right arm, the neck and lower jaw, the epigastric area, or the back between the scapulae. Aside from the retrosternal location, anginal attacks can develop in any of these locations, separately or in combination. Although "atypical angina" has been used to describe attacks in nonretrosternal locations, it has also been used to describe atypical characteristics of the anginal pain or discomfort, and the term should not be used as a descriptor. Anginal equivalents refer to nonpressure sensations such as nausea, vomiting, fatigue, diaphoresis, eructation, dyspnea, and anxiety that may reflect autonomic or hemodynamic changes occurring with ischemia in the absence of angina itself.

Silent Ischemia

Silent ischemia (the absence of any symptom relevant to ischemia) develops in up to 60 per cent of patients with coronary artery disease and exertional angina. It commonly occurs with ischemia in patients with coronary artery disease. The prevalence of silent myocardial ischemia increases from 2 per cent in the fifth and sixth decades of life to 15 per cent in the ninth decade of life. It is more likely to occur if neuropathy is present (diabetics and hemodialysis patients). The time between the onset of angina and ischemic ST-segment depression is prolonged in diabetics, especially in those with abnormal heart rate responses to the Valsalva maneuver. In patients who are not diabetics and who exhibit silent ischemia, there is a general hyposensitivity to pain stimuli. In nondiabetics, there is no relationship between the anginal perception threshold and either the autonomic function or the somatic pain threshold. Hypertensive patients, who also have increased anginal thresholds, are also more likely to have silent ischemia. (At least 15 per cent of myocardial infarctions are also silent.) Some patients without angina periodically display ST depression on ambulatory electrocardiograph monitors. The significance of these changes with regard to myocardial ischemia is not clear, especially in women in whom the changes develop only during exercise. Totally asymptomatic populations with characteristic ST depressions on ambulatory monitoring have a prevalence of angiographically documented coronary artery disease of 2.5 to 10 per cent. This suggests a low probability of coronary artery disease unless episodes of angina are also present. Plasma concentrations of beta-endorphin and met-enkephalin do not appear to correlate with angina or silent myocardial ischemia.

Classic Angina Pectoris

The traditional concept underlying angina is that myocardial ischemia occurs when increased myocardial demand cannot be met. This is typically due to a fixed stenosis that prevents CBF from increasing enough to balance the increased demand. According to this concept, a balance between myocardial oxygen demand and supply exists in nonischemic periods, but during increasing demand the reduced coronary reserve in the presence of a fixed obstruction proximal to dilated coronary arteries prevents blood flow and oxygen supply from increasing sufficiently. Myocardial oxygen demand is conceptualized as a rate-pressure product involving heart rate, systolic wall tension, and myocardial contractility. Oxygen supply is determined by myocardial blood flow and the oxygen-carrying capacity of hemoglobin. Exercise testing is frequently employed to determine the anginal threshold for a fixed coronary stenosis. The response to exercise is reproducible in many individuals and provides an excellent physiologic assessment of stenosis severity. Because angina pectoris is caused by ischemia that is related to the degree of coronary artery stenosis, worsening angina should presage progression of coronary artery disease. Yet, there is no convincing correlation of the severity of angina with the presence or degree of coronary artery stenosis. This suggests that pathophysiologic mechanisms other than progression of stenosis strongly influence symptoms.

Variant Angina (Prinzmetal's Angina)

Variant angina occurs when demand remains constant but supply is diminished because of coronary vasospasm in patients with normal exercise tolerance. Angina at rest may occur with unstable angina, but it can also be seen in variant or Prinzmetal's angina. The latter term refers to angina that develops without atheromatous obstruction and is associated with epicardial coronary artery spasm. It differs in several ways from classic angina in that ST elevations rather than depressions are seen, marked ventricular ectopy is present, the heart rate and blood pressure may not change, and no chest discomfort or electrocardiographic changes may develop during exercise. Its periodicity varies with changes in frequency of anginal events over months or years. Ergot alkaloids or hyperventilation can induce spasm. Greater than 50 per cent of ECG-identified coronary artery spasm is not associated with chest discomfort, and spontaneous arrhythmias may occur in 10 per cent of those silent episodes of ischemia. Heart rate reduction and atrioventricular (AV) block also occur frequently.

Coronary artery spasm has been associated with life-threatening arrhythmias in some patients, with both variant angina and silent ischemia; the only constant is often ST elevation on the electrocardiograph monitor. These malignant dysrhythmias (usually polymorphic ventricular tachycardia) may develop during reperfusion after the spasm-induced ischemia. Coronary artery spasm can cause rupture of an atheromatous plaque, leading to thrombus formation and unstable angina or infarction. Repeated episodes of spasm can also lead to intimal disruption and the eventual development of an atheromatous plaque.

Mixed Angina

Secondary angina results from myocardial demand that exceeds a fixed stenotic supply capacity, whereas primary angina is due to increased vascular tone producing decreased CBF. Mixed angina may be conceptualized as resulting from the variable contribution of fixed and dynamic coronary stenosis. This is manifested clinically when patients demonstrate both fixed and variable thresholds capable of inducing anginal attacks. These patients typically recognize a level of exercise that will produce anginal attacks, but they also have anginal episodes with little activity. Others may experience episodes of rest angina as a result of coronary spasm. Patients with mixed angina may have diurnal variations in their anginal pattern, during which varying amounts of exercise can provoke angina.

Angina Pectoris Without Epicardial Coronary Artery Disease (Syndrome X)

Syndrome X refers to typical angina pectoris with characteristic ST depressions on the ECG during ischemia but with normal coronary arteriograms and evidence of impaired coronary flow reserve based on increased concentration of lactate in the coronary sinus and increased coronary resistance before and after dipyridamole administration. An abnormal vasoconstrictive response of the epicardial coronary vessels to low doses of acetylcholine can also be seen. Microvascular disease has been suggested as the possible cause (Table 4). Hypertensive patients often demonstrate these findings. Silent ischemia may be present in up to 85 per cent of episodes of ischemic ST depression during ambulatory electrocardiographic monitoring. Many of these hypertensive patients have decreased coronary flow reserve. The absence of significant coronary artery disease is noted in 10 to 20 per cent of patients with anginalike chest pain undergoing coronary arteriography. Common associated findings in syndrome X are severe and prolonged pain and marked variability in the development of symptoms by exercise testing as well as variability of response to anti-ischemic medication.

Table 4. Diseases of the Small Coronary Arteries

Arteritis	Polyarteritis
	Systemic lupus erythematosus
	Whipple's disease
Mural thickening	Scleroderma
	Idiopathic fibromuscular hyperplasia
	Friedreich's ataxia
Endothelial lesions	Congenital homocystinuria
Medial necrosis	Marfan's syndrome
Emboli	Cardiac surgery
	Mitral or aortic valvulitis
	Percutaneous transluminal coronary angioplasty (PTCA)
	Tumor metastases
	Fat or air emboli

These patients often have evidence of gastroesophageal acid reflux and esophageal motility problems, and many have noncardiac causes for their anginalike pain. About 50 per cent are found to have an esophageal functional abnormality (see article on disorders of the esophagus). Of these, approximately half have nutcracker esophagus, with normal peristaltic sequence but abnormal duration and amplitude. Almost 40 per cent have an abnormal motility disorder, 10 per cent have diffuse esophageal spasm, and 2 per cent have evidence of achalasia. Esophageal evaluation should include endoscopy, manometry, 24-hour pH monitoring, and/or a Bernstein acid infusion test (see article on chest pain).

PHYSICAL EXAMINATION

The physical examination with the patient at rest is rarely, if ever, confirmatory of ischemia, but evanescent signs during an anginal episode can suggest reversible ischemia. These signs include the development of a systolic pulsation over the precordium, suggesting focal left ventricular dyskinesia; a fourth heart sound gallop, associated with changes in left ventricular diastolic stiffness; rarely a third heart sound gallop; paradoxical splitting of the second heart sound with changes in systolic performance; and an apical systolic murmur due to transient mitral valve regurgitation as a result of papillary muscle ischemia. These findings can persist with stunned or hibernating myocardium or after a myocardial infarction. Although increases in heart rate and blood pressure are typical of ischemia with exertion, they are nonspecific.

Other causes of chest discomfort or nonanginal pain may be evaluated by the physical examination. The pain of pericarditis is positional and relieved by sitting up. A two- or three-component friction rub may be heard over the precordium. Aortic dissection may be accompanied by the decrescendo diastolic murmur of aortic regurgitation. Hypertrophic cardiomyopathy with obstruction often presents as a bifid carotid pulse and an early to midsystolic murmur over the base that increases with the Valsalva maneuver. Aortic stenosis or regurgitation must be evaluated as a possible cause of angina. The presence of significant coronary artery disease may correlate with findings suggestive of atheromatous disease elsewhere. Tendinous or tuberous xanthomas or xanthelasmas over the eyelids suggest lipid abnormalities.

DIAGNOSTIC STUDIES

All patients with suspected ischemic heart disease should have a resting ECG and a chest film. The chest radiograph is of little assistance in diagnosing ischemia, but it is useful in evaluating heart size, vascular redistribution typical of congestive heart failure, a dilated ascending aortic shadow that may suggest dissection or aneurysm, and calcification of the aortic valve and coronary arteries.

The resting ECG may be entirely normal between attacks in a patient with classic angina. The ECG can also provide evidence of previous infarction and other cardiac causes of angina or chest discomfort. Prior infarction may be diagnosed by the presence of appropriate Q waves. Voltage and ST-T criteria for left ventricular hypertrophy may support the diagnosis of target organ damage from hypertension or aortic valve disease, both of which predispose to myocardial ischemia. Diffuse ST elevation and electrical alternans may support the diagnosis of pericardial effusion or pericarditis as a cause of chest discomfort. Ambulatory electrocardiographic monitoring can be used to evaluate ST-segment changes during usual daily activity.

Additional Diagnostic Tests

The history, physical examination, resting ECG, and ambulatory ECG can detect more than 80 per cent of the diagnoses of myocardial ischemia. When required, further noninvasive evaluation may include exercise stress testing using electrocardiography, thallium-201 (^{201}Tl) or technetium-99m sestamibi (^{99m}Tc-sestamibi) nuclear imaging and echocardiography or resting studies using dipyridamole or dobutamine. These studies can help diagnose ischemia and define coronary artery disease according to location and severity.

This additional testing is primarily used to assess vulnerability to myocardial infarction and risk for sudden cardiac death based on the severity of coronary artery disease and the extent of ischemia. The presence of previous damage due to prior myocardial infarction and the compromise of left (and right) ventricular function can also be assessed. Exercise stress testing in some form is often used to evaluate patients for major noncardiac surgery (including carotid, aortic, and peripheral arterial surgery) by excluding significant coronary artery disease. A patient without a history of angina or myocardial infarction who has a normal resting ECG probably needs no further study.

Electrocardiographic Stress Testing

The basis of an abnormal ECG is ST depression in relation to the PR segment in the same cardiac cycle. Various criteria are used, but the most accepted includes (1) J-point depression of at least 1 mm following the QRS complex and (2) a relatively flat ST segment with at least 1-mm depression at 60 to 80 msec after the J-point. The estimated sensitivity and specificity of electrocardiographic treadmill testing is 60 per cent and 85 per cent, respectively. Nuclear imaging, which demonstrates exercise-induced perfusion defects that are reversible with rest, has a sensitivity of 80 per cent and a predictive value of 90 per cent. The usefulness of these tests depends on the pretest likelihood of coronary artery disease.

Patients with symptomatic exercise-induced ischemia have a higher prevalence of severe coronary artery disease than do those without angina during exercise testing. However, in patients without prior myocardial infarction, ST-segment depression is a better predictor of significant coronary artery disease. The heart rate may affect the degree of ST depression in response to ischemia. Normalization is obtained by dividing ST-segment change by heart rate change. The best sensitivity (93 per cent) for significant coronary artery disease is provided by measurement of the normalized ST depression at 60 msec after the J-point compared with normalized ST measurements at 0, 20, 40, and 80 msec after the J-point.

The time course evaluation of ST depression during and after exercise testing also shows that electrocardiographic changes observed during recovery are helpful in predicting coronary artery disease. In addition, electrocardiographic changes occurring during exercise and continuing well into recovery are associated with more significant coronary artery disease than are changes occurring during exercise and reverting rapidly during recovery.

Nuclear Imaging With Exercise Stress Testing

^{201}Tl myocardial imaging studies can demonstrate regional myocardial perfusion imbalance with exercise and thereby provide evidence of significant epicardial coronary artery disease. ^{201}Tl is a potassium analogue that functions as a marker for myocardial perfusion and viability, because only intact myocardial membranes retain the tracer. ^{201}Tl stress images reflect relative perfusion modified by myocardial extraction, which is, in turn, dependent on regional blood flow. In necrotic tissue, even with adequate flow, the tracer is not retained by the tissue and appears as a filling defect. Usually two scans are performed, one at the time of peak exercise just after intravenous injection of ^{201}Tl and another 3 to 4 hours later. Absence of ^{201}Tl uptake during the exercise phase, with filling in during the rest phase, indicates ischemia. A defect present in both phases suggests myocardial infarction of unknown age. If myocardial stunning or hibernation has occurred, redistribution takes from 18 to 72 hours. To visualize these areas, a second injection of ^{201}Tl can be performed after the delayed image scan; reperfusion can be seen in up to 50 per cent of patients with apparent fixed defects before the second injection.

Images can be obtained using both planar and single-photon emission computed tomography (SPECT) techniques. The former approach obtains images in three views, and individual coronary artery beds are superimposed on one another. SPECT technology acquires images in a 180-degree arc around the patient, with reconstruction of the heart in three dimensions. The radioisotope uptake is then evaluated by tomographic slices in three orientations, separating individual coronary tributaries. Increased ^{201}Tl uptake by the lung suggests ischemic left ventricular dysfunction and is found in about one third of patients with ST depression on the ECG. It is also seen in 14 per cent of those without ST depression.

^{99m}Tc-sestamibi nuclear stress studies have the advantage of shortening the time of a nuclear stress test because the radiotracer does not redistribute after injection. Regional artifacts are less common with ^{99m}Tc than with ^{201}Tl and images can be gated to assess regional wall motion and myocardial thickness. The studies are accomplished by a rest-stress sequence in which the rest injection is given followed in 60 to 90 minutes by a scan. The second injection is then given during exercise followed by a second scan 60 to 90 minutes later. Alternatively a stress-rest protocol can be followed; if the stress image is normal, the rest study need not be performed. Differentiating hibernating myocardium from infarcted myocardium is difficult with this study. ^{99m}Tc stress studies show a sensitivity of 90 per cent for detecting 50 per cent stenosis and 95 per cent for detecting 70 per cent stenosis. Unfortunately, the specificity rate is only between 75 and 82 per cent.

^{99m}Tc-sestamibi can also be used to evaluate patients at the time of spontaneous chest pain. The sensitivity for detecting significant coronary artery disease is more than 95 per cent, but the specificity is less than 80 per cent, indicating frequent false-positive results. The perfusion defect, when present, correlates closely with the location of significant coronary artery disease. In unstable angina, perfusion defects are frequently found at rest with or without chest pain or electrocardiographic evidence of ischemia.

Nuclear Imaging With Pharmacologic Stress Testing

For patients who cannot perform exercise, pharmacologic stress testing may be performed with dobutamine, dipyridamole, and adenosine. Dobutamine increases contractility, heart rate, systolic blood pressure, and $M\dot{V}O_2$. It is infused in graded doses from 5 to 40 μg/kg per minute over 5-minute periods, with injection of radioisotope at the time of maximal dose infusion.

Pharmacologic stress tests using dipyridamole do not depend on an increased heart rate–blood pressure product but on an absolute decrease in the arterial supply to a region of myocardium. Dipyridamole acts indirectly by inhibition of cellular uptake of endogenous adenosine. Increasing CBF by vasodilatation creates a "steal" from constricted vessels, producing a perfusion defect in myocardium supplied by the constricted vessel. In collateral-dependent coronary arteries, the blood flow is diverted into the normal vessels. Perfusion defects seen by radioisotope scan are due to (1) limited vasodilator reserve in a noncollateralized vessel or (2) stenosis proximal to the collateralized vessel. Maximal pharmacologic effect develops 4 minutes after completion of the dipyridamole infusion and lasts for 20 to 40 minutes. ^{99m}Tc-sestamibi SPECT imaging with dipyridamole has provided a sensitivity for detection of significant coronary artery disease as high as 95 per cent, with close to 80 per cent identification of the diseased coronary arteries.

Echocardiographic Stress Testing

The principle of echocardiographic stress testing is based on ischemia-induced regional degradation of left ventricular myocardial performance. The technique permits a choice between treadmill stress testing and pharmacologic studies at rest. With exercise stress echocardiography, four tomographic views are obtained at rest and immediately after treadmill exercise. As with pharmacologic nuclear stress imaging, dobutamine, dipyridamole, or adenosine can be used, but dobutamine stress echocardiograms are most common. Pharmacologic studies are performed with the same dosing as is used in nuclear studies. A relative decrease in regional wall motion or the absence of increased contraction with increasing dobutamine dosage constitutes a positive test. Exercise echocardiographic testing is superior to electrocardiography in the diagnosis of myocardial ischemia in patients with an abnormal baseline ECG, with sensitivities ranging from 63 to 100 per cent and specificities ranging from 64 to 100 per cent. The sensitivity and specificity for dobutamine stress echocardiography is comparable to that for nuclear imaging studies in two- and three-vessel coronary artery disease. It is less sensitive for single-vessel coronary artery disease. Dobutamine can be used in conjunction with dipyridamole. The concordance of both tests is in the range of 80 to 85 per cent. The sensitivity for detecting significant coronary artery disease increases from 70 to 75 per cent for each agent individually to more than 90 per cent when used in combination, with a specificity of 90 per cent.

The Role of Cardiac Catheterization

Cardiac catheterization is employed to make a definitive diagnosis in patients with chest pain of uncertain cause, inconclusive noninvasive testing, or suspected coronary artery disease. Although most patients with chest pain can be diagnosed with reasonable certainty using the history, physical examination, and noninvasive testing (see Table 3), the results in some patients may be equivocal. This group includes those with inadequate heart rate response to exercise or the presence of factors associated with false-positive test results.

Patients with severe stable angina pectoris or unstable angina refractory to medications are candidates for surgical vascularization, and angiography is necessary to define the coronary anatomy. Although knowledge of coronary anatomy is used to develop management strategies, events such as myocardial infarction cannot be reliably predicted on the basis of angiographic findings. However, left ventricular ejection fraction, the number of major epicardial vessels with greater than 50 per cent stenosis, and age constitute the most powerful predictors of mortality in coronary artery disease. In general, patients with left main stenosis or three-vessel coronary artery disease are candidates for bypass surgery, and those with single-vessel disease are best treated with drugs, angioplasty, or atherectomy. Patients with two-vessel disease and selected patients with three-vessel disease may be candidates for either coronary intervention or surgical bypass.

DIAGNOSIS OF RECURRENT CHEST PAIN FOLLOWING PERCUTANEOUS INTERVENTIONAL PROCEDURES

Up to 80 per cent of patients experience restenosis following balloon angioplasty, atherectomy, and laser procedures within the first 6 months after the procedure. Stents may diminish the incidence of restenosis or merely delay its recurrence. When patients experience symptoms (especially within the first 6 months) similar to those present before intervention, the likelihood of restenosis is sufficiently high that coronary angiography should be performed without unnecessary delay. When the symptoms are less clear, or when the possibility of medical management rather than a repeat procedure is contemplated, a stress test may be useful to (1) determine the likelihood of restenosis, (2) assess exercise tolerance and symptom severity, and (3) evaluate the amount of myocardium at risk. These data provide an estimate of the likelihood of response to medical therapy and prognosis without revascularization. In patients with multivessel disease, the difficulty of assessing recurrent symptoms is further complicated, and a stress echocardiogram may be the most useful test to assist in determining whether restenosis has occurred.

ACUTE MYOCARDIAL INFARCTION

By Laura L. Bilodeau, M.D.
Denver, Colorado

Ischemic heart disease is a continuum ranging from reversible myocardial injury (stable angina and unstable angina) to acute myocardial infarction (AMI), an irreversible injury that is characterized by several cellular and nuclear changes. These changes include nuclear pyknosis and karyorrhexis, the disruption of cellular membranes and subsequent influx of free radicals and calcium ions. The dissolution of intracellular lysosomal membranes with the release of enzymes into the cytoplasm leads to enzymatic digestion of cellular components and the ultimate replacement of nonviable tissue with fibrotic, noncontractile scar tissue. AMI is caused by complete occlusion of a coronary artery with cell death in the distribution of that arterial system. The most common cause of coronary artery occlusion is the rupture of an atherosclerotic plaque and subsequent thrombus formation that blocks blood flow. Thrombolytic therapy has enabled clinicians to impede the development of the acute thrombus and therefore significantly decrease morbidity and mortality from such an event.

The patient with acute chest pain, who is usually admitted to "rule out AMI," is one of the leading causes of emergency department visits in the United States, and missing the diagnosis is a leading cause of medical malpractice expenditures. Establishing the diagnosis of AMI quickly and using triage to direct patients to the proper level of care—whether it be immediate therapy, inpatient monitoring, or outpatient evaluation—is crucial for appropriate patient care and efficient use of resources. The diagnosis of AMI is based on World Health Organization (WHO) criteria, which includes the following: (1) characteristic, prolonged chest pain, (2) diagnostic electrocardiographic changes, and (3) serial determinations of cardiac enzymes to document a rise and fall in serum activity. At least two of these criteria are needed to establish the diagnosis. The clinical manifestations of AMI can be extremely deceptive, with subtle electrocardiographic changes, silent ischemia, or small changes in serial enzymes that might go unnoticed. Ordering more laboratory tests and procedures will not necessarily help make the diagnosis of AMI, but increased awareness of the subtlety of the criteria and knowledge of the risk factors (see article on cardiovascular risk factors) can guide the clinician to the correct diagnosis.

HISTORY AND PHYSICAL EXAMINATION

A brief but focused history is essential for distinguishing myocardial infarction from the four disorders that can be immediately life-threatening and often mimic the clinical presentation of AMI. These include aortic dissection, pneumothorax, acute pericarditis with tamponade, and pulmonary embolism. The duration of symptoms, the quality of pain, a history of similar pain, related symptoms, and a review of risk factors all should be documented as quickly as possible. Myocardial infarction pain typically has a duration of minutes to hours (usually 30 minutes or more), rather than seconds to minutes. It is classically described as crushing and substernal in location and can be severe (usually described as a 10 on a scale of 0 to 10). The pain may radiate to the jaw or down the left arm. The patient may not be able to identify an exact location because the myocardium is visceral rather than somatic in origin. The pain is not relieved by positional changes; rest; or medications such as aspirin, antacids, or nitroglycerin alone. Many patients have a prior history of angina or other myocardial events that can increase the likelihood of another cardiac event; however, a negative history does not exclude the diagnosis. Related symptoms, including shortness of breath, nausea, vomiting, diaphoresis, or weakness, should be elicited, but they usually do not aid the diagnosis. At least one quarter of all patients in the United States with AMI are incorrectly diagnosed, and about 50 per cent of these diagnostic errors are due to atypical or subtle presentations.

On physical examination, vital signs (e.g., pulse and blood pressure symmetry) that are important in making the diagnosis of aortic dissection should be noted. Fever and tachypnea may be present. The patient may be tachycardic or bradycardic or the pulse may be normal, just as the blood pressure may be increased, decreased, or normal. Particular attention must be directed to examination of the heart, noting rhythm (atrial fibrillation, heart block), rubs (possible pericardial effusion), murmurs (valvular regurgitation secondary to papillary muscle rupture or the development of a ventricular septal defect), or gallops (S_3 gallop commonly heard in congestive heart failure). Breath sounds should be equal; unilateral absence of breath sounds suggests pneumothorax. The presence of crackles or rales may result from pulmonary edema from congestive heart failure or atelectasis from pulmonary emboli. The abdominal examination can help differentiate AMI from intra-abdominal causes of chest pain such as peptic ulcer disease, perforated viscus, or gastroesophageal reflux. Neck veins should be examined for jugular venous distention that may suggest right ventricular dysfunction or pulmonary hypertension. The entire history and physical examination can be completed in the emergency department within a few minutes (Table 1).

Table 1. Differential Diagnosis of Acute Myocardial Infarction

Life-Threatening
Aortic dissection
Pulmonary embolism
Acute pericarditis-tamponade
Pneumothorax
Non–Life-Threatening
Pneumonia
Chest wall pain–costochondritis
Esophageal dysmotility-reflux
Peptic ulcer disease
Perforated viscus
Renal stones
Cholecystitis

ELECTROCARDIOGRAPHY

One of the WHO criteria consists of diagnostic electrocargiographic changes. A 12-lead electrocardiogram (ECG) is used to evaluate the conduction system and to identify the site of a conduction abnormality based on differences from the usual electrical axis of the heart. Aside from clinical history and physical examination, the ECG provides the most important data required for determining whether the patient requires immediate treatment. The sensitivity of the ECG is greatly enhanced if previous ECGs can be reviewed for comparison; however, this is a luxury that is not always possible. Four characteristic electrocardiographic phases are seen in AMI; the changes of the hyperacute phase appear early in coronary artery occlusion. The amplitude of the T waves is increased in the leads affected by the ischemic area: leads II, III, and aVF for inferior injury; V_1 and aVL for high lateral injury; and leads V_1 through V_6 for lateral injury. These T waves may resemble the "peaked" T waves seen in hyperkalemia. The next phase is the acute phase, which also occurs early after arterial occlusion. This phase is characterized by ST-segment elevation in the leads affected by the injured myocardium (see preceding discussion). During this phase, Q waves may also begin to appear. The presence of Q waves does not aid in estimating the time or extent of infarction because they may appear several hours into the infarction sequence. Therefore, the presence or absence of Q waves should not be used as a criterion for determining which patients are eligible for immediate treatment with thrombolytic agents or angioplasty. The subacute phase of injury shows inverted T waves over the affected areas of myocardium, and the ST segments begin to return to baseline. In the chronic phase, the ECG stabilizes to its new "baseline," often with Q waves, T-wave inversion, or slight ST-segment elevation. Unfortunately, more patients present with "nondiagnostic" electrocardiographic changes than present with "classic" findings.

BIOCHEMICAL MARKERS OF INFARCTION

Traditionally, serial enzyme testing for AMI involved time-consuming, laborious methods that could not be used for immediate testing, in either the emergency department or the coronary care unit. These tests were typically performed by electrophoresis (creatine kinase-MB [CK-MB] and lactate dehydrogenase [LD] isoenzymes), and results were not available for several hours. Serum markers for AMI have undergone a methodologic and utilization revolution over the past decade. With the advent of more rapid methods employing immunochemical methods and random-access analyzers, laboratories can perform testing in "real time" rather than batching samples together over several hours. This revolution has also led to the development of markers that are more specific for myocardial injury, decreasing the number of false-positive results due to skeletal muscle disorders. In addition to older tests such as total CK, CK-MB, and LD isoenzymes, today we have myoglobin, CK isoforms, myosin light chains (MLCs), troponin T (TnT), and troponin I (TnI). At this writing, MLCs have not been approved by the Food and Drug Administration (FDA) for use in the United States.

Total CK and CK-MB provide the current gold standard for the laboratory diagnosis of AMI. Total CK is composed of three cytoplasmic isoenzymes: MM, which is found predominantly in skeletal muscle and also in myocardium; MB, which is more specific for myocardium than is MM but is still found in skeletal muscle; and BB, which is found in the brain and genitourinary tract. The traditional testing sequence for total CK and CK-MB is at admission and then every 8 to 12 hours over the course of 24 hours to detect any increase above the upper limit of the reference range (3 to 8 hours) and to estimate peak serum activity (12 to 24 hours). The rise and fall of total CK usually mirrors that of CK-MB. The sensitivity of a single CK-MB result can vary greatly, depending on the time elapsed after the onset of symptoms (17 to 62 per cent at time zero and 92 to 100 per cent at 3 hours). Previous statements that CK-MB requires 4 to 8 hours to increase to above the upper limit of the reference range were based on methodology (electrophoresis measuring enzyme activity) that lacked the analytic sensitivity of the current methods (immunoassay measuring mass concentration). The new immunoassays can also be performed on an immediate basis with results generally available within 10 to 20 minutes. The use of the relative index (CK-MB ng/mL mass concentration/total CK IU/L enzyme activity $\times$ 100) helps distinguish cardiac injury from skeletal muscle injury in patients whose total CK is very high. In severe skeletal muscle injury, the relative index is less than 2 to 3 per cent, whereas in AMI, the relative index is typically greater than 10 per cent. The WHO criteria emphasize the importance of serial enzyme determinations with a classic rise-and-fall pattern of enzyme activity, rather than a single CK-MB determination or relative index.

LD is present in the cytoplasm of most tissues, including skeletal muscle, myocardium, liver, red blood cells, kidney, lung, and spleen. Electrophoresis demonstrates that there are five LD isoenzymes: LD_1, LD_2, LD_3, LD_4, and LD_5. The various isoenzymes are composed of four subunit peptides designated M (for muscle) and H (for heart). LD_1 (H_4) is composed entirely of H peptides, whereas LD_5 (M_4) is made up entirely of M peptides (Table 2). The isoenzyme of interest in AMI is LD_1, which is found in myocardium, kidney, and red blood cells. After AMI, there is a rise in the LD_1 isoenzyme, peaking between 72 and 144 hours and remaining increased in the serum for 10 days. The so-called flipped pattern ($LD_1 > LD_2$) has a sensitivity of 75 per cent in patients with suspected AMI and a specificity of 85 to 90 percent; however, timing is crucial because most clinicians order LD isoenzyme determinations at the time of admission and during the first 24 hours as they monitor CK and CK-MB. Obviously by drawing LD isoenzymes during the acute phase, very few "positives" will be seen, and even these may reflect another disease process (renal infarction or more likely a hemolyzed sample). Also, the diagnostic utility of LD isoenzymes is zero when a rise-and-fall pattern for CK-MB or classic electrocardiographic changes have been documented. LD isoenzyme determinations should be used only in patients who seek medical attention more than 24 hours after the onset of chest pain or in patients whose earlier AMI is suspected only after the acute changes in CK-MB and the ECG have occurred.

Myoglobin is an oxygen-carrying heme protein found in both cardiac and skeletal muscle. It has a low molecular weight (17,800 daltons) and is rapidly cleared from the circulation by glomerular filtration. It is located within the cytoplasm of muscle cells and is released into the blood with skeletal muscle or cardiac injury. However, its lack of tissue specificity prevents myoglobin from distinguishing between myocardial infarction and skeletal muscle trauma. Myoglobin typically rises above the reference range within 1 hour after AMI and reaches peak concentration in the blood by 4 hours, making it the earliest marker available for AMI. The sensitivity of myoglobin to AMI is in the range of 90 to 100 per cent, but specificity is poor, ranging from 60 to 95 per cent. The problem of low specificity has been addressed by measuring both myoglobin and carbonic anhydrase III (CA III). Following AMI, CA III levels remain unchanged, but myoglobin levels increase above the reference range. With severe skeletal muscle injury, both myoglobin and CA III levels are increased. Unfortunately, no FDA-approved test for CA III is available at this time.

Electrophoresis of total CK demonstrates that CK-MM and CK-MB have several isoforms. CK-MM has three isoforms: MM_1, MM_2, and MM_3. The latter is released into the circulation, where it undergoes a time-dependent post-translational hydrolysis, giving rise to MM_2 and MM_1. CK-MB has two isoforms: MB_1 and MB_2. The latter is released into the circulation and undergoes a similar post-translational modification, giving rise to MB_1. An increase in the ratio of CK-MM_3 to CK-MM_1 is consistent with AMI early

Table 2. Lactate Dehydrogenase Isoenzymes

LD_1 (HHHH)
Hemolytic-megaloblastic anemia
Renal cortical infarction
AMI
LD_2 (HHHM)
LD_3 (HHMM)
LD_4 (HMMM)
LD_5 (MMMM)
Hepatitis
Cirrhosis
Skeletal muscle trauma-disease

LD = lactate dehydrogenase; AMI = acute myocardial infarction.

in the course of infarction. However, MM isoforms are also present in skeletal muscle, and therefore the test lacks tissue specificity. The MB_2:MB_1 ratio shows improved, although not absolute, tissue specificity for myocardium and is increased early in AMI, with a time frame similar to the release of myoglobin into the circulation. Isoforms may also be increased following severe skeletal muscle trauma or strenuous exercise, further limiting specificity. A range of sensitivities has been reported for CK isoforms (MB_2:MB_1 ratio), ranging from 67 per cent at 1 to 3 hours to 87 per cent at 3 to 6 hours. The method is an electrophoretic assay that measures enzyme activity. It is labor-intensive and lacks the analytic sensitivity of a mass concentration immunoassay.

Myosin is a myofibrillary structural protein with isoforms found in myocardium and skeletal muscle. Two MLCs are attached to each amino terminal end of the myosin heavy chain molecule. Although two MLCs can be differentiated by monoclonal antibodies, the skeletal muscle and cardiac forms cannot be distinguished using current methods. MLCs are released into the blood 3 to 5 hours after the onset of myocardial damage and persist in the circulation for 10 to 14 days. No automated methods are available for the detection of MLCs, and the manual assay is not specific for the cardiac form, limiting the clinical utility of the test.

Troponin is one of the contractile proteins of the myofibril. It is actually a complex of three proteins: TnT (the tropomyosin-binding component), TnI (the inhibitory component), and troponin C (the calcium-binding component). The troponin complex is present both in the myocardium and in skeletal muscle. The skeletal muscle and cardiac muscle forms of troponin C are identical; however, cardiac-specific forms of TnI and TnT have been identified. Cardiac TnI has an additional 31 amino acid sequence at its amino terminal end, whereas TnT has an 11 amino acid sequence that confers its cardiac specificity.

The biggest misconception about the troponins is that they are early markers of AMI. The release of TnT from infarcted myocardium mirrors that of CK-MB, reaching peak concentrations at approximately 12 hours following infarction. TnT has clinical sensitivities similar to those of CK-MB for the detection of AMI. One advantage of TnT is that it remains increased for 7 to 10 days rather than returning to baseline after 2 to 3 days as does CK-MB. TnT remains increased in the circulation because the initial release of the cytoplasmic pool of TnT is followed by release of the myofibril-bound TnT. For this reason, TnT could help replace several of the cardiac markers (CK-MB and LD isoenzymes) currently used in the diagnosis of AMI. Unfortunately, issues of specificity persist. Some investigators suggest that measurable TnT is released after minor myocardial damage (small infarcts, unstable angina), whereas others conclude that the antigenic difference between the cardiac muscle form and the skeletal muscle form is too small to allow adequate tissue specificity. Clearly more study is necessary if the issue is to be resolved.

An immunoassay for TnI has recently been approved by the FDA and is currently being studied as a marker for AMI in the United States. Like TnT, TnI levels begin to rise above the upper limit of the reference range 4 to 6 hours after infarction, paralleling the rise of CK-MB, and peaking at 12 to 24 hours after the onset of symptoms. TnI has a biphasic release like that of TnT and remains increased for 7 to 10 days. In studies comparing TnI with CK-MB in patients with skeletal muscle injury only, CK-MB reached activity close to 30 times the upper limit of normal, whereas TnI remained essentially undetectable, suggesting nearly complete tissue specificity. These studies have been corroborated in marathon runners, in patients with chronic myopathy (e.g., Duchenne muscular dystrophy), and in patients with renal failure who are receiving chronic dialysis. Perioperative AMI was more accurately diagnosed with the use of TnI because it is more specific for myocardium than is CK-MB or TnT.

Table 3. Patterns of Cardiac Enzyme Release Into the Circulation

Early markers (increase within 1 to 3 hr of occlusion)
CK isoforms
Myoglobin
Intermediate markers (increase within 3 to 8 hr of occlusion)
CK-MB
TnT
TnI
MLC
Late markers (increase >8 hr after occlusion)
LD isoenzymes (LD_1)

CK = creatine kinase; TnT = troponin T; TnI = troponin I; MLC = myosin light chain; LD = lactate dehydrogenase.

A single biochemical test is not sufficient because none of the currently available markers answers all the clinical questions. No one marker has adequate cardiac specificity (Table 3) and sensitivity for early (1 to 4 hours) and late (past 3 days) detection of AMI. The combination of an early myocardial marker such as myoglobin or CK isoforms with CK-MB, or an early marker with either TnT or TnI, is likely to replace the traditional CK-MB and LD isoenzymes for the diagnosis of AMI.

THROMBOLYTIC AGENTS AND ANGIOPLASTY

The treatment of choice for AMI is reperfusion of the occluded coronary artery with either thrombolytic agents or angioplasty. Thrombolytic therapy has been shown to decrease morbidity and mortality in patients with AMI; however, many patients do not meet the criteria for this intervention. The four main reasons for exclusion are (1) advanced age, (2) nondiagnostic electrocardiographic changes, (3) specific contraindications for thrombolytic therapy itself (e.g., history of cerebrovascular accident or gastrointestinal hemorrhage), and (4) delay in treatment (time really *is* myocardium) either by the patient prior to admission or in the hospital while awaiting evaluation or test results. When thrombolytic agents or angioplasty is used, the success of the therapy must be assessed. The clinician traditionally relied on nonspecific clues, such as evidence of new cardiac arrhythmias on the ECG, the diminution of chest pain, or the return to a normal or baseline ECG. The gold standard has been the use of an invasive procedure, such as coronary catheterization, which may be contraindicated in the patient who is receiving thrombolytic agents because it carries a much higher risk of complication and bleeding.

Noninvasive methods for determining successful reperfusion employ many of the same markers as used for the diagnosis of AMI. In general, successful reperfusion causes an earlier and greater release of enzymes into the circulation known as the "washout" effect. During times of arterial occlusion (AMI), the enzymes are released and slowly enter the lymphatic and circulatory systems. When the artery is reopened (with thrombolytic agents or angioplasty), accumulated enzymes from the surrounding injured tissue are suddenly released directly into the circulation. This leads to an early and more marked increase of the cardiac markers in the blood than is seen with unsuccessful reperfusion or no therapy at all. By monitoring the patient every 30 to 60 minutes, the changes in these markers are detected. Following thrombolytic therapy, a twofold or greater increase in CK-MB occurs within 90 minutes of successful reperfusion, and the rate of increase of CK-MB within the first 4 hours after treatment differentiates nonreperfused from reperfused patients. CK isoform ratios (MM_3:MM_1, MB_2:MB_1) also show the washout effect. As expected from the tissue distribution, the MB_2:MB_1 ratio is a more specific marker for myocardial reperfusion. The MB_2:MB_1 ratio peaks much earlier (<2.5 hours) and detects successful reperfusion within 1 hour of initiating thrombolytic therapy. TnT has also been proposed as a noninvasive marker for evaluating reperfusion. Patients with successful reperfusion generally show peak TnT concentrations within 24 hours, whereas those in whom reperfusion fails show a more gradual, prolonged rise in TnT concentration. TnI shows similar peaks and rates of rise in successful reperfusion and may even surpass those of CK-MB, showing changes as early as 30 to 60 minutes following reperfusion. Myoglobin shows a fivefold increase in the first 2 hours following successful reperfusion and peaks three times earlier with successful reperfusion.

CONCLUSION

AMI is a major health care concern and a cause for many patients to present to an emergency department. The diagnosis is based on the triad of clinical history, which may be noncontributory; electrocardiographic changes, which may be nondiagnostic; and laboratory values, which are not always available or not always tissue-specific. To prevent tissue necrosis from AMI, however, urgent treatment, such as with thrombolytic agents or angioplasty, must be started within several hours of coronary artery occlusion. Unfortunately, this therapy is not without risk and cannot be used indiscriminately in all patients with chest pain. Understanding the ancillary tests available, the laboratory tests, and the ECG, as well as their limitations, interpretations, and general principles, is crucial not only for establishing the diagnosis of AMI but also for efficiently using health care resources and managing the cost of medicine without sacrificing the quality of patient care.

CARDIOVASCULAR RISK FACTORS

By Donald A. Smith, M.D.
New York, New York

Everyone can be placed on some scale of risk of experiencing clinical coronary heart disease (CHD)—from as low as less than 1 per cent per 10 years when young without risk factors, to 21 per cent per 10 years in those older than 65 years of age, to as high as 40 to 50 per cent per 10 years in older persons with many risk factors. The role of the clinician is to assess individual risk and to suggest ways of reducing it.

Table 1. Risk Factors Associated With the Onset of Coronary Heart Disease (CHD)

Age	Increased relative weight
Male gender	Left ventricular hypertrophy
Total cholesterol	Nonspecific ST-T wave changes or intraventricular block on ECG
Hypertension	
Cigarette smoking	

The Framingham Study, begun in 1948, developed the concept of coronary risk by measuring possible risk factors for CHD at baseline and biennially in a healthy population of 5127 adults aged 30 to 60 years. In the first 10 years of follow-up several risk factors were clearly associated with the onset of CHD (Table 1). Through the years, various prospective population studies have identified other factors associated with increased risk of CHD (Table 2).

The primary difficulty with the coronary risk concept is the tendency of the clinician to be overwhelmed by the sheer number of risk factors (nearly 250 have been suggested). As the list grows, clinicians are challenged not only to educate patients about the concept of risk factor reduction but also to quantitate the benefit from such reduction and to prioritize the risks amenable to change.

Fortunately, logistic regression equations predicting CHD risk over 5- and 10-year periods (with the use of a string of risk factors measured in the original Framingham population and the Framingham offspring cohort) can measure baseline risk and changes in risk following modification of risk factors in Americans aged 30 to 74 years of age who are free from cardiovascular disease. These equations have been reduced to a point score algorithm to demonstrate the concepts of baseline risk and risk reduction in patients. By knowing age, gender, systolic blood pressure (average of 2 sitting values), total cholesterol, high-density lipoprotein (HDL) cholesterol, the presence or absence of cigarette smoking (within the past year), diabetes mellitus (under treatment or fasting blood glucose greater than 140 mg/dL), and left ventricular hypertrophy (LVH) on electrocardiogram (ECG) (increased R-wave amplitude in leads reflecting potentials from the left ventricle associated with ST-segment depression and T-wave flattening or inversion), the clinician may attempt to predict baseline risk over 10 years and reduction in risk if such risk factors are modified. A simple, computerized program called Life-style Change Tool (distributed by the Upjohn Company) can be easily installed; or the clinician can use a manual system (Circulation 1991; 83:361) to predict risk.

Because many risk factors are related to each other, such as obesity, hypertriglyceridemia, low HDL cholesterol,

Table 2. Other Factors Associated With Increased Risk of CHD

Diabetes mellitus
Increased LDL cholesterol
Decreased HDL cholesterol
Lipoprotein (a)
Increasing weight, obesity, weight gain since age 25 years, waist-to-hip ratio
Fibrinogen levels and other measures of increased thrombotic or decreased fibrinolytic activity
Psychoemotional factors, including measures of personality type, depression, etc.

increased blood pressure, and increased glucose levels, one risk factor may lose much of its power as a predictor when other risk factors are taken into account. For example, obesity becomes an insignificant predictor of risk of CHD when the associated variables listed above are placed into the equation. As a result, obesity has been dropped as a risk factor in the National Cholesterol Education Program's Adult Treatment Panel II guidelines because its short-term risk can be explained by associated increases in blood pressure, serum glucose, and serum triglyceride, and decreases in HDL cholesterol. This removal of obesity as a risk factor is unfortunate because weight control simultaneously improves several of the associated risk factors.

DIAGNOSIS OF DYSLIPIDEMIAS

The diagnosis and management of atherogenic dyslipidemias is fundamental in both the primary and the secondary prevention of cardiovascular disease. In societies with lower circulating low-density lipoprotein (LDL) cholesterol, hypertension and smoking do not increase the risk of CHD. In the United States, diagnosis and management of LDL cholesterol has become the cornerstone of risk reduction for CHD.

The diagnosis is based on serum total and HDL cholesterol in CHD-free individuals. When total cholesterol is less than 200 mg/dL and HDL cholesterol is 35 mg/dL or more, or when total cholesterol is 200 to 239 mg/dL, HDL cholesterol is 35 mg/dL or more, and the patient has less than two risk factors, a lipid profile is not necessary. For other patients, especially those with higher risk or known CHD, a complete lipid profile (total cholesterol, triglycerides, HDL cholesterol, and LDL cholesterol) is required. The guidelines set goals for LDL cholesterol that depend on the severity of the risk for a first or further clinical coronary event. The severity of risk is based on the presence of CHD (high risk) or other independent risk factors for CHD. Zero or one risk factor means mild risk; two or more risk factors mean moderate risk (Table 3).

Although some may question these goals (Is it really necessary to achieve an LDL cholesterol below 130 mg/dL for secondary prevention?) or the list of risk factors (Shouldn't obesity or lack of physical activity be added?), this basic approach to the diagnosis and management of lipid disorders maintains its focus as different approaches to lipid management are instituted, and it avoids the excessive use of lipid-lowering pharmacologic agents in primary prevention while it aggressively manages those with CHD who are at high risk for secondary events.

An LDL cholesterol measurement for each patient is required in this system because goals are better defined by LDL cholesterol than by total cholesterol. After triglyceride and HDL cholesterol have been determined, changes in total cholesterol typically reflect changes in LDL cholesterol, and clinicians may use the less expensive total cholesterol as a surrogate test for LDL cholesterol. A few laboratories report only the total cholesterol, triglycerides, and HDL cholesterol in their lipid profile. In this case, LDL cholesterol must be calculated using the Friedewald formula: total cholesterol = LDL cholesterol + HDL cholesterol + VLDL cholesterol.

The very low density lipoprotein (VLDL) particle is the only particle in the fasting state that contains triglycerides. The concentration of triglycerides to cholesterol within the particle is 5 to 1. To calculate VLDL cholesterol, the fasting triglyceride concentration is divided by 5; this calculated value correlates well with the concentration of VLDL cholesterol measured after laborious separation of lipoproteins by ultracentrifugation. Most laboratories perform and report this LDL cholesterol calculation automatically. The formula does not work as well when triglyceride concentrations exceed 400 mg/dL; calculated LDL cholesterol values underestimate measured values by 5 to 10 per cent.

Table 3. CHD Risk Factors and LDL Cholesterol Goals

No. of Risk Factors	Goal LDL Cholesterol (mg/dL)	Concentration of LDL Cholesterol to Institute Drug Therapy (mg/dL)
0, 1	160	190
2 or more	130	160
Presence of CHD	100	130

The following example details the use of the Adult Treatment Panel guidelines to determine goal LDL cholesterol for a specific patient. The patient S.Z. is a 44-year-old female whose parents are alive and healthy at 76 years of age. She smokes one pack of cigarettes per day and is unwilling to stop. She has no history of diabetes or hypertension, but she is 15 pounds over ideal weight. Her recent lipid profile results are as follows: total cholesterol, 261 mg/dL; triglycerides, 100 mg/dL; HDL cholesterol, 56 mg/dL; LDL cholesterol, 185 mg/dL.

First count the number of risk factors according to Table 4. Because smoking appears to be the only risk factor, her goal LDL cholesterol should be 160 mg/dL. This patient is within 30 mg/dL of her goal, so lipid-lowering agents are not indicated, but she should be advised to lose weight and to lower fat and cholesterol in her diet.

Twelve years later, S.Z. reappears, still smoking but now menopausal. She does not take hormones, and her LDL cholesterol is 205 mg/dL. According to Table 4, she now has 2 coronary risk factors (smoking and postmenopausal status without hormone replacement). Thus, her goal LDL cholesterol is 130 mg/dL, and pharmacologic lipid-lowering therapy may be required. However, if she stops smoking or takes estrogen, her LDL cholesterol goal may remain 160 mg/dL, and she may reach the 160 to 190 mg/dL range for LDL cholesterol with proper diet alone.

Table 4. Revised Risk Factors for CHD

Positive
Age, yr
Men ≥45
Women ≥55 or premature menopause without estrogen replacement therapy
Family history of premature CHD (father, brother <55 yr; mother, sister <65 yr)
Cigarette smoking
Hypertension (≥140/90 or taking antihypertensive medication)
HDL cholesterol <35 mg/dL (0.9 mmol/L)
Diabetes mellitus
Negative
HDL cholesterol ≥60 mg/dL (1.6 mmol/L)

Modified from Summary of the Second Report of the National Cholesterol Education Program (NCEP) Expert Panel on Detection, Evaluation, and Treatment of High Blood Cholesterol in Adults (Adult Treatment Panel II). JAMA, 269:3015–3023, 1993, with permission.

Hypertriglyceridemia

In some patients, hypertriglyceridemia may be atherogenic. The Framingham Study reported increased risk of CHD when triglyceride concentrations exceeded 140 mg/dL and HDL cholesterol measured less than 40 mg/dL in both men and women. In Sweden, a 20-year follow-up indicates that serum triglyceride predicts later CHD in both males and females, but total serum cholesterol does not. A German trial suggests an increased incidence of CHD when serum triglyceride exceeds 200 mg/dL and the total cholesterol–to–HDL cholesterol (TC/HDL-C) ratio is greater than 5.0. The Helsinki Trial placebo group demonstrated a relative risk of 5.0 in those with triglycerides greater than 200 mg/dL and an LDL-C/HDL-C ratio greater than 5.0. CHD decreased by 31 per cent in the total group treated with gemfibrozil for 5 years. By contrast, the subgroup treated with gemfibrozil with increased triglycerides and LDL-C/HDL-C experienced a 71 per cent decrease in CHD. Therefore, a triglyceride concentration above 200 mg/dL should be considered a risk factor for CHD when the family history indicates premature CHD, HDL cholesterol measures less than 40 mg/dL, the LDL/HDL cholesterol ratio is 5.0 or greater, or the LDL cholesterol exceeds 200 mg/dL.

The mechanism by which hypertriglyceridemia contributes to atherogenesis is not clear. Although small, dense LDL particles begin to appear when the serum triglyceride level exceeds 150 mg/dL, hypertriglyceridemia is also associated with abnormalities of clotting or impaired fibrinolysis, including hyperfibrinogenemia and plasminogen activator inhibitor (PAI-1) antigenemia. In multivariate analysis that controls for the high blood pressure, obesity, insulin resistance, and low HDL cholesterol that accompany hypertriglyceridemia, the triglyceride concentration often loses its predictive significance. However, the newer prospective studies mentioned earlier have analyzed the predictive risk of hypertriglyceridemia stratified on HDL cholesterol. In the presence of lowered HDL cholesterol, hypertriglyceridemia maintains its predictive importance. Because familial combined hyperlipidemia (phenotypes IIa, IIb, and IV) is the most common lipid disorder in persons with myocardial infarction, hypertriglyceridemia should not be ignored in those with CHD or in those with a family history of CHD. However, despite the possibility that gemfibrozil may lower triglycerides and enhance primary prevention of CHD, gemfibrozil and other agents have not yet proved beneficial in secondary CHD prevention.

HDL Cholesterol

In the United States, average HDL cholesterol concentrations in the serum of white males and females are 45 and 55 mg/dL, respectively. Decreased HDL cholesterol concentrations are linearly related to increased CHD risk. Concentrations below 35 mg/dL are considered independent risk factors by the National Cholesterol Education Program. Nevertheless, when total cholesterol measured less than 150 mg/dL, Framingham residents did not experience CHD, even in the presence of decreased HDL cholesterol. As total cholesterol exceeds 150 mg/dL in the presence of low HDL cholesterol the risk for CHD steadily rises. For these patients, clinicians should advise that serum cholesterol not exceed 200 mg/dL. Finally, because low HDL cholesterol is often accompanied by increased serum triglycerides, HDL cholesterol concentrations are best interpreted in the context of serum triglycerides and LDL cholesterol measurements.

Other Lipid Measurements

Lipoprotein Electrophoresis

Historically, lipoprotein separation by electrophoresis facilitated assignment of a lipid phenotype to a patient with abnormal lipids. Lipoprotein electrophoresis is no longer done because it does not add significantly to the information from a standard lipid profile. It is reasonable to presume the presence of chylomicrons in the serum when triglyceride concentrations exceed 1000 mg/dL. This condition should be treated to avoid pancreatitis.

Apolipoproteins

Immunoassays for apolipoprotein A (found in HDL) and apolipoprotein B (found in VLDL and LDL cholesterol in the fasting state) have not added significantly to cardiovascular risk assessment. The measurements are difficult to standardize, and the results do not guide or influence therapy.

Non-HDL cholesterol (total cholesterol minus HDL cholesterol) in the fasting state generally reflects cholesterol in VLDL and LDL particles. Non-HDL cholesterol may provide not only a surrogate for apolipoprotein B but also a means of setting lipid goals in persons with high triglycerides and incalculable LDL cholesterol. Goal non-HDL cholesterol values are set 30 mg/dL higher than LDL cholesterol values. Table 5 compares LDL cholesterol goals with non-HDL cholesterol goals, which can be adopted when triglyceride concentrations are too high to calculate LDL cholesterol. Importantly, the accuracy and clinical utility of this approach for predicting CHD has not been empirically tested.

Lipoprotein Subtypes

Low-density lipoprotein particles may be separated on the basis of size and charge via gradient gel electrophoresis. Pattern B, which contains smaller and denser LDL particles, may be more atherogenic, but as yet there is no clinical utility for such analyses. That the prevalence of type B LDL subgroups increases as the serum triglyceride level exceeds 150 mg/dL supports the hypothesis that triglyceride levels exceeding 150 to 200 mg/dL may be associated with increased atherogenic risk.

High-density lipoprotein particles may be separated into HDL_2 and HDL_3 particles. Increased HDL_2 particles may be found in women and in persons who perform heavy exercise, while HDL_3 particles are increased with increasing alcohol consumption. As yet there is no conclusive evidence that one HDL particle protects better than the other, and there is no clinical utility in separating and quantitating HDL particles. Those containing apolipoprotein A-I may be more protective than those containing both apolipoprotein A-I and apolipoprotein A-II, but there is currently no clinical significance to this observation.

Lipoprotein (a) [Lp(a)] is an LDL particle whose apo B-100 is attached to a surrounding apolipoprotein (a) through disulfide bridges. High concentrations of this lipoprotein have been associated with increased risk of CHD, of closure

Table 5. Comparison of LDL Cholesterol Goals With Non-HDL Cholesterol Goals

No. of Risk Factors	LDL Goal (mg/dL)	Non-HDL Goal (mg/dL)
0, 1	160	190
2 or more	130	160

of saphenous vein bypass grafts, of stroke, and of intimal-medial thickening of the carotid arteries. Concentrations of Lp(a) within atherosclerotic plaques are substantially higher than those in serum. Apolipoprotein (a) is homologous with plasminogen but does not have the enzymatic protease to lyse fibrin and clots. Apolipoprotein (a) and plasminogen compete for binding to fibrin, a competition that suggests interference with fibrinolysis as a plausible mechanism for increased risk of atherogenesis. Lp(a) values in the upper quintile of the population have been associated with increased risk of CHD. In whites in the United States, this upper quintile begins at 25 mg/dL. Values that exceed 25 mg/dL are associated with a two-fold increase in the relative risk of CHD. Although ingestion of niacin may reduce Lp(a), there is no evidence that independent reduction of Lp(a) provides clinical benefit.

HYPERTENSION

Systolic blood pressure of 160 mm Hg or greater or diastolic pressure of 95 mm Hg or greater increases the risk of CHD two to three fold and of stroke seven fold. Systolic pressure of 140 to 159 mm Hg or diastolic pressure of 90 to 94 mm Hg increases the risk of CHD by 50 per cent and of stroke three fold.

Meta-analysis of 14 prospective intervention trials indicates substantial reductions in stroke (35 to 40 per cent) and CHD (10 to 15 per cent) when diastolic blood pressure is reduced by 5 to 6 mm Hg over 5 years. In the Systolic Hypertension in the Elderly Project (SHEP), persons older than 60 years with diastolic pressures less than 90 mm Hg and systolic pressures exceeding 160 mm Hg had 36 per cent fewer strokes and 25 per cent fewer coronary events with the use of chlorthalidone and/or atenolol over 4 to 5 years. Thus, consistent increases in sitting, resting blood pressure should be treated. Physicians must also acknowledge hypertension associated with the "white coat syndrome," where increased blood pressure is detected more often in young persons and women when readings are obtained by physicians. This problem of overdiagnosis may be ameliorated by recording blood pressures at home or in the clinic over 6 to 12 months or by applying an ambulatory monitor that automatically and repeatedly measures and records blood pressure throughout the day. When average ambulatory systolic pressure is less than 130 mm Hg and diastolic pressure is less than 85 mm Hg, the chances of increased left ventricular mass or diastolic filling abnormalities on echocardiography are small. (For further discussion of the diagnosis of hypertension, see the article on hypertension.)

SMOKING

Cigarette smoking is associated with a two-fold increased risk of myocardial infarction, ischemic and hemorrhagic stroke, peripheral vascular disease, and death from coronary artery disease—but not of angina pectoris. An increased risk of myocardial infarction and sudden cardiac death has been demonstrated at levels of 1 to 4 cigarettes per day for men in Sweden, and at levels of 1 to 14 cigarettes per day in the Nurses' Health Study. The risk of coronary death almost doubled in the Framingham Study as daily consumption increased from less than 20 to more than 20 cigarettes per day. This increased risk of myocardial infarction and CHD death is found in cigarette smokers of both genders and at all ages.

For those with CHD, smoking increases the incidence of silent myocardial ischemia; moreover, the recurrent myocardial infarction and mortality rates of those who continue to smoke after myocardial infarction are double those of patients who quit. Passive smoking also increases the risk of CHD. Men in the Multiple Risk Factor Intervention Trial with wives who smoked doubled their risk of both fatal and nonfatal coronary events. Pipe and cigar smoking did not increase the risk of cardiovascular disease in Framingham; however, it did produce a risk lower than that for cigarette smokers but greater than that for nonsmokers in Scandinavia.

The contribution of cigarette smoking to increased risk of CHD may be short-lived in some patients who stop smoking. Many studies, however, suggest that increased risk is cut in half in the first 5 years after cessation and is generally gone at 10 years, but may remain increased for up to 15 years in persons who originally smoked more than 20 cigarettes per day. The Northwick Park Study indicates that serum fibrinogen levels decreased by 50 per cent during the first 5 years after cessation of smoking and completely normalized in the next 5 years. The effect of smoking on CHD risk may therefore be related to its procoagulant effects, such as increased serum fibrinogen and increased platelet aggregation. Other proposed mechanisms of risk include nicotine-stimulated increases in epinephrine and norepinephrine, which increase heart rate, blood pressure, cardiac output, cardiac workload, and oxygen consumption, leading to cardiac ischemia in patients with fixed coronary obstruction.

OBESITY AND FAT DISTRIBUTION

Excess adipose tissue, especially increased intra-abdominal fat, is clearly associated with changes most likely due to increased resistance to insulin-mediated glucose disposal. Such changes include increased blood pressure, increased levels of serum triglycerides, and decreased circulating HDL cholesterol, increased fasting concentrations of insulin and glucose, and increased serum fibrinogen levels. Definitions of overweight and obesity are often stated in terms of a relative weight, actual weight divided by an ideal weight and multiplied by 100. Ideal weight becomes 100, overweight 110 to 119, and obesity 120 or more. In examining the risk of CHD associated with excessive weight, the Framingham Study used Metropolitan Life Insurance relative weight, which is actual weight divided by the midpoint of the ideal weight range for medium frame by height. As baseline relative weight increased from less than 110, to 110 to 129, to 130 or more, the 26-year incidence of cardiovascular disease, CHD, sudden-death congestive heart failure in males and females, and stroke in females increased two to three fold. The relative risks were even greater in persons younger than 50 years of age at baseline. All the increased risk derived from weight gain starting at age 25 years and could not be explained by other baseline risk factors. These findings were corroborated for women in the Nurses' Health Study, in which a 20-kg weight gain beyond 18 years of age predicted a three- to six-fold increase in risk of CHD over a 14-year follow-up.

One recognized marker of excessive weight is the amount of intra-abdominal fat, which can be estimated from the percentage area of intra-abdominal fat in a computed tomography scan of the abdomen at the level of L3–L5. The clinician can also obtain a waist-to-hip ratio using a tape measure. Waist circumference is measured at the smallest circumference between the lowest rib and the iliac crests, or at the level of the umbilicus with the patient standing or supine. Hip circumference is measured at the level of the maximum protrusion of the buttocks while standing, or at the level of the symphysis pubis while supine. The upper 10th percentile ratio in women is 0.85 and above, and in men is 0.95 and above. When waist-to-hip ratios exceed these thresholds, the relative risk for obesity-related diseases, such as diabetes, increases in white women from 3.7 to 10.3. Confirmation of an increased waist-to-hip ratio may increase the patient's motivation for losing weight.

DIABETES AND IMPAIRED GLUCOSE TOLERANCE

The Multiple Risk Factor Intervention Trial included 5000 middle-aged diabetic men among the more than 350,000 participants. These men with diabetes had a three- to five-fold increased risk of coronary mortality compared to men without diabetes. In Framingham, CHD risk associated with diabetes was much greater in women than in men. In the Nurses' Health Study 15,000 diabetic nurses had a five-fold increased incidence of CHD compared with nurses without diabetes. The mechanisms by which diabetes increases the risk of CHD may include the following: (1) dyslipidemias and insulin resistance, (2) procoagulant states with increased activity of factors VII and X with increased platelet aggregation, (3) decreased fibrinolysis with increased tissue plasminogen activator inhibitor (PAI), and (4) glycation of proteins such as collagen, which increases their avidity for LDL cholesterol. Increased glycohemoglobin may also be associated with increased risk of CHD in the diabetic elderly. There are some data showing that impaired glucose tolerance as well as overt diabetes is a risk factor for coronary heart disease.

Diabetes mellitus must be considered whenever a fasting plasma or serum glucose greater than 140 mg/dL is observed. The fasting plasma glucose is not very sensitive, so the 2-hour glucose tolerance test has been used to detect persons who are normoglycemic when fasting but have 2-hour glucose concentrations of 200 mg/dL or more (diabetes) or 140 to 199 mg/dL (impaired glucose tolerance) following the ingestion of 75 g of glucose. The oral glucose tolerance test is more likely to be abnormal when fasting plasma glucose measures 115 to 139 mg/dL, age is greater than 65, relative body weight is greater than 120, there are first-degree relatives with diabetes, or the patient has a history of giving birth to a baby that weighed more than 9 pounds.

PHYSICAL INACTIVITY

Low levels of habitual physical activity are associated with a 1.5- to 2.4-fold increase in risk of CHD, a relative risk comparable to that seen with other CHD risk factors, such as hypertension, smoking, and hypercholesterolemia. A two- to three-fold increase in the incidence of CHD was noted in Harvard alumni with the lowest level of physical activity, with increasing protection from CHD as levels of activity increased. Exercise training may improve some metabolic parameters associated with increased risk of CHD. Exercise may increase HDL cholesterol; reduce weight and serum triglycerides; reduce blood pressure; increase insulin sensitivity, thereby reducing glucose intolerance; enhance fibrinolysis; decrease platelet aggregation; and reduce the risk of ventricular arrhythmias, perhaps by desensitizing the myocardium to the effects of catecholamines.

Recommendations for the year 2000 are to increase to 30 per cent the number of people who engage regularly, and hopefully daily, in at least 30 minutes of light to moderate physical activity. Currently, only 22 per cent of the population meets this standard; another 24 per cent do not exercise at all, and the remaining half fall somewhere in between. In the Behavioral Risk Factor Surveillance System from 1987, the percentage of persons involved in less than 20 minutes of leisure time activity three times per week ranged from 47.2 per cent in Montana to 73.5 per cent in New York state with a national median of 59 per cent. Clearly, physicians must encourage their patients to increase their physical activity.

The total time devoted to physical activity of moderate intensity correlates with decreased risk of CHD. This total time can be segmented so that 10 minutes three times per day improves maximal oxygen uptake and HDL cholesterol as well as one 30-minute session. Thus, clinicians need not ask patients how much exercise they get per week, but rather should gauge the types and duration of physical activity (Table 6), including activities at home, at work, and while commuting. Clinicians should encourage short spurts of moderate activity, such as lunchtime walks, stair climbing in lieu of taking the elevator, and light stationary cycling while watching television. Recurrent assessment of physical activity is required to convince a sedentary patient that increased physical activity is beneficial and important.

PSYCHOSOCIAL FACTORS

Coronary heart disease is more prevalent in the lower socioeconomic strata of Western societies. For example, the 5-year mortality rate in symptomatic middle-aged whites with one-vessel stenosis of 75 per cent or greater and annual incomes less than $10,000 was double that of similar patients with incomes of $40,000 or more.

Lack of social support is another major risk factor. Both men and women have increased risk of CHD mortality for several months after the death of a spouse. Single persons have in-hospital mortality rates following myocardial infarction that are 40 to 50 per cent higher than those of married persons. Five-year mortality rates in white middle-aged symptomatic patients with at least one 75 per cent coronary stenosis were tripled in persons who were unmarried and did not have a confidant compared with those who either were married or had a confidant.

Psychological traits have also been related to increased risk of CHD. Type A personality, a term that refers to driven, hostile, rarely relaxed persons, was originally associated with a doubling of the risk of CHD over an 8.5-year follow-up. At 22 years, however, the relationship no longer held. Moreover, the link between type A personality and CHD was not confirmed in the Multiple Risk Factor Intervention Trial over a 9-year period. The type A interview apparently contained too many behavioral characteristics; among them, hostility and cynicism (measured by the Minnesota Multiphasic Personality Inventory [MMPI]) correlate best with the risk of CHD. The Western Electric Study of 1877 middle-aged male employees reported that MMPI hostility scores (independent of other risk factors) predicted myocardial infarction and CHD death over 10 years and CHD and total death over 20 years. The hostile personality has been described as cynical and untrusting, with

Table 6. Examples of Common Physical Activities for Healthy U.S. Adults by Intensity of Effort

Light (<3.0 METs or <4 kcal-min^{-1})	Moderate (3.0–6.0 METs or 4–7 kcal-min^{-1})	Hard or Vigorous (>6.0 METs or >7 kcal-min^{-1})
Walking slowly (strolling 1–2 mph)	Walking briskly (3–4 mph)	Walking briskly uphill or with a load
Cycling, stationary (<50 W)	Cycling for pleasure or transportation (≤10 mph)	Cycling, fast or racing (>10 mph)
Swimming (slow treading)	Swimming (moderate effort)	Swimming (fast treading or crawl)
Conditioning exercise (light stretching)	Conditioning exercise (general calisthenics)	Conditioning exercise (stair ergometer, ski machine)
—	Racket sports, table tennis	Racket sports (singles tennis, racquetball)
Golf (power cart)	Golf (pulling cart or carrying clubs)	—
Bowling	—	—
Fishing (sitting)	Fishing (standing/casting)	Fishing in stream
Boating (power)	Canoeing leisurely (2–3 mph)	Canoeing (rapidly, ≥4 mph)
Home care (carpet sweeping)	Home care (general cleaning)	Moving furniture
Mowing lawn (riding mower)	Mowing lawn (power mower)	Mowing lawn (hand mower)
Home repair (carpentry)	Home repair (painting)	—

Modified from Pate, R.R., Pratt, M., Blair, S.N., et al.: Physical activity and public health: A recommendation from the Centers for Disease Control and Prevention and the American College of Sports Medicine. JAMA, 273:402–407, 1995, with permission.

negative emotional reactions to others and overt anger when faced with frustrations and problems.

Major depression has a significant impact on CHD outcome. Persons discharged from the hospital after myocardial infarction with a diagnosis of major depression (as defined by a psychiatric interview schedule including depressed mood; changes in appetite and sleep patterns; fatigue; problems with concentrating; feelings of guilt, shame, and decreased self-esteem; and thoughts of death or suicide) had a mortality rate in the first 6 months that was five times greater than that of patients who did not have this diagnosis.

PROCOAGULANT AND ANTIFIBRINOLYTIC RISK

The Northwick Park Heart Study of men in London aged 40 to 54 years at entry examined the prospective relationship between the incidence of CHD and both procoagulant and low fibrinolytic activity. Fibrinogen and factor VII concentrations as well as antifibrinolytic activity measured by longer clot lysis times showed strong independent associations with CHD, especially during the first 5 years of follow-up. The Framingham Study suggested a two-fold increased risk of CHD and stroke over 14 years of follow-up for both males and females in the top one third versus the bottom one third of fibrinogen concentrations. Fibrinogen increases with advancing age, smoking, excess body weight, menopausal status, and physical inactivity, which partially but not totally explains its contribution to the risk of CHD. The European Concerted Action on Thrombosis (ECAT) and Disabilities Angina Pectoris Study followed 3000 patients with angina for 2 years. Persons in the upper quintile of fibrinogen concentration had a three-fold increased risk of myocardial infarction or sudden death compared with those in the lowest quintile. Increasing cholesterol concentrations predicted coronary events only in those in the upper two thirds of fibrinogen concentrations, a fact that suggests an important permissive effect of increased fibrinogen on CHD risk associated with increasing serum cholesterol. Perhaps increased fibrinogen is a marker for endothelial perturbation, which makes these cells more susceptible to the effects of hypercholesterolemia. It is not yet clear whether fibrinogen is a causal risk factor or a surrogate marker for "active" or inflammatory coronary artery disease.

Decreased fibrinolytic activity in the Northwick Park Heart Study was associated with increased risk of CHD. In the Physicians' Health Study, increased tissue plasminogen activator (t-PA) antigen was associated with increased risk of CHD. These two findings seem contradictory until one realizes that t-PA antigen and tissue plasminogen activator inhibitor (PAI-1) measurements are positively correlated. Hence, t-PA antigen measurements include t-PA bound to PAI-1 and therefore may actually and perversely be a measure of higher PAI-1 concentrations and thus of decreased fibrinolytic activity. The ECAT study (see above) demonstrated a two-fold increased risk of CHD events over a 2-year follow-up in those with angina who were in the highest quintile versus the lowest for t-PA antigen. Increased PAI-1 antigen may contribute to increased risk of CHD in patients with diabetes. Although fibrinogen, factor VII, t-PA antigen, and PAI-1 are proven markers for increased risk of CHD, the role of thrombosis and fibrinolysis in CHD remains to be determined.

CONGESTIVE HEART FAILURE

By Evan Loh, M.D.,
and Joseph R. McClellan, M.D.
Philadelphia, Pennsylvania

Congestive heart failure (CHF) afflicts 3 to 4 million patients in the United States, with more than 400,000 new diagnoses made each year. The National Hospital Discharge Survey listed CHF as the primary diagnosis on 643,000 hospital discharge records in 1989, nearly a doubling of hospitalization rates since 1973. As the population ages and the incidence rates of CHF for both men and women double each decade after the age of 45 years, these numbers will only increase.

PATHOPHYSIOLOGY OF CONGESTIVE HEART FAILURE

Heart failure is defined pathophysiologically as the inability of the heart to provide adequate cardiac output to meet the perfusion and oxygenation requirements of the tissues. The signs and symptoms of CHF result mainly from body mechanisms that compensate for reduced cardiac output. The major adaptation expands intravascular volume to restore resting cardiac output. However, increased diastolic volume and pressure are transmitted to the atria and the pulmonary and systemic venous circulation, resulting in pulmonary and systemic edema. In addition, other compensatory mechanisms can impair cardiac effectiveness. For example, catecholamines can augment contractility and heart rate, thereby increasing myocardial oxygen consumption and precipitating myocardial ischemia. By increasing peripheral resistance, catecholamines can also increase left ventricular afterload, further depressing cardiac function. The clinician must understand these mechanisms and the heart's responses to formulate appropriate treatment strategies for patients with heart failure.

Left Ventricular Pressure-Volume Relationships

Length-Tension Basis of Cardiac Contraction

The myocardium is composed of individual striated muscle cells (fibers). Each fiber contains the fundamental unit of muscle contraction, the sarcomere. These sarcomeres contain overlapping thick (myosin) and thin (actin) filaments that interact via cross-bridging, an energy-consuming process requiring adenosine triphosphate (ATP) and calcium, which binds to troponin C and promotes actin-myosin cross-bridging. The force of contraction depends on an optimal "overlap" length of these filaments at the start of contraction; that is, the force of contraction diminishes in direct proportion to any decrease in overlap between actin and myosin filaments. The sensitivity of the force of contraction to calcium is also regulated by fiber length. The relationship between initial muscle length and developed force defines the Frank-Starling relation. Therefore, an increase in the volume (pressure) of the heart results in an increased force of ventricular contraction. This fundamental relationship defines Starling's law of the heart.

Normal Left Ventricular Pressure-Volume Relationship

The normally contracting left ventricle ejects blood under pressure. The relationship between left ventricular pressure generation and ejection can be expressed in a plot that relates developed left ventricular pressure to volume (Fig. 1). At end-diastole (point A in the figure), the fibers have an optimal stretch or length, which is determined by the resting force. This distending force (or preload) is a function of chamber pressure and compliance. After depolarization, the ventricle generates pressure isovolumically until the ventricular pressure exceeds aortic pressure, opening the aortic valve with ejection of blood (point B in the figure). The peak systolic pressure achieved is related to the force generated by the myocardium and is a function of both chamber pressure and volume (point C in the figure). During ejection, the heart must also develop enough force to overcome the resistance and capacitance of the circulatory vasculature, that is, the afterload. At end-systole (point C in the figure), the aortic valve closes, followed by isovolumic relaxation as left ventricular pressure falls. When intraventricular pressure falls below left atrial pressure, the mitral valve opens and left ventricular diastolic filling begins (point D in the figure).

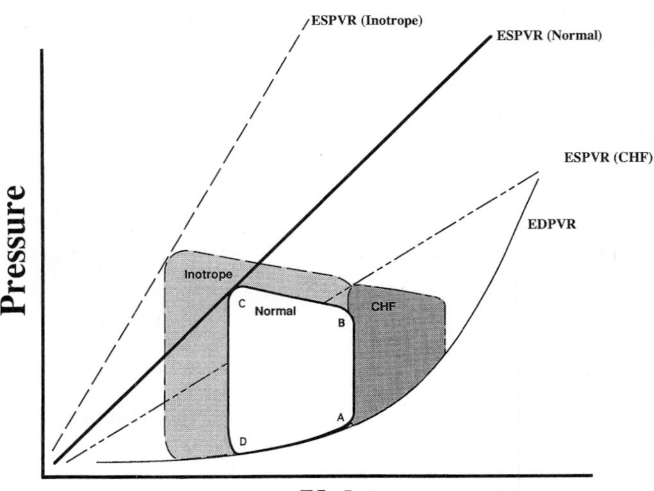

Figure 1. Left ventricular pressure-volume relationships in patients with normal contractility, heart failure, and following treatment with positive inotropic agents. ESPVR = end-systolic pressure-volume relationship. EDPVR = end-diastolic pressure-volume relationship; CHF = congestive heart failure.

The three major determinants of the left ventricular stroke volume and performance are the preload (venous return and end-diastolic volume), myocardial contractility (the force generated at any given end-diastolic volume), and the afterload (aortic impedance and wall stress).

PRELOAD. Frank and Starling established the relationship between ventricular end-diastolic volume (preload) and ventricular performance (stroke volume, cardiac output, and/or stroke work). Subsequent studies have shown that the isovolumetric force at any contractile state is a function of the degree of end-diastolic fiber stretch. As end-diastolic volume and fiber length are increased, there is a linear increase in developed force. The left ventricle normally functions on the ascending limb of this force-length relationship.

CONTRACTILITY. The stroke volume at any given fiber length is a function of the contractile properties of the myocardium. Each myocardial cell can vary the amount of tension during contraction. The tension is related to the amount of calcium bound to regulatory sites on the troponin complex of the myofilaments. The amount of intracellular calcium delivery and removal is determined by the effects of cyclic adenosine monophosphate (cAMP) on calcium channel function. Pharmacologic agents that alter the sensitivity of these elements and/or the delivery of calcium can influence the contractile properties of the heart. For example, the administration of norepinephrine stimulates adrenergic receptors and increases cyclic adenosine monophosphate, which, in turn, increases intracellular calcium and enhances contractility. Accordingly, the ventricle can develop a greater force from any equivalent fiber length (see Fig. 1).

AFTERLOAD. Ventricular performance is also a function of the afterload or impedance to ejection. The afterload on the contracting fibers is the force per unit area that acts in the direction in which these fibers are arranged in the ventricular wall. This constitutes the wall stress and can be estimated by applying LaPlace's law ($\delta = (P \times a)/2h$ where δ = circumferential wall stress, P = intraventricular pressure, a = radius of the chamber, and h = wall thickness). In the heart with normal contractility, stroke volume is only minimally altered by changes in afterload. The failing ventricle, however, is highly afterload-dependent, and small changes may result in large changes in stroke volume. Afterload can also help regulate myocardial contractility. For example, an increase in stroke volume leads to an increase in aortic impedance. The increase in aortic impedance produces a reduction in stroke volume that results in a greater end-systolic and end-diastolic chamber volume. As a consequence of the increase in preload, stroke volume can be restored to original levels.

Left Ventricular Pressure-Volume Relationship in Heart Failure

In the presence of a primary abnormality in myocardial contractility or excessive hemodynamic stresses, the heart relies on three major adaptive mechanisms to maintain cardiac output: (1) the Frank-Starling mechanism, in which an increase in preload from salt and water retention helps sustain cardiac performance; (2) neurohormonal adaptations designed to maintain arterial pressure and vital organ perfusion through activation of the adrenergic nervous system (norepinephrine), the adrenal medulla, and the renin-angiotensin-aldosterone system; and (3) myocyte hypertrophy and increased left ventricular mass with or without chamber dilatation.

The pressure-volume relationships of heart failure are illustrated in Figure 1. With decreased forward stroke volume and contractility, the slope of the relation between initial length and developed force is less, that is, the curve shifts downward and to the right. Renal salt and water retention produces an expansion of blood volume that elevates end-diastolic volume and pressure to restore stroke volume.

Left ventricular hypertrophy (LVH) develops, which unloads individual muscle fibers and allows enhanced contraction. The hypertrophy reduces wall stress (LaPlace relationship), and the dilatation lengthens sarcomeres to optimize overlap of thick and thin myofilaments, which enhances contractility and preserves stroke volume. Further left ventricular remodeling and compensatory dilatation result in increased wall stress, which damages myocytes and induces further fibrosis and abnormalities in diastolic compliance. Each decrement in the developed force-length relation attenuates the ability of the heart's diastolic reserve to restore stroke volume; the increment in force (or shortening) that is possible with chamber dilatation (i.e., greater fiber length) becomes less. As systolic heart failure progresses, there evolves a family of Starling curves that reflects overall reductions in cardiac performance and a fall in the maximal cardiac output generated for any given filling pressure (Fig. 2).

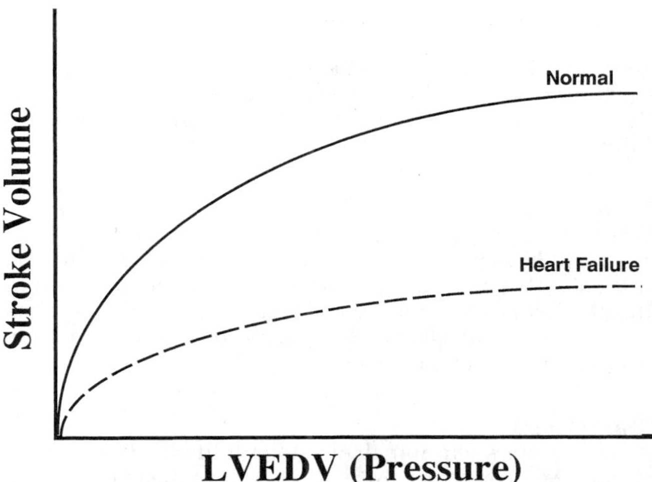

Figure 2. The Starling relationship between left ventricular end-diastolic volume (LVEDV) and stroke volume in the patient with normal contractility and with systolic heart failure.

SYSTOLIC VERSUS DIASTOLIC CONGESTIVE HEART FAILURE

There are two major mechanisms contributing to the pathophysiology of heart failure: (1) *systolic dysfunction,* in which there is impaired cardiac contractility, and (2) *diastolic dysfunction,* in which resting contractility is normal, but decreased compliance of the heart impairs ventricular filling. In both of these abnormalities, there is almost always decreased forward cardiac output either at rest (systolic heart failure) or with exertion (systolic and diastolic heart failure).

Systolic Heart Failure

Systolic heart failure is the classic form in which impaired contractility leads to a reduction in cardiac output. The most common causes of systolic dysfunction include coronary artery disease, hypertension, valvular heart disease, and idiopathic dilated cardiomyopathy. The original Framingham data determined that hypertension was the most common cause of systolic heart failure. However, more effective treatment and earlier detection of hypertension have changed the pattern so that coronary artery disease is now more prevalent, accounting for nearly 50 per cent of cases of systolic dysfunction. Less common causes include drugs (such as the anthracyclines), metabolic disorders (such as hypothyroidism), and infectious myocarditis (as with coxsackievirus B or echovirus infection).

Diastolic Heart Failure

With pure diastolic failure, left ventricular end-systolic volume and stroke volume are preserved. There is, however, an abnormal increase in left ventricular diastolic pressure at any given volume. This indicates a decrease in left ventricular diastolic distensibility (decreased compliance), with a higher diastolic pressure required to achieve the same diastolic volume, impairing ventricular filling. Diastolic dysfunction may occur alone or in association with systolic dysfunction. However, patients presenting with chronic heart failure secondary to ischemia, hypertension, and valvular abnormalities with primary systolic dysfunction almost always have an additional component of diastolic dysfunction that contributes to the elevation in filling pressures.

Etiology

The major causes of primary or pure diastolic dysfunction include ischemia (usually transient), systemic hypertension with LVH, coronary artery disease and myocardial fibrosis, hypertrophic obstructive cardiomyopathy, and restrictive cardiomyopathy. Sixty per cent of these patients have chronic systemic hypertension.

Pathogenesis

Three factors can impair diastolic filling in the absence of valvular heart disease: (1) excessive tachycardia, in which the duration of diastole is diminished; (2) impaired relaxation, which is an active, energy-requiring process; and (3) decreased diastolic compliance, in which hypertrophy or fibrosis impairs passive stretching of the ventricle. The summated effect is a greater increase in left ventricular diastolic pressure for any given left ventricular volume. The major clinical consequence of diastolic dysfunction is an abrupt rise in end-diastolic pressure, leading to pulmonary and/or peripheral congestion with symptoms of shortness of breath and fatigue.

ACUTE MYOCARDIAL ISCHEMIA. This condition produces transient diastolic dysfunction by altering the relaxation of myocardial cells, which may acutely increase left ventricular end-diastolic filling pressure. Patients can present with sudden ("flash") pulmonary edema, as an "anginal equivalent" without a prodrome of progressive volume overload.

LEFT VENTRICULAR HYPERTROPHY. This condition can produce diastolic dysfunction early in the course of hypertension. It is manifested as symptomatic cardiac failure in the absence of systolic functional impairment and is especially common in the elderly.

HYPERTROPHIC OBSTRUCTIVE CARDIOMYOPATHY. This condition may be idiopathic or familial. It is characterized by a nondilated, hypertrophied heart with disproportionate thickening of the interventricular septum in the absence of another cardiac or systemic disease, which causes LVH. Histologic examination reveals cellular disarray with short, thick, fragmented muscle fibers in whorls throughout the myocardium, particularly within the core of the ventricular septum.

RESTRICTIVE CARDIOMYOPATHY. This condition is characterized by decreased ventricular compliance secondary to infiltrative diseases of the myocardium such as amyloidosis, eosinophilic cardiomyopathy, endocardial fibroelastosis, and hemochromatosis. The clinical characteristics include a nondilated, nonhypertrophied heart with stiff ventricular walls that restrict diastolic relaxation and normal filling.

NEUROHORMONAL ADAPTATIONS IN HEART FAILURE

The principal compensatory neurohormonal systems involved in heart failure include (1) the adrenergic nervous system, (2) the renin-angiotensin-aldosterone system, and (3) the arginine-vasopressin system. These compensatory mechanisms include (1) maintenance of blood pressure with vasoconstriction (norepinephrine, endothelin, angiotensin II), (2) restoration of cardiac output by stimulation of myocardial contractility (norepinephrine), and (3) expansion of extracellular fluid volume (renin, vasopressin), which augments stroke volume (Starling's law).

Adrenergic Nervous System

One of the first responses to a decrease in cardiac output (sensed as a fall in blood pressure) is activation of the adrenergic nervous system through the baroreceptors. Regulation of baroreceptors includes both negative and positive feedback limbs. For example, an increase in blood pressure and cardiac contractility leads to withdrawal of sympathetic tone, whereas hypotension, poor cardiac contractility, and left ventricular chamber dilatation result in sympathetic activation. Net sympathetic tone is determined by a combination of inhibitory and stimulator signals. Under normal circumstances, increased left atrial pressure stimulates atrial stretch receptors and atrial natriuretic peptide release and inhibits renal efferent sympathetic nerve activity. Initially, reflex inhibition of adrenergic activity diminishes extracellular fluid volume, restoring normal atrial pressure. In CHF, however, chronic stimulation of these atrial stretch afferent fibers leads to desensitization of atrial and arterial baroreceptors, with blunting of these inhibitory reflexes, as sympathetic stimulation of the heart and vasculature continues unabated. The resultant increase in plasma norepinephrine levels (produced by increased release and decreased uptake of norepinephrine at adrenergic nerve endings) is a barometer of the severity of the syndrome and correlates negatively with survival in patients with CHF. Increased adrenergic activity is characterized by peripheral vasoconstriction, increased venous tone, increased myocardial contractility, and increased heart rate. Progressive augmentation of ventricular contractility is important in the early phases of heart failure, but as the ventricle dilates, contractility eventually reaches a plateau (see Fig. 2). An increased heart rate then becomes the major mechanism by which activation of the sympathetic nervous system helps maintain cardiac output (cardiac output = stroke volume × heart rate). Finally, chronic adrenergic stimulation of the heart can also lead to calcium overload, hypertrophy, increased myocardial oxygen requirements, and contraction band necrosis of the myocardium.

Renin-Angiotensin System

The major physiologic stimuli to renin secretion include renal hypoperfusion (via baroreceptors in the wall of the afferent arteriole and the macula densa of the distal tubule) and increased sympathetic activity (from increased neural activity and circulating catecholamines that stimulate β_1-adrenergic receptors). The afferent arteriole of each glomerulus contains specialized cells, the juxtaglomerular cells, which synthesize the precursor prorenin. This substance is cleaved to renin, which is stored and released from secretory granules. Renin catalyzes the cleavage of a decapeptide, angiotensin I, from renin substrate (angiotensinogen), an α_2-globulin produced in the liver. Angiotensin I is then converted to an octapeptide, angiotensin II, which is an extremely potent vasoconstrictor. This reaction is catalyzed by an enzyme called angiotensin-converting enzyme, which is located in the lung, the luminal membrane of vascular endothelial cells, the glomerulus itself, and other organs.

Although the concentration of angiotensin-converting enzyme is highest in the lung, angiotensin II can be synthesized at various sites, including the kidney, vascular endothelium, adrenal gland, and brain. Measurement of the plasma renin activity or angiotensin II concentration therefore underestimates the tissue activity of this system. Angiotensin-dependent renal vasoconstriction may occur in early or stable CHF with normal levels of renin. Renal vasoconstriction (mediated by both the sympathetic nervous system and angiotensin II) occurs primarily at the efferent arteriole and produces an increase in the filtration fraction. This, in turn, enhances proximal tubular reabsorption of sodium. In addition, there are direct stimulatory effects of the sympathetic nervous system on proximal sodium transport. The enhanced reabsorption of sodium and the increase in venous tone serve to increase the effective central blood volume and preload of the ventricle.

Angiotensin II has three important effects in CHF, which are mediated by binding to specific angiotensin II receptors: (1) production of arteriolar vasoconstriction and increased systemic vascular resistance, (2) stimulation of myocyte hypertrophy, and (3) promotion of renal sodium reabsorption, leading to expansion of the extracellular volume. Sodium reabsorption is enhanced by (1) preferential constriction of the efferent glomerular arteriole, which increases the filtration fraction and proximal tubular sodium reabsorption; (2) stimulation of aldosterone secretion from the adrenal cortex; and (3) direct stimulation of thirst and the secretion of vasopressin.

Vasopressin

Increased concentrations of vasopressin also contribute to the increased systemic vascular resistance in patients with CHF. The mechanisms responsible for increased vasopressin secretion include both baroreceptor stimulation and increased concentrations of angiotensin II. The combination of increased proximal tubular sodium reabsorption from the actions of the sympathetic nervous system and angiotensin II (see previous discussion) and vasopressin-enhanced water reabsorption in the collecting duct can severely decrease free water excretion, producing hyponatremia. The severity of the defect in water excretion tends to parallel the severity of heart failure, and the presence of hyponatremia suggests a poor prognosis in patients with heart failure.

Atrial Natriuretic Peptide

Atrial natriuretic peptide (ANP) is released primarily from the atria in response to volume expansion, which appears to be sensed as an increase in atrial stretch. Ventricular cells may also secrete ANP and brain natriuretic peptide (BNP), an analogous peptide, in response to stretch. These agents have multiple actions that counter the effects of the volume-conserving hormones norepinephrine and angiotensin II. Accordingly, ANP is a potent vasodilator that inhibits the secretion of renin and aldosterone and also has natriuretic properties. Plasma ANP concentrations rise early in the course of CHF. Little is known at present about the role these peptides play in the pathophysiology of CHF, but it is possible that increased concentrations help balance the effects of the other neurohumoral systems by reducing both afterload and preload. High concentrations of ANP also indicate a poor prognosis.

Other Hormone Mediators

Substances produced by the vascular endothelium also contribute to the regulation of vascular tone and peripheral resistance in CHF. Endothelin, an extremely potent vasoconstrictor, is increased in patients with symptomatic heart failure. By contrast, nitric oxide, the endothelium-derived relaxing factor (EDRF), is a potent vasodilator whose effects are mediated by stimulation of guanylate cyclase. Deficient release or production of nitric oxide from the vascular endothelium may contribute to the vasoconstricted state observed in patients with heart failure.

CLINICAL FEATURES

The signs and symptoms of CHF can vary depending on the underlying cause. Impaired cardiac output and fluid retention are responsible for many of the observed clinical abnormalities. The final common pathway is decreased cardiac output that is inadequate to meet peripheral metabolic demands, leading to the retention of salt and water distributed along pressure gradients in multiple tissue beds.

Dyspnea

Dyspnea is the uncomfortable sensation of difficult or labored breathing. The exact pathophysiology of breathlessness remains unclear. Most persons with normal cardiac function and exercise capacity experience the sensation of dyspnea at high workloads. However, patients with CHF have reduced exercise capacity, with a sensation of dyspnea occurring at low workloads. In patients who experience rapidly worsening heart failure with pulmonary edema and interstitial-alveolar fluid accumulation, there is a reduction in overall lung compliance. Patients with chronic heart failure also have a disproportionate increase in dead space ventilation both at rest and during exercise when compared with patients who have a normal exercise capacity. Reduced cardiac output also produces impairment in perfusion of skeletal muscle, especially the respiratory muscle apparatus. In other patients with heart failure, dyspnea occurs because of an increase in the work of breathing. However, this increase in ventilation and work of breathing appears to be independent of left atrial or pulmonary capillary wedge pressure. Some perception of dyspnea may occur because of activation of j or stretch receptors in the lung interstitium, which are activated by increased lung water. In the absence of pulmonary edema, other mechanisms are more likely. In any event, dyspnea increases as the work of breathing increases. As the CHF syndrome worsens, dyspnea also progresses until it is present at rest.

Orthopnea

Orthopnea is the presence of dyspnea when the patient assumes the supine position. When the patient reclines and elevates the legs, venous return is increased. This increase in central blood volume leads to an increase in pulmonary venous pressure followed by extravasation of fluid into the interstitial and alveolar spaces, which initiates the dyspneic sensation. In the recumbent position, the diaphragm is also elevated, resulting in further impairment in diaphragm excursion. Typically, patients with advanced heart failure prefer a position in which the upper torso is elevated to minimize these symptoms. Another frequent symptom is trepopnea, in which patients with heart failure experience symptoms on assuming the lateral decubitus position. Often, patients with heart failure will note that they are uncomfortable lying on the left side.

Paroxysmal Nocturnal Dyspnea

Paroxysmal nocturnal dyspnea is the occurrence of sudden dyspnea that awakens the patient from sleep and is associated with advanced heart failure. On assuming the supine position, there is slow but progressive reabsorption of third space fluid accumulated throughout the day. This reabsorption is redistributed into the lungs, resulting in interstitial and peribronchiolar edema that reduces total lung volume. Bronchospasm and wheezing often accompany this sensation of acute dyspnea. Cough is frequent in patients with advanced heart failure and occurs from an increase in bronchiolar and prebronchial fluid or frank alveolar transudation with excessive mucus production.

A common manifestation of CHF is easy fatigability. A chronic reduction in cardiac output and stroke volume leads to impaired skeletal muscle function. As the heart failure syndrome progresses, skeletal muscle function declines, and patients experience a persistent inability to perform exercise. Improvement in the skeletal muscle dysfunction may occur only with restoration of good cardiac output and continued rehabilitation and aerobic training. Patients with profoundly impaired cardiac output can progress to a full state of cardiac cachexia in which there is obvious generalized muscle wasting and profound weight loss. The cachexia syndrome may also result in part from abnormal gastrointestinal absorption combined with increased metabolic demands produced by excessive work of breathing.

Other symptoms of CHF include nocturia, abdominal discomfort, and mental confusion. When patients sleep or assume the supine position, blood flow requirements for skeletal muscle diminish. Renal blood flow is improved, with enhanced urine production. Abdominal complaints are a common feature of the heart failure syndrome. Congestion of the liver and spleen and entire gastrointestinal (GI) tract may lead to sensations of abdominal fullness, right upper quadrant discomfort, and loss of appetite. As heart failure progresses and cardiac output becomes increasingly impaired, inadequate cerebral perfusion may result in somnolence and/or decreased mentation.

PHYSICAL EXAMINATION

The initial diagnostic approach to patients with heart failure includes a careful and complete physical examination. A great deal of information can be obtained from the general physical examination. However, the focus for recognizing and determining the cause of CHF is the cardiovascular examination.

Vital Signs

Blood Pressure

Blood pressure may be normal, low, or increased in the patient with heart failure. Reduction in cardiac output may lead to intense peripheral vasoconstriction, which may "overcompensate," causing increased systemic blood pressure. The clinician should determine the pulsus paradoxus (the difference in blood pressure during expiration and inspiration). Initially, inflate the cuff pressure above the Korotkoff sounds and then slowly lower the pressure until the sounds are heard only in expiration. Note the pressure and release the cuff further until Korotkoff sounds are heard throughout the respiratory cycle. Note this pressure and calculate the difference between the two pressures. This difference is known as the pulsus paradoxus and is normally less than 10 mm Hg. An increase in the pulsus paradoxus may occur in advanced CHF in which alterations in venous return are important to the subsequent stroke volume. The pulsus paradoxus can also be increased in patients with pericardial tamponade or during marked increases in pleural pressure during inspiration, for example, in severe asthma. The occurrence of a significant pulsus paradoxus in patients with left ventricular dysfunction suggests severe CHF.

Pulse

Tachycardia is a common feature of the CHF syndrome. It is a response to increased sympathetic outflow, thereby compensating for reduced stroke volume. As cardiac output is improved and stroke volume increases, sympathetic tone is withdrawn and the heart rate decreases. Cardiac dysrhythmias, such as atrial fibrillation or ventricular tachycardia, are often seen in patients with severe impairment of ventricular function, and they may first be recognized from palpation of the pulse. Another hallmark finding of CHF is pulsus alternans. This is perceived as a beat-to-beat variation in the intensity of the pulse pressure. Pulsus alternans is associated with severe, advanced CHF. It suggests a marked reduction in ventricular function and is invariably associated with a third heart sound.

Respiratory Rate

The development of CHF and extravasation of fluid into the interstitial and intra-alveolar spaces produces decreased compliance in the lung, with resulting tachypnea. In addition, altered respiratory patterns may occur. In Cheyne-Stokes breathing, for example, progressive increases in the depth and rate of inspiration are followed by apneic periods. The duration of the apneic period increases in proportion to the circulation time and severity of impairment of cardiac output. Cheyne-Stokes respirations are the result of decreased sensitivity of the respiratory center to arterial $Paco_2$. Prolongation of the circulation time from the lung to the brain in patients with severe heart failure also contributes to the pathophysiology of Cheyne-Stokes breathing.

Cardiovascular Examination

The cardiovascular examination is essential in the recognition and diagnosis of CHF. Characterization of the jugular venous pressure and pulse, the arterial pulse, and the left ventricular apical impulse, as well as careful auscultation, can facilitate recognition of cardiovascular causes of the heart failure syndrome.

Jugular Venous Pulse and Pressure

Increased jugular venous pressure and abnormalities in the venous wave form are significant signs of CHF. Sympathetic nervous system activation leads to relative venoconstriction with reduced venous capacity in combination with volume overload. This is reflected and observed as increased venous pressure. The jugular venous pressure is measured as the vertical distance above the sternal angle. In virtually every position, the sternal angle is about 5 cm H_2O above the left atrium, and the height of the column above the sternal angle can be added to produce the estimated venous pressure, which is normally less than 10 cm H_2O. Place the patient in a comfortable position and observe the meniscus, or the top of the venous pressure column. Determine the vertical distance above the sternal angle and estimate venous pressure. Analysis of the wave form may also provide important information regarding the cause of the heart failure syndrome. An increased v wave suggests tricuspid regurgitation and an increased a wave suggests an abnormality in right ventricular compliance or obstruction at the tricuspid valve level. In addition, the analysis of the x and y descent can provide clues to the presence of pericardial disease. Repeated assessments of the venous pressure may be helpful in following the patient's response to diuretics.

Palpation

Palpation of the left ventricular apical impulse can define its location, size, and character as well as the presence or absence of a thrill. The apical impulse is best discerned by visual inspection followed by palpation. The ventricular impulse should be palpated with the patient in the left lateral position. The normal apical impulse usually occupies a discrete area on the chest of approximately 1 cm width in the midclavicular line at the fourth or fifth intercostal space. Cardiac enlargement displaces the apical impulse both laterally and downward, often moving to the sixth or seventh intercostal space in the anterior or midaxillary line. In addition, the duration of the apical impulse is increased, and it tends to be diffuse, occupying a larger area on the precordium. With careful palpation, one can recognize the presence of a presystolic impulse that occurs in patients with an abnormality of left ventricular compliance. This presystolic distention corresponds to the presence of an audible fourth heart sound. Similarly, an early diastolic filling wave can also be appreciated with palpation. This represents an abnormality in compliance during early diastole that corresponds to the presence of a third heart sound on auscultation. A thrill can also be identified in patients with severe mitral regurgitation, and a diastolic rumble can be palpated in patients with mitral stenosis. Also, a palpable thrill may be sensed in the aortic area with aortic stenosis. Precordial palpation should be performed on other portions of the chest wall, including the pulmonic area, where increased pulmonary pressure or pulmonary dilatation can be appreciated. Right ventricular palpation is usually performed in the subxiphoid area. With right ventricular pressure or volume overload, the examiner can appreciate a prominent, sustained right ventricular impulse moving downward. Right ventricular events can also be appreciated by placing the left hand over the spine and the right hand over the anterior sternum. One can then sense the displacement of the right ventricular impulse between the hands.

Auscultation

The hallmark finding of CHF on cardiac auscultation is the presence of a third heart sound or S_3 gallop. A third heart sound is normal in childhood and in young adults but is pathologic in patients older than 40 years of age. It occurs during the rapid passive filling phase of diastole and represents cardiac decompensation in this age group. A third heart sound can also be heard with intense volume overload, as in severe mitral regurgitation. The third heart sound gallop can occur from the right ventricle and is recognized by an increased intensity during inspiration when there is augmentation of venous return to the right side of the heart. The left ventricular third heart sound is often ideally heard directly over the apical impulse in the left lateral position. Frequently, this is the only place it is audible. It is a low-frequency sound best detected by the bell of the stethoscope. Improvement or resolution of the third heart sound often occurs with improved ventricular function or reduction in volume overload.

Careful cardiac auscultation can also enhance the understanding of the pathophysiology of the heart failure syndrome. Typically, the intensity of the first heart sound is decreased. The reduction of compliance in the left ventricle and increased left ventricular and right ventricular end-diastolic pressure produce partial closure of the mitral and tricuspid valves prior to the onset of systole. Hence, the vibrations generated during early systole are diminished and the first heart sound is less prominent. The intensity of the second heart sound may be increased, reflecting increased pulmonary venous and arterial pressures with prolongation of right ventricular electrical-mechanical systole, delayed pulmonic closure, and increased intensity of the pulmonic component. The second heart sound may also be paradoxically split when there is profound impairment of left ventricular function and marked prolongation of left ventricular systole that delays aortic closure until after pulmonic closure.

A fourth heart sound is also common in many conditions that lead to CHF. The fourth heart sound reflects abnormalities in left or right ventricular compliance that produce increased vibrations during atrial contraction. A fourth heart sound is often noted in hypertension, aortic valve disease, and both idiopathic and hypertrophic cardiomyopathy. At increased heart rates, the third and fourth heart sounds may merge in mid-diastole, producing a summation gallop.

Frequently, patients with left ventricular dysfunction of any cause will experience "functional" mitral regurgitation due to left ventricular dilatation and altered geometry of the mitral valve annulus and papillary muscles. However, the mitral regurgitation murmur may decrease in intensity following treatment that reduces left ventricular end-diastolic volume and pressure.

General Examination

Patients with heart failure may have pleural effusions that are usually bilateral. These can be detected by eliciting basilar dullness to percussion, reduced breath sounds, and decreased fremitus in the area of the effusion. Pulmonary crackles due to alveolar fluid and expiratory wheezes due to peribronchial edema may be prominent. Abdominal examination often reveals tender hepatomegaly and hepatojugular reflux, which reflects increased jugular venous pressure following compression of the midabdomen. Hepatojugular reflux is often difficult to detect because cessation of breathing or a Valsalva maneuver may also increase jugular venous pressure. Abdominal distention, shifting dullness, and a palpable fluid wave suggest ascites, which typically reflects severely increased venous pressure most often seen with impaired right ventricular structure or function. Dependent edema indicates extravasation of fluid and sustained venous pressure elevation, primarily in the feet and legs while the patient is standing and in the presacral region in the patient who is chronically bedridden or supine. Chronic venous stasis and peripheral edema often produce superficial skin changes that range from acute inflammation to chronic hyperpigmentation and induration. Finally, clubbing and cyanosis suggest congenital heart disease, whereas tender xanthomas often reflect hyperlipidemia associated with coronary artery disease.

DIAGNOSTIC EVALUATION

Noninvasive Testing

In the evaluation of the patient with CHF, noninvasive diagnostic modalities that often provide complementary information include electrocardiography, exercise testing, echocardiography, nuclear angiocardiography, computed tomography (CT), and magnetic resonance imaging (MRI). Selection of the right test at the right time depends on the outcome sought. For example, the clinician may wish to define the cause of heart failure in patients with early symptoms or assess the functional limitation and/or progress in patients with advanced disease.

Electrocardiography

The electrocardiogram (ECG) may provide important information about the cause of ventricular dysfunction and the severity of impairment. The presence of Q waves and an "infarct" pattern on the ECG does not always reflect coronary artery disease or a myocardial infarction. Pathologic Q waves are seen in patients with idiopathic cardiomyopathy or with secondary cardiomyopathy characterized by infiltration and replacement of myocardium. For example, Q waves have been described in patients with sarcoid, amyloidosis, tumor infiltration, scleroderma, and various neuromuscular diseases. (By contrast, acute myocardial infarction with regional wall motion abnormalities, in the absence of segmental coronary artery stenosis, has been well documented in patients with active myocarditis.) Patients with hypertrophic cardiomyopathy also frequently have Q waves that mimic anterior and inferior infarction ("pseudoinfarction"). Abnormal Q waves may accompany LVH from any cause and may also be seen with chronic airway disease, pulmonary embolism, and spontaneous pneumothorax.

In patients with coronary artery disease and previous myocardial infarction, the ECG may help quantitate the severity of ventricular dysfunction. Patients with a normal R-wave voltage in the precordial leads (V_1 through V) usually have limited impairment in ventricular function; their ejection fractions typically exceed 40 per cent. A normal ECG argues strongly against coronary artery disease as a cause of severe ventricular dysfunction.

Electrocardiographic evidence of LVH may also help determine the cause of ventricular dysfunction. The ECG may show increased electrical voltage (either from right ventricular hypertrophy or from LVH), left axis deviation, prolongation of electrical activation, and left atrial enlargement. In more than half of the patients in whom these electrocardiographic changes develop, chronic hypertension precedes the development of CHF. Valvular and congenital diseases with resultant pressure and volume overload of the left ventricle also produce electrocardiographic evidence of LVH.

Electrocardiographic abnormalities frequently detected in patients with idiopathic cardiomyopathy include low limb lead voltage, precordial criteria for LVH, left bundle branch block, impaired atrioventricular (AV) conduction, ventricular and atrial dysrhythmias, ST-segment and T-wave abnormalities, evidence of chamber enlargement and hypertrophy, abnormal Q waves, and generalized low voltage.

Cardiopulmonary Exercise Testing

In patients with heart failure, cardiopulmonary testing is employed to assess the severity of functional impairment, to follow the response to therapy, and to evaluate patients for heart transplantation. During cardiopulmonary testing, ventilation and inspiratory and expiratory oxygen and carbon dioxide concentrations are measured during a graded exercise test. From this direct measurement, oxygen consumption, carbon dioxide production, and the anaerobic threshold (AT) can be calculated. Oxygen consumption directly reflects cardiac output, whereas the AT is reached when oxygen delivery to the tissues becomes inadequate to maintain aerobic metabolism in skeletal muscle. Normal patients can exercise well beyond the AT, which typically occurs halfway to the maximal exercise capacity. At this point, the rate of carbon dioxide production increases and the respiratory quotient (ratio of carbon dioxide production to oxygen consumption) rises. Maximal exercise occurs when cardiac output can no longer increase in the face of increasing workload, thereby defining the maximal cardiac output obtainable.

The primary abnormality in heart failure is the inability to augment cardiac output. Thus, the maximal uptake of oxygen is impaired. Patients with heart failure often cannot exercise much beyond the AT. This inability to exercise may be exacerbated by skeletal muscle dysfunction and coexistent pulmonary disease. In general, patients with the lowest maximal oxygen uptake have the worst prognosis.

Doppler Echocardiography

The echocardiogram with analysis of Doppler flow patterns and velocities also helps the clinician define the cause of heart failure and the severity of impairment of ventricular function. Echocardiograms are widely used as the initial noninvasive test in patients with heart failure. Abnormalities of valvular function can be identified and quantified with measurement of flow velocities across the valves. Congenital abnormalities also can be accurately characterized. Hypertrophic and infiltrative myopathies produce distinctive echocardiographic tissue patterns. In addition, ventricular volumes and mass can be calculated. Finally, both systolic and diastolic function can be quantitated.

DIASTOLIC DYSFUNCTION. Doppler echocardiography is uniquely valuable in the assessment of diastolic function because it measures blood flow velocity noninvasively. Mitral, tricuspid, pulmonary, and vena caval flow patterns can be used to quantitate alterations in left and right ventricular diastolic function. Many of these changes depend on myocardial loading conditions and are most useful in serial evaluations. The normal Doppler mitral inflow pattern provides information regarding the velocity and timing of left ventricular filling. Several values can be obtained, including the velocities of flow, which represent the driving force across the mitral valve. After the mitral valve opens, there is rapid passive filling of the left ventricle, and the peak velocity of flow—the E point—is reached. Flow then decreases until atrial contraction occurs, with another increase in velocity of flow across the mitral valve—the A point. Doppler studies also measure timing intervals. The first is the isovolumic relaxation time, which measures the interval from the closure of the aortic valve to the opening of the mitral valve. By contrast, after mitral opening and the E point (maximal velocity), there is a linear decrease in velocity of flow, which is extrapolated to the baseline. The time from the E point to the intersection with the baseline is the deceleration time.

Abnormalities in diastolic function can be detected by analysis of these velocities and intervals. Impaired relaxation of the ventricle reduces the E velocity, prolongs the isovolumic relaxation period, and increases the deceleration time. The velocity often exceeds the E velocity. The increased A:E ratio has been widely used as an index of abnormal ventricular compliance. However, this ratio depends on loading conditions. The driving force that creates the peak velocity during rapid passive filling is dependent on left atrial volume. If the preload is low, the resultant E velocity will also be decreased, even if ventricular relaxation is normal. Coexisting abnormalities such as valvular heart disease and cardiac dysrhythmias can also influence these parameters, and they must be integrated into a comprehensive analysis of the echocardiogram.

Venous inflow patterns from the venae cavae, hepatic veins, and pulmonary veins can be analyzed during transthoracic or transesophageal echocardiography. Doppler recordings of pulmonary venous flow patterns demonstrate antegrade flow in systole and diastole, with minimal retrograde flow during atrial contraction (flow reversal). With abnormalities in left ventricular compliance, the flow stops abruptly and atrial reversal increases. As the disease worsens, systolic filling decreases, and most of the antegrade flow occurs during diastole. Similarly, right-sided venous flow patterns can be used to detect abnormalities in right-sided heart filling.

VOLUME AND MASS. Two-dimensional techniques accurately measure ventricular volumes that correlate well with values obtained by angiographic and radionuclide techniques ($r = 0.8$ to 0.9). Among the various two-dimensional methods used to determine ventricular volumes, the best correlations are obtained with biplane analysis and the application of Simpson's rule. In this method, the ventricle is sliced into 1-cm pieces in two views, the apical two-chamber and parasternal short-axis views. From these views, the area for each 1-cm slice is obtained, and the sum of the areas equals the volume. Calculations for both systole and diastole are used to determine the cardiac output and ejection fraction. A modification of these techniques allows for the accurate measurement of left ventricular mass. Again using Simpson's rule with two views, the total left ventricular volume, which includes the walls, and the left ventricular cavity volume are obtained. The difference between these volumes multiplied by the specific gravity of muscle equals the mass. Studies using these techniques have demonstrated excellent correlation with the mass obtained from direct postmortem measurements.

LEFT VENTRICULAR SYSTOLIC FUNCTION. The ejection fraction can be accurately determined from two-dimensional echocardiography. The ejection fraction remains the single most important prognostic indicator for patients with cardiac disease. However, the ejection fraction depends on loading conditions. Other measures derived from the echocardiogram, such as velocity of circumferential fiber shortening, are also useful in defining ventricular contractility. This ejection index represents the difference between the end-diastolic and end-systolic circumference divided by the end-diastolic circumference multiplied by the duration of ejection. This is a more sensitive indicator of intrinsic contractility and is independent of preload but significantly influenced by afterload.

Echocardiography is also an excellent method for evaluation of regional wall motion and thickening. Coronary artery disease produces segmental abnormalities in ventricular function initially characterized by a decrease in endocardial motion and wall thickening. Later thinning of the myocardial segment will be accompanied by endocardial thickening. These changes can be recognized with two-dimensional echocardiography, and the extent of impairment in regional function can be quantitated. Global ventricular dysfunction suggests a myopathy.

RIGHT VENTRICULAR FUNCTION. The right ventricle is a complex geometric structure that has been more difficult to characterize and quantitate than the left ventricle. However, two-dimensional echocardiographic techniques are available to analyze and measure right ventricular function. Similar but more complex models than those used for analysis of left ventricular function have been developed. These models produce accurate measurement of right ventricular volume, ejection fraction, and regional function. As described, Doppler techniques are available for analysis of right ventricular diastolic function. The peak velocity of the tricuspid regurgitation jet on continuous-wave Doppler can also be used to estimate pulmonary artery pressure by using a modification of the Bernoulli equation, which relates flow to changes in intravascular pressure. The formula is $p\ (pressure) = 4V(velocity)^2$. Adding this value to the estimate of venous pressure in the right atrium provides an accurate estimate of pulmonary artery pressure.

Nuclear Cardiology—Radionuclide Angiography and Myocardial Perfusion Imaging

Nuclear techniques, using first-pass analysis or gating of image acquisition to the ECG to acquire summated images throughout the cardiac cycle, are valuable in determining systolic and diastolic volumes. The left and right ventricular volume and ejection fraction measurements are reproducible, accurate, and comparable to data obtained by conventional angiography. Nuclear images summate information from the entire blood pool and hence are more accurate than two-dimensional techniques. Radionuclide angiography can also be performed during exercise to measure the ejection fraction, regional wall motion, and ventricular volumes before and after stress. However, determination of precise chamber size and analysis of valvular function are best obtained by echocardiography.

Diastolic function can be analyzed from the time-activity curves, which reflect the volume in the ventricle as a function of time over the cardiac cycle. Various measurements from the time-activity curve can help characterize diastolic function. These measurements include the peak filling rate, which is the most rapid change in ventricular volume; the time-to-peak filling, which is the interval from time of lowest ventricular volume (end-systole) to the time the peak filling rate occurs; and the first-half filling fraction, or the fraction of total volume that enters the ventricle in the first one half of diastole. Diastolic dysfunction is characterized by a reduced peak filling rate, a delay in the time to peak filling, and a decreased first-half filling fraction.

Myocardial perfusion imaging is typically performed to evaluate coronary artery disease and resultant abnormalities in blood flow or myocardial cellular function. The extent of fixed defects (representing previous myocardial infarction or "scar") correlates with the severity of impairment of ventricular function and ejection fraction. Newer techniques using technetium-based radiopharmaceuticals and tomographic image processing allow gating of the perfusion images to define wall thickening and motion during systole. Regional wall motion and global ventricular function can be analyzed, and correlations of perfusion and function can be made. These techniques will enhance the role of perfusion-function imaging in the evaluation of ventricular function.

Magnetic Resonance Imaging and Computed Tomography

MRI and CT are important tools for evaluating abnormalities in heart structure. With MRI, accurate measurement of right and left ventricular mass and cardiac volumes can be achieved, and ejection fractions can be calculated. MRI produces excellent spatial resolution with precise definition of heart structures, and electrocardiographic gating allows evaluation of cardiac wall motion. Similarly, CT with gating to the ECG permits evaluations of cardiac function. Accurate volume, ejection fraction, and regional wall motion measurements can be obtained, especially in machines (ultrafast) modified for this purpose. However, MRI appears to be undergoing much more rapid development, with wider cardiovascular applications. A newer approach to MRI analysis of wall motion employs an overlying magnetic grid that produces very precise measurement of regional wall motion and systolic thickening. Other uses of magnetic imaging include characterization of myocardial tissue, visualization of the coronary arterial tree, and evaluations of pericardial thickness and motion. With the development of more powerful magnets and enhanced capabilities, this technique holds great promise for precise characterization of the wide range of cardiac abnormalities associated with CHF.

Invasive Testing—Cardiac Catheterization and Angiography

Cardiac catheterization has been an extremely important tool for assessing overall cardiac performance. The initial characterization of ventricular function and concepts of myocardial performance were achieved with information obtained at cardiac catheterization. Often, information obtained during catheterization is critical to the diagnosis and successful management of patients with the heart failure syndrome. This technique is invasive, however, and carries a small but real risk of complications and procedure-related mortality and should be applied judiciously.

Hemodynamic Assessment

Intracardiac pressures, stroke volume, and cardiac output can be precisely determined with right-sided cardiac catheterization. From these data, the cardiac preload (with pressure often used as a surrogate for volume determination) and afterload are calculated, and the relationships between loading conditions and overall cardiac function may be characterized. Hemodynamic techniques can also be employed to define the severity of stenotic and regurgitant valvular lesions, which may contribute to the heart failure syndrome.

Angiography

Coronary angiography allows precise analysis of the presence, extent, and severity of coronary artery disease. With ventriculography, left ventricular systolic and diastolic volumes are measured, and both global and regional ventricular function can be assessed. In addition, the relationships between pressure and volume are important in the analysis of both systolic and diastolic dysfunction, as discussed in the section on the pathophysiology of congestive heart failure.

SUMMARY

An extensive array of diagnostic techniques is available to the physician confronted with a patient with heart failure. In an era characterized by increased concern for cost containment and the judicious application of expensive and potentially harmful technology, how does the clinician choose the tests that are most appropriate for the diagnosis and treatment of a patient with CHF?

The first goal is to carefully identify the important clinical question. For example, will more precise diagnosis alter therapeutic strategy? If a reasonably accurate diagnosis has been secured, is better information required for risk stratification and prognosis? Is careful anatomic delineation of a complex congenital abnormality most important? Prior to the performance of other tests, the physician should ensure that critical information that is often easily obtained during a careful history and physical examination is not overlooked. Frequently, the history, physical examination, and ECG are sufficient for diagnosis and therapy, especially in the patient with severe, long-standing hypertension and insidious development of heart failure. Next, other considerations, including diagnostic accuracy and range of information, relative risk, patient comfort, ease of performance, utility for serial observations, and cost, are factored into the decision regarding the chosen diagnostic approach. Not surprisingly, echocardiography has become the most popular initial noninvasive test performed in many centers. Occasionally, cardiac catheterization with hemodynamic measurements and angiography will suffice for diagnosis and initiation of treatment. Nevertheless, each of the testing modalities discussed has potential important applications as either the initial or adjunctive diagnostic maneuver. A thoughtful and cost-effective strategy should be employed to provide the maximal degree of information required for the safe and effective care of the patient with heart failure.

CARDIAC ARRHYTHMIAS

By Bruce Perlman, M.D.,
and Boaz Avitall, M.D., Ph.D.
Chicago, Illinois

Cardiac arrhythmias, especially tachyarrhythmias, are an important cause of morbidity and mortality and occur in patients with or without overt intrinsic cardiac disease. The signs and symptoms can range from barely noticeable to incapacitating, and the prognosis does not always parallel the morbidity. Patients with relatively benign arrhythmias may have lifestyle-limiting symptoms, and patients with a predisposition to a dangerous arrhythmia may be unaware of their risk. A clinician may be asked to evaluate a known or suspected arrhythmia or to assess the risk of developing an arrhythmia in the future. The treatment of cardiac arrhythmias requires an accurate diagnosis of the arrhythmia and knowledge of its underlying mechanism. Acquiring this information often involves a combination of history, physical examination, surface electrocardiogram (ECG), and other noninvasive tests for evaluating cardiac function and for identifying the presence of an arrhythmogenic substrate (e.g., ischemia). Noninvasive analysis can provide adequate information to guide appropriate treatment. Invasive electrophysiologic studies (EPS) are the "gold standard" for defining the mechanisms of cardiac arrhythmias, estimating prognosis, and guiding the selection of effective therapy. The purpose of this article is to discuss the noninvasive evaluation of arrhythmias and the appropriate reasons for performing invasive studies. A brief discussion of cardiac electrophysiology has been included to help illustrate the underlying mechanisms of arrhythmias.

Figure 1. The phases of a cardiac action potential from a Purkinje fiber.

Phase 0	Rapid depolarization Rapid sodium influx, slow calcium influx (SN and AVN only) Conduction speed
Phase 1	Rapid repolarization - not seen in all cells
Phase 2	Plateau - maintained by slow inward calcium and sodium Duration of action potential
Phase 3	Slow repolarization - potassium efflux Recovery (refractoriness)
Phase 4	Resting State - slow depolarization in pacemaker cells only Automaticity

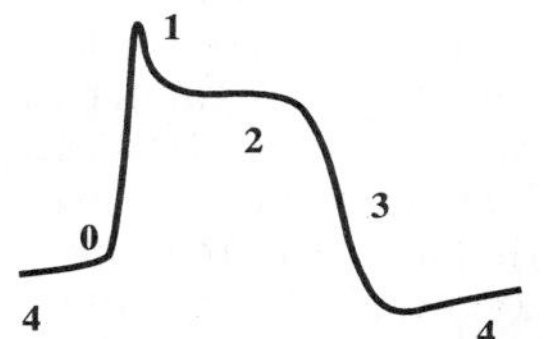

MECHANISMS OF NORMAL RHYTHMS

Understanding the relationship between arrhythmias and the cardiac conduction system is facilitated by knowledge of the anatomy and electrophysiology of its various components.

Simplified Cellular Electrophysiology

One possibly confusing aspect of cellular electrophysiology is that the electrophysiologic characteristics of different regions vary according to function. The sinus node (SN) and atrioventricular node (AVN) are the dominant pacemaker regions, producing spontaneous impulses, or automaticity, and conducting them slowly. The His-Purkinje system conducts impulses rapidly with less automaticity than the SN and AVN. The atrial and ventricular myocardia have a moderate conduction speed with the least automaticity. These functional differences are reflected in the action potentials found in these regions. The phases of myocardial electrical activity include the resting (polarized), active (depolarized), plateau, and recovery (repolarization) phases. The relationships between these states and the phases of the action potential are shown in Figure 1.

Normal Automaticity

A resting myocardial cell is polarized with a large negative charge. This charge corresponds with phase 4 of the intracellular action potential. Phase 0 (rapid depolarization) occurs when the cell's membrane potential reaches the "threshold" voltage. At threshold, in the atrial and ventricular myocardia, the fast sodium channels open. In the AVN and SN, the slow calcium channels open. The sodium and calcium cations stream into the cell, along their concentration gradients, reversing the membrane potential from negative to positive. This change in membrane potential is called depolarization. The voltage reversal induces neighboring cells to depolarize via cell-to-cell connections or by changes in the extracellular voltage.

In cells with inherent automaticity, the membrane potential in phase 4 slowly decreases toward threshold. This tendency means that given enough time, the membrane potential will eventually reach threshold on its own, initiating an action potential. The higher the slope of a cell's phase 4 depolarization, the faster the cell reaches threshold. Therefore, the phase 4 slope is proportional to the automaticity of a cell (and its intrinsic rate). The SN has the highest rate of spontaneous depolarization and is the normal pacemaker of the heart. The AVN has the next highest intrinsic automaticity, followed by the cells in the His-Purkinje system. Normally, atrial and ventricular myocardia have flat phase 4 slopes and little intrinsic automaticity. Automaticity increases with increased sympathetic tone but decreases with parasympathetic tone.

Normal Conduction

Spontaneous depolarization does not occur in most cells, because they are depolarized by neighboring cells before they reach threshold. Normal impulses originate in the SN, which is located near the junction of the superior vena cava and the high right atrium (Fig. 2). The size and exact location of the SN vary, especially in patients with congenital anomalies. This variation poses an increased risk of damage during surgical procedures. The SN spontaneously depolarizes without nervous stimulation, as shown by either pharmacologic or surgical autonomic blockade (intrinsic automaticity). There is no specific pacemaker region, but there are preferential areas for impulse formation that shift location and rate, depending on the autonomic tone. The impulse exits the SN and spreads throughout both atria, entering the AVN near the septal leaflet of the tricuspid valve.

The AVN performs three important functions: (1) it varies the PR interval, with changes in autonomic tone, maximizing AV synchrony; (2) it controls the maximal ventricular response to supraventricular arrhythmias (e.g., atrial fibrillation) by loss of 1:1 AV conduction at excessive heart rates (HRs); and (3) it is a subsidiary pacemaker in the event of SN failure. The bundle of His (HIS) is the direct continuation of the AVN. It enters the membranous ventricular septum, bifurcating into the left and right bundle

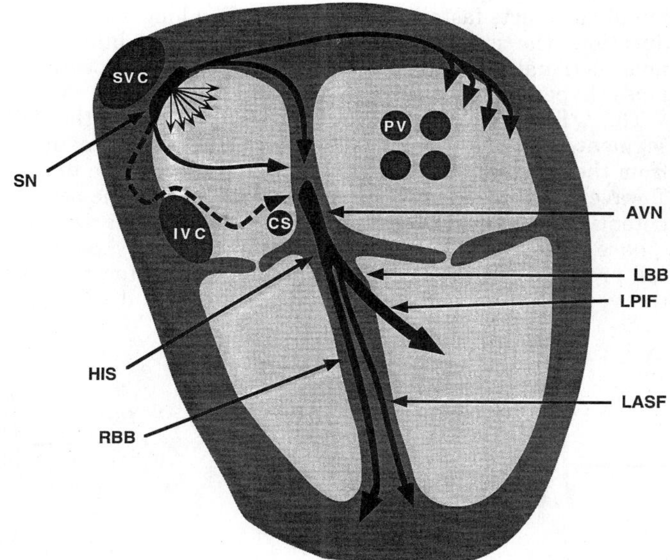

Figure 2. The cardiac conduction system. SN = sinus node; AVN = atrioventricular node; RBB = right bundle branch; LBB = left bundle branch; LASF = left anterosuperior fascicle; LPIF = left posteroinferior fascicle; SVC = superior vena cava; IVC = inferior vena cava; PV = pulmonary veins; CS = coronary sinus; HIS = bundle of His.

branches (LBB and RBB). The left bundle divides into a broad band called the left posterior inferior fascicle and also into a group of fibers collectively called the left anterior superior fascicle. The right and left bundles' fascicles terminate in a network of Purkinje fibers that conduct impulses directly to the myocardium.

Both the His-Purkinje system and the AVN may conduct in both an antegrade (atrium-to-ventricle) and a retrograde (ventricle-to-atrium) direction. Antegrade conduction is usually stronger. Retrograde conduction is absent in 20 per cent of people and is seen most often with premature ventricular beats or ventricular pacing.

Relationship of the Surface ECG to Intracardiac Electrograms

The surface ECG reflects global cardiac electrical activity. Its major components are the PR and QT intervals, the P wave, the QRS complex, and the PR and JT (ST) segments. The P wave duration estimates the time for the depolarization wave from the SN to reach all atrial tissue. This wave increases with atrial disease, especially enlargement of the left atrium. Because the terminal portion of the P wave normally reflects left atrial depolarization, the P wave is not always prolonged by enlargement of the right atrium. Atrial repolarization usually falls within the QRS and is not normally seen. The PR interval consists of three separate conduction intervals (Fig. 3): the time for depolarization to spread (1) from the SN through the right atrium to the AVN (P-A); (2) from the AVN to the bundle of His (A-H); and (3) from the proximal bundle of His to the ventricular tissue (H-V). The QRS duration reflects the time it takes to depolarize all ventricular tissue. The QRS is normally narrow because conduction to both the right and the left ventricles occurs simultaneously through the Purkinje networks. The Purkinje fibers conduct electrical impulses much faster than ventricular cell-to-cell conduction. The QRS is prolonged (widened) by anything that disrupts the synchronous activation of both ventricles or slows down cell-to-cell conduction. A bundle branch block (BBB) morphology seen on a surface ECG implies that one bundle conducts faster than the other. The longer the QRS duration, the greater the likelihood that the bundle is nonfunctional, not just impaired. Increased myocardial mass (hypertrophy) also widens the QRS complex.

The QT interval consists of the QRS duration, the JT segment, and the T wave. The JT segment is measured from the junction of the ST segment and the S wave to the T wave and correlates with the plateau phase of the action potential. The T wave represents ventricular repolarization (phase 3) and reflects the ventricular refractory periods. QT prolongation implies a dispersion of refractoriness in the ventricles. This means that toward the end of the T wave, some ventricular cells have regained the ability to conduct, whereas others are still refractory. This situation predisposes to arrhythmias involving re-entry or triggered activity. The QT interval has an inverse relationship to the HR. Slow HRs increase the QT, whereas fast HRs shorten the QT interval. This is why formulas were developed to correct the QT interval for changes in the HR. Women have a longer QT interval, corrected for rate, and an increased risk of related arrhythmias.

ARRHYTHMIA MECHANISMS

What Is an Arrhythmia?

The conduction of electrical impulses through the heart is not analogous to an electrical circuit, in which current flows in a continuous loop. A normal impulse originates from the SN, reaches the AVN, and then depolarizes the ventricular myocardium. There is no circular motion involved. The wave terminates when the last area of myocardium has been depolarized. The myocardium then repolarizes, awaiting the next spontaneous discharge from the SN. An arrhythmia is said to exist when the discharge rate of the SN is abnormally fast or slow, the conduction of an impulse from the SN to the ventricle is impaired, or the rhythm originates from a location or mechanism other than normal SN automaticity. Bradyarrhythmias involve either the lack of normal impulse formation (depressed automaticity) or impaired impulse conduction (block). Re-entry accounts for 70 to 75 per cent of all tachyarrhythmias. Less common are automaticity and triggered activity, accounting for 25 and less than 2 per cent, respectively.

Re-entry

Normally, a depolarization wave spreads throughout the myocardium and ceases only when all excitable tissue has been depolarized. In sustained re-entry, the wave never encounters refractory tissue and continues propagating in a circular fashion. Most episodes of re-entry are initiated and terminated by premature depolarizations (Figs. 4 and 5*A*). Occasionally, there is a mild warm-up phenomenon during the first few beats. Re-entrant supraventricular tachycardia (SVT) is usually very regular, while ventricular tachycardia (VT) may be slightly irregular. Termination is abrupt, without significant slowing down. There are several types of re-entry, but they all follow this general scheme.

Re-entrant circuits may be static or dynamic. Static re-entry involves either prior myocardial damage (e.g., scar from myocardial infarction) or a congenital re-entrant loop (e.g., Wolff-Parkinson-White syndrome). Dynamic re-entry involves the formation or modification of re-entrant circuits

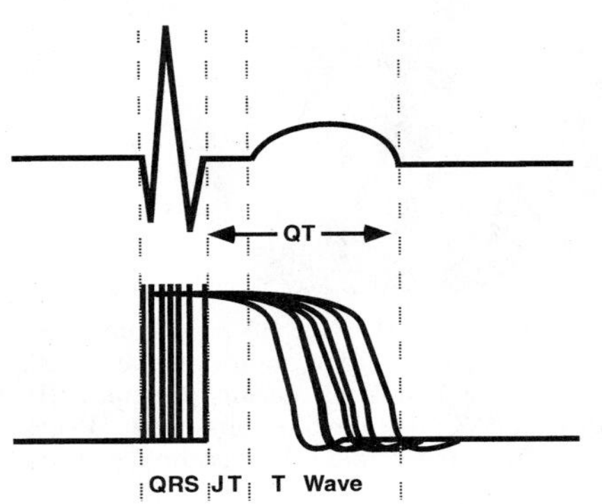

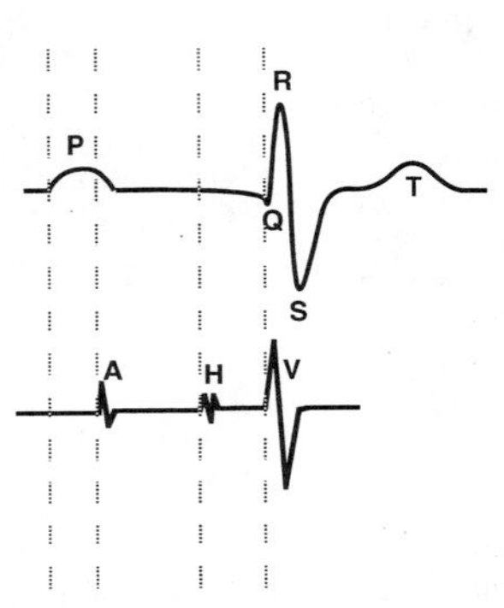

Figure 3. The relationship of the surface ECG to ventricular action potentials *(left)* and atrioventricular conduction intervals *(right)*.

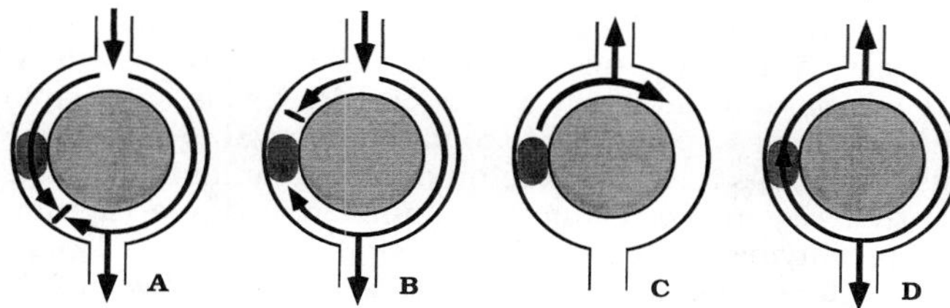

Figure 4. Re-entry requires the presence of two depolarization pathways. Under normal conditions an impulse conducts down both pathways and terminates when they collide *(A)*. A premature depolarization blocks in one pathway *(B)*. It conducts down the other pathway and up the pathway that had initially blocked *(C)*. It continues as a circus movement re-entrant tachycardia *(D)*.

due to acute ischemia, autonomic imbalance, or electrolyte abnormalities. A re-entrant arrhythmia is named for the location of the circuit. Occasionally, it is confined to one area, as in intra-atrial re-entry (e.g., atrial flutter); more commonly it spans several tissues, as in AV re-entry.

Automaticity

An automatic cell has an inherent rate of spontaneous depolarization at which it will fire unless it is suppressed by a faster rhythm. Automatic tachycardias are caused by cells depolarizing faster than their normal intrinsic rates. Abnormal automaticity involves cells that do not normally have significant automaticity (atrial, ventricular). Enhanced normal automaticity occurs in cells with baseline automaticity (AVN).

The most frequent automatic arrhythmias are simple premature atrial or ventricular depolarizations. Sustained automatic rhythms usually begin at a certain rate and slowly increase to the maximal rate (warm-up phenomenon). The HR during the tachycardia tends to fluctuate mildly (see Fig. 5*B*). Termination is usually spontaneous, often with prodromal slowing (cool-down).

All cells may have increased automaticity under pathologic conditions, such as marked bradycardia, hypokalemia, myocardial injury, and high sympathetic tone. Drugs that increase automaticity include catecholamines, theophylline, digoxin, amrinone, and all agents that either decrease parasympathetic or increase sympathetic tone.

Suppression of spontaneous depolarization causes a cell to fire below its intrinsic rate, leading to an automatic bradycardia. Normal automaticity may be depressed by intrinsic disease, electrolyte or metabolic abnormalities (especially severe hyperkalemia), autonomic influence (vagal stimulation), or drugs (e.g., beta-blockers, calcium antagonists).

Triggered Activity

Triggered activity is an uncommon arrhythmia mechanism that acts like a cross between automaticity and re-entry. Two types of triggered activity have been well documented in cellular (in vitro) and animal (in vivo) experiments. Neither has been conclusively shown to be a cause of sustained human arrhythmias. The clinical course of and therapy for arrhythmias differ significantly between the two types of afterdepolarizations.

Most triggered arrhythmias involve early afterdepolarizations. This type of afterdepolarization is seen in conditions that prolong the QT interval, such as electrolyte abnormalities (hypokalemia, hypomagnesemia), ischemia, and bradycardia, and with the use of antiarrhythmics. The most common arrhythmia believed to be caused by early afterdepolarizations is a type of polymorphic ventricular tachycardia called torsade de pointes (see Fig. 5*C* and *D*).

Arrhythmias due to delayed afterdepolarizations are very uncommon. They may be involved in some of the arrhythmias related to digoxin intoxication (bidirectional VT) or extremely high catecholamine states. Digitalis-related arrhythmias are more common in patients with concurrent hypokalemia or hypercalcemia. Delayed afterdepolarizations are increased by tachycardia—not bradycardia.

Conduction Block

The recovery time that a cell requires after depolarization, before it is able to conduct another impulse, is called its refractory period. Impulses that fall within the refractory period will be "blocked" and will not cause the cell to depolarize. Normal (physiologic) block occurs when a tissue is depolarized faster than its usual maximal rate. In atrial flutter, the atrial rate is approximately 300 BPM. Even in an adolescent, the AVN rarely conducts faster than 200 BPM. The first flutter wave will conduct, but the second will fall within the refractory period and block. By the time the third depolarization wave reaches the AVN, it has recovered and will conduct. This leads to an alternating pattern of conduction and block called 2:1 atrioventricular (AV) conduction. This type of block occurs in all myocardial tissues. The atria and ventricles can conduct at the highest HR, followed by the His-Purkinje system. The conduction

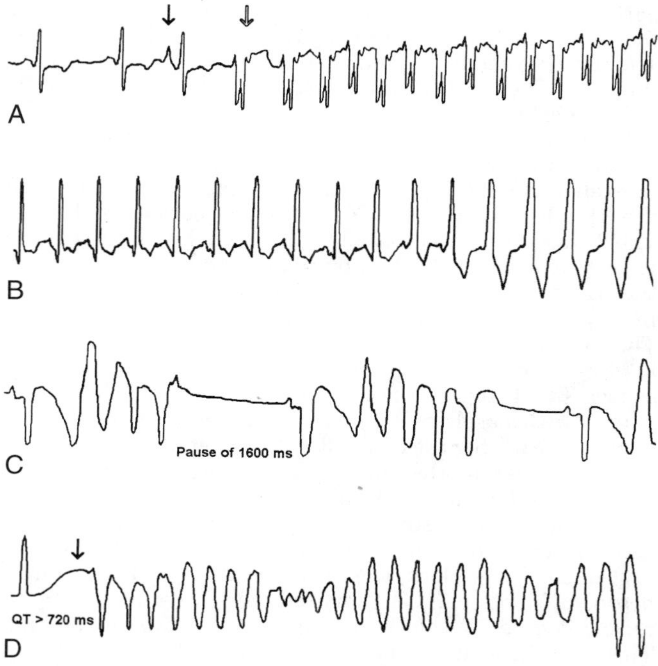

Figure 5. Mechanisms of tachycardia. *A*, The onset of AVN re-entry with an atrial premature depolarization *(solid arrow)*. Retrograde P waves are seen in the ST segment *(open arrow)*. *B*, An example of isorhythmic AV dissociation between sinus tachycardia and an accelerated idioventricular rhythm (due to abnormal automaticity). *C* and *D*, Examples of triggered activity due to early afterdepolarizations. The bursts of tachycardia are pause dependent, occur in the middle of giant T waves, and are polymorphic. The pause after each run induces another burst of activity. *D*, From a patient with tachy-brady syndrome and atrial fibrillation who was started on quinidine as an outpatient. More than 100 episodes occurred over 24 hours, predominantly during periods of bradycardia. The longest episode was more than 4 minutes, with HRs ranging from 130 to 260 BPM.

velocity of waves traveling through these tissues remains stable until just below the rate at which block occurs.

The SN and AVN have conduction characteristics different from those of the rest of the myocardium. They block at lower heart rates than do the atria, ventricles, or His-Purkinje cells. These differences are more clinically apparent in AVN function, through visible changes in the PR interval. Changes in SN function have a more subtle effect on the surface ECG.

The PR interval changes with autonomic tone. It decreases with sympathetic stimulation and increases with parasympathetic. At any level of autonomic tone, a premature atrial complex (PAC) will reach the AVN earlier than expected. The AVN will not be ready to conduct normally and will either block completely, or conduct slower than usual, with a prolonged PR interval. This is called decremental conduction and occurs in both the SN and the AVN but is not normally seen in other cardiac tissues. The amount of time between the onset of a QRS complex and a PAC is called the RP interval. It estimates the amount of time the AVN has had to recover from a conducted beat before the arrival of the PAC. The shorter the RP interval, the sooner the AVN encounters that P wave, and the longer the induced conduction delay and PR interval of the PAC. If the RP is shorter than the AVN refractory period, the beat will block altogether.

Wenckebach periodicity is a manifestation of the PR-RP relationship. This periodicity may occur in the SN but is more common in the AVN. In AV nodal Wenckebach periodicity, the P waves occur in a regular fashion, but there is progressive PR prolongation and, eventually, block. The first P wave in a group conducts with the shortest PR interval. The next P wave has an RP interval that is much shorter than that of the prior P wave, causing PR prolongation. The third P wave, coming at its usual time, will necessarily have an even shorter RP interval, leading to even more PR prolongation. This cycle continues until the RP falls within the AVN's refractory period and blocks. The dropped beat leads to a long RP, and the first PR in the next cycle shortens back to baseline. The largest change in the RP interval occurs with the second conducted P wave in a cycle, leading to the largest change in the PR interval. The successive RP intervals shorten less and less, resulting in only marginal lengthening of the PR interval. This causes the R-to-R intervals in a cycle to shorten. In a person with baseline PR prolongation, a reverse RP phenomenon with paradoxical PR shortening after a PAC can occur, because of the increased RP interval following a premature atrial or ventricular complex.

First-degree (1°) sinoatrial and AVN block involve an increase in conduction time, rather than actual block. In first-degree AVN block, the PR interval is prolonged. First-degree SN block can be diagnosed only by detailed EPS. In second-degree (2°) block, single impulses fail to conduct. This failure results in conduction ratios of 2:1, 3:2, 4:3, and so forth. Second-degree block has two subtypes, which differ in etiology and mechanism. Type I second-degree block (Mobitz I) manifests Wenckebach periodicity with a progressive increase in conduction time. Type II (Mobitz II) has fixed conduction intervals. Higher levels of block (e.g., 3:1, 5:2) are called advanced or high-grade block. Total lack of conduction is called third-degree (3°) or complete block.

CARDIAC RHYTHMS

Escape Versus Premature Depolarization

During a regular rhythm, a ventricular or atrial depolarization is considered to be early when it comes before the next native complex was expected. When such depolarization comes after the next complex was expected, or when the rate is unusually slow (40 to 50 BPM), it is an escape beat. For an escape beat, the coupling interval to the previous complex is related to the inherent rate of automaticity for that region. For example, a junctional escape rhythm has an intrinsic rate of 40 to 55 BPM. The expected coupling interval for a junctional escape beat is between 1.1 and 1.5 seconds.

Ectopy

Ectopy is the general term for any depolarization that does not stem from normal SN automaticity. Several terms are used to describe premature ectopy, including premature beat or contraction, and premature depolarization or complex. The majority of premature depolarizations involve abnormal automaticity and are categorized by their site of origin, frequency, and morphology. Nearly all premature depolarizations are atrial (PAC), ventricular (PVC), or junctional (PJC).

Isolated monomorphic complexes are the most commonly seen form. Noncomplex ectopy consists of isolated monomorphic beats or runs lasting two to three beats. Two consecutive premature depolarizations is called a couplet, and three a triplet. Bigeminy describes a rhythm in which normal beats alternate with single premature beats. Figure 6*A* shows examples of isolated monomorphic PVCs, Figure 6*C* and *D* demonstrates ventricular couplets, and Figure 6*E* illustrates ventricular bigeminy. The specific terms describing bigeminy in which an isolated premature beat occurs after two or three normal impulses are trigeminy and quadrigeminy. Bigeminy during sinus rhythm, with atrial or junctional premature depolarizations, may mimic SN or AVN conduction abnormalities. Ectopy is considered complex when an episode lasts for more than three beats, or when the complexes have multiple morphologies (multifocal). Nonsustained episodes are longer than four beats but less than sustained episodes, and are without hemodynamic compromise. The definition of sustained tachycardia depends on its location. Supraventricular tachycardia (SVT) must last for at least 2 minutes to be considered sustained, whereas VT needs to last only 30 seconds. Regardless of duration, both are considered to be sustained when they are hemodynamically unstable. Hemodynamic instability is defined as syncope, chest pain, severe near-syncope, congestive heart failure, or overt decrease in cerebral or renal perfusion.

The Regularity of an Arrhythmia

An arrhythmia may be completely regular, or it may be irregular. Irregular rhythms may be regularly irregular, in which grouped beating occurs, as in ventricular bigeminy, or with Wenckebach periodicity. They may also be irregularly irregular, as in atrial fibrillation or multifocal atrial tachycardia.

Concealed Conduction

A premature stimulus may partially conduct into the AVN or His-Purkinje system and then block. Concealed conduction, the presence of altered AV conduction that occurs after a blocked beat, is caused by induction of refractoriness in the AV conduction system by the premature stimulus. This alteration in conduction may present as AV block (AVB), prolonged conduction time, or BBB, depending on the timing of the premature depolarization and the location of the initial block. Two episodes of retrograde

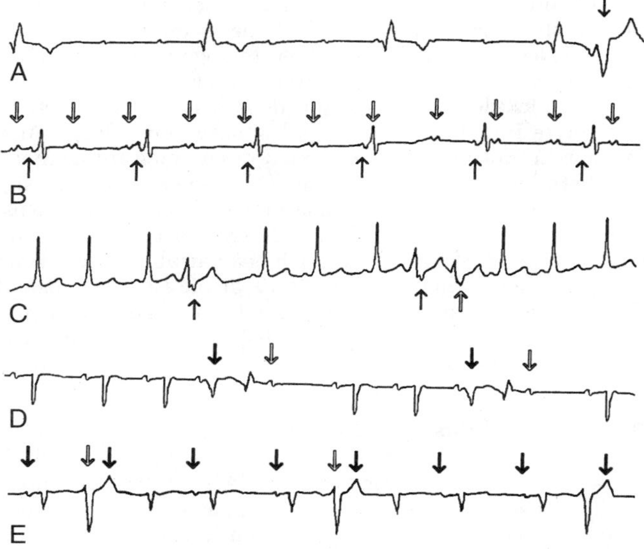

Figure 6. AV block (AVB) and pseudo-AVB. *A,* Complete AVB with a ventricular escape rhythm and one PVC *(arrow). B,* An example of pseudo-AVB in a patient after an orthotopic cardiac transplant. The rhythm of the transplanted heart is sinus bradycardia at 50 BPM *(solid arrows).* The other P waves are in sinus rhythm at 90 BPM from his retained right atrium *(open arrows). C,* PVCs with manifest retrograde conduction and inverted P waves at end of S wave *(solid arrows).* The second PVC in the couplet does not conduct, and no P wave is seen *(open arrow).* That is why the subsequent sinus P wave occurs so closely to the ventricular couplet. *D* and *E,* Concealed retrograde conduction. In strip D, the second PVC in each couplet *(solid arrow)* conducts retrograde into the AVN, but not all the way to the atrium. The P wave seen after the PVC *(open arrow)* does not conduct because of this "concealed" conduction. *E,* Sinus rhythm *(solid arrows)* with ventricular bigeminy (quadrigeminy). Concealed retrograde conduction of the PVC *(open arrows)* causes the PR of the next sinus beat to be markedly prolonged. The PR interval shortenings seen after the episodes of concealed conduction in strips C and D are examples of the PR-RP phenomenon.

concealed conduction are depicted in Figure 6*D* and *E.* Some kinds of concealed conduction can be documented only with EPS.

Proarrhythmia

Antiarrhythmic drugs affect automaticity, conductivity, and refractoriness in both normal and abnormal tissues. Paradoxical worsening of an established arrhythmia or presentation of a new arrhythmia during antiarrhythmic therapy is called proarrhythmia. Drug-induced changes in conduction and/or refractoriness may result in new reentrant arrhythmias or may make the previous arrhythmia slower but more incessant. The dispersion of refractoriness with an antiarrhythmic drug (especially class Ia) may predispose the patient to torsade de pointes (see Fig 5*D*) or other unstable polymorphic rhythms. The risk of proarrhythmia and the severity of its effects increase as left ventricular function worsens. This is unfortunate, because the incidence of and mortality from VT also increase with heart failure. Thus, the person who may derive the largest benefit from an antiarrhythmic agent also has the greatest risk of proarrhythmia. Paradoxical acceleration of SVT may occur during therapy with class I (e.g., quinidine, flecainide) or class III (amiodarone, sotalol) antiarrhythmics. These agents affect intra-atrial conduction and may slow the atrial rate of the tachycardia. For example, a 2:1 atrial flutter with an atrial rate of 300 BPM often conducts at 150 BPM (2:1 AVB). An antiarrhythmic (e.g., quinidine) can slow the atrial rate to 200 BPM. This slower tachycardia may conduct 1:1, with an apparent increase in the ventricular response to the flutter from 150 to 200 BPM. Bradycardic events, including drug-induced SN dysfunction or AVB, are also types of proarrhythmia.

Autonomic Tone

The heart has direct parasympathetic (vagus nerve) and sympathetic (thoracic ganglia) innervation. Stimulation of one system inhibits the other. When both systems are maximally stimulated, the parasympathetic usually predominates. The heart is also affected by circulating catecholamines (epinephrine) from the adrenal gland. The effects of sympathetic stimulation or sympathomimetic agents include enhanced automaticity of all tissues, PR interval shortening, and increased maximal rate of AVN conduction. Parasympathetic stimulation or the use of cholinergic drugs (e.g., edrophonium) leads to decreased automaticity, decreased maximal AVN conduction rate, and increased PR interval. Sympathetic stimulation tends to diminish sinoatrial and AV nodal blocks, with parasympathetic stimulation worsening them. Circadian variation in the risk of cardiac events (e.g., myocardial infarction, sudden death) corresponds to the usual diurnal peaks of sympathetic activity. The proarrhythmic effects of exercise appear to be mediated by increases in sympathetic tone.

Parasystole

Parasystole describes an uncommon and usually benign arrhythmia caused by the presence of an automatic focus outside of the SN that is not suppressed by the faster sinus rate. The focus continues to fire at its intrinsic rate but rarely captures the myocardium because it usually fires when the myocardium is refractory. The diagnosis requires that one analyze the intervals between premature depolarizations to see whether the rate at which they occur is a multiple of a number that turns out to be the cycle length of the parasystolic focus. For example, premature beats that occur with intervals of 1400, 2100, and 3500 msec imply the presence of a parasystolic focus with an intrinsic cycle length of 700 msec. Most parasystole is ventricular or atrial. Sinus node parasystole has been described, but it cannot be distinguished from atrial parasystole by surface electrocardiography alone.

SINUS ARRHYTHMIAS

Common Sinus Rhythms

A "normal" sinus rhythm is regular, with a rate between 60 and 100 BPM. Sinus bradycardia is a regular sinus rhythm between 40 and 59 BPM. Rates below 40 BPM are uncommon in the absence of medications or SN dysfunction. People with high vagal tone (especially athletes) have a tendency toward sinus bradycardia (40 to 55 BPM). Sinus tachycardia has a range from 101 to 180 BPM. The maximal predicted heart rate (MPHR) is related to age and approximated by the formula: MPHR = 220 − age. The MPHR for men tends to be 5 to 10 BPM higher than that for women. Sinus tachycardia without evidence of increased sympathetic tone is deemed inappropriate. It is a frequent reason for consultation, especially after surgery. Most episodes are secondary to occult infection, discomfort, anemia, medications, endocrine disorders (especially hy-

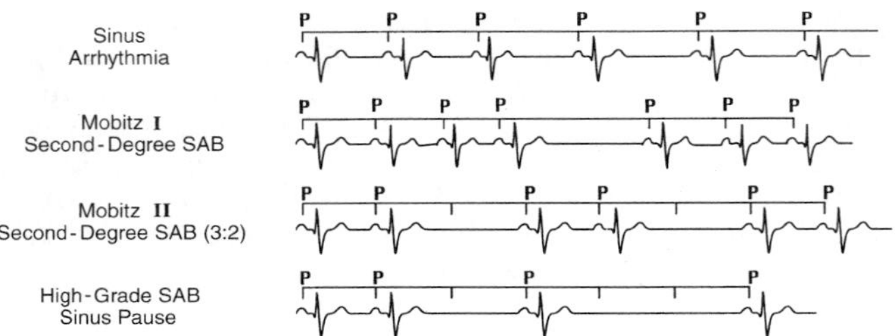

Figure 7. Examples of sinoatrial block (SAB) and sinus arrhythmia.

perthyroidism), or other conditions that elevate sympathetic tone. The uncommon causes include an atrial tachycardia (AT) with a P wave morphology similar to sinus, 2:1 atrial flutter with one P wave hidden in the QRS or T wave, and sinoatrial re-entrant tachycardia (SART).

Sinus Arrhythmia

Phasic shortening and lengthening of the P-P interval (with the longest interval being greater than the shortest by at least 0.16 second) is called sinus arrhythmia (Fig. 7). Occasionally, the change from short to long is abrupt, mimicking Wenckebach block in the SN. The P wave morphology, following the longer intervals, may change from normal and round to tall and peaked. The variant seen in younger people without intrinsic heart disease is caused by normal respiratory changes in vagal tone. The nonrespiratory variant is more common in older patients with intrinsic heart disease and is often due to increased sympathetic tone.

Premature depolarizations arising from within the SN have been described but are impossible to distinguish with ECG from PACs arising near the SN. The diagnosis of SART requires documentation of the rapid onset and end of the tachycardia, which is usually induced with a single premature atrial depolarization. It may terminate spontaneously, with another premature complex, or with vagal maneuvers (e.g., carotid massage).

Sick Sinus Syndrome

The terms sick sinus syndrome and bradycardia-tachycardia (tachy-brady) syndrome are often used interchangeably. Technically, sick sinus syndrome is the combination of sinoatrial arrest or block (SAB), chronotropic incompetence, and the bradycardia-tachycardia syndrome. Sick sinus syndrome often coexists with significant AVN conduction abnormalities. The bradycardia-tachycardia syndrome is characterized by an inappropriately low baseline sinus rate, episodic bradycardia, and tachycardia. The episodes of bradycardia may be associated with SN or AVN conduction abnormalities. The most commonly seen tachycardias are atrial fibrillation (AF) and AT. Ventricular tachycardia may occur if the bradycardia is severe (see Fig. 5*C* and *D*). Tachycardia is facilitated by the periods of bradycardia and may be suppressed by permanent atrial pacing. Sick sinus syndrome is a progressive (often familial) disorder that usually requires placement of a permanent pacemaker.

Sinus Node Dysfunction

Sinus node dysfunction is usually extrinsic—not intrinsic. Intrinsic dysfunction implies impaired impulse formation due to aging, medications, or trauma. With extrinsic SN dysfunction, impulse formation is normal, but conduction to the surrounding atrial tissue is impaired. This is called SN exit block (SAB). It is analogous to AVN block and uses the same grading system (see Fig. 7). The causes of SAB include pharmacologic depression of conduction, electrolyte imbalance, and vagal suppression. Drugs such as digoxin, antiarrhythmics, calcium channel antagonists, and beta-blockers rarely cause SAB, unless there is significant underlying SN disease or the dosages are excessive. Acute ischemic intrinsic SN dysfunction is uncommon. Occlusion of the SN artery has a variable effect owing to anastomotic blood flow or dual blood supply. Most of the episodes of sinus bradycardia seen during an acute myocardial infarction reflect vagal hyperactivity—not the direct effects of ischemia.

Sinus Pauses, Block, and Arrest

Sinus block (SAB) manifests as missing (dropped) P waves (see Fig. 7). Second-degree SAB implies the intermittent absence of isolated SN impulses—not consecutive. Mobitz I second-degree SAB (SA Wenckebach block) is uncommon and difficult to prove. There is a progressive shortening of P-P intervals before each dropped P wave. Mobitz I SAB may be difficult to differentiate from sinus arrhythmia, which can also show periodic loss of P waves but usually shows lengthening (as opposed to shortening) of the P-P interval before the longest P-P interval. Sinus node Wenckebach block is sometimes seen in young people with heightened vagal tone. Digoxin intoxication may cause a combination of SA and AVN Wenckebach block. Mobitz II second-degree SAB is more common and is easier to diagnose. It is characterized by the loss of P waves without a change in the P-P intervals. The block is usually 2:1 and mimics sinus bradycardia. Third-degree SAB is difficult to differentiate from primary SN failure, since both show reduction in spontaneous P waves, long pauses, and occasionally no SN activity at all. Benign sinus pauses are common during sleep because of heightened vagal tone and rarely require therapy unless they are excessively long or are associated with symptoms. Long sinus pauses are often seen during apneic episodes (especially nocturnal) in severe sleep apnea. Pseudo-SAB is caused by blocked PACs, which are not seen because they lie in the T wave or ST segment (concealed conduction). These PACs may reset the SN or cause exit block that results in pauses even though SN function is normal.

Chronotropic incompetence is defined as an impaired ability of the SN to appropriately increase the HR with a rise in sympathetic tone. In AF, chronotropic incompetence may present as an inability to raise the HR by enhancing AVN conduction. Secondary chronotropic incompetence may be caused by medications.

ATRIAL ARRHYTHMIAS

Atrial Escape

The inherent automaticity of atrial myocardium is less than that of the SN and AVN. The intrinsic rate is usually 30 to 45 BPM. The P wave morphology varies, depending on the location of the ectopic focus and the spread of the impulse through the atria. The PR interval during an atrial escape rhythm depends on the proximity of the focus to the AVN and the AVN conduction time. A 2:1 AVB with a hidden P wave may mimic an atrial escape rhythm.

Between the coronary sinus and the crista terminalis is a region that may contain cells histologically similar to

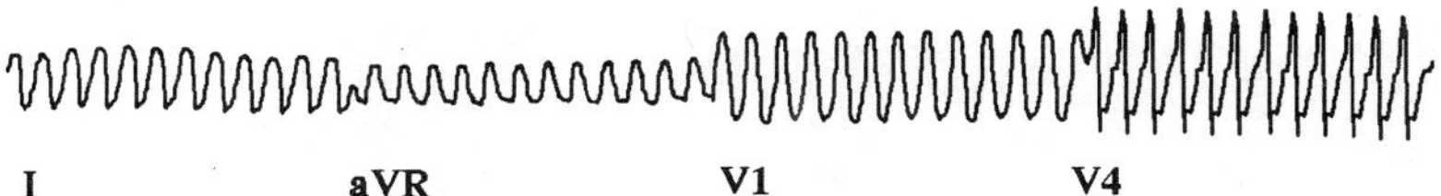

Figure 8. WPW. Atrial flutter conducting 1:1 over an AP at 300 BPM. Compare this with the VT in Figure 14. This tachycardia satisfies morphologic criteria for VT.

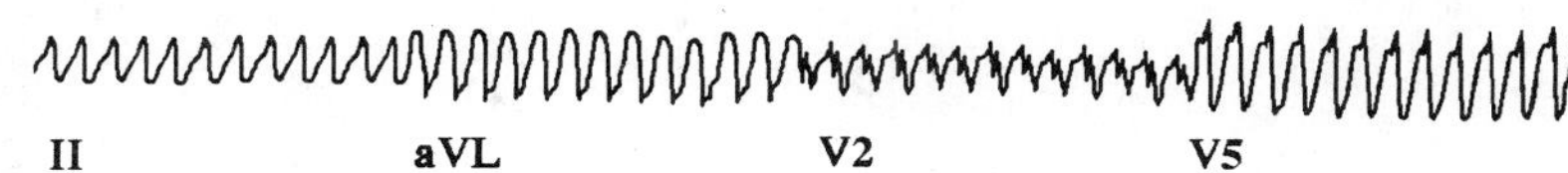

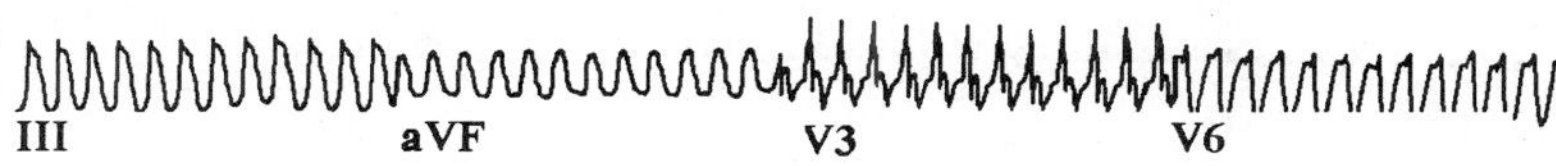

automatic SN cells. These cells can produce a benign automatic rhythm seen primarily in younger people during periods of high vagal tone. This rhythm is called a low atrial or coronary sinus rhythm and has a slow or normal rate (50 to 85 BPM). The rhythm has a shorter PR interval than sinus with a retrograde (inverted) P wave morphology. A low atrial rhythm may compete with a sinus rhythm for dominance.

Ectopic Atrial Tachycardia

These rhythms are typically referred to as paroxysmal atrial tachycardia (PAT). Overlap in the presentation and response to therapy among the different types of PATs makes it difficult to determine the mechanism. The automatic tachycardias may occur in any location. However, most foci arise near the SN, the crista terminalis, the right and left atrial appendages, and the pulmonic veins. Reentrant PAT circuits often involve the venous inlets of both atria (superior and inferior vena cavae, coronary sinus, pulmonary veins) as well as both appendages. People who have myocardial injury or surgery may develop re-entry around the scars or suture lines. Localizing the site of the tachycardia by ECG criteria alone is often difficult. Reentry can also occur in damaged atria without the use of an orifice. Usually, PAT has a rate between 90 and 180 BPM (except for atrial flutter), often with physiologic AVB. Classically seen with digoxin intoxication are PAT with AV conduction block and ventricular rates of 80 to 100 BPM.

Multifocal Atrial Rhythms

The terms multifocal atrial tachycardia (MAT), chaotic atrial rhythm, and wandering atrial pacemaker describe rhythms with irregular P-P intervals, multiple P wave morphologies (at least three), and PR intervals (at least three). They each involve multiple automatic ectopic foci vying for predominance. The result is an almost beat-to-beat shift in the location of the dominant atrial focus. A wandering atrial pacemaker has a benign nature, with a relatively slow rate (55 to 80 BPM), and relatively long P-P intervals. It may be seen in hypervagal states. MAT has very short P-P intervals, resulting in a rapid irregular tachycardia that may be difficult to distinguish from AF and ranges from 120 to 190 BPM. MAT is often associated with pulmonary disease and/or hypoxia. Some physicians believe that MAT involves triggered activity, but this has not been conclusively proved. Chaotic atrial rhythm describes a rhythm that is slower than MAT, but faster and less benign than a wandering atrial pacemaker.

Atrial Flutter

Atrial flutter is the most common re-entrant AT. There are two types of atrial flutter. Type I has a negative sawtooth pattern in the inferior leads and an atrial rate of 240 to 300 BPM and utilizes a macrore-entrant circuit located in the right atrium. Physiologic AVB is the rule, in AF or atrial flutter, except in the presence of medications that slow the flutter rate or an accessory pathway (Fig. 8). Other than sinus tachycardia, atrial flutter is the most common cause of regular SVT with a rate between 140 and 150 BPM. Often one of the flutter waves will be buried in the QRS, leading to a pseudo-RBBB pattern in lead V_1 (Fig. 9). In older patients, 4:1 conduction is common, but 3:1 AVB is uncommon. Type II atrial flutter occurs less frequently than type I. Its P waves are positive in the inferior leads, with a faster atrial rate of 320 to 360 BPM. Type II usually originates from a focus near the pulmonic vein orifices in the left atrium. Atrial flutter is associated with pulmonary disease and congenital heart disease (uncorrected and corrected), but most atrial flutter is idiopathic.

Atrial Fibrillation

Atrial fibrillation is the most common sustained cardiac arrhythmia, with a 0.4 per cent prevalence in the United States population. Its incidence increases with age, reaching an estimated 2 to 4 per cent of persons older than 60 years of age. In the 1990s, there are more than one million people with AF in the United States. This number is expected to rise as the population grows older over the next 20 years. The causes of AF include valvular disease (especially mitral stenosis and regurgitation), hypertension, ischemic atrial damage, cardiomyopathy, and pulmonary disease. The complications of AF are related to the underlying cardiac disease and increase with age. In younger patients, underlying cardiac or metabolic disorders are seldom found, and these people suffer fewer complications (lone AF). The most feared complication is thromboembolism, which is facilitated by the pooling of blood (which leads to hypercoagulability) and by the impaired antithrombotic activity of the atrial endocardial surface due to disease. During AF, the atria contract too fast to allow for adequate filling. They contract in a disorganized fashion, with loss of AV synchrony. This loss is especially important in people with diastolic dysfunction who require the atrial kick. Inappropriate elevation of the heart rate can also cause destabilization, leading to episodes of ischemia or congestive heart failure.

Atrial fibrillation is caused by intra-atrial re-entry—not

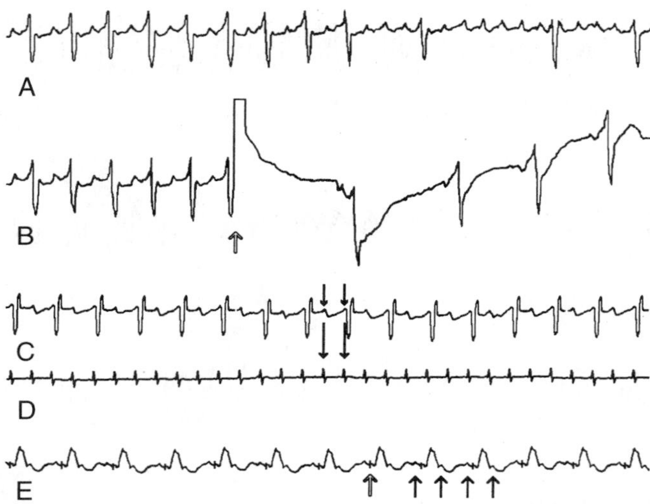

Figure 9. Strips *A* to *C* show 2:1 atrial flutter masquerading as a long PR interval and incomplete RBBB. The first two strips come from the same patient and demonstrate loss of R′ with adenosine and cardioversion *(open arrow)*. In strip *C*, the initial small R wave is a flutter wave. This was proved by obtaining an atrial electrogram *(D)*. The flutter waves correlated with the atrial electrograms *(arrows)*. *E*, From a patient with a dual-chamber pacemaker admitted for heart failure. The rhythm was thought to be sinus tachycardia, but was shown to be atrial flutter. Every other flutter wave falls within the atrial refractory period and is not sensed, mimicking 2:1 AVB.

true chaotic atrial electrical activity. In AF, there are multiple re-entrant foci in both atria vying for dominance. The result on the surface ECG is an irregular, often chaotic, appearance. The marked interpatient variability in rate and regularity is due to the number, location, and rates of the individual circuits. Atrial fibrillation may be coarse or fine, depending on the state of the atrial myocardium and the amount of myocardium depolarized by the individual circuits. A patient with few foci, each capturing a large portion of the atrial tissue, may look similar to one with MAT. The rate and regularity of AV conduction depend on the autonomic tone. Atrial fibrillation with a ventricular response that regularizes during digoxin therapy may represent complete heart block with a junctional escape.

Atrial Standstill

True lack of atrial electrical activity (atrial quiescence or standstill) occurs in three settings: severe ischemic disease of the atria, end-stage atrial disease from chronic AF, and infiltrative disease, such as amyloidosis. The loss of electrical activity is often patchy. The findings during EPS include an inability to obtain atrial electrograms or capture at maximal output settings. Severe hyperkalemia can cause atrial and ventricular standstill.

Holiday Heart Syndrome

The association of alcoholic binges and cardiac arrhythmias, predominantly atrial, has been recognized for many years. In the United States, Thanksgiving and the Fourth of July are the holidays most frequently associated with this syndrome. The arrhythmias usually begin 24 to 48 hours after the binge and resolve within several days. The most commonly seen arrhythmias are frequent unifocal and multifocal PACs, and AF. Treatment is supportive, primarily with beta-blockers and digoxin.

ATRIOVENTRICULAR NODE (AV JUNCTION) ARRHYTHMIAS

Automatic Junctional Rhythms

A junctional escape rhythm is regular with a rate between 40 and 55 BPM. The P waves are usually inverted in the inferior leads and may occur before (with a short PR), inside, or after the QRS (ST segment). If the P wave falls within the QRS, atrial activity may not be discernible. A junctional escape can be differentiated from a low atrial rhythm by the shorter PR interval and slower HR. Junctional escape rhythms are often seen during bradycardic episodes of any etiology, including cardioinhibitory or vagal episodes. An accelerated junctional rhythm has a rate between 60 and 100 BPM, and junctional tachycardia (JT) has a rate above 100 BPM. These rhythms are usually associated with high sympathetic tone, drugs that enhance automaticity, or AVN inflammation. People with congenital third-degree AVB may have rapid junctional rhythms with exertion. Junctional tachycardia is frequently seen after damage to the AVN from surgery or catheter ablation. This typically subsides within 24 to 48 hours. The accelerated junctional rhythms seen with digoxin intoxication are usually within the 80 to 100 BPM range.

Junctional Re-entry

Several arrhythmias use the AVN as a requisite part of their re-entrant circuit. The AVN must conduct for these rhythms to continue. If block is induced with drugs or a vagal maneuver, the tachycardia must terminate. Most of the re-entry involving the AVN is due to atrioventricular nodal re-entrant tachycardia (AVNRT), which presents with rates between 120 and 240 BPM. The common type of AVNRT has a very long PR, with the P wave usually buried in the QRS or proximal ST segment (Fig. 10). The uncommon form of AVNRT has a normal PR, usually less than 180 msec. The P wave morphology with both of these is usually inverted (retrograde). Atrioventricular re-entrant tachycardia and paroxysmal JT also involve the AVN.

Physiologic and Pathologic Atrioventricular Block

The AVN serves as a filter by manifesting physiologic block when the atrial rate is excessive (e.g., atrial flutter or fibrillation). The rate at which physiologic block occurs is dynamic. It increases with sympathetic stimulation (exercise) and decreases with parasympathetic (rest). It also decreases with age and with many medications. Physiologic block may manifest as Mobitz type I, Mobitz type II, or high-grade AV block. There are four types of pathologic block (Fig. 11). Atrioventricular block may occur either in the AVN or in the His-Purkinje system. Mobitz type I block is usually located in the AVN, while Mobitz type II block is infranodal. Infranodal block is often associated with

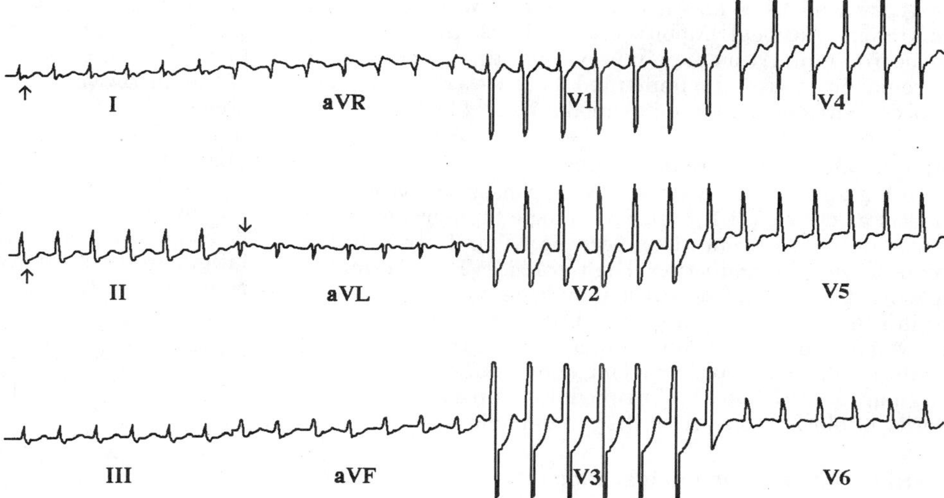

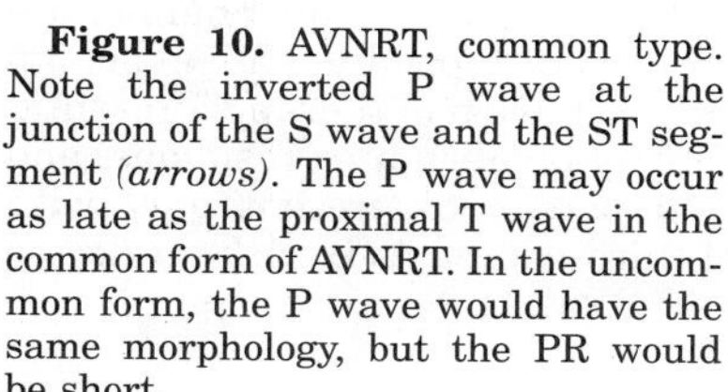

Figure 10. AVNRT, common type. Note the inverted P wave at the junction of the S wave and the ST segment *(arrows)*. The P wave may occur as late as the proximal T wave in the common form of AVNRT. In the uncommon form, the P wave would have the same morphology, but the PR would be short.

BBB with the conducted beats. Often, AVN block shows a narrow QRS with first-degree AVB with the beats that conduct. Intranodal AVB is often improved with the administration of atropine or sympathomimetics. Paradoxical worsening of AVB occurs more frequently with infranodal AVB. A 2:1 AVB may be caused by Mobitz type I or II block. Electrocardiographic criteria alone do not always differentiate these types reliably.

First-Degree Atrioventricular Block

The most common type of AVB is prolongation of the AV conduction time—not true block. It is defined as a PR interval greater than 210 msec. It has a benign prognosis and rarely progresses to higher block without pharmacologic help or further damage or degeneration. An exception is a new first-degree AVB that occurs in patients with endocarditis. Mild to moderate first-degree AVB is not associated with significant hemodynamic effects. Severe first-degree AVB (PR ≥.32) may impair AV synchrony. The PR normally decreases with an increase in sympathetic tone, and an interval of .20 is abnormal with sinus tachycardia.

Second-Degree Atrioventricular Block Type I

Mobitz type I AVB presents with regular or irregular bouts of grouped beating (see Fig. 11). Physiologic Wenckebach block occurs at high HRs. Abnormal Wenckebach block occurs at lower HRs and may be idiopathic or drug-induced or may be secondary to enhanced vagal tone. Vagally mediated AVB is usually preceded by slowing of the sinus rate before block. It may coexist with Mobitz type I SAB, especially during an acute inferior wall myocardial infarction or with digoxin intoxication. Mobitz type I AVB implies block in the AVN but may occur with infranodal block. It has a benign prognosis and infrequently progresses to third-degree AVB. When it does progress, the junctional escape is preserved. No therapy is usually required unless the person is symptomatic or evidence of infranodal disease is found in an EPS. Mobitz type I AVB that occurs in an inferior wall myocardial infarction may be due to direct AVN damage, or marked vagal stimulation, and frequently improves over time.

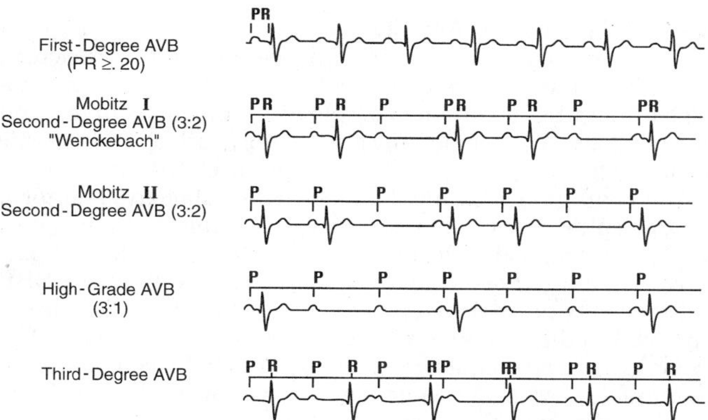

Figure 11. Examples of atrioventricular block (AVB).

Mobitz Type II Atrioventricular Block

Second-degree AVB with a constant PR interval on the conducted beats is called Mobitz type II. It is less common than Mobitz type I and has a different ECG appearance, etiology, and prognosis. The P-P intervals should be regular (no PACs), and there is no significant variation in the PR interval. The R-R intervals are regular except for the dropped beat. As with Mobitz type I AVB, fixed-ratio grouped beating is often seen. The conducted beats may show a normal QRS, but Mobitz type II is typically seen with concomitant BBB, bifascicular block, or nonspecific intraventricular conduction delay. Occasionally, the first interval after the blocked beat has a shorter PR than the subsequent ones because of the longer RP interval. This difference is much smaller than those seen with Wenckebach block. Mobitz type II has a less benign prognosis than that of Mobitz type I because the block is usually distal to the AV junction and proximal to the bundle of His. When it progresses to third-degree AVB, the escape rhythm, when present, is ventricular or fascicular in origin, slow, wide-complex, and irregular. Hemodynamic compromise may be caused by the lack of a reliable escape rhythm. This type of block usually does not respond to atropine or sympathomimetics and may paradoxically worsen. Mobitz type II block may be induced or worsened by drugs and by abnormal vagal stimulation. This type of block is usually seen in an acute anterior wall myocardial infarction but may be seen during an acute inferior wall myocardial infarction in those who have had a prior anterior wall myocardial infarction. Although Mobitz type II block from an acute myocardial infarction may improve over time, a permanent pacemaker is usually implanted because of the serious consequences of complete infranodal heart block.

High-Grade Atrioventricular Block

In high-grade (or advanced) AVB, consecutive atrial impulses block (e.g., 3:1, 5:3). Physiologic high-grade AVB is normally seen in conditions such as AT and atrial flutter with 3:1 or 4:1 conduction. High-grade AVB at normal or low heart rates implies severe impairment of the AVN and/or infranodal conduction system because of drugs, disease, or vagal stimulation. Junctional or ventricular escape beats commonly appear in long, nonconducted intervals. High-grade AVB may be intranodal or infranodal. The severity of block often varies with autonomic tone.

Third-Degree Atrioventricular Block

Complete heart block may be transient or persistent. It is a form of AV dissociation where the supraventricular rhythm is faster than the ventricular rhythm, and P waves occur in places where they should be conducted but are not. There should be no evidence for AV conduction. The treatment and prognosis depend on the etiology of the block, level of the block, effect on hemodynamics, and symptomatology.

Pseudo-Atrioventricular Block

Atrioventricular block may be mimicked by closely coupled PACs that do not conduct. Analyze closely the T wave and ST segment of the beat preceding the block for morphologic differences (e.g., asymmetric T waves) between beats. PVCs can cause AV block by retrograde concealed conduction (see Fig. 6*B*).

Atrioventricular Dissociation

Atrioventricular dissociation describes conditions in which there are independent rhythms above the AVN (atria) and below the AVN (ventricles). The atrial rhythm is frequently sinus. The rhythm below the AVN may be ventricular, junctional, or ventricularly paced. Third-degree AVB requires AV dissociation, but dissociation may occur without third-degree AVB. Any rhythm with a ventricular rate that is faster than the atrial rate may be dissociated. For example, if the underlying rhythm is sinus at 70 BPM and a ventricular pacemaker is set at a rate of 90 BPM, the ventricular impulses may or may not be conducted retrograde back to the atrium. If they are, the SN will be overdriven. If they are not, the SN will continue with its intrinsic rhythm at 70 BPM. In the latter case, the ECG would show AV dissociation, with P waves marching independently of the paced rhythm. There is no evidence for antegrade AVB. Isorhythmic AV dissociation describes the presence of two competing rhythms at approximately the same rate vying for dominance (see Fig. 5*B*). Occasionally, isorhythmic AV dissociation mimics normal conduction, especially when the QRS is narrow, as may be seen with the AV dissociation between sinus and junctional rhythms. In this instance, respiratory variation is often seen in the sinus rate, without a similar change in the junctional rate, altering the PR interval.

Degenerative Atrioventricular Block

Senile degeneration of the AVN may occur with or without concomitant SN disease. It is more common in the elderly, but there exist familial forms that have onset earlier in life. The pathologic changes include loss of functional cells, fatty and fibrous infiltration, and/or calcification. The latter may accompany overt cardiac calcification of the mitral valve annulus. The most common conduction abnormality is first-degree AVB, seen most often in patients treated with sympatholytics or calcium channel antagonists. The first-degree AVB typically has a benign course that does not require cessation of therapy. Presentation of this acquired AVB may be abrupt or insidious, and it is not uncommon for a person to present only with fatigue in the presence of third-degree AVB with an escape rhythm and HR of 35 to 40 BPM.

Atrioventricular Block in Endocarditis

The AVN-His complex runs from near the septal leaflet of the tricuspid valve under the noncoronary cusp of the aortic valve passing close to the anterior leaflet of the mitral valve. Aortic valve endocarditis has the highest incidence of AVB, typically because of abscess formation near the noncoronary cusp. The development of first-degree AVB during acute aortic endocarditis is an indication for acute intervention because the AVB may progress to complete AVB.

Unusual Causes of Atrioventricular Block

Kearns-Sayre ophthalmoplegia is a rare syndrome associated with progressive infranodal AVB. Other forms of muscular dystrophy are also associated with an increased risk of conduction abnormalities or AVB. Sarcoidosis, rheumatic heart disease, Lyme disease, and Chagas' disease all cause acquired AVB in specific populations. Tricuspid, mitral, and aortic valve surgery and the repair of some types of atrial and ventricular septal defects are associated with AVB.

Congenital Complete Atrioventricular Block

Heart block is an uncommon finding in childhood and adolescence and usually has a relatively benign course unless the patient reports impaired exercise tolerance. There is usually a fully functional junctional pacemaker that responds better to exercise than the usual junctional pacemaker. Exertional HRs of up to 180 BPM have been documented. The incidence of sudden death and the requirement for a pacemaker appear to decrease with age in this group.

VENTRICULAR ARRHYTHMIAS

Ventricular Ectopic Activity

The term used to describe all spontaneous ventricular electrical activity is ventricular ectopic activity. It is categorized by rate, duration, complexity, clinical course, and morphology. With monomorphic ectopy, all of the ectopic complexes, with the possible exception of the first one to three beats in a run, have a similar morphology. The term polymorphic describes ectopy with multiple morphologies. Left ventricular depolarizations usually have a RBBB pattern, whereas those from the right ventricle have a LBBB pattern. Ventricular ectopy is also described by its axis, as in left bundle left axis or right bundle normal axis. The complexity and frequency of ectopy should be considered in conjunction with left ventricular function and underlying cardiac disease. Frequent PVCs are often a sign of high sympathetic tone (e.g., congestive heart failure).

Ventricular Escape

Escape beats from the His-Purkinje system and from the ventricular myocardium cannot be distinguished by ECG alone. Owing to normal phase 4 automaticity, escape rhythms that arise from Purkinje cells are faster and more stable than those that arise from ventricular cells. A ventricular escape rhythm is usually 20 to 40 BPM and irregular, while a Purkinje escape rhythm is 35 to 45 BPM (see Fig. 6*A*). Ventricular escape beats are facilitated by underlying bradycardia or high catecholamine states. An agonal rhythm is an extremely slow (5 to 20 BPM) ventricular escape rhythm (QRS usually more than 160 msec) seen just before cardiac standstill, most commonly during respiratory arrest or the terminal portion of electromechanical dissociation.

Accelerated Idioventricular Rhythm

Two types of accelerated idioventricular rhythm are seen under similar clinical circumstances, but they differ in prognosis and need for treatment. They are most often seen during reperfusion after acute ischemia. Type I is relatively slow (50 to 110 BPM), is regular, and is due to automaticity (see Fig. 5*B*). It rarely degenerates directly into unstable rhythms unless the rate causes further ischemia. Type II is faster (100 to 140 BPM), irregular, and often polymorphic. It has a more malignant course, with a higher risk of degeneration. It should be viewed as a slow VT and treated appropriately.

Monomorphic Ventricular Tachycardia

Most clinical sustained VT is monomorphic (Figs. 12 to 14). Untreated monomorphic VT is usually 120 to 200 BPM, but faster rates are occasionally seen. The onset of the tachycardia may help delineate its mechanism. Re-entrant VT often starts with a PVC that has a morphology different from that of the monomorphic VT. Automatic VT usually has a single morphology without a preceding PVC.

The most common mechanism of monomorphic VT is re-entry that uses fixed areas of ischemic scar. Ventricular aneurysms, from ischemia (or, in other countries, Chagas' disease), predispose to re-entrant VT. Dilated cardiomyopathies predispose to monomorphic VT through high catecholamine levels and stretch-induced conduction abnormalities, in addition to fixed scar. Dilated cardiomyopathy has a higher proportion of automatic and possibly triggered arrhythmias than does ischemic VT. This predominance explains some of the differences involved in the diagnosis and treatment of VT in these two groups. There are several forms of idiopathic monomorphic VT that often present in younger people without overt cardiac disease, including VT from the right ventricular outflow tract and from the inferoseptal aspect of the left ventricle. The idiopathic right ventricular outflow tract VT frequently has a left bundle–right axis morphology and often occurs with exertion. The inferoseptal VT usually has a right bundle–left axis or right bundle–right superior axis morphology, and echocardiography may reveal a "false tendon" in the left ventricle. These two idiopathic VTs often respond both acutely and chronically to verapamil, and each has a good long-term prognosis. The outflow tract VT can be distinguished from VT secondary to right ventricle dysplasia with echocardiography, ventriculography, and cardiac magnetic resonance imaging.

Ischemic Ventricular Tachycardia

Monomorphic VT during acute ischemia is either re-entrant or automatic. Ventricular tachycardia during either reperfusion or the first 48 hours after a myocardial infarction is most frequently caused by abnormal automaticity or triggered activity. Accelerated idioventricular rhythms are common during reperfusion and usually do not require therapy. Re-entry is the most common mechanism for VT after 48 hours. The initial VT episode may occur anywhere from days after a myocardial infarction to 20 years later (see Fig. 14). The late re-entrant arrhythmias are due to the ischemic scar and do not require active coronary disease. Rapid polymorphic VT and ventricular fibrillation (VF) are associated with acute coronary vasospasm. The R-on-T phenomenon is the propensity for a PVC occurring during the terminal portion of the T wave (vulnerable period) to induce VF. Although this vulnerability exists in all people, it is uncommon for VF to be induced by this method without ischemia.

Right Ventricular Dysplasia

The idiopathic syndrome known as right ventricular dysplasia presents initially with monomorphic VT (often rapid), later with polymorphic VT, and occasionally VF. Its cause is unknown, and it is sometimes related to the partial or complete absence of the right ventricular pericar-

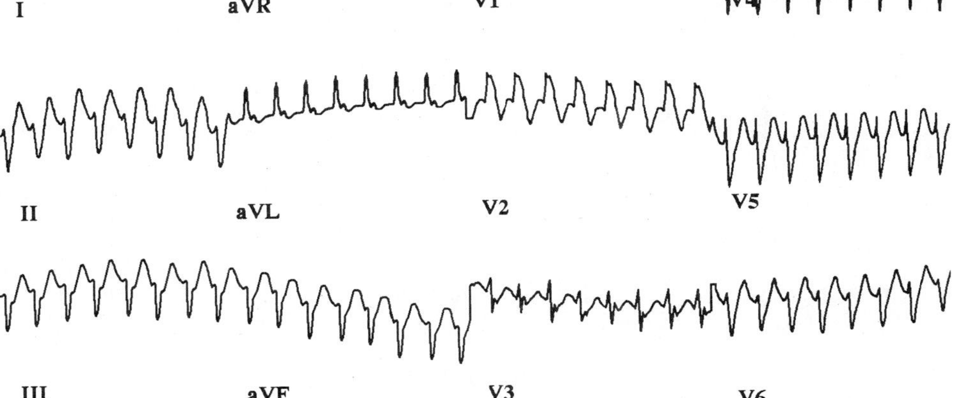

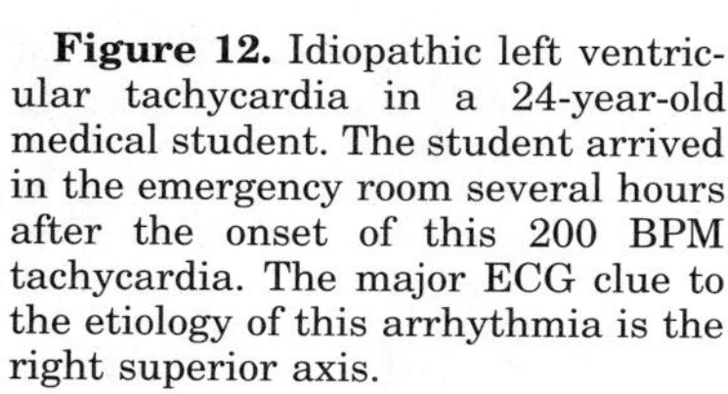

Figure 12. Idiopathic left ventricular tachycardia in a 24-year-old medical student. The student arrived in the emergency room several hours after the onset of this 200 BPM tachycardia. The major ECG clue to the etiology of this arrhythmia is the right superior axis.

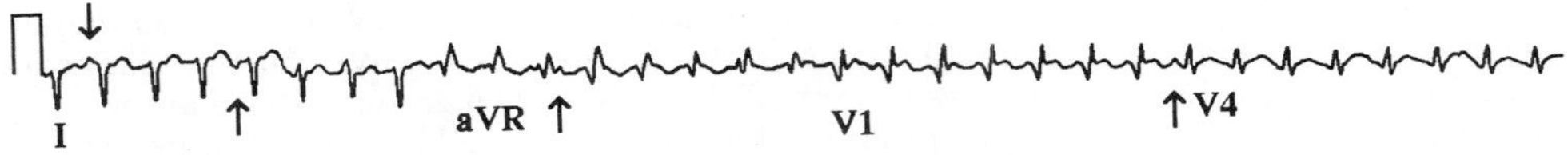

Figure 13. Narrow QRS ventricular tachycardia. A 40-year-old woman had this tachycardia 1 week after a large anterior wall MI. Adenosine was ineffective. She then received 5 mg of verapamil, decompensated, and required resuscitation. The tachycardia was mapped to the ventricular septum during bypass surgery and was successfully cryoablated. AV dissociation is implied by the irregular baseline. Note the possible P waves *(arrows)*.

dium (Uhl's anomaly). The ECG usually shows a right ventricular strain pattern with large inverted T waves in V_1 to V_3. A terminal upward deflection in the T wave called the epsilon wave is sometimes seen. Pharmacologic, surgical, and electrical therapies for the arrhythmic aspects of this condition have been successful in patients with good right ventricular function. The prognosis is worse when the right heart dysfunction progresses to overt failure.

Fascicular Tachycardia

Fascicular tachycardia is an uncommon form of VT that arises next to or inside a fascicle of the left bundle. It often exhibits a narrow QRS complex because of partial conduction over the His-Purkinje system. It is of interest because of its occasional termination with carotid massage and its ability to mimic SVT.

Polymorphic Ventricular Tachycardia

There are several types of polymorphic VT that differ in presentation and mechanism. All are unstable and may degenerate into VF. The polymorphic VT with the best prognosis is an idiopathic catecholamine-dependent tachycardia that occurs with exercise. Seen in younger patients with normal heart function, it is suppressed by beta-blockers or calcium channel antagonists. Patients with active coronary ischemia are subject to an extremely rapid (200 to 250 BPM) nonsustained polymorphic VT. The episodes usually last for only a few beats but may degenerate into VF. A subset of patients with mitral valve prolapse have an elevated risk of sudden death associated with polymorphic VT. Episodes of polymorphic VT may degenerate into VF. The idiopathic and acquired long QT syndromes are associated with a specific form of polymorphic VT called torsades de pointes.

Torsades de Pointes

The most infamous form of polymorphic VT is called torsade de pointes (see Fig. 5*C* and *D*). Its name means "twisting of the points " and describes the tendency of QRS polarity to vary from positive to negative. It is a highly unstable rhythm that frequently reverts to sinus rhythm after only a few beats. Although the episodes are usually short, longer episodes occur. They may last for up to several minutes, leading to syncope, or, in extreme cases, sudden death. Episodes often show a bigeminal pattern (short-long-short sequence) at the onset of tachycardia (see Fig. 5*C*). The episodes may be so frequent that the polymorphic tachycardia becomes the dominant rhythm, with interspersed isolated sinus beats. In a person with normal

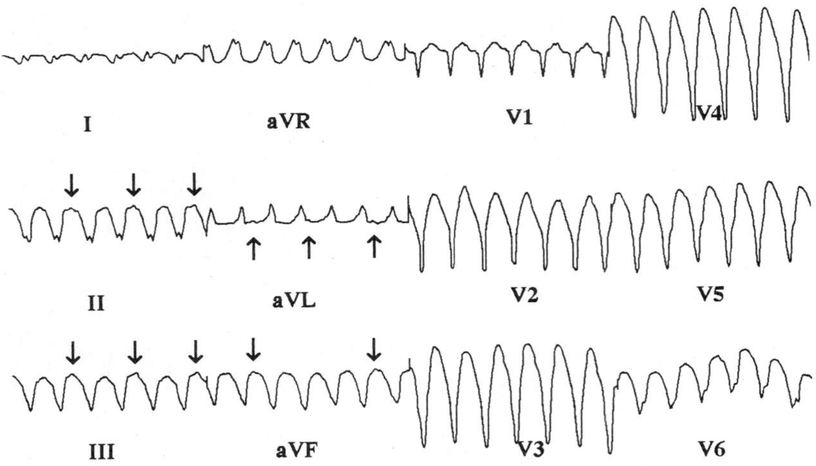

Figure 14. Ventricular tachycardia. From a 65-year-old man with coronary disease who presented with palpitations and chest discomfort. The tachycardia satisfies many of the criteria mentioned in the text for distinguishing VT from SVT with aberrancy. There is negative concordance (no R wave in precordium). AV dissociation can be seen in the inferior leads *(arrows)*. The tachycardia also satisfies the morphology criteria. The RS duration does not apply due to the lack of R wave.

cardiac function, fewer than 1 per cent of episodes degenerate into VF. However, a patient may have several hundred episodes in a day. The risk of VF is related to the underlying heart dysfunction, especially active ischemia, and the severity of the condition that predisposed to the arrhythmia.

Torsades de pointes is the only clinical ventricular arrhythmia thought to be due to early afterdepolarizations. Early afterdepolarizations and torsades are facilitated by bradycardia and conditions that prolong the QT interval, including both the idiopathic and the acquired forms of the long QT syndrome (Table 1). The idiopathic long QT syndrome includes both the Romano-Ward and the Jervell and Lange-Nielsen syndromes, which differ in genetic and clinical but not arrhythmic characteristics. The Romano-Ward syndrome is autosomal dominant. The Jervell and Lange-Nielsen syndrome is autosomal recessive and is associated with congenital deafness.

Autonomic imbalance is considered to be a major factor in the genesis of the arrhythmias in these syndromes. The location of the abnormality responsible for the imbalance is unknown. Sympathetic blockade and left stellectomy are used in therapy. Sudden death in the idiopathic long QT syndrome often occurs during exercise.

Many drugs and conditions associated with QT prolongation predispose to arrhythmias, including torsades. Most antiarrhythmic agents, especially the class Ia and III antiarrhythmics, cause marked QT prolongation. Quinidine is most likely the antiarrhythmic with the highest incidence of torsades. The less commonly known causes include antibiotics (erythromycin), antihistamines (terfenadine), and psychiatric medications (haloperidol, desipramine). Starvation (especially during refeeding), diuretics, and low-protein diets may cause electrolyte abnormalities, which may lead to torsades.

Ventricular Flutter

Most episodes of VT have sustained rates below 220 BPM. An exception is ventricular flutter, which is an electrically (but not hemodynamically) stable ventricular rhythm with rates between 260 and 320 BPM. After a short period, often seconds, the arrhythmia induces ischemia and degenerates into VF.

Ventricular Fibrillation

Ventricular fibrillation is defined as an extremely rapid polymorphic and irregular ventricular rhythm with rates between 250 and 350 BPM. Primary VF, without prodromal symptoms or arrhythmias, is uncommon. It may be induced by closely coupled PVCs (R-on-T wave phenomenon), especially during active ischemia. VF episodes are usually sustained and result in death unless witnessed and treated appropriately. The majority of sudden death episodes begin as monomorphic VT, which degenerates into VF. It can be difficult to distinguish VF from AF conducting rapidly over an accessory pathway (therefore wide complex) in a person with a pre-excitation syndrome. ECG lead dislodgement and/or motion artifact often mimic VF.

Bundle Branch Re-entry

The circuit in bundle branch re-entry includes both bundle branches and the intervening myocardium. It occurs in people who have some measure of infranodal conduction disease, as evidenced by BBBs or intraventricular conduction delays on baseline ECG. Bundle branch re-entry is the cause of between 2 and 5 per cent of clinical monomorphic VT and is more common in dilated than ischemic cardiomyopathies. Its diagnosis requires invasive EPS to document that the arrhythmia does involve the bundle branches. This arrhythmia runs from 180 to 240 BPM and is often hemodynamically unstable.

Bidirectional Ventricular Tachycardia

A very rare form of bimorphic VT is seen only in digoxin intoxication. The cause of the arrhythmia is considered to be abnormal automaticity or triggered activity involving the fascicles of the left bundle and, occasionally, the right bundle. The QRS complexes alternate morphologies in a bigeminal pattern and are often classically right bundle–

Table 1. Medications and Conditions Associated With Torsades de Pointes

	Antihistamines		
	Astemizole	Terfenadine	
	Antibiotics and Antifungals		
Bactrim (trimethoprim-sulfamethoxazole) Pentamidine	Clarithromycin Quinine derivatives	Erythromycin	Ketoconazole
	Antiarrhythmics		
Almokalant Disopyramide Lidocaine (rare) Propafenone Tocainide	Ajmaline Digoxin (rare) Mexiletine Quinidine	Amiodarone (rare) Dofetilide NAPA (*N*-acetylprocainamide) Sematilide	Aprindine Encainide Procainamide Sotalol (d or d/l)
	Antidepressants and Neuroleptics		
All tricyclic antidepressants	Chloral hydrate	Lithium	Phenothiazines
	Other Cardiovascular Agents		
Bepridil	Indapamide	Ketanserin	Probucol
	Miscellaneous		
Bradycardia Hypomagnesemia Myocardial infarction or ischemia	Central nervous system events Hypothermia Mitral valve prolapse	Exercise Liquid diets Myocarditis	Hypokalemia Long QT syndrome

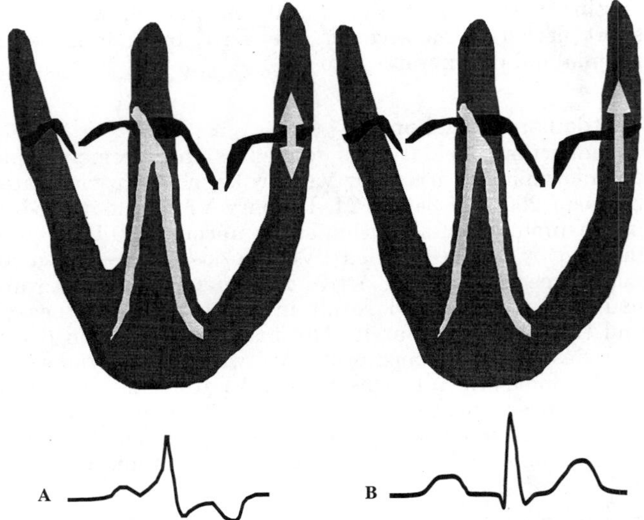

Figure 15. Manifest *(A)* versus concealed *(B)* conduction during sinus rhythm in WPW.

left posterior fascicular block and right bundle–left anterior fascicular block.

WOLFF-PARKINSON-WHITE (WPW) AND THE PRE-EXCITATION SYNDROMES

Pre-excitation

The AVN conducts much slower than myocardium but is the only normal electrical AV connection. In WPW there are myocardial bridges across the AV groove. These extra AV connections are called accessory pathways (APs) or bypass tracts. Conduction over an AP is extremely rapid compared with the AVN. Like the AVN, APs may conduct antegradely and/or retrogradely. Pre-excitation is defined as antegrade or retrograde conduction that is faster than normal AVN conduction and/or occurs away from the normal conducting system.

During sinus rhythm, AV conduction may then occur down the AVN, the AP, or both. The PR interval of a sinus impulse, conducted only over the AP, is dependent on its location. APs on the right side of the heart usually receive the impulse faster than left-sided APs, resulting in a shorter PR. Conduction over an AP results in a wide QRS because the ventricles are excited from an abnormal site, and conduction occurs from cell to cell, rather than via the Purkinje network. With intact AVN conduction, the ECG reflects a fusion of normal (narrow) and pre-excited (wide) conduction over the AP. The initial slurred portion of the QRS, due to local conduction at the ventricular insertion of the AP, is called a delta wave. Pre-excitation may be mild or marked, depending on the proximity of the AP to the SN and the underlying autonomic tone that affects AVN, but not AP, conduction. Left-sided APs sometimes have normal PR intervals and minimal delta waves, because conduction over both the AVN and the His-Purkinje system has occurred before the impulse from the SN reached the AP. Higher sympathetic tones predispose to faster AVN conduction and diminished pre-excitation, whereas the opposite holds true for rest and sleep and parasympathetic tone. If pre-excitation is lost with exertion, it may be due to enhanced AVN conduction or a weakly conducting AP.

WPW and Arrhythmias

Manifest pre-excitation is defined as a short PR interval and a wide QRS with a delta wave (Figs. 15 and 16). When there is retrograde but no antegrade pre-excitation (see Fig. 15), no evidence for pre-excitation is seen on the surface ECG. This is called concealed pre-excitation. Retrograde pre-excitation can be proved only by EPS. In orthodromic atrioventricular re-entrant tachycardia, conduction proceeds antegradely over the normal conduction system and retrogradely via the AP. The QRS complex is narrow unless aberrancy is present (Figs. 17 and 18). Tachycardia conducting in the opposite direction is called antidromic atrioventricular re-entrant tachycardia. In antidromic tachycardia, antegrade conduction is via the AP and is always wide-complex (see Fig. 17). Antidromic tachycardia is much less common than orthodromic and is associated with the presence of multiple APs. An AP may also serve as a "bystander tract" in which it is not part of the arrhythmia mechanism but rather a passive conduit for many types of SVT, including AF (Fig. 19), atrial flutter (see Fig. 8), and AT. Antegrade conduction over APs (wide-complex) may be very rapid because they can conduct at rates much faster than those of the AVN. Atrial fibrillation or 1:1 atrial flutter at rates of 300 BPM can occur and are a cause of sudden death in young people with WPW because they can degenerate into VF. The incidence of AF in patients with WPW is much higher than that of the general population (10 per cent of young people with WPW). Sudden death is less common in patients with concealed APs or with weakly conducting manifest pathways. The P-wave morphology in the orthodromic tachycardia is dependent on the location of the AP, with a long PR interval because of conduction over the AVN. In antidromic tachycardia, the P-wave morphology should be retrograde (inverted), with a very short PR interval. There is a strong association between

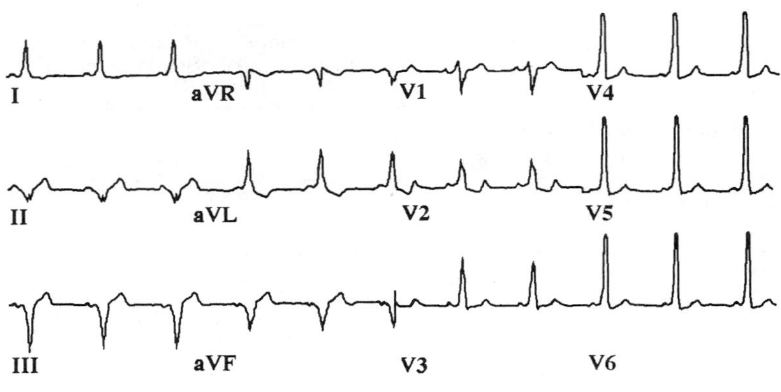

Figure 16. WPW: right-sided accessory pathway mimicking an inferior wall MI pattern. The PR interval is not short because of concomitant Ebstein's anomaly.

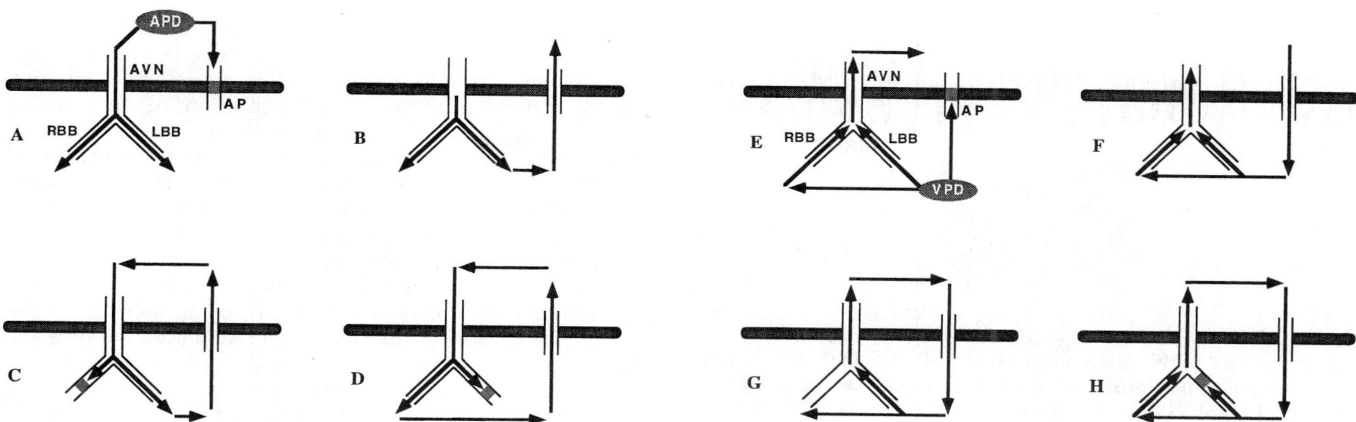

Figure 17. Atrioventricular re-entry: orthodromic *(A* to *D)* and antidromic *(E* to *F)* AVRT. Orthodromic occurs with both manifest and concealed WPW, while antidromic occurs only with manifest. Both arrhythmias are induced by premature depolarizations *(A* and *E)*. The wavefront blocks in the AP *(B* and *F)*, conducting through the AVN. It then "re-enters" through the AP *(C* and *G)* resulting in AVRT. Bundle branch block ipsilateral to the AP during tachycardia (*D* and *H*) increases the circuit size, slowing the tachycardia.

Ebstein's anomaly and right-sided APs (often multiple). The accessory pathways in Ebstein's anomaly may conduct slowly, giving a longer PR interval (normal duration) than that of most other pathways (see Fig. 16). Patients with Ebstein's anomaly usually have a baseline RBBB on their ECGs without pre-excitation. There may be a weak association between left-sided APs and mitral valve prolapse.

Localization of Accessory Pathways

In addition to the 12-lead ECG, several modalities have been used for the localization of APs, with partial success. Echocardiography, cardiac magnetic resonance imaging, and radionuclide ventriculography may reveal eccentric cardiac contraction. Intricate ECG algorithms and body surface mapping can predict location with a 70 to 90 per cent accuracy, depending on the true location and the specific algorithm. APs located in the posteroseptal region are often difficult to localize even with some of the newer, more complicated algorithms. The only reason for predicting the location of an AP is to decide about the use of catheter or surgical ablation because the risk-versus-benefit ratios vary by location. Intracardiac localization during EPS is

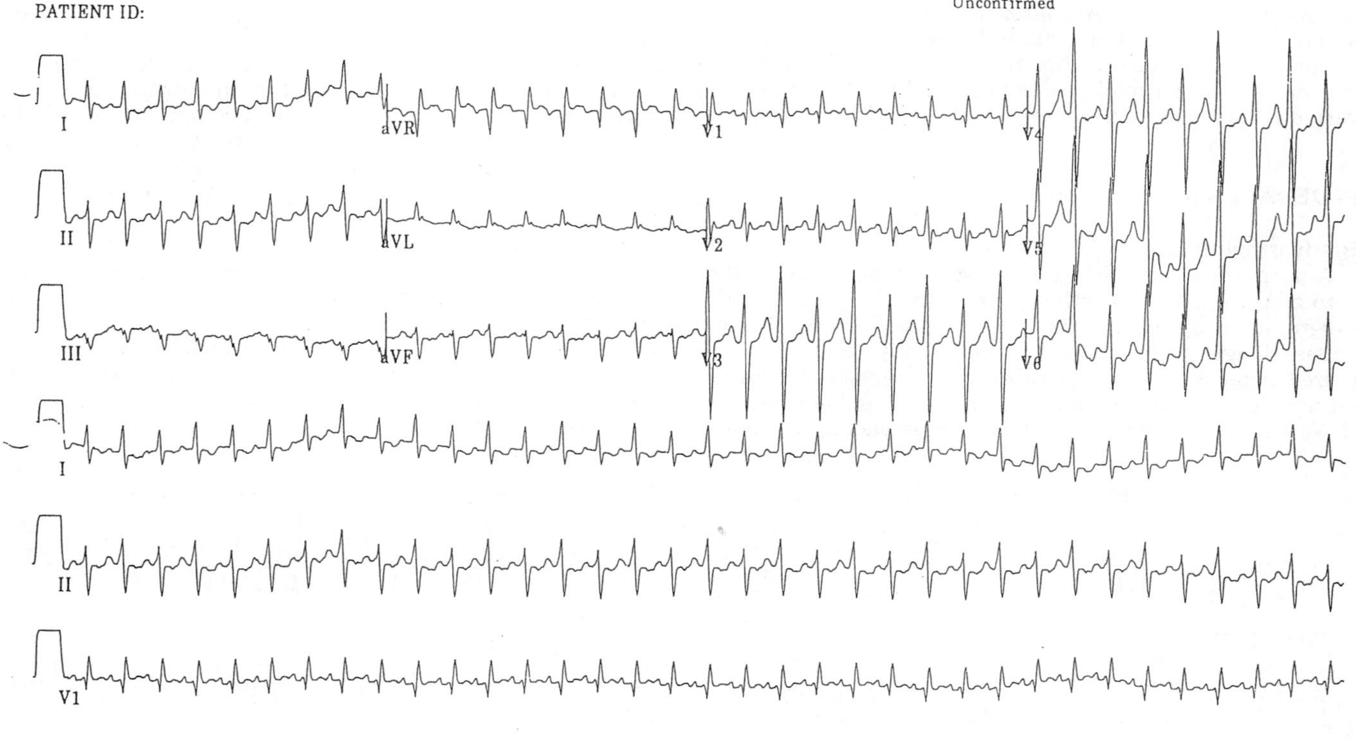

Figure 18. AVRT, orthodromic: The P-wave morphology is upright, rather than inverted, and occurs after the T wave. This patient had a concealed left lateral AP (WPW).

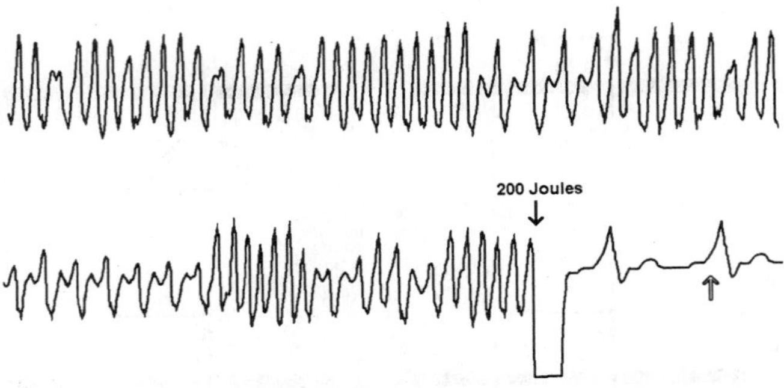

Figure 19. WPW. Extremely rapid polymorphic tachycardia consisting of atrial fibrillation conducting rapidly down an AP at rates up to 350 BPM interspersed with episodes of either orthodromic AVRT or conduction of the atrial fibrillation via the AV node. The patient was cardioverted during the bottom strip *(arrow)*. This tachycardia may resemble both ventricular fibrillation and torsade de pointes. Note the pre-excitation of the sinus beats after cardioversion *(open arrow)*.

the gold standard and may show the presence of multiple APs, especially in patients with Ebstein's anomaly. Occasionally large negative delta waves in the anteroseptal and/or inferior leads may mimic a Q-wave infarct (see Fig. 16).

Other Pre-excitation Syndromes

Lown-Ganong-Levine syndrome describes the combination of a short PR interval, normal QRS duration, and palpitations. The arrhythmia in this syndrome is similar to AVNRT except that it involves the use of a rapidly conducting AP and may have a faster rate. Nodofascicular, nodoventricular, and atriofascicular re-entrant arrhythmias occur rarely and present as LBBB morphology tachycardias. Paroxysmal junctional re-entrant tachycardia is an uncommon form of pre-excited tachycardia with inverted P waves located midway between QRS complexes.

PACEMAKER ARRHYTHMIAS

Bradyarrhythmia

A pacemaker should begin to pace the heart when the rate of the intrinsic rhythm falls below the pacemaker's programmed pacing interval. Paced HRs slower than, or pauses longer than, the set interval may be due to impaired sensing, failure to capture, hysteresis, or device failure. If a pacemaker senses electrical signals not due to R waves, it may inappropriately inhibit pacing. Common causes include oversensing of skeletal myopotentials, T waves, P waves, and electromagnetic interference. Failure of the pacemaker to capture may be caused by lead fracture, lead displacement, loss of insulation, or an increase in the pacing threshold. The pacing threshold may increase with a myocardial infarction involving the myocardium at the lead tip, use of medications that raise the pacing threshold (especially amiodarone), or electrolyte or metabolic abnormalities (especially hyperkalemia). When a pacemaker battery becomes depleted, the internal circuitry recognizes the drop in voltage and (depending on the device) usually decreases the paced rate automatically. Device failure is rarely due to battery depletion unless the patient refused standard follow-up. Some devices can revert to back-up modes or can become inoperative after electrical cardioversion. Hysteresis is a programmable function used to extend battery life by decreasing the frequency of pacing. In hysteresis mode, two rates are set; the pacing interval, and the minimal unpaced rate. The minimal unpaced rate is the HR at which pacing occurs, but the rate is at the programmed pacing interval. For example, with a hysteresis rate of 50 BPM and a paced rate of 70 BPM, no pacing would occur if the HR remained above 50 BPM. Below 50 BPM, however, the pacemaker would pace at 70 BPM. This is especially useful in patients with carotid hypersensitivity, in whom abrupt drops in HR may occur and faster paced rates may be required to maintain cardiac output.

Tachyarrhythmia

Tachycardia in a patient with a pacemaker may be paced or nonpaced. If tachycardia is nonpaced, evaluation should be similar to that in patients without pacemakers. The classic form of pacemaker-mediated tachycardia is similar in mechanism to orthodromic AVRT, except that the pacemaker itself is the retrograde limb of the circuit. The tachycardia begins when a PVC conducts retrogradely to the atrium. This conduction is sensed by the atrial lead of the pacemaker. The pacemaker cannot tell that this sensed P wave is not sinus, and it paces the ventricle. The ventricular depolarization conducts back up to the atrium, and a re-entrant loop is formed (Fig. 20). This can occur only with dual-chamber pacemakers. The rate of the pacemaker-mediated tachycardia is never faster than the upper rate limit for the pacemaker. Newer dual-chamber devices have innate and programmable features to avoid this arrhythmia. Other potential causes of paced tachycardias include rate-responsive pacemakers, and the tracking of SVT by dual-chamber pacemakers. The highest HRs in any of these arrhythmias will be at or below the programmed maximal tracking rate.

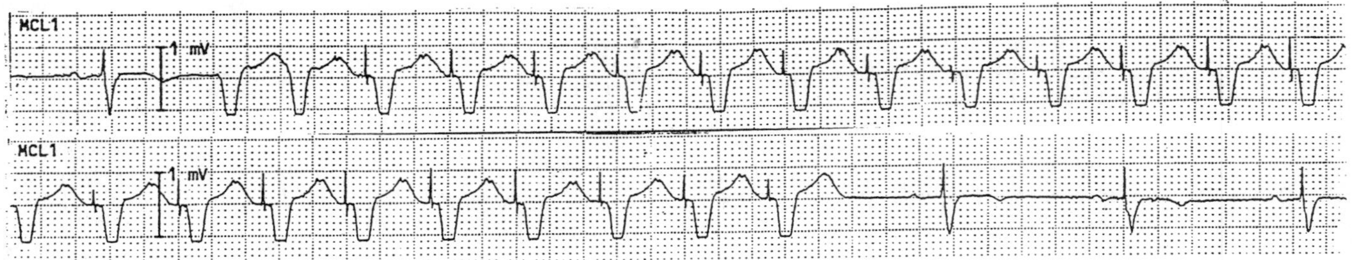

Figure 20. Pacemaker-mediated tachycardia (PMT): A ventricular couplet conducts retrogradely and is sensed by the atrial lead of a DDD pacemaker. It paces the ventricle, "thinking" it is tracking sinus rhythm. Further retrograde conduction perpetuates the tachycardia (the notch in the T wave is a P wave). The bottom strip shows the spontaneous termination of the tachycardia when retrograde block occurs (loss of notch in T wave).

Pacemaker Wenckebach

When the first dual-chamber pacemakers were implanted, the upper rate limits were set by refractory periods. If the atrial refractory period was set at 120 BPM, the ventricle would be paced for every sensed P wave, up to an atrial rate of 120 BPM. If the HR increased to 130 BPM, every other P wave would fall into the sensing refractory period, and the ventricular rate would fall to 65 BPM. This drop could result in impaired exercise tolerance or induce exertional syncope. The newer DDD pacemakers avoid this problem with the use of the maximal tracking rate. P waves coming faster than the tracking rate will be sensed, but the ventricle will not be paced with the normally programmed AV delay. Instead, the pacemaker lengthens the AV delay to keep the V-V interval at or below the maximal tracking rates interval. Successive P waves occur earlier, further increasing the AV delays until a P wave falls inside the atrial refractory period and is not conducted. This is called pacemaker Wenckebach block, and is often seen during exertion when the HR is above the maximal tracking rate and during regular AT. Thus, atrial rates faster than the atrial sensing refractory period conduct similar to Mobitz type II AVB, while slower rates, between the maximal tracking rate and the refractory period, conduct like Mobitz type I AVB.

PRESENTATION OF ARRHYTHMIAS

History

There is significant individual variability in the presentation and severity of symptoms associated with arrhythmic episodes. It is not uncommon to see a person walk into an emergency room in a rapid tachycardia with a rate of 220 BPM and only moderate symptoms. Another person with similar cardiac function may have syncope with a slower tachycardia at 170 BPM. There is variability in the response of the same person to different arrhythmia episodes of similar rate. Some of the factors, other than the rate of the arrhythmia, known to influence the severity of symptoms and hemodynamic stability include the presence or absence of AV synchrony, underlying myocardial disease (ischemia, ventricular dysfunction, and valvular disease), cerebrovascular disease, intravascular volume, vasomotor tone, and autonomic tone. Vasovagal (neurocardiogenic) reactions may occur with the onset or termination of arrhythmias, resulting in frank or near syncope. Episodes initiated by changes in position or turning of the head are often vagally mediated and include carotid hypersensitivity, neurocardiogenic syncope, orthostatic volume depletion, and benign positional vertigo. Obtaining a proper history is a crucial step in appropriate diagnosis and therapy.

Frequency, Duration, and Timing

Determine how many events there have been, how often they occur, and how long they last. Symptoms lasting for a few seconds may be caused by simple isolated ectopy, whereas those lasting for long periods may involve sustained arrhythmias. Ask the patient whether there has been a change in frequency, duration, or severity. Recent worsening of an arrhythmia should lead to a more aggressive approach. A relationship with menstrual cycles, circadian rhythms, meals, micturition, coughing, or defecation may indicate the presence of a hormonal or an autonomic imbalance. Episodes that occur at rest may not have the same etiology or may not respond to the same therapy as those for episodes that occur with exertion. For example, many exertional arrhythmias, irrespective of location or mechanism, are often suppressed by beta-blockers.

Symptoms

Thoroughly discuss with the patient the symptoms involved with the episodes (see below). Symptoms that begin before an arrhythmia may indicate a secondary cause, such as ischemia. Symptoms that begin after an episode, especially when they do not occur with every episode, imply that they are an epiphenomenon. Most arrhythmias are worsened by exertion, including bradyarrhythmias. Rest and recumbence usually improve the symptoms of arrhythmias. If a person feels better when he or she stands or moves, this may point to either orthopnea or anxiety. Many people (most frequently those with re-entrant SVT) are able to initiate or terminate their arrhythmias with the use of vagal and nonvagal maneuvers.

Documentation

If any episodes have been documented, obtain the records, including ECGs, Holter monitors, and EPS. "History" of a condition is not documentation. It is common for patients to have a history of arrhythmias that have never been diagnosed by EPS or, in some cases, have never been documented at all. If a witness is available, ask them what happened; often the patient will have amnesia or altered perceptions of the event. Pseudoseizures and volitional fainting rarely are associated with significant trauma, whereas true syncope often is.

Medications

Obtain a list of all medications, dosages, and schedules. Examine the list for drugs that may induce bradyarrhythmia, tachyarrhythmia, hypotension, or torsades de pointes. Recent changes or additions to medications are very important. Ask specifically about over-the-counter medications, herbal remedies or teas, and oral contraceptives. Some Chinese herbal remedies contain cardiac glycosides, and many energy supplements contain sympathomimetic agents. Discuss drug allergies and intolerance.

General

Evaluate the patient for noncardiac medical problems that could explain episodes or complicate therapy, such as thyroid or pulmonary disease.

Definitions of Symptoms

The variability in the perception of symptoms is matched by the variability in description. Most people do not know the true definitions of the words often used to describe their symptoms. When a patient presents to a physician and reports symptoms, it is important to discuss the symptoms using the patient's language, and not medical terms, to avoid misunderstanding. For instance, a patient may complain of "falling out," which may mean dizziness to the patient but syncope to the doctor. Below is a partial list of common complaints often, but not exclusively, associated with arrhythmias.

Palpitations

The most commonly described symptom of arrhythmia is palpitations. They are defined as an unusual, often unpleasant, sensation of one's heart beating. The definition does not imply either bradycardia or tachycardia, nor does it describe regularity or irregularity, both of which should be determined. The most common causes are sinus tachycardia for regular palpitations, and simple premature beats for irregular palpitations. Atrial fibrillation is a common cause of sustained irregular palpitations. Many patients with palpitations are found to be in a regular sinus rhythm without any rhythm abnormalities. Documenting the presence of an arrhythmia is paramount to further evaluation or therapy. It is important to classify palpitations as regular or irregular. Regular palpitations have only mild beat-to-beat variability. There are two types of irregular palpitations; regularly irregular palpitations have repetitive grouped beating as in bigeminy, and irregularly irregular palpitations have no set pattern, as in AF. Tapping examples of these rhythms on a table for the patient is often helpful.

Syncope and Near-Syncope

Syncope is defined as an actual loss of consciousness with or without observation. The presence of physical signs, such as trauma, is supportive. Seizure activity, tongue biting, and/or incontinence do not rule out a cardiac cause of syncope, although they do increase the likelihood of a primary neurologic event. Seizures can occur in any condition that decreases cerebral blood flow, including vasovagal events, bradycardia, or nonsustained rapid tachyarrhythmias. One should be able to differentiate syncope from near-syncope and aborted sudden-death episodes (cardiopulmonary resuscitation [CPR] survivors). The majority of people experience some amnesia with their syncopal episodes. The symptoms prior to syncope may be the clue to its etiology. Syncope without prodromal symptoms appears to be more common in bradyarrhythmic events than in tachyarrhythmic ones. Directly question witnesses whenever possible to assess the patient's symptoms just prior to the event. A history of physical activity, the time of day, fluid intake, mental stress, and positional changes are important. The uncommon causes of syncope should also be considered. Syncope associated with postmicturition syndrome, post-tussive syndrome, pulmonary embolism, and pheochromocytoma all present with bradycardia and hypotension (vagal). Near-syncope describes severe episodes of dizziness, lightheadedness, or fatigue that impair activity (the person must sit or lie down) but do not result in loss of consciousness. Ask the patient to describe their symptoms, for example, "What do you mean by dizziness?"

Angina, or Chest Pain

Many people complain of chest discomfort during rapid tachycardia without underlying coronary disease or ventricular dysfunction. Discomfort secondary to ischemia often results in infarct if the ischemia is prolonged and goes untreated. It is uncommon for someone with critical coronary disease to tolerate a very rapid tachycardia for an extended period of time, without degenerating into VF. Hemodynamic stability in an episode of rapid tachycardia (HR $\geq$180) is often a sign of less severe disease. Chest discomfort prior to the onset of an arrhythmia may indicate that the arrhythmia was secondary to ischemia, whereas symptoms starting after the arrhythmia imply that the ischemia is secondary.

Dyspnea

Dyspnea is defined as an unpleasant awareness of one's breathing. It does not require respiratory insufficiency or true shortness of breath. Hyperventilation is usually associated with dyspnea. To avoid miscommunication, the physician should attempt to classify the symptoms as dyspnea on exertion, periodic shortness of breath, postural nocturnal dyspnea, or orthopnea.

Diaphoresis

Diaphoresis is defined as hot or cold sweats. Cardiogenic diaphoresis is usually described as cold. It is a manifestation of vagal tone that may occur during ischemic, arrhythmic, or neurocardiogenic events. Try to obtain estimates of body temperature at the time of the diaphoresis to exclude an infectious etiology. Many hormonal disturbances, most notably hyperthyroidism, pheochromocytoma, and the carcinoid syndrome, are associated with diaphoresis.

Sudden Cardiac Death

Sudden death may be due to primary respiratory failure, massive stroke, primary bradycardia, pulmonary embolism, electromechanical dissociation, or cardiac arrhythmias. For all causes of death, the final heart rhythm is either VF or asystole (or agonal). Sudden cardiac death (SCD) applies only to those patients in whom the arrhythmia was the primary cause of death. The term should be used to describe only those patients with known aborted sudden death episodes (resuscitated arrhythmias, not syncope). The incidence is approximately 400,000 episodes per year, with 80 per cent due to coronary artery disease. (Fifty per cent of these die from tachyarrhythmias.) In one fourth of patients, SCD is the primary manifestation without prior symptoms. In those who are resuscitated, 20 per cent are shown to have had an acute myocardial infarction. The risk of SCD recurrence in 1 year is 25 per cent when SCD was not associated with an acute myocardial infarction, but only 4 per cent when SCD was accompanied by an acute myocardial infarction. Many people with aborted SCD without myocardial infarction have mildly increased myocardial enzymes, possibly related to CPR or defibrillation. Only those episodes with symptoms of ischemia prior to the SCD, or those with massive increases in enzymes, can be ascribed to myocardial infarction. Evaluation should include cardiac catheterization unless coronary anatomy is known. Usually, EPS are performed when SCD was not a complication of an acute myocardial infarction.

Sudden cardiac death is divided into several categories based on the presence and duration of symptoms prior to the episode. For example, a patient with absolutely no prodromal symptoms is different from one that has an episode preceded by anginal discomfort. Most SCD appears to be sustained monomorphic VT that degenerates into VF—primary VF is much less common. Occasionally, SCD follows bradycardia and asystole. The noncardiac causes of SCD include primary respiratory failure and pulmonary embolus. The most common cause of SCD is ischemic heart disease. The causes in younger people include WPW, hypertrophic cardiomyopathy, long QT syndrome, malignant mitral valve prolapse, sarcoidosis, anomalous coronary arteries, and dilated cardiomyopathies. Hypokalemia rarely causes fatal arrhythmias in the absence of underlying cardiac disease or other metabolic derangements.

EVALUATION OF KNOWN OR SUSPECTED ARRHYTHMIA

Unfortunately, not all patients present with ECGs of their arrhythmias in hand; a work-up is usually required. Sometimes a person at high risk will undergo an evaluation to quantify the risk of developing an arrhythmia in the future. Some of the tests used to evaluate complaints of, or risk of, arrhythmias include:

Electrophysiologic Studies (EPS)

The gold standard for the evaluation of re-entrant arrhythmia is EPS. It is the only way of confirming the presence of certain arrhythmias, such as bundle branch reentry or concealed WPW, and it is the most sensitive test for evaluating monomorphic VT in patients at risk (especially those with coronary artery disease). Although EPS are invasive, significant complications from EPS are very infrequent. The sensitivity of EPS is more than 90 per cent for VT in a patient with a prior myocardial infarction but only 60 per cent in one with an idiopathic dilated cardiomyopathy. The sensitivity of EPS for conduction system disease is about 70 per cent. In general, the indications for EPS include the following:

1. Unknown syncope or sudden death, to determine the mechanism
2. Suspected or known VT or SVT, to determine appropriate treatment or quantify risk, especially when catheter ablation of the arrhythmia or cardiac defibrillator implantation is under consideration
3. Known VT or SVT, to test the efficacy of, or proarrhythmia from, a treatment
4. Testing or programming of an implantable cardiac defibrillator
5. Evaluation of SN or AVN function or the level of AVB, if the need for a pacemaker has not been demonstrated by other means
6. Evaluation of SN or AVN function, if a pacemaker is needed, but the optimal pacemaker type or mode cannot be determined by other means

Event Recorder

The earliest event recorders were attached to leads or placed directly on the chest during an event. They had no memory, and the transmission of the single-lead ECG had to be accomplished during the event. Newer models, including smaller, lighter devices about the size of a beeper, use telemetry or Holter-type lead systems as well as wrist recorders on watchbands that do not require separate leads. Some devices can store many events in memory, whereas others can store only one. A person can trigger the recorder during an arrhythmia and can later send the recording to a doctor's office or central station transtelephonically for evaluation. Looping recorders document cardiac electrical events for as long as 45 to 90 seconds. When the device is triggered, those data are placed in permanent storage along with a rhythm strip of 30 to 60 seconds after the trigger. This will often record the onset of an arrhythmia, thereby facilitating the diagnosis. Some devices have programmable alarms for tachycardia and bradycardia; others record asymptomatic events or events during sleep. The usual duration of monitoring is 3 to 4 weeks. Many patients may not wear the lead systems for this length of time because of discomfort (itch) or visibility. Many patients try to attach the leads only when an arrhythmia occurs. Typically, the arrhythmia resolves before the leads are in place. The watch-based devices are the easiest to use, but they may not have the same recording quality as the lead systems and are not compatible with the looping technologies at this time. The weakness of event recorders is that they record single events only. They do not allow for quantification of arrhythmia frequency, and they do not record most asymptomatic rhythms. A negative study does not exclude the possibility of an arrhythmia, especially when no significant symptoms are recorded in the diary. However, if during a recording, a person complains of symptoms similar to their presenting symptoms, and the recordings are normal (sinus rhythm or tachycardia with or without PACs), the likelihood of significant arrhythmia is low.

Holter Monitor

Much of what we know about electrocardiography, including the evidence that tachyarrhythmias, primarily monomorphic VT degenerating into VF, are responsible for most SCD episodes came from Holter recordings. Both the monitors and the analysis software have undergone continuous advancement since Holter designed the original heavy, semiportable monitors. Modern devices record 24 to 48 hours of continuous surface ECG, using either analog or digital acquisition. Most recorders can acquire two or three leads simultaneously. The analysis packages have improved algorithms for differentiating normal depolarizations from premature ones and can often deduce the site of the depolarization. These monitors often have difficulty in analyzing aberrancy and artifact; confirmatory reading by qualified personnel is essential. The advantages of a Holter monitor are its ease of use and ability to record both symptomatic and asymptomatic rhythms. The weakness of these monitors is that they require an arrhythmia to be quite frequent (at least once a day) to enhance the probability of capturing the arrhythmia. The false negativity of a Holter monitor is quite high (fewer than one third of initial Holter recordings are positive) and is a reason for obtaining multiple recordings, using an event recorder, or (in selected cases) proceeding directly to EPS. The clinician must correlate symptoms with the presence or lack of ECG findings. The ability of these monitors to quantify arrhythmia encourages their use in managing some patients with antiarrhythmic therapy. Day-to-day variability in ectopy requires that at least two 24-hour or one 48-hour recording be performed to quantify changes in ectopy. The definitions of adequate ectopy suppression vary considerably.

The indications for use of a Holter as opposed to EPS in the management of arrhythmias provide an ongoing controversy in electrophysiology. In general, re-entrant arrhythmias are better followed with EPS, while those due to automaticity or triggered activity may be followed with Holter monitoring. For re-entrant arrhythmias, only one PVC is needed to initiate a tachycardia. Changes in the frequency of isolated PVCs may not reflect changes in the re-entrant circuit but may indicate changes in triggered activity or automaticity. Holter monitors do not replace hospital-based telemetry for high-risk patients with overt arrhythmias or for the initiation of antiarrhythmic therapy in those with structural heart disease. Some packages allow other forms of analysis, including heart rate variability, signal-averaged ECG (SAECG), and ST-segment analysis.

Signal-Averaged Electrocardiogram

An SAECG looks for evidence of slow ventricular conduction that could be involved in re-entrant VT. This slowed conduction may manifest at the end of a QRS complex as "fractionated late potentials." The SAECG uses the Frank orthogonal (X, Y, Z) lead system. Many QRS complexes are analyzed, and those that match a template QRS complex (designated as the normal QRS by the operator) are then "averaged." This process retains all recurring electrical signals in the QRS but filters out signals made by equipment, environment, or motion artifact, which constitute the background noise seen on surface ECGs. All three leads are summed into an "average" lead, on which further analysis is performed. The physician evaluates three parameters on the SAECG in the "time domain analysis," looking for these late potentials. The filtered QRS duration (which is different from a 12-lead QRS) may be prolonged, there may be an abnormally long period of low-amplitude signal, or the terminal portion of the QRS complex may be of abnormally low amplitude. These last two parameters reflect delayed conduction in an area of myocardium, which may be a substrate for intraventricular re-entry. Conduction system disease (BBB or intraventricular conduction delay) with a widened QRS adversely affects the sensitivity and specificity of time domain analysis. The demarcation between normal and borderline-normal, and borderline-normal and abnormal, must be set for each parameter. Few tests are abnormal in all three parameters. Studies in which only one parameter is abnormal, or in which several parameters are borderline, are difficult to interpret.

Although the SAECG is easy to perform and relatively inexpensive, the lack of consistent parameters for positive-versus-negative SAECG, and moderate sensitivity coupled with low specificity, have hampered the general acceptance of this procedure. No study that used SAECG alone has demonstrated value in stratifying patients according to their risk for sudden death or VT. However, the use of SAECG, in conjunction with Holter monitoring and left ventricular function testing of patients after myocardial infarction, shows promise.

Much of the recent SAECG literature concerns "frequency domain analysis." Impulses moving through regions of impaired conduction have a different electrical frequency spectrum. This is analogous to the change in the speed and character of a sound when it changes from one conduction medium (air) to another (water). Frequency analysis of an SAECG could involve the entire QRS, not just the terminal portion, and could potentially increase the sensitivity. It would be less affected by conduction abnormalities, including RBBB, where SAECG evaluation by time domain analysis is not possible. These theoretical possibilities are intriguing, but have not yet been proved clinically. The predictive accuracy of frequency domain analysis is now under investigation.

Head-Up Tilt Testing

This test is usually employed in the work-up of neurocardiogenic syncope, which is not truly an arrhythmia. Neurocardiogenic syncope reflects abnormal hyperactivity of both the sympathetic and the parasympathetic systems. In most who suffer from this disorder, there is an initial increase in sympathetic tone followed by an excessive parasympathetic overshoot. This overshoot is characterized by severe depression of blood pressure and/or HR. Sinus bradycardia and junctional escape rhythms are common during such episodes. When a person is tilted into the upright position, cardiac output falls as a result of the normal drop in venous return. This drop in cardiac output causes a reflex sympathetic surge. In susceptible people, the surge in sympathetic outflow induces an excessive parasympathetic overshoot that mimics a clinical event. A positive test should reproduce the patient's clinical symptoms. Isoproterenol and other agents are sometimes used to enhance sympathetic tone and to increase the sensitivity of the test, but these agents also decrease the specificity of the test. Appropriate pretest screening decreases the likelihood of a false-positive test result. Interpretation of the literature regarding tilt-testing for syncope is difficult because there is no consensus regarding the optimal protocol or interpretation of the results.

Carotid Massage

The clinician should listen for carotid bruits before performing carotid massage, because there is a small risk of stroke after massage. Massage is performed by rhythmically depressing a carotid sinus for 5 to 10 seconds and then releasing it. The usual response to carotid massage is slowing of the sinus rate and pauses of less than 3 seconds. Junctional escape beats or rhythm is common and normal. A positive carotid massage (consistent with carotid hypersensitivity) is defined as induced pauses of more than 3 seconds without escape beats, and it should correlate with symptoms. The classic response in carotid hypersensitivity is decreased HR plus vasodilatation with a marked drop in blood pressure. Either response alone occurs in about 25 per cent of persons with carotid hypersensitivity. Thus, blood pressure as well as HR should be measured during the massage. A positive test should be correlated with clinical symptomatology. Carotid hypersensitivity alone is not an indication for therapy. Carotid massage may also be used to help diagnose or treat tachycardia (Table 2). Many arrhythmias that involve either the SN or the AVN terminate with carotid massage or other vagal maneuvers. Others may reveal themselves through increased AVB. Carotid massage may also increase retrograde block during VT, causing AV dissociation.

Heart Rate Variability

Heart rate varies with shifts in autonomic tone. Rapid (high-frequency) variations in rate are normally caused by respiratory changes in parasympathetic tone. Longer-lasting (low-frequency) changes in rate are related to alterations in sympathetic tone. Computer-aided analysis of the beat-to-beat variability in HR can distinguish the relative contributions of low-, middle-, and high-frequency variations. Loss of high-frequency variability is seen in high-catecholamine states as well as autonomic dysfunction. Although decreased high-frequency HR variability may be associated with an increased risk of cardiac events, includ-

Table 2. Effect of Vagal Maneuvers on Common Arrhythmias

Sinus tachycardia	Transient slowing of HR, increased AVB, or no response
SART	Termination, increased AVB, or no response
Atrial tachycardia	No response, increased AVB, occasional termination, or rare increase in atrial rate
Atrial fibrillation or flutter	Increased AVB, or no response
PJRT	Termination, increased AVB, or no response
Junctional tachycardia	No response or increased AVB
Ventricular tachycardia	No response, rare termination, may increase AVB
WPW (AVRT)	Termination or no response
AVNRT	Termination or no response
Parasystole	Usually no response

AVNRT = atrioventricular nodal re-entrant tachycardia; PJRT = premature junctional re-entrant tachycardia; SART = sinoatrial re-entrant tachycardia; WPW (AVRT) = Wolff-Parkinson-White syndrome (atrioventricular re-entry tachycardia).

ing arrhythmia and sudden death, not all studies have been reproduced. Investigators do not yet agree on the appropriate definitions for the various frequency components and their physiologic counterparts. Data acquisition and analysis have not yet been standardized, and the reliability of HR variability in people with frequent ectopy needs further study. Heart rate variability may become a useful tool for screening of patients who may be at high risk for cardiac events, but the lack of standardization in data acquisition and analysis limits its current applicability.

Stress Testing

Exercise testing is used to provoke arrhythmias, test therapeutic efficacy, or test for a proarrhythmic response to drugs (especially with class Ic antiarrhythmic agents). It can be used to maximize rate-responsive pacemaker function. The exertional change in HR may reveal chronotropic incompetence or help set the rate cutoffs for an antitachycardia pacemaker or implantable defibrillator. Stress testing may also be used to look for an inducible arrhythmogenic substrate, such as ischemia.

Pharmacologic Testing

Propranolol and atropine may be used to create pharmacologic autonomic block. This block permits evaluation of SN and AVN function without autonomic influence. Adenosine has been used to evaluate SN function and to detect weakly conducting APs. Isoproterenol, epinephrine, and phenylephrine all have been used to induce catecholamine-sensitive arrhythmias with or without invasive EPS.

DIAGNOSIS OF MANIFEST ARRHYTHMIA

Nonelectrocardiographic Diagnosis of Arrhythmias

History

A prior history of arrhythmia is helpful but should not be considered an absolute diagnosis. It is not uncommon for a person to have multiple arrhythmias. For example, there is an association between atrial flutter and both AF and AVNRT. People with a prior history of myocardial infarction, age above 35 years, or congestive heart failure are more likely to present with VT than SVT with aberrancy.

If a patient has a well-documented history of SVT or VT, and the ECG tracings are similar to previous ones or consistent with the previous diagnosis, the rhythms are probably the same. Remember, however, that the previous diagnosis may not have been correct, and there are frequent reports of VT mimicking the morphology of a preexisting SVT. A history of WPW increases the likelihood of AVRT (orthodromic with aberrancy or antidromic) as the cause of a wide-complex tachycardia.

Some forms of congenital heart disease, corrected or uncorrected, have been associated with cardiac arrhythmias. Ebstein's anomaly of the tricuspid valve is associated with both WPW and VT. Patients with tetralogy of Fallot are subject to both VT and atrial flutter. Familial arrhythmias and/or SCD is associated with the congenital long QT syndromes, hypertrophic cardiomyopathy, and WPW.

Physical Examination

The physical examination may be helpful in arrhythmia diagnosis. It can supplement a history in an unconscious patient. Regular cannon A waves in the jugular venous pulse, caused by the right atrium contracting against a closed tricuspid valve, may be due to SVT or VT if there is a consistent block (e.g., 2:1, 3:1). However, the irregular occurrence of such waves is a sign of AV dissociation and points toward a diagnosis of VT (or rarely junctional tachycardia). In the absence of an irregular rhythm, only mild respiratory variability is seen with S_1 during a supraventricular rhythm, except when there is an underlying process that accentuates the respiratory variability, such as pericardial tamponade or restriction. Variability is commonly seen when the rhythm is irregular or when atrial depolarization is intermittent, as in VT with retrograde AVB.

Vagal Maneuvers

There are several nonpharmacologic methods for enhancing vagal (parasympathetic) tone that will often terminate tachycardias involving the SN and AVN (see Table 2). These maneuvers occasionally terminate other rhythms but usually result in increased AVB. An ECG rhythm strip should be obtained during vagal maneuvers (pharmacologic or nonpharmacologic) to document any changes in rhythm.

Nonpharmacologic Maneuvers

The two most common maneuvers, the Valsalva maneuver and carotid sinus massage, are often performed by patients themselves, to terminate their tachycardia episodes. The Valsalva maneuver is performed by taking a breath and bearing down as if to defecate. The effects of the maneuver are usually seen several seconds later in phase IV of the Valsalva maneuver. (Carotid sinus massage is described in an earlier section of this article.) Often, the response to carotid massage is enhanced by concurrently performing the Valsalva maneuver. The diving reflex is elicited by placing a plastic bag filled with ice water on the face. The cough or gag response, which is typically elicited with a tongue depressor, causes direct vagal stimulation. Pressing indirectly on the eyeball through gauze and a closed lid often causes significant vagal response, but this maneuver should be avoided in the elderly, diabetics, or people who suffer from glaucoma. The Müller maneuver is performed by taking a deep inspiration against a closed glottis, often with a straw.

Pharmacologic Maneuvers

There are two pharmacologic agents commonly used to enhance vagal tone: edrophonium and adenosine. Edrophonium enhances cholinergic activity in the heart. Its effects are similar to those of the vagal maneuvers. Adenosine has several modes of action in the heart, but its primary antiarrhythmic effects, and on both SN and AVN function, involve activation of the same acetylcholine receptor that is stimulated by the vagus. The effects of adenosine are therefore similar to those of edrophonium but are more pronounced and of shorter duration. Degeneration of arrhythmias and hemodynamic compromise requiring resuscitation have been documented with the use of adenosine.

Electrocardiographic Diagnosis of Arrhythmias

There are no perfect algorithms for arrhythmia analysis. The following method of analysis is useful but may not be effective in every situation. With some patients, it is easier for the physician to determine the dominant rhythm by analyzing P waves. With others, the rhythm of the QRS complex is more important. Automated ECG analysis is useful but is notably weak in the evaluation of rapid tachycardias and rhythms with marked first-degree AVB. ECGs with P waves buried in QRS complexes, or that cause pseudo-BBB, may defy automated or manual analysis. At the outset, the clinician must determine the amount of time available for analysis. Do not analyze a complex arrhythmia with only one lead unless absolutely necessary. A 12-lead ECG is preferred, and on most telemetry systems, the lead can easily be switched among limb leads and some of the precordial leads.

Alternative ECG Leads

The standard 12-lead ECG is often not sufficient for detection of P waves or analysis of their rhythm. The unipolar electrodes of the precordial leads may be used to search for P waves by moving them around the chest (Lewis leads). The clinician may obtain atrial recordings with the use of an esophageal electrode or epicardial pacing wires (post–cardiac surgery patient), or intra-atrial recordings from an intravascular pacing electrode. These electrodes can be attached to any precordial lead, such as V_1 or V_2. Sometimes, the best recordings are obtained by attaching the electrodes to the right and left arm leads. A 2:1 A:V ratio implies that the rhythm is SVT with 2:1 AVB. The reverse is true for VT. Carotid massage or pharmacologic AVB should be used when a 1:1 A-V relationship is seen. Complex arrhythmias that involve multiple morphologies, levels of block, and competing foci are difficult to diagnosis. To simplify this process, first attempt to discern the dominant rhythm, then diagnose the irregularities.

Evaluate the ECG

Obtain a 12-lead ECG to confirm that an arrhythmia exists in multiple leads. Artifact can mimic almost any arrhythmia. Frequently impersonated arrhythmias include AF, atrial flutter, VT (monomorphic or polymorphic VT), asystole, AVB, and VF. Clues that abnormalities are due to artifact include an arrhythmia seen in only one lead, rhythmic electrical activity that does not alter the underlying rhythm, impossibly short spike-to-spike intervals, and lack of a T wave after spike. Most artifact is confined to only a few leads and does not affect an entire 12-lead ECG. A notable exception is the pseudo–atrial flutter wave associated with Parkinson's disease. ECG machines can run at speeds other than 25 mm per second. At 50 mm per second, most rhythms appear to be narrow-complex tachycardia.

Evaluate P Waves

1. If P waves are present, check the rate and regularity of P-P intervals
2. P wave morphology—sinus or ectopic, unifocal or multifocal
3. Search for hidden P waves in T wave, ST segment, flutter waves in QRS (pseudo-RBBB); any regular rhythm between 100 and 150 BPM may be atrial flutter with 2 or 3:1 AVB

Evaluate QRS Complex

1. QRS rate and regularity
2. QRS morphology—bundle branch and/or fascicular block, intraventricular conduction delay, Q waves, hypertrophy, electrolyte abnormalities, drug effects
3. QRS duration (normal $\leq$0.10, narrow $\leq$0.12, wide $>$0.12, very wide $\geq$0.16)

Evaluate AV Conduction

1. Mark all P wave and QRS complexes; determine atrial and ventricular rates, PR and RP intervals (are they constant?)
2. Is there AV association? PR intervals consistent with AV conduction; determine AV conduction ratio, A = V, AVB (A > V), VAB (V > A), AV dissociation
3. Is pre-excitation present? PR interval (short), QRS (delta wave, BBB)
4. Look for concealed conduction

Evaluate Premature Depolarizations

1. QRS Width
   Narrow = PAC or PJC
   Wide = PVC or aberrant PAC or PJC
2. Is there a P wave before the premature complex? Also look at T-wave contour.
   "No" = PJC or PVC
   "Yes"
   PR ≥ baseline rhythm, most likely PAC
   PR < baseline but > 0.12, PAC if QRS is narrow, PVC if QRS is wide
   PR < 0.12, PJC or PVC is present
3. Frequency (per hour) and complexity of premature complexes

Narrow-Complex Tachycardia

Tachycardia (Greater Than 100 BPM)

Regular Tachycardia

Evaluate the P-wave morphology and relationship to the QRS. Sinus tachycardia is the most common reason for narrow-complex tachycardia. Atrial flutter with 2:1 AVB is the most common nonsinus rhythm in the range of 140 to 150 BPM (see Fig. 9*A* to *D*). In the common form of AVNRT, the P wave is inverted in the inferior leads and is often inside the QRS or at the beginning of the ST segment (see Fig. 10). In orthodromic AVRT, the P-wave morphology is variable, depending on the AP location, and may be seen in the late ST segment or T wave (see Fig. 18). In PJRT, there is a retrograde P wave midway between QRS complexes. In the uncommon form of AVNRT, there is a retrograde P wave less than 200 msec before the QRS. In AT, any P-wave morphology is possible, although it is usually upright in most leads, with a variable relationship to the conducted QRS. Rare episodes of VT are narrow-complex (see Fig. 13).

Regularly Irregular Tachycardia

Most likely this is a regular SVT (AT, atrial flutter) with AVB. It cannot be a macrore-entrant arrhythmia involving the AVN (AVRT or AVNRT).

Irregularly Irregular Tachycardia

Most likely this is AT with rapid ventricular response. If multiple P-wave morphologies are present, consider MAT.

Wide-Complex Tachycardia

Causes

The most common form of aberrancy, especially at younger ages, is BBB. Right bundle branch block is more common than left bundle branch block, because the right bundle has a higher refractory period than the left and blocks at a lower rate. An intraventricular conduction delay is commonly seen in patients with cardiomyopathies, ventricular hypertrophy, or ischemic scar. This type of aberrancy occurs only at very rapid rates, just before a rhythm degenerates. WPW causes wide complexes only when conduction is over the AP, and not the AVN, unless there is concomitant BBB (see Fig. 8). The other causes of QRS prolongation include acute ischemia, hyperkalemia, and drug effects. Some antiarrhythmics, such as flecainide, may cause marked QRS widening, leading to misdiagnosis of SVT as VT.

Tachycardia (Greater Than 100 BPM)

Regularly Irregular Tachycardia

This is most likely atrial flutter or atrial tachycardia with AVB.

Irregularly Irregular Tachycardia, Monomorphic

Typically, this represents AF with a rapid ventricular response and aberrancy or conduction over an accessory pathway (see Fig. 16). This is an important rhythm to diagnose appropriately, as the usual medications for rapid AF may destabilize patients with WPW, leading to VF. Degeneration of AF to VF in WPW has been documented with the use of digoxin, verapamil, and adenosine. Ventricular fibrillation is faster than other rhythms and should be self-evident.

Irregularly Irregular Tachycardia, Polymorphic

Atrial fibrillation may present as a rapid polymorphic wide-complex tachycardia when there is intermittent aberrancy, or in WPW syndrome with competing conduction between the AP and either the AVN or other APs. Polymorphic VT may be due to torsade de pointes or ischemia or may be idiopathic. It is sometimes difficult to distinguish WPW with AF from torsades with a short ECG strip. However, the tendency of torsades to self-terminate is usually apparent in a longer recording (see Figs. 5*D* and 16). Torsades are usually slower (140 to 220 BPM) than the other types of polymorphic VT (180 to 300 BPM). All types of polymorphic VT may be induced with closely coupled PVCs, but torsades have a stronger association with bradycardia and bigeminal patterns (short-long-short sequences). Rarely, one can see AV dissociation with AF in the upper chambers, and VT in the ventricles. The AF may intermittently conduct down the AVN, making the rhythm polymorphic and irregular. It may be misdiagnosed as either AF alone or polymorphic VT.

Regular Tachycardia

Physicians have been attempting to define ECG criteria that will quickly and reliably differentiate between VT and SVT with aberrancy or pre-excitation (WPW). Criteria have been developed by many cardiac electrophysiologists, including Marriott, Wellens, Josephson, Kindwall, and Brugada, that can have a high accuracy if used appropriately (Fig. 21). The failure of ECG criteria is due, in small part, to the ability of various SVTs to mimic VT, or vice versa, but is primarily due to physicians' lack of knowledge concerning the criteria and how to implement them. All of the standard ECG criteria are flawed because they have not been tested in patients with pre-existing conduction abnormalities, medications that alter conduction, or WPW. The atrial flutter in Figure 19 satisfies at least two of the criteria for VT listed below. Information gathering may be time-consuming and is not always helpful. *When in doubt treat the condition as VT and diagnose it at a later time.* Treating an SVT as though it were VT is much less dangerous than treating VT as SVT. Use of a drug such as procainamide will be effective in most cases of VT and many cases of SVT. This type of drug is also safe and effective in the treatment of wide-complex arrhythmias in WPW. *Use of verapamil results in hemodynamic compromise that requires resuscitation in more than 40 per cent of patients with VT.*

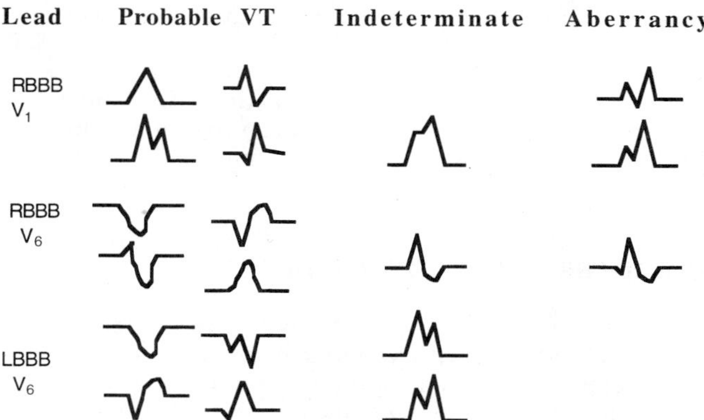

Figure 21. Morphologies associated with ventricular tachycardia and aberrancy. (Modified from Wellens, H.J., Marriott, H.J.L.) See text for explanation.

If Any of the Following Criteria Are Met, There Is a Strong Likelihood of VT

1. Concordance (also known as absence of RS complex) is loss of the normal transition of the QRS from downgoing to upright as it marches across the precordium. The QRS complexes are either all upright (only R wave) or all downgoing (QS complex; see Fig. 14). Pre-excited tachycardia in WPW is never associated with negative concordance.

2. Impaired ventricular conduction, as demonstrated by an RS of 0.10 or more (from start of R wave to nadir of S wave) in any precordial lead. Less specific is the use of absolute criteria for QRS duration, such as criteria of 0.14 or more for RBBB-morphology and 0.16 or more for LBBB-morphology tachycardias. Impulses conducted down an AP in WPW may be extremely wide and bizarre.

3. AV dissociation is extremely rare with SVT with aberrancy and is the most specific criterion for VT (see Figs. 12 to 14). There is often a problem finding P waves during tachycardia. Sometimes the VT has VA-associated conduction retrogradely up the AVN, which becomes the dominant atrial rhythm. Complete VA block is common and allows the atrial rhythm to remain sinus. When there is complete VA block, occasional supraventricular impulses may conduct down the AVN, resulting in fusion complexes. Therefore, these complexes are a sign of AV dissociation. Be wary of PVCs occurring during VT, mimicking supraventricular fusion beats. Often the VA conduction is not 1:1 but rather 2:1 or may manifest a retrograde Wenckebach block. When a patient is stable, and one is having difficulty in finding P waves on a standard ECG, consider obtaining atrial recordings, as described under the section on alternative ECG leads. In VT, when the QRS complexes occur more frequently than the atrial ($V > A$), the diagnosis is VT. When the atrial complexes are more frequent ($A > V$), the diagnosis is likely to be SVT. When they are equal, it can be either. The use of vagal maneuvers or adenosine may help by increasing antegrade or retrograde AVB.

4. Morphologic criteria for differentiating VT from SVT with aberrancy have been used for many years. Unfortunately, they have been evaluated only in patients for whom there were no baseline intraventricular conduction delays (WPW, Q wave myocardial infarction, antiarrhythmics, etc.). Figure 21 shows the classic morphologies arranged as probable VT, indeterminate, and probable aberrancy. A RBBB tachycardia that satisfies only morphology criteria in only one lead should be considered indeterminate. The morphology criteria should be used with caution because of low specificity.

5. Fusion beats are occasional narrow (narrower) complex beats that occur during a tachycardia and may represent intermittent AV conduction. PVCs can cause narrow fusion complexes when they originate on the side of the BBB.

6. Any patient who cannot be proven to have SVT should be treated as if he or she had VT (see Fig. 13).

CONCLUSION

A patient may present with a manifest arrhythmia or with history or symptoms of an arrhythmia or to ascertain the risk of developing an arrhythmia. Evaluation of patients with symptoms referable to an arrhythmia depends on the specific symptoms, and the patient's underlying heart disease. Clinicians should aggressively evaluate syncope, to avoid a risk of sudden death. Those with lesser symptoms, and no underlying cardiac disease, are at lower risk for severe arrhythmia. A negative Holter recording does not exclude the presence of significant arrhythmia. Event recorders may be helpful, but they can be difficult to use and usually record only symptomatic arrhythmias. Invasive electrophysiologic studies are the most sensitive and specific tests for re-entrant tachycardias but are less sensitive for automatic and triggered arrhythmias. Risk stratification for the development of cardiac arrhythmias is performed primarily in patients with dilated or ischemic cardiomyopathies or with familial arrhythmia syndromes or as part of routine post–myocardial infarction care. Stratification includes the estimation of myocardial function and coronary artery patency. The presence of abnormal ventricular conduction may be evaluated with the use of single-averaged ECG or with EPS. Holter monitors can be used to quantify ventricular ectopy in patients with cardiomyopathies.

When a patient is hemodynamically stable and without significant symptoms, analysis of a manifest arrhythmia may be undertaken at a leisurely pace to maximize accuracy. However, when the patient is symptomatic or hemodynamically unstable or may decompensate if the arrhythmia persists, then treatment should be initiated with only a cursory triage evaluation to guide therapy. If the patient's condition is stable, additional information may be gleaned from the history and physical examination, which may confirm or modify the initial diagnosis.

Significant changes have occurred in the diagnosis of and therapy for arrhythmias over the past 10 years. Pharmacologic therapy, which was once the mainstay of treatment, has decreased in popularity. This decline contrasts with a rise in the use of catheter ablation, implantable defibrillators, and arrhythmia surgery. Although empirical antiarrhythmic therapy is difficult to justify at this time, guided therapy can be both safe and effective in selected populations for specific arrhythmias.

VALVULAR HEART DISEASE

By Thomas M. Bashore, M.D.,
Steven E. Hearne, M.D.,
and J. Kevin Harrison, M.D.
Durham, North Carolina

Valvular heart disease remains a formidable challenge in cardiovascular medicine despite many recent advances in both medical and surgical therapy. Younger patients with valvular heart disease often face a lifetime of medical and/or surgical procedures involving significant risks. In women of childbearing age, issues regarding the use of warfarin sodium (Coumadin), angiotensin-converting enzyme inhibitors, and other drug therapies complicate pregnancy. This contrasts with the problems experienced by the elderly—valve repair or replacement puts these patients at high risk for substantial morbidity or mortality, which is often related to comorbid problems that accompany the aging process. It is especially critical to identify patients with valvular disease before irreversible myocardial injury or endocarditis intervenes. Advances in echocardiography have substantially refined the diagnosis of patients with valvular disease, and many new therapeutic options are now available. This article focuses on modern concepts of identifying and following patients with valvular disease.

GENERAL CONCEPTS

There are several general concepts that clinicians should keep in mind when assessing the patient with valvular heart disease.

- Patients typically become symptomatic only when atrial pressures increase. These pressures generally increase because of diastolic dysfunction. In most patients, therefore, symptoms are due to diastolic failure.
- In stenotic valvular disease, diastolic failure typically occurs first and causes symptoms prior to loss of systolic function.
- In regurgitant valvular disease, systolic failure generally precedes diastolic failure. Therefore, symptoms may be a late phenomenon, occurring only after systolic dysfunction is manifested.

These clinical tenets provide a guide for following patients with either stenotic or regurgitant valvular disease. In aortic stenosis or mitral stenosis, diastolic failure means an increase in pulmonary venous pressure. This occurs when left ventricular diastolic dysfunction accompanies the outflow obstruction imposed by the stenotic aortic valve or when there is progressive mitral valve obstruction. Symptoms emerge in almost all patients before any loss of systolic function occurs.

In the case of regurgitant valvular disease, the problem is that left ventricular systolic failure will usually precede the loss of diastolic dysfunction. This means that left ventricular systolic function may be declining while the patient has few if any complaints. Thus, the clinician must look for markers other than symptoms to appreciate the decline of systolic function and to avoid delay in referral for valve replacement. The single best parameter to follow in patients with regurgitant valvular disease is the left ventricular end-systolic volume (or dimension by echocardiography) because the ejection fraction (EF) and other common measures of systolic function are maintained in the face of altered loading conditions despite the loss of contractile function.

PRINCIPLES OF HEMODYNAMICS

A few basic concepts of hemodynamics are critical in evaluating patients with valvular heart disease. They are best explained by using the pressure-volume relationship defined in a simplified and clinically useful manner.

Figure 1 shows a pressure-volume loop. It represents a single heartbeat. Note several key features. The loop rotates counterclockwise. The mitral valve closes (MC on the

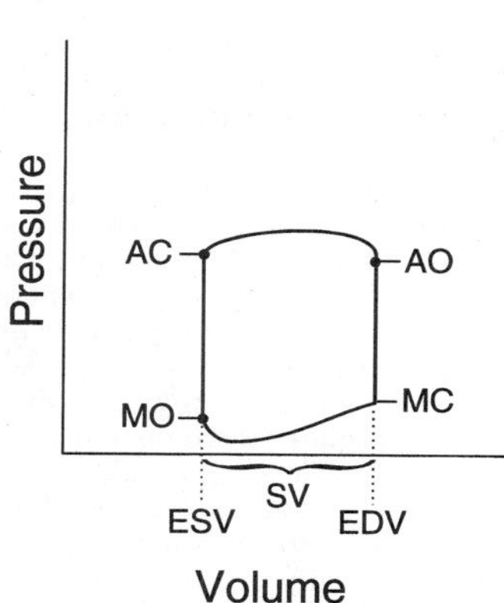

Figure 1. *The normal pressure-volume relationship.* A single heartbeat is represented. When systole is initiated, the mitral valve closes (MC), isovolumic contraction occurs and, finally, the aortic valve opens (AO). The heart ejects blood until diastole results in aortic valve closure (AC) followed by isovolumic relaxation and mitral valve opening (MO). Diastolic filling then occurs until systole is again initiated. Note that the limits of the loop are the end-systolic volume (ESV) and the end-diastolic volume (EDV), respectively. The difference (width of the loop) equals the stroke volume. The width (stroke volume) divided by the end-diastolic volume defines the ejection fraction.

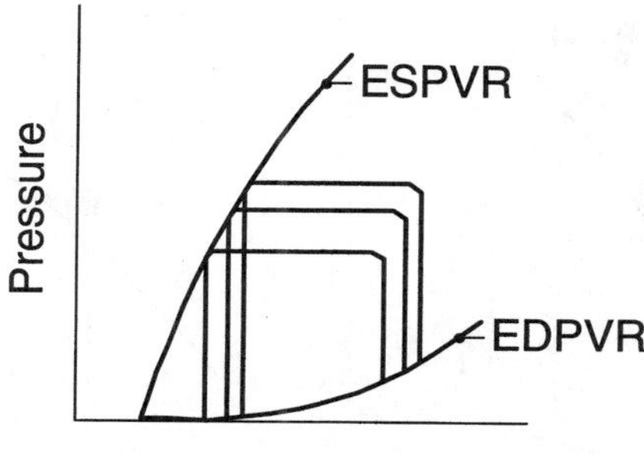

Figure 2. *Definitions of systolic and diastolic function.* Altering loading conditions results in a series of consecutive loops of progressively smaller size. Isochronous lines can be drawn at intervals, with each line representing elastance. Eventually a maximal slope is achieved. An upper limit represented by the end-systolic pressure-volume points derived from these series of loops can be used to define systolic function. A line connecting the end-diastolic point of each loop can be used to represent diastolic function. Each heartbeat must occur within these boundaries of intrinsic systolic function (the end-systolic pressure-volume relationship [ESPVR]) and diastolic function (the end-diastolic pressure-volume relationship [EDPVR]).

figure) at the beginning of systole, and an isovolumic period occurs prior to aortic valve opening (AO on the figure). The heart then ejects blood until diastole ensues. Aortic closure (AC on the figure) then occurs, followed by an isovolumic phase until the mitral valve opens (MO on the figure). The heart then fills, initially rapidly and then gradually, during diastole until systole resumes and the whole process begins anew. Looking carefully at the loop that is created, note that the boundaries of the loop along the x-axis represent the *end-systolic volume* and the *end-diastolic volume,* respectively. The width of the loop is therefore the *stroke volume*. The ratio of the stroke volume to the end-diastolic volume is therefore the more commonly expressed EF.

To understand what happens at different loading conditions, an expression of systolic and diastolic function must first be understood. If either preload or afterload alone is altered quickly, the heart volumes and pressures will change predictably. For example, if preload is suddenly dropped, each successive pressure-volume loop will change as shown in Figure 2. A series of ever smaller pressure-volume loops are thus drawn, each representing a beat with less preload. If one draws a line connecting the 10-msec point on each loop, the 20-msec point on each loop, and so forth, a series of lines can be drawn and connected as shown. The slope of these lines represents elastance. Eventually a maximal slope is reached (the maximal elastance or Emax), which roughly connects the end-systolic pressure-volume points of all the loops. This maximal slope can be thought to represent ventricular contractility, as it is relatively independent of loading conditions. If one similarly connects the end-diastolic pressure-volume points, a line emerges that effectively represents the diastolic limits for the ventricle. At any one time, the pressure-volume loop of the heart is virtually trapped within these boundaries of systolic contraction and diastolic compliance.

This is similarly emphasized in Figure 3. When an afterload is applied to the heart, the pressure-volume loop gets taller and the width of the loop narrows. This means that applying an afterload to the heart reduces stroke volume (the width of the loop) and consequently the EF. This occurs with no change in contractility (no change in the maximal line of contractility) or diastole (no change in the end-diastolic compliance line). In aortic stenosis, the EF may thus be reduced, yet contractility and diastolic

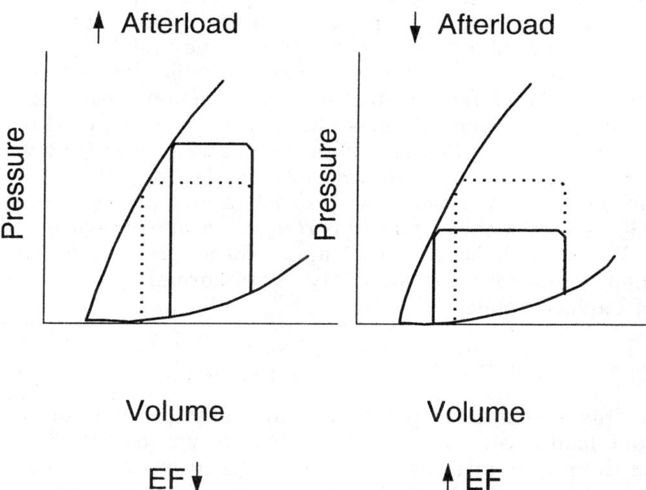

Figure 3. *The effects of loading conditions on measures of cardiac function.* The normal heart can be thought to operate within the boundaries of the end-systolic and end-diastolic pressure-volume lines. In the left panel, increased afterload (such as occurs in aortic stenosis) results in increased pressure and a decrease in the stroke volume (and the ejection fraction) without altering contractility or diastolic function. Reduced afterload is shown in the right panel (such as in mitral regurgitation), where an increase in the stroke volume (and the ejection fraction [EF]) occurs but there is no intrinsic alteration in systolic or diastolic function. Valvular disease produces hemodynamic overload that alters commonly used measures of heart function such as the EF.

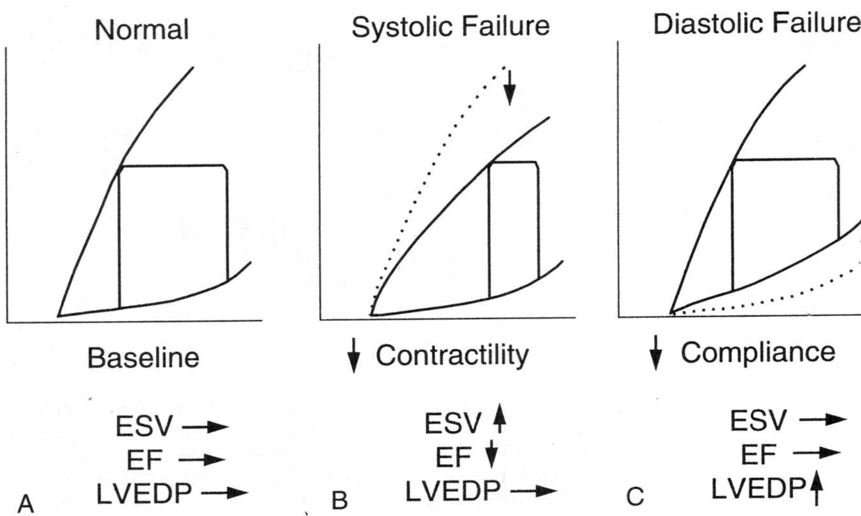

Figure 4. *The result of pure systolic or diastolic failure. A,* The normal heart is represented within the confines of the end-systolic pressure-volume line (representing systolic function) and the end-diastolic pressure-volume line (representing diastolic function). If contractility declines *(B),* the line of contractility (end-systolic pressure-volume relationship) falls. This results in both a reduced EF and an increase in the end-systolic volume. If diastolic dysfunction occurs *(C),* the end-diastolic pressure-volume relationship curve rises more steeply, and diastolic pressures are higher for any given left ventricular volume (the compliance is reduced). These changes can occur together or separately. Thus, systolic failure can occur without diastolic failure and vice versa. ESV = end-systolic volume; EF = ejection fraction; LVEDP = left ventricular end-diastolic pressure.

function remain intact. In mitral regurgitation, the opposite occurs. In this condition, there is afterload reduction, and the stroke volume is increased as the ventricle ejects more blood and the end-systolic volume becomes smaller. This means the EF is increased. Again, however, this occurs with no actual change in contractility or diastolic function of the heart.

Now suppose that systolic function actually does worsen. This will be reflected by a decline in the slope of the end-systolic pressure-volume relationship (Fig. 4). This results in two important changes to the pressure-volume loop. First, the EF will decrease and, second, the end-systolic volume will increase. These are critical observations that will be discussed later. For instance, in chronic aortic insufficiency or mitral regurgitation, an EF that exceeded the normal value (see Fig. 3) may decrease but still be within normal limits when the patient is initially seen. However, there is an obligatory increase in the end-systolic volume when contractility worsens. This observation becomes the clue to appreciating when systolic dysfunction is occurring.

On the flip side, the diastolic pressure-volume relationship may worsen (become more steep) and systolic function may be unaffected, as shown in Figure 4. This latter situation is seen in patients with heart failure and a normal EF, especially those with hypertrophic cardiomyopathy.

When the heart is placed under these afterload or preload stresses from related valvular abnormalities, the law of Laplace applies:

$$\text{Wall Tension} \propto \frac{\text{Pressure} \times \text{Radius}^3}{\text{Wall Thickness}}$$

This means that whenever an increased pressure or volume load is placed on the heart, the response of the myocardium is to increase mass. Since the heart cannot make more myocytes after birth, it responds to *systolic* stress by laying down sarcomeres side-by-side within the myocyte. Thus, under a pressure overload, the walls become thickened and this reduces wall stress. Conversely, the heart responds to increased volume by laying down sarcomeres end-to-end. This difference is a function of the *diastolic* nature of the *stress* in volume overload conditions, in which the heart becomes much larger in volume and mass but the walls thicken only slightly. The stimulus for hypertrophy of the myocytes under systolic or diastolic stress also stimulates collagen hypertrophy. (There are, in fact, many more collagen cells [fibroblasts] than myocytes in the heart, although they are small relative to muscle cells.) Collagen hypertrophy then contributes to the resulting myocardial stiffness that occurs. The hypertrophied myocyte is also dysfunctional in both its systolic and diastolic performance. In summary, the stimulus for hypertrophy is the abnormal pressure or volume stress placed on the heart by valvular disease.

These two types of hypertrophic responses cause rather different hemodynamic responses (and different pressure-volume loops). As shown in Figure 5, pressure hypertrophy leads to markedly thickened walls, whereas the diastolic pressure-volume loop rises dramatically when compared with that in normal individuals. A small change in cardiac volume creates symptoms resulting from a more rapid rise in diastolic filling pressure than would otherwise be expected.

In acute regurgitation, the sudden increase in volume in the heart chamber that has yet to compensate causes a marked rise in diastolic pressure as shown in Figure 5. In chronic regurgitation, however, the heart compensates by laying sarcomeres end-to-end, and a flat diastolic pressure-volume curve results. In this case, the increased volume is handled well without a rise in filling pressure. Patients with chronic regurgitation may therefore survive for pro-

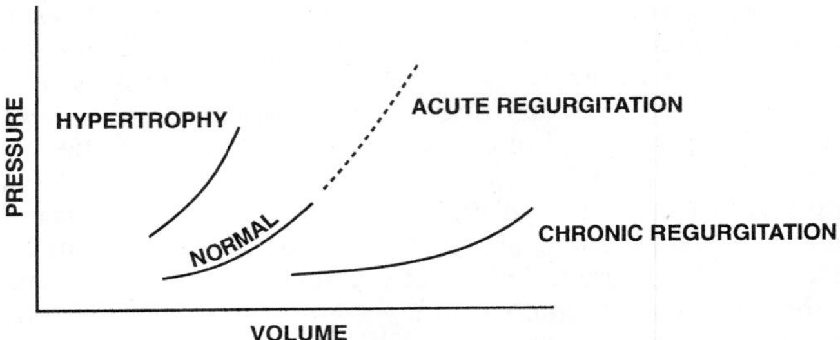

Figure 5. *The effect of valvular disease on the diastolic pressure-volume curve.* In myocardial hypertrophy, with its inherent reduction in left ventricular compliance, the diastolic pressure-volume curve is steeper. This is common in aortic stenosis. In acute regurgitation, the left ventricle has had insufficient time to adapt, and the diastolic pressures rise sharply following the same diastolic curve the heart had been using. In chronic regurgitation, the diastolic pressure-volume curve is flattened. Thus, considerable volume can be present within the heart without increasing diastolic pressure (see text for explanation).

longed periods before congestive symptoms emerge. The clinical result is that diastolic failure may occur much later in regurgitant valvular disease than in stenotic valvular disease.

WHEN TO OPERATE

How does the clinician decide that surgery is appropriate in a patient with valve disease? Recall that symptoms are primarily a function of a rise in diastolic pressure. In *stenotic valvular disease,* the problem is diastolic failure. This can be a direct result of a compromised valve (as in mitral stenosis) or a consequence of the hypertrophy that occurs secondary to valve obstruction (as in aortic stenosis). In both situations, surgery or valvuloplasty should be considered when symptoms emerge. It should be emphasized that symptoms are more important than valve gradients or valve areas in guiding decisions about surgery. This is clinically reasonable because, essentially, diastolic failure always precedes systolic failure in stenotic disorders.

In chronic regurgitant disease, the left ventricular volumes are high, but diastolic pressures are often normal (see Fig. 5). In these diseases (such as aortic insufficiency or mitral regurgitation), symptoms may be minimal for long intervals. Diastolic failure may not become evident until late in the course of disease and long after systolic dysfunction has occurred. Thus, the decision for surgery should be based on *any* evidence of systolic dysfunction in these patients. As noted in Figure 4, once contractility declines, the EF also declines and the end-systolic volume must rise. Because the baseline EF may be higher than normal at the outset in aortic insufficiency or mitral regurgitation, the EF may still be in a normal range (>50 per cent) despite loss of contractility. Serial measures of the EF and the end-systolic volume (or dimensions) provide the clue as to when to operate in chronic mitral or aortic insufficiency. Since the clinician may not have access to serial data when such a patient is first seen, Tables 1 and 2 outline commonly used dimensions and parameters for operating on patients with aortic insufficiency and chronic mitral regurgitation, respectively. The key is not to focus on symptoms or on the EF alone but rather to follow the end-systolic dimensions. As noted previously, as contractility falls, there is an obligatory increase in the end-systolic dimensions. Once end-systolic dimensions reach the 5.0 cm range by echocardiography, the patient with aortic insufficiency or mitral regurgitation should undergo surgery even if no symptoms exist.

Table 1. Valvular Heart Disease: Aortic Insufficiency and No Symptoms—When to Operate

Reduced exercise capacity
Pulmonary hypertension on examination
Chest film-to-cardiothoracic ratio ≥0.60
Echocardiography
  EDDI ≥38 mm/m²
  ESD >50 mm
  EF <60%
  Fractional shortening <25%
Catheterization
  Elevated LVEDP
  Pulmonary hypertension
  EF <50%
  ESVI >60 mL/m²
RNA—? reduced exercise EF response

EDDI = end-diastolic dimension–body surface area; ESD = end-systolic dimension; EF = ejection fraction; LVEDP = left ventricular end-diastolic pressure; ESVI = end-systolic volume index; RNA = radionuclide angiography.

Table 2. Valvular Heart Disease: Chronic Mitral Regurgitation and No Symptoms—When to Operate

Reduced exercise capacity
Abnormal exercise RNA
Pulmonary hypertension on examination
Echocardiography
  ESD >50 mm
  ESD >26 mm/m²
  Fractional shortening <31%
Catheterization
  Elevated LVEDP
  Elevated pulmonary pressure
  Increased RVEDP
  ESVI >60 mL/m²
  EF <50%

ESD = end-systolic dimension; LVEDP = left ventricular end-diastolic pressure; RVEDP = right ventricular end-diastolic pressure; EF = ejection fraction; RNA = radionuclide angiography.

CLINICAL RECOGNITION OF VALVULAR HEART DISEASE

Aortic Stenosis

Natural History and Etiology

Obstruction of the outflow from the left ventricle may occur above the aortic valve (supravalvular), below the valve (discrete or hypertrophic subaortic stenosis), or within the valve itself. Congenital valvular lesions are primarily unicuspid or bicuspid in nature. It has been postulated that in the elderly a tricuspid valve with cusps of unequal size causes abnormal turbulence, which over time results in calcium deposition in the valve cusps because of recurrent valvular injury. Thus, much of the degenerative valvular aortic stenosis seen in the elderly may have begun in a trileaflet valve with cusps of unequal size that existed even when the patient was a child. Rheumatic aortic stenosis can also occur, but it is much less common in the United States and is usually accompanied by aortic insufficiency. In adults, aortic stenosis is primarily related to either a congenitally bicuspid valve or, more frequently, to calcific degeneration of a tricuspid aortic valve. In the adult population, aortic stenosis is generally associated with minimal aortic regurgitation. In calcific aortic stenosis, diabetes and hypercholesterolemia are thought to be risk factors.

Patients with aortic stenosis may be relatively asymptomatic for many years. Those with bicuspid valves typically note symptoms beginning at age 50 to 65 years. Classically, survival averages 2 years once heart failure symptoms emerge, 3 years once syncope is present, and 5 years once angina occurs. More recent experience in the elderly, however, suggests that *any* symptom enhances the risk of accelerated mortality. One symptom may be no more or less important than another in the octagenarian with aortic stenosis.

Symptoms

Symptoms of aortic stenosis are primarily related to the effect of the stenotic aortic valve on the myocardium. As previously noted, when systolic stress is placed on the left ventricle, hypertrophy occurs. This hypertrophy is characterized by the laying down of sarcomeres in a side-to-side manner with the walls becoming markedly thickened. This thickening reduces wall stress but results in a shift in the diastolic pressure-volume curve upward and to the left. Small increases in volume therefore result in large increases in the diastolic pressure. This is reflected clinically as pulmonary congestion.

Initially, symptoms in aortic stenosis almost always occur with exertion. Congestion is not only prominent but angina also occurs because of underperfusion of the endocardium. It is clear that the marked wall thickness results in endocardial underperfusion and a reduction in coronary flow reserve as well as angina that is often indistinguishable from that seen with coronary artery disease. Most patients with angina due to aortic stenosis experience only moderate exertional angina. In addition, patients with aortic stenosis may exhibit presyncope or syncope that is most likely related to stimulation of left ventricular baroreceptors. With exertion, the rise in left ventricular pressure stimulates the baroreceptors to lower peripheral resistance. The decreased afterload results in an increase in cardiac output that causes the left ventricular pressure to rise again. The left ventricular baroreceptors then turn on reflexively, causing further peripheral vasodilatation, and the cycle repeats itself. Without a stenotic aortic valve, the peripheral vasodilatation would reduce left ventricular pressure, and the baroreceptors would be turned off. With the stenotic aortic valve present, however, the peripheral vasodilatation results in increased cardiac output that increases the left ventricular systolic pressure, and the baroreceptors are turned on again. The cycle of baroreceptor stimulation and peripheral vasodilatation eventually produces systemic hypotension, and syncope or presyncope is the result. Occasionally, syncope can also be related to atrial or ventricular arrhythmias, in part because the calcium in the stenotic valve may progress to calcium invasion of the conduction system. Sinus rhythm must be maintained in these hypertrophic ventricles because atrial contribution to cardiac output may be greater than 25 per cent. Thus, atrial fibrillation may lead to considerable reduction in cardiac output and hypotension.

Physical Examination

The normal left ventricle may generate pressures as high as 340 mm Hg. Therefore, the observation of systolic hypertension in a patient with aortic stenosis does not exclude significant aortic valvular disease. In the younger patient, the examination should begin by noting the carotid pulse. Because of the loss of the percussion wave in the carotid pulse, it may appear to rise slowly and be sustained (pulsus parvus et tardus). In the elderly, the upstroke may appear more normal because of reduced compliance of the ascending aorta as elastin is lost with age. As aortic stenosis increases in severity, the carotid pulse pressure may be dramatically decreased because of reduced stroke volume. At times, systolic vibrations resulting from marked turbulence are readily noted in the carotid pulse, the so-called carotid shudder. The jugular venous pulse is typically normal until late in the course of the disease, when right-sided heart failure complicates the picture. Prominent A waves in the jugular venous pulse most likely reflect decreased right ventricular compliance due to ventricular interdependence (especially the sharing of the hypertrophied interventricular septum). The apical examination usually reveals a sustained left ventricular impulse with a readily palpable A wave (the palpable fourth heart sound). Systolic thrills may be felt along the aortic outflow tract.

On auscultation, the first heart sound is usually normal. If the valve is mobile, an early ejection sound may precede the diamond-shaped aortic outflow murmur. The ejection sound is lost once severe aortic stenosis is established. The ejection murmur is generally pronounced, and there is a correlation between the timing of its peak and the severity of stenosis. The later peaking murmur correlates with a greater gradient occurring later in systole (see discussion of invasive findings further on). In most patients, the second heart sound provides a better clue than does the murmur to the severity of aortic stenosis. With an immobile valve, the second heart sound will be markedly diminished or absent. A normal second heart sound virtually excludes severe aortic stenosis. The intensity of the murmur reflects output and poorly reflects severity. Paradoxical splitting of the second heart sound is difficult to detect clinically but is another indication of severe stenosis. An auscultatory fourth heart sound is extremely common, whereas an auscultatory third heart sound should suggest left ventricular failure, except in children.

Because of the known association of a bicuspid valve with aortic coarctation, the clinician should examine the pulses in both arms and relate the brachial pulse to the femoral artery. The loss of the percussion wave in the femoral artery results in a delay in the upstroke of the femoral artery pulse relative to the brachial artery and confirms coarctation.

To help distinguish the murmur of aortic stenosis from that of hypertrophic subaortic stenosis, several maneuvers can be employed. Perhaps the easiest and most reliable is the Valsalva maneuver. During this maneuver, as the left ventricular volume decreases, the murmur of aortic stenosis will decline, whereas the murmur of hypertrophic cardiomyopathy will increase.

Certain high-pitched components of the aortic stenosis murmur are often transmitted to the apex (the Gallaverdin phenomenon), and the murmur sounds like that of mitral regurgitation. To distinguish this murmur from mitral regurgitation, note the presence of an "auscultatory gap" between the first and second heart sounds and the systolic murmur. As shown in Figure 6, an aortic stenosis murmur begins after the first heart sound and ends prior to the second heart sound. These gaps represent the isovolumic contraction and relaxation periods, respectively. In contrast, mitral insufficiency murmurs begin immediately with closure of the mitral valve (first heart sound) and run through the second heart sound until mitral opening occurs. With loss of diastolic performance, eventual pulmonary congestion and finally pulmonary hypertension and signs of right-sided heart failure may ensue. Although severe pulmonary hypertension has been observed rarely in patients with aortic stenosis, this complication is much more common in mitral stenosis.

Noninvasive Evaluation

ELECTROCARDIOGRAM. Although the electrocardiogram (ECG) is not particularly sensitive, 85 per cent of individuals with significant aortic stenosis will meet the criteria for left ventricular hypertrophy. A representative ECG is shown in Figure 7. Progression of ST-T wave abnormalities and the loss of anterior forces (the pseudoinfarction pattern) have been correlated with progression in the severity of the disease. Left atrial enlargement may also occur. Atrial fibrillation generally occurs late. With the loss of the atrial contribution, a drop in cardiac output occurs. Calcific invasion from the valve into the conduction system may cause varying degrees of atrioventricular as well as interventricular conduction block.

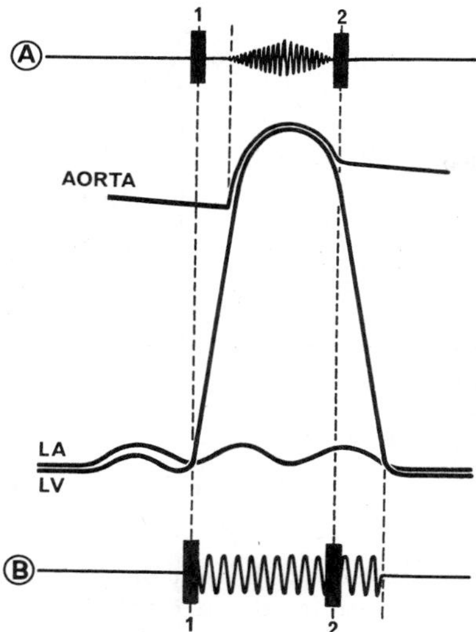

Figure 6. *Aortic stenosis versus mitral regurgitation.* Distinguishing the aortic stenosis murmur *(A)* from the mitral regurgitation murmur *(B)*. Note the auscultatory gap before and after the murmur of aortic stenosis, whereas the murmur of mitral regurgitation begins with the first heart sound and moves through the second heart sound. LA = left atrium; LV = left ventricle.

CHEST FILM. A representative chest film is shown in Figure 8. In aortic stenosis, the heart size is usually normal or only mildly increased. In patients with a bicuspid aortic valve, the aortic jet is often asymmetric, and post-stenotic dilatation of the aorta is commonplace. This may not be seen, however, in elderly patients with a tricuspid stenotic aortic valve and a more centrally directed aortic jet. Calcification can occasionally be detected in the aortic valve. The amount of visible calcification in this valve correlates poorly with the degree of obstruction. As the disease progresses, the left atrium may enlarge and venous hypertension becomes evident.

ECHOCARDIOGRAPHY. This modality provides essentially all the important data needed to make a decision regarding the severity of aortic stenosis (Fig. 9). In patients with aortic stenosis, the aortic valve systolic opening is reduced. Echocardiography can usually distinguish the number of cusps present. The presence of calcium deposition is also obvious. Doppler echocardiography allows the calculation of the left ventricle–aortic pressure gradient with a high degree of accuracy. The maximal gradient described by echocardiography represents the peak instantaneous gradient, which should not be confused with the peak-to-peak gradient or the mean gradient typically reported at catheterization. Using a modified Bernoulli equation, an estimate of the aortic valve area by Doppler and echocardiographic measurements can be made. In most hands, this latter determination is rather gross and not always reliable. The equation relies on measurement of the velocity and area both above and below the aortic valve and the "outflow" area below the valve. The area measurements below the valve are often difficult to define by echocardiography and can result in significant errors in determination of the valve area. The estimated aortic *gradient* itself is more reliable clinically. Color flow or pulsed Doppler reveals turbulence across the valve but adds little except evidence for the coexistence of aortic insufficiency. Echocardiography also provides data regarding aortic root size and the systolic and diastolic status of the left ventricle. Transesophageal echocardiography is most useful if endocarditis is present. It can better define vegetations and help exclude a ring abscess.

OTHER STUDIES. Magnetic resonance imaging (MRI) and other imaging studies have yet to provide clinically

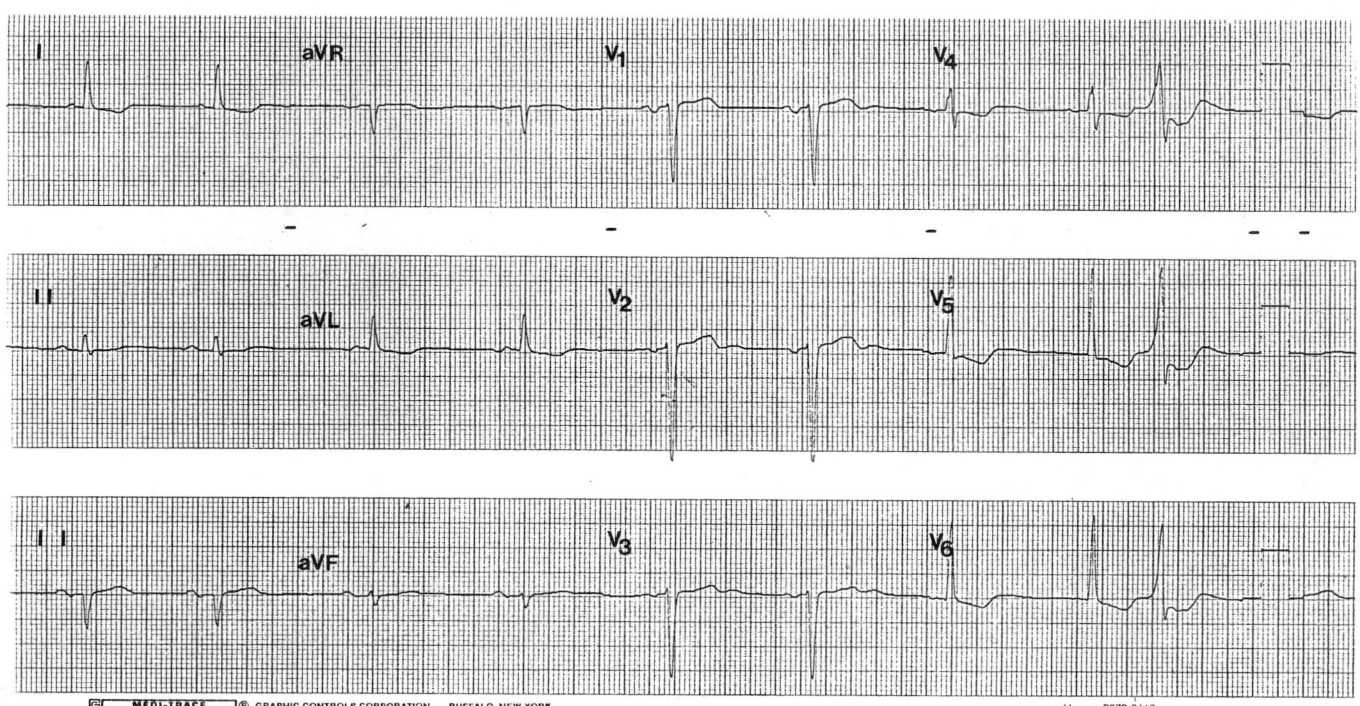

Figure 7. *Representative electrocardiogram (ECG) in aortic stenosis.* Left ventricular hypertrophy is evident with delayed R-wave progression.

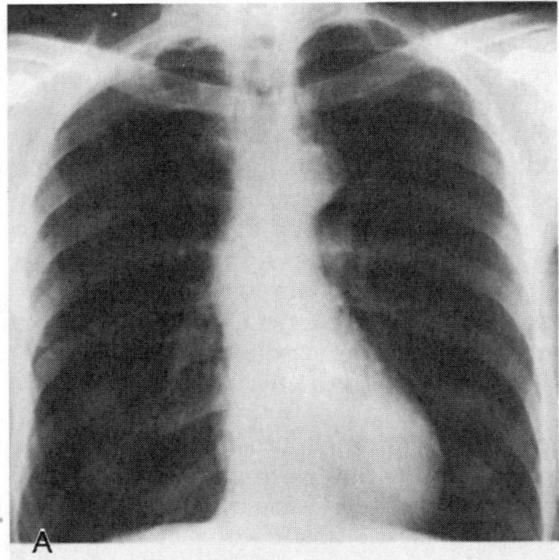

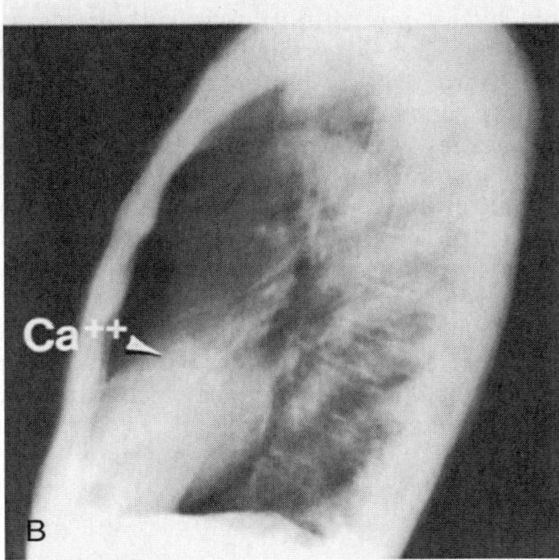

Figure 8. *Representative chest film in aortic stenosis.* The posteroanterior (PA) view is shown in *A* and the lateral view is seen in *B*. Note the presence of valvular calcium (Ca^{2+}) on the lateral view. The aortic root is moderately dilated and the overall heart size only modestly enlarged, which is consistent with left ventricular pressure overload.

useful data not obtainable by other methods. Myocardial perfusion scanning can be useful, however. Low-level bicycle exercise stress or pharmacologic stress can be performed safely in patients with aortic stenosis. Exercise treadmill testing, however, may initiate the spiral of hypotension related to baroreceptor stimulation, as noted previously and should not be done.

Invasive Evaluation

As shown in Figure 10, when obstruction occurs at the aortic valve, a gradient is present across the valve itself. As the stenosis worsens, the gradient increases. The loss of the percussion wave in the aorta becomes more evident, reducing the upstroke of the aortic pressure, As a result, the murmur peaks later and produces the delayed upstroke in the carotid artery. There are actually three gradients that are often measured in aortic stenosis. As shown in the figure, the maximal gradient occurs on the upslope of the aortic pressure and is referred to as the peak instantaneous gradient. This is the gradient reported as the peak echocardiographic gradient. The peak-to-peak aortic gradient has no real significance physiologically; however, it is commonly reported at catheterization because of the ease by which it is obtained. The mean gradient is calculated by using a planimeter to measure the gradient over time. This mean gradient can then be used in various formulas to calculate an estimated valve orifice area. For example:

$$\text{Aortic Valve Area} = \frac{\text{Cardiac Output}}{\sqrt{\text{Mean Gradient}}}$$

This formula, commonly referred to as the "Hakki" formula, provides a reasonable estimate of the valve area. By contrast, the more commonly used Gorlin formula assumes laminar flow and requires a gravitational constant as well as a determination of how many seconds in a minute the heart is in systole:

$$\text{Aortic Valve Area} = \frac{\text{Cardiac Output / (SEP) (HR)}}{44.3\ \sqrt{\text{Mean Gradient}}}$$

where SEP = systolic ejection period; HR = heart rate; 44.3 = gravitational constant.

These formulas perform poorly at high and low cardiac outputs and actually are not true constants. They are, however, the best estimates of disease severity available,

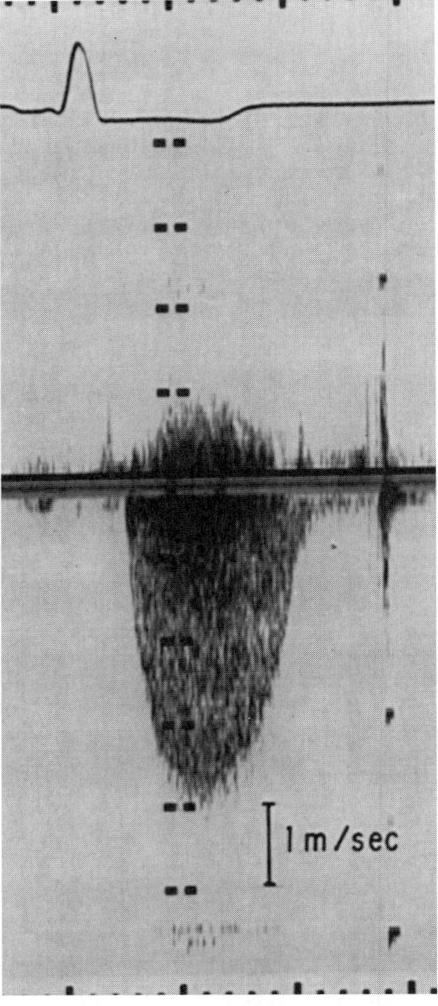

Figure 9. *Doppler in aortic stenosis.* Continuous-wave Doppler is shown with a peak instantaneous aortic valve gradient (P) of 64 mm Hg. ($P = 4V^2$, where V = peak velocity in m/sec, which is 4 m/sec in this example.)

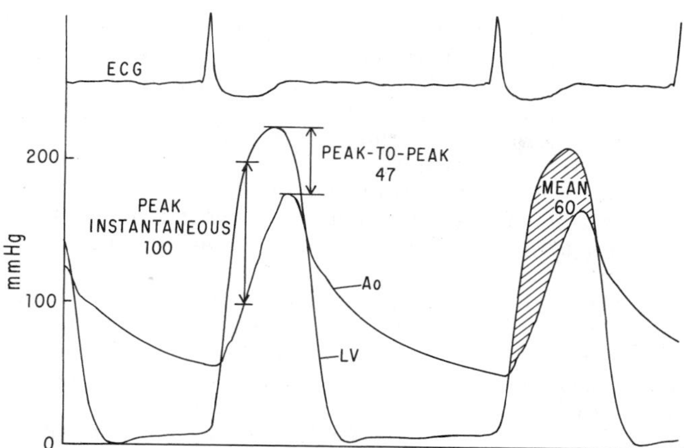

Figure 10. *Representative pressure gradient between the aorta and left ventricle in aortic stenosis.* Note that there are three gradients measured: the peak instantaneous, the peak-to-peak, and the mean gradient (see text for explanation). ECG = electrocardiogram; Ao = aorta; LV = left ventricle.

and they have withstood the test of time. A clinically significant relationship can be derived from the valve area, aortic flow, and the aortic gradient. In Figure 11, as the valve area approaches 0.8 cm^2, the curves relating cardiac output to the valve gradient tend to flatten. This means that minor additional increases in the cardiac output are accompanied by much greater increases in the aortic gradient. Thus, patients who have an aortic valve area of 0.8 cm^2 or less may have changes sufficient to produce exertional symptoms.

When to Operate

Aortic stenosis produces symptoms once diastolic dysfunction becomes evident. Diastolic dysfunction generally precedes systolic dysfunction and results in both angina and congestive symptoms. Although syncope may not be strictly related to diastolic failure, syncope is rarely seen without preceding or concomitant symptoms of congestion or angina. Patients with aortic stenosis should, therefore, undergo surgery when symptoms develop and the aortic valve area equals or falls to less than 0.8 cm^2. Evidence of pulmonary hypertension or an elevated pulmonary capillary wedge pressure also implies diastolic dysfunction that warrants a surgical approach. Despite the excellent correlation between the gradient or the valve area and symptoms in aortic stenosis, patients may experience significant aortic stenosis for rather long periods before symptoms emerge. In general, symptoms should guide the clinician.

The impact of valve replacement on other organ systems and the quality of life a patient may experience after valve replacement must always influence the decision to operate. Patients are not made smarter after cardiopulmonary bypass, and many patients may not have a significantly improved quality of life. As with all decisions regarding major surgery, comorbid factors must be carefully considered, and stringent cutoff values for operability are to be used as guidelines only.

Mitral Stenosis

Natural History and Etiology

Mitral stenosis in adults is still largely attributed to rheumatic fever. In the United States, isolated pockets of mitral stenosis persist despite a marked decline in the incidence of acute rheumatic fever. The role of other microbes has never been completely determined. Mitral stenosis in children is usually congenital and is characterized by fusion of the commissures, abnormal displacement of papillary muscles toward each other, total fusion of papillary muscle with formation of the parachute mitral valve, and redundancy of mitral valve tissue with commissural fusion or an associated membrane within the mitral orifice. Mitral stenosis has been reported rarely with systemic lupus erythematosus, rheumatoid arthritis, amyloidosis, methysergide therapy, or carcinoid. In the elderly adult, calcification of the mitral annulus can invade the mitral valve and result in significant mitral stenosis—often with accompanying mitral regurgitation.

Rheumatic fever may cause commissural fusion, thickening of the valve leaflets, chordal fusion, and eventually calcification. The extent of these individual lesions is used to aid the decision regarding commissurotomy (either surgical or percutaneous balloon commissurotomy) and valve replacement. One common scoring system rates each of these four factors on a scale of 0 to 4, with total scores of more than 8 correlating with less improvement after percutaneous commissurotomy when compared with scores less than or equal to 8. Mitral stenosis tends to be much more common in women (two thirds of all patients with rheumatic mitral stenosis are female) and tends to follow a more malignant course in Third World countries, where recurrent bouts of rheumatic fever pose additional risk. Symptoms often present in the third and fourth decades of life, and mitral stenosis can complicate pregnancy.

Symptoms

There are two syndromes that classically occur in patients with mitral stenosis. As shown in Figure 12, these syndromes are distinguished by the development of secondary stenosis in the pulmonary arterioles. In patients with moderate mitral stenosis, the first symptom is often pulmonary congestion with modestly increased pulmonary systolic pressures (in the 45 mm Hg range). Some patients, however, progress through this stage and experience significant pulmonary arteriolar hypertrophy and profound

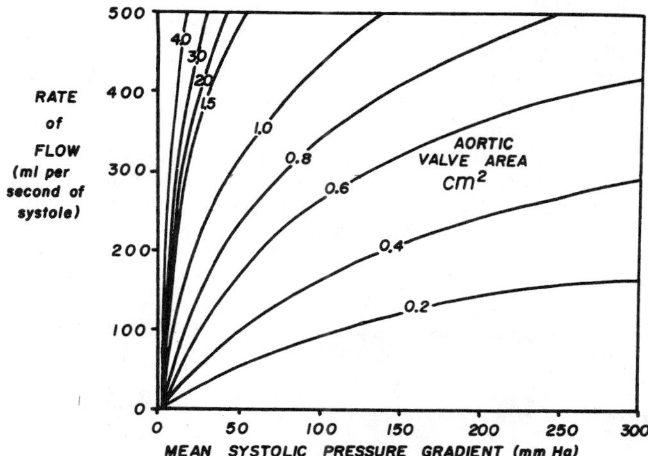

Figure 11. *The relationship between cardiac output and valve gradient with the aortic valve area.* Note that the aortic valve area curves tend to flatten at a valve area of about 0.8 cm^2. This means that minor increases in output result in large increases in the gradient as the valve area is less than or equal to 0.8 cm^2. The usually accepted cutoff for the implication of severe aortic stenosis is 0.8 cm^2.

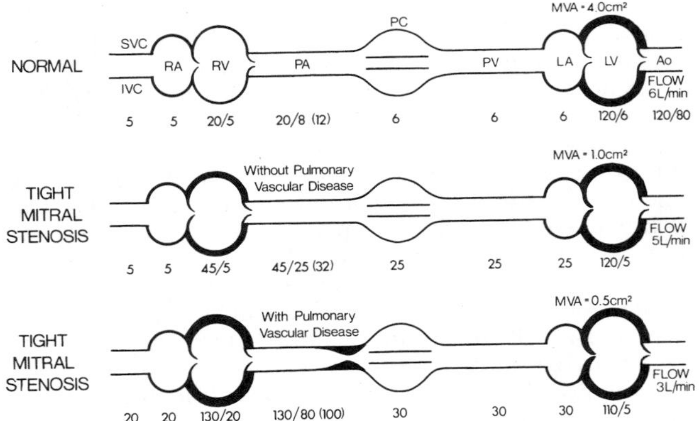

Figure 12. *The two syndromes in patients with mitral stenosis.* The top line represents normal pressures. The middle line represents moderate mitral stenosis with evidence of moderate pulmonary hypertension. Patients at this stage often experience pulmonary congestion with exertion. The bottom line represents the patient with mitral stenosis who has a secondary stenosis at the pulmonary arteriolar level. Patients in this latter category often present with low-output symptoms rather than congestion. SVC = superior vena cava; IVC = inferior vena cava; RA = right atrium; RV = right ventricle; PA = pulmonary artery; PC = pulmonary capillaries; PV = pulmonary vein; LA = left atrium; LV = left ventricle; MVA = mitral valve area. (From Grossman, W.: Profiles in valvular heart disease. *In* Bain, D.S., and Grossman, W. (eds.): Cardiac Catheterization, Angiography and Intervention, 5th ed. Baltimore, Williams & Wilkins, 1996, p. 737, with permission.)

pulmonary hypertension. Pulmonary pressures may equal systemic pressures in this latter group. When secondary stenosis is present, symptoms are often purely of low output and then eventually of right-sided heart failure. If the clinician waits for congestive symptoms, worsening pulmonary hypertension may not be detected. The secondary stenosis of pulmonary arterioles tends to "protect" the lungs from congestion, and patients may not experience orthopnea or paroxysmal nocturnal dyspnea (PND); rather, they note profound low output and fatigue and demonstrate evidence of right-sided heart failure.

The primary symptom in mitral stenosis is dyspnea with exertion, which results from the reduced compliance in the lungs because of increased pulmonary capillary wedge pressure associated with mitral obstruction. PND and orthopnea are common unless secondary stenosis of pulmonary arterioles has occurred. Because the mitral valve gradient is related to heart rate and output, symptoms are typically precipitated by exercise, stress, or atrial fibrillation. Rarely, a patient may present with hemoptysis when thin-walled bronchial veins rupture. Chest pain is unusual, but its presence has been attributed to right ventricular hypertension with right ventricular subendocardial underperfusion. Coronary arteriosclerosis is not common in patients with mitral stenosis.

At times, the left atrium can become quite enlarged. Compression of the left recurrent laryngeal nerve by a huge left atrium or dilated pulmonary artery may cause hoarseness (Ortner's syndrome). Patients with mitral stenosis are also particularly susceptible to emboli from the mitral valve itself or from the enlarged left atrium. This is especially true once atrial fibrillation ensues. Increased right-sided heart pressures may result in tricuspid regurgitation and an increased propensity to venous thromboembolism. The presence of mitral stenosis and a patent foramen ovale or a true atrial septal defect defines Lutembacher's syndrome, which is characterized by symptoms of profound right ventricular volume overload.

Physical Examination

The patient with mitral stenosis may exhibit a "mitral facies" characterized by pink patches on both cheeks. The arterial pulses are usually normal until cardiac output is markedly reduced. The jugular venous pulse often exhibits a prominent A wave because of the poorly compliant right ventricle. During ventricular systole, expansion of the jugular venous pulse suggests tricuspid regurgitation (the CV wave). Atrial fibrillation may alter the wave forms and occasionally make the diagnosis of tricuspid regurgitation more difficult. Hepatojugular reflux is common.

Palpation of the precordium often reveals a palpable first heart sound, indicating stiffened but mobile mitral leaflets. When pulmonary hypertension occurs, the second heart sound may be palpable along the left sternal border. A right ventricular lift may occur when right ventricular hypertrophy is present. Rarely the intensity of diastolic rumble may be felt in the left lateral recumbent position.

On auscultation, the first heart sound is often markedly accentuated if the valve is pliable. The timing relationship between the second heart sound (aortic valve component) and the opening snap provides a clinical clue regarding severity. As the left atrial pressures rise, the opening snap moves closer to the aortic second heart sound. A short aortic second heart sound–opening snap interval therefore implies significant mitral stenosis (Fig. 13). When mitral stenosis becomes more severe, the intensity of the first heart sound will be reduced, and the second heart sound may appear almost single. Physiologic splitting of the second heart sound becomes reduced when the resistance of

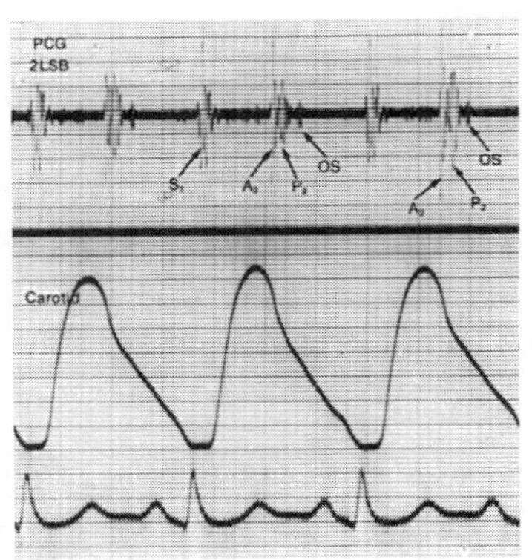

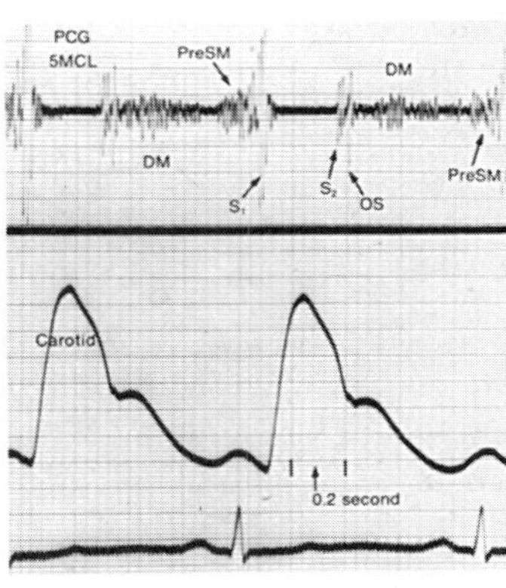

Figure 13. *The heart sounds in mitral stenosis.* Mild mitral stenosis *(left panel)* is contrasted with severe mitral stenosis *(right panel)*. Note that as the severity of mitral stenosis increases, the aortic second heart sound–opening snap (OS) interval declines, the diastolic murmur (DM) becomes louder and now has presystolic accentuation (PreSM). PCG = phonocardiogram; 2LSB = second interspace along the left sternal boarder *(left panel)*; 5MCL = fifth interspace in the midclavicular line *(right panel)*.

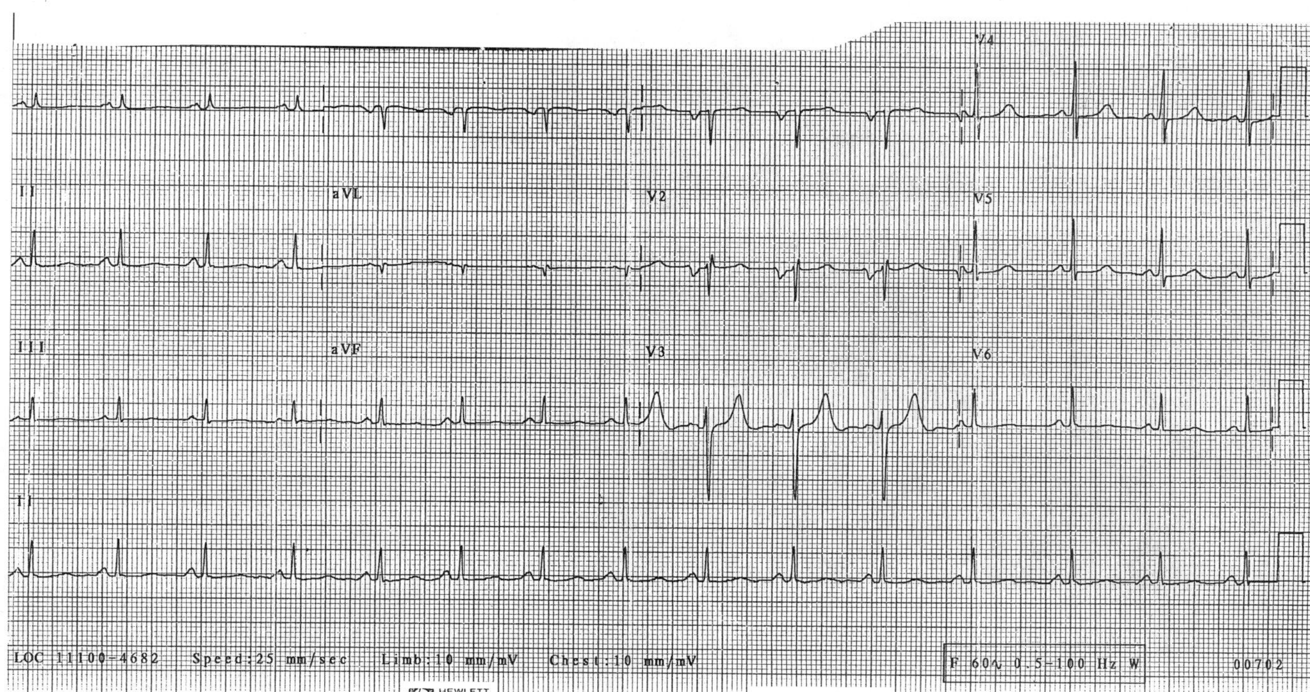

Figure 14. A representative ECG in mitral stenosis.

the pulmonary circuit worsens and begins to equal that of the systemic circuit.

The rumble of mitral stenosis is best heard with the bell of the stethoscope at the left ventricular apex and the patient in the left lateral position. The intensity of the rumble can often be enhanced by asking the patient to perform sit-ups to increase the heart rate and cardiac output. Often a presystolic component can be heard even in the presence of atrial fibrillation. The greater the mitral gradient, the more evident the murmur. With pulmonary hypertension, pulmonic insufficiency (the Graham Steell murmur) may be audible. A third and/or fourth heart sound of right-sided origin may also be audible. These gallops may be heard in the neck. When severe pulmonary hypertension ensues, a pulmonic valve component will be dramatically increased, and associated tricuspid insufficiency may reflect worsening right ventricular function. Hepatic congestion, ascites, and edema ensue in the latter stages of the disease.

Noninvasive Evaluation

ELECTROCARDIOGRAM. Figure 14 shows a representative ECG from a patient with mitral stenosis. The ECG reflects right ventricular hypertrophy in association with left atrial enlargement. Atrial fibrillation is a common associated finding.

CHEST FILM. The radiographic findings in mitral stenosis reveal significant left atrial enlargement. Occasional calcification along the annulus and/or within the valve can be seen. The size of the left ventricle is generally normal, whereas the right ventricle and pulmonary arteries are enlarged (Fig. 15). The presence of a large left atrium, with evidence of pulmonary venous hypertension, a redistribution of the venous pattern, associated Kerley B lines of edema, and pulmonary artery enlargement, is relatively classic for pure mitral stenosis.

ECHOCARDIOGRAM. The echocardiogram in mitral stenosis reveals thickening of the stenotic rheumatic valve with fusion of the commissures. Chordal fusion, calcification, valvular thickening, and anterior leaflet mobility are all used as part of the echocardiographic scoring system described earlier. The mitral orifice can also be measured by planimeter to approximate the valve orifice area. Doppler echocardiography is especially useful, and the mitral valve area can be estimated from the pressure half-time measurements. Echocardiography also provides chamber dimensions and evidence of associated aortic or other val-

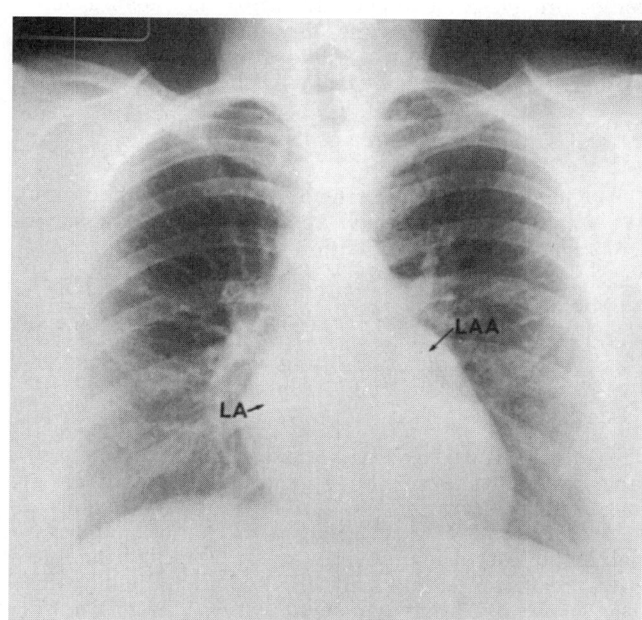

Figure 15. *A representative chest film in mitral stenosis.* Note the left atrial (LA) double density and the prominent left atrial appendage *(arrow on right).* Vascular redistribution to the upper lobes is also present.

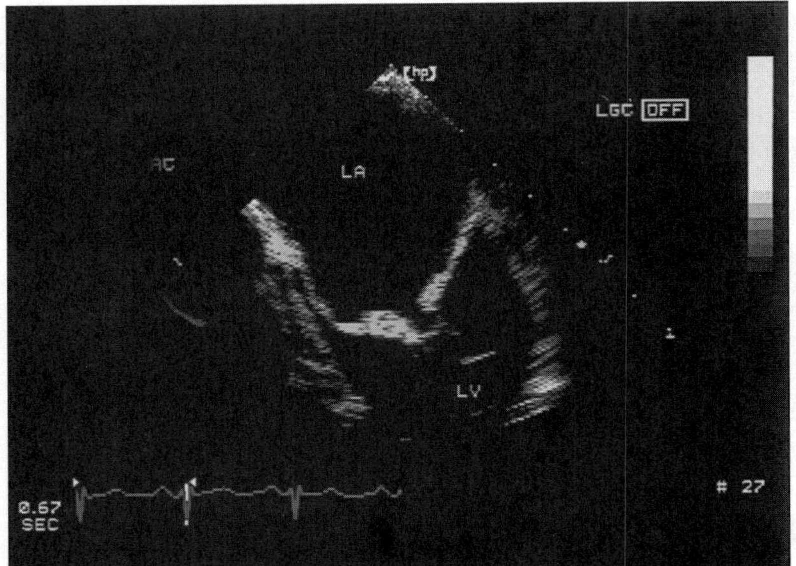

Figure 16. *Echocardiography in mitral stenosis.* The thickened mitral leaflets are well seen in this transesophageal echocardiogram. LA = left atrium; LV = left ventricle.

vular disease. Younger patients can undergo surgery based on the echocardiogram only. Transesophageal echocardiography (Fig. 16) may reveal atrial thrombi in patients with mitral stenosis. This observation may influence the performance of percutaneous balloon commissurotomy because the catheters must traverse the left atrium.

Invasive Evaluation

Comparing either the pulmonary capillary wedge pressure or the left atrial pressure to the left ventricular diastolic pressure, a diastolic gradient occurs when there is obstruction to the mitral valve. This is shown in Figure 17. The magnitude of the gradient depends on heart rate and output as well as the severity of the stenosis. Invasive studies provide a means of calculating the mean gradient and, using the Gorlin or other formula as noted previously, an estimate of the mitral valve area can be derived. A "ballpark estimate" can be made by the following:

$$\text{Mitral Valve Area} = \frac{\text{Cardiac Output}}{\sqrt{\text{Mean Gradient}}}$$

The Gorlin formula uses the amount of time in a minute that flow is traversing the valve during diastole, a gravitational constant, and a correction factor.

$$\text{Mitral Valve Area} = \frac{\text{Cardiac Output / (DFP) (HR)}}{44.3\ (0.85)\sqrt{\text{Mean Gradient}}}$$

where DFP = diastolic filling period; HR = heart rate; 44.3 = gravitational constant; 0.85 = correction factor.

Figure 18 reveals the relationship among the mitral valve area, cardiac output, and the gradient in mitral stenosis. These curves tend to flatten around a valve area of 1.5 to 1 cm^2. With these valve areas, minor increases in the cardiac output lead to dramatic increases in the mitral valve gradient. Most persons with symptomatic mitral stenosis have valve areas approaching 1 cm^2. Angiography at catheterization simply demonstrates other lesions or related mitral regurgitation. Catheterization indicates the extent of pulmonary hypertension and the presence of associated tricuspid valve disease.

When to Operate

In general, patients with exertional symptoms and appropriate anatomy (valve area < 1.5 cm^2) should undergo either surgical intervention or percutaneous balloon commissurotomy.

Because diastolic failure is created by the stenotic mitral valve, surgery is appropriate whenever symptoms emerge resulting from increased left atrial pressure. The presence of atrial fibrillation may imply that the left atrial pressures are increasing, but atrial fibrillation can also result from primary rheumatic involvement of the atrial myocardium. Left ventricular dysfunction can also be present in patients with mitral stenosis without associated mitral regurgitation, a phenomenon that appears more common in men than in women. The combination of poor left ventricular function and mitral stenosis may precipitate earlier symptoms. The retraction of chordae can result in regional left ventricular wall motion abnormalities as well. It does not appear, however, that associated left ventricular dysfunction should dissuade one from considering percutaneous balloon commissurotomy or valve replacement in these patients.

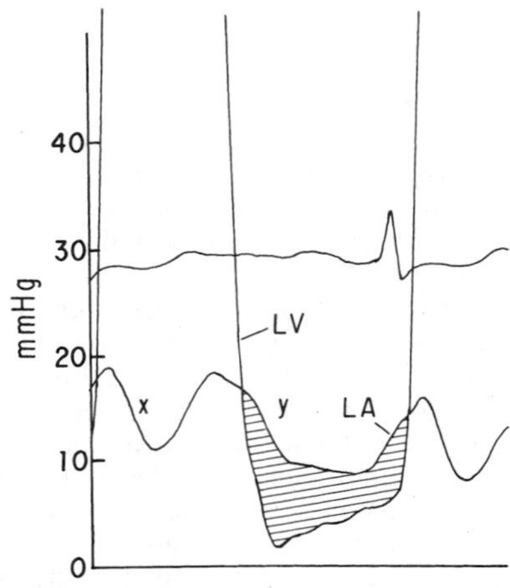

Figure 17. *The hemodynamic gradient in mitral stenosis.* A diastolic gradient between the left atrium (LA) and the left ventricle (LV) is noted.

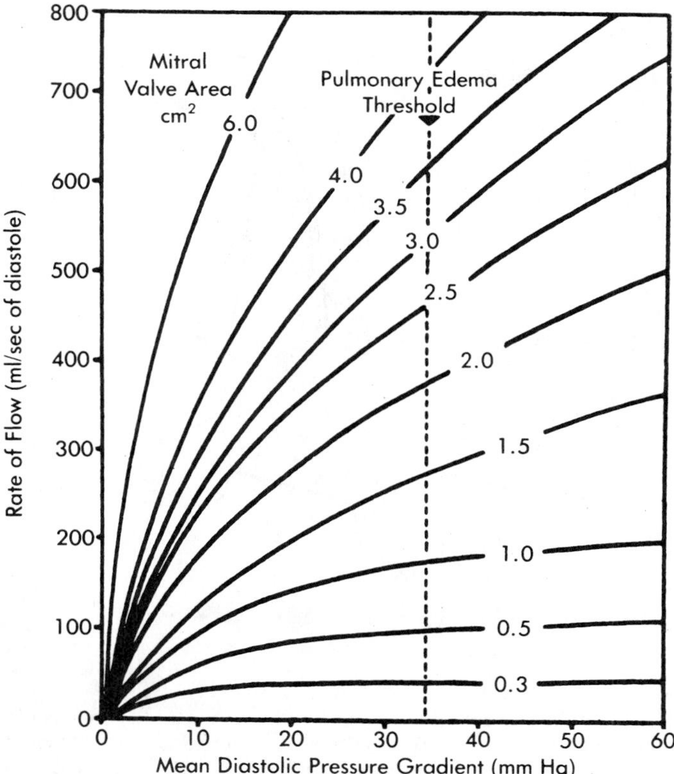

Figure 18. *The relationship of cardiac output and valve gradient to the mitral valve area.* Note that the curves tend to flatten between a mitral valve area of 1.5 to 1 cm^2. This means the gradient rises rapidly with minor changes in cardiac output at this level. The cutoff used for proceeding toward intervention in symptomatic patients with mitral stenosis is often 1.5 to 1 cm^2.

Aortic Regurgitation

Natural History and Etiology

Many patients with aortic insufficiency experience a prolonged period of relatively few symptoms. Aortic insufficiency can be caused by abnormalities of the valvular tissue, the aortic annulus, or the aorta itself. Rheumatic fever can lead to fibrosis and scarring of the aortic valve with resultant insufficiency. Infective endocarditis can destroy the valve or cause perforations. The bicuspid aortic valve may also become incompetent. Occasionally, bicuspid leaflets may prolapse into the left ventricle. A membranous ventricular septal defect (VSD) may compromise commissural integrity and lead to prolapse of a leaflet into the VSD. With prolapse, the murmur of the VSD may decrease or disappear, whereas the murmur of the aortic insufficiency becomes evident. Progressive regurgitation is also seen in patients with disease of the aortic root, including those with Marfan's syndrome, cystic medial necrosis of the aorta (annuloaortic ectasia), Ehlers-Danlos syndrome, and other diseases of connective tissue. Inflammatory processes associated with aortic insufficiency include systemic lupus erythematosus, rheumatoid arthritis, ankylosing spondylitis, Whipple's disease, Crohn's disease, and Jaccoud's arthropathy. In years past, syphilis was a common cause of aortic insufficiency. Other disorders that primarily affect the aortic root include Reiter syndrome, giant cell arteritis, psoriasis, osteogenesis imperfecta, and Behçet's syndrome. Aortic dissection can also lead to loss of aortic valve integrity and severe aortic insufficiency.

Symptoms

In acute aortic insufficiency, the ventricle cannot tolerate the sudden increase in volume, so the pressures rise dramatically along the normal myocardial diastolic pressure-volume curve. This leads to cardiovascular collapse, congestive heart failure, severe dyspnea, and hypotension. The systolic pulse pressure may not be wide. Because there may be little difference between the aortic diastolic pressure and the left ventricular diastolic pressure, the murmur of aortic insufficiency may be difficult to hear.

In chronic aortic insufficiency, symptoms usually develop in the fourth or fifth decade of life and classically include orthopnea, PND, and exertional dyspnea. In contrast to aortic stenosis, syncope is rare, as is angina. Mild angina can be present, however, and can be unrelated to coronary artery disease. In patients with significant aortic insufficiency, the wide pulse pressure leads to a pounding sensation that may be detected by the patient. As the disease progresses, pulmonary hypertension and right-sided heart failure ensue. In chronic aortic insufficiency, dyspnea may occur gradually, and considerable loss of systolic function occurs before symptoms emerge.

Physical Examination

ACUTE AORTIC REGURGITATION. The physical examination in a patient with acute aortic regurgitation reflects the sudden increase in left ventricular diastolic pressure and the resultant pulmonary venous hypertension (Fig. 19). The patient typically appears anxious and dyspneic. Pulmonary edema is evident, but the peripheral signs of chronic aortic insufficiency generally are not present. Jugular venous pulsation may be normal unless pulmonary hypertension has caused pressures on the right side of the heart to increase. The carotid artery examination may also be unremarkable, and the ventricular impulse may only be more vigorous. On auscultation, a short aortic insufficiency murmur may be all that is heard as the diastolic gradient between the aorta and LV is confined to early diastole. The rapid rise in left ventricular diastolic pressure leads to early closure of the mitral valve even before ventricular systole is initiated. Thus, the first heart sound may be very soft or absent. Occasionally the first heart sound (mitral closure sound) can be heard in mid-diastole. Mitral regurgitation may also occur in diastole because of the rapid increase in the left ventricular diastolic pressure. A third heart sound is often present. If pulmonary hypertension is present, the pulmonic second heart sound may be accentuated.

CHRONIC AORTIC REGURGITATION. The examination is dramatically different in chronic aortic insufficiency (see Fig. 19). The most impressive findings are due to the wide pulse pressure. As the reflected wave from the extremities summates with the exaggerated pulse pressure moving toward the extremities, the pulse pressure rises further in the legs compared with the arms. This difference may exceed 40 mm Hg (Hill's sign). Retrograde flow into the left ventricle during diastole produces "pistol shots" or Corrigan's pulse that tend to be rapid in upstroke and end abruptly. Pistol shot sounds over the femoral artery are referred to as Traube's sign. Retrograde flow into the left ventricle can be detected by partially compressing the femoral artery with the edge of the stethoscope's diaphragm; with this maneuver, a to-and-fro murmur may be heard (Duroziez's sign). Compression of the skin of the face or hands with a glass slide or light compression or illumination of the nail beds can also reveal the pulsatile nature (intermittent flushing) of the capillary bed (Quincke's sign).

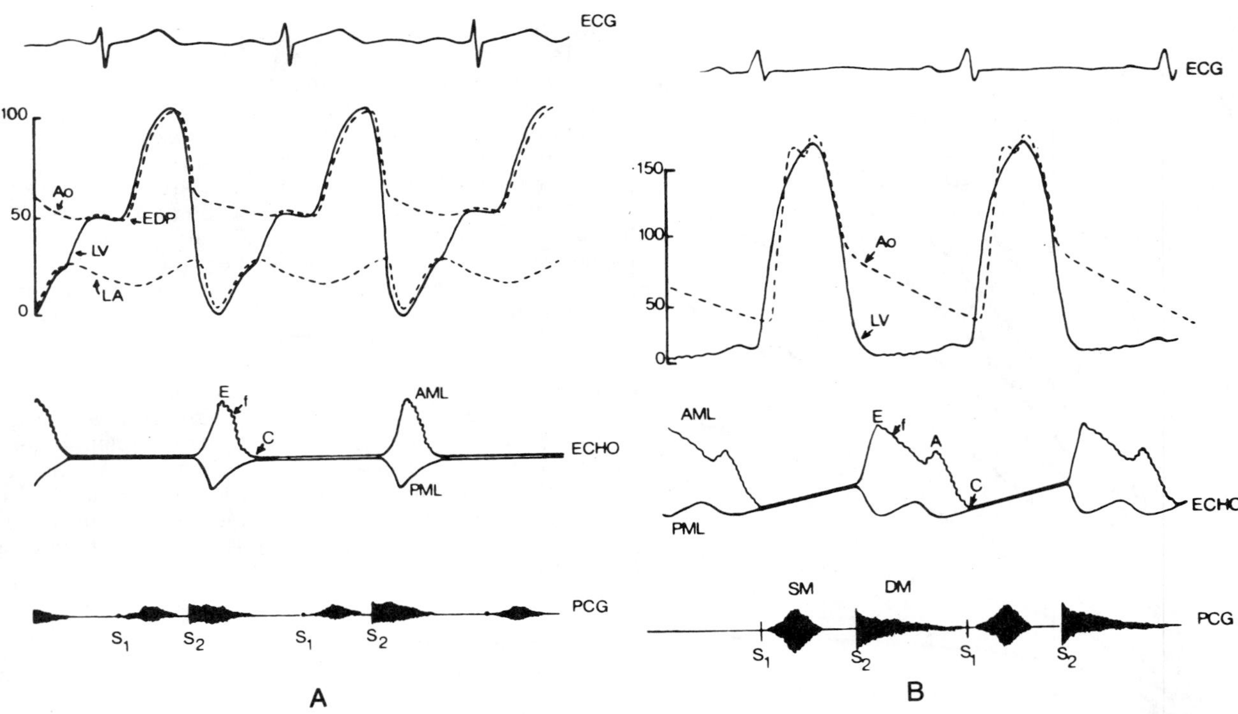

Figure 19. *Representative pressures in acute versus chronic aortic insufficiency.* In *acute aortic insufficiency (A),* left ventricular diastolic pressures are dramatically high. Mitral preclosure occurs and the aortic pulse pressure is relatively narrow. In *chronic aortic insufficiency (B),* the diastolic pressures remain normal for long periods and the pulse pressure is quite wide. Many of the peripheral signs of aortic insufficiency are a reflection of this widened pulse pressure. ECG = electrocardiogram; ECHO = echocardiogram; PCG = phonocardiogram; Ao = aorta; EDP = end-diastolic pressure; LV = left ventricle; LA = left atrium; AML = anterior mitral leaflet; PML = posterior mitral leaflet; f = flutter of anterior mitral valve leaflet; SM = systolic murmur; DM = diastolic murmur; C = closure point of mitral valve. (From Morganroth, J., Perloff, J.K., Zeldis, M., et al.: Acute severe aortic regurgitation. Ann. Intern. Med. 87:223–232, 1977, with permission.)

The high pulse pressure may cause bobbing of the head (de Musset's sign), the uvula (Müller's sign), the liver (Rosenbach's sign), the spleen (Gerhardt's sign), and even the cervix. When the patient crosses the legs while sitting, the foot will often bob (Baker's sign).

The jugular venous pulse is typically normal in aortic insufficiency unless significant right-sided heart failure develops. The carotid pulse may be rapid and bounding; occasionally it may have a bisferiens quality, especially if there is associated aortic stenosis. The point of maximal impulse (PMI) is markedly enlarged and hyperdynamic. The clinician may palpate both an A wave (correlating to the fourth heart sound) and a rapid filling wave (correlating with a third heart sound). A systolic thrill is not uncommon, even with minimal associated aortic stenosis. The thrill may be palpated throughout the precordium and up into the carotid arteries. The most prominent feature on auscultation is the loud diastolic blowing murmur along the left sternal border. If the murmur is heard loudest along the *right* sternal border, the aortic root may be dilated. The first heart sound is typically soft because of rapidly rising pressures toward the end of diastole. The aortic second heart sound is frequently soft as well. Paradoxical splitting is occasionally noted. A third heart sound gallop and a fourth heart sound are often detected. An aortic systolic ejection sound may be present if the valve is mobile.

The aortic insufficiency murmur is often best heard at end-expiration with the patient leaning forward. Occasionally, with the patient on hands and knees, a soft murmur of aortic insufficiency will be revealed when no other maneuver works. The murmur may have a high-pitched, musical ("cooing dove") quality that implies a narrow jet of regurgitant blood. An aortic insufficiency murmur is noted most often in endocarditis and with eversion of one of the cusps. Premature closure of the mitral valve may produce the Austin Flint murmur of relative mitral stenosis. The absence of a mitral opening snap and the softness of the first heart sound help to distinguish the Austin Flint murmur from that of actual mitral stenosis.

Noninvasive Evaluation

ELECTROCARDIOGRAM. The ECG in chronic aortic insufficiency typically reveals left ventricular hypertrophy. Intraventricular conduction defects are relatively common. In acute aortic insufficiency, the ECG may reveal only sinus tachycardia with nonspecific ST-segment changes.

CHEST FILM. The chest film in acute aortic insufficiency may reveal a relatively normal-sized heart with marked pulmonary congestion. In chronic aortic insufficiency, the heart is often markedly enlarged. The left atrium is typically unremarkable in the absence of associated mitral valve disease. The ascending aorta may be markedly dilated. Figure 20 shows a chest film from a patient with chronic aortic sufficiency.

ECHOCARDIOGRAPHY. This modality remains one of the best tools for the detection and characterization of insufficiency. Echocardiography enables the clinician to follow those cardiac dimensions that are critical in the decision to operate. Echocardiography reveals the size of the aortic root, the status of the leaflets themselves, and the presence of associated vegetations or calcium. Color

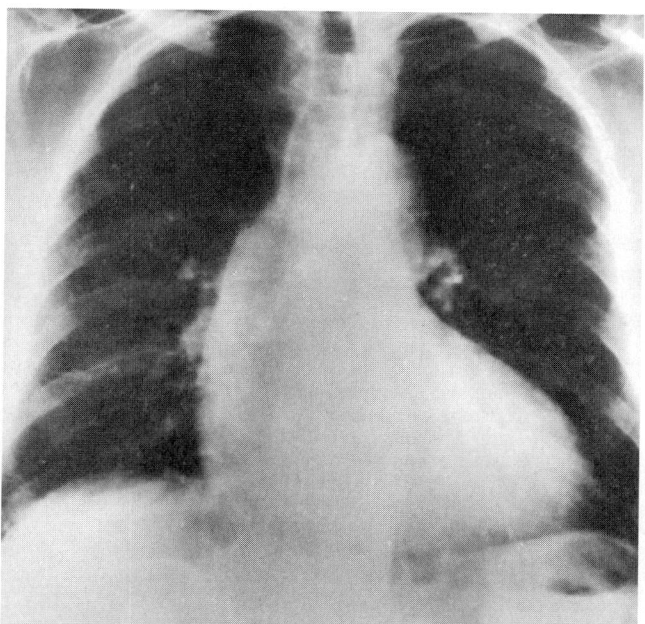

Figure 20. *Representative chest film in a patient with chronic aortic insufficiency.* Note the volume-overloaded left ventricle with dilatation of the aortic root. (From Alpert, J.S.: Chronic aortic regurgitation. *In* Dalen, J.E., and Alpert, J.S. [eds.]: Valvular Heart Disease, 2nd ed. Boston, Little, Brown, 1987, p. 296, with permission.)

flow Doppler detects aortic insufficiency of even a minor degree. In acute aortic insufficiency, the echocardiogram may confirm the presence of mitral valve preclosure (before systole begins). This finding implies that surgery will likely be required.

In chronic aortic insufficiency, the echocardiogram provides crucial data regarding chamber sizes. Whenever the end-systolic dimension exceeds 5 cm, surgery may be required regardless of symptoms. Transesophageal echocardiograms are especially useful for the detection of abscesses and vegetations.

OTHER STUDIES. Stress radionuclide angiography has been used to determine serial EFs and to uncover those patients with aortic insufficiency and limited cardiac reserve. The exercise hemodynamics in aortic insufficiency are quite complex, however. The degree of aortic insufficiency per beat is a function of the heart rate. Since diastolic time decreases more than systolic time as the heart rate increases, the diastolic time may be markedly reduced with exercise stress. Thus, the resulting aortic insufficiency per beat actually declines during higher heart rates. This contrasts with other disorders in which left ventricular end-diastolic volumes rise during stress. This abnormal loading makes interpretation of stress radionuclide angiography in aortic insufficiency difficult.

Invasive Evaluation

Cardiac catheterization provides useful information as well. Aortography helps define the extent of aortic dilatation or the presence of dissection. Calcium deposition within the valves and the degree of aortic insufficiency can be judged by contrast angiography and compared with that from color flow and continuous- or pulsed-wave Doppler. Contrast angiography often provides a better measure of the degree of aortic insufficiency than does echocardiography and Doppler. Aortic insufficiency is graded using a scale of 0 to 4+. A score of 3+ means that at some point during aortography the opacity of the left ventricle equals that of the aorta. A score of 4+ means that at some point, the left ventricular contrast is greater than that of the aorta. A score of 2+ means that aortography contrast density is less than that of the left ventricle throughout the run, and a score of 1+ implies that only a minor amount of aortic insufficiency exists. Clinical evidence of diastolic dysfunction, increased left ventricular end-diastolic pressures, end-diastolic and end-systolic volumes, and evidence for associated pulmonary hypertension can also be confirmed at catheterization. Figure 19 shows representative pressure data from both acute and chronic aortic insufficiency patients. The hemodynamics are obviously quite disparate.

When To Operate

In patients with acute aortic insufficiency, urgent surgery should be recommended if symptoms of congestion are present. This is most often seen in aortic dissection or endocarditis. Incomplete medical treatment for endocarditis should not delay surgery if congestive symptoms are present.

In chronic aortic insufficiency, symptoms typically occur late in the course of disease. Thus, the clinician should obtain serial EF and end-systolic dimension data. If the end-systolic dimensions appear to be increasing over time, systolic function is most likely declining. An end-systolic dimension exceeding 5 cm should prompt serious consideration of valve replacement even in a patient with minimal or no symptoms. By contrast, if the end-systolic dimension is normal (less than 4 cm), the clinician can follow the patient and prescribe pharmacologic afterload reduction, if necessary.

Mitral Insufficiency

Mitral Apparatus

The mitral apparatus is shown in Figure 21. It is a complex of structures that must all work in concert if mitral insufficiency is to be avoided. The important structures include the papillary muscles and the associated myocardium, the chordae tendineae, the leaflets themselves, and the mitral annulus. Note that chordae from both leaflets attach to both papillary muscles. Note also that the mitral annulus is a dynamic structure that during contraction can reduce the overall mitral orifice by 20 to 40 per cent.

Activation of the endocardium results in contraction of the papillary muscles. As chordae from both the posteromedial and anterolateral papillary muscles are attached to both leaflets, the mitral valve is pulled toward the endocardium and aligns the anterior and posterior leaflets. As systole continues, the left ventricular pressure rises. The two leaflets converge, eventually abutting each other. The interventricular pressure helps hold the leaflets together. This latter function has been described as the "keystone effect" because it mirrors the physical events seen with a keystone in the middle of an archway. The mitral annulus then contracts.

If the papillary muscles are dysfunctional or displaced; if the chordae are too short or too long, fractured, or malpositioned; if the leaflets are too redundant, too stiff, perforated, or cleft; or if the annulus itself is dysfunctional and does not contract properly, mitral insufficiency may result.

There are many causes of mitral insufficiency. Abnormalities of the papillary muscle are generally related to ischemia, scar, or displacement of the muscles themselves when

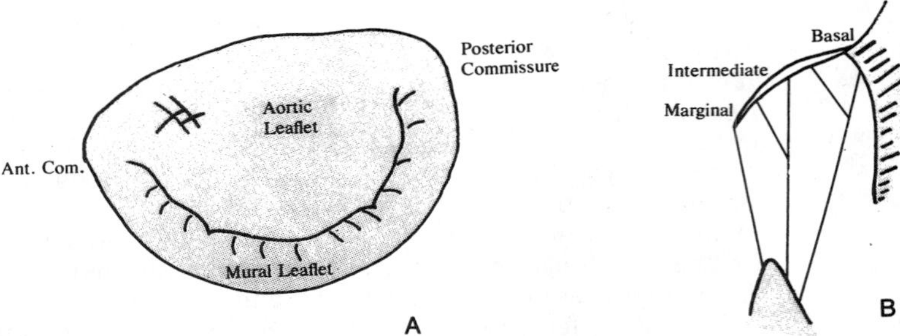

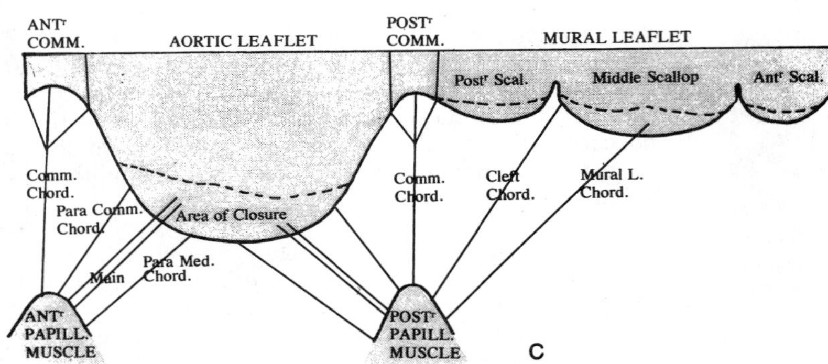

Figure 21. *The mitral apparatus. A,* View from left atrium. *B,* Cross-sectional view showing site of insertion of the chordae on the leaflet. *C,* Mitral apparatus opened, showing the various components. (From Carpentier, A., Guerion, J., Deloche, A., et al.: Pathology of the mitral valve: Introduction to plastic and reconstructive surgery. *In* Kalmanson, D. [ed.]: The Mitral Valve. Acton, MA, Publishing Sciences Group, 1976, p. 66, with permission.)

the left ventricle dilates. Ischemia may lead to rupture of one or more of the papillary muscle heads as well. Congenital malposition of the papillary muscles can occur. The papillary muscles can be altered by infiltrative processes such as amyloidosis and sarcoidosis.

The chordae can rupture either spontaneously, as is often seen in myxomatous mitral valve disease, or from trauma, rheumatic fever, or infection. Because the chordae branch out progressively as they approach the valvular leaflets, the consequence of ruptured chordae depends on the amount of valvular tissue supplied downstream by the ruptured chord. Abnormalities can occur in the valvular leaflets themselves, either from cleft valves or from scarring and rigidity related to rheumatic fever, trauma, endocarditis, or connective tissue disease. Redundant mitral valve leaflets are commonly seen in the mitral valve prolapse syndrome, and this redundancy may result in loss of valvular integrity during systole and subsequent mitral regurgitation. Finally, the annulus can be markedly dilated when left ventricular (and occasionally marked left atrial) dilatation is present. In the elderly, calcification of the mitral annulus also results in loss of annular contraction; associated mitral insufficiency is common. It is noteworthy that this calcium can actually invade the mitral valve itself and create stiffness of the leaflets as well. Mitral annular calcification is more prominent in patients with systemic hypertension, aortic stenosis, diabetes, hypertrophic cardiomyopathy, Marfan's syndrome, and chronic renal failure with secondary hyperparathyroidism.

Symptoms

There are two distinct syndromes of mitral insufficiency. *Acute mitral insufficiency* most often arises from ruptured mitral chordae, endocarditis, or ischemia. Because the left atrium has not dilated in the acute setting, the extra supply of blood presented to it during ventricular systole causes left atrial pressure to rise dramatically. Pulmonary congestion is common. In *chronic mitral insufficiency,* the left atrium typically has dilated to the point that substantial mitral insufficiency is easily tolerated without a marked increase in the left atrial pressure. The accompanying volume load on the heart, however, eventually results in a cardiomyopathy of volume overload much as that seen in aortic insufficiency.

The symptoms described in mitral insufficiency depend on the speed of evolution of the process and relate to the chamber compliance of the left atrium. In acute mitral insufficiency, pulmonary edema develops quickly, and cardiovascular collapse may occur. In chronic mitral insufficiency, the patient may tolerate the regurgitation for many years as the atrium enlarges. However, the enlarged left atrium is susceptible to atrial fibrillation and thrombus formation. Symptoms often occur late in the course of chronic mitral insufficiency. The presence of any reduction in left ventricular systolic performance, as measured by the serial EF or end-systolic dimension, should trigger referral for valve repair or replacement. Symptoms in mitral regurgitation are initially related to the high pulmonary capillary wedge pressure and eventually to low output. When right-sided heart failure intervenes, hepatic congestion, edema, and ascites can occur. Angina is uncommon and is usually not considered part of the chronic mitral regurgitation syndrome.

Physical Examination

The jugular venous pulse is frequently normal until later in the course of mitral insufficiency, when an increased A wave and the CV wave of tricuspid regurgitation may become obvious. The carotid pulse is usually normal, but a rapid decline related to regurgitation into the left atrium is occasionally noted. The left ventricular apex is typically hyperdynamic and displaced to the left. A palpable filling wave, A wave, and systolic thrills can occasionally be felt.

On auscultation, the predominant murmur is the blowing holosystolic murmur. In acute mitral insufficiency, the systolic murmur might actually end before the second heart sound as equilibration of the left atrial and left ventricular pressures occurs. A third heart sound is extremely common in such patients. In chronic mitral insufficiency, the murmur begins with the first heart sound and generally obscures the second heart sound. The radiation of the murmur varies considerably and may fool the clinician who looks only for apex-to-axilla radiation. Its differentiation from aortic stenosis has been explained earlier (see Fig. 6). In mitral valve prolapse, for instance, prolapse of the posterior leaflet may result in anterior radiation of the murmur and radiation up the aorta itself. Anterior prolapse may cause the murmur to radiate posteriorly and even be heard up the spine and occasionally on top of the head. The murmur of mitral regurgitation is usually high-pitched and typically loudest at the apex in the left lateral position. In contrast to aortic outflow murmurs, the intensity of mitral insufficiency murmurs does not significantly change during atrial fibrillation.

In mitral valve prolapse, the murmur may be positional, that is, it may be louder with any maneuver that reduces left ventricular volume. For example, the murmur usually moves earlier in systole when the patient stands. Thus, in mitral valve prolapse, it is not uncommon to hear a midejection click followed by a late systolic murmur when the patient is supine, with the click and murmur moving more toward the first heart sound with the patient upright. This relationship, however, is inconsistent, and once significant mitral regurgitation is present, these traditional changes may be less evident. The murmur of acute mitral insufficiency in patients with acute myocardial infarction may be distinguished from a ventricular septal rupture by noting its radiation and the lack of the associated thrill along the left sternal border.

Noninvasive Evaluation

ELECTROCARDIOGRAM. Electrocardiographic findings in mitral insufficiency most often relate to left atrial enlargement and/or atrial fibrillation. At times, left ventricular hypertrophy is present. When pulmonary hypertension is noted, the criteria for right ventricular hypertrophy may also be fulfilled.

CHEST FILM. Cardiomegaly is common in patients with mitral insufficiency. There is little correlation, however, between atrial size and pressure. Atrial size correlates better with chronicity. Interstitial pulmonary edema and Kerley B lines are seen in the acute phase but are rarely present in chronic mitral regurgitation until later in the course of disease. When mitral annular calcium is present, the calcium forms a C-hook configuration, as the mitral valve shares a common annulus with the aortic valve and calcium usually spares this shared portion. The cardiac silhouette can be dramatically enlarged when there is associated pulmonary hypertension and tricuspid regurgitation.

ECHOCARDIOGRAPHY. This modality can help determine the cause of mitral regurgitation, and it may also provide a rough estimate of its severity. Each of the structures of the mitral apparatus can be examined for abnormalities. The effect of mitral regurgitation on left ventricular mass and its systolic and diastolic function can be assessed. The echocardiogram is very sensitive to mitral regurgitation but is less helpful in quantitating the amount present.

OTHER STUDIES. Radionuclide angiography can define the resting EF. Sometimes an enlarged left atrium may overlap the left ventricle in the left anterior oblique position; this must be carefully considered when EF data are obtained. Exercise radionuclide angiography is particularly valuable for identifying patients in whom ventricular function is marginal. A fall in the EF of more than 5 per cent during stress is considered significant.

Invasive Evaluation

Figure 22 shows relatively acute mitral insufficiency with the presence of a very large V wave in the pulmonary capillary wedge tracing that is even reflected in the pulmonary artery pressure. The height of the V wave in the left atrium is a function of atrial compliance and atrial volume. Large V waves can be seen even without mitral insufficiency in some patients, so the absolute height of the V wave may not correlate with severity. For instance, patients with chronic renal insufficiency receiving dialysis often have a noncompliant left atrium (commonly due to long-standing systemic hypertension). The high output associated with the renal shunt combined with this poorly compliant left atrium can result in a large V wave that is

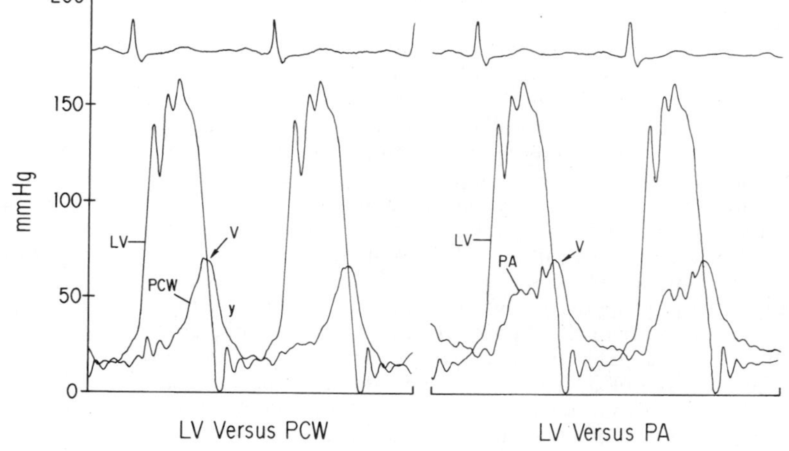

Figure 22. *The hemodynamics of mitral regurgitation.* The large V wave is seen in the pulmonary capillary wedge (PCW) on the left. It can even occasionally be reflected into the pulmonary artery (PA) pressure (shown on the right). LV = left ventricle.

unrelated to mitral insufficiency. The height of the V wave, therefore, is a function not only of mitral insufficiency but also of atrial compliance and the amount of flow through the atrium. In acute mitral insufficiency, therefore, the regurgitant V wave can be dramatic with only moderate mitral regurgitation, whereas the V wave may be only mildly elevated despite severe mitral regurgitation in a patient whose left atrium is markedly dilated.

When to Operate

Patients with mitral insufficiency are especially difficult to monitor because they frequently feel well for long periods, even after systolic dysfunction begins. However, once there is any evidence of decreased systolic function as reflected in serial reductions in the EF, or the presence of increasing end-systolic dimensions, surgery should be considered (see Table 2). When either of these events is obvious, there is loss of contractile reserve. Stress radionuclide angiography in patients with mitral regurgitation is particularly useful in defining the marginal ventricle with limited cardiac reserve because it is not limited by the complexity of hemodynamic changes seen in aortic insufficiency.

Mitral Valve Prolapse Syndrome

Patients who have mitral valve prolapse deserve particular mention because of the high frequency, especially in women, of what has been described as the "mitral valve prolapse syndrome."

Anatomically, many of these patients demonstrate myxomatous (floppy) mitral valve tissue and elongated chordae. Mitral valve prolapse has been associated with a wide variety of symptoms and signs. The tensing of the chordae, and perhaps the popping of the redundant leaflet scallops, cause one or more systolic clicks. Loss of apposition of the mitral leaflets contributes to the mitral insufficiency. Mitral valve prolapse has been described in patients with Marfan's syndrome, coronary artery disease, cardiomyopathy, inflammatory diseases, Ehlers-Danlos syndrome, pseudoxanthoma elasticum, straight back syndrome, and various congenital heart diseases.

A unique feature in some patients with mitral valve prolapse is an associated hyperadrenergic syndrome. The clinician should approach these patients with sincerity and compassion. They frequently experience fatigue, palpitations, symptoms suggestive of autonomic dysfunction, angina, migraine headache, and so on. These patients should be told that these symptoms are not related to the prolapsing mitral valve. Do not focus on the mitral valve prolapse because many patients will experience a cardiac neurosis relative to the valve itself.

Mitral insufficiency progresses in about 15 per cent of mitral valve prolapse patients. It is not known why progression appears to be more common in men than in women. Although cerebral emboli occasionally occur and aspirin prophylaxis has been recommended, the only prophylactic regimen in routine use is the prevention of endocarditis. Because auscultation is a dying art in the United States, the clinician should use endocarditis prophylaxis in all patients with mitral valve prolapse.

Catecholamine excess in some of these patients helps explain the propensity toward arrhythmias and the intermittent attacks of chest pain, dizziness, and psychosomatic discomfort. In most women, these symptoms tend to abate after the age of 50 years. Aerobic exercise programs that improve conditioning can reduce the cathecholamine excess that may affect some patients. Beta-blocking agents are also useful and can be given prophylactically if the patient can identify stress periods ahead of time.

Tricuspid Regurgitation

Natural History and Etiology

Tricuspid regurgitation is extremely common in patients with valvular heart disease. This is because the tricuspid valve does not have discrete papillary muscles attaching it to the right ventricular endocardium but rather chordae that attach throughout the right ventricular wall. Any disease that increases the size of the right ventricle can cause displacement of these chordae and tricuspid regurgitation. Once tricuspid regurgitation occurs, the increased volume overload further dilates the right ventricle and the tricuspid annulus, and a vicious cycle is begun. Most tricuspid insufficiency is related to pulmonary hypertension or right ventricular dilatation. Occasionally, direct tricuspid valvular changes are noted in patients with Marfan's syndrome (when prolapse or annular dilatation is present) or Ebstein's anomaly (with displacement of the tricuspid valve). Rheumatic fever can involve the tricuspid valve. This is more frequent in Third World countries than in the United States. Endocarditis can also involve the tricuspid valve. In drug addicts, the mitral valve is the most common site of endocarditis. In the United States, most tricuspid valve endocarditis is seen in drug abusers. Carcinoid plaque, myxoma, tumors, and other inflammatory diseases can also involve the tricuspid valve.

Symptoms

Tricuspid insufficiency leads to peripheral congestion with hepatomegaly, ascites, and occasionally massive edema. Systolic pulsations of the eyeballs and the neck have been described. With reduced forward output, symptoms of fatigue and weakness are common. Bowel edema may reduce appetite and decrease the absorption of medications such as furosemide.

Physical Examination

Tricuspid regurgitation can usually be diagnosed by careful examination of the neck veins. In the normal individual, the *X* descent of the jugular venous pulse occurs during ventricular systole, as shown in Figure 23. This can be timed by palpating the opposite carotid artery while observing the jugular venous pulse wave forms. In a patient with tricuspid regurgitation, there is systolic expansion—the CV wave—that occurs during ventricular systole. If the jugular venous pulse reveals a pulsation in concert with the systolic pulsation of the carotid artery, tricuspid insufficiency should be presumed present. The neck vein is generally markedly distended. If after completing the observation of the neck vein, one is unsure of the presence of tricuspid regurgitation, it is often difficult to support the diagnosis by any other physical finding. A systolic venous thrill is occasionally heard in the presence of severe tricuspid regurgitation. The right ventricular impulse is often hyperdynamic and thrusting. The liver is often congested and may be pulsatile with systole. On auscultation, a right-sided third heart sound may be heard. This is often audible in the neck (where left-sided gallops are rarely heard). If pulmonary hypertension is present, the pulmonic second heart sound is accentuated. The murmur of tricuspid insufficiency increases with inspiration (the Carvallo sign), but this is an inconsistent finding. Occasionally in severe tricuspid regurgitation, an associated diastolic rumble across the tricuspid valve is audible.

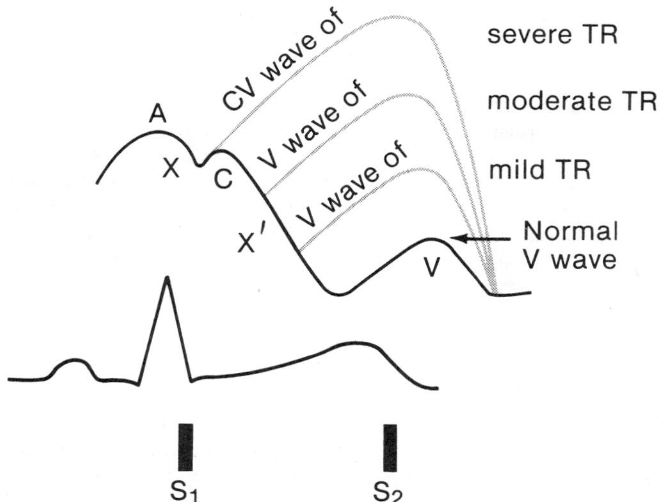

Figure 23. *The jugular venous pulse in tricuspid regurgitation.* The jugular venous pulse wave normally drops during ventricular systole. As tricuspid regurgitation (TR) becomes more severe, the CV wave becomes more obvious during ventricular systole.

Noninvasive Evaluation

ELECTROCARDIOGRAM. The ECG is rather nonspecific in tricuspid regurgitation. Atrial fibrillation is observed in some patients with tricuspid regurgitation and an enlarged right atrium.

CHEST FILM. Cardiomegaly is generally seen when the right ventricle enlarges. With increased right atrial pressure, there is reduced drainage of the pleural space and pleural effusions are common. The diaphragms are often displaced upward if ascites is present. Pulmonary arterial and venous hypertension is common. Enlargement of the superior vena cava and azygos vein is also frequently seen. Figure 24 shows PA and lateral chest films of a patient with tricuspid regurgitation.

ECHOCARDIOGRAPHY. In patients with tricuspid regurgitation secondary to a dilated tricuspid annulus, the right atrium, right ventricle, and tricuspid annulus are all markedly enlarged. Paradoxical motion of the interventricular septum is common. The echocardiogram also reveals anatomic abnormalities in the tricuspid valve itself. Color flow Doppler may reveal systolic pulsation of blood into the inferior vena cava. There may be loss of normal inferior vena caval collapse with a rapid sniff. The maximal velocity of the tricuspid Doppler jet reflects right ventricular systolic and consequently pulmonary artery systolic pressure.

Invasive Evaluation

At catheterization, the right atrial and right ventricular pressures are frequently increased in tricuspid regurgitation. When the right side of the heart becomes markedly enlarged, myocardium exceeds pericardium and the hemodynamics of constrictive pericarditis can occasionally be observed. If pulmonary systolic pressure is less than 40 mm Hg, primary tricuspid regurgitation should be considered. When pulmonary pressures exceed 40 mm Hg, tricuspid regurgitation is more likely secondary.

When to Operate

Although the criteria for the use of chamber sizes based on pressure-volume data are now emerging for mitral and aortic insufficiency, no such data exist for tricuspid regurgitation. However, there is a growing trend toward the use of tricuspid annuloplasty whenever there is significant tricuspid insufficiency, especially when it exists in association with other valvular disease. If the right ventricular systolic pressure is less than 40 mm Hg, tricuspid repair or replacement is generally indicated if tricuspid regurgitation is severe. In rare cases of endocarditis, the tricuspid valve can be excised in its entirety for short periods (1 to 3 months) to facilitate cure of the endocarditis. This is not, however, a viable long-term solution.

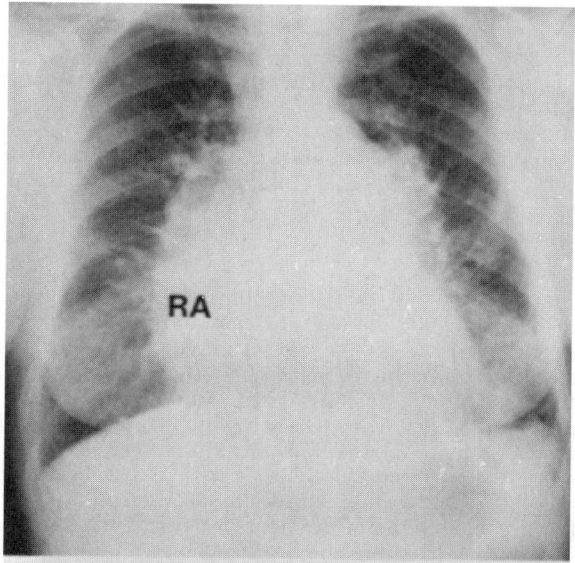

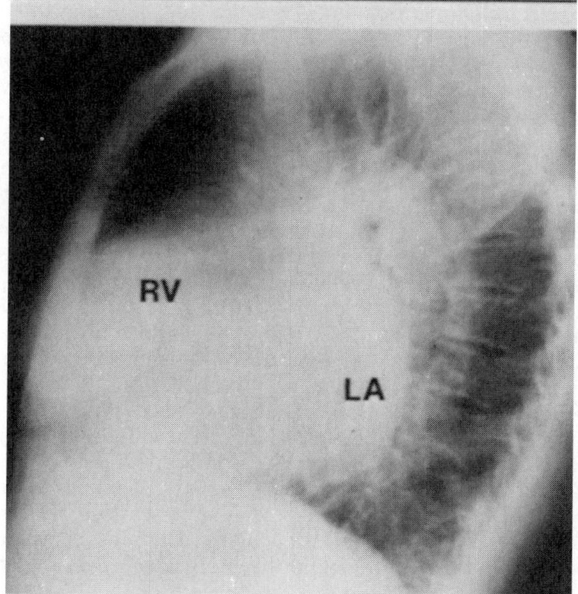

Figure 24. *Representative chest films in chronic tricuspid regurgitation.* PA above, lateral below. The patient also had mitral stenosis and pulmonary hypertension. There is enlargement of all four chambers and dilated pulmonary arteries. RA = right atrium; RV = right ventricle; LA = left atrium. (From Ockene, I.S.: Tricuspid valve disease. *In* Dalen, J.E., and Alpert, J.S. [eds.]: Valvular Heart Disease, 2nd ed. Boston, Little, Brown, 1987, p. 366, with permission.)

Tricuspid Stenosis

Natural History and Etiology

Tricuspid stenosis is uncommon in the United States. Most patients with tricuspid stenosis have rheumatic heart disease, but the carcinoid syndrome can produce plaques that narrow the tricuspid valve. Right atrial tumors and congenital tricuspid hypoplasia or atresia are less frequent causes of obstruction. Rheumatic tricuspid stenosis is almost never present as an isolated lesion. As with mitral stenosis, tricuspid stenosis is more common in women. Frequently, tricuspid stenosis is associated with significant tricuspid regurgitation. Left unattended, tricuspid stenosis can present with evidence of marked right atrial hypertension.

Symptoms

Tricuspid stenosis generally presents with fatigue and symptoms of hepatomegaly, ascites, and anasarca. Low-output symptoms are also common. Giant A waves can be seen in the jugular venous pulse, and the patient may become aware of them. Pulmonary congestion is rarely seen.

Physical Examination

Tricuspid stenosis usually accompanies rheumatic mitral stenosis. Tricuspid stenosis is commonly overlooked because of the focus on the mitral valve or aortic valve in chronic rheumatic heart disease. In the presence of sinus rhythm, the jugular venous pulse should be carefully observed for a giant A wave. Occasionally, a presystolic pulsation in the liver or the lack of *Y* descent in the neck vein may be appreciated. The right ventricle may not be markedly enlarged unless associated tricuspid regurgitation is present. Signs of pulmonary hypertension are usually absent. A diastolic thrill during inspiration has been described.

A tricuspid opening snap is best heard along the left sternal border. The diastolic murmur, which is also best heard along the left sternal border, often exhibits a prominent presystolic component during the A wave. As with most right-sided events, the opening snap and murmur are augmented by inspiration.

Noninvasive Evaluation

The ECG is relatively nondescript. Atrial fibrillation is actually uncommon. Marked right atrial enlargement out of proportion to the degree of right ventricular hypertrophy has been described. The chest film reveals the marked right atrial enlargement, which extends into a dilated superior vena cava and azygos vein but without dilatation of the pulmonary artery.

Echocardiographic changes in the tricuspid valve are similar to those in the rheumatic mitral valve, with thickened leaflets, reduced motion of the chordae due to commissural fusion, and calcification of the leaflets and/or annulus. Diastolic doming of the leaflets caused by fusion of their tips is a characteristic feature. Doppler assessment reveals the tricuspid gradient, and associated tricuspid regurgitation is common.

Invasive Evaluation

Tricuspid stenosis is documented by simultaneous measurement of the right atrial and right ventricular pressures. Right atrial angiography reveals the limited excursion of contrast into the right ventricle. The inflow pattern of contrast from the right atrium resembles a triangular orifice. A tricuspid valve area can be determined, but its clinical relevance is poorly documented.

When to Operate

Surgical replacement should be considered for tricuspid stenosis that results in a mean diastolic gradient exceeding 5 mm Hg. Percutaneous balloon commissurotomy and surgical commissurotomy have both been performed with mixed results. Tricuspid insufficiency frequently follows either of these procedures. For that reason, replacement of the valve with a porcine prosthesis is usually recommended.

Pulmonic Regurgitation

Natural History and Etiology

The right ventricle performs its pump function like a bellows against the interventricular septum and is designed to handle a volume load. Pulmonic insufficiency can be tolerated well over many years in both congenital and noncongenital cardiac disorders. For example, repair of tetralogy of Fallot often leaves the pulmonic valve insufficient, but only late in the course does volume overload result in right ventricular dysfunction. The most common nonsurgical cause of pulmonic insufficiency is dilatation of the valve ring secondary to pulmonary hypertension. Enlargement of the pulmonary artery itself may also occur in connective tissue disorders or with idiopathic dilatation of the pulmonary artery. Other less common lesions that result in valvular insufficiency include the carcinoid syndrome, syphilis, and trauma. Rheumatic disease of the pulmonic valve is exceptionally rare. The pulmonic valve is subjected to the least hemodynamic stress of all the valves. Right ventricular systolic pressures of 25 mm Hg open the valve, and the pulmonary artery diastolic pressure averages 15 mm Hg.

Symptoms

Pulmonic insufficiency causes right ventricular volume overload. In general, symptoms are minimal and the discovery of pulmonic insufficiency incidental. Only rarely does right ventricular failure occur. Those patients who tolerate pulmonic insufficiency poorly have associated disease of the right ventricle, such as previous hypertrophy from tetralogy of Fallot or prior VSD. As patients with repaired tetralogy of Fallot increasingly reach adulthood, the number of such individuals needing pulmonary valve replacement has increased.

Physical Examination

Pulmonic insufficiency causes right ventricular hypertrophy as well as dilatation. If significant pulmonary hypertension is present, the pulmonary artery may be palpated along the second intercostal space. The pulmonic closure sound may be palpable as well. Pulmonic insufficiency in the presence of pulmonary hypertension is referred to as the Graham Steell murmur. It is typically high-pitched, begins immediately after the pulmonic second heart sound, and is heard along the left parasternal region in the second to fourth interspace. The Graham Steell murmur can be distinguished from the murmur of aortic insufficiency by its association with pulmonary hypertension. With inspiration, the pulmonic insufficiency murmur increases and conversely decreases during a Valsalva maneuver.

In patients with primary pulmonary valvular insufficiency, the gradient between the right ventricle and the pulmonary artery may be small. Thus, even with substan-

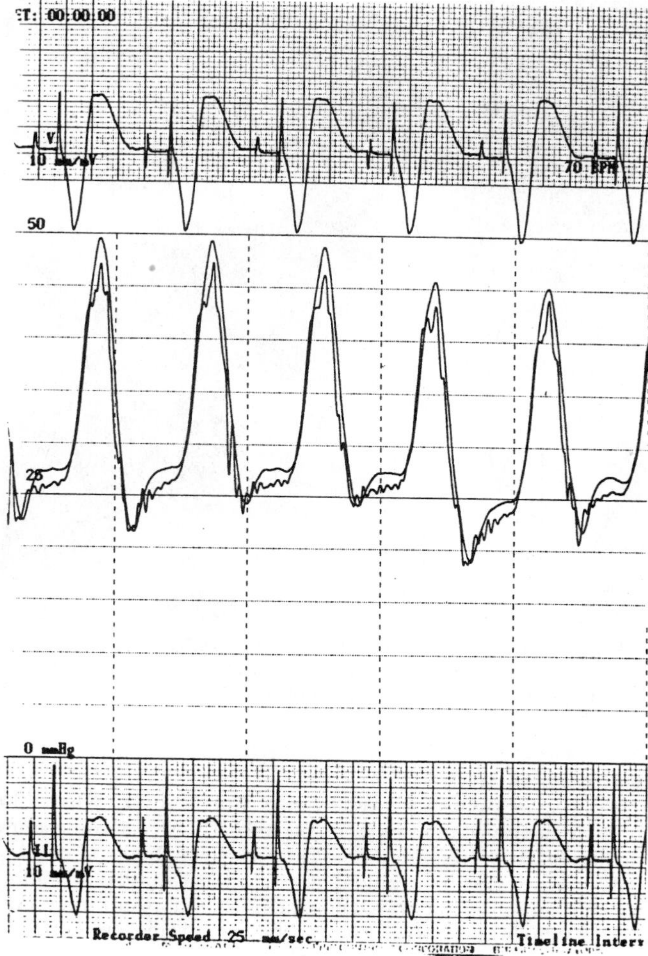

Figure 25. *The hemodynamics of pulmonic insufficiency.* Note the minimal diastolic gradient present between the pulmonary artery and right ventricle in this patient with pulmonary valve insufficiency but without significant pulmonary hypertension.

tial pulmonic insufficiency, little murmur may be audible. As shown in Figure 25, primary pulmonic insufficiency can result in a pulmonary artery pressure that is almost superimposable on the right ventricular pressure. It is this minimal gradient that explains why the murmur may be quite soft. Pulmonary insufficiency due to pulmonary hypertension results in a much louder murmur that is often heard throughout diastole.

Noninvasive Evaluation

The ECG in pulmonary insufficiency is nonspecific. In the absence of pulmonary hypertension and associated right ventricular pressure overload, right ventricular hypertrophy is only occasionally present. Radiographically, both the pulmonary artery and the right ventricle are usually enlarged. The echocardiogram provides good evidence for pulmonic insufficiency, but even the echocardiogram may underestimate the severity of pulmonic insufficiency, as the gradient during diastole is often trivial. Doppler echocardiography is useful in diagnosing pulmonary hypertension, in estimating pulmonary artery systolic pressure, and in distinguishing primary from secondary pulmonic insufficiency.

Invasive Evaluation

Contrast in the pulmonary artery can document dramatic pulmonic insufficiency in patients who lack auscultatory or echocardiographic evidence of pulmonary insufficiency. The clinician should anticipate this situation if the right ventricle appears excessively dilated with clinical pulmonic insufficiency as the only observable lesion.

When to Operate

Primary pulmonic insufficiency may not require surgical intervention unless evidence for right-sided heart failure ensues. Symptoms of fatigue and exercise intolerance predominate. At that time, valve replacement can be pursued. Pulmonic insufficiency due to pulmonary hypertension is usually considered a secondary lesion, and therapy (if possible) for the pulmonary hypertension is the usual practice.

Pulmonic Stenosis

Natural History and Etiology

Pulmonic stenosis is typically congenital. Its severity ranges from complete atresia to various dysplastic forms to simple commissural fusion. Rheumatic inflammation is extremely uncommon and, essentially, rheumatic involvement always involves other valves as well. Carcinoid plaques may cause an acquired form of pulmonic stenosis. Tolerance of pulmonic stenosis depends on its severity. For example, severe congenital pulmonic stenosis may reduce pulmonary flow and require early intervention. Because the right ventricle is designed to perform volume—not pressure—work, right ventricular dysfunction may emerge in patients with significant pulmonic stenosis.

Symptoms

In general, pulmonic stenosis is asymptomatic until right ventricular failure ensues. At that time, venous distention, ascites, and anasarca can emerge. Tricuspid regurgitation invariably accompanies right ventricular failure.

Physical Examination

The jugular venous pulse often reveals an increased A wave consistent with reduced right ventricular compliance. The carotid artery is normal. The apical examination may reveal mild right ventricular enlargement. Poststenotic dilatation of the pulmonary artery may result in a palpable pulmonary artery along the second intercostal space. The first heart sound is usually normal. The second heart sound shows wide splitting resulting from delayed pulmonic valve closure. If poststenotic dilatation of the pulmonary artery is considerable, the respiratory variation of the second heart sound may be diminished.

A pulmonic ejection sound is often present. *As opposed to all other auscultatory events on the right side of the heart, the pulmonic ejection sound becomes quieter with inspiration* because of premature opening of the pulmonic valve with inspiration. Premature opening occurs because the pulmonary artery diastolic pressure is frequently similar to that of the right ventricular diastolic pressure. Because of the low pulmonary pressures and high right ventricular diastolic pressure (as a consequence of right ventricular hypertrophy), the atrial A wave contribution to the right ventricular volume increases pressure in the right ventricle to such an extent that premature opening of the pulmonic valve occurs. The intensity of the opening sound (click) depends on pulmonic valve motion. The greater the premature opening of the valve, the less distance it travels during ventricular systole. This decrease

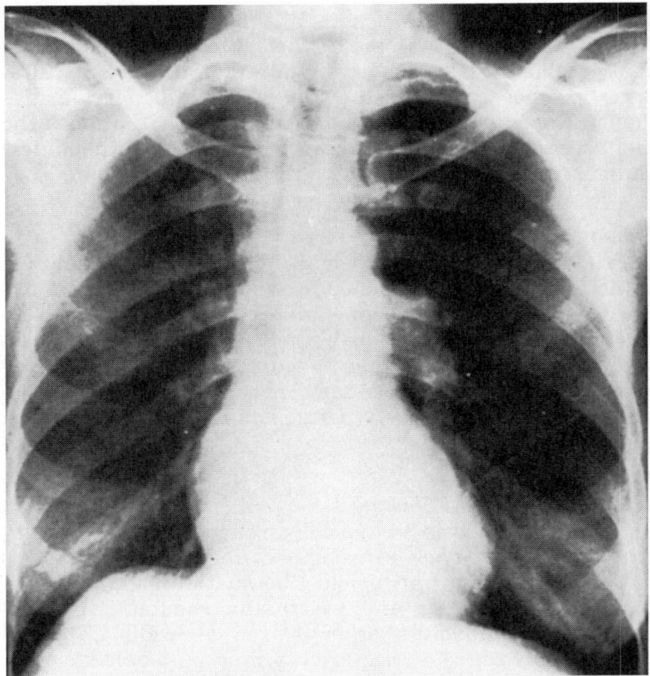

Figure 26. *A representative chest film in pulmonic stenosis.* Because of the direction of flow, the left pulmonary artery tends to be larger than the right pulmonary artery. (From Perloff, J.K.: The Clinical Recognition of Congenital Heart Disease, 4th ed. Philadelphia, W.B. Saunders, 1994, p. 222, with permission.)

in valve motion causes the pulmonic ejection sound to be reduced. In a dysplastic pulmonic valve, the ejection sound is usually absent. The murmur of pulmonic stenosis is an ejection murmur heard along the left sternal border with frequent radiation toward the left lung. The murmur increases with inspiration. In severe pulmonic stenosis, a thrill may be palpable.

Noninvasive Evaluation

The ECG reveals evidence of right ventricular hypertrophy. The chest film reveals enlargement of the right ventricle. Poststenotic dilatation of the pulmonary artery can occasionally be dramatic. There is preferential flow of blood to the left lung, and enlargement of the left lower lung vessels in comparison with the right lower lung vessels has been reported (Fig. 26). The echocardiogram reveals right ventricular hypertrophy and doming of the pulmonic valve (in nondysplastic valves). Continuous-wave Doppler can define the magnitude of the gradient across the pulmonic valve. Color flow Doppler provides evidence for turbulence into the pulmonary artery.

Invasive Evaluation

In pulmonary stenosis, a gradient between the right ventricle and right atrium appears across the pulmonic valve. Once this gradient exceeds 50 mm Hg, significant pulmonary stenosis is felt to be present. Pulmonary angiography and right ventricular angiography can define the pulmonary anatomy. Figure 27 shows the classic doming of the pulmonic valve during right ventricular angiography. The pressure gradient is shown in Figure 28. Percutaneous balloon valvuloplasty is effective in reducing the gradient.

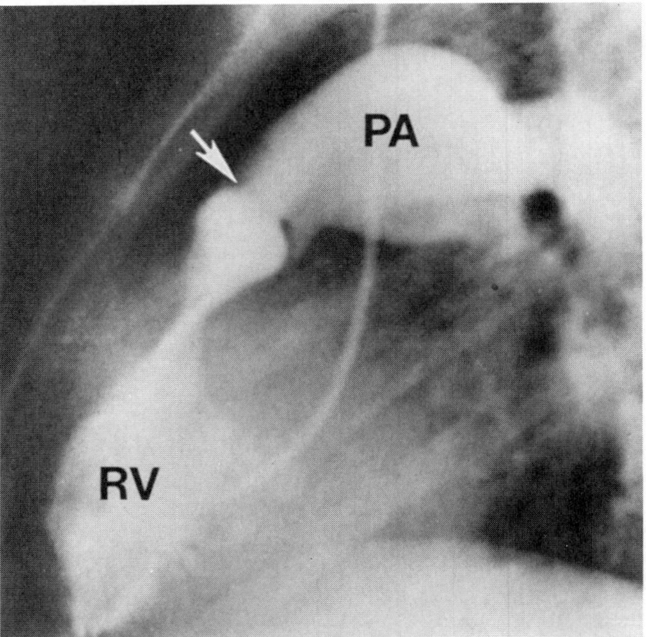

Figure 27. *Pulmonic valve stenosis by right ventricular angiography.* The doming of the pulmonic valve is well seen *(arrow).* Subpulmonic stenosis is also evident. PA = pulmonary artery; RV = right ventricle.

When to Operate

Pulmonic stenosis may require intervention when the peak-to-peak gradient exceeds 50 mm Hg. Echocardiography is helpful in screening. For patients who have a doming valve, percutaneous valvuloplasty is almost universally effective. Other surgical approaches include commissurotomy, outflow patch enlargement and, rarely, valve replacement.

SUMMARY

In summary, valvular heart disease remains a continuing challenge to all physicians. New diagnostic and thera-

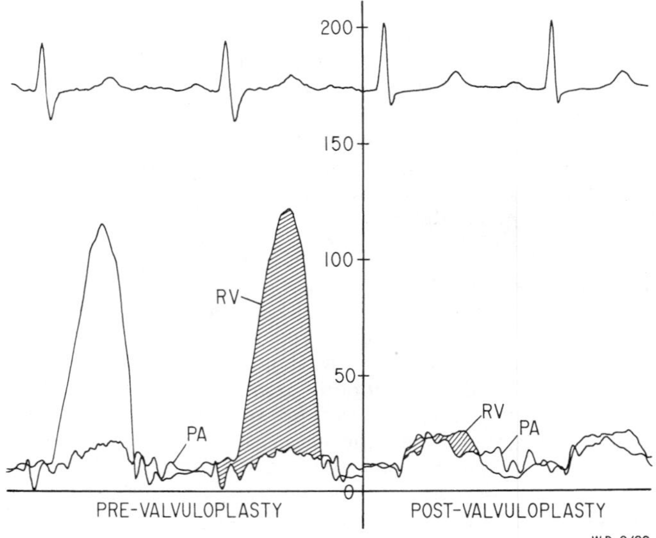

Figure 28. Pulmonary pressure in pulmonic stenosis before and after percutaneous valvuloplasty. RV = right ventricle; PA = pulmonary artery.

peutic approaches emphasize the importance of accurate diagnosis early in the patient's clinical course. With the advent of two-dimensional echocardiography, Doppler, color flow Doppler, and transesophageal echocardiography, anatomic descriptions of valvular disease can be readily obtained. Echocardiography is usually superior to the physical examination in defining valvular disease, but proper patient selection for echocardiography still requires the performance of an adequate physical examination. Because the art of auscultation has received waning attention over the last 20 years, physicians are more likely than ever to miss important diagnostic clues. Catheterization provides useful additional information in most but not all patients.

The decision to refer the patient for valvuloplasty, surgical repair, or valve replacement should focus on symptoms in patients who have right-sided lesions, mitral stenosis, or aortic stenosis. In left-sided regurgitant valvular disease, including aortic insufficiency and mitral insufficiency, the clinician must follow the patient with serial measurements of the EF and the end-systolic volume or dimension to avoid unnecessarily delayed surgery. It is unfortunate that surgical techniques and prosthetic valve complications have yet to reach a stage that morbidity and mortality are such rare occurrences that prophylactic valve replacement or repair could be offered to every patient with valvular disease.

ACUTE RHEUMATIC FEVER

By William A. Alto, M.D.,
and Michael E. Clark, M.D.
Waterville, Maine

Acute rheumatic fever is the most serious nonsuppurative sequela of upper respiratory tract infection with group A streptococcus *(Streptococcus pyogenes)*. The incidence of acute rheumatic fever had been declining in the United States for years, but the recent unexplained resurgence in the 1980s has renewed interest in the disease.

Acute rheumatic fever was traditionally considered a disease of poor and/or minority children living in unhygienic and overcrowded conditions. However, recent clusters have been reported in both white middle-class groups and adults. Although certain populations (Samoans), areas (Salt Lake City, Utah), and families appear to be at increased risk, no group is spared. Acute rheumatic fever has been reported in children as young as 2 years of age and in adults in their mid-40s. Older children and adolescents, however, make up the bulk of patients who acquire the disease.

The diagnosis of acute rheumatic fever can be difficult because there is no specific symptom, sign, or laboratory test to confirm the clinician's impressions. In 1944, Jones first proposed guidelines to facilitate the diagnosis. The criteria have undergone several revisions over the years. The last update was published in 1992 by the American Heart Association (Table 1). Each revision has been driven by the need to incorporate new knowledge as well as new laboratory and technical procedures. The desire to decrease the false-positive diagnosis rate has also influenced recent revisions of the Jones criteria, which are intended to support the diagnosis of the initial attack of acute rheumatic fever. The Jones criteria have been divided into five major and a number of minor clinical signs, symptoms, and laboratory findings. Two major or one major and two minor criteria are required for making the diagnosis of acute rheumatic fever. In addition, supporting evidence of a preceding group A streptococcal infection is required except in special circumstances, as explained further on. The Jones criteria are guidelines and do not supersede clinical judgment in the diagnosis of acute rheumatic fever.

Table 1. Jones Criteria, 1992 Update: Guidelines for the Diagnosis of Acute Rheumatic Fever

Major Manifestations	Minor Manifestations
Carditis	Clinical findings
Polyarthritis	Arthralgia
Chorea	Fever
Erythema marginatum	Laboratory findings
Subcutaneous nodules	Elevated acute-phase reactants
	Erythrocyte sedimentation rate
	C-reactive protein
	Prolonged PR interval
Supporting Evidence of Antecedent Group A Streptococcal Infection	
Throat culture	
Streptococcal antibody test	
Exceptions to the Jones Criteria	
Chorea	
Indolent carditis	
Recurrent attack	

CARDITIS

Of the major manifestations of rheumatic fever, carditis is the most serious and most common. Carditis is defined clinically as a new or changed audible heart murmur of valvulitis. The most common murmur is that of mitral regurgitation (apical, high-pitched, blowing, and holosystolic), which radiates to the axillae with or without aortic regurgitation (diastolic, basal, high-pitched, blowing, and decrescendo). New-onset aortic regurgitation *with* a mitral regurgitation murmur is often acute rheumatic carditis. Isolated aortic murmurs, especially those occurring in systole, are rarely indicative of the acute disease. Mitral regurgitation predominates over aortic regurgitation murmurs by a 3:1 ratio. Mitral murmurs of acute rheumatic carditis must be differentiated from the midsystolic click, late systolic murmur of mitral valve prolapse, and functional murmurs accentuated by febrile tachycardia or anemia, Still's murmur, and other congenital murmurs. Pulmonary or tricuspid murmurs are rarely found, especially in the absence of mitral disease.

Echocardiography is frequently helpful in sorting out the origins and severity of valvular disease. Color flow Doppler studies have detected clinically silent mitral disease in a number of patients. However, valvulitis identified by echocardiography alone does not fulfill a major criterion. Only the auscultation of a typical murmur may be used in meeting the Jones criteria.

Myocarditis, pericarditis, and congestive heart failure may accompany acute rheumatic valvulitis. Tachycardia, increased cardiac enzyme levels, and conduction delays in the electrocardiogram suggest myocarditis. Isolated myocarditis without other signs of valvulitis is unusual. Pericarditis with chest pain, a friction rub, electrocardiographic changes, and an effusion is also uncommon (incidence of less than 5 per cent). Pericarditis rarely occurs as the sole manifestation of rheumatic carditis. A chest film, electrocardiogram, and echocardiogram should be obtained when acute rheumatic fever is suspected.

ARTHRITIS

Arthritic acute rheumatic fever is polyarticular, migratory, and more frequently observed in adults. The knees, ankles, elbows, and wrists are most frequently involved, often simultaneously, and the patient typically has a fever. Isolated arthritis in the hands or feet is unusual and should suggest another diagnosis. Rheumatic arthritis is sudden in onset and reaches a maximum intensity in hours to days. The involved joints are hot, swollen, tender, and red, and motion is limited. Arthrocentesis may be required to exclude other causes of arthritis. Joint fluid is typically clear, with increased protein and cell counts. Polyarthritis generally resolves by 3 to 4 weeks without sequelae.

CHOREA

Sydenham's chorea may present insidiously as weakness, moodiness, clumsiness, tics, and emotional lability progressing over several weeks to bilateral involuntary and purposeless ataxia. Rarely, the onset may be explosive. Chorea is often the sole manifestation of acute rheumatic fever, or it may occur weeks to months following a more typical presentation of carditis. When chorea occurs in isolation, serologic evidence of a previous streptococcal infection may have waned. More common in preteen girls, chorea usually resolves in 2 to 6 months. Unusual neurologic problems found in less than 5 per cent of patients include meningoencephalitis, encephalitis, seizures, hemiparesis, papilledema, diplopia, and acute psychosis.

ERYTHEMA MARGINATUM

Erythema marginatum occurs in less than 10 per cent of patients with acute rheumatic fever. This pink-to-red, macular, confluent rash on the trunk and proximal extremities is almost never seen on the face. Fever or the application of heat increases its prominence, and the lesion blanches on pressure. The rash is nonpruritic, evanescent, migratory, and typically observed in patients with severe manifestations of rheumatic fever. Erythema marginatum may easily be missed in dark-skinned patients, and it is seldom an isolated major criterion of acute rheumatic fever.

SUBCUTANEOUS NODULES

Found in fewer than 3 per cent of patients with rheumatic fever, subcutaneous nodules occur most often in persons with chronic carditis. The nodules are 2 to 20 mm in diameter, symmetrical, painless, and freely movable. They are most frequently found over the extensor surfaces of the elbow, knee, wrist, and ankle and the spinous processes of the vertebrae.

MINOR CRITERIA

Minor criteria for the diagnosis of rheumatic fever are relatively nonspecific and are used to support the diagnosis when only a single major criterion is present. Fever exceeding 38°C (100.4°F) is present in almost all patients with acute rheumatic fever. This is an early finding and may not be present in patients with pure chorea or late-onset carditis. Arthralgia is pain in the joints without evidence of inflammation. Arthralgia may be counted as a minor criteria only if arthritis is not present.

Laboratory data are also nonspecific. The erythrocyte sedimentation rate (ESR) and C-reactive protein (CRP) are almost always increased in patients with polyarthritis or acute carditis. However, they are often normal in patients presenting with chorea. A decreased ESR and C-reactive protein level may indicate that an acute phase of rheumatic fever has subsided. Electrocardiographic changes are frequently present. Prolongation of the PR interval (first-degree heart block) is most commonly seen. Other changes include sinus tachycardia and the Wenckebach phenomenon. Electrocardiographic changes may be either transient or permanent. Isolated prolongation of the PR interval does not prove the presence of active carditis.

EXCEPTIONS TO THE JONES CRITERIA

There are three circumstances in which rheumatic fever can be diagnosed without strictly adhering to the Jones criteria. The diagnosis remains presumptive, however, until other potential causes are excluded. First, chorea may be a delayed and sole manifestation of rheumatic fever that presents when laboratory data are unremarkable. Second, carditis can also be the only manifestation in patients who seek medical attention at a time when all other signs of rheumatic fever have abated. Furthermore, carditis is often discovered for the first time when the sole presenting feature of rheumatic fever is chorea. Lastly, a presumptive diagnosis of recurrent rheumatic fever can be made in a patient with a known previous episode of rheumatic fever and a single major or several minor criteria. Patients with a past history of rheumatic fever remain at high risk for infections with group A streptococci.

OTHER SIGNS AND SYMPTOMS

Additional findings that are not part of the Jones criteria but are frequently reported include fatigue, irritability, abdominal pain, and chest pain. Epistaxis, resting tachycardia, and normochromic normocytic anemia are also common. Mild renal involvement (incidence of 51 to 65 per cent) with microhematuria, proteinuria, and transient azotemia as well as abnormal liver function tests (incidence of 64 per cent) have also been reported. There appears to be a familial predisposition to the development of rheumatic fever.

DIFFERENTIAL DIAGNOSIS

It is unusual for a patient with acute rheumatic fever to present with three or more major criteria. The most common presentations are, in decreasing order of frequency, carditis, chorea, and carditis with arthritis. Skin manifestations are rare and usually accompany carditis with polyarthritis. The weakest combination of signs and symptoms that meet the Jones criteria are monoarticular arthritis with fever, an increased ESR, and a single increased streptococcal antibody test result. Many of these patients will have another disease such as septic arthritis, rheumatoid arthritis, systemic lupus erythematosus, Lyme disease, serum sickness, a drug reaction, leukemia, or tuberculosis. Juvenile rheumatoid arthritis is the disorder most frequently confused with acute rheumatic fever. Adequate salicylate treatment rapidly and dramatically resolves the fever and arthritis of acute rheumatic fever, usually within 48 hours.

The isolated carditis of rheumatic fever can be confused with viral myocarditis and subacute bacterial endocarditis. Chorea may be the only manifestation of acute rheumatic fever, or it may appear months after asymptomatic carditis has cleared. Echocardiographic evidence of silent mitral valve incompetence may suggest the diagnosis. Other causes of chorea are unusual in children and adolescents, but Huntington's disease, Wilson's disease, systemic lupus erythematosus, and adverse reactions to phenothiazines, oral contraceptives, isoniazid, or lithium should be considered.

The physician should remember that appropriate treatment of streptococcal pharyngitis does not preclude the development of rheumatic fever. Fewer than one third of patients with acute rheumatic fever recall an antecedent episode of pharyngitis. Because the clinical diagnosis is unreliable, scarlet fever is no longer considered proof of recent streptococcal infection. Rising titers of antistreptococcal antibodies provide better evidence of recent infection, especially in patients who exhibit only arthritis as a major criterion. The exceptions to this rule are Sydenham's chorea and indolent rheumatic carditis.

To avoid overdiagnosis, the clinician may have to follow the untreated patient's vague symptoms for several days to weeks, avoiding the use of salicylates or steroids, which can mask one or more of the criteria required for accurate diagnosis. It is always prudent to seek the advice of a physician experienced in the protean manifestations of rheumatic fever.

INFECTIVE ENDOCARDITIS

By Rosemary A. Kearney, M.D.,
and Judith E. Wolf, M.D.
Philadelphia, Pennsylvania

Infective endocarditis is, by definition, an infection of the endothelial lining of the heart. Since the time of Osler, it has remained a disease of varied presentation and often perplexing diagnosis. Most commonly, the infection occurs in valvular tissue, but it may also occur in areas of mural endocardium, congenital malformations, septal defects, surgically constructed shunts, or intracardiac prosthetic material, such as heart valves. Clinically, the manifestations of infected arteriovenous shunts, coarctation of the aorta, and patent ductus arteriosus are similar and are included under the heading of infective endocarditis. Although infective endocarditis was formerly referred to as bacterial endocarditis, it is widely known that fungi as well as rare organisms such as rickettsiae, mycoplasma, and spirochetes can cause this disease. The role of viruses is unknown. Infective endocarditis had previously been classified as acute, subacute, or chronic, depending on the duration of clinical illness. These classifications became largely arbitrary, however, as clinicians realized that certain organisms that cause the disease can have varied presentations and clinical courses.

The incidence of infective endocarditis ranges from 0.16 to 5.4 cases per 1000 hospital admissions, with at least 60 per cent of patients being male. In the last 30 years, the elderly have become increasingly affected by infective endocarditis, primarily because of a longer life span associated with an increased likelihood of invasive procedures and intravascular devices. Despite advances in prevention, diagnosis, and treatment, infective endocarditis remains prevalent and is associated with significant morbidity and mortality.

PREDISPOSING FACTORS

It is widely known that most patients with infective endocarditis have an identifiable predisposing lesion. However, as many as 30 to 40 per cent of infections may occur in apparently normal endocardium. The latter cases are usually associated with more virulent infections and typically present with a more aggressive clinical course.

The most frequent predisposing factor in adult infective endocarditis is mitral valve prolapse with an associated systolic murmur. Certain degenerative valvular lesions, such as aortic stenosis, mitral stenosis, and calcified mitral annulus, are also common, accounting for a large percentage of cases in the elderly. Other degenerative lesions that are not necessarily valvular in nature may become infected, including calcific nodular lesions secondary to atherosclerosis and thrombi occurring after myocardial infarction. Rheumatic heart disease, formerly a common cause of acquired valvular disease, has rapidly declined over the past several decades. Hence, there has been an associated dramatic drop of infective endocarditis in this population. Congenital cardiovascular lesions such as tetralogy of Fallot, ventricular septal defect, bicuspid aortic valve, pulmonic stenosis, and coarctation of the aorta also predispose patients to infective endocarditis. Hypertrophic cardiomyopathy (idiopathic hypertrophic subaortic stenosis [IHSS]) and syphilitic aortic valvular disease may be affected as well, the latter being much more rare. In idiopathic hypertrophic subaortic stenosis, infective endocarditis is more common in patients with severe hemodynamic alterations. Patients with Marfan's syndrome, another condition with anatomic abnormalities, are also at risk for infection. The often redundant and myxomatous mitral valve is at significant risk for the development of infection. Although the aortic valve and proximal aorta are also typically abnormal in Marfan's syndrome, they rarely become infected.

Nosocomial acquisition of infective endocarditis does occur and is the most common predisposing factor to infective endocarditis in the elderly. Patients typically are severely ill and compromised, subjected to long-term therapies or hyperalimentation requiring multiple intravascular catheters or procedures. Infective endocarditis originating in other intravascular devices such as permanent cardiac pacemakers rarely occurs. Patients with prosthetic valves, both mechanical and bioprosthetic, are a large population predisposed to endocarditis. Another large and seemingly growing population at high risk for infective endocarditis is intravenous drug users, including human immunodeficiency virus (HIV)-positive patients. The overwhelming majority of valvular infections in intravenous drug users involve the tricuspid valve, followed by the aortic and the mitral valves. Right-sided endocarditis often occurs in normal valves, whereas left-sided infections in this population usually occur in previously damaged or abnormal valves. HIV-positive intravenous drug users usually have a more fulminant clinical course and higher mortality than those without HIV disease. Finally, intravenous drug users are at greatest risk for recurrent endocarditis, but any patient with a history of prior endocarditis is at risk for the development of future infection.

CLINICAL MANIFESTATIONS

Infective endocarditis is wide-ranging and varied, involving every body system to some extent. Hence, this entity is part of many differential diagnosis lists. Systemically, patients may present with nonspecific symptoms of weight loss, fatigue, malaise, night sweats, and anorexia. Fever is also a common complaint, although it rarely occurs with shaking chills except in extremely acute and virulent presentations. In addition, fever is an almost universal finding in infective endocarditis, with few exceptions, which include the elderly as well as those with renal failure, congestive heart failure, or severe debility. In these subsets of patients, presenting signs and symptoms may include only shortness of breath or a change in mental status, for example, requiring a low threshold of clinical suspicion for the diagnosis of infective endocarditis.

Musculoskeletal symptoms such as myalgia and arthralgia occur in more than half of patients and are usually seen early in the course of disease. Myalgias are diffuse, whereas arthralgias are typically proximal and oligo- or monarticular in nature. Lower extremity oligo- or monarticular arthritis also occurs, although less commonly than arthralgias. Severe low back pain, a common general complaint, may be difficult to discern from typical musculoskeletal problems. Interestingly, the back pain typically resolves with treatment and may be associated with actual infection of the vertebra, disk space, or sacroiliac joint.

Clinically evident embolization is frequent and depends on the side of the heart affected. Embolization of a portion or all of the vegetation of right-sided lesions may prompt patients to complain of shortness of breath, pleuritic chest pain, or other symptoms associated with pulmonary emboli. Pneumonia, effusion, and sometimes empyema develop. Evidence of peripheral embolization from left-sided lesions, such as stroke or extremity ischemia, also occurs. Central nervous system embolization typically is in the distribution of the middle cerebral artery. Peripheral embolization causing ischemia of the extremities can be dramatic and devastating. Mycotic aneurysms of the central nervous system or peripheral vascular system, which were the most common presenting finding for infective endocarditis in the preantibiotic era, are still seen. Clinically, they are silent until rupture occurs, or they may be associated with persistent headache prior to rupture. The aneurysms are typically located at points of vessel bifurcation, with viridans streptococcus being the most frequently diagnosed organism implicated in their formation.

Neurologic complaints may present diagnostic confusion as an initial presentation of infective endocarditis. Beyond stroke and aneurysm rupture, manifestations can include signs and symptoms of space-occupying lesions and elevated intracranial pressure due to abscesses or cerebritis. Both cerebral abscesses and cerebritis are uncommon with endocarditis, although they are typically associated with fulminant *Staphylococcus aureus* infection. Meningeal signs may also be manifested either from aseptic meningitis or, less commonly, from true infection.

PHYSICAL EXAMINATION

Many physical findings can provide clues to the diagnosis of infective endocarditis, although most are nonspecific and often associated with other diseases. The diagnosis of infective endocarditis should always be entertained in any patient with fever, heart murmur, and anemia. Although seen less commonly, embolic phenomena and splenomegaly are also noted. Virtually all patients have a heart murmur throughout the course of disease, either episodically or continuously. This may not be a prominent finding, however, in patients with acute infections or right-sided heart disease, such as intravenous drug users. Suspicion of infective endocarditis should be strongly entertained in any febrile intravenous drug user with persistence of fever beyond 1 week without any other source of infection. The traditional description of a changing murmur is actually noted in less than 5 to 10 per cent of patients. A new murmur in a febrile patient, especially if consistent with aortic insufficiency, is a major criterion for diagnosing infective endocarditis. The presence of a regurgitant murmur may signal the development of congestive heart failure. Pericarditis with a pericardial rub is uncommon. Tachycardia is often seen, as with other systemic infections.

Peripheral and cutaneous manifestations are probably the most classic physical findings seen in infective endocarditis. Although nonspecific and often associated with other disease states, they are noted in about half of infective endocarditis patients. Earlier diagnosis has decreased the incidence of these findings over the years, as they are typically found in illness of longer duration. Petechiae are the most common cutaneous manifestation in infective endocarditis and are most frequently located on the conjunctivae, palate, buccal mucosa, extremities, and skin above the clavicle. Osler nodes, occurring in less than a quarter of patients, are small, subcutaneous, tender nodules, typically found on the finger or toe pads, which may persist for several days. Janeway lesions are nontender hemorrhagic macular lesions seen in less than 5 per cent of patients, usually in association with acute staphylococcal endocarditis. Splinter hemorrhages, especially if located in the proximal nail bed, are also suggestive of but not diagnostic for infective endocarditis. Clubbing is now an uncommon finding, but when present it suggests prolonged illness.

Roth spots are the most common ophthalmologic finding in infective endocarditis. These pale-centered, oval retinal hemorrhages occur in less than 5 per cent of patients. Other findings include retinal artery occlusion due to embolism, cotton-wool spots, endophthalmitis, and hemorrhage without pale centers. Papilledema may be present in the patient with a brain abscess or intracerebral hemorrhage.

Arthritis, arthralgias, and myalgias may mimic certain rheumatologic disorders. However, true septic arthritis is uncommon. Another physical finding that may be evident is splenomegaly, which is found in less than one third of patients. Acute septic arthritis develops after a prolonged period of infection and is rarely noted with acute disease. Embolization to the spleen is common, although often it is not clinically detectable. Renal embolization also occurs frequently but is usually noted only on laboratory studies.

Neurologic findings such as those seen with stroke, intracerebral hemorrhage, or space-occupying lesions may be present. Neurologic complications occur in approximately one third of patients, contributing significantly to the morbidity and mortality associated with infective endocarditis. Peripheral embolization to the extremities with decreased pulses, ischemia, pallor, and coolness is uncommon with bacterial endocarditis. Fungal infection with associated large, friable vegetations may, however, cause occlusion of a major systemic artery associated with often drastic findings and complications.

INFECTING MICROORGANISMS

Alhough a wide variety of organisms can be seen, the majority of episodes of infective endocarditis are caused by a fairly limited number of organisms. Underlying patient conditions and the presence of a prosthetic valve both affect the type of infecting organism. The most common causative organisms are streptococci, occurring in more than half of infections overall. Viridans streptococci such as *Streptococcus mitis, S. sanguis*, *S. milleri* and *S. mutans* represent the largest group, most commonly inhabiting the oral cavity. *Enterococcus* as well as group D streptococcus, namely *S. bovis*, are also common. Both are found in the gastrointestinal tract, with *Enterococcus* also residing in the genitourinary tract. *S. pneumoniae* is a less common cause, typically affecting the diabetic and alcoholic populations. Its presentation is usually fulminant. Group A, group B and group G streptococci may also be implicated in infective endocarditis.

Staphylococci are the second largest group of infecting organisms, accounting for approximately one quarter of infections. *Staphylococcus aureus* occurs most commonly, is an important organism afflicting prosthetic valves, and may cause complications such as valve ring abscess. Previously normal valves may be infected, and peripheral stigmas are common. Coagulase-negative staphylococci may infect abnormal native valves but are the most common cause of prosthetic valvular endocarditis. *Staphylococcus epidermidis* is seen most frequently, with rare infections due to *Staphylococcus saprophyticus* and *Staphylococcus capitis*.

Infective endocarditis in intravenous drug abusers is usually due to *Staphylococcus aureus*, but the most common gram-negative organism causing disease in this population is *Pseudomonas aeruginosa*. *Pseudomonas*, like staphylococci, can invade apparently normal valves and typically produces a virulent, rapidly progressive course. *Serratia marcescens* endocarditis also occurs. Two other groups at risk for acquiring gram-negative infection are patients with cirrhosis and those with prosthetic valves. Gram-negative bacteria cause less than 5 per cent of infective endocarditis cases overall, despite a high frequency of positive blood cultures in the hospitalized population.

Salmonella species and other Enterobacteriaceae such as *Escherichia coli*, *Klebsiella*, *Enterobacter*, *Proteus,* and *Citrobacter* species have been implicated. Unusual gram-negative bacteria, including *Neisseria* species as well as the HACEK group of organisms (*Haemophilus* species, *Actinobacillus actinomycetemcomitans*, *Cardiobacterium hominis*, *Eikenella* species, and *Kingella* species) may also cause clinical illness. Many other bacteria have been described as causing infective endocarditis, including species of *Corynebacterium*, *Listeria*, *Bacillus*, *Bacteroides*, *Acinetobacter*, *Brucella*, and *Yersinia*. Other microorganisms implicated include *Coxiella*, *Spirillum*, *Chlamydia*, and *Mycoplasma*. Polymicrobial endocarditis is uncommon. *Candida* and *Aspergillus* species are the most common causes of fungal endocarditis and are typically seen in drug abusers, prosthetic heart valve patients, or chronically ill and debilitated patients receiving prolonged therapy that requires intravenous catheterization.

LABORATORY FINDINGS

It is a difficult task to make the diagnosis of infective endocarditis by presenting signs and physical findings alone. Elderly patients may not present with fever, for example, and intravenous drug users may not have a murmur. Treatment of congestive heart failure or a cerebrovascular accident may initially overshadow the underlying diagnosis.

The hallmark of infective endocarditis is bacteremia, with the blood culture being the most important laboratory test available. The bacteremia in infective endocarditis is typically continuous and low grade. No particular time or body temperature is required for optimal culture yield, and arterial blood offers no advantage over usual venous sampling. The diagnosis rests on persistently positive blood cultures, with cultures being positive in more than 95 per cent of patients with infective endocarditis.

Previous antibacterial therapy is the most common cause for negative blood cultures, occurring in up to 25 per cent of patients who receive prior therapy. Therefore, treatment should be delayed, if possible, until multiple blood cultures are obtained from various venipuncture sites. Other possibilities of negative cultures include unusual organisms such as *Legionella*, *Chlamydia*, *Coxiella*, *Mycoplasma,* or *Rochalimaea*. The HACEK group of fastidious organisms requires long incubation periods and may be difficult to culture. Therefore, all blood cultures should be held at least 3 weeks to promote the growth of fastidious organisms. Another cause of negative blood cultures is fungal infection, with greater than 50 per cent of *Candida* species producing negative cultures. Infections with other fungi such as *Aspergillus* and *Histoplasma* are rarely culture-positive. Since large embolizations may occur more commonly with fungi, culture of the embolus may be diagnostic. Lysis-centrifugation culture methods may have a higher yield for fungal cultures than do traditional culture methods.

Certain laboratory values may be abnormal, although none is diagnostic. Most patients have a mild normochromic, normocytic anemia that is consistent with chronic disease and that worsens with the duration of the illness. The leukocyte count may be increased, especially in more acute forms of the illness. Although a decreased leukocyte count may be seen, it is uncommon and usually associated with splenomegaly. Thrombocytopenia may also be present. The erythrocyte sedimentation rate and C-reactive protein level are usually increased, with a normal sedimentation rate considered evidence against the diagnosis of infective endocarditis. Exceptions include patients with congestive heart failure, renal failure, and disseminated intravascular coagulation.

Tests of renal function are abnormal in most patients. Urinalysis reveals protein in more than 50 per cent, hematuria in one to two thirds, and renal casts in more than 10 per cent of patients. Increased creatinine levels occur in 5 to 15 per cent of patients. Microscopic pyuria also occurs. Hypocomplementemia may be present, reflecting an increased incidence of renal involvement, especially glomerulonephritis.

Hypergammaglobulinemia and a positive rheumatoid factor test result may also be seen, the latter being present in up to one half of patients. A false-positive rapid plasma reagin (RPR) test for syphilis is uncommon. High concentrations of immune complexes may be noted and may be helpful in the diagnosis of culture-negative or right-sided endocarditis. These complexes, as well as other serologic markers, can be followed because they decrease with treatment. Resurgence in values as well as recurrence of positive blood cultures should forewarn about relapse or a metastatic focus of infection such as an abscess. Electrocardiography may provide useful information about baseline heart disease. In addition, the development of conduction abnormalities such as right and left bundle branch blocks, second-degree atrioventricular block, and complete heart block suggest extension of infection into surrounding perivalvular tissue affecting the His bundle or the area of the atrioventricular node.

IMAGING STUDIES

Chest films may reveal signs of congestive heart failure, pleural effusions, or fluffy or wedge-shaped infiltrates and are abnormal in more than 70 per cent of intravenous drug users. Echocardiography has markedly enhanced the diagnosis of infective endocarditis in the past two decades. Advances with color flow Doppler and two-dimensional imaging now permit determination of vegetations as small as approximately 3 mm. Echocardiographic demonstration of vegetations typically indicates higher morbidity and mortality rates when compared with the clinical syndrome of infective endocarditis without obvious vegetations. This is based on a higher rate of regurgitant valvular disease, congestive heart failure, and the possibility of surgical intervention in patients with echocardiographically determined vegetations. Thus, echocardiography should be performed on every patient with suspected endocarditis (including patients at risk for endocarditis in whom bacteremia develops or patients without an obvious source for bacteremia).

In the appropriate clinical setting, positive echocardiographic findings can confirm the diagnosis. False-positive results are extremely rare. A negative study, however, does not eliminate the possibility of infective endocarditis. This is because of the variable specificity of transthoracic echocardiography. For example, previously diseased valves and frequent degenerative changes as seen in the elderly are typically affected by endocarditis, sometimes making it difficult to distinguish true vegetations from "normal" findings in a particular patient. In addition, limitations in the use of transthoracic echocardiography include poor resolution in patients with devices such as prosthetic valves and a limited sensitivity in diagnosing perivalvular extension such as abscess formation.

Transesophageal echocardiography (TEE) has recently enhanced the field of echocardiography, remarkably increasing the sensitivity and specificity of endocarditis determination, particularly that occurring with prosthetic valve disease. In addition, it is now the procedure of choice in evaluating perivalvular extension of disease, as in abscess formation with aortic valve endocarditis as well as other complications of infective endocarditis. Although invasive, it is associated with minimal risk and is typically well tolerated. It is therefore warranted in all patients in whom there is a clinical suspicion of infective endocarditis but in whom transthoracic echocardiography produced negative results. Normal TEE makes the diagnosis of infective endocarditis less likely.

Other imaging techniques occasionally used in the diagnosis of infective endocarditis include radionuclide imaging, computed tomography (CT), and magnetic resonance imaging (MRI). Because of low sensitivities, indium- and gallium-labeled scans are of limited value in diagnosing endocarditis. CT scanning may provide some information in conjunction with other methods, such as in patients with large aortic aneurysms. Experience with MRI has been limited, but it may be superior to CT scanning, especially in the patient with suspected multivalvular involvement. MRI can be performed in patients with cardiac valve disease and may also provide valuable information when difficult lesions such as aortic root abscesses cannot be confirmed with echocardiography. Lastly, cardiac catheterization and angiography can be of value in the management of patients with endocarditis, especially if surgical intervention is considered. It is, however, an invasive procedure, and extra caution should be used when it is performed in the presence of aortic insufficiency and congestive heart failure.

COMPLICATIONS

Morbidity and mortality from infective endocarditis remains high, with congestive heart failure resulting from valvular insufficiency being the most common contributing complication. Other cardiac complications include myocardial abscess with or without fistula formation or rupture, conduction abnormalities, myocarditis, myocardial infarction, and pericarditis. Relapse after a usual course of treatment does occur. Valvular stenosis may develop as a long-term consequence of the infection. Extracardiac complications are highlighted by embolic phenomena, sometimes resulting in mycotic aneurysms, metastatic foci of infection, central nervous system abnormalities, renal disease, or peripheral ischemia and musculoskeletal abnormalities. The type and degree of complications that occur can affect the course of treatment, often influencing the need for surgical intervention versus medical therapy alone.

CONCLUSION

Infective endocarditis remains a serious disease that is often difficult to diagnose and treat despite marked advances over the years. The presentation may vary from patient to patient, requiring a low threshold of suspicion by the clinician. Current criteria are expanding to use echocardiography, including TEE, to assist in the initial diagnosis as well as to identify hemodynamic and anatomic complications of the disease. In addition, intravenous drug use is now a widely recognized risk factor regardless of other known predisposing conditions. Symptoms such as persistent fever, prolonged bacteremia, recurrent embolic events, and the development of conduction abnormalities or hemodynamic alterations during an appropriate course of treatment should prompt a thorough investigation for complications of infective endocarditis.

CARDIOMYOPATHY

By Richard A. Lange, M.D.,
Ellen C. Keeley, M.D.,
William C. Daniel, M.D.,
and L. David Hillis, M.D.
Dallas, Texas

Cardiomyopathy is a primary disorder of heart muscle. Patients with this condition have impaired systolic and/or

Table 1. Classification of Cardiomyopathies

Dilated (or congestive) cardiomyopathy
Hypertrophic cardiomyopathy
Restrictive cardiomyopathy

diastolic cardiac function that is not the result of ischemic, hypertensive, valvular, or congenital heart disease. Based on clinical manifestations and pathophysiologic mechanisms, the cardiomyopathies may be classified into three major categories (Table 1).

DILATED (CONGESTIVE) CARDIOMYOPATHY

Definition

Dilated cardiomyopathy is characterized by impaired systolic function and dilatation of the left ventricle. Usually, but not invariably, right ventricular systolic dysfunction and dilatation are present. The majority of cases have no definable cause and are termed idiopathic; occasionally, however, a cause is found. The most common identifiable causes are listed in Table 2. Of these, ethanol abuse is the most common cause of dilated cardiomyopathy in the Western hemisphere. Conversely, in South and Central America, chronic infection with the protozoan *Trypanosoma cruzi* (Chagas' disease) is the most common cause of this condition.

Presenting Signs and Symptoms

The patient with dilated cardiomyopathy usually complains of fatigue, dyspnea on exertion, orthopnea, paroxysmal nocturnal dyspnea, and/or ankle edema. Less commonly, palpitations and/or chest pain similar in character to angina pectoris is noted. On occasion, the patient may come to medical attention after a syncopal episode or a neurologic event caused by systemic arterial embolization of a left atrial or ventricular thrombus. Rarely, this condition is discovered when a patient is incidentally noted to have an enlarged cardiothoracic silhouette on a chest radiograph or a conduction abnormality on a routine electrocardiogram.

Physical Examination

On physical examination, the patient with dilated cardiomyopathy often has resting tachycardia and a narrow pulse pressure. Jugular venous distention is usually present, and there may be prominent V waves in the jugular venous contour (reflective of tricuspid regurgitation). Moist rales over the lung fields are usually present but may be absent even with radiologic evidence of pulmonary congestion. Evidence of unilateral or bilateral pleural effusions may be present. There is generalized cardiomegaly with a laterally displaced point of maximal impulse, and a left and/or right ventricular lift may be appreciated. Third heart sounds from the right and left ventricles are frequently audible, and murmurs of tricuspid and mitral regurgitation (due to annular dilatation from ventricular enlargement) are often present. If tricuspid regurgitation is severe, the patient may have an enlarged, tender, and pulsatile liver. In some patients, the clinical features of right-sided heart failure may predominate, with the presence of hepatomegaly, ascites, and peripheral edema.

Table 2. Common Causes of Dilated Cardiomyopathy

Idiopathic
Infectious
Viral (coxsackievirus, echovirus, adenovirus, rhinovirus, influenza, human immunodeficiency virus [HIV])
Bacterial (diphtheria)
Protozoal (*Trypanosoma cruzi* [Chagas' disease], toxoplasmosis)
Parasitic (*Borrelia burgdorferi* [Lyme disease])
Toxins (alcohol, cocaine, cobalt, doxorubicin, arsenic)
Nutritional deficiencies (scurvy, pellagra, beriberi, selenium deficiency)
Peripartum (probably immunologic)
Endocrine (hyperthyroidism, hypothyroidism, diabetes, pheochromocytoma)
Inherited (X-linked)

Clinical Course and Prognosis

With dilated cardiomyopathy, a disparity may exist between the patient's symptoms and the magnitude of left ventricular dysfunction. Some patients with a markedly depressed left ventricular ejection fraction (<20 per cent) may be incapacitated, whereas others are virtually asymptomatic. Thus, the left ventricular ejection fraction is not a particularly useful indicator of symptoms or prognosis. In contrast, the symptomatic status of the patient and the severity of hemodynamic derangement (e.g., elevated pulmonary capillary wedge or right atrial pressures) are predictive of survival. The best predictor, however, is maximal oxygen consumption—an objective measure of systemic oxygen delivery (or consumption) at peak exercise levels. Patients with marked cardiac dysfunction are unable to increase their cardiac output—and hence, oxygen delivery to tissues—during exercise. Individuals with markedly reduced maximal oxygen consumption have a poor prognosis.

The patient who presents with dilated cardiomyopathy and the onset of symptoms of congestive heart failure has about a 50 per cent chance of being alive 5 years later. In an occasional patient, partial or complete resolution of left ventricular systolic dysfunction and congestive symptoms may occur, with a resultant good long-term prognosis. The same may occur when a cause can be identified (i.e., hypothyroidism, pheochromocytoma, high cardiac output) and corrected early in the course of disease. In most patients, however, left ventricular dysfunction is progressive. The patient with severe symptoms of congestive heart failure despite maximal medical therapy has only a 50 per cent chance of being alive 1 year later. About 40 per cent of these deaths occur suddenly, with most attributed to ventricular arrhythmias. Progressive heart failure and thromboembolic events in the pulmonary or systemic circulation account for most of the remainder.

Common Complications

Dizziness, lightheadedness, palpitations, syncope, and even sudden death are common because of the high incidence of atrial and ventricular tachyarrhythmias in these patients. Occasionally, progressive cardiac dilatation and stretching of the conduction system leads to advanced heart block and Stokes-Adams (syncopal) attacks. Symptoms of congestive heart failure are usually progressive and may eventually become refractory to medical therapy. In such patients, an invasive hemodynamic evaluation—including measurement of right-sided cardiac and pulmonary capillary wedge pressures and cardiac output—can be used to assess the severity of cardiac dysfunction and to direct therapy. Patients with dilated cardiomyopathy have a high incidence of cerebrovascular and/or pulmonary embolic events from atrial or ventricular thrombi.

Laboratory Evaluation

The chest film demonstrates moderate to severe cardiomegaly with pulmonary vascular congestion; in addition, pleural effusions may be present. The 12-lead electrocardiogram often demonstrates sinus tachycardia with atrial or ventricular ectopy and nonspecific ST-T wave abnormalities. Left atrial enlargement and ventricular hypertrophy are common, and 10 to 15 per cent of patients have Q waves in the anterior or inferior leads in the absence of previous myocardial infarction (a so-called pseudoinfarction pattern).

When dilated cardiomyopathy is due to an identifiable cause, the history and physical examination most often reveal the cause (i.e., peripartum, alcohol-induced, infectious, diabetic, and so on). Occasionally, specific blood or urine analyses may be needed to identify the cause (i.e., endocrine abnormalities, toxin ingestion, nutritional deficiencies). Most commonly, a cause is not found, and the dilated cardiomyopathy is termed idiopathic. Many examples of so-called idiopathic dilated cardiomyopathy are thought to be viral in origin, since many of these patients have a prodromal upper respiratory tract infection 2 to 4 weeks before the onset of symptoms of cardiac dysfunction. A fourfold rise between acute and convalescent viral antibody titers may confirm the presence of a recent viral illness; however, it does not establish definitively that virus is the causative agent of the cardiomyopathy.

Useful Imaging Procedures

When dilated cardiomyopathy is suspected, echocardiography or equilibrium multigated [MUGA] blood pool scintigraphy confirms the diagnosis best by demonstrating dilated and poorly contractile ventricles. Atrial or ventricular thrombi may be visualized with two-dimensional echocardiography, and Doppler echocardiography frequently reveals mitral and tricuspid valve regurgitation. Right- and left-sided cardiac catheterization demonstrates elevated filling pressures and diminished cardiac output. Cineangiography will show an enlarged left ventricular chamber with impaired systolic function so that the ejection fraction is depressed (<50 per cent). Some degree of mitral regurgitation is usually present.

Diagnostic Procedures That May Not Be Helpful

Endomyocardial biopsy is frequently performed in patients with idiopathic dilated cardiomyopathy in an attempt to identify active inflammation of the heart (so-called myocarditis). In general, the diagnostic yield of endomyocardial biopsy in such patients is low. Inflammatory myocarditis is most likely to be found in patients with a preceding viral illness in whom the biopsy is performed within 1 month of the onset of cardiac symptoms; those with chronic symptoms of heart failure (>6 months' duration) are unlikely to demonstrate histologic evidence of inflammation. Additionally, there are no convincing data that treatment with immunosuppressive agents is beneficial in patients with active myocarditis.

Potential Errors and Pitfalls

In addition to primary disorders of heart muscle, other conditions may lead to ventricular dilatation and impaired systolic function. Silent (or symptomatic) myocardial ischemia or infarction should be excluded, as patients with these conditions may benefit from coronary artery revascularization. Valvular stenosis or regurgitation may also lead to cardiac dilatation and congestive heart failure. Although careful cardiac auscultation usually identifies a valvular abnormality, the murmur of mitral stenosis may be barely audible and overlooked. In the patient with a dilated cardiomyopathy and mitral or aortic valve regurgitation, it may be difficult to establish whether the valvular insufficiency was the cause or result of the ventricular dilatation. Congenital heart conditions that result in left-to-right shunting of blood (i.e., atrial septal defect, ventricular septal defect, or patent ductus arteriosus) may also lead to cardiac dilatation and dysfunction. Finally, in the patient who presents with pulmonary congestion or edema, noncardiac causes—such as renal failure, infection, hypersensitivity reaction, or vasculitis—should be considered.

HYPERTROPHIC CARDIOMYOPATHY

Definition

Hypertrophic cardiomyopathy is characterized by an increased left ventricular wall thickness in the absence of an apparent cause (i.e., hypertension or aortic valve stenosis). In this condition, systolic (contractile) function is normal, but diastolic function is severely impaired, since the left ventricle is hypertrophied, stiff, and noncompliant. Although the hypertrophy may be diffuse and concentric, it is typically asymmetrical, with the septum, apex, or lateral wall being more involved. Hypertrophic cardiomyopathy may be *obstructive* or *nonobstructive,* depending on whether there is asymmetrical septal hypertrophy with obstruction to left ventricular outflow and a resultant pressure gradient between the left ventricular cavity and aorta. Both types exhibit marked restriction to left ventricular filling as a result of increased wall thickness and impaired ventricular relaxation.

The nonobstructive type accounts for approximately 75 per cent of all patients with hypertrophic cardiomyopathy. Only 25 per cent of cases are the obstructive type, which is also known as idiopathic hypertrophic subaortic stenosis (IHSS) or asymmetrical septal hypertrophy (ASH). This form is characterized by a variable and dynamic obstruction to left ventricular outflow due to (1) a markedly thickened and asymmetrical septum, (2) abnormal movement of the anterior mitral valve leaflet during ventricular systole, and (3) cavity obliteration during ventricular systole. The obstruction is dynamic in that it is worsened when the left ventricular cavity decreases in size (e.g., after a Valsalva maneuver or nitrate administration) or when left ventricular contractility increases. Conversely, the obstruction is reduced when the left ventricular cavity increases in size (e.g., after squatting orperformance of an isometric hand grip) or when ventricular contractility decreases.

Presenting Signs and Symptoms

The most common symptom is dyspnea, which results from increased left ventricular pressure during diastole, with increased left atrial and pulmonary venous pressures. In addition, other symptoms of pulmonary congestion—orthopnea and paroxysmal nocturnal dyspnea—are frequently present. Angina, palpitations, and syncope commonly occur in patients with hypertrophic cardiomyopathy. Angina may be due to atherosclerotic coronary artery disease or inadequate microvascular flow to the thickened myocardium. Ventricular or atrial arrhythmias often occur and may cause palpitations, dizziness, or syncope. Syncope or near syncope may also occur during exercise as a result of worsening outflow tract obstruction in patients with the obstructive form of this disorder. In rare circumstances, sudden cardiac death from an arrhythmia is the initial manifestation of the disease. In fact, hypertrophic cardiomyopathy is the leading cause of sudden death in young athletes.

Physical Examination

The carotid upstrokes are brisk and may demonstrate a bisferiens (bifid) configuration in the patient with an obstructive form of this disorder. The jugular venous pulse is usually normal. On palpation, the apical cardiac impulse is often laterally displaced and abnormally forceful. A prominent fourth heart sound may be palpable, resulting in a double apical impulse. With dynamic outflow tract obstruction, a systolic thrill can be palpated along the left sternal border. The first and second heart sounds are typically normal, and a prominent fourth heart sound is audible. In patients with the obstructive form of this condition, a harsh crescendo-decrescendo systolic murmur is audible along the left sternal border. In contrast to the murmur of aortic stenosis, it radiates to the base of the heart, is not well appreciated in the carotid arteries, and is devoid of a systolic ejection click. In addition, the murmur (1) increases in intensity with any physiologic or pharmacologic maneuver that reduces left ventricular cavity size or increases contractility and (2) diminishes in intensity with any maneuver that increases left ventricular cavity volume or decreases contractility. In addition to the murmur of left ventricular outflow tract obstruction, many patients with obstructive hypertrophic cardiomyopathy have an apical holosystolic murmur of mitral regurgitation.

Clinical Course and Prognosis

The clinical course of patients with hypertrophic cardiomyopathy is varied. Symptoms remain absent or mild throughout life in many patients and are slowly progressive in others. Likewise, the degree of left ventricular hypertrophy may remain stable in many patients and increase markedly in others, especially children. Although the percentage of patients with severe symptoms increases with age, the annual mortality rate is highest in children (6 per cent in children versus 3 per cent in adults). The risk of sudden death is particularly increased in individuals with a history of syncope, a family history of sudden death, or evidence of ventricular arrhythmias. Since sudden death often occurs during exercise, these patients should be advised to avoid strenuous exertion. Interestingly, the severity of symptoms and risk of sudden death are not related to the presence or severity of left ventricular outflow tract obstruction.

Common Complications

Worsening symptoms in a patient with hypertrophic cardiomyopathy may be due to (1) increased hypertrophy, (2) the development of atrial fibrillation, or (3) worsening mitral regurgitation. An echocardiogram and electrocardiogram should be obtained to distinguish these possibilities. In 10 to 15 per cent of patients, the left ventricular wall thins, with progression to dilated cardiomyopathy. When nonexertional syncope occurs, it is most likely due to ventricular or atrial arrhythmias and warrants careful evaluation with ambulatory electrocardiographic monitoring and/or invasive electrophysiologic testing. Infective endocarditis occurs in 5 per cent of patients and is usually due to viridans streptococci infection of the aortic valve. Less commonly, the mitral valve or the area of the intraventricular septum that it contacts may be infected.

Laboratory Evaluation

On routine chest film, the cardiac silhouette is of normal size and shape. The 12-lead electrocardiogram usually demonstrates left ventricular hypertrophy. About 10 to 15 per cent of patients have a "pseudoinfarct pattern" of poor R-wave progression across the precordium. Prominent Q waves caused by septal hypertrophy are common in the inferior and lateral limb leads. Giant negative (inverted) T waves in the precordial leads are characteristic of the hypertrophic cardiomyopathy, which is principally localized to the apex.

Useful Imaging Procedures

The cardinal feature of this disease, left ventricular hypertrophy, is best seen with two-dimensional echocardiography: Normal systolic function with near obliteration of the cavity during systole is observed. Although asymmetrical left ventricular hypertrophy of the interventricular septum is the classic finding, other left ventricular segments may be involved, such as the lateral or apical regions, and occasionally the process is symmetrical. With asymmetrical septal hypertrophy, the ratio of septal thickness to posterior wall thickness is at least 1.3:1, and the left ventricular outflow tract is narrowed by the septal hypertrophy and the anterior movement of the anterior mitral valve leaflet during ventricular systole. An estimate of the outflow tract gradient can be obtained by Doppler echocardiography. In some patients with marked exertional symptoms, the outflow tract gradient may be small at rest but increase substantially with the infusion of an inotropic agent (e.g., isoproterenol). Magnetic resonance imaging and computed tomography have been used to assess left ventricular mass and asymmetrical hypertrophy. When adequate echocardiographic images cannot be obtained, these techniques should be considered.

Other Useful Diagnostic Procedures

Cardiac catheterization is not generally required to establish the diagnosis of hypertrophic cardiomyopathy. If performed, it usually demonstrates diminished left ventricular compliance (markedly increased pressure during diastole) and normal left ventricular systolic function. In the obstructive form of hypertrophic cardiomyopathy, a dynamic pressure gradient can be demonstrated between the body of the ventricle and the ascending aorta, and the effects of pharmacologic or physiologic maneuvers on the gradient can be assessed. If cineangiography of the left ventricle is performed, it typically shows nearly complete obliteration of the cavity during systole. The left ventricle often has a characteristic shape, which has been described as banana-shaped in patients with asymmetrical septal hypertrophy or spade-shaped in those with the apical form of the disease.

Potential Errors and Pitfalls

In the patient with obstructive hypertrophic cardiomyopathy, the left ventricular outflow tract murmur may be mistaken for valvular aortic stenosis. These entities can easily be distinguished from each other by assessing the response of the murmur to physiologic maneuvers, such as the Valsalva maneuver, squatting, and the isometric hand grip. In elderly hypertensive patients, echocardiography frequently demonstrates left ventricular hypertrophy and a "knob" of tissue just below the aortic valve. This condition should not be confused with asymmetrical septal hypertrophy: It causes minimal outflow tract obstruction, is usually not associated with cardiac symptoms, and carries a good prognosis.

RESTRICTIVE CARDIOMYOPATHY

Definition

Of the three types of cardiomyopathy, the restrictive form is the least common. In this condition, a variety of disease processes (Table 3) infiltrate the myocardium, leading to excessive rigidity of the right and left ventricles and marked impairment of diastolic filling. Normal ventricular systolic function and wall thickness distinguish it from dilated and hypertrophic cardiomyopathies. Amyloidosis, hemochromatosis, and sarcoidosis are the most common causes of restrictive cardiomyopathy in the United States (of note, amyloid and sarcoid may also cause dilated cardiomyopathy). In tropical and temperate regions of the world, eosinophilic infiltration of the heart, with subsequent endocardial fibrosis (i.e., endomyocardial fibrosis and Löffler's endocarditis), is a leading cause of restrictive cardiomyopathy. Carcinoid tumors that invade the liver secrete vasoactive substances that cause fibrosis of the right side of the heart; the left side of the heart is not involved unless there are pulmonary metastases. There are also inherited forms of restrictive cardiomyopathy, including those associated with glycogen or lipid storage diseases and those associated with a poorly characterized skeletal myopathy. Finally, in some individuals, restrictive cardiomyopathy occurs without an identifiable cause and is, therefore, termed idiopathic.

Presenting Signs and Symptoms

Because of the abnormally increased right atrial and ventricular filling pressures, the cardiac output is diminished, and the clinical manifestations are predominantly right-sided. Fatigue, especially with exertion, and peripheral edema are the most common complaints. Dyspnea on exertion (due to diminished cardiac output and not to pulmonary vascular congestion) and abdominal discomfort (due to hepatic congestion) may also be noted. Pulmonary congestion is unusual because the impediment to right ventricular filling prevents an excessive amount of the intravascular volume from reaching the pulmonary vasculature. The infiltrative process also involves the cardiac conduction system, so atrial fibrillation or heart block may be the initial manifestation of this disease in an occasional patient.

Table 3. Causes of Restrictive Cardiomyopathy

Causes
Amyloidosis
Sarcoidosis
Hemochromatosis
Eosinophilic causes
Endomyocardial fibrosis
Löffler's endocarditis
Carcinoid (metastatic to liver)
Inherited causes
Fabry disease
Gaucher disease
Myopathic (skeletal)
Mediastinal irradiation
Idiopathic causes

Physical Examination

Findings of right-sided heart failure, including jugular venous distention, hepatomegaly, and peripheral edema, are evident, and an inspiratory increase in jugular venous distention (Kussmaul's sign) is often present. The apical cardiac impulse and heart sounds (first and second heart sounds) are typically unremarkable. In patients with endomyocardial fibrosis or Löffler's endocarditis, fibrosis of the atrioventricular valve leaflets and subvalvular apparatus may cause mitral and/or tricuspid regurgitation. In carcinoid heart disease, marked thickening of the pulmonary valve leaflets can occur and may lead to pulmonary valve stenosis or, rarely, pulmonary insufficiency.

Course and Prognosis

The prognosis in most individuals with restrictive cardiomyopathy—regardless of its cause—is extremely poor, with most patients dying within 1 to 2 years of diagnosis. Death usually occurs as a result of progressive right-sided heart failure (with resultant decreasing cardiac output), heart block, or refractory ventricular arrhythmias.

Common Complications

Atrial fibrillation and ventricular arrhythmias are common and usually respond poorly to medical therapy. Since digoxin binds to amyloid fibrils in the heart, patients with cardiac amyloidosis are extremely sensitive to digoxin and may experience toxicity at low serum concentrations. Involvement of the conduction system frequently leads to bundle branch or complete heart block. Thromboembolic events are common as a result of atrial fibrillation, a low-output state, and endocardial fibrosis.

Laboratory Procedures

The routine chest film usually demonstrates a normal-sized or minimally enlarged heart. Pulmonary venous congestion is not prominent, but pleural effusions may be present. The electrocardiogram often demonstrates diffuse low voltage, and atrioventricular and rhythm disturbances are common. Blood should be assayed for elevated concentrations of serotonin, ferritin, immunoglobulin, and eosinophils in the patient suspected of having restrictive cardiomyopathy. Assays for specific glycogen or lipid pathway enzymes may be performed on circulating lymphocytes or tissue if the patient is suspected of having a previously undiagnosed genetic defect.

Useful Imaging Procedures

Two-dimensional echocardiography is helpful in establishing that left and right ventricular systolic function is normal, the ventricles are of normal size, and the ventricular walls are not hypertrophied. Enlarged atria and intracardiac thrombi may also be seen on the echocardiogram. A "ground-glass" appearance of the myocardium on two-dimensional echocardiography was once thought to be helpful in identifying cardiac amyloid, but subsequent studies have failed to confirm its utility. In patients with advanced amyloidosis, myocardial scintigraphy may reveal diffuse uptake of technetium-99m pyrophosphate. Characteristic pressure tracings can be obtained during right- and left-sided cardiac catheterization. The atrial pressures are increased and equal, with a prominent Y descent. The ventricular pressure tracings demonstrate a "square root sign"—a deep and rapid early decline at the onset of diastole followed by a rapid rise to a plateau (so-called dip and plateau). Cardiac output is diminished despite the fact that the left ventricular systolic function and ejection fraction are normal.

Other Useful Diagnostic Procedures

In contrast to the other types of cardiomyopathy, endomyocardial biopsy may be extremely useful in the patient suspected of having restrictive cardiomyopathy. In addition to establishing the diagnosis of restrictive cardiomyopathy, it often reveals the cause. Endomyocardial biopsy is particularly important in the patient with restrictive physiology in whom constrictive pericardial disease is a consideration, because a normal endomyocardial biopsy in such a patient makes constrictive pericardial disease more likely.

Potential Errors and Pitfalls

The clinical and hemodynamic features of restrictive cardiomyopathy closely resemble those of chronic constrictive pericarditis. Accordingly, an assessment of pericardial thickness with echocardiography, magnetic resonance imaging, or computed tomography may be indicated. Pulmonary hypertension, regardless of the cause, also produces signs and symptoms of right-sided heart failure. In contrast to the patient with restrictive cardiomyopathy, the echocardiogram in these patients typically demonstrates a markedly dilated and poorly contractile right ventricle.

PERICARDIAL DISEASE

By Paul Schoenfeld, M.D.
La Crosse, Wisconsin

The pericardium consists of the membranous structures surrounding the heart. Closely adherent to the myocardium is a layer of serosal cells called the visceral pericardium. This combination is referred to as the epicardium, which is in apposition to the parietal pericardium. The parietal pericardium is frequently referred to as the "pericardium" and consists of another fine layer of serosal cells inside a fibrous membrane that constitutes the mediastinum in the region of the heart. Between the two serosal membranes is a potential space that normally contains 15 to 30 mL of pericardial fluid derived from the lymphatic drainage of the myocardium. This fluid reduces friction between the serosal surfaces and may have an immunologic function as well. The pressure in this potential space is usually subatmospheric and reflects the pleural pressure.

ACUTE PERICARDITIS

Acute pericarditis is inflammation of these membranes surrounding the heart. It gives rise to fairly typical symptoms and physical findings. The electrocardiogram and echocardiogram often support the diagnosis. During pericardial inflammation, the smooth frictionless motion of the surfaces against each other is disrupted, causing pain and a friction rub. The inflammatory process leads to the accumulation of fluid in the space and thickening of the membranes, which may be detected by echocardiography. Pericarditis falls into the differential diagnosis of chest pain. In this age of aggressive interventional therapy for acute myocardial infarction, it is important to recognize acute pericarditis, which generally responds to conservative therapy. The clinician should also be alert for complications of acute pericarditis, such as cardiac tamponade and hemodynamic collapse.

Chest pain is the most common complaint. Although it is typically retrosternal or affects the left precordium, it may radiate to the jaw, neck, or left arm as ischemic pain does. The pain from pericarditis is pleuritic in nature, tends to last as long as several days, and is made worse by lying supine or on the left side. It is improved by sitting up and by leaning forward. It is not relieved by nitroglycerin.

The most revealing finding is a pericardial friction rub, which sounds like creaking leather through the stethoscope. The rub may have one, two, or three components produced by the roughened pericardial surfaces abrading each other during atrial systole, ventricular systole, and ventricular diastole. Since the friction rub can be transient, frequent auscultation improves detection. It often helps to listen during forced expiration so that rubs are not confused with bronchial breath sounds. Sometimes the rub is heard better when the patient leans forward. A pleural friction rub sounds similar but occurs only with the respiratory cycle, not with the cardiac cycle. The clinician should press the diaphragm of the stethoscope firmly against the skin to decrease potentially confusing adventitial skin sounds. Other physical findings include fever, tachycardia, and tachypnea.

The electrocardiogram is usually abnormal and may help distinguish acute infarction and acute pericarditis. With pericarditis, the electrocardiogram progresses through four stages. The first stage involves ST-segment elevation that is concave upward in all leads except aVR and V_1. The ST-segment elevation of acute infarction is convex upward and tends to be localized in groups of leads, with the opposite groups showing reciprocal ST-segment depression. In the second stage, the ST segment becomes isoelectric. This may occur within the first few days and tends to occur before T-wave inversion begins. During infarction, the T waves begin to invert before the ST segment becomes isoelectric. In the third stage, the T waves begin to invert, and in the final stage the electrocardiogram returns to normal. Abnormal Q waves do not develop. Other electrocardiographic findings include depression of the PR segment in any leads with ST-segment elevation. This can be a subtle but helpful finding. Arrhythmias are uncommon.

The echocardiogram is the most important diagnostic imaging method for acute pericarditis as well as its complications. The presence of a pericardial effusion supports the diagnosis of pericarditis, although effusion can occur with congestive heart failure, hypothyroidism, hypoalbuminemia, and pregnancy. The chest film may reveal an enlarged cardiac silhouette with a "water bottle" configuration. The chest film should raise suspicion of pericardial disease when there is no pulmonary congestion despite a rapidly enlarging or enlarged heart. Left or bilateral pleural effusions are commonly seen. Associated conditions such as malignancy, tuberculosis, or pulmonary infection may be apparent on the chest film.

Acute pericarditis presents as a chest pain syndrome requiring differentiation from acute myocardial infarction, pulmonary embolism, dissecting aortic aneurysm, bronchial pneumonia, mediastinal emphysema, and pleurisy. The cause of acute pericarditis and associated conditions

Table 1. Etiology of Pericarditis and Associated Conditions

Idiopathic cause
Malignancy
Uremia
Diagnostic procedures
Connective tissue disease
Dissecting aortic aneurysm
Anticoagulant therapy
Bacterial infection
Postpericardiotomy syndrome
Trauma
Radiation
Myxedema
Tuberculosis
Post–myocardial infarction syndrome
Chylopericardium
Fungal infection
Age-related pericarditis

include uremia, malignancy, connective tissue disease, anticoagulant therapy, complications of diagnostic procedures, postpericardiotomy syndrome, trauma, tuberculosis, myxedema, dissecting aortic aneurysm, and treatment with hydralazine or procainamide (Table 1). Commonly the cause is not identified. Laboratory studies should seek to establish a cause or the presence of associated conditions. An increased leukocyte count may indicate infection. An increased erythrocyte sedimentation rate is sensitive for connective tissue disease but is not specific. Rheumatoid factor determinations and tests for lupus erythematosus are usually positive only after rheumatoid arthritis and lupus are already apparent clinically. Creatine kinase (CK) as well as the CK-MB fraction may be mildly increased. Screening tests for renal and thyroid disease, skin tests for tuberculosis and fungi, and acute and convalescent viral titers may be revealing.

Acute idiopathic or viral pericarditis is usually self-limited to 1 or 2 weeks. Occasionally there may be a recurrence of symptoms over months or years. Rarely a patient has a refractory course that flares whenever therapy is tapered or discontinued. Depending on the cause of the pericarditis, other complications such as cardiac tamponade or constrictive pericarditis may develop.

Table 2. Useful Laboratory Tests

Pericardial Fluid

- Cultures: bacterial and fungal
- Gram stain
- Cytologic studies
- Antinuclear antibody (ANA) test
- Glucose concentration (low in tuberculosis, rheumatoid arthritis, and bacterial infection)
- Protein levels greater than 3 g/dL in infection, tuberculosis, malignancy, and irradiation

Other Laboratory Tests

- Leukocyte count
- Serum creatinine, urea nitrogen
- Thyroid-stimulating hormone (TSH)
- Erythrocyte sedimentation rate (ESR)
- Rheumatoid factor
- Serum antinuclear antibody (ANA) test
- Tuberculin and fungal skin tests
- Serial viral neutralizing antibody titers
- Cardiac enzymes (creatine kinase [CK], CK-MB, lactate dehydrogenase [LD], LD isoenzymes)

PERICARDIAL EFFUSION

The normal pericardial space contains 15 to 30 mL of a clear fluid that is similar to lymph. It originates from the subepicardial lymphatics that drain the heart to the mediastinum and the cavities of the right side of the heart. It is likely that some degree of effusion occurs in all patients with acute pericarditis, but this fluid is not detectable on chest film until 250 mL has accumulated. It is more readily detectable by echocardiography when 100 mL has accumulated. Pericardial effusion can occur without hemodynamic compromise. The most important aspect of pericardial effusion is the potential threat of hemodynamic collapse resulting from cardiac tamponade. This requires careful observation of the patient until the problem is resolved.

There are no exact data for the incidence of pericardial effusion, but it is certainly not an unusual finding in a busy echocardiographic laboratory. The causes of pericardial effusion are essentially the same as those of acute pericarditis. There are no symptoms specific to the presence of pericardial effusion unless cardiac tamponade is present.

On examination, the left border of cardiac dullness may be displaced laterally. There may or may not be a friction rub. There may be dullness to percussion at the angle of the left scapula, along with egophony and bronchial breath sounds, which result from compression of lung tissue by a large pericardial effusion.

It is possible to obtain pericardial fluid for laboratory analysis. In acute pericarditis, however, the diagnostic yield from pericardiocentesis may be low. Because of this, routine pericardiocentesis for diagnostic purposes is generally not recommended in the absence of specific indications. Such indications may include suspicion of purulent pericarditis, metastatic carcinoma, or hemopericardium. Aspiration is unlikely to be helpful when the clinical diagnosis is viral pericarditis, postirradiation pericarditis, connective tissue disease, or uremia. If pericardial fluid is aspirated, the tests listed in Table 2 may be helpful.

Echocardiography is sensitive and the most practical procedure for making the definitive diagnosis of pericardial effusion. It may reveal a very small effusion that is only seen posterior to the heart, or it may reveal the entire heart swinging in a massive pericardial effusion. A loculated effusion with local hemodynamic effects can be detected. The fluid itself, however, cannot be well characterized, and it is not possible to distinguish serous fluid from hemorrhagic, chylous, or purulent effusion. An effusion can be present without pericarditis in patients with congestive heart failure, hypoalbuminemia, hypothyroidism, or uremia, as well as in those who are pregnant or in whom the effusion is secondary to certain drugs (Table 3). Most patients who have had recent cardiac surgery have a detectable pericardial effusion. Serial echocardiograms may help gauge the risk of tamponade. Echocardiographic guidance of pericardiocentesis is now standard practice.

The natural history of a pericardial effusion depends on the underlying cause of the pericarditis. Most of the time, there is resolution without further complications. Occa-

Table 3. Drugs Associated With Pericarditis and Effusion

Hydralazine	Dantrolene
Procainamide	Cromolyn sodium
Minoxidil	Anticoagulants
Methysergide	Phenytoin

sionally there will be a chronic effusion; rarely there will be progression to constrictive or effusive constrictive pericarditis. The most frequent and potentially devastating complication is the development of cardiac tamponade.

CARDIAC TAMPONADE

Cardiac tamponade is the impairment of diastolic filling caused by an abnormal increase in intrapericardial pressure. When this pressure is modest, there may be little more than a compensatory increase of venous pressure. When the intrapericardial pressure is high, there can be circulatory collapse. Thus, tamponade is a life-threatening complication of pericardial effusion that requires urgent or emergent relief.

The patient is likely to present with dyspnea, fatigue, tachycardia, hypotension, and increased central venous pressure. There may be chest pressure or pain. A friction rub may be heard. A patient may present with Beck's triad: a small, quiet heart; jugular venous distention; and hypotension. This should be an important signal indicating tamponade.

Pulsus paradoxus can also be a helpful physical finding. This is a normal physiologic finding that is exaggerated in conditions such as tamponade, constrictive pericarditis, restrictive cardiomyopathy, bronchial asthma, and chronic obstructive pulmonary disease (COPD). Normally there is a minor decrease in systolic blood pressure during inspiration, followed by an increase of systolic blood pressure during expiration. When the difference between these two pressures exceeds 10 mm Hg, it is likely that there is pericardial tamponade in the presence of pericarditis (see Table 4 for a method of identifying pulsus paradoxus).

The echocardiogram provides useful information in cardiac tamponade. When the intrapericardial pressure exceeds the cavitary pressure of the right ventricle, the right ventricular free wall will invert or collapse. This effect is readily observed on two-dimensional echocardiography. The right atrium can also be seen to collapse for the same reasons. The right ventricle and left ventricle change dimensions in a reciprocating fashion during respiration. Inspiration causes right ventricular enlargement; expiration causes left ventricular enlargement. Inspiration also causes decreased Doppler flow velocities on the left but increased flow velocities on the right. It should be noted, however, that small increases in pericardial effusion occurring acutely, such as with trauma, may lead to a tamponade physiology without the preceding echocardiographic changes. It should also be noted that loculated pericardial effusion causing localized compression of the right ventricle, right atrium, or right ventricular outflow track may not produce typical changes.

Since the patient's presentation may suggest congestive heart failure, it is critical to appreciate conditions associated with cardiac tamponade that might lead to the correct diagnosis. This is important because tamponade can be readily relieved with aspiration of even a small amount of pericardial fluid.

Table 4. Determination of Pulsus Paradoxus

Be able to observe gentle but visible respiratory motion
Determine systolic blood pressure during expiration
Set the manometer 10 mm Hg lower
If systolic blood pressure sounds are still heard only during expiration, there is abnormal pulsus paradoxus
Lower manometer to the level that systolic blood pressure is heard in both expiration and inspiration
The difference between these two readings is the amount of pulsus paradoxus

CONSTRICTIVE PERICARDITIS

Constrictive pericarditis is marked by compression of the heart resulting from fibrotic thickening of the pericardial membranes. Compression interferes with normal diastolic filling of the right and left ventricles. Thickening of both the visceral and the parietal pericardial membranes frequently leads to obliteration of the pericardial space. An effusive-constrictive pericarditis is the result of fibrotic thickening with residual fluid remaining in portions of the pericardial space. Constrictive pericarditis can affect people of all ages but tends to increase in frequency after the third decade of life. It can occur following any cause of acute pericarditis but is rare following myocardial infarction or rheumatic fever. Typically, the cause is unknown or it is a consequence of idiopathic pericarditis. Other possible causes include irradiation, surgery, connective tissue disease, sarcoidosis, tuberculosis, trauma, neoplasm, and uremia. Constrictive pericarditis should be considered when a patient who seems to have congestive heart failure does not respond to adequate treatment. This is even more likely in the absence of ischemic, hypertensive, or valvular heart disease.

The earliest symptoms of this condition are dyspnea on exertion and fatigue, followed by abdominal swelling and pedal edema. Symptoms tend to progress slowly over years. Late in the process, muscle wasting, weakness, anorexia, and weight loss occur. Chest pain, orthopnea, and paroxysmal nocturnal dyspnea are unusual symptoms.

Patients present with tachycardia and normal or low blood pressure. Atrial fibrillation and atrial dysrhythmias are more common than with acute pericarditis. There is jugular venous distention and Kussmaul's sign, which persists despite good diuresis. Pulsus paradoxus is not commonly present. Heart sounds are soft or normal. There are no murmurs, and the precordial pulsations are normal. There may be a pericardial knock, which is an early diastolic sound due to sudden deceleration of ventricular filling. The sound may be palpable and augmented in the squatting position. The liver is enlarged, firm, tender, and nonpulsatile. Ascites is usually more prominent than pedal edema.

Echocardiographic findings of a thickened pericardium correlate poorly with both anatomy and the presence of constriction. Some Doppler findings reflect the inspiratory decrease of pulmonary venous and left atrial pressure. When compared with apnea, there is a decrease of the mitral E-wave velocity and the aortic flow velocity that is seen during the first beat following inspiration.

Cardiac catheterization will demonstrate elevation and equalization of the diastolic pressures of the right and left ventricles, mean pulmonary capillary wedge pressure, and mean right atrial pressure. These tend to be within 4 to 5 mm Hg of each other and increased to the range of 12 to 30 mm Hg. Left ventricular filling is accelerated in early diastole. The ejection fraction is normal. The pulmonary artery pressure is usually less than 40 mm Hg. The electrocardiogram tends to show low voltage with intra-atrial conduction defects or atrial fibrillation. Other electrocardiographic changes are nonspecific.

Pericardial thickening is a hallmark of this process and is helpful in differentiating constrictive pericarditis from restrictive cardiomyopathy, which tends to have similar hemodynamic findings. Ultrafast computed tomography (CT), conventional CT, and magnetic resonance imaging are all capable of detecting pericardial thickening in excess of 5 mm, which strongly supports the diagnosis of constrictive pericarditis. On chest film, almost half of the patients may exhibit calcification. The heart size is variable but tends to be smaller than might otherwise be expected for the degree of edema and ascites. The pulmonary artery is not enlarged, the lung fields are clear, and there may be a pleural effusion.

The important differential diagnosis is between restrictive cardiomyopathy and constrictive pericarditis. Until the advent of magnetic resonance imaging and CT scanning, this was a confounding diagnosis to make. The findings of a thickened pericardium are helpful. Ascites and cachexia may also suggest advanced liver disease.

The natural history is a slow progressive course occurring over years. Occasionally the process may progress more rapidly in the space of months. Once the diagnosis is confirmed, early surgery is generally recommended because of a lower mortality rate when compared with later surgery.

ANEURYSMS OF THE AORTA

By Robert J. Rizzo, M.D.,
and Lawrence H. Cohn, M.D.
Boston, Massachusetts

The aorta is "the greatest artery," and an aneurysm is a widening, or dilatation, of the wall of a blood vessel or the heart. Thus, an aortic aneurysm is a widening, or dilatation, of the greatest artery of the body. When the amount of dilatation is small, the aorta may be termed ectatic, rather than aneurysmal. The phrase "annuloaortic ectasia" has been used to describe ascending aortic aneurysms that involve the aortic root and valve annulus, which are also associated with aortic valve regurgitation. The condition in which the aorta is diffusely aneurysmal has been termed "aortomegaly," and the presence of multiple separate aneurysms has been called "aneurysmosis."

Aortic dissection, also known as "dissecting aortic aneurysm," occurs when an intimal tear allows circulating blood to penetrate into the aortic wall and create a false channel within the media, which may extend longitudinally and circumferentially for variable distances along the aorta. At first, aortic dissection may not result in significant dilatation of the aortic wall and thus initially may not deserve to be called an aneurysm. However, aortic dissection does damage the aorta and results in a weakened aortic wall that may become aneurysmal. Aortic dissection may also develop as a complication of an aortic aneurysm. Aortic dissection is termed "acute" when the onset has occurred within the past 2 weeks and "chronic" when a longer time has elapsed.

In the early 1960s, DeBakey defined dissections that involve the ascending aorta and more distal aorta as type I, those that involve only the ascending aorta as type II, and those that involve the descending aorta as type III. In 1970, the Stanford group defined dissections that involve the ascending aorta as type A and those that do not involve the ascending aorta as type B. The Stanford classification was based on the difference in management recommended for the two groups, which is still appropriate today.

Emergency surgery is recommended for patients with acute type A dissection because devastating, early, and frequent complications ensue without surgery. These complications include intrapericardial aortic rupture with tamponade, aortic valve regurgitation, and organ ischemia. The resulting mortality rate of 50 per cent within 2 days of onset of the dissection with nonoperative therapy is significantly reduced with operative repair. However, initial management with antihypertensive medical therapy is recommended for patients with type B dissection, because fewer early complications occur, and surgery is reserved only for patients who present with or develop signs of impending aortic rupture, organ ischemia, or aneurysmal degeneration.

CLASSIFICATIONS

Aortic aneurysms can be classified according to location, type, shape or form, or etiology. The location may be in the ascending aorta, the aortic arch or descending thoracic aorta, or the abdominal segments of the aorta. Aneurysms that extend from the descending thoracic aorta, through the diaphragm, and into the abdominal aorta are classified as thoracoabdominal aortic aneurysms. The aneurysm may be true, in which case the aortic wall has actually dilated, or false, in which case the aortic wall itself has not dilated, but has perforated and allowed blood to extravasate and to be contained by the surrounding tissues. False aneurysms, also called "pseudoaneurysms," usually occur following spontaneous or iatrogenic trauma or infection. The shape of an aortic aneurysm may be saccular, with only a portion of the circumference of the aortic wall dilated so that a bubble or sac developed on the side of a vessel of otherwise normal caliber, or an aortic aneurysm may be fusiform, with a larger portion of the circumference of the aortic wall dilated, creating a more generalized widening of the involved aortic segment. Short, fusiform aneurysms appear globular in shape, but those that involve longer segments of the aorta result in a typical spindle or cylindrical shape.

The etiology of aortic aneurysms may be classified as congenital, traumatic, inflammatory, or degenerative, although etiology may be related to several of these categories and abnormal hemodynamic stress may contribute to many. Congenital defects fall into two groups, those in which a developmental abnormality creates a focal abnormality in the circulatory system, resulting in abnormal hemodynamic stress (as in coarctation or aortic arch anomalies), and those in which an inherited disorder results in a diffuse weakening of the aortic wall (as in Marfan's and Ehlers-Danlos syndromes). Aortic aneurysms of traumatic etiology include those that follow blunt trauma, such as deceleration injury. Those that follow penetrating trauma may occur as a consequence of catheter-based or surgical interventions. Aortic aneurysms of inflammatory etiology include those associated with Takayasu's disease, giant cell arteritis, rheumatic arthritis, or infections such as syphilis, salmonellosis, and mycosis. The term "mycotic aneurysm" now applies to aneurysms that result from either a fungal or a bacterial infection. Some atherosclerotic abdominal aortic aneurysms also exhibit an inflammatory component, but they are usually classified in the degenerative category. Aortic aneurysms of degenerative origin may be related to atherosclerosis, dissection, myxomatous degeneration as in annuloaortic ectasia, toxin exposure, or abnormal hemodynamic stress.

Hypertension and poststenotic turbulence are the most common conditions that increase the hemodynamic stress on the aortic wall, but aberrant circulatory patterns associated with anomalous aortic arches, aortic reconstructions, and arteriovenous fistulae can alter hemodynamic stress and may contribute to aneurysmal degeneration or aortic dissection. Poststenotic turbulence may cause aneurysmal dilatation or aortic dissection and may be related to congenital or acquired lesions. Congenital lesions capable of producing poststenotic turbulence include bicuspid aortic valve stenosis, coarctation, and pseudocoarctation. Acquired lesions include calcific tricuspid aortic valve stenosis and stenotic implanted aortic grafts or valves.

Aortic dissection typically occurs in patients with predisposing factors, such as atherosclerosis, myxomatous degeneration, iatrogenic trauma, and abnormal hemodynamic stress of either congenital or acquired origin. Aortic dissection may develop without any pre-existing aneurysm and is usually related to hypertension, which may, in turn, be due to exposure to a drug such as cocaine. Aortic dissection can also develop in patients with pre-existing aneurysms with the intimal tear occurring at the aortic aneurysm or elsewhere.

CLINICAL MANIFESTATIONS

In general, the clinical manifestations of aortic aneurysms are related to aortic rupture, compression of adjacent structures, ischemia, or infection. Aortic rupture may be contained by adjacent tissues, thereby allowing for hemodynamic stability, or may be free, in which case circulatory collapse results. Aneurysms of the ascending aorta typically rupture into the pericardium, causing tamponade, electromechanical dissociation, and sudden death. Rupture of aneurysms of the aortic arch and descending thoracic aorta may be temporarily contained within the mediastinum or retropleural spaces, but if untreated they eventually rupture into the pleural spaces, causing hemothorax, dyspnea, and hemorrhagic shock. Ruptured abdominal aortic aneurysms may be temporarily contained within the retroperitoneum. If untreated they typically rupture into the peritoneal cavity, causing hemoperitoneum, abdominal distention, and hemorrhagic shock. A tender, pulsatile abdominal mass may be palpable in the abdomen or flank. Aortic rupture is usually heralded by the acute onset of pain that is localized to the anterior chest with ascending aortic rupture; superior chest and back with arch aortic rupture; midscapular and central back with descending thoracic aortic rupture; and lower back, flank, abdomen, groin, or lower extremities with abdominal aortic rupture.

Aortic rupture may also occur into adjacent organs, creating fistulous communications with the heart, great veins, tracheobronchial tree and lungs, or gastrointestinal system. The ascending aorta may rupture into the right atrium, superior vena cava, or lung. Rupture of the arch and descending thoracic aorta may occur into the esophagus, tracheobronchial tree, or lung, and rupture of the abdominal aorta may communicate with the duodenum, inferior vena cava, or left renal vein. Aortoatrial and aortocaval fistulae present with high-output congestive heart failure, venous hypertension, and swollen extremities. Auscultation may reveal a continuous murmur, which when located in the abdomen in combination with a pulsatile mass and acute congestive heart failure is diagnostic for an abdominal aortocaval fistula. Typically, aortoenteric fistulae present with hematemesis, hematochezia, or melena, and aortobronchopulmonary fistulae present with hemoptysis. A short initial hemorrhage, often termed a "sentinel bleed," serves as a warning sign that a more catastrophic hemorrhage may ensue.

The compression of adjacent structures caused by progressive expansion of aortic aneurysms is responsible for many of the chronic symptoms of aortic aneurysm disease. In general, once patients become symptomatic from aortic aneurysms, their average survival is limited to less than 1 year, with death often resulting from aortic rupture. Chronic pain is often described as a dull ache but may have a gnawing or pulsating character and may gradually worsen in intensity and frequency over time. The pain probably arises from compression of, or erosion into, adjacent musculoskeletal structures. Ascending and proximal arch aortic aneurysms tend to press against the underside of the manubrium, sternum, and costochondral cartilages and produce anterior chest pain; sometimes, a pulsation can be palpated. Distal aortic arch and descending thoracic aortic aneurysms press against the thoracic vertebrae, posterior ribs, and intercostal muscles, producing posterior chest pain in the midscapular area or lower, depending on the location of the aneurysm. Abdominal aortic aneurysms impinge on the lumbar vertebrae and psoas and iliac muscles, producing lower back pain. Palpation of the abdomen may reveal a pulsatile mass in the epigastrium, between the xiphoid process and the umbilicus near the location of the aortic bifurcation. When it appears that the superior aspect of the pulsatile mass does not decrease in size at the xiphoid level, this is a sign that the abdominal aneurysm may extend into the chest and may actually be a thoracoabdominal aneurysm.

Aortic root aneurysms may cause aortic valve insufficiency and congestive heart failure by pushing apart the aortic valve commissures or by dilating the annulus. Ascending aortic aneurysms may also cause compression of the superior vena cava or innominate vein and produce venous obstruction with upper extremity swelling. Aortic arch aneurysms can cause hoarseness, weak cough or voice, or aspiration due to stretch injury of the left recurrent laryngeal nerve, with resultant left true vocal cord paralysis, or dyspnea due to left phrenic nerve palsy. Arch and descending aortic aneurysms may also cause dysphagia from esophageal compression, or obstructive respiratory symptoms, such as wheezing, stridor, cough, and pneumonitis due to compression of the tracheobronchial tree. Abdominal aortic aneurysms can cause compression of the inferior vena cava or iliac veins, with resultant swelling of the lower extremities. Compression of the nerves within the retroperitoneum, such as the femoral nerves, results in pain, paresthesias, or weakness of the thigh and knee.

Ischemia caused by aortic aneurysms may be secondary to thrombosis, embolization, or dissection. Thrombosis of aortic aneurysms most commonly occurs in the infrarenal abdominal aortic segment and is a form of aortoiliac occlusive disease. Indeed, patients with a thrombosed aortic aneurysm often have associated atherosclerotic occlusive disease or aneurysm disease in other arterial segments and may present with an acute or a chronic lower body ischemic syndrome. Signs of acute ischemia include pain, pallor, paresthesias, absence of pulse, paralysis, and poikilothermy or coldness. Chronic ischemia may present as claudication, rest pain, or gangrene. Either acute or chronic thrombosis of the abdominal aorta usually results in loss of palpable pulses in the lower extremities, unless large collaterals have developed.

Embolization of atherothrombotic debris from within aortic aneurysms may present with small, blue or black lesions on the toes, the so-called blue toe syndrome of chronic atheroembolism, or as a catastrophic event associated with all the signs of acute ischemia, including livedo reticularis (a reddish-blue netlike mottling of the skin). This type of ischemic presentation, along with palpable pedal pulses, is classic for embolization; however, a single large embolism or multiple chronic emboli may cause loss of pedal pulses. Thus, absence of a pedal pulse does not rule out this mechanism. Acute renal failure may develop owing to either direct embolization to the kidneys or the toxic effects of myonecrosis and myoglobinuria. Embolization to the bowel should be suspected when abdominal pain with hematochezia or melena is present. Either mucosal or transmural ischemia may be responsible.

Aortic dissection may cause ischemia, because as the false lumen advances, enlarges, and extends, it can progressively limit flow through the true lumen of the aorta or any aortic branch vessel. Thus, aortic dissection can cause ischemic dysfunction of many organ systems, including those perfused by the coronary, carotid, subclavian, spinal, visceral, renal, iliac, and femoral arteries. Peripheral pulses may be weak, absent, or intermittent in the regions of ischemia.

Infection is another means by which aortic aneurysms may manifest clinically. Infected aneurysms usually are painful and tender to palpation (when in a palpable location, such as the abdomen) and are associated with fever, tachycardia, and other clinical signs of systemic infection. Chronic, noninfected aneurysms may become infected during an episode of bacteremia, or a previously normal aorta may become infected from an adjacent organ, such as an infected lymph node or a lung abscess. Peripheral signs consistent with systemic embolization of infected microemboli may be present, such as splinter and conjunctival hemorrhages, Osler nodes, dermal infarcts, and palatal petechiae. Infective endocarditis may coexist, and then the central signs of endocarditis may also be present, including murmurs, gallops, rales, and the electrocardiographic signs of progressive heart block.

Thoracic Aortic Aneurysms

Thoracic aortic aneurysms are caused most frequently by aortic dissection and atherosclerosis, followed by myxomatous degeneration, which includes both Marfan's syndrome and annuloaortic ectasia. Less frequent causes include aortitis, trauma, poststenotic dilatation, and infection. Aneurysms caused by myxomatous degeneration or aortitis tend to involve the aortic root and valve, typically resulting in aortic valve regurgitation. Traumatic aortic aneurysms most commonly result from blunt deceleration injuries sustained in motor vehicle accidents and falls and most frequently involve the proximal descending thoracic aorta. Aneurysms of poststenotic etiology often involve the ascending aorta as a result of aortic valve stenosis, or the proximal descending aorta related to coarctation.

Patients with aortic aneurysms caused by aortic dissection typically report a history of chest and/or back pain and are more likely to develop aortic rupture than are patients who do not have dissection. The classic pain of acute aortic dissection is described as acute in onset and severe (not crescendo, as in myocardial ischemia) with a tearing or ripping quality that migrates along with the course of the dissection. Acute aortic dissection may present as acute myocardial ischemia, congestive heart failure, cerebrovascular accident, syncopal attack, acute abdomen, spinal injury, of limb ischemia. However, when the patient is able to communicate and the presentation has been caused by aortic dissection, typical severe tearing pain in the chest or back at the onset of the acute illness is nearly always reported.

Abdominal Aortic Aneurysms

Abdominal aortic aneurysms are caused by, or at least associated predominantly with, atherosclerosis. Because atherosclerosis is often a systemic disease, patients may have a history of symptoms or signs of atherosclerotic occlusive or aneurysm disease at other sites. Associated coronary artery, cerebrovascular, chronic mesenteric, renovascular, and peripheral vascular disease may be present. False aneurysms at old aortic graft anastomoses and infected aneurysms may be found in the abdomen. Some thoracic aortic atherosclerotic aneurysms and dissections extend into the abdomen, creating thoracoabdominal aneurysms.

Patients with abdominal aneurysms are often asymptomatic, and the aneurysms may be diagnosed on routine physical examination. Some patients notice an abnormal pulsation when resting a book on their abdomen when recumbent. Because abdominal aneurysms are often asymptomatic, are relatively common, and typically rupture at a smaller size, they are more likely to present with aortic rupture than are thoracic aneurysms. Screening programs that use abdominal ultrasonography have been developed for use in patients with other risk factors for atherosclerotic disease or a family or personal history of aneurysm disease.

DIAGNOSTIC EVALUATION

History

Helpful information obtained in the history includes age, sex, and race. Atherosclerotic and giant cell aneurysms and dissections related to hypertension are more likely to occur in patients older than 40 years of age, but younger patients are more likely to have aneurysms or dissections related to myxomatous degeneration or congenital abnormalities. Takayasu's arteritis tends to occur in young women and may occur in any race. Blacks are more likely to develop aortic dissection than atherosclerotic aneurysms.

The evaluation of symptoms should include the location, character, severity, and acuity of onset of pain, because acute onset and severe pain usually imply an emergency situation. Cardiopulmonary signs and symptoms may include presyncope or syncope, diaphoresis, dyspnea, anginal pain, hemoptysis, cough, wheeze, or pneumonitis. Gastrointestinal signs and symptoms of dysphagia, hematemesis, or hematochezia may be present. Neurologic and musculoskeletal signs and symptoms may include syncope, limb paresthesias, pain, paresis or paralysis, hoarseness, or incontinence.

The past medical history should include an assessment of atherosclerotic risk factors, including hypertension and tobacco use in particular. Tobacco use appears to accelerate elastic tissue destruction and thus is thought to be an important contributing factor to the development of aneurysms and emphysema, and perhaps hernias. A history of congenital abnormalities of the circulation or connective tissues or any history of systemic or vascular inflammatory disease may provide helpful clues. Any history of significant trauma, such as a fall or a motor vehicle accident, or prior cardiac or vascular surgery should be obtained. Even the obstetric history is important because the rare aortic and splenic aneurysms found in young women usually occur during pregnancy, perhaps related to a temporary systemic weakening and relaxation of connective tissue complicated by hypertension. Exposure to illicit drugs, such as cocaine, may explain an aortic dissection. Even exposure to lathyrogenic toxins that weaken connective tissue, such as beta-aminopropionitrile, found in sweet peas, or dimethyl hydrazine, an industrial chemical, may lead to aneurysms.

Physical Examination

Assessment of vital signs is first and foremost, because patients with aortic aneurysms can be acutely ill and in shock. Hypertension may be present, and renovascular ischemia should be considered as a cause.

Patients with tamponade from an acute ascending aortic dissection or rupture may be hypotensive, with neck vein distention, pulsus paradoxus, and a pericardial rub. Murmurs and gallops consistent with aortic or mitral valve regurgitation or aortic valve stenosis or coarctation are often heard in association with thoracic aortic aneurysms or dissection.

A rapid assessment of the general appearance can provide important clues. The elderly, tobacco-smoking, barrel-chested patient with excessively wrinkled skin is likely to have atherosclerosis, emphysema, and probably hypertension. The younger patient who is particularly tall and thin, with long, slender fingers and toes (arachnodactyly) is likely to have annuloaortic ectasia or dissection. Closer examination of the patient with Marfan's syndrome may reveal dislocation of the lens, pectus deformities, scoliosis, high-arched palate, and murmurs of aortic and possibly mitral valve regurgitation. Other conditions with inherited disorders of connective tissue and a tendency to develop aneurysms or dissection include pseudoxanthoma elasticum, Ehlers-Danlos syndrome, and osteogenesis imperfecta.

Abdominal aortic and peripheral pulses all should be evaluated for strength, character, width, bruits, and tenderness. Weak or absent pulses may reflect acute or chronic conditions, but the absence should be assumed to be acute and critical until proven otherwise. Broad or widened and prominent pulses usually represent aneurysms. If pulses are palpable, they are most commonly felt in the abdominal aorta and femoral and popliteal arteries. Peripheral aneurysms often accompany abdominal aneurysms and are often bilateral. The absence of a pulse may be consistent with the presence of a thrombosed aneurysm. Abdominal palpation may result in the incorrect diagnosis of an abdominal aortic aneurysm when the aortic pulsation is being transmitted through an abdominal mass, such as a tumor that is adjacent to the aorta, or when the aorta is very tortuous. A continuous midabdominal bruit is typically heard in the presence of an aortocaval fistula, and swollen extremities and dilated veins may also be present.

Laboratory Examination

The laboratory evaluation should include serial complete blood counts in patients with acute presentations. A falling hematocrit and platelet count are consistent with hemorrhage, provided that correction is made for dilution from resuscitative fluids. Patients with type B dissection may lose blood within a thrombosing false lumen, without actually hemorrhaging outside of the aortic wall. Leukocytosis and increased erythrocyte sedimentation rate (ESR) are often seen in the acute conditions or those related to aortitis. If the results of these tests are much higher than usual, active infection should be considered, and blood cultures for bacteria and fungi should be obtained downstream from the aneurysm. Creatine kinase (CK) levels may be increased owing to skeletal, cardiac, or smooth muscle ischemia that can originate from the aortic wall with dissection. Urea nitrogen, creatinine, and potassium may be increased as the result of muscle damage and/or renal ischemia or failure. Tests for autoimmune disease may be appropriate in patients who have arthritis-associated aortitis, and syphilis serology may help detect patients with possible syphilitic aortitis. A screen for illicit drugs should be considered, especially in young patients with aortic dissection.

Imaging Studies

The aorta can be evaluated for the presence of aneurysms with many modalities, including plain abdominal and chest films, ultrasonography, computed tomography, magnetic resonance imaging, and aortography. These techniques have various advantages and disadvantages, including availability, degree of invasiveness, speed of acquisition of data, quality of image, cost, operator dependence, patient or situation compatibility, and risk. Some of these issues may also vary between hospitals.

The evaluation of aortic diameter can be falsely exaggerated with the use of any cross-sectional imaging technique when the longitudinal axis of the aorta is not perpendicular to the plane of the image. The aorta has natural curves, especially across the arch, and it becomes more tortuous with age and disease, especially just above the diaphragm. This is a real limitation of tomographic imaging techniques and may lead to misinterpretation. When the longitudinal axis is not perpendicular to the cross-sectional image, the aorta appears elliptical, usually in locations prone to tortuosity. The absence of an intraluminal thrombus, which is often present within significantly dilated segments of aorta, may also serve as a clue that a significant aneurysm is not present. The use of oblique cross-sectional imaging perpendicular or parallel to the longitudinal axis of the aorta can avoid misrepresentation of the aortic diameter and is most easily obtained noninvasively with ultrasonography or magnetic resonance imaging.

Plain Roentgenography

Plain roentgenography is a readily available, simple, and inexpensive technique that may provide enough information to establish the diagnosis of either thoracic or abdominal aortic aneurysms. Thoracic aortic aneurysms can often be detected on the posteroanterior or anteroposterior views by mediastinal widening, and arch aneurysms can cause deviation of the trachea toward the right with depression of the left mainstem bronchus. Rupturing aneurysms are suggested by a globular-shaped heart in cases of tamponade, or by apical caps or pleural effusions when blood is leaking into the mediastinum or pleural spaces. Aneurysms or acute transections secondary to blunt trauma may have other signs of trauma, such as sternal, rib, or vertebral fractures. The lateral chest film helps differentiate anterior from posterior aneurysms and provides a better estimation of size.

Abdominal aortic aneurysms are suggested on the plain abdominal film by a separation between the calcified edges of the aortic wall. If one side is obscured by overlying vertebral calcification, this sign is of limited value, and lateral films may help.

Ultrasonography

Transthoracic echocardiography and abdominal ultrasonography are noninvasive methods that can usually establish the presence and size of ascending and infrarenal abdominal aortic aneurysms, respectively. Transesophageal echocardiography is more invasive and requires patient cooperation, but it provides an excellent view of the ascending and descending thoracic aorta, as well as the heart. Imaging of the aortic arch is obscured by the air within the tracheobronchial tree, and imaging of the proximal abdominal aorta can be obscured by bowel gas. All the ultrasonic imaging techniques are relatively operator dependent, and availability depends on the cardiology and vascular services. However, these ultrasonic imaging techniques can provide a rapid and definitive diagnosis of thoracic and abdominal aortic aneurysm disease and dissection. Short- and long-axis views are available, and intraluminal thrombus and atherosclerotic debris are well visualized. All the ultrasonographic techniques have the advantage of providing rapid results at the patient's bedside, which is particularly helpful in the unstable patient.

Transesophageal echocardiography appears to be more reliable and more sensitive than transthoracic echocardiography as a method of definitively diagnosing acute aortic dissection. Cardiac valvular and left ventricular function can also be assessed, and pericardial effusions are easily seen. If an evolving acute aortic rupture or dissection is clinically suspected, further stress to the patient can be avoided by immediately moving the patient to the operating room, where transesophageal echocardiography can be performed with ready access to anesthesia and surgical intervention.

Computed Tomography and Magnetic Resonance Imaging

Both computed tomography and magnetic resonance imaging can provide an accurate assessment of the thoracic and abdominal aorta, including the presence of intraluminal thrombus, debris or dissection, wall thickness, aortic size, and any signs of aortic rupture, such as periaortic hematoma, pericardial effusion, pleural effusion, and retroperitoneal hematoma. The ability to measure wall thickness is extremely helpful for establishing the presence of inflammatory aortic aneurysms. Inflammatory aneurysms are often densely adherent to adjacent structures, requiring different surgical approaches.

Both computed tomography and magnetic resonance imaging also provide accessory information about adjacent organs, anatomic abnormalities, and unrelated diseases. The diagnosis of a horseshoe kidney, a retroaortic left renal vein, or a mass consistent with tumor may alter the clinical approach.

Computed tomography requires more exposure to radiation and intravenous injection of contrast material when intraluminal detail is required. However, calcification is more easily visualized, and this visualization can help differentiate an acute from a chronic process. Because data acquisition is rapid, image quality is good, and hemodynamic monitoring can be performed when needed, computed tomography is particularly useful for evaluation of the acutely ill but hemodynamically stable patient.

Magnetic resonance imaging does not require radiation, but sometimes an injection of gadolinium is used for contrast. Data acquisition time is longer, and it is more difficult to monitor acutely ill patients. Patients often complain of claustrophobia and may require sedation. Patients with pacemakers or certain implanted metallic devices cannot be studied. Multiplanar views can be readily obtained, including oblique sagittal views that clearly illustrate the aortic arch and areas of tortuosity. Information about tissue characteristics allows differentiation between bloody and serous effusions, and between flowing and stagnant blood. Magnetic resonance imaging is most useful for the evaluation of the complicated aortic problem in the asymptomatic, hemodynamically stable patient.

Aortography

Aortography is an invasive imaging technique that requires a room lined with lead and specially equipped for arterial puncture, aortic catheterization, and contrast administration by trained personnel, such as a cardiologist or a radiologist. Often, aortography is not readily available and is associated with more risks. However, when a qualified catheterization team is available, the procedure can be completed swiftly and safely, with an overall complication rate of less than 1 to 2 per cent. Aortography provides excellent detail of the lumen of the aorta and major branch vessels, as well as any intimal irregularities or stenoses. True aortic diameter may be underestimated when an intraluminal thrombus is present. Aortic dissection is identified with visualization of an intimal tear or double lumen and a characteristically narrowed lumen on aortography. If the false lumen is thrombosed and the true lumen is not characteristically narrowed, the dissection may be missed. A practical advantage of aortography is that when the coronary arteries also need to be evaluated, selective coronary angiography can be performed through the same puncture site during the procedure.

Diagnostic and Therapeutic Procedures

When the patient is hemodynamically unstable, as the result of acute ascending aortic dissection or rupture of the aorta in any location, the definitive diagnosis may need to be made in the operating room via exploratory sternotomy, thoracotomy, or laparotomy.

Pericardiocentesis, thoracentesis, and paracentesis can be performed preoperatively to determine whether effusions or ascites are present and, if so, whether they are bloody or serous. Unfortunately, when the tap is traumatic these methods may be misleading, and when fluid is not present there is a greater risk of puncturing underlying organs. Limited exploration of the pericardium via a subxiphoid incision, of the pleural space via tube thoracostomy or thoracoscopy, and of the peritoneum via minilaparotomy or laparoscopy may provide safer, more reliable and effective diagnostic information than that obtained with the percutaneous needle techniques. Upper gastrointestinal endoscopy is useful during the evaluation of possible aortoenteric fistula.

The diagnosis of patients with aortic aneurysm disease should proceed quickly and efficiently, especially in unstable patients with acute onset of symptoms or worsening symptoms. A missed or delayed diagnosis or referral for surgery may result in an unnecessary fatality. The goals of the diagnostic evaluation in the acute situation should be (1) to consider the possibility that an acute aortic problem may exist; (2) to rapidly define the nature, location, and extent of the aortic problem as completely as the clinical situation allows; and (3) to move the patient to the operating room for surgical repair without delay.

CHRONIC ARTERIAL OCCLUSIVE DISEASE OF THE LOWER EXTREMITY

By Bartholomew O'Beirne Woods, M.D.
Burlington, Massachusetts

Patients with chronic arterial occlusive disease of the lower extremities (CAODLE) or arteriosclerosis obliterans (ASO) are reported to have a life span 10 years shorter than that of the general population. Compared with patients who have no evidence of arterial disease, the risk of premature death is doubled for patients with intermittent claudication and more than tripled for patients with coexistent coronary heart disease and peripheral arterial disease. The principal causes of death in these patients are coronary heart disease and cerebrovascular disease.

GENERAL CONSIDERATIONS

Atherosclerosis is the most common cause of CAODLE. This degenerative condition most commonly involves the abdominal aorta and the carotid, coronary, iliac, and femoral arteries. Occasionally, the tibial vessels are involved, especially in diabetics. In older patients who develop arteriosclerosis with calcification of the media, the arteries feel hard and can be visualized readily with radiographs of the soft tissues. Clinically, the temporal artery is most often abnormal, but the radial, brachial, and femoral arteries should also be palpated. This medial calcific sclerosis, by itself, does not cause obstruction, but atherosclerosis often coexists. In addition, risk factors, such as age, diabetes mellitus, continued cigarette smoking, systemic hypertension, hypercholesterolemia, low-serum high-density lipoprotein (HDL) cholesterol, and increased ratio of total cholesterol to plasma HDL, contribute to the development of CAODLE.

As a major cause of occlusive vascular disease, atherosclerosis often occurs segmentally, especially at major arterial bifurcations and at points of arterial angulation, such as the superficial femoral artery in Hunter's canal. Less commonly involved, except in diabetics, are the deep femoral artery, the midpopliteal artery after the point of flexion of the knee joint, and the popliteal trifurcation, including proximal portions of the tibial and peroneal vessels.

The patient with CAODLE may be totally asymptomatic, symptomatic only with exercise (intermittent claudication), or symptomatic at rest (ischemic pain at rest). These clinical variations reflect the hemodynamic principle that reduction of vascular lumen diameter does not lead to decreased blood flow or pressure until "critical narrowing" is reached, which at rest is approximately 85 to 95 per cent of the diameter of the original lumen. Exercise of the affected limb or limbs can "unmask" arterial obstruction in patients with lesser degrees of stenosis during evaluation at the bedside or in the noninvasive vascular laboratory. In the presence of CAODLE, collateral circulation typically feeds arteries distal to the stenosis or occlusion. Daily exercise in patients with CAODLE stimulates the development of collateral flow and increases walking distance and time to claudication during peripheral vascular rehabilitation.

INCIDENCE AND PREVALENCE

Many patients with CAODLE remain asymptomatic for years. The most common initial symptom is intermittent claudication; 1.5 per cent of men younger than 49 years of age and 5 per cent of men older than 50 years develop intermittent claudication during their lifetime. Women have a similar incidence, but the onset typically occurs 10 years later and generally follows a benign course. About 25 per cent of patients eventually require reconstructive surgery, and fewer than 5 per cent require a major amputation. The onset of symptoms usually occurs between 50 and 70 years of age; when symptoms occur in patients younger than 50 years of age, the disease runs a more aggressive course. Heavy cigarette smoking and a strong family history of atherosclerosis further increase the risk of premature death in patients younger than 40 years of age who have symptomatic arterial occlusive disease of the lower extremities.

CAODLE is a significant risk factor for premature death caused by myocardial infarction or stroke. When compared with age-matched control subjects, the mortality rate for men with chronic lower extremity ischemia is doubled or tripled after 5 years. Approximately 50 per cent of deaths are attributed to myocardial infarction, 15 per cent to stroke, and 10 per cent to vascular disease in the abdomen.

SYMPTOMS

A careful history and physical examination can be particularly useful in the diagnosis of vascular disease. The extremities are easy to examine, and the experienced observer can often detect subtle abnormalities by meticulous inspection, palpation, and auscultation of the affected limb. However, because peripheral vascular changes may be caused or aggravated by disorders arising elsewhere in the body, the clinician must also systematically search for dissection of the aorta, emboli from the heart or aneurysms of more proximal vessels, diabetes mellitus, hyperlipidemia, hypertension, gout, obesity, coronary artery disease, and cerebrovascular disease.

Intermittent Claudication

The primary symptom of CAODLE is intermittent claudication. Patients typically describe calf pain, discomfort, or disability associated with exertion. Atypical symptoms include heaviness, fatigue, numbness, coolness, or changes in the color of the limbs. The incidence of intermittent claudication is substantially greater in patients younger than 70 years of age, whereas gangrene is more frequent in patients older than 70. Therefore, in an evaluation of the elderly, the clinician is challenged to identify patients at risk for gangrene even though ischemic symptoms may not be experienced prior to irreversible injury. Patients with aortoiliac disease typically have claudication of the buttock or thigh, characterized by aching discomfort and weakness. However, a considerable number also complain of calf claudication, characterized by severe, crampy muscle pain. Severe bilateral aortoiliac occlusive disease may also be associated with erectile impotence in men (Leriche syndrome).

Ischemic claudication of the foot is uncommon and may occur independent of claudication of the calf. Claudication of the foot is more often noted in thromboangiitis obliterans (Buerger's disease) than in arteriosclerosis obliterans because of the typically more distal distribution of occlusive lesions in Buerger's disease, which is more frequently seen in young men who are heavy smokers and who may have associated superficial thrombophlebitis or Raynaud's phenomenon, or both. Claudication of the foot typically occurs only with advanced arterial insufficiency and thus may be associated with ischemic pain in the foot at rest.

Ischemic Pain at Rest

Ischemic pain at rest typically presents as severe, diffuse, nocturnal discomfort distal to the metatarsals. Occasionally, the pain is localized sharply to the vicinity of an ischemic ulcer or a gangrenous toe. Opiate analgesia does not always relieve the pain, but partial relief may follow placement of the affected limb in a dependent position. Few conditions produce such demoralizing pain, and the careful clinician should also look for dependent rubor as well as involvement of multiple arterial segments. Approximately 20 per cent of those who have experienced intermittent claudication for 5 or more years progress to ischemic pain at rest.

SIGNS

Ischemic Ulcers

Ischemic nocturnal foot pain at rest is often associated with ischemic ulcers. Some of these lesions may have irregular margins; others have a "punched-out" appearance. Ischemic ulcers most often develop on the dorsum of the foot or toes, but pretibial lesions also occur. Ischemic ulcers must be distinguished from shallower stasis ulcers, which typically arise near the medial malleolus and have a moist, granulating base surrounded by a zone of stasis dermatitis. Stasis ulcers invariably accompany underlying venous disease. Chronic gangrene, which may arise following minor trauma such as nail trimming, begins at the tips of the toes in contact with pressure points. By the time tissue necrosis occurs, the patient's ability to walk is usually severely limited. Five to ten per cent of patients who develop intermittent claudication progress to amputation due to limb ischemia.

Additional Signs

Following palpation and auscultation of the arterial pulses, the examiner should look for trophic signs of ischemia, such as diminished hair growth, thickened brittle toenails, subcutaneous atrophy, blue toes, changes in skin color or temperature, and small petechial lesions that may indicate microemboli.

The blood pressure and blood flow of the limb should also be evaluated. A systolic pressure of 60 to 75 mm Hg is required to keep a foot warm and pink when it is raised upright from the supine position for at least 1 minute. Blood pressure in the limb can be measured just as it is measured in the arm. Buerger's posture test can also be performed. With the patient supine, raise the leg about 60 to 75 degrees from the horizontal, keeping the knee straight. Support the legs of the patient while he or she flexes and extends the ankles and toes to the point of mild fatigue. When the arterial blood supply to the limb is deficient, the sole of the foot reveals a cadaveric pallor, and prominent veins on the dorsum of the foot become empty. By contrast, when the feet remain warm and pink, it is highly unlikely that the patient requires immediate intravascular intervention to prevent ischemic necrosis, gangrene, ulceration, or amputation. As the feet are lowered, and the patient is returned to a sitting posture, the clinician should also determine how long it takes for the color to return or for reactive dependent rubor to develop, and how long it takes for the veins to become distended over the dorsum of the foot (venous filling time). Color should return within 10 seconds, and venous filling should require no more than 15 seconds of dependency. In patients with moderate ischemia, return of color should take less than 25 to 30 seconds, and venous filling should be complete within 30 seconds. When the patient's feet require more than 30 to 40 seconds to show return of color and development of venous filling, inadequate collateral perfusion should be strongly suspected. However, the venous filling time becomes unreliable in the patient with severe venous disease or with incompetent venous valves that permit retrograde filling of the veins regardless of the status of their arterial circulation.

PHYSIOLOGIC TESTING

Physiologic testing provides quantitative data that may help determine the severity of ischemia and the location of obstructive lesions. Such testing is accomplished most easily with a portable, hand-held Doppler ultrasonographic flow probe. This instrument is widely available, inexpensive, and easy to use. This probe should be used with a standard sphygmomanometer to evaluate the dorsalis pedis, posterior tibial, and brachial arteries. Decreased systolic pressure may indicate a degree of arterial stenosis somewhat less than that required to decrease blood flow or to eliminate a palpable pulse. Systolic pressure in the ankle is usually equal to or greater than the brachial systolic pressure. When systolic pressure of the ankle measures less than 97 per cent of the brachial pressure, arterial occlusive disease is likely to be present. Patients with moderate to severe claudication typically have ankle pressures between 50 and 80 per cent of arm pressures. Ischemic pain at rest is usually associated with ankle pressure measuring less than 30 per cent of the brachial pressure. Patients with mild intermittent claudication may have slightly abnormal ankle pressures at rest; detection of appreciably abnormal pressures may require repeated measurements during exercise or during reactive hyperemia testing. Patients with diabetes mellitus may have calcified arteriosclerotic arteries that are difficult to compress with the blood pressure cuff. Therefore, abnormally high (falsely normal) ankle systolic pressures can be measured in patients with diabetes.

SEGMENTAL PRESSURE MEASUREMENT

Segmental pressures can be measured by placing blood pressure cuffs at the high thigh, calf, and ankle level to determine the site of occlusive disease. This examination is usually performed in combination with segmental volume plethysmography or analysis of Doppler-derived pulse waveforms. Vascular stress testing with walking exercise or reactive hyperemia produces increased arterial blood flow in an extremity and can be used to unmask subcritical stenosis or marginally significant stenotic lesions. Treadmill exercise provides a functional evaluation of the patient's symptoms. Standard stress measurements such as a modified Bruce protocol are typically employed for 5 minutes. The time-to-claudication and the maximum walking time are obtained and postexercise ankle pressures are recorded at 2 minutes, 5 minutes, and 10 minutes.

TRANSCUTANEOUS OXYGEN MEASUREMENT

Transcutaneous oximetry provides another noninvasive means of evaluating CAODLE. Oximetry measures oxygenation of the skin of the foot or at the level of a proposed amputation. The ratio of peripheral to central transcutaneous oxygen tension provides a measure of local tissue perfusion. This regional perfusion index averages 0.9 or greater in normal subjects. Some authorities suggest that oximetry can predict the likelihood of successful healing of an ulcer or an amputation site.

DUPLEX ULTRASONOGRAPHY

Duplex ultrasonography has also been used to evaluate CAODLE. This method can assess both arterial anatomy and physiology. Spectral analysis looks at the hemodynamic effect of localized stenosis, and velocity profiles are compared before and after balloon angioplasty, atherectomy, stent placement, or peripheral vascular bypass surgery.

ANGIOGRAPHY

Angiography does not define the physiologic significance of stenotic lesions. Thus, angiographic confirmation of CAODLE is best reserved for patients who are candidates for percutaneous transluminal angioplasty or for reconstructive vascular surgery. Complete arteriography of the abdominal aorta, runoff vessels, and pedal arches in both lower extremities should be obtained. Oblique views may enhance evaluation of the iliac or femoral bifurcation. The complications of arteriography include arterial puncture, peripheral embolism, and renal failure associated with administration of contrast media.

MAGNETIC RESONANCE IMAGING

Because magnetic resonance imaging provides images of the entire arterial wall, this technique can help identify intraluminal thrombus as well as the surrounding musculoskeletal structures. Magnetic resonance imaging has been most valuable in characterizing aneurysm, entrapment, and cystic adventitial degeneration in the popliteal fossa. The disadvantages of magnetic resonance imaging are its limited resolution and its high cost. Patients with pacemakers, metallic heart valves, or intracerebral metallic clips should not be evaluated by magnetic resonance imaging, although patients with metal-joint prostheses have been safely evaluated. While images of major intra-abdominal arteries and veins are easily obtained, images of smaller, more peripheral arteries have more limited definition and resolution. The ability of magnetic resonance imaging to characterize blood flow may prove useful in assessing hemodynamics in vivo, but further research with magnetic resonance imaging is required before it can become a practical clinical tool for evaluating vascular disease.

PROGNOSIS

Many elderly patients who lead an inactive life have occlusion of limb vessels and remain asymptomatic until they die. In patients who are still active, claudication may remain static or may improve. Many surveys have established the course of the disease and the effect of various factors on prognosis. Nearly 60 per cent of patients improve considerably, even up to 3 years after the onset of symptoms. In a series involving almost 4000 patients, approximately 10 per cent required amputation of the limb in a 5-year follow-up. The factors known to increase the likelihood of amputation include diabetes and the failure to stop smoking. Among patients with intermittent claudication who seek medical attention, the likelihood of surgical intervention is approximately 20 to 30 per cent. However, in large epidemiologic studies that include patients with intermittent claudication who have not sought medical advice, the likelihood that these patients will require surgical treatment is 10 per cent. Similarly, the likelihood of eventual amputation is approximately 5 per cent in surgical series. Coexisting coronary and cerebrovascular occlusive disease is a major concern in patients with CAODLE and should be sought meticulously during evaluation of the patients with peripheral vascular disease.

NONATHEROSCLEROTIC OBSTRUCTIVE ARTERIAL DISEASES

Obstructive arterial diseases other than atherosclerosis may produce claudication, pain at rest, and ischemic ulceration. Thromboangiitis obliterans (Buerger's disease), Takayasu's arteritis, giant cell arteritis, and fibromuscular dysplasia are the best-known examples. The renal and carotid arteries are most frequently involved in fibromuscular dysplasia, which may also affect the mesenteric, coronary, subclavian, and iliac arteries. The clinical manifestations in the arteritides and dysplasia are similar to those of atherosclerosis. Both surgical reconstruction and percutaneous angioplasty have been employed in the management of fibromuscular dysplasia.

Adventitious cysts and vascular tumors of the arterial wall may produce clinically significant obstruction by mass effect or as a result of superimposed thrombosis. Neurovascular compression due to anatomic relationships of muscular, tendinous, or bony structures may be associated with popliteal artery entrapment, which is found in males younger than 30 years of age and is bilateral in 20 per cent of patients. The symptoms progress in severity, and ultimately arterial thrombosis may occur. This syndrome should be distinguished from intrinsic vascular disease.

PERIPHERAL VENOUS DISEASE

By William G. Jamieson, M.D.
London, Ontario, Canada
and William Z. Borer, M.D.
Philadelphia, Pennsylvania

Venous disease is extremely common. Venous stasis ulcers affect 500,000 individuals in the United States each year. Chronic venous stasis with ulcer is the second most common cause of absence from work in the United Kingdom (after the common cold), and it costs the National Health System between 3 million and 1.2 billion dollars per year. A knowledge of the pathogenesis, diagnosis, and management of these problems is necessary to manage the conditions efficiently.

TELANGIECTASIAS

Telangiectasias, or "spider veins," are dilated venules in the skin. They are blue or red and no more than 1 mm in diameter. They occur in one of two patterns: a linear arrangement or a starburst configuration. Telangiectasias do not blanch on elevation. They are usually asymptomatic, but occasionally they are associated with a mild burning sensation, especially during menses.

SUPERFICIAL VENOUS INSUFFICIENCY (VARICOSE VEINS)

Varicose veins are dilated, distended, tortuous superficial veins that usually become obvious in the legs when the patient stands motionless for a few moments. About 20 to 25 per cent of adults have varicose veins, and of these individuals, 60 to 70 per cent are women. Although varicosities can occur virtually anywhere in the body, the saphenous veins and their tributaries are common sites of involvement. These veins lie on the deep fascia, and they can become dilated and tortuous. In obese patients there may be few obvious signs on physical examination. If the veins can be localized, a Doppler flow examination can document incompetence of the venous valves. However, duplex ultrasonography (combining imaging ultrasound and Doppler) and venography are the most helpful studies. Varicose veins are usually apparent on physical examination.

Most patients with varicose veins are asymptomatic, but some describe leg fullness, heaviness, or aching. A "bursting feeling" may be associated with edema. Symptoms are typically relieved when the legs are elevated. Patients with varicose veins should feel no discomfort just before rising in the morning because a night in bed relieves the venous hypertension and, with it, the symptoms. Pain is not associated with uncomplicated varicose veins.

CHRONIC DEEP VENOUS INSUFFICIENCY

This chronic condition is the result of venous obstruction (e.g., deep vein thrombosis) and/or incompetent deep venous valves leading to venous hypertension and reflux of venous blood down the legs. Patients report aching, heavy, swollen legs often associated with pruritus, hyperpigmentation, or ulcers on the ankles. Edema is typically not present in the morning, but it develops gradually during the day with either ambulatory or sedentary activity. The ulcers usually occur above either the medial or the lateral malleolus and are often surrounded by areas of brown, thickened skin (lipodermatosclerosis). Symptoms are relieved by leg elevation, but relief is not immediate as with varicose veins. About half of patients with chronic venous insufficiency can recall an attack of phlebitis. Physical examination, duplex ultrasonography, impedance plethysmography, and ascending and descending venography can be used to determine whether the cause is obstruction or primary valvular insufficiency.

VENOUS THROMBOSIS AND THROMBOPHLEBITIS

Venous thrombosis refers to the development of an intraluminal thrombus usually within one or more of the superficial or deep veins of the leg. The thrombus is typically composed of fibrin and platelets with entrained erythrocytes; it is attached to the vessel wall and propagates in the direction of blood flow. The term "thrombophlebitis" includes a reference to the inflammatory process that may involve the vein and surrounding tissue. The severity of the phlebitis is not necessarily proportional to the severity of the disease process. It is clinically useful to distinguish between superficial thrombophlebitis and deep vein thrombosis.

Superficial Thrombophlebitis

Uncomplicated thrombophlebitis of the superficial veins of the legs is rarely, if ever, associated with pulmonary embolism or chronic venous insufficiency. Predisposing factors include varicose veins, indwelling intravenous catheters, deep vein thrombosis, and local trauma. Patients with superficial thrombophlebitis have pain, swelling, and often redness along the course of the vein or veins affected. On physical examination, the phlebitic veins are localized, tender, and palpable (venous cord). Diffuse calf or thigh swelling is usually *not present* with uncomplicated superficial thrombophlebitis. Septic thrombophlebitis may present with systemic signs of infection such as fever, chills, and leukocytosis and is often associated with needle puncture.

The differential diagnosis of superficial thrombophlebitis includes cellulitis and lymphangitis. If the thrombus is close to a major perforating vein (e.g., the saphenous-femoral junction or the short saphenous-popliteal junction), the evaluation should include duplex venous ultrasonography or venography to exclude an extension of the thrombus to the deep veins. If extension to the deep venous system is confirmed, anticoagulation may be indicated to prevent further propagation of the thrombus and pulmonary embolism (see article on pulmonary embolism).

Deep Vein Thrombophlebitis

Deep vein thrombosis is a common disorder associated with a number of predisposing conditions (Table 1). Immobility, recent thoracic or abdominal surgery, and the presence of malignancy are important risk factors that should be elicited in the history to help assess the probability of venous thrombosis. Deep vein thrombosis is more common in women, the elderly, and the critically ill. The clinical importance of deep vein thrombosis lies in its potential sequelae: acute pulmonary embolism and chronic venous insufficiency. Thrombi that form in the deep veins of the calf are often silent and undergo spontaneous lysis. Up to 30 per cent of these thrombi extend above the knee, making embolism more likely, because lysis of proximal thrombi is usually incomplete if left untreated.

When present, the physical findings are usually nonspecific. They include localized swelling, discoloration, and/or tenderness involving the calf, thigh, or inguinal area. The skin color may vary from red with inflammation to white if edema is the primary feature. A warm, swollen, bluish purple limb with engorged collateral veins in the thigh is typical of the obstruction to venous outflow seen with iliofemoral thrombosis. When the calf is affected, pain can be elicited by squeezing the gastrocnemius muscle or by dorsiflexing the foot (Homans' sign). If the thrombus involves only the calf, the sulci just lateral to the patella are

Table 1. Conditions Associated With an Increased Risk of Development of Venous Thrombosis

Surgery
  Orthopedic, thoracic, abdominal, and genitourinary procedures
Cancer
  Pancreas, lung, ovary, testis, urinary tract, breast, stomach
Trauma
  Fractures of spine, pelvis, femur, tibia
Immobilization
  Acute myocardial infarction, congestive heart failure, stroke, postoperative convalescence, prolonged travel by air or automobile
Pregnancy
Estrogen therapy
  Replacement or contraception
Hypercoagulable states
  Deficiencies of antithrombin III, protein C, or protein S
  Presence of anticardiolipin antibodies, myeloproliferative disorder, dysfibrinogenemia; disseminated intravascular coagulation
Venulitis
  Thromboangiitis obliterans, Behçet's disease, homocysteinuria
Previous deep vein thrombosis

Adapted from Creager, M.A., and Dzau, V.J.: Vascular diseases of the extremities. *In* Isselbacner, K.J., Braunwald, E., Wilson, J.D., et al. (eds.): *Harrison's Principles of Internal Medicine*, 13th ed., New York, McGraw-Hill, 1994, with permission.

concave and not swollen. The differential diagnosis includes infection (cellulitis, lymphangitis, fasciitis, or myositis), muscle trauma (ruptured plantaris or gastrocnemius muscle, hematoma, or cramp), ruptured Baker cyst, superficial thrombophlebitis, chronic venous insufficiency, bone malignancy, herniated lumbar disk, and external venous compression.

Imaging Studies

Because the clinical signs of deep vein thrombosis are variable and nonspecific, objective evidence of thrombosis is required before committing the patient to a course of anticoagulant therapy. *Venography* has traditionally been the benchmark imaging study, and it is still the most accurate diagnostic modality. Unfortunately, this test is invasive, technically demanding, expensive, and painful, and it can induce thrombophlebitis. *Impedance plethysmography* (IPG) is a noninvasive test that detects changes in blood volume by measuring changes in electrical impedance (or resistance) of the tissues, which are produced by respiratory maneuvers or a pneumatic pressure cuff. The technique is used to detect decreased blood flow in the large veins of the thigh. It does not determine the cause of the reduced flow, nor is it useful in detecting obstruction in the small veins of the calf or thigh. *Venous ultrasonography (duplex ultrasonography)* has become the noninvasive method of choice, with reported sensitivities and specificities approaching 95 per cent. Duplex scanning combines real-time imaging with a pulsed and color-coded Doppler study that permits identification of the involved veins. A single duplex scan has a sensitivity of about 50 per cent for the detection of thrombi in calf veins and small thigh veins. If the initial scan is normal, however, a second study performed 7 days later can detect thrombi that have extended since the initial scan. Negative sequential duplex scans effectively exclude significant extension of thrombi to the proximal veins.

VENOUS DISEASE OF THE UPPER EXTREMITIES

Venous disease in the upper extremities is uncommon. It is now seen most often as a complication of vascular trauma induced by chronic indwelling venous catheterization and administration of chemotherapeutic drugs. Superficial phlebitis in the arm is self-limited and typically resolves without sequelae. Embolization is rare. Intravenous drug abuse predisposes to chemical as well as septic phlebitis and sepsis. Signs include localized swelling, erythema, and pain associated with fever and leukocytosis. Evidence of needle tracks and a history of drug abuse confirm the diagnosis.

Axillary or subclavian vein thrombosis presents as the sudden onset of edema, cyanosis, and collateral venous distention in the shoulder, arm, and deltoid region accompanied by pain in the axilla. It can be seen as a complication of chronic intravenous catheterization or as a sequela of mastectomy with or without localized radiotherapy. It also can occur in healthy, muscular individuals within 24 hours after strenuous exercise of the affected arm. Diagnostic imaging studies include venography and duplex ultrasonography, although the latter can be confusing because of the extensive collateral circulation around the shoulder. Deep vein thrombosis of the upper extremity can embolize and should be treated accordingly.

Section Six

BLOOD AND BLOOD-FORMING ORGANS

ANEMIAS CAUSED BY DECREASED ERYTHROCYTE PRODUCTION

By Munsey S. Wheby, M.D.,
and S. Kirk Payne, M.D.
Charlottesville, Virginia

An absolute decrease in the production of erythrocytes by the bone marrow characterizes the hypoproliferative anemias. As a consequence, an anemia develops accompanied by an inappropriately low reticulocyte count. The impaired marrow function may be due to a hematopoietic factor deficiency, inadequate stimulation by erythropoietin, intrinsic marrow defects, or extrinsic injury or infiltration of the marrow. Table 1 lists the anemias caused by decreased erythrocyte production.

ANEMIA OF RENAL INSUFFICIENCY

Anemia secondary to renal insufficiency primarily reflects inadequate erythroid production caused by inappropriately low erythropoietin production. Other factors that may contribute include blood loss, decreased red blood cell survival, and the toxic effects of uremia.

Pallor of mucous membranes, weakness, listlessness, fatigue, and easy bruising characterize chronic renal insufficiency.

Table 1. Differential Diagnosis of Anemias Caused by Decreased Erythrocyte Production

Decreased marrow erythroid stimulation
- Anemia of renal insufficiency
- Anemia associated with endocrinopathies
- Anemia of chronic disease

Primary marrow erythroid failure
- Pure red cell aplasia
- Hypoplastic anemia

Ineffective erythropoiesis
- Myelodysplastic syndromes
- Thalassemia trait*
- Megaloblastic anemia*
  - Folate deficiency
  - Vitamin B_{12} deficiency

Myelophthisic (marrow replacement) anemias
- Agnogenic myeloid metaplasia*
- Marrow infiltrative disorders (malignancy, infection, and so on)

*Iron deficiency anemia**

*Indicates topics discussed in other articles.

The anemia is usually normocytic and normochromic with a normal or slightly decreased reticulocyte count. Occasionally, acanthocytes, echinocytes, and schistocytes may be seen on the peripheral smear with normal leukocytes and platelets. Bone marrow examination typically shows normal myeloid and erythroid maturation. Erythropoietin concentrations are inappropriately low for the degree of anemia.

A microcytic anemia in the presence of renal insufficiency suggests the coexistence of either aluminum toxicity of the marrow secondary to antacids or dialysate, or iron deficiency anemia. Hyperparathyroidism with marrow fibrosis (osteitis fibrosa) further compromises marrow production of erythrocytes. Finally, chronic dialysis introduces the aggravating factor of blood loss and may result in folic acid deficiency because this vitamin is removed by dialysis.

A trial of recombinant erythropoietin, 50 to 100 U/kg given subcutaneously three times per week, should prompt a reticulocytosis followed by an increase in the hematocrit.

ANEMIAS SECONDARY TO ENDOCRINE ABNORMALITIES

Anemia may occur secondary to hypothyroidism, hyperthyroidism. hypogonadism. hypopituitarism, adrenal insufficiency, and hyperparathyroidism, illustrating the important role of hormones in the regulation of erythropoiesis. Although these anemias are usually mild, they may be the presenting sign of these disorders. Correction of the endocrine abnormality results in resolution of the anemia.

Anemia secondary to endocrine abnormalities is usually mild and therefore asymptomatic. Any abnormal signs or symptoms are usually attributable to the underlying endocrine disorder. The degree of anemia often correlates with the severity of the endocrinopathy.

Hematologic laboratory values are neither sensitive nor specific for these anemias, which are usually normocytic. The anemia of hypothyroidism is usually normocytic but may be macrocytic. When the anemia is macrocytic, a vitamin B_{12} deficiency must be ruled out with serum assay. Hypochromic microcytic indices with hypothyroidism may reflect iron deficiency anemia.

Decreased plasma volume may obscure the diagnosis of anemia in adrenal insufficiency, hypothyroidism, and hypopituitarism. Intercurrent iron or vitamin B_{12} deficiency (pernicious anemia) may contribute to the anemia of hypothyroidism.

ANEMIA OF CHRONIC DISEASE

Synonyms for anemia of chronic disease include anemia of chronic disorders, anemia of infection, anemia of malignancy, simple chronic anemia, anemia of defective iron utilization, and sideropenic anemia with reticuloendothelial siderosis.

Anemia of chronic disease occurs with chronic infections, inflammatory diseases, and malignancies. These conditions cause increased release of cytokines, particularly interleukin-1 and tumor necrosis factor. These cytokines bring about a decreased erythroid response to erythropoietin, which is present at inappropriately low concentrations for the degree of anemia. In addition, the supply of iron for erythropoiesis is limited by inadequate release of iron from reticuloendothelial cells. Treatment or control of the underlying illness ameliorates the anemia.

Because of the mildness of the anemia, symptoms and signs often reflect the underlying infectious, malignant, or inflammatory disease process. Rarely, the anemia may become severe enough to produce dyspnea, weakness, and pallor of mucous membranes, conjunctiva, and nail beds. The anemia usually becomes apparent after the first month of the underlying illness, and the degree of anemia may roughly correlate with the severity of the underlying disease process. The mild to moderate severity of the anemia rarely produces symptoms or requires intervention.

The anemia is usually normochromic and normocytic, but it may be microcytic in up to 25 per cent of patients. Although the reticulocyte percentage may be normal or slightly elevated, the absolute reticulocyte count is low, reflecting inadequate erythroid production. In 20 per cent of patients, the hematocrit may be less than 25 per cent. Decreased serum iron, decreased serum iron-binding capacity (transferrin), and decreased transferrin saturation, together with normal or increased serum ferritin, are hallmarks of this anemia. Although not required for the diagnosis, bone marrow aspirates demonstrate increased iron storage and decreased sideroblasts (erythroid precursors with visible iron granules). Coupled with decreased serum iron levels, these findings strongly support the diagnosis of anemia of chronic disease.

The characteristic serum iron pattern must be present to make the diagnosis of anemia of chronic disease. Any clinical clues suggesting other causes of the anemia must be investigated before accepting this diagnosis. Iron deficiency anemia may occur concurrently with anemia of chronic disease. Although a serum ferritin level greater than 60 μg/L makes iron deficiency unlikely, bone marrow aspirate staining for the presence of iron stores may be required to rule out iron deficiency.

PURE RED CELL APLASIA

Synonyms for pure red cell aplasia include erythroblastic hypoplasia, erythroblastopenia, erythroid hypoplasia, red cell agenesis, and chronic erythrocytic hypoplasia. Chronic hypoplastic anemia, Diamond-Blackfan anemia, and erythrogenesis imperfecta refer to congenital forms of the disorder.

Pure red cell aplasia may result from a transient or permanent depression of erythrocyte production. Transient red cell aplasia manifests itself clinically as an anemia only in those patients in whom the red cell life span is short because of a pre-existing hemolytic process such as sickle cell anemia or hereditary spherocytosis. Conditions associated with pure red cell aplasia include chronic lymphocytic leukemia, large granular lymphocyte syndrome, thymoma, autoimmune disorders including systemic lupus erythematosus and rheumatoid arthritis, exposure to drugs and toxins, and infections due to parvovirus B-19 and Epstein-Barr virus.

Presenting symptoms include weakness, fatigue, and shortness of breath, often following a mild febrile or upper respiratory tract infection. Pallor of the skin and mucous membranes is common. The liver and spleen are normal in size. Children with Diamond-Blackfan anemia may present with poor appetite, listlessness, congestive heart failure, hepatomegaly, and splenomegaly.

Resolution of the inciting infection or removal of the offending toxin usually results in correction of the anemia over several weeks or months. Chronic aplasia may undergo spontaneous remission or respond to immunosuppression with prednisone, antithymocyte globulin, or cyclosporine. Patients unresponsive to immunosuppression require multiple transfusions, which may lead to organ dysfunction secondary to iron overload. Progression to aplastic anemia and acute granulocytic leukemia occurs rarely.

Anemia is usually normochromic and normocytic with an absolute reticulocyte count less than 50,000 cells/μL (reticulocyte % × red blood cell). Platelet and leukocyte counts are usually normal. Bone marrow examination shows normal myeloid and megakaryocytic maturation with near absence of erythroblasts. Large pronormoblasts are frequently seen on marrow examination when parvovirus B-19 is involved. Other laboratory findings that may suggest the cause of the aplasia include rheumatoid factor, antinuclear antibody (ANA), parvovirus B-19 titers, and abnormal liver studies consistent with hepatitis.

Thymic enlargement in the anterior mediastinum may be seen on chest film or computed tomography (CT) scan. Thymectomy is recommended in patients with an enlarged thymic gland, as this may produce clinical improvement in up to one third of patients.

Maturation abnormalities of the bone marrow may occasionally present with dysplastic changes limited to the erythroid cell line.

MYELOPHTHISTIC ANEMIA

Infiltration of bone marrow by tumor cells, infectious processes, or granulomatous diseases can significantly impair hematopoiesis, thus producing a myelophthistic anemia. Metastases from lung, prostate, and breast cancer, as well as lymphoma, leukemia, and multiple myeloma may crowd out and replace normal marrow elements.

Along with the usual symptoms of anemia, including pallor, fatigue, and weakness, systemic signs and symptoms of the underlying disease process may include fever, weight loss, anorexia, and bone pain.

The peripheral smear often shows a leukoerythroblastic process characterized by nucleated red blood cells and immature myeloid cells. The anemia is usually normochromic and normocytic with poikilocytosis and occasional teardrop-shaped cells. Leukoerythroblastic findings should always be evaluated with a bone marrow biopsy and aspirate.

MYELODYSPLASTIC SYNDROMES

Myelodysplastic syndromes are a heterogeneous group of bone marrow disorders believed to result from neoplastic transformation at the earliest hematopoietic stem cell level. Thus, they are considered to be clonal disorders. Some cases follow radiation or chemotherapy, but most lack an identifiable cause. Marrow cytogenetic abnormalities are frequently associated with this syndrome, which is most often seen in the elderly.

Synonyms include refractory anemia, refractory anemia

with ringed sideroblasts, refractory anemia with excess blasts, refractory anemia with excess blasts in transformation, and chronic myelomonocytic leukemia. Other synonyms include smoldering leukemia, preleukemia, oligoblastic leukemia, and idiopathic refractory sideroblastic anemia.

Symptoms are related to the degree of anemia, with moderate to severe anemia causing pallor, weakness, and exertional dyspnea. Petechiae, ecchymoses, and infectious complications may complicate the decrease in platelets and neutrophils.

The anemia is usually macrocytic, but it may be normocytic with a peripheral smear showing anisocytosis, poikilocytosis, acanthocytosis, tear drops, basophilic stippling, and nucleated red blood cells. More than half of the patients have a decreased number of neutrophils, and one fourth have a mild to moderate thrombocytopenia. Neutrophils are often hyposegmented and hypogranulated with sticklike projections protruding from the nucleus. Platelets are often abnormally large and agranular. Bone marrow examination typically shows abnormal maturation of all cell lines. It is important to distinguish the myelodysplastic syndrome from megaloblastic anemia caused by folate or vitamin B_{12} deficiency.

PERNICIOUS ANEMIA AND OTHER MEGALOBLASTIC ANEMIAS

By Rajiv K. Pruthi, M.D.,
and Ayalew Tefferi, M.D.
Rochester, Minnesota

Megaloblastic anemias result from various disorders that have in common macrocytosis of the erythroid lineage. With increasing use of automated cell counters, increased mean corpuscular volume (MCV) is frequently the first clue to the presence of macrocytosis. The normal range of the MCV of erythrocytes varies slightly among laboratories; however, an MCV of 100 fL or more generally establishes the presence of macrocytosis. Review of a peripheral blood smear is essential in evaluating an increased MCV to determine the morphology of the macrocytes (Table 1) and to exclude spurious causes of macrocytosis. Mild degrees of macrocytosis may be overlooked by even an experienced observer. However, if an increased MCV is found on a hematologic profile, the cause should be determined because macrocytosis per se is not a diagnosis, and, more important, it may be the harbinger of a treatable disorder, such as pernicious anemia (PA), or an ominous disease, such as one of the dysmyelopoietic syndromes. The differential diagnosis of macrocytosis is outlined in Table 1.

The most common causes of macrocytosis are the megaloblastic anemias, which are typically caused by altered cobalamin (Cbl) and folate metabolism. The use of cytotoxic chemotherapeutic agents for malignant and nonmalignant conditions may also cause megaloblastosis. The causes of megaloblastic anemias are outlined in Table 1. Megaloblastic hematopoiesis is partly the result of impaired DNA synthesis, which leads to maturation arrest in the development of the nucleus. This arrested development produces characteristic morphologic changes that are not restricted to the hematologic elements but to all rapidly dividing cells in the body. Impaired DNA synthesis results from perturbation of enzymatic DNA repair or synthetic pathways. Decreased enzyme activity may be caused by either a deficiency or an inhibition of the activity of a cofactor. The latter mechanism is exploited in cancer chemotherapy. Two of the cofactors required for DNA synthesis are Cbl and folate. Knowledge of Cbl and folate metabolism and their interrelationship is essential to understanding the mechanisms of megaloblastic anemia and forming a rational diagnostic approach to these disorders.

Table 1. Differential Diagnosis of Macrocytosis

Spurious
Hyperglycemia
Cold agglutinins
Hyperleukocytosis
Regenerative
Reticulocytosis
Physiologic
Pregnancy
Fetal and neonatal
Megaloblastic
Vitamin B_{12} deficiency (oval macrocytosis)
Folate deficiency (oval macrocytosis)
Drug-induced (oval macrocytosis)
Congenital disorders
Dysmyelopoietic syndromes (oval macrocytosis)
Nonmegaloblastic
Liver disorders (round macrocytosis)
Alcohol effect (round macrocytosis)
Hypothyroidism (round macrocytosis)

COBALAMIN METABOLISM

Vitamin B_{12}, a corrinoid, consists of a corrin nucleus (four reduced pyrrole rings linked in a planar configuration) with a central cobalt atom. The addition of various ligands above and below the plane of the nucleus produces different compounds such as the cobalamins (Cbls), which have in common a 5,6-dimethylbenzimidazole group below the plane of the nucleus. The addition of various anionic group ligands, such as cyanide (CN), methyl (Me), adenosyl (Ado), and hydroxyl (OH), above the plane of the nucleus results in the formation of cyano-Cbl (CN-Cbl), methyl-Cbl (Me-Cbl), adenosyl-Cbl (Ado-Cbl), and hydroxyl-Cbl (OH-Cbl), respectively.

Although Cbl and its analogues are synthesized by the natural flora of the large bowel, they are not absorbed; thus, animal products such as meat (OH-Cbl, Ado-Cbl) and dairy products (OH-Cbl, Me-Cbl) are the primary dietary sources of Cbl for humans. The daily requirement is 1 μg, and a typical diet in the Western Hemisphere provides 5 to 15 μg daily. After ingestion, the protein-bound Cbls are broken down in the acidic gastric environment and preferentially bind to R proteins rather than to intrinsic factor (IF). The R proteins, so-named because of their rapid movement on electrophoresis, occur in saliva and gastric juice. The holo-R protein (Cbl–R protein complex) and the apo-R protein (unbound R protein) pass into the duodenum. Intrinsic factor is a glycoprotein produced by the gastric parietal cells. Of the volume secreted daily, only 20 per cent is needed for absorption of the daily requirement of vitamin B_{12}. In the second part of the duodenum, pancreatic proteases degrade the R proteins and release the Cbl, allowing it to bind to IF. The Cbl-IF complex moves into the terminal ileum, where about 70 per cent of the ingested Cbl is absorbed in the presence of IF. In the absence of IF, less than 2 per cent of the ingested Cbl is absorbed. At the ileal mucosal surface, the receptor for the Cbl-IF complex facilitates its transport into enterocytes, where the complex is dissociated and Cbl is released. The vitamin then is transported into the portal circulation, where it binds with transcobalamin II (TCII), the most important transport protein. At the sites of its use, the TCII-Cbl complex is taken up into cells through receptor-mediated endocytosis. The complex is dissociated intracellularly, and Cbl is transformed to its active coenzyme forms, namely Me-Cbl and Ado-Cbl (see below).

FOLATE METABOLISM

Folic acid (pteroylglutamic acid [PGA]) consists of a pteridine moiety linked to a para-aminobenzoic acid residue attached to the glutamate side chain. Unlike the case with Cbl, the dietary sources of folate include both animal products and leafy vegetables, where folate exists as polyglutamates (PGA_n); the synthetic vitamin is a monoglutamate (PGA_1). The adult daily requirement of folate is about 200 μg, but the recommended amount increases during pregnancy and lactation.

The glutamate side chains of the ingested folyl polyglutamates are hydrolyzed at the surface of the jejunal brush border by folate hydrolase (a deconjugase) to the monoglutamate form (PGA_1), which is required for transport across cell membranes. Within the enterocytes, PGA_1 is again polyglutamated to its active coenzyme forms. The resynthesis of polyglutamates helps maintain a concentration gradient for the uptake of monoglutamates. Before release into the portal circulation, the folyl polyglutamates are reduced to monoglutamates and methylated to form methyltetrahydrofolate ($MeTHF_1$). No specific transport protein has been isolated. At the sites of its use, folate interacts with folate receptors prior to cell entry.

INTRACELLULAR COFACTOR ACTIVITIES OF COBALAMIN AND FOLATE

The target cell (e.g., an erythrocyte precursor) is provided with $MeTHF_1$ and a Cbl derivative. Coparticipation of these two compounds in intermediary metabolic pathways leads to effective DNA synthesis. Although these pathways have not been characterized precisely, available data provide a framework within which reasonable postulates can be constructed and discussed.

The primary intracellular function of folate analogues is to transfer one-carbon (1-C) units, in the form of methyl ($-CH_3$), methylene ($-CH_2-$), or formyl (HCO) groups, to facilitate DNA synthesis. To act as coenzymes, the folate analogues must exist in both a reduced and a polyglutamated form (THF_n).

The primary function of Cbl is to act as a coenzyme for the synthesis of methionine and succinyl coenzyme A (CoA). For this function, the Cbl derivatives must be converted to Me-Cbl or to Ado-Cbl, and the Cbl molecule must exist in a reduced state for optimal enzyme binding.

In DNA synthesis, the formation of methionine is a key reaction. Both Cbl and folate are required for this reaction to occur. Me-Cbl is the cofactor for methionine synthase, which methylates homocysteine to methionine. The original methyl donor for the reaction is Me-THF, in either the monoglutamate form ($Me\text{-}THF_1$, obtained primarily from the diet) or the polyglutamate form ($Me\text{-}THF_n$, obtained primarily from intracellular recycling of folate intermediates). The methyl group is first transferred from Me-THF to the enzyme-bound Cbl to form Me-Cbl, which then transfers the methyl group to homocysteine to generate methionine. This central reaction provides two products essential for DNA synthesis: THF_n for 1-C unit transport and methionine, which some believe may facilitate availability of the appropriate folate intermediary in the process.

DIAGNOSIS OF COBALAMIN DEFICIENCY

The pursuit of suspected Cbl deficiency begins with a review of the hematologic indices of the patient and a peripheral blood smear. With progressive Cbl deficiency, there is often worsening macrocytosis and, eventually, anemia. Of 100 consecutive patients with confirmed Cbl deficiency, 64 per cent had an MCV of more than 100 fL. Hence, a substantial proportion of cases of Cbl deficiency will not be detected if the sole criterion is the MCV value. Even with a normal MCV, further testing should proceed if clinically indicated. Conversely, 17 per cent of patients had an MCV of less than 90 fL. The presence of concomitant conditions that predispose to microcytosis, such as iron deficiency, thalassemia trait, and anemia associated with chronic inflammation, results in a falsely normal MCV. Thus, peripheral blood smears should be examined for the presence of microcytosis.

Anemia is not consistently present when Cbl deficiency is first detected. In the 100 patients mentioned above, the median concentration of hemoglobin was 13 g/dL (range, 4 to 17 g/dL), and only 29 per cent of the patients had a concentration less than 12 g/dL. The hemoglobin concentration and the MCV may be normal despite the presence of neurologic manifestations of Cbl deficiency. Occasionally, leukopenia and thrombocytopenia are observed. More consistently, an increased red blood cell distribution width and an increased number of hypersegmented neutrophils may be seen. Because of ineffective erythropoiesis, indirect hyperbilirubinemia and increased lactate dehydrogenase may be detected. In the plasma, approximately 20 per cent of Cbl is bound to TCII, which has a half-life of 6 to 9 minutes in the circulation. The remainder of the Cbl is bound to TCI and TCIII (R binders); the R binder–bound Cbl has a slow turnover. Traditionally, serum concentrations of Cbl were measured with microbiologic assays in which the microorganisms were fastidious for the corrinoids in the growth media. The amount of Cbl present in serum was determined by comparing a standard bacterial growth curve prepared with a known concentration of Cbl with a curve prepared with the unknown sample. This method was laborious and inaccurate; however, it was quite specific, because Cbl analogues would not support the growth of these organisms.

Later assays for serum Cbl concentrations were based on competitive inhibition (by serum Cbl) of the binding between radiolabeled Cbl and Cbl-binding proteins. The first generation of assay methods were even more inaccurate than microbial methods, because binding proteins in the commercial kits contained R proteins, which can bind Cbl analogues other than cyano-Cbl, yielding falsely normal values. With the introduction of purified IF radioisotope dilution assay kits, more reliable results were obtained. Nonisotopic methods have been developed, but their use is not widespread.

Despite the development of generally accurate assay methods for Cbl, serum concentrations may nevertheless be falsely low, as in late pregnancy, multiple myeloma, folate deficiency, and TCI deficiency and in patients taking high doses of ascorbic acid. The presence of other radioisotopes (e.g., gallium administered for scanning) interferes with the assay (just as the presence of antibiotics interfered with the microbiologic assay systems). The release of Cbl binders in the myeloproliferative diseases and liver disease leads to falsely increased serum concentrations of Cbl. Importantly, a subset of patients have clinical evidence of Cbl deficiency but normal serum concentrations of Cbl.

To overcome these pitfalls in the diagnosis of Cbl deficiency, assays based on the intermediary metabolism of Cbl and folate have been developed. Cobalamin is essential in the (folate-dependent) conversion of homocysteine to methionine and the (folate-independent) conversion of methylmalonyl CoA (MMA) to succinyl CoA. Therefore, Cbl deficiency results in the accumulation of both homocysteine and MMA, whereas folate deficiency results in the accumulation of only homocysteine. Thus, increased urinary concentrations of MMA more accurately reflect Cbl deficiency and are not invalidated by the presence of heterozygous methylmalonicacidemia. In one series of patients, 40 per cent had increased urinary MMA but normal serum Cbl; however, on follow-up evaluation, they had clinical or laboratory evidence of Cbl deficiency. Thus, normal serum concentrations of Cbl do not rule out Cbl deficiency.

Subsequent refinement of assay systems for serum MMA and homocysteine not only have increased the sensitivity and specificity for detecting Cbl deficiency but also have helped in the early diagnosis of Cbl deficiency, despite normal serum concentrations of Cbl. Of the patients with Cbl deficiency, 95 per cent have increased serum MMA and homocysteine. In comparison, fewer than 2 per cent of patients with folate deficiency have increased serum MMA. In contrast, only 60 to 70 per cent of patients with Cbl deficiency have decreased serum Cbl. The MMA concentrations may be falsely increased by renal failure, dehydration, or gut floral metabolism. In general, serum values of MMA seem to be more sensitive than those for homocysteine in the diagnosis of Cbl deficiency. However, the sensitivity is increased by measuring the concentrations of both compounds.

The most important transport protein, TCII binds about 20 per cent of serum Cbl. Unlike TCI and TCIII, TCII normally does not bind Cbl analogues. With the progression of Cbl deficiency, Cbl-bound TCII (holo-TCII) in the serum progressively decreases and is the earliest indicator of Cbl deficiency in patients with acquired immunodeficiency syndrome (AIDS).

The deoxyuridine suppressant test, which measures the uptake of tritium-labeled thymidine, estimates the ability of bone marrow cells to convert deoxyuridine to deoxythymidine using the 1-C unit from 5,10-methylenetetrahydrofolate. Deficiency of either folate or Cbl increases the uptake of the labeled thymidine, which is corrected by the addition of the deficient element. This laborious test is not cost-effective for routine clinical use.

CAUSES OF COBALAMIN DEFICIENCY

Gastric Defects

Pernicious Anemia

Currently, PA is considered the most common disorder involving vitamin B_{12} deficiency. The clinical manifestations are attributed to a deficiency of Cbl. Because intracellular Cbl is required for effective DNA synthesis, PA affects tissues with rapid turnover of cells, especially the bone marrow and the mucosa of the intestinal and genitourinary tracts. Through the years, the clinical features of PA have been tempered by increased clinical acumen and early diagnosis of the disorder. Initially, patients with PA may report wide-ranging symptoms that reflect involvement of various organ systems, or they may be entirely asymptomatic and referred for assessment of macrocytosis detected with an automated cell counter. Symptoms may be due to the anemia per se or to other manifestations of Cbl deficiency. In general, lassitude and fatigue are the dominant complaints. Cardiopulmonary signs and symptoms include dyspnea on exertion, palpitation, angina, and heart failure (in severe cases). These symptoms often depend on the rapidity of onset and the severity of the anemia. Occasionally, patients may be entirely asymptomatic and still have severe anemia, reflecting the insidious development of the disorder.

Skin changes include premature gray or white hair, a sallow appearance of the skin, and frank jaundice, depending on the degree of ineffective intramedullary erythropoiesis. Vitiligo may occur. Glossitis may present as a painful, red, beefy tongue devoid of papillae or, more commonly, as a pale, smooth, clean-appearing tongue with loss of papillae on the lateral and superior surfaces. Anorexia may be attributed to glossitis, to intrinsic gastric disorders, or to anemia and heart failure. Malabsorption and episodic diarrhea may result from megaloblastic changes in the epithelium of the gastrointestinal tract. Atrophy of the gastric parietal cells causes decreased secretion of IF and hydrochloric acid. Infiltration of the mucosa with lymphocytes implies a possible immune basis for the pathogenesis of PA.

About 40 per cent of patients with Cbl deficiency have neurologic symptoms. The most common symptom is paresthesia or numbness (or both). Of these patients, about one fifth have unremarkable neurologic examinations. Other symptoms include gait disturbance, memory deficits, and, occasionally, psychosis. Conversely, of the patients with abnormal findings on neurologic examination, about 30 per cent have no neurologic symptoms. The most common neurologic sign is impaired proprioception and vibratory sensation, with loss of perception of higher frequency vibration (256 Hz) before that of lower frequency vibration (128 Hz). Also seen are loss of deep tendon reflexes, long-tract signs, limb weakness, spasticity, and altered mental status. The underlying pathologic changes include demyelination and axonal destruction in the posterior and lateral columns of the spinal cord (subacute combined degeneration). The frequency of neuropathy is influenced by early diagnosis and the specialty interest of the referral center.

The results of neurologic tests are nonspecific and include decreased conduction velocity and, occasionally, evidence of axonal damage. In about 10 to 15 per cent of patients with neurologic findings, anemia and macrocytosis are not detected. However, the bone marrow almost always shows megaloblastic changes.

Diagnosis of Pernicious Anemia

Between 31 and 76 per cent of patients with PA have type I IF antibodies in their serum. These antibodies block the binding of Cbl to IF, while type II antibodies react with ileal IF receptors. Both types of antibodies may be found in gastric secretions and in urine. The presence of IF antibody is a fairly specific indication of PA; however, testing for this antibody lacks sensitivity because 40 per cent of PA patients do not have detectable antibody. In addition, IF antibody may be found in patients with Graves' disease and atrophic gastritis. Conversely, as many as 90 per cent of patients with PA have parietal cell antibodies, which are less specific than IF antibodies.

The Schilling test measures the absorption of orally ingested radiolabeled crystalline cyano-Cbl (1 μg) without (stage I) and with (stage II) IF. The radiolabeled Cbl is administered orally before or with the flushing parenteral dose of nonradioactive vitamin B_{12} (1 mg), and a complete 24-hour urine specimen is collected to measure the excreted radiolabeled Cbl, which should be 7 per cent or less of the ingested dose. Administration of IF (stage II) with radiolabeled Cbl should result in correction of the malabsorption and excretion of more than 7 per cent of the ingested dose. This test reveals the mechanism of Cbl deficiency but provides no information about the Cbl status of the patient.

The physician should exercise caution in interpreting the results of the Schilling test. The patient with PA always has an abnormal stage I result, and for the same patient, a normal stage II result typically confirms the diagnosis. By contrast, decreased excretion of radiolabeled Cbl at both stages suggests malabsorption not related to IF. However, spuriously abnormal stage I results may occur because of incomplete urine collection or the presence of renal insufficiency (inadequate renal excretion rather than malabsorption). Occasionally, a spuriously low urinary excretion during stage II Schilling testing in patients with PA may result during the acute stage of the disease due to intestinal malabsorption attributed to megaloblastoid epithelial changes. The advantages of the Schilling test are that the results are independent of the Cbl status of the patient and that the test can be performed even after treatment, which may be imperative in patients with neurologic symptoms.

Importantly, a normal stage I result and a low serum concentration of Cbl do not exclude malabsorption of Cbl. The radioactive Cbl used as the oral dose in the Schilling test is the unbound crystalline variant, and hypochlorhydric patients may have malabsorption of food-bound Cbl due to inadequate dissociation of the Cbl from protein. This problem is overcome by performing the egg yolk Cbl absorption test, in which the radioactive Cbl used as the oral dose is bound to egg yolk; the test is performed in the same manner as the Schilling test.

The chief cells in the gastric fundal mucosa produce two immunologically distinct groups of pepsinogens (PG): PG I and PG II (PG II is also produced by the glands in the pyloric mucosa and Brunner's glands in the proximal duodenum). The serum concentrations of PG I are higher than those of PG II despite the apparent greater cell mass responsible for the secretion of PG II. Serum PG is decreased in patients with gastric atrophy. In patients with PA, low serum PG I and a PG I–to–PG II ratio of less than 3 were found in 92 per cent and 82 per cent of patients, respectively. At least one of these abnormalities was present in 97 per cent of the patients. The reversal of the PG I–to–PG II ratio can be explained by the origins of the enzymes and the characteristic histopathology in patients with PA, including atrophy of the fundic gland mucosa, preservation of the pyloric gland mucosa, and extensive pyloric gland metaplasia of the proximal stomach. In screening studies of relatives of patients with PA, serum PG I concentration is predictive of atrophic gastritis. Serum concentrations of gastrin, which may be increased in 62 to 95 per cent of patients with PA, are not commonly used to aid diagnosis.

Gastrectomy

Due to the minute daily requirements, large liver stores, and enterohepatic circulation of Cbl, it takes 3 to 5 years for Cbl deficiency to develop after gastrectomy.

However, with lifelong administration of Cbl after gastrectomy, Cbl deficiency rarely occurs. In fact, folate deficiency is probably more common after gastrectomy. Due to concomitant malabsorption of iron, an increased MCV may not be observed. Although stage I of the Schilling test will be abnormal and corrected with IF, the test need not be performed after gastrectomy.

Hypochlorhydria

As mentioned earlier, some hypochlorhydric patients with low serum Cbl have a normal Schilling test (stage I). The inability to dissociate food-bound Cbl results in malabsorption of Cbl. Yet, the crystalline Cbl used in the Schilling test is normally absorbed. The egg yolk Cbl test should aid in the diagnosis.

Zollinger-Ellison Syndrome

In the Zollinger-Ellison syndrome, excessive gastrin production causes increased gastric acid secretion. The acidic environment of the duodenum does not facilitate neutralization of gastric acid by pancreatic secretions; thus, Cbl cannot dissociate from the R proteins for transfer to IF. Patients typically have long-standing symptoms that suggest peptic ulcer disease. Measurement of gastric acidity and serum gastrin can lead to the diagnosis, which should be confirmed with the appropriate imaging study (e.g., computed tomographic scan of the abdomen).

Intestinal Defects

Intestinal defects that may lead to Cbl malabsorption are outlined in Table 2. Removal of the terminal part of the ileum leads to Cbl malabsorption. Thus, the extent of any bowel resection should be well documented. Overgrowth of bacteria in a blind loop (due to stricture, diver-

Table 2. Etiology of Cobalamin Deficiency

Defects in Intake
- Strict vegetarians

Defects in Absorption
- Gastric
  - Intrinsic factor deficiency (pernicious anemia)
  - Gastrectomy or bypass
  - Achlorhydria
  - Zollinger-Ellison syndrome
- Intestinal
  - Ileal resection
  - Inflammatory bowel disease
  - Fish tapeworm
  - Blind loop
  - Megaloblastic changes in epithelium
  - Tropical sprue
- Pancreatic insufficiency
- Drugs

Congenital Defects
- Defects in absorption
  - Intrinsic factor
  - Imerslund-Graesback syndrome
- Defects in transport
  - Transcobalamin II deficiency
- Defects in cellular metabolism
  - Defects in coenyzme synthesis

ticula, surgical blind loop, or amyloidosis) results in Cbl malabsorption. Barium studies of the small intestine may suggest bacterial overgrowth, but culture of microorganisms from a small bowel aspirate is required for confirmation. In regional ileitis, especially when it involves the terminal ileum, the Cbl-IF complex is not adequately absorbed. Exogenous IF in the Schilling test does not correct the Cbl malabsorption. Barium small intestinal series can lead to the correct diagnosis. Rarely, a history of travel to an area endemic for the fish tapeworm *(Diphyllobothrium latum)* is elicited; endoscopic biopsy is necessary to confirm the diagnosis. Megaloblastic transformation of the intestinal epithelium may perpetuate Cbl deficiency due to malabsorption; this malabsorption, in turn, may lead to malabsorption of other nutrients, such as folate. Tropical sprue usually results in combined malabsorption of folate and Cbl. The xylose absorption test is typically abnormal, barium studies reveal thickened mucosa and flocculation of the barium, and intestinal biopsy shows villous atrophy.

Pancreatic Defects

Patients with chronic exocrine pancreatic insufficiency lack pancreatic proteases and are unable to dissociate the Cbl from R binders; thus, the Cbl-IF complex does not form and Cbl malabsorption occurs in as many as 40 per cent of patients. However, Cbl malabsorption rarely causes overt megaloblastic anemia. The results of the Schilling test (stages I and II) are typically abnormal. The defect is corrected with administration of pancreatic enzyme preparations.

Drugs

Mild Cbl malabsorption has been described in patients treated with para-aminosalicylic acid for tuberculosis. The defect is corrected by stopping the drug. Other agents implicated in Cbl malabsorption are colchicine, neomycin, and ethanol. Prolonged inhalation of nitrous oxide, as in patients with tetanus, may cause megaloblastic anemia. Nitrous oxide converts cob(I)alamin to cob(II)alamin, thereby inactivating methionine synthetase, which requires cob(I)alamin for optimal activity. Demethylation of folate is inhibited, leading to functional folate deficiency.

Congenital Defects

Congenital defects in Cbl metabolism are rare but well documented. Clinicians should also ensure that mothers are not supplying Cbl-deficient breast milk to their infants.

Defects in Absorption

Children with IF abnormalities have delayed developmental milestones and manifestations of PA. Serum concentrations of Cbl are low, but antibodies to IF are absent and the gastric mucosa is histologically unremarkable. Addition of IF to the diet corrects the defect, which may be the absence of IF or the presence of a nonfunctional IF.

Patients with Imerslund-Graesback syndrome have features of PA with normal gastrointestinal function and normal IF. These patients have a specific defect in the absorption of the Cbl-IF complex, and they may have proteinuria.

Defects in Transport

Deficiency of TCII can be distinguished from absorptive defects because the former typically presents in the first few months of life with failure to thrive and other manifestations of Cbl deficiency. Serum Cbl is often within the reference range because most serum Cbl is carried by TCI and R binders. Serum MMA is increased in some but not all patients, indicating the presence of an alternative pathway of Cbl metabolism.

Defects in Cellular Metabolism

These disorders involve deficient synthesis of the metabolically important coenzyme forms of Cbl (Ado-Cbl, Me-Cbl). The defects appear in the first few months of life and are clinically severe. The patients have increased serum MMA and homocysteine, at concentrations exceeding those found in the aforementioned congenital disorders.

DIAGNOSIS OF FOLATE DEFICIENCY

The microbiologic methods for measuring serum folate have the same problems as those for measuring Cbl. Over the years, these methods have been largely replaced by radioisotopic dilution assays. In a folate-deficient patient, the serum folate can be falsely increased if blood is sampled soon after a meal containing adequate folic acid. Other causes of falsely increased concentrations include hemolysis and Cbl deficiency. Conversely, low serum folate with no evidence of megaloblastosis is seen in pregnancy, in anorexia, and in patients taking anticonvulsant medications. Because serum folate concentration is exquisitely dependent on dietary folate, assay for red blood cell folate is a more reliable indicator of folate deficiency. In the presence of Cbl deficiency, however, excess intracellular folate, which is not used, leaks out of the cell, producing low red blood cell folate and increased serum concentrations of folate.

Formiminoglutamic acid (FIGLU) is an intermediate in the conversion of histidine to glutamate, which requires the transfer of the formimino group from FIGLU to tetrahydrofolate. This transfer forms the basis of the FIGLU excretion test, in which an oral dose (15 g) of histidine is administered, urine is collected for 8 hours, and the concentrations of FIGLU (normal, 1 to 17 mg) are measured. The sensitivity and specificity of the test are not ideal. In patients with folate deficiency, FIGLU excretion usually is not increased until a load of histidine is administered. However, 25 to 50 per cent of hospitalized patients have increased excretion of FIGLU. Other conditions in which FIGLU excretion is increased include congestive heart failure, hemolytic anemia, Hodgkin's disease, and other tumors. The administration of the histidine load itself has potentially serious consequences in patients with liver impairment and may precipitate coma. Increased concentrations of FIGLU in the urine are not always correlated with depleted tissue stores, and most patients with Cbl deficiency have increased amounts of FIGLU (these amounts may not be as high as in folate deficiency).

A more reliable means for assessing folate deficiency is the measurement of serum MMA and homocysteine. Although folate-deficient patients have increased serum homocysteine, fewer than 2 per cent have increased serum MMA. The deoxyuridine suppression test is seldom employed.

CAUSES OF FOLATE DEFICIENCY

The cause of folate deficiency is often apparent from a detailed dietary history. The most common cause is poor nutritional intake, typically associated with excess alcohol

Table 3. Etiology of Folate Deficiency

Inadequate intake
Increased requirement
  Pregnancy and lactation
  Infancy
  Hemolytic anemias
  Exfoliative dermatitis
Malabsorption
  Inflammatory bowel disease
  Tropical or nontropical sprue
Congenital
  Hereditary malabsorption of folate

consumption (Table 3). In contrast with Cbl, folate reserves in the liver last only 3 to 4 months. Thus, with inadequate intake, folate deficiency occurs relatively more rapidly than Cbl deficiency. Elderly persons who live alone and do not prepare nutritious meals for themselves, and patients with psychiatric illness are at risk for folate deficiency.

In pregnancy, chronic hemolysis, and exfoliative dermatitis, the increased demand for folate may not be met, especially in less developed parts of the world. Pregnancy is a particular clinical challenge because the serum concentrations of folate normally decrease and physiologic macrocytosis and dilutional anemia typically develop following changes in the intravascular volume. In view of these difficulties, and because folate administration most likely decreases the incidence of neural tube defects, the diet of pregnant women should be routinely supplemented with folic acid.

Celiac sprue (nontropical sprue) can lead to severe malabsorption of folate. Small bowel biopsy often confirms the diagnosis, and restriction to a gluten-free diet improves absorption. Regional ileitis can cause malabsorption of folate, as with Cbl.

DRUGS THAT CAUSE MEGALOBLASTIC ANEMIA

Chemotherapeutic agents have an expanded role in the treatment of malignant and nonmalignant conditions. Not surprisingly, the incidence of drug-induced megaloblastic hematopoiesis is clinically significant. Methotrexate and aminopterin block dihydrofolate reductase, causing megaloblastic anemia. Other antifolates include pyrimethamine, trimethoprim, and sulfasalazine. Hydroxyurea induces reversible megaloblastosis within a few days of initiating treatment. Other agents that cause megaloblastosis include 5-fluorouracil, 6-mercaptopurine, 6-thioguanine, and cytarabine (cytosine arabinoside).

Anticonvulsants (phenytoin, phenobarbital) occasionally cause megaloblastosis in association with low serum folate, but the mechanism remains unknown.

CONGENITAL DISORDERS THAT CAUSE MEGALOBLASTIC ANEMIA

Hereditary Oroticaciduria

Hereditary oroticaciduria, an inherited defect in pyrimidine metabolism, causes megaloblastic anemia and orotic acid crystalluria.

Lesch-Nyhan Syndrome

Lesch-Nyhan syndrome results from a deficiency in purine metabolism. The disorder is characterized by hyperuricemia, choreoathetosis, spasticity, mental retardation, and self-mutilation.

Thiamine-Responsive Megaloblastic Anemia

Although the pathophysiology of this condition is not known, patients have severe megaloblastic anemia, sensorineural deafness, and diabetes mellitus.

IRON DEFICIENCY ANEMIA

By Malcolm L. Brigden, M.D.
Victoria, British Columbia, Canada

Synonyms for iron deficiency anemia include iron lack anemia and anemia of chronic blood loss. Iron deficiency is not necessarily synonymous with iron deficiency anemia. The symptoms associated with iron deficiency may occur in the absence of anemia in the early stages of iron deficiency and may also be present in patients who are truly anemic secondary to advanced iron deficiency.

DEFINITION AND PREVALENCE

The definition of iron deficiency anemia is quantitative. It is based on a reduction of the hemoglobin concentration in grams per deciliter secondary to a lack of iron for erythropoiesis to at least two standard deviations below the mean adjusted for age, sex, and altitude of residence. Normal hemoglobin values increase in proportion to the elevation above sea level and also in cigarette smokers. For women of childbearing age, normal hemoglobin values are 10 per cent lower than those in men.

Frank iron deficiency anemia represents the last stage in the progression of iron deficiency. The progression of iron deficiency can be divided into three stages, each of which can be identified by laboratory testing. In the first stage, which is characterized by depletion of iron stores, stainable iron is absent from the bone marrow and the serum ferritin concentration is low. The second phase is known as iron-deficient erythropoiesis or iron deficiency without anemia. In this phase, in addition to the absence of stainable marrow iron and decreased serum ferritin concentrations, the serum iron is decreased and the total iron-binding capacity (TIBC) is increased (such that the per cent transferrin saturation as calculated by dividing the serum iron by the TIBC is usually decreased to less than 15 per cent) and free erythrocyte protoporphyrin is high. In the third phase, which is iron deficiency with anemia, anisocytosis is the earliest recognized morphologic change. As the iron deficiency progresses further, there is often a mild normochromic anemia with hemoglobin concentrations less than 11 g/dL and microcytosis so that the mean corpuscular volume (MCV) is less than 80 fL. At this point, the red cell distribution width (RDW), which is an index of red cell variability in size, starts to increase. With further evolution, hemoglobin concentration, erythrocyte count, MCV, and mean erythrocyte hemoglobin concentration all decline together. Lastly, hypochromia may be noted on stained blood films. It is important to realize that hypochromia is the last evolutionary change seen,

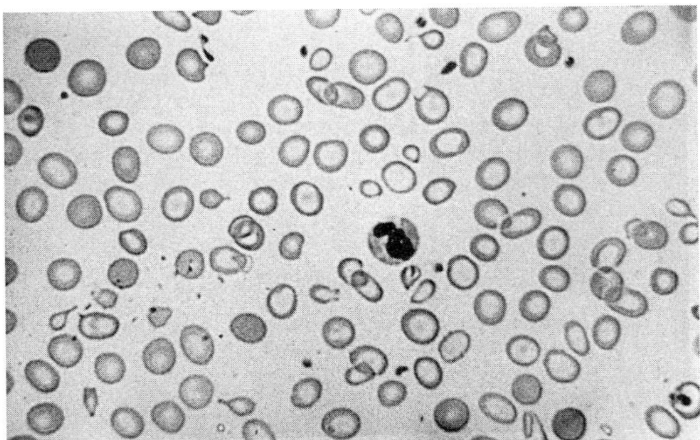

Figure 1. The classic appearance of microcytosis, anisocytosis, and hypochromia on peripheral blood smear. It is important to realize that hypochromia is a relatively late finding in iron deficiency.

appearing only after anisocytosis and microcytosis. Even the most skilled morphologists may experience difficulty in reliably recognizing hypochromia until the hemoglobin concentration decreases to less than the 8 to 9 g/dL range (Fig. 1).

Iron deficiency is widespread throughout the world, affecting persons of all ages and economic groups. Data from the World Health Organization show that worldwide, approximately 43 per cent of preschool children, 37 per cent of school-aged children, and 51 per cent of pregnant women are anemic, with iron deficiency by far being the most common cause. In parts of the world where there is a high frequency of intestinal parasitemia and the population subsists on an iron-poor diet, iron deficiency anemia may be the norm. Iron deficiency anemia is more common in the very young, in adolescents (especially during the growth spurt), in women between menarche and menopause (particularly those who are pregnant or have a history of menorrhagia), and in those with poor diets. Even in a developed country like the United States, iron deficiency has a high prevalence. The United States National Health and Nutrition Examination Survey (NHANES II) found that 5.7 per cent of infants, 5.9 per cent of teenage girls, 5.8 per cent of young women, and 4.4 per cent of elderly men could be classified as anemic (hemoglobin less than 95 per cent reference range for sex and age). Iron deficiency anemia was documented in 0.2 per cent of men, 2.6 per cent of premenopausal women, and 1.9 per cent of postmenopausal women. Iron deficiency, and to a lesser extent iron deficiency anemia, is being recognized more commonly in endurance athletes. As many as 82 per cent of female and 29 per cent of male elite Canadian distance runners had a low serum ferritin level (less than 25 ng/mL). Overt iron deficiency was found in 3 to 7 per cent of endurance runners.

ETIOLOGY

The average North American diet is well fortified with iron, and in the absence of unusual iron losses, dietary iron deficiency is uncommon. Iron availability in food is determined by whether dietary iron is present in the heme form in meat, fish, or poultry or as elemental iron. Much dietary iron is in the elemental form in plants, dairy products, and other non–heme-containing proteins. Heme iron is efficiently absorbed (15 to 35 per cent), with the avidity of absorption inversely proportional to body iron stores. Although the majority of dietary nonheme iron is less efficiently absorbed, (2 to 20 per cent), the presence of ascorbic acid in the diet can facilitate the absorption of nonheme iron by aiding the conversion of ferric iron to the ferrous form. Grains, cereals, and corn contain phytates and neutral detergent fibers that may form insoluble complexes with iron, inhibiting absorption. Tea is known to contain tannin and other substances that may block inorganic iron absorption. Calcium supplements such as those prescribed for the prevention of osteoporosis may retard iron absorption by as much as 50 per cent, so such therapy should always be taken at an alternative time when oral iron supplements are also consumed.

Iron is absorbed primarily in the duodenum where the stomach's acidity facilitates reduction of iron from the ferric form to the better absorbed ferrous form. Thus, nonheme iron is poorly absorbed if achlorhydria is present secondary to chronic gastritis, prior gastric surgery, or the use of drugs such as cimetidine or omeprazole, which inhibit the production of hydrochloric acid by the stomach. The dilemma of trying to treat concomitant peptic ulcer and iron deficiency anemia may be resolved by using cimetidine in low dosage (i.e., 400 mg at bedtime) or, alternatively, it may be necessary to treat the peptic ulcer first and the iron deficiency after the ulcer has healed or become asymptomatic. Malabsorption of iron rarely causes iron deficiency except in patients who have undergone partial gastrectomy or those with malabsorbtive syndromes such as sprue. Approximately 50 per cent of patients who have undergone partial gastrectomy (Billroth procedures) ultimately experience iron deficiency, often up to 10 years later. However, such patients are able to absorb oral iron salts.

Potential causes of iron deficiency anemia are outlined in Table 1. In infancy, iron deficiency with significant anemia is often secondary to the exclusive consumption of milk products. Infants who are exclusively breast- or bottle-fed for 18 months or longer are at significant risk. In early childhood, adolescence, and pregnancy, daily iron requirements are increased, but dietary deficiency alone is usually not the only cause of significant iron deficiency anemia. Children with iron deficiency anemia may also have a history of prematurity, low birth weight, or unsupplemented milk feeding. In pregnancy, there is a significant loss of iron secondary to an increase in maternal red cell mass as well as fetal needs. At delivery, additional red cell loss often occurs, resulting in further depletion of iron. Overall, pregnancy can result in a net loss of iron of up to 400 mg, with an additional ongoing loss of 0.5 mg of iron per day secondary to lactation.

Menstrual blood loss is the most common cause of iron deficiency and iron deficiency anemia in women between the ages of 15 and 45 years. The amount of blood lost with menses varies from woman to woman and is frequently difficult to evaluate by routine questioning. Although the average menstrual blood loss is about 50 mL per cycle, the volume of blood lost in the course of one menstrual cycle may be as large as 500 mL in women who do not regard their menstrual blood flow as excessive. An adequate menstrual history should determine the number of pads used, whether they are completely soaked through (approximately 50 mL of blood is required to soak through one pad), if large clots are passed with urination, and if there is ever blood on the bedsheets. Heavy menstrual blood loss is frequently defined as greater than 300 mL per menstrual

Table 1. Potential Causes of Iron Deficiency Anemia

Infants and Children
- Growth demands
- Inadequate nutrition
- Gastrointestinal hemorrhage
- Malabsorption syndromes
- Meckel's diverticulum

Adolescents
- Growth spurt
- Menstruation

Women of Childbearing Age
- Excessive menstrual blood loss
- Pregnancy
- Lactation

Men and Postmenopausal Women

Decreased Absorption
- Partial gastrectomy
- Malabsorption syndromes

Gastrointestinal Blood Loss
- Drugs (salicylates, NSAIDS, and so on)
- Peptic ulcer disease
- Diaphragmatic hiatal hernia
- Infection, inflammation, malignancy
- Telangiectasia
- Long-distance runner's anemia
- Parasitic infections

Respiratory Blood Loss
- Pulmonary hemosiderosis
- Infection, inflammation, malignancy

Genitourinary Blood Loss
- Intravascular hemolysis
- Infection, inflammation, malignancy

Phlebotomy
- Blood donor
- Diagnostic phlebotomy
- Polycythemia
- Surreptitious (self-inflicted)

NSAIDs = nonsteroidal anti-inflammatory drugs.

period or the use of more than 10 tampons or pads per menstrual period.

In males and postmenopausal women, iron deficiency is most commonly caused by gastrointestinal blood loss. In asymptomatic individuals, chronic unsuspected gastrointestinal blood loss should be the first consideration, and stool testing for occult blood should always be performed. At least six stool samples should be obtained over several days because bleeding may be intermittent. False-positive reactions with occult blood testing may occur from various kinds of meat in the diet as well as peroxidase-containing foods such as bananas, horseradish, broccoli, and turnips. Liquid stool specimens may also give false-positive results, whereas dried stools and aged specimens may produce false-negative results, as may vitamin C ingestion. Ulcerating lesions secondary to peptic ulcer disease, hiatal hernias with mucosal trauma, drug-associated mucosal blood loss (from aspirin, nonsteroidal anti-inflammatory agents, glucocorticoids, or enteric-coated potassium supplements) parasitic infections, and inflammatory or malignant states are only a few of the potential causes.

The documentation of blood in the stool always mandates a work-up to identify the source. Site-specific symptoms are predictive of abnormality in the corresponding portion of the gastrointestinal tract, so initial evaluation should be directed by the location of symptoms. If no localizing gastrointestinal symptoms are present, the lower gastrointestinal tract should be studied first, preferably by colonoscopy. Although hemorrhoids are the most common cause of lower gastrointestinal bleeding, blood loss from hemorrhoids is rarely sufficient to explain iron deficiency anemia. In the elderly, angiodysplasia and neoplasm are common causes of lower gastrointestinal bleeding. The incidence of colon cancer increases 40-fold between the ages of 40 and 80 years. If investigation of the lower bowel is unrewarding, investigation of the upper gastrointestinal tract should be pursued with esophagoscopy and gastroscopy. Some data suggest that synchronous gastrointestinal lesions are rare. However, one study of elderly patients with iron deficiency and benign upper gastrointestinal lesions discovered via endoscopy (which could have accounted for their anemia) detected coexistent malignant lower tract lesions by concomitant colonoscopy or barium enema in 7 of the 44 patients.

Percutaneous retrograde angiography of celiac or mesenteric arteries may localize the site of active gastrointestinal bleeding when the rate of blood flow into the intestinal lumen is 0.5 mL per minute or more. This procedure should be considered for any patient who is actively bleeding from the gastrointestinal tract and in whom the site of blood loss has not been established by other methods, including endoscopy, and for whom surgery is contemplated. Meckel's diverticulum is one of the most common causes of obscure gastrointestinal bleeding in children. These diverticula often contain ectopic gastric mucosa that concentrates pertechnetate following intravenous injection.

Other less common nongastrointestinal forms of blood loss include genital, urinary, and respiratory conditions. The use of extracorporeal dialysis for the treatment of chronic renal disease may cause iron deficiency, which is often superimposed on anemia of chronic renal disease. A diagnosis of idiopathic pulmonary hemosiderosis should be strongly considered in any patient, especially a child, who is found to have interstitial pulmonary infiltrates accompanied by iron deficiency anemia.

Other common but often overlooked causes of iron deficiency anemia are excessive blood donations and frequent phlebotomies, especially in hospitalized patients. One unit of blood represents an iron loss of approximately 250 mg, and although donors are screened with hematocrit testing, they are not evaluated for iron stores. Intravascular hemolysis, prosthetic heart valves, or other mechanical cardiac causes may produce iron deficiency secondary to increased urinary loss of hemosiderin. Paroxysmal nocturnal hemoglobinuria may also result in chronic intravascular iron loss and iron deficiency anemia. Besides drugs that may lead to iron deficiency anemia secondary to mucosal ulceration, a number of other agents may be associated with altered hemostasis and blood loss, such as warfarin, heparin, and various antiplatelet agents (acetylsalicylic acid, dipyridamole, nonsteroidal anti-inflammatory drugs). Finally, fictitious iron deficiency anemia due to self-inflicted bleeding may present a formidable diagnostic and therapeutic problem. These patients are most frequently women with a history of receiving blood transfusions for an iron deficiency of obscure cause who have also been subjected to numerous nondiagnostic radiographic and endoscopic examinations.

PRESENTING SIGNS AND SYMPTOMS

Symptoms Common to All Anemia

Iron deficiency anemia can result in a low concentration of hemoglobin with an associated decreased oxygen-carrying capacity and drop in work output. The effect of mild iron deficiency on work output of a nonanemic person is more controversial. However, animal investigations suggest that a partial repletion of iron deficiency can increase work output. Although acute blood loss can produce dramatic symptoms, the progression of iron deficiency anemia is frequently insidious. With chronic, slow blood loss, otherwise healthy patients may exhibit hemoglobin concentrations as low as 4 to 5 g/dL and still function well. However, below this concentration (or at higher concentrations when there is associated cardiac or pulmonary disease), the low hemoglobin and associated decreased oxygen-carrying capacity result in weakness, fatigue, lassitude, exertional dyspnea, pallor, and an increased heart rate. A few patients may present with headaches as the initial symptom. Obviously, these signs and symptoms are not specific for iron deficiency anemia and may be seen in association with anemia of any cause.

Symptoms More Specifically Related to Iron Deficiency Anemia

Depletion of iron-containing enzymes is probably responsible for many symptoms relating to the gastrointestinal tract and epidermal structures. In past years, a disease complex known as the Plummer-Vinson syndrome was frequently associated with iron deficiency. This syndrome is manifested by dysphagia accompanied by the presence of esophageal webs but is now rarely seen.

The angular stomatitis often seen in normal edentulous patients may also be associated with iron deficiency as a nonspecific finding. Pica, as defined by the habitual ingestion of nonfood substances or an unusual craving for a single food item, is noted in more than half of patients with iron deficiency anemia. The diagnosis of pica is frequently missed by clinicians, since they fail to ask about this symptom and patients are often reluctant to admit bizarre dietary habits. Pica for soil is known as geophagia, pica for starch is amylophagia, and pica for ice is pagophagia. In the United States, ice eating is the most common form of pica, but different preferences exist in different cultures. African Americans in the southern United States favor laundry starch and clay. Hispanics along the United States and Mexico border favor earth in the form of adobe fragments. In Mexico, earth is actually pressed into hand-sized cakes imprinted with an image of Christ for sale to iron-deficient children to suck on.

Dysfunction of the nervous system may also occur with iron deficiency. As the body becomes depleted of iron, changes occur in many tissues, including a decrease in the activity of various tissue enzymes, such as succinic dehydrogenase and xanthine oxidase, and brain γ-aminobutyric acid. Because fatigue, irritability, abnormal mentation, and poor memory may predate the presence of anemia, these observations suggest that many of the associated neurologic symptoms are caused by the impaired function of iron-containing enzymes or proteins other than hemoglobin. Similarly, headache, paresthesia, and a burning sensation involving the tongue are also symptoms of iron deficiency anemia that do not result from the anemia but are likely secondary to deficiency of iron within tissue cells. In infants, iron deficiency may be associated with poor attention span, poor responses to sensory stimuli, and a retardation in developmental achievements, even in the absence of anemia. School-aged children with iron deficiency anemia who receive iron treatment have better academic achievement than those who do not, but some degree of intellectual and motor impairment may persist for life. Cold intolerance in women may be an early symptom of iron deficiency and iron deficiency anemia.

Symptoms Relating to Loss of Blood or Iron

By definition, occult blood loss is not associated with any signs or symptoms. Any history of abnormalities involving the gastrointestinal tract detected in the review of systems is especially important in establishing the cause of iron deficiency anemia. Food fads leading to strict prohibition of certain food types may directly explain a nutritional iron deficiency anemia. If the individual is a strict vegetarian, the use of iron, vitamins, and other mineral supplements and their presence in the diet should be established, as well as any history of pica. A history of ingestion of agents known to be associated with an increased risk of gastrointestinal bleeding or a history of cigarette smoking, which is a major risk factor for peptic ulcer disease and cancer, should be sought. Symptoms of peptic ulcer disease, gastroesophageal reflux, or hiatal hernia suggest occult gastrointestinal blood loss. Patients with inflammatory bowel disease almost invariably give a history that quickly leads to a suspicion of iron deficiency as a cause of anemia. In elderly persons, symptoms of peptic ulcer disease may include less pain but more weight loss, nausea, and vomiting. Dysphagia may indicate the presence of an esophageal web associated with chronic iron deficiency anemia or esophageal neoplasm, or both, as a primary source of blood loss. Details regarding weight loss, diarrhea, melena, hematochezia, or changes in the caliber of stool may provide important clues to the diagnosis of an underlying gastrointestinal disease responsible for iron deficiency. A history of hemorrhoids by itself should never suffice as an explanation for iron deficiency unless other causes have been ruled out.

A careful genitourinary history may also prove useful. A history of excessive vaginal blood loss may be invaluable in explaining the cause of iron deficiency anemia. Multiple pregnancies may explain an iron deficiency anemia because uncompensated loss to the fetus, the need for increased maternal red cell mass, and lack of pre-existing iron stores may all contribute. Women with postmenopausal bleeding, particularly those with a history of postmenopausal estrogen use or obesity, should be promptly evaluated for the presence of endometrial cancer and associated iron deficiency anemia. A history of hematuria may be of considerable importance, whether it is macroscopic and massive or asymptomatic and microscopic. A primary genitourinary malignancy may rarely present with sufficient hematuria to cause iron deficiency anemia.

Physical Signs

Physical signs that are the result of iron deficiency anemia include pallor, koilonychia, and cheilosis. A careful examination of the mucous membranes and nail beds often documents pallor. Pallor of the palmar creases correlates with the degree of anemia. When the color of the palmar creases is as pale as the surrounding skin, the hemoglobin level is usually less than 7 g/dL. Glossitis, atrophy of the lingual papillae, and angular stomatitis may also be noted with severe iron deficiency anemia. Retinal hemorrhage may occasionally accompany acute severe iron deficiency. A rare patient may present with the clinical picture of pseudotumor cerebri with visual disturbances, sixth cranial nerve palsy, and associated papilledema. Cardiovascular physical signs include a widened systolic pressure usually noted when the hemoglobin level is less than 7 g/dL, as well as an increased pulse rate. The widened pulse pressure is frequently accompanied by a systolic flow murmur. Ten per cent of patients with iron deficiency may have splenomegaly, which has been attributed to hemolysis of iron-deficient red blood cells.

Physical signs that may be associated with the cause of iron deficiency anemia include cutaneous or mucosal telangiectasias, suggestive of hereditary hemorrhagic telangiectasia, or punctate melanin spots on the lips and buccal mucosal that may signify the Peutz-Jeghers syndrome, which is characterized by hamartomatous gastrointestinal polyps, gastrointestinal bleeding, and iron deficiency anemia. Dark velvety lesions of acanthosis nigricans found in the axillae of patients may suggest gastrointestinal or pulmonary malignancy. Inspection of the abdomen may reveal flank ecchymoses with the red-purple or green-brown discoloration of Turner's sign, resulting from retroperitoneal hemorrhage, or blue discoloration of the periumbilical region, resulting from intraperitoneal hemorrhage (Cullen's sign). Abdominal ascites and a dilated superficial venous pattern may correlate with the presence of alcoholic liver disease and a multifactorial anemia, including iron deficiency. Abdominal masses may represent neoplastic lesions of the colon or abdominal aortic aneurysms, both of which are potential causes of blood loss and iron deficiency anemia.

Table 2. Confirmatory Tests for the Diagnosis of Iron Deficiency

Test	Expected Result
Storage iron	
Bone marrow examination	Absent
Serum ferritin	<12 μg/L
Total iron-binding capacity	>400 mg/dL
Functional iron	
Mean cell volume (MCV)	<80 fL
Anemia–hemoglobin	<13 g/dL (men) <12 g/dL (women) <11 g/dL (pregnancy)
Serum iron	<35 μg/dL
Per cent transferrin saturation	<15 per cent
Free erythrocyte protoporphyrin	>70 μg/dL RBC
Therapeutic trial of iron	
2–3 mg iron/kg per day	Reticulocytosis in 10–14 days Hemoglobin increase 2 to 3 g per month Normal hemoglobin in 3 to 4 months

RBC = red blood cell.

Other Complications

When iron deficiency anemia becomes severe, cardiovascular adaptation may no longer compensate, and weakness and tachycardia may ensue. In patients with underlying coronary artery disease, there may be an exacerbation of angina pectoris. The effects of iron deficiency anemia on immune function and increased susceptibility to infection remains controversial. Although some authors have claimed multiple defects in immune function, including cell-mediated immunity and defective phagocytosis, others have been unable to duplicate these findings.

LABORATORY DIAGNOSIS

Initial laboratory investigations in an anemic patient allow classification into one of three morphologic categories: microcytic, normocytic, and macrocytic. This requires several basic studies, including a complete blood count (hemoglobin, hematocrit, red cell count, and the red cell indices—MCV, mean corpuscular hemoglobin, mean corpuscular hemoglobin concentration, RDW), a Wright-Giemsa–stained peripheral blood smear, and a reticulocyte count. The differential diagnosis of a microcytic anemia includes iron deficiency, a thalassemic syndrome or other hemoglobinopathy, sideroblastic anemia, lead toxicity, and copper deficiency, as well as the most common alternative consideration, anemia of chronic disease. Of the various confirmatory tests, the most useful in the diagnosis of iron deficiency are the hemoglobin concentration, the MCV, the serum ferritin level, the serum iron level and TIBC, and bone marrow examination for stainable iron (Table 2).

MORPHOLOGIC CHANGES

In early iron deficiency, microscopic examination of the red cells can provide little information beyond that given by the hemoglobin concentration and the MCV. This is because the morphologic changes, including hypochromia, are relatively poor indicators of early iron deficiency, and the evaluation of such changes is hampered by subjectivity and inconsistency among examiners. Similarly, although both mean corpuscular hemoglobin and mean corpuscular hemoglobin concentration decrease in iron deficiency anemia, they provide little relevant information beyond that supplied by the MCV. Measurement of the heterogeneity of red cell size distribution (the RDW as supplied by newer analyzers) may play some role in the diagnosis of iron deficiency. The RDW tends to be increased in iron deficiency and normal in thalassemia minor or anemia of chronic disease. Numerous exceptions occur, however, and an increased RDW has been reported in up to 50 per cent of patients with anemia of chronic disease and in a significant number of patients with thalassemia. If the RDW is normal, it militates against the presence of iron deficiency anemia.

Careful examination of the various features of the peripheral smear can help to differentiate iron deficiency anemia from the other microcytic anemias when the anemia is severe and the morphologic features are classic (Table 3). In severe iron deficiency, the blood film should show anisopoikilocytosis, hypochromia, and microcytosis with an obvious undercrowding of red blood cells (see Fig. 1). Cigar-shaped cells and bizarre microcytes can also be seen. The reticulocyte count is usually normal, and a mild thrombocytosis may be present. In thalassemia minor, there is less anisopoikilocytosis, but red cell targeting and basophilic stippling are usually present. The cells appear hypochromic because they are thinner than normal, but the mean corpuscular hemoglobin concentration is usually normal. Many of the other heterozygous hemoglobinopathies resemble thalassemia trait morphologically, showing a similar microcytosis and hypochromia. Sideroblastic anemias may demonstrate a dimorphic red cell population with normochromic and hypochromic cells. Pernicious anemia is frequently associated with iron deficiency; in this instance, the peripheral smear is often dimorphic, showing hypochromic microcytic cells with some oval macrocytes. Although the overall indices and MCV may be in the normal range secondary to the averaging of the two cell populations, hypersegmented neutrophils usually are detectable.

Table 3. Typical Test Results Differentiating Iron Deficiency From Other Anemias

Condition	Smear Morphologic Features	Red Cell Distribution Width	Ferritin	Serum Iron	Total Iron-Binding Capacity	Per Cent Transferrin Saturation	Free Erythrocyte Protoporphyrin	Hemoglobin A_2	Marrow Iron (Prussian Blue Stain)
Iron deficiency anemia	Anisocytosis Microcytic Hypochromia (late)	↑	↓	↓	↑	<15%	↑	N	None
Anemia of chronic disease	Microcytic or normocytic	N or ↑ (50% cases)	N or ↑	↓	N or ↓	N or ↓ (usually not <15%)	↑	N	N or ↑
Thalassemia trait	Microcytic Target cells Basophilic stippling Hypochromia with normal MCHC	Frequently N	N or ↑	N	N	N	N	↑ β-thalassemia N α-thalassemia	N or ↑
Sideroblastic anemia	Dimorphic (hypochromia and normochromia)	Frequently N	N or ↑	N or ↑	N or ↑	N or ↑	N	N	↑ Ring sideroblasts present

N = normal; ↑ = increased; ↓ = decreased; MCHC = mean corpuscular hemoglobin concentration.

The bone marrow examination in iron deficiency usually shows an erythroid hyperplasia with normoblasts displaying poor hemoglobinization with scanty, often vacuolated cytoplasm. Bone marrow examination remains the "gold standard" for confirming iron deficiency anemia, and the presence of any iron stainable with Prussian blue rules out a diagnosis of iron deficiency anemia. In anemia of chronic disease, bone marrow iron storage is increased, and the iron is redistributed into the reticuloendothelial cells instead of the normoblasts. In sideroblastic anemia, ringed sideroblasts are seen.

SERUM IRON

The normal values for serum iron range from approximately 50 to 200 mg/dL. Values are usually higher in men than in women. There is also a diurnal variation in serum iron, with the concentrations being 10 to 40 mg/dL lower in the evening. Oral iron therapy should be discontinued 24 hours before measuring serum iron levels. Parenteral iron therapy may cause increases in the serum iron concentration for weeks after administration. Serum iron is typically low in iron deficiency anemia and anemia of chronic disease but normal or high in thalassemia, other hemoglobinopathies, and the sideroblastic anemias. The TIBC reflects the transferrin concentration in the blood. The per cent transferrin saturation is calculated by dividing the serum iron value by the value for the TIBC. At any one time in a normal adult, approximately one third of the transferrin-binding sites are occupied by iron, giving a per cent saturation of around 30 per cent. Usually the TIBC rises in response to iron deficiency anemia, so the per cent transferrin saturation is less than 15 per cent. Sometimes in iron deficiency anemia, however, the serum iron level and iron-binding capacity are both low. This combination commonly occurs in anemia of chronic or inflammatory disease. In summary, a per cent saturation of less than 15 per cent is strongly suggestive of iron deficiency, especially if the TIBC is increased. If the per cent saturation is in the range of 15 per cent, however, iron deficiency cannot be reliably differentiated from anemia of chronic disease, especially if the TIBC is normal or decreased.

SERUM FERRITIN

Mean values for serum ferritin are 35 μg/L in women and about 100 μg/L in men. In healthy persons whose serum ferritin is greater than 12 μg/L, one may estimate tissue iron stores by multiplying the numeric value for the serum ferritin by 10. For example, a healthy man with a serum ferritin value of 100 μg/L should have 1000 mg of tissue iron stores. The serum ferritin level is a sensitive measure of total tissue iron in that a serum ferritin level less than 12 μg/L indicates the absence of body iron. However, ferritin is also an acute-phase reactant so that in iron deficiency anemia, the serum ferritin concentration can still be greater than 12 μg/L when inflammation is present. Thus, in the setting of coexistent inflammatory states, cellular damage, or malignancy, individual serum ferritin values must be interpreted with caution.

Patients with inflammatory conditions and anemia of chronic disease with serum ferritin concentrations in the lower portion of the normal range, that is, 50 to 100 μg/L, may or may not have iron deficiency. Those with inflammatory conditions and ferritin concentrations of approximately 12 to 50 μg/L are likely to have iron deficiency. For instance, in a group of 67 patients with active rheumatoid arthritis, a serum ferritin concentration less than 60 μg/L had a positive predictive value of 83 per cent for iron deficiency anemia. A bone marrow examination with evaluation of marrow iron stores may ultimately be necessary in some instances of suspected anemia of chronic disease when the ferritin level is in the 10 to 100 μg/L range.

It may be possible to correct the ferritin concentration for the degree of inflammation present using the sedimentation rate, thus potentially avoiding a bone marrow examination. A nomogram in Figure 2 shows that when an inflammatory condition is manifested by an increased sedimentation rate, a serum ferritin level greater than 100 μg/L suggests that iron deficiency is highly unlikely. With a ferritin level of 20 to 100 μg/L, the likelihood of iron deficiency depends on the sedimentation rate. These same caveats for interpreting ferritin values when inflammation is present also apply for the diagnosis of iron deficiency in the postoperative state or during recovery from acute infection, with liver cell–associated necrosis, or acute or chronic liver disease. For instance, a serum ferritin concentration as high as 150 μg/L has been reported in an iron-depleted alcoholic. Similarly, the serum ferritin level may also be normal or increased in marrow iron–depleted patients who are being treated with maintenance hemodialysis.

FREE ERYTHROCYTE PROTOPORPHYRINS AND SERUM TRANSFERRIN RECEPTORS

Measurement of free erythrocyte protoporphyrin may also be useful in screening for iron deficiency anemia when iron is lacking or lead interferes with the incorporation of iron into heme and zinc substitutes as a ligand. This test is relatively simple, reliable, and accurate, especially when iron deficiency is severe. When iron deficiency or lead intoxication is mild, however, the test is subject to procedural difficulties that may limit reliability.

A relatively new assay involves the measurement of serum transferrin receptors via monoclonal antibodies. Following depletion of iron stores, serum transferrin receptors are shown to increase and to correlate with the degree of

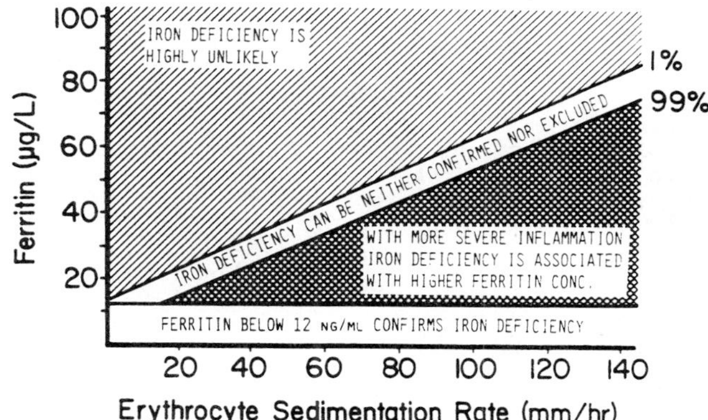

Figure 2. Nomogram used to determine the presence or absence of iron deficiency by correlating serum ferritin level with degree of inflammation, as indicated by erythrocyte sedimentation rate (ferritin level <12 μg/L). (Adapted from Witte, D.L., Angstadt, D.S., Davis, S.H., et al.: Predicting bone marrow iron stores in anemic patients in a community hospital using ferritin and erythrocyte sedimentation rate. Am. J. Clin. Pathol. 90:85–87, 1988, with permission.)

serum iron deficiency. Thus this test appears to provide an excellent measure of tissue iron deficiency, although its precise role in the diagnosis and management of iron deficiency has yet to be elucidated.

INTEGRATED LABORATORY APPROACH

Figure 3 and Table 3 summarize and integrate the most useful diagnostic parameters. When microcytosis is present in association with a low iron level and increased iron-binding capacity and a low ferritin level, iron deficiency is likely present. In this instance, the RDW is frequently increased to greater than 16 per cent. If the iron concentration is low and the TIBC is low (such that the per cent saturation is in the range of 15 per cent) in association with a normal or high ferritin level, the picture is suggestive of anemia of chronic disease. Iron deficiency cannot be excluded by these data, and using the ferritin erythrocyte sedimentation rate nomogram may be helpful. Alternatively, a bone marrow examination to evaluate the iron stores remains the gold standard for diagnosing iron deficiency anemia. The clinical condition in which this diagnostic dilemma most commonly occurs is in patients with active rheumatoid arthritis who are being treated with anti-inflammatory drugs that could be inducing chronic gastrointestinal blood loss, causing iron deficiency. When the iron concentration is normal and is associated with a normal TIBC and a normal ferritin level, another cause for microcytosis, such as a hemoglobinopathy, should be sought. In this instance, the RDW often is normal. With thalassemia, the peripheral blood film should demonstrate little anisopoikilocytosis with associated basophilic stippling and target cells (see Table 3). Hemoglobin electrophoresis may show an increased hemoglobin A_2 in the case of beta-thalassemia minor, and hemoglobin H inclusions may be present on supravital stain in patients with alpha-thalassemia minor. If the serum iron and/or ferritin levels are high, the possibility of sideroblastic anemia exists. In this case, ring sideroblasts should be present on bone marrow examination.

THERAPEUTIC TRIAL

Some physicians or patients may not have access to all the studies described for the diagnosis of iron deficiency anemia. In these situations, response to iron therapy may serve as proof of the correctness of the diagnosis of iron deficiency anemia. Iron administration for a therapeutic trial should take place via the oral route only. If the cause of anemia is iron deficiency, adequate iron therapy should result in a reticulocytosis, with a peak occurring approximately 10 days to 2 weeks after the start of therapy. When the anemia is mild, the reticulocyte response may be minimal. However, a significant increase in hemoglobin concentration should be evident within 3 to 4 weeks (2 to 3 g/dL), and the hemoglobin concentration should become normal after 3 to 4 months of therapy. Unless there is evidence of continued sustained blood loss, the absence of such a response must be taken as evidence that iron deficiency is not the cause of the anemia. A therapeutic trial of iron uses the same dosing of iron as that used to treat iron deficiency. In adults, this is 300 mg of non–enteric-coated non–sustained-release ferrous sulfate (each tablet contains 60 mg of elemental iron) taken one to three times daily. In children, the dosage is 1.5 to 2.0 mg/kg of elemental iron three times daily.

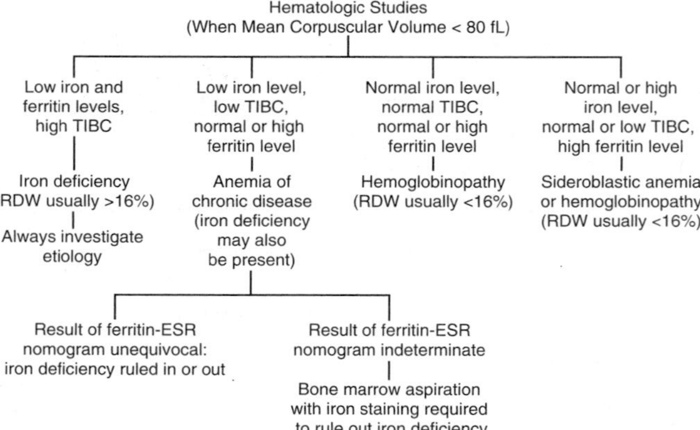

Figure 3. Flow chart for evaluation of microcytic anemia (i.e., mean corpuscular volume <80 fL). ESR = erythrocyte sedimentation rate; RDW = red cell distribution width; TIBC = total iron-binding capacity.

PITFALLS IN DIAGNOSIS

In taking the medical history, the two most common errors are failure to elicit a prior history of gastric surgery and failure to take an adequate menstrual history. Iron deficiency anemia may develop 10 to 15 years after gastric surgery, and many women who think they have scant periods actually experience significant menstrual blood loss.

No single test is diagnostic in complex cases suggestive of iron deficiency anemia. When microcytosis is present, the primary differential diagnosis is usually between iron deficiency and anemia of chronic disease or thalassemia. Although thalassemia can usually be distinguished via the features outlined in Table 3, distinguishing iron deficiency from anemia of chronic disease may be more difficult. Analysis of the combination of serum ferritin with iron and iron-binding capacity results may be helpful, but in some instances, bone marrow examination with iron staining may ultimately be required to diagnose or exclude iron deficiency.

The most potentially serious pitfall in diagnosis is to treat iron deficiency as a disease rather than a symptom by giving iron therapy without adequately determining why the iron deficiency anemia developed in the first place. Another common mistake in the diagnosis of iron deficiency anemia is to assume the patient cannot be iron-deficient because of the failure to respond to a trial of oral iron therapy. The most common reason for failure to respond is failure to take the iron medication. When iron tablets are not taken with food and the dosage is not built up slowly (initially one pill at mealtime with no increase until gastrointestinal tolerance develops), almost all patients experience some dyspepsia and frequently stop the medication in disgust. Problems with bioavailability constitute the second most common reason for failure to respond to oral iron therapy. This can usually be traced to the use of enteric-coated or sustained-release iron preparations. Such iron preparations provide a false sense of security, turning the stools black but often not dissolving until reaching the jejunum and thus providing little or no iron delivery to the duodenal absorptive site. Many pharmacists are unaware of the bioavailability status of individual iron preparations, so a strategy of writing "non–enteric-coated, non–sustained-release" on prescriptions for iron will not necessarily be successful. To circumvent this problem, physicians should prescribe a brand-name iron preparation with which they are familiar and add "no substitution" to the prescription. Patients with malabsorption syndromes, such as unsuspected sprue, may fail to respond to oral iron therapy, as may individuals with unsuspected mixed deficiencies such as an iron deficiency and folate and/or vitamin B_{12} deficiency.

Finally, and most importantly, individuals who are losing blood continuously or intermittently may not absorb enough oral iron to overcome ongoing iron losses, and their anemia will not be corrected. For instance, patients who are iron-deficient and regular blood donors who receive replacement iron therapy only until the hemoglobin level is normal will soon experience recurrent iron deficiency anemia. The iron therapy must be continued for at least 6 months beyond the time that the hemoglobin level returns to normal so that bone marrow iron stores are actually replenished. Patients who have a clear-cut iron deficiency and show only a partial response or an initial response to iron therapy followed by relapse must be re-evaluated because unsuspected cancers often produce intermittent bleeding.

HEMOGLOBINOPATHIES

By Andrew J. Fishleder, M.D.
Cleveland, Ohio

The term hemoglobinopathies can be broadly defined to include those inherited defects in hemoglobin synthesis that result in the production of structurally abnormal hemoglobin molecules (e.g., hemoglobin S [Hb S]) or in the decreased production of normal hemoglobin (thalassemia). This article focuses on the diagnosis and clinical implications of the structural hemoglobinopathies. Thalassemia is discussed in a subsequent article.

The structural hemoglobinopathies have in common the presence of some genetic defect that results in an alteration of the amino acid sequence of the globin chain component of hemoglobin. Many of these alterations have little or no impact on hemoglobin function or red blood cell (RBC) survival and therefore are of minimal importance to the practitioner. Several, however, result in hemolytic anemia or an alteration of hemoglobin oxygen affinity. The more common, clinically significant abnormal hemoglobins are addressed in this article.

SICKLE CELL DISEASE

The most frequently encountered hemoglobinopathy in the United States is Hb S, which is present in approximately 8 per cent of African Americans. Hb S results from an amino acid substitution in the beta-globin chain of hemoglobin. When an individual inherits a normal beta-globin gene from one parent and a beta-S gene from the other, they produce both hemoglobin A (Hb A) and Hb S, resulting in the condition known as sickle cell trait (hemoglobin AS [Hb AS]). In contrast, the term sickle cell disease refers to those inherited disorders in which the defective sickle gene is coinherited with another abnormal beta-globin gene, resulting in anemia, hemolysis, and tissue injury (e.g., hemoglobin SS [Hb SS] or hemoglobin SC [Hb SC]). Sickle cell anemia refers to the most common type of sickle cell disease in which an individual inherits two beta-S genes (Hb SS).

The clinical abnormalities that are encountered in sickle cell disease result from the tendency of Hb S to polymerize within the RBC during deoxygenation, with consequent formation of a deformed, sickle-shaped cell. In sickle cell trait, the amount of Hb A in the RBC protects against this polymerization under normal oxygenation so that this condition is clinically silent. In sickle cell disease, however, RBC sickling occurs under physiologic conditions. The deformed RBC is readily damaged in the microcirculation, resulting in hemolysis and anemia, and can cause ischemic tissue damage by clogging small blood vessels because of its poor deformability. Clinical conditions such as hypoxia, acidosis, dehydration, and fever that shift the RBC toward deoxygenation result in increased RBC sickling with its attendant complications.

The clinical severity of sickle cell disease varies with the tendency of the RBC to sickle. Hb SS, hemoglobin SO (Hb SO), and hemoglobin SD (Hb SD) cells all sickle readily and can produce severe disease. Hb SC disease is a more moderate sickling disorder. In contrast, Hb S in combination with many other hemoglobins, such as hemoglobin G (Hb G), hemoglobin E (Hb E), and hemoglobin N (Hb N), is similar to sickle cell trait without clinically significant sickling. Hemoglobin F (Hb F) is also known to protect against sickling, and individuals with Hb S and hereditary persistence of fetal hemoglobin (Hb S-HPFH) are clinically normal. Finally, thalassemia has a moderating effect on sickling, presumably because of the lower RBC mean corpuscular hemoglobin concentration (MCHC) in that condition. Additional genetic factors can also influence RBC sickling, particularly in sickle cell anemia, so that disease severity can vary significantly from one family to another.

SICKLE CELL ANEMIA

The clinical manifestations of sickle cell anemia result primarily from vascular occlusion and chronic extravascular hemolysis. Patients typically present in infancy or early childhood with moderate to severe anemia and painful crises due to tissue ischemia. Infants may present with fever and swelling of the hands and feet—a vaso-occlusive condition known as "hand-foot" syndrome. Splenic dysfunction also develops in infancy and predisposes these children to life-threatening infection by encapsulated bacteria, such as pneumococci. This has prompted recommendations for prophylactic penicillin therapy until at least 2 years of age.

As children with sickle cell anemia grow older, their symptoms primarily result from painful vaso-occlusive episodes. Musculoskeletal pain is encountered most frequently, and avascular necrosis of the femoral head is a particularly serious complication. Abdominal pain, chest pain, and pain from organ infarcts are also common. "Autosplenectomy" in early childhood from recurrent splenic infarcts invariably develops. In males, recurrent, painful priapism is also common.

Ischemic damage to many organ systems eventually ensues, although the clinical course is extremely variable among patients. Neurologic deficits resulting from recurrent strokes are relatively common, and subarachnoid hemorrhages occur with increased frequency in adults. Renal dysfunction with hematuria and salt-losing nephropathy may be seen. Pulmonary dysfunction with reduced lung capacity commonly develops and can exacerbate heart failure. Hepatomegaly and liver function abnormalities are frequent, and cholelithiasis from chronic hemolysis develops in many patients. Chronic skin ulcers, typically on the lower leg, are common and may be sites for secondary infection. Lastly, ocular dysfunction due to retinal infarcts, intraocular hemorrhages, and/or proliferative retinopathy eventually is seen in many patients.

In addition to the chronic, progressive clinical morbidity of sickle cell anemia, several distinct syndromes are encountered and need to be recognized. They include acute chest syndrome, abdominal crisis, splenic sequestration crisis, and aplastic crisis. The acute chest syndrome is a potentially life-threatening condition characterized by the sudden onset of pleuritic chest pain, fever, and shortness of breath, typically associated with a chest film that reveals pulmonary infiltrates. Often, this is preceded by bone pain. The differential diagnosis includes small pulmonary infarcts versus bacterial pneumonia; frequently both are present. *Pneumococcus*, *Haemophilus influenzae*, and *Staphylococcus aureus* are commonly implicated infectious agents. Although the cause in some patients is uncertain, in many instances the associated hypoxia results in severe sickling that may cause bone marrow infarcts with subsequent bone marrow emboli. Early recognition and treatment may be critical. Abdominal crises are characterized by acute pain, marked increases in liver enzyme levels, and increased serum bilirubin. The differential diagnosis includes hepatitis, cholelithiasis, and intrahepatic sickling. Acute splenic sequestration crisis is a life-threatening complication that typically occurs in young children whose spleens have not yet become infarcted. Patients present with a rapidly enlarging spleen caused by a massive accumulation of blood from splenic outflow obstruction. Severe anemia and hypovolemic shock may rapidly ensue and result in death unless aggressively treated. Recurrence during early childhood may occur, and mortality is high. Lastly, an aplastic crisis characterized by severe, progressive anemia with reticulocytopenia is common in sickle cell anemia as in other chronic hemolytic diseases. This complication is associated with parvovirus B-19 infection, which causes aplasia of RBC precursors in the bone marrow. Anemia rapidly develops because of the reduced RBC survival in sickle cell anemia. The patient may present with fever, vomiting, and fatigue, but the presentation of severe anemia without a reticulocyte response helps establish the diagnosis. Supportive therapy is sufficient if the patient's immune function is intact because the viral infection will be self-limited.

OTHER SICKLING DISORDERS

Chronic hemolysis and intravascular sickling are encountered with other forms of sickle cell disease. Clinical manifestations in Hb SO_{Arab} and Hb SD diseases may be as severe as in sickle cell anemia. In contrast, Hb SC disease differs in its clinical severity. Overall, Hb SC results in a milder disease with less hemolysis and therefore higher hemoglobin concentrations and a lower incidence of cholelithiasis and leg ulcers than occurs in sickle cell anemia. In addition, RBCs may be mildly microcytic. Painful crises are less frequent but are still common. Autosplenectomy is less frequent, although fatal pneumococcal sepsis has been reported. In fact, because of persistent splenic function, splenic sequestration crises in adults have been reported, a problem that is rare in sickle cell anemia. In contrast, when compared with sickle cell anemia, patients with Hb SC disease have a higher incidence of renal papillary necrosis, retinopathy, avascular necrosis of the femoral head, and thromboembolic complications. In addition, almost 50 per cent of Hb SC patients have been reported to have splenomegaly. Although differences in clinical manifestations can help distinguish these disorders, simple laboratory tests (see further on) readily distinguish sickle cell anemia from other sickle cell diseases.

HEMOGLOBIN C–RELATED DISORDERS

Hemoglobin C (Hb C) is the second most commonly encountered abnormal hemoglobin in the United States, with an incidence of 3 per cent in African Americans. Individuals with Hb C trait (Hb AC) are asymptomatic, although they may have mildly reduced RBC survival (without anemia) and increased numbers of target-shaped RBCs. In contrast, patients with Hb C disease (Hb CC) have mild chronic hemolysis and an associated increased incidence of cholelithiasis. Patients may present with intermittent bouts of abdominal pain or jaundice. Anemia is of mild to moderate severity, with numerous target cells and mild microcytosis. Hemolysis is probably related to the decreased solubility of Hb C, with Hb C crystals visible on peripheral blood smears.

HEMOGLOBIN E–RELATED DISORDERS

Hb E is less common than Hb C in the United States but is the second most prevalent abnormal hemoglobin worldwide, with a high incidence in individuals of Southeast Asian descent. Because of immigration of Southeast Asians to the United States, Hb E–related disorders are being encountered with greater frequency. Hb E trait (Hb AE) is associated with microcytosis and mild erythrocytosis but is clinically silent. Hb E disease is likewise typically asymptomatic, although RBC microcytosis is more prominent and slight anemia may be present because Hb E is somewhat unstable. In contrast, Hb E–beta-thalassemia is a moderately severe disorder with significant anemia. Clinical and hematologic features resemble thalassemia intermedia or thalassemia major (see article on thalassemia).

UNSTABLE HEMOGLOBINS

Many abnormal hemoglobins that are "unstable" have been identified and characterized. Although the list is long, all are relatively uncommon. In the heterozygous state, these hemoglobins result in hemolytic anemia that spans a broad range of clinical severity. (Homozygous conditions are probably incompatible with life.) Most unstable variants cause mild chronic hemolysis with compensatory reticulocytosis that may result in little or no anemia. Others, however, can cause moderate to severe hemolytic anemia and present early in life. Splenomegaly is commonly encountered with the unstable hemoglobinopathies, as is cholelithiasis. Acute hemolytic crises that exacerbate chronic hemolysis may be presenting features and can be precipitated by fever associated with acute infection or drugs. Sulfa-containing medications or other drugs causing oxidative stress are commonly implicated. Patients may have intermittent jaundice and dark urine. As with other causes of chronic hemolysis, aplastic crises caused by parvovirus B-19 infection may result in transient severe anemia; however, this should be self-limited in the context of normal immune function.

In addition to causing instability, the structural defects in unstable hemoglobins commonly involve sites on the hemoglobin molecule that affect its oxygen affinity. Decreased or increased oxygen affinity can independently result in anemia or erythrocytosis, respectively, so that the patient's clinical symptoms may not correlate with the severity of the unstable hemolytic anemia. For example, some unstable hemoglobins with mild hemolysis but low oxygen affinity may produce mild to moderate anemia without clinical symptoms because of enhanced oxygen delivery to tissues. In contrast, unstable hemoglobins with moderate hemolysis but high oxygen affinity may produce milder anemia than expected because of compensatory erythrocytosis. These individuals still have chronic hemolysis and its potential complications. Others with comparable hemoglobin instability and hemolysis but normal oxygen affinity have more moderate to severe anemia with associated clinical symptoms. The unstable hemoglobins with their associated hemolytic anemia must be differentiated from other forms of acquired hemolysis including RBC enzyme defects such as glucose-6-phosphate dehydrogenase deficiency, RBC membrane defects such as hereditary spherocytosis, and acquired forms of hemolytic anemia.

HEMOGLOBINS WITH ALTERED OXYGEN AFFINITY

As indicated earlier, the inherited amino acid defect in some hemoglobinopathies can alter the ability of the heme portion of hemoglobin to bind oxygen. Although some of these abnormal hemoglobins are also unstable, many are not. The resultant clinical and laboratory abnormalities in this latter group reflect the physiologic response to altered oxygen delivery. In patients with increased oxygen affinity, the reduced oxygen delivery results in a compensatory increase in erythropoietin production and consequent polycythemia. This must be differentiated from other causes of primary and secondary polycythemia, including, for example, myeloproliferative disorders, thalassemia, congenital heart disease, and chronic pulmonary disease. Other abnormal hemoglobins have reduced oxygen affinity with associated facilitated tissue delivery of oxygen. This results in a blunting of erythropoietin production and consequent "anemia," although the patients are physiologically normal. Although these hemoglobinopathies should be considered in the differential diagnosis of polycythemia and anemia, respectively, they are low on the differential list, as both high- and low-oxygen affinity hemoglobins are rarely encountered. Unfortunately, many of these abnormal hemoglobins are indistinguishable from normal Hb A by routine laboratory procedures so that their identification in many instances becomes one of exclusion unless more sophisticated testing of hemoglobin function is performed.

LABORATORY DIAGNOSIS

The identification of the clinically significant hemoglobinopathies can typically be achieved by several simple laboratory tests. Performance of a complete blood count with review of RBC morphologic features should always be performed as part of the evaluation except when simple screening for Hb S is desired (see discussion of solubility testing). The presence of anemia, reticulocytosis, target cells, sickle cells, Howell-Jolly bodies, Hb C crystals, or "bite cells" provides clues to the diagnosis prior to any other laboratory tests.

When an abnormal hemoglobin is suspected, the best method for screening is cellulose acetate electrophoresis at pH 8.6 (or isoelectric focusing in some laboratories). This simple procedure uses electrophoretic migration to separate proteins by their charge and thereby differentiates many of the clinically significant hemoglobinopathies from normal Hb A. Hb S, Hb C, Hb E, Hb D, Hb G, Hb O, and others can be differentiated from Hb A by this method because their amino acid mutations change the charge of the hemoglobin molecule. However, many hemoglobinopathies have amino acid substitutions that do not alter their charge or, therefore, their electrophoretic migration. These cannot be distinguished from Hb A by electrophoresis and require more sophisticated laboratory tests for specific identification. Most, however, are clinically insignificant. Those unstable hemoglobins that migrate like Hb A on cellulose acetate can still be identified as unstable by other tests (see further on), even though the specific abnormal hemoglobin may be difficult to identify.

In addition to identifying many of the clinically significant hemoglobinopathies, cellulose acetate electrophoresis also differentiates Hb A from Hb F and Hb A_2. Increases in Hb F can be seen in HPFH and thalassemia as well as in a variety of acquired conditions such as myeloproliferative diseases, erythroleukemia, aplastic anemia, and pregnancy. HB F concentrations are also high in newborns but are reduced to normal adult values (approximately 1 per cent of total hemoglobin) by age 1 to 2 years. Hb A_2 normally represents approximately 2 to 3 per cent of total hemoglobin but is increased to as high as 10 per cent in beta-thalassemia. Hb A_2 concentrations are decreased, however, in delta beta–thalassemia as well as in iron deficiency. The latter may obscure the expected increase of Hb A_2 in beta-thalassemia, making diagnosis more difficult.

Once the presence of an abnormal hemoglobin is noted by cellulose acetate electrophoresis, specific identification of the abnormal hemoglobin requires follow-up electrophoresis on citrate agar at pH 6. The laboratory should reflexively perform this step when an abnormality is encountered because several hemoglobinopathies of differing clinical significance migrate in similar positions on cellulose acetate. For example, Hb S migrates in the same position as Hb D and Hb G, and Hb C migrates in the same position as Hb O and Hb E. Cellulose acetate electrophoresis patterns that look like sickle cell trait therefore could be Hb D trait, for example, and patterns resembling Hb SC disease could be Hb SE, a clinically innocuous condition. Citrate agar electrophoresis separates Hb S from Hb D and Hb G, and Hb C from Hb O and Hb E, allowing specific identification of Hb S and/or Hb C, the two most clinically important hemoglobinopathies.

An additional test, globin-chain electrophoresis, can be used to further separate Hb D from Hb G and Hb E from Hb O, if necessary. In some circumstances, family studies may be useful, particularly when an abnormal hemoglobin is identified in a newborn or infant. This may be required because of the normally high amount of Hb F in newborns.

The sickle solubility test is another simple method for rapidly identifying the presence of Hb S; however, it does not specifically characterize the hemoglobinopathy present. The presence of Hb S with or without other abnormal hemoglobins gives the same result. This test is based on the reduced solubility of deoxygenated Hb S in a phosphate buffer with resultant increased turbidity of the solution; therefore, it is purely qualitative. Sickle cell trait (Hb AS), sickle cell anemia (Hb SS), Hb SC disease, and Hb SE, for example, all yield positive solubility tests that are indistinguishable, even though clinically they have differing tendencies to sickle. For this reason, although the solubility test can be used as a rapid screen for the presence of Hb S, it should not be used to diagnose a specific hemoglobinopathy and should always be followed by, at least, cellulose acetate electrophoresis. Conversely, the solubility test can be used to confirm the presence of apparent sickle cell trait (Hb AS) that has been previously identified by cellulose acetate electrophoresis. Because other abnormal hemoglobins that migrate in the Hb S position do not sickle, a positive solubility test would confirm the identity of presumed sickle cell trait seen on cellulose acetate. The solubility test can also be useful in differentiating other unusual abnormal hemoglobins, such as hemoglobin Hasharon, that migrate like Hb S on both cellulose acetate and citrate agar; however, this is not routinely necessary.

The sickle solubility test may yield false-negative results under certain conditions, most notably in severe anemia and instances in which the Hb S percentage is low. In the case of severe anemia, at hemoglobin concentrations less than 7 g/dL the decreased Hb S solubility may not yield a sufficient increase in solution turbidity to be visible simply because of a dilutional effect and the test will therefore appear negative. False-negative results due to a low percentage of Hb S (less than approximately 25 per cent Hb S) result from the same inability of a small amount of Hb S to increase the turbidity of a solution to visually detectable levels. This can be important in transfused patients in whom the percentage of Hb S can be substantially diluted by normal RBCs. This is also the reason that the solubility test cannot be used as a screening test in newborns, who normally have high levels of Hb F (70 to 75 per cent) at birth. Newborns with sickle cell trait (Hb AS) only have 10 to 15 per cent Hb S, and even newborns with sickle cell anemia (Hb SS) may have only 25 per cent Hb S. For this reason, electrophoretic screening or isoelectric focusing must be used to diagnose newborn blood samples.

When an unstable hemoglobin is suspected, additional laboratory tests may be useful. The isopropanol denaturation test (Carrell test) and heat instability test both demonstrate positive results by precipitation of unstable hemoglobins in a hemolysate. A Heinz body stain to identify denatured hemoglobin in intact RBCs can also be used. This latter test is less useful, however, because other conditions such as glucose-6-phosphate dehydrogenase deficiency with certain oxidant drugs can yield a positive result. In addition, normal splenic function may remove denatured hemoglobin (Heinz bodies) from red cells, resulting in a false-negative result even in the presence of an unstable hemoglobin.

NEWBORN SCREENING

Evidence that active intervention in the care of infants with sickle cell anemia reduces morbidity and mortality has prompted a proliferation of newborn hemoglobinopathy screening programs throughout the United States. Twice-daily oral penicillin given prophylactically significantly reduces morbidity and mortality from pneumococcal infection in Hb SS children and should be initiated by 2 months of age. Prompt recognition of infection and potential splenic sequestration crises is equally important. The ability to initiate these interventions obviously requires diagnosis of sickle cell disease at the time of birth.

Cellulose acetate electrophoresis (or isoelectric focusing) is the method of choice for hemoglobinopathy screening. This can be accomplished from filter paper samples, such as those routinely collected for metabolic disease screening or, preferably, from anticoagulated umbilical cord blood samples (3 to 5 mL). Although filter paper screening is convenient, it is limited by sample size and commonly requires follow-up testing for confirmation of abnormal results. Umbilical cord blood samples provide sufficient volume for accurate hemoglobinopathy characterization but are less convenient in terms of specimen shipping and handling. Cord blood samples have the added disadvantage of potential maternal blood contamination; however, this should be recognizable on electrophoresis by the presence of Hb A_2. Newborns do not yet produce Hb A_2, and therefore its presence suggests maternal contamination and warrants repeat evaluation if an abnormal hemoglobin is also identified. This is particularly important in infants with sickle cell anemia in whom electrophoresis patterns may be misread as sickle cell trait because of maternal Hb A. Maternal contamination is obviously not a problem with heel-stick filter paper samples. As discussed previously, solubility testing has no place in newborn screening because of the high percentage of Hb F and low percentage of Hb S in neonates.

Even with adequate samples, sickle cell anemia cannot be definitively identified in newborns because its electrophoretic pattern is identical to Hb S-HPFH and Hb S–beta-thalassemia. Newborns with only Hb S and Hb F, however, should be considered to have presumptive sickle cell anemia until proved otherwise. Family studies, in most instances, should enable distinction between these conditions and are recommended if possible.

PRENATAL DIAGNOSIS

Advances in molecular biology have broadened our understanding of the hemoglobinopathies and enable the specific identification of mutations responsible for abnormal hemoglobins by DNA analysis. This technique provides the physician and family with the opportunity to detect specific hemoglobinopathies such as sickle cell anemia from a fetal tissue sample. DNA extracted from a chorionic villous biopsy or amniotic fluid cells can allow diagnosis of Hb SS and other abnormal hemoglobins in the first and second trimesters of pregnancy, respectively. Various thalassemia disorders can also be identified. This information can then be used by families to help make informed decisions regarding pregnancy. The procedure for sample collection does carry some risk, however, so prescreening of parents' blood is critical to ensuring that an infant is truly at risk for disease, and the implications of a positive result should be carefully considered prior to testing.

THALASSEMIA

By Jane Chen Huang, M.D.,
and LoAnn Peterson, M.D.
Chicago, Illinois

Thalassemia is a hereditary disorder of hemoglobin production with decreased or absent synthesis of structurally normal globin chains. It is a quantitative disorder, in contrast with structural hemoglobinopathies, such as sickle cell anemia. Thalassemias are complex and heterogeneous and are classified according to the type of globin chain that is deficient. Synthesis of α chains is decreased or absent in α-thalassemias, and the production of β chains is impaired

Table 1. Composition of Hemoglobins

Hb A ($\alpha_2\beta_2$)
Hb A_2 ($\alpha_2\delta_2$)
Hb F ($\alpha_2\gamma_2$)
Hb Bart's (γ_4)
Hb H (β_4)
Hb^{CS} ($\alpha_2{}^{CS}\beta_2$)*
Hb Lepore ($\alpha_2[\delta\beta]_2$)†
Hb E ($\alpha_2\beta_2{}^{26Glu\rightarrow Lys}$)

*CS = Constant Spring.
†[δβ] refers to fused globin chain with parts of δ and β chains.

in β-thalassemias. Gamma- and delta-thalassemias also exist, but are much less common. Furthermore, combined thalassemias also occur (i.e., δβ-thalassemia).

The word thalassemia is derived from the Greek term for "sea in the blood," referring specifically to the Mediterranean Sea. The Mediterranean region, including Italy, Greece, and Sicily, has a high prevalence of thalassemia. Thalassemia is also very common in Africa and Asia. These tropical and subtropical regions of the world are also endemic for malaria. The thalassemic trait may confer protection against the *Plasmodium* parasites.

The $\alpha^0\beta^0$ designations represent total absence of α or β globin chain production from the corresponding gene, and the α^+/β^+ symbols refer to decreased synthesis. Anemia in thalassemias is caused by two basic mechanisms. First, there is a production problem, with decreased synthesis of the various globin chains and, hence, decreased synthesis of hemoglobin. The decreased amount of hemoglobin in the red blood cells causes hypochromia and microcytosis, resulting in a thalassemic blood picture. Second, an excess of globin chains results from the normal globin genes. The amount of excess, unpaired globin chains is the major determinant in the severity of the clinical disease. The unpaired chains aggregate and precipitate within the cells, cause membrane damage, and lead to premature destruction of erythroid precursors within the bone marrow and hemolysis of the red blood cells. The end result is ineffective erythropoiesis and peripheral hemolysis.

β-THALASSEMIAS

The β globin gene cluster, located on the short arm of chromosome 11, consists of two γ (A_γ and G_γ), one β, and one δ gene. The resulting non-α chains determine the various types of hemoglobin (Hb) that are observed (Table 1). Normal adults have approximately 96 per cent Hb A, 3 per cent Hb A_2, and 1 per cent Hb F. In contrast, newborns have predominantly Hb F (80 per cent) and about 20 per cent Hb A. The switch from γ to β chain synthesis occurs just before birth, and normal adult hemoglobin composition is reached by 6 months of life.

Most of the molecular defects underlying β-thalassemias are point mutations in the β gene. Various terms have been used to refer to the degree of clinical severity. Thalassemia minor/trait usually does not cause symptoms, and affected individuals are only mildly anemic. Thalassemia major is the most severe clinical expression of this disorder, in which the patients are transfusion-dependent. Thalassemia intermedia is intermediate in clinical severity; affected persons are moderately anemic and are not transfusion-dependent but may require transfusions in certain "stressful" conditions, such as infections. These terms do not designate any specific genetic mutation.

β-Thalassemia Trait

In β-thalassemia trait, only one β gene is mutated, and the other β gene is normal. Although individuals with thalassemia trait are mildly anemic at most, the identification and diagnosis of such a disorder is clinically important. Such individuals can receive genetic counseling to determine the potential risk of thalassemia in future offspring, and repeat iron studies or iron therapy will be avoided. Affected persons are usually detected by a routine complete blood count (CBC). A typical CBC in thalassemia trait includes a hemoglobin concentration no lower than 10 g/dL, a normal or increased red blood cell count, a mean corpuscular volume (MCV) usually less than 70 fL, and a normal red cell distribution width (RDW).

The main differential diagnosis is iron deficiency anemia (Table 2). Comparison of the various red cell indices provides clues to the correct diagnosis. In thalassemia trait, the decreased MCV is out of proportion with the degree of anemia, which is characteristically very mild. A hemoglobin concentration less than 9 or 10 g/dL makes thalassemia trait unlikely. The RDW, a measure of the degree of anisocytosis, is increased in iron deficiency but is normal or only slightly increased in thalassemia trait. Likewise, the extent of anisopoikilocytosis in the peripheral smears is greater in iron deficiency than in thalassemia trait. In iron deficiency states, elliptocytes and hypochromic microcytes are commonly seen. Target cells and coarse basophilic stippling are typically observed in peripheral blood smears of persons with thalassemia trait. The basophilic stippling represents the aggregated, unpaired α chains in β-thalassemia.

Ultimately, iron studies including serum iron, total iron-binding capacity (TIBC), and serum ferritin may be needed to exclude iron deficiency. In iron deficiency, serum iron is decreased; TIBC is increased; transferrin saturation is depressed (usually less than 15 per cent); and serum ferritin levels are below the reference range. However, a coexistent inflammatory state may cause a spuriously normal ferritin level, because ferritin is an acute-phase reactant. Storage iron in thalassemia is usually increased, with increased ferritin, normal or increased serum iron, decreased or normal TIBC, and increased or normal transferrin satu-

Table 2. Comparison of Laboratory Features of Thalassemia Trait and Iron Deficiency

	Thalassemia Trait	Iron Deficiency
Red blood cell count	Normal or increased	Decreased
Hb/Hct	Slightly decreased	Decreased
MCV	Significantly decreased	Decreased
RDW	Normal	Increased
Blood smear	Slightly hypochromic microcytes	Hypochromic microcytes
	Target cells	Elliptocytes
	Basophilic stippling in β-thalassemia	Anisopoikilocytosis

ration. However, superimposed iron deficiency can occur in thalassemic patients.

The red cell indices and peripheral blood picture may be highly suggestive of thalassemia trait, but they cannot differentiate among β-thalassemia trait, δβ-thalassemia trait, α-thalassemia trait, and thalassemic hemoglobinopathies such as hemoglobin E (Hb E). Following Hb S, Hb E is the second most common hemoglobinopathy in the world; it is especially common in Southeast Asia. The abnormal β^E gene also causes decreased synthesis of the abnormal β chains, and this can result in a blood picture that is indistinguishable from thalassemia. Individuals with Hb E trait are not anemic but show microcytosis and hypochromia in the peripheral blood. Hb E disease (homozygous state) causes a mild microcytic anemia. Therefore, additional tests are needed to confirm β-thalassemia trait. Hemoglobin electrophoresis can exclude structural hemoglobinopathies. Hb E comigrates with Hb C on cellulose acetate at alkaline pH and comigrates with Hb A on citrate agar at acid pH.

Quantitative Hb A_2 and F concentrations should be obtained; β-thalassemia trait causes an increase in Hb A_2 ($\alpha_2\delta_2$) and a slight increase in Hb F ($\alpha_2\gamma_2$). Hb A_2 ranges from 1.5 to 3.5 per cent in normal persons but is increased in β-thalassemia trait, usually more than 3.5 per cent, but not exceeding 6 per cent. Hb F is usually less than 1 per cent in normal adults but is mildly increased to 2 or 3 per cent in about half the patients with β-thalassemia trait. The decreased production of β chains results in a compensatory, increased synthesis of δ and γ chains. Densitometric scanning of hemoglobin electrophoresis gels only provides a rough estimation of the relative proportions of the various hemoglobins. A quantitative Hb A_2 level by chromatography is needed to detect the relatively mild elevation of Hb A_2 in β-thalassemia trait. Quantitative Hb F levels can be determined by the alkali denaturation test, in which all hemoglobins except F are denatured by a strong alkaline solution. The remaining alkali-resistant Hb F is measured spectrophotometrically.

Not all individuals with β-thalassemia trait have increased Hb A_2. A concomitant iron deficiency results in a normal or decreased concentration. In δβ-thalassemia trait with deletion of both the δ and the β genes on one chromosome, Hb A_2 is normal or decreased, but Hb F is increased to an extent greater than that seen in β-thalassemia trait, in the 5 to 10 per cent range. The γδβ-thalassemia trait involves deletion of the γ, δ, and β genes on the same chromosome; therefore, no compensatory rise in Hb A_2 or F occurs.

The relative percentages of the various hemoglobins in persons with the α-thalassemia trait remain the same as in nonthalassemic individuals; therefore, neither Hb A_2 nor Hb F is increased. The diagnosis of α-thalassemia trait is primarily one of exclusion, after other causes of hypochromic, microcytic anemia (e.g., iron deficiency and β-thalassemia trait) have been eliminated. If necessary, the diagnosis can be confirmed by globin chain synthesis studies or DNA analysis.

β-Thalassemia Major

Thalassemia major usually results from mutations of both β genes. Individuals afflicted with this disease are transfusion-dependent for life. It is also known as "Cooley's anemia" after the pediatrician who first described the condition in children of Italian and Greek immigrants in Detroit in 1925. The diagnosis is made early in life, between 6 months and 2 years of life. These infants present with pallor, failure to thrive, severe anemia, and massive hepatosplenomegaly. Inadequately transfused infants develop "chipmunk facies" from bone marrow expansion of the skull and maxilla and are susceptible to fractures from thinned cortices. In addition to the spleen and liver, extramedullary hematopoietic masses may develop in the chest and paraspinal region.

At presentation, the infant is severely anemic with a hemoglobin concentration of 3 to 4 g/dL, but the reticulocyte response is not commensurate with the degree of anemia. The peripheral smear shows striking anisopoikilocytosis with nucleated erythroid precursors, hypochromia, target cells, variable basophilic stippling, microcytes, and red cell fragments. Inclusion bodies full of excess α chains can be seen best with the use of supravital stains. Hemoglobin electrophoresis shows increased proportions of Hb F, ranging from less than 10 per cent to more than 90 per cent. The Kleihauer-Betke stain (see below) shows a heterogeneous distribution of Hb F. Laboratory evidence of hemolysis is manifested by increased indirect bilirubin and lactate dehydrogenase, but decreased haptoglobin.

Study of family members and DNA analysis are needed to confirm a diagnosis of thalassemia major. DNA testing is simplified by the observation that only three to five mutations account for most of the thalassemic genetic defects for a particular ethnic group. With the availability and ease of polymerase chain reaction for DNA amplification, restriction enzyme analyses and dot and reverse-dot hybridization assays that use specific oligonucleotide probes are able to detect specific, known mutations. Southern blotting and direct sequence analysis are also available.

With hypertransfusion regimens, the characteristic facies recedes, and some restoration of normal growth occurs. Besides the maintenance of an adequate hemoglobin level in these patients, adequate iron chelation therapy is of utmost importance in the effort to decrease the morbidity and mortality that results from this disease. Diffuse iron overload is a major problem because of all the blood products these individuals receive on a regular basis and the increased iron absorption by the gastrointestinal tract. Excessive iron deposition in the heart can cause cardiac enlargement and hypertrophy, congestive heart failure, and arrhythmias. Treatment currently consists of chelation regimens that use deferoxamine. Newer forms of therapy, including bone marrow transplantation, drugs for augmenting Hb F production, and gene therapy, appear to be promising, but they are still in the experimental stages.

β-Thalassemia Intermedia

Individuals with thalassemia intermedia usually have a moderate degree of hemolytic anemia but are not transfusion-dependent. The clinical severity is determined by the degree of chain imbalance, which, in turn, can be decreased by three basic mechanisms. Homozygosity or compound heterozygosity for mild β-thalassemia mutations results in thalassemia intermedia instead of thalassemia major, because the mutations are so mild that a relatively high production of β chains is maintained. Second, coinheritance of α-thalassemia mutations causes decreased synthesis of α chains and, therefore, fewer unpaired α chains. Last, conditions that augment γ chain synthesis allow the excess α chains to combine with the increased γ chains to form Hb F. Homozygosity for δβ-thalassemia or Hb Lepore results in mostly Hb F. Hb Lepore is also another thalassemic hemoglobinopathy. It is a structurally abnormal hemoglobin with an abnormal non-α chain composed of a portion of a δ globin chain at the N-terminal end and part of a β globin chain at the C-terminal end. Hb Lepore results from an unequal crossover between δ and β genes on opposite chromosomes; the end result is the absence of normal δ and β genes on the chromosome with the Hb Lepore gene, similar to δβ-thalassemia. It is thalassemic because expression of the Lepore fusion gene is decreased, relative to the normal β gene. Coinheritance of hereditary persistence of fetal hemoglobin also leads to increased Hb F production (see below).

The clinical phenotype of thalassemia intermedia encompasses a wide spectrum. At the mild end, hemoglobin concentrations of 10 to 12 g/dL are maintained. At the opposite end of the spectrum, the individual barely maintains a hemoglobin concentration of 6 g/dL without regular transfusion, and stunted growth and development with skeletal abnormalities are typical with severe disease. The peripheral blood picture also varies, depending on the clinical severity. The smear may show target cells, basophilic stippling, and hypochromia with slight anisopoikilocytosis, or it may show nucleated red blood cells with marked anisopoikilocytosis, red cell fragments, target cells, and large, hypochromic red cells. Hemoglobin electrophoresis may show variable degrees of increased Hb A_2 and F. If the patient has Hb Lepore, an abnormal band comigrating with Hb S on cellulose acetate and with Hb A on citrate agar may be present. Blood transfusions may be required if the patient becomes infected, hypersplenic, or folic acid deficient. These patients also have problems with iron overload from increased gastrointestinal absorption. Splenectomy may be indicated in hypersplenism or symptomatic splenomegaly.

HEREDITARY PERSISTENCE OF FETAL HEMOGLOBIN

As stated earlier, hereditary persistence of fetal hemoglobin (HPFH) is another condition in which Hb F is increased. There are various types of HPFH, deletion-versus-nondeletion and pancellular-versus-heterocellular types. The deletion form of HPFH involves deletion of both the δ and the β genes, which is very similar to δβ-thalassemia, but γ chain synthesis is more efficient. Heterozygous states usually have 20 to 30 per cent Hb F without any hematologic abnormalities. Homozygous individuals have 100 per cent Hb F with a thalassemic blood picture and decreased MCV. Homozygous δβ-thalassemia also has 100 per cent Hb F, but the clinical phenotype is that of thalassemia intermedia. Another potential way of differentiating between HPFH and δβ-thalassemia is to perform a Kleihauer-Betke stain, given that the HPFH is of the pancellular type. The Kleihauer-Betke test is an acid elution test in which all hemoglobins except Hb F are solubilized and eluted in an acidic solution. The aggregated Hb F stays within the red blood cells and picks up the eosin stain. Only red blood cells with Hb F stain red-pink, and normal adult red cells appear as ghosts. In the pancellular form of HPFH, all red blood cells stain. In contrast, the red blood cells in δβ-thalassemia show a "heterocellular" distribution of Hb F in which only a portion of the red blood cells stain. This test is not helpful in certain forms of nondeletion type of HPFH that show a "heterocellular" or uneven distribution of Hb F.

α-THALASSEMIAS

In contrast with β-thalassemias, in which most genetic defects are due to point mutations, most mutations in α-thalassemias are secondary to deletions of the α genes. The α globin gene complex is located on the short arm of chromosome 16 and includes two α genes. The α_2 gene is the dominant gene on the 5′ end, and the α_1 gene is the minor gene on the 3′ end. The expression of the α_2 gene is three times that of the α_1 gene. The less common nondeletional types of α-thalassemic mutations almost always involve the dominant α_2 gene.

Alpha-thalassemias are further classified according to the number of α genes deleted (Table 3). The loss of one α gene results in the silent carrier state; deletion of two genes leads to α-thalassemia trait/minor. Deletion of three α genes causes Hb H (β_4) disease, and loss of all four α genes is incompatible with life, producing Hb Bart's (γ_4) hydrops fetalis. The lack of α globin chains leads to the synthesis of Hb H in adults and Hb Bart's in infants. Hb H is composed of a tetramer of excess β chains, and Hb Bart's is a tetramer of γ chains. The carrier state involves the deletion or mutation of one α gene without any hematologic abnormalities. Normal infants at birth have little or no Hb Bart's (γ_4), but infants who are α-thalassemic carriers contain 1 to 2 per cent Hb Bart's in their peripheral blood.

Alpha-thalassemia trait has been described earlier, in the differential diagnosis of β-thalassemia trait. It can be due to two gene deletions or mutations from one chromosome or one gene deletion or mutation from each of the two chromosomes. In persons of African descent, the inheritance of an α^0 chromosome with both α genes deleted from the same chromosome is virtually never seen; therefore, α-thalassemia trait in such individuals is characterized by the $(-\alpha/-\alpha)$ genotype. In contrast, Asians and people of Mediterranean descent can also have the genotype with both α genes from the same chromosome deleted $(--/\alpha\alpha)$. Analysis of cord blood in these individuals usually reveals 5 to 6 per cent Hb Bart's. In adults, hemoglobin electrophoresis is normal, and definitive diagnosis, if necessary, would require globin chain synthesis studies and/or DNA analysis. Globin chain synthesis studies measure the relative synthetic rates of each chain by utilizing high-pressure liquid chromatography to separate and quantitate the various globin chains. A decreased α-to-β ratio can confirm the diagnosis of α-thalassemia trait with two α gene deletions, or the carrier state with one gene deletion. DNA analysis has largely replaced the globin chain synthesis studies.

In most cases of Hb H disease, three α genes are nonfunctional due to deletion or mutation. It is most commonly seen in Southeast Asia, and it is extremely rare in Africa and in African Americans, because the α^0 haplotype is essentially nonexistent in the latter ethnic group. Hb H (β_4) is very unstable and easily oxidized, causing peripheral hemolysis. It also has a high affinity for oxygen and does not deliver oxygen efficiently.

Table 3. Alpha-Thalassemias

No. of α Genes Affected	Genotype	Clinical Phenotype
1	$-\alpha/\alpha\alpha$	Silent carrier
2	$--/\alpha\alpha$ $-\alpha/-\alpha$	Alpha-thalassemia trait
3	$--/-\alpha$ $--/\alpha^{CS}\alpha$*	Hb H disease
4	$--/--$	Hb Bart's Hydrops fetalis

*CS = Constant Spring.

The clinical severity of Hb H disease is variable, with hemoglobin concentrations ranging from as low as 3 g/dL to as high as 13 g/dL. Splenomegaly and bony changes are variable. The peripheral blood smear shows hypochromia and anisopoikilocytosis with target cells and red cell fragments, depending on the degree of hemolysis. With use of the brilliant cresyl blue stain, pale blue Hb H inclusions are seen in most red blood cells. Hemoglobin electrophoresis demonstrates a fast moving band representing Hb H on cellulose acetate. A small amount of Hb Bart's, which is also fast moving, may also be present. Hb H and Hb Bart's may be missed when the bands are faint and when the interpreter does not specifically look for these bands. In fact, they may be so fast moving that the bands may migrate off the electrophoresis gel. Hb H constitutes 5 to 30 per cent of the circulating hemoglobin, with Hb A the major hemoglobin component. Cord blood in infants with Hb H disease contains 20 to 40 per cent Hb Bart's.

In about 40 per cent of the cases of Hb H disease in Southeast Asia, the mutated α gene for Hb Constant Spring is inherited in conjunction with two other deleted α genes. This hemoglobin constitutes only about 2 per cent of the circulating hemoglobin. A point mutation in the stop codon of the α gene in Hb Constant Spring results in an abnormal, elongated α chain with 172 amino acids instead of the usual 141 amino acids. Hb Constant Spring is represented by a faint, slow moving band on cellulose acetate, migrating between carbonic anhydrase and Hb A_2. A large amount of hemolysate is recommended in the hemoglobin electrophoresis of Asian patients because Hb Constant Spring is common in this ethnic group but is present in low concentrations that are difficult to detect.

Heterozygosity for Hb Constant Spring ($\alpha^{CS}\alpha/\alpha\alpha$) does not cause any hematologic abnormality, and the hemoglobin electrophoresis is normal except for a faint, slow moving band representing Hb Constant Spring. A clinical phenotype similar to Hb H disease is seen in the homozygous state ($\alpha^{CS}\alpha/\alpha^{CS}\alpha$) with 5 to 6 per cent Hb Constant Spring, a small amount of Hb Bart's, a normal concentration of Hb A_2, and Hb A constituting the remainder of the circulating hemoglobin with no Hb H. Red cell indices are not characteristic of thalassemia, and no hypochromia or microcytosis is seen. Acquired forms of Hb H disease have been described in patients with myeloproliferative disorders and have been associated with mental retardation.

Deletion of all four α genes results in Hb Bart's hydrops fetalis. It is almost exclusively seen in Southeast Asia, where the prevalence of the α^0 haplotype is high. This condition is incompatible with life; affected infants are stillborn and appear edematous and pale with massive hepatosplenomegaly. They are severely anemic with mostly Hb Bart's and small amounts of Hb H, but no Hb A or Hb F. The peripheral blood smear shows numerous nucleated red blood cells and large, hypochromic red cells with marked anisopoikilocytosis.

INTERACTION OF THALASSEMIAS WITH HEMOGLOBINOPATHIES

Coinheritance of thalassemias and hemoglobinopathies is common in areas that have a high prevalence of both disorders. The most common hemoglobinopathies associated with β-thalassemia include Hb S, C, and E. Double heterozygosity for HbS/β-thalassemia results in a clinical picture similar to that of sickle cell disease, especially when the thalassemic defect is β^0. The amount of Hb S in this condition is more than what is seen in sickle cell trait; such an individual may have 60 to 90 per cent Hb S, 0 to 30 per cent Hb A, increased Hb A_2, and 5 to 15 per cent Hb F. The peripheral smear shows some sickled cells, along with the usual thalassemic features. Hb C/β-thalassemia is seen mainly in blacks and causes a mild hemolytic anemia with splenomegaly. The electrophoretic pattern depends on the severity of the β-thalassemia, but the amount of Hb C is more than Hb C trait alone. The peripheral blood smear contains numerous target cells, which are characteristically seen in Hb C disorders along with other thalassemic features. Hb E/β-thalassemia is most common in Thailand and Southeast Asia. Most often a β^0-thalassemia is inherited together with Hb E, resulting in severe clinical disease, similar to thalassemia major. About 50 per cent Hb F and 50 per cent Hb E with no Hb A are typically found in the hemoglobin electrophoresis. Findings in peripheral blood include anisopoikilocytosis, hypochromia, microcytosis, target cells, and nucleated red blood cells.

Compound heterozygosity for Hb S and α-thalassemia results in less Hb S than sickle cell trait because the abnormal β^S chains cannot compete as efficiently as the normal β chains for the decreased numbers of α chains. Thalassemic red blood cell indices and peripheral blood findings remain the same. Coinheritance of α^0-thalassemia with α chain variants such as Hb $G^{Philadelphia}$ and Hb Q usually results in Hb H–like disease in which the circulating hemoglobin consists of the abnormal hemoglobin and Hb H.

HEMOLYTIC ANEMIA CAUSED BY ERYTHROCYTE ENZYME DEFICIENCY

By Imad A. Tabbara, M.D.,
and Chitra Venkatraman, M.D.
Washington, D.C.

During the process of maturation, the erythrocyte loses its capacity for protein synthesis and oxidative phosphorylation. As a result, the mature red blood cell (RBC) generates energy through anaerobic glycolysis via the Embden-Meyerhof (EM) pathway, through oxidative glycolysis via the hexose monophosphate (HMP) shunt, and through nucleotide salvage pathways. Several enzyme deficiencies that influence these pathways have been reported to cause hereditary hemolytic anemia (Table 1). These enzymopathies are typically inherited as autosomal recessive disorders except for X-linked glucose-6-phosphate dehydrogenase (G-6-PD) deficiency and X-linked phosphoglycerate kinase (PGK) deficiency (Table 2).

Most of the RBC adenosine triphosphate (ATP) is synthesized through the EM pathway (Fig. 1), and about 90 per cent of RBC glucose is converted to lactate via this pathway. Thus, an enzyme deficiency that affects this pathway causes decreased RBC ATP. The ATP-deficient RBCs are rigid and are removed from the circulation by the spleen. The HMP shunt is the major source of reduced nicotinamide-adenine dinucleotide (NADH) in RBCs, and about 10 per cent of the glucose consumed is metabolized via this pathway. On exposure to certain oxidants, normal RBCs increase the amount of glucose metabolized through the

Table 1. Hereditary Hemolytic Disorders

Erythrocyte Membrane Defects

Hereditary spherocytosis
Hereditary pyropoikilocytosis
Hereditary elliptocytosis

Erythrocyte Enzyme Defects

Defects in Glucose Metabolism

Enzymopathies of the Embden-Meyerhof (EM) pathway
- Hexokinase
- Phosphofructokinase
- Glucose phosphate isomerase
- Triosephosphate isomerase
- Phosphoglycerate kinase
- Pyruvate kinase

Enzymopathy of the hexose monophosphate pathway
- Glucose-6-phosphate dehydrogenase (G-6-PD)

Defects in Glutathione Metabolism

Glutathione reductase
Glutathione peroxidase
Glutathione glutamyl cysteine synthetase
Glutathione synthetase

Defects in Nucleotide Metabolism

Adenylate kinase
Adenosine deaminase
Pyrimidine 5′-nucleotidase

Erythrocyte Na^+/K^+ Pump Defects

Hereditary stomatocytosis
Hereditary xerocytosis

Hemoglobinopathies

Sickling disorders
Thalassemias
Unstable hemoglobin hemolytic diseases

shunt. This regenerates the reduced glutathione that protects erythrocytes against oxidant insult. In patients with enzyme deficiency of the HMP shunt (see Fig. 1), the RBCs cannot make sufficient reduced glutathione. As a result, the sulfhydryl groups of hemoglobin are oxidized, hemoglobin is precipitated, and Heinz bodies are formed.

HISTORY AND PHYSICAL FINDINGS

Knowledge of the duration of hemolysis is helpful in the differential diagnosis of hemolytic anemia. Lifelong hemolysis suggests an inherited disorder, whereas a history of episodic hemolysis associated with ingestion of certain drugs or foods or physiologic stresses such as surgery and infections is typically seen in patients with G-6-PD deficiency. A thorough family history can determine the mode of inheritance of certain enzyme deficiencies. Because most enzyme deficiencies of the EM pathway display an autosomal recessive pattern of inheritance, screening of family members can be valuable. By contrast, adenosine deaminase (AD) deficiency is transmitted as an autosomal dominant trait with clinical manifestations in successive generations and in both sexes. In patients with chronic hemolysis, icteric sclerae and splenomegaly are commonly present, whereas the physical examination may be normal in patients with enzyme deficiencies that are manifested clinically as episodic hemolysis.

LABORATORY EVALUATION

The diagnosis of hemolytic anemia caused by the RBC enzyme deficiencies typically requires exclusion of other causes of hemolysis. The presence of spherocytes, elliptocytes, acanthocytes, or schistocytes in the peripheral smear suggests that the hemolytic process is not secondary to RBC enzyme deficiencies, which are usually manifested by macrocytic and spiculated RBCs on peripheral smear. Basophilic stippling is seen in pyrimidine 5′-nucleotidase (P5N) deficiency as well as in lead poisoning.

Patients with enzyme deficiencies affecting the EM pathway have a congenital, nonspherocytic hemolytic anemia. The peripheral smear shows normocytic, normochromic RBCs and reticulocytosis. The osmotic fragility of fresh RBCs is normal; however, fragility increases when these cells are incubated. Increased unconjugated serum bilirubin, low or absent serum haptoglobin, increased serum lactate dehydrogenase (LD), and erythroid hyperplasia of the bone marrow are commonly noted. Severe intravascular hemolysis causing hemoglobinemia, hemoglobinuria, and hemosiderinuria is rare but has been documented in patients with severe hemolysis secondary to G-6-PD deficiency.

The clinical characteristics of a patient undergoing hemolysis provide insufficient information for a diagnostic evaluation. Thus, if hemolysis is acquired, a direct antiglobulin (Coombs') test should be performed as an initial

Table 2. Red Cell Enzyme Deficiencies

Enzyme	Inheritance	Frequency	Anemia	Clinical Features
Hexokinase	Autosomal recessive	Rare	Mild to severe	None
Glucose phosphate isomerase	Autosomal recessive	Unusual	Moderate to severe	None
Phosphofructokinase	Autosomal recessive	Rare	Mild	Myopathy
Aldolase	Autosomal recessive	Very rare	Moderate to severe	Mental retardation
Triosephosphate isomerase	Autosomal recessive	Rare	Moderate to severe	Cardiomyopathy and neuropathies
Phosphoglycerate kinase	X-linked	Rare	Mild to severe	Myoglobinuria and mental retardation
Pyruvate kinase	Autosomal recessive	Rare	Mild to severe	None
Glucose-6-phosphate dehydrogenase	X-linked	Common in certain ethnic groups	Moderate to severe	None
Glutathione reductase	—	Very rare	Mild	None
Glutathione synthetase	Autosomal recessive	Rare	Mild	Mental retardation, 5-oxoprolinuria
Pyrimidine 5′-nucleotidase	Autosomal recessive	Rare	Mild	? Mental retardation
Adenosine deaminase (excess)	Autosomal dominant	Rare	Mild	None

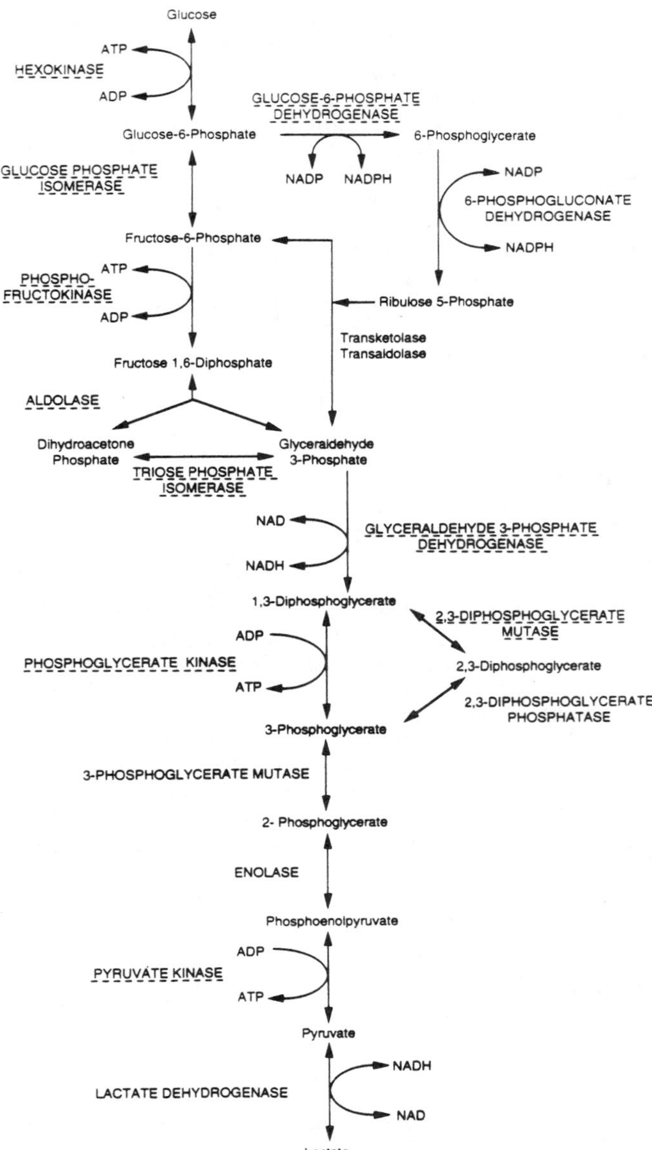

Figure 1. The Embden-Meyerhof (EM) and hexose monophosphate (HMP) (pentose shunt) pathways. It has been reported that deficiencies of the underlined enzymes cause hemolytic anemia.

screening measure. If hemolysis is congenital, initial testing should include hemoglobin electrophoresis, measurement of osmotic fragility, and analysis of G-6-PD and pyruvate kinase (PK) activities. If these tests do not reveal the cause of hemolysis, screening for other enzyme deficiencies can be performed in highly specialized laboratories. The yield, however, is usually limited. Most of the RBC enzyme assays employ spectrophotometric measurement of the rate of change in the absorbance of ultraviolet light at 340 nm by NADH or reduced nicotinamide-adenine dinucleotide phosphate (NADPH).

ENZYME DEFICIENCIES OF THE EMBDEN-MEYERHOF PATHWAY

Hexokinase Deficiency

Because it is the first enzyme in the glycolytic pathway, HK is a major determinant of glucose consumption. HK activity decreases quickly as the erthrocyte matures. Decreased HK activity may result from a quantitative defect in a normal enzyme or the inheritance of a functionally abnormal enzyme. Since young RBCs have increased activity, normal HK activity can be seen with increased reticulocytosis. Thus, to avoid a false-positive test result, HK activity should always be corrected for the extent of reticulocytosis. The degree of hemolytic anemia can vary from mild to severe, and periodic transfusions may be required. RBC morphologic features are typically unremarkable except for reticulocytosis, polychromatophilia, and a few spherocytes. The enzyme assay links the HK reaction with G-6-PD–catalyzed reduction of NADP to NADPH, causing an increase in optical density at 340 nm.

Glucosephosphate Isomerase Deficiency

Glucosephosphate isomerase (GPI) deficiency is the third most common hemolytic enzymopathy after G-6-PD and PK deficiencies. Although this enzyme is produced in all cells, hemolytic anemia of variable severity is most often the only clinical manifestation because mature RBCs are the only cells unable to accelerate synthesis of the enzyme to maintain a steady state. In these rare patients, in whom glucosephosphate isomerase deficiency is severe and generalized, hemolysis is accompanied by myopathy, ataxia, and mental retardation. The peripheral smear typically reveals poikilocytosis, anisocytosis, marked polychromatophilia, and extreme reticulocytosis.

Phosphofructokinase Deficiency

Phosphofructokinase (PFK) is a tetrameric enzyme that contains one or more of three distinct subunits known as M (muscle), L (granulocytes), and F (fibroblasts, platelets). Erythrocyte PFK is a tetramer of L subunits. The clinical manifestations of PFK deficiency reflect the variable expression of subunits in different tissues. PFK deficiency may be associated with myopathy alone, hemolysis alone, or a combination of the two. The hemolysis is usually mild and often compensated. A fresh blood sample should be used for PFK assay because the activity of the enzyme decreases rapidly if blood is not stored at 4°C in ethylenediamine tetraacetic acid (EDTA), heparin, or acid-citrate-dextrose.

Triosephosphate Isomerase Deficiency

Triosephosphate isomerase (TPI) is coded by a single structural gene on chromosome 12 and is present in all tissues. TPI deficiency is associated with autosomal recessive inheritance and may lead to a progressive multisystem syndrome. Hemolytic anemia and hyperbilirubinemia occur in early life, and affected patients may require frequent blood transfusions. Within the first year of life, spasticity, paresthesia, weakness, and mental retardation may develop. Cardiac arrhythmias and recurrent systemic infections have been reported and can be fatal. A provisional diagnosis can be made using a spot test. Prenatal diagnosis is made by measuring the stability of the enzyme in cultured fibroblasts and amniocytes. In this enzyme assay, the rate of decline in absorbance of NADH is measured by linking the TPI reaction with the α-glycerophosphate dehydrogenase reaction.

Phosphoglycerate Kinase Deficiency

PGK deficiency is the only X-linked enzyme deficiency affecting the RBC-EM pathway. PGK-deficient males develop normally until age 4 to 5 years, when behavioral aberrations, motor regression, and cerebellar tremors become apparent.

Pyruvate Kinase Deficiency

PK deficiency is the most common enzyme deficiency involving the EM pathway. It has a worldwide, multiracial distribution, with several hundred patients reported. PK catalyzes the conversion of phosphoenolpyruvate (PEP) to pyruvate, and during this process ATP is generated. PK deficiency results in impaired glycolysis and diminished capacity to produce ATP. Clinical expression is highly variable and ranges from severe hemolytic anemia in neonates to fully compensated hemolysis in adults. As a rule, anemia or jaundice, or both, are recognized in infancy or early childhood.

The clinical and hematologic features of PK deficiency are nonspecific. The peripheral smear shows a significant number of spiculated RBCs, tailed poikilocytes, and acanthocytes. The screening test is based on the fluorescence of NADH under ultraviolet light. The patient's blood is first mixed with PEP, LD, and NADH and is then incubated. This mixture is then spotted on filter paper so that fluorescence can be measured. If the spot test is abnormal, an assay for the enzyme may confirm the diagnosis.

The enzyme assay is performed on hemolysate freed of leukocytes because white blood cells (WBCs) possess 300 times the PK activity of normal RBCs. In this test, PEP is used as the substrate for PK. The rate of formation of pyruvate is measured by linking it to the oxidation of NADH to NAD when pyruvate is converted to lactate by LD. The decrease in optical density resulting from the oxidation of NADH is measured. This assay should employ two substrate concentrations (high and low) because some mutations are associated with formation of an enzyme that displays near-normal activity at high substrate concentration but reduced activity at low substrate concentration.

DEFECTS OF NUCLEOTIDE METABOLISM

Pyrimidine 5′-Nucleotidase Deficiency

Ribosomal RNA of reticulocytes is degraded to 5′-nucleotides such as cytidine, thymidine, and uridine monophosphate by the pyrimidine 5′-nucleotidase (P5N) enzyme. In P5N deficiency, these nondiffusible catabolites form large aggregates, which are seen as basophilic stippling on Wright-stained blood smears. In the screening test for P5N activity, RBCs are mixed with perchloric acid to extract purine and pyrimidine. The extract is then analyzed by spectrophotometry for pyrimidine accumulation. The absorption wavelength for pyrimidine nucleotides is 270 nm, and normal RBCs show no peak at this wavelength, since 5′-nucleotides are dephosphorylated by P5N. In P5N deficiency, a large peak representing abnormal pyrimidine is observed at 270 nm.

Adenylate Kinase Deficiency

Adenylate kinse (AK) catalyzes the formation of ATP and adenosine monophosphate (AMP) from 2 molecules of adenosine diphosphate (ADP). This is a rare enzymopathy, and hemolytic anemia of moderate severity has been described in few subjects. In this enzyme assay, the AK reaction is linked to PK and LD reactions, with end point measurement of the decrease in optical density at 340 nm resulting from oxidation of NADH to NAD.

Hyperactivity of Adenosine Deaminase

AD catalyzes the deamination of adenosine to inosine. AD deficiency has been associated with immune deficiency states, and a 40- to 70-fold increased activity of the enzyme has been associated with chronic hemolytic anemia. This enzyme is transmitted by autosomal dominant genes. The enzyme activity is measured by the decrease in optical density at 265 nm resulting from the conversion of adenosine to inosine.

ENZYME DEFICIENCIES OF THE HEXOSE MONOPHOSPHATE SHUNT

Glucose-6-Phosphate Dehydrogenase Deficiency

G-6-PD deficiency is the most prevalent inborn error of erythrocyte metabolism in the world. The enzymatically active form of G-6-PD is either a dimer or a tetramer. There is only one structural gene for G-6-PD in the human genome, and it is located on the long arm of the X chromosome (band Xq28).

Many G-6-PD variants have been detected and distinguished on the basis of electrophoretic mobility, biochemical characteristics, the ability to use the substrate analog, the K_m for NADP and G-6-PD, the pH activity profile, and thermal stability. The normal enzyme is designated G-6-PD-B and is seen in more than 99 per cent of whites and 70 per cent of African Americans. More than 180 variants have been described, but only a few are clinically significant. G-6-PD-A+ is the most frequent African American variant and is seen in 20 per cent of this population. G-6-PD-A+ has normal activity but increased electrophoretic mobility. G-6-PD-A− is seen in 10 per cent of African Americans and has the same electrophoretic mobility as G-6-PD-A+ but only 5 to 15 per cent activity. G-6-PD Mediterranean variant is seen in Mediterranean, Indian, and Southeast Asian populations. Its prevalence among Greeks, Sardinians, and Sephardic Jews ranges from 5 to 50 per cent. Other G-6-PD variants are seen in Asian populations.

G-6-PD deficiencies have been divided into five classes based on clinical severity and the degree of enzyme deficiency. Class 1 variant is characterized by chronic hemolysis without precipitating causes. Class 2 and 3 variants make up 90 per cent of G-6-PD deficiency states. These two groups of patients experience acute hemolysis when they are exposed to oxidant drugs, physiologic stresses, or certain foods such as fava beans. The Mediterranean variant is the most prevalent class 2 deficiency state. In this condition, the enzyme is synthesized in subnormal amounts and is also unstable. In African Americans with the G-6-PD-A− variant, the half-life of the enzyme is about 50 per cent of normal. Following a hemolytic episode, the remaining young RBCs may have near-normal amounts of G-6-PD, and as a result, hemolysis will stop in African Americans with G-6-PD-A− even if oxidant exposure continues. However, in whites with G-6-PD Mediterranean variant, almost all RBCs are oxidant-sensitive and hemolysis may be fatal. Class 4 and 5 variants are clinically harmless.

The classic manifestations of G-6-PD deficiency include neonatal jaundice and acute hemolytic anemia. Neonatal jaundice secondary to G-6-PD deficiency differs from the classic Rh-related neonatal jaundice in that its peak incidence occurs between days 2 and 3, and the jaundice is more pronounced compared with the anemia.

Available screening tests for G-6-PD deficiency include the dye decolorization test, the methemoglobin reduction test, and the fluorescence test. All are semiquantitative and essentially define a blood sample as normal or deficient. Every abnormal screening test should be confirmed by a spectrophotometric assay. Testing should be performed in a steady state rather than in posthemolytic periods because young RBCs have substantially higher G-6-PD activity than do aged RBCs. However, in patients with the Mediterranean variant, the assay can be performed at any stage because even the youngest RBCs have limited G-6-PD activity. The G-6-PD assay measures the rate of increase in absorbance caused by the formation of NADPH. The hemolysate must be free of leukocytes because they have a very high concentration of G-6-PD. In normal RBCs, the range of G-6-PD activity measured at 30°C is 7 to 10 IU/g hemoglobin.

DEFECTS IN GLUTATHIONE METABOLISM

Glutathione Reductase Deficiency

The activity of glutathione is dependent on riboflavin in the diet. Patients with riboflavin deficiency have low enzyme activity that can be restored to normal with administration of riboflavin. Genetically determined glutathione reductase deficiency has been reported in only a few patients. The fluorescent spot test can be used as a screening method.

Glutathione Peroxidase Deficiency

Glutathione peroxidase (GSH-Px) catalyzes the oxidation of reduced glutathione by peroxides such as hydrogen peroxide and organic hydroperoxides. This enzymopathy results in mild hemolytic anemia. Acquired deficiency of this enzyme has been reported in patients with iron and selenium deficiencies, cirrhosis of the liver, and Glanzmann's thrombasthenia. The enzyme assay links the glutathione peroxidase reaction to the glutathione reductase reaction and measures decreased absorbance resulting from the oxidation of NADPH.

γ-Glutamyl Cysteine Synthetase Deficiency

γ-Glutamyl cysteine synthetase catalyzes the formation of γ-glutamyl cysteine. Deficiency of this enzyme causes a mild congenital hemolytic anemia associated with myopathy, neuropathy, spinocerebellar degeneration, and psychosis developing in early adulthood.

Glutathione Synthetase Deficiency

Glutathione formation is catalyzed by glutathione synthetase (GSH synthetase). Severe GSH deficiency has been reported to cause a syndrome characterized by mild hemolytic anemia, metabolic acidosis, cerebral and cerebellar degeneration, mental retardation, and 5-oxoprolinuria. Episodes of hemolysis can be precipitated by consumption of fava beans. In the screening test for this enzyme deficiency, GSH concentration in RBCs is assayed.

ENZYME DEFICIENCIES OF DOUBTFUL CLINICAL SIGNIFICANCE

Congenital deficiencies of the RBC enzymes 2-3 diphosphoglycerate mutase, glyceraldehyde-3-phosphate dehydrogenase, enolase, aldolase, lactate dehydrogenase, and adenosine triphosphatase (ATPase) have been reported in association with chronic hemolytic anemia. However, a causal relationship between these enzymes deficiencies and hematologic abnormalities has not been established.

Acquired deficiency of the preceding enzymes is more prevalent than the inherited form and is seen in patients with myelodysplastic and myeloproliferative syndromes and acute leukemias.

ANTENATAL DIAGNOSIS

Antenatal diagnosis can be achieved by measuring fetal RBC enzyme activity as early as the 17th week of pregnancy. Gene probes are available for many RBC enzymopathies. Lestas and colleagues characterized the normal activities of at least 12 glycolytic enzymes in fetal RBCs at 17 to 24 weeks of gestation, and these reference values can be used in screening for RBC enzymopathies.

SUMMARY

Erythrocyte enzyme deficiencies are one of the common causes of hereditary hemolytic anemia. More than 150 million individuals have G-6-PD deficiency, which is the most common cause of hereditary hemolysis. Enzyme deficiencies affecting the glycolytic pathway are rare with PK deficiency, accounting for 95 per cent of cases. Although improved assays for RBC enzymes are available, some of the hemolytic disorders remain difficult to diagnose. However, progress in molecular biology and gene therapy may improve the accuracy and frequency of diagnosis and enhance the possibility of useful treatment.

The authors thank Connie Ghazal for her technical expertise in preparing the manuscript.

HEREDITARY SPHEROCYTOSIS, HEREDITARY ELLIPTOCYTOSIS, AND RELATED DISORDERS

By Patrick G. Gallagher, M.D.
New Haven, Connecticut

HEREDITARY SPHEROCYTOSIS

Hereditary spherocytosis (HS) refers to a group of disorders characterized by spherical, doughnut-shaped erythrocytes in the peripheral blood. HS affects approximately 1 in 4000 to 5000 individuals in the United States and England. It is the most common inherited anemia in individuals of northern European ancestry and is much more common in whites than in African Americans. This group of disorders is characterized by clinical, laboratory, and genetic heterogeneity. Inheritance is autosomal dominant in approximately three quarters of patients. In the remaining patients, HS is the result of a de novo mutation or an autosomal recessive pattern of inheritance.

Pathophysiology

The primary defect in HS is the loss of erythrocyte membrane surface area, resulting in decreased cellular deformability. Splenic destruction of these abnormal erythrocytes is the primary cause of the hemolysis experienced by HS patients. Physical entrapment of erythrocytes in the splenic microcirculation and ingestion by phagocytes have been proposed as mechanisms of destruction. Furthermore, the splenic environment is hostile to erythrocytes. Low pH, low glucose and adenosine triphosphate (ATP) concentrations, and high local concentrations of toxic free radicals produced by adjacent phagocytes all contribute to membrane damage. The loss of surface area is the basis for laboratory diagnosis of this condition (see further on).

The loss of erythrocyte membrane is due to defects in several membrane proteins, including α-spectrin, β-spectrin, ankyrin, band 3 (the anion transporter), and pallidin. Qualitative and/or quantitative defects of one or more of these membrane proteins lead to membrane instability, which, in turn, leads to membrane loss. In some cases, the precise molecular defects have been identified. Like the clinical and laboratory manifestations of HS, the genetic defects are heterogeneous; multiple genetic loci are implicated and various abnormalities, including gene deletions, point mutations, and mRNA processing defects, have been described.

Signs and Symptoms

The clinical manifestations of HS are variable. The classic triad of anemia, jaundice, and splenomegaly is found in about two thirds of HS patients. Jaundice is intermittent and is less pronounced in childhood. Uncommon manifestations include chronic ankle skin ulceration, gout, and chronic leg dermatitis. Very rare accompanying manifestations include cardiomyopathy, spinal cord dysfunction, movement disorders, and extramedullary hematopoietic tumors. In severe untreated HS, poor growth and findings attributable to extramedullary hematopoiesis (such as skull and hand deformities) may be found.

In general, affected individuals of the same kindred experience similar degrees of disease. Rarely, members of the same kindred will experience varying degrees of hemolysis.

Course and Outcome

Many HS patients are rarely symptomatic and are diagnosed during evaluation for unrelated conditions. Although most HS patients have red blood cells with a life span of 20 to 30 days (normal = 120 days), they often compensate adequately for hemolysis by increased erythropoiesis. It is only when complications occur, usually related to anemia or chronic hemolysis, that these patients seek medical attention.

The markedly shortened life span of the HS erythrocyte predicts that symptoms will develop if anemia occurs. These anemic episodes have been described as "crises" because the severity of anemia may require intensive medical therapy. Aplastic crises often follow virally induced bone marrow suppression and present with anemia, jaundice, fever, and vomiting. The most common cause of aplastic crisis in HS patients is parvovirus B-19. Parvovirus selectively invades erythrocyte progenitor cells, leading to a 7- to 10-day period of red cell aplasia. This infection is tolerated without a significant drop in hematocrit in normal individuals, whereas individuals with HS may experience a life-threatening illness with sudden onset of severe anemia and reticulocytopenia. "Family outbreaks of HS," in which entire HS kindreds have come to medical attention because of a household epidemic of parvovirus B-19 infection, are well documented.

Hemolytic crises, typically associated with viral illness and occurring before 6 years of age, are usually mild and present with jaundice, increased spleen size, and a drop in hematocrit. Some of these patients may actually be in the recovery phase of an aplastic crisis. A third, preventable crisis is the megaloblastic crisis that occurs in HS patients with increased folate demands (e.g., pregnant patients, growing children, or patients recovering from an aplastic crisis).

Chronic hemolysis leads to the formation of bilirubinate gallstones, the most frequently reported complication in HS patients. Although gallstones have been observed in infancy, most appear in adolescents and young adults. Routine management should include interval ultrasonography to detect gallstones because many patients with cholelithiasis and HS are asymptomatic. Typically, an HS patient presents with sudden onset of unusually severe jaundice accompanied by indirect and direct hyperbilirubinemia. In these patients, a bilirubinate gallstone has migrated out of the liver and is entrapped in the biliary tree.

Finally, HS may escape detection until old age. With senescence, bone marrow function wanes. The previously well compensated hemolysis becomes more apparent, and anemia develops. This anemia is aggravated by folate deficiency in some elderly patients.

Laboratory Findings

As in the clinical presentation of HS, laboratory findings in HS are heterogeneous. Erythrocyte morphologic characteristics are variable. Typical HS patients have blood smears with easily identifiable spherocytes lacking central pallor (Fig. 1). Less commonly, patients present with only a few spherocytes on peripheral smear or, at the other end of the spectrum, with numerous small, dense spherocytes and bizarre erythrocyte morphologic features with anisocytosis and poikilocytosis. Specific morphologic findings, including pincered erythrocytes, ovalocytic and stomatocytic spherocytes, and acanthocytes may be correlated with specific membrane protein defects. Because spherocytes are a common artifact in peripheral smears, the erythrocytes must be well separated, and the field of examination must contain some red cells with central pallor.

The mean corpuscular hemoglobin concentration (MCHC) is increased (35 to 38) because of relative cellular dehydration. The mean corpuscular volume (MCV) is usually normal or slightly decreased.

In the normal erythrocyte, a redundancy of cell membrane gives the cell its characteristic discoid shape and abundant surface area. In spherocytes, a decrease in surface area relative to cell volume produces the abnormal

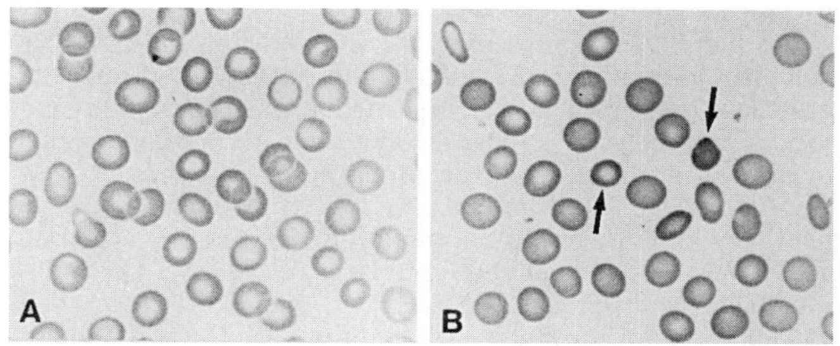

Figure 1. Peripheral blood smears. *A,* Normal. *B,* Typical hereditary spherocytosis. Characteristic spherocytes lacking central pallor are seen (*arrows*).

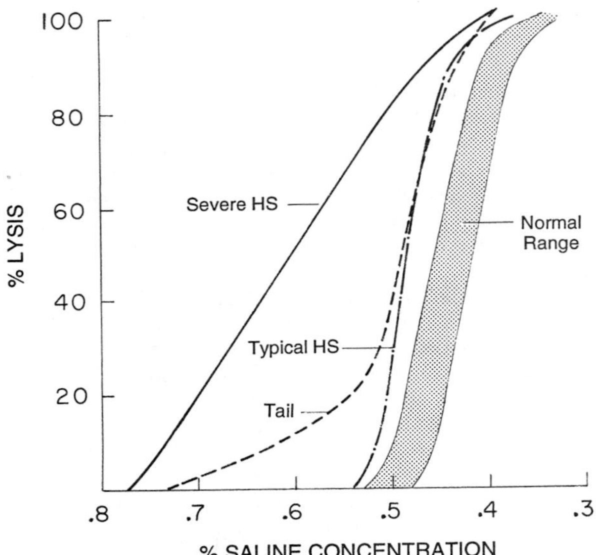

Figure 2. Osmotic fragility curves in hereditary spherocytosis. The shaded area is the normal range. Results representative of both typical and severe spherocytosis are shown. A "tail," representing very fragile erythrocytes that have been conditioned by the spleen, is common in many HS patients prior to splenectomy.

shape and increased osmotic fragility found in these cells. Osmotic fragility is examined by adding increasingly hypotonic concentrations of saline to red cells (Fig. 2). The normal erythrocyte is able to increase its volume by swelling, but spherocytes, which are already at maximal volume for surface area, burst at higher than normal saline concentrations. Approximately one quarter of individuals with HS will have normal osmotic fragility on freshly drawn red blood cells, with the osmotic fragility curve approximating the number of spherocytes seen on peripheral smear. However, after incubation at 37°C for 24 hours, HS red cells lose membrane surface area more readily than normal because their membranes are leaky and unstable. Thus, incubation accentuates the defect in HS erythrocytes, making incubated osmotic fragility the standard test in diagnosing HS. When the spleen is present, a subpopulation of very fragile erythrocytes that have been conditioned by the spleen form the "tail" of the osmotic fragility curve. This tail disappears after splenectomy. Unfortunately, the osmotic fragility test suffers from poor sensitivity, with as many as 20 per cent of mild cases of HS missed after incubation. The osmotic fragility test is unreliable in patients who have small numbers of spherocytes, including those who have undergone recent transfusion. It is also abnormal in other conditions in which spherocytes are present as well as in bacterial sepsis.

Autohemolysis of erythrocytes after 48 hours at 37°C is normally less than 5 per cent in the absence of glucose or less than 1 per cent in the presence of glucose. Autohemolysis of spherocytes is increased to 15 to 45 per cent in the absence of glucose. In HS, the degree of autohemolysis is reduced by the addition of glucose, whereas in acquired disorders such as immune-mediated anemias, the degree of autohemolysis is not reduced. Thus, if positive, the autohemolysis test suggests an intrinsic red cell abnormality, whereas a negative test result is noncontributory. Although this differentiation may be helpful, the autohemolysis test is time-consuming, cumbersome, highly variable, and rarely performed today.

The acidified glycerol test is based on the rate rather than the extent of hemolysis. Its accuracy increases if the samples to be tested are incubated for a day prior to testing. Its results are positive in pregnancy and renal failure, and it suffers from interlaboratory variability. A modification of the original glycerol lysis test, the "Pink test," is claimed to be more accurate that the original test. Neither test enjoys widespread use.

Other laboratory abnormalities in HS are manifestations of ongoing hemolysis. Increased serum bilirubin levels, increased urinary and fecal urobilinogen concentrations, and decreased serum haptoglobin levels reflect increased erythrocyte destruction. Haptoglobin may be decreased or absent in neonates and thus is an unreliable marker of hemolysis in the newborn.

Specialized testing is available if additional information is desired. Potentially useful tests include erythrocyte membrane protein quantitation, limited tryptic digestion of spectrin, spectrin self-association studies, and ion transport. Membrane rigidity and fragility may be examined with an ektacytometer When a molecular diagnosis is desired, cDNA and genomic DNA analyses are available.

Members of the family of an HS patient should be examined for the presence of HS. Identification of HS can be of great epidemiologic importance, particularly for very old and very young patients.

Differential Diagnosis

Acquired spherocytic anemias may easily be confused with the HS syndromes because both groups of disorders have spherocytes on peripheral blood smears (Table 1) and abnormalities of osmotic fragility. The most common cause of an acquired spherocytosis syndrome is an autoimmune process with circulating, warm-reacting IgG (or less commonly, IgA) autoantibodies. This condition, frequently referred to as autoimmune hemolytic anemia, may be associated with an underlying disorder affecting the immune system, such as chronic lymphocytic anemia, non-Hodgkin's lymphoma, or systemic lupus erythematosus. In most patients, antibodies on the erythrocyte membrane can be detected by the direct antiglobulin test or other, more sensitive detection methods. Clues to the diagnosis may be obtained from the history, including sudden onset later in life, recent prescription of various medications such as methyldopa, or other symptoms attributable to malignancy or connective tissue disease.

Pitfalls in Diagnosis

Disorders that increase the surface area–to–volume ratio of red cells may actually mask the abnormal shape, high mean corpuscular hemoglobin concentration, and increased osmotic fragility of HS red cells. These disorders include

Table 1. Disorders With Spherocytes in the Peripheral Blood

Hereditary spherocytosis
Autoimmune hemolytic anemias (warm-reacting antibodies)
Liver disease
Thermal injuries
Microangiopathic and macroangiopathic hemolytic anemias
Clostridial septicemia
Transfusion reactions with hemolysis
Poisoning with certain snake, spider, and Hymenoptera venoms
Severe hypophosphatemia
ABO incompatability (in neonates)
Heinz body anemias

deficiencies of iron, vitamin B_{12}, or folate; beta-thalassemia; obstructive jaundice; or hemoglobin SC disease. After correction of the underlying condition (e.g., treatment of iron deficiency, relief of obstructive jaundice), the typical abnormalities in osmotic fragility return.

Summary

Patients with HS may present at any age, usually with anemia or an abnormal blood smear. Initial evaluation should include a thorough history and physical examination. Particular attention should be paid to the possibility of infection, toxin exposure, medications and, most importantly, family history. The latter should include questions about anemia, jaundice, gallstones, and splenectomy. Initial laboratory investigation should include a complete blood count with a peripheral smear, reticulocyte count, direct antiglobulin test (Coombs' test), and serum bilirubin determination. The differential diagnosis of hemolytic anemia is long and includes hemoglobinopathies, red cell enzyme deficiencies, and immune-mediated hemolysis. When the peripheral smear or family history is suggestive of HS, an incubated osmotic fragility specimen should be obtained. Rarely, additional, specialized testing is required to confirm the diagnosis.

HEREDITARY ELLIPTOCYTOSIS

Hereditary elliptocytosis (HE) is characterized by the presence of elliptical or oval, cigar-shaped erythrocytes on peripheral blood smears of affected individuals. The worldwide incidence of HE has been estimated at 1 in 2000 to 1 in 4000 individuals. The true incidence of HE is unknown because its clinical severity is heterogeneous, and many patients are asymptomatic. It is common in African Americans and inidividuals of Mediterranean ancestry, presumably because elliptocytes confer some resistance to malaria. In parts of Africa, the incidence of HE approaches 1 in 100. HE is inherited in an autosomal dominant pattern with rare cases of de novo mutations.

Pathophysiology

The principal defect in HE is mechanical weakness or fragility of the erythrocyte membrane skeleton. Qualitative and quantitative defects in a number of red cell membrane proteins have been described in HE. These include α-spectrin, β-spectrin, protein 4.1, and glycophorin C. The majority of defects occur in spectrin, the principal structural protein of the erythrocyte membrane skeleton. Spectrin is composed of heterodimers of the homologous, but nonidentical, proteins αβ-spectrin, which, in turn, self-associate into tetramers and higher order oligomers. These tetramers and oligomers are critical for erythrocyte membrane stability and erythrocyte shape and function. Most spectrin defects in HE impair the ability of spectrin dimers to self-associate into tetramers and oligomers, thereby disrupting the membrane skeleton. Structural and functional defects of protein 4.1 appear to disrupt the spectrin-actin contact in the membrane skeleton. Glycophorin C variants are also deficient in protein 4.1. The precise pathobiologic features of elliptocyte formation in these syndromes is unclear.

Genetically, HE is heterogeneous. Various mutations have been described in the α-spectrin, β-spectrin, protein 4.1, and glycophorin C genes, including point mutations, gene deletions and insertions, and mRNA processing defects. Distinct mutations have been identified in persons of similar genetic background, suggesting a "founder effect" for these mutants.

Course and Outcome

The clinical presentation of HE is heterogeneous, ranging from asymptomatic carriers to patients with severe, life-threatening anemia. The overwhelming majority of patients with HE are asymptomatic. Approximately 12 per cent of patients with HE will become symptomatic because of anemia at some time during their lives. Typically, patients are diagnosed incidentally during testing for unrelated conditions. It is also possible to identify asymptomatic carriers with normal peripheral smears who possess the same molecular defect as an affected HE relative. The erythrocyte life span, which is normal in most patients, may be decreased in 10 per cent of patients with HE. It is this subset of patients with decreased red cell life span who experience hemolysis, anemia, splenomegaly, and intermittent jaundice. Many of these patients have parents with typical HE and thus are homozygotes or compound heterozygotes for defects inherited from each of the parents. Symptoms may vary among members of the same family and may also vary in the same individual.

Although presentation in the newborn period is uncommon, anemia and jaundice may be seen. In infants who become symptomatic, anemia often appears around 4 to 6 months of age. Occasionally, severe forms of HE may present with severe hemolysis, anemia, and jaundice requiring blood transfusions. In many severely affected infants, the hemolysis abates by 1 to 2 years of age, and the patient goes on to develop typical HE with mild anemia.

Laboratory Diagnosis

The hallmark of HE is the presence of cigar-shaped elliptocytes on the peripheral blood smear (Fig. 3). These normochromic, normocytic elliptocytes may number from a few to 100 per cent; the degree of hemolysis does not correlate with the number of elliptocytes present. Ovalocytes, spherocytes, stomatocytes, and fragmented cells may also be seen. Elliptocytes also may be present in megaloblastic anemias, hypochromic microcytic anemias (iron deficiency anemia and thalassemia), myelodysplastic syndromes, and myelofibrosis. However, elliptocytes typically make up less that one third of red cells in these conditions. History and additional laboratory testing usually clarify the diagnosis of these disorders. Pseudoelliptocytosis is an artifact of blood smear preparation. Pseudoelliptocytes are found only in certain areas of the smear, usually near its tail, and the long axes of pseudoelliptocytes are parallel, whereas the axes of true elliptocytes are distributed randomly.

Osmotic fragility is abnormal in severe HE and in the related condition, hereditary pyropoikilocytosis (HPP; see further on). Other laboratory findings in HE are similar to those found in other hemolytic anemias and are nonspecific markers of increased erythrocyte production and destruction. The reticulocyte count usually is less than 5 per cent but may be higher when hemolysis is severe. Increased serum bilirubin, increased urinary urobilinogen, and decreased serum haptoglobin levels reflect increased erythrocyte destruction. Haptoglobin may be decreased or absent in neonates and thus is an unreliable marker of hemolysis in the newborn. Specialized tests such as erythrocyte membrane protein quantitation, ektacytometry, spectrin self-association studies, limited tryptic digestion of spectrin, and cDNA–genomic DNA analyses may prove diagnostically useful in selected patients.

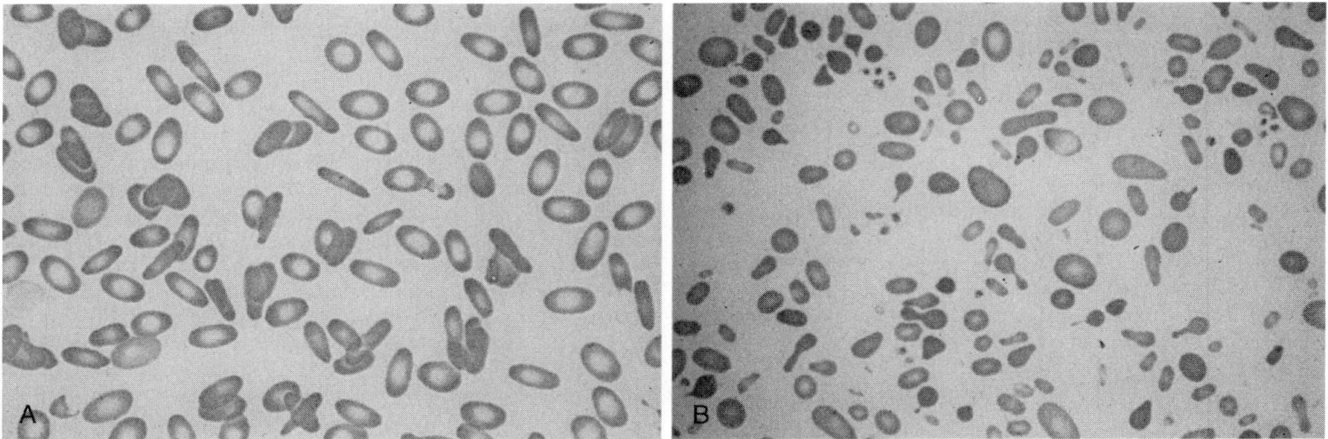

Figure 3. Peripheral blood smears. *A,* Typical hereditary elliptocytosis. Smooth, cigar-shaped elliptocytes are seen. *B,* Hereditary pyropoikilocytosis. Pronounced microcytosis, poikilocytosis, fragmentation of erythrocytes, and elliptocytes are seen.

HEREDITARY PYROPOIKILOCYTOSIS

HPP is a rare cause of severe hemolytic anemia, with erythrocyte morphologic characteristics reminiscent of those seen in patients with severe burns. Red blood cells from these patients possess abnormal thermal sensitivity compared with normal erythrocytes. HPP occurs predominantly in patients of African descent. There is a strong relationship between HPP and HE. Approximately one third of parents or siblings of patients with HPP have typical HE. Many patients with HPP demonstrate a clinical and laboratory course compatible with typical mild HE. Patients with HPP tend to experience severe hemolysis and anemia in infancy that gradually improves, evolving toward typical elliptocytosis later in life.

HPP erythrocytes are characterized by bizarre shapes, elliptocytes, fragmentation, and budding. Microspherocytosis is common and the mean corpuscular volume is frequently decreased (50 to 65 fL). Pyknocytes are prominent in smears of neonates with HPP. Osmotic fragility in HPP is abnormal.

SOUTHEAST ASIAN OVALOCYTOSIS

Southeast Asian ovalocytosis (SAO) is characterized by the presence of oval erythrocytes with a central longitudinal slit or transverse bar in the peripheral blood smears of affected individuals. It is common in parts of the Philippines, Indonesia, Malaysia, and New Guinea and is inherited in an autosomal dominant fashion. SAO erythrocytes are resistant to invasion by malarial parasites. Remarkably rigid, these erythrocytes possess a defective band 3 protein, the anion transporter. Patients with SAO are asymptomatic, with little or no evidence of hemolysis. Osmotic fragility is normal. The finding of characteristic ovalocytes in the peripheral blood of an asymptomatic individual from one of the previously mentioned ethnic backgrounds is highly suggestive of the diagnosis. Biochemical and DNA diagnostic techniques are available to detect this condition.

ACQUIRED HEMOLYTIC ANEMIA

By Michael B. Dabrow, D.O.,
and Thomas G. Gabuzda, M.D.
Wynnewood, Pennsylvania

Acquired hemolytic anemia is typically caused by factors extrinsic to the red cell. Accurate identification of the factors causing a specific patient's hemolysis can be enhanced by proper selection of the tests most often used to establish the presence of hemolysis.

The most useful tests initially are the serum lactate dehydrogenase (LD) activity level, the reticulocyte production index (RPI), the serum haptoglobin concentration, and the serum unconjugated bilirubin concentration. Serum LD activity provides an excellent screen for hemolysis. LD isozymes LD_1 and LD_2 are typically increased; their activity in serum is especially high during mechanical cardiac hemolysis. Accelerated destruction of red cells typically leads to erythroid hyperplasia and an increased reticulocyte count (RC) in the peripheral blood. The RC should be corrected for the degree of anemia and expressed as an index that compares the production of reticulocytes in the patient to that in a normal person. The RPI may be considered a "normalized" RC, expressed as:

$$\text{RPI} = \text{RC} \times [\text{patient Hct/normal Hct}] \times 1/\text{y}$$

where RC is the measured reticulocyte count, Hct is hematocrit, and y represents the altered reticulocyte maturation time varying with the degree of anemia as follows:

Hct (%)	45	35	25	15
y (days)	1.0	1.5	2.0	2.5

The reticulocyte maturation time is derived from measurements of marrow production at varying hematocrit values and correlates with the increased time required for circulating reticulocytes to lose their reticulum. The RPI is the best indicator of a normal marrow response to anemia, with a baseline value of 1 increasing to a maximum of 8 to 10 with progressively severe anemia. This index may be low during hemolysis if erythropoiesis is arrested because of infection, autoantibodies, or deficiency of vitamin B_{12}, folate, or iron.

A decrease in the serum haptoglobin concentration is seen with intravascular or extravascular hemolysis as free hemoglobin is released into the plasma. This is a sensitive test for detecting hemolysis. The haptoglobin-hemoglobin complex is rapidly cleared from the circulation by the liver. Even when hemolysis is primarily extravascular within the confines of macrophages, the hemoglobin released into the plasma is often sufficient to reduce the haptoglobin concentration. However, the decline from hemolysis may be masked because haptoglobin is an acute-phase reactant, and baseline concentrations can rise significantly in acute illness. By contrast, spuriously low concentrations of haptoglobin may be transiently observed after a blood transfusion, resulting from small numbers of lysed red cells in the transfused product. When hemolysis is predominantly intravascular, the hemoglobin-binding capacity of haptoglobin and the other heme-binding plasma proteins (hemopexin and albumin) is readily exceeded. Hemoglobin is then filtered by the glomerulus and reabsorbed in the renal tubule, where it is degraded. The heme iron is converted to ferritin and hemosiderin. The hemosiderin-laden renal tubular cells are shed into the urine, where they may be detected with an iron stain.

The serum bilirubin concentration, which may be normal or increased, is not a sensitive indicator of hemolysis. Importantly, bilirubin concentrations exceeding 5 mg/dL typically indicate obstructive jaundice, intrinsic liver disease, or disorders other than or in addition to hemolysis. Pigment (bilirubin) gallstones should be suspected in any patient with chronic hemolysis.

IMMUNE HEMOLYTIC ANEMIA

The *direct antiglobulin* or *Coombs' test* identifies antibodies and/or the third component of complement bound to the red cell surface. In immune hemolytic anemia, the direct Coombs' test is almost always positive. The *indirect Coombs' test* detects antibodies in the patient's serum. If the indirect Coombs' test is positive, the detected antibodies may be autoantibodies (associated with autoimmune hemolytic anemia) or alloantibodies (directed at specific red cell antigens), or both. Nonspecific warm reactive autoimmune antibodies typically react (most actively at 37°C in vitro) with all red cells except Rh null cells lacking Rh antigens. A positive indirect Coombs' test not only routinely aids the diagnosis of immune hemolytic anemia but also reminds the clinician that virtually all transfused red blood cells are incompatible when an autoantibody is present.

The most common form of immune hemolysis involves *warm reacting antibodies* on the surface of the red blood cell. The direct Coombs' test identifies IgG antibodies on the red blood cell surface and may be positive or negative for complement. Occasionally, autoimmune hemolysis occurs with a negative direct Coombs' test if the offending antibody is of the IgA class or if fewer than 200 IgG molecules are bound to each red cell. Coombs'-negative autoimmune hemolysis is most often seen in patients with lymphoma or chronic lymphocytic leukemia. A Coombs'-negative spherocytic anemia, however, is presumed to result from hereditary spherocytosis until proved otherwise.

Warm antibodies do not cause agglutination, but they do bring about premature destruction of red blood cells, especially in the spleen, which often becomes enlarged. The Fc receptors on splenic macrophages recognize the Fc portion of the bound antibody. This enables the macrophages to pinch off red cell membrane fragments producing spherocytes (Fig. 1). Sphered erythrocytes are then entrapped and engulfed by the macrophage. The hemolysis is primarily extravascular, and hemosiderin is not found in the urine sediment. As the marrow attempts to compensate for the early destruction of red cells, reticulocytes (seen as polychromatophilic cells on the peripheral smear) give rise to a macrocytic subset of red cells. These larger reticulocytes plus the smaller spherocytes increase the *red cell distribution width* (RDW) reported on most automated blood counters. As cells are destroyed, LD and, to a lesser degree, aspartate aminotransferase are released into the plasma. Heme is converted to unconjugated bilirubin, which is also released into the plasma bound to albumin. The constellation of a positive Coombs' test, an increased RPI, macrocytosis, a diminished haptoglobin level, an increased RDW, and an increased serum LD level, with or without a rise in the indirect fraction of bilirubin, should alert the clinician to the possibility of an immune hemolytic anemia.

Fifty per cent of immune hemolytic anemias caused by warm antibodies are idiopathic. About 20 per cent are associated with lymphoproliferative diseases, such as chronic lymphocytic leukemia, and 10 per cent are associated with connective tissue or other autoimmune disorders. The remaining warm immune hemolytic anemias are drug-induced.

Drug-induced hemolysis occurs via three distinct mechanisms. First, a drug such as penicillin may initially bind to the red blood cell surface. An antibody to the cell-bound drug (or hapten) then binds, thereby sensitizing the cell for destruction. Hapten-induced hemolysis rapidly stops when the drug is withdrawn. In the second, or innocent bystander, mechanism of hemolysis, the initial binding of drug to IgM antibody occurs in the serum, and the complex then binds to the red blood cell surface. The amount of IgM is enough to promote the binding of complement to the red cells, giving a positive Coombs' test for the C3 complement component, whereas the Coombs' test for IgG is negative. The cold agglutinin titer in this IgM-mediated process is also negative. Re-exposure to the offending drug may cause dramatic hemolysis with hypovolemic shock and acute renal failure. In the third mechanism, drugs such as methyldopa induce a true autoantibody to a red cell antigen. This insidious mechanism of hemolysis often requires

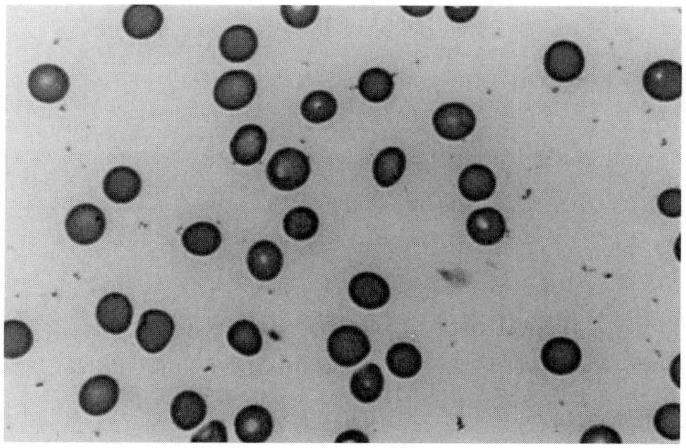

Figure 1. Spherocytes—small round red cells with absence of central pallor.

at least 3 to 4 months of exposure to the drug, and the antibody may persist for months following discontinuation of the medication. Although 10 to 30 per cent of patients who take methyldopa have a positive direct Coombs' test, hemolysis actually develops in only 1 per cent. In addition, agents such as the cephalosporins can cause nonimmune absorption to red cells and a positive Coombs' test, but no hemolysis. Hence, not all patients with a positive Coombs' test have hemolysis. A list of drugs commonly associated with the various mechanisms of warm antibody immune hemolysis is presented in Table 1.

Cold agglutinin disease is typically associated with IgM antibodies that bind to red blood cells with increasing avidity as the temperature is reduced below that of body temperature. Agglutination and complement fixation occur in the superficial vessels; on warming in the central circulation, the IgM molecule is released, leaving complement and a positive Coombs' test for C3 only. The clinician must specifically ask the laboratory to perform a cold agglutinin titer to detect this antibody effect at low temperature. This test measures the ability of serial dilutions of the patient's serum to agglutinate compatible red cells at 4°C in vitro. The hemolysis is often mild, chronic, and seasonal. Ischemic signs in exposed body parts, such as the digits, nose, and ears, may be seen. The thermal amplitude is the highest temperature at which these antibodies cause detectable agglutination. The thermal amplitude, not the cold agglutinin titer, determines the severity of the hemolysis.

Most cold immune hemolytic IgM molecules bind red cells only at depressed temperatures and rapidly elute as body temperature is approached. This allows time to activate the complement cascade to the C3b stage only. C3b receptors on the macrophage surface bind C3b, leading to extravascular hemolysis. Alternatively, C3b on the cell surface may be degraded by C3b inactivator to C3d. If C3b can be degraded to C3d prior to phagocytosis, the red cells are released from the receptor and are free to circulate unimpeded once again. By contrast, cold agglutinins only rarely activate the lytic complement sequence C5 through C9. However, those IgM molecules with a thermal amplitude that allows binding to erythrocytes closer to 37°C are more prone to promote in vivo complement activation and a more severe hemolysis. About 95 per cent of cold agglutinin antibodies are specific for the I antigen in red cells. The most common stimuli for acute cold agglutinin production are infectious mononucleosis and infection with *Mycoplasma pneumoniae.* Chronic production of cold agglutinins is typically associated with B-cell neoplasms. Lymphocytoid plasma cells may be observed in the marrow, and IgM monoclonal bands are occasionally seen on serum protein electrophoresis. Splenomegaly, which is commonly observed in warm antibody immune hemolytic anemia, may also be seen in cold agglutinin disease. Splenectomy, however, is of little benefit. Cold agglutinins must be distinguished from cryoglobulins, which are serum proteins that self-associate and precipitate or gel in the cold.

In a few patients, the immune hemolytic anemia involves both warm and cold antibodies. The clinical picture is primarily that of warm antibody hemolytic anemia. The cold agglutinins are of low titer but high thermal amplitude. Table 2 summarizes the use of the Coombs' test and cold agglutinin titer in distinguishing the warm immune hemolytic anemias from cold agglutinin disease.

Paroxysmal cold hemoglobinuria is an entity rarely seen in syphilis; it is more commonly observed in children after a viral illness. The antibody can be identified in the serum with the Donath-Landsteiner test. The IgG antibody binds to the red cell at 4°C and fixes complement. Hemolysis becomes evident with warming to about 20°C. The direct Coombs' test is usually negative, but it may be transiently positive during acute attacks.

NONIMMUNE HEMOLYSIS

Destruction of red cells by nonimmune mechanisms should be suspected when the peripheral smear of the anemic patient shows altered red blood cell morphologic characteristics and the Coombs' test is negative (Table 3). Fragmented red blood cells are common markers of intravascular nonimmune hemolysis; the schistocyte is the characteristic cell seen on the peripheral smear (Fig. 2). An acute intravascular nonimmune hemolysis causes hemoglobinemia, hemoglobinuria, and pink or red plasma. By contrast, a more chronic process may be identified by detecting hemosiderin in the urine.

The incidence of hemolytic anemia caused by mechanical damage to erythrocytes has increased as the frequency of prosthetic heart valve implantation has increased. In the past, defective surgical techniques or valve design most often caused hemolysis. Today, most hemolysis is attributed to worn-out valves. The damage is caused by high flow rates through small apertures, especially those associated with perivalvular leaks and artificial surfaces. Clinically insignificant hemolysis may nevertheless be sufficient to reduce the serum haptoglobin concentration because the hemolysis is entirely intravascular. Native but severely stenosed aortic valves may cause minimal or mild hemolysis, whereas severe hemolysis occurs only in the presence of defective prosthetic valves. The serum LD concentration is extraordinarily high, and urine hemosiderin is consistently identified with the use of an iron stain on the spun sediment. Loss of iron in the urine may lead to iron deficiency, which limits the ability of the marrow to compensate. The platelet count is normal in cardiac hemolysis. Mechanical damage to erythrocytes also occurs during ex-

Table 1. Drugs Associated With Warm Antibody Immune Hemolysis

Hapten	Innocent Bystander	Autoimmune	Uncertain Cause
Penicillin	Quinidine	Methyldopa	Omeprazole
Ampicillin	Quinine	Procainamide	Sulindac
Methicillin	Hydrochlorothiazide	Ibuprofen	5-Fluorouracil
Cephalothin	Rifampin	Diclofenac	
Cephaloridine	Isoniazid	Thioridazine	
Carbenicillin	Acetaminophen	Mefenamic acid	
	Hydralazine		
	Chlorpromazine		
	Probenecid		

Table 2. Use of the Coombs' Test to Distinguish Warm Immune Hemolytic Anemia and Cold Agglutinin Disease

	Coombs' Test			Cold Agglutinin
	Polyspecific	*IgG*	*C3*	
Warm immune hemolytic anemia	+	+	+/−	Negative
Warm immune hemolytic anemia–drug				
Hapten	+	+	+/−	Negative
Innocent bystander	+	−	+	Negative
Autoantibody	+	+	−	Negative
Cold agglutinin disease	+	−	+	High titer
Mixed warm-cold	+	+	+	Positive

tracorporeal circulation for cardiac surgery, but the hemolysis that occurs is not a significant clinical problem. March hemoglobinuria was first observed in a soldier after strenuous marching. This phenomenon is observed in distance runners and is most likely related to damage to red cells as they pass through vessels in the soles of the feet.

Microangiopathic hemolytic anemia refers to red cell damage associated with occlusive processes in the microcirculation. Erythrocytes rupture when they are "clotheslined" by aberrant fibrin strands. Disorders characterized by microangiopathic hemolysis include thrombotic thrombocytopenic purpura (TTP), hemolytic uremic syndrome (HUS), intravascular coagulopathy, and the HELLP (*h*emolysis, *e*levated *l*iver enzymes, *l*ow *p*latelet) syndrome. Clinicians must recognize TTP because treatment dramatically improves prognosis and changes the natural history of what was once typically a fatal disease. The examination of the peripheral smear is crucial. The appearance of helmet cells, burr cells, spherocytes, triangulated and other fragmented forms, polychromatophilic macrocytes, reduced platelets, and increased granulocytes should always suggest the diagnosis of TTP. Because of the emergent nature of TTP, the inaccessibility of tissues for biopsy, and the fear of bleeding, diagnosis from tissue is often not feasible. However, bone marrow biopsies or gingival biopsies occasionally reveal arterioles occluded by hyaline deposits of fibrin and platelets. The inciting factor may be an endothelial abnormality that incites platelet deposition in arterioles in various tissues. This triggers a multisystem disorder with signs of hemolysis, including an increased LD level and reticulocyte index, along with renal failure, neurologic signs, cardiac conduction abnormalities, and pancreatitis. The clinical expression of these latter signs may be delayed, and early clinical decisions may rely primarily on the hematologic picture.

Table 3. Nonimmune Hemolysis

Mechanical Hemolysis
- Cardiac hemolysis
- March hemoglobinuria
- Microangiopathic hemolysis with low platelets
  - TTP-HUS-HIV-drug-induced—mitomycin C, cyclosporine
  - Intravascular coagulation
    - disseminated
    - localized vascular malformations
  - Carcinoma
  - Malignant hypertension
  - HELLP syndrome
  - Severe vasculitis—SLE, other CVD, Wegener's granulomatosis

Other Physical Injury
- Thermal burns
- Osmotic hemolysis—fresh water drowning

Oxidative Hemolysis
- Indirect oxidants—phenazopyridine, sulfapyridine, sulfasalazine
- Direct oxidants—chlorate, perchlorate, permanganate, arsenate

Membrane Defects
- PNH
- Spur cell anemia

Infections
- RBC invasion-adhesion—malaria, bartonellosis, babesiosis
- Hemolytic toxins—*Clostridium welchii*

Hypersplenism

TTP = thrombotic thrombocytopenic purpura; HUS = hemolytic uremic syndrome; HIV = human immunodeficiency virus; HELLP = hemolysis, elevated liver enzymes, low platelet; SLE = systemic lupus erythematosus; CVD = collagen vascular disease; PNH = paroxysmal nocturnal hemoglobinuria; RBC = red blood cell.

HUS resembles TTP in pathogenesis but is dominated by renal dysfunction. The hematologic picture and morphologic changes in renal arterioles are similar. However, HUS is not particularly responsive to infusions of normal plasma, and hemodialysis is often required. The HELLP syndrome occurs in late pregnancy, can lead to disseminated intravascular coagulopathy or hepatic rupture, and may occur in the absence of eclampsia. Treatment includes prompt delivery of the fetus. Other microvascular disorders that can cause microangiopathic hemolysis are disseminated cancer with occluded small vessels, malignant hypertension, and severe vasculitis as can be seen in systemic lupus erythematosus, Wegener's granulomatosis, or other autoimmune disorders. Mitomy-

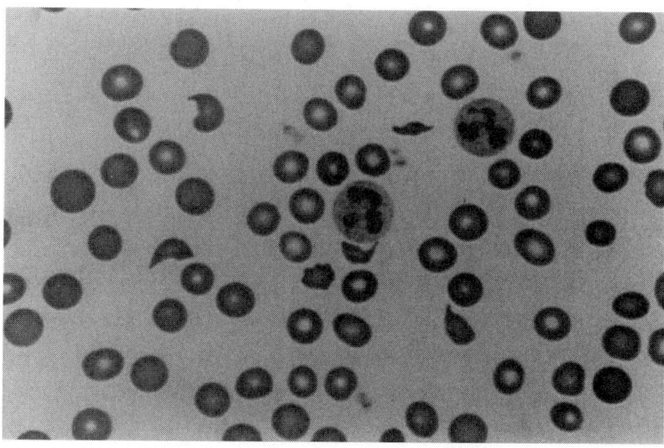

Figure 2. Schistocytes—fragmented red blood cells of varying shapes.

cin C and cyclosporine may also cause microangiopathic anemia that resembles TTP or HUS.

Patients deficient in glucose-6-phosphate dehydrogenase (G-6-PD) may develop hemolysis following exposure to oxidant drugs. Even in patients who are not G-6-PD–deficient, hemolysis may result from drug-induced production of reactive oxygen species. Patients who are not G-6-PD–deficient are typically females taking phenazopyridine (Pyridium) for urinary symptoms. Other drugs associated with oxidative hemolysis include sulfasalazine (Azulfidine), sulfones, and sulfapyridine. Chlorate, perchlorate, permanganate, and arsenate can also cause direct oxidation, leading to hemolysis. The morphologic changes of oxidative hemolysis are similar to those of microangiopathic hemolysis. However, the platelet count is normal in oxidative hemolysis. The methemoglobin concentration may be slightly increased, but Heinz bodies are rarely detected unless the spleen is absent or hemolysis is relatively brisk and testing is performed during or shortly after administration of the offending agent.

Paroxysmal nocturnal hemoglobinuria (PNH) is a stem cell disorder in which hemolysis is acquired as a result of increased sensitivity of red cells to lysis by complement components C5 through C9. Both decay-accelerating factor (DAF) and membrane antigen CD59, which normally limit C3 deposition and function on cell membranes, are absent from the cell surface in PNH. The primary defect in PNH is a failure to synthesize the glycosylphosphatidylinositol anchor because of abnormalities in the X-linked pig-A gene. This defect blocks the integration of decay accelerating factor into the cell membrane. Pancytopenia, slight or modest splenomegaly, and arterial or venous thrombosis are typically observed. The diagnosis is made by demonstrating hemosiderinuria, a positive sugar water test, and/or a positive acid hemolysis test (Ham test). The latter tests measure increased sensitivity to complement-mediated lysis. The leukocyte alkaline phosphatase score is reduced. As in cardiac hemolysis, urinary iron losses may be sufficient to cause iron deficiency.

The spur cell anemia of cirrhosis reflects severe hemolysis associated with end-stage liver disease. The enlarged spleen is the primary site of erythrocyte destruction, but splenectomy is not indicated in view of the poor prognosis. The key to diagnosis is the large number of spur cells, or acanthocytes, which are densely stained red cells with multiple irregular spiny and knobby projections extending out from the membrane (Fig. 3). Acanthocyte formation is most likely the result of excessive accumulation of free (unesterified) cholesterol in the red cell membrane.

Parasitic invasions of erythrocytes may also cause hemolysis. The most prominent of these is malaria, which should be suspected in patients with cyclic fevers and a history of travel or recent transfusion. Babesiosis is most common along the northeast coast of the United States, especially on Nantucket Island. The infection is especially severe in splenectomized individuals. The erythrocyte damage in *Bartonella* infection is caused by adherence of the organism to the erythrocyte exterior. The diagnosis of these infections is made by examination of the blood film, which reveals the presence of the organism in or on the

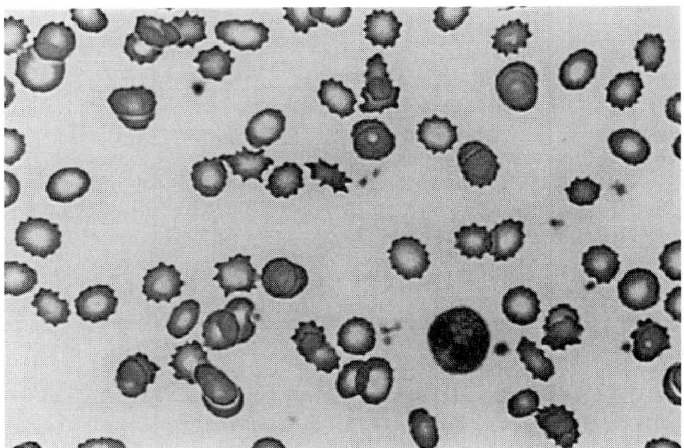

Figure 3. Spur cells—red blood cells with multiple irregular projections.

erythrocyte. The toxin of *Clostridium welchii* causes degradation of the red cell membrane. This occurs in patients with severe obstetric or biliary infection. The hemolysis is overwhelming and often fatal. The autoimmune hemolytic anemia that occurs following viral infections (Ebstein-Barr virus, cytomegalovirus, human immunodeficiency virus) or *Mycoplasma pneumoniae* has already been discussed. HUS may follow in the wake of infection with a rare serotype of *Escherichia coli*.

Splenomegaly of any cause may bring about premature destruction of red cells. The degree of premature destruction depends on the particular circulatory pathway followed by the erythrocytes, which may course slowly through the splenic cords or more directly into the venous sinusoids draining the spleen. The increased plasma volume of splenomegalic states adds a factor of dilutional anemia. A summary of the use of the laboratory in the diagnosis of acquired hemolytic anemia is presented in Table 4.

Table 4. Laboratory Evaluation of Acquired Hemolytic Anemia

Initial Evaluation
Reticulocyte production index
Haptoglobin
Lactate dehydrogenase
Bilirubin
Peripheral blood smear
Look for macrocytosis, polychromatophilia, spherocytes, schistocytes, spur cells, parasites
Direct Coombs' test
Further Evaluation
Cold agglutinin titer (if Coombs' test is negative)
Urinary hemosiderin (if cardiac hemolysis or PNH is suspected)
Sugar water test, leukocyte alkaline phosphatase, Ham acid hemolysis test (if pancytopenia is present)

QUANTITATIVE DISORDERS OF GRANULOCYTES

By Starr P. Pearson, M.D., and Stanley J. Russin, M.D.
Philadelphia, Pennsylvania

Abnormal numbers of circulating granulocytes (i.e., neutrophils, basophils, eosinophils, and monocytes) may indicate a primary disorder of production, maturation, or utilization of cells or a secondary response to a disease process or toxin. Granulocytosis and granulocytopenia should always be interpreted in the context of the patient's age, since the distribution of granulocytes, or "differential," undergoes specific developmental changes as well as variations that reflect disease states. This chapter focuses on *abnormal* increases and decreases in the number of mature granulocytes.

NEUTROPENIA

Neutropenia is typically defined as a neutrophil count of fewer than 1500 cells/mm^3. However, there is well-documented variation by age and race. In neonates, a predominance of neutrophils persists until the second or third week of life, when lymphocytes begin to predominate. By age 5 years, the neutrophil again becomes, and remains, the most abundant leukocyte. The absolute neutrophil count (ANC) is calculated as ANC = WBC × (% bands + % mature neutrophils) × 0.01. Neutrophils less mature than bands are not included in the calculation. In neutropenic patients, a propensity for infection is directly related to the ANC. This relationship is strongest for processes that result in decreased neutrophil production. Since the relationship of frequency and type of infection to the ANC is inexact, the neutropenic syndromes discussed here are primarily described according to their clinical manifestations. Mild neutropenia (ANC of 1000 to 1500 cells/mm^3) typically produces no significant risk of infection. Neutrophil counts in the range of 500 to 1000 cells/mm^3 may cause an increased susceptibility to infection, while counts of fewer than 500 cells/mm^3 correlate with a substantial risk of infection.

CLINICAL COURSE

The severity, chronicity, and etiology of the neutropenia determine the frequency and type of infections encountered. Neutropenia secondary to decreased production can persist for weeks in otherwise immunocompetent adults without serious infectious sequelae. When pyogenic infection does occur, it is most often caused by gram-positive cocci involving the skin, oropharynx, bronchi, anal canal, or vagina. Similarly, children with chronic benign neutropenia of infancy and childhood may have neutrophil counts of fewer than 200 cells/mm^3 for months or years, yet have no serious infections. Many neutropenic patients present with an associated monocytosis. The fact that monocytes function as phagocytes may explain the lack of correlation between neutrophil counts and the risk of infection in certain patients. However, neutrophils have much greater motility and phagocytic capability than monocytes. Hence, the presence of monocytes offers only marginal protection against pyogenic infections in the severely neutropenic patient. It appears that humoral and cell-mediated immunity and the tissue macrophage system also play a pivotal role in the prevention of infection in these individuals. In addition, tissue delivery of neutrophils in chronic neutropenias may be greater than in neutropenias of equal severity induced by chemotherapy. Thus, it is possible that peripheral counts may not always accurately reflect neutrophil availability.

In contrast, when the patient is debilitated, is receiving chemotherapy or glucocorticoids, or is ingesting excessive alcohol, the frequency and severity of infection are substantially greater. *Staphylococcus aureus, Pseudomonas aeruginosa, Escherichia coli,* and *Klebsiella* species are common causes of infection in such patients. Patients with less severe chronic neutropenias (ANC >300 cells/mm^3) or immune neutropenia may experience recurrent sinusitis, stomatitis, perirectal abscesses, and gingivitis but rarely develop septicemia.

The clinician must recognize that there is a decrease in pus formation in the severely neutropenic patient. This failure to suppurate can be misleading and can delay identification of the site of infection because of minimal physical and radiographic findings. For example, a lack of pneumonic consolidation is characteristic of pneumonia in granulocytopenic patients. Exudate, swelling, calor, and regional adenopathy all are less prevalent. However, fever, local pain, tenderness, and erythema are common despite the marked decrease in neutrophils.

DISORDERS OF GRANULOPOIESIS

Kostmann's Syndrome (Infantile Agranulocytosis)

This disorder presents in early infancy with severe, recurrent infections, including otitis, gingivitis, pneumonia, enteritis, peritonitis, and bacteremia. The neutrophil count is often fewer than 200 cells/mm^3, but eosinophilia and monocytosis may also be present. Inheritance may be autosomal dominant or recessive. Immunoglobulin levels are usually normal or increased. The bone marrow typically shows myeloid hypoplasia, with an arrest at the promyelocyte stage. Mild splenomegaly is common. Because there is no specific diagnostic test for this disorder, it may be difficult to distinguish from other severe and sometimes reversible causes of neutropenia, such as agranulocytosis of early childhood. Rarely, patients survive into adolescence and develop myelogenous leukemia.

Reticular Dysgenesis

This autosomal recessive congenital syndrome of agranulocytosis, thymic aplasia, and lymphoid hypoplasia is associated with low serum IgM and IgA concentrations and deficiencies of both T and B cells. Severe neutropenia and lymphopenia lead to extreme susceptibility to fatal bacterial and viral infections in infancy.

Myelokathexis and Lazy Leukocyte Syndrome

Patients with this rare disorder are severely neutropenic with peripheral counts of fewer than 500 cells/mm^3. The marrow, however, contains abundant neutrophil precursors and some mature neutrophils. Myelokathexis may arise from a defect in neutrophil mobility that impairs release from the marrow. Morphologic abnormalities, especially in the marrow, include hypersegmentation, cytoplasmic vacuoles, and abnormal nuclei. The lazy leukocyte syndrome is similar to myelokathexis, with ample marrow precursors and mature neutrophils, but very few circulating cells.

Shwachman-Diamond-Oski Syndrome

This presumed autosomal recessive disorder is characterized by dwarfism, pancreatic exocrine insufficiency, and neutropenia (ANC <500 cells/mm^3) without reciprocal monocytosis. These patients usually present as neonates with steatorrhea and various infections. A lack of gastrointestinal symptoms, however, does not exclude the diagnosis. The physical examination reveals strabismus, cleft palate, syndactyly, and microcephaly. Twenty-five per cent of patients have metaphyseal dysplasia. Thrombocytopenia is present in 70 per cent, and a mild megaloblastic anemia in 10 per cent. The bone marrow is typically hypoplastic, but it can also be normal. Sweat chloride testing is normal. Unlike cystic fibrosis, this disorder is not associated with chronic pulmonary disease. However, as with other constitutional marrow failure disorders, there is an increased risk of leukemia.

Chédiak-Higashi Syndrome

This rare autosomal recessive disorder is characterized by oculocutaneous albinism, neutropenia, progressive neurologic impairment, and giant cytoplasmic granules in neutrophils, monocytes, and lymphocytes. Patients with this syndrome exhibit an increased susceptibility to infection because of defects in neutrophil chemotaxis, degranulation, and bactericidal activity.

Dyskeratosis Congenita

This X-linked disorder is associated with leukoplakia, nail dystrophy, mild neutropenia, and reticulated hyperpigmentation of the skin. The marrow may be hypocellular. The majority of patients live into adulthood without serious infections.

Cartilage-Hair Hypoplasia Syndrome

In this autosomal recessive disorder, individuals exhibit short-limbed dwarfism, hyperextensible digits, fine hair, moderate neutropenia, and an increased predilection for infection. An accompanying defect in cellular immunity also makes these patients susceptible to viral infections, especially varicella-zoster.

Benign Ethnic Neutropenia

This autosomal dominant disorder is characterized by total leukocyte counts in the range of 2100 to 2600 cells/mm^3, with neutrophil counts generally between 1000 and 1200 cells/mm^3. These individuals are not at increased risk for infection. The bone marrow is normocellular. Several ethnic populations have an increased incidence of this disorder, including American and African blacks, Yemenite Jews, and West Indians. This condition represents an unusual variant of normal neutrophil proliferation and kinetics. Increased neutrophil margination has also been seen in some of these individuals. Not surprisingly, the epinephrine stimulation test, which produces a normal or supernormal circulating neutrophil count in these patients through recruitment of marginated neutrophils, may be helpful in distinguishing this entity from other congenital neutrophil disorders.

Cyclic Neutropenia

This is a rare autosomal dominant disorder with variable penetrance, affecting children and adults. It is characterized by regularly (cyclic) recurring episodes of severe neutropenia (ANC <200 cells/mm^3) occurring every 21 days and lasting for 3 to 6 days. There are also regular oscillations of lymphocytes, monocytes, reticulocytes, and platelets. The disorder may involve a stem cell regulatory defect. About 80 per cent of cases are diagnosed in children by age 5 years. Thirty per cent of these children have a family history of neutropenia. In a small number of patients, the disorder can present first in adulthood.

The diagnosis is established through serial differential counts, obtained at least three times per week for a minimum of 6 weeks, which reveal the typical "cycling." The bone marrow is usually hypoplastic, with myelocyte arrest during periods of neutropenia. Most patients survive to adulthood, but they can have associated recurrent fever, pharyngitis, stomatitis, and other bacterial infections. However, the disease tends to be benign, and symptoms tend to lessen after puberty.

Chronic Idiopathic Neutropenia

This diagnosis is applied to a constellation of findings that do not fit well into other categories of neutropenia. Onset can occur from infancy to late adulthood, and the presentation is variable. Neutrophil counts can fall to as low as 200 cells/mm^3, but typically they are greater than 500 cells/mm^3. Bone marrow examination reveals normal to increased numbers of myeloid precursors with maturation arrest. Peripheral monocytosis is often associated with this disorder. The physical examination of these patients is normal.

Essentially, chronic idiopathic neutropenia is a diagnosis of exclusion. There should be no infectious, inflammatory, or malignant processes to which the neutropenia can be attributed. No individual diagnostic test is pathognomonic. Generally, these patients have a benign course in spite of the severity of neutropenia. This benign course is due to the associated monocytosis and a normal marrow reserve, as demonstrated by increased neutrophil counts in response to a hydrocortisone stimulation test. These individuals can more effectively mobilize neutrophils to the tissues than patients with acute drug-induced neutropenia of equal degree. Antineutrophil antibodies, as well as other immunologic abnormalities, including circulating immune complexes, can be seen in some patients. Other than administration of antimicrobials during episodes of confirmed infection, these patients require no specific therapy. Evolution to acute leukemia or aplastic anemia is a very rare complication of this disorder.

Nutritional Deficiencies

Neutropenia is an early and consistent feature of anemias associated with vitamin B_{12}, folate, and copper deficiencies. Mild thrombocytopenia may also be present. These neutropenias are characterized by ineffective myelopoiesis and megaloblastic changes in the marrow. Similar findings have been seen in the hereditary form of vitamin B_{12} deficiency. Neutropenia and megaloblastosis have also been associated with sideroblastic anemia in the diabetes insipidus, diabetes mellitus, optic atrophy, and deafness syndrome (DIDMOAD). Copper deficiency typically is seen in patients receiving parenteral nutrition without adequate replacement of trace metals. Mild neutropenia can also be seen in some patients with anorexia nervosa.

Neutropenia Associated with Immunologic Abnormalities

A number of immunologic abnormalities are associated with neutropenia. These patients typically present in childhood with frequent bacterial infection, hepatosplenomegaly, and failure to thrive. Some die in the first few years of life. Hypergammaglobulinemia and hypogammaglobulinemia, T cell defects, and natural killer cell abnormalities have been observed. Many affected individuals have a positive family history of neutropenia. The bone marrow in these disorders is normocellular, with an arrest at the myelocyte stage and an increase in lymphocytes.

DISORDERS OF ACCELERATED DESTRUCTION

Autoimmune Neutropenia

Autoimmune neutropenia has been observed as an isolated phenomenon, in association with bacterial infections, in response to drugs, and secondary to other autoimmune diseases. Furthermore, cases previously considered idiopathic are now being recognized as immune-mediated because of more sophisticated testing. Immune neutropenia may be associated with idiopathic thrombocytopenic purpura and immune-hemolytic anemia in adults, but infrequently in children. Patients with autoimmune neutropenia have moderate to severe neutropenia, usually associated with monocytosis. Marrow cellularity is increased. The risk of infection correlates only moderately with the degree of neutropenia. Hepatosplenomegaly is seen in half of these patients. The initial clinical presentation varies from early childhood to old age.

Neutrophil antibodies have been identified through various assays, including leukoagglutination, opsonization of random donor neutrophils by the patient's sera, direct and indirect immunofluorescence assays that identify IgG and IgM (rarely IgA) on the surface of neutrophils, complement activation, and direct quantitation of surface-bound IgG using staphylococcal protein A or anti-human IgG monoclonal antibodies. Because of a lack of readily available known antigens, most assays detect only the presence of neutrophil-associated antibody. Discovery of these antibodies is helpful in establishing the diagnosis of immune neutropenia, but a negative result does not exclude the diagnosis. The degree of neutropenia is related to the specificity of the antibody, as well as its titer. In addition, circulating immune complexes (CIC) are found in one third of these patients. Although CIC can cause a positive indirect immunofluorescence test result, negative antineutrophil antibody tests have also been reported.

Therapy for autoimmune neutropenia depends on the severity of the neutropenia-related symptoms and the underlying disease, if present. Given the usual benign nature of the disease, therapy solely to increase the neutrophil count is not indicated. If recurrent or severe infections develop in the setting of significant neutropenia (ANC $<$500 cells/mm^3), high doses of immunoglobulin or steroids may be used. Splenectomy provides only transient correction of the neutropenia and results in a subsequent increased risk of infection.

Isoimmune (Alloimmune) Neonatal Neutropenia

This disorder is a transient cause of neonatal neutropenia due to the transplacental transfer of maternal IgG antibodies, analogous to Rh hemolytic disease. Prenatal maternal sensitization to neutrophil antigens occurs and results in the production of antibodies. The incidence of this disorder is estimated at 2 to 1000 live births.

Isoimmune neonatal neutropenia may present with sepsis or may be asymptomatic. Bone marrow examination shows normal cellularity with a late myeloid arrest. Diagnosis is made by identification of antineutrophil antibodies in infant and maternal sera that show specificity for paternal neutrophils. Cutaneous infections are most common, typically involving *Staphylococcus aureus, E. coli,* or beta-hemolytic *Streptococcus.* Although the neutropenia usually resolves within 12 to 16 weeks, patients with neutropenia persisting for up to 6 months have been cited. The resolution of the neutropenia corresponds to the half-life of maternal IgG.

Drug-Induced Neutropenia

Idiosyncratic reactions due to various therapeutic agents are a frequent cause of neutropenia. The mechanisms of such reactions vary greatly. Most drug-induced neutropenias are due to dose-dependent bone marrow suppression, in which myeloid precursors seem to be exquisitely sensitive to agents that interfere with protein synthesis or cell replication. Phenothiazines, nonsteroidal anti-inflammatory agents, histamine blockers, antineoplastic agents, and antithyroid medications are commonly implicated. This form of neutropenia exhibits a latency period of 20 to 40 days after exposure to the drug and is often detected incidentally on a routine blood test.

Some drugs induce neutropenia through an allergic or immune mechanism. Serving as haptens, these drugs stimulate antibody formation, causing accelerated neutrophil destruction. Neutropenia occurs abruptly at 7 to 14 days after the initial exposure to the drug or immediately after re-exposure. A wide array of drugs can cause this effect, including aminopyrine derivatives, penicillins, and gold. Women are affected more often than men, older patients are affected more often than young, and patients with a history of allergies, including those to drugs, are more frequently affected. Fever, malaise, chills, sore throat, and frank prostration can occur. Rashes or other allergic-type symptoms are unusual.

The bone marrow exhibits a varied appearance in drug-induced neutropenia, from hypocellular to hypercellular, and myeloid precursors may be absent, normal, or increased. The rate of recovery can be roughly predicted from the degree of marrow hypoplasia noted. On withdrawal of the offending drug, patients with sparse marrow neutrophils, but normal precursor cells (promyelocytes and myelocytes), will have neutrophils reappear in the blood in about 4 to 7 days. Frequently, a rise in the monocyte count heralds marrow recovery, with an associated marked neutrophilia, including peripheral blasts that may simulate a leukemic state. When early precursor cells are severely depleted, recovery may take considerably longer.

Patients with drug-induced neutropenia present a diagnostic challenge for any clinician. A high level of suspicion and a careful review of the clinical history are crucial to identifying the offending agent. The differential diagnosis should include acute viral infections, particularly infectious mononucleosis and hepatitis, and acute bacterial sepsis. If other hematologic abnormalities are also present, acute leukemia and aplastic anemia should be considered.

Neutropenia Associated With Infectious Diseases

Neutropenia can result from acute or chronic viral, bacterial, parasitic, or rickettsial diseases through several mechanisms. Viral infections commonly cause neutropenia, especially in children. The onset of neutropenia is typically within a few days of onset of the infection, and the neutropenia lasts several weeks. Counts usually return to normal as the infection resolves. Viral diseases known to cause neutropenia include varicella, rubella, hepatitis A and B, human immunodeficiency virus (HIV) infection, measles, infectious mononucleosis, influenza, and Kawasaki disease. The mechanism of the neutropenia involves decreased production, redistribution, and increased destruction of cells. A virus-induced antibody may also cause protracted immune neutropenia. More than 70 per cent of patients with acquired immunodeficiency syndrome (AIDS) develop leukopenia, which may be associated with hypersplenism and antineutrophil antibodies. The marrow is usually hypercellular, with a late myeloid arrest.

Staphylococcus aureus, Rickettsia, Mycobacterium tuberculosis, Brucellosis, and *Francisella tularensis* can cause moderate neutropenia. With overwhelming gram-negative bacterial infections, severe neutropenia can be seen paradoxically. This neutropenia may be due to increased adherence of cells to the endothelium in response to C5a, a neutrophil activator, as well as exhaustion of the marrow reserve pool at the site of infection. This phenomenon is most commonly seen in debilitated adults and newborns.

Neutropenia Associated With Autoimmune Diseases

Antineutrophil antibodies of the IgG type have been found in patients with *systemic lupus erythematosus.* About half of patients with lupus are neutropenic, although few have counts low enough to result in increased susceptibility to infection, unless they are taking immunosuppressive drugs. Anemia is present in about 75 per cent of patients with the disease. Thrombocytopenia, a positive Coombs' test, and splenomegaly can be seen in these patients. Neutropenia may also be related to decreased granulopoiesis in some patients with lupus.

Felty's syndrome (rheumatoid arthritis, splenomegaly, and neutropenia) has been associated with the presence of antineutrophil antibodies. This autoimmune disorder exhibits diminished neutrophil survival and production. By contrast, leukopenia is unusual in uncomplicated rheumatoid arthritis (<3 per cent). Improvement of the neutropenia and decreased antineutrophil antibody concentrations often accompany methotrexate treatment, providing support for the autoimmune theory of Felty's syndrome. The incidence of bacterial infection in patients with Felty's syndrome is low when the neutrophil count does not fall below 200 cells/mm^3.

Sjögren's syndrome (keratoconjunctivitis sicca, xerostomia, and rheumatoid arthritis or another connective tissue disease) causes leukopenia in as many as 30 per cent of patients. While mild to moderate neutropenia can be seen in this condition, severe neutropenia with recurrent infections is rare.

Other autoimmune neutropenias, presumed to arise through mechanisms similar to those in lupus and Felty's syndrome, have been infrequently associated with Hodgkin's disease, chronic autoimmune hepatitis, and Crohn's disease. Severe neutropenia associated with thymoma and hypogammaglobulinemia has been labeled *pure white cell aplasia.*

Metabolic Neutropenia

Neutropenia can be seen in patients with diabetic ketoacidosis and in conjunction with glycogen storage disease type Ib. Numerous qualitative defects in neutrophils have been noted in these disorders, which are frequently complicated by recurrent infections. The bone marrow is normocellular or hypercellular.

MALDISTRIBUTION OF NEUTROPHILS

Neutropenia Due to Complement Activation (Increased Margination)

Complement activation during or in association with cardiopulmonary bypass, hemodialysis, and bacterial sepsis can result in acute and chronic neutropenia and is associated with pulmonary dysfunction. Production of C5a activates neutrophils, causing increased adherence, aggregation, and entrapment of neutrophils in the pulmonary vasculature. Patients experiencing burns or transfusion reactions have also exhibited complement-mediated neutropenia because of shifts in the neutrophil pool. Because pulmonary infiltrates have been noted in some of these patients, the neutrophil has been considered as a possible factor in the pathophysiology of the adult respiratory distress syndrome (ARDS). However, the lack of severe neutropenia and pulmonary neutrophilic infiltration in some patients with ARDS suggests mechanisms in addition to direct damage by neutrophils.

Reticuloendothelial Sequestration (Hypersplenism)

Neutropenia as a consequence of hypersplenism is well established. Often anemia and thrombocytopenia are present. The degree of neutropenia is typically not severe, unless it is associated with an antineutrophil antibody, such as in Felty's syndrome.

A DIAGNOSTIC APPROACH TO NEUTROPENIA

The clinical approach to the patient with neutropenia should be guided by the history and physical examination, as well as the duration and severity of the neutropenia. An extensive laboratory evaluation is not always required. Symptomatic patients with acute neutropenia frequently have fever and infection involving the skin or mucous membranes or have a readily apparent metabolic derangement, such as hyperglycemia or ketosis. Acute neutropenia presents an urgent clinical problem requiring panculture for microbes, broad-spectrum antibiotics, and other appropriate supportive measures. In the absence of recent hospitalization and antibiotic use, surface bacteria sensitive to numerous agents are usually the cause of infection. However, the astute clinician should also consider overwhelming infection as a cause of acute neutropenia in individuals who lack characteristic signs and symptoms of inflammation, since neutropenic patients often do not have enough cells to generate suppuration and local inflammatory signs.

During the initial evaluation of the neutropenia patient, special emphasis should be placed on eliciting a history of fever, night sweats, weight loss, and anorexia as well as exposure to medications associated with neutropenia. Although a thorough physical examination is necessary in all patients, the clinician should focus on the identification of existing lymphadenopathy, splenomegaly, and bone tenderness that would greatly increase the risk of associated infection or malignancy. Review of a complete blood count (CBC), differential, and peripheral blood smear is essential in all patients. In younger patients, especially children, consider obtaining serial CBC and differential counts three times per week for 4 to 6 weeks to identify the typical cycling seen in cyclic neutropenia. Asymptomatic neutropenia with a normal physical examination and CBC and peripheral blood smear would be an unusual presentation for a serious underlying disease.

Acute symptomatic neutropenia, neutropenia associated

with an abnormal peripheral smear, and any neutropenia associated with either anemia or thrombocytopenia warrant a bone marrow aspiration with biopsy to further classify the neutropenia. A marrow with normal or increased cellularity and normal morphologic features would favor abnormalities in neutrophil distribution, such as splenic sequestration or reduced neutrophil survival due to an autoimmune process. These patients should be evaluated for the presence of splenomegaly, and testing for sedimentation rate, antinuclear antibodies, rheumatoid factor, and antineutrophil antibodies should be undertaken. Hypocellular marrow suggests a primary marrow defect and may be the first clue to an unsuspected congenital defect in myelopoiesis. Maturation arrest and megaloblastic changes on the biopsy should prompt testing for vitamin B_{12} and folate deficiencies, while other morphologic abnormalities may warrant chromosomal analysis to aid the diagnosis of myelodysplastic syndromes. Hydrocortisone stimulation testing can provide an indication of storage pool size and predict the clinical course of congenital neutropenias. Epinephrine stimulation testing, neutrophil kinetic studies, and bone marrow culture are of little discriminatory value and do not alter the approach to treatment. Typically, when neutropenia is associated with connective tissue and other nonhematologic diseases, the clinical presentation is readily apparent and severe. Occasionally, however, the disease may be occult, presenting with serologic abnormalities and minimal clinical findings. Chronic neutropenia is rarely caused by infection or nutritional deficiencies, which, if present, are also most often readily apparent. If evaluation has been nondiagnostic, consider HIV and quantitative immunoglobulin testing.

LEUKOCYTOSIS AND LEUKEMOID REACTIONS

Leukocytosis is defined as an increase in the absolute number of circulating leukocytes. The usual upper limit of normal for the total adult leukocyte count is 10,000 cells/mm^3. Significantly higher counts are normal in the neonate (38,000 cells/mm^3 at 12 hours), but leukocyte counts steadily approach adult values by 1 week of age. Until age 5 years, the differential exhibits a predominance of lymphocytes. The term "neutrophilia" refers to an increase in the absolute blood neutrophil count and is calculated by multiplying the total white cell count by the percentage of neutrophilic granulocytes. *Granulocytosis* is a less specific term that refers to increased numbers of neutrophils, basophils, eosinophils, and monocytes.

The term "leukemoid reaction" refers to a reactive increase in circulating leukocytes, including early precursor forms. The total white cell count frequently exceeds 50,000 cells/mm^3. The differential shows a marked "left shift" with increased percentages of myelocytes, metamyelocytes, and band forms. Promyelocytes may be observed in severe reactions. Leukemoid reaction can easily be confused with leukemia. However, unlike leukemia, proliferation of all normal myeloid elements is observed in the bone marrow. A leukemoid reaction is further distinguished from chronic myelogenous leukemia (CML) because most CML patients exhibit a low leukocyte alkaline phosphatase score. In addition, 85 per cent of CML patients harbor the Philadelphia chromosome on karyotypic analysis of the bone marrow. Leukemoid reactions due to infections may display toxic granulations, Döhle's bodies, and cytoplasmic vacuoles in the neutrophils on the peripheral blood smear.

Leukemoid reactions have also been associated with numerous congenital anomalies, including tetralogy of Fallot, dextrocardia, absent radii, and rudimentary little toes. Infants with Down's syndrome may have a transient leukemoid reaction that resembles congenital leukemia and can have an exaggerated leukemoid response to stress during childhood. Leukemoid reactions are also commonly associated with overwhelming infection, primary nonhematologic malignancy invading the marrow, heat stroke, hepatic or renal failure, diabetic ketoacidosis, excess production of adrenocorticotropic hormone or glucocorticoids, eclampsia, and thyroid storm.

When the marrow is directly invaded by fibrosis, fungi, tumor, or granulomas, neutrophilia associated with immature granulocytes and nucleated or teardrop-shaped red blood cells may be seen in the peripheral blood, often accompanied by thrombocytosis. This is termed a "leukoerythroblastic response." A bone marrow biopsy to search for granulomas or fibrosis and a marrow culture to exclude fungus and tuberculosis are generally indicated in these patients.

NEUTROPHILIA

Neutrophilia in adults is defined as an absolute blood neutrophil count of more than 7500 cells/mm^3. In the neonate, the upper limit of normal is 13,000 cells/mm^3, with a rapid decline to adult levels over the first few weeks of life. Leukocyte kinetic studies utilizing radioactive labels have been a very useful tool in delineating the pathophysiology of neutrophilia.

The sudden onset of neutrophilia is typically caused by an acute stimulus or in response to infection, toxins, drugs, or acute inflammation. Several mechanisms have been described. Severe emotional stress, hypoxia, strenuous exercise, or extreme temperature can precipitate neutrophilia as a result of demargination of the endothelial pool of neutrophils into the circulation. This reaction occurs within minutes of the stimulus, lasts from 4 to 24 hours, and is thought to be induced by catecholamines. Glucocorticoid infusion or endotoxin-producing infections produce neutrophilia by mobilizing neutrophils from the marrow storage pool. Glucocorticoids also impede the egress of neutrophils from the circulation into the tissues. The increase in lymphocytes and monocytes that accompanies simple demargination is not seen in the neutrophilia produced by glucocorticoids or endotoxins. Finally, acute neutrophilia may be triggered by the onset of labor, the induction of general or epidural anesthesia, acute subarachnoid hemorrhage, major trauma, or severe burns. The mechanisms, however, remain poorly understood.

Chronic neutrophilia may result from increased granulopoiesis following inhibition of marrow feedback mechanisms. Chronic infection or inflammation and prolonged lithium or glucocorticoid administration are commonly associated with chronic neutrophilia. The neutrophilia can persist for days to weeks, or occasionally months, after resolution of the associated illness or withdrawal of the offending agent. Chronic leukocytosis can also occur in otherwise healthy individuals. An entity termed "chronic idiopathic neutrophilia" has been identified in asymptomatic patients with leukocyte counts between 11,000 and 40,000 cells/mm^3 who were followed for more than 20 years. Bone marrow examination, leukocyte alkaline phosphatase, and the remainder of the hematologic profile were normal in these patients.

Neutrophilia may also accompany hematologic disorders such as hemolytic anemia or immune thrombocytopenia. For example, patients with sickle cell anemia commonly have leukocyte counts in the range of 12,000 to 15,000 cells/mm^3 and have an exaggerated rise in the total white cell count in response to infection. This response may be augmented by functional asplenia. Finally, leukocytosis, fever, urticaria, rash, and muscle and skin tenderness on exposure to cold are seen in infants with *familial cold urticaria.* This is an autosomal dominant disorder with onset of symptoms in the delivery room. Urticaria is followed by fever at about 7 hours after exposure. The leukocytosis, often as high as 35,000 cells/mm^3, begins about 10 hours after cold exposure and begins to wane within 12 to 14 hours. In contrast with other urticarial disorders, the rash is characterized by marked infiltration of neutrophils.

EOSINOPHILIA

Eosinophil counts exhibit diurnal variation in normal individuals that correlates inversely with adrenal glucocorticoid output. The circulating count tends to be highest late at night, decreases in the morning, and begins to rise at midafternoon.

Eosinophilia is defined as an absolute eosinophil count of more than 450 cells/mm^3. Worldwide, parasitic infection is the most common cause of eosinophilia. It is the granulomatous reaction of tissue that occurs when the parasites attach to mucosal surfaces—and not the parasites themselves—that produces the eosinophilia. Thus, eosinophilia is more common in helminthic than protozoal infections. In children, ascariasis and toxocariasis are the most common parasitic infections, and differential cell counts may reveal 80 to 90 per cent eosinophils and total white cell counts as high as 100,000 cells/mm^3. Anemia and hypergammaglobulinemia may also be present. Clinically, these children may present with fever, cough, and wheezing. The course may be complicated by seizures, myocarditis, encephalitis, and retinal lesions that can resemble retinoblastoma.

Allergic disorders are the most common cause of eosinophilia in industrialized countries. The degree of eosinophilia does not correlate closely with the severity of symptoms. However, marked eosinophilia is most frequently seen in bronchial asthma, drug reactions, eczema, atopic dermatitis, pemphigus, acute urticaria, and toxic epidermal necrolysis. Patients with ulcerative colitis, chronic hepatitis, connective tissue disorders, Hodgkin's disease, IgA deficiency, and vasculitis, those on chronic hemodialysis, and 40 per cent of individuals receiving radiation therapy for an intra-abdominal neoplasm may also exhibit eosinophilia.

Idiopathic hypereosinophilic syndrome (IHES) is a rare disorder in which marked eosinophilia ($>$1500 cells/mm^3) persists for more than 6 months with otherwise unexplained organ system dysfunction. Although children are occasionally affected, most of the patients are young adult males. Increased numbers of peripheral blood and marrow eosinophils and diffuse eosinophilic infiltration of the liver and spleen are found in 80 per cent of individuals with IHES. In the past, the term "eosinophilic leukemia" was used in the absence of diagnostic criteria for acute or chronic leukemia to describe what would currently be called IHES. Because patients with IHES may progress to end-stage endomyocardial fibroelastosis with congestive heart failure, early treatment designed to lower the eosinophil count should be undertaken in all patients with IHES who display eosinophilic organ infiltration and dysfunction.

MONOCYTOSIS

Variation in the number of circulating monocytes is commonly seen in clinical practice. Although the total count is higher in the first 2 weeks of life, monocytes typically constitute up to 9 per cent of peripheral blood leukocytes. Monocytosis is defined as a total count of more than 500 cells/mm^3 in adults. The blood monocyte and tissue monocyte-macrophage system play an important role in defending against bacterial and fungal pathogens. However, there is no clear association between the number of circulating monocytes and the risk of infection.

Monocytosis is frequently associated with malignant or premalignant hematologic disorders, such as acute and chronic nonlymphocytic leukemia, Hodgkin's and non-Hodgkin's lymphoma, myeloproliferative syndromes, and histiocytoses. In many of these patients, abnormal circulating monocytes cannot be distinguished from normal cells by light microscopy. Also associated with monocytosis are nonhematologic malignancies, tuberculosis, syphilis, subacute bacterial endocarditis, fever of unknown origin, systemic lupus erythematosus, rheumatoid arthritis, temporal arteritis, polyarteritis, myositis, inflammatory bowel disease, and sarcoidosis.

Finally, monocytosis has been observed in primary neutropenic states such as cyclic neutropenia, chronic idiopathic neutropenia, and Kostmann's syndrome. In addition, a relative monocytosis occurs with secondary neutropenia, such as marrow recovery after chemotherapy and in hyposplenic states.

BASOPHILIA

The normal blood basophil count is difficult to define precisely. The typical absolute count lies between 20 and 80 cells/mm^3, or 0.5 per cent of the total leukocyte count. Basophilia is commonly associated with hypersensitivity reactions of the immediate type, often accompanied by increased concentrations of IgE. Drug and food allergies, inhaled irritants, and urticaria are examples of such hypersensitivity reactions.

The number of basophils may also be increased in juvenile rheumatoid arthritis and ulcerative colitis. However, most inflammatory conditions that cause leukocytosis are associated with basophilopenia. Diabetes mellitus, myxedema, estrogen administration, radiation exposure, and iron deficiency anemia infrequently exhibit basophilia. Infectious causes of basophilia include chickenpox, influenza, smallpox, and tuberculosis. The concentration of blood basophils is slightly increased in polycythemia vera, idiopathic myelofibrosis, and primary thrombocythemia, and increased absolute basophil counts may provide a useful marker of early myeloproliferative disease. In CML, an increase in the absolute basophil count occurs in virtually all patients. Therefore, the clinician must distinguish CML from other nonmalignant causes of basophilia.

A DIAGNOSTIC APPROACH TO LEUKOCYTOSIS (GRANULOCYTOSIS)

Patients with leukocytosis or leukemoid reactions may have quite variable clinical presentations, reflecting the diversity of underlying diseases that cause these hematologic abnormalities. As always, a careful, detailed history and physical examination often provide essential clues to the diagnosis. Signs and symptoms of infection, malignancy, or autoimmune disease must be thoroughly evaluated.

Laboratory testing should begin with a CBC to determine which cell lines are involved. Review of the peripheral smear is essential for ascertaining the differential cell count, the degree of leukocyte atypia or maturity, and the red cell morphology. Furthermore, the presence of toxic granulations or Döhle bodies in the leukocytes may suggest an infectious process.

A bone marrow aspiration and biopsy are indicated when malignancy cannot be excluded by less invasive techniques. Marrow cultures should be considered when other foci of infection have been excluded. To distinguish a leukemoid reaction from CML, marrow cytogenic studies for the Philadelphia chromosome are of value, given the often similar appearance of the peripheral smear and marrow aspirate in these two entities. A low leukocyte alkaline phosphatase further supports the diagnosis of CML.

Patients with eosinophilia should be evaluated for parasite infestation and allergic disorders. Hepatosplenomegaly, unexplained organ failure, and marked eosinophilia persisting for more than 6 months in a young adult male suggest the diagnosis of the idiopathic hypereosinophilic syndrome, a disorder with a grave prognosis. The presence of immature eosinophils and normoblasts in the peripheral smear is consistent with a diagnosis of eosinophilic leukemia. The finding of monocytosis warrants an evaluation for an underlying hematologic, chronic inflammatory, infectious, or granulomatous disorder. Basophilia should spark an evaluation for hypersensitivity reaction or a myeloproliferative disorder such as CML.

Finally, the clinician should be aware of the common pitfalls in the evaluation of the patient with leukocytosis. To prevent unnecessary work-ups, age-related normal variations in the total and differential leukocyte count must be recognized, especially in infants and young children. Clinicians should also be aware that most episodes of leukocytosis in otherwise healthy individuals appear to be self-limited and benign; therefore, close follow-up with serial counts may be the best approach in many patients. Finally, physicians must distinguish leukemoid reaction from leukemia. This distinction, which can usually be made on the basis of the patient's clinical presentation and the results of the leukocyte alkaline phosphatase, can save many patients the discomfort and expense of a bone marrow aspiration and biopsy.

MYELODYSPLASTIC SYNDROMES AND SIDEROBLASTIC ANEMIAS

By Michael B. Streiff, M.D.,
and Chi Van Dang, M.D., Ph.D.
Baltimore, Maryland

MYELODYSPLASTIC SYNDROMES

The myelodysplastic syndromes are a collection of clonal acquired bone marrow failure disorders characterized by refractory cytopenias and a tendency to degenerate into acute myelogenous leukemia (AML). Prior to their official designation as the myelodysplastic syndromes by the French-American-British cooperative group (FAB) in 1976, these disorders were known by various labels, including the preleukemic syndrome, preleukemia, smoldering leukemia, refractory anemia (RA), preleukemic anemia, and the herald state of leukemia.

Pathogenesis

The exact molecular details underlying the pathogenesis of the myelodysplastic syndromes have yet to be elucidated. Most investigators believe, however, that they result from a series of mutational events in the pluripotent stem cell compartment that disrupts normal growth and differentiation. When sufficient mutations accumulate, transformation to AML occurs.

History

The myelodysplastic syndromes are typically diseases of elderly individuals, with greater than 50 per cent of patients being 70 years of age or older. Nevertheless, they can occur in young adults and even in children. Most patients present with asymptomatic bicytopenia or pancytopenia that is refractory to treatment with standard hematinics (vitamin B_{12}, folate, pyridoxine, and iron).

Symptomatic patients usually complain of exertional dyspnea or fatigue attributable to anemia, which is almost always present. A history of hemorrhage or recurrent infections is unusual. About 15 per cent of patients present with rheumatologic complaints or experience such symptoms during the course of the illness.

Physical Examination

The physical examination generally does not reveal any dramatic abnormalities. Occasionally pallor, petechiae, splenomegaly (10 to 20 per cent of patients); hepatomegaly (5 to 25 per cent of patients); or lymphadenopathy (5 to 10 per cent of patients) is noted. An exception to this characterization is chronic myelomonocytic leukemia (CMML), a subtype of the myelodysplastic syndromes in which splenomegaly (in 30 to 50 per cent of patients) and other evidence of extramedullary involvement (hepatic, skin, peritoneal, pleural, or pericardial implants) is common.

Laboratory Abnormalities

Anemia (hemoglobin <12 g/dL) at presentation is almost universal in patients with the myelodysplastic syndromes. The anemia is usually macrocytic or normocytic and hypoproliferative (low reticulocyte count), although a high reticulocyte count may be encountered with sideroblastic anemia. Poikilocytosis, anisocytosis, basophilic stippling, and rare nucleated red blood cells are often seen on the peripheral smear.

Leukocytes are generally mildly to moderately reduced in number, except in CMML, which is characterized by monocytosis (>1000 monocytes/μL) and often a neutrophilic leukocytosis. White blood cell morphologic abnormalities include nuclear hypolobulation (pseudo–Pelger-Huët anomaly), chromatin clumping, and hypogranulation of polymorphonuclear leukocytes. Circulating immature myeloid precursors, including blasts, are occasionally seen, particularly in refractory anemia with excess blasts (RAEB), CMML, and refractory anemia with excess blasts in transformation (RAEBT). Functional abnormalities of leukocytes are common and contribute to the patient's increased susceptibility to infection.

Thrombocytopenia is present in 25 to 60 per cent of patients. In general, advanced stages of the myelodysplastic syndromes (RAEB, RAEBT) are more frequently associated with significant thrombocytopenia. Although thrombocytopenia is usually due to impaired production, immune-mediated destruction has been demonstrated in occasional patients. Hypo- or hypergranulation of platelets as well as giant platelets is commonly noted on peripheral blood smears. Functional platelet abnormalities have been documented in a number of patients.

Bone marrow aspiration and biopsy are essential parts of the diagnostic evaluation of the myelodysplastic syndromes. The bone marrow is typically hypercellular or normocellular, reflecting the ineffective hematopoiesis that characterizes these disorders. Nevertheless, the diagnosis of a myelodysplastic syndrome should not be discarded on the basis of cellularity alone, since 10 per cent of patients have hypocellular marrow. Characteristic morphologic abnormalities are outlined in Table 1. Bone marrow iron stores are typically normal or increased, and marrow fibrosis is not unusual.

Bone marrow cytogenetic studies are often helpful and should be performed in any patient suspected of having a myelodysplastic syndrome. Karyotypic abnormalities are present in approximately 50 per cent of patients with the myelodysplastic syndromes and provide important prognostic information. The most common abnormalities include monosomy 7, 7q−, monosomy 5, 5q−, trisomy 8, and 20q−.

Specific Myelodysplastic Syndrome Subtypes and Their Clinical Course

The myelodysplastic syndromes have been subdivided into five separate types on the basis of peripheral blood and bone marrow morphologic features (Table 2).

Table 1. Characteristic Morphologic Abnormalities in the Peripheral Smear and Bone Marrow in the Myelodysplastic Syndromes

Peripheral Smear

Red blood cells—macrocytosis, anisocytosis, poikilocytosis, acanthocytosis, basophilic stippling, nucleated red blood cells

White blood cells–hypolobulated and/or hypogranular polymorphonuclear leukocytes, including the pseudo–Pelger-Huët anomaly, chromatin clumping, myeloblasts with or without Auer rods, atypical monocytosis

Platelets—large platelets, hypogranular or hypergranular platelets

Bone Marrow

Normocellular to hypercellular

Erythroid precursors—dyserythropoiesis—bizarre multilobulated nucleated erythroid precursors, binucleated erythroblasts, ringed sideroblasts

Megaloblastoid erythropoiesis—nuclear-cytoplasmic maturation dyssynchrony, Howell-Jolly bodies

White blood cell precursors—left shift in the myeloid precursors characterized by an increased number of myeloblasts, abnormal localization of immature myeloid precursors (ALIP)

Megaloblastoid myelopoiesis—giant juvenile cells

Megakaryocytes—hypolobulated micromegakaryocytes

Iron stores—abundant

Refractory Anemia

RA is characterized by mild to moderate marrow dysplasia and peripheral cytopenias. Bone marrow myeloblasts are present in normal or minimally elevated numbers(<5 per cent). Cytogenetic findings are usually normal or demonstrate prognostically favorable abnormalities such as 5q−. Correspondingly, patients with this subtype enjoy long, stable clinical courses or ones characterized by gradually worsening cytopenias, with few progressing to acute leukemia.

Refractory Anemia With Ringed Sideroblasts

Although morphologically similar in many respects to RA, refractory anemia with ringed sideroblasts (RARS) is distinguished by the presence of numerous bone marrow sideroblasts (>15 per cent of all erythroid precursors). These cells are easily identified by the presence of Prussian blue–stained iron granules (iron-laden mitochondria) that partially or completely encircle the nucleus of developing erythroblasts. By definition, sideroblasts must contain at least six abnormally large iron granules that stretch at least one third of the distance around the nucleus.

Unlike other sideroblastic disorders, RARS is characterized by sideroblasts in all stages of erythroid maturation. Although the exact cause is unknown, it is theorized that sideroblasts result from acquired defects in heme biosynthesis. The peripheral smear in these patients may reveal hypochromic microcytes and macrocytes as well as normochromic red blood cells and rare siderocytes. Like patients with RA, RARS patients often have long, favorable clinical courses that rarely progress to acute leukemia.

Refractory Anemia With Excess Blasts

RAEB is characterized by more pronounced trilineage dysplasia and severe cytopenias. By definition, myeloblasts are present in increased numbers in the peripheral blood(<5 per cent) and bone marrow (5 to 20 per cent). Cytogenetic findings are often abnormal, and unfavorable karyotypes are common. Not surprisingly, mortality from hemorrhage, infections, and leukemic transformation is much greater in this subtype than in the previous two subtypes discussed.

Refractory Anemia With Excess Blasts in Transition

The most unfavorable type of myelodysplastic syndrome, RAEBT is defined by the presence of greater than 5 per cent peripheral blood blasts or 20 to 30 per cent bone marrow blasts. The presence of Auer rods has also been considered sufficient for inclusion in this category. Recent studies, however, do not support this practice, since Auer rods appear to have a positive impact on prognosis. Unfavorable karyotypic abnormalities and severe trilineage dysplasia are routinely seen. These patients have a dismal prognosis, with more than 60 per cent of cases progressing to acute leukemia, and many of the remaining patients succumbing to infection or hemorrhage.

Chronic Myelomonocytic Leukemia

CMML is unique in myelodysplastic syndromes because of the presence of monocytosis (>1000 monocytes/μL) and often a neutrophilic leukocytosis. Marrow fibrosis and extramedullary disease (hepatosplenomegaly, skin and central nervous system [CNS] involvement, as well as pleural, pericardial, or peritoneal serositis with or without effusions) are common. Male patients predominate. Trilineage

Table 2. The French-American-British Classification of the Myelodysplastic Syndromes

Myelodysplastic Syndrome Type	Peripheral Blood Blasts	Bone Marrow Blasts	Auer Rods	Monocytosis (1000/μL)	Ringed Sideroblasts (>15%)	Progress to Acute Myelogenous Leukemia	Median Survival (mo)
Refractory anemia	≤1%	≤5%	–	–	–	10–15%	50
Refractory anemia with ringed sideroblasts	≤1%	≤5%	–	–	+	10%	51
Refractory anemia with excess blasts	<5%	5–20%	–	–	–	30%	12
Refractory anemia with excess blasts in transformation	>5%	20–30%	+	–	–	60%	6
Chronic myelomonocytic leukemia	<5%	≤20%	–	+	–	20–30%	16

dysplasia is common, and bone marrow blasts vary between 1 and 20 per cent.

Because of its similarities to myeloproliferative disorders, especially chronic myelogenous leukemia, CMML is the most controversial category of the myelodysplastic syndromes and is considered by some to be a separate entity midway between the myelodysplastic syndromes and the myeloproliferative disorders. Nevertheless, the bulk of the evidence supports CMML's continued inclusion in the myelodysplastic syndromes.

Given the vast range of blast counts that are included in this subtype, it is not surprising that the clinical outcome of CMML patients is variable. A small subset of CMML patients with few bone marrow blasts do relatively well, similar to patients with RA or RARS. Unfortunately, a large percentage of CMML patients have higher blast counts and typically behave much like patients with RAEB. The overall median survival of patients with CMML is 1 to 2 years.

Unique Subsets of the Myelodysplastic Syndromes

5q− Syndrome

A specific subgroup of RA patients have the 5q− syndrome, in which there is an isolated deletion in the long arm of chromosome 5. Characteristic features of this entity include macrocytic anemia with erythroid hyperplasia, normal or elevated platelet counts, and nonlobulated micromegakaryocytes. Females outnumber males by a 2:1 ratio. Patients typically enjoy long, stable clinical courses and have a low risk of subsequent leukemic transformation. Loss of a putative tumor suppressor gene such as IRF-1 (interferon regulatory factor 1), which is present on the long arm of chromosome 5, has been proposed as a cause.

Therapy-Related or Secondary Myelodysplastic Syndromes

Although morphologically indistinguishable from primary myelodysplastic syndrome, secondary myelodysplatic syndrome represents a biologically unique subset because of its uniformly dismal prognosis and often rapid progression to AML. The principal risk factors for secondary myelodysplastic syndrome are previous exposure to alkylating agents or epipodophyllotoxins. Radiation appears to be associated with a smaller risk of subsequent myelodysplastic syndrome. Older patients (>40 years of age) and heavily treated patients are at especially high risk. The peak incidence of the myelodysplastic syndromes occurs 3 to 4 years after exposure.

In comparison to the primary myelodysplastic syndromes, secondary myelodysplastic syndrome is more often associated with karyotypic abnormalities (90 per cent versus 50 per cent) and unfavorable cytogenetics (monosomy 7 in 60 per cent of patients). Given the limited therapeutic options and grim prognosis in these patients, it behooves all physicians to carefully consider the use of cytotoxic therapy and limit its duration whenever possible.

Prognosis

Although bone marrow blast percentage (as reflected in the FAB classification) is the most important prognostic indicator, several other independent variables can provide additional prognostic information. These factors include the severity of peripheral cytopenias, cytogenic abnormalities, the presence or absence of abnormal localization of immature myeloid precursors, and age (older or younger than 60 years of age).

Given that infections and hemorrhage are the most common causes of death in the myelodysplastic syndromes, it is intuitive that the severity of cytopenias should be an important prognostic factor. Equally apparent is the prognostic impact of cytogenetic findings, since the myelodysplastic syndromes are thought to represent a disorder of genetically damaged bone marrow stem cells. Because the myelodysplastic syndromes may result from cumulative genetic damage in bone marrow stem cells, it is understandable that cytogenetic changes should have a profound effect on prognosis. In general, a normal karyotype is better than an abnormal karyotype, and simple abnormalities are better than complex or multiple karyotypic abnormalities. Favorable cytogenetic findings include a normal karyotype and an isolated deletion of the long arm of chromosome 5 (5q−). Monosomy 7 or monosomy 5 and chromosome 11q abnormalities (typical of secondary MDS due to epipodophyllotoxins) predict a poor prognosis, whereas trisomy 8 portends an intermediate outcome. The effect of many other karyotypic abnormalities on prognosis has yet to be established.

Abnormal localization of immature myeloid precursors (ALIP) refers to the shift of granulocytopoiesis from its normal paratrabecular location to a central intertrabecular site typical of the myelodysplastic syndromes. The presence of ALIP predicts a significantly higher incidence of leukemic evolution and shorter survival. Although not universally accepted as a prognostic indicator, ALIP nonetheless is an important sign of myelodysplastic bone marrow involvement.

Older patient age appears to confer an increased risk of death from infection and bleeding, although not all studies are in agreement on this point. No effect on leukemic transformation has been demonstrated.

Common Complications

The most common complications associated with the myelodysplastic syndromes are infections, hemorrhage, and transformation to acute myeloid leukemia. Infections are principally bacterial, but fungal and mycobacterial infections can be seen in rare patients. Because granulocyte and platelet function is impaired in the myelodysplastic syndromes, even mild or moderately pancytopenic individuals may be at risk for bleeding or infection. Standard preventive health care (pneumococcal vaccination and annual influenza vaccines) and prompt evaluation and treatment with antibiotics are critical to limiting infectious morbidity and mortality.

The ineffective erythropoiesis that characterizes these disorders can often be so severe that transfusion support is required. In these patients, routine assessment of total body iron burden (ferritin) should be performed to determine the need for chelation therapy. In general, chelation therapy should be considered when ferritin values are consistently elevated. Sudden declines in cell counts are not uncommon during the long-term follow-up of patients with the myelodysplastic syndromes and should be promptly evaluated. Culprits include pure red cell aplasia (due to parvovirus infection or the underlying myelodysplasia) and the emergence of acute leukemia.

Splenomegaly, a common finding in CMML (30 to 50 per cent of patients), should be treated only when symptomatic. Chemotherapy, splenic irradiation, and splenectomy have all been used with varying success. Skin involvement (usually pruritic papules) in CMML also has been managed successfully with oral etoposide. A number of reports have suggested an increased incidence of autoimmune disorders in association with the myelodysplastic syndromes.

Differential Diagnosis and Diagnostic Pitfalls

Although many patients with the myelodysplastic syndromes fit the textbook description, it is always important to consider alternative hematologic entities that may present in a similar fashion. A list of these disorders and tests that may help to distinguish among them is presented in Table 3.

Table 3. Differential Diagnostic Considerations in Hematologic Disorders

Aplastic Anemia

Little or no peripheral blood or bone marrow dysplasia
Hypocellular marrow
No increase in myeloblasts

Acute Leukemia

Greater than 30% bone marrow blasts

Megaloblastic Anemia

Low serum vitamin B_{12} or red cell folate
Positive Schilling test and anti-intrinsic factor antibodies
Hypersegmented polymorphonuclear neutrophils
Megaloblastic bone marrow morphologic characteristics

Alcoholism

Characteristic history and presentation
Concomitant folate deficiency common
Vacuolated early erythroblasts in bone marrow
Sideroblasts in late erythroid progenitors
Prompt recovery with nutritional support and abstinence

Myelofibrosis

More prominent leukoerythroblastic peripheral blood picture and more numerous teardrop-shaped red blood cells than typically present in fibrotic MDS
More prominent marrow fibrosis and splenomegaly than MDS, less marrow dysplasia than MDS

Chronic Myelogenous Leukemia

More prominent neutrophilic leukocytosis, basophilia, and eosinophilia than CMML, less monocytosis, presence of t(9;22) or BCR-ABL gene rearrangement

Hypersplenism

Prominent splenomegaly, normal bone marrow morphologic characteristics

Paroxysmal Nocturnal Hemoglobinuria

Hyperproliferative anemia with hyper- to hypocellular bone marrow, absent marrow iron stores, less marrow dysplasia than MDS, positive sucrose hemolysis test and urine hemosiderin, low leukocyte alkaline phosphatase score and absence of CD55 and CD59 cells on flow cytometric studies

Recent Cytotoxic Therapy

History of recent chemotherapy, self-limited pancytopenia

Intramedullary Tumor

Leukoerythroblastic blood picture, tumor present in bone marrow biopsy

MDS = myelodysplastic syndromes; CMML = chronic myelomonocytic leukemia.

PRIMARY HEREDITARY SIDEROBLASTIC ANEMIA AND SECONDARY TOXIN-ASSOCIATED SIDEROBLASTIC ANEMIA

Unlike primary acquired sideroblastic anemia (RARS), primary hereditary sideroblastic anemia and secondary toxin-associated sideroblastic anemia are not panmyelopathies. Instead, they represent disorders of heme biosynthesis and iron utilization that result in ineffective erythropoiesis and iron overload. Although the precise pathogenesis remains to be elucidated, it is generally believed that inherited or acquired defects in the heme biosynthetic pathway are responsible for the accumulation of mitochondrial iron in developing erythroblasts. The resulting increased intramedullary cell death precipitates a vicious cycle of enhanced intestinal iron absorption and further sideroblast generation.

Hereditary sideroblastic anemia is usually inherited in an X-linked fashion, although rare instances of autosomal recessive inheritance have been described. Although typically only males are affected, mildly symptomatic female carriers have been documented occasionally. Both male hemizygotes and female carriers appear to be at increased risk for iron overload. Patients usually present in childhood with moderate to severe anemia; however, isolated examples of diagnosis in early adulthood have been described. Splenomegaly is noted in 50 per cent of patients.

Laboratory abnormalities include a microcytic hypochromic anemia with a low reticulocyte count and an increased red cell distribution width (RDW). Serum iron, transferrin saturation, and ferritin are increased, reflecting iron overload. The peripheral smear reveals two distinct red cell populations, one microcytic and hypochromic and the other normocytic and normochromic. Basophilic stippling is common.

The definitive diagnostic procedure is a bone marrow aspirate, which characteristically is normo- or hypercellular and, in contrast to RARS, contains numerous ring sideroblasts, predominantly in late erythroblasts. Abundant bone marrow iron is routinely seen. The principal therapy for hereditary sideroblastic anemia is pyridoxine (200 mg/

day) to which as many as 50 per cent of patients respond. Phlebotomy (if tolerated) or chelation therapy to reduce iron stores can also improve the hematocrit in some patients.

Not surprisingly, the most common complication for these patients is symptomatic iron overload (endocrinopathies including diabetes, hypopituitarism, or hypogonadism as well as cirrhosis, heart failure, and arthritis). This complication generally can be avoided with periodic assessment of total body iron burden (ferritin) and judicious phlebotomy or chelation therapy.

Secondary or Toxin-Associated Sideroblastic Anemia

A large number of toxins have been associated with the development of secondary sideroblastic anemia (Table 4). The most common culprits are alcohol and antituberculous agents such as isoniazid. The typical patient is a poorly nourished alcoholic who presents with a mild to moderate macrocytic or normocytic anemia. Macrocytosis and hypersegmentation of polymorphonuclear leukocytes are seen often in these patients because of concomitant folate deficiency.

In contrast, isoniazid toxicity produces a microcytic anemia without megaloblastic changes. In general, the typical morphologic changes associated with hereditary sideroblastic anemia are less impressive in the secondary types. Red cell changes are mild, and modest numbers of sideroblasts, principally late erythroid precursors, are noted in the bone marrow. Alcohol-induced vacuolation of early erythroblasts is common. Significant iron overload is unusual. Withdrawal of the offending agent is the primary form of therapy. Administration of pyridoxine with isoniazid can prevent sideroblastic changes from occurring.

Differential Diagnosis and Pitfalls in Diagnosis

The principal diagnostic considerations in hypochromic microcytic anemia (iron deficiency, thalassemia) rarely are confused with sideroblastic anemia. Unlike iron deficiency, sideroblastic anemia is not associated with pica and is characterized by increased iron indices (increased serum iron, transferrin saturation, ferritin, and bone marrow iron). Thalassemias are often associated with positive family histories in select ethnic groups (Mediterranean and African American ancestry). Increased fetal hemoglobin and hemoglobin A_2 concentrations are often helpful in confirming the diagnosis of beta-thalassemia.

Table 4. The Classification of Sideroblastic Anemias

- Primary hereditary
  - X-linked
  - Autosomal recessive
- Primary acquired (refractory anemia with ringed sideroblasts)
- Secondary (toxin-associated)
  - Alcohol
  - Isoniazid
  - Pyrazinamide
  - Cycloserine
  - Chloramphenicol
  - Zinc
  - Copper deficiency

ADULT ACUTE LEUKEMIA

By Jorge E. Cortes, M.D.,
and Hagop Kantarjian, M.D.
Houston, Texas

Acute leukemias are clonal disorders of hematopoietic precursors. They are characterized by a dysregulated proliferation of cells with an arrest in maturation at some step of their differentiation pathway. This arrested maturation distinguishes acute leukemias from chronic leukemias, in which the dysregulated proliferation affects cells with a normal or near-normal differentiation pattern. The arrested maturation can affect cells of either lymphoid or myeloid lineage, giving rise to the two major types of acute leukemia, acute lymphoblastic leukemia (ALL) and acute myelogenous leukemia (AML; also known in the old literature as acute nonlymphoblastic leukemia). Initially, leukemias were classified based solely on morphologic criteria. With newer techniques for the identification of immunophenotypic, cytogenetic, and molecular markers of lineage differentiation, the classification has become more complex. Adequate identification of the type of leukemia is important because it has major prognostic and therapeutic implications. A more detailed study of the characteristics of the leukemias has also provided useful information about the cause of acute leukemias.

CLINICAL CHARACTERISTICS

The initial symptoms of acute leukemia reflect the inability of the bone marrow to proceed with normal hematopoiesis. Patients usually present with signs of anemia, including pallor, weakness, easy fatigability, palpitations, and lethargy. Hemorrhagic signs and symptoms are also frequent as a consequence of thrombocytopenia and include easy bruising, petechiae, subconjunctival hemorrhage, and bleeding from mucosal surfaces (e.g., epistaxis, gum bleeding). Fever without identifiable infection may be seen at presentation and in 10 to 20 per cent of patients, often as a consequence of neutropenia and neutrophil dysfunction. Acute leukemia is frequently diagnosed during evaluation of an infectious process in a previously healthy individual. Bone pain and arthralgias can be seen at presentation—more frequently in ALL than in AML and more often in children than in adults.

On physical examination, signs of anemia and hemorrhage are common. Splenomegaly and hepatomegaly are seen in fewer than 20 per cent of patients with AML but in at least 50 per cent of patients with ALL. Moderate lymphadenopathy is common in ALL but is seldom observed in AML.

Signs and symptoms of tissue infiltration can be seen in both AML and ALL, and certain patterns of infiltration suggest a specific type of leukemia. Central nervous system (CNS) involvement is seen in 5 to 10 per cent of patients with ALL at presentation. Without adequate prophylaxis, however, CNS leukemia will eventually occur in more than 50 per cent of patients with ALL. CNS involvement frequently presents with signs and symptoms of meningeal infiltration, with headache and neck stiffness. Papilledema represents increased intracranial pressure caused by obstruction to the outflow of the cerebrospinal fluid. Cranial nerve involvement is also common, affecting more commonly cranial nerves II, IV, VI, and VII. Parenchymal CNS involvement is less common. In general, AML is infrequently associated with CNS involvement. However, monocytic phenotypes (AML-M4 and AML-M5) may spread to the CNS; acute myelomonocytic leukemia with dysplastic eosinophils (M4Eo), associated with an inversion of chromosome 16 [inv(16)], is particularly prone to CNS involvement.

Testicular infiltration is also a feature of ALL, primarily in children. It is uncommon at presentation, but testicular relapses in children represent 5 to 10 per cent of treatment failures after a first complete remission (CR) is achieved. Clinically significant testicular involvement presents as painless, firm swelling of the testes that is often asymptomatic. Therefore, when one testis is involved, the other should be biopsied to rule out bilateral infiltration. Routine testicular biopsies in children who achieve complete remission are frequently advocated.

Other signs and symptoms of tissue infiltration can be seen in patients with AML. Granulocytic sarcomas, also known as chloromas, are tumors composed of myeloblasts and a few normal granulocytes in different stages of differentiation. These sarcomas can infiltrate the skin, bones, CNS, soft tissues, and other organs. They are frequently misdiagnosed as lymphoma, and special staining with chloroacetate esterase or antilysozyme immunoperoxidase can aid in the diagnosis. These lesions occur in approximately 20 per cent of patients with AML and rarely may precede the hematologic manifestations of the disease. Skin infiltration can also take the form of leukemia cutis, which is seen in up to 15 per cent of patients with AML but is uncommon in ALL. It usually presents as a skin rash or multiple small skin tumors. There is a strong association of leukemia cutis with meningeal involvement. This entity must be distinguished from Sweet's syndrome, which is characterized by painful erythematous skin lesions that show infiltration by mature neutrophils on skin biopsy. This is also seen in association with AML, but in more than 80 per cent of patients, the lesions are idiopathic or associated with other malignancies. Gum infiltration is characteristic of acute myelomonocytic or acute monocytic leukemia, and is usually manifested by painless hypertrophy of the gums.

LABORATORY FEATURES

The leukocyte counts are increased in approximately 50 per cent of patients with acute leukemia. Counts higher then 100 $\times$ 10^9/L can be seen in 10 to 20 per cent of patients with AML but are less common in ALL. Extreme leukocytosis in ALL is more frequently associated with a T-cell immunophenotype. In ALL, the neutrophil count is usually decreased. Anemia and thrombocytopenia are common in both AML and ALL.

Coagulation abnormalities are frequently seen. Acute promyelocytic leukemia (APL; AML-M3) is typically associated with disseminated intravascular coagulation (DIC), either at diagnosis or after the start of chemotherapy. However, other subtypes of AML, particularly those with monocytic phenotypes, and even ALL, frequently show evidence of DIC, although in most patients it is subclinical.

Other laboratory abnormalities seen at diagnosis include hyperuricemia and electrolyte imbalance, with hyperkalemia, hyperphosphatemia, and hypocalcemia. After initiation of therapy, a tumor lysis syndrome can be observed with hyperkalemia, hyperphosphatemia, hypercalcemia, hyperuricemia, and renal failure. This is seen more frequently in ALL than in AML.

CLASSIFICATION

The French-American-British (FAB) group proposed a classification for both AML and ALL nearly 20 years ago, and it is still widely used. The updated classification of 1985 and an expanded version are shown in Tables 1 and 2, with modifications for recently recognized categories. It provides a good guide for uniform criteria in the diagnosis of the subtypes of acute leukemia. However, the original FAB classification had several problems, which included the difficult distinction between some cases of ALL and immature cases of AML, the poor reproducibility of the classification when based on morphologic data alone, and the fact that it does not consider biphenotypic cases. More importantly, the immunophenotypic and cytogenetic changes that provide a biologically relevant classification of acute leukemia are not considered in the FAB classification. A flow chart integrating the available procedures for classification is presented in Figure 1. This provides alternatives for diagnosis when cytochemical studies are not sufficient for classification.

DIAGNOSIS

The diagnosis of acute leukemia requires the identification of 30 per cent or more blasts in a bone marrow aspirate. The bone marrow is frequently hypercellular, but it is sometimes normocellular. Occasionally, acute leukemia, particularly ALL, can present as pancytopenia with hypoplastic bone marrow containing 30 per cent or more blasts. Once the diagnosis of acute leukemia is made, a complete work-up is required to classify the leukemia as AML or ALL of a particular subtype. This is of the utmost importance because therapeutic decisions depend on the appropriate identification of the acute leukemia. A complete work-up is suggested in Table 3 and is described more extensively further on.

Table 1. French-American-British Group Classification for Adult Acute Lymphoblastic Leukemia

Type	Incidence (%)	Cellular Characteristics	Complete Remission (%)	3-Year Survival (%)
L1	30	Small, homogeneous cells; round nucleus; nucleolus inconspicuous or not seen; scanty cytoplasm	85	40
L2	60	Large, heterogeneous cells; irregular nucleus, clefted or indented; nucleolus; often abundant cytoplasm	75	35
L3	10	Large, homogeneous; regular oval or round nucleus; prominent nucleolus; vacuolated, basophilic cytoplasm; Burkitt's leukemia	65–90	10–50

Table 2. French-American-British Classification for Acute Myelogenous Leukemia

Type	Name	Incidence	Observations
M0		Unknown	Myeloid differentiation evident only by immunophenotyping or electron microscopy
M1	Without maturation	15–20%	Morphologic features similar to ALL
M2	With maturation	25–30%	t(8;21) in 25%
M3	Promyelocytic, APL	5–15%	Young, low-normal WBC count t(15;17) DIC
	Microgranular variant (M3V)	1–2%	Morphologically similar to M5
M4	Myelomonocytic, AMML	10–15%	Tissue involvement frequent
	M4Eo	2–3%	Dysplastic eosinophils inv(16) CNS involvement frequent Good prognosis
M5	Monocytic, AMoL	2–10%	M5a = poorly differentiated, M5b = well differentiated Tissue involvement: gingival hyperplasia, skin involvement, CNS, liver, spleen, lymph nodes High WBC count
M6	Erythroleukemia, Di Guglielmo	2–5%	Erythroblasts ≥50% of bone marrow nucleated cells, blasts ≥30% of bone marrow nonerythroid cells Old age Rheumatic, immunologic findings Preceding "erythemic myelosis"
M7	Megakaryocytic	3–5%	Low WBC count Hepatosplenomegaly Marrow fibrosis ("dry tab")

APL = acute promyelocytic leukemia; AMML = acute monomyelocytic leukemia; AMoL = acute monocytic leukemia; ALL = acute lymphoblastic leukemia; WBC = white blood cell; DIC = disseminated intravascular coagulation; CNS = central nervous system; M4Eo = acute myelomonocytic leukemia with dysplastic eosinophils.

Morphologic Features

The initial step in the diagnosis and classification of acute leukemia is the morphologic analysis of the Wright-Giemsa–stained bone marrow aspirate slides, with quantification of the percentage of blasts. For this purpose, the FAB group has proposed recognition of two types of blasts. Type I blasts are immature cells with uncondensed chromatin, a high nuclear-to-cytoplasmic (N:C) ratio, absence of a Golgi area, frequently prominent nucleoli, and no granules in the cytoplasm. Type II blasts have similar features but a lower N:C ratio and the presence of a few azurophilic granules. Recently a type III blast has been recognized, which is characterized by numerous azurophilic granules and is often seen in patients with AML-M2 with a translocation t(8;21).

Distinction of AML from ALL by morphologic features alone can de difficult and often erroneous. Lymphoblasts are usually smaller than myeloblasts, have a higher N:C ratio, and have no cytoplasmic granules. The chromatin is characteristically clumped and distributed irregularly, but it is more prominent along nuclear and nucleolar membranes, which makes the nucleoli appear prominent. Myeloblasts, in contrast, have a more abundant cytoplasm, frequently with granules, and fine chromatin, with indistinct nuclear and nucleolar membranes. Some features can also suggest the lineage more specifically. They include (1) the presence of Auer rods, seen only in myeloid leukemias, but present in less than 30 per cent of patients; (2) vacuolated basophilic cytoplasm, suggestive but not pathognomonic of mature B-cell ALL; and (3) "hand mirror" morphologic features, suggestive of ALL. However, these and other morphologic features are not definitive and require further identification of lineage.

Cytochemistry

Several cytochemical stains are useful in the diagnosis and classification of acute leukemia. Those among the more widely used are discussed in the following paragraphs.

Myeloperoxidase

Myeloperoxidase (MPO) is an enzyme found in the azurophilic granules of cells of granulocyte and monocyte lineage. The free oxygen liberated by the peroxidase reacts with the benzidine dye used in this test and stains cells dark brown. This is a key test to distinguish AML from ALL: When 3 per cent or more of blasts stain positive for MPO, a diagnosis of AML is made. Importantly, the counting of blasts must not include neutrophils, because they show a positive MPO stain regardless of the lineage of the leukemia. Cells in the monocytic series show weak staining with MPO, whereas lymphoid and erythroid precursors are MPO-negative.

Sudan Black B

Sudan Black B (SBB) stains phospholipids and other lipids and occasionally nonlipid cellular components. It usually parallels MPO staining, but a few cases of MPO-negative AML (e.g., in subjects with MPO deficiency) stain with SBB, whereas as many as 2 per cent of ALL can be SBB-positive. The threshold for diagnosis of acute myeloid leukemia is also 3 per cent or more positive cells.

Esterase

Two different esterase tests can be used. Nonspecific esterase (NSE) staining uses α-naphthyl butyrate (ANB) or α-naphthyl acetate (ANA) as substrates for the esterase

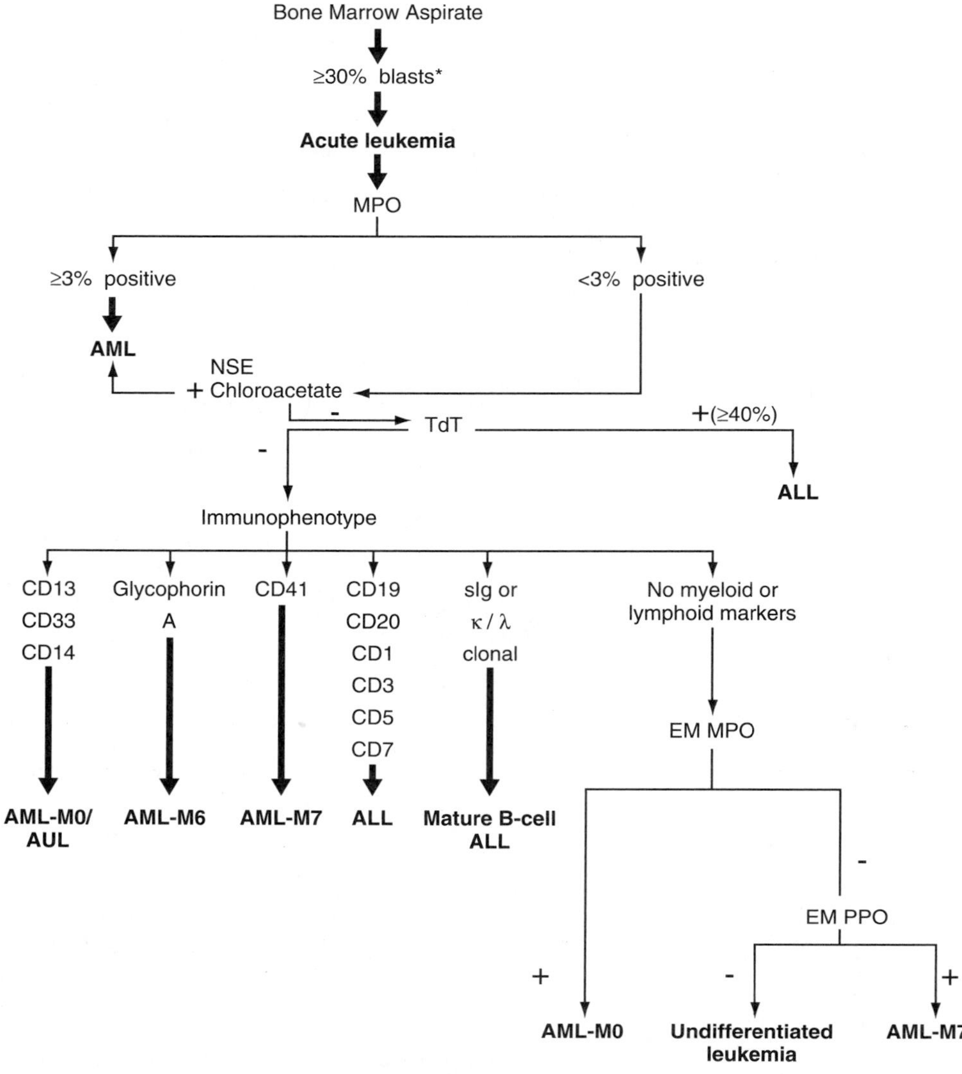

Figure 1. Flow chart for differentiation of lineage in acute leukemia. AML = acute myelogenous leukemia; ALL = acute lymphoblastic leukemia; AUL = acute undifferentiated leukemia; MPO = myeloperoxidase; TdT = terminal deoxynucleotidyl transferase; NSE = nonspecific esterase; EM MPO = myeloperoxidase by electron microscopy; PPO = platelet peroxidase by electron microscopy. Asterisk (*) indicates that total blast count may be less than 30 per cent when red cell precursors are greater than or equal to 50 per cent and the blast count is greater than or equal to 30 per cent of nonred cells; this suggests AML-M6.

cleavage of a naphthyl group, which is then allowed to react with a diazo dye. This reaction is strongly positive in cells of monocytic lineage and weak in granulocyte precursors. Furthermore, when cells are pretreated with sodium fluoride, the activity is inhibited in monocytic but not in granulocytic precursors. Therefore, nonspecific esterase is a useful stain for the identification of AML with monocytic differentiation when results are positive in 20 per cent or more of blast cells. Naphthol AS-D chloroacetate esterase (NASD) gives a strong positive azo dye staining to cells of neutrophilic lineage but is only weak or negative in monocyte precursors. Some early granulocyte cells are negative, however, and this test is therefore less sensitive than MPO or SBB.

Terminal Deoxynucleotidyl Transferase

Terminal deoxynucleotidyl transferse (TdT) is a nuclear enzyme present in normal cortical thymocytes and in some normal bone marrow cells but not in peripheral blood lymphocytes. It allows the template-independent addition of deoxynucleotides onto DNA chains at the recombination junction. It can be detected in most patients with ALL, although it is noticeably absent in mature B-cell ALL (Burkitt's leukemia, ALL-L3). TdT is not lineage-specific, however, and it can be detected in some patients with AML, although the incidence of this phenomenon varies with the threshold used to define positivity. Patients with fewer than 3 per cent MPO-positive blasts and 40 per cent or more TdT-positive blasts have ALL.

Periodic Acid–Schiff Reaction

The periodic acid–Schiff (PAS) reaction identifies cellular glycogen. Lymphoblasts have positive coarse granules or blocks, whereas myeloblasts, when positive, show a fine, diffuse pattern. In most cases of erythroleukemia (AML-M6), erythroid precursors also show coarse granular or diffuse cytoplasmic staining with PAS.

Immunophenotype

The work-up for acute leukemia should include identification of antigenic markers on the cell surface and in the cytoplasm using monoclonal antibodies. One theory of leukemogenesis suggests that an arrest in maturation with proliferating advantage occurs at some point during the normal differentiation pathway of hematopoietic cells. The stages of differentiation are better defined in ALL, both

Table 3. Suggested Evaluation for Acute Leukemia

Routine

- History and physical examination
  - Signs and symptoms of anemia
  - Bleeding
  - Infections
  - Lymphadenopathy
  - Liver and/or splenic enlargement
  - CNS involvement
  - Other organ infiltration
- Laboratory tests
  - Leukocyte count with differential count
  - Electrolytes
  - DIC profile (PT, PTT, Fibrinogen, FSP, D-dimer)
  - Liver function tests
  - Renal function tests
- Bone marrow aspirate and biopsy
  - Morphologic analysis (cell count)
  - Cytochemical studies
  - Immunophenotyping
  - Cytogenetics
- Lumbar puncture when clinical suspicion of CNS involvement, unless part of treatment strategy (e.g., in some ALL programs)
  - Cell count

Optional

- Electron microscopy
- Molecular analysis
- FISH

CNS = central nervous system; DIC = disseminated intravascular coagulation; PT = prothrombin time; PTT = partial thromboplastin time; FSP = fibrin split products; ALL = acute lymphocytic leukemia; FISH = fluorescent in situ hybridization.

with B-cell and T-cell phenotypes. The immunophenotypic classification of ALL is presented in Table 4. Identifying these subgroups of ALL is important, because the prognosis of various stages may be different. Leukemic cells show the same immunophenotypic characteristics of normal cells at the stage of differentiation at which the arrest occurred. Although this is true in many patients, exceptions exist. Antigenic markers characteristic of different stages of differentiation may occur simultaneously, producing phenotypes that do not correspond to any normal stage known. In other situations, markers from different lineages occur in the same leukemic cells (i.e., ALL with myeloid markers, AML with lymphoid markers) in what has been called "lineage infidelity." The exact clinical and biologic significance of this phenomenon is not known. Immunophenotype can also identify some subtypes of acute leukemia in which morphologic and cytochemical criteria are not well defined.

Table 5. Suggested Panel of Antibodies for Immunophenotyping

- B-cell markers
  - CD19
  - CD20
  - Cytoplasmic immunoglobulin (cIg)
  - Surface immunoglobulin (sIg)
- T-cell markers
  - CD1
  - CD3
  - CD5
  - CD7
  - CD4
  - CD8
- Myelomonocytic markers
  - CD13
  - CD33
  - CD14 (monocyte only)
- Others
  - CD34 (early progenitor cells)
  - CD41 (megakaryocytes)
  - CD56 (NK cells)
  - CD10 (common ALL)
  - Glycophorin A (erythroid precursors)

ALL = acute lymphoblastic leukemia.

These include erythroleukemia (AML-M6), which characteristically expresses glycophorin A; megakaryocytic leukemia (AML-M7), which expresses the platelet- and megakaryocytic-specific markers CD41 (GP IIb/IIIa) and CD42 (GP Ib); AML-M0, which lacks evidence of myeloid differentiation by morphologic or cytochemical techniques but expresses myeloid-specific antigens; undifferentiated leukemia, which has no cytochemical or immunophenotypic characteristics of AML or ALL; and ALL-L3, in which phenotyping requires identification of surface immunoglobulins.

The study of the immunophenotypic characteristics of acute leukemia requires a minimal panel of antibodies that can identify some of the most relevant antigenic markers for classification purposes. A suggested panel is shown in Table 5. This panel allows characterization of most acute leukemias.

Cytogenetic Studies

The study of the chromosomal content and structure in leukemic cells provides invaluable information for the understanding of the biology of acute leukemia. With regular banding cytogenetic techniques, 50 to 60 per cent of patients with acute leukemia have chromosomal abnormal-

Table 4. Immunophenotype in Acute Lymphoblastic Leukemia: Expression of Differentiation Markers

B-Lineage	HLA-DR	CD19	CD24	CD10	CD20	CD21	CD22	CD23	cIg	sIg
Early pre-B	+	+	+	+	±	−	Cyt	−	−	−
Pre-B	+	+	+	+	+	+	+	−	+	−
Transitional B	+	+	+	±	+	+	+	−	+	+μ*
Mature B	+	+	+	−	+	+	+	+	−	+
T-Lineage	**CD7**	**CD2**	**CD5**	**CD1**	**CD4**	**CD8**	**CD3**			
Early	+	+	+	−	−	−	−			
Intermediate	+	+	+	+	±	±	−			
Mature	+	+	+	−	+	+	+			

*μ heavy chains but no light chains.

ities. These can be classified as numeric (hyperdiploidy, hypodiploidy), and structural, most frequently including translocations, inversions, deletions, and isochromosomes. Some of the most common cytogenetic abnormalities in acute leukemia are shown in Table 6. Cytogenetic abnormalities constitute one of the most important prognostic factors in acute leukemia. Patients with AML with t(8;21) or inv(16) have a distinctly good prognosis, with complete remission rates near 90 per cent and long-term disease-free survival rates of 40 to 50 per cent. In contrast, those with monosomies or deletions of chromosomes 5 and/or 7 have a very poor prognosis. A similar scenario exists in ALL: Patients with a hyperdiploid karyotype (>50 chromosomes) have the best prognosis, whereas patients with a t(9;22) have a high incidence of relapse. Some cytogenetic changes are characteristic of specific subtypes of acute leukemia. One example is the translocation t(15;17), which is seen in nearly all patients with APL (AML-M3) and is not present in any other subtype. Another example includes the translocations involving chromosome 8, t(2;8), t(8;14), and t(8;22), which are a feature in patients with B-cell ALL. In many situations, therapeutic decisions can be influenced by the presence of cytogenetic abnormalities. Patients with ALL and t(9;22), or the Philadelphia chromosome, do not benefit from maintenance chemotherapy, in contrast with most other patients with ALL.

There is some correlation among morphologic, immunologic, and cytogenetic characteristics of acute leukemias. Although not universally accepted, a new classification of ALL called MIC (morphologic, immunologic, cytogenetic) has been proposed and provides some information about the associations most frequently seen in ALL.

Other Diagnostic Procedures

Several other techniques are available for patients in whom the routine work-up is still equivocal as to the nature of the acute leukemia. Some of the most frequently used are discussed in the following paragraphs.

Electron Microscopy

In approximately 5 per cent of patients with acute leukemia, the diagnosis can be finally defined by electron microscopy (EM). In some acute leukemias without myeloid markers by morphologic criteria, MPO is negative by regular cytochemical technique, but EM can demonstrate MPO positivity. These acute leukemias can then be classified as AML-M0. Electron microscopy can also identify platelet peroxidase reactivity, which is a very sensitive marker for acute megakaryocytic leukemia (AML-M7).

Molecular Studies

Several techniques are now available for identifying chromosomal changes at the molecular level. These techniques allow the identification of genetic abnormalities with greater sensitivity than with regular cytogenetic analysis. They include (1) Southern blot and (2) polymerase chain reaction (PCR). In Southern blot, DNA is extracted from cells in the sample to be analyzed and digested with restriction endonucleases. The fragments are separated by gel electrophoresis and transferred to a membrane. The membrane is then hybridized with labeled probes that are short fragments of DNA with a sequence complementary to the gene of interest. This technique's main use is for the identification of rearrangements of lineage-specific genes

Table 6. Some Common Cytogenetic Abnormalities in Acute Leukemia

Acute Lymphoblastic Leukemia	Frequency (%)	Comments
Numeric Abnormalities		
Hyperdiploidy	10–20	Good prognosis, especially when 47 to 50 chromosomes
Hypodiploidy	5–10	Intermediate prognosis
Diploidy	25–35	Intermediate prognosis; most common
Structural abnormalities		
t(9;22)(q34;q11) (Philadelphia chromosome)	15–25	Poor prognosis
t(8;14), t(8;2), t(8;22)	5–10	B-cell phenotype; need short-term dose-intensive therapy
t(4;11)(q21;q23) and others involving 11q23	5	Very common in infants; poor prognosis
t(1;19)	<5	Pre-B phenotype; poor prognosis
14q11 abnormalities	5–10	T cell
7q35 abnormalities	<5	T cell
Others	5–15	Most common 6q, 12p
Acute Myelogenous Leukemia	**Frequency (%)**	**Comments**
Numeric abnormalities		
Trisomy 8	15	Associated with AHD; poor prognosis
Monosomy 7	20 (Monosomy 7 and Monosomy 5 combined)	Associated with AHD; poor prognosis
Monosomy 5 (and del(5q))		Associated with AHD; poor prognosis
Diploid	30	Intermediate prognosis
Others	<5	Most common trisomy 21
Structural abnormalities		
t(8;21)(q22;q22)	5	Good prognosis; frequently M2
t(15;17)(q22;q11)	5–10	M3; DIC, good prognosis
inv(16)	5	Good prognosis; M4Eo; CNS involvement
11q23 abnormalities	5	Poor prognosis; frequent after prior exposure to topoisomerase II–reactive drugs
Others	5–10	

AHD = antecedent hematologic disorder; DIC = disseminated intravascular coagulation; CNS = central nervous system; M4Eo = acute myelomonocytic leukemia with dysplastic eosinophils.

(e.g., immunoglobulin or T-cell receptor genes). PCR is a very sensitive technique that allows the amplification of low copy numbers of a gene of interest up to a million times. It uses small sequences of DNA, called primers, that are complementary to flanking regions of the gene of interest; a heat-stable DNA polymerase; and repeated cycles of denaturation of DNA double-strands, annealing of primers, and chain elongation.

These techniques can be used for several purposes. In cases of uncertainty about the lineage, molecular analysis can aid in the classification of leukemias. During the initial steps of differentiation of lymphocytes, they undergo rearrangements of the immunoglobulin (B cells) or T-cell receptor (T cells) genes. These rearrangements can be identified by molecular techniques and define lymphoid lineage involvement. Myeloid lineage molecular markers are not so widely used.

Molecular analysis also provides a more sensitive way to look for chromosomal aberrations in acute leukemia. This is particularly useful when morphologic or cytochemical data suggest a diagnosis that is not confirmed by regular cytogenetic analysis. One example is the patient with a morphologic diagnosis of APL who has no evidence of t(15;17) by cytogenetic analysis. Molecular analysis can document rearrangement of the retinoic acid receptor alpha (RAR-α) and PML, the genes involved in this translocation.

Finally, molecular analysis can be used to monitor residual disease. When a specific abnormality is detected at diagnosis, sequential analysis after treatment can document complete disappearance of all detectable disease or persistence of some evidence of disease. Recurrence can sometimes be identified by this method before clinical evidence of recurrence. Although these techniques are not routinely used in most centers, and no standard therapeutic guidelines exist for patients with minimal residual disease at different points in the therapy for acute leukemia, they are frequently used in a research setting, and information derived from them will aid in designing more rational therapy for acute leukemia.

Fluorescent In Situ Hybridization

Regular cytogenetic analysis is a time-consuming technique that is limited to the analysis of a few cells (usually 20 to 25) during metaphase. Thus, only dividing cells can be analyzed. Furthermore, the origin of chromosomal fragments in some complex translocations might not be identified with a regular cytogenetic analysis. Fluorescent in situ hybridization (FISH) allows detection of specific gene sequences in metaphase or interphase nuclei and is therefore not dependent on cell division. The technique involves heating cells in a conventional cytogenetic slide preparation to denature the DNA, followed by hybridization with the probe of interest labeled with a marker that can be identified by color. The probe can be specific for centromeres of specific chromosomes to identify numeric chromosomal abnormalities or for certain genes to detect structural changes in that gene. This technique allows simultaneous analysis of several hundred cells, thus increasing the sensitivity. Furthermore, cytogenetic findings can be correlated with cell morphologic features.

POLYCYTHEMIA VERA AND OTHER POLYCYTHEMIA SYNDROMES

By Richard T. Silver, M.D.
New York, New York

Polycythemia may be defined as an increase in the volume of circulating red cells per kilogram of body weight or, equivalently, an increase in the red blood cell mass. Clinically, this is expressed as an absolute increase in the number of red cells, usually but not always accompanied by corresponding increases in the hemoglobin and hematocrit. Polycythemia may occur as a primary disease of unknown cause, polycythemia vera, or as a secondary manifestation of other illnesses. The diagnosis of polycythemia vera is often an exclusionary diagnosis.

The terms erythremia and erythrocytosis are often used to refer to primary and secondary polycythemia, respectively. Others use erythremia as a classification for patients whose only abnormality is an increased red cell volume. Both terms are superfluous and confusing and therefore are not recommended. The term "relative" polycythemia is also a misnomer, and its use should be discontinued. A better term is "false" polycythemia, which is not polycythemia because the red cell volume per kilogram of body weight is normal. In this instance, the increased hematocrit is related to a decrease in plasma volume. In true polycythemia, the plasma volume may be increased, normal, or decreased. Other terms referring to false or relative polycythemia include stress polycythemia, stress erythrocytosis, pseudopolycythemia, and benign polycythemia. In addition, probably some of the patients diagnosed as having Gaisböck's syndrome have false polycythemia. The determination of red cell volume per kilogram of body weight separates both primary and secondary polycythemia from false polycythemia, and polycythemia vera can be differentiated from secondary polycythemia by other means (to be described) but not by blood volume determination as has sometimes been implied.

PRESENTING SIGNS AND SYMPTOMS

Polycythemia vera is twice as common in men as in women. It is usually a disease of middle age, but its range extends broadly from 20 to 60 or 70 years. The development of symptoms is insidious and those related to increased red cell mass and whole blood viscosity include easy fatigue, weakness, shortness of breath, dizziness, tinnitus, bone pain, visual disturbances, headaches, pounding in the ears, and pruritus. The pruritus increases in intensity after a tub bath and less often after showering. It is worse when the temperature of the water is warm rather than cool. Burning or throbbing pain in the legs, feet, or hands, accompanied by a mottled redness, may occur.

Minor wounds may cause an unusual loss of blood. The most common source of major hemorrhage is the upper gastrointestinal tract, where peptic ulcer may be seen in about 10 per cent of patients with polycythemia vera. Thus,

This study was supported by grants from the United Leukemia Fund and the Cancer Research and Treatment Fund.

iron deficiency may distort the overall picture because of anemia, hypochromia, and microcytosis. Sometimes iron deficiency occurs in a previously polycythemic woman owing to menometrorrhagia, producing the same distorted picture. In these instances, the nature of the underlying polycythemia is revealed only when hemorrhage is controlled and the anemia has been treated with iron.

Incompletely understood abnormalities of coagulation responsible for the hemorrhagic tendency paradoxically contribute to thrombotic episodes, which may also be the presenting manifestations of polycythemia vera. Most often these episodes result from qualitative and quantitative platelet abnormalities. Patients referred for the evaluation of vascular thromboses of unknown cause in small vessels in the hands or feet may suffer from polycythemia and in particular thrombocythemia. Thromboses of larger vessels may involve the arterial and venous circulations of the heart, brain, liver, spleen, gastrointestinal tract, and lung. Thrombophlebitis is common. Acute gouty attacks may accompany excess production of uric acid.

In the early stage of polycythemia vera, the conjunctivae are injected. The liver is palpable in about 50 per cent of patients, and the spleen is enlarged in more than 75 per cent. The size of the spleen depends on the stage of the illness and ranges from barely palpable below the left costal margin to filling the left half of the abdomen. Spleen size is not a simple function of blood volume. Extremely large spleens may herald the future development of myelofibrosis and myeloid metaplasia.

HEMATOLOGIC MANIFESTATIONS

Red cell counts of 7 to 10 million cells/mm^3, hematocrits of 55 to 70 per cent, and hemoglobin concentrations of 18 to 24 g/dL are commonly observed. Often the hemoglobin is not increased as much as the red cell count, and thus the hematocrit may be slightly reduced in proportion to the erythrocyte count. If there has been hemorrhage, the hemoglobin content of the red blood cells is reduced more than their size, and the red cells may appear hypochromic and microcytic. In general, however, the individual erythrocytes appear normocytic and normochromic. A rare normoblast may be found. The number of reticulocytes is usually normal except after hemorrhage.

In about one half of patients, there is a moderate increase in the peripheral leukocyte count, ranging from 10,000 to 30,000 cells/mm^3. Values greater than 50,000 cells/mm^3 have been reported. Metamyelocytes may be seen in the peripheral blood smear. An increase in the absolute basophil count may be seen and may be related to certain features of polycythemia vera, such as peptic ulcer and pruritus.

The number of blood platelets is increased in about one third of patients at the time of diagnosis. Typically the increase is modest, the platelet count ranging between 500,000 and 1 million cells/mm^3. In some patients, the initial platelet count may be more than 1 million cells/mm^3, accompanied by only a modest elevation of the hematocrit. Of great importance is the fact that the platelet count may increase substantially after spontaneous bleeding or phlebotomy. The association of increased platelet counts and hemorrhage or thrombosis usually occurs at counts of 1 to 2 million cells/mm^3.

The bone marrow in patients with polycythemia vera is hypercellular, and marrow fat is reduced, findings particularly well recognized in biopsy sections. Although each of the three developmental series typically participates in the hyperplasia, erythroid hyperplasia is paramount. (In contrast, the hyperplasia in secondary polycythemia is typically confined to the erythroid series.) There is no abnormality in maturation, and orthochromic normoblasts predominate. There may be a slight shift to the left in the neutrophilic series. Eosinophils and basophils may also be common.

Bone marrow examination by itself cannot unequivocally distinguish primary and secondary polycythemia. However, an immature and hyperplastic granulocyte series and an increase in megakaryocytes favors polycythemia vera. Also, marrow iron stores are depleted more often in primary than in secondary polycythemia. This difference may be of diagnostic importance. However, since secondary iron deficiency is so common in women, it is doubtful that the absence of marrow iron can be of significant differential diagnostic value, at least in the female patient.

Normally, reticulin fibers extend throughout the marrow and provide a supporting stroma for hematopoietic tissue. In disease states, two different patterns of the reticulin network can be recognized. The first consists of an increased prominence of the normal network, which probably occurs in response to an increase in functioning hematopoietic tissue. It is a nonspecific change, since it is found in various hematologic disorders. The second, or "fibroblastic" pattern, consists of coarsening of the network, resulting from the formation of fibers that are thicker than normal. These thick fibers tend to form bundles or fascicles that follow a waving or swirling course. The fibroblastic pattern has been seen in patients with polycythemia vera and other myeloproliferative diseases.

HYPERURICEMIA

Hyperuricemia, a characteristic of all myeloproliferative diseases, occurs in most patients with polycythemia vera. A good correlation between serum urate concentration and red and white cell counts has not been demonstrated. The incidence of gout in patients with polycythemia vera has ranged from 5 to 10 per cent. Although gout may precede the development of polycythemia vera, it usually occurs 5 to 10 years after the onset of polycythemia. Thus, gout and excessive uric acid excretion appear in the later stages of polycythemia vera, often when there is evidence of myelofibrosis and myeloid metaplasia.

Increased urate production and excretion may result in the precipitation of uric acid in the kidneys, causing stones or uric acid nephropathy. Renal colic is an unusual presenting manifestation of patients with polycythemia vera, but it has been observed. Although serum uric acid may be increased in secondary polycythemia, it is rare to find the same high concentrations that occur in the primary disease.

NATURAL HISTORY

An appreciation of the natural course of polycythemia vera is required because a patient may be observed during a stage when the disease is in transition. Polycythemia vera is an illness of reasonably long duration, usually ranging from 10 to 20 years. Although phlebotomy and other treatment modalities influence the course of the disease and its clinical manifestations, after a number of years the hemoglobin concentration gradually falls and anemia develops. The spleen (and sometimes the liver) progressively enlarges and may fill the entire abdomen. Splenic infarcts, causing mild to severe left upper quadrant pain, may mimic an acute abdominal crisis or renal colic. Rarely, the enormous spleen may cause large bowel obstruction. Erythrocytes of variable size and shape, teardrop forms, nucleated red cells, and immature granulocytes appear in the peripheral blood. The white blood cell count, often normal or moderately increased throughout the early phase of the illness, continues to rise. Blood platelets may increase or decrease in number. Bone marrow examination at this time reveals a prominent "fibroblastic" reticulin network, myelofibrosis, and osteosclerosis. Although the degree of extramedullary hematopoiesis (myeloid metaplasia) generally is proportional to the duration of the disease, some patients display features of it early in the course of the illness and even relatively early during the polycythemic phase. Without an antecedent history of polycythemia vera, it may appear that the patient is suffering from primary myelofibrosis with myeloid metaplasia (MMM). Sometimes the clinical and hematologic picture resembles chronic granulocytic leukemia. Nevertheless the histochemical, biochemical, and cytogenetic findings remain more consistent with polycythemia vera than with typical chronic myeloid leukemia. The Philadelphia chromosome, the hallmark of chronic myeloid leukemia, is never present in polycythemia vera. The terminal picture of acute myeloid leukemia is indistinguishable from that seen in end-stage myelofibrosis with myeloid metaplasia or blast-phase chronic granulocytic leukemia.

DIAGNOSTIC TESTS

Hematocrit

Polycythemia is first suspected most commonly from the hematocrit. However, the extent of reliance on the hematocrit for the *diagnosis* of polycythemia is the source of much confusion both at the bedside and in published texts. Despite reasonably good correlation between the hematocrit and the circulating total red cell volume over a wide range of hematocrit determinations, the value of a single hematocrit measurement for predicting total red cell volume is poor. For hematocrit readings ranging from 50 to 60 per cent, the total red cell volume may range from normal to a maximum of twice normal. Furthermore, red cell volume cannot be accurately predicted by measuring plasma volume. Hence, red cell volume must be measured directly to ascertain whether or not it is increased. To compare total red cell volume from one individual to another, it is best to express it in terms of cubic centimeters per kilogram of body weight, since the use of volume alone does not provide a basis for comparison between persons of different body mass. A satisfactory and widely used method for determining red cell volume is the direct tagging of red cells with radioactive chromium (chromium-51). The method is easy to perform and is reproducible. The coefficient of variation is only 1.5 per cent. The red cell mass in a normal man differs from that in a normal woman. As measured by ^{51}Cr-labeled erythrocytes, a red cell mass greater than 36 cc/kg body weight is considered increased in a man and one greater than 32 cc/kg body weight is considered increased in a woman. It should be noted that a normal red blood cell mass may occur on occasion in patients with polycythemia vera. This is usually associated with recent bleeding, typically gastrointestinal, and evidence of iron deficiency.

Arterial Oxygen Saturation

Causes of secondary polycythemia can be classified for clinical use as (1) those related to oxygen delivery that does not meet tissue needs and (2) those that are not so related. These are summarized in Table 1. It is helpful to define the following terms: "Hypoxia" means inadequate tissue oxygenation. It may result from an increased demand for or a decreased supply of oxygen. "Hypoxemia" refers to decreased oxygen content in the blood. It implies decreased arterial oxygen tension or decreased oxygen saturation, or both. "Arterial oxygen tension" (Po_2) is the partial pressure of oxygen in arterial blood measured in millimeters of mercury. Because of the shape of the oxyhemoglobin dissociation curve, arterial oxygen tension may be reduced without any reduction in arterial oxygen saturation. "Arterial oxygen saturation" is the percentage of hemoglobin saturated with oxygen in the arterial blood. Customarily an arterial oxygen saturation of 92 per cent or more has been considered characteristic of polycythemia vera, whereas a lower saturation has been regarded as strong evidence of polycythemia related to hypoxemia. Recent studies have cast doubt on the usefulness of arterial oxygen saturation measurements in differentiating primary and secondary polycythemia, even when the latter is related to impaired arterial oxygen supply.

Some patients with pulmonary disease have respiratory alkalosis due to hyperventilation. Because of the influence of pH on the oxyhemoglobin dissociation curve, oxygen saturation in these patients may be normal even though arterial oxygen tension is significantly reduced. To illustrate, at pH 7.4, an abnormal oxygen tension (Po_2) of 65 mm Hg results in an abnormal saturation of about 91.5 per cent. At pH 7.45, however, the saturation is 93.5 per cent for the same Po_2. Changes in pH of this magnitude may even result from hyperventilation induced by an arterial puncture, especially the "single-stick" type.

The frequency with which misleading normal arterial oxygen saturation determinations are recorded is unknown. It is even less well known and appreciated that polycythemia vera uncomplicated by cardiac or pulmonary disease may in itself cause arterial oxygen undersaturation. The cause of hypoxemia in polycythemia vera uncomplicated by cardiac or pulmonary disease is not well understood. The arterial undersaturation is not related to abnormal hemoglobin function, the high hematocrit, or in-

Table 1. Clinical Classification of Polycythemia

Secondary polycthemia
- Related to inadequate oxygen delivery to tissues with respect to need
  - Due to decreased arterial oxygen tension
    - With physiologic or anatomic cardiopulmonary abnormalities
      - Abnormalities of lungs, chest bellows, or ventilatory control mechanisms
      - Right-to-left vascular shunts
    - Without physiologic or anatomic cardiopulmonary abnormalities
      - Low oxygen tension, i.e., high altitudes
      - Impaired oxygen-carrying capacity of hemoglobin
  - Due to increased blood flow—congestive heart failure
- Unrelated to inadequate oxygen delivery and need and associated with benign or malignant lesions of
  - Kidney—cysts, hydronephrosis, adenoma, hypernephroma, sarcoma
  - Cerebellum—hemangioblastoma
  - Uterus—myoma
  - Liver—hepatoma, hamartoma
  - Other—adrenal (pheochromocytoma), lung

Primary polycythemia (polycythemia vera)

creased blood volume per se. In general, patients with polycythemia vera have normal ventilatory function, alveolar ventilation, and distribution of ventilation. Controversy still exists, however, about diffusion measurements and ventilation-perfusion relationships. It is not known whether hypoxemia is an integral feature of the disorder or a nonspecific finding. In polycythemia vera, hypoxemia may represent the combined effects of age, associated and unrelated pulmonary disease, and possibly vascular abnormalities of the pulmonary microcirculation.

The limited usefulness of an arterial oxygen saturation measurement in the differential diagnosis of polycythemia stems from its lack of discriminatory value, except in patients who have moderately severe arterial undersaturation, that is, less than 88 per cent. Mild undersaturation (90 to 94 per cent) is commonly found in primary polycythemia and in some forms of secondary polycythemia.

Erythropoietin

A readily available test for measuring erythropoietin has become important in the diagnosis of the polycythemias. Decreased arterial oxygen tension typically leads to increased red cell production, presumably mediated by erythropoietin. A major exception is in patients with emphysema who have diminished arterial oxygen tension but normal red cell mass. An increase in erythropoietin has nevertheless been demonstrated in some of these patients, implying that the absence of polycythemia does not depend on an inability to produce erythropoietin. Chronic infection, seen commonly in obstructive pulmonary disease, has been offered as one explanation for the suboptimal increase in red cell mass observed in these hypoxemic patients.

Polycythemia unrelated to tissue hypoxia may be due to autonomous erythropoietin production by benign or malignant tumors. Biologically active erythropoietic substances, which have been demonstrated in plasma, urine, and tissue extracts from such patients, are not subject to physiologic control mechanisms and are independent of the red cell mass. The causal relationship between polycythemia and tumor is indicated by the fact that in many patients remission of the polycythemia has occurred following removal of the tumor. This type of polycythemia has been most frequently associated with renal abnormalities, especially neoplasms and benign cysts. Erythropoietin can be detected in cyst fluid or kidney extracts from some patients, but increased concentrations of erythropoietin have not been observed consistently in plasma or urine. Whether the tumor or cyst is directly related to the increased production of erythropoietin has not been demonstrated; for example, the tumor or cyst may cause local changes in the kidney by compressing blood vessels and thus may lead to increased elaboration of erythropoietin.

In contrast to the observations in polycythemia secondary to anoxia and tumors, the polycythemia of polycythemia vera is not oxygen-dependent and is not associated with increased erythropoietin in plasma or urine. In fact, erythropoietin output is less than normal, implying both that red cell production by the marrow is autonomous and that erythropoietin output has been suppressed by the increased red cell mass.

The relation between erythropoietin and polycythemia may be summarized as follows:

1. Increased, but regulated, erythropoietin production is proportional to the stimulus in secondary hypoxemic polycythemia.
2. Autonomous erythropoietin production irrespective of red cell mass is observed in secondary polycythemia accompanying tumors.
3. Autonomous erythropoiesis by the marrow, irrespective of erythropoietin concentrations, is seen in polycythemia vera.

Vitamin B_{12} and Its Binding Proteins

Abnormalities of the serum concentrations of vitamin B_{12}, total vitamin B_{12}–binding capacity (TBBC), and unsaturated vitamin B_{12}–binding capacity (UBBC) indicate that vitamin B_{12} metabolism is altered in myeloproliferative diseases, including polycythemia vera.

In polycythemia vera (and in chronic granulocytic leukemia), concentrations of serum vitamin B_{12} and vitamin B_{12}–binding capacity are increased to greater than normal, paralleling the degree of leukocyte proliferation. Serum vitamin B_{12} tends to be modestly increased in polycythemia vera and greatly increased in chronic granulocytic leukemia. A similar, but more striking, relative increase occurs in the UBBC.

An increase in the UBBC can aid in the differential diagnosis of polycythemia vera and false (relative) polycythemia. In one series, UBBC exceeded 2000 pg/mL in 24 of 27 patients with active polycythemia vera. By contrast, only 4 of 28 normal patients and 3 of 17 patients with false polycythemia demonstrated similar values. The mean UBBC values in the three groups were 3516 pg/mL, 1667 pg/mL, and 1857 pg/mL, respectively. Corresponding mean serum vitamin B_{12} levels were 894 pg/mL, 472 pg/mL, and 305 pg/mL.

Leukocyte Alkaline Phosphatase

Because some patients with polycythemia vera may have a significant increase in the leukocyte count, the leukocyte alkaline phosphatase (LAP) stain can help distinguish polycythemia vera from chronic granulocytic leukemia. The principle of the LAP staining method is based on the amount and staining intensity of a dye precipitated at presumed sites of enzyme activity within mature and band neutrophils, which are the only granulocytes with significant LAP activity in the peripheral blood or bone marrow. Usually peripheral blood is scored semiquantitatively; 100 neutrophils are graded 0 to 4+. The total score may thus range from 0 to 400.

Abnormally low or absent LAP activity is observed in chronic granulocytic leukemia and in some patients with myelofibrosis with myeloid metaplasia. A marked increase both in LAP activity and in the number of neutrophils showing such activity may be seen in polycythemia vera, idiopathic thrombocytopenia, leukemoid reactions, and patients with myelofibrosis with myeloid metaplasia.

The normal LAP score ranges from 25 to 50. In leukemoid reactions and in polycythemia vera, it may rise to more than 200, whereas in chronic granulocytic leukemia it is usually less than 25. In general, LAP values in uncomplicated secondary polycythemia are normal. However, because so many factors may increase the LAP (e.g., infection, fever, hemorrhage), and since the LAP may be normal in primary polycythemia, this test may lose its discriminatory value in the individual patient.

DIFFERENTIAL DIAGNOSIS OF POLYCYTHEMIA VERA

In most patients with secondary polycythemia due to hypoxemia, the structural abnormalities of the heart and lung are sufficiently apparent to indicate the underlying cause of the polycythemia. However, occasional patients may have obscure pulmonary or neuromuscular disease or an inapparent right-to-left shunt in which reduced arterial oxygen saturation can significantly aid diagnosis. Furthermore, other abnormalities of primary polycythemia, such as splenomegaly, deranged serum vitamin B_{12} concentrations and LAP values, or increased platelet and white cell counts, typically do not occur.

Tissue hypoxia may be found in patients with familial high-affinity hemoglobins. In these patients, the partial pressure of oxygen at which the hemoglobin is half-saturated with oxygen (P50) is reduced. The diagnosis is relatively easy because most of these patients have a positive family history, and abnormal hemoglobins may be found on electrophoresis. Similarly, a low concentration of 2,3-diphosphoglycerate (2,3-DPG) inhibits oxygen unloading of hemoglobin. Sometimes blood carboxyhemoglobin concentrations are increased in patients who smoke. Carboxyhemoglobin measurements should be made at the end of the day when levels are highest.

It deserves emphasis that moderate arterial undersaturation does not rule out the diagnosis of polycythemia vera. However, if the arterial saturation is greater than 92 per cent, the clinician can confidently exclude hypoxemic polycythemia, although not the secondary polycythemia associated with tumors or polycythemia vera. Remember that in the polycythemia accompanying tumors, there may be increases in the platelet and white cell counts and even splenomegaly and that some patients with primary polycythemia may not have some or most of the expected characteristics in addition to the increased red cell mass. To confound the situation even more, the coexistence of primary and secondary polycythemia (e.g., polycythemia vera and chronic pulmonary disease) is not uncommon.

Although it is easy to list the common characteristics that occur in groups of patients with various types of polycythemia, the clinician at the bedside who is faced with a single patient with an increased red cell mass, cannot rely on group statistics or a fixed set of criteria that must be satisfied to arrive at a diagnosis for the individual. Therefore, each case of polycythemia must be evaluated thoroughly with the laboratory studies previously outlined and summarized in Table 2. The results must then be interpreted within the limitations discussed. Clearly, the diagnosis of "mild" polycythemia vera must be made only after excluding all known possible causes of secondary polycythemia.

Table 2. Evaluation of the Patient with Polycythemia

- History
- Physical examination, including neurologic and pelvic examinations
- Complete blood count, reticulocyte count, platelet count
- Urinalysis
- Red blood cell volume
- Leukocyte alkaline phosphatase determination
- Hemoglobin electrophoresis
- Serum uric acid and potassium determinations
- Plasma cortisol determination
- Serum erythropoietin level
- Serum vitamin B_{12} and vitamin B_{12}–binding capacity
- Arterial oxygen tension and saturation determinations
- Bone marrow biopsy with stains for iron, reticulin, and collagen
- Chest x-ray

Table 3. Polycythemia Vera Study Group Criteria

A_1 Increased red blood cell mass	B_1 Thrombocytosis, platelets >600,000 cells/mm^3
A_2 Arterial oxygen ≥92%	B_2 White blood cell count ≥12,000/mm^3 in absence of fever
A_3 Hypercellular bone marrow	B_3 Elevated leukocyte alkaline phosphatase >100
A_4 Splenomegaly	B_4 Elevated serum vitamin B_{12} (>900 pg/mL) or elevated unsaturated vitamin B_{12} binding capacity >2200 pg/mL

The diagnosis is acceptable if one of the two following combinations are present:

(1) $A_1 + A_2 + A_3 + A_4$

or in the absence of splenomegaly,

(2) $A_1 + A_2 + A_3$ + any two items from category B

For nearly 30 years, the criteria of the Polycythemia Vera Study Group (PVSG) have been clinically useful, but they must be used carefully (Table 3). Occasionally, a patient may seem to fulfill the PVSG criteria but does not have polycythemia vera. For example, a patient with splenomegaly secondary to cirrhosis or liver cancer may have leukocytosis or thrombocytosis and yet not have polycythemia. Patients who smoke and have other myeloproliferative disorders similarly may be diagnosed incorrectly. Conversely, there are some patients with bona fide polycythemia vera who do not exactly meet the PVSG criteria. This is particularly true of patients with borderline elevated red cell masses of 32 to 34 cc/kg. Importantly, the PVSG criteria of 36 cc/kg was chosen to assure that patients randomized to the study did in fact have a significantly increased red cell mass.

COMPLICATIONS RESULTING FROM THERAPY

In the PVSG data, thrombotic and hemorrhagic complications occurred during the first few years of therapy in the phlebotomy-only group. Conversely, it was clearly demonstrated that patients treated with chlorambucil and radioactive phosphorus (32-phosphorus) had a higher incidence of acute leukemia. Malignancy of the gastrointestinal tract and skin occurred more frequently in patients treated with chlorambucil. By contrast, hydroxyurea is now the most commonly used myelosuppressive agent. This drug is also associated with a small but definite increase in acute leukemia. Myelodysplastic syndromes and malignant lymphoma have also been described following treatment with hydroxyurea. Thus, the effects of chemotherapy may further complicate diagnostic considerations in patients with polycythemia vera.

Acknowledgment

The capable secretarial assistance of Ms. Helen Zurawinsky is gratefully acknowledged.

AGNOGENIC MYELOID METAPLASIA AND ESSENTIAL THROMBOCYTHEMIA

By Bong H. Hyun, M.D., D.Sc.,
and Gene L. Gulati, Ph.D.
Philadelphia, Pennsylvania

Agnogenic myeloid metaplasia (AMM) and essential thrombocythemia, along with polycythemia vera (PV) and chronic granulocytic leukemia (CGL), represent a group of conditions generally referred to as chronic myeloproliferative disorders. These clinical entities are characterized by clonal proliferation of one or more cell lineages in the bone marrow, spleen, and liver. The proliferation of hematopoietic elements at sites other than bone marrow is described as extramedullary hematopoiesis. Myeloproliferative disorders share many clinical and laboratory features. Transitional forms that are difficult to categorize may occur. One form of myeloproliferative disease may evolve into another during the course of illness, often terminating in acute leukemia. These disorders may last many years and are typically encountered with equal frequency in men and women older than 50 years of age. The cause or causes of myeloproliferative disorders remain unclear.

AGNOGENIC MYELOID METAPLASIA

AMM has many synonyms. Some of the commonly used names include myelofibrosis (MF), primary myelofibrosis, chronic myelofibrosis, myelofibrosis with myeloid metaplasia (MMM), and myelosclerosis (MS). AMM is an uncommon disorder with an incidence approximately one third that of CGL. Extramedullary hematopoiesis occurs in the spleen, liver, lymph nodes, and occasionally other tissues. Extramedullary hematopoiesis (primarily in the spleen) is frequently associated with an increased number of stem cells in the peripheral circulation. Early in its course, AMM is characterized by generalized overactivity of hematopoietic stem cells, but hematopoiesis tends to be ineffective. In the marrow, myelofibrosis is the predominant finding. Although hematopoietic proliferation is of clonal origin, the myelofibrosis is reactive and most likely due to megakaryocytic hyperplasia. Platelets and their precursors secrete platelet-derived growth factor (PDGF), which has been shown to stimulate the proliferation of fibroblasts.

Clinical Features

AMM is a disorder primarily of middle-aged and elderly persons. More than two thirds of these patients are 50 to 70 years of age. The onset is insidious, and morphologic abnormalities may precede symptoms by several years. Symptoms related to anemia (weakness, fatigue, anorexia, night sweats) and abdominal discomfort (sense of fullness, pain, indigestion, loss of appetite) are common complaints at presentation. Hemorrhagic manifestations due to quantitative or qualitative defects in platelets may be noted late in the course in 50 per cent of patients with AMM. Splenomegaly is the chief physical finding and is noted in virtually all patients. Hematopoietic hyperplasia, fibrosis, and exaggerated red cell pooling all contribute to massive splenomegaly. Hepatomegaly develops in about two thirds of patients. Although extramedullary hematopoiesis also occurs in lymph nodes, it rarely leads to significant nodal enlargement. As the disease progresses, patients may experience weight loss, skin and mucous membrane bleeding, and bone pain. Other complications include gout, autoimmune hemolytic anemia, and jaundice.

Peripheral Blood Findings

A mild normocytic normochromic anemia (hemoglobin 9 to 13 g/dL) is almost always found at presentation. It is attributed to ineffective erythropoiesis and hypersplenism. The reticulocyte count is frequently increased early in the course of disease, and megaloblastic changes may develop because of folate deficiency during the early hyperproliferative phase. Microcytic hypochromic anemia develops in patients with bleeding varices or peptic ulcer. The anemia grows worse as the disease advances. The leukocyte and platelet counts are usually increased initially, but leukopenia and thrombocytopenia ensue as the disease progresses. Ineffective hematopoiesis, marrow fibrosis, and hypersplenism all contribute to the pancytopenia. The peripheral smear reveals leukoerythroblastosis characterized by immature granulocytes (from metamyelocyte to blast form) and nucleated red blood cells (NRBCs) (Fig. 1*A*). Teardrop-shaped red cells (dacrocytes) are found in numbers unmatched in any other hematologic or nonhematologic disorder (see Fig. 1*B*). Basophilia, eosinophilia, megakaryocytes, denuded megakaryocytes (megakaryocyte nuclei or nuclear fragments), and giant platelets may also appear. Megaloblastic changes and dysplastic features, such as hypolobation of neutrophils (pseudo–Pelger-Huët cells), hypogranularity of neutrophils and platelets, bizarre platelets, and mononuclear megakaryocytes, may also be seen.

Ancillary findings include increased serum vitamin B_{12} and vitamin B_{12}–binding capacity, increased urate concentration, and increased serum activities of lactate dehydrogenase (LD) and hydroxybutyrate dehydrogenase. Serum and red cell folate concentrations are typically decreased.

Bone Marrow Findings

Attempts at bone marrow aspiration yield a dry tap in more than 90 per cent of patients even when the marrow is very cellular. When the aspirate is obtained, the smears may show primarily neutrophils and dysplastic megakaryocytes. Trephine biopsy, readily performed at the posterior iliac crest, may reveal a hypercellular marrow with panmy-

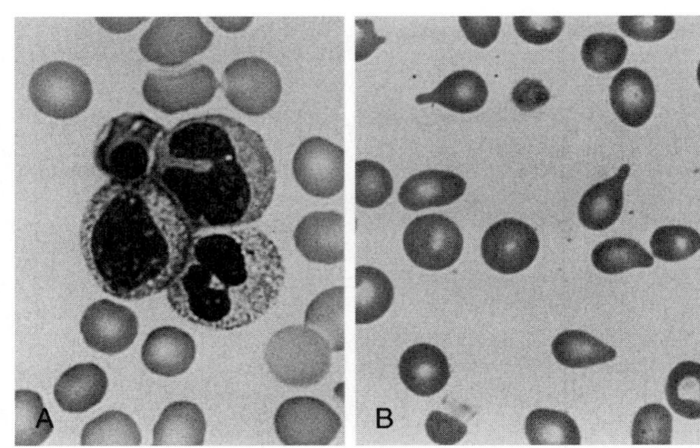

Figure 1. Peripheral blood, agnogenic myeloid metaplasia. *A,* Leukoerythroblastosis. *B,* Teardrop cells.

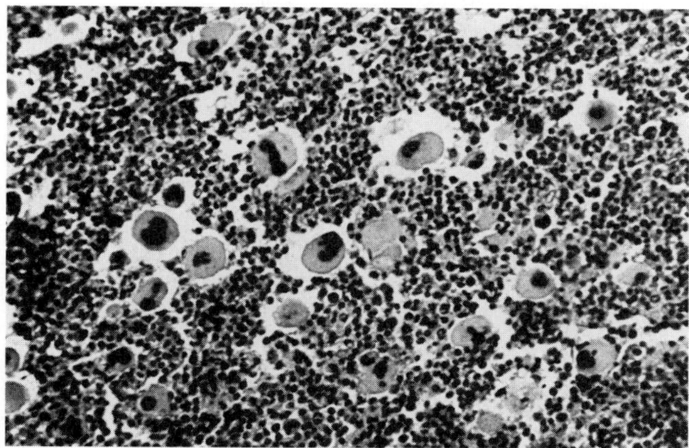

Figure 2. Bone marrow biopsy, cellular phase of agnogenic myeloid metaplasia. Panhyperplasia (100 per cent cellularity).

elosis in the early phase of disease (Fig. 2). The most striking feature is the increased number of morphologically abnormal megakaryocytes. The megakaryocyte nuclei may be small and hypolobated or hyperchromic and hyperlobated. Immature forms and micromegakaryocytes are prevalent. Clustering of megakaryocytes is common, and some of these cells are found close to the endosteum. Marrow sinusoids may be distended and contain foci of hematopoietic cells. The interstitium may show increased numbers of lymphocytes, plasma cells, mast cells, and macrophages. Reticulin stain (silver stain) is required to detect early myelofibrosis, which may be patchy. If one biopsy produces negative results, a second biopsy at another site should be performed when there is strong clinical suspicion of AMM. Variability in fibrotic changes, with one intertrabecular space showing hypercellular marrow and another showing dense fibrosis, is often present. Type III collagen is a major constituent of the fibrotic tissue. An early mild increase in reticulin progresses to a marked increase in the later stages of disease. In severely fibrotic marrow, increased osteoblastic activity with new bone formation may be observed. Osteosclerosis, which may also be detected radiographically, accompanies myelofibrosis in roughly 50 per cent of patients (Fig. 3).

Flow cytometry, cytogenetic studies, and molecular studies seldom, if ever, aid the initial diagnosis of AMM. However, a search for the Philadelphia chromosome and for a BCR/ABL gene rearrangement may be required to distinguish AMM from CGL. Flow cytometry may confirm leukemic transformation.

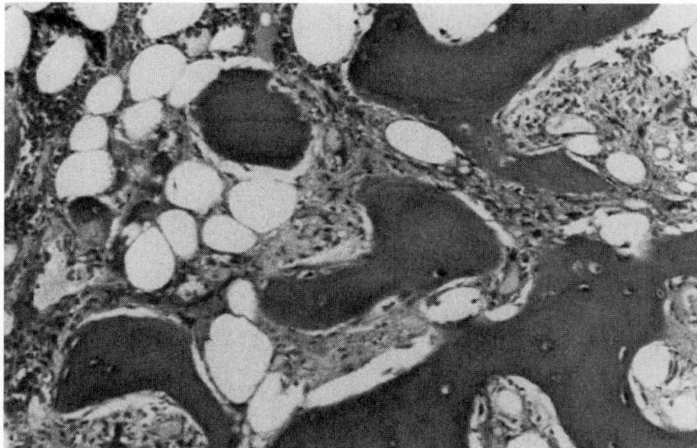

Figure 3. Bone marrow biopsy. Agnogenic myeloid metaplasia; advanced osteosclerosis and myelofibrosis.

Prognosis

Duration of survival in AMM is difficult to predict because the time of onset of the disease is difficult to determine. Acute leukemic transformation of AMM, which is seen in 10 to 20 per cent of patients, is marked by a sudden drop in hemoglobin and platelet count and a rapid increase in the size of the spleen. Occasionally, AMM may transform into CGL.

By contrast, acute myelofibrosis presents with marked pancytopenia, insignificant red cell poikilocytosis, minimal or no splenomegaly, and marrow fibrosis with a preponderance of megakaryocytes. The course is rapid and usually fatal within 6 months. Acute myelofibrosis is often indistinguishable from acute granulocytic leukemia—M7 type. In fact, it is considered by some to be identical to or a variant of acute granulocytic leukemia—M7 (acute megakaryoblastic leukemia).

ESSENTIAL THROMBOCYTHEMIA

Essential thrombocythemia (ET), also known as idiopathic thrombocythemia (IT), hemorrhagic thrombocythemia, primary thrombocytosis, and primary thrombocythemia, primarily afflicts middle-aged and elderly persons. ET has the lowest incidence among the chronic myeloproliferative disorders. This clonal proliferation of hematopoietic stem cells is characterized by a massive increase in circulating platelets (typically more than 1 million cells/mm^3) and a preponderance of megakaryocytes in the bone marrow.

Clinical Features

Approximately 20 per cent of patients are asymptomatic when first seen. They are discovered incidently when blood counts are obtained as part of a routine check-up or for some unrelated illness. The remaining 80 per cent of patients with ET present with recurrent episodes of hemorrhage and/or thrombosis. Hemorrhagic episodes, which may be spontaneous or related to trauma, are seen in 60 per cent of symptomatic patients. Typical lesions include hematomas and bleeding in the skin or mucous membranes. Thrombotic events, which are seen in 40 per cent of symptomatic patients, may involve arteries or veins, or both. Localized platelet aggregates or platelet emboli cause microvascular occlusion, resulting in transient ischemic symptoms, stroke, or digital ischemia. In fact, general symptoms attributable to small vessel obstruction (headache, dizziness, visual disturbances, and parasthesias) are not uncommon. Venous thrombosis may involve superficial or deep veins, including portal, splenic, hepatic, and renal veins. Myocardial infarction and the Budd-Chiari syndrome are among the severe thrombotic events occasionally seen in the course of ET. The pathogenesis of these hemorrhagic and thrombotic events is poorly understood.

Mild to moderate splenomegaly is present at diagnosis in about 70 per cent of patients, and hepatomegaly is seen in approximately 20 per cent. Although uncommon, splenic atrophy may develop because of blockade of the splenic microcirculation resulting from marked thrombocytosis. Symptoms related to anemia are noted in patients with iron deficiency secondary to blood loss through the gastrointestinal or genitourinary tract.

Peripheral Blood Findings

The prominent finding in the peripheral blood is a marked and sustained increase in the platelet count, which typically reaches 1 to 3 million cells/mm^3. The leukocyte count is normal or moderately increased (typically fewer than 30,000 cells/mm^3), primarily from neutrophilia. Mild to moderate normocytic normochromic or microcytic hypochromic anemia is often noted, the latter in patients who have suffered recurrent hemorrhagic episodes. Platelet morphologic features are usually unremarkable, but a few giant forms (platelets larger than normal red cells), abnormally shaped (bizarre) platelets, platelet aggregates, and megakaryocytic fragments (denuded nuclei) may be seen in the blood smear (Fig. 4*A* and *B*). Neutrophilic leukocytosis may be accompanied by a few immature granulocytes (usually myelocytes and metamyelocytes) and absolute basophilia in some patients. The presence of Howell-Jolly bodies, target cells, acanthocytes, spherocytes, and/or nucleated red blood cells indicates hyposplenism associated with splenic atrophy. Platelet function, as studied by platelet aggregation with adenosine diphosphate (ADP), epinephrine, and collagen, is often found to be impaired. However, these studies are not routinely performed or required. Ancillary findings include increased serum concentrations of lactate dehydrogenase, alkaline phosphatase, muramidase, vitamin B_{12}–binding protein, potassium, calcium, and phosphorus.

Bone Marrow Findings

The bone marrow is usually hypercellular but may be normocellular. Panmyelosis is frequent, but megakaryocytic hyperplasia predominates (Figs. 5 and 6). The degree of megakaryocytic hyperplasia does not correlate with the platelet count in the peripheral blood. Megakaryocytes in ET are generally large and hyperploid, whereas megakaryocytes in reactive thrombocytosis are small and euploid. In ET, large masses of platelets may be present. Clusters of megakaryocytes are especially common, and some megakaryocytes may lie close to the endosteum. Emperipolesis (other hematopoietic cells wandering in and out of megakaryocytes) and mitotic figures are increased. A mild increase in reticulin, which often is focal (patchy myelofibrosis), is seen in some patients.

Flow cytometry, cytogenetic studies, and molecular diagnostic studies do not significantly aid the initial diagnosis. However, chromosome analysis for the Philadelphia chromosome and gene rearrangement (BCR/ABL) studies may help distinguish ET from CGL, and flow cytometry may confirm acute leukemic transformation.

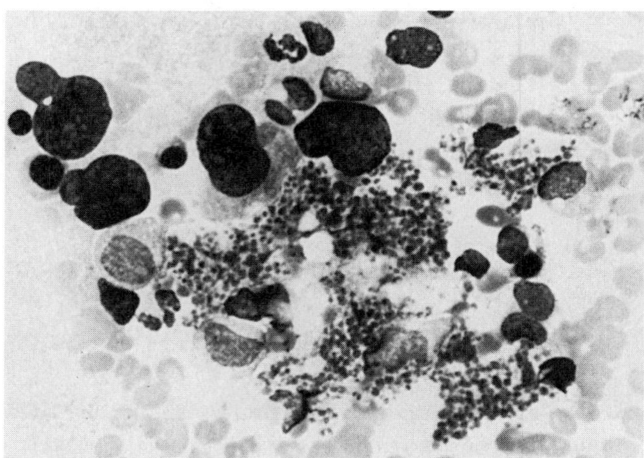

Figure 5. Bone marrow aspirate smear. Essential thrombocythemia and marked megakaryocytosis with active platelet production.

Prognosis

ET usually runs a chronic and sometimes benign course, lasting 3 to 5 years, particularly in younger patients. Fewer than 10 per cent of cases transform into other chronic myeloproliferative disorders (CGL, PV, AMM) or acute leukemia. The acute leukemic transformation may be myeloblastic, lymphoblastic, or megakaryoblastic.

DIFFERENTIAL DIAGNOSIS

The foremost consideration in the differential diagnosis of AMM is to exclude other conditions associated with myelofibrosis, especially chronic myeloproliferative disorders such as CGL, PV, or ET (Table 1). The absence of significant splenomegaly essentially excludes the diagnosis of AMM. CGL can be excluded in the absence of both the Philadelphia chromosome and the BCR/ABL gene rearrangement. PV is characterized by an increased red cell

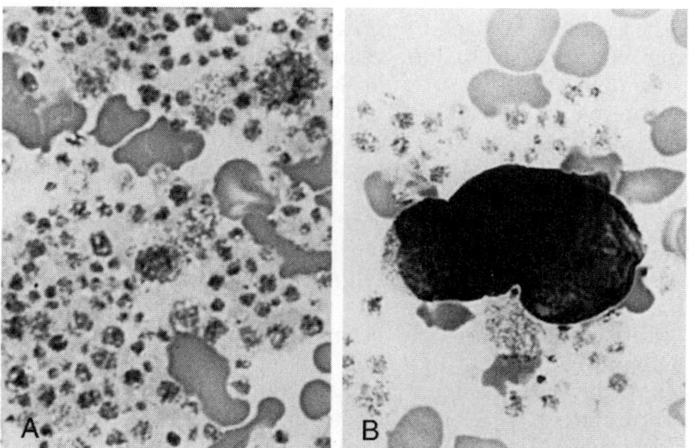

Figure 4. Peripheral blood, essential thrombocythemia. *A,* Marked increase in platelets and giant platelets. *B,* Marked increase in platelets and a megakaryocyte nucleus.

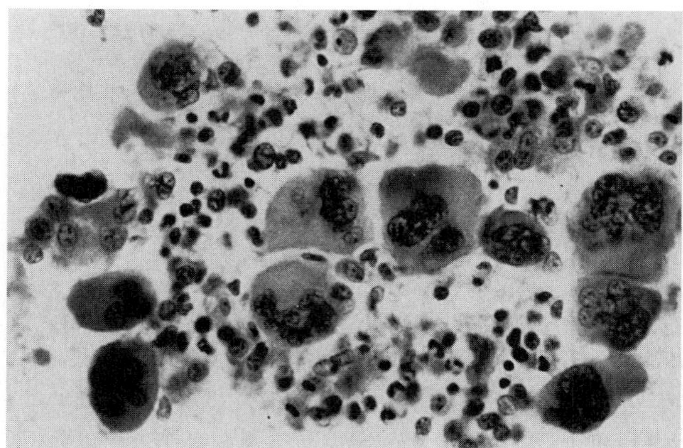

Figure 6. Bone marrow aspirate section. Essential thrombocythemia and panhyperplasia of marrow with marked megakaryocytosis.

Table 1. Differential Diagnostic Features of Chronic Myeloproliferative Disorders

	Agnogenic Myeloid Metaplasia	Essential Thrombocythemia	Chronic Granulocytic Leukemia	Polycythemia Vera
Splenomegaly	Moderate to marked	Mild or absent	Moderate	Mild or absent
Peripheral Blood				
Hemoglobin	Decreased	Normal or decreased	Decreased	Increased
Leukocyte count ($x10^9$/L)	Variable (<30)	Variable (<30)	>50	<30
Platelet count	Variable	Increased	Variable	Normal or increased
Immature granulocytes	Present	Rare	Many	Rare
Eosinophilia-basophilia	Present	May be present	Present	May be present
Red blood cell morphologic characteristics	Teardrop	Normal or microcytic hypochromic	Normal	Normal or microcytic hypochromic
Nucleated red blood cells	Common	Rare	Rare	Rare
Leukocyte alkaline phosphatase	Increased or normal	Increased or normal	Decreased or absent	Increased
Megakaryocyte-fragments	May be present	Present	May be present	Rare
Red blood cell mass	Decreased	Decreased or normal	Decreased	Increased
Bone Marrow				
Aspirate	Hypercellular (panmyelosis) Fibrosis Dry tap	Hypercellular (panmyelosis)	Granular hyperplasia	Hypercellular (panmyelosis) Fibrosis
Stainable iron	Normal or increased	Decreased or normal	Normal	Decreased or absent
Megakaryocytosis	Moderate	Marked	Mild	Moderate
Dysplasia	Common	Uncommon	Uncommon	Uncommon
Fibrosis	Mild to moderate	Mild or absent	Mild to moderate	Mild to moderate
Philadelphia chromosome or BCR/ABL gene rearrangement	Absent	Absent	Present	Absent

mass, whereas ET is usually defined by a platelet count in excess of 1 million cells/mm^3 of blood, a finding almost never approached in any of the other myeloproliferative disorders. Furthermore, significant myelofibrosis is uncommon in ET.

Differentiation of AMM from the spent phase of PV is sometimes difficult, but the behavior of colony-forming cells (CFC) cultured in the presence or absence of exogenous erythropoietin can be evaluated. In PV (spent phase or otherwise), most of the progenitor cells (CFC-erythroid, burst-forming cells-erythroid [BFC-E]) do not require exogenous erythropoietin for erythroid colony formation, whereas in AMM they do. Finally, the clinician should attempt to exclude all the other known causes of secondary myelofibrosis, such as acute leukemias, metastatic carcinoma, disseminated tuberculosis, sarcoidosis, histoplasmosis, and exposure to environmental agents such as benzene.

By contrast, the foremost consideration in the differential diagnosis of ET is to exclude various causes of secondary thrombocytosis, including infections, severe hemorrhage, severe hemolysis, iron deficiency, malignancy, splenectomy, connective tissue disease such as rheumatoid arthritis, trauma, and the postoperative state.

CHRONIC MYELOGENOUS LEUKEMIA

By David L. Porter, M.D.,
and Joseph H. Antin, M.D.
Boston, Massachussetts

Chronic myelogenous leukemia (CML) is also referred to as chronic myeloid, chronic myelocytic, and chronic granulocytic leukemia. It is one of the myeloproliferative disorders and results from neoplastic transformation of the pluripotent hematopoietic stem cell. Therefore, although the predominant hematologic feature of the disease is leukocytosis, all hematopoietic lineages, including erythroid, megakaryocytic, and occasionally lymphoid cells, may be affected. There are typically three clinical phases of CML (Table 1). Most patients present in the *chronic phase,* which typically lasts 3 to 4 years and is manifested primarily by increased blood cell counts and minimal symptoms. Eventually patients enter the *accelerated phase*, which is associated with rapidly rising blood cell counts and progressive constitutional symptoms; the accelerated phase often evolves into the terminal phase or *blast crisis.* This phase of CML resembles acute leukemia and is usually

Table 1. Classification of Chronic Myelogenous Leukemia

Chronic Phase
Asymptomatic after therapy
No features of accelerated phase or blast crisis
Accelerated Phase
Leukocyte count increasingly difficult to control with standard therapies
Increased blast percentage
>10% in blood or bone marrow
>20% blasts plus promyelocytes in blood or bone marrow
>20% basophils plus eosinophils in blood
Progressive anemia or thrombocytopenia
New cytogenetic abnormalities, especially a second Ph chromosome or trisomy 8
Worsening constitutional symptoms
Progressive splenomegaly
Development of myeloblastomas or myelofibrosis
Blast Crisis
>30% blasts plus promyelocytes in blood or bone marrow

refractory to therapy, leading to death, often within 26 months. Myeloid blast crisis develops in approximately 70 per cent of patients, whereas lymphoid blast crisis develops in 30 per cent of patients. Some patients proceed directly from the chronic phase to blast crisis CML without an obvious period of acceleration.

The sine qua non of CML is the finding of the Philadelphia (Ph) chromosome in cells of hematopoietic origin. The Ph chromosome (a truncated chromosome 22) results from a translocation between chromosomes 9 and 22 and is found in more than 90 per cent of patients with CML (Fig. 1). The small number of patients who do not have this translocation on normal karyotypic analysis typically carry the translocation at the molecular level. The translocation juxtaposes the putative oncogene c-*ABL* on chromosome 9 to the *BCR* gene on chromosome 22. The novel chimeric *bcr/abl* protein has tyrosine kinase activity that is postulated to have a major pathogenic role in CML. If the *BCR/ABL* fusion cannot be detected by molecular analyses, the diagnosis of CML should be questioned.

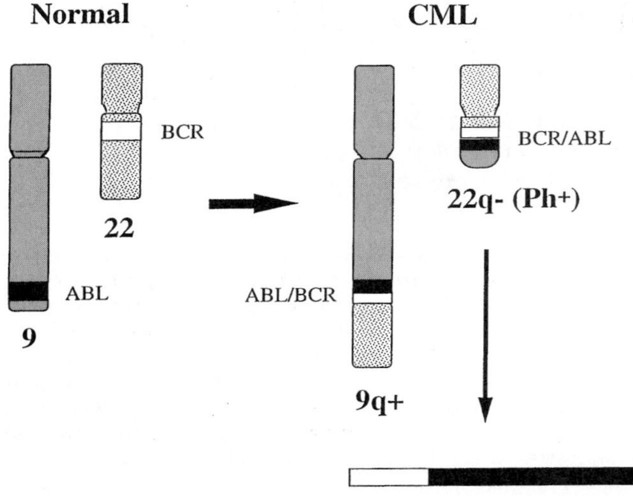

Figure 1. Schematic representation of the chromosomal translocation found in chronic myelogenous leukemia. A reciprocal translocation from the long arm of chromosome 9 to the long arm of chromosome 22 results in a shortened chromosome 22, referred to as the Philadelphia (Ph) chromosome. This translocation results in the production of a novel fusion *BCR/ABL* gene product.

SIGNS AND SYMPTOMS

The hallmark of CML is an increased leukocyte count. It is becoming increasingly common to diagnose asymptomatic patients with CML following routine blood testing for other reasons. The peripheral blood film typically shows all stages of myeloid maturation with a distinct shift toward immature myeloid cells such as myelocytes and metamyelocytes. Basophilia and eosinophilia are common, whereas the morphologic characteristics of the myeloid cells appear relatively normal. A small number of peripheral blasts can be seen in chronic-phase CML. When clinical signs and symptoms develop, they are often referable to abnormalities in the blood cell counts or functions. If the leukocyte count is extremely high (>200,000 to 500,000 cells/μL), symptoms associated with leukostasis may occur. Patients may present with symptoms of anemia or may experience easy bruising or bleeding because of platelet dysfunction. Hypermetabolic symptoms may develop because of the rapid proliferation of myeloid cells; some patients may present with symptoms related to splenomegaly, which results from extramedullary hematopoiesis. Common presenting signs and symptoms are shown in Table 2.

Accelerated-phase CML is often associated with worsening constitutional symptoms; progressive splenomegaly, with or without adenopathy; or the occurrence of isolated myeloblastomas. The leukocyte count becomes difficult to control with standard therapy and there is a greater shift toward earlier myeloid precursors in the peripheral blood and bone marrow, including up to 10 per cent blasts. Marked eosinophilia or basophilia may develop. Additional cytogenetic abnormalities may be acquired, such as a second Ph chromosome or trisomy 8.

The accelerated phase heralds a transformation to blast crisis, which is associated with a worsening of symptoms, splenomegaly, and peripheral blood and bone marrow findings that resemble acute leukemia with a predominance of blasts and promyelocytes. Signs and symptoms may progressively worsen during blast crisis, and patients may experience severe constitutional symptoms, anemia, bleeding, bone pain resulting from a rapidly expanding myeloid cell compartment, massive splenomegaly, and other complications.

LABORATORY EVALUATIONS

Complete Blood Count and Peripheral Blood Examination

The complete blood count (CBC) and peripheral blood examination are the most important diagnostic tests. The leukocyte count is almost always increased and may vary between 15,000 and 500,000 cells/μL. Early in the course of disease, many patients have a normal hematocrit or present with only mild anemia. The anemia may be more pronounced in patients with significant splenomegaly or higher white cell counts. Mild or moderate thrombocytosis is common, but platelet counts may exceed 1 million cells/μL in some patients; occasionally, CML presents with thrombocytopenia, especially in the more advanced phases.

The peripheral blood smear is characteristic. The mor-

Table 2. Presenting Signs and Symptoms in Chronic Myelogenous Leukemia

Asymptomatic elevation in the leukocyte count	None
Anemia	Fatigue, lethargy, shortness of breath, angina, or other symptoms of anemia. Pallor on examination
Platelet dysfunction	Easy bruising, mucosal bleeding, phlebitis Petechiae, ecchymoses, or evidence of thrombosis
Hyperviscosity (due to elevated leukocyte count, typically >300,000 cells/μL)	Central nervous system abnormalities including lethargy, visual changes, seizures; rarely, shortness of breath caused by pulmonary leukostasis, angina, priapism
Hypermetabolic state	Night sweats, weight loss; rarely fevers unless accelerated phase or blast crisis; hyperuricemia with gout; rarely kidney stones, renal failure
Splenomegaly (extramedullary hematopoiesis)	Increasing abdominal girth, early satiety, left upper quadrant pain
Increased myeloid mass	Bone pain

phologic features of the red blood cells, platelets, and leukocytes are relatively normal. An increased number of myeloid cells is apparent, with the presence of both mature and immature myeloid forms readily noted. Frequent basophils or eosinophils may be seen, and the number of monocytes and lymphocytes may be decreased.

Bone Marrow Evaluation

A bone marrow evaluation is not strictly necessary to make the diagnosis of CML; leukocytosis with the finding of Ph+ metaphases on cytogenetic evaluation of the peripheral blood is sufficient, but examination of the bone marrow often provides important supportive and prognostic information. Furthermore, cytogenetic studies performed on the bone marrow are more likely to yield results than those performed on the peripheral blood. The marrow morphologic features are characteristic of a myeloproliferative syndrome, but there are few changes specific for CML. An aspirate smear demonstrates hypercellular spicules, with a relative increase in myeloid progenitors, including an increase in the percentage of blasts and promyelocytes, as well as more mature myeloid cells. The percentage of blasts and promyelocytes may have prognostic significance and is useful for identifying patients who are entering the accelerated phase. The megakaryocytes may be increased in number and dysplastic in appearance. Erythroid maturation is typically normal, but due to myeloid expansion, a proportionate decrease in erythroid precursors is noted. The bone marrow biopsy specimen is frequently hypercellular, with almost complete obliteration of fat spaces. Mild fibrosis may be evident, and clustering of megakaryocytes is most apparent on examination of the biopsy specimen.

Cytogenetics and Molecular Genetics Studies

Detection of the Ph chromosome, representing the translocation between chromosomes 9 and 22 (t(9:22)), on cytogenetic analysis of the blood or bone marrow is diagnostic of CML and is found in approximately 95 per cent of patients. Some patients suspected of having CML will not have an obvious Ph abnormality. In these patients, the translocation of a portion of the *ABL* gene from chromosome 9, to the *BCR* gene on chromosome 22 can be readily detected at the molecular level. Southern blot analysis of restriction enzyme–digested chromosomal DNA reveals the typical DNA rearrangement. Alternatively, reverse transcription followed by the polymerase chain reaction (PCR) can be used to identify the presence of the chimeric *BCR*/*ABL* mRNA transcript. The diagnosis of CML should be questioned if cytogenetic and molecular studies are normal.

Other Supportive Laboratory Tests

Several laboratory abnormalities are frequently associated with CML and lend support to the diagnosis, but none is diagnostic. In chronic-phase CML, the leukocyte alkaline phosphatase (LAP) activity in neutrophils is typically low. An LAP score is determined by staining peripheral blood neutrophils for LAP activity and estimating the stain intensity. The LAP score is characteristically low in chronic-phase CML but may be normal or even increased in the accelerated phase or in blast crisis.

The intense metabolic activity resulting from the increased hematopoietic cell turnover frequently results in lactate dehydrogenase (LD) and uric acid increases. Vitamin B_{12} and vitamin B_{12}–binding protein concentrations tend to be increased in CML, presumably due to the release of these products from large numbers of granulocytes in the phlebotomy tube. The same artifact may also cause "pseudohyperkalemia," causing release of potassium into the serum.

IMAGING PROCEDURES

Imaging procedures are usually not required in CML. Abdominal ultrasound can accurately measure spleen size, which may have prognostic implications for patients with CML. Radiologic procedures are otherwise obtained only to evaluate specific symptoms.

DIFFERENTIAL DIAGNOSIS

In most patients, the diagnosis of CML is obvious from the presenting signs and symptoms and the characteristic peripheral blood smear. However, before results are available from the appropriate cytogenetic and/or molecular tests, a limited differential diagnosis can be generated. Nonmalignant inflammatory disorders that result in a "leukemoid reaction" can be confused with CML and may present with similar signs and symptoms, such as fever and splenomegaly. These conditions include infections such as subacute bacterial endocarditis, tuberculosis, and other chronic infectious or inflammatory diseases. Patients with acute physiologic stress from sepsis, severe burns, or hemorrhage may have a slightly increased leukocyte count and increased numbers of immature myeloid cells in the peripheral blood; these diagnoses are usually obvious, and the leukocyte count returns to normal after treatment of the underlying disorder. Any process resulting in myelophthisis (replacement of the bone marrow), such as metastatic cancer, can present with an increased leukocyte count and left shift, mild anemia, and thrombocytopenia or thrombocytosis resembling early CML. In all of these situations, the white blood cell count is usually only mildly increased and the left shift of the myeloid series is less prominent than in CML. The basophil count and LAP score are normal, and the underlying disorder is usually readily apparent.

Any of the myeloproliferative disorders (polycythemia vera, essential thrombocythemia, agnogenic myeloid metaplasia with myelofibrosis [see articles on these topics]) can present with features of CML, but the Ph chromosome is rarely detected. Finally, a rare disorder classified as a "myelodysplastic syndrome" or chronic myelomonocytic leukemia (CMML) can be confused with CML. Chronic myelomonocytic leukemia is distinguished, however, by a significant increase in monocytes, trilineage marrow dysplasia, and lack of the Ph chromosome.

PROGNOSIS

The median survival for patients with CML is approximately 3.5 to 4 years from the time of diagnosis; the risk of entering the accelerated phase is approximately 20 per cent per year. Ultimately, most patients who cannot be cured die of the complications of blast crisis CML, which include inanition, infections associated with neutropenia, or bleeding due to thrombocytopenia. Myeloid blasts are found in approximately 70 per cent of patients with blast crisis; aggressive chemotherapy successfully induces a second chronic phase in only 5 to 10 per cent of these patients. By contrast, 30 per cent of patients experience a lymphoid blast crisis, and 30 per cent of these patients enter a second chronic phase following chemotherapy. However, even those patients who achieve a second chronic phase typically re-enter blast crisis rapidly, and most patients die within 2 to 6 months without further therapy.

The prognosis for CML patients is determined primarily by the phase of the disease. A low leukocyte count and a small spleen size suggest a good prognosis that is most likely related to a low leukemia cell burden or slow proliferation of leukemic cells. Other factors that may be associated with a good prognosis include young age, normal platelet count at diagnosis, a low percentage of basophils, and a low percentage of blasts in the bone marrow.

The only available curative therapy for CML is allogeneic bone marrow transplantation (BMT). Approximately 60 per cent of patients who undergo allogeneic BMT in the chronic phase enjoy long-term disease-free survival, whereas results are less impressive for patients who undergo transplantation in the advanced stages of disease. It is also clear that BMT performed within the first year of diagnosis is associated with a significantly better outcome than if BMT is delayed. Thus, for appropriate patients, once the diagnosis of CML is made, a timely search for a suitable donor should be initiated.

CHRONIC LYMPHOCYTIC LEUKEMIA

By Susan O'Brien, M.D.,
and Michael J. Keating, M.B., B.S.
Houston, Texas

Chronic lymphocytic leukemia (CLL) is a hematopoietic neoplasm characterized by a clonal expansion of small lymphocytes. In the earlier stages of the disease, these lymphocytes are present in bone marrow and peripheral blood; with disease progression, they accumulate in lymph nodes, liver, and spleen, this accumulation causing lymphadenopathy, hepatomegaly, and splenomegaly. Later in the disease evolution, bone marrow failure occurs. In more than 95 per cent of patients, the cells are B cells, as evidenced by cell surface phenotyping and DNA rearrangement studies.

DIAGNOSTIC CRITERIA

Two working groups, the National Cancer Institute Working Group (NCI-WG) and the International Workshop on CLL (IWCLL), have submitted recommendations for diagnosis, evaluation of response, and indications for commencement of therapy. Both require a sustained lymphocytosis in the peripheral blood and the bone marrow. A minimum threshold for blood lymphocytes is 5×10^3 cells/μL for the NCI-WG and 10×10^3 cells/μL for the IWCLL. In the latter, lower lymphocyte counts are accepted when lymphocyte phenotyping demonstrates a typical pattern of CD5-positive B cells. Both groups require more than 30 per cent lymphocytes on bone marrow differential; the NCI-WG study requires bone marrow to be normocellular or hypercellular, but this criterion is not used by the IWCLL. The lymphocyte immunophenotype should demonstrate cells positive for CD19 or CD20 and coexpression of CD5 in the absence of other pan-T cell markers. Light chain expression is restricted to kappa or lambda, and surface immunoglobulin (sIg) has low cell-surface-density expression.

CLINICAL FEATURES

Many patients with CLL are asymptomatic at the time of initial diagnosis. This lack of symptoms is becoming more common, because the disease is detected by blood tests used in evaluating other conditions or in preoperative screening. Lymphocytosis may be the first abnormality seen; although lymphocyte counts may range from 5×10^3 to 500×10^3 cells/μL, hyperviscosity is uncommon. The rarity of hyperviscosity may be a result of the small size of CLL cells.

The most common symptom reported by patients is related to enlarged lymph nodes in the neck, axilla, or groin. Some patients complain of left upper quadrant discomfort and early satiety related to splenomegaly. Fever, sweats, and loss of weight (B symptoms) occur in fewer than 2 per cent of patients at diagnosis, and fewer than 5 per cent of patients have had a serious infection. Anemia (hemoglobin < 11g/dL) is also uncommon at diagnosis; when present, it may result in symptoms of fatigue, shortness of breath, headache, and dizziness. Thrombocytopenia (platelet count $< 100 \times 10^3$ cells/μL) at diagnosis is noted in fewer than

5 per cent of patients. Symptoms of purpura, ecchymosis, or bleeding are rare. Pure red cell aplasia and immune neutropenia have been described in CLL. An exaggerated reaction to insect bites is an ill-understood feature that occurs in 2 to 5 per cent of patients with CLL at the time of initial diagnosis.

The characteristic feature of CLL on clinical examination is lymphadenopathy that may involve a single site, most commonly the cervical area, but may also involve all lymph node–bearing areas. Nodes are firm, discrete, freely mobile, and nontender. As the disease progresses, the lymph nodes become larger; they may become confluent and matted but usually remain freely movable. The development of tender, hard, or fixed nodes is an indication for an evaluation with needle aspiration or biopsy to assess the possible development of a large cell lymphomatous (Richter's) transformation, metastatic cancer from another site, or associated infection. Marked enlargement of the liver is uncommon, but moderate to marked splenomegaly is not infrequent. When present as a dominant feature in the absence of lymphadenopathy, splenomegaly should raise the possibility of a mantle zone lymphoma, splenic lymphoma with villous lymphocytes, or prolymphocytic leukemia.

A small percentage of patients develop a variety of skin rashes that are often nonspecific in type. Biopsies may illustrate lymphocytic infiltration but are usually not characteristic. Infiltration of the ocular area, salivary glands, gastrointestinal tract, or lungs raises the possibility of mucosal-associated lymphoid tissue (MALT) lymphoma. Clinically significant involvement of other organs, such as the heart, lungs, and kidneys, is uncommon, particularly early in the disease, and central nervous system infiltration is very uncommon in CLL. As the disease progresses, lymph nodes can become massive but rarely cause obstruction of ducts or viscera. In addition, despite massive lymphadenopathy, lymphedema is a very infrequent feature. Some patients develop ascites and pleural effusions late in their illness, and this is a poor prognostic sign.

LABORATORY FINDINGS

As noted earlier, the sine qua non of CLL is lymphocytosis in the peripheral blood and bone marrow. The cells are morphologically mature lymphocytes. The majority of patients have leukocytosis much greater than that required to establish a diagnosis. The height of the white blood cell count increases with the clinical stage of the disease, varying from 10×10^3 cells/μL to 250×10^3 cells/μL, with the lymphocyte proportion of the white cell differential count ranging from 50 to 99 per cent. Extremely high white cell counts are uncommon in early disease. The hemoglobin concentration varies with the stage of disease and the degree of prior therapy; only a small percentage of patients are anemic or thrombocytopenic at diagnosis. The direct antiglobulin (Coombs') test result is positive at some stage in 15 to 20 per cent of patients with CLL, but it is positive in fewer than 5 per cent at the time of diagnosis.

Characteristically, CLL B cells express the pan-B cell markers CD19 and CD20 and coexpress CD5. Immunophenotypic studies, in addition to confirming the pan-B cell and CD5 expression, typically demonstrate a clonal excess of membrane-bound kappa or lambda light chains. Surface immunoglobulin shows low-intensity expression with either sIgM or sIgD, or a combination of both. Less commonly, sIgG is present.

Morphologically, the cells are small, with a narrow rim of cytoplasm, and the nuclear chromatin is dense. Nucleoli are not visible. Peripheral blood smears may disrupt CLL lymphocytes during preparation of the blood film and cause smudge cells. A bone marrow examination is not essential for establishing a diagnosis of CLL, because in most patients with sustained peripheral lymphocytosis a bone marrow aspirate demonstrates more than 30 per cent lymphocytes. The percentage of lymphocytes in the bone marrow increases with stage of disease at diagnosis, and the pattern of marrow infiltration varies. The patient may have intertrabecular foci or nodules of mature lymphocytes, an interstitial infiltrate, a combination of these patterns, or a diffuse infiltration. The nodular patterns are more common in early-stage disease, and the diffuse pattern becomes more prominent as the disease progresses or with advanced stage at diagnosis. Lymph node biopsies are usually not performed, but when they are done, the normal lymph node architecture is typically effaced by small well-differentiated lymphocytes. Small foci of atypical lymphocytes may be found occasionally. Pseudonodules can also be seen in the lymph node biopsy.

Blood chemistry testing is not usually helpful in CLL. Occasionally, patients have an increase in serum lactate dehydrogenase (LD), bilirubin, or uric acid. These features tend to be more common as the disease progresses. Rarely patients are hypercalcemic at the time of diagnosis, and some patients develop hypercalcemia as a poor prognostic feature later in the illness.

DIFFERENTIAL DIAGNOSIS

A variety of monoclonal antibodies against surface antigens can be applied to the evaluation of patients with CLL. Cell surface markers that are useful in confirming the diagnosis and differentiating between the less common subvarieties of the CLLs are described later. In reactive lymphocytosis from infections such as pertussis and toxoplasmosis and viral infections such as infectious mononucleosis and cytomegalovirus infection, the lymphocytes are usually large and activated. They are mostly T cells, with some polyclonal B cells. The characteristic feature of CLL is that lymphocytes are CD5-positive B cells, the lymphocytosis is sustained, and cells can be demonstrated to be monoclonal by the use of light chain restriction on the surface and immunoglobulin gene rearrangement pattern. The most important differential diagnosis is between prolymphocytic leukemia (PLL), hairy cell leukemia (HCL), splenic lymphoma with circulating villous lymphocytes (SLVL), leukemic phase of non-Hodgkin's lymphoma (L-NHL), and Waldenström's macroglobulinemia (WM). In PLL, the phenotype differs from CLL by showing more intense expression of surface immunoglobulins, low mouse rosette formation, low CD5 expression, and greater positivity for FMC7. Prolymphocytes differ morphologically from typical CLL cells by larger size, prominent nucleoli, and lower nuclear-to-cytoplasmic ratio. Patients with PLL typically have a high white cell count with splenomegaly disproportionate to the degree of lymph node involvement. Some patients have a mixture of typical CLL cells and prolymphocytes (PLL/CLL). This mixture is more common as the disease evolves into a prolymphocytic transformation than at diagnosis. Hairy cell leukemia is seldom a difficult diagnosis because these patients usually present with splenomegaly and pancytopenia. In some patients, however, there is a high white cell count in the range of 10,000 to 30,000 cells/μL. These cells can be distinguished by the presence of hairy projections, a positive reaction to tartrate-resistant acid phosphatase (TRAP) staining, and a high rate of positivity for CD25, CD11c, and HC2 with a lack of CD5 positivity. Atypical variants of HCL have morphologic features intermediate between HCL and PLL and are often TRAP negative. Patients with splenic lymphoma and circulating villous lymphocytes usually present with massive splenomegaly, moderate leukocytosis (10 to 25 × 10^3 cells/μL), serum or urine monoclonal immunoglobulin bands in half to two thirds of patients, and lymphocytes characterized by cytoplasmic villous projections. The membrane markers resemble those of PLL.

Some patients with non-Hodgkin's lymphoma, usually follicular or diffuse small cleaved cell types, develop a leukemic phase (not usually a feature at the time of initial diagnosis). The cells are typically cleaved and pleomorphic. Lymph node biopsy often demonstrates a prominent follicular pattern. The histology of the bone marrow is also follicular. The immunologic features that distinguish these patients from those with CLL are strong surface immunoglobulin expression, a low percentage of mouse rosette–positive cells, positivity for FMC7 and CD10, and negativity for CD5. Patients with Waldenström's macroglobulinemia (WM) usually have modest lymph node and spleen enlargement and moderate lymphocytosis. The few circulating lymphocytes generally have plasmacytoid features, and IgM paraprotein is seen in the serum. Although a monoclonal gammapothy occurs in 10 per cent of CLL cases, the immunoglobulin is usually IgG. A combination of clinical features, morphology, immunophenotyping, protein electrophoresis, special stains, and occasionally cytogenetic information can be useful in separating these chronic lymphoid leukemias.

PROGNOSIS

The commonly used CLL staging systems are the ones proposed by Rai and by Binet (Table 1). Both systems evaluate the tumor burden in terms of lymphadenopathy, hepatosplenomegaly, and bone marrow failure (anemia and thrombocytopenia). The Rai system originally included five stages, which were later reduced to three (modified Rai system) by joining stages 1 with 2 and 3 with 4. The former stage 0 remained unchanged and was labeled "low risk." Stages 1 and 2 were considered "intermediate," and stages 3 and 4 high-risk stages. The Binet staging system comprises three categories: A, B, and C (see Table 1). Although both systems correlate with survival in several series, they do not identify which patients in a given stage will have disease progression. This drawback may result from the fact that these systems estimate disease burden rather than disease aggressiveness.

Table 1. The Rai and Binet Staging Systems for Chronic Lymphocytic Leukemia

Rai Stage	Clinical Characteristics	Median Survival (yr)
0	Lymphocytosis only, in blood (≥15,000 cells/μL) and bone marrow ≥40%)	>10
1	Lymphocytosis + lymphadenopathy	>8
2	Lymphocytosis + splenomegaly +/− hepatomegaly	6
3*	Lymphocytosis + anemia (hemoglobin <11 g/dL)	2
4*	Lymphocytosis + thrombocytopenia (platelets <100,000 cells/μL)	2
Binet Stage		
A	No anemia, no thrombocytopenia, <3 involved nodal areas	†
B	No anemia, no thrombocytopenia, ≥3 involved nodal areas	7
C	Anemia (hemoglobin <10 g/dL) and/or thrombocytopenia (platelets <100,000 cells/μL)	2

*Stages III and IV may or may not include lymphadenopathy, splenomegaly, or hepatomegaly.

†Survival equivalent to that of age- and sex-matched (French) population.

The term "smoldering CLL" has been proposed for a subgroup of patients who belong to Binet stage A and who have a lymphocyte count less than 30 × 10^3 cells/μL, a lymphocyte doubling time (LDT) greater than 12 months, a hemoglobin concentration greater than 13 g/dL, and a nondiffuse pattern of bone marrow infiltration. This group has a 5 per cent chance of progression after 3 years, compared with a 32 per cent chance for other patients in stage A. Similar criteria for a diagnosis of smoldering CLL have been proposed by the French Cooperative Group on CLL. In one study, smoldering CLL accounted for 20 per cent of all patients and for 46 per cent of stage A patients.

Examination of a bone marrow biopsy specimen can also yield prognostic information. A diffuse pattern of bone marrow involvement indicates a worse prognosis than does other types of CLL marrow infiltration (interstitial, nodular, or mixed), particularly in early-stage disease. As in acute leukemia, cytogenetic analysis appears to provide promising information regarding differences in survival in various groups; further validation of the early studies is needed.

AUTOIMMUNE COMPLICATIONS

When autoantibodies are present in CLL patients, they are preferentially targeted against hematopoietic cells. Autoimmune hemolytic anemia, immune thrombocytopenia, immune neutropenia, pure red cell aplasia, and aplastic anemia all have been reported with CLL. The incidence of autoantibodies directed at hematopoietic cells in CLL ranges from 10 to 75 per cent. The incidence of a positive Coombs' test increases significantly with disease stage.

TRANSFORMATION

Although most patients with CLL demonstrate a stable histology throughout the clinical course, a small percentage may evolve to more aggressive disease forms, including Richter's syndrome, prolymphocytoid transformation, and rarely, acute leukemia.

Richter's transformation occurs in about 3 to 10 per cent of CLL patients and represents a change to a large-cell lymphoma (LCL) histology. Symptoms at transformation include progressive lymphadenopathy and systemic symptoms in the majority of patients. Extranodal involvement and paraproteinemia are noted in about 40 per cent of patients. The most frequent clinical feature is increased lactate dehydrogenase activity. Median survival is short (5 months), although responders to chemotherapy live longer than nonresponders.

THE LYMPHOMAS

By Peter McLaughlin, M.D.
Houston, Texas

The lymphoid or lymphoreticular neoplasms are divided into two broad categories, Hodgkin's disease and the malignant lymphomas (non-Hodgkin's lymphoma, or NHL). These diseases typically arise in and involve lymph nodes, the spleen, or the bone marrow. Extranodal presentations are not unusual, however, especially for diffuse NHLs.

Classification of the lymphomas is a process that continues to evolve, along with increasing sophistication in immunologic and molecular biologic information. Even the traditional distinction between Hodgkin's disease and NHL is not rigid: it is becoming clear that many patients with lymphocyte predominant Hodgkin's disease have B-cell gene rearrangement. Of the four histologic subtypes of Hodgkin's disease, the nodular sclerosis and mixed cellularity types are by far the most common. Together they constitute about 90 per cent of Hodgkin's disease cases (Table 1). For the NHLs, the Working Formulation (Table 2) has been widely used in North America since 1982, in large part due to its clinical relevance. Even at its inception the Working Formulation did not incorporate immunologic concepts. During the past decade, a number of pathologic entities have been more clearly defined, which has recently led to a proposal for a revised European-American lymphoma ("REAL") classification (Table 3) that largely recapitulates the Kiel system used widely in Europe. The reproducibility, comprehensiveness, and clinical relevance of this REAL scheme have not yet been established, but the clear definition of distinct immunologic and biologic entities is appealing.

The definition of subtypes of small lymphocytic lymphoma illustrates the utility of biologic insights in the classification of the lymphomas. Most small cell lymphomas can be characterized by their expression of the following antigens: CD10, the common acute lymphoblastic leukemia–associated antigen, which is often present in follicle center cells but absent in follicle mantle lymphomas; CD5, a pan–T cell antigen that is usually aberrantly expressed in chronic lymphocytic leukemia and small lymphocytic lymphoma; and CD23, a B-cell activation antigen. Small lymphocytic lymphoma typically is CD5-positive, CD10-negative, and CD23-positive. Mantle cell lymphoma is CD5-positive, most often CD10-negative, and CD23-negative. Follicle center lymphomas are CD5-negative, most often CD10-positive, and most often CD23-negative. Marginal zone lymphomas are CD5-negative, CD10-negative, and most often CD23-negative.

Table 1. Hodgkin's Disease: Stage According to Histologic Subtype

Histologic Subtype	No. of Patients	Stage (%) I–II	III	IV
Lymphocyte predominant	55	76	22	2
Nodular sclerosis	628	60	35	5
Mixed cellularity	215	44	47	9
Lymphocyte depleted	21	19	62	19

Adapted from Desforges, J. F.: Hodgkin's disease. N. Engl. J. Med., 301:1212–1222, 1979.

Table 2. Working Formulation

Grade	Category	% of Cases	Median Survival (yr)
Low	A. Small lymphocytic (SL)	3.6	5.8
	B. Follicular small cleaved cell (FSC)	22.5	7.2
	C. Follicular mixed small cleaved and large cell (FM)	7.7	5.1
Intermediate	D. Follicular large cell (FLC)	3.8	3.0
	E. Diffuse small cleaved cell (DSC)	6.9	3.4
	F. Diffuse mixed small and large cell (DM)	6.7	2.7
	G. Diffuse large cell (DLC)	19.7	1.5
High	H. Large cell immunoblastic (IBL)	7.9	1.3
	I. Lymphoblastic (LB)	4.2	2.0
	J. Small noncleaved cell (SNC)	5.0	0.7
	Miscellaneous		
	Composite; mycosis fungoides; histiocytic; extramedullary plasmacytoma; unclassified	12.0	

Adapted from Rosenberg, S. A., et al.: The Non-Hodgkin's Lymphoma Pathologic Classification Project: National Cancer Institute Sponsor Study Classification of Non-Hodgkin's Lymphomas: Summary and description of a working formulation for clinical usage. Cancer, 49:2112–2135, 1982, with permission.

Table 3. Comparison of Two Non-Hodgkin's Lymphoma Classifications

Revised European-American Lymphoma Classification	Corresponding Working Formulation Category(ies)*
B-Cell	
Precursor B-lymphoblastic	LB
B-CLL or small lymphocytic	SL
Lymphoplasmacytoid	**SL,** DM
Mantle cell	**DSC,** SL, FSC, DM, DLC
Follicle center, follicular	**FSC, FM,** FLC
Marginal zone	**SL,** DSC, DM
Hairy cell leukemia	—
Plasmacytoma or myeloma	—
Diffuse large cell	**DLC,** IBL, DM
Burkitt's	SNC
T-Cell and Putative NK-Cell	
Precursor T-lymphoblastic	LB
T-CLL	**SL,** DSC
Large granular lymphocyte leukemia	**SL,** DSC
Mycosis fungoides or Sézary syndrome	(Miscellaneous)
Peripheral T-cell	**DM, IBL,** DSC, DLC
Angioimmunoblastic	**DM, IBL,** DLC
Angiocentric	**DM, IBL,** DSC, DLC
Intestinal	**IBL,** DSC, DM, DLC
Adult T-cell lymphoma/leukemia	**DM, IBL,** DSC, DLC
Anaplastic large cell	IBL

*See Table 2 for abbreviations; bold letters indicate the predominant corresponding Working Formulation category.

Adapted from Harris, N. L., Jaffe, E. S., Stein, H., et al.: A Revised European-American classification of lymphoid neoplasms: A proposal from the International Lymphoma Study Group. Blood, 84:1361–1392, 1994, with permission.

Mantle cell lymphoma, in particular, emerges as a distinct entity that heretofore had been difficult to categorize (see Table 3). In addition to its characteristic phenotype, mantle cell lymphoma also has a distinctive cytogenetic finding, t(11;14) (q13;q32), resulting in rearrangement of the bcl-1 locus and overexpression of a nuclear protein, cyclin D1, which is encoded by the *PRAD1* gene.

PRESENTING SIGNS AND SYMPTOMS

For Hodgkin's disease and the low-grade follicular lymphomas, the most common presenting sign is painless lymph node enlargement. Hodgkin's disease (especially the nodular sclerosis type) is typically a disease of the young, with about 80 per cent of patients between the ages of 15 and 40 years. The male-to-female ratio is roughly equal for nodular sclerosis Hodgkin's disease, in contrast with most other lymphomas, which have a male predominance. Hodgkin's disease is usually localized at presentation, especially the lymphocyte predominant and nodular sclerosis types (see Table 1). Young females classically present with nodular sclerosis Hodgkin's disease, mediastinal involvement, and stage I to II disease. Male patients and those with mixed cellularity cell type are more likely to have abdominal involvement.

The follicular NHLs usually present in middle age with slowly progressive, widespread adenopathy, and frequently with splenomegaly and bone marrow involvement. The male-to-female ratio is nearly equal in follicular lymphoma. For the diffuse intermediate grade NHLs, onset can occur at any age, and about one third of patients have localized disease that can involve extranodal sites. The intermediate grade and especially the high grade lymphomas can grow rapidly and cause pain at involved sites. More than half of childhood lymphomas are high grade (lymphoblastic and small noncleaved cell). Lymphoblastic lymphoma is often associated with a mediastinal mass, and the superior vena cava syndrome can occur. Small noncleaved cell lymphoma often presents with abdominal masses with or without gastrointestinal tract involvement, and especially in children there can be a role for debulking surgery.

In extranodal presentations of NHL, symptoms relate to the specific site. The gastrointestinal tract is the most common extranodal site, particularly if Waldeyer's ring is included, so symptoms can be those of a gastric ulcer or a sore throat. The variety of extranodal sites makes lymphoma, at times, a diagnostic challenge; lymphoma presenting in the testis, bone, skin, or central nervous system can be symptomatically indistinguishable from other tumors at these sites. Thus, adequate biopsy material is crucial. An interesting group of extranodal presentations is the subset of marginal zone lymphomas known as "MALT" (mucosa-associated lymphoid tissue) lymphomas, which were probably largely dismissed in the past as "pseudolymphoma." These most commonly involve the stomach and predominantly occur in women.

Constitutional ("B") symptoms include unexplained fever higher than 38°C, sweats, or weight loss greater than 10 per cent of body mass in the preceding 6 months. These symptoms are less frequent in low grade lymphomas than in Hodgkin's disease and the intermediate and high grade lymphomas. Pruritus can also be present, especially in Hodgkin's disease, and alcohol-induced pain at the sites of masses is another classic but uncommon manifestation of Hodgkin's disease.

CLINICAL COURSE

Hodgkin's disease is potentially curable. For early-stage disease, treatment is based on radiotherapy, whereas advanced-stage disease requires chemotherapy. Combined-modality approaches are often employed. For patients whose disease relapses, salvage therapy can be effective and even curative, particularly when relapse occurs after radiotherapy only or when it occurs late (more than a year after chemotherapy). Relapse following chemotherapy often occurs in sites of initial disease. Conversely, following radiotherapy, relapse is usually outside the treated field.

Low grade lymphomas are indolent, but, with rare exception, they are considered incurable with current therapy. Only 10 to 20 per cent of patients have stage I to II disease at diagnosis; about half of stage I to II patients may be curable with radiation-based treatment. Patients with advanced-stage disease typically respond to chemotherapy, but control is temporary, and progressively shorter remissions are achieved over a course that can span a decade or more. During the disease course, there are often periods during which it is feasible to monitor asymptomatic patients without therapy. Spontaneous waxing and waning of adenopathy can occur. Ultimately, transformation to a histologically more aggressive phase is common, such as evolution from follicular small cleaved cell to diffuse large cell lymphoma, which is usually an ominous development.

Many intermediate grade lymphomas are potentially curable with appropriate front-line therapy, which virtually always is chemotherapy based. The majority of patients who achieve complete remission and remain in remission for 2 years are cured. Prognostic models such as the International Index (see below) provide a framework for selecting intensive or innovative therapy based on the risk of failure with standard therapy. If relapse occurs, durable subsequent remissions are rare, so optimal primary therapy is crucial.

One of the high grade lymphoma categories, large cell immunoblastic, is similar to diffuse large cell lymphoma in its course and appropriate therapy. But the other two high grade categories, lymphoblastic and small noncleaved cell lymphoma, have important highly distinctive features. Both can present with, or evolve into, an overt leukemic phase, and chemotherapy programs for these diseases are commonly modeled on programs for acute lymphoblastic leukemia. Both carry a substantial risk of central nervous system disease. These diseases are potentially curable, and the response to therapy is often brisk.

COMMON COMPLICATIONS AND HOW TO IDENTIFY THEM

Complications can relate to specific organ involvement, such as upper gastrointestinal tract bleeding in gastric lymphoma. Bulky or strategically located lymph nodes can cause obstructive jaundice, hydronephrosis, lymphedema, or other local symptoms. Mediastinal disease can cause subtle airway impingement, resulting in a cough or wheeze, or it can produce the superior vena cava syndrome. Serosal involvement can cause ascites or pleural effusions, and lymphatic obstruction can result in chylous effusions. Meningeal disease can cause cranial nerve palsies, headache, or other global neurologic signs. Nerve entrapment can cause plexopathies. More urgently, spinal cord compression can cause loss of sphincter control or sensory or motor dysfunction; but in fact these are usually late manifestations of spinal cord compression, and recognizing early symptoms such as back pain or subtle sensory abnormalities can lead to early intervention, thus avoiding a neurologic emergency. In addition to focal symptoms, there can be cytopenias due to marrow infiltration, autoimmunity, hypersplenism, or chronic disease. Hypercalcemia is infrequent, except in adult T-cell lymphoma/leukemia.

Infection is a common cause of problems and one of the most common causes of death in lymphoma. Opportunistic infections are notable in acquired immunodeficiency syndrome (AIDS)-related lymphoma and are also being seen in patients receiving purine nucleoside analogues. One of the most dramatic complications of therapy is the tumor lysis syndrome. This complication is typically seen in highly proliferative lymphomas (e.g., small noncleaved cell lymphoma), when the tumor burden is high, and when aggressive therapy is employed. When sudden massive cell lysis occurs, metabolic complications can include hyperkalemia, hyperuricemia, hyperphosphatemia with reciprocal hypocalcemia, and renal failure; serious associated clinical problems include life-threatening arrhythmias and oliguria.

The combination of a young patient population and effective therapy creates the potential for the emergence of late complications as a consequence of success. Infertility after therapy can be anticipated, so sperm banking should be considered when appropriate. Because xerostomia results from radiotherapy to the neck (e.g., in the mantle field), preventive dental care should be employed. Also, after neck radiotherapy, monitoring for hypothyroidism is appropriate. Although staging laparotomy with splenectomy is performed less often now than in the past, when it is done, especially in children, it entails a subsequent risk of infection with encapsulated organisms (e.g., *Streptococcus pneumoniae).* Cardiac complications can include cardiomyopathy from anthracyclines, and radiation-induced damage to the pericardium, myocardium, or coronary arteries. Second malignancies are also sobering late complications. Following therapy, particularly when combined-modality therapy is employed or when specific drugs such as procarbazine are included, the risk of acute leukemia increases, especially for the first decade following therapy. Beyond about 7 years the leukemia risk decreases, but the risk for other second malignancies, that is, solid tumors, continues to rise. In the Hodgkin's disease population, one notable type of second malignancy is NHL; thus, an apparent late "relapse" is another setting, like the initial diagnosis, in which an adequate biopsy is important for proper classification and planning of treatment.

EXPECTED AND UNUSUAL FINDINGS ON PHYSICAL EXAMINATION

When localized, Hodgkin's disease is much more frequently found in upper torso sites than in the lower torso. Occasionally, infraclavicular adenopathy can be present, and extensive mediastinal and internal mammary adenopathy may be associated with a palpable parasternal mass.

In low grade lymphoma, widespread adenopathy can include sites that are unusual in other lymphomas, such as epitrochlear and occipital nodes. The characteristic slow pace of growth can result in surprisingly large asymptomatic abdominal masses or splenomegaly. The various MALT lymphoma presentations can be challenging and can include not only disease in the stomach but also the parotid, conjunctiva, thyroid, bronchi, and breast.

Intermediate and high grade lymphomas are highly variable. Some distinctive presentations include skin involvement in anaplastic large cell lymphoma, and B-symptoms, skin rash, and polyclonal hypergammaglobulinemia in angioimmunoblastic T-cell lymphoma. Other notable manifestations of particular sites of involvement include cranial nerve palsies in the setting of meningeal disease, brain or other unusual extranodal sites in AIDS-related lymphoma, superior vena cava syndrome in lymphoblastic lymphoma, jaw involvement in young children with endemic (African) Burkitt's lymphoma, and abdominal masses in those with nonendemic Burkitt's lymphoma. Mycosis fungoides can present with multiple skin plaques or with cutaneous nodules. Erythroderma is characteristic of the Sézary syndrome.

DIAGNOSTIC PROCEDURES AND STAGING

Recommended staging procedures are outlined in Table 4. An adequate biopsy is crucial for proper classification of disease, which in turn is crucial to management. Increasingly, ancillary tests on biopsy specimens are important, especially phenotyping; molecular genetic or cytogenetic analyses; and measures of proliferation such as staining for the nuclear antigen Ki-67. After the diagnosis is established, much of the subsequent work-up is focused on properly assigning stage and characterizing other known prognostic factors.

The Ann Arbor staging system (Table 5) was initially developed for Hodgkin's disease. It stratifies meaningful subsets of patients with Hodgkin's disease and is an excellent conceptual framework for planning the radiotherapy that is a key element in treating patients with stage I to II and even stage III Hodgkin's disease. But the Ann Arbor staging system has limitations for NHL: NHL does not follow as predictable a pattern of contiguous nodal spread as does Hodgkin's disease; in some categories of NHL such

Table 4. Recommended Staging Procedures

1. History, with attention to B-symptoms, performance status, and antecedent autoimmune or other immunologic disorders
2. Physical examination, with attention to nodal sites, liver, spleen, and Waldeyer's ring
3. Adequate surgical biopsy (when possible, a whole node); phenotyping*
4. Laboratory tests, including complete blood count, differential, and platelets; serum chemistry panel including lactate dehydrogenase, liver and renal function, albumin, calcium, uric acid; β_2-microglobulin;* erythrocyte sedimentation rate†
5. Bilateral bone marrow aspirate and biopsy
6. Radiologic evaluation: chest radiograph; computed tomography of abdomen and pelvis; bipedal lymphangiogram†
7. Additional considerations under special circumstances:
   - Computed tomography of chest (if x-ray film suspicious or equivocal)
   - Computed tomography of the head and neck
   - Gallium scan
   - Technetium bone scan
   - Ultrasonography (e.g., of equivocal spleen or liver lesions)
   - Magnetic resonance imaging (e.g., of spine)
   - Lumbar puncture (if symptoms present, or for high grade non-Hodgkin's lymphoma)
   - Endoscopy (if symptoms present, or if primary in Waldeyer's ring)
   - Staging laparotomy† or laparoscopy
   - Peripheral blood and/or bone marrow lymphocyte surface marker studies*

*More relevant for non-Hodgkin's lymphomas.
†More relevant for Hodgkin's disease.

Table 5. Ann Arbor Staging System

Stage I

A single lymph node region, or a single extralymphatic organ or site (IE)

Stage II

Two or more lymph node regions on the same side of the diaphragm, or a localized extralymphatic site plus one or more lymph node regions on the same side of the diaphragm (IIE)

Stage III

Lymph node regions on both sides of the diaphragm, with or without localized involvement of an extralymphatic site (IIIE) or the spleen (IIIS)

Stage IV

Disseminated involvement of one or more extralymphatic organs

A or B

Denotes absence (A) or presence (B) of unexplained weight loss >10% of body weight in the previous 6 months; unexplained fever >38°C; or night sweats

as low grade lymphoma, bone marrow involvement is so common that Ann Arbor staging does not result in much stratification; and nonanatomic variables such as serum level of lactate dehydrogenase (LD) are of major prognostic importance. As a result, other prognostic models have been devised, particularly the International Index, developed mainly for intermediate grade lymphoma but also relevant for low grade lymphoma. For the aggressive lymphomas (i.e., diffuse mixed, diffuse large cell, and immunoblastic), Table 6 depicts the strong correlation of outcome with the presence of one or more of five adverse risk factors: age more than 60 years; serum LD level above normal; Eastern Cooperative Oncology Group (ECOG) performance status greater than 2; Ann Arbor stages III to IV; and two or more extranodal sites. Separate staging schemes exist for lymphoblastic and small noncleaved cell lymphoma.

The importance of serum LD in NHL is illustrated by its prominence in the International Index. Serum β_2-microglobulin is another widely recognized and important factor; caveats include unreliability in the setting of renal failure or human immunodeficiency virus (HIV) infection. In addition to those listed in Table 4, laboratory tests of occasional value are: Coombs' test; antiplatelet antibody assay; serum protein electrophoresis, especially when plasmacytoid features are evident on biopsy or when the total serum protein concentration is increased; and spinal fluid analysis, including spinal fluid β_2-microglobulin.

Computed tomography (CT) is the most important abdominal imaging technique, providing information on the retroperitoneum, the mesentery, the spleen, liver, and other organs. Lymphangiography remains a key imaging procedure in Hodgkin's disease. In NHL, it is probably most useful in low grade lymphoma when the CT scan shows only small or borderline lymph nodes. If lymphangiography is to be done, CT scanning can be limited to the abdomen and exclude the pelvis. Gallium scanning has a role in Hodgkin's disease and the intermediate grade lymphomas, but it is of limited value in low grade lymphoma. It is particularly useful as a baseline procedure against which to compare follow-up studies. Reversion to negative on gallium scanning suggests that residual abnormalities on other radiographs (e.g., CT scans) represent "scar" rather than active disease. Staging laparotomy should be performed selectively. It warrants consideration if the findings would change the treatment approach.

ERRORS AND PITFALLS IN DIAGNOSIS

Some categories of lymphoma have a deceptively slow course. The use of empiric antibiotic treatment for adenopathy is common, but if there is no clear infection or other explanation for the nodes and if the nodal enlargement persists, the diagnosis of lymphoma should be considered. Similarly, abdominal complaints can be nonspecific. Despite the availability of CT scanning, it is still true that many abdominal presentations of lymphoma are diagnosed only when the adenopathy is quite bulky.

After the decision to biopsy has been made, attention to details maximizes the amount of information obtained. First, an excisional biopsy of an intact lymph node offers the best chance for accurate classification. Second, Sutton's law—to go where the money is—dictates that the biggest node or mass is the most informative to biopsy, even when it is not technically the most accessible. Third, the biopsy material should be handled with attention to the almost routine need for surface marker studies and the foreseeable increasing need for molecular genetic analysis. Fourth, expertise in hematopathology is required; in difficult cases, consultation may be necessary.

Because architecture and adequacy of material are crucial, fine-needle aspiration (FNA) is not optimal for making the initial diagnosis. However, FNA can be useful, especially if morphologic, phenotypic, and kinetic data all are assessed on the material obtained and are taken into account. Also, FNA is helpful for confirming the persistence of disease after therapy or relapse, and it can be useful in staging (e.g., confirming disease on the opposite side of the diaphragm) or in assessing areas that would otherwise require major surgery. For example, when there is a known diagnosis of low grade lymphoma in a peripheral lymph

Table 6. International Index for Aggressive Non-Hodgkin's Lymphoma

Risk Group	No. of Risk Factors*	% Complete Remission	% Relapse-Free		% Survival	
			2 Yr	*5 Yr*	*2 Yr*	*5 Yr*
Low	0–1	87	79	70	84	73
Low–intermediate	2	67	66	50	66	51
High–intermediate	3	55	59	49	54	43
High	4–5	44	58	40	34	26

*Risk factors include age; serum lactate dehydrogenase level; performance status; stage; number of extranodal sites (see text).

Adapted from Shipp, M. A., et al.: A predictive model for aggressive non-Hodgkin's lymphoma. N. Engl. J. Med, 329:987–994, 1993.

node, FNA can be used to assess an abdominal mass for the possibility of transformation to large cell lymphoma.

After the diagnosis has been made, conscientious staging is important, with attention to relevant prognostic features such as LD and β_2-microglobulin. Interaction and collaboration between the pathologist, the diagnostic radiologist, the radiotherapist, and the oncologist is extremely helpful in planning treatment.

MULTIPLE MYELOMA AND OTHER PLASMA CELL DISORDERS

By Mohamad A. Hussein, M.D., *and* Ronald M. Bukowski, M.D.
Cleveland, Ohio

Multiple myeloma is the prototype of a group of conditions known as plasma cell neoplasms. These neoplasms are a group of related disorders, each of which is associated with proliferation and accumulation of immunoglobulin-secreting cells that are derived from the B-cell series of immunocytes. Monoclonal components occur both in the malignant plasma cell disorders, such as multiple myeloma, Waldenström's macroglobulinemia, solitary bone plasmacytoma, extramedullary plasmacytomas, osteosclerotic myeloma (POEMS syndrome [polyneuropathy, organomegaly, endocrinopathy, monoclonal protein and skin changes]), amyloidosis, and heavy chain disease, and in the clinically unclear monoclonal gammopathy of undetermined significance or "smoldering" multiple myeloma (SMM).

PRESENTING SIGNS AND SYMPTOMS

The clinical features of multiple myeloma result from tissue damage by multiple bone tumors, complications from the monoclonal protein, and an increased vulnerability to infection due to decreased concentrations of normal immunoglobulins. These complications provide the first clues to the diagnosis and form the basis for defining the stage and prognosis.

Subjective Symptoms

Bone pain is the most common symptom resulting from pathologic fractures. Compression fractures of the thoracic and lumbar vertebral bodies usually result in severe muscle spasms and back pains. Multiple compression fractures may culminate in painless dorsal kyphosis and a loss of as much as 6 inches (15 cm) of height. Pleuritic pain from pathologic rib and clavicular fractures is also common and is associated with marked local tenderness. Destruction of the proximal bones of the extremities is less frequent, and distal bones of the extremities are rarely affected. Bandlike or radicular pain should alert the clinician to impending spinal cord compression, a serious complication representing an emergency requiring immediate diagnosis and treatment. Nausea, confusion, polyuria, and constipation are common symptoms secondary to hypercalcemia. Easy fatigability or dyspnea on exertion are usually secondary to anemia. When immunoglobulins are present in concentrations greater than 5 g/dL in serum, selected IgG or IgA monoclonal proteins can produce features of hyperviscosity syndrome. Lassitude, confusion, headache, transient disturbances of vision, and increased bleeding tendency are part of this syndrome. Recurrent bacterial infections are a major cause of illness and are the most common cause of death in patients with advanced myeloma. Systemic amyloidosis with or without multiple myeloma can present with weakness, weight loss, ankle edema, dyspnea, paresthesias, lightheadedness, or syncope. Aching in the hands, particularly at night, can result from median nerve compression associated with carpal tunnel syndrome caused by amyloid infiltration of the transverse carpal ligament.

Objective Findings

No specific physical abnormalities may be detected. Most patients with symptomatic myeloma have tenderness with pressure over an involved bone, kyphosis, or a pathologic fracture to indicate the site of bone lesions. In approximately 15 per cent of patients, firm plasma cell tumors arise in areas of underlying bone destruction and may be palpated on the skull, sternum, clavicles, and ribs, where the affected bone is close to the skin. Fundus examination, especially in patients with suspected hyperviscosity syndrome, may reveal segmental dilatation of the retinal veins with retinal hemorrhages. Examination of the neck and oropharynx occasionally reveals extramedullary plasmacytomas that may develop in the oral cavity or paranasal sinuses. Signs of lobular pneumonia may be detected on auscultation and palpation of the chest. In rare instances in which pleural effusions develop from plasmacytoma and plasmacytosis, these effusions can be detected clinically and radiologically. Cardiac examination may reveal ventricular gallop as a sign of heart failure secondary to severe anemia, hypercalcemia, or amyloid heart disease. Neurologic signs caused by spinal cord or nerve root compression, sensory motor peripheral neuropathy, or myelomatosis meningitis are frequent. Spinal examination can reveal kyphosis and, on palpation, tenderness at the area of fracture or plasmacytoma. Palpation may also trigger radiculopathy, which can help localize the site of imminent cord compression. Upper extremities may show signs of carpal tunnel syndrome. Skin plaques or joint effusions secondary to amyloid deposits may be presenting features. Generalized edema secondary to nephrotic syndrome and/or congestive heart failure may be found on physical examination.

DISEASE COURSE

The median survival of patients with multiple myeloma who receive symptomatic treatment is only 7 months. Since the introduction of chemotherapy, the median survival has improved to 36 to 48 months. Cure, however, is rare in this disease. Several clinical and laboratory parameters provide important prognostic information that is extremely valuable in evaluating disease progression and the effects of different treatment regimens. The staging system of Durie and Salmon, which is based on hemoglobin, serum calcium, and monoclonal protein concentrations as well as the characteristics of the bone survey, classifies patients into three stages that correlate with myeloma cell mass. Serum β_2-microglobulin uncorrected for serum creatinine predicts survival remarkably well in myeloma patients. Karyotypic abnormalities occur in 30 per cent of individuals with myeloma. Irrespective of the treatment status, patients with an abnormal karyotype have a significantly shorter median survival than do those with a normal karyotype. The plasma cell labeling index powerfully and independently predicts survival. Also, it is a useful tool for distinguishing between monoclonal gammopathy of undetermined significance and multiple myeloma. Serum interleukin-6, C-reactive protein, serum interleukin-2, and serum interleukin-6 receptor concentrations appear to be other factors that can assist in predicting the course of disease and/or response to therapy. Secondary acute leukemia develops in approximately 2 per cent of patients who survive 2 years, which is 50 to 100 times more frequent than in normal individuals. Fewer than 5 per cent of patients with multiple myeloma have acute leukemia at diagnosis or acquire the disease within several months after starting chemotherapy. The frequency of solid tumors in multiple myeloma patients is no higher than in persons of similar age or sex.

COMPLICATIONS

Bone Destruction

Approximately 20 per cent of patients with multiple myeloma have bone demineralization only. At least 30 per cent of bone calcium must be lost before radiographic changes are evident. In 1.4 per cent of patients, an osteoblastic reaction is present, which suggests the POEMS syndrome.

Renal Failure

Renal failure occurs in approximately 25 per cent of patients, more frequently in patients with extensive disease. Most patients with mild azotemia have no symptoms; however, easy fatigability, nausea, vomiting, and confusion can occur with severe renal insufficiency. The pathogenesis of this complication is multifactorial, but more than 90 per cent of patients with renal failure have light chains in their urine (Bence-Jones proteinuria) and/or hypercalcemia.

Infection

Recurrent bacterial infections are a major cause of morbidity and are the most frequent cause of death in patients with advanced myeloma. Infections result primarily from the marked depression of the production of normal immunoglobulins, which occurs in more than 75 per cent of patients. *Streptococcus pneumoniae* and *Haemophilus influenzae* are the most common pathogens in previously untreated myeloma patients and in non-neutropenic patients who respond to chemotherapy. However, in neutropenic patients and in those with refractory disease, *Staphylococcus aureus* and gram-negative bacteria are the predominant organisms. Pneumococcal vaccination may be worth trying; however, most multiple myeloma patients respond poorly to bacterial antigenic stimulation. Herpes zoster occurs in patients with multiple myeloma and is more common in patients with renal failure.

Hyperviscosity Syndrome

Symptoms and signs of hyperviscosity syndrome generally are not seen unless the relative serum viscosity is greater than 4 U (reference range 1.4 to 1.8 U), and the classic syndrome usually is not observed unless the viscosity is greater than 5 U. The signs and symptoms include lassitude, confusion, blurred vision, dizziness, vertigo, diplopia, and an increased tendency to bleed, especially oronasal bleeding.

Neurologic Complications

Thoracic or lumbosacral radiculopathy is the most frequent neurologic complication. Root pain results from compression of the nerve by the vertebral lesion or the collapsed bone itself. Spinal cord or cauda equina compression from an extradural plasma cell tumor results in back pain with radicular features, weakness, or paralysis in which immediate diagnosis and treatment are necessary. Occasionally, patients with multiple myeloma experience peripheral neuropathy that may be severe. Electromyographic studies suggest that this complication occurs more frequently than is clinically recognized. Although the pathogenesis is unclear, the neuropathy may be caused by associated amyloidosis in some patients. Severe motor neuropathy occurs more frequently in younger patients with localized or osteosclerotic myeloma.

Hypercalcemia

At diagnosis, one fourth of patients have serum calcium concentrations greater than 11.5 mg/dL after correction for serum albumin. Some hypercalcemic patients may not show bone destruction on radiographs. Nausea, confusion, polyuria, and constipation are common symptoms.

LABORATORY PROCEDURES

Routine laboratory screening tests such as complete blood count, serum biochemistry studies, urinalysis, and chest radiography are usually not diagnostic; however, they are extremely helpful in choosing additional diagnostic procedures. Anemia is present in most patients and provides a major diagnostic clue. Several factors account for anemia, such as bone marrow infiltration by plasma cells, renal failure, and chronic disease. Decreased serum vitamin B_{12} concentrations may occur without signs of functional vitamin B_{12} deficiency. However, in our experience, careful evaluation by clinical examination, reviewing the peripheral blood film, and obtaining serum methylmalonic acid and homocysteine detect a significant number of early asymptomatic, functional vitamin B_{12}–deficient patients. High concentrations of IgA or IgG frequently increase the plasma volume, and the hematocrit may be 6 per cent less than the value expected from the measured red cell volume. Thrombocytopenia is uncommon at the time of diagnosis and when present reflects a marked degree of bone marrow replacement by plasma cells. Mild granulocytopenia occurs frequently for reasons that are unclear and may persist throughout the clinical course.

Increased total globulins, hypoalbuminemia, or overall hypoproteinemia secondary to nephrotic syndrome is also observed. Hypercalcemia, hyperuricemia, and increased serum creatinine secondary to multiple myeloma and/or renal failure are frequent. Increased lactate dehydrogenase (LD) is noted in 10 to 15 per cent of patients and usually signifies a poor prognosis. The serum alkaline phosphatase is usually normal but may be increased in patients with healing pathologic fractures or osteosclerotic lesions. Proteinuria is detected in approximately 65 per cent of patients. The chest film may reveal osteolytic lesions in the clavicles, scapulae, or ribs, or it may show a pleural effusion. Cardiomegaly may be seen in patients with cardiac amyloidosis. When plasma cell dyscrasia is suspected, the tests discussed in the following paragraphs should be performed to confirm the diagnosis, detect complications, assist in the staging of the disease, and establish baseline values for following the progress of treatment.

Myeloma Proteins

Serum and urine protein electrophoresis demonstrates a peak or localized band in 80 per cent of patients, hypogammaglobulinemia in 10 per cent, and no apparent abnormalities in the remainder. In multiple myeloma patients with hypogammaglobulinemia, a monoclonal light chain protein in the urine is usually present. Immunoelectrophoresis and immunofixation are rather expensive; however, they are very sensitive when compared with protein electrophoresis, which may not detect 15 per cent of monoclonal gammopathies. In 99 per cent of patients, a monoclonal protein in the serum or the urine, or both, is detected, and in 1 per cent of patients, no monoclonal protein is found. In these cases, the diagnosis of nonsecretory multiple myeloma is made. This finding is believed to be secondary to a defect in the synthesis or assembly of the light or heavy chains of the immunoglobulin molecule.

Bone Marrow Aspirate and Biopsy

Performing bone marrow aspiration and biopsy is helpful in evaluating the different causes of cytopenias and is crucial in the diagnosis of multiple myeloma. Additionally, it provides evaluation of cell morphologic features and plasma cell biologic features that may be useful in determining prognosis. Bone marrow plasmacytosis may be spotty, but an increase in the bone marrow plasma cells is typically demonstrable. Reactive plasmacytosis secondary to connective tissue disorders, liver disease, viral and bacterial infections, and carcinoma can be distinguished from the monoclonal plasma cell proliferation of multiple myeloma or monoclonal gammopathy of unknown significance by performing immunohistochemical studies. If available, a plasma cell labeling index on the bone marrow can add important prognostic information and possibly aid in planning patient management. A labeling index of less than or equal to 0.8 per cent usually indicates a good prognosis. Cytogenetic abnormalities occur in 30 per cent of multiple myeloma patients, and their presence usually indicates a shorter median survival. Numeric anomalies occur most often in chromosome 11, and structural aberrations occur most often in chromosomes 1, 11, and 14.

Urinalysis

Proteinuria is detected in approximately 65 per cent of patients. The recognition of light chain protein (Bence-Jones protein) depends on the demonstration of the monoclonal light chain by immunoelectrophoresis or immunofixation. A 24-hour urine collection for protein quantitation supplemented by urine protein electrophoresis is essential for following the response to therapy.

Imaging Procedures

A complete radiographic bone survey is an essential part of the evaluation of monoclonal gammopathies. The skeletal survey should include the skull, ribs, complete spine, pelvis, and long bones of the arms and legs. Radiographs of the axial skeleton, which must include both femurs, will support the diagnosis of multiple myeloma in approximately 70 per cent of patients. Punched-out lesions are best seen on lateral skull radiographs. Ten per cent of patients have a normal skeletal survey at the time of diagnosis. Computed tomography (CT) and magnetic resonance imaging (MRI) techniques may be more sensitive and are especially useful in determining the extent of extramedullary soft tissue lesions. Magnetic resonance imaging of the lumbar spine and pelvis may detect more advanced disease in patients with an apparently localized plasmacytoma or with asymptomatic indolent multiple myeloma that may require chemotherapy.

Other Useful Diagnostic Procedures

Serum β_2-microglobulin is part of the major histocompatibility complex of the cell membrane. Increased concentrations are found in patients with active multiple myeloma. A close relationship exists between the serum β_2-microglobulin (uncorrected for serum creatinine) and measured myeloma cell mass. Concentrations greater than 6 mg/dL are predictive of a large tumor burden and poor prognosis. C-reactive protein may also be an important prognostic factor because its concentration is controlled in vivo by interleukin-6, and therefore it may be a convenient and direct indicator of interleukin-6 production.

Technetium-99m bone scans are inferior to conventional radiographs for detecting lesions in patients with multiple myeloma and are rarely indicated.

DIFFERENTIAL DIAGNOSIS

Lytic bone lesions can be seen in metastatic carcinoma, connective tissue diseases, chronic infections, or lymphoma. Patients with multiple myeloma must be distinguished from those with monoclonal gammopathy of undetermined significance and SMM. Asymptomatic patients with an M-component less than 3 g/dL, fewer than 10 per cent bone marrow plasma cells, no osteolytic lesions, anemia, hypercalcemia, or renal function impairment have monoclonal gammopathy of unknown significance (MGUS). Asymptomatic patients who have an M-component greater than 3 g/dL or more than 10 per cent but less than 20 per cent bone marrow plasma cells fulfill the criteria for SMM. These patients do not have anemia, renal failure, hypercalcemia, osteolytic bone lesions, or other clinical manifestations related to the monoclonal protein. Clinically and biologically they are closer to monoclonal gammopathy of undetermined significance than to overt multiple myeloma. The recognition of these patients is extremely important because they should not be treated with chemotherapy until progression occurs. There is no particular laboratory parameter or clinical factor that can distinguish patients with MGUS and SMM from those with overt multiple myeloma. The decreased concentrations of uninvolved immunoglobulins are not a useful criterion for distinction because 30 to 40 per cent of patients with MGUS also have a decrease in normal immunoglobulins. Although the presence of Bence-Jones proteinuria is suggestive of multiple myeloma, it is not unusual to find small amounts of monoclonal light chains in the urine of patients with MGUS. Lytic bone lesions in the skeletal survey strongly suggest the diagnosis of multiple myeloma. In patients with recently diagnosed MGUS, serum electrophoresis should be repeated after 3 months to exclude an early myeloma; if results are stable, the test should be repeated in 6 months and then, if stable, once or twice yearly. Patients should be aware that the evolution of MGUS to multiple myeloma can be abrupt, and therefore they should be re-examined promptly if the clinical condition deteriorates.

MULTIPLE MYELOMA VARIANTS

Solitary Bone Plasmacytoma

Solitary bone plasmacytoma (SBP) is an uncommon type of tumor occurring in 3 to 5 per cent of patients with plasma cell neoplasms. The disease occurs predominantly in males and affects any age group, with the median age of diagnosis being 55 plus or minus 5 years, slightly younger than in patients with multiple myeloma. The most common mode of presentation is pain at the site of a skeletal lesion. Neurologic dysfunction in the form of nerve root compression or cord compression is another presenting symptom occurring predominantly in patients with SBP in the vertebral column. In more than half of patients with skeletal SBP, the presentation is in the axial skeleton, with the remainder occurring in the appendicular skeleton. The essential diagnostic criteria for solitary plasmacytoma is the presence of a solitary bone lesion with a normal skeletal survey; histologically proven plasmacytoma by biopsy of the tumor; a normal bone marrow aspirate with less than 5 per cent plasma cells; absence of anemia, hypercalcemia, or renal dysfunction; and the presence of a low or undetectable concentration of monoclonal protein by immunoanalytic assay. Criteria that are nonessential for the diagnosis of SBP, but could shed some light on the prognosis, include the disappearance of the monoclonal protein after surgery and/or radiation therapy and normal immunoglobulin concentrations after the therapeutic procedure. Progression to multiple myeloma occurs in approximately 55 per cent of patients with SBP.

Extramedullary Plasmacytoma

Extramedullary plasmacytoma (EMP) is a rare primary soft tissue plasma cell tumor. These tumors are known to originate in a variety of anatomic sites, although more than 90 per cent have been reported in the head and neck area, and most of these arise in the upper respiratory passages, including the nasopharynx and the paranasal sinuses. Metastases to regional lymph nodes occur in 8 to 15 per cent of patients. Progression to multiple myeloma is reported in 0 to 40 per cent of patients.

POEMS Syndrome

POEMS syndrome is characterized by the clinical complex of polyneuropathy, organomegaly, endocrinopathy of various forms, and skin changes with a monoclonal protein. All these symptoms are considered secondary to a plasma cell dyscrasia, with most patients demonstrating a monoclonal protein. Electromyography and nerve biopsy demonstrate a variety of abnormalities, ranging from demyelination to axonal degeneration. Nerve deposits of immunoglobulins are usually absent. Organomegaly may include splenomegaly, hepatomegaly, and enlarged lymph nodes. Endocrinopathy ranges from overt diabetes mellitus to amenorrhea, hyperprolactinemia, hyperestrogenemia, and hypothyroidism. The latter is usually present in 40 to 60 per cent of patients. All M-proteins have a λ light chain. The skin changes can include local or general hyperpigmentation that is not related to adrenal insufficiency. Thrombocytosis is noted in about 40 per cent of these patients, and polycythemia is seen in approximately 20 per cent. Bone marrow examination usually demonstrates less than 5 per cent plasma cells, and the amount of serum M-protein is modest.

Amyloidosis

Amyloid is a substance with a homogeneous, amorphous appearance under the light microscope that stains pink with hematoxylin and eosin. Amyloidosis results from the interplay of many factors, including excessive deposition of amyloid and deranged degradation of amyloid fibrils. The clinical diagnosis is usually delayed either because the underlying mechanism is unclear or because the signs and symptoms of the primary disease mask or are similar to those produced by the deposition of amyloid itself. Amyloidosis should be suspected with the insidious onset of unexplained proteinuria or renal failure, hepatomegaly, splenomegaly, macroglossia, peripheral neuropathy, malabsorption, or cardiomyopathy. Weakness, fatigue, and weight loss are the most frequent symptoms. Dyspnea, pedal edema, angina pectoris, arrhythmia, syncope, and lightheadedness occur secondary to congestive heart failure, and orthostatic hypotension often develops during the course of the disease. The initial diagnostic procedure is abdominal fat aspiration, since this is positive for amyloid in more than 80 per cent of patients. A bone marrow aspirate and biopsy specimen should be obtained to determine the degree of plasmacytosis. The bone marrow specimen stains for amyloid are positive in slightly more than 50 per cent of patients. If the abdominal fat and bone marrow biopsies are normal, a rectal biopsy with submucosa should be performed. These biopsy results are positive in approximately 80 per cent of patients. If the results from all these biopsy sites are negative, tissue should be obtained from a clinically involved organ. Approximately 10 per cent of patients with multiple myeloma experience amyloidosis, and 15 to 20 per cent of patients with primary amyloidosis actually have multiple myeloma.

OTHER PLASMA CELL DYSCRASIAS

Heavy Chain Disease

Heavy chain disease represents a proliferative process of B cells characterized by the production of incomplete heavy chains devoid of light chains. These monoclonal proteins are present in the serum, urine, or both. Gamma, alpha, mu, and delta heavy chain diseases have been described.

Gamma Heavy Chain Disease

Gamma heavy chain disease is a serologically determined entity. Although a lymphomalike illness has been considered characteristic of γ heavy chain disease, it does not represent a specific pathologic process but is a biochemical expression of a mutant B-cell clone. The median age at diagnosis is almost the same as that for multiple myeloma and primary amyloidosis—approximately 60 years. However, the disease may occur in children or very young adults and has been diagnosed before the age of 20 years in several patients. In contrast to the uniformity of findings associated with α heavy chain disease, patients with γ heavy chain disease have variable clinical and pathologic features. A specific pathologic pattern corresponding to γ heavy chain disease does not exist. Gamma heavy chain disease most often presents as a lymphoproliferative disorder. Lymphadenopathy and constitutional symptoms are the most common presenting features. The duration of the symptoms before diagnosis can range from a few weeks to more than 20 years. Generalized peripheral lymphadenopathy with prominent cervical involvement is present in approximately 55 per cent of patients. Waxing and waning of lymphadenopathy may occur. Edema of the uvula and palate occurs in about 20 per cent of patients, presumably from lymphatic obstruction with involvement of Waldeyer's ring. Splenomegaly is present in approximately 60 per cent of patients. Isolated splenomegaly may be the presenting feature of γ heavy chain disease. Autoimmune disorders associated or unassociated with an underlying lymphoproliferative disorder are frequent in patients with γ heavy chain disease. The serum protein electrophoretic pattern is extremely variable and usually does not suggest a monoclonal gammopathy.

Pseudogamma Heavy Chain Deposition Disease

Patients with pseudo–γ heavy chain disease may present with acute renal failure. Renal biopsy typically reveals dense granular deposits associated with a linear pattern of IgG4 heavy chain deposition in vascular, tubular, and glomerular basement membranes. Neither circulating nor cellular free γ chains are detectable. The immunohistologic findings may best be explained by a change in the three-dimensional conformational structure of the protein after entrapment and binding to the basement membrane, rendering the light chain antigenic sites inaccessible to antibody reagent and thereby undetectable.

Alpha Heavy Chain Disease

In α heavy chain disease, anemia is frequent and usually normochromic, normocytic, and moderate except in patients with autoimmune hemolytic anemia. Bone marrow aspiration and biopsy reveal increased plasma cells, lymphocytes, or plasmacytoid lymphocytes similar to the bone marrow findings in Waldenström's macroglobulinemia. The bones usually appear normal radiographically. Lymph node pathologic characteristics have no consistent morphologic features. This is the most frequent of the heavy chain diseases. Most reported cases of α heavy chain disease have originated in the Mediterranean region or the Middle East. The incidence is slightly greater in males than in females and is highest in the third decade of life. A common denominator in these patients is low social economic status and poor hygiene, resulting in repeated acute infectious diarrhea and chronic parasitic infections. In approximately one half of patients, serum protein electrophoresis shows no evidence of an abnormal protein. In the remainder, an abnormal broad band is seen in the αβ globulin region. The diagnosis depends on the recognition of a monoclonal α heavy chain in the serum or in the gastrointestinal contents. The clinical pattern of α heavy chain disease in its "digestive form" is remarkably uniform, with diarrhea, steatorrhea, weight loss, abdominal pains, and vomiting being the most common presenting symptoms. Hepatosplenomegaly and peripheral lymphadenopathy are uncommon findings. Pathologically, α heavy chain disease is divided into three stages depending on the depth and degree of cellular atypia of intestinal infiltrate. Mesenteric lymph nodes are usually involved in the "digestive" form of α heavy chain disease. On the basis of the cellular type of the infiltrate and on the degree of obliteration of the nodal architecture, three histologic stages equivalent to those described in small intestine can be identified. The characteristic pathologic features usually extend throughout the small bowel without intervals of normal mucosa. Alpha heavy chain disease may also be confined to the respiratory tract, but the respiratory form is rare.

Mu Heavy Chain Disease

Mu heavy chain disease is rare, with a median age of 57.5 years at the time of diagnosis. An associated B-cell lymphoproliferative disorder (chronic lymphocytic leukemia, lymphoma, Waldenström's macroglobulinemia, and myeloma) is common in these patients. Splenomegaly and hepatomegaly are common physical findings, and lymphadenopathy is less frequent. Bone marrow lymphocytosis and plasmacytosis are common findings. Lytic bone lesions are rare but have been described occasionally.

Delta Heavy Chain Disease

One case of possible δ heavy chain disease has been described. The patient presented with renal insufficiency and features of multiple myeloma.

Macroglobulinemia

Patients with IgM paraprotein can be divided into individuals with Waldenström's macroglobulinemia, lymphoma, chronic lymphocytic leukemia, IgM myeloma, amyloidosis, or monoclonal gammopathy of uncertain significance of the IgM type. The incidence of MGUS in this category is 56 per cent; the incidence of Waldenström's macroglobulinemia is 31 per cent; the incidence of lymphoma is 7 per cent; the incidence of chronic lymphocytic leukemia is 5 per cent; and the incidence of amyloid is 1 per cent. IgM myeloma constitutes less than 1 per cent of cases. In patients with Waldenström's macroglobulinemia, extensive bone marrow infiltration with lymphocytes, lymphocytoid plasma cells, and plasma cells is seen. Lymphomas are diagnosed in patients who, on lymph node biopsy, show a predominance of lymphoid features in the area of infiltration, destruction of architecture, extension of cellular infiltrate through the capsules, and predominance of one cell type with a minimal expression of lymphocytoid plasma cells and plasma cells. Chronic lymphocytic leukemia is usually characterized by bone marrow infiltration with small, round lymphocytes and a peripheral lymphocytosis. The diagnosis of IgM myeloma is reserved for patients who have lytic bone lesions that on biopsy are found to be exclusively composed of plasma cell infiltrates. Symptoms are similar to those seen in multiple myeloma except that the hyperviscosity syndrome including bleeding or visual disturbances occurs in 10 to 30 per cent of patients. Hepatosplenomegaly and lymphadenopathy occur in 30 and 40 per cent of patients, respectively. Hepatomegaly without splenomegaly is relatively uncommon.

MYCOSIS FUNGOIDES AND SEZARY SYNDROME

By Susan M. Zurowski, M.D.
Columbia, Missouri

Mycosis fungoides (MF) and Sézary syndrome (SS) are part of a group of malignant lymphoproliferative disorders known as the cutaneous T-cell lymphomas (CTCL). These diseases are the most common T-cell lymphomas that present in the skin. CTCL is used synonymously for MF and SS, although the latter are more specific terms.

MF and SS are clonal proliferations of mature helper T cells, although rarely suppressor T cells are reported. The disease is most common in middle-aged adults and is seen only rarely in children and adolescents. A history of chronic dermatitis for 10 years or more is usual; males are affected twice as often as females, and blacks more often than whites. The annual incidence in the United States is 4 per million, with an estimated prevalence of 40,000 to 50,000 cases nationwide. These statistics suggest a doubling of the disease over the last 10 years, and in some medical centers the incidence is now approximating that of Hodgkin's disease.

The clinical stages of MF have been recognized for more than a century. The majority of patients with classic MF move through three stages of skin disease: patch, plaque, and tumor. The disease can progress to involve peripheral and central lymph nodes. Visceral organ involvement occurs late, with advanced disease most commonly affecting the spleen, liver, and lungs. When the disease presents with total erythematous skin involvement, lymphadenopathy, and abnormal circulating T cells, it is known as Sézary syndrome.

PRESENTING SIGNS AND SYMPTOMS

The patch stage represents early skin involvement with variable numbers of scaly, erythematous, flat patches. These lesions usually begin on skin not exposed to the sun, such as that on the buttocks, thighs, and breasts. The plaque stage is characterized by more infiltrated, thicker, palpable lesions. Plaques may arise de novo or from existing patches. The disease takes its name from the ulcerated tumors or "fungoid" lesions that appear late. Lesions on the face may accentuate normal skin lines, this accentuation giving the patient a "leonine facies."

Patients presenting with classic SS actually have systemic disease from the onset. They have an exfoliative erythroderma, lymphadenopathy, and, frequently, leukemic manifestations. Severe pruritus is the most prevalent symptom of SS and can predate the visible skin eruption by several months. Fever generally develops in patients with underlying infection, rather than as a result of their lymphoma.

Other clinical variants of MF can occur. The "tumeur d'emlee" form begins suddenly as tumors without pre-existing patches and may be mistaken for deep fungal or mycobacterial infections. Some patients may present with disease located only on the palms or soles mimicking eczema or psoriasis. Hypopigmented MF, discoid lupus–like, and alopecialike MF have also been described.

Pagetoid reticulosis, or Woringer-Kolopp disease, is a rare localized form of MF that is usually limited to one or several lesions on an extremity. It seems to have a more benign course. Several chronic benign skin diseases may be precursors of MF. These disorders include large plaque parapsoriasis, poikiloderma atrophicans vasculare, and lymphomatoid papulosis. Mycosis fungoides and Hodgkin's lymphoma are seen together and sequentially in some patients. The exact relationship between these two lymphomas is unclear.

COURSE

The natural history of MF is highly variable among individuals. There have been reports of indolent disease present for more than 30 years, as well as aggressive fulminant disease with rapid demise of the patient in a few weeks. Treatment may reverse or delay progression by decreasing the numbers of abnormal T cells. Eventually, there may develop more malignant subpopulations of T cells that become less responsive to therapy. Mycosis fungoides can also undergo transformation into a large cell lymphoma, which can then have a much worse prognosis. The prognosis depends on the degree and extent of skin involvement, the presence or absence of lymphadenopathy, and the involvement of blood and visceral organs.

In the early patch stage, with disease confined to less than 10 per cent of the skin and no node involvement, the median survival is greater than 12 years. The median survival rate drops to 5 years in patients with plaque disease, erythroderma, and cutaneous tumors. Patients with visceral involvement have a median survival of only 2.5 years. Other factors that adversely affect prognosis include advancing age, black race, prior malignancy, and the presence of SS.

COMMON COMPLICATIONS

As MF progresses to the tumor or erythrodermic stage, bacterial, viral, and fungal infections can occur with increasing frequency. Pyodermas, cellulitis, and secondary infections of ulcerated tumors are most common. With the decline in the immune status, opportunistic infections can occur. The most probable causes of death are infections with sepsis from organisms such as *Staphylococcus* and *Pseudomonas*. Patients with MF are more likely to develop herpes varicella-zoster, which can be severe and disseminated. Herpes simplex infections may become generalized or chronic.

In SS, the patient has an exfoliative erythroderma that involves the whole body surface. As with all erythrodermas, the widespread disruption in the skin barrier leads to chills from poor temperature regulation as well as significant protein and water loss. High-output cardiac failure may ensue.

PHYSICAL EXAMINATION

Early skin involvement with MF begins as chronic recurrent dermatitis with erythematous, annular, scaly patches. The surface may look atrophic, a subtle but characteristic finding. Lesions may take on a more bizarre configuration, with arcuate, circinate, or serpiginous borders. Tumors have the appearance of "squashed tomatoes," and they may ulcerate and become malodorous. The clue to diagnosis is the chronicity of each lesion and slow progression, which is enough to request consultation.

In SS, the extensive involvement of the skin gives a shiny "varnishlike" appearance. Involvement of the palms and soles results in thick, hyperkeratotic, fissured skin associated with dystrophic nails. Lymphadenopathy can occur during any skin stage but is more common with advanced skin involvement. Hepatosplenomegaly is uncommon except in advanced MF or in SS. Other visceral involvement may be inapparent except at autopsy.

LABORATORY DIAGNOSIS

Biopsy is the most useful laboratory tool for making the diagnosis of MF. The process is challenging and fraught with pitfalls. Lesion selection is important, and several biopsies may be required for diagnosis. If patients have been using topical corticosteroids, it is best to discontinue their use 2 weeks prior to biopsy, as these medications may mask the epidermal nature of the infiltrate. Even so, early disease may be difficult to diagnose, and several biopsies may be necessary. Expert advice is usually required.

The histologic examination of early MF reveals atypical

cerebriform, or convoluted, lymphocytes within the epidermis or involving the papillary dermis. Pautrier's microabscesses, which are collections of atypical cells within the epidermis with little intercellular edema, are pathognomonic for MF. As the disease progresses to thicker plaques and nodules, the histology reveals involvement of the deeper dermis, with loss of the epidermal component. The histologic diagnosis is more apparent with diseases at the plaque and tumor stages, since there is generally a dense infiltrate of atypical lymphocytes.

Studies with electron microscopy (EM), DNA flow cytometry, and immunophenotyping can be helpful diagnostic tools. Electron microscopy can assess the nuclear contour of the lymphocytes and give a quantitative measure with the high values typical of this disease. DNA flow cytometry is used to distinguish benign atypical lymphocytes from malignant ones. Immunophenotyping characterizes the cell surface markers, which in the case of MF or SS are CD4+ helper T cells. Characteristic deficiency of cell markers such as CD7 in the cutaneous infiltrate or lymph node may support the diagnosis of MF.

Immunogenotyping is a very sensitive study and allows determination of T-cell receptor gene rearrangements in skin, blood, and lymph nodes. It is more sensitive than light microscopy; however, in early disease false-negative results can occur.

All routine blood, chemistry, and urine examinations are normal in early disease. A complete blood count and Sézary prep are useful baseline studies. The Sézary cell prep of the peripheral blood identifies atypical lymphocytes that have a characteristic cerebriform nucleus. Counts greater than 15 per cent are typical of leukemic involvement.

When there is palpable adenopathy, a lymph node biopsy is useful for staging the lymphoma. Histopathologic classification of the extent of lymph node involvement has prognostic value. The most frequent abnormal finding is dermatopathic lymphadenopathy (DL), which is present in early disease and reveals small numbers of atypical lymphocytes with paracortical expansion. As the disease progresses, the most common extracutaneous site of involvement is the lymph node, and once effacement of the node architecture occurs, median survival drops from 90 months with DL to 30 months with total node effacement.

RADIOLOGIC EVALUATION

A chest radiograph and computed tomography or magnetic resonance imaging are useful for determining central node enlargement, especially in patients with more advanced cutaneous disease and peripheral adenopathy. Lymphography contributes little. Bone scans, liver-spleen scans, and gallium scans are not particularly useful.

ERRORS AND PITFALLS IN DIAGNOSIS

Because MF is difficult to diagnose in the early skin stages, one must have a high index of suspicion in chronic dermatitides that resemble MF. Long-term follow-up and repeat biopsy by a skilled observer is necessary. Response to topical therapies such as emollients, steroids, or ultraviolet A or B light should not entirely influence the decision of whether a dermatitis is benign or malignant. The key is the biopsy of untreated plaques early in the disease.

Benign conditions such as chronic allergic contact dermatitis, tinea corporis, and drug eruptions can be mistaken for MF. Patch testing for contact allergens and potassium hydroxide preparation for identifying dermatophytes are essential for excluding benign conditions that mimic MF. If the tests are negative, then multiple biopsies and the use of more sensitive technology with cell surface markers and T-cell receptor gene rearrangements may be necessary in difficult cases. MF is a chronic lymphoma with a small potential for cure, but diagnosis and early therapeutic intervention may induce a clinical remission and prevent disease progression.

DISEASES OF THE SPLEEN

By Nadine M. Tung, M.D.,
and Stephen H. Robinson, M.D.
Boston, Massachusetts

The spleen has several functions. First, as the largest lymphoid organ in the body, it plays an important role in antibody production. Second, it acts as a filter that sequesters and removes microorganisms and immature blood cells from the circulation and "pits" material such as iron granules and nuclear debris from early red blood cells recently released from the bone marrow. Third, the spleen is a source of hematopoiesis during embryogenesis, and in pathologic conditions such as agnogenic myeloid metaplasia with myelofibrosis, this organ can be reactivated as a site of extramedullary hematopoiesis.

Most disorders affecting the spleen are manifested by splenic enlargement, and this article primarily addresses the diagnostic approach to splenomegaly. A few conditions can be associated with splenic hypofunction, and these are discussed briefly. A normal spleen is usually not palpable on physical examination. However, it may be palpable in normal young children and in some healthy young adults. In the latter, the splenomegaly may be due to recent inapparent viral infection (e.g., infectious mononucleosis). The normal spleen is less than 12 cm in length and 7 cm in width, with a total volume of less than 250 cm^3. Minimal splenomegaly, with a spleen size exceeding these limits, is sometimes not detectable by physical examination but can be discerned with imaging techniques. Thus, if a finding of splenomegaly would help contribute to a diagnosis and the spleen is not palpable on physical examination, an imaging study should be done. An abdominal ultrasound study is the least expensive and easiest procedure, although a computed tomography (CT) scan or liver-spleen scan can sometimes yield additional information regarding lymphadenopathy or portal hypertension, respectively.

The disorders that are often associated with splenomegaly are listed in Table 1. A general approach to the workup of the patient with splenomegaly is offered in this article, with reference to specific diseases when appropriate. The details of these diseases are to be found in other articles.

GENERAL APPROACH

The evaluation of the patient with splenomegaly should begin with a careful history, physical examination, complete blood count including reticulocyte count, and liver function tests. A history of fever and systemic symptoms

Table 1. Causes of Splenomegaly

I. Diseases That Cause Portal Hypertension
  A. Prehepatic
    1. Portal vein or splenic vein thrombosis
  B. Hepatic
    1. Cirrhosis—alcoholic or viral in origin
    2. Schistosomiasis
    3. Infiltrative diseases (rarely)*
  C. Posthepatic
    1. Hepatic vein occlusion (Budd-Chiari syndrome)
    2. Constrictive pericarditis or chronic right-sided failure
II. Infiltrative Disorders
  A. Malignant
    1. Acute and chronic leukemia
    2. Lymphoma
    3. Myeloproliferative disorders
    4. Metastatic solid tumors (rarely)*
  B. Benign
    1. Storage diseases (Gaucher's and Niemann-Pick diseases)
    2. Amyloidosis (rarely)*
III. Work Hypertrophy
  A. Hemolytic anemia
IV. Infectious Diseases
  A. Infectious mononucleosis (Epstein-Barr virus, cytomegalovirus)
  B. Disseminated fungal diseases
  C. Leishmaniasis
  D. Trypanosomiasis
  E. Splenic abscess
  F. Subacute bacterial endocarditis
  G. Malaria
  H. Viral hepatitis
  I. Typhoid fever
  J. Miliary tuberculosis
V. Inflammatory Diseases
  A. Rheumatoid arthritis or Felty's syndrome
  B. Systemic lupus erythematosus
  C. Serum sickness
  D. Sarcoidosis
VI. Other Causes
  A. Splenic cysts
  B. Splenic hemorrhage

*Rare causes of splenomegaly.

suggests infection, malignancy, or an inflammatory disorder. Moderate to marked anemia with reticulocytosis often indicates that splenomegaly is related to hemolysis. A high leukocyte count or abnormal leukocytes in the peripheral smear suggests leukemia or lymphoma, whereas the presence of many atypical lymphocytes suggests a viral disease, such as infectious mononucleosis. An enlarged liver or abnormal liver function test results suggest splenomegaly associated with portal hypertension and liver disease.

HEMATOLOGIC ASSESSMENT

A hematocrit, leukocyte count, differential count, platelet count, and reticulocyte count should be obtained in all patients with splenomegaly. Many patients with enlarged spleens, of whatever cause, demonstrate "hypersplenism," with a decrease in the white blood cell, red blood cell, and platelet counts, although sometimes only one or two of these counts are reduced, due to increased sequestration and/or destruction of these cells in the enlarged spleen. The degree of depression of the cell counts is mild to moderate and is typically accompanied by a mild reticulocytosis.

The leukocyte count is increased, often markedly, in patients with chronic lymphocytic or chronic myelogenous leukemia. In the former disorder, the differential count shows many mature lymphocytes; in the latter, many neutrophils and some immature granulocytic forms are seen. An uncommon, usually aggressive disease, prolymphocytic leukemia can evolve from chronic lymphocytic leukemia or can present de novo. This disorder is typically found in older patients, who often have marked splenomegaly but no lymphadenopathy. The clinician can make the diagnosis by observing typical prolymphocytes in the peripheral smear and by confirming their presence with flow cytometry. The leukocyte count may be high, normal, or low in patients with acute leukemia; however, in almost all of these patients, characteristic blast cells can be found in the peripheral blood. Rarely, a bone marrow examination is required to discern the leukemic blasts. Hairy cell leukemia is an unusual disorder in which the white cell count, hematocrit, and platelet count all are typically low. The peripheral smear usually contains variable numbers of characteristic "hairy" lymphocytes. A bone marrow examination is usually required to confirm the diagnosis. Patients with non-Hodgkin's lymphoma may have circulating lymphoma cells that provide a clue to the underlying diagnosis; a definitive diagnosis requires biopsy of a lymph node or the bone marrow. The presence of many atypical lymphocytes suggests a diagnosis of infectious mononucleosis, viral hepatitis, or cytomegalovirus infection.

Invasion of the bone marrow by metastatic cancer, granulomatous disease, or fibrosis often causes a so-called leukoerythroblastic reaction, with the peripheral smear revealing immature white blood cells, nucleated and teardrop-shaped red blood cells, and megakaryocyte fragments or giant platelets. When such a leukoerythroblastic or myelophthisic smear is seen in a patient with splenomegaly, the most likely diagnosis is agnogenic myeloid metaplasia with myelofibrosis, otherwise called idiopathic myelofibrosis. This disorder is one of the four classic myeloproliferative disorders. (The others are polycythemia vera, essential thrombocythemia, and chronic myelogenous leukemia.) Although splenomegaly is common in all of these diseases, it occurs least often in essential thrombocythemia. The peripheral blood in patients with polycythemia vera characteristically reveals increased numbers of red blood cells, leukocytes, and platelets. In essential thrombocythemia there is a moderate to marked increase in the platelet count, often accompanied by abnormalities in platelet morphology.

Patients with significant anemia and increased reticulocyte counts may have splenomegaly due to hemolysis. Some patients with ongoing hemolysis have splenomegaly but are not anemic. In the latter group, erythroid hyperplasia of the bone marrow is sufficient to compensate for the decreased life span of red cells. Such patients are said to have "compensated hemolysis." Evidence of hemolysis includes increased serum unconjugated bilirubin and lactate dehydrogenase (LD), decreased serum haptoglobin concentration, and increased reticulocyte counts. The peripheral smear typically contains abnormal red blood cells with morphology that may implicate a specific type of hemolytic anemia. However, red cell morphology may be virtually normal in some forms of hemolytic anemia, e.g., paroxysmal nocturnal hemoglobinuria. Patients with hereditary spherocytosis show many spherocytes, some quite small ("microspherocytes"), in the peripheral blood; the presence of spherocytes can be confirmed by demonstrating increased osmotic fragility of the red blood cells. The diagnosis of hereditary elliptocytosis requires a preponderance of elliptical or oval cells in the blood smear. Most patients with this disorder have little or no hemolysis; a minority have splenomegaly and a clinical picture similar to that of hereditary spherocytosis. Patients with hemoglobinopathies, such as hemoglobin CC disease, SC disease, and S-thalassemia, may have splenomegaly. In most patients with homozygous SS disease (sickle cell anemia) and in some patients with S-thalassemia or severe SC disease, the spleen atrophies because of repeated episodes of infarction during the first few years of life. The hemoglobin C disorders are associated with the presence of numerous target cells in the peripheral smear, while the sickle hemoglobin syndromes are associated with sickle cells. The latter may be difficult to find in patients with SC disease, in whom "boat-shaped" red blood cells are more common.

The hereditary disorders associated with splenomegaly include the hemolytic anemias described above and the thalassemias, which are more accurately viewed as defects in hemoglobin synthesis than as true hemolytic anemias. Splenomegaly may also be associated with acquired forms of hemolytic anemia, especially autoimmune hemolytic anemia, in which IgG and/or the third component of complement are found on the red cell membrane. The peripheral smear usually reveals many spherocytes, and the Coombs' test is positive. By contrast, in an analogous disorder of platelets known as idiopathic or immune thrombocytopenic purpura (ITP), the spleen is characteristically not enlarged. Thus, the patient with severe thrombocytopenia and splenomegaly should be evaluated for lymphoma, infectious mononucleosis, or other disorders that may lead to both of these abnormalities.

EXAMINATION OF THE BONE MARROW

In the patient with splenomegaly who has one or more of the peripheral blood changes mentioned above, bone marrow biopsy and aspiration are often required for the definitive diagnosis of acute or chronic leukemia, myeloproliferative disorders, granulomas, or metastatic cancer.

Granulomas containing characteristic mycobacterial or fungal organisms are observed in a bone marrow biopsy. Identification of the specific organism requires appropriate cultures of the marrow specimen. In the era of human immunodeficiency virus (HIV) infection, patients with opportunistic infection may present with pancytopenia as well as splenomegaly. A bone marrow examination may be helpful in such patients.

In some patients, the cause of splenomegaly may not be clear following initial assessment of the peripheral blood and liver function. In these patients, a bone marrow biopsy should be performed because the bone marrow, like the spleen, is part of the reticuloendothelial system and may demonstrate lymphoma, granulomatous disease, or other disorders characterized clinically by splenomegaly. Primary splenic lymphoma refers to a heterogeneous group of lymphomas initially confined to the spleen; on occasion, microscopic involvement of the bone marrow may provide a clue to the diagnosis.

ASSESSMENT OF LIVER DISEASE OR PORTAL HYPERTENSION

The splenic veins drain through the portal vein; as a result, splenomegaly is often a complication of portal hypertension. The most common cause of portal hypertension is liver cirrhosis; other causes are listed in Table 1. The work-up includes evaluation of liver function tests and, if appropriate, liver biopsy. The liver-spleen scan is sometimes a useful test for portal hypertension. The diagnosis of thrombosis of the portal, splenic, or hepatic vein can be confirmed with a magnetic resonance imaging-angiogram or Doppler study.

IMAGING STUDIES

Imaging techniques may be useful in evaluating the patient with splenomegaly. If a lymphoma is suspected, a CT scan of the torso (chest, abdomen, and pelvis) may reveal internal lymph node enlargement in the absence of peripheral lymphadenopathy on physical examination. Computed tomography–guided biopsy may then establish the diagnosis. Abdominal CT scan may demonstrate pancreatitis or pancreatic malignancy associated with splenic vein thrombosis and splenomegaly. A CT scan may also reveal focal abnormalities in an enlarged spleen consistent with lymphoma, simple splenic cysts, or subcapsular hemorrhage.

ROLE OF SPLENECTOMY

In some patients, careful diagnostic evaluation fails to reveal a cause of the splenomegaly. At this point, clinical judgment may dictate removal of the enlarged spleen to facilitate a histologic diagnosis. Some patients may have an indolent primary splenic lymphoma that does not require treatment for many years. Thus, the clinician may simply follow the patient with periodic CT scans, looking for further spleen and lymph node enlargement. By contrast, if the patient is ill or the blood counts are significantly decreased, the spleen should be removed and the abdomen explored to arrive at a diagnosis and institute proper therapy.

Decreased splenic function, or hyposplenism, may be due to several causes. Changes in the peripheral blood that are commonly seen in such patients with hyposplenism include the following: a mild increase in the platelet count and occasionally in the leukocyte count; an increase in the mean corpuscular volume (MCV) of the red blood cells; target cells, acanthocytes, nucleated red blood cells, immature white blood cells, and large platelets in the peripheral blood smear; and the presence in red blood cells of debris produced during red blood cell maturation, including Howell-Jolly bodies (nuclear remnants) and Pappenheimer bodies (iron inclusions). Hyposplenic conditions include the postsplenectomy state, autosplenectomy in patients with severe sickle cell syndromes, and functional hyposplenism in a patient with an anatomically intact spleen. The last has been reported to occur during the neonatal period and in rheumatic disorders, amyloidosis, inflammatory bowel disorders, and sarcoidosis.

BENIGN AND MALIGNANT HISTIOCYTIC AND DENDRITIC CELL DISORDERS

By Bruce A. Woda, M.D.,
and John L. Sullivan, M.D.
Worcester, Massachusetts

The benign and malignant histiocytic and dendritic cell disorders represent a group of diseases characterized by a localized or systemic proliferation of cells of the dendritic cell lineage or derived from the mononuclear phagocyte. The differential diagnosis of the systemic forms of these diseases can be difficult owing to appreciable overlap of clinical and pathologic features.

INFECTION-ASSOCIATED HEMOPHAGOCYTIC SYNDROME

The synonyms for this disorder include virus-associated hemophagocytic syndrome and histiocytic medullary reticulosis.

Clinical Features

The term virus-associated hemophagocytic syndrome (VAHS) originally described a disorder characterized by viral infection, a benign systemic proliferation of histiocytes, and marked hemophagocytosis. However, various nonviral microbial agents have also been linked to the induction of hemophagocytosis. Hence, the use of the term infection-associated hemophagocytic syndrome (IAHS) has increased (Table 1).

Patients with this disorder present with fever, myalgias, and malaise. Physical examination typically reveals hepatosplenomegaly and generalized lymphadenopathy. Pancytopenia, abnormal liver function tests, and an unexpectedly severe coagulopathy are commonly reported. IAHS has been most frequently observed in patients with underlying immunosuppression, especially allograft recipients, patients with leukemia, and individuals treated with corticosteroids for connective tissue disorders.

The X-linked lymphoproliferative syndrome (XLP) is a form of VAHS linked to the Epstein-Barr virus (EBV). Nearly 75 per cent of males with XLP die with a systemic proliferation of histiocytes. In addition, non-Hodgkin's lymphoma and infiltrations of B and T immunoblasts are seen in at least 25 to 30 per cent of patients with XLP.

Table 1. Infection-Associated Hemophagocytic Syndrome

Viral
Epstein-Barr virus (EBV)
Cytomegalovirus (CMV)
Herpes simplex virus (HSV)
Varicella-zoster virus (VZV)
Adenovirus
Parvovirus B19
Bacterial
Enteric gram-negative rods
Haemophilus influenzae
Streptococcus pneumoniae
Staphylococcus aureus
Brucella abortus
Babesia microti
Mycoplasma pneumoniae
Fungal
Histoplasma capsulatum
Candida albicans
Cryptococcus neoformans
Mycobacterial
Mycobacterium tuberculosis
Rickettsial
Coxiella burnetii
Parasitic
Leishmania donovani

Modified from Sullivan, J.L., and Woda, B.A.: Lymphohistiocytic disorders. *In* Nathan, D.G., and Oski, F.A. (eds): Hematology of Infancy and Childhood, 4th ed. Philadelphia, W.B. Saunders, 1993, p. 1362, with permission.

Pathologic Features

In VAHS, the sinusoids of the lymph nodes, liver, and spleen are infiltrated by benign-appearing histiocytes that may exhibit erythrophagocytosis. The pathologic features of VAHS evolve during the course of the disease. Initially, the bone marrow may be hypercellular with few infiltrating histiocytes. Erythrophagocytosis may be difficult to recognize in the biopsy, but careful examination of an aspirate smear typically demonstrates this phenomenon. Later in the disease, the bone marrow shows markedly decreased hematopoiesis and substantial infiltration by histiocytes. Early in the disease, lymph nodes show few histiocytes but may exhibit an intense proliferation of immunoblasts with partial effacement of nodal architecture. As the disease evolves, lymphoid depletion supervenes, and a massive sinusoidal infiltration by benign, erythrophagocytic histiocytes may ensue. Liver biopsy reveals substantial portal infiltrates of lymphocytes, immunoblasts, and histiocytes, with erythrophagocytosis typically seen in hepatic sinusoids.

Few studies of the immune system of patients during VAHS have been reported. As noted above, VAHS is most often associated with EBV infection. Compared with patients who recover spontaneously after acute EBV infection, patients with VAHS have fewer circulating atypical lymphocytes and activated CD8 cells. Thus, immunodeficiency or immunosuppression may play a role in the pathogenesis of VAHS. Immunoregulatory disturbances may also lead to cytokine release by activated T cells that elicits the proliferation and activation of histiocytes.

FAMILIAL ERYTHROPHAGOCYTIC LYMPHOHISTIOCYTOSIS

The synonyms for this disorder include familial erythrophagocytic lymphohistiocytosis, familial hemophagocytic reticulosis, generalized lymphohistiocytosis of infancy, and familial lymphohistiocytic syndrome.

Clinical Features

In 1963, MacMahon and colleagues* described a narrow but distinct category of uncommon familial diseases of infancy and childhood that they termed familial erythrophagocytic lymphohistiocytosis (FEL). Typically developing in infancy, this syndrome is characterized by fever, failure to thrive, hepatosplenomegaly, and anemia. Distinguishing FEL from systemic malignant histiocytosis or IAHS can be difficult. Patients with FEL may have lymphoid, pulmonary, central nervous system, pericardial, bone, soft tissue, and gastrointestinal involvement. Circulating atypical or bizarre-appearing mononuclear cells are frequently observed. Leukopenia and coagulation disturbances may be present. Laboratory abnormalities include hypercholesterolemia, hypertriglyceridemia, and increased serum transaminases.

The onset of illness in patients with FEL may be abrupt or insidious. The duration of disease is extremely variable;

*MacMahon, H. E., Bedizel, M., et al.: Familial erythrophagocytic lymphohistiocytosis. *Pediatrics,* 32:868, 1963.

survival for months to years has been reported. The distinguishing features of FEL are the early age at onset, with most patients presenting during the first 3 months of life, and the familial pattern of disease, indicating an autosomal recessive mode of inheritance.

Pathologic Features

The most consistent histopathologic abnormality is the widespread proliferation of histiocytes. Virtually all reticuloendothelial organs are infiltrated, and central nervous system involvement is frequently noted. Histiocytic infiltration is often accompanied by profound lymphoid depletion of lymph nodes, thymus, spleen, and bone marrow.

The cellular immune defects include depressed lymphocyte proliferation, mitogenic and antigenic anergy, and loss of delayed cutaneous hypersensitivity. Plasma from patients with FEL tends to inhibit the antigen-induced proliferation of normal lymphocytes in vitro. Exchange transfusion may reduce the concentration of this inhibitory factor. Cell-mediated cytotoxicity, including monocyte and natural killer (NK) cell activity, is severely depressed in the majority of patients with FEL.

Extensive studies of hemophagocytic syndromes have increasingly revealed similarities between FEL and IAHS. Because immune dysfunction and viral infection have been demonstrated in infants who meet the criteria for the diagnosis of FEL, it is possible that FEL represents a primary immunodeficiency that predisposes to IAHS.

Differential Diagnosis

The definitive diagnosis of FEL and XLP requires a well-documented family history of such disorders. In the absence of a clear family history, the overlapping clinical and pathologic features of VAHS, FEL, and XLP make precise diagnosis difficult. The degree of histiocytic proliferation varies and, by itself, cannot be used to distinguish VAHS, FEL, and XLP. However, the histiocytic proliferation in XLP typically is not as intense as that seen in the most florid cases of FEL and VAHS. By contrast, necrosis of the splenic white pulp and lymph node follicles, although seen most often in XLP and VAHS, may also be seen in FEL. Thymic atrophy is found in all three of these diseases, while severe progressive hepatitis is commonly seen in patients with XLP. Immunologic studies may be helpful in distinguishing FEL, XLP, and VAHS. In FEL, generalized defects in mitogen responses and deficiencies in NK and monocyte-killing activities are usually present. In XLP, NK cell activity is normal or increased, and substantial alloreactive killer cell activity is present. Immunologic studies show normal natural killing in EBV-induced VAHS, whereas alloreactive killing is decreased.

SINUS HISTIOCYTOSIS WITH MASSIVE LYMPHADENOPATHY

The synonyms for this disorder include Rosai-Dorfman disease.

Clinical Features

Described by Rosai and Dorfman, this syndrome is characterized by fever, leukocytosis, increased erythrocyte sedimentation rate, hyperglobulinemia, and chronic benign massive enlargement of cervical lymph nodes. Sinus histiocytosis with massive lymphadenopathy (SHML) is most commonly seen during the first decade of life. More than 90 per cent of patients present with cervical lymph node enlargement, which is usually bilateral and painless. Rarely is a single node involved. Extranodal sites, including the skin, sinonasal region, soft tissues, orbit, bone, salivary glands, and central nervous system, are infiltrated by histiocytes in approximately 40 per cent of cases.

Low-grade fever (less than 38°C) is frequently present. The patient may have mild normochromic, normocytic or hypochromic, microcytic anemia. The peripheral leukocyte count is normal, but a reversed CD4:CD8 ratio may be seen. The erythrocyte sedimentation rate is typically greater than 50 mm per hour. Many patients with SHML develop polyclonal hyperglobulinemia; some have hemolytic anemia associated with red blood cell antibodies.

Pathologic Features

Lymph nodes removed from patients with SHML are markedly enlarged. Capsular fibrosis may be seen. The sinuses are distended by characteristic histiocytes with bland nuclei and abundant pink cytoplasm. Many of these cells exhibit emperipolesis, or the presence of small lymphocytes within their cytoplasm. Increased numbers of plasma cells may also be seen within the sinuses and within the lymph node medulla. The histiocytes present in SHML have unique phenotypic features. These cells express the macrophage-associated proteins CD68, lysozyme, alpha$_1$-antitrypsin, and alpha$_1$-antichymotrypsin. CD30, a member of the tumor necrosis factor receptor family that is expressed on immunoblasts, is seen in some of these patients. SHML histiocytes express the dendritic cell–associated marker S-100 but do not express the dendritic cell antigen CD1. An etiologic agent has not been identified in SHML. Increased titers of antibodies to EBV and measles virus have been repeatedly observed, but evidence to incriminate these viruses as etiologic agents is lacking.

Differential Diagnosis

The differential diagnosis of SHML includes other disorders that affect lymph node sinuses. The histologic and immunophenotypic features of SHML are typically so distinct, however, that reaching the correct diagnosis is not difficult. For example, the histiocytes in SHML exhibit emperipolesis and express S-100. These features are not usually observed in other sinusoidal disorders, such as metastatic tumors, sinusoidal lymphomas, malignant histiocytosis, and benign localized sinus histiocytosis.

LANGERHANS' CELL HISTIOCYTOSIS

The synonyms for this disorder include histiocytosis X, HX, eosinophilic granuloma, Hand-Schüller-Christian disease, and Letterer-Siwe disease.

Clinical Features

Langerhans' cell histiocytosis (LCH) represents a disorder that may be present as a single lesion or as a multifocal, multisystem disease. Although LCH is primarily a pediatric disorder, single lesions may also present in adults. Single lesions, often called eosinophilic granulomas, have a predilection for lung, lymph node, and bone, especially skull, femur, and rib. Multifocal disease (Hand-Schüller-Christian disease) is usually seen in young children, whereas systemic disease (Letterer-Siwe disease) is seen in infants and young children. The prognosis varies with the amount of disease present and the number of organs involved. In general, organ dysfunction is associated with poor outcome.

In children, LCH can present in newborns as well as in adolescents as old as 15 years of age. The median age at onset is 2 to 3 years. At the time of diagnosis, approximately 80 per cent of patients have lytic bone lesions; 50 to 60 per cent have adenopathy, skin lesions, or hepatomegaly; 30 to 40 per cent have otitis and fever; and about 20 per cent have diabetes insipidus or pulmonary involvement.

The typical skin lesions are vesicular, pustular, and hemorrhagic and are seen on the scalp, axillae, postauricular areas, hands, and feet. Head and neck manifestations are common and include external otitis, destructive mandibular lesions, and gum involvement leading to pain, swelling, and loss of teeth. Multifocal LCH typically involves the lung. By contrast, isolated lung involvement is occasionally observed in adults but is usually not seen in childhood. Chest films in patients with LCH may reveal reticular or micronodular opacities, large nodules, and honeycombing, while clinical manifestations include tachypnea, dyspnea, cough, cyanosis, pneumothorax, alveolar or interstitial infiltrates, and/or pleural effusion.

Hepatomegaly and liver dysfunction are also observed in LCH. Objective evidence of liver disease includes edema, ascites, hypoproteinemia (less than 5.5 g/dL total protein, and/or less than 2.5 g/dL albumin), and/or hyperbilirubinemia (greater than 1.5 mg/dL total and not attributed to hemolysis). Evidence of marrow dysfunction in disseminated LCH includes hemoglobin less than 10 g/dL, neutrophil count of fewer than 1500 cells/mm^3, white blood cell count of fewer than 4000 cells/mm^3, or platelet count of fewer than 100,000 cells/mm^3. Twenty to fifty per cent of patients with multifocal LCH have diabetes insipidus. Skull films may be abnormal, and light microscopic evaluation of tissue may reveal parapituitary infiltration by LCH.

Pathologic Features

In LCH, one or more organs are infiltrated by large mononuclear cells. The nuclei of these cells are bland and folded and often contain a central groove. The chromatin is usually finely dispersed, small nucleoli may be present, and some cells display pleomorphism and hyperchromatism. The typical cells of LCH are accompanied by various numbers of histiocytes, lymphocytes, eosinophils, and neutrophils. The number of eosinophils tends to increase as the lesions age, and increased numbers of eosinophils are associated with the presence of necrosis. Occasionally, giant cells may be seen. Late lesions may undergo xanthomatous and fibrotic changes.

In lymph nodes, the infiltrates of LCH are typically sinusoidal, and partial or total effacement of the lymph node architecture may be seen. Histologic evidence of LCH should be confirmed with ultrastructural, enzymatic, or, more often, immunophenotypic studies of Langerhans' cells. Electron microscopy can demonstrate the Birbeck granule, a pentalaminar organelle whose function remains obscure. Enzymatic studies may reveal nonspecific esterase, acid phosphatase, and adenosine triphosphatase activity characteristic of dendritic cells.

The typical mononuclear cells of LCH can also be characterized by immunoperoxidase studies of frozen or paraffin sections. Langerhans' cells and the cells of LCH express class I and class II histocompatibility proteins, CD1, CD4, CD14, S100, CD74, and vimentin. The cells of LCH also may express CD25, interferon-γ (IFN-γ), CD11b (CR3), CD35 (CR1), and CD21 (CR2) receptors. By contrast, LCH cells do not express macrophage-associated lysozyme or alpha$_1$-antitrypsin. Although the pathogenesis of LCH is not well understood, recent application of X-linked polymorphic DNA probes suggests that most patients with LCH have a clonal neoplastic disease.

Differential Diagnosis

The pathologic features of LCH occasionally overlap those of metastatic carcinoma, sinusoidal lymphoma, SHML, sinus histiocytosis, or dermatopathic lymphadenitis. In most patients, the presence of eosinophils and the characteristic mononuclear cells facilitates the diagnosis of LCH. However, when specimens are poorly fixed or exhibit extensive necrosis, the characteristic cytologic features may be obscured, and diagnoses such as reactive granuloma and Hodgkin's disease may be considered. Establishing the diagnosis of LCH in these patients usually entails the identification of Birbeck granules or documentation of the expression of S-100 or CD1 protein.

MALIGNANT HISTIOCYTOSIS

The synonyms for this disorder include histiocytic medullary reticulosis.

Clinical Features

Malignant disorders of mononuclear phagocytes represent uncommon forms of lymphoma. In 1966, Henry Rappaport introduced the term malignant histiocytosis to describe a systemic disease characterized by the malignant proliferation of cytologically atypical histiocytes within lymphoid organs. Although these disorders are seen predominantly in adults, they occur in all age groups. Localized forms are usually classified as true histiocytic lymphoma (THL), whereas systemic forms that infiltrate the reticuloendothelial system are classified as malignant histiocytosis (MH).

Both THL and MH can involve the skin. Bluish-red tumor masses are seen in THL, while disseminated papulonodular lesions are found in patients with MH. The clinical features of MH in the blood-borne phase overlap those of acute monoblastic leukemia.

Pathologic Features

Historically, the diagnosis of MH was considered when lymph node sinusoids were infiltrated by large tumor cells with abundant cytoplasm. Recent phenotypic, genotypic, and virologic studies of these disorders indicate that most are T-cell or null-cell malignancies that often express CD30. These tumors are often referred to as Ki-1 lymphoma or anaplastic large cell lymphoma. Benign disorders with these morphologic features usually fall into the category of IAHS; therefore, MH is a rare disorder.

To establish the rare diagnosis of MH, sinusoids of the spleen, liver, and lymph nodes should contain noncohesive clusters of large tumor cells with abundant cytoplasm and lobulated nuclei. In cytologic preparations, many of the cells should exhibit cytoplasmic vacuoles.

The malignant histiocytes exhibit cytologic atypia that can vary from minimally atypical cells to anaplastic forms that resemble pleomorphic large cell lymphomas. When the cells are well differentiated, some of them may contain ingested erythrocytes or leukocytes. The anaplastic cells, by contrast, do not often reveal phagocytosis. In the description of MH by Rappaport, phagocytosis was an essential criterion in establishing the diagnosis. In the 1990s, however, the diagnosis of MH does not require the identification of phagocytosis when the tumor cells have the appropriate phenotypic features.

A definitive diagnosis of MH requires documentation of the lineage of the tumor cells. MH cells do not exhibit the phenotypic characteristics of B or T lymphocytes, and clonal rearrangement of the immunoglobulin or T-cell receptor is not detected. On the other hand, the tumor cells often possess nonspecific esterase activity, and variable expression of monocyte-associated proteins, such as CD4, CD11, CD13, CD14, CD33, and CD68, has been reported.

Differential Diagnosis

The disease that may pose the greatest challenge in the differential diagnosis of MH is VAHS. The clinical features of VAHS (i.e., fever, cytopenias, lymphadenopathy, hepatosplenomegaly, liver dysfunction, and coagulopathy) are similar to those of MH. VAHS is more common than MH, and many previously reported cases of MH were actually VAHS. The distinction between MH and VAHS is important because VAHS is an acute, life-threatening, but potentially reversible disease and chemotherapy may be contraindicated in VAHS.

The clinician who must distinguish VAHS from MH should remember that VAHS is associated with documented viral infection, severe cytopenias, and a coagulopathy. Skin lesions have not been reported in VAHS. The lymph node sinusoidal infiltrate in VAHS is morphologically distinct from the destructive, cytologically malignant infiltrate seen in MH. Total effacement of lymph node architecture is usually not seen in VAHS.

In patients who present with the VAHS or MH syndrome, an aggressive work-up includes bone marrow biopsy, lymph node biopsy, and, possibly, liver biopsy and splenectomy. Tissues are processed for virologic and cytogenetic studies. The distinction between MH and pleomorphic T-cell lymphomas associated with phagocytic histiocytes or systemic hemophagocytosis requires histochemical, immunophenotypic, and genotypic studies. Malignant histiocytosis must also be distinguished from reactive disorders such as SHML. The histiocytes in SHML are cytologically benign and show prominent leukophagocytosis, and most patients with SHML manifest limited distribution of disease. Finally, MH can be distinguished from LCH by its cytologic atypia and lack of cells with dendritic features.

HEMOPHILIA AND OTHER INHERITED HEMOSTATIC DISORDERS

By Evan Vosburgh, M.D.
Boston, Massachusetts

Clinical bleeding disorders can be divided broadly into defects of primary hemostasis and disorders of coagulation and fibrinolysis (secondary hemostasis). Disorders of primary hemostasis involve the early events in clot formation, are associated with mild to moderate mucocutaneous bleeding following trauma or surgery, and are often associated with a prolonged bleeding time. Disorders of coagulation and fibrinolysis involve later events in clot formation; are associated with more serious bleeding, including deep tissue hemorrhage; and are often associated with prolongation of the partial thromboplastin time (PTT), prothrombin time (PT), and/or the thrombin time (TT).

It is only by chance that the two most common congenital bleeding disorders (von Willebrand's disease [vWD] and hemophilia A) which serve as paradigms of these two broad categories of bleeding, involve components of the same plasma protein complex–the factor VIII complex.

The factor VIII complex is composed of two distinct glycoproteins; the von Willebrand factor (vWF) and the factor VIII coagulant (antihemophilia protein, F-VIII). The two proteins are encoded on separate genes, inherited by different mechanisms, synthesized in separate sites, and become associated only after they have been secreted into the circulation. Table 1 provides an annotated list of the International Committee on Thrombosis and Haemostasis, which attempts to demystify the terminology for the structural and functional components of the factor VIII complex.

For decades, vWD and hemophilia were thought to represent different ends of a spectrum of a single inherited deficiency, and vWD was earlier referred to as "pseudohemophilia" or "vascular hemophilia." However, detailed study of the biology of the distinct proteins within the factor VIII complex has permitted a clear separation of the clinical and laboratory features of these bleeding disorders.

VON WILLEBRAND'S DISEASE

In 1926, Eric von Willebrand reported the first patient with vWD—a girl who died of hemorrhage during her fourth menstrual cycle. von Willebrand described a "platelet defect," which was shown in later experiments to be corrected by normal plasma and, years later, to be corrected by a specific plasma fraction enriched in the factor VIII complex. Critical experiments demonstrated the correction of the "platelet defect" in vWD patients by a similar plasma fraction obtained from patients with classic hemophilia, demonstrating that these two syndromes were caused by defects in different plasma factors. In the 1970s, the two main components of the factor VIII complex were characterized as separate proteins, leading to an explosion in the investigation of the genetics, biosynthesis, structure, and function of these molecules.

vWF is a high molecular weight glycoprotein synthesized by endothelial cells and megakaryocytes. The biosynthesis of vWF involves transformation of pro-vWF monomers, which rapidly form dimers via disulfide bonds. The pro-vWF dimers are linked head-to-tail via additional disulfide bonds to form a series of *multimers* with a wide range of molecular weights.

The mature vWF multimers have several fates after synthesis. Endothelial cells secrete vWF constitutively (without stimulation) and after exposure to physiologic (thrombin, fibrin, histamine) and pharmacologic (DDAVP [desmopressin acetate]) secretagogues. Constitutive secretion is the primary source of circulating vWF, which is present in the plasma at a concentration of 7 to 10 μg/mL and consists of a full range of multimers with molecular weights ranging from 500,000 to 20×10^6. Stimulated release of vWF occurs from a specific storage organelle, the Weibel-Palade body. Contained within the Weibel-Palade body is vWF rich in the higher molecular weight multimers. The vascular subendothelium is also rich in vWF, presumably secreted adluminally by endothelial cells. Megakaryocyte biosynthesis of vWF is similar to that of

Table 1. Terminology Used in Reference to Factor VIII and von Willebrand Factor

Terminology	Abbreviation	Structure/Function	Tests Used
General Term Factor VIII (antihemophiliac factor)	F-VIII (AHF)	Plasma protein deficient in patients with severe classic hemophilia (hemophilia A); reduced but not absent in mild to moderate hemophilia	
Immunologic Identity Factor VIII antigen	F-VIII antigen	Antigenic determinant (or determinants) on F-VIII	Immunoassays employing human or monoclonal antibodies
Functional Identity Factor VIII:C	F-VIII:C	Coagulant property of F-VIII (often used interchangeably with F-VIII)	Standard coagulation assays
General Term von Willebrand factor	vWF	Large, multimeric glycoprotein necessary in vitro for normal platelet adhesion and in vivo for normal bleeding time	
Immunologic Identity von Willebrand factor antigen	vWF antigen	Antigenic determinant (or determinants) on vWF; previously called F-VIII–related antigen (F-VIIIR:Ag), AHF-like antigen, F-VIII antigen, or AHF antigen	Immunoassays employing heterologous antibodies to the F-VIII–vWF complex
Functional Identity Ristocetin cofactor activity	RCoF activity	Ability of normal plasma to induce agglutination of washed or fixed normal platelets on exposure to the antibiotic ristocetin	Ristocetin cofactor assay (quantitative measure of vWF activity)

endothelial cells except that there is no constitutive release from the megakaryocyte or the mature platelet. The vWF is stored in the alpha granule and released only on platelet activation.

vWF has two principal functions. First, it acts as an intracellular bridge between platelet glycoprotein receptors and the vascular subendothelium—a function critical to the adhesion of platelets to the site of vascular injury. The platelet-subendothelial and platelet-platelet interactions involve the unique shear rate dependence of vWF behavior, a property that resides primarily in the higher molecular weight forms of vWF. A second function of vWF is to act as a carrier protein for F-VIII. vWF thereby prolongs the half-life of F-VIII and delivers it to sites of vascular injury. The binding of F-VIII to vWF to form the factor VIII complex explains (1) the long recognized and once confusing parallel decrease in vWF and F-VIII concentrations, (2) the mild and clinically insignificant prolongation of the PTT found in many patients with vWD, and (3) the clinical overlap between classic hemophilia and severe vWD that is seen when vWF levels (and therefore F-VIII levels) are less than 10 per cent of the reference range.

Clinical Presentation

vWD represents a heterogeneous group of bleeding disorders characterized by a variable decrease in the quantitative or functional level of vWF. The mode of inheritance is generally thought to be autosomal dominant with variable penetrance. The heterogeneity makes estimates of the prevalence difficult, but vWD is clearly the most common inherited disorder of hemostasis, with estimates ranging from 1 per 100 to 3 per 100,000 individuals. The variability of clinical manifestations and laboratory features applies to single patients over time and within a family of known vWD patients, and is further influenced by age, exercise, estrogen status (or therapy), and thyroid function. The variability in vWD highlights the need for a careful family and patient history.

vWD is typically a mild to moderate bleeding disorder that can escape diagnosis despite clinical symptoms. The most common symptom is mucocutaneous bleeding: epistaxis in 60 per cent of patients, easy bruising in 40 per cent of patients, menorrhagia in 35 per cent of females, and gingival bleeding in 35 per cent of patients. Post-traumatic and postsurgical bleeding is also common, and a history of significant bleeding following dental extractions often provides a critical clue to the diagnosis. Intrapartum and postpartum bleeding are less common because of the ameliorating effects of estrogen. Neonatal diagnosis is often obscured by the temporary increase of vWF levels secondary to the stress of delivery.

Only in the presence of a dramatic decrease in the levels of vWF, as seen in less than 1 per cent of vWD patients, will deep tissue hematomas, hemarthroses, or spontaneous central nervous system (CNS) hemorrhage develop. Death from vWD is rare.

vWD patients require accurate diagnosis to guide appropriate therapy, which currently emphasizes limited exposure to plasma products. (Unfortunately, numerous vWD patients were infected with the human immunodeficiency virus [HIV] virus prior to the availability of screening assays in the mid-1980s.) vWF levels tend to rise with age, accounting for a decreased prevalence after the second or third decade. vWF levels also rise when estrogen increases; thus, the diagnosis of vWD may be difficult to make and the disorder may be clinically silent during pregnancy.

Laboratory Diagnosis of von Willebrand's Disease

The bleeding time is an important test in the diagnosis of vWD and in fact was the first laboratory abnormality demonstrated by von Willebrand in his original report.

Although there is a parallel decrease in vWF and factor VIII coagulant activity (F-VIII:C), the decrease in F-VIII:C is most often to levels at which the sensitivity of the PTT does not support its use as a reliable screening test.

The vWF antigen can be measured by various techniques, including Laurel rocket immunoelectrophoresis and the enzyme-linked immunosorbent assay (ELISA). Meanwhile, vWF activity can be determined semiquantitatively by ristocetin-induced platelet aggregation and quantitatively by the ristocetin cofactor (RCoF) assay. The first assay involves platelet aggregation of the patient's platelet-rich plasma in the presence of ristocetin. The test result is abnormal in more than 50 per cent of vWD patients. The RCoF assay uses fixed or lyophilized donor platelets in an assay in which the only variable is the quantity of patient vWF. Using dilutions of control plasma, a standard curve can be generated that allows the quantitation of vWF activity in the patient. The RCoF assay is the single most sensitive and specific test for the diagnosis of vWD.

Qualitative abnormalities of vWF can be evaluated by crossed immunoelectrophoresis or sodium dodecyl sulfate (SDS)–agarose electrophoresis. In the first method, a precipitin arc forms. The amplitude (intensity) of the arc depends on the quantity of vWF, and the shape of the arc depends on the distribution of multimer forms. SDS-agarose electrophoresis provides linear separation of multimers and may identify subtle or fine structural abnormalities.

Clinical Subtypes of von Willebrand's Disease

The explosion of information concerning vWF structure and function has been accompanied by the clinical description of close to 30 subtypes. A recent proposal for a simplified classification of vWD subtypes emphasizes a division into two broad categories: a quantitative defect (type 1 and type 3) or a qualitative defect (type 2) of vWF.

Type 1 vWD is seen in 70 per cent of all vWD patients and is characterized by a decrease in the amount of vWF without identifiable functional abnormality in the protein itself. There is a parallel decrease in the levels of RCoF, vWF antigen, and F-VIII. Electrophoresis demonstrates a full range and normal distribution of multimers. Type 3 vWD is a rare disorder in which proteins have little or no detectable vWF, and a resultant decrease in factor VIII. It may represent the homozygous state or type 2 vWB in some patients. The bleeding time and PTT are both prolonged, and the values of vWF, RCoF, F-VIII:C all are less than 5 per cent. The bleeding manifestations include mucocutaneous and deep-tissue hemorrhage, and are often severe.

Type 2 vWD accounts for approximately 20 per cent of vWD patients and is characterized by the absence of multimers of large to intermediate size in both the plasma and platelets. Because RCoF activity is concentrated in the higher molecular weight multimers, there is a disproportionate decrease in the RCoF activity relative to the values of vWF antigen and F-VIII. Patients with type 2A vWD have an absence of intermediate to high molecular weight multimers due to rapid proteolysis following their release from endothelial cells. The bleeding time is often increased, and the clinical manifestations are mild to moderate. Patients with type 2B vWD have a loss of the higher molecular weight multimers in the plasma, with a demonstrated paradoxical enhancement of platelet aggregation in the presence of low concentrations of ristocetin. Patients with type 2B vWD demonstrate an absence of large molecular weight multimers in the plasma due to the spontaneous binding of circulating vWF to the platelet surface. Spontaneous binding of vWF to platelets may account for the association of type 2B vWD with mild thrombocytopenia. The bleeding time is often prolonged, and the bleeding manifestations are moderately severe. Both type 2A and type 2B have been linked to changes within the vWF gene that lead to structural changes in the mature vWF protein.

The subclassification of vWD currently defines therapy. Types 1 and 2A are treated with DDAVP, a synthetic vasopressin analog that causes the release of vWF from endothelial cells. By contrast, DDAVP is ineffective in type 3 vWD may be contraindicated in patients with type 2B vWD.

HEMOPHILIAS

The hemophilias represent the most common congenital disorders of coagulation. The dramatic clinical consequences (often fatal prior to modern replacement therapy), the historical impact on the royal descendants of Queen Victoria, and the devastation of the hemophiliac community by HIV transmission via blood-derived products have all contributed to the persistent notoriety of these unusual disorders.

Hemophilia A

Synonyms for hemophilia A include classic hemophilia and factor VIII deficiency. It is an X-linked recessive disorder seen in approximately 1 in 10,000 males. Seventy-five per cent of these males have a clear family history of a deficiency of the factor VIII coagulant protein (F-VIII:C). F-VIII serves as a cofactor that accelerates the cleavage of factor X by activated factor IX. F-VIII is probably synthesized by the liver and circulates in plasma noncovalently bound to vWF, an association that protects F-VIII from proteolysis and delivers it to sites of vascular injury when vWF binds to subendothelium. Factov VIII need only be present at 20 per cent of the normal level to provide its function. This explains why the decreased levels seen in most patients with vWD are more than adequate to support normal coagulation.

The frequency and sites of bleeding vary substantially among patients with hemophilia A. Beyond the need to manage acute bleeding episodes, the clinician should recognize that the chronic sequelae of the bleeding as well as its therapy create physical, psychosocial, and economic hardships because of loss of function and time lost from school or work.

The clinical severity of hemophilia A is closely correlated with the plasma activity of F-VIII:C and is classified as mild, moderate, or severe (Table 2). The F-VIII:C activity and associated clinical manifestations tend to be constant within a family. Female carriers with approximately 50 per cent F-VIII:C rarely bleed unless they experience major trauma or surgery.

Although cephalohematoma has been reported after traumatic delivery, newborns with hemophilia A typically have no problems at birth. Thus, vaginal delivery of affected males is reasonable. During the first year of life, bleeding is typically limited to that occurring after circumcision and perhaps after venipuncture. Lip or tongue trauma may cause excessive or prolonged bleeding, perhaps due to increased fibrinolysis in the oral mucosa. Once

Table 2. Classification of Hemophilia A

	Factor VIII Coagulant Activity (%)	Bleeding Sites and Frequency
Severe	<1	Presents in first year of life, occasionally with bleeding at time of circumcision; hemarthroses and deep tissue bleeding occurs spontaneously; CNS hemorrhage may occur without trauma
Moderate	1–5	Presents in childhood with hemorrhage after trauma; spontaneous hemarthroses and deep tissue bleeding are less common; CNS hemorrhage only after trauma
Mild	5–20	Presents in childhood or in adults with hemorrhage after trauma, surgery, or dental extraction

CNS = central nervous system.

children begin to ambulate, the clinician begins to observe the more classic and serious bleeding manifestations that are the hallmark of hemophilia A. The typical sites of hemorrhage are the joints (hemarthroses) and muscles (deep hematomas), with potentially fatal hemorrhage occurring after trauma or surgery.

Hemophilia A patients typically have no problems with cuts and abrasions because platelet function and vWF activity are unaffected, allowing normal early hemostasis. By 3 to 4 years of age; almost all patients with severe or moderate hemophilia A have had a significant bleeding episode. Although sites of bleeding do not correlate with F-VIII:C activity, inciting factors and frequency of bleeding often do. Patients with a severe defect (<1 per cent) have frequent spontaneous bleeding. Patients with a moderate defect (2 to 5 per cent) may not bleed spontaneously but bleed readily after trauma or surgery. Patients with a mild defect (>5 per cent) have rare spontaneous bleeding but do bleed after trauma or surgery. Normal primary hemostasis in hemophilia A limits the amount of mucosal bleeding and accounts for the delay in onset of hemorrhage after the initial trauma or surgery. This delay fortunately provides an opportunity for early treatment prior to significant hemorrhage.

Hemarthroses

Acute and chronic joint disease is the most important cause of morbidity in hemophilia A. Severely affected patients have early acute hemarthroses and may experience debilitating joint disease before the age of 20 years. The joints most commonly involved (in decreasing order of frequency) are the knees, elbows, ankles, wrists, and hips. Bleeding in the joints of the hands and in the spine is rare. Many patients experience early symptoms of "tingling" and joint discomfort with each acute episode. Early administration of appropriate therapy may prevent further bleeding, thereby reducing the significant pain that follows. Young children may manifest only irritability, guarding, and lack of movement of an affected joint. Radiologic examination is not helpful unless fracture is suspected and only leads to delays in appropriate therapy. The joint should be immobilized immediately. Once appropriate therapy has been undertaken, the joint should be mobilized within the first several days to prevent more long-term sequelae.

Chronic Hemophilic Arthritis

Repeated bleeding into a joint induces synovial hypertrophy. The friable synovium only bleeds more easily, creating "target joints." This vicious cycle leads to further destruction of the articular cartilage as well as the surrounding bone and soft tissues. Recurrent and/or improperly treated hemarthroses invariably lead to loss of movement, flexion contractures, and muscle atrophy. Management requires a comprehensive program of physiotherapy, joint splinting, minor orthopedic procedures, synovectomy and, in advanced cases, arthrodesis or arthroplasty.

Hematomas

Depending on the severity of the hemophilia, bleeding into muscle or subcutaneous tissues occurs either spontaneously or following trauma. Bleeding into the pharyngeal or retropharyngeal areas may cause airway obstruction. Retroperitoneal hematomas cause abdominal pain and flexion deformity of the hip and may lead to neurovascular compromise. Hematomas, however, most often involve muscles of the upper and lower limbs. These hematomas present as a painful expanding mass that may compress adjacent nerves, blood vessels, and other structures. Many hematomas are self-limited and superficial and can be managed without factor replacement. All other hematomas are managed with factor replacement, analgesia, and other conservative measures. Aspiration of lesions should not be undertaken unless infection is suspected in order to avoid continued hemorrhage or the creation of a sinus. Pseudotumors and bone cysts are rare complications of severe hemophilia that often arise at the site of previous hematomas. They occur most commonly in the femur, pelvis, and tibia and are manifested as a painless, expanding mass. These lesions can lead to further bleeding, bone fracture, infection, or neurovascular compromise. Surgical excision is often required.

Hematuria

Hematuria is relatively common in hemophiliacs and may be a presenting feature of previously undiagnosed disease. Greater than 90 per cent of severely affected hemophiliacs have at least one significant episode of hematuria during a lifetime. Fortunately, most episodes are of short duration and of no long-term consequence. Anemia can result from significant gross hematuria, and factor replacement may be required if bleeding persists for several days. Because the extravasated blood may clot in the urinary tract, the use of fibrinolytic inhibitors (aminocaproic acid [Amicar] and transexamic acid) is contraindicated.

Intracranial Bleeding

Intracranial bleeding that occurs spontaneously or follows head trauma remains a significant cause of morbidity and mortality in hemophilia. Prior to the acquired immunodeficiency syndrome (AIDS) epidemic intracranial bleeding accounted for approximately 25 per cent of deaths in patients with hemophilia. Half of these intracranial catastrophes were associated with head trauma. A patient with known hemophilia and a history of head trauma and even simple signs of head injury should be treated immediately with factor replacement and undergo radiologic evaluation (computed tomography [CT] scan or magnetic resonance imaging [MRI]). In a patient with a history of head trauma without any signs of trauma or neurologic deficits, a decision for treatment is less clear. If in doubt, provide factor replacement first, then decide on further management.

Lacerations

Superficial abrasions and lacerations can be managed conservatively, often without the use of factor replacement.

Tooth Extraction

With appropriate planning, tooth extractions and other dental work can be performed with little risk in the outpatient setting. Use of DDAVP in documented DDAVP-responders can limit the amount of exposure to factor replacement. The use of fibrinolytic inhibitors can also contribute to the maintenance of hemostasis following procedures.

Complications of Hemophilia Therapy

Following the discovery of concentrated factor VIII in plasma cryoprecipitate, a revolution occurred in the therapy of hemophilia. This was followed by the development of plasma concentrates of increasingly higher purity and specific activity. Widespread use of factor VIII concentrates revolutionized the care of hemophiliacs, allowing home therapy, maintenance of a nearly normal lifestyle, and improvement in the median life expectancy. Unfortunately, the ease of therapy with Factor VIII concentrates, prepared from a large number of donors, led to an increasing incidence of hepatitis A, B, and nonA-nonB. Efforts were under way in the early 1980s to reduce viral contamination when the first multitransfused hemophiliacs with AIDS were reported. In the United States, the percentage of hemophiliacs estimated to test positive for antibodies to HIV varies from 33 to 90 per cent for patients who received pooled plasma–derived products prepared prior to the advent of HIV screening of blood products in 1985. The AIDS epidemic in hemophiliacs crushed the growing optimism that had developed in the previous two decades. The current availability of heat-treated, affinity chromatography–purified, and now recombinant factor VIII concentrates, however, has substantially decreased the risk of exposure to hepatitis and HIV. Parvovirus, hepatitis A, and other unknown viruses remain a concern in nonrecombinant products. All newly diagnosed and seronegative hemophiliacs should receive hepatitis B vaccination.

Inhibitors to Factor VIII

Approximately 10 to 15 per cent of patients with hemophilia A acquire antibodies against the "foreign protein" following initial exposure to factor concentrates. The presence of the inhibitor does not change the clinical manifestations of hemophilia but greatly complicates treatment. Presence of an inhibitor can be detected by a rising PTT following exposure to factor VIII concentrates. Low-titer inhibitors can often be managed with increasing doses of factor VIII concentrates. High-titer inhibitors, often rising shortly after exposure to factor VIII concentrates, often cause therapy with factor VIII concentrates to fail. Alternative measures include factor IX concentrates, porcine factor VIII, recombinant factor VIIa, and other less established therapies such as immunoglobulin, plasmapheresis, and the staphylococcal A column.

Hemophilia B

Synonyms for hemophilia B include Christmas disease and factor IX deficiency. Hemophilia B is an X-linked disorder that is clinically indistinguishable from hemophilia A. Laboratory evaluation reveals a prolongation of the PTT, normal F-VIII:C activity, and decreased factor IX. Hemophilia B is less common than hemophilia A and occurs in approximately 1 per 30,000 males. As for hemophilia A, DNA probes are available for the detection of carriers and sometimes for prenatal diagnosis. Replacement therapy can often be accomplished with fresh frozen plasma and, if necessary, factor IX concentrates. The use of fresh frozen plasma has somewhat reduced the incidence of hepatitis and HIV infection in the hemophilia B population when compared with the hemophilia A population. Nevertheless, more than 50 per cent of the patients who received factor IX concentrates prepared before 1985 have tested positive for HIV. Newer forms of heat-treated and affinity chromatography–purified concentrates have now markedly reduced viral contamination.

OTHER INHERITED HEMORRHAGIC DISORDERS

Quantitative or qualitative deficiencies have been described for just about every plasma coagulation factor. Several of the factors are involved in the early stages or in the intrinsic pathway (contact factors), and although they lead to marked prolongation of the PTT assay, they are not associated with any hemorrhagic tendency. They include factor XII deficiency (Hageman trait), plasma prekallikrein deficiency (Fletcher trait), and high molecular weight kininogen deficiency (Fitzgerald-Williams-Flaujeac). The remaining deficiencies are all quite rare, together composing less than 2 per cent of inherited hemorrhagic disorders. They are described briefly in the following paragraphs and summarized in Table 3.

Factor XI Deficiency

A synonym for factor XI deficiency is plasma thromboplastin antecedent (PTA). More than 200 individuals have been identified with a deficiency in factor XI. In this autosomal recessive disorder, homozygotes tend to have excessive bleeding, whereas heterozygotes have mild bleeding. There is no direct correlation between the severity of bleeding and the level of factor XI. Diagnosis is suggested

Table 3. Less Common Hereditary Hemorrhagic Disorders

Factor	Inheritance	Type of Bleeding	Diagnostic Tests
Factor I (fibrinogen)	Autosomal recessive	Variable, deep tissue hemorrhage	Prolonged PT, low fibrinogen level
Factor II (prothrombin)	Autosomal recessive	Epistaxis, hemarthrosis, ecchymoses, menorrhagia	Prolonged PT, assay factor II
Factor V (parahemophilia)	Autosomal recessive	Postoperative and spontaneous bleeding	Prolonged PTT, PT, assay factor V
Factor VII (proconvertin)	Autosomal recessive (only homozygotes bleed)	Epistaxis, hemarthrosis, ecchymoses, menorrhagia	Prolonged PT, normal PTT, assay factor VII
Factor X (Stuart-Prower)	Autosomal recessive (only homozygotes bleed)	Epistaxis, hemarthrosis, ecchymoses, menorrhagia	Prolonged PT, PTT, assay factor X
Factor XI (plasma thromboplastin antecedent deficiency)	Autosomal recessive	Less severe than hemophilia A or B	Prolonged PTT, assay factor XI
Factor XII (Hageman trait)	Autosomal recessive	None	Prolonged PTT, assay factor XII
Factor XIII (fibrin-stabilizing factor)	Not clear	Umbilical bleeding, post-traumatic and late postoperative bleeding, impaired wound healing, keloid formation	Clot solubility in 5M urea or 1% monochloracetic acid, assay factor XIII

PT = prothrombin time; PTT = partial thromboplastin time.

by a long activated partial thromboplastin time (APTT) and confirmed by a specific factor XI assay.

Afibrinogenemia

Approximately 150 cases of this autosomal recessive disorder have been reported. Homozygotes experience variable clinical manifestations; some patients have very mild bleeding despite extremely low serum fibrinogen concentrations. Laboratory testing reveals a normal or prolonged bleeding time and prolongation of the APTT, PT, and TT. Fibrinogen is decreased in functional as well as immunologic assays.

Dysfibrinogenemia

Dysfibrinogenemia includes numerous qualitative defects in the fibrinogen molecule. Clinically, the bleeding tends to be mild, typically arising from mucous membranes. Epistaxis, menorrhagia, and excess bleeding following trauma or surgery have been reported. Laboratory evaluation reveals a variable prolongation of the PT and APTT and a consistent and marked prolongation of the TT.

Factor XIII Deficiency

Synonyms for factor XIII deficiency include fibrin-stabilizing factor deficiency and plasma transglutaminase precursor deficiency.

Factor XIII is the precursor of the enzyme transglutaminase that is responsible for cross-linking fibrin monomers. Patients classically present with a history of lifelong bleeding starting with hemorrhage from the umbilicus and followed by bleeding after trauma or surgery. The bleeding characteristically starts 1 day or more following initial hemostasis. Impaired wound healing and the keloid development are also characteristic. Laboratory testing demonstrates a normal bleeding time, PT, PTT, TT, and serum fibrinogen concentration. The deficiency can be detected by clot lysis in 5M urea or 1 per cent monochloracetic acid. Both substances dissolve fibrin that has not been cross-linked. Diagnosis is confirmed by direct assays for factor XIII.

THE PURPURAS: VASCULAR AND PLATELET DISORDERS AS CAUSES OF BLEEDING

By Angelina Carvalho, M.D., *and* Nancy J. Freeman, M.D.
Providence, Rhode Island

To contain red blood cell extravasation and restore vascular integrity after trauma, normal hemostasis requires a finely tuned equilibrium and interaction between the vessel wall, the platelets, and the coagulation and fibrinolytic systems. Bleeding may result from congenital or acquired vascular abnormalities, thrombocytopenia, defects in platelet function, or abnormal coagulation. Vascular purpuras and bleeding from platelet disorders are manifested primarily by superficial and mucosal bleeding, specifically petechiae (pinpoint hemorrhages smaller than 2 mm), ecchymoses (2 mm to 1 cm), and purpura (larger than 1 cm).

The cornerstone of diagnosis in patients with vascular- or platelet-related purpuras is the bleeding time (BT), which serves as an indicator of platelet number and function as well as vascular integrity. In addition to the BT and platelet count, the evaluation of a bleeding patient should also include the prothrombin time (PT) and activated partial thromboplastin time (APTT), which are necessary for investigating blood coagulation defects. Bleeding from thrombocytopenia is atypical when platelet counts are greater than 50,000 cells/mm^3, unless platelet dysfunction coexists. Platelet counts less than 10,000 cells/mm^3 have been associated with spontaneous hemorrhage, the most ominous of which is central nervous system bleeding. When platelet dysfunction is suspected, platelet aggregation studies can provide another means of establishing an appropriate diagnosis. The purpuras are classified according to vascular or platelet disorders in Table 1.

BLEEDING SECONDARY TO VASCULAR DISORDERS

Vascular purpura (Table 2) result from abnormalities of either the perivascular connective tissues or the vessel wall. These disorders are heterogeneous and are characterized by a tendency to bruise easily and spontaneous bleeding from small vessels. Petechiae and ecchymoses are common, as is mucosal bleeding. In these diseases, the parameters of hemostasis, including platelet number and

Table 1. The Purpuras: Vascular and Platelet Disorders as Causes of Bleeding—an Overview

Vascular Disorders

- Congenital
  - Connective tissue disorders
  - Vascular abnormalities
- Acquired
  - Nonpalpable purpuras
    - Disorders resulting from increased transmural pressure
    - Disorders due to alteration of the integrity of the vessel wall
    - Disorders resulting from trauma
    - Disorders of which the nature of the defect is unknown
  - Palpable purpuras
    - Vasculitides
    - Dysproteinemias

Quantitative Platelet Disorders

- Thrombocytopenias
  - Congenital
    - Decreased production of megakaryocytes
    - Normal to increased numbers of megakaryocytes
  - Acquired
    - Decreased production of megakaryocytes
    - Normal to increased numbers of megakaryocytes
      - Ineffective thrombopoiesis
      - Increased peripheral destruction of platelets
        - Immune
        - Nonimmune
    - Abnormal platelet distribution
- Thrombocytosis
  - Primary myeloproliferative disorders
  - Secondary (no bleeding diathesis)

Qualitative Platelet Disorders

- Congenital disorders of platelet function
- Acquired disorders of platelet function

Table 2. Bleeding Secondary to Vascular Disorders

Congenital Vascular Disorders

Connective tissue disorders
- Ehlers-Danlos syndrome
- Pseudoxanthoma elasticum
- Marfan's syndrome
- Osteogenesis imperfecta

Vascular abnormalities
- Giant cavernous hemangioma (Kasabach-Merritt syndrome)
- Hereditary hemorrhagic telangiectasia (Rendu-Osler-Weber syndrome)

Acquired Vascular Disorders

Nonpalpable purpuras
- Disorders due to increased transmural pressure
  - Facial petechiae with Valsalva-like maneuvers
  - Chronic stasis of the lower extremities
  - High altitude
- Disorders due to alteration of the mechanical integrity of the vessel wall and supporting structures
  - Senile purpura
  - Steroid excess
  - Scurvy (vitamin C deficiency)
  - Amyloidosis
  - Diabetes mellitus
  - Acquired angiodysplasia
  - Purpura simplex
- Disorders due to trauma
  - Physical injury
  - Ultraviolet radiation
- Infectious, allergic, inflammatory causes
- Embolic or thrombotic causes
- Neoplastic disorders
- Disseminated intravascular coagulation (DIC)
- Antiphospholipid antibody syndrome
- Paroxysmal nocturnal hemoglobinuria
- Drugs
  - Warfarin
- Purpuras without known vascular defects
  - Factitious purpura

Palpable purpuras
- Vasculitides
  - Henoch-Schönlein purpura
  - Collagen vascular disorders
  - Paraneoplastic disorders
  - Hypersensitivity vasculitis (including drugs)
  - Autoerythrocyte sensitivity
- Dysproteinemias
  - Cryoglobulinemia or cryfibrinogenemia
  - Hyperglobulinemia

function, PT, and APTT, are typically normal. The BT may be elevated.

Congenital Vascular Disorders

The congenital connective tissue disorders (Ehlers-Danlos syndrome, pseudoxanthoma elasticum, Marfan's syndrome, and osteogenesis imperfecta) result from inborn errors of collagen biosynthesis. Vascular abnormalities, such as giant cavernous hemangioma (Kasabach-Merritt syndrome), present at birth (usually with a mass of tortuous dilated blood vessels), occur in superficial or visceral locations, and may be associated with thrombocytopenia and disseminated intravascular coagulation (DIC). Occurring in 1 in 50,000 births, hereditary hemorrhagic telangiectasia (HHT; Rendu-Osler-Weber syndrome) is a rare autosomal dominant hereditary disorder characterized by widespread telangiectasias in the viscera, mucosa, and skin. The vascular lesions blanch with pressure, and localized bleeding results in purpura. The number and size of the lesions progress with age, and bleeding from the nose, gastrointestinal and genitourinary tracts, and lungs may occur, although gastrointestinal and nasal bleeds are the most common. Iron deficiency anemia frequently develops.

Acquired Vascular Disorders

The acquired vascular disorders are best categorized into those that cause nonpalpable purpura and those that result in palpable purpura.

Nonpalpable Purpuras

Activities that increase intrathoracic pressure, such as Valsalva-like maneuvers, can, in turn, increase transmural pressure across the vessel wall and cause acute facial, neck, and upper chest petechiae. Patients who have chronic venous stasis of the lower extremities can also develop purpura, particularly after minimal local injuries. Several clinical conditions in which the mechanical integrity of the vessel wall and supporting tissues is compromised lead to extravasation of red blood cells and purpura. These disorders include senile purpura, glucocorticoid excess, vitamin C deficiency, amyloidosis, diabetes, acquired angiodysplasia, and purpura simplex.

In elderly individuals, patches of senile purpura may be found on all aspects of the upper and lower extremities. The skin is thin and fragile, and the lesions are bright red. Shearing stress is a typical precipitating factor. Clinically similar to senile purpura, the lesions seen with glucocorticoid excess result from the use of parenteral, oral, or inhaled steroids. After 2 or 3 months of insufficient intake of ascorbic acid, scurvy develops, with skin changes that include follicular keratosis (keratinous plugs of the follicular orifices), perifollicular purpura, corkscrew hairs, petechiae, and hemorrhage from mucosal surfaces.

Mucocutaneous hemorrhage, particularly after trauma, is a feature of amyloidosis, a condition in which light chain deposits of amyloid infiltrate vessel walls, this infiltration leading to vascular fragility. "Pinch purpura" results from minimal trauma, and petechiae develop after an increase in transmural pressure. Subendothelial small vessel connective tissue abnormalities as well as purpura can occur in diabetes mellitus. Acquired angiodysplasia, distinguished by gastrointestinal lesions and bleeding, has been reported in association with aortic insufficiency, mitral valve prolapse, uremia, and von Willebrand's disease. Purpura simplex (female easy-bruising syndrome), and its association with phases of the menstrual cycle, may be due to hormonal effects on small vessels and surrounding tissues. Patients develop purpuric and ecchymotic lesions with minimal trauma.

Various types of trauma to the vessel wall may cause hemorrhage, purpura, and ecchymosis. Physical injury can cause skin hemorrhage. The lesions are typically well demarcated, although the morphologic pattern varies, depending on the specific etiology. Ultraviolet radiation (sunburn) can present with a petechial component if the injury is sufficiently severe. Infections of all types—bacterial, viral, protozoal, parasitic, and rickettsial—can produce petechiae, purpura, hemorrhagic bullae, ulcers, and ecchymoses with ischemic infarction of the skin (purpura fulminans). The pattern can be characteristic and may result from direct invasion, toxic effects, immune complex vasculitis, or thrombocytopenia. Embolic phenomena from infectious organisms can generate both palpable and nonpalpable purpuras, and infections without embolism may result in palpable purpura as well. In allergic and/or inflammatory conditions, such as serum sickness from drugs

Table 3. Drug-Related Nonthrombocytopenic Purpuras

Acetaminophen	Meclofenamate sodium
Alclofenac	Mefenamic acid
Alcohol	Mercury
Allopurinol	Methanol
Apronalide	Morphine
Aspirin	Naproxen
Atropine	Nifedipine
Belladonna	Nitrofurantoin
Bismuth	Penicillamine
Carbamazepine	Penicillin
Carbimazole	Phenacetin
Chloral hydrate	Phenytoin
Chlordiazepoxide	Piperazine
Cimetidine	Piroxicam
Desipramine	Pyrazolone derivatives
Disopyramide	Quinidine
Doxepin	Quinine
Fenbufen	Suldinac
Gold salts	Sulfonamides
Indomethacin	Thiouracils
Iodides	Tolmetin
Isoniazid	

or infections, morbilliform or urticarial eruptions have been described, as have petechiae, palpable purpura, and erythema multiforme. Irritant contact dermatitis represents another cause of purpuric eruptions.

Cholesterol *emboli,* most frequently reported in older men receiving anticoagulation therapy or after invasive vascular procedures, produce an array of cutaneous abnormalities, including acral petechiae and purpura, livedo reticularis, nodules, ulcers, cyanosis, and gangrene. A specific syndrome in these cases, the "blue-purple toe syndrome," has been defined and is characterized by bluish-purple discoloration of the first and fifth toes on and across the plantar surface of the foot, with or without necrosis. Fat emboli occurring a few days after trauma cause upper body petechiae, fever, respiratory distress, pulmonary infiltrates, and varied neurologic symptoms.

Skin infiltrates in many *malignancies* form papules, which should be differentiated from purpura. Thrombotic phenomena from multiple etiologies—DIC, warfarin, skin necrosis, paroxysmal nocturnal hemoglobinuria (PNH), and the antiphospholipid antibody (APA) syndrome—can effect cutaneous changes, including petechiae, purpura, and ecchymoses. In paroxysmal nocturnal hemoglobinuria, the lesions are often palpable.

Petechial and purpuric reactions have been observed after the administration of a wide variety of *drugs* (Table 3) or after toxin exposure, perhaps as the result of an allergic hypersensitivity reaction or direct injury. Some purpuras, such as factitious purpura, which raises the question of self-inflicted injury, occur without clear evidence of a specific vascular defect or platelet abnormality.

Palpable Purpuras

Vasculitides

A myriad of clinical conditions produce vasculitis, which may be systemic. The resultant cutaneous findings include petechiae, papules, ecchymoses, hemorrhagic bullae, and splinter and periungual hemorrhages.

Henoch-Schönlein purpura, presumably an immune-complex hypersensitivity reaction with deposition of IgA, IgG, and C3 in the small vessels of the skin, gastrointestinal tract, joints, and kidneys, is a syndrome characterized by leukocytoclastic vasculitis. Henoch-Schönlein purpura is seen predominantly in children between the ages of 2 and 10 years, often following an infection and particularly during the winter months. In addition to palpable purpuric lesions, abdominal cramping (50 per cent), hematuria and proteinuria (40 per cent), and arthralgias of the knees and ankles (more than 95 per cent) are described. Cardiac, pulmonary, and central nervous system lesions may occur as well. In more than 50 per cent of patients, skin manifestations consisting of urticarial papules and plaques, purpura, and hemorrhagic bullae develop acutely and symmetrically over the legs and buttocks and can progress to larger necrotic lesions. Fifty per cent of patients have an IgA rheumatoid factor; IgA-containing immune complexes have also been observed. On direct immunofluorescence of a skin biopsy, a stippled pattern of IgA in the dermal blood vessels is typical. The disease is self-limiting, although chronic renal failure may ensue (10 to 20 per cent).

Patients with collagen vascular disorders and systemic vasculitis exhibit the cutaneous changes delineated previously as well as nonpalpable purpura, ulcers, nodules, livedo reticularis, erythema, plaques, and telangiectasias. Paraneoplastic vasculitis has been reported in association with hairy cell leukemia (HCL), other lymphoproliferative and myeloproliferative disorders, and solid tumors. The lesions include petechiae, palpable purpura, urticaria, ulcers, maculopapular lesions, and erythema multiforme.

Hypersensitivity vasculitis is a disease in which palpable purpura with histologic leukocytoclastic vasculitis is evident. Numerous drugs (Table 4) have been implicated, as have subacute bacterial endocarditis, hepatitis B and C, tuberculosis, and human immunodeficiency virus (HIV). Autoerythrocyte sensitivity (psychogenic purpura) is a syndrome of recurrent ecchymoses in women. The hypothesis that the cause is an allergic reaction to red blood cells or DNA is not fully accepted. Self-inflicted trauma is suspected.

Dysproteinemias

Single-component cryoglobulinemia (idiopathic, or in Waldenström's macroglobulinemia, multiple myeloma, or lymphoma) or mixed-component cryoglobulinemia (idiopathic, or that found in a variety of subacute or chronic disorders) can cause intermittent acral hemorrhagic necrosis, palpable purpura, livedo reticularis, subungual hemorrhages, urticaria, leg ulcers, Raynaud's phenomenon, and erythema multiforme–like lesions.

Cryofibrinogenemia, characterized by an abnormal cold-precipitable protein in the blood, may be primary (essen-

Table 4. Drug-Induced Hypersensitivity Vasculitis (Leukocytoclastic Vasculitis)

Acebutolol	Iodides
Amiodarone	Nifedipine
Amphetamine	Ofloxacin
Anistreplase	Penicillin
Aspirin	Phenacetin
Captopril	Phenothiazines
Cefoxitin	Procainamide
Chlorthalidone	Propranolol
Cimetidine	Propylthiouracil
Ciprofloxacin	Quinidine
Diltiazem	Rifampin
Ethacrynic acid	Streptokinase
Furosemide	Sulfonamides
Hydralazine	Tamoxifen
Hydrochlorothiazide	Tartrazine
Interferon	Warfarin

Table 5. Disorders That May Simulate Purpuras

Disorders with telangiectasias
- Hereditary hemorrhagic telangiectasia
- CREST syndrome
- Chronic actinic telangiectasia
- Chronic liver disease
- Pregnancy-related telangiectasia
- Ataxia-telangiectasia

Cherry angiomas
Kaposi's sarcoma
Fabry disease
Neonatal extramedullary hematopoiesis
Angioma serpiginosum

CREST = calcinosis, Raynaud's phenomenon, esophageal motility disorders, sclerodactyly, and telangiectasia.

tial) or secondary (due to malignancy, thromboembolism, or infections). The latter form is usually associated with DIC. Skin lesions, appearing on the distal extremities, buttocks, nose, and ears, include purpura, livedo reticularis, cyanosis, ulcers, erythema, urticaria, gangrene, and Raynaud's phenomenon.

In collagen vascular disorders, myeloma, thymoma, sarcoidosis, or multiple sclerosis, a polyclonal increase in globulins may occur and is termed hyperglobulinemic purpura of Waldenström (benign hyperglobulinemic purpura). Macular or papular, discrete or confluent purpuric lesions with hemosiderin staining have been observed and frequently commence as crops of petechiae on the lower legs and ankles of young women. Disorders with telangiectasias and cherry angiomas demonstrate lesions that simulate purpura (Table 5).

BLEEDING DUE TO QUANTITATIVE PLATELET DISORDERS

Congenital Thrombocytopenias

Several rare congenital and hereditary conditions that involve a paucity of megakaryocytes and thrombocytopenia are listed in Table 6.

Isolated thrombocytopenias associated with normal to increased production of megakaryocytes (occasionally with other features, such as large platelets) may not be rare and have been described in many families, inherited as either an autosomal dominant or recessive trait. Patients are frequently discovered as adults. Bleeding is unusual, and these patients are often misdiagnosed as having immune thrombocytopenia. Alport's syndrome, inherited in an autosomal dominant pattern, is associated with giant platelets, severe thrombocytopenia, hereditary nephritis, and deafness. Patients are often diagnosed as adults, and some are misdiagnosed as having immune thrombocytopenia. May-Hegglin syndrome is defined by an autosomal dominant inheritance of giant platelets, moderate thrombocytopenia, a glycoprotein CD34 defect, and Döhle-like inclusion bodies in leukocytes. Most patients are asymptomatic and are identified incidentally.

Acquired Thrombocytopenias with Decreased Megakaryocyte Production

The many diseases and toxins known to induce direct bone marrow damage with thrombocytopenia include viruses, toxins, radiation, alcohol, drugs, and bone marrow replacement with fibrosis or neoplasia. Amegakaryocytic aplasia or hypoplasia is a rare immune-related cause of acquired thrombocytopenia. Patients usually present with thrombocytopenia with or without other cytopenias. Re-

Table 6. Bleeding Due to Quantitative Bleeding Disorders

Thrombocytopenias

Congenital

- Decreased numbers of megakaryocytes
  - Megakaryocytic thrombocytopenia
  - Fanconi's anemia
  - Thrombocytopenia with absent radius
  - Bernard-Soulier syndrome
  - Gray platelet syndrome
- Normal to increased numbers of megakaryocytes
  - Alport's syndrome
  - May-Hegglin syndrome
  - Wiskott-Aldrich syndrome

Acquired

- Decreased numbers of megakaryocytes
  - Megakaryocytic aplasia
  - Viral infection
  - ETOH, toxins, radiation
  - Bone marrow replacement
    - Fibrosis
    - Neoplasia
  - Drugs
- Normal to increased numbers of megakaryocytes
  - Ineffective thrombopoiesis
    - Myelodysplastic syndromes
    - Nutritional causes
      - Vitamin B_{12}
      - Folate
      - Iron
    - Paroxysmal nocturnal hemoglobinuria
- Increased peripheral destruction of platelets
  - Immune
    - Immune thrombocytopenia
      - Primary idiopathic
      - Secondary (see text)
    - Drugs
    - Neonatal
    - Post-transfusion purpura
  - Nonimmune
    - Disseminated intravascular coagulation
    - Thrombotic thrombocytopenic purpura, hemolytic-uremic syndrome
    - Pregnancy-associated thrombocytopenias
    - Incidental: HELLP syndrome (see text)
      - Infectious
      - Drugs
      - Vascular damage: ARDS
      - Cardiopulmonary bypass
- Abnormal platelet distribution
  - Hypersplenism
  - Pseudothrombocytopenia
  - Dilutional thrombocytopenia

Thrombocytosis

Acquired

- Primary myeloproliferative disorders
- Secondary (see text)

ARDS = adult respiratory distress syndrome; ETOH = ethanol; HELLP = hemolysis, elevated liver enzymes, and low platelet count.

duced platelet survival is typical. Other signs and symptoms depend on the specific condition involved.

The peripheral blood smear shows diminished numbers of generally small platelets, and bone marrow evaluation demonstrates a lack of megakaryocytes. Peripheral smears that reveal teardrop-shaped cells, nucleated red blood cells, and early white blood cells, the so-called leukoerythroblastic picture, constitute evidence of a myelophthistic marrow or a bone marrow that has been overtaken by an alternative process (e.g., myelodysplasia). Other bone marrow findings, such as fibrosis with reticulin staining, or morphologic changes typical of alcoholism, may pinpoint a more specific diagnosis.

Viral-induced thrombocytopenia is probably the most common cause of a mild transient thrombocytopenia. Mumps, varicella, Epstein-Barr virus, rubella, rubeola, dengue fever, cytomegalovirus, and parvovirus infections all have been implicated. A decreased platelet count, which remains unnoticed in most situations, may become evident if the patient also has an underlying thrombocytopenia from other causes (e.g., immune thrombocytopenia). The platelet count should return to normal within a month.

Thrombocytopenia in alcoholics is multifactorial, with direct toxic effects, hypersplenism from cirrhosis, and folic acid deficiency representing contributing factors. One needs to ingest alcohol for 5 to 10 consecutive days to sustain direct toxic injury with diminished megakaryocytes and shortened platelet survival. Bone marrow findings also include hypogranulation of the myeloid line and vacuoles in both red and white blood cell precursors. On the peripheral smear, leukocyte hypogranulation is typical. After the alcohol ingestion has been discontinued, the platelets usually recover within 5 to 21 days, occasionally with a transient thrombocytosis. Platelet counts may plunge further for about 2 days after the patient has been admitted to the hospital; thereafter, platelet counts stabilize and then increase.

Radiation therapy directed at prime bone marrow–bearing areas, such as the pelvis, can result in a mild transient thrombocytopenia. A long-term effect of radiation is marrow fibrosis after which permanent thrombocytopenia may ensue. Drugs and toxins depress platelets by marrow suppression or by immune or nonimmune mechanisms. Drugs that directly damage megakaryocytes include thiazide diuretics, diethylstilbestrol (DES), granulocyte-macrophage colony-stimulating factor (GM-CSF), and oral contraceptives. When the offending agent is removed, recovery usually occurs within days to weeks, but the time course ultimately depends on the half-life of the drug.

Acquired Thrombocytopenias With Normal to Increased Megakaryocyte Production

In the thrombocytopenias resulting from nutritional deficiencies or the myelodysplastic syndromes, the marrow exhibits normal to increased numbers of megakaryocytes with ineffective thrombopoiesis. Both cyanocobalamin (vitamin B_{12}) and folic acid are required for the proper construction of DNA and the subsequent development and proliferation of hematopoietic cells. Thrombocytopenia occurs in patients with megagloblastic anemia from deficiencies of both vitamin B_{12} (20 per cent) and folic acid (more than 20 per cent). Concentrations of vitamin B_{12} and folic acid should be measured in the evaluation of thrombocytopenia, regardless of whether other cytopenias are present. A bone marrow biopsy may be useful in confirming megaloblastosis and the presence of megakaryocytes and in excluding other etiologies of the reduced platelet count. Concentrations of red blood cell folate can be measured for up to 2 weeks after folate replacement in patients whose plasma concentration of folate has returned to normal. After a transfusion of red blood cells, however, neither red blood cell folate nor plasma folate concentrations will be accurate. Although thrombocytosis is fairly common in iron deficiency, a mild thrombocytopenia has also been reported. Iron deficiency may impair the utilization of folate and vitamin B_{12}, or a concurrent deficiency of vitamin B_{12} or folate may have to be present for thrombocytopenia to develop.

Myelodysplastic syndromes encompass refractory anemia (RA), refractory anemia with ringed sideroblasts (RARS), refractory anemia with excess blasts (RAEB), refractory anemia with excess blasts in transformation (RAEB-T), and chronic myelomonocytic leukemia. Although cytopenias can occur in one or more cell lines, the symptoms that develop depend on the cell lines that are involved and the severity of the cytopenia. In each of these entities, bone marrow biopsy is essential and generally shows hyperplasia with both ineffective hematopoiesis and dysplasia in one or more cell lines. The peripheral smear can also reveal dysplasia.

Paroxysmal nocturnal hemoglobinuria is characterized by an abnormal sensitivity of cells to complement, pancytopenia, positive Ham's test and sucrose lysis test results, iron deficiency anemia, and a hypercoagulable state. The bone marrow is frequently hypoplastic with reduced numbers of megakaryocytes but can be normal with ineffective thrombopoiesis. The primary cause of the thrombocytopenia, however, may be complement-mediated lysis.

Acquired Thrombocytopenias With Peripheral Destruction of Platelets (Immune)

Idiopathic thrombocytopenic purpura (immune or autoimmune thrombocytopenic purpura, Werlhof's disease), probably best termed immune thrombocytopenic purpura, is an acquired disorder characterized by thrombocytopenia with or without evidence of purpura. In adults, chronic immune thrombocytopenic purpura usually has an insidious onset and rarely remits spontaneously (less than 10 per cent). Acute immune thrombocytopenic purpura in adults, with the abrupt onset of superficial and mucosal bleeding, is less common. The incidence of immune thrombocytopenic purpura is estimated at 66 new cases per 1 million population per year. The idiopathic variety is more common in women.

Patients typically present with petechiae in dependent areas, recurrent epistaxis, ecchymoses, hypermenorrhea (menorrhagia), or gingival bleeding or are discovered incidentally by way of routine blood counts ordered for other reasons. The remainder of the history and physical examination are normal in those with the idiopathic variety; a palpable spleen is evidence that idiopathic thrombocytopenic purpura does not exist. In patients with secondary immune thrombocytopenic purpura from conditions such as collagen vascular disorders, lymphoproliferative disorders, HIV infection, and drugs (e.g., gold and procainamide), the clinical situation should reflect the primary disorder.

The hallmarks of immune thrombocytopenic purpura include decreased numbers of large platelets (larger than 2.5 μm) on the peripheral smear and normal to increased numbers of megakaryocytes in the bone marrow; the megakaryocytes are frequently young, with one or two lobes. When sensitive techniques are used, 80 per cent of patients are found to have platelet-associated IgG (some IgM), and

50 per cent to have increased activity of platelet-associated C3. Antibody concentrations in the plasma are not as consistent. Positive antibody test results may indicate the presence of antibody-mediated platelet destruction, but a negative test result does not exclude immune thrombocytopenic purpura. When platelet counts decrease below 100,000 cells/mm^3, the antibody tests are more likely to be positive.

One third of patients with idiopathic thrombocytopenic purpura have platelet counts of more than 30,000 cells/mm^3 and a benign course. The overall mortality is estimated at 5 per cent. Older patients may have more bleeding complications and a greater mortality. Overall, however, intracranial, abdominal, or retinal hemorrhages are rare. In patients with secondary immune thrombocytopenic purpura, when the underlying condition is in remission or the offending agent has been removed, the thrombocytopenia ultimately resolves.

Drug-induced thrombocytopenia can result from a wide variety of drugs (Table 7). Thrombocytopenia and purpura can occur hours to months after drug ingestion. These idiosyncratic reactions are generally dose-independent and immune in nature. Increased platelet-associated IgG and normal to increased numbers of marrow megakaryocytes are typical. Usually, the platelet count returns to normal within several weeks after discontinuation of the drug in question. The thrombocytopenia develops via the formation of a hapten (penicillin) or by the induction of a neoantigen on the platelet surface that is recognized by antibodies only in the presence of the drug (quinines). Purpuric lesions that are palpable should raise the possibility of a hypersensitivity vasculitis rather than immune thrombocytopenic purpura.

Heparin-induced thrombocytopenia (HIT) occurs in as many as 5 per cent of patients who receive bovine heparin and as many as 1 per cent who receive pork heparin. This condition can result from any heparin preparation, delivered by any route (e.g., heparin flushes of indwelling catheters in doses as low as 100 U per day). The incidence appears to be dose-related. HIT should be suspected when the platelet count falls below 150,000 cells/mm^3 in patients who originally had normal counts, or when a 40 per cent decrease occurs with a platelet count greater than 150,000 cells/mm^3. Petechiae and purpura typically occur with more severe thrombocytopenia, and some patients show evidence of arterial thrombosis (HIT with thrombosis). Heparin-dependent antibodies mediate platelet aggregation and can be detected in the laboratory, although with difficulty, by several techniques.

The average time of onset for HIT is 6 to 12 days in patients who have never received heparin, but onset may occur within 24 hours in those previously exposed. Although severe thrombocytopenia is possible, it is not the rule. The decision to discontinue heparin in the setting of a dropping platelet count is difficult, particularly if the need for heparin is critical. Mild thrombocytopenia is not of clinical consequence, and many patients recover spontaneously, even if the heparin is continued. Some clinicians recommend suspending the heparin immediately in all cases, whereas others suggest doing so when the platelet count dips below 50,000 cells/mm^3 or decreases by 20 per cent (after the elimination of other causes of platelet reduction, such as DIC or infection). After heparin therapy has been interrupted, platelet counts typically improve within several days. Twenty per cent of patients with HIT develop evidence of arterial thrombosis resulting from immune-related platelet stimulation. The mortality in these patients is estimated at 50 per cent, and heparin is contraindicated.

Table 7. Common Causes of Drug-Induced Thrombocytopenia

Heparin	Cimetidine
Gold salts	Noraminopyrine
Quinidine	Carbamazepine
Quinine	Phenytoin
Sulfonamides	Chlorthalidone
Indomethacin	Furosemide
Allylisopropylacetylurea	Chloroquine
Arsenical antiluetics	Chlorothiazide
Aspirin	Digitoxin
Rifampin	Interferon
Valproic acid	Procainamide
Amrinone	Ranitidine
Heroin	Vinyl chloride

Post-transfusion purpura (PTP) is an unusual entity that develops 1 week after a blood transfusion. It is characterized by the emergence of platelet-specific alloantibodies directed most frequently against the Pl^{A1} antigen (more than 90 per cent of the population is Pl^{A1}-positive), resulting in severe thrombocytopenia (fewer than 10,000 cells/mm^3) and bleeding. The antibody, for reasons not well understood, successfully destroys autologous platelets, which are Pl^{A1}-negative, as well as Pl^{A1}-positive platelets from the transfused blood. Most patients are multiparous women receiving their first transfusion. Although spontaneous recovery occurs within 1 to 6 weeks, fatal intracranial hemorrhage has been reported in 10 per cent of cases.

Acquired Thrombocytopenia With Peripheral Destruction of Platelets (Nonimmune)

Disseminated intravascular coagulation is associated with a multitude of common clinical conditions (e.g., malignancy, infection, and acidosis) that cause widespread intravascular coagulation with platelet consumption. (See the article on bleeding due to intravascular coagulation and fibrinolysis.) Clotting with microthrombi in the vessels of all organs, and secondary fibrinolysis, lead to ischemia, necrosis, and hemorrhage. The bleeding diathesis results from the combination of thrombocytopenia, dysfunctional platelets, lack of blood coagulation factors (factors V, VIII, II, and XIII and fibrinogen), and excessive fibrinolysis. The severity of DIC and the rate at which it develops vary, depending on the initiating condition, with the clinical manifestations ranging from laboratory abnormalities only to significant bleeding with dysfunction of multiple organs.

Progressive thrombocytopenia is a consistent laboratory feature of active acute DIC. In a patient who does not have decreasing platelet counts, the diagnosis of DIC should be reconsidered. Chronic but stable thrombocytopenia is seen in chronic DIC. In acute DIC, prolongation of the PT and APTT and increases in fibrin and fibrinogen degradation products (FDPs) and/or D-dimer concentrations with decreasing fibrinogen concentration help support the diagnosis. In chronic DIC, thrombocytopenia and a high FDP titer are typical, while the PT, APTT, and fibrinogen concentration remain normal.

Thrombotic thrombocytopenic purpura (TTP, thrombohemolytic purpura, Moschcowitz's disease) and the hemolytic-uremic syndrome (HUS, Gasser syndrome, Morbus Gasser syndrome) are considered to represent different expressions of the same disease process and are often referred to as TTP-HUS (TTP will be used here to encompass both). This condition may be idiopathic (more frequently in women) or may be seen with pregnancy, specific infections (verotoxin-producing *Escherichia coli* and *Shigella dysenteriae* type 1), metastatic cancer, specific cancer chemotherapeutic agents (mitomycin C, cisplatin), immunosuppressive agents (cyclosporine), quinine, bone marrow transplantation, rheumatic diseases, and HIV infection. A familial occurrence has also been reported.

Patients often present with a clinical pentad of fever, thrombocytopenia (severe) with hemorrhage (cutaneous purpura, epistaxis, hematuria, gastrointestinal bleeding, hypermenorrhea), microangiopathic hemolytic anemia, neurologic abnormalities (headache, confusion, paresis, dysphasia, seizures, visual problems), and renal involvement (proteinuria, hematuria, casts, azotemia) but not all patients present with each of these features. Some criteria require only the dyad of microangiopathic hemolytic anemia and thrombocytopenia for establishing the diagnosis. Neurologic and renal manifestations are seen in approximately 60 per cent of patients, fever in 24 per cent, and bleeding in 44 per cent. Abdominal pain is prominent in many series (35 per cent), as is nausea, vomiting, and diarrhea. These signs and symptoms have not been explained by pancreatitis or other specific abdominal pathology. In classic hemolytic-uremic syndrome, neurologic symptoms are lacking.

In patients with thrombocytopenia and red blood cell fragmentation on peripheral smear (multiple fragments in each high-power field), the diagnosis of TTP must be immediately entertained. Disseminated intravascular coagulation is in the differential diagnosis but can be excluded by demonstrating that the PT, APTT, and fibrinogen and D-dimer concentrations are normal. Some patients with TTP have slightly increased concentrations of FDPs—but not to the concentrations seen with DIC. As a result of the microangiopathic hemolytic anemia, lactate dehydrogenase (LD) activity is increased, as is the indirect bilirubin concentration. The LD activity is a superb marker for monitoring the efficacy of therapy. White blood cell counts are typically increased as well. If organ biopsies are obtained, the characteristic lesion of eosinophilic, granular (hyaline) material in the lumina of arterioles and capillaries can be observed. This material is composed mostly of platelets and fibrin.

Although as many as 6 per cent of women develop an incidental thrombocytopenia (rarely fewer than 75,000 cells/mm^3) late in the third trimester of pregnancy, thrombocytopenia occurs in 10 to 35 per cent of women with preeclampsia and fewer than 5 per cent develop counts below 50,000 cells/mm^3. It is thought that thrombocytopenia results from accelerated platelet destruction by nonimmune mechanisms. Ten per cent of patients with preeclampsia develop what is referred to as the HELLP syndrome, which includes microangiopathic **H**emolysis, **El**evated **L**iver function tests, and **L**ow **P**latelet counts. The signs and symptoms of liver dysfunction predominate. Treatment requires delivery of the fetus and, if this is not feasible, plasma exchange.

Thrombocytopenia, which can complicate any infectious process, is the result of marrow suppression (viral diseases), DIC (bacterial sepsis), immune mechanisms, aggregation on endotoxin-stimulated monocytes, neutrophil activation and cosequestration of platelets, direct damage, direct aggregation, and vasculitis with platelet adhesion. The direct interaction of certain drugs (ristocetin, protamine, bleomycin) with platelets causes destruction by a nonimmune mechanism. In patients who have extensive vascular damage (adult respiratory distress syndrome [ARDS], burns), platelets are activated, and the result is thrombocytopenia. Patients who undergo cardiopulmonary bypass develop thrombocytopenia from hemodilution and direct damage from the bypass procedure.

Thrombocytopenia From Abnormal Platelet Distribution

The spleen normally contains approximately one third of the platelet mass. With splenomegaly, from virtually any cause, as much as 90 per cent of the total platelet mass can be sequestered within the spleen. Although the total number of platelets in circulation is normal, the peripheral count may be reduced to 20 per cent of normal. Mild to moderate thrombocytopenia is the rule, and bleeding is uncommon.

The clinical signs and symptoms generally reflect the underlying disease (e.g., cirrhosis) that has produced the splenomegaly. When the spleen becomes palpable on physical examination, it is probably at least twice its normal size. However, a nonpalpable spleen does not exclude the possibility of splenomegaly, especially in an obese patient or one with ascites or if the spleen is posteriorly displaced. If splenomegaly is a real diagnostic possibility, ultrasound studies, a liver-spleen scan, or computed tomography should be considered.

In splenomegaly, the platelet count rarely drops below 50,000 cells/mm^3. Thrombocytopenia below this number requires a search for other or additional causes (alcohol, drugs, infection, DIC, and immune thrombocytopenic purpura). The patient may also have an associated anemia and/or leukopenia. In alcoholics who have chronic liver disease, portal hypertension, and splenomegaly, platelet counts range from 60,000 to 120,000 cells/mm^3.

When thrombocytopenia is first identified, the peripheral smear must be examined to ensure the accuracy of the low platelet count. Reduced numbers of small platelets suggest bone marrow suppression, while reduced numbers of large platelets should raise one's suspicion for a process involving peripheral destruction, such as immune thrombocytopenic purpura. A smear showing clumps of platelets (misidentified by automated counting as white blood cells), or platelets surrounding leukocytes (platelet satellitism), confirms the diagnosis of pseudothrombocytopenia, which is a laboratory artifact. These patients have autoagglutinins that clump platelets in the presence of some anticoagulants, such as ethylenediaminetetraacetic acid (EDTA), and the reaction may be temperature-dependent. Evaluating a second blood sample with the use of a different anticoagulant (e.g., heparin) frequently corrects this in vitro artifact.

Transfusion of packed red blood cells may be accompanied by thrombocytopenia. The total number of units transfused, as well as splenic factors (platelet release) and other underlying clinical conditions (platelet consumption), ultimately determines the final platelet count. Patients who receive 15 U of red blood cells within 24 hours often develop thrombocytopenia with platelet counts of 47,000 to 100,000/mm^3, and those who receive 20 U may have platelet counts as low as 25,000 to 61,000 cells/mm^3. Patients who receive 2 to 4 U of red blood cells may have platelet counts that decrease by 20,000 to 40,000 cells/mm^3, and this decrease is more obvious in those who have pre-existing thrombocytopenia or other medical problems (e.g., infection).

Thrombocytosis

Thrombocytosis is a condition that may be primary, as with the myeloproliferative disorders, or occur secondary to other clinical conditions (reactive thrombocytosis). The platelets in secondary thrombocytoses (occurring with splenectomy, malignancies, infections, iron deficiency, hemolysis, or inflammation) function normally and do not cause bleeding diatheses. In contrast, the platelets in myeloproliferative disorders are dysfunctional, and bleeding and/or thrombosis is common.

BLEEDING DUE TO QUALITATIVE PLATELET DISORDERS

In patients with mucocutaneous bleeding, the combination of a normal platelet count, PT, and APTT with a prolonged BT suggests the presence of an inherited or acquired qualitative platelet disorder. In some of these conditions, thrombocytopenia coexists, and the BT is prolonged out of proportion to the degree of thrombocytopenia. The inherited platelet function disorders usually represent defects in one aspect of platelet function, such as the inability of platelets to adhere, aggregate, and release their contents, or their inability to provide procoagulant activity to the blood coagulation system. The detailed study of these inherited platelet conditions has led to the diagnosis of a variety of bleeding diatheses and has provided the basis for our understanding of platelet physiology. The inherited qualitative platelet disorders are classified by their primary site of platelet dysfunction (Table 8).

Inherited Disorders of Platelet Function

Inherited Defects in Platelet Membrane

Bernard-Soulier syndrome (BSS, giant platelet syndrome, macrothrombocytopenic thrombocytopathy) is a rare inherited autosomal recessive platelet disorder, but an autosomal dominant form has also been described. The syndrome is a mucocutaneous bleeding diathesis characterized by variable thrombocytopenia, giant platelets, and markedly impaired platelet–vessel wall interaction due to deficiencies in platelet membrane glycoproteins (GPIb, GPIb-IX complex, and GPV).

Table 8. Inherited Disorders of Platelet Function

Platelet Membrane Defects

Reduced platelet–vessel wall interaction (platelet adhesion defects)
- Glycoprotein (GP) abnormalities
  - Bernard-Soulier syndrome
  - Platelet-type pseudo–von Willebrand's disease
  - Wiskott-Aldrich syndrome
  - Deficiency in GPIa or IIa
  - Deficiency in GPIV or GPVI
  - von Willebrand factor plasma abnormalities—von Willebrand's disease

Defects in platelet-to-platelet interaction (platelet aggregation defects)
- Glanzmann's thrombasthenia
- Afibrinogenemia

Platelet Secretion and Signal Transduction Defects (Platelet Release Defects)

Abnormalities of platelet granules
- Storage pool deficiency
  - Delta granule deficiency
  - Alpha and delta granule deficiencies
  - Alpha granule deficiency (gray platelet syndrome)
- Defects in arachidonic acid (AA) metabolism
  - Impaired liberation of AA
  - Deficiency of cyclooxygenase
  - Deficiency of thromboxane synthase
- Signal transduction defects (primary secretion defects)
  - Defects in calcium mobilization and responsiveness
  - Defects in phosphatidylinositol metabolism
  - Defects in myosin phosphorylation

Platelet Procoagulant Activity Defects

Scott syndrome (defect in factor Va-Xa interaction on platelets)

Purpura, epistaxis (70 per cent), ecchymoses (58 per cent), menometrorrhagia (44 per cent), gingival hemorrhage (42 per cent), and gastrointestinal bleeding (22 per cent) are the common clinical features. Spontaneous deep visceral bleeding and hemarthrosis have not been reported. Considerable variability in bleeding symptoms occurs between patients and even between members of the same family. The bleeders are usually homozygous for the trait, with consanguinity observed in most kindreds. Heterozygous subjects have no bleeding symptoms, and their platelet counts are normal, but the platelets are large and have low (less than 50 per cent) levels of GPIb-GPIX complex. The causes of bleeding in Bernard-Soulier syndrome are thrombocytopenia, reduced or absent platelet interaction with von Willebrand factor (vWF; i.e., impaired platelet adhesion), abnormal platelet interactions with thrombin, and reduced platelet coagulant activity.

The platelet count is variably decreased, and giant platelets are observed in most patients with Bernard-Soulier syndrome. On the peripheral smear, the platelets may be larger than lymphocytes (greater than 15 μm), and they may be vacuolated. The BT is prolonged out of proportion to the thrombocytopenia. In Bernard-Soulier syndrome, platelets fail to aggregate in response to ristocetin or botrocetin, both of which require the vWF-GPIb interaction. Platelet aggregation is normal in response to ADP, epinephrine, collagen, or thrombin (high concentrations), but it is decreased in response to low thrombin concentrations. Additional tests showing normal vWF antigenic concentration and functional activity can separate Bernard-Soulier syndrome from von Willebrand's disease. Confirmatory tests for the syndrome include electron microscopy of platelets (Swiss-cheese appearance), and establishing the absence of or a reduction in GPIb, GPIb-IX complex, or GPV.

An autosomal dominant disorder, platelet-type (pseudo-) von Willebrand's disease (GPIb, IX qualitative defect, platelet type von Willebrand's disease) includes a heterogeneous group of patients with mild to moderate mucocutaneous bleeding, variable platelet counts, enlarged platelets, and reduced concentrations of high-molecular-weight vWF multimers in plasma. The key platelet membrane defect is a qualitatively abnormal GPIb-IX receptor that binds selectively to high-molecular-weight vWF multimers in plasma, thereby decreasing the concentration of high-molecular-weight vWF in plasma. A characteristic finding in platelet-type von Willebrand's disease is enhanced platelet aggregation to low doses of ristocetin or botrocetin. Patients do well when precautions are taken to avoid treatments (e.g., 1-deamino, 8-D-arginine vasopressin [DDAVP, desmopressin] or cryoprecipitate) that increase plasma vWF activity. Von Willebrand's disease, characterized by congenital or acquired deficiencies of vWF or abnormal structure of vWF in the plasma, is discussed in the article on hemophilia and other inherited coagulation disorders.

Wiskott-Aldrich syndrome (CD34 deficiency) is an X-linked disorder characterized by small platelets, thrombocytopenia, platelet dysfunction, mucocutaneous bleeding, recurrent infections, T-cell dysfunction, and eczema. In addition to CD34 platelet membrane deficiency, the platelets also have reduced δ granule content, leading to impaired platelet aggregation and secretion. The prognosis is poor.

The thrombocytopenia improves with splenectomy, but the subsequent risk of overwhelming infections with encapsulated organisms is greatly enhanced.

Glycoprotein Ia-IIa deficiency is a syndrome distinguished by the tendency to bruise easily and excessive postoperative bleeding. Laboratory findings include prolonged BT, normal platelet morphology and number, and lack of the platelet aggregation response to collagen. The concentration of GPIa is reduced to 15 to 25 per cent of normal, and the GPIIa concentration is reduced as well.

A deficiency in platelet membrane GPIV (CD36) occurs in 3 per cent of the Japanese population and 0.3 per cent of the United States population. GPIV is involved in platelet interaction with collagen, thrombospondin, and monocytes. Individuals who lack platelet GPIV can develop antibodies against GPIV after a transfusion, or they can become sensitized during pregnancy.

Patients with a deficiency in platelet membrane GPVI have a bleeding tendency caused by impaired platelet-collagen interaction. An acquired case of autoantibody production against GPVI associated with bleeding has been reported.

An autosomal recessive bleeding disorder, Glanzmann's thrombasthenia (GT, hereditary hemorrhagic thrombasthenia, Glanzmann's disease, thrombasthenia) is rare except in populations in which inbreeding is common. Consanguinity occurs in 67 per cent of the cases reported.

Bleeding occurs only in homozygous patients. Purpura, petechiae, and subconjunctival hemorrhage (86 per cent) may be the first symptoms in neonates and infants. Epistaxis (73 per cent) in childhood is frequent and sometimes life-threatening, but this symptom diminishes with age. Hypermenorrhea is the most frequent symptom in women (98 per cent). Gastrointestinal bleeding (49 per cent) occurs intermittently and results in iron deficiency anemia. Bleeding into the central nervous system or deep visceral hematomas are rare (2 per cent). Women with Glanzmann's thrombasthenia typically do not bleed during pregnancy, but they do bleed excessively during the postpartum period. Minor surgical procedures and dental extractions are also associated with bleeding when prophylactic measures are not taken.

Platelets are normal in number and morphology. The BT is markedly prolonged. The whole-blood clot retraction is absent or reduced. Primary platelet aggregation (primary wave) is absent or reduced in response to all agonists except ristocetin and botrocetin. Both quantitative and qualitative deficiencies in GPIIb and/or GPIIIa have been reported. The differential diagnosis of Glanzmann's thrombasthenia includes all inherited platelet disorders with normal platelet counts, prolonged BTs, and defective platelet aggregation. Acquired Glanzmann's thrombasthenia can occur in patients with acute promyelocytic leukemia, myelodysplastic syndromes, and multiple myeloma, in whom chromosome abnormalities may have disrupted the GPIIb and GPIIIa genes.

Beginning at birth, bleeding in Glanzmann's thrombasthenia varies in severity from mild to severe. Correlation is poor between the degree of platelet biochemical defects and the severity of clinical bleeding. Overall, survival is good in spite of severe bleeding, which can be unpredictable. Preventive measures should be carried out in all patients prior to minor surgical procedures.

Afibrinogenemia is a rare inherited disorder resulting from the lack of plasma fibrinogen, which is required for platelet-to-platelet interaction. Afibrinogenemia leads to a severe bleeding diathesis. An extrinsic platelet defect, this disorder is treated with plasma infusion.

Platelet Secretion and Signal Transduction Defects (Platelet Release Defects)

Platelet granule defects or storage pool deficiency (SPD) comprises a heterogeneous group of patients born with deficiencies in either platelet dense granules (δ-SPD), α granules (α-SPD or gray platelet syndrome), or α,δ granules (α,δ-SPD). Clinically, most patients exhibit mild to moderate mucocutaneous bleeding.

Inherited as an autosomal dominant trait, δ-storage pool deficiency constitutes approximately 10 to 15 per cent of all congenital platelet disorders. Bleeding results from a lack of platelet-to-platelet interaction. Dense granules normally contain ADP, Ca^{2+}, and serotonin, all of which are agonists involved in secondary platelet aggregation (secretion). In δ-storage pool deficiency, platelets fail to undergo the secondary wave of aggregation in response to all agonists. Variable deficiencies in δ granules have also been reported in inherited disorders involving multiple organs, such as Hermansky-Pudlak syndrome, Chédiak-Higashi syndrome, Wiskott-Aldrich syndrome, and thrombocytopenia with absent radius syndrome.

The most common manifestations of δ-storage pool deficiency are a tendency to bruise easily, epistaxis, and bleeding following tooth extractions and surgical procedures. These symptoms are augmented by the intake of antiplatelet agents. In Hermansky-Pudlak syndrome, bleeding is severe or even fatal. Platelet size and appearance are normal. The BT is markedly prolonged. Platelet aggregation and secretion are impaired. Electron microscopy shows an absence of or a reduction in δ granules. Some families with δ-storage pool deficiency have monosomy of chromosome 7 and a predisposition to hematologic malignancies.

Gray platelet syndrome (α-SPD) is an autosomal recessive condition in which platelets are devoid of α granules and contain, instead, α-granule membranes that form abnormal vesicular structures. In contrast with δ-storage pool deficiency, the number of platelets can be moderately to severely decreased (fewer than 50,000 cells/mm^3). The platelets are larger than normal, oval, and "grayish" and lack granules. The platelet secretion response to thrombin and collagen is impaired, but the response to ADP and epinephrine is normal or slightly reduced. Electron microscopy confirms the selective absence of α granules, with preservation of δ granules. A similar acquired α-granule deficiency has been recognized in patients who have undergone cardiopulmonary bypass. The bleeding diathesis is generally mild, although some patients who have sustained head trauma can hemorrhage severely.

α,δ-Storage pool deficiency is defined by moderate to severe defects in both α and δ granules. The defects of the δ granules are more pronounced than those of the α granules. The clinical and laboratory features are similar to those of δ-storage pool deficiency. In some patients, decreases in platelet alpha$_2$-adrenergic receptors and increases in GPIV have been found. An association between α,δ-storage pool deficiency and a predisposition to hematologic malignancies has also been reported. Platelet defects in arachidonic acid (AA) metabolism occur in approximately 20 per cent of all congenital platelet disorders. Liberation of arachidonic acid from platelet membrane phospholipids and subsequent enzymatic conversion to thromboxane A_2 (TXA_2) are essential steps in platelet activation. Inherited platelet defects in arachidonic acid metabolism include (1) impairment of arachidonic acid release from platelet membrane phospholipids; (2) deficiency in cyclooxygenase (the enzyme required to convert arachidonic acid to the prostaglandins PGH_2 and PGG_2 prior to TXA_2 formation); and (3) deficiency in thromboxane synthase. The clinical aspects and management of these defects are similar to those of the other platelet secretion defects.

The complex process of platelet activation involves binding of the stimuli to the membrane receptor, signal transduction, phosphoinositol metabolism that results in calcium mobilization and phosphorylation of proteins, arachidonic acid metabolism leading to TXA_2 production, and release of platelet granule contents. Congenital defects in any of these steps result in impaired platelet-to-platelet aggregation and secretion. Abnormalities of signal transduction pathways usually produce only mild clinical bleeding tendencies. Therapy is generally not required.

Defects in Platelet Procoagulant (Scott Syndrome)

In contrast to patients with other congenital platelet disorders, patients with Scott syndrome do not have a tendency to bruise easily and do not bleed after small incisions, but they can bleed severely after tooth extractions or develop hypermenorrhea, postpartum bleeding, or even spontaneous pelvic hemorrhages.

The laboratory diagnosis of Scott syndrome requires the demonstration of impaired platelet factor 3, with normal platelet aggregation, platelet secretion, and BT. The patient's platelets fail to facilitate thrombin generation in vivo. Abnormalities in translocation of phosphatidylserine to the platelet outer membrane result in impaired binding of activated factors (Va, Xa, and IXa).

Acquired Platelet Disorders

Acquired qualitative platelet defects are far more common than the inherited qualitative platelet disorders. Platelet dysfunction occurs with the intake of multiple medications, foods, and food additives (Table 9) and in association with a wide variety of acquired clinical conditions (Table 10). Unlike the case with inherited platelet disorders, in which a single platelet function is affected, in the acquired platelet disorders, multiple platelet functional defects are found. In some disorders, the nature of the defect is unclear.

Systemic Disorders

Uremia (uremic bleeding, uremic hemostatic defect, acquired platelet dysfunction in uremia) is associated with frequent and sometimes fatal bleeding. Its incidence has declined with improved treatment of the underlying disorders, dialysis, and avoidance of antiplatelet agents. However, in patients undergoing invasive and surgical procedures, bleeding can still be a serious problem. The major hemostatic defects are thought to be dysfunctional platelets and impaired platelet–vessel wall interaction. Other factors that occur infrequently in uremia but that may

Table 9. Drugs and Foods That Can Cause Platelet Dysfunction

Drug	Mechanism
Aspirin, nonsteroidal anti-inflammatory agents	Inhibition of cyclooxygenase
Dazoxiben	Inhibition of thromboxane synthase
Ticlopidine	Interference with glycoprotein IIb-IIIa receptor
Omega-3 fatty acids	Competition with arachidonate
Dipyridamole, methylxanthines	Phosphodiesterase inhibition, ↑ cAMP
Prostaglandins I_2, D_2, and E	Adenylate cyclase activators, ↑ cAMP
Penicillins, cephalosporins	Interference with agonist receptor interactions, ↓ TXA_2 and inhibition of Ca^{2+} mobilization
Nitrofurantoin	Signal transduction inhibition (?)
Hydroxychloroquine	Signal transduction inhibition (?)
Thrombolytic therapy (streptokinase, urokinase, tissue plasminogen activator)	Proteolysis of platelet membrane GP, inhibition of TXA_2
Anticoagulants (heparin)	Interference with platelet aggregation receptor
Beta-blockers	Inhibition of AA release, ↓ TXA_2, competition with serotonin uptake
Calcium channel blockers	Interference with Ca^{2+} flux
Nitroglycerin	↑ PGI_2, ↑ nitric oxide
Nitroprusside	↑ cGMP
Quinidine	Interference with agonist receptor
Tricyclic antidepressants	(?) Interference with agonist receptors
Anesthetics (halothane)	↓ platelet aggregation; mechanism unclear
Chemotherapeutic agents (daunorubicin, BCNU, mitomycin)	Inhibition of aggregation and secretion; (?) mechanism
Dextrans	Interference with GP receptors, ↓ Platelet factor 3
Lipid-lowering agents (Lopid [gemfibrozil], clofibrate)	Competitive inhibitor with membrane agonist receptors
ϵ-Aminocaproic acid	Mechanism unknown
Antihistamines	Competitive inhibition of agonist receptor (?)
Ethanol	↓ AA metabolism
Vitamin E	↓ AA metabolism
Radiographic contrast agents	Inhibition of intracellular Ca^{2+} flux, inhibition of signal transduction receptor (?)
Foods and food additives	
Chinese black tree fungus	Inhibition of AA metabolism
Onion, cumin, tumeric, garlic	Inhibition of AA metabolism

BCNU = *bis*-chloroethyl-nitrosourea, carmustine; cAMP = cyclic adenosine monophosphate; cGMP = cyclic guanosine monophosphate; AA = arachidonic acid.

Table 10. Conditions Associated With Acquired Qualitative Platelet Disorders

Systemic Disorders
Uremia
Cardiopulmonary bypass
Acquired storage pool disorders
Antiplatelet antibodies
Liver disease
Miscellaneous
Hematologic Disorders
Myeloproliferative disorders
Essential thrombocytosis
Polycythemia vera
Chronic myelogenous leukemia
Agnogenic myeloid metaplasia
Acute leukemias
Myelodysplastic syndromes
Dysproteinemias
Acquired von Willebrand's disease

contribute to bleeding include reduction in blood coagulation factors and thrombocytopenia. The prolongation in BT correlates with clinical bleeding. Bleeding into skin and mucous membranes (gastrointestinal or genitourinary tracts) is frequent, while intracranial, pericardial, deep visceral, and retroperitoneal hemorrhages are rare.

Multiple platelet abnormalities are recognized. Platelet production can be defective (low megakaryocyte ploidy). Decreased platelet factor 3, prolonged BT, and flawed platelet adhesion are consistent defects. Other irregularities include impairment of platelet aggregation and secretion to various agonists, storage pool disease, and interference with intracellular Ca^{2+} mobilization. Results of vWF measurements in plasma are variable and include normal to high concentrations and a multimeric pattern that is either normal or defective in high-molecular-weight multimers. Interactions between platelet membrane GPIIb-IIIa and vWF are reduced. Prostacyclin production by endothelial cells is increased, this increase adding to the platelet dysfunction. The anemia of renal failure represents yet another factor contributing to clinical bleeding. The causes of the "uremic platelet defects" are complex, but strong evidence exists that uremic retention "toxins" directly affect platelets as well as the vessel wall.

Patients undergoing cardiopulmonary bypass (CPB) develop a consistent coagulopathy characterized by thrombocytopenia, platelet dysfunction, reduced plasma coagulation factors, and, occasionally, excessive fibrinolysis. Platelet dysfunction, however, represents the major hemostatic defect responsible for the excessive bleeding that occurs in 5 per cent of postoperative patients. Intraoperative bleeding occurs from multiple sites, but postoperative hemorrhage is seen primarily from chest tubes and surgical incisions.

Platelet counts drop by 50 per cent during CPB in most patients and may not return to preoperative levels for several days. The causes of the thrombocytopenia are hemodilution, retention of platelets in the bypass circuitry, and platelet activation followed by rapid platelet clearance. Cardiopulmonary bypass causes prolongation of the BT out of proportion to the thrombocytopenia, and impairment of platelet aggregation in response to ristocetin. The severity of the platelet defects correlate with the duration of the CPB, and the defects typically resolve on completion of the procedure.

Depletion of platelet granules (α, δ) has been reported in association with a variety of clinical conditions, including steroid therapy, systemic lupus erythematosus, chronic immune thrombocytopenia, DIC, thrombotic thrombocytopenic purpura, hemolytic-uremic syndrome, renal transplant rejection, myeloproliferative disorders, hairy cell leukemia, acute myelogenous leukemia, and severe cardiac valvular disease, and in patients with Dacron aortic grafts and those undergoing cardiopulmonary bypass. The clinical and laboratory features and management are identical to those of the congenital storage pool disorders described above.

Although platelets contain IgG in their α granules, binding of an autoantibody or alloantibody to platelet membrane receptors (GPIb, GPIIb, GPIIIa, and GPIV) leads to impairment of platelet response to various stimuli and/or to platelet destruction. Platelet activation also occurs. The overall impact of antiplatelet antibodies is an acquired bleeding diathesis secondary to both thrombocytopenia and platelet dysfunction. These disorders include acute and chronic immune thrombocytopenic purpura that is either idiopathic or secondary to other diseases, such as lymphoproliferative disorders, Graves' disease, lupus, collagen vascular disorders, or HIV infection. The BT is generally normal in acute immune thrombocytopenic purpura and is prolonged in the chronic form. Impaired platelet aggregation to ADP, epinephrine, collagen, arachidonic acid, and ristocetin occurs in both. Because antiplatelet antibodies cause platelet dysfunction, a BT should be performed in patients undergoing surgical procedures, even if the platelet count exceeds 50,000 cells/mm^3.

Liver disease of various causes is often associated with a bleeding diathesis attributable to many factors, such as deficiency of blood coagulation factors, increased fibrinolysis and decreased fibrinolytic inhibitors, thrombocytopenia, and platelet dysfunction.

The qualitative platelet defects in liver disease include prolongation of the BT out of proportion to the platelet number, reduced platelet aggregation, impaired platelet adhesion, decreased platelet factor 3, and diminished platelet survival. Platelet TXA_2 is altered owing to a defect in the release of free arachidonic acid from platelet membrane phospholipids. A dialyzable factor present in the plasma of cirrhotic patients has been shown to interfere with platelet aggregation. Excessive plasmin formation in the circulation may alter platelet membrane glycoproteins and phospholipids and explain the platelet defects.

In DIC, patients exhibit abnormal platelet aggregation and storage pool disorders owing to platelet activation in vivo by thrombin and other agonists. The low plasma fibrinogen activity may account, in part, for the reduction in platelet aggregation. Excess plasmin production or increased FDPs may also alter the platelet receptors. Qualitative platelet defects have been detected in many disorders, including infectious mononucleosis, adult respiratory distress syndrome, cyanocobalamin (vitamin B_{12}) deficiency, eosinophilia, allergies, asthma occurring with hay fever, Bartter's syndrome, congenital heart disease, and hypothyroidism.

Hematologic Disorders

A bleeding tendency, thromboembolic complications, and qualitative platelet defects are found in all myeloproliferative disorders, including essential thrombocytosis, polycythemia vera, chronic myelogenous leukemia, and agnogenic myeloid metaplasia or myelofibrosis myeloid metaplasia. These complications are a significant cause of morbidity and mortality. Mortality in the myeloproliferative disorders is estimated to be 10 per cent from bleeding and 40 per cent from thrombosis.

Essential thrombocytosis (ET, essential thrombocythemia, idiopathic thrombocythemia, hemorrhagic thrombocythemia) is a myeloproliferative disorder characterized by autonomous proliferation of an abnormal clone of megakaryocytes that are unresponsive to the normal control mechanisms of platelet production. This disorder affects both sexes and occurs predominantly in middle-aged to older individuals. The paradox of bleeding and thrombosis can occur simultaneously. The bleeding occurs predominantly from mucocutaneous sources. The thromboembolic phenomena consist of transient ischemic attacks, stroke, myocardial infarction, hepatic and mesenteric vein thrombosis, and microvascular occlusion involving the digits (erythromelalgia, digital syndrome). Splenomegaly occurs in 80 per cent of patients.

Platelet counts in essential thrombocytosis range from 500,000 cells/mm^3 to more than 1 million. The platelets on the peripheral smear show clumps and bizarre forms, with occasional fragments of megakaryocytes. Patients develop mild iron deficiency anemia owing to gastrointestinal bleeding, and a mild leukocytosis is typical. Bone marrow biopsy shows a marked increase in the megakaryocytic mass, which may be dysplastic, as well as eosinophilia and basophilia. Leukocyte alkaline phosphatase (LAP), serum uric acid, and vitamin B_{12} concentrations all are increased. Pseudohyperkalemia is common because of in vitro loss of potassium from platelets clumping in the test tube. The BT may be prolonged or normal and has no predictive value for bleeding. Platelet aggregation is impaired. The most consistent and characteristic defect in essential thrombocytosis is the absence of or a marked reduction in epinephrine-induced platelet aggregation (absence or reduction of primary wave) due to a deficiency of platelet alpha$_2$-adrenergic receptors. Deficiencies in platelet membrane glycoproteins and defects of platelet secretion (α,δ-granule deficiency) have been reported, as has increased TXA_2 production. The concentration of platelet factor 3 is increased in patients with thromboembolic complications but is decreased in those with bleeding. The platelet defects described above result from the "abnormal clone" of megakaryocytes.

Essential thrombocytosis must be differentiated from secondary thrombocytosis (from causes such as collagen vascular disorders and malignancies). The diagnosis is facilitated by the clinical association of bleeding and thrombotic complications, both of which are absent in secondary thrombocythemia. In asymptomatic patients, demonstration of persistent thrombocytosis and absence of epinephrine-induced platelet aggregation support the diagnosis of essential thrombocytosis.

In polycythemia vera, thromboembolic events, both arterial and venous, are far more common than bleeding complications. However, patients undergoing surgical procedures are at a high risk for developing both thrombotic and hemorrhagic problems. The factors involved include hyperviscosity, blood stasis, intravascular coagulation, and qualitative platelet defects.

The most consistent platelet function defect is hypoaggregation in response to ADP, epinephrine, and collagen, which occurs in fewer than half of the patients. Reduced platelet adhesion is seen in 18 per cent. Prolongation of the BT is infrequent. By electron microscopy, 80 per cent of patients with polycythemia vera have decreased platelet density. The decreased platelet survival reported in patients with thromboembolic complications suggests in vivo platelet activation. Activation of the blood coagulation system has also been observed in asymptomatic patients with hematocrits ranging from 40 to 45 per cent. Whether activation of the coagulation system and platelets is the cause or an effect of the thrombotic events is unclear. Other platelet abnormalities in polycythemia vera include defects in platelet membrane glycoproteins, storage pool abnormalities, and acquired von Willebrand's disease (or vWD) due to IgG inhibitors of vWF.

In comparison to the other myeloproliferative disorders, bleeding and thrombosis occur less frequently in chronic myelogenous leukemia. When bleeding is present, it has the characteristic features of a qualitative bleeding disorder. During the chronic phase of chronic myelogenous leukemia, platelet counts are normal, but when patients enter the accelerated phase or a blastic crisis, thrombocytopenia is present and contributes to the bleeding diathesis. The qualitative platelet defects include impaired adhesion and aggregation, prolonged bleeding time, storage pool abnormalities, decreased platelet secretion (TXA_2), acquired von Willebrand's disease, and decreased plasma factor V activity (possibly due to absorption of factor V by platelets and leukocytes). The bone marrow biopsy in chronic myelogenous leukemia reveals megakaryocytes unable to develop high ploidy.

The platelets in patients with myelofibrosis myeloid metaplasia are the most hypofunctional of all the myeloproliferative disorders. Bleeding in patients with thrombocytosis is common, but thromboembolic complications are rare. Prolonged BT and impaired platelet adhesion are more pronounced in myelofibrosis myeloid metaplasia than in all the other myeloproliferative disorders. Bizarre, vacuolated, and degranulated platelets, including fragments of megakaryocytes, are observed in the peripheral smear. Platelet aggregation, platelet factor 3, and platelet secretion are markedly impaired in 68 per cent of patients.

In acute leukemia and myelodysplastic syndromes, the most common cause of bleeding is thrombocytopenia. Patients with normal or increased platelet counts, however, may also have a mucocutaneous bleeding diathesis. Acquired platelet defects associated with bleeding are found in acute leukemias, hairy cell leukemia, and myelodysplastic syndromes. Laboratory findings include decreased aggregation (in response to ADP, epinephrine, and collagen), reduced platelet secretion, acquired storage pool abnormalities (δ granules), decreased platelet factor 3 activity, and acquired vWF-like defect in hairy cell leukemia. In acute leukemias and myelodysplastic syndromes, the bone marrow biopsy reveals dysplastic megakaryocytes that, in some patients, are decreased in number. In myelodysplastic syndromes, the platelets have a balloonlike appearance and are devoid of δ granules. The qualitative platelet abnormalities may result from defective platelet production in the marrow.

Qualitative platelet defects occur in 33 per cent of patients with IgA multiple myeloma and Waldenström's macroglobulinemia, in 15 per cent of patients with IgG multiple myeloma, and infrequently in patients with monoclonal gammopathy of unknown significance. Bleeding results from thrombocytopenia, altered blood coagulation factors, inhibitors of blood coagulation factors (factors V and VIII), and hyperviscosity. The BT is prolonged. Platelet factor 3 production and platelet adhesion, aggregation, and secretion all are impaired. The mechanism of these defects involves binding of the paraprotein to glycoproteins (GPIIIa and GPIb) and subsequent interference with platelet stimulation and secretion. An acquired von Willebrand's disease has been reported as well.

Acquired von Willebrand's disease occurs in individuals

older than 40 years of age who do not have a previous history of mucocutaneous bleeding. The associated disorders include collagen vascular disorders, myeloproliferative disorders, lymphoproliferative disorders, monoclonal gammopathies, gastrointestinal angiodysplasia, congenital cardiac defects, and Wilms' tumor. The typical laboratory evaluation reveals a prolonged BT, a normal or increased platelet count, and a prolonged APTT. Factor VIII, vWF antigen, and vWF function (ristocetin cofactor) all are decreased. Ristocetin-induced platelet aggregation is impaired. Multimeric analysis of vWF shows absence of high-molecular-weight multimers and an abnormal multimer "triplet" pattern. Some patients with acquired von Willebrand's disease have autoantibody production against vWF. In patients with lymphoproliferative disorders, the abnormal lymphocytes either produce an inhibitor or accelerate the clearance of vWF.

Drug-Induced Platelet Dysfunction

Drug-induced platelet defects represent a major cause of acquired platelet disorders. Although many drugs (see Table 9) alter platelet function in vitro, relatively few cause prolongation of the BT or clinical bleeding. The mechanisms by which many drugs affect platelet function are still largely unknown.

Aspirin (ASA) is the most common and relevant cause of platelet dysfunction in clinical medicine today, because it is so widely used. Aspirin inhibits platelets by acetylating and irreversibly inhibiting the enzyme cyclooxygenase. The effect lasts 5 to 7 days. Inhibition of cyclooxygenase prevents synthesis of cyclic endoperoxides (PGH_2 and PGG_2) and TXA_2. The latter is necessary for contraction of the platelet tubular system, mobilization of Ca^{2+}, and secretion of platelet granule contents. Thus, after ingestion of aspirin (325 mg), platelet prostaglandin synthesis is blocked, this block causing prolongation of the BT and impairment of secondary platelet aggregation and secretion. Because aspirin has an additive effect, ingestion of 80 mg/day for 3 days or 40 mg for 5 days can achieve the same platelet inhibition as 325 mg given once. Although these small doses of aspirin inhibit both platelet and endothelial cell cyclooxygenase irreversibly, the effect endures only in the platelets because the endothelial cells are able to resynthesize cyclooxygenase. Aspirin prolongs the BT in normal individuals (males and females) by one to two times, but the effect can be much more profound in patients who have underlying congenital or acquired platelet defects. After aspirin is discontinued, the BT may be prolonged for up to 4 days, but platelet aggregation remains abnormal for the entire life span of the platelets.

Nonsteroidal anti-inflammatory agents (e.g., indomethacin) inhibit cyclooxygenase reversibly, and the effect is usually short-lived (less than 24 hours). Piroxicam is an exception, because it has a long half-life. Drugs such as ibuprofen, suldinac, and phenylbutazone have been used in the management of arthritis in hemophiliacs, apparently without causing abnormal bleeding. However, ibuprofen should be avoided in hemophiliacs with HIV who are receiving zidovudine (AZT) because it causes severe bleeding.

Ticlopidine differs from aspirin in its mechanism of antiplatelet action. It prolongs the BT more than aspirin by two to five times, and the effects of both drugs are additive. Ticlopidine's effects on platelet aggregation and BT occur within 24 to 48 hours after intake, are maximal at 6 days, and persist for 4 to 10 days after discontinuation of the drug. Ticlopidine impairs fibrinogen binding to platelet GPIIb-IIIa and thus causes abnormal platelet adhesion, a prolonged BT and inhibition of platelet stimulation by various agonists (decreased platelet aggregation and secretion).

Most penicillins cause a dose-dependent prolongation of the BT and clinical bleeding. These drugs include carbenicillin, penicillin G, ticarcillin, ampicillin, nafcillin, cloxacillin, mezlocillin, and piperacillin. The antiplatelet effect takes 2 to 3 days to become apparent and lasts from 3 to 10 days after the drug is discontinued. Cephalosporins likewise impair platelet function.

The only cardiovascular agents that can prolong the BT mildly are nitroprusside at infusion rates of 6 to 8 μg/kg per minute and inhalation of nitric oxide. Calcium channel blockers, beta-blockers, and nitroglycerin impair platelet aggregation and secretion slightly but do not cause prolongation of the BT. Quinidine at high concentrations can prolong the BT and potentiate the effect of aspirin. The mechanism of the antiplatelet effect is largely unknown. Beta-blockers appear to interfere with platelet membrane receptors, compete with serotonin uptake, inhibit the release of arachidonic acid from phospholipids, and reduce TXA_2 synthesis.

Heparin predisposes to bleeding through its anticoagulant effect, by causing thrombocytopenia, and also by impairing platelet function. Bleeding during fibrinolytic therapy results from multiple mechanisms involving the effect of plasmin on blood coagulation factors and platelets and from dissolution of hemostatic plugs at areas of vascular abnormality or breach. Plasmin formation in vivo causes platelet activation, degradation of platelet membrane GPIb, inhibition of TXA_2 production, and disaggregation of platelet plugs. ε-Aminocaproic acid at high doses (greater than 24 g/day) prolongs the BT.

Infusions of dextrans cause clinical bleeding with prolongation of the BT, and impairment of platelet factor 3 production, and platelet adhesion, aggregation, and secretion. Dextrans are absorbed to platelet membranes and alter platelet interaction with adhesive proteins and agonists. Fish oils, rich in omega-3 fatty acids, cause slight prolongation of the BT by reducing the arachidonic acid content of platelets and competing with arachidonic acid for cyclooxygenase.

BLEEDING DUE TO INTRAVASCULAR COAGULATION AND FIBRINOLYSIS

By Martin D. Phillips, M.D.
Houston, Texas

The term disseminated intravascular coagulation (DIC) is used to describe the end result of a variety of severe derangements in the coagulation and fibrinolytic systems. Owing to the diverse causes and clinical manifestations, no single term is sufficient to describe the imbalance that develops between the initiation of blood coagulation, the failure of normal control mechanisms, and the breakdown of the resulting thrombi. Other terms that describe certain aspects of DIC are consumption coagulopathy, which refers to the hemorrhage that results chiefly from the consumption of platelets and fibrinogen; defibrination syndrome, which is self-explanatory; and purpura fulminans—acute necrosis of patches of skin, which may result from DIC, some infections, "loading" doses of warfarin, or congenital deficiencies of protein C or S. DIC may also be acute or chronic. Chronic DIC is also called compensated DIC.

DIC is a clinical syndrome that results from overactivation of the factors that initiate blood coagulation. Two axioms guide the diagnosis and therapy of DIC: (1) DIC is a thrombotic disorder, although paradoxically the manifestations of DIC are hemorrhagic, and (2) DIC is not a primary hemostatic disorder but is almost always secondary to another disease process (Table 1).

All of these diseases have in common the capacity to initiate coagulation. Coagulation is typically activated by the exposure of blood to thrombogenic surfaces such as subendothelium or smooth muscle, or by the activation of monocytes or macrophages and the expression of tissue factor on their surfaces. With snakebites, or rarely cancer, proteases that directly activate the coagulation factor proenzymes may be introduced. When the stimulus to initiate coagulation exceeds the capacity of the local controlling mechanisms, activated clotting factors are released into the circulation, and generalized or disseminated coagulation reactions follow. They may result in hemorrhage due to the consumption of coagulation factors and platelets or may lead to thrombosis of veins or arteries.

PRESENTATION

Acute DIC most commonly presents as a hemorrhagic disorder, although thrombosis of superficial or deep veins or distal arteries (acral cyanosis or thrombosis) is not infrequent. Typical presentations include oozing of blood from venipuncture sites, intravenous catheter sites, or surgical wounds; petechiae, purpura, or ecchymoses; a decreasing platelet count; or a prolongation of the prothrombin time (PT) or activated partial thromboplastin time (APTT). Bleeding from mucous membranes, the respiratory tract, or the gastrointestinal tract may also occur. Paradoxically, a coagulopathy can coexist with deep venous thrombosis (with or without pulmonary embolism) or arterial thrombosis (typically of small distal arteries such as digital arteries). Thrombi can develop even when the patient appears to have undergone therapeutic anticoagulation. Rarely, the PT, APTT, or thrombin time is shorter than the normal control values owing to circulating activated clotting factors.

The spectrum of diseases that can be complicated by acute DIC is wide (see Table 1). Most common are bacteremia, with or without sepsis syndrome, due to gram-positive or gram-negative bacteria; fungemia; obstetric complications including abruptio placentae, amniotic fluid embolism, or retained products of conception with infection or tissue necrosis; snakebite; and trauma. Brain tissue is exceptionally thrombogenic; therefore, head trauma or destructive lesions within the central nervous system are potent initiators of DIC. Circulatory shock is associated with many of the conditions that cause DIC, and in a few patients it is the only discernible causative factor. Extensive intravascular hemolysis also has been implicated.

Chronic, or compensated, DIC most commonly presents with signs or symptoms of thrombosis. The "compensation" is tenuous, so hemorrhage may ensue at any point. Chronic DIC may complicate certain malignancies, especially adenocarcinomas (Trousseau's syndrome); certain vascular lesions such as cavernous hemangiomas (the Kasabach-Merritt syndrome) or an aneurysm with a false lumen; or an incomplete abortion with retained products of conception.

Table 1. Conditions Associated with Disseminated Intravascular Coagulation

Usually Acute
Sepsis (bacteria, fungi)
Trauma, burns
Obstetric complications
Abruptio placentae
Amniotic fluid embolism
Retained products of conception
Snakebites
Infections: *Rickettsia,* viruses, malaria
Acute leukemia (especially promyelocytic)
Acute hemolytic transfusion reaction
Peritoneovenous shunt
Intravenous infusions
Prothrombinase complexes, factor VIIa
Factor IX (older formulations)
Lipid suspensions
Shock, anaphylaxis
Usually Chronic
Cancer (particularly adenocarcinoma)
Giant hemangiomas (Kasabach-Merritt syndrome)
Vascular aneurysms or dissection, vascular grafts
Vasculitis

COURSE

Because DIC is not one entity but is virtually always a complication of another primary disease, the course is dictated by the progress of the underlying disorder. If the primary disorder is readily treated (such as the delivery of a fetus whose placenta has begun to separate or the surgical replacement of an aortic aneurysm), complete correction of the DIC will follow immediately. However, in massive trauma or septic shock, the derangements of coagulation may be progressive and improve only slowly with supportive care and treatment of the underlying disease. For unknown reasons, the manifestations of DIC can change from hemorrhage to thrombosis, or both may coexist.

PHYSICAL EXAMINATION

The physical examination should document the sites and extent of hemorrhage, searching for evidence of venous or arterial thrombosis and elucidating any underlying illness that could cause DIC. Close attention should be paid to hemorrhage from surgical wounds, intravenous or catheterization sites, mucous membranes, or skin.

LABORATORY TESTING

There is no one test or battery of tests that makes or excludes the diagnosis of DIC. The finding of increased fibrin(ogen) degradation products (FDPs, formerly called fibrin(ogen) split products [FSPs]), including D-dimers, on occasion is equated with DIC, but this is an oversimplification. A constellation of abnormal coagulation test results in an appropriate clinical situation comprises the syndrome of DIC. Serial testing may be helpful because a single "snapshot" may not accurately reflect a dynamic process.

Platelets, fibrinogen, and some coagulation factors are acute-phase reactants; that is, the physiologic stress associated with the illness that initiated the DIC can also cause the concentrations of these factors to be increased in the absence of DIC. Therefore, a value within the reference range may be the product of an acute phase reaction with superimposed DIC.

The most helpful tests are the PT, APTT, platelet count, fibrinogen concentration, and FDPs (Table 2). As noted previously, typically the PT and APTT become prolonged and may be mildly to markedly so, depending on the stage of the illness. In a few patients, either or both may be shorter than the control range, reflecting the activation of the coagulation system in vivo. This is neither sensitive nor specific but may be a clue to the diagnosis.

The platelet count decreases commensurate with the degree of DIC but is rarely less than 20,000/μL. The fibrinogen concentration will also decrease, typically to 50 to 150 mg/dL. Again, serial measurements may be helpful. Both platelets and fibrinogen are "acute-phase reactants," so their plasma concentrations may be increased in some stressful situations, and a single normal value may indicate that a significant decline is in progress.

Fibrin(ogen) degradation products are the hallmark of DIC. A specific fibrin degradation product, the D-dimer, is becoming more widely used, because the assay is technically simpler than the latex bead agglutination test for FDPs and can be performed on a standard citrated blood sample. Note that FDPs and D-dimers are physiologically increased when a thrombus is being remodeled (e.g., less than 10 days postoperatively or after an episode of venous thrombosis) or pathologically increased in severe liver or renal dysfunction. Rarely, some abnormal fibrinogen molecules can cause a falsely positive FDP (but not D-dimer) result. Most D-dimer assays are less sensitive than the FDP assay but are still sufficiently sensitive for most clinical applications.

Chronic DIC can exhibit any of these laboratory abnormalities. Typically, the platelets and fibrinogen are in the lower end of the reference range, and the PT can be slightly prolonged. The FDPs and D-dimers are usually moderately increased.

Schistocytes can be observed on the blood film in about one fourth of patients with acute DIC. They are nearly always present in chronic DIC; however, the difficulty in quantitation and the lack of specificity of this finding limit its usefulness. The finding of prominent schistocytosis, thrombocytopenia, and microvascular thrombosis should raise the possibility of thrombotic thrombocytopenic purpura (see further on).

The thrombin time is frequently prolonged. This test is dependent on fibrinogen; as the fibrinogen concentration decreases to less than 100 mg/dL, the thrombin time becomes prolonged. Also, FDPs can interfere with the polymerization of fibrin in vitro. The thrombin time is sensitive to even small increases in the concentration of FDP. Once the diagnosis of DIC is established, the thrombin time usually is not helpful.

Antithrombin III (AT-III) is frequently consumed in DIC. Studies are in progress to determine whether the replacement of AT-III will alter the course of DIC. AT-III measurements are not helpful in the diagnosis of DIC and should be obtained only if AT-III replacement is being considered.

It is possible to measure the plasma concentration of the peptides released by the activation of prothrombin to thrombin ("F_{1+2}") or of fibrinogen to fibrin ("fibrinopeptides A and B"). Although these are useful research assays to measure the degree of activation of the coagulation system, they add nothing to the clinical diagnosis of DIC. Soluble or circulating fibrin monomer also has been proposed to distinguish DIC from "primary fibrinolysis." If the latter does exist as a separate entity, the pathogenesis and current treatment are the same as those for DIC, and the clinical distinction is not important.

Tests that clearly are not indicated are bleeding time and platelet autoantibodies. FDPs can inhibit platelet function and prolong the bleeding time. However, the bleeding time is prolonged in any thrombocytopenic state, is variably prolonged with anemia or hypofibrinogenemia, and will not affect either the diagnosis or management of any of these conditions. Platelet autoantibodies are sometimes measured in an attempt to discern the cause of thrombocytopenia. However, this test is unreliable as performed in most clinical laboratories and should not be used in the decision to alter treatment. This test should not be confused with the test for heparin-associated antibodies. The latter have the capacity to aggregate platelets and are the cause of the heparin-induced thrombocytopenia syndrome (see further on). The test for heparin-associated antibodies is sensitive and specific, and is useful in the appropriate situation.

Table 2. Tests for Disseminated Intravascular Coagulation

Tests
Very Useful
Platelet count: decreasing
PT, APTT: usually prolonged, occasionally shortened
Fibrinogen: decreasing
FDP, D-dimer: present
Schistocytosis
Less Useful
Thrombin time
AT-III
F_1+_2, FpA and B
Fibrin monomer
Factors VIII and V
No Value
Bleeding time
Platelet autoantibodies

DIC = disseminated intravascular coagulation; PT = prothrombin time; APTT = activated partial thromboplastin time; FDP = fibrinogen degradation products; AT-III = antithrombin III; F_1+_2 = activation of prothrombin to thrombin; FpA and B = fibrinopeptides A and B.

PITFALLS IN DIAGNOSIS

Some diseases with apparent similarities to DIC are compared in Table 3. The most difficult distinction to be made clinically is distinguishing fulminant hepatic failure from DIC. Both conditions are associated with coagulopathy, prolongation of the PT and APTT, increased FDP and D-dimers, and decreased fibrinogen concentration. The liver is the site of synthesis of all coagulation factors and is also a site for the clearance of FDPs from the plasma. In addition, some abnormal fibrinogen molecules made by a diseased liver can cause a falsely increased FDP (but not D-dimer) assay. Many of the conditions that are complicated by DIC, such as sepsis or trauma, may also be associated with liver dysfunction and thrombocytopenia. Therefore, in a seriously ill patient, it can be difficult to determine the cause of a prolonged PT and/or APTT, a low fibrinogen level, modestly elevated FDPs, thrombocytopenia, and abnormal liver function. Various surrogate

Table 3. Diagnostic Considerations

	PT, APTT, TT	Platelets	Fibrinogen	FDP, D-Dimer	Schistocytes
DIC	Usually prolonged May be shortened	Decreasing	Decreasing	Present	May be present
Liver failure	Prolonged	May be low	May be low	May be present	May be present
TTP	Usually normal	Low	Normal	Absent early	Present
ITP	Normal	Low	Normal	Absent	Absent
Heparin-induced thrombocytopenia	Normal, unless prolonged by heparin	Decreasing	Normal	Absent early	Absent

PT = prothrombin time; APTT = activated partial thromboplastin time; TT = thrombin time; FDP = fibrinogen degradation products; DIC = disseminated intravascular coagulation; TTP = thrombotic thrombocytopenic purpura; ITP = idiopathic thrombocytopenic purpura.

markers have been used: factor VIII (high in liver disease), factor V (low in DIC), or schistocytes (variably observed in DIC but also observed in splenic dysfunction); however, none of these is reliable in clinical practice. In fact, the distinction may be more semantic than clinically important. In either case, the patient would be very ill, underlying disorders would be actively sought and treated, and supportive measures for hemorrhage would be provided. The clinical finding that is distinctive is thrombosis, which is not associated with simple hepatic failure and is treated with anticoagulation and/or fibrinolytic agents.

Other disorders that have some similar features are thrombotic thrombocytopenic purpura (TTP), which causes thrombocytopenia, schistocytosis, and hemolytic anemia, and multiple organ dysfunction. The principal diagnostic difference is that the humoral coagulation system is not primarily affected in TTP. The PT, APTT, fibrinogen, FDP, and D-dimer assays are usually normal in TTP.

Heparin-induced thrombocytopenia is caused by antibodies directed against heparin complexed with platelet surface molecules, probably platelet factor 4. Acute heparin-induced thrombocytopenia presents clinically with a falling platelet count and paradoxical thrombosis. The thrombosis usually involves one or more large arteries, resulting in limb or myocardial ischemia in a patient being treated with heparin. Trace amounts of heparin, including subcutaneous prophylaxis or catheter flush doses are sufficient to induce this syndrome. In this disorder, as in TTP, the PT, fibrinogen, and FDP levels are likely to be normal. The APTT is prolonged only as a function of the concentration of heparin in the plasma. This disorder should be suspected in any patient in whom the platelet count decreases substantially or in whom arterial thrombosis develops while even trace amounts of heparin are being administered. The diagnostic laboratory test, called either "heparin-associated (platelet) antibodies" or "heparin platelet aggregation," is 75 per cent sensitive and 100 per cent specific.

Rare cases of congenital dysfibrinogenemia may cause thrombosis, a prolonged APTT, and an increased FDP assay (but not D-dimers). Typically, the antigenic fibrinogen assay is normal, but functional assays are slightly decreased. In the chronic setting, the history and lack of physical disorders are inconsistent with DIC. Acutely and in combination with other disorders the distinction is difficult. A history of previous thrombosis or a family history of dysfibrinogenemia is helpful.

HEMORRHAGIC DISEASES DUE TO CIRCULATING ANTICOAGULANTS

By Jeffry B. Lawrence, M.D.
Indianapolis, Indiana

Circulating anticoagulants are molecules, endogenous or exogenous in origin, that interfere with one or more components of the blood coagulation system. Circulating anticoagulants are observed in one of three clinical settings. Most commonly, circulating anticoagulants are observed in patients *without any clinical evidence of pathologic hemorrhage or thrombosis.* In these patients, abnormal results are observed in tests performed as part of coagulation screening (often before an invasive procedure). In hospitalized patients, the most frequent cause of this finding is probably heparin contamination of the blood sample, whereas the so-called lupus anticoagulant (LA) is most commonly detected in outpatients. In addition, patients without a previous history of coagulopathy may present with the *new onset of hemorrhage or thrombosis attributable to a circulating anticoagulant.* Among these conditions, an acquired antibody to factor VIII is the most commonly encountered specific coagulation factor inhibitor responsible for a hemorrhagic diathesis. Fibrin or fibrinogen degradation products (FDPs), observed in disseminated intravascular coagulation (DIC), and certain paraproteins are among the common acquired circulating anticoagulants that lead to bleeding, given the incidence of DIC and plasma cell dyscrasias. By contrast, the LA is the best recognized cause of an acquired thrombotic tendency. Finally, patients with an inherited coagulation factor deficiency may *acquire antibodies directed against the deficient protein in response to replacement therapy.* Hemophilia A is the most important example, and acquired factor VIII inhibitors can greatly complicate the clinical management of these patients.

A thorough clinical history and complete physical examination are essential for the evaluation of patients suspected of having circulating anticoagulants. Since many patients overlook diagnostically important hemorrhagic manifestations, whereas others overemphasize the importance of insignificant bleeding, the physician must explore any hemorrhagic events in detail. Ask the patient about petechiae, bruising, epistaxis, joint or muscle bleeds, and gingival, gastrointestinal, or genitourinary hemorrhage.

Obtain a detailed menstrual and obstetric history. Assess previous hemostatic challenges faced by the patient. Determine whether bleeding has occurred in response to minor trauma. Document major surgery and minor operative procedures, such as circumcision, tonsillectomy, and dental extractions. Detail any operative or postoperative hemorrhage, including the duration of bleeding after the procedure and whether blood transfusions were required. Compare present hemorrhagic (or thrombotic) manifestations with the patient's past medical and family history so that inherited conditions may be distinguished from acquired coagulopathies. Seek historical evidence of autoimmune disorders, malignancy, drug reactions, and recent use of medications. During the physical examination, carefully evaluate current hemorrhagic or thrombotic manifestations and seek evidence of the systemic disorders mentioned earlier.

LABORATORY EVALUATION

Careful, nontraumatic phlebotomy, use of plastic or siliconized glass tubes, and rapid processing of the patient's citrated blood sample are essential for the diagnostic evaluation of patients suspected of having circulating anticoagulants. Patients typically demonstrate a prolongation of the activated partial thromboplastin time (APTT) or prothrombin time (PT), or both. A mixing study is then employed to distinguish prolongation due to coagulation factor deficiency in the intrinsic (APTT) or extrinsic (PT) coagulation pathways from the presence of an inhibitor, or circulating anticoagulant, in the patient's plasma. A 1:1 mix is prepared, with equal volumes of the patient's plasma and normal plasma, and the previously prolonged coagulation test is repeated with the 1:1 mixture. If the latter assay is still prolonged, an inhibitor is implicated as the cause, whereas correction of the test with a 1:1 mix indicates a factor deficiency. When the coagulation test is minimally prolonged, differentiation between inhibitors and deficiency states can be difficult. However, such ambiguous studies are typically observed in asymptomatic patients in whom further diagnostic evaluation is not required. Nevertheless, when detection of weak inhibitors is clinically useful, detection can be enhanced by performing the mixing study at various ratios of normal to patient plasma. Some circulating anticoagulants (e.g., factor VIII inhibitors described further on) are time-dependent, requiring 1 to 2 hours of incubation at 37°C to demonstrate maximal in vitro inhibition. Thus, in patients with a prolonged APTT, the 1:1 mixing study should include APTT assays performed both immediately after preparing the mixture and after the mixture has been incubated for 1 or 2 hours. To control for deterioration of coagulation factor activity, the APTT result observed with prolonged incubation should be compared with a control consisting of a 1:1 mix prepared after the patient's plasma and normal plasma have been incubated separately for the same time and then mixed immediately prior to performing the APTT.

After the screening and 1:1 mixing studies, other coagulation tests are often required for appropriate evaluation of circulating anticoagulants. The thrombin time (TT) is determined by adding exogenous thrombin to the patient's citrated plasma and measuring the time required for conversion of fibrinogen to fibrin. The TT is prolonged in hypofibrinogenemia and dysfibrinogenemias. The presence of heparin or FDPs also prolongs the TT. A normal reptilase time plus a prolonged TT suggests the presence of a heparinlike inhibitor, since reptilase clots fibrinogen but is not inhibited by heparin. Coagulation factor assays using deficient substrate plasma are employed to establish the specificity of a circulating anticoagulant.

COAGULATION PROTEIN INHIBITORS

Inhibitors of Factors VIII and IX

The development of inhibitors to factor VIII and factor IX in transfused patients with hemophilia A and B, respectively, is discussed in the article on hemophilia. Spontaneously acquired factor VIII inhibitors are the most common clinically significant circulating anticoagulants other than FDP and paraproteins. These inhibitors are usually IgG antibodies (most commonly of the IgG4 subtype) directed at factor VIII, and they typically present with the dramatic onset of hemorrhage, often spontaneous massive bruising, or a hematoma. Inhibitors are most common in the elderly, with a peak incidence in the seventh decade of life. In about half of the patients, this circulating anticoagulant is associated with an underlying condition such as autoimmune disorders (including systemic lupus erythematosus [SLE], rheumatoid arthritis, inflammatory bowel disease, asthma, temporal arteritis, exfoliative dermatitis, psoriasis, dermatitis herpetiformis, erythema multiforme, or pemphigus), drug reaction (particularly penicillin, phenytoin, sulfa drugs, nitrofurazone, and phenylbutazone), malignancy (especially plasma cell dyscrasias), or the postpartum state. Most commonly, postpartum factor VIII inhibitors occur after the birth of the first child, and usually there is hemorrhage within weeks to months after delivery following an otherwise normal pregnancy. The postpartum circulating anticoagulants differ from other spontaneous factor VIII inhibitors in that most disappear spontaneously after 12 to 18 months. After resolution, anamnestic responses in subsequent pregnancies are uncommon.

Because of the complex kinetics governing their interaction with factor VIII, spontaneously acquired factor VIII inhibitors may incompletely neutralize factor VIII activity in vitro and still cause severe, life-threatening hemorrhage at factor activity levels that rarely cause spontaneous bleeding in uncomplicated hemophilia (i.e., 0.04 to 0.19 U/mL). Patients with acquired factor VIII inhibitors present with a prolonged APTT and a normal PT and TT. As discussed earlier, these antibodies typically require a 1- to 2-hour incubation at 37°C to maximally inhibit factor VIII activity in vitro. The diagnosis is confirmed by incubating a dilution of the patient's plasma with an equal volume of normal plasma and measuring residual factor VIII activity in samples removed after 2 hours. This Bethesda assay is used for quantifying the inhibitor, with 1 Bethesda unit/mL of plasma defined as the concentration of inhibitor necessary for reducing residual factor VIII activity by 50 per cent after a 2-hour incubation. Spontaneously acquired factor IX inhibitors are rare. The clinical settings in which they occur are similar to those associated with spontaneous anti–factor VIII circulating anticoagulants.

Inhibitors of von Willebrand Factor

Inhibitors of von Willebrand factor (vWF) are IgG antibodies directed against the vWf protein, which circulates in plasma in association with factor VIII and mediates platelet adherence to subendothelium. Although these antibodies may develop in response to replacement therapy in patients with severe von Willebrand's disease, most reported vWF inhibitors have arisen in patients who do not have this hereditary disorder. Acquired vWF inhibitors may develop in previously healthy individuals, or they may occur in patients with lymphoma, myeloproliferative disorders, plasma cell dyscrasias, autoimmune diseases, or hypothyroidism. In most patients, bleeding is mild to moderate, with epistaxis, bruising, and operative hemorrhage the most frequent manifestations. Laboratory studies typically demonstrate roughly parallel reductions in ristocetin cofactor activity, von Willebrand antigen levels, and factor VIII activity, along with a prolonged bleeding time. The patient's plasma impairs ristocetin cofactor activity of normal plasma, but such assays are difficult to standardize. In some patients, the best diagnostic test may be infusion of cryoprecipitate or a factor VIII concentrate rich in high molecular weight vWF multimers, followed by measurement of vWF parameters and the bleeding time. In patients with severe von Willebrand's disease, development of an inhibitor is heralded clinically by the loss of hemostatic response to cryoprecipitate or vWF-rich concentrate infusions.

Inhibitors of Factor XI

Approximately 30 cases of acquired factor XI inhibitors have been described in patients without factor XI deficiency, and approximately half that number have been described in factor XI–deficient patients. In each report, the inhibitor was an IgG antibody. Among the patients with spontaneous inhibitors, most were female, one third had SLE, and others had rheumatoid arthritis. Nearly all the affected males had either SLE or a procainamide-induced SLE-like syndrome. Just as in factor XI deficiency without inhibitors, clinical manifestations vary in severity, with most bleeding patients showing mild mucosal hemorrhage. Patients exhibit a prolonged APTT and a normal PT and TT, abnormal mixing studies, and depressed factor XI activity in mixing study samples.

Inhibitors of Factor V

Of the approximately 30 patients with factor V inhibitors reported in the literature, only 2 had factor V deficiency. The circulating anticoagulants appeared postoperatively in half of the reported patients, often in association with blood transfusions, whereas others were associated with drugs such as streptomycin, gentamicin, and penicillin as well as with tuberculosis, pancreatic disease, and malignancy, particularly myeloproliferative disorders. The hemorrhagic tendency associated with these circulating anticoagulants varies in severity, perhaps because of variability in the accessibility of platelet factor V to the factor V antibody. Some patients show significant hemostatic response to platelet transfusion therapy, even in the presence of a strong inhibitor; this may aid diagnosis. Most factor V inhibitors have been IgG antibodies; typically they are transient, disappearing in less than 6 months with or without immunosuppressive therapy. The APTT and PT are prolonged, whereas the TT is normal. The abnormal test results are not correctable in mixing studies, and demonstration that a mixture of the patient's plasma and normal plasma specifically lacks factor V procoagulant activity is required for definitive diagnosis. Some patients with chronic myeloid leukemia and acquired factor V deficiency have been reported to demonstrate in vivo unresponsiveness to fresh-frozen plasma infusions despite normal mixing studies.

Inhibitors of Factor XIII

Inhibitors of factor XIII are invariably associated with bleeding, which is usually severe. At least six deaths have been reported. Only 1 of the nearly 20 published examples occurred in an individual who was congenitally deficient in factor XIII. Nearly half of the reported examples were associated with isoniazid, but penicillin, phenytoin, and practolol have also been linked to this circulating anticoagulant. In patients with drug-associated inhibitors, discontinuation of the drug frequently results in disappearance of the anticoagulant. Since coagulation screening tests are normal in these patients (as is also observed in patients congenitally deficient in factor XIII), demonstration of impaired clot stability in urea in the absence of previous history of hemorrhage, suggesting congenital factor XIII deficiency, is presumptive evidence for an acquired factor XIII inhibitor. The urea clot stability test is a qualitative assay, and thus mixing studies are unlikely to be helpful. By contrast, measurement of factor XIII activity requires assays of transglutaminase performed only in research laboratories. Nevertheless, infusion of fresh-frozen plasma, with measurement of factor XIII recovery and survival, may be required for establishing a definitive diagnosis of an anti–factor XIII circulating anticoagulant.

Inhibitors of Fibrinogen and Fibrin Polymerization

The terminal phase of blood coagulation is characterized by thrombin-induced cleavage of fibrinopeptides A and B from fibrinogen to form fibrin monomers, spontaneous polymerization of these monomers, and cross-linking of polymerized fibrin by activated factor XIII. In addition to the factor XIII inhibitors described previously, rare examples of spontaneous inhibitors to each of the other terminal-phase coagulation reactions have been described, as have inhibitors complicating transfusion therapy in hereditary afibrinogenemia. In some patients, the spontaneous IgG inhibitors have been associated with SLE, chronic active hepatitis, ulcerative colitis, or Down syndrome. Moreover, monoclonal paraproteins, abnormal fibrinogens associated with liver disease, and FDPs arising from DIC can impair fibrinopeptide cleavage and/or fibrin polymerization, leading to friable clots that exhibit poor clot retraction. Except in DIC, patients with these circulating anticoagulants usually have either a mild hemorrhagic diathesis or no bleeding. Patients typically exhibit a prolonged APTT, PT, TT, and reptilase time. Mixing studies may demonstrate prolongation of the TT of normal plasma.

Inhibitors of Prothrombin and Thrombin

Except for the prothrombin antibody associated with the LA (see further on), spontaneous inhibitors of this protein are rare. The few patients reported have most frequently had SLE. Use of topical bovine thrombin during surgery has been associated with the development of anti–bovine thrombin antibodies that may cross-react with human thrombin. Some of these preparations also contain appreciable amounts of bovine factor V and other factors that have elicited similar cross-reacting antibodies. In some of these patients, severe hemorrhage may occur because of the acquired thrombin and/or factor V inhibitors. These patients exhibit prolonged APTT and PT assays that are uncorrectable in mixing studies.

Inhibitors of Factors VII, X, and XII

Only very rare examples of inhibitors directed against these coagulation factors have been described. A single example of a factor VII inhibitor has been reported in a patient with a pulmonary neoplasm who showed minor bleeding. Two poorly characterized examples of factor X inhibitors in leprosy have been described in patients without clinical bleeding. More commonly, however, an acquired factor X deficiency is observed in patients with systemic amyloidosis, some of whom have a hemorrhagic diathesis. Although such patients lack a circulating factor X inhibitor, the amyloid fibrils have been shown to selectively bind factor X and remove it from the circulation. Acquired factor XII antibodies have been observed in SLE, Waldenström's macroglobulinemia, and glomerulonephritis. Though lacking demonstrable circulating anticoagulants, some patients with angioimmunoblastic lymphadenopathy have been reported as developing an acquired factor XII deficiency. The factor XII inhibitors have not been associated with hemorrhage; however, one patient had thrombosis.

Heparinlike Anticoagulants

Spontaneously acquired heparinlike coagulation inhibitors have been described in patients with neoplasms, most commonly plasma cell malignancies, and in patients treated with suramin for adrenocortical carcinoma. Nearly all these patients had a severe hemorrhagic disorder accompanied by a prolonged APTT and PT and a markedly prolonged TT that does not correct in mixing studies but does correct after addition of protamine sulfate, toluidine blue, or heparinase to the patient's plasma. The reptilase time is normal.

LUPUS ANTICOAGULANTS AND ANTIPHOSPHOLIPID ANTIBODIES

The LA is an antibody (usually IgG or IgM but occasionally IgA) that prolongs phospholipid-dependent coagulation reactions by binding to anionic phospholipids, such as phosphatidylserine and phosphatidylinositol. Although this inhibitor was first described in patients with SLE, the term is a misnomer because the inhibitor is most frequently observed in patients who do not have lupus and is associated with thrombosis rather than abnormal bleeding. The antibody does not inhibit the activity of specific coagulation factors. Rather, it is detected by the prolongation it causes in phospholipid-dependent coagulation tests, such as the APTT, dilute Russell's viper venom time (DRVVT), the kaolin clotting time (KCT), the dilute phospholipid APTT, the dilute tissue thromboplastin inhibition test, and, to a lesser extent, the PT.

When the APTT is used for its detection, the LA is found in approximately 10 per cent of patients with SLE. However, with a more sensitive assay that uses less exogenous phospholipid, such as the DRVVT or KCT, the prevalence of LA in SLE is greater than 50 per cent. The LA is also observed in patients with other autoimmune disorders, human immunodeficiency virus (HIV) infection, acute viral syndromes, pregnancy, various neoplasms, and monoclonal gammopathies, and it has been associated with phenothiazine (especially chlorpromazine), hydralazine, and quinidine therapy. It is also very commonly observed as an incidental finding in coagulation screening tests performed in patients with no history of abnormal bleeding or thrombosis. Patients with the LA often have a biologic false-positive test result for syphilis related to the anticardiolipin antibodies (ACA) that frequently accompany the LA, as discussed further on.

Most patients with the LA do not experience abnormal bleeding. However, as many as 25 per cent of these patients have acquired hypoprothrombinemia caused by antiprothrombin antibodies that bind to prothrombin without neutralizing its in vitro procoagulant activity. The prothrombin antigen-antibody complexes are cleared, eventually leading to depressed plasma prothrombin concentrations. In addition, a number of patients with the LA experience thrombocytopenia, including as many as 40 per cent of SLE patients who have this circulating anticoagulant. Thus, patients with the LA are at risk for hemorrhage if they also have hypoprothrombinemia and/or thrombocytopenia.

By contrast, thrombosis has been reported in 25 to 60 per cent of patients with the LA, with an average incidence of 33 per cent in published reports. Thrombosis may be either arterial or venous, and recurrent spontaneous abortion due to placental thrombosis and infarcts is an important clinical complication associated with the LA. The risk of thrombosis is believed to be highest in patients with IgG LA antibodies, in patients with SLE, and in those with high-titer ACAs (see further on).

In most patients with the LA, the APTT is prolonged. This is not correctable in mixing studies, and incubation is not required for demonstrating the APTT prolongation in 1:1 mixtures. In fact, the clotting time of the mixture is often longer than that of the patient's plasma alone (cofactor effect). The PT is either normal or minimally to moderately prolonged. In patients in whom the APTT prolongation is equivocal, the more sensitive assays with dilute phospholipid, such as the DRVVT or KCT, demonstrate significant prolongation. To confirm the presence of the LA, it is necessary to demonstrate correction of the prolonged clotting tests after addition of exogenous phospholipid, for example, freeze-thawed platelets, liposomes containing phosphatidylserine, or rabbit brain phospholipid. Additional evidence in support of the diagnosis is the observation of low values for several clotting factors in one-stage assays based on the APTT, accompanied by increasing apparent values for the clotting factors with increasing dilutions of the test plasma in the assay system.

As noted previously, most patients with the LA harbor other antiphospholipid antibodies, including antibodies directed against cardiolipin, a normally sequestered antigen localized to the inner mitochondrial membrane. ACAs are measured by enzyme-linked immunosorbent assay (ELISA), and their presence is a risk factor for thrombosis, fetal wastage, and/or thrombocytopenia independent of the presence of the LA. Although most patients with the LA have elevated titers of ACA, some patients lack ACA, and some ACA-positive patients fail to demonstrate the LA.

HYPERCOAGULABLE STATES

By Houria I. Hassouna, M.D., Ph.D.
East Lansing, Michigan

The hypercoagulable state is a condition that places an individual at risk for thrombosis but does not, in and of itself, invariably lead to thrombosis. Diagnosis and management require an understanding of the mechanisms of the hypercoagulable state that enhance and maintain the production of thrombin in circulating blood while preventing progression to thrombosis. These mechanisms include (1) reactions that produce thrombin from prothrombin, (2) feedback loop mechanisms that affect the rate of thrombin production from prothrombin, and (3) the inactivation of thrombin in blood. The fibrinolytic system is involved in clot lysis—but not in thrombin production and inactivation. Fibrinolysis disorders relate to hypercoagulability through mechanisms discussed in the article on intravascular coagulation and fibrinolysis.

The hypercoagulable state has been defined as having the potential to develop thrombosis in association with hereditary and nonhereditary genetic mutations (Table 1). The most commonly encountered include (1) heterozygote antithrombin, protein C, and protein S nonsense mutation defects associated with both decreased protein concentrations and anticoagulant activity; (2) abnormal clotting factor V, which resists proteolytic degradation by protein C; (3) heterozygote antithrombin, protein C, and protein S missense mutation defects associated with normal protein concentrations and decreased anticoagulant activity; (4) inherited regional fibrinogen variants that decrease the rate of fibrin polymerization (the physiologic pathway for thrombin inactivation is via specific binding to fibrin and incorporation into the fibrin clot; fibrin produced from variant forms of fibrinogen does not effectively incorporate thrombin into clots); and (5) vascular malformations and congenital heart disease. Other genetic disorders with associated risk factors include diabetes, polycythemia rubra vera, sickle cell anemia, thalassemia, increased concentrations of lipoproteins, homocystinemia, hypertriglyceridemia, and paroxysmal nocturnal hemoglobinuria.

Acquired risk factors include (1) physiologic conditions, such as neonatal and postpartum states and pregnancy; (2) acquired coagulation and platelet disorders (thrombocytosis, fibrinogen variants, lupus anticoagulant, antiphospholipid antibodies, antithrombin deficiency, protein C deficiency, protein S deficiency), (3) cardiovascular diseases and procedures (mitral valve prolapse, heart failure, prosthetic heart valves, atrial fibrillation, hypertension with increased angiotensin II, injured vessel wall, valvular insufficiency, abdominal aortic surgery, angioplasty, coronary bypass, central venous catheters, other indwelling vascular access devices, cardiopulmonary bypass), (4) medical therapy (oral contraceptives, androgens, L-asparaginase, low warfarin anticoagulation, thrombolytic therapy, factor IX concentrates), (5) surgical intervention (hepatic resections, gynecologic surgery, hip replacements, laparoscopic cholecystectomy), (6) malignancy (acute promyelocytic leukemia, pancreatic and prostate cancers, metastatic tumors), (7) infection (gram-negative sepsis, acute pancreatitis), (8) nephrotic syndrome, and (9) cerebral infarcts.

The most intriguing aspect of hypercoagulable states is the low frequency with which they are associated with thrombosis. For example, in pregnancy and other acquired and inherited hypercoagulable states, the calculated incidence of associated thrombosis, although slightly higher than in the general population, is much less than 10 per cent. The low incidence of thrombosis in association with hypercoagulable states has not received deserved attention and is reviewed in this article with the intent of providing a basis of information necessary for establishing both a diagnosis and a plan of management for the hypercoagulable patient.

Table 1. Genetic Disorders Associated with Hypercoagulability

Hemostatic System	Other Systems
Antithrombin	Diabetes
Protein C	Polycythemia rubra vera
Protein S	Sickle cell anemia
Abnormal clotting factor V	Congenital heart disease
Fibrinogen variants	Thalassemia
	Elevated lipoprotein (a)
	Homocystinemia
	Hypertriglyceridemia
	Paroxysmal nocturnal hemoglobinuria

REGULATORY SYSTEMS THAT GOVERN THE HEMOSTATIC STATE

In contrast to hemostatic clots that form at the site of injury, hypercoagulability and thrombosis develop in circulating blood. The enzyme thrombin has a central regulatory role in hemostasis, and its participation in the pathology of hypercoagulability and thrombosis is well documented. Thrombin clots blood, slows the rate by which it is produced from prothrombin, and initiates the reaction by which it is irreversibly inactivated by antithrombin. In both hemostasis and thrombosis, thrombin enables the clotting of blood by limited proteolysis of two peptides from fibrinogen molecules, permitting spontaneous assembly to form a polymerized fibrin monomer network. It then catalyzes a step necessary for insolubilizing the polymerized fibrin network by proteolytic activation of factor XIII in the presence of calcium ions. It autoregulates its own generation so that more thrombin is produced at a faster rate through feedback loops that include (1) activation of nonenzymatic cofactors—factors V and VIII—and (2) binding of specific platelet receptors that unmask platelet phospholipid coagulant activity and initiate assembly and sequential activation of vitamin K–dependent factors. Finally, thrombin initiates platelet aggregation and its own entrapment in the fibrin network. Evidence exists that the balance between excess blood fluidity and hypercoagulability in the hemostatic state or basal state is governed by multigene interactions (thrombin-independent mechanisms) and that deregulation of these pathways can result in hypercoagulability.

REGULATION OF THE RATE OF PROTHROMBIN CONVERSION

The rate of formation of the clotting activity of thrombin is a function of the velocity of prothrombin conversion. If coagulation is triggered with identical amounts of tissue thromboplastin in the blood of two groups of individuals—one healthy and the other receiving oral anticoagulants—the velocity of prothrombin conversion is much greater in the group of healthy individuals. Similarly, with coagulation factor deficiencies or severe thrombocytopenia, the velocity of prothrombin conversion is decreased. Physiologic reactions that have a positive influence on the velocity of prothrombin conversion are listed in Table 2. Entry into the circulating blood of substances with pronounced tissue factor activity, such as placental or malignant tissues or certain bacteria, greatly enhances the velocity of prothrombin conversion.

Acquired or genetic factor deficiencies as well as thrombocytopenia and mechanical hindrance of complex assembly by antibodies directed against specific factor activities or against micelle phospholipids (antiphospholipid antibodies or lupuslike inhibitors) decrease the rate of prothrombin conversion. Antithrombin anticoagulant mechanisms (antithrombin, heparin cofactor II, histidine-rich glycoprotein) do not directly alter the rate of prothrombin conver-

Table 2. Reactions That Alter the Rate of Prothrombin Conversion in Blood

Reaction	Reaction Site	Reaction Components	Coagulation Factors Involved
Release	Cell membrane	Tissue factor*	Factor III
Activation	Platelets	Cell membrane phospholipids	Platelet factor 3 (procoagulant activity)
	Blood	Extrinsic pathway	Factor VII/factor VIIa
	Blood	Intrinsic pathway	Factor XIa, factor IXa
	Activated endothelial and mononuclear cells	Factor VIIa–tissue factor complex	Factor VIIa, factor X, Ca^{2+}, factor III,
		Tissue factor pathway inhibitor	Tissue factor pathway inhibitor
Complex formation	Platelet cell membrane phospholipids	Prothrombinase complex	Factor X, factor IXa, factor VIIIa, platelet factor 3, Ca^{2+}
	Platelet cell membrane phospholipids	Prothrombin complex	Factor Xa, factor Va, prothrombin, platelet factor 3, Ca^{2+}
Carboxylation	Microsomal membranes of hepatocytes and other cells	Vitamin K, glutamate residues of inactive vitamin K–dependent factors	Prothrombin, factor VII, factor IX, factor X, protein C, protein S

*Tissue factor previously known as tissue thromboplastin.

sion (Table 3). Factor XI and the factors of the contact phase of plasma activation function in the hemostatic state at different levels. A role for thrombin as the major activator of factor XI has been recently determined, removing the contact system from the intrinsic pathway. Three proteins (factor XII, prekallikrein, and high molecular weight kininogen) function in the generation of bradykinin and activation of coagulation on artificial surfaces and interaction with blood and vascular cells, including platelets, neutrophils, monocytes, and endothelial cells.

ATTENUATION OF THE RATE OF PROTHROMBIN CONVERSION

The tissue factor pathway inhibitor (TFPI) and the protein C pathway are physiologic mechanisms by which the rate of prothrombin conversion is attenuated. TFPI, a serine protease, acts by reversible competitive inhibition of factor X and the extrinsic pathway. Protein C, a serine protease, inactivates nonenzymatic activated cofactors factors V and VIII. Free protein S, also a nonenzymatic cofactor, enhances the protein C–mediated degradation of factor Va by forming a complex with protein C on lipid surfaces. Neither of those two inhibitors is capable of directly inhibiting the clotting activity of thrombin, although protein C is classified as an anticoagulant. TFPI decreases the rate of prothrombin conversion after factor Xa has been generated. In clotting blood after fibrin formation, activated protein C inhibits thrombin amplification mechanisms and reduces the rate of prothrombin conversion and the clot (thrombus) mass. An additional role may exist for protein C in host defense reactions that occur during intravascular sepsis.

INACTIVATION OF THROMBIN IN BLOOD

The antithrombin pathway includes (1) two forms of antithrombin, which are both 58,000-d glycoproteins but differ in their carbohydrate content and their affinity for heparin; (2) heparin stored in the secretory granules of mast cells; (3) heparan sulfate and dermatan sulfate found on the surface endothelial cells and in the extracellular matrix; (4) heparin cofactor II, a dermatan sulfate–dependent protease inhibitor; (5) histidine-rich glycopro-

Table 3. Factors That Alter the Rate of Prothrombin Conversion

	Increase Rate	Decrease Rate	No Influence
Tissue factor pathway	Tissue factor Factor VII–factor VIIa Factor IXa Factor Xa	Tissue factor pathway inhibitor	
Prothrombinase complex	Thrombin Prothrombin Factor Va Factor VIIIa Platelet phospholipid 3		
Protein C pathway		Protein C Protein S Thrombomodulin Thrombin	
Antithrombin III pathway			Antithrombin Heparin cofactor II Histidine-rich glycoprotein

tein and platelet factor 4 that competitively inhibit antithrombin binding to heparin; and (6) thrombin incorporation into clots. The concentration of antithrombin in circulation exceeds the potential for thrombin generation in blood; however in the absence of heparin, thrombin inhibition occurs slowly. Thrombin is inactivated by antithrombin 1000 times faster when heparin is added to plasma.

Antithrombin binds thrombin in an irreversible equimolar complex that requires a thrombin-mediated cleavage of a small peptide from antithrombin before thrombin is proteolytically inactivated. Antithrombin-thrombin complexes circulate with a half-life of a few minutes and are probably degraded and cleared by hepatocytes. The role of heparin cofactor II as an antithrombin has not been established. Because the placenta is rich in dermatan sulfate, heparin cofactor II may function as an inhibitor of coagulation within the placenta. Histidine-rich glycoprotein and platelet factor 4, a protein released from platelet alpha granules, bind heparin in blood with high avidity. Platelet factor 4 is thought to act at the site of injury by blocking the binding of antithrombin to heparin sulfate. Another pathway of thrombin inactivation is by thrombin incorporation into clots and thrombi. Clot-bound thrombin is inaccessible to large molecules (e.g., antithrombin) that cannot penetrate clots.

MOLECULAR MARKERS

Molecular markers related to the hemostatic system consist of proteins or peptides that are produced during an ongoing physiologic or pathophysiologic process related to clot formation, thrombosis, vascular damage, or drug effect. Molecular markers are currently quantitated by means of specific antibodies prepared against them. The list of hemostatic molecular markers is growing rapidly, and most of the assays developed for their measurement are used primarily for research purposes. Molecular markers of coagulation activation and inactivation are directly related to hypercoagulability.

Markers of Coagulation Activation

Coagulation occurs with the sequential activation by limited proteolysis of a precursor factor by a procoagulant enzyme. With the exception of the factors of the contact phase of plasma activation and factor VII, activation peptides released during the clotting process have been isolated, purified, and used to develop antibodies in animals. Activation peptides are also interchangeably called "markers of coagulation activation." In the emerging field of markers of coagulation activation, it is convenient to divide the clotting process into three phases. Each phase, although not distinctly demarcated from the others, is identified by its own set of specific markers.

Prothrombin Conversion Phase

The prothrombin conversion stage is an early phase of clotting that occurs before solid clots form. Activation peptides released by reactions involving prothrombin conversion are markers of hypercoagulability. Antibodies have been developed against markers of hypercoagulability that include prothrombin fragment 1.2, factor X activation peptide, factor IX activation peptide, and other miscellaneous prothrombin fragments. The antibodies are then used to detect these activation peptides in plasma, providing measurements that reflect the extent of prothrombin conversion. Antibodies against prothrombin fragment 1.2 are used in the enzyme-linked immunosorbent assay (ELISA), which is commercially available. Other antibodies are used primarily for research.

Conversion of Fibrinogen by Thrombin

The process of conversion of fibrinogen by thrombin occurs during clot or thrombus formation; its reaction products are markers of early thrombosis. It involves thrombin proteolysis of fibrinogen with release of two fibrinopeptides. Antibodies that specifically target fibrinopeptide A are markers of thrombosis.

Inactivation of Thrombin by Antithrombin

The final phase of the clotting process is the inactivation of thrombin by antithrombin, which results from the feedback loop generated by thrombin that enhances and later slows the conversion of prothrombin. It generates thrombin-antithrombin complexes, as well as protein C activation markers that indicate a well-established thrombotic event. Antibodies against thrombin-antithrombin complex (TAT) are used in commercially developed ELISA kits to detect this molecular marker in plasma. Assays for protein C activation peptides are primarily research tools.

Molecular Markers of Fibrinolysis, Vascular Damage, or Drug Effect

Markers of fibrinolysis are detected by antibody assays that are commercially available. These include measurements of D-dimer and fibrin degradation products. A more recent development involves the plasmin–α_2-antiplasmin complex. A novel coagulation activation marker, free γ-carboxyglutamic acid, was measured in 11 patients with disseminated intravascular coagulation (DIC) and in 9 patients hospitalized for leg pain. The marker was increased in the patients with disseminated intravascular coagulation but not in 19 normal subjects or in the patients hospitalized for leg pain. A significant decrease in γ-carboxyglutamic acid was noticed during vitamin K antagonist therapy.

Thrombomodulin (TM) is a marker of endothelial cell integrity. Plasma TM concentrations in patients with atheromatous arterial disease suggest that increased shedding of TM into the plasma occurs with endothelial cell damage. Other specific markers of endothelial cell activation include prostacyclin, tissue plasminogen activator, and plasminogen activator inhibitor-1.

Evaluation of the Hemostatic System by Molecular Markers

Exercise-induced activation of coagulation factor VIII:C, von Willebrand factor, and an antithrombin coagulation activation marker (TAT) were studied in healthy individuals and in patients with uncomplicated non–insulin-dependent diabetes. In neither group was the activation marker TAT increased above baseline. Tissue factor released perioperatively during total hip replacement caused sequential intrapulmonary and systemic activation of coagulation and fibrinolysis. Markers of prothrombin activation appeared during preparation of the bone, and activation of fibrinolysis followed almost immediately.

The extent of neutralization of thrombin by antithrombin was studied in spontaneously clotting whole blood. The effects of adding heparin and of antithrombin deficiency were also examined by markers of prothrombin coagulation activation, antithrombin-thrombin complex, and fibrinopeptide A. Both markers were significantly increased, suggesting that large amounts of fibrin had formed. Plasma antithrombin alone was not sufficient to neutralize thrombin, but the addition of heparin resulted in virtually complete suppression of thrombin formation in normal blood as well as in antithrombin-deficient blood.

The effect of the Hickman catheter and the influence of blood sampling on the assessment of activation fragments has shown that blood from the Hickman catheter provides reliable results for determination of activation markers of coagulation and fibrinolysis in patients with hematologic malignancies. In clinical practice, however, aberrant results may be seen because of frequent heparin contamination. Prothrombin activation marker fragment 1.2, thrombin-antithrombin complexes, and D-dimer measurements by the ELISA method were performed in plasma from normal individuals and from patients deficient in antithrombin, protein C, and protein S using (1) sodium citrate, (2) acid-citrate-dextrose–ethylenediaminetetraacetic acid–adenosine heparin (ACD-EDTA-adenosine heparin), and (3) EDTA-aprotinin. Antithrombin-thrombin complex measurements gave a different pattern from the other markers. The findings also showed that the use of vacuum tubes with sodium citrate were reliable for the measurement of prothrombin activation markers as well as for D-dimer markers.

Severe inherited homocystinemia, an autosomal recessive metabolic disorder, is the result of cystathione β-synthase deficiency. In the acquired condition, increased blood concentrations of homocysteine, an intermediate sulfhydryl amino acid, results from cobalamin, folate, and pyridoxine deficiency. Homocysteine is also a marker for vascular disease and thrombosis. The effect of homocysteine on vascular hemostatic activities promoting thrombosis include tissue factor expression, enhanced factor V activity, suppression of thrombomodulin activity, and decreased fibrinolysis. The pattern linking atherogenesis and thrombosis with this condition is markedly heterogeneous.

The effect of oral contraceptives on increased whole blood coagulability was reversed by aspirin. In flowing whole native human blood, a prothrombotic effect of leukocyte products enhanced shear-induced platelet thrombus formation on collagen fibers. A less pronounced effect promoting clot lysis also was noted.

The Sienco Sonoclot Analyzer and thromboelastography were used to assess abnormal hemostasis in whole blood obtained from patients with solid tumors. There was no indication of hypercoagulability in patients with benign tumors, whereas colon and breast cancer caused an increased incidence of blood clots.

The effectiveness of heparin, oral anticoagulants, and compression stockings in maintaining blood fluidity and preventing extension of venographically proven deep vein thrombosis (DVT) was compared in 90 patients. The effect of anticoagulation versus nonanticoagulation was verified by venography 30 days following initiation of treatment in 29 of the anticoagulation group and 30 of the nonanticoagulation group. No effect on the progression of deep vein thrombosis was observed in either group.

HYPEREOSINOPHILIC SYNDROME

By Peter F. Weller, M.D.,
and Glenn J. Bubley, M.D.
Boston, Massachusetts

Idiopathic hypereosinophilic syndrome (HES) is a leukoproliferative disorder, likely of multiple etiologies, marked by a sustained overproduction of eosinophils. In addition to the marked eosinophilia, this syndrome is noted for its predilection for damaging specific organs, including the heart. The cardiac pathology associated with HES may also develop with other eosinophilic diseases that have identifiable causes. Not all patients with hypereosinophilia, however, develop the organ damage characteristic of HES. No specific tests are diagnostic of HES; rather, the syndrome is defined by the combination of unexplained prolonged eosinophilia and evidence of organ involvement.

To diagnose HES, three criteria must be met. First, the patient must have sustained blood eosinophilia of more than 1500 cells/mm^3 present for longer than 6 months. Second, other apparent etiologies of eosinophilia, such as parasitic infections and allergic diseases, must be absent. In addition, the clinician must also exclude patients with eosinophilic syndromes that are clinically distinct from HES, whether they have apparent etiologies, such as the L-tryptophan–associated eosinophilia-myalgia syndrome, or remain idiopathic, such as eosinophilic pneumonia. Third, patients must have signs and symptoms of organ involvement. This last criterion excludes patients who have clinically benign eosinophilia. These patients, who may be underrepresented among the eosinophilic patients studied at referral centers, can remain asymptomatic for decades.

MANIFESTATIONS

Hypereosinophilic syndrome is more common in men than women (9:1) and typically occurs between the ages of 20 and 50 years, although a few cases have been reported in children. Clinically, HES is a heterogeneous disease with variable manifestations. Not only is the cause of HES unknown, but also it is likely to include a range of diseases. A possible multiplicity of etiologies may contribute to the clinical heterogeneity of HES.

The presenting manifestations of HES may be due to sudden cardiac or neurologic complications, but they are typically more insidious and chronic. About one in eight patients with HES has eosinophilia that is detected incidentally. Other presenting symptoms include tiredness (26 per cent), cough (24 per cent), breathlessness (16 per cent), muscle pains or angioedema (14 per cent), rash or fever (12 per cent), and retinal lesions (10 per cent). Sweating and pruritus are quite common, and patients with HES may experience fevers, which are usually low grade. Patients with HES do not have a propensity for developing complicating bacterial or other infections and are not anergic. Weight loss or cachexia is not seen, unless there is secondary malnutrition or end-stage congestive heart failure. Some HES patients experience alcohol intolerance, with abdominal pain, flushing, nausea, weakness, or diarrhea. Hypereosinophilic syndrome has developed in patients with human immunodeficiency virus type 1 (HIV-1) infections, and eosinophilia can occur with human T-cell lymphotropic virus type II (HTLV-II).

Hematologic Manifestations

The defining hematologic abnormality is sustained eosinophilia. Total leukocyte counts are often less than 25,000 cells/mm^3, with between 30 and 70 per cent eosinophils, but extremely high leukocyte counts (more than 90,000 cells/mm^3) develop in some patients and are associated with a poor prognosis. Eosinophils in the blood may be mature; less commonly, they can include numbers of eosinophilic myeloid precursors. Eosinophils often exhibit morphologic abnormalities, including decreases in granule numbers and sizes, cytoplasmic vacuolation, and nuclear hypersegmentation. No specific morphologic abnormalities distinguish HES from secondary causes of eosinophilia.

Many patients with HES also have an absolute neutrophilia along with their eosinophilia, further contributing to increases in the white blood cell count. Band forms and less mature neutrophilic precursors, at times with dysplastic features, may be present in the peripheral blood. However, myeloblasts, as may be found in acute leukemia, are uncommonly present. Basophilia, usually mild, is seen in some patients with HES. Leukocyte alkaline phosphatase activities may be abnormal, but these measures are as likely to be increased as decreased. Concentrations of serum vitamin B_{12} and vitamin B_{12}–binding proteins may be normal or increased.

Platelet numbers may be increased or decreased. Anemia is present in about 50 per cent of patients with HES, and teardrop and nucleated erythrocytes can be found in the peripheral blood. Bone marrow findings demonstrate increased numbers of eosinophils, often 30 to 60 per cent, with a shift to the left in eosinophil maturation. Increased numbers of myeloblasts are not usually seen. Myelofibrosis is encountered in a minority of patients.

Chromosome studies are normal in most patients who have HES. In the HES patients who do have chromosomal abnormalities, no consistent abnormality is found. Occasionally, a Philadelphia chromosome is found, but the commonest abnormality is aneuploidy in a minority of mitoses.

Splenomegaly is found in about 40 per cent of individuals (Table 1). Patients with splenomegaly may experience hypersplenism, which contributes to their thrombocytopenia and anemia, and infarction of the spleen can lead to diminution of the hypersplenism. Splenic pain, due to capsular distention and/or infarcts, is common in those with enlarged spleens.

Clinical Manifestations

Cardiac Manifestations

Cardiac disease, frequent in HES (see Table 1), is a major cause of morbidity and mortality, the latter especially occurring in previous decades. Damage to the heart, ranging from early necrosis to subsequent thrombosis and fibrosis, occurs with the same pathogenesis whether the eosinophilia is due to HES or other causes, such as eosinophilic leukemia, eosinophilia with carcinomas or lymphomas, and eosinophilia from drug reactions or parasites. While diverse eosinophilic diseases can cause identical forms of cardiac disease, some patients with sustained eosinophilia never develop cardiac disease.

Eosinophil-mediated heart damage evolves through three stages. The first is an acute necrotic stage seen in patients who have eosinophilia of short duration (mean of 5.5 weeks). The second is a later thrombotic stage found in those with a mean 10-month duration of eosinophilia, and the third stage is a late fibrotic stage encountered in those who have had eosinophilia for about 2 years. The early necrotic stage of cardiac disease is usually not recognized when it occurs with HES. During this stage, damage to the endocardium occurs, and the myocardium is infiltrated by eosinophils and lymphocytes. The histopathologic findings include myocardial necrosis, eosinophilic degranulation, and eosinophilic microabscesses. A similar acute eosinophilic myocarditis can develop, with hypersensitivity reactions. In patients with HES and acute-stage myocardial necrosis, splinter hemorrhages may be prominent, but clinical cardiac findings are often absent. Rarely, deaths due to acute progressive cardiac disease can occur. Echocardiography and angiography typically detect no abnormalities during this stage, and endomyocardial biopsy, usually from the right ventricle, is needed to make the diagnosis.

The second stage of heart disease involves formation of thrombi along the damaged endocardium of either or both ventricles and, occasionally, the atrium. Outflow tracts near the aortic and pulmonic valves are usually spared. In the final fibrotic stage, progressive scarring ensues and may lead to entrapment of chordae tendineae, with the development of mitral and/or tricuspid regurgitation, and to endomyocardial fibrosis, producing a restrictive cardiomyopathy. Patients with HES often present at the later thrombotic and fibrotic stages. The common manifestations include dyspnea, chest pain, signs of left and/or right ventricular congestive heart failure, murmurs of mitral regurgitation, cardiomegaly, and T-wave inversions. Two-dimensional echocardiography is valuable in detecting intracardiac thrombi and the manifestations of fibrosis, which include thickening of the posterior mitral valve leaflet and its attachment to a thickened posterior wall as well as increases in intensities of endomyocardial echoes in areas of endomyocardial fibrosis. Cardiac catheterization demonstrates increased right and left ventricular end-diastolic pressures, and angiography can demonstrate valvular incompetence as well as delineate apical obliteration or irregularities. Cardiac biopsies confirm the diagnosis, although with intense fibrosis in late disease biopsy instruments may fail to obtain samples.

The risks of developing cardiac disease are not related to the extent of eosinophilia or the duration of HES. Rather, those who develop evident cardiac disease are more likely to be male and HLA-Bw44 positive, and they are likely to have splenomegaly, thrombocytopenia, increased serum concentrations of vitamin B_{12}, hypogranular or vacuolated eosinophils, and abnormal early myeloid precursors in their blood. The HES patients free from cardiac disease tend to be female and have angioedema, hypergammaglobulinemia, increased concentrations of IgE, and circulating immune complexes in their serum.

HES heart disease can also present as a dilated cardiomyopathy. Variant angina with normal coronary arteries,

Table 1. Frequency of Organ Involvement in HES

Organ System	Percentage
Hematologic	100
Cardiovascular	58
Cutaneous	56
Neurologic	54
Pulmonary	49
Splenic	43
Hepatic	30
Ocular	23
Gastrointestinal	23

Adapted from Weller, P.F., and Bubley, G.J.: The idiopathic hypereosinophilic syndrome. Blood, 83:2759–2779, 1994, with permission.

asymmetrical septal hypertrophy, and constrictive pericarditis have been reported rarely with HES.

Neurologic Manifestations

Neurologic complications, also frequent in HES (see Table 1), may be of three forms. The first form of neurologic disease is due to thromboemboli. With the propensity for intracardiac thrombus formation, thromboemboli usually originate in the left ventricle. Patients can experience embolic strokes or episodes of transient ischemia, either of which can be multiple and recurrent. Such thromboembolic episodes may develop before cardiac disease is demonstrable with echocardiography and can be the presenting manifestation of HES.

The second form of HES-associated neuropathy is primary central nervous system dysfunction. Patients exhibit signs of a distinct encephalopathy that produces behavioral changes, confusion, ataxia, memory loss, and upper motor neuron signs with increased muscle tone and deep tendon reflexes, and a positive Babinski sign. Impaired cognitive abilities may persist for months. Seizures, intracranial hemorrhages, dementia, and organic psychoses occur less frequently. The anatomic or pathologic basis of this form of diffuse central nervous system disease remains unknown. Eosinophilic meningitis has been noted only uncommonly with HES; infiltration of eosinophils into the brain or meninges is more suggestive of eosinophilic leukemia than of HES.

The third form of neurologic dysfunction in HES is peripheral neuropathy, which occurs in about half of HES patients who have neurologic manifestations. Symmetrical or asymmetrical sensory polyneuropathies manifested by sensory deficits, painful paresthesias, or mixed sensory and motor deficits are common, although pure motor neuropathies have been noted. Mononeuritis multiplex occurs with HES, as do radiculopathies and muscle atrophy due to denervation. Biopsies of affected nerves generally show an axonal neuropathy with varying degrees of axonal loss and no evidence of vasculitis or direct or contiguous eosinophil infiltration.

Cutaneous Manifestations

The skin is one of the most frequently involved organs in HES, with cutaneous manifestations occurring in more than 50 per cent of patients (see Table 1). The commonest skin manifestations are of two types, either angioedematous with urticarial lesions or erythematous with pruritic papules and nodules. Patients who experience angioedema and urticaria are likely to have benign courses without cardiac or neurologic complications. Either they do not require systemic therapy, or they respond to prednisone alone. Some patients with angioedema and eosinophilia are now recognized as having a syndrome (episodic angioedema and eosinophilia) that is distinct from HES.

In HES patients with papular or nodular lesions, dermal biopsies usually show a mixed cellular infiltrate that is not solely eosinophilic and is devoid of vasculitis. Perivascular infiltration with eosinophils and mild-to-moderate perivascular neutrophilic and mononuclear infiltrates are found. These lesions usually improve in proportion to the response to systemic therapy for HES. Also reported to occur with HES are blistering skin lesions and small bowel necrosis due to dermal microthrombi and mesenteric thrombi and vasculitis, lesions due to cutaneous microthrombi, vesiculobullous lesions, ulcerations with dermal arteriolar microthrombi, generalized erythroderma, and erythema annulare centrifugum. Particularly incapacitating mucocutaneous manifestations of HES are mucosal ulcers that may be early or late manifestations of HES. These ulcers can occur in the mouth, nose, pharynx, penis, esophagus, stomach, and anus. Biopsies demonstrate only a nonspecific mixed cellular infiltrate without a prominence of eosinophils and no evidence of vasculitis or microthrombi. Mucocutaneous disease can flare independently of other hematologic or clinical manifestations of HES.

Pulmonary Manifestations

Pulmonary involvement is reported in about 40 per cent of HES patients (see Table 1). The commonest respiratory symptom in patients with HES is a chronic, persistent, generally nonproductive cough. The basis for this symptom may be sequestration of eosinophils in pulmonary tissues. Most of these symptomatic individuals have clear chest films. Although bronchospasm has been reported in some patients with HES, asthma is rare. Pulmonary symptoms may be secondary to congestive heart failure or pulmonary emboli originating from right ventricular thrombi, or they may reflect primary infiltration of the lungs by eosinophils. Chest films may reveal abnormalities associated with each of these processes. With frank congestive heart failure, pleural effusions are the commonest abnormality. While these are transudative, rarely an eosinophil-containing exudative pleural effusion may occur.

Pulmonary infiltrates are seen in 14 to 28 per cent of HES patients. The infiltrates may be diffuse or focal without a predilection for any specific region of the lung, in contrast to the often peripheral infiltrates in chronic eosinophilic pneumonia. Biopsies of the infiltrates in HES reveal eosinophilic parenchymal accumulations and, occasionally, infiltration and cuffing of small pulmonary arteries. These infiltrates may improve with prednisone administration. Pulmonary fibrosis may develop over time, especially in those with cardiac fibrosis. Bronchoalveolar lavage may recover large numbers of eosinophils in HES, but this finding does not distinguish HES from other eosinophilic pneumonias that also may yield large numbers of eosinophils in the lavage fluid.

Ocular Manifestations

Visual symptoms, most commonly blurring, can be experienced by patients with HES. Even in those who do not have visual symptoms, fluorescein angiography demonstrates that more than 50 per cent of HES patients have choroidal abnormalities, including patchy and delayed filling, and retinal vessel abnormalities. While retinal arteritis can develop with HES, most of the ocular abnormalities are presumed to be due to microemboli or local thrombosis.

Rheumatologic Manifestations

Arthralgias and large joint effusions can occur with HES. Long-standing rheumatoid arthritis or nonerosive polyarthritis involving large joints and causing a synovial fluid eosinophilia has been noted. Patients with HES may experience cold-induced Raynaud's phenomenon and can develop digital necrosis of the fingers or toes. The reported cases have occurred in those with HES alone and in a patient with eosinophilia and acquired immunodeficiency syndrome (AIDS) who had arteriographic evidence of digital vasculitis. Although myalgias are frequent, HES with focal myositis or polymyositis occurs uncommonly.

Digestive System Manifestations

Gastrointestinal tract involvement can accompany HES, and 20 per cent of patients may at some time have diarrhea. Eosinophilic gastritis, enterocolitis, or colitis may develop. Pancreatitis and sclerosing cholangitis occur rarely. Hepatic involvement with HES can include chronic active hepatitis and the Budd-Chiari syndrome from hepatic vein obstruction.

Immunologic Manifestations

The variability of associated immunologic abnormalities suggests the heterogeneity of HES. About a third of HES patients have extremely high IgE concentrations. This subgroup with increased IgE usually requires no therapy or responds well to prednisone, so increased IgE concentrations are a good prognostic factor and suggest the existence of a distinct subgroup of HES patients.

DIFFERENTIAL DIAGNOSIS OF HES

In patients with an eosinophilia of more than 1500 cells/mm^3 sustained for more than 6 months, the diagnosis of HES must be considered. Because no specific diagnostic test exists for this disorder, evaluation must be guided by the organ system involvement and deliberate exclusion of other disparate diseases that may be associated with eosinophilia. Many of the eosinophilic syndromes and diseases are of unknown etiology; therefore, distinctions between these and HES must be made on clinical and pathologic bases. Eosinophilic syndromes limited to specific organs, such as eosinophilic pneumonia and eosinophilic gastroenteritis, characteristically do not extend beyond the target organ and, hence, lack the multiple organ involvement often found with HES. They do not have the predilection for developing secondary eosinophil-mediated cardiac damage, for reasons that are not known. Individual patients may occasionally present with overlapping features that confound classification.

In the differential diagnosis of HES, the major vasculitis that is associated with eosinophilia is the Churg-Strauss syndrome. This syndrome is characterized by a history of asthma, migratory pulmonary infiltrates, blood eosinophilia of more than 10 per cent, paranasal sinus abnormalities, mononeuropathy or polyneuropathy, and a blood vessel biopsy demonstrating extravascular eosinophils. Biopsies showing necrotizing vasculitis of small arteries and veins with extravascular granulomas are characteristic of the Churg-Strauss syndrome, but not all patients exhibit these pathologic features. Asthma, peak eosinophilia of more than 1500 cells/mm^3, and systemic vasculitis of two or more extrapulmonary organs help identify this syndrome. Neurologic, pulmonary, and, less commonly, paranasal involvement may occur with HES, but asthma is uncommon. In individual patients, clear-cut distinction between HES and Churg-Strauss syndrome may not be possible.

For those with cutaneous involvement and eosinophilia, angiolymphoid hyperplasia with eosinophilia or Kimura's disease, eosinophilic cellulitis (Wells' syndrome), eosinophilic fasciitis, and eosinophilic pustular folliculitis can be distinguished from HES on the basis of the histopathology of the biopsied lesions. The eosinophilia-myalgia syndrome due to ingestion of contaminated L-tryptophan should be excluded. Another syndrome, episodic angioedema with eosinophilia, is characterized by recurring episodes of angioedema, urticaria, fever, and marked blood eosinophilia. The clinical course of this disease with its prominent periodic occurrences of angioedema and eosinophilia and its lack of association with cardiac damage distinguish it from HES.

Eosinophilia may also accompany some malignancies. Prior to the recognition that most patients with hypereosinophilia did not have a truly malignant disease, patients with HES were diagnosed as having eosinophilic leukemia. Acute eosinophilic leukemia, a rare subtype of acute nonlymphocytic leukemia, can be distinguished from HES by a marked increase in the number of immature eosinophils or myeloblasts in the blood and/or marrow. Also, eosinophilic leukemia has a clinical course similar to that of other acute leukemias, including pronounced anemia and thrombocytopenia and susceptibility to infections. The cardiac and neurologic complications of HES can develop in acute eosinophilic leukemia, as in other eosinophilic diseases, and are not distinguishing clinical features.

Although chromosomal abnormalities can occur with eosinophilia due to HES or leukemias, eosinophilic leukemia is often associated with those abnormalities described in other acute nonlymphocytic leukemias, including trisomy 1, 8:21, and 10p + 11q − translocations. Eosinophilic leukemia has also been described as a variant of the M-4 phenotype of acute myelomonocytic leukemia with typical chromosome 16 abnormalities. Eosinophilic leukemia with abnormalities of chromosomes 5 or 7 has been reported after treatment with alkylating agents. While eosinophilia may accompany some lymphomas, including Hodgkin's disease, T-cell lymphoblastic lymphoma, and adult T-cell leukemia/lymphoma, this eosinophilia is usually modest. Several patients with the typical clinical and hematologic features of HES have later developed T-cell lymphomas or acute lymphoblastic leukemia.

Some patients with HES exhibit features common to myeloproliferative disorders, including increased vitamin B_{12} concentrations, abnormal leukocyte alkaline phosphatase scores, splenomegaly, cytogenetic abnormalities, myelofibrosis, anemia, erythrocyte abnormalities, myeloid dysplasia, and basophilia. Patients with these features are less likely to respond to prednisone and more likely to require cytotoxic therapy. However, HES patients rarely have expansions of cell lines other than eosinophils to the extent seen in myeloproliferative disorders, and they do not develop myelofibrosis severe enough to cause pancytopenia.

The diagnosis of HES also requires that eosinophilias with identifiable etiologies be excluded. These include allergic diseases, such as allergic rhinoconjunctivitis ("hayfever") and asthma as well as eosinophil-eliciting parasitic infections, which, with the exceptions of two enteric protozoans, *Isospora belli* and *Dientamoeba fragilis,* are due to helminthic parasites. Those more likely to elicit prolonged eosinophilia in adults include filarial infections and strongyloidiasis. Trichinosis may cause an acute, marked eosinophilia, but this eosinophilia does not persist unless reinfection occurs. It is especially important that the clinician exclude infection with *Strongyloides stercoralis,* which may be difficult to diagnose solely by stool examination. Such infection may cause marked eosinophilia mimicking HES, and it can also develop into a disseminated, often fatal, disease (hyperinfection syndrome) in patients receiving immunosuppressive corticosteroids. Indeed, HES has been misdiagnosed in patients with unsuspected strongyloidiasis. Serial stool examinations and a serologic test for *Strongyloides* should be performed. An ELISA serology has proved valuable in detecting strongyloidiasis, even when aggressive examinations of stool samples have been unrevealing. Some helminthic infections not detectable by stool examinations that can cause marked eosinophilia include filarial infections, trichinosis, and visceral larva migrans. In children, visceral larva migrans due to *Toxocara canis* is a potential etiology for sustained eosinophilia, especially if reinfection is occurring (see the articles on helminthic and other parasitic diseases).

Thus, the presence of a persistently increased blood eosinophilia not associated with allergic or parasitic diseases or with other diseases or disease syndromes that may be associated with eosinophilia suggests the diagnosis of HES. To distinguish benign, asymptomatic eosinophilia from HES, by definition, the clinician must find evidence of organ involvement. Evaluation of the specific organs that may be involved is guided by the patient's presenting symptoms but should include echocardiography to detect possible endomyocardial fibrosis and thrombosis that may be clinically occult at presentation.

TRANSFUSION REACTIONS

By Holly Dastghaib, M.D., *and* Ira A. Shulman, M.D.
Los Angeles, California

A transfusion reaction is any adverse effect of blood component therapy. Although transfusion is usually safe, the risks should be weighed against the expected benefits prior to its initiation. Transfusion reactions can be divided into two broad categories—acute and delayed—which, in turn, can each be subdivided into immune- and non–immune-mediated groups. Table 1 lists the various kinds of transfusion reactions.

ACUTE TRANSFUSION REACTION

Immune-Mediated Reaction

Acute Hemolytic Transfusion Reaction

DEFINITION. When transfused red blood cells interact with the recipient's antibodies or, less commonly, when transfused antibodies interact with the recipient's red blood cells, hemolysis may occur in the vascular space—that is, intravascular hemolysis. Most severe acute hemolytic transfusion reactions (HTRs) are due to transfusion of ABO-incompatible red blood cells.

CLINICAL PRESENTATION. Symptoms of acute HTR may occur after infusion of as little as 10 to 15 mL of incompatible red blood cells. The most common presenting symptoms are fever and chills. Other symptoms include back, chest, and abdominal pain; hypotension; dyspnea; hemoglobinuria; oliguria; and generalized bleeding. In anesthetized patients, the only manifestation of acute HTR may be bleeding at surgical sites (due to disseminated intravascular coagulation [DIC]), hypotension, or hemoglobinuria.

CLINICAL COURSE. The red blood cell–antibody interaction may activate many systems that mediate the diverse clinical manifestations of an acute HTR. The activation of the clotting system can result in DIC; in turn, activation of factor XII produces bradykinin and hypotension. Release of catecholamines causes vasoconstriction in the renal, pulmonary, splanchnic, and cutaneous vascular beds. Finally, cytokine release may also contribute to the fever, hypotension, and activation of T and B cells.

DIAGNOSTIC PROCEDURES. Once an acute HTR is suspected, stop the transfusion immediately. Check all labels, forms, and patient identification to ascertain that the transfused unit was intended for the patient. Submit the donor unit, administration set, accompanying intravenous solutions, forms, labels, and a postreaction blood sample to the clinical laboratory.

A diagnosis of intravascular hemolysis can be made by visual examination of a postreaction specimen. Pink or red discoloration of the serum or plasma may indicate free hemoglobin. In addition, a direct antiglobulin test (DAT) should be performed on an ethylenediaminetetraacetic acid (EDTA) anticoagulated post-transfusion specimen. A pretransfusion DAT may also be performed for comparison; if all the transfused incompatible red blood cells have not been destroyed, the postreaction DAT result may be positive.

Other useful laboratory tests include ABO and Rh determinations on pre- and postreaction specimens as well as on blood from the transfused unit. Also, an antibody screen and urinalysis as well as hemoglobin and hematocrit, serum haptoglobin, bilirubin, lactate dehydrogenase (LD), and urine hemosiderin determinations may be performed. Visual inspection of supernatant from a centrifuged specimen of urine may show red discoloration consistent with hemoglobinuria.

Serum haptoglobin may decrease in a post-transfusion specimen because of binding with hemoglobin. Serum bilirubin (primarily unconjugated) may increase and peak in 3 to 6 hours and disappear within 24 hours of the hemolytic event; serum LD (primarily LD_1) increases because of release from red blood cells. Urine hemosiderin may be detected 2 to 7 days after hemolysis and can be helpful if an initial evaluation of hemoglobin was not performed. A coagulation panel for evaluation of DIC as well as serum urea nitrogen and creatinine determinations to monitor renal function may also aid diagnosis.

POTENTIAL ERRORS AND PITFALLS

1. Hemoglobin in the serum or plasma due to hemolysis caused by the phlebotomy procedure may lead to an incor-

Table 1. Transfusion Reactions

Acute Reaction		Delayed Reaction	
Immune	*Nonimmune*	*Immune*	*Nonimmune*
Hemolytic	Circulatory overload	Alloimmunization and hemolytic	Iron overload
Febrile nonhemolytic	Hemolytic	Platelet transfusion refractoriness	Infection
Urticaria	Septic	Graft-versus-host disease	
Anaphylactic	Metabolic	Immunomodulation	
Transfusion-related acute lung injury	Air embolism		

rect diagnosis; hemoglobinuria should not be present in phlebotomy-associated hemolysis.

2. Hemoglobinemia and hemoglobinuria may occur in nonimmune hemolysis resulting from exposure of red blood cell units to excess heat (via a blood warmer), inadvertent freezing, inadequate deglycerolization of the red blood cell unit, or use of roller pumps (used in cardiac bypass), pressure cuffs, or small-bore needles. Nonimmune hemolysis of red blood cells may also follow the addition of drugs or hypotonic solutions to the blood container during transfusion or secondary bacterial contamination of the red blood cell unit.

3. A negative DAT result may occur in immune-mediated hemolysis if the postreaction blood sample is collected several hours after the hemolysis and all (or most) antibody-coated and/or complement-coated erythrocytes are destroyed.

Febrile Nonhemolytic Transfusion Reaction

SYNONYM. Fever without hemolysis is another name for febrile nonhemolytic transfusion reaction (FNHTR).

DEFINITION. An increase in temperature of more than 1°C in association with transfusion therapy constitutes FNHTR. The required temperature rise varies from 0.5 to 2°C among experts in the field. FHTRs occur in about 1 per cent of transfusions.

CLINICAL PRESENTATION. The temperature rise can occur early in the course of the transfusion or several hours after its completion. FNHTRs are thought to result primarily from an interaction between the recipient's antibodies and the membrane antigens of donor lymphocytes, granulocytes, or platelets.

COURSE AND OUTCOME. The majority of these reactions are benign. The chills usually resolve within 1 hour of onset, and the fever is gone within 8 to 12 hours of onset.

DIAGNOSTIC PROCEDURES. Since fever may be the presenting symptom in an acute HTR or septic reaction, the initial laboratory evaluation for a FNHTR should be the same as that for an acute HTR. When acute HTR and bacterial contamination of the transfused unit are excluded, the diagnosis of FNHTR becomes one of exclusion.

POTENTIAL ERRORS AND PITFALLS

1. A chill may be perceived by a patient because of a cool room, intravenous solution, or infusion of medication (e.g., amphotericin B) close to the time of transfusion.

2. A patient may have onset of fever because of infection, or a rise in temperature may occur in a febrile patient during or shortly after transfusion therapy. The latter should be referred to as probable FNHTR.

Urticaria

SYNONYM. Hives is another name for urticaria.

DEFINITION. Urticaria is a reaction characterized by rash and/or hives and itching that is typically without fever or other adverse effects. Urticaria complicates about 1 per cent of transfusions. The reaction is thought to result from allergy to a soluble substance in the plasma of the transfused blood component.

COURSE AND OUTCOME. Urticarial reactions are usually mild, and the majority resolve after administration of antihistamines. The transfusion may be stopped during treatment; once the urticaria resolves, the transfusion of the same unit may be restarted to avoid the risks of infection that may be associated with a replacement unit.

DIAGNOSTIC PROCEDURES. The diagnosis of urticaria is clinically evident. Since urticaria is rarely related to hemolysis, an extensive laboratory evaluation to exclude hemolysis is rarely indicated.

POTENTIAL ERRORS AND PITFALLS. Urticaria may be secondary to drug reactions. Attention to the temporal relationship among the urticaria, drug administration, and transfusion therapy may help distinguish transfusion reaction from adverse drug reaction.

Anaphylactic Reaction

DEFINITION. Anaphylaxis refers to a severe hypersensitivity reaction following the transfusion of various components of plasma. Anaphylaxis may occur after the administration of only a few milliliters of blood. Some patients may have an IgA deficiency and anti-IgA antibodies stimulated by previous transfusions or pregnancy; other patients have no previous alloimmunizing event. Other mechanisms of anaphylactic reactions include severe allergic reactions to soluble plasma antigens or drugs (e.g., penicillin) accompanying the transfusion of blood components. Although IgA deficiency is relatively common (1 in 700 persons), anaphylactic reactions are fortunately rare, since the reaction requires the presence of anti-IgA. IgA-deficient individuals can have antibodies to the IgA α heavy chain (i.e., class-specific antibodies) or antibodies to other heavy chain subclass specificities (i.e., type-specific antibodies). Individuals with normal IgA levels have only type-specific antibodies.

CLINICAL PRESENTATION. The anaphylactic reaction is usually characterized by cough, bronchospasm, respiratory distress, and vascular instability. Other signs and symptoms may include nausea, abdominal cramps, diarrhea, and loss of consciousness. Fever is conspicuously absent.

CLINICAL COURSE. Most reactions occur within seconds or minutes of the start of the transfusion and may progress rapidly to shock, syncope, and death within 15 minutes of onset.

DIAGNOSTIC PROCEDURES. Anaphylactic reactions are diagnosed on the basis of signs and symptoms; there are no laboratory tests, except in the case of IgA deficiency, in which the IgA concentration can be measured after the treatment of the acute episode.

POTENTIAL ERRORS AND PITFALLS. Other acute medical conditions such as asthma, myocardial infarction, pulmonary embolism, and vasovagal syncope may occur in the same temporal relationship to the transfusion as an anaphylactic reaction.

Transfusion-Related Acute Lung Injury

SYNONYM. Noncardiogenic pulmonary edema and pulmonary hypersensitivity reaction are synonyms for transfusion-related acute lung injury.

DEFINITION AND CLINICAL PRESENTATION. Transfusion-related acute lung injury is characterized by acute respiratory insufficiency and/or radiographic findings consistent with pulmonary edema in the absence of cardiac failure. The volume of blood transfused is usually too small to cause respiratory distress secondary to hypervolemia. The reaction may also be accompanied by fever, chills, tachycardia, and hypotension. Several mechanisms have been proposed, including the following:

1. A reaction between donor anti-HLA or antineutrophil antibodies and recipient leukocytes may occur, causing an alteration in pulmonary microcirculation permeability,

which leads to pulmonary edema. In the case of granulocyte transfusions, the reverse occurs; recipient antileukocyte antibodies interact with transfused granulocytes, leading to severe pulmonary edema, especially in patients with pre-existing lung infection or alloimmunization to HLA antigens present on the donor leukocytes.

2. Activation of complement with release of C3a and C5a may occur, leading to release of histamine and serotonin from basophils and platelets. These processes alter the pulmonary microcirculation, and edema may ensue.

CLINICAL COURSE. In the majority of patients, acute symptoms resolve within 24 hours, and pulmonary infiltrates clear in 4 days. However, the reaction may be fatal in compromised patients.

DIAGNOSTIC PROCEDURES. The chest film in transfusion-related acute lung injury reveals the typical pattern of pulmonary edema with a normal cardiac silhouette. The pulmonary capillary wedge pressure in a monitored patient is typically normal. Laboratory evaluation reveals antigranulocyte antibodies in the donor's blood component or the recipient's plasma.

POTENTIAL ERRORS AND PITFALLS. This is a diagnosis of exclusion that is made when other causes of pulmonary edema, such as cardiac failure and hypervolemia, are excluded.

Non–immune-Mediated Reaction

Circulatory Overload

DEFINITION. Overload is defined as cardiac failure and pulmonary edema resulting from the transfusion of large volumes of blood components. Patients with cardiac or pulmonary compromise or with chronic anemia and expanded plasma volumes are at particular risk for this complication.

CLINICAL PRESENTATION. Patients may present with dyspnea, orthopnea, tachycardia, nonproductive cough, cyanosis, and heart failure 1 to 2 days after transfusion. Physical examination may reveal bilateral rales at the bases of the lungs and distended jugular veins.

DIAGNOSTIC PROCEDURES. The diagnosis is usually clinically apparent. The chest film reveals bilateral pulmonary infiltrates and cardiac enlargement. In a monitored patient, central venous pressure is typically elevated.

Acute Hemolytic Transfusion Reaction (Non–immune-Mediated)

DEFINITION. In vitro hemolysis of transfused red blood cells (either in the blood container or in the infusion tubing) causes hemoglobinemia and hemoglobinuria in the presence of a negative DAT result.

CLINICAL PRESENTATION. Patients may exhibit only hemoglobinuria and hemoglobinemia with rapid resolution, or a severe reaction may develop with hypotension, shock, and renal dysfunction.

DIAGNOSTIC PROCEDURES. A laboratory evaluation identical to that for an immune-mediated HTR is usually indicated. The results for bilirubin, LD, haptoglobin, and urine hemosiderin and urobilinogen are similar in both situations. Hemoglobinuria and hemoglobinemia are often present; however, the serologic evaluation reveals negative DAT and antibody screening results and no evidence of ABO-Rh incompatibility. If a nonimmune HTR is suspected, the blood remaining in the container and infusion tubing should be examined for evidence of hemolysis. If a hypotonic solution is used in conjunction with the unit of red blood cells, hemolysis will be present in both the blood container and the tubing. In the case of a faulty roller pump, however, hemolysis will be present only in the tubing.

Transfusion-Induced Septic Reaction

DEFINITION. Bacterial contamination of transfused blood components may result in septic shock if the unit is heavily contaminated; however, only mild symptoms may occur with a lesser degree of contamination.

CLINICAL PRESENTATION. Reactions may include fever, rigors, cardiopulmonary collapse, hemoglobinuria, hemoglobinemia, DIC, and renal failure. These conditions can occur within minutes to hours of the start of the transfusion, depending on the degree of contamination of the unit.

CLINICAL COURSE. A transfusion-induced septic reaction may range from mild to severe to fatal, depending on the bacterial load of the transfused unit.

DIAGNOSTIC PROCEDURES. If bacterial contamination is suspected, the unit should be examined for abnormal appearance, including purple-brown or murky discoloration, or for the presence of clots. A portion of the transfused unit should be sent for Gram stain and culture. In addition, blood cultures and routine post-transfusion specimens should be obtained from the patient.

POTENTIAL ERRORS AND PITFALLS. Septic transfusion reactions should be distinguished from immune anaphylaxis or HTR. Therefore, a laboratory evaluation to exclude intravascular hemolysis should be initiated.

Metabolic Reaction

DEFINITION. Metabolic reaction is a broad category that refers to complications that may occur following massive transfusions. Among these, coagulopathies and metabolic abnormalities are particularly important. Although dilutional coagulopathy may occur as a direct complication of massive transfusions, coagulopathy may be present in a critically ill patient prior to transfusion or may occur following inadequate resuscitation. A range of metabolic derangements may occur, including hypothermia from transfusion of refrigerated blood, citrate toxicity due to large volumes of blood components transfused at rates exceeding 100 mL per minute, and hypo- or hyperkalemia in a hypotensive patient.

CLINICAL PRESENTATION. Coagulopathy is clinically evident as bleeding abnormalities (e.g., oozing from surgical sites in a postoperative patient). Citrate toxicity is manifested as hypocalcemia; the clinical symptoms of hypocalcemia are more apparent in patients with liver dysfunction, patients undergoing aphresis procedures, patients in shock, and neonates undergoing exchange transfusion. Hypothermia may cause ventricular arrhythmia; this is more likely to occur when cold blood is administered through a central line in close proximity to the conduction system. Hypothermia also increases the cardiac toxicity of hypocalcemia and hyperkalemia. Transfusion-induced hyperkalemia is an unusual event because excess potassium is rapidly cleared if the patient's renal function is intact. In fact, transfusion-associated hypokalemia is much more common because the red blood cells take up a considerable amount of potassium once transfused. In addition, transfused citrate is metabolized to bicarbonate, causing alkalosis and exacerbating hypokalemia in these patients.

Air Embolism

DEFINITION. Air embolism may occur if blood is transfused under pressure using an open system or if air enters the infusion set or blood container. Presenting symptoms may include cough, dyspnea, chest pain, and shock.

DELAYED TRANSFUSION REACTION

Immune-Mediated Reaction

Alloimmunization and Hemolytic Transfusion Reaction

DEFINITION. The incidence of transfusion-associated alloimmunization to red blood cell antigens (other than D) is 1 to 1.6 per cent per unit of red blood cells transfused. Alloimmunization may also occur to leukocyte, platelet, and plasma antigens. In the case of red blood cell transfusion, alloantibodies may be detected within a few hours of transfusion, but sometimes they are not detected for several weeks to months. If red blood cell antibodies develop shortly after transfusion, they may react with transfused red blood cells and cause a delayed hemolytic transfusion reaction. A significant delayed hemolytic reaction can occur in a previously alloimmunized recipient who experiences an anamnestic response to transfused red blood cell antigens. A delayed serologic reaction occurs when an alloantibody is detected by the laboratory in the absence of clinical signs and symptoms of hemolysis.

CLINICAL PRESENTATION AND COURSE. The patient may present with an unexpected decrease in hemoglobin a few days after the transfusion; the DAT result and/or the antibody screen is usually positive. The patient may experience mild jaundice and fever; rarely, renal failure occurs.

DIAGNOSTIC PROCEDURES. The DAT and antibody screening results are usually positive in patients undergoing a delayed HTR. At the outset of a delayed HTR, the DAT result may be positive before the antibody screen turns positive. As the reaction runs its course, the antibody screen invariably turns positive, and the DAT eventually produces negative results. Although the DAT results are typically negative within days to weeks, the antibody screen may remain positive for years after a delayed HTR. The hemoglobin and hematocrit, serum bilirubin, and urine hemosiderin determinations can be obtained along with urea nitrogen and creatinine evaluations to monitor renal function.

Platelet Transfusion Refractoriness

DEFINITION. Platelet transfusion refractoriness is defined as repeatedly poor incremental increases in platelet number after suitable doses of platelets have been administered. Platelet refractoriness may result from immune or nonimmune causes. Immune refractoriness can be caused by auto- or alloantibodies; the latter may be directed against platelet antigens, ABO antigens, or class I HLA antigens present on the surface of platelets. Nonimmune mechanisms include splenomegaly, drugs, and accelerated platelet destruction. Identifying the cause of platelet refractoriness can be extremely difficult.

Transfusion-Associated Graft-Versus-Host Disease

DEFINITION. Graft-versus-host disease (GVHD) is caused by viable, transfused T lymphocytes in blood components. Except for fresh-frozen plasma and cryoprecipitate, all blood components contain sufficient viable lymphocytes to initiate GVHD in a susceptible recipient. Several factors increase a recipient's risk for the development of GVHD; they include immune status, degree of similarity between donor and recipient, and number of viable lymphocytes transfused.

CLINICAL PRESENTATION AND COURSE. GVHD may be divided into acute and chronic forms. Acute GVHD occurs 4 to 30 days following transfusion and can present with fever, dermatitis, hepatitis, enterocolitis, pancytopenia, and immunosuppression. Acute GVHD has a mortality rate of 90 per cent. Chronic GVHD usually begins 100 days after transfusion and presents with a sclerodermalike illness; sicca syndrome, bronchitis, and diarrhea may follow.

Post-transfusion Purpura

DEFINITION. Post-transfusion purpura (PTP) is a rare event characterized by a rapid decrease in platelets, producing generalized purpura about a week after a blood transfusion. It occurs almost exclusively in multiparous women. Patients acquire a platelet-specific alloantibody, anti-HPA-1a. HPA-1a has a prevalence of 98.3 per cent in the population; therefore, only 1.7 per cent of the patients undergoing transfusion are at risk for the development of anti-HPA-1a. Interestingly, both transfused HPA-1a–positive and autologous HPA-1a–negative platelets are destroyed in post-transfusion purpura. The mechanism for the latter event remains under investigation.

Immunomodulation by Transfusion

Transfusion has been implicated in modulating the immune response; for example, there have been reports of improved renal allografts in transfused patients. Transfusion modulation of the immune response may also contribute to increased rates of solid tumor recurrence and postoperative bacterial infection.

Non–immune-Mediated Reactions

Iron Overload

A unit of red blood cells contains about 200 mg of iron. In chronically transfused patients (e.g., individuals with thalassemia), after about 100 transfusions, continued accumulation of iron in vital organs can lead to cardiac, hepatic, and endocrine dysfunction.

Infection

The most significant infectious risk of transfusion therapy is the transmission of hepatitis C virus (HCV). The current per unit risk is 1 in 4000. Other important infections that can be transmitted by blood transfusion include human immunodeficiency virus (HIV; risk of 1 in 460,000), and hepatitis B virus (HBV; risk of 1 in 200,000). The transmission of these infectious agents is prevented by careful blood donor screening and testing, and by avoiding unnecessary blood transfusions.

Section Seven

GASTROINTESTINAL TRACT

FUNCTIONAL DISORDERS OF THE GASTROINTESTINAL TRACT

By James R. Curtiss, M.D.,
and Jack A. DiPalma, M.D.
Mobile, Alabama

Functional disorders of the gastrointestinal (GI) tract are a group of syndromes that frequently frustrate both patient and physician because of the chronicity of symptoms and the lack of objective findings. Symptoms range from vague descriptions of bodily discomfort to precise, elegant reports of discomfort or pain with knowledge of the inciting event. Many patients, including those whose illness may be psychogenic, have altered reflex responses in various regions of the GI tract, with an inappropriate, heightened perception of these physiologic events. Functional disorders continue to be among the most common reasons for referral of patients from primary care providers to gastroenterologists.

CLASSIFICATION

Disorders of the GI tract are typically classified into three groups: (1) structural disorders, (2) functional disorders, and (3) psychogenic disorders. The symptoms in the structural disorders group are most often related to an anatomically distorted organ in the GI tract. The distortion may be macroscopic or microscopic and intrinsic or extrinsic. In functional disorders, symptoms are typically derived from an aberration of physiologic function in the absence of a structural abnormality. Symptoms of psychogenic disorders are secondary to underlying unconscious mechanisms, without alteration of normal physiology or anatomy. Malingering, in which a patient's symptoms are contrived for secondary gain (attention-seeking behavior, drug-seeking behavior, and so on), is not unique to the practice of gastroenterology and should probably be considered a behavioral disorder.

APPROACH TO THE PATIENT WITH A FUNCTIONAL DISORDER

History

Patients with functional bowel disorders typically have a long history of symptoms, but a focused, detailed inquiry may be required to elicit the history accurately. Many patients will have been evaluated by several physicians and will have undergone numerous diagnostic procedures, but it remains important to obtain a detailed history even if this requires more than one office visit. A communicative patient-physician relationship is essential for optimal diagnosis and management of patients with functional disorders.

Symptoms of functional GI tract disorders are typically vague and include complaints of nonspecific abdominal pain, abdominal fullness or bloating, nausea, poor appetite, weakness, fatigue, and feelings of incomplete defecation. These symptoms may be long-standing and often have an erratic pattern, with periods of quiescence interrupted by exacerbations. By contrast, any change in a patient's typical symptom complex or the onset of fever, weight loss, hematochezia, melena, or vomiting associated with the aforementioned complaints may suggest a structural disorder warranting a different approach to diagnosis.

Physical Examination

Although older age can be associated with functional GI disorders, most patients are middle-aged or younger. The physical examination often reveals little more than poorly localized tenderness, usually in the lower quadrants. By contrast, objective physical findings of point tenderness, organomegaly, or occult GI blood loss warrant additional evaluation. Functional disorders may be attributed to the esophagus, stomach, small and large intestines, rectum, and biliary system. Some of the more common functional disorders are listed in Table 1 and deserve specific attention.

ESOPHAGUS

Psychogenic Dysphagia

Also known as globus sensation, and previously known as globus hystericus, the patient with psychogenic dysphagia usually complains of a "lump" or "fullness" in the

Table 1. Specific Functional Disorders

Esophagus
Psychogenic dysphagia (globus sensation)
Rumination (merycism)
Esophageal dysmotility
Stomach
Aerophagia
Gastroparesis
Nonulcer dyspepsia
Small Intestine
Pseudo-obstruction
Large Intestine and Rectum
Irritable bowel syndrome
Constipation
Pruritus ani
Proctalgia fugax
Pseudo-obstruction
Biliary System
Sphincter of Oddi dysfunction

throat. The sensation is often constant and does not interfere with the swallowing of solids or liquids. Globus may be temporarily relieved by deglutition. Symptoms of globus may accompany a structural disorder, and a diagnosis of globus should not be made until gastroesophageal reflux, hypertensive upper esophageal sphincter, neuromuscular disorders, and abnormalities of the pharynx and larynx have been excluded. As the previous name of globus hystericus implies, globus has been considered a symptom of a hysterical personality trait or disorder. However, globus has been reported to be more common in patients with obsessive-compulsive disorders and depression and somewhat rare in hysterics.

Rumination

The rumination syndrome is an eating disorder in which patients regurgitate small amounts of food immediately after swallowing, rechew, and then reswallow the bolus. Although there is no associated psychiatric diagnosis, the syndrome is more commonly observed in institutionalized patients and in children or adolescents with emotional disorders or intellectual impairment. There are generally three groups of patients with rumination. In the first and most common group, rumination develops as a maladaptive, learned habit in response to conscious or unconscious stressors. Patients may complain of vomiting, reflux symptoms, halitosis, weight loss, or dental caries. In the second group, rumination is associated with bulimia, which may or may not have been previously recognized. The third group includes emotionally or intellectually deprived adults or adolescents whose behavior has been observed by a health care worker. The clinical diagnosis of rumination can be made in the absence of an underlying organic or emotional pathologic condition. Although esophageal manometry may reveal a distinctive pattern, extensive testing is not necessary.

Esophageal Dysmotility

Esophageal dysmotility has been described with hypertensive and hypotensive lower esophageal sphincter, diffuse esophageal spasm, nutcracker esophagus, achalasia, irritable bowel syndrome (IBS), and nonspecific motility disorders. Reported symptoms reflect this diversity and may include chest pain, dysphagia, reflux symptoms, chronic cough or hoarseness, nausea, vomiting, and odynophagia.

The clinician should document the duration of symptoms, alleviating or exacerbating factors, presence of dysphagia with solids or liquids, degree of the progression of symptoms, amount and duration of tobacco and ethanol use, family history, use of medication, and history of diabetes, connective tissue disease, thyroid disorders, hypertension, and amyloidosis. If the symptoms are located in the cervical esophagus or are characterized by the inability to transport food from the mouth to the esophagus, the possibility of a cerebrovascular accident or neuromuscular disorder should be considered.

In the absence of extensive underlying malignancy or connective tissue disease, physical examination and laboratory evaluation are typically unremarkable. The initial evaluation of the patient with presumed esophageal dysmotility should include a barium esophagram or esophagogastroduodenoscopy (EGD). Esophagrams can reveal structural abnormalities, including achalasia, and esophagogastroduodenoscopy can detect fine mucosal abnormalities, including evidence of reflux. Neither technique, however, will confirm motor disorders of the esophagus. Manometry can measure esophageal motor function, but contraction abnormalities are found in only 28 per cent of patients with suspected motor dysfunction. Ice water challenge, balloon distention, edrophonium administration, 24-hour pH determination, and motility testing may slightly increase the rate of positive diagnosis.

STOMACH

Aerophagia

Aerophagia, or swallowing of air, normally accompanies ingestion of solids and liquids. The ingested air can then be voluntarily or involuntarily released from the stomach through the oral cavity. There are, however, a number of conditions in which the swallowed air is excessive and produces symptoms that may not be initially attributed to the upper GI tract.

Aerophagia is seen in association with the hyperventilation syndrome, gastroesophageal reflux disease, and noncardiac or anginalike chest pain. Patients with aerophagia frequently have a history of bloating, chronic belching, excessive flatus, or other vague abdominal complaints. The magenblase syndrome is a sharp, fleeting chest pain in the left anterior chest or left hypochondrium that may radiate to the neck or shoulder. This syndrome is related to gastric distention by air and is exacerbated by deep breathing, bending, or other maneuvers that increase pressure on the distended stomach or on the diaphragm. Eructation of the air relieves the pain. The diagnosis is often made by history alone, but the possibility of myocardial ischemia must always be kept in mind. Radiographic evidence of gastric distention and positive maneuvers on physical examination support the diagnosis.

Ingested air not released through the oral cavity continues through the GI tract and is released as flatus. Air can be trapped at the splenic flexure, leading to the splenic flexure syndrome. Patients with this syndrome complain of aching or pressure in the left upper abdomen or left precordium with occasional radiation to the neck or shoulders. Radiographic evidence of gaseous distention near the splenic flexure and exacerbation of the pain during palpation further support the diagnosis. Defecation or passage of flatus provides relief.

Finally, aerophagia may be a part of the hyperventilation syndrome seen in patients with panic disorders, phobias, situational anxiety, and cardiac or respiratory disorders. Patients present with chest pain with or without associated lightheadedness, dyspnea, paresthesias, palpitations, and anxiety. The chest pain has been attributed to mechanical discomfort from hyperinflated lungs, a distended stomach from aerophagia, musculoskeletal sources in the chest wall, forceful myocardial contractions from heightened sympathetic tone, and myocardial ischemia due to coronary vasoconstriction and altered oxygen supply (Bohr effect).

Physical examination may reproduce or exacerbate pain from a mechanical or musculoskeletal source, but myocardial ischemia or infarction may present with chest wall pain as well. Confounding the diagnosis of hyperventilation syndrome is the fact that hyperventilation itself may cause electrocardiographic changes consistent with ischemia.

Gastroparesis

Gastroparesis is a motility disorder in which gastric emptying of solids or liquids is delayed. Gastroparesis typically accompanies a pre-existing illness or condition, but an idiopathic form exists. Common causes of gastroparesis include diabetes mellitus; connective tissue disease, including scleroderma and dermatomyositis; hypokalemia; hypothyroidism; drugs, such as opiates, anticholinergics, and psychotropics; pregnancy; viral or bacterial gastroenteritis; and previous gastric surgery that included vagotomy. Patients with delayed gastric emptying have nausea, vomiting, bloating, reflux symptoms, early satiety, anorexia, and weight loss.

Because the symptom complex is ubiquitous and not pathognomonic for gastroparesis, the history of a gastroparetic patient should exclude or elicit secondary causes of slowed gastric emptying. Important aspects of the history include timing of the symptoms (i.e., immediately versus hours after meals), frequency, duration, amount and consistency of emesis; dysphagia; constipation; diarrhea; and fecal incontinence. The physical examination is unrevealing except for the possible presence of a "succussion splash," which is a splashing noise caused by stasis of liquids or semiliquids that is heard with or without a stethoscope on shaking of the abdomen. A succussion splash may also be heard with adynamic ileus if large volumes of gas and liquid are present.

The evaluation of gastroparesis should exclude metabolic and mechanical causes of slowed gastric emptying. Appropriate laboratory testing should exclude hypokalemia, hyper- and hypocalcemia, hypothyroidism, syphilis, and pregnancy, whereas an upper GI series with small bowel follow-through can exclude mechanical obstruction. If these tests are normal or if there is evidence of gastric stasis due to retained food particles or bezoar, gastric emptying can be evaluated directly by administration of a radiolabeled test meal and measurement of the degree of retention. If a diagnosis of gastroparesis still cannot be made, the clinician should consider empirical treatment with a prokinetic agent or referral to a center that performs gastric manometry or electrogastrography.

Nonulcer Dyspepsia

Nonulcer dyspepsia refers to those functional gastrointestinal disorders whose symptoms suggest an upper tract source. Many of the symptoms, including epigastric pain, postprandial bloating, nausea, and vomiting, overlap with known GI disorders previously termed idiopathic, including IBS. As more sophisticated diagnostic modalities become available, it is likely that underlying pathologic causes will be detected. Possible diagnoses, many of which are discussed in this article, include motor dysfunction of the stomach, small bowel, and biliary system. *Helicobacter pylori*, a microbe that contributes to antritis and peptic ulcer disease, probably does not play a role in functional dyspepsia.

SMALL INTESTINE

Pseudo-obstruction

Primary small intestinal pseudo-obstruction is a rare syndrome characterized by recurrent episodes of small bowel obstruction in the absence of a mechanical lesion. The primary forms are subdivided into familial visceral myopathy with degeneration of enteric smooth muscle and familial visceral neuropathy with degeneration of the myenteric plexus. Secondary causes of pseudo-obstruction include drugs (tricyclic antidepressants, clonidine, opiates), connective tissue disorders, endocrine disorders (diabetes mellitus, hypothyroidism), and neurologic disorders (Parkinson's disease).

Patients have a long history of nausea, vomiting, abdominal pain, distention, constipation, diarrhea, and/or urinary problems. These symptoms may be part of a generalized visceral neuromyopathy syndrome in which all hollow viscera have hypomotility. Patients often have experienced multiple diagnostic procedures, including laparotomy. A thorough history should detect any symptoms suggesting a secondary cause of pseudo-obstruction or a family history of similar symptomatology. Physical examination may show abdominal distention, and if the pseudo-obstruction is severe, a succussion splash may be present.

In the absence of endocrine diseases, serum chemistry panels are normal. Radiographic changes, however, are not uncommon and may provide clues to the cause of the underlying defect. Patients with visceral myopathy typically display an enlarged duodenum, dilated colon with loss of haustral folds, and poor to absent contractions. Visceral neuropathy and secondary causes of pseudo-obstruction are associated with nonspecific radiographic findings of increased intestinal gas and air-fluid levels.

The diagnosis of intestinal pseudo-obstruction is difficult. The clinician must be aware of the syndrome and must eliminate structural causes using barium radiography and endoscopy. If these studies produce normal results or evidence of a motor disorder, an investigation of intestinal motor function is warranted. In properly selected patients, abnormalities of intestinal motor activity have been shown in 85 per cent of cases. Such testing, however, requires referral to a tertiary center with experience in performing the procedure.

LARGE INTESTINE AND RECTUM

Irritable Bowel Syndrome

IBS is a common functional bowel disorder, and represents the most common condition seen by gastroenterologists. Although most individuals with IBS do not seek medical care, it is a specific disorder and not a diagnosis of exclusion. Criteria for the diagnosis of IBS are based on symptoms that are present in most persons but are seen in greater degree in IBS patients. These symptoms include abdominal pain, altered bowel habits, a sensation of incomplete defecation, passage of mucus with the stool, flatus, bloating, and relief of discomfort with defecation. Indicators of organic disease such as significant weight loss, anemia, gastrointestinal blood loss, or onset after 40 years of age are not part of IBS; these indicators warrant an independent investigation.

The history in patients with possible IBS should focus not only on the presence of typical symptoms for at least 3 months but also on defined criteria such as those supported by the International Congress of Gastroenterology (Table 2). The dietary history should elicit symptoms of lactose maldigestion or food intolerance. The use of medication should be reviewed, and symptoms of organic disease such as fever, weight loss, and nocturnal symptoms should be excluded. Although the relationship of psychosocial factors to symptoms should be explored, the clinician should recognize that a diagnosis of IBS does not carry a concomitant diagnosis of psychiatric illness. Although it is true that patients with symptoms of IBS who seek medical care have a higher prevalence of psychiatric diagnoses than do those who do not seek care, it is also true that patients with psychiatric illness or psychosocial dysfunction are more likely to seek medical attention for nongastrointestinal illnesses as well. Psychosocial factors are important in IBS as far as how the patient's discomfort is perceived but

Table 2. International Congress of Gastroenterology Criteria for the Irritable Bowel Syndrome

Continuous or recurrent symptoms for at least 3 months
Abdominal pain or discomfort that is relieved with defecation and/or is associated with a change in frequency and/or consistency of stool
An irregular (varying) pattern of defecation at least 25% of the time (two or more of the following):
Altered stool frequency (>3 bowel movements per day or <3 bowel movements per week)
Altered stool form (lumpy or hard or loose or watery stool)
Altered stool passage (straining or urgency or a feeling of incomplete evacuation)
Passage of mucus
Bloating or feeling of abdominal distention

not as a cause of the symptoms. Theories regarding the pathophysiology of IBS include alterations in gut motility, autonomic nervous system dysfunction, and increased perception and awareness of gut distention.

The physical examination is generally normal, with nonspecific abdominal tenderness to palpation elicited most frequently. Objective abnormalities such as visceromegaly, ascites, or modified guiac test (Hemoccult)–positive stools are not consistent with IBS and should lead away from the diagnosis. Routine laboratory studies are frequently normal, but reasonable screening tests include a complete blood count, chemistry panel, and lactose hydrogen breath testing for lactose maldigestion. Some centers advocate erythrocyte sedimentation rates, stool studies for ova and parasites, thyroid profiles, and flexible sigmoidoscopy in the initial evaluation, but recent studies have not demonstrated the clinical utility of this approach. Structural evaluations using flexible sigmoidoscopy, barium enema, radiography, or colonoscopy should be performed as dictated by symptoms and age-related risks of colon cancer.

Constipation

Constipation is a common subjective complaint. Objectively, constipation is defined as fewer than three bowel movements per week or straining to pass a stool during 25 per cent or more of the total weekly number of bowel movements. The evaluation of constipation begins with a complete history. Inquiries should focus on the confirmation of true constipation, the onset and duration of symptoms, amount of physical activity, genitourinary symptoms, fiber intake, frequency of laxative use, and evidence of depression or other affective disorders. Medications may cause or aggravate constipation, which is not a natural phenomenon of the aging process. Thus, elderly individuals should not be evaluated any less aggressively than younger patients with the same complaint. The physical examination of the constipated patient should search for evidence of secondary causes of constipation and should include a neurologic examination and inspection of the perineum, rectum, and anus to evaluate for rectal prolapse, abnormal location of the anus, anal stenosis, and rectosphincteric dyssynergia.

Diagnostic evaluation of the constipated patient is focused initially on exclusion of organic disease. Laboratory testing should include thyroid-stimulating hormone (TSH) determinations to detect hypothyroidism. Flexible sigmoidoscopy and colonoscopy may reveal melanosis coli or intraluminal obstruction. Barium radiographs may indicate obstructing lesions or retention of stool, and they can be used to evaluate the efficacy of cathartics in fecal impaction. These studies, however, are not helpful in assessing anorectal and colonic motor function or transit time. Colonic transit studies using either radiopaque markers or radioactive isotopes can document slow or normal transit time and further direct the evaluation. Patients with abnormal transit studies typically fall into two categories: those with colonic inertia and those with outlet obstruction.

Patients with colonic inertia have a hypomotile colon with decreased phasic activity and increased compliance. These patients should undergo anorectal manometry to detect abnormalities of rectal sensation, rectal elasticity, and internal anal sphincter function. Patients with abnormalities by anorectal manometry should be considered for evaluation of more widespread GI motor dysfunction. Thus, esophageal, gastric, and small intestinal motility studies may be warranted. Patients with outlet obstruction have a more localized abnormality and should be evaluated with anorectal manometry and defecography.

Pruritus Ani

Pruritus ani refers to anal itching, frequently attributed to poor hygiene or nonspecific, short-lived conditions. Seventy-five per cent of patients with pruritus ani, however, have underlying anorectal or colon abnormalities such as hemorrhoids, anal fissures, and rectal carcinoma. Pruritus ani occurs in 1 to 5 per cent of the population and shows 4:1 preponderance in males. The primary event of itching or burning causes an itch-scratch cycle, which can ultimately abrade the perianal skin and induce a local inflammatory response with worsening edema and itching.

The history should elucidate the onset and duration of symptoms, previous symptomatology, previous diagnostic tests results, radiation or other treatments to the pelvis, new personal hygiene products, laundry detergents and soaps, proctalgia, hematochezia, diet, sexual habits, and exposure to children. The risk of underlying neoplasia is increased in those older than 50 years of age whose symptoms have been present longer than 7 weeks.

The physical examination should note the degree of perianal irritation, fecal spillage, lesions of the anal outlet, and abnormalities on digital rectal examination.

The diagnosis of pruritus ani may be made by history and physical examination alone, but skin scrapings for parasites such as *Enterobius vermicularis* may be helpful. Those cases that prove refractory to conservative management should be evaluated with endoscopy and biopsies, if appropriate, to exclude secondary causes of pruritus ani.

Proctalgia Fugax

Proctalgia fugax is a condition of unknown cause that is characterized by sudden, brief episodes of severe rectal pain that last less than 1 minute. Proctalgia fugax occurs fewer than six times a year. The condition has been attributed to anal internal sphincter spasm, spasm of the pelvic floor musculature, and accumulation of rectal gas. Although many persons with proctalgia fugax do not seek medical attention, those who do describe a sharp midline pain above the anus lasting seconds to minutes without reproducible associated symptoms. Results of physical examination, serum chemistry panels, radiographs, and endoscopy are unremarkable.

Pseudo-obstruction

Acute Colonic Pseudo-obstruction (Ogilvie's Syndrome)

Acute colonic pseudo-obstruction is typically seen in patients with severe illness or injury and is characterized by acute nonmechanical dilatation of the distal colon. Patients complain of nausea, vomiting, difficulty with feedings, abdominal pain, and abdominal distention. The physical examination reveals absent to decreased bowel sounds and tympanitic percussion notes. Radiographs reveal segmental colonic distention (9 to 18 cm), especially in the cecum. Because cecal perforation is better correlated with the duration of colonic dilatation than with the diameter of the colon, close observation may be warranted in some patients.

Chronic Colonic Pseudo-obstruction

Chronic colonic pseudo-obstruction is a motility disorder of the colon of unknown cause that is typically part of a diffuse GI motor disorder but can occur in isolated form. Most patients complain of recurrent postprandial abdominal pain and distention; a few present with nausea and vomiting. The history should determine the age of onset, duration of symptoms, family history of similar symptoms, presence of weight loss, dietary habits, previous surgeries, constipation, use of laxatives, and symptoms of diabetes, thyroid disorders, and connective tissue disease.

In asymptomatic patients with chronic colonic pseudo-obstruction, the results of the physical examination are nonspecific or unremarkable. By contrast, examination during a period of abdominal pain or distention may reveal a tympanitic abdomen that is painful to palpation but does not display rebound or guarding. Radiographic studies are also most informative when obtained during an episode of pain. Plain radiographs may reveal a distended colon with little small intestinal gas, whereas barium enema studies may reveal megacolon. Upper GI barium radiographs and small intestinal motility studies are unremarkable. Anorectal manometry should be performed to exclude adult presentations of Hirschsprung's disease.

BILIARY SYSTEM

Sphincter of Oddi Dysfunction (Biliary Dyskinesia)

The sphincter of Oddi is the portion of the bile duct that extends from the junction of the common bile duct and pancreatic duct and drains bile into the duodenum through an orifice in the papilla of Vater. The sphincter of Oddi is usually 10 to 15 mm in length, and its physiologic function includes regulation of the flow of bile into the duodenum, diversion of hepatically formed bile into the gallbladder, and prevention of reflux of duodenal contents into the common bile duct.

Patients with sphincter of Oddi dysfunction almost always present after cholecystectomy (1 to 37 years previously) with continued or renewed upper abdominal pain of pancreaticobiliary origin. Sphincter of Oddi dysfunction is more common in middle-aged women who present with sharp epigastric or right upper quadrant pain with radiations to the left shoulder or right shoulder blade areas. Fever, chills, and jaundice are not common, but nausea and vomiting may be present. The physical examination is typically unremarkable, but right upper quadrant or epigastric pain may be elicited.

The diagnosis of sphincter of Oddi dysfunction requires a combination of abnormal laboratory tests results and abnormalities on endoscopic retrograde cholangiopancreatography (ERCP) and is divided into three categories. Type I patients have mild elevations of aspartate aminotransferase (AST) and alkaline phosphatase with delayed drainage of ERCP contrast material (>45 minutes and a common bile duct dilatation of greater than 12 mm). Biliary manometry is not required for diagnosis in this group. Type II patients have the same pain characteristics as type I patients, but only one or two of the laboratory or ERCP criteria; biliary manometry that demonstrates a high sphincter of Oddi resting pressure is necessary for diagnosis. Type III patients have only the pain syndrome and no laboratory or ERCP abnormalities, and manometry is required for diagnosis.

DYSPHAGIA, ESOPHAGEAL OBSTRUCTION, AND ESOPHAGITIS

By Michael K. Koehler, M.D.,
and Gregory S. Cooper, M.D.
Cleveland, Ohio

Dysphagia is a symptom related to the hindrance of food passing from the mouth to the stomach and can be secondary to esophageal obstruction or a variety of neuromuscular disorders. Patients frequently state that food gets "caught" or "stuck." Pain with swallowing or odynophagia is rare and is most often associated with esophageal mucosal disease. True dysphagia is pathologic and indicative of an organic esophageal abnormality. Therefore, it is warranted to distinguish true dysphagia from other swallowing sensations (i.e., globus sensation) with a thorough medical history. Dysphagia can be characterized in many different ways, but difficulty in swallowing both solids and liquids implies an abnormality in peristalsis (motility disorder), whereas progression of dysphagia from solids to liquids suggests a mechanical esophageal obstruction. Dysphagia can also be classified on a structural basis—an abnormality affecting striated muscle (oropharyngeal dysphagia) or affecting smooth muscle (esophageal dysphagia). Investigating dysphagia in either situation requires a multidisciplinary approach of radiologic, endoscopic, and manometric evaluation. An algorithm for the evaluation of patients with dysphagia is presented in Figure 1.

OROPHARYNGEAL DYSPHAGIA

Oropharyngeal dysphagia is due to an abnormality in the striated muscle of the mouth, oropharynx, and/or proximal esophagus. There are many causes of oropharyngeal dysphagia, but neuromuscular disorders account for a majority (approximately 80 per cent). It is most prevalent in the elderly and frequently indicates a poor prognosis. The history is most important in localizing the abnormality. During attacks, patients repeatedly attempt to swallow and localize the difficulty at the suprasternal notch and/or retrosternal area. The sensation typically occurs immediately after swallowing and may be associated with difficulty in transferring food into the proximal esophagus. The patient may also report nasal regurgitation or aspiration at meals and, in severe cases, drooling while not eating. Associated findings include dysarthria, facial paralysis, hoarseness, muscle weakness, fatigue, and weight loss.

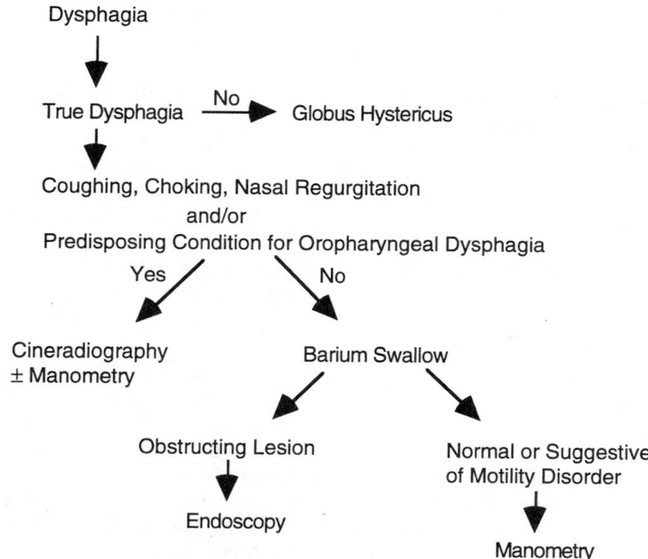

Figure 1. Algorithm for evaluation of dysphagia.

The history and physical examination highlight a systemic neuromuscular disorder in many patients. Diagnosis of oropharyngeal dysphagia is made by cineradiography and manometry. Cineradiography is usually chosen because it provides a videotape of the patient's complete swallowing mechanism from the oropharynx to the proximal esophagus. The consistency of the bolus can be varied during the examination for both diagnostic and therapeutic benefits in planning treatment. Manometry is less helpful, but it can be used to characterize the upper esophageal sphincter (UES) with respect to tone, relaxation, and coordination. Endoscopic evaluation has the most limited role but is helpful in excluding luminal distal obstruction with symptoms referred to the proximal esophagus.

Neurologic Disorders

Stroke or any neurologic insult affecting the swallowing center or the cranial nerves involved in swallowing (cranial nerves V, VII, IX, X, and XII) can result in oropharyngeal dysphagia. Cerebrovascular accident (CVA) is one of the most common causes of oropharyngeal dysphagia, but most deficits resolve over a short time. Computed tomography (CT) and magnetic resonance imaging (MRI) scans frequently reveal multiple brain lesions. Isolated hemispheric lesions, however, can cause oropharyngeal dysphagia as well, most likely secondary to brain stem edema. On initial presentation, most patients display other abnormalities on physical examination. Oropharyngeal dysphagia as an initial presenting symptom of an acute CVA is rare. Some patients do have persistent swallowing dysfunction following an acute CVA. These patients may benefit from speech therapy to learn various maneuvers that aid in swallowing. In patients with amyotrophic lateral sclerosis (ALS), weakening of both the tongue and pharyngeal muscles results in oropharyngeal dysphagia. Other, less common causes include chronic bulbar and pseudobulbar palsies, which are secondary to degeneration of the upper and lower motor neuron tracts, respectively. Parkinson's disease, which is secondary to degeneration of the substantia nigra of the midbrain, can also affect the swallowing center in the brain stem. Patients with Parkinson's disease present in a heterogeneous fashion; some have no symptoms, whereas others have oropharyngeal dysphagia with life-threatening aspiration. They typically have other parkinsonian features on evaluation, including resting tremor, blank facies, and balance disturbances. Cineradiography reveals pharyngeal stasis with poor food transfer and aspiration. Approximately 35 per cent of patients with multiple sclerosis have oropharyngeal dysphagia. Abnormalities in food bolus transfer, proximal esophageal tone, and UES tone all have been described. Disorders of the peripheral nervous system secondary to toxic agents such as botulism, tetanus, lead, or alcohol can also produce oropharyngeal dysphagia.

Muscular Disorders

Polymyositis and dermatomyositis are diseases of the striated muscle that frequently involve the proximal esophagus. Although 60 to 70 per cent of patients demonstrate esophageal abnormalities on radiologic and manometric investigation, only 50 per cent complain of dysphagia. Cineradiography typically reveals poor pharyngeal contraction, pooling and retention of barium in the oropharynx, and a disorganized emptying pattern. Manometry usually shows both decreased proximal muscle contraction and UES tone. Both dermatomyositis and polymyositis have also been associated with paraneoplastic syndromes (Eaton-Lambert syndrome), which most commonly occur in the setting of small cell carcinoma. Manometry is characteristic, showing esophageal contractions that increase with repetitive activity.

Myasthenia gravis (MG) is a prototypic motor end-plate disorder that can involve the proximal esophagus. Patients may begin eating normally, but throughout the meal, dysphagia progresses resulting from fatigue with activity. On cineradiography, normal swallowing can occur initially, but as the test continues, poor bolus transfer may become apparent. Manometry typically confirms the same swallowing pattern, as esophageal contraction amplitude diminishes with repetitive activity. A Tensilon test confirms the diagnosis by using an anticholinesterase inhibitor such as edrophonium.

Oropharyngeal dysphagia has also been associated with two types of muscular dystrophy: (1) myotonic dystrophy and (2) oculopharyngeal dystrophy. Myotonic dystrophy is a familial disease of young men that produces dysphagia in 50 per cent of cases. Cineradiography shows impaired oropharyngeal emptying, and manometry reveals both decreased UES and proximal esophageal tone. Oculopharyngeal dystrophy is a rare autosomal dominant disease seen in elderly patients with ptosis followed by oropharyngeal dysphagia. Dysphagia is due to pharyngeal muscle weakness manifested by an inability to transfer food into the proximal esophagus. Unlike myotonic dystrophy, manometric studies of the proximal esophagus and UES produce normal results.

Upper Esophageal Sphincter Disorders

"Cricopharyngeal hypertension" is a term used for higher than normal UES tone seen in the setting of dysphagia. This abnormality has been associated with gastroesophageal reflux, the postlaryngectomy state, globus hystericus, and the rare Plummer-Vinson syndrome (esophageal web and iron deficiency anemia). Cricopharyngeal hypotonia refers to low UES tone and is most commonly seen in the setting of neuromuscular disorders and in postlaryngectomy patients.

Abnormal UES relaxation can also produce oropharyngeal dysphagia and is due to incomplete relaxation (cricopharyngeal achalasia), delayed relaxation, or premature closure. Cricopharyngeal achalasia is seen most often in newborns and less frequently in adults. Cineradiography may reveal incomplete relaxation of the UES with a cricopharyngeal bar at C6–C7. Delayed relaxation of the UES has been associated with autosomal recessive dysautonomia (Riley-Day syndrome). Zenker's diverticula are also frequently seen in the setting of premature closure of the UES.

ESOPHAGEAL DYSPHAGIA

Esophageal dysphagia is due to an abnormality affecting the lower two thirds of the esophagus (smooth muscle). A variety of causes exist, and they can be most conveniently classified into those causing a neuromuscular (motility) defect or mechanical obstruction of the esophagus. Symptoms may be poorly localized to the sternum or retrosternal notch or referred to the neck and shoulder, mimicking cardiac angina. Neuromuscular disorders frequently result in dysphagia with both solids and liquids, whereas mechanical obstruction, such as carcinoma or peptic stricture, results in progressive dysphagia from solids to include liquids. Therefore, the clinical history is the most valuable tool for distinguishing the cause of the dysphagia by eliciting the type of food causing the symptoms and determining the location and duration of the dysphagia as well as other associated symptoms such as weight loss, regurgitation, heartburn, or nocturnal cough. As with oropharyngeal dysphagia, evaluation requires a multidisciplinary approach using radiology, endoscopy, and manometry.

Neuromuscular Disorders

Idiopathic achalasia is an esophageal motility disorder due to a defect in the innervation of the esophagus and lower esophageal sphincter (LES). The cause remains unknown, but there is a degeneration of ganglion cells at Auerbach's plexus, with resulting aperistalsis of the esophageal body and obstruction at the gastroesophageal junction. Clinically, this results in progressive dysphagia of solids and liquids with regurgitation of food. Patients present most commonly between the ages of 20 and 40 years with long-standing symptoms, and men and women are affected equally. Patients may complain of odynophagia early in the course, but rarely heartburn, because the increased LES pressure seems protective against reflux. Typical findings on chest film include mediastinal widening secondary to a dilated esophagus, evidence of recurrent aspiration pneumonia, and the absence of a gastric air bubble. The barium esophagram shows a characteristic "bird-beaked" appearance with a dilated fluid-filled esophagus tapered at the distal end. The diagnosis is further substantiated by typical manometric findings, including (1) aperistalisis of the esophageal body, (2) incomplete relaxation of the LES, (3) increased LES pressure, and (4) increased esophageal pressure relative to gastric pressure. The diagnosis is not confirmed until the endoscopic evaluation is complete, however, because secondary achalasia or pseudoachalasia may occur from infiltration of the gastroesophageal junction by primary or metastatic cancer (e.g., bronchogenic, breast, or pancreatic) or lymphoma with clinical symptoms that can mimic idiopathic achalasia.

Symptomatic diffuse esophageal spasm is a motility disorder of unknown cause characterized by chest pain and dysphagia. Chest pain is present in 80 to 90 per cent of patients and dysphagia in 30 to 60 per cent, and patients most often present for evaluation after a normal cardiac evaluation. Chest pain is often provoked by hot or cold liquids, carbonated beverages, or even stress. Women are affected more often than men and the disease occurs most commonly in middle age. The barium esophagogram reveals simultaneous, nonperistaltic contractions in a segmental fashion, resembling a "rosary bead" or, in extreme cases, there is a "corkscrew" appearance. The diagnosis rests on characteristic clinical symptomatology with abnormal manometric findings. These findings include increased simultaneous nonperistaltic contractions (>10 per cent wet swallows) with intermittent normal peristalsis and, occasionally, repetitive wave peaks (>2 peaks per wave), increased duration and amplitude of contractions, and fewer esophageal sphincter defects.

Progressive systemic sclerosis (PSS), or scleroderma, is a systemic disorder characterized by the replacement of smooth muscle by fibrosis secondary to a small vessel vasculitis. The cause remains unclear, but an autoimmune mechanism is favored. The esophagus is involved in 80 to 90 per cent of cases and is characterized by abnormal esophageal motility with progressive dysphagia with solids and liquids. A majority of patients have symptoms consistent with Raynaud's phenomenon, but they also have characteristic joint complaints and taut skin changes of fingers, hands, and face. Heartburn is common because of severe gastroesophageal reflux. The barium esophagogram reveals absent to poor peristalsis in the lower two thirds of the esophagus. In contrast to patients with achalasia, reflux of barium at the gastroesophageal junction is seen frequently. Manometry reveals aperistalsis or low-amplitude contractions in the smooth muscle esophagus similar to those seen in achalasia. However, in contrast to the increased LES pressure seen in achalasia, the LES pressure in progressive systemic sclerosis is abnormally low (<15 mm Hg), accounting for frequent symptoms of esophageal reflux. Upper endoscopy frequently reveals severe erosive esophagitis and in extreme cases a peptic stricture.

ESOPHAGEAL OBSTRUCTION

Diseases that cause esophageal obstruction, including esophageal cancer and peptic stricture, typically present with dysphagia to solids. This symptom generally does not manifest until the luminal diameter is reduced from a normal size of 20 mm to less than 12 mm. With further obstruction, patients may subsequently experience symptoms with semisolid foods or liquids. Patients may experience dysphagia localized to a specific point in the chest, but this point is often proximal to the actual site of obstruction.

Esophageal Cancer

Esophageal carcinoma is an important cause of obstruction. Approximately 12,000 new cases are diagnosed annually in the United States, and the high rate of metastatic disease at presentation results in almost 11,000 fatalities. Specific risk factors include black or Hispanic race, male gender, and tobacco and alcohol use, with a relative risk of more than 150-fold in patients who consume large quantities of both carcinogens. Less common predisposing conditions are tylosis, an autosomal dominant condition with thickening of the skin of the palms and soles; long-standing achalasia; and a prior history of lye-induced stricture. Although most carcinomas have squamous histologic characteristics, there has been an increasing incidence of esophageal adenocarcinoma over the past several years. These tumors are presumably related to underlying Barrett's esophagus (see further on). In addition to dysphagia, symptoms include dull midsternal pain, sometimes radiating to the back and usually reflecting local extension; weight loss; cough due to aspiration or tracheoesophageal fistula; hoarseness secondary to recurrent laryngeal nerve involvement; and hiccoughs resulting from phrenic nerve irritation. Rarely, primary malignancies of the esophagus may be due to spindle cell carcinoma (with histologic features of sarcomas), adenosquamous carcinoma, melanoma, oat cell carcinoma, and carcinoid tumors. Metastatic cancer to the esophagus is rare and is usually due to melanoma or breast carcinoma. The most common benign tumor of the esophagus is a leiomyoma, which presents as a smooth, rounded mass and is usually asymptomatic; dysphagia and retrosternal pain may develop in some patients.

Benign Strictures

Benign strictures are usually due to reflux esophagitis (see further on). Less common causes are previous caustic ingestion, radiation treatment, and associated bullous skin diseases. Strictures develop in about 10 to 20 per cent of patients who have ingested a caustic substance; they typically occur 4 to 8 weeks after ingestion and are usually associated with more severe acute injury. These strictures are characteristically dense and are commonly located near the tracheal bifurcation. Bullous disease, including pemphigus vulgaris, bullous pemphigoid, and epidermolysis bullosa, are disorders that affect squamous epithelium of the esophagus as well as the skin and produce symptoms from blistering and stricture formation. These benign conditions typically present with dysphagia but usually have a longer course of development.

Other Causes

The esophagus may also undergo extrinsic compression with resultant obstruction. Cardiovascular abnormalities (including an enlarged left atrium, aortic arch aneurysm or, rarely, anomalous right subclavian artery [dysphagia lusoria]), lung cancer, mediastinal tumors, or adenopathy; cervical osteophytes; thyromegaly; and mediastinal fibrosis all may produce external compression or displacement of the esophagus.

A lower esophageal or Schatzki's ring is a diaphragmlike structure that results from hyperplasia of both mucosa and submucosa at the gastroesophageal junction. It may be congenital or, more likely, a result of gastroesophageal reflux disease. Generally, these rings are manifested in patients older than 40 years of age. Although most rings are asymptomatic, they classically produce intermittent dysphagia, particularly with large boluses of meat ("steakhouse syndrome"). Mucosal webs are thin membranes of squamous epithelium, usually in the upper or midesophagus. Their prevalence increases with age. Most webs are asymptomatic, but intermittent dysphagia with solids is sometimes present. When associated with iron deficiency anemia (Plummer-Vinson syndrome), there is an increased risk of the development of cervical esophageal and pharyngeal cancer.

Diverticula are saclike protrusions of one or more layers of the wall. The most common type is Zenker's diverticulum, in which the posterior hypopharyngeal mucosa protrudes between the fibers of the inferior pharyngeal constrictor and cricopharyngeal muscles. This disorder is thought to result from poor compliance of the upper esophageal sphincter, with a resultant increase in hypopharyngeal pressure. Symptoms, which include dysphagia with solids and liquids, regurgitation of undigested food, cough, and halitosis, typically begin after age 50 years and are present from weeks to years before diagnosis. Diverticula may also develop in the middle or distal (epiphrenic) esophagus and are rarely symptomatic. Although these diverticula may result from traction by contiguous structures, most are thought to be due to motility disorders.

Evaluation

In patients with suspected esophageal obstruction, most clinicians use a barium study rather than endoscopy as the first diagnostic test. Radiography excludes lesions such as Zenker's diverticulum, which could potentially be perforated with passage of an endoscope. It also provides information about location, length, and luminal caliber around the mechanical lesion, which could influence the choice of endoscope and accessories. Moreover, radiography may be more sensitive than endoscopy for detecting strictures and rings, particularly if their caliber is larger than that of the endoscope. However, if a Schatzki's ring is suspected, the sensitivity of barium studies is even higher if a full-column technique or barium marshmallow is used instead of a double-contrast study. Although radiographic features (i.e., smooth versus irregular caliber, associated mass) are often suggestive of a benign versus malignant process, all strictures should undergo endoscopy with biopsy for definitive diagnosis. In addition, endoscopic dilation of lesions is generally performed at the same time.

Esophageal cancer is recognized radiographically in its early stage by disruption or loss of the normal mucosal pattern, irregularity or stiffness of the wall, or small ulcerations. Advanced lesions usually are polypoid intraluminal masses, and less frequently they infiltrate the submucosa with loss of distensibility with or without luminal narrowing. The gold standard for the diagnosis of esophageal cancer is endoscopy with biopsy, which has an accuracy of up to 95 per cent, particularly if multiple biopsy specimens are taken. Brush cytology studies via endoscopy are positive in 70 to 90 per cent of cases. Although computed tomography is useful for evaluating the presence of regional metastasis for suspected or known carcinoma, endoscopic ultrasound is probably the most accurate method for staging.

ESOPHAGITIS

Esophagitis, or inflammation of the esophagus, is due to a multitude of causes, including acid peptic disease, infection, or medication use, among others. Gastroesophageal reflux disease (GERD) accounts for the majority of cases of esophagitis, particularly in the immunocompetent host.

Gastroesophageal Reflux Disease

Gastroesophageal reflux, in which stomach contents migrate into the esophagus, occurs in both normal individuals and those with esophagitis and may or may not evoke symptoms. Conversely, the acronym GERD suggests clinical and/or histologic sequelae of reflux. Laymen often equate hiatal hernia with GERD. However, hiatal hernia refers to herniation of part of the stomach into the mediastinum through an incompetent diaphragmatic hiatus and can occur in individuals with or without objective evidence of esophageal reflux. The true prevalence of GERD is difficult to estimate, since most patients have intermittent or mild symptoms and do not seek medical attention. In telephone surveys, 44 per cent of adults said they experienced symptoms at least monthly, 5 to 10 per cent reported daily symptoms, and 13 per cent used over-the-counter antacids at least twice weekly. The disorder is even more common in pregnancy, with up to 80 per cent of women experiencing daily symptoms.

The cardinal symptom of GERD is heartburn or pyrosis, which is described as upward-moving, retrosternal burning pain, occasionally radiating to the throat. Symptoms are often postprandial, resulting from increased intragastric pressure, and are especially provoked by spicy foods, citrus fruits, fatty food, chocolate, and alcohol. Symptoms are also induced by vigorous exercise, especially running; tight fitting clothing; or increases in external pressure on the stomach, for example, bending, coughing, obesity, and ascites. Less common symptoms are regurgitation, in which gastric contents traverse both the lower and upper esophageal sphincters; belching, due to swallowing saliva and air brought on by esophageal reflux; waterbrash, which is the sudden appearance in the mouth of excess saliva secreted in response to intraesophageal acid exposure; and odynophagia, which is suggestive of significant mucosal injury. It is now recognized that GERD, rather than esophageal dysmotility, represents the most common cause of noncardiac chest pain and is due to the common innervation of the heart and esophagus. In addition, medications such as progesterone, nitrates, calcium channel blockers, anticholinergics, alpha-adrenergic antagonists, beta-2–agonists, and methylxanthines all may reduce lower esophageal sphincter tone and exacerbate esophageal injury.

In some series, as many as 25 per cent of patients with GERD exhibit only head and neck manifestations, which are thought to be due to pharyngeal reflux of acid. Patients may present to ear, nose, and throat specialists with symptoms that include chronic cough, sore throat, hoarseness, postnasal drip, otalgia, and the sensation of a "lump in the throat" that is unrelated to swallowing (globus hystericus). Suggestive physical findings include loss of the glistening appearance of the pharyngeal mucosa, heaped-up granularity of lymphoid follicles in the posterior pharynx, and erythema or edema of the vocal cords, which is termed "acid posterior laryngitis."

A subset of patients with GERD may present with primary pulmonary symptoms resulting from either microaspiration of gastric contents or a vagally mediated reflex arc. Approximately 50 to 70 per cent of asthmatics have acid reflux symptoms, independent of the use of predisposing medications (i.e., bronchodilators) and, conversely, 3 to 46 per cent of patients with GERD have asthma. As many as 50 per cent of patients with pulmonary fibrosis have evidence of GERD, and 4 per cent of those with GERD have fibrosis.

Complications of GERD include peptic stricture, which develops in as many as 10 per cent of patients during the course of disease. Typical symptoms include dysphagia with solids, especially boluses of meat, followed by semisolid foods, and lastly, liquids. Symptoms typically develop insidiously over months and are due to mucosal edema and spasm as well as fibrous scarring. Strictures are typically 2 to 4 cm in length and are usually located in the distal esophagus. A subset of patients either may have no antecedent heartburn or may have improvement in pyrosis once the stricture develops and an acid barrier is established.

Barrett's esophagus, or replacement of the squamous mucosa of the esophagus by columnar epithelium, is present in 5 to 12 per cent of patients with reflux symptoms, 33 per cent of patients with esophagitis, and nearly 50 per cent of patients with peptic strictures. As many as one third of patients have no antecedent history of reflux, raising the question of acid insensitivity. Adenocarcinoma, the most important sequela of Barrett's esophagus, is found in 7 to 15 per cent of patients at the first diagnosis of Barrett's esophagus, and the subsequent risk of cancer is between 1 in 80 and 1 in 450 per year. Overt gastrointestinal hemorrhage is an uncommon manifestation of esophagitis, and esophagitis accounts for only 2 to 6 per cent of all upper gastrointestinal bleeding episodes. Patients typically have diffuse ulcerative esophagitis.

Evaluation

Diagnosis of GERD is usually made by clinical symptoms as well as relief of symptoms by over-the-counter antacids or H_2-receptor antagonists. The so-called alarm symptoms that should warrant early evaluation include dysphagia, odynophagia, aspiration, wheezing, weight loss, and anemia. Barium studies are insensitive, particularly for mild esophagitis, and are not useful for assessing the presence or severity of reflux. The major use of barium studies is in evaluating the anatomy of patients with dysphagia associated with reflux. Esophageal manometry is also not recommended in the evaluation because there is significant overlap in findings (e.g., decreased LES pressure and abnormal contractions) between patients and controls. The Bernstein test, in which acid is infused into the esophagus, induces symptoms in 80 per cent of patients but is not routinely recommended because it does not correlate with severity of symptoms.

Esophagogastroduodenoscopy (EGD) is generally indicated for all patients with symptoms that persist after empirical therapy with H_2 antagonists or for those who relapse following discontinuation of therapy. EGD has several roles, including confirmation of the diagnosis by biopsy and exclusion of other diagnoses, assessment of disease severity and complications, and prediction of the likelihood of recurrence and the need for aggressive therapy. Histologic criteria include hyperplasia of the basal layer of the mucosa, with more than 15 per cent of the entire epithelial thickness, and elongation of dermal papillae close to the surface. The presence of inflammatory cells is neither sensitive nor specific. Esophagitis is usually graded endoscopically as 0 (normal), 1 (friability caused by thinning of the mucosa, erythema, or edema), 2 (isolated round or linear erosions with white exudate surrounded by red halos of erythema), 3 (confluent erosions or ulcerations extending around the entire circumference), and 4 (deep ulcerations, stricture, and/or Barrett's esophagus). Patients with grade 3 to 4 disease usually require more aggressive and long-term therapy. Grossly, Barrett's esophagus is recognized by pink mucosa that replaces the normal pale squamous epithelium, but biopsy is needed for definitive diagnosis and detection of dysplastic changes. Most patients found to have Barrett's esophagus are placed in an endoscopic surveillance program given the high risk of adenocarcinoma. Peptic strictures are usually recognized endoscopically and are often dilated at the time of the procedure.

The gold standard for diagnosis of GERD is a 24-hour pH monitor, using a probe placed 5 cm above the LES. The probe records both frequency and duration of acid reflux (defined as pH <4), and associated symptoms are recorded in a diary. The procedure has a sensitivity and specificity of about 90 per cent and is reserved mainly for patients with atypical and persistent symptoms associated with a normal EGD result.

Other Causes of Esophagitis

Drug-induced esophagitis is due to local irritation and occurs typically in the proximal or midesophagus. Drugs most commonly implicated are potassium chloride, quinidine, tetracycline, and nonsteroidal anti-inflammatory drugs. Specific risk factors include a structural esophageal abnormality (including left atrial enlargement) that increases mucosal contact time, use of sustained-release preparations, and advanced age.

Infectious esophagitis usually develops in immunocompromised hosts with conditions such as human immunodeficiency virus (HIV) infection or hematopoietic malignancy; those undergoing cancer chemotherapy and/or chest radiotherapy, or corticosteroid therapy; those with poorly controlled diabetes mellitus; and those undergoing solid organ or bone marrow transplantation. In general, such patients with dysphagia and/or odynophagia should undergo endoscopy promptly to identify the disease process and obtain biopsy and culture specimens. The only exception is the HIV-positive patient with dysphagia and oral thrush, who may be treated with empirical antifungals for presumed candidal esophagitis.

Esophageal candidiasis is recognized endoscopically by raised white or yellow plaques. Herpes simplex esophagitis is often associated with constant retrosternal chest pain and generally lacks systemic symptoms. Early on, there are rounded 1- to 3-mm vesicles, which progress to sharply demarcated ulcers with a yellow-gray base. Cytomegalovirus esophagitis is frequently associated with nausea, vomiting, and abdominal pain reflecting involvement of other organs as well. Lesions typically consist of shallow ulcerations in the mid- or distal esophagus. Acute or established HIV infection can result in multiple small or large undermining esophageal ulcers that are typically diagnosed by exclusion with negative cultures and failure to respond to empirical antiviral therapy. Radiation- or chemotherapy-induced mucositis, which is usually characterized by dysphagia, odynophagia, and/or chest pain, typically occurs from 1 to 4 weeks following initiation of exposure. Because these entities are clinically indistinguishable from infectious esophagitis, endoscopy with biopsy and culture should be performed. Strictures resulting from fibrosis may develop from 4 months to 5 years following radiation injury.

GASTRITIS

By Linda K. Green, M.D.,
and Bhupinderjit S. Anand, M.D.
Houston, Texas

The term gastritis means different things to different individuals. It is currently accepted to be any diffuse lesion of the gastric mucosa that shows inflammation on histologic examination. To the lay public, and indeed most physicians, gastritis suggests an inflamed gastric mucosa accompanied by symptoms of epigastric burning or discomfort, nausea or vomiting, and anorexia caused by overeating, excessive ethanol intake, spices, or the use of medications, especially nonsteroidal anti-inflammatory drugs (NSAIDs). In reality, gastritis rarely causes any of these symptoms, and most of the factors listed have little or no role in its pathogenesis.

Some clinicians have applied the term gastritis to conditions with vague upper gastrointestinal symptoms and endoscopically abnormal gastric mucosa or conditions that produce abnormal radiographic studies. However, without confirmation of inflammatory infiltrates on histologic examination of the gastric mucosa, the term gastritis is misused. To the endoscopist, gastritis implies hyperemia and erosions of the gastric mucosa whether or not there are accompanying histologic abnormalities. To the pathologist, it indicates the presence of increased inflammatory cellular infiltrate in the gastric mucosa, with or without damage to glandular elements.

TYPES OF GASTRITIS

Gastritis is a common condition that is often found in the elderly but may be seen at any age. Understanding the various causes of gastritis is necessary for directing appropriate diagnostic testing. The causes of gastritis are often multifactorial and may include infections, immunologic abnormalities, drug or alcohol use, systemic diseases, vascular abnormalities, bile reflux, gastric wall infiltrates, or ingestion of irritants. Currently, the most widely accepted histologic classification system of gastritis is that of the Sidney group, which sensibly classifies gastritis into acute, chronic, and special forms. Chronic gastritis can be further divided into (1) *Helicobacter pylori*–associated, (2) autoimmune (gastric atrophy), (3) drug-associated, and (4) idiopathic. *H. pylori* has been found in more than 90 per cent of patients with gastritis and is the causative agent in most forms of acute and chronic gastritis.

Another classification system used by clinicians is based on pathogenesis and associated clinical conditions (Table 1). Clinically, the most useful and simplest approach is to combine the endoscopic and histologic findings (Table 2).

PRESENTING SIGNS AND SYMPTOMS

The onset of gastritis can be insidious, with few clinical manifestations until complications such as pernicious anemia or carcinoma develop. If symptoms do appear, the patient typically presents with complaints of diffuse epigastric burning that lacks the periodicity of a duodenal ulcer. This pain is likely to increase after a large meal because the inflamed, thickened gastric wall is being stretched. Nonspecific symptoms can include nausea, vomiting, anorexia, weight loss, dysphagia, dyspepsia, weakness, hematemesis, and melena. The patient may abruptly present with an unheralded massive gastrointestinal bleeding episode or melena caused by erosive or hemorrhagic gastritis. Less frequently, there may be chronic blood loss, with the development of iron deficiency anemia and the presence of a positive stool guaiac test. Such a presentation is often seen in patients receiving chronic NSAID therapy. With ingestion of corrosive fluids, patients present with severe epigastric pain, retching, vomiting of blood-stained material, and hematemesis as the result of necrosis of the gastric wall. If disease has progressed to atrophic gastritis and pernicious anemia, the patient may have a burning tongue, paresthesias, and neurologic abnormalities. Bile reflux gastritis may cause bilious or green-yellow, watery vomitus. A young patient with eosinophilic gastritis may present with recurrent attacks of pain and vomiting due to pyloric outlet obstruction. Patients with phlegmonous gastritis, an extremely rare form of gastritis, present with fever, severe abdominal pain, and vomiting. The vomitus contains blood, pus, sloughed-off gastric mucosa, and even a "cast" of the stomach.

The clinical history should include a complete list of all types and dosages of medications being used, especially

Table 1. Classification of Gastritis

Erosive and Hemorrhagic	Nonerosive Nonspecific	Specific and Distinctive Forms
Stress	**Infectious**	**Infectious**
Organ system failure, burns, CNS trauma	(*Helicobacter pylori*)	Bacterial (tuberculosis, syphilis)
Drugs	**Reactive gastropathies**	Viral (CMV, herpes)
Aspirin, NSAIDs, alcohol, corrosive agents, iron, potassium chloride, hepatic arterial chemotherapy	Postgastrectomy	Fungal
Trauma	**Autoimmune**	Parasites
Nasogastric tube, retching, foreign body ingestion, endoscopic hemostasis	Pernicious anemia, lymphocytic gastritis	**Gastritis with generalized gastrointestinal disease**
Radiation	**Associated with adenocarcinoma**	Crohn's disease
Vascular	**Idiopathic or unexplained**	Eosinophilic gastritis
Ischemia due to thrombosis, vasculitis		**Gastritis with a systemic disease**
Reflux injury		Sarcoid
Uremia		Graft-versus-host disease
Idiopathic		Chronic granulomatous disease
		Unknown causes
		Ménétrier's disease

CNS = central nervous system; NSAIDs = nonsteroidal anti-inflammatory drugs; CMV = cytomegalovirus.

nonsteroidal anti-inflammatory agents, the amount of alcohol consumed, recent swallowing of corrosive substances (acid or alkali), previous abdominal surgical procedures, recent radiation or gastroendoscopic procedures, and past gastrointestinal illnesses.

The physical examination is frequently noncontributory. There may be epigastric tenderness or pallor and weakness secondary to anemia. A "smooth" tongue or glossitis (autoimmune gastritis), paresthesias, or melena on rectal examination may be found on rare occasion.

USEFUL LABORATORY OR DIAGNOSTIC PROCEDURES

Useful laboratory information may include the presence of anemia with hypochromic features due to the loss of iron via bleeding or macrocytic features due to vitamin B_{12} deficiency. Hypoproteinemia may occur as a result of exudation from the gastric mucosa. The severity of protein loss can be determined by measuring the amount of chromium-51 in the stool after intravenous administration of ^{51}Cr-labeled albumin. In pernicious anemia, vitamin B_{12} malabsorption is documented by an abnormal Schilling test and low serum vitamin B_{12} concentration. Cultures of gastric contents may be helpful for gastritis secondary to infections. Serum gastrin concentrations with atrophic gastritis can help determine whether a gastrinoma is present (Zollinger-Ellison syndrome). Gastric analysis with detection of bile or acid production is of limited value. Tests of gastric function are rarely performed, but normal gastric secretion makes a diagnosis of gastritis unlikely.

H. pylori can be detected by many methods, including gastric biopsy with special stains for identification of the organism, a culture of the gastric biopsy specimen, an enzyme-linked immunosorbent assay (ELISA) for *H. pylori*, a rapid urease test during endoscopy, a urea carbon breath test using carbon-13– or carbon-14–labeled urea, or polymerase chain reaction (PCR) tests of gastric biopsy specimens. Histologic studies with a routine hematoxylin and eosin (H and E) stain of an endoscopic biopsy specimen is the "gold standard" for diagnosis and helps not only in detecting the bacteria but also in determining the extent and severity of the gastritis. Recently, a rapid office-based blood test has become available. The main limitation of serologic testing is that the antibody concentration declines slowly after treatment, and the test cannot be used to assess cure.

Imaging Studies

Upper gastrointestinal radiography with contrast barium ingestion is of limited value. In atrophic gastritis, a "bald fundus" with thin, flat rugae can be seen, representing gastric atrophy. On double-contrast studies, varioliform gastritis shows typical halolike erosions. In Ménétrier's disease (giant hypertrophic gastritis), imaging studies disclose a markedly thickened gastric wall with prominent rugae so bizarre as to suggest the possibility of carcinoma. In phlegmonous gastritis, imaging studies, such as computed tomography (CT), are helpful and may show thick-

Table 2. Endoscopic and Histologic Findings

Nonerosive	Erosive or Hemorrhagic	Specific
Autoimmune	Damaging agents	Large folds
Helicobacter pylori	(NSAIDs, ethanol, corrosives, potassium)	(Ménétrier's disease, Zollinger-Ellison syndrome, lymphoma)
	Stress	Infections
	(Multiorgan failure, burns, CNS trauma)	(Bacterial, viral, fungal, parasitic)
	Local trauma	Eosinophilic infiltrate
	(Nasogastric tube, foreign body, endoscopic)	(Submucosal, muscular, subserosal)
	Ischemic	Granulomatous
	(Vascular, volvulus)	(Tuberculosis, Crohn's disease, sarcoid)

NSAIDs = nonsteroidal anti-inflammatory drugs; CNS = central nervous system.

ening of the wall of the stomach with pockets of pus and air (emphysematous gastritis).

Endoscopic Findings

In acute gastritis, the only reliable diagnosis is provided by endoscopy, which reveals erosions, superficial ulcerations, or sometimes a diffuse oozing of blood. Varioliform gastritis is recognized by the appearance of multiple umbilicated mounds in the gastric mucosa, usually surmounting the gastric folds. Acute erosive gastritis typically shows diffuse hyperemia or erosions of the gastric mucosa. Early endoscopy can assess the extent of injury but carries the risk of perforation. Erosions are defined as superficial breaks in the mucosal lining less than 0.5 mm in diameter. Acute erosions have a red base, often with a red halo. In some patients, the mucosa may be diffusely hyperemic, with or without discrete erosions. If evidence of active bleeding is seen, hemorrhagic gastritis is diagnosed. In Ménétrier's disease, gastric folds are observed along the greater curvature, with conspicuously increased height and thickness often accompanied by superficial ulcerations of the mucosa. In phlegmonous gastritis, endoscopy can be performed safely before transmural spread of infection and gangrene has occurred. The gastric mucosa is diffusely involved with ulcerations and necrosis. In emphysematous gastritis, submucosal gas-containing blebs can be seen. In eosinophilic gastritis, endoscopic findings range from normal-appearing gastric mucosa to thickened, nodular mucosal folds and superficial ulcerations. The antrum may be deformed with narrowing of the pyloric opening, which may not allow passage of the endoscope. Biopsy specimens should be obtained with "jumbo" forceps to obtain deeper tissue for histologic examination. In granulomatous gastritis, there may be mucosal ulcerations, nodularity, and a "cobblestone" pattern. In nonerosive gastritis, endoscopic findings are nonspecific, and random well-fixed biopsies of lesions from multiple sites are necessary.

Findings on Endoscopic Biopsy

Autoimmune gastritis (type A gastritis) involves the body and fundus of the stomach and progresses from chronic superficial gastritis to chronic atrophic gastritis and finally to gastric atrophy. There is a gradual decrease in the size and number of gastric glands, with loss of parietal and chief cells and replacement by mucus-secreting cells (pyloric metaplasia) and intestinal cells (intestinal metaplasia). Infiltration by lymphocytes and plasma cells is also seen.

H. pylori gastritis predominantly involves the antrum but may spread to involve the entire stomach. The organism—a comma-shaped gram-negative bacterium—is responsible for the most common form of gastritis, type B or *H. pylori*–associated gastritis. Nearly 50 per cent of the population in the United States is infected with *H. pylori*, and the infection rate may be greater than 90 per cent in developing countries. Histologically, there is an increase in the number of acute and chronic inflammatory cells, which is initially superficial. Eventually the infection extends deeper into the gastric pits, resulting in a variable degree of gastric atrophy and intestinal metaplasia.

Erosive-hemorrhagic gastritis is primarily an endoscopic diagnosis that despite the severity at endoscopy reveals only superficial epithelial abnormalities with little or no inflammatory cell infiltration. Gastric biopsy may provide clues to some forms of chemical gastritis. Bile (alkaline) reflux gastritis is associated with mucosal edema, foveolar (pit) hyperplasia, and a typical corkscrew appearance of the gastric glands. NSAID-induced gastritis is also characterized by foveolar hyperplasia accompanied by extension of muscle fibers into the mucosa between the gastric glands.

On biopsy, Ménétrier's disease reveals elongation and tortuosity of the foveolar part of the gastric glands, which may form cystic dilatations, with cysts often extending deep into the mucosa. The parietal and chief cells are reduced in number and are replaced by mucous glands. As a result, hypochlorhydria is usually present, and the pentagastrin-stimulated peak acid output is in the neighborhood of 10 mmol per hour.

Phlegmonous gastritis due to an acute bacterial infection reveals acute inflammation and necrosis and is diagnosed by biopsy and culture. The most common infecting organism is alpha-hemolytic *Streptococcus*, which is isolated in greater than 50 per cent of patients. If the infection is caused by a gas-forming organism such as *Clostridium perfringens*, air may be seen within the wall (emphysematous gastritis).

Gastric infections secondary to specific organisms are being recognized with increasing frequency in patients with human immunodeficiency virus (HIV) infection and acquired immunodeficiency syndrome (AIDS). The most common infecting agents are cytomegalovirus (CMV), herpes simplex, *Candida albicans, Cryptococcus*, and *Cryptosporidium*. In addition, the stomach may be involved as part of a systemic disease process such as disseminated *Mycobacterium tuberculosis*, histoplasmosis, and secondary syphilis. Special stains and cultures may be required to identify the infection.

Eosinophilic gastritis is often part of a more generalized disease of the gastrointestinal tract characterized by the presence of sheets or clumps of eosinophils in the gastric mucosa. Histologically, three forms of eosinophilic gastritis are recognized: predominantly mucosal disease, predominantly muscle layer involvement, and predominantly serosal involvement. In patients with involvement of the muscle layer or serosa, a full-thickness biopsy is required for confirmation of the diagnosis.

Granulomatous gastritis reveals infiltrates of chronic inflammatory cells and granulomas of the gastric mucosa. In the absence of an infectious cause (tuberculous or fungal), the differential diagnosis may include Crohn's disease or sarcoidosis. In Crohn's disease, lesions in other parts of the gastrointestinal tract should be sought by barium studies and endoscopy. There is no specific test for sarcoidosis, and the diagnosis is based on the presence of disease elsewhere, particularly in the lungs.

COMPLICATIONS OF GASTRITIS

Complications associated with long-term gastritis include mucosal atrophy and malignancies. Autoimmune gastritis results in atrophy, leading to pernicious anemia. An important sequela is the associated intestinal metaplasia or dysplasia that may be a precursor for adenocarcinoma. *H. pylori* gastritis is usually asymptomatic, and its clinical importance lies in its association with duodenal and gastric ulcers and gastric malignancies (adenocarcinoma and lymphoma). In phlegmonous gastritis, the infection may spread through the full thickness of the stomach wall, resulting in gangrene or perforation.

PEPTIC ULCER DISEASE

By Thomas R. Viggiano, M.D.
Rochester, Minnesota

Peptic ulcers are defects in the gastric or duodenal mucosa that result from an imbalance between the digestive activity of acid and pepsin in gastric juice and the host's protective mechanisms for resisting mucosal digestion. Acid peptic disease includes defects superficial to the muscularis mucosae, termed "erosions," and defects that penetrate the muscularis mucosae, called "ulcers." Recent advances in the understanding of peptic ulcer pathogenesis have caused a modification of the presumption that idiopathic acid hypersecretion is a major causative factor. Newer classifications of peptic ulcers categorize ulcers by their association with three possible causative factors: (1) *Helicobacter pylori*, (2) nonsteroidal anti-inflammatory drugs (NSAIDs) or aspirin, or (3) miscellaneous causes. Miscellaneous causes include ulcers caused by hypersecretion from gastrinomas (Zollinger-Ellison syndrome), ulcers due to idiopathic hypersecretion, and ulcers secondary to duodenogastric reflux of gastric mucosal barrier-breaking agents such as bile salts or lysolecithin. Recent reports estimate that fewer than 5 per cent of ulcers are due to miscellaneous causes. Thus, at least 95 per cent of peptic ulcers are due to either *H. pylori* or NSAIDs. The most common cause of duodenal ulcer is *H. pylori*, and the most common cause of gastric ulcer is NSAIDs.

ETIOLOGIC FACTORS

Helicobacter Pylori

H. pylori is a gram-negative bacillus that resides beneath and within the mucous layer of the gastric mucosa. This organism produces multiple enzymes, including a urease that protects the organism from the acid environment and serves as the basis for diagnostic tests. *H. pylori* causes a persistent gastric infection that exists for the life of the patient unless treated.

In the United States, *H. pylori* has an age-related prevalence; it occurs in 10 per cent of the general population younger than 30 years of age and in 60 per cent of the population older than 60 years of age. *H. pylori* is prevalent in 40 to 50 per cent of the United States population overall, but it is more prevalent in African Americans and Latinos, poorer socioeconomic groups, and institutionalized persons.

In humans, *H. pylori* produces a chronic active gastritis. An important concept is that *H. pylori*–induced gastritis is the basic disease and that duodenal ulcers, gastric ulcers, or malignancy develops as a complication of the chronic gastritis. *H. pylori* is found in 90 to 95 per cent of patients with duodenal ulcer and in 80 per cent of patients with gastric ulcer; eradication of *H. pylori* decreases the relapse rates for duodenal ulcers and gastric ulcers. There are also reports that associate *H. pylori* with chronic atrophic gastritis and the development of noncardiac gastric adenocarcinoma and with primary B-cell lymphoma of the stomach. Further investigation is needed to determine the exact role that this organism plays in the development of gastric adenocarcinoma and lymphoma. There is no convincing evidence that *H. pylori* plays a significant role in gastroesophageal reflux disease or in nonulcer dyspepsia.

Nonsteroidal Anti-inflammatory Drugs

Gastric prostaglandin production plays a major role in determining mucosal cytoprotection because prostaglandins are involved in gastric mucus secretion, bicarbonate production, and mucosal blood flow. NSAIDs inhibit gastroduodenal prostaglandin synthesis, which results in decreased secretion of mucus and bicarbonate, decreased mucosal blood flow, and disruption of the gastric mucosal barrier. Acute gastric erosions develop within 2 weeks in more than 80 per cent of patients taking NSAIDs daily. When NSAID use is discontinued, NSAID ulcers typically heal and do not recur. The risk of peptic ulcer disease with NSAID use is maximal in the first 3 months of treatment, and elderly patients and patients with a previous history of peptic ulcer disease are at highest risk.

The risk of peptic ulcer disease with NSAIDs is dose-dependent. However, there are different dose-response relationships for the analgesic and the anti-inflammatory properties of NSAIDs. The maximal analgesic effect plateau is much lower than effective anti-inflammatory doses. Low doses of aspirin or NSAIDs give pain relief but have little anti-inflammatory activity. Increased doses improve the anti-inflammatory effect and predispose to ulceration (prostaglandin inhibition) but do not increase the analgesic effect. Many patients take NSAIDs for pain relief of noninflammatory conditions such as degenerative arthritis and do not need the anti-inflammatory properties of NSAIDs. The newer NSAIDs have been marketed with more convenient (less frequent) dosing intervals and in doses that have marked anti-inflammatory activity. Thus, use of newer NSAIDs subjects the patient to an increased risk of ulceration without providing increased analgesia. The clinician must decide whether simple analgesic treatment (e.g., acetaminophen) can be substituted for NSAIDs. If the anti-inflammatory properties of NSAIDs are required, an attempt should be made to use the lowest possible dose. The prostaglandin analogue misoprostol has been shown to protect the gastroduodenal mucosa effectively from NSAID injury. H_2-receptor antagonists, antacids, and sucralfate have not been shown to protect the gastroduodenal mucosa effectively from NSAID injury.

SYMPTOMS

Dyspepsia is a common symptom that occurs in up to 26 per cent of the population, yet it is difficult to define precisely. Dyspepsia literally means *bad digestion*, and the traditional definition is *intestinal symptoms related to eating*. Recently, experts have proposed a newer definition: persistent or recurrent abdominal discomfort centered in the upper abdomen or epigastrium. Patients use the term indigestion to refer to various nonspecific symptoms related to eating. Clinicians often use the term dyspepsia to refer to a combination of symptoms, including epigastric discomfort, nausea, anorexia, vomiting, distention, bloating, early satiety, and flatulence. The most important characteristics of the symptom complex of dyspepsia are its relationship to eating, its localization to the upper abdomen, and the absence of lower intestinal symptoms. Clinicians must distinguish organic causes of dyspepsia, such as peptic ulcer, cholelithiasis, and pancreatitis, from functional causes, such as nonulcer dyspepsia and irritable bowel syndrome.

The symptoms of duodenal ulcer and gastric ulcer are similar, but they are neither sensitive enough nor specific enough to distinguish peptic ulcer disease from other causes of dyspepsia. Many patients who present with dyspepsia do not have peptic ulcer disease. Approximately 80 per cent of patients with peptic ulcers present with epigastric discomfort, but as many as 20 per cent of patients are free from pain. These painless or silent ulcers occur most commonly in the elderly and in patients receiving NSAIDs. Peptic ulcer symptoms frequently are relieved before ulcer healing occurs, but approximately 25 per cent of patients have persistent epigastric discomfort despite documented ulcer healing. Experienced clinicians accurately diagnose the cause of dyspepsia by history alone in fewer than 50 per cent of cases. Some features of dyspepsia make a diagnosis of peptic ulcer disease more likely.

Character and Location

The pain of uncomplicated peptic ulcers is a vague midline epigastric discomfort consistent with its visceral origin. Patients describe the discomfort as burning, gnawing, dull, aching, or a hunger pain. The pain is frequently relieved by ingesting food or antacids, and the pain of an uncomplicated peptic ulcer typically does not radiate.

Rhythmicity and Periodicity

Rhythmicity refers to the fluctuating intensity or waxing and waning of peptic ulcer pain throughout the day and night. Patients with regular eating habits frequently report that their pain begins 1 to 3 hours after eating. Approximately 50 per cent of ulcer patients experience nocturnal awakening (midnight to 3 AM) from pain; however, pain in the morning before breakfast is rare. Although rhythmicity is sometimes helpful, many patients with peptic ulcer disease deny the presence of these rhythmic temporal features of their pain. Most patients with peptic ulcers observe discrete episodes of pain that last for days to weeks followed by symptom-free periods of weeks to months.

Associated Symptoms

Often, other symptoms associated with dyspepsia suggest a possible complication of peptic ulcer disease or help distinguish peptic ulcer disease from other causes of dyspepsia. Nausea and anorexia occur more commonly in patients with gastric ulcers than in those with duodenal ulcers. Minor weight loss (<5 to 10 pounds) may also occur, but more significant weight loss is unusual in uncomplicated peptic ulcer disease and should raise suspicion of malignancy or partial gastric outlet obstruction. Intermittent vomiting occasionally occurs, but persistent vomiting or vomiting of undigested food after meals suggests a mechanical gastric outlet obstruction or a gastric motility disorder. Flatulence, belching, bloating, and fatty or spicy food intolerance may occur in peptic ulcer disease, but these are nonspecific symptoms and occur in irritable bowel syndrome and other intestinal disorders. A burning substernal pain that ascends the chest suggests gastroesophageal reflux disease. Cholelithiasis most commonly presents as severe episodic colicky right upper quadrant abdominal pain that may radiate to the back. Acute pancreatitis is a severe illness that is not commonly mistaken for dyspepsia.

PHYSICAL EXAMINATION

The findings of physical examination are often normal in uncomplicated peptic ulcer disease. Epigastric tenderness to deep palpation may be present, but it is neither sensitive nor specific for peptic ulcer disease. Special attention should be paid to the hemodynamic status, and the stool should be tested for occult blood.

ROUTINE LABORATORY TESTS

The results of routine laboratory studies in patients with uncomplicated peptic ulcer disease are usually normal. Anemia may indicate chronic intestinal blood loss from a bleeding ulcer and should be sought especially in elderly patients taking NSAIDs. In patients with *H. pylori*–negative ulcers who are not taking NSAIDs, an increased serum calcium concentration suggests the possibility of a gastrinoma related to a multiple endocrine neoplasia, type I syndrome (pituitary, parathyroid, and islet cell tumors).

Increased values on liver function tests are rare in peptic ulcer disease and suggest gallstones or other hepatobiliary disorders. Leukocytosis is unusual and is either unrelated or suggests penetration or perforation of an ulcer. In patients with severe pain, increased amylase activity suggests acute pancreatitis or penetration of an ulcer posteriorly into the pancreas.

COURSE

Benign peptic ulcers usually measure 2 cm or less and usually heal completely within 6 weeks with an adequate treatment program. Occasionally, larger benign ulcers occur and may require up to 12 weeks to heal completely. The natural history of peptic ulcer disease can be summarized in one word—recurrence. Recent reports, however, have shown a dramatic reduction in the recurrence of *H. pylori*–associated gastric and duodenal ulcers after eradication of the bacteria.

COMPLICATIONS

Approximately 10 to 20 per cent of patients with peptic ulcer disease experience a complication some time during the course of the disease. The elderly, especially those taking NSAIDs, often have painless or silent ulcers that appear as complications at presentation.

Hemorrhage

Of patients who present with upper gastrointestinal (GI) hemorrhage, 50 per cent have bleeding from a peptic ulcer. Overall, 15 to 20 per cent of ulcer patients bleed at some time during the course of their disease. Hematemesis or melena, or both, are seen in 95 per cent of patients, and 80 per cent of patients relate a history of previous ulcer symptoms. Postural hypotension is an important physical finding because it indicates clinically significant hemorrhage even early in the course of bleeding when the hematocrit may be normal as a result of volume contraction.

Perforation

Perforation occurs in approximately 1 per cent of patients with ulcer disease. The incidence of gastric perforation appears to be increasing in elderly patients taking NSAIDs. The most common presentation is the sudden onset of severe epigastric pain, which spreads rapidly throughout the abdomen. The patient appears acutely and seriously ill, lying immobile with shallow respirations. Patients usually have tachycardia, fever, and progressive hypotension. Signs of acute peritonitis include abdominal guarding, rebound tenderness, and absent bowel sounds. Often, leukocytosis and a mild increase in amylase activity are noted. The diagnosis may be confirmed by the presence of free intraperitoneal air on chest film or flat and upright abdominal films.

Penetration

Penetration of an ulcer refers to erosion of the ulcer through the full thickness of the intestinal wall without leakage of digestive contents into the peritoneal cavity. The incidence of penetration is unknown because it can be diagnosed only at operation. Surgical series indicate that approximately 20 per cent of patients who require operation for peptic ulcer disease have penetration into a contiguous structure, such as the pancreas, liver, biliary tree, colon, and omentum. Classically, a patient's typical ulcer pain becomes more severe but loses the periodicity and rhythmicity. Pain often radiates into the back. Laboratory studies may produce normal results or show leukocytosis and a mild increase in amylase activity (less than five times the upper limit of normal), which helps distinguish penetration from the higher amylase activities found in acute pancreatitis.

Obstruction

Gastric outlet obstruction develops in approximately 2 per cent of all ulcer patients. Ninety per cent of patients present with recurrent vomiting of partially digested or undigested food. Significant weight loss, nausea, and early satiety are often present. Physical examination typically reveals evidence of dehydration in 20 per cent of patients and a succussion splash in greater than 25 per cent of patients.

DIAGNOSTIC EVALUATION

The ideal strategy for the evaluation of dyspepsia would be both cost-effective and precise so that a specific diagnosis could be made and a specific treatment instituted. Unfortunately, dyspepsia is very common and is composed of a vague nonspecific symptom complex that may be caused by several different organic or functional disorders. It is neither cost-effective nor desirable to investigate every patient. An accurate diagnosis first requires a history that carefully characterizes the patient's symptoms and their duration. Diagnostic studies are usually unnecessary in patients with transient or short-lived symptoms. In patients younger than 45 years of age with mild symptoms and no evidence of systemic symptoms or possible complications, a trial of empirical therapy with antacids and H_2-receptor antagonists may be appropriate. If a therapeutic trial in a previously uninvestigated patient fails to relieve the symptoms or if the symptoms recur shortly after the trial, a diagnostic evaluation is recommended.

Early diagnostic evaluation should be performed if the patient has not been previously evaluated and if one or more of the following are present: (1) age older than 45 years; (2) clinical evidence of organic disease (including significant weight loss, bleeding, anemia, pain radiating to the back, recurrent vomiting, jaundice, dysphagia, or a palpable abdominal mass); (3) history of the use of NSAIDs or aspirin, excessive alcohol intake, or excessive cigarette smoking; or (4) a strong family history of documented peptic ulcer disease or gastric cancer. The preceding clinical features are associated with an increased risk of organic disease in patients with dyspepsia. It is also reasonable to investigate patients who, in the judgment of the physician, may have a functional illness but would not be sufficiently reassured unless definitive tests have eliminated the possibility of serious underlying disease. Patients with more chronic symptoms who have associated psychologic disorders and are heavy users of the health care system are usually not reassured by repeated investigations. Therefore, diagnostic studies in these patients should be performed to evaluate new symptoms or objective clinical findings.

A careful clinical evaluation may identify some clinical situations in which a trial of empirical therapy is preferred to initial evaluation. Patients with dyspepsia of recent onset coinciding with the use of NSAIDs and without anemia or other alarming symptoms do not require evaluation. Patients whose major symptom complex suggests gastroesophageal reflux disease can be given a therapeutic trial of acid suppression therapy. Although 20 to 40 per cent of patients with ulcers may also have some refluxlike symptoms, it is important for physicians to remember that gastroesophageal reflux disease is due to abnormal motility (incompetence) of the lower esophageal sphincter and is not associated with NSAID use or *H. pylori* infection (see article on esophageal disease).

The term nonulcer dyspepsia describes a condition in a large group of patients with chronic dyspepsia in whom a clinical evaluation, including upper GI endoscopy, is normal. In the United States, 15 per cent of middle-aged men and women have nonulcer dyspepsia. Most patients have symptoms that mimic either a motility disorder or peptic ulcer disease.

Dyspepsia that is aggravated by food and is associated with postprandial fullness, abdominal bloating, and early satiety without weight loss suggests dysmotilitylike nonulcer dyspepsia. Many of these patients also have irritable bowel syndrome. Younger patients who present with dysmotilitylike symptoms who are not taking NSAIDs and are not infected with *H. pylori* have a low probability of organic findings at endoscopy. A gastric motility study should be considered in patients with dysmotilitylike symptoms associated with weight loss, recurrent vomiting, or other symptoms of organic disease.

The other common form of nonulcer dyspepsia includes well-localized epigastric discomfort that occurs before meals or when the patient is hungry and is relieved by eating. This syndrome has been referred to as ulcerlike nonulcer dyspepsia. Patients with *H. pylori*–positive ulcerlike nonulcer dyspepsia do not consistently respond to either acid suppression or antibiotic treatment. If psychological factors contribute to the problem, these patients should be evaluated and treated. Many patients benefit from the reassurance of a thorough clinical evaluation, including endoscopy and dietary restrictions of alcohol, coffee, or other specific foods that precipitate symptoms.

Prior to our understanding that eradication of *H. pylori* greatly reduced ulcer recurrence rates, there was considerable debate as to whether it was more cost-effective for a patient with dyspepsia to undergo an endoscopic examination or to have empirical treatment with an H_2-receptor antagonist. A recent cost-effective analysis used a decision analytic model to estimate cost per ulcer cured for five different management strategies for patients with dyspepsia. The estimated costs per ulcer cured for each strategy were (1) endoscopy with biopsy, $8,045; (2) endoscopy without biopsy, $6,984; (3) serologic test for *H. pylori*, $4,541; (4) empirical antisecretory therapy, $952; and (5) empirical antisecretory therapy with antibiotics to eradicate *H. py-*

lori, $818. This study and another one concluded that the cost savings and lower recurrence rate justify initial empirical antisecretory therapy with antibiotics. However, the cost-effective advantage of noninvasive strategies diminishes as the probability of recurrent symptoms (?nonulcer dyspepsia) in the population increases, as the prevalence of *H. pylori* in the population decreases, and as the cost of serologic tests for *H. pylori* and endoscopy decreases. Future developments, including rapid inexpensive serologic tests, decreased fees for endoscopy, and simple and effective antibiotic regimens, will determine which diagnostic strategy is most cost-effective in evaluating the many patients with such a vague symptom complex as dyspepsia.

Special Diagnostic Studies

Clinicians should understand the diagnostic accuracy and cost of special diagnostic studies to evaluate dysphagia. There is some debate as to whether upper GI radiography or upper GI endoscopy is the diagnostic procedure of choice. Radiologists argue that the sensitivity of radiography approaches that of endoscopy and that it is safer, more comfortable, and only one third the cost of endoscopy. Endoscopists argue that gastroscopy is superior to radiography and has the capability of making a biopsy diagnosis of *H. pylori* infection or malignancy.

Upper Gastrointestinal Radiography

Upper GI radiographs detect 80 to 90 per cent of ulcer craters. Clinical situations that compromise diagnostic accuracy include antral or duodenal bulb deformity and previous peptic ulcer operation. Radiography is less sensitive for the detection of erosions, gastritis, or duodenitis. Upper GI radiography has a false-negative rate of more than 18 per cent and a false-positive rate between 13 and 35 per cent. Upper GI radiographs correctly identify gastric malignancy 80 to 85 per cent of the time.

Upper Gastrointestinal Endoscopy

Endoscopy correctly identifies greater than 95 per cent of gastroduodenal ulcers. Endoscopy is more sensitive for the diagnosis of superficial inflammation such as reflux esophagitis or gastroduodenal erosions, and endoscopy has both biopsy and therapeutic capabilities. Endoscopy combined with biopsy correctly identifies 95 per cent of gastric malignancies.

Symptomatic patients with previous scarring on upper GI radiographs should undergo endoscopy to determine whether active inflammation is present. Patients with long-standing abdominal pain that is refractory to medical treatment or those with previous normal radiographs should undergo endoscopy. Patients suspected of having gastric ulcers or those in whom a gastric ulcer has been documented by radiography should undergo endoscopy and biopsy to eliminate the possibility of malignancy. Patients with giant or unusual ulcers should undergo endoscopy. Finally, endoscopy is the preferred test in patients who present with acute or chronic bleeding.

Tests for *Helicobacter Pylori*

Almost all patients in whom an ulcer develops and who are not taking aspirin or NSAIDs are *H. pylori*–positive. There is controversy as to whether *H. pylori* testing is necessary in these ulcer patients. Experts currently recommend routine testing for *H. pylori* in these ulcer patients. However, many practicing physicians treat ulcers not related to NSAIDs empirically for *H. pylori*.

Several tests are available to detect *H. pylori*. Serologic studies and breath tests are noninvasive, whereas a biopsy urease test, histologic examination, and culture require endoscopy. The clinician should understand the usefulness, effectiveness, and cost of these tests.

Serologic Studies

H. pylori produces not only a local immune response but also a systemic immune response. Current methods detect antibodies of the IgG, IgA, and IgM classes. Serologic studies are the most cost-effective, noninvasive methods for diagnosing primary *H. pylori* infection, but serologic methods remain positive over time, which limits their usefulness in follow-up evaluation. Sensitivity is 95 per cent and specificity is 90 to 95 per cent.

Breath Test

A radiolabeled dose of urea is given orally. If *H. pylori* is present, the urease splits the urea so that radiolabeled carbon dioxide is exhaled. The advantage of this test is that it is quick and easy to perform and does not require endoscopy. As the availability of the breath test increases, it will be the test of choice for follow-up evaluation. Sensitivity is 95 to 98 per cent, and specificity is 95 to 98 per cent.

Biopsy Urease Test

A biopsy specimen is impregnated into agar that contains urea and a pH indicator. As the urea is split, the pH of the medium changes the color of the agar from yellow to red. The test is positive if *H. pylori* is present (bacterial urease is present), and the greater the number of organisms, the more rapidly the test becomes positive. Sensitivity is 95 per cent and specificity is 98 per cent.

Histologic Examination

An advantage of histologic examination is the opportunity to examine the underlying inflammatory reaction site. *H. pylori* can be seen on a Gram stain, a hematoxylin and eosin stain, a Giemsa stain, and the Warthin-Starry stain (a silver stain). Sensitivity is 98 per cent and specificity is 98 per cent.

Culture

Culturing *H. pylori* is tedious and expensive and should be reserved for special circumstances such as investigation of antibiotic resistance or virulence. Sensitivity is 90 to 95 per cent, and specificity is 100 per cent. Because many symptomatic patients undergo endoscopy to determine whether the symptoms are due to reflux esophagitis, nonulcer dyspepsia, or an ulcer, histologic or biopsy urease tests are most commonly used in the initial evaluation.

Serum Gastrin

All patients who present with *H. pylori*–negative ulcers and are not taking NSAIDs should have serum gastrin concentrations measured to eliminate the possibility of a hypersecretory state (Zollinger-Ellison syndrome). Other clinical situations that suggest the possibility of hypersecretion and in which serum gastrin concentration should be checked include multiple ulcers (especially in a postbulbar location), intractable ulcers, recurrent ulcers postoperatively, ulcers associated with hypercalcemia, ulcers associated with diarrhea, ulcers in patients with a strong family history of ulcer disease, and ulcers in patients with known multiple endocrine neoplasia syndrome. Finally, many experts advocate measurement of the serum gastrin concentration before any surgical procedure to manage ulcer disease.

Gastric Analysis

Gastric analysis has limited clinical usefulness. Most experts agree that gastric analysis studies are helpful only for the preoperative evaluation of patients with suspected Zollinger-Ellison syndrome or in patients who have had ulcer surgery and in whom recurrent ulcers develop.

SUMMARY

Recent advances have revolutionized our understanding of the pathogenesis of peptic ulcer disease. Traditionally, peptic ulcer disease was a chronic recurrent illness of unknown cause. However, we now know that 95 per cent of ulcers have a specific cause (*H. pylori* or NSAIDs), and recurrence can be prevented. Many patients have dyspepsia from other causes, such as reflux esophagitis, nonulcer dyspepsia, and hepatobiliary or pancreatic disorders. History, physical examination, and routine laboratory studies are often nonspecific and of limited usefulness in establishing a correct diagnosis. Endoscopy is more expensive than upper GI radiography, but it is more sensitive and specific for establishing a diagnosis, and it has biopsy and therapeutic capabilities. Patients with ulcers who take NSAIDs should discontinue this medication or taper it to the lowest possible dose. Almost all patients who acquire an ulcer without taking aspirin or NSAIDs are infected with *H. pylori*. Controversy exists as to whether *H. pylori* testing is necessary or if these patients should be treated empirically for *H. pylori*. Outcome analysis studies are needed to develop a cost-effective strategy for the evaluation of patients with dyspepsia.

NEOPLASMS OF THE STOMACH

By Timothy A. Woodward, M.D.
Jacksonville, Florida

Gastric adenocarcinoma is the second most common cancer worldwide. In 1995, 22,800 Americans were diagnosed with gastric cancer, with 14,000 eventually dying of the disease. This article reviews the classifications of various stomach neoplasms, focusing on gastric adenocarcinoma and its diagnosis, staging, and treatment.

GASTRIC POLYPS

Gastric polyps are uncommon, accounting for fewer than 1 per cent of tumors at autopsy. They almost always are asymptomatic and are discovered incidentally on endoscopy or radiographically. The overwhelming majority of gastric polyps are hyperplastic, accounting for 75 per cent of all gastric polyps. Hyperplastic polyps do not have malignant potential and are usually small (<15 mm). Adenomatous polyps have the potential for malignant degeneration and account for approximately 20 per cent of gastric polyps. Adenomatous polyps should be removed. Fundic gland polyps consist of dilated and distorted fundic glands. They are usually small (<10 mm) and occur in large numbers (from 10 to more than 100); they are located in the fundus and generally do not give rise to any symptoms other than epigastric discomfort.

LEIOMYOMA

Leiomyomas are benign submucosal tumors that arise from the smooth muscle of the gastric wall. They account for fewer than 5 per cent of gastric neoplasms and are usually asymptomatic. Leiomyomas may be difficult to distinguish from their malignant counterpart leiomyosarcomas. The benign and malignant neoplasms are distinguished principally by the number of mitoses seen on pathologic examination.

LEIOMYOSARCOMA

Leiomyosarcomas account for 1 per cent of gastric malignancies. Clinically they are distinguished by their predisposition to gastrointestinal hemorrhage. Endoscopically they are generally pedunculated, large, and ulcerated. With resection, there is a 50 per cent chance of cure.

GASTRIC CARCINOIDS

Most gastric carcinoids occur in the body of the stomach, with this organ representing the location of 3 per cent of all carcinoids. Being of foregut origin, gastric carcinoids may secrete 5-hydroxyindoleacetic acid (5-HIAA), which produces the classic flushing syndrome. However, most gastric carcinoids are asymptomatic and are found incidentally. Carcinoids occur more frequently in patients with pernicious anemia and atrophic gastritis with achlorhydria.

GASTRIC LYMPHOMA

The stomach is the most common primary site of extranodal non-Hodgkin's lymphomas. The majority of gastric lymphomas are the large cell type of B-cell lineage. Primary small cell gastric lymphomas are less frequent and are usually localized. Recent data have suggested that these small cell lymphomas originate from mucosa-associated lymphoid tissue (MALT). Dull epigastric pain, anorexia, and weight loss are common symptoms. Endoscopically, certain findings favor the diagnosis of lymphoma over carcinoma. These findings include total stomach involvement, proximal stomach involvement, extension of tumor into the duodenum, and the presence of volcano crater–like ulcers on polypoid lesions. Recent studies suggest a causative role for *Helicobacter pylori* as a risk factor for gastric lymphoma.

CARCINOMA OF THE STOMACH

The incidence of gastric cancer varies widely among countries and, in the United States, among racial groups. China, Japan, South America, and eastern Europe have the highest incidence of gastric cancer worldwide. In the

United States, the overall incidence rates for gastric cancer have dropped over the past 50 years. However, African Americans, Native Americans, and Hispanic Americans are 1.5 to 2.5 times more likely to acquire gastric cancer than are white Americans. For white males in the United States, over the past 20 years there has been a steady increase in the incidence of adenocarcinoma involving the proximal stomach and gastroesophageal junction, whereas the incidence of distal cancers has slightly decreased.

Conditions that predispose to carcinoma of the stomach include adenomatous polyps larger than 2 cm; chronic atrophic gastritis, pernicious anemia, hypertrophic gastropathy (Ménétrier's disease); Billroth II gastric remnants and anastomoses; and Barrett's esophagus, which is associated with tumors of the gastroesophageal junction.

Symptoms of Gastric Carcinoma

The clinical features of gastric cancer are vague and nonspecific until late in the course of the disease. As the disease progresses, anemia may develop secondary to gastrointestinal bleeding; luminal obstruction or motor involvement may cause early satiety, postprandial fullness, or dyspepsia. Vomiting is typically a late sign suggesting outlet obstruction or diffuse involvement of the gastric wall. Dysphagia suggests tumor involving the gastric cardia.

In the United States, where the incidence of gastric carcinoma is relatively low, screening may be considered for high-risk patients who have chronic atrophic gastritis, pernicious anemia, gastric adenomatous polyps, or long-standing previous peptic ulcer surgery. Patients with late-onset hypogammaglobulinemia (also known as common variable immunodeficiency) are at high risk for the development of pernicious anemia and gastric cancer. The detection of gastric cancer in a relatively young patient should raise the suspicion of a familial cancer syndrome, especially a Lynch II kindred.

Physical Signs of Gastric Carcinoma

There are no pathognomonic physical features that suggest early gastric cancer. Weight loss and anemia are usually later manifestations of the disease. Signs of local or metastatic disease include Virchow's sentinel node (left supraclavicular node), Blumer's rectal shelf, Sister Mary Joseph's node (infiltration of the umbilicus), and Krukenberg's ovarian tumor.

Infrequently, certain paraneoplastic conditions may be associated with gastric cancer. Examples include microangiopathic hemolytic anemia, membranous nephropathy, sudden onset of seborrheic keratoses (the Leser-Trélat sign), and acanthosis nigrans.

Diagnostic Procedures

Laboratory Tests

No tumor markers are known to facilitate early diagnosis of cancer of the stomach. Carcinoembryonic antigen (CEA) concentrations are increased in up to 40 per cent of patients with metastatic gastric cancer. However, only 10 per cent of patients with increased CEA have resectable tumors. Thus, the main application of CEA in gastric cancer may be as a marker of recurrence if concentrations return to normal following resection. Alpha-fetoprotein is increased in nearly 30 per cent of patients with gastric carcinoma. Like CEA, however, alpha-fetoprotein increases are typically seen in patients with metastatic disease.

Noninvasive markers of chronic atrophic gastritis may be useful as indirect markers of gastric carcinoma in select high-risk groups. Decreased serum pepsinogen I and increased serum gastrin concentrations have been reported in patients with atrophic gastritis with achlorhydria, a condition associated with carcinoma of the stomach.

Radiographic Studies

When stomach cancer is suspected, an upper gastrointestinal (GI) series is often the first test performed. The accuracy of a single-contrast upper GI series in the detection of gastric cancer is nearly 80 per cent. Suspicious abnormalities on barium studies include lack of distensibility of the stomach, enlarged gastric folds, an ulcerated mass, or a large ulcer with heaped borders. The major goal in radiographic evaluation of gastric ulcers, however, is to distinguish benign from malignant lesions.

When gastric ulcers are evaluated by endoscopy with biopsy, fewer than 3 per cent are malignant. Therefore, a competent clinical strategy involves demonstration of complete healing of a radiographic ulcer on a second barium study. Endoscopy and biopsy should be performed if a lesion seen on upper GI examination has not healed in 6 weeks. Computed tomography (CT) of the abdomen is useful primarily as a staging modality. Unfortunately, CT scans often underestimate the extent of disease within lymph nodes and the omentum.

Endoscopy

The diagnostic accuracy of endoscopy with regard to cancer is reportedly as high as 95 per cent. Accuracy increases with the number of biopsies. Thus, a minimum of eight biopsies is recommended. Cytologic brushings of the biopsy site may further increase the yield. During preoperative assessment, endoscopy provides information about the proximal and distal extent of tumor. Gastroparesis suggests vagal infiltration, especially by lesions in the cardia.

Endoscopic ultrasound can be used preoperatively to determine the depth of primary tumor and, to a lesser extent, nodal involvement. Several studies suggest ultrasound may be superior to CT as a sensitive preoperative diagnostic tool. Laparoscopy can be a useful adjunct in assessing tumor stage. Up to 37 per cent of patients initially viewed as operative candidates have occult peritoneal seeding or hepatic metastases when staged laparoscopically.

INTESTINAL OBSTRUCTION

By Andrew M. Davidoff, M.D.,
and Perry W. Stafford, M.D.
Philadelphia, Pennsylvania

Intestinal obstruction is a condition in which the intestinal luminal contents fail to progress in the normal aboral direction. The admitting diagnosis for more than one fifth of all surgical admissions, intestinal obstruction is one of the most common surgical emergencies. Early recognition and appropriate treatment of this condition is essential because it still carries a significant mortality.

Several definitions can help provide an understanding of the pathophysiology of intestinal obstruction. Mechanical obstruction occurs when a complete or partial physical barrier occludes the intestinal lumen. Such occlusion can be due to obturation of the lumen or to intrinsic or extrinsic encroachment on the bowel lumen. In simple mechanical obstruction, only the lumen is occluded, whereas in strangulated obstruction, the mesenteric blood flow is impaired. A closed-loop obstruction exists when the intestinal lumen is occluded in two places; this condition is frequently associated with strangulation. Ileus, although synonymous with intestinal obstruction, more commonly refers to conditions in which a functional obstruction prevents the passage of succus entericus down the gastrointestinal tract. This impaired transit is generally due to dysfunctional propulsive motility of the bowel (adynamic or paralytic ileus).

A careful history and thorough physical examination are essential for the prompt diagnosis and appropriate management of intestinal obstruction. Assessing the degree of the obstruction and the etiology are crucial to appropriate management. During the patient evaluation, the critical question to be answered is whether the obstruction is a complete mechanical obstruction with strangulated bowel, because such a condition is a surgical emergency.

HISTORY

Presenting Symptoms

The classic presentation for a patient with intestinal obstruction is crampy abdominal pain, nausea and vomiting, abdominal distention, and obstipation (the failure to pass feces or gas via the rectum). Unfortunately, many patients do not present with classic symptoms, so the presence of any one of these symptoms should raise the question of intestinal obstruction. The pain is due to distention of the bowel as it attempts to propel luminal contents past an obstruction. Early on, the pain is typically intermittent, diffuse, and crampy and coincides with the peristaltic waves. These paroxysms occur about every 5 minutes in a proximal bowel obstruction but less frequently in a more distal obstruction. The pain typically becomes localized, based on the embryonic segment of the gut involved; that is, epigastric pain implies foregut localization; periumbilical pain, midgut; and hypogastric pain, hindgut. The transition to constant, localized pain suggests progression to bowel necrosis and peritonitis. Pain associated with ileus is due strictly to distention in association with decreased peristalsis and therefore is usually less severe, more constant, and less crampy.

Vomiting, although occasionally reflex in nature, is often due to the accumulation of bowel fluid proximal to an obstruction. Therefore, proximal bowel obstruction leads to the earlier onset of vomiting. Patients with distal bowel obstruction can rarely present with vomiting. The feculent emesis seen in patients with distal bowel obstruction is due to bacterial overgrowth in stagnant, proximally sequestered small bowel fluid—not to regurgitated feces. Conversely, abdominal distention is seen more often in patients with distal bowel obstruction.

Distention is due to the accumulation of intraluminal fluid from intestinal hypersecretion, and gas consisting primarily of swallowed air. Gas may also be produced secondary to bacterial fermentation proximal to a luminal obstruction. This distention results in progressive venous congestion with edema of the bowel wall and, eventually, arterial compromise and intestinal ischemia. If left uncorrected, this process results in intestinal necrosis, perforation, and diffuse peritonitis. Distention may also be seen in generalized ileus. Patients with a colonic obstruction and a competent ileocecal valve do not develop diffuse abdominal distention, but they may develop massive colonic distention that can ultimately result in cecal perforation. This condition, like other closed-loop obstructions, is particularly prone to strangulation and perforation, because the progressively distending bowel cannot become decompressed by any other route.

Obstipation heralds a complete intestinal obstruction. This symptom usually occurs relatively late, however, because luminal contents distal to a complete bowel obstruction frequently continue to be passed until the distal bowel is empty. Cramping pain followed by explosive diarrhea often accompanies partial intestinal obstruction.

Past Medical History

The age of the patient influences the list of possible etiologies of intestinal obstruction and, therefore, management of the condition. Vomiting in a neonate is most often due to simple formula intolerance or gastroesophageal reflux, conditions treated with conservative management. However, bilious emesis in a newborn should be considered a surgical emergency until malrotation with midgut volvulus has been excluded. Other congenital anomalies, such as intestinal atresia, meconium ileus, and Hirschsprung's disease, are also on the list of possibilities in the differential diagnosis; in a child up to 2 years of age, intussusception can occur. These diseases are almost never seen in adults. Bilious emesis in an adult with a history of prior surgery is usually due to adhesive bowel disease, and if the obstruction is partial it can often be successfully managed with nasogastric tube decompression alone. Other possibilities include obstruction due to hernia (internal, inguinal, or ventral), carcinoma, or an inflammatory process (Crohn's disease or diverticulitis). The vast majority of patients who have previously undergone laparotomy have adhesions as the cause of the bowel obstruction, especially if they have had previous operations for adhesions.

Other medical conditions can suggest possible causes of obstruction, such as a history of Crohn's disease, hernias, abdominopelvic irradiation, cholelithiasis, or malignancy. Based on this information, different treatment plans can be formulated. However, even if the history is positive for one of these conditions, other causes of obstruction should be considered until a definitive etiology is documented. For example, almost half of the patients with malignancy and a bowel obstruction have a benign cause of the obstruction. The other conditions that may be associated with adynamic ileus include sepsis or intraperitoneal inflammation; retroperitoneal hematoma; spinal fracture; mesenteric ischemia; metabolic abnormalities, such as hyponatremia, hypokalemia, and hypomagnesemia; and drugs such as narcotics, anticholinergics, and antipsychotics.

PHYSICAL EXAMINATION

A careful and thorough physical examination must be performed on all patients with possible bowel obstruction to help determine the cause, to exclude adynamic ileus, and to assess the patient's fitness for surgery. Vital signs are extremely important and should always be recorded. Tachycardia and hypotension often occur in patients with severe dehydration, sepsis, and peritonitis. Although nonspecific, these signs reflect a patient's general condition. Other signs of dehydration include dry mucous membranes, poor skin turgor, and concentrated urine. Fever often accompanies sepsis and, in patients with suspected intestinal obstruction, should raise the possibility of bowel strangulation.

The abdominal examination should always note the presence and location of surgical scars from prior operations. This knowledge helps predict the likelihood of adhesions; in the absence of an accurate history, the location of the scars may be useful in determining the nature of the prior surgery. A careful search should be made for incarcerated hernias in the inguinal region and at other sites on the abdominal wall; manual reduction should be attempted. The detection of ventral hernias in obese patients may be difficult. Abdominal distention can be assessed and distinguished from ascites by tympany to percussion and the absence of shifting dullness or a fluid wave. Occasionally, ascites may develop secondary to intestinal obstruction, and therefore these conditions may occur concurrently.

Auscultation of the abdomen in the presence of a simple mechanical obstruction typically reveals loud, high-pitched rushes or "tinkles" of peristalsis associated with crampy abdominal pain. Progression to obstruction with strangulation usually produces gradual loss of bowel sounds. Bowel sounds are usually present in adynamic ileus, although they are typically diminished in frequency and intensity. Mild, diffuse tenderness to palpation is common in simple obstruction and may be more severe with muscle guarding during a colic attack. Localized tenderness with peritoneal signs, such as guarding and rebound tenderness, suggests bowel strangulation or perforation. Palpation of the abdomen may also reveal the presence of a mass, which could represent a fixed, distended, obstructed loop of bowel, a carcinoma, or a localized inflammatory process.

A rectal examination must be performed. This examination can help identify the lesion responsible for a distal bowel obstruction, or it may suggest the presence of a complete proximal obstruction if no stool is detected in the rectal vault. The detection of gross or occult blood suggests the presence of a mucosal lesion associated with carcinoma, intussusception, or intestinal infarction.

LABORATORY DATA

Laboratory data are typically nonspecific and insensitive to the presence or cause of intestinal obstruction. Nevertheless, certain laboratory abnormalities are often found in patients with intestinal obstruction. Early third-space fluid losses may be extensive but are usually isotonic. Therefore, the only abnormal laboratory data are those that reflect general dehydration, such as an increased hematocrit or urea nitrogen concentration. In addition, the urine specific gravity is increased. Even these laboratory values are not always reliable. For example, the hematocrit may actually be decreased because of occult blood loss from an obstructing carcinoma, or the urea nitrogen increased owing to chronic renal insufficiency or the presence of intraluminal blood in the gut. Thrombocytopenia can be seen in cases of intestinal obstruction or ischemia, especially in neonates, but this finding is nonspecific. Similarly, leukocytosis can be seen in intestinal obstruction, but it also occurs in general conditions such as stress and sepsis. An extremely increased white blood cell count, in the appropriate clinical setting, strongly suggests a strangulated intestinal obstruction or even a primary mesenteric occlusion. Hyperamylasemia can also occur in intestinal obstruction and may complicate the distinction of this condition from acute pancreatitis.

With persistent dehydration and intestinal obstruction, intracellular sodium-free water is mobilized during cell catabolism in an attempt to restore intravascular volume, this mobilization resulting in hyponatremia and hypochloremia. These conditions may be exacerbated by profuse vomiting and the resultant loss of hydrochloric acid. Hypokalemia also develops as the body tries to correct the alkalosis associated with vomiting by sequestering total body potassium stores. Alternatively, a metabolic acidosis may be generated from starvation and ketosis or may consist of lactic acid generated from ischemic bowel. Respiratory acidosis may occur when abdominal distention is so great that it compromises diaphragmatic excursion and ventilation.

IMAGING STUDIES

Abdominal Films

Both supine and erect abdominal films should be obtained to assess the bowel gas pattern in the search for other causes of the presenting symptoms. The classic radiographic findings in bowel obstruction consist of dilated bowel filled with both fluid and air. The bowel may have a "stepladder" appearance that is best seen on the erect or decubitus film, because the dependent fluid provides a sharp demarcation at the air-fluid interface. The site of obstruction may be inferred by the amount of air-filled bowel seen and by certain characteristic features of the dilated bowel. The small intestine is distinguished by the valvulae conniventes or plicae circulares that traverse the entire circumference of the bowel. The colon is identified by the haustral markings that incompletely traverse the bowel wall. Bowel dilatation is classically defined on standard radiographs as small bowel diameter greater than 3 cm, and colon diameter greater than 6 cm or cecum diameter greater than 9 cm.

Typically, no air is observed distal to the point of complete obstruction. The absence of dilated air-filled bowel may also be observed in proximal obstruction, and the distention may not be detected if the bowel is filled with fluid instead of gas. Closed-loop obstruction associated with colonic volvulus has a typical appearance in which a large loop of dilated bowel has an apex that points to the location of the volvulus. The radiographic appearance of the abdomen in a patient with adynamic ileus may also show distended loops of bowel with air-fluid levels. A distinguishing feature of ileus is the presence of air throughout the entire small and large bowel and into the rectum. Chest films should also be included among the initial studies to check for the presence of free intra-abdominal air and to exclude pneumonia as a cause of sepsis and associated ileus. A left-lateral decubitus film may be substituted for the erect film if a patient cannot stand or sit upright, as pneumoperitoneum should still be detectable around the smooth, solid contour of the liver.

Contrast Radiography

The role of contrast radiography in the diagnosis of intestinal obstruction is controversial. Nevertheless, it has some clinical utility when the diagnosis is unclear. A contrast enema may define the site of a colonic obstruction or exclude obstruction if contrast material passes freely into the terminal ileum. Reflux into a collapsed terminal ileum against a background of distended unopacified bowel suggests the presence of a more proximal small bowel obstruction. If the terminal ileum is distended, ileus is more likely. Contrast enemas should be used with great caution if bowel perforation is a possibility. Barium peritonitis carries a significant morbidity. Additionally, barium can cause perforation of an inflammatory process, such as diverticulitis and appendicitis, and water-soluble contrast agents should be used instead.

A contrast upper gastrointestinal (GI) series with small bowel follow-through or primary tube enteroclysis may be used when a partial obstruction is suspected—but not if complete obstruction is a possibility. Many surgeons object to the use of a barium upper GI series even in partial obstruction, fearing that inspissated barium will convert a partial obstruction to a complete one. Such conversion may also occur with barium enema performed for a partially obstructing colon lesion. Nevertheless, a contrast upper GI series can be helpful in distinguishing a partial obstruction from ileus, especially in the postoperative period. Contrast material should eventually pass unimpeded (albeit slowly) into the colon with ileus. The role of other radiographic modalities, such as ultrasound, computed tomography, magnetic resonance imaging, and arteriography, is limited in the setting of suspected intestinal obstruction.

SMALL BOWEL TUMORS

By Geronimo Sahagun, M.D.,
and M. Brian Fennerty, M.D.
Portland, Oregon

Tumors of the small intestine are uncommon compared with malignancies of the esophagus, stomach, and colon. Neoplasms of the small intestine represent 6 per cent of benign tumors and 2 per cent of malignant tumors in the gastrointestinal tract. The factors that may account for the decreased incidence of small bowel tumors include a neutral or alkaline pH in the lumen, low luminal bacterial counts, rapid intestinal transit, and increased cellular and humoral immune mechanisms.

As a group, small bowel tumors exhibit diversity that reflects both epithelial and mesenchymal components. Tumors of the small intestine are often asymptomatic and clinically insignificant. When symptoms do arise, the location of the tumor is not suggested by its presenting features. Therefore, the early detection and correct diagnosis of these tumors require experience and a high level of suspicion on the part of the clinician.

TUMOR CHARACTERISTICS

Malignant tumors of the small intestine become symptomatic and are usually fatal, whereas the majority of benign tumors of the small intestine remain asymptomatic. Not surprisingly, more epidemiologic data are available for malignant tumors than for benign tumors. In 1990, there were approximately 2800 new cases of, and 900 deaths from, malignant small bowel tumors in the United States. The incidence of malignant small bowel neoplasms is slightly higher in men than in women, and these lesions typically occur in the sixth decade of life.

Benign small bowel tumors are derived from smooth muscle, epithelium, and connective tissue. More than 35 types of benign tumors of the small bowel have been described.

Leiomyomas arise from the smooth muscle in the intestine and are often lobulated. Leiomyomas originate from either the muscle coat or the blood vessel and constitute 20 per cent of all benign small bowel tumors. Leiomyomas may extend to the lumen or serosa and histologically consist of bundles of smooth muscle cells.

Connective tissue tumors include fibromas, lipomas, and vascular lesions, such as hemangiomas and lymphangiomas. Neurofibromas and other benign tumors derived from neural elements account for fewer than 5 per cent of tumors in this category.

Benign epithelial tumors include villous adenomas, Brunner's gland adenomas, and other adenomatous polyps. Of these, villous adenomas of the small bowel are similar to those of the large bowel, but those in the small bowel may have higher potential for malignancy. Villous adenomas larger than 5 cm in diameter have a 50 per cent incidence of malignancy.

Malignant tumors of the small intestine include adenocarcinoma, carcinoid, primary lymphoma, leiomyosarcoma, neuroendocrine tumors, and metastatic tumors. More than 80 per cent of these malignant small bowel tumors become symptomatic. The most common malignant small bowel tumor, adenocarcinomas account for 50 per cent of tumors within this category. Histologically, they are similar to other gastrointestinal adenocarcinomas and are usually well differentiated. The majority of adenocarcinomas are found in the proximal bowel and typically occur in the duodenum near the ampulla, but they can also be found in the jejunum and ileum. These tumors spread via lymphatics or blood vessels and by direct extension into adjacent structures.

Malignant carcinoid tumors of the small bowel most frequently arise in the ileum and account for 39 per cent of small intestine malignancies. Carcinoid tumors are currently viewed as neuroendocrine or amine precursor uptake and decarboxylation (APUD) tumors. Patients often present with a combination of tumor-related symptoms and signs and bizarre endocrine syndromes. Hematogenous spread may lead to hepatic metastases and the carcinoid syndrome, characterized by flushing, diarrhea, hypotension, and vasoconstriction. Histologically, the tumor is composed of small cells that have hyperchromatic nuclei. A distinguishing feature of these tumors is the production of polypeptides and 5-hydroxyindoleacetic acid (5-HIAA), which may be detected in body fluids or demonstrated by immune staining or electron microscopy.

In the United States, primary small bowel lymphomas (PSBLs) typically present as localized tumors. In Middle Eastern and developing countries, the presentation is typically more diffuse and is called immunoproliferative small intestine disease (IPSID). Almost all PSBLs are non-Hodgkin's lymphomas, and PSBLs represent about 2 per cent of malignant tumors of the small bowel. Histologically, most PSBLs and IPSID-related tumors are of B-cell origin, but rare forms of T-cell lymphomas have been reported in patients with celiac sprue. The primary lesion typically develops in the ileum but has been found in the jejunum and in the duodenum. In contrast, IPSID, or Mediterranean lymphomas, usually infiltrates the proximal bowel and may involve entire segments of the intestine. The clinical features of IPSID differ considerably from those of PSBLs, and IPSID usually presents earlier—in the second or third decade of life. The signs and symptoms of IPSID include diarrhea, abdominal pain, anorexia, weight loss, and increased serum concentrations of the IgA α heavy chain.

Leiomyosarcomas account for 9 per cent of small bowel malignant tumors. Liposarcomas, angiosarcomas, and neurofibrosarcomas occur more rarely. Leiomyosarcomas commonly arise in the jejunum and ileum and spread primarily via lymphatics. Leiomyosarcomas are submucosal or subserosal growths that typically produce symptoms of obstruction or abdominal pain. Rarely, mucosal extension and subsequent ulceration lead to hemorrhage as the presenting sign.

Neurogenic tumors, which constitute fewer than 1 per cent of small bowel malignancies, arise from neural elements, including nerve sheath cells (neurilemomas), sympathetic ganglia (ganglioneuromas), and neural connective tissue (neurofibromas). These lesions can produce abdominal pain, melena, and intussusception. Histologically, it can be difficult to distinguish neurogenic tumors from leiomyosarcomas by light microscopy. Thus, electron microscopy and immunoperoxidase staining for S-100 protein may be necessary to confirm the diagnosis.

Tumors that metastasize to the small intestine include melanoma; lung, breast, renal, uterine, ovarian, and biliary tumors; and other gastrointestinal malignancies. Sixty per cent of metastatic malignant tumors of the small bowel are melanomas. Most of these tumors arise from hematogenous or lymphatic seeding of the submucosa, but they can also arise from direct contiguous spread. The clinical presentations can include bleeding, obstruction, and/or intussusception.

ETIOLOGY

The mechanisms responsible for the development of tumors of the small bowel have not been well characterized. As mentioned earlier, a number of pathophysiologic mechanisms are thought to protect against carcinogenesis. No particular dietary, chemical, or toxic process has been unequivocally implicated as a causal factor. The etiology almost certainly varies with the type of tumor, and certain factors may predispose to more than one kind of neoplasm.

Hereditary factors cannot be implicated in most patients, but adenomas of the small intestine may be present in patients with genetic varieties of colonic polyposis, such as Gardner's syndrome or familial polyposis. These adenomatous polyps have significant malignant potential and are most common in the periampullary region of the proximal small intestine. The risk of malignancy is greatest in lesions with a diameter exceeding 1.0 cm.

An increased risk of small bowel adenocarcinoma seems to exist in patients with celiac sprue and Crohn's disease. These tumors usually appear in the distal ileum. The carcinogenic mechanism is unclear, but histologic examination of the small intestine reveals dysplasia adjacent to these tumors, suggesting that chronic inflammation may be a key factor in the pathway to malignancy.

Acquired immunodeficiency syndrome (AIDS) has been associated with an increased incidence of non-Hodgkin's lymphoma and Kaposi's sarcoma of the small bowel. The causative mechanism of this association is not known, but recent reports suggest that surgery is performed more frequently for abdominal complications in AIDS patients with these small bowel tumors. Typically, patients present with bleeding, perforation, or obstruction.

PRESENTING SIGNS AND SYMPTOMS

Because the majority of tumors of the small bowel grow intraluminally or cause extrinsic compression, they usually lead to obstruction or hemorrhage. Obstruction may be partial or complete and is usually associated with abdominal pain. Bleeding can be occult and occur over many years, or it can be severe or even life-threatening. Bleeding usually occurs as the slowly expanding tumor mass compresses and erodes overlying mucosa. A benign tumor is rarely detected as a palpable abdominal mass on physical examination. In contrast, malignant tumors are usually symptomatic and present with abdominal pain, small intestinal obstruction, gastrointestinal bleeding, and/or weight loss in more than 80 per cent of patients. In patients with chronic iron-deficiency anemia who have had negative colonic, esophageal, and gastric examinations, the clinician should consider small bowel tumors in the differential diagnosis. Occult gastrointestinal blood loss has been reported in more than half of all patients with benign and malignant tumors of the small bowel.

The majority of periampullary tumors are malignant and associated with a poor prognosis. These tumors usually cause jaundice or are found during screening of susceptible patients. Other lesions in the duodenum, especially adenocarcinomas, may be confused with peptic ulcer disease when they cause nausea, epigastric pain, and vomiting. About one third of patients with malignant small bowel tumors develop partial or complete small bowel obstruction. Distal tumors in the jejunum and ileum are sometimes difficult to distinguish from more common causes of obstruction.

Other nonspecific symptoms such as flushing, diarrhea, and abdominal pain may be helpful in suggesting the carcinoid syndrome, but they rarely occur unless liver metastases are present. Benign small bowel neoplasms tend to remain asymptomatic until they have attained large size. In contrast, malignant tumors are usually symptomatic. In general, physical examination is rarely helpful because specific physical findings are few. For the majority of small bowel tumors, endoscopy and radiographic examinations appear to be essential for diagnosis.

DIAGNOSTIC TESTS

Various radiographic and endoscopic procedures are useful in the diagnosis of small bowel neoplasms. The diagnostic study of choice depends on the suspected location of the lesion. In the past, the standard diagnostic study for neoplasms of the small intestine had been the barium small bowel series. Unfortunately, routine barium studies often fail to demonstrate tumors.

The more accurate and specific small bowel enteroclysis study is performed by passing a tube through the stomach and beyond the ligament of Treitz. The gut is rendered relatively atonic by administration of glucagon or a potent anticholinergic agent, and increments of barium mixed with air are used to distend the gut. The distention with dilute barium gives excellent visualization of the intestinal mucosa. The greatest advantage of this test is the increased ability to detect small mucosal abnormalities. A modified version of this study is hypotonic duodenography, which has been used to distinguish infiltrative from inflammatory lesions of the duodenum. While the accuracy and sensitivity of enteroclysis are unknown, it appears to be superior to standard barium radiography of the small bowel in the detection of small bowel tumors.

Endoscopic evaluation of the small intestine has increased in popularity. The two methods used differ in the degree of skill required of the endoscopist and in the level of patient comfort. Push small bowel enteroscopy, the more common method, involves the use of a longer special endoscope or a pediatric colonoscope to examine the small intestine beyond the ligament of Treitz. Push enteroscopy allows direct visualization of the small bowel and has the advantage of utilizing standard endoscopic instruments to biopsy or snare abnormal areas. Sonde enteroscopy, a newer technique, uses a 5-mm endoscope (up to 9 feet in length) with two internal channels, each 1 mm in diameter. One channel is used to inflate a balloon along the side of the endoscope. This balloon permits peristalsis to carry the scope distally in the small intestine over time. The other channel is used to pass air into the small intestine. Unlike push enteroscopy, sonde enteroscopy does not permit routine biopsies or other standard endoscopy instruments to pass through the channel.

Push enteroscopy provides a substantial diagnostic yield in patients with small bowel tumors but negative barium studies. As this procedure becomes more available, proximal small intestinal lesions should be detected earlier. In the past, push enteroscopy had been used primarily for the diagnosis of obscure small intestinal bleeding, such as angiodysplasia, but its role now includes the evaluation of suspected small bowel tumors. Endoscopic examination of the ileum with push enteroscopy is rarely achieved, but during operative endoscopy clinicians are now able to reach the terminal ileum routinely using a modified technique in which the surgeon slides the intestine over the endoscope. Unfortunately, this technique and expertise are not widely available. The sensitivity of enteroscopy for small bowel tumors has not been determined, but it appears to be superior to that of standard barium studies.

Angiography can demonstrate small bowel tumors indirectly by detecting actively bleeding intraluminal tumors that extravasate contrast material, or directly by demonstrating intraluminal or extraluminal tumor that displays abnormalities of blood vessels. Another radiographic test used for localization of bleeding sites is the technetium-99m(^{99m}Tc)–labeled red blood cell study. In this study, an aliquot of the patient's blood is drawn, and the red blood cells are labeled with the nuclear marker ^{99m}Tc. Following reinjection of the labeled autologous red blood cells, serial scans demonstrate accumulation of nucleotide near the tumor in the small intestine. Unlike angiography, a ^{99m}Tc study can detect a rate of hemorrhage of less than 0.5 mL per minute. Both procedures are usually performed for the evaluation of obscure gastrointestinal hemorrhage despite a lack of specificity for the diagnosis of small bowel tumors.

Computed topography has been used in patients with abdominal pain due to small bowel tumors, but its efficacy has been limited in the early detection of small bowel tumors. Unlike barium studies, computed tomography can accurately define not only malignant and larger benign lesions in the small bowel but also adjacent changes associated with malignant tumors. Computed tomography is most useful in the detection of tumor infiltration of the bowel wall or adjacent mesentery.

Refinements in endoscopic ultrasonography (EUS) equipment should allow definitive evaluation of mucosal and submucosal lesions within reach of an enteroscope. This method may become the preferred means of staging accessible lesions.

APPENDICITIS

By James F. Flaherty, M.D.,
and Giles F. Whalen, M.D.
Farmington, Connecticut

Appendicitis is the most common cause of "acute abdomen," an abdominal condition for which operation is required. In the United States, approximately 6 per cent of the population will develop appendicitis during their lifetimes. Fewer than 10 per cent of the cases will occur after age 60 years or before age 10. Appendicitis is an affliction of young adults, with the incidence rising through the teen-age years and peaking in the mid-20s. In this age group, men are affected twice as commonly as women. The morbidity and mortality that attend appendicitis come from peritonitis and sepsis as consequences of appendiceal gangrene and rupture. Resolution of this abdominal crisis and avoidance of patient morbidity require diagnosis and intervention prior to gangrene and rupture. Because rupture does not usually occur before 36 hours after the onset of symptoms and because most patients seek medical attention within 12 hours after the onset of symptoms, ample opportunity exists for the astute clinician to make a timely diagnosis.

Gratifyingly, in this era of "high-tech" medicine, a timely diagnosis of appendicitis still depends on a careful history, skillful physical examination, and mature judgment—and little on laboratory evaluation or imaging studies. Fortunately, a classic clinical picture typically evolves. However, because appendicitis is so common, most clinicians occasionally encounter it presenting in an atypical fashion. Therefore, appendicitis should be included in the differential diagnosis for any patient seeking medical attention for new abdominal pain. In the setting of acute abdominal pain that may indicate appendicitis, the physician attending the stricken patient should be animated by a sense of diagnostic urgency and a willingness to contemplate surgical intervention before the symptoms and signs of rupture make diagnosis easier.

ANATOMY AND PATHOPHYSIOLOGY

The vermiform appendix is a true diverticulum of the colon. A 6- to 12-cm tubular structure, it is lined by intestinal mucosa and has a muscular wall and an orifice at the cecum, generally below the ileocecal valve. The other end of this hollow muscular tube usually lies in the right iliac fossa (right lower quadrant of the abdomen), but it may lie in a variety of other locations, including the pelvis, the right upper quadrant, and a retroperitoneal location behind the cecum and right colon.

An attack of appendicitis probably begins with obstruction of the appendiceal lumen. The obstructing agent may be inspissated mucus, a fecalith, or a swelling from the rich lymphoid follicles near the mouth of the appendix. However, many other causes of appendiceal obstruction have been described, including mechanical kinking, carcinoid, adenocarcinoma of the appendix or cecum, metastatic disease, foreign bodies, worms, and other parasites. After obstruction has occurred, continued secretion of mucus by the appendiceal epithelium leads to a rise in the intraluminal pressure and ultimately to distention of the appendix. As with other hollow muscular tubes in the body (e.g., the bile duct, gallbladder, ureter, and bowel), the increased intraluminal pressure and distention are experienced as visceral pain. This primitive type of pain is characteristically intense but poorly localized. Classically, the patient experiences the pain more or less in the midline, with "midgut" pain from the appendix felt around the umbilicus. However, patients often relate that their pain exists in a wide band across the middle abdomen, or that it is "all over" the abdomen without localization. Pain that occurs early in an attack of appendicitis causes patients to feel restless with a sense that their severe "gas pain" will diminish if they can have a bowel movement or pass flatus.

Palpation of the abdomen at this juncture does not typically reveal tenderness, although if the examiner can press on the distended appendix and increase the intraluminal pressure, the patient's sense of discomfort increases.

With time, bacteria in the obstructed lumen multiply exponentially and intraluminal pressure eventually exceeds the capillary perfusion pressure and produces appendiceal ischemia. The visceral pain worsens, and protective reflexes of the gut cause the patient to become anorectic or nauseous. Finally, bacteria and inflammatory cells migrate into the wall of the ischemic appendix.

Between 8 and 20 hours after the onset of pain, the inflammation that develops in the wall of the appendix is sufficient to irritate the periappendiceal parietal peritoneum, which is supplied by somatic afferent nerve fibers. These fibers detect touch and chemical irritation (visceral fibers do not), and the patient experiences the pain as sharp and precisely localized to the point of irritation. Now, for the first time since the inception of the attack, palpation will reveal an area of localized tenderness. The patient may even be able to say that the pain has moved to a location or that he or she can point to the area with a finger. Classically, this area is defined as McBurney's point, a point one third of the distance along the line between the anterior iliac spine and the umbilicus. However, point tenderness is confined to the location of the appendix. For example, if the appendix is found in the pelvis, no localized abdominal pain or tenderness may be detected. Instead, tenderness on pelvic or rectal examination can be elicited. Similarly, if the appendiceal tip extends into the right upper quadrant, tenderness may be found there. Over the next several hours, appendiceal and periappendiceal inflammation worsens, and the signs of local inflammation become more pronounced. The patient typically lies still and assumes a "flexed-thigh" position. Inside the abdominal cavity, omentum and surrounding tissues can encapsulate the appendix. The signs of systemic inflammation (i.e., low-grade temperature and leukocytosis) appear during this phase of the attack, and a localized ileus develops.

Ultimately, 24 to 72 hours after the onset of pain, the appendix becomes gangrenous. If it has been walled off by this time, a phlegmon or abscess develops. If the appendix has not been encapsulated, generalized peritonitis ensues. The appendix can also be partially walled off, with peritonitis and abscesses confined to, for example, the right lower abdomen and the pelvis. Whichever of these occurs, the patient usually will have become toxic and febrile, with obvious physical findings. In the absence of treatment, the infection will be walled off, with slow recovery (typically with complications such as abscess, ileus, and small bowel obstruction), or sepsis and death will ensue.

DIAGNOSIS

The diagnosis of appendicitis becomes more obvious as the disease progresses. Historically, institutions that have the lowest rates of false-positive diagnoses of appendicitis (percentage of appendices that are histologically normal when removed during surgery for "appendicitis") also have the highest rates of perforated appendices. In the most common diagnostically challenging group, women of childbearing age, a threefold to fivefold increased risk of tubal infertility follows perforated—but not nonperforated—appendicitis. As a result, false-positive rates in the range of 20 per cent for the diagnosis of appendicitis are accepted as the price of keeping the perforation rate low. The mortality rate for appendectomy with a normal appendix is zero, and the morbidity rate is less than 2 per cent.

Without appropriate diagnostic discipline, unnecessary appendectomy rates can rise as high as 45 per cent in adolescent and young adult women. When the diagnosis is uncertain, hospital admission with conscientious and repeated examination over 4 to 8 hours is both safe and cost effective. Imaging studies such as computed tomography (CT) and ultrasound of the appendix probably add little to the management of these patients. Some studies have found that experienced surgeons can reduce false-positive appendectomy rates to the range of 5 to 10 per cent without increasing perforation rates. No single symptom, sign, or laboratory abnormality is diagnostic of appendicitis. Instead, an evolving constellation of physical and laboratory findings that fit into a progressing historical narrative will ultimately provide the diagnosis.

History

Antecedent illnesses, such as Crohn's disease, sickle cell disease, and vasculitis, can mimic the presentation of acute appendicitis. Any patient who has had abdominal or pelvic surgery (particularly gynecologic operations) may have had the appendix removed incidentally. The patient often knows whether it was. In women, a menstrual and reproductive history is mandatory. A history of dietary indiscretions and any symptoms immediately preceding the attack can be helpful. An overt prodrome of chills, rigor, headaches, or muscle pain is distinctly unusual in appendicitis. Occasionally, a history of vague malaise immediately before the attack is elicited.

The cardinal historical feature of appendicitis is the temporal order in which the symptoms and signs occur. The first symptom experienced is a poorly localized midabdominal pain that develops over an hour or two or wakes the patient up from sleep. It may be described as cramping but is more commonly described as steady. The next symptom is typically anorexia, nausea, retching, or vomiting. The third symptom is more localized pain, usually in the right lower quadrant of the abdomen. This pain is often exacerbated by movement, such as walking to the bathroom or riding in the car to the emergency room. Fever and the awareness of a worsening illness then ensue.

Patients may relate a history of "constipation" or "diarrhea" at any point after the onset of pain. The inflamed appendix can lie against the sigmoid colon or rectum and cause irritation of these structures, leading to tenesmus. Similarly, the inflamed appendix may lie against the bladder, causing urinary urgency, or against the genitofemoral nerve, leading to testicular discomfort. These symptoms can result in misdiagnosis of primary urinary tract disease (infection or stones). The symptoms that are *atypical* of appendicitis include nausea or vomiting *prior* to the onset of abdominal pain, high fever (greater than 38.7°C, 101.7°F) and/or rigors early in an attack, abdominal pain that *begins* in the right lower quadrant, the passage of large volumes of liquid stool, and the complete absence of associated gastrointestinal symptoms. A history of any of these argues against the diagnosis of appendicitis.

Virtually every intra-abdominal condition, and some extra-abdominal conditions, such as right lower lobe pneumonia and the abdominal pain associated with diabetic ketoacidosis, have been misdiagnosed at some time as appendicitis. Consequently, the list of possibilities in the differential diagnosis is long and includes some exotic conditions, such as typhoid, tuberculosis, and amebiasis. More common causes of diagnostic uncertainty are variants of gastroenteritis, "food poisoning," urinary tract infections, passage of ureteral stones, mesenteric adenitis, flares of inflammatory bowel disease, and perforated duodenal ulcer (leaking down along the right colic gutter). Also misdiagnosed as appendicitis, but less frequently, are variants of small bowel obstruction (e.g., intussusception, adhesions, and incarcerated inguinal hernias), cholecystitis, pancreatitis, sigmoid diverticulitis, cecal cancer, cecal ulcers and typhlitis, or cecitis (especially in immunocompromised patients), ischemic bowel, omental torsion and infarction, shingles (before the cutaneous lesions appear), abdominal wall bruises, and rectus sheath hematomas. The cause of the abdominal pain is never found in as many as one third of patients who undergo appendectomy. The diagnosis may also be complicated by a variety of gynecologic conditions, such as a ruptured ovarian cyst (often follicular), salpingitis (pelvic inflammatory disease), endometriosis, torsion of the ovary, ovarian cyst, and ectopic pregnancy. Recalling that appendicitis is independent of the menstrual cycle, the physician can find clues to the correct diagnosis by establishing the relationship of the attacks of abdominal pain to the menstrual cycle.

Physical Examination

Determination of the chronology and duration of the physical findings is crucial to arriving at the correct diagnosis. Few abdominal signs are expected early in an attack, but after 36 hours of pain they are. The location of the appendix determines the site of localizing tenderness; if the appendix lies in the pelvis or behind the right colon and cecum, localized tenderness may be absent on abdominal examination. If the appendix lies on the left side, tenderness may be localized to the left lower quadrant, and if it lies next to the uterus and fallopian tubes, tenderness may be elicited with movement of the cervix during pelvic examination. In addition to abdominal examination, careful attention to chest (diaphragm), rectal and pelvic examinations should be routine. Similarly, the diagnosis of appendicitis must not be excluded simply because the tenderness has localized to an area other than the right lower quadrant.

A gentle approach to a painful abdomen yields the best results. Auscultation of the heart and lungs with a warm stethoscope prior to examination of the abdomen may relax the patient. If the patient presents early in the course, bowel sounds are typically normal. If peritonitis is present, bowel sounds are usually hypoactive or absent. Before beginning abdominal palpation, the physician should ask the patient to cough. Localized abdominal pain with a small cough usually indicates peritoneal irritation at that site. The physician can also elicit this finding with a firm strike on the heels of a supine patient or by asking the patient to drop from toes to heels if he or she is able to stand up. Light percussion of all four quadrants of the abdomen is another accurate and subtle way of demonstrating localized peritoneal irritation.

Superficial palpation of the abdomen should begin in an area away from the site of greatest pain. Tenderness referred to the right lower quadrant on palpation of other parts of the abdomen may occur with localized peritoneal irritation associated with appendicitis. Voluntary guarding refers to tensing of the abdominal muscles in anticipation of the examination. Patients can often be distracted from voluntary guarding, especially when there is no peritoneal irritation, by conversational chatter that diverts attention from this part of the examination. Involuntary guarding occurs when local inflammatory changes become so advanced that a spasm is induced in the abdominal wall muscles, causing failure of relaxation on expiration. Deep palpation of the most painful quadrant, combined with sudden, reverberating release of the abdomen may elicit so-called rebound tenderness. Such palpation is a less reliable way of determining localized peritonitis than the other maneuvers and can cause excruciating pain.

The posterior abdominal wall can be partially evaluated with maneuvers such as extension of the hip joint while the patient is in the left lateral decubitus position, thus stretching the psoas muscle. If the peritoneum overlying the psoas is inflamed by adjacent retroperitoneal appendicitis, it is painful (psoas sign). Similarly, the obturator sign demonstrates inflammation of the obturator internus fasciae in the posterolateral pelvis from adjacent appendicitis. The clinician elicits this sign by flexing the patient's hip and knee while rotating the hip joint.

The pelvic sidewalls are best evaluated by rectal or vaginal examination. Bimanual examination of the pelvic viscera is also useful because it may suggest an alternative diagnosis. Visualization of the cervix with a speculum may reveal a discharge, suggesting salpingitis, or blue engorgement, suggesting early pregnancy.

Laboratory Tests

No specific laboratory test will secure a diagnosis of appendicitis. Like physical findings, laboratory findings evolve over the course of an attack. Leukocytosis is expected but may be absent early in an attack, and approximately half the patients who will be found to have nonsurgical conditions will have a white blood cell count (WBC) of more than 10,000 cells/mm^3. The differential WBC may be more helpful; a percentage of granulocytes of 85 per cent or more with more than 7 per cent bands is more consistent with appendicitis. The WBC rarely exceeds 20,000 cells/mm^3 unless the appendix has already ruptured. Urinalysis is performed to exclude urinary tract infection or ureteral calculi. Appendiceal irritation of the ureter or bladder can result in both leukocytes and erythrocytes in the urine, although it is unusual for this condition to result in more than 10 cells per high-power field (hpf). Other blood tests that are frequently obtained—glucose, electrolytes, serum urea nitrogen, creatinine, amylase, and beta-human chorionic gonadotropin (HCG; pregnancy test)—serve chiefly to alert the clinician to other problems or complications.

Imaging

For the patient in whom appendicitis is suspected, the physician often orders a plain film of the abdomen and occasionally a chest film is taken in the emergency room. No plain film findings are pathognomonic for appendicitis. As the attack progresses, radiologic evidence of localized inflammation may develop: loops of small intestine containing increased amounts of air in the right lower quadrant or increased air in the cecum (local ileus), or loss of the fat stripe (due to edema) marking the psoas margin in retroperitoneal appendicitis. Appendicoliths, visualized as isolated radiographic densities in the right lower quadrant must be distinguished from vascular calcifications and ureteral calculi. Appendiceal concretions occur in approximately 2 per cent of the normal population and are seen on 10 per cent of the films taken when appendicitis is suspected. In the latter cases, an appendicolith is a highly suggestive finding and, unfortunately, is associated with a greater likelihood of a gangrenous appendix. However, the greatest value of plain films in appendicitis is probably their ability to suggest or exclude other possibilities in the differential diagnosis. For example, free air on the chest film is almost never due to appendicitis—even perforated appendicitis.

Barium enema has been used in the management of the patient suspected of having acute appendicitis. Complete filling in of the appendix on a barium enema study virtually guarantees that the patient does not have appendicitis, and the study may even suggest another diagnosis (e.g., intussusception, cancer, diverticulitis, or ischemic colitis). Failure to fill in the appendix is taken as indirect evidence of appendicitis or, at least, of some obstructive problem at the appendiceal orifice that could cause appendicitis. However, the false-positive rates for this procedure are not known, and most clinicians are concerned about introducing barium to an intraperitoneal site that may rupture. The mixture of barium and stool free in the peritoneal cavity can be lethal. Also, modern imaging techniques with ultrasound and CT are more sensitive, safer, and less cumbersome in an emergency setting. Consequently, today barium enema is rarely used as a diagnostic aid for acute appendicitis. This procedure may still have some utility in the diagnosis of recurrent or chronic appendicitis.

Transvaginal ultrasound is frequently and usefully employed in women to evaluate the possibility of nonappendiceal pelvic pathologic conditions. Transabdominal ultrasound using "graded compression" for making a specific diagnosis of appendicitis is being employed with increasing frequency and accuracy, especially in children. Ultrasonographic diagnosis of early appendicitis depends on demonstrating an intraluminal appendicolith or an appendix that does not compress to less than 7 mm in diameter along its entire length. More subtle findings, such as loss of the normal submucosal echo pattern, may also be helpful. As an attack advances, periappendiceal edema or even abscess may also be found ultrasonographically. Finally, other pathologic conditions accounting for the attack, such as gallstones or intussusception, may be seen by the competent ultrasonographer. The accuracy of ultrasonographic testing is greatly dependent on the skill of the examining ultrasonographer. Transabdominal ultrasound has not yet been shown to be more accurate than the clinical diagnosis of appendicitis. In expert hands, ultrasound has a false-negative rate of approximately 20 per cent and a false-positive rate of about 10 per cent in patients for whom surgical consultation has been obtained and for whom an initial therapeutic decision has been made. Ultrasound is not necessary in the majority of patients, but it may be helpful in diagnostically challenging cases when ultrasonographic expertise is available.

Computed tomography of the abdomen may diagnose even relatively early appendicitis with surprising accuracy, but it is unnecessary in the majority of patients. Again, as the localized inflammation progresses, the diagnostic accuracy of CT increases. Computed tomography is probably superior to ultrasonography as an imaging modality because increasing bowel gas may limit the ultrasound examination. Other advantages of CT include an excellent view of other peritoneal and retroperitoneal structures and a relative lack of dependence on the skill of the person who performs the test. The major drawbacks are the expense, the radiation, and the usual need for oral and intravenous contrast media to achieve the best evaluation. Occasionally, a surprise diagnosis of appendicitis is made with a CT scan obtained for evaluating what is suspected of being another condition. Computed tomography adds little new information when the clinical diagnosis of acute appendicitis is firm, but it can be useful in guiding the appropriate management of a patient who presents late with a right lower quadrant mass.

Laparoscopy

The application of laparoscopy to the diagnosis of appendicitis has become especially popular recently. Its chief advantage is an accuracy at diagnosing appendicitis that equals that of open appendectomy. The appendix can be removed via a laparoscopic approach as safely as it can be through an incision. Using laparoscopy, the physician can also visualize other pelvic and abdominal organs. The major disadvantage of laparoscopy is that the patient must be anesthetized in the operating room and undergo a procedure that is as invasive as a McBurney muscle-splitting incision. The decision to perform laparoscopy contributes nothing to the preoperative diagnosis of appendicitis and must be made with the same information that the physician would use in deciding to perform an open appendectomy.

Diagnostic Pitfalls

Although 10 to 20 per cent of attacks of appendicitis are "atypical," appendicitis is usually misdiagnosed because a history of the cardinal symptoms and their temporal order is not accurately obtained. Misdiagnosis can also occur when the examiner fails to appreciate the variability of the location of the appendix and the consequences of that variability on the development of localized tenderness. However, in certain circumstances, the typical evolution of appendicitis is masked, or the multiplicity of diagnostic possibilities in a particular case may draw attention away from the correct diagnosis. Finally, some attacks of appendicitis do not progress inexorably to gangrene and rupture. These cases improve spontaneously and then recur (recurrent appendicitis), or progress to chronic right lower quadrant pain (chronic appendicitis). These syndromes are unusual and typically present an elective diagnostic problem rather than an immediate clinical threat.

Retrocecal Appendicitis

Appendicitis that occurs in an appendix situated behind the cecum and right colon is notoriously difficult to diagnose. The patient may experience the typical initial pain, which is vague and ill defined, as being more lateral. More important, the pain frequently never localizes but remains ill defined. The cecum and colon mask the inflammatory process from the abdominal wall. If the appendix is in juxtaposition to the psoas muscle, an examiner may find that either the psoas sign can be elicited on physical examination or that the psoas margin has disappeared on abdominal plain film. An appendix located behind the cecum and right colon can be difficult to visualize on ultrasound because of the overlying bowel gas. In this case, CT scan may be helpful. However, the most valuable diagnostic aid is a high index of suspicion.

Steroids, Antibiotics, and Pain Medication

The evolution of the signs of local inflammation and of systemic inflammation may be masked in a patient receiving steroids. There is no simple solution to this problem if the diagnosis is unclear. Even greater emphasis on the clinical history is necessary, and imaging studies may be helpful. Frequently, however, the clinician must be prepared to proceed with appendectomy if the patient fails to improve after a brief period of observation. Appendicitis may follow an atypical course in patients who have received antibiotic therapy. Most commonly, a diagnosis of urinary tract infection will have been made several days previously. Similarly, a patient being treated with analgesic medication for abdominal pain may not have as much localized tenderness as expected or may not feel that the pain is worsening. The physician can usually resolve this problem by stopping the pain medication. These clinical situations present diagnostic pitfalls primarily for the unwary; the clinician can best deal with them by inquiring about the use of medications early in the evaluation.

Appendicitis in the Young
Key historical features may not be obtainable, especially in very young children. Those younger than 4 years of age may not be able to convey a coherent account of the order of their symptoms, and they frequently present late and are ill with perforation. The physical findings are consonant with that stage of the disease. In this age group particularly, abdominal ultrasound may be a useful aid for making an earlier diagnosis. However, in any sick young child with abdominal pain and tenderness, a high index of suspicion is the primary requisite for diagnosis.

Appendicitis in the Old
The diagnosis is also often delayed in older patients. Appendicitis is unusual in patients older than 60 years of age, but this group accounts for more than 50 per cent of the deaths due to appendicitis. The reasons for the increased mortality include the infirmity of age and a delay in diagnosis, but the reasons for the delay are a matter of conjecture. The symptom complex in the elderly may seem more vague, and the findings on physical examination not impressive. Such elderly patients may not develop leukocytosis or fever as readily as younger patients. In addition, medical problems other than appendicitis may seem to the examiner to be a more likely cause of the patient's symptoms.

Appendicitis in Pregnancy
Appendicitis in the pregnant patient has an incidence of about 1 in 1500 births. Nausea, vomiting, and vague abdominal symptoms are common during pregnancy. Also, because a fetus is present, physicians avoid, if possible, interventions that either may be teratogenic or may increase the risk of premature labor. Consequently, the diagnosis is often delayed. The most common abdominal surgical emergency of pregnancy, appendicitis frequently has a typical course. On physical examination, the position of the cecum and appendix may shift, often to the right upper quadrant, as the uterus enlarges. One can attempt to differentiate intra-abdominal pain from uterine pain by positioning the patient with her left side down. Persistence of tenderness in the right lower quadrant as the uterus falls away suggests some source of abdominal pain other than the uterus. In questionable cases, ultrasound may be helpful. To avoid the low but measurable incidence of maternal as well as fetal mortality, one must occasionally be willing to proceed to appendectomy without a certain diagnosis.

Human Immunodeficiency Virus (HIV)
HIV-positive patients usually have a fairly typical early clinical course and do not always develop leukocytosis. However, the range of possibilities in the differential diagnosis is wider than usual, with the addition of opportunistic intra-abdominal infections. Once again, these diagnostic possibilities tend to distract the examiner and to delay the diagnosis. In questionable situations, laparoscopic evaluation is recommended. Appendectomy performed in these patients prior to perforation results in no increase in morbidity or mortality.

CHRONIC DIARRHEA AND MALABSORPTION

By Frank J. Aberger, M.D.
LaCrosse, Wisconsin

CHRONIC DIARRHEA

Diarrhea, often described by patients as an abnormal loosening and/or increased frequency of the stools, is an extremely common symptom. Many patients who report diarrhea do not, however, have true medically defined diarrhea, which is an increase in stool weight to more than 200 g per day associated with an increase in stooling frequency to at least two or three bowel movements per day. Although 72-hour stool collections to quantitate and document diarrhea can certainly be useful in certain circumstances, such a collection is not always practical, and the clinician usually relies simply on the patient's description of symptoms in deciding on further evaluation. Diarrhea is defined as chronic when it persists for more than 3 weeks.

Four major mechanisms are recognized as producing diarrhea:

1. Osmotic diarrhea due to poorly absorbable osmotic solutes in the gut lumen (e.g., lactose malabsorption secondary to lactase deficiency, ingestion of magnesium-containing cathartics or antacids)
2. Secretory diarrhea due to intestinal ion secretion or failure to absorb ions (e.g., cholera, VIPoma, carcinoid syndrome)
3. Inflammatory diarrhea due to inflammatory mucosal changes (e.g., inflammatory bowel disease)
4. Abnormal intestinal motility (e.g., irritable bowel syndrome)

History and Physical Examination

The medical history can provide many helpful clues regarding the cause of chronic diarrhea and help direct further work-up. A history of large-volume diarrhea suggests a small bowel or right colon lesion, whereas small-volume diarrhea implies a left colonic or rectal cause. Tenesmus with associated small-volume diarrhea suggests a rectosigmoid lesion. Nocturnal diarrhea suggests an organic cause, arguing against the diagnosis of irritable bowel syndrome.

Hematochezia implies inflammation (i.e., inflammatory bowel disease, infection), neoplasia, or perianal disease, such as hemorrhoids or anal fissures. Blood observed on the toilet paper only, or blood noted to be dripping into the toilet water or the underpants after a bowel movement, implies a perianal source. Pus in the stools is observed with inflammation of the intestinal mucosa, and mucus in the stools occurs with irritable bowel syndrome, but these two symptoms may be confused by the patient. Large, bulky stools suggest malabsorption, especially if oil droplets are observed. The location of any associated pain may also prove helpful (e.g., right lower quadrant pain in Crohn's disease). Fasting usually causes osmotic diarrhea to cease, but secretory diarrhea typically persists through a fast.

A dietary history can be invaluable in providing clues to the cause of diarrhea. Lactose intolerance occurs in nearly 50 million American adults and in the majority of the African American, North American Indian, Mexican American, Jewish American, and Asian American adult populations. It is least common among northern European descendants. Common symptoms include flatulence, bloating, abdominal pain, and diarrhea. Alcohol; caffeine; fructose in corn syrup; and sorbitol in diet products, sugarless gums, and mints can also lead to chronic diarrhea. Raw milk ingestion suggests the possibility of brainerdiasis, a prolonged, but usually self-limiting diarrhea that is probably caused by an infectious agent in nonpasteurized milk. The ingestion of well water or stream water may implicate giardiasis as a cause of diarrhea. A wide variety of medications can also cause or aggravate diarrhea (e.g., magnesium-containing antacids, cisapride, misoprostol, beta-blockers, and antibiotics).

The results of physical examination may vary from normal to revealing a seriously ill, dehydrated, and/or cachectic patient. Physical signs can suggest the correct diagnosis (e.g., dermatitis herpetiformis, with sprue; perirectal fistulas, with Crohn's disease; goiter, with hyperthyroidism). The finding of blood or pus in the stool mandates a search for an organic cause of the diarrhea.

Evaluation

The initial step in the evaluation of chronic diarrhea (Fig. 1) is to check the stool for occult blood (Hemoccult) and white blood cells (Wright's stain) unless obvious blood or pus is found on physical examination. (Many laboratories check for white blood cells as part of the parasitology examination.) A Sudan stain of a stool specimen for fat globules suggests malabsorption if the result is positive, but it is an insensitive test and may be negative in low-grade steatorrhea. Sodium hydroxide alkalization testing to check stool for phenolphthalein can be performed in the office and is evidence of phenolphthalein laxative abuse (e.g., Ex-Lax). Other types of laxatives are not detected with this test. Stool pH less than 5.3 is diagnostic of carbohydrate (e.g., lactose) intolerance.

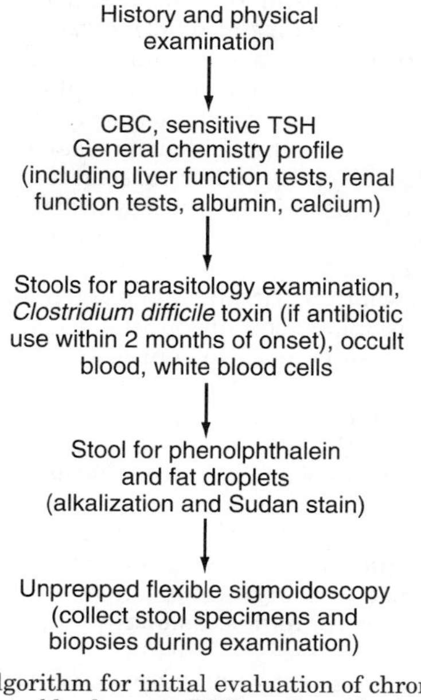

History and physical examination
↓
CBC, sensitive TSH
General chemistry profile
(including liver function tests, renal function tests, albumin, calcium)
↓
Stools for parasitology examination, *Clostridium difficile* toxin (if antibiotic use within 2 months of onset), occult blood, white blood cells
↓
Stool for phenolphthalein and fat droplets
(alkalization and Sudan stain)
↓
Unprepped flexible sigmoidoscopy
(collect stool specimens and biopsies during examination)

Figure 1. Algorithm for initial evaluation of chronic diarrhea. CBC = complete blood count; TSH = thyroid-stimulating hormone.

Stools collected for bacterial culture and sensitivity, parasitology examination, and analysis for *Clostridium difficile* toxin can be helpful in the appropriate setting. In the United States, the most common parasite found as a cause of chronic diarrhea is *Giardia lamblia*. Approximately 50 per cent of the stool specimens from patients with giardiasis are negative for the parasite, and several specimens may be required for making the diagnosis. An enzyme-linked immunosorbent assay for giardia in the stool can provide more than 90 per cent sensitivity. Stools collected for testing for *C. difficile* toxin are very helpful in making the diagnosis of antibiotic-induced colitis, especially in patients with normal flexible sigmoidoscopy examination (as many as one third of patients with antibiotic-induced colitis have involvement limited to the right colon). This diagnosis should be suspected in any patient with diarrhea who has received antibiotics within 6 to 8 weeks prior to the onset of the diarrhea.

Flexible sigmoidoscopy provides a view of the rectosigmoid mucosa that may suggest the cause of the diarrhea (i.e., pseudomembranes, melanosis coli, carcinoma, colitis). Stools can be obtained through the scope and examined for white cells, ova and parasites, *C. difficile* toxin, phenolphthalein, and fat droplets with the use of Sudan stain. Biopsies can also be obtained. Initially, an unprepped examination is preferred to avoid trauma from the enema tip and artifact leading to either endoscopic or histologic misinterpretation. If too much solid stool is present for adequate examination at the time of the unprepped sigmoidoscopy, two Fleet enemas can be given and the examination repeated.

Laboratory Evaluation

Laboratory studies for the initial evaluation of chronic diarrhea include a complete blood count (CBC), sensitive thyroid-stimulating hormone (TSH), and a general chemistry profile that includes liver function tests, renal function tests, serum albumin, and serum calcium. If malabsorption is in the differential diagnosis, prothrombin time, serum carotene, vitamin B_{12} and folate, and iron studies are indicated.

If the diagnosis remains unclear, colonoscopy and/or air contrast barium enema may be used to evaluate the colon. Biopsies of apparently normal mucosa at the time of colonoscopy can reveal granulomas (Crohn's disease), melanosis coli (laxative abuse), or microscopic or collagenous colitis. The latter two conditions are characterized by normal-appearing mucosa on radiographs and endoscopy, but the mucosa is histologically abnormal.

Upper endoscopic examination can also be helpful in the evaluation because it permits the performance of small bowel biopsies. Duodenal secretions may be obtained through the scope for examination for parasites (particularly useful in cases of giardiasis in which stool specimens are negative for parasites).

Upper gastrointestinal series with small bowel follow-through can be used to better evaluate the small bowel mucosa beyond the range of the standard upper endoscope. Barium studies of the gastrointestinal tract are often complementary to the endoscopic evaluation. Parasitology examinations must be performed prior to any barium studies, because barium interferes with the visualization of parasites such as *Entamoeba histolytica*. Small bowel antero-grade enteroclysis can better define subtle small bowel mucosal changes than can standard small bowel contrast films, but it is more cumbersome and uncomfortable and requires nasoenteric intubation. Ultrasound and/or computed tomography may be helpful in detecting tumors, inflammatory masses, bowel wall thickening, or pancreatic calcifications.

Empirical therapeutic trials are often useful in the diagnosis of the cause of the diarrhea. A 3-week trial of a lactose-free diet may be helpful in diagnosing lactose intolerance if symptoms improve. Unfortunately, inadvertent lactose ingestion can confound the diagnosis. Although milk products are obvious lactose sources, the sugar may be present in a wide variety of other foods, including hot dogs, salad dressings, breads, candies, and processed meats. The lactose-hydrogen breath test is a noninvasive procedure that is more sensitive in making the diagnosis of lactose intolerance. An empirical trial of metronidazole can be used if giardiasis, small bowel bacterial overgrowth, or *C. difficile* colitis is suspected. There is, however, a risk of adverse drug side effects induced by metronidazole.

A 24-hour stool collection for stool weight and fecal fat measurement can provide true quantitative data, but it is a cumbersome, aesthetically unpleasant test for both the patient and laboratory personnel. A stool weight greater than 200 g per day defines diarrhea, and a stool fat greater than 7 g per day (with the patient on a diet of 100 g of fat per day) defines steatorrhea. Some chronic watery diarrheas, however, can induce low-grade steatorrhea. Consequently, a fecal fat content of 7 to 14 g per day may or may not signify a true malabsorptive diarrhea. Fecal fat excretion greater than 14 g per day does, however, define a true malabsorptive diarrhea (i.e., celiac sprue, chronic pancreatitis).

Although an analysis of stool electrolyte content and measurement of fecal osmotic gap may provide helpful information, it is not practical for most clinicians and laboratories. Initially, the osmolality of normal feces approximates that of plasma (290 mOsm/kg). With storage of the stool, osmolality increases significantly because of bacterial fermentation of nonabsorbed carbohydrates. Therefore, for the purpose of calculating the stool osmotic gap, the stool osmolality is assumed to be 290 mOsm/kg, and actual measurement of the stool osmolality is not usually done. Osmotic diarrheas are characterized by stool osmolality as it leaves the rectum (290 mOsm/kg) greater than twice the sum of the sodium and potassium content of the stool (stool osmolality $> 2 \times [Na^+ + K^+]$). In osmotic diarrhea, the unmeasured osmotically active substances in the stool account for this gap. An osmotic gap of 50 mOsm/kg or more is considered significant. Secretory diarrheas are not characterized by an osmotic gap, and the stool osmolality is equal to the sum of the stool sodium and potassium content multiplied by 2 (stool osmolality $= 2 \times [Na^+ + K^+]$). Osmotic diarrheas (lactose intolerance) are characterized by an abatement of the diarrhea with fasting, whereas secretory diarrheas (VIPoma) are generally characterized by persistence of the diarrhea despite fasting.

If the diagnosis remains elusive, a number of other studies may provide useful clues. Urine can be checked for the presence of laxatives (e.g., bisacodyl, anthraquinones, and phenolphthalein) and diuretics. Measurable magnesium and phosphate in the stool is consistent with laxative abuse, which is the most common cause of diarrhea of undetermined origin. These patients usually deny laxative ingestion and may require psychiatric consultation. Fasting serum gastrin concentrations may be helpful, because approximately 7 per cent of patients with Zollinger-Ellison syndrome present with diarrhea without obvious ulcer disease. Massive secretory, watery diarrhea greater than 1 L per day, especially with associated hypokalemia, suggests VIPoma (see article on endocrine disease of the gastrointestinal tract).

Small intestinal aspirates for culture or hydrogen breath testing to confirm small bowel bacterial overgrowth can be helpful in selected patients. Small bowel bacterial overgrowth can present as a watery chronic diarrhea or as a malabsorptive syndrome with steatorrhea and vitamin B_{12} deficiency. Any condition that causes small bowel stasis or hypochlorhydria can lead to small bowel bacterial overgrowth.

Other tests that may rarely be of use in the evaluation of unexplained diarrhea include a serum calcitonin measurement (medullary thyroid carcinoma), immunoglobulin electrophoresis (hypogammaglobulinemia), and a 24-hour urine collection for 5-hydroxyindoleacetic acid (carcinoid syndrome), vanillylmandelic acid, catecholamines, and metanephrines (pheochromocytoma).

Irritable bowel syndrome is not an uncommon cause of diarrhea of undetermined origin. Factors favoring irritable bowel include the *absence* of the following: nocturnal symptoms, significant weight loss (more than 5 kg), blood or pus in the stools, anemia or other baseline laboratory abnormalities. A long duration of symptoms is also a factor favoring irritable bowel syndrome. Endocrine disorders, such as hyperthyroidism and diabetes, can also cause chronic diarrhea. Chronic diarrhea for which no etiology can be found despite exhaustive evaluation is termed chronic idiopathic diarrhea. Fortunately, with the passage of time (often months or years) most cases of chronic idiopathic diarrhea eventually resolve. Symptomatic therapy (e.g., Imodium) usually provides adequate relief.

MALABSORPTION

Malabsorption is defined as impaired absorption of nutrients. A history of extensive small bowel resection or radiation therapy suggests a short bowel syndrome or radiation enteritis, respectively. A history of large, bulky, malodorous stools perhaps with oil droplets is typical of malabsorption. Malabsorptive stools can be sticky and difficult to flush down the toilet. A history of floating stools does not indicate malabsorption, but excess gas produced by bacteria. The physical examination in malabsorption may be completely normal, or it may reveal a variety of abnormalities, including glossitis (vitamin B deficiencies), ecchymoses (vitamin K malabsorption), pallor (associated with anemia), or signs of hypocalcemia (Trousseau's sign or Chvostek's sign). Laboratory studies (Fig. 2) may reveal a positive Sudan stain of the stool or an increased 72-hour fecal fat content in association with fat malabsorption. Low serum iron concentrations in the absence of blood loss, hypocalcemia, hypoalbuminemia, hypoprothrombinemia, and/or low serum carotene concentration are consistent with small bowel malabsorption. Malabsorption of iron alone or calcium alone without other mineral, nutrient, or fat malabsorption can occur in proximal small bowel disease (e.g., celiac sprue) and either can be the sole presenting manifestation of this disorder. Decreased serum vitamin B_{12} concentrations suggest terminal ileal disease, but they may also be seen in pernicious anemia, in small bowel bacterial overgrowth, and occasionally in pancreatic insufficiency.

Small bowel radiographs may reveal strictures, multiple jejunal diverticula, or blind surgical loops, conditions conducive to small bowel bacterial overgrowth and subsequent

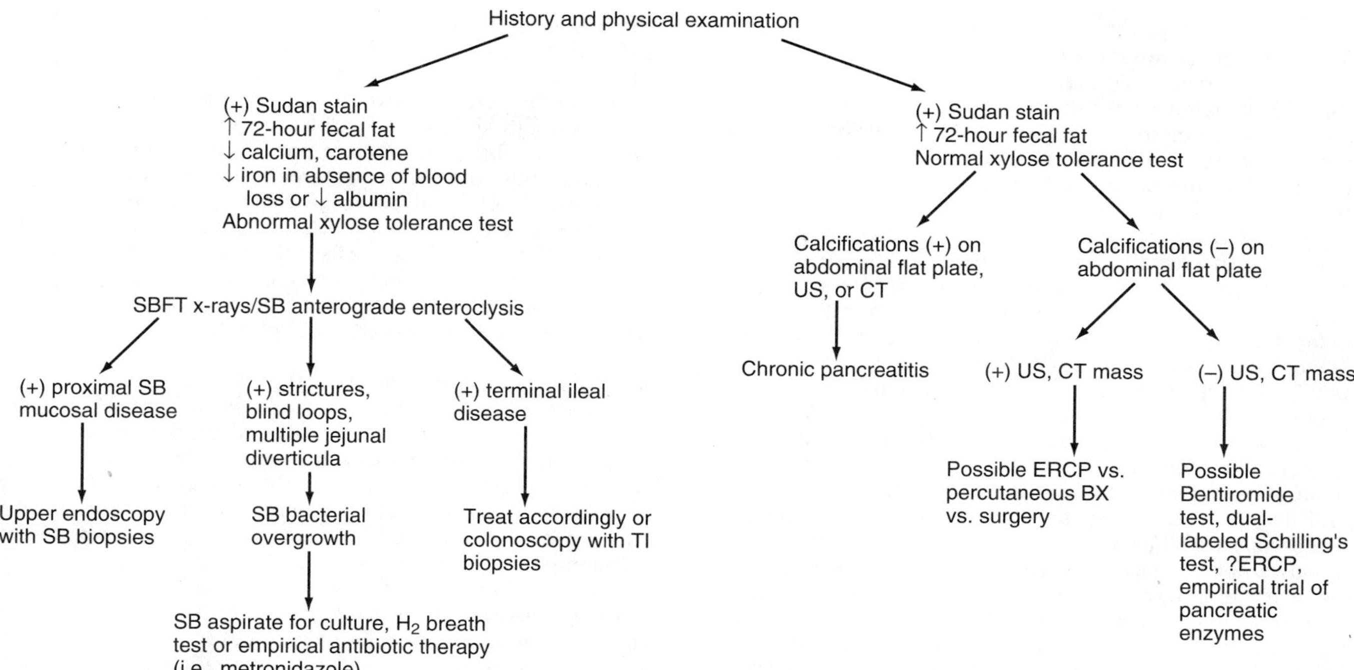

Figure 2. Malabsorption evaluation. BX = biopsy; CT = computed tomography; TI = terminal ileum; SB = small bowel; US = ultrasound; ERCP = endoscopic retrograde cholangiopancreatography; SBFT = small bowel follow-through.

malabsorption. Hypochlorhydria (seen in association with aging, pernicious anemia, pharmacologic acid suppression) and small intestinal motility disorders (e.g., scleroderma, intestinal pseudo-obstruction) also predispose to small bowel bacterial overgrowth. Small bowel radiographs may also show intestinal dilatation (sprue, giardiasis), nodularity (lymphoma), thickening, edema, or terminal ileal disease (Crohn's disease). Small bowel films may be completely normal in small bowel mucosal malabsorptive diseases. If the small bowel x-ray series suggests proximal small bowel disease or if proximal small bowel disease is suspected despite negative x-ray findings, upper endoscopy with small bowel biopsies should be done.

In celiac sprue, endoscopy may reveal flattened or scalloped-appearing folds in the postbulbar duodenum. Biopsies of the proximal duodenal mucosa in celiac sprue can show various degrees of villous atrophy, but this finding is nonspecific and can be found in a variety of other conditions (e.g., nontropical sprue, viral gastroenteritis, small intestinal bacterial overgrowth, small intestinal lymphoma). The villous atrophy in celiac sprue, unlike that seen with other conditions, responds to a gluten-free diet. The proximal small bowel is always involved in celiac sprue, and a normal proximal small bowel biopsy virtually excludes the diagnosis. Eosinophilic gastroenteritis is characterized by infiltration of the mucosal lining with eosinophils and peripheral eosinophilia on the complete blood count. Whipple's disease is rare and is diagnosed by the observation of abundant macrophages in the lamina propria that stain positive with periodic acid–Schiff (PAS) stain and demonstration of *Tropheryma whippelii* (Whipple's bacillus) on electron microscopy. Small bowel biopsy can also be useful in diagnosing several other small bowel disorders, including but not limited to giardiasis, collagenous sprue, abetalipoproteinemia, and small intestinal lymphoma.

Diseases that affect the small bowel in a patchy fashion (i.e., lymphoma) may be missed by small bowel biopsy. Terminal ileal disease can be detected by examination of the terminal ileum during colonoscopy if the small bowel follow-through (or barium enema with terminal ileal reflux) is not helpful.

Pancreatic exocrine insufficiency also causes malabsorption and is usually secondary to chronic pancreatitis, but it may be due to other causes (e.g., pancreatic carcinoma, cystic fibrosis). A history of alcohol abuse suggests chronic pancreatitis as the cause of malabsorption. Pancreatic calcifications on an abdominal flat plate are occasionally seen in chronic pancreatitis. Both ultrasound and computed tomography are more sensitive in detecting pancreatic calcifications and may also reveal an irregularly shaped pancreas, pancreatic pseudocysts, pancreatic ductal dilatation, or a pancreatic mass. Ultrasound and computed tomography may be completely normal in chronic pancreatitis, and occasionally endoscopic retrograde cholangiopancreatography (ERCP) is necessary. ERCP may reveal the classic dilated chain-of-lakes appearance to the pancreatic duct or may help distinguish between chronic pancreatitis and pancreatic carcinoma, but ERCP can be normal in chronic pancreatitis and the examination carries the risk of inducing acute pancreatitis. ERCP is usually abnormal in pancreatic carcinoma, because most pancreatic carcinomas are ductal in origin. Pancreatic insufficiency can be very difficult to diagnose and may require additional testing that is not readily available (e.g., bentiromide test, dual-labelled Schilling's test, aspiration and analysis of pancreatic secretions after intravenous secretin). Problems persist, however, with the sensitivity and specificity of these tests. If chronic pancreatitis is suspected as a cause of steatorrhea, an empirical trial of pancreatic enzymes may be useful.

The xylose tolerance test can be used to distinguish between a malabsorptive diarrhea secondary to a mucosal gastrointestinal tract abnormality (e.g., celiac sprue) and a pancreatic cause (e.g., chronic pancreatitis). Poor absorption of xylose suggests a mucosal cause, whereas normal absorption is typically observed in chronic pancreatitis. More reliable results are obtained if serum xylose concentrations are measured rather than urine xylose concentration. False-negative results may be observed in mild small bowel disease or distal disease of the small bowel. Cholestatic disorders can also cause malabsorption owing to a deficiency of bile acids delivered to the intestinal lumen, but associated jaundice is usually obvious.

The patient with acquired immunodeficiency syndrome (AIDS) with chronic diarrhea and/or malabsorption may have several pathogens simultaneously responsible for the diarrhea. The list is long, and it includes bacteria (*Salmonella, Campylobacter, Clostridium difficile, Shigella, Mycobacterium avium*), viruses (cytomegalovirus, herpes simplex, adenovirus, human immunodeficiency virus [HIV]), protozoa (*Giardia, Entamoeba, Cryptosporidium, Microsporidium, Isospora* and *Cyclospora*). The evaluation of chronic diarrhea and malabsorption in the AIDS patient usually begins with stool cultures, a *C. difficile* toxin assay, and at least three stool specimens for ova and parasites. Endoscopy with biopsies (e.g., flexible sigmoidoscopy, colonoscopy, upper endoscopy with small bowel biopsies) is indicated if the diarrhea is persistent or large in volume and especially if it is accompanied by significant weight loss. Electron microscopy of biopsy specimens may also prove helpful. In approximately 15 to 25 per cent of AIDS patients, no pathogen is found, and symptomatic therapy for diarrhea and/or malabsorption must be provided for patient comfort.

ENDOCRINE DISORDERS OF THE GASTROINTESTINAL TRACT

By Robert T. Jensen, M.D.,
and Fathia Gibril, M.D.
Bethesda, Maryland

Endocrine disorders of the gastrointestinal tract include the gastroenteropancreatic (GEP) tumor syndromes and multiple endocrine neoplasias. Gastric carcinoid tumors are included in this section because, although they do not cause endocrine disorders, they are frequently the result of hypergastrinemia. Diagnosis of these disorders is important because patients have symptoms due to the effects of the ectopically released hormone and because the tumors are frequently malignant. Because these uncommon conditions often masquerade as more common disorders, the diagnosis is frequently missed; for example, with Zollinger-Ellison syndrome (ZES), the delay in diagnosis is typically 6 years. Early diagnosis allows effective treatment of the hormonal symptoms and the tumors, which can greatly extend survival.

MULTIPLE ENDOCRINE NEOPLASIAS

The multiple endocrine neoplasia (MEN) syndromes are inherited disorders that are autosomal dominant with variable penetrance. They are characterized by hyperplasia or tumors of multiple endocrine organs. The two major types include MEN type I (MEN-I, Wermer's syndrome) and MEN type II (MEN-II, Sipple's syndrome). MEN-II has been subdivided into two subtypes: MEN-IIA and MEN-IIB (also called MEN-III). MEN-I syndrome involves, in decreasing relative frequency, parathyroid, pancreas, pituitary, adrenal, and gastric enterochromaffin-like cells (ECL cells). MEN-IIA involves, in decreasing relative frequency, the thyroid, adrenal medulla, and parathyroids. MEN-IIB involves the thyroid more often than the adrenal medulla; is associated with the occurrence of multiple mucosal neuromas, marfanoid features, and bony abnormalities; and does not involve the parathyroid glands.

Multiple Endocrine Neoplasia Type I

Almost all (90 to 99 per cent) patients with MEN-I develop hyperplasia of the parathyroid glands, causing hyperparathyroidism. Functional pancreatic endocrine tumors (60 to 100 per cent) typically develop later. Pituitary tumors occur in 54 to 80 per cent, adrenal abnormalities in 27 to 36 per cent, and lung carcinoid tumors and gastric ECLomas in a lower percentage of patients.

The initial manifestation of the disease is usually hyperparathyroidism manifesting as nephrolithiases, usually in the third or fourth decade of life. Later, pancreatic endocrine tumor syndromes and pituitary adenomas are seen, and late in the course, pulmonary carcinoids and gastric ECLomas may develop. The most common pancreatic endocrine tumor syndromes are pancreatic polypeptide–releasing tumors (PPomas) or nonfunctional tumors (80 to 100 per cent), gastrinomas (54 per cent), insulinomas (21 per cent), glucagonomas (3 per cent), and VIPomas secreting vasoactive intestinal peptide (1 per cent). Of the functional pituitary tumors, prolactinomas (70 per cent) occur more often than growth hormone–releasing adenomas causing acromegaly and corticotropin-releasing adenomas causing Cushing's disease.

The diagnosis of MEN-I should be suspected in any patient with nephrolithiases, especially in a patient with a family history of nephrolithiases or endocrinopathies. Because the most common functional pancreatic endocrine syndrome is ZES, any patient with the syndrome and an endocrinopathy, especially hyperparathyroidism, or with a family history of peptic ulcer disease or peptic ulcer disease with hypercalcemia should be suspected of having MEN-I. Pituitary tumors may manifest with symptoms caused by the tumor (e.g., headaches, visual field defects) or by the endocrine manifestations of the tumor (e.g., galactorrhea, acromegaly, Cushing's disease).

The genetic abnormality in MEN-I is on chromosome 11q12-13 near the *PYGM* locus, but the exact genetic alteration is unknown, and there is no genetic test that allows all patients to be identified. If the diagnosis is clinically suspected, the initial screening study is measurement of serum calcium and plasma parathyroid hormone concentrations. Some patients present with gastrinomas or insulinomas that are diagnosed by performing a fasting gastrin concentration and secretin test or fasting insulin, proinsulin, and glucose measurements, respectively. For the patient with a suspected pituitary tumor, assessment requires a magnetic resonance imaging (MRI) scan of the sella turcica and measurement of plasma prolactin and growth hormone concentrations and urinary free-cortisol excretion.

Multiple Endocrine Neoplasia Type II

MEN-IIA is characterized by medullary thyroid carcinoma (MTC), pheochromocytomas in 20 to 40 per cent (bilateral in 70 per cent), and primary hyperparathyroidism in 20 to 60 per cent of patients. The onset of MEN-IIA is variable, but the MTC usually develops by the first to third decade and may vary in how aggressively it metastasizes. All MEN-IIB patients develop MTC, and 60 per cent have pheochromocytomas (70 per cent bilateral), but they do not have parathyroid disease. In patients with MEN-IIB, the characteristic multiple mucosal neuromas, with puffy lips, marfanoid habitus, and bony abnormalities (e.g., pes cavus, prominent jaw) frequently are the initial abnormalities of the disease. MEN-IIB typically manifests by the first decade of life, and the MTC is often virulent, with patients presenting with regional or distant metastases.

Until recently, the mainstay for establishing the diagnosis of MTC, which is the earliest presenting endocrine abnormality in patients with MEN-IIA or MEN-IIB, was measurement of fasting calcitonin and pentagastrin-stimulated calcitonin concentrations (i.e., provocative calcitonin test) in serum. MTC is a disorder of the calcitonin-secreting cells (C cells) within the thyroid in which hyperplasia, followed by neoplasia, occurs. All patients with MTC develop increased fasting serum calcitonin concentrations or have abnormal provocative calcitonin test results. The pentagastrin provocative test is performed by administering 0.5 μg/kg of pentagastrin in a rapid intravenous infusion after taking a control serum sample for a serum calcitonin concentration. Blood samples are obtained at 1, 5, 10, and 15 minutes after injection. The test is considered positive when there is an absolute increase in the serum calcitonin concentration above the upper limit of the reference range. MEN-IIA is caused by mutations on chromosome 10 in exons 10 or 11 of the *RET* proto-oncogene, and MEN-IIB results from a mutation in exon 16 of the *RET* proto-oncogene. A genetic test for these mutations is based on their direct detection. Pheochromocytomas can be diagnosed by measuring urinary excretion of catecholamines, vanillylmandelic acid, and metanephrines.

GASTROENTEROPANCREATIC ENDOCRINE TUMOR SYNDROME

Functional GEP endocrine tumor syndromes usually produce initial symptoms due to the hormone excess state and, late in the course of the disease, symptoms due to the tumor itself. The functional GEP tumor syndromes include ZES, insulinoma, glucagonoma, somatostatinoma, VIPoma, and GRFoma (which secretes growth factor–releasing hormone). PPomas are functional in that pancreatic polypeptide is released, but this hormone causes no symptoms. PPomas resemble nonfunctional pancreatic endocrine tumors in that they cause symptoms only due to the tumor itself.

Zollinger-Ellison Syndrome

Zollinger-Ellison syndrome is characterized by severe peptic ulcer disease due to gastric acid hypersecretion that is secondary to autonomous release of gastrin by a duodenopancreatic tumor (i.e., gastrinoma). The annual incidence of ZES is 1 to 3 new cases per million persons. Except for the few patients presenting late in the course of the disease, all the presenting symptoms are caused by severe gastric acid hypersecretion. More than 95 per cent of the patients have the gastrinoma located in the duodenum or pancreas. Twenty per cent of patients with ZES have MEN-I, and ZES is the most common symptomatic GEP endocrine tumor in patients with MEN-I.

Table 1. Clinical or Laboratory Findings That Suggest Zollinger-Ellison Syndrome

- In a patient with peptic ulcer disease
  - Diarrhea
  - History of recurrent ulcers after treatment or surgery
  - Duodenal ulcers that do not heal with treatment of *H. pylori* or standard doses of antisecretory medication
  - Family history of peptic ulcer disease
  - Personal or family history of other endocrinopathies, particularly hyperparathyroidism
  - Multiple peptic ulcers or peptic ulcers in unusual locations
  - Lack of *H. pylori*
  - Peptic ulcer disease severe enough to require surgery
  - Associated with complicated disease (e.g., perforation, bleeding, obstruction, penetration)
  - Severe, resistant esophageal reflux disease
  - Laboratory findings of hypercalcemia
- Gastric rugal hypertrophy on upper gastrointestinal radiographs or endoscopy
- Hypergastrinemia
- Peptic ulcer disease in a patient with multiple endocrine neoplasia type I

Presenting Symptoms and Signs

ZES is slightly more common in males (60 per cent), and the mean age at presentation is 45 years; however, the range is wide, from infancy to 75 years of age. The principal symptom is abdominal pain (90 to 95 per cent) due to peptic ulcer disease. The abdominal pain cannot be clinically distinguished from that of a patient with idiopathic peptic ulcer disease. Important clinical clues in patients with ZES that often differ from those in most patients with idiopathic peptic ulcer disease and should suggest ZES are summarized in Table 1. With idiopathic peptic ulcer disease, diarrhea is uncommon now that antacids are rarely used in large amounts. In some studies, as many as 73 per cent of patients with ZES have diarrhea alone or with pain, and 18 per cent have only diarrhea as the initial symptom. The diarrhea can be secretory and severe but is most frequently three to four loose bowel movements per day, especially in the morning, associated with abdominal pain or heartburn. Severe esophageal reflux disease should also suggest the diagnosis of ZES, with 61 per cent of patients initially having endoscopic evidence of reflux disease. In general, the peptic ulcer disease is more severe and persists in patients with ZES; therefore, any patient with complications of peptic ulcer disease, refractory disease, recurrent disease, multiple peptic ulcers, or ulcers in unusual locations should be suspected of having ZES.

In some studies, 90 to 95 per cent of patients with duodenal ulcers due to idiopathic peptic ulcer disease had evidence of *Helicobacter pylori*. In contrast, fewer than 50 per cent of patients with ZES have *H. pylori* infection. Consequently, a patient with duodenal ulcer disease who does not have evidence of *H. pylori* or who fails to heal with effective *H. pylori* treatment should be suspected of having ZES.

Hypochlorhydria or achlorhydria is the most common cause of hypergastrinemia; however, these patients rarely have peptic ulcers unless they are caused by salicylates or nonsteroidal anti-inflammatory agents (Table 2). In any patient with peptic ulcer disease and hypergastrinemia, ZES should be suspected. Chronic hypergastrinemia encourages growth of the gastric mucosa, and any patient with peptic ulcer disease with prominent gastric folds should be suspected of having ZES (see Table 1).

Table 2. Conditions That Cause Hypergastrinemia

Associated with hypochlorhydria or achlorhydria
Atrophic gastritis
Pernicious anemia
Postvagotomy
Gastric acid antisecretory drugs (particularly H^+,K^+-ATPase inhibitors, such as omeprazole and lansoprazole)
H. pylori infection
Chronic renal failure
Associated with gastric acid hypersecretion
H. pylori infection
Zollinger-Ellison syndrome
Chronic renal failure (rarely)
Gastric outlet obstruction
Massive small bowel resection
Retained gastric antrum syndrome
Antral G-cell hyperfunction or hyperplasia

Diagnosis

The diagnosis of ZES requires the demonstration of inappropriate hypergastrinemia (i.e., increased fasting gastrin concentration) in the presence of normal or increased gastric acid secretion. The initial study is assessment of the fasting serum gastrin concentration. If this is normal on two occasions, the diagnosis of ZES is very unlikely, because more than 99 per cent of patients with ZES have increased concentrations under such conditions. If the fasting serum gastrin concentration is increased, the increase may be secondary to hypochlorhydria or achlorhydria, which can be confirmed by measuring gastric fluid pH and basal acid output. If the serum gastrin is greater than 1000 pg/mL (normal <100 pg/mL) and the gastric pH is less than 2.5 (30 per cent of patients with ZES), the patient almost certainly has ZES, and no additional diagnostic studies are needed. Only the retained gastric antrum syndrome gives similar values (see Table 2) and can be excluded by a history negative for a Billroth II resection.

Several conditions are associated with moderate fasting hypergastrinemia (100 to 999 pg/mL) and normal to increased gastric acid secretion; these must be distinguished from ZES (see Table 2). Seventy per cent of patients with ZES have this degree of hypergastrinemia. For these patients, a direct measurement of gastric acid basal secretory rate and a secretin provocative test should be performed. Basal acid output characteristically exceeds 15 mmol per hour in patients with ZES who have not had previous gastric acid–reducing surgery. Those who have undergone such a procedure typically have a basal gastric acid output that is less than 5 mmol per hour. The secretin test is performed by measuring the baseline serum gastrin concentration twice, then administering secretin-KABI (2 clinical units/kg) by intravenous bolus, and taking blood samples at 2, 5, 10, 15, and 20 minutes for serum gastrin measurements. An absolute increase of more than 200 pg/mL over the mean of the two basal values constitutes a positive result and is observed in 87 per cent of patients with ZES and fasting gastrin concentrations less than 1000 pg/mL. No false-positive results have been reported, except in patients with achlorhydria, who can be excluded by measuring gastric fluid pH.

Each patient with ZES has a gastrinoma, which is malignant in 60 to 90 per cent of cases. Localization of the gastrinoma and determination of its extent are essential to subsequent disease management. Abdominal computed tomography (CT) scanning and isotope scanning after injection of ^{111}In-DTPA-DPhe^{1}octreotide (i.e., somatostatin receptor scintigraphy) are the preferred localization methods. All patients should be evaluated for the presence of MEN-I, as described previously, because MEN-I affects 20 per cent of patients with ZES.

Insulinomas

Insulinomas are insulin-secreting tumors that are almost always located in the pancreas and cause symptoms due to hypoglycemia. Insulinomas have an annual incidence of 1 to 2 new cases per million persons, and they differ from other GEP endocrine tumors in that only 5 to 16 per cent are malignant.

Clinical Features and Course

The peak incidence occurs between 40 and 45 years of age, and 60 per cent are found in females. Symptoms are caused by hypoglycemia and are typically associated with fasting or delay of a meal. Most symptoms (Table 3) result from neuroglycopenia, the insufficient availability of glucose to the central nervous system. Neuroglycopenic symptoms include visual disturbances, confusion, altered consciousness, abnormal behavior, coma, and seizures. Symptoms can also be caused by catecholamine release (i.e., adrenergic symptoms) secondary to the hypoglycemia and include anxiety, palpitations, weakness, and fatigue (see Table 3). Patients frequently learn to avoid symptoms by eating frequently.

Diagnosis of Insulinomas

Hypoglycemia can be classified as postprandial (reactive) or fasting hypoglycemia. Insulinoma is only one of the causes of fasting hypoglycemia, which include hepatic enzyme deficiencies and decreased hepatic glucose output (e.g., glycogen storage diseases or diffuse liver disease). Other causes include exogenous hypoglycemic agents (e.g., surreptitious insulin use, hypoglycemic agents) and functional hypoglycemia due to autoantibodies. Reactive hypoglycemia is distinguished from fasting hypoglycemia by a 72-hour fast, with insulin and glucose concentrations sampled every 2 hours or at any time the patient becomes symptomatic. Seventy-five per cent of fasting patients with insulinomas develop symptoms and serum glucose concentrations less than 40 mg/dL within 24 hours; 92 to 98 per cent develop symptomatic hypoglycemia within 48 hours;

Table 3. Common Symptoms in Patients With Insulinomas

Symptoms	Frequency (%)
Neuroglycopenic	
Visual disturbances (diplopia, blurred vision)	59
Confusion	51
Altered consciousness	38
Weakness	32
Transient motor defects, hemiplegia	29
Dizziness	28
Inappropriate behavior	27
Speech difficulty	24
Seizure	23
Syncope	21
Adrenergic	
Sweating	43
Tremulousness	23
Hunger	12
Palpitations	10

Modified from Jensen, R. T., et al.: *In* Sleisinger, M. H., and Fordtran, J. S. (eds.): *Gastrointestinal Diseases,* 5th ed. Philadelphia, W.B. Saunders, 1993, p. 1698, with permission.

and nearly 100 per cent become symptomatic and hypoglycemic within 72 hours. The test is considered positive in nonobese patients if the plasma insulin (in μU/mL) to glucose (in mg/dL) ratio is greater than 0.3. Some obese patients may have insulin resistance, and the ratio will be increased; however, the fasting glucose remains normal and does not decrease with fasting, as it does with insulinomas.

Because a variety of conditions other than insulinoma can cause fasting hypoglycemia, several other tests are used, including plasma proinsulin, C-peptide, and sulfonylurea concentrations and antibodies to insulin. Plasma proinsulin concentration is increased in 80 to 90 per cent of patients with insulinoma to greater than 22 per cent of the plasma insulin concentration. In patients who surreptitiously use insulin or hypoglycemic agents, the proinsulin concentration is normal. C peptide is secreted in quantities equimolar to insulin, into the plasma. In patients with insulinoma or surreptitious use of sulfonylurea, the C-peptide concentration is increased or normal, but it is low with surreptitious use of insulin.

After the diagnosis of insulinoma has been established, tumor localization studies are needed. More than 90 per cent of insulinomas are smaller than 2 cm in diameter and can be difficult to detect. CT scanning, MRI, and ultrasound detect fewer than 30 per cent of insulinomas. Selective abdominal angiography visualizes 50 to 80 per cent and is best coupled to selective intra-arterial injection of calcium with hepatic venous insulin sampling for functional localization. Endoscopic ultrasound also has a high sensitivity, but somatostatin receptor scintigraphy has a lower sensitivity for insulinomas than for other GEP endocrine tumors because insulinomas frequently lack or have a low density of somatostatin receptors.

Glucagonomas

Glucagonomas, tumors that secrete excessive amounts of glucagon, are located in the pancreas and cause a distinct syndrome characterized by a specific dermatitis, weight loss, glucose intolerance, and anemia. In contrast to insulinomas, most glucagonomas are large at the time of diagnosis, with an average diameter of 5 to 10 cm. Glucagonomas are about 20 times less common than insulinomas or gastrinomas. The pathophysiology of the syndrome is related to the known actions of glucagon. Glucagon causes an increase in blood glucose (i.e., through gluconeogenesis, glycogenolysis, and lipolysis), alters gut physiology, and has catabolic effects.

Clinical Features and Course

Glucagonomas usually occur in middle-aged persons or in the elderly and are slightly (55 per cent) more common in females. The most common clinical and laboratory features are listed in Table 4. Necrolytic migratory erythema (64 to 90 per cent) is the most common finding. This dermatitis typically starts as an erythematous area around periorificial or intertriginous areas, such as the groin and buttocks, and spreads laterally. The lesions become raised with superficial, central blistering, followed by healing in the center with the development of hyperpigmentation. This dermatitis is commonly misdiagnosed as pemphigus, pemphigoid, vasculitis, acrodermatitis enteropathica, psoriasis, or contact dermatitis. Glucose intolerance occurs in 83 to 90 per cent, with 42 per cent requiring oral hypoglycemics and 24 per cent requiring insulin. Weight loss is a prominent feature, occurring in 56 to 96 per cent of patients. Thromboembolic phenomena such as venous thrombosis and pulmonary emboli occur in 12 to 35 per cent, and anemia occurs in 44 to 85 per cent of cases. Diarrhea is reported by 14 to 15 per cent of patients, and hypoaminoacidemia occurs in 26 to 100 per cent.

Table 4. Frequency of Clinical Symptoms and Laboratory Abnormalities in Glucagonoma

Findings	Frequency (%)
Clinical Symptom	
Dermatitis	64–90
Glucose intolerance	83–90
Weight loss	56–96
Diarrhea	14–15
Thromboembolic disease	12–35
Laboratory Abnormality	
Anemia	44–85
Hypoaminoacidemia	26–100

From Jensen, R. T., et al.: *In* Sleisenger, M. H., and Fordtran, J. S. (eds.): *Gastrointestinal Diseases,* 5th ed. Philadelphia, W.B. Saunders, 1993, p. 1702, with permission.

Diagnosis

The distinctive character of the rash often provides the first clue to the diagnosis, which is then established by measuring fasting plasma glucagon concentrations. A value greater than 1000 pg/mL is virtually diagnostic. Hyperglucagonemia occurs in chronic renal insufficiency, diabetic ketoacidosis, prolonged starvation, acute pancreatitis, acromegaly, hyperadrenocorticism, severe burns, hepatic insufficiency, and familial hyperglucagonemia, most of which are easily excluded by laboratory studies or clinical data. Plasma glucagon is usually less than 500 pg/mL in these conditions. Patients with familial hyperglucagonemia may be difficult to exclude. Fractionation of plasma glucagon immunoreactivity can be helpful in diagnosing these patients because they have an increased percentage of high-molecular-weight plasma glucagon.

The size and location of the glucagonoma can be best determined by CT scanning and somatostatin receptor scintigraphy. These tumors are often large at the time of presentation, and 95 per cent have metastases. The location and extent of metastases are important, because these patients may benefit from surgical debulking of the tumors.

VIPomas

VIPomas, neuroendocrine tumors usually located in the pancreas in adults, release vasoactive intestinal peptide (VIP), which causes a syndrome characterized by severe secretory diarrhea, hypochlorhydria, and hypokalemia. The syndrome is also called the Verner-Morrison syndrome or pancreatic cholera and is also known by the acronym WDHA, for watery diarrhea, hypokalemia, and achlorhydria. VIPomas are one tenth as common as insulinomas or gastrinomas. In children younger than 10 years of age, the VIPoma syndrome is frequently caused by a ganglioneuroma or ganglioneuroblastoma. In adults, 80 to 90 per cent of VIPomas are pancreatic, 5 to 10 per cent are ganglioneuromas, and rare cases are VIP-producing small intestinal carcinoids or pheochromocytomas.

Clinical Features and Course

The mean age in adults at the time of diagnosis is 50 years, with a slight female predominance (60 per cent).

The mean age in children is 2 to 4 years. The cardinal clinical feature of VIPomas is severe secretory diarrhea (100 per cent), associated with hypokalemia (100 per cent), and dehydration (90 to 100 per cent). The diarrhea is typically large in volume and persists during fasting. Stool volume less than 700 mL per day has been proposed as a criterion for excluding the diagnosis of VIPoma. Cramping, abdominal pain, or colic (63 per cent) is common with the diarrhea. Weight loss is almost always present (90 to 100 per cent). Flushing occurs in 21 per cent of patients, usually over the head and trunk area. Hypercalcemia and hyperglycemia are occasionally observed (41 and 8 per cent, respectively).

Diagnosis

The volume and nature of the diarrhea should suggest the diagnosis. All patients with VIPoma have stool volumes greater than 700 mL per day, and 80 to 85 per cent have more than 3 L per day. The diarrheal fluid is typical of secretory diarrhea, and the stool osmolality can be estimated by twice the sum of the sodium and potassium concentrations. Malabsorption usually does not occur in patients with VIPomas, and a daily fecal fat content of greater than 15 g per day should suggest some other diagnosis. Severe secretory diarrhea can also be caused by gastrinomas, by chronic laxative abuse, and, in some cases, by a pseudo-VIPoma syndrome of unknown origin. To distinguish VIPoma from these other conditions, a reliable measurement of plasma VIP concentration is required. In most laboratories, a value of 0 to 170 pg/mL is normal, and almost every VIPoma patient has an increased plasma VIP concentration. Localization and determination of the extent of the VIPoma can be assessed best with CT scanning and somatostatin receptor scintigraphy. Because 63 to 90 per cent of VIPomas are associated with metastases, careful evaluation of the extent of the disease is important.

Somatostatinomas

Somatostatinomas are GEP tumors that usually originate in the small intestine or pancreas. They typically release large amounts of somatostatin and cause a distinct clinical syndrome characterized by diabetes mellitus, gallbladder disease, diarrhea, and weight loss. Somatostatinomas are the least common GEP endocrine tumor syndrome; fewer than 50 cases have been reported.

Clinical Features

The mean age at presentation is 51 years, with a female predominance (66 per cent). Between 65 and 75 per cent of somatostatinomas occur in the pancreas, and the remainder originate in the small intestine (95 per cent in the duodenum and 5 per cent in the jejunum). The clinical features depend on location (Table 5). Diabetes mellitus occurs in 55 per cent of patients; however, it is much more common in patients with pancreatic somatostatinomas than those with small intestinal somatostatinomas (95 versus 21 per cent). The diabetes is usually mild, ketoacidosis is uncommon, and blood glucose can be controlled in most patients with oral hypoglycemic agents or low doses of insulin. Gallbladder disease occurs in 65 per cent of patients with somatostatinomas and is more common in patients with pancreatic than those with small intestinal somatostatinomas. Gallbladder disease includes cholelithiasis and gallbladder dilatation. Diarrhea and steatorrhea occur in 70 per cent of patients with somatostatinomas, most often in those with pancreatic tumors. Other features of the somatostatinoma syndrome include hypochlorhydria (70 per cent of patients), weight loss (33 per cent), and anemia (67 per cent).

Table 5. Clinical and Laboratory Findings in Patients With the Somatostatinoma Syndrome

Finding	Pancreatic Tumor (%)	Small Intestinal Tumor (%)
Clinical Symptom		
Diabetes mellitus	95	21
Gallbladder disease	94	43
Diarrhea	97	36
Weight loss	90	44
Laboratory Abnormality		
Steatorrhea	83	12
Hypochlorhydria	86	17

Modified from Jensen, R. T., et al.: Endocrine tumors of the pancreas. *In* Sleisenger, M. H., and Fordtran, J. S. (eds.): *Gastrointestinal Diseases,* 5th ed. Philadelphia, W.B. Saunders, 1993, p. 1709, with permission.

Diagnosis

Somatostatinomas are usually found by accident. The tumors are often large (mean, 5 cm in diameter), and the typical presentation is a patient with metastases of a GEP tumor to the liver or with a large pancreatic tumor that is diagnosed at surgery. Somatostatinomas can also be found at the time of cholecystectomy. Somatostatinomas, especially those in the duodenum, are associated with neurofibromatosis.

The diagnosis is usually established by immunocytochemical analysis of the resected tumor demonstrating the endocrine nature of the tumor with increased numbers of D-like cells, positive somatostatin immunoreactivity, or an increased plasma somatostatin concentration. Like PP, glucagon, insulin, and gastrin, somatostatin is commonly found in many GEP tumors. However, it is not associated with any clinical syndrome or even increased plasma hormone concentration in many cases. The diagnosis of somatostatinoma should not be made unless an increased plasma somatostatin concentration is found and the clinical syndrome is present.

More than 80 per cent of somatostatinomas have evidence of metastatic spread at the time of presentation. Metastases are usually found in the liver (75 per cent) and lymph nodes (31 per cent). Tumor localization with the use of CT scanning, MRI, and angiography is essential for establishing the location and extent of the somatostatinoma.

GRFomas

GRFomas are tumors that secrete large amounts of growth hormone–releasing factor (GRF), which causes acromegaly. This GEP endocrine tumor syndrome was first described in 1982. The true incidence of these tumors is unknown. Pancreatic GRFomas occur frequently in patients with MEN-I (33 per cent of all GRFomas in some studies); 40 per cent of patients have Cushing's syndrome, and as many as 40 per cent have ZES. Only 33 per cent of all GRFomas are in the pancreas, 53 per cent are in the lung, 10 per cent are in the small intestine, and 7 per cent are found at other sites.

Clinical Features

The mean age at diagnosis is 38 years, with a female predominance (75 per cent). The clinical features are typical of acromegaly. The acromegalic features are indistinguishable from those of classic acromegaly and include enlargement of the hands and feet, facial changes, headache, skin changes, and peripheral nerve entrapment.

Diagnosis

The diagnosis should be suspected in any patient with clinical features of acromegaly *and* a pancreatic, pulmonary, or small intestinal tumor. GRFomas are frequently associated with Cushing's syndrome, ZES, and MEN-I; these tumors should be suspected particularly when acromegaly is also present. GRFomas are uncommon causes of acromegaly. One report of 177 patients with acromegaly found only three with GRFomas.

The diagnosis of acromegaly is established by demonstrating an increased fasting growth hormone concentration (>5 ng/mL in males, 10 ng/mL in females). The diagnosis of GRFoma is confirmed by measuring GRF concentration in plasma. A number of dynamic tests of growth hormone stimulation have been described, such as oral glucose loading to suppress physiologic growth hormone secretion, intravenous administration of thyroid-releasing hormone to increase growth hormone secretion, and the use of dopamine agonists or gonadotropin-releasing hormone. However, all dynamic tests have been found to produce the same responses as those seen in patients with classic acromegaly.

Metastatic disease to the liver occurs in 30 per cent of patients with pancreatic GRFomas and in two thirds of those with intestinal GRFomas. Because GRFomas have been reported with lung carcinomas, sympathetic neuronal tumors, and pheochromocytomas, detailed imaging studies establishing tumor location and extent are essential. Somatostatin receptor scintigraphy, CT scanning, and MRI are the preferred modalities. MRI or CT scans of the sella turcica should be used to address the possibility of a pituitary tumor and to estimate the size of the pituitary.

PPomas and Nonfunctional Pancreatic Endocrine Tumors

A PPoma is a tumor, usually of the pancreas, that releases excessive amounts of pancreatic polypeptide, and the clinical symptoms are due to local effects of the tumor itself, not to the actions of PP. A nonfunctioning pancreatic endocrine tumor is a tumor of the pancreas that has the typical histologic features of a GEP endocrine tumor and is not associated with increased plasma concentrations of any known peptide. All symptoms are caused by the local effects of the tumor itself. Infusions of PP into humans and animals have numerous biologic effects, including alteration of the secretion of water and electrolytes in the small intestine; inhibition of pancreatic fluid and enzyme secretion; effects on esophageal, gastric, intestinal, and gallbladder motility; and metabolic effects such as decreased somatostatin or insulin release. It is unclear why patients with high circulating plasma PP concentrations have no symptoms specifically due to the PP. In various studies, nonfunctional or PPomas account for 15 to 30 per cent of all pancreatic endocrine tumors removed at surgery.

Clinical Features

Because these endocrine tumors do not secrete a hormone that causes symptoms, all of the clinical symptoms represent the effects of the tumor or the effects of metastases of the tumor. The tumors usually manifest late and are large, with a mean diameter of 5 cm. The mean age at diagnosis is 51 years, and the incidence is equal in both sexes. Almost one half of the patients present with abdominal pain, 30 per cent have jaundice, 20 per cent are incidentally diagnosed at surgery when an abdominal mass is found, and the remaining patients have a variety of symptoms related to the tumor mass.

Diagnosis

The main diagnostic challenge is to distinguish these GEP endocrine tumors from a pancreatic nonendocrine tumor and to determine whether the patient has another type of GEP endocrine tumor with an incidental accompanying increase in plasma PP concentration. Plasma PP concentration is increased in 22 to 70 per cent of patients with other pancreatic endocrine tumor syndromes and exceeds 1000 pg/mL in 32 per cent of gastrinomas, 21 per cent of insulinomas, 60 per cent of glucagonomas, 25 per cent of VIPomas, 33 per cent of somatostatinomas, and 45 per cent of carcinoid tumors. These other functional pancreatic endocrine tumors must be excluded. A PPoma is also difficult to distinguish from a nonendocrine tumor. However, in one study of 53 patients with adenocarcinoma of the pancreas, none had an increased plasma PP concentration. Conversely, increased plasma PP concentrations have been reported in several other conditions, including old age, bowel resection, alcohol abuse, infection, chronic noninfective inflammatory disorders, acute diarrhea, chronic renal failure, diabetes mellitus, and chronic pancreatitis. Because an increased plasma PP concentration is not diagnostic of a PPoma, an atropine suppression test has been proposed to improve the specificity. Atropine (1 mg intramuscularly) does not alter the plasma concentration of PP in patients with pancreatic PPomas, but the drug decreases the hormone concentration by 50 per cent or more in patients who do not have tumors. The metastasis rate for PPomas is 60 to 90 per cent, and CT scanning, MRI, or somatostatin receptor scintigraphy should be used to establish the location and extent of the tumor.

GASTRIC CARCINOIDS

Gastric carcinoids constitute 3 of every 1000 gastric neoplasms. In older studies, these tumors were reported to be frequently multifocal and metastatic (40 to 60 per cent of cases). Later, gastric carcinoids were shown to develop as a result of chronic hypergastrinemia. These tumors originate from gastric ECL-like cells and are called ECLomas. ECLomas characteristically react with argyrophil stains and chromogranin A antibodies, and results are negative when they are stained for gastrin or somatostatin. Gastric carcinoids have been reported in chronic hypergastrinemic states, including pernicious anemia (5 per cent of patients), atrophic gastritis, and ZES. ECLomas are at least 30 times more common in ZES patients with MEN-I than in those without MEN-I.

Gastric carcinoids occurring in patients with hypergastrinemia are reported to have a more benign course than those occurring in patients who do not have hypergastrinemia. Only 9 per cent of patients with ECLomas develop metastases, mostly to lymph nodes, with only 2 per cent developing liver metastases. In patients without hypergastrinemia, 55 per cent have metastases, and 24 per cent have distant metastases to liver or bone.

Foregut carcinoids, which include carcinoids of the stomach, occasionally produce the carcinoid syndrome. They occasionally secrete 5-hydroxytryptophan, corticotropin, and a variety of hormones, including tachykinins (e.g., substance P, neuropeptide K, substance K) and neurotensin. Skin flushing differs from that in the usual carcinoid syndrome, which is caused by a midgut carcinoid. The flushing is reddish and patchy in distribution on the face and neck and has central clearing. It may also be pruritic.

Diagnosis

Gastric carcinoids generally produce no symptoms due to the release of hormonally active agents. They are usually found at upper gastrointestinal endoscopy or suspected after an upper gastrointestinal x-ray study. The diagnosis is established by biopsy or after removal of a polypoid lesion and chromogranin A stains are performed. The presence or absence of hypergastrinemia should be documented, because the prognosis is different for patients with and without hypergastrinemia. Rarely, a gastric carcinoid produces the carcinoid syndrome typically seen with a foregut carcinoid.

ULCERATIVE COLITIS AND CROHN'S DISEASE

By James H. Reichheld, M.D.,
and Mark A. Peppercorn, M.D.
Boston, Massachusetts

The inflammatory bowel diseases (IBDs) constitute a group of chronic inflammatory conditions of unknown cause that manifest themselves primarily in the gastrointestinal tract. They are divided into two types, ulcerative colitis (UC) and Crohn's disease, on the basis of clinical and histologic distinctions. Despite characteristic findings, the inflammatory bowel diseases remain diagnostic challenges because they have variable presentations and often unanticipated clinical courses marked by potentially devastating complications.

In ulcerative colitis, the rectum is virtually always involved, and the colon may also be involved to a variable extent. Disease limited to the rectum is referred to as proctitis, while disease involving the rectosigmoid is termed proctosigmoiditis. The entire large bowel may be affected, and, although the small bowel is not involved in ulcerative colitis, right-sided colitis may be associated with mild ileal inflammation, referred to as backwash ileitis. Involvement of the entire large bowel is termed pancolitis.

Crohn's disease may involve large or small bowel. Large bowel disease is simply termed Crohn's disease of the colon or Crohn's colitis, while disease of the small bowel is commonly referred to as regional enteritis. Ileocolitis refers to Crohn's disease involving both the ileum and large bowel. Granulomatous colitis is a synonym for Crohn's disease of the colon, alluding to the granulomas characteristic of tissue biopsy in Crohn's disease. The granulomas are found only sporadically, however.

PRESENTATION AND COURSE

Ulcerative Colitis

Ulcerative colitis involves the rectum in more than 95 per cent of cases. Disease may be limited to the rectum, or it may extend proximally and continuously and involve part or all of the colon. Bloody diarrhea and abdominal pain are the most common presenting symptoms in ulcerative colitis. More severe disease may be marked by fever (usually low grade), weight loss, volume depletion, and fatigue. Involvement of the rectum is associated with tenesmus. If disease is limited to the rectum, the patient may present with constipation instead of diarrhea. Less commonly, fever and weight loss may dominate the clinical picture instead of intestinal symptoms, and, rarely, an extraintestinal symptom, such as arthralgias, may be the primary presenting symptom.

The physical examination may not show distinct findings. The abdomen may be distended and mildly tender, but an absence of physical findings is common. More severe disease can be marked by fever and signs of volume depletion. The extraintestinal signs of the disease may include skin lesions, jaundice, arthritis, and others discussed below. Laboratory studies may show anemia secondary to iron deficiency or chronic disease. Diarrhea can result in hypokalemia, and mucosal protein loss may cause hypoalbuminemia. In more severe disease, there may be leukocytosis with left shift and an increased erythrocyte sedimentation rate. Associated hepatobiliary disease can result in increased alkaline phosphatase and transaminase activity.

The course of ulcerative colitis can vary. Most patients have moderate disease with acute flares (relapses) and can be managed medically as outpatients. Recurrence is typical of this chronic disease, and the initial attack is commonly followed by relapse within 1 year. Effective medical management includes treatment with sulfasalazine, 5-aminosalicylic acid (5-ASA) compounds, corticosteroids, and immunosuppressive agents. A subset of patients with ulcerative colitis, however, may have a more severe course, developing fulminant disease with the potential for dilatation of the inflamed bowel (toxic megacolon) and intestinal perforation. Emergent surgical intervention is indicated in this setting and, barring other complications, is curative. Patients with ulcerative colitis are at higher risk than the general population for both severe dysplasia and colonic malignancy.

Crohn's Disease

Unlike ulcerative colitis, the inflammation of Crohn's disease most commonly spares the rectum and does not extend continuously. Instead, Crohn's disease is marked by skip lesions, areas of inflamed tissue that may appear anywhere along the intestinal tract but are separated by normal, uninvolved bowel. Unlike ulcerative colitis, even early inflammation is commonly transmural and predisposes the patient to perforation, abscesses, fistulas, and strictures. Patients typically present with diarrhea that is *not* bloody. Fever may be present. Large bowel disease can cause tenderness over the colon, while small bowel disease typically involves the ileum and may present with intermittent cramps or constant right lower quadrant pain. Associated anorexia, nausea, and vomiting may occur. More rarely, extraintestinal symptoms may predominate. Elderly patients and children may present with subtle symptoms, including fever of unknown origin and weight loss without a clear cause. Uncommon presentations include malabsorption, initial presentation with small bowel obstruction, and urinary infection or pneumaturia with enterovesical fistula.

On physical examination, patients may be febrile and typically have abdominal tenderness localized to the region of inflammation, such as the right lower quadrant with ileitis. A palpable mass suggests inflamed, matted loops of small bowel (phlegmon) or abscess. While the rectum is frequently spared, perianal involvement may be complicated by tags, fissures, fistulas, or abscesses, which may be evident on examination well before the development of colitis. Laboratory examination often reflects inflammation, with leukocytosis, an increased erythrocyte sedimentation rate, and anemia.

The course of Crohn's disease, like that of ulcerative colitis, is marked by recurrent attacks of acute inflammation that are usually manageable with medical treatment. Complications such as obstruction, perforation, and fistulas may require surgical intervention, but, unlike the case with ulcerative colitis, resection of affected bowel is not typically curative. The rate of recurrence after resection approaches 80 per cent by 7 to 10 years.

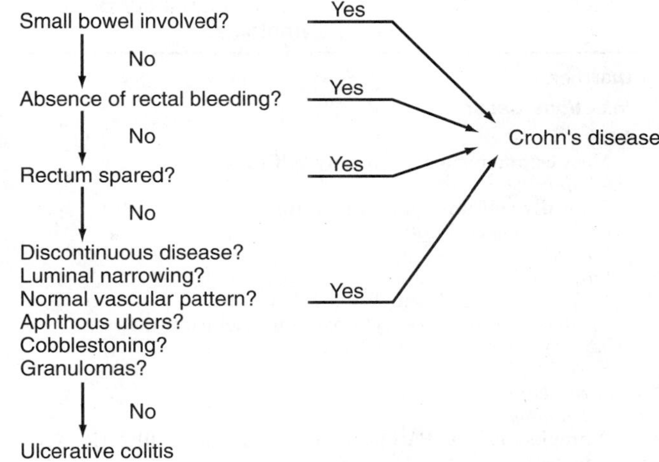

Figure 1. Distinguishing ulcerative colitis from Crohn's disease.

DIAGNOSIS

The clinical presentation and course of Crohn's disease and ulcerative colitis may vary significantly, and there are no pathognomonic findings that ensure accurate diagnosis of either disease. However, the history and physical examination, along with laboratory, radiographic, and endoscopic findings, can provide a strong clinical impression and, collectively, a diagnosis (Tables 1 and 2; Fig. 1).

History

Demographics can suggest the risk for developing inflammatory bowel disease. Whites are at significantly higher risk than blacks or Asians. Jews of northern European (Ashkenazic) origin are three to six times more likely to develop inflammatory bowel disease than are non-Jews or Jews of Middle Eastern or Mediterranean (Sephardic) origin. The peak incidence is between 15 and 40 years of age, but onset can occur at virtually any age. While estimates vary, the incidence and prevalence of ulcerative colitis and Crohn's disease have become similar, as the incidence of Crohn's disease has risen over several decades. The incidence of ulcerative colitis is 5 to 8 per 100,000, and the prevalence 50 to 150 per 100,000. Crohn's disease has an incidence of 2 to 5 per 100,000 and a prevalence of 20 to 50 per 100,000.

Table 1. Findings in Ulcerative Colitis and Crohn's Disease

	Ulcerative Colitis	Crohn's Disease
Demographics and history	Cigarette smoking may be protective Watery, bloody diarrhea Tenesmus	Cigarette smoking exacerbates disease Watery diarrhea, typically without blood Tenesmus only if rectum involved, cramps with small bowel disease Malabsorption, steatorrhea
Physical examination	Fever, volume loss Variable tenderness Peritoneal signs suggest perforation Extraintestinal disease may be evident	Fever, volume loss Oral ulcerations, perianal disease Tenderness common Abdominal mass: abscess, phlegmon Peritoneal signs suggest perforation Extraintestinal disease may be evident
Laboratory findings	Leukocytosis, with left shift Elevated erythrocyte sedimentation rate Iron-deficiency anemia Hypokalemia, hypomagnesemia	Same findings as those in ulcerative colitis plus: hypocalcemia (vitamin D loss), hypoalbuminemia, vitamin B_{12} deficiency
Radiographic and endoscopic evaluation	Continuous disease, involving the rectum, no small bowel disease	Discontinuous disease, skip lesions, rectum often spared, small bowel usually involved, large bowel also commonly involved
	Fine ulcerations, loss of haustral markings, shortened and thickened bowel, stricture	Aphthous ulcerations, cobblestoning, often multiple strictures
	No granuloma formation	Granulomas on microscopy
	No fistulas	Fistulas occur as complication
	Abnormal vascular pattern; friable mucosa	Vascular pattern adjacent to ulcerations may be normal; mucosa not friable
	Toxic dilatation	Toxic dilatation more rare
	Carcinoma frequent	Carcinoma of the colon may be as frequent

Table 2. Differential Diagnosis of Inflammatory Bowel Disease by Symptoms

Diarrhea

Infectious Causes

Viral
- Most common cause, typically self-limited

Bacterial
- Typically self-limited and identifiable on stool culture
- *Campylobacter jejuni*
- *Shigella*
- *Salmonella*
- *Yersinia enterocolitica*
- *Clostridium difficile*—cytotoxin on stool examination
- Enterotoxigenic *Escherichia coli*
- *E. coli* 0157:H7
- *Aeromonas*
- *Plesiomonas*
- Whipple bacillus: PAS-positive macrophage infiltration on biopsy
- *Mycobacterium tuberculosis:* acid-fast stain biopsy

Parasitic
- Identifiable on examination of stool for ova and parasites
- *Entamoeba histolytica*
- *Giardia lamblia*

HIV-Related (in addition to the above)
- *Isospora*
- Microsporida
- *Cryptosporidium*
- *Mycobacterium avium-intracellulare*
- Cytomegalovirus
- HIV

Noninfectious Causes
- Lymphoma
- Pancreatic disease
- Collagenous colitis
- Lymphocytic colitis
- Malabsorption syndromes
- Medication effects

Hematochezia
- Hemorrhoids—diagnosis of exclusion
- Diverticular disease
- Adenomatous polyps
- Carcinoma
- Arteriovenous malformation
- Radiation proctitis
- Infectious proctitis
  - HIV-related proctitis (herpes simplex virus)
  - Proctitis acquired sexually *(Neisseria gonorrhoeae, Chlamydia trachomatis)*

Abdominal Pain
- Irritable bowel syndrome
- Ischemic bowel
- Nonabdominal cause
  - Myocardial ischemia
  - Psychiatric condition
  - Seizure producing abdominal pain
  - Porphyria

HIV = human immunodeficiency virus; PAS = periodic acid–Schiff stain.

The principal symptoms of inflammatory bowel disease include diarrhea, abdominal pain, and fever. In both ulcerative colitis and Crohn's disease, diarrhea is described as watery. In ulcerative colitis, it is typically profuse and bloody and accompanied by tenesmus. Isolated ulcerative proctitis may present deceptively as constipation. The diarrhea of Crohn's disease frequently presents without gross evidence of blood. When blood is present, its character may suggest the distribution of disease. Bright red blood can result from inflammation of the rectum, sigmoid, or descending colon, while melena, though rare, suggests disease of, or proximal to, the ascending colon. Rarely, bright red blood in Crohn's disease may be found with brisk bleeding of an inflamed area within the upper gastrointestinal tract. Tenesmus in Crohn's disease is less common than in ulcerative colitis. In severe Crohn's disease, malabsorption may result in steatorrhea. When inflammation involves the anal sphincter, patients may become incontinent of stool.

Abdominal pain is more common and typically more severe in Crohn's disease than in ulcerative colitis. Pain in ulcerative colitis is mild and dominated by tenesmus secondary to inflammation of the rectum. The inflammation of Crohn's disease can cause narrowing of the bowel lumen, resulting in marked cramps or constant pain that may be accompanied by anorexia, nausea, or vomiting. Right lower quadrant pain is typical of ileitis, while more proximal small bowel disease may present with periumbilical pain. Bilateral lower quadrant pain suggests colonic inflammation, while tenesmus is characteristic of rectal involvement. Pain near the anus in Crohn's disease may be secondary to fissures, fistulas, or abscesses. Pain, nausea, and vomiting without passage of flatus or stool suggest obstruction, while urinary symptoms—particularly, pneumaturia—are associated with enterovesical fistula.

Fever is found more frequently in Crohn's disease than in ulcerative colitis; therefore, fever in ulcerative colitis should alert the clinician to complications such as perforation and colonic dilatation. High fever in either Crohn's disease or ulcerative colitis suggests complication. Fever of unclear cause may be the only presenting symptom of Crohn's disease in the elderly and children.

The history should include a review for the signs and symptoms of extraintestinal disease. Arthritis is the most common extraintestinal symptom, affecting from 4 to more than 20 per cent of patients with inflammatory bowel disease. The arthritis may be peripheral, asymmetrical, and migratory and involve primarily the knees, hips, ankles, wrists, and elbows. This arthritis tends to wax and wane with the patient's intestinal inflammation. Approximately 5 per cent of patients are affected by ankylosing spondylitis, with progressive lower back pain worse in the morning and relieved with activity. Most of these patients are HLA-B27 positive and may present with arthritis well before the onset of intestinal symptoms. Sacroiliitis may be found on radiograph but is typically asymptomatic.

Other extraintestinal manifestations of inflammatory bowel disease, including skin lesions, oral ulcerations (particularly in Crohn's disease), and ocular disease, may prompt patients to seek medical attention. While uveitis is less common than episcleritis, uveitis may predate intestinal symptoms and is marked by acutely blurred vision and headaches. Jaundice may be the primary indication of hepatobiliary disease. A history of thromboembolic disease is uncommon but is not rare in inflammatory bowel disease. Thromboembolic disease usually presents as deep venous thrombosis or pulmonary embolus. Arteritis has also been associated with inflammatory bowel disease and may present as cerebrovascular disease or as acute monocular symptoms in the setting of temporal giant cell arteritis. Rarely, presentation with characteristic chest pain leads to the diagnosis of inflammatory bowel disease–associated pericarditis. While many other extraintestinal associations with inflammatory bowel disease exist, they are less likely to be identified from the history.

Other significant points in the medical history include cigarette smoking, which is strongly associated with exacerbation of Crohn's disease but, in contrast, may actually help quell flares of ulcerative colitis. A familial component to inflammatory bowel disease exists, with concordance of identical twins occurring more commonly than that of fraternal twins in Crohn's disease. Relatives are affected by inflammatory bowel disease in 10 to 25 per cent of patients with ulcerative colitis and Crohn's disease. The risk factors for diarrhea due to other causes may be elicited in the history, including recent antibiotic use, lactose intolerance, recent travel, and human immunodeficiency virus (HIV) risk factors. An association exists between psychological stress and inflammatory bowel disease. A direct causal relationship has not been established, but a history of recent stress can be associated with the onset and recurrence of disease.

Physical Examination

Vital signs are typically notable for fever, more common in Crohn's disease and suggestive of complications such as perforation when high grade. Perforation must be considered when fever is high in either ulcerative colitis or Crohn's disease and, in Crohn's disease, may be complicated further by fistula or abscess formation. Orthostasis and tachycardia are proportional to volume loss and are typically more marked when diarrhea is profuse.

The physical findings are few in ulcerative colitis. Tenderness over the colon may be found when the disease extends proximally from the rectum, or abdominal fullness may be observed. The abdominal examination may be unremarkable when disease is limited to the rectum. Peritoneal signs suggest advanced inflammation with perforation and can occur as a complication of toxic megacolon.

Because Crohn's disease may involve any part of the intestinal tract, the physical findings can include aphthous ulcerations of the mouth or pharynx, abdominal findings, or perianal disease. Abdominal fullness and tenderness are common. The location and degree of tenderness suggest the distribution and severity of the inflammation. Right lower quadrant tenderness suggests ileal disease, inflammation of the proximal small bowel frequently presents with periumbilical discomfort, and tenderness over the large bowel is typical of colonic disease. Inflammation may result in loops of matted bowel, known as a phlegmon, palpable as a mass typically in the right lower quadrant. Abscess formation secondary to perforation should always be considered in the differential diagnosis of a mass found on examination in the setting of inflammatory bowel disease, especially when associated with fever or leukocytosis. While Crohn's disease spares the rectum in half of the cases, the perianal examination may reveal tags, fissures, fistulas, or abscesses that predate proctitis.

The examination should always include a thorough search for extraintestinal manifestations of inflammatory bowel disease (Table 3), which may present before the onset of intestinal disease. Arthritis, the most common manifestation of extraintestinal inflammatory bowel disease, may be detected as inflammation of the knees, hips, ankles, elbows, or wrists. More rarely, distal joints of the hands or feet are involved. While this peripheral form of inflammatory bowel disease–associated arthritis most often presents concurrently with intestinal inflammation, a central spondylitis with inflammation of the hips, shoulders, or knees may instead be found when intestinal disease is quiescent and may even predate the diagnosis of inflammatory bowel disease. Clubbing is sometimes found in patients with ulcerative colitis and more commonly in Crohn's disease secondary to associated hypertrophic osteoarthropathy.

Table 3. Extraintestinal Manifestations of Inflammatory Bowel Disease

Musculoskeletal
- Arthritis
  - Peripheral—asymmetrical and migratory
  - Central
    - Ankylosing spondylitis
    - Sacroiliitis
- Osteomalacia (Crohn's disease)
- Hypertrophic osteoarthropathy

Ophthalmologic
- Uveitis
- Episcleritis
- Cataracts

Skin
- Erythema nodosum
- Pyoderma gangrenosum

Hepatobiliary
- Primary sclerosing cholangitis
- Cholangiocarcinoma
- Cholelithiasis (Crohn's disease)
- Cirrhosis
- Fatty infiltration of the liver

Vascular
- Deep venous thrombosis
  - Pulmonary embolus
- Arteritis—giant cell (temporal) arteritis, Takayasu's arteritis, cerebrovascular accident

Hematologic
- Anemia—folate and vitamin B_{12} deficiency (Crohn's disease), iron deficiency

Pulmonary
- Bronchiectasis
- Abnormal pulmonary function tests without underlying disease

Renal
- Nephrolithiasis
  - Urate stones
  - Calcium oxalate stones (Crohn's disease)
- Ureteral obstruction by inflammation, abscess, or phlegmon (Crohn's disease)
- Enterovesical fistula (Crohn's disease)
- Amyloidosis

Nutritional
- Protein-wasting enteropathy
  - Hypoalbuminemia
- Vitamin deficiencies (Crohn's disease)
- Delayed growth and sexual development

Other extraintestinal findings include those of ophthalmologic disease with uveitis, episcleritis, and cataracts, each associated with active intestinal inflammation. Erythema nodosum is found on the pretibial surface of the lower extremities or the anterior surface of the arms and appears as tender red nodules. Deep skin ulcerations of the anterior tibia or other locations may represent pyoderma gangrenosum, most often described in patients with ulcerative pancolitis and, less commonly, in patients with Crohn's disease. Both lesions are typically related to active bowel disease and occasionally predate the diagnosis of inflammatory bowel disease.

Jaundice may develop in inflammatory bowel disease–associated hepatobiliary disease. In Crohn's disease of the terminal ileum, gallstones are common and can cause biliary colic or cholecystitis with or without jaundice. Primary sclerosing cholangitis, most commonly associated with ulcerative colitis, may present as jaundice preceded by weight loss and pruritus. More often in ulcerative colitis than Crohn's disease, weight loss and right upper quadrant pain may be followed by jaundice, heralding carcinoma of the bile duct. Pancolitis can also be associated with cirrhosis, which may be asymptomatic but observed on examination as stigmata of chronic liver disease.

Vasculitis in inflammatory bowel disease typically involves the deep veins and may present on examination as a swollen, often painful extremity. Association with acute tachypnea should raise suspicion of pulmonary embolism. Deteriorating pulmonary function in a chronic setting can be caused by bronchiectasis or chronic bronchitis associated with inflammatory bowel disease. Renal complications, including calculi and ureteral obstruction, are commonly associated with inflammatory bowel disease, although they are not usually detected on physical examination. Adolescents with Crohn's disease and, less commonly, ulcerative colitis may lag behind their peers in growth and sexual development.

Laboratory Findings

Laboratory findings are helpful in assessing the presence or severity of inflammation or hemorrhage and in further refining the differential diagnosis. Leukocytosis is common, and the degree of left shift can correlate with the severity of inflammation, this correlation suggesting the possibility of associated infection or perforation. The erythrocyte sedimentation rate is often used as an index of disease activity. Anemia is common and, in inflammatory bowel disease, typically develops over time secondary to chronic disease, vitamin B_{12} deficiency, or iron deficiency from chronic blood loss. Even moderate diarrhea may result in hypokalemia or hypomagnesemia, and electrolytes may reflect a non–anion gap acidosis with more profound diarrhea.

Crohn's disease of the small bowel may have associated laboratory findings consistent with malabsorption. Decreased absorption of vitamin D can result in low calcium concentrations, and mucosal loss of protein may cause hypoalbuminemia. Ileal disease may produce decreased concentrations of vitamin B_{12}, but a discrete macrocytic anemia is rare.

Centesis of arthritic joints reveals an inflammatory effusion. Hepatobiliary disease may result in increased alkaline phosphatase activity owing to sclerosing cholangitis, with bilirubinemia appearing later. Fatty liver related to malnutrition can result in increased transaminase and alkaline phosphatase activity. Renal calculi commonly cause hematuria, and rarely proteinuria can occur with inflammatory bowel disease–associated renal amyloidosis. Pulmonary function tests can be abnormal even without symptoms of pulmonary disease. Stool for bacterial culture, ova and parasites, and *Clostridium difficile* toxin should always be obtained in patients presenting with diarrhea of unclear etiology. Serology may be helpful if amebiasis is suspected.

Radiographic Findings

Flat plate (plain film) of the abdomen may provide useful information regarding the extent and severity of inflammatory bowel disease. Signs of colonic inflammation include loss of crisp mucosal outlines, absence of fecal residue, and loss of haustral markings. Luminal narrowing in chronic ulcerative colitis may result in a short, thickened colonic segment with a characteristic lead-pipe appearance. Dilatation of the colon suggests toxic megacolon. Intestinal pneumatosis (air in the bowel wall) presages imminent perforation, and free air under the diaphragm on upright abdominal plain film is observed with perforation of bowel viscus. In patients with Crohn's disease, dilated loops of small bowel accompanied by abdominal pain, vomiting, and lack of flatus suggest small bowel obstruction. Loss of the psoas shadow in patients with Crohn's ileitis suggests abscess formation.

Double-contrast barium enema (BE), an excellent method for evaluation of the mucosa, can help distinguish between ulcerative colitis and Crohn's disease and can demonstrate the distribution of disease or the presence of complications, such as stricture, fistula, or carcinoma. Early in the course of ulcerative colitis, the evacuation air-contrast film typically shows fine continuous ulcerations extending proximally from the rectum. Progressive disease demonstrates a rough and irregular mucosa with deeper ulcerations. In chronic ulcerative colitis, a shortened, thickened bowel with loss of haustral markings may be seen. Strictures are seen as concentric segments, in contrast with the eccentric luminal narrowing seen with carcinoma. Crohn's disease on double-contrast barium enema shows isolated patches of inflammation (skip lesions), sparing the rectum in more than half of patients. Longitudinal ulcerations and strictures may accompany more advanced disease. Barium enema alone cannot always distinguish ulcerative colitis from Crohn's disease, but reflux of barium into the ileum can strengthen the diagnosis by showing mucosal changes consistent with Crohn's disease. Although barium enema can demonstrate dilatation of the colon, the procedure is contraindicated when severe disease is suspected, because it may precipitate dilatation and subsequent perforation. Barium enema is not helpful in evaluating disease limited to the rectum.

Upper gastrointestinal series (UGIS) is less sensitive than endoscopy for the evaluation of upper intestinal symptoms. Still, it can be useful for identifying mucosal abnormalities from the esophagus to the duodenojejunal flexure in some patients. Patients with ulcerative colitis or Crohn's disease of the colon or small bowel who develop upper intestinal symptoms may benefit from UGIS to detect or exclude disease of the upper intestinal tract. Early findings in Crohn's disease include ulcerations that later may coalesce; concurrent development of cobblestoning and thickening of mucosal folds are typical. The stomach and duodenum are most commonly involved, and stomach and duodenum disease is found in approximately 10 per cent of patients with ileocolic disease.

Small bowel follow-through (as an extension of the UGIS) is usually less sensitive than large-volume barium examination of the small bowel. The greater amount of barium can facilitate visualization of loops of small bowel. The mucosa of the small bowel can also be evaluated with enteroclysis in which barium is infused directly into the small bowel via an oral catheter advanced to the jejunum. Enteroclysis can also show the presence and distribution of Crohn's disease, including obstruction and fistula formation. Findings in Crohn's disease of the small bowel are analogous to those observed in the colon and include progressive mucosal thickening, ulceration, and cobblestoning.

Computed tomography is useful for evaluating complications of Crohn's disease and may differentiate phlegmon from abscess. Perianal disease may also be observed on computed tomography scan, but the technique is not as sensitive as barium studies for detection of mucosal abnormalities. Marked thickening of the bowel wall in either Crohn's disease or ulcerative disease can result in a characteristic "target lesion," with rings of concentric inflammation involving the mucosa, submucosa, and muscularis surrounding a narrowed lumen.

Endoscopic Evaluation

Endoscopy provides the opportunity for direct visualization, biopsy, and histopathologic examination of the bowel. Esophagogastroduodenoscopy is the most sensitive technique for detecting mucosal involvement of the stomach, the duodenum, and, rarely, the esophagus by Crohn's disease. The rectum is involved in at least 95 per cent of patients with active ulcerative colitis. Therefore, proctoscopy with biopsy is essential for initial evaluation of patients with suspected ulcerative colitis. Because the rectum is spared in more than 50 per cent of patients with Crohn's disease, proctoscopy may be normal. However, inspection of the perianal area can reveal changes typical of Crohn's disease, including fissures, abscesses, and fistulas.

The initial evaluation of ulcerative colitis should include flexible sigmoidoscopy. While barium enema is often interpreted as normal in early or mild disease, flexible sigmoidoscopy can demonstrate even subtle mucosal changes that can be easily biopsied. Colonoscopy is preferred in chronic ulcerative colitis, but complete colonoscopy is not indicated in acute ulcerative colitis because it may cause unnecessary discomfort and because it carries a significant risk of provoking colonic dilatation or perforation. The goal of flexible sigmoidoscopy is to establish the presence of disease, but it can also reveal the extent of disease and thus be of prognostic and therapeutic value. For example, if inflammatory changes extend beyond 30 to 50 cm, it is less likely that the patient will respond to topical treatment alone and systemic therapy may be needed.

Colonoscopy is useful in the initial evaluation of suspected Crohn's disease unless prohibited by severe perianal or rectal disease. This method permits examination of the terminal ileum, which is useful because about one third of patients have disease limited to the small bowel and another 40 to 50 per cent have ileocolic disease. The distribution of disease is often incorrectly predicted from the physical examination, but colonoscopy permits mucosal biopsy and surveillance for dysplasia. Therefore, colonoscopy is of value in the management of chronic ulcerative colitis as well as Crohn's disease.

Gross and Microscopic Pathology

In ulcerative colitis, endoscopy early in the course of the disease typically shows erythema and friable mucosa. With more severe disease, superficial ulcerations are seen and a bloody, purulent exudate may be observed. Chronic colitis produces granular mucosal changes with a loss of vascularity; inflammatory pseudopolyps may develop, consisting of raised, edematous mucosa surrounded by ulceration. Later, strictures may develop. The histologic findings in ulcerative colitis show diffuse inflammation with infiltration of crypts by neutrophils, resulting in crypt abscesses that may converge in chronic disease. While inflammation is widespread, it does not penetrate to the serosa unless disease activity becomes severe and results in thinning of the bowel wall, dilatation, and ultimately perforation. Over time, carcinoma can develop from progressive dysplastic transformation of the epithelium.

The findings in Crohn's disease of the small bowel and of the large bowel are similar. Aphthous ulcerations are common and may coalesce to form large ulcerations. The mucosa is not usually friable or granular; cobblestoning is typical and is consistent with submucosal inflammation. Areas of luminal narrowing may be observed, and edema frequently extends through the submucosa to involve the mesentery and surrounding lymph nodes. This transmural inflammation can lead to the development of abscesses and fistulas, classic complications of Crohn's disease. Granulomas are found in 30 to 50 per cent of biopsy specimens and are a hallmark of Crohn's disease.

Seventy to eighty per cent of patients with Crohn's disease have some small bowel involvement. Of the 20 to 30 per cent with isolated large bowel involvement, the diagnosis of ulcerative colitis is far less likely if rectal bleeding is absent. Radiographic, endoscopic, and histologic findings help establish the diagnosis of Crohn's disease by documenting the presence of discontinuous disease, aphthous ulcers, cobblestoning, granulomas, and a normal vascular pattern adjacent to areas of involved bowel (skip lesions). Systematically approached, a specific diagnosis of ulcerative colitis or Crohn's disease can be mde in all but 10 to 15 per cent of patients (see Fig. 1).

COMPLICATIONS

The extraintestinal complications associated with inflammatory bowel disease are discussed above, and are outlined in Table 3.

Perforation

Perforation can occur in either ulcerative colitis or Crohn's disease. Severe disease in any bowel segment predisposes to perforation—even when dilatation is not present. Toxic dilatation of the colon (toxic megacolon) occurs more commonly in ulcerative colitis. Thinning of the bowel wall and loss of neuromuscular tone result in a flimsy, dilated bowel predisposed to perforation. Toxic dilatation can be induced by barium studies, antimotility drugs, and endoscopy. Toxic megacolon typically presents with fever and abdominal pain in an ill-appearing patient. Diarrhea may actually decrease secondary to loss of colonic neuromuscular tone. Signs of peritoneal inflammation and volume depletion may be observed if perforation has occurred. Plain film may show colonic dilatation, free air, or pneumatosis intestinalis. Toxic megacolon is a medical emergency; the mortality rate with perforation is over 30 per cent. Perforation of the small bowel in Crohn's disease is typically more subtle, and early diagnosis may be difficult. Abscess formation is presumed to occur as a result of microperforation and seeding of the peritoneum with bowel flora.

Cancer

Both ulcerative colitis and Crohn's disease carry a risk of cancer that is increased over that of the general population. The risk of cancer in ulcerative colitis is well known but may be similar in Crohn's colitis, given the same extent and duration of disease. The incidence of cancer increases proportionally to the extent of disease. Patients with pancolitis are at higher risk than those with proctosigmoiditis, and patients with disease limited to the rectum have no increased risk of carcinoma. Cancer risk further increases with the duration of disease. In patients who have had chronic ulcerative colitis for 10 years, the risk of developing carcinoma increases by 0.5 to 1 per cent per year.

The diagnosis of colon cancer can be difficult in ulcerative colitis. Symptoms secondary to carcinoma may be similar to those of typical inflammatory bowel disease (changes in bowel habits, rectal bleeding, abdominal pain, weight loss) and may be difficult to identify on radiographic and endoscopic examination in the setting of acute and chronic changes of colitis. Furthermore, neoplasms in ulcerative colitis are more likely to occur distally, to be multiple, and to be of a higher malignant grade. Carcinoembryonic antigen (CEA) is *not* a useful index of colon cancer in ulcerative colitis because it may be increased nonspecifically. Therefore, routine endoscopic surveillance has become the standard of care for detecting carcinoma; dysplasia serves as the primary histologic marker for malignant change. The frequency of surveillance varies with the extent and duration of ulcerative colitis and with the degree of dysplasia previously observed. As many as 50 per cent of patients with high-grade dysplasia may have underlying malignancy. Therefore, high-grade dysplasia is an indication for colectomy that removes both the inflammatory process and the malignant potential.

The incidence of carcinoma of the biliary tract is significantly increased in inflammatory bowel disease, particularly in ulcerative colitis. Patients are more commonly male and present in the fourth or fifth decade with right upper quadrant pain and progressive jaundice that may actually predate the onset of colitis. Most patients, however, have had a protracted course of inflammatory bowel disease, and carcinoma can develop even years after colectomy.

WHIPPLE'S DISEASE (INTESTINAL LIPODYSTROPHY)

By Robert J. Quinet, M.D.
New Orleans, Louisiana

Whipple's disease is a rare, chronic, relapsing infection caused by a rod-shaped, gram-positive actinomycete, *Tropheryma whippelii.* This multisystem disease is gratifyingly responsive to appropriate antibiotic therapy but can be fatal if untreated. Persons most commonly affected are middle-aged (40 to 60 years), white (more than 90 per cent), and male (more than 90 per cent).

SYMPTOMS

Diarrhea, weight loss, fever, and polyarthritis are the symptoms at presentation. Typically, the arthritis precedes the other symptoms by years or even decades. The arthritis is usually migratory, transient, symmetrical, and polyarticular and predominantly affects large joints, such as the knees, ankles, wrists, and elbows. Active arthritis may be present in the absence of bowel or other symptoms. Sacroiliitis and spondylitis with backache may occur in 10 to 20 per cent of patients. Without a strong clinical suspicion, it is extremely difficult to make the diagnosis when arthritis is the only symptom. However, in a middle-aged white man with seronegative polyarthritis, particularly if it has a migratory pattern and is poorly responsive to antirheumatic therapies, Whipple's disease should be strongly considered. Fever is usually low grade and is often present for several years before diagnosis. Whipple's disease is a rare cause of fever of unknown origin (FUO). Diarrhea may start gradually but eventuates in malabsorption and steatorrhea, with consequent weight loss that may be profound. Associated symptoms of malaise, fatigue, and generalized weakness are invariably present by this time. Vague abdominal pain, discomfort, cramping, bloating, and distention are frequently, but not invariably, present (approximately 50 per cent of patients). Hematochezia may occur but is unusual.

Personality change, confusion, memory loss, and apathy resulting in a dementialike state are not unusual. Less common neurologic problems include myoclonus, supranuclear ophthalmoplegia, cranial neuropathies, and chronic meningitis. Neurologic symptoms are characteristically present in relapses of Whipple's disease if antibiotics that fail to penetrate the central nervous system (CNS) have been used in previous treatment.

PHYSICAL EXAMINATION

Lymphadenopathy (axillary more often than cervical) and hyperpigmentation (generalized) are present in 50 per cent of patients. Weight loss can be documented. Occasional palpable abdominal lymph nodes, abdominal distention, ascites, or a palpable liver or spleen may be present. Hypotension, peripheral edema, and signs of malnutrition and vitamin deficiency such as muscle wasting, cheilitis, glossitis, and purpura may be seen in advanced cases with malabsorption and steatorrhea. Clubbing may also be seen. Examination of the joints may reveal redness, warmth, swelling, and limited motion in affected joints, such as the knees, ankles, wrists, elbows, and shoulders, and sometimes the small finger joints. Chest expansion and lumbar flexion may be limited, and the sacroiliac joints tender in patients with spondylitis. Neurologic examination may reveal decreased memory on mental status assessment, ataxic gait, spastic paresis, peripheral neuropathy, ophthalmoplegia, nystagmus, papilledema, optic neuritis with disk pallor, uveitis, and decreased hearing. Cardiac auscultation rarely can reveal a pericardial rub or systolic murmurs. Chest examination may reveal cough, pleural rub, effusion, or consolidation.

LABORATORY DATA

A mild normocytic and normochromic or hypochromic anemia is typical but may be severe (hemoglobin concentration less than 8 g). An associated iron, folate, or vitamin B_{12} deficiency anemia can develop because of blood loss and/or malabsorption. The erythrocyte sedimentation rate is moderately increased in 70 per cent of patients. The white blood cell count is usually normal, but leukocytosis may occur, and, rarely, leukopenia. Hypoalbuminemia and low-serum carotene concentrations are present in more than 90 per cent of patients. Urinalysis results may be abnormal in 60 per cent of patients and are characterized by proteinuria, pyuria, or, rarely, microhematuria. A prolonged prothrombin time and a low cholesterol concentration are present in 50 per cent of patients. One third of patients may have increased transaminase and alkaline phosphatase activity or hypokalemia. Hypocalcemia is rare. A finding of 24-hour fecal fat is abnormal in more than 90 per cent of patients, as is the D-xylose concentration in about 80 per cent of patients, confirming malabsorption and steatorrhea.

RADIOGRAPHY

Chest films may show interstitial infiltrates, pleural thickening, and rarely effusions, as well as incidental findings. Small bowel studies, although not diagnostically helpful, typically show nonspecific coarsening of duodenal and jejunal folds, sometimes with dilatation, which is consistent with a malabsorption pattern. Abdominal ultrasound and especially computed tomography (CT) may reveal evidence of retroperitoneal, mesenteric, para-aortic, or other intra-abdominal lymphadenopathy. Whipple's disease has been diagnosed by CT-guided percutaneous needle biopsy of intra-abdominal nodes. Abdominal imaging is nonspecific, however, and a biopsy specimen is more easily, safely, and definitively obtained from the small bowel. Cranial magnetic resonance imaging (MRI) and CT may show nonspecific abnormalities in Whipple's disease patients with CNS symptoms based on findings in a few case reports. Scintigraphy using granulocytes labeled with technetium-99m hexamethyl propyleneamine oxime (HM-PAO) may be a way of determining the extent of the disease, but findings are still preliminary. Limited data suggest that bone radiographs commonly reveal osteoporosis, and joint films may rarely demonstrate erosions and evidence of sacroiliitis or spondylitis.

DIAGNOSIS

Definitive diagnosis is best made by peroral biopsy of the duodenojejunal region of the small bowel. Esophagogastroduodenoscopy (EGD) results are often normal but may reveal thickened mucosal folds that may be yellow-white and granular, resembling shag carpet. Biopsy of these areas often produces abnormal results. Multiple biopsy specimens should also be obtained of normal-appearing mucosa; these specimens should be stained with periodic acid–Schiff (PAS), even if the results of hematoxylin and eosin (H&E) staining are normal.

The classic light microscopic findings include (1) abundant, foamy macrophages containing PAS-positive granules (diastase-resistant) in the lamina propria; (2) free bacilli in the lamina propria; (3) distorted villi; and (4) dilated lymphatics. Staining with Ziehl-Neelsen stain should always be performed to exclude *Mycobacterium avium-intracellulare* because this organism can be PAS-positive and can cause a syndrome virtually identical to Whipple's disease, especially in the population with acquired immunodeficiency syndrome (AIDS). The PAS granules within macrophages likely represent remnants of the innermost polysaccharide-containing portion of the bacterial cell wall contained within lysosomes.

Electron microscopy invariably reveals rod-shaped bacillary bodies (approximately 1 to 2.5 μm × 0.25 μm) lying free in the mucosa and submucosa or within macrophages. The electromicroscopic findings are pathognomonic and are not present in mycobacteriosis. In biopsies of rectum or lymph nodes, PAS-positive macrophages may be found in benign conditions as well as in normal persons, and specific diagnosis depends on visualizing bacillary bodies by light microscopy or electron microscopy. Besides the small bowel, the PAS-positive macrophages have been found in many other tissues, including lymph nodes, bone marrow, synovium, brain, skin, subcutaneous nodules, cerebrospinal fluid, pericardium, endocardium (heart valves), lung, liver, spleen, pancreas, esophagus, stomach, colon, muscle, and adrenal glands.

Whipple's disease may also be diagnosed by polymerase chain reaction (PCR) analysis of bacterial DNA isolated from peripheral blood to identify the novel bacterial 16S rRNA gene sequence of *T. whippelii*. This may become the diagnostic test of choice in the near future.

ERRORS AND PITFALLS IN DIAGNOSIS

Arthritis and arthralgia typically precede other manifestations, including fever, weight loss, and diarrhea, by years. As a result, middle-aged white men have carried diagnoses of seronegative rheumatoid arthritis, palindromic rheumatism, systemic lupus erythematosus, and ankylosing spondylitis for years before diagnosis.

Fever may be present for months to years before the other symptoms appear, making Whipple's disease a cause of fever of unknown origin. Lymphadenopathy, weight loss, and anemia can suggest lymphoma, leukemia, or infection with human immunodeficiency virus (HIV). Hyperpigmentation, hypotension, and fever may suggest Addison's disease. The finding of noncaseating granulomas in lung, liver, or lymph nodes may suggest tuberculosis or sarcoidosis if PAS staining is not performed. *Mycobacterium avium-intracellulare* infection of the intestine can cause identical symptoms and requires Ziehl-Neelsen staining or electron microscopy of the biopsy material to distinguish it from Whipple's disease. Pulmonary involvement including pleuritis, hilar adenopathy, and interstitial disease may mimic sarcoidosis.

COURSE AND OUTCOME

Treatment with appropriate antibiotic therapy results in dramatic improvement with resolution of fever within days, diarrhea within a week, and joint symptoms within several weeks. All other symptoms improve within several months. Appropriate therapy requires a 12-month course of an oral antibiotic (e.g., trimethoprim-sulfamethoxazole) that penetrates the CNS. Many would advise an initial 10- to 14-day course of parenteral penicillin and streptomycin preceding oral treatment.

A relapse may be a recurrence of the original clinical (joint and gastrointestinal) symptoms or it may occur as CNS involvement, including dementia, confusion, personality change, ataxia, ophthalmoplegia, and so on. However, there have been no documented CNS relapses with the use of either of the preceding antibiotic regimens. Relapses are easily treatable except for neurologic manifestations. Relapses may be preceded by recurrence of bacilli in the small intestine and documented by a repeat small bowel biopsy. Diagnosis of isolated CNS relapse can be supported by clinical context, biopsy of small bowel or lymph nodes, noninvasive cranial imaging with magnetic resonance imaging or CT, and lumbar puncture with cerebrospinal fluid analysis, including examination for PAS-positive macrophages and bacillary bodies. Such evidence may justify an empirical trial of CNS-active antibiotics as an alternative to a brain biopsy. Patients who have an equivocal response to therapy could undergo a repeat small bowel biopsy in 3 months to determine whether the bacilli have been eradicated, but routine follow-up biopsies are not necessary. The PAS-positive macrophages often remain for months to years, but the bacilli disappear within 2 to 3 months with appropriate antibiotic therapy. Whipple's disease is invariably fatal without such therapy.

CELIAC SPRUE

By Jerry S. Trier, M.D.
Boston, Massachusetts

Celiac disease, gluten-sensitive enteropathy, and gluten-induced enteropathy as used in the current literature are synonymous with celiac sprue. The term "nontropical sprue" was often used to refer to celiac sprue in older literature 20 or more years ago.

Celiac sprue is a chronic disease in which wheat gliadins (the alcohol-soluble fractions of wheat gluten) and equivalent rye, barley, and oat prolamins cause damage to the small intestine, producing a characteristic, though not specific, mucosal lesion. Although the entire length of the small intestine is at risk, a proximal-to-distal gradient of involvement is typical. Often, the damage is limited to the proximal small intestine. Impaired absorption of dietary nutrients results, although the degree of malabsorption varies and correlates with the extent and severity of the intestinal lesion. Withdrawal of the offending cereal grains from the diet results in reversal of the mucosal damage with improvement of nutrient absorption and diminished symptoms. The response to gluten withdrawal is a crucial aspect of the diagnosis, as the clinical and pathologic features of a number of other diseases closely resemble those of celiac sprue, but these disorders do not respond to a gluten-free diet.

Epidemiologic studies from Europe suggest that prevalence rates among most white populations range from 1 in 1000 to 1 in 2000, although rates as high as 1 in 300 have been observed in western Ireland. The disease is rare in native Africans, African Americans, and Asians, but well-documented cases among natives of India and Pakistan have been reported.

The exact pathogenesis of celiac sprue is not fully understood, but considerable evidence implicates both genetic factors and immune mechanisms. Approximately 10 per cent of first-degree relatives are affected, many with latent, virtually asymptomatic disease. The HLA antigens DR3 and DQw2 are closely linked to the disease. Most patients who lack DR3 are DR5/DR7 heterozygotes. These haplotypes share a specific HLA-DQ α-β heterodimer that may be important in the presentation of toxic gluten peptides to mucosal T cells, triggering immunologically mediated mucosal damage. However, the majority of individuals with the DR3 and DR5/DR7 haplotypes do not have celiac sprue, and discordance for celiac sprue among 30 per cent of identical twins has been reported. Hence, other triggers, including an as yet undefined susceptibility gene or an environmental factor, may be essential.

PRESENTING SYMPTOMS AND PHYSICAL SIGNS

Clinical manifestations of celiac sprue may begin at any age, but they have been observed most frequently in infants and young children at the time of introduction of cereals into the diet and in adults during the third, fourth, and fifth decades. The spectrum of symptoms and signs is broad and depends on the extent and severity of intestinal involvement.

If much of the small intestine is damaged, gastrointestinal symptoms caused by generalized malabsorption predominate. These symptoms include diarrhea with bulky to watery steatorrheic stools; weight loss, often in the setting of normal or increased caloric intake; flatulence; and abdominal distention. Extraintestinal manifestations vary from patient to patient.

Anemia is common. If mucosal damage is confined to the duodenum and proximal jejunum, anemia caused by iron deficiency, folate deficiency, or both may be the sole clinical manifestation. Hence, the anemia can be microcytic, macrocytic, or dimorphic. Food iron and folate are absorbed most avidly by the proximal intestine.

Symptoms related to osteopenia, such as back pain, may be prominent and can overshadow gastrointestinal symptoms. Pathologic fractures can occur. Hypoproteinemia caused by protein-losing enteropathy may produce edema. Amenorrhea and impotence may reflect nutritionally related pituitary suppression. Cheilosis, stomatitis, peripheral neuropathy, and night blindness indicate specific nutritional deficiencies.

CLINICAL COURSE

If the disease goes untreated, the clinical course may vary widely. When the diagnosis is missed during infancy and childhood, most patients' symptoms improve somewhat even without specific treatment during late adolescence and early adulthood. When the disease presents in adulthood, the symptoms may wax and wane for years if the diagnosis is missed, or they may progress relentlessly. Ultimately, severe cachexia, malnutrition, and even death may ensue in the severely afflicted patient whose condition goes undiagnosed.

On the other hand, the response to complete withdrawal of gluten from the diet of patients with flagrant symptoms is prompt and dramatic. Diarrhea and steatorrhea rapidly improve within a few days to several weeks. Secondary manifestations, such as anemia and endocrine symptoms, may require a longer period before reversion to normal is complete. Severe osteopenic bone disease can be irreversible but is usually arrested as intestinal absorption normalizes.

The most frequent cause of no response or an incomplete response to dietary gluten withdrawal is intentional or inadvertent poor compliance. Gluten is ubiquitous in the Western diet, and the patient must eliminate all hidden sources of gluten, such as wheat extenders added to processed foods, ice cream, bouillon cubes, and so forth. Such innocent-sounding additives as hydrolyzed vegetable protein, dextrin, and emulsifiers may be derived from wheat and thus could be rich in gluten. The principles of gluten withdrawal are simple enough, but strict adherence to the diet is difficult and requires an informed and motivated patient who has been thoroughly counseled by both a knowledgeable physician and a dietitian. On a rigid gluten-free diet, nearly all patients remain well indefinitely. Only a small percentage develop complicating disease directly associated with celiac sprue.

COMPLICATIONS

Major extraintestinal complications resulting from protracted malabsorption were described above. In a very small subgroup of patients with celiac sprue, symptoms recur after an initial response to gluten withdrawal despite continued strict adherence by patients to a gluten-free diet. Patients who experience recurrence of symptoms must be carefully evaluated for intestinal lymphoma, which occurs at increasing frequency in patients with celiac sprue. When lymphoma has been excluded and no other cause found, these patients are classified as having evolved to refractory sprue, a syndrome not responsive to gluten withdrawal. Some of these patients respond to corticosteroids or other immunosuppressive agents, but many do not and face a dismal prognosis. The scarcity of available epidemiologic data suggests that some other malignancies, including extraintestinal lymphoma and carcinoma of the oropharynx, esophagus, small intestine, and breast, occur with somewhat greater frequency among adults with celiac sprue. Small intestinal strictures and ulcers, occasionally with perforation, have rarely been observed in patients with celiac sprue, but rigorous study of such individuals often reveals underlying intestinal lymphoma. Among the many diseases reported to occur in concert with celiac sprue, convincing evidence has emerged of associations with dermatitis herpetiformis, type I diabetes mellitus, autoimmune thyroid disease, and selective IgA deficiency.

LABORATORY STUDIES

An algorithm detailing the approach to the diagnosis of celiac sprue is shown in Figure 1. The clinician establishes the diagnosis by using biopsy to document the presence of the characteristic mucosal lesion of the small intestine and by noting a response to gluten withdrawal. The changes in mucosal architecture associated with the characteristic lesion consist of shortened or absent villi and hyperplastic crypts. The number of mitotic figures in the crypts is strikingly increased. Absorptive cells, which are usually columnar, are decreased in height and appear cuboidal or even squamoid, with attenuation of the brush border and, often, cytoplasmic vacuolation. The cellularity of the lamina propria is increased, predominantly by increased numbers of plasma cells, lymphocytes, and macrophages, but scattered neutrophils, eosinophils, and mast cells are also present. Finally, the ratio of intraepithelial lymphocytes to epithelial cells is strikingly increased.

If the index of suspicion for celiac sprue is high because of the history, the physical findings, and routine laboratory studies, the evaluation can proceed directly to small intestinal biopsy without incurring costs for other special tests. However, the clinical features are often nonspecific. In such instances, it is helpful to determine whether steatorrhea is present. Steatorrhea can be assessed qualitatively by microscopic examination of stool stained with Sudan III. Quantitative assessment of stool for steatorrhea is more accurate but also more expensive and somewhat cumbersome. It requires a 3- to 4-day pooled stool collection that is submitted for quantitative fat content. The patient ingests a fixed amount of fat (80 to 100 g/day). The stool must be kept refrigerated until assay to prevent the bacteria in the stool from metabolizing some of the excreted fat. Significant steatorrhea is present if stool fat excretion exceeds 10 per cent of estimated dietary intake. Low concentrations of serum cholesterol and carotene also suggest fat malabsorption, but these measurements are neither sensitive nor specific.

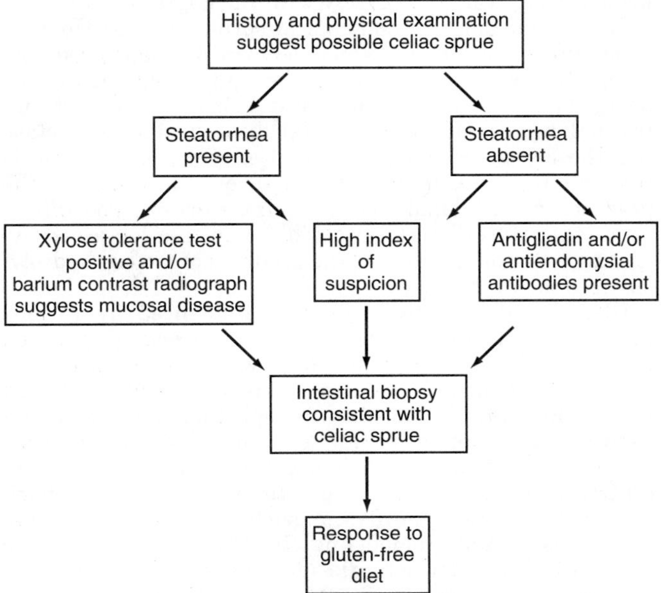

Figure 1. Approach to the diagnosis of celiac sprue.

If it is unclear whether steatorrhea is caused by intestinal mucosal disease, such as celiac sprue, or pancreatic insufficiency, further tests are necessary for selecting appropriate patients for intestinal biopsy. A xylose absorption test is often useful. Xylose absorption is decreased in most patients with primary mucosal disease of the proximal small intestine, such as celiac sprue, but the test result is normal in most patients with pancreatic disease. If stool fat was quantitated and stool mass was determined, stool fat concentration can be calculated. In diffuse mucosal diseases, fluid secretion and malabsorption dilute the stool, whereas in pancreatic insufficiency, fluid absorption is less severely perturbed. A low fecal fat concentration (less than 9 g/100 g) suggests mucosal disease, such as celiac sprue, but a high fat concentration (more than 10 g/100 g) suggests pancreatic disease. In celiac sprue, barium contrast studies of the small intestine frequently reveal effacement and coarsening of mucosal folds, luminal dilatation, and dilution of barium by unabsorbed and secreted fluids. Conversely, pancreatic insufficiency shows barium contrast studies of the small intestine that typically reveal a normal mucosal pattern.

If steatorrhea is absent, but the index of suspicion for proximal mucosal disease is high, as in patients with unexplained iron or folate deficiency, the next appropriate step is intestinal mucosal biopsy. If the index of suspicion is low, for example, in a patient who is not anemic and has nonspecific symptoms consistent with irritable bowel syndrome but has a family history of celiac sprue, measurement of circulating antigliadin and antiendomysial antibodies is useful. If antibody studies are negative in such a patient, the likelihood of celiac sprue is very low, and more costly and uncomfortable mucosal biopsy can be avoided. Antiendomysial IgA is the most definitive of the available serum antibody tests, with reported specificities ranging from 90 to 100 per cent. Antigliadin IgA and IgG antibodies are less specific, but because selective IgA deficiency is increased in association with celiac sprue, antigliadin IgG may be the only detectable antibody. Concomitant measurement of serum IgA facilitates interpretation of these serologic tests.

Determination of circulating antiendomysial IgA is also useful in patients thought to have celiac sprue but who fail to improve with gluten withdrawal. The specificity of this serum antibody test is so high that a positive test result should prompt a search for inadequate dietary compliance; conversely, a negative test result calls into question the presumptive diagnosis. Most patients with refractory sprue and other mucosal diseases that mimic celiac sprue lack circulating antiendomysial IgA. In most patients, strict adherence to a gluten-free diet results in a decrease in and the eventual disappearance of circulating antiendomysial IgA.

IMAGING PROCEDURES

In long-standing malabsorption, bones may show evidence of osteopenia, including pseudofractures and pathologic fractures. In patients who develop recurrent symptoms after an initial response to gluten withdrawal, contrast studies of the small intestine should be obtained to search for possible lymphoma or other intestinal disease (see above). Enteroclysis, if available, is particularly useful. Abdominal-pelvic computed tomography should be performed in the search for evidence of lymphoma in patients who develop recurrent symptoms after an initial response to a gluten-free diet.

PITFALLS IN DIAGNOSIS

Because the spectrum of clinical manifestations in celiac sprue is so broad, the diagnosis is often unduly delayed. Timely diagnosis requires a high index of suspicion for patients with more subtle presentations, such as unexplained iron or folate deficiency, osteopenic bone disease, and intestinal symptoms when the caloric intake appears excessive in relation to the patient's weight. The lack of specificity of the mucosal histology of the small intestine may also lead to diagnostic confusion. The mucosal lesions observed in tropical sprue, refractory sprue, eosinophilic enteritis, lymphoma-associated enteropathy, Crohn's disease of the proximal intestine, and, in the pediatric population, viral enteritis and milk or soy protein allergy can be indistinguishable from the mucosal lesion of celiac sprue. Since viral gastroenteritis and milk or soy protein allergy may improve in concert with institution of a gluten-free diet, a gluten challenge associated with a rise in circulating antigliadin and antiendomysial antibody titers can confirm the diagnosis in the pediatric population if necessary.

INTESTINAL DISACCHARIDASE DEFICIENCY

By Louis N. Aurisicchio, M.D.,
and C.S. Pitchumoni, M.D.
Bronx, New York

In the United States, the average diet derives 50 per cent of the total daily caloric intake from the digestion and absorption of carbohydrates. Dietary carbohydrate consists predominantly of complex polysaccharides, such as starch, while the remainder is composed of disaccharides, such as sucrose and lactose, as well as a small amount of monosaccharides (e.g., fructose). Starch must undergo hydrolysis by pancreatic amylase to yield oligosaccharides, principally maltose, maltotriose, and limit dextrins. These oligosaccharides and dietary disaccharides then undergo hydrolysis by enzymes (disaccharidases) at the level of the intestinal brush border membrane, yielding monosaccharide components. The monosaccharides are absorbed by either active transport (e.g., glucose and galactose) or facilitated diffusion (e.g., fructose).

Intestinal disaccharidases are components of enzyme complexes and can be classified as either α-glycosidases (maltase, sucrase-isomaltase, trehalase) or β-glycosidases (lactase). The distribution of enzyme activity within an intestinal villus is such that little or no disaccharidase activity exists in the basal crypt, while enzyme activity reaches maximum in the middle to upper third of the villus then falls off slightly toward the tip. A considerable concentration gradient of disaccharidase activity also occurs from the proximal to distal segments of the small intestine. All disaccharidase activities are lowest in the proximal duodenum, peak in the upper jejunum, and decrease in the terminal ileum. Maltase is an exception, since its activity remains persistently high, even in the distal terminal ileum.

The deficiency of an intestinal disaccharidase causes malabsorption of its corresponding disaccharide, resulting in carbohydrate malabsorption. This discussion focuses primarily on lactase deficiency, then briefly describes deficiencies of sucrase-isomaltase and trehalase. Isolated deficiency of maltase is not discussed, since maltase activity occurs in any of several α-glycosidase complexes.

LACTASE DEFICIENCY

Physiology

Lactose, a water-soluble disaccharide found in milk products, must undergo hydrolysis by an intestinal disaccharidase (lactase) to yield absorbable monosaccharides (glucose and galactose). Lactase activity appears in the fetal gut by the 10th week of gestation and increases until just prior to birth, when there is a "burst" in synthesis. During the first year of life, intestinal activity declines to 50 per cent of that present at birth. This pattern of synthesis, surge, and decline in lactase activity occurs similarly in all mammals.

Lactase activity is fairly stable over the 5-day life span of an enterocyte as the result of a balance between lactase synthesis and degradation. Certain conditions may lead to enterocyte injury, with the result that intestinal disaccharidase activity varies inversely with the degree of intestinal injury. Celiac disease (nontropical sprue) and kwashiorkor exemplify disorders in which lactase deficiency can develop. In comparison to the other intestinal disaccharidases, lactase is the enzyme most vulnerable to gastrointestinal injury. Of the intestinal disaccharidases, lactase has the lowest baseline intestinal enzyme activity and is the first to decrease and last to revert to normal in the presence of any small bowel injury. Lactase also differs from other intestinal disaccharidases in that lactase activity can be autoregulated by the products of lactose hydrolysis (feedback inhibition).

Disaccharidase activity may be influenced by various intraluminal factors, including pancreatic enzyme activity, intestinal pH, and bacterial overgrowth. Pancreatic proteolytic enzymes (primarily elastase), as well as bile acids and lysolecithin, are responsible for splitting and degrading α-glycosidase complexes into subunits. In patients with pancreatic exocrine insufficiency, decreased degradation of α-glycosidase complexes results in increased disaccharidase activity. β-Glycosidases, such as lactase, undergo post-translational remodeling by "intrinsic enterocyte peptidases," so their activities are generally unaffected by pancreatic exocrine insufficiency. The activity of intestinal lactase is optimal at pH 6.0; thus, a decrease in enzymatic activity occurs during acid-hypersecretory states, despite adequate concentrations of intestinal lactase. Finally, bacterial overgrowth can result in increased degradation of intraluminal enzymes, particularly intestinal disaccharidases.

Definitions and Terminology

The term lactose intolerance should not be used synonymously with lactase deficiency. A clinician determines that lactose intolerance is present by assessing the symptomatic response of an individual to a standard load of lactose. For example, a lactase-deficient individual may be able to tolerate the lactose load in one glass of milk, yet may not be able to tolerate higher lactose loads. Although milk and dairy products are the principal dietary sources of lactose, lactase deficiency is also not synonymous with milk intolerance. Milk intolerance may result from intolerance to any one of several components of milk: malabsorption of lactose, defective absorption of glucose-galactose, hypersensitivity to milk protein (principally casein), or intolerance to fat.

Classification

Lactase deficiency may result from any one of several disorders in which diminished intestinal lactase activity can lead to symptoms of lactose intolerance. Congenital lactase deficiency is an extremely rare inborn error of metabolism, with an autosomal recessive mode of inheritance. At birth, affected infants have no detectable activity of intestinal brush-border enzyme (alactasia). They present with severe diarrheal illness, dehydration, and failure to thrive when fed breast milk or lactose-containing milk products. If congenital lactase deficiency is diagnosed early, the physician can avoid these complications by placing the affected infant on a lactose-free diet.

Secondary lactase deficiency can arise from either an acute process (infectious gastroenteritis, medication-induced mucosal injury) or a chronic disorder (celiac sprue, regional enteritis, enteropathy associated with human immunodeficiency virus [HIV] infection). In either situation, damage to the intestinal villi results in a decreased reserve of lactase. After acute episodes of gastrointestinal disease (notably infectious gastroenteritis in children), a relative deficiency of lactase may persist for several weeks to months. In this situation, a lactose-reduced diet would be prudent throughout the infectious and early convalescent periods. Chronic disorders may, however, require lifelong adherence to a lactose-reduced diet.

Primary lactase deficiency is an autosomal recessive disorder that results in a postweaning loss of lactase activity. The disorder generally presents by 5 years of age, when intestinal lactase activity declines to 5 to 10 per cent of that present at birth. However, the onset of the clinical disorder may be delayed until adolescence or early adulthood. It appears that the genetic mechanism for the development of primary lactase deficiency involves production of an abnormal allele by an autosomal recessive gene. This defect can result in either a decrease in mRNA synthesis or a block in post-translational processing of the lactase complex. Regardless of whether an individual develops primary lactase deficiency, the structure of the lactase complex is homogeneous. No defect occurs in the structural genes responsible for lactase production.

Epidemiology

The prevalence of primary lactase deficiency varies worldwide according to ethnic background. The most commonly affected groups are Asians, Africans, and Asian Indians. The prevalence among these groups may approach 80 to 100 per cent of the population. This predominance contrasts sharply with whites of northern European and American ancestry, in whom the prevalence comprises only 5 to 15 per cent of the population. The geographic variation in lactase activity is believed to have arisen as the result of a selective mutation (culture-historic hypothesis). After the herding of domesticated animals was established by ancient humans, dairy products provided a potential source of subsistence. As a consequence, natural selection may have favored the development of a persistence of intestinal lactase activity, which is inherited as an autosomal dominant trait. This genetic drift enabled herding cultures to consume milk products, the consumption of which provided adults with an inherent survival advantage during times when other foods were limited.

Pathophysiology of Lactose Intolerance

A deficiency of intestinal lactase prevents hydrolysis of lactose, resulting in the presence of free, unabsorbable lactose within the intestinal lumen. The presence of unabsorbable lactose results in an osmotic gradient, leading to a flux of water and electrolytes into the intestinal lumen, further providing a stimulus for intestinal peristalsis (independent of hormonal control). The increase in intestinal water can exceed the "critical ileal flow rate," with fluid, electrolytes, and lactose then being dumped into the large intestine. Most of the fluid and electrolytes are salvaged by the colon, but the unabsorbed lactose is fermented by colonic bacteria to yield various gases (hydrogen, methane, carbon dioxide) and fatty acids. The combination of increased fecal water, intestinal peristalsis, gas formation, and the presence of fatty acids in the colon can cause a wide array of gastrointestinal complaints. Bloating, abdominal cramps, and borborygmi can result from the osmotic effect of unabsorbable lactose within the small intestine. Symptoms typically occur within 30 minutes of lactose ingestion, while additional symptoms of diarrhea and flatulence usually occur 1 to 2 hours later. Intolerance for lactose can also arise from a variety of conditions that cause impaired digestion and absorption of carbohydrates. These conditions include postgastric resection (Billroth type II), bacterial overgrowth, short-bowel syndrome, and congenital glucose-galactose malabsorption (a defect in the active transport of the monosaccharide components of lactose).

In primary lactase deficiency, the defect is rarely absolute, with enzyme activity remaining at roughly 5 to 10 per cent of that present at birth. As a result, the majority of individuals with lactase deficiency have enough lactase activity to tolerate small amounts of lactose-rich foods (e.g., 12 g of lactose in 1 cup of milk) without experiencing any symptoms following lactose ingestion (physiologic load). Therefore, clinically significant lactose intolerance may actually occur in a rather small percentage of individuals from lactase-deficient ethnic groups. Lactose malabsorption can also occur in individuals with fixed lactase activity (nonadaptability) when an increased physiologic load of lactose is ingested, because lactose feeding fails to induce lactase activity in these patients.

Diagnosis

In the majority of patients with suspected lactase deficiency, exclusion of milk and dairy products for a trial period of several weeks can lead to the resolution of symptoms. The recurrence of symptoms following milk challenge may provide sufficient evidence to support the diagnosis of lactase deficiency. The following tests may be utilized to confirm the presence of lactase deficiency.

Lactose Tolerance Test

This test measures the serum glucose response to an oral lactose challenge. After obtaining a baseline fasting serum glucose concentration, an oral loading dose of 1 g/kg of aqueous lactose (maximum 50 g) is administered. Serial measurements of serum glucose are obtained at intervals (15, 30, 60, 90, and 120 minutes) over 2 hours following lactose ingestion. Failure of the serum glucose to increase by 20 mg/dL over baseline within 2 hours is considered a "flat response." Ideally, a flat response should be accompanied by symptoms of intolerance. A combination of a flat response and intolerance supports the diagnosis of lactase deficiency in 80 to 100 per cent of subjects. However, a false-positive lactose tolerance test result can occur in other disorders that cause accelerated gastric emptying or small bowel malabsorption.

The lactose tolerance test is simple and inexpensive to perform. Unfortunately, the 50-g lactose load is a nonphysiologic dose and can cause symptoms not only in lactase-deficient individuals but also in 20 per cent of subjects with adequate intestinal lactase levels. Unfortunately, this phenomenon may lead to the false assumption that smaller physiologic loads, which are usually well tolerated, can also cause symptoms.

Hydrogen Breath Test

In the presence of lactase deficiency, unabsorbed lactose freely enters the colon, where bacterial degradation produces various gases, especially large quantities of hydrogen. Only bacteria are able to hydrolyze unabsorbed carbohydrates and generate hydrogen. (Humans lack the enzyme systems capable of producing hydrogen.) The hydrogen is then absorbed by the colon, diffuses into the blood, and subsequently is eliminated via the respiratory system over several hours (breath hydrogen).

The hydrogen breath test is routinely performed by administering a 10 per cent aqueous solution of lactose (e.g., 50-g aliquot of lactose in 500 mL of water). After obtaining a baseline breath sample, additional samples are obtained at intervals of 15 minutes for up to 4 hours. Breath samples are analyzed for hydrogen content with the use of gas chromatography, and concentration is expressed in parts per million (ppm). Most often, a rise in breath hydrogen above baseline of more than 20 ppm provides presumptive evidence of lactase deficiency.

The hydrogen breath test is accurate, relatively easy to perform, and noninvasive. It assesses malabsorption of lactose more reliably than does the lactose tolerance test, and thereby provides greater specificity. The clinician can also perform hydrogen breath testing in infants and young children, utilizing a mid- to end-expiratory nasal prong technique for collection of breath samples. Before beginning the hydrogen breath test, subjects should be instructed to abstain from oral intake (NPO) and cigarette smoking for 8 hours prior to testing. In addition, patients should not receive antibiotic therapy for 1 week before the hydrogen breath test, because antibiotics can alter the quantity and composition of bacterial flora in the colon.

Fecal pH

Unabsorbed lactose is fermented by colonic bacteria and yields gases and short-chain fatty acids. Following a standard lactose load of 50 g, detection of a fecal pH below 6.0 suggests malabsorption of ingested lactose. The sensitivity for fecal pH assay is low, because colonocytes absorb and metabolize short-chain fatty acids. Fecal assays utilizing radiolabeled carbohydrate (^{13}C) may provide increased specificity but are costly.

Intestinal Biopsy

Measurement of lactase activity in small bowel biopsies provides the most sensitive and specific means of diagnosing lactase deficiency. Utilizing standard endoscopic forceps, the physician obtains multiple small bowel mucosal biopsies from the region just proximal to the ligament of Treitz. A homogenate of biopsy samples can then be assayed for lactase activity, which is expressed as units per gram of mucosal wet weight. Deficiency is defined as a reduction in activity by 2 standard deviations from the reference mean (i.e., less than 0.7 units/g mucosal wet wt). Small bowel biopsy is performed mostly for research purposes and is rarely necessary in clinical practice, unless clinical data and the results of diagnostic tests are inconclusive.

Management

Diagnosis of lactase deficiency requires detailed history taking and physical examination, coupled with a high index of suspicion, especially in individuals who have nonspecific gastrointestinal symptoms. The majority of patients are aware of their intolerance for milk and dairy products and may have modified their diet to avoid symptoms prior to seeking medical advice.

Dietary management focuses on having the patient restrict lactose intake to one serving at a time (12-g equivalent), and preferably ingest dairy products with solid foods to slow gastric emptying. Consumption of any product that contains milk, lactose, dry milk solids, or whey should be limited. Total lactose elimination (lactose-free diet) is not necessary except in those rare patients with congenital lactase deficiency or severe primary lactase deficiency. Particular emphasis should be given to the management of lactase deficiency in children, adolescents, and postmenopausal women, since mere dietary avoidance will deny these individuals the benefits of the calcium contained in dairy products.

Dairy products prehydrolyzed with β-galactosidase (bacteria-derived lactase) are available in food markets. These products provide an average 70 per cent reduction in total lactose content, contributing to a significant reduction in the symptoms of intolerance compared with an equivalent amount of a nonhydrolyzed product. In addition, caplets containing lactase can be taken within 30 minutes of anticipated ingestion of dairy products. Generally, two caplets are needed to ensure sufficient hydrolysis of an 8-oz equivalent of whole milk (12 g of lactose).

Skim milk is not an appropriate substitute for whole milk, because these products contain an equivalent lactose content and differ only in fat content. On the other hand, yogurts with "live and active cultures" (more than 10 million live bacteria/g) provide an excellent milk substitute. The bacteria found in active cultures release β-galactosidase when degraded by gastric secretions and thereby "autodigest" the lactose contained within the yogurt.

SUCRASE-ISOMALTASE DEFICIENCY

The sucrase-isomaltase complex is a heat-labile glycoprotein containing both sucrase and isomaltase activity. Sucrase is essential for hydrolyzing sucrose into glucose and fructose, while isomaltase is capable of digesting 1,6 linkages of starch, producing oligosaccharides. Sucrase activity is present solely within the sucrase-isomaltase complex, whereas isomaltase activity may also exist in other disaccharidase complexes (e.g., maltases).

Sucrase-isomaltase deficiency is a congenital disaccharidase deficiency inherited in an autosomal recessive pattern. The disorder is rare, except among Canadian Indians and native Greenlanders, in whom 10 per cent of the population are affected. Infants generally present with chronic watery diarrhea and failure to thrive when fed sucrose-containing formula.

The clinician can make the diagnosis by performing an oral tolerance test or hydrogen breath test, utilizing a sucrose-based substrate. Small intestinal biopsy for assay of mucosal sucrase activity can also be performed. Treatment consists of eliminating sucrose-based products and substituting fructose, since there is no defect in absorption of constituent monosaccharides.

TREHALASE DEFICIENCY

Trehalose is a disaccharide present in insects as well as young mushrooms. Trehalase deficiency is a rare disorder, which may also occur in about 10 per cent of native Greenlanders. Trehalase deficiency may present as an intolerance for mushrooms; however, overt deficiency is extremely uncommon because trehalose is contained in only a fraction of the average diet.

DIVERTICULAR DISEASE OF THE COLON

By Lawrence J. Cheskin, M.D.,
and Robert Lamport, M.D.
Baltimore, Maryland

Diverticular disease of the colon refers to the full range of possible manifestations of an acquired anatomic deformity of the colonic wall, diverticulosis. The abnormality usually consists of a number of small pseudodiverticula, herniations of the mucosal and submucosal layers of the colonic wall through the muscular layer so that balloon-shaped sacs lie below the serosa. The presence of diverticula does not imply symptoms. Symptomatic diverticular disease may manifest as painful diverticular disease without perforation or inflammation, diverticulitis (i.e., perforation and inflammation), or diverticular bleeding.

About 50 per cent of persons older than 70 years in developed countries have colonic diverticulosis. About 80 per cent of persons with this anatomic lesion remain asymptomatic. The lesions are typically incidental findings at laparotomy, endoscopy, or contrast radiographic study of the lower gastrointestinal (GI) tract, with no symptoms, physical findings, or laboratory abnormalities. The diverticula may be few, multiple but limited to one area (typically the sigmoid colon), or multiple and scattered throughout the colon. Plain abdominal films, a contrast barium enema, computed tomography (CT), ultrasound, angiography, and nuclear scanning all may be useful modalities for diagnosing diverticular disease in the appropriate clinical setting. Although some asymptomatic patients suffer later complications, it is probably not a useful exercise to attempt to make this diagnosis when the disease is still asymptomatic. The clinician's role in asymptomatic cases should be to urge adoption of a high-fiber diet, which in epidemiologic studies is correlated with a low prevalence of all manifestations of this disorder. No evidence of an independent increase in the risk of colorectal carcinoma in diverticular disease has been reported, although a diet low in fiber is a risk factor for both diseases.

PAINFUL DIVERTICULAR DISEASE

Presenting Signs and Symptoms

The presence of pain attributable to diverticula without evidence of peridiverticular inflammation, perforation, or abscess formation defines this condition. The usual manifestation of painful diverticular disease (PDD) is in middle-aged or elderly men and women with a history of recurrent abdominal pain, often with alterations in bowel habits, bloating, distention of the abdomen, or flatulence. The painful episodes are often crampy, vary in intensity from mild to severe, and last for minutes to hours. The pain is most often located in the left lower quadrant, overlying the sigmoid colon; less commonly, it is more generalized. The painful episodes can be discrete or even solitary, or they can continue intermittently for days. The pain is rarely continuous. With time, the painful episodes tend to occur with greater frequency. No consistent relationship with diet or stress has been observed, although some patients may notice an association after the fact. The alteration in bowel habits may be constipation, diarrhea, or an alternation between the two, although constipation alone is most common.

Pitfalls in Diagnosis

Painful diverticular disease can be very difficult to distinguish from the most common forms of chronic abdominal pain, the irritable bowel syndrome (IBS), and functional bowel disease (i.e., motility disorders). Although PDD and IBS have similar colonic motility patterns and presenting symptoms, they are usually clinically distinguishable. The age at onset for IBS is typically in the young-adult to middle-age groups, but episodes of painful diverticular disease rarely occur before middle age and are most common after 60 years of age. Pain due to IBS is more clearly precipitated by stress or diet, and symptoms may affect the upper GI or lower GI tract.

In distinguishing IBS from PDD, the clinician should recall that the processes may not be mutually exclusive. The prevalence of asymptomatic diverticular disease with increasing age is so high in developed countries that the presence of diverticula may be a diagnostic red herring. The presence of diverticula in the setting of abdominal pain is not necessarily evidence for diverticula causing the abdominal pain.

One important differential diagnosis is between PDD and adenocarcinoma of the colon. Patients with the latter may also present with colicky abdominal pain, particularly after meals and associated with constipation or diarrhea. The age groups for both diseases overlap completely. Inquiring about carcinoma-associated symptoms such as weight loss and weakness is helpful, because these are not typical features of PDD. Colonoscopy or a barium contrast study is required to exclude carcinoma and should be performed in the initial evaluations of elderly patients with a clinical picture suggestive of PDD. In patients with previous abdominal or pelvic surgery (e.g., total hysterectomy), adhesions may mimic PDD. Pelvic diseases such as ovarian cysts, torsion of an ovary, or uterine fibroids must also be considered. For women with possible pelvic disease, abdominal or transvaginal ultrasonography is likely to be the most helpful initial imaging study.

Course

Most cases of PDD have a benign course, although these patients may suffer repeated attacks of pain. The frequency of attacks varies greatly among patients. A single attack and continuous attacks are uncommon. The site of involvement and the constellation of symptoms seen during a patient's first attack of PDD are often repeated with little variation during subsequent episodes. The complication rate of painful diverticular disease appears to be no higher than that of asymptomatic disease.

Physical and Laboratory Findings

The physical examination may reveal nothing unusual during an attack of PDD, but it most often shows a firm area of tenderness in the left lower quadrant that overlies the affected loop of colon (i.e., "palpable cord"). The examination is otherwise unremarkable, with no signs of peritoneal irritation, such as rebound tenderness, that can be seen with complicated diverticular disease. To make the diagnosis of uncomplicated painful diverticular disease, the total leukocyte count, erythrocyte sedimentation rate, and body temperature all should be normal, and the stool should contain no occult blood, pathogens, or fecal leukocytes.

Diagnostic Procedures

If PDD is suggested, confirmation of the diverticula is necessary. Diagnostic studies are more useful for excluding other bowel lesions as the cause of the pain than for definitively diagnosing PDD. In patients with all forms of diverticular disease, except diverticulitis, plain abdominal radiography is typically normal and is thus of limited diagnostic value. Its utility is in its rapid availability and usefulness in detecting other causes of abdominal pain. For example, mucosal "thumbprinting" suggests ischemia of the bowel; air-fluid levels suggest an ileus; and air under the diaphragm suggests a perforated viscus.

The single-contrast barium enema is most commonly used to document the presence of diverticula or other lesions that can cause pain. Diverticula appear on the barium enema as contrast-filled, mushroomlike protrusions of the colonic lumen. Postevacuation films may be the most dramatic in appearance, because the contrast is retained in the diverticula. Error rates as high as 50 per cent can occur in the diagnosis of concomitant lesions such as neoplasms in a diverticula-bearing segment of the colon by barium enema. A double-contrast study, multiple views, compression spot films, and postevacuation films can greatly improve the accuracy of this study. The number and distribution of diverticula usually correlate poorly with the clinical picture. The barium enema is also useful for diagnosing carcinoma of the colorectum, inflammatory bowel disease, and ischemic colitis.

Lower GI endoscopy is less helpful than contrast radiography for identifying diverticula, because the lesions are difficult to quantitate and the surrounding tissues cannot be visualized. The utility of endoscopy, both sigmoidoscopy and colonoscopy, lies in its accuracy in identifying other colonic lesions. Barium enema is the preferable procedure in most cases, particularly if the patient has pain. When the barium enema reveals abnormalities other than or in addition to diverticula, endoscopy permits visualization of the lesion and biopsy. If the patient does not have pain at the time of presentation, colonoscopy may be preferable to barium enema.

DIVERTICULITIS

Diverticulitis, the second most common complication of diverticular disease, affects perhaps 10 to 25 per cent of patients with diverticulosis. Despite the name, the inflammation is probably secondary, preceded by microperforation of the weakened wall of a diverticulum due to increased intraluminal pressure.

Presenting Signs and Symptoms

Diverticulitis progresses through four stages, each representing more advanced disease and a poorer prognosis. The first stage after microperforation is pericolic abscess, with inflammation involving the mesentery of the affected segment. This may progress to a pelvic abscess requiring open or percutaneous drainage. More advanced stages include generalized peritonitis after rupture of a pelvic abscess and free perforation with feces spilling into the peritoneum. The latter two stages are surgical emergencies, and occur uncommonly.

Clinically, diverticulitis is distinguished by abdominal pain and fever, usually low grade. The disease usually involves the sigmoid colon; symptoms are typically left lower quadrant in location, often with extension to the back. Rarely, right-sided diverticulitis occurs and can mimic acute appendicitis. The pain is usually distinguished from PDD, because it tends to be more severe, acute in onset, localized, and more persistent. Other symptoms can include chills, nausea, vomiting, anorexia, dysuria, and changes in bowel function that may range from constipation to diarrhea. The frequency of these secondary symptoms is typically related to the stage and severity of the diverticulitis.

On physical examination, the bowel sounds may be hyperactive, normal, decreased, or absent, depending on the stage of the process. Findings usually include left lower quadrant tenderness, with involuntary guarding if peritoneal inflammation exists. A tender, nonmobile mass, classically described as "sausagelike," is usually found in this area. Digital rectal examination may reveal tenderness and induration due to the inflammation adjacent to the sigmoid colon. As many as one fourth of patients have some colonic bleeding that is typically occult. Occasionally, mild hematochezia occurs, but massive bleeding is not a feature of diverticulitis.

Laboratory evaluation in the immunocompetent patient almost invariably reveals an increase in the total leukocyte count, with increased numbers of immature cells. In the elderly or immunocompromised patient, even severe acute diverticulitis may not manifest with an increased leukocyte count or fever, and pain may be muted. For these patients, a high index of suspicion is required to make an early diagnosis before generalized peritonitis ensues.

Course and Complications

The clinical course of diverticulitis can vary greatly. Factors that affect the clinical course include age, immune status, and whether the initial microperforation is contained. A small, well-contained diverticular abscess may resolve spontaneously. Most cases, however, progress to a stage that requires medical and/or surgical intervention, including intravenous antibiotics, percutaneous drainage, or staged surgical resection. In order of frequency, fistulas, free perforation with intra-abdominal abscess, and obstruction are the most common complications of diverticulitis. They occur when the acute inflammation accompanying diverticular perforation is not contained locally.

Fistulas

Fistulas are probably the most common complication, occurring in 10 to 25 per cent of patients. Although fistulas may form between the colon and any of a number of organs, the most common is the bladder (i.e., colovesical fistula). Other sites of fistula formation include the vagina, uterus, small bowel, skin (e.g., perineum, scrotum, buttock, abdominal wall), ureter, and portal system, and other parts of the colon. Colovesical fistulas occur less frequently in women, because the uterus and broad ligaments lie between the sigmoid colon and the bladder.

A colovesical fistula should be suspected when recurrent or refractory urinary tract infection, pneumaturia, or fecaluria occurs. These findings in the presence of suspected diverticulitis require cystoscopy to make the diagnosis. Colonoscopy, cystography, intravenous pyelography, and barium enema are unlikely to reveal the fistula itself, but they may be useful in excluding other diseases that can cause fistulas.

Passage of stool and gas through the organ to which the fistula has formed is often the first sign of fistula development. In the case of coloenteric or colocolonic fistulas, diarrhea and steatorrhea occur instead. Confirmation of the clinical suspicion of a fistula is often difficult. For skin fistulas, a fistulogram can be performed, and contrast radiography or CT can be useful in detecting colovesical fistulas. Other fistulas are less likely to be diagnosed by contrast studies, perhaps because of their small diameters.

Fistulas are unlikely to respond to antibiotic treatment and are an indication for surgery. However, colovesical fistulas in elderly patients who are poor surgical risks may be best treated medically.

Perforation

All diverticulitis is probably caused by at least microperforation of a diverticulum, but gross perforation with spillage of intraluminal contents is less common. Frank perforation should be suspected when there is persistent spiking fever despite antibiotics and a persistent mass on abdominal or rectal examination. The diagnosis can be confirmed and the process followed by abdominal CT, which may reveal matted bowel loops, fluid or pus collections, and elevation and fixation of the diaphragm. Plain upright abdominal films are useful for detecting free air under the diaphragm, but free air is not always present. If frank perforation is suspected, barium enema and lower endoscopy are best avoided.

Obstruction

Obstruction occurs in about 2 per cent of patients with diverticulitis. Small bowel obstruction is more common than colonic obstruction and occurs when loops of small bowel adjacent to the site of recurrent inflammation become involved in the acute process or the subsequent adhesions. This complication often manifests as a paralytic ileus with obstructive symptoms such as crampy pain, abdominal distention, and nausea. Colonic obstruction differs from typical small bowel obstruction in that altered bowel habits (i.e., severe constipation or diarrhea from leakage and secretion around the obstructed area) predominate. Plain supine and upright abdominal films can often establish the diagnosis and site of obstruction.

Useful Imaging and Diagnostic Procedures

Patients with uncomplicated diverticular disease typically have normal abdominal films. Diverticulitis, however, may cause a localized ileus adjacent to the inflamed sigmoid colon or an irregularity, a narrowing, or an extrinsic compression of the sigmoid colon. If free perforation has occurred, pneumoperitoneum may be seen on upright or lateral decubitus films.

A barium enema is contraindicated for the diagnosis of acute diverticulitis, because it can exacerbate the acute attack. The pressure used to perform the procedure can cause frank perforation and bacterial or chemical (barium) peritonitis. Sigmoidoscopy or colonoscopy also is best deferred until after the acute process has resolved.

Computed tomography is the procedure of choice for the diagnosis of diverticulitis. It is also used to follow the progression and resolution of the acute process and to detect complications such as abscesses or fistulas. Bowel opacification with oral contrast, such as 12 mL of Gastrografin in 500 mL of fluid the evening before scanning, plus one half as much just before the examination, helps avoid mistaking unopacified bowel loops for extracolonic abscesses, phlegmon, or colonic wall thickening. If diverticulitis exists, CT reveals diverticula and usually inflammatory infiltration of the pericolic fat; abscesses and fistulas can also be observed. Also, CT is useful in distinguishing acute diverticulitis from perforated colorectal carcinoma, other intra-abdominal causes of abscess or perforation, and pelvic inflammatory diseases. Overall, CT is the diagnostic procedure of choice for acute diverticulitis and its complications. It is the least invasive and the best at detecting early disease and its complications and can be done repeatedly, when needed, to follow the patient's course.

Pitfalls in Diagnosis

The diagnosis of acute diverticulitis can be difficult to make on purely clinical grounds, because the presenting symptoms and signs are not specific. In the elderly, the process can be muted so that few clinical clues are available. An early imaging procedure, especially abdominal CT, can confirm the presence of diverticula with evidence of inflammation or perforation, and it can exclude some of the conditions that have a similar clinical presentation.

DIVERTICULAR BLEEDING

Diverticular bleeding is caused by rupture of the vasa recta vessels at the antimesenteric margin of a single diverticulum. Bleeding is not typically associated with diverticulitis, but intimal thickening and medial thinning are often observed. Bleeding occurs most frequently at a mean age of 68 to 74 years. The right side of the colon is the site of 70 per cent of major diverticular bleeds, in contrast to the predominance of left-sided locations for PDD and diverticulitis. Although as many as 10 to 30 per cent of patients with diverticular disease may have some evidence of bleeding during the course of their disease, only 3 to 5 per cent experience a severe bleed. Diverticular bleeding and angiodysplasias are the two most common causes of life-threatening lower GI hemorrhage in the older age groups, though.

Presenting Signs and Symptoms

The prevalence of asymptomatic diverticular disease is high, and 16 per cent of diverticular bleeds are the initial presenting sign of diverticular disease. The typical event is the painless passage of bright red or maroon blood per rectum; with slower bleeding, melena may be observed. The typical patient is an elderly man or woman, usually with no previous history of bowel problems or perhaps with known but uncomplicated diverticulosis, who notices the sudden onset of rectal urgency, sometimes with mild cramping and followed soon after by bleeding. Except in those with rapid hemorrhage, the signs and symptoms of hypovolemia or shock are often absent. The blood loss may be continual or intermittent over several days. Seventy to eighty per cent of patients stop bleeding with conservative medical management. The 10-year incidence of recurrent bleeding is 20 to 25 per cent after the initial episode and about 50 per cent after a second episode. The physical examination is often unremarkable. Auscultation of the abdomen usually reveals normal active bowel sounds; the abdomen is soft, nontender, and without guarding or rebound tenderness.

Laboratory Findings

The hematocrit, depending on the rate of bleeding and the time since its onset, may or may not be significantly decreased. After volume repletion has occurred, the hematocrit more accurately reflects the true extent of blood loss. Normal red cell indices (e.g., mean corpuscular hemoglobin concentration, mean corpuscular volume, red cell distribution width) reflect acute blood loss. Thrombocytosis may be observed, reflecting the acute loss of blood volume; this may be accompanied by prerenal azotemia or an increasing serum sodium concentration. The total leukocyte count is usually normal but may be slightly elevated because of stress-induced demargination.

Diagnostic Studies

All cases of apparently lower GI hemorrhage must exclude the possibility of a brisk upper GI bleed proximal to the ligament of Treitz. This can be accomplished by passing a nasogastric tube into the stomach to sample the gastroduodenal contents. The aspiration of clear or bile-stained fluid without gross blood provides a 90 per cent probability that the source of bleeding is distal to the ligament of Treitz. After this simple test has been performed, other diagnostic procedures can be directed exclusively at evaluating the lower GI tract.

Evaluation of the lower GI tract is initiated by performing (preferably flexible) proctosigmoidoscopy to exclude nondiverticular causes of bleeding, especially hemorrhoids and severe ulcerative proctitis. Little or no bowel preparation is necessary, and the procedure can be done quickly. If the site of bleeding has not been identified, the next diagnostic procedure is chosen based on the rate of bleeding and the patient's clinical status.

If the rate of bleeding is rapid (1 mL per minute or about 3 units of blood loss over a 24-hour period if sustained), the procedure of choice is angiography, which identifies the source of bleeding in 60 to 90 per cent of cases. Angiography does not show diverticular bleeding if the vessel is not actively bleeding at the moment of the dye injection, but it can reveal other potential or actively bleeding sources, such as vascular malformations. The procedure begins with injection of contrast medium into the superior mesenteric artery, because this vessel supplies the right colon, which is the usual site of diverticular hemorrhage. If contrast material extravasates into the bowel lumen, the procedure is discontinued unless interventional radiographic techniques are to be employed. If the results are negative or equivocal, the inferior mesenteric artery and the celiac axis are canulated to study the rest of the GI tract.

When bleeding is slower or a less invasive procedure is preferred, a ^{99m}Tc-labeled red blood cell scan can be performed. This study is less precise in localizing the source of bleeding, especially if frequent scans are not performed. Only the location of blood loss—not its cause—can be determined, and the average time required for preparation and performance of the test is usually more than 2 hours. Its advantage is that a very slow and/or intermittent bleed can be detected when images are obtained repeatedly over a 24-hour period.

Colonoscopy can be useful if results of the imaging studies are negative or if the rate of bleeding is slow. Adequate bowel preparation is needed for an optimal study. Barium enema is an alternative procedure, although it is not useful in detecting vascular malformations. After bleeding has ceased, even if the source has been tentatively identified, colonoscopy or barium enema is performed to exclude other potential causes of bleeding, such as polyps, cancer, hemorrhoids, and colitis. These lesions were detected in one third of elderly patients with known diverticular disease and GI bleeding in one large study.

POLYPS AND TUMORS OF THE COLON

By John H. Bond, M.D.
Minneapolis, Minnesota

COLORECTAL POLYPS

A colorectal polyp is a tissue growth that projects above the mucosal surface of the large bowel. Varying in size, some benign polyps are almost microscopic, whereas others are larger than 8 cm in diameter. Benign polyps are grossly described as either pedunculated or sessile, depending on whether they contain a discrete stalk. As polyps grow, they can ulcerate and cause rectal bleeding. Very rarely, large distal polyps cause symptoms of partial, intermittent bowel obstruction. The great majority of polyps, however, are asymptomatic lesions that are detected by screening studies or as the result of diagnostic examinations performed for other reasons. The main importance of polyps is the relationship of neoplastic polyps (adenomas) to colorectal cancer. Colorectal polyps are common, being reported in more than 30 per cent of postmortem examinations of persons older than 60 years of age in western countries.

Histologically, polyps are classified as either neoplastic (adenomas) or non-neoplastic (Table 1). Non-neoplastic polyps have no premalignant potential and include hamartomas, inflammatory polyps, lymphoid aggregates, and hyperplastic polyps. Neoplastic polyps or adenomas have measurable malignant potential and are subclassified as tubular, tubulovillous, or villous, depending on the presence and the fraction of the polyp that is composed of

Table 1. Classification of Large Bowel Polyps

Non-neoplastic
Hamartomas: juvenile, Peutz-Jeghers polyps
Hyperplastic polyps
Inflammatory polyps
Lymphoid aggregates
Neoplastic (Adenomas)
Tubular adenomas
Tubulovillous adenomas
Villous adenomas

villous tissue. Tubular adenomas contain straight or branched tubules of dysplastic tissue. Villous adenomas contain long, fingerlike projections of dysplastic epithelium. Of polyps removed from adult patients at colonoscopy, approximately 70 per cent are adenomas; 75 to 85 per cent of these adenomas are classified according to the World Health Organization (WHO) criteria as being tubular (0 to 25 per cent villous tissue), 10 to 25 per cent as being tubulovillous (25 to 75 per cent villous tissue), and less than 5 per cent as being villous (75 to 100 per cent villous tissue).

NON-NEOPLASTIC POLYPS

Non-neoplastic polyps constitute about 30 per cent of all polyps resected at colonoscopy. About 50 per cent of all polyps that are 5 mm in diameter or smaller are non-neoplastic.

Hyperplastic Polyps

Hyperplastic polyps are small protrusions that arise from the mucosal surface and have a slightly altered histologic architecture, which consists of a characteristic serrated histologic pattern due to infolding of the normal columnar epithelium. The surface cells appear otherwise normal, without the cellular crowding, pseudostratification, and hyperchromatism that is characteristic of adenomas. Cellular proliferation is confined to the basal zone of the crypts. Endoscopically, hyperplastic polyps are usually small, round, sessile growths smaller than 5 mm in diameter with a color that is similar to the surrounding mucosa. They are most commonly seen in the distal left colon, increase with age, and are more common in males than in females.

Hyperplastic polyps virtually never cause symptoms. They are typically diagnosed by screening flexible sigmoidoscopy or by colonoscopy performed for other reasons. Larger ones may be detected by barium enema radiographic studies. Endoscopic biopsy is needed to reliably distinguish hyperplastic polyps from adenomas.

Hyperplastic polyps have no premalignant potential per se. A number of retrospective uncontrolled series, however, have suggested that a hyperplastic polyp found in the lower left colon during screening flexible sigmoidoscopy is predictive of an increased prevalence of proximal adenomas and therefore is an indication for full colonoscopy. However, at least three prospective studies, performed in asymptomatic patients at average risk for cancer and including comparison with an appropriate control group, failed to confirm this relationship. Current practice guidelines therefore do not recommend colonoscopy for the finding of a hyperplastic polyp during screening flexible sigmoidoscopy.

When a small polyp (5 mm or smaller) is found during sigmoidoscopy, it should be biopsied to determine whether it is a hyperplastic polyp or an adenoma. Most patients with adenomas require colonoscopy (discussed further on). If nothing other than a hyperplastic polyp or polyps is found, colonoscopy is not indicated. Because 70 to 85 per cent of polyps larger than 5 mm found at sigmoidoscopy are adenomas, a more cost-effective approach in these patients may be to proceed to colonoscopy directly without biopsy during sigmoidoscopy to save the cost of an additional pathology fee. For smaller polyps, biopsies performed during sigmoidoscopy are cost-effective because they obviate the need for subsequent colonoscopy in about half of patients.

Juvenile Polyps

Juvenile polyps are hamartomatous mucosal growths that consist mainly of retention cystic glands rather than a proliferation of epithelial cells as seen in hyperplastic and adenomatous polyps. Juvenile polyps are acquired lesions that are most commonly found in children between 2 and 10 years of age, rarely being seen in the first year of life. They usually either slough or regress spontaneously, although they are occasionally found in young adults. Most juvenile polyps are solitary and pedunculated and are located in the sigmoid colon or rectum. The stroma of these polyps has a generous vascular supply, and the most common presenting complaint is rectal bleeding. Occasionally, low rectal juvenile polyps may prolapse from the anus during defecation. Because of the high risk of bleeding, juvenile polyps should usually be endoscopically resected when detected.

Familial juvenile polyposis is a rare autosomal, dominantly inherited condition in which multiple hamartomas occur in the colon and, in some kindreds, throughout the gastrointestinal tract. The different familial patterns are believed to be due to variable mutations of a single gene, perhaps related to the familial adenomatous polyposis (FAP) gene. Although the juvenile polyps in these families are not premalignant, the condition is associated with an increased risk of adenomatous polyps and of colorectal cancer. This cancer risk mandates that all colorectal polyps found in these patients be resected. No reports have appeared linking upper gastrointestinal tract carcinoma to this genetic condition.

Peutz-Jeghers Syndrome

The Peutz-Jeghers syndrome is an autosomal, dominantly inherited genetic condition consisting of mucocutaneous pigmentation and gastrointestinal hamartomatous polyps. The condition is rare, occurring about one-tenth as frequently as FAP. The gastrointestinal polyps are most common in the small intestine, but they also occur in the colon and stomach. Acute and chronic gastrointestinal bleeding is a common early presenting manifestation of the disease; later, as the polyps grow, intussusception or intestinal obstruction may occur. Mucocutaneous pigmentation occurs in more than 95 per cent of affected patients. These melanin deposits are most commonly found around the mouth, nose, lips, buccal mucosa, hands, and feet.

Patients with Peutz-Jeghers syndrome have an increased risk of both intestinal tract and extraintestinal cancer. Gastric and duodenal cancers are most common, but cancers are also reported in the distal small bowel and colon. Whether special screening measures would be beneficial in affected families has not yet been determined.

NEOPLASTIC COLORECTAL POLYPS: THE POLYP-CANCER SEQUENCE

Epidemiologic, pathologic, and genetic studies indicate that most colorectal cancers arise in previously benign, neoplastic polyps or adenomas. Some degree of dysplasia exists in all adenomas. Dysplasia is classified as being either low grade or high grade. The latter term includes previously used designations of superficial carcinoma or carcinoma in situ, terms that have now been abandoned clinically because they connote an incorrect impression of clinical malignancy, often leading to overtreatment. Approximately 5 to 7 per cent of adenomas exhibit high-grade dysplasia, and 4 to 7 per cent show invasive carcinoma (carcinoma penetrating through the muscularis mucosa layer) at the time of resection. The likelihood of high-grade dysplasia increases with polyp size and villous component. Adenomas are monoclonal, being derived from a single stem cell mutation, perhaps involving the FAP gene. The cause of colorectal adenomas appears to involve both inherited genetic factors and acquired environmentally induced genetic alterations. Most simple small tubular adenomas appear to remain static, whereas a few grow and develop villous changes and high-grade dysplasia. As these advanced adenomas grow, a series of acquired genetic mutations and chromosome deletions occur, leading to invasive carcinoma.

Although the adenoma-to-carcinoma sequence can probably never be directly proved, compelling indirect evidence supports the relationship, including the following observations:

1. The prevalence of adenomas in different countries parallels that of colorectal carcinoma; the average age of patients with adenomas is 5 to 7 years younger than that of patients with carcinoma.
2. Benign adenomatous tissue is frequently found contiguous with small cancers, and in western countries small carcinomas without adenomatous components are rare.
3. As adenomas grow, they exhibit increasing signs of malignant transformation, including villous change, high-grade dysplasia, and acquired genetic mutations and chromosome deletions.
4. Carcinomas arising in the FAP and hereditary nonpolyposis colorectal cancer syndromes are preceded by histologically typical adenomas.
5. The anatomic location of adenomas and cancers in the large bowel is virtually identical in both sporadic cancers and the familial cancer syndromes.
6. Synchronous adenomas are found in 30 to 40 per cent of patients with colorectal cancer, and following curative resection, metachronous adenomas develop in a similar fraction.

Primary Prevention of Adenomas and Cancer

If most colorectal cancers arise in neoplastic polyps, preventing or resecting these polyps should reduce the incidence and mortality of colorectal cancer. Epidemiologic studies and studies of migrating populations clearly indicate that environmental factors, especially dietary substances, influence the incidence of the disease. Several dietary components have been implicated including excessive fat consumption and insufficient intake of fruits, vegetables, and fiber. Also, several vitamins (A, E, C, and folate), minerals (calcium, selenium), and drugs (aspirin and other nonsteroidal anti-inflammatory agents) may protect against the development of colorectal cancer.

Increasing the ingestion of vegetables, fruits, and fiber and reducing fat intake are likely to improve the overall quality of an individual's diet. However, specific recommendations about vitamins and other micronutrients cannot yet be made pending the results of controlled chemoprevention trials.

Secondary Prevention of Cancer

Secondary prevention of colorectal cancer results from the detection and resection of colorectal adenomas. Colonoscopy is the procedure of choice for both the diagnosis and the treatment of colorectal adenomas. It is much more accurate than barium enema for the detection of small polypoid lesions, even when high-quality, double-contrast techniques are employed for radiographic studies. The entire large bowel can be thoroughly examined by experienced endoscopists, with minimal discomfort, in more than 95 per cent of patients. The most important advantage of colonoscopy is the opportunity to biopsy suspicious lesions directly and to resect most polyps of the colon. A simple examination, which usually takes 30 minutes or less to complete, can thus be both diagnostic and therapeutic.

Major complications of bleeding and perforation, although rare, occur more commonly with colonoscopy (0.1 to 0.2 per cent) than with barium radiographic studies (0.02 per cent) or flexible sigmoidoscopy (0.01 to 0.04 per cent). In addition, the cost of colonoscopy at present is significantly greater than the cost of barium enema plus flexible sigmoidoscpy. Although these cost and risk comparisons seem to favor the initial strategy of performing barium enema plus flexible sigmoidoscopy, one must consider the need to perform subsequent colonoscopy in patients found to have a cancer or polyp. Because this can occur in 30 to 40 per cent of high-risk patients or in patients with an abnormal screening test result, the two strategies are, on average, equally expensive and risky.

Because most adenomas are asymptomatic, they are usually found during screening flexible sigmoidoscopy or are incidental findings made during patient evaluations performed for other reasons. In the United States, a fundamental change has occurred in the way most of these lesions are initially diagnosed. In the past, a large fraction of patients were referred for colonoscopy because a barium radiographic study had detected a polypoid filling defect. Today, the majority of patients referred for possible colon disease undergo primary colonoscopy without a prior barium enema. The reasons for this change are the increasing awareness that colonoscopy is substantially more accurate than radiography and that it is safe and well tolerated when performed by experienced examiners. In addition, it can now be performed at an average cost equal to the alternate strategy of performing barium enema plus proctosigmoidoscopy if one factors in the cost of false-positive results on barium enema and the need to do colonoscopy anyway whenever abnormal findings are detected. The added convenience to the patient of having both diagnosis and perhaps treatment accomplished at one examination with a single preparation also has influenced the shift in management of these patients.

Today, a large fraction of adenomas are detected as the result of a screening test (proctosigmoidoscopy or fecal occult blood tests) for colorectal cancer. Although screening flexible sigmoidoscopy using a conventional 60-cm endoscope is theoretically capable of diagnosing 60 to 70 per cent of all colorectal neoplasms, in practice the average sensitivity for all adenomas is 50 to 60 per cent. Screening fecal occult blood tests, which can be highly sensitive for detecting colorectal cancers, are not very sensitive for detecting adenomas. Most small polyps diagnosed as the result of fecal occult blood screening are detected incidently. Reports from large trials indicate that this method can detect 20 to 40 per cent of adenomas larger than 1 cm.

Cohort and case-controlled studies of the effect of proctosigmoidoscopy suggest that removing all adenomas in the distal large bowel substantially reduces both the incidence of and the mortality from rectal and rectosigmoid cancer. A recent landmark report from the United States National Polyp Study showed that removing all adenomas from a large group of patients with these lesions, plus follow-up colonoscopy surveillance every 3 years for an average of about 6 years, reduced the expected total incidence of colorectal cancer by 76 to 90 per cent.

Management of Malignant Polyps

A malignant polyp is one that appears benign during colonoscopy but is then found to have malignant cells that invade the submucosa. The clinician must then decide whether further surgical resection is required or whether the likelihood of residual cancer or adjacent lymph node spread is insufficient to warrant the risk of surgery. A large number of outcome studies are now available to confirm that the risk of residual cancer after colonoscopic polypectomy of a malignant polyp is less than the risk of surgery if a number of criteria are favorable. Favorable criteria include the following: The endoscopist is confident that polypectomy was complete, the cancer invasion does not extend to the margin of cautery and resection, the cancer is not poorly differentiated, and there is no histologic evidence of vascular or lymphatic invasion. Patients with these favorable prognostic criteria should have follow-up colonoscopy in 3 months to check for residual polyp tissue at the resection site, especially if the malignant polyp was sessile. If the results of this early follow-up examination are normal, subsequent surveillance is the same as that recommended for patients with benign adenomas.

Patients with malignant polyps and unfavorable prognostic criteria should usually be referred for surgical colectomy. In patients who are poor risks for surgery, or in those with low rectal polyps that would require an abdominoperineal resection, the risk of further treatment may not exceed the relatively low risk of residual cancer.

Follow-Up Surveillance After Polypectomy

Most patients who have undergone resection of one or more colorectal adenomas have an increased subsequent risk of recurrent adenomas and of colorectal cancer and may benefit from long-term colonoscopic follow-up surveillance. Several recent studies stress that all patients are not at equal risk after undergoing initial polypectomy. Surveillance recommendations must be structured in a cost-effective way to address the specific risks and needs of each patient. The stakes are high because more than 800,000 patients undergo colonoscopic polypectomy in the United States each year. If we err regarding the type and frequency of follow-up, patients will be placed at unnecessary risk for subsequent cancer, or precious medical resources will be wasted. For example, the cost of follow-up for patients found to have polyps represents 30 to 40 per cent of the overall cost of colorectal cancer screening. If adequate resources are to be devoted to screening, postpolypectomy surveillance must be performed in a cost-effective manner.

Studies have shown that patients with only single, small (1 cm or less) tubular adenomas have no measurable subsequent increased risk of colorectal cancer. However, patients with larger or multiple adenomas, or adenomas with villous changes or high-grade dysplasia, have an appreciable risk of later cancer unless careful surveillance is performed. Recent data from the National Polyp Study indicate that the presence of a strong family history of large bowel cancers or adenomas also increases the subsequent risk of cancer in patients undergoing polypectomy.

New polyps develop and grow slowly. It is estimated that, on average, it takes 10 to 12 years for a polyp to develop in a grossly normal-appearing colon, grow to a clinically significant size, and then degenerate into a life-threatening cancer. Therefore, follow-up surveillance does not have to be performed frequently provided that accurate methods such as colonoscopy are employed. The National Polyp Study found that colonoscopy performed 3 years after the initial polypectomy was adequate to protect patients with adenomas from advanced lesions.

Based on all available data, recommendations for post-polypectomy surveillance have been made by the major digestive disease societies. Widespread adoption of these recommendations should substantially reduce the cost of postpolypectomy surveillance as currently practiced and at the same time provide adequate protection for this high-risk group. The recommendations are as follows:

1. Complete colonoscopy is performed at the time of polypectomy to detect and resect all synchronous adenomas. Additional clearing examinations may be required after resection of a large sessile adenoma or of multiple adenomas to ensure complete resection.
2. Repeat colonoscopy to check for missed synchronous and for metachronous adenomas is performed in 3 years for most patients with a single adenoma, or only a few adenomas, provided that they have had a high-quality initial examination.
3. Selected patients with multiple adenomas or those who have had a suboptimal initial clearing examination might require colonoscopy at 1 and 4 years.
4. After one normal 3-year follow-up examination, subsequent surveillance intervals may be increased to 5 years.
5. The presence of severe or high-grade dysplasia in a resected polyp does not, per se, modify recommendations 1 through 4.
6. If complete colonoscopy is not possible, flexible sigmoidoscopy plus double-contrast barium enema is an acceptable alternative.
7. Because patients undergoing resection of a single, small, tubular adenoma (<1 cm) do not have an increased subsequent risk of cancer, follow-up surveillance may not be indicated.
8. Surveillance should be individualized according to the age and comorbid conditions present in the patient and should be discontinued when it appears unlikely that continued follow-up is capable of prolonging life expectancy.

MALIGNANT TUMORS OF THE COLON AND RECTUM

Colorectal adenocarcinomas compose nearly 99 per cent of all large bowel malignancies. The disease is common (more than 160,000 new cases in the United States annually) and lethal (more than 65,000 annual deaths), yet it is readily curable when detected at an early stage (overall 5-year survival rate about 50 per cent). Complete surgical resection of all malignant tissue offers the only reasonable chance for cure, and postsurgical survival is roughly proportional to the anatomic extent of the tumor at the time

Table 2. Five-Year Survival After Resection of Colorectal Cancer

Dukes Stage	Five-Year Survival (%)
A	84–95
B	60–70
C	36–45
D	1–3

of resection (Table 2). When detected prior to the development of symptoms, most colorectal cancers are localized to the bowel wall (Dukes A and B cancers), and the 5-year survival rate averages about 80 per cent. By the time most colorectal cancers cause symptoms, however, the majority have spread to lymph nodes or beyond, and the chance of cure is less than 40 per cent.

Epidemiology, Etiology, and Pathogenesis

As described earlier in the discussion of adenomas, there is considerable geographic variation in the incidence of the disease, which appears to be environmental rather than genetic. Populations migrating from low-risk to high-risk countries (Japan to Hawaii, American- versus African-born blacks) experience a marked increase in the rate of colorectal cancer. Table 3 lists environmental factors that have been associated with an increased incidence. Recently, inherited genetic factors have also been implicated in the pathogenesis of colorectal cancer. Table 4 lists the three types of genetic and familial patterns currently recognized.

Familial Polyposis

The familial polyposis syndromes, including FAP and Gardner's syndrome, account for about 1 per cent of all cases of colorectal cancer. The disease is caused by an inherited autosomal dominant germ line mutation of a complex gene on chromosome 5 called the *APC* gene. The mutated gene results in the production of an abnormal truncated protein that leads to the proliferation of colonic epithelial cells and the formation of hundreds to thousands of colorectal adenomas. As the result of additional acquired mutations and chromosomal deletions, virtually all affected individuals experience colon cancer by age 40 years if a colectomy is not performed first.

Polyps begin to appear in late childhood. The disease is diagnosed by pedigree analysis, screening flexible sigmoidoscopy, and by recently developed genetic DNA tests employing blood lymphocyte analyses. Both the genetic tests and the flexible sigmoidoscopy should be performed at about age 10 to 12 years in all FAP family progeny. If the genetic test gives positive results, flexible sigmoidoscopy is repeated annually to determine when polyps emerge, indicating the need for colectomy. In persons with negative

Table 3. Environmental Factors Associated With Colorectal Cancer

Diet, especially animal fat
Low fiber intake
Low calcium intake
Elevated serum cholesterol concentration
Sedentary activity
Tobacco and alcohol use
Possible protective factors: vitamins A, C, E, selenium, nonsteroidal anti-inflammatory drugs

Table 4. Hereditary Risk of Colorectal Cancer

Adenomatous polyposis syndromes: familial adenomatous polyposis, Gardner's syndrome
Hereditary nonpolyposis colorectal cancer, site-specific colorectal cancer, cancer family syndrome
Genetic risk for sporadic colorectal cancer

results on genetic testing, flexible sigmoidoscopy should be performed about every 3 years until these tests prove to be 100 per cent accurate. Genetic tests are not recommended at earlier ages because there is no clinical need for them to protect the patient from cancer, and the results can interfere with complex parental-child and sibling social bonding and acceptance.

Gardner's syndrome consists of the same intestinal phenotype as FAP but is accompanied by a variety of benign extraintestinal growths, including osteomas, soft tissue tumors, dental abnormalities, and odontomas.

Hereditary Nonpolyposis Colorectal Cancer Syndromes

Hereditary nonpolyposis colorectal cancer (HNPCC) is an autosomal, dominantly inherited germ line mutation in which affected individuals develop a few adenomas with a high predisposition to cancer. The condition makes up 5 to 6 per cent of all colorectal cancer cases. Two variants are currently recognized: site-specific colorectal cancer and cancer family syndrome, which are synonymous with Lynch syndromes I and II, respectively. Colon cancers tend to occur at a young age (average 45 years), are often multiple, and are located in the right colon. The cancer family syndrome differs from site-specific colorectal cancer in that affected women also experience uterine, ovarian, and occasionally breast cancer at an increased rate. Four different genetic mutations have now been linked to different families with HNPCC. The mutations appear to interfere with the cells' normal ability to repair DNA replication errors.

HNPCC is currently diagnosed by pedigree analysis. The presence of three closely related individuals with colorectal cancer is highly suggestive, especially if a cancer has occurred before age 50 years. All progeny in HNPCC families should undergo colonoscopy every 2 years beginning at age 25 years, or 5 years younger than the earliest age at which the colorectal cancer was diagnosed in the family. With the identification of the abnormal genes responsible for HNPCC, reliable genetic tests should also soon be available.

Genetic Risk of Sporadic Cancers

One of the most intriguing and potentially important discoveries of recent years is the likelihood that a sizable fraction of sporadic cancers, which were previously believed to be environmentally induced, may have an underlying genetic predisposing cause. Epidemiologic studies show a threefold increased risk of colorectal cancer for individuals with one first-degree relative with the disease, and pedigree studies of adenoma incidence patterns suggest that at least 50 per cent of sporadic cancers may ultimately be due to a genetic predisposition to the disease. Whether a given individual acquires a cancer may depend on the combination of the genetic trait plus superimposed environmental factors.

The discovery of these inherited risk patterns indicates that individuals who have first-degree relatives with colorectal cancers or advanced adenomas should be screened.

The likelihood of inherited risk is greater when the affected relative acquired the disease at a younger age. Current recommendations are for colonoscopy surveillance every 5 years beginning at age 40 years for first-degree relatives (parents, siblings, children) of individuals with colorectal cancer or advanced adenomas diagnosed before the age of 65 years.

Other Risk Factors for Colorectal Cancer

Besides a family history of colorectal cancer, the three main risk factors for the disease are age older than 50 years, a personal past history of colorectal adenomas (discussed earlier), a personal past history of colorectal cancer (discussed further on), and chronic inflammatory bowel disease.

Carcinoma of the colon and rectum occurs much more frequently in patients with chronic ulcerative colitis than in the general population. Histologic dysplasia often precedes or occurs with the malignant transformation in the mucosa, and colonoscopic surveillance with multiple mucosal biopsies therefore has the potential to identify those persons at greatest risk.

Clinically, the risk of cancer is strongly related to both the duration and the extent of disease. Patients with pancolitis appear to have minimal risk until after 8 to 10 years of disease activity. Thereafter, the risk increases rapidly to more than 20 times that of the general population by 20 years of disease and to more than 30 times the risk of the general population by 30 years. Patients with left-sided colitis are also at increased risk; however, cancers tend to develop about 10 years later in these persons than in patients with universal colitis. Persons with ulcerative colitis limited to the rectum and sigmoid colon appear to have no appreciably increased risk. In ulcerative colitis, the distribution of cancer is uniform throughout the colon and at times is multifocal.

Carcinoma of the colon also occurs more frequently in patients with long-standing Crohn's disease. However, the risk appears to be less than that seen in ulcerative colitis, and because it may not be as consistently associated with mucosal dysplasia, surveillance is not currently recommended.

Although no controlled study has proved the efficacy of colonoscopic surveillance for patients with chronic ulcerative colitis, considerable indirect evidence supports its use. Colonoscopy with multiple biopsies is recommended every 2 years beginning 8 years after the onset of pancolitis, or 15 years after the onset of left-sided colitis. High-grade dysplasia confirmed by an expert pathologist or persistent low-grade dysplasia is an indication for colectomy in a patient who is a good surgical risk. Fewer than 10 per cent of patients under this type of surveillance program acquire dysplastic changes prompting consideration of surgery.

Symptoms and Diagnosis of Colorectal Cancer

Patients with symptoms or signs of colorectal cancer are *not* candidates for screening (see further on) but require prompt complete examination of the colon. The main early signs and symptoms of this disease are a change in bowel movement pattern, abdominal discomfort, rectal bleeding (gross or occult), or unexplained microcytic hypochromic anemia. Late signs and symptoms include colon obstruction, perforation, a palpable abdominal mass, and weight loss.

Colonoscopy is the primary diagnostic procedure of choice for patients suspected of having a colorectal cancer because of a positive screening test result, signs or symptoms of colorectal cancer, or the presence of special risk factors. A recent study from Indiana shows comparable accuracy of colonoscopy and barium enema for detecting cancers (96 per cent and 85 per cent, respectively). Colonoscopy also has the distinct advantage of allowing immediate biopsy of possible cancers and resection of most synchronous polyps. If colonoscopy is incomplete or suboptimal, the combination of double-contrast barium enema and flexible sigmoidoscopy is an acceptable alternative.

Screening for Colorectal Neoplasia

For the following reasons, colorectal cancer is ideally suited to detection by screening.

1. It is sufficiently common and lethal to warrant expenditure of health care resources.
2. It has a long, curable preclinical phase.
3. Safe and accurate diagnostic tests are available.
4. Early detection leads to prolonged survival.

Currently, only two screening tests that are capable of satisfying the WHO criteria for a screening test are available for colorectal cancer. They are the fecal occult blood test and flexible sigmoidoscopy. The WHO criteria require a screening test to be effective, improving both mortality and function. The test must be simple and therefore generally available and acceptable. Benefits must outweigh detriments, and the test should have a favorable cost-benefit relationship.

Flexible sigmoidoscopy performed by experienced, well-trained examiners is safe, well-tolerated, accurate, and reasonably inexpensive, and it is capable of detecting 50 to 70 per cent of all colorectal neoplasias. Everything known about the procedure suggests that its widespread use in the average-risk population should reduce mortality from colorectal cancer. However, screening efficacy remains unproved because a definitive randomized, controlled trial has never been performed. Long-term descriptive studies using rigid proctoscopy suggest that screening examinations of the rectum can greatly reduce the incidence and mortality of rectal cancer. Recent case-controlled studies suggest that screening with flexible sigmoidoscopy every 10 years or less might reduce mortality from cancer of the distal colon and rectum by 60 to 70 per cent. A large National Cancer Institute–funded multicenter trial using flexible sigmoidoscopy is currently under way.

Annual fecal occult blood test screening of average-risk (older than 50 years of age, no high-risk factors), asymptomatic individuals, followed by colonoscopy for all positive test results, has been shown in long-term trials to reduce mortality from colorectal cancer by 33 to 43 per cent. All current randomized controlled trials report that this approach detects a high percentage (70 to 90 per cent) of cancers, that the diagnosed cancers are at an early favorable stage, and that survival after diagnosis is prolonged.

Based on the preceding studies, current screening guidelines promulgated by the American Cancer Society, the WHO, and the National Cancer Institute recommend annual fecal occult blood test screening and flexible sigmoidoscopy every 5 years for average-risk individuals beginning at age 50 years. Screening should be continued until it is no longer likely that further screening is capable of prolonging useful life. Depending on each individual's health and comorbid conditions, screening can usually be discontinued at about age 75 years, especially if previous screens have had normal results.

Follow-Up Surveillance After Surgical Resection of Colorectal Cancer

The goals of surveillance after curative resection of a colorectal cancer are to detect treatable recurrences, missed synchronous cancers or adenomas, and new metachronous neoplasia. Except in a few selected patients, curative treatment of recurrent large bowel cancer is rarely possible at present, and palliation for unresectable recurrent cancer is not very effective. Furthermore, little evidence exists that palliative treatment is more effective applied early in comparison with when recurrences cause symptoms. Therefore, the main objectives of follow-up surveillance in most patients are to detect curable synchronous and metachronous adenomas and carcinomas. The incidence of synchronous cancers and polyps in the colon of a patient with a known cancer is reported to be 2 to 7 per cent and 25 to 45 per cent, respectively. Metachronous cancers and adenomas are reported in 2 to 5 per cent and 20 to 40 per cent of patients, respectively.

Based on available data, the following is presented as a perioperative management plan for patients with potentially curable colorectal cancer. Compared with traditional follow-up practices still used in many centers, this program consists of more accurate studies performed less frequently and directed primarily at reducing mortality from the disease.

1. Colonoscopy is performed during the perioperative period to clear the colon of synchronous neoplasia, preferably preoperatively so that cancers and large polyps can be included in the resection. If precluded before surgery by an obstructing left colon cancer, clearing colonoscopy is performed 3 to 6 months postoperatively if no distant metastases are found at surgery.
2. Postoperative visits are scheduled as needed to educate the patient about symptoms of early recurrence, check for postsurgical complications or problems, and provide medical and emotional support.
3. Repeat colonoscopy is performed every 3 years to detect metachronous neoplasia.
4. Serial rectal evaluation (digital, proctoscopy) is reserved for selected patients undergoing sphincter-sparing, low anterior resection of rectal cancers (see further on).

Treatable Recurrent Colorectal Cancer

With modern surgical techniques, anastomotic (suture line) recurrences of cancers of the abdominal colon (above the rectum) are rare. Resection of these few recurrences rarely results in long-term survivors. Thus, nearly all recurrences of proximal colon cancer occur outside the bowel and are not detected by follow-up surveillance examinations of the colon. A few suture line recurrences are found, but this rarely leads to curative therapy.

Local recurrences in the area of the anastomosis do, of course, often occur after anterior resection of Dukes B or C rectosigmoid cancers. Since these recurrences are amenable to radiation, or sometimes second surgical resections, these patients should be followed more closely with flexible sigmoidoscopy every 3 to 6 months for a period of 2 years.

Long-term survival has been reported in patients who have undergone surgical resection of solitary hepatic and, less commonly, pulmonary metastases. Some report that about 20 per cent of patients who have undergone curative resection of colorectal cancers will acquire isolated hepatic metastases; about 20 per cent of these metastases are ultimately resectable, with a 5-year survival rate of about 20 per cent. Thus, the total number of patients with a favorable outcome is very small and may not justify routine intensive surveillance for all patients. Rather, selected patients whose health is good enough to tolerate hepatic or pulmonary resection, and who have colorectal cancers with a substantial likelihood of metastasis (Dukes B or C), might be offered special intensive surveillance.

Because the majority of solitary metastases occur in the first 2 years after colon resection, this surveillance usually should not be prolonged beyond that interval. Surveillance for this select group (which composes only 15 to 20 per cent of all colorectal cancer patients) includes serial chest films every 3 to 6 months and serum carcinoembryonic antigen determinations every 2 months. Routine surveillance with either abdominal or pelvic computed tomography scans has not proved cost-effective, and liver function tests are insufficiently sensitive to be of value.

ANORECTAL AND PERIANAL DISORDERS

By Bertram A. Portin, M.D.,
Ronald F. Teitler, M.D.,
and Fred E. Boehmke, M.D.
Buffalo, New York

An appropriate history, inspection, and palpation constitute the cornerstone of the physical diagnosis of perianal and anorectal diseases. To utilize these techniques properly, the clinician must have a thorough understanding of the anatomy of this region and the pathologic conditions that affect it.

TERMINOLOGY AND ANATOMY

Although anorectal anatomy is constant, the terminology is often variable, confusing, and conflicting. Three general areas are included in the anatomic description. The *perianal area* is limited medially by the anal verge and laterally by an arbitrary distance of 2 to 3 inches. The verge is the external portion of the anal opening. The entire area is covered by skin (like any other epidermal area). The external sphincters lie subcutaneously and surround the verge. Lateral to the sphincters are subcutaneous potential spaces that are significant in the development of localized abscesses and fistulas.

The *anal canal* is the terminal portion of the digestive tract. Proximally, it begins at the anorectal line. This line marks the junction between intestinal mucosa and the squamous epithelium of the anal canal. The first centimeter is a transitional zone similar to that found in other body areas where mucosa meets skin; it is the site of the anal crypts and columns that are important in the development of the common cryptogenic abscess. Distally, the anal canal ends at the anal verge.

The third region is the *rectum*, a mucosal tube whose proximal border lies at about the level of the third sacral vertebra. The rectum descends along the hollow of the sacrum for about 10 to 15 cm and ends at the anorectal line. The course of the rectum is in an anterocaudal direction until the last 4 or 5 cm, where there is approximately a 90-degree angulation to a more posterocaudal direction. This angulation is the result of traction by the puborectal muscle in an anterior direction.

Muscles

The *levator muscles* are a striated series of support slings that extend from the bony pelvis to the region of the lower rectum. The iliococcygeal and pubococcygeal muscles support the lower rectum in a vertical plane, and the puborectal muscle supports it in a horizontal plane. The puborectal muscle is responsible for creating and maintaining the anorectal angle. Its integrity is vital for fecal continence.

The *internal sphincter muscle* is a thickening of the most distal portion of the circular smooth muscle layer of the rectum. Its lowest portion actually lies about 1 cm below the anorectal line. Hypertrophy, spasm, and fibrosis of this portion of the internal sphincter are related to the pathogenesis of chronic anal fissure.

The circular rings of skeletal muscle surrounding the anus and anal canal are the *external sphincters*. In reality, they are extensions of the levator ani muscles and are involved with continence and the control of defecation.

Blood Vessels and Lymphatics

The blood supply of the anorectum is important, because the most common disease of this region, hemorrhoids, is a vascular condition. The *superior hemorrhoidal veins* drain into the portal system via the inferior mesenteric venous system. Thus, portal cirrhosis may be associated with hemorrhoidal disease owing to the restricted outflow caused by portal hypertension. The middle and inferior hemorrhoidal veins drain into the systemic circulation via the internal iliac system. The lymphatic drainage of the anorectum follows the vascular pattern. Perianal and anal canal lymphatics drain to the inguinal lymph nodes. The more proximal lymphatic drainage is cephalad toward the inferior mesenteric and internal iliac nodes.

Innervation

The external sphincters, levators, and sensory portion of the anal canal are supplied by somatic nerves. The autonomic nervous system provides sensation (distention and pressure), both stimulatory and inhibitory types, through motor innervation of the internal sphincter and the more proximal intrinsic muscles of the rectum. These muscles control propulsion and participate in the defecatory reflex.

PATIENT HISTORY

As with many diseases, the diagnosis can frequently be made by proper history alone. Therefore, an important part of the diagnostic process is knowing what to ask and knowing what the answers indicate. Bleeding, pain, itching, control problems, stool abnormalities (constipation, diarrhea, foul-smelling stools, frothy stools, acholic stools), and abdominal cramping constitute the major symptoms of this region. However, it is not sufficient to elicit a history of pain. Its location, intensity, character, time relationship, and relationship to defecation and swelling are important factors that differentiate its nature. Constipation means different things to many people. Some confuse irregularity with constipation; others do not appreciate that the diarrhea of fecal impaction is primarily a constipation problem. Therefore, careful questions bordering on tedious attention to minute detail may be rewarding in establishing a diagnosis in a difficult case.

PHYSICAL EXAMINATION

Good illumination, appropriate diagnostic instruments, patient relaxation and comfort, and examiner comfort are the essentials of a good anorectal examination. Either the lateral Sims' position or the knee-chest position is satisfactory. In noting pathology, the clinician should remember that the position of examination may vary and that it is necessary to have a standard reference point. Reference should be made to right and left or posterior and anterior, rather than to positions on the face of a clock.

Inspection

Inspection is the appropriate first step in the physical examination. Most patients are apprehensive about rectal examinations. Embarrassment, expected discomfort, and fear of the diagnosis all contribute to apprehension. Patience, gentleness, and conversation may help allay fear and divert the patient's attention.

The perianal area should be inspected for the various dermatoses; idiopathic pruritus ani is the most common. Differentiation from secondary pruritus, psoriasis, lichen sclerosus, basal cell cancer, or Bowen's or Paget's disease may require a trial of nonspecific therapy, hygienic measures, or even biopsy.

Inspection often provides the diagnosis of para-anal or ischiorectal abscess, external hemorrhoids, thrombotic hemorrhoids, fistula, hidradenitis suppurativa, condylomata acuminata, or fissure. The pilonidal area should be inspected for the telltale intergluteal dimple or sinus. During inspection, the clinician can glean valuable information by having the patient bear down. Levator weakness, hemorrhoidal prolapse, or even complete rectal procidentia, cystocele, rectocele, or uterine prolapse may become evident with this maneuver.

Palpation

Tactile examination is done both by palpation of the perianal area and by digital rectal examination. Direct palpation to elicit tender areas can detect such diseases as early deep abscess or coccygodynia. Gentle lateral separation of the anus by stretching the buttocks may elicit pain that provides presumptive evidence of anal canal spasm and an associated anal fissure.

Careful digital examination is a valuable diagnostic measure. All too often the examination is done rapidly and solely for the purpose of ruling out a large rectal cancer. Far more information is available beyond the palpation for a mass lesion. It is helpful to develop a habit of circumferential examination that begins and ends at the same point. A well-lubricated, gloved index finger gently inserted while the patient is straining allows easy access to the anal canal. The state of the sphincters, both external and internal, and the state of pliability or rigidity of the soft tissues of the anal outlet provide information about sphincter spasm, stricture, and sphincter incompetence. Reassurance and diversion help relax the patient. Additional questions about the patient's history can provide this diversion.

On insertion of the examining finger, a gentle and sequential examination of the rectum and adjacent organs is done. The prostate gland (and sometimes the seminal vesicles), levator muscles, rectovaginal septum, cervix, uterus, cul-de-sac, coccyx, and sacrum can be evaluated by the examining finger. The diagnosis of internal hemorrhoids cannot be made by digital examination alone. The venous plexus is collapsed by digital pressure, and even large hemorrhoids can escape detection. With digital examination, the clinician can diagnose thrombosed hemorrhoids, hypertrophied anal papillae, neoplasms, rectovaginal fistulas, and submucosal, intermuscular, and supralevator abscesses. If a deep chronic anal ulcer, fissure, or other lesion is present, a digital examination may be much too painful to pursue without anesthesia. Topical anesthetic ointments generally are of little use. A few milliliters of a local anesthetic infiltrated into the painful area offers pain relief, and immediate sphincter relaxation allows both digital and anoscopic evaluation.

ANOSCOPY

After the initial digital examination, a well-lubricated anoscope is gently introduced into the anal canal. The pliability and distensibility of the anal sphincter assessed during digital examination determine the selection of an instrument of the proper diameter. During digital examination, the physician should be alert to the presence of anal canal pathology that needs to be visualized or that may make the introduction of an instrument too painful for the patient to tolerate. The entire circumference of the anal canal is now visualized through the anoscope. The lining of the canal and lower rectum is examined for changes in color, consistency, and vascular pattern suggestive of lesions or inflammatory bowel disease. As the anoscope is slowly withdrawn, the internal hemorrhoidal complexes come into view. The patient is asked to strain, and a determination is made of the extent of enlargement and prolapse. The area of the anal crypts and dentate line is examined for lesions as the instrument is further withdrawn. A primary fistulous opening in the base of an anal crypt may be seen, as may hypertrophic anal papillae, anorectal inflammatory disease, or anal canal neoplasm. As the area just distal to the crypt is traversed, anal fissures, if present, can be visualized.

LOWER INTESTINAL ENDOSCOPY

Although this article deals primarily with the diagnosis of anorectal pathology, subsequent evaluation of the lower intestinal tract to exclude additional disease processes is part of the complete colorectal evaluation. Several diagnostic modalities exist, and the appropriate choice depends on the experience of the examiner and the clinical situation.

Rigid Sigmoidoscopy

The 25-cm rigid sigmoidoscope provides visual access to the lower rectum and rectosigmoid colon. With the patient in either the knee-chest or the left Sims' position, the instrument is gently introduced transanally. This maneuver is accompanied by verbal reassurance from the physician. The sigmoidoscope is passed proximally into the rectum, and, if possible, the rectosigmoid angle is negotiated to gain further visualization. Introduction of the rigid sigmoidoscope involves careful manipulation to reduce discomfort to the patient. Most of the examination of the lower colon is accomplished on gradual withdrawal of the instrument, occasionally aided by the insufflation of small quantities of air. It is not always possible to advance the rigid sigmoidoscope to its full 25 cm. Too vigorous an attempt to do so may cause the patient undue pain and increase the risk of perforation of the bowel. The rigid sigmoidoscope allows an excellent view of the lower rectum and rectal ampulla; biopsy of pathology and endoscopic polypectomy can be readily performed. The limited diagnostic capability of the rigid sigmoidoscope, however, must be appreciated.

Flexible Sigmoidoscopy

While the diagnostic yield with the rigid sigmoidoscope (cancer, polyps) is approximately 35 per cent, the flexible fiberoptic sigmoidoscope (FFS), 60 cm in length, has increased the diagnostic capability of the examiner to 70 to 80 per cent. Flexible sigmoidoscopy is slightly more time-consuming and requires greater technical expertise. However, when properly performed, the examination is well accepted by patients. The visualization of the colonic mucosa is unparalleled. The superior diagnostic yield of the FFS suggests it as the instrument of choice when sigmoidoscopy is indicated. With this instrument, the clinician can detect lesions in the tortuous sigmoid colon that are unidentifiable on barium enema examination. This ability to achieve an early and accurate diagnosis has allowed more rapid institution of appropriate and effective therapy in a variety of disease conditions. The preoperative confirmation of disease and radiographically suspicious areas of the sigmoid colon can prevent unnecessary surgical procedures.

Flexible sigmoidoscopy is a diagnostic tool. Therapeutic procedures should not be performed in an office setting. If bleeding or perforation occurs, the sequelae can be extremely hazardous. Such electrosurgical procedures should be performed only in locations where immediate surgical intervention is possible.

Total Colonoscopy

Flexible fiberoptic sigmoidoscopy is never a substitute for total colonoscopy when the latter examination is indicated. Undiagnosed sources of bleeding in the colon require further investigation with total colonoscopy, as do unresolved symptoms and radiographically suspicious areas beyond the reach of the FFS. The electrosurgical removal of polyps, when detected, may be safely accomplished at the time of colonoscopy.

RADIOGRAPHY

Evaluation of the colon may necessitate barium enema examination to exclude undetected pathology beyond the reach of the sigmoidoscope. The choice between standard barium enema examination and an air-contrast enema depends on the facilities and skill of the radiologist and the information required. Specialized studies, such as angiography, may be indicated in the diagnosis of obscure sources of colonic bleeding. The appropriate combination of endoscopic and radiographic techniques provides optimal diagnostic certainty.

LABORATORY STUDIES

Hematologic evaluation is occasionally part of the colorectal examination. Determination of the hemoglobin and hematocrit may provide information regarding the extent and duration of colonic bleeding. Liver function tests can provide information about the presence of intercurrent disease, the surgical risk, or the presence of metastatic disease. Carcinoembryonic antigen (CEA) determinations aid in the evaluation and follow-up of cancer of the colon. In the evaluation of patients with anal and perianal condylomata acuminata, serologic studies for syphilis are indicated, because the coexistence of these diseases is not uncommon. Recently, coexistence of hepatitis B in patients with condylomata acuminata has also been noted. Liver function tests and possibly hepatitis B antigen studies should be performed prior to surgical intervention.

In the evaluation of patients with intractable diarrhea, stool and serologic studies for ova and parasites and stool culture for bacterial overgrowth provide information that can lead to the appropriate choice of treatment. Testing of the stool for occult blood can detect the presence of occult neoplasms of the colon. In the presence of intercurrent anal canal pathology, false-positive results may occur; treatment of such pathology, followed by repetition of the occult blood testing, may be considered prior to further extensive work-up. The examiner also must be aware that a negative result for stool occult blood does not definitively exclude colon carcinoma or polyps with any degree of certainty when compared with properly combined endoscopic and radiographic evaluation.

PERIANAL AND ANAL CANAL DISEASES

Pruritus Ani

Perianal itching, burning, and irritation are common complaints of the patient with a colorectal condition. What begins as a slight tickle, sometimes following a bowel movement, may progress to severe unremitting itching that is often worse at night. Scratching and other attempts to alleviate the situation only tend to make the problem worse. Questioning of the patient regarding dietary habits may reveal the excessive intake of substances such as spicy foods, beer, tomatoes, chocolate, coffee, tea, and cola drinks. The history may also suggest the presence of pinworms, diabetes mellitus, or allergic reactions to dyes, chemicals, or drugs. On examination, the perianal area is moist and the skin is thickened with a whitish, lichenified appearance. Corrugated, thickened folds extend radially from the anal verge. Superimposed excoriation from vigorous wiping or scratching may be present and may have caused the patient to observe blood on the toilet paper. Occasionally, superinfection with fungus is noted. In the female patient, any excessive vaginal discharge should be noted.

Bowen's Disease

This condition, manifested by plaquelike thickening and redness of the perianal skin, may mimic pruritus ani. Failure of the condition to respond to antipruritic measures should raise the suspicion of malignancy. Biopsy is necessary to make the diagnosis of this slow-growing carcinoma in situ. The high association of systemic malignancy with Bowen's disease indicates the necessity for further work-up.

Paget's Disease

A patient with this lesion may present with a complaint of perianal pruritus that is unresponsive to antipruritic measures. Examination reveals erythema, eczematoid changes, and either a moist and weeping lesion or a dry and scaly lesion of the perianal skin. Paget's disease is neoplastic. Diagnosis is made by biopsy of the lesion.

Squamous Cell Carcinoma of the Anus

The patient with squamous cell carcinoma of the anus most frequently presents with a complaint of bleeding and pain in the anal region. The assumption that the symptoms are caused by other benign conditions may delay the proper diagnosis. Squamous cell carcinoma may appear as a hard, grayish nodule in the perianal region or as an indolent anal canal ulceration with raised, rolled, pearl-gray borders. Careful examination and biopsy of suspicious lesions can lead to the appropriate treatment of this malignancy.

Anal Fissure or Ulcer

The patient with an anal fissure reports of a tearing or knifelike pain on defecation. This pain is frequently accompanied by bright red rectal bleeding. The pain may persist for hours following a bowel movement. As the disease progresses, the pain becomes severe and unremitting. An anal fissure may be accompanied by either marked constipation or diarrhea. Gentle spreading of the buttocks reveals the presence of a fissure, most commonly in the posterior midline or sometimes the anterior midline. Often there is an associated external edematous skin tag (sentinel pile). In the presence of marked spasm, the clinician should utilize local anesthesia to avoid causing severe pain during digital examination. Treatment should be instituted prior to more extensive evaluation. If spasm and pain are not severe, digital examination is done to detect the presence of any additional anal canal pathology. Anoscopy, when possible, reveals the anal fissure with fibromuscular tissue in its base. Just proximal to the fissure, a hypertrophic anal papilla may be seen. An atypical location of an anal fissure (off the midline) should lead to the suspicion of Crohn's disease, squamous cell carcinoma, or anal canal trauma.

Condylomata Acuminata

Condylomata acuminata, or venereal warts, appear as raised, tufted, pedunculated collections of pinkish or purplish lesions at the anal verge or within the anal canal. They may be accompanied by excessive moisture, a foul odor, or maceration of the adjacent skin. Other associated symptoms include itching and pain. Because of the possible sexual transmission of the virus associated with these lesions, an appropriate history should be taken. Also, appropriate serologic studies are indicated prior to treatment.

Hemorrhoidal Disease

Hemorrhoids are varicose dilatations of the superior and/or inferior hemorrhoidal venous plexuses. Dilatations of the superior hemorrhoidal plexuses, called internal hemorrhoids, originate above the anorectal line. Dilatations of the inferior venous plexuses, called external hemorrhoids, appear at the anal verge, where they are covered by modified anal skin. Increased hydrostatic pressure in the hemorrhoidal veins causes progressive weakening of the fibromuscular attachments of the musculus submucosae ani and results in progressive, saccular, serpiginous dilatation of the venous plexus. This dilatation causes prolapse of the venous plexus with its mucosal covering into the distal anal canal with defecation.

The etiologic factors in hemorrhoidal disease include a hereditary propensity, straining at stool, constipation, diarrhea, and pregnancy. A more obscure etiology, such as portal vein hypertension, uncompensated heart failure, pelvic tumors, and carcinoma of the rectum, must be excluded as well. The cardinal symptoms of internal hemorrhoids are bleeding and prolapse. Prolapse may lead to the patient's reporting the discharge of a foul-smelling, fecally stained, mucoid material from the anal canal, accompanied by secondary perianal irritation. Pain is not a symptom of internal hemorrhoids. If this complaint is present, its cause should be sought elsewhere.

Bleeding from internal hemorrhoids is almost always

bright red and ranges from a scant streaking of blood on the stool in the early stages of disease to spontaneous hemorrhage unrelated to defecation in the advanced stages. This bleeding can reach such significant proportions that a secondary anemia develops in some individuals.

The prolapse associated with internal hemorrhoids is progressive in nature. Initially, patients note that the hemorrhoids spontaneously reduce themselves after defecation. In advanced stages of the disease, the prolapse may require manual reduction after a bowel movement. Prolapse may occur spontaneously with exercise and may eventually become constant. In the latter stage of the disease, the patient is exposed to the risk of acute strangulation of the prolapsing hemorrhoids. On inspection, the clinician may note the presence of enlarged or possibly thrombosed external hemorrhoids, skin tags at the site of previous external thromboses, and possibly prolapsed internal hemorrhoids. Digital examination is usually noncontributory.

The diagnosis of internal hemorrhoids is made during anoscopy. With the anoscope inserted, and with the patient bearing down, the bulbous internal hemorrhoids are easily seen. If the patient continues to strain as the instrument is gently withdrawn, the size of the hemorrhoids and the degree of prolapse may be assessed. Sometimes an actual bleeding site can be identified.

Fistulous Abscess

Fistula in ano is the legacy of an anorectal abscess. In its simplest form, it is a chronic granulating tract connecting two epithelium-lined surfaces: an external opening on the skin and an internal opening originating in the mucosa of the anal canal, usually at the level of an anal crypt.

Cryptogenic abscesses may progress in several directions: (1) downward to form a para-anal abscess, (2) laterally to form an ischiorectal abscess, (3) submucosally to form a submucosal abscess, (4) proximally to form a supralevator abscess, and (5) intersphincteric, between the internal and the external sphincters. The site of the abscess, its point of origin, and the secondary opening or point of decompression combine to produce a fistulous tract that may be categorized as a low intrasphincteric, a transsphincteric, or a suprasphincteric fistula.

A para-anal abscess appears as a red, tender, ovoid swelling in the para-anal area. If left untreated, it eventually leads to skin necrosis and spontaneous decompression of the abscess. The findings from digital examination are usually normal except for some tenderness in the area immediately adjacent to the abscess. An ischiorectal abscess also causes severe pain in the para-anal area. As the disease progresses, a diffuse, brawny swelling develops over the ischiorectal fossa and even farther out on the buttock. Rectal examination reveals tenderness but rarely extension of the septic process into the rectum, a situation always found in intersphincteric and submucosal abscesses, which can be palpated only by digital rectal examination.

In the evaluation of abscesses of the para-anal area, it is important to exclude abscesses arising from other causes, such as periprostatic or periurethral glands (occurring in the male) or Bartholin's gland abscesses (occurring in the female). Also, postanal abscesses must be distinguished from pilonidal abscesses that can occur at the same site.

An anal fistula may occur spontaneously, with no antecedent abscess having been noted by the patient. The patient then presents with a history of discharge and perianal irritation. A fistula is painless, although the patient may develop a secondary pruritus from the continual discharge or episodic pain from small, recurrent, spontaneously draining abscesses. Inspection of the anal region should reveal one or more external openings at the distal site of the fistula. The secondary opening may be healed over and marked by a raised area of granulation or scar tissue. The skin surrounding this secondary opening may be red and thickened, and irritation from the chronic seepage may be noted. On palpation, it may be possible to express pus from the secondary opening of the fistulous tract or to palpate the tract as a thickened cord and trace it back toward its primary opening in the anal canal. Sometimes a fine silver probe can be gently passed along the tract to determine its course back to the anal canal. Digital examination may reveal induration at the site of the primary opening. On anoscopy, the clinician may identify the primary opening either by noting a small amount of purulent material escaping from it or by direct visualization of the opening and passage of a hooked probe into it.

It is important to exclude underlying pathology, such as Crohn's disease, colloid (mucinous) carcinoma of the rectum, and lymphogranuloma venereum, all of which may be associated with fistula formation. Also, the clinician should remember that carcinoma can arise from a longstanding fistula.

Crohn's Disease

The most common lesion of Crohn's disease of the anal canal is an atypical fissure. This fissure is distinguished by being a broad-based ulceration that occurs as frequently anteriorly or laterally as it does posteriorly. Multiple simultaneous fissures may be present. The skin tags associated with these fissures are edematous. The ulcers themselves are indolent and undermined and often exude a watery, purulent material from the base. The fistulas associated with Crohn's disease are extensive and complicated with undermined edges. They exude purulent material when palpated, and the entire area surrounding them takes on a brawny induration and dusky purplish discoloration. Rectal examination of the patients may show normal findings but often reveals a secondary stenosis of the anal canal due to the extensive inflammatory changes surrounding the fistula. In many instances, biopsy of the ulcer or fistula can be extremely helpful in establishing the differential diagnosis.

RECTAL DISEASES

Inflammatory Bowel Disease and Carcinoma

In the evaluation and diagnosis of the patient with anal pathology, the clinician must always be alert to the possibility of the simultaneous presence of rectal pathology. Thus, in the case of the patient presenting with hemorrhoids and rectal bleeding, the clinician should not assume that the bleeding is coming from the hemorrhoids. A thorough and complete investigation is required to exclude the possibility of proctitis or rectal carcinoma existing simultaneously.

Inflammatory bowel disease is characterized by a wide spectrum of symptoms ranging from slight looseness of bowel movements and passage of blood, to severe diarrhea with the passage of liquid fecal material, blood, mucus, and pus. This disease may also be associated with symptoms of colicky abdominal pain, lethargy, anemia, and pyrexia.

Inspection of the anal area may reveal signs of local complications of the disease, such as abscess, fissure, and fistula. Digital examination may indicate the presence of a stenosis or a granular texture of the mucosa. Sigmoidoscopic examination is important for defining the extent of the disease above the anal verge and also for assessing the severity of the disease by evaluating the degree of granularity and friability of the colonic mucosa and the presence of ulcerations, exudate, or inflammatory polyps. The mucosal biopsy is often a valuable diagnostic aid for the dual purpose of confirming the diagnosis and evaluating the progression or remission of the disease process over a period of time. This procedure also serves an important role in checking for the dysplastic changes that may herald the development of carcinoma.

Carcinoma of the rectum is characterized primarily by rectal bleeding associated with a change in bowel habits. Secondary symptoms, such as anorexia, weight loss, and rectal or abdominal pain, are usually late features of this disease. Digital examination may show blood on the fingertip, and palpation of the rectal wall may reveal induration or the raised edge of an ulcerated tumor. Digital examination may also reveal a nodular, friable mass extending into the lumen or an annular constricting lesion of the rectum that will not permit the passage of a fingertip through it. In performing the digital examination, the clinician must ascertain the location of the tumor, its size, the extent of its invasiveness, and whether the lesion is fixed or mobile. Sigmoidoscopic examination permits direct visualization of the lesion and assessment of its size, its location, and the degree of obstruction. The microscopic characteristics of the lesion can be assessed with biopsy. Endoscopy can exclude synchronous lesions and the possibility of adenomatous polyps in adjacent areas of the colon. Barium enema or colonoscopy, performed either preoperatively or postoperatively, is important for excluding the presence of more proximal synchronous pathology.

Foreign Bodies

Foreign bodies may be divided into two broad categories: those that are ingested and those that are inserted. Ingested foreign bodies may be fragments of bone, eggshells, seeds, pits, toothpicks, or food materials swallowed either deliberately or inadvertently by the patient. Patients on psychiatric wards have been known to ingest nails, screws, needles, and thermometers.

Inserted foreign bodies include such mundane objects as rectal thermometers and enema tips, as well as more unusual items—lightbulbs, bottles, vibrators, and the like. The main concern is that inserted objects can lacerate or cause necrosis of the lining of the anal canal or rectum.

Because of the patient's embarrassment, the history is often sketchy or misleading. Schizophrenic patients also fail to provide adequate histories. Therefore, diagnosis may occur accidentally during an abdominal radiographic, digital, or endoscopic examination performed for other reasons.

Removal of foreign objects by the transanal route, with consequent avoidance of laparotomy, should be attempted first. The specific technique of extraction must be individualized, depending on the nature of the object encountered. The mechanics involved often tax the imagination and ingenuity of the physician. Because of the complexity of this problem, removal should be attempted only by experienced personnel.

MESENTERIC VASCULAR DISEASES

By Ronald N. Kaleya, M.D.,
and Scott J. Boley, M.D.
Bronx, New York

Mesenteric vascular diseases (MVDs) are caused by insufficient flow of blood to all or part of the intestines. The causes of the ischemic insult vary, while the end result for all ischemic intestinal injuries is a spectrum of bowel injury ranging from completely reversible alterations of intestinal function to transmural hemorrhagic necrosis of the intestinal wall. The clinical syndromes associated with MVD depend on the degree of ischemic injury as well as the site and length of intestine affected by the injury. Thus, the symptoms and signs of MVDs vary considerably and can obscure their diagnosis.

Ischemic disorders of the intestine can be divided into those caused by a transient decrease of blood flow and those caused by more permanent interruption of mesenteric vascular supply. Mesenteric vascular disease can be further categorized as acute or chronic and of arterial or venous origin. While the viability of the intestine is not compromised in the chronic forms, the blood flow may be insufficient to support the functional demands of the intestine. In contrast, the viability of the intestine is endangered in the acute forms of mesenteric ischemia. Atherosclerotic narrowing or occlusion of the mesenteric arteries, producing intestinal angina, and gradually evolving mesenteric venous thrombosis (MVT) are the common forms of chronic ischemia. Acute mesenteric ischemia is more common than chronic, and arterial ischemia occurs more frequently than venous disease. The arterial forms of acute mesenteric ischemia include superior mesenteric arterial embolus (SMAE), nonocclusive mesenteric ischemia (NOMI), superior mesenteric artery thrombosis (SMAT), and focal segmental ischemia (FSI) due to local atherosclerotic emboli or vasculitides. Acute mesenteric venous thrombosis (AMVT) and FSI caused by strangulation obstruction of the small intestine or by localized venous thrombosis constitute the venous forms of acute mesenteric ischemia. Colonic ischemia is almost always the result of acute but transient arterial insufficiency.

ISCHEMIC DISORDERS OF THE COLON

Colonic ischemia (CI) refers to a general pathophysiologic process that leads to varied clinical outcomes. The spectrum of CI includes (1) reversible ischemic colonopathy (submucosal or intramucosal hemorrhage), (2) reversible or transient ischemic colitis; (3) chronic ischemic ulcerative colitis, (4) ischemic colonic stricture, (5) colonic gangrene, and (6) fulminant universal colitis.

Clinical Manifestations

Presentation

The diagnosis of CI is usually made after the period of ischemia has passed and blood flow to the affected segment of colon has been restored. Many episodes of transient or reversible ischemia are probably missed because the condition resolves before medical attention is sought or because a barium enema or colonoscopy is not performed early in the course of the disease. Furthermore, many cases of CI are misdiagnosed as infectious colitis or inflammatory bowel disease. Thus, the precise incidence of CI is difficult to determine. Although CI has no significant sex predilection, 90 per cent of patients are older than 60 years of age and have other evidence of systemic atherosclerosis. In younger individuals, CI has been associated with vasculitis (especially systemic lupus erythematosus), medications (estrogens, danazol, vasopressin, gold, psychotropic drugs), sickle cell anemia, coagulopathies (thrombotic thrombocytopenic purpura, protein C and protein S deficiencies, antithrombin III deficiency), competitive long-distance running, and cocaine abuse.

Colonic ischemia typically presents with the sudden onset of mild, crampy abdominal pain, usually localized to the left lower quadrant. Less commonly the pain is severe, or, conversely, the description of pain can be elicited only retrospectively, if at all. An urgent desire to defecate frequently accompanies the pain, and is followed, within 24 hours, by the passage of either bright red or maroon blood in the stool. The bleeding is not vigorous, and blood loss requiring transfusion is so rare that it should suggest an alternative diagnosis. Physical examination may reveal mild to severe abdominal tenderness at the site of the involved segment of bowel.

Natural History of Colonic Ischemia

Despite similarities in the initial presentation of most episodes of CI, the outcome cannot be predicted at the time of onset unless the initial physical findings unequivocally indicate an intra-abdominal catastrophe. The ultimate course of an ischemic insult depends on many factors, including (1) the cause, that is, occlusive or nonocclusive; (2) the caliber of an occluded vessel; (3) the duration and degree of ischemia; (4) the rapidity of onset of the ischemia; (5) the condition of the collateral circulation; (6) the metabolic requirements of the affected bowel; (7) the presence and virulence of bowel flora; and (8) the presence of associated conditions, such as colonic distention.

Symptoms must commonly subside within 24 to 48 hours, and clinical, roentgenographic, and endoscopic evidence of healing is seen within 2 weeks. More severe but still reversible ischemic damage may take 1 to 6 months to resolve. Most patients with reversible disease exhibit only colonic hemorrhage or edema; one third develop transient colitis. With more severe yet reversible ischemia, the entire mucosa may occasionally slough as a tube. In half of the patients with CI, the ischemic damage does not heal, and irreversible disease ultimately develops. In two thirds of these patients, CI follows a protracted course, leading to chronic segmental ulcerative colitis or ischemic stricture. The remaining one third develop signs and symptoms of intestinal gangrene with or without perforation. This intra-abdominal catastrophe typically evolves within hours of the initial presentation.

Patients who develop CI as a complication of shock, congestive heart failure, myocardial infarction, or severe dehydration have a particularly poor prognosis. These patients are typically older individuals who take digitalis preparations that may act as potent splanchnic vasoconstrictors, further compromising colonic circulation. In one series, these factors were present in one quarter of the patients with CI, and 12 of 13 patients who presented in shock did not survive.

Because the outcome of an episode of CI is often unpredictable, patients must be examined serially for evidence of peritonitis, rising temperature, leukocytosis, or worsening symptoms. Patients with diarrhea or bleeding that persists beyond 10 to 14 days often go on to perforation or, less frequently, a protein-wasting enteropathy. Strictures may develop over weeks to months and may be asymptomatic or produce progressive bowel obstruction. Some of the asymptomatic strictures resolve spontaneously over many months.

Diagnosis

Early and appropriate diagnosis of CI requires serial radiographic and/or colonoscopic evaluation of the colon as well as repeated clinical evaluations of the patient. More severe episodes of CI may be difficult to distinguish from acute mesenteric ischemia, whereas less severe episodes may be confused with acute or chronic idiopathic ulcerative colitis, Crohn's colitis, infectious colitis, or diverticulitis. A combination of radiographic, colonoscopic, and clinical findings may be necessary for establishing the diagnosis of CI.

In the patient with suspected CI, if abdominal films are nonspecific, sigmoidoscopy is unrevealing, and no signs of peritonitis are found, a gentle barium enema or colonoscopy should be performed in the unprepared bowel within 48 hours after the onset of symptoms. The most characteristic finding on barium enema is "thumbprinting" or "pseudotumors." Hemorrhagic nodules seen at colonoscopy represent bleeding into the submucosa and are equivalent to the "thumbprints" seen on barium enema. Segmental distribution of these lesions, with or without ulceration, strongly suggests CI, but the diagnosis of CI cannot be made conclusively with a single study. In fact, persistence of the thumbprints suggests a diagnosis other than CI (e.g., lymphoma and amyloidosis).

Close observation of the clinical course and repeated radiographic or endoscopic examinations of the colon are often necessary for confirming the diagnosis of CI. Segmental colitis associated with a tumor or other potentially or partially obstructing lesions is also characterized by ischemic disease. In contrast, radiographic evidence of universal colonic involvement, loss of haustrations, and pseudopolyposis is more typical of chronic idiopathic ulcerative colitis, whereas the presence of skip lesions, linear ulcerations, or fistulas suggests Crohn's disease.

The clinician must obtain radiographs early in the course of the disease because thumbprinting disappears within days, as the submucosal hemorrhages are either resorbed or evacuated into the colon when overlying mucosa ulcerates and sloughs. Barium enema or colonoscopy performed 1 week after the initial study should reflect the evolution of the disease, either by a return to normal or by the replacement of the thumbprints with a pattern of segmental ulcerative colitis.

If colonoscopy is chosen as the initial study, caution is indicated. Distention of the bowel with air to pressures greater than 30 mm Hg diminishes colonic blood flow, shunts blood from the mucosa to the serosa, and causes a progressive decrease in the arteriovenous oxygen difference. Because intraluminal pressure exceeds 30 mm Hg during routine endoscopic examination of the colon, colonoscopy can potentially induce or exacerbate CI. This risk can be decreased with insufflation of carbon dioxide, which increases colonic blood flow at similar pressures. Furthermore, carbon dioxide is rapidly absorbed from the colon, this absorption thereby decreasing the duration of distention and increased intraluminal pressure.

Biopsies of nodules or bullae identified endoscopically early in the course of CI reveal submucosal hemorrhage, while biopsies of the surrounding mucosa typically show nonspecific inflammation. Histologic evidence of mucosal infarction, though rare, is pathognomonic of ischemia. Angiography seldom reveals significant occlusion or other abnormalities and is not indicated in patients suspected of having CI. Computed tomography (CT) may show thickening of the bowel wall but this finding is not specific for CI.

When the clinical presentation does not clearly distinguish CI from acute mesenteric ischemia, and plain films of the abdomen do not show the characteristic thumbprinting pattern of CI, an "air enema" is performed by gently introducing air into the colon under fluoroscopic observation. The submucosal edema and hemorrhage that produce the thumbprinting pattern of CI can be accentuated and identified in this manner.

After the provisional diagnosis of CI has been made, a gentle barium enema is performed to determine the site and distribution of the disease as well as to determine any carcinoma, stricture, or diverticulitis that predisposed to the episode of ischemia. If thumbprinting is not observed and the air enema does not suggest the diagnosis of CI, a selective mesenteric angiogram is immediately performed to exclude the diagnosis of acute mesenteric ischemia. Because this condition progresses rapidly to an irreversible outcome and optimal diagnosis and treatment of this condition require angiography, the diagnosis of acute mesenteric ischemia must be established or excluded prior to a barium study. Residual barium from a contrast study of the colon may obscure the mesenteric vessels and therefore preclude an adequate angiographic examination and intervention.

Late Manifestations of Colonic Ischemia

Chronic Segmental Ulcerative Colitis

Colonic ischemia may be asymptomatic during the acute insult but nevertheless produce chronic segmental ulcerative colitis. Patients with this form of CI are frequently misdiagnosed if not seen during the acute episode. Barium enema may show a segmental colitis pattern, a stricture simulating a carcinoma, or even an area of pseudopolyposis. At this stage of the disease, the clinical course is often indistinguishable from that of other causes of colitis or stenosis unless the patient has been followed from the time of the acute episode. Although crypt abscesses and pseudopolyposis are usually considered histologically diagnostic of chronic idiopathic ulcerative colitis, they can also be seen in ischemic colitis. Nevertheless, the de novo occurrence of a segmental area of colitis or stricture in an elderly patient should be considered most likely ischemic and treated accordingly. Thus, the natural history of noninfectious segmental colitis in the elderly is that of ischemic colitis; the involvement remains localized, resection is not followed by recurrence, and the response to steroid therapy is usually poor.

Ischemic Strictures

Patients with asymptomatic segmental ulcerative colitis may develop a stenosis or stricture of the colon. Strictures that produce no symptoms should be observed and some of these will return to normal over a period of 12 to 24 months without therapy. However, if symptoms of obstruction develop, segmental resection is required.

Specific Clinical Problems Associated With Colonic Ischemia

Colonic Ischemia Complicating Abdominal Aortic Surgery

Mesenteric vascular reconstruction is not indicated in most patients with CI, but it may be required for preventing CI during and after aortic reconstruction. Following elective aneurysmectomy, 3 to 7 per cent of patients develop colonoscopic evidence of CI. The incidence of CI following repair of ruptured aortic aneurysms has been reported as high as 60 per cent. Clinical evidence of this complication occurs in only 1 to 2 per cent of patients, but its occurrence is responsible for approximately 10 per cent of the deaths following aortic replacement. The factors contributing to postoperative CI include rupture of the aneurysm, hypotension, operative trauma to the colon, hypoxemia, arrhythmias, prolonged cross-clamping time, and improper management of the inferior mesenteric artery (IMA) during aneurysmectomy.

The diagnostic challenge and significant mortality associated with postoperative CI mandate that postoperative colonoscopy be performed in high-risk patients. Individuals at high risk for the development of postoperative CI following aortic reconstruction are those with ruptured abdominal aortic aneurysms, prolonged cross-clamping time, a patent IMA on preoperative aortography, nonpulsatile flow in the hypogastric arteries during surgery, and postoperative diarrhea. In these patients, colonoscopy is routinely performed within 2 or 3 days after the operation, and if CI is identified, treatment is begun before major complications develop. Clinical deterioration with progression of the ischemic insult to transmural necrosis necessitates reoperation.

Fulminating Universal Colitis

A rare fulminating form of ischemia involving all or most of the colon and rectum has been recently identified. These patients experience the sudden onset of toxic universal colitis with bleeding, fever, severe diarrhea, abdominal pain and tenderness, and frequent signs of peritonitis. The clinical course is rapidly progressive.

Lesions Mimicking Colon Carcinoma

Ischemic colitis can present with lesions that appear to be colon carcinoma on barium enema and colonoscopy. Colonoscopy may distinguish malignancy from ischemic cicatrization; colonoscopy should be performed if an annular lesion is identified on barium enema.

Ischemic Colitis Associated With Colon Carcinoma

Acute colitis in patients with carcinoma of the colon has been recognized for years. The colitis typically occurs proximal to the tumor, with or without clinical obstruction. Patients may present with the symptoms of CI or with tumor-related symptoms such as bleeding, acute obstruction, and chronic cramping. Most patients, however, experience the sudden onset of mild to moderate abdominal pain, fever, bloody diarrhea, and abdominal tenderness.

Colonic Ischemia as a Manifestation of Acute Mesenteric Ischemia

Ischemia localized to the ascending colon may be a manifestation of acute mesenteric ischemia. If colonoscopy or thumbprinting suggests isolated right colonic ischemia, angiography of the superior mesenteric artery (SMA) is indicated. A partially or completely obstructed SMA may require revascularization.

ACUTE MESENTERIC ISCHEMIA

Acute mesenteric ischemia refers to a wide spectrum of injury to bowel within the distribution of the superior mesenteric vessels. The changes associated with acute mesenteric ischemia range from reversible alterations in bowel function to transmural necrosis of the bowel wall. Acute mesenteric ischemia may result from an SMA embolus, thrombosis of the superior mesenteric artery or vein, or NOMI. The various clinical presentations ultimately depend on the degree and duration of ischemia and the length of bowel that is compromised.

Clinical Manifestations

Presentation

In the past 25 years, acute mesenteric ischemia has been increasingly diagnosed, but its exact incidence is difficult to determine. The increased incidence has been attributed to the aging of the population, since acute mesenteric ischemia primarily occurs in geriatric patients, especially those with cardiovascular and systemic disorders. The widespread use of intensive care has salvaged patients who previously would have rapidly died of cardiovascular conditions, but who now survive to develop acute mesenteric ischemia as a delayed consequence of their primary disease.

Together, SMAE and NOMI account for 70 to 80 per cent of patients with acute mesenteric ischemia. A recent decline in the incidence of nonocclusive ischemia has been attributed to increased use of systemic vasodilators in coronary intensive care units. These agents may protect the mesenteric vascular beds from vasospasm and decrease the period of profound hypotension associated with acute myocardial events. In addition, the increased use of left ventricular assist devices in the treatment of cardiogenic shock has decreased the period of profound hypotension associated with left ventricular failure and, presumably, has attenuated its effect on the mesenteric circulation.

Arterial Causes of Acute Mesenteric Ischemia

Superior mesenteric artery emboli are responsible for 40 to 50 per cent of the episodes of acute mesenteric ischemia. The emboli usually originate from a left atrial or ventricular mural thrombus that is dislodged or fragmented during a period of dysrhythmia or following cardiac catheterization. Many patients with SMAE have a history of previous peripheral artery embolism, and approximately 20 per cent have synchronous emboli in other arteries.

Nonocclusive mesenteric ischemia causes 20 to 30 per cent of the episodes of acute mesenteric ischemia. This condition is thought to result from splanchnic vasoconstriction caused by vasoactive drugs or decreased cardiac output secondary to dysrhythmias, myocardial depression, or hypovolemia. The vasoconstriction may persist despite elimination or correction of the precipitating cause. The factors that predispose to NOMI include acute myocardial infarction, congestive heart failure, aortic insufficiency, liver disease, and kidney disease, especially in patients requiring hemodialysis and major cardiac or intra-abdominal surgery. Frequently, an immediate cause of NOMI, such as acute pulmonary edema, cardiac arrhythmia, and shock, is well documented. Intestinal ischemia, however, may not be clinically evident until hours or days later.

Superior mesenteric artery thrombosis occurs at sites of severe atherosclerotic narrowing, most often at the origin of the SMA. The acute ischemic episode is commonly superimposed on chronic mesenteric ischemia; 20 to 50 per cent of patients with SMAT have a history of abdominal pain with or without evidence of malabsorption and weight loss during the weeks to months preceding the acute episode. Furthermore, most patients with SMAT have severe and diffuse atherosclerosis with a history of coronary, cerebrovascular, or peripheral arterial insufficiency.

Venous Causes of Acute Mesenteric Ischemia

Mesenteric venous thrombosis (MVT) may present as an acute, a subacute, or a chronic process. Mesenteric venous thrombosis accounts for fewer than 5 per cent of all patients with acute mesenteric ischemia and is discussed later in this chapter.

Clinical Response to Acute Mesenteric Ischemia

The response to decreased intestinal blood flow is complex. Occlusion of the SMA initially results in a marked increase in bowel activity. Increased motor function causes rapid bowel evacuation and increased intestinal oxygen demand. Shortly thereafter, bowel motility ceases owing to massive sympathetic discharge or local factors associated with the ischemia itself. Within hours, the bowel becomes hemorrhagic and edematous as capillary integrity is compromised. As edema and hemorrhage increase, intramural hydrostatic pressure rises. In normal bowel, this increased intramural pressure is often well tolerated, but as perfusion pressure to the edematous bowel decreases, the edema can further compromise an already marginal blood flow. In addition, bacterial utilization of a marginally adequate intestinal oxygen supply and production of toxic metabolites may exacerbate the ischemic injury.

The shift of intravascular volume into the bowel wall causes severe hemoconcentration and hypovolemic shock. Vasoactive mediators and bacterial endotoxins are released from the ischemic bowel into the peritoneal cavity and absorbed into the general circulation, this absorption causing cardiac depression, septic shock, and acute renal failure. These effects may contribute to the death of the patient even before the development of complete necrosis of the bowel wall.

Diagnosis

Early identification of acute mesenteric ischemia requires a high index of suspicion fueled by recognition of the significant risk factors associated with this disease. Acute mesenteric ischemia occurs most frequently in patients older than 50 years of age who have congestive heart failure that is poorly controlled with diuretics or digitalis. Cardiac arrhythmias (especially atrial fibrillation), recent myocardial infarction, and hypotension due to burns, pancreatitis, or hemorrhage all predispose to acute mesenteric ischemia. Previous or synchronous arterial emboli increase the likelihood of an acute SMA embolus. The sudden onset of abdominal pain in a patient with any of these risk factors suggests the diagnosis of acute mesenteric ischemia.

Presentation

Acute abdominal pain that varies in severity, nature, and location occurs in 75 to 98 per cent of patients with intestinal ischemia. A history of postprandial abdominal pain in the weeks to months preceding the acute onset of severe abdominal pain occurs primarily in the small fraction of patients with acute mesenteric ischemia caused by SMAT. In early acute mesenteric ischemia, the pain experienced by the patient is markedly out of proportion to the physical findings. Therefore, sudden severe abdominal pain accompanied by rapid and often forceful bowel evacuation and minimal or no abdominal signs strongly suggests an acute arterial occlusion in the mesenteric circulation.

Unexplained abdominal distention or gastrointestinal bleeding may be the only indication of acute intestinal ischemia, especially in nonocclusive disease, since pain is absent in as many as 25 per cent of patients with acute mesenteric ischemia. Patients who survive cardiopulmonary resuscitation only to develop culture-proven bacteremia and diarrhea without abdominal pain should be suspected of having NOMI. Although absent early in the course of mesenteric ischemia, distention is often the first sign of impending intestinal infarction. The stool contains occult blood in 75 per cent of patients, and this bleeding may precede other symptoms of ischemia. Right-sided abdominal pain associated with the passage of maroon or bright red blood in the stool, though characteristic of CI, also suggests the diagnosis of acute mesenteric ischemia.

Although abdominal findings are absent early in the course of intestinal ischemia, as infarction develops, increasing tenderness, rebound tenderness, and muscle guarding reflect the progressive loss of intestinal viability and the presence of transmural gangrene. Significant abdominal findings strongly indicate the presence of infarcted bowel. Nausea, vomiting, hematochezia, hematemesis, massive abdominal distention, back pain, and shock are other late signs of compromise of bowel viability.

Laboratory Signs

Leukocytosis exceeding 15,000 cells/mm^3 occurs in 75 per cent of patients with acute mesenteric ischemia, while metabolic acidemia develops in 50 per cent. Increased amylase and phosphate in the serum, and increased alkaline phosphatase and phosphate in peritoneal fluid have been described, but the sensitivity and specificity of these markers for intestinal ischemia have not been established. Leukocytosis out of proportion to the clinical findings, increased hemoglobin and hematocrit due to hemoconcentration, and blood-tinged peritoneal fluid with increased amylase activity are not specific for acute mesenteric ischemia but do suggest advanced intestinal necrosis and sepsis.

Radiographic Signs

Before infarction occurs, plain abdominal films are usually normal. As mesenteric ischemia progresses, an abdomen without gas, a pattern of adynamic ileus, or a small bowel pseudo-obstruction can be seen. Late in the course of ischemia, formless loops of small intestine or small intestinal "pinkieprinting" can suggest the diagnosis of acute mesenteric ischemia. Less commonly, isolated thumbprinting of the right colon may be the only indication of acute mesenteric ischemia. Ischemia confined to the right colon may be caused by disease in the main SMA, rather than by local interference with colonic blood flow. Rare findings that accompany all types of bowel infarction include pneumatosis or gas in the portal venous circulation.

Upper gastrointestinal series can show dilated loops of small intestine with thickened folds, mucosal ulceration, or a scalloped bowel border. These findings, however, are more characteristic of focal segmental ischemia. Duplex scanning may aid the identification of portal and superior mesenteric venous thrombosis and, less often, SMA occlusion. Computed tomography has also been used to identify arterial and venous thromboses and ischemic bowel, but only in the late stages of the disease. In the future, magnetic resonance imaging and positron emission tomography may be helpful in the diagnosis of mesenteric ischemia.

Laparoscopy

Laparoscopy may be useful in patients whose clinical status precludes angiography. However, because laparoscopic examination of the bowel is limited to the serosal surface, this procedure is unreliable for diagnosing the early mucosal necrosis that precedes any grossly visible changes in the serosa.

Angiography

Historically, angiography primarily identified arterial occlusions by embolus or thrombus. Currently, selective angiography is the mainstay of diagnosis and initial treatment of both occlusive and nonocclusive forms of acute mesenteric ischemia. Regarding NOMI, four reliable angiographic criteria for the diagnosis of mesenteric vasoconstriction have been identified: (1) narrowing of the origins of multiple branches of the SMA, (2) alternate dilatation and narrowing of the intestinal branches (string-of-sausage sign), (3) spasm of the mesenteric arcades, and (4) impaired filling of intramural vessels.

While mesenteric vasoconstriction occurs in hypotensive patients and in those with pancreatitis, its presence in patients with suspected intestinal ischemia who are not in shock, do not have pancreatitis, and are not receiving vasopressors is diagnostic of NOMI. Therefore, if angiography is performed sufficiently early in the course, patients with occlusive and nonocclusive AMI can be identified before the development of clinical and radiographic signs of bowel infarction.

Any patient at increased risk for acute mesenteric ischemia who suddenly develops abdominal pain lasting more than 2 hours and requiring the attention of a physician should be suspected of having acute mesenteric ischemia. Less absolute indications for mesenteric angiography include unexplained abdominal distention, colonoscopic evidence of isolated right-sided colonic ischemia, and acidosis without identifiable cause. Because the presence of diagnostic clinical or nonangiographic radiographic signs usually indicates irreversible intestinal injury, broad patient selection criteria are essential if early diagnosis and successful treatment are to be achieved. Some negative angiograms must be accepted in the process of identifying and salvaging patients who do have acute mesenteric ischemia.

MESENTERIC VENOUS THROMBOSIS

Mesenteric venous thrombosis is an infrequent but distinct form of intestinal ischemia. Thrombosis of the superior mesenteric vein can develop slowly with no symptoms, subacutely with pain but no intestinal infarction, or acutely with the classic presentation.

Clinical Manifestations

The number of conditions associated with MVT, as well as the number of patients with those conditions who also develop MVT, has increased over the years. Hypercoagulable states, oral contraceptives, sclerotherapy, and deficiencies of antithrombin III, protein S, and protein C all have been causally linked to MVT.

Natural History of Mesenteric Venous Thrombosis

The location of the initial thrombus in the mesenteric veins varies with the cause. Superior mesenteric vein thrombosis (SMVT) secondary to cirrhosis, neoplasm, or surgical injury clearly starts at the site of obstruction and extends peripherally. Thromboses caused by hypercoagulable states tend to start in smaller venous branches and propagate into the major trunks. Infarction of the intestine rarely occurs unless the branches of the peripheral arcades and the vasa recta are involved, even when the junction of the portal and superior mesenteric vein is occluded. Inferior mesenteric vein thrombosis (IMVT) leading to infarction has been reported in fewer than 6 per cent of patients with MVT.

When collateral circulation is inadequate and venous drainage from a segment of bowel is compromised, congestion increases in the involved intestine. The bowel becomes edematous, cyanotic, and thickened with intramural hemorrhages. Ultimately, similar changes occur in the subjacent mesentery. Serosanguineous peritoneal fluid accompanies early hemorrhagic infarction. Arterial vasoconstriction can be intense, but pulsations persist up to the bowel wall. Late in the process, transmural infarction occurs, and the physician may find it impossible to distinguish venous from arterial occlusion.

Presentation

Superior mesenteric vein thrombosis can present with a sudden acute onset, a subacute onset over weeks to months, or a chronic onset that typically is asymptomatic until late complications occur. As many as 60 per cent of patients have a history of deep venous thrombosis of the extremities.

Acute Superior Mesenteric Venous Thrombosis

The symptoms and signs of acute SMVT (the form of the disease classically described) are both varied and nonspecific, and SMVT has long been known as the "great imitator" of other abdominal disorders. In series that predate angiography and imaging studies, a correct preoperative diagnosis was made infrequently. Except for abdominal pain, which is present in more than 90 per cent of patients, no symptoms point to the diagnosis of MVT. Even the duration, nature, severity, and location of the pain vary widely. Typically, however, the pain is out of proportion to the physical findings. The mean duration of pain prior to admission ranges from 5 days to more than 1 month. Patients with pain of long duration may have the increasingly recognized subacute form of SMVT.

Nausea and vomiting are reported by more than half of the patients with SMVT. Lower gastrointestinal bleeding or bloody diarrhea in as many as 15 per cent of patients, and hematemesis in as many as 13 per cent are indications of bowel infarction. The presence of hematemesis or bleeding per rectum should alert the physician to the possibility of a mesenteric ischemic catastrophe. Occult blood is present in the stools of more than half of the patients.

The initial physical findings in acute SMVT vary greatly, this diversity reflecting different stages and degrees of ischemic injury. Although most patients present with abdominal tenderness, distention, and decreased bowel sounds, only two thirds manifest clear signs of peritonitis. Guarding and rebound tenderness develop later in the course, as bowel infarction evolves. Most patients with SMVT have temperatures greater than 38°C, but only 25 per cent present with clinical signs of septic shock.

Laboratory studies for the diagnosis of all forms of intestinal ischemia have a low specificity or a low sensitivity. In the authors' series of 22 patients, only a white blood cell count of more than 12,000 cells/mm^3 and an increase in the proportion of polymorphonuclear cells were observed in more than two thirds of the patients. At present, these laboratory tests can suggest—but cannot confirm or exclude—the diagnosis of intestinal ischemia.

Patients who have a personal or family history of deep venous thrombosis or other thrombotic episodes and who present with symptoms consistent with mesenteric ischemia should be evaluated for the presence of a hypercoagulable state. The work-up should include measurement of antithrombin III, protein S, and protein C concentrations and a routine coagulation profile.

Subacute Superior Mesenteric Venous Thrombosis

The term subacute superior mesenteric venous thrombosis is used to describe the condition of patients who have had abdominal pain for several weeks to months without intestinal infarction. This presentation can be attributed either to extension of the thrombotic process at a rate rapid enough to cause pain, but slow enough to allow collateral circulation to develop before infarction occurs, or to acute thrombosis of only a few veins permitting recovery from ischemic injury. Most often, the diagnosis has been made serendipitously on imaging studies performed for evaluating other suspected diagnoses, and the pain has subsided spontaneously or after the initiation of anticoagulant therapy.

Typically, pain is the only symptom, although some patients have nausea or diarrhea. The findings on physical examination and the laboratory test results are normal. In a few patients, the pain is related to meals, but in most it is nonspecific in site and nature. Some patients who initially have this type of presentation do ultimately develop intestinal infarction; hence, the distinction between the acute and the subacute forms of SMVT may become blurred. The late occurrence of infarction may be the result of recurrent SMVT. Histologically new and old thromboses have been found at autopsy in nearly half of the cases with major vein thromboses. Moreover, some patients with subacute onset, in whom the symptoms subside, may later develop the problems seen with asymptomatic chronic SMVT.

Chronic Mesenteric Venous Thrombosis

The term chronic mesenteric venous thrombosis (CMVT) has been applied to patients who have no symptoms during the period when the thrombosis occurs. These patients may never develop problems related to the SMVT, but in those that do, gastrointestinal bleeding from esophageal or intestinal varices occurs. Most have bleeding esophageal varices, and all of these patients have associated thrombosis of the portal or splenic vein. If the portal veins are involved, the physical findings of CMVT are those of portal hypertension. However, when only the superior mesenteric veins are involved, no abnormal findings may be observed. Laboratory studies with portal or splenic vein involvement may also show secondary hypersplenism with pancytopenia or simple thrombocytopenia.

Diagnosis

Acute Mesenteric Venous Thrombosis

The absence of any reliable specific symptoms, signs, or laboratory studies makes a preoperative diagnosis of acute mesenteric venous thrombosis (AMVT) very difficult. Moreover, the variability in the course of the disease—with some patients having an indolent course of days to weeks and others having a relatively acute onset and progressive course—further obscures the diagnosis. The continuing difficulty in diagnosing MVT was graphically described by

Anane-Sehaf and Blair in this statement, "Perhaps the best overall finding was an uneasy feeling on the part of the examining physician that his patient looks sick but that he could not say why or from what."* Hence in the past, in 90 to 95 per cent of patients the correct diagnosis has been made only at laparotomy. In more recent series in which the newer diagnostic modalities have been used, the majority of patients have been diagnosed without, or prior to, surgery.

Radiographic and other imaging studies can establish the definitive diagnosis of MVT before intestinal infarction occurs. Plain films of the abdomen, if abnormal, almost always reflect the presence of infarcted bowel, and the changes, when present, rarely permit differentiation of the venous and arterial forms of ischemia. In the authors' series, 75 per cent of the patients had abnormal plain films, but 50 per cent showed only a nonspecific ileus pattern. In only 25 per cent of these patients did the study suggest the presence of some form of acute mesenteric ischemia. Gas in the wall of the bowel or in the portal vein and free air in the peritoneal cavity, all late signs of intestinal infarction, may be seen on plain films.

Barium enemas are of little value, since MVT rarely involves the colon. Some authors report that small bowel studies are both specific and sensitive. Characteristic findings include (1) marked thickening of the bowel wall and valvulae conniventes due to congestion and edema, (2) separation of loops due to mesenteric thickening, (3) a long transition zone between involved and uninvolved bowel with progressive narrowing of the lumen by the thickened wall, and (4) thumbprints or pseudotumors.

Selective mesenteric arteriography can establish a definitive diagnosis before bowel infarction, differentiating between venous thrombosis and arterial forms of ischemia and providing access for the administration of intra-arterial vasodilators if relief of an associated arterial vasoconstriction is deemed therapeutically important. The angiographic findings of MVT have been determined experimentally and clinically and include (1) demonstration of a thrombus in the superior mesenteric vein with partial or complete occlusion, (2) failure to visualize the superior mesenteric or portal vein, (3) slow or absent filling of the mesenteric veins, (4) arterial spasm, (5) failure of arterial arcades to empty, and (6) a prolonged blush in the involved segment. In addition, the angiogram may show reconstitution of venous blood flow above the thrombus, which can be an important factor in selecting therapy.

Ultrasonography, CT, and magnetic resonance imaging all have been used to demonstrate thrombi in the superior mesenteric and portal veins before bowel infarction. Ultrasonography is of less value in pure SMVT because overlying gas may prevent adequate visualization of the vein, but the study can be used as a quick screening test in problem cases. Thickening of the bowel wall and free peritoneal fluid are ultrasonographic findings suggestive of intestinal ischemia.

Abdominal CT can establish the diagnosis in more than 90 per cent of patients with MVT by demonstrating the thrombus, venous collateral circulation, and involved intestine. Specific findings include thickening and persistent enhancement of the bowel wall, enlargement of the SMV, a central lucency in the lumen of the vein representing a thrombus, a sharply defined vein wall with a rim of increased density, and dilated collateral vessels in a thickened mesentery. These finding may be more consistent with the chronic form of MVT, because most of the patients undergo CT for another indication and the mesenteric thrombosis is found serendipitously. Some authors believe that when a diagnosis of MVT is made on the basis of CT findings, little is gained by performing a subsequent selective mesenteric angiogram. However, the better delineation of thrombosed veins, and the access for administration of intra-arterial vasodilators provided by this study, may make it of value in selected patients.

No firm evidence attests to the value of performing angiography and CT in the patient with AMVT. A small number of patients diagnosed just with imaging techniques, and without abdominal findings, have been treated successfully without angiography or surgery. Magnetic resonance imaging has also been used to diagnose MVT in a few patients, but its only apparent advantage is that it avoids the use of ionizing radiation. Isolated cases of MVT have been diagnosed with various endoscopic methods. Routine gastroduodenoscopy and colonoscopy rarely are of value, because the duodenum and colon are infrequently involved, but examination of the proximal jejunum with a long endoscope can suggest the diagnosis if that portion of the bowel is involved. Laparoscopy may be useful when the diagnosis is uncertain. Scintillation angiography has been diagnostic of MVT; however, it has not proved clinically reliable.

The diagnosis of MVT is usually made at laparotomy. The hallmarks of MVT are serosanguineous peritoneal fluid, dark-red to blue-black edematous bowel, striking thickening of the mesentery, good arterial pulsations in the involved segment, and thrombus in cut mesenteric veins; at this stage, some degree of intestinal infarction has invariably occurred. Thus, as with the other forms of acute mesenteric ischemia, improved survival can be achieved only through earlier diagnosis. If patients with suspected acute mesenteric ischemia have factors that suggest MVT, such as a history of deep venous thrombosis or a family history of an inherited coagulation defect, the first imaging study ordered should arguably be a contrast-enhanced CT scan. Following prompt resuscitation, selective mesenteric angiography is more appropriately reserved for the patients who have no factors suggesting venous thrombosis.

Chronic Mesenteric Venous Thrombosis

Since CMVT is asymptomatic or presents as gastrointestinal bleeding, the evaluation is directed toward determining the source of the hemorrhage. Upper and lower gastrointestinal endoscopy and the same imaging studies used for AMVT should establish the diagnosis of CMVT, the extent of the thrombosis, and the site of the bleeding. Transhepatic splenoportography can be used to better define the extent of the thromboses and varices if necessary, but papaverine-enhanced selective SMA angiography is a better study if the portal vein is occluded.

FOCAL INTESTINAL ISCHEMIA

Ischemic insults localized to short segments of the small intestine produce a broad spectrum of clinical features without the life-threatening systemic consequences associated with damage to more extensive portions of the gut. The most frequent causes are atheromatous or small thrombotic emboli, strangulated hernias, blunt abdominal trauma, and segmental venous thrombosis.

*Anane-Sehaf, J.C., and Blair, E.: Primary mesenteric venous occlusive disease. Surg. Gynecol. Obstet., 141:740–742, 1975.

Clinical Manifestations

Focal intestinal ischemia usually occurs in the presence of adequate collateral circulation, which prevents transmural hemorrhagic infarction. Typically, the lesions are infected infarcts that follow partial necrosis of the bowel wall and secondary invasion by the intestinal bacteria. Limited tissue necrosis may result in complete healing, a chronic enteritis simulating Crohn's disease, or a stricture with partial or complete intestinal obstruction. Transmural necrosis with perforation or localized peritonitis can follow a severe local insult.

Presentation

Patients with short-segment ischemic bowel injury present differently, depending on the severity of the infarct. In the acute presentation, seen with transmural necrosis, the onset of abdominal pain is sudden and often simulates acute appendicitis. These patients manifest clinical signs of peritonitis and sepsis. Another common presentation is that of chronic enteritis, with crampy abdominal pain, diarrhea, occasional fever, and weight loss. This clinical picture is indistinguishable from Crohn's disease of the small intestine. The most common presentation, however, is that of chronic small bowel obstruction, with or without a history of some antecedent episode of trauma, pain, or hernia incarceration. Intermittent abdominal pain, distention, and vomiting are the direct results of obstruction, and bacterial overgrowth in the dilated loop proximal to the obstruction may lead to the metabolic and clinical derangements (e.g., anemia, diarrhea, and steatorrhea) that are usually associated with the blind loop syndrome. A preoperative diagnosis of focal ischemia is difficult to make. A previous episode of transient pain, trauma, or incarcerated hernia or a known systemic illness can suggest the correct diagnosis.

PERITONITIS AND INTRA-ABDOMINAL ABSCESSES

By Hiram C. Polk, Jr., M.D.,
and Walid Abou-Jaoude, M.D.
Louisville, Kentucky

PERITONITIS

Definition

Peritonitis is defined as inflammation of the peritoneum. Its causes are multiple, and many overlapping subclassifications have been devised to characterize its etiology, including septic or aseptic, bacterial or viral, primary or secondary, localized or diffuse, and acute or chronic. Peritonitis is most commonly attributed to bacterial contamination of the sterile peritoneum after trauma to or perforation of the gastrointestinal tract (secondary peritonitis). Less commonly, peritonitis is caused by hematogenous or genital tract spread of bacteria to the peritoneum (primary peritonitis).

Primary peritonitis occurs without perforation of a viscus and usually develops in patients with conditions that predispose to infection of the peritoneal cavity (Table 1). Rarely, primary bacterial peritonitis develops in apparently normal infants and young children. Impaired immunologic function and the administration of steroids increase the risk of peritonitis in children with nephrotic syndrome and ascites. Similarly, immunologic impairment and portal hypertension in patients with cirrhosis increase the permeability of the gut wall, facilitating bacterial migration into ascitic fluid. Finally, the spread of genital tract bacteria from the fallopian tube along the paracolic gutter to the subphrenic area leads to the Fitz-Hugh–Curtis syndrome in patients with pelvic inflammatory disease.

Table 1. Subgroups of Patients Who Acquire Primary Peritonitis

Apparently normal infants and young children
Children with nephrotic syndrome
Patients with cirrhosis (usually associated with ascites)
Immunocompromised hosts
Women with pelvic inflammatory disease

Conditions that lead to loss of bowel integrity and secondary peritonitis (Table 2) include bowel perforation secondary to appendicitis, peptic ulcer, diverticulitis, cholecystitis, necrotic tumor, salpingitis, or postoperative anastomotic leak; operative injury; or external trauma. Aseptic peritonitis is attributed to irritation of the peritoneum by nonbacterial agents, such as bile, blood, meconium, gastric or pancreatic juice, barium, and glove powders containing talc or starch. Although aseptic peritonitis may begin as a noninfectious process, superinfection frequently supervenes. Tuberculous peritonitis, fungal and parasitic peritonitis, drug-related (beta-blocker) peritonitis, peritonitis associated with connective tissue disease, and peritonitis associated with familial Mediterranean fever have also been reported.

Presenting Signs and Symptoms

The onset of peritonitis varies; it may be sudden in patients with perforation or insidious in nonoperative patients and in certain postoperative patients. Most patients present with abdominal pain unless it is masked by medication, altered mental status, or the presence of a fresh surgical wound. Sudden onset of pain may accompany a

Table 2. Causes of Secondary Peritonitis

Viscus Perforations Secondary to Disease
Appendicitis
Gastric or duodenal ulcer
Meckel's diverticulum
Suppurative cholecystitis
Acute pancreatic necrosis
Inflammatory bowel disease
Volvulus
Intussusception
Tumor
Diverticulitis
Salpingitis
Traumatic Injuries
External trauma
Operative injury
Induced abortion or trauma during parturition
Postoperative Causes
Anastomotic leak
Retained foreign body in the peritoneal cavity
Contamination of the peritoneum

perforated viscus, whereas gradual onset of pain is often due to inflammation of an intra-abdominal organ.

The intensity of the pain, like the onset, varies. Sometimes the pain is severe and unremitting; at other times it is reported as a dull ache. Abdominal pain is typically most intense at the spreading edge of the *parietal* peritoneal inflammation. With either localization or resolution of the *peritoneal* inflammation, the pain decreases or shifts to a specific area of the abdomen. Shifting of pain is classically seen in patients with acute appendicitis. The pain originates in the periumbilical region and then localizes to the appendix.

Anorexia and nausea are frequently present in patients with peritonitis and may be accompanied by vomiting. In acute peritonitis, pain virtually always precedes vomiting. In the early stages of peritonitis, vomiting is forcible; later, it is caused by paralytic ileus. The vomitus results initially from the emptying of the stomach contents; later, it is brownish and bile-stained. Finally, when obstruction is complete, it is dark and feculent.

The patient's temperature varies according to the presentation. The temperature may be normal in patients with acute viscus perforation, but it gradually increases as peritonitis develops. By contrast, hypothermia may occur in severely ill patients with high cardiac output and peripheral vasodilation.

The pulse rate often indicates the true course of peritonitis. As the disease process advances, the rate and strength of the pulse increase steadily; later, the pulse becomes faster and weaker. Respirations typically are rapid and shallow because of the greater oxygen demand and immobility of the diaphragm. Most patients with peritonitis are constipated. A few patients with pelvic peritonitis may have diarrhea.

Physical Examination

The diagnosis of acute peritonitis is suggested by the early symptoms and is confirmed by physical examination. The characteristic appearance of a patient with advanced peritonitis was described by Hippocrates: The face is masklike, the eyes are hollow, the lips are blue, and the tongue is brown and dry. Although this classic description of the hippocratic facies applies to patients in the preterminal state, patients can appear seriously ill even in the early stage of the disease. Fever, tachycardia, shallow respirations, and signs of hypovolemia (reduced skin turgor, diminished peripheral pulse volume, hypotension, oliguria) are characteristic findings. The patient often lies quietly supine in bed, with the knees flexed to limit motion that would exacerbate the abdominal pain and to relieve tension on the abdominal muscles.

The abdomen is distended, quiet to auscultation, and exquisitely tender to palpation. Maximal tenderness is usually noted over the causative focus; in some patients, it is found over the advancing edge of inflammation. Rebound tenderness is pain caused by the sudden release of pressure by the examining hand. It is elicited by either direct palpation or percussion. Referred tenderness is pain experienced over the involved area from pressure exerted in an uninvolved portion of the abdominal wall. Rebound tenderness and referred tenderness are strong indicators of perotonitis. However, rigidity of the abdominal muscles is the most reliable sign. Initially, rigidity is the product of voluntary guarding and reflex muscle spasm caused by inflammation of the parietal peritoneum. As peritonitis advances, the reflex spasm becomes so severe that boardlike abdominal rigidity develops. Intestinal sounds are decreased at the onset and disappear entirely as gas in the adynamic, distended intestine is easily noted with percussion of the abdomen.

Rectal and pelvic examinations are important in assessing the degree of involvement of the pelvic peritoneum as well as in confirming the presence of inflammation in the uterus and fallopian tubes. A positive iliopsoas or obturator sign may also suggest retroperitoneal or pelvic inflammation. Serial examinations by the same examiner are invaluable in establishing the diagnosis, providing evidence of disease progression, and determining the need for surgical intervention.

Laboratory Tests

Leukocytosis with neutrophilia and increased band forms is common in peritonitis. However, the leukocyte count may be normal in early peritonitis as leukocytes are mobilized to the diseased area. Pyuria with bacteriuria suggests urinary tract infection, whereas sterile pyuria may indicate inflammation near the ureter or bladder. Blood cultures, hematocrit, serum electrolyte determinations, and urine specific gravity can also be useful tests in the diagnosis as well as management of peritonitis.

Diagnostic Tests

Lavage of the peritoneal cavity may confirm the diagnosis of peritonitis when the patient cannot provide a history or when the physical examination is unreliable because of altered sensorium, immune system compromise, or the presence of drugs. Recovery of blood, pus, or bowel contents is abnormal, and the presence of bilirubin, amylase, at least 100,000 erythrocytes/mm^3, or at least 500 leukocytes/mm^3 constitutes a positive lavage result. Lavage is sensitive but is not specific for the diagnosis of peritonitis.

Paracentesis is a useful tool for the clinician attempting to make a diagnosis of spontaneous bacterial peritonitis (SBP). In patients with cirrhosis, SBP has been classically defined by the presence of at least 250 neutrophils/mm^3 of ascitic fluid or by the culture of pathogenic bacteria from the ascitic fluid. The measurement of interleukin-6, tumor necrosis factor-alpha, and other mediators of inflammation in ascitic fluid may, in the future, aid the diagnosis or monitoring of treatment in cirrhotic patients with SBP.

Imaging Studies

Extensive imaging studies are not required for confirming clinical evidence of peritonitis. An upright chest film not only confirms the diagnosis of peritonitis preoperatively when free intraperitoneal air is present but also may exclude other intrathoracic and intraperitoneal causes of abdominal pain. Abdominal films may reveal biliary and renal calculi, fecaliths, air in the biliary tree, or abnormal bowel gas patterns suggesting either paralytic ileus or mechanical bowel obstruction. Rarely, air in the superior mesenteric or portal vein (a sign of advanced intestinal necrosis) may be seen. Obliteration of the psoas shadow and perinephric fat line suggests retroperitoneal inflammation.

Barium contrast studies can aid the diagnosis of volvulus, intestinal obstruction, or intussusception. However, because extravasation of barium alone can cause aseptic peritonitis, its use must be avoided if viscus perforation is strongly suspected. Water-soluble contrast medium is preferred for the confirmation or exclusion of perforation in patients whose radiographs do not show free intraperitoneal air.

Ultrasound can be used to detect cholelithiasis, cholecystitis, bile duct dilatation, intraperitoneal fluid, and pancreatic, intra-abdominal, and pelvic masses. Increasingly, ultrasonography should be used as part of the basic physical examination by the clinician. Computed tomography (CT) is the test of choice if an abscess is suspected.

Differential Diagnosis

The differential diagnosis is the same as that for the acute abdomen. In fact, many conditions—appendicitis, intussusception, peptic ulcer—may progress to peritonitis if left untreated. Early in the course of peritonitis, the signs and symptoms may overlap with other conditions in which abdominal pain is present. As peritonitis progresses, continuous abdominal pain, vomiting, abdominal tenderness, rigidity, and increasing distention make the diagnosis more obvious. Intrathoracic conditions such as lower lobe pneumonia and pleurisy may present with abdominal pain that is referred along the intercostal nerves, mimicking peritonitis. There is little or no abdominal rigidity, however, and the results of chest examination may be abnormal. Peritonitis and pulmonary disease may also coexist or present simultaneously. Patients with pericarditis and coronary thrombosis may complain of epigastric pain, suggesting a diagnosis of perforated peptic ulcer, cholecystitis, or acute pancreatitis. In these patients, the history of the pain and the results of the chest examination can help elucidate the diagnosis.

Intra-abdominal conditions that cause severe pain and mimic peritonitis include torsion of the ovary, torsion of a uterine fibroid, psoas abscesses, and intraperitoneal hemorrhage caused by trauma. Acute pyelonephritis usually causes severe flank pain on the side of the affected kidney, but associated ileus may contribute to diffuse abdominal discomfort. Systemic illnesses that cause abdominal pain include diabetic ketoacidosis, acute porphyria, and sickle cell crisis. Spinal cord tumors that compress nerve roots can also cause abdominal pain.

Course and Complications

The course of peritonitis depends on the speed of onset, the causative agent, and the site and extent of involvement. Every episode of peritonitis initiates a sequence of primary responses of the peritoneal membrane, the bowel, and body fluid compartments, which, in turn, produce secondary endocrine, cardiac, respiratory, renal, metabolic, and immunologic responses. The peritoneal membrane responds to insult with hyperemia and edema, followed by exudation of interstitial fluid (rich in fibrin) into the peritoneal cavity. In most patients, the fibrinous exudate absorbs without a trace. In some patients, the exudate distributes throughout the peritoneal cavity, disseminating the infection and causing sepsis. In other patients, the exudate remains localized, with resultant abscess formation and agglutination of loops of bowel and other viscera. Other complications include intestinal obstruction secondary to adhesions.

Peritoneal inflammation initially causes hypermotility of the bowel, which is followed by hypomotility and ultimately adynamic ileus. Fluid secretion into the bowel lumen is enhanced during ileus, and further sequestration of fluid occurs with overwhelming sepsis. As hypovolemia develops, venous return is decreased, cardiac output is diminished, and the heart compensates by increasing its rate. Hypovolemia, reduced cardiac output, and increased secretion of aldosterone and antidiuretic hormone act synergistically to decrease renal blood flow. In untreated patients, tubular necrosis and ultimately acute renal failure may occur. Metabolic acidosis is enhanced by decreased tissue perfusion, impairment of renal function, and bacterial infection. Pulmonary dysfunction is common in patients with peritonitis. Abdominal distention due to ileus and restricted diaphragmatic and intercostal respiratory movements due to pain result in atelectasis and predispose the patient to pulmonary infection. Inadequately treated peritonitis progresses to septicemia, disseminated intravascular coagulation, adult respiratory distress syndrome, multiple organ system failure, and death.

INTRA-ABDOMINAL ABSCESSES

Definition

An intra-abdominal abscess is a collection of infected material (fibrin, blood clots, pus) within the abdominal cavity. Solitary or multiple abscesses may occur in the peritoneal cavity, retroperitoneum, or abdominal viscera. Intraperitoneal abscesses commonly result from gastrointestinal perforations or inflammation (appendix, gallbladder, colon), operative complications (anastomotic leak or retained foreign body), penetrating trauma, genitourinary tract infections (pelvic inflammatory disease, septic abortion), or generalized peritonitis. Retroperitoneal abscesses are uncommon and result from either primary or secondary infection of tissue in the retroperitoneal space. Visceral abscesses typically arise from hematogenous spread.

Signs and Symptoms

The signs and symptoms of an intra-abdominal abscess include persistent spiking fever, tachycardia, anorexia, weight loss, and abdominal tenderness. Symptoms may be masked, especially in postoperative, chronically ill, or diabetic patients as well as in those receiving antibiotics, analgesics, or immunosuppressive drugs. In these patients, fever, tachycardia, and pain may be mild or even absent. Patients with an abscess located deep within the abdomen may present with fever only. Frequently, symptoms are related to irritation of contiguous structures by the abscess. A subphrenic abscess may irritate the diaphragm, causing shoulder or chest pain, hiccups, and dyspnea. Pelvic abscesses may impinge on the bowel and bladder, causing diarrhea or urinary urgency.

Physical Examination and Laboratory Findings

On physical examination, patients with intra-abdominal abscesses classically have spiking fevers, a high pulse rate, and abdominal tenderness. An abdominal mass is not usually palpable, and tenderness localized to the site of the abscess is not found consistently. Vaginal and digital rectal examinations are helpful in detecting a pelvic fluid collection, mass, cervical motion tenderness, or tubo-ovarian mass.

The complete blood count often shows a persistent leukocytosis. If the abscess is not contained, septicemia and multisystem organ failure may ensue, accompanied by leukocytosis or leukopenia, abnormal results on liver function tests, and metabolic acidosis. In septic patients, blood cultures are typically positive. The diagnosis of intra-abdominal abscess should be suspected in any patient with a predisposing condition and in any postoperative patient with intermittent fever who fails to recover in a reasonable time frame.

Diagnostic Tests

Plain films of the abdomen and chest are frequently helpful but are nonspecific for the diagnosis of intra-abdominal abscesses. An elevated, immobile, poorly defined diaphragm; basilar atelectasis; and pleural effusion suggest the presence of a subphrenic abscess. Air-fluid levels, extraluminal gas, loss of soft tissue density, and displacement of intra-abdominal organs may be seen on plain abdominal films. Despite low diagnostic sensitivity, oral and rectal contrast studies may confirm the extraintestinal location of an abnormal gas collection. These studies may also reveal a perforation, leak, or obstruction or displacement of genitourinary structures in the presence of a retroperitoneal abscess.

Ultrasonography provides rapid, noninvasive bedside evaluation of the abdomen and may well become a standard part of the physical examination. The classic ultrasound image of an abscess is a sonolucent mass with thick irregular margins, a hypoechogenic cavity, distal acoustic enhancement, and a thin peripheral halo. Sometimes the fluid collections are echogenic if particulate matter or septa are present in the abscess cavity. Ultrasound is highly sensitive in detecting abscesses in the right upper quadrant, retroperitoneum, and pelvis. This study is very technician-dependent. Interpretation is adversely influenced by excessive adipose tissue or bowel gas or the presence of ostomies, drains, and abdominal bandages. Limitations of transcutaneous ultrasonography can be overcome using direct endosonography via the gastrointestinal lumen. The transgastric route enhances detection of abscesses in the lesser sac, the left subphrenic area, the subhepatic spaces, and the liver parenchyma. A combined transgastric and transduodenal approach provides accurate visualization of the entire pancreas, whereas a transrectosigmoid approach aids detection of deep pelvic abscesses.

Similarly, intraoperative ultrasonography can avoid some of the disadvantages of percutaneous ultrasound. It is valuable in localizing abscesses prior to tissue dissection, confirming or excluding the diagnosis of an abscess suspected preoperatively, identifying important adjacent structures such as major blood vessels and pancreatic and biliary ducts, and guiding the needle for aspiration of fluid collections.

Computed tomography (CT) is currently the "gold standard" test for detecting intra-abdominal abscesses. It is fast and probably cost-effective. When compared with conventional scans, CT offers a slight increase in diagnostic accuracy at the expense of a higher dose of radiation. Oral ingestion of diluted, water-soluble contrast medium is needed to opacify the bowel; otherwise it is mistaken for an abscess. When a pelvic abscess is suspected, rectal contrast medium is administered. A CT scan with intravenous administration of contrast medium enhances the rim of an abscess because of the hyperthermia that typically surrounds the lesion. Classically, abscesses on CT scans appear as well-defined, low-density masses that are round or ellipsoid, with inappropriate extraluminal gas pockets, air-fluid levels, and thickening of fascial planes.

CT and ultrasound are not entirely specific for the diagnosis of intra-abdominal abscesses. Tumors, hematomas, cysts, bile, and urine collections cannot always be distinguished from abscesses. Hence, the radiographic findings must be correlated closely with clinical findings, physical examination, and supporting laboratory data and must be confirmed by CT-guided needle aspiration. Percutaneous needle aspiration may permit rapid identification of pathogenic organisms via Gram stain and culture of the aspirate as well as placement of a percutaneous drain through the pre-existing needle tract.

Radioisotope scanning is occasionally useful when focal symptoms are absent and occult sepsis or fever of unknown origin is present. Available techniques include a gallium-67 citrate scan, a technetium-99m (^{99m}TC) sulfur colloid liver-spleen scan, a combined liver-lung scan, and indium-111 oxinate–labeled leukocyte scan. ^{67}Ga-citrate isotope is relatively inexpensive and has the greatest clinical applicability. After intravenous administration, ^{67}Ga-citrate strongly binds to plasma proteins and to neutrophil membranes. Imaging is performed at 48, 72, or 96 hours. ^{67}Ga-citrate scanning is highly sensitive in localizing intra-abdominal abscesses; however, ^{67}Ga-citrate tends to accumulate in neoplastic tissues, fresh surgical scars, colostomies, surgical drain sites, fractures, and myocardial and cerebral infarcts. Physiologic uptake of gallium by the liver and spleen renders this type of scanning nonspecific for diagnosis of an upper abdominal abscess. Because a considerable amount of the injected isotope is excreted through the gut, its distribution must be evaluated within 48 hours of administration.

^{111}In-labeled neutrophil scanning is a relatively expensive and elaborate technique based on the hypothesis that leukocytes migrate to areas of inflammation or abscess formation. Hence, false-positive results may be found in chronically walled-off abscesses or fungal and parasitic abscesses. Like ^{67}Ga-citrate, ^{111}In uptake is nonspecific, and this radioisotope can localize in tumors as well as in normal liver, bone marrow, and spleen. Because the amount of radiation required for visualizing these organs is relatively large, especially in the spleen, the amount of injectable isotope is limited. Other disadvantages of ^{111}In are the bowel preparation required prior to scanning and the lack of specificity in diagnosing upper abdominal inflammation. Administration of steroids and antibiotics that inhibit neutrophil function may interfere with the sensitivity of the test. Because ^{111}In-labeled leukocytes do not typically accumulate in the gut, the examination is usually completed in 24 hours.

In general, the specificity of the ^{111}In scan is reported to be slightly better than that of ^{67}Ga-citrate. When combined with a ^{99m}Tc-sulfur colloid liver-spleen scan and subtraction imaging, ^{67}Ga-citrate leukocyte scans and ^{111}In-labeled leukocyte scans are highly specific for detecting an upper abdominal abscess. A combined ^{99m}Tc liver-lung scan is used occasionally for the demonstration of right-sided subphrenic abscesses. Radioisotope studies are time-consuming and require the patient to be able and willing to lie motionless for several minutes.

Magnetic resonance imaging (MRI) affords delineation in multiple planes and provides information about the presence of fluid or tissue inflammation at improved resolution when compared with a CT scan. Magnetic resonance imaging is highly accurate in detecting intra-abdominal abscesses but does have certain limitations; it is a time-consuming technique hindered by respiratory motion. Moreover, MRI is difficult to accomplish in the presence of respiratory support and monitoring equipment. Finally, MRI is difficult to interpret and probably should not be undertaken in patients with heart-assist and other ferromagnetic devices.

VIRAL HEPATITIS

By Brent A. Neuschwander-Tetri, M.D.,
and Bruce R. Bacon, M.D.
St. Louis, Missouri

Viral hepatitis continues to be a major cause of acute disability, chronic illness, and death despite both an improved understanding of the causative agents and progress in the development of therapeutic options. Preventing the spread of viral hepatitis and treating infected patients appropriately requires timely identification of the cause as well as appropriate patient education. Liver injury caused by the hepatotropic viruses typically leads to symptoms and serum biochemical changes that are also found in many other causes of acute and chronic liver injury (Tables 1 and 2). To identify a viral cause, a number of serologic and molecular tests are available. Interpretation of the results of these tests is not always straightforward, however, and diagnostic accuracy remains suboptimal. Nevertheless, this article details various strategies that help distinguish viral hepatitis from other causes of liver injury.

HEPATITIS A VIRUS

Infection by the hepatitis A virus (HAV) causes an acute, self-limited illness that results in permanent immunity to reinfection.

Clinical Findings

The clinical course of hepatitis A depends on the patient's age and the presence or absence of pre-existing liver disease. For example, infected children often have clinically silent or unrecognized illness, whereas older children experience diarrhea, abdominal pain, malaise, and fever that may suggest a nonspecific viral syndrome. Jaundice occurs in a small fraction of children, and death from fulminant liver disease in children is extremely rare.

Table 1. Causes of Clinically Significant Acute Liver Injury

Clinical Characteristics

Rise of aminotransferase levels (ALT and AST), often to >1000 U/L, over days to weeks
Possible complications: fulminant hepatic failure, persistence as chronic hepatitis

Most Common Causes

Alcohol*
Autoimmune hepatitis
Biliary obstruction (acute)
Drugs: acetaminophen
Infections: HAV, HBV, HCV
Shock liver

Less Common Causes

Drugs: chlorpromazine, halothane, isoniazid, phenytoin, sodium valproate
Fulminant Wilson's disease
Infections: HEV, CMV, coxsackievirus, EBV (infectious mononucleosis), HSV, toxoplasmosis
Metastatic disease to the liver: solid tumors, lymphoma
Right-sided congestive heart failure (severe)
Toxins: *Amanita* mushrooms

*Acute alcoholic hepatitis is rarely associated with an AST activity greater than 500 U/L. The AST activity is typically two times higher than the ALT activity.

AST = aspartate aminotransferase; ALT = alanine aminotransferase; HAV = hepatitis A virus; HBV = hepatitis B virus; HCV = hepatitis C virus; HEV = hepatitis E virus; CMV = cytomegalovirus; EBV = Epstein-Barr virus; HSV = herpes simplex virus.

Table 2. Causes of Clinically Significant Chronic Liver Injury

Clinical Characteristics

Persistent increased aminotransferase activities, usually <1000 U/L, for months to years
Normal or nearly normal aminotransferase activities in some diseases (e.g., hemochromatosis, HCV infection)
Possible complications: cirrhosis, hepatocellular carcinoma

Most Common Causes

Alcohol
Autoimmune hepatitis
Drugs: α-methyldopa, amiodarone, nitrofurantoin, vitamin A
Hemochromatosis
Infections: HBV and HCV infection
Steatohepatitis in nonalcoholic patients

Less Common Causes

α_1-Antitrypsin deficiency
Carbohydrate and glycogen storage disorders
Cholestatic diseases: malignant obstruction, primary biliary cirrhosis, primary sclerosing cholangitis
Chronic venous congestion
Infections: delta hepatitis
Protein and amino acid metabolic disorders
Schistosomiasis (common in endemic areas)
Vascular obstruction: veno-occlusive disease, Budd-Chiari syndrome
Wilson's disease

HCV = hepatitis C virus; HBV = hepatitis B virus.

Adults infected with HAV typically present with a more severe illness. Malaise, jaundice, and fever are characteristic and can persist for several weeks. Fulminant hepatitis, leading to death or liver transplantation, occurs more frequently than in the pediatric population but is still unusual. Pre-existing liver disease probably increases the likelihood of fulminant hepatitis and may explain many of the deaths caused by HAV.

Laboratory Evaluation

Compared with the evaluation of other types of viral hepatitis, the laboratory evaluation of HAV is relatively straightforward. At the time of presentation, serum aminotransferase concentrations are increased, often exceeding 1000 U/L. The total serum bilirubin concentration rises, and most of it is conjugated ("direct reacting"), reflecting the capacity of the injured liver to conjugate but not excrete bilirubin. With severe liver injury, the prothrombin time is prolonged as a result of immediately impaired synthetic capacity. Changes in prothrombin time and factor V concentrations are especially useful in the setting of acute liver injury. The dehydrated patient or the patient with a prothrombin time that is prolonged more than several seconds requires hospitalization until a reversal of these trends is observed.

Establishing the diagnosis of acute HAV infection relies entirely on the serologic evaluation (Table 3). Part of the immediate immune response to HAV infection is the production of IgA, IgM, and IgG antibodies directed toward viral capsid antigens. As with most acute infections, the IgM response is transient and generally becomes unmeasurable within 6 months, although measurable persistence of detectable IgM can occur for up to 12 months. Thus, in

Table 3. Serologic Findings in Hepatitis A Infection

Test	When to Order	Positive Interpretation	Negative Interpretation
Anti-HAV IgM	Acute illness with increased ALT or AST activities Recent (<6 mo) icteric illness	HAV infection within preceding 6 mo	No HAV infection within preceding 12 mo
Anti-HAV, total	Identify vaccine candidates? Attempt to diagnose an earlier (>6 mo) icteric illness	HAV infection or vaccine during lifetime (recent or remote) Immune globulin prophylaxis within preceding 2 mo	No previous HAV infection

Anti-HAV IgM = IgM antibody to hepatitis A virus; ALT = alanine aminotransferase; AST = aspartate aminotransferase; HAV = hepatitis A virus; anti-HAV, total = total antibody to hepatitis A virus (IgA, IgG, and IgM).

acute liver injury, the presence of HAV IgM usually implicates this virus as the causative organism. The second test for the diagnosis of HAV infection is the measurement of total antibody to the virus (anti-HAV) (see Table 3). A positive total anti-HAV test result reflects the presence of IgG antibody when the IgM assay is negative. Anti-HAV IgG is lifelong and confers protection against reinfection. Measurement of total antibody has value primarily in epidemiologic studies and perhaps in identifying potential candidates for vaccination.

Liver Biopsy

Liver biopsy generally is not required for the management of a patient with HAV infection. The serologic findings are definitive and the clinical course is characteristic, leaving little doubt as to the diagnosis. Occasionally, patients with HAV infection experience a prolonged cholestatic illness. In these patients, a liver biopsy can exclude other causes of intrahepatic cholestasis if the extrahepatic biliary tree is normal as seen by sonography and/or endoscopic retrograde cholangiopancreatography (ERCP).

Differential Diagnosis

Serologic evaluation for acute HAV infection typically follows the recognition of increased aminotransferase activity in serum with or without hyperbilirubinemia. Until serologic test results are available, the search for mononucleosis, drugs (e.g., acetaminophen), toxins (e.g., mushrooms), compromised blood flow (e.g., transient hypotension, right-sided heart failure), and other less common causes of acute liver injury (see Table 1) should continue. Because HAV IgM determinations can remain positive for up to 12 months after acute infection, a positive finding of anti-HAV IgM may be due to an earlier subclinical episode of HAV infection. The rate at which the increased serum aminotransferase concentrations return to normal may distinguish an infectious cause of liver injury from a toxic or ischemic insult. Because the latter causes of liver injury are typically limited to hours or a few days, the recovery phase after injury is characterized by normalization of aminotransferase activity in serum at rates that correspond to their respective circulating half-lives (aspartate aminotransferase [AST] about 12 hours; alanine aminotransferase [ALT] about 24 to 36 hours). In contrast, following acute viral injury, the normalization of aminotransferase activity takes place over weeks.

HEPATITIS B VIRUS

Although dramatic progress has been achieved in eliminating the hepatitis B virus (HBV) from blood products and preventing infection with HBV by vaccination, about 200,000 individuals are still infected with the virus yearly in the United States. Dominant modes of transmission are heterosexual exposure and intravenous drug abuse. As many as 10 per cent of these new infections lead to chronic infection, adding to the roughly 750,000 carriers of this virus in the United States. Two questions should be asked when evaluating any patient with evidence of HBV.

1. Is this acute or chronic infection with HBV?
2. If this is chronic infection with HBV, what is the degree of ongoing viral replication?

Clinical Findings

Acute infection with HBV is evident clinically by symptoms associated with most other causes of acute liver injury: anorexia, fatigue, nausea, and vomiting followed within days by the development of jaundice. These symptoms typically persist for several weeks. In patients with chronic HBV, the severity of symptoms ranges from nonexistent to debilitating. Patients with low viral replication ("healthy carriers") are asymptomatic, whereas patients with active viral replication experience fatigue and manifest extrahepatic complications of immune complex deposition, including rashes, arthralgias, and renal impairment.

Laboratory Evaluation

The clinician caring for a patient with HBV infection faces a daunting array of laboratory tests to aid evaluation and management (Table 4). Physicians must understand what each test means and when it should be used for diagnosis and/or therapy.

Hepatitis B surface antigen (HBsAg) is the major viral coat protein. HBsAg is detectable in hepatocytes and in the serum (up to 10^{13} particles/mL) of patients with active viral replication. A minute fraction (<1 per cent) of HBsAg detected in serum represents intact virus. HBsAg is often detectable at the time of presentation in patients with acute HBV infection, but in some patients it may already have been diminished by an effective immune response.

Antibody to HBsAg (anti-HBs) develops in 90 per cent of patients infected with the virus and reflects effective clearance of the viral infection. HBsAg may become undetectable several weeks before the appearance of measurable anti-HBs. This "window" period probably reflects the inability of many assays to detect low concentrations of antigen and antibody during this period of seroconversion. Anti-HBs also develops in response to HBV vaccination. Both HBsAg and anti-HBs are detected in a few patients. In this case, the antibody is not protective and the patient should be considered to have active HBV infection. Although the development of anti-HBs indicates resolution of infection, the presence of this antibody following viral

Table 4. Serologic Findings in Hepatitis B Infection

Test	When to Order	Positive Interpretation	Negative Interpretation
HBsAg	Evaluate increased serum aminotransferase activity Risk factors for HBV (sexual, intravenous drug abuse, vertical transmission)	Acute, unresolved HBV infection Chronic HBV infection	Does not fully exclude acute or chronic HBV infection
Anti-HBs	Question of prior HBV infection Known prior HBV infection, question of seroconversion Evaluate response to vaccine	Prior HBV infection, seroconverted Prior HBV vaccine (Generally not seen following administration of hepatitis B immune globulin)	No seroconversion
Anti-HBc, total	Screen blood donors	Prior HBV infection, acute or chronic	No prior HBV infection
Anti-HBc, IgM	Evaluate increased serum aminotransferase activity Distinguish acute from chronic HBV infection (only if a low titer IgM is considered negative)	Acute HBV infection (if IgM titer is high) Chronic HBV infection (usually low IgM titer)	
HBeAg	Determine replicative activity in a patient with known HBV infection	HBV in a high replicative state (acute or chronic)	If previously positive, reflects either seroconversion or conversion to a low replicative state
Anti-HBe	Determine replicative activity in a patient with known HBV infection	Recent acute HBV infection Chronic HBV infection in a low replicative state	High replicative state if HBsAg determination positive
HBV DNA	Determine replicative activity in a patient with known HBV infection	High concentrations signify active viral replication	

HBsAg = hepatitis B surface antigen; anti-HBs = antibody to HBsAg; anti-HBc, total = total antibody to hepatitis B core antigen; anti-HBc, IgM = antibody to hepatitis B core antigen IgM; HBeAg = hepatitis Be antigen; anti-HBe = antibody to HBeAg; HBV DNA = hepatitis B virus DNA.

infection does not imply complete clearance of the virus from the host. Residual virus may exist in extrahepatic tissues (lymphocytes, bone marrow, spleen, pancreas), and resurgence of clinically severe hepatitis can occur in such patients after immune suppression (e.g., cancer chemotherapy).

Another clinically important viral protein is hepatitis B core antigen (HBcAg), which is not detectable in serum but generates an antibody response measured as anti-core IgM (anti-HBc IgM) and total anti-core antibody (anti-HBc total). The IgM response is detected in patients with acute HBV and is thus useful in diagnosing patients in the window period that can occur after HBsAg has become undetectable and before anti-HBs has appeared. Anti-HBc IgM can help distinguish acute from chronic HBV infection in patients with increased aminotransferase activity and detectable HBsAg. Patients with acute HBV infection have relatively high titers of anti-HBc IgM, whereas patients with chronic HBV infection typically have low titers of anti-HBc IgM. Test manufacturers define the cutoff point between a positive and a negative test result to exclude low titers from being interpreted as positive results. Defining a positive and negative result in this way generally distinguishes between patients with acute and chronic disease. Some overlap exists, however, with a few patients with chronic HBV infection exhibiting concentrations of anti-HBc IgM high enough to be interpreted as a positive result.

In managing the individual patient, measuring anti-HBc total is less helpful. Because anti-HBc total detects the presence of anti-HBc IgM, this test result is positive whenever the IgM test gives positive results. The IgG response occurs in patients with chronic HBV infection as well as in patients who have cleared the infection. Anti-HBc total is therefore useful in screening blood donors for prior HBV exposure. Anti-HBs and anti-HBc generally persist indefinitely. A small fraction of patients may lose anti-HBs over decades, leaving an isolated anti-HBc IgG. Unfortunately, undetectable HBsAg can develop in patients with low-level viral replication over many years as well. This is especially true for chronic hemodialysis patients. Thus, an isolated anti-HBc total (with a negative anti-HBc IgM result) indicates prior HBV exposure but does not allow the important distinction between the patient in whom immunity has developed and the patient with low-grade chronic infection.

Another viral protein, the hepatitis B e antigen (HBeAg), is an extended and modified form of HBcAg, with a leader sequence that destines this protein for export into the blood. The presence of HBeAg signifies active viral replication, in either acute or chronic HBV infection. The antibody response to HBeAg is detectable as antibody to HBeAg (anti-HBe). Patients with suppressed viral replication that occurs following mother-to-child (vertical) transmission or seroconversion in the course of chronic HBV infection typically have detectable antibody but no antigen. Conversely, patients with active viral replication have detectable antigen but no antibody. Seroconversion occurs in about 10 per cent of patients with chronic HBV infection yearly and may not be permanent. It is usually associated with a symptomatic flare of the hepatitis and substantial increases in serum aminotransferase activity. HBeAg and anti-HBe testing is best used to identify patients who show active replication and might be candidates for interferon therapy or to evaluate patients during flares of disease. Establishing the infectivity of patients with HBV infection based on the presence or absence of HBeAg is no longer a valid use of the test because of the potential infectivity of all patients with chronic HBV infection.

Supplanting the detection of HBeAg as a means of establishing active viral replication is the direct measurement of serum HBV DNA. The DNA detected is in the form of intact virions, which in chronic HBV infection can be present in concentrations up to 10^9 particles/mL of blood. The test is useful primarily in predicting and evaluating the response to interferon treatment.

Liver Biopsy

Blood tests are usually adequate to establish the diagnosis of acute and chronic HBV. Nonetheless, a liver biopsy contributes to management decisions by establishing the degree of inflammation and fibrosis. The progression to cirrhosis, which occurs in about one quarter of patients with chronic HBV infection, is associated with a poor prognosis.

A wide spectrum of inflammatory changes is found in the liver in chronic HBV infection. The patient with active viral replication has portal and lobular lymphocyte-predominant inflammatory cell infiltrates, whereas a minimal or absent inflammatory response is characteristic of the quiescent "healthy carrier" without evidence of viral replication. Both HBsAg and HBcAg are detectable in scattered hepatocytes by immunohistochemical techinques when there is doubt as to the diagnosis.

Differential Diagnosis

Similar to the other forms of viral hepatitis, the diagnostic considerations during the period of acute hepatitis are broad (see Table 1). Because HBsAg and anti-HBc IgM can be found occasionally in chronic HBV infection as well as in acute HBV infection, the presence of these markers does not establish HBV as a cause of acute liver injury with certainty. The other potential causes of liver injury should be excluded in all patients by history and laboratory evaluation.

HEPATITIS C

Acute infection with the hepatitis C virus (HCV) is rarely recognized. Infection with this virus typically persists, and chronic HCV infection has become one of the most common causes of chronic liver disease. Fully 1.4 per cent of the population in the United States has serologic evidence of HCV infection, and cirrhosis caused by chronic HCV infection is currently one of the leading indications for liver transplantation. Although exposure to infected blood by transfusion or intravenous drug abuse accounts for a significant portion of HCV transmission, about 40 per cent of patients have acquired the infection "sporadically" without an identifiable parenteral source. Sexual transmission of HCV occurs but is much less frequent than the sexual transmission of human immunodeficiency virus (HIV) or HBV and is presumed to account for only a small fraction of cases.

Clinical Findings

Most patients with acute HCV infection have a mild and clinically unrecognized illness. Twenty-five per cent of acutely infected patients have an overt illness that is indistinguishable from acute HAV or HBV. The symptoms resolve within several weeks of the onset of symptoms, leaving most patients (>80 per cent) with sustained viremia and chronic low-level hepatitis. Fatigue can remain a debilitating symptom in patients with chronic HCV infection whose hepatic synthetic reserve is otherwise adequate.

The likelihood of chronic HCV infection progressing to cirrhosis is unresolved. Studies of several large groups of patients with HCV infection have not demonstrated significantly increased mortality from liver-related causes over one to two decades. However, the patients who come to medical attention invariably have some degree of inflammation seen on liver biopsy, and fibrosis is frequently observed. The subset of patients with chronic HCV infection that come to medical attention may reflect important differences in either viral or host factors that predispose to the development of liver disease.

Laboratory Evaluation

The history of laboratory diagnosis of HCV is short. Following the discovery of the virus in 1989, a test for the presence of antibodies to one viral antigen known as c100-3 was released in May 1990. Although this first-generation enzyme immunoassay (EIA-1) greatly improved the safety of the blood supply, it was not particularly sensitive or specific. The second-generation test (EIA-2) improved the sensitivity, especially early after acute infection, by identifying antibodies against three viral epitopes (c100-3, c33c, and c22-3). The EIA-2 has adequate specificity for reliably testing patients with identifiable risks, but in those with a low pretest probability of HCV infection, the significant risk of a false-positive result continues to require confirmatory testing.

There are at least two confirmatory tests for HCV infection (Table 5). The second generation recombinant immunoblot assay (RIBA-2) identifies antibodies to four specific viral antigens (c100-3, c33c, c22-3, 5-1-1) and at least two of the four antibodies must be present to consider the result positive. Detecting viral RNA in the blood directly by the polymerase chain reaction (PCR) is the other diagnostic option. Usually the two tests agree with each other and are more than 90 per cent sensitive and specific. Many clinicians rely on the RIBA-2 as a confirmatory test and use PCR to sort out the occasional indeterminate RIBA-2 result.

False-positive EIA-2 test results for HCV infection are problematic in selected groups of patients. Patients with autoimmune hepatitis (AIH) can have a positive EIA-2 result without demonstrable viral infection seen by PCR or RIBA-2. The response of these patients to corticosteroid therapy confirms the diagnosis of AIH in retrospect, but this distinguishing characteristic is of little help to the clinician when the diagnostic options are being weighed prospectively. In general, patients with AIH are more symptomatic and jaundiced than are patients with HCV. Much of the concern about misdiagnosing patients was raised before the availability of PCR testing for HCV. If the autoimmune serologic tests (antinuclear, anti–smooth muscle, and anti–liver-kidney-microsomal [anti-LKM] antibodies) raise the possibility of AIH and the liver biopsy is not characteristic for AIH or HCV, the positive EIA-2 result can be confirmed or negated using PCR.

The high prevalence of positive EIA-2 test results in alcoholic patients has been confirmed by the more specific tests. Although alcoholic patients could have a high false-positive rate of HCV infection by EIA-2 testing due to hyperglobulinemia or other factors, it appears more likely that these individuals have a greater risk of acquiring HCV or that alcoholic patients infected with HCV have a greater likelihood of acquiring liver disease that requires medical attention.

False-negative EIA test results for HCV can be a significant problem. False-negative results occur early in the

Table 5. Serologic Findings in Hepatitis C Infection

Test	When to Order	Positive Interpretation	Negative Interpretation
HCV EIA-2 (ELISA)	Increased aminotransferase activity Dialysis patients	HCV infection (likely with risk factors and increased aminotransferase activity) False-positive result (about 50 per cent chance in the absence of risk factors and normal aminotransferase activity)	No HCV infection Too early in the course of acute HCV infection to detect False-negative result (dialysis, immunosuppression)
HCV RIBA-2	Positive EIA-2 without risk factors	HCV infection	HCV infection unlikely False-negative result (dialysis)
HCV RNA by PCR	Indeterminate findings on RIBA-2 Negative EIA-2 and/or RIBA-2 with high index of suspicion	HCV infection	No HCV infection

HCV = hepatitis C virus; EIA-2 = second-generation enzyme immunoassay; ELISA = enzyme-linked immunosorbent assay; RIBA-2 = second-generation recombinant immunoblot assay; PCR = polymerase chain reaction.

course of a recently acquired infection or in patients who are immunosuppressed or receiving dialysis. Although no large studies have been conducted using PCR as a gold standard, limited reports suggest that the EIA-2 misses up to one third of those with HCV infection, or even more in dialysis patients. When the index of suspicion is high and the EIA-2 results are negative, further testing for HCV infection using PCR to detect viral RNA directly is warranted. Unfortunately, the index of suspicion is not always high, and the progression to significant liver disease occurs silently. The advance to EIA-2 from EIA-1 testing did reduce the chance of failure to diagnose HCV infection earlier in its course because the newer test can detect antibodies to c22c and c33c, which may develop earlier than the antibodies to c100-3. Despite this improvement, a delay of up to 6 months after infection can occur before antibodies are detected by the EIA-2.

Although patients with chronic HCV infection can have normal serum aminotransferase activities, the typical patient has aminotransferase activities ranging from barely above normal to four times the upper limit of normal. A pattern of cholestatic injury (increased bilirubin concentration and alkaline phosphatase activity) is not typically found in patients with HCV infection. In the final stages of liver failure, the serum bilirubin concentration increases, but this is accompanied by obvious complications of end-stage liver disease (wasting, ascites, encephalopathy, variceal hemorrhage). Mixed cryoglobulinemia is a recently recognized complication of chronic HCV infection and is manifested by arthralgias, weakness, and palpable purpura. Serum is obtained from warm whole blood and then cooled to identify this entity.

Liver Biopsy

The number of patients with chronic liver disease of unknown cause shrank considerably when HCV was discovered. The distinction between chronic persistent hepatitis and chronic active hepatitis has now been abandoned in favor of a classification system based on the likely cause (HCV), the degree and location of inflammation (mild, moderate, or severe), and the presence and severity of fibrosis. The characteristic histologic findings of chronic HCV infection include hepatocellular steatosis, mixed inflammatory cell infiltrates and occasional lymphoid aggregates in the portal region, and varying degrees of portal fibrosis. The presence of fibrosis is worrisome as a possible progenitor of cirrhosis. However, the prognosis of the varying degrees of inflammation is uncertain and may reflect host factors as well as the viral subtype.

A liver biopsy is warranted in most patients with HCV infection and increased aminotransferase activity in the serum. An argument can also be made for performing a liver biopsy in patients with normal aminotransferase activity because the serum markers do not predict liver histopathologic findings, and 30 to 50 per cent of these patients will have varying degrees of chronic hepatitis. For the latter group, biopsy is typically used to assess prognosis.

Differential Diagnosis

Other than blood transfusion or intravenous drug abuse, there is nothing in the clinical history that would enhance suspicion of HCV as a cause of acute or chronic hepatitis (see Tables 1 and 2). Thus, the diagnosis of HCV infection relies primarily on serologic tests. The liver biopsy may help identify the role of HCV infection as a cause of liver injury when other likely causes are clinically relevant. These other causes typically include transplant rejection, AIH, and drug-induced injury.

HEPATITIS D (DELTA) VIRUS

The delta hepatitis virus is an unusual cause of liver disease in the United States. As a copathogen with HBV, delta infection primarily occurs in the urban intravenous drug user.

Clinical Findings

Delta infection occurs either as an acute coinfection with HBV or as a secondary superinfection in patients with preexisting chronic HBV infection. Delta infection is not a consideration in patients who do not have active HBV infection. The presentation of coinfection with delta virus is similar to that of acute HBV infection, and establishing the additional presence of delta virus cannot be made on clinical grounds alone. Coinfection with delta virus does not diminish the 90 per cent chance that acute HBV infection will be cleared and not persist as chronic hepatitis. Acute delta virus infection in the patient with pre-existing chronic HBV (superinfection) can have similar clinical manifestations as a flare of HBV infection. However, delta virus infection in the patient with chronic HBV infection can cause fulminant hepatic failure and also accelerates the progression to end-stage liver disease despite the suppression of HBV replication.

Table 6. Serologic Findings in Delta Virus Infection

Test	When to Order	Positive Interpretation	Negative Interpretation
Anti-HDV	Acute hepatitis B (+ anti-HBc IgM) Chronic hepatitis B (measure once in everyone) Chronic hepatitis B with a clinical flare of liver disease	HDV infection; with acute HBV = coinfection with chronic HBV = superinfection	No HDV infection Too early in course (retest later)

Anti-HDV = antibodies to delta hepatitis; anti-HBc IgM = antibody to hepatitis B core antigen IgM; HDV = hepatitis delta virus; HBV = hepatitis B virus.

Laboratory Evaluation

An antibody response to the delta virus is detected within 6 to 8 weeks after infection coincident with or shortly after the onset of symptoms (Table 6). Patients with delta virus infection usually have detectable HBsAg, although occasionally patients with acute coinfection do not have measurable HBsAg and the only indication of possible viral infection is the presence of anti-HBc IgM. Thus, the rational sequence of serologic studies in patients with clinical evidence of hepatitis is first to perform the relevant HBV tests (HBsAg and anti-HBc IgM) and then to test any patient with HBsAg for delta virus at least once by measuring total antibody to delta antigen (anti-delta). Patients also should be retested during flares of disease if risk factors for delta virus transmission persist. Secondary infection with delta virus is typically associated with a reduction of HBV replication. This is documented serologically by the loss of HBeAg and the development of anti-HBe.

Liver Biopsy

Delta antigen is easily detected by immunohistochemical staining of the biopsy specimen. Thus delta virus infection may be detected in patients even when antibody is not detectable. Delta antigen testing is usually unnecessary in patients who have both HBsAg and anti-delta.

Differential Diagnosis

Diagnosing delta virus infection requires testing for anti-delta in all patients presenting with acute HBV infection or an exacerbation of chronic HBV infection. The failure to consider delta virus as a coinfecting agent may cause the physician to underestimate the rate of progression of disease or the chance of fulminant liver failure developing.

HEPATITIS E VIRUS

The hepatitis E virus (HEV) is transmitted by the oral-fecal route and is associated with epidemics in developing nations. Infection in the United States has been reported only in travelers from endemic areas, and there have been no cases of secondary infection of other individuals.

Clinical Findings

Typical symptoms of acute HEV infection develop 4 to 6 weeks after exposure and lead to a fully resolved illness within several weeks. Patients in large outbreaks in endemic areas have been uniformly jaundiced, although this may reflect a bias caused by the degree of illness that leads to medical evaluation. Lifelong immunity develops following infection, and progression to chronic disease is not a feature of HEV infection. A unique feature of HEV infection, when compared with the clinically similar disease of acute HAV infection, is the risk of fulminant hepatitis leading to a nearly 20 per cent mortality rate in pregnant women. The basis for this unusual presentation is not known.

Laboratory Evaluation

Serologic tests for the presence of IgM and IgG antibodies to HEV have been developed using recombinant peptides (Table 7). The IgM is detectable in the serum at the time of presentation or within several weeks thereafter. The IgM response becomes undetectable after several months and is replaced by IgG. The availability of serologic testing to establish the diagnosis of HEV infection makes the need for liver biopsy less urgent. Cholestatic injury is a prominent histologic feature in most cases. HEV infection should be suspected in patients presenting with an acute icteric illness after exposure in an endemic region. Until the serologic evaluation is complete, the differential diagnosis includes all forms of acute hepatitis (see Table 1).

SUMMARY

Diagnosing viral hepatitis requires an understanding of each of the known viral causes as well as the diseases they can mimic. HAV, HBV, and HCV—the most common causes of viral hepatitis—should be considered as possible causes of acutely increased serum aminotransferase activities, especially when the activities of these enzymes exceed 20 times the upper limit of normal. When such increases are encountered, the diagnostic considerations should also include AIH, acute biliary obstruction, drug toxicity, ischemia, and the less common causes of acute liver injury (see Table 1). Although each of the hepatotropic viruses can cause acute hepatitis, only HBV and HCV cause chronic

Table 7. Serologic Findings in Hepatitis E Infection

Test	When to Order	Positive Interpretation	Negative Interpretation
Anti-HEV IgM	Acute hepatitis with recent (4–6 wk) travel to area of poor sanitation	Acute HEV infection	No HEV infection Too early in course (retest later)

Anti-HEV IgM = antibodies to hepatitis E virus IgM; HEV = hepatitis E virus.

hepatitis (fewer than 10 per cent and more than 80 per cent, respectively) with persistently increased aminotransferase activities and progression to cirrhosis. The aminotransferase increases of chronic HBV and HCV infection are commonly 1 to 10 times the upper limit of normal. When nearly normal to moderately increased aminotransferase activities are present, causes of chronic liver disease other than viral hepatitis should also be considered. These causes include liver disease in alcoholic patients, AIH, drug toxicity, hemochromatosis, steatohepatitis in nonalcoholic individuals, and other less common diseases (see Table 2). Because effective treatments are available for some types of liver disease (e.g., AIH, Wilson's disease, hemochromatosis, congestive hepatopathy) and essential risk reduction measures are available for contacts of patients with viral hepatitis (e.g., vaccination, immune globulin), establishing the cause of acute or chronic liver injury should not be deferred in favor of observing the clinical course. A logical approach to evaluating all patients with acute or chronic hepatitis should be pursued at the time of presentation using available laboratory tests. This strategy will usually lead to a timely diagnosis and foster a discussion of prognosis and treatment options with the patient.

CIRRHOSIS OF THE LIVER

By Rebecca E. Rudolph, M.D.,
and Kris V. Kowdley, M.D.
Seattle, Washington

Cirrhosis can be defined as a widespread, irreversible alteration of normal hepatic architecture caused by chronic injury to the hepatic parenchyma. Diffuse fibrosis and structurally abnormal hepatic nodules are invariably present. Cirrhosis is the final common pathway of a large number of chronic hepatic diseases (Table 1). Many of these diseases produce unique clinical manifestations that enable the astute clinician to identify cirrhosis early in its course. In many cases, treatment directed toward the specific cause of cirrhosis can slow or halt its progression. If the underlying cause of cirrhosis is left untreated, portal hypertension and hepatic insufficiency eventually develop. Increased resistance to blood flow at the level of the hepatic sinusoids is thought to be the main cause of portal hypertension. The increased resistance is due to sinusoidal narrowing from perisinusoidal deposition of collagen in Disse's space. Compression of the central veins by regenerative nodules may also increase resistance to blood flow. Finally, arteriovenous anastomoses in fibrous scars may increase hydrostatic pressure directly by adding a component of arterial pressure.

Portal hypertension is the primary cause of the development of varices, portal hypertensive gastropathy, splenomegaly, and hypersplenism in patients with cirrhosis. Portal hypertension also contributes to the development of ascites, hepatic encephalopathy, and hepatorenal syndrome. Cirrhosis is not the sole cause of portal hypertension. Noncirrhotic causes include hepatic veno-occlusive disease, portal vein occlusion, and schistosomiasis. The morbidity and mortality due to cirrhosis are not limited to the complications of portal hypertension. As shown in Table 2, cirrhosis can lead to pathologic changes in every organ system of the body. In addition, cirrhosis is a major risk factor for primary hepatocellular carcinoma. As will be discussed in detail further on, hepatocellular carcinoma is a common cancer worldwide and is associated with a high mortality rate.

Table 1. Causes of Cirrhosis

Causes of Cirrhosis
Common Causes
Alcohol
Chronic hepatitis B
Chronic hepatitis C
Cryptogenic causes
Hereditary hemochromatosis
Primary biliary cirrhosis
Uncommon Causes
Biliary Obstruction
Biliary atresia
Biliary strictures
Cystic fibrosis
Primary sclerosing cholangitis
Drugs and Toxins
Amiodarone
Chlorpromazine
Dimethylnitrosamine
Methotrexate
Methyldopa
Vitamin A (hypervitaminosis A)
Other drugs
Metabolic Causes
Alpha_1-antitrypsin deficiency
Galactosemia
Glycogen storage disease
Hereditary fructose intolerance
Hereditary tyrosinemia
Secondary hemochromatosis
Wilson's disease
Other metabolic disorders
Vascular Causes
Chronic right-sided cardiac failure
Hepatic vein obstruction
Hepatic veno-occlusive disease
Miscellaneous Causes
Chronic autoimmune hepatitis
Hereditary hemorrhagic telangiectasia
Indian childhood cirrhosis
Jejunoileal bypass
Nonalcoholic steatohepatitis
Other chronic hepatitis
Sarcoidosis
Syphilis

The cause of cirrhosis should be determined even in advanced disease for several reasons:

1. The prognosis of the patient is affected not only by the severity of portal hypertension and hepatic insufficiency but also by the underlying cause of cirrhosis.
2. Medical therapy can be helpful in some forms of cirrhosis (e.g., hereditary hemochromatosis) even late in the course of disease.
3. The success rate of liver transplantation varies significantly with the cause of cirrhosis. For example, patients with cirrhosis due to hepatitis B infection often have poor outcomes.

This article reviews the clinical manifestations observed in cirrhosis of all causes and then reviews the laboratory and imaging tests as well as the tests of function used in

Table 2. Complications of Cirrhosis

Constitutional
Anorexia
Fatigue
Fever
Malnutrition
Weight loss
Cardiopulmonary
Hepatopulmonary syndrome
Hypertrophic pulmonary osteoarthropathy
Hypoxia
Low blood pressure
Primary pulmonary hypertension
Resting tachycardia
Dermatologic
Edema
Jaundice
Palmar erythema
Prominent superficial abdominal veins
Scleral icterus
Spider angiomas
Endocrine
Amenorrhea
Diabetes mellitus
Gynecomastia
Impotence
Secondary hyperaldosteronism
Gastrointestinal
Ascites
Calcium bilirubinate stones
Decreased liver size
Gastroesophageal reflux disease
Hepatocellular carcinoma
Hepatomegaly
Peptic ulcer disease
Portal hypertensive gastropathy
Spontaneous bacterial peritonitis
Varices
Hematologic
Anemia
Coagulopathy
Hypersplenism
Leukopenia
Splenomegaly
Thrombocytopenia
Metabolic
Hypoalbuminemia
Hypokalemia
Hyponatremia
Neurologic
Acute hepatic encephalopathy
Chronic hepatic encephalopathy
Renal
Acute hepatorenal syndrome

the evaluation of patients with cirrhosis. It then concludes with a discussion of the epidemiology and clinical manifestations of cirrhosis due to alcohol ingestion, chronic viral hepatitis, primary biliary cirrhosis, and hereditary hemochromatosis.

COMPLICATIONS OF PORTAL HYPERTENSION

Variceal Hemorrhage

Elevated hydrostatic pressure in the portal system is directly responsible for the formation of varices (i.e., dilated veins) in the esophagus, stomach, rectum, and other parts of the gastrointestinal system. Rupture of varices can quickly result in life-threatening hemorrhage. The most common sites of severe variceal hemorrhage are the esophagus and proximal stomach. Rectal varices also occasionally cause significant hemorrhage. Rarely, major hemorrhage may arise from duodenal, mesenteric, or gallbladder varices. Major risk factors for variceal bleeding in the esophagus are a previous esophageal variceal bleed, recent diagnosis of esophageal varices (less than 1 year previously), large varix diameter, and continued alcohol use. Less well documented risk factors are the presence of "cherry red" spots on varices and simultaneous gastric varices. Patients with esophageal or proximal gastric varices usually present with hematemesis. Occasionally, the first sign of variceal hemorrhage is hematochezia or melena. Upper gastrointestinal hemorrhage in a patient with known or suspected cirrhosis may also be due to esophagitis, gastritis, a Mallory-Weiss tear, portal hypertensive gastropathy, or peptic ulcer disease. Upper endoscopy is the preferred diagnostic modality because it can establish the cause of hemorrhage and can be used to perform sclerotherapy if esophageal varices are the source of hemorrhage. Lower endoscopy should be used to evaluate severe hematochezia.

Ascites

Ascites may be defined as excess fluid in the peritoneal cavity. Several physiologic changes found in patients with cirrhosis are thought to promote the formation of ascites.

- Increased hydrostatic pressure (portal hypertension)
- Decreased oncotic pressure (due to impaired albumin production by a diseased liver)
- Excess retention of sodium and water (as a result of activation of the renin-angiotensin-aldosterone system, the sympathetic nervous system, and antidiuretic hormone [ADH] production)
- Increased intrahepatic lymph production (as a result of leakage of lymph from the hepatic capsule into the peritoneal space)

Risk factors for the development of ascites include gastrointestinal bleeding, bacterial infection of any kind (especially spontaneous bacterial peritonitis [SBP]), excess salt intake, noncompliance with diuretic medication, advancement of underlying liver disease, continued alcohol ingestion, and development of hepatocellular carcinoma or portal vein thrombosis. The onset of ascites in a patient with cirrhosis is a poor prognostic sign. Approximately 50 per cent of such patients will die within 2 years unless liver transplantation is performed.

Patients with ascites often present with complaints of weight gain or increased abdominal girth. However, ascites is often first detected on physical examination. Several physical examination techniques have been developed for the detection of ascites. The most sensitive is evaluation for shifting dullness. Even with this test, 1.5 L of ascites must be present to achieve a positive result. The average specificity of the test (when compared with the "gold standard" of ultrasonography) is in the range of 50 to 60 per cent. The false-positive rate is particularly high in obese patients. Because an even larger amount of ascitic fluid must be present, the fluid wave test has a lower sensitivity than does examination for shifting dullness. However, the specificity of the fluid wave test is higher (80 to 90 per cent) than that for shifting dullness.

Cirrhosis is by far the most common cause of ascites.

Less common causes are massive liver metastases, peritoneal carcinomatosis, congestive heart failure, tuberculosis, pancreatic disease, nephrotic syndrome, hemodialysis, iatrogenic (as in peritoneal dialysis), a ruptured abdominal viscus, the Budd-Chiari syndrome, and connective tissue disease. Because therapy and prognosis vary, the precise cause of ascites must be established in all patients. The diagnostic tests used to determine the cause of ascites are ultrasonography and peritoneal fluid analysis. An ultrasound not only can confirm the presence of ascites but also can evaluate for hepatic vein obstruction (Budd-Chiari syndrome), portal vein thrombosis, or hepatocellular carcinoma. Peritoneal fluid should be evaluated for albumin concentration and a cell count with differential and should be cultured. Optional tests include total protein determination, Gram stain; amylase, glucose, triglyceride, and lactate dehydrogenase [LD] measurements; acid-fast bacilli [AFB] staining and culture; and cytologic examination. Albumin in the ascitic fluid is used to determine the serum ascites albumin gradient (SAAG). The SAAG is calculated by subtracting albumin in the ascitic fluid from the serum albumin. An SAAG greater than 1.1 g/dL is consistent with ascites due to portal hypertension (e.g., cirrhosis). The causes of a low SAAG include peritoneal carcinomatosis, tuberculous peritonititis, pancreatic ascites, serositis from connective tissue disease, and nephrotic syndrome.

Because of the high prevalence of infection even in asymptomatic patients, ascitic fluid should be sent for a cell count with differential and culture. If the differential cell count shows a predominance of lymphocytes in the setting of a low SAAG or if clinical suspicion is high, fluid should be sent for an acid-fast bacillus stain and culture and cytologic examination. Ascitic fluid to be sent for routine bacterial culture should be inoculated into blood culture bottles at the bedside. Recent studies have shown that inoculating at least 10 mL of ascitic fluid into each blood culture bottle substantially increases the sensitivity of bacterial culture. Gram staining of ascitic fluid can be helpful for early identification of the pathogen causing SBP but has a sensitivity of only about 10 per cent. Some authors recommend measurement of ascitic fluid total protein as a way to predict the patient's risk for the development of SBP. If total protein is less than 1 g/dL, the patient is at higher risk for SBP. Classification of the fluid into categories of transudate or exudate using pleural fluid criteria has not been shown to be helpful. If pancreatic disease is suspected, ascitic fluid amylase concentration should be measured.

Spontaneous Bacterial Peritonitis

SBP is an infection of ascitic fluid in the absence of any obvious intra-abdominal source such as bowel perforation. SBP is thought to be due to translocation of normal intestinal bacteria into the bloodstream with subsequent seeding of the ascitic fluid. The majority of cases of SBP are caused by a single pathogen. *Escherichia coli, Streptococcus* species, and *Klebsiella* species are the causative agents in greater than two thirds of cases. Polymicrobial SBP should raise suspicion of bowel perforation. Clinical manifestations of SBP may include fever, chills, abdominal pain, decreased bowel sounds, rebound tenderness, and/or hypotension. Less commonly, diarrhea, encephalopathy, renal insufficiency, or hypothermia may signal the onset of SBP. Many patients with SBP are asymptomatic. Diagnostic paracentesis should be performed on all patients with symptoms suggestive of ascites, new-onset ascites, ascites on admission to the hospital, or clinical deterioration during a hospitalization.

The classic criteria for SBP include an ascitic fluid neutrophil count greater than 250 cells/mm^3, a positive ascitic fluid culture, and absence of an obvious intra-abdominal source of infection. The neutrophil count is particularly useful in the early diagnosis of SBP. An ascitic fluid neutrophil count of greater than 250 cells/mm^3 has a sensitivity and specificity greater than 80 per cent. An ascitic fluid total leukocyte count greater than 10,000 cells/mm^3, however, is suggestive of peritonitis caused by a perforated viscus. Surgical consultation should be obtained in such cases. Blood and urine cultures should also be obtained prior to the initiation of antibiotic therapy. Results of such cultures can be particularly useful if ascitic fluid cultures are negative.

Variants of SBP include culture-negative neutrocytic ascites and bacterascites. Criteria for culture-negative neutrocytic ascites are met when ascitic fluid cultures remain negative despite an initial neutrophil count greater than 250 cells/mm^3, no antibiotic therapy within 30 days, and no obvious intra-abdominal source of infection. Lack of bacterial growth in culture could be due to poor culture technique or recent resolution of SBP. Patients with culture-negative neutrocytic ascites should be treated in the same manner as those who meet the classic criteria for SBP. Positive blood and/or urine cultures can be used to guide antibiotic therapy. If all cultures are negative, the sensitivity patterns of the usual causative agents of SBP can be used to help select an appropriate antibiotic. The diagnosis of bacterascites (also known as monomicrobial non-neutrocytic bacterascites) is made when ascitic fluid culture yields growth of a single organism, but the initial ascitic fluid neutrophil count is less than 250 cells/mm^3. The presence of bacteria in ascitic fluid culture may represent contamination or the transient residence of these bacteria. Patients with bacterascites who do not manifest any symptoms or signs consistent with SBP do not require treatment.

Hepatorenal Syndrome

Hepatorenal syndrome is characterized by the development of oliguria, markedly decreased urine sodium excretion, and progressive azotemia. Hepatorenal syndrome is the result of severe underlying liver dysfunction rather than intrinsic renal disease. The functional (i.e., nonorganic) nature of the renal insufficiency is suggested by the following:

- Normal renal histologic features are present.
- Kidneys from patients with hepatorenal syndrome that have been transplanted to patients with chronic renal failure function immediately.
- Hepatorenal syndrome is reversible with liver transplantation.

Hepatorenal syndrome often occurs coincident with other complications of cirrhosis, for example, hepatic encephalopathy, bacterial infections, and gastrointestinal bleeding. In addition, acute hepatorenal syndrome may be caused by intravascular depletion after overuse of diuretics or large-volume paracentesis without colloid infusion.

In hepatorenal syndrome, serum urea nitrogen and serum creatinine concentrations rapidly increase and oliguria develops within a few days. In addition to renal failure, patients often have ascites, hyponatremia, jaundice, relative hypotension, and hepatic encephalopathy. Since the mortality rate of hepatorenal syndrome is greater than 90 per cent without liver transplantation, other causes of acute renal failure must be excluded. The criteria pre-

Table 3. Diagnostic Aids for the Evaluation of Acute Renal Failure in Patients With Cirrhosis

	Hepatorenal Syndrome	Prerenal Azotemia	Acute Tubular Necrosis
Fractional excretion of sodium (%)	<1	<1	>1
Urine sediment	Normal	Normal	Muddy brown casts
Response to intravenous fluid	No improvement	Improved renal function	No improvement

sented in Table 3 are useful for distinguishing among the most common causes of acute renal failure in patients with cirrhosis: acute tubular necrosis (ATN), prerenal azotemia, and hepatorenal syndrome. Other diagnoses to consider include nephropathy related to intravenous contrast material or the use of nonsteroidal anti-inflammatory medication, papillary necrosis, or glomerulonephropathies associated with some liver diseases (e.g., hepatitis B–related membranous or membranoproliferative glomerulonephritis, or hepatitis C–related membranoproliferative glomerulonephritis).

Hepatic Encephalopathy

Acute hepatic encephalopathy is a functional and often reversible alteration of the central nervous system that appears in patients with acute and chronic liver disease. In contrast, chronic hepatic encephalopathy (also known as acquired hepatocerebral degeneration) is a progressive and irreversible alteration in the central nervous system that appears only in the setting of chronic liver disease. Hepatic encephalopathy is thought to be due to increased serum concentrations of neurotoxins that are normally produced and/or absorbed by the intestine and metabolized in the liver. In the setting of cirrhosis, decreased hepatic clearance of these neurotoxins may occur as a result of hepatocyte impairment or portal-systemic shunting. Putative neurotoxins include ammonia, mercaptans, phenols, short- and medium-chain fatty acids, false neurotransmitters derived from aromatic amino acids, and γ-aminobutyric acid (GABA)–related substances. Neurotoxins may facilitate their own penetration into the central nervous system by increasing the permeability of the blood-brain barrier.

Acute hepatic encephalopathy is usually caused by one or more of the following: dietary protein overload, gastrointestinal bleeding, infection, constipation, electrolyte imbalance, drugs (e.g., diuretics, sedatives, opiates), or alcohol binges. Chronic hepatic encephalopathy often follows several episodes of acute hepatic encephalopathy. The psychiatric and neurologic abnormalities associated with acute hepatic encephalopathy are nonspecific. The differential diagnosis includes hypercapnia, hypoglycemia, drug overdose, subdural hematoma, Wernicke's encephalopathy, meningitis, encephalitis, and encephalopathy following a seizure. The neuropsychiatric changes observed in acute hepatic encephalopathy have been classified into four stages:

Stage I: Mild confusion, euphoria, depression, irritability, insomnia
Stage II: Drowsiness, lethargy, inappropriate behavior, mild disorientation
Stage III: Somnolent but arousable, disoriented behavior in regard to time and place, marked confusion, amnesia, and incomprehensible speech
Stage IV: Coma

Asterixis (also known as "liver flap") is often present in patients with acute hepatic encephalopathy. It is defined as a nonrhythmic, nonsustained, asymmetric lapse in the voluntary sustainability of position of extremities, head, or trunk. To demonstrate asterixis, the patient should be asked to extend the arms horizontally, dorsiflex the wrists, and spread the fingers widely for at least 15 seconds. If asterixis is mild, brief intermittent flexion of individual fingers with a rapid return to their original position will be observed. In more severe asterixis, the flexion is observed at the wrist or even at the shoulder. Because the demonstration of asterixis requires that the patient sustain a position voluntarily, some authors feel that it cannot be demonstrated in the comatose patient. However, others consider clonus in the comatose patient to be equivalent to asterixis in the cooperative patient. Additional findings of neuromuscular dysfunction observed in acute hepatic encephalopathy include difficulty with writing or drawing geometric figures, variable rigidity of the trunk and limbs, hyperreflexia, and (rarely) seizures.

No diagnostic test is pathognomonic for hepatic encephalopathy. Serum ammonia concentrations are often used in clinical practice to assess whether a patient has hepatic encephalopathy; however, 10 per cent of patients with hepatic encephalopathy have normal serum ammonia concentrations. In severe hepatic encephalopathy, cerebrospinal fluid concentrations of glutamine (synthesized by astrocytes from ammonia) are often increased. A simple psychometric test called the number connection test is useful in the initial diagnosis and follow-up of mild hepatic encephalopathy. The test requires the patient to connect the numbers 1 to 25 (scattered randomly on a page) in sequence from lowest to highest as rapidly as possible. As hepatic encephalopathy resolves, the time to completion of the test diminishes. An electroencephalogram (EEG) can help support the diagnosis of hepatic encephalopathy. As with the tests already described, however, findings are nonspecific. In mild to moderate hepatic encephalopathy, a decrease in wave frequency and an increase in wave amplitude are observed. In more severe hepatic encephalopathy, bilateral, synchronous delta waves (characteristically triphasic) are seen. In hepatic coma, progressive flattening of waves is noted.

Common findings in chronic hepatic encephalopathy include dysarthria; mild ataxia; a wide-based, unsteady gait; choreoathetosis of the face, neck, and shoulders; a coarse rhythmic tremor of the arms; and dementia. Less frequent signs are muscular rigidity, nystagmus, asterixis, and myoclonus. Findings characteristic of acute hepatic encephalopathy may also be present in chronic hepatic encephalopathy. The full syndrome evolves gradually over months to years.

Other Complications of Portal Hypertension

Additional complications of portal hypertension include splenomegaly, hypersplenism, portal hypertensive gastropathy, and prominent superficial abdominal vasculature. Splenomegaly is a common finding in patients with portal hypertension. Because splenomegaly generally does not produce symptoms, it is usually detected by physical examination, laboratory findings, or imaging studies. The development of splenomegaly can be associated with increased intrasplenic destruction of erythrocytes, platelets, or leukocytes and can lead to anemia, thrombocytopenia, or leukopenia. The diagnosis of hypersplenism is made when evidence of destruction of at least one peripheral blood cell line accompanies splenomegaly.

Portal hypertensive gastropathy is a condition in which the gross appearance of the gastric mucosa has been altered by the effects of portal hypertension. The mucosal appearance may be categorized as mild or severe. Mild mucosal findings include a scarlatinalike rash, superficial erythema on the surface of rugae, or a mosaic pattern in which areas of raised pink mucosa are separated by a fine white reticular pattern. Severe mucosal findings include cherry red spots and diffuse hemorrhagic gastritis. Portal hypertensive gastropathy is an uncommon cause of acute, severe hemorrhage in patients with cirrhosis. Patients with acute hemorrhage from portal hypertensive gastropathy usually present with melena, but hematemesis can occur. A more common manifestation of portal hypertensive gastropathy is anemia due to chronic gastrointestinal blood loss.

Prominent superficial abdominal veins are a minor but frequent manifestation of portal hypertension. The veins characteristically radiate outward from the umbilicus. The term caput medusae (i.e., head of Medusa) has been applied to this finding.

HEPATOCELLULAR CARCINOMA

Hepatocellular carcinoma is a common complication of cirrhosis. An estimated 60 to 90 per cent of hepatocellular carcinomas arise in cirrhotic livers. The risk of hepatocellular carcinoma is known to be particularly high in cirrhosis due to chronic hepatitis B infection or hereditary hemochromatosis. In the United States, the annual incidence of hepatocellular carcinoma is about 2.5 cases per 100,000 persons. In regions where hepatitis B is endemic (e.g., Asia, Africa), the annual incidence is greater than 20 cases per 100,000 persons. Male gender appears to be an independent risk factor for hepatocellular carcinoma. The male-to-female ratio is estimated to be 4:1. The male predominance cannot be fully explained by increased rates of cirrhosis or chronic hepatitis B infection. Other independent risk factors for hepatocellular carcinoma include chronic infection with hepatitis B in the *absence* of coexisting cirrhosis, older age and, possibly, exposure to aflatoxins. These substances are mycotoxins produced by *Aspergillus* that are known to contaminate some types of grain.

Hepatocellular carcinoma usually remains asymptomatic until late in the course of disease. Common symptoms at the time of diagnosis include malaise, anorexia, and abdominal pain. Weight loss, ascites, a palpable mass, nausea, vomiting, jaundice, fever, leg edema, hematemesis, and melena may also be reported at the time of presentation. Occasionally, patients present with acute abdominal pain caused by rupture of the tumor and hemoperitoneum. Physical findings observed primarily in patients with large tumors include a palpable mass in the right upper quadrant, arterial bruit or friction rub over the mass, and an elevated right hemidiaphragm. Signs of gastrointestinal hemorrhage, hepatomegaly, ascites, splenomegaly, and/or jaundice may also be present as a result of tumor invasion or underlying cirrhosis. The possibility of hepatocellular carcinoma should always be considered in any patient with cirrhosis who has symptoms or signs of clinical deterioration. Diagnostic paracentesis often yields blood-tinged ascitic fluid, but tumor cells are rarely present. A rapidly decreasing hematocrit may be due to gastrointestinal hemorrhage or bleeding of the tumor into the peritoneal cavity. A few patients may have erythrocytosis or hypercalcemia due to paraneoplastic syndromes known to occur in hepatocellular carcinoma.

Concentrations of alpha-fetoprotein, a glycoprotein produced in the fetal yolk sac, liver, and intestine, are often increased in patients with hepatocellular carcinoma. The majority of symptomatic patients with hepatocellular carcinoma have serum alpha-fetoprotein concentrations greater than 500 ng/mL (normal is <20 ng/mL). However, normal or slightly increased alpha-fetoprotein concentrations may be observed in some patients. An increased serum alpha-fetoprotein concentration is not specific for hepatocellular carcinoma. Patients with chronic hepatitis or cirrhosis may have concentrations as high as 500 ng/mL. Because alpha-fetoprotein determination is a nonspecific test, it is usually combined with abdominal ultrasound when used in screening for hepatocellular carcinoma. Screening has been recommended for high-risk patients such as those with chronic hepatitis B infection or cirrhosis resulting from any chronic liver disease.

Tumors as small as 3 cm can be detected by abdominal ultrasonography or computed tomography (CT). The differential diagnosis of hepatocellular carcinoma includes regenerating nodules, adenomas, focal nodular hyperplasia, metastases from another site, or liver abscess. Thus, a firm diagnosis of hepatocellular carcinoma can be made only by obtaining a sample of tumor for histopathologic examination. A tissue sample can be obtained by percutaneous biopsy guided by CT or ultrasonography. Alternatively, surgical procedures such as laparoscopy or laparotomy may be used.

The prognosis for patients with hepatocellular carcinoma is usually poor. The overall 5-year survival rate is about 4 per cent. Most patients die within several months of diagnosis. The only curative treatment is surgical resection. Unfortunately, most tumors are not resectable because of size, involvement of critical structures such as the porta hepatis, metastatic disease, or severity of underlying cirrhosis. Because the outcome for most patients with asymptomatic hepatocellular carcinoma is poor, current medical efforts are being directed toward prevention through vaccination for hepatitis B and screening of high-risk groups with alpha-fetoprotein determinations and abdominal ultrasonography.

Other Complications of Cirrhosis

Constitutional Problems

Anorexia, weight loss, malnutrition, weakness, and fatigue are common complications of cirrhosis. Malnutrition may occur as a result of anorexia, gastrointestinal distress, substitution of alcohol for other sources of calories, or an increased resting metabolic rate. A poor nutritional status increases susceptibility to infection and contributes to ascites and edema by depressing serum albumin concentration. Low-grade fever often occurs in the context of decompensated cirrhosis. Whenever fever is present, however, careful evaluation for an infectious cause is warranted.

Hematologic Problems

The major hematologic manifestations of cirrhosis are hypocoagulability and cytopenias. The majority of coagulation factors are produced by hepatocytes. Thus, impaired coagulation is observed in all forms of advanced cirrhosis.

Of the routine laboratory tests available, the prothrombin time most closely reflects the degree of hypocoagulability. The partial thromboplastin time may also be prolonged. Hypersplenism contributes to anemia, thrombocytopenia, and leukopenia. Gastrointestinal blood loss, folate deficiency, iron deficiency, and occasionally vitamin B_{12} deficiency are other causes of anemia in cirrhosis. Hypersplenism can cause platelet counts to fall as low as 30,000 cells/mm^3.

Gastrointestinal Problems

The deleterious effects of cirrhosis on the gastrointestinal system are not limited to variceal hemorrhage and portal hypertensive gastropathy. Peptic ulcer disease, cholelithiasis, gastroesophageal reflux disease, and hepatomegaly all occur at increased frequency in patients with cirrhosis. The possibility of peptic ulcer disease exists in any patient with cirrhosis and upper gastrointestinal hemorrhage or epigastric pain. Calcium bilirubinate stones (but not cholesterol stones) occur at higher frequencies in patients with cirrhosis. The increased bilirubin load generated by the chronic hemolytic anemia associated with hypersplenism is thought to be responsible for the higher rates of calcium bilirubinate stones. Although such stones have the potential to cause cholecystitis or common bile duct obstruction, they appear to do so at a lower frequency than do cholesterol stones. An increased frequency of gastroesophageal reflux appears to be limited to patients with cirrhosis and ascites. Increased intra-abdominal pressure is thought to be responsible for the higher incidence of acid reflux in such patients. Liver size in patients with cirrhosis may be large, small, or normal. Percussion can be used to estimate the size of the liver but is imprecise when compared with measurement by CT or ultrasonography. Hepatomegaly is commonly seen in early alcoholic liver disease, acute alcoholic hepatitis, congestive heart failure, primary biliary cirrhosis, hemochromatosis or other storage diseases. Small livers are often found in advanced cirrhosis due to chronic alcohol abuse or chronic hepatitis.

Endocrine Problems

Common endocrinologic complications of cirrhosis are gynecomastia, a change in body hair patterns, amenorrhea, diabetes mellitus, and secondary hyperaldosteronism. Conversion of weakly androgenic steroids to estrogens in the skin, adipose tissue, muscle, and bone occurs at low rates in all persons. These androgenic steroids are normally destroyed by the liver. Portal-systemic shunting in advanced cirrhosis leads to decreased intrahepatic destruction of these hormones and thus increased production of estrogens in peripheral tissues (e.g., the skin). The increased serum concentration of estrogens may result in gynecomastia and loss of the male escutcheon.

Amenorrhea is probably due to a combination of malnutrition and the stress of chronic illness. The pathophysiologic characteristics of diabetes mellitus in cirrhosis are not completely understood. Increased peripheral insulin resistance due to hyperglucagonemia and hypersomatotropism is thought to contribute to this form of diabetes. Diabetes mellitus induced by cirrhosis can usually be controlled with diet or oral hypoglycemic agents. If insulin is required, the patient most likely has type II diabetes mellitus. Secondary hyperaldosteronism contributes to hypokalemia, ascites, edema, and hepatorenal syndrome.

Cardiopulmonary Problems

As cirrhosis progresses, many patients experience increased cardiac output and decreased peripheral vascular resistance. The clinical manifestations of these physiologic changes are mild resting tachycardia and low blood pressure. Pulmonary complications include hypoxia, primary pulmonary hypertension, and hypertrophic pulmonary osteoarthropathy. Hypoxia is primarily due to ventilation-perfusion mismatch and intrapulmonary arteriovenous shunting. A small number of patients with intrapulmonary shunting experience orthodeoxia, which refers to arterial deoxygenation with a change from a supine to an upright position. Patients who experience dyspnea with this change in posture are said to have platypnea. Because vascular shunts tend to be located in the lung bases, a change to the upright position induces hypoxia by causing more blood to flow through the shunts. Primary pulmonary hypertension occurs in less than 1 per cent of patients with cirrhosis but is six times more common in such patients than in normal persons. Clinical findings include exertional dyspnea, a murmur at the left upper sternal border, cardiomegaly, right ventricular hypertrophy on electrocardiography, and prominent pulmonary arteries on chest roentgenogram. Hypertrophic pulmonary osteoarthropathy is an uncommon complication of cirrhosis. Patients with primary biliary cirrhosis are more likely to suffer from this complication than are those with other types of cirrhosis. Manifestations of this disorder include pain and tenderness in the distal long bones of the forearms and legs and clubbing of the fingers. The cause of hypertrophic pulmonary osteoarthropathy in cirrhosis has yet to be defined.

Dermatologic Problems

Patients with cirrhosis often manifest jaundice, scleral icterus, spider angiomas, and palmar erythema. Jaundice and scleral icterus are due to bilirubin staining of elastic tissue. Scleral icterus is a more sensitive indicator of hyperbilirubinemia than is yellowing of the skin. It is observed when bilirubin concentrations rise to 2 to 3 mg/dL. The scleral icterus is most apparent laterally. The frenulum of the tongue also becomes icteric at low concentrations of hyperbilirubinemia. Long-standing jaundice can produce a greenish discoloration of the skin that is due to the metabolism of bilirubin to biliverdin. Jaundice does not correlate well with severity of liver disease and is not specific for cirrhosis. Spider angiomas are also known as spider angiomata or spider telangiectasias. A single spider angioma is composed of several precapillary vessels radiating from a central arteriole. The angioma can be made invisible by application of pressure to the central arteriole. When pressure is released, blood flows rapidly into the central portion of the angioma and then diffuses radially. Spider angiomas are generally distributed over the face, neck, upper extremities, and upper trunk. Angiomas are rarely seen on the lower trunk or extremities. Large numbers of angiomas can be observed in cirrhosis, acute hepatitis, and pregnancy. Normal individuals rarely have more than two angiomas. Palmar erythema is distributed on the distal finger pads, the thenar and hypothenar eminences, and occasionally on the periungual surfaces of the fingers. Palmar erythema can also be seen in rheumatoid arthritis, pregnancy, and thyrotoxicosis.

DIAGNOSTIC TESTS USED IN CIRRHOSIS

Diagnostic tests in cirrhosis can be classified into tests of liver anatomy and those of liver function. Imaging tests of the liver that delineate hepatic architecture are generally classified as tests of structure. Tests of liver function include either tests that actually measure hepatic synthetic or metabolic activity or those that provide a "snapshot" of hepatic inflammation or enzyme activity. The tests commonly used to examine liver structure and function and the most appropriate indication for their use are discussed in the following paragraphs.

Tests of Liver Structure

A number of diagnostic modalities are available to assess liver architecture, including transcutaneous ultrasonography, CT, magnetic resonance imaging (MRI), nuclear medicine scintigraphic techniques, cholangiography, liver biopsy, laparoscopy, and mesenteric and portal angiography.

Ultrasonography

Ultrasonography is performed by evaluation of reflected sound waves transmitted from a probe placed on the patient's abdomen. This diagnostic modality is extremely useful for evaluating the caliber of intrahepatic and extrahepatic bile ducts and cystic liver lesions and for examining the gallbladder. Ultrasonography has a sensitivity of more than 90 per cent for detection of gallstones. It is also useful in evaluating patency and direction of flow in the portal vein. In addition, ultrasonography can be used to follow hepatic masses prospectively. Because cirrhosis and fatty infiltration have characteristic ultrasonographic appearances, such imaging may be a valuable adjunct to standard diagnostic tests in patients with these disorders. Ultrasonography is not sensitive for lesions in the common bile duct or pancreas. The sensitivity of ultrasonography for choledocholithiasis is about 25 per cent. Ultrasonography is invaluable in the management of patients after liver transplantation because it may detect biliary dilatation, intra-abdominal fluid collections, thrombosis in the hepatic artery, and occlusion of portal or hepatic veins. Occasionally, ultrasonography can identify cystic liver lesions, fatty infiltration, or metastases.

Computed Tomography and Magnetic Resonance Imaging

Computed tomography and MRI are relatively expensive but occasionally useful. The introduction of the double-spiral technique in CT scanning has improved the identification of liver tumors and increased the accuracy of hepatic artery imaging. Thus, mesenteric angiography is typically not required for patients undergoing evaluation for orthotopic liver transplantation. The various densities observed on a CT scan also help distinguish among the possible causes of cirrhosis. For example, although increased density is seen in hemochromatosis, decreased density is observed in fatty liver. Computed tomography is superior to other modalities for detection and follow-up of focal liver abnormalities and may be diagnostic in diseases such as hemangioma.

Magnetic resonance imaging offers some advantages over CT. It can examine structures in multiple planes and is especially useful in distinguishing among types of tissues. Furthermore, MRI does not expose patients to ionizing radiation and may be particularly helpful in defining vascular structures in patients who cannot tolerate the administration of intravenous contrast material. In addition, MRI has been used to assess hepatic iron concentration. This technique is not widely available for clinical use, however, and may be insensitive in patients with minimal iron overload.

Nuclear Medicine Scintigraphy

A number of nuclear medicine techniques are available to evaluate the hepatobiliary system. Technetium-labeled colloids (such as sulfur colloid) are taken up by the reticuloendothelial cells in the liver. This technique can be used to characterize the presence of cirrhosis (wherein the liver uptake is heterogenous, with increased uptake in the spleen and redistribution to the bone marrow) and to identify focal liver lesions that may appear as filling defects. Currently, these liver-spleen scans (as they are commonly known) are rarely used. They may be useful in the rare patient in whom cirrhosis is suspected clinically but in whom a liver biopsy cannot be performed and ultrasonography or CT scans are nondiagnostic. Certain radioactive tracers are actively taken up by the liver and secreted into the biliary tree. These tracers can be used to define cystic or common bile duct obstruction and bile leaks such as may occur after laparoscopic cholecystectomy.

Cholangiography

The two methods used to visualize the biliary tree are transhepatic cholangiography and endoscopic retrograde cholangiopancreatography (ERCP). ERCP has largely replaced transhepatic cholangiography as the initial method of choice to both visualize and intervene therapeutically in the biliary tree. Transhepatic cholangiography involves passage of a needle into the liver until a bile duct can be located under a fluoroscope. Guidewires and catheters can then be passed into the bile ducts to obtain cholangiograms and place stents or other devices. Transhepatic cholangiography is associated with more patient discomfort and can be particularly difficult in patients with small-caliber bile ducts. ERCP is associated with minimal patient discomfort and has the advantage of being intraluminal (i.e., no external stents are needed to achieve biliary drainage). The disadvantage of ERCP is a small but definite risk of pancreatitis. This risk is greater if endoscopic sphincterotomy of the biliary sphincter or biliary manometry (used in the diagnosis of sphincter of Oddi dysfunction in patients with unexplained biliary type pain) is performed. Transhepatic cholangiography and ERCP are invaluable in evaluating patients with cholestatic disorders, especially when there is evidence of obstruction. In such cases, either transhepatic cholangiography or ERCP can be used to establish the diagnosis and relieve the obstruction.

Liver Biopsy

Liver biopsy is the gold standard for the diagnosis of many liver diseases. It can definitively establish the diagnosis of liver disease and detect cirrhosis. Liver biopsy is relatively inexpensive and is associated with relatively minimal risk. The major complications are infrequent but include hemorrhage, bile leak, pneumothorax, or hemothorax. Biopsy is now an outpatient procedure, with patients usually being discharged after 4 to 8 hours.

Laparoscopy

Despite its widespread use in other settings, laparoscopy is used infrequently by gastroenterologists and hepatologists. Laparoscopy is useful in evaluating gross liver architecture, finding metastatic lesions, and evaluating the peritoneum in patients with exudative ascites.

Tests of Liver Function

Functional liver tests are generally designed to study the metabolic activity of the liver or blood flow to the liver, or both.

Monoethylglycine Xylidide

Monoethylglycine xylidide (MEGX) is a first-pass metabolite of lidocaine. Since lidocaine is almost completely taken up from the blood and metabolized by the liver (cytochrome P-450 system), the rate of MEGX formation can be used to determine liver function. MEGX determination has proved useful in examining organ viability in potential liver donors and in predicting prognosis in patients with severe hepatic insufficiency.

Other tests of hepatic blood flow and metabolic activity include the galactose elimination test, the aminopyrine breath test, and indocyanine green clearance. Organic anion dyes have been used for many years to study liver function. The rate at which these dyes are excreted into bile can be used to evaluate liver function. The sulfobromophthalein (BSP) test is one such study.

Liver Enzymes

The term liver function test as used to describe liver enzyme activity is actually a misnomer because the measurement of serum enzymes released by hepatocytes does not provide information about liver function (such as synthetic activity, metabolic activity, or blood flow). However, these tests are frequently the first biochemical abnormalities detected in patients with liver dysfunction. Serum albumin, prothrombin time, and bilirubin concentrations are better measures of liver function.

Liver enzymes commonly measured in serum include the following:

- Aminotransferases: alanine aminotransferase (ALT), previously known as serum glutamic-pyruvic transaminase (SGPT), and aspartate aminotransferase (AST), previously known as serum glutamic-oxaloacetic transaminase (SGOT).
- Other enzymes: γ-glutamyltransferase (GGT), alkaline phosphatase, and 5′-nucleotidase

Increased "cholestatic enzymes" (both alkaline phosphatase and GGT) are generally due to increased activity or synthesis of these enzymes. In contrast, increases in serum concentrations of "hepatocellular enzymes" (ALT, AST) reflect leakage of these enzymes from damaged hepatocytes into the systemic circulation. The degree and pattern of liver enzyme abnormalities can therefore be used to evaluate the nature and severity of liver disease.

COMMON CAUSES OF CIRRHOSIS

Alcohol Abuse

In North America and Europe, chronic alcohol abuse is the cause of cirrhosis in approximately 60 to 75 per cent of cases. The likelihood that an individual will acquire cirrhosis is related to the amount and duration of alcohol use. Cirrhosis tends to develop in women with substantially less daily intake than required in men. The minimal amount of daily alcohol use required for the development of cirrhosis has been estimated as 20 g per day for women and 60 g per day for men. (For reference, 12 oz of beer, 5 oz of wine, or 1.5 oz of "hard liquor" each contains 13 g of alcohol.) This level of daily consumption must be sustained for at least 10 to 15 years. The risk for cirrhosis clearly rises as daily consumption increases. Approximately three quarters of patients who consume 160 g of alcohol (e.g., a pint of whiskey) a day will acquire cirrhosis. Because only 10 to 30 per cent of individuals who consume the requisite quantity of alcohol acquire cirrhosis, other causative factors are thought to play a role. Such factors may include genetic predisposition to the development of alcoholic cirrhosis or decreased catabolism of acetaldehyde (a hepatotoxic by-product of alcohol metabolism).

Alcoholic cirrhosis is thought to progress through recurrent episodes of clinical or subclinical alcoholic hepatitis. The clinical presentation of alcoholic hepatitis is highly variable. Patients can have no symptoms; mild, nonspecific illness; or fatal hepatic insufficiency. Common symptoms of alcoholic hepatitis are anorexia, nausea, vomiting, malaise, weight loss, abdominal pain, jaundice, and fever. Fever can be as high as 40°C (104°F) and may persist for weeks. On examination, patients often have right upper quadrant tenderness and hepatomegaly. Splenomegaly, ascites, peripheral edema, or encephalopathy may occur.

Laboratory results usually show leukocytosis in the range of 10,000 to 20,000 cells/mm^3, but even higher concentrations can be seen. Mildly increased concentrations of AST and ALT are common in patients with alcoholic hepatitis. If aminotransferase concentrations are found to be greater than 15 times the upper limit of normal, however, alcoholic hepatitis is an unlikely diagnosis. Alkaline phosphatase and bilirubin concentrations can be normal or increased to a degree that suggests extrahepatic biliary obstruction. Biopsy shows hepatocellular necrosis, "ballooning" of hepatocytes, and polymorphonucleocyte infiltration, particularly around injured hepatocytes and alcoholic hyalin. Alcoholic hyalin (i.e., Mallory bodies) is perinuclear eosinophilic material that is suggestive of the diagnosis of alcoholic liver disease but is nonspecific. Biopsy may also show deposition of collagen around the central vein and in perisinusoidal areas. This pattern of collagen deposition, known as central hyaline sclerosis, is thought to be a precursor to cirrhosis. A prolonged prothrombin time, greatly increased bilirubin concentration, rising serum creatinine concentration, ascites, encephalopathy, and/or infection are poor short-term prognostic signs. The long-term prognosis is affected by the severity of the initial episode of alcoholic hepatitis and by the drinking habits of the patient after recovery. Up to 40 per cent of patients who continue heavy alcohol use will acquire cirrhosis within 5 years. Some patients will acquire cirrhosis after alcoholic hepatitis even with total abstinence.

The diagnosis of alcoholic cirrhosis is difficult because the clinical presentation varies greatly among patients. Some patients will have had one or more documented episodes of alcoholic hepatitis. Others will present with nonspecific complaints such as anorexia, loss of muscle mass, fatigue, weight loss, abdominal discomfort, or diarrhea. Still others will present with a complication of portal hypertension. In a minority of cases (about 10 to 20 per cent), the cirrhosis is first discovered at laparotomy or autopsy. Some physical findings are more common in alcoholic cirrhosis than in other forms of cirrhosis, but none are pathognomonic. Patients with alcoholic cirrhosis tend to have more florid palmar erythema and greater numbers of spider angiomas than do patients with other forms of cirrhosis. Dupuytren's contractures, parotid enlargement, gynecomastia, and testicular atrophy are considered to be more common in alcoholic cirrhosis than in nonalcoholic cirrhosis. Of note, testicular atrophy arises from the direct toxic effects of alcohol on the testes rather than from the underlying liver disease. Neurologic findings may include the Wernicke-Korsakoff syndrome, alcoholic dementia, alcohol withdrawal seizures or delirium tremens. Again, these findings are not due to cirrhosis but instead arise from the toxic effects of alcohol or malnutrition, or both.

No laboratory abnormality is unique to alcoholic cirrhosis. An increased mean corpuscular volume (MCV) is suggestive of alcohol use. Moderately increased aminotransferase concentrations with an AST-to-ALT ratio of 3:1 supports a diagnosis of alcoholic liver disease but is not pathognomonic. Liver biopsy shows bridging fibrosis with greatest collagen deposition near the central vein. In addition, the biopsy may show features of alcoholic hepatitis and steatosis (i.e., fatty liver).

Many patients with a history of chronic alcohol abuse also have nonalcoholic liver disease. In one study, 25 per cent of patients with presumed alcoholic cirrhosis were found to have an additional cause of cirrhosis on the basis of liver biopsy findings. Some patients are initially unwilling to share the extent of their alcohol use. If alcoholic cirrhosis is suspected on clinical grounds, however, the history should be pursued further. Possible approaches include questioning close family members or friends, using standardized questionnaires such as CAGE, or gently confronting the patient with your suspicions. The prognosis of patients with alcoholic cirrhosis can be improved significantly by the cessation of alcohol use. The average 5-year survival rate is less than 40 per cent in those who continue to drink but is greater than 60 to 70 per cent in abstinent patients.

Chronic Viral Hepatitis

Chronic viral hepatitis is the cause of cirrhosis in about 10 to 15 per cent of cases in the United States. Chronic hepatitis is usually defined as persistent increases of aminotransferase concentrations for greater than 6 months. In countries where hepatitis B infection is endemic (e.g., Asia, Africa), the prevalence of cirrhosis related to chronic viral hepatitis is significantly higher than in the United States. Hepatitis B and hepatitis C viruses can produce chronic hepatitis that leads to cirrhosis. In addition, coinfection with the hepatitis D virus (i.e., the delta hepatitis agent) can cause chronic hepatitis B infection to progress more quickly to cirrhosis. Moreover, the incidence of cirrhosis arising from chronic infection with hepatitis B appears to be much higher in patients coinfected with the hepatitis D virus. This latter virus cannot cause acute or chronic hepatitis by itself because it requires the assistance of hepatitis B for replication. Hepatitis A and hepatitis E do not cause chronic hepatitis.

Hepatitis B

In countries with a low prevalence of hepatitis B infection, such as the United States, the virus is usually acquired in adulthood. Modes of transmission include parenteral drug use, sexual intercourse, needlestick injuries in the health care setting, and rarely, renal dialysis. The risk of transmission by sexual intercourse is greater for homosexuals than for heterosexuals. Institutionalized patients such as mentally retarded children are also at higher risk for infection. In regions with high carrier rates, such as the Far Fast and Africa, neonatal exposure to infected maternal serum during birth is the most common mode of transmission. Hepatitis D is transmitted primarily through parenteral routes. Vertical transmission of the hepatitis D virus has also been reported.

Overall, about 2 to 10 per cent of adults in the United States acquire chronic hepatitis as a result of infection with the hepatitis B virus. Neonates, patients with Down's syndrome, chronic hemodialysis patients, symptomatic human immunodeficiency virus (HIV)–positive patients, as well as other immunosuppressed patients are at much higher risk for the development of chronic hepatitis B than are normal immunocompetent hosts. The annual probability that patients with chronic hepatitis B infection will acquire cirrhosis is 1 to 12 per cent. Major risk factors for progression to cirrhosis are the presence of bridging hepatic necrosis on a biopsy specimen and persistence of hepatitis B virus DNA in the serum. Bridging hepatic necrosis is defined as at least one confluent area of necrosis connecting a portal vein to a central vein.

Patients with hepatitis B infection are frequently asymptomatic. In symptomatic patients, the most common complaint is fatigue. Some patients with chronic hepatitis B infection experience episodes of jaundice, anorexia, fatigue, and low-grade fever during times of greater disease activity. A small percentage of patients may experience extrahepatic complications such as arthritis, leukocytoclastic vasculitis, mixed cryoglobulinemia, membranous or membranoproliferative glomerulonephritis, or polyarteritis nodosum. These complications are caused by the deposition of immune complexes in other organs. As hepatitis progresses, liver size may decrease.

Aminotransferase concentrations do not correlate with the severity of chronic hepatitis or cirrhosis. The concentrations frequently fluctuate in the range of 100 to 1000 U/L but can be normal. Patients are seropositive for hepatitis B surface antigen and hepatitis B core antibody. Although some patients have low concentrations of hepatitis B surface antibody, most are seronegative. The median survival of patients with cirrhosis due to chronic hepatitis B is 5 years. Most patients die of a complication of portal hypertension or severe hepatic insufficiency.

Hepatitis C

Because the serologic test for hepatitis C has been available for only a few years, the mode of transmission and the incidence of cirrhosis secondary to chronic infection is less well defined than that for hepatitis B. Hepatitis C is thought to be acquired most commonly through parenteral drug use and blood transfusions. Prior to the implementation of effective screening of blood products in the United States, hepatitis C caused 85 to 95 per cent of cases of post-transfusion hepatitis. Hepatitis C is also thought to be spread at low rates through sexual contact, maternal-neonatal routes, needlestick injury, and nonpercutaneous routes. A significant percentage of patients with hepatitis C infection acquire chronic hepatitis. Of those with chronic hepatitis C infection, it is estimated that 40 to 50 per cent will develop cirrhosis.

Initial infection with hepatitis C is often subclinical. Many patients continue to be asymptomatic during the chronic phase of illness. In patients who are symptomatic, fatigue and weakness are common complaints. Jaundice is an unusual finding early in the course of disease. Extrahepatic manifestations include polyarteritis nodosum, mixed cryoglobulinemia, membranoproliferative glomerulonephritis, autoimmune thyroiditis, and sialadenitis resembling that seen in Sjögren's syndrome. Again, these manifestations are thought to be immune-mediated and are unusual complications of chronic infection with hepatitis C. Liver size may decrease as cirrhosis evolves. Most patients with chronic hepatitis C infection have increased aminotransferase concentrations, but concentrations higher than 800 U/L are uncommon. The aminotransferase concentrations tend to fluctuate significantly and do not correlate with level of disease activity.

The combination of persistent elevation of aminotransferases and a positive hepatitis C antibody test is highly suggestive of chronic hepatitis due to hepatitis C infection.

However, false-positive results for hepatitis C antibody are seen in some patients with chronic autoimmune hepatitis. If the diagnosis of chronic autoimmune hepatitis is suspected, polymerase chain reaction (PCR) techniques can be used to establish the presence or absence of hepatitis C virus RNA in the serum. Progression to cirrhosis may take many years. Once cirrhosis develops, patients are at risk of death from hepatocellular dysfunction or a complication of portal hypertension. However, patients with cirrhosis due to hepatitis C infection can be treated effectively with liver transplantation.

Primary Biliary Cirrhosis

Cirrhosis is due to intrahepatic or extrahepatic biliary disease in approximately 5 to 10 per cent of cases. The most common of this group of diseases is primary biliary cirrhosis. This condition is an autoimmune disorder characterized by the destruction of small and medium-sized intrahepatic bile ducts over many years. Although all races can be affected by primary biliary cirrhosis, the disease is most frequent in whites. In England, the estimated prevalence is 54 cases per million persons. Greater than 90 per cent of patients are female. The typical age at disease onset is 30 to 65 years.

Primary biliary cirrhosis is diagnosed during the asymptomatic period in up to 60 per cent of patients. Increased alkaline phosphatase and aminotransferase concentrations, hepatomegaly, or other physical signs of liver disease are the usual reasons that primary biliary cirrhosis is detected in the asymptomatic period. The most common early symptoms are pruritis due to cholestasis, malaise, and fatigue. Even though bilirubin concentrations do not rise until later in the disease course, 10 to 40 per cent of patients are jaundiced at the time of initial diagnosis. Some patients also present with weight loss or right upper quadrant pain. Other autoimmune disorders such as Sjögren's syndrome, CREST (calcinosis, Raynaud's phenomenon, esophageal motility disorders, sclerodactyly, and telangiectasia), scleroderma, autoimmune thyroiditis, rheumatoid arthritis, psoriatic arthritis, and pernicious anemia are associated with primary biliary cirrhosis. Of these associated autoimmune diseases, Sjögren's syndrome, CREST, scleroderma, and autoimmune thyroiditis are the most common. Renal tubular acidosis and hypertrophic pulmonary osteoarthropathy are also seen.

The most common physical findings in primary biliary cirrhosis are excoriations. Patients often have hyperpigmentation in areas of heavy scratching. As the disease progresses, many patients experience hepatomegaly, splenomegaly, clubbing of the fingers, and xanthelasmas. The xanthelasmas tend to arise at the inner canthus of the eye and spread laterally. Less frequently, xanthomas are found in locations such as the elbow, palms, buttocks, knees, back, and chest. Xanthelasmas and xanthomas are the result of sustained increases in serum cholesterol concentration.

More than 90 per cent of patients have antimitochondrial antibody (AMA), and many will also have increased IgM concentrations. As expected in cholestatic liver disease, alkaline phosphatase, GGT, and 5′-nucleotidase concentrations are increased in the vast majority of patients. Aminotransferase concentrations may be slightly increased or normal. As the disease progresses, bilirubin concentrations begin to rise and can reach greater than 30 mg/dL. Increased cholesterol concentrations are seen throughout the disease course. Elevations in low-density lipoprotein (LDL) tend to be greater in later stages of disease. The histologic features of the liver vary with progression of primary biliary cirrhosis. In early disease, dense infiltrates of inflammatory cells are present around partially necrotic small and medium-sized bile ducts. Later, bile ducts disappear and cirrhosis becomes apparent.

Major complications of advanced disease include malabsorption of fat-soluble vitamins and osteoporosis. The malabsorption of fat-soluble vitamins is due to decreased secretion of conjugated bile acids into the intestine. Deficiency of vitamin A can result in night blindness. Less commonly, vitamin E deficiency can produce a neurologic syndrome characterized by ataxia, ophthalmoplegia, areflexia, proprioceptive impairment, and paresthesias. Osteoporosis predisposes patients to vertebral compression fractures and rib fractures. Complications of portal hypertension may also occur in advanced disease.

No cure exists for primary biliary cirrhosis. Some studies have shown, however, that disease progression can be slowed if treatment is initiated before the development of frank cirrhosis. Medications currently under study include colchicine, ursodiol, and low-dose methotrexate.

Hereditary Hemochromatosis

Hereditary hemochromatosis is a disorder characterized by accumulation of excess iron in the liver, heart, pancreas, pituitary gland, adrenal glands, skin, and synovium. Increased intestinal iron absorption over the life of the patient is thought to be the cause of iron overload. Hereditary hemochromatosis has been estimated to be the cause of cirrhosis in about 5 per cent of patients with cirrhosis. This condition is an autosomal recessive disease that is most common among persons of European origin. Heterozygotes may accumulate iron but do not develop end-organ damage. Among white persons, the frequency of homozygotes vary between 1 in 200 and 1 in 600 persons. The proportion of homozygotes who acquire cirrhosis caused by hemochromatosis is unclear. Factors leading to clinical disease may include iron content of food, age, sex, alcohol use, and a coincident liver disease such as chronic hepatitis. Accumulation of enough iron to cause disease takes many years. Thus, the typical age at onset of disease is 40 to 60 years. Women lose iron through menstruation and therefore tend to acquire the disease later in life or not at all. The male-to-female ratio for clinically apparent disease is about 8:1. Alcohol may promote symptomatic hemochromatosis through its direct hepatotoxic effect, stimulation of intestinal iron absorption, or both.

Hereditary hemochromatosis is often detected before the onset of symptoms because of the appearance of hepatomegaly or elevated aminotransferase concentrations. Common presenting symptoms are weakness, lethargy, chronic abdominal pain, arthralgias, decreased libido, impotence, and complaints related to diabetes or congestive heart failure. The first, second, and third metacarpophalangeal joints and the proximal interphalangeal joints of the hands are the most common sites of arthralgia. Joint involvement is usually symmetrical. As the disease progresses, degenerative arthritis often arises in these joints. In some patients, degenerative arthritis also develops in the knees, hips, shoulders, and lower back. Pseudogout may affect large joints such as the knee. Frequent physical findings at presentation are hepatomegaly and abnormal skin pigmentation. Bronze skin pigmentation is due to increased melanin production. The bronze color is most noticeable in sun-exposed areas, scars, and mucous membranes. Because it results from iron deposition in the basal epidermis and sweat glands, the slate-gray discoloration is more noticeable late in the disease course. Other physical findings include joint enlargement or deformity, signs of cardiac failure, or testicular atrophy. Hypogonadism in hereditary hemochromatosis arises from iron deposition in the pituitary gland. Occasionally, patients present with infections caused by organisms that grow preferentially in the setting of excess iron. These organisms include *Yersinia enterocolitica, Pasteurella pseudotuberculosis,* and *Vibrio vulnificus.*

Concentrations of AST, ALT, alkaline phosphatase, and/or bilirubin may be increased but are nondiagnostic in hereditary hemochromatosis. The best screening tests are serum iron concentration, per cent transferrin saturation, and serum ferritin concentration. A transferrin saturation of greater than 60 per cent or a ferritin concentration greater than 200 μg/L for females or 300 μg/L for males is consistent with hereditary hemochromatosis. In the appropriate clinical setting, an abnormally high transferrin saturation or ferritin concentration is an indication for liver biopsy. The definitive test for hereditary hemochromatosis is determination of the concentration of iron in liver tissue. The result is often stated as the hepatic iron index, that is, the hepatic iron concentration (in micromoles per gram dry weight) divided by age in years. The value for homozygotes is nearly always greater than 1.9. (The only false-negative results have occurred in homozygotes with a long-term source of blood loss.) Inclusion of age in the index makes it possible to identify patients with homozygous hereditary hemochromatosis early in life. The index has been found to be reliable over the age range of 15 to 80 years. The biopsy specimen should also be examined for the presence or absence of cirrhosis because this will clearly have an impact on prognosis.

Quantitation of iron in liver tissue does not enable one to distinguish hereditary hemochromatosis from other forms of hemochromatosis. Fortunately, clinical findings and routine laboratory results usually allow one to differentiate primary from secondary hemochromatosis. Secondary hemochromatosis may occur as a result of anemias associated with ineffective erythropoiesis (e.g., thalassemia major), increased oral intake of iron (e.g., African iron overload), transfusional iron overload, parenteral iron overload, and neonatal iron overload.

The diagnosis of hereditary hemochromatosis has the potential to be of great benefit to the patient and his or her family. Treatment with phlebotomy can result in decreases in hepatomegaly, abdominal discomfort, malaise, lethargy, weakness, abnormal skin pigmentation, and glucose intolerance. Congestive heart failure may also improve. Unfortunately, arthropathy may progress, and hypogonadism does not improve. All first-degree relatives should be screened for hereditary hemochromatosis with serum iron, transferrin saturation, and ferritin determinations. If iron stores as estimated by serum studies are sufficiently high, liver biopsy should be performed. Relatives with a hepatic iron index greater than 1.9 should be treated with phlebotomy. Patients who are treated before the onset of cirrhosis appear to have a normal life expectancy. Because patients with secondary hemochromatosis due to ineffective erythropoiesis or transfusional iron overload cannot tolerate phlebotomy, they are treated with iron chelation therapy using deferoxamine rather than with phlebotomy.

UNCOMMON CAUSES OF CIRRHOSIS

Other causes of cirrhosis are less frequent. Because a significant number of patients with Wilson's disease, $alpha_1$-antitrypsin deficiency, autoimmune hepatitis, cystic fibrosis, primary sclerosing cholangitis, glycogen storage disease, and sarcoidosis will acquire these diseases before the age of 40 years, young persons with progressive liver disease should be evaluated carefully for these disorders. In 10 to 15 per cent of patients, no cause of cirrhosis can be identified. Patients with cirrhosis of unknown cause are said to have cryptogenic or idiopathic cirrhosis.

DISORDERS OF THE GALLBLADDER AND BILE DUCTS

By Robert V. Rege, M.D.,
and David L. Nahrwold, M.D.
Chicago, Illinois

Biliary tract disorders account for 500,000 operations and billions of dollars in health care costs each year. Laparoscopic cholecystectomy, which has been rapidly and widely accepted by patients and surgeons, has nevertheless sparked controversy concerning the treatment of asymptomatic gallstones, proper preoperative evaluation of suspected bile duct stones, and correct treatment of ductal stones after detection. Although less common, other disorders of the gallbladder and bile ducts present interesting diagnostic and therapeutic challenges to the clinician. To ensure appropriate treatment, these disorders must be distinguished from gallstone disease. This article emphasizes issues important in the diagnosis of biliary tract disease, but treatment is also addressed when diagnostic and therapeutic approaches are linked.

GALLSTONES

Gallstones typically arise in the gallbladder and are found in approximately 10 per cent of patients in the United States. The presence of stones in the gallbladder is called cholelithiasis. Choledocholithiasis refers to stones in biliary ducts. Most stones in the ducts arise in the gallbladder (i.e., secondary stones), but primary ductal stones may form in the bile ducts, typically proximal to bile duct strictures. Seventy-five to eighty per cent of gallbladder gallstones in Western societies are composed primarily of cholesterol. About 20 per cent of cholesterol stones with calcified centers or rims can be seen on abdominal films. Twenty to twenty-five per cent of gallbladder gallstones contain black pigment mixed with the carbonate, phosphate, and bilirubinate salts of calcium. Eighty per cent of black stones are visible on abdominal films. Primary ductal stones are typically orange-brown, appearing "muddy" when wet, and "earthy" when dry. Ductal stones contain calcium bilirubinate, free fatty acids, and less than 10 per cent cholesterol.

Epidemiology and the Natural History of Gallstones

The incidence of gallstones increases with age. Gallstones are also more common in women, especially after multiple pregnancies. However, gallstones have been reported at all ages and are quite common in men. Others at increased risk for gallstones include obese persons, diabetics, patients who have undergone prolonged periods of fasting with or without parenteral nutrition, individuals who lose weight rapidly, cirrhotics, and patients with ileal dysfunction due to inflammatory bowel disease, ileal bypass operations, or surgical resection of the ileum. Pigment gallstones are more common in patients with hemolytic anemia. Heredity also contributes to the development of gallstones; the incidence is increased in some ethnic groups. For example, 90 per cent of Pima Indian women develop gallstones. Some drugs, including exogenous estrogen and octreotide (the somatostatin analogue), may cause gallstones. In general, gallstones are quite common, and most patients have no predisposing factors. Gallstone disease should be considered in the diagnosis of any patient who exhibits classic signs and symptoms.

Most gallstones cause no symptoms, and most remain silent for many years. Fewer than 10 per cent of patients with asymptomatic gallstone disease develop symptoms during 5-year follow-up; only 18 per cent manifest symptoms after 20 years. Each year, 1 million patients develop symptoms of gallstone disease; one half of these patients require cholecystectomy. Most patients with gallstones develop symptoms before serious complications occur. The risk associated with observation of asymptomatic gallstones is similar to the risk associated with prophylactic surgery. However, after symptoms have developed, they tend to recur with increased frequency and/or intensity. The incidence of complications increases until observation has a greater risk of complication than does surgery. The current approach is to operate on patients with symptomatic, but not asymptomatic, gallstones. The same reasoning applies to laparoscopic cholecystectomy, which reduces postoperative pain and time to complete recovery but does not reduce the morbidity and mortality of cholecystectomy.

Clinical Signs and Symptoms

Postprandial pain, the most common symptom of gallstone disease, is most often felt in the right upper quadrant of the abdomen, but it can also occur in the midepigastrium. Although an attack of pain is commonly called biliary colic, the term is a misnomer. The pain is usually steady, rather than colicky, and often radiates into the back or is referred to the right shoulder. It typically begins 15 to 60 minutes after a meal, is associated with nausea and vomiting, and can be quite severe. Some patients also complain of flatulence, bloating, and epigastric fullness, and they may relate the onset of pain to ingestion of greasy or fatty foods, milk products, cabbage, or onions. Pain can last 15 to 30 minutes or as long as several hours and typically resolves spontaneously. Specific interventions, other than pain medication, are usually ineffective. The pain is thought to be caused by intermittent obstruction of the cystic duct by a stone. Although gallstones may cause nausea, bloating, flatulence, and indigestion without pain, these symptoms are nonspecific and may be caused by many other gastrointestinal disorders. Gallstones are considered symptomatic only if they cause the classic pattern of pain previously described. Gallstones associated with nonspecific symptoms should be classified as asymptomatic, and patients in this category do not require cholecystectomy.

Physical examination during an attack of biliary colic may reveal a patient in severe distress, although without significant abdominal tenderness. The gallbladder is not palpable, and Murphy's sign, jaundice, and scleral icterus are absent. The patient is afebrile. Pain lasting more than several hours or associated with significant physical findings suggests other disorders of the liver, biliary tract, or gastrointestinal tract or complications of gallstones including acute cholecystitis, obstructive jaundice, cholangitis, or gallstone pancreatitis. Patients with intermittent symptoms attributable to gallstones are classified as having chronic cholecystitis.

Diagnostic Studies

The leukocyte count, serum amylase, serum aspartate aminotransferase (AST), serum alkaline phosphatase, and total serum bilirubin values are usually unremarkable during an attack of biliary colic. Transient increases may be observed if the patient passes a stone through the bile duct. Persistent abnormalities of laboratory tests suggest complications of gallstones. Abdominal films rarely reveal gallstones and have little value in establishing the diagnosis of cholelithiasis, but films may exclude perforated peptic ulcer and other upper gastrointestinal problems that mimic gallstone disease.

Ultrasonography, the diagnostic study of choice in patients with chronic cholecystitis, is safe, noninvasive, and extremely reliable in detecting gallstones, but it can be limited by intestinal gas. A typical history of biliary colic and demonstration of gallstones by ultrasonography provide sufficient indication for cholecystectomy; further testing is not required. During ultrasonography, gallstones are detected by the presence of echogenic filling defects in the gallbladder lumen, which produce characteristic sonographic shadows. Gallstones move when the patient changes position. During ultrasonography of the gallbladder, the clinician should examine the liver and measure the diameter of the bile duct. A diameter exceeding 7 mm suggests the presence of common duct stones. The pancreas should also be examined, but it is frequently obscured by bowel gas. Although the presence of gallstones is a sufficient indication for cholecystectomy in patients with typical symptoms, patients with atypical symptoms may require further testing to exclude peptic ulcer or other disorders of the bowel, liver, and kidneys.

Ultrasonography does not establish the diagnosis of gallstones in all patients. Small stones may be missed, and overlying intestinal gas may obscure the gallbladder. Moreover, some patients without gallstones have typical biliary colic. In some patients, oral cholecystography (OCG) may be helpful when ultrasonography is not. The patient ingests tablets of iopanoic acid the night before examination, because contrast agent must be absorbed from the intestine, extracted by the liver, and excreted into bile. Bile containing iopanoic acid enters a normal gallbladder through a patent cystic duct. The gallbladder is seen on abdominal films when bile is concentrated by the gallbladder. Thus, OCG detects gallstones as filling defects in the gallbladder lumen and evaluates cystic duct patency and gallbladder absorptive function. OCG is essential in screening patients for oral dissolution therapy and biliary lithotripsy. Nonvisualization of the gallbladder after two doses of iopanoic acid (i.e., a positive test) is accurate in 98 per cent of patients when compared with surgical findings. However, several pitfalls may result in false-positive test results. Patients must take the tablets as directed without vomiting, and they cannot have intestinal malabsorption or significant liver disease. OCG is not accurate if the patient has a total serum bilirubin exceeding 3 mg/dL.

COMPLICATIONS OF GALLSTONES

Acute Cholecystitis

Acute inflammation of the gallbladder, or acute cholecystitis, occurs in 10 to 20 per cent of patients with gallstones.

Acute cholecystitis is usually caused by persistent obstruction of the cystic duct by a stone. Pain is unremitting and often accompanied by fever and abdominal tenderness. Acute cholecystitis requires prompt treatment, because inflammation may progress to gangrene with subsequent pericholecystic abscess, free perforation into the peritoneal cavity, and/or sepsis. Most patients with acute cholecystitis have gallstones, but about 5 per cent have acute acalculous cholecystitis. Cystic duct obstruction exists in most of these patients. Sometimes, acute calculous or acalculous cholecystitis is caused by *Salmonella* infection. This complication occurs in about 1 per cent of patients with salmonellosis.

Acute cholecystitis does not develop in every gallbladder with an obstructed cystic duct. In some cases, bile is absorbed from the lumen. The gallbladder then fills with clear, mucoid material. Known as hydrops of the gallbladder, this complication leads to a distended, nontender gallbladder.

Clinical Signs and Symptoms

Most patients with acute cholecystitis have had previous symptoms. Pain with acute cholecystitis begins like biliary colic, but it does not resolve. The pain progressively worsens and localizes in the right upper quadrant of the abdomen or epigastrium. The pain may radiate into the back or right shoulder, and it is often associated with loss of appetite, nausea, and vomiting. Most patients have a low-grade fever and, sometimes, chills. High fever suggests another problem or a complication of acute cholecystitis.

Abdominal examination demonstrates well-localized right upper quadrant tenderness directly over the gallbladder. Tenderness increases with inspiration when the abdominal wall is palpated directly over the gallbladder. This physical finding, known as Murphy's sign, occurs when the inflamed gallbladder moves below the costal margin and contacts the examiner's hand. Murphy's sign specifically refers to localized tenderness and must be distinguished from the generalized tenderness along the entire edge of the liver that occurs with acute right heart failure and acute hepatitis. A distended gallbladder is sometimes palpable just below the costal margin.

The leukocyte count commonly increases, and there is a shift to immature forms. Although liver function tests and serum amylase activity are most often normal, mild to moderate increases in serum amylase, AST, alkaline phosphatase, and total bilirubin may occur in some patients. Increased serum bilirubin usually ranges between 1.5 and 3.0 mg/dL and rarely exceeds 5 mg/dL.

Patients with acalculous cholecystitis present with the same signs and symptoms as those of calculous acute cholecystitis, but the disease seems to progress more rapidly, and patients are more likely to develop gangrene. Patients with *Salmonella* cholecystitis usually have profuse diarrhea and a history of travel to an endemic area.

Diagnostic Studies

Ultrasonography and radionuclide cholescintigraphy (HIDA scan) are useful in establishing a diagnosis of acute cholecystitis. Ultrasonography usually confirms the diagnosis by detecting gallstones in a patient with typical symptoms, but the presence of gallstones alone is not specific for this disorder. More specific signs of gallbladder inflammation, such as gallbladder wall thickening, a positive sonographic Murphy's sign, and the presence of pericholecystic fluid, are less often present. Ultrasonography can accurately detect acute cholecystitis in 90 to 95 per cent of patients with acute cholecystitis, but it sometimes demonstrates stones in patients with pain from other causes. Specificity has been reported to range from 75 to 95 per cent.

Cholescintigraphy with a radiolabeled derivative of iminodiacetic acid is sensitive and specific for acute cholecystitis. Iminodiacetic acid and its derivatives are extracted from serum and excreted into bile within 5 minutes. If the cystic duct is patent, bile enters the gallbladder and can be visualized within 15 minutes to 1 hour, although 3 to 4 hours may be required for a chronically diseased gallbladder. Cholescintigraphy detects cystic duct obstruction and, when the gallbladder is not visualized for 4 hours, is accurate in 98 per cent of patients with acute cholecystitis. About 2 per cent of patients have acalculous cholecystitis without cystic duct obstruction. Cholescintigraphy results are normal for these patients. Indeterminate scans occur in patients with liver disease and acute cholangitis. These conditions manifest by poor uptake of radioisotope, delayed excretion of radioisotope into the ductal system, and visualization of radioisotope in the renal collecting systems. If the diagnosis of acute cholecystitis is not clear with one of these tests, the other test is usually helpful. Both tests should be necessary for only 10 to 20 per cent of patients.

Complications of Acute Cholecystitis

To decrease morbidity and mortality, several complications of acute cholecystitis, including empyema of the gallbladder, emphysematous cholecystitis, gallbladder perforation, and pericholecystic abscess, must be promptly recognized. Empyema of the gallbladder occurs when the gallbladder fills with pus and essentially becomes an abscess. A distended gallbladder is palpable, although abdominal guarding may obscure this finding. There is no specific test for the diagnosis of empyema of the gallbladder, but this disorder is often characterized by a distended, markedly thickened gallbladder on ultrasonography or computed tomography (CT) of the abdomen. Emphysematous cholecystitis occurs in a gallbladder infected with gas-forming bacteria *(Clostridium* species and *Escherichia coli)*. Gas in the gallbladder lumen and/or wall on abdominal film or CT scan confirms the diagnosis. Gallbladder perforation results in diffuse peritonitis or, if contained, in a pericholecystic abscess that can be detected with ultrasonography or CT of the abdomen.

Patients with complications of acute cholecystitis present with signs and symptoms similar to those observed in patients with uncomplicated acute cholecystitis. However, fever is usually greater, pain more severe, and the leukocyte count markedly higher. Patients can also present with diffuse peritonitis and signs of sepsis, including hypotension and mental confusion. When patients have peritonitis and/or sepsis, it may be difficult to distinguish gallbladder disease from other causes of the acute abdomen. Acute cholangitis, perforated viscus, vascular compromise or obstruction of the small or large bowel, and acute pancreatitis must be considered.

Cholecystoenteric Fistula and Gallstone Ileus

A fistula between the gallbladder and the duodenum, stomach, or colon develops when a gallstone erodes through the wall of the gallbladder into an adjacent organ. Symptoms specific to the fistula are rare; fistulas are often found incidentally when air is seen in the biliary tract on abdominal films or, rarely, when barium enters the biliary tract during an upper gastrointestinal series. Although most gallstones eventually pass through the gastrointestinal tract, stones eroding directly into it may be quite large and may cause intestinal obstruction, a condition known as gallstone ileus. The point of obstruction is most often at a narrowing in the gastrointestinal tract, usually the ileocolic valve or the sigmoid colon. Gallstone ileus should be suspected when abdominal films show classic signs of small or large intestinal obstruction and air in the biliary tract. Occasionally, a radiopaque gallstone is seen at the point of obstruction.

OTHER DISORDERS OF THE GALLBLADDER

Congenital Defects

Although variants of ductal and vascular anatomy of the biliary system are well described, congenital anomalies of the gallbladder are rare. Congenital absence, duplication, intrahepatic gallbladder, and "floating" gallbladder (i.e., gallbladder with a complete mesentery) have been reported. Ultrasonography may diagnose or suggest each of these anomalies. Floating gallbladder can result in torsion of the gallbladder.

Porcelain Gallbladder

A calcified or porcelain gallbladder is easily seen on an abdominal film as a gallbladder outlined by a rim of calcium. Porcelain gallbladder is a significant finding, because gallbladder cancer is found in 20 to 60 per cent of these patients. Cholecystectomy is definitely indicated, but laparoscopic cholecystectomy is contraindicated, because seeding of trochar sites with tumor has been reported for cases of gallbladder cancer.

Benign Tumors and Pseudotumors

Benign neoplasms of the gallbladder occur in fewer than 3 per cent of patients undergoing cholecystectomy. A list of benign tumors and pseudotumors is given in Table 1. These lesions may cause symptoms, but symptoms most often result from gallstones. Patients experience episodes of right upper quadrant or epigastric pain, but most often have nonspecific symptoms such as dyspepsia, flatulence, nausea, and vomiting. Benign lesions can be detected by ultrasonography, oral cholecystography, and CT of the upper abdomen and are usually less than 1 cm in diameter, are closely associated with the mucosa, do not move when the patient changes position, and do not produce sonographic shadows. Localized adenomyomatous hyperplasia, most common in the gallbladder fundus, is typically identified by a characteristic sessile defect with central opaque indentation on OCG. Ultrasound sometimes reveals a filling defect with anechoic cystic spaces.

Table 1. Benign Tumor and Pseudotumors of the Gallbladder

Benign Tumors
Adenoma
Papillary
Nonpapillary
Hemangioma
Lipoma
Leiomyoma
Granular cell tumor
Carcinoid
Pseudotumors
Adenomyosis
Ectopic tissue
Liver
Pancreas
Gastric or intestinal mucosa
Gallbladder polyps
Cholesterol
Inflammatory

Cholecystectomy is indicated for tumors and pseudotumors associated with symptoms. Growths that are asymptomatic may be observed if the diagnosis is certain and the size of the lesion is less than 1 cm. Studies should be repeated at 3 and 6 months after diagnosis to exclude a significant increase in the size of the lesion.

Cholesterolosis

In cholesterolosis, cholesterol esters accumulating in the gallbladder mucosa produce a yellow, reticular pattern. In 80 per cent of patients, accumulation of cholesterol is confined to the mucosa, and in the remainder, a cholesterol polyp is also present. Patients with cholesterolosis, especially those with polyps, develop symptoms similar to those in patients with gallstones. Cholesterolosis is a difficult clinical diagnosis to make. On ultrasound, the polyps appear as nonshadowing filling defects in the gallbladder lumen that do not move when the patient changes position. OCG may reveal a luminal filling defect and decreased concentration of contrast medium. Gallbladder emptying may be impaired if the patient is given cholecystokinin or a fatty meal to empty the gallbladder.

Gallbladder Cancer

Gallbladder cancer is usually associated with gallstones, but the risk of developing gallbladder cancer if gallstones are present is less than 1 per cent over a period of 20 years. Early gallbladder cancer is asymptomatic, or the symptoms are vague and nonspecific. Advanced disease causes symptoms by invading into adjacent structures, and patients present with weight loss and malaise, an abdominal mass, acute cholecystitis when the cystic duct is obstructed by tumor, or jaundice if the tumor involves the bile duct. Although gallbladder cancer may be detected with ultrasonography or CT, it is often missed and the diagnosis is not made before surgery. This is especially true for early stages (stage I, only mucosal involvement; stage II, involvement of the mucosa and muscularis), which have the best prognosis when properly treated. The surgeon should open and examine the gallbladder at the time of cholecystectomy. When a diagnosis of gallbladder cancer is established, CT and sometimes angiography are useful in staging the tumor. CT is particularly accurate for detection of tumor extension into the liver.

Gallstone Pancreatitis

Gallstone, or biliary, pancreatitis is caused by passage of gallstones through the common bile duct. Pancreatitis is thought to result from acute obstruction of the duct, but the exact pathogenesis of gallstone pancreatitis is not completely understood. Pancreatitis can range from mild, transient episodes to a severe, fulminant disease that can cause death. Pain begins suddenly, and patients describe steady epigastric discomfort with radiation into the back. Most patients have nausea and vomiting. Physical findings vary with the severity of the attack of pancreatitis; many patients have tachycardia and/or tachypnea, and some have epigastric tenderness. Peritoneal signs are usually absent, but with severe pancreatitis, the patient may present with all the features of an acute abdomen.

Serum amylase is increased in more than 90 per cent of patients with gallstone pancreatitis. Amylase values typically exceed those seen in alcoholic pancreatitis. Although the degree of increase of serum amylase does not correlate with the severity of the attack, the higher the activity of serum amylase, the more likely the diagnosis of pancreatitis. Other disorders associated with increased serum amylase usually cause only mild to moderate increases. Serum lipase, which may be more specific for pancreatic inflammation, may also be increased.

Abdominal films show signs of intestinal ileus in one half of patients with gallstone pancreatitis. These films can also be used to exclude perforated viscus and bowel obstruction as causes of pain. A localized, distended loop of colon or small intestine directly over the pancreas, called a sentinel loop, suggests inflammation in the pancreas. Ultrasonography detects gallstones in the gallbladder, but it rarely demonstrates common duct stones. Dilatation of the common bile duct may be present, but it is frequently absent despite acute obstruction. In one third of these patients, the pancreas and retroperitoneum cannot be adequately evaluated by ultrasound, but CT allows reasonable visualization of the inflamed pancreas. Diffuse enlargement of the gland, loss of peripancreatic fat planes, and peripancreatic fluid are demonstrated early. Late findings include pancreatic pseudocyst and abscess.

DISORDERS OF THE BILE DUCTS

Most diseases of the bile ducts cause partial or complete obstruction of the biliary tract. Patients with diseases of the biliary ducts present with obstructive jaundice or acute cholangitis. Less commonly, a patient with liver or biliary tract disease presents with bleeding into the biliary tract, called hemobilia. The differential diagnosis of bile duct obstruction includes choledocholithiasis, benign bile duct strictures, bile duct cancer, extrinsic compression of the bile duct by metastatic cancer, and infestation of the ducts with parasites (Table 2). The presentations of all these disorders of the bile duct are similar and are discussed together in the following sections. Specific features of choledocholithiasis and benign and malignant strictures are also reviewed.

Obstructive Jaundice

Acute bile duct obstruction presents with pain, jaundice, and dark urine. Some patients may have symptoms of chronic cholecystitis, but choledocholithiasis also can be the initial presentation of gallstone disease. Pain is present in 80 per cent of patients, is felt in the right upper abdomen or epigastrium, and may radiate to the back or right shoulder. The intensity of pain may range from mild to severe. Nausea and vomiting are common. If bile is colonized with bacteria, cholangitis with its characteristic symptoms may ensue.

The degree of abdominal tenderness varies, but patients do not exhibit peritoneal signs. Jaundice, scleral icterus, and dark urine occur simultaneously with pain or may follow as long as 48 hours later. The liver may be tender on palpation. The gallbladder is usually not palpable unless acute cholecystitis also exists. The serum bilirubin concentration increases, but it rarely exceeds 10 mg/dL. The serum alkaline phosphatase activity is significantly increased, and serum AST and lactate dehydrogenase concentrations are only moderately increased. However, the patterns of abnormalities of serum enzymes cannot distinguish intrahepatic from extrahepatic bile duct obstruction. The blood leukocyte count may be increased or normal.

In bile duct obstruction due to chronic disease, pain and tenderness are less common, the gallbladder may be palpable, and the patient may have a history of weight loss. Nausea and vomiting are less frequent, and the development of jaundice may be more insidious. The serum bilirubin concentration is often increased; concentrations exceeding 15 mg/dL suggest benign or malignant bile duct strictures. Liver function tests are abnormal, and the blood leukocyte count is normal unless cholangitis complicates the disease. Patients with chronic obstructive jaundice exhibit coagulation defects due to vitamin K deficiency. A prothrombin time should be measured, and defects corrected before invasive testing. Patients with obstructive jaundice also have circulating factors that influence vascular tone and depress cardiac function. The presence of these factors significantly increases the risk of renal failure and cardiac collapse during invasive procedures, especially if radiographic contrast agents are administered or if complications such as bleeding or bile peritonitis ensue. Fortunately, most detrimental effects of biliary obstruction can be corrected with fluid and electrolytes.

In acute and chronic types of obstruction, ultrasonography and CT reveal dilatation of the intrahepatic and extrahepatic biliary tract. These tests rarely demonstrate a common duct stone or bile duct stricture, but they may reveal a malignant mass lesion of the bile duct or pancreas, a metastatic lesion and enlarged periductal nodes, or enlargement of the pancreas and calcifications characteristic of pancreatitis. Cholangiography is required to define the cause and the level of the obstruction. Endoscopic retrograde cholangiopancreatography (ERCP) provides the safest approach, especially in the absence of bile duct dilatation. ERCP can be accomplished in 90 to 95 per cent of patients. Gallstones can be removed after sphincterotomy, and bile duct strictures can be dilated. Ampullary lesions can be directly visualized, biopsy can be performed, and strictures can be brushed for cytologic diagnosis. Malignant lesions can be treated palliatively, if appropriate, with biliary stents placed over a guidewire from below. Unfortunately, adequate cholangiograms may be difficult to obtain in patients with duodenal diverticula, low ductal obstructions, or previous gastric surgery with Billroth II reconstruction. As with ERCP, percutaneous transhepatic cholangiography (PTC) is also successful in more than 90 per cent of patients with dilated ducts. PTC, however, has a greater rate of complications, including bile peritonitis and intra-abdominal bleeding. Nevertheless, PTC provides ex-

Table 2. Causes of Extrahepatic Bile Duct Obstruction

Choledocholithiasis
- Secondary bile duct stones (form in gallbladder)
- Primary ductal stones

Cancer
- Cholangiocarcinoma
- Gallbladder cancer
- Metastatic disease (extrinsic compression)
- Tumor emboli (hepatoma)

Benign Bile Duct Strictures
- Postoperative
- Inflammatory (sclerosing cholangitis)
- Chronic pancreatitis (Snape's syndrome)
- Caroli's disease

Parasites
- *Ascariasis lumbricoides*
- *Clonorchiasis sinensis*

cellent visualization of the proximal biliary tract and allows external drainage of bile. Palliative placement of stents through malignant lesions is simpler with PTC than with ERCP.

Acute Cholangitis

Bacteriobilia refers to colonization of bile with bacteria. Mere colonization frequently occurs without sequelae. Acute cholangitis refers to clinically significant bacterial infections of the biliary tract. Toxic cholangitis is a term that describes patients with severe cholangitis who exhibit signs of sepsis and shock. The onset of acute cholangitis requires bile contaminated with bacteria and obstruction of the bile duct with increased bile duct pressure or injury to biliary epithelium from indwelling catheters or instrumentation of the duct during ERCP or PTC.

The presenting symptoms of patients with acute cholangitis vary from mild and transient to life threatening, with evidence of septic shock. The signs and symptoms of acute cholangitis are similar to those of other serious upper gastrointestinal disorders. The medical history can be helpful in distinguishing acute cholangitis from other maladies. Previous attacks of biliary colic suggest gallstone disease and its complications. Shaking chills are characteristic of acute cholangitis, and a recent history of ERCP, PTC, or surgical manipulation of the bile ducts implies iatrogenically induced cholangitis. Three signs and symptoms described by Charcot (i.e., right upper quadrant abdominal or epigastric pain, jaundice, and fever) are highly specific for acute cholangitis. Unfortunately, all three features of Charcot's triad are present in fewer than 60 per cent of patients with acute cholangitis. Fever is the most consistent sign and is present in 90 per cent of patients. The fever is frequently intermittent and spiking because of transient episodes of bacteremia. Jaundice and abdominal pain, usually without severe tenderness, are present in two thirds to three fourths of patients. When hypotension and mental confusion accompany Charcot's triad, the symptom complex is called Reynold's pentad. This pentad is characteristic of toxic cholangitis, but only a minority of patients with toxic cholangitis manifest all five signs and symptoms.

Liver function test results are uniformly abnormal, reflecting damage caused by bacteria refluxing into periductal tissues. The serum total bilirubin concentration is less than 2 mg/dL in one fifth of patients. The leukocyte count can be increased, but it may be suppressed in critically ill patients. The serum amylase activity may also be increased in acute cholangitis, but the increase does not necessarily indicate that the patient has pancreatitis. Abnormal serum electrolytes, serum urea nitrogen, and creatinine may reflect severe volume contraction or renal failure. Coagulation studies may be abnormal because of vitamin K deficiency or sepsis-related disseminated intravascular coagulation.

Patients with acute cholangitis are seriously ill. Fluid and electrolyte imbalances and coagulation defects must be corrected before invasive or radiographic studies are undertaken. The physician should initiate empirical antibiotic therapy immediately to cover organisms typically found in bile and obtain blood and bile cultures and tailor antibiotics to the specific organisms isolated. Patients who stabilize with medical treatment should undergo prompt, elective testing to determine the cause of cholangitis, which should then be treated promptly to avoid recurrent episodes of the disorder.

Patients who do not respond to antibiotics or who present with toxic cholangitis require urgent decompression of the biliary tract. Identification of patients at highest risk for complications is now possible. Risk factors that correlate with morbidity and mortality include concomitant medical problems, especially renal failure and cardiovascular disease, serum pH less than 7.4 on presentation or during initial treatment, serum total bilirubin greater than 5.3 mg/dL, platelet count of fewer than 150,000 cells/mm^3, and albumin less than 3.0 g/dL. Choice of diagnostic and therapeutic procedures depends on the condition of the patient. Highest-risk patients are best treated with decompression of the duct; definitive treatment of the biliary duct problem can be undertaken days to weeks later. Low-risk patients are candidates for definitive therapy from the outset.

Urgent evaluation and decompression of the biliary tract is most efficiently and safely accomplished with ERCP, limited papillotomy, and placement of a nasobiliary tube. Elective, definitive treatment of the biliary obstruction by endoscopic or surgical means is undertaken later, when the patient is stable. When ERCP is not possible, percutaneous drainage can adequately relieve biliary pressure, but morbidity and mortality rates are greater than with the endoscopic approach. Emergency surgical decompression of the biliary tract is reserved for patients who do not respond to medical, endoscopic, and percutaneous therapy. It is usually unwise to proceed with definitive therapy at surgery and the operation is usually limited to placement of a T-tube.

Hemobilia

Hemobilia refers to bleeding into the biliary ductal system. Hemobilia is characterized by upper gastrointestinal hemorrhage, most often manifested as melena, without an identifiable cause in the esophagus, stomach, or duodenum. Usually, passage of clots through the common bile duct causes right upper quadrant abdominal pain and intermittent obstruction with jaundice. Hemobilia most commonly results after trauma to the liver and biliary tract. In the past, the classic patient had a history of severe penetrating or blunt trauma to the abdomen, but iatrogenic trauma to the liver and biliary tract during percutaneous and endoscopic procedures has become the most common cause of hemobilia. Hemobilia may also be caused by gallstones, benign and malignant tumors of the liver and biliary tract, parasitic infections, and rupture of a hepatic artery aneurysm. Angiography is the diagnostic study of choice because it demonstrates the arterial– or venous–bile duct fistula and facilitates concomitant therapeutic embolization.

SPECIFIC DISORDERS OF THE BILE DUCTS

Choledocholithiasis

Bile duct stones may be completely asymptomatic. About 4 per cent of patients have unsuspected bile duct stones on cholangiography performed routinely at the time of cholecystectomy. Most patients with symptomatic common bile duct stones present with obstructive jaundice or acute cholangitis. Although acute pancreatitis is caused by passage of stones through the bile duct, only one third of biliary pancreatitis patients have common bile duct stones at the time of cholecystectomy.

Common bile duct stones may be detected with ultrasonography and CT scan, but cholangiography is the most reliable diagnostic test. Cholangiography may be performed endoscopically in a retrograde manner (i.e., ERCP), percutaneously (i.e., PTC), or intraoperatively, depending on the therapeutic approach chosen for the patient. Preoperative ERCP is preferred in patients in whom common bile duct stones are strongly suspected. Bile duct stones can be removed in more than 90 to 95 per cent of patients through papillotomy performed after radiographic films are obtained, allowing the patient to undergo laparoscopic cholecystectomy. Routine ERCP in patients at low or moderate risk for common bile duct stones is not cost effective. Small stones found with intraoperative cholangiography in these patients can be removed laparoscopically, with an open bile duct exploration, or postoperatively using ERCP and papillotomy.

Benign and Malignant Biliary Strictures

Most benign bile duct strictures are caused by traumatic injury to the bile duct, often after cholecystectomy. Strictures may also result from choledocholithiasis and distal bile duct stricture may be caused by chronic pancreatitis with enlargement of the pancreatic head, a condition called Snape's syndrome. Sclerosing cholangitis is a diffuse disease of the ductal system resulting in fibrosis and scarring of bile ducts. Sclerosing cholangitis usually results in multiple intrahepatic strictures, but it can affect the extrahepatic biliary system, sometimes without intrahepatic involvement. Seventy-five per cent of patients with sclerosing cholangitis have inflammatory bowel disease. Early symptoms of benign bile duct strictures, which develop slowly, include pruritus, unexplained increases in alkaline phosphatase, and mild jaundice. Late presentations include symptoms of obstructive jaundice and acute cholangitis. ERCP and PTC are the most useful tests for diagnosis and characterization of the stricture. Brushing of the stricture for cytologic examination can usually be performed with ERCP or PTC after the stricture has been characterized. Thin-needle biopsy of the pancreas using CT guidance may also be useful if there is enlargement of the pancreatic head. A positive brushing or needle biopsy result is highly specific for tumor, but negative findings do not exclude tumor. Diagnosis of malignant strictures may be difficult, and surgery may be required for definitive diagnosis and for treatment.

ACUTE AND CHRONIC PANCREATITIS

By Giuseppe Aliperti, M.D.
St. Louis, Missouri

Whether acute or chronic, inflammatory diseases of the pancreas have many causes, but only two main clinical presentations. Acute pancreatitis can occur in patients who do not have a prior history, or it can present as an event superimposed on chronic pancreatitis. The latter condition, which is a smoldering inflammatory process, results in irreversible structural damage to the pancreas, glandular tissue loss and fibrosis, and decreased secretory function. Both diseases can result in local or systemic complications, ranging in severity from mildly symptomatic to rapidly fatal. Acute pancreatitis can resolve without sequelae and without recurrence if the cause is eliminated. However, its course may be devastating if complications occur. The initial clinical manifestations of chronic pancreatitis may present after repeated subclinical injury has resulted in extensive structural damage.

Pancreatitis has a wide variety of causes. Gallstones and chronic alcohol abuse are the leading causes of acute and chronic pancreatitis, respectively. Together they are responsible for more than two thirds of cases in the United States. The precise microenvironmental events leading to pancreatitis remain unclear. The activation of potent digestive enzymes produced by the pancreas probably occurs within the gland itself rather than after release into the small intestine, resulting in damage to parenchymal tissue and inflammation. The activated enzymes released from dying cells into lymphatics and veins can then damage neighboring and distant organs.

ACUTE PANCREATITIS

Acute pancreatitis can present as a mild, self-limited illness or a devastating disease resulting in a prolonged hospital stay and high mortality rates. The medical treatment of this condition is mostly supportive and concentrates on the prevention and early management of complications. Close monitoring of the patient and the diagnostic acumen of the clinician are of the utmost importance. An important goal is the removal of the cause, if one can be identified, in an attempt to prevent recurrence.

Gallstones are the single most common cause of acute pancreatitis. A small gallstone can become lodged within the sphincter of Oddi and prevent drainage of biliary and pancreatic secretions in the approximately 30 to 40 per cent of patients with a common channel. Microorganisms from refluxed bile may be responsible for the activation in situ of pancreatic enzymes and may start an inflammatory cascade. Pancreatitis is associated with the use of certain drugs (e.g., thiazide diuretics, sulfonamides, and antimetabolites) and with hyperlipidemia and hypercalcemia. Other events associated with pancreatitis include trauma to the abdomen, endoscopic retrograde cholangiopancreatography (ERCP), cardiac or abdominal surgery, and organ transplantation. Peptic ulcer penetrating into the pancreatic bed, hypotensive episodes, atheromatous emboli, vasculitis, and infectious agents such as mumps and coxsackievirus, or parasites (e.g., *Ascaris* and *Clonorchis sinensis*) may cause pancreatitis. Annular pancreas, choledochal cyst, and duodenal duplication cyst represent congenital risk factors. Although controversial, pancreas divisum (nonfusion of dorsal and ventral pancreatic ducts occurring in 2 to 5 per cent of otherwise healthy individuals) may be associated with pancreatitis. Acute pancreatitis remains idiopathic in 10 to 20 per cent of patients. Those with recurrent idiopathic pancreatitis should be evaluated for microlithiasis (in which transient obstruction is caused by small stones that evade radiographic detection) and for sphincter of Oddi dysfunction.

Clinical Manifestations

The most common initial symptom of acute pancreatitis, occurring in 98 per cent of patients, is abdominal pain in the epigastrium or the left upper quadrant. The pain reaches its maximal intensity over 15 minutes to an hour and radiates to the back in half of patients. Position appears to aggravate the perception of pain, and most patients are more uncomfortable in a supine position. Resolution of pain is usually slow and may not occur for days.

Nausea and vomiting occur in 80 per cent of patients in the first day or two. On physical examination, intense abdominal tenderness is rarely associated with signs of peritoneal irritation such as rebound or guarding, attesting to an entirely retroperitoneal process. Low-grade fever is frequent and can be prolonged. The differential diagnosis includes biliary colic, renal colic, peptic ulcer with or without perforation, mesenteric ischemia, intestinal obstruction, salpingo-oophoritis, and ectopic pregnancy. Laparotomy is necessary on rare occasions for excluding diseases requiring urgent operative management, such as mesenteric infarction, small bowel volvulus, or intestinal perforation.

Patients with pancreatitis can undergo subtle deterioration, and complications are difficult to reverse once they occur. For this reason, frequent clinical evaluation is necessary for detecting early signs of deterioration. A rigid and distended abdomen with peritoneal signs occurs only in more severe cases in which there is extension of the inflammatory process into the small intestinal and colonic mesentery, inducing chemical peritonitis or hemorrhagic pancreatitis and intra-abdominal bleeding. Tachycardia and hypotension occur in one third of patients and indicate clinically significant hypovolemia. Fluid may be removed from the intravascular space by plasma exudation into the retroperitoneum, fluid accumulation in an atonic intestine, vomiting, hemorrhage, and increased vascular permeability with third-spacing, or peripheral vasodilation. In most patients, oliguria and azotemia reflect hypovolemia, but they may also be due to direct renal toxicity. Dyspnea can result from adult respiratory distress syndrome (ARDS), atelectasis, or pleural effusions. Encephalopathy is usually an effect of systemic illness (e.g., infection or cerebral hypoperfusion) but it can also reflect direct neurologic damage. Fever with a septic curve suggests an infection complicating the basic process. Infection of necrotic tissue or fluid collections, pneumonitis, cholangitis, and cholecystitis are all diagnostic considerations in patients with spiking fever or confusion. Rapid diagnosis and treatment of infectious complications can be lifesaving in patients with severe pancreatitis because sepsis and mortality are closely associated in these patients. Loss of ionized calcium within areas of fat necrosis may induce tetany, a rare event with poor prognosis. Continued pain and increased enzyme activity or recurrent pain after attempts at oral feeding are typical of pseudocyst development. Dissection of peripancreatic bleeding into subcutaneous tissue is very rare and may lead to discoloration of the flanks (Grey Turner's sign) or of the periumbilical region (Cullen's sign).

Laboratory Tests

Increases in amylase and lipase activity in the serum are commonly associated with acute pancreatitis, and their release into the bloodstream follows cell death resulting from the inflammatory process. The magnitude of increases in enzyme activity should not be used to predict disease severity or duration because they often reflect only the condition of the pancreas prior to the attack. A healthier, more cellular pancreas may have more parenchyma to be destroyed during the first attack than does a gland already damaged by chronic disease or repeated attacks. In self-limited episodes, serum amylase activity usually returns to normal within 4 to 5 days, whereas lipase activity is typically slower in returning to baseline levels. Hyperlipemic serum may falsely decrease amylase activity unless the laboratory uses a method to clear the lipemia. Other conditions are associated with elevated activity of both these enzymes. Increased serum amylase activity can result from intestinal injury caused by ischemia or obstruction or from tubo-ovarian disease. Acute parotitis and alcoholic binges can also precipitate the release of salivary-type isoamylases, with increased activity of total serum amylase. In macroamylasemia, several molecules of amylase aggregate in a large macromolecule that cannot undergo efficient glomerular filtration, leading to increased serum amylase activity in the absence of pancreatic or renal disease. Serum lipase activity remains normal in all these conditions. In patients with renal failure, activity of both serum amylase and lipase is increased because of the reduced glomerular filtration of both proteins. In such cases, urinary amylase activity is usually low, which can be a clue to the correct diagnosis.

Other laboratory values should be monitored in patients with acute pancreatitis. The white blood cell count often parallels disease activity and remains increased during the acute stages of the inflammatory process. Supervening infection, a severe and potentially lethal complication, must be strongly considered in patients with leukocytosis in whom severe pancreatitis develops. Serum creatinine and serum urea nitrogen concentrations and the hematocrit value are important indicators of intravascular volume and must be monitored closely. If all three values begin to increase, prompt early fluid resuscitation is required to prevent the development of clinical consequences of hypovolemia. Measurement of arterial blood gases helps monitor oxygen exchange and allows an early diagnosis of ARDS. Abnormal liver function test results point to gallstones as a potential cause of pancreatitis. Modest decreases in serum calcium concentrations are not uncommon and parallel the loss of serum albumin to the third space. Treatment of hypocalcemia is usually not necessary until the ionized serum calcium concentration is reduced or symptoms of impending tetany occur. Hyperglycemia occurs in half of the patients with acute pancreatitis and more commonly in those with underlying chronic pancreatitis. When this abnormality is observed during an acute attack in patients without underlying chronic pancreatitis or diabetes, the prognosis becomes poor. Diagnostic paracentesis is of minimal value except to diagnose infection. Sterile pancreatic ascites is straw-colored and usually has concentrations of amylase greater than 10,000 U/L.

Imaging Studies

Chest and abdominal radiographs are obtained early to confirm the presence of ileus and to detect radiographic signs of pancreatitis such as the sentinel loop and the colon cutoff sign. These studies are also helpful to exclude perforation and other processes in the differential diagnosis of an acute abdomen. Ultrasound is essential for detecting stones within the gallbladder, where its accuracy is approximately 95 to 98 per cent. Ultrasound is less useful for the evaluation of bile duct stones in the acute stages, during which a normal ultrasound examination does not exclude gallstones as the cause of pancreatitis. Detection of gallbladder stones or a dilated common bile duct is sufficient evidence to support this as a cause of pancreatitis in an appropriate clinical setting. Computed tomography (CT) is a valuable tool in the diagnosis and management of acute pancreatitis, but during the earliest stages of disease, it rarely adds important new information. This study is most valuable when used in two different modes. Urgent evaluation of patients with an unstable clinical presentation can establish inflammatory involvement of the organs surrounding the pancreas and the presence of fluid collections or necrotic tissue. Follow-up of these complications at intervals is used to guide further therapy in patients who fail to respond. Dynamic CT can identify the presence and extent of tissue necrosis by quantifying contrast enhancement of pancreatic tissue. This technique relies on the difference in contrast uptake between viable and necrotic tissue, and CT-guided needle aspiration with Gram staining and culture is invaluable in guiding the management of septic patients.

ERCP is an important study in patients with acute as well as chronic pancreatitis. This study is usually unnecessary in patients with mild gallstone pancreatitis in whom direct cholangiography to exclude common duct stones can be obtained at the time of cholecystectomy. ERCP is an essential urgent procedure in patients with severe gallstone pancreatitis in whom early identification and removal of obstructing stones is associated with a significant reduction in complications. ERCP is also the procedure of choice for the diagnosis and removal of common bile duct stones in patients with gallstone pancreatitis and without a gallbladder. Its usefulness in the absence of gallstones lies in the identification of other causes of pancreatitis such as sphincter disease, ampullary neoplasms, and congenital anomalies. Manometric assessment of the sphincter region during ERCP can diagnose sphincter disease, which is usually treatable with sphincterotomy. Bile specimens obtained during ERCP directly from the biliary tree or from the duodenum after injection of cholecystokinin can provide specimens for microscopic detection of microlithiasis.

Clinical Course and Complications

Mortality rates in acute pancreatitis vary from less than 5 per cent in patients with mild disease to 30 per cent in patients with severe disease; they increase dramatically (from 2 to 56 per cent) when organ systems beyond the pancreas are involved. Several risk factors have been identified to predict mortality (Table 1). Mortality rates range from less than 1 per cent in patients with up to 2 risk factors to 80 per cent for patients with 9 to 11 risk factors; more than 5 risk factors are rarely found, even in very severe illness. One disadvantage of this system is that fewer than half of the risk factors are present at the time of admission, and those that appear later may be affected by treatment. Some clinicians use increases in serum urea nitrogen and glucose concentrations as the the two most important early criteria of severity.

Systemic complications of acute pancreatitis include hypovolemic shock from reduced blood volume or intra-abdominal bleeding from erosion into abdominal vessels, diabetic ketoacidosis or hyperosmolar coma (due to decreased insulin production), and disseminated intravascular coagulation. Tetany can result from severe hypocalcemia due to complexing of calcium with disrupted fat, stimulation of thyrocalcitonin release by released glucagon, or inadequate parathyroid hormone (PTH) release in response to low calcium concentrations. Infection from intestinal sources, fluid collections, and phlegmonous or necrotic tissue may occur with few systemic clues; these can be further obscured by the use of antibiotics that fail to penetrate secluded and scantily perfused areas. Pulmonary complications are a major source of morbidity and mortality, and include pleural effusions caused by the passage of peripancreatic fluid through permeable diaphragmatic lymphatics, atelectasis from abdominal distention and pain, and ARDS. Acute tubular necrosis due to shock or direct renal toxicity can lead to renal failure.

Fluid leaking from the injured pancreas can collect throughout the peritoneal cavity or organize into collections called pseudocysts. These encapsulated collections of enzyme-containing fluid and necrotic debris lack epithelial lining and often maintain communication with the pancreatic duct. Pseudocysts are detected radiographically in 10 to 20 per cent of patients and by physical examination in 2 to 4 per cent of patients with pancreatitis. They can dissect into the midabdomen, chest, pelvis, a hollow viscus, or major vessels, causing intra-abdominal hemorrhage. Pseudocysts can leak slowly into the abdomen, causing ascites, or into the chest, causing pleural effusions, and can become infected. Although small pseudocysts formed during acute pancreatitis often disappear without specific therapy, those that are present for more than 6 weeks and are larger than 5 cm in diameter usually require treatment. Obstruction at different locations can be caused by edema, phlegmon, or fluid collections. Compression of the common bile duct produces obstructive jaundice, whereas compression of the duodenum results in gastric outlet obstruction. Fibrosis with healing can make the process irreversible, requiring surgical decompression.

Table 1. Risk Factors That Predict Mortality in Acute Pancreatitis

Age greater than 55 yr
White blood cell count greater than 16,000 cells/mm^3
Serum glucose greater than 200 mg/dL
Serum lactate dehydrogenase greater than 350 IU/L
Aspartate aminotransferase (AST) greater than 250 IU/L, or developing during the first 48 h
Hematocrit fall greater than 10 per cent after hydration
Serum urea nitrogen increased by more than 5 mg/dL
Arterial P_{O_2} less than 60 mm Hg
Base deficit greater than 4 mEq/L
Serum calcium level less than 8 mg/dL
Estimated fluid sequestration greater than 6 L

Modified from Ranson, J.H.C.: Etiological and prognostic factors in human acute pancreatitis: A review. Am. J. Gastroenterol., 77:633, 1982, with permission.

Diagnosing the Cause of Acute Pancreatitis

The search for a cause of pancreatitis is crucial but must be carried out urgently *only* when gallstones are suspected. Early diagnosis and treatment of gallstone pancreatitis can actually improve the prognosis. Early re-establishment of drainage with urgent stone removal by ERCP significantly reduces complications in patients with severe disease and three or more of the risk factors listed in Table 1. The presence of cholecystolithiasis on ultrasonography is not always sufficient for a clinical diagnosis because gallstones are common. Clinical and laboratory predictors for gallstone pancreatitis include age greater than 50 years, female gender, amylase activity greater than 4000 U/L, aspartate aminotransferase concentrations (AST) greater than 100 U/L, and alkaline phosphatase concentrations greater than 300 U/L. Gallstone pancreatitis occurs in 5 per cent of patients with one predictor, 50 per cent of patients with two predictors, and 90 per cent of patients with three or more predictors. Increases in serum amylase and lipase activity are less pronounced in alcohol-induced pancreatitis, perhaps because of the subclinical tissue destruction that occurred prior to the attack. Transabdominal ultrasonography is an appropriate initial study in patients with gallbladders, but it is usually not necessary in patients who have undergone prior cholecystectomy or in those in whom ERCP is planned for simultaneous diagnosis and treatment. Most patients with gallstone pancreatitis suffer self-limited episodes with early resolution because 70 to 90 per cent of impacted stones pass spontaneously into the intestine. Once gallstones are confirmed as the cause of pancreatitis in patients with gallbladders and self-limited disease, further diagnostic studies are usually unnecessary. Intraoperative cholangiography at the time of cholecystectomy is used to demonstrate that the bile ducts are free from stones. Cholecystectomy is usually curative under these circumstances.

After excluding gallstones, further investigation is required to identify causes that are treatable in order to prevent recurrence. This investigation can usually be performed electively. Careful review of the history, medical record, and medications often detects conditions missed during the initial interview. Laboratory abnormalities such as hypercalcemia and hypertriglyceridemia are easily detected and investigated, but serum calcium concentrations can be transiently decreased and serum triglyceride concentrations transiently increased during the acute episode. Both of these analytes should be rechecked electively. Unexplained pancreatitis in older patients who do not have gallstones may suggest the presence of neoplasia. Patients who have systemic disease known to be associated with pancreatitis should also undergo further investigation. Some local obstructive complications of pancreatitis, such as pancreatic duct strictures, stones, and obstructing pseudocysts or tumors, can often worsen symptoms and the disease course, increasing the frequency of hospital admissions.

CHRONIC PANCREATITIS

Alcohol is the main cause of chronic pancreatitis in the United States. Protein and bicarbonate precipitate, forming plugs and stones in the presence of increased sphincter tone; this is probably the main pathogenetic mechanism. These events cause local inflammation with reactive fibrosis, obstruction, and destruction of the occluded lobules. This chronic, subclinical process then leads to irreversible structural damage to the pancreas. Histologically, predominant fibrosis can be observed with small discrete areas of acute pancreatitis. Calcification of protein plugs and stones occurs in alcoholic pancreatitis, in some cases of hereditary pancreatitis, and in calcific pancreatitis of the tropics, a disease of unknown cause. Chronic pancreatitis can develop after recurrent bouts of acute pancreatitis from any cause. Cystic fibrosis, hyperparathyroidism, and perhaps pancreas divisum represent other risk factors. The pathophysiology of hereditary pancreatitis, an autosomal dominant disease, remains unknown.

Clinical Manifestations

Patients with chronic pancreatitis can present with chronic pain, recurrent acute attacks, or clinical sequelae of impaired pancreatic function and mechanical complications. Chronic abdominal pain radiating to the back and reduced by leaning forward is a common presentation. This pain often becomes severe and unremitting, frequently requiring narcotics for adequate control. Exocrine insufficiency is manifested clinically by chronic diarrhea with steatorrhea, weight loss, and malabsorption; this syndrome typically occurs after the loss of more than 90 per cent of pancreatic function. Endocrine insufficiency may result from islet cell destruction by the fibrotic process, leading to brittle diabetes. Acute clinical attacks can be superimposed on the chronic process, usually when obstruction of the main pancreatic duct becomes complete. This complication can cause increased pain, pseudocyst formation with rupture or infection, and fistula formation. Obstructive jaundice occurs with entrapment of the intrapancreatic common bile duct in fibrosing and contracting pancreatic tissue. Duodenal obstruction can result from a similar process. Bleeding from a peripancreatic source, such as a splenic artery aneurysm or a pseudocyst wall, can be channeled into the intestine via the pancreatic duct, causing massive gastrointestinal hemorrhage. The diagnosis may be challenging and may require a multimodality approach. Gastric varices induced by splenic vein thrombosis can be diagnosed by endoscopy or angiography.

Laboratory Tests and Pancreatic Function Studies

Measurement of serum amylase activity in chronic pancreatitis usually adds little to clinical management unless the patient complains of new pain or a different pattern of pain. The increases are usually modest, but persistent when superimposing obstruction occurs. The most reliable study of pancreatic exocrine function is the secretin test, but it is rarely used because it requires intubation of the duodenum. Bicarbonate concentrations are measured in the pancreatic secretions collected after stimulation with intravenous secretin. The bentiromide test is a noninvasive screening test of pancreatic insufficiency based on the hydrolysis of a synthetic peptide linked to para-aminobenzoic acid (PABA) by chymotrypsin. Renal excretion of the liberated para-aminobenzoic acid is measured in the urine. The sensitivity of this test is low in early disease, and it requires good intestinal absorption, renal function, and diuresis. Fecal fat analysis measures fat excretion in stool and cannot distinguish between small bowel disease and pancreatic insufficiency.

Imaging Studies

Plain films and CT of the abdomen are useful for visualizing calcifications of the pancreatic ducts. Transabdominal ultrasonography can also provide information regarding dilatation of ducts, fluid collections, and gallstones. Abnormalities such as a dilatated main pancreatic duct, pseudocysts, biliary dilatation, pleural effusions, ascites, and splenic vein thrombosis can be detected with a single CT study and easily compared with prior or subsequent studies. Endoscopic ultrasonography is used in some centers to distinguish between fibrosis and tumors. Fibrosis has increased echogenicity, whereas tumors are usually hypoechogenic. The gold standard for anatomic delineation of the pancreatic duct is ERCP, which is used to assess irregularities of main duct and secondary ductules, to detect strictures and stones, to allow tissue sampling for malignancy, and to provide therapeutic intervention when appropriate.

PANCREATIC CYSTS AND NEOPLASMS

By Virginia Rhodes, M.D.,
and Richard Pazdur, M.D.
Houston, Texas

The differential diagnosis of space-occupying lesions of the pancreas poses a difficult challenge to the physician because these defects vary in terms of etiology, clinical presentation, and malignant potential. Pancreatic lesions are of two main types: cystic lesions and neoplasms (or solid tumors). The most common pancreatic cystic lesions include postinflammatory lesions and cystic neoplasms. Among the pancreatic neoplasms, ductal adenocarcinomas (nonendocrine) are the most common type. Other pancreatic neoplasms include islet cell (endocrine) tumors and lymphomas. The advent of new diagnostic techniques, including radiolabeled octreotide imaging and high-resolution computed tomography (CT) scanning, has improved the ability to distinguish these lesions and localize them by noninvasive means. Endocrine tumors, for example, are often easy to diagnose because they present with characteristic syndromes; the diagnostic challenge arises in localization of these often small tumors.

CYSTIC LESIONS

Pancreatic cystic lesions encompass a diverse group of disorders, each with its own pathogenesis and natural history. These lesions may be classified into five groups: postinflammatory cystic lesions, cystic neoplasms, congenital true cysts, parasitic cysts, and extrapancreatic cystic disorders that mimic true pancreatic cystic lesions.

Postinflammatory Cystic Lesions

Postinflammatory lesions, with a cystic cavity that lacks an epithelial lining, account for 70 to 75 per cent of all cystic lesions and are thus the most common type. Included in this group of lesions are (1) pancreatic pseudocysts (the most frequently occurring of the postinflammatory lesions), which are fluid collections of pancreatic exocrine secretions arising from pancreatic ductal disruption; (2) pancreatic sequestra, which are areas of pancreatic or peripancreatic (fat) necrosis that have undergone cystic degeneration, may or may not have a ductal communication, and are characterized by the presence of necrotic material within the fluid collection; and (3) lesions that mimic pseudocysts and are made up of inflammatory collections of serous fluid that do not communicate with the pancreatic ductal system.

The causes of cystic lesions include pancreatitis of all causes, pancreatic necrosis, trauma, ischemia, vasculitis, drug-induced injury, and neoplastic obstruction of the pancreatic duct. Pancreatic pseudocysts may arise within the pancreas or in one of the potential spaces that separate the pancreas from adjacent viscera. Rarely, pseudocysts may arise in the mediastinum by dissecting through the esophageal or aortic hiatus of the diaphragm or in the inguinal canal by traversing the pericolic gutter. Five to 15 per cent of patients with pancreatic pseudocysts have multicentric lesions.

Pancreatic pseudocysts occur in 5 to 15 per cent of patients with acute pancreatitis. Most lesions have a defined fibrous wall that usually requires several weeks to develop. However, lesions that do not communicate with the ductal system and that contain only serous fluid lack a well-defined fibrous wall and occur early in the history of acute pancreatitis. Such early lesions occur in 30 to 50 per cent of patients with acute pancreatitis.

The most common presenting symptom in patients with pancreatic pseudocysts is persistent or recurrent upper abdominal pain (seen in 90 per cent of patients). Other symptoms include nausea and vomiting (70 per cent of patients), weight loss (35 per cent of patients), jaundice (10 to 15 per cent of patients), fever (5 to 20 per cent of patients), early satiety, and symptoms of gastroduodenal obstruction. Less frequently, patients can present with sepsis, variceal bleeding from splenic or portal vein obstruction, pruritus from common bile duct obstruction, or abdominal hemorrhage. Physical examination typically reveals upper abdominal tenderness, but a palpable mass is detected in only 25 to 40 per cent of patients with pseudocyts.

Laboratory findings in patients with pancreatic pseudocysts are usually nonspecific. Sixty to 70 per cent of patients have increased serum amylase activity; fewer (20 to 57 per cent) have liver function abnormalities. Other findings include mild leukocytosis (in 8 to 70 per cent of patients), hypoalbuminemia, and mild anemia.

The diagnostic imaging modality of choice is CT scanning of the abdomen, with sensitivity and specificity rates approaching 100 per cent and an overall accuracy rate greater than 90 per cent. CT allows evaluation of the entire pancreas and provides information about other abdominal conditions, such as biliary occlusion. Ultrasound is a less accurate diagnostic method (sensitivity, 88 to 100 per cent; specificity, 92 per cent; overall accuracy, 87 per cent), and its results can be difficult to interpret as a result of overlying bowel gas; however, ultrasound is recommended as a follow-up procedure for patients who are known to have pseudocysts. Magnetic resonance imaging provides a diagnostic accuracy similar to that of CT but has no distinct advantage over CT. Endoscopic retrograde cholangiopancreatography (ERCP) is a safe technique in patients with pseudocysts and can define ductal abnormalities in that population; ERCP findings are abnormal in 50 to 95 per cent of patients with pseudocysts. It is most useful for planning appropriate interventions rather than for making the initial diagnosis.

Patients with lesions for which imaging results are equivocal may benefit from analysis of cystic fluid aspirate. Analysis of fluid and cytologic specimens using the tumor markers carcinoembryonic antigen (CEA) and CA-125 has proved valuable for detecting malignant lesions, whereas the use of CA 19-9 has been nondiagnostic. Results of cystic fluid amylase and lipase determinations are variable but can generally discriminate pseudocysts from cystic neoplasms. Amylase activity in pseudocysts can vary from 50 to greater than 2 million U/L, with median values between 500 and 20,000 U/L. Cytologic analysis is also beneficial, with the presence of epithelial elements suggesting malignancy.

The clinical course of pseudocysts varies with the size of the cyst, the intensity of symptoms, and the development of complications. The use of CT imaging has allowed better selection of patients whose lesions can be managed expectantly; approximately 20 to 50 per cent of pseudocysts resolve spontaneously. Factors that predict a lesion that will not resolve in this manner include pseudocyst size, chronicity, multiplicity, and traumatic origin.

Complications of pancreatic pseudocysts include infection, hemorrhage, obstruction, and rupture. The incidence of all complications increases from the time of diagnosis. Although past series have reported the incidence of infection to be as high as 20 per cent, recent series have reported incidences in the range of 5 per cent. Pseudocysts may become contaminated or colonized with bacteria and should be distinguished from true infected pseudocysts that contain purulent material (abscesses). Aspiration and culture are the diagnostic procedures of choice for evaluation of infection.

Arterial hemorrhage, reported in 7 per cent of patients

with pseudocysts, results from erosion of the cyst into major vessels and has a mortality rate approaching 50 per cent. Patients present with an abrupt onset of abdominal pain and hypovolemia. This complication is observed most commonly in patients with alcoholic pancreatitis. In cases of arterial hemorrhage, arteriography can be both diagnostic and therapeutic using selective embolization. Contrast-enhanced dynamic CT scanning can also localize the bleeding site.

Enlarging pseudocysts may cause mechanical obstruction of the duodenum, stomach, jejunum, colon, esophagus, or urinary tract. Pseudocysts may also externally compress the portal system or the vena cava, resulting in portal hypertension or edema of the lower extremities.

Spontaneous rupture can occur in 3 per cent of patients with pseudocysts. Some patients may be asymptomatic, and pancreatic ascites or pleural effusions may subsequently develop. In other patients, severe abdominal pain or other symptoms mimicking an acute surgical abdomen can develop. Spontaneous rupture must be distinguished from intracystic hemorrhage as a cause of acute abdominal pain; this is accomplished by appropriate abdominal imaging. The diagnosis of pancreatic ascites or pleural effusions requires demonstration of increased protein concentrations and amylase activity in the cystic fluid; diagnostically indicative amylase concentrations frequently exceed 1000 U/L and protein concentrations exceed 3.0 g/dL.

Cystic Neoplasms

Primary cystic neoplasms represent the second most common cystic disorder of the pancreas, accounting for 5 to 15 per cent of pancreatic cystic lesions. However, these neoplasms represent fewer than 5 per cent of all pancreatic tumors and only 1 per cent of all pancreatic malignancies. Cystic neoplasms are rare and arise from serous or mucinous cells of the pancreatic ducts. (Several other malignancies that can also present as slow-growing cystic lesions include acinar cell cystadenocarcinoma, cystic choriocarcinoma, cystic teratoma, papillary-cystic neoplasms, and angiomatous neoplasms.)

Serous cystadenomas arise from the centroacinar cell and are usually benign. They are characterized on CT by a microcystic (cysts <2 cm in diameter) and honeycomb appearance. These tumors have a vascular stroma that may be calcified, resulting in a central stellate scar seen on CT in up to 38 per cent of patients. Serous cystadenomas, which have a predilection for the head of the pancreas, are usually asymptomatic. The cystic fluid aspirate may contain CEA or mucin. Malignant transformation is rare, with only four cases reported in the literature.

In contrast, mucinous cystic neoplasms have greater malignant potential. Located within the tail or body of the pancreas, these are macrocystic lesions with cysts greater than 2 cm in diameter. Mucinous cystic neoplasms demonstrate patchy peripheral or eggshell calcification on CT in 16 per cent of patients. These tumors can be mistaken for pseudocysts on CT, a misdiagnosis that can delay appropriate therapy. The epithelium of mucinous neoplasms is often discontinuous and variable in appearance (columnar or cuboidal to flat); thus, random biopsies of the cyst wall may fail to yield the correct diagnosis. Complete evaluation must involve multiple biopsies from different areas of the cyst wall; this is best accomplished with an open surgical procedure.

Patients likely to have pancreatic cystic neoplasms include older individuals (over 50 years), nonalcoholic patients, women, patients without a history of pancreatitis or abdominal trauma, patients with recurrent pseudocysts after surgery, or patients in whom CT or ultrasound demonstrates a mixed solid and cystic mass. The clinical presentation involves signs and symptoms related to the mass effect of the lesion. Importantly, patients lack symptoms of jaundice, weight loss, malaise, fatigue, and pain characteristic of ductal cancer of the pancreas.

Computed tomography and ultrasound are reliable for distinguishing serous from mucinous cystadenomas, but these methods are less reliable for distinguishing cystadenomas from complex pancreatic pseudocysts, cystic islet neoplasms, or other cystic neoplasms. Computed tomography is also unreliable for distinguishing mucinous cystadenomas from their overtly malignant mucinous cystadenocarcinoma counterparts. Other imaging modalities do not provide additional discriminatory value. ERCP may be useful for demonstrating ductal involvement that is characteristic of pseudocysts, but not of cystic neoplasms. Percutaneous aspiration of cystic fluid can distinguish cystic neoplasms from pseudocysts by demonstrating increased amylase activity and the absence of mucin, CEA, and CA 19-9 in the latter.

Mucinous ductectatic cystadenoma, a cystic lesion usually located in the uncinate process of the pancreas, represents a cystic dilatation of a side branch of the pancreatic duct that contains mucinous secretions. The diagnostic test of choice for this lesion is ERCP, which demonstrates the abnormality of the pancreatic duct with filling defects representing the mucinous secretions.

True Cysts

True epithelial-lined cysts of the pancreas are unusual; they may be congenital or may be seen as part of the spectrum of hereditary disorders such as polycystic liver, kidney, or pancreas disease; cystic fibrosis; or von Hippel-Lindau disease. These lesions usually require no treatment, but sometimes they require biopsy or excision to distinguish them from mucinous cystadenomas.

Retention cysts are enlargements of pancreatic ducts that arise from obstructive processes such as chronic pancreatitis, pancreatic duct stones, or pancreatic duct strictures. Retention cysts, which are usually smaller than pseudocysts, rarely exceed 5 cm in diameter. Patients with retention cysts may be asymptomatic or may have chronic pain suggestive of chronic pancreatitis. Symptoms of nausea, vomiting, early satiety, and obstruction occur less frequently than with pseudocysts. Palpable masses are rarely detected in these lesions, which have a longer natural history (often exceeding 6 months) than do pseudocysts. Congenital pancreatic cysts may be single or multiple and unilocular or multilocular. These cysts are usually located in the body or tail of the pancreas and are rarely symptomatic.

Von Hippel-Lindau disease is an autosomal dominant inherited disease characterized by cerebellar, spinal, medullary, or cerebral hemangioblastomas; retinal hemangioblastomas; multiple renal cysts (59 per cent of patients) or renal adenocarcinoma; cysts of the liver (17 per cent of patients), spleen (7 per cent of patients), or lung (3 per cent of patients); pancreatic cysts, cystadenocarcinoma, or islet cell tumors; pheochromocytoma; or epididymal cystadenomas. Diagnosis requires a specific lesion in at least one of these areas in a family in which at least one relative has a central nervous system or eye lesion, renal cyst, or adenocarcinoma. Screening tests should be performed in all family members and should include ophthalmologic evaluation, with fluorescein angiography of suspicious lesions; measurement of urinary catecholamine and metanephrine concentrations; CT or ultrasound scan of the abdomen; magnetic resonance imaging or CT scan of the brain; and chromosome studies.

Another true epithelial cystic lesion of the pancreas is the recently described lymphoepithelial cyst. Histologically, these lesions resemble branchial cleft cysts and are lined by stratified squamous epithelium with dense lymphoid tissue in the walls. Lymphoepithelial cysts have also been described in the parotid and thyroid glands. Percutaneous needle aspiration can correctly identify this lesion as a true cyst.

Parasitic Cysts

Parasitic cysts, composed of organisms such as *Echinococcus* or *Taenia solium*, must be included in the differential diagnosis of cystic lesions if the patient resides in or has visited a geographic region where these organisms are endemic. Multiple internal septations and occasional calcification are characteristic findings on CT. Parasitic cysts are typically seen in association with hydatid disease of the liver.

Extrapancreatic Cystic Disorders

Extrapancreatic cystic lesions that mimic pancreatic lesions may arise from retroperitoneal structures proximal to the pancreas. These lesions arise from the left adrenal gland, spleen, mesentery, or retroperitoneum and may be difficult to distinguish from cystic neoplasms. Extrapancreatic cysts may require intervention for diagnosis or for treatment if excessive size and/or symptoms develop.

NEOPLASMS (SOLID TUMORS)

Nonendocrine Epithelial Tumors

Adenocarcinomas of ductal origin account for 75 to 90 per cent of all solid pancreatic cancers and are the fourth most common cause of deaths from cancer in the United States. An increased incidence of pancreatic adenocarcinoma exists in patients who smoke, in patients who have had a gastrectomy previously, and, possibly, in those who have a history of chronic pancreatitis.

The clinical features of pancreatic cancer are nonspecific and insidious. Symptoms usually precede the diagnosis by 3 to 6 months. Weight loss (in 90 to 100 per cent of patients), epigastric or back pain (66 per cent of patients), and jaundice (75 per cent of patients) are the usual presenting symptoms. Pruritus may accompany the jaundice. Less frequent symptoms include nausea, vomiting, diarrhea, anorexia, acute pancreatitis, or gastrointestinal bleeding. In 10 to 15 per cent of patients, glucose intolerance may herald the diagnosis of pancreatic cancer.

Jaundice is the most common physical finding. A palpable distended gallbladder (Courvoisier's sign) suggests malignant obstruction of the common bile duct and may be present in 25 per cent of patients. Patients with advanced disease may present with ascites, cervical adenopathy (Virchow's node), or a periumbilical mass (Sister Mary Joseph nodule).

Laboratory studies in patients with pancreatic adenocarcinoma characteristically reveal evidence of extrahepatic obstructive jaundice, with increased bilirubin and alkaline phosphatase and mildly increased aminotransferase in the serum. Mild anemia, coagulopathy, or pancreatic endocrine and exocrine insufficiency may also be present. The tumor markers CEA and alpha-fetoprotein are not useful in confirming the diagnosis of pancreatic cancer due to low sensitivity and cross-reactivity with other tumors. New tests for mucin antigens such as CA 19-9, although not exclusive to pancreatic cancer, have a sensitivity and specificity approaching 85 per cent. However, no tumor markers are sufficiently sensitive or specific to serve as screening tests.

Computed tomography of the abdomen is the diagnostic imaging modality of choice for a jaundiced patient with a suspected pancreatic malignancy; this method is as effective as ultrasonography in defining biliary structures and is superior in defining small tumors, peripancreatic nodal involvement, and small metastases (accuracy of CT is 96 per cent versus 84 per cent for ultrasonography). Dynamic CT with contrast injection can also assess vascular involvement. Magnetic resonance imaging provides no additional benefit despite its increased cost.

When a CT scan demonstrates biliary obstruction, ERCP may be used to distinguish tumors of the pancreaticobiliary junction and to obtain a tissue diagnosis from brushings or washings of the pancreatic duct. Although the ultimate role of endoscopic ultrasonography is yet to be defined, this method is used increasingly to detect small tumors and to aid in tumor staging because it allows assessment of portal vein involvement. The use of angiography to delineate vascular anatomy and invasion is controversial and should be reserved for selected patients. It has little role in the routine preoperative evaluation of patients with pancreatic cancer.

Because percutaneous fine-needle biopsy has been demonstrated to result in seeding along the needle tract and has increased the rates of intraperitoneal spread of disease, this method (sensitivity 57 to 96 per cent) is recommended routinely only for patients who are not operative candidates or in situations in which histologic confirmation of malignancy is required before nonsurgical palliative therapy is initiated. All operative candidates should undergo surgery for tissue diagnosis and definitive therapy.

In pancreatic cancer patients treated with the Whipple procedure with preservation of the tail of the pancreas (10 per cent of patients), postoperative complications include anastomotic leaks, the dumping syndrome, and pancreatic exocrine or endocrine insufficiency. Complications in patients with unresectable disease (90 per cent) include obstructive jaundice, pain, and duodenal obstruction; both operative and nonoperative techniques exist for palliation. Other pancreatic ductal tumors include a mucin-producing tumor (noncystic) and intraductal papillary tumors, which are low-grade, slow-growing malignancies. These tumors secrete mucin, which can cause ductal occlusion and result in chronic pancreatitis, leading patients to seek medical attention. Rare squamous cell carcinomas and mixed adenosquamous carcinomas that behave clinically like ductal adenocarcinomas also have been reported.

Nonductal pancreatic tumors include acinar cell carcinoma and pancreaticoblastoma; they are characterized by immunocytochemical demonstration of pancreatic enzymes and by the absence of CEA and CA 19-9. The acinar tumors release lipase, which can cause disseminated subcutaneous fat necrosis, polyarthralgia, and peripheral blood eosinophilia. Pancreaticoblastoma is a tumor that may produce alpha-fetoprotein and is seen in children younger than 7 years of age.

Endocrine Tumors (Islet Cell Tumors)

Neoplasms that produce gastrointestinal regulatory peptides can be found throughout the gastroenteropancreatic axis, but the majority are located within the pancreas. Most of these tumors are malignant and may be either functional or nonfunctional. Functional tumors present as distinct clinical syndromes resulting from hypersecretion of peptides. Immunoreactive assays have allowed early detection and treatment of these lesions.

These tumors tend to be slowly growing but they can metastasize. Histologic characteristics do not readily separate malignant lesions from benign ones, and the only reliable indicator of malignancy is the presence of metastases. Pancreatic endocrine tumors may be either sporadic or familial. The familial syndrome is well described as multiple endocrine neoplasia type I (MEN I), including pancreatic islet cell tumors, parathyroid tumors, and pituitary tumors.

The recommended sequence of imaging studies for tumor localization is an initial CT scan and selective angiography. If no tumor is found, selective venous sampling (success rate of 84 per cent) should be performed. Tumors that are still not detected should be subjected to operative exploration and intraoperative ultrasound. Iodine-labeled octreotide binds to somatostatin receptors on islet cell tumors; this technique has been used with increasing success to localize tumors. Recent studies have reported localization of primary tumors and previously unrecognized metastases in 80 to 86 per cent of patients with endocrine tumors. A positive octreotide scan also predicts a favorable response to octreotide therapy. Five major tumors of the pancreatic islets have characteristic clinical syndromes based on the predominant secreted peptide: (1) insulinoma, (2) glucagonoma, (3) somatostatinoma, (4) gastrinoma, and (5) VIPoma.

Insulinoma

Insulinomas are the most prevalent functioning endocrine tumors; in contrast to the other tumor types, 80 to 90 per cent of insulinomas are benign adenomas. Multiple tumors occur in 10 per cent of patients and are usually associated with the MEN I syndrome. Clinically, patients present with a long history of periodic attacks of hypoglycemia that become more frequent and more severe with time. Symptoms of hypoglycemia typically occur at night or in the early morning before breakfast and are provoked by fasting or exercise. Common symptoms include headache, confusion, blurred vision, drowsiness, sweating, trembling, weakness, palpitations, and irritability. Some of the symptoms can be life-threatening. The diagnosis is established by the demonstration of hypoglycemia in the presence of an inappropriately increased insulin concentration in plasma during prolonged fasting. Insulinoma is strongly suggested if hypoglycemia is associated with a plasma insulin concentration of greater than 15 mU/L. Most patients experience hypoglycemia (<40 mg/dL) in 24 to 36 hours. The diagnosis is also established by demonstrating an inappropriately high ratio (>0.3) of plasma insulin (mU/L) to plasma glucose (mg/dL) during fasting. Patients with insulinoma also demonstrate increased proinsulin concentrations. Because of the reliability of fasting determinations, provocative tests to stimulate insulin release with tolbutamide, calcium, glucagon, and L-leucine are no longer recommended. In patients who fail to demonstrate hypoglycemia with fasting, disease can be assessed with insulin or C peptide suppression tests.

The differential diagnosis of insulinoma-induced hypoglycemia includes factitious hypoglycemia caused by insulin or sulfonylurea abuse, extrapancreatic tumors, B-cell hyperplasia (nesidioblastosis), hypopituitarism, Addison's disease, alcohol-induced hypoglycemia, liver disease, or autoantibodies to insulin or insulin receptors. Diagnostic testing can readily exclude the possibility of these conditions.

Glucagonoma

The glucagonoma syndrome is characterized by dermatitis, diabetes mellitus, weight loss, anemia, hyperglucagonemia, and an A (alpha) cell tumor of the pancreas. The majority of these tumors are malignant (60 to 80 per cent). The skin rash, necrolytic migratory erythema, occurs in approximately 70 per cent of patients and is characterized by remissions and exacerbations. Skin lesions initially appear as a red papule or pale brown macule on the face, abdomen, groin, perineum, or extremities. The lesions then become bullous and heal with residual brown pigmentation in a confluent manner.

Other features of the syndrome include painful glossitis, angular stomatitis, weight loss, mild diabetes, anemia, psychiatric disorders, hypoaminoacidemia, and thromboembolic problems. Intermittent diarrhea, ileus, and constipation occur in some patients. Venous thrombosis and pulmonary emboli occur in up to 30 per cent of patients.

The differential diagnosis of glucagonoma includes renal failure, hepatic insufficiency, and familial hyperglucagonemia. However, these conditions all lack the skin rash of glucagonoma. Diagnosis requires the demonstration of increased concentrations of glucagon (>1000 pg/mL or 10 to 20 times the upper limit of the reference range). Provocative or inhibitory tests are rarely required when increased serum glucagon concentration is documented.

Somatostatinoma

Somatostatinomas may be found in either the gut or the pancreas. The majority of patients who have this tumor in the pancreas are symptomatic, whereas those with gut tumors tend to be asymptomatic. Somatostatinomas are highly metastatic and virulent. Clinical features of the syndrome include diabetes mellitus, gallbladder disease, diarrhea, steatorrhea, hypochlorhydria, and weight loss. These symptoms are due to the inhibitory action of somatostatin.

Diagnosis requires demonstration of increased somatostatin concentrations in plasma or tissue and identification of D (delta) cells in tumor tissue by immunocytochemical studies. Because plasma somatostatin concentrations are often nearly normal, provocative testing with tolbutamide can be used to demonstrate an increase.

Gastrinoma

Gastrinoma, which is metastatic in 50 to 60 per cent of patients at diagnosis, is the second most commonly diagnosed type of pancreatic islet cell tumor. The Zollinger-Ellison syndrome of gastric acid hypersecretion with fulminant peptic ulcer disease is characteristically found in patients with gastrinomas. Ninety per cent of patients experience epigastric pain. Up to one third of patients also have severe diarrhea. The duration of the symptoms may be months to years.

The diagnosis of gastrinoma is established by gastric acid analysis and determination of fasting serum gastrin concentrations by radioimmunoassay. The diagnosis is suggested by a basal acid output greater than 15 mEq per hour and by hypergastrinemia (>200 pg/mL). Regardless of the serum gastrin concentration, the diagnosis must be confirmed by provocative testing with secretin (2 U/kg as an intravenous bolus), which will increase the fasting serum gastrin in gastrinoma patients to more than 200 pg/

mL (or a 100 per cent increase in serum gastrin concentrations) within 5 to 10 minutes. Intra-arterial injection of secretin may also be helpful in localizing these tumors by identifying which of the three feeding arteries to the pancreas supplies the tumor.

VIPoma

VIPomas are tumors of immature endocrine cells of the pancreas that produce vasoactive intestinal peptide (VIP). They are malignant in 50 to 80 per cent of cases. The watery diarrhea–hypokalemia-achlorhydria (WDHA) syndrome (also known as pancreatic cholera or the Verner-Morrison syndrome) is characteristic of VIPoma. Since concentrations of other peptides are often increased in the plasma of patients with the watery diarrhea–hypokalemia-achlorhydria syndrome, the role of VIP as the sole cause of the diarrhea in these patients is less well established.

Patients present with large-volume secretory diarrhea exceeding 3 L per day. The stool is isotonic, and the diarrhea persists during fasting or nasogastric suctioning. Laboratory studies reveal hypokalemia and acidosis, with large losses of potassium and bicarbonate in the stool. Achlorhydria or hypochlorhydria is observed in all patients, and 50 per cent of individuals have hypercalcemia or glucose intolerance. Physical examination may reveal flushing. The differential diagnosis includes islet cell hyperplasia; catecholamine-producing lesions such as ganglioneuroma, neuroblastoma, or pheochromocytoma; neurofibromatosis; and laxative abuse.

Provocative or inhibitory studies to confirm the diagnosis of VIPoma do not exist. The VIP concentrations are increased in the majority, but not all, patients. Diagnosis rests on the clinical presentation of diarrhea with large stool volumes, isotonic stool, persistence of diarrhea during fasting, and achlorhydria.

Other Tumors

Other uncommon pancreatic endocrine tumors include neurotensinoma, pancreatic polypeptidoma, atypical carcinoid tumors, and tumors that produce ectopic adrenocorticotropic hormone, growth hormone or growth hormone–releasing factor, or parathyroid hormone. These tumors have in common an increased frequency of malignancy (90 to 100 per cent).

Multiple Endocrine Neoplasia Type I

The MEN syndromes are disorders characterized by familial autosomal dominant inheritance of specific endocrine tumors. MEN I (Werner's syndrome) consists of parathyroid hyperplasia, pituitary tumors, and pancreatic islet cell tumors. The most common manifestation of MEN I is primary hyperparathyroidism with hypercalcemia (in 95 per cent of cases). The parathyroid glands are usually hyperplastic rather than neoplastic. Pituitary tumors are the least commonly observed tumors in 30 per cent of patients. The tumors can produce prolactin, corticotropin, or growth hormone or they may be nonfunctional.

Pancreatic endocrine tumors occur in approximately two thirds of patients with the MEN I syndrome. Gastrinomas are the most frequently reported tumor type (67 per cent of patients) followed by glucagonoma (11 per cent of patients), insulinoma (9 per cent of patients), insulinoma and glucagonoma (6 per cent of patients), and undefined tumors (6 per cent of patients). VIPomas are rare. Pancreatic neoplasms are symptomatic in 50 per cent of patients. Multiple pancreatic tumors can occur, and tumors can express multiple peptides. Clinical syndromes observed are those caused by the polypeptides produced; the Zollinger-Ellison syndrome is the most frequently observed syndrome.

Clinical diagnosis of MEN I in the index patient of the cohort requires recognition of at least two lesions associated with the syndrome. Recognition of any single lesion is diagnostic in family members. Screening studies should include measurement of parathyroid hormone, serum calcium, prolactin, somatomedin C, blood glucose, insulin, proinsulin, pancreatic polypeptide, glucagon, and gastrin concentrations. The localization of the causative gene to chromosome 11q13 and the identification of allelic loss at chromosome 11 have made it possible to screen family members and identify gene carriers by restriction fragment-length polymorphism.

Lymphoma

Lymphomas of the pancreas are rare and account for less than 0.2 per cent of pancreatic malignancies. The incidence of pancreatic involvement is highest in large cell lymphoma and nonendemic Burkitt's lymphoma. It is often difficult to distinguish peripancreatic nodal disease from intrinsic pancreatic lymphoma due to the absence of a capsule around the pancreas.

The clinical presentation resembles that of pancreatic ductal carcinoma, with pain, weight loss, jaundice, and nausea and vomiting. It is not possible to distinguish lymphoma from pancreatic adenocarcinoma with the use of clinical and radiographic techniques; such distinction requires histologic diagnosis of percutaneous or surgical biopsy specimens. This distinction is crucial because lymphoma is much more responsive to therapy and generally has a better prognosis.

Tumors Metastatic to the Pancreas

Only 3 per cent of patients with advanced remote primary malignancies are reported to have metastases to the pancreas. Involvement is usually by direct extension from a contiguous organ or involved peripancreatic nodal group. Less frequently, spread is by the hematogenous route. Tumors that are most frequently metastatic to the pancreas include melanoma (37.5 per cent), breast carcinoma (19 per cent), and bronchogenic carcinoma (8.4 per cent). Other malignancies reported to metastasize to the pancreas include ovarian, prostatic, gastric, hepatocellular, colonic, esophageal, biliary, renal, and cervical carcinomas as well as various sarcomas.

HERNIAS OF THE ABDOMINAL WALL

By Lisa Chen, M.D.,
and Ronnie Ann Rosenthal, M.D.
New Haven, Connecticut

Abdominal wall hernia is a common surgical problem that is typically diagnosed by history and physical examination. Occasionally, however, the presence of the hernia or the nature of its contents may not be immediately apparent. Under these circumstances, additional diagnostic modalities must be employed. An accurate approach to the diagnosis of abdominal wall hernia depends on a thorough understanding of the definitions and epidemiology of each of the various types of hernia.

An abdominal wall hernia is defined as a defect in the abdominal wall through which intra-abdominal contents may protrude. Such hernias are usually identified according to location and are classified as either congenital (resulting from a developmental abnormality) or acquired (resulting from increased intra-abdominal pressure). Hernias also can be defined based on the characteristics of the contents of the hernial sac. Reducible hernias are those in which the contents move freely in and out of the defect, whereas incarcerated hernias are those in which the contents become trapped, usually by the fibrotic neck of the hernial sac. Although some incarcerated hernias can exist without sequelae for years, most progress rapidly to cause compromise of the blood supply to the incarcerated organ. A hernia in which the blood supply of the contents is impaired is referred to as strangulated. An incarcerated hernia containing bowel most often involves the entire bowel circumference, and intestinal obstruction is the obvious sequela. In Richter's hernia, however, only one wall of a bowel loop becomes incarcerated. Strangulation, therefore, often results without signs of obstruction, thereby making Richter's hernia particularly hazardous.

On occasion, a portion of an abdominal organ may comprise the posterior wall of the actual hernia sac in the inguinal canal. This type of hernia is referred to as a sliding hernia. The organs typically involved are the ovary in female infants and the sigmoid colon in adults. Although sliding hernias are frequently associated with significant bowel dysfunction, particularly in older men, they rarely become incarcerated.

Hernia repair is historically the most common general surgical procedure in the United States, the majority being performed for inguinal hernia. Herniation into the inguinal canal occurs four to eight times more commonly in men than in women. In infants and young persons, greater than 90 per cent of inguinal hernias are congenital or indirect. These hernias result from failure of fusion of the processus vaginalis. With increasing age, the incidence of acquired inguinal hernias increases so that 35 per cent of hernias in men older than 65 years of age are direct, resulting from an acquired defect in the transversalis fascia that constitutes the floor of the inguinal canal.

Hernias through the femoral canal are less common than inguinal hernias in both genders but are more common in women than in men. They are often difficult to diagnose because the groin pain they produce tends to be poorly localized. In addition, the hernial mass, typically located inferior to the inguinal ligament, is frequently too small to palpate. Often, the first sign of a femoral hernia is incarceration, and strangulation is 8 to 10 times more common than with an inguinal hernia. Approximately one quarter to one third of incarcerated femoral hernias are of the Richter's type, making the diagnosis even more difficult.

Umbilical hernia is the second most common congenital abdominal wall hernia, occurring in approximately 20 per cent of live births. In the United States, the incidence is eight times higher in African American infants than in white infants. Additional predisposing factors for umbilical hernia include prematurity and low birth weight. Herniation occurs through the patent umbilical ring, and although most resolve by 2 years of age, a small percentage persist into adulthood. Most umbilical hernias in adults are acquired, however. Incarceration rarely occurs in children, but in adults the risk is significant and repair is warranted.

Incisional hernia is the next most common acquired hernia. Disruption of a previous operative incision can result from several factors. When wound infections progress to fasciitis with muscle necrosis, subsequent dehiscence is common. Excessive tension on the repair also contributes to the pathogenesis of incisional hernia and can occur as a result of surgical technique or because of increased intra-abdominal pressure secondary to obesity, ascites, or prolonged ventilatory support. Factors that cause impairment of nutrition or metabolic functions, for example, steroid administration, also cause impaired wound healing. Recurrences after repair of an incisional hernia are common and usually occur as a result of persistent or recurrent wound infection, difficulty exposing sufficient intact fascia for closure, and closure under excessive tension. Other less common hernias include epigastric and linea alba, spigelian, lumbar, and obturator hernias. These hernias may be particularly challenging to diagnose and are given special consideration later in this article.

REDUCIBLE HERNIAS

Clinical Presentation

The clinical presentation of most uncomplicated abdominal wall hernias is clear. Although some hernias are asymptomatic, most patients have been aware of the bulge produced by protruding intra-abdominal contents for varying periods. It is not uncommon for patients to recall the specific incident that caused the bulge. Frequently, they can relate a history of a reducible bulge that recurs with coughing, heavy lifting, straining to defecate, or other maneuvers associated with increased intra-abdominal pressure. Herniation is often associated with some degree of pain or discomfort, and many patients wear a truss or limit their physical activity to avoid these symptoms.

A detailed history with special attention to pre-existing conditions that may cause increased intra-abdominal pressure is essential. These conditions include smoking, asthma, and chronic cough; chronic constipation or a change in bowel habits or stool caliber; urinary hesitancy, urgency, frequency, or change in stream; a history of alcoholism or liver disease; a recent increase in abdominal girth or unexplained weight loss; obesity; and pregnancy. Some clinicians advocate routine screening colonoscopy in all patients older than 55 years of age prior to elective hernia repair. Although the incidence of neoplastic lesions found on screening in this age group is *not* higher in patients with hernia than in those without, the 15 to 20 per cent incidence of abnormalities appears to justify the cost of screening.

Physical Examination

For uncomplicated hernias, vital signs should be within normal limits in the absence of concomitant disease processes. A complete physical examination should be conducted in a standard fashion. The abdomen is typically soft and nondistended, with normoactive bowel sounds. In addition, the abdominal examination should include a thorough search for predisposing factors for hernia development, such as obesity, previous surgical scars, intra-abdominal mass, and ascites. As always, a rectal examination should be performed to exclude a rectal mass, prostate enlargement, and occult blood.

The examiner should then look specifically for a hernia by trying to find a visible bulge or palpable defect. At this point in the examination, the patient should be relaxed. Physical findings may vary, depending on the contents of the hernial sac. A sac containing omentum may present an ill-defined mass, whereas a sac containing bowel is soft and deformable and perhaps crepitant if the loop of bowel contains gas. A herniated solid organ is palpable as a firmer, movable mass with more definite borders. Gentle reduction of the herniated mass can be attempted at this time but should be abandoned once resistance is met.

Next, the examination should be repeated in the presence of increased intra-abdominal pressure. In the supine position, a cough increases intra-abdominal pressure transiently. Sustained increased intra-abdominal pressure, however, is often more effective for eliciting herniation. The patient can achieve this by straining during a Valsalva maneuver or by lifting the head and shoulders off the bed, thus contracting the abdominal muscles. In the erect position, intra-abdominal pressure is increased when the former maneuvers are repeated. Gravity also causes a slightly increased pressure of the intraperitoneal contents on the anterior abdominal wall.

For hernias of the groin, a bulge or defect is best palpated inside the inguinal canal. This can be achieved by inserting the index finger along the cord structures from the scrotum toward the external inguinal ring. When gentle pressure is applied so that the overlying skin and subcutaneous tissue is invaginated over the examiner's index finger into the canal, the hernia usually can be palpated accurately. By determining whether the hernia is medial or lateral to the inferior epigastric artery pulse, the examiner can attempt to determine whether the hernia is direct (medial) or indirect (lateral). This technique is sometimes misleading, however, because the hernial contents may track along a course within the superficial abdominal wall.

Femoral herniation typically occurs inferior to the inguinal ligament and medial to the femoral vessels. Although the hernial sac is often too small to palpate, occasionally these hernias can become large. Unfortunately, however, the sac of a large femoral hernia tends to protrude over the inguinal ligament and is commonly misdiagnosed as an inguinal hernia. The examination for a femoral hernia should begin with palpation of the groin below the inguinal ligament, just medial to the femoral pulse. When the patient is asked to cough, increased intra-abdominal pressure is transmitted into the sac, and the impulse produced is palpable over the hernial mass. Pressure transmitted into the femoral vein, however, can sometimes be misinterpreted as a hernia impulse in the absence of an actual hernia.

Laboratory Values

The diagnosis of uncomplicated hernia is usually clinical, made on the basis of a consistent history confirmed by physical examination. Laboratory values and plain films of the abdomen are typically within normal limits and are therefore of limited value.

Special Considerations

Not all reducible hernias are easy to diagnose, especially in certain subsets of the population. Hernias are common in children, and frequently an observant parent notices a lump that appears when the child cries. Unfortunately, the lump often disappears when the child stops crying, sometimes with no discernible or palpable abdominal wall defect.

Young athletic males frequently experience musculoskeletal groin pain that can be difficult to distinguish from pain caused by a hernia. The presence of well-developed musculature in the groin region also makes palpation of a defect difficult. Pain that is musculoskeletal usually worsens with manipulation of the affected joint, muscle, or bone. Therefore, testing whether certain movements reproducibly produce pain can help focus the differential diagnosis.

Elderly patients often have recurrent hernias, and blurring of the normal anatomy by previous surgical repairs and the presence of palpable scar obscures the diagnosis. When the diagnosis is unclear, other diagnostic modalities may be necessary. These are discussed later in this article.

INCARCERATED HERNIAS

Clinical Presentation

The particular course of any given hernia depends on several factors, including the size of the anatomic defect, the location of the hernia, and the lifestyle of the patient. Hernias with a narrow neck, characterized by a tight, constricting ring of tissue at the site of the defect, are more prone to incarceration, strangulation, and obstruction than are wide-necked hernias. Generally, the smaller the anatomic defect, the more likely the hernial contents are to become incarcerated and hence strangulated. Several types of hernias more commonly have narrow necks; incarceration is particularly common in men with indirect hernias and in women with femoral hernias. Some lifestyle factors, such as occupations that involve heavy lifting, increase the risk of protrusion of hernial contents and subsequent incarceration, strangulation, or obstruction.

Patients with incarcerated hernias frequently notice when a previously reducible lump is no longer freely movable. Pain that is usually transient in a reducible hernia becomes constant with incarceration and is often associated with significant tenderness. These patients often recall previous episodes of incarcerated hernia that resolved spontaneously.

Physical Examination

Early in the course, the physical examination is significant for normal temperature, blood pressure, and heart rate, although the latter can be slightly increased if the patient is uncomfortable or anxious. Generally, an irreducible lump is present, which may be tender to palpation. The mass does not exhibit transillumination but may contain bowel sounds. Laboratory values and plain films for a simple incarcerated hernia are typically within normal limits.

Clinical Course

Chronic Incarceration

Some incarcerated hernias resolve spontaneously or after manual reduction. Alternatively, hernias with wide necks, whose contents are fixed in the sac only by adhesions, often remain chronically incarcerated without progression of symptoms. Such hernias are often found incidentally or during autopsy.

Obstruction

An incarcerated hernia can cause closed-loop obstruction by compression of an edematous, herniated loop of bowel or volvulus around a fixed point. Conversely, in Richter's hernia, the intestinal lumen is preserved because only a part of the bowel circumference is involved, and patients typically present without obstruction.

Strangulation

Compromise of the blood supply to the contents of the hernial sac can occur either acutely or subacutely. Acute strangulation results from torsion of the hernial contents around their vascular pedicle; acute arterial obstruction subsequently progresses rapidly to tissue necrosis. More often, strangulation occurs more insidiously. The initial incarceration leads to mild venous and lymphatic outflow obstruction with resulting bowel wall edema. As obstruction progresses and luminal pressure increases, there is further compromise of venous outflow and increased edema in the tissues. Finally, when the interstitial fluid pressure exceeds arteriolar pressure, intestinal ischemia and bowel necrosis follow.

Physical examination is often significant for fever, hypotension, and tachycardia. Local cellulitis, characterized by erythema, and tenderness over the hernia are signs of bowel compromise. Abdominal tenderness and peritoneal signs are ominous indicators of bowel necrosis and possible perforation.

Laboratory Values

Once an incarcerated hernia has been diagnosed, the degree to which the bowel is acutely threatened usually can be ascertained on physical examination. In some cases, however, physical examination may be insufficient to distinguish uncomplicated incarceration from strangulation and intestinal ischemia. A straightforward method of detecting bowel ischemia would be invaluable in this circumstance.

Unfortunately, at this time, standard laboratory tests have been of extremely limited value. Although the leukocyte count and differential may reflect inflammation, and routine chemistry screening may reflect dehydration secondary to restriction of oral intake, third-space fluid sequestration, and emesis, these findings are completely nonspecific.

Many biochemical constituents have been evaluated in the search for a marker for intestinal ischemia, but unfortunately no clinically practical predictor of bowel compromise has been found. Studies with animal models have demonstrated increases in blood concentrations of serum urea nitrogen (SUN), phosphorus, aminotransferases, creatine kinase, hexosaminidase, porcine ileal peptide, and alkaline phosphatase and decreases in serum maltase concentrations associated with intestinal infarction. In addition, increased concentrations of diamine oxidase have been found in serum, lymph, and intestinal lumina of rats in a model of intestinal ischemia produced by superior mesenteric artery occlusion.

In humans, plasma malondialdehyde concentrations thought to represent a measure of lipid peroxidation were significantly increased in patients with strangulated obstruction when compared with simple obstruction alone. Other potential markers include lactate dehydrogenase (LD), amylase, oxidized glutathione, and D-lactate.

Although these indices reproducibly reflect varying degrees of intestinal ischemia, especially transmural necrosis, they universally lack specificity and early sensitivity for damage. Promising studies measuring intestinal fatty acid–binding protein (I-FABP), a normal constituent of small intestinal mucosa in humans and rats, have shown increased concentrations of I-FABP following ischemia and reperfusion in a rat model (as early as 15 minutes in serum and 60 minutes in urine). Thus, I-FABP appears to be a specific and sensitive marker of intestinal ischemia in rats. I-FABP is currently under study as a potential future marker for ischemia in humans.

Radiographic Findings

Plain films of the abdomen can be consistent with obstruction and localized inflammation, demonstrating distended loops of bowel with air-fluid levels and paucity of air in the large intestine. On rare occasions, free air can be visualized on a plain film after perforation has occurred, although the volume of intraperitoneal air is usually too small to be seen. Most commonly, plain films are unremarkable and thus may be misleading.

Special Considerations

Although the presentation of a strangulated hernia is usually dramatic, with most patients appearing quite ill, the diagnosis of strangulated hernia is not always straightforward, especially early in the pathophysiologic process. Compromised bowel may be difficult to identify on physical examination in elderly or immunocompromised patients who have an impaired immune response and therefore may not show the early signs of fever, localized erythema, and tenderness. Forced reduction of the hernial contents through the abdominal wall defect may result in “en masse” reduction of the compromised bowel, still within its constricting hernial sac, into the abdominal cavity. There, the ischemic process continues unrecognized until perforation, peritonitis, and sepsis develop. In these circumstances, forced reduction can have catastrophic consequences and should be avoided. In addition, these patients are often sicker than they appear initially, and delays in treatment are common. Such delays lead to bowel necrosis and perforation, necessitating bowel resection with its additional associated risks.

DIFFERENTIAL DIAGNOSIS

Although the diagnosis of hernia is generally straightforward, it is important to recognize that other conditions occasionally produce a similar defect or mass that may confuse the diagnosis.

Umbilical Defects

Omphalocele

In some neonates, spontaneous closure of the umbilical defect is incomplete. Although this developmental abnormality more frequently results in umbilical hernia, it can also lead to omphalocele so that the abdominal contents are covered only by peritoneum at the umbilicus. Careful visual inspection usually easily differentiates the two.

Persistent Omphalomesenteric Duct

The omphalomesenteric duct connects the small intestine to the yolk sac in the normal embryo. Occasionally, this vitelline duct is lined with bowel epithelium and, if it persists, can exist as a draining enterocutaneous fistula around which volvulus can occur, with subsequent obstruction. A history of antecedent drainage from the umbilicus usually distinguishes this condition from umbilical hernia.

Persistent Urachal Sinus

The urachal sinus, a tract from the umbilicus to the bladder, can also persist as a remnant of the cephalic portion of the embryonic bladder. Like the persistent omphalomesenteric duct, persistent urachal sinus usually differs from hernia in that it has a history of drainage.

Abdominal Wall Mass

Abscess

Although both abdominal wall abscess and hernia typically present with mass, tenderness, and fluctuance, it is generally easy to distinguish one from the other. Abdominal wall abscesses are relatively rare in the absence of preceding trauma, surgery, or a foreign body. They also typically cause fever, shaking chills, local tenderness, and erythema. Unlike hernia, the mass is not reducible and contains no bowel sounds, and there are no signs or symptoms of bowel obstruction. Occasionally, however, an abscess may be difficult to distinguish from a strangulated hernia, particularly in the groin area. In these cases, other diagnostic modalities may be necessary.

Benign Tumors

Lipoma is a common benign tumor that can arise at any position on the anterior abdominal wall. The mass of a lipoma differs from that of a hernia in that it is nontender, less fixed to adjacent structures, and relatively uniform on palpation. Other less common benign tumors of the abdominal wall include fibroma, hemangioma, neurofibroma, and the locally invasive desmoid tumor.

Malignant Tumors

Although primary malignancies, such as skin cancer and soft tissue sarcomas, can arise from the abdominal wall, metastatic nodules are the most common tumors of the anterior abdominal wall. Metastatic involvement of an umbilical lymph node, typically by pancreatic or gastric carcinoma, is classically known as a Sister Marie Joseph's nodule and is frequently misdiagnosed as an umbilical hernia. Factors distinguishing malignant masses from hernias include a history of malignancy, slow growth of the mass over time, the presence of multiple nodules, a firm consistency, and absence of pain or tenderness.

Rectus Sheath Hematoma

A hematoma can form in the rectus sheath as the result of bleeding from a ruptured epigastric artery or vein. Conditions that can cause this bleeding are varied and range from the minor strain of a cough or sneeze to seizure or direct trauma. Rectus sheath hematoma can occur spontaneously in patients who have undergone anticoagulation or who have other underlying conditions such as typhoid fever, collagen vascular diseases, blood dyscrasias, or pregnancy.

Although most rectus sheath hematomas are self-limited, presentation can be dramatic, and therefore they can be confused with almost every other cause of an acute abdomen, including incarcerated hernia. Typically, patients present with sharp pain that is severe, progressive, and localized. Often the pain is associated with anorexia, nausea, tachycardia, low-grade fever, and a mildly elevated white blood cell count. Emesis is rare. Physical examination can narrow the diagnosis, especially if the mass is still palpable when the rectus abdominis muscle is tensed (Fothergill's sign) and if the bluish tinge of the hematoma is visible. However, the majority of rectus hematomas are diagnosed correctly only with the aid of ultrasound or computed tomography (CT) on which the mass is seen to be limited to the rectus sheath.

Inguinal Mass

Lymphadenopathy

Inguinal and femoral lymphadenopathy in response to infection or malignancy may produce a palpable mass in the groin that is difficult to distinguish from a hernia. Features that are useful in differentiating enlarged lymph nodes from hernias include local infection or trauma in areas drained by these nodes, a history of malignancy, palpable lymph nodes in the contralateral groin, or fixation of the mass to adjacent tissues. Occasionally, a patient presents with a single, enlarged, tender lymph node that may be difficult to distinguish from an inguinal or femoral hernia without operative exploration.

Undescended Testis

In approximately 5 per cent of infants, the normal descent of the testicle into the scrotum does not progress completely. The undescended testicle can reside in the posterior abdomen, internal inguinal ring, inguinal canal, or external ring. When the testicle lies in the inguinal canal, it is usually palpable but differs from a hernial mass because it is firmer and nontender. In addition, inspection of the scrotum should reveal the absence of a palpable testicle on the ipsilateral side.

Hydrocele

Hydrocele, an accumulation of fluid around the testicle or cord structures, can arise independently or in association with an inguinal hernia. Hydroceles can be primary or secondary and communicating or noncommunicating. In a primary or idiopathic hydrocele, the accumulation of fluid can be large and may occasionally cause symptoms. Secondary hydrocele results from the production of serous fluid, most commonly as a result of epididymitis, tuberculosis, trauma, or mumps. Occasionally, testicular tumors can cause acute hydrocele as well.

Communicating hydrocele results when the processus vaginalis remains patent. Therefore, the size of the mass can vary with position, movement, or changing intra-abdominal pressure. One clue that a communicating hydrocele may exist instead of, or in conjunction with, a hernia is that the size of the mass often increases during the day and decreases with sleep. A noncommunicating hydrocele remains confined to the scrotum or the inguinal canal. Hydroceles of the cord are commonly misdiagnosed as incarcerated hernias. Hydrocele differs from hernia in that most are painless. Most importantly, a light shining through a hydrocele produces a characteristic transillumination that clearly distinguishes it from most hernias.

Varicocele

Dilatated veins of the pampiniform plexus may appear as swellings around the cord and as a visible mass in the scrotum. These varicoceles occur more commonly on the left side because the left spermatic vein and pampiniform plexus drain into the renal vein, which enters the inferior vena cava higher than the right spermatic vein. Unlike hernia, varicocele characteristically resembles a "bag of worms" both on inspection and palpation. In addition, the mass of a varicocele typically disappears spontaneously when the patient is placed supine.

Synovial Cyst

Although synovial cysts typically occur in the spine and upper extremities, on rare occasion they have been described in the groin region and should be included in the differential diagnosis of an inguinal mass. Synovial cysts are usually firmer than other groin masses and appear to be firmly fixed to the underlying tissues.

ADJUNCTIVE DIAGNOSTIC MODALITIES

The data provided by a thorough history and physical examination generally are sufficient to confirm the suspicion of abdominal wall hernia. When it is particularly difficult to elucidate the cause of a patient's nonspecific symptoms, poorly localized pain, or palpable mass, other diagnostic modalities can be used to aid in the diagnosis.

Ultrasonography

Ultrasonography is particularly useful for characterizing the nature of a palpable abdominal wall or groin mass. By ascertaining whether the mass is solid or cystic, fluid-filled, or is undergoing peristalsis, the astute clinician can often distinguish herniated intestine from neoplasm, rectus sheath hematoma, and hydrocele. Ultrasound also can be useful in demonstrating disruption of the normal anatomy. It is particularly useful in the diagnosis of spigelian hernias when a defect in the transversus abdominis aponeurosis or internal oblique muscle can be demonstrated. In epigastric hernias, a defect in the linea alba can often be visualized as well. Often, the position of the mass relative to abdominal wall muscle layers can be discerned, although considerable tracking of hernial contents from the anatomic defect sometimes occurs within the abdominal wall. In cases that remain unclear, tangential radiographs can be performed to demonstrate air or feces in herniated bowel more clearly.

Although it has the potential to be a powerful diagnostic tool in experienced hands, ultrasonography is severely limited in that it is extremely operator-dependent and requires familiarity with the normal ultrasonographic appearance of local anatomy. It is not uncommon for the interpretation of a study by an inexperienced ultrasonographer to contribute to misdiagnosis, and the experience level of the interpreter should always be considered when evaluating a clinical situation (Fig. 1).

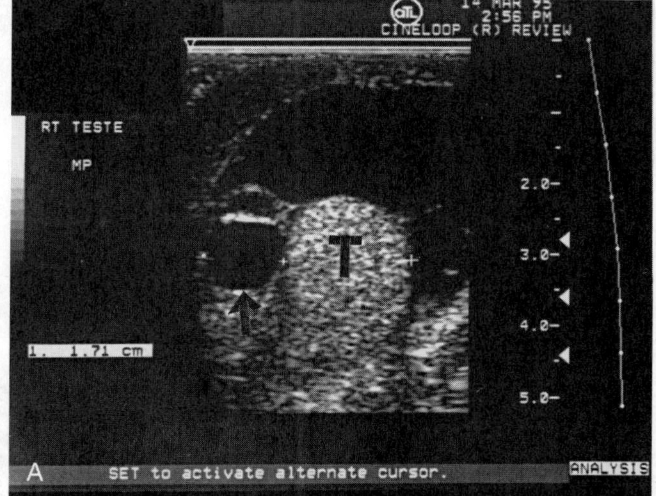

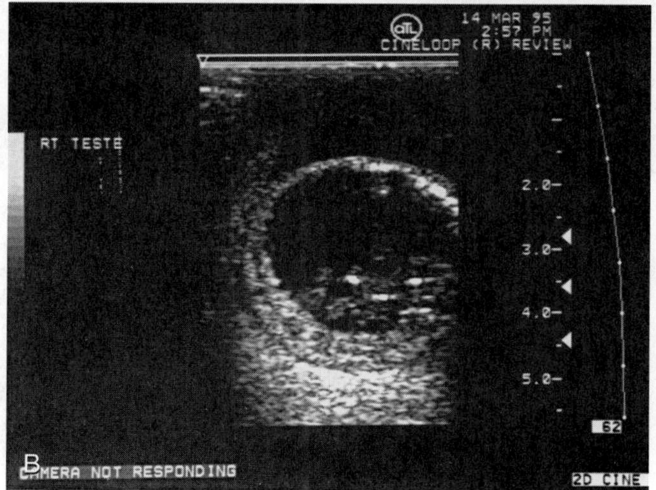

Figure 1. Scrotal ultrasound in a patient with inguinal hernia. *A,* Several simple fluid-filled pockets *(arrow)* in the scrotum surrounding the testis (T), an appearance characteristic of hydrocele. *B,* A different ultrasonographic view of the same patient, clearly demonstrating debris in the fluid-filled spaces, which is more consistent with intestinal contents within the lumen of the herniated small intestine. Thus, ultrasonography is not a definitive diagnostic procedure and has the potential to be misleading, especially in inexperienced hands.

Computed Tomography

Unlike ultrasound, CT is less operator-dependent; however, familiarity with the anatomic appearance of each region on CT requires a certain level of expertise. In addition, CT scans are generally easier for most clinicians to interpret because, unlike ultrasound, the patient's position relative to the axis of the scanner is constant.

Computed tomography can provide information about the contents of a mass, its location relative to the abdominal wall, and whether it is contiguous with adjacent structures (Fig. 2). It has the additional advantage of providing more precise anatomic information about surrounding structures. For example, CT is particularly useful for visualizing the estimated 1 to 4 per cent of adult inguinal hernias that are associated with bladder herniation. Some clinicians advocate the routine use of preoperative CT or cystoscopy for all male patients older than 50 years of age with inguinal hernias and symptoms of urinary outlet obstruction or prostatism. Further, unlike ultrasound, CT can be used reliably in obese patients. CT is also particularly useful for the expedient diagnosis of obturator hernias (see further on).

Laparoscopy

Recent advances in minimally invasive surgical techniques have provided a new tool for both the diagnosis and treatment of abdominal wall hernia. The laparoscopic approach to inguinal hernia is particularly useful when persistent localized groin pain is present in the setting of previous hernia repair, especially when no defect is easily palpable. It offers the additional advantage of concomitant therapeutic intervention as well.

RARE HERNIAS

Although many clinicians may never encounter several of the following types of hernias, familiarity with the characteristics of spigelian, lumbar, obturator, linea alba, and epigastric hernias is necessary to minimize the delays in diagnosis that typically lead to unfortunate outcomes in patients with these rare hernias.

Spigelian Hernia

Spigelian hernias compose less than 1 per cent of all hernias. They affect men and women with equal frequency,

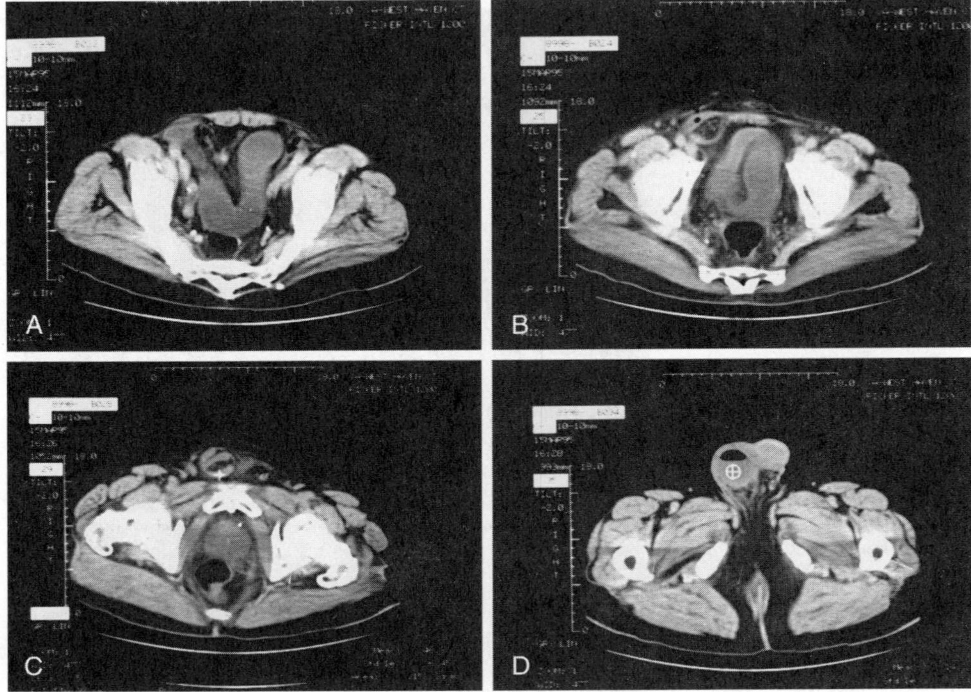

Figure 2. Computed tomogram of the abdomen and pelvis in a patient with inguinal hernia. *A,* The radiolucent mass pressing on the anterior abdominal wall is clearly contiguous with small intestine. *B,* Herniation of the intestine through the anterior abdominal wall is seen, with visualization of air and intestinal contents within the lumen. *C,* The herniated intestine can be seen within the inguinal canal. *D,* Air is seen in the lumen of the herniated intestine in the scrotum.

and their peak incidence is at 50 years of age. The anatomic defect occurs in the transversus abdominis aponeurosis lateral to the rectus muscle at the level of the linea semicircularis. Spigelian hernias are difficult to diagnose because they present with poorly localized pain, often in the absence of a palpable mass. Because the anatomic defect is characteristically composed of a narrow neck of stiff aponeurotic fascia, these hernias have an extremely high incidence of incarceration and strangulation.

Lumbar Hernia

Lumbar hernias are also extremely rare, with approximately 300 reported cases in the literature. The more common superior lumbar hernia occurs through the triangle of Grynfeltt and Lessgaft, whose boundaries include the 12th rib superiorly and the internal oblique muscle anteriorly. Inferior lumbar hernias occur through Petit's triangle, which is formed by the external oblique muscle anteriorly, the iliac crest inferiorly, and the latissimus dorsi muscle posteriorly. The origin of these hernias can be congenital, spontaneous, incisional, or traumatic.

Obturator Hernia

Obturator hernias are extremely rare, with fewer than 550 reported cases and a female-to-male preponderance of 9:1. They typically occur in frail, elderly, multiparous women in the seventh to eighth decade of life who often have a history of chronic constipation, pulmonary disease, or weight loss. They occur where the neurovascular bundle exits the pelvis between the obturator foramen and the suprapubic ramus. The cause has been linked to relaxation of the pelvic musculature, loss of extraperitoneal fat, and increased intra-abdominal pressure. Most involve small bowel, predominantly ileum, and Richter's-type involvement is not infrequent.

Pain along the medial aspect of the thigh radiating to the knee, known as the Howship-Romberg sign, is present in 50 per cent of patients. The pain is caused by the pressure of the hernial sac contents on the obturator nerve. This pain is exacerbated by extension, abduction, and internal rotation of the hip. Pressure on the nerve can also cause the absence of the adductor reflex. This is know as the Hannington-Kiff sign and may occur even in the absence of a positive Howship-Romberg sign. In nearly 20 per cent of patients, a mass may be felt lateral to the abductus longus tendon in the proximal medial thigh. In another 10 to 20 per cent of patients, a rectal or vaginal examination may reveal a lateral mass.

Obturator hernias can be particularly insidious because they usually have no external signs; therefore, diagnosis typically is delayed for days. Only 11 to 33 per cent are diagnosed preoperatively and as a result, up to 50 per cent of patients require bowel resection because of strangulation. The subsequent operative mortality is estimated to be as high as 10 to 20 per cent (Fig. 3).

Hernias of the Linea Alba

Hernias of the linea alba occur in the abdominal midline. Epigastric hernias refer to the more common subset located superior to the umbilicus, which typically affect men in the third and fourth decades of life. Their incidence has been estimated at 5 per cent in the general population, but because they are usually small and asymptomatic, they are often diagnosed only at autopsy. Occasionally, however, they cause pain that characteristically worsens when the patient reclines, causing traction on the incarcerated tissue, often the omentum. A mass usually can be palpated subcutaneously in the linea alba, although the hernia is occasionally too small to be felt.

SUMMARY

Although the majority of abdominal wall hernias can be diagnosed with a thorough history and physical examination, certain hernias present particular diagnostic challenges, especially in pediatric and elderly age groups and in young athletic men. Rare abdominal wall hernias, such

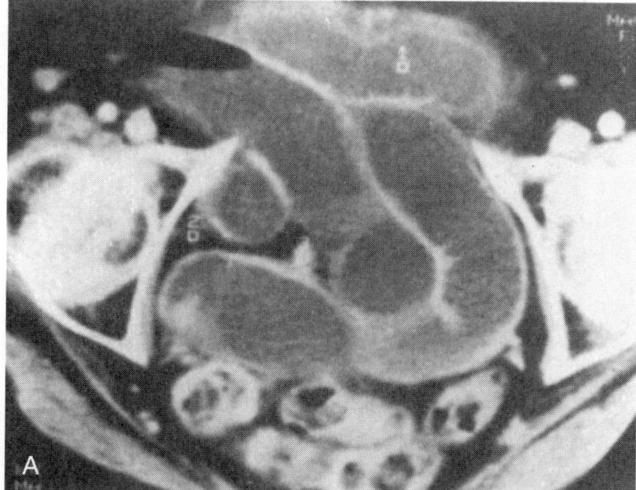

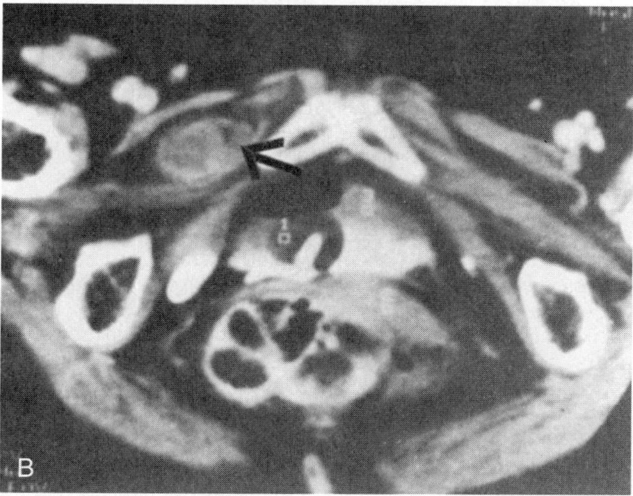

Figure 3. Abdominal and pelvic CT in a patient with an incarcerated obturator hernia. *A,* Dilated loops of intestine consistent with small bowel obstruction. *B,* The herniated intestine can be seen in the obturator canal *(arrow).* (From Emory, R.E., and LaPorta, A.J.: Obturator hernia. Surg. Rounds, January 1993, p. 43, with permission.)

as the femoral, epigastric, obturator, and spigelian hernias, are likewise difficult to diagnose because of low clinical suspicion combined with nonspecific presentation and obscure physical findings. In addition, many conditions have presentations similar to that of abdominal wall or groin hernias. When the diagnosis is unclear, ultrasonography, CT, and laparoscopy can be extremely useful modalities to help reduce or eliminate the delays in diagnosis.

DIAPHRAGMATIC HERNIAS

By Jeffrey H. Peters, M.D.,
and Tom R. DeMeester, M.D.
Los Angeles, California

With the advent of clinical radiology, it became evident that a hiatal hernia was a relatively common abnormality and was not always accompanied by symptoms. Three types of esophageal hiatal hernias were identified: (1) the sliding hernia (type I), which is characterized by an upward dislocation of the cardia in the posterior mediastinum (Fig. 1); (2) the rolling, or paraesophageal, hernia (type II), which is characterized by an upward dislocation of the gastric fundus alongside a normally positioned cardia (Fig. 2); and (3) the combined sliding-rolling, or mixed, hernia (type III), which is characterized by an upward dislocation of both the cardia and the gastric fundus (Fig. 3). Pure type II hernias are rare. Most paraesophageal hernias have a component of a sliding hiatal defect on careful examination. The end stage of a type I or type II hernia occurs when the whole stomach migrates up into the chest by rotating 180 degrees around its longitudinal axis with the cardia and pylorus as fixed points. In this situation, the abnormality is usually referred to as an intrathoracic stomach (Fig. 4).

Most hiatal hernias in adults are acquired. Structural deterioration of the phrenoesophageal membrane occurs over time and leads to the development of the hernia (Fig. 5). These changes involve thinning of the upper fascial layer of the membrane (supradiaphragmatic continuation of the endothoracic fascia) and loss of elasticity in the lower fascial layer (infradiaphragmatic continuation of the transversalis fascia). Consequently, the membrane yields to stretching in the cranial direction because of persistent intra-abdominal pressure. The upper fascial layer is formed by loose connective tissue only and is of little importance. The lower fascial layer is thick, stronger, and more important. It divides into an upper and a lower leaf about 1 cm before attaching intimately to the esophageal adventitia. Because of stretching in the cranial direction from intra-abdominal pressure, the attachment of the lower leaf protrudes upward and can frequently be identified in the thoracic cavity. These observations suggest that the development of a hiatal hernia appears to be a phenomenon related to age and is secondary to repetitive upward stretching of the phrenoesophageal membrane. This stretching occurs as the membrane is subjected to the

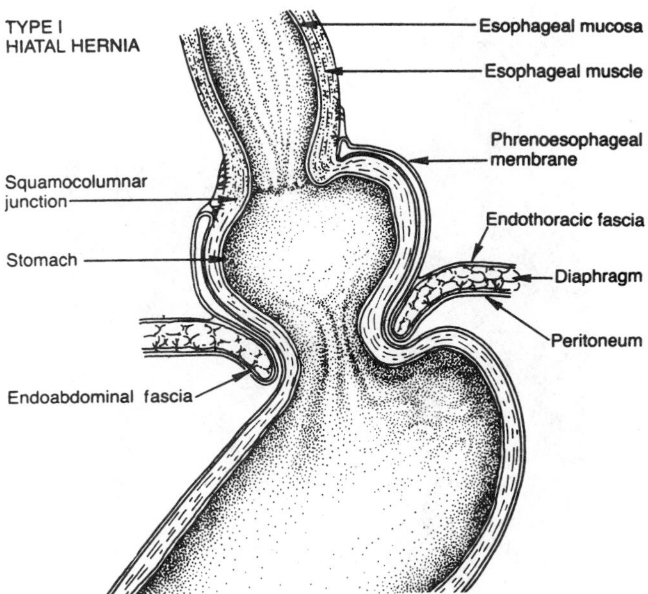

Figure 1. Schematic diagram of a type I sliding hiatal hernia. (From Skinner, D.: *In* Sabiston, D.C., Jr. [ed.]: *Textbook of Surgery,* 13th ed., Philadelphia, W.B. Saunders, 1986, p. 756, with permission.)

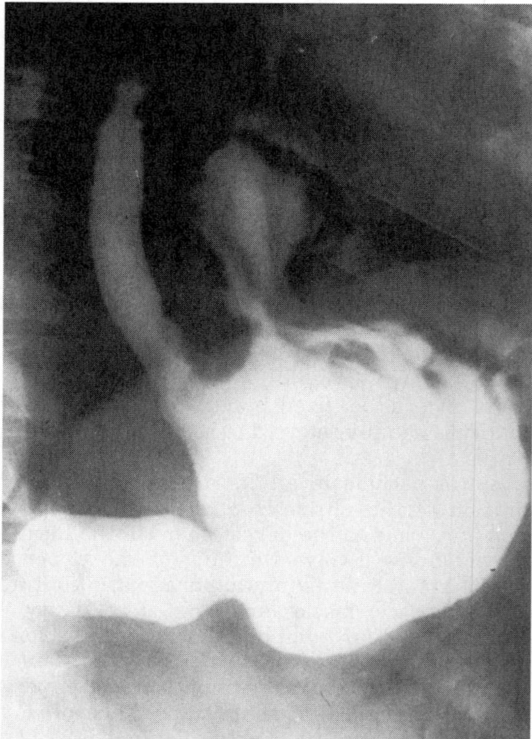

Figure 2. Radiograph of a type II rolling or paraesophageal hernia.

repetitive up-and-down movements of the esophagus during swallowing and the upward push of intra-abdominal pressure. A paraesophageal hernia—rather than a sliding hernia—develops when there is a defect, perhaps partly congenital, in the esophageal hiatus anterior to the esophagus. The persistent posterior fixation of the cardia to the preaortic fascia and the median arcuate ligament is the only essential difference between a sliding hernia and a paraesophageal hernia. When an anterior defect in the hiatus occurs in association with a loss of fixation of the cardia, a mixed, or type III, hernia develops.

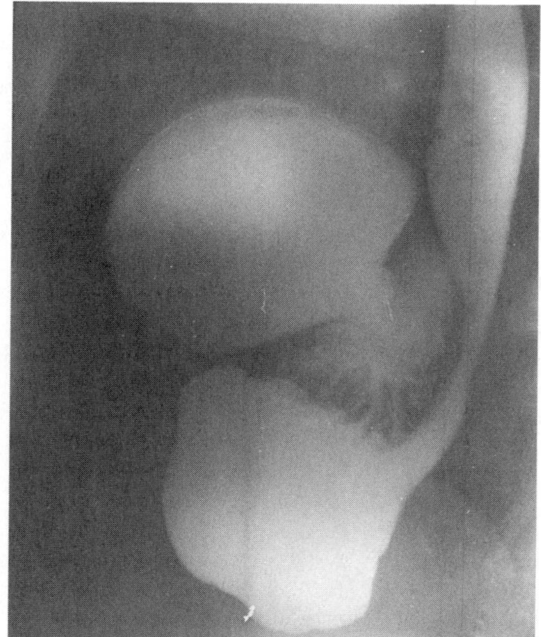

Figure 3. Radiograph of a type III combined sliding-rolling, or mixed, hernia.

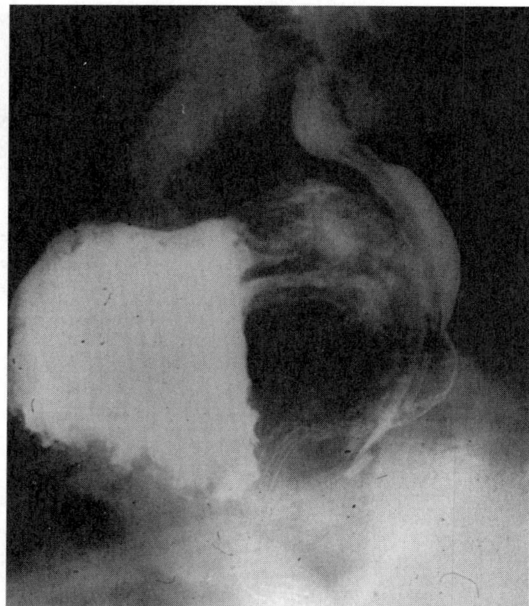

Figure 4. Radiograph of an intrathoracic stomach. This is the end stage of a large hiatal hernia regardless of its initial classification. Note that the stomach has rotated 180 degrees around its longitudinal axis with the cardia and pylorus as fixed points.

INCIDENCE AND ETIOLOGY

The true incidence of hiatal hernia in the overall population is difficult to determine because of the absence of symptoms in a large number of persons. When radiographic examinations are performed in response to gastrointestinal symptoms, a hiatal hernia is identified in as many as 15 per cent of patients. Sliding hiatal hernias are found approximately seven times more frequently than are paraesophageal hernias. The age distribution of patients with paraesophageal hernias is significantly different from that observed in sliding hiatal hernias. The former has a median age of 61 years, whereas the median age of the latter is 48 years. Paraesophageal hernias are more likely to occur in women, by a ratio of 4:1.

SYMPTOMS AND SIGNS

The symptoms of sliding hiatal hernias are usually due to functional abnormalities associated with gastroesophageal reflux and include heartburn, regurgitation, and dysphagia. Many patients have a mechanically defective lower esophageal sphincter, giving rise to reflux of gastric juice and symptoms of heartburn and regurgitation. Dysphagia occurs from the presence of mucosal edema, Schatzki's ring, stricture, or the inability to organize peristaltic activity in the body of the esophagus as a consequence of severe reflux disease. Some patients with hiatal hernias unassociated with reflux have dysphagia without obvious endoscopic or manometric explanation. Video barium radio-

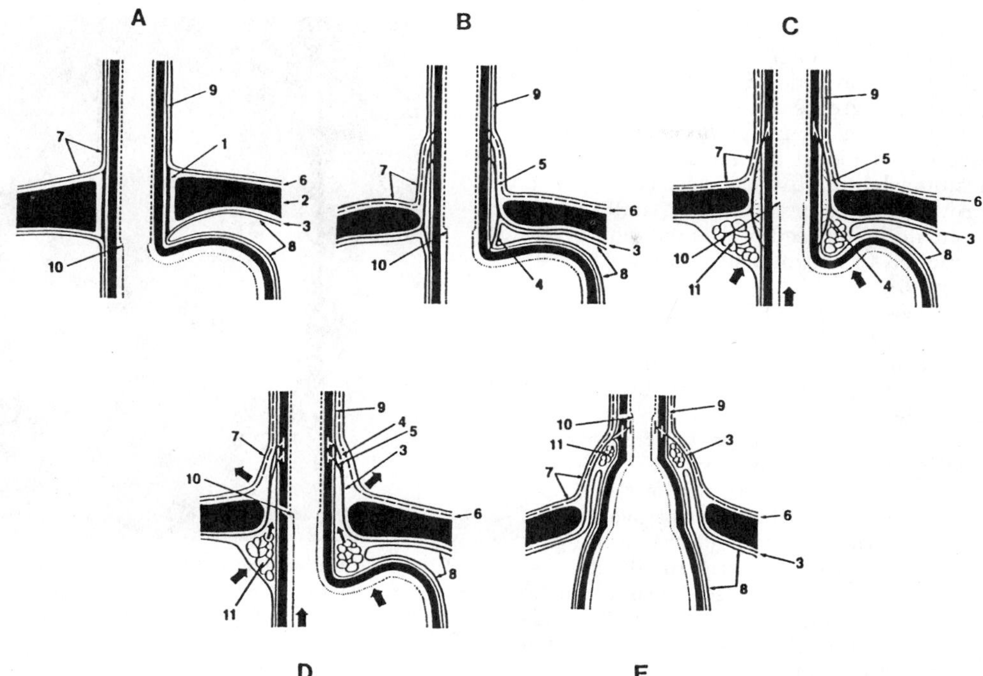

Figure 5. Changes in the anatomy of the phrenoesophageal membrane over time based on the dissection of 163 human cadavers from the fetal period to age 75 years. *A,* Fetus. *B,* Newborn and small infants and young adults 20 to 30 years of age. *C,* Old adults 55 to 70 years of age. *D,* Old adults in transition to a hiatal hernia. *E,* Old adults with hiatal hernia. In the fetus, the membrane is closely attached to the adventitia of the esophagus. In neonates, children, and young adults, the membrane is slightly stretched. In old adults, loose connective tissue develops in the lower fascial layer. In old adults in transition to hiatal hernia, the lower fascial tissue is pushed cranially to form the developed hernia shown in *E.* Broad arrows indicate direction of stretch owing to intra-abdominal pressure and movement of the esophagus during swallowing. 1, Phrenoesophageal membrane; 2, diaphragmatic crus; 3, lower fascial tissue; 4, lower leaf of lower fascial layer; 5, upper leaf of lower fascial layer; 6, upper fascial layer; 7, pleura; 8, peritoneum; 9, esophageal adventitia; 10, gastroesophageal epithelial junction; 11, subperitoneal fat.

graphs have shown the cause of dysphagia in these patients to be obstruction to the passage of the swallowed bolus by diaphragmatic impingement on the herniated stomach. These patients usually have a mechanically competent sphincter, but the impingement of the diaphragm on the stomach can propel the contents of the supradiaphragmatic portion of the stomach up the esophagus and into the pharynx and result in regurgitation and aspiration, which is often confused with typical gastroesophageal reflux disease. Surgical reduction of the hernia results in relief of the dysphagia in 91 per cent of these patients.

The clinical presentation of a paraesophageal hiatal hernia differs from that of a sliding hernia. There is usually a higher prevalence of dysphagia and postprandial fullness with paraesophageal hernias, but the typical symptoms of heartburn and regurgitation that are present in sliding hiatal hernias can also be seen. Both are caused by gastroesophageal reflux secondary to an underlying mechanical deficiency of the cardia. The symptoms of dysphagia and postprandial fullness in patients with a paraesophageal hernia are explained by the compression of the adjacent esophagus by a distended cardia or twisting of the gastroesophageal junction by the torsion of the stomach that occurs as it becomes progressively displaced in the chest.

About one third of patients with paraesophageal hernia complain of hematemesis due to recurrent bleeding from ulceration of the gastric mucosa. Respiratory complications are frequently associated with paraesophageal hernia. Dyspnea may occur from mechanical compression of the dilated intrathoracic stomach, and recurrent pneumonia and pulmonary fibrosis may occur from repetitive aspiration. Intermittent esophageal obstruction can develop in patients with an intrathoracic stomach owing to the rotation that has occurred as the organ migrates into the chest. Conversely, many patients with paraesophageal hiatal hernia are asymptomatic or complain of minor symptoms.

Physical examination and laboratory findings are normal in most patients with sliding hiatal hernia. Patients with paraesophageal hernia may manifest decreased breath sounds and/or bowel sounds over the left lower chest. As many as one third of patients are found to be anemic on presentation.

Diaphragmatic hernia is life-threatening in one fifth of patients in that the hernia can lead to sudden catastrophic events, such as excessive bleeding or volvulus with acute gastric obstruction or infarction. With mild dilatation of the stomach, the gastric blood supply can be markedly reduced, causing gastric ischemia, ulceration, perforation, and sepsis.

DIAGNOSTIC APPROACH

Patients who do not respond to simple behavior and/or lifestyle modifications or primary medical therapy, patients who require long-term (more than 1 year) antisecretory agents, and those in whom surgery is contemplated should undergo a thorough diagnostic evaluation. This includes upper endoscopy, video barium radiography, manometry, and 24-hour pH studies. A chest film taken with the patient in the upright position can diagnose a hiatal hernia if it shows an air-fluid level behind the cardiac shadow

(Fig. 6). This finding is usually caused by a paraesophageal hernia or an intrathoracic stomach. The accuracy of the upper gastrointestinal barium study in detecting a paraesophageal hiatal hernia is greater than it is for a sliding hernia because reduction can occur spontaneously in the latter. The paraesophageal hiatal hernia is a permanent herniation of the stomach into the thoracic cavity, so a barium swallow provides the diagnosis in virtually every patient. Attention should be focused on the position of the gastroesophageal junction to distinguish it from a type II hernia (see Figs. 2 and 3).

Fiberoptic esophagoscopy is useful in the diagnosis and classification of a hiatal hernia because the scope can be retroflexed. With the scope in this position, a sliding hiatal hernia can be identified as a gastric pouch lined with rugal folds extending above the impression caused by the crura of the diaphragm or by measuring at least 2 cm between the crura (identified by having the patient sniff) and the squamous columnar junction on withdrawal of the scope. A paraesophageal hernia is identified on retroversion of the scope by noting a separate orifice adjacent to the gastroesophageal junction into which gastric rugal folds ascend (Fig. 7). A sliding-rolling, or mixed, hernia can be identified by noting a gastric pouch lined with rugal folds above the diaphragm, with the gastroesophageal junction entering about midway up the side of the pouch.

It has long been assumed that a sliding hiatal hernia is associated with an incompetent distal esophageal sphincter, whereas a paraesophageal hiatal hernia constitutes a pure anatomic entity and is not associated with an incompetent cardia. Over the past 3 decades, there has been an increased interest in the physiology of the gastroesophageal junction and its relationship to the various types of hiatal hernias. Physiologic testing with 24-hour esophageal pH monitoring has shown increased esophageal exposure to acid gastric juice in 60 to 70 per cent of patients with paraesophageal hiatal hernia, which is nearly identical to the 71 per cent incidence observed in patients with sliding hiatal hernia. No relation was found between the symptoms experienced by the patients with paraesophageal hernia and the competency of the cardia (Table 1). Thus, it is now recognized that paraesophageal hiatal hernia can be associated with pathologic gastroesophageal reflux.

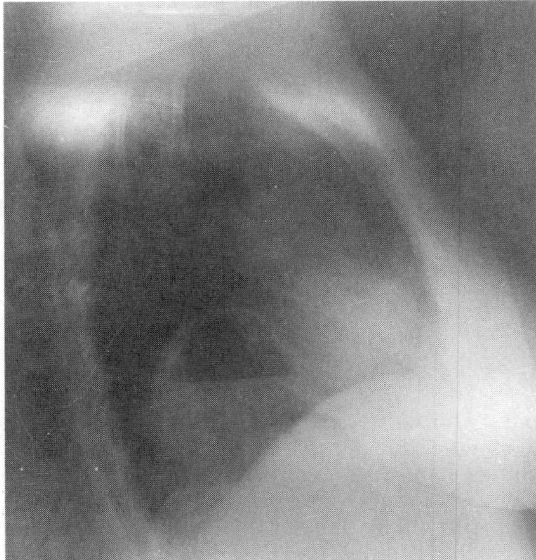

Figure 6. Lateral chest film showing a posterior mediastinal air-fluid level in a gas bubble, indicating the presence of a paraesophageal hernia.

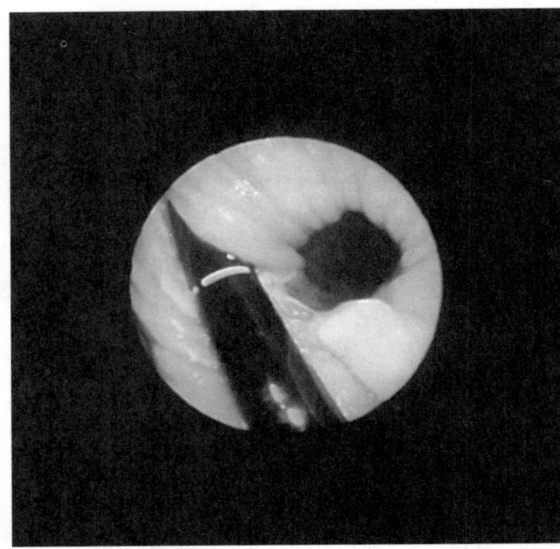

Figure 7. Endoscopic view through a retroflexed fiberoptic gastroscope showing the shaft of the scope coming down through the gastroesophageal junction adjacent to a separate orifice of the paraesophageal hernia into which the gastric rugal folds ascend.

Physiologic studies have shown that the competency of the cardia depends on an interrelationship of distal esophageal sphincter pressure, the length of the sphincter exposed to the positive pressure environment of the abdomen, and the overall length of the sphincter. A deficiency in any one of these manometric characteristics of the sphincter is associated with incompetency of the cardia whether or not a hernia is present. Patients with paraesophageal hernia and an incompetent cardia have been shown to have a distal esophageal sphincter with normal pressure but a shortened overall sphincter length and displacement of the sphincter outside the positive pressure environment of the abdomen. In a sliding hernia, even though the sphincter appears to be within the chest on a radiographic barium study, it still can be exposed to abdominal pressure because of the surrounding hernial sac that functions as an extension of the abdominal cavity (Fig. 8). A high insertion of the phrenoesophageal membrane into the esophagus provides an adequate length of distal esophageal sphincter exposed to abdominal pressure. A low insertion provides an inadequate length. The importance of the anatomic length of esophagus within the hernial sac has been emphasized by Bombeck, Dillard, and Nyhus* in their careful dissections of the hiatus. In 55

*Bombeck, T.C., Dillard, D.H., and Nyhus, L.M.: Muscular anatomy of the gastroesophageal junction and role of the phrenoesophageal ligament. Ann. Surg., 164:643, 1966.

Table 1. Symptoms in 15 Patients With Paraesophageal Hernia Compared With Results of 24-Hour Esophageal pH Monitoring

Status	Positive	Negative
Heartburn	6 of 9	4 of 6
Regurgitation	6 of 9	3 of 6
Dysphagia	6 of 9	4 of 6
Postprandial fullness	8 of 9	3 of 6
Bleeding	4 of 9	1 of 6

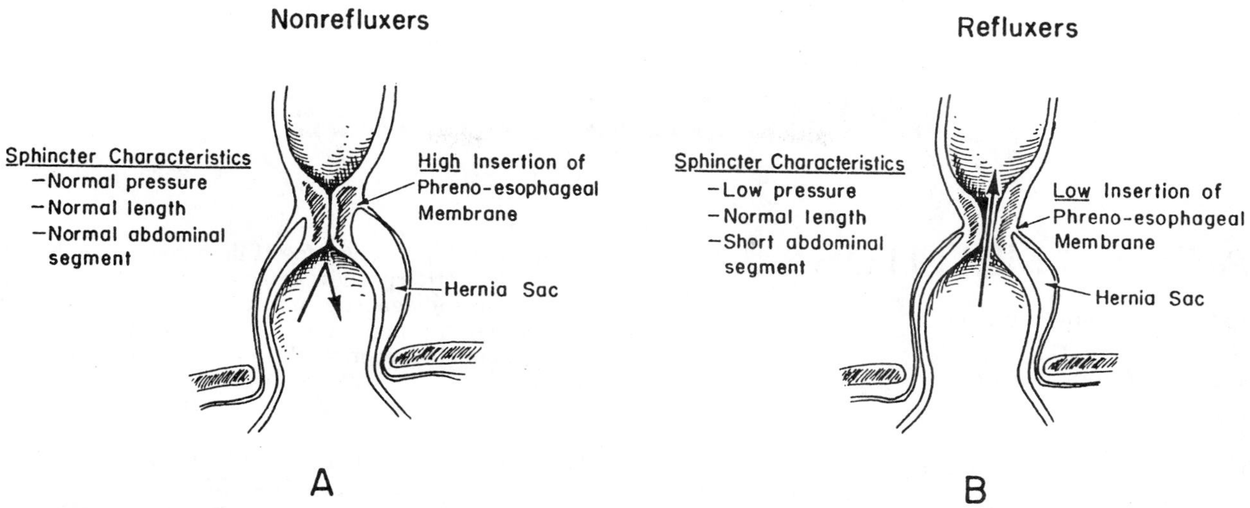

Figure 8. Schematic diagram of the anatomic and manometric differences between patients without a sliding hiatal hernia with reflux *(A)* and those with one *(B)* based on 24-hour esophageal pH monitoring.

patients who underwent postmortem dissection, 8 persons had a hiatal hernia and 5 of these 8 individuals had no evidence of esophagitis. In these five patients, the phrenoesophageal membrane inserted 2 to 5 cm, with a mean of 3.6 cm, above the gastroesophageal junction. The other three patients had evidence of esophagitis and therefore an incompetent cardia. In these patients, the membrane inserted 0 to 1 cm, with a mean of 0.5 cm, above the gastroesophageal junction. This difference was significant and emphasized the importance of an adequate length of intra-abdominal esophagus in maintaining competency of the cardia even in the presence of a hiatal hernia.

In contrast to a paraesophageal hernia in which the sphincter remains fixed in the abdomen, in a mixed type III hernia, the sphincter moves extraperitoneally into the thorax through the widened hiatus, along with a portion of the lesser curvature of the stomach and cardia, and forms part of the wall of the hernial sac. Consequently, the lower esophageal sphincter lies outside the abdominal cavity and is unaffected by its environmental pressures. The loss of normal esophageal fixation that occurs in a type I sliding hernia or a type III mixed hernia results in the body of the esophagus being less able to carry out its propulsive function. This contributes to a greater exposure of the distal esophagus to refluxed gastric juice when components of an incompetent cardia are present.

Section Eight

METABOLIC DISEASE

DIABETES MELLITUS

By Rose Mary Fair-Covely, D.O.,
and José F. Caro, M.D.
Philadelphia, Pennsylvania

Diabetes mellitus is a chronic disorder that is characterized by hyperglycemia or by plasma glucose levels that are above defined limits during oral glucose tolerance testing and by major alterations in carbohydrate, fat, and protein metabolism. Diabetes is associated with an increased propensity to develop specific forms of nephropathy, retinopathy, neuropathy, and premature cardiovascular disease. The resulting abnormalities occur primarily from a deficiency in the synthesis, secretion, or function of insulin.

Approximately 15 million persons, or 6 per cent of the population, have diabetes in the United States. Unfortunately, one half of the patients with diabetes remain undiagnosed. Type II diabetes accounts for 90 to 95 per cent of the cases of diagnosed diabetes and almost 100 per cent of the undiagnosed cases. The prevalence of diabetes increases with age, with one half of all cases in persons older than 55. Almost 17 per cent of the U.S. white population (65 to 74 years old) have diabetes. The prevalence of diabetes tends to be higher in women than in men, especially in black Americans. There is an increased prevalence of type II diabetes among blacks, Latinos, and Mexican Americans.

The prevalence of type I diabetes by the age of 20 years is approximately 0.26 per cent, and the lifetime prevalence approaches 0.9 per cent. The disease can occur at any age, with a small midlife peak in incidence. Type I diabetes has a lower incidence among persons of Asian or Native-American heritage.

Persons with diabetes face a decreased life expectancy and an impaired quality of life. Diabetes causes 50 per cent of all nontraumatic amputations, 15 per cent of all blindness, and 35 per cent of all end-stage renal disease. Diabetes is one of the four major risk factors for cardiovascular disease. Diabetes mellitus is the seventh leading cause of death in the United States. Mortality caused by diabetes represents about 2 per cent of total U.S. mortality. This number underestimates the true mortality due to diabetes, because diabetes is under-reported on death certificates.

Diabetes costs the nation annually more than 100 billion dollars, or one of each seven dollars spent on health care. A major issue is that type II diabetes is underdiagnosed and therefore undertreated (Fig. 1). The undiagnosed stage is not a benign condition, and it is estimated to last about 10 years. It is imperative that diabetes and its complications be properly diagnosed so that therapeutic strategies can be implemented to alter the natural course of the disease.

This article reviews the World Health Organization's diagnostic criteria for diabetes; the classification of diabetes and other forms of glucose intolerance; the differential diagnosis of type I and type II diabetes using clinical and biochemical criteria; how to screen for early diagnosis of diabetes; the diagnostic indicators of long-term glycemic control; how to diagnose the acute complications of diabetes; and how to recognize the chronic complications of diabetes.

DIAGNOSIS OF DIABETES MELLITUS AND IMPAIRED GLUCOSE TOLERANCE

The World Health Organization has set up criteria to assist in the diagnosis of diabetes mellitus and impaired glucose tolerance in nonpregnant and pregnant adults and in children. Table 1 summarizes the criteria used for the diagnosis.

Oral glucose tolerance testing is unnecessary if the criteria of No. 1 or No. 2 under the diagnostic criteria for diabetes mellitus found in Table 1 are met. If these set criteria are not met, an oral glucose tolerance test may be needed to confirm or exclude the diagnosis. The state of impaired glucose tolerance is defined as a glycemic response to a glucose challenge intermediate between normal and diabetic and therefore can be determined only by an oral glucose tolerance test.

Increased fasting plasma glucose and impaired glucose tolerance can be produced by trauma, burns, pregnancy, endocrinopathies, and various drugs. Physical inactivity and a restricted diet (<150 g of carbohydrates/day) may produce abnormal glucose tolerance. For this reason, an increased fasting plasma glucose or an abnormal glucose tolerance test must be demonstrated on at least two occasions before the diagnosis is established. The protocol for

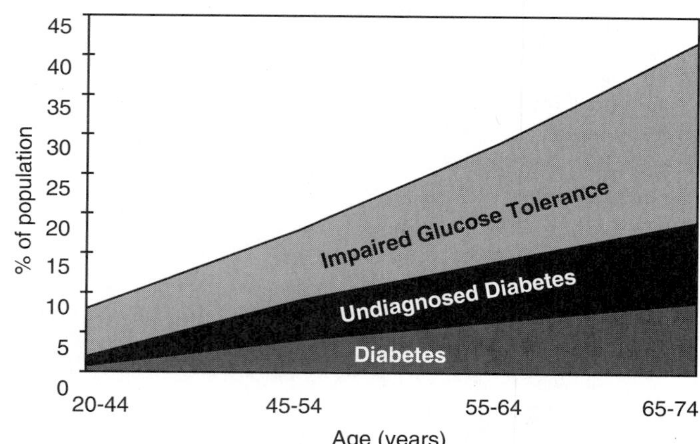

Figure 1. Prevalence of diagnosed and undiagnosed diabetes and impaired glucose tolerance in the U.S. population. Data generated by the Second National Health and Nutrition Examination Survey (NHANES II) by performing demographic and medical history interview (n = 7688), physical examination (n = 5901), and 75-g oral glucose tolerance test (n = 5826) in a representative sample of the U.S. population. The study was conducted by the National Center for Health Statistics (NCHS).

Table 1. Diagnostic Criteria for Diabetes Mellitus, Impaired Glucose Tolerance and Normal Glucose Tolerance

Diabetes Mellitus Criteria; At Least One of the Following:

1. Random plasma glucose of 200 mg/dL or greater together with classic symptoms of diabetes mellitus (polydipsia, polyuria, polyphagia, weight loss)
2. Fasting plasma glucose ≥140 mg/dL on more than one occasion
3. Fasting plasma glucose level <140 mg/dL and two 75-g OGTT with a 2-hour plasma glucose ≥200 mg/dL

Impaired Glucose Tolerance Criteria; All of the Following:

1. Fasting plasma glucose <140 mg/dL
2. Two 75-g OGTT with a 2-hour plasma glucose between 140 and 199 mg/dL

Normal Glucose Tolerance Criteria; All of the Following:

1. Fasting plasma glucose <140 mg/dL
2. Two 75-g OGTT with a 2-hour plasma glucose <140 mg/dL

the performance of oral glucose tolerance testing (OGTT) is detailed in Table 2.

To establish glucose intolerance during pregnancy, the World Health Organization (WHO) recommends the use of the 75-g 2-hour glucose tolerance test and follows the same criteria used in nonpregnant subjects. One study compared the WHO and National Diabetes Data Group (NDDG) procedures in the detection of diabetes during pregnancy. The standard WHO criteria were more likely to predict abnormal outcomes in pregnant women than the more cumbersome two-step NDDG test. The NDDG criteria had a number of drawbacks including the need for blood samples at four times, a test duration of 3 hours, a high glucose load that is often unpalatable to pregnant women, and no comparability with the 75-g test that is done post partum. The NDDG test also requires that women with abnormal screening tests have a diagnostic test. The WHO test requires no repeat testing and has the added advantage of being directly comparable with the standard glucose test used in nonpregnant women and with postpartum testing.

Diabetes mellitus in children usually presents with severe symptoms, very high blood glucose levels, heavy glucosuria, and ketonuria. In most children, the diagnosis can be confirmed without delay with blood glucose measurements, and treatment (i.e., insulin injections) is initiated immediately and is often a lifesaving measure. OGTT is neither necessary nor appropriate for most patients. In general, the diabetes diagnostic criteria for children are the same as those recommended for adults (see Table 1).

Table 2. Standardized Protocol for Performance of an Oral Glucose Tolerance Test

1. Should be performed only on stable ambulatory patients
2. Perform only on those patients whose fasting plasma glucose is more than 140 mg/dL
3. Perform on patients who have had unrestricted activity and carbohydrate intake of at least 150 g/day for 3 days before testing
4. If possible, discontinue for 3 days all medications that may influence test results
5. Have the patient fast 10–14 hours before the study, preferably from 6 PM the night before to 8 or 9 AM on the day of the test
6. Oral glucose load should be 75 g for nonpregnant and pregnant adults and 1.75 g/kg of ideal body weight for children up to a maximum of 75 g. Ingestion of the glucose load should be complete within 5 minutes. The test begins with the first swallow of the glucose load. Nausea and vomiting rarely occur, but if they do occur, the test should be terminated
7. Subjects should be seated during the test. They should not smoke, nor should they ingest caffeine
8. A venous plasma glucose concentration should be measured before and 2 hours after the ingestion of glucose

CLASSIFICATION OF DIABETES MELLITUS

The WHO system of classification contains three major clinical classes: diabetes mellitus, gestational diabetes mellitus, and impaired glucose tolerance. The clinical class of diabetes mellitus is divided into four subtypes: type I diabetes (previously called juvenile-onset or insulin-dependent diabetes mellitus); type II diabetes (previously called maturity-onset diabetes or NIDDM); malnutrition-related diabetes mellitus; and secondary diabetes mellitus associated with certain conditions and syndromes. The classification also includes statistical risk classes in which patients have a normal glucose tolerance but a substantially increased risk of developing diabetes. Table 3 is a summary of the WHO classification of diabetes mellitus and allied categories of glucose intolerance. Most diabetics have diabetes mellitus, gestational diabetes, or impaired glucose tolerance.

Patients with type I diabetes are ketosis prone secondary to insulin deficiency due to islet cell loss. Diabetes mellitus type I can occur at any age and is common in youth. It usually appears before the age of 30 years. It is often associated with specific human leukocyte antigen types on chromosome 6, with a predisposition to viral insulinitis or autoimmune phenomena. Because of the acute nature of its symptoms, type I diabetes usually does not remain undetected for very long.

Patients with type II diabetes are ketosis resistant under basal conditions. However, if sufficiently stressed, these patients can develop ketosis. Type II diabetes is more common in adults but occurs at any age. Measured insulin concentrations may be normal, increased, or depressed. The patient is typically symptom free for many years, and the onset and progression of symptoms can be slow. About 80 per cent of type II diabetic patients are obese. The incidence of type II diabetes approaches 90 per cent of all diagnosed cases of diabetes. Because of the subtle and slow progression of diabetes, most unidentified cases of diabetes are type II diabetes, and the main focus of screening is asymptomatic individuals with type II diabetes.

Gestational diabetes mellitus (GDM) is a disorder that is first recognized during pregnancy. GDM occurs in 3 per cent of pregnancies. GDM symptoms generally are mild and are not life threatening. However, hyperglycemia is associated with increased fetal morbidity, and therefore, maintenance of normal serum glucose concentrations is required. The diagnosis of GDM is an important aspect of prenatal care. Post partum, some women whose glucose intolerance is first recognized in pregnancy revert to normal glucose tolerance, but others may continue to have impaired glucose tolerance or type II diabetes. The women who revert to normal have a high likelihood of developing gestational diabetes again in a subsequent pregnancy and have a high risk of developing diabetes, estimated at a rate of 5 per cent per year.

Impaired glucose tolerance (IGT) occurs when the glycemic response to glucose loading is abnormal but does not meet the criteria for diabetes mellitus on standardized glucose testing. Impaired glucose tolerance is associated with an increased rate of progression to type II diabetes.

Table 3. Classification of Diabetes Mellitus and Other Categories of Abnormal Glucose Metabolism

Clinical Classes	Distinguishing Characteristics
Diabetes mellitus	
Type I diabetes insulin-dependent diabetes mellitus (IDDM)	Patients may be of any age, are usually thin, and usually have an abrupt onset of signs and symptoms of insulinopenia before the age of 30. These patients also have strongly positive urine ketone tests in association with hyperglycemia and are dependent on insulin therapy to sustain life.
Type II diabetes mellitus non–insulin-dependent (NIDDM)	Patients are usually older than 30 years of age at diagnosis and have relatively few classic symptoms. They can be subgrouped into obese or nonobese subtypes. They are not prone to ketoacidosis except during periods of stress. They are not dependent on exogenous insulin for survival. However, they may require it for adequate control of hyperglycemia.
Malnutrition-related diabetes mellitus	Patients are usually young (between 10 and 40 years old), are usually symptomatic, and are not prone to ketoacidosis, but many require insulin therapy.
Secondary and other types of diabetes	Patients with secondary and other types of diabetes mellitus conditions or syndromes; examples include diabetes mellitus secondary to pancreatic disease, endocrinopathies, drugs and other chemical agents. Patients also may develop diabetes mellitus or impaired glucose tolerance secondary to insulin receptor abnormalities, genetic syndromes, polycystic ovaries, or other conditions.
Gestational diabetes mellitus	Glucose intolerance is discovered during pregnancy.
Impaired glucose tolerance (IGT), obese or nonobese	Patients with impaired glucose tolerance have positive glucose levels that are higher than normal, but not diagnostic for diabetes mellitus.
Statistical risk classes	
Previous abnormality to glucose tolerance	Persons in this category have normal glucose tolerance and a history of transient diabetes mellitus or impaired glucose tolerance.
Potential abnormality of glucose tolerance	Patients in this category have never experienced abnormal glucose tolerance but have a greater than normal risk of developing diabetes. Individuals who are at a risk for type I include (in decreasing order of risk) persons with islet cell antibodies, monozygotic twin of a type I diabetic, sibling of a type I diabetic (especially one with identical HLA haplotypes), and offspring of a type I diabetic. Individuals who are at an increased risk for type II diabetes include (in decreasing order of risk) monozygotic twin of a type II diabetic, first-degree relative to a type II diabetic (this includes siblings, parent, and offspring), mother of a neonate weighing more than 9 lb, obese individuals, and members of a racial ethnic group who have a higher prevalence of diabetes. The degree of risk for any of these categories is not firmly established.

The rate has been estimated at 1.5 to 4 per cent per year over a 10-year period in most populations. About 25 per cent of the patients with IGT eventually develop diabetes. Patients who meet this criteria are then subdivided by weight (obese and nonobese). Patients with IGT do not have an increased risk of microvascular complications of diabetes, but in certain subsets of the population, patients with IGT have an above-average risk of atherosclerotic disease that is attributed to risk factors such as hypertension, decreased high-density lipoprotein, and increased serum triglycerides.

DIFFERENTIAL DIAGNOSIS OF TYPE I AND TYPE II DIABETES MELLITUS

The correct classification of diabetic subjects at the time of diagnosis is often difficult, but clearly important in clinical practice. Before therapy is initiated, the patient must have a complete medical evaluation and be classified appropriately.

A complete personal and family history enables the physician to assign a classification. The patient should not be classified on the basis of age, body weight, or use of insulin. Although all patients with type I diabetes receive insulin, most patients with type II diabetes also require insulin after years of disease. A history of ketoacidosis or excessive urinary ketones is the most useful indication of type I diabetes. The clinician should document episodes of ketosis to confirm the diagnosis of type I diabetes. The most important clinical characteristics that distinguish type I from type II diabetes are presented in Table 4. The same table demonstrates the usefulness of basal C-peptide measurement in distinguishing between type I diabetes and type II diabetes.

Proinsulin, the precursor of insulin, is produced in the pancreas and is split into insulin and C-peptide. Unlike insulin, C-peptide is not metabolized in the liver. Its serum concentration reflects insulin secretion. A C-peptide measurement is a valid assay of pancreatic secretion in a diabetic, because the clearance rate of C-peptide is similar in diabetics and nondiabetics. The assay of C-peptide is not valid in patients with renal failure, because the primary site of C-peptide metabolism is the kidney. Abnormal renal function often leads to a false increase in the C-peptide concentration in serum. Measurement of C-peptide may help the clinician decide whether to withdraw or initiate insulin therapy in selected patients whose diabetic classification is uncertain.

Patients with a basal C-peptide value above 0.5 nmol/L should be considered to have type II diabetes, and patients with a value below 0.2 nmol/L should be considered to have

Table 4. Clinical Characteristics of Type I and Type II Diabetes Mellitus

Characteristics	Type I	Type II
Age of onset	Usually <30 yr	Usually >40 yr
Ketosis	Common	Rare
Body weight	Nonobese	Obese (80% of patients)
Prevalence	0.5%	4–5%
Proportion of diabetes mellitus	10–20%	80–90%
Complications	Frequent	Frequent
Rate of appearance of symptoms	Acute or subacute	Slow
Seasonal trend	Fall or winter	None
HLA association	Yes	No
Beta cell function	Decreased	Variable
Insulin antibodies	Yes	No
Fasting C peptide	<0.2 nmol/L	>0.5 nmol/L
Sustacal-stimulated C peptide	<0.5 nmol/L	>1 nmol/L

type I diabetes (see Table 4). Patients with intermediate values should be further evaluated. Low C-peptide concentrations should be interpreted with caution, especially during episodes of hypoglycemia, because hypoglycemia inhibits C-peptide secretion.

A more precise determination of endogenous insulin reserve can be accomplished by the Sustacal stimulation test. Table 5 shows the Sustacal-stimulated C-peptide protocol, and Table 4 interprets results. In general, the Sustacal stimulation test can differentiate type I from type II diabetics. However, type II diabetics of long duration and type I diabetics are not invariably separated by measurement of Sustacal-stimulated C-peptide because of a significant overlap of C-peptide concentrations in these two populations.

SCREENING FOR EARLY DIAGNOSIS OF DIABETES

Because one half of the patients with diabetes are undiagnosed, it is appropriate to seek the disease in the population. An effective screening protocol requires that the clinically silent stage of the disease is not considered benign, therapy is available to modify the natural course, and diagnostic methods are not harmful or expensive (favorable cost-benefit ratio). Employing these criteria, screening for diabetes is mandatory in every pregnant woman; targeted screening for type II diabetes is indicated in the high-risk population; and screening for type I diabetes is not indicated.

Table 5. Protocol for Sustacal-Stimulated C-Peptide Test

1. Fasting overnight
2. Withhold morning insulin injection
3. As soon as the patient arrives, blood glucose should be checked. If blood glucose value is >400 mg/dL or if the blood glucose value is <240 mg/dL and moderate or greater ketonuria is present, the test should be rescheduled.
4. A 10-mL blood sample should be obtained by venipuncture in a red top tube for measurement of C peptide and glucose. Immediately after collection of the blood sample, the patient should ingest the test meal within 10 min. The test meal consists of a commercial mixed meal, Sustacal. The amount to be ingested should be 3 mL of Sustacal per kilogram of body weight, with a maximum of 360 mL.
5. Blood sample is obtained 90 min after ingestion of the test meal. It should consist of 10 mL of blood placed in a red-topped tube and handled as in step 4.
6. Immediately after the second blood sample, the patient takes his or her usual morning insulin dosage and returns to his or her usual diabetes care regimen.

Early Diagnosis of Diabetes in Pregnancy

All pregnant women should be screened for glucose intolerance, because selective screening based on clinical features or past obstetric history is inadequate. Pregnant women who have not been identified as glucose intolerant before the 24th week of gestation should have an oral glucose tolerance test. (Venous plasma glucose is measured before and 2 hours after the patient ingests 75 g of glucose.) Testing is best performed between the 24th and the 28th weeks of pregnancy.

All patients with GDM are at risk for having children with fetal macrosomia. The risk of neonatal hyperglycemia, hypoglycemia, polycythemia, and hyperbilirubinemia is also increased. The offspring of mothers who have experienced fasting (≥105 mg/dL) and postprandial (>120 mg/dL) hyperglycemia are at greatest risk for intrauterine death or neonatal mortality. Mothers in this category must undergo careful antepartum fetal surveillance.

Risk factors for GDM include glycosuria, a family history of diabetes in a first-degree relative, maternal obesity, a previous "heavy" baby, a previous fetal abnormality, a previous stillbirth or spontaneous abortion, high maternal age, and parity of five or more. The presence of one or more of these risk factors increases the risk of gestational diabetes mellitus.

Early Diagnosis of Type II Diabetes

Among the 7 million persons with undetected diabetes mellitus, there is an increased prevalence of hypertension (61 per cent), hypercholesterolemia (49 per cent), low-density lipoprotein cholesterol greater than 160 mg/dL (40 per cent), hypertriglyceridemia (20 per cent), obesity (50 per cent in males and 82 per cent in females), and cigarette smoking (32 per cent). When coupled with the frequent delay (of many years) in the diagnosis of diabetes mellitus, these risk factors increase the probability that microvascular and macrovascular abnormalities are already present at the time of initial diagnosis of type II diabetes. Not surprisingly, prospective studies document similar death rates in diagnosed and undiagnosed type II diabetics. The death rate for diagnosed and undiagnosed diabetics is approximately twice the death rate for nondiabetic individuals.

Many clinicians advocate targeted screening for diabetes in individuals older than 40 years of age. They recommend measurement of fasting plasma glucose followed by a 2-hour oral glucose tolerance test for specified persons at risk for diabetes mellitus type II. Figure 2 summarizes a diagnostic algorithm for diabetes type II. Step 1 consists of a fasting plasma glucose (FPG) in all individuals older than 40 years of age with appropriate follow-up, and step 2 reviews a 2-hour plasma glucose after a 75-g OGTT for persons at risk for diabetes mellitus. The risk factors (in the algorithm) for developing diabetes include a family history of diabetes; obesity; Native-American, Latino, or African-American heritage; and a history of GDM or giving birth to babies weighing more than 9 lb.

In theory, the early identification of individuals with impaired glucose tolerance, or with newly diagnosed type II diabetes but without severe hyperglycemia, could in-

Step 1: FPG in all adults > 40 years of age

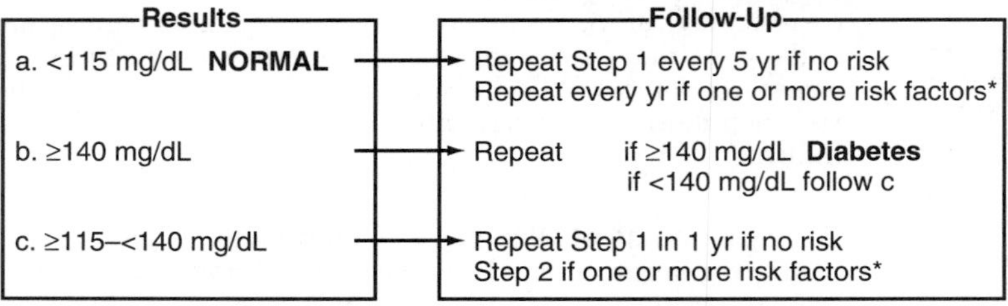

Step 2: 2-hr FPG after 75-g OGTT in people at risk* with FPG ≥115–<140 mg/dL

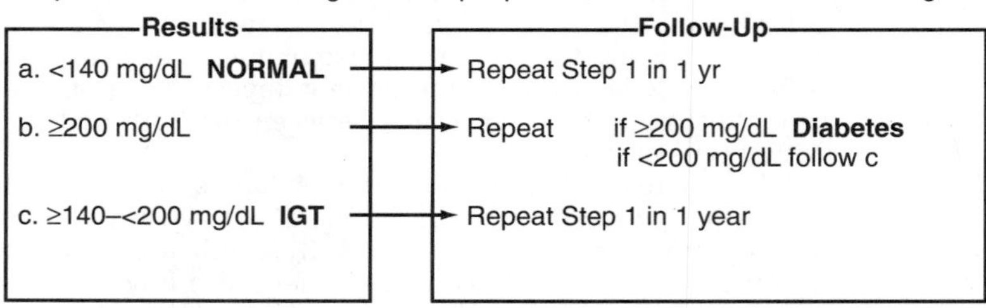

Figure 2. Diagnostic algorithm for diabetes. *, Risk factors for developing diabetes include family history of diabetes; obesity; Native American, Latino, or African American heritage; history of gestational diabetes or giving birth to babies weighing more than 9 lb. FPG = fasting plasma glucose; IGT = impaired glucose tolerance; OGTT = oral glucose tolerance test.

crease the frequency of timely and aggressive treatment designed to decrease the prevalence of complications. However, patients may not benefit from early diagnosis and treatment of diabetes without concomitant aggressive treatment of coronary artery disease risk factors such as hypertension, hyperlipidemia, cigarette smoking, and obesity. Between 60 and 70 per cent of deaths in undiagnosed cases of diabetes mellitus result from coronary artery disease.

Early Diagnosis of Type I Diabetes

Using a combination of laboratory tests, it may be possible to identify first-degree relatives most likely to develop type I diabetes within 10 years of the analyses. Test results that may predict type I diabetes include high cytoplasmic islet cell antibodies (>40 JDF units), insulin autoantibody titer greater than 1:1000, and first-phase insulin release of less than 1 per cent after intravenous glucose. These markers may assist in the early detection of individual susceptibility to type I diabetes, but they will not help in the early diagnosis of type I diabetes.

Early targeted screening is not useful in diagnosing type I diabetes, because type I diabetes manifests with acute or subacute signs and symptoms that require immediate treatment; complications of type I diabetes are usually absent at the time of diagnosis; and no practical therapy is available to alter the progression from prediabetes to type I diabetes. However, prevention trials are in progress, and the results should be available within 10 years.

DIAGNOSTIC INDICATORS OF LONG-TERM GLYCEMIC CONTROL

Goals for long-term glycemic control should consider the patient's capacity to carry out treatment, the risk of severe hypoglycemia, and other factors that may increase or decrease the benefits of tight control of plasma glucose concentrations. The use of intensive control of blood glucose is supported by the results of the Diabetes Control and Complications Trial (DCCT), which conclusively demonstrated that the risk of progression of retinopathy, nephropathy, and neuropathy in type I diabetics is reduced 50 to 75 per cent by intensive treatment compared with conventional treatment. An average hemoglobin A_{1C} of 9.0 per cent in the conventional treatment group was reduced to an average hemoglobin A_{1C} of 7.2 per cent in the intensively treated group. The reduced risk of progression of diabetic complications correlated continuously with the reduction in hemoglobin A_{1C} produced by intensive treatment. The nondiabetic reference range for hemoglobin A_{1C} in the DCCT was 4.0 to 6.0 per cent. Because glycohemoglobin values differ in various laboratories, the reference range should be adjusted for local differences in methodology. Table 6 outlines the indicators of glycemic control and desired end points for persons with diabetes.

During intensive treatment, glucose should be measured at least three or four times each day; during less intensive regimens, glucose should be measured two to three times each day. Glucose targets to be monitored by the patient should be individually adjusted, especially if the patient has an increased risk of severe hypoglycemia.

No randomized clinical trial has unequivocally confirmed the DCCT. Considerable evidence, however, documents that a relation between microvascular disease and hyper-

Table 6. Biochemical Indices of Metabolic Control

Characteristic	Normal	Goal	Acceptable	Poor
Fasting plasma glucose (mg/dL)	115	<120	140	>200 mg/dL
2-hr postprandial glucose (mg/dL)	140	<160	200	>240 mg/dL
Hemoglobin A_{1c} (%)	4–6	<7	8	>9
Total cholesterol (mg/dL)	<200	<200	200–240	>240 mg/dL
Fasting LDL cholesterol (mg/dL)	0–130	<130	130–159	≥160
Fasting HDL cholesterol (mg/dL)	≥35	>35		≤35
Fasting triglyceride (mg/dL)	150	150–199	200	>250 mg/dL

HDL = high-density lipoprotein; LDL = low-density lipoprotein.

glycemia similar to that of type I diabetes occurs in type II diabetes. Therefore, it is reasonable to employ the same glycohemoglobin and blood glucose goals as described in Table 6 for type II diabetes.

Measurement of hemoglobin A_{1C} is the most reliable way of assessing blood glucose control over the previous 1 to 2 months. For detailed adjustment of insulin therapy, hemoglobin A_{1C} testing does not replace self-monitoring of blood glucose. Glycohemoglobin testing verifies the reliability of self-monitored blood glucose determinations.

DIAGNOSIS OF ACUTE COMPLICATIONS IN DIABETES

The two major types of acute complications of diabetes are metabolic abnormalities, and infections.

Metabolic Complications

In type I diabetes, the major acute complications are ketoacidosis and hypoglycemia, and in type II diabetes, they are hyperosmolar hyperglycemic nonketotic coma and hypoglycemia (Table 7).

Diabetic ketoacidosis (DKA) is a life-threatening but reversible complication of type I diabetes that requires intensive medical care. DKA is caused by an absolute or relative insulin deficiency. DKA occurs more often in type I diabetics than in type II diabetics. The arterial pH in DKA typically falls below 7.2, the plasma bicarbonate concentration is less than or equal to 15 mmol/L, blood glucose usually exceeds 250 mg/dL, and ketones are detected in blood and urine. The circulating concentrations of glucagon, catecholamines, cortisol, and growth hormones are increased. These substances collectively antagonize the biologic effects of insulin and exacerbate the metabolic abnormalities of DKA. Hyperglycemia results from increased production and decreased metabolism of glucose. Severe hyperglycemia causes osmotic diuresis that results in dehydration. Hyperlipidemia reflects increased lipolysis, and high anion gap acidosis reflects increased production of acetoacetate and β-hydroxybutyrate (Table 8).

Diabetic ketoacidosis may be confused with alcoholic ketoacidosis or starvation ketosis, because all these conditions lead to acidosis and ketonemia. Blood glucose less than 250 mg/dL usually excludes DKA unless there has been partial correction of the patient's condition with insulin and intravenous fluids or caloric intake has been restricted.

Table 7. Initial Laboratory Findings in Severe Diabetic Decompensation

Characteristic	Diabetic Ketoacidosis	Hyperosmolar Coma
Glucose (mmol/L [mg/dL])	26 (475)	65 (1166)
Sodium (mmol/L)	132	144
Potassium (mmol/L)	4.8	5
Bicarbonate (mmol/L)	<10.0	17
Serum urea nitrogen (mmol/L [mg/dL])	9 (25)	31 (87)
Acetoacetate (mmol/L)	4.8	ND
β-Hydroxybutyrate (mmol/L)	13.7	ND
Free fatty acids (mmol/L)	2.1	0.73
Lactate (mmol/L)	4.6	ND
Osmolarity (mmol/kg)	310	384
pH	<7.2	>7.3

Table 8. Conditions With High Anion Gap Acidosis

Metabolic acidosis with increased "anion gap"
1. Renal failure
2. Diabetic ketoacidosis
3. Lactic acidosis
4. Exogenous poisons (e.g., ethylene glycol, salicylates, methanol, paraldehyde)

The initial signs and symptoms of DKA are polyuria, polydipsia, hyperventilation, and dehydration. Alterations of mental status range from drowsiness to frank coma, and the breath may reveal the fruity odor of ketones. Young patients may present with abdominal pain, slight leukocytosis, and increased serum amylase concentrations that typically resolve with therapy. If severe abdominal pain persists, the possibility of appendicitis, bowel perforation, or bowel infarction should be excluded.

Factors that may precipitate DKA include infections, trauma, myocardial infarction, or stroke. The patient may have deliberately or inadvertently omitted insulin therapy. Many patients withhold insulin if they are vomiting and unable to eat, because they fear that insulin administration will cause hypoglycemia and further vomiting. Counseling the patient about sick day management is important in preventing further episodes of DKA.

Hyperosmolar hyperglycemic nonketotic coma (HHNC) is common in older patients with type II diabetes and can be life threatening. HHNC sometimes occurs spontaneously in patients with undiagnosed diabetes or in patients with long periods of uncontrolled hyperglycemia. Common precipitating events include the use of hyperglycemic drugs (e.g., potassium-wasting diuretics, alcohol, corticosteroids), acute and chronic conditions (especially infections), and myocardial infarction. Most patients present with severe hyperglycemia (>600 mg/dL and generally between 1000 and 2000 mg/dL), and many develop a slight degree of ketosis. Hyperosmolarity (>340 mOsm/kg of water) with profound dehydration is the rule. Patients often develop altered sensorium with coma, confusion, severe dehydration, shallow respirations, and excessive thirst.

Hypoglycemia occurs in type I and type II diabetic patients. Hypoglycemia is precipitated by administration of excess insulin, oral hypoglycemic agents, decreased food intake, excess exercise, alcohol, and other drugs. Hypoglycemia should be suspected in patients with altered mental status and symptoms of adrenergic overdrive and neuroglycopenia. Typical adrenergic responses include tachycardia, palpitations, increased sweating, and hunger. Symptoms of neuroglycopenia range from mild confusion to frank coma. Hypoglycemia is confirmed by plasma glucose values of less than 50 to 60 mg/dL in a patient with appropriate symptoms.

Infections

Infections are the major cause of metabolic abnormalities leading to diabetic coma. Infections require rapid diagnosis and treatment. Common infections in diabetic patients include furunculosis, carbuncles, vulvovaginitis, and cellulitis alone or in combination with vascular ulcers of the lower extremities.

Patients with diabetes are prone to urinary tract infections; up to 20 per cent have asymptomatic bacteriuria. Serious urinary tract infections require hospitalization, with identification and susceptibility testing of the offending organisms. Treatment is mandatory for diabetics with pyelonephritis.

Pneumonia is one of the most common infections in diabetics. Among the various microbial causes of pneumonia in diabetics, *Streptococcus pneumoniae* is identified most frequently. Diabetic patients also develop ear infections. Malignant external otitis is seen most often in elderly diabetics with chronic drainage from an ear and sudden onset of severe pain. *Pseudomonas aeruginosa* is the most common ear pathogen in diabetics. Without timely administration of appropriate antibiotics and, if indicated, surgical debridement, the mortality rate of malignant external otitis approaches 50 per cent in diabetics.

DIAGNOSIS OF CHRONIC COMPLICATIONS IN DIABETES

The major complications of diabetes include microvascular disease (e.g., retinopathy, nephropathy, neuropathy) and macrovascular disease (e.g., peripheral, cerebral and coronary artery disease). These complications lead to severe consequences such as blindness, renal failure, amputations, stroke, myocardial infarction, and a shortened life span. Definitive evidence that intensive treatment of diabetes can delay onset or progression of many of these complications has been provided by the DCCT. Intensive treatment can delay the onset and slow the progression of diabetic neuropathy, kidney disease, and retinopathy.

Microvascular Complications

Diabetic Retinopathy

Retinopathy occurs in all forms of diabetes. Clinical evaluation requires ophthalmoscopic examination, and if indicated, slit-lamp examination and fluorescein angiography of the retina. In the initial stages of nonproliferative retinopathy, small but visible microaneurysms (<100 μm) arise from terminal capillaries of the retina. The escape of erythrocytes from the microaneurysms causes dot-blot hemorrhages. Many retinal vessels develop increased permeability and leak serous fluid. Hard exudates eventually form. The presence of hard exudates, microaneurysms, and dot-blot hemorrhages is called nonproliferative retinopathy. The danger of visual loss derives from the development of nonproliferative retinopathy near the maculae, resulting in macular edema.

The stage known as preproliferative retinopathy occurs when vessels become occluded and ischemia compromises the nerve fiber layer of the retina. Soft, "cotton-wool" exudates form, and new vessels develop in a process known as neovascularization. The development of new vessels heralds the onset of proliferative retinopathy. These weak new vessels can proliferate onto the retinal surface and into the vitreous space. Hemorrhage into the vitreous can result in obstructed vision that typically resolves in 1 to 3 months. Fibroproliferative changes that follow may cause traction and detachment of the retina, leading to permanent loss of vision.

Proliferative retinopathy is subdivided into neovascularization of the disk (if this occurs within one disk diameter of the disk) and neovascularization elsewhere because the risk of loss of vision varies with the size and location of the lesions. Table 9 summarizes the characteristics of retinal lesions that require laser therapy. This table describes lesions that warrant referral to an ophthalmologist who specializes in laser treatment of diabetic retinopathy. Appropriate laser therapy has decreased the loss of vision associated with asymptomatic macular edema and proliferative retinopathy.

Table 9. Characteristics of Retinal Lesions Requiring Laser Therapy

Proliferative Retinopathy

Neovascularization greater than a quarter of the disk area and within one disk diameter of the disk

or

Any neovascularization of the disk within one disk diameter of the disk and associated with vitreous or preretinal hemorrhage

or

Neovascularization elsewhere greater or equal to one half of the disk area and associated with hemorrhage

Clinically Important Macular Edema

Retinal thickening within 50 μm of center of macula or hard exudates within 500 μm of macular center if associated with thickening of adjacent retina

or

Zone of retinal thickening greater or equal to one disk area, any part of which is within one disk diameter of the macular center

One half of adult diabetics are not appropriately screened for retinopathy. Direct ophthalmoscopy is not very sensitive, especially if there are few retinal lesions. If the pupils are not dilated, a considerable amount of proliferative retinopathy is not detected. Patients with type I diabetes should be examined annually by an ophthalmologist after the fifth year. Patients with type II diabetes should be examined at the time of diagnosis and annually thereafter.

Diabetic Neuropathy

Diabetic neuropathy refers to peripheral, somatic, or autonomic nerve damage attributable solely to diabetes mellitus. Other causes of neuropathy, including lumbar spinal root disease, advanced peripheral vascular disease, nondiabetic neuropathy, and psychological disorders, should be excluded before making the diagnosis of diabetic neuropathy.

The evaluation of neuropathy typically includes an assessment of sensation, motor function, reflexes in the upper and lower extremities, cranial nerve function, and autonomic nerve function. Family history of nondiabetic peripheral nerve disease should be sought, and the possibility of toxic, metabolic, mechanical, and vascular causes of nerve disease should be explored. Nutritional deficiency, connective tissue disease, malignancy, tabes dorsalis, and drug or toxin exposure should be specifically addressed.

The electrodiagnostic examination can help the clinician distinguish mononeuropathy, mononeuritis multiplex, plexopathy, polyradiculopathy, and sensorimotor neuropathy. Nerve conduction studies typically reflect the functional status of large, myelinated, sensory and motor nerve fibers in the upper and lower extremities. Normal results, however, do not exclude neuropathy.

Electromyography (EMG) may provide evidence of partial denervation of intrinsic foot muscles; EMG may be the most sensitive indicator of motor axonal degeneration.

The most common form of diabetic neuropathy is peripheral, symmetrical, sensorimotor neuropathy. Other forms of diabetic neuropathy include cranial and peripheral motor neuropathies and autonomic neuropathies.

Sensorimotor Neuropathy

Distal, symmetrical sensorimotor neuropathy usually develops in the lower extremities. Motor deficits and upper extremity involvement are less common. The Achilles reflex is frequently absent, and this can be documented at the time of diagnosis, along with decreased vibratory sensations. Symptoms include paresthesias, numbness, tingling, and burning that may intensify at night. A few patients may report extremely severe lancinating or lightning pain in the extremities. Depression and anorexia may supervene; patients should be told that the pain is not permanent and will subside spontaneously within months to years as the involved neurons die.

As the neuropathy progresses, hyperesthesia is replaced by hypoesthesia, placing the patient at increased risk for trauma and foot ulcers. Altered pedal architecture and mechanics plus the loss of sensation in the foot creates a formidable clinical challenge. Ultimately, with progression of neuropathy, there may be a loss of all sensation (e.g., light touch, pain, position) in a stocking-and-glove distribution. When sensory loss due to polyneuropathy is severe, secondary changes due to unrecognized trauma may develop in the lower extremities. Neuropathic ulcers typically occur in areas of callous formation. Charcot joints (i.e., neuropathic arthropathy) may develop in the ankle or the foot at the metatarsal or metatarsophalangeal joint; patients may present with unilateral pain, swelling, and erythema of the ankle, foot, or both. Joint instability, disruption of articular surfaces, and bone demineralization may be detected on physical or radiographic examination.

Motor Neuropathy

Focal motor (cranial and peripheral) compression neuropathies and mononeuritis multiplex are less common than the sensorimotor neuropathies. Radiculopathies that mimic disk disease may occur. Mononeuropathies are symmetrical and abrupt in onset. Paralyses of extraocular muscles supplied by the third and sixth nerves are well-known signs of cranial mononeuropathies. Patients can also develop palsies involving the median nerve, the ulnar nerve, and various cranial nerves. The mononeuropathies usually resolve spontaneously in 6 weeks to 6 months. Carpal tunnel syndrome and other compression neuropathies are more common in diabetics, and these conditions may require surgical decompression.

Autonomic Neuropathy

Abnormalities of the autonomic nervous system occur in long-standing diabetes, particularly in patients with peripheral polyneuropathy. The effects of autonomic neuropathy can be seen in gastrointestinal motility, erectile function, bladder function, vascular tone, and cardiovascular function (Table 10). Approximately 5 to 10 years after the onset of diabetes, some clinical changes can be documented by testing the autonomic nervous system. Abnormal gastric contraction, loss of variation in sinus rhythm with respirations, and resting tachycardia greater than 100 beats/min may reflect autonomic dysfunction.

Gastroparesis may alter absorption and cause nausea and early satiety. In patients with suspected diabetic gastroparesis, the clinician should assess glycemic control and medication history and determine whether the patient has used ganglionic blocking agents or psychotropic drugs. The clinician should perform gastroduodenoscopy to exclude pyloric or other mechanical obstruction and optimize glycemic control, and perform a solid-phase gastric study to document delayed gastric emptying time. The delayed absorption of meals may adversely influence metabolic control and predispose the patient to episodes of hyperglycemia or hypoglycemia.

Autonomic dysfunction may cause orthostatic hypotension, a condition in which renin is not released and normal vasomotor tone is lost when the patient assumes an upright position. Autonomic dysfunction may also lead to decreased sweating in the lower extremities and excess sweating in the upper part of the body. Episodes of excessive sweating may occur shortly after food ingestion.

Table 10. Functional Changes Associated With Autonomic Failure

Systems Involved	Manifestations
Cardiovascular	Resting tachycardia, impaired exercise-induced cardiovascular responses, cardiac denervation, orthostatic hypotension, heat intolerance, impaired vasodilation, impaired venoarteriolar reflex (dependent edema)
Ocular	Decreased diameter of dark-adapted pupil (dark-adapted miosis)
Gastrointestinal	Esophageal enteropathy, gallbladder atony, impaired colonic motility (diarrhea, constipation), anorectal sphincter dysfunction (incontinence)
Genitourinary	Neurogenic vesical dysfunction (decreased bladder sensitivity/incontinence/retention), sexual dysfunction (male: penile erectile failure and retrograde ejaculation; female: defective lubrication)
Sudomotor	Anhidrosis/hyperhidrosis (heat intolerance), gustatory sweating
Endocrine	Hypoglycemia-associated autonomic failure

The development of "hypoglycemic unawareness" can make the control of blood glucose very difficult. Hypoglycemic unawareness typically does not occur until diabetes has been present for approximately 10 to 15 years. Patients with hypoglycemic unawareness, particularly type I diabetics, typically lose adrenergic warning signs and proceed directly to signs and symptoms of neuroglycopenia. Adrenergic signs and symptoms include sweating, nervousness, tremors, tachycardia, and palpitations, but the neuroglycopenic symptoms that follow are distinctly different and can progress from mild confusion to frank coma.

Autonomic dysfunction can also affect the motility of the lower gastrointestinal tract. Diabetics may experience diarrhea, constipation, and incontinence. Diarrhea is characteristically worse at night and may be associated with fecal incontinence. Diarrhea caused by such autonomic dysfunction is diagnosed only by exclusion of other causes and requires confirmation of the presence of autonomic neuropathy. Constipation in a diabetic warrants a digital examination to evaluate rectal sphincter tone. Other causes of constipation should be excluded.

Diabetic autonomic failure is defined as impaired function of the peripheral autonomic nervous system. A simple bedside test of parasympathetic function involves measuring the heart rate response to deep breathing by comparing the longest RR interval in expiration with the shortest during inspiration. With the patient breathing at six breaths/min, a difference in heart rate (maximal versus minimal) of more than 15 beats/min is considered normal, and a difference of less than 10 beats/min is considered abnormal. Computerized electrocardiographic techniques for assessing RR variability relative to respiration are available. Heart rate response can also be determined while the patient stands up or performs the Valsalva maneuver. Testing of blood pressure control mainly evaluates the sympathetic nervous system. When the patient stands up, a decrease in systolic pressure of more than 20 mmHg accompanied by signs and symptoms of orthostasis is usually viewed as evidence of sympathetic failure.

With increased duration of diabetes, there is initially an increase, followed by a slowing, and finally a fixed heart rate. In normal individuals, the heart rate increases and RR variation decreases predictably with age. Furthermore, parasympathetic activation is reduced in obese individuals. In diabetics, however, RR variation decreases early and rapidly after the diagnosis of diabetes has been established.

Almost one half of all men with diabetes experience impotence, the most common symptom of autonomic neuropathy. Diabetic males also experience retrograde ejaculation, urinary incontinence, and difficulty in emptying their bladder fully. Patients with a dilated and fully contractile bladder are predisposed to urinary tract infections. The diagnosis of diabetic penile neuropathy can be reached only after exclusion of other causes of erectile dysfunction. Impotence can be determined by history and analysis of nocturnal penile tumescence or sleep-related erections. Serum concentrations of total testosterone, free testosterone, luteinizing hormone, follicle-stimulating hormone, and prolactin should be obtained before evaluation of the response to intracavernosal vasodilators (such as prostaglandin E_1). If the nocturnal penile tumescence test is abnormal but the hormonal profile is normal and the patient develops a full erection in response to vasodilators, significant vascular disease is excluded. If the patient does not respond to intracavernosal injections, vascular dysfunction (arterial or venoocclusive disease) with or without associated neuropathy becomes the most likely diagnosis.

Diabetic Nephropathy

Diabetic nephropathy is one of the most devastating complications of diabetes mellitus. More than one third of type I diabetics and almost one fourth of type II diabetics experience renal disease. The number of diabetics requiring treatment for end-stage renal disease has increased at an annual rate of 11 per cent since 1980. More than one third of new cases of end-stage renal disease are caused by diabetic nephropathy. End-stage renal disease is more common in African-American, Latino, and Native-American populations than in the white population.

Clinical diabetic nephropathy is defined as albuminuria greater than 300 μg per 24 hours or an albumin to creatinine ratio of greater than 0.2. This definition is used for patients without clinical or laboratory evidence of other diseases of the kidney or urinary tract who have had type I diabetes for more than 5 years with evidence of diabetic retinopathy.

Compared with type I diabetics who do not have clinical evidence of nephropathy, type I diabetics with progressive nephropathy have higher mean blood pressures, higher hemoglobin A_{1C} values, and a higher incidence of proliferative retinopathy. In addition, cigarette smoking is more commonly observed among type I diabetics with persistent albuminuria.

The natural history of albuminuria in type II diabetes has not been fully documented. Renal disease can be documented in at least 5 to 10 per cent of type II diabetics approximately 20 years after diagnosis. Clinical evidence of diabetic kidney disease or increased urinary albumin excretion may be found at the time of diagnosis of type II diabetes. This may reflect the typically longer period of hyperglycemia that is present before the diagnosis of type II diabetes is made.

Nephropathy tends to progress through several defined stages. The first sign of kidney disease is the excretion of more than 40 mg of albumin in a 24-hour urine specimen. As diabetic kidney disease progresses, clinical proteinuria (>300 mg of albumin per 24 hours) develops. Eventually, nephrotic range (>3.5 g of albumin per 24 hours) proteinuria develops, followed by a decreased glomerular filtration rate (GFR), an increased serum creatinine, and progression to end-stage renal disease (Table 11).

Microalbuminuria is a predictor of mortality in type II diabetics. Microalbuminuria is also a significant risk factor for cardiovascular mortality in diabetics.

The National Kidney Foundation has recommended the following screening and follow-up measures for patients with diabetes and associated kidney disease:

- Albumin should be measured annually in all patients who have had type I diabetes for at least 5 years and in all subjects with type II diabetes. If urinary albumin excretion is abnormal, three additional urine albumin measurements over 6 months will confirm the diagnosis before specific intervention. Serum creatinine or creatinine clearance should be measured at least annually, and other diseases of the kidney and urinary tract should be excluded.
- Blood pressure should be measured frequently (at least once each year). If initial systolic blood pressure is greater than 140 mm Hg or diastolic blood pressure is greater than 90 mm Hg, two readings of blood pressure should be obtained over 1 month. If initial readings are substantially increased or if there is evidence of organ damage, treatment with antihypertensive drugs that avoid serious side effects or further renal impairment should be initiated.
- Glycemic control and protein consumption should be maintained within American Diabetes Association guidelines.
- Attempts should be made to ameliorate risk factors for coronary heart disease, such as hypercholesterolemia and cigarette smoking.
- An evaluation of the retina should be performed annually.
- Patients with impending renal failure (serum creatinine greater than 2.0 mg/dL or GFR less than 70 mL/min)

Table 11. Typical Clinical Course of Diabetic Nephropathy

Years After Onset of Diabetes, Approximate	Clinical Course
0	Enlarged kidneys, supernormal function, microalbuminuria reversed by meticulous insulin treatment
2	Thickening of glomerular basement membrane and increase in mesangial matrix
10–15	Silent period: no overt proteinuria; microalbuminuria may be present especially after exercise (>30 μg/min indicative of future proteinuria)
10–20	Proteinuric period intermittent at first, then persistent (>0.5 g/24 hr); meaning that a relentless decline in glomerular function has begun
>15	Azotemic period begins, on average, 17 yr after onset
20	Uremic period: diabetic retinopathy, hypertension, and nephrotic syndrome

and patients with poorly controlled hypertension or hypercalcemia require thorough evaluation by a nephrologist.

The rate of decrease of GFR can be slowed by antihypertensive treatment, aggressive amelioration of risk factors, and improved glycemic control. Among the beneficial effects of glycemic control demonstrated by the DCCT was a decrease in the incidence and severity of microalbuminuria and clinical grade albuminuria. It is also important to eliminate or reduce the risk factors that lead to diabetic kidney disease. Factors known to precipitate renal insufficiency include hypertension, neurogenic bladder, infection, urinary obstruction, and nephrotoxic agents (e.g., nonsteroidal anti-inflammatory drugs, radiocontrast dyes).

Macrovascular Complications

The major risk factors for atherosclerosis in the diabetic population are the same as those for the nondiabetic population: hyperlipidemia, hypertension, obesity, and cigarette smoking. Amelioration of these risk factors may delay or prevent macrovascular complications in diabetes.

Diabetics have an increased prevalence of premature cardiac, cerebral, and peripheral vascular disease. There is a sevenfold increase in macrovascular disease that occurs at an earlier age and with greater frequency than in nondiabetic individuals. Macrovascular complications are responsible for 80 per cent of the mortality in diabetic adults. Cardiovascular complications occur three to four times more frequently in type II diabetic women than in nondiabetic women. Diabetic women may lose the proposed protective effect of estrogen. Ulceration and amputation of the lower extremities are among the most important complications of diabetes. Neuropathy and macrovascular disease often occur together and synergistically cause limb-threatening complications.

Physicians should be alert to signs and symptoms of accelerated atherosclerosis among diabetic patients. Evaluation of complications is critical so that treatment can be instituted. Most patients have the same symptoms of coronary, cerebral, and peripheral vascular disease as nondiabetics. However, neuropathic factors may alter these symptoms in the diabetic patient. For example, a diabetic may have no or atypical symptoms of angina. Cerebral signs and symptoms of hypoglycemia may mimic transient ischemic attacks, and symptoms of neuropathy must be differentiated from signs and symptoms of intermittent claudications.

The management of type I and type II diabetics should include control of dyslipidemias and control of hyperglycemia and hypertension. Diabetics should be tested annually for lipid disorders with fasting serum cholesterol, triglycerides, and low-density lipoprotein, and high-density lipoprotein cholesterol determinations. The control of hypertension dramatically reduces the rate of progression of retinopathy, nephropathy, cardiovascular disease, and cerebrovascular disease. Blood pressure should be measured in all patients with diabetes mellitus, including children and adolescents at each physical examination or at least every 6 months. Blood pressure should be maintained at less than 140/90 mm Hg in adults or less than the 95th percentile for age- and sex-adjusted norms.

The patient should be asked about signs and symptoms of cerebrovascular disease. A neurologic examination should be done to exclude manifestations of cerebrovascular disease. Noninvasive procedures, including Doppler ultrasound, may significantly aid the diagnosis. Exercise tolerance testing, exercise thallium studies, and gated blood pool scans may help establish the diagnosis of myocardial ischemia.

Peripheral vascular disease should be suspected when patients complain of buttock, calf, or thigh pain that occurs during exercise and is relieved with rest. The diagnosis of peripheral vascular disease can be established with noninvasive Doppler studies. The American Heart Association has recommended regular assessment of ankle/brachial indices in type I diabetics older than 35 years of age. However, sclerotic vessels may lead to falsely increased systolic blood pressure and indeterminate or invalid results. Patients with a decreased index have peripheral vascular disease and coronary artery disease.

HYPOGLYCEMIA

By Richard J. Comi, M.D.
Lebanon, New Hampshire

DEFINITION

Patients think of hypoglycemia as a symptom complex relieved by eating, but the clinician must utilize a definition that identifies pathologic conditions. Clinical hypoglycemia is best defined as a reduction in circulating concentrations of glucose that results in central nervous system dysfunction. In general, clinical hypoglycemia (as defined above) is not seen at glucose concentrations greater than 50 mg/dL. From these considerations, the clinician can derive an updated version of Whipple's classic triad that now defines hypoglycemia as (1) blood glucose less than 50 mg/dL with (2) symptoms of central nervous system dysfunction (confusion, aberrant behavior, drowsiness, coma, seizure) and (3) relief from symptoms after ingestion of nutrients or simple carbohydrates, such as glucose.

INITIAL HISTORY

In practice, the suspicion of clinical hypoglycemia is based on a history of transient episodes of central nervous system dysfunction relieved by food or administration of glucose. These episodes vary from slurred speech and confusion to obtundation and are rapidly relieved by ingesting nutrients. Patients often modify their diet to ward off further episodes; thus, weight gain is common in patients with insulinoma or other chronic hypoglycemic disorders.

Patients often attribute autonomic symptoms, such as palpitations, tachycardia, anxiety, tremulousness, pallor (adrenergic), and sweating (parasympathetic), to hypoglycemia. However, hypoglycemia is only one of several causes of these autonomic symptoms, which are seldom diagnostic.

DETAILED HISTORY AND EXAMINATION

The three basic diagnostic categories of hypoglycemia (see Tables 1 to 3) are (1) drug-induced, (2) postprandial, and (3) preprandial (fasting) hypoglycemia. These categories are distinguished by the history; the physical examination is of limited value in the differential diagnosis of hypoglycemia. Examination of the liver may reveal signs of fulminant hepatitis (tenderness and hepatomegaly), acute

Table 1. Drug-Induced Hypoglycemia

Frequently associated
Insulin
Sulfonylureas
Pentamidine
Toxins
Alcohol
Rodenticides (Vacor)
Occasionally associated
Beta-blockers
Aspirin
Antimalarial agents

hepatic congestion due to congestive heart failure (hepatojugular reflux and hepatomegaly), or metastatic liver disease.

DRUG-INDUCED HYPOGLYCEMIA

Insulin

Medications, especially insulin, are the most common causes of clinical hypoglycemia (Table 1). Attempts to achieve a near-euglycemic state in the treatment of diabetes cause a significant number of cases of hypoglycemia. In the Diabetes Complications and Control Trial (DCCT), the annual incidence of hypoglycemia that required intervention was 19 episodes per 100 patients attempting to achieve conventional control (average blood glucose around 200 mg/dL) and 62 episodes per 100 patients trying to achieve excellent glycemic control (average glucose 120 mg/dL). Hypoglycemic events due to insulin therapy are typically caused by mismatching the kinetics of subcutaneous insulin with the timing of diet and exercise. Common scenarios include the injection of preprandial insulin followed by delayed ingestion of a meal, participation in unplanned strenuous exercise after a large dose of intermediate or long-acting insulin, or failure to increase nutrient intake in the hours following strenuous exercise. Accidental intramuscular or intravenous injection of insulin may cause rapid absorption of an intermediate-acting dose and rapid onset of hypoglycemia. Finally, patients who use insulin obtained from animals may have the kinetics of insulin action altered. The binding of animal insulin to circulating antibodies may prolong its duration of action and render insulin pharmacokinetics less predictable, this unpredictability increasing the risk of hypoglycemia.

Patients who maintain excellent glycemic control may have decreased ability to detect hypoglycemic symptoms. Many patients find that their warning symptoms are altered when they switch from animal to human insulin, but there is no convincing evidence that human insulin induces hypoglycemia unawareness. Rarely, patients with autonomic neuropathy from diabetes do not detect hypoglycemia until symptoms are quite severe (true hypoglycemia unawareness).

Early-morning (2 AM) hypoglycemia may occur if intermediate insulins (NPH insulin and Lente insulin) are injected at 5 PM. Since hypoglycemia induces a hormonal response that raises the blood glucose concentration (glucagon, catecholamines, cortisol, and growth hormone), and patients with diabetes cannot secrete insulin to modulate the counter-regulatory response, a hyperglycemic overshoot may follow a hypoglycemic episode. For example, one sign of nocturnal hypoglycemia is increased morning glycemia despite increased doses of evening insulin. This has been called the Somogyi effect.

Sulfonylureas

Sulfonylureas increase the amount of insulin released in response to a given stimulus to insulin secretion. In large doses, especially with prolonged fasting, simultaneous alcohol use, or exercise, these medications may cause hypoglycemia.

Alcohol

In the fasting state, the liver is the sole supplier of glucose to the circulation. To synthesize glucose, the enzymes of the hepatocyte require nicotinamide-adenine dinucleotide (NAD). NAD is also used in the metabolism of alcohol and may be depleted by acute use of alcohol, which, in turn, impairs hepatic glucose production. Severe hypoglycemia, manifested by coma, may accompany acute alcohol ingestion, especially in the malnourished state. Malnourished alcoholics may present with coma resulting from profound, prolonged hypoglycemia.

Other Drugs

Pentamidine, in the intravenous or aerosolized forms, is used for prophylaxis and treatment of *Pneumocystis carinii* infections. Pentamidine is toxic to beta islet cells, and as many as 33 per cent of patients receiving pentamidine may experience hypoglycemia due to insulin leakage from these damaged beta cells. Antimalarial agents also cause hypoglycemia. The rodenticide Vacor is a notorious islet cell poison that causes a biphasic pattern of hypoglycemia followed by hyperglycemia. Other commonly used drugs occasionally associated with hypoglycemia include beta-blocking agents and aspirin.

POSTPRANDIAL HYPOGLYCEMIA

If drug-induced hypoglycemia is unlikely, the clinician should determine the longest fasting period of the day. If symptoms do not occur at the end of that period, the patient's symptoms are considered postprandial in timing. Many patients describe feelings of lassitude, sleepiness, weakness, or mild confusion as well as loss of consciousness within 4 hours of a meal. These symptoms are often relieved by eating and constitute a postprandial syndrome (Table 2). However, this syndrome has only rarely been associated with hypoglycemia. Postprandial hypoglycemia most often occurs in patients with prior gastric resection or bypass. In these patients, rapid transit of simple carbohydrates to the jejunum may cause excessive release of insulin.

Although hypoglycemia is unlikely, the postprandial syndrome should be carefully investigated. Disability, poor job performance, and risk of injury may result from the postprandial syndrome. Most patients believe that the syndrome is due to hypoglycemia, and they can be most effec-

Table 2. Causes of the Postprandial Syndrome

Chronic gastritis
Peptic ulcer disease
Dumping syndromes after intestinal surgery
True postprandial hypoglycemia (very rare)
After gastric bypass
Billroth type II
Bariatric surgery
During a 75–100 g oral glucose tolerance test
Idiopathic

tively counseled and treated if the diagnosis is considered. The most useful diagnostic test is a meal tolerance test. The patient should consume a meal that typically brings on the symptoms. Blood glucose should be measured every 30 minutes for 4 hours. Fingerstick glucose measurements are appropriate for concentrations greater than 60 mg/dL, but the patient should be observed throughout the test period. A blood sugar less than 50 mg/dL, with recurrence of the patient's symptoms, is diagnostic, but the diagnosis should be confirmed by glucose measurement in a standard laboratory. A liquid mixed meal (e.g., Sustacal) may also be administered. The possibility of hypoglycemia should *not* be evaluated with an oral glucose tolerance test. Ingestion of 75 to 100 g of glucose is not relevant to typical mealtime carbohydrate ingestion, and as many as 16 per cent of asymptomatic individuals have a hypoglycemic response to oral glucose loading.

An alternative approach to postprandial syndrome is to reassure patients and treat them first with frequent small meals. This approach may be more appropriate for the patient who values relief from symptoms more than a specific diagnosis. Virtually all cases of postprandial syndrome respond well to frequent small feedings containing moderate amounts of fat.

The postprandial syndrome may accompany peptic ulcer disease or chronic gastritis. Many of these patients have a prior history of peptic ulcer, and a trial of an H_2-blocking agent may provide total relief.

FASTING HYPOGLYCEMIA

Symptoms of neuroglycopenia that occur more than 6 hours after the last ingestion of food should raise the suspicion of fasting hypoglycemia (Table 3). Neuroglycopenic symptoms indicate an interruption of the glucose supply to the brain and are virtually always associated with a clinically significant condition. There are rare reports of hypoglycemia following very strenuous exercise in otherwise normal individuals, but this must be a diagnosis of exclusion. The two major pathophysiologic mechanisms that render hepatic gluconeogenesis inadequate are intrinsic hepatic dysfunction and excessive insulin effect on the liver.

Hepatic Dysfunction

Generalized hepatic dysfunction can result from fulminant hepatitis or severe passive hepatic congestion due to right-sided heart failure. Enzyme defects that impair the ability of the liver to release glucose are associated with hypoglycemia in children. A more subtle cause is an acquired decrease in the concentrations of the enzymes required for gluconeogenesis. The enzymes are regulated to some degree by growth hormone, thyroid hormone, and cortisol, and severe or multiple deficiencies may result in the inability of the liver to meet the glucose requirements of the brain.

Table 3. Causes of Fasting Hypoglycemia

- Hepatic dysfunction
  - Acute general hepatic dysfunction
    - Fulminant hepatitis
    - Acute right-sided congestive heart failure
  - Inborn errors of gluconeogenesis
  - Combined or severe endocrine deficiencies
- Excessive insulin effect
  - Insulinoma
  - Surreptitious insulin use
  - Surreptitious sulfonylurea use
  - Tumor-associated hypoglycemia
  - Agonistic antibodies to the insulin receptor

Excessive Insulin Effect

Insulin is an important inhibitor of hepatic gluconeogenesis. Excessive insulin effect in the liver may result from high concentrations of endogenous insulin released from an insulinoma, high concentrations of exogenous insulin (in the absence of diabetes therapy) due to factitious use of insulin, or the actions of insulinomimetic antibodies or other substances that bind to and activate the insulin receptor. The autoantibody syndromes are exceedingly rare and are usually associated with other autoimmune diseases, such as systemic lupus erythematosus. Tumors may synthesize insulinomimetic hypoglycemic factors, usually insulin-like growth factor 2 (IGF-2). These tumors are rare, typically sarcomas, and often very large.

The evaluation of fasting hypoglycemia consists of (1) documenting clinical hypoglycemia in the fasting state, (2) demonstrating that inappropriate insulin is or is not present at the time of hypoglycemia, and, if insulin is present, (3) determining whether the insulin is exogenous or endogenous.

The determination of the source of inappropriate insulin is best accomplished by an observed fast in which hypoglycemia with neuroglycopenic symptoms is produced and a study of insulin and C peptide is undertaken. C peptide is a marker for endogenous insulin secretion because this peptide is cleaved from proinsulin during insulin synthesis but is retained and secreted in the same secretory granule as insulin. The clinician should have the patient begin the fast at the time of day that symptoms are most likely to occur. Most patients can readily identify this timing. In general, perform the test in the hospital under controlled conditions. Ninety to ninety-five per cent of insulinomas can be detected by symptomatic episodes within 48 hours. At the start of the fast, measure serum glucose and insulin and perform a baseline neurologic examination, with documentation of an easily tested cognitive task, such as serial sevens or counting backward. Repeat the blood tests every 4 hours, or until the serum glucose concentration falls below 50 mg/dL. At that point, measure the blood glucose concentration and perform simple cognitive testing hourly until neuroglycopenia is documented and the blood glucose concentration is less than 40 mg/dL. At that point, obtain at least two blood samples for glucose, insulin, and C peptide measurement. Then terminate the fast.

The data from the observed fast can help the clinician sort out the differential diagnosis in a logical sequence (Table 4). Interpretation is based on the fact that the patient has spontaneously developed symptoms as well as a blood glucose concentration less than 40 mg/dL. Data from this pathologic state can be interpreted directly. Inappropriate insulin secretion is always due to islet cell tumor; there are no documented cases of ectopic insulin secretion. If the serum insulin value is greater than 6 μU/mL, the differential diagnosis is insulinoma or factitious hypoglycemia. If the insulin value is increased but the C peptide concentration is suppressed, the patient has injected exogenous insulin. If the insulin and C peptide values are increased, the patient most likely has an insulinoma. This approach is summarized in Table 4. If the serum insulin value is less than 6 μU/mL, insulinoma is typically excluded and hepatic disease or rare syndromes of autoanti-

Table 4. Interpretation of Test Results of the Observed Fast Terminated for Glucose <40 mg/dL or at 48 Hours

	Diagnosis				
	No Fasting Hypoglycemia	***Possible Insulinoma, Repeat Fast for 72 Hours***	***Insulinoma***	***Surreptitious Insulin Injection***	***Insulin-Like Substance (Tumor-Associated or Antibody)***
Glucose	Never <40 mg/dL	40–50 mg/dL	<40 mg/dL	<40 mg/dL	<40 mg/dL
Insulin	<6 μU/mL	<6 but detectable	>6 μU/mL	>6 μU/mL	<6 μU/mL
Insulin trend*	Progressive decline	Initial decline, then stable for hours	Initial decline, stable for hours	Sudden increase, slow decline	Progressive decline
C peptide	Below lower limit of normal	Normal range	Greater than normal range	Below lower limit of normal	Below lower limit of normal

*The pattern of insulin concentrations over the time of the fast.

bodies or tumor-associated hypoglycemia should be considered. On occasion, the pattern of insulin secretion while the blood sugar is falling is helpful; the insulin and glucose concentrations normally fall in parallel, whereas in insulinoma the insulin concentrations are maintained while glucose decreases.

There are several other tests for the diagnosis of insulinoma. In the C-peptide suppression test, C peptide is measured in serum, then insulin is injected (0.2 U/kg) to induce a rapid fall in blood glucose to less than 50 mg/dL. The serum C-peptide concentration is measured again, and intravenous glucose is given to avoid symptomatic hypoglycemia. Suppression of C peptide by more than 50 per cent eliminates insulinoma as a cause of hypoglycemia. Increased serum concentrations of proinsulin after an overnight fast or during a hypoglycemic event also suggest insulinoma, but these measurements are not diagnostic. The tolbutamide tolerance test, in which tolbutamide, a sulfonylurea, is given intravenously to stimulate excessive insulin release from an insulinoma, is a sensitive and specific test in experienced centers, but the risk of precipitous hypoglycemia exists.

Factitious hypoglycemia must *always* be considered during these evaluations. This condition, usually due to surreptitious insulin injection, can be evaluated by measuring serum insulin and C-peptide concentrations. In the past, antibodies to animal insulins were measured, but the increased use of human insulins has decreased the usefulness of antibody measurements. Rarely, high concentrations of insulin and C peptide at the time of hypoglycemia are due to surreptitious sulfonylurea ingestion. When such suspicion is high, the urine should be screened for specific sulfonylurea compounds. The important risk factors for factitious hypoglycemia are a history of depression, a history of diabetes or a family member with diabetes, a background in the health professions, or employment in a medical setting.

After the diagnosis has been made, insulinomas must be localized to avoid the risks of extensive surgical exploration of the pancreas. Insulinomas are multicentric in 10 per cent of cases and malignant in another 10 per cent. The size of the tumor does not correlate with the severity of the hypoglycemic syndrome, and the tumors are frequently quite small.

Pancreatic subselective arteriography identifies the location of an insulinoma in 90 per cent of patients. If the tumor is not identified, regional calcium infusions can be given at the time of arteriography, with collection of venous drainage in the hepatic vein. A dramatic increase in insulin concentration after infusion of a region with calcium indicates that the insulinoma is in that region. Finally, subselective transhepatic portal venous sampling can identify the region of the pancreas that harbors an insulinoma in 95 per cent of patients.

Multiple endocrine neoplasia type I is a syndrome in which parathyroid adenomas, islet cell tumors, and pheochromocytomas all may occur. In these patients, the insulinomas are often multicentric. Careful palpation of the entire pancreas at the time of surgery is important for identifying multicentric tumors in these patients and should be done in all cases.

In many ways, the evaluation of hypoglycemia is a paradigm for clinical logic based on detailed pathophysiology. When an organized approach is coupled with effective communication, the evaluation should be rewarding to both physician and patient.

HYPERURICEMIA AND GOUT

By Daniel J. McCarty, M.D.,
and Geraldine M. McCarthy, M.D.
Milwaukee, Wisconsin

Hyperuricemia refers to an increased serum urate concentration, typically measured by the specific uricase method. In many laboratories, hyperuricemia refers to urate concentrations that exceed an established mean by more than two standard deviations. The mean urate concentration for men typically exceeds that for women. Conversely, some clinicians prefer to define hyperuricemia as any concentration that exceeds the solubility of urate in plasma, which at pH 7.4 and 37°C is 0.4 mmol/L. This definition fits all ages and both genders. The term asymptomatic hyperuricemia describes the state in which the serum urate concentration is abnormally high but symptoms have not occurred. Hyperuricemia is not gout. Gout is a syndrome resulting from tissue deposition of monosodium urate crystals. This condition is characterized by hyperuricemia; recurrent attacks of acute arthritis; monosodium urate crystals in synovial fluid; accumulation of potentially destructive crystalline aggregates in tissue, called tophi; uric acid urolithiasis; and, less frequently, renal impairment (gouty nephropathy). Synonyms include crystalline arthritis and podagra (from the Greek, meaning foot seizure). Importantly, the term podagra has also been applied to disorders such as calcific periarthritis or pseudogout.

Excessive production and/or diminished renal excretion of uric acid contributes to the development of hyperuricemia and resultant crystal deposition. Patients with gout have one or both of these abnormalitites in primary and secondary hyperuricemia. The vast majority of patients with gout exhibit defective renal tubular secretion of uric acid.

The term primary hyperuricemia refers to increased serum urate concentrations caused by abnormal uric acid metabolism not associated with another acquired disorder. Gout in such cases is called primary gout. Rare patients with gout have specific genetic defects that cause overactivity of phosphoribosylpyrophosphate synthetase or the absence of hypoxanthine guanine phosphoribosyltransferase(HGPRTase), leading to uric acid overproduction. When HGPRTase deficiency is complete, the Lesch-Nyhan syndrome occurs in childhood and is characterized by spasticity, choreoathetosis, mental retardation, and compulsive self-mutilation. Individuals with partial deficiency of HGPRTase do not typically experience neurologic problems but may experience gout and/or uric acid urolithiasis at a young age.

Secondary hyperuricemia arises when a primary disease or process produces hyperuricemia. Individuals with symptoms of gout under these circumstances are said to have secondary gout. This type of gout most often occurs in the myeloproliferative diseases associated with increased cell and nucleic acid turnover, particularly polycythemia rubra vera and multiple myeloma. Secondary gout occurs less commonly with chronic leukemia, hemolytic anemia, and lymphoma. It can also occur in psoriasis, sarcoidosis, Down syndrome, and glycogen storage disease as well as after strenuous exertion or strict dieting. Lead-induced toxic nephropathy causes markedly diminished renal tubular urate secretion. Lead-associated arthritis is called saturnine gout. In some parts of the United States, moonshine liquor produced with a makeshift still containing lead solder is the leading cause of gout. Chronic diuretic use as well as low doses of aspirin, nicotinic acid, pyrazinamide, ethambutol, and cyclosporine have the potential to reduce renal excretion of uric acid and may result in gout. Consumption and metabolism of quantities of absolute ethanol in excess of 60 mL per day causes increased blood lactate concentrations, which blocks renal uric acid excretion and increases purine nucleotide production by the liver. Finally, intense cellular destruction by cytotoxic agents or radiation therapy may lead to overproduction of uric acid and symptoms of gout.

Epidemiologic studies have confirmed associations between both hyperuricemia and gout and hypertension, atherosclerosis, obesity, hyperlipidemia, and calcium urolithiasis. Patients with gout frequently have a family history of gout.

PRESENTING SYMPTOMS AND SIGNS

Acute arthritis is the most common early clinical manifestation of gout. Gouty arthritis typically occurs in middle-aged men, with a peak incidence in the fourth to sixth decades of life. The metatarsophalangeal joint of the first toe is involved most often and is affected at some time in 75 per cent of patients. The ankle, midfoot, and knee are also commonly involved. Wrist or finger joints are less often the site of early attacks. Heberden's nodes may develop superimposed gouty arthritis. The shoulder, hips, and joints of the axial skeleton are seldom involved with acute gouty synovitis but may be the sites of attack in patients with advanced tophaceous gout and, for reasons that remain unclear, in gout associated with organ transplantation. Post-transplant gouty arthritis is often provoked by cyclosporine therapy, which irreversibly inhibits renal tubular secretion of urate. The temporomandibular joint is least likely to be involved in gout.

The first episode of acute gouty arthritis typically involves the first metatarsophalangeal joint and often occurs during the night. The patient awakens with dramatic, unexplained joint pain and swelling. Pain is often first noticed when the patient's foot is placed on the floor on arising from bed. A vague discomfort or "premonitory twinge" at the site often precedes the acute attack by 2 to 24 hours. Such twinges may be helpful in diagnosis and may help the patient initiate therapy. Pain typically becomes so intense that the weight of even a bed sheet on the affected joint is intolerable. There may be associated chills and low-grade fever. The skin over the affected joint is typically warm, red, and tender. Joint motion is exquisitely painful. The diffuse periarticular erythema is often confused with cellulitis or thrombophlebitis. Early attacks tend to subside spontaneously over 3 to 10 days. The swollen, red skin over the affected joint often desquamates after the acute attack begins to subside. Between acute attacks, the involved joints are usually grossly normal and functional. Because the inflammatory response to monosodium urate crystals is dose-related, less painful "petite" attacks of arthritis occur.

Polyarticular inflammation occurs in 10 to 15 per cent of patients having their first attack, but most patients with more than one inflamed joint have had more prolonged disease and suboptimal management. Although gout is less common in women and its occurrence prior to menopause is rare, women have a higher incidence of polyarticular onset of gout and subsequent polyarticular attacks. Diuretic therapy has a high correlation with gout in postmenopausal women, particularly with the development of tophaceous deposits in osteoarthritic interphalangeal joints of the hands with relatively minor or no inflammation ("impostumous gout").

Acute attacks of gout may have no apparent precipitating cause or may be triggered by a specific recognizable event such as trauma (often trivial), alcohol, drugs, surgical stress, or acute medical illness. Swings in the concentration of serum urate may precede episodes of acute gouty arthritis, especially following treatment with allopurinol, diuretics, or uricosuric drugs. The rapid decrease in serum urate concentrations after an increase caused by consumption of a high purine meal with or without alcohol may also provoke acute gouty arthritis.

COURSE

Four stages can be identified in the evolution of the disease: asymptomatic hyperuricemia, acute gouty arthritis, intercritical gout, and chronic tophaceous gout. Asymptomatic hyperuricemia is a biochemical abnormality that may be noted in the teenage years and continuing thereafter. Documentation of increased uric acid is not, by itself, sufficient reason to begin treatment. The uric acid concentration varies with age, sex, diet, and genetic predisposition. Hyperuricemia can be detected in at least 5 per cent of asymptomatic Americans on at least one occasion during adulthood. An incidence of 13 per cent has been reported in hospitalized adult men. However, fewer than 20 per cent of hyperuricemic individuals develop symptomatic urate crystal deposition. The relatively infrequent occurrence of gout in this population is at least in part due to relatively mild increases in serum urate concentrations in the majority of hyperuricemic individuals and to transient hyperuricemia occurring in response to changes in diet or to ingestion of certain drugs.

The major sources of uric acid in the body are purines derived from de novo synthesis and from metabolism of nucleic acids. The most important stage of purine metabolism leading to the synthesis of uric acid is the final stage, in which the oxidation of hypoxanthine to xanthine and then to uric acid is catalyzed by the enzyme xanthine oxidase.

Serum uric acid concentrations reflect the uric acid miscible pool, which is normally 600 to 1000 mg. This pool turns over once every 24 hours. One third of uric acid is eliminated from the body via the intestinal tract (approximately 150 to 300 mg per day on a low-purine diet). Renal excretion accounts for the other two thirds, usually 300 to 600 mg per day on a low-purine diet. Adding the approximately 300 mg of uric acid consumed daily with an ordinary diet produces a normal urinary excretion of 600 to 900 mg daily. Following complete filtration of urate at the glomerulus, about 98 per cent is resorbed in proximal tubules. Urate is then secreted by the distal tubules, and finally there is postsecretory resorption. Toxic agents, drugs, or disease will alter the renal handling of uric acid. Allopurinol inhibits xanthine oxidase and accelerates the conversion of phosphoribosylpyrophosphate to its ribonucleotide. (Phosphoribosylpyrophosphate drives the first step of de novo purine synthesis.) Probenecid blocks postsecretory resorption of uric acid.

There is no typical pattern of subsequent attacks following the onset of acute gouty arthritis. A second attack may occur many years after the first. In general, the greater the degree of hyperuricemia, the greater the frequency of acute attacks and the development of tophi. Approximately 50 to 60 per cent of untreated patients have tophi within 15 years of their first attack of gout. The passage of uric acid stones precedes the initial attack of acute arthritis in 20 to 25 per cent of patients. Fewer than 1 per cent of patients have tophi at the time of the first attack.

Not all gout is preceded by hyperuricemia. Monosodium urate crystal deposition is temperature-dependent, which is why tophi form in the great toe (temperature 31°C) or in the pinna of the ears, tips of the olecranon, and back of the fingers. At 31°C and a sodium concentration of 140 mmol/L, urate is saturated at 0.27 mmol/L. Acute attacks correlate with a decrease in serum urate concentrations. As many as 25 per cent of patients have normal serum urate concentrations at the time of the acute attack. Some patients with gout never have hyperuricemia if hyperuricemia is defined as any serum concentration of urate exceeding 0.4 mmol/L.

The intervals between attacks constitute the intercritical stage of gout. Initially, the intercritical periods are typically without symptoms or abnormal physical findings. Even during an asymptomatic period, monosodium urate crystals can often be aspirated from previously involved joints or from joints that have never been overtly affected. Monosodium urate crystals have been found in up to 97 per cent of synovial fluid from previously inflamed asymptomatic joints and in 22 per cent of knees that have never been inflamed in patients with untreated hyperuricemia.

Clinically evident subcutaneous tophi are generally first noted after the onset of clinical gout, which is, on the average, about 10 years after the first episode of arthritis. Tophi may eventually occur in as many as 50 per cent of inadequately treated patients. Subcutaneous tophi tend to be apparent only in advanced gout, although microtophi may be present in the synovial membrane even at an early stage. Bony tophi, seen as sharply "punched-out" defects on radiographs, always precede subcutaneous tophi. Bony tophi are generally associated with more frequent and severe episodes of inflammation.

Deforming arthritis can develop from the erosion of cartilage and subchondral bone caused by deposition of monosodium urate crystals and chronic, smoldering inflammation. White, chalky tophaceous material occasionally extrudes spontaneously through the overlying skin. This material can be analyzed by compensated polarized light microscopy for the presence of monosodium urate crystals, or the tophus can be pricked with a needle. *A tophus is never a tophus until its contents have been characterized microscopically and/or chemically.*

PHYSICAL EXAMINATION

The patient with gout is typically an obese, plethoric, garrulous, bibulous, and gluttonous middle-aged man who is unable to bear weight on the involved foot. Initially, the involved joint is only slightly puffy and tender, but within several hours it becomes erythematous and swollen. In a few days, the skin may become purplish and dusky. Motion of the involved joint is unbearable. The patient may have cut a pair of shoes or slippers to relieve the pressure. Articular effusion may be readily detectable in larger joints such as the knee. Redness and swelling extend beyond the anatomic confines of the joint, mimicking cellulitis. The acute attack may last from 2 to 3 weeks, but the site becomes gradually less painful, less swollen, and less sensitive. The skin overlying the site desquamates as the attack subsides. Follow-up attacks are frequently in the same joint or in its contralateral mate.

The olecranon and prepatellar bursae may become enlarged, red, warm, and tender. The adjoining elbow or knee joints move without too much discomfort, whereas gouty or septic arthritis of the elbow or knee joint is markedly painful with joint motion. Once the inflammation subsides, the joint is completely functional and can be used in a normal manner. Frequent recurrences of acute attacks of gout over time may result in persistent joint effusion and reduced range of motion.

COMMON COMPLICATIONS

The most serious musculoskeletal disability is associated with progressive chronic gouty arthritis. Patients with chronic, recurring, acute, or subacute attacks of gout often have persistent joint pain that may be mistaken for pseudogout, calcific periarthritis, septic arthritis, rheumatoid arthritis, inflammatory osteoarthritis, or other forms of joint disease. Avascular necrosis of bone, especially of the head of the femur, occurs more frequently in gout; some episodes relate to chronic excess alcohol consumption.

The most important extraskeletal complication is renal damage. Renal parenchymal disease and renal stones may occur in patients with gout. Some gouty kidneys contain interstitial monosodium urate crystal deposits that may cause sterile inflammation. However, nephropathy seen in patients with gout is associated chiefly with intrinsic renal disease or hypertension. Gout per se rarely causes depression of renal function. Proteinuria and hypertension have been reported in 20 to 40 per cent of patients with gout.

More severe forms of renal disease with nephrosclerosis or reduced renal function are usually associated with aging, more severe hypertension, diabetes mellitus, renal calculi, pyelonephritis, lead nephropathy, or primary overproduction of uric acid. Intrinsic renal disease is itself a cause of hyperuricemia and may account for some cases of gout early in life.

The risk of urolithiasis is increased in gout, and the frequency of stone formation parallels the increase in serum uric acid, the acidity of the urine, and the concentration of urinary uric acid. The prevalence of urolithiasis increased from 11 per cent in patients with urinary uric acid excretion of 300 mg per day to 50 per cent in patients with values greater than 1100 mg per day.* Uric acid stones are usually radiolucent and white or pink, but they sometimes contain sufficient calcium salts to become radiopaque. They are often associated with uric acid gravel. Pink gravel can mimic hematuria ("brick dust urine"). The incidence of calcium stones is also increased in patients with gout, perhaps because calcium oxalate becomes nucleated on sodium urate crystals.

Marked increases in serum urate concentrations, as high as 2.3 to 3.5 mmol/L, may occur in patients with leukemia or lymphoma due to the rapid release of nucleic acids from cells killed by corticosteroids, irradiation, or alkylating agents. Uric acid precipitation in the renal tubules of these patients may lead to urinary obstruction with prolonged oliguria. This phenomenon can be prevented or reversed by the administration of allopurinol.

LABORATORY FINDINGS

Monosodium urate crystals must be demonstrated in joints, bursae, or tophi to establish the diagnosis of gout. Even during asymptomatic periods, monosodium urate crystals can be recovered from many joints. A single drop of fluid is sufficient for the detection of intra- or extracellular rod- or needle-shaped (3 to 20 μm) crystals, which are best seen with a polarizing microscope using a first-order red plate compensator. Monosodium urate crystals are negatively birefringent, appearing bright yellow when their long axis is aligned parallel to the direction of slow vibration of light (marked on the compensator) and blue when their long axis is perpendicular to this direction. Monosodium urate crystals are more frequently detected in fresh joint fluid. In acute attacks, most monosodium urate crystals are seen within neutrophilic leukocytes.

The number of synovial fluid leukocytes, predominantly neutrophils, increases to 8 to 40,000 (mean approximately 20,000) cells/mm^3 in acute gouty arthritis. Rarely, leukocyte counts exceed 50,000 cells/mm^3. Effusions appear cloudy because of the high concentration of cells. Occasionally, masses of crystals produce a thick, pasty, white joint fluid. Infection can coexist with urate crystals; thus, joint fluid cultures should also be obtained if clinically indicated.

The value of serum uric acid measurements in the diagnosis of gouty arthritis is limited. Although more than 95 per cent of patients with gout eventually experience hyperuricemia, serum uric acid concentrations are often normal during attacks of acute gouty arthritis. By contrast, serum urate measurements are useful in following the treatment of hyperuricemia. However, most patients with elevated serum urate concentrations do not have gout.

The leukocyte count is increased in many patients, and the erythrocyte sedimentation rate (ESR) is increased in nearly all patients with acute gout. The erythrocyte sedimentation rate increases 48 to 72 hours after the acute attack has begun. Nearly 10 per cent of patients have a positive test for IgM rheumatoid factor despite a strong negative association between rheumatoid arthritis and gout. The reason for this observation is unknown.

Measurement of uric acid and creatinine in urine collected over 24 hours is valuable in assessing the risk of renal stones, in elucidating the cause of hyperuricemia, and in determining the best treatment. Excretion in urine of more than 900 mg of uric acid per day (on a regular diet) suggests overproduction of uric acid. Diuretics, aspirin, alcohol, or radiographic contrast dyes can alter uric acid excretion for a few days; therefore, these agents should be avoided before and during collection. Colchicine and indomethacin do not interfere with urate excretion. The urine pH is often low (5 to 5.5). This is particularly important in patients in whom renal stones form; an alkaline urine is optimal for uric acid solubility in these patients. Albuminuria occurs in 20 to 40 per cent of patients with gout.

Renal function can be assessed by measuring serum creatinine concentrations and creatinine clearance. Liver function tests should be performed because many antigout medications are hepatotoxic, particularly nonsteroidal anti-inflammatory agents and allopurinol. Liver function should be monitored initially and then monthly during therapy with allopurinol and yearly once the optimal stable dose has been determined.

Finally, the ratio of uric acid to creatinine in urine may suggest a deficiency of HGPRTase. In the complete deficiency syndrome, this ratio exceeds 2; in the partial expression of the abnormality, values exceed 0.75.

DIAGNOSTIC IMAGING PROCEDURES

Gout cannot be definitively diagnosed by radiographs, and they are of no value during the acute attack, showing only soft tissue swelling surrounding the affected joint. However, radiographs can help exclude some conditions that clinically resemble acute gouty arthritis, including septic changes, chondrocalcinosis, and calcific periarthritis. The periarticular tophi of chronic gout produce irregular asymmetric soft tissue swelling.

Intra-articular or periarticular bony erosions may occur in chronic disease. They may be round or oval and surrounded by a sclerotic margin. A thin "overhanging edge" of bone may be seen. Punched-out subcortical cysts may also be seen. Joint spaces (cartilage) are preserved until late in the disease. Scintigraphy using bone-seeking radionuclides shows a marked local increase in uptake by periarticular bone at the site of inflammation induced by monosodium urate crystals. Renal calculi may be demonstrated radiographically in 6 per cent of patients with gout; however, because uric acid stones are radiolucent, contrast dye is required. There is also an increased incidence of radiopaque calcium oxalate stones in patients with gout.

THERAPEUTIC RESPONSE TO COLCHICINE AS AN AID TO DIAGNOSIS

Acute joint inflammation is suppressed in 80 to 90 per cent of patients who receive a full therapeutic dose of colchicine. This drug should be given as early as possible after the acute attack begins. An experienced patient should start treatment within the first hour of the onset of an attack.

*Yu, T.-F., and Gutran, A.B.: Uric acid nephrolithiasis in gout: Predisposing factors. Ann. Intern. Med., 67:1133–1148, 1967.

Despite clinical efficacy, the therapeutic oral administration of colchicine causes gastrointestinal toxicity in nearly all patients. Nausea, vomiting, diarrhea, dehydration, and cramping abdominal pain may be severe. Symptomatic relief is typically noted 6 to 12 hours after the complete therapeutic dose of colchicine is given and progresses over the next 24 to 48 hours. Oral colchicine is usually administered as 0.5-mg tablets taken hourly until one of three end points is reached: (1) relief of pain and inflammation, (2) gastrointestinal toxicity, or (3) the administration of a maximal total dose of 8 mg, assuming normal renal and hepatic function.

Intravenous administration of colchicine avoids gastrointestinal toxicity and is therefore useful in the postoperative patient for whom oral intake is restricted. Following a dose of only 1 mg, blood concentrations of 10^{-6}M are reached. These concentrations are tenfold higher than those achieved by a full therapeutic (and toxic) oral dose. Some patients may experience significant relief of symptoms within 30 minutes of intravenous administration. The drug is intensely irritating locally. Side effects of intravenous colchicine include thrombophlebitis if the drug is not diluted properly and skin sloughing if it is extravasated.

The improper use of colchicine, particularly the intravenous form, has caused serious systemic toxicity and fatality. Excessive colchicine may cause bone marrow suppression, renal failure, disseminated intravascular coagulation, hypocalcemia, cardiopulmonary failure, seizures, and death. Used chronically to prevent acute attacks, oral colchicine is effective in doses of 0.5 to 1.5 mg daily but has been associated with myopathy or peripheral neuropathy. These effects are reversible when the drug is stopped. All reported cases of death, severe toxicity, or neuromuscular disease involved unusually high doses of colchicine, renal insufficiency, advanced age, or the use of both oral and intravenous preparations over a short period.

A single intravenous dose of colchicine should not exceed 2 mg, and the total cumulative dose for an attack should not exceed 4 mg in a 24-hour period. Patients should receive no more colchicine by any route for 7 days after a full intravenous dose. The dose should be reduced by half in the presence of renal or hepatic disease and in patients older than 70 years of age, even in those with apparently normal renal function. Use of intravenous colchicine is contraindicated in the presence of combined renal and hepatic disease, a glomerular filtration rate of less than 10 mL per minute, or extrahepatic biliary obstruction. Intravenous colchicine should never be given if the patient has been taking the drug by mouth.

Patients suffering from pseudogout respond to intravenous colchicine just as patients with gout do; the response of acute attacks of pseudogout to oral colchicine is less predicable than is the response of acute gout.

PITFALLS IN DIAGNOSIS

A clinician may be tempted to think of gout when hyperuricemia is detected and the patient has musculoskeletal symptoms. However, hyperuricemia may be found in many other conditions, and there are many causes of musculoskeletal symptoms besides gout.

Radiocontrast agents may temporarily reduce the serum urate concentration and increase its excretion for 5 to 6 days. Calcium pyrophosphate dihydrate crystal deposition disease (pseudogout) is often associated with episodes of acute arthritis that most often occur in the knees but may involve smaller joints. This condition usually occurs in older patients (more than 70 years). There may be evidence of chronic polyarticular disease. The diagnosis may be suggested by radiographic evidence of chondrocalcinosis and may be confirmed by the presence of calcium pyrophosphate crystals in the synovial fluid aspirated from the inflamed joint. These rhomboidal crystals exhibit weakly positive birefringence under compensated polarized light. Gout and pseudogout may coexist.

Acute attacks of palindromic rheumatism (focal fibrin deposition) causing para- or periarticular inflammation, with associated severe pain, may mimic acute gout. These attacks usually last less than 4 days, disappear completely, and are not associated with hyperuricemia. Joint fluid is rarely present, and if it is obtained crystals are not found.

In a few patients without a history of clinical gout, monosodium urate crystal tophi have been found. Olecranon bursitis in patients with rheumatoid arthritis and rheumatoid nodules may occasionally require differentiation from gout by biopsy or aspiration.

Septic arthritis or cellulitis or acute thrombophlebitis near a joint may suggest acute gouty arthritis, particularly in a patient with a history of gout. Patients with septic arthritis usually have an acutely swollen, painful joint. Joint aspiration with Gram stain and culture should be performed to reveal the causative organism. If there is a question of bacterial infection and gout affecting the same joint concurrently, the joint should be treated as septic until proved otherwise. Acute joint destruction from sepsis, or even death, can thereby be avoided. Traumatic arthritis may be confused with gout, but usually the degree of injury and the history identify the cause.

A recurrence of gouty arthritis often follows inadequate therapy of the acute attack or failure to continue daily prophylactic colchicine or nonsteroidal anti-inflammatory drugs following an acute attack. The initiation of a uricosuric drug (probenecid or sulfinpyrazone) or xanthine oxidase inhibitor (allopurinol) without prophylaxis with colchicine or a nonsteroidal anti-inflammatory drug results in acute gout in most patients. Chronic pain and joint deformity result from chronic gouty arthritis. Such cases may be confused with other chronic forms of arthritis, particularly rheumatoid arthritis, especially if treatment with prednisone is prolonged.

Urate crystals dissolve in formalin, so tissue samples should be fixed in absolute ethanol in preparation for microscopic analysis. After making a crystal-proven diagnosis of gout, at least three intercritical serum urate and creatinine measurements should be obtained. A 24-hour collection of urine from a patient consuming a regular diet should be examined for uric acid and creatinine concentrations. Treatment of hyperuricemia is intended to continue for life and should not be taken lightly. Common associated abnormalities such as obesity, hypertension, alcoholism, hypertriglyceridemia, and hypercholesterolemia should be identified and treated as well.

IRON STORAGE DISORDERS

By James C. Barton, M.D.
Birmingham, Alabama

SYNONYMS OF IRON STORAGE DISORDERS

Synonyms of hemochromatosis include hereditary hemochromatosis, familial hemochromatosis, idiopathic he-

This work was supported by Southern Iron Disorders Center and Southeastern Chapter of Iron Overload Diseases Association, Inc., Birmingham, AL.

mochromatosis, and HLA-linked autosomal recessive iron loading. A synonym for African iron overload is Bantu siderosis. Synonyms for neonatal hemochromatosis include neonatal iron storage disease and perinatal hemochromatosis. A synonym for cerebrohepatorenal syndrome is Zellweger syndrome. A synonym for hereditary tyrosinemia is hypermethioninemia.

HEMOCHROMATOSIS

Definition

Hemochromatosis is a disorder of metabolism that increases intestinal iron absorption beyond that required to replace the body's unavoidable losses of iron. Physiologic excretory mechanisms for iron are limited, and the increased iron absorption in hemochromatosis continues even after body iron content becomes increased. Consequently, hemochromatosis causes the accumulation of excess iron in the liver, synovium and cartilage, heart, pancreas, anterior pituitary gland, skin, and many other organs and tissues. Hemochromatosis is an inherited disorder that is transmitted as an autosomal recessive trait. The hemochromatosis gene (or genes) has been mapped through linkage analysis to the human leukocyte antigen (HLA) class I region (near the HLA-A locus) on the short arm of chromosome 6. However, the hemochromatosis gene and its abnormal product have not been identified. The clinical expression of hemochromatosis is largely due to iron overload, with consequent organ damage, and usually occurs only in homozygotes. Further, most homozygotes eventually exhibit manifestations of iron overload. However, occasional heterozygotes may also have an increased body iron burden.

Frequency

The frequency of homozygosity for the hemochromatosis allele in the general white population is about 5 in 1000 persons. Approximately 13 per cent of whites are heterozygotes for the hemochromatosis gene. Thus, hemochromatosis is among the most common autosomal recessive disorders in humans.

Signs and Symptoms

Most patients who are ascertained to be hemochromatosis homozygotes are diagnosed in routine clinical practice. In these persons, symptoms are common and are almost entirely attributable to iron overload. The most common of these symptoms include weakness or lethargy (62 per cent of patients); arthralgias (52 per cent of patients); abdominal pain (37 per cent of patients); palpitations or heart failure (33 per cent of patients); impotence, loss of libido, or premature menopause (32 per cent of patients); and weight loss greater than 10 per cent of normal body weight (30 per cent of patients). When hemochromatosis homozygotes are identified by routine screening of apparently healthy individuals, more than three quarters of them are asymptomatic. This high fraction of asymptomatic persons is due to the ability of screening iron parameters to identify hemochromatosis in younger persons, before iron overload occurs.

In routine clinical practice, hepatomegaly is the most common abnormal physical finding (47 per cent of patients) in homozygotes. Others include arthropathy (51 per cent of patients), particularly of the second and third metacarpophalangeal joints and knees; cutaneous hyperpigmentation (60 per cent of patients), usually of a tan or gray hue due to excess melanin production and iron deposition, respectively; cardiac arrhythmia or congestive heart failure (16 per cent of patients); testicular atrophy (29 per cent of patients); and decreased facial hair. Men with hemochromatosis have, on average, two and a half times more iron stores than do female homozygotes. Consequently, men who are hemochromatosis homozygotes often have more prominent symptoms and physical abnormalities from iron overload than do women. Abnormal physical findings are unusual in hemochromatosis homozygotes who have been identified as part of population screening studies.

Laboratory Diagnosis

Serum Tests of Iron Stores

Three measures of body iron stores are readily available in most clinical laboratories. They are the serum iron concentration, the per cent saturation of transferrin (serum iron concentration ÷ total serum iron binding capacity), and the serum ferritin concentration. Although normal values for these parameters vary among laboratories, typically the serum iron concentration is less than 32 μmol/L; transferrin saturation is less than 50 per cent; and, in adults, serum ferritin concentration is less than 325 μg/L in men and less that 125 μg/L in women. The diagnosis of hemochromatosis and the relative degree of iron overload can be determined by measuring these parameters.

Transferrin Saturation

Increased saturation of transferrin is the earliest indicator of the abnormal homozygous genotype and is nearly always due to increased serum iron concentrations. Increased transferrin saturation is often detected in young homozygotes (including children) prior to accumulation of excessive body iron. A transferrin saturation greater than 60 per cent strongly suggests the diagnosis of hemochromatosis. A second transferrin saturation above 60 per cent makes the diagnosis of hemochromatosis even more likely. More than 90 per cent of hemochromatosis homozygotes have repeated transferrin saturation values greater than 60 per cent in males or greater than 50 per cent in females. Occasionally, homozygotes have normal (or subnormal) serum iron concentrations and transferrin saturation values during prolonged fasting, iron deficiency, or acute or chronic infectious, inflammatory, or neoplastic illnesses associated with an increased erythrocyte sedimentation rate. Children and young adults tested prior to the accumulation of excess body iron may also have a normal serum iron concentration and transferrin saturation.

Serum Ferritin Concentration

Approximately 70 to 80 per cent of adults with homozygous hemochromatosis identified in routine clinical practice have increased serum ferritin concentrations. In young homozygotes who are followed for several years, the serum ferritin concentration usually rises to greater than normal. In patients of all ages, the serum ferritin concentration correlates well with hepatic iron stores measured by atomic absorption spectrometry or semiquantified by histologic grading of Prussian blue–stained biopsy specimens.

Liver Enzyme Studies

Increased serum concentrations of aspartate aminotransferase (AST, serum glutamic-oxaloacetic transaminase [SGOT]) and alanine aminotransferase (ALT, serum glutamic-pyruvic transaminase [SGPT]) are frequently noted in patients with hemochromatosis. Although the enzyme concentrations may be 2 to 10 times greater than normal values, the concentrations are only slightly increased in many patients and do not correlate with the extent of hepatic iron overload. The serum concentrations of alkaline phosphatase, γ-glutamyl transferase, and bilirubin are typically unremarkable but may be increased in a few patients with advanced hepatic iron overload. When end-stage renal failure accompanies hemochromatosis, jaundice, hyperbilirubinemia, hypoproteinemia, hypoprothrombinemia, and ascites appear.

Liver Biopsy

Percutaneous liver biopsy should be performed when there is a markedly increased transferrin saturation and serum ferritin concentration accompanied by hepatomegaly and/or increased serum concentrations of hepatic enzymes. Liver tissue can then be studied microscopically to assess its general architecture (hematoxylin-eosin stain), fibrosis or cirrhosis (trichrome stain), hepatocellular necrosis or parenchymal collapse (reticulin stain), and ferric iron content (Prussian blue stain–Perks stain–acid ferrocyanide stain). Whenever sufficient liver tissue is available, its iron content should be measured by atomic absorption spectrometry (see hepatic iron index further on). Iron in hepatocytes is graded microscopically on a scale of 0 to 4+ (normal, 0 to 1+). Additional iron may also be visualized in Kupffer's cells and bile ductule cells. Adult hemochromatosis homozygotes nearly always have stainable iron of 2+ to 4+ in hepatocytes. Cirrhosis is present in many homozygotes if clinical symptoms are present at diagnosis and may be expected more frequently in persons with heavy ethanol consumption or evidence of hepatitis B or C infection. Some young homozygotes have normal stainable iron (grade 0 to 1+) in hepatocytes but may accumulate an excessive amount of iron over a period of years. Therefore, in patients with a persistent, unexplained increased transferrin saturation who do not have evidence of hepatopathy, the value of liver biopsy in the diagnostic evaluation is less certain. The diagnosis of hemochromatosis in these patients should be accepted without liver biopsy and therapeutic phlebotomy initiated.

Hepatic Iron Index

When the quantitative hepatic iron content is adjusted for age, a clinically useful index results:

$$\text{hepatic iron index} = (\mu\text{mol Fe/g dry weight}) \div \text{age in years}$$

Typically, normal individuals have an index of 1.1 or less; those with alcoholic liver disease have an index of 1.7 or less; hemochromatosis heterozygotes have an index of 1.9 or less; and hemochromatosis heterozygotes have an index of 1.9 or greater. Diagnostic use of the index is valid only for white individuals without significantly increased dietary, medicinal, or transfusional iron intake. The index may give misleading results in persons who have other genetic or acquired disorders that increase iron absorption independent of the hemochromatosis gene or in hemochromatosis homozygotes who have lost significant quantities of blood from community blood donation, therapeutic phlebotomy, menstruation, childbearing, lactation, or pathologic blood loss.

HLA Immunophenotyping

One or more HLA-A3 alloantigens is detectable in approximately 60 to 75 per cent of hemochromatosis patients. However, histocompatibility antigen testing is not required for diagnosis or population screening, and the specific HLA haplotypes present in hemochromatosis pedigrees vary from family to family. The test is expensive in most laboratories. In a few families, HLA typing can be useful within a family study to identify very young siblings who have the same two HLA haplotypes as the affected sibling and thus will experience iron overload in the future. However, the critical diagnostic information can be obtained by repeated analysis of serum transferrin and serum ferritin concentrations in the siblings of hemochromatosis patients at age 15 years, 20 years, 25 years, and so on. This type of methodical, orderly follow-up will help the physician make the diagnosis of hemochromatosis and iron overload in family members at increased risk.

Molecular Genetic Testing

Because hemochromatosis is a genetic disorder in which the approximate chromosomal location of the mutation is known (short arm of chromosome 6 near the HLA loci), cloning of the gene (or genes) and identification of its structure should eventually lead to a valid test for the abnormal DNA responsible for this disorder.

Such testing would permit precise identification of homozygotes and heterozygotes, identification of hemochromatosis gene variants and, possibly, the development of nongenetic tests for the hemochromatosis gene product. Although microsatellite probes show promise as molecular genetic reagents for hemochromatosis, this type of evaluation for hemochromatosis has not achieved sufficient reliability for routine clinical practice.

Radiographic Detection of Iron Overload

The physical properties of iron deposited in certain iron-loaded organs permit visualization of this iron burden in some patients by appropriate computed tomography (CT) or magnetic resonance imaging (MRI) techniques. This phenomenon is especially pronounced in the liver and the anterior pituitary gland, but it is occasionally observed in the thyroid gland, pancreas, synovium, or other locations. However, these radiographic methods are relatively insensitive to mild or moderate degrees of iron overload, may yield false-positive or false-negative results in coexisting disease states, and may provide little histologic and quantitative data (e.g., those obtained by liver biopsy). Altogether, these radiographic techniques should be reserved for special circumstances in selected patients rather than employed as routine evaluation tools.

Complications Associated With Hemochromatosis

Hepatic Cirrhosis

Approximately 20 per cent of hemochromatosis homozygotes who are identified in routine clinical practice have hepatic cirrhosis. This complication is almost always accompanied by other common manifestations of iron overload and induces physical and laboratory findings common to hepatic cirrhosis of many causes. In patients with obvious evidence of portal hypertension, liver biopsy is relatively contraindicated. Other findings characteristic of hemochromatosis and iron overload should be sought in these patients to establish the cause of cirrhosis and provide a rational basis for treatment. Hemochromatosis homozygotes who exhibit heavy ethanol intake or active hepatitis B or C infection commonly acquire hepatic cirrhosis at an earlier age and with less hepatic iron burden than do other hemochromatosis homozygotes.

Hepatoma

Primary liver cancer (hepatocellular carcinoma, primary intrahepatic cholangiocarcinoma) develops commonly in advanced iron overload associated with hemochromatosis and is nearly always associated with hepatic cirrhosis. Approximately 1 per cent of hemochromatosis homozygotes who are diagnosed in routine clinical practice present with primary liver cancer. Approximately one third of homozygotes with hepatic cirrhosis will eventually acquire primary liver cancer. These malignancies, which are often multifocal, are commonly heralded by rapid worsening of malaise, weight loss, progressive hepatomegaly, abdominal pain, loss of muscle mass, jaundice, hyperbilirubinemia, and ascites. The occurrence of portal vein thrombosis is sometimes the initial indicator of the presence of hepatoma. Approximately 40 per cent of these primary liver cancers produce relatively large amounts of alpha-fetoprotein. However, multicentric hepatomas often do not cause a marked increase in plasma alpha-fetoprotein concentrations and may be difficult to detect by computed tomography.

Diabetes Mellitus

Diabetes mellitus, either insulin-dependent or independent, is present in approximately one quarter of symptomatic homozygotes but usually does not result from heavy iron overload of the pancreatic islet cells alone. First, diabetes mellitus and hemochromatosis segregate independently as genetic traits. Second, patients with hemochromatosis who have a relative with diabetes mellitus are much more likely to acquire diabetes mellitus than are patients without a positive family history. End-organ vascular and neurologic complications typical of diabetes mellitus occur in some patients with hemochromatosis.

Hypogonadism

Hypogonadism occurs in approximately one third of symptomatic men with hemochromatosis but is much less frequent in women. The usual cause of hypogonadism is iron infiltration and fibrosis of the anterior pituitary gland with destruction of gonadotrophin-secreting cells. This results in decreased plasma concentrations of luteinizing hormone, follicle-stimulating hormone, testosterone, and dihydrotestosterone (secondary hypogonadotrophic hypogonadism). In males, testicular atrophy and hypotestosteronemia occur consequent to the loss of gonadotrophic hormones. Impotence frequently develops. Midline structures that are sensitive to stimulation by plasma dihydrotestosterone (midline facial hair, pubic hair, and the prostate gland) undergo atrophic or involutional changes, including loss of moustache and beard, a loss in pubic hair density and distribution, and shrinkage of the prostate gland. In females, amenorrhea, atrophy of breasts and genitals, and loss of pubic hair occur.

Thyroid Disease

Hypothyroidism or hyperthyroidism occurs in about 5 per cent of hemochromatosis homozygotes. In some cases, thyroid-stimulating hormone concentrations are low, implying an effect of iron deposition in the anterior pituitary gland. In other cases, excessive deposition of iron occurs in the thyroid gland itself.

Panhypopituitarism

Diffuse pituitary failure caused by iron overload occurs in approximately 3 per cent of individuals with symptomatic hemochromatosis. This causes a loss of multiple trophic hormones such as gonadotrophins, thyroid-stimulating hormone, and adrenocorticotrophic hormone. The diagnosis of panhypopituitarism can be verified by finding markedly decreased plasma concentrations of the trophic hormones, serum thyroxine, plasma testosterone, fasting plasma cortisol as well as decreased amounts of plasma 11-deoxycortisol following administration of metyrapone.

Syndrome of Cardiomyopathy and Endocrine Failure

A catastrophic syndrome of rapidly progressive cardiomyopathy and hypogonadism occurs in some young homozygotes, usually between the ages of 15 and 35 years. Caused by massive iron overload, this syndrome is usually fatal unless the diagnosis of iron overload is made, and aggressive, prolonged phlebotomy is started soon after the symptoms and signs of illness occur. The same syndrome can occur in patients who undergo chronic transfusion with massive iron overload.

Arthritis

Arthropathy occurs in two thirds of symptomatic patients. Radiographs of the metacarpophalangeal joints show decreased joint space, periarticular mineral loss, and subperiosteal bone resorption or cyst formation. The second and third metacarpophalangeal joints and proximal interphalangeal joints are most commonly affected, and this involvement is usually more pronounced on the dominant hand. Involvement of these or other joints in the hand sometimes suggests the diagnosis of rheumatoid arthritis, but the rheumatoid factor assay is nearly always normal. Radiographs of knees, hips, or other diarthrodial joints sometimes reveal chondrocalcinosis, and acute episodes of pseudogout can occur, especially in the knees. The shoulders, wrists, ankles, and temporomandibular joints are infrequently involved with hemochromatotic arthropathy. The expression of hemochromatotic arthropathy may be more pronounced in patients who have an independently inherited tendency to develop Heberden's and/or Bouchard's nodes or in those in whom certain occupational or avocational maneuvers increase joint trauma. In a patient thought to have "seronegative rheumatoid arthritis" with enlarged metacarpophalangeal joints or in persons with degenerative arthritis of the hip or knee (with or without chondrocalcinosis), hemochromatosis should be considered as a diagnostic possibility. Although synovial biopsy is not routinely advocated as a diagnostic procedure, the Prussian blue staining of synovium obtained at the time of hip or knee replacement for degenerative arthropathy may reveal the true nature of the arthropathy in previously undiagnosed and untreated subjects with iron overload. An accelerated form of degenerative arthropathy including osteoporosis that typically affects the thoracic and lumbar spine may occur in some patients with hemochromatosis and iron overload, particularly those with hypogonadism.

Prognosis

Three circumstances correlate well with decreased survival in hemochromatosis: (1) the presence of hepatic cirrhosis, (2) the presence of diabetes mellitus, and (3) the failure of the patient to achieve thorough iron depletion by repeated phlebotomies (usually within 1 year). Early diagnosis and aggressive iron depletion before symptoms occur can prevent end-organ complications and premature death.

Family Studies

Because hemochromatosis is inherited in an autosomal recessive mode, approximately 25 per cent of full siblings of index patients with hemochromatosis will be found to have hemochromatosis also. The relatives of a patient with hemochromatosis who are most likely to be affected are the siblings (25 per cent have abnormal findings) because of the autosomal recessive mode of transmission. About 13 per cent of hemochromatosis homozygotes marry hemochromatosis heterozygotes (13 per cent of the general population are heterozygous for the hemochromatosis allele). Relatives should be contacted and tested for hemochromatosis (all siblings, parents, and offspring of hemochromatosis patients) using serum iron concentration, transferrin saturation, and serum ferritin concentration. Individuals with increased values should undergo liver biopsy. If hepatic iron overload is found, frequent phlebotomy therapy should be started. Regardless of their iron parameters, full siblings who are HLA-identical with hemochromatosis probands are assumed to be homozygous for the hemochromatosis gene.

Screening

The routine systematic evaluation for hemochromatosis and iron overload in persons in a large segment of the general population is now cost-effective because of the frequency of hemochromatosis, the relatively low cost of ascertaining the diagnosis of hemochromatosis homozygosity, and the improved cost-to-benefit ratio associated with early diagnosis and therapy. In screening healthy individuals for hemochromatosis, the transferrin saturation value is the most useful measurement, but the serum ferritin concentration can also be helpful. If the transferrin saturation is greater than 60 per cent, liver biopsy is indicated, as is a pedigree study in which the transferrin saturation is measured in family members (particularly in siblings). The screening of diabetic patients in diabetes clinics has yielded twofold to threefold the fraction of persons who are homozygotes for hemochromatosis usually observed in the general population.

OTHER DISORDERS ASSOCIATED WITH IRON OVERLOAD

Hemochromatosis, African iron overload, African American iron overload, atransferrinemia, porphyria cutanea tarda, sideroblastic anemia, ineffective erythropoiesis, alcoholic liver disease, chronic viral hepatitis, chronic pancreatic insufficiency, hemolytic anemia, medicinal iron overload, transfusional iron overload, perinatal iron overload, and localized iron storage disorders are also associated with iron overload.

African Iron Overload

Progressive iron overload has been commonly documented among natives of sub-Saharan Africa. Affected individuals typically ingest large quantities of iron contained in homemade beer brewed in iron and steel vessels. This iron, which is largely in the ferrous state, is readily absorbed. Early in the course of African iron overload, the iron accumulates predominantly in macrophages in the liver, spleen, and marrow; deposits of Prussian blue–reactive iron are less prominent in hepatocytes and other parenchymal cells. The serum iron concentration, degree of transferrin saturation, and serum ferritin concentration may be normal or minimally increased, especially before the development of hepatic cirrhosis. In advanced cases, the occurrence of hepatic cirrhosis, cardiomyopathy, arthropathy, diabetes mellitus, and various endocrinopathies appears to be related to parenchymal iron deposits in the corresponding organs. Laboratory parameters of iron in florid patients reveal consistently high concentrations of serum iron, increased transferrin saturation, and hyperferritinemia. Hereditary anemias are common among many African populations with African iron overload, but the role of anemia in contributing to excessive iron absorption has not been systematically evaluated. Unlike hemochromatosis in whites, African iron overload does not exhibit linkage to HLA immunophenotypes, and recent studies indicate that an autosomal recessive allele not localized to chromosome 6 is, in part, responsible for this disorder. Therefore, African iron overload appears to represent a relatively common form of iron storage disorder in sub-Saharan African natives in whom the dietary factors of increased iron and ethanol intake and a hereditary factor or factors are necessary for full expression of the disorder.

African American Iron Overload

Iron overload unexplained by dietary or medicinal iron excess, transfusion, or sideroblastic anemia occurs in Americans of African descent. Although infrequently described in the medical literature, African American iron overload may be a relatively common disorder that has a hereditary basis, at least in part. The serum iron concentration and transferrin saturation values are often (but not invariably) increased. By definition, the serum ferritin concentration is elevated and is attributable to iron overload. Some individuals exhibit heavy ethanol use. Clinical abnormalities observed include weakness and fatigue, decreased libido and/or impotence, hepatopathy, arthropathy, hyperglycemia and/or diabetes mellitus, hypogonadotrophic hypogonadism, hypopituitarism, hyperpigmentation, and cardiomyopathy. Hepatic parenchymal cell iron deposits are sometimes present, but Kupffer's cell iron deposits are prominent in most patients. Macrophages in other sites such as the spleen and bone marrow also contain increased quantities of histochemically demonstrable iron. Iron overload is verified by liver iron quantification and/or therapeutic phlebotomy. As among African Americans in general, α- or β-thalassemia minor or hemoglobin S and C traits are common, but the role of these forms of mild anemia in contributing to the iron overload is unclear. Unlike hemochromatosis in white persons, HLA-A3 positivity is uncommon. Iron overload in African Americans is usually less severe than in African natives, but in many other respects it is more similar to African iron overload than to classic hemochromatosis in whites.

Atransferrinemia

Persons with the rare congenital defect of atransferrinemia lack the iron transport protein transferrin. Classic signs of severe iron deficiency occur because of a lack of transferrin, which is necessary for delivery of iron to erythroblasts and other tissues. In contrast to iron deficiency, however, transferrin measured by total iron-binding capacity or by specific immunologic methods is virtually absent. Iron absorption is markedly increased, and erythrocyte transfusion administered to alleviate the anemia may exacerbate the iron overload. Marked iron deposition occurs in the liver, pancreas, heart, endocrine organs, and kidneys, but little or no Prussian blue–stainable iron is observed in the bone marrow and spleen.

Porphyria Cutanea Tarda

The majority of patients with the sporadic type of porphyria cutanea tarda have a modestly or moderately increased per cent saturation of transferrin, an increased serum ferritin concentration, and increased liver iron stores in the range commonly seen in hemochromatosis heterozygotes. However, a few individuals with sporadic porphyria cutanea tarda have massive hepatic iron overload compatible with homozygosity for the hemochromatosis gene. The clinical expression of sporadic porphyria cutanea tarda may depend in part on the presence of one or more hemochromatosis alleles.

Individuals who have porphyria cutanea tarda often complain of photosensitive dermatitis (especially noticeable on the dorsal surfaces of the hands) or increased temporal hair growth. They have subnormal activity of hepatic uroporphyrinogen decarboxylase and excrete excessive amounts of 8-carboxyl and 7-carboxyl porphyrins in urine; a 24-hour urine collection shows excessive amounts of uroporphyrin I to support the diagnosis. In about half the patients with porphyria cutanea tarda, the enzymatic defect is due to a dominantly transmitted mutation at the uroporphyrinogen decarboxylase locus on chromosome 1 (familial porphyria cutanea tarda). In the remaining patients, there is no clear evidence of genetic transmission (sporadic porphyria cutanea tarda).

Sideroblastic Anemia

Myelodysplasia with ringed sideroblasts (idiopathic refractory type of sideroblastic anemia), which is typically seen in older individuals, is characterized by a modestly or moderately elevated per cent saturation of transferrin, an increased serum ferritin concentration, and increased liver iron stores in the range commonly seen in hemochromatosis heterozygotes. Some patients have massive hepatic iron overload consistent with hemochromatosis homozygosity. Myelodysplasia with ringed sideroblasts is usually unresponsive to drug therapy, and patients often require transfusion therapy, which may exacerbate iron overload. Hereditary forms of sideroblastic anemia (X-linked and autosomal recessive patterns of inheritance) are less common but are often associated with iron loading due to the effects of increased erythropoiesis, abnormal iron and heme metabolism in the erythron, and/or erythrocyte transfusion therapy. Some of these patients may have one (or two) genes for hemochromatosis. Sideroblastic anemia associated with the use of certain drugs (e.g., isoniazid, cycloserine) or with exposure to certain chemicals (e.g., ethanol, lead) are usually not associated with iron overload and resolve after removal of the offending agent and with appropriate ancillary therapy. Regardless of the cause of sideroblastic anemia, the peripheral blood erythrocytes are usually hypochromic and microcytic, sometimes with dimorphic morphologic characteristics, and contain Prussian blue–positive Pappenheimer bodies. Microscopic examination of a bone marrow aspirate stained by Prussian blue technique demonstrates the sine qua non of sideroblastic anemias: erythroblasts that contain iron-laden mitochondria surrounding the nucleus (ringed sideroblast).

Iron Overload Associated With Ineffective Erythropoiesis

Increased absorption of dietary iron may cause iron overload in patients with severe, long-standing erythroid hyperplasia with ineffective erythropoiesis. In many cases, excessive intestinal iron absorption unrelated to the presence of hemochromatosis alleles appears to cause the iron loading. In a few individuals, however, the presence of one or two hemochromatosis genes can be demonstrated by family studies and HLA typing. These disorders include thalassemia major and intermedia (both α- and β-thalassemia), hemoglobin E–β-thalassemia, congenital dyserythropoietic anemia, pyruvate kinase deficiency, hereditary spherocytosis, and certain sideroblastic anemias. α-Thalassemia major (Cooley's anemia) and β-thalassemia major, transmitted as an autosomal recessive disorder, are commonly diagnosed on the basis of the following abnormalities: severe anemia; markedly decreased mean corpuscular volume and hemoglobin concentration of peripheral red blood cells; hypochromia, microcytosis, anisocytosis, poikilocytosis, and basophilic stippling of peripheral red blood cells; and a family history of anemia. β-Thalassemia is readily distinguished from α-thalassemia by the occurrence of target cells (leptocytosis), a decreased percentage of hemoglobin A, and increased amounts of hemoglobin A_2 and hemoglobin F. These patients usually receive many transfusions but may also have markedly increased intestinal absorption of iron, accounting for iron overload. Children with thalassemia who receive a large number of transfusions may eventually experience heart failure, multiple endocrinopathies, and/or liver failure due to massive organ iron overload.

Coincidental Liver Disease

Individuals with liver disease due to alcoholism or viral hepatitis may have increased iron stores on blood testing or increased amounts of stainable iron in a liver biopsy specimen. The amount of stainable iron in these conditions usually is grade 0 to 2+ (normal 0 to 1+ on a scale of 0 to 4+). Alcoholic patients who have a heavy liver iron burden (grade 3 to 4+) may possess one or two hemochromatosis alleles. The hepatic iron index may be helpful in distinguishing individuals with coincidental liver disease who have also inherited hemochromatosis alleles.

Chronic Pancreatic Insufficiency

Occasional individuals with chronic pancreatic insufficiency experience mild iron overload, particularly apparent in the liver, which is often attributed to increased iron absorption due to the lack of bicarbonate from pancreatic secretions. However, some of these persons may have increased liver and body iron concentrations from increased ethanol consumption and/or the independent inheritance of one or two hemochromatosis genes.

Medicinal Iron Overload

Some persons who take oral medicinal iron supplements for many years experience iron overload. Often, it is not apparent whether these individuals undergo iron loading solely because of the quantity of iron ingested or whether they possess one or more hemochromatosis alleles. Many patients have a coexistent mild form of anemia (e.g., thalassemia minor, mild hereditary spherocytosis) for which chronic iron therapy was inadvertently prescribed. Published cases typically describe cardiomyopathy, hepatic cirrhosis, diabetes, and other grave complications of severe, long-standing iron overload. Laboratory iron parameters in these patients are indistinguishable from those of advanced hereditary hemochromatosis. However, some patients with similar degrees of iron overload have been surprisingly free of target organ injury. In routine clinical practice, lesser degrees of oral medicinal iron overload are relatively common. These patients often have moderate hyperferritinemia without increased serum iron concentrations and transferrin saturation values. Percutaneous liver biopsy specimens reveal increased iron in both hepatocytes and Kupffer's cells, and bone marrow aspirates reveal increased macrophage iron. Although serum hepatic enzyme concentrations are often increased in these mildly affected persons, hepatic cirrhosis is uncommon, as is injury to other major organs. Uncommonly, iron overload may occur from the repeated, erroneous treatment of chronic anemia with injectable iron dextran. The laboratory and clinical picture of this disorder is similar to that for oral iron excess.

Transfusional Iron Overload

Iron overload is expected following chronic transfusion in patients who have anemia that is not due to blood loss. Typically, these patients have sickle cell disease, severe thalassemia, and other severe hereditary hemolytic anemias; the Blackfan-Diamond syndrome; myelodysplasia; and congenital atransferrinemia. More recently, some patients successfully treated for acute leukemia have acquired iron overload from erythrocyte transfusions given during induction therapy. Unlike patients who undergo transfusion for the management of chronic anemia, patients with acute leukemia that is in remission can be treated with postremission therapeutic phlebotomy.

Perinatal Iron Overload

Perinatal iron overload is rare and usually fatal and is presumed to be due to abnormal fetal iron metabolism or fetal-maternal iron balance. Neonatal hemochromatosis is associated with hepatic cirrhosis, a threefold to fourfold increase in hepatic iron content, and iron deposition in the parenchymal cells of the liver, heart, and endocrine organs. However, iron excess is not observed in the bone marrow or spleen. Cerebrohepatorenal syndrome, transmitted through an autosomal recessive pattern of inheritance, is associated with abnormal facies, hypotonia, and polycystic kidneys. Parenchymal iron deposits are found in liver, spleen, kidney, and lung. In hereditary tyrosinemia, there is moderate iron excess in a cirrhotic liver; abnormalities of the pancreatic islet cells are also present.

Localized Iron Storage Disorders

In some conditions, excessive quantities of iron may accumulate in certain organs or tissues in the absence of a more generalized disorder of iron metabolism. In idiopathic pulmonary hemosiderosis, repeated intra-alveolar hemorrhage leads to the development of excessive iron content demonstrable by Prussian blue staining of lung tissue obtained by biopsy. However, other parameters of iron metabolism often reveal evidence of iron deficiency. In disorders characterized by chronic hemoglobinuria—for example, paroxysmal nocturnal hemoglobinuria—progressive renal iron deposition is usually not associated with a decrement in renal function. However, some patients experience iron deficiency because of the constant loss of iron through the urine. In sickle cell disease, repeated infarction of the renal medulla may lead to significant iron deposition in the kidneys. More importantly, however, many patients with sickle cell disease who require repeated transfusion for severe anemia and various complications of intravascular sickling experience iron overload due to excessive transfusion. Hallervorden-Spatz disease, a degenerative neurologic disease transmitted in an autosomal recessive pattern, causes progressive motor abnormalities, dementia, and optic atrophy in childhood. Marked iron deposits in the globus pallidus and in the reticular zone of the substantia nigra occur in these cases, but their relationship to the neurologic deficits is undetermined.

THE SPHINGOLIPIDOSES

By Donald F. Farrell, M.D.
Seattle, Washington

The sphingolipidoses constitute a group of rare genetic disorders that affect primarily the central and peripheral nervous systems. Some forms affect the reticuloendothelial system, and one disorder affects the vascular endothelial system. The sphingolipidoses are a subgroup of the lysosomal storage diseases, which also include the mucopolysaccharidoses, oligosaccharidoses, and one of the glycogen storage disorders. Table 1 is a summary of the sphingolipid storage disorders. A systematic approach to the diagnosis of these disorders requires knowledge of a few principles.

BIOCHEMICAL NOMENCLATURE OF THE SPHINGOLIPIDOSES

The classification of this group of genetic disorders is based on the complex structure of lipids that contain the amino alcohol sphingosine. In each of the chemical species that accumulate in this series of disorders, the sphingosine moiety is linked through the amino group of the acidic component of a fatty acid, forming a lipid known as a ceramide. The fatty acid composition varies according to the site of synthesis. For example, ceramides synthesized in neurons have a preponderance of C_{16} and C_{18} saturated fatty acids, and those synthesized by oligodendrocytes are enriched in C_{24} or longer-chain fatty acids that have a high percentage of hydroxyl groups in the alpha position of the fatty acid. All the sphingolipidoses contain a ceramide linked through the alcohol component to a single sugar, a modified sugar, or a series of sugars. Some of these sugars are linked to a sialic acid (i.e., neuraminic acid). The exception to this rule is sphingomyelin, in which the ceramide is linked to a phosphorylcholine moiety. When ceramide is linked to a simple sugar, it is known as cerebroside. In the nervous system, cerebrosides contain the sugar galactose; in other organs, cerebrosides contain glucose. Two major cerebrosides are found in the body: galactosylcerebroside and glucosylcerebroside. A ceramide linked to a complex series of sugars plus one or more neuraminic acids forms a ganglioside. The sequence of sugars establishes the name of the ganglioside. Many species of ganglioside exist, but only two are associated with diseases.

To simplify the nomenclature of the gangliosides, a shorthand has been developed to identify the different chemical forms. The upper case G stands for ganglioside; the subscripted small capital M stands for mono and signifies that the ganglioside has a single neuraminic acid attached to the first galactose in the sugar chain; and the subscripted numeral 1 or 2 signifies the structure of the sugar chain. Subscript 1 denotes a series of four sugars linked to ceramide: glucose-galactose-*N*-acetylhexosamine-galactose. The subscript 2 structure contains three sugars: glucose-galactose–*N*-acetylhexosamine. The two diseases associated

Table 1. The Sphingolipidoses

Sphingolipid	Disease	Enzyme
Ceramide-galactose	Globoid cell leukodystrophy	Cerebroside β-galactosidase
Ceramide-galactose sulfate	Metachromatic leukodystrophy	Arylsulfatase A
Ceramide-glucose-galactose (sialic acid) hexosamine-galactose	G_{M1} gangliosidosis	β-Galactosidase
Ceramide-glucose-galactose (sialic acid) hexosamine	G_{M2} gangliosidosis	β-Hexosaminidase A or A and B
Ceramide-glucose	Gaucher disease	β-Glucosidase
Ceramide-phosphorylcholine	Niemann-Pick disease	Sphingomyelinase
Ceramide-glucose-galactose-galactose	Fabry disease	α-Galactosidase
Ceramide	Farber disease	Ceramidase

with gangliosides are known as G_{M1} and G_{M2} gangliosidoses.

CLINICAL FORMS OF THE SPHINGOLIPIDOSES

The sphingolipidoses can be divided into two classes. Disorders that affect primarily the myelin membrane are known as leukodystrophies. Disorders that affect neurons are known as neuronal storage diseases. The sphingolipid neuronal disorders can be further divided clinically by the presence or absence of hepatomegaly, splenomegaly, or both conditions. The amount of organomegaly can be useful in diagnosing a specific disorder.

The basic problem in the sphingolipidoses is the abnormal storage of various lipids in lysosomes. These lysosomes contain lipid-degrading enzymes that are structurally and functionally defective. In a given storage disorder, the specific enzyme deficiency is found in every tissue of the body. However, each of these disorders is also characterized by disproportionate, if not exclusive, synthesis and abnormal storage of sphingolipid in specific cell types. For example, in the leukodystrophies, the sphingolipids stored (i.e., galactosylceramide and sulfogalactosylceramide) are synthesized almost exclusively by oligodendrocytes, and the complex sphingolipids that cause the neuronal storage diseases are synthesized primarily in neurons.

In the various types of sphingolipidoses, a number of clinical variants exist. Each disorder may have two or three different clinical forms based on the age at onset. The typical clinical presentation in one age group may be quite different from that in another age group. Additional clinical variation occurs when the mutant enzyme is made up of multiple subunits. A mutation affecting one subunit causes one form of disease, and a mutation affecting a second subunit causes a different disorder. In some variants, the primary lysosomal enzyme is normal, and the sphingolipid storage disease results from a mutation that alters a low-molecular-weight "activator" protein. These activator proteins are required for the catabolism of one or more specific sphingolipids. The specific developmental patterns of each of the variants are discussed as each specific disorder is considered.

GENETICS OF THE SPHINGOLIPIDOSES

Except for Fabry disease, all the sphingolipidoses are inherited as autosomal recessive disorders. With this type of inheritance, the clinician expects to find individual patients or affected siblings only. Typically, no family history of a similar disorder is obtained. Fabry disease is inherited as an X-linked recessive disorder. In Fabry disease, affected males are the rule, and a careful history of maternal relatives is particularly important. If the family is large enough, the clinician should attempt to document or identify afflicted maternal uncles. As with other X-linked disorders, an occasional female with a milder form of the disorder is clinically recognized.

THE LEUKODYSTROPHIES

Among the leukodystrophies, only a few are categorized as sphingolipidoses. In this section, only two disorders, globoid cell leukodystrophy and metachromatic leukodystrophy, are discussed. Each disorder has been associated with infantile, juvenile, and adult clinical variants, and advances in brain imaging, especially the widespread use of magnetic resonance imaging (MRI), have increased the likelihood of identifying these variants. Although MRI findings are not very specific for a given leukodystrophy, they may help define the nature and scope of further diagnostic testing. Enzyme tests are the most powerful tools used for establishing a specific diagnosis.

Globoid Cell Leukodystrophy

Globoid cell leukodystrophy (GLD), also known as Krabbe's disease or cerebroside lipidosis, was the first of the leukodystrophies to be identified as a specific disorder because of the characteristic pathologic changes in the nervous system (Fig. 1).

Infantile Form

The most frequent clinical form is the infantile form. Children with this variant usually present between 3 and

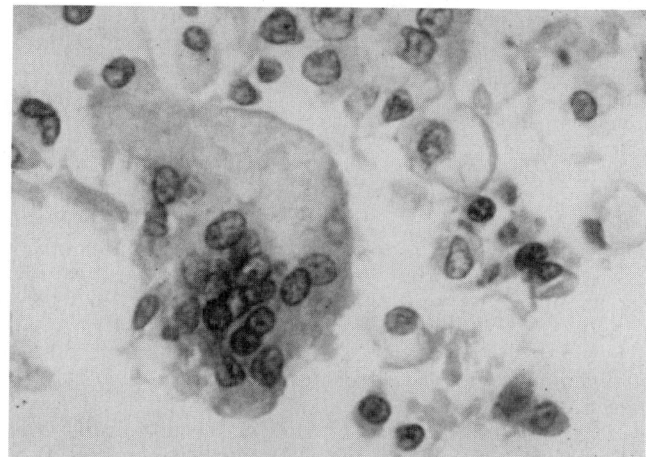

Figure 1. Multinucleated giant cell (globoid cell) in the white matter of a child who died of globoid cell leukodystrophy.

6 months of age, but examples of this disorder have been recognized shortly after birth. Before the onset of the disease, the developmental profile of the infant may be normal or only slightly delayed. These infants may present with failure to thrive or feeding difficulties leading to weight loss and muscle wasting. For the parents, an especially distressing feature of this disorder is the extreme irritability of the infant. Comforting by the parents does not reduce the almost constant crying and screaming. Typical parental attempts to soothe the infant may instead increase the irritability. Central and peripheral nerve functions are affected in this disorder. Some GLD infants may present with body stiffening (i.e., spasticity) or, more rarely, floppiness. The most common feature is early spasticity with a mild peripheral neuropathy. Myoclonic, tonic, and other types of seizures occur frequently, as does uncontrolled vomiting. Many of these infants suffer from fevers of unknown origin, and an infectious cause is seldom found.

The course of the infantile form of GLD is relentlessly progressive. The slightest auditory or tactile stimuli may trigger prolonged bouts of crying and screaming. Increased motor tone (i.e., severe spasticity) to the point of complete extension of the neck and spine (i.e., opisthotonus) frequently occurs, and deep tendon reflexes are almost always increased. As the disorder progresses, the peripheral neuropathy worsens, eventually obliterating the signs of central nervous system long fiber tract involvement. In the later stages, hypotonia and decreased to absent deep tendon reflexes are typically observed. Virtually all infants with GLD develop blindness and have pale optic disks, and many become deaf. Combined malnutrition and muscle atrophy lead to emaciation in the terminal stages. Most infants with GLD die within months to a couple of years after the onset of their illness.

Routine laboratory studies are of little help in establishing the clinical diagnosis. The cerebrospinal fluid protein concentration is typically increased. The electroencephalogram is often abnormally slow and shows epileptiform activity, but the findings are not specific for GLD. Nerve conduction velocities may be abnormal, but these tests have been supplanted by modern enzyme analysis. The typical infantile form is the most common presentation of GLD and is readily recognized. The diagnosis of GLD is confirmed by enzyme analysis, a topic that is addressed later.

Late-Infantile and Juvenile Forms

After discovery of the enzyme defect in GLD, several noninfantile variants of the disorder were reported. A number of children have been reported with the onset of clinical symptoms between 2 and 10 years of age. These variants have been subdivided into late-infantile forms and juvenile forms, depending on the age at onset. These variants may be caused by different mutated forms of the defective enzyme, but they are diagnosed by demonstrating a severe deficiency of cerebroside β-galactosidase. The clinical presentation and course of these disease variants differ rather substantially from that described for the infantile form. For example, only some of the younger infants (1 to 3 years of age) are irritable. The older children show no signs of irritability, and none of the age-at-onset variants have unexplained fevers. Seizures are found in a much smaller percentage of the patients.

In the late-infantile form of GLD, children typically present with a disturbance of gait. Juveniles, by contrast, typically present with a decline in school performance. Gait disturbances tend to be spastic or ataxic. Younger children often progress rapidly during the early phases of the illness, but then the course slows and appears to be nonprogressive for variable periods of time. Progressive paralysis of the extremities ensues early in the course; it often begins as a hemiparesis but rapidly progresses to spastic quadriparesis. Blindness, optic atrophy, and progressive pseudobulbar palsy are common. Signs of peripheral nerve involvement are more prominent in the younger patients, but slowed nerve conduction velocities may be found in the late-infantile and juvenile forms of GLD. Some of the juvenile patients present with ataxia, but the remainder of their disease progression is similar to other patients with GLD. The younger-onset forms tend to have a much shorter life expectancy (2 to 3 years), and some of the older children may live into their midteens or older. The MRI scan is particularly helpful in confirming that the principal problem is a leukodystrophy, but the demyelinating pattern is not specific for GLD. As will be recognized in the later discussion of metachromatic leukodystrophy, the older variants of GLD are not clinically distinct disorders, and the final diagnosis is established by enzyme analysis.

Adult-Onset Form

Only a handful of patients have been reported with the onset of GLD beyond the age of 10 years. A description of a typical clinical profile is not possible; most patients have presented with paralysis and spasticity of a single limb, most commonly one leg. The spread of the disease process varies, but the progressive nature of the illness is soon apparent, with the upper limb on the same side as the affected leg becoming more involved than contralateral limbs. Spastic quadriparesis eventually develops with associated reflex hyperactivity and Babinski's signs. A pes cavis deformity of the foot has been documented in most of these patients. Speech and swallowing difficulties are attributed to bulbar or pseudobulbar palsy. Intellect remains intact in some patients, but an equal number show signs of dementia. Optic disk pallor is common. Early in the course of this form of GLD, nerve conduction velocities are normal, but they decrease with progression of the disease. MRI may provide an early clue to the diagnosis of leukodystrophy.

Like the late-infantile and juvenile forms of GCL, the onset and course of the adult form can be seen in other leukodystrophies; thus, a definitive diagnosis requires enzyme analysis.

Enzymatic Diagnosis

Enzymatic diagnosis is accomplished by measuring the activity of the enzyme cerebroside β-galactosidase, using radiolabeled galactosylcerebroside as substrate. The galactose moiety of the brain cerebroside is labeled with tritium, and the assay measures the enzymatic release of water-soluble radiolabeled galactose. Several cellular sources provide adequate enzyme for analysis. Leukocytes can be isolated by dextran sedimentation, with contaminating erythrocytes eliminated by hypotonic disruption and centrifugation. Although leukocytes are the least expensive and most easily obtained cells, cultured skin fibroblasts and amniotic fluid cells are also excellent sources of enzyme. All forms of GLD have been associated with severe deficiencies of cerebroside β-galactosidase activity. Most patients have enzyme activities in the range of 1 to 2 per cent of controls or less. Rarely, a patient may have a residual enzyme activity as high as 10 to 20 per cent of the control value. The validity of those values, however, should probably be challenged. The various age-at-onset forms do not show significant differences in the amount of residual enzyme activity measured in vitro. However, the different forms of GLD will soon be determined by direct analysis of control and mutant DNAs.

Metachromatic Leukodystrophy

Metachromatic leukodystrophy (MLD) is also known as sulfatide lipidosis or Greenfield's disease. The name of this disorder is based on specific neuropathologic alterations. Metachromatic leukodystrophy is characterized by metachromatic-staining material in the nervous system or kidneys. This change in the expected color (from violet to brown) of an acidic dye such as cresyl violet led to the recognition of this specific leukodystrophy. Metachromatic leukodystrophy is a more common disorder than GLD. Several age-at-onset variants are recognized, but additional genetic forms have also been described.

Late-Infantile Form

The late-infantile form of MLD typically presents during the second year of life. In most patients, the first indication of the disorder is loss or regression of a previously learned motor skill. The most frequent early problem is loss of the ability to walk, but approximately one third of affected children never learn to walk or encounter great difficulty in learning to walk. Ataxia, staggering gait, and frequent falls are common. When examined at this early stage, most infants demonstrate hypotonia and decreased to absent deep tendon reflexes. Rapid progression of symptoms in the early stages of MLD is typically followed by a plateau in which little change occurs over a number of years. During the rapid phase of the illness, children with MLD develop additional motor disabilities, including weakness of the upper extremities, difficulty in speaking and swallowing (i.e., bulbar and/or pseudobulbar palsies), nystagmus, and blindness with pale optic disks (i.e., optic atrophy). Intellectual decline occurs, but is difficult to measure because of severe motor deficits. Most parents know whether their child can recognize family members, and parents also have a better understanding of what is happening in their environment than can be documented by testing. Terminal children with MLD become spastic, dystonic, emaciated, and irritable, and they may have seizures. Life expectancy for those with the late-infantile form of the illness is usually 2 to 3 years, but at least one patient has survived to the age of 19. Late-infantile MLD may be confused clinically with the older-onset forms of GLD. However, late-infantile MLD patients present with hypotonia and areflexia, and infants with the same age at onset of GLD are spastic and have increased pathologic reflexes.

Juvenile-Onset Forms

The age at onset for juvenile MLD ranges from about 5 to 10 years. Children in this group typically present with "school problems." Previously good or adequate students begin to perform at lower levels, and their grades begin to suffer. Many become uncooperative or confused or develop other behavioral abnormalities. The child with juvenile-onset MLD may be described as "off in another world." Progression typically occurs rapidly, and these children develop a cerebellarlike ataxia or other gait disturbance secondary to weakness of the legs. Dysarthria and dysphagia result from bulbar or pseudobulbar palsies; demyelination of central and peripheral nerves contributes to abnormalities on clinical examination. Patients with juvenile MLD almost always develop blindness with optic atrophy and spastic quadriparesis with Babinski's signs, because the course in this age group is typically longer than the course in the late-infantile group.

Adult-Onset Forms

In the adult forms of MLD, symptoms may begin as early as the teenage years or as late as the seventh decade of life. Some adults present with a decline in general intellectual performance (i.e., dementia) manifested by altered personality, apathy, emotional lability, confusion, and/or loss of memory. Others present with behavioral abnormalities, such as depressed affect, schizophreniclike thought processes, and mania. Still others present with combined intellectual and behavioral disturbances that may be complicated by chronic alcoholism. A few adult-onset patients present with cerebellar ataxia or, very rarely, peripheral neuropathy. Like the earlier age-at-onset variants, the progression of this disorder is quite variable. Patients who experience a protracted course eventually develop spastic quadriparesis with hyperactive reflexes and Babinski's signs and blindness with optic atrophy. Terminal patients are bedridden, blind, and unable to move voluntarily. They must be fed through a nasogastric tube or feeding gastrostomy.

Many of the older-onset leukodystrophies are initially recognized by MRI studies of the brain. Widespread demyelination of the subcortical white matter is readily identified by standard weighted images. In many patients, the U-fibers immediately beneath the cortical ribbon appear intact. In some individuals, the frontal white matter may be more heavily damaged, but in others, the damage affects the parieto-occipital region. Computed tomography (CT) scans may also be diagnostic, but MRI is more sensitive in identifying adult-onset MLD. Nerve conduction velocities continue to be of value in establishing a diagnosis of leukodystrophy, because peripheral demyelination is often subclinical. Metachromatic staining of urine sediment or nerve biopsy material is no longer recommended.

Enzymatic Diagnosis

The variants of MLD mentioned previously are caused by a failure of the enzyme arylsulfatase A to degrade the myelin-associated lipid sulfatide (ceramide-galactose-3-sulfate). Although various methods have been devised to measure the activity of arylsulfatase A, the most popular test is a colorimetric assay that uses 4-nitrocatechol sulfate as substrate. When the 4-nitrocatechol sulfate assay was compared with an assay that uses radiolabeled natural substrate to measure cerebrosulfatidase activity, the correlation was excellent. The use of a fluorometric substrate such as 4-methylumbelliferyl sulfate requires that arylsulfatase A activity be separated from the other arylsulfatases by electrophoresis or by various ion exchange methods before assay. Arylsulfatase A can be measured in polymorphonuclear leukocytes, cultured skin fibroblasts, or amniotic fluid cells. There are no significant differences in residual arylsulfatase A activity among the various forms of MLD. In most MLD patients, the enzyme activity approaches zero. Occasionally, arylsulfatase A activity in the range of 1 to 2 per cent of control values may be detected.

The measurement of human arylsulfatase A activity is tricky, because a mutation unrelated to the disease process decreases the activity of the enzyme when measured in the test tube. This mutation is relatively common, occurring in as many as 25 per cent of the population. The presence of this mutation must always be considered, but when an infant, child, or adult has an appropriate clinical presentation, widespread demyelination on MRI, and arylsulfatase A activity less than 1 to 2 per cent of the control, the clinician can be confident that the correct diagnosis has been made. The arylsulfatase A pseudoallele has greater impact on heterozygote detection and antenatal diagnosis, on which its presence can have devastating results if not correctly identified.

Other Genetically Unrelated Forms

Two other genetically unrelated forms of MLD occur. The first is MLD with normal arylsulfatase A activity. This disorder is rare and results from a deficiency of sphingolipid activator protein-1 (SAP-1). This low-molecular-weight protein is required for the catabolism of sulfatide by the enzyme cerebrosulfatidase. This form of MLD is detected with specific DNA probes or by sequencing a portion of the mutant gene.

The second of these unrelated forms is known as multiple sulfatase deficiency. Although this rare disorder has some features of late-infantile MLD (arylsulfatase A deficiency) it usually manifests earlier, and the infants also have features of a mucopolysaccharidosis (arylsulfatase B deficiency) with hepatosplenomegaly, coarse facial features, bony abnormalities, and excretion of both dermatan sulfate and heparan sulfate in the urine. Congenital ichthyosis (arylsulfatase C deficiency) appears after a number of months. All of the measurable arylsulfatases are deficient in this rare disorder.

NEURONAL STORAGE DISEASES

Four major groups of disorders are covered in this section. Whereas the leukodystrophies result from storage of sphingolipids primarily in oligodendrocytes, the neuronal storage diseases result from storage of different sphingolipids in neurons of the brain and spinal cord. A high percentage of the infants and children with neuronal storage diseases reveal a "cherry-red spot macula" on examination of the retina (Fig. 2). The frequency of this diagnostic finding varies with the specific storage disorder. Another distinctive feature of this group of disorders (except for the various age-at-onset forms of G_{M2} gangliosidoses that result from hexosaminidase A deficiency) is the presence of hepatosplenomegaly. Organomegaly varies from moderate enlargement to severe enlargement, in which the spleen is palpated well beneath the pelvic brim. In many of these disorders, organomegaly is less pronounced when the patient has a later onset of symptoms. In addition to age-related variants attributed to different mutations at the same locus, several rare variants arise from different genetic mechanisms that cause phenotypically similar disorders.

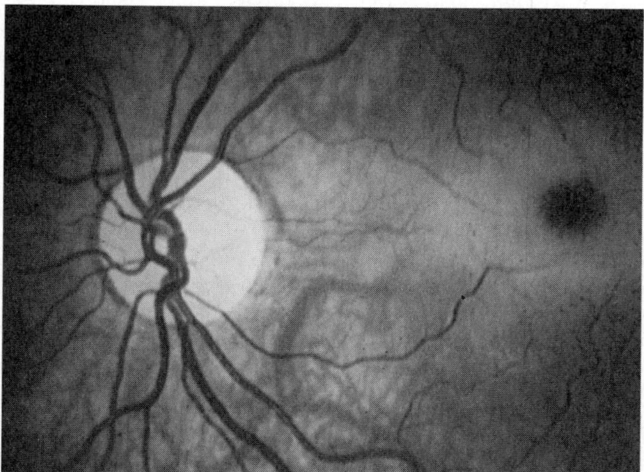

Figure 2. Funduscopic photograph showing an excellent example of a cherry-red spot macula. This important physical finding may be seen in a number of different sphingolipid neuronal storage diseases.

G_{M1} Gangliosidosis

Other names for the infantile form of this disorder include generalized gangliosidosis or Landing's disease. G_{M1} gangliosidosis was the second of the ganglioside storage disorders to be recognized. (Tay-Sachs disease was the first.) This disorder has three age-at-onset variants: infantile, juvenile, and adult. The primary defect in all three variants is a severe deficiency of the β-galactosidase that removes the terminal galactose from G_{M1} ganglioside.

Infantile Form

Severe impairment of psychomotor development occurs during the first few months of life. Many infants develop symptoms and/or signs of gangliosidosis at or shortly after birth. The literature documents failure to thrive, little interest in feeding, poor sucking, and subnormal growth rates. Early in the course, many β-galactosidase–deficient infants have decreased tone (i.e., hypotonia) and are hypoactive. The face or the entire body may be edematous. Signs of facial dysmorphism include a depressed nasal bridge, frontal bossing, low-set ears, and tongue enlargement. Infants whose symptoms begin a little later in life may not demonstrate these dysmorphic features. At funduscopy, almost 50 per cent of β-galactosidase–deficient infants demonstrate a cherry-red spot macula. Neurologic development is severely delayed in most of these children, and some fail to learn to roll over, crawl, or sit unassisted. Hepatosplenomegaly usually is noticeable by 6 months of age but is never as severe as that seen in Gaucher disease or Niemann-Pick disease. Stiff joints, spinal curvatures, and contractures frequently develop, and generalized major motor seizures (tonic-clonic) typically begin around 1 year of age. These seizures may not respond to treatment with anticonvulsants. Between 1 and 2 years of age, these infants progress to quadriparesis, with decerebrate posturing and an inability to feed. Most patients must be fed by nasogastric tube or by feeding gastrostomy. Death occurs around 2 years of age.

Skeletal radiographs frequently reveal dystosis multiplex similar to that found in many of the mucopolysaccharidoses. By contrast, CT and MRI are not useful in the diagnosis of infantile G_{M1} gangliosidosis. Although many β-galactosidase–deficient infants have vacuolated lymphocytes in the peripheral smear, this finding is not specific for gangliosidosis.

Juvenile-Onset Form

The term juvenile onset is a misnomer, because most children in this group first demonstrate clinical symptoms between 1 and 2 years of age. The term juvenile is actually more descriptive of the longer life expectancy in this group: survival to the age of 10 years or more is common. Dysmorphic features are generally absent, and bony abnormalities are so minimal that they are not helpful in establishing a diagnosis. Early development is normal or near normal, with attainment of expected developmental milestones. Between 1 and 2 years of age, however, there is an arrest in further development. Many of these patients lose fine motor skills and develop strabismus. Movement disorders, including cerebellar-like ataxia or even choreoathetosis, soon become apparent. Examination at this time typically reveals hyperactive deep tendon reflexes, Babinski's signs, and scissoring of the lower extremities (i.e., spasticity). Organomegaly is generally not found in β-galactosidase–deficient juveniles. Major motor seizures are common and often unresponsive to anticonvulsant therapy. Intellectual decline occurs early, and unlike patients with leukodystrophies, these children may not respond with familiarity to their families. Progressive intellectual and motor loss is relentless, terminating in decerebrate rigidity with an inability to feed or interact with the environment. During these later stages, an increased startle reflex is common. Blindness is a late finding and a cherry-red spot macula is not found in this form. Most of the children die by 10 years of age. As in the earlier-onset form, vacuolated lymphocytes are commonly present. Juvenile-onset G_{M1} gangliosidosis is difficult to distinguish clinically from some of the other forms of gangliosidoses; a definitive diagnosis requires enzyme analysis.

Adult-Onset Form

An increasing number of adult-onset forms of G_{M1} β-galactosidase deficiency are being reported in the literature. Unfortunately, there is no typical pattern, but the most present with a movement disorder or amyotrophy during the teenage years. Adult patients do not develop organomegaly or cherry-red spots. Vacuolated lymphocytes are not present on peripheral smear. The movement disorders may mimic early-onset parkinsonism or one of the spinal cerebellar degenerations. Progressive dystonia eventually leads to incapacitation. The amyotrophic form may mimic amyotrophic lateral sclerosis or juvenile-onset spinal muscular atrophy. Seizures are decidedly rare. Intelligence varies greatly and is frequently normal early in the course of the disorder. Many of these patients have completed high school, and some have been successful in a college career. This form of G_{M1} gangliosidosis cannot be distinguished clinically from the adult form of G_{M2} gangliosidosis. Definitive diagnosis requires enzyme analysis.

Enzymatic Diagnosis

The primary biochemical defect in G_{M1} gangliosidosis is a deficiency of β-galactosidase. These patients cannot remove the terminal galactose moiety from G_{M1} ganglioside. The β-galactosidase responsible for this disorder is not related to the cerebroside β-galactosidase responsible for GLD. Several artificial substrates have been used to measure G_{M1} β-galactosidase activity. The most common is 4-methylumbelliferyl β-galactoside, a sensitive, specific, and reliable fluorometric substrate. All age-at-onset forms of G_{M1} gangliosidosis have severe deficiencies of β-galactosidase activity ranging from zero to 2 per cent of control values; thus, the various forms cannot be differentiated by routine enzyme analysis. Isolated leukocytes, cultured skin fibroblasts, or amniotic fluid cells provide the best sources of enzyme.

Several disorders have been associated with secondary deficiencies of β-galactosidase activity. These disorders include I-cell disease, mucolipidosis III, galactosialidosis, and some of the mucopolysaccharidoses. In I-cell disease and mucolipidosis III, multiple enzyme deficiencies are detected only in cultured skin fibroblasts, but enzyme activities are normal in isolated leukocytes. Clinically, galactosialidosis is virtually identical to infantile G_{M1} gangliosidosis. Before galactosialidosis was recognized, some individuals with that disorder were most likely diagnosed as having G_{M1} gangliosidosis. Patients with galactosialidosis excrete excessive amounts of oligosaccharides containing sialic acid (e.g., neuraminic acid) in their urine, and patients with mucopolysaccharidoses excrete various types of specific mucopolysaccharides in their urine.

G_{M2} Gangliosidoses

In the G_{M2} gangliosidoses, neurons store excessive amounts of the normally minor ganglioside G_{M2}. This group of disorders is the most complex among the sphingolipidoses because mutations may lead to abnormalities in either of two distinct subunits making up hexosaminidase A. Abnormalities of the alpha subunit lead to deficient hexosaminidase A activity, and abnormalities of the beta subunit cause deficiencies of hexosaminidase A and B. A nonallelic variant of G_{M2} gangliosidosis results from deficiency of G_{M2} ganglioside activator protein. In this form of the illness, the hexosaminidase enzymatic activities are normal. The infantile G_{M2} gangliosidosis secondary to hexosaminidase A deficiency is known as Tay-Sachs disease, and the infantile G_{M2} gangliosidosis associated with combined hexosaminidase A and B deficiency is known as Sandhoff's disease.

Hexosaminidase A Deficiency

Infantile Form

Infants with hexosaminidase A deficiency, also called Tay-Sachs disease, are typically normal at birth and develop normally during the first 3 to 4 months of life. The earliest sign of a problem is the onset of muscle weakness and hypotonia. Within weeks to months, an exaggerated startle response is recognized. Any sharp sound may elicit a myoclonic-like extension (jerk) of the body. Weakness and hypotonia progress. Loss of previously acquired head control ensues, and the infant's response to the parents and environment decreases. Acquired developmental milestones are soon lost. Blindness develops early but may remain unrecognized for weeks to months. Erratic, wandering, nystagmoid eye movements, however, may provide an early clue to the loss of vision. Virtually all infants with Tay-Sachs disease have a cherry-red spot macula; most Tay-Sachs infants also have signs of upper and lower motor neuron dysfunction, with hyperactive deep tendon reflexes and marked atrophy of the muscles of the trunk and limbs. Seizures typically occur by 1 year of age. During the later stages of Tay-Sachs disease, the patient's head size increases. Macrocephaly from ganglioside accumulation and diffuse gliosis is common. The development of decerebrate posturing, inability to feed, and unresponsiveness to all stimuli eventually leads to death by the age of 2 or 3 years.

If the parents of the infant are of Ashkenazi Jewish descent, Tay-Sachs disease is readily suspected clinically and confirmed by enzyme analysis. To identify heterozygotes for this disorder, a worldwide screening program for persons of Ashkenazi descent has been available for many years. As a result, the worldwide incidence of Tay-Sachs disease has been reduced by up to 90 per cent. However, the incidence of this disorder in non-Jewish populations has not changed. Phenotypically, this form of G_{M2} gangliosidosis is identical in both Jewish and non-Jewish populations. The presence of a cherry-red spot macula without organomegaly should alert the clinician to include Tay-

Sachs in the differential diagnosis and to request the appropriate enzyme analyses.

Juvenile Form

The juvenile form of hexosaminidase A deficiency is very rare. These children typically develop normally until age 2 to 6 years. They present with a gait disturbance (i.e., ataxia), and progressive intellectual loss (i.e., dementia) ensues early. Progressive motor weakness with spasticity is common and eventually leads to spastic quadriparesis. Seizures become a prominent feature late in the course of the illness. Not all patients develop blindness, and cherry-red spot maculas are rare. Optic atrophy and pigmentary retinopathy are more frequently encountered than the cherry-red spot macula, and the former explains the visual loss when it occurs. These children become decerebrate and usually die during the teenage years.

A chronic variant form with onset in this age group has also been described in which intelligence remains normal, but emotional lability (pseudobulbar palsy) or a maniclike state becomes a prominent part of the clinical picture. Spinocerebellar ataxia in combination with amyotrophy is common, and these individuals may live into their third or fourth decade.

Adult-Onset Form

The adult form of hexosaminidase A deficiency may be difficult to distinguish from the chronic juvenile-onset form. Many of the adults have had nonspecific neurologic problems earlier in life, and occasionally these symptoms have not been related to the current neurologic or psychiatric condition. Although presenting symptoms vary, they tend to fall into two major categories. One group presents with spinocerebellar degeneration that is frequently associated with amyotrophy. A second group presents with psychosis. Schizophrenic symptoms, manic states, or severe depression are common. As many as 30 per cent of patients have a major behavioral component to their illness. Most frequently, patients manifest both motor and behavioral symptoms, but some individuals present with a behavioral disorder unaccompanied by motor signs. Intellectual performance can remain normal for years. Clinically, the adult form of hexosaminidase A deficiency is virtually identical to the adult form of G_{M1} gangliosidosis. Definitive diagnosis requires enzyme analysis.

Hexosaminidase AB Deficiency

Infantile Form

The infantile form of this disorder is clinically similar to Tay-Sachs disease. However, infants with Sandhoff disease have organomegaly and may have bony abnormalities similar to those found in the infantile form of G_{M1} gangliosidosis. Essentially all of these infants have cherry-red spot maculas, but the genetic abnormality is not more prevalent in Ashkenazi Jews. Thin-layer chromatographic analysis of the urine may identify the presence of oligosaccharides containing *N*-acetylglucosamine, but enzyme analysis is easy, available, and more reliable.

Juvenile Form

Only a few individuals have been reported with the juvenile form of hexosaminidase AB deficiency. These patients have presented between 3 and 10 years of age with cerebellar ataxia, slurred speech, and progressive psychomotor retardation. Blindness and cherry-red spot maculas have not been observed. Relentless progression leads to spastic tetraparesis and dementia. Death results after a few years. Clinically, this disorder cannot be specifically distinguished from the other juvenile-onset gangliosidoses, and the clinician must establish the diagnosis with appropriate enzymatic analysis.

G_{M2} Ganglioside Activator Deficiency

There is nothing specific about the clinical features of G_{M2} ganglioside activator deficiency. Only infantile-onset patients with phenotypes of Tay-Sachs disease or Sandhoff disease have been reported. This disorder is biochemically distinct, however, because standard enzyme analysis indicates normal hexosaminidase A and B activities in these patients.

Enzymatic Analysis of Hexosaminidase A and B

Serum, isolated leukocytes, cultured skin fibroblasts, and amniotic fluid cells are used for analysis of hexosaminidase A and B. Standard assays use colorimetric or fluorometric artificial substrates. In most laboratories, assays using the fluorometric substrate 4-methylumbelliferyl β-*N*-acetylglucosaminide are considered reasonably sensitive and specific. Hexosaminidase A is typically measured indirectly under standardized conditions. The assay takes advantage of the fact that hexosaminidase A is heat-labile at pH 4.4, while hexosaminidase B is heat-stable. One series of reaction tubes is held on ice, and another series of reaction tubes undergoes heat treatment at 50°C for 1, 2, and 3 hours. Total hexosaminidase is measured in the unheated tubes, while hexosaminidase B activity is measured in the 1-, 2-, and 3-hour heat-treated tubes. Activity in the 1-, 2-, and 3-hour heat-treated tubes should be the same to guarantee that hexosaminidase A has been fully inactivated. The difference between total hexosaminidase activity and hexosaminidase B activity is reported as hexosaminidase A activity. In general, Tay-Sachs patients have no measurable hexosaminidase A activity. The juvenile and adult forms of G_{M2} gangliosidosis generally have some residual hexosaminidase A activity, but only in the range of 3 to 4 per cent of controls. Sandhoff disease has an almost complete deficiency of both hexosaminidase A and B. The juvenile form of Sandhoff disease may have residual hexosaminidase B activity of less than a few per cent of controls. Other methods are available for confirming the results of standard enzyme assays. For example, hexosaminidase A and B isoenzymes can be separated by ionic exchange chromatography, and each fraction analyzed individually. The isoenzymes can also be separated by various types of electrophoreses, including separations in cellulose gels, starch gels, or by isoelectric focusing. Radiolabeled G_{M2} ganglioside is sometimes used as a substrate, but it is not commercially available. Assays using this natural substrate fail to diagnose the form of G_{M2} gangliosidosis secondary to an activator deficiency. In general, most assays using the natural substrates employ various detergents to solubilize the sphingolipid substrate in an aqueous environment. Detergents bypass the need for the activator protein during the enzymatic reaction. One successful approach to this problem has been to feed the patient's cultured skin fibroblasts radiolabeled G_{M2} ganglioside and demonstrate that affected cells do not hydrolyze the substrate. Addition of purified activator protein should correct the deficit. These types of studies are typically performed in research laboratories and are not generally available without prior consultation with the laboratory director.

Gaucher Disease

Gaucher disease, or glucosylceramide lipidosis, is by far the most common of the sphingolipidoses. The disorder occurs in three clinical forms. The most common form (type 1) does not affect the nervous system. The remaining two types (types 2 and 3) affect the central nervous system but differ in severity and their effects on life expectancy. A severe deficiency of glucosylceramide β-glucosidase activity is found in all three forms. Nonallelic forms of the disorder affecting the central nervous system have been attributed to a deficiency of SAP-2, a small-molecular-weight activator protein genetically related to SAP-1, the activator protein deficient in rare forms of metachromatic leukodystrophy.

Type 1, or Adult-Onset Form

Gaucher disease (type 1) is a clinically diverse disorder with great variability in the age at onset and severity. Type 1 Gaucher disease may begin early in infancy, when it is impossible to predict involvement of the nervous system. On the other hand, the diagnosis of type 1 Gaucher disease may be delayed until the eighth or ninth decade of life. Most patients are diagnosed in their late teens or early twenties.

The clinical symptoms vary greatly. Organomegaly is the most common presenting sign. Typically, a very large spleen provokes a diagnostic search for the cause of organomegaly. Many patients with type 1 Gaucher disease are asymptomatic, and the organomegaly is discovered on routine physical examination. Some patients, however, present with symptoms of a bleeding diathesis. Easy bruisability is common and results from hypersplenism. Low platelet counts are particularly common, but all blood elements may be decreased. Physical examination may reveal mild to moderate diffuse lymphadenopathy. The enlarged nodes are nontender and freely movable.

Many patients with this form of Gaucher disease develop significant bone disease. This results from the excessive storage of Gaucher cells (i.e., macrophages loaded with glucosylceramide) in the bone marrow and erosion of bone. Osteopenia often develops, and minor trauma may cause fractures. Bone pain is frequently reported in and around large joints such as the hips, knees, shoulders, and spine. The severity of osteopenia may be less, and its onset may be delayed in patients whose spleens have not been removed. The liver is frequently enlarged, and liver function tests may be abnormal owing to glucosylceramide storage in reticuloendothelial cells. Liver failure is decidedly uncommon. The nervous system is not affected, even in patients who have had their illness for decades. Life expectancy is normal.

Type 2, or Acute Infantile Neuronopathic Form

Unlike type 1, Gaucher disease type 2 has a predictable, almost stereotypical presentation and course. Birth and the first 3 months of life are typically unremarkable. The clinician recognizes a protuberant abdomen and detects massive hepatosplenomegaly but cannot find a cherry-red spot macula in a 3-month-old child. At 6 months of age, the child has documented severe neurologic disability, including severe spasticity of the trunk, marked extension of the neck and spine, strabismus, and pseudobulbar palsy. The deep tendon reflexes are hyperactive, and pathologic reflexes are observed. A few months later, seizures develop, and the relentless downward course of the illness ensues. Within a few months to a year, the infant becomes apathetic and has no voluntary movements. Death generally occurs by the age of 2 years. The clinician should not make a diagnosis of this form of Gaucher disease in the absence of early and severe nervous system involvement.

Type 3, or Subacute Neuronopathic Form

In Gaucher disease type 3, the initial presentation with hepatosplenomegaly may precede the development of neurologic symptoms by several years. The neurologic presentation is quite variable but may include dementia, progressive supranuclear palsy, or gait disturbances secondary to cerebellar ataxia or spastic paraparesis. Major motor (tonic-clonic) or complex partial (psychomotor) seizures are common. This author has evaluated two siblings with a prolonged history of hepatomegaly who developed cerebellar ataxia at 9 years of age. Over the next 10 years, both patients progressed from wheel chair confinement to bed confinement to death in a state of dementia and paralysis.

Gaucher Disease With Normal β-Glucosidase Activity

Several patients have been reported with Gaucher disease in which the typical and expected enzyme deficiency was not found. These infants and children had a clinical course indistinguishable from the acute infantile neuronopathic form (type 2) and the subacute neuronopathic form (type 3). Glucosylceramide β-glucosidase cannot hydrolyze its substrate in the absence of a low-molecular-weight activator protein, known as SAP-2. A deficiency of this activator protein causes a phenotypically identical disorder that cannot be distinguished clinically from the more common forms of Gaucher disease. Special biochemical tests required to measure the activity of SAP-2 are not generally available at this time.

Enzymatic Analysis

The enzyme deficiency responsible for Gaucher disease is glucosylceramide β-glucosidase. With appropriate conditions, the fluorometric substrate 4-methylumbelliferyl-β-glucoside can be used to diagnose all forms of the disorder. In general, the residual enzyme activity in all forms of Gaucher disease is less than 2 per cent of control values. Enzyme analysis alone cannot differentiate the various forms of the disorder. Therefore, great care must be taken in counseling parents concerning the future of their affected infant. Many patients (especially type 1) continue to be diagnosed without the aid of enzyme analysis. A bone marrow aspirate with routine histologic demonstration of Gaucher cells is helpful, but it may be incorrect. Electron microscopy of the same aspirate can be diagnostic if it reveals the typical crystalline inclusions of stored glucosylceramide in lysosomes. In the future, various forms of Gaucher disease are likely to be distinguished by characterization of the various DNA mutations that cause the disorder.

Niemann-Pick Disease

Niemann-Pick disease is also known as sphingomyelin lipidosis. The classification is complicated because disorders are incorporated into this group that are unrelated to sphingomyelinase deficiency. Only those disorders resulting from a deficiency of sphingomyelinase are reviewed in this section. Some of the disorders frequently grouped with Niemann-Pick disease have a nonspecific increase of sphingomyelin along with increased cholesterol, glycosphingolipids, and bis-(monoacylglyero)phosphate. The latter compound is a valuable marker for lysosomes and is increased in all disorders characterized by lysosomal proliferation. Some reports indicate that type A Niemann-Pick disease results from sphingomyelinase deficiency and type B Niemann-Pick results from other biochemical mechanisms that are not understood. Niemann-Pick disease has a number of age-related variants. These include acute infantile, subacute juvenile, and chronic adult forms.

Type A Niemann-Pick Diseases

Acute Infantile Form

Development is generally normal for the first 3 to 4 months of life. Massive hepatosplenomegaly is recognized between 6 months and 1 year of age. Increased serum AST and ALT concentrations suggest liver cell injury in some patients with type A disease. Early in life, these infants present with failure to thrive. Severe feeding problems, vomiting, and diarrhea are commonly present. Attainment of developmental milestones usually halts before acquisition of the ability to sit. Progressive loss of motor skills and the ability to interact with the environment (i.e., dementia) is prominent during the period between 6 months and 1 year of life. Cherry-red spot macula occurs in approximately 50 per cent of affected infants. A chest film frequently demonstrates a diffuse granular infiltrate in the lung fields. Spastic tetraparesis, pseudobulbar palsy, and severe dementia typically ensue, and the child often dies in an emaciated state despite adequate nutrition provided via a nasogastric tube or feeding gastrostomy. Death occurs before 5 years of age.

Juvenile-Onset Form

Significant clinical variation occurs within this group. Many patients present with splenomegaly, followed by hepatomegaly. However, they do not develop symptoms or signs of nervous system dysfunction for many years. Others present in the same manner, but between the ages of 10 and 20, they develop a constellation of neurologic signs, including cerebellar ataxia, dementia (i.e., mental retardation), extrapyramidal movement disorders, and progressive supranuclear palsy. Combinations of these neurologic symptoms occur frequently. Asthma, recurrent respiratory infection, and granular infiltrates seen on the chest film are also reported. Observation of a cherry-red spot macula is rare, but pigmentary maculopathy may be present.

Adult Form

One form of Niemann-Pick is recognized during the adult years. Patients typically present with hepatosplenomegaly, sometimes found on routine physical examination. Many of these individuals remain asymptomatic for years. Some develop signs and symptoms of hypersplenism, including anemia, leukopenia, and thrombocytopenia. Rare individuals have been reported with biliary cirrhosis. After many years, a few adult patients develop cerebellar ataxia and changes in intellectual functioning. A cherry-red spot macula has been observed in some individuals. The adult form of Niemann-Pick cannot readily be distinguished from the juvenile-onset form. Delayed diagnosis may account for some of the patients included in this group. Some have a normal life expectancy, and others have their lives shortened by one or more of the complications of the disorder.

Enzymatic Diagnosis

Although a bone marrow aspirate may aid the diagnosis of Niemann-Pick disease, the histopathology is not entirely specific. Therefore, suspected cases of Niemann-Pick should have the benefit of enzyme analysis so that genetic counseling can be provided to the patient or the family.

The forms of Niemann-Pick disease discussed here are the result of a marked deficiency of acid sphingomyelinase activity. Sphingomyelinase activity can be measured colorimetrically, but radiolabeled ^{14}C-sphingomyelin has been the most widely used commercially available substrate. Acid sphingomyelinase normally releases phosphorylcholine from sphingomyelin. In the variants of Niemann-Pick disease discussed previously, residual enzyme activity is typically less than 5 per cent of normal control values. Isolated leukocytes, cultured skin fibroblasts, and amniotic fluid cells remain the most popular sources of sphingomyelinase.

MISCELLANEOUS SPHINGOLIPIDOSES

Fabry Disease

Fabry disease is also known by the stored product, ceramide trihexosidosis, or by the older clinical name, angiokeratoma corporis diffusum. Fabry disease is a systemic disorder with variable clinical manifestations that result from the storage of the sphingolipid ceramide trihexoside in vascular endothelial cells. Although most patients with this X-linked disorder are male, female carriers with severe forms of the disease have been reported.

Although many organs can store ceramide trihexoside, the accumulation of this sphingolipid in the vasculature of skin, oral mucosa, and cornea can be helpful in establishing the diagnosis of Fabry disease. The typical skin lesion is the angiokeratoma (Fig. 3). Clusters of these vascular lesions can be found on the abdomen, buttocks, scrotum, and shaft of the penis. Biopsy reveals small vessels with lipid-laden endothelial cells that narrow the lumen. Vascular lesions of the oral mucosa, conjunctiva, and vermilion border of the lip are also common. Infiltrates of the cornea (Fig. 4) are found in most affected males and in many heterozygous females. These infiltrates can be seen with the ophthalmoscope, but they are better appreciated during a slit-lamp examination.

Fabry disease may remain relatively silent for years or may cause vascular insufficiency in vital organs. The kidneys, heart, and brain are especially vulnerable to the vascular insufficiency caused by this disease. Renal insufficiency progressing to complete renal failure, myocardial ischemia, transient ischemic attacks, and recurrent strokes are well documented. Retinal infarction has been observed.

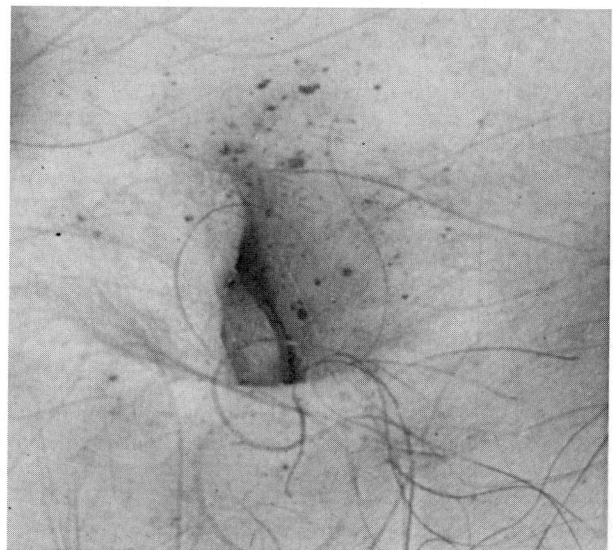

Figure 3. Typical angiokeratoma of the periumbilical region in a patient with Fabry disease. Other common sites of this lesion include the buttocks, scrotum, penis, and upper thighs.

Pain is probably the most common debilitating symptom. Some patients describe chronic burning and paresthesias of the feet or, less often, the hands. The pain is similar to the "burning neuropathy" associated with diabetes mellitus. Physical examination may reveal decreased light touch, decreased vibration sense, and other sensory abnormalities. Other patients describe pain that lasts for minutes to days and is characterized by excruciating, sharp, stabbing discomfort that may start in the hands or feet but quickly spreads up the extremity to involve the abdomen and other parts of the body. Some descriptions of these events may remind the clinician of the painful crises of sickle cell anemia. Although repeated bouts of ischemic damage to important organs are characteristic of Fabry disease, some patients never experience life-threatening vascular compromise.

Enzymatic Diagnosis

In Fabry disease, a deficiency of α-galactosidase results in failure to remove the terminal galactose from ceramide trihexosamide. Colorimetric substrates, fluorometric substrates, and radiolabeled natural substrates all have been used to measure α-galactosidase activity. The most sensitive and specific assay uses 4-methylumbelliferyl α-galactoside as the substrate. α-Galactosidase activity in young males with Fabry disease is less than 5 per cent of control values. Sources of enzyme include leukocytes, cultured skin fibroblasts, amniotic fluid cells, isolated platelets, and hair root cells obtained by plucking hairs from the scalp.

Farber Disease

Farber disease, also known as Farber lipogranulomatosis, results from a deficiency of ceramidase, an acid hydrolytic enzyme that catalyzes the cleavage of ceramide to fatty acid and sphingosine. This exceedingly rare disorder begins at 1 to 4 months of age with painful swelling of joints followed by hoarseness. Generalized swelling of the extremities is also an early finding, but the swelling soon subsides. Affected joints develop flexion contractures that are difficult to manage with physical therapy because movement induces severe pain. As the disease progresses, subcutaneous nodules develop around the interphalangeal, wrist, elbow, and ankle joints. Subcutaneous nodules also develop over typical pressure points, including the back of the head and the lower spine. Fevers may occur. Swelling of the larynx and epiglottis produces difficulty in swallowing and breathing. Respiratory insufficiency with bronchospasm is common. Involvement of the nervous system is variable; about one third of these patients have developmental delays. Peripheral neuropathy is common and leads to hypotonia and muscular atrophy. Granulomas may also form in the heart, liver, lymph nodes, and eyes. Death typically occurs before the age of 20 years.

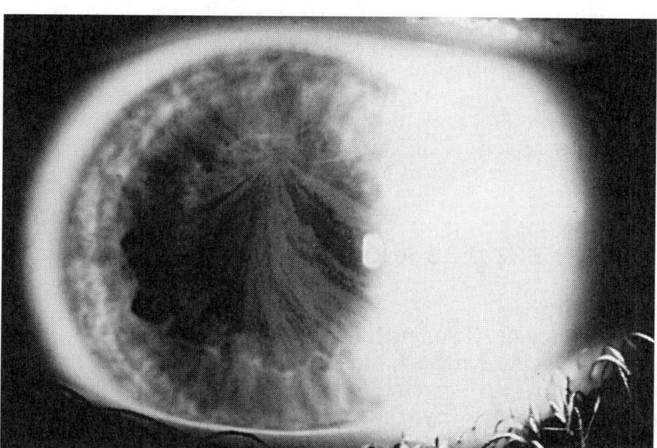

Figure 4. Slit-lamp photograph demonstrating the typical corneal infiltrate of ceramide trihexoside. This physical finding is seen in most males with Fabry disease and in a high percentage of female carriers of the disorder.

Milder Forms of Farber Disease

A few individuals with milder forms of Farber disease have been reported. These patients also have subcutaneous nodules, joint deformities, and laryngeal involvement, but many of those with milder forms of Farber disease have survived past the age of 20 years.

Enzymatic Diagnosis

This rare disorder is readily confirmed by enzyme analysis using isolated leukocytes or cultured skin fibroblasts. Acid (lysosomal) ceramidase activity is measured in the presence of radiolabeled natural substrate and a detergent at pH 4.8. In all patients with Farber disease, ceramidase activity ranges from 1 to 5 per cent of control values.

THE PORPHYRIAS

By David A. Paslin
Oakland, California

OVERVIEW

Many vital functions in living systems are the result of electron transfer by metal ions. To function as electron donors, these metals are chelated to porphyrins. In plants, the metal ion is magnesium, forming chlorophyll. In animals, the metal ion is iron, forming heme. The chelation of iron to porphyrins permits the gain, transfer, and release of energy. The iron porphyrins, or hemes, are coupled, as prosthetic groups, to protein. Various heme proteins are used for many cellular functions. For example, hemoglobin supports oxygen transport; microsomal cytochromes promote oxidative reactions and mixed metabolic functions; peroxidases catalyze the decomposition of hydrogen peroxide and the oxidation of substrates; catalases promote the decomposition of hydrogen peroxide and the generation of free oxygen; and mitochondrial cytochromes facilitate the transport of electrons for the generation of adenosine triphosphate (ATP).

Living systems tend to form complex products by variably assembling simple and ubiquitous starting materials. In bacteria and animals, assembly of complex porphyrins begins with the simpler molecules of glycine and succinate. These starting materials are transformed along a pathway of eight enzymatic steps to form heme. The first and rate-limiting enzyme of the pathway is δ-aminolevulinic acid (ALA) synthase. Deficiencies in each of the seven subsequent enzymes cause the seven porphyrias. The diagnoses of the heterozygous and homozygous forms of these disorders are reviewed in this article. The classification of the porphyrias is given in Table 1.

Table 1. Classification of the Porphyrias

Disorder	Synonyms	Enzyme Defect	Acute Attack (AA) and/or Skin Expression (SE)	Organ of Porphyrin Production
ALA dehydrase porphyria	ALADP Plumboporphyria Porphobilinogen synthase porphyria Hereditary δ-aminolevulinic aciduria	ALA dehydrase (ALA-D)	AA	Liver
Acute intermittent porphyria	AIP Swedish porphyria Pyrroloporphyria	PBG deaminase (PBG-D)	AA	Liver
Congenital erythropoietic porphyria	CEP Günther's disease Erythropoietic porphyria	Uroporphyrinogen III synthase (uro III-S)	SE	Red blood cells
Porphyria cutanea tarda	PCT Symptomatic porphyria Chronic hepatic porphyria	Uroporphyrinogen decarboxylase (uro-D)	SE	Liver
Hereditary coproporphyria	HCP	Coproporphyrinogen oxidase (coprox)	AA SE	Liver
Variegate porphyria	VP Mixed porphyria South African porphyria	Protoporphyrinogen oxidase (protox)	AA SE	Liver
Erythropoietic protoporphyria	EPP Erythrohepatic protoporphyria Protoporphyria	Ferrochelatase	SE	Red blood cells Liver

THE PATHWAY

The porphyrias represent a sequence of enzymatic impairments in the pathway to heme; thus, a rational approach to diagnosis requires an understanding of that pathway (Fig. 1).

The pathway begins with the ancient organelle, the mitochondrion, which resembles a primitive miniature cell containing nucleic acids, porphyrins, and cytochromes able to generate energy by electron and oxygen transfer. In the mitochondria, glycine combines with pyridoxal phosphate and succinyl coenzyme A (succinyl CoA) to form the postulated intermediate α-amino-β-ketoadipic acid. This intermediate is rapidly decarboxylated to ALA in a reaction catalyzed by ALA synthase.

ALA diffuses from the mitochondria into the cytosol. In a reaction catalyzed by ALA dehydrase, two molecules of ALA condense to form the monopyrrole ring porphobilinogen (PBG). In the presence of the cytosolic enzyme porphobilinogen deaminase, the monopyrrole rings of PBG are sequentially deaminated and attached by methylene bridges in the sequence of ring A, B, C, and then D to form the putative straight-chained tetrapyrrole intermediate hydroxymethylbilane. In the absence of the cytosolic enzyme, uroporphyrinogen III synthase (uro III-S), hydroxymethylbilane spontaneously cyclizes to uroporphyrinogen I. In the presence of uro III-S, as ring D is about to attach to ring A, ring D reverses position to form the III isomer of uroporphyrinogen. In the III isomer, the acetic acid group of ring D is juxtaposed to the acetic acid group of ring A, and the propionic acid group of ring D is juxtaposed to the propionic acid group of ring C.

Uroporphyrinogen decarboxylase (uro-D) in the cytosol decarboxylates the four acetic acid groups of both the I and III isomers of uroporphyrinogen to produce the four methyl groups of coproporphyrinogen. The sequence of decarboxylations appears to proceed from ring D, to A, to B, and finally to C.

Coproporphyrinogen diffuses from the cytosol into the mitochondria, where coproporphyrinogen III oxidase, by oxidation and decarboxylation, catalyzes the stepwise conversion of the propionic acid groups of rings A and B of coproporphyrinogen III to vinyl groups. The monovinylporphyrinogen, harderoporphyrinogen, is an intermediate between coproporphyrinogen III and protoporphyrinogen IX. As the name implies, coproporphyrinogen III oxidase does not oxidize porphyrinogens of the I isomer series. Coproporphyrinogen I is a dead end.

The remaining enzymes in the heme synthetic pathway are also mitochondrial. Protoporphyrinogen oxidase converts protoporphyrinogen IX to protoporphyrin IX (protoporphyrin), which, in the presence of ferrochelatase, traps ferrous iron to form heme. The reduction of ferric ions in the cytosol to ferrous ions in the mitochondria appears to enhance the sequential oxidations of the 4, 3, and 2 carboxylic acid porphyrinogens. Heme, formed in the mitochondria, represses the activity of mitochondrial ALA synthase. If the concentration of mitochondrial heme falls, as typically occurs in the porphyrias, then ALA synthase becomes derepressed, and porphyrin synthesis accelerates with increased production of the substrates in the pathway to heme.

PATHWAY ENZYMES AND RESULTING DISEASES

ALA Synthase

Deficiency of ALA synthase (synonyms: ALA-S, 5-aminolevulinic acid synthase, δ-aminolevulinic acid synthase, and succinyl CoA glycine C-succinyl transferase) does not cause porphyria. (Synthase, not synthetase, is used because the former denotes an enzyme that does not require ATP in the reaction.) Instead, ALA synthase deficiency is typically associated with the sideroblastic anemias, a group of diseases characterized by impaired ferrochelatase activity and impaired utilization of iron to form heme.

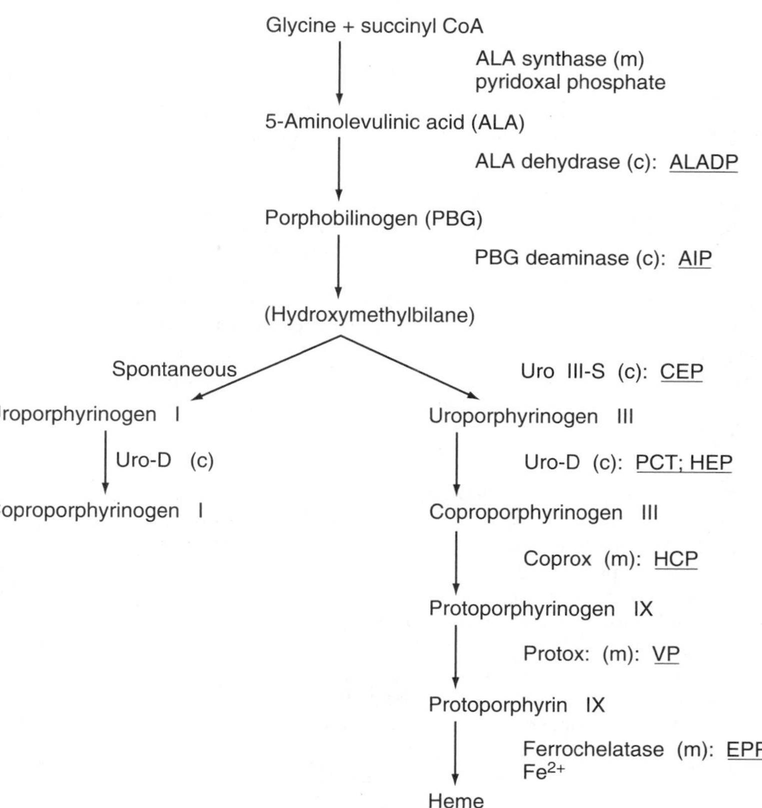

Figure 1. The pathway to heme. Deficiencies of the enzymes permit expression of the corresponding porphyrias (underlined). ALADP = 5-aminolevulinic acid dehydrase porphyria; AIP = acute intermittent porphyria; CEP = congenital erythropoietic porphyria; PCT = porphyria cutanea tarda; HEP = hepatoerythropoietic porphyria; HCP = hereditary coproporphyria; VP = variegate porphyria; EPP = erythropoietic protoporphyria. Note that HEP is the homozygous or compound heterozygous expression of a defect in uroporphyrinogen decarboxylase. (m) = in mitochondria; (c) = in cytosol.

Rarely, the sideroblastic anemias are accompanied by photosensitivity and increased levels of protoporphyrin, and less often coproporphyrins and uroporphyrins. Both the genetic and the acquired forms of sideroblastic anemia are characterized by accumulation of excess iron in the mitochondria, ringed sideroblasts in the marrow, heavy deposits of hemosiderin in the marrow, and iron granules in siderocytes in the peripheral blood.

ALA synthase is the rate-limiting enzyme in the pathway to heme. The activity of ALA synthase is normally low because heme decreases the stability of pro-ALA synthase messenger ribonucleic acid (mRNA) translation, slows the translocation of pro-ALA synthase into mitochondria, and directly inhibits the catalytic activity of the enzyme.

In the porphyrias, by contrast, the activity of ALA synthase is typically increased. Two forms of ALA synthase, linked to genes on separate chromosomes, have been identified. The 59.5-kd erythroid form is the product of a gene on the X chromosome, while the housekeeping, or regulating, 64.6-kd hepatic form is a product of a gene on chromosome 3. The activity of ALA synthase in hepatocytes is also increased by the administration of lipophilic porphyrinogenic drugs and steroids. These agents induce the terminal oxidase in the microsomes, cytochrome P-450, which requires heme as its prosthetic group. The high affinity of cytochrome P-450 for heme draws heme out of mitochondria, and ALA synthase activity is derepressed.

ALA Dehydrase

ALA dehydrase (synonyms: ALA-D, 5-aminolevulinic acid dehydrase, 5-aminolevulinate hydrolase, porphobilinogen synthase, plumboporphyria synthase) is usually present in great excess in the cytosol. Thus, a mutation in one of the alleles of the ALA dehydrase gene typically does not produce disease. However, homozygous or compound heterozygous mutations produce ALA dehydrase porphyria (ALADP), a condition that typically presents in childhood. ALADP and congenital erythropoietic porphyria (CEP) (see later) are the two recessively transmitted porphyrias. A second genetic form of ALADP is encountered in patients with hereditary tyrosinemia type I. Decreased fumarate acetoacetate-hydrolase activity leads to increased concentrations of 4,6-dioxoheptanoic acid, an inhibitor of ALA dehydrase. Succinylacetone, which also inhibits ALA dehydrase, can be detected in the urine of patients with hereditary tyrosinemia. If no succinylacetone is found, the diagnosis of hereditary tyrosinemia can be excluded. ALADP can also be acquired during poisoning with lead, styrene, bromobenzene, and alcohol, meaning not only ethanol, but also propanol, butanol, and amyl alcohol found at high concentrations in scotch and red wine.

PBG (Porphobilinogen) Deaminase

PBG deaminase (synonyms: PBG-D, uroporphyrinogen I synthase, hydroxymethylbilane synthase, porphobilinogen ammonia lyase polymerizing) is the second rate-limiting enzyme in the pathway to heme. Humans possess two isozymes of PBG deaminase, an erythroid enzyme and a nonerythroid enzyme. Their activities differ. In rat liver, the ratio of PBG deaminase activity to ALA synthase activity is 2:1, whereas in rat erythroid cells, the ratio is 6:1. Thus, PBG deaminase is a potential rate-limiting enzyme in liver, but not in erythroid cells.

PBG deaminase deficiency permits expression of acute intermittent porphyria (AIP), yet only 10 percent of persons with known deficiency of PBG deaminase become symptomatic. In a family with 17 individuals heterozygous for PBG deaminase deficiency, only 2 had increased urine

PBG, and only 1 developed an acute attack of porphyria over 15 years of follow-up. Some drugs precipitate attacks of AIP by derepressing ALA synthase, while others (e.g., carbamazepine and sulfonamides) precipitate attacks by inhibiting hepatic PBG deaminase.

Uroporphyrinogen III Synthase

Abnormalities of uroporphyrinogen III synthase (synonyms: uro III-S, uro III synthase, uroporphyrinogen III cosynthase) produce disease only in patients with homozygous or compound heterozygous defects. Congenital erythropoietic porphyria is a rare and mutilating disorder characterized by uro III-S activity that ranges from 2 to 20 per cent of that seen in individuals who do not have the genetic defect. Total absence of enzyme activity is incompatible with life.

Uroporphyrinogen Decarboxylase

Both the hereditary and the acquired forms of uroporphyrinogen decarboxylase (synonym: uro-D) deficiency have been reported. Acquired deficiency produces porphyria cutanea tarda (PCT) type I, whereas hereditary deficiency leads to PCT types II and III. In acquired PCT, uro-D activity is decreased primarily in hepatocytes. Although total body iron stores increase, iron deposition is most prominent in hepatocytes. Familial PCT (type II) is characterized by decreased uro-D activity in both hepatocytes and erythrocytes, whereas the less common familial PCT (type III) reveals decreased uro-D activity only in liver cells. Homozygous or compound heterozygous mutations cause disease that begins in childhood and involves both liver and red blood cells (hepatoerythropoietic porphyria [HEP]).

As in other hepatic porphyrias, ALA synthase is derepressed, and abundant ALA enters the heme pathway. However, in contrast to other hepatic porphyrias, PCT is not associated with acute attacks of porphyria because PCT patients have increased red cell PBG deaminase activity in symptomatic and asymptomatic cases and in sporadic and familial forms of the disease. Increased hepatic PBG deaminase activity has also been reported in PCT. The mechanism by which PBG deaminase activity increases in PCT is unknown, but the effect appears to be post-translational.

Coproporphyrinogen III oxidase catalyzes the oxidative decarboxylation of 5-carboxylic acid porphyrinogen III to form dehydroisocoproporphyrinogen, which, in turn, is converted to isocoproporphyrinogen, a form of 4 carboxylic acid porphyrin III diagnostic of PCT.

Coproporphyrinogen III Oxidase

Coproporphyrinogen III oxidase (synonyms: coproporphyrinogen oxidase, coprox) catalyzes the oxidation and decarboxylation of isomers of the III series only. Deficiency of coproporphyrinogen III oxidase causes hereditary coproporphyria (HCP), an autosomal dominant condition. When the genetic defect is homozygous or compound heterozygous, harderoporphyria results from the accumulation of 3 carboxylic acid harderoporphyrins.

Protoporphyrinogen Oxidase

Variegate porphyria (VP) is an autosomal dominant disorder associated with deficiency of protoporphyrinogen oxidase (protox).

Both HCP (coproporphyria) and VP are characterized by acute attacks and sporadically increased ALA and PBG. The same stimuli that derepress ALA synthase in AIP operate in HCP and VP, but in HCP and VP derepression of ALA synthase is not sufficient to produce acute attacks of porphyria. Rather, experiment has shown inhibition of PBG deaminase by coproporphyrinogen III and protoporphyrinogen IX. Activity of PBG deaminase was impaired in sonicates of Epstein-Barr virus–transformed lymphocytes from subjects with VP, but not from control subjects. However, activity of PBG deaminase became impaired in sonicates from control subjects after addition of protoporphyrinogen IX or coproporphyrinogen III to the mix. Removal of endogenous porphyrinogens from VP sonicates restored PBG deaminase kinetics to normal. Since uroporphyrinogen had no effect and since coproporphyrinogen III had less effect than protoporphyrinogen IX, enzyme inhibition increases as the number of carboxylic acid groups in the tetrapyrrole ring decreases. Protoporphyrinogen IX inhibits coproporphyrinogen oxidase. Therefore, patients with VP accumulate not only protoporphyrinogen but also coproporphyrinogen.

Ferrochelatase

Ferrochelatase (synonyms: heme synthase, protoheme-ferrolyase) deficiency is transmitted as an autosomal dominant trait and expressed as erythropoietic protoporphyria (EPP). Various point or splice site mutations have been documented, and exon deletions may be observed. Ferrochelatase deficiency is expressed in hepatocytes as well as erythrocytes. Red blood cells contribute about 80 per cent, and hepatocytes about 20 per cent of protoporphyrin overproduction.

SUBSTRATE ACCUMULATION

The correct diagnosis of porphyria typically requires identification of the substrates that accumulate in response to enzyme deficiency. For example, ALA accumulates in patients with rare homozygous or compound heterozygous inheritance of ALA dehydrase deficiency. Other causes of increased ALA must be excluded, however.

PBG deaminase deficiency leads to accumulation of PBG and ALA. In patients with AIP, HCP, and VP, marked PBG and ALA accumulation is typically seen during acute attacks. However, PBG and ALA may also mildly accumulate in some asymptomatic patients with AIP and marginally accumulate in some asymptomatic patients with HCP and VP. Slightly increased uroporphyrins, coproporphyrins, and protoporphyrins also may be identified in patients with AIP, but accumulation of these compounds seldom leads to cutaneous signs or symptoms.

In CEP, the loss of activity of uro III-S ranges from 80 to 98 per cent. Shunting of substrate along the I isomeric pathway leads to marked accumulation of uroporphyrin I and coproporphyrinogen I. Smaller amounts of the III isomers also accumulate. Increased PBG deaminase activity in patients with CEP may produce sufficient hydroxymethylbilane to cause a mass effect, thereby enhancing its processing by whatever uro III-S is available in the cytosol.

Patients with PCT predictably generate increased concentrations of uroporphyrin III, uroporphyrin I, and coproporphyrin I. By contrast, the preponderance of I isomers is less predictable and may depend on the degree of inhibition of uro III-S by accumulated uroporphyrinogen III. In PCT, uroporphyrins I and III are present in greater quantity than coproporphyrins. Also, 7, 6, and 5 carboxylated porphyrins accumulate. Oxidative decarboxylation of 5 carboxylic acid porphyrinogen by coprox generates isocoproporphyrin, a compound seldom detected in any other porphyria.

Hereditary coproporphyria is distinguished chiefly by accumulation of coproporphyrin III in urine and stool. In the homozygous variant, harderoporphyria, the tricarboxylic harderoporphyrin accumulates in feces.

In VP, protoporphyrinogen and coproporphyrinogen accumulate. Gut flora oxidize these substrates to protoporphyrins and coproporphyrins in the feces. X-porphyrins, representing hydrophilic porphyrin peptide complexes, are also found in the feces of patients with VP. Although X-porphyrins often partition with fractions harvested for recovery of uroporphyrin, the X-porphyrins seen in VP can be chromotographically distinguished from the porphyrins seen in PCT. During acute attacks of HCP and VP, ALA and PBG accumulate in urine (as is true in acute attacks of AIP).

Erythropoietic protoporphyria is characterized by accumulation of protoporphyrin. In patients with liver involvement, increased coproporphyrin, heptacarboxylic acid porphyrin, and uroporphyrin may be found in urine.

SITE OF SUBSTRATE EXCRETION

The presence of carboxylic acid groups increases the water solubility and urinary excretion of porphyrins. Those molecules with fewer carboxylic acid groups are more fat soluble and are excreted in feces. The water-soluble compounds include ALA, PBG, uroporphyrinogen, and the 7, 6, and 5 carboxylic acid porphyrins. Intermediate solubilities characterize the 4 carboxylic acid porphyrins, coproporphyrinogen, and isocoproporphyrinogen, and these compounds are found in both urine and feces. With only 2 carboxylic acid groups, protoporphyrinogen IX is water insoluble and almost exclusively found in feces.

ALA Dehydrase Porphyria

ALA is markedly increased, and PBG, uroporphyrinogen III, and coproporphyrinogen III are moderately increased in the urine of patients with genetically transmitted ALADP. In lead poisoning, by contrast, both ALA dehydrase and ferrochelatase are inhibited. Therefore, not only are ALA and uroporphyrin found in urine, but also protoporphyrin is found in red blood cells (bound as zinc protoporphyrin), and both protoporphyrin and coproporphyrin may be found in feces.

Acute Intermittent Porphyria

Both ALA and PBG are markedly increased in urine during acute attacks and may or may not be mildly increased during latency in patients with AIP. Uroporphyrin and coproporphyrin in urine and protoporphyrin in feces are often mildly increased during acute attacks.

Congenital Erythropoietic Porphyria

In CEP, uroporphyrin I and coproporphyrin I are markedly increased in urine and in feces. Coproporphyrin I in urine is the product of renal clearance of coproporphyrinogen, not of coproporphyrin. By contrast, the liver clears coproporphyrinogen less rapidly than coproporphyrin. Uroporphyrin I, coproporphyrin I, and zinc protoporphyrin are increased in erythrocytes. The protoporphyrin in CEP is entirely chelated by zinc, whereas that in EPP is not. Increased zinc protoporphyrin in red blood cells is also found in iron deficiency anemia, but the concentrations are not sufficient to provoke photosensitivity.

Porphyria Cutanea Tarda

Increased concentrations of uroporphyrin I and III, coproporphyrin I, and isocoproporphyrin are found in urine and feces in patients with PCT. The urinary ratio of uroporphyrin to coproporphyrin approximates 5:1, and this ratio is one of the features that distinguishes PCT from VP. In the homozygous or, more likely, the compound heterozygous form of PCT known as HEP, the excretory patterns (but not the concentrations) of substrates are similar to those of acquired PCT. However, elevated concentrations of protoporphyrin in red blood cells and feces are also seen in HEP. This finding suggests that high levels of HEP substrates may inhibit ferrochelatase.

Hereditary Coproporphyria

Markedly increased concentrations of coproporphyrin III are found in the feces of patients with HCP, while moderately increased levels are found in urine. Protoporphyrin levels are normal, a feature that distinguishes HCP from VP. During acute attacks, ALA and PBG are increased in urine. ALA and PBG may be marginally increased during latency in HCP (or VP) so that HCP (or VP) cannot be reliably distinguished from AIP by such measurements.

Variegate Porphyria

Protoporphyrin IX is markedly increased and coproporphyrin III is moderately increased in the feces of patients with VP. Meanwhile coproporphyrin III and uroporphyrin III are detected in urine. During acute attacks of VP, ALA and PBG are increased in urine.

Erythropoietic Protoporphyria

Patients with EPP typically demonstrate a 50- to 100-fold increase in free (unbound) protoporphyrin IX in red blood cells. The concentration of protoporphyrin IX is also markedly increased in plasma, bile, and feces. Young red blood cells contain most of the protoporphyrin, which soon leaks from erythrocytes into the plasma. A small amount of coproporphyrin may be found in feces. However, patients with protoporphyin-induced cirrhosis produce markedly increased amounts of coproporphyrin (mostly isomer I) in urine, while fecal excretion decreases with advancing liver failure.

INITIAL MANIFESTATIONS OF PORPHYRIA

Most patients with porphyria experience the first clinical manifestation during puberty. Signs and symptoms typically develop when patients with predisposing hormonal milieus are exposed to a porphyrinogenic drug. Less commonly, children with latent enzyme deficiencies of the porphyrin pathway develop clinically apparent porphyria when exposed to a porphyrinogenic drug. Rarely, children may produce excessive amounts of porphyrinogenic hormones, such as pregnanetriol due to 21-hydroxylase deficiency in the adrenogenital syndrome. The porphyrias that are typically expressed in children are the erythropoietic porphyrias (CEP and EPP), where markedly increased production of porphyrins occurs chiefly in erythroid cells. The signs and symptoms of the erythropoietic porphyrias do not require the induction of hepatic enzymes by porphyrinogenic endogenous hormones or exogenous drugs. Yet,

EPP is not purely erythropoietic, since the liver is responsible for as much as 20 per cent of the protoporphyrin overproduction. By contrast, the amount and the significance of the hepatic contribution to the overproduction of uroporphyrin I and coproporphyrin I in CEP is less clear. Importantly, the hepatic porphyrias (ALADP, AIP, PCT, HCP, and VP), when transmitted as homozygous or compound heterozygous disorders, may also present in children.

The hepatic porphyrias that are transmitted as heterozygous, autosomal dominant disorders typically show themselves clinically when porphyrinogenic drugs are administered to patients who produce physiologic amounts of porphyrinogenic adrenal and gonadal steroids. When produced in excess, some of the more potent endogenous steroids have porphyrinogenic capacity equivalent to that of barbiturates. These steroids include pregnanolone, pregnanediol, pregnanetriol, pregnanedione, androsterone, etiocholanolone, etiocholandiol, and etiocholandione. Moderately porphyrinogenic steroids include DHEA, 17-OH-pregnanolone, and androstenedione. Pregnanediol is the major metabolite of progesterone, and pregnanetriol is the major metabolite of 17-OH-progesterone. Luteal-phase increases in these hormones may account for the premenstrual attacks of AIP seen in some women. Androsterone and etiocholanolone are the major metabolites of androstenedione and testosterone. Also porphyrinogenic are 11-hydroxyetiocholanolone and 11-keto-etiocholanolone, both minor metabolites of cortisol. Estrogens are not directly porphyrinogenic; instead, they decrease excretion of porphyrins in bile and increase release of porphyrins into the general circulation via the hepatic vein.

Drugs and hormones that have been strongly associated with the clinical manifestations of the hepatic porphyrias are *italicized* in Table 2. This table also provides a list of unsafe drugs, contentious drugs, and drugs believed to be safe for use in patients with porphyria. For example, while most benzodiazepines are considered unsafe, temazepam is reported to be safe for use in persons at risk for porphyria, lorazepam is probably safe, and the safety of diazepam is disputed.

Several mechanisms have been proposed to explain the influence of drugs and hormones on the synthesis of ALA and heme. Phenobarbital increases the concentration of porphyrinogenic steroids by increasing the synthesis of the apoprotein of cytochrome P-450 and impairing 5-α-reductase activity. Griseofulvin destroys heme and inhibits ferrochelatase. Alcohol (ethanol) blocks the synthesis of heme, increases its utilization, and inhibits ALA dehydrase. Estrogens by mouth adversely influence processing of porphyrins by the liver during first-pass metabolism (see above); estrogens by patch do not. In the absence of other factors, pregnancy is rarely complicated by abdominal attacks or by photosensitivity in patients at risk for porphyria.

PUTATIVE MECHANISMS IN THE PORPHYRIAS

Enzyme deficiencies in the porphyrias are typically observed in all tissues. Organ and cellular specialization, however, create differences in the response to inducing agents, leading to differences in disease expression. For example, the loss of mitochondrial enzymes (including heme-pathway enzymes) in mature red blood cells explains the accumulation of protoporphyrins in younger red blood cells in patients with EPP. The striking accumulation of substrates in red blood cells in the erythropoietic porphyrias occurs because nearly 80 to 85 per cent of porphyrins in the body are synthesized in erythroid cells. The biotransformation of hormones and drugs in the liver accounts for the nonerythrocytic expression of the acute hepatic porphyrias because these same agents do not cause similar changes in red blood cells.

Acute Porphyrias

Many of the acute porphyrias manifest similar symptoms, signs, biochemical abnormalities, and clinical presentations. Neuropathologic mechanisms that may account for all or almost all the symptoms and signs of an acute attack include neuronal heme deficiency; depletion of substrates, such as glycine, pyridoxal phosphate, and zinc; and neurotoxicity of ALA, PBG, and/or metabolites of accumulated substrates (e.g., porphobilin).

Cutaneous Porphyrias

Photosensitivity, the hallmark of the cutaneous porphyrias, results from interaction of the Soret band of light (400 to 410 nm) with porphyrins in the skin. The severity of the photosensitivity directly correlates with the amount of porphyrin in the skin, while the type of photosensitivity depends on the water and lipid solubilities of the accumulated porphyrins. Lipid-soluble porphyrins induce the acute cutaneous porphyrias (especially EPP), while the water-soluble porphyrins induce chronic cutaneous porphyrias (especially PCT). Although acute photosensitivity is also reported in plumboporphyria (lead poisoning), HEP, VP, and even CEP, HEP, VP, and CEP more commonly present with the PCT-like findings of the chronic cutaneous porphyrias.

The lipid-soluble porphyrins (especially protoporphyrin) concentrate in mitochondria and inhibit succinate dehydrogenase, an enzyme bound to the lipoproteins of mitochondrial inner membranes. Photo-oxidation of mitochondrial enzymes impairs oxidative phosphorylation and ATP synthesis. In patients with EPP, young red blood cells retain substantial amounts of protoporphyrin IX; what is not retained leaks into the plasma, where it is bound to albumin and hemopexin prior to clearance by the liver. Dermal red blood cells and capillaries sustain significant injury following exposure to Soret-band light as the protoporphyrins generate short-lived, high-energy singlet oxygen states mediating photodynamic reactions, tissue damage, and cell death. Photohemolysis causes mildly decreased hemoglobin concentrations, while dermal edema and purpura are associated with perivascular mast cell degranulation and destruction of endothelial cells of the dermal capillaries. These mechanisms are associated with acute redness, burning, stinging, and swelling of the light-exposed skin in patients with EPP.

By contrast, uroporphyrin and the 7, 6, and 5 carboxylic acid porphyrins concentrate in the cytosol and lysosomes. Following exposure to Soret-band light, lysosomal enzymes are released, cell membranes are disrupted, and water-soluble porphyrins leak into the interstitium. Further tissue injury leads to reduplication of basal laminae at the dermoepidermal junction (DEJ) and around dermal vessels. Because of the redundant and defective DEJ, minor trauma causes separation of epidermis from dermis, forming the subepidermal blisters and subsequent scarring characteristic of the chronic cutaneous porphyrias.

The small dermal vessels in both the acute and the chronic cutaneous porphyrias are marked by deposition of eosinophilic, amorphous, proteinaceous periodic acid–Schiff–positive material, containing in part glycoproteins, lipids, immunoglobulins, and complement.

Table 2. Drugs and the Hepatic Porphyrias

Believed to Be Unsafe	Contentious	Believed to Be Safe	
Aminophylline	Allopurinol	Acetazolamide	Ketoprofen
Androgens and metabolites, including androsterone and etiocholanolone	Alprazolam	Acetaminophen	Loperamide
Barbiturates	Amidopyrine	ACTH	Lorazepam
Bemegride	Amiodarone	Acyclovir	Mefenamic acid
Benzodiazepines, most, including chlordiazepoxide	Articaine	Amethocaine	Meperidine
Bromobenzene	Bretylium	Amitriptyline	Methadone
Carbamazepine	Bromocriptine	Amoxicillin	Metoclopramide
Chloramphenicol	Bupivacaine	Amphotericin B	Midazolam
Chlorpropamide	Captopril	Aspirin	Morphine
Danazol	Carisoprodol	Atropine	Naloxone
Disopyramide	Cimetidine	Bromazepam	Naproxen
Enflurane	Clomiphene	Carpipramine	Neostigmine
Ergotamine tartrate	Clonidine	Chloral hydrate	Nitroprusside
Estrogens, orally	Diazepam	Chloroquine (a little)	Nitrous oxide
Ethanol	Diltiazem	Chlorpheniramine	Norepinephrine
Etomidate	Erythromycin	Chlorpromazine	Norfloxacin
Eucalyptol	Etidocaine	Clomipramine	Organon
Glutethimide	Fenofibrate	Clorazepate (a little)	Oxazepam
Griseofulvin	Halothane	Codeine	Oxybate sodium
Halothane	Hydralazine	Corticosteroids	Oxybuprocaine
Hydantoins	Hydroxyzine	Curare	Pancuronium
Imipramine	Isoniazid	Cyclopropane	Paracetamol
Ketamine	Lidocaine	Dexchlorpheniramine	Paraldehyde
Ketoconazole	Lignocaine	Diazoxide	Penicillins
Mepivacaine	Loprazolam	Diclofenac	Pentamethonium
Meprobamate	Mephenesin	Dicoumarol	Perhexiline
Methsuximide	Methyclothiazide	Diethylene ether	Phenothiazines
Methyldopa	Mexiletine	Digoxin	Piracetam
Metronidazole	Nitrazepam	Diphenhydramine	Piroxicam
Miconazole	Oxazepam	Dipyridamole	Prazosin
Nifedipine	Pargyline	Droperidol	Probucol
Nikethamide	Pentoxifylline	EDTA	Procainamide
Pentazocine	Phenoxybenzamine	Epinephrine	Procaine
Phenazone	Prilocaine	Estazolam	Promazine
Phensuximide	Primidone	Flucytosine	Promethazine
Phenylbutazone	Probenecid	Flumazenil	Propanidid
Progesterone and metabolites	Propantheline	Flunitrazepam	Propofol
Progestogens	Pyrrocaine	Fluphenazine	Propoxyphene
Pyrazinamide	Quinine	Furosemide	Propranolol
Sulfonamides	Ranitidine	Gentamicin	Proxymetacaine
Tolbutamide	Rifampicin	Glucagon	Reserpine
Troxidone	Spironolactone	Guanethidine	Salbutamol
Valproate	Tamoxifen	Haloperidol	Sulindac
Verapamil	Tinidazole	Heparin	Temazepam
	Trazodone	Hydrochlorothiazide	Tetracyclines
	Triazolam	Indomethacin	Triamterene
	Trimipramine	Insulin	Verapamil
			Vitamins A, B, C, D, and E

Adapted from Bonkovsky H. L. The Porphyrias. In Conn, R. B. (ed.): Current Diagnosis 8. Philadelphia, W. B. Saunders, 1990, p. 800; and Harrison, G. G., Meissner, P. N., and Hift, R. J.: Anesthesia for the porphyric patient. Anaesthesia, 48:417–421, 1993, with permission.

CLINICAL DIAGNOSIS

Although the history and the physical examination may lead the clinician to suspect porphyria, additional testing is usually necessary for proving the diagnosis, for determining which porphyria is present, and for excluding other disease states that share clinical features of the porphyrias.

Qualitative screening tests may be performed at the bedside. Urine, feces, and/or blood should be sent to an appropriate clinical laboratory for measurement of porphyrins and porphyrin precursors. Assays of the activities of enzymes in the pathway to heme are occasionally useful in challenging cases, but these tests are performed only in a handful of research laboratories. Defective genes may be amplified and sequenced to identify sites and types of mutation which, in turn, determine the degree of enzyme impairment. Such testing is also not readily available.

The diagnosis of the porphyrias depends primarily on clinical recognition supported by qualitative laboratory screening and quantitative laboratory confirmation. Many people with defects of enzymes in the pathway to heme do not have clinical disease. Therefore, demonstration of enzyme deficiency or a genetic defect is not sufficient for diagnosing clinically significant porphyria. Rather, diagnosis most frequently depends on standard assays of accumulated porphyrins and porphyrin precursors.

Clinical Presentation

Acute Porphyrias

Severe cramping lower abdominal pain is the initial symptom in 85 per cent of patients with acute porphyrias.

Autonomic abnormalities produce intestinal spasm and dilation. Constipation is frequent, nausea and vomiting common, and impaction occasional. Acute attacks may mimic an acute surgical abdomen, but rebound tenderness is usually lacking. Tachycardia, severe anxiety, confusion, and overt psychosis have been described. Peripheral motor and sensory neuropathy, cranial nerve impairment, and seizures may accompany acute attacks.

Neuropathy is usually reversible, but some patients experience residual flaccid paralysis. Respiratory paralysis is a leading cause of coma and death in untreated acute porphyria. These patients may also experience postural hypotension, labile hypertension, sweating, vascular spasms of retinal and cutaneous vessels, and incontinence or retention of urine. Occasionally, low-grade fever may be related to increased concentrations of etiocholanolone. Epinephrine and norepinephrine production may be episodically increased.

Hyponatremia may accompany hypothalamic injury and inappropriate secretion of antidiuretic hormone. Acute attacks of porphyria occur more often in women than in men typically in the luteal phase of the menstrual cycle. The leukocyte count is usually normal. Serum transaminases may be slightly increased.

Acute Cutaneous Photosensitivity

Acute cutaneous photosensitivity is a characteristic feature of EPP, the most common of the childhood porphyrias. The first episode of photosensitivity typically occurs prior to 6 years of age. Burning, itching, redness, and swelling of sun-exposed skin develop within minutes of exposure to sunlight. Blisters and purpura may be superimposed, but hirsutism and hyperpigmentation are unusual. Objective findings may be limited to a cobblestone appearance of the knuckles. In the absence of physical findings, the patient may be dismissed as hypochondriacal.

Gallstones, consisting largely of protoporphyrin, are present in about 12 per cent of patients with EPP. Liver biopsy often shows porphyrin deposits in hepatocytes, Kupffer's cells, and bile canaliculi. Under polarized light, yellow-to-green, granular, "Maltese-cross" fluorescence is seen. Early hepatic involvement is accompanied by increased serum aminotransferases and bilirubin as well as increased coproporphyrin in urine. Liver biopsy should be performed early in the course of EPP because 65 per cent of these patients show hepatic protoporphyrin deposition and 25 per cent show hepatic fibrosis without clinical evidence of liver disease. Increasing concentrations of red blood cell protoporphyrin also suggest liver involvement; erythrocyte protoporphyrin concentrations closely correlate with γ-glutamyl transferase (GGT) concentrations in serum. As liver disease worsens, biliary excretion of protoporphyrin into feces decreases, reflecting damage to the canalicular secretory apparatus. Inspissated bile and cholestatic jaundice may ensue. As protoporphyrin in feces decreases (<300 nmol/g), coproporphyrin (mostly isomer I) excretion in urine increases (>400 nmol/L). Uncoupling of oxidative phosphorylation and disruption of mitochondria lead to hepatocellular necrosis, periportal fibrosis, cirrhosis, and death.

Chronic Cutaneous Photosensitivity

The cutaneous manifestations of PCT, HCP, and VP are virtually identical and generally appear during, after, or long after (PCT) puberty. The cutaneous findings in CEP and HEP are similar but more severe. Approximately 100 patients with CEP have been reported; most of them presented early in childhood. The initial finding is often a pink stain of diapers by urine and meconium. Infants may scream when placed in sunlight. Photophobia is later accompanied by keratoconjunctivitis, which may lead to blindness. Hemolytic anemia is almost always present and often requires transfusion. Blistering is severe, and onycholysis is common. Hirsutism is marked by heavy lanugo and terminal hair covering the sun-exposed areas. Synophrys may occur. Scarring may cause alopecia and ectropion, and patients may prevent closure of the lips that pull back. Mutilating loss of ears, nose, fingertips, and toes has been described. Uroporphyrin binds to calcium phosphate in the teeth and bones as they are formed, generating an orange-red fluoresence of these calcified structures as well as of meninges, brain, heart, lungs, liver, gallbladder, kidneys, intestines, and skin, as demonstrated at the autopsy of a 14-year-old boy with CEP. Iron deposition in the liver and spleen is frequent, and splenomegaly is common.

Like CEP, HEP is characterized by severe photosensitivity from birth. Children with HEP develop hypertrichosis, hyperpigmentation, conjunctivitis, photophobia, scleromalacia perforans, and scarring. The scarring may progress to mutilation. Children with HEP, however, lack the erythrodontia, hemolytic anemia, and splenomegaly seen in children with CEP.

The chronic cutaneous manifestations of PCT, HCP, and VP include blistering, skin fragility, milia, scarring, hirsutism, and melasmalike hyperpigmentation of sun-exposed skin. PCT is the most common of the porphyrias, with an incidence of 1 in 25,000 in the United States. Seventy-five per cent of these cases are sporadic. Alcohol or estrogen ingestion commonly triggers clinical manifestation of the disease, and iron appears to be one of several factors that inactivate uroporphyrinogen decarboxylase. In PCT, skin signs predominate, but significant liver disease may also be present. In PCT, abnormalities of liver function tests, of serum iron, and of ferritin are often found. Patients may have increased hemoglobin and hematocrit, and glucose tolerance may be abnormal. Antibodies to hepatitis B, hepatitis C, and/or human immunodeficiency virus (HIV) are often detected in the sera of patients with PCT.

PCT-like states are occasionally associated with porphyrin-producing hepatic tumors and may be seen in chronic dialysis patients. Pseudoporphyria in dialysis patients resembles PCT, but porphyrin concentrations are normal. Photosensitivity reactions that mimic PCT may ensue from the interaction of light (usually in the UVA range) with various drugs. Among the more common photosensitizers are the tetracyclines (excluding minocycline), sulfonamides, sulfones, nonsteroidal anti-inflammatory drugs, fluoroquinolones, and vitamin A analogues.

HCP is distinctly uncommon, whereas VP is found in South Africa at an incidence of 1 in 400 persons of European (especially Dutch) descent. HCP and VP patients may present with skin changes similar to those of PCT. However, only 30 per cent of patients with HCP have skin abnormalities, while as many as 80 per cent of persons with VP have skin involvement. Enzymatic, biochemical, and clinical abnormalities in PCT are exacerbated by iron loading and are improved by iron removal. These changes are not observed in either HCP or VP.

Assays of Porphyrins and Porphyrin Precursors

Acute Porphyrias

When they are positive, the quick "bedside" tests for the presence of porphyrin precursors (ALA and PBG) are considered reliable. The bedside tests for porphyrins may indicate the presence of porphyrins but do not reveal the quantity of porphyrins or the type of porphyrins in the solution. Porphyrin precursors are usually detected with the Watson-Schwartz test. The concentrations of PBG found in acute attacks of AIP, HCP, and VP are sufficient to generate a positive Watson-Schwartz test following butanol extraction. By contrast, patients who are between attacks or who are genetic carriers typically do not produce enough porphyrin precursors to generate a positive Watson-Schwartz test.

Occasionally, patients with increased concentrations of ALA in urine may have a positive Watson-Schwartz test in the absence of increased PBG in urine. The test must be performed on freshly obtained urine. When urine is allowed to stand, especially at acidic pH, PBG may oxidize to porphobilin and polymerize to uroporphyrin. Butanol extraction removes the non-PBG Ehrlich reactors. These reactors include urobilinogen, indoles, pyrrole mono- and dicarboxylic acids, phylloerythrinogen, and metabolites of methyldopa, levomepromazine (methotrimeprazine), and cascara sagrada bark extract.

To perform the Watson-Schwartz test with butanol modification, 0.7 g of Ehrlich's reagent (*p*-dimethylaminobenzaldehyde [DMAB] in HCl) is dissolved in 150 mL of concentrated HCl plus 100 mL of water. One mL of this solution is added to 1 mL of the patient's urine. The mixture turns red if PBG is present. Then, 2 mL of saturated sodium acetate is added to the mixture, which is then extracted with 4 mL of butanol. If PBG is present, the pink color remains in the lower aqueous phase. For a positive result, at least 5 mg/L of PBG must be present in the urine. In acute attacks of porphyria, the concentration of PBG almost always exceeds 10 mg/L.

A second quicker test is the Hoesch test, where a single drop of the patient's urine is added to 1 mL of Ehrlich's reagent (2.0 g of DMAB in 100 mL of 6M HCl). PBG is present if a cherry-red color quickly forms at the surface as the drop hits the reagent.

Chronic Cutaneous Porphyrias

Spectrofluorometry

As described by Poh-Fitzpatrick, direct spectrofluorometry of diluted red blood cells and plasma provides a rapid means of distinguishing among some of the porphyrias. CEP red blood cells have an excitation maximum of 425 nm and fluoresce strongly with a main band at 620 nm; PCT red blood cells excite at 425 nm and fluoresce weakly at 595 nm; EPP red blood cells excite at 397 nm and fluoresce at 634 nm. CEP and PCT plasma share excitation maxima at 398 nm and fluorescence at 619 nm; VP excites at 400 nm and fluoresces sharply at 626 nm. EPP plasma has a excitation maximum at 405 nm and fluoresces at 634 nm.

Table 3 records de Salamanca's modification of the method of Poh-Fitzpatrick. The modification relies on excitation at 405 nm for all patient samples. Note that 405 nm is the excitation maximum for uroporphyrin and 405 nm also lies roughly midway between the 394-nm excitation maximum of coproporphyrin and the 411-nm excitation maximum of protoporphyrin.

Quantitative Methods

The acetone extraction technique of Hart and Piomelli permits quantitation of free and zinc-bound protoporphyrins. Red blood cell protoporphyrin is extracted into acetone and water (80/20 by vol.). Free protoporphyrin enters the solution, whereas zinc-bound protoporphyrin does not. Fluorometry measures the total red blood cell protoporphyrins before extraction and the zinc-bound red blood cell protoporphyrins after extraction, thereby providing the concentrations of zinc-bound and free.

Table 3. Spectrofluorometric Scanning of Plasma Porphyrins

Disorder	Absorption Excitation Band (nm)	Emission Excitation Band (nm)
CEP	405	618–622
PCT	405	618–622
HCP	405	618–622
VP	405	626–628
EPP	405	636

Emission excitation bands of control standards when incubated with control plasma: uroporphyrin, 620 nm: coproporphyrin, 619 nm; and protoporphyrin, 633 nm. The distinct emission excitation band of VP is due to protein binding of the X-porphyrins.

Quantitative testing is preferred for both porphyrins and porphyrin precursors. Reverse-phase high-performance liquid chromatography (HPLC) can separate and quantitate urinary porphyrins and isomers. Isocratic ion-pair HPLC measures urinary coproporphyrins and their isomers. Although HPLC is preferred for initial measurements of protoporphyrin, quantitative cytofluorometry can be used to measure changes in erythrocyte protoporphyrin over time.

CAVEAT. No method is free from pitfalls, particularly interference from drugs. For example, dipyridamole obscures the concentrations of coproporphyrin III and protoporphyrin IX on HPLC because of similar retention times in the column. Similarly, overlapping emission spectra are found for porphyrins and ofloxacin, norfloxacin, and ciprofloxacin, resulting in falsely increased porphyrin concentrations.

Summation of Clinical Laboratory Methods as Applied to Patient Diagnosis

Urinary ALA and PBG can be measured qualitatively (Watson-Schwartz or Hoesch test) and quantitatively (HPLC) in patients with acute porphyria (ALADP, AIP, dHCP, and VP). If cutaneous manifestations of porphyria are present, ALADP and AIP can be excluded. HCP may be distinguished from VP by spectrofluorometry of plasma and by quantitative assay of feces for coproporphyrins and protoporphyrins. HCP plasma has an emission excitation band of 618 to 622 nm, whereas VP plasma is excited at 626 to 628 nm. During the acute attacks of HCP, concentrations of fecal coproporphyrin typically exceed those of protoporphyrin. Conversely, in VP, the concentrations of fecal protoporphyrin usually exceed those of coproporphyrin. Between attacks, coproporphyrin concentrations in urine are typically higher in HCP than in VP, while coproporphyrin levels in feces are about the same in both disorders. Between attacks, fecal protoporphyrin concentrations are normal in HCP but are slightly increased in VP. If X-porphyrins are detected in feces, the diagnosis is usually VP. X-porphyrins, however, may also be found in the feces of patients with PCT. The X-porphyrins of PCT may be chromatographically distinguished from those detected in VP.

If cutaneous manifestations are not observed during acute childhood attacks of porphyria, homozygous or compound heterozygous forms of the acute porphyrias should be considered. Homozygous HCP can be identified by detecting harderoporphyrins in feces. If acute attacks occur after puberty, ALADP is less likely. Urine concentrations of ALA and PBG are increased in all four of the acute porphyrias. In ALADP, however, the ratio of ALA to PBG is very high. In acute attacks of ALADP and AIP, fecal coproporphyrin is normal. During acute attacks of HCP and VP, fecal coproporphyrin is high. During acute attacks, red blood cell protoporphyrins are increased only in patients with ALADP.

In patients with cutaneous porphyria (CEP, PCT, HEP, HCP, VP, and EPP), porphyrins are measured by spectrofluorometry and by chromatography (usually HPLC). If signs and symptoms of acute porphyria are also present, the diagnosis is either HCP or VP. In the absence of a clinical history of acute attacks of porphyria, PCT and HCP may be distinguished from VP and EPP with the use of excitation emission spectra. EPP may also be identified when erythrocyte concentrations of protoporphyrin (but not uroporphyrin or coproporphyrin) are significantly increased. EPP, however, is not the only porphyria in which red cell protoporphyrins are consistently increased. Increased erythrocyte protoporphyrin can also be documented in the rare homozygous and compound heterozygous porphyrias. The mechanism for the increased red blood cell protoporphyrin in these disorders has not yet been explained. In EPP, liver biopsy may reveal characteristic granular, yellow-to-green Maltese-cross fluorescence, canalicular damage, and fibrosis, while the urine may contain increased concentrations of coproporphyrin I.

In PCT, urine concentrations of uroporphyrin and heptacarboxylic acid porphyrin exceed those of coproporphyrin. In HCP, urine concentrations of coproporphyrin exceed those of uroporphyrin and heptacarboxylic acid porphyrin. In PCT (but not HCP), uroporphyrins are typically found in feces. In addition, isocoproporphyrins are characteristically found in feces in PCT, but not in other porphyrias. In PCT, the urinary ratio of uroporphyrin to coproporphyrin approaches 5:1; in VP, coproporphyrins usually predominate.

CEP is characterized by early age at onset, severe mutilating disease, increased urinary coproporphyrin, and increased uroporphyrin in urine, feces, and erythrocytes. HEP clinically resembles CEP, but red blood cell uroporphyrin and coproporphyrin are normal.

In rare patients, the specific diagnosis remains elusive despite careful assessment of clinical features and assays of porphyrin and porphyrin precursors. In these patients, assays of enzyme activity may be necessary.

Assays of Enzyme Deficiencies

Measurement of enzyme activity can not only aid diagnosis in difficult cases but also identify carriers of clinically silent porphyric traits. Many patients with impaired enzyme activity have no clinical illness and may have little risk of developing clinical manifestations of disease. For example, persons with ALA dehydrase deficiency rarely develop ALADP, and the clinical expression of AIP occurs in only 10 per cent of those who are heterozygous for PBG deaminase deficiency. The clinician who requests an enzyme assay must consider the site of enzyme production and the activity of the enzyme in a particular tissue. For example, the gene that governs production of PBG deaminase is spliced at different loci in erythroid and nonerythroid tissues. In most cases of AIP, abnormalities of PBG deaminase may be identified in red blood cells. In some patients, however, abnormal PBG deaminase activity is found only in nonerythroid cells.

HCP, VP, and EPP are disorders that result from abnormalities of mitochondrial enzymes. Mature red blood cells lack mitochondria. Therefore, enzymes relevant to HCP, VP, and EPP should not be measured in the erythrocytes of patients who are being evaluated for these disorders. Instead, heme-pathway enzyme activity should be measured in the patient's fibroblasts or in lymphoid cells transformed by the Epstein-Barr virus.

Identification of Genetic Defects

Determination of genetic defects in the porphyrias may be diagnostically useful in several settings. Genetic techniques permit prenatal diagnosis so that fetuses with homozygous or compound heterozygous disease may be identified. In a case whose clinical features and enzyme activities fell between those of HEP and PCT, nucleotide sequencing revealed two separate missense mutations, each on a separate allele of the cDNAs of uroporphyrinogen decarboxylase, establishing a diagnosis of HEP. Unlike prior patients with HEP whose enzymatic activity levels were less than 10 per cent of normal, in this patient the levels were subnormal but substantial because the loci of their mutations interfered less with enzymatic structure and activity than in cases previously reported.

Variations in the severity of clinical manifestations of CEP have been correlated with five missense mutations, a partial gene deletion, and abnormalities of uro III-S mRNA. A proband with CEP had 10 per cent, the father 70 per cent, and the mother 50 per cent of normal uroporphyrinogen III synthase activity. The father had one missense mutation for the enzyme, while the mother had a different missense mutation. Although the proband was a compound heterozygote, he developed a mild form of CEP because inheritance of the father's mutation permitted partial yet substantial synthesis of functional enzyme.

By 1992, genetic analyses of patients with AIP had identified at least seven point mutations in the PBG deaminase gene by direct sequencing of amplified complementary deoxyribonucleic acid (cDNA). Of these seven mutations, three were silent, and four caused amino acid substitutions. By early 1993, 14 different mutations in the PBG deaminase gene had been reported, and by late 1993, 20 such mutations were known. In 1994, 11 new mutations were reported with the use of denaturing gradient gel electrophoresis (dgge). Dgge exploits the instability of heteroduplex (point) mutations. These points of mutation have the lowest melting domain within the altered amplified fragment. This physicochemical characteristic allows the mutated fragment to be separated from normal and more stable fragments prior to sequencing.

No combination of the methods of genetic analysis (e.g., dgge, restriction fragment length polymorphisms, single-strand conformation polymorphisms) has enabled identification of all family members with asymptomatic AIP or all carriers of other porphyrinogenic diseases. Caution is required because many mutations are biochemically silent and cause no disease. The clinician and laboratory must identify the patients whose mutations result in amino acid substitutions. The position of the amino acid substitution determines the degree of impairment. For example, a child with compound heterozygosity for ALADP inherited one allele from the father that coded for some functional enzyme. By contrast, the allele inherited from the mother coded for an amino acid substitution that decreased the ability of substrate to bind to ALA dehydrase. Because the mutation on the father's allele did not involve the substrate binding site, enzyme activity was less drastically altered. The rates of turnover of enzymes formed from each allele also vary. In the case of the child with ALADP, the enzyme derived from the mother turned over at a normal rate, whereas that of the father turned over and was lost more quickly. These factors may be measured by transfecting mutant human cDNA into Chinese hamster ovary cells and then measuring enzyme activity in those cells.

HEPATOLENTICULAR DEGENERATION (WILSON'S DISEASE)

By George J. Brewer, M.D.
Ann Arbor, Michigan

Although Wilson originally proposed the name progressive lenticular degeneration, the important synonyms for this disease are hepatolenticular degeneration and Wilson's disease. Copper is an essential nutrient, but the amount in the diet is about 25 per cent more than is required. The normal mechanism for eliminating excess dietary copper is excretion in the bile and subsequent loss in the stool. In patients with Wilson's disease, this excretory mechanism is abnormal. As a result, small amounts of copper accumulate daily and are stored in the liver until its storage capacity is exceeded and copper toxicity develops. By the time of diagnosis, the liver is invariably damaged. When the storage capacity of the liver is exceeded, copper accumulates in other parts of the body. The next most sensitive tissues are those parts of the brain that coordinate movement. Other parts of the body are less commonly affected.

CLINICAL MANIFESTATIONS

Wilson's disease manifests, in about equal numbers, as a hepatic or neurologic or psychiatric disorder. The hepatic form may be one of liver failure, hepatitis, or chronic cirrhosis. If the patient presents in liver failure, it may be severe, with a rapid downhill course that leads to death in the absence of liver transplantation. However, the failure may be mild and protracted, with hypoalbuminemia, ascites, pedal edema, mild hyperbilirubinemia, and mild reduction in clotting factors. The clinical picture of hepatitis in Wilson's disease is similar to that of other causes. Serologic test results are usually negative, but a Wilson's disease patient may occasionally test positive for viral antigens, reflecting past exposure or coexisting disease. Hepatitis in Wilson's disease may wax and wane and prompt a diagnosis of chronic active hepatitis. Alternatively, the patient may develop hypersplenism, with thrombocytopenia and leukopenia, and cirrhosis, with complications such as bleeding varices. Cirrhosis due to Wilson's disease cannot be clinically distinguished from cirrhosis due to other causes. The age at first presentation of Wilson's liver disease may be as young as 6 years, particularly if the patient presents with acute fulminant hepatic failure. However, the liver disease may manifest at any time from early childhood through adulthood. Most patients typically present with hepatitis or cirrhosis in their late teens or early twenties.

The peak age at which patients present with neurologic Wilson's disease is about 21 years. However, the disease can manifest in the teenage years or as late as the fifties. Copper toxicity affects primarily those parts of the brain that coordinate movement; thus, neurologic Wilson's disease is a movement disorder. Abnormalities of speech are found in more than 90 per cent of patients who present with neurologic Wilson's disease. The speech is variably described as slurred, hypokinetic, and ataxic, and the disorder may progress to anarthria. Difficulties in controlling fine movements of the hand are common and lead to abnormalities of handwriting. Patients often write micrographically, perhaps in an unconscious effort to avoid the clumsy, sloppy handwriting that would otherwise occur. Difficulties in controlling the hands progress to difficulties in controlling arm and leg movements, posture, and facial expression. Drooling is common. Dystonia frequently evolves to rigidity and contractures. Some patients appear parkinsonian, and neurologic Wilson's disease has occasionally been mistaken for parkinsonism. Dysphagia is common. A significant tremor occurs in about one third of these patients. There is no sensory deficit.

Behavioral abnormalities are the earliest manifestations in about one third of patients with Wilson's disease. Psychiatric diagnoses are common, and behavioral symptoms may precede the onset of obvious neurologic signs and symptoms by as many as 4 to 5 years. The psychiatric symptoms vary, but one of the most common problems is decreased performance at school or work. Patients have difficulty in concentrating and performing normal tasks efficiently. Rapid deterioration of marks in high school or college is common, and patients may lose the ability to focus mentally in the workplace. Actual cognitive changes, if any, are probably minor. Depression is common, and the patient may develop suicidal ideation. Loss of emotional control, temper tantrums, and unreasonable demands by the patient are frequently observed. Spouses of such patients leave or consider leaving. Insomnia, hyperactivity, and delusions are reported. Sexual exhibitionism is common, as is loss of sexual inhibitions.

The simultaneous occurrence of hemolysis and liver disease in a relatively young patient almost always means Wilson's disease. This combination is precipitated by acute hepatic necrosis that releases sufficient copper into the blood to initiate red cell destruction.

Many clinical events caused by Wilson's disease may precede the diagnosis by months to years, but they are not distinctive enough to suggest the diagnosis. These include cholelithiasis, abnormal renal tubular function, renal stones, amenorrhea, chronic abortion, myocarditis, pancreatic disease, hypoparathyroidism, sunflower cataracts, and arthritis, typically in the knees.

In the early, presymptomatic phase of Wilson's disease, the only manifestation that may come to the attention of a physician is an increase in liver-derived serum transaminases. In the absence of other known causes of hepatic inflammation, increased liver-derived serum enzymes should always prompt the physician to consider Wilson's disease. Importantly, each full sibling of a diagnosed patient has a 25 per cent risk of having the disease in the presymptomatic state, and they should be vigorously evaluated for abnormalities of copper excretion.

The gene responsible for Wilson's disease has been cloned. This gene codes for a membrane-bound, copper-binding ATPase that transports copper across membranes. At least 23 different mutations in this gene have been described in fewer than 100 patients with Wilson's disease, demonstrating that this autosomal recessive disorder manifests great allelic heterogeneity.

COURSE OF THE DISEASE

Wilson's disease is progressive and fatal if it goes untreated. In patients with primarily liver manifestations, multiple bouts of hepatitis and/or the development of cirrhosis gradually leads to death from liver failure. Most untreated patients are dead before the age of 30 years.

Similarly, patients with neurologic disease have progressive loss of control of movement until they are wheelchair-bound or bedridden. The dystonia may lead to contractures and an inability to move the extremities. Ultimately, such patients die of the complications of severe neurologic disease. Dysphagia may lead to chronic aspiration and chronic pulmonary disease, unless a gastrostomy or nasogastric tube is employed. With or without aspiration, many patients develop bronchopneumonia or other infection that contributes to their demise. Patients with psychiatric disease, if undiagnosed and untreated, eventually develop the neurologic manifestations and complications described.

COMMON COMPLICATIONS

One of the most common complications of Wilson's disease is hypersplenism due to portal hypertension. Some degree of cirrhosis almost always exists in this disease, and many patients exhibit hypersplenism, even if they have presented with neurologic problems or have been diagnosed before the onset of symptoms. The most common manifestations of hypersplenism in these patients are leukopenia and thrombocytopenia. The most dangerous complication of portal hypertension is bleeding from esophageal or gastric varices. Some patients who present with liver disease have a history of bleeding varices or may first present with variceal bleeding. This history is less likely for a patient presenting with neurologic disease and unlikely for a presymptomatic patient.

DIAGNOSIS

Physical Examination

The neurologic examination typically reveals the most striking physical abnormalities in patients with Wilson's disease. Slow or slurred speech, uncoordinated movement, tremor, dysphagia, dystonia, abnormal facial expression, drooling, progressive micrographia, and sloppy handwriting have been documented.

The small and often cirrhotic liver is seldom appreciated as abnormal on physical examination, but the edge of the spleen can often be palpated. Deposits of copper in the cornea, known as Kayser-Fleischer rings, may be seen with a flashlight. Kayser-Fleischer rings are typically viewed as bluish green discolorations of the upper and lower limbus of the cornea. These rings are most reliably detected by slit-lamp examination.

Useful Laboratory Procedures

A serum ceruloplasmin determination is the most commonly requested and most easily obtained laboratory test for the diagnosis of Wilson's disease. In 9 of 10 patients with Wilson's disease, the serum ceruloplasmin concentration falls below the reference range. However, the serum ceruloplasmin concentration is normal in 10 per cent of Wilson's disease patients, including as many as one half of those who present with liver disease. Ceruloplasmin is an acute-phase reactant, and its concentration in serum may increase as a result of active hepatitis in a patient who would otherwise show a low value. Similarly, patients on birth control pills may have a normal serum ceruloplasmin concentration even though they have Wilson's disease. Ten per cent of carriers of the Wilson's disease gene have a low ceruloplasmin concentration but they never develop clinical manifestations of the disease. Carriers are 400 times more frequent in the population than affected individuals; thus, decreased serum ceruloplasmin in heterozygotes is 40 times more common than decreased ceruloplasmin in homozygotes for Wilson's disease. A decreased serum ceruloplasmin concentration should increase the index of suspicion for Wilson's disease, but it should never provide the basis for a definitive diagnosis.

Measurement of copper in a 24-hour collection of urine is a more reliable diagnostic aid. Normal individuals excrete less than 50 μg of copper in 24 hours, but patients with symptomatic Wilson's disease typically excrete more than 100 μg in a 24-hour urine sample. If specimens are carefully collected in metal-free containers, the 24-hour urine copper determination is an excellent, noninvasive screening test for Wilson's disease. There are two situations, however, in which the urine copper may not be diagnostic. In presymptomatic homozygotes, the 24-hour urine copper concentration may fall between 50 and 100 μg, and in heterozygotes, urine copper may reach 65 μg in a 24-hour urine sample. It may not be possible to differentiate presymptomatic homozygotes from heterozygous carriers using urine copper concentrations. The amount of urine copper can also be misleading in patients with long-standing obstructive liver disease, because copper may accumulate in the liver, leading to increased copper excretion. However, the serum alkaline phosphatase concentration in Wilson's disease rarely exceeds 400 IU/L, but in obstructive liver disease, the alkaline phosphatase frequently exceeds 400 IU/L.

The gold standard for diagnosis remains percutaneous liver biopsy with quantitation of hepatic copper. The normal hepatic copper concentration rarely exceeds 50 μg per gram of dry weight of tissue. In Wilson's disease, hepatic copper typically exceeds 200 μg/g of dry weight of tissue. Intermediate levels of 100 μg/g of tissue are often measured in heterozygous carriers.

There are at least three situations in which hepatic copper content is not diagnostic of Wilson's disease. First, in obstructive liver disease, the hepatic copper content may equal that seen in Wilson's disease. Second, chronic treatment with anticopper agents may reduce the hepatic copper content below 200 μg/g of liver. Third, a vegetarian diet may influence the accumulation of copper and the presentation of Wilson's disease. Copper in vegetables is much less bioavailable, and the hepatic copper in vegetarian patients with Wilson's disease may theoretically drop below the diagnostic value of 200.

Useful Imaging Procedures

Magnetic resonance imaging and computed tomography of the brain are useful imaging procedures in diagnosing Wilson's disease. In patients who have presented with neurologic disease, both typically show abnormalities of the basal ganglia, putamen, and related structures. The abnormalities on these images are not specific for Wilson's disease but are sometimes helpful in making the diagnosis of a puzzling neurologic disorder.

The slit-lamp examination remains an important procedure in the diagnosis of Wilson's disease. In patients with neurologic or psychiatric symptoms, the absence of corneal copper deposits (Kayser-Fleischer rings) is strong evidence against the diagnosis of Wilson's disease.

Less Useful Diagnostic Procedures

Radiocopper tests for the diagnosis of Wilson's disease involve the oral or intravenous administration of radiocopper and the determination of a second blood radiocopper peak, usually at 24 hours or 48 hours after the administration of the original radiocopper. The second blood peak follows hepatic incorporation of copper into ceruloplasmin and secretion of the labeled ceruloplasmin into the blood. In Wilson's disease, this second peak is always decreased compared with normal individuals. Unfortunately, this peak is also low in many heterozygotes. False-positive radiocopper tests are common and can lead to an inappropriate diagnosis of Wilson's disease.

Another procedure with questionable clinical value is the penicillamine challenge. In this test, penicillamine is administered, and the amount of copper excreted over a period (e.g., 24 hours) is determined. Copper excretion can be documented in normal and heterozygous patients and in homozygotes with Wilson's disease. There are, however, no standards or consensus urine copper values that distinguish among the three types of patients.

Errors and Pitfalls in Diagnosis

Perhaps the greatest diagnostic challenge is to distinguish the patient with Wilson's disease from the patient with biliary or other obstructive liver disease. In a patient with markedly increased alkaline phosphatase or other evidence of obstructive liver disease, the clinician should make the diagnosis of Wilson's disease with great caution. A decreased serum ceruloplasmin suggests Wilson's disease, and the patient should improve with 1 to 2 years of anticopper treatment. However, it is possible that obstructive or other liver disease could also improve during that period. The development of a genetic DNA test may alleviate this diagnostic dilemma.

Serum ceruloplasmin and urine copper concentrations do not always distinguish the carrier state from the presymptomatic state. A liver biopsy remains essential for accurate classification.

The clinician must develop a high index of suspicion for Wilson's disease in patients who present with liver disease or behavioral abnormalities. Screening tests are appropriate because Wilson's disease is a treatable disorder. In the future, DNA testing will attempt to identify specific mutations that are causing Wilson's disease in a particular family. These tests will be used to study and counsel family members. In addition, clinically applicable tests that screen for 30 or more mutations are likely to be developed.

THE AMYLOIDOSES

By Robert A. Kyle, M.D.,
and Morie A. Gertz, M.D.
Rochester, Minnesota

Although amyloid appears homogeneous and amorphous under the light microscope, it actually consists of rigid, linear, nonbranching, aggregated fibrils that are 7.5 to 10 nm wide and of indefinite length. The unique staining and optical features are due to arrangement of the fibrils in antiparallel or crossed β-pleated sheet configuration. Congo red is considered the most specific stain; when viewed with a polarized light source, it produces apple-green birefringence. Amyloid also stains with metachromatic dyes such as methyl violet or crystal violet. Electron microscopy reveals the fibrillar ultrastructure. The amyloid fibrils that are deposited typically resist proteolytic digestion. This leads to disorganization of tissue architecture and the loss of normal tissue elements.

All types of amyloid appear the same on Congo red staining as well as on electron microscopy. However, the fibrils in primary amyloidosis (AL) consist of the variable portion of a monoclonal light chain (κλ); the fibrils of secondary amyloidosis (AA) consist of protein A, a nonimmunoglobulin; the fibrils of familial amyloidosis are composed of a mutated transthyretin (prealbumin); the fibrils of senile systemic amyloidosis consist of normal transthyretin; and amyloid associated with long-term dialysis consists of β_2-microglobulin (Tables 1 and 2).

Supported in part by a grant from the National Institutes of Health CA 62242.

PRESENTING SIGNS AND SYMPTOMS

Primary Amyloidosis

The median age at diagnosis of AL is 64 years, which is similar to that in multiple myeloma. Weakness or fatigue and weight loss are the most frequent initial symptoms. The median weight loss is more than 20 lb; some patients lose 40 to 50 lb without apparent cause. Purpura, particu-

Table 1. Classification of Amyloidosis

Classification	Amyloid Type	Major Protein Component
Primary: no evidence of preceding or coexisting disease except multiple myeloma or macroglobulinemia	AL	κ or λ light chains
Secondary: coexistence with other conditions such as rheumatoid arthritis and other inflammatory diseases	AA	Protein A
Familial		
Neurologic	AF	Transthyretin (prealbumin)
Nephropathic		
Familial Mediterranean fever	AA	Protein A
Ostertag (renal)		Fibrinogen
Cardiopathic		
Danish	AF	Transthyretin (Met 111)
Appalachian	AF	Transthyretin (Ala 60)
Senile		
Senile systemic amyloidosis	SSA	Transthyretin (normal)
Dialysis-associated	A β_2-M	β_2-microglobulin

AL = amyloid light chain protein; AA = amyloid A protein; AF = familial amyloidosis; SSA = serum amyloid A protein; A β_2-M = dialysis-associated amyloidosis.

Modified from Kyle, R.A., and Greipp, P.R.: Amyloidosis: Clinical and laboratory features in 229 cases. Mayo Clin. Proc. 58:665–683, 1983. Used by permission.

Table 2. Immunohistochemical Identification of Amyloid

	Congo Red	κ or λ	Serum Amyloid A	β_2-Micro-globulin	Transthyretin (Prealbumin)
Primary (AL)	+	+	−	−	−
Secondary (AA)	+	−	+	−	−
Familial Mediterranean fever (AA)	+	−	+	−	−
Dialysis (A β_2-M)	+	−	−	+	−
Familial (AF)	+	−	−	−	+
Senile systemic (SSA)	+	−	−	−	+

β_2-M, = β_2-microglobulin; AF = familial amyloidosis; SSA = serum amyloid A protein.

larly in the periorbital and facial areas, is present in 15 per cent of patients. Dyspnea and pedal edema are frequent in patients with congestive heart failure. Paresthesias, lightheadedness, and syncope are often prominent features in patients with peripheral neuropathy or autonomic neuropathy. Impotence is a common problem. Hoarseness or weakness of the voice often occurs. The liver is palpable at diagnosis in one fourth of patients, whereas splenomegaly is present initially in only 5 per cent. Macroglossia occurs in approximately one tenth of patients.

Malabsorption occurs in fewer than 5 per cent of patients. Decreased motility of the small bowel may resemble mechanical obstruction but actually represents pseudo-obstruction, for which surgical treatment is ineffectual and contraindicated. Gastrointestinal bleeding may occur. Ascites is not uncommon. The skin is often fragile. Generalized lymphadenopathy is infrequent. Signs of congestive heart failure, nephrotic syndrome, peripheral neuropathy, carpal tunnel syndrome, and orthostatic hypotension must be sought during the history and physical examination. Nephrotic syndrome or renal insufficiency is the presenting symptom in more than one fourth of patients, and carpal tunnel syndrome is a presenting feature in one fifth of patients. Congestive heart failure is the major feature at diagnosis in one sixth of patients, and peripheral neuropathy is the major manifestation in one sixth of patients (Fig. 1). The presence of one of these syndromes and a monoclonal protein (M protein) in the serum or urine is a strong indication of the presence of AL and requires appropriate biopsies for diagnosis.

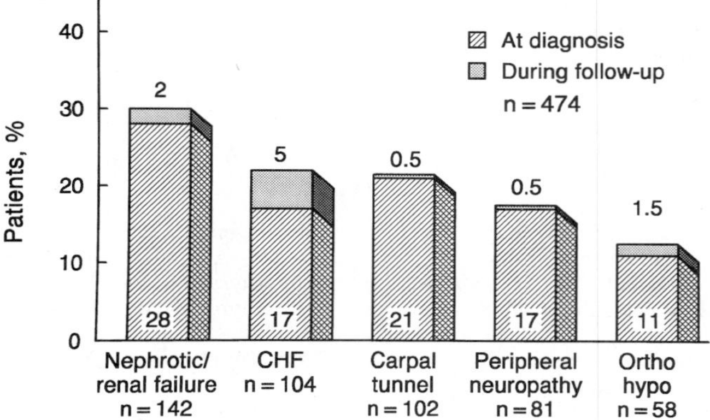

Figure 1. Frequency of amyloid syndromes at diagnosis of primary systemic amyloidosis. CHF = congestive heart failure; Ortho hypo = orthostatic hypotension. (From Kyle, R.A., and Gertz, M.A.: Primary systemic amyloidosis: Clinical and laboratory features in 474 cases. Semin. Hematol., 32:45–59, 1995, with permission.)

Secondary Amyloidosis

AA presents as renal insufficiency or nephrotic syndrome in 90 per cent of patients. In contrast to AL, the heart and peripheral nerves are rarely involved. In the western world, the most common causes of AA are rheumatoid arthritis and its variants, such as ankylosing spondylitis or juvenile rheumatoid arthritis. Crohn's disease and bronchiectasis may also produce AA. In the Middle East, familial Mediterranean fever is characterized by recurrent episodes of abdominal pain and the appearance of proteinuria or renal insufficiency.

Familial Amyloidosis

Familial amyloidosis is most commonly manifested by a sensorimotor peripheral neuropathy that begins in the lower extremities, as well as autonomic dysfunction, disturbances of gastrointestinal and bladder function, and carpal tunnel syndrome. The diagnosis is easily overlooked because many patients do not have a positive family history and may have a "late onset," with symptoms first occurring in the sixth or seventh decade of life. In some families, the heart is the major organ of amyloid deposition, whereas in other families, renal insufficiency or nephrotic syndrome is the presenting symptom.

Senile Systemic Amyloidosis

Senile systemic amyloidosis most often presents with congestive heart failure or atrial fibrillation. Echocardiography reveals findings consistent with amyloidosis, and an appropriate biopsy shows amyloid consisting of normal transthyretin.

Dialysis-Associated Amyloidosis

Amyloidosis associated with dialysis often presents with pain involving the shoulders, hands, wrists, hips, and knees as well as a carpal tunnel syndrome. Radiolucencies from deposition of amyloid are often seen in the bones. This amyloidosis may occur with either long-term hemodialysis or peritoneal dialysis.

COURSE AND OUTCOME

AL is a progressive disease in which the median survival is 13 months. Only 7 per cent of patients survive for 5 years or more, and 1 per cent of individuals are alive at 10 years. Survival depends on the clinical manifestations. In patients presenting with congestive heart failure, the median survival is 4 months. Patients presenting with peripheral neuropathy but no evidence of cardiac or renal involvement have a median survival of 2 years. Death is attributed to cardiac involvement from congestive heart failure or arrhythmias in at least one half of patients. The actual number of cardiac deaths is likely higher because many patients whose death is ascribed to "amyloidosis" have a terminal arrhythmia. Infection and renal failure are also important causes of death.

Survival in AA is approximately 2 years. Death usually occurs within 10 years for patients with familial amyloidosis. In senile systemic amyloidosis, the median survival is 5 years, even in the presence of congestive heart failure.

USEFUL LABORATORY PROCEDURES

In AL, anemia is not a prominent feature unless the patient has renal insufficiency, multiple myeloma, or gastrointestinal bleeding. The leukocyte and differential counts are usually normal. Thrombocytosis (platelet count, more than 500 × 10^9/L) occurs in nearly 10 per cent of patients. Howell-Jolly bodies may be seen in the peripheral blood smear and are an indication of massive splenic amyloid deposits. Renal insufficiency is present in nearly one half of patients at diagnosis, and about 20 per cent of individuals have a serum creatinine concentration of 176.8 μmol/L or more. The serum cholesterol and triglyceride concentrations are frequently increased, mainly because of the nephrotic syndrome. Malabsorption manifested by decreased serum carotene or vitamin B_{12} concentrations occurs in 5 per cent of patients. The serum alkaline phosphatase concentration is increased in one fourth of patients. Hyperbilirubinemia is uncommon, but when present it indicates a short survival. The serum albumin concentration is frequently reduced. The prothrombin time is prolonged in about 15 per cent of patients. The thrombin time is prolonged in 40 per cent of individuals, whereas an isolated deficiency of factor X occurs in about 10 per cent of patients. These coagulation abnormalities are rarely the cause of bleeding.

In AL, the serum protein electrophoretic pattern shows a localized band or spike in about one half of patients, but its size is modest (median, 10.4 g/L). Hypogammaglobulinemia is present in one fifth of patients. Immunoelectrophoresis or immunofixation shows a serum M protein in 70 per cent of patients. One fourth of patients have only a free monoclonal light chain (Bence Jones proteinemia). About 70 per cent have a λ light chain, which is the reverse of the finding in multiple myeloma. The urine contains a monoclonal light chain in about 70 per cent of patients. An M protein is found in the serum or urine at the time of diagnosis in almost 90 per cent of patients with AL.

The bone marrow in AL is characterized by a monoclonal proliferation of plasma cells. However, 60 per cent of patients have fewer than 10 per cent bone marrow plasma cells, and less than one fifth have 20 per cent or more bone marrow plasma cells. About 15 per cent of patients presenting with AL also have multiple myeloma. In AA, 90 per cent of patients present with proteinuria, which usually reaches nephrotic concentrations. Renal insufficiency is common.

DIAGNOSTIC PROCEDURES

The diagnosis of amyloidosis depends on the histologic demonstration of amyloid deposits in tissue. The most universally accepted stain is Congo red, which produces an apple-green birefringence under polarizing light. If the results are equivocal, electron microscopy demonstrates typical amyloid fibrils.

A bone marrow aspirate should be obtained and biopsy should be performed initially to determine the number of plasma cells and if they are monoclonal (producing κλ light chains). Ninety-eight per cent of patients with AL have an M protein in the serum or urine or a monoclonal population of plasma cells in the bone marrow. The bone marrow biopsy specimen should be stained for amyloid because it is positive in more than one half of patients. Abdominal fat aspiration should be carried out because it is positive in almost 80 per cent of patients. It must be stained carefully with Congo red because overstaining and incorrect decolorization may produce inaccurate results. Interpretation by a pathologist experienced with the staining technique is essential. Nearly 90 per cent of patients with AL have amyloid in the fat aspirate or in the bone marrow at diagnosis.

If the results of bone marrow examination and the subcutaneous fat aspiration are normal, obtain a biopsy of the rectum or a suspected involved organ such as the kidney, liver, heart, or sural nerve. The mucosa and submucosa must be included in a rectal biopsy. Renal biopsy results are almost always abnormal in systemic amyloidosis with proteinuria or renal insufficiency, but occasionally the renal abnormality may be from an unrelated kidney disorder. The risk of hematuria or other complications is no higher than that in renal biopsy of patients without amyloidosis. Small amounts of amyloid may be overlooked with light microscopy, and electron microscopy is then required. Biopsy of the liver often produces positive results, and bleeding is not a frequent problem. Tissue obtained at carpal tunnel decompression is usually positive. In patients with peripheral neuropathy, sural nerve biopsy results are usually abnormal. A sural nerve biopsy should not be performed unless the patient has severe peripheral neuropathy because the procedure produces numbness in the distribution of the sural nerve. Endomyocardial biopsy is associated with a minimal risk of complications, and results are almost always positive in patients with AL involving the heart.

The finding of amyloid in any tissue and the presence of an M protein in the serum or urine or a monoclonal proliferation of bone marrow plasma cells confirms the diagnosis of AL. The presence of a family history of peripheral neuropathy (autosomal dominant transmission) is strong evidence of familial amyloidosis. Patients with familial amyloidosis have no monoclonal plasma cells or M protein. However, as many as one half of patients with familial amyloidosis do not have a positive family history at diagnosis. Immunohistochemical staining will give a positive result with transthyretin antisera. In older patients with congestive heart failure or arrhythmias, senile systemic amyloidosis must be considered in the differential diagnosis. When transthyretin is found immunohistochemically in amyloid deposits, leukocyte DNA must be examined for a transthyretin mutation. More than 50 mutations of transthyretin have been recognized. Recognition of familial amyloidosis is essential because liver transplantation is beneficial.

Iodine I 123–labeled human serum amyloid P component is useful for locating and monitoring the extent of systemic amyloidosis because the P component is present in all types of amyloid. Small deposits of amyloid, such as in carpal tunnel ligaments, can be visualized. Uptake by the heart and kidney may be obscured by the increased blood flow in these organs.

OTHER USEFUL DIAGNOSTIC PROCEDURES

The electrocardiogram in cardiac amyloidosis characteristically shows low voltage in the limb leads or features consistent with anteroseptal infarction (loss of anterior forces), but affected patients have no evidence of myocardial infarction at autopsy. Arrhythmias, including atrial fibrillation, atrial or junctional tachycardia, ventricular premature contractions, or bundle branch block, are also common electrocardiographic features.

Echocardiography is a valuable technique for the detection and evaluation of amyloid cardiac disease. The diagnosis of amyloidosis was first recognized with echocardiographic findings in 10 per cent of our patients. The major features are increased thickness of the left and right ventricular walls, abnormal myocardial texture (granular sparkling), normal or small left ventricular cavity size with normal or decreased left ventricular systolic function, abnormal ventricular diastolic function, increased thickness of the cardiac valves (often associated with mild valvular regurgitation), atrial enlargement, and pericardial effusion. In advanced cases this pattern is distinctive, but in milder cases the echocardiographic appearance may be difficult to distinguish from that of left ventricular hypertrophy. The electrocardiographic voltage can be helpful, however, because amyloidosis is associated with decreased voltage in the presence of increased ventricular mass.

Early cardiac amyloidosis is characterized by abnormal relaxation, whereas advanced involvement (mean wall thickness of 15 mm or more) is characterized by restrictive hemodynamics. The most typical diastolic abnormality is a short deceleration time consistent with restriction in the advanced stages of the disease. An echocardiographic abnormality is found in two thirds of patients at the time of diagnosis. The ejection fraction is normal in most patients, but when reduced it is associated with a short survival. Amyloid involvement must be distinguished from left ventricular hypertrophy due to hypertension or hypertrophic obstructive cardiomyopathy. Constrictive pericarditis may be difficult to distinguish from AL.

DIAGNOSTIC PROCEDURES THAT OFTEN ARE NOT HELPFUL

Biopsy of the gum is rarely performed because of the ease and high probability of positive results from subcutaneous fat aspiration and bone marrow biopsy. Congo red produces an apple-green birefringence under polarizing light, but after pretreatment with potassium permanganate, AA amyloid loses its affinity for Congo red, whereas amyloid in AL, senile, familial, and localized amyloidosis is resistant to potassium permanganate. Exceptions occur, however, and the technique is unreliable. Treatment of amyloid deposits with alkaline guanidine may facilitate identification of a specific type of amyloid fibril. Amyloid in AA loses its affinity for Congo red after incubation with alkaline guanidine for 1 minute, whereas amyloid in AL loses its affinity for Congo red after 2 hours. By contrast, amyloid in familial amyloidosis does not lose its affinity for Congo red after alkaline guanidine incubation for 2 hours. This finding has not been confirmed. Increased uptake of technetium Tc 99m pyrophosphate has also been reported, but false-negative and false-positive results are not infrequent. Increased uptake of gallium-67 citrate is often found in renal amyloid, but increased uptake is also found in the kidneys of patients with nephrotic syndrome due to other causes. Examination of the urine sediment for the presence of amyloid fibrils is an unreliable technique. The Paunz test (Congo red) is no longer used because it is not accurate, and anaphylactic reactions may occur.

PITFALLS IN DIAGNOSIS

The performance of Congo red staining and its interpretation may be difficult. Overstaining with Congo red may lead to erroneous results. Not infrequently, results of staining with Congo red are initially interpreted as positive but are found to be negative on re-evaluation with other diagnostic procedures. Electron microscopy can be diagnostic in amyloidosis, but amyloid fibrils must be distinguished from the larger fibrils of immunotactoid glomerulopathy.

The clinical features of amyloid conditions are useful in avoiding errors in diagnosis. The presence of periorbital purpura, macroglossia, and submandibular swelling are manifestations of AL rather than AA or familial amyloidosis. The presence of a nephrotic syndrome, congestive heart failure, carpal tunnel syndrome, sensorimotor peripheral neuropathy, or orthostatic hypotension in conjunction with an M protein in the serum or urine is a strong indication of AL. The presence of nephrotic syndrome or renal insufficiency in a patient with rheumatoid arthritis or Crohn's disease should alert the clinician to the possibility of AA. The presence of peripheral neuropathy or cardiomyopathy in the family points toward familial amyloidosis, but many patients have a negative family history at diagnosis. Senile systemic amyloidosis should be considered in the differential diagnosis when there is no M protein in the serum or urine and no evidence of extracardiac manifestations such as renal insufficiency, nephrotic syndrome, peripheral neuropathy, orthostatic hypotension, macroglossia, or purpura.

If immunohistochemical staining is positive for transthyretin (prealbumin), one must distinguish between late-onset familial amyloidosis and senile systemic amyloidosis. The demonstration of a mutation in transthyretin by DNA studies establishes the diagnosis of familial amyloidosis.

The clinician usually suspects AL and searches for an M protein in the serum and urine. When no M protein is detected, many physicians conclude that the patient has nonsecretory AL, which occurs in 10 per cent of patients with AL. Immunohistochemical staining of the biopsy specimen with antisera to transthyretin, κλ light chains, and amyloid A is necessary for accurate classification. If the results of staining for transthyretin are positive, the patient has either familial or senile amyloidosis, and DNA must be examined for a transthyretin mutation. Precise classification of the patient's amyloidosis is critical because the management and survival of patients with familial and senile amyloidosis differs substantially from that of patients with nonsecretory AL.

Section Nine

ENDOCRINE SYSTEM

HYPOPITUITARISM

By Mary Lee Vance, M.D.
Charlottesville, Virginia

Hypopituitarism is defined as the loss of target endocrine gland function secondary to failure of pituitary secretion of a stimulatory hormone or hormones. Hypopituitarism may be partial or complete, involving one, more than one, or all of the anterior and/or posterior pituitary hormones. The most common cause of pituitary failure is a lesion in the pituitary gland, usually an adenoma. Regardless of the cause of hypopituitarism, physiologic hormone replacement is indicated and the dose must be tailored to each patient's needs.

CLINICAL DIAGNOSIS

For practical purposes, the diagnosis of pituitary failure can be made without admission of the patient to a hospital; however, if hypoadrenalism or hypothyroidism are diagnosed, treatment should begin immediately. The symptoms and signs of pituitary failure vary with the hormone or hormones that are deficient and the severity of the deficiency or deficiencies.

The most common deficiencies are those of growth hormone (GH) and the gonadotropins, luteinizing hormone (LH) and follicle-stimulating hormone (FSH). Although acquired GH deficiency in adults is rarely assessed, GH deficiency contributes to increased body adipose mass and decreased muscle mass compared with age- and sex-matched normal subjects; patients with GH deficiency may report a diminished sense of well-being and fatigue despite adequate replacement of other hormones.

The symptoms of adrenal insufficiency are often nonspecific and include fatigue, a general sense of not feeling well, diminished appetite, decreased ability to concentrate, and, in some patients, weight loss, headache, nausea, vomiting, or abdominal pain. The physical findings include orthostatic hypotension and diminished axillary and pubic hair in postmenopausal women due to loss of adrenal androgen production. Importantly, in hypopituitarism with secondary adrenal insufficiency, serum sodium and potassium concentrations are often normal. By contrast, hyponatremia and hyperkalemia typically occur in primary adrenal failure because of a loss of aldosterone production.

Symptoms of hypothyroidism include nonspecific complaints of decreased energy, constipation, weight gain, difficulty in losing weight, "puffiness," and, occasionally, decreased mental alertness. Women may experience increased volume of menstrual flow if gonadotropin function remains intact. Signs of hypothyroidism are also nonspecific, including periorbital "puffiness," yellowish "doughy" skin, a thyroid gland of normal size, and either delayed or "deliberate" relaxation of the deep tendon reflexes.

The symptoms of gonadal failure in women include amenorrhea, oligomenorrhea, regular menstrual cycles with infertility, decreased libido, hot flashes, vaginal dryness, and dyspareunia. Postmenopausal women do not have change in menses as a "marker" and therefore most often come to medical attention because of headache or loss of vision from a large pituitary tumor. The symptoms of gonadal failure in men may not be recognized because the patient does not report symptoms or because the physician does not ask appropriate specific questions. Decreased libido is not always attributable to "aging" or "stress." Sexual dysfunction in men may be "psychogenic," but this is a diagnosis of exclusion. An organic basic for sexual dysfunction must be excluded before concluding that the cause is psychogenic. The absence of early morning erections, an involuntary event, suggests an organic cause of gonadal sexual dysfunction.

Loss of posterior pituitary function results in diabetes insipidus and is most frequently caused by a metastatic lesion, a craniopharyngioma, or sarcoidosis. Patients experience urinary frequency, including nocturia, and polydipsia. Urination may occur hourly, even at night. Patients often report that only cold water relieves the thirst.

BIOCHEMICAL DIAGNOSIS

Clinically significant hormone deficiencies can be identified in the outpatient clinic. Table 1 lists the suggested screening tests for defining pituitary and target organ function. Blood samples should be taken in the morning to optimize analysis of adrenal cortisol production. A morning serum cortisol concentration of less than 5 μg/dL indicates adrenal insufficiency. However, a normal morning cortisol concentration does not exclude partial pituitary corticotropin deficiency, and the clinician should request a stimulation test such as insulin-induced hypoglycemia or a metyrapone test to determine the integrity of the hypothalamic-pituitary-adrenal axis. Such a test can be delayed if clinically appropriate. Table 2 summarizes two dynamic tests of the hypothalamic-pituitary-adrenal axis. If the

Table 1. Results of Screening Hormone Studies for a Patient With Suspected Hypopituitarism

Hormone or Test	Levels in Hypopituitarism
Morning cortisol (0800–0900 hr)	Normal or low
Thyroxine (T_4), T_3 resin uptake	Low
Thyroid-stimulating hormone	"Normal"* or low
Luteinizing hormone, follicle-stimulating hormone	"Normal" or low
Testosterone (men)	Low
Estradiol (premenopausal women)	Normal or low
Insulin-like growth factor-1	Low
Urine osmolality	Low

*"Normal": Value within the reference range, but inappropriate for the target organ hormone level.

Table 2. Dynamic Tests of Hypothalamic-Pituitary-Adrenal Function

Test	Method	Normal Response
Overnight metyrapone	Metyrapone, 2 g at midnight (given with a snack)	Cortisol >7.5 μg/dL, 0800 hr
Insulin-hypoglycemia*	Regular insulin, 0.15 U/kg	Glucose <40 mg/dL Cortisol ≥20 μg/dL
Water deprivation test†	NPO after 0600 hr; measure urine osmolality and weight every hour until osmolality <20% variance; administer DDAVP 1 μg SC	Increase in osmolality after DDAVP, indicates central diabetes insipidus

*Test performed under the supervision of a physician; it should not be performed in patients with seizure disorders, coronary artery disease, or generalized debility. Accurate serum glucose results must be obtained immediately to assess the adequacy of the insulin dose.
†Test performed under the supervision of a physician in a hospitalized patient.
DDAVP = desmopressin; NPO = nothing by mouth; SC = subcutaneously.

morning cortisol concentration is low, give the patient steroids immediately to prevent an adrenal crisis. Meanwhile, direct stimulation of the adrenal glands with synthetic corticotropin (Cortrosyn) can also be used to diagnose adrenal insufficiency. Cortrosyn administration provides a valid test of adrenal responsiveness but can result in a normal cortisol response if corticotropin deficiency is only partial or of such recent onset that the adrenal glands have not yet atrophied. A normal cortisol response to corticotropin may not accurately reflect the function of the hypothalamic-pituitary-adrenal axis. However, the metyrapone test assesses the function of the entire hypothalamic-pituitary-adrenal axis.

In assessing thyroid function in hypopituitarism, measurement of serum thyroid-stimulating hormone (TSH) only is not reliable, because a "normal" TSH may accompany a decreased serum thyroxine (T_4). If a patient is found to be hypothyroid, adrenal function must be determined, and steroids must be administered before initiating thyroid hormone replacement. Administration of thyroid hormone to a patient with unrecognized and untreated adrenal insufficiency is likely to precipitate an acute adrenal crisis.

Assessment of gonadal function in men should include measurement of serum LH, FSH, and testosterone. A normal LH and FSH with subnormal serum testosterone indicates hypothalamic-pituitary dysfunction. In premenopausal women, the best indicator of gonadal function is the menstrual cycle history. Serum LH and FSH are usually normal or low. Estradiol concentrations may vary, but with long-standing amenorrhea, estradiol is typically decreased. In pituitary insufficiency, gonadotropin (e.g., LH, FSH) concentrations in postmenopausal women are usually inappropriately normal or low. In any man or woman with symptoms of gonadal dysfunction, serum prolactin should be measured, because prolactin-producing pituitary adenomas are the most common types of secretory pituitary tumors.

The diagnosis of GH deficiency is usually made with a stimulation test, but in a well-nourished patient of normal body weight, measurement of serum insulin-like growth factor-1 (IGF-1) provides an appropriate screening test. The results must be interpreted with comparison to age- and sex-matched normal subjects, because GH secretion declines with age and differs by gender. Obesity reduces GH secretion and may lead to a decreased concentration of circulating IGF-1.

The biochemical diagnosis of diabetes insipidus (DI) may be difficult if the patient's fluid intake matches urinary loss. Serum sodium and serum osmolality are typically normal if the patient is ingesting enough fluid to balance the urinary excretion. Urinary osmolality is reduced because of the inability of the kidney to concentrate urine. Definitive diagnosis of DI is made with a water deprivation test (see Table 2), which should be performed in a hospital under physician supervision.

ANATOMIC STUDIES

Magnetic resonance imaging (MRI) scanning with gadolinium enhancement provides the best method for imaging the hypothalamic-pituitary region. If MRI is unavailable, a properly performed computed tomography (CT) scan provides adequate visualization of the hypothalamic-pituitary anatomy. The request for CT scans should specify thin, 1.5-mm sections through the pituitary, preferably in the coronal plane. Although the CT scan does not provide an image of the optic chiasm, a microadenoma (<10 mm) or macroadenoma (>10 mm) of the pituitary is readily demonstrated. If suprasellar extension of the lesion is documented or strongly suspected, the clinician should obtain visual acuity and visual field examinations using automated perimetry (Goldmann, Humphries-Octopus) to determine the effect of the lesion on the visual system.

PITFALLS IN THE DIAGNOSIS

To establish the source of hormone deficiency, the clinician must interpret serum pituitary hormone concentrations in conjunction with serum concentrations of target gland hormones. For example, interpretation of serum TSH without serum thyroxine (T_4) may be misleading, because TSH may be normal while T_4 is subnormal. It is the combination of normal TSH and low T_4 that suggests hypothalamic-pituitary dysfunction. Similarly, in men, proper interpretation of serum testosterone requires a serum LH; normal LH with subnormal testosterone indicates hypothalamic-pituitary dysfunction and warrants an imaging study to exclude a pituitary lesion. Simultaneous measurement of serum corticotropin and cortisol is more problematic, because corticotropin is often detected in the serum of patients with hypopituitarism. The best way of excluding significant adrenal insufficiency is to measure serum cortisol concentration in the morning. A normal morning cortisol indicates at least modest adrenal function; a subnormal morning cortisol indicates the need for immediate glucocorticoid (e.g., hydrocortisone, prednisone) replacement to avoid the crisis of adrenal insufficiency. In premenopausal women, the best indicators of significant hypogonadism are a change in menstrual function, oligomenorrhea, or amenorrhea. The serum LH and FSH in these patients are in the normal range, and the serum estradiol may be normal or decreased. In postmenopausal women with pituitary insufficiency, serum LH and FSH are usually in the "normal" range, but these concentrations are inappropriately reduced for the postmenopausal state. The diagnosis of diabetes insipidus may not be obvious if the patient is ingesting adequate fluid to maintain normal fluid balance, normal serum osmolality, and normal serum sodium. Even if these measurements fall within the reference ranges, the urine osmolality or specific gravity may nevertheless be decreased.

SUMMARY

The diagnosis and treatment of hypopituitarism is straightforward and can usually be accomplished in the outpatient setting. The diagnosis of this potentially life-threatening disorder requires awareness that nonspecific clinical symptoms may indicate hormone deficiency. A thorough history and serum quantitation of appropriate hormones can define the scope of clinically significant deficiencies. Anatomic studies are indicated to exclude a mass in the hypothalamic-pituitary region. Hormone replacement is instituted according to the specific deficiency.

DIABETES INSIPIDUS

By Kellie L. Faulk, M.D., M.P.H.,
and K. Patrick Ober, M.D.
Winston-Salem, North Carolina

Diabetes insipidus (DI) is a disorder manifested by the inability to conserve water, resulting in polyuria and polydipsia. Polyuria has been defined as urinary volumes above 30 mL/kg per day, with most patients becoming aware of symptoms of polyuria at volumes greater than 3 to 4 L per day. Hypertonicity (i.e., hypernatremia) may also be a manifestation of DI, but this condition occurs only if the patient has an impaired thirst mechanism, an impaired state of responsiveness, or limited access to water.

DIFFERENTIAL DIAGNOSIS OF POLYURIA

For the patient with polyuria, the clinician should first consider the possibility of osmotic diuresis. Diuresis may be triggered by physiologic solutes such as glucose (in diabetes mellitus) and urea (in postobstructive diuresis) or by pharmacologic solutes such as mannitol.

Exclusion of an osmotic diuresis leads to consideration of hypotonic polyuria, defined as increased urine volume accompanied by decreased urine osmolality (<300 mOsm/kg). The three causes of hypo-osmolar polyuria are inadequate secretion of antidiuretic hormone (ADH), referred to as central or neurogenic DI; impaired renal responsiveness to ADH, referred to as nephrogenic DI; and increased water intake, also called primary polydipsia. In all three disorders, urine volume is increased, urine osmolality is decreased, and plasma osmolality is typically within the reference range at the time of presentation.

CLINICAL FEATURES

In adults, the symptoms of DI include frequent, large-volume urination, excessive thirst, and increased fluid intake. Infants and children may present with chronic dehydration, fever, failure to thrive, enuresis, or sleep disturbances. Additional manifestations usually are related to the underlying disease process itself.

The severity of symptoms in DI varies widely, and the manifestation of milder forms is often delayed. Urine volumes range from 2 to 20 L per day, with fluid ingestion as high as 15 L or more per day. DI occurs at any age and in both sexes.

PHYSIOLOGIC DIAGNOSIS OF DIABETES INSIPIDUS

The most easily recognized patients with DI are hypertonic and hypernatremic, with hypotonic urine at the time of presentation. These findings immediately exclude primary polydipsia, and the inappropriately dilute urine indicates a defect in ADH secretion or action. The patient's response to exogenous arginine vasopressin usually discriminates between central and nephrogenic DI.

Standard Dehydration and Vasopressin Injection Test

Even with profound disorders in ADH function, most patients maintain plasma osmolality within the reference range as long as they have a normal thirst mechanism and access to water. In such patients, the standard evaluation includes a dehydration test. The aim of the test is to produce hypertonicity (>295 mOsm/kg) and hypernatremia (>145 mEq/L) so that the adequacy of ADH secretion and function can be readily assessed. If a patient is already hypertonic and hypernatremic, the dehydration test is unnecessary and should not be undertaken.

Several variations of the dehydration test have been used. Measure the patient's weight, urine volume, plasma and urine osmolality, and serum sodium concentration as often as every hour. Terminate the test if weight decreases by more than 5 per cent to avoid severe volume depletion. Terminate fluid restriction when two consecutive hourly urine samples have osmolalities that differ by less than 10 per cent after the patient has lost at least 2 per cent of body weight. Diagnostic discrimination improves, however, if dehydration is continued until serum sodium exceeds 145 mEq/L.

Patients with full-blown DI typically maintain a urine osmolality of less than 200 mOsm/kg. Primary polydipsia is excluded if the urine osmolality remains less than 300 mOsm/kg with dehydration, and the differential diagnosis becomes central versus nephrogenic DI. These disorders are differentiated by subcutaneous injection of aqueous vasopressin (5 U) or desmopressin acetate (1 μg), with subsequent monitoring of urine volume and osmolality at 30, 60, and 120 minutes. If urine osmolality increases by 50 per cent, severe hypothalamic DI is likely. If the increase is less than 50 per cent, severe nephrogenic DI is the probable diagnosis.

For many patients, the classic dehydration test cannot provide a specific diagnosis. Chronic polyuria of any cause washes out the renal medullary concentration gradient and thus prevents the attainment of maximal urine osmolalities of 900 mOsm/kg or greater; instead, the maximal urine osmolality may reach no more than 450 to 800 mOsm/kg. If maximal concentrating ability is impaired, the ADH status is no longer the limiting factor for maximal urine osmolality, and the impaired response to exogenous vasopressin cannot lead to a single definitive conclusion regarding ADH status. Many patients with central or nephrogenic DI have an incomplete defect and maintain a moderate ability to concentrate urine after depletion or vasopressin administration; it may be impossible to distinguish these individuals from the patient who has a "flushed out" concentration gradient.

Despite its shortcomings, the standard water deprivation test remains a useful tool for distinguishing severe central DI from severe nephrogenic DI. The test is less useful in patients with partial central DI, partial nephrogenic DI, or primary polydipsia.

Antidiuretic Hormone Measurements

Measurement of plasma ADH may increase the accuracy of diagnosis of DI. However, the reliability and validity of ADH values varies with the quality of commercially available assays, and analysis may not be necessary for the patient with a classic response to the standard water deprivation test. Importantly, the well-defined relationships of ADH concentrations to plasma and urine osmolality require that ADH values be interpreted not as an isolated value, but in the context of simultaneously measured urine and plasma osmolality values. These interpretations are most reliable as part of a standard water deprivation test. With a dilute urine, increased ADH concentrations indicate nephrogenic DI. Decreased ADH concentrations cannot be interpreted in a well-hydrated patient. With volume depletion and development of hypertonicity, an ADH concentration below that expected for the patient's serum osmolality indicates deficient ADH production (i.e., central DI).

Hypertonic Saline Infusion

The infusion of hypertonic saline (3 per cent saline at 0.1 mL/kg per minute) provides an alternative to the water deprivation test, especially when fluid deprivation is not feasible or when attempted dehydration does not produce serum osmolality above 295 mOsm/kg and a serum sodium concentration over 145 mEq/L. Hypertonic saline is typically infused for 1 to 2 hours; the goal is to establish a hypertonic state during which the adequacy of ADH production and renal responsiveness to ADH can be readily evaluated. The results are interpreted using the same criteria as during the dehydration test. Hypertonic saline is contraindicated in patients with severe congestive heart failure.

Therapeutic Trial With Antidiuretic Hormone

A less satisfactory approach to the diagnosis of DI involves the administration of ADH or an analogue. A decrease in urine volume after treatment with ADH excludes nephrogenic DI. Reduction of polyuria and polydipsia suggests central DI, and reduced urinary output with continuing fluid ingestion strongly suggests primary polydipsia that may lead to severe hyponatremia and water intoxication. Therapeutic trials of ADH are not preferred, because they do not yield a definitive diagnosis. Moreover, severe water intoxication may also occur after administration of ADH to patients with true central DI who have become accustomed to drinking large volumes of water prophylactically.

ETIOLOGIC DIAGNOSIS OF DIABETES INSIPIDUS

Central Diabetes Insipidus

After central DI has been documented by appropriate testing, the clinician must determine the specific cause. In developed countries, neurosurgery and trauma are the most common causes of DI. Intracranial tumors and infiltrative processes are less common causes, and some patients are categorized as "idiopathic" despite thorough evaluation.

Central DI associated with trauma may be transient or permanent, depending on the location of injury. Because ADH is synthesized in the hypothalamus, damage to the pituitary or lower pituitary stalk frequently produces temporary DI, and lesions in the higher stalk or hypothalamus often produce permanent DI.

Postsurgical or Post-traumatic Causes

Three distinct patterns of DI follow neurosurgery or trauma. At least one half of these patients experience the acute onset of polyuria, typically within 24 hours of the initial insult, with resolution within 3 to 5 days or occasionally longer. This pattern is most often seen after resection of a pituitary adenoma. The second most common pattern is permanent DI. These patients typically have damage to the more proximal pituitary stalk or the hypothalamus. The least common pattern is the "triphasic response," which can be difficult to manage. The first phase is that of typical DI of abrupt onset. This is followed within several days by cessation of brisk diuresis for up to 2 weeks, a phase presumably related to increased release of ADH from injured neurohypophyseal tissue. Although this second phase has been described as a normal interphase, this period is marked by an inappropriate release of ADH. During this stage, the patient is at risk of hyponatremia and water intoxication with the excessive administration of hypotonic fluids that may be used to treat the initial phase. After the phase of antidiuresis, DI eventually returns, reflecting progressive death of magnocellular neurons by means of retrograde axonal degeneration.

Hypopituitarism

Anterior pituitary hypofunction is not uncommon in patients who have experienced severe head trauma or pituitary surgery. For example, adrenal insufficiency has been reported in 36 per cent of patients with post-traumatic DI. Because cortisol is required for excretion of maximally dilute urine, DI can be masked in the patient with adrenal insufficiency. The administration of glucocorticoids to these patients can rapidly unmask the DI.

Hereditary Forms

DI may occur in the absence of trauma or surgery. Hereditary DI is relatively uncommon; it can occur alone or with diabetes mellitus, optic atrophy, and nerve deafness in the so-called DIDMOAD syndrome.

Associated Central Nervous System Disorders

DI may be associated with central nervous system tumors such as craniopharyngiomas, pinealomas, meningiomas, or dysgerminomas and occasionally with very large pituitary tumors. Metastatic tumor is an important cause of DI that must be evaluated radiographically before a patient is labeled as having idiopathic DI. Patients with breast cancer develop DI late in the course of the malignancy; DI is rarely a presenting feature of breast cancer, and patients almost uniformly have widespread disease by the time DI occurs.

Other causes of DI include infiltrative hypothalamic diseases such as sarcoidosis, histoplasmosis, and Wegener's granulomatosis. Histiocytosis X (Langerhans' cell histiocytosis) causes DI in children, especially those with multisystemic involvement. Intracranial defects, including septo-optic dysplasia, and infections of the central nervous system can also cause DI in children. Vascular disorders, including infarctions and aneurysms, occasionally produce DI.

Pregnancy

Transient DI has been associated with pregnancy, and it resolves after delivery. Although failure of these patients to respond to large doses of ADH suggests a type of nephrogenic DI, the DI of pregnancy has been linked to excessive degradation of ADH by vasopressinase, which is produced by the placenta. DI in pregnancy responds well to desmopressin acetate, which is not degraded by vasopressinase.

Idiopathic Forms

Idiopathic DI accounts for 25 to 30 per cent of all patients with DI. The possibility that idiopathic DI is an autoimmune disorder has been suggested by an unconfirmed report of circulating antibodies to hypothalamic ADH-secreting neurons in one third of these patients. Thoughtful radiographic evaluation (preferably magnetic resonance imaging) is important in these individuals, who may have unsuspected malignant or infiltrative processes. Abnormal cell counts, increased protein concentrations, or the presence of tumor markers (e.g., human chorionic gonadotropin, alpha-fetoprotein) in the cerebrospinal fluid may also suggest occult disease of the central nervous system.

No standard has been established for the frequency of reinvestigation of the patient with apparent idiopathic DI. In a large series of children followed for up to 20 years, some patients with initially negative results developed positive results with follow-up tests; after 4 years, however, no new anatomic diagnoses were established with repeated routine testing. No comparable study of adults has been performed.

Nephrogenic Diabetes Insipidus

Nephrogenic DI may be inherited (sex-linked recessive) but can also be caused by hypokalemia, hypercalcemia, lithium, demeclocycline, sickle cell disease, sarcoidosis, polycystic kidney disease, amyloidosis, or pyelonephritis. Nephrogenic DI has also been associated with metastatic leiomyosarcoma as a paraneoplastic phenomenon.

Primary Polydipsia

Primary polydipsia is usually considered to be idiopathic. Psychogenic polydipsia is a mental illness that involves an irrational faith in the therapeutic value of water. There is a "dipsogenic" form of primary polydipsia in which the osmotic threshold for thirst is lower than that for ADH secretion (i.e., a reversal of the normal relationship). These patients exhibit chronic thirst, polydipsia, and polyuria. Compulsive water drinking combines features of mental illness with abnormally increased thirst.

Owing to the proximity of the hypothalamic thirst center to the hypothalamic ADH-producing neurons, virtually any process that causes DI may also cause thirst disorders. Polydipsia may accompany infiltrative hypothalamic disease or structural lesions in the presumed thirst center; the clinician should therefore evaluate patients with primary polydipsia for biochemical or structural disorders.

PITFALLS IN DIAGNOSIS

Many patients with central or nephrogenic DI have incomplete defects and maintain moderate abilities to concentrate urine after volume depletion or vasopressin administration. Chronic polyuria of any cause washes out the renal medullary concentration gradient and prevents the attainment of maximal urine osmolalities of 900 to 1200 mOsm/kg. Concurrent adrenal insufficiency masks DI until steroids are replaced.

SYNDROME OF INAPPROPRIATE ANTIDIURETIC HORMONE SECRETION

By Gregory W. Rutecki, M.D.,
and Frederick C. Whittier, M.D.
Canton, Ohio

As a group, hyponatremic disorders constitute a substantial segment of the electrolyte disturbances encountered in clinical practice. Recent figures for hyponatremia highlight an incidence and prevalence of 1 and 2.5 per cent, respectively. In many patients, hyponatremia is associated with increased morbidity and mortality. Sick-cell syndrome accompanied by a decrease in sodium (Na^+) concentration is an example of more severe disease. In fact, certain susceptible populations—especially females and the elderly—may sustain irreversible brain injury as a direct result of hyponatremia irrespective of the primary etiology.

The syndrome of inappropriate antidiuretic hormone secretion (SIADH) is a well-established and common cause of decreased serum Na in hospitalized patients. However, the diagnosis of SIADH remains one of exclusion. Thus, as the number of diseases complicated by hyponatremia continues to increase, a systematic approach to the diagnosis and etiology of hyponatremia, in general, and SIADH, in particular, is essential.

Hyponatremia can be simply defined as an excess of total body water for available body solute—essentially a pathologic state of intracellular as well as extracellular hypotonicity. In the context of this definition of hyponatremia, SIADH may be further characterized as hypotonicity-hyponatremia in the euvolemic to slightly hypervolemic (nonedematous) patient who has (1) a urine osmolality higher than plasma osmolality; (2) a spot urine Na^+ concentration greater than 20 mEq/L; and (3) persistent, inappropriate ADH release that is not suppressed by the presence of hypotonicity. In patients with SIADH, serum Na concentration increases with water restriction. A firm diagnosis of SIADH should always presuppose the exclusion of other conditions associated with hyponatremia. These conditions include renal disease or other causes of salt loss, hypothyroidism, hypoadrenalism, cardiac failure, cirrhosis, and nephrosis. To exclude other causes of hyponatremia during the diagnostic evaluation for SIADH, knowledge of the medical history, physical examination, and laboratory studies is necessary (Fig. 1).

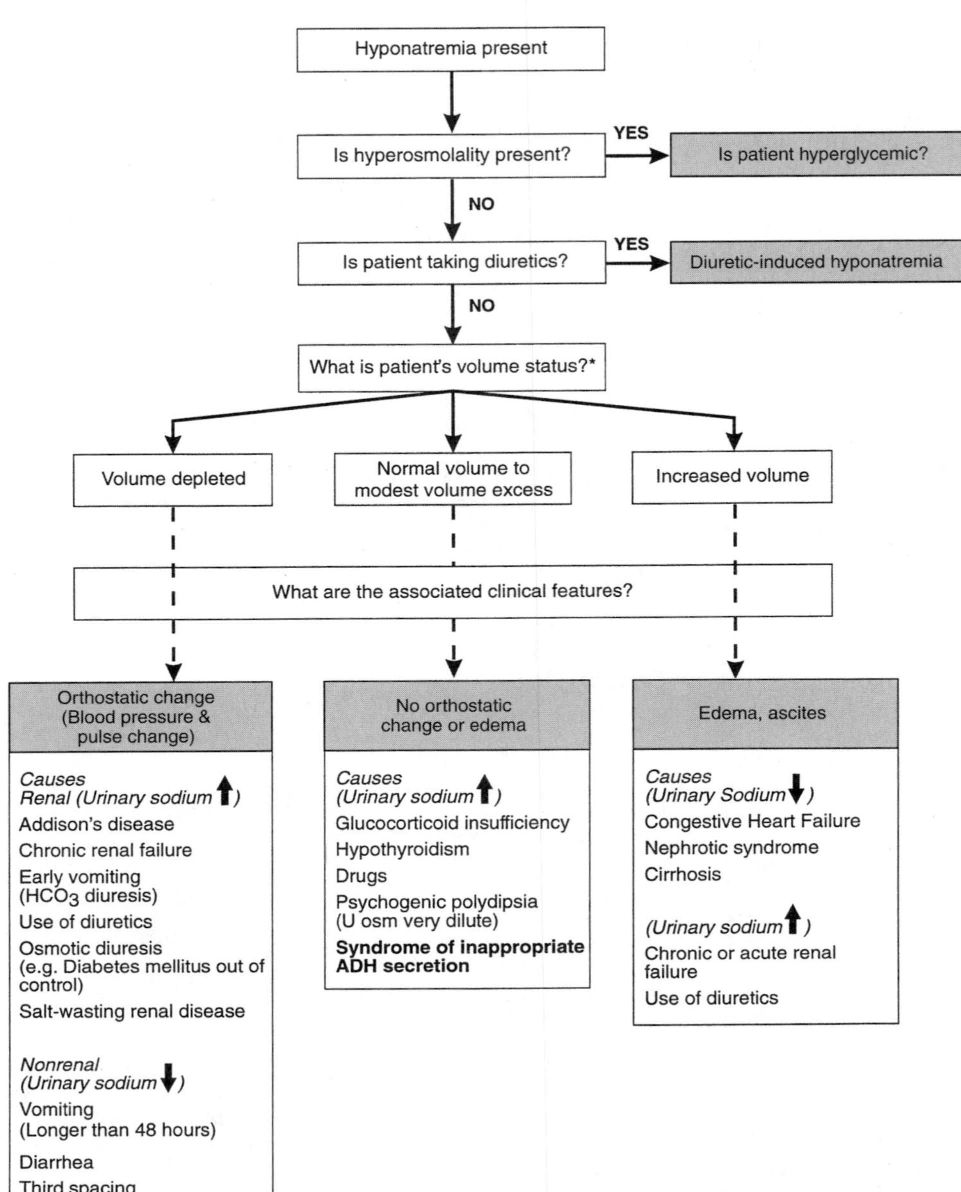

Figure 1. Algorithm for categorizing hyponatremia.

HYPONATREMIA WITH VOLUME CONTRACTION

Hyponatremia and volume contraction occur via a wide variety of pathophysiologic mechanisms. These include gastrointestinal fluid loss accompanied by plasma hypotonicity (vomiting and/or diarrhea); diuretic-induced volume loss; Addison's disease (combined mineralocorticoid and glucocorticoid deficiency); renal salt wasting (chronic renal disease or renal tubular disorders); and osmotic diuresis (e.g., hyperglycemia) or third spacing of volume (e.g., during pancreatitis) with a relative excess of water in the presence of a decrease in total body Na content.

The medical history and physical examination provide information about the medication history, gastrointestinal symptoms, renal disease, and orthostatic blood pressure and pulse changes. The spot urine Na^+ helps distinguish between the two subgroups within this category. A low urine Na^+ ($\leq$20 mEq/L) occurs when the kidney is capable of responding to the stress of volume contraction with Na^+ retention. Conversely Na^+ wasting (>20 mEq/L) suggests an inappropriate renal response to volume contraction and implicates renal tubular abnormalities, diuretics, or mineralocorticoid deficiency as possible causes of hyponatremia. If the urine Na^+ concentration is very high ($\geq$70 mEq/L)—especially in the setting of combined volume contraction, hyponatremia, hyperkalemia, and prerenal azotemia—Addison's disease must be considered. A spot urine osmolality is measured simultaneously and often shows moderate concentration ($\geq$500 mOsm/kg of H_2O) unless the patient is receiving diuretics or has renal disease. Hyponatremia with volume contraction during vomiting or nasogastric suction can be accompanied by either increased or low urine Na^+ concentration, depending on whether the clinical situation represents early (<48 to 72 hours) or prolonged upper gastrointestinal tract fluid loss. Early vomiting is associated with substantial bicarbonate diuresis, resulting in increased urine Na^+ concentration to maintain electroneutrality. The urine chloride concentration is markedly decreased (<10 mEq/L) and is essential to the diagnosis. Both urine Na^+ and Cl^- concentrations are decreased after 48 to 72 hours of vomiting or nasogastric suction; the urine bicarbonate concentration is also decreased because the renal tubules begin to absorb bicarbonate more efficiently.

HYPONATREMIA WITH VOLUME OVERLOAD

Hyponatremia with volume overload occurs in patients with low serum Na concentrations and ankle edema, anasarca, or ascites. The history and physical examination of this group is directed at underlying cardiac (congestive heart failure), renal (nephrotic syndrome, chronic renal failure), and hepatic (cirrhosis) diseases alone or in combination.

The spot urine Na^+ concentration can help distinguish two further subgroups: higher and lower Na^+ excretion. Higher Na^+ excretion (>30 mEq/L) can occur either when diuretics are given to patients with heart or liver disease or when renal insufficiency is present. A tendency toward more severe degrees of hyponatremia occurs whenever thiazide or metolazone diuretics are prescribed. The lower spot urine Na^+ concentration subgroup (<20 mEq/L) occurs with heart and liver disease as well as nephrotic syndrome when these disorders are accompanied by intact renal function without diuretics. Ineffective circulating volume is the stimulus for the renal Na^+ and H_2O retention, leading to hyponatremia and decreased urine Na^+ concentration. This condition is accompanied by an appropriate increase in ADH secretion in response to the ineffective circulation. The urine osmolality in this group is usually greater than the plasma osmolality (≥400 mOsm/kg of H_2O) unless diuretics are used or renal disease is simultaneously present.

HYPONATREMIA WITH EUVOLEMIA

Volume excess may be present in this group, but it is too subtle to measure clinically. When compared to patients on the volume depletion end of the spectrum, these patients do not have orthostatic blood pressure changes or pulse deficits, and physical examination does not reveal congestive heart failure, nephrosis, cirrhosis, peripheral edema, or ascites. Spot urine Na^+ concentration is typically greater than 20 mEq/L unless volume depletion is superimposed, and urine osmolality is usually moderately concentrated compared to plasma (400 to 700 mOsm/kg of H_2O). Certain drugs cause hyponatremia by either stimulating central ADH release or increasing renal tubular ADH sensitivity (Table 1). Symptoms or signs of hypothyroidism or glucocorticoid deficiency (including excessively rapid tapering of chronic glucocorticoid therapy) also provide important diagnostic clues. Psychogenic polydipsia presents with a typical history and is unique to this category, because the spot urine osmolality is usually less than 100 mOsm/kg of H_2O and is often maximally dilute (50 mOsm/kg of H_2O). Ancillary tests that assist with the diagnosis of disorders of this category include a thyroid-stimulating hormone (TSH) test even when signs and symptoms are equivocal for hypothyroidism.

SIADH: THE DIAGNOSIS OF EXCLUSION

A clinical diagnosis of SIADH as the cause of hyponatremia is considered only when all the criteria are satisfied. First, volume depletion is either absent or corrected. Second, edema and ascites secondary to cardiac, renal, and liver disease are excluded. Third, endocrine disorders are absent (especially thyroid and adrenal insufficiency). Fourth, associated drugs (especially diuretics) are not being administered (Table 1). An algorithm (Fig. 1) is helpful in developing a stepwise approach to hyponatremic disorders. After the diagnosis of SIADH has been established, the next step is identification of the cause of SIADH.

Secretion of ADH is physiologically suppressed when the plasma osmolality drops below 280 mOsm/kg of H_2O. Normal individuals who undergo water loading are capable of excreting between 15 and 20 L of H_2O per day or 20 mL/kg during a 4-hour period. The osmotic suppression of ADH at or below 280 mOsm/kg of H_2O may be overridden during two separate pathophysiologic settings. First, the nonosmotic stimulus of volume contraction or ineffective circulating volume via a baroreceptor-dependent mechanism stimulates continued ADH release despite the development of hypotonicity. Under circumstances of volume depletion or ineffective circulation, the retention of H_2O despite hypotonicity is fundamentally important for preventing further volume loss. Such a survival release of ADH despite hypotonicity can also be seen during stress, because the maintenance of volume takes precedence over the risks of hypotonicity. Second, water retention and hyponatremia can develop secondary to autonomous secretion of ADH, producing SIADH. Diseases that cause the unregulated release of ADH are classified as shown in Table 2.

Of the neoplasms associated with SIADH, bronchogenic carcinoma and, more specifically, oat or small cell carcinoma are most frequently associated with ectopic production of ADH by the neoplasm. SIADH may be clinically present months before the tumor itself is obvious. Another pathophysiologic mechanism of SIADH associated with neoplasms is a reset osmostat variant reported in gastric carcinoma and tuberculosis. The features of the reset osmostat variant of SIADH include normal volume hyponatremia, exclusion of other diseases associated with hyponatremia (see above), the ability to concentrate the urine when plasma osmolality is higher that the reset level of osmolality, normal diluting capacity with water loading, and a retained ability to maintain Na^+ balance with variations in Na^+ intake.

Even though the malignancy that initiates SIADH is usually clinically apparent, SIADH may precede the diagnosis of the neoplasm by months. In smokers with SIADH, chest films may reveal a small cell carcinoma. If the chest film is negative and the clinical suspicion for small cell

Table 1. Drugs Associated With Hyponatremia and the Mechanism Leading to SIADH

Chlorpropamide (central and renal tubular)
Chemotherapeutic agents: vincristine (central) and cyclophosphamide (central and renal tubular)
Carbamazepine (central)
ADH analogues, such as desmopressin (renal tubular)
Clofibrate (central)
Narcotics (central)
Major tranquilizers: haloperidol (?central); fluphenazine (?central); thioridazine (?central)
Antidepressants: amitriptyline (?central); fluoxetine (?central)
Anaglesics: nonsteroidals (renal tubular) and acetaminophen (renal tubular)
Diuretics (central and renal tubular) especially thiazide and Zaroxolyn (metolazone) group agents

Table 2. Diseases and Disorders Associated With SIADH

Neoplasms

- Small cell cancer of the lung
- Other bronchogenic carcinomas
- Gastrointestinal malignancies, including gastric, duodenal, pancreatic, and colonic
- Lymphomas, including Hodgkin's disease
- Leukemia
- Urinary tract malignancies, including bladder, ureteral, and prostate cancer
- Carcinoids
- Thymoma
- Ewing's sarcoma
- Mesothelioma
- Olfactory neuroblastoma

Pulmonary Diseases

- Infections: pneumonias, tuberculosis, lung abscess, bronchitis or bronchiolitis, and cavitary disease
- Trauma: pneumothorax, barotrauma
- Other: cystic fibrosis, asthma, chronic obstructive lung disease

Central Nervous System Causes

- Infections: meningitis, abscess, viral encephalitis, rickettsial disease (Rocky Mountain spotted fever)
- Trauma, including subdural hematoma and trauma occurring after neurosurgery
- Vascular disorders: subarachnoid hemorrhage, thromboses, stroke
- Specific diseases: Guillain-Barré syndrome, multiple sclerosis, temporal arteritis, vasculitis
- Psychosis (see drug list as well as Pitfalls in Diagnosis no. 2)
- Epilepsy
- Hydrocephalus
- Metastases or primary central nervous system malignancy
- Delirium tremens

Miscellaneous

- Hypopituitarism
- Acute intermittent porphyria
- Anorexia nervosa
- Acquired immunodeficiency syndrome (AIDS)

cancer remains high, bronchoscopy is considered next. Tests based on strong clinical suspicion are appropriately pursued, but an undirected search for malignancy in the patient with SIADH in the absence of other symptoms and signs is not indicated. A wide variety of pulmonary diseases (see Table 2) is associated with SIADH, and these disorders are clinically apparent concurrently with the presence of hyponatremia. SIADH that occurs during the course of central nervous system diseases may involve increased intracranial pressure (due to subarachnoid hemorrhage or hydrocephalus) or alterations in neurotransmitters (due to delirium tremens or psychoses), leading to autonomous ADH release. As many as one half of hospitalized patients with acquired immunodeficiency syndrome (AIDS) may experience hyponatremia. Hyponatremia in AIDS can result from various causes, such as hypoadrenalism, drugs (especially narcotics for pain relief), renal failure, hypothyroidism, and infections (*Pneumocystis carinii* pneumonia, cryptococcal meningitis, lung abscess). The development of SIADH significantly increases the mortality in AIDS patients, as it does in those with other associated diseases. Idiopathic SIADH is usually related to increasing age and is sufficiently rare that other causes—especially neoplasm—must be excluded before the diagnosis is made. Drugs associated with SIADH (see Table 1) must be reviewed in each patient who develops the syndrome.

The symptoms and signs of SIADH may reflect the effects of hyponatremia, its treatment, or the primary disease causing the inappropriate release of ADH. Any increase in total body water content (hyponatremia or, more correctly, hypotonicity) can lead to brain volume expansion within the rigid confines of the skull. Even a modest (5 per cent) increase in brain cell volume—especially if acute—with hyponatremia can cause herniation. The central nervous system signs and symptoms of hyponatremia typically progress from normal mentation to confusion, disorientation, obtundation, coma, seizures, paralysis, and eventually death if they go unchecked.

Autopsy studies of patients who die with hyponatremic brain damage reveal three types of pathologic lesions. Diffuse cerebral edema often leads to cerebral herniation. This finding is most common in hyponatremic patients with anoxia who die soon (within 48 hours) after a respiratory arrest. Cerebral edema with diffuse demyelination and occasionally cerebral infarction occurs in another subset of patients with fatal hyponatremia. A third group undergoes diffuse demyelination with associated focal injuries, such as oculomotor nerve damage and pituitary damage. The lesion described as central pontine myelinolysis is not common in hyponatremic patients unless a hyponatremic patient is also alcoholic or has serious underlying liver disease. Hyponatremic demyelination is often associated with ischemic injury, and it affects the basal ganglia, the cerebellum, subcortical white matter, and, less commonly, the pons. It can also develop after overly vigorous correction of the hypotonicity.

LABORATORY DIAGNOSIS

Occult endocrine disease must always be excluded in suspicious clinical settings. The possibility of underlying cardiac, renal, and hepatic pathology may require echocardiography or ultrasonography for further evaluation. Serum urate and urea nitrogen concentrations may be decreased, possibly owing to increased fractional excretion of urate and urea. The term pseudohyponatremia has been used to describe the apparent decrease in serum Na^+ concentration with normal or increased serum osmolality seen in patients with hyperchylomicronemia or hyperproteinemia. This artifact has been eliminated in most laboratories by the use of ion-specific electrodes for electrolyte measurement.

Water loading has been recommended for diagnosing the reset osmostat variety of SIADH. This test is rarely, if ever, indicated and runs the risk of water intoxication in sensitive patients. If considered at all, it should not be performed unless the serum Na^+ is above 130 mEq/L and the patient is carefully supervised during water loading.

PITFALLS IN DIAGNOSIS

The following pitfalls should be considered in the differential diagnosis of SIADH.

1. SIADH should never be accepted as the specific diagnosis for hyponatremia unless all other diagnoses are excluded. SIADH is hyponatremia accompanied by euvolemia or slight volume excess in the absence of diseases associated with volume depletion; cardiac, renal, and hepatic diseases; endocrine disorders (hypothyroidism

and hypoadrenalism); and drugs that lead to water retention. The failure to exclude all these disturbances can lead to a mistaken diagnosis of SIADH.

2. Patients with psychiatric disorders may develop hyponatremia from various causes including psychogenic polydipsia, water intoxication, effects of antipsychotic drugs, concomitant thiazide use, concurrent disease (see above), downward resetting of the osmostat, increased thirst, and SIADH.
3. A diagnosis of so-called idiopathic SIADH is rare and typically occurs only in the elderly.
4. A specific syndrome of salt wasting with a secondary increase in ADH occurs acutely in postoperative neurosurgical patients (termed cerebral salt-wasting syndrome [CSWS]) and may be mistaken for SIADH. The treatment of SIADH (water restriction) and CSWS (salt replacement) differ enough that the diagnosis is important. Although no test is completely specific, the clinical setting of CSWS raises the clinical index of suspicion that salt wasting and volume depletion are likely to be responsible for the development of hyponatremia—rather than SIADH.
5. Hyponatremia accompanied by decreased serum urate, urea, and creatinine concentrations that correct with water restriction suggests SIADH. Only the reset osmostat variant of SIADH does not correct with water restriction.
6. Spot urine osmolality in SIADH needs only to be relatively concentrated in relation to plasma and does not have to be absolutely concentrated to corroborate the presence of SIADH.
7. Urine Na^+ excretion in a patient with SIADH who is secondarily volume depleted may be low, and this does not exclude the presence of SIADH. Urine Na^+ concentration should be rechecked after Na^+ repletion.
8. Some malignancies (especially small cell cancer of the lung) may be preceded by SIADH for a period of months before the primary diagnosis becomes apparent. Chest film and bronchoscopy may be warranted for early diagnosis.

ACROMEGALY

By Vivien Herman, M.B., Ch.B.,
and Shlomo Melmed, M.B., Ch.B.
Los Angeles, California

Acromegaly, or hypersomatotropism, results from sustained hypersecretion of pituitary growth hormone (GH) and its target hormone, insulin-like growth factor I (IGF-I). The annual incidence of the disorder is estimated to be 3 per million, with a prevalence in the population of 50 to 70 per million.

Pituitary GH secretion is dually regulated by the hypothalamic stimulatory polypeptide growth hormone–releasing hormone (GHRH) and an inhibitory hormone, somatostatin (SRIF). The resultant secretory bursts of GH stimulate hepatic IGF-I production from the liver. More than 95 per cent of the cases of acromegaly are due to a pituitary tumor, arising from GH-secreting (somatotroph) cells (Fig. 1). A small number of acromegalic patients have extrapituitary tumors that secrete either ectopic GHRH or GH (Table 1). Ectopic GHRH secretion results in somatotroph hyperplasia, detectable on magnetic resonance imaging (MRI) as an enlarged pituitary gland.

Table 1. Causes of Hypersomatotropism

Pituitary
Eutopic
Densely or sparsely granulated GH-cell adenoma
Mixed GH-cell and PRL-cell adenoma
Mammosomatotroph-cell adenoma
Acidophil stem-cell adenoma
Plurihormonal adenoma
Albright's syndrome
Ectopic
Sphenoid sinus or parapharyngeal GH-cell adenoma
Extrapituitary
Ectopic GH-secreting tumor of pancreas, breast, or lung
Excess GHRH secretion
Eutopic
Hypothalamic hamartoma
Ectopic
Bronchial and intestinal carcinoid tumors
Pancreatic islet-cell tumors
Acromegaloidism

GH = growth hormone; GHRH = growth hormone–releasing hormone; PRL = prolactin.

About one third of acromegalic patients harbor GH-secreting adenomas that co-secrete prolactin; rarely, the tumor may be plurihormonal, producing thyroid-stimulating hormone (TSH) and/or adrenocorticotropic hormone (ACTH; corticotropin) in addition to the alpha-subunit of the glycoprotein hormones.

SIGNS AND SYMPTOMS

The clinical manifestations of acromegaly can be divided into local tumor effects, somatic effects, and endocrine-metabolic effects (Table 2). Younger patients generally present with more aggressive tumors. Local mass effects caused by the expanding pituitary tumor may compress the optic chiasm superiorly and invade the cavernous sinus laterally. Compression of adjacent or surrounding normal pituitary tissue may cause hypopituitarism by impairing trophic hormone secretion. Symptoms associated with the locally enlarging tumor mass correlate well with tumor size and invasiveness. At diagnosis, 15 per cent of GH-cell adenomas are microadenomas ($<$10 mm in diameter), and about 85 per cent are macroadenomas ($>$10 mm in diameter). One third of the macroadenomas exhibit sellar erosion, and about 20 per cent have suprasellar extension. Fifty to sixty per cent of acromegalic patients experience headaches. No correlation exists between tumor size or extrasellar extension and the frequency or severity of headaches. These last two may, in fact, be directly related to minimally increased intracranial pressure.

Hypopituitarism secondary to the expanding tumor mass has several clinical consequences. Fifty to seventy per cent of premenopausal acromegalic females have amenorrhea, and a similar percentage of males have decreased libido and impotence. This central hypogonadism may be due to associated hyperprolactinemia or to impingement on the gonadotroph cells by the macroadenoma. Decreased adrenal reserve or rarely, frank hypoadrenalism can occur secondary to decreased ACTH secretion. Hypothyroidism may result from decreased TSH secretion.

The somatic effects of acromegaly result from GH excess.

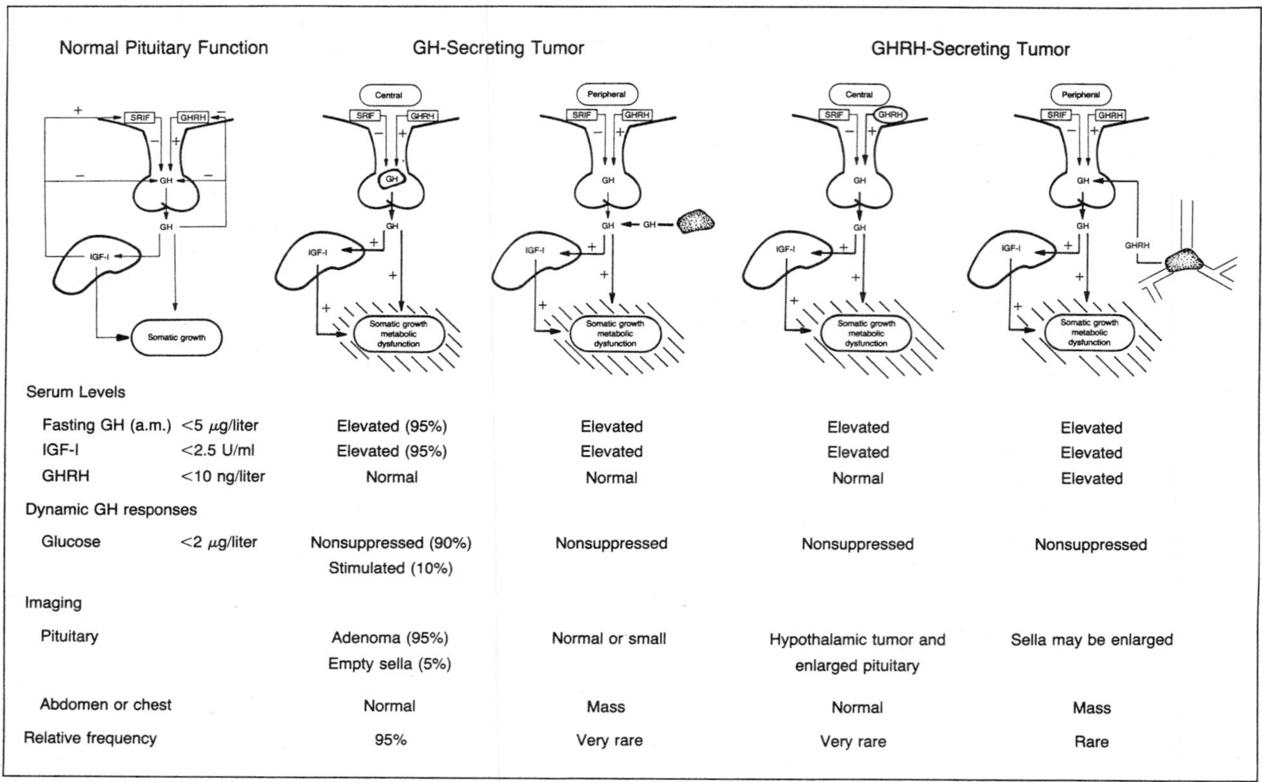

	Normal	GH-Secreting Tumor (Central)	GH-Secreting Tumor (Peripheral)	GHRH-Secreting Tumor (Central)	GHRH-Secreting Tumor (Peripheral)
Serum Levels					
Fasting GH (a.m.)	<5 μg/liter	Elevated (95%)	Elevated	Elevated	Elevated
IGF-I	<2.5 U/ml	Elevated (95%)	Elevated	Elevated	Elevated
GHRH	<10 ng/liter	Normal	Normal	Normal	Elevated
Dynamic GH responses					
Glucose	<2 μg/liter	Nonsuppressed (90%) Stimulated (10%)	Nonsuppressed	Nonsuppressed	Nonsuppressed
Imaging					
Pituitary		Adenoma (95%) Empty sella (5%)	Normal or small	Hypothalamic tumor and enlarged pituitary	Sella may be enlarged
Abdomen or chest		Normal	Mass	Normal	Mass
Relative frequency		95%	Very rare	Very rare	Rare

Figure 1. Pathophysiology and diagnosis of four types of acromegaly. Although only hepatic production of insulin-like growth factor I (IGF-I) is depicted, IGF-I is produced and appears to be locally bioactive in a number of extrahepatic tissues, including cartilage. Most of the growth-promoting activity of growth hormone (GH) appears to be mediated by IGF-I. GHRH = growth hormone–releasing hormone; SRIF = somatostatin; plus signs = stimulated secretion; minus signs = suppressed secretion. (From Melmed, S.: Acromegaly. N. Engl. J. Med., 322:966–977, 1990, with permission.)

Growth hormone acts on the liver to increase IGF-I synthesis. Plasma IGF-I concentrations are increased in acromegaly, where IGF-I is the primary mediator of changes in cartilage and bone. Circulating IGF-I acts as a classic endocrine hormone, whereas IGF-I released locally acts as a paracrine hormone. Growth hormone also acts directly to influence the function of differentiated cells. Moreover, GH may modulate cell proliferation via binding to specific receptors in extrahepatic tissues. Excessive soft-tissue growth results in characteristic coarsening of facial features, with prognathism, rhinophyma, macroglossia, and enlarged frontal bones and facial sinuses. Glove and ring size and shoe width increase. Characteristic skin changes include thickening, development of skin tags (which may be associated with colonic polyps), oiliness, excessive sweating, and acanthosis nigricans. Acral changes and changes in cartilage result in arthralgias and arthropathy. Musculoskeletal changes cause nerve entrapment syndromes, including carpal tunnel syndrome, cauda equina syndrome, and radiculopathies. Bony changes cause prognathism with dental malocclusion, loosening of incisors, widening of the spaces between the incisors, hypertrophy of frontal bones, and enlargement of facial sinuses. Acromegalic patients have a threefold to eightfold increased risk of colon cancer or premalignant polyps. Colonic polyps occur more frequently in older (>50 years) male patients with a family history of colon polyps who harbor more than three skin tags.

Cardiac disease is common in acromegaly and occurs in about one third of patients. As many as 80 per cent of patients may demonstrate echocardiographic abnormalities, including asymmetrical septal hypertrophy, concentric left ventricular wall thickening, and reduced ventricular ejection fraction. Only half of patients with echocardiographic abnormalities develop clinically significant heart failure. Abnormal resting electrocardiograms are frequently documented, including ST-segment and T-wave abnormalities, conduction defects, and arrhythmias. About 20 per cent of patients have symptomatic heart problems due to coronary artery disease, angina pectoris, myocardial infarction, arrhythmias, or congestive cardiac failure. Hypertension of unknown mechanism, which is present in a third of acromegalic patients, rarely improves when GH levels return to normal after treatment.

Respiratory disturbances manifest as upper airway obstruction due to deformities of the jaw, hypertrophied epiglottis, and enlarged tongue. Sixty per cent of acromegalic patients, usually males, have sleep apnea that is both obstructive and central in origin.

The third category of disorders in acromegaly comprises the endocrine-metabolic disturbances. Menstrual disturbances are caused by hyperprolactinemia or by gonadotroph destruction secondary to the enlarging GH-cell macroadenoma. GH-cell adenomas can secrete prolactin as well as GH, or the GH-cell macroadenoma may interrupt dopaminergic inhibitory control of prolactin secretion, resulting in secondary hyperprolactinemia. The hyperprolactinemia can also cause galactorrhea. Males with hyperprolactinemia and/or hypogonadotropism manifest decreased libido and impotence. Although carbohydrate intolerance occurs

Table 2. Clinical Features of Acromegaly

Local Tumor Effects

Pituitary enlargement
Visual field defects
Cranial nerve palsy
Headache
Hypopituitarism

Somatic

Acral Enlargement

Spadelike hands and feet
Increased heel pad thickness
Enlarged nose and lips

Musculoskeletal

Hypertrophic arthropathy
Osteoarthritis
Prognathism
Malocclusion of jaw
Arthralgias
Carpal tunnel syndrome
Acroparesthesias
Proximal myopathy
Hypertrophy of frontal bones
Enlarged sinuses

Skin Hyperhidrosis

Seborrhea
Skin tags
Acanthosis nigricans

Colon Polyps

Carcinoma

Cardiovascular

Left ventricular hypertrophy
Asymmetrical septal hypertrophy
Hypertension
Congestive heart failure
Arrhythmias

Respiratory

Upper airway obstruction
Sleep apnea
Narcolepsy

Visceromegaly

Tongue
Thyroid
Salivary gland
Liver
Spleen
Kidney

Neurologic

Carpal tunnel syndrome
Radiculopathy
Cauda equina syndrome

Endocrine-Metabolic

Reproduction

Menstrual abnormalities
Galactorrhea
Decreased libido, impotence
Decreased sex hormone–binding globulin

Multiple Endocrine Neoplasia (I)

Hyperparathyroidism
Pancreatic islet-cell tumors

Carbohydrate

Impaired glucose tolerance
Insulin resistance
Hyperinsulinemia
Diabetes mellitus

Lipids

Hypertriglyceridemia

Mineral

Hypercalciuria, increased 1,25-dihydroxyvitamin D_3
Increased urinary hydroxyproline

Electrolyte

Decreased renin
Increased aldosterone

Thyroid

Decreased thyroxine-binding globulin

in about half of acromegalic patients, only 10 to 25 per cent experience overt diabetes mellitus. Hypertriglyceridemia occurs in 20 to 45 per cent of acromegalic patients.

DISEASE COURSE

The very gradual progression of changes in physical features or tumor size often results in a delayed diagnosis. The delay has been estimated to average 12.5 years. Most patients are diagnosed in the fourth or fifth decade of life. Common presenting features include menstrual disturbances in females, changes in appearance, acral growth, and headaches. Acromegalic patients have an increased mortality rate that is ameliorated by effectively suppressing GH concentrations.

The death rate in acromegalics is twofold to threefold higher than the normal rate, and 50 per cent of untreated acromegalic patients die prematurely. Excess mortality is associated with cardiovascular, malignant cerebrovascular, and respiratory disease in acromegalic patients. Acromegalic patients with overt diabetes mellitus experience twice the mortality rate of nondiabetic acromegalic patients. Early treatment may reverse the soft-tissue changes, diabetes, cardiovascular diseases, sleep apnea, and neuromuscular disease. Decreased morbidity and mortality correlates with the degree of GH suppression attained with treatment. Attainment of a normal GH concentration decreases mortality to the expected age-matched rate. Whether early and effective treatment averts neoplasia is currently unclear, and patients should continue to be screened for colon polyps. Hypopituitarism may be present at initial presentation owing to compression of normal pituitary tissue by the expanding tumor mass, or it may develop after radiotherapy or surgery.

PHYSICAL EXAMINATION

Because of the gradual and often clinically subtle progression of the physical features of acromegaly over 5 to 10 years, the clinician should examine serial photographs of the patient, noting the increase in size of the nose, lips, and skin folds. In many patients, the physical examination reveals the classic features of prominent supraorbital ridges, enlarged nose, downward and foreward growth of the mandible leading to prognathism, and widely spaced teeth. In acromegalic patients, the facial features are coarse, and facial and infraorbital puffiness occurs. Soft-tissue growth of the hands and feet results in large, broad, blunt, spadelike fingers and toes.

The skin is thickened, oily, and sweaty. Hypertension and cardiomegaly (secondary to hypertension, atherosclerosis, or cardiomyopathy) may be present. Visual field defects, predominantly bitemporal hemianopia, may be due to impingement of an enlarging tumor mass on the optic chiasm. Hypopituitarism may cause hypogonadism (small testes and loss of pubic and axillary hair in males), hypoadrenalism, and hypothyroidism. Galactorrhea occurs in about 15 per cent of patients. Although acromegaly may be associated with multiple endocrine neoplasia type I (MEN-I), it is unusual to find accompanying hyperparathyroidism or a pancreatic islet-cell tumor.

COMPLICATIONS

Several years of excessive GH secretion produce late complications such as progressive cosmetic disfigurement, hypertrophic arthropathy, and osteoarthritis leading to disabling degenerative arthritis, which may require surgical intervention. When GH hypersecretion is present for several years, mortality rates are increased threefold owing to cardiovascular and cerebrovascular atherosclerosis and respiratory disease. Colonic and esophageal neoplasia is more common and has been associated with the risk factors mentioned earlier. Local effects of the progressively expanding tumor mass may cause headache and visual impairment. Growth hormone hypersecretion induces insulin resistance and glucose intolerance in 30 to 40 per cent of acromegalic patients and overt diabetes mellitus in 10 to 20 per cent.

LABORATORY INVESTIGATIONS

The clinical features of acromegaly are very characteristic. Examination of serial photographs over the preceding 5 to 10 years is helpful in confirming a clinical suspicion. However, the diagnosis must be confirmed by laboratory assessment of GH hypersecretion. Other conditions associated with paradoxical GH hypersecretion, which must be considered in the differential diagnosis, include type I diabetes mellitus, anxiety, exercise, protein-calorie malnutrition, acute illness, chronic renal failure, and cirrhosis. Patients with these conditions do not have clinical features of acromegaly, but they demonstrate abnormal GH suppressibility by glucose and, often, an abnormal GH response to thyrotropin-releasing hormone (TRH).

Measurement of random serum GH concentration is of limited value in the diagnosis of acromegaly, because GH secretion occurs episodically, and because other conditions, mentioned earlier, as well as physical and emotional stress also increase serum GH concentrations. Increased basal GH concentrations alone are therefore not diagnostic. A new ultrasensitive GH chemiluminescence assay is available. Compared with conventional radioimmunoassay (RIA) and immunoradiometric assay (IRMA), the chemiluminescence assay detects very low concentrations of GH. The detection limit of the ultrasensitive assay is approximately 0.002 μg/L (2 ng/L).

Suppression of increased serum GH with oral glucose is the classic and most specific dynamic test for establishing the diagnosis of acromegaly. In normal individuals, oral administration of 100 g of glucose reduces serum GH to less than 2 ng/mL at 120 minutes. By contrast, acromegalic patients may show no GH response to oral glucose; or they may show a partial decrease of GH concentrations, but not to below 2 ng/mL; or they may develop a paradoxical increase of serum GH after 30 and 60 minutes. This lack of suppressibility of serum GH after oral glucose establishes the diagnosis of acromegaly. As mentioned earlier, IGF-I is synthesized in several tissues, with the highest concentration and synthetic rate occurring in the liver. Growth hormone is the primary regulator of IGF-I synthesis, and circulating IGF-I concentrations reflect integrated GH secretion over the preceding days. Serum IGF-I is increased in active acromegaly. Importantly, IGF-I concentrations are relatively stable (even in acromegalics), whereas GH concentrations fluctuate during the course of the day and are increased by stress. Thus, a single measurement of serum IGF-I correlates well with disease activity and is a useful and precise screening test.

Growth hormone concentrations in the serum of acromegalic patients may increase paradoxically following the administration of TRH or luteinizing hormone–releasing hormone (LHRH). Serum GH is not altered in normal subjects given TRH, whereas nearly 50 per cent of acromegalic patients demonstrate a paradoxical increase of GH. The increment may exceed either 50 per cent of the basal value or 6 ng/mL following a bolus dose of 200 to 500 μg of intravenous TRH. Intravenous administration of LHRH (100 μg) increases serum GH and prolactin concentrations after 15 to 30 minutes; circulating concentrations of these hormones return to normal by 90 minutes in 15 per cent of acromegalic subjects. A positive GH response to LHRH may predict a positive response to subsequent treatment with a somatostatin analogue. By contrast, levodopa, converted centrally and peripherally to dopamine, stimulates GH secretion in normal subjects but suppresses GH concentrations in some acromegalic patients. The ingestion of 500 mg of levodopa by fasting acromegalics reduces GH concentrations by 50 per cent at 120 minutes in 75 per cent of these patients. Importantly, the aforementioned tests need be employed only in rare patients with acromegaly in whom normal or mildly increased GH concentrations are detected or in patients with equivocal GH responses to an oral glucose load. Finally, GH hypersecretion may cause hyperinsulinemia, glucose intolerance (frank diabetes occurs in only 15 per cent of acromegalics), hypercalciuria, hyperphosphatemia, and increased urinary hydroxyproline, but these biochemical abnormalities have no specificity for the diagnosis of acromegaly.

Following biochemical confirmation of GH hypersecretion, radiographic localization of the source of excessive GH must be undertaken. Most acromegalic patients harbor GH-secreting pituitary adenomas. Magnetic resonance imaging has superseded computed tomography as the imaging procedure of choice. Imaging studies should be performed only after biochemical confirmation of excessive GH secretion because 25 per cent of the normal population harbor nonfunctioning, asymptomatic pituitary microadenomas that may be seen with sensitive MRI. The pituitary and hypothalamus are visualized in both sagittal and coronal planes at intervals of 1.5 to 2 mm during MRI. Lesions as small as 2 mm can be seen by this technique. Administration of the contrast agent gadolinium allows clearer delineation of small adenomas from normal pituitary tissue. Ninety per cent of tumors in acromegalic patients are larger than 1 cm in diameter, and MRI may document extension of intrapituitary lesions. Larger tumors compress normal surrounding pituitary tissue, displace the pituitary stalk, or extend into the suprasellar space, compressing the optic chiasm and displacing it dorsally.

Less commonly, lateral extension into the cavernous sinus can be visualized. If diffuse pituitary enlargement without a discrete mass is detected with MRI, ectopic GHRH production by an extrapituitary lesion should be suspected. Hypothalamic hamartomas can be visualized with MRI and bronchial, intestinal, or thymic carcinoid tumors or pancreatic islet-cell tumors can be localized by appropriate imaging of the chest or abdomen. If a normal pituitary is documented with MRI, ectopic GH secretion should be suspected. This rare event is typically associated with pancreatic, breast, or lung tumors.

After the diagnosis of a GH-secreting macroadenoma has been established, biochemical evidence of hypopituitarism should be excluded. Serum TSH, serum testosterone (in males), and serum estradiol (in females) concentrations should be measured, and a Cortrosyn (cosyntropin) stimulation test should be completed. These tests determine the integrity and function of the ACTH, TSH, and gonadotropin-dependent axes.

Acromegaly is a disorder of protean somatic and biochemical manifestations. Diagnosis is not difficult in advanced cases, but early in the disease, when physical changes are subtle, the diagnosis is often not considered by the patient, family, or treating physician. Clinicians must suspect GH excess early in the disease, prior to the onset of irreversible acromegalic features and complications.

HYPERPROLACTINEMIA

By Mark E. Molitch, M.D.
Chicago, Illinois

PROLACTIN SECRETION

Prolactin (PRL) is secreted episodically. Thirteen to 14 peaks per day, with an interpulse interval of 93 to 95 minutes, can be documented in healthy young adults. An increase in the amplitude of PRL secretory pulses begins about 60 to 90 minutes after the onset of sleep; the amplitude increases with non–rapid eye movement (REM) sleep and decreases prior to the next period of rapid eye movement sleep. Small increments in PRL during the afternoon and evening have been attributed to the central action of dietary amino acids, especially phenylalanine, tyrosine, and glutamic acid.

Basal serum PRL concentrations gradually increase during pregnancy owing to the stimulation of pituitary lactotrophs by estrogens. The number of pituitary lactotrophs gradually increases during pregnancy, and by term basal serum PRL has typically increased tenfold, often exceeding 200 μg/L. Increased PRL at term prepares the breast for lactation. The tumor cells of a prolactinoma may also be stimulated by the hormonal milieu of pregnancy.

During the first 4 to 6 weeks postpartum, basal PRL concentrations remain high in lactating women, and each suckling episode triggers increased synthesis and rapid release of PRL. Over the next 4 to 12 weeks, as the suckling frequency decreases, basal PRL concentrations gradually fall to normal and the lactotroph response to suckling diminishes. If intense nursing behavior is maintained, basal PRL remains increased, ovulation does not occur, and postpartum amenorrhea persists.

PROLACTIN REGULATION

The hypothalamus primarily regulates PRL secretion through one or more PRL inhibitory factors that reach the pituitary via the hypothalamic-pituitary portal vessels. Importantly, the hypothalamus produces PRL-releasing factors as well. Disruption of the pituitary stalk typically causes increased secretion of PRL and decreased secretion of the other pituitary hormones.

Dopamine is the predominant physiologic PRL inhibitory factor. Stimuli that cause an acute release of PRL typically cause an acute decrease in portal vessel dopamine concentrations. Blockade of endogenous dopamine receptors by various drugs, including phenothiazines and butyrophenones, increases PRL. The axons responsible for release of dopamine into the median eminence originate in perikarya in the arcuate ventromedial nuclei of the hypothalamus. The dopamine that traverses this pathway binds to the D_2 class of dopamine receptors on the lactotroph plasma membrane. The neurotransmitter γ-aminobutyric acid (GABA) can also inhibit PRL secretion, but its physiologic significance is not clear.

Thyrotropin-releasing hormone (TRH) causes a rapid release of PRL from cultured pituitary cells and in humans after intravenous injection. However, the physiologic role of TRH as a PRL releasing factor in humans has not yet been clarified. Passive immunization studies, analysis of thyroid-stimulating hormone (TSH) concentrations during lactation, and examination of PRL concentrations in various thyroid conditions suggest, at best, a minor role for TRH as a physiologic PRL releasing factor.

Vasoactive intestinal peptide (VIP) selectively stimulates PRL release. Passive immunoneutralization with anti-VIP antisera partially inhibits the PRL response to suckling, stress, and other stimuli. Peptide histidine methionine, which is a fragment of the 170 amino acid precursor of VIP, may also stimulate PRL secretion. The precise roles of hypothalamic VIP versus pituitary VIP, and peptide histidine methionine versus other PRL releasing factors remain to be determined.

DEFINITION OF HYPERPROLACTINEMIA

Hyperprolactinemia is defined as a basal PRL concentration that exceeds 20 to 25 μg/L. Serum PRL concentrations are 3 to 7 μg/L higher in women than in men. When PRL concentrations are borderline, multiple sampling may be required to establish the presence of sustained hyperprolactinemia. Samples should be obtained at least 60 minutes after stimulation of the breasts or ingestion of a high-protein meal.

PRESENTING SIGNS AND SYMPTOMS OF HYPERPROLACTINEMIA

In humans, PRL primarily acts to prepare the breast for postpartum lactation. High PRL concentrations may also influence other organs, but the role of physiologic concentrations of PRL in nonmammary tissues remains speculative.

Galactorrhea

High circulating concentrations of estrogen, progesterone, prolactin, and placental lactogen stimulate development of the lobular, alveolar breast tissue during pregnancy. Once the breast is fully developed and hormonally primed, PRL stimulates the production of milk proteins and other components. Prior to term, increased estrogen concentrations suppress the effects of high PRL on milk production. After delivery the rapid decrease in circulating estrogens allows milk production to proceed.

Clinically, nonpuerperal galactorrhea is viewed as a sign of possible hyperprolactinemia. The presence of even minute amounts of milk that can be expressed from one or both breasts justifies the diagnosis of galactorrhea. Inappropriate lactation is defined as the persistence of galactorrhea for more than 1 year after normal delivery and cessation of breast-feeding or as the occurrence of galactorrhea in the absence of pregnancy. If the material expressed from the nipple looks like milk, it probably is milk. When there is doubt, the diagnosis of galactorrhea can be confirmed by staining of fat globules with Sudan IV.

The incidence of galactorrhea in normal women ranges from 1 to 45 per cent of patients tested. This variability probably results from differences in techniques used to express milk from the breast and in classifications of nonmilky secretions. Inappropriate lactation may provide an important clue to the presence of pituitary-hypothalamic disease, especially if lactation is accompanied by amenorrhea. Galactorrhea is found in 5 to 10 per cent of normally menstruating women, but basal PRL concentrations are increased in no more than 5 to 10 per cent of women with galactorrhea.

Amenorrhea, Anovulation, and Infertility

The effect of physiologic PRL concentrations on gonadotropin secretion is not well understood. However, hyperprolactinemia influences many steps in the reproductive axis. Importantly, hyperprolactinemia suppresses the pulsatile secretion of gonadotropin-releasing hormone (GnRH) and the pulsatile secretion of the gonadotropins. In castrated men or menopausal women, hyperprolactinemia often prevents the expected rise in gonadotropins; normalization of PRL concentrations with bromocriptine may lead to increased gonadotropin secretion and hot flashes. Hyperprolactinemia in women has also been associated with loss of positive estrogen feedback on gonadotropin secretion.

The role of PRL in normal human ovarian function is not well established. Hyperprolactinemia can suppress ovarian secretion of progesterone and estrogen by antagonizing both the stimulation of aromatase activity by follicle-stimulating hormone (FSH) and the stimulation of androgen synthesis by luteinizing hormone (LH), thereby depriving the ovary of the substrate for conversion to estrogen.

Nearly 75 per cent of women in whom galactorrhea and amenorrhea (or oligomenorrhea) develop have hyperprolactinemia. Although the amenorrhea caused by excess prolactin is typically secondary, it can also be primary if the onset of the hyperprolactinemia predates the onset of puberty. In patients with primary amenorrhea due to hyperprolactinemia, estrogen deficiency and the failure of normal secondary sexual characteristics to develop may be the presenting problem. The frequency and intensity of galactorrhea are difficult to predict because the breast may not have been appropriately primed with estrogen and progesterone. Patients with primary amenorrhea harbor pituitary macroadenomas more commonly than do patients with secondary amenorrhea. Hyperprolactinemia is common in women with a short luteal phase; conversely, a short luteal phase may provide early evidence that hyperprolactinemia interferes with the normal menstrual cycle.

Patients with hyperprolactinemia may present with infertility, especially when gonadotropins are suppressed. Conversely, about one third of women presenting with infertility are found to have hyperprolactinemia. Many of these women also present with oligo/amenorrhea, often associated with galactorrhea.

In response to specific questioning, most women with hyperprolactinemia and amenorrhea will report reduced libido and orgasmic dysfunction. Normalization of prolactin restores normal libido and sexual function in most of these women. Although plasma dehydroepiandrosterone (DHEA), DHEA sulfate (DHEAS), and free testosterone concentrations are increased in about half of women with hyperprolactinemia, the correlation with hirsutism is poor.

Impotence and Male Infertility

The role of PRL in normal testicular function is unclear. Ninety per cent of males with chronic hyperprolactinemia experience impotence and decreased libido. Other findings of hypogonadism, including decreased beard growth and strength, are less common. Galactorrhea has been reported in 10 to 20 per cent of males with hyperprolactinemia; galactorrhea in males is virtually pathognomonic of a prolactinoma. The pulsatile secretion of LH and FSH is blunted, and testosterone concentrations are low or low normal in males with hyperprolactinemia. The stimulation of testosterone secretion with human chorionic gonadotropin (hCG) may be normal or suppressed. In patients with decreased responses to hCG, reduction of PRL concentrations with bromocriptine may improve the response. If there is sufficient normal pituitary tissue, normalization of serum PRL usually normalizes testosterone concentrations. Testosterone therapy for men with hyperprolactinemia does not usually correct impotence until PRL concentrations are significantly reduced. A significant role for decreased dihydrotestosterone production in men with hyperprolactinemia has not been verified directly. Sperm counts and motility are decreased, abnormal forms are increased, and histologic studies reveal abnormal seminiferous tubule walls and an altered Sertoli cell ultrastructure. The semen may remain abnormal even if serum PRL and testosterone concentrations return to normal.

Five to 25 per cent of males with impotence have hyperprolactinemia. However, only 1 to 5 per cent of men with infertility have hyperprolactinemia. Despite these relatively low frequencies, the cost of measuring prolactin is low, and hyperprolactinemia is generally easy to treat. Thus, measurement of PRL is well advised in the routine investigation of any man complaining of infertility or impotence.

Osteoporosis

Women with hyperprolactinemia have decreased bone mineral density. Correction of hyperprolactinemia usually results in an increase in bone mass. However, women with hyperprolactinemia who do not have amenorrhea and hypoestrogenemia have normal bone mineral density, confirming the hypothesis that estrogen deficiency mediates the bone mineral loss. A similar, androgen-dependent loss of bone mineral in men with hyperprolactinemia is reversible with correction of the hypoandrogenic state.

DIFFERENTIAL DIAGNOSIS OF HYPERPROLACTINEMIA (Table 1)

Medications

Psychotropic Agents

The neuroleptics (phenothiazines and butyrophenones) increase PRL concentrations (28 to 140 μg/L) within a few

Table 1. Differential Diagnosis of Hyperprolactinemia

Pituitary Disease	Neurogenic Causes	Medications
Prolactinomas Acromegaly Empty sella syndrome Lymphocytic hypophysitis Cushing's disease Pituitary stalk section	Chest wall lesions Spinal cord lesions Breast stimulation	Phenothiazines Butyrophenones Monoamine oxidase inhibitors Tricyclic antidepressants Reserpine Methyldopa Metoclopramide Amoxepin Verapamil Cocaine
Hypothalamic Disease	**Other**	
Craniopharyngioma Meningioma Dysgerminoma Clinically nonfunctioning pituitary adenoma Other tumors Sarcoidosis Eosinophilic granuloma Neuraxis irradiation Vascular causes	Pregnancy Hypothyroidism Renal failure Cirrhosis Pseudocyesis **Idiopathic Disease**	

From Molitch, M.E.: Management of prolactinomas. Annu. Rev. Med., 40:225–232, 1989. With permission from the Annual Review of Medicine, © 1989, by Annual Reviews Inc.

hours of administration. These increased concentrations of PRL persist with chronic (long-term) use of neuroleptics. These agents most likely increase PRL by blocking dopamine receptors in the hypothalamus and on the plasma membrane of pituitary lactotrophs. PRL concentrations typically normalize within 48 to 96 hours of discontinuing neuroleptic therapy. Tricyclic antidepressants and monoamine oxidase inhibitors also cause modest hyperprolactinemia in about 25 per cent of recipients. The mechanism or mechanisms by which these drugs increase circulating PRL are not certain. Chronic abuse of opiates has been associated with mild hyperprolactinemia and menstrual dysfunction. Cocaine abuse has also been associated with chronic, mild hyperprolactinemia.

Antihypertensive Drugs

α-Methyldopa causes moderate hyperprolactinemia by (1) inhibiting L-aromatic amino acid decarboxylase, the enzyme that converts L-dopa to dopamine and (2) acting as a false neurotransmitter to decrease dopamine synthesis. Reserpine causes hyperprolactinemia by interfering with the storage of hypothalamic catecholamines in secretory granules. Verapamil increases basal PRL secretion and may cause galactorrhea and/or amenorrhea owing to a decrease in hypothalamic dopamine synthesis.

Renal Disease

Hyperprolactinemia occurs in about 75 per cent of women and 50 per cent of men with end-stage renal disease. Although degradation of PRL is delayed in renal failure, there is also increased production because of disordered hypothalamic regulation of PRL secretion. About one quarter of individuals with renal insufficiency not requiring dialysis (serum creatinine concentration 176.8 to 1060.8 μmol/L) have PRL concentrations ranging from 25 to 100 μg/L. When such patients take methyldopa, metoclopramide, or other medications known to alter hypothalamic regulation of PRL, serum concentrations may exceed 2000 μg/L. Correction of renal failure with transplantation causes PRL concentrations to return to normal. Hyperprolactinemia is one of several causal factors in the hypogonadism of chronic renal failure.

Cirrhosis

Basal PRL concentrations are increased in 10 to 20 per cent of patients with cirrhosis and may be partially responsible for the hypogonadism of cirrhosis. The mechanism most likely involves disordered regulation of central catecholamines and may involve altered estrogen-to-androgen ratios.

Hypothyroidism

Although primary hypothyroidism is associated with modestly increased PRL concentrations in 40 per cent of patients, concentrations exceed 25 μg/L in only 10 per cent. Proposed mechanisms include increased TRH production, increased sensitivity of lactotrophs to TRH, and increased pituitary VIP synthesis. Many patients with long-standing hypothyroidism may have signs and symptoms of pituitary enlargement, hyperprolactinemia, galactorrhea, and/or amenorrhea and thus may be erroneously thought to have a prolactinoma. Treatment with L-thyroxine will normalize serum PRL and reduce pituitary size.

Adrenal Insufficiency

Glucocorticoids suppress PRL gene transcription and PRL release. Hyperprolactinemia seen in patients with adrenal insufficiency has been corrected by the administration of glucocorticoids.

Neurogenic Causes of Prolactinemia

Breast stimulation and suckling cause reflex release of PRL mediated by afferent neural pathways coursing through the spinal cord. Irritative chest wall and cervical cord lesions may also lead to hyperprolactinemia and galactorrhea via stimulation of these pathways. Similar chronic increases in PRL concentrations have been reported after mastectomy and thoracotomy.

Ectopic Prolactin Secretion

Ectopic production of PRL is exceedingly rare. In a series of 215 patients with various malignancies, serum PRL was increased in only 14. Hyperprolactinemia in 12 patients could be explained by the use of medications, prior irradiation to the chest wall or head, or chest wall involvement by the cancer. Symptomatic hyperprolactinemia has been attributed to ectopic PRL production from a renal cell carcinoma, a gonadoblastoma, and ectopic pituitary tissue in two ovarian teratomas. In general, a search for an ectopic source of PRL secretion is not warranted because prolactinomas, "idiopathic hyperprolactinemia," and medications are significantly more frequent causes of excessive prolactin production.

Hypothalamic–Pituitary Stalk Disease

Lesions of the hypothalamus and pituitary stalk may decrease the amount of dopamine that reaches the pituitary. In these patients, increased serum PRL typically does not exceed 100 μg/L and almost never exceeds 250 μg/L. Distinguishing prolactinomas from "clinically nonfunctioning" pituitary adenomas or other lesions (e.g., craniopharyngioma, Rathke's cleft cyst, lymphocytic hypophysitis) is clinically important because, following administration of dopamine agonists, the former will frequently get smaller and the latter will rarely change in size. Hyperprolactinemia has been reported in patients with infiltrative hypothalamic lesions caused by sarcoidosis, histiocytosis X, or tuberculosis. Distortions of the pituitary stalk that accompany the partially empty sella syndrome may also cause hyperprolactinemia that may be complicated by varying degrees of hypopituitarism and diabetes insipidus.

Neuraxis Irradiation

Nearly half of all patients who receive pituitary or whole brain irradiation experience hyperprolactinemia. When the secretion of other anterior pituitary hormones is also impaired, radiation injury of the hypothalamic region has most likely occurred.

Idiopathic Hyperprolactinemia

Hyperprolactinemia of uncertain cause has been designated as idiopathic. Many patients with idiopathic hyperprolactinemia probably harbor prolactinomas that are too small for detection by current imaging techniques. In some patients, idiopathic hyperprolactinemia may be the result of hypothalamic regulatory dysfunction, but no dysfunction specific to idiopathic hyperprolactinemia has been definitively elucidated. Long-term follow-up of patients with idiopathic hyperprolactinemia indicates that in one third, PRL concentrations return to normal; in one sixth, serum PRL increases; and in the other half, PRL concentrations do not change. Follow-up over 2 to 6 years leads to detection of microadenomas in 15 per cent of individuals. Patients with unremarkable magnetic resonance imaging (MRI) scans should undergo repeat MRI every other year for 6 years to rule out developing infiltrative or mass lesions.

Prolactinomas

Prolactinomas are classified by size as microadenomas (<10 mm in diameter), macroadenomas (>10 mm in diameter), and macroadenomas with extrasellar extension. In general, serum PRL concentrations parallel the size of the tumors. Patients with microadenomas followed for up to 8 years without treatment show an incidence of progression to macroadenoma of 7 per cent. Both micro- and macroadenomas are commonly treated with dopamine agonists; transsphenoidal resection of adenoma is undertaken in selected cases.

Mixed Pituitary Tumors

Forty per cent of patients with acromegaly have tumors that cosecrete growth hormone (GH) and PRL. Occasionally, such patients will complain of amenorrhea and/or galactorrhea with minimal signs and symptoms of acromegaly. Less commonly, patients harbor tumors that secrete PRL as well as other hormones, including adrenocorticotropic hormone (ACTH), LH, FSH, and α-subunit.

DIAGNOSTIC STUDIES

Prolactin Measurement

PRL is secreted episodically, and some PRL concentrations during the day may exceed the upper limit of the reference range established in a particular laboratory. Thus, a slightly increased serum PRL concentration must be confirmed in several samples. A variety of conditions may be associated with hyperprolactinemia that typically does not exceed 250 μg/L. A careful history and physical examination will exclude many of these causes.

Stimulation and suppression tests with TRH, hypoglycemia, chlorpromazine, and L-dopa yield nonspecific results and have been largely abandoned as tools in the differential diagnosis of hyperprolactinemia.

Additional Laboratory Assessment

In patients with mild hyperprolactinemia (<250 μg/L), renal insufficiency and liver disease should be excluded. Thyroxine and TSH determinations will exclude hypothyroidism, and a serum hCG determination will exclude pregnancy. Serum cortisol and adrenocorticotropic hormone need only be measured if there is clinical evidence of adrenal insufficiency or Cushing's disease. If there is any evidence of acromegaly, serum insulin-like growth factor I (IGF-I) should be measured.

Patients found to have macroadenomas, hypothalamic disease, or empty sella syndromes should undergo evaluation of the sufficiency of their other anterior and posterior pituitary hormones. LH and FSH can be evaluated only when PRL concentrations return to normal. If menses resume in women and libido and potency are restored in men, normal gonadotropin function can be presumed. Measurement of serum estradiol or testosterone may also be helpful, but stimulation with gonadotropin-releasing hormone is rarely useful. Simple measurement of thyroxine and TSH will determine whether TSH is deficient. TRH testing is rarely necessary. However, stimulation of the hypothalamic-pituitary-adrenal axis with insulin-induced hypoglycemia or metyrapone is often appropriate to ensure that this axis is capable of responding to stress. Because therapy with GH in adults is not indicated at present, testing is rarely performed. In children with these lesions, testing for GH deficiency is clearly indicated. However, GH testing in the presence of gonadal insufficiency may be misleading, and such testing should be deferred until PRL concentrations return to normal and/or gonadal function is at least transiently normalized. Assessment for diabetes insipidus may include measurement of the urinary concentration and plasma vasopressin responses to dehydration or hypertonic saline infusion.

Diagnostic Imaging

When there is no obvious cause of hyperprolactinemia discerned from the screening outlined earlier, imaging of the hypothalamic-pituitary area is required to exclude a mass lesion. Imaging is necessary, even in patients with mild hyperprolactinemia. The most frequently employed procedures are MRI with gadolinium enhancement, and computed tomography (CT) with intravenous contrast enhancement and direct coronal views. MRI is generally preferred because it provides better delineation of structures in the cavernous sinus, vascular structures, and optic chiasm. It is very important to distinguish between a large nonsecreting tumor causing modest PRL elevations (usually <250 μg/L) from a PRL-secreting macroadenoma (PRL concentrations usually >250 μg/L), as the therapy may be quite different.

False-positive CT or MRI scans have been reported. The observation of a "microprolactinoma" on a scan in a patient with hyperprolactinemia may ulitmately prove to be a cyst, infarct, or incidental nonsecreting tumor at the time of biopsy or surgery.

Visual Fields

Visual fields (Goldmann perimetry) should be assessed in patients whose tumors are adjacent to or pressing on the optic chiasm (as visualized on MRI). If only CT is available for imaging, patients with suprasellar extension require visual field assessments.

Bone Mineral Density Studies

Dual x-ray absorptiometry (DEXA) scans may be indicated in some patients to document the degree of osteoporosis. For some patients, the presence of significant osteoporosis may influence decisions about therapy.

SUMMARY OF DIAGNOSTIC EVALUATION

Patients usually present because of reproductive dysfunction, galactorrhea, or evidence of a mass lesion. PRL concentrations exceeding 250 μg/L are almost always caused by a prolactinoma. PRL concentrations less than 250 μg/L have many causes, and a careful history, physical examination, routine chemistry panel, a pregnancy test, and a TSH determination will usually suffice to exclude most of these causes. If this evaluation is unremarkable, diagnostic imaging with MRI or CT is mandatory in all patients to determine the presence of a mass lesion and its anatomic extent. Some patients with tumors that have extended above the sella turcica require visual field assessments to determine the presence of chiasmal compression. In addition, patients with macroadenomas and/or hypothalamic disease should be evaluated for hypopituitarism or diabetes insipidus.

HYPERTHYROIDISM

By Neena Natt, M.B., B.Chir.,
and Ian D. Hay, M.B., Ph.D.
Rochester, Minnesota

Hyperthyroidism, also called thyrotoxicosis, is a complex clinical syndrome that develops when body tissues are exposed to excess circulating thyroid hormone. In most patients, thyroxine (T_4) and triiodothyronine (T_3) are increased in the serum, but isolated increases in T_4 and T_3, so-called T_4- and T_3-toxicosis, are also recognized. In individual patients, the clinical manifestations may range from subtle to florid; the intensity of symptoms and signs depends on the degree and duration of hormonal excess, the age of the patient, the underlying cause of the hyperthyroidism, and the presence of concomitant disease.

Hyperthyroidism can have many underlying causes (Table 1). Graves' disease, characterized by diffuse enlargement and hyperactivity of the thyroid gland, accounts for most cases. This disorder can occur at any age, including the neonatal period, but typically affects women in the third through fourth decades of life. The pathogenesis of the hyperthyroidism involves the formation of thyroid-stimulating immunoglobulins that bind to thyrotropin receptors in the thyroid cell membrane and directly stimulate the growth and activity of the gland. Graves' disease can be clinically distinguished from other forms of hyperthyroidism by the presence of unique extrathyroidal manifestations, including infiltrative ophthalmopathy, infiltrative dermopathy (i.e., pretibial myxedema), and thyroid acropachy. All of these associated features may precede, accompany, or follow the onset of hyperthyroidism, and they tend to run clinical courses that are largely independent of one another.

Table 1. Etiology of Hyperthyroidism

Autonomous Thyroid Overactivity
Graves' disease
Toxic multinodular goiter
Solitary toxic adenoma
Hormonal Discharge During Thyroiditis
Granulomatous thyroiditis
Subacute lymphocytic thyroiditis
Pituitary Thyroid-Stimulating Hormone Hypersecretion
Pituitary adenoma
Selective pituitary resistance syndromes
Extrathyroidal Source of Thyroid Hormone
Iatrogenic or factitious hyperthyroidism
Functioning metastatic follicular thyroid carcinoma
Struma ovarii (i.e., functioning thyroid tissue in ovarian teratoma)

Toxic multinodular goiter, or Plummer's disease, typically affects the older patient with a history of long-standing multinodular goiter. The hyperthyroidism typically develops insidiously as multiple areas within the gland gradually assume autonomous function. In the less common situation of solitary toxic follicular adenoma, the hyperfunctioning tissue is limited to a single nodule, with subsequent functional suppression of extranodular thyroid tissue.

A spontaneously remitting form of thyrotoxicosis can develop in either the acute phase of granulomatous (painful) or subacute (painless) lymphocytic thyroiditis, and is caused by the release of substantial amounts of stored hormone from the inflamed thyroid gland. The thyrotoxicosis is typically transient, lasting a few weeks to months until hormone stores are depleted, and it may be followed by a brief period of hypothyroidism before the thyroid gland recovers function. The important feature of this type of thyrotoxicosis is that the disease tends to be self-limiting and only rarely requires more than symptomatic treatment.

Most cases of thyrotoxicosis are caused by intrinsic thyroid disease; excessive thyroid-stimulating hormone (TSH) secretion by the pituitary gland is rare. Exogenous hyperthyroidism, in which the source of excess hormone is outside of the thyroid gland, is usually the result of inadvertent overdose with thyroid hormone preparations or surreptitious ingestion of excess thyroid hormone. Other rare forms of exogenous hyperthyroidism are listed in Table 1 and are not discussed further in this section.

PRESENTING SYMPTOMS

The variety of complaints with which a hyperthyroid patient may present reflects the multiple sites of action of thyroid hormone. In the classic patient, a well-recognized symptom complex evolves that is related to the increased catabolic and sympathetic activity associated with hormonal excess. Often, however, the thyrotoxic patient seeks medical advice by virtue of only one or two of these symptoms but, on direct questioning, usually admits to noticing the characteristic thyroid-mediated effects on the cardio-

Table 2. Clinical Features of Hyperthyroidism

General
Fatigue
Heat intolerance
Increased perspiration
Cardiovascular
Palpitations, dyspnea
Angina pectoris
Sinus tachycardia or atrial fibrillation
Cardiac failure
Neuromuscular or Psychiatric
Nervousness, agitation
Emotional lability
Tremor
Proximal muscle weakness
Gastrointestinal
Weight loss despite good appetite
Increased stool frequency
Ocular
Lid retraction, lid lag
Pain or sensation of grittiness, increased lacrimation*
Periorbital or conjunctival edema*
Proptosis*
Ophthalmoplegia, diplopia*
Papilledema, loss of visual acuity*

*Features of Graves' disease only.

vascular, gastrointestinal, and neuromuscular systems (Table 2).

Heat intolerance, described as an inordinate sense of warmth and preference for cooler weather, is a common symptom in hyperthyroidism. Patients often admit to turning the thermostat down or reducing the number of covers on the bed at night, even in the winter. Sweating is particularly noticed by the female patient, who may also complain of brittle nails and friable hair that does not retain a permanent wave.

Cardiovascular symptoms are frequently the major manifestations of hyperthyroidism. Patients typically complain of palpitations due to sinus tachycardia or, in the case of the elderly patient, atrial fibrillation. The older patient is also at risk of developing symptoms of high output cardiac failure, although reduced exercise tolerance and dyspnea with activity may also be noticed by thyrotoxic patients who do not have cardiovascular disease. Angina may appear for the first time or be exacerbated in a patient with pre-existing coronary artery disease.

The neuropsychiatric features of hyperthyroidism are diverse. Patients tend to be irritable and restless and may complain of difficulty in concentration. The patient may at one moment be jovial and laughing and at another, for no apparent reason, be depressed and tearful. Many thyrotoxic persons experience tiredness and easy fatiguability, but some are never tired and find it impossible to stop and relax.

The most common neuromuscular manifestation of thyrotoxicosis is nonspecific fine tremor, particularly noticeable during purposeful movements of the hands that may interfere with writing and use of utensils. Weakness can be general, but it is characteristically more prominent in the proximal limbs, evident as difficulty in climbing stairs, rising from a chair, shaving, and combing hair. In some patients, the weakness is so profound that it may initially be mistaken for myasthenia gravis, which may coexist with Graves' disease. Hyperthyroidism has also been known to unmask hypokalemic periodic paralysis, especially in males of Asian descent.

Weight loss, despite a normal or increased appetite, is characteristic, although a small percentage of young patients may actually gain weight owing to excessive appetite stimulation. Conversely, the elderly patient may complain of anorexia. Gastrointestinal motility is enhanced, but the passage of soft stools is more frequent than frank diarrhea.

Ocular symptoms are typically limited to the patient with Graves' disease, who may complain of a "gritty" sensation in the eyes, excessive tearing, photophobia, and in more severe cases, blurred or double vision. In some individuals, the disease may start as itching of the eyelids, with subsequent conjunctival irritation that may be diagnosed erroneously as allergic conjunctivitis.

Less common symptoms of hyperthyroidism include oligomenorrhea or amenorrhea in females, and reduced libido and gynecomastia in males.

CLINICAL FINDINGS

Other than the aforementioned extrathyroidal phenomena specific for Graves' disease, the physical findings of thyroid hormone excess are common to all forms of hyperthyroidism, regardless of the underlying cause. The variety of clinical signs reflects the vulnerability of different organ systems to the effects of excess thyroid hormone and depend on the rate of onset and severity of the disease. Signs that apparently show a high correlation with thyrotoxicosis include weight loss, thyroid enlargement, hyperkinesis, fine tremor of the fingers, and tachycardia or atrial fibrillation.

The patient's general appearance may be the first clue that hyperthyroidism is present. The typical patient is fidgety and cannot keep still; speech is often rapid, and the facial features convey a look of apprehension. The skin is characteristically warm and moist, has a velvety texture, and lacks wrinkles. An increase in cutaneous blood flow may give rise to facial telangiectasia and palmar erythema. Onycholysis, in which the distal nail plate separates from the nail bed, may also be evident.

The clinical characteristics of the thyroid gland itself often provide a clue to the cause of the hyperthyroidism. In most patients with Graves' disease, the thyroid enlargement is typically symmetrical and may vary from a barely palpable normal size gland (15 to 20 g) to an enlargement of five times (100 g) or, rarely, even more. A bruit is frequently audible over the gland owing to a markedly increased blood flow. Patients with multinodular goiter usually have a large, irregular gland with at least one distinctly palpable nodule. The solitary toxic adenoma is typically more than 3 cm in diameter and sometimes represents the only palpable thyroid tissue due to involution of adjacent thyroid parenchyma. An exquisitely tender goiter associated with constitutional symptoms and a preceding viral illness often indicates subacute granulomatous thyroiditis. The thyroid gland in subacute lymphocytic thyroiditis is typically painless; this condition occurs more frequently in the postpartum period and has a tendency to recur in subsequent pregnancies. The absence of a goiter in a hyperthyroid patient is unusual but does not exclude the diagnosis. This clinical picture should, however, lead the physician to consider exogenous causes of thyrotoxicosis. Approximately 30 per cent of elderly patients with Graves' disease do not have palpable goiters. Thyroid enlargement may be missed during examination because of a shortened neck or, in the case of a multinodular goiter, because of retrosternal extension.

A resting sinus tachycardia is invariably the most frequent cardiovascular finding. Atrial fibrillation is particularly common in the elderly patient and may dominate the clinical picture; thyrotoxicosis should always be considered in the differential diagnosis of an elderly patient with unexplained atrial fibrillation or congestive cardiac failure. Other recognized cardiac features include bounding peripheral pulses, reflecting the widened pulse pressure and increased cardiac output induced by hyperthyroidism; a prominent apical impulse; and a nonspecific systolic flow murmur heard over much of the precordium.

Examination of the neuromuscular system usually reveals a fine tremor, best demonstrated with the hands outstretched, and brisk deep tendon reflexes. Proximal muscular weakness is detected in most patients and, in the more severe case, is accompanied by muscular atrophy.

The ocular findings of hyperthyroidism are classified as: noninfiltrative and infiltrative ophthalmopathic features. Noninfiltrative features are associated with all types of hyperthyroidism and are most likely caused by increased sympathetic activity. Infiltrative ophthalmic phenomena are peculiar to Graves' disease and are related to specific pathologic changes in the orbit and its contents.

The noninfiltrative features include retraction of the upper lid, allowing the sclera to be visible above the iris. This results in the characteristic "stare" or "bright-eyed" look of hyperthyroidism, which may initially give the false impression of proptosis. Other common findings are lid lag, elicited by asking the patient to slowly gaze downward; infrequent blinking; and a widened palpebral fissure.

Infiltrative ophthalmopathic findings are considered pathognomonic of Graves' disease. Basic features include periorbital edema, conjunctival injection with chemosis, and weakness of the extraocular muscles with decreased ability to converge or to perform extreme movements of gaze. Diplopia, strabismus, papilledema, and optic atrophy are more severe manifestations of disease. Proptosis with forward protrusion of the globe is caused by infiltration and swelling of retrobulbar tissues and extraocular muscles by glycosaminoglycans and mononuclear inflammatory cells. Exophthalmos is usually bilateral but may be asymmetrical or even unilateral. The Krahn exophthalmometer allows accurate measurement of the distance between the anterior surface of the globe and the lateral orbital rim. Normal measurements in Caucasians are 18 to 20 mm or less, and up to 3 mm of asymmetry is considered within normal limits.

Examination of the extremities may reveal the characteristic infiltrative dermopathy seen in approximately 5 per cent of patients with Graves' disease. Pruritic, well-demarcated peau d'orange plaques are most commonly found on the anterior surface of the lower legs and occasionally, on the dorsum of the feet. An even rarer finding in a minority of patients with Graves' disease is thyroid acropachy, which in its fully developed form consists of clubbing of the digits, periosteal new bone formation principally involving the phalanges, and soft tissue swelling, particularly overlying the affected bones.

COMMON COMPLICATIONS

Complications of hyperthyroidism are usually the consequence of prolonged exposure of organ systems to excessive concentrations of thyroid hormone and may include high-output cardiac failure; arrhythmias, particularly atrial fibrillation; and rarely, severe myopathy. Proptosis with increased exposure of the globe may lead to corneal ulceration and panophthalmitis, and proptosis with compression or traction at the optic foramen may cause injury to the optic nerve. Loss of vision has been documented.

The most severe complication of hyperthyroidism is thyrotoxic crisis or "thyroid storm." This condition is most likely to occur if thyroid hormone excess remains unrecognized or is inadequately managed. Fortunately, with better diagnosis and treatment of thyroid disease, this life-threatening syndrome is a rare occurrence, accounting for only 1 per cent of hospital admissions for hyperthyroidism. Patients still at risk include those with concurrent medical illness or those with unrecognized hyperthyroidism undergoing anesthesia and surgery. Clinically, the syndrome is characterized by exaggerated manifestations of thyrotoxicosis, including fever, usually higher than 39°C; profuse diaphoresis; tachycardia out of proportion to the fever; and mental status changes such as agitation, delirium, stupor, and coma. Despite appropriate medical management, the mortality rate of this condition approaches 10 to 15 per cent.

LABORATORY DIAGNOSIS

Although the diagnosis of hyperthyroidism is essentially a clinical one, confirmatory laboratory tests are recommended, because the hyperthyroid state may be mimicked by certain medical and psychiatric conditions. The disease manifestation can be so subtle that it is impossible to exclude the diagnosis solely on the basis of clinical findings. There are several readily available laboratory tests to assess a patient's thyroid status. To develop a cost-effective approach to the laboratory diagnosis of hyperthyroidism, the clinician must recognize the limitations of each of these tests.

The development of highly sensitive TSH assays has greatly facilitated the diagnosis of hyperthyroidism; the investigation of any suspected case of thyroid hormone excess should begin with this test (Fig. 1). A normal value provides convincing evidence against the diagnosis of hyperthyroidism, except in the rare patient with TSH-induced hyperthyroidism. A suppressed TSH concentration, although consistent with a state of hyperthyroidism, does not in itself establish the diagnosis and should therefore be correlated with an estimate of the free thyroxine (FT_4) concentration. The combination of a suppressed TSH and increased FT_4 confirms the presence of hyperthyroidism. If the TSH concentration is suppressed but the FT_4 is normal, serum T_3 should be measured, because T_3 toxicosis accounts for nearly 5 per cent of all cases of hyperthyroidism. T_3 toxicosis is most often seen in patients with solitary toxic adenoma or in patients with Graves' disease that has relapsed after treatment. Suppressed TSH with normal FT_4 and T_3 suggests subclinical hyperthyroidism, a condition whose management depends largely on the clinical situation. When TSH or FT_4 is used alone in the diagnosis of hyperthyroidism, the results in some circumstances can be misleading. Low TSH values may be encountered in hospitalized patients with nonthyroidal illness or with the use of certain medications (e.g., dopamine, glucocorticoids). A spuriously increased FT_4 may be seen in some clinically euthyroid patients with familial dysalbuminemic hyperthyroxinemia, a syndrome characterized by a variant serum albumin with a preferential affinity for T_4.

After the diagnosis of hyperthyroidism has been confirmed, the clinician must determine the underlying cause.

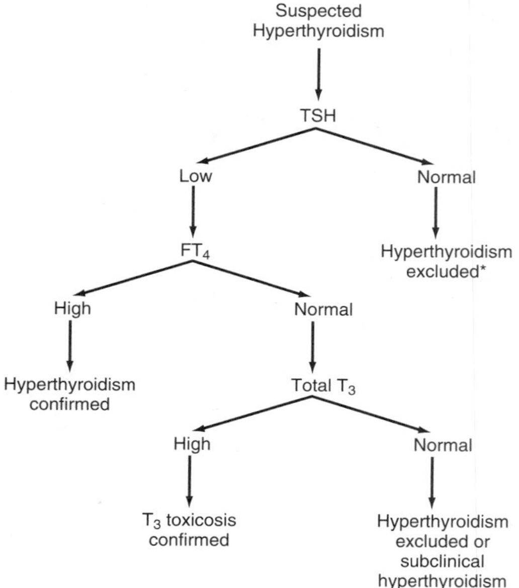

Figure 1. Diagnostic approach to suspected hyperthyroidism.
*Except in rare cases of TSH-producing pituitary tumor or selective pituitary resistance syndromes.

If the cause is not obvious from the history and physical examination, a 24-hour radioiodine uptake (RAIU) may help to clarify the clinical picture. A relatively high 24-hour RAIU (>12 to 15 per cent) is associated with hyperthyroidism caused by Graves' disease, toxic multinodular goiter, solitary toxic adenoma, or a TSH-producing pituitary adenoma. A low 24-hour RAIU (<3 per cent) is characteristic of inflammatory thyroiditis or thyrotoxicosis caused by an extrathyroidal source of thyroid hormone. Although the RAIU provides a functional assessment of the thyroid gland, this test should not be used to determine whether a patient is hyperthyroid. RAIU may, however, be useful in demonstrating satisfactory iodine trapping before administration of a therapeutic dose of radioiodine. Thyroid scanning procedures with ^{99m}Tc, ^{123}I, or ^{131}I assess the distribution of functioning tissue within the thyroid gland and may be indicated to confirm a clinical suspicion of toxic multinodular goiter or toxic solitary adenoma as a cause of hyperthyroidism. These scans do not measure thyroid function and therefore are of no value in establishing a clinical state of thyroid hormone excess.

Serum Total Thyroxine

Before the advent of highly sensitive TSH assays, the serum T_4 concentration was the most widely used test in the laboratory evaluation of suspected hyperthyroidism. The major disadvantage of T_4 is that almost all the measured hormone is bound to thyroid hormone–binding proteins, principally thyroid-binding globulin (TBG). An increased value may be caused by increased TBG and not represent true hyperthyroidism. Elevations of TBG can be inherited or induced by the hyperestrogenic state associated with pregnancy, estrogen therapy, or liver disease. In these circumstances, some form of measurement of TBG is essential before making a diagnosis of hyperthyroidism on the basis of an increased T_4.

Thyroid-Binding Proteins and Free Thyroxine Index

The T_3-resin uptake test provides an indirect estimate of the concentration of plasma TBG by measuring the equilibrating uptake of radiolabeled T_3 into a nonspecific resin that competes with the more specific binding proteins of the patient's serum. The T_3 uptake by the resin varies inversely with the number of unoccupied thyroid binding sites in the patient's serum. When there are excess binding sites in the patient's serum owing to a high TBG level, the T_3 uptake (by the resin) is low. With fewer binding sites owing to TBG deficiency or thyrotoxicosis with consequent saturation of sites, the T_3 uptake is high. A specific radioimmunoassay (RIA) for TBG is available. The TBG RIA may be useful in evaluating the thyroid status of a patient with an inappropriately high serum T_4 who may have inherited or acquired alterations in the plasma concentration of TBG. Abnormal thyroid-binding proteins can also be characterized by using thyroid-binding protein electrophoresis on polyacrylamide gel.

The free thyroxine index (FT_4I) is derived from the product of the serum T_4 and T_3-resin uptake and is commonly expressed as a thyroid hormone–binding ratio. In theory, this index is proportional, but not equal, to the FT_4 concentration and is a means of correcting total T_4 levels for variations that may be present in the patient's binding proteins. The FT_4I must be interpreted with caution for patients with severe nonthyroidal illness or when there are severe abnormalities of binding proteins, as in patients with familial dysalbuminemic hyperthyroxinemia.

PITFALLS IN DIAGNOSIS

Classically, the diagnosis of hyperthyroidism is suggested by the general appearance and demeanor of the patient. In some patients, however, the manifestations of hyperthyroidism may be atypical or extremely subtle. The resulting diagnostic confusion may delay treatment and cause significant morbidity and mortality. "Masked hyperthyroidism" refers to the patient in whom many of the common features of hyperthyroidism are absent or easily overlooked because of the predominance of one symptom. Atrial fibrillation or congestive cardiac failure may at first be inappropriately attributed to a primary cardiac or pulmonary process. Characteristically, these cardiac features are refractory to conventional treatments if the underlying hormonal disturbance is not recognized. Weight loss may initially suggest an occult neoplasm, and the diagnosis of hyperthyroidism is missed entirely or only considered after extensive evaluation fails to yield a diagnosis. A rare form of hyperthyroidism, called apathetic hyperthyroidism, is observed in some elderly patients who lack the hyperkinetic and adrenergic symptoms characteristic of thyrotoxicosis; instead, the combination of lethargy, inactivity, and flat affect may be misdiagnosed as depression, prompting inappropriate referral to a psychiatrist.

True hyperthyroidism must be distinguished from conditions that increase serum thyroid hormone levels without affecting clinical status. Euthyroid hyperthyroxinemia is most often encountered in patients with anomalies of thyroxine-binding proteins. The laboratory diagnosis of hyperthyroidism also becomes more difficult in the hospitalized patient with acute or chronic nonthyroidal illness for whom thyroid function tests may be abnormal despite the absence of clinical evidence of hyperthyroidism. The preferred approach to these patients is to repeat the laboratory investigation after the illness has resolved. Diagnostic confusion may likewise arise with conditions that mimic hyperthyroidism, including anxiety disorders or the hypermetabolic state of pheochromocytoma. The best protection against an incorrect diagnosis of hyperthyroidism is to perform a meticulous history and physical examination, with particular attention to current medications and past or concurrent illnesses; to obtain thyroid function tests for a hospitalized patient only when a clinical suspicion of hyperthyroidism exists; and to rely on a combination of tests rather than a single test for the definitive diagnosis of hyperthyroidism.

HYPOTHYROIDISM

By Gary W. Cushing, M.D.
Burlington, Massachusetts

Hypothyroidism occurs when the cells of the body suffer from insufficient availability of thyroid hormone. In most patients, hypothyroidism is caused by failure of the thyroid gland to produce sufficient amounts of thyroid hormone to meet the needs of tissues. Rarely, cells can be resistant to thyroid hormone to such a degree that hypothyroidism results. The most common cause of inadequate production of thyroid hormone is disease of the thyroid gland itself (i.e., primary hypothyroidism). Infrequently, decreased production of thyroid hormone is caused by insufficient stimulation of the gland by thyroid-stimulating hormone (TSH). This condition, which is usually the result of disease in the anterior pituitary gland or, less commonly, the hypothalamus, is referred to as central hypothyroidism.

ETIOLOGY

The causes of hypothyroidism are shown in Table 1. In areas of the world where iodine is present in sufficient amounts in the diet, hypothyroidism most commonly results from damage to or destruction of the thyroid gland. In the absence of iodine deficiency, lymphocytic thyroiditis is the most common cause of spontaneously occurring hypothyroidism. This autoimmune disorder is more common in women and can manifest with goiter (i.e., Hashimoto's thyroiditis) or atrophy. The atrophic form can be caused by complete destruction of the gland or by antibodies that block the binding of TSH to its receptor.

Many cases of permanent hypothyroidism are iatrogenic.

Table 1. Causes of Hypothyroidism

- Primary hypothyroidism
  - Damaged or absent thyroid gland
    - Agenesis or hypoplasia of thyroid gland
    - Thyroiditis
      - Chronic autoimmune (i.e., Hashimoto's thyroiditis)
      - Transient: subacute, postpartum, painless
    - Thyroidectomy
    - Therapeutic irradiation: ^{131}I therapy, external beam
    - Thyroidal infiltration: amyloidosis, cystinosis, sarcoidosis, hemochromatosis, systemic sclerosis
  - Defective synthesis of thyroid hormone
    - Iodine deficiency or excess
    - Inherited enzymatic defects
    - Ingestion of drugs
- Central hypothyroidism
  - Pituitary: tumor, surgery, infiltrations
  - Hypothalamic disease
- Resistance to thyroid hormone

Hypothyroidism develops in most patients treated with radioiodine for Graves' disease or toxic nodular goiter. Total or subtotal thyroidectomy for neoplasia, Graves' disease, or nodular goiter may also lead to inadequate reserves of thyroid hormone. Hypothyroidism develops in about one third of patients who receive external beam irradiation for lymphoma or carcinoma of the neck. Congenital athyreosis and acquired infiltrative diseases are distinctly uncommon causes of permanent hypothyroidism.

Transient spontaneous hypothyroidism occurs in three distinct conditions: subacute (painful, de Quervain's) thyroiditis, postpartum thyroiditis, and silent (painless) thyroiditis. Damage to the thyroid gland initiates the release of thyroid hormone, causing a brief thyrotoxic phase, followed by hypothyroidism that usually resolves within weeks to months.

In the intact thyroid gland, decreased synthesis of thyroid hormone due to iodine deficiency is the most common cause of hypothyroidism worldwide. In developed countries, iodine deficiency is rarely seen; rather, ingestion of medication causes most of the acquired biosynthetic defects in the production of thyroid hormone. Paradoxically, iodine excess may cause hypothyroidism in developed countries. For example, substantial amounts of iodine are present in cough syrups and the antiarrhythmic drug amiodarone. Importantly, lithium can act as a goitrogen, and phenytoin and carbamazepine can accelerate hepatic catabolism of thyroid hormone. Rare, inherited enzymatic defects cause dyshormonogenesis and can induce goiter and hypothyroidism.

Central hypothyroidism results when secretion of TSH is inadequate to stimulate a normal thyroid gland. Insufficient TSH may be related to pituitary macroadenoma, previous pituitary surgery or irradiation, or infiltrative diseases (e.g., sarcoidosis). Similar lesions in the hypothalamus decrease the secretion of TSH-releasing hormone (TRH) and reduce the production of TSH. Taken together, pituitary and hypothalamic causes account for a small fraction of all hypothyroidism. Moreover, other features of panhypopituitarism almost always exist concomitantly, making the diagnosis less difficult.

CLINICAL PRESENTATION

Congenital Hypothyroidism

The clinical presentation of hypothyroidism depends on the age of onset and the degree of thyroid hormone insufficiency. In congenital hypothyroidism, the unique aspects of the clinical presentation involve the central nervous system (CNS). In utero and during the first year of life, the CNS requires thyroid hormone for proper development. Maternal thyroid hormone crosses the placenta and can prevent some of the deficiency in the hypothyroid fetus. Most infants with congenital hypothyroidism appear normal at birth. If the mother is also hypothyroid (most often caused by endemic goiter), the severe combined deficiency of hormone can cause irreversible brain damage to the infant (i.e., cretinism). More often, the condition of the hypothyroid infant born to a euthyroid mother is difficult to diagnose at birth. Early signs may include prolonged jaundice, feeding difficulties, somnolence, and constipation. In the absence of timely diagnosis and treatment, the infant gradually develops the typical features of mental and physical retardation, including hoarse cry, late-closing fontanels, poor linear growth with short arms and legs, puffy eyelids, thick tongue, coarse hair, dry skin, protuberant abdomen, umbilical hernia, weak muscles, decreased reflexes, delayed motor milestones, and significantly subaverage general intellectual functioning. Treatment in the first weeks to months of life can abort this progression and prevent mental retardation. In the United States, all neonates must undergo blood testing for thyroid function. Moreover, the physician should not hesitate to test any infant who presents with symptoms consistent with congenital hypothyroidism.

Childhood and Adolescent Hypothyroidism

The most common causes of hypothyroidism in the child or adolescent are mild enzymatic defects, autoimmune thyroiditis, ablation of all or part of the thyroid gland, and medications. Signs and symptoms are similar to those seen in adults. Growth and sexual development are impaired, and the classic finding is short stature. When thyroid hormone is deficient, the secretion of growth hormone is reduced; together, these deficiencies retard bone growth. A falloff in the child's growth curve that crosses height percentiles is a warning sign. The bone age is delayed. Weight may be maintained or even increased. Delayed puberty is an additional feature. Much less commonly, precocious puberty may be seen in the patient with primary hypothyroidism and is thought to be caused by the concomitant oversecretion of TSH and the pituitary gonadotropins that stimulate gonadal function. Early menarche and the development of breasts in girls and testicular and penile enlargement in boys warrant investigation with tests that measure the functioning of the thyroid gland.

Adult Hypothyroidism

In adults, hypothyroidism presents a spectrum of findings, depending on the severity of the hormone deficiency and the rapidity of onset. In overt hypothyroidism with a significant decline in the concentration of thyroid hormone, classic signs and symptoms ensue (Table 2). Fatigue, lethargy, or generalized weakness are common but nonspecific complaints. Changes in skin and hair are often observed, and the nails become dry, coarse, and brittle. Hair loss may bring a person to the physician. The patient may experience intolerance to cold temperatures, require extra clothing or bedding, and to the dismay of household members, may keep the thermostat turned up. Complaints of constipation and weight gain are common. However, weight gain is usually modest; hypothyroidism is rarely the cause of obesity. Neurologically, the patient may experience paresthesias, especially of the median nerve, causing carpal tunnel syndrome; muscle stiffness or cramps, often in the calves at night; and less frequently, hearing loss. Limited capacity for exercise, with shortness of breath and even chest discomfort, can be elicited in the history, sometimes erroneously provoking the diagnosis of myocardial ischemia. Menorrhagia and iron deficiency anemia may develop in women. Conversely, hypothyroidism may induce hyperprolactinemia leading to amenorrhea and galactorrhea.

On examination of the patient with frank hypothyroidism, the pulse is slow and the pulse pressure narrowed. Diastolic blood pressure may be increased. The affect may be dull. The skin is pale, cool, and dry. Myxedema results from the accumulation of hyaluronic acid and water in the dermis, producing periorbital and facial swelling and nonpitting edema of the extremities. In severe cases, macroglossia is accompanied by slow or hoarse speech. A goiter may be present or absent. Distant heart sounds may indicate pericardial effusion. The deep tendon reflexes exhibit a delayed relaxation phase, but percussion of the muscle body may evoke pseudomyotonia. When most or all of these features are present, the diagnosis of hypothyroidism is straightforward. Many patients, however, present with a milder degree of hypothyroidism. The symptoms may be nonspecific, and the examination may reveal fewer abnormalities. For these patients, laboratory testing is required to confirm the diagnosis.

Table 2. Clinical Features of Hypothyroidism

Fatigue
Dry skin
Coarse hair
Decreased sweating
Intolerance to cold temperatures
Skin pallor
Impaired memory
Facial edema
Constipation
Hair loss
Weight gain
Paresthesias
Muscle cramps
Dyspnea
Deepened voice
Menorrhagia
Chest pains
Deafness

COURSE AND COMPLICATIONS

Undiagnosed and untreated congenital hypothyroidism leads to the disastrous result of cretinism, with permanent mental and physical retardation. In the adult with hypothyroidism, the course varies. In subacute and postpartum thyroiditis, the hypothyroidism can be transient. However, women with postpartum thyroiditis are more likely to experience permanent hypothyroidism in the future. Mild hypothyroidism caused by chronic thyroiditis may persist in many patients for years. A few patients may experience remission. Most patients progress slowly from mild hypothyroidism to the full-blown picture previously described. If the deficiency of hormone is severe and long-standing, predisposing factors such as infection, CNS events, hypothermia, or sedative-hypnotic medications may plunge the patient into myxedematous coma, a rare complication characterized by hypothermia, stupor, hypopnia, and hypercapnia. The mortality rate is high.

Hyperlipidemia commonly accompanies hypothyroidism and has been implicated in the doubling of the incidence of atherosclerotic cardiovascular disease. Other unusual complications of hypothyroidism include sleep apnea, toxic megacolon, cerebellar ataxia, pleural and pericardial effusions, and bleeding diathesis. The syndrome of inappropriate antidiuretic hormone (SIADH) can also be seen.

LABORATORY DIAGNOSIS

Thyroxine (T_4) is the major hormone produced and secreted by the thyroid gland. When the gland first fails, the level of T_4 begins to decline, but serum concentrations may remain within the reference range. In primary hypothyroidism, the release of inhibition of TSH secretion increases the concentration of TSH in the blood. At this stage, symptoms may be subtle. The combination of a low-normal T_4 concentration and a high TSH concentration in the minimally symptomatic patient has been called subclinical hypothyroidism. Increased secretion of TSH helps to maintain the secretion of thyroid hormone. Triiodothyronine (T_3), the active hormone at tissue receptors, is produced preferentially when the thyroid gland begins to fail. T_3 concentrations are also maintained by an increased peripheral conversion of T_4 to T_3. With further decrease in the function of the thyroid gland, the level of T_4 declines below the reference range, followed by a decrease in the serum concentration of T_3. At this stage, overt signs and symptoms are usually observed. In central hypothyroidism, peripheral concentrations of hormones are low, with a correspondingly low or inappropriately normal concentration of TSH.

Serum T_4 and T_3 Measurements

T_4 and T_3 concentrations can be accurately measured in serum by radioimmunoassay, enzyme immunoassay, or immunoradiometric assay. More than 75 per cent of laboratories use nonisotopic immunoassays that rely on high-affinity anti-T_4 and anti-T_3 antibodies. Endogenous T_4 released from serum binding proteins competes with enzyme-labeled T_4 for a limited number of antibody-binding sites. An assortment of photometric, fluorescent, and luminescent substrates are available for monitoring the activity of the enzyme-labeled hormone. Alternatively, T_4 can be labeled with fluorescent or chemiluminescent molecules rather than enzymes. In hypothyroidism, the measurement of T_4 is a more useful test because the concentration of T_3 is preserved until late in the disease process. Thyroid hormones circulate highly bound to T_4-binding globulin (TBG), albumin, and transthyretin (T_4-binding prealbumin). Only the free hormones, representing less than 1 per cent of the total, are available to influence cellular metabolism. In general, the concentrations of free hormones parallel total concentrations, but exceptions occur. Free T_4 measured directly by equilibrium dialysis remains the gold standard for T_4 analysis. However, the procedure is labor intensive, time consuming, and expensive.

An estimate of the concentration of free T_4 is almost always clinically useful. One such estimate, called the free T_4 index (FT_4I), is calculated as the product of the total T_4 and the T_3-resin uptake (T_3RU). The T_3RU reflects inversely the number of empty binding sites on the thyroid-binding proteins. In true hypothyroidism, the total concentration of T_4 is low, as is the T_3RU, reflecting empty protein-binding sites. Therefore, the product, FT_4I, is also low. A decreased concentration of total T_4 with an increased T_3RU suggests decreased binding proteins as the cause of hypothyroxinemia and not true hypothyroidism. The FT_4I value is normal. Hypoproteinemia, generalized illness, and inherited deficiency of TBG are all causes of decreased thyroid-hormone binding proteins. Some laboratories report the T_3RU as a ratio of the patient value to a pooled normal sera value and call this the thyroid-hormone binding ratio. The FT_4I is calculated similarly as the product of T_4 and the thyroid-hormone binding ratio.

Direct free-T_4 assays provide an alternative estimate of free T_4. These assays use an analogue of T_4 that binds minimally to TBG and can therefore compete with the free T_4 of the patient in radioimmunoassays or chemiluminescent radiometric assays. Although some authorities are not convinced that these assays measure true free T_4, the results correlate well with FT_4I determinations and equilibrium dialysis values in a wide range of patients, including those with disturbances of protein binding. The use of free-T_4 assays has therefore become more widely accepted.

Determinations of Serum Thyroid-Stimulating Hormone

The immunoradiometric (IRMA) double-antibody assays for TSH are highly sensitive and specific. The combination of increased TSH and decreased free T_4 is sufficient to confirm the diagnosis of primary hypothyroidism. Transiently increased TSH that is not caused by permanent hypothyroidism can be seen during the recovery of sick patients from nonthyroidal illness and in acute adrenal insufficiency. Resolution of the underlying illness or treatment of the adrenal insufficiency with corticosteroids typically normalizes the TSH concentration. Most commercial kits have eliminated the problem of falsely increased TSH values in the unusual person with antibodies to the mouse immunoglobulins used in the assay. In pituitary hypothyroidism, the concentration of TSH typically is decreased but may be normal or slightly increased. The latter observation is consistent with immunologically active but biologically inactive TSH.

Ancillary Tests for Differential Diagnosis

The most common cause of spontaneous hypothyroidism remains autoimmune thyroiditis. Circulating antibodies to thyroid antigens can serve as a marker of this condition. The most prevalent of these antibodies are the antimicrosomal and antithyroglobulin antibodies, which occur in more than 90 per cent of patients. The antigen for the antimicrosomal antibody is a thyroid peroxidase. Specific antithyroid peroxidase antibody assays are available and may offer slightly improved sensitivity at a greater cost. These antibody tests may help the clinician to predict which women are more likely to experience postpartum thyroiditis and to stratify the risk for development of overt hypothyroidism in patients with subclinical hypothyroidism, especially the elderly.

The clinical utility of the TRH stimulation test has declined with the advent of the improved TSH assays. The assessment of TSH response to injected TRH does not reliably distinguish pituitary causes from hypothalamic causes of central hypothyroidism.

The radioactive iodine uptake (RAIU) is seldom useful in the evaluation of the patient with hypothyroidism and should be avoided. The abundant intake of iodine in the United States causes significant overlap of the lower limit of normal RAIU with the low values typically found in patients with significant hypothyroidism. In early-stage hypothyroidism, the RAIU value may be normal or slightly increased because of stimulation by TSH. In the unusual instance of a metabolic defect in hormonogenesis, the RAIU result may be frankly increased, and the uptake can be discharged by the administration of perchlorate as part of a test for defects in organification.

Associated Biochemical Abnormalities

Hypothyroidism causes a number of biochemical abnormalities whose documentation may support the diagnosis. Hypercholesterolemia and hypertriglyceridemia are the most common abnormalities. Serum creatine kinase, lactate dehydrogenase, and transaminases may be increased. Anemia, often macrocytic, may be present with or without vitamin B_{12} or folate deficiency. Increases in serum prolactin are usually mild. Hypercarotenemia may be suspected when yellowing of the skin is observed.

Electrocardiography may reveal bradycardia, T-wave inversion or flattening, and low voltage caused by pericardial effusion or by a primary myocardial abnormality. Pericardial effusion may enlarge the cardiac silhouette, and a chest film may also reveal pleural effusions.

Screening Approaches

Avoidance of the devastating effects of untreated congenital hypothyroidism has provided an important reason to support standardized screening of neonates for thyroid disorders. Initially, screening programs obtained serum T_4 concentrations. Serum TSH was measured in the samples with low T_4 concentrations. More recently, screening has relied solely on measurement of TSH. Importantly, both approaches detect congenital hypothyroidism with a frequency of about 1 in 4000 live births.

An incidence of hypothyroidism of less than 5 per cent in the adult population does not seem to justify the cost of routine screening. However, testing should be requested for patients with goiter, a history of surgery or irradiation of the thyroid gland, or nonspecific symptoms compatible with hypothyroidism. Screening also may be warranted in members of families with a strong history of autoimmune disease of the thyroid gland, women in the postpartum period, patients who are older than 65 years of age, and patients with other autoimmune diseases (e.g., Addison's disease, type I diabetes, pernicious anemia, and premature gonadal failure).

The traditional paradigm for testing began with a determination of total or free T_4. Later algorithms employ the serum TSH as the first-line test because of its higher sensitivity in detecting mild insufficiency of the thyroid gland. This approach should not be used if central hypothyroidism is suspected in a patient with features of hypopituitarism or a history of pituitary tumor, neurosurgery, or radiation therapy, because the concentrations of TSH may be normal or decreased.

DIAGNOSTIC CHALLENGES

Subclinical Hypothyroidism

An increased TSH concentration is the earliest detectable serum abnormality in primary hypothyroidism. Serum TSH is frequently increased for months before the free-T_4 concentration falls below the reference range. When this occurs in the absence of overt symptoms, the term subclinical hypothyroidism has been applied. Abnormalities in the metabolism of lipids and water and in parameters of myocardial contractility suggest that subclinical hypothyroidism reflects a real, albeit mild, deficiency in thyroid hormone for which the increase in TSH does not completely compensate. In randomized studies of patients treated with T_4 for subclinical hypothyroidism, careful questioning indicates appreciable improvement in symptoms. If a patient presents with symptoms that may be associated with thyroid hormone deficiency, a therapeutic trial of T_4 is warranted.

Euthyroid Sick Syndrome

Acute or chronic nonthyroidal illness is often associated with abnormalities of thyroid hormone tests that must be differentiated from true disturbances in the metabolism of thyroid hormone. The most common finding is a decrease in serum T_4, typically related to a decline in T_4-binding proteins. The T_3RU is increased accordingly. Free-T_4 estimates remain normal initially but can decline as the severity of illness progresses. Measurement of free T_4 by dialysis techniques reflects euthyroidism most accurately. However, free-T_4 analysis is seldom required, because the TSH concentration typically remains normal. On occasion, mild increases in serum TSH can be seen, especially in the recovery phase. Observation is the prudent path, unless the TSH concentration exceeds 20 μU/mL. Conversely, low concentrations of TSH occur in a fraction of ill patients, but they do not imply pituitary deficiency.

Laboratory Testing During Treatment

In the treatment of primary hypothyroidism, the goal is relief of symptoms without induction of iatrogenic hyperthyroidism. This goal is best achieved by assessing the patient receiving T_4, normalizing the serum TSH and avoiding oversuppression. The long half-life of T_4 (the most commonly prescribed agent) requires the clinician to allow the patient 4 to 6 weeks to reach therapeutic equilibrium. Doses should not be changed, nor should TSH be measured before this much time has elapsed. Frequently, a problem arises in the patient who has been treated with thyroid hormone for many years for questionable indications or without a clear diagnosis. A practical approach is to halve the dose of T_4 and reassess the patient after 4 to 6 weeks. If the patient truly has primary hypothyroidism, the serum concentration of TSH will be increased by this time, and medication can be resumed. The degree of hypothyroidism sustained with this approach is usually minimal. If the concentrations of TSH and free T_4 are normal, the hormone can be discontinued entirely, and the patient may be retested after another 4- to 6-week interval.

THYROIDITIS

By Roland Sakiyama, M.D.
Los Angeles, California

Thyroiditis encompasses a spectrum of diseases that differ in their cause and clinical course, but they share common histologic findings of inflammation, fibrosis, or lymphocytic infiltration. Clinically, the most useful classification of thyroiditis distinguishes the onset of signs and symptoms, the duration of inflammation, and the persistence of thyroid abnormalities. Thyroiditis can be approached as an acute, a subacute, or a chronic process.

ACUTE THYROIDITIS

Etiology

Acute thyroiditis, also known as bacterial suppurative, or pyogenic thyroiditis, is a rare infection caused by bacteria, fungi, mycobacteria, or parasites. Various microbes may reach the thyroid through lymphatic spread from areas of pharyngitis or mastoiditis. Other routes of infection include hematogenous seeding from distant sites and local spread from piriform sinus fistulas. The most common pathogens are *Staphylococcus aureus, Streptococcus pyogenes,* and *Streptococcus pneumoniae,* with Enterobacteriaceae, *Haemophilus influenzae,* and anaerobic bacteria less commonly found. Unusual pathogens that may infect the thyroid include *Mycobacterium tuberculosis, Treponema pallidum, Aspergillus, Coccidioides immitis,* cytomegalovirus, and *Pneumocystis carinii.* Microscopic evaluation reveals neutrophil infiltration with small or large abscess formation. Fistulous tracts may also develop in more indolent cases.

Clinical Presentation and Course

Acute thyroiditis more commonly affects women than men. Most cases develop between the ages of 20 and 40 years, but infants and the elderly may also be infected. More than 60 per cent of patients have a pre-existing thyroid disorder. Individuals with acute thyroiditis typically present with the abrupt onset of anterior neck pain and swelling, pharyngitis, fever, dysphagia, and dysphonia (Table 1). Examination typically reveals a toxic, febrile patient with a warm, erythematous, tender thyroid and enlarged cervical lymph nodes. One or both lobes of the thyroid may be infected. Coexisting infections of the pharynx or mastoid may be observed. Patients with acute thyroiditis typically are not thyrotoxic or hypothyroid.

Laboratory Findings

Patients with acute thyroiditis typically develop leukocytosis with immature cells, (i.e., a "shift to the left"). Thyroid hormone concentrations are usually normal, but extensive inflammation may disrupt and release follicular stores of thyroxine (T_4) and triiodothyronine (T_3). Anti-thyroid antibody tests are typically unremarkable, but thyroglobulin (Tg) concentrations are increased. Radioiodine uptake (RAIU) is variable, but radioiodine thyroid imaging reveals a "cold" area corresponding to the infected tissue. Ultrasonography or computed tomography may delineate large abscesses. Fine-needle aspiration provides cytologic confirmation of the diagnosis and culture material for identification of the etiologic agent.

Diagnosis

The diagnosis of acute or pyogenic thyroiditis must be considered for any patient who presents with the acute onset of fever, anterior neck pain, and dysphagia. A leukocyte count, thyroid hormone concentrations, blood cultures, and a fine-needle aspiration of the thyroid should be obtained. Normally, radioiodine imaging is not helpful, but ultrasonography may identify large abscesses that require surgical drainage. Other causes of acute thyroid pain include subacute thyroiditis, hemorrhage into a thyroid adenoma or cyst, and anaplastic thyroid carcinoma. Although patients with these diseases present with thyroid tenderness, it is usually less severe, and fever and leukocytosis are absent. Fine-needle aspiration of the thyroid provides the most direct method for diagnosis of a carcinoma, adenoma, or hemorrhagic cyst.

SUBACUTE THYROIDITIS

Subacute thyroiditis can be caused by subacute granulomatous thyroiditis (i.e., de Quervain's thyroiditis or painful thyroiditis) and by painless thyroiditis (i.e., silent thyroiditis or painless subacute lymphocytic thyroiditis).

SUBACUTE GRANULOMATOUS THYROIDITIS

Etiology

Subacute granulomatous thyroiditis is the most common cause of anterior neck pain. Symptoms frequently follow a respiratory infection or viral prodrome and most cases occur in the summer and fall. Viruses are thought to be the cause of subacute granulomatous thyroiditis. Adenovirus, coxsackievirus, influenza virus, echovirus, and enteroviruses are most commonly implicated. The presence of antithyroid antibodies in many patients suggests that autoimmunity contributes to the course of the disease. Autoantibodies may be associated with the sensitization

Table 1. Features of Thyroiditis

Disease	Etiology	Presentation	Laboratory
Acute thyroiditis	Bacterial; *S. aureus, S. pyogenes, S. pneumoniae*	Anterior neck pain, tender thyroid, erythema, fever, pharyngitis, or mastoiditis	WBC increased with left shift; T_4 and T_3 normal; ultrasonography to define abscesses; fine-needle aspiration for culture
Subacute granulomatous thyroiditis	Viral; adenovirus, coxsackievirus, influenza, echovirus, enterovirus	Viral prodrome, low-grade fever, anterior neck pain, tender thyroid; may have thyrotoxicosis symptoms, later hypothyroidism	ESR increased; Tg increased; in 50% of patients with thyrotoxicosis, T_4 and T_3 increased, RAIU $< 5\%$; hypothyroid phase: T_4 decreased, TSH high or normal
Subacute, painless and postpartum thyroiditis	Autoimmune	Thyrotoxicosis symptoms; later may have hypothyroid symptoms, no neck pain, 50% with goiter	T_4 and T_3 increased initially; Tg increased; RAIU $< 5\%$; ESR normal; hypothyroid phase: T_4 decreased, TSH high or normal
Hashimoto's thyroiditis	Autoimmune	Asymptomatic goiter or hypothyroid symptoms, firm bosselated goiter; associated autoimmune diseases	T_4 and TSH normal; if hypothyroid, T_4 decreased and TSH increased; antithyroid peroxidase antibody increased
Riedel's thyroiditis	Unknown	Anterior neck pressure, neck pain; stony hard goiter fixed to surrounding structures	WBC mildly elevated; ESR mildly elevated; TSH, T_4 and T_3 normal; antithyroid peroxidase antibody positive in 50%; open biopsy often needed

ESR = erythrocyte sedimentation rate; RAIU = radioiodine uptake; T_3 = triiodothyronine; T_4 = thyroxine; Tg = thyroglobulin; WBC = white blood cells.

of T lymphocytes to thyroid antigens released during the inflammatory process. After the inflammation has abated, antithyroid antibodies typically disappear. Patients who develop subacute granulomatous thyroiditis often carry the HLA-Bw35 haplotype, which may render these individuals more susceptible to certain viral infections and presumably increase their risk of developing this form of thyroiditis.

The viral invasion causes thyroid inflammation with microscopic evidence of giant cells, granulomas, and follicular disruptiom. In 50 per cent of patients, the disruption of follicles releases sufficient thyroid hormone into the circulation to cause thyrotoxicosis.

Clinical Presentation and Course

Patients with subacute granulomatous thyroiditis are usually 40 to 50 years old. Women experience this disorder four times more commonly than men. Patients often report a viral prodrome with myalgias, low-grade fever, lassitude, sore throat, and dysphagia. Anterior neck pain is characteristically abrupt in onset, unilateral or bilateral, and can radiate to the ear, mandible, or occiput. In the subset of patients in which there is release of thyroid hormone, thyrotoxic symptoms of diaphoresis, tachycardia, palpitations, tremor, or weight loss may be found. Physical examination reveals a low-grade fever and a firm to hard, tender thyroid with occasional overlying erythema. Cervical lymphadenopathy is usually absent. Although uncommon, pronounced thyroid swelling may produce obstructive symptoms of the airway or esophagus.

In the initial phase of thyroid inflammation, pain and thyrotoxicosis usually last 3 to 6 weeks. As thyroid hormone stores are depleted, serum T_4 and T_3 concentrations fall to normal, and a euthyroid phase ensues. If damage to the thyroid is extensive, a hypothyroid phase may occur until disrupted follicular cells fully recover. Hypothyroidism develops in about one third of patients and persists for several weeks to months. Patients with significant hypothyroid symptoms may benefit from temporary thyroid hormone replacement.

After a period of hypothyroidism, most patients recover and return to a euthyroid state. The clinician must remember to stop T_4 replacement at this time and to re-evaluate the patient's thyroid status. Permanent hypothyroidism may develop in 5 per cent of patients. Many of these individuals have coexistent autoimmune thyroid disease, such as Hashimoto's thyroiditis (i.e., chronic lymphocytic thyroiditis). It is prudent to perform periodic thyroid hormone testing in all patients after recovery.

Laboratory Findings

Laboratory findings include mild anemia and a normal to slightly increased leukocyte count. An increased erythrocyte sedimentation rate (ESR), usually greater than 50 mm/hour, is so commonly present that a normal ESR should lead the clinician to consider an alternative diagnosis. Increased serum T_4 and T_3 in one half of these patients is attributed to inflammation and damage to thyroid follicles, with subsequent release of stored thyroid hormone. Serum T_4 is disproportionately higher than serum T_3, reflecting the higher intrathyroidal concentration of T_4 than T_3. Thyroid-stimulating hormone (TSH) is invariably suppressed if T_4 and T_3 are increased. Thyroglobulin (Tg) is also released in response to thyroid inflammation, and serum Tg concentrations are invariably increased.

The inflammation and destruction of thyroid follicular cells results in an inability of the thyroid to trap iodine; therefore, the RAIU is suppressed to less than 5 per cent. The suppression of the RAIU, high T_4 and T_3 concentrations, and thyroid pain are hallmarks of subacute thyroiditis. Ultrasound examination may reveal multiple hypoechogenic areas in the thyroid parenchyma.

In the patient with increased T_4 and T_3 the hormone values will gradually decrease until normal serum concentrations are achieved. In this euthyroid phase, TSH may remain suppressed, but it slowly normalizes in most patients. One third of patients develop transient hypothyroidism with increased TSH and normal to low T_4. These hypothyroid individuals should have periodic monitoring of serum T_4 and TSH until a euthyroid state is reached. Complete recovery is the rule, and only 1 per cent of patients with subacute granulomatous thyroiditis develop permanent hypothyroidism.

Diagnosis

The diagnosis of subacute granulomatous thyroiditis in the patient presenting with a viral prodrome and neck pain is usually confirmed by documenting a tender thyroid, an increased ESR, and an increased serum Tg. If T_4 is increased, RAIU should be performed. Suppression of the RAIU to less than 5 per cent is consistent with the diagnosis of subacute thyroiditis. An elevated RAIU value indicates Graves' disease, toxic adenoma, or toxic multinodular goiter as the cause of the thyrotoxicosis.

Other causes of thyroid tenderness include acute pyogenic thyroiditis, hemorrhage into a thyroid adenoma or cyst (often manifesting as a discrete nodule with normal ESR and Tg), Hashimoto's thyroiditis (i.e., normal ESR with markedly increased antithyroid antibodies), or extensive infiltrating carcinoma of the thyroid (i.e., invasion of surrounding structures, diagnosis confirmed with fine-needle aspiration).

For the 50 per cent of patients who develop thyrotoxicosis, other causes of high T_4 and suppressed RAIU that should be considered include silent thyroiditis (i.e., no thyroid pain or tenderness and a normal ESR), thyrotoxicosis factitia or the surreptitious ingestion of thyroid hormone (i.e., low Tg and a normal ESR), Graves' disease with iodine excess (i.e., history of iodine ingestion or recent iodine-diagnostic study), ectopic thyroid tissue (i.e., struma ovarii or pelvic mass), or iodine excess (i.e., history of iodine ingestion).

For the one third of patients who develop hypothyroidism, serial measurements of TSH and T_4 are appropriate. Radioiodine imaging and ultrasonography are not helpful. For the occasional patient with persistent hypothyroidism, measurement of antithyroid antibodies may help establish the diagnosis of Hashimoto's thyroiditis.

PAINLESS THYROIDITIS AND POSTPARTUM THYROIDITIS

Etiology

Painless thyroiditis (i.e., silent thyroiditis or painless subacute lymphocytic thyroiditis) can present sporadically or in the postpartum period. The sporadic form of painless thyroiditis accounts for 5 to 33 per cent of patients presenting with thyrotoxicosis. Nearly 90 per cent of cases are reported from the Great Lakes region. In other parts of the United States, painless thyroiditis accounts for 1 to 5 per cent of newly diagnosed cases of thyrotoxicosis. Postpartum thyroiditis may be found in 4 to 8 per cent of postpartum women screened 4 to 12 weeks after delivery.

Painless and postpartum forms of thyroiditis have been

associated with autoimmune events. Antithyroid antibodies are found in 50 per cent of patients with painless thyroiditis and in 80 per cent of women with postpartum thyroiditis. A high prevalence of HLA-DR3, HLA-DR4, and HLA-DR5 haplotypes has been reported in these patients, and lymphocytic infiltration of thyroid tissue is the most common histologic abnormality.

The inflammation in painless and postpartum thyroiditis causes follicular damage, with the release of T_4 and T_3 into the circulation. After follicular stores of thyroid hormone are depleted, peripheral T_4 and T_3 fall to normal or, in some cases, subnormal concentrations.

Autoimmune events and lymphocytic infiltration are also documented in chronic lymphocytic thyroiditis (i.e., Hashimoto's). However, subacute thyroiditis lacks the fibrosis or Hürthle cell changes seen in chronic lymphocytic thyroiditis. Complete recovery is the rule for patients with painless or postpartum thyroiditis, but clinical progression is common in Hashimoto's thyroiditis.

Clinical Presentation and Course

Most patients with painless thyroiditis are 30 to 40 years of age, and almost 80 per cent are female. Patients with painless thyroiditis present with symptoms of thyrotoxicosis rather than neck pain. Occasionally, patients may present later in the disease course with symptoms of hypothyroidism. Women with postpartum thyroiditis may present with thyrotoxicosis, generally 6 to 12 weeks after delivery, or with symptoms of hypothyroidism, typically 3 to 6 months after delivery. Postpartum depression appears to be more common in women with postpartum thyroiditis, but postpartum thyroiditis is not the cause of most episodes of postpartum depression.

Physical examination reveals a small, slightly firm, nontender goiter in 50 per cent of patients. The absence of anterior neck pain and tenderness clinically distinguishes painless thyroiditis from subacute granulomatous (painful) thyroiditis. Painless thyroiditis is more difficult to distinguish from Graves' disease, but the clinician must make the distinction, because treatment for these two disorders is not the same.

The clinical course of painless or postpartum thyroiditis is similar to that of subacute granulomatous thyroiditis and consists of roughly three phases: an initial thyrotoxic phase, a hypothyroid phase (one third of patients), and a recovery phase. Patients may not exhibit all of these phases, and although most patients typically present in the thyrotoxic phase, they may also present during the hypothyroid period.

Although total recovery is the rule for patients with painless and postpartum thyroiditis, up to 50 per cent develop persistent goiter, antithyroid antibodies, or both. As many as 6 per cent of these patients develop permanent hypothyroidism. The clinician should request a TSH measurement annually, because permanent hypothyroidism may develop years after an episode of painless thyroiditis.

Laboratory Findings

Patients who present in the thyrotoxic phase of painless thyroiditis typically have increased T_4 and T_3 and suppressed TSH in the serum. The RAIU value is typically suppressed to less than 5 per cent during this thyrotoxic phase. In the hypothyroid phase, the T_4 is low, and the TSH is usually increased. Occasionally, serum TSH can be normal or low. If the pituitary is still suppressed from the recently increased T_4 and T_3 concentrations, thyrotrophs may not be able to increase TSH secretion in response to low T_4 and T_3. In some patients, the RAIU value may also show residual suppression; in other patients, the RAIU value may be normal or increased if the thyroid is replenishing its iodine stores. Serum thyroglobulin may be increased, but the leukocyte count and ESR are usually unremarkable.

Diagnosis

Patients presenting with a small goiter and thyrotoxicosis may have painless thyroiditis or Graves' disease. Patients with Graves' disease typically have an insidious onset of thyrotoxic symptoms, but patients with painless thyroiditis often have an abrupt onset of symptoms. Infiltrative ophthalmopathy (i.e., proptosis and limitation of extraoccular movements) is exclusive to Graves' disease and is not seen in patients with painless thyroiditis. In the absence of Graves' ophthalmopathy, the RAIU value is the most reliable way to distinguish Graves' disease (elevated RAIU) from painless thyroiditis (RAIU < 5 per cent). Thyroid-stimulating immunoglobulin is present in 80 per cent of patients with Graves' disease and is not found in those with painless thyroiditis. The importance of separating the thyrotoxicosis of Graves' disease and painless thyroiditis lies in the approach to treatment. Thyrotoxicosis due to Graves' disease is treated with antithyroid drugs (i.e., propylthiouracil or methimazole) or with radioiodine. Both of these modalities are ineffective and inappropriate treatment for the thyrotoxicosis of painless thyroiditis. The latter disorder is managed with expectant observation and selective use of beta-adrenergic receptor antagonists.

Patients with Hashimoto's thyroiditis may present with a small goiter and hypothyroidism and may be confused with patients in the hypothyroid phase of their painless thyroiditis. High titers of antithyroid antibodies and persistent hypothyroidism are commonly observed in Hashimoto's thyroiditis.

HASHIMOTO'S THYROIDITIS

Hashimoto's thyroiditis, or chronic lymphocytic thyroiditis, was first described by the Japanese physician Hashimoto in 1912. Chronic lymphocytic thyroiditis is the most common cause of noniatrogenic hypothyroidism and has been found in up to 2 per cent of women at autopsy. Markedly increased titers of antithyroid antibodies, a small to modest goiter, and hypothyroidism are the classic findings of Hashimoto's thyroiditis.

Etiology

Hashimoto's thyroiditis is an autoimmune disorder that is typically associated with the presence of antibodies to thyroid peroxidase (antithyroid peroxidase or antimicrosomal) and thyroglobulin (antithyroglobulin). Antibodies to colloid antigens, T_4, T_3, and the TSH receptor have also been reported. Hashimoto's thyroiditis is associated with HLA-DR5 and occurs with increased frequency in patients with Down and Turner's syndrome. The family history may be positive for Hashimoto's disease, goiter, or hypothyroidism. Coexisting autoimmune disorders, including Graves' disease, primary adrenal insufficiency, diabetes mellitus, autoimmune oophoritis, systemic lupus erythematosus, rheumatoid arthritis, and pernicious anemia may be present in the proband or family members. Histologic findings include lymphocytic infiltration, obliteration of thyroid follicles, and fibrosis. Lymphocytes may form typical lymphoid follicles with germinal centers.

Clinical Presentation and Course

Although the disease may occur in any age group, up to 95 per cent of patients with Hashimoto's thyroiditis are women, usually between the ages of 30 and 50 years. A small to medium-sized goiter is the outstanding clinical feature of this disease. Its appearance is insidious, its growth is gradual, and the goiter is often discovered as an incidental finding. About 20 per cent of patients present with hypothyroid symptoms. In patients who are euthyroid at presentation, hypothyroidism may develop over the ensuing years. Rarely, patients may present with hyperthyroidism, although this is thought to indicate the coexistence of Graves' disease or, if the thyrotoxicosis is transient, the presence of painless thyroiditis.

Physical examination may reveal findings of hypothyroidism, but typically only a diffuse, mild to modest enlargement of the thyroid is found. The gland is firm, with a lobulated or bosselated surface. Discrete, palpable nodules are unusual. Regional lymphadenopathy may be present, along with enlargement of the pyramidal lobe. Rarely, the goiter may be large enough to compress surrounding structures and cause dysphagia or recurrent laryngeal nerve dysfunction.

Laboratory Findings

Depending on the stage of the disease, the results of hormonal evaluation are variable. In the 20 per cent of patients who present with hypothyroidism, increased TSH and low T_4 are commonly found. Some patients may have increased TSH with a normal T_4, or so-called subclinical hypothyroidism. Antithyroid antibodies (i.e., antithyroid peroxidase and antithyroglobulin) are present in 90 per cent of patients. Antithyroid peroxidase antibodies are more sensitive and specific and are the preferred antibody test. Antithyroid peroxidase antibodies may be present in other thyroid diseases (e.g., Graves' disease, painless thyroiditis); however, high antibody titers are characteristic of Hashimoto's thyroiditis.

RAIU and thyroid scan are not indicated in most patients with Hashimoto's; however, if performed, the RAIU result is variable, and the scan typically reveals a diffuse, patchy uptake pattern. Fine-needle aspiration reveals the presence of lymphocytes, scant colloid, and occasional plasma cells.

Diagnosis

For most patients, the presence of a firm, bosselated goiter and antithyroid peroxidase antibodies is sufficient for the diagnosis of Hashimoto's thyroiditis. Fine-needle aspiration is indicated only if there is a coexisting thyroid nodule for which neoplasm must be excluded. Routine fine-needle aspiration may generate confusion, because the cytologic features of Hashimoto's thyroiditis and neoplasm can overlap. Thyroid RAIU or imaging is not routinely required but may be useful in the evaluation of coexisting thyroid nodules, Graves' disease, or subacute thyroiditis.

Distinguishing Hashimoto's thyroiditis from diffuse nontoxic goiter can be difficult. The consistency of a diffuse nontoxic goiter is typically softer than that of a Hashimoto's gland, and antithyroid peroxidase antibodies are absent or present at low titers in a diffuse nontoxic goiter. However, the clinician must be cautious in diagnosing adolescents, because Hashimoto's thyroiditis in this age group may not be accompanied by the high antibody titers seen in adults. Multiple, well-defined thyroid nodules in an older adult suggests the presence of a nontoxic multinodular goiter.

The differentiation of Hashimoto's thyroiditis from a thyroid carcinoma can usually be made clinically. Thyroid cancer typically presents as a dominant nodule with normal surrounding thyroid tissue. Diagnostic difficulties occur in the asymmetrically enlarged Hashimoto's gland, which may be mistaken for a large thyroid nodule or for a thyroid neoplasm that has developed in the presence of Hashimoto's thyroiditis. Regional lymphadenopathy, which is unusual in Hashimoto's thyroiditis, may indicate a neoplastic process. High titers of antithyroid peroxidase antibodies favor the diagnosis of Hashimoto's thyroiditis. Thyroid scintiscanning may reveal a hypofunctioning or "cold" area for the neoplastic lesion, and a diffuse, patchy pattern is typical of Hashimoto's disease. Direct cytologic examination of tissue from fine-needle aspiration can help exclude a neoplastic process.

RIEDEL'S THYROIDITIS

Etiology

Riedel's thyroiditis (i.e., Riedel's struma, invasive fibrous thyroiditis, or chronic sclerosing thyroiditis) is a rare disorder that primarily occurs in middle-aged or elderly women. The underlying process is a sclerosing fibrosis that is diffuse in 70 per cent and partial in 30 per cent of patients. Eventually, the fibrosis transforms the thyroid into a woody or stony-hard mass that is fixed to surrounding structures. As the disease progresses, the trachea, esophagus, or recurrent laryngeal nerve may be obstructed or compressed. Many patients may also develop retroperitoneal fibrosis and, less commonly, fibrosis in the orbits, liver, lungs, and mediastinum. Although the cause of Riedel's thyroiditis is unknown, some authorities think that fibrosis of the thyroid is one component of a more generalized disorder characterized by proliferation of fibrous tissue.

Clinical Presentation and Course

Patients complain of anterior neck pressure, dysphagia, and dyspnea due to tracheal compression. The thyroid is enlarged and attached to surrounding structures. The consistency of the gland is described as woody or stony hard. Hypothyroidism may develop in 30 to 40 per cent of patients with Riedel's thyroiditis.

Laboratory Findings

Laboratory evaluation may reveal a mildly increased leukocyte count and ESR. Serum TSH, T_4 and T_3 concentrations are normal until extensive destruction of the gland has occurred and hypothyroidism has ensued. Antithyroid peroxidase antibodies are detected in 40 to 50 per cent of patients, typically in titers lower than those seen in Hashimoto's thyroiditis. The diagnosis of Riedel's thyroiditis is difficult with fine-needle aspiration; open surgical biopsy is usually required.

Diagnosis

The stony-hard texture of the thyroid and low-titer or absent antithyroid peroxidase antibodies usually distinguish Riedel's thyroiditis from Hashimoto's thyroiditis. However, the stony-hard texture and invasion of surrounding structures may suggest invasive thyroid carcinoma. Attempts at fine-needle aspiration or an open surgical biopsy usually establish the correct diagnosis. Occasionally, surgical excision is required to exclude carcinoma and to treat the invasive Riedel's thyroiditis.

THYROID NODULES AND GOITER

By Silvio E. Inzucchi, M.D.,
and Gerard N. Burrow, M.D.
New Haven, Connecticut

THYROID NODULES

Nodular disease of the thyroid is a common clinical problem. The causes of thyroid nodules are listed in Table 1. Estimates of the prevalence of thyroid nodules vary and depend on the method of detection. By physical examination, thyroid nodules are palpated in up to 5 to 10 per cent of individuals. By ultrasonography, detection rates approach 50 per cent in some groups. Despite the striking frequency of thyroid nodules, the mean incidence of malignancy in all patients with nodules does not exceed 5 per cent. In addition, with the exception of anaplastic carcinoma, mortality rates for thyroid cancers are relatively low when compared with rates for nonthyroidal malignancies. Thus, the chief responsibility of the physician evaluating patients with thyroid nodules is to distinguish that small minority with malignant neoplasms from the vast majority with benign conditions. The evaluation must be accurate, cost-effective, and performed with minimal risk to the patient.

Clinical Presentation

Thyroid nodules are most commonly detected on routine physical examination. They may also be discovered fortuitously during radiographic procedures that image the neck, such as chest films, computed tomography (CT) of the thorax, and carotid ultrasound. Patients may complain of a cosmetically apparent mass, an ill-defined discomfort in the anterior neck, or symptoms of local compression, such as dysphagia, hoarseness, chronic cough, or dyspnea. However, because of their slow growth, even sizable thyroid nodules are usually well tolerated by patients, and most are clinically silent.

Table 1. Causes of Thyroid Nodules

Benign
Follicular adenoma (microfollicular adenoma)
Colloid adenoma (macrofollicular adenoma)
Hürthle cell adenoma
Embryonal adenoma
Fetal adenoma
Papillary cystadenoma
Nodular autoimmune thyroiditis
Multinodular goiter
Marine-Lenhart nodule (in Graves' disease)
Simple cyst
Malignant
Papillary carcinoma
Follicular carcinoma
Mixed papillary-follicular carcinoma
Hürthle cell carcinoma
Medullary carcinoma
Anaplastic carcinoma
Lymphoma
Sarcoma
Metastatic cancer to the thyroid

Thyroid nodules typically present in the fourth through sixth decades of life. They are more likely to be malignant in the young (<20 years of age) and when newly discovered after the age of 60 years. The majority of thyroid cancers occur in women. However, because thyroid nodules in general are much more common in women and because the great majority are benign, an individual nodule is more likely to be malignant in men. Certain clinical features, such as size, growth rate, and associated local symptoms increase the risk of malignancy, although there remains a significant degree of overlap with benign lesions. Larger nodules are more likely to be malignant, particularly those larger than 3 to 5 cm. Increasing size is accompanied by a greater frequency of local compressive symptoms resulting from invasion or impingement of various structures in the neck, such as the trachea, esophagus, ipsilateral recurrent laryngeal nerve, and jugular vein. Progression to the point of airway obstruction is unusual, although it is occasionally seen in highly aggressive neoplasms and in large multinodular goiters. Pain in the cervical region or radiating to the jaw or ears may also be seen in thyroid cancer if extracapsular invasion has occurred with involvement of local neural structures. Neck pain is unusual with benign nodules unless acute expansion occurs from hemorrhagic degeneration. Benign lesions are characterized by stability of size, although slow growth (years) or regression is not uncommon. Rapid growth (hours to days) may also occur, but this usually indicates hemorrhage into an adenoma or cyst. In contrast, thyroid cancer demonstrates an intermediate growth rate (months), although two forms—anaplastic carcinoma and thyroid lymphoma—can grow faster (weeks). With distant metastases from a thyroid malignancy, symptoms referable to a focally destructive process in a particular tissue may become evident, such as bone pain from skeletal deposits. In widely metastatic disease, there may be generalized symptoms such as weight loss.

Abnormal thyroid function is the exception in nodular thyroid disease. Indeed, the discovery of either hyperthyroidism or hypothyroidism usually indicates a benign process. In patients with autonomous toxic nodules, which compose a small minority of all nodules in iodine-replete regions of the world, features of hyperthyroidism may dominate the clinical picture. As in other causes of thyrotoxicosis, symptoms may include weight loss, heat intolerance, palpitations, anxiety, emotional lability, tremor, muscular weakness, and fatigue. Circulating levels of thyroid hormones are, on average, not as high as in Graves' disease, and symptoms are typically not as severe. However, as is the case with other forms of hyperthyroidism, there is no direct correlation between thyroid hormone levels and the degree of clinical symptoms. Some individuals with toxic nodules are diagnosed with subclinical hyperthyroidism, that is, suppression of pituitary secretion of thyroid-stimulating hormone (TSH) but normal circulating levels of thyroid hormones. Although subtle physiologic aberrations have been measured in this condition, as its name implies, patients have no apparent symptoms. However, affected older individuals may be at risk for cardiovascular complications. Rarely, nodules representing focal areas of hyperplasia occur in Graves' disease. Hypothyroidism and its accompanying symptoms are occasionally discovered during the evaluation of a patient with a thyroid nodule. This most commonly represents a nodular variant of autoimmune thyroiditis. In such patients, the entire gland is enlarged, with discrete nodules resulting from focal lymphocytic infiltration or from the creation of pseudonodules by the intraparenchymal retraction of bands of fibrous tissue.

In medullary carcinoma of the thyroid, flushing and diarrhea associated with hypercalcitoninemia may occur. Paraneoplastic phenomena (e.g., ectopic adrenocorticotropic hormone [ACTH] secretion) have also been described. In cases of medullary carcinoma of the thyroid associated with multiple endocrine neoplasia type IIA and IIB (MEN IIA, IIB), there may be features of coexisting hyperparathyroidism and/or pheochromocytoma.

Most prior medical conditions have little impact on the nature of a thyroid nodule. Previous therapeutic radiation of the head or neck, however, is associated with an increased risk of both benign and malignant nodules. The dosage of radiation appears to be important. Therapeutic low-dose radiotherapy was a popular treatment in the 1940s and 1950s for thymic enlargement, recurrent tonsillitis, acne, and other skin conditions. Impressive rates of thyroid malignancies have been reported decades later in those who were irradiated. Doses greater than 20 Gy have been associated with follicular cell destruction and consequent hypothyroidism and thus have not been as commonly implicated in the development of subsequent neoplasia.

A family history of benign nodules or goiter typically predicts a similarly benign process in the patient. By contrast, members of kindreds affected by MEN IIA and MEN IIB are clearly at increased risk for the development of medullary carcinoma of the thyroid. Familial medullary carcinoma of the thyroid without neoplasia of other endocrine glands has also been described. In general, however, thyroid malignancies are not strongly associated with any genetic predisposition.

Physical Examination

The thyroid gland lies in the anterior neck anterior to the trachea at the level of the second tracheal ring just below the cricoid cartilage. Two lobes extend posterolaterally from an adjoining isthmus toward the tracheoesophageal recesses. Each lobe measures approximately 1 to 2 cm in thickness, 2 to 3 cm in width, and 4 to 5 cm in length, and normally weighs 20 to 25 g in adults. The right lobe is characteristically larger than the left. Occasionally, and most commonly in goitrous conditions, a small pyramidal lobe projects cephalad from the isthmus. Examination of the thyroid gland should begin with simple observation of the neck before and during swallowing. Frequently, masses, generalized enlargement, or abnormalities of contour can be seen. Next, palpation is best accomplished with both hands as the examiner stands behind the patient, feeling each lobe in turn. Having the patient consume small sips of water will aid in the palpation, as the thyroid slides upward over the cricoid cartilage during deglutition. Thyroid nodules, unless located posteriorly, substernally, under the sternocleidomastoid muscle, or beneath large deposits of adipose tissue, can usually be felt when they are larger than 1 cm. Whenever possible, the size of the nodule should be carefully measured by ruler or traced on paper to facilitate follow-up.

Nodule consistency ranges from soft and smooth to rock-hard and irregular, as may be seen in papillary carcinoma. Most nodules, however, including colloid adenomas, follicular adenomas, and follicular carcinoma, have an intermediate firm texture. Benign nodules tend to be well circumscribed, clearly distinguishable from surrounding normal tissue, and freely mobile. These characteristics also apply to most well-differentiated thyroid cancers. Several distinct nodules or diffuse nodularity suggests multinodular goiter, a benign process. The presence of cervical adenopathy increases the suspicion of malignancy, but adenopathy is also occasionally seen in autoimmune thyroiditis. Induration of overlying skin, fixation to underlying structures, dysphonia, and evidence of jugular vein compression suggest aggressive local disease. Thyroid lymphoma has a characteristic bulky and rubbery texture, and there may be associated cervical or generalized lymphadenopathy. In anaplastic carcinoma, the goiter is firm to hard and often asymmetric, with frequent evidence of local or metastatic spread. Areas of bony tenderness or deformity suggest skeletal metastases of thyroid cancer. In toxic thyroid nodules, the usual features of thyrotoxicosis, such as hyperkinesia, diaphoresis, tachycardia, stare, tremulousness, and hyperreflexia, may be noted. In addition, when a toxic nodule secretes enough thyroid hormone to suppress TSH, the remainder of the thyroid gland may be involuted. However, symptoms specific to Graves' disease (e.g., orbitopathy, pretibial myxedema) are absent. Increased arterial pressure may be noted in medullary carcinoma of the thyroid associated with MEN IIA or IIB due to coexisting pheochromocytoma. In addition, mucosal neuromas in the oral cavity may be seen in MEN IIB.

Unfortunately, in the absence of a strikingly hard and fixed nodule or impressive lymphadenopathy, the physical examination typically is not of sufficient predictive value to detect or exclude malignancy. Thus, further diagnostic testing is virtually always required.

Laboratory Procedures

Following a complete history and physical examination, the evaluation of a thyroid nodule proceeds to the clinical laboratory. Routine hematology and chemistry panels are rarely helpful. Anemia may be documented in widely metastatic thyroid cancer. Various hematologic indices may be abnormal in patients with lymphoma. In medullary carcinoma of the thyroid associated with MEN IIA, the concentration of serum calcium may be increased due to coexisting hyperparathyroidism. Calcium concentrations are also occasionally increased in thyrotoxicosis induced by an autonomous thyroid nodule. Concentrations of alkaline phosphatase, a marker of enhanced bone turnover, may also increase with hyperthyroidism. Leukopenia and other laboratory signs of Graves' disease typically are not seen in patients with thyroid nodules.

Of greater utility in the evaluation of thyroid nodules are routine thyroid function tests and TSH. If serum TSH concentrations are within the reference range, the measurement of total thyroxine (T_4), triiodothyronine (T_3) resin uptake or thyroid-binding capacity, and a calculated estimate of free T_4 add little new information. If TSH is suppressed, however, thyroid function should be evaluated. If the TSH concentration is low and the estimate of free T_4 is normal, total T_3 should be measured. Preferential production of T_3 is not uncommon in autonomous nodules (T_3 toxicosis). Once hyperthyroidism is documented, the clinician should request scintigraphy to evaluate autonomous function. If TSH is increased, a diagnosis of primary hypothyroidism is made. Autoimmune thyroiditis is the most common cause of hypothyroidism in North America and may present as nodular disease of the thyroid. Although the diagnosis of autoimmune thyroiditis may not appreciably alter the initial work-up of a suspicious thyroid nodule, this information is helpful when interpreting cytologic descriptions from fine needle aspirates and when considering the use of thyroid hormone suppression. Increased titers of thyroid autoantibodies (antithyroglobulin Ab and antimicrosomal Ab) provide evidence of underlying autoimmune thyroiditis. The laborious and expensive direct measurements of free T_4 and free T_3 and more elaborate dynamic testing, such as thyrotropin-releasing hormone (TRH) stimulation, are not usually indicated. Thyroglobulin concentrations generally are not helpful in the initial evaluation of the thyroid nodule. However, once thyroid cancer is diagnosed, thyroglobulin may be used as a tumor marker. Finally, serum calcitonin concentrations, either basal or after calcium or pentagastrin stimulation, are frequently increased in medullary carcinoma of the thyroid and can be invaluable in evaluation of this condition.

Radiographic Procedures

The use of some imaging studies in the evaluation of thyroid nodules has decreased as the use of fine needle aspiration (FNA) biopsy has increased.

Plain Radiographs

Routine radiography is not recommended. Large nodules may displace or narrow the trachea (Fig. 1). Fine stippling of calcium that correlates with the pathognomonic psammoma bodies of papillary carcinoma may be seen in the neck region of the plain film. In patients with widespread malignant disease, a chest film may demonstrate pulmonary lesions, and a bone survey may reveal skeletal metastases.

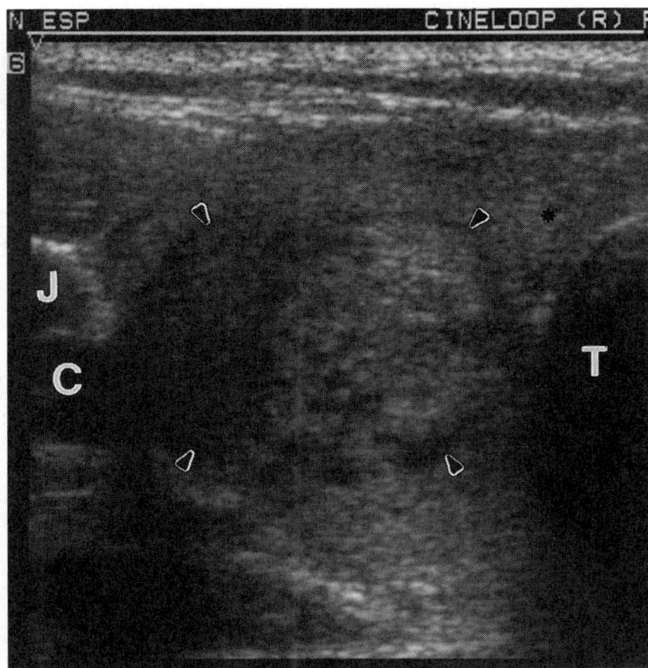

Figure 2. Ultrasound examination of the thyroid, showing a 3.5-cm hypoechoic, well-circumscribed nodule in the right lobe *(arrowheads).* Normal thyroid parenchyma is noted with an asterisk. FNA revealed this to be a colloid nodule. C = carotid artery; J = internal jugular vein; T = trachea.

Ultrasound

Most thyroid nodules are well circumscribed and hypoechoic when compared with normal thyroid parenchyma (Fig. 2). Sonography can delineate the size and extent of thyroid nodules. Ultrasound is valuable when a nodule is suspected but not definitively confirmed by physical examination. In some patients with multinodular goiter, only one nodule may be appreciated by the examiner, whereas ultrasound may delineate the presence and size of otherwise unrecognized lesions. Despite recent dispute, an individual nodule in multinodular goiter is less likely to be malignant than is a solitary nodule. Therefore, the finding of other nodules, especially if they are of similar size, is frequently reassuring. Sonography is most helpful in the diagnosis of simple cysts, which are almost always benign but exceedingly rare. By contrast, ultrasound does not provide distinguishing information on solid lesions, which are much more common. Thus, ultrasound is not justified as a routine study in the diagnostic evaluation of solitary thyroid nodules. However, in long-term follow-up, the measurement of nodule size is more precise and reproducible with ultrasound, especially when the nodule is not easily or completely palpable.

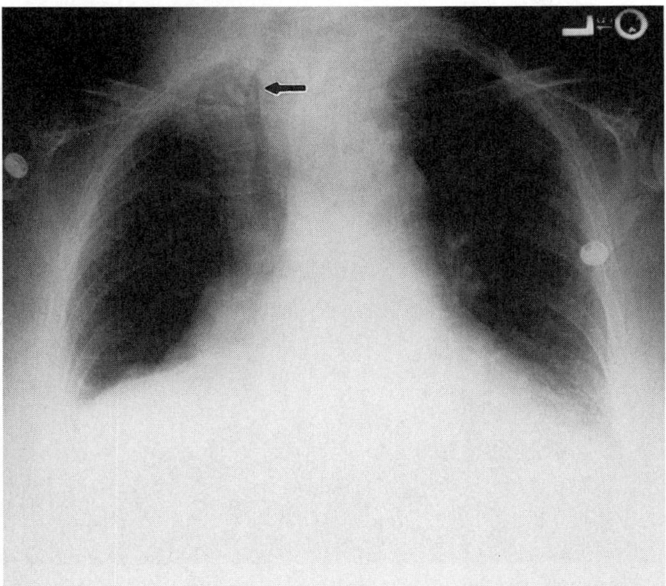

Figure 1. Chest radiograph of a patient with a large multinodular goiter. Note significant tracheal deviation *(arrow).*

Scintigraphy

In contrast to ultrasound, radioisotope imaging of the thyroid yields both anatomic and functional information (Fig. 3). The uptake of radiotracer correlates with the degree of trapping and/or organification of iodine by thyroid tissue. Nodules are described as cold (i.e., photopenic, nonfunctioning), warm (i.e., uptake equivalent to surrounding normal parenchyma), or hot (i.e., intense uptake, secondarily diminishing uptake in the rest of the gland). Technetium Tc 99m (^{99m}Tc), the most commonly used tracer, is widely available to nuclear medicine departments. This isotope is trapped by thyroid follicles but not organified. Iodine-123 (^{123}I) provides more information, as it is both trapped and organified. In general, nodules that demonstrate increased or decreased activity with ^{99m}Tc will have a similar appearance with ^{123}I. Thyroid malignancies that are warm on ^{99m}Tc scanning but cold on ^{123}I imaging occur rarely. Iodine-131 (^{131}I) by contrast, has a greater cost, longer half-life, and higher energy. Thus, ^{131}I is reserved for radioablation and for imaging after surgery for thyroid cancer.

Most thyroid nodules, including most malignant thyroid

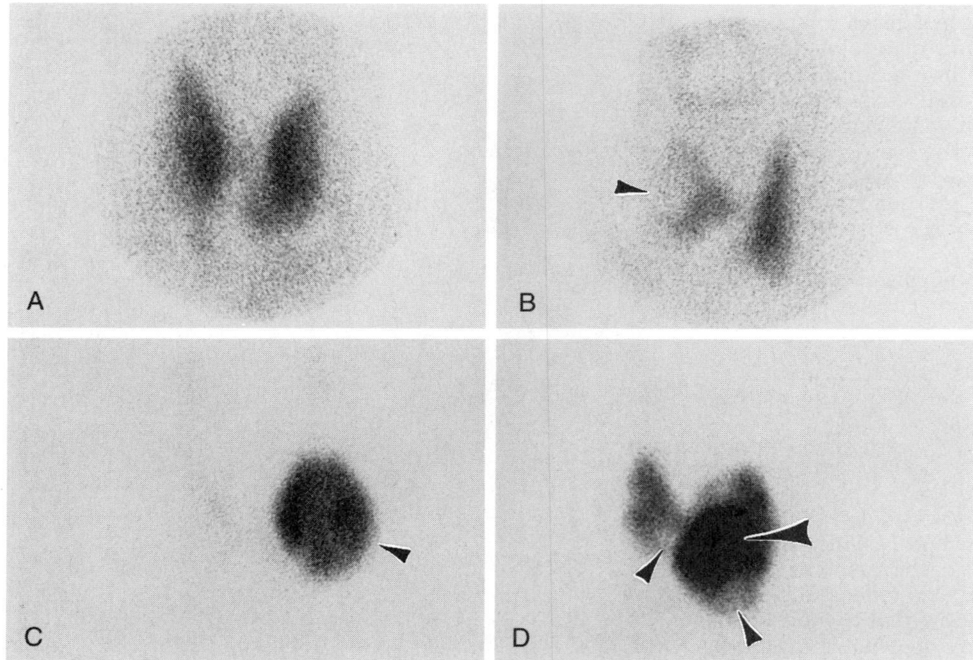

Figure 3. ^{99m}Tc thyroid scintigraphy in four patients: *A,* Normal scan. *B,* Cold, 2-cm nodule (colloid nodule by FNA) in the midlateral aspect of the right lobe *(arrowhead). C,* Hot, 5-cm nodule in the left lobe *(arrowhead),* with suppression of tracer activity in the rest of the thyroid. *D,* Multinodular goiter (same patient as in Fig. 1) with various areas of increased *(large arrowhead)* and decreased activity *(small arrowheads).*

nodules, are cold by scintigraphy. Thus, isotope scanning cannot reliably distinguish thyroid cancer from benign lesions. By contrast, because almost all hot nodules represent benign autonomously functioning adenomas, this intense uptake essentially rules out malignancy, with few exceptions. Although the discovery of a warm nodule also typically indicates autonomous tissue, further investigation is required. The possibility of a cold nodule hidden by adjacent functioning follicles should be excluded. In such patients, scintigraphy should be repeated after 4 to 6 weeks of levothyroxine treatment at a dose sufficient (150 to 175 μg per day) to suppress endogenous TSH secretion. With this maneuver, an autonomous nodule will be more easily identified because normal thyroid parenchyma will no longer take up tracer. Once function is demonstrated in a nodule, the patient can simply be followed. If thyrotoxicosis develops, radioablation or surgery should be considered. However, as most thyroid nodules in North America are cold, scintigraphy does not prevent a significant number of patients from requiring further evaluation. In this light, the cost-effectiveness of radioisotope studies has been questioned. Scintigraphy may be most logically employed in patients who have cytologic evidence of follicular neoplasm by FNA. Virtually all functioning nodules will be included in this group. Finally, in regions of the world where iodine supply is deficient or marginal, a greater percentage of nodules are functioning. Here, scintigraphy can more efficiently exclude individual patients from further investigation. Although nonscintigraphic iodine uptake measurements are valuable in the diagnosis of hyperthyroidism, they are not useful in the evaluation of nodular disease.

Computed Tomography and Magnetic Resonance Imaging

CT and magnetic resonance imaging (MRI) can reveal nodules of sufficient size, but these techniques are less sensitive than ultrasound or scintigraphy. When malignancy is suspected, however, both are ideal for delineating the degree of local invasion as well as the presence of cervical lymph node metastases. This information may be useful to those planning an operative approach. In addition, CT and magnetic resonance imaging may help in determining the degree of tracheal luminal narrowing (Fig. 4) in a patient with a large thyroid mass and local symptoms of airway compression.

Other Diagnostic Tests

Fine Needle Aspiration

FNA is the most useful test in the evaluation of thyroid nodules and has gained increased popularity over the past decade. Although the technique is relatively simple to

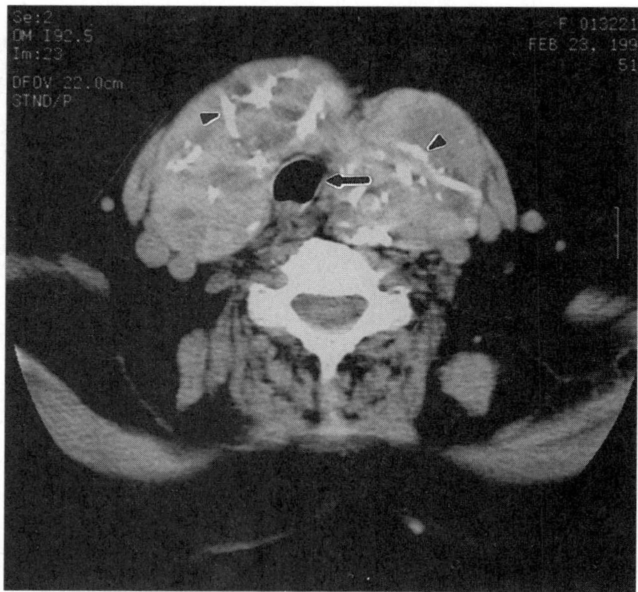

Figure 4. CT scan of large multinodular goiter, with mild deviation of the trachea *(arrow).* Note prominent calcium deposition *(arrowheads).*

learn, a thorough understanding of its indications and the implications of various cytologic interpretations is required. *An experienced cytopathologist familiar with thyroid aspirates is essential for the successful use of this important procedure.* Biopsy with large-bore cutting needles provides more generous specimens that are easier to interpret, but this technique is more difficult to learn, is associated with greater morbidity, and is not currently favored.

TECHNIQUE. To prevent alterations of clotting parameters, the patient should not ingest aspirin for 7 to 10 days prior to FNA. In addition, the clinician should exclude any history of bleeding diathesis or allergy to local anesthesia. With the patient supine, palpate the nodule and mark its position with a pen. Swab the neck with antiseptic solution, drape the neck, and inject lidocaine. Fix the nodule between two fingers. Introduce a No. 22- to No. 27-gauge needle attached to a 10-ml syringe into the lesion. Apply suction and move the syringe repetitively in the same plane until a small amount of aspirate, typically red-orange, enters the hub. Withdraw the needle and release suction before exiting the skin. Prepare cytologic slides and rapidly immerse them in 95 per cent alcohol. Two to six passes are recommended to assure adequate sampling. In larger nodules, try to enter various regions of the mass. Occasionally, cystic fluid or colloid will be aspirated. Drain the lesion as completely as possible and send the fluid for analysis. Reaspirate any residual nodule. Following aspiration, apply direct pressure to the site of entry and observe the patient for 15 minutes. Some patients may experience discomfort for 1 to 3 days, especially on swallowing. The procedure is usually well tolerated, and clinical significant adverse effects are distinctly rare.

RESULTS. Cytologic results of FNA specimens are classified into four groups:

1. In 5 to 10 per cent of patients with nodules, the specimen is diagnostic of or suspicious for malignancy. These aspirates are typically cellular and demonstrate cytologic features of papillary carcinoma or, less commonly, aggressive follicular carcinoma, medullary carcinoma, anaplastic carcinoma, or lymphoma. The rate of false-positive aspirates can approach 20 to 30 per cent. However, unless operative risk is extraordinarily high, thyroidectomy should be advised.

2. In 50 to 60 per cent of patients, the specimen is clearly benign. The aspirate typically reveals groups of cytologically bland epithelial cells in a follicular distribution, with a moderate to large amount of colloid. Occasionally, lymphocytes or Hürthle cells (follicular cells with granular, eosinophilic cytoplasm) may be seen. If substantial lymphocytic infiltration is noted, a diagnosis of autoimmune thyroiditis may be made, especially if thyroid autoantibody titers are increased. Thyroidectomy is not indicated for this group of individuals, and patients can be followed safely with simple observation or thyroid hormone suppression of the gland. False-negative rates are in the range of 1 to 2 per cent.

3. In 15 to 20 per cent of patients, the specimen is described as a follicular neoplasm or a microfollicular lesion. These highly cellular specimens with a paucity of colloid are indeterminate because they may represent either follicular adenomas or follicular carcinomas. Unfortunately, unless marked cellular atypia is noted, the diagnosis of follicular carcinoma cannot be made by FNA. Instead, direct visualization of capsular or vascular invasion in tissue sections is required for a diagnosis of malignancy. If such a nodule is cold on radioisotope scan, the risk of malignancy approaches 20 per cent. At this juncture, surgical excision or careful follow-up with thyroid hormone suppression is advisable. Various clinical considerations should contribute to this decision, including patient age, the size and growth history of the neoplasm, the presence of associated local symptoms, comorbid disease and operative risk, and the degree of certainty that is required by the patient. Most well-differentiated thyroid cancers are not particularly aggressive; thus, delayed diagnosis following a period of observation rarely influences the clinical outcome.

4. In 10 to 15 per cent of cases, the specimen contains excessive blood and too few cells for adequate cytologic analysis. FNA should be repeated in these persons.

Levothyroxine Suppression

The use of levothyroxine for the suppression of thyroid nodules is controversial. Although it makes intrinsic sense that thyroid tissue should respond with involution to a decrease in pituitary secretion of TSH caused by exogenous thyroid hormone administration, the response of individual nodules at best varies. Autonomous lesions typically do not respond. Indeed, levothyroxine will simply augment thyroid hormone levels. In nonfunctioning nodules, most prospective trials show response rates no greater than 30 to 50 per cent and any decrease in size is usually minor. Chronic high-dose levothyroxine therapy may be associated with long-term side effects, including osteoporosis and left ventricular hypertrophy. Thus, the questions of whether to use thyroid hormone suppression, to what degree, and to what endpoint remain difficult to answer. Although documented reduction in nodule size following administration of levothyroxine argues against malignancy, this result is not diagnostically definitive because occasional thyroid cancers temporarily regress during suppression. When levothyroxine is administered, the dose should be sufficient to suppress TSH into the low-normal (but not undetectable) range (0.1 mU/L). Patients should be monitored for signs of hyperthyroidism. Follow-up examination with or without ultrasound is recommended 3 to 6 months after the start of treatment. To suppress the growth of residual tumor, levothyroxine is routinely administered after surgery for thyroid cancer.

Recommended Evaluation

An algorithm for the evaluation of thyroid nodules is provided in Figure 5. Within this framework, an individualized approach is required for each patient.

GOITER

The precise distinction between thyroid nodular disease and goiter is somewhat arbitrary. In multinodular goiter, the entire gland is enlarged *because* of multiple nodules. The term goiter is often used to describe any increase in thyroid volume. However, the term is best reserved for enlargement of the entire thyroid in the absence of nodules. The causes of goiter are listed in Table 2. The frequency of goiter varies throughout the world; it is most common in regions where the diet is deficient in iodine (endemic goiter). In North America, where the average iodine intake is high, thyroid enlargement that is nontoxic and unassociated with disorders of autoimmunity is termed sporadic goiter. The histologic features of endemic and sporadic goiter overlap. These entities are therefore primarily distinguished on the basis of the local iodine

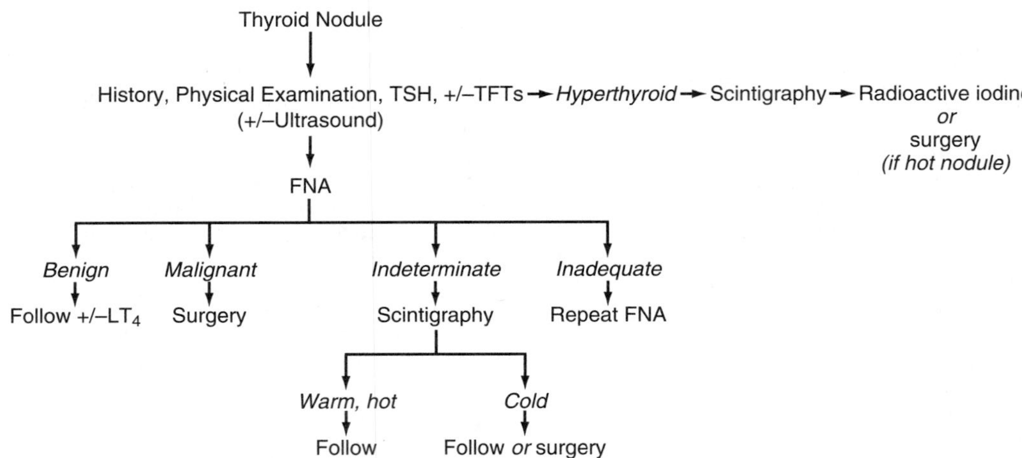

Figure 5. Diagnostic approach to thyroid nodules. (FNA-fine-needle aspiration; LT_4-levothyroxine; TFTs-thyroid function tests.)

supply. In endemic goiter, thyroid growth is primarily under TSH control. In sporadic goiter, which is a continuum from an early diffuse stage to a later nodular stage, growth factors that are as yet undefined may also play a significant role. The pathogenesis of the more common causes of goiter, including Graves' disease, autoimmune thyroiditis (Hashimoto's disease), and subacute thyroiditis (de Quervain's disease) are better understood. In almost all forms of goiter, the family history is frequently positive.

The most important task in the evaluation of goiter is the initial determination of thyroid function. Abnormalities of thyroid function are more likely to occur in patients with goiter than in those with solitary nodules. Conversely, the risk of thyroid malignancy is lower in patients with goiter than in patients with solitary nodules.

Clinical Presentation

Goiter is most commonly discovered incidentally during routine physical examination. It is also frequently detected during the evaluation of thyroid dysfunction. Occasionally, a patient may complain of swelling in the neck or symptoms of local compression. As with thyroid nodules, larger goiters are associated with more symptoms. Most goiters grow slowly, if at all. More rapid growth (weeks) is occasionally seen in patients with anaplastic carcinomas or lymphomas that may diffusely involve the thyroid.

Table 2. Causes of Goiter

- Endemic goiter (iodine deficiency goiter)
- Sporadic goiter
  - Diffuse nontoxic goiter
  - Multinodular goiter
- Diffuse toxic goiter (Graves' disease)
- Thyroiditis
  - Autoimmune (Hashimoto's disease)
  - Subacute
  - Silent
  - Postpartum
  - Suppurative
- Defects of thyroid hormone biosynthesis
- Dietary and environmental goitrogens
- Drugs (thionamides, iodide, lithium)
- Diffuse malignancy
  - Lymphoma
  - Anaplastic carcinoma
- Infiltrative diseases
  - Riedel's thyroiditis
  - Sarcoidosis
  - Amyloidosis

Goiter is commonly associated with abnormal thyroid function, especially when goiter accompanies Graves' disease, autoimmune or subacute thyroiditis or, rarely, a defect in thyroid hormone biosynthesis. In these forms of goiter, features stemming from the overproduction or underproduction of thyroid hormone tend to dominate the clinical picture. Patients with Graves' disease present with thyrotoxicosis, manifested by palpitations, heat intolerance, tremor, weakness, and weight loss. Diplopia, proptosis, and symptoms of corneal irritation may result from orbital involvement. Without treatment, Graves' disease may take years or even decades to remit, with gradual involution of the gland. Untreated Graves' disease is often accompanied by atrial fibrillation that may lead to hypotension, cardiac failure, or cerebral or systemic embolization. Prolonged thyrotoxicosis has also been associated with left ventricular hypertrophy and osteopenia. In rare cases, thyroid storm may develop. This clinical syndrome, manifested by tachycardia, fever, and altered mental status, carries a high mortality rate. Graves' disease during pregnancy may be complicated by increased fetal loss and fetal or neonatal hyperthyroidism. With autoimmune thyroiditis, primary hypothyroidism frequently results, and symptoms include weight gain, fatigue, edema, and cold intolerance. A small to moderate goiter may occur; as in Graves' disease, the thyroid may eventually involute. Unlike Graves' disease, autoimmune thyroiditis has a slower progression. Patients with hypothyroidism may experience cardiac dysfunction, cognitive deficits, and premature atherogenesis. In subacute thyroiditis, thyroid pain, sometimes experienced as a sore throat, is a cardinal feature. The granulomatous inflammation typically follows a viral illness. In the early phase, mild transient thyrotoxicosis is common, whereas in a later stage, hypothyroidism may develop. In most patients with subacute thyroiditis, however, normalization of thyroid function is the ultimate outcome.

In contrast, sporadic goiter is usually *not* associated with abnormal circulating thyroid hormone concentrations. Toxic nodules (Plummer's disease), however, may be seen in up to 20 to 30 per cent of patients with multinodular sporadic goiter. Toxic multinodular goiter is classically seen in elderly patients, particularly after large iodine loads, as found in radiocontrast agents (Jod-Basedow effect). Symptoms of local compression are more common in sporadic goiter, especially the nodular variety. Progression to airway obstruction may rarely occur especially if there is substernal extension. Acute hemorrhage into a degenerating nodule may cause neck pain and increased mass effect. Rarely, mild to moderate goiter is associated with an inherited deficiency in one of the enzymes responsible for thyroid hormone biosynthesis.

Physical Examination

In Graves' disease, the thyroid is diffusely enlarged and soft. Subtle lobulation may be noted, and the gland may be doubled, tripled, or even quadrupled in size. A bruit and/or thrill is sometimes appreciated over the gland because of increased blood flow. Patients with Graves' disease also demonstrate other physical signs, such as tachycardia, tremor, hyperkinesia, and hyperreflexia. Extrathyroidal manifestations include orbitopathy and pretibial myxedema. Physical signs may include those of other associated autoimmune conditions (e.g., myasthenia gravis and vitiligo). By contrast, the goiter of autoimmune thyroiditis is smaller than that of Graves' and is typically enlarged by only 50 to 100 per cent. The texture is diffusely firm and grainy, with occasional asymmetry. During an acute phase of autoimmune thyroiditis, the gland may be somewhat tender. Other clinical signs may include bradycardia, periorbital edema, dry skin, and coarse hair. In atypical cases, an initial phase of hyperthyroidism may be observed. Sporadic diffuse goiters are typically two to three times larger than the normal thyroid, with a variably soft to firm texture. Multinodular glands are composed of nodules in various stages of growth and degeneration. These nodules range in size from several millimeters to several centimeters. Gland enlargement ranges from moderate to dramatic, with frequent compression of adjacent neck structures, leading to hoarseness or stridor. Multinodular goiter may also be associated with thyrotoxicosis due to one or more autonomously functioning nodules. In subacute thyroiditis, the goiter is small, soft, and tender to palpation. Goiters resulting from biosynthetic defects are diffuse and small to medium in size. Clinical signs of hypothyroidism are usually absent because these patients produce sufficient amounts of thyroid hormone, albeit at the expense of an enlarged, inefficient gland. One type of dyshormonogenesis, Pendred's syndrome, is associated with deafness.

Laboratory Procedures

Routine chemistry and hematology panels are not helpful in the evaluation of goiter. Mild hypercalcemia, leukopenia, and increased serum alkaline phosphatase concentrations may be seen in Graves' disease. Lipid abnormalities are frequently detected, and mild anemia may be seen in any condition associated with hypothyroidism.

Biochemical evaluation of thyroid function is of greater importance. TSH is suppressed in patients with hyperthyroidism due to Graves' disease, toxic multinodular goiter, and thyroiditis. Serum T_4 and T_3 concentrations are increased or, in subclinical hyperthyroidism, measure in the high-normal range. Titers of thyrotropin receptor antibodies (thyroid-stimulating immunoglobulin [TSI]) are commonly increased in Graves' disease. Titers of thyroid autoantibodies may also be increased in this condition. In autoimmune thyroiditis, autoantibodies are measured in even higher titers. When primary hypothyroidism has developed, TSH is increased, and T_4 and T_3 concentrations are low or low-normal. There are no distinguishing laboratory features of multinodular goiter or goiters caused by defects in hormone synthesis. The erythrocyte sedimentation rate is always increased in subacute thyroiditis.

Radiographic Procedures

Plain films may reveal tracheal deviation or obstruction. In large glands with substernal extension, a mediastinal mass may be seen on chest film. Irregular, calcific deposits are frequently seen on plain films in patients with multinodular goiter. Osteopenia may be noted in skeletal series of patients with goiter associated with long-standing hyperthyroidism. Ultrasonography will distinguish diffuse goiters, which have a homogeneous echotexture, from multinodular glands, which are heterogeneous with a variable number of hypoechoic foci representing distinct nodules in various stages of growth and degeneration. Glands with autoimmune thyroiditis reveal a heterogeneous echotexture, and areas of subtle nodularity may be observed.

Radioiodine uptake measurements may help in distinguishing the two main causes of hyperthyroid goiters. Uptake is increased in Graves' disease but low or absent in subacute thyroiditis. Uptake is variable in autoimmune thyroiditis and multinodular goiter. Trapping is normal in patients with organification defects; thus, iodine uptake will be high after 1 to 2 hours but low at 24 hours. The rarely used perchlorate discharge test takes advantage of this phenomenon and facilitates diagnosis of biosynthetic blocks as obscure causes of goiter. Perchlorate displaces trapped iodine from follicles, and radioiodine uptake will fall several hours after administration of perchlorate to patients with biosynthetic defects. Thyroid scanning is not particularly useful in the evaluation of goiter. Scans may demonstrate diffuse and enhanced radiotracer uptake in Graves' disease and little or no image in subacute thyroiditis. The pattern of uptake in autoimmune thyroiditis is often reduced and heterogeneous. In multinodular goiter, scattered areas of increased and decreased uptake are usually seen. CT delineates the degree of airway obstruction in very large goiters.

Other Diagnostic Procedures

FNA is rarely performed in the evaluation of goiter, unless a dominant nodule in a multinodular goiter requires further attention. Cytologic examination is nonspecific in Graves' disease. FNA may be diagnostic in autoimmune thyroiditis, but immunologic testing is much easier and less costly to perform. In rare cases, spirometry is required to document the degree of physiologic airway obstruction in large goiters.

PRIMARY HYPERPARATHYROIDISM

By Jeffrey T. Kirchner, D.O.
Lancaster, Pennsylvania

Primary hyperparathyroidism (PHPT) is a disorder of calcium metabolism caused by excessive secretion of parathyroid hormone (PTH). In 80 to 90 per cent of patients, PTH excess is caused by a single hyperfunctioning gland or benign adenoma. The overall incidence of PHPT is about 27 cases per 100,000, but in persons older than 60, this increases to about 200 cases per 100,000 persons. Women are affected three times more frequently than men. Primary hyperparathyroidism is rare in children younger than 10 years of age.

Chief cell hyperplasia is the second most common cause of PHPT, with all four parathyroid glands involved. Distinguishing hyperplasia from adenoma by gross or histologic examination of a single gland remains controversial. In the traditional description, a rim of normal tissue surrounds the tumor or nodule of an adenoma. Unfortunately, this rim of normal parathyroid tissue cannot always be found by the pathologist viewing a single gland. DNA studies have identified genetic differences between adenomas and multiglandular hyperplasia. The origin of adenomas is primarily monoclonal and is associated with the loss of a PTH gene on chromosome 11. Glandular hyperplasia is polyclonal, reflecting the genetic predisposition of the parathyroid cell to react to environmental stimuli. A small number of adenomas have been associated with a history of local ionizing radiation to the head and neck.

The least common cause of primary disease is parathyroid cancer, which accounts for about 1 per cent of all patients with PHPT. Parathyroid carcinoma is characterized by excessive PTH secretion and a more severe degree of hypercalcemia.

A small subset of patients with PHPT have one of the two familial syndromes of multiple endocrine neoplasia (MEN I or MEN II). The type I disorder includes parathyroid hyperplasia, pancreatic islet-cell tumors, and pituitary adenoma. MEN type II includes parathyroid hyperplasia, thyroid carcinoma, and pheochromocytoma.

SIGNS AND SYMPTOMS

Most patients with primary hyperparathyroidism are asymptomatic at the time of diagnosis. Early diagnosis has been attributed, at least in part, to the detection of hypercalcemia through multiphasic screening tests. When patients are evaluated clinically, the symptoms are often vague and may include only fatigue, malaise, mild depression, or weakness. Symptoms are sometimes discovered retrospectively after hypercalcemia is found in an otherwise healthy person or in a patient being evaluated for an unrelated medical problem. In the era before multiphasic screening, the diagnosis of PHPT often was not made before the onset of osteitis fibrosa cystica, spontaneous pathologic fractures, vertebral collapse, shortening of stature, and other evidence of severe bone disease.

In the past, renal manifestations of PHPT were diverse, but only 5 per cent of patients today present with nephrolithiasis. Nephrocalcinosis (i.e., metastatic deposition of calcium in the renal parenchyma) can lead to decreased glomerular filtration and ultimate renal failure in the absence of treatment. Hypercalcemia may induce mild nephrogenic diabetes insipidus, with excessive thirst, polyuria, and polydipsia.

Gastrointestinal symptoms resulting from PHPT are diverse and nonspecific. They include abdominal pain, nausea, vomiting, anorexia, dyspepsia, peptic ulcer disease, and constipation. The incidence of acute and chronic pancreatitis is also increased in patients with PHPT.

Musculoskeletal disorders include myopathy, neuropathy, and nonspecific weakness. Associated joint problems may be related to gout, pseudogout, and/or periarticular calcification. The association between gout and PHPT has prompted some experts to recommend that all patients with gout be screened for the possibility of PTH excess.

Although a causal connection between PHPT and hypertension has been suggested, available data do not yet support this hypothesis. In particular, there are few or no data documenting the surgical cure of hypertension after parathyroidectomy (Table 1).

Table 1. Clinical Features of Primary Hyperparathyroidism

System Affected	Clinical Features
Renal	Calculi, nephrocalcinosis, reduced glomerular filtration, polyuria, polydipsia
Skeletal	Bone pain, cystic bone lesions, demineralization, spontaneous fractures
Neurologic	Weakness, fatigue, apathy, depression
Articular	Gout, pseudogout, periarticular calcification
Gastrointestinal	Abdominal pain, anorexia, constipation, peptic ulcer disease, pancreatitis
Cardiovascular	Arrhythmias, hypertension (?)
Ophthalmologic	Corneal calcifications (band keratopathy)

COURSE

The clinical course of patients with primary hyperparathyroidism is unpredictable and the subject of some debate. Many patients remain asymptomatic, but others more rapidly develop some of the signs and symptoms previously discussed. No long-term randomized, controlled trial has adequately assessed the progression of complications. Over the years, diagnosis and management of PHPT has focused on morbidity and not on mortality. Asymptomatic patients older than 50 years with mildly increased serum calcium concentrations are traditionally followed with close medical surveillance.

COMPLICATIONS

Because of early detection of PHPT, serious complications are rarely encountered. Among the more serious problems are nephrolithiasis and nephrocalcinosis that can lead to renal failure. Demineralization of bone with cystic changes and vertebral fractures may occur. Less common complications include cardiac arrhythmias, pancreatitis, insulin resistance, and an increased incidence of gastrointestinal malignancies. Hypercalcemic crisis (defined as volume depletion, encephalopathy, and a serum calcium exceeding 14 mg/dL) is an infrequently encountered complication of PHPT.

PHYSICAL EXAMINATION

The physical examination of most patients with primary hyperparathyroidism is unremarkable. A few patients may present with joint pain and swelling. Band keratopathy due to calcium deposition in the cornea is occasionally observed in late-stage disease. Mild to moderate muscle weakness occurs in many patients, although frank atrophy is rare. Depressive symptoms and memory impairment may be detected with a mental status examination. Skin necrosis induced by hypercalcemia is rarely seen.

LABORATORY PROCEDURES

The most useful test for the diagnosis of primary hyperparathyroidism is the measurement of the total serum calcium concentration (Table 2). In 96 per cent of patients

Table 2. Differential Diagnosis of Hypercalcemia

Primary hyperparathyroidism
Malignancy
Medications (e.g., lithium, thiazides, estrogens)
Familial hypocalciuric hypercalcemia
Granulomatous disease (e.g., sarcoidosis, tuberculosis, histoplasmosis)
Acute and chronic renal disease
Immobilization
Nonparathyroid endocrine disorders (e.g., thyrotoxicosis, pheochromocytoma, acute adrenal insufficiency)

with PHPT, the total serum calcium exceeds the normal range of 8.5 to 10.4 mg/dL. The upper limit of the reference range may vary slightly among laboratories, but it should never exceed 10.6 mg/dL.

All patients with fasting hypercalcemia on screening must have at least one or two repeat fasting calcium determinations. Appropriate correction of total serum calcium is required when the serum albumin concentration is decreased. One gram of albumin per deciliter of serum binds about 0.8 mg of calcium. Thus, 0.8 mg/dL should be added to or subtracted from the calcium concentration for every 1.0 g/dL of serum albumin greater than or less than 4.0 g/dL. Alternatively, the clinician may request measurement of the ionized calcium concentration in serum. Ionized calcium determinations are seldom required in the absence of complex abnormalities of plasma proteins or changes in acid-base status.

The definitive diagnosis of PHPT is established by measuring circulating immunoreactive parathyroid hormone (iPTH). Parathyroid hormone is a single-chain polypeptide of 84 amino acids. The serum iPTH concentration is increased in 90 per cent of patients with PHPT; the remaining 10 per cent typically have values in the high-normal range when serum is analyzed by the double-antibody (two-site) immunoradiometric assay or the immunochemiluminometric assay. These tests measure abnormally increased concentrations or the intact bioactive fragment of parathyroid hormone with a sensitivity of 90 per cent. These assays also distinguish PTH values that typically fall below the reference range when hypercalcemia is associated with malignancy.

Another advantage of two-site assays is their reliability in the presence of inactive, middle, and carboxyterminal PTH fragments that accumulate in patients with renal insufficiency. However, thiazide diuretics and lithium may spuriously increase serum calcium and PTH concentrations. These drugs should be discontinued before measuring PTH. All serum PTH analyses should be accompanied by concurrent measurement of serum calcium.

The oral calcium-loading test is occasionally used to diagnose hyperparathyroidism. After a baseline PTH determination, the patient ingests 1 g of elemental calcium, and serum PTH is measured at 30, 60, and 120 minutes after ingestion. In the truly hyperparathyroid patient, the PTH decreases to about 20 per cent of the baseline value. This test may help to confirm the diagnosis of PHPT in patients with intermittently or minimally increased serum calcium and a normal baseline PTH.

Measurement of urinary or nephrogenous cyclic AMP is a nonspecific test that is not considered cost effective in light of the newer PTH immunoassays.

OTHER BIOCHEMICAL MARKERS

The serum phosphorus concentration in PHPT is typically decreased, and the serum chloride often exceeds 102 mEq/L. The hypophosphatemia is a response to PTH-induced renal bicarbonate loss, which produces mild metabolic acidosis, decreased serum carbon dioxide content, and increased serum chloride concentration. However, serum phosphorus may be normal if blood samples are not obtained in the fasting state, because many foods contain phosphates. Renal insufficiency may also result in a normal or high serum phosphorus concentration.

Increased serum alkaline phosphatase secondary to increased osteoblastic activity may be seen in about 10 per cent of patients with PHPT. This is a nonspecific finding that occurs with various hypercalcemic conditions characterized by bone resorption, including malignancy and Paget's disease.

Hypercalciuria is common in PHPT. Although the physiologic effect of PTH on the kidney is to decrease calcium clearance, the filtered load is increased in PHPT, resulting in an excess of calcium in the urine. However, the degree of hypercalciuria in PHPT is typically less than that seen in other hypercalcemic conditions. A 24-hour measurement of urinary calcium excretion can supplement the evaluation of patients with PHPT, especially those with recurrent renal calculi. A 24-hour urine calcium determination can also aid the diagnosis of familial hypocalciuric hypercalcemia (FHH), an uncommon, autosomal dominant syndrome characterized by asymptomatic hypercalcemia. The pathophysiology is not fully understood. Some of these patients may also have increased PTH in the serum. The urinary calcium excretion in familial hypocalciurics is usually less than 150 mg/day, but patients with PHPT lose 300 to 350 mg/day.

RADIOLOGIC EVALUATION

Routine films are typically normal and therefore not very helpful in the evaluation of patients with PHPT. Chondrocalcinosis, articular erosions, and subchondral fractures may be seen in symptomatic patients. Diffuse osteopenia may be associated with a loss of cortical bone in the appendicular skeleton. Abdominal radiographs may show calcifications consistent with nephrocalcinosis or renal calculi. These findings usually warrant further investigation by intravenous urogram.

Measurement of bone density of the forearm with single-photon densitometry or with dual-energy x-ray absorptiometry has been recommended for following asymptomatic patients for the progression of disease. The routine use of these tests in following individual patients remains to be determined.

OTHER DIAGNOSTIC PROCEDURES

Several procedures have been evaluated in an attempt to improve preoperative localization of parathyroid adenomas. The tests include ultrasonography, computed tomography, magnetic resonance imaging, and thallium-technetium scanning. Invasive methods such as selective venous sampling and arteriography are also available. Most authorities indicate that these studies are not required for initial localization of the parathyroid glands. They may have a role in recurrent disease if a second surgery is required.

ERRORS IN DIAGNOSIS

The availability of sensitive and specific assays for iPTH has made the diagnosis of PHPT easier. Ectopic PTH production from ovarian and small cell carcinoma has been reported only rarely. With increased availability of reliable measurements of PTH-related protein, the hypercalcemia of malignancy will be more readily distinguished from PHPT.

The syndrome of FHH may be initially misdiagnosed as PHPT. However, these patients do not respond to surgery. An appropriate family history and a decreased 24-hour urine calcium are typically more than sufficient to distinguish FHH from PHPT.

HYPOPARATHYROIDISM

By Victor R. Lavis, M.D.,
and Herbert L. Fred, M.D.
Houston, Texas

Hypoparathyroidism encompasses a group of disorders characterized by deficiency of or resistance to parathyroid hormone (PTH). These disorders are outlined in Table 1.

The most common cause of deficient PTH secretion is the inadvertent removal of or damage to parathyroid tissue during thyroidectomy or surgery for hyperparathyroidism. The idiopathic type of hypoparathyroidism usually begins in childhood, but new cases occur even in the elderly. In this presumed autoimmune condition, the parathyroid glands are absent or atrophied. The DiGeorge syndrome is a congenital disorder in which the interrupted development of the third and fourth pharyngeal pouches results in parathyroid and thymic hypoplasia. In polyglandular endocrine failure type I, the onset of hypoparathyroidism usually occurs around age 7 to 9. Magnesium depletion, when severe, inhibits PTH secretion and blocks the normal stimulatory effect of hypocalcemia. The resultant state of physiologic hypoparathyroidism is readily reversed by magnesium repletion, although not by calcium supplementation alone. Rarely, hypoparathyroidism results from ^{131}I treatment of thyrotoxicosis, from siderosis of the parathyroids in patients with thalassemia, or from metastases to the parathyroids.

Chronic renal insufficiency may be viewed as a state of acquired resistance to PTH. Such resistance has two components. One is inadequate renal 1-hydroxylation of 25-hydroxyvitamin D, which leads to impaired gastrointestinal absorption of calcium; the other is retention of phosphate. Both of these mechanisms depress ionized calcium concentrations, resulting in compensatory secretion of PTH. Pseudohypoparathyroidism includes several heritable syndromes characterized by resistance to the phosphaturic action of PTH. Some of these patients have increased bone resorption; others have no bone disease.

SIGNS AND SYMPTOMS

Hypocalcemia, the cardinal feature of hypoparathyroidism, gives rise to a variety of clinical manifestations (Table 2). Any of these manifestations, if not otherwise explained, should prompt measurement of serum calcium, because most of them improve or disappear with calcium supplementation.

The neuromuscular instability of latent tetany can be elicited by testing for Trousseau's sign (i.e., carpal spasm appearing within 2 minutes after a blood pressure cuff applied to the arm is inflated above systolic pressure). Chvostek's sign (i.e., ipsilateral contraction of facial muscles after tapping the facial nerve below the zygomatic process) is less helpful, because it occurs in some normal individuals.

Seizures, papilledema, or both may signal idiopathic or

Table 1. Causes of Hypoparathyroidism

Deficiency of Parathyroid Hormone

- Surgery
- Idiopathic
- Congenital maldevelopment of derivatives of third and fourth pharyngeal pouches (DiGeorge syndrome)
- Polyglandular endocrine failure, type 1: mucocutaneous candidiasis, hypoparathyroidism, and Addison's disease
- Hypomagnesemia
- Irradiation (external beam or ^{131}I)
- Siderosis of parathyroids
- Cancer metastatic to parathyroids

Resistance to Parathyroid Hormone

- Pseudohypoparathyroidism
  - Type 1 (classic)
    - High circulating PTH concentration; low urinary cAMP; no phosphaturia or increase of urinary cAMP in response to injection of purified PTH
    - Resistance to other hormones, such as high concentrations of circulating thyrotropin, reduced serum prolactin, hypogonadism
    - Albright's hereditary osteodystrophy
    - Deficiency of the stimulatory guanine nucleotide-binding regulatory protein in erythrocytes and other tissues
  - Type 2
    - High circulating PTH concentration; injection of purified PTH elicits a normal increase of urinary cAMP, but no phosphaturia

PTH = parathyroid hormone; cAMP = cyclic adenosine monophosphate.

Table 2. Clinical Manifestations of Hypocalcemia

Neuromuscular Features

- Paresthesias (e.g., circumoral, fingers, toes)
- Tetany, overt or latent
- Laryngospasm with inspiratory stridor

Neuropsychiatric Features

- Seizures, generalized or focal
- Dementia
- Mental retardation
- Psychosis
- Calcifications in basal ganglia and cerebellum
- Movement disorders

Ectodermal Features

- Dry hair and skin
- Brittle nails with transverse bridging
- Defective tooth enamel
- Maleruption of teeth

Ocular Features

- Cataracts
- Blepharospasm
- Keratoconjunctivitis
- Papilledema, with and without raised intracranial pressure

Cardiac Features

- Dilated cardiomyopathy
- Congestive heart failure
- Electrocardiographic changes (e.g., prolonged Q-T interval; heart block)

postoperative hypoparathyroidism. Long-standing hypocalcemia may cause calcifications in the basal ganglia and cerebellum. These calcifications may be asymptomatic or produce neurologic syndromes such as parkinsonism, choreoathetosis, dystonic spasms, and dementia. Defects in enamel formation occur only in individuals whose hypocalcemia precedes or coincides with dental development.

LABORATORY TESTS

Normally, about 55 per cent of circulating calcium is tightly bound to organic or inorganic anions and is unavailable for bone formation or regulation of neuromuscular excitability. The physiologically relevant *ionized* fraction varies inversely with blood pH and plasma protein concentration. Ionized calcium can be measured directly with a calcium-specific electrode, and the typical reference range is 1.0 to 1.5 mmol/L (1 mmol/L = 4 mg/dL).

To determine the role of PTH in the pathogenesis of hypocalcemia, the clinician should request serum phosphorus and PTH determinations. PTH evokes phosphaturia, and the combination of hyperphosphatemia and hypocalcemia in a patient with normal renal function suggests that PTH is lacking or ineffective. Other than hypoparathyroidism, the only other situations characterized by hypocalcemia and hyperphosphatemia involve administration of exogenous phosphate (e.g., intravenous infusion, enema) or release of intracellular phosphate, as might occur with rhabdomyolysis, malignant hyperthermia, or the tumor lysis syndrome.

The most useful assay for PTH is the highly specific two-site immunoradiometric assay. Because hypocalcemia is a strong stimulus of PTH secretion, the finding of hypocalcemia together with a PTH concentration that does not exceed the reference range of 10 to 65 ng/L indicates inadequate parathyroid response. The combination of hypocalcemia, hyperphosphatemia, and increased serum PTH indicates inadequate renal response (i.e., resistance) to PTH.

DIAGNOSTIC APPROACH

To evaluate hypocalcemia, the clinician should inquire about paresthesias, muscle cramps, movement disorders, and seizures; test for Trousseau's sign; examine the teeth; and search for the somatic characteristics of Albright's hereditary osteodystrophy, such as short stature, obesity, round facies, mental retardation, and short fourth or fifth metacarpals. Clinicians should also obtain an electrocardiogram and measure circulating concentrations of total and ionized calcium, magnesium, phosphate, urea nitrogen, creatinine, albumin, and total protein. If the patient has hyperphosphatemia and ionized hypocalcemia, the serum concentration of PTH should be determined by two-site immunoradiometric assay. If the results indicate resistance to the action of PTH despite normal renal function, additional studies of the renal response to PTH may be appropriate (see Table 1).

ACUTE ADRENAL INSUFFICIENCY

By Sandra S. Hsu Werbel, M.D., *and* Robert Chin, Jr., M.D.
Winston-Salem, North Carolina

Acute adrenal insufficiency is a rare disorder associated with a high morbidity and mortality if unrecognized and allowed to progress. Acute adrenal insufficiency may result from primary glandular failure (e.g., autoimmune destruction, infectious or tumorous infiltration, hemorrhage, drug inhibition of steroidogenesis) or secondary glandular failure due to dysfunction of the hypothalamic-pituitary-adrenal (HPA) axis. A high index of suspicion is needed in diagnosing this disorder. Timely and accurate recognition of the specific form of adrenal insufficiency is an important determinant of the course and the treatment of this life-threatening disorder.

CLINICAL PRESENTATION

The clinical presentation of adrenal insufficiency depends on the degree of loss of the three major adrenal hormones: glucocorticoids, mineralocorticoids, and androgens. Glucocorticoids are essential for survival. These compounds influence carbohydrate, lipid, and protein metabolism; regulate immune, circulatory, and renal function; and influence growth, development, bone metabolism, and central nervous system activity. Glucocorticoid production is regulated by the HPA axis, an autoregulatory feedback loop. Varying concentrations of cortisol, the primary adrenal glucocorticoid end product, causes reciprocal and inverse changes in the output of corticotropin releasing factor from the hypothalamus and adrenocorticotropic hormone (ACTH) from the pituitary, maintaining cortisol within a normal range. However, other stimulatory input from stress and/or cytokines can also influence the HPA axis and increase the resting cortisol concentration. Mineralocorticoids primarily act to maintain intravascular volume by conserving sodium and eliminating potassium and hydrogen ions. Mineralocorticoid activity is regulated primarily by the renin-angiotensin-adrenal axis. Adrenal androgens exert their clinical effects primarily through conversion to active androgens or estrogens (e.g., testosterone or estradiol). These compounds contribute to the physiologic development of pubic and axillary hair during normal puberty. Although corticotropin (ACTH) is a potent stimulator of adrenal androgens, its precise role in androgen regulation is not clear, because other, unidentified factors have also been implicated in normal adrenal androgen secretion. The complexity of adrenocortical biochemistry leads to significant variation in the manifestation of acute adrenal insufficiency. Primary glucocorticoid deficiency is characterized by abnormalities in carbohydrate metabolism (e.g., hypoglycemia) and asthenia, but primary mineralocorticoid deficiency manifests predominantly as electrolyte disorders (e.g., hyperkalemia, hyponatremia) and intravascular volume depletion (e.g., systemic arterial hypotension). Isolated androgen deficiency in females is revealed by a loss of body hair but can go undetected in males owing to the greater contribution of gonadal testosterone to the total androgen pool. Primary adrenal insufficiency due to destruction of the adrenal glands manifests with symp-

Table 1. Clinical Findings in Adrenal Insufficiency

Symptoms and Signs	Isolated Hypo-aldosteronism	Secondary Adrenal Insufficiency *(Primary Glucocorticoid Deficiency)*	Primary Adrenal Insufficiency *(Mixed Glucocorticoid and Mineralocorticoid Deficiency)*
Asymptomatic	X		
Weakness or fatigue		XX	XX
Anorexia		X	X
Nausea or emesis		X	X
Malaise		X	X
Myalgias		X	X
Personality changes		X	X
Salt craving			X
Abdominal discomfort			X
Weight loss		XX	XX
Postural hypotension	X	X	X
Hypotension		XX	XX
Shock			X
Hyperpigmentation			X
Vitiligo			X
Loss of body hair (females)			X

X = can be seen.
XX = found in >50% of patients.

toms and signs of combined glucocorticoid, mineralocorticoid, and adrenal androgen deficiencies. Secondary adrenal insufficiency results from interruption of the normal HPA axis' function and, thus, presents with mainly signs and symptoms of glucocorticoid and androgen deficiency; the former being more clinically relevant. The cardinal features of both primary and secondary acute adrenal insufficiency in most patients are fatigue, weakness, and weight loss.

Adrenal insufficiency often is expressed gradually over a period of days in patients who are not acutely stressed. However, this disorder may also be revealed by sudden decompensation over a period of minutes to hours in a patient who is stressed by acute trauma, illness, or surgery. Symptoms often begin with nausea, vomiting, fatigue, weakness, myalgias, anorexia, and weight loss (Table 1). Gastrointestinal symptoms (e.g., anorexia, nausea, vomiting, abdominal pain, diarrhea) are common, as are psychiatric symptoms, including depression, apathy, or confusion. Symptoms of hypoglycemia are uncommon in fed patients, but confusion and stupor may occur in fasting individuals, children, and patients with panhypopituitarism with a deficiency of counter-regulatory hormones. Any history of autoimmune disorders, fungal disorders, tuberculosis, meningococcemia, human immunodeficiency virus infection, metastatic tumor, or exposure to drugs that decrease steroid synthesis (e.g., aminoglutethimide, etomidate, ketoconazole) may suggest the possibility of adrenal insufficiency and prompt further investigation.

Clinical signs tend to vary with the cause of the acute adrenal insufficiency. Patients with acute exacerbations of chronic primary adrenal insufficiency may show hyperpigmentation due to high serum concentrations of ACTH, especially over the extensor surfaces, hand creases, dental gingival margin, lips, or buccal mucosa. Hypotension may predominate, especially if mineralocorticoid deficiency exists. Increased cardiac output is frequently accompanied by normal wedge pressure and low systemic resistance. Patients with acute primary adrenal insufficiency can rapidly develop severe hypotension and hypovolemic shock. Acute adrenal hemorrhage in patients with fulminant meningococcemia (Waterhouse-Friderichsen syndrome) classically manifests with abdominal, flank, back, or chest pain, followed by fever, cyanosis, purpura, hypotension, and shock. Bilateral adrenal hemorrhage has also been reported in critically ill patients who present with fever, abdominal or flank pain, and a precipitous drop in the hemoglobin concentration.

Secondary adrenal insufficiency may be characterized by hypotension and, occasionally, fever. Hyperpigmentation typically is not present. In panhypopituitarism, hair loss often accompanies the signs of various pituitary hormone deficiencies. It is important to obtain a careful history of the patient's glucocorticoid use during the previous year. Some patients experience secondary adrenal insufficiency after withdrawal from prolonged use of exogenous steroids. Moon facies, buffalo hump, or cutaneous atrophy often indicate prior use of exogenous glucocorticoids, and the onset of symptoms of adrenal insufficiency indicates the need for supplemental or stress doses of steroids in the event of major surgery, trauma, or illness. Mineralocorticoid deficiency is not typically seen in secondary adrenal insufficiency, because aldosterone production is regulated through the renin-angiotensin-adrenal axis.

Isolated hypoaldosteronism is most often associated with the specific enzyme deficiencies described in the adrenogenital syndrome. Hyporeninemic hypoaldosteronism usually accompanies mild renal insufficiency, diabetes mellitus, or prolonged heparin therapy. Laboratory testing reveals hyperkalemia and occasional hyperchloremic metabolic acidosis.

The course of acute adrenal insufficiency ultimately leads to death if the disorder is not correctly recognized and treated. If the diagnosis is suspected, identified, and appropriately treated, significant morbidity and mortality can be avoided.

LABORATORY ABNORMALITIES

Eosinophilia is found in 10 to 20 per cent of patients with Addison's disease. Hyponatremia, hyperkalemia, increased urea nitrogen, and increased serum creatinine result from glucocorticoid and mineralocorticoid deficiencies. Anemia and reversible neutropenia are rarely reported in cases of adrenal insufficiency, but anemia may be prominent when adrenal hemorrhage occurs. Hypercalcemia and hypoglycemia can also be seen in acute adrenal insufficiency (Table 2).

Table 2. Laboratory Findings in Acute Adrenal Insufficiency

Laboratory Assessments	Isolated Hypo-aldosteronism	Secondary Adrenal Insufficiency	Primary Adrenal Insufficiency
Hyperkalemia	XX		XX
Hyponatremia	XX	XX	XX
Prerenal azotemia			X
Hypoglycemia		X	X
Anemia		X	X
Eosinophilia		X	X

X = can be seen.
XX = found in >50% of patients.

DIAGNOSTIC EVALUATION

The diagnosis of acute adrenal insufficiency requires a high index of suspicion. Patients with primary adrenal insufficiency typically have low serum cortisol and markedly increased ACTH. Patients with secondary adrenal insufficiency usually have low serum concentrations of cortisol and ACTH. The radioimmunoassay for ACTH has been notoriously unreliable, but some of the commercial laboratories specializing in endocrine assays now perform ACTH immunoassays of greater accuracy, sensitivity, and specificity. Serum cortisol concentrations normally exhibit a circadian pattern that is lost in response to stress.

However, basal ACTH and cortisol concentrations do not reflect the adequacy of HPA function, especially in partial adrenal insufficiency. Several provocative and imaging tests have been employed in the diagnosis of acute adrenal insufficiency (Table 3).

Initial assessment of the HPA axis is usually accomplished with the rapid synthetic ACTH stimulation test. A 250 μg dose of synthetic ACTH is injected intravenously or intramuscularly. Cortisol concentrations are measured before and after the administration of ACTH. In normal patients, the peak cortisol concentration at 30 minutes equals or exceeds 18 μg/dL. Alternatively, an increment (at 30 minutes) of 10 μg/dL over baseline is also considered within normal limits. When initial results are borderline or equivocal, repetition of the rapid ACTH test does not improve accuracy. A significant number of false-positive results can be seen, and the rapid ACTH stimulation test should be used primarily for screening, with a peak postinfusion cortisol equal to or greater than 20 μg/dL indicating normal adrenal function.

Aldosterone concentrations may also be used to distinguish primary from secondary forms of acute adrenal insufficiency. A normal aldosterone response with circulating concentrations greater than 4 ng/mL indicates secondary adrenal failure. Concentrations that fail to reach 4 ng/mL indicate primary adrenal failure. The patient must remain supine during testing, because plasma aldosterone concentrations vary greatly with changes in posture.

Occasionally, a prolonged ACTH stimulation test (lasting 48 to 72 hours) is required to distinguish primary from secondary adrenal failure. In primary adrenal insufficiency, cortisol concentrations remain subnormal despite prolonged ACTH stimulation.

The corticotropin-releasing hormone (CRH) stimulation test is used to distinguish pituitary from hypothalamic causes of secondary adrenal insufficiency. However, CRH is not readily available, and CRH stimulation testing is seldom warranted because treatment and patient outcomes are seldom influenced by this test.

Other tests that evaluate the stress response of the HPA axis include the insulin tolerance test and the metyrapone test. The insulin tolerance test is considered the gold standard for evaluation of chronic adrenal insufficiency; the metyrapone test has a similar sensitivity. Both tests involve exposure of the patient to a stress (hypoglycemia in the former, or cortisol depletion in the latter), followed by measurement of the cortisol response. Importantly, these tests are risky in patients with acute adrenal insufficiency. Both have precipitated adrenal crisis with fatalities, especially in unstable patients or those who could not tolerate significant stress.

After the diagnosis of acute adrenal insufficiency is made, appropriate imaging studies are required. Magnetic resonance imaging of the pituitary should be performed in the evaluation of secondary adrenal insufficiency to distinguish tumor from hemorrhage from an empty sella syndrome. Abdominal computed tomography should be performed in the evaluation of primary adrenal insufficiency to distinguish autoimmune adrenalitis from adrenal hemorrhage or infiltration.

Table 3. Diagnostic Testing for Adrenal Insufficiency

Characteristic	Serum Cortisol Concentration
Baseline; nonstressed	5–23 μg/dL or 138–635 nmol/L
Short ACTH stimulation test	30 min, 18–20 μg/dL 60 min, >18 μg/dL
2- to 3-day ACTH stimulation test	Day 1, 2, or 3, >20 μg/dL Increase in the 17-OHCS urinary excretion to 15 mg/24 hr

17-OHCS = 17-hydroxycorticosteroid.

CHRONIC ADRENAL INSUFFICIENCY

By Jesse C. Krakauer, M.D.
Birmingham, Michigan

and Sheldon S. Stoffer, M.D.
Southfield, Michigan

Chronic adrenal insufficiency, the state of relative hypofunction of the adrenal cortex, may be primary, resulting from adrenocortical disease (Addison's disease), or secondary, owing to lack of appropriate adrenocorticotropic hormone (ACTH) stimulation (pituitary-hypothalamic dysfunction). Adrenocortical steroid production from cholesterol proceeds along three principal pathways. Glucocorticosteroid (cortisol) and, most likely, adrenal androgen production are exclusively dependent on ACTH, while mineralocorticoid (aldosterone) production is regulated primarily by the potassium-renin-angiotensin system. In primary adrenal insufficiency, plasma aldosterone concentrations are low or undetectable and unresponsive to ACTH, while in secondary adrenal insufficiency, aldosterone concentrations are normal and the aldosterone response to ACTH is preserved. Therefore, the aldosterone status can be quite helpful in distinguishing primary from secondary adrenal insufficiency.

With the advent of specific hormone replacement therapy in the 1950s and increased understanding of adrenal physiology in the 1960s, mortality from adrenal disorders declined dramatically and the need for accurate diagnosis of adrenal insufficiency was clear. Since the 1970s, administration of α^{1-24}-cosyntropin, a synthetic subunit of ACTH, has provided a simple, highly reliable test for glucocorticoid reserve. Development of abdominal computed tomography (CT) improved the imaging of gross anatomic abnormalities, but CT may also have contributed to the "incidentaloma epidemic." In the 1980s and 1990s, assays of aldosterone and ACTH have largely displaced the cumbersome, time-consuming, and potentially hazardous tests still promoted in many textbooks. Idiopathic atrophy, presumably an autoimmune disorder, is now recognized as the most common etiology of Addison's disease. Cosyntropin testing and measurement of adrenal antibodies may be clinically useful in presymptomatic patients who are likely to develop autoimmune adrenal insufficiency. However, there has been little recent interest in the diagnostic evaluation and monitoring of therapy in established adrenal insufficiency. The recommendations in contemporary sources for empirical one-dose-for-all therapy, adjusted by clinical response, are little changed over the last 30 years. As one patient, first diagnosed in 1954, recently wrote: "Other Addisonians, along with me, all seem to have the same complaint. Doctors are not too interested in us. I guess we're not a challenge, as basically there is only one treatment." By contrast, significant, well-justified attention is given to ensuring physiologic thyroid replacement in hypothyroidism and to normalizing the glucose profile in diabetes mellitus. Similarly, diagnostic assessment of therapy in chronic adrenal insufficiency is also feasible with the use of readily available tests.

CAUSES

Primary Adrenal Insufficiency (Table 1)

Although autoimmunity is currently the most common cause of adrenal failure in Western clinical practice, the rising incidence of tuberculosis may result in a resurgence of tuberculous adrenal insufficiency. In addition, many cases of primary adrenal insufficiency are being reported in patients with advanced acquired immunodeficiency syndrome (AIDS), including cryptococcal, mycobacterial, cytomegaloviral, histoplasmosis, and *Pneumocystis carinii* infections; Kaposi's sarcoma; lymphoma; and adrenal hemorrhage. Adrenal enzyme inhibition by ketoconazole and accelerated cortisol clearance by rifampin may also contribute to adrenal insufficiency in AIDS patients. Finally, steroid substrate deficiency may be associated with profound hypocholesterolemia.

Adrenocortical antibodies can be detected in 60 to 80 per cent of patients with idiopathic adrenal atrophy. These antibodies may be the sole manifestation of autoimmunity. Some of these antibodies are specific for 21-hydroxylase, a cytochrome P-450 enzyme that may be found in the serum of addisonian patients. The polyglandular autoimmune syndrome refers to a relatively rare group of disorders, often divided into three types. Type I is characterized by the onset of candidiasis and hypoparathyroidism in childhood, followed by Addison's disease in the teens. Most cases are sporadic, with no gender preference and with autosomal recessive inheritance in some families. Addison's disease associated with autoimmune thyroid disease and/or insulin-dependent diabetes mellitus defines type II, or Schmidt's, syndrome, which has also been associated with gonadal failure and hypophysitis with diabetes insipidus. Nonendocrine diseases associated with Schmidt's syndrome include myasthenia gravis, idiopathic thrombocytopenic purpura, rheumatoid arthritis, Sjögren's syndrome, vitiligo, alopecia, and premature graying of the hair. Autoimmune thyroid disease and Addison's disease have also been reported following immunotherapy for cancer with interleukin-2 plus tumor-infiltrating lymphocytes. Type II presents most often in young adults, especially women (3:1). Type II is typically a familial, autosomal dominant disorder with variable penetrance and linkage to HLA subtypes B8, DR3, and DR4. The same syndrome in the absence of, or prior to, the development of adrenal failure is termed type III.

Tumor metastases and a number of systemic diseases (sarcoidosis, amyloidosis, and hemochromatosis) can involve the adrenals and occasionally present as adrenal insufficiency. Adrenal function may also be destroyed by hemorrhage due to anticoagulation, disseminated intravascular coagulation (DIC), or the Waterhouse-Friderichsen syndrome or infarction due to adrenal vein thrombosis or shock.

Disorders of lipid metabolism (e.g., adrenoleukodystrophy and adrenomyeloneuropathy), classic 21-hydroxylase deficiency (congenital adrenal hyperplasia), and familial adrenal hypoplasia may also present with adrenal failure.

Bilateral adrenalectomy or treatment with mitotane, suramin, metyrapone, or aminoglutethimide can result in adrenal insufficiency. Rifampin increases the hepatic metabolism of cortisol, while phenytoin increases the hepatic metabolism of fludrocortisone. Phenytoin has precipitated mineralocorticoid deficiency in patients with chronic Addison's disease. Hypoaldosteronism with normal cortisol production may complicate long-term heparin therapy or diabetic nephropathy.

Table 1. Causes of Chronic Adrenal Insufficiency

Causes
Primary Adrenal Insufficiency
Intrinsic Adrenocortical Pathologies
Autoimmune ("idiopathic" atrophy, polyglandular)
Infectious (tuberculosis, fungal, viral, AIDS associated)
Hemorrhage (anticoagulation, DIC, shock)
Metastatic
Adrenalectomy
Exogenous or Hormone Pathway Mediated
Severe congenital adrenal hyperplasia
Enzyme inhibitors (ketoconazole, aminoglutethimide)
Adrenal cytotoxics (mitotane)
Accelerated steroid metabolism (phenytoin, rifampin)
ACTH receptor defects (familial, blocking antibodies)
Secondary Adrenal Insufficiency
Pituitary-Hypothalamic Disease
Pituitary necrosis–stalk section (Sheehan's syndrome, trauma)
Neoplasm (pituitary tumor, craniopharyngioma, metastatic)
Infiltration-granulomatous (sarcoidosis, histiocytosis X)
Infection (tuberculosis, fungus)
Autoimmune (lymphocytic hypophysitis)
Pituitary-Hypothalamic Suppression
Exogenous corticosteroids
Endogenous corticosteroid excess (adrenal tumor or adenomatous hyperplasia, ectopic ACTH)

Secondary Adrenal Insufficiency (see Table 1)

In the absence of panhypopituitarism, ACTH secretion is preserved in most patients with pituitary disease. Isolated ACTH deficiency, and selective loss of hypothalamic corticotropin-releasing hormone, have been reported, but these deficiencies are associated most frequently with sustained hypercortisolism, regardless of its cause. "Peripheral" glucocorticoid insufficiency is seen in patients treated with the steroid antagonist mifepristone (RU 486) and in syndromes associated with glucocorticoid receptor defects. ACTH receptor defects may lead to syndromes that mix the characteristic hyperpigmentation of primary adrenal insufficiency with the intact renin-aldosterone axis typical of secondary adrenal insufficiency. High doses of Megace (megestrol acetate) and other progestational agents may cause secondary adrenal suppression after prolonged administration to patients.

Adrenal insufficiency has occurred after the surgical removal of clinically "silent" adrenal adenomas, with subtle endogenous hypercortisolism only suspected in retrospect. The risk and duration of hypothalamic-pituitary suppression from corticosteroid therapy varies with the specific pharmacologic agent, its dose, and its duration of use. For chronic use, alternate-day dosing with a relatively short-acting agent such as prednisone, administered as a single morning dose, is not likely to cause secondary adrenal insufficiency. Daily or split-dose therapy typically leads to adrenal atrophy and disruption of ACTH release, but adrenal suppression is rarely of clinical significance unless the duration of therapy extends beyond 2 weeks. In patients who withdraw from long-term corticosteroid therapy, recovery of adrenocortical responsiveness to ACTH precedes return of the capacity to release ACTH following stress. Inadequate central ACTH release and the increased risk of stress-induced adrenal crisis can be seen up to 1 year after the complete withdrawal of chronic corticosteroid therapy.

CLINICAL FEATURES

The diagnosis of adrenal insufficiency should always be considered in patients who report weight loss, anorexia, salt craving, nausea, altered bowel habits, syncope, weakness, dizziness, arthralgias, fatigue, depression, and altered cognition. Accurate statistics are not available on the frequency of these signs and symptoms in patients with adrenal insufficiency. The National Addison's Disease Foundation (Great Neck, NY) cites a survey in 1960 showing a prevalence of 39 cases diagnosed per million population in London, England.

The succinct description of adrenal insufficiency by Addison in 1855 remains clinically useful nearly 150 years later: "Anemia, general languor and debility, remarkable feebleness of the heart's action, irritability of the stomach, and a peculiar change of color in the skin." Adrenal insufficiency may still go undiagnosed for years after the onset of symptoms. A recent patient whose symptoms eluded diagnosis for 7 years poignantly stated: "I was branded as a malingerer and goldbrick, because of the inability of . . . doctors to analyze this malady. I almost lost my career, reputation and life as a result." In long-standing Addison's disease, the stimulation of melanocytes by ACTH and co-released β-lipotropin causes easy or persistent tanning as well as hyperpigmentation of the palmar creases, elbows, knees, lips, and buccal mucosa. Concurrent vitiligo is common. Calcified pinnae, or "stone ears," have been described. Many of the clinical manifestations of adrenal insufficiency have been attributed to the loss of antagonism of insulin effects and to the loss of glucocorticoid effect on cardiac inotropism and the vascular response to beta-agonists. Addisonian anemia is normochromic and normocytic and is usually associated with neutropenia. Unexplained lymphocytosis or eosinophilia may occasionally provide a sentinel diagnostic clue. Depression, irritability, and restlessness are frequent symptoms. The electroencephalogram may show generalized slowing and reduced amplitude. Altered taste, olfaction, and hearing are reversible with replacement therapy. Axillary and pubic hair may be decreased in women.

In both primary and secondary adrenal insufficiency, mild hyponatremia frequently occurs and is often associated with increased serum concentrations of arginine vasopressin. In Addison's disease, mineralocorticoid deficiency and sodium loss contribute to hyponatremia, which, in turn, may lead to dehydration, hyperkalemia, and acidosis. Mild to moderate hypercalcemia is a frequent finding that may contribute to the symptomatic presentation of adrenal insufficiency.

DIAGNOSTIC TESTING IN SUSPECTED ADRENAL INSUFFICIENCY (Table 2)

The 30-minute cosyntropin test should be performed whenever adrenal insufficiency is a consideration. The administration of 250 μg of cosyntropin typically induces a serum cortisol increment of at least 7 μg/dL, with a peak cortisol response exceeding 18 μg/dL. The cosyntropin test is quick and safe and can be done without regard to time of day, patient status, or patient age. Some maximally stressed patients show little or no increment in cortisol concentrations that are already *well above* the reference range. Clearly, however, such patients should not be confused with addisonian patients. It is most often expedient to obtain a baseline serum ACTH and cortisol as well as baseline and postcosyntropin aldosterone concentrations. Normally, the aldosterone concentration increases by more than 5 ng/dL. An increased ACTH concentration with a low serum cortisol is diagnostic of Addison's disease, but these results should be confirmed by demonstrating the absence of stimulation of cortisol and aldosterone production by cosyntropin. A low or an inappropriately normal concentration of ACTH in a cortisol-deficient patient showing normally responsive aldosterone concentrations is diagnostic of secondary adrenal insufficiency. Although the aldosterone response may be somewhat attenuated in secondary adrenal insufficiency compared with normal control values, it is nearly always greater than the response in primary adrenal insufficiency. Plasma renin activity is also typically normal in secondary adrenal insufficiency while distinctly increased in primary adrenal insufficiency.

Intermediate cortisol responses to cosyntropin (plasma cortisol concentration fails to increase by 7 μg/dL or to exceed 18 μg/dL within 30 to 60 minutes) indicate impaired adrenal function and may merit stress steroid coverage or a therapeutic trial of replacement therapy in selected patients. Following a borderline cortisol response, some experts always perform intravenous infusion of cosyntropin (0.25 mg) over 6 to 8 hours, with plasma cortisol measurements at 4, 6, and 8 hours. The cortisol concentration normally rises above 35 μg/dL and usually peaks between 40 and 80 μg/dL. Others, however, have not performed such testing routinely; instead, they closely monitor patients for progressive adrenal insufficiency. Further diagnostic studies are undertaken when appropriate, and repeat cosyntropin testing is performed at least annually, especially in patients with polyglandular syndromes or de-

Table 2. Diagnostic Testing in Adrenal Insufficiency

Adrenal insufficiency suspected from history, physical examination, or laboratory studies

Proceed to next steps

1. Measure baseline ACTH if Addison's disease is suspected
2. Measure baseline cortisol and aldosterone
3. Administer cosyntropin, 250 μg IV or IM*
4. Measure 30-minute cortisol and aldosterone

Normal responses to cosyntropin stimulation:
Cortisol increment > 7 μg/dL, peak > 18 μg/dL
Aldosterone increment > 5 ng/dL

IM = intramuscularly; IV = intravenously.

*In suspected secondary adrenal insufficiency, a 1-ng dose may be more sensitive. In some cases, an 8-hour cosyntropin infusion test may be needed.

tectable adrenal antibodies. Some have advocated adrenal antibody testing and clinical assessment annually in patients with type III polyglandular autoimmunity (who, on diagnosis of adrenal insufficiency, are reclassified as type II) and also in the first-degree relatives of patients with type II and III polyglandular autoimmunity syndromes. Those high-risk patients with adrenal antibodies or previous borderline cortisol responses could undergo cosyntropin testing to achieve early diagnosis in advance of acute symptomatic adrenal insufficiency. An alternative approach to the diagnosis of mild secondary adrenal insufficiency is the low-dose (1-μg) cosyntropin test, which may be more sensitive in detecting secondary adrenal insufficiency than the standard 250-μg infusion. Recently, four patients with secondary adrenal insufficiency have been described who had normal responses of cortisol with the standard 250-μg cosyntropin 30-minute test, but clearly abnormal responses to metyrapone as well as to 8-hour cosyntropin infusion in two of two patients tested. Therefore, in suspected secondary adrenal insufficiency, a normal 30-minute 250-μg standard cosyntropin test cannot be relied on and must be confirmed by other tests.

AUXILIARY TESTING (Table 3)

In the sick patient who may have adrenal insufficiency, steroid coverage for stress should not be withheld pending the results of initial diagnostic studies. High resolution CT is now the preferred adrenal imaging procedure. Computed tomography–guided adrenal biopsy in patients with primary adrenal insufficiency may help the physician distinguish tuberculosis and metastasis in the gland. Chest films should be reviewed for signs of tuberculosis or other granulomatous diseases, and tuberculin skin testing should be performed. Evaluation of secondary adrenal insufficiency not due to corticosteroid therapy usually includes magnetic resonance imaging or CT of the pituitary as well as testing for other pituitary hormone deficiencies.

The initial laboratory characterization should include a complete blood count and differential as well as measurement of serum electrolytes, creatinine, and calcium. Thyroid function should be evaluated with a serum thyroid-stimulating hormone (TSH) test and a free thyroxine estimate. Tests for thyroid antibodies may provide evidence for autoimmunity. Adrenal antibody testing is increasingly available and may be more widely used for screening in the future. In males, screening for hypogonadism with serum total and/or free testosterone may be appropriate. In women with menstrual irregularities, infertility, or changes in sexual hair growth, antiovarian antibodies may be detected.

Table 3. Auxiliary Laboratory Tests in Adrenal Insufficiency

Primary Adrenal Insufficiency
CBC, differential
Biochemical profile (electrolytes, calcium)
Thyroid testing (TSH, thyroxine index, thyroid antibodies)
Gonadal function (if hypogonadism suspected)
Adrenal antibodies
Adrenal imaging and biopsy (computed tomography, magnetic resonance imaging)
Chest radiograph–PPD tuberculin skin testing
Secondary Adrenal Insufficiency
Pituitary function testing (possible role for ovine corticotropin-releasing hormone)
Pituitary hypothalamic imaging and biopsy (magnetic resonance imaging, computed tomography)

CBC = complete blood count; PPD = purified protein derivative; TSH = thyroid-stimulating hormone.

The management of patients whose diagnosis of adrenal insufficiency has not been confirmed may present a significant clinical challenge. Without endocrine testing, the clinician cannot logically decide to discontinue possibly unnecessary steroid therapy. The following vignette demonstrates the clinical utility of aldosterone measurements in a patient receiving replacement corticosteroids:

A 34-year-old woman had received prednisone, 5 mg twice daily, for possible adrenal insufficiency following delivery of her first child 3 years previously. On examination, the patient was 5 feet 3 inches tall and weighed 113 pounds. Her blood pressure was 95/60 mm Hg. Pubic and axillary hair growth was normal. Adrenal studies were done at 4:00 PM, 8 hours after the last dose of prednisone. Baseline cortisol was 3 μg/dL (normal 3 to 13 μg/dL), and aldosterone 5 ng/dL (normal 2 to 5 ng/dL). A half hour after Cortrosyn injection, the serum aldosterone concentration increased to 39 ng/dL (normal increase >5 ng/dL), but the serum cortisol was only 5 μg/dL. From these results, physicians concluded that the patient did not have primary adrenal insufficiency. Based on prior normal results of pituitary magnetic resonance imaging and history of a subsequent second full-term pregnancy with resumption of normal menses, physicians further concluded that her blunted cortisol response to Cortrosyn was likely the result of prednisone therapy. After 2 months of prednisone, 5 mg as a single morning dose, the baseline serum cortisol concentration 24 hours after the last dose of prednisone was 13 μg/dL and increased to 24 μg/dL 30 minutes after Cortrosyn. While the patient continued to receive prednisone, 2.5 mg each morning, she experienced increasing joint discomfort, and it was thought that the previous higher-dose prednisone therapy had likely been masking an underlying arthritic condition. Indeed, on further testing, HLA-B27 antigen was found to be positive. However, while the patient received prednisone, 2.5 mg daily, the serum cortisol concentration was 14 μg/dL at 11:00 AM, and she was assured that she did not have either primary or secondary adrenal insufficiency and that prednisone therapy could be discontinued.

DIAGNOSTIC CAVEATS

A number of older but still frequently mentioned diagnostic tests do not have a role in the contemporary assessment of adrenal insufficiency. Among these are biochemical stress testing of adrenal function with metyrapone (an inhibitor of the conversion of 11-deoxycortisol to cortisol, not currently available in the United States) and insulin-induced hypoglycemia. The accuracy and reliability of the two-site IRMA (immunoradiometric assay) for ACTH have greatly diminished the need for "standard" tests of glucocorticoid reserve with 24-hour ACTH infusions and 24-hour urine collections for steroid determinations. However, do not measure ACTH immediately after cosyntropin administration, because one-site binding will occur and will falsely lower the ACTH IRMA result. Further, plasma ACTH declines rapidly, and accurate measurements require special collection containers, rapid centrifugation, and freezing. Some experts have proposed that in appropriate clinical circumstances, the sensitive IRMA ACTH assay be used to screen for adrenal insufficiency. Ovine corticotropin-releasing hormone (CRH) is available in some facilities for direct testing of corticotroph responsiveness, but CRH offers no clear advantage as an agent for the assessment of secondary adrenal insufficiency.

Urinary 17-hydroxy and keto steroid determinations are no longer made in most commercial laboratories. These measurements have been supplanted by urinary cortisol, serum aldosterone, and specific steroid hormone assays. Most patients with adrenal insufficiency have decreased 24-hour urine cortisol, but some may have values in the low-normal range. Therefore, urinary cortisol is not a useful test in the initial evaluation of adrenal insufficiency.

Although hypothyroidism is commonly encountered and diagnosed in daily practice, the physician should always consider the possibility of underlying adrenal insufficiency in patients beginning therapy for hypothyroidism. Adrenal crisis has been reported with the initiation of thyroid hormone replacement in patients with previously undiagnosed adrenal insufficiency.

DIAGNOSTIC TESTING IN PATIENTS WITH ESTABLISHED ADRENAL INSUFFICIENCY (Table 4)

Patients with Addison's disease describe low energy levels, lethargy, weakness, morning depression, abdominal pain, arthralgias, and muscle cramps. As illustrated by the following vignette, "standard" replacement therapy may not prevent periods of severe, symptomatic adrenal insufficiency from occurring on a daily basis for years:

A 28-year-old white male presented with abdominal pain, lethargy, weakness, and marked salt craving. He was hyperpigmented and had lost 20 pounds. Primary adrenal insufficiency was diagnosed. The patient recalls feeling better after replacement treatment with cortisone acetate, 25 mg at 8:00 AM and 12.5 mg at 5:00 PM, along with Florinef 0.1-mg tablets, half a tablet daily. Despite adherence to this regimen over the next 5 years, the patient never returned fully to his normal healthy state. He was hospitalized for adrenal crisis during a bout of the flu 18 months prior to evaluation. Antiadrenal antibodies were positive at 2 U (normal undetectable). Urine for cortisol was 10 μg per 24 hours (normal 25 to 50 μg). At 8:00 AM, the serum ACTH was 2790 pg/mL (normal 9 to 52 pg/mL). The simultaneous serum cortisol was 2 μg/dL (normal 8 to 24 μg/dL). The ACTH drawn at 5:00 PM was 750 pg/mL, with a simultaneous serum cortisol of 3 μg/dL (normal 2 to 17 μg/dL). After reclining 1 hour from 4:00 PM to 5:00 PM, the plasma renin was 7.6 ng/mL per hour (normal less than 10 ng/mL). The serum aldosterone was less than 1 ng/dL (normal 2 to 9 ng/dL). The patient was asked to discontinue cortisone acetate and begin treatment with hydrocortisone, 15 mg at 6:00 AM, 15 mg at 2:00 PM, and 10 mg at 10:00 PM. Because the patient lived 1500 miles away, he could not return for short-term follow-up studies. However, on two phone calls he reported feeling much better, with more energy and less need for sleep. His muscle strength improved, he resumed regular jogging, and he considered training for a marathon. At 9 months, the 24-hour urine cortisol was 115 μg. Subsequently, the hydrocortisone prescription was tapered to 15 mg at 6:00 AM, 10 mg at 2:00 PM, and 10 mg at 10:00 PM. The repeat urinary cortisol was 53 μg per 24 hours (normal 25 to 50 μg).

Table 4. Diagnostic Testing in Established Adrenal Insufficiency Patients Receiving Hydrocortisone Therapy (Ambulatory Protocol)

Collect urine sample to measure 24-hour urinary excretion of cortisol on day before initiating protocol.

Patient maintains usual medication and as much of daily routine as possible.

8 AM: Measure serum cortisol and corticotropin levels.

12 NOON: Measure serum cortisol and corticotropin levels.

4–5 PM: Have patient recline for 1 hour.

5 PM: Measure blood pressure and plasma renin, serum electrolytes, aldosterone,* cortisol, and corticotropin levels.

*Omit aldosterone testing, if aldosterone confirmed to be deficient on prior testing.

In the absence of endocrine testing, chronic symptoms may be difficult to interpret, as may the results of dosing adjustments. The testing protocol can often provide objective evidence of periods of cortisol excess and deficiency in the same patient on a less-than-optimal regimen. The 24-hour urine cortisol assay is particularly useful during efforts to find the dose that maintains most patients within or just above the reference range. Plasma renin provides a guide to the need for and appropriate dosing of mineralocorticoid replacement with fludrocortisone. A plasma renin of less than 10 ng/mL per hour is probably adequate for most patients, and overtreatment with fludrocortisone (biologic half-life 36 to 72 hours) may be complicated by hypertension and hypokalemia. The following case demonstrates that excessive corticosteroid therapy can be hazardous, yet the patient may be subject to symptomatic adrenal insufficiency in the course of the day because of the poor timing of administered doses:

A 74-year-old woman was diagnosed with Addison's disease 12 years ago. The patient recalls lethargy, hyperpigmentation, and improvement of symptoms after starting on hydrocortisone replacement. She underwent surgery for chronic pancreatitis 14 years ago and subsequently had two further episodes of pancreatitis, the last some 2 years ago. (Chronic abdominal pain attributed to recurrent pancreatitis has previously been reported in Addison's disease.) The patient developed primary hypothyroidism and began replacement therapy with daily levothyroxine, 0.1 mg. Two years ago, she fell and fractured her left hip and continues to have chronic hip and back pain. Bone densitometry studies showed severe osteopenia, with values 78 per cent of normal age expectation at the unfractured right hip and 66 per cent for the cortical radius. The patient was taking 40 mg of hydrocortisone daily; 15 mg at 8:00 AM, 15 mg at NOON, and 10 mg at 5:00 PM. With this regimen, 8:00 AM serum ACTH was 176 pg/mL (normal 9 to 52 pg/mL), and serum cortisol was 3.0 μg/dL (normal 5 to 25 μg/dL), confirming the diagnosis of primary adrenal insufficiency. At noon, the serum ACTH was 10 pg/mL (normal 9 to 52 pg/mL), and serum cortisol was 21 μg/dL. At 5:00 PM, the serum ACTH was 7 pg/mL (normal 7 to 52 pg/mL), and the serum cortisol was 16 μg/dL (normal 3 to 13 μg/dL). The patient reclined from 4:00 PM to 5:00 PM. Serum renin activity was 6.9 ng/mL per hour (normal <10 ng/mL), and serum aldosterone was less that 2.5 ng/dL (normal 4.0 to 16 ng/dL). Adrenal antibodies were positive at 1:80 (normally undetectable). While on the total dose of 40 mg of hydrocortisone a day, 24-hour urine cortisol was 63 μg (normal 25 to 50 μg). With the daily hydrocortisone reduced to 30 mg, administered as 10 mg every 8 hours, 24-hour urinary cortisol was 55 μg. Owing to concerns about adverse corticosteroid effects on bone mass, the hydrocortisone dosing was decreased to 10 mg at 7:00 AM, 10 mg at 3:00 PM, and 5 mg at 11:00 PM. The patient seemed to be feeling quite well on the new regimen, and she felt that she had more energy. Repeat 24-hour urine cortisol was 32 μg.

Reassessment of patients during treatment can be done frequently with selected tests. The full-day outpatient protocol can be repeated at 1- to 2-year intervals to monitor changing requirements.

SUMMARY

The diagnosis of chronic adrenal insufficiency is important and is readily demonstrated by measuring cosyntropin-stimulated serum cortisol and aldosterone concentrations. Modern hormone assays allow efficient diagnosis and may also be utilized in ongoing diagnostic assessment of patients with established adrenal insufficiency.

CUSHING'S SYNDROME

By James W. Findling, M.D.
Milwaukee, Wisconsin

Cushing's syndrome is an endocrinopathy reflecting the biologic effects of glucocorticoid excess. Although the source of corticosteroid excess may be either endogenous or exogenous, the clinical manifestations are similar and well appreciated by all clinicians. Endogenous hypercortisolism is an unusual disorder (annual incidence of 10 to 15 new cases per million population per year), but its clinical features—in particular, weight gain, hypertension, and glucose intolerance—are seen in the daily practice of primary care physicians. The clinical diagnosis of Cushing's syndrome does not depend on any one specific clinical feature, but on a constellation of features. The disorder usually evolves insidiously, with the duration of illness often exceeding 4 to 5 years. The appreciation of subclinical Cushing's syndrome in some patients with incidentally discovered adrenal masses has provided evidence that mild hypercortisolism is as difficult to appreciate as subclinical hypothyroidism or hyperthyroidism. The diagnosis can be achieved only with a high index of suspicion and the use of simple biochemical screening studies.

CLINICAL FEATURES

Endogenous hypercortisolism may affect virtually every organ system, and its severity is usually a function of the duration and magnitude of the excessive cortisol secretion. Table 1 summarizes prominent clinical findings and their prevalence in patients with Cushing's syndrome.

The most apparent clinical manifestation of Cushing's syndrome is typically obesity. Although cortisol is actually a catabolic hormone, glucocorticoid excess results in insulin resistance and stimulation of appetite. Patients usually gain weight with a truncal distribution, and have a characteristic body habitus and facial appearance. One of the most reliable physical findings is the presence of significant supraclavicular fullness. These patients may often be indistinguishable from patients with the syndrome of insulin resistance (syndrome X), emphasizing again how frequently Cushing's syndrome should be a common diagnostic consideration in clinical practice. Although obesity is considered a hallmark of Cushing's syndrome, some patients, particularly those with ectopic adrenocorticotropic hormone (ACTH) and severe hypercortisolism, do not gain weight. Depression resulting from cortisol excess may even lead to weight loss. A few patients have presented with anorexia nervosa.

Table 1. Clinical Features of Cushing's Syndrome (% Prevalence)

General		Neuropsychiatric	85
Obesity	90	Gonadal dysfunction	
Hypertension	85	Menstrual disorder	70
Skin		Impotence, decreased libido	85
Plethora	70	Metabolic	
Hirsutism	75	Glucose intolerance, diabetes	75, 20
Striae	50	Hyperlipidemia	70
Acne	35	Polyuria	30
Bruising	35	Kidney stones	15
Musculoskeletal			
Osteopenia	80		
Weakness	65		

Cutaneous wasting from thinning of the epidermis and underlying connective tissue causes the thin skin, plethoric facial appearance, and easy bruisability that is characteristic of this disorder. Acne may result from hyperandrogenism. Characteristic violaceous striae are usually depressed and wide (>1 cm), in contrast with the pinkish white striae seen with pregnancy or rapid weight changes. Striae may occur on the abdomen, hips, buttocks, thighs, and axilla and are typically found only in patients younger than 40 years of age. Acanthosis nigricans due to hyperinsulinism and insulin resistance may also be found in patients with Cushing's syndrome. In women, hirsutism due to adrenal androgen excess is typically manifested as excessive terminal hair; increased lanugo facial hair is also seen in some patients.

Cushing's syndrome often causes profound muscular atrophy and weakness, especially in the proximal muscles of the lower extremities. Myopathy may be less prominent in well-conditioned patients because exercise decreases glucocorticoid-induced muscular atrophy. Cortisol excess may also cause significant osteopenia. Patients may present with frequent unexplained fractures, typically of the feet, ribs, or vertebrae. Metabolic bone disease may be the major feature of Cushing's syndrome in some patients; indeed, unexplained osteopenia in any young or middle-aged adult should always prompt an evaluation for Cushing's syndrome, even if there are no other signs or symptoms of cortisol excess. Although avascular necrosis of bone is a well-appreciated complication of exogenous glucocorticoid administration, this problem is rarely observed in patients with endogenous hypercortisolism. Cortisol excess impairs renal tubular absorption of calcium. Secondary hyperparathyroidism then results from decreased hepatic hydroxylation of vitamin D and inhibition of vitamin D–dependent absorption of calcium from the intestine. Impaired renal tubular absorption of calcium leads to hypercalciuria and nephrolithiasis in patients with Cushing's syndrome.

Neuropsychiatric manifestations are common in Cushing's syndrome. Frequently reported symptoms include depressed mood, crying, decreased mental concentration, impaired memory, insomnia, and decreased libido. Euphoria and even manic behavior may occur. In untreated patients with Cushing's syndrome, depression may lead to suicide. Children with Cushing's syndrome typically perform well in school. However, treatment of the disorder may be associated with some deterioration in that performance. Neurologic manifestations of hypercortisolism include pseudotumor cerebri and spinal lipomatosis producing spinal cord or nerve root compression.

Increased blood pressure can be documented in most patients with Cushing's syndrome, and hypertension may occur even though salt intake is restricted. Hypertension, hyperlipidemia, and diabetes in patients with Cushing's syndrome substantially increase their risk of developing atherosclerotic cardiovascular disease.

Excessive cortisol stimulates the production of very low density lipoprotein (VLDL), low density lipoprotein (LDL), and triglycerides. Hypercortisolism also antagonizes the effects of insulin, but frank diabetes mellitus occurs in only 10 to 20 per cent of patients with Cushing's syndrome. In the absence of glucosuria, many patients still experience polyuria due to inhibition of vasopressin (antidiuretic hormone) secretion and the direct enhancement of renal free water clearance by cortisol.

Gonadal hypofunction often accompanies hypercortisolism, especially in patients with longer duration of symptoms. Hypercortisolemia as well as hyperandrogenemia may suppress the hypothalamic-pituitary-gonadal axis, causing oligomenorrhea or amenorrhea with infertility. Occasionally, however, patients with Cushing's syndrome become pregnant. Male patients typically have a decreased libido as well as impotence associated with a decrease in the serum testosterone concentration.

Glucocorticoids also have a profound effect on the immune system. Hypercortisolism may suppress both humoral and cell-mediated immunity, leading to increased risk of superficial fungal infections of the skin (e.g., tinea versicolor or pityriasis) as well as poor wound healing. Patients with profound hypercortisolism (serum cortisol concentration >70 μg/dL [>1900 nmol/L]) are at increased risk for opportunistic infections, especially *Pneumocystis carinii* pneumonia, nocardiosis, and cryptococcosis.

Routine laboratory studies are rarely helpful, and all the abnormalities are nonspecific. The hemogram may provide clues with high-normal values of hemoglobin, hematocrit, and red cell count. Leukocytosis with lymphopenia may also be present, along with hyperglycemia and hyperlipidemia. Electrolyte abnormalities are typically observed only in patients with profound hypercortisolism (urine free cortisol concentration >1500 μg per day [4140 nmol/24 h]). The presence of hypokalemia or metabolic alkalosis from hypercortisolism strongly suggests either the ectopic ACTH syndrome or an adrenal carcinoma.

SCREENING FOR CUSHING'S SYNDROME

Some of the clinical features of Cushing's syndrome, including obesity, hypertension, menstrual irregularities, hirsutism, and mood changes, are nonspecific and commonly seen in general practice. To diagnose Cushing's syndrome in patients with these problems, the clinician must look for features of Cushing's syndrome that are seen less often in the typical patient with upper body obesity. Clinically useful findings include significant supraclavicular fullness, ecchymoses, facial plethora, proximal myopathy, metabolic bone disease, hypertension, and leukocytosis (>11,000 cells/mm^3). Examination of serial photographs to verify progressive physical changes can also be helpful. Earlier recognition of Cushing's syndrome has increased awareness of the varied and subtle presentations of this disorder. Timely diagnosis requires a thoughtful clinician with a high index of suspicion. Fortunately, there are simple, sensitive, inexpensive, and easily performed studies that should confirm the presence or absence of Cushing's syndrome.

BIOCHEMICAL DIAGNOSIS OF CUSHING'S SYNDROME

The clinical diagnosis of Cushing's syndrome requires biochemical verification of cortisol excess. In addition, a determination of the cause of the disorder is required for timely and appropriate treatment. The clinician should always assess the potential contribution of other illnesses, drugs, alcohol, or neuropsychiatric problems to the patient's current condition. In general, the biochemical analyses and the differential diagnosis of Cushing's syndrome can be undertaken without hospitalizing the patient.

Dexamethasone Suppression Tests

The overnight dexamethasone suppression test is the most valuable screening tool for evaluating patients with suspected hypercortisolism. This study requires the administration of 1 mg of dexamethasone at bedtime (11:00 PM) with determination of plasma cortisol concentrations early the following morning. Normal individuals should undergo suppression of plasma cortisol to less than 3 μg/dL (80 nmol/L) following the overnight 1-mg dexamethasone suppression test. Traditionally, a plasma cortisol concentration of less than 5 μg/dL had been considered normal; however, several false-negative results have been observed with the use of this criterion. These results have been attributed to the occasional intermittent nature of hypercortisolism and to the exquisite sensitivity of some patients with pituitary ACTH-dependent Cushing's syndrome (Cushing's disease) to the negative feedback action of glucocorticoids. In addition, both normal persons and obese individuals (body mass index greater than 30 kg/m^2) undergo suppression of plasma cortisol to less than 2.5 μg/dL (70 nmol/L) following the overnight 1-mg dexamethasone suppression test. Although the new criterion has improved the sensitivity of the overnight 1-mg dexamethasone suppression test (i.e., false-negative results are rare), it has also increased the number of false-positive results and decreased the specificity of the test. The overnight suppression test should be employed *only* as a screening tool; biochemical confirmation of Cushing's syndrome must rely on urine free cortisol excretion. False-positive results following the overnight 1-mg dexamethasone suppression test may be recorded in patients receiving drugs that accelerate dexamethasone metabolism (phenytoin, phenobarbital, rifampin), in patients receiving estrogen therapy or tamoxifen (due to increases in corticosteroid-binding globulin), in patients suffering from endogenous depression, or in patients undergoing a stressful event or serious illness. Overnight dexamethasone suppression is most useful in the ambulatory setting and should not be used for hospitalized patients.

The low-dose dexamethasone suppression test, in which urinary 17-hydroxycorticosteroid and free cortisol concentrations are measured during the oral administration of 0.5 mg dexamethasone every 6 hours for 2 days, has been in use for more than 35 years. A urinary 17-hydroxycorticosteroid concentration greater than 4 mg per 24 hours (14.6 μmol/24 h) on the second day of dexamethasone administration supports the diagnosis of Cushing's syndrome. This test, however, does not reliably exclude the diagnosis of Cushing's syndrome. Many patients with mild hypercortisolism due to pituitary ACTH-dependent Cushing's syndrome may undergo suppression of urine steroid secretion to undetectable ranges with even low doses of dexamethasone. Furthermore, as many as 15 to 25 per cent of patients with pseudo-Cushing states may have false-positive test results. In patients with mild hypercortisolism, the low-dose dexamethasone suppression test has an accuracy of only 70 per cent and a poor sensitivity of 55 per cent. In light of the expense and cumbersome nature of consecutive urine collections and frequent dexamethasone administration, continued use of this test cannot be justified.

Urine Free Cortisol

The most useful clinical study for the confirmation of Cushing's syndrome is the measurement of free cortisol in a 24-hour urine specimen. Most commercial laboratories analyze cortisol by radioimmunoassay of a solvent extract of urine. The upper range of normal in this type of assay is typically 80 to 100 μg (200 to 270 nmol) of cortisol per 24 hours. High-performance liquid chromatography provides a more specific analysis of free cortisol. With this methodology, normal subjects typically excrete less than 50 μg (140 nmol) cortisol per 24 hours. Regardless of the method employed, urine free cortisol excretion in most patients with Cushing's syndrome exceeds 100 μg (270 nmol) per 24 hours. However, because of the occasional intermittent nature of endogenous hypercortisolism as well as the mild subclinical autonomous cortisol secretion from some adrenal adenomas, urine free cortisol measurement may be within the normal range in as many as 5 to 10 per cent of patients with true Cushing's syndrome.

Urine free cortisol determinations usually provide a clear discrimination between patients with hypercortisolism and obese patients without Cushing's syndrome. In 10 to 15 per cent of obese patients, increased urinary 17-hydroxycorticosteroid concentrations may lead to an erroneous diagnosis of Cushing's syndrome. By contrast, less than 5 per cent of obese persons have slightly increased urine free cortisol concentrations. Unfortunately, in pseudo-Cushing states (e.g., alcoholism and neuropsychiatric disorders), the urine free cortisol concentration may be indistinguishable from that in patients with true Cushing's syndrome, and additional testing may be required.

Diurnal Rhythm

The absence of diurnal rhythm has been considered a hallmark of the diagnosis of Cushing's syndrome. Normally, cortisol is secreted episodically with a diurnal rhythm paralleling the secretion of ACTH. Plasma concentrations are usually highest early in the morning and decrease gradually throughout the day, reaching their nadir late in the evening. The reference (normal) range for plasma cortisol is rather broad; thus, the concentrations found in Cushing's syndrome often may be normal. Documenting the presence or absence of diurnal rhythm is rather tedious because single determinations obtained in the morning and evening often cannot be interpreted because of the pulsatility of pathologic and physiologic ACTH and cortisol secretion. Nevertheless, a plasma cortisol concentration exceeding 7 μg/dL (190 nmol/L) at midnight in a nonstressed patient is reasonably specific for the diagnosis of Cushing's syndrome. However, some patients with spontaneous Cushing's syndrome have cortisol concentrations less than 7 μg/dL (190 nmol/L) at midnight. In these patients, measurement of cortisol in saliva may provide a simple, convenient, and practical means of probing nighttime cortisol secretion. Patients with Cushing's syndrome have midnight salivary cortisol concentrations that typically exceed 0.4 μg/dL (11 nmol/L) (normal range of 0.5 to 5.0 nmol/L).

Problems in Diagnosis

Many factors may confound the biochemical evaluation of patients with suspected Cushing's syndrome. Dexamethasone administration may result in a wide range of actual dexamethasone concentrations due to wide variability in the metabolic clearance of this synthetic steroid. In patients receiving anticonvulsants or other drugs that induce hepatic microsomal drug-metabolizing enzymes, accurate interpretation of the dexamethasone suppression test may occasionally require measurements of both cortisol and dexamethasone. The diagnosis of endogenous hypercortisolism in patients with renal failure is difficult. Urine collections are either unavailable or unreliable, the overall absorption of dexamethasone is erratic, and plasma cortisol determinations may be spuriously increased in chronic renal failure because of accumulation of interfering substances structurally related to unconjugated glucocorticoids.

Distinguishing patients with mild Cushing's syndrome from those with mild physiologic hypercortisolism due to pseudo-Cushing's syndrome is a major diagnostic problem. Patients with alcoholism, withdrawal from ethanol intoxication, anorexia, bulimia, or the depressed phase of affective disorder may have biochemical features of Cushing's syndrome with increased concentrations of urine free cortisol, disruptions of the normal diurnal pattern of cortisol secretion, and lack of suppression of cortisol after the overnight 1-mg dexamethasone suppression test. Although the history and physical examination may provide specific clues to the appropriate diagnosis, definitive biochemical confirmation may be difficult and requires repeated testing. If the clinical findings are equivocal and repeated measurements of urine free cortisol concentrations and the overnight 1-mg dexamethasone suppression test yield inconclusive results, referral to a center with expertise in pituitary-adrenal disorders may be appropriate.

The most definitive study currently available for distinguishing mild Cushing's syndrome from pseudo-Cushing conditions is the use of dexamethasone suppression followed by corticotropin-releasing hormone (CRH) stimulation of the pituitary gland. CRH is the primary hypothalamic factor that stimulates ACTH secretion. This test relies on the overt sensitivity of patients with Cushing's syndrome to both dexamethasone and CRH. The oral administration of dexamethasone (0.5 mg) every 6 hours for eight doses is followed immediately by the intravenous administration of 100 μg of ovine CRH 2 hours after completion of low-dose dexamethasone suppression. A plasma cortisol concentration exceeding 1.4 μg/dL (38 nmol/L) 15 minutes after the administration of CRH correctly identifies the majority of patients with Cushing's syndrome. The dexamethasone-CRH study requires special expertise and the availability of a sensitive and specific assay for plasma cortisol.

The algorithm in Figure 1 provides a simple and cost-effective means of evaluating patients with suspected Cushing's syndrome.

DIFFERENTIAL DIAGNOSIS OF CUSHING'S SYNDROME

The accurate differential diagnosis of Cushing's syndrome is required for appropriate and effective treatment. Since Cushing's initial description of basophilic pituitary adenomas, many other causes of hypercortisolism have been identified. The differential diagnosis of Cushing's syndrome is outlined in Table 2.

Causes of Cushing's Syndrome

The majority of patients with spontaneous Cushing's syndrome have an ACTH-secreting neoplasm. ACTH-dependent Cushing's syndrome causes bilateral adrenal hyperplasia or sometimes nodular adrenal hyperplasia. Adrenal gland nodules ranging in size from 1 to 4 cm may occasionally be seen in patients with ACTH-secreting neoplasms and are a source of diagnostic confusion. As Cushing initially recognized, most patients with ACTH-dependent hypercortisolism do have a pituitary tumor, and this form of Cushing's syndrome is referred to as Cushing's disease. These ACTH-secreting tumors (corticotroph adenomas) are seen in 90 per cent of patients with ACTH-

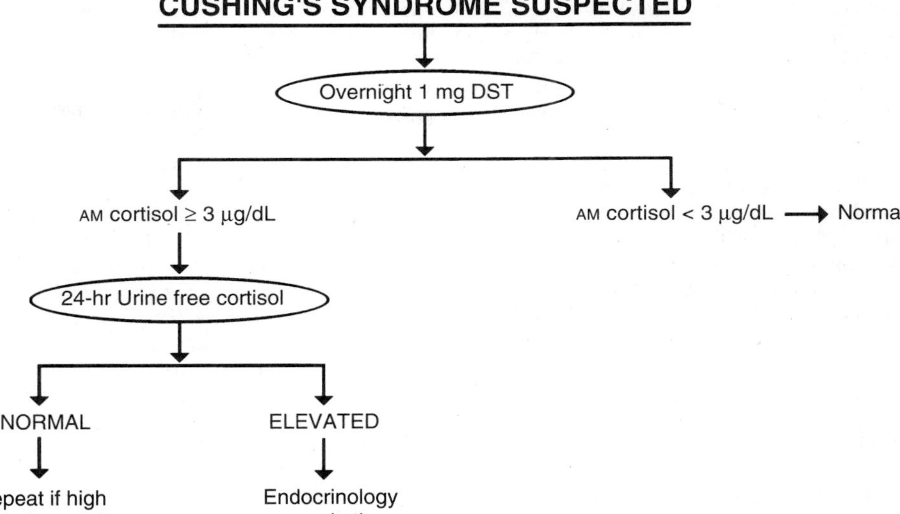

Figure 1. Algorithm for evaluating patients with suspected Cushing's syndrome. (DST = dexamethasone suppression test.)

dependent Cushing's syndrome. By contrast, various nonpituitary ACTH-secreting tumors (the ectopic ACTH syndrome) make up the other 10 per cent of lesions causing this form of Cushing's syndrome. Specifically, neuroendocrine carcinoma or small cell carcinoma of the lung may be associated with ACTH production and severe hypercortisolism. Patients with ACTH-secreting small cell carcinoma typically present with various catabolic effects of glucocorticoid excess, including severe myopathy, weight loss, hypertension, hyperglycemia, and hypokalemic metabolic alkalosis. This well-appreciated paraneoplastic syndrome portends a poor prognosis and a mean survival of less than 1 month.

Patients with the occult ACTH syndrome may be difficult to distinguish clinically and biochemically from patients with ACTH-secreting pituitary tumors. Some nonpituitary ACTH-secreting tumors are radiographically occult and may not be recognized clinically until many years after Cushing's syndrome has been diagnosed. Most of these tumors are bronchial carcinoids, but islet cell tumors, thymic carcinoids, pheochromocytoma, and medullary carcinoma of the thyroid have also been reported.

Some patients with Cushing's syndrome have ACTH-independent glucocorticoid excess. Most of these patients have iatrogenic Cushing's syndrome from oral or parenteral use of synthetic corticosteroids. Megestrol acetate, a potent progestational agent used in the management of patients with malignancies and acquired immunodeficiency syndrome (AIDS), may also cause iatrogenic Cushing's syndrome. Megestrol acetate binds to glucocorticoid receptors and may suppress the endogenous hypothalamic-pituitary adrenal axis. Most patients with noniatrogenic, ACTH-independent Cushing's syndrome harbor an adrenal neoplasm secreting cortisol autonomously. Most of these tumors are benign adrenocortical adenomas (usually <5 cm in diameter and easily identified with computed tomography [CT]) and less commonly represent adrenocortical carcinoma (usually >5 cm in diameter).

Table 2. Differential Diagnosis of Cushing's Syndrome

ACTH-dependent
Pituitary adenoma (Cushing's disease)
Nonpituitary neoplasm (Ectopic ACTH)
ACTH-independent
Iatrogenic (glucocorticoids, megestrol acetate administration)
Adrenal neoplasm (adenoma-carcinoma)
Nodular adrenal hyperplasia
Primary pigmented nodular adrenal disease
Massive macronodular, adrenonodular hyperplasia
Food-dependent (GIP-mediated)
Factitious

ACTH = adrenocorticotropic hormone; GIP = gastric inhibitory polypeptide.

There are some rare forms of adrenal-dependent Cushing's syndrome categorized as nodular adrenal hyperplasia. These entities have been identified as morphologic consequences of several unique pathophysiologic disorders. Primary pigmented nodular adrenal disease presents in adolescents or young adults and is a familial autosomal dominant disorder that may be associated with myxomas (cardiac, cutaneous, mammary), spotty skin pigmentation (lentigines and blue nevi), endocrine overactivity (sexual precocity and acromegaly), and schwannomas. The adrenal glands in primary pigmented nodular adrenal disease are often small or normal and have multiple black and brown nodules with intranodular cortical atrophy. This disorder may be caused by adrenal-stimulating immunoglobulins that bind to the ACTH receptor in the adrenal cortex, provoking adrenal steroid biosynthesis. Another type of nodular adrenal hyperplasia has been characterized as massive macronodular adrenal hyperplasia. This adrenal-dependent cause of Cushing's syndrome is characterized by large bilateral nodules (3 to 6 cm in diameter). This disorder is rarely familial and its cause has not been determined. Rare patients with massive macronodular adrenal hyperplasia have been reported with food-dependent hypercortisolism. The adrenal cortex in these patients expresses abnormal receptors for gastric inhibitory peptide (GIP). Food consumption, therefore, stimulates GIP, which, in turn, binds the adrenal cortex, thereby stimulating adrenal growth and steroid biosynthesis. Finally, factitious Cushing's syndrome has been reported and characterized. Surprisingly, this condition is uncommon despite the widespread use of exogenous glucocorticoid preparations.

Biochemical and Radiologic Differential Diagnosis

The differential diagnosis of Cushing's syndrome may be difficult, and endocrinologic consultation is always warranted. The CRH stimulation test with sampling of the inferior petrosal sinus for ACTH, a specific and sensitive immunoradiometric assay for ACTH, and CT and magnetic resonance imaging (MRI) of the pituitary and adrenal glands have improved the accuracy of diagnosis over the past 10 to 15 years.

The initial step in the differential diagnosis of Cushing's syndrome is to distinguish ACTH-dependent Cushing's syndrome (pituitary or nonpituitary ACTH-secreting neoplasm) from ACTH-independent hypercortisolism. The best way of distinguishing these two types of Cushing's syndrome is with the measurement of plasma ACTH by immunoradiometric assay (ACTH-IRMA). The development of this assay has provided a remarkable degree of sensitivity and specificity for the analysis of this anterior pituitary hormone. ACTH is consistently and reliably suppressed by immunoradiometric assay in patients with ACTH-independent Cushing's syndrome (Fig. 2). ACTH concentrations do not exceed 5 pg/mL (1.1 pmol/L) and exhibit a blunted response to CRH (peak concentration does not exceed 10 pg/mL [2.2 pmol/L]) in patients with cortisol-producing adrenal neoplasms, autonomous bilateral nodular adrenocortical hyperplasia, and factitious Cushing's syndrome.

A major challenge in the differential diagnosis of ACTH-dependent hypercortisolism is identifying the source of the ACTH-secreting tumor. Because the vast majority of these patients (90 per cent) have a pituitary tumor, whereas the others harbor a nonpituitary tumor, diagnostic studies needed to distinguish these two entities must provide nearly perfect sensitivity, specificity, and accuracy. Although plasma concentrations of ACTH by immunoradiometric assay tend to be higher in patients with ectopic ACTH than in those with pituitary ACTH-dependent Cushing's syndrome, there is considerable overlap between these two groups. As mentioned, many of the ectopic ACTH-secreting tumors are radiologically occult and may not become clinically apparent for many years after the initial diagnosis of Cushing's syndrome. With the introduction of pituitary microsurgery as the treatment of choice in patients with Cushing's disease, an accurate differential diagnosis is essential.

In the presence of ACTH-dependent Cushing's syndrome, MRI of the pituitary gland with gadolinium enhancement will identify an adenoma in 50 to 60 per cent of patients. If the patient has classic clinical and laboratory findings of ACTH-dependent hypercortisolemia, and an unequivocal adenoma of the pituitary gland is seen on MRI, the likelihood of Cushing's disease (pituitary ACTH-dependent hypercortisolism) is 98 to 99 per cent. However, it must be remembered that up to 10 per cent of the population in the 20- to 50-year age group will have incidental tumors of the pituitary gland demonstrable by MRI. Therefore, patients with ectopic ACTH will rarely have radiographic evidence of a pituitary adenoma.

Traditionally, high-dose dexamethasone suppression testing has been used in the differential diagnosis of Cushing's syndrome. In the classic test, 2 mg of dexamethasone are administered orally every 6 hours for 2 days with collections of urine for steroid analysis. This high-dose test immediately follows the low-dose test as previously described as well as 2 days of basal urine steroid measurements. A decrease in urine steroid excretion of more than 50 per cent on day 2 of the high-dose dexamethasone suppression test is considered diagnostic of pituitary disease, whereas an absence of suppression suggests primary adrenal disease or ectopic ACTH. Unfortunately, these criteria cannot reliably distinguish pituitary from ectopic ACTH-secreting tumors, nor can they distinguish ACTH-dependent from ACTH-independent Cushing's syndrome. The diagnostic accuracy of the procedure is only 70 to 80 per cent, which is much less than the pretest probability of Cushing's disease, which is 90 per cent. More recent criteria for this test have yielded better specificity, sensitivity, and accuracy. A decrease in urine free cortisol concentrations of more than 90 per cent and a decrease in 17-hydroxycorticosteroid secretion of more than 64 per cent following the traditional high-dose dexamethasone suppression test yielded a 100 per cent diagnostic specificity for Cushing's disease in one series. However, the overall diagnostic accuracy of the test is still only 86 per cent, and reports of false-positive test results persist even with these new criteria.

An overnight 8-mg dexamethasone suppression test has also been used for distinguishing pituitary from nonpitu-

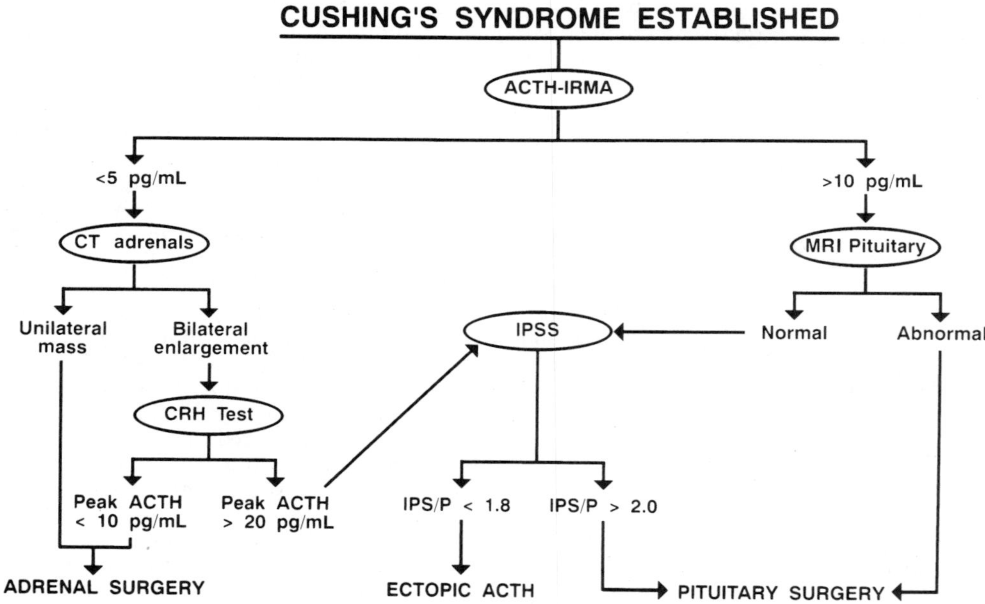

Figure 2. Algorithm for the differential diagnosis of Cushing's syndrome. IPSS = inferior petrosal sinus sampling; IPS/P = inferior petrosal sinus-to-peripheral ACTH ratio.

itary ACTH-dependent Cushing's syndrome. This simpler and certainly more cost-effective outpatient procedure involves the ingestion of 8 mg of dexamethasone at bedtime (11 PM) and measurement of plasma cortisol concentrations the following morning. The suppression of plasma cortisol concentrations to less than 50 per cent of baseline is most consistent with pituitary-dependent Cushing's syndrome. This overnight test provides nearly the same accuracy as the 2-day high-dose dexamethasone suppression test and is preferred by most clinicians even though false-positive and false-negative results are not uncommon. Dexamethasone suppression tests in the differential diagnosis of Cushing's syndrome must be interpreted cautiously and with careful consideration of the clinical presentation and the results of other biochemical and radiographic studies.

The most definitive means of accurately and reliably distinguishing pituitary from nonpituitary ACTH-dependent Cushing's syndrome is bilateral, simultaneous inferior petrosal sinus sampling (IPSS) following CRH stimulation. This procedure takes advantage of the route by which anterior pituitary hormones such as ACTH reach the systemic circulation. Blood leaves the anterior lobe of the pituitary gland and drains into the cavernous sinuses, which empty into the inferior petrosal sinus which, in turn, feeds the jugular bulb and vein. Simultaneous sampling of the inferior petrosal sinus and peripheral blood (for ACTH measurements) before and after CRH stimulation can reliably confirm the presence or absence of an ACTH-secreting pituitary tumor. An inferior petrosal sinus–to–peripheral ACTH (IPS-to-P) ratio of greater than 2.0 is consistent with a pituitary ACTH-secreting tumor and an IPS-to-P ratio less than 1.8 supports the diagnosis of ectopic ACTH. Because each petrosal sinus receives venous drainage from the ipsilateral side of the pituitary gland with little intercavernous mixing, ACTH-secreting tumors located laterally should secrete ACTH primarily into the corresponding petrosal sinus. Interpetrosal sinus gradients have been used for preoperative localization of corticotroph adenomas. Bilateral IPSS with CRH stimulation requires a skilled invasive radiologist, but in experienced hands the procedure has yielded a diagnostic accuracy of almost 100 per cent in the differential diagnosis of ACTH-dependent Cushing's syndrome.

The search for occult ectopic ACTH-secreting tumors may be difficult. Because most of these lesions are in the thorax, high-resolution CT of the chest may be helpful; however, MRI of the chest appears to have even better sensitivity in finding the typical small bronchial carcinoid tumor. Some ectopic ACTH-secreting tumors have somatostatin receptors; thus, a radiolabeled somatostatin analog scan (octreotide acetate scintigraphy) may also be used to find these tumors.

Patients with ACTH-independent Cushing's syndrome are easily identified by the suppressed plasma ACTH seen by immunoradiometric assay (less than 5 pg/mL [1.1 pmol/L]). Patients with suppressed plasma ACTH concentrations should undergo CT of the adrenal glands. When Cushing's syndrome is due to an autonomously functioning adrenal adenoma, a unilateral mass (always 2 cm or larger) will be seen. The uninvolved ipsilateral and contralateral adrenal glands will become normal or less commonly atrophic. CT of the adrenal glands in patients with ACTH-dependent hypercortisolism due to a pituitary adenoma or an ectopic ACTH-secreting pituitary tumor is often associated with bilaterally hyperplastic glands, with or without adrenal gland nodules. However, in at least a third of patients with proven Cushing's disease, the adrenal glands actually appear normal. Nodular adrenal hyperplasia is present in 10 to 15 per cent of patients with ACTH-dependent hypercortisolism. When a large nodule involves a single gland, it can be confused with autonomously functioning adrenal adenoma and lead to the inappropriate diagnosis of a cortisol-producing adenoma.

In summary, technologic advances in the past few years have greatly improved the diagnosis and differential diagnosis of Cushing's syndrome. The clinical features, the biochemical evaluation, and the radiographic findings must be interpreted together to establish the correct diagnosis.

PRIMARY ALDOSTERONISM

By Michael L. Tuck, M.D.,
and Pongamorn Bunnag, M.D.
Sepulveda, California

Primary aldosteronism (PA) is a secondary form of hypertension caused by excessive production of aldosterone. Aldosterone is the major mineralocorticoid hormone produced by the zona glomerulosa of the adrenal cortex. The other zones of the adrenal cortex cannot normally produce aldosterone, because they lack aldosterone synthase (CYP11B2), an enzyme that catalyzes the conversion of corticosterone to aldosterone.

Aldosterone accounts for 50 to 60 per cent of all mineralocorticoid activity. Weaker mineralocorticoid hormones include corticosterone, deoxycorticosterone, 18-hydroxycorticosterone, and 18-hydroxy-deoxycorticosterone.

Aldosterone promotes sodium reabsorption and potassium and hydrogen excretion in the distal tubules and cortical collecting ducts of the kidneys. The principal regulator of aldosterone secretion is the renin-angiotensin system; increased angiotensin II stimulates aldosterone secretion. Corticotropin (ACTH) also increases aldosterone secretion, but its effect is short lived (<24 hours). Potassium stimulates aldosterone production, and aldosterone is an important regulator of potassium excretion. Dopamine and atrial natriuretic peptide are the major inhibitors of aldosterone secretion.

Patients with hypertension caused by excessive aldosterone production account for fewer than 1 per cent of all hypertension. However, with the introduction of better detection, the prevalence may be higher than previously thought. In general, the duration and severity of hypertension caused by PA cannot be distinguished from essential hypertension. Hypokalemia is the single most useful clue to the diagnosis of PA and is detected in more than 60 to 80 per cent of these patients. Hypokalemia in PA is accompanied by inappropriate loss of potassium in the urine (>30 mEq/day). Any hypertensive patient with spontaneous hypokalemia should be vigorously investigated for PA. The use of diuretics that may induce hypokalemia should be excluded before the investigation. Other "inappropriate" hypertension (e.g., hypertension in patients younger than 20 years of age, hypertension with strong family history suggesting autosomal dominant transmission, hypertension resistant to conventional drug treatment) should also prompt an evaluation for PA.

The diagnosis of PA is based on the demonstration of excessive and autonomous production of aldosterone. Because the production of aldosterone can be influenced by

Table 1. Duration of Discontinuation of Antihypertensive Drugs Before Establishing the Diagnosis of Primary Aldosteronism

Drug	Discontinuation Period (wk)
Spironolactone	6
Diuretics	4
Angiotensin-converting enzyme inhibitors	2
Sympathetic inhibitors	1
Calcium channel blockers	1
Vasodilators	1

serum potassium and by drugs that affect the renin-angiotensin system, hypokalemia should be corrected and various antihypertensive drugs (e.g., diuretics, beta-blockers, angiotensin-converting enzyme inhibitors) discontinued at least 2 to 3 weeks before the investigation (Table 1).

Measurement of plasma renin activity (PRA) should be the first step in the evaluation. PRA is suppressed (<1 ng/mL per hour) in most patients with PA. However, low PRA is also seen in as many as 30 per cent of patients with essential hypertension, and PRA varies widely with sodium intake and posture. A single value of PRA is difficult to interpret. Plasma and urinary aldosterone concentrations in PA also overlap with those seen in patients with essential hypertension, and basal values of aldosterone cannot reliably distinguish patients with PA from patients with other causes of hypertension. Simultaneous measurements of PRA and plasma aldosterone concentrations, as expressed in aldosterone-renin ratios (ARR), are less disturbed by sodium intake or posture and are more reliable than single values alone. An ARR of 30 or greater is considered a distinguishing, or threshold, value. Since the introduction of ARR as a screening test, the number of patients with PA, including those with normokalemic hyperaldosteronism, has increased considerably.

The captopril test has also been recommended as a useful screening test. Captopril, the angiotensin-converting enzyme inhibitor, rapidly blocks the conversion of angiotensin I to angiotensin II. This blockade results in decreased angiotensin II and aldosterone secretion and decreased negative feedback inhibition of renin release. Captopril increases the PRA in normal subjects and in essential hypertensive patients. In primary aldosteronism, however, aldosterone secretion is not decreased by captopril because its secretion does not depend on the renin-angiotensin system. PRA remains low owing to the continued negative feedback of volume expansion due to excessive concentrations of aldosterone. The captopril test can be performed by administering 25 or 50 mg of captopril orally and measuring PRA and plasma aldosterone 1 to 2 hours later. After captopril blockade, an aldosterone-to-renin ratio of 50 or greater is considered a positive test result.

The recommended screening tests for PA are shown in Table 2. The definitive diagnosis of PA requires demonstration of nonsuppressible aldosterone production after volume expansion. The adequacy of volume expansion should be documented as urinary sodium excretion exceeding 250 mEq/day. Volume expansion to suppress aldosterone production can be accomplished by normal saline infusion, by fludrocortisone administration, or by 5 days of a high-salt diet (i.e., adding 12 g of sodium chloride to the patient's daily intake). Saline loading is done by infusion of normal saline (25 mL/kg) over 4 hours each day for 3 days. In patients with PA, urinary aldosterone content exceeds 14 μg/24 hours; in other forms of hypertension, the values are much lower. Alternatively, fludrocortisone acetate (0.1 mg) can be administered every 6 hours for 4 days. In normal persons, plasma aldosterone concentrations are suppressed on days 3 and 4 to less than 5 ng/dL. By contrast, this suppression typically does not occur in patients with PA.

Table 2. Screening Tests for Primary Aldosteronism

Serum potassium (K^+ <3.5 mEq/L)
Urine potassium (K^+ >30 mEq/day)
Aldosterone/plasma renin activity ratio (>30–50)
Captopril suppression test (ARR >30)

Table 3. Causes of Primary Aldosteronism

Cause	Percentage of Diagnoses
Aldosterone-producing adenoma	65
Idiopathic hyperaldosteronism	30
Primary adrenal hyperplasia	<1
Aldosterone-producing carcinoma	<1

Most patients with PA have an aldosterone-producing adenoma (APA) or idiopathic hyperaldosteronism (IHA; Table 3). Several tests can be used to distinguish APA from IHA (Table 4). Hypertension tends to be more severe in APA than in IHA, but these two disorders cannot be distinguished on clinical grounds alone. Hypokalemia is documented more often in APA (>90 to 95 per cent) than in IHA (40 to 60 per cent). Serum K^+ of less than 2.5 mEq/L is rarely observed in IHA. The procedure most commonly used to distinguish between APA and IHA is the postural test. In IHA, PRA and aldosterone concentrations tend to increase after 4 hours of upright posture, suggesting some degree of dependence on the renin-angiotensin system. In APA, however, there is a slight fall, the so-called anomalous aldosterone response, in plasma aldosterone concentrations related to the circadian rhythm. Serum concentrations of 18-hydroxycorticosterone, the biosynthetic precursor of aldosterone, typically exceed 100 ng/dL in APA but not in IHA.

Two other surgically correctable subsets of PA are aldosterone-producing renin-responsive adenoma (AP-RA) and primary adrenal hyperplasia (PAH). In AP-RA, the biochemical test results resemble IHA, but a unilateral tumor is found, and the hypertension can be cured by surgical removal of the tumor. In PAH, the biochemical test results are similar to those for APA, but no tumor can be found, and the gland is unilaterally or bilaterally hyperplastic. Surgical removal of 75 per cent of the gland can produce long-term remission. AP-RA and PAH account for fewer than 5 per cent of all patients with PA.

Computed tomography (CT) scanning can localize the APA in most patients. With high-resolution CT, tumors as

Table 4. Tests for Distinguishing Aldosterone-Producing Adenoma From Idiopathic Hyperaldosteronism

Computed tomography scan
Posture response
Plasma 18-hydroxycorticosterone
Adrenal scintigraphy
Adrenal venous aldosterone sampling

small as 5 to 7 mm are readily detected, and diagnostic accuracy approaches 80 per cent. However, CT does not always distinguish APA from the nonfunctioning adrenal mass, and biochemical diagnosis of PA should precede the visualization of adrenal lesions by CT. Iodocholesterol scanning is no more sensitive than CT, but it can determine the functional activity of the tumor. Occasionally, the clinician may have to refer the hypertensive patient to a facility that specializes in catheterization of adrenal veins. Measurement of aldosterone concentrations in adrenal venous blood remains the gold standard for localizing APAs. The diagnostic accuracy for APA approaches 95 per cent. Aldosterone concentrations on the side of the lesion are typically 10 times greater than those on the uninvolved side.

GLUCOCORTICOID-REMEDIABLE ALDOSTERONISM

Glucocorticoid-remediable aldosteronism (GRA) is a unique subset of PA with an autosomal dominant mode of transmission. In many of these patients, hypertension begins in childhood and is accompanied by a family history of stroke in the young. The production of aldosterone in GRA is under the control of corticotropin (ACTH). Dexamethasone, by suppressing ACTH secretion, can correct hypokalemia and hypertension in GRA. Patients with GRA produce two hybrid steroids of the C-18 oxidation pathway: 18-hydroxycortisol and 18-oxocortisol. Increased circulating concentrations of these steroids may reflect ectopic aldosterone synthase activity in the zona fasciculata. The molecular genetics of GRA reveals chimeric gene duplication of a segment spanning the 5′ regulatory sequence of 11β-hydroxylase *(CYP11B1)* and the distal coding sequence of aldosterone synthase *(CYP11B2)*. This chimeric gene *(CYP11B1/B2)* has been detected by blood DNA analysis in all GRA patients. For DNA analysis phone the International GRA Registry at (800)–GRA–2262.

MANAGEMENT OF PRIMARY ALDOSTERONISM

Unilateral adrenalectomy is the treatment for APA but is contraindicated for IHA. Resection of tumor normalizes serum potassium concentrations in most of the patients with APA; surgery normalizes blood pressure in about 70 per cent of the patients. An acquired postoperative syndrome of hyporeninemic hypoaldosteronism may persist for weeks to months, and serum potassium should be carefully monitored during this period.

Medical therapy is indicated for patients with IHA and patients with APA who do not respond to surgery or have contraindications to surgery. Spironolactone (100 to 400 mg/day) is the most widely used drug. The higher dose of spironolactone is usually associated with more side effects, especially antiandrogenic effects. The use of diuretics in PA may help control blood pressure, because PA is a form of volume-dependent hypertension. Hydrochlorothiazide or furosemide can be used in combination with potassium-sparing diuretics (e.g., amiloride, triamterene). Serum potassium should be carefully monitored during treatment. Calcium channel blockers and other antihypertensive drugs may also be required for controlling hypertension in some patients.

CONGENITAL ADRENAL HYPERPLASIA

By Maria I. New, M.D.,
and Patricia Schram, M.D.
New York, New York

Congenital adrenal hyperplasia (CAH) comprises a group of inherited (inborn) errors of steroidogenesis. Each of the major variants of CAH is caused by a specific deficiency of one of the enzymes necessary for cortisol synthesis. The enzymes most frequently affected are (1) steroid 21-hydroxylase (21-OH), (2) steroid 11β-hydroxylase (11β-OH), and (3) 3β-hydroxysteroid dehydrogenase (3β-HSD) (Table 1).

Cortisol production by the adrenal cortex is stimulated by the pituitary peptide adrenocorticotropic hormone (ACTH). Regulation occurs at the level of the hypothalamus and pituitary by negative feedback mechanisms in which high cortisol inhibits and low cortisol promotes ACTH release. When less cortisol is produced owing to an enzymatic defect, secretion of ACTH by the pituitary is abnormally increased at all levels of cortisol demand. Cycling of ACTH is also exaggerated. Hyperplasia of the adrenal cortex is the consequence of chronic overstimulation by ACTH.

The multiple interconnections of the pathways of steroid biosynthesis result in specific steroid compounds being produced inadequately or excessively in patients with inborn errors of steroidogenesis (Fig. 1). Steroids proximal to the block are generated in excess and are released into the circulation, or they spill over into unimpeded pathways to increase adrenal output of other hormones. Each particular enzyme defect in CAH is expressed biochemically by a distinct pathophysiologic combination of steroids and their metabolites in serum and urine. The clinical picture for each of the forms of CAH depends on the sum of hormonal effects of the specific steroids produced inadequately or excessively. These hormonal effects are developmental and metabolic.

EXTERNAL GENITAL AMBIGUITY

Development of the external genitalia is a steroid-dependent process, and ambiguous genital formation in genetic females from excess adrenal androgen secretion occurs in 21-hydroxylase deficiency and 11β-hydroxylase deficiency. Genetic males with either of these enzyme deficiencies show no abnormality at birth. The genitals of an affected female may be markedly masculinized in appearance, and sex misassignment as a male is known to occur. In addition to these two virilizing forms, CAH due to 3β-hydroxysteroid dehydrogenase (3β-HSD) deficiency can produce genital ambiguity in genetic females as a result of massive adrenal overproduction of dehydroepiandrosterone (DHEA). The virilizing effects are limited because the androgenic activity of this steroid is low, and because further conversion of DHEA to more potent adrenal androgens is impeded. The enzyme 3β-HSD is also expressed in the gonads; therefore genetic males are incompletely masculinized as a result of defective testicular steroidogenesis. The remaining two enzymes of cortisol synthesis, (4) steroid 17α-hydroxylase/17,20-lyase and (5) the cholesterol side chain-cleavage enzyme (cholesterol desmolase), are only

Table 1. Major Forms of Adrenal Hyperplasia

Deficiency	Syndrome	Ambiguous Genitalia	Postnatal Virilization	Salt Metabolism	Steroids Increased (Serum)	Steroids Decreased (Serum)	Enzyme (Protein or Activity)	Chromosomal Location (Cloned Genes)	Frequency
21-Hydroxylase									1 in 12,000
	Salt wasting	Females	Yes	Salt wasting	17-OHP, Δ^4-A	Aldo, cortisol	Cytochrome P-450c21	6p (HLA-B40; HLA-Bw47, DR7)	75%
	Simple virilizing	Females	Yes	Normal	17-OHP, Δ^4-A	Cortisol	P-450c21	6p (HLA-B5)	25%
	Nonclassic	No	Yes	Normal	17-OHP, Δ^4-A	—	P-450c21	6p (HLA-B14; DR1)	0.1–1% (3% in European Jews)
11β-Hydroxylase	Classic	Females	Yes	Hypertension	DOC, 11-deoxycortisol(s)	Cortisol, ± aldo	P-450c11	8q	1 in 100,000 (increased in Moroccan and Tunisian Jews)
	Nonclassic	No	Yes	Normal	11-deoxycortisol ± DOC	—	P-450c11	8q	More frequent
3β-OH-steroid dehydrogenase	Classic	Males	Yes	Salt wasting	DHEA, 17-OH-pregnenolone	Aldo, T, cortisol	3β-OH-steroid dehydrogenase	1q	Rare
	Nonclassic	No	Yes	Normal	DHEA, 17-OH-pregnenolone	—	3β-OH-steroid dehydrogenase	?	Common

Aldo = aldosterone; T = testosterone; Δ^4-A = Δ^4-androstenedione; DHEA = dehydroepiandrosterone, DOC = 11-deoxycorticosterone; 17-OHP = 17α-hydroxyprogesterone.

rarely deficient, but they are also required in gonadal steroid production. In CAH from either of these deficiencies, synthesis of androgens is compromised, and males are born with ambiguous genitalia.

ELECTROLYTE ABNORMALITIES

In addition to cortisol and androgens, the adrenal cortex produces the potent sodium-conserving hormone aldosterone. The synthesis of aldosterone, although dependent on the tonic stimulus of adrenal steroidogenesis by ACTH, is under the primary control of the renin-angiotensin system, which regulates plasma volume and plasma electrolyte balance. Low plasma volume reduces renal perfusion pressure, stimulating specialized cells in the afferent arterioles of the juxtaglomerular apparatus to release stores of renin. Renin acts in the circulation to generate the peptide angiotensin I, which is cleaved from a much larger plasma globulin precursor called angiotensinogen or renin substrate. The peptide angiotensin II is further split from angiotensin I by the action of angiotensin-converting enzyme (ACE). The drop in renal perfusion pressure is corrected by vasoconstriction acting immediately to reduce the total intravascular space, compensating for the reduced plasma volume, and by stimulating aldosterone synthesis and secretion by the adrenal cortex. Aldosterone promotes the transport of sodium ions across the epithelium of the distal and collecting renal tubules to the extracellular fluid space. This increased reabsorption of sodium from the renal filtrate slowly increases the total plasma sodium, which, in turn, corrects the total plasma volume. The sodium transport mechanism promoted by aldosterone involves H^+ or K^+ ion exchange, and aldosterone synthesis is also stimulated directly by elevated serum potassium concentration to regulate electrolyte balance. In three of four cases of steroid 21-hydroxylase deficiency, in most cases of 3β-HSD deficiency, and in cholesterol desmolase deficiency, aldosterone synthesis is also impaired, resulting in salt-wasting owing to inadequate reabsorption of sodium manifested by increased urinary sodium excretion, hyperkalemia and hyponatremia, and reduced plasma volume with increased plasma renin activity (PRA). Uncorrected salt wasting may lead to life-threatening adrenal crisis, especially in conjunction with stress of unusual exertion, trauma, or infection.

CLINICAL FEATURES OF THE SPECIFIC ENZYME DEFECTS

Classic 21-Hydroxylase Deficiency

The steroid 21-hydroxylation step is the most common defect in CAH. 21-hydroxylase defects cause accumulation of steroid precursors and adrenal overproduction of androgens whose synthesis does not involve the enzyme. When the deficiency is severe, the diagnosis is made early in life (classic disease), but when the defect is mild, signs and symptoms occur later (nonclassic). The primary presenting feature of classic disease, caused by exposure to increased androgens in fetal life, is virilization of the external genitalia in newborn females. 21-hydroxylase deficiency is the most common cause of female pseudohermaphroditism, though the internal genitalia in even the most severely virilized of these genetic or gonadal females is entirely compatible with conception and childbearing.

Hyperkalemia can be marked in salt-wasting 21-hydroxylase deficiency, and patients can develop serum potassium concentrations above 8 mEq/L and sodium concentrations below 120 mEq/L. First-born genetic males are at high risk because the genitalia are not ambiguous, and the diagnosis is easily missed. Statistics show a steady rise over the past few decades in the incidence of salt wasting in 21-hydroxylase deficiency CAH, possibly because in the past many patients died in infancy with their condition undiagnosed.

Virilization in females is variable in either clinical form (i.e., simple virilizing or salt wasting), and the finding of less extreme genital ambiguity is no guarantee that the salt wasting form will be mild or absent. Males with either form have normal genitalia and show no signs of disease for the first few days of life. Simple virilizing males may show the first signs of virilization by the end of the first year or even later in life. Salt wasting usually does not appear until the seventh day of life. Thus, the firstborn male may have an adrenal crisis at home, since discharge from the nursery occurs before the onset of adrenal insufficiency.

Deficiency of 21-hydroxylase is inherited as a monogenic autosomal recessive trait that is closely linked to the HLA major histocompatibility complex (MHC) located on the short arm of chromosome 6. In addition to linkage of the 21-hydroxylase locus with the HLA-B and HLA-DR antigen loci, 21-hydroxylase deficiency alleles are found in linkage disequilibrium with HLA antigen genes in configurations known as haplotypes. The salt-wasting form is associated with the extended haplotype HLA-AcBw47, DR7, and the nonclassic disease is associated with the haplotype HLA-B14, DR1.

The structural gene encoding the adrenal cytochrome P-450 specific for 21-hydroxylation (P-450c21) is named *CYP21* and contains 10 exons. This gene and a 98 per cent identical pseudogene, *CYP21P* (nonactive), are located in close proximity in the HLA complex. During meiosis, a gene conversion apparently occurs that transfers deleterious point mutations from the *CYP21P* gene to the *CYP21* gene. Large gene rearrangements (large gene conversions or gene deletions) also occur as a result of unequal crossover.

Mutations (large gene conversions, gene deletions, and R356W) shown to result in complete inactivation of 21-hydroxylase activity have been associated with the salt-wasting phenotype. Gene deletions account for 10 to 39 per cent of the reported cases. Gene conversions are responsible for the 65 to 90 per cent of the disease haplotypes in which deletional mutations were not identified. Nine mutations are the result of transferral of normal sequences of the *CYP21P* pseudogene into the active *CYP21* gene; they have adverse effects at any of the stages of gene suppression.

Nonclassic 21-Hydroxylase Deficiency

The degree of androgen excess in nonclassic 21-hydroxylase deficiency causes no genital abnormality, but signs of hormonal imbalance may appear at any time. Clinical symptoms vary widely and may change with age in the same individual. Similar biochemical values are observed in patients with nonclassic 21-hydroxylase deficiency and frank androgenic signs, in mildly symptomatic patients,

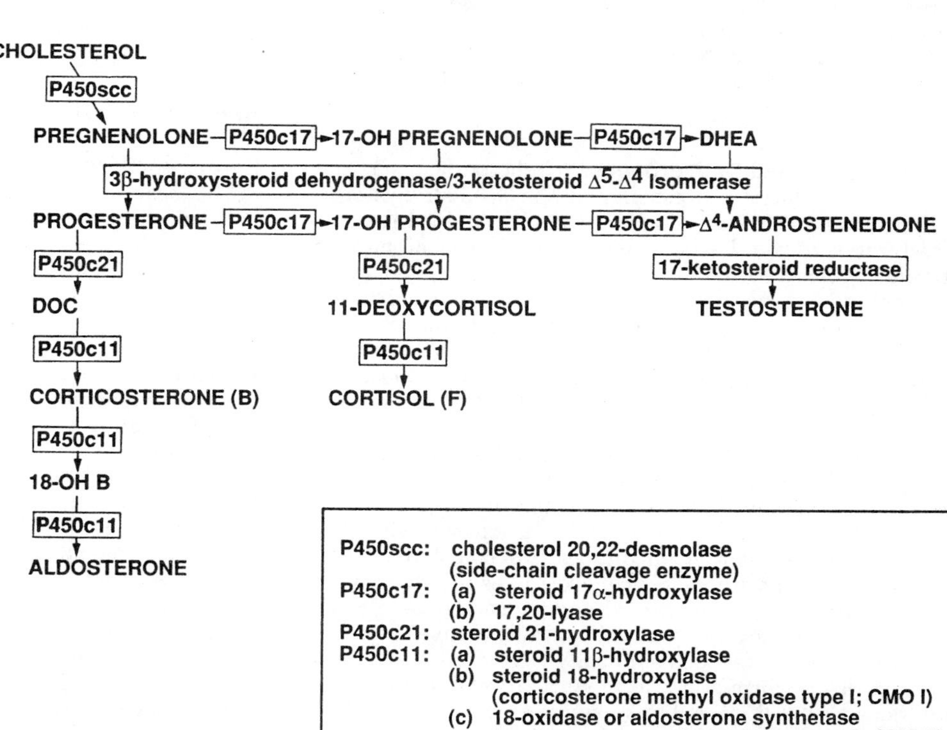

Figure 1. Adrenal steroidogenesis. Conversions are catalyzed by the enzyme protein or activity shown in the boxes. The key at lower right lists multiple activities for cytochromes P-450c17 and P-450c11. In addition to the four cytochromes P-450 with functions in the cortisol pathway, a fifth steroidogenic P-450 carries out aromatization of androgens to estrogens (P-450aro, not shown here). The two remaining enzyme activities, named 3β-hydroxysteroid dehydrogenase (3β-HSD) and 17-ketosteroid reductase (also 17β-hydroxysteroid dehydrogenase) are not cytochromes P-450. The enzyme activity 3-ketosteroid-$\Delta^{5,4}$-isomerase is closely associated with 3β-HSD.

and even in asymptomatic affected individuals. In addition to the common symptoms of mild androgen excess in females (menstrual irregularity, hirsutism, acne, balding), oligospermia, and infertility have been found in men. Growth may be affected, even in individuals who are otherwise asymptomatic. A discernible trend toward short adult height, to a lesser degree than that seen in classic CAH, is roughly proportional to the degree of androgen excess. The partial deficiencies of the steroid 21-hydroxylase enzymes (cytochrome P-450c21), which cause nonclassic 21-hydroxylase deficiency, are known to stem from allelic variants at the same structural gene locus (CYP21).

11β-Hydroxylase Deficiency

Excessive production of adrenal androgens with consequent signs of virilization (as described for defective 21-hydroxylase) also results from 11β-hydroxylase deficiency. In this disorder, however, the excess adrenal prehormones exert net mineralocorticoid agonist activity and cause sodium retention and volume expansion. Variable consequences include suppressed PRA, potassium depletion, and clinical hypertension. 11-Deoxycorticosterone (DOC), secreted in very small amounts by the normal adrenal cortex and markedly increased in the sera of patients with 11β-hydroxylase deficiency, has sodium-retaining activity and is the presumed hypertension-producing steroid in this form of CAH. Excess DOC—or even excess mineralocorticoid effect of steroid(s)—does not account entirely for the abnormality, however, because the values of serum potassium, plasma DOC concentration, and plasma renin activity (PRA) correlate poorly with each other and with elevated blood pressure.

Nonclassic forms of 11β-hydroxylase deficiency have been reported and may represent allelic variants. Investigators have been unable to demonstrate a consistent biochemical defect in obligate heterozygotes (parents) for mild 11β-hydroxylase deficiency, either in the baseline state or with ACTH stimulation.

Ten mutations have been identified in the *CYP11B1* gene on chromosome 8q22, where the 11β-hydroxylase enzyme is encoded.

3β-Hydroxysteroid Dehydrogenase Deficiency

The classic form of deficiency of the 3β-hydroxysteroid dehydrogenase enzyme (3β-HSD, 3β-ol) results in diminished rates of synthesis of all three classes of adrenal steroids, glucocorticoid (cortisol), mineralocorticoid (aldosterone), and androgens. Greatly increased concentrations of all precursors proximal to the action of the 3β-HSD–catalyzed steps are detected in the sera of patients with severe deficiency of the enzyme. These steroids, biochemically 3β-hydroxy-5-ene compounds, termed Δ^5-steroids (delta-5, equivalent to 5-ene), have low physiologic activity, and severely affected patients exhibit frank adrenal insufficiency and have a poor prognosis. In affected males, the impaired secretion of cortisol, aldosterone, and testosterone results in male pseudohermaphroditism with life-threatening salt wasting in infancy. Affected females can present at birth with mild virilization resulting from the effect of the Δ^5 androgen dehydroepiandrosterone (DHEA) converted peripherally to Δ^4 (biologically active) steroids. Variant forms have been clinically described, such as a non–salt-losing form and a form with adrenal insufficiency but normal onset of puberty, suggesting that DHEA is converted to more active androgens and, subsequently, estrogens.

The nonclassic 3β-HSD deficiency is being identified with increasing frequency as an underlying basis of hyperandrogenism in females, either in preadolescent girls with premature adrenarche or in adolescents and young adults with hirsutism and oligomenorrhea as a syndrome that resembles polycystic ovarian disease (PCO). The presentation of 21-hydroxylase and 3β-HSD deficiencies can be distinguished from other forms of PCO by the adrenal hormone profile observed in sera following ACTH stimulation testing.

All salt-losing and non–salt-losing forms of classic 3β-HSD deficiency studied so far are caused by one or more point mutations in the type II 3β-HSD gene, located on chromosome 1, leading to the expression of a truncated or mutant 3β-HSD protein. No genetic defects have been reported in the nonclassic 3β-HSD deficiency.

Rare Adrenal Enzyme Defects

Defects of cholesterol desmolase or steroid 17α-hydroxylase/17,20-lyse, the early enzymes in the cortisol synthetic pathway, are found only rarely. Complete cholesterol desmolase deficiency precludes the formation of any steroids whatsoever, clearly a very grave condition. The hyperplastic response to sustained ACTH elevation in this form of CAH typically produces an extremely abnormal appearance of the adrenocortical tissue due the accumulation of cholesterol esters in intracellular storage, a condition called lipoid adrenal hyperplasia.

Steroid 17α-hydroxylase deficiency permits adrenal production of 17-deoxysteroids. Since DOC (see 11β-hydroxylase deficiency above) is included among these intermediates, hypertension is also a feature of this form of CAH. The 17-deoxysteroid corticosterone (compound B) exhibits marginal glucocorticoid activity. Increased concentrations of compound B in the sera suppress the hypothalamus-pituitary axis, resulting in less severe plasma ACTH increases than those seen in other forms of CAH. In addition, 17β-hydroxylase deficiency patients seem better able to respond to infection and other types of stress.

APPROACH TO DIAGNOSIS

Hormonal Measurements

The best approach to the diagnosis of 21-hydroxylase deficiency is to measure the morning serum concentration of 17α-hydroxyprogesterone (17-OHP), which is markedly increased in 21-hydroxylase deficiency. Neonatal screening based on dried capillary blood 17-OHP (obtained by heelprick and spotted on filter paper) taken on days 3 to 5 of life is a reliable and cost-effective procedure. Routine screening improves detection of all cases and reduces morbidity and mortality from severe salt wasting in males and prevents wrong sex assignment of females.

The two index serum steroids for detection of the steroid 11β-hydroxylase deficiency are DOC and 11-deoxycortisol (compound S). Increased concentrations of these steroids in serum are reflected by increases in the excreted amounts of the corresponding tetrahydro (TH) compounds (3α-hydroxy, 5β-hydro reduced forms), THDOC and THS in the urine. Suppressed renin is also observed in this condition.

A high ratio of 3β-hydroxy, 5-ene to 3-oxo, 4-ene steroids in the serum or urine is evidence of the presence of a 3β-hydroxysteroid dehydrogenase enzyme defect. Absolute serum concentrations of 5-ene (Δ^5-) steroids pregnenolone, 17α-hydroxypregnenolone, and DHEA are increased in 3β-HSD deficiency, and urinary excretion of the metabolites (Δ^5-) pregnenetriol is increased. Plasma renin is increased,

Table 2. Diagnosis of the Forms of 21-Hydroxylase Deficiency

Indications for Testing

The following clinical signs and symptoms should lead the physician to consider the diagnosis of 21-hyroxylase deficiency:

In the Neonate

Ambiguity of the genitalia in the genetic female, including clitoromegaly, fusion of the labia majora or minora, and urogenital sinus
History of a previously affected member of the family
Cryptorchid testes, not responsive to human chorionic gonadotropin (HCG)

In Childhood

Advanced stature or advanced bone age
Precocious appearance of sexual hair
Seborrhea or acne; oily hair
Recession (frontal or temporal) of the hairline
Enlarged clitoris, fusion (posteroanterior) of the labia in genetic females
Enlarged penis relative to the size and volume of the testes in males
Early onset of puberty

At Pubertal Age and After Puberty

Short stature with history of early end of growth
Excessive hair on the face, abdomen, inner thighs, or arms
Enlarged or enlarging clitoris in the female
Severe acne
Loss of scalp hair
Excessively deep voice in the female
Amenorrhea or irregular menses in the female
Infertility in either sex

Testing

Give Cortrosyn (synthetic $ACTH_{1-24}$) 0.25 mg IV bolus at 8 AM.
Obtain blood at the time of Cortrosyn administration (0 minutes) and again after 60 minutes.
Separate serum samples (and freeze if necessary). Submit serum for 17α-hydroxyprogesterone measurement.
Compare values with those shown on the nomogram (see Fig. 3) and score for indicated 21-hydroxylase genotype.

Interpretation of Results

The coordinates of the baseline and ACTH-stimulated values form a regression line, and subjects aggregate into groups around the regression line. Patients with classic CAH have the most severe 21-hydroxylase deficiency. Patients with the symptomatic or asymptomatic nonclassic forms have a less severe deficiency, while heterozygotes for all three forms have an even milder deficiency that is unmasked only with ACTH stimulation. Those members of the general population who are in the heterozygote range may be carriers of a gene for 21-hydroxylase deficiency (see Fig. 3).

reflecting the decreased synthesis of mineralocorticoid and sodium wasting in this condition. The diagnosis is always made by an ACTH stimulation test. The results are compared with the diagnostic criteria described for each of the enzyme deficiencies (Tables 2 and 3).

Table 3. Assessment of Adrenal 3-Hydroxysteroid Dehydrogenase Activity in Pubertal and Postpubertal Women by Serum Steroid Concentrations/Ratios on ACTH Testing

Indications for Testing

Same as for diagnosis of 21-hydroxylase deficiency (see Table 2)

Testing Procedure

Same as for 21-hydroxylase deficiency

Interpretation of Results

Deficiency of adrenal 3β-hydroxysteroid dehydrogenase is diagnosed when all of the following ACTH stimulated hormone concentrations or ratios are found to be more than 2 standard deviations above the reference mean.

1. Δ^5-17-Hydroxypregnenolone
2. Δ^5-17-Hydroxypregnenolone/17α-hydroxyprogesterone
3. Δ^5-17-Hydroxypregnenolone/cortisol
4. Dehydroepiandrosterone (DHEA)

Optional

5. DHEA/Δ^4-androstenedione

Prenatal Diagnosis of 21-Hydroxylase Deficiency

Prenatal diagnosis by hormone measurement during the second trimester has been used for two decades in pregnancies known to be at risk. Currently, cultured fetal cells from either the amniotic fluid or chorionic villus sampling (CVS) provide DNA and allow early genetic diagnosis (at 9 to 10 weeks of gestation with the use of CVS) and the possibility for intervention. The administration of dexamethasone (20 μg/kg/day) to pregnant women to suppress the fetal adrenal has been done, with good results. The greatest experience in prenatal diagnosis and treatment has been with 21-hydroxylase deficiency CAH. Treatment is started as soon as the pregnancy is confirmed by increased human chorionic gonadotropin (HCG) concentration in the maternal serum (Fig. 2) when a couple is at genetic risk for having an affected offspring. Hormonal treatment, regardless of the gender or affected status of the fetus, consists of dexamethasone given orally to the mother. Using the cells from CVS, karyotype and DNA analysis are performed. If the fetus is male, the dexamethasone can be stopped immediately. If the fetus is female, treatment continues until the results of DNA analysis are obtained. If the fetus is unaffected, the dexamethasone is discontinued, but if 21-hydroxylase CAH is diagnosed, treatment is continued to term. If CVS is not an option for the family or if its results are not conclusive, similar studies at 15 to 18 weeks on cells obtained by amniocentesis should be performed. The current recommendation is to continue the therapy uninterrupted until delivery, not sus-

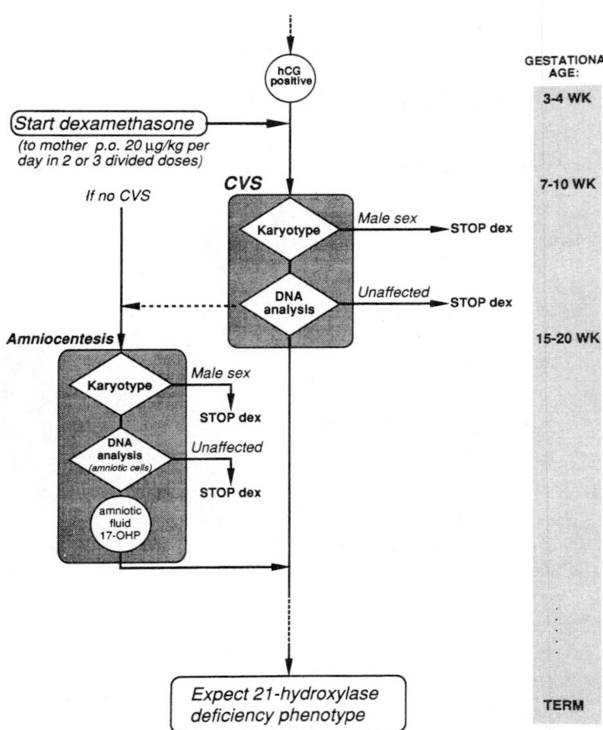

Figure 2. Algorithm for prenatal diagnosis and treatment of congenital adrenal hyperplasia. (Modified from Speiser, P.W., et al.: First trimester prenatal treatment and molecular genetic diagnosis of congenital adrenal hyperplasia [21-hydroxylase deficiency]. J. Clin. Endocrinol. Metab., 70:838–848, 1990, © by The Endocrine Society.)

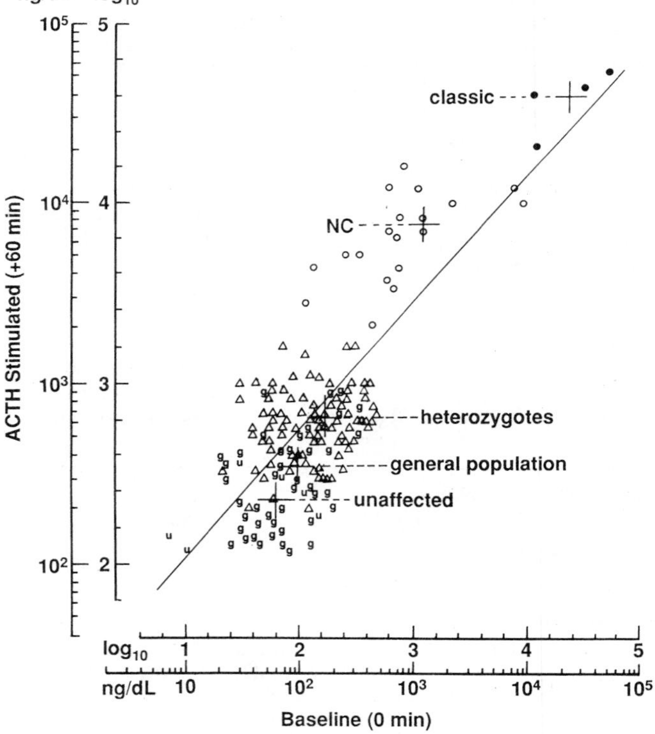

Figure 3. Nomogram relating baseline to ACTH-stimulated serum concentrations of 17α-hydroxyprogesterone. Scales are logarithmic. A regression line for all data points is shown. (Datapoints from New, M.I., et al.: Genotyping steroid 21-hydroxylase deficiency: Hormonal reference data. J. Clin. Endocrinol. Metab., 57:320–326, 1983; data collected from 1982–1991 at Department of Pediatrics, The New York Hospital–Cornell Medical Center.)

pending it prior to amniocentesis, as was done earlier when only hormonal testing was available.

ACTH Testing in the Evaluation for Classic and Nonclassic CAH

See Tables 2 and 3 and Figure 3.

ENDOCRINE PARANEOPLASTIC SYNDROMES

By José S. Subauste, M.D.,
and David E. Schteingart, M.D.
Ann Arbor, Michigan

The clinical manifestations of endocrine paraneoplastic syndromes result from the secretion of hormones and other factors by tumors arising in tissues that normally do not secrete them. Manifestations of the paraneoplastic syndrome may precede the diagnosis of the tumor, and the hormonal effect of the tumor may be more deleterious to the patient than the neoplasm itself. Therefore, prompt and accurate diagnosis is crucial to improving the clinical course and survival of these patients. Coexisting endocrine disease, drug toxicity, or other disorders must be considered in the differential diagnosis of paraneoplastic syndromes in a cancer patient.

MALIGNANCY-ASSOCIATED HYPERCALCEMIA

Malignancy is the cause of two thirds of the cases of hypercalcemia seen in hospitalized patients. Eighty per cent of malignancy-associated hypercalcemia demonstrates little or no skeletal involvement by the tumor, and this condition is known as humoral hypercalcemia of malignancy (HHM). The HHM syndrome is mediated by the production of parathyroid hormone–related protein (PTHRP) by the tumor, which binds to the PTH receptor and mimics many of the actions of PTH. Malignant neoplasms associated with PTHRP production include the following: squamous cell carcinoma (lung, esophagus, cervix, vulva, skin, head, and neck), lymphoma, carcinomas of the kidney, bladder, and ovary. Rarely, in some cases of Hodgkin's and B-cell lymphoma and human T-cell lymphotropic virus (HTLV-I)–associated T-cell lymphoma-leukemia, the hypercalcemia is mediated by the production of 1,25-dihydroxyvitamin D_3 by these tumors.

In the remaining 20 per cent of malignancy-associated hypercalcemia, also termed local osteolytic hypercalcemia (LOH), bone metastasis causes extensive destruction mediated by several cytokines, interleukin-1 (IL-1), IL-6, lymphotoxin, tumor necrosis factor-α (TNFα), and transforming growth factor-α (TGFα). LOH is seen in multiple myeloma and breast carcinoma. Essentially all patients with multiple myeloma develop extensive bone destruction, but only 20 to 40 per cent of them develop hypercalcemia at some point during the course of the disease. Hypercalcemia in breast carcinoma is almost always associated with bone metastasis, but in some instances it is mediated by PTHRP.

Clinical Manifestations

The symptoms of altered mental status often predominate in the hypercalcemia due to malignancy and can vary from poor mental concentration to depression, confusion, and coma. Gastrointestinal symptoms, such as anorexia, nausea, vomiting, and constipation, are frequent, and muscle weakness is common. Polyuria, due to impaired ability of the distal nephron to concentrate urine, is common and accompanied by polydipsia. The combination of vomiting and polyuria may lead to dehydration. Cardiac arrhythmias, particularly sinus bradycardia and atrioventricular block can be seen, with shortening of QT interval on electrocardiogram (ECG) due to an increase in the rate of cardiac repolarization. Nephrolithiasis, band keratopathy, and pruritus, which are long-term complications of hypercalcemia, are rarely observed in malignancy-associated hypercalcemia.

Laboratory Evaluation

Hypercalcemia due to malignancy tends to progress rapidly, with total calcium concentrations frequently greater than 12 mg/dL. On the other hand, the majority of patients with primary hyperparathyroidism are asymptomatic and have relatively mild hypercalcemia for months to years, with concentrations within 1 mg/dL above the upper limits of normal and usually below 12 mg/dL. Three fractions of calcium occur in serum: ionized calcium (50 per cent), protein-bound calcium (40 per cent), and calcium that is complexed with phosphate and citrate (10 per cent). The total serum calcium concentration may be misleading in patients with malignancy-associated hypercalcemia, because these patients commonly have hypoalbuminemia, which causes lower total serum calcium concentrations. Other patients, particularly those with multiple myeloma, may have abnormal proteins that bind calcium avidly and increase the total calcium concentration. Therefore, in any clinical setting where a calcium-binding protein disorder is suspected, measurement of ionized calcium is recommended.

The most important combination of tests for evaluating patients with hypercalcemia is the measurement of the intact PTH concentration by two-site immunoradiometric assay (IRMA) together with the determination of the serum calcium concentration. The intact PTH concentration is increased in more than 90 per cent of patients with primary hyperparathyroidism. In all other causes of hypercalcemia, including malignancy, intact PTH is typically suppressed because it does not cross-react with PTHRP. Currently, several assays for detecting different regions of PTHRP are available. The most sensitive of these assays is IRMA, which measures large N-terminal regions by using monoclonal antibodies, with detection limits of 0.1 pmol/L and no cross-reactivity with PTH. However, not all patients with increased PTHRP concentrations have a malignant tumor. Increased N-terminal PTHRP can be seen in nonmalignant pheochromocytoma, mammary hypertrophy, and lymphedema, and C-terminal PTHRP can be increased in renal failure (creatinine clearance below 30 mL per minute). PTHRP is not stable in plasma samples owing to rapid degradation by proteases. This could account for false-negative results in patients with malignancy. Therefore, the addition of protease inhibitors (leupeptin and aprotinin) is recommended for stabilizing PTHRP in blood samples.

The serum phosphate concentration is usually decreased in malignancy and primary hyperparathyroidism and is increased in hypervitaminosis D. But overall, the serum phosphate concentration is not very useful in the evaluation of a patient with hypercalcemia, because it is influenced by dietary intake, diurnal variations, and renal function. Also, patients with severe hypercalcemia from any cause can have a low serum phosphate concentration.

Classically, hypercalcemia in malignancy is associated with metabolic alkalosis, whereas primary hyperparathyroidism is associated with metabolic acidosis. However, overlap is significant and blood pH and carbon dioxide concentrations are not useful for the differential diagnosis. Similarly, serum alkaline phosphatase activity is not helpful in the differential diagnosis of hypercalcemia because it is a marker of bone formation and is typically normal in patients with lytic lesions, such as multiple myeloma, and in most patients with primary hyperparathyroidism.

Increased 1,25-dihydroxyvitamin D_3 concentrations are seen in granulomatous diseases, vitamin D intoxication, and primary hyperparathyroidism. With the exception of some lymphomas, patients with malignancy-associated hypercalcemia have low 1,25-dihydroxyvitamin D_3 concentrations in their sera.

A 24-hour urine collection for calcium is particularly helpful for ruling out familial hypocalciuric hypercalcemia, a benign autosomal dominant disorder that is usually asymptomatic. In this condition, the ratio of calcium clearance to creatinine clearance is below 0.01, whereas in all other causes of hypercalcemia it is above 0.01. Malignancy-associated hypercalcemia typically causes a marked increase in urinary calcium excretion.

Imaging Studies

Neither skeletal radiographs nor radionuclide bone scans detect all bone metastasis. Skeletal radiographs are particularly useful for the evaluation of lytic lesions (e.g., multiple myeloma), whereas bone scans are superior for blastic lesions (e.g., metastatic carcinoma of the prostate). The subperiostal resorption sometimes seen in primary hyperparathyroidism does not occur in malignancy-associated hypercalcemia.

Pitfalls in Diagnosis

Approximately 10 per cent of patients with malignancy have coexisting primary hyperparathyroidism. This condition should be suspected when a cancer patient has mild hypercalcemia with an indolent course; the diagnosis is confirmed on finding an increased intact PTH concentration in the serum. Ectopic PTH production by the tumor is extremely rare. Other potential causes of hypercalcemia in patients with malignancy include drugs (e.g., tamoxifen, thiazides, lithium, estrogens), immobilization, renal failure, adrenal failure (possibly due to extensive metastasis to the adrenal glands), hyperthyroidism, and excessive vitamin A or D or calcium supplements. Hypercalcemia due to malignancy is a poor prognostic factor; 75 per cent of these patients die within 3 months.

ECTOPIC ACTH SYNDROME

Ectopic adrenocorticotropic hormone (ACTH) syndrome (EAS) represents 15 per cent of patients with Cushing's syndrome. A variety of nonpituitary tumors can secrete ACTH and/or corticotropin-releasing hormone (CRH). In early reports, small cell lung carcinoma (SCLC) was the leading cause of EAS. But more recent studies show that thoracic carcinoids are the most common cause of EAS, representing as many as 46 per cent of all patients, while SCLC is responsible for fewer than 20 per cent of patients with this syndrome. Other tumors associated with ectopic ACTH production include pancreatic carcinoma, pheochromocytoma, medullary thyroid carcinoma, neurogenic tumors, and carcinomas of the ovary, prostate, and kidney. ACTH-dependent Cushing's syndrome in a male is most likely caused by a nonpituitary tumor, whereas in a female, ACTH-secreting pituitary neoplasms are a more frequent cause of ACTH-dependent Cushing's syndrome.

Clinical Presentation

Small cell lung carcinoma is an example of an overt ACTH-secreting tumor. The history of symptoms is short, usually less than 3 months, with an aggressive course. Most patients are older than 45 years of age, and cushingoid habitus is usually absent. Hypokalemic metabolic alkalosis is seen in as many as 100 per cent of patients owing to excessive secretion of deoxycorticosterone acetate (DOCA) and/or cortisol. Hypertension, peripheral edema, glucose intolerance, weight loss, hyperpigmentation, and proximal weakness are also common.

Occult ACTH-secreting tumor is represented by bronchial and thymic carcinoids and some pancreatic tumors. These slow-growing neoplasms have a duration of symptoms ranging from 6 months to several years. The indolent course of these tumors often results in the development of classic cushingoid features. Hypokalemic metabolic alkalosis is seen in more than 75 per cent of patients with occult EAS, but it occurs in fewer than 10 per cent of patients with pituitary-dependent Cushing's syndrome.

Laboratory Evaluation

A 24-hour urinary collection for free cortisol (UFC) and the 1-mg overnight dexamethasone suppression test are excellent screening tests for the initial evaluation of Cushing's syndrome. Patients with a high 24-hour UFC and a lack of suppression of the morning cortisol level to less than 5 μg/dL after the 1-mg overnight dexamethasone suppression test should undergo the 2-day low-dose (0.5 mg every 6 hours) dexamethasone suppression test, which is the most accurate test in establishing the diagnosis of Cushing's syndrome. A suppression of the 24-hour UFC to less than 20 μg/dL or plasma cortisol to less than 5 μg/dL is a normal response and excludes Cushing's syndrome as a cause.

After establishing the diagnosis of Cushing's syndrome, a morning plasma ACTH concentration should be measured. Plasma ACTH concentrations above 400 pg/mL are typically observed in patients with overt ectopic ACTH-secreting tumors. But patients with occult ACTH-secreting tumors may have ACTH concentrations (50 to 400 pg/mL) indistinguishable from patients with pituitary-dependent Cushing's syndrome.

A series of dynamic tests can help distinguish between pituitary-dependent Cushing's syndrome and EAS.

Standard 2-Day High-Dose Dexamethasone Suppression Test (2 mg Every 6 Hours)

A reduction in 24-hour UFC to more than 50 per cent below baseline supports the diagnosis of pituitary-dependent Cushing's syndrome. However, 13 per cent of patients with pituitary-dependent Cushing's syndrome fail to suppress; moreover, as many as one third of patients with EAS, particularly those with occult tumors, suppress 24-hour UFC to more than 50 per cent. If we use a stricter criteria with 90 per cent or greater suppression of UFC, none of the patients with EAS has a positive test.

Overnight High-Dose (8-mg) Dexamethasone Suppression Test

A reduction in morning plasma cortisol concentration to less than 50 per cent of baseline value indicates pituitary-dependent Cushing's syndrome. Because this test is easier to perform and has a greater sensitivity and specificity than the traditional 2-day high-dose dexamethasone test, it is the preferred screening test for evaluating the cause of Cushing's syndrome.

Metyrapone Test

A twofold to threefold increase above baseline in 24-hour urinary 17-hydroxycorticosteroid excretion or an 8 AM plasma 11-deoxycortisol concentration of 7 to 22 μg/dL or more indicates pituitary-dependent Cushing's syndrome. Unfortunately, this test has a low specificity, and one third of patients with EAS secondary to occult tumors have a positive response.

Ovine CRH Stimulation Test

A rise of more than 20 per cent in plasma cortisol and an increase of more than 50 per cent in ACTH after intravenous administration of CRH are observed in pituitary-dependent Cushing's syndrome. This test has a sensitivity and specificity of more than 90 per cent, but some EAS secondary to occult neoplasms can show a positive response. The occult tumors that respond to dexamethasone and metyrapone and exhibit CRH stimulation are probably those that produce CRH without associated ACTH.

Inferior Petrosal Venous Sampling

Inferior petrosal venous sampling is probably the best test for diagnosing pituitary-dependent Cushing's syndrome versus EAS. A measurement of ACTH concentrations from the inferior petrosal sinus (IPS) bilaterally and the peripheral veins (PV) is obtained in the basal state and after CRH stimulation. Basal IPS-to-PV ratios greater than 2.0 and greater than 3.0 after CRH stimulation indicate pituitary-dependent Cushing's syndrome. This test has a sensitivity and specificity near 100 per cent, and it is particularly useful in the differential diagnosis of occult forms of EAS, which are often clinically indistinguishable from pituitary ACTH-dependent Cushing's syndrome by the usual steroid dynamic tests and scanning procedures.

Imaging Studies

Routine chest film can usually detect SCLC with overt Cushing's syndrome and some thymic tumors but is negative in 70 per cent of bronchial carcinoids. Computed tomography (CT) of the chest detects most thymic tumors and 83 per cent of bronchial carcinoids. Magnetic resonance imaging (MRI) of the chest can visualize bronchial carcinoids not seen on CT. Indium-111 somatostatin analogue scintigraphy detects 85 per cent of carcinoid tumors and predicts an inhibitory effect of octreotide on circulating ACTH and cortisol concentrations. CT of the abdomen detects two thirds of pancreatic neuroendocrine tumors; MRI of the abdomen gives no additional information and is therefore not recommended. Once the diagnosis of EAS has been established, CT of the chest should be performed first. If the finding is negative, abdominal CT should be performed. If neither study is able to localize the tumor, an MRI scan of the chest and/or indium-111 octreotide scan is obtained.

Pitfalls in Diagnosis

Obesity, stress, diuretic use, and high salt administration can cause a mild increase in 24-hour UFC excretion, whereas renal failure causes unreliably low 24-hour UFC. Anorexia nervosa and stress can be associated with a lack of suppression in the low-dose overnight dexamethasone test. Drugs such as phenytoin and phenobarbital can enhance the clearance of dexamethasone and can cause false-positive results in dexamethasone suppression tests. Therefore, measurement of 8 AM cortisol and dexamethasone concentrations in blood improves the diagnostic accuracy. Estrogens increase the plasma cortisol by increasing corticosteroid binding globulin (CBG) concentration, but 24-hour UFC is within normal limits. Patients with severe depression can have increased 24-hour UFC and may show lack of suppression with the low-dose dexamethasone test. However, patients with depression lack the physical findings of Cushing's syndrome, their circadian rhythm for cortisol is preserved, and they show blunted response after CRH stimulation test.

Alcoholism is also associated with an elevated 24-hour UFC and is indistinguishable from Cushing's syndrome by physical findings, standard dynamic tests, and circadian rhythm for cortisol. Therefore, if equivocal the tests are repeated after several weeks of alcohol abstinence.

HYPOGLYCEMIA

Neoplasms associated with hypoglycemia are located in the abdomen in two thirds of cases (peritoneal or retroperitoneal areas), and the remainder are found in the thorax. Approximately 45 per cent of these tumors are of mesenchymal origin (fibromas, sarcomas, mesotheliomas). Hepatoma and adrenal carcinoma account for 20 and 10 per cent of the cases, respectively. Other neoplasms associated with hypoglycemia include carcinomas of the stomach, pancreas, and colon in addition to cholangioma and carcinoids.

The hypoglycemia is mediated by the production of insulin-like growth factor-II (IGF-II) by these tumors. IGF-II can cause hypoglycemia by a dual mechanism: increasing glucose utilization as a consequence of insulin-like actions and inhibiting growth hormone secretion with a subsequent decrease in hepatic glucose production.

Clinical Manifestations

These tumors are typically large, slow-growing, and bulky, weighing as much as several kilograms. They present with fasting hypoglycemia that must satisfy the Whipple triad: symptoms consistent with hypoglycemia, measured low blood glucose concentration (i.e., below 50 mg/dL in males and below 45 mg/dL in females) at the time of the symptoms, and relief of the symptoms by the administration of glucose or food. The symptoms of neuroglucopenia are similar to those of insulinoma, with poor mental concentration, confusion, visual disturbances, seizures, and coma more prominent than symptoms of adrenergic activity.

Laboratory Evaluation

A prolonged supervised fast, up to 72 hours, has been the mainstay of the evaluation of fasting hypoglycemia. The patient is kept active, ingesting only noncaloric fluids. Plasma glucose, insulin, C-peptide, and cortisol concentrations are measured every 6 hours and with the development of symptomatic hypoglycemia. In most patients, symptomatic hypoglycemia develops during the first 24 hours of fasting. In tumor-induced hypoglycemia, insulin and C-peptide concentrations are typically suppressed to less than or equal to 2 mU/L and 0.1 nmol, respectively. If by 72 hours no symptomatic hypoglycemia has occurred, 30 minutes of exercise is performed. Fewer than 2 per cent of patients with organic fasting hypoglycemia have a normal 72-hour fasting test. If the diagnosis of fasting hypoglycemia is established, other causes must be excluded (Table 1).

The utility of determining plasma IGF-II concentrations in the diagnosis of tumor-induced hypoglycemia is still unclear. Increased IGF-II supports the diagnosis, but often the values are normal. Under these circumstances, a concomitant measurement of IGF-I can be helpful. Typically, a decreased plasma IGF-I concentration is associated with a decreased plasma IGF-II concentration; thus, a normal IGF-II value in the presence of a low plasma IGF-I value supports a diagnosis of tumor-induced hypoglycemia in patients with insulin-independent, nonketotic fasting hypoglycemia. Artifactual hypoglycemia can be observed in patients with leukemia or hemolysis if the cells are not separated from serum within 1 hour. Alternatively, an antiglycolytic agent can be added to the whole blood specimen.

SYNDROME OF INAPPROPRIATE ANTIDIURETIC HORMONE

The syndrome of inappropriate antidiuretic hormone (SIADH) consists of autonomous release of ADH that is unresponsive to either osmotic or nonosmotic stimuli. The diagnosis of SIADH requires (1) presence of hyponatremia with hypo-osmolality in the presence of inappropriately concentrated urine; (2) absence of edema or volume depletion; (3) absence of renal failure, adrenal insufficiency, and hypothyroidism, all of which can impair water excretion and present with a clinical picture identical to SIADH; and (4) absence of several drugs that can cause water retention by stimulating ADH release and/or by potentiating ADH action in the kidney; chemotherapeutic agents (cyclophosphamide, vincristine, and vinblastine) and narcotics have especially been implicated in SIADH. Conditions such as severe pain, emesis, and stress (e.g., postoperative state), frequently seen in cancer patients, are also physiologic stimuli for ADH secretion and can therefore mimic SIADH.

Bronchogenic carcinoma, especially SCLC, is by far the most frequent malignant cause of SIADH. Clinical SIADH occurs in 20 to 40 per cent of patients with SCLC, although as many as 88 per cent of patients with extensive SCLC have increased circulating ADH levels. Other tumors associated with ectopic production of ADH include carcinomas of the bladder, ureter, prostate, duodenum, and pancreas; lymphoma; mesothelioma; thymoma; and Ewing's sarcoma.

Table 1. Differential Diagnosis of Hypoglycemia

Drugs
Insulin, sulfonylureas, alcohol, salicylates, quinine, pentamidine, $beta_2$-agonists, disopyramide, and propranolol
Insulin-Independent Conditions
Liver and renal failure, sepsis
Cortisol, adrenocorticotropic hormone (ACTH), and/or growth hormone deficiency
Autoimmune disorders (IgG antibodies against insulin or insulin receptors)
Insulin-Dependent Conditions
Insulinoma, nesidioblastosis

Clinical Manifestations

Most patients are asymptomatic. When symptoms occur, the serum sodium concentration is typically below 120 mEq/L. The severity of symptoms also depends on the rate at which the serum sodium concentration decreases. In addition, children and the elderly are most likely to become symptomatic. The symptoms of hyponatremia are manifested by a deterioration of central nervous system function that includes irritability, lethargy, disorientation, psychosis, seizures, and coma. Gastrointestinal symptoms can be seen, particularly in the early stages of the disease.

Laboratory Evaluation

Patients with SIADH have decreased plasma osmolarity (<280 mOsm/kg). Urine osmolality is higher than that of plasma and is frequently over 300 mOsm/kg. Serum urea nitrogen and uric acid concentrations are low in SIADH. In the vast majority of cases, urinary sodium excretion is greater than 20 mEq/L but could be lower if patients are placed on a low salt diet (see article on SIADH).

PHEOCHROMOCYTOMA

By Jong-Yoon Yi, M.D.,
and George L. Bakris, M.D.
Chicago, Illinois

Pheochromocytoma is also known as chromaffinoma and paraganglioma.

DEFINITION AND ETIOLOGY

Rarely, pheochromocytoma can cause hypertension characterized by variable clinical presentations. The failure to diagnose pheochromocytoma can be fatal in certain clinical situations, such as surgery, anesthesia, and delivery. Named after their tendency to turn a dusky (pheo) color (chromo) when exposed to dichromate, pheochromocytomas have an estimated incidence of 6 per 100,000 hypertensive patients per year in the United States. The estimated incidence is even lower in other countries. This tumor is more common in whites than in African Americans. No sex or age predominance has been recognized in any group. Ten per cent of these tumors are bilateral or multiple in the adrenals, 10 per cent are extra-adrenal, 10 per cent occur in children, 10 per cent are malignant, and 10 per cent secrete epinephrine. Computed tomography (CT) and magnetic resonance imaging (MRI) have increased the number of incidental findings of adrenal masses. The evaluation of these masses has led to a differential diagnosis of functionally active or malignant masses, including pheochromocytoma. Many clinicians seek guidance on cost-effective ways of diagnosing pheochromocytoma; this article offers one reasonable approach to the problem.

Cells that make up the sympathetic nervous system arise from the primitive neural crest. Stem cells (sympathogonia) from this neural crest differentiate into several cell lines that have the potential to degenerate into tumors (e.g., neuroblasts form neuroblastomas, ganglion cells degenerate to ganglioneuromas, and chromaffin cells yield pheochromocytomas). The latter are catecholamine-releasing tumors that may arise anywhere in the sympathoadrenal system. All neural crest tumors share histologic and biologic characteristics. Neuroblastomas and ganglioneuromas, however, occur primarily in childhood and are typically more aggressive than pheochromocytomas.

EVALUATION

To secure the diagnosis of pheochromocytoma, the clinician must have a strong clinical suspicion that is confirmed by imaging studies and biochemical tests of urine or plasma. If biochemical testing is inconclusive, pharmacologic studies should be undertaken. Overproduction of norepinephrine can be documented in 90 per cent of pheochromocytomas. Other neurochemical and peptide products, however, can be released from the tumor.

Clinical Manifestations

Patients with pheochromocytoma classically present with *headache, tachycardia,* and *sweating.* Tachycardia and sweating are most commonly associated with epinephrine-secreting tumors. Alternatively, patients may present with *hypertension, headache, hyperglycemia, hyperhidrosis,* and a *hypermetabolic state.* The more infrequent symptoms and signs (Table 1) are attributed to dopa, dopamine, and epinephrine, which have more vasodilatory effects than norepinephrine. Secretion of physiologically active peptide hormones (e.g., corticotropin, somatostatin, vasoactive intestinal peptide, calcitonin, neuropeptide Y, opioid peptides, human growth hormone–releasing factor, insulin-like growth factor II, erythropoietin, and parathyroid hormone–related protein) also contributes to the development of the symptoms and signs listed in Table 1.

Seventy-five per cent of patients with pheochromocytoma experience weekly episodes of symptoms that last for an hour in 80 per cent of cases. However, the frequency, duration, and severity of episodes vary with the size of tumor and the turnover rate of catecholamine metabolites. Clinically apparent episodes can be induced or provoked by physical or emotional stimuli, including exercise, urination, defecation, bending over, or smoking. The ingestion of corticosteroids, histamine, opiates, tricyclic antidepressants, or beta-blockers, the administration of radiocontrast media, or the induction of anesthesia can also induce an "episode" by increasing the synthesis and release and decreasing the reuptake of catecholamines. *Hypertension* is the most consistent feature of pheochromocytoma, and its positive predictive value is estimated at more than 95 per cent. Thus, if the patient has clinical manifestations suggestive of pheochromocytoma without hypertension, the chances that these clinical manifestations are due to pheochromocytoma are less than 5 per cent.

Table 1. Symptoms and Signs of Pheochromocytoma

Symptoms*	Frequency (%)
Headaches	40–96
Diaphoresis	40–74
Palpitations	45–70
Pallor	40–45
Nervousness and/or anxiety	22–43
Tremulousness	29–31

*Infrequent symptoms: flushing, Raynaud's phenomenon, nausea, seizures, dizziness, dyspnea, and abdominal, chest, or arm pain.

Signs†	Frequency (%)
Hypertension	>90
Sustained	50–60
Intermittent	2–50
Paroxysms	50
Weight loss (hypermetabolic state)	80
Funduscopic changes	50–70
Orthostatic hypotension	40–70

†Infrequent signs: acrocyanosis, bradycardia, fever, and glucose intolerance.

Table 2. Medical Conditions and Physical Findings Associated With Pheochromocytoma

Medical Conditions	Physical Findings
Neurofibromatosis	Café au lait spots, mucosal neuromas on lips, eyelids
Sturge-Weber syndrome	Facial hemangioma in trigeminal nerve distribution
Tuberous sclerosis	Adenoma sebaceum
von Hippel–Lindau disease	Hemangioblastomas in the retina
Multiple endocrine neoplasia (MEN) syndrome II	

A number of conditions may result from periodic surges or persistent increases of catecholamines. The cardiovascular conditions include stroke, renal damage, hypertensive retinopathy, intracranial hemorrhage, myocardial infarction, arrhythmia, catecholamine cardiomyopathy, pulmonary embolism, and sudden cardiac death. Other clinical conditions include gallstone formation, hyperfunction or hypofunction of the adrenal gland, diabetes, renovascular hypertension, polycythemia, and rhabdomyolysis. The latter conditions are associated primarily with mechanical or neurohormonal effects of atypical pheochromocytomas. Finally, some individuals are at higher risk for the development of pheochromocytoma. The conditions that carry a higher risk are listed in Table 2. In short, the presence of the following clinical features should lead to a heightened suspicion of pheochromocytoma: (1) at least two findings from the "triad," particularly in a paroxysmal pattern; (2) new-onset hypertension or symptoms in patients with MEN type II or familial neurocutaneous syndromes; (3) orthostatic hypotension in nondiabetic untreated hypertensive patients younger than 65 years of age; (4) an unexplained sudden rise in, or difficulty in controlling, blood pressure during surgery, parturition, or anesthesia.

Physical Examination

In general, patients with pheochromocytoma are thin and appear anxious, agitated, or diaphoretic, especially during the "episode." Vital signs typically show tachycardia, high blood pressure with or without orthostatic hypotension, and slight fever. No specific physical findings distinguish pheochromocytoma patients from other hypertensive subjects. However, the physical findings associated with certain familial syndromes are helpful (see Table 2).

Laboratory Tests

In patients with pheochromocytoma, the leukocyte count, hemoglobin, and/or hematocrit may be increased owing to hemoconcentration. Hyperglycemia, hypercalcemia, or hypokalemic alkalosis may also be observed. Increased serum glucose and calcium concentrations are typically seen with concomitant secretion of neurohormones in patients with MEN syndromes. When the clinical presentation supports a reasonable suspicion of pheochromocytoma, biochemical assays of urine and plasma can help establish the diagnosis in more than 95 per cent of patients.

Measurements of plasma concentrations of norepinephrine and epinephrine (or their metabolites) are *not* useful in screening patients for pheochromocytoma. Plasma assays generate significantly more false-positive results than urine assays because many factors influence plasma catecholamine concentrations, including emotional and physical stress, old age, and volume depletion. Moreover, as many as 15 per cent of patients with essential hypertension show increased plasma catecholamine concentrations.

Assays of urine typically measure dopamine, norepinephrine, epinephrine, metanephrine (MN), normetanephrine (NMN), and vanillylmandelic acid (VMA). The results of spot urine tests for MN correlate well with those of 24-hour urine MN determinations, which have the greatest sensitivity (96 per cent) and least susceptibility to drug interferences.

Various drugs and foods may interfere with the assays and lead to significant numbers of false-positive and false-negative test results. Exposure to caffeine, bananas, acetaminophen, aspirin, labetalol, tetracycline, nasal sympathomimetic preparations, or methyldopa may cause a false-positive result. By contrast, false-negative results are seen in patients exposed to propranolol, clonidine, methyldopa, monoamine oxidase (MAO) inhibitors, or radiocontrast media. Occasionally, increased concentrations of dopamine and its metabolite, homovanillic acid (HVA), with normal concentrations of norepinephrine and its metabolites, VMA and MN, indicate the presence of a malignant pheochromocytoma (Page's syndrome) with deficient dopamine-β hydroxylase (dopamine β-monooxygenase), the enzyme that oxidizes dopamine to norepinephrine. Malignant pheochromocytoma can be diagnosed only when metastases to nonchromaffin organs (e.g., liver, lungs, lymph nodes, and bones) are documented.

The combination of history, physical examination, and quantitation of urinary catecholamine concentrations establishes the diagnosis in more than 60 per cent of patients with pheochromocytoma. The accuracy of diagnosis exceeds 90 per cent when urine samples are obtained during an "episode." When biochemical confirmation cannot be achieved, a provocative and/or suppression test can be helpful.

A provocative test should be considered when urinary catecholamine concentrations are normal or slightly increased. Glucagon (1 to 2 mg intravenously) is the agent most commonly used to stimulate norepinephrine secretion. A positive response is defined as a threefold or greater increase over baseline concentrations, or a plasma concentration of norepinephrine exceeding 2000 pg/mL 1 to 3 minutes after injection of glucagon. To avoid a hypertensive crisis, provocative tests should not be performed in patients with moderate to severe hypertension.

Suppression tests are safer than provocative tests because norepinephrine release is inhibited rather than stimulated. Suppression is achieved with clonidine, a well-known antihypertensive medication. Pheochromocytomas overproduce catecholamines in the periphery. Therefore, inhibition of central release of catecholamines by clonidine should *not* influence the amount of catecholamine produced by a pheochromocytoma. By contrast, clonidine reduces the normal production of catecholamines. Unfortunately, catecholamine plasma concentrations must have already reached the upper end of the reference range to achieve a meaningful result. The sensitivity of the clonidine suppression test may be as high as 81 per cent, and the specificity may reach 97 per cent. The suppression test eliminates the diagnosis of pheochromocytoma when plasma concentrations of norepinephrine plus epinephrine do not exceed 500 pg/mL 2 to 3 hours after the oral administration of 0.3 mg of clonidine.

Imaging Studies

If the diagnosis of a pheochromocytoma is strongly suspected, the site of the tumor must be determined. Most pheochromocytomas (97 to 99 per cent) are intra-abdominal, and most (50 to 70 per cent) are found within the adrenal gland. Localization of the tumor can be accomplished with computed tomography (CT), magnetic resonance imaging (MRI), and adrenal scintigraphy using ^{131}I or ^{123}I-metaiodobenzylguanidine (MIBG) and ^{131}I-6β-iodomethylnorcholesterol (NP-59). Most pheochromocytomas exceed 2 cm and are usually discrete, rounded, or oval homogeneous masses. Thus, most tumors can be easily detected with CT or MRI.

Magnetic resonance imaging may be slightly more specific than CT for the diagnosis of pheochromocytoma. Both imaging techniques are highly sensitive (greater than 90 to 95 per cent). The use of MRI avoids unnecessary radiation exposure of pregnant patients. Typically, MRI shows hyperintensity ("shining") in T2-weighted images in patients with pheochromocytoma.

Adrenal scintigraphy with MIBG or NP-59 relies on the selective uptake of these radioiodine-labeled substances into chromaffin cells. The selective uptake of MIBG has been attributed to structural similarities between norepinephrine and the guanidine compound in MIBG. Positive imaging with NP-59 has been attributed to the affinity of this substance for the specific low-density lipoprotein receptor on adrenal cell membranes. The MIBG and NP-59 scans have the highest specificity (almost 100 per cent) among the imaging studies. These studies are particularly useful in patients with suspected multiple or extra-adrenal masses, or adrenal masses measuring less than 1 cm.

When biochemical assays are abnormal but imaging studies are normal, the patient most likely does not have a pheochromocytoma. In these patients, the clinician must consider the conditions that mimic a pheochromocytoma, including baroreceptor dysfunction, drug interaction, withdrawal or ingestion of sympathomimetic drugs (e.g., cocaine, amphetamines, MAO inhibitors), neurosis, other endocrine syndromes, and central nervous system abnormalities (e.g., cerebrovascular disease, brain tumors, seizure disorder). These conditions may involve activation of the sympathoadrenal system, surges of catecholamines from sources other than a pheochromocytoma, or decreased metabolism of catecholamines. An algorithm that incorporates these concepts is shown in Figure 1.

Pitfalls in Diagnosis

Factors that should be considered during an evaluation for pheochromocytoma include (1) absence of a typical paroxysm, (2) presence of other causes of hypertension, (3) biochemical assays performed in patients taking certain drugs or having conditions that may produce false-positive test results, (4) imaging studies performed without biochemical test confirmation, and (5) conditions simulating pheochromocytoma. Only 50 per cent of patients with pheo-

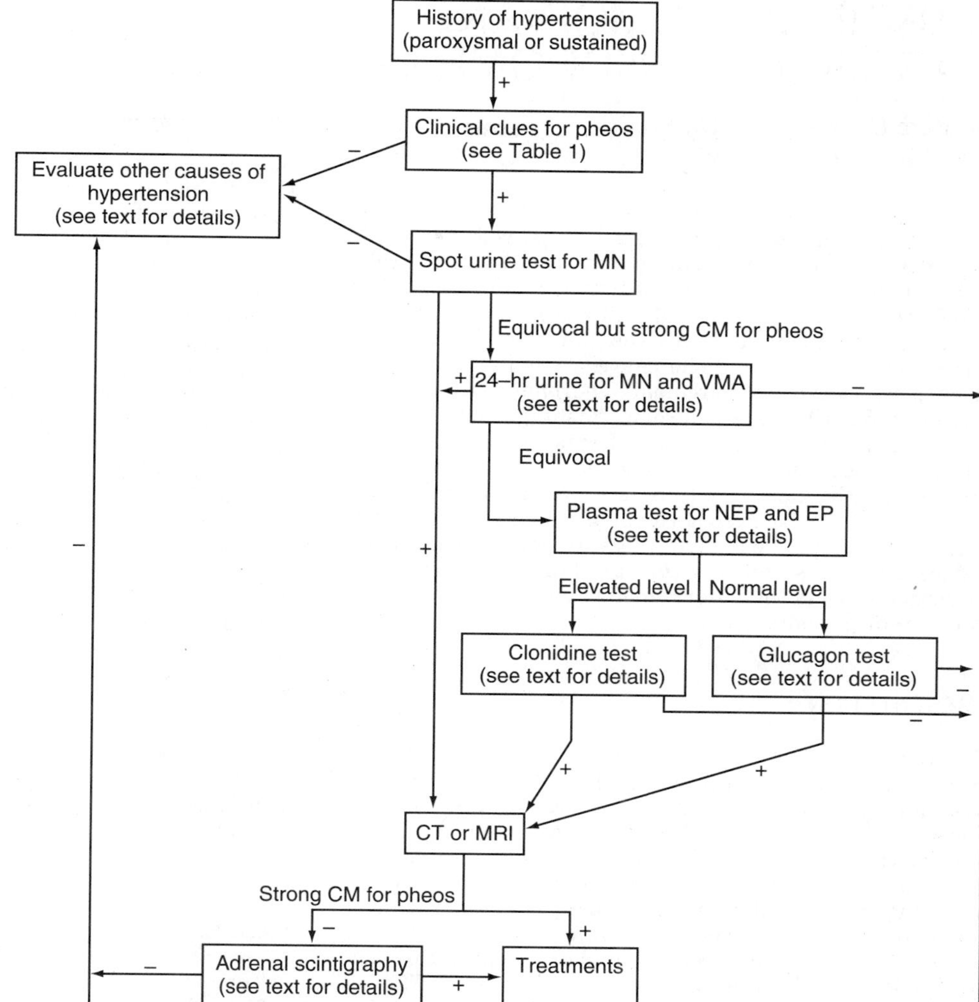

Figure 1. Algorithm for evaluation of pheochromocytoma. pheos = pheochromocytoma; CM = clinical manifestations; MN = metanephrine; VMA = vanillylmandelic acid; NEP = norepinephrine; EP = epinephrine; CT = computed tomography scan; MRI = magnetic resonance imaging; + = positive laboratory test (more than two to three times normal value) or present; equivocal = less than two times normal laboratory value; − = normal laboratory test or not present.

chromocytoma present with the typical triad of headache, tachycardia, and sweating. Twenty per cent do not report paroxysmal episodes. Thus, the clinician cannot ignore the diagnosis of pheochromocytoma in patients who do not present with typical signs and symptoms.

The concomitant presence of other causes of hypertension may confuse the diagnostic evaluation. (Renal artery stenosis and bilateral adrenal hyperplasia may also cause hypertension.) Pheochromocytomas that go unrecognized can cause disasters during diagnostic evaluation of secondary hypertension. For example, the administration of radiocontrast medium during renal angiography may provoke a hypertensive crisis if a pheochromocytoma is present. To avoid this problem, a step-by-step diagnostic evaluation is recommended (see Fig. 1).

To avoid unnecessary laboratory tests, the clinician should know the frequency of each clinical manifestation of pheochromocytoma as well as the sensitivity and specificity of each biochemical assay and imaging study. A spot or 24-hour urine metanephrine measurement is the screening test of choice, with high sensitivity and specificity, lower cost, and the least susceptibility to drug influences. Plasma catecholamine assays should not be used as primary screening tests owing to the lability of analytes, the higher cost, and many false-positive results. When urine screening tests show equivocal data, provocative studies can help establish the diagnosis. If plasma catecholamine concentrations are slightly increased, a clonidine suppression test may be useful. The use of clonidine to suppress catecholamine production is considered safer and more physiologic than the use of glucagon to stimulate catecholamine release.

For the diagnosis of pheochromocytoma, imaging studies without biochemical tests are expensive and of low yield. A CT scan is the imaging method of choice after positive biochemical assays. However, MRI has several advantages, including a higher specificity, unique imaging (hyperintensity in T2-weighted imaging) for pheochromocytoma, and decreased radiation hazard. Adrenal scintigraphy is not widely available but has a role in the diagnosis of small (<1 cm), extra-adrenal, and multiple lesions. If imaging studies are normal after positive biochemical tests, the clinician must consider conditions that simulate pheochromocytoma. These conditions include withdrawal states from drugs (e.g., heroin, cocaine, clonidine), neurosis, central nervous system abnormalities (brain tumors, seizure), and Page's syndrome.

CARCINOID TUMOR AND CARCINOID SYNDROME

By Marc D. Basson, M.D., Ph.D.
New Haven, Connecticut

Carcinoid tumors are neuroendocrine cell neoplasms (i.e., derived from enterochromaffin or Kulchitsky cells) that secrete a spectrum of bioactive peptides, many of which remain uncharacterized. They are most often found in the gastrointestinal tract, the lungs (embryologically part of the foregut), and the ovaries, but they may occur elsewhere. Classically, carcinoid syndrome is composed of secretory diarrhea and episodic flushing, sometimes in combination with valvular heart disease or bronchospasm, but the clinical picture may vary widely. Although serotonin released by carcinoid tumors was once believed to be the cause of the symptom complex called carcinoid syndrome, it is now clear that these tumors release many different peptides and that the variability of the carcinoid syndrome reflects the heterogeneous mix of these peptides in different patients.

PRESENTATION

Carcinoid tumors are frequently classified by the embryonic origin of the organ in which they are found, and this nosology often correlates with differences in tumor biology. Foregut tumors are located in the lungs, stomach, or first part of the duodenum. Midgut tumors are located from the second part of the duodenum through the right colon, including the appendix and the pancreas. Hindgut tumors originate in the transverse or left colon or the rectum. Midgut carcinoids most commonly cause classic carcinoid syndrome, usually after metastasis to the liver. The appendiceal carcinoid is an exception. It rarely causes systemic symptoms, because appendiceal obstruction usually occurs early in its course, prompting early diagnosis and therapy. Foregut carcinoids and hindgut carcinoids cause systemic symptoms less frequently than the midgut carcinoid, and they often manifest with local symptoms or with atypical systemic symptoms. This difference probably reflects differences in tumor biology that alter the mix of peptides secreted. Midgut carcinoid metastasizes chiefly to the liver, but foregut and hindgut carcinoid usually metastasizes to bone.

Carcinoid tumors typically manifest with one of two distinct patterns. The first involves the local mass effect of the tumor itself. A bronchial carcinoid may mimic a lung lesion on chest radiography or may cause wheezing or postobstructive pneumonia. A carcinoid tumor of the stomach or intestine can cause abdominal pain or bleeding as it erodes through the overlying mucosa, or rarely, it may obstruct the bowel directly. A carcinoid of the pancreas, ovary, or retroperitoneum or hepatic metastasis may cause local symptoms referable to a mass in any of these locations. Bone metastasis may also cause pain in patients with disseminated disease. The diagnosis of carcinoid tumor is rarely suspected until histologic analysis becomes available, but the diagnostic evaluation is usually straightforward, focusing on the radiographic characterization of the mass and then on obtaining tissue by percutaneous, endoscopic, or surgical means.

The more diagnostically challenging patients are those in whom an occult tumor causes symptoms by its bioactive secretions. Any one of the symptoms of the carcinoid syndrome symptom complex may be exhibited, and the disease should be considered in instances of inexplicable episodic diarrhea or steatorrhea, flushing, or bronchospasm. One third of patients with increased serotonin concentrations may fail to exhibit diarrhea or flushing. Depending on the character of the tumor secretions, carcinoid tumors (particularly bronchial carcinoids) may also manifest as Cushing's syndrome or glucose intolerance. Patients with otherwise minimal symptoms may present with telangiectasias over the face and anterior chest from a chronic "carcinoid flush." Much has been written about distinguishing different types of carcinoid tumors by the characteristics of the flushing, but the reliability of these inferences has not been confirmed. The induction of flushing by ethanol or caffeine ingestion should raise the question of a carcinoid flush. Another important detail is a history of lacrimation that occurs simultaneously with the flushing.

A problematic presentation involves the systemic fibrosis that can be associated with some carcinoid tumors. This may cause retroperitoneal fibrosis (e.g., ureteral obstruction) or intra-abdominal fibrosis and bowel obstruction. The correct diagnosis can be difficult to make in such cases without a high index of suspicion, because the surgeon's differential diagnosis of obstructive disorders generally focuses on the site of the obstruction rather than an occult cause.

Physical findings can be few. Signs of a local mass effect may be observed in large, biologically "silent" tumors, and intermittent flushing may result in telangiectasias. If valvular heart disease or bronchospasm are present, the physical findings characteristic of these disease entities are observed rather than carcinoid syndrome per se.

LABORATORY STUDIES

Tumors with bioactive secretions must be approached differently from other malignancies. Suspicion of neoplasm generally leads to a series of imaging procedures in an attempt to localize a tumor, followed by an attempt to secure tissue to make a diagnosis and characterize the neoplasm. In the case of neuropeptide-secreting tumors such as carcinoids, however, biochemical characterization should precede imaging studies. Reversal of the standard sequence is advantageous for several reasons. First, many small tumors can be missed by conventional imaging modalities, or a more aggressive search may be prompted by biochemical confirmation that the tumor exists. Second, biochemical confirmation permits the physician to treat the patient's symptoms with octreotide while a search for the primary tumor is being performed. Third, manipulation of the tumor during invasive imaging tests such as angiography may precipitate a carcinoid crisis that could be averted by pretreatment with octreotide.

The first biochemical test generally used for the diagnosis of a carcinoid tumor is the 24-hour urinary 5-hydroxyindoleacetic acid (5-HIAA) determination. 5-HIAA is a metabolite of serotonin and is therefore increased in patients with serotonin-secreting tumors (Table 1). Excretion of 5-HIAA in the urine normally ranges from 2 to 8 mg/24 hours, and it is highly specific but has a sensitivity of only about 75 per cent. A qualitative urinary 5-HIAA test in a single spot urine sample is less sensitive, because it is positive only when the urinary 5-HIAA concentration exceeds 30 mg/24 hours. Patients should be cautioned to avoid foods with high serotonin contents, including nuts

Table 1. Reference Ranges for a Carcinoid Diagnostic Evaluation

Determination	Reference Range
Plasma serotonin	5–100 pmol/mL
Plasma substance P	<10 pg/mL
24-hr urine 5-HIAA	2–10 mg/24 hr
Spot urine 5-HIAA	0 (test is less sensitive than 24-hr urine 5-HIAA)

and fruits. Medications that increase urinary 5-HIAA levels include reserpine, phenothiazines, Lugol's solution, guaifenesin (common in many over-the-counter antitussives), acetaminophen, and cyclobenzaprine hydrochloride (Flexeril). Patients with severe dumping syndrome after subtotal gastrectomy can also have increased urinary and plasma serotonin and urinary 5-HIAA. Salicylates and levodopa therapy decrease urinary 5-HIAA. Plasma or urinary serotonin concentrations can be measured in patients with equivocal urinary 5-HIAA concentrations. Plasma substance P concentrations may also be increased or may become so during pentagastrin provocative testing. Radioimmunoassays for plasma concentrations of other neuropeptides such as neurotensin, chromogranins, or alpha-human chorionic gonadotropin can be useful for selected patients.

If biochemical tests are unrevealing but clinical suspicion is high, provocative testing should be performed. Provocation with epinephrine or norepinephrine is neither sensitive nor specific and is only of historical interest. Pentagastrin provocation (Table 2) is the pharmacologic test most likely to stimulate carcinoid symptoms. This test should be performed in a monitored hospital setting with octreotide available to treat an acute carcinoid crisis if it occurs. Pentagastrin does not stimulate serotonin secretion directly by the carcinoid tumor; it appears to act by stimulating adrenal release of catecholamine and dopamine, which secondarily stimulate tumor peptide secretion. The sensitivity of this provocative test can be improved by measuring plasma substance P concentrations during pentagastrin stimulation. Plasma substance P concentrations are normally less than 10 pg/mL, but patients with carcinoid tumors typically show an increase in plasma substance P concentrations to more than 25 pg/mL at some point during provocation testing. This occurs most commonly within the first 5 to 10 minutes after pentagastrin infusion and requires several timed samples shortly after infusion. Some patients with idiopathic flushing syndrome have exhibited plasma substance P concentrations of 25 to 50 pg/mL. Careful questioning may demonstrate that the patient's symptoms are postprandial or follow the ingestion of ethanol or coffee; reproduction of the symptoms in such a manner may also permit simultaneous phlebotomy and biochemical demonstration of the tumor.

Table 2. Steps for Pentagastrin Provocation Testing

Patient must fast overnight before the test.
Intravenous access must be established with monitoring of vital signs.
Octreotide (100 μg IV) must be available to treat carcinoid crisis.
Draw baseline plasma samples 30, 15, and 0 minutes before the test.
Administer pentagastrin (0.6 μg/kg IV) over 5 to 10 seconds.
Monitor for carcinoid symptoms.
Draw plasma samples at 1, 3, 5, 7, 10, 15, 20, 30, 45, 60, 90, and 120 minutes.
Draw all blood into cold EDTA tubes, spin immediately, and store at −20°C.

PHARMACOLOGIC BLOCKADE

Patients for whom biochemical testing has demonstrated evidence of a carcinoid tumor should be treated with the long-acting somatostatin analogue octreotide while the remainder of the diagnostic evaluation is completed. The relief of symptoms with octreotide may itself help to confirm the diagnosis of a neuroendocrine tumor, although diarrhea from many different causes may respond to octreotide, but carcinoid bronchospasm is often resistant. Tumor manipulation during diagnostic testing can stimulate massive release of bioactive secretions from the tumor and precipitate a carcinoid crisis characterized by profound hypotension or bronchospasm.

Given subcutaneously before an intervention such as endoscopic biopsy or angiography 100 to 400 μg of octreotide prevents carcinoid crisis. Patients with frequent symptoms should receive continuous octreotide treatment during the diagnostic evaluation. Starting at 100 μg subcutaneously twice daily, the dose may be titrated upward to 1500 μg per day in divided doses. Pentagastrin stimulation testing can also be used to determine the adequacy of octreotide blockade before invasive procedures in severely symptomatic patients.

IMAGING PROCEDURES

The choice of imaging procedures should be guided by any clinical suspicion about tumor location. Carcinoids of the hollow organs are best imaged by endoscopy or bronchoscopy or by radiographic contrast studies (i.e., upper or lower gastrointestinal series or enteroclysis), and pancreatic carcinoid tumors require computed tomographic scanning. Because of the submucosal location of carcinoid tumors of the hollow organs, endoscopy may demonstrate a mass lesion, but the biopsy may be negative if only the overlying mucosa has been sampled. Double-bite or needle biopsy techniques may be useful in such instances. Increasing experience with endoscopic ultrasound suggests that it may be used to define small submucosal lesions that are not readily visualized by standard endoscopic visualization or by radiographic contrast studies.

Metastases are most commonly detected by computed tomography. Some reports suggest that magnetic resonance imaging is more sensitive with appropriately weighted image processing. Radionuclide liver and spleen scans may be more sensitive than computed tomography for hepatic metastases, but they cannot demonstrate metastases elsewhere. The technetium bone scan is useful for demonstrating osseous metastases.

If biochemical characterization has demonstrated an active carcinoid tumor, but no site can be identified, statistical parameters are needed to guide the search for the tumor. The midgut is the most common site of a carcinoid tumor, and this probability rises if the tumor has manifested with systemic symptoms. A barium enema, an upper gastrointestinal series with small bowel follow-through, and an abdominal computed tomography scan are performed sequentially. Although less statistically likely to yield a positive result, a chest film is also obtained at this time.

Two novel imaging modalities have been used to localize

occult carcinoid tumors. These are scanning with ^{123}I-iodinated octreotide and ^{131}I-metaiodobenzylguanidine. Each of these has been reported to have high sensitivity. As experience with these tests increases, they will probably replace the contrast studies previously described for the initial localization of the occult carcinoid. The choice between these tests is determined by local availability.

Arteriography is not useful in the diagnosis of carcinoid of unknown origin, because there is little to guide the angiographer. It may however, play a role in the localization of pancreatic lesions or in aggressive evaluation of the abdomen in patients with positive ^{123}I-iodinated octreotide or ^{131}I-metaiodobenzylguanidine scans. Tumor manipulation by angiographic dye injection may provoke a carcinoid crisis that can be avoided by prophylactic octreotide blockade.

OTHER DIAGNOSTIC PROCEDURES AND THERAPEUTIC TESTS

Selective vein sampling and assay for carcinoid products can help localize the occult tumor that has been biochemically demonstrated but not visualized radiographically. Exploratory laparotomy may be necessary in extreme cases when the presence of a carcinoid tumor is strongly suspected clinically and confirmed biochemically but cannot be localized by any of the techniques described. Conversely, a "silent" or locally symptomatic carcinoid tumor may be identified and localized by conventional imaging or surgical techniques without any clinical suspicion of its neuroendocrine nature, and histologic analysis gives the first clue about the true nature of the lesion. Confirmation of carcinoid histology on frozen section is not likely, but the demonstration of a homogeneous tumor with multiple, small, rounded cells organized in clusters suggests the diagnosis. This is further supported by argentaffin or argyrophil staining. Foregut and hindgut carcinoid tumors usually are argyrophilic positive and argentaffin negative, and midgut carcinoids usually exhibit positive staining by both techniques. Argentaffin staining is specific for carcinoids, but other neuroendocrine tumors may also be argyrophilic.

PITFALLS IN DIAGNOSIS

The most devastating consequence during diagnosis is the carcinoid crisis. Manipulation of the tumor may induce catastrophic hypotension or bronchospasm when bioactive peptides are released. This can be avoided by pharmacologic blockade with a stable somatostatin analogue such as octreotide before invasive testing of patients in whom the carcinoid syndrome is suspected. The adequacy of blockade can be confirmed by the loss of a positive pentagastrin stimulation test result in selected cases with extreme symptoms. The intravenous administration of 100 μg of octreotide may substantially ameliorate a carcinoid crisis that has been precipitated in an unblocked or unsuspected case.

A second problem of diagnosis and therapy involves the propensity of some carcinoid tumors to induce collagen deposition and fibrosis, which may lead to small bowel or ureteral obstruction or to mesenteric vascular compromise. The failure to recognize fibrosis can impede diagnosis and may compromise treatment. The surgeon may resect an unnecessarily long segment of bowel if the mesenteric shortening and kinking of the compromised bowel is not recognized and dissected from viable bowel.

Carcinoid tumors may be synchronous or metachronous with other carcinomas. A patient with a new lesion after resection of a carcinoid or with more than one site of tumor at surgery should not be assumed to have metastatic carcinoid. The identification of a second primary tumor of a different histologic type may substantially alter the management of these patients.

An overly aggressive search for an unknown primary tumor is not necessary in a patient with widespread hepatic metastases. The primary lesion should be sought in a patient with isolated and resectable hepatic metastases, but a primary tumor that remains occult after standard imaging studies and laparotomy is unlikely to become clinically significant if the hepatic metastases dominate the clinical picture.

MULTIPLE ENDOCRINE NEOPLASIA

By Jeffrey A. Norton, M.D.
St. Louis, Missouri

MULTIPLE ENDOCRINE NEOPLASIA TYPE I

Multiple endocrine neoplasia type I (MEN-I) is an inherited endocrine disorder that includes tumors of the parathyroid gland, pancreatic islets, anterior pituitary gland, and occasionally other glands and tissues. It is an autosomal dominant genetic disorder.

Genetic Abnormalities

Cases are caused by a mutation in one gene, the *MEN1* gene, which has been mapped to the long arm of chromosome 11. Genetic linkage analysis can be used to determine whether an individual of a family with MEN-I carries the disease gene. The exact genetic defect in patients with MEN-I has not been identified. Screening for the presence of MEN-I in individuals from affected families should begin during the teenage years. Screening is best done by measuring concentrations of calcium, glucose, prolactin, gastrin, and pancreatic polypeptide in serum. Individuals at risk should be questioned and examined for kidney stones, lipomas, Cushing's syndrome, hypoglycemia, peptic ulcer disease, headaches, acromegaly, and visual field defects.

Parathyroid Disease

Primary hyperparathyroidism is the most common expression of MEN-I. The clinical features of primary hyperparathyroidism in MEN-I include asymptomatic hypercalcemia, nephrolithiasis, and decreased bone density. The prevalence of primary hyperparathyroidism increases with age, approaching 100 per cent after 50 years of age. The age at onset of primary hyperparathyroidism in patients with MEN-I occurs approximately 25 years earlier than in the general population. The diagnosis of primary hyperparathyroidism is made by the detection of increased serum concentrations of total calcium and intact parathyroid hormone. The type of primary hyperparathyroidism in MEN-I patients is always parathyroid hyperplasia or multiple gland disease.

Primary hyperparathyroidism exacerbates the expression of Zollinger-Ellison syndrome in MEN-I patients. Cure of the primary hyperparathyroidism in MEN-I patients can decrease the drug dosage requirement for antisecretory drugs and cause remission of the biochemical features of Zollinger-Ellison syndrome.

Pancreatic Islet Cell Tumors

Patients with MEN-I also develop pancreatic or duodenal islet cell tumors. More than 95 per cent of MEN-I patients who develop pancreatic islet cell tumors already have primary hyperparathyroidism at the time of diagnosis. Islet cell tumors may be nonfunctional, or they may produce hormones with associated clinical syndromes. The most common functional hormone-secreting pancreatic or duodenal islet cell tumor in patients with MEN-I is gastrinoma. Virtually any islet cell tumor can occur in patients with MEN-I, including gastrinoma, insulinoma, glucagonoma, VIPoma, GRFoma, somatostatinoma, PPoma, and carcinoid tumor. Some of the islet cell tumors in MEN-I patients can be malignant.

Symptoms of gastrinoma are related to gastric acid hypersecretion and include peptic ulcer disease, secretory diarrhea, and esophagitis. The diagnosis of Zollinger-Ellison syndrome in patients with MEN-I is made by detection of increased gastric acid output and increased fasting serum gastrin concentration. For the diagnosis, the clinician should discontinue all acid antisecretory medication and measure the fasting serum gastrin concentration and amount of gastric acid output. Patients with a fasting serum gastrin concentration greater than 100 pg/mL and a basal acid output greater than 15 mEq/hour have evidence of Zollinger-Ellison syndrome. A secretin stimulation test can be performed to confirm the diagnosis. Two units of secretin per kilogram is given intravenously, and the serum gastrin concentration is measured at 0, 2, 5, 10, 15, and 20 minutes. If the serum gastrin concentration increases by more than 200 pg/mL over the basal concentration after the administration of secretin, the patient also has confirmatory evidence of Zollinger-Ellison syndrome. Approximately 85 per cent of patients with Zollinger-Ellison syndrome have this response to secretin.

Patients with insulinoma have neuroglycopenic symptoms during a period of fasting. These symptoms can include personality changes, drowsiness, altered mental status, coma, and seizures. Insulinoma is diagnosed by a supervised fast. Patients undergo a hospitalized, observed 72-hour fast to evoke symptoms of hypoglycemia. When neuroglycopenic symptoms develop, the fast is terminated, and serum concentrations of glucose, insulin, C peptide, and proinsulin are measured. Patients who have glucose concentrations less than 45 mg/dL, insulin concentrations greater than 5 μU/mL, and increased concentrations of C peptide and proinsulin have insulinomas.

Patients with glucagonoma have a characteristic rash called necrolytic migratory erythema and an increased plasma concentration of glucagon (>500 pg/mL). They also have cachexia, hypoaminoacidemia, anemia, type II diabetes mellitus, weight loss, and thromboembolic disease.

Patients with VIPoma have severe watery diarrhea, dehydration, hypochloremia, hypercalcemia, and hypokalemia. The diagnosis is made by detecting increased plasma concentrations of vasoactive intestinal polypeptide.

Radiologic studies are performed to localize the islet cell tumor. Some patients with biochemical evidence for an islet cell tumor may have no tumor identified. This commonly occurs in patients with MEN-I and Zollinger-Ellison syndrome. Radiologic studies include computed tomography (CT), endoscopic ultrasound, octreotide scan, angiogram, secretin angiogram or calcium angiogram, and portal venous sampling for hormone concentrations.

Pituitary Tumors

Tumors of the anterior pituitary are also associated with MEN-I. The most common pituitary tumor is the prolactinoma. Increased serum concentrations of prolactin are diagnostic for a prolactinoma and can be used as a screening study in patients with MEN-I. Pituitary tumors can also secrete other hormones, including corticotropin (ACTH), growth hormone, and thyroid-stimulating hormone (TSH). Patients are evaluated by measuring serum concentrations of the appropriate hormones when the diagnosis is suspected clinically. A magnetic resonance (MR) or CT scan of the sella and visual field examination are obtained. Bitemporal hemianopsia can occur if very large tumors compress the optic chiasm.

MEN-I patients with Cushing's syndrome may have hypercortisolism caused by a pituitary adenoma, an ectopic ACTH-producing carcinoid or islet cell tumor, or an adrenal cortical tumor. Complete evaluation is necessary for determining the precise cause of the hypercortisolism. Studies include dexamethasone suppression test, petrosal sinus sampling, and imaging studies of the pituitary, adrenals, and CT or MR scans of the chest and pancreas if ectopic ACTH secretion is suspected.

Other Tumors

Other tumors in patients with MEN-I include bronchial or thymic carcinoid tumors, intestinal carcinoid tumors, gastric carcinoid tumors, benign adenomas of the thyroid gland, benign adrenal cortical adenomas, and rarely, adrenocortical carcinomas. Cortical adenomas of the thyroid gland and benign cortical adenomas of the adrenal cortex usually require no treatment unless evidence exists of excessive hormonal function. Patients with MEN-I may also have multiple subcutaneous lipomas. Each of these more rare tumors in MEN-I patients should be diagnosed and treated as they would be in a sporadic occurrence.

MULTIPLE ENDOCRINE NEOPLASIA TYPE IIA, IIB, AND FAMILIAL MEDULLARY THYROID CARCINOMA

Multiple endocrine neoplasia type IIA (MEN-IIA) is an inherited disease syndrome that is characterized by medullary thyroid carcinoma (MTC), pheochromocytoma, and parathyroid hyperplasia. Multiple endocrine neoplasia type IIB (MEN-IIB) is an inherited disease syndrome that is characterized by MTC, pheochromocytoma, mucosal neuromas, marfanoid habitus, intestinal ganglioneuromas, and corneal nerve hypertrophy. Parathyroid disease is not part of MEN-IIB. Familial MTC is characterized by MTC that occurs without any other endocrine abnormality. The pattern of inheritance in all three syndromes is autosomal dominant with a high degree of penetrance and variable expression.

Medullary Thyroid Carcinoma

MTC originates in the parafollicular calcitonin-producing C cells of the thyroid gland. Patients with MTC have increased serum concentrations of calcitonin, especially in response to provocative agents such as calcium, pentagastrin, or a combination of both. Screening of patients at risk for familial MTC in the setting of MEN-IIA, IIB, or familial MTC has been accomplished by measuring serum concentrations of calcitonin in response to provocative agents. In patients with MEN-IIA, the biochemical manifestations of MTC typically appear between the ages of 5 and 25 years, before the onset of pheochromocytoma or parathyroid hyperplasia.

The gene for MEN-IIA is located at the pericentromeric region of chromosome 10. Studies have detected mutations in the *RET* proto-oncogene in all individuals with MEN-IIA. Because 100 per cent of individuals with MEN-IIA develop MTC, total thyroidectomy is advocated when *RET* mutations are detected. Similarly, individuals with MEN-IIB and familial MTC also have mutations in the *RET* oncogene. When the diagnosis of MEN-IIA, MEN-IIB, or familial MTC is confirmed by the presence of a mutation in the *RET* oncogene, total thyroidectomy and median lymph node dissection is indicated. Pheochromocytoma must be excluded in individuals from kindreds with MEN-II by measuring 24-hour urinary excretion of vanillylmandelic acid (VMA), metanephrines, and total catecholamines.

Patients with MTC in the setting of MEN-IIB have a characteristic phenotype that includes prognathism, puffy lips, poor dentition, mucosal neuromas, corneal nerve hypertrophy, and multiple bony abnormalities. Bony abnormalities include a marfanoid habitus, talipes equinovarus, pectus carinatum, and pectus excavatum. The diagnosis of MEN-IIB is also suggested by corneal nerve hypertrophy on slit-light examination. MEN-IIB patients develop medullary thyroid carcinoma at an early age. Although this trait is inherited in an autosomal dominant pattern, most patients first develop the disease as a sporadic mutation. MEN-IIB patients usually do not have large kindreds, because the MTC is more lethal. Most have tumor-positive lymph nodes at the time of diagnosis. Individuals with familial MTC have the best prognosis. In these patients, MTC commonly occurs at an older age, and cure is more likely with surgery. Death due to metastatic MTC is atypical. Although the same oncogene is affected, the virulence of the MTC is different. The most lethal form is MEN-IIB, the intermediate form is MEN-IIA, and the least virulent is familial MTC. Total thyroidectomy is indicated for each of the familial types of MTC, because both lobes of the gland are involved.

Pheochromocytoma

Patients with MEN-IIA or MEN-IIB can develop bilateral pheochromocytomas. These tumors are always located within the adrenal medulla and are usually not malignant. The diagnosis of pheochromocytoma is made by confirming increased 24-hour urinary excretion of VMA, metanephrines, or total catecholamines. Imaging studies are used to identify which adrenal gland is involved with tumor. CT, MR, and metaiodobenzylguanidine scan have each been used by some groups. MR scan has some specificity for pheochromocytoma because the tumor appears bright on the T2-weighted image. MR and CT scans can reliably detect intra-adrenal pheochromocytomas as small as 1 cm in diameter. Bilateral adrenal medullary hyperplasia is detected in 70 per cent of individuals.

Parathyroid Disease

Some patients with MEN-IIA develop primary hyperparathyroidism that is typically caused by multiple gland disease or parathyroid hyperplasia. The diagnosis of parathyroid hyperplasia in these patients is confirmed by detection of increased concentrations of calcium and parathyroid hormone in the serum.

Gastrointestinal Manifestations

Some patients with MEN-IIA have Hirschsprung's disease, which is associated with *RET* mutations. Individuals with MEN-IIB can develop constipation, megacolon, and diverticular disease due to intestinal ganglioneuromas and abnormal peristalsis. MTC can secrete a wide variety of peptide hormones that cause diarrhea. Patients who have metastatic MTC frequently develop secretory diarrhea.

Section Ten

NERVOUS SYSTEM

MIGRAINE HEADACHES

By Howard S. Derman, M.D.
Houston, Texas

A migraine headache is an idiopathic recurring headache with attacks lasting 4 to 72 hours. The typical characteristics of this headache include a unilateral location, a pulsating quality, moderate or severe intensity, aggravation by routine physical activity, and association with nausea, photophobia, and phonophobia.

The prevalence of migraine in the adult population ranges from 0.5 to 2 per cent. The sex distribution in children is 1:1, but in adults, women represent 75 per cent of patients. About 40 per cent of men and 50 per cent of women who report headaches to the physician actually have migraine headaches. Approximately 18 million women and 5.5 million males older than 12 years of age suffer from migraine. Although migraine was initially thought to affect individuals of higher socioeconomic groups, recent studies suggest no association with any socioeconomic group.

Forty per cent of migraineurs report one attack or fewer per month, 35 per cent experience one to three attacks per month, and 25 per cent report more than four attacks per month. This frequency is constant in both males and females.

The annual impact of migraine on society is significant. Ninety per cent of migraineurs worked 6 days a month at half their usual level of productivity, and 50 per cent of migraineurs missed an average of 2.2 work days a month. Yearly lost labor costs are estimated to reach $6864 per working man and $3600 per working woman.

CLINICAL SYMPTOMS

Migraine should be considered a three-stage syndrome consisting of a preheadache phase, a headache phase, and a postheadache phase. The preheadache phase is often heralded by premonitory symptoms (prodrome), followed at times by an aura. In some patients, the postheadache phase may last as long as 36 hours. Migraine without aura is present in 75 per cent of migraine sufferers, whereas 25 per cent of migraineurs report an aura associated with the headache.

Prodrome

Most migraineurs report a prodrome consisting of a group of nonspecific phenomena that may occur days, but more often hours, before the head pain occurs. These complaints may be mental (e.g., depression, irritability, and euphoria) or constitutional (e.g., increased defecation, urination, anorexia, and fluid retention). Patients also report phonophobia, photophobia, and hyperosmia. Migraineurs can often anticipate their headaches when these premonitory symptoms appear. Patients often report that the migraine prodrome may be more disabling than the period of actual head pain.

Aura

Migraine with aura is seen in 25 per cent of all migraine attacks. The aura precedes the headache by an average of 5 to 30 minutes. It usually occurs before the actual head pain, although some migraineurs may have aura without subsequent head pain. Visual auras are most common and include scotoma, teichopsia, fortification spectra, distortion of images, and photopsia. Sensory auras are next in occurrence, but aphasia and hemiparesis can also occur (Table 1).

Headache Pain

The actual pain of migraine is unilateral in the majority of attacks (60 per cent). The pain is typically periorbital and may extend to the cheek and ear unilaterally or bilaterally (40 per cent). Migraine pain can occur in any area in the head and neck region. Typical head pain may last as long as 4 hours, but in some patients it may last longer. The intensity of the pain is variable; in some patients it is mild, whereas in others it is severe. It usually has a pulsating character with associated symptoms sometimes occurring, including nausea and vomiting and photophobia. Any of the features mentioned in the prodrome can also occur with the actual head pain.

Postdrome

Following the actual head pain, patients may describe fatigue, listlessness, and generalized achiness. They may also describe a dull headache that is frequently a secondary muscle contraction headache. This postdrome period may be as short as 1 to 2 hours or as long as 36 hours.

CLASSIFICATION OF MIGRAINE AND VARIATIONS

The formal classification by the International Headache Society is helpful in evaluating migraineurs (Table 2).

Migraine Variations

Hemiplegic Migraine

Hemiplegic migraine can be both sporadic and familial, with a male predominance. It may begin in children as young as 1 to 2 years. The hemiplegia may be part of the aura or may remain during the headache and at times

Table 1. Characterization of Migraine Aura

Visual	Motor	Sensory	Basilar
Teichopsia	Monoplegia	Dysesthesias	Diplopia
Fortification spectra	Hemiplegia	Paresthesia	Vertigo
Scotomas	Language deficits		Dysphagia
			Ataxia

Table 2. International Headache Society Classification of Migraine

Migraine without aura
Migraine with aura
Migraine with typical aura
Migraine with prolonged aura
Familial hemiplegic migraine
Basilar migraine
Migraine with acute-onset headache
Ophthalmoplegic migraine
Retinal migraine
Childhood periodic syndrome
Benign paroxysmal vertigo of children
Alternating hemiplegia of childhood
Complications of migraine
Status migrainosus
Migrainous infarction

outlast the headache. An associated cerebrospinal fluid (CSF) pleocytosis may be observed.

Basilar Migraine

A basilar migraine is preceded by an aura that suggests involvement of the basilar or brain stem territory. It is usually seen in younger patients, and symptoms include diplopia, ataxia, visual field loss, dysarthria, tinnitus, and bilateral sensory loss. A subgroup of basilar migraineurs can have drop attacks or trancelike states associated with the headache.

Migraine Aura Without Headache—Migraine Equivalent

Patients may have a full-blown migraine aura, including basilar symptoms, without the subsequent onset of headache. Diagnosis is made after the patient has been thoroughly evaluated for other illnesses, including collagen vascular disorders, transient ischemic attacks, and coagulopathy. A group of patients with late-life migraine, a condition also called transient migraine accompaniments, has been reported to have attacks of episodic neurologic events after age 50 years with the absence of headache. These attacks can last as long as 72 hours.

Ophthalmoplegic Migraine

Ophthalmoplegic migraine constitutes a variant of migraine that typically consists of migraine headache associated with a paresis of one or several extraocular muscles. The pupil may or may not be dilated. The ophthalmoplegia can last days or even weeks after the headache abates. Other diagnostic possibilities include Tolosa-Hunt syndrome, intracerebral aneurysm (especially a posterior communicating aneurysm), diabetic neuropathy, and glaucoma. Imaging by magnetic resonance imaging (MRI) or computed tomography (CT) may be necessary for excluding aneurysm.

Retinal Migraine

Retinal migraine is characterized by repeated headache attacks associated with visual impairment or blindness involving one eye. The visual loss may last up to 1 to 2 hours before a headache ensues. The patient must be evaluated for ischemic optic neuropathy, transient ischemic attacks, and other organic causes of visual loss.

Cluster Headache

Episodic cluster attacks (typical cluster headaches) are seen primarily in male patients, with a male-to-female incidence of 5:1. The onset is in the third to fifth decades of life, but some patients can have the initial headache as late as 70 years. Typically, a cluster attack lasts 2 to 3 months and can occur as often as every 4 months or as infrequently as every 3 to 4 years. The average period of recurrence is 12 to 18 months.

The pain of cluster headaches is somewhat different from migraine in that there is no aura associated with the headache. The head pain is almost always unilateral and periorbital in nature. The pain is usually more severe than migraine pain and has a boring quality that can last from 30 to 45 minutes. Patients can have several attacks during a 24-hour period, often without nausea or vomiting. Ipsilateral lacrimation, ptosis, and miosis as well as conjunctival injection typically occur on the side of the periorbital pain. Alcohol and certain medications can often precipitate a single attack of cluster headache, but not a full-blown series of headaches that lasts the full 4 to 6 weeks.

Chronic cluster headaches differ from classic cluster headaches by the absence of a long remission period between headaches. Chronic cluster headaches can occur as frequently as every 2 weeks, similar to the periodicity of typical migraine. The head pain is similar to that seen in typical episodic cluster headache.

Complications of Migraine

Status migrainosus is a migraine attack that lasts 72 hours or more with only a 4-hour pain-free interval. These attacks can even last 1 to 2 weeks and are often associated with debilitating nausea and vomiting as well as dehydration. The condition can be difficult to treat, and hospital admission is often necessary.

Rarely, patients suffering from migraine with aura experience a permanent neurologic abnormality accompanied by a focal lesion on an imaging study. This condition is typically seen in migraineurs who have a long history of migraine with aura. Visual field abnormalities and hemiplegia are the most frequently encountered deficits, and these patients should be evaluated for other causes of cerebral infarction, for example, a hypercoagulable state, collagen vascular disease, and so on.

EVALUATION OF THE PATIENT WITH MIGRAINE

History

A thorough history of headache, including frequency of attack, location of pain, age at onset, type and severity of pain, precipitating factors, and associated symptoms, should be obtained. The headache can then be distinguished and categorized according to its characteristics (Table 3). Also important are autonomic disturbances that can accompany migraine and affect a variety of organ systems.

Patients with migraine often complain of anorexia and intolerance to food odors as early symptoms in their prodrome. Nausea and vomiting are common not only during the prodrome-aura phase but also during the head pain stage. Diarrhea can also occur with the migraine attack. The presence of abdominal pain as a manifestation of migraine is controversial, but some childhood migraine patients have stomach pain with a migraine attack.

Systemic hypertension secondary to extreme pain and hypotension due to bradycardia with associated syncope can occur with migraine. Distention of the superior temporal artery during a severe attack of head pain has been reported. Patients often complain of a cold, clammy feeling

Table 3. Distinguishing Among Headache Types

Characteristic	Migraine	Typical (Episodic) Cluster	Tension-Type Headache
Onset	Teenage to age 40 yr; occurs anytime during day	Ages 25–40 yr; often occurs at night, waking patient	Adolescence, adulthood, and old age
Location of pain	Half of face Frontal, usually in or around eye or cheek	Periorbital, behind eye	Bandlike; temporal region, occipital
Precipitating factor	Fatigue, stress; hypoglycemia; diet (tyramine, alcohol); sunlight; hormonal change (menstruation)	Alcohol, vasodilator (i.e., nitroglycerin)	Fatigue, stress, or no precipitant
Frequency of attack	2–4 per mo or sporadically; may be cyclic with menstruation	One or two cycles of daily headache per year; may be 4 per day; 4- to 8-wk cycles, may be seasonal	Insidious onset; continuous for weeks, months, or years
Sex distribution	70% female, 30% male	90% male, 10% female	Slight majority female
Duration of attack	Head pain 4 hr; aura to postdrome 24–36 hr	Minutes to hours; usually 30–45 min; many attacks within 24 hr (rarely)	Continuous, persistent
Pain type and severity	Begins as dull ache, progresses to stabbing pain; intense	Deep, burning, excruciating, stabbing pain; pain so extreme that patients may be suicidal	Dull, nagging ache with occasional exacerbations of severe pain
Associated symptoms	Nausea and vomiting; photophobia, obscured vision	Nasal stuffiness, rhinorrhea; redness of eye ipsilateral to head pain, miosis, ptosis	Neck stiffness, shoulder ache

associated with skin pallor and cold extremities. Facial edema involving the temporal and periorbital regions is often seen. Piloerection (goose bumps) is also troublesome to the patient, as is facial redness and flushing. Rarely, excessive sweating is encountered. Extreme yawning can be a presenting sign in migraine, as can hyperventilation and increased sighing. Rhinorrhea and nasal congestion are seen more often in patients with cluster headaches.

Physical Examination

A thorough physical and neurologic examination is crucial in all headache patients; the examination is normal in most of these patients. A carotid, cardiac, and pulmonary auscultatory examination is equally important. Special attention is given to the neck area to assess nuchal rigidity and focal areas of tenderness, especially in the occipital nerve exit zone. Equally important is palpation and observation of the cranium, jaw, neck, and ears. The mental status examination is crucial, as is an ophthalmologic examination including visual fields, extraocular movements, funduscopic examination, and pupillary response.

TRIGGERS TO MIGRAINE

Several clear triggers to migraine include the monthly menstrual cycle, alcohol, certain foods, missed meals, and an irregular sleep pattern. Migraineurs benefit greatly from regular meals and a structured sleep schedule. They should eat three meals a day at 5- to 6-hour intervals, and they should sleep 7 to 8 hours per night, awaking at the same time, give or take 1 hour. Migraineurs should be educated regarding foods that may trigger their headaches. A list of foods to avoid (Table 4) may be helpful in educating patients. The goal is not to eliminate all foods on the list but to have the patient check the list for possible offending foods with the intent of avoiding them in the future.

Women with menstrual cycle–related migraine should be identified to provide medical therapy prior to the beginning of their cycle. Judicious use of vitamin supplements, magnesium, and other elements may be helpful as adjunct therapy in this subgroup of patients.

DIAGNOSTIC TESTING AND IMAGING STUDIES

Neurodiagnostic testing is not necessary for establishing a diagnosis of migraine. Ancillary studies may be needed to exclude other causes of headache and include imaging studies (CT and MRI), lumbar puncture, electroencephalography, and blood studies.

Magnetic Resonance Imaging and Computed Tomography

Imaging studies are ordered when the patient has an abnormal neurologic examination or if the history strongly suggests an organic lesion as a cause of the headaches. An MRI or a CT examination may be helpful in excluding subarachnoid hemorrhage in a patient who presents with acute onset of headache associated with nausea, vomiting, and stiff neck. A CT scan is as acceptable as an MRI scan in excluding subarachnoid hemorrhage or a structural lesion, but MRI may be more helpful if the clinician is also considering inflammatory or demyelinating disease or ischemic brain disease. Also, if the clinician is considering an Arnold-Chiari malformation or is trying to visualize the pituitary fossa, MRI is the preferable study. Finally, for

Table 4. Diet Modification (Foods to Be Avoided)

Foods rich in tyramine
Foods containing monosodium glutamate (MSG)
Foods containing nitrites
Anything pickled, marinated, or fermented
Alcoholic beverages
Caffeinated beverages

some patients an imaging study is the only acceptable reassurance to allay fears of a serious organic cause of headache.

Lumbar Puncture

A lumbar puncture is useful in excluding subarachnoid hemorrhage, meningitis, or increased intracranial pressure. If lumbar puncture is included as part of a headache evaluation, an imaging study should be performed prior to the lumbar puncture. Spinal fluid should be sent for a cell count; protein and glucose determinations; and various microbiologic studies including a Gram stain, an acid-fast bacillus stain, culture and sensitivity tests, and cryptococcal antigen determination. An accurate opening and closing pressure must be recorded, and if the CSF is bloody or blood-stained, it must be centrifuged to see whether the fluid is xanthochromic. If it is, blood has not been introduced through a traumatic tap, and a true subarachnoid hemorrhage exists.

Electroencephalography

An electroencephalogram (EEG) is not helpful in the evaluation of migraine because 80 per cent of migraineurs have abnormal EEGs, including sharp waves. The EEG may be helpful if loss of consciousness or a confusional state is associated with the headache.

Blood Studies

Blood studies are usually normal in migraineurs and are not recommended in a routine evaluation of migraine. In selected patients, a urine drug screen, thyroid panel, glucose tolerance test (GTT), and follicle-stimulating hormone (FSH) and prolactin measurements may be indicated. Finally, in patients 50 years of age or older who present with constitutional symptoms and visual complaints, an increased erythrocyte sedimentation rate suggests a diagnosis of temporal arteritis.

DIFFERENTIAL DIAGNOSIS OF MIGRAINE

Before the clinician makes a diagnosis of migraine headache, several points must be addressed. First, migraine headaches are seen in a younger population, typically from the teenage years to 40 years of age. Migraines can be encountered after 40 years of age, but middle-aged migraineurs usually give a history of headaches as a child with a quiescent period before recurrence in middle age. Late-life migraine (also known as transient migraine accompaniments) can occur, but usually without head pain (see earlier discussion). Many neurologic problems are associated with headache and must be included in the differential diagnosis of migraine (Table 5).

Table 5. Differential Diagnosis of Migraine

Subarachnoid hemorrhage
Intracerebral hemorrhage
Meningitis, encephalitis
Sinusitis
Temporal arteritis
Benign intracranial hypertension
Intracerebral tumor
Acute glaucoma
Carotid dissection
Facial pain—typical and atypical
Severe hypertension
Transient ischemic attacks
Cortical and venous thrombosis
Temporomandibular joint dysfunction
Subdural hematoma

Subarachnoid Hemorrhage

Blood in the subarachnoid space can occur from either trauma or rupture of an arteriovenous malformation (AVM) or an aneurysm. An MRI or a CT scan shows this blood, and the CSF is grossly bloody. The headache is acute and is usually associated with nausea, vomiting, and stiff neck. Focal neurologic deficits including pupillary asymmetry, extraocular movement abnormalities, and hemiplegia may be observed. Altered mental status is common.

Intracerebral Hemorrhage

Intracerebral hemorrhage may present as a subarachnoid hemorrhage if blood dissects from the brain parenchyma to the subarachnoid space. Signs of increased intracranial pressure, stiff neck, nausea, vomiting, and altered mental status are common. An imaging study will document blood in the intracerebral space.

Cerebrospinal Fluid Infection

Both viral and bacterial meningitis can present with headache, photophobia, and nuchal rigidity. Early on, this central nervous system (CNS) infection can be confused with migraine. Certainly, bacterial meningitis takes a more fulminant course characterized by stiff neck, high fever, and altered mental status. Viral meningitis can be confused with migraine, and pleocytosis in the spinal fluid may be the only distinguishing point. If lumbar puncture is considered in the evaluation of headache, a CT or an MRI study should be performed to exclude mass effect or document the presence of blood in the CSF or parenchyma.

Sinusitis

Acute sinusitis as a cause of headache is uncommon, and patients and clinicians often confuse pain under and above the eye with sinus pain when, in fact, the majority of these patients have migraine. Chronic sinusitis may or may not cause headache. Surgical intervention as a definitive treatment of chronic sinusitis with the hope of relief of head pain is strongly discouraged.

Granulomatous Cranial Arteritis

Temporal arteritis presents with generalized symptoms of malaise, myalgias, arthralgias, and headache and possible visual loss. This condition is a diagnostic consideration for new onset of headaches in patients older than 50 years of age, and an increased erythrocyte sedimentation rate strongly suggests the diagnosis in these patients.

Pseudotumor Cerebri

Pseudotumor cerebri (benign intracranial hypertension) presents as increased intracranial pressure with no evidence of intracranial malignancy. Patients with benign intracranial hypertension often have headaches and obscured vision. Patients with pseudotumor are more often female with menstrual irregularities and are usually obese. An MRI study shows slitlike ventricles without evidence of structural lesion. The CSF pressure is increased, visual field examination may show enlargement of the blind spot, and funduscopic examination reveals disk edema. The headaches of pseudotumor cerebri are associated with transiently increased intracranial pressure.

Headaches may be worse in the morning, and the diagnosis is confirmed by detecting increased CSF pressure during lumbar puncture.

Brain Tumor

Headaches associated with brain tumors can easily be confused with tension or migraine headaches. These headaches are typically frequent and can occur on a daily basis, often awakening the patient from sleep. Neurologic examination can show papilledema as well as focal neurologic findings. Headaches occur as the initial symptom of brain tumor in 40 per cent of patients. They can be exacerbated by altered positions, coughing, and exertion.

Acute Glaucoma

Acute glaucoma often presents with sudden orbital pain associated with nausea and vomiting. The pain may follow the use of anticholinergic drugs. Increased intraocular pressure is diagnostic of acute angle-closure glaucoma.

Carotid Dissection

Unilateral headache, usually in the orbital, frontal, or neck region, accompanied by neurologic findings suggestive of carotid disease, can be the initial presentation of internal carotid artery dissection. Horner's syndrome may develop. Carotid dissection usually follows trauma to the neck region or occurs after extreme manipulation of the head and neck.

Facial Pain

Either typical facial pain (tic douloureux) or atypical facial pain can be confused with migraine headache, especially if the pain mainly involves the sensory distribution of the second branch of the fifth cranial nerve. Cluster headaches often have symptoms that are indistinguishable from those of facial pain. The age at onset and the periodicity of cluster pain can be helpful in distinguishing between the two.

CEPHALIC NEURALGIAS

By David A. Keith, B.D.S., D.M.D.,
and Steven J. Scrivani, D.D.S.
Boston, Massachusetts

TRIGEMINAL NEURALGIA

Trigeminal neuralgia (tic douloureux) is an excruciating, sharp pain experienced in one of the divisions of the trigeminal nerve. The pain is probably the worst known, and patients who have experienced this pain live in fear of it returning. The pain is described as a stabbing, knifelike, electric shock sensation that can be triggered by moving or touching any part of the sensory distribution of the trigeminal nerve. Patients frequently have difficulty in swallowing, eating, talking, brushing the teeth, washing the face, or applying lipstick. Although any of the sensory branches of the trigeminal nerve can be affected, the usual areas are the second and third divisions. The pain lasts a few seconds, and then the patient is pain-free until the next attack. After several weeks or several months, the pain typically goes into remission, only to return again at a later time. In the majority of patients, the cause is undetermined (primary trigeminal neuralgia), but occasionally the neuralgia is due to a demyelinating condition (multiple sclerosis) or a blood vessel pressing on the nerve. The diagnosis is made predominantly by obtaining a history. Physical examination may detect a trigger area, but the rest of the sensory examination is usually within normal limits. Laboratory tests are not helpful, but a magnetic resonance imaging (MRI) scan is an appropriate part of the evaluation for excluding detectable lesions. When a pathologic condition is identified (e.g., cysts or tumors at the cerebellopontine angle or multiple sclerosis), a secondary neuralgia is diagnosed. The drug of choice for medical management is carbamazepine (Tegretol); if it does not relieve the symptoms, the diagnosis must be questioned.

Differential Diagnosis

Trigeminal neuralgia with characteristic features can be readily diagnosed by the history alone. Atypical features raise the possibility of an associated pathologic condition mimicking the neuralgialike pain. Occasionally, postsurgical or post-traumatic neuralgias present in a similar way. The condition is said not to occur in younger patients; patients with neuralgialike trigeminal pain who are younger than 40 years of age must be carefully evaluated for other neurologic diseases. Occasionally, cluster headache or chronic paroxysmal hemicrania presents with intense paroxysmal facial pain, but the history and associated features usually distinguish it from a true trigeminal neuralgia.

Glossopharyngeal Neuralgia (Vagoglossopharyngeal Neuralgia)

Glossopharyngeal neuralgia is 100 times less common than trigeminal neuralgia but has the same sharp, shooting, lancinating features confined to the sensory distribution of the ninth or tenth cranial nerves. The pain may be experienced in the ear, larynx, base of tongue, and tonsillar pillar, and it can be stimulated by swallowing or eating. Because this pain is seen in a predominantly older age group, a meticulous search for occult tumors of the nasopharynx is required. Because the pain is frequently referred to the ear and jaw area and may be associated with mandibular motion, it can be confused with a temporomandibular disorder. The lancinating character of the pain in the absence of joint or muscle tenderness or dysfunction usually distinguishes the two conditions. A variety of other symptoms can accompany the attacks of glossopharyngeal neuralgia and include hiccups, coughing, seizures, syncope, bradycardia, hypertension, and even cardiac arrest. These symptoms are believed to be mediated through the carotid sinus, with resulting increased vagal tone.

Atypical Trigeminal Neuralgia

A whole host of atypical neuralgic pains can be experienced in the mouth and the face, usually as a result of surgical intervention or trauma. Surgical interventions include all types of dental and oral and maxillofacial surgery, head and neck surgery, plastic surgery, and otolaryngologic surgery. These pains are less intense and more constant than a true trigeminal neuralgia. The pain is invariably described as aching, burning, and constant; only occasionally do sharp stabs of pain occur. Because these pains are chronic, they may be accompanied by myofascial and vascular components and psychogenic comorbidity. If a history of surgery or trauma is elicited, a careful neurologic examination usually uncovers subtle sensory changes in the skin or mucous membranes of the affected area. The nature of these problems often attracts litigation or workmen's compensation issues that can frequently compound the complex clinical picture. Damage to one of the major branches of the third division of the trigeminal nerve (i.e., the inferior alveolar and lingual nerves) as a result of the removal of a third molar is seen in a small percentage of patients. Depending on the extent of the damage, microneurosurgical repair may be possible with some return of sensation and alleviation of pain, provided that the repair is performed within the first few months.

Atypical Odontalgia (Atypical Periodontalgia, Phantom Tooth Pain)

Atypical odontalgia is an unusual trigeminal neuralgia that is characterized by pain in the teeth or supporting structures. It can be described as pressure or dull toothache, but it does not respond to extensive dental treatment. Typically, the diagnosis is made retrospectively in a patient who gives a history of toothache treated by dental fillings, root canal, surgical apicoectomy, extraction, or curettage of the bone. Characteristically, the pain returns and may even escalate after each surgical intervention, finally spreading to adjacent teeth. The problem may not be recognized until the patient has been rendered edentulous in the area of neuralgia. Because the attention of the patient and the dentist has been focused on the dental origin of the pain, these patients are often fixated on dental problems rather than on recognizing the likely neurologic basis. Some reports have suggested that these pains are of deafferentation origin.

Burning Mouth Syndrome (Glossodynia)

Burning mouth syndrome is a condition typically affecting older women and was once thought to be of hormonal or psychogenic origin. The pain is described as burning and may primarily affect the tongue, or it may involve the oral mucosa, lips, and oropharyngeal mucosa. The pain is aggravated by hot and spicy foods and may be ameliorated by cold liquids. Frequently, patients make drastic changes to their diets to accommodate their discomfort. Most patients complain bitterly of the personal and social disability that results, and indeed the incidence of depression in these patients is high. Typically, the patient may be relatively pain-free on wakening, but the pain can increase as the day progresses. The cause is unknown. Patients with clinically significant iron deficiency anemia, diabetes, or other deficiency diseases can acquire this condition, but virtually all results of laboratory tests, including biopsy and imaging are within normal limits. A neurologic basis has been suggested for this disorder because some patients have a subtle neuropathy involving thermal sensitivity in the tongue.

Atypical Facial Pain

Atypical facial pain is characterized by a poorly defined pain complex involving the mouth and face. It is described in vague terms that change over time, and it is highly associated with psychogenic comorbidity. The patients (invariably female) bitterly describe a constant and fluctuating pain in the mouth and face. Despite the patients' accounts of the impact that the pain has on their lives, they seem to function normally. The pain may change in character and intensity over time and may be described in various areas of the mouth and face. Associated vascular and myofascial pain is typical.

Temporomandibular Disorders

The most common facial pain complaint arises from a group of conditions generically termed temporomandibular disorders. They are defined as pain and dysfunction of the temporomandibular joints and muscles of mastication. Patients complain of head, face, jaw, and throat pain that is usually aggravated by moving the jaw. A sense of fatigue and limitation of jaw motion with clicking and popping sounds in the joint are typical. Examination reveals tenderness in the muscles of mastication, including the temporalis, masseter, and pterygoid muscles, and tenderness can be elicited over both temporomandibular joints. Mandibular range of motion may be restricted. A click or pop of the temporomandibular joint can frequently be heard or palpated. Sensory loss, swelling, and adenopathy are not associated with this condition. Although various causes have been suggested, this condition is probably a complex neuropsychologic condition accompanied by muscle pain and joint capsulitis resulting from noxious jaw habits. The predominant habit is bruxism or grinding of the teeth, but clenching of the teeth and posturing of the jaw may also be involved. Certain occupational factors, such as the playing of a wind instrument and scuba diving, may be identifiable. Predisposing factors include structural problems, such as hypermobility syndrome and malocclusion. The precipitating factors may be unrecognized but could include minor trauma to the jaw, opening wide to bite into food, routine dental treatment, or intubation for general anesthesia. Perpetuating factors usually include continuing noxious jaw habits, sleep disruptions, and associated depression.

Signs and symptoms of temporomandibular disorders are frequent and equally distributed throughout both genders and all ages. A small proportion of afflicted individuals consider these symptoms to be abnormal, and only 5 to 15 per cent require treatment. Initial laboratory and imaging studies are nearly always normal. The condition is self-limited, and symptoms typically resolve with recognition of the nature of the problem. Symptoms in some patients may progress to severe mandibular limitation and continuous pain caused by internal derangement of the temporomandibular joint. This derangement can eventually lead to an arthritic condition within the joint. Eventually, the typical patient returns to a functional level of pain-free motion, and at this time the mandibular condyles can show extensive remodeling. The joints must be evaluated for other uncommon disorders such as systemic arthritides, growth abnormalities, and tumors.

Temporal Arteritis

Temporal (cranial) arteritis is an inflammatory condition involving the cranial blood vessels. It is uncommon in individuals younger than 55 years of age. The patient complains of pain in the temple associated with chewing and jaw motion. The temporal arteries are nonpulsatile, tender, and rigid. The clinical presentation can be confused with that of temporomandibular dysfunction and temporalis muscle spasm, but the findings related to the temporal artery should distinguish the two. Any suspicion of this diagnosis should trigger an immediate request for an erythrocyte sedimentation rate determination. If the results are increased, an immediate referral for an ophthalmologic evaluation is indicated because the central retinal artery can be involved, causing blindness.

Cluster Headache

Cluster headache is an excruciating pain located behind or around the eye with radiation to the maxillary teeth, upper jaw, cheek, or temporal region. The headaches persist for minutes to hours and occur in clusters lasting several weeks. The pain may awaken the patient at the same time each time each night (alarm clock headache). Associated features include ptosis, rhinorrhea, conjunctival injection, unilateral sweating, facial flushing, and nasal congestion. Cluster headache is considerably less common than migraine, but its exact prevalence has not been determined. It is more common in males and generally begins in the second or third decade of life. The pain can be so severe that patients are unable to remain still and frequently pace the floor. When in extreme distress they may bang their heads against a wall or hit their heads. The differential diagnosis of cluster headache is made by eliciting the history of characteristic symptoms. The diagnosis is often confused with trigeminal neuralgia, but cluster headache pain has many associated features not seen in trigeminal neuralgia; it lasts much longer and does not usually have the sharp, shooting, electric shock–like character of trigeminal neuralgia.

Occipital Neuralgia

Occipital neuralgia is sharp pain arising from the superior occipital line and spreading to the vertex of the head. It can be spontaneous or related to pressure over the back of the head or to head motion. Associated disorders include cervical myofascial pain, ankylosing spondylitis, and cervical arthritis. Sensory changes in the scalp may cause patients to complain of pain or hypersensitivity when they brush or wash their hair. In extreme cases, patients may have their hair shaved or cut short to avoid further discomfort. Local anesthetic blocks usually relieve the pain, but occasionally surgical interventions are necessary.

Postherpetic Neuralgia

The acute phase of postherpetic neuralgia is characterized by a vesicular eruption, usually in the distribution of ophthalmic division of the trigeminal nerve. It is extremely painful and may become chronic. A typical description is a constant burning pain with an occasional stabbing quality. The affected skin is usually hypersensitive to all types of stimuli. Older patients appear to have more pain. The diagnosis is made on the basis of the clinical description and the preceding attack of herpes zoster.

DIZZINESS AND VERTIGO

By Athanasios Katsarkas, M.D.
Montreal, Quebec, Canada

Vision, proprioception, and vestibular function are the main sensory contributors to space orientation. Dizziness can be defined as the distortion of space orientation, frequently leading to a sensation or illusion of motion and loss of postural control. Vertigo is a particular type of dizziness characterized by a sensation or illusion of rotation of the surroundings or of the self. Dizziness is due to the reception of abnormal information from the sensory organs or abnormal processing of sensory information by the central nervous system (CNS), or both. Conditions inducing dizziness can be classified according to those that (1) directly affect the sensory organs, (2) directly affect the CNS, (3) indirectly affect the sensory organs or the CNS (e.g., cardiovascular disorders or side effects of non–CNS acting drugs), or (4) are functional with no known anatomic localization, such as phobias, somatization, stress, or anxiety.

The vestibular end-organ in the inner ear responds to rotational (semicircular canals) and/or linear (otoliths) head movements and detects gravitational orientation. Vestibular signals to the oculomotor muscles contribute to gaze control during head movements via the vestibulo-ocular reflex (VOR). Similar signals to the spinal motor neurons provide postural control via the vestibulospinal reflexes (VSRs).

Sudden unilateral peripheral vestibular dysfunction induces a sensation of rotation, loss of postural control, nystagmus, nausea, and vomiting. These symptoms subside with time and, if the vestibular function does not recover, their disappearance is due to central compensation. By a similar mechanism, symptoms of acute vestibular dysfunction may never appear if the vestibular function fails slowly. Under certain conditions, the initial symptoms of acute vestibular dysfunction can reappear in compensated patients. This is called decompensation. In general, the absence of vertigo does not exclude vestibular involvement and the presence of vertigo does not always indicate peripheral vestibular disease. Loss of bilateral vestibular function is a major handicap inducing severe postural instability with little, if any, tendency for compensation.

MEDICAL HISTORY

The medical history remains the most important diagnostic tool in dizziness, despite recent technologic developments. Details frequently lead to the diagnosis, but they must be elicited by meaningful questions. As patients relate the history, they may be unable to decide on the importance of symptoms or they may suffer from more than one type of dizziness, which can further complicate the clinical picture. After listening to the patient's story, the following details must be carefully described and documented.

The Principal Sensation

Dizziness may be described as lightheadedness, fainting (blackout), fatigue, "empty head," pressure on or around the head, the room being unstable, the road being tilted, or a vague sensation of motion. If dizziness affects postural control, imbalance may become a prominent feature portrayed as not feeling solid on the feet, unable to walk straight, walking as if drunk, walking on foam, bumping into objects, being dragged toward either side, and off balance but walking straight. Dizziness may also be described as a sensation of rotation of self or surroundings, and patients frequently have no difficulty in defining the direction of rotation. If patients are able to stand, they may also point to the direction of falling.

Organic syndromes, affecting vestibular function in the end-organ or the brain stem, usually induce more clear and precise sensations. Conversely, patients with compensated vestibular dysfunction may describe vague events, although they often have a history of acute vertigo. A well-defined sensation of rotation increases the likelihood that organic disease probably also affects the vestibular function. Sustained postural instability, usually aggravated by darkness, crowded areas, or head movements, indicates organic disease. Patients with such instability frequently recall an earlier experience of acute vertigo.

Patients with functional conditions may also complain of persistent postural instability that is aggravated by inconsistent or even contradictory circumstances. These patients may describe sensations (e.g., the surroundings moving as a pendulum or dizziness and instability induced by noise, loud voices, or intense light) that cannot be attributed to known organic syndromes. Patients with functional diseases can also recall the previous experience of organic disease and report it as part of the present illness. Fainting (blackout), real or imaginary, suggests a functional disease. There are patients, however, who have the tendency to faint, and in rare cases, acute severe vertigo can induce fainting like any other intense sensory stimulus. Epilepsy or circulatory problems obviously must be excluded. The history becomes more confusing when patients suffer from two types of dizziness, such as Ménière's disease and paroxysmal positional vertigo (PPV) or vestibular neuronitis and functional disease.

Duration of Dizziness

Persistence of the initial symptoms in acute vestibular dysfunction can indicate lack of compensation. This raises the possibility of brain stem disease. Whether the dizziness was or is episodic or sustained for the reported period must also be clarified. This differentiates between syndromes inducing either acute sustained vestibular dysfunction (e.g., vestibular neuronitis) or episodic vestibular dysfunction (e.g., PPV). Furthermore, if episodic vertigo is triggered by certain head positions, the vertigo may subside within seconds or may persist as long as the provocative head position is maintained (see further on).

Dizziness as First Episode or Recurrence

Most frequently, recurrences indicate an end-organ disorder. Diseases such as transient ischemic attacks (TIAs) or acute exacerbations of multiple sclerosis can recur over long periods. If dizziness recurs, the question is whether the sensation in previous events was similar to the present illness. Patients with PPV, for instance, may experience similar dysfunction in the other ear, or subsequent similar episodes may be attributable to brain stem TIAs.

Conditions at the Onset of Dizziness

Physical exertion can induce a TIA with additional focal symptoms usually accompanying the dizziness. Physical exertion, sneezing, scuba diving, or difficult delivery can cause inner ear fistula, which is usually accompanied by unilateral hearing loss and tinnitus. Vague dizziness or feeling weak or faint after exertion may be related to cardiovascular disease.

Conditions That Change the Dizziness

In patients with compensated vestibular dysfunction, head movements or fast-moving visual targets (e.g., traffic, shopping centers) can cause short periods of instability and/or hazy vision. Patients suffering from positional vertigo may feel worse in the supine than in the upright position.

Concomitant Symptoms

If the history suggests episodes of acute vertigo, all symptoms of acute vestibular dysfunction must be substantiated. These symptoms are aggravated by rapid head movements. Patients may not recall all details, and the absence of several symptoms does not exclude acute vestibular dysfunction. The symptoms and the sequence of their appearance depend on the degree of loss and the speed with which the vestibular function was lost. Imbalance accompanies severe vertigo and can persist after the vertigo subsides; nausea usually follows other symptoms of vestibular dysfunction, but it may simply accompany a mild degree of imbalance, as with advanced Ménière's disease or inner ear fistulas. If many symptoms of acute vestibular dysfunction are absent, nonvestibular syndromes must be considered.

If hearing loss and/or tinnitus are present, their relationship to the dizziness must be established or excluded. Patients with hearing loss and tinnitus from noise exposure or presbycusis can be misdiagnosed as suffering from Ménière's disease if they complain of vertigo. In Ménière's disease, acute vertigo is accompanied or preceded by increased tinnitus and decreased hearing.

Headaches can induce dizziness that is usually described as lightheadedness. Some diseases, such as cerebrovascular disease and migraine, cause both headaches and dizziness. Migraine affecting the posterior circulation can induce true vertigo and, in rare cases, nystagmus. Patients suffering from true vertigo quickly learn that head movements aggravate the condition. Attempting to keep the head steady, these individuals contract the neck muscles, inducing occipital headaches.

A multitude of symptoms that are unrelated to each other suggest a functional condition. Conversely, organic nonvestibular symptoms accompanying the dizziness can help define the nature of organic disease. Vertebrobasilar TIA can cause symptoms of unilateral facial numbness and/or weakness, hemiparesis, slurred speech, or diplopia. The latter is an important symptom, but patients frequently confuse this with the visual haziness caused by nystagmus and the sensation of rotation during vertigo. With true diplopia, most patients are able to describe the relative position of the two objects.

Other Diseases (Nonvestibular, Non–Central Nervous System)

Dizziness can occasionally be due to direct cochleovestibular involvement. In autoimmune diseases, for example, inner ear dysfunction can occur as one of the initial symptoms. Cardiovascular diseases, neuropathies, vision deficits, muscular weakness, and reduced motor abilities are associated with various sensations often described by patients as dizziness.

Medication

Dizziness may be a side effect of many drugs. It is occasionally accompanied by nausea, a sense of imbalance, or lightheadedness. In patients with compensated vestibular dysfunction, some drugs induce dizziness due to either reduced mental alertness or decompensation. A typical example of decompensation is the intolerance to even small amounts of alcohol reported by many patients with compensated loss of vestibular function.

CLINICAL EXAMINATION

Clinical assessment focuses on the brain stem functions and includes testing of postural control, the search for and identification of nystagmus, and detection of other oculomotor deficits. Hearing is also clinically tested with tuning forks (usually 0.5, 1, and 4 kHz) using the Weber and Rinne tests.

Postural Control

Romberg's test and tandem gait with eyes open and closed give rough estimates of postural control. Past-pointing is also helpful in acute cases. In Romberg's position with the arms extended forward and eyes closed, patients tend to shift toward the direction of the slow phase of nystagmus. Postural instability during clinical testing may be "voluntary," and patients with functional disorders can sway in this manner. Occasionally, the distinction between voluntary sway and pathologic postural instability is difficult.

Nystagmus

The fast phase is the most prominent clinically observed component and defines the nystagmus. Horizontal nystagmus is observed with the fast phase toward the patient's right (right beating) or left (left beating); vertical nystagmus denotes nystagmus with the fast phase toward the patient's forehead (upbeat) or feet (downbeat), regardless of the body position in space. Clinically observed nystagmus may be spontaneous, positional, or evoked (e.g., with headshaking). It can also be persistent or paroxysmal, depending on its duration. With a few exceptions, such as congenital or endpoint nystagmus, clinically observed nystagmus is always pathologic.

Spontaneous Nystagmus

Nystagmus that appears in patients in an upright position without subjecting them to provocative maneuvers immediately preceding the examination is called spontaneous nystagmus. It may be torsional (rotatory) or linear, or both, depending on the trajectory the eye is observed to describe. This trajectory is defined by the pathologic process inducing the nystagmus and/or the position of the eye in the orbit. Direction fixed or direction changing are terms used to describe whether the direction of the fast phase remains constant or changes when the gaze changes direction.

Horizontal direction fixed nystagmus usually includes torsional and linear components and shows no change in the direction of the fast phase with changes in gaze direction. It is more obvious when the gaze is in the direction of the fast phase and becomes less obvious in the opposite direction. This nystagmus is usually a sign of peripheral disease if other oculomotor deficits are absent. Rarely, this nystagmus may be unidirectional gaze paretic. The fast phase of gaze paretic nystagmus changes direction according to the direction of gaze. Thus, during gaze to the patient's right, the fast phase is toward the right and during leftward gaze, the fast phase is toward the left. Gaze paretic nystagmus is a sign of CNS disease usually due to dysfunction of the cerebellum or its brain stem connections. Gaze paretic nystagmus in all four directions is frequently a sign of a lesion near the fourth ventricle. Horizontal gaze paretic nystagmus can occasionally be observed during the early hours after acute unilateral end-organ vestibular dysfunction. This nystagmus quickly becomes direction fixed. Vertical direction fixed nystagmus appears when the eyes are in midposition. Vertical nystagmus that appears only during upward or downward gaze is gaze paretic. Vertical nystagmus is always a sign of CNS disease, that is usually localized in the midline of the brain stem. Downbeat nystagmus, for example, can be induced by a lesion of the cerebellar vermis or by Arnold-Chiari malformations in which cerebellar structures and connections are compressed by a herniation in the spinal canal.

Positional Nystagmus

Positional nystagmus is the nystagmus that appears or the nystagmus that is greatly enhanced in head positions other than the upright. Positional nystagmus can be either paroxysmal if it subsides while the provocative head position is still maintained or persistent if it continues as long as the provocative head position is maintained. Paroxysmal positional nystagmus can be of short (less than 10 to 15 seconds) or long (more than 1 or 2 minutes) duration; the latter may be confused with the persistent type. It must be observed in two opposite directions of gaze, which is difficult if the nystagmus is of short duration. A typical example is the nystagmus observed during an episode of PPV. To elicit it, the patient is brought quickly from the sitting to the provocative head position. Usually after a short delay nystagmus appears and is mainly torsional with a fast phase toward the lowermost ear during gaze in this direction. It then becomes upward linear oblique during gaze in the opposite direction. This nystagmus is consistent with excitation of the posterior semicircular canal of the lowermost ear. In rare cases, the nystagmus of PPV may be purely linear horizontal, remaining unchanged when the gaze changes direction. This nystagmus is consistent with excitation of the horizontal semicircular canal of the lowermost ear. Persistent positional nystagmus usually has torsional and linear components and may be horizontal or vertical. Clinically it must be observed while the patient is supine and the head is in a midline, lateral, or hyperextended position. Nystagmus appearing in a lateral head position with a fast phase toward the lowermost ear is called geotropic; if the fast phase is in the opposite direction, it is termed apogeotropic. Persistent positional nystagmus does not change direction when the gaze changes direction while holding the same head position. If it does, it is gaze paretic. It may appear in one or both lateral head positions and may be of the same type in both or geotropic in one and apogeotropic in the other. Both types have been encountered in inner ear disease (e.g., inner ear fistulas) or brain stem disease (e.g., intra-axial tumors, multiple sclerosis). The apogeotropic type is more frequently associated with a brain stem pathologic condition than is the geotropic type. The vertical type is always due to brain stem disease. Alcohol also induces similar nystagmus, called positional alcoholic nystagmus (PAN). Shortly after alcohol ingestion, this nystagmus is geotropic (PAN I); a few hours later, it becomes apogeotropic (PAN II).

Headshaking (Evoked) Nystagmus

In patients with unilateral loss of vestibular function, regardless of location, nystagmus appears following an oscillation of the head to the patient's right and left. The direction of nystagmus depends on the speed of oscillation, the fast phase being usually toward the healthy side.

Other Oculomotor Deficits

Pursuit eye movements are clinically tested by instructing the patient to follow a slowly moving visual target in front of the eyes. Normally the eyes, remaining continuously on target, execute a smooth movement. A jerky type of pursuit can be caused by inattention, drugs, or brain stem disease. It is never a sign of inner ear disease unless caused by the presence of nystagmus. Saccadic eye movements are clinically tested by instructing the patient to move the eyes quickly, first from a midpoint to a point located on the right side and then from a midpoint to the left side. Normally, the eyes execute one quick movement from the original to the final point. In conditions such as inattention, drug use, brain stem disease, or Parkinson's disease, the eyes may develop saccadic dysmetria. If they undershoot and slide slowly to the target, it is called hypometria; if they overshoot the target and return, it is termed hypermetria. Saccadic dysmetria is never associated with inner ear disease.

Vestibular nystagmus can be suppressed or greatly diminished by fixing the eyes on a visual target. To test this visual-vestibular interaction, the patient is asked to fix the eyes on a forward-extended index finger while sitting on a chair that can be rotated. As the chair oscillates from side to side, the patient with peripheral dysfunction, even in the presence of nystagmus, can successfully accomplish this task, suppressing the nystagmus as the chair oscillates back and forth. However, if an interruption of the visual-vestibular interaction has occurred, the nystagmus is poorly suppressed, or the eyes may develop a jerky movement, usually as a result of cerebellar (floccular) disease. Inattention and certain drugs can also induce jerky eye movements during such testing.

LABORATORY TESTS

Laboratory tests are typically used to confirm or "fine-tune" the clinical impression. "Battery tests," performed before the clinical assessment, are frequently useless. Imaging techniques may also be required.

Oculomotor Function

Various methods are used to record eye movements in light or dark. Electronystagmography (electroculography) records changes of the corneoretinal potential by the use of surface electrodes. Other methods include the use of infrared sensors placed in front of the eyes or tiny metallic coils in contact lenses that record eye movements in a magnetic field. Accurate measurements of eye movements are possible with these sensors, permitting a precise diagnosis (see further on). As with all laboratory data, they must be interpreted in the context of the observed clinical condition.

Vestibular Function

The eye response is recorded by any of the methods described previously, and vestibular stimulation is induced by either caloric stimulation or rotation. Caloric testing permits the comparison of the excitability of one ear over the other and is performed by irrigating the ear with water of a temperature above or below 37°C (98.6°F). The maximum velocity of the slow phase of the induced nystagmus is compared with its counterpart obtained under the same conditions from the other ear. The bithermal caloric testing uses two irrigations—with water above and below body temperature—for each ear. Rotational tests are performed with the patient sitting on a rotating chair with the head fixed during continuous, rapid, sinusoidal, or random movements. Similar data can be obtained with the patient performing specific active head movements while seated on a fixed chair.

Postural control (VSR) is tested by the H-reflex, elicited by an electrode around the calf, while the patient is linearly accelerated on a sled. The evoked electric responses reflect the vestibular function. Posturography measures body sway while the patient stands on a computerized platform. Posturography is static or dynamic, depending on whether the platform is rigid or movable.

Otolith function can be tested using movements on parallel swings or long radius centrifuges by rotations off the vertical axis. However, the preferred clinical methods are the H-reflex (see preceding discussion) or recording of eye counter-rolling. When the head tilts toward one side, the eyes roll in the opposite direction. This is a measurable manifestation of the eye-otolith reflex, although the angle of eye counter-rolling in humans is small.

Auditory Function

The standard hearing test consists of the audiogram, which shows the behaviorally defined pure tone thresholds measured in decibels in the audible range of frequencies measured in hertz. This is achieved by the use of audiometers. Supplementary methods to assess the auditory function are tympanometry (testing the mobility of the middle ear structures), brain stem auditory evoked responses (testing the "electric conductivity" of the central auditory pathways), otoacoustic emissions and cochleography (testing the electric activity of the inner ear), and so on.

Other laboratory tests useful in selected cases include electromyography, and the recording of various evoked potentials such as somatosensory, visual, and others.

Imaging Techniques

Diagnostic capabilities in the temporal bone and the CNS have been revolutionized by imaging techniques. Occasionally such techniques may miss the pathologic condition if the clinician fails to provide sufficient information to the radiologist. This is especially relevant in pathologic conditions of the posterior fossa, where lesions of the lower brain stem can be missed.

COMMON SYNDROMES INDUCING DIZZINESS

Peripheral Syndromes

PPV is by far the most common syndrome of peripheral origin. Probably caused by deposits in the semicircular canals, it occurs when the head is tilted to the provocative position. During the following short paroxysm, patients tend to fall backward or forward because the posterior semicircular canal is usually affected. PPV may be idiopathic or may appear following head injuries, and the diagnosis is suspected from the history and is confirmed by observing the nystagmus during the paroxysm (see preceding discussion). Epidemic vertigo and vestibular neuronitis are apparently viral syndromes that cause acute vertigo not accompanied by hearing loss. The acute symptoms of epidemic vertigo disappear quickly, and vestibular function recovers. In vestibular neuronitis, the loss of function is permanent and the acute symptoms last longer and resolve after central compensation. Ménière's disease produces a sensation of fullness in the ear, tinnitus, usually low-frequency hearing loss, and acute episodes of vertigo. The relationship of these symptoms is essential in establishing the diagnosis. Ménière's disease is apparently due to inner ear hydrops of unknown cause, although a number of causes have been suggested, such as malformations of the inner ear, trauma, immune reactions, and allergies. The differential diagnosis includes sudden hearing loss of unknown etiology, inner ear fistulas and, rarely, acoustic neuromas. The history, an audiogram, vestibular testing, and imaging studies all may be required for confirming the diagnosis. Two other Ménière's-like syndromes include fluctuation of hearing without vertigo and episodes of vertigo without hearing loss (recurrent vestibular neuronitis). Inner ear fistulas are created when the round or oval window membrane breaks from excessive pressure. The inner ear then loses perilymph, inducing symptoms similar to those of Ménière's disease. The differential diagnosis between the two conditions can be difficult or even impossible. Geotropic positional nystagmus is sometimes induced when the affected ear assumes the lowermost position. Autoimmune diseases may cause cochleovestibular dysfunction, which can be the first manifestation of the disease. In Cogan's syndrome, the loss of auditory and vestibular function is usually profound. Most cases are accompanied by an interstitial keratitis. Bilateral loss of vestibular function is characterized by profound postural instability that remains uncompensated. It is not accompanied by vertigo, is usually due to ototoxicity, and has been encountered in other situations, such as in patients receiving chronic dialysis. Sudden unilateral hearing loss is apparently due to viruses; rare cases can result from vascular events or tumors. Hearing loss is frequently accompanied by vertigo that subsides within days. If the hearing does not improve concomitantly, a space-occupying lesion must be excluded by imaging techniques. Patients with permanent loss of vestibular function may be misdiagnosed as having Ménière's disease.

Peripheral sensory neuropathies are occasionally accompanied by loss of vestibular function and severe postural instability. Whiplash injury can induce a mild postural instability during head movements that usually subsides within weeks. Chronic dizziness is not caused by such injuries. Viral cranial polyneuritis is a syndrome with multiple cranial nerve involvement. The diagnosis is one of exclusion, and tumors and demyelinating disease must be excluded. Multifactorial postural instability in aging is due to a combination of factors, such as diminished vision, loss of proprioception, vestibular dysfunction, and reduced motor abilities. Drop attacks cause patients to lose postural control suddenly and fall without loss of consciousness. This can be a symptom of either inner ear disease or brain stem TIA; the latter is usually accompanied by additional symptoms of brain stem dysfunction. Acoustic neuromas usually induce tinnitus and progressive high-frequency sensorineural hearing loss. These symptoms are accompanied or followed by postural instability. An early sign of brain stem compression is Bruns' nystagmus, which is a combination of gaze paretic and vestibular nystagmus with coarser and slower beats during gaze toward the side of the lesion and finer and faster beats during gaze in the opposite direction. Imaging techniques provide the diagnosis.

Central Nervous System Syndromes

In most patients with dizziness due to CNS disease, additional symptoms of brain stem dysfunction are evident. In acute vertigo, persistence of symptoms with lack of compensation suggests brain stem disease. Intra-axial tumors may present with vertigo and positional nystagmus in the supine position (see earlier discussion). Additional symptoms of brain stem dysfunction often appear early. Tumors of the fourth ventricle can induce both horizontal and vertical gaze paretic nystagmus. Slowly progressive cerebellar and/or brain stem degeneration causes imbalance and clumsiness but not vertigo. Gaze paretic nystagmus, failure of visual-vestibular interaction (see previous discussion), or other oculomotor pathologic condition may be present. In subacute cases, vertigo may be one of the initial prominent symptoms. Vascular disease involving the brain stem can induce dizziness or even true vertigo. The type and duration of dizziness depend on the extent and location of vascular involvement. Permanent extensive ischemia (e.g., Wallenberg's syndrome) results in severe dysfunction including serious vestibulo-oculomotor deficits. Brain stem TIAs or aneurysms of the vertebrobasilar system can cause acute vertigo. Additional signs of brain stem dysfunction usually establish the diagnosis. In rare cases, vertigo accompanied by nystagmus suggestive of brain stem disease may be the only symptom. Imaging techniques may help establish the diagnosis. Demyelinating disease can cause dizziness, depending on the location of the lesions; true vertigo may be the prominent symptom during the acute onset or acute exacerbations. The persistence of symptoms and the presence of nystagmus or other oculomotor deficits (e.g., internuclear ophthalmoplegia) help establish the diagnosis, which is usually confirmed by magnetic resonance imaging. Postconcussion syndrome can be accompanied by some vague dizziness and must be differentiated from symptoms due to focal lesions or post-traumatic PPV. Fear of heights accompanied by dizziness is similar to other phobias, with no known organic vestibular component or CNS localization. Many other pathologic CNS conditions are associated with dizziness. Arnold-Chiari malformations induce imbalance and downbeat nystagmus; Parkinson's disease, syringomyelia, and spinal cord disease are frequently accompanied by imbalance, but not vertigo. Patients with familial periodic ataxia report intermittent imbalance, and progressive supranuclear palsy can induce postural instability, especially with rapid head movements. Dizziness may or may not be related to other pre-existing CNS disease. For example, patients with epilepsy may experience dizziness as part of the disease, as an adverse effect of the medication, or as a manifestation of another syndrome.

CEREBROVASCULAR DISEASE

By Robert D. Brown, Jr., M.D.
Rochester, Minnesota

Stroke persists as one of the most significant causes of mortality and morbidity in the United States in the late 20th century, resulting in more than 100,000 deaths and leaving thousands with varying levels of disability. In the United States, between 500,000 and 600,000 people have a stroke each year. One third of these die within 1 month, making stroke the third leading cause of death. Two thirds of survivors have a permanent disability. The diagnosis and treatment of cerebrovascular diseases have drastically changed in the last 20 years, and it appears that the next decade will be met with even more significant changes. Evaluation of patients with cerebrovascular disorders requires a knowledge of the anatomy and pathophysiology of the cerebral vasculature, the signs and symptoms of the various stroke syndromes, the differential diagnosis of ischemic and hemorrhagic stroke, and a logical evaluation of the patient following a transient ischemic attack (TIA) or stroke.

A detailed history is the most important aspect of the evaluation for potential cerebrovascular disease. One must first consider whether the signs and symptoms are vascular in nature. Features of the history that are important in clarifying the cause include the time of onset, temporal profile of symptom onset and progression, type of deficit associated with the symptoms, presence of other symptoms occurring either simultaneously or following the symptoms, and knowledge of any precipitating event.

Stroke is a generic term that covers a range of disorders characterized by the relatively acute onset of symptoms and signs secondary to dysfunction of the cerebral circulation. Stroke can be broken down into three large categories, including (1) nonhemorrhagic or ischemic infarction, (2) intracerebral hemorrhage, and (3) subarachnoid hemorrhage. The basic distinction between ischemic stroke and hemorrhagic stroke carries great significance, because the problems that they present are diametrically opposed. By far the most common type and causing about 80 per cent of all strokes is nonhemorrhagic or ischemic infarction resulting from a lack of blood supply to an area of the brain for a period of time leading to nerve cell ischemia and death. Ischemic infarction can include thrombotic strokes that result from a locally decreased blood supply due to a blockage formed within an artery. Alternatively, an embolic stroke refers to blockage caused by a "plug" of material that has broken free from a more proximal site. Lacunar infarctions are usually caused by a thrombosis of one of the small penetrating branch arteries that has been affected by a specific pathologic process commonly associated with hypertension.

Classifying stroke into one of the main subgroups, determining the area of brain affected by ischemia or hemorrhage, and delineating the site of arterial blockage are the most important features of the evaluation. Distinguishing the type of stroke requires knowledge of the presence of stroke risk factors; the clinical presentation, including the onset and course; neuroanatomy; accompanying symptoms, such as headache and vomiting; any change in the level of consciousness; and the results of imaging and vascular studies.

Table 1. Hemorrhagic Cerebrovascular Disorders

Location	Causes
Epidural hematoma	Head trauma, meningeal artery tear
Subdural hematoma	Head trauma, bridging vein tear
Subarachnoid hemorrhage	Saccular aneurysm, arteriovenous malformation, trauma, bleeding dyscrasia, anticoagulant use, mycotic aneurysm, neoplastic aneurysm, dissecting aneurysm, hypertension, primary or metastatic tumors, vasculitis, illicit drug use, venous sinus thrombosis
Intraparenchymal hemorrhage	Hypertension, arteriovenous malformation, cavernous malformation, venous angioma, saccular aneurysm, amyloid angiopathy, venous thrombosis, bleeding dyscrasia, primary and metastatic tumors, vasculitis, moyamoya disease, arterial dissection, tissue plasminogen activator, antiplatelet or anticoagulant use, hemorrhage into cerebral infarction, illicit drug use
Intraventricular hemorrhage	Extension from intraparenchymal hemorrhage or subarachnoid hemorrhage, saccular aneurysm, arteriovenous malformation, primary or metastatic neoplasm

HEMORRHAGIC STROKE

Epidural and Subdural Hemorrhage

Intracranial hemorrhage can be categorized by the site of bleeding, starting with the most superficial site (Table 1). Epidural hemorrhage occurs between the skull and the dura, usually following head trauma and skull fracture resulting in arterial bleeding from the middle meningeal artery. The event is characterized by transient loss of consciousness, followed by a lucid interval lasting minutes to hours. Worsening headache, often with nausea or vomiting, is typical, and the level of consciousness decreases with progressive hemorrhage and increased intracranial pressure. Far more common is subdural hemorrhage caused by mild trauma that may seem trivial at the time of occurrence. Venous bleeding from bridging veins crossing the subdural space is the cause and is most common in older individuals. Clinical presentations include subtle cognitive dysfunction, headache, focal neurologic deficits, seizures, and transient episodes that can mimic TIAs.

Subarachnoid Hemorrhage

Subarachnoid hemorrhage (SAH) causes about 5 to 10 per cent of strokes and is often heralded by the abrupt onset of a severe headache. However, less severe headache with or without loss of consciousness, nausea, and vomiting can occur, and mild SAH may be dismissed as a benign syndrome. Typically, no focal abnormalities are detected on examination, although cranial nerve deficits can suggest aneurysm at specific sites. Unilateral third or sixth nerve palsy suggests a posterior communicating aneurysm. Optic nerve compression may be caused by a supraclinoid internal carotid artery (ICA) or ophthalmic aneurysm, and optic chiasm compression causing visual loss can be seen with either anterior cerebral artery or supraclinoid ICA lesions. Cranial neuropathies localizing to the cavernous sinus suggest an internal carotid artery aneurysm. Other brain stem or cranial nerves may also be involved, including upper brain stem compression with basilar or posterior cerebral lesions. The former often present with facial pain from trigeminal nerve involvement or facial weakness caused by facial nerve impingement. Aneurysms in vertebral segments may cause deficits related to lower brain stem mass effect or compression of medullary-level cranial nerves in the subarachnoid space. Other focal signs may suggest an intracerebral hemorrhage, such as abulia and lower extremity weakness from a frontal hemorrhage caused by an anterior communicating artery lesion. Speech dysfunction with evidence of temporal, frontal, or parietal lobe hematoma can be seen with a middle cerebral artery aneurysm. On ophthalmologic examination, subhyaloid hemorrhages, well-circumscribed preretinal hemorrhages (due to an abrupt increase in intracranial pressure), suggest subarachnoid hemorrhage.

If the clinical symptoms or signs suggest possible SAH, computed tomography (CT) is indicated. Computed tomography is about 90 per cent sensitive for hemorrhage in the subarachnoid space if performed within 24 to 48 hours (Fig. 1). If the CT scan is unremarkable and the clinical suspicion remains high, a lumbar puncture is performed to search for blood in the cerebrospinal fluid. Blood from a

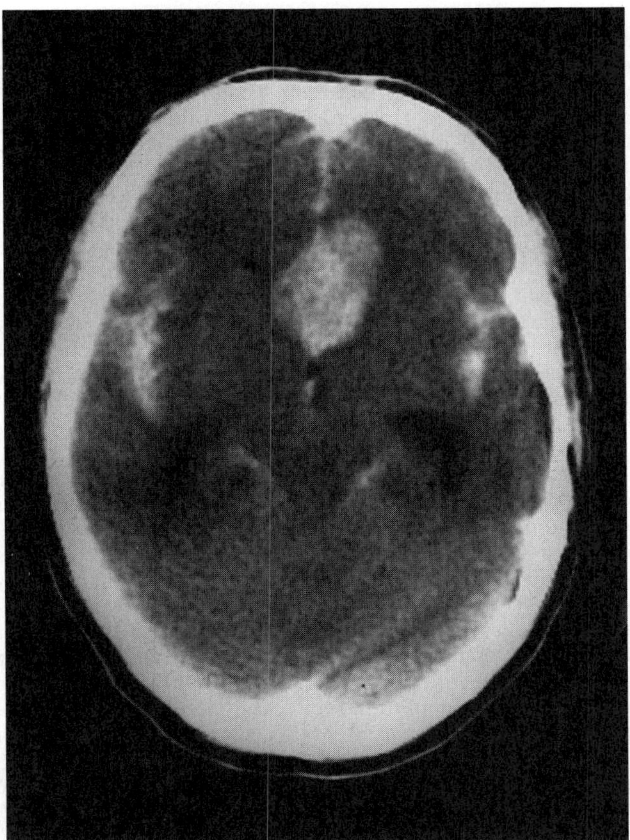

Figure 1. Head computed tomography demonstrates subarachnoid hemorrhage in the sylvian fissures bilaterally, in the interhemispheric fissure, and surrounding the upper brain stem, with a focal area of hemorrhage anteriorly. The hemorrhage was caused by an anterior communicating artery aneurysm.

traumatic tap clears as successive samples of cerebrospinal fluid are obtained. Xanthochromia appears in the cerebrospinal fluid within a few hours of the hemorrhage and persists for 3 to 4 weeks.

The most common nontraumatic cause of SAH is a ruptured saccular aneurysm, and less common causes include arteriovenous malformations, bleeding dyscrasia, anticoagulant use, dissecting aneurysms, and mycotic aneurysms (see Table 1). Cerebral angiography is considered early in the evaluation to define the cause of the hemorrhage. If the cause remains obscure, repeat angiography is appropriate in 10 to 14 days. Patients with negative initial angiography and hemorrhage localized only to the perimesencephalic region have a more benign prognosis than patients with abnormal angiography revealing an aneurysm as the cause of the hemorrhage, or those with negative angiography but abnormal CT showing hemorrhage extending into the interhemispheric fissure or sylvian fissures.

Saccular aneurysm as a cause of SAH occurs in about 30,000 people each year in the United States and has a 40 per cent short-term case mortality rate. Aneurysms were once considered to be congenital, but it is now apparent that most aneurysms are acquired. About 3 to 5 per cent of the population may harbor an intracranial saccular aneurysm. People with intracranial arteriovenous malformations have intracranial aneurysm in about 10 to 15 per cent of cases. Other disorders associated with intracranial aneurysms include polycystic kidney disease, Marfan's syndrome, Ehlers-Danlos syndrome, pseudoxanthoma elasticum, neurofibromatosis, tuberous sclerosis, Sturge-Weber syndrome, coarctation of the aorta, hereditary hemorrhagic telangiectasia, moyamoya disease, and fibromuscular dysplasia.

Intraparenchymal Hemorrhage

Intraparenchymal hemorrhage causes about 10 per cent of all strokes. Hypertension associated with fibrinoid necrosis, lipohyalinosis, and microaneurysms is the most common cause of intracranial hemorrhage, but other causes include hematologic disorders, anticoagulant use, vascular malformations, inflammatory angiopathies, and infections. The most common sites of intracranial hemorrhage caused by hypertensive vascular disease are the basal ganglia (60 per cent), thalamus and internal capsule (10 per cent), pons (10 per cent), and cerebellum (10 per cent). Metastatic neoplasms can undergo hemorrhagic change and include hypernephroma, lung cancer, malignant melanoma, and choriocarcinoma; primary neoplasms such as glioma, pituitary adenoma, and hemangioblastoma can also hemorrhage (see Table 1).

Venous sinus thrombosis and cortical venous thrombosis can produce hemorrhage with focal neurologic deficit, seizures, headache due to intracranial hypertension, and cavernous sinus syndrome. The clinical signs of an intracranial hemorrhage are usually straightforward. Typically, intracranial hemorrhage is associated with the acute onset of a focal neurologic deficit with some mental status alteration, headache, vomiting, and seizures. The deficit often crosses arterial territories, unlike that caused by ischemic infarctions. Computed tomography scan reveals the focal collection of blood (Fig. 2). Intraventricular hemorrhage usually occurs as a result of extension from an intraparenchymal or a subarachnoid site.

CEREBROVASCULAR ISCHEMIA

Transient Ischemic Attack

Transient ischemic attack (TIA) is a focal cerebral ischemic event lasting less than 24 hours and leaving no apparent permanent neurologic deficit. Typically, the temporal profile of an ischemic event is one of acute onset with rapid evolution to maximal deficit. Not all transient neurologic symptoms or deficits are ischemic in nature. Focal ischemic episodes often last 2 to 30 minutes, and most TIAs last less than 6 hours. While "negative" phenomena with some type of neurologic deficit are considered the hallmark of a TIA, occasionally transient episodes of "positive" phenomena, such as rhythmic appendicular shaking, tingling, scintillations, and hallucinations, may be ischemic in nature. Episodes that are very brief, lasting less than a few seconds, spells of unconsciousness without other vertebrobasilar symptoms such as diplopia, ataxia, limb weakness, vertigo, dysarthria, and dysphagia, and episodes that exhibit a slow progression of symptoms over many minutes usually are not caused by transient cerebral ischemia.

The differential diagnosis of TIA always includes seizures, which may evolve slowly over 1 to 2 minutes and include "positive" phenomena; migrainous phenomena, which evolve over a longer period, approximately 15 minutes, frequently followed by a severe headache; generalized or global ischemia; and a labyrinthine source of vertigo unassociated with impairment of sensory or motor function. Intracranial tumors, vascular malformations, and

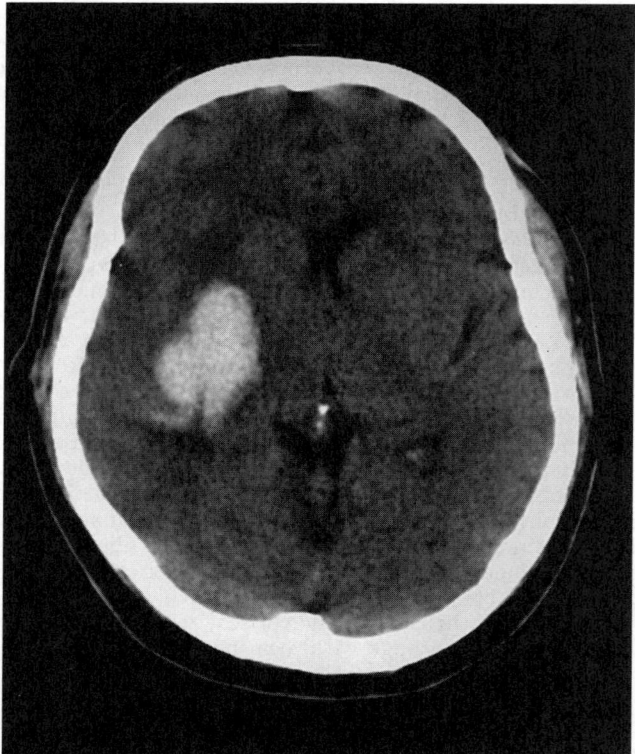

Figure 2. Head computed tomography demonstrates a right basal ganglia hemorrhage caused by hypertensive vascular disease.

intracranial hemorrhage, including subdural hematoma, epidural hematoma, and intracerebral hemorrhage, all can mimic TIA. Drop attacks are characterized by a sudden loss of strength and muscle tone occurring in both legs unassociated with loss of consciousness or other focal symptoms. Transient global amnesia, presumably related to temporal lobe ischemia, usually lasts from many minutes to nearly 24 hours, and presents with an isolated, transient amnesic syndrome. Demyelinating disorders must also be considered, particularly in younger patients, although symptoms usually present subacutely, and the deficit typically lasts longer than 24 hours. Paroxysmal symptoms seen in multiple sclerosis are often associated with "positive" phenomena and are unlikely to be confused with a TIA. Metabolic disorders, such as hypoglycemia, can also cause transient focal symptoms and must be excluded, particularly in persons with a history of diabetes.

Cerebral Infarction

A reversible ischemic neurologic deficit (RIND) is a cerebral infarction subtype that consists of a focal cerebral ischemic event with a deficit lasting longer than 24 hours but resolving in less than 3 weeks. A completed stroke refers to an acute cerebral ischemic event with persistent focal neurologic deficit, lasting longer than 24 hours. Progressive stroke, or stroke in evolution, denotes that the deficit is not stable or improving but, instead, is worsening in either a stuttering or a slowly progressive way. Most progression occurs within 24 hours in the carotid circulation, or within 72 hours in the vertebrobasilar circulation. Ischemic strokes are then further subdivided by etiology and size.

Ischemic stroke is the most common type and accounts for 70 to 80 per cent of all strokes. Thrombotic stroke due to a blockage in a "larger" vessel is accompanied by a variety of risk factors, including smoking, coronary artery disease, diabetes, peripheral vascular disease, and hypertension. Thrombotic stroke is preceded by TIAs in about 40 per cent of cases. The deficit progresses unevenly over time and is specifically related to the occluded vessel. Computed tomography scan reveals an area of decreased attenuation in the distribution of the blocked vessel, although the study may be normal within the first 24 to 48 hours (Figs. 3 and 4). Embolic strokes are associated with similar risk factors. They are less likely to be preceded by TIAs, and their onset is sudden with the maximal deficit occurring within minutes of the occlusion. Circulation to the brain can be blocked by an embolus originating either at the site of atherosclerosis or from another source, such as the heart.

The term lacunar infarct refers to a small lesion (less than 20 mm in diameter) in the deep part of the brain or brain stem. This infarct is often associated with hypertension, and the type of deficit it produces usually permits clinical distinction from a larger ischemic stroke. Many syndromes have been specifically related to lacunar infarcts; these include pure motor stroke (internal capsule or base of the pons), pure sensory stroke (ventroposterior nucleus of the thalamus), clumsy-hand dysarthria (the pons), and ataxic hemiparesis (the pons). This type of stroke is never associated with aphasia, apraxia, loss of consciousness, isolated alteration in cognition, or hemianopia. Rarely, a lacunar infarct causes paresis of a single limb.

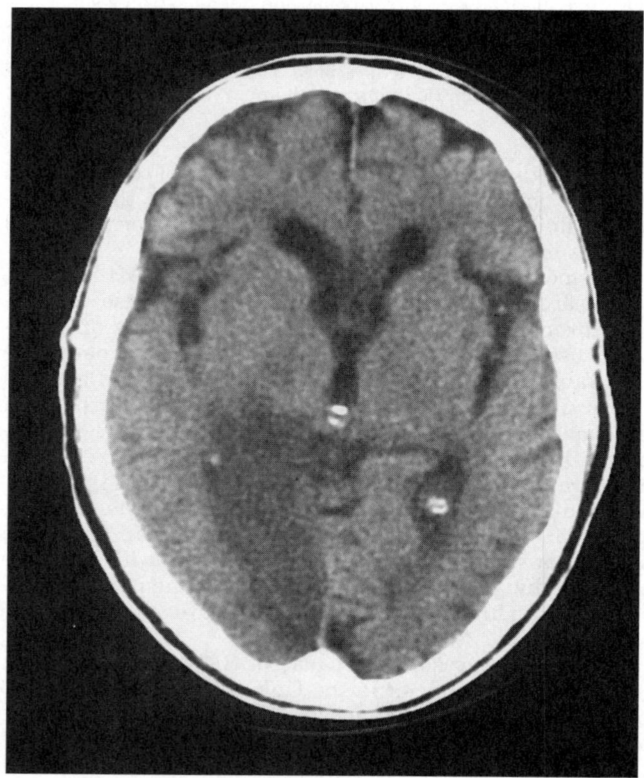

Figure 3. Computed tomography performed 48 hours after the onset of symptoms demonstrates decreased attenuation in the distribution of the right posterior cerebral artery consistent with an area of cerebral infarction.

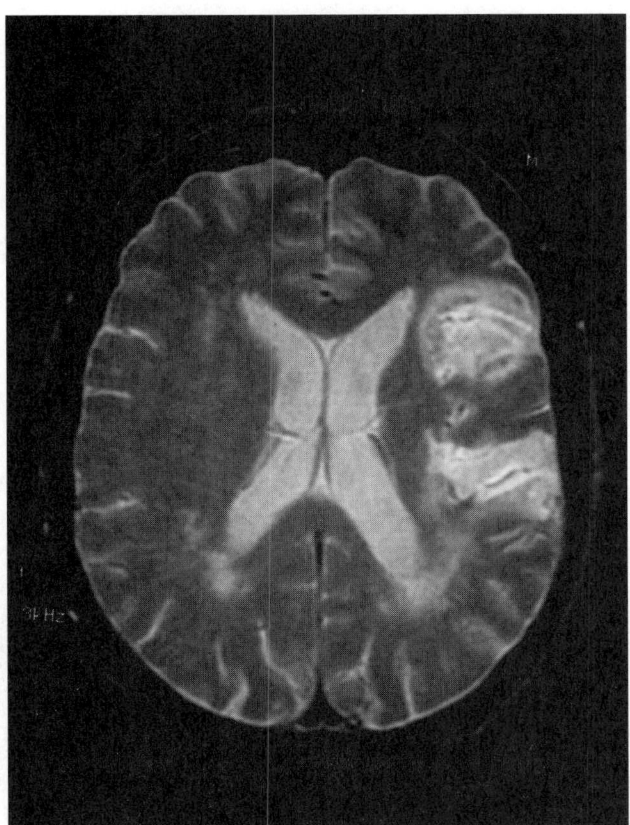

Figure 4. Magnetic resonance imaging of the head demonstrates a large area of subacute cerebral infarction involving the left middle cerebral artery distribution.

The mechanisms of an ischemic event can be classified based on the source or cause of cerebral arterial obstruction (Table 2). Nonarterial factors include venous thromboses and paradoxical emboli. Some cardiac sources are known to produce emboli (Table 3), while others are suspected or putative cardiac sources of emboli (Table 4).

Anatomy and Clinical Correlations

A basic knowledge of the functional anatomy of the cerebral circulation is necessary for correlating the area of the brain involved with a clinical syndrome. The aortic arch is usually the origin of (1) the innominate artery on the right, which subsequently branches into the subclavian artery and the right common carotid artery, (2) the left common carotid artery, and (3) the left subclavian artery. The common carotid arteries variably bifurcate into the internal carotid and the external carotid arteries at the level of the thyroid cartilage, and the vertebral arteries are branches of the right and left subclavian arteries.

The internal carotid artery has no branches in its cervical segment. At the base of the skull, the internal carotid artery enters the petrous bone, bends anteromedially, assumes a horizontal course before exiting anteriorly near the apex of the petrous bone (petrous segment), and then forges ahead intracranially via the foramen lacerum before passing into the cavernous sinus (cavernous segment). At this level, the internal carotid artery lies in close relation to cranial nerves III, IV, and VI and the ophthalmic and maxillary divisions of the trigeminal nerve. The first major branch of the internal carotid artery, arising at the level of the anterior clinoid process, is the ophthalmic artery, which courses anteriorly through the optic canal and then enters the orbit. Clinically, the most important ophthalmic branches are the central retinal artery (the typical site of occlusion in transient monocular blindness, or amaurosis fugax) and the anterior and posterior ciliary arteries (the site of involvement in visual loss from temporal arteritis). Subsequent important branches of the internal carotid artery include the posterior communicating artery, allowing connection to the posterior cerebral artery and contributing the posterior extension of the circle of Willis. The anterior choroid artery is the next significant branch, traveling posteriorly to supply the optic tract and, variably, the inferior and medial aspects of the posterior limb of the internal capsule, globus pallidus, lateral geniculate body, and portions of the temporal lobe. The supraclinoid segment of the internal carotid artery concludes with bifurcation into the anterior and middle cerebral arteries.

Following the origins of the vertebral arteries from the subclavian arteries, the vertebral arteries course through the lateral neck anteriorly to the anterior scalene muscles before entering the transverse foramina of the cervical spine at about C6 and continuing to C2, where the arteries exit through the transverse foramen of the atlas and pass posteriorly behind the articular process of the atlas before piercing the dura and traversing the foramen magnum. Anteriorly to the lower brain stem, the arteries join to form the basilar artery, which continues its course along the ventral aspect of the brain stem and eventually divides into a pair of posterior cerebral arteries at the level of the interpeduncular cistern.

Symptoms in Cerebrovascular Ischemia

Recognition of the patterns of symptoms and signs permits identification of the vessel involved in cerebral ischemia (Table 5). The clinician must attempt to clarify whether the anterior (carotid) or posterior (vertebrobasilar) systems are involved (Tables 6 and 7). Typically, anterior cerebral artery occlusion leads to contralateral weakness and sensory loss, primarily in the leg. Middle cerebral artery syndromes depend, in large part, on the branch vessels occluded and the location of the ischemia with respect to the dominant hemisphere. Usually, contralateral weakness and sensory loss, which is maximal in the face and arm, occurs along with possible speech and language disorder (aphasia), difficulty in reading, writing, or calculating, and homonymous hemianopia. Nondominant hemisphere symptoms may include left visual neglect, contralateral weakness and sensory loss, contralateral sensory neglect, confusion, denial of deficit, and spatial disorientation. Marked impairment of consciousness is unusual in the acute phase following a unilateral ischemic stroke; if such impairment is present, bilateral ischemia, brain stem ischemia, increased intracranial pressure, hemorrhage, global hypoxia, and seizure all must be considered.

Vertebrobasilar distribution symptoms are usually related to brain stem cerebellar and occipital lobe ischemia (see Table 7). The symptoms typically occur in combination and include diplopia, dysarthria, ataxic gait or ataxic limbs, unilateral or bilateral visual changes, facial sensation change or weakness, vertigo, and unilateral or bilateral sensorimotor changes.

Ischemic Stroke and Transient Ischemic Attack

In 33 per cent of patients who have experienced TIA, stroke occurs within 5 years. Of these strokes, 20 per cent occur within the first month, and 50 per cent occur during

Table 2. Ischemic Cerebrovascular Disorders

Ischemia Source	Entity
Cardiac	1. Venous source with right-to-left shunt: patent foramen ovale, atrial septal defect, ventricular septal defect, pulmonary arteriovenous fistulas, pulmonary vein thrombosis
	2. Intracardiac thrombus: atrial fibrillation, sick sinus syndrome, recent myocardial infarction, akinetic left ventricle segment, dilated cardiomyopathy
	3. Cardiac mass lesions: atrial myxoma, cardiac papillary fibroelastoma
	4. Valve disease: prosthetic valve, infective endocarditis, rheumatic heart disease, calcified mitral annulus, nonbacterial thrombotic endocarditis, mitral valve prolapse, calcific aortic stenosis, Libman-Sacks endocarditis
Large vessel disease	1. Atherosclerosis: aortic arch, carotid, vertebrobasilar system, major intracranial branches
	2. Dissection, fibromuscular dysplasia
	3. Infection: syphilis, fungal infection such as mucormycosis and aspergillosis, tuberculosis, herpes zoster; basal meningitis: cryptococcosis, histoplasmosis, coccidioidomycosis
	4. Other: Takayasu's disease, homocystinuria, moyamoya disease, Fabry disease, vasospasm, pseudoxanthoma elasticum, Sneddon's syndrome
Small vessel disease	1. Atherosclerosis, hypertension
	2. Infections: malaria, Lyme disease, HIV, syphilis, trichinosis, schistosomiasis, cysticercosis, bacterial meningitis
	3. Noninfection arteritis: systemic lupus erythematosus; polyarteritis nodosa; sarcoidosis; rheumatoid arthritis; Churg-Strauss syndrome (allergic granulomatosis angiitis); Sjögren's syndrome; Wegener's granulomatosis; temporal arteritis; isolated central nervous system angiitis; Behçet's disease; systemic sclerosis (scleroderma); microangiopathy of the brain, ear, and retina; Degos' syndrome (malignant atrophic papulosis); illicit drug use (especially heroin, cocaine, and amphetamines)
	4. Migraine, hypertensive encephalopathy, subarachnoid hemorrhage
	5. Neoplastic angioendotheliomatosis, lymphomatoid granulomatosis
	6. MELAS (mitochondrial myopathy, encephalopathy, lactic acidosis, strokelike episodes)
Hematologic	1. Polycythemia, thrombocytosis, leukemia
	2. Thrombotic thrombocytopenic purpura, sickle cell disease and other hemoglobinopathies, disseminated intravascular coagulation (DIC)
	3. Protein C and protein S deficiencies, antithrombin III deficiency, lupus anticoagulant positivity, anticardiolipin antibodies
	4. Oral contraceptives, pregnancy, malignancies, heparin-induced antibodies
	5. Multiple myeloma, Waldenström's macroglobulinemia, cryoglobulinemia
Other	1. Air emboli
	2. Fat emboli
	3. Cortical vein thrombosis
	4. Hypotension

HIV = human immunodeficiency virus.

the first year. After the first month, the risk of stroke accrues at about 5 per cent per year, which is five times the incidence for a group of similar age who have not had a TIA.

After a hemispheric TIA, amaurosis fugax, or an ischemic stroke, the history and neurologic examination followed by a few laboratory studies help localize the area of ischemia and suggest a possible cause. The initial evaluation includes a complete blood count, prothrombin time (PT) and activated partial thromboplastin time (APTT), erythrocyte sedimentation rate, chemistry and lipid profiles, chest film, and electrocardiogram. Other studies that must be considered include lumbar puncture if an SAH is suspected and the CT scan is negative, arterial blood gases if the patient appears hypoxic, and electroencephalogram if seizures are a concern.

Examination of the patient who presents with a probable stroke must be carried out with specific regard to the patient's condition and should include airway, breathing, and circulation. A brief neurologic examination is performed with a neurovascular examination including auscultation of the heart, neck, cranium, and orbits. A carotid bruit reflects turbulence at that site, but it is a relatively poor predictor of a carotid stenosis. A carotid bruit is detected in 66 per cent of patients with stenosis greater than 50 per cent; however, 10 per cent of those with less than 50 per cent stenosis also have an audible bruit. In patients with carotid distribution ischemia, the positive predictive value of a carotid bruit for an underlying moderate or severe stenosis is about 80 per cent. The presence of a diastolic component to the bruit is an unusual finding, but it is a better predictor of a high-grade stenosis. Palpation

Table 3. Proven Cardiac Risk Factors for Cerebral Ischemia

Atrial fibrillation
Mechanical valve
Dilated cardiomyopathy
Recent myocardial infarction
Intracardiac thrombus
Intracardiac mass

Table 4. Putative Cardiac Risk Factors for Cerebral Ischemia

Sick sinus syndrome
Patent foramen ovale
Thoracic aorta atherosclerotic debris
Spontaneous echo contrast
Previous myocardial infarction, 2 to 6 months following event
Hypokinetic or akinetic left ventricular segment
Mitral annulus calcification

Table 5. Clinical Syndromes in Cerebral Ischemia

Vessel	Structures Supplied	Symptoms and Signs If Vessel Occluded
Internal carotid artery	Frontal, parietal, temporal lobes	Contralateral hemiparesis, homonymous hemianopia, hemianesthesia, aphasia (DH), neglect (NDH)
Ophthalmic artery	Orbit	Ipsilateral monocular blindness (amaurosis fugax)
Anterior choroidal artery	Optic tract, posterior limb of internal capsule, lateral geniculate body	Pure motor (PLIC) or sensory stroke (thalamic), may cause homonymous hemianopia, mild language disorder
Anterior cerebral artery	Medial cerebrum, superior frontal and parietal lobes	Contralateral weakness in leg greater than arm, behavioral changes such as abulia
Middle cerebral artery	Lateral cerebrum, deep structures of frontal and parietal lobes	Contralateral hemiplegia, hemianesthesia, homonymous hemianopia, aphasia (DH), visuospatial defect (NDH)
Posterior cerebral artery	Occipital lobe, inferior and medial portion of temporal lobe	Contralateral homonymous hemianopia or quadrantanopia, visual hallucinations, agnosias
Penetrating thalamogeniculate branches	Posterior thalamus	Déjérine-Roussy syndrome: contralateral sensory loss, dysesthesias
Basilar artery	Pons, midbrain, cerebellum (ends in posterior cerebral artery territory)	Wide-ranging symptoms, depending on level of involvement, branch vessel
Weber syndrome: penetrating posterior cerebral artery branches	Midbrain, third-nerve nucleus, cerebral peduncle	Third-nerve palsy, contralateral hemiparesis
Benedikt syndrome: penetrating posterior cerebral artery branches	Midbrain, third-nerve nucleus, red nucleus	Third-nerve palsy, contralateral ataxia, athetosis
Basilar artery, paramedian branches	Base of pons	Locked-in syndrome, with quadriparesis, may be able to move eyes vertically
Wallenberg's syndrome: posterior inferior cerebellar artery	Lateral medulla	Ipsilateral facial sensory loss, contralateral body sensory loss, vertigo, ataxia, dysarthria, dysphagia, Horner's syndrome

DH = dominant hemisphere; NDH = nondominant hemisphere; PLIC = posterior limb of internal capsule.

of the carotid artery is not useful and has the potential for dislodging emboli. Palpation of the temporal arteries provides some information regarding collateral supply from the external carotid artery, and the presence of external carotid artery disease (e.g., temporal arteritis and external carotid artery occlusion).

A complete neuro-ophthalmologic examination is also necessary. Useful findings can include cholesterol and fibrin platelet emboli that are consistent with advanced atherosclerotic disease. Venous stasis retinopathy is a result of high-grade stenosis in the ipsilateral carotid arterial system. It has the appearance of diabetic retinopathy, but also includes venous engorgement, retinal hemorrhages, and microaneurysms. Papilledema suggests increased intracranial pressure, and subhyaloid hemorrhage may accompany SAH. Nuchal rigidity, which can be caused by intracranial or subarachnoid hemorrhage or infection, is evaluated if cervical spine injury can be excluded.

Most patients presenting with a possible ischemic or hemorrhagic stroke should receive early CT imaging. The study is a rapid and safe method of excluding the presence of a significant hemorrhage (subarachnoid, intraparenchy-

Table 6. Clinical Symptoms of Ischemia of the Anterior Circulation

1. Motor dysfunction of contralateral extremities and/or face:
   - Clumsiness
   - Weakness
   - Paralysis
   - Slurred speech
2. Visual loss in ipsilateral eye
3. Contralateral homonymous hemianopia or quadrantanopia
4. Language deficit if dominant hemisphere involved, may include problems with expressive speech, comprehension, calculation, reading, naming, or writing
5. Visuospatial deficit, inattention, denial of deficit, or hemineglect if nondominant hemisphere involved
6. Sensory deficit of contralateral extremities and/or face:
   - Numbness or loss of sensation
   - Paresthesias

Table 7. Clinical Symptoms of Ischemia of the Posterior Circulation

1. Motor dysfunction of any combination of extremities and/or the face:
   - Clumsiness
   - Paralysis
   - Ataxia
   - Bilateral or alternating symptoms suggest the posterior circulation. Other brain stem symptoms (see no. 4) are often associated.
2. Loss of vision of one or both homonymous visual fields. Bilateral visual field deficit suggests posterior circulation involvement.
3. Sensory deficit of extremities and/or face:
   - Numbness or loss of sensation
   - Paresthesias
   - Bilateral or alternating symptoms suggest the posterior circulation. Other brain stem symptoms (see no. 4) are often associated.
4. The following symptoms typically occur but are not diagnostic if they occur in isolation:
   - Ataxic gait, ataxic extremities
   - Vertigo
   - Diplopia
   - Dysphagia
   - Dysarthria

mal, subdural, or epidural) and, thereby, directs appropriate treatment. A normal CT scan does not exclude the presence of stroke—a CT scan may be normal for 48 hours following the onset of an ischemic stroke—but the exclusion of hemorrhage is crucial. Subtle findings of ischemic stroke may be observed early on CT scan; they include relative unilateral hypodensity, loss of gray matter–white matter junction, and flattening of sulci, indicating early edema.

Magnetic resonance imaging (MRI) is more sensitive to ischemic stroke during the first several hours, with infarction typically detected within 4 to 8 hours. However, acute hemorrhage can be difficult to distinguish on an MRI scan. Also, the relatively long period needed to perform an MRI scan may make it impossible. Lack of patient cooperation also leads to poor magnetic resonance images, particularly of the posterior fossa, cerebellum, and brain stem.

Patients with recent multiple TIAs, changing neurologic deficit, coma, seizures, significant fixed neurologic deficit of recent onset, or CT revealing intracranial hemorrhage require hospitalization for observation, aggressive evaluation, and appropriate treatment. Hospitalization may not be necessary for patients who are seen for the first time a week or more after the onset of a stable minor deficit, or those who experienced a TIA more than 2 weeks before presentation. However, hospitalization must be strongly considered for patients who have had more than four episodes in 2 weeks, a possible cardioembolic source of a stroke (see Tables 3 and 4), a diastolic-systolic bruit over the ipsilateral carotid artery, a clinical setting for embolism, or a severe deficit during a transient event.

Ischemia of the Anterior Circulation

An effective, noninvasive, and safe method for detecting extracranial carotid artery stenosis is duplex carotid ultrasound, utilizing Doppler flow studies to evaluate blood flow and real-time B-mode imaging to visualize the vessel in cross-section. The overall accuracy of ultrasound studies in estimating the degree of carotid stenosis compared with conventional angiography is 80 to 95 per cent. Oculoplethysmography (OPG) can also be used as an initial screening study. This noninvasive test is sensitive (93 per cent) for the detection of a hemodynamically significant carotid stenosis from the carotid origin to the cavernous segment of the internal carotid artery at the ophthalmic artery branch, but it does not localize the stenosis or occlusion.

Magnetic resonance angiography (MRA) can noninvasively visualize the extracranial and proximal intracranial arterial and venous circulations. Its advantages over standard angiography include imaging without the need for administration of contrast medium and elimination of the risks associated with arterial puncture and catheterization. The overall accuracy of MRA compared with conventional angiography is about 90 per cent, and another recent study has demonstrated a good rate of detection for severe stenosis. The sensitivity of the technique for mild to moderate degrees of stenosis is lower, and MRA distinguishes poorly between occlusion and high-grade stenosis. Magnetic resonance angiography is limited in its ability to quantitate carotid arterial stenosis and to evaluate the intracranial circulation. MRI in combination with MRA is also useful for detecting intracranial saccular aneurysms larger than 4 mm, small arteriovenous malformations, venous angiomas, and cavernous malformations.

Transcranial Doppler ultrasound (TCD) noninvasively examines intracranial segments of the proximal anterior and middle cerebral arteries, the distal internal carotid artery, and, in the posterior circulation, the distal intracranial segments of the vertebral arteries and, at least proximal segments of the basilar artery. By measuring the velocity of blood flow in the main intracranial arteries and by listening for abnormal acoustic properties, TCD can be used to evaluate the intracranial hemodynamic effects of extracranial carotid arterial occlusive disease and the presence and evolution of hemodynamically significant intracranial major vessel stenoses. Also, TCD can detect proximal intracranial stenosis that may alter the treatment approach.

If carotid ultrasound and oculoplethysmography detect carotid stenosis on the side appropriate to symptoms, conventional angiography is usually performed and a surgical procedure planned, depending on the angiographic findings. This strategy, of course, implies that the patient is an appropriate surgical candidate. Cerebral angiography is used to delineate a stenotic lesion in the extracranial or intracranial segments of the internal carotid artery. This diagnostic technique also provides evaluation of the intracranial circulation for simultaneously occurring distal lesions and is the most sensitive method for detecting intracranial saccular aneurysms. Unfortunately, standard angiography is not without the potential for complication. The risk of stroke with the procedure is less than 1 per cent. Other uncommon complications include infection or hemorrhage at the puncture site and renal failure from the angiographic dye.

Ischemia of the Posterior Circulation

Ischemia in a vertebrobasilar distribution typically leads to symptoms related to the brain stem, cerebellum, or occipital lobe. The distal vertebral and basilar arteries may be noninvasively evaluated with TCD, which has a sensitivity of 75 per cent for detecting hemodynamically significant stenosis. Magnetic resonance angiography provides an alternative method of noninvasively evaluating the same segments. The ability of MRA to detect stenosis in the vertebrobasilar system is not known with certainty, but its sensitivity is probably between 70 and 85 per cent. Extracranial vertebral segments can be evaluated with vertebral Doppler studies, which indicate the direction of flow, providing indirect evidence of a more proximal stenosis or occlusion.

Although treatment options can be made based on abnormal results of the noninvasive studies, cerebral angiography may be necessary in patients with inconclusive TCD or MRA results. A more proximal stenosis must be considered in these patients, especially if they continue to have posterior circulation ischemic episodes.

A normal electrocardiogram, chest film, past cardiac history, and cardiac examination make the detection of a cardiac source of emboli unlikely. Cardiac imaging studies should be reserved for patients with ischemic events involving multiple vascular distributions, younger patients (less than 40 years old), and patients with negative noninvasive or angiographic studies. Holter monitoring is indicated in some patients to detect permanent or episodic atrial arrhythmias, especially in younger patients who do not have an alternative cause of the ischemic events. Many less common causes of cerebral ischemia are listed in Table 2.

COMPLICATIONS OF ISCHEMIC STROKE

The complications following an acute ischemic stroke can be classified as either neurologic or medical. Cerebral edema, which occurs in about 10 to 15 per cent of patients typically reaches a maximum at 3 to 5 days following the event. Hemorrhagic transformation is a common occurrence in the setting of embolic infarcts. Petechial hemorrhages noted on an MRI scan are usually not clinically relevant. Seizures during the first few hours and days following stroke are not uncommon, but frequency of seizures is not high enough to recommend prophylactic use of anticonvulsants.

An infarction that has a carotid distribution typically progresses over 24 hours after the initial onset of symptoms, and progression is observed in an even higher percentage of vertebrobasilar distribution infarctions. Any metabolic derangement may lead to apparent worsening of symptoms, and in cases of thrombotic infarction, propagation of the arterial thrombus can produce further symptoms. Recurrent embolization can occur in patients with cardioembolic or other embolic events.

Twenty per cent of patients die within 30 days of a cerebral infarction, and one half of these deaths are related to medical causes. A major area of concern is the prevention of pulmonary embolism and pneumonia. Both hypertension and myocardial infarction can occur and must be treated appropriately. Other sites of complications include the skin, with decubitus ulcer formation; ocular disease in those who may lack muscle tone to close the eye completely; and urinary tract disorders, including incontinence, retention, and urinary tract infection, particularly if an indwelling catheter is present. Gastrointestinal complications include vomiting, acute peptic (stress) ulcers, and fecal incontinence or constipation. Nutrition is often a problem following the event; pain and restlessness may also occur. Seizures are not uncommon following all types of stroke.

STROKE PREVENTION

Irreversible risk factors for stroke are age, family history, male gender, and race. Treatable risk factors include systolic and diastolic increase in blood pressure, cigarette smoking, diabetes, hyperlipidemia, pre-existing cardiovascular disease (e.g., coronary artery disease, cardiac failure, or intermittent claudication), atrial fibrillation, left ventricular hypertrophy, and excessive alcohol intake. The relative contribution of each of the risk factors has been studied, and high blood pressure has emerged as the major risk factor for stroke. Stroke incidence is indeed proportional to the degree of blood pressure increase. Isolated systolic hypertension is also a significant risk factor, and the incidence of stroke decreases when it is treated. The duration of cigarette smoking may be the most important predictor of carotid atherosclerosis, followed by hypertension, diabetes, and age. Fortunately, medical therapy or behavioral modification is possible for both hypertension and cigarette smoking. Aggressive treatment of hyperglycemia is useful for reducing stroke in diabetics, and cholesterol-lowering therapy is also associated with a reduced risk of stroke. The effects of regular moderate exercise and a diet low in fat on stroke are currently under investigation.

ACUTE BACTERIAL MENINGITIS

By Jack L. LeFrock, M.D.
Sarasota, Florida

Acute bacterial meningitis can be a rapidly devastating illness associated with significant neurologic morbidity and mortality. Nowhere has the impact of antimicrobial therapy been more dramatically demonstrated than in bacterial meningitis. Fifty years ago, the mortality rate for bacterial meningitis exceeded 90 per cent, and most of the survivors were neurologically devastated. When effective antibiotic therapy became available, the mortality rate declined to a range of 10 to 20 per cent, where it has remained essentially unchanged during the past 15 years. Despite the remarkable advances in specific antimicrobial therapy and various rehabilitative measures, bacterial meningitis remains one of the most serious infectious diseases and should always be regarded as a medical emergency.

The major task presented to the clinician by patients with meningitis is rapid identification of the infecting organism, which is the basis for selection of effective antimicrobial therapy. Examination of a Gram stain of spinal fluid often defines the causative agent, but this is not always possible. The value of bacterial cultures is limited by the time required (24 to 48 hours or more) for the results to become positive, which is an unacceptable delay in initiating treatment. Experience has clearly demonstrated that early treatment of pyogenic meningeal infection results in a higher survival rate and a lower incidence of potentially fatal complications.

EPIDEMIOLOGY AND ETIOLOGY

Since 1960, the incidence of meningitis (based on community hospital studies) has ranged between 5 and 10 cases per 100,000 persons per year. It is age related; approximately 15 per cent of cases occur in infants younger than 1 month of age, 37 per cent of cases occur before 1 year of age, and 75 per cent of cases occur in patients less than 15 years of age. In the United States, approximately 25,000 cases are diagnosed per year; of these, nearly 2200 patients die and 4000 to 5000 survive with significant residual complications. This incidence has remained fairly constant over the past 40 years. Mortality also varies with age and is highest in the first year of life. It decreases during the middle years and rises again after 50 years of age.

A variety of factors predispose individuals to bacterial meningitis, including otitis media, mastoiditis, sinusitis, recent neurosurgical procedures, head trauma, respiratory infections, immunologic defects, and sickle cell anemia. *Haemophilus influenzae, Neisseria meningitidis,* and *Streptococcus pneumoniae* are the most common pathogens, accounting for about 80 per cent of all reported cases. The causative organism is clearly related to the patient's age (Table 1).

Meningitis due to gram-negative bacilli (excluding *H. influenzae*) is relatively uncommon in adults. However, the proportion of cases caused by these organisms has increased significantly in the past two decades. After the neonatal period, gram-negative bacillary meningitis occurs

Table 1. Common Pathogens of Acute Bacterial Meningitis

Age Group	Organisms
Newborn to 2 mo	Enteric bacilli *(Escherichia coli, Klebsiella, Enterobacter, Proteus)* group B streptococci, *Listeria monocytogenes, Streptococcus pneumoniae, Haemophilus influenzae, Neisseria meningitidis, Pseudomonas aeruginosa, Staphylococcus aureus*
2 mo to 10 yr	*H. influenzae, N. meningitidis, S. pneumoniae*
10 to 50 yr	*S. pneumoniae, N. meningitidis*
Older than 50 yr	*S. pneumoniae, N. meningitidis,* miscellaneous gram-negative bacilli, *Staphylococcus aureus,* streptococci, *L. monocytogenes, H. influenzae*

primarily in patients whose anatomic defenses against central nervous system (CNS) infection have been compromised. The most common predisposing factor is cranial trauma, either neurosurgical or accidental. Gram-negative bacillary meningitis can also occur as a rare complication of bacteremia in hospitalized patients with diabetes, urinary tract infection, cancer, cirrhosis, or advanced age. *S. pneumoniae* is by far the most frequent cause of recurrent meningitis.

CLINICAL SETTINGS AND FEATURES

The clinical features of bacterial meningitis are the same regardless of the causative agent; however, specific bacteria may be suspected under certain circumstances.

1. Meningitis associated with acute otitis media, mastoiditis, or sinusitis is most likely caused by *S. pneumoniae.* If the patient is 2 months to 3 years of age, *H. influenzae* must also be considered.
2. Meningitis associated with pneumonia is most likely pneumococcal.
3. A petechial or purpuric skin rash or the presence of shock suggests infection with *N. meningitidis.*
4. Meningitis developing within 3 days of a nonpenetrating, nondepressed head injury is almost always pneumococcal.
5. Delayed-onset post-traumatic meningitis or meningitis that follows penetrating skull or spinal wounds can be caused by a variety of organisms, including *S. pneumoniae, Staphylococcus aureus,* and gram-negative bacilli (e.g., *Escherichia coli, Proteus, Pseudomonas*).
6. Recurrent bacterial meningitis is most commonly due to *S. pneumoniae* and, occasionally, *H. influenzae.*
7. Meningitis occurring in young children with sickle cell anemia is most likely pneumococcal.
8. Meningitis that follows neurosurgical procedures often results from gram-negative bacilli and *Staphylococcus aureus.* The infection may be polymicrobial.
9. Shunt-associated meningitis (ventriculoatrial) is usually due to coagulase-negative staphylococci. Less commonly, coagulase-positive staphylococci, gram-negative bacilli, diphtheroids, and enterococci are involved. Ventriculoperitoneal shunts have a greater chance of becoming infected with enteric bacilli than do ventriculoatrial shunts. Meningitis associated with shunts may show local signs of inflammation along the subcutaneous course of the shunt as well as prolonged postoperative fever.
10. Meningitis in patients with leukemia or lymphoma or in individuals taking immunosuppressive drugs is likely to be due to *E. coli, P. aeruginosa, Staphylococcus aureus, Listeria monocytogenes,* or *S. pneumoniae.*
11. Seizures may be present at the onset of disease in adults with meningitis due to *L. monocytogenes.*

The typical manifestations of infection—fever, chills, malaise, generalized aching, varying degrees of prostration, and leukocytosis—are present in nearly all adults and children with bacterial meningitis. The specific manifestations of meningeal infection are headache, vomiting, nuchal rigidity, and positive Kernig's and Brudzinski's signs. The headache is often described as generalized and severe beyond anything previously experienced. The vomiting, which is more common in children, occurs without abdominal pain or other gastrointestinal symptoms. Marked irritability, manic behavior, wild delirium, confusion, drowsiness, stupor, coma, seizures (focal or generalized), cranial nerve palsies, and paresis of one or more of the extremities may occur.

The pathophysiologic bases for the disordered neurologic function are (1) inflammation of the arteries and veins that traverse the subarachnoid space, resulting in ischemia and infarction of the cerebral tissue; (2) cerebral edema and increased intracranial pressure; and (3) entrapment of cranial nerves by thick basilar exudate.

Extremes of age or immunocompromised states can alter the clinical symptoms at presentation of meningeal disease. In one series only 28 per cent of elderly patients presented with neck pain or stiffness. The most commonly observed symptoms in this population were confusion, headache, and nausea.

In infants less than 2 months of age, signs of meningeal irritation are usually absent. A high-pitched cry, irritability, vomiting, or poor feeding may be the only complaints described by parents. Fever is often absent, and temperature may be below normal. The only sign of meningitis may be fullness or bulging of the fontanelles, and this may be absent if the infant is dehydrated from vomiting.

RECURRENT BACTERIAL MENINGITIS

Repeated episodes of bacterial meningitis usually indicate a communication between the subarachnoid space and the outside. Frequently a history can be elicited of cranial trauma resulting in a skull fracture with dural tear and the development of a cerebrospinal fluid (CSF) fistula that serves as a portal of entry for organisms. The common fracture sites are the cribriform plate, the base of the skull, and the petrous bone. The associated dural tear provides a communication between the subarachnoid space and paranasal sinuses or the middle ear. Previously undetected skull fractures, often related to minor trauma in the distant past, are usually responsible. Dural defects with CSF fistula can also occur after neurosurgical procedures. *S. pneumoniae* is by far the most frequent cause of recurrent meningitis in all these cases; rarely, *H. influenzae* may be involved.

Less commonly, recurrent bacterial meningitis is due to communication between the subarachnoid space and the skin through congenital defects along the craniospinal axis, such as midline dermal sinuses, meningomyeloceles, and dermoid cysts that are usually evident before adult life. The causative agents in these cases are typically gram-negative bacilli and occasionally *S. aureus.*

Chronic infections of the paranasal sinuses and the middle ear can also lead to recurrent meningitis but are more commonly associated with relapsing meningitis. Recurrent meningitis has also been reported in patients with impaired host defense mechanisms such as agammaglobulinemia, multiple myeloma, leukemia, and lymphoma.

In all cases of recurrent or post-traumatic meningitis, an anatomic defect should be sought using polytomography of the frontal and mastoid regions. During the acute phase of meningitis, CSF rhinorrhea may not be present. After inflammation subsides, however, CSF rhinorrhea typically returns. It can be most easily elicited by having the patient lean forward in a sitting position. Demonstration of glucose in nasal secretions with glucose oxidase tape (Tes-Tape) suggests CSF rhinorrhea. Confirmatory evidence can be obtained by injecting indigo carmine or radioiodine-labeled albumin into the lumbar sac and examining nasal packs for the presence of dye or radioactivity. Surgical closure of CSF fistulas is necessary for preventing recurrence of meningitis. CSF rhinorrhea following acute head injury usually subsides spontaneously in about 2 weeks. If it persists more than 6 weeks, neurosurgical intervention is indicated, but even surgery does not ensure cessation of rhinorrhea.

GRAM-NEGATIVE BACILLARY MENINGITIS IN ADULTS

Gram-negative bacillary meningitis occurs mostly in patients whose anatomic defense against CNS infection has been compromised. The most common predisposing factor to gram-negative bacillary meningitis is cranial trauma, either neurosurgical or accidental. Approximately two thirds of all cases follow neurosurgical procedures. This type of infection may also occur as a rare complication of bacteremia, usually in hospitalized patients with diabetes, cirrhosis, urinary tract infection, cancer, or advanced age. Whenever hospitalized patients with serious underlying disease acquire bacterial meningitis, the suspicion of gram-negative bacillary meningitis should be high. Chronic otitis media and mastoiditis have also been associated with this type of meningeal infection. The most common gram-negative agents are *Klebsiella* (40 per cent); *E. coli* (15 to 30 per cent); and *P. aeruginosa* (10 to 20 per cent).

The typical signs and symptoms of meningitis can be diminished in elderly and debilitated patients with gram-negative bacillary meningitis. Changes in mental status can present without headache or nuchal rigidity. Furthermore, these patients often have cervical osteoarthrosis, and the signs of meningeal inflammation can be difficult to elicit.

DIAGNOSIS

Successful treatment of bacterial meningitis depends on early diagnosis. Blood for culture is obtained for every patient who is suspected of having meningitis. The causation pathogens can also be isolated from the blood in nearly 60 to 70 per cent of patients with documented bacterial meningitis. The key to the diagnosis is a thorough examination of the CSF. If meningitis is suspected and the patient does not have papilledema or focal neurologic deficits, prompt lumbar puncture is imperative; the procedure should not be delayed until computed tomography (CT) is performed.

When signs and symptoms of meningitis have been present for less than 24 hours and are rapidly progressive, a bacterial cause is most likely. If bacterial meningitis is strongly suspected, antibiotic therapy is started immediately. No more than 30 minutes should elapse between the diagnostic lumbar puncture and the initiation of therapy.

The physician's responsibilities do not end with the lumbar puncture. The fluid must be delivered immediately to the technologists who perform the cell counts, chemistry tests, and cultures. A detailed procedure note listing the tests ordered should be entered into the patient's record.

Lumbar puncture should not be performed in patients with suspected brain abscess or parameningeal infections. In these patients, CSF findings are nonspecific, organisms are usually absent, and the loss of CSF that occurs through the defect produced by the spinal fluid can precipitate brain herniation and death in 10 to 20 per cent of patients within a few hours of the procedure. If at all possible, lumbar puncture should be avoided in patients with severe thrombocytopenia or abnormalities of clotting function until the coagulation disorder can be temporarily reversed. Persistent bleeding at the lumbar puncture site can result in local hematoma and nerve root compression causing permanent neurologic deficit. Cisternal and high cervical (C2) approaches are occasionally used in cases of chronic meningitis when previous attempts to recover organisms from lumbar CSF have been unsuccessful.

CSF pressure is always measured (opening and closing pressures). Normal opening CSF pressure in the adult ranges between 50 and 195 mm CSF (3.8 to 15 mm Hg). Values less than 150 mm CSF are normal, and those greater than 200 mm are abnormal. CSF pressure can be spuriously increased by Valsalva maneuvers, and falsely low readings are possible if the patient is hyperventilating.

Normal CSF is colorless and clear. It may become turbid if as few as 200 leukocytes/mm^3 or 400 red blood cells/mm^3 are present. CSF will be visibly bloody if 6000 or more red blood cells/mm^3 are present. Yellowish discoloration (xanthochromia) of the CSF supernatant after centrifugation is usually due to breakdown of red blood cells or to protein. Xanthochromia may develop within 1 to 2 hours in vitro if uncentrifuged fluid from a traumatic lumbar puncture is allowed to sit. Xanthochromia due to protein usually indicates a protein concentration greater than 1.5 g/L.

In addition to the Gram stain, the CSF cell count (including differential), glucose concentration (with simultaneous serum glucose determination), and protein concentration should be obtained.

Cell counts and concentrations of protein and glucose in the CSF do not firmly establish a bacterial cause because the range for these values in bacterial meningitis overlaps the range in viral, tuberculous, and fungal meningitis. However, if the values are markedly abnormal in the direction of a purulent profile—that is, more than 1000 polymorphonuclear leukocytes, protein concentration greater than 150 mg/dL, and CSF glucose concentration less than 50 per cent of the blood glucose concentration—the diagnosis of bacterial meningitis is very likely to be correct.

In most patients, antibiotics have little effect on CNS total and differential cell counts or protein or glucose concentrations during the first 2 to 3 days of therapy. In occasional patients, however, antibiotic therapy may convert the CSF response to a predominantly lymphocytic pleocytosis. Prior antibiotic therapy can reduce the diagnostic yield of a Gram stain by 20 per cent and of culture by 30 per cent.

Cerebrospinal Fluid Findings in Bacterial Meningitis

CSF in bacterial meningitis is characterized by polymorphonuclear pleocytosis, decreased glucose concentrations, and increased protein concentrations. Cell counts may vary from a few cells to many thousands, but they are usually between 1000 and 10,000 cells. Glucose concentration is typically less than 40 mg/dL, and the CSF-to-blood glucose ratio is usually less than 0.4. Protein is increased to 100 to 500 mg/dL in most patients and can be considerably higher in the presence of severe inflammation.

In a few patients, CSF changes may be atypical. A lymphocytic pleocytosis is present in up to 14 per cent of patients and is particularly common in neonatal gram-negative meningitis and in meningitis due to *L. monocytogenes.* Normal CSF cell counts and protein concentrations may be seen in specimens obtained at the onset of meningitis, in some cases of neonatal meningitis, and in severely immunocompromised patients. In 9 per cent of cases of bacterial meningitis, the CSF glucose concentration is normal.

Cerebrospinal Fluid Findings in Tuberculous Meningitis

Typical findings in tuberculous meningitis are a pleocytosis of between 100 and 400 cells, a differential count that shows varying degrees of lymphocytic predominance on serial examinations, a decreased glucose concentration, and an increased protein concentration. In approximately 27 per cent of patients, polymorphonuclear leukocytes compose more than 50 per cent of cells. In severe cases, the cell count may be as high as 1000 to 1200 cells/mm^3. Pleocytosis may be minimal or absent in patients with acquired immunodeficiency syndrome (AIDS) or other conditions of impaired host response. Glucose concentrations are usually 30 to 45 mg/dL but may occasionally be less than 10 mg/dL and are within normal limits in 17 per cent of patients. Protein concentrations are 100 to 500 mg/dL in 65 per cent of patients and may reach 1000 mg/dL or more if treatment is delayed.

Cerebrospinal Fluid Findings in Fungal and Other Chronic Meningitides

CSF findings in fungal meningitis are similar to those described in tuberculous meningitis, with predominantly lymphocytic pleocytosis and increased protein and decreased glucose concentrations. As in tuberculous meningitis, the CSF may be acellular in severely immunocompromised patients, including those with AIDS. Morphologic identification of fungi in Gram or silver stains of CSF sediment is usually not successful, although *Cryptococcus neoformans, Blastomyces dermatidis, Coccidioides immitis,* and *Candida albicans* may occasionally be detected. *C. neoformans* can be detected on India ink preparation in about 50 per cent of cases, although material from several lumbar punctures may need to be examined before organisms are found. In AIDS patients with cryptococcal meningitis, the India ink preparation is positive in about 75 per cent of patients. Table 2 summarizes the characteristic findings in infectious meningitis.

Cerebrospinal Fluid Findings in Lyme Disease With Meningeal Involvement

In Lyme disease, CSF changes are typically those of a mild lymphocytic pleocytosis, a modest increase in protein concentration, and a normal glucose concentration. In some cases, however, CSF may be normal or it may show changes identical to those seen in bacterial meningitis. Detection of antibody to *Borrelia burgdorferi* in CSF is strongly suggestive of CNS involvement by the Lyme agent. However, not all patients with neurologic involvement by *Borrelia* acquire CSF antibody, and the presence of antibody in CSF is not essential for diagnosis. Accuracy and reliability of serologic tests for Lyme disease vary widely among laboratories, and positive values reported by laboratories unfamiliar to the physician should be approached with caution.

PITFALLS IN DIAGNOSIS

Distinguishing between pyogenic meningitis of bacterial origin and aseptic meningitis syndrome is of primary importance to the clinician making therapeutic decisions. The overlap of characteristic CSF abnormalities demonstrates the difficulty in differentiating some cases. For stable patients whose CSF parameters suggest a nonbacterial origin, withholding therapy and repeating the lumbar puncture in 6 to 12 hours may facilitate the diagnosis. The CSF profile associated with a viral or nonpyogenic cause remains stable or demonstrates conversion to a lymphocytic pleocytosis, whereas CSF in bacterial meningitis becomes more purulent, polymorphonuclear with neutrophils predominating. Any acute deterioration in clinical status mandates more rapid re-evaluation and a reconsideration of antibiotic therapy.

If a viral infection or chronic meningitis is suspected, CSF and serum specimens should be frozen for subsequent culture and serologic investigation. Pneumococcal, meningococcal, and cryptococcal capsular polysaccharides may be detected, and, when present, are diagnostic. They should be sought when the CSF examination is inconclusive, but epidemiologic and clinical evidence suggests these organisms.

Staining CSF fluid with acridine orange stain (AOS) can demonstrate organisms in 100 per cent of patients with untreated culture-positive bacterial meningitis. The Gram stain is less sensitive for detecting intracellular bacteria than is the AOS. The AOS is positive in 96 per cent of partially treated patients and is more useful in detection of persisting intracellular pathogens.

Rapid diagnostic studies, such as counterimmunoelectro-

Table 2. Typical Cerebrospinal Fluid Findings in Infectious Meningitis

Type	Pressure	Leukocytes/mm^3	Differential Count	Glucose Concentration	Protein Concentration
Bacterial	Normal to increased	500–20,000	Mostly polymorphs	Decreased, usually <2.8 mmol/L	Increased
partially treated	Normal to increased	Usually <1000	Variable	Normal	Increased
Viral	Usually normal	Usually <1000	Polymorphs early, mostly mononuclear cells later	Normal	Normal to increased
Tuberculous	Increased	Usually <500	Mostly mononuclear cells	Decreased	Increased
Fungal	Increased	Usually <500	Mostly mononuclear cells	Decreased	Increased

Table 3. Laboratory Methods for Diagnosis of Meningitis

Organism	Laboratory Tests
Bacteria	Blood cultures
	Gram stain of CSF
	Culture of CSF
	Antigen detection in CSF
	Endotoxin assay of CSF
	Cell count of CSF
	Chemistry tests of CSF
Viruses	Serologic tests of serum
	Culture of CSF
Mycobacteria	Acid-fast bacillus smear of CSF
	Culture of CSF
	Antigen detection in CSF by serologic determination
Fungi	Blood cultures
	Culture of CSF
	Serology tests on CSF
	India ink test on CSF

CSF = Cerebrospinal fluid.

phoresis (CIE), the latex particle agglutination test (LPA), and the enzyme-linked immunosorbent assay (ELISA) are now available. These tests detect bacterial antigen in the CSF of patients with *H. influenzae* type b; meningococcal serogroup A, B, C or Y; group B streptococci; and pneumococcal disease. The latex agglutination test appears to be more sensitive than counterimmunoelectrophoresis; it has been reported to detect antigen in 80 to 90 per cent of culture-proven cases of bacterial meningitis. Detection of antigen in the serum or urine of patients with bacterial meningitis has not yet been shown to be a sensitive diagnostic method.

Other tests have been used to distinguish bacterial from aseptic meningitis. An increased concentration of CSF lactate is a good indicator of untreated bacterial meningitis but is not specific. It occurs in fungal meningitis, brain abscess, CNS ischemia, infarction, or tumor and is less sensitive in partially treated bacterial meningitis. C-reactive protein (an acute-phase reactant) in the CSF has also been measured in an attempt to distinguish bacterial from aseptic meningitis. The problem with this test is that its sensitivity and specificity have varied widely.

Specimens for blood and nasopharyngeal cultures should be obtained concomitantly with CSF specimens before antibiotics are given. Cultures of sputum, urine, and aspirate (joint, abscess, pleural fluid, and so on) are also obtained if appropriate. When petechiae are present, a Gram-stained specimen of exuded material often demonstrates the infecting organism with leukocytes. Table 3 summarizes the laboratory methods for the diagnosis of meningitis.

BRAIN ABSCESS

By James P. Chandler, M.D.,
and Robert M. Levy, M.D., Ph.D.
Chicago, Illinois

Brain abscesses develop when microorganisms seed necrotic areas of the brain parenchyma. They typically develop as solitary lesions; however, multiple brain abscesses are not uncommon. Although they can occur in any age group, brain abscesses are most common in the first three decades of life. Nearly a third of all brain abscesses are seen in children younger than 15 years of age.

The microorganisms causing brain abscesses enter the brain through trauma, the direct extension of local infection, or hematogenous spread from a distant site of infection. Infections of the paranasal sinuses, middle ear, and mastoid are the most common local events leading to brain abscess formation. Brain abscesses arising secondary to paranasal sinus infection tend to occur in the frontal or temporal lobes by retrograde thrombophlebitis of the diploic veins. Osteomyelitic involvement of the frontal sinus can extend directly into anterior and basal frontal lobes, whereas middle ear infections can extend directly via the transpetrous or translabyrinthine route to produce temporal lobe abscesses. Mastoid infections can extend directly into the temporal lobe or cerebellum or can produce abscesses by retrograde thrombophlebitis of the emissary veins within the temporal bone.

Unlike abscesses arising from direct extension, which are usually solitary, metastatic brain abscesses arise from the hematogenous spread of microorganisms from a distant site of infection and tend to be multiple. Included most often are infections of the skin, lungs, bone, oral cavity, and heart valves. Although abscesses originating from sinusitis or otitis are typically superficial, metastatic abscesses tend to occur at the corticomedullary junction. Their distribution follows that of cerebral blood flow; thus, regions of the frontal and parietal lobes supplied by the middle cerebral artery are most frequently involved. Less commonly, these abscesses are found in the thalamus, brain stem, and cerebellum. Interestingly, transient bacteremia does not appear to cause brain abscesses; this probably results from resistance to infection by the blood-brain barrier.

Congenital heart disease in which cardiac malformations result in right-to-left shunting is another condition that predisposes to brain abscess formation. Bypassing the pulmonary capillary bed, where filtration normally occurs, bacteria can seed the brain and cause abscesses. This is exacerbated by the associated hypoxemia, polycythemia, and increased blood viscosity that may lead to brain microinfarction and establish conditions conducive to bacterial growth and abscess formation.

Penetrating head trauma is another major cause of brain abscess, which tend to develop soon after the trauma, although they may occur years later. Inoculation of the brain usually occurs from retained contaminated bone fragments and debris; bullets, heat-sterilized during their firing, tend not to cause brain contamination. Basilar skull fracture is another post-traumatic cause of infection; subsequent cerebrospinal fluid leak and meningitis may lead to brain inoculation with microorganisms. Prior craniotomy can result in the formation of brain abscesses when microorganisms may be inadvertently introduced during surgery or by direct spread from wound or osteomyelitic infections of the cranial bone flap. In these cases, the infected bone flap must be removed to cure the infection.

Finally, immune system compromise, from immunosuppressive drug administration, the administration of cytotoxic chemotherapeutic agents, or human immunodeficiency virus (HIV) infection, can predispose to the development of brain abscesses from opportunistic organisms. These opportunistic infections can be fungal, protozoal, or viral and arise from the reactivation of latent infection rather than from new infection with these pathogens.

The causative microorganism of brain abscesses can often be related to the initial site of infection. Thus, otitic and dental infections lead to anaerobic bacterial abscesses. Infections from sinusitis give rise to *Staphylococcus aureus,* aerobic streptococcal, and *Haemophilus influenzae* abscesses. More than half of patients are coinfected with anaerobic bacteria. Metastatic abscesses are typically caused by anaerobic bacteria. Pulmonary infections can give rise to a variety of offending organisms, whereas cardiac infection may result in streptococcal brain abscesses. Patients with acquired immunodeficiency syndrome (AIDS) or other immunocompromised states can acquire fungal abscesses (*Candida albicans*) and parasitic abscesses (*Toxoplasma gondii*). In as many as 30 per cent of patients, the primary source of infection is not identified.

PRESENTING SIGNS AND SYMPTOMS

About 80 per cent of patients with brain abscesses have a known clinical factor predisposing to the development of the abscess. Other specific clinical features are not common. Although brain abscesses occur as a result of infection, only about 50 per cent present with fever, which is usually low grade. Fevers greater than 38.5°C (101°F) suggest concomitant meningitis or systemic infection. The symptoms related to brain abscesses depend largely on their size and location and are often indistinguishable from those caused by other space-occupying lesions. Symptoms related to increased intracranial pressure are common. Thus, headache is a significant feature in more than 70 per cent of patients, and nausea and vomiting occur in 25 to 50 per cent of patients. Alterations of consciousness occur in two thirds of patients with brain abscesses. Focal neurologic deficits, the nature of which is related to the location of the infection, occur in 60 per cent of patients. They include hemiparesis, dysphasia, visual field defects, ataxia, and nystagmus. Seizures occur in 30 to 50 per cent of patients. The timing of symptoms and their progression may help distinguish brain abscesses from other intracranial processes such as tumors. Thus, symptoms related to brain abscesses tend to be of rapid onset and progression; they are usually present less than 2 weeks prior to medical evaluation. In the immunocompromised patient, however, symptoms may be of insidious onset and slowly progressive.

DIAGNOSIS

Laboratory tests are of little value in the diagnosis of brain abscesses. The peripheral leukocyte count is usually less than 15,000 cells/mm^3; only 30 per cent of patients have leukocyte counts greater than 11,000 cells/mm^3. Fewer than 10 per cent of patients have leukocyte counts greater than 20,000 cells/mm^3; this reflects the presence of concomitant systemic infection or meningitis. In 90 per cent of patients, the erythrocyte sedimentation rate is increased to an average of about 50 mm per hour. Cerebrospinal fluid (CSF) examination is usually unhelpful in making the diagnosis of brain abscess. Reflecting increased intracranial pressure, the opening pressure is often increased. Unless complicated by meningitis, brain abscesses are associated with only a mild cerebrospinal fluid pleocytosis, with a leukocyte count typically less than 100 cells/mm^3. Protein concentrations in the CSF are usually only mildly increased (<100 mg/dL), and glucose concentrations are often normal. Cultures of the CSF are usually negative. In light of the nonspecific findings of CSF evaluation, and the danger of herniation from elevated intracranial pressure, lumbar puncture should usually be avoided in these patients.

Plain films of the skull are usually normal; however they can demonstrate separation of sutures in children and increased convolution markings, displacement of pineal calcification, enlargement of the sella turcica, or thinning of the clinoid process in adults. These are nonspecific findings. The electroencephalographic findings are equally nonspecific and are similar to those present in other cases of space-occupying lesions. Angiography and pneumoencephalography permit detection of intracranial mass lesions. In the case of a brain abscess, angiography reveals displaced blood vessels and may demonstrate capsule vascularity. These studies are now considered obsolete.

Computed tomography (CT) has significantly improved our ability to diagnose and treat brain abscesses. CT permits accurate localization of the abscess, estimation of its evolutionary stage, and serial assessment of its size during the course of therapy. During the early cerebritis stage, CT demonstrates an ill-defined lesion of low density, consistent with necrosis and often associated with patchy peripheral contrast enhancement. Subsequently, a thin enhancing ring with a hypodense center develops. This ring becomes increasingly more defined, and surrounding edema develops. Primary or metastatic tumors, radiation necrosis, hematomas, and infarctions can have a similar computed tomographic appearance.

Magnetic resonance imaging (MRI) provides detailed imaging of abscess-related white matter changes and internal abscess structure. Posterior fossa and brain stem lesions are better visualized by MRI than by CT. Additionally, the greater sensitivity of MRI can demonstrate cerebritis and early abscesses undetectable by CT scan. T1-weighed MRI images reveal a central region of marked low intensity surrounded by a discrete ring that is isointense to mildly hyperintense. This is surrounded by a region of mild hypointensity. These regions correlate with the necrotic center, the abscess capsule, and surrounding brain edema. T2-weighted MRI images reveal a central region of iso- to hyperintensity and a discrete ring of hypointensity surrounded by a zone of hyperintensity.

Technetium Tc 99m brain scans are sensitive in detecting brain abscesses; however, CT and MRI provide superior localization and size determination. Similarly, Indium-111–labeled leukocyte scintography can identify or confirm a focus of inflammation but provides little additional information. These tests may be of adjunctive value in difficult cases.

A number of different intracranial processes must be considered in the differential diagnosis of brain abscesses, including malignant brain tumors, subdural and extradural empyemas, sinus thrombosis, meningitis, mycotic aneurysms, and encephalitis. The diagnosis of brain abscess is suggested, but not confirmed by the presence of an asymmetric capsule, multiple lesions, the location of the lesion or lesions at the corticomedullary junction, and associated leptomeningeal enhancement. Ultimately, aspiration and biopsy are often necessary for confirming the diagnosis of brain abscess. Using image-based stereotactic techniques, aspiration and biopsy of brain abscesses can be performed with a high degree of precision and with little morbidity.

As with all infectious diseases, the choice of antibiotic therapy for the treatment of brain abscess should be based on the results of culture and sensitivity testing. When direct culture results are pending or when they are impossible to obtain, empirical antibiotic therapy is based on the presumed pathogenesis of the brain abscess. Thus, abscesses resulting from sinusitis frequently contain streptococci and obligate anaerobes; therefore, agents effective against these bacteria should be chosen. Abscesses of otitic origin often contain mixed aerobic and anaerobic bacteria, whereas metastatic abscesses can involve a wide variety of organisms; thus, multiple broad-spectrum antibiotics are needed for empirical therapy. Post-traumatic brain abscesses usually involve *S. aureus,* requiring therapy with vancomycin or a semisynthetic penicillinase-resistant penicillin.

OUTCOME

Although the classic literature reports an overall mortality of 50 per cent, there has been a significant reduction in mortality with advances in the diagnosis and treatment of brain abscesses. In one series, the mortality rate fell from 41 per cent between 1970 and 1974 to 9 per cent between 1975 and 1980. Improvement in microbiologic isolation techniques, more effective antibiotics, and the advent of neuroimaging techniques such as CT and MRI have resulted in earlier diagnosis and more effective treatment at stages when patients are relatively well neurologically.

The most significant predictor of response to therapy is the neurologic condition of the patient on presentation. Those who are awake and alert tend to do well, whereas patients who are stuporous or in a coma at presentation have high mortality. Patients with slowly progressive symptoms typically do better than those with a rapidly deteriorating course. Abscesses of otitic origin or those from sinusitis tend to respond better than those of metastatic origin, presumably because the latter tend to be multiple and involve deep brain structures. Recurrence of brain abscesses occurs in 5 to 10 per cent of patients despite apparently adequate therapy. Reasons for recurrence can include the use of inappropriate or insufficient antibiotic therapy, the failure to aspirate or excise large abscesses, the presence of retained contaminated foreign bodies, and the failure to fully treat distant sites of infection. The long-term morbidity associated with successful therapy includes seizures, cognitive dysfunction, and focal neurologic deficits. Seizures occur in 30 to 50 per cent of patients, fully half of patients have permanent neurologic deficits, and 35 per cent have hemiparesis related to the parietal location of many abscesses.

SUMMARY

Brain abscess is an acute life-threatening illness. Early diagnosis and treatment has resulted in significant improvements in morbidity and mortality. Recent advances in diagnostic techniques and antibiotic therapy have reduced mortality rates from 40 to 60 per cent in the era before CT to 0 to 10 per cent now with the widespread availability of CT and MRI. Patients with neurologic complaints and symptoms consistent with brain abscess should undergo immediate CT or MRI with infusion. If a focus of cerebritis or abscess is suspected, stereotactic image-guided aspiration should be considered, especially for any abscess resulting in symptomatic mass effect or greater than 2.5 cm in diameter. Craniotomy with excision of the entire abscess or repeat aspiration may be necessary in some instances. Empirical antibiotic therapy should be initiated immediately and then modified based on culture results. Serial neuroimaging to assess response to therapy should be performed. Sequelae of brain abscess may include residual focal neurologic deficits and seizures. With early diagnosis and aggressive treatment, potential morbidity and mortality from brain abscesses can be significantly reduced.

ACUTE VIRAL ENCEPHALITIS AND MENINGITIS

By Suzanne Maxson, M.D.,
and Richard F. Jacobs, M.D.
Little Rock, Arkansas

Encephalitis and meningitis describe inflammations of the brain and the meninges, respectively. Viral encephalitis and meningitis are relatively common pediatric illnesses, but they are often diagnostic challenges because they are difficult to distinguish from other treatable forms of encephalitis and aseptic or bacterial meningitis. Timely diagnosis is important, because treatment differs according to the patient's age and the associated cerebrospinal fluid (CSF) findings. The prognosis for enteroviral meningitis, which is the most common cause of viral meningitis, is generally excellent, and complications are rare. However, some viral infections of the central nervous system (CNS), such as eastern equine encephalomyelitis virus, rabies, and herpes simplex encephalitis, can be devastating. The common and usually self-limiting causes of viral encephalitis and meningitis are discussed below.

VIRAL AGENTS

Herpes simplex virus, arboviruses, and lymphocytic choriomeningitis virus account for the largest number of cases of acute viral encephalitis. Although some arboviruses are more frequently encountered in certain geographic sections of the country (e.g., eastern equine encephalomyelitis virus in the Atlantic and Gulf states, California encephalitis virus in the upper Midwest states, and western equine encephalomyelitis virus in states west of the Mississippi River), most viruses that cause acute encephalitis and meningitis are distributed nationwide. Enteroviruses account for approximately 15 to 20 per cent of all proven cases of viral encephalitis. Encephalitis occurs in 0.1 to 0.2 per cent of patients who have varicella-C zoster virus infection. Mumps virus, measles virus, human immunodeficiency virus (HIV), rabies virus, adenoviruses, cytomegalovirus, and Epstein-Barr virus can also cause acute viral encephalitis.

Enteroviruses cause 85 per cent of the cases of viral meningitis. In the prevaccine era, mumps virus accounted for most cases of viral meningitis, and even today mumps virus is a common cause in the United Kingdom. Now that vaccines against mumps virus are available, the most common specific causes of viral meningitis in the United States are coxsackievirus B5 and echovirus types 4, 6, 9, and 11. A new variant of echovirus, type 30, is also associated with viral meningitis. Arboviruses account for about 5 per cent of all cases of aseptic meningitis in North America, with St. Louis encephalitis virus being the most common arboviral cause. Other agents account for the remaining 10 per cent of cases of viral meningitis. Adenoviruses have been implicated, and about 1 per cent of persons infected with the wild type of poliovirus contract meningitis. Central nervous system involvement has been associated with infection with rhinovirus, influenzavirus, parainfluenza virus, rotavirus, coronavirus, cytomegalovirus, Epstein-Barr virus, lymphocytic choriomeningitis virus, rabies virus, herpes simplex virus, and HIV. Among patients with HIV infection, a clinical picture consistent with aseptic meningitis occurs in 5 to 10 per cent, according to some retrospective adult studies.

DIAGNOSTIC APPROACH

The initial evaluation of patients with acute encephalitis or meningitis must exclude bacterial meningitis, herpes simplex virus encephalitis, varicella-zoster meningoencephalitis, tuberculous meningitis, fungal meningitis, and *Mycoplasma* meningoencephalitis. All these entities require specific therapy that must be given as early as possible to improve outcome. For most cases of viral encephalitis and viral meningitis, a specific etiology is never determined. However, specific viral agents should be sought with the use of appropriate cultures and other diagnostic tests, listed below. If a cause is found, the search for a diagnosis can end and prognostic information can then be given to the patient and family.

The diagnostic approach to acute viral encephalitis and meningitis begins with the exclusion of treatable causes, followed by the establishment of a specific diagnosis. Much of this process depends on the clinical presentation of the patient. Important historical aspects include contacts with sick persons, recent vaccinations, exposures, travel history, and recent use of medications. The physical examination is equally important, and special attention must be paid to CNS symptoms, rashes, tick or animal bites, and pharyngitis or conjunctivitis. Finally, other aids to establishing a definitive diagnosis encompass laboratory results, including CSF findings, culture results, and other tests, such as polymerase chain reaction (PCR), brain biopsy, electroencephalograms, and radiologic imaging studies.

CLINICAL PRESENTATION

Encephalitis is characterized by alterations in consciousness. Lethargy can be the initial finding, which then can progress to confusion, stupor, and coma. In addition to these changes in mental status, patients with viral encephalitis usually have signs and symptoms of meningeal inflammation, such as headache, fever, and nuchal rigidity. Focal neurologic signs usually develop, and seizure activity is common. Motor weakness, accentuated deep tendon reflexes, and extension plantar reflexes may be observed. If the spinal cord is involved, flaccid paralysis, depression of deep tendon reflexes, and paralysis of the bowel and bladder may occur. Increased intracranial pressure can cause papilledema and third and sixth cranial nerve palsies. When the hypothalamic-pituitary area is involved, severe hypothermia or poikilothermy, diabetes insipidus, and inappropriate antidiuretic hormone secretion may occur.

In herpes simplex encephalitis, the infection often localizes in the temporal lobe. Following a brief clinical influenzalike prodrome, bizarre behavior, hallucinations, and aphasia may ensue. Other signs include partial motor seizures, hemichorea, and acute cerebellar ataxia. Focal encephalitis can also be caused by certain enteroviruses, particularly group A coxsackieviruses. Rabies often begins with local paresthesia at the site of the initial animal bite. A history of an animal bite (e.g., a bat bite) or exposure to bat dung may be elicited, although most patients in the United States never give such a history. Acute contralateral hemiparesis may occur after herpes zoster ophthalmicus related to a localized cerebral angiitis, and lead to frontal lobe infarction. A parkinsonian syndrome is common in Japanese encephalitis. Rashes can be helpful clues to diagnosis in varicella or herpes zoster encephalitis. An exanthem is also occasionally seen in coxsackievirus and echovirus infections, and viral infection may be subacute in children. Adenoviral and enteroviral encephalitis can present as acute disease in immunologically healthy individuals and as subacute disease in immunologically compromised individuals. Prolonged enteroviral infection of the CNS can occur in patients with hypogammaglobulinemia. Although encephalitis is usually present in arboviral infections of the CNS, with both St. Louis and California encephalitis in children, the illness is usually benign and findings typical of encephalitis may be absent. However, with eastern equine encephalomyelitis virus infection, neurologic sequelae occur in 70 per cent of those who recover and include mental retardation, behavior changes, convulsive disorders, and paralysis. Seizures are more common in arboviral infections than in enteroviral infections of comparable severity.

Viral meningitis is most common in children between the ages of 1 and 10 years. Its duration is variable, and disability due to neurologic involvement usually lasts 1 to 2 weeks. Since most cases of viral meningitis are enteroviral, the incidence of the disease peaks in the summer and early fall. Enteroviruses are spread directly from person to person, with an incubation period of approximately 4 to 6 days. The clinical presentation of enteroviral infections is similar to that of other forms of viral meningitis, and children usually present with the acute onset of fever, headache, nausea, and vomiting. Occasionally, signs and symptoms are preceded by several days of a nonspecific acute febrile illness with general malaise and anorexia. Young children may be irritable and resist being handled. Older children may report myalgia, photophobia, and headache. Approximately 3 per cent of children ranging from newborns to 6 month olds have nuchal rigidity with aseptic meningitis, versus 79 per cent of patients older than 19 months. Convulsions are rare in patients who do not have a pre-existing seizure disorder. Other manifestations of enteroviral infections include pharyngitis, exanthem, pleurodynia, pericarditis, myocarditis, and conjunctivitis. Mumps is typically associated with salivary gland, gonadal, and pancreatic involvement.

Adenoviral infections tend to be more severe than enteroviral infections. Mumps and varicella-zoster virus infections are usually associated with encephalitis. Herpes simplex virus type 2 infections of the CNS can be devastating in infants, but in adults and adolescents with primary genital infections, a relatively benign aseptic meningitis syndrome is typical. Acute aseptic meningitis or encephalopathy may be the initial manifestation of primary HIV infection; it presents with fever, headache, and meningeal signs as well as cranial nerve involvement, most often involving the fifth, seventh, and eighth cranial nerves. Other treatable and nontreatable opportunistic infections must be excluded, including CNS cytomegalovirus, toxoplasmosis, and cryptococcosis even if infection with HIV is diagnosed.

LABORATORY FINDINGS

Peripheral white blood cell (WBC) counts are generally not helpful in the diagnosis of CNS infections because leukopenia, leukocytosis, or normal WBC counts may occur. Atypical lymphocytosis, however, is consistent with Epstein-Barr virus or cytomegalovirus infection, and mumps can be accompanied by increased serum amylase activity. Pulmonary infiltrates can be seen in lymphocytic choriomeningitis virus infection.

The most important diagnostic test is analysis of the CSF. Viral illnesses are typically associated with a mononuclear pleocytosis of 10 to 1000 WBCs/mm^3, and as many as 4000 WBCs/mm^3 have been reported. Infections of the CNS may also be associated with no pleocytosis or, even, an initial polymorphonuclear neutrophil leukocyte (PMN) predominance. However, lumbar punctures performed more than 24 hours after the onset of clinical illness in patients with enteroviral meningitis typically contain fewer than 50 per cent PMNs, and most of the cells are monocytes. With herpes simplex and arboviral meningoencephalitides, WBC counts can exceed 1000 WBCs/mm^3, and red blood cells are more commonly seen.

The CSF protein concentration is frequently increased, and in chronic infections an increased proportion of this protein is IgG. During convalescence, plasma cells may produce specific IgG within the CNS, as observed with mumps, herpes simplex, and varicella-zoster encephalitis. If antibody to a particular pathogen is seen at a comparable or higher concentration in CSF than in serum and the CSF protein is only moderately elevated, CNS infection with that agent is probable. The CSF glucose concentration is usually normal but may be decreased in 20 per cent of patients.

A CSF sample should be refrigerated and transported immediately to a viral diagnostic laboratory for viral culture and for detection of viral antigens. The common enteroviruses can be grown in viral culture of the CSF. Arboviruses and herpes simplex viruses are not usually recovered from older patients with encephalitis. Enteroviruses generally grow in 4 to 7 days from CSF, but more rapid diagnostic methods are being evaluated. A solid-phase reverse immunosorbent test (SPRIST) and an enzyme immunoassay (EIA) for the detection of enterovirus-specific IgM antibodies in the serum have been evaluated for use in the serologic diagnosis of enteroviral meningitis. These tests are not particularly sensitive or specific, and they are not widely available. The PCR has also been used in serum, CSF, and urine to diagnose enteroviral infection. Herpes simplex virus may be diagnosed with PCR in the CSF.

Serologic confirmation of infection with the use of IgM and IgG is available for La Crosse virus, California encephalitis virus, eastern and western equine encephalomyelitis viruses, mumps virus, lymphocytic choriomeningitis virus, St. Louis encephalitis virus, herpes simplex virus types 1 and 2, and measles virus. Complement fixation tests are available for adenovirus, influenzavirus types A and B, varicella-zoster virus, coxsackievirus types A and B, and echovirus. The clinician can save the serum drawn at initial presentation and compare it with that obtained 3 to 4 weeks later, looking for a fourfold rise in specific antibody titer. Serum is collected on presentation for all patients with aseptic meningitis or encephalitis. In this manner, the clinician can preserve information that may change with time, while avoiding expensive laboratory tests that may be unnecessary if another procedure in the initial evaluation yields a diagnosis.

Brain biopsy, the "gold standard" for diagnosis of encephalitis, is useful in cases where the patient presents with significant illness with no pathognomonic clinical signs. The specimen can be sent for histopathology, special stains such as fluorescent antibody studies, and cultures. The diagnosis of rabies virus encephalitis can be made from examination of a skin biopsy taken at the nape of the neck by direct fluorescent antibody technique.

Brain imaging with computed tomography (CT) or magnetic resonance imaging (MRI) is seldom diagnostic in cases of viral meningitis or encephalitis. However, in cases of herpes simplex infection, focal findings in the frontal or temporal lobes can aid in the diagnosis. These studies are also useful to detect brain abscesses or the basilar enhancement associated with tuberculous meningitis. The magnetic resonance imaging scan allows better visualization of the spinal cord, is a sensitive indicator of demyelination, and allows detection of the edematous changes that can be an early feature of encephalitis. The electroencephalogram is often diffusely abnormal in viral encephalitis. In herpes simplex virus infection, however, it commonly shows a focal abnormality with frequent localization to the frontal or temporal lobes.

DIFFERENTIAL DIAGNOSIS

Partially Treated Bacterial Meningitis

Anyone with CSF abnormalities who has received oral or parenteral antibiotics or has parameningeal infection (e.g., sinusitis or otitis media) should be evaluated for partially treated bacterial meningitis, which may be clinically indistinguishable from aseptic meningitis. In bacterial meningitis, the CSF typically shows a higher WBC count (400 to 100,000 WBCs/mm^3) with a high percentage of PMNs. The protein concentration is usually increased (up to 500 mg/dL), and the glucose concentration is usually low. Although Gram stain is often negative, the culture is positive in as many as 50 per cent of cases. Latex agglutination tests for selected bacterial antigens may also be positive, but the clinical utility of these tests is questionable. The sensitivity and specificity of these tests depend on the antigen and are as follows: *Neisseria meningitidis,* 83 and 100 per cent; *Streptococcus pneumoniae,* 66 and 100 per cent; *Haemophilus influenzae* type b, 89 and 99 per cent; and *Streptococcus agalactiae,* 100 and 100 per cent.

In patients with bacterial meningitis who have received an oral antibiotic, the CSF findings are not significantly different from those in untreated patients with bacterial meningitis. In a study comparing patients who had received oral antibiotics (from one dose to several days of treatment) before lumbar puncture with untreated patients, the culture and Gram stain of the CSF were negative in treated patients more often than in untreated patients, but the differences were not statistically significant. Patients who have been treated with parenteral ceftriaxone can still present with evidence of meningitis. In one study, lumbar puncture was performed before and then 4 to 12 hours after ceftriaxone was given; 43 per cent of the second set of cultures were still positive. In other studies, lumbar puncture was done before and then 24 hours after ceftriaxone administration; 98 to 100 per cent of the cultures and 65 to 95 per cent of the Gram stains of the CSF from the second lumbar puncture were negative. The WBC count, percentage of PMNs, and protein and glucose concentrations were unchanged between the initial and the second lumbar punctures regardless of whether the patient had received oral or parenteral antibiotics.

Tuberculous Meningitis

Typically, tuberculous meningitis occurs 3 to 6 months after the primary infection and is found most commonly in children younger than 4 years of age. Because the pathologic features take several months to develop, the disorder is very uncommon in infants younger than the age of 4 months. Although the onset may be abrupt or insidious, tuberculous meningitis typically has three clinical stages. The first stage is characterized by fever, headache, malaise, irritability, and drowsiness and can last 1 to 2 weeks. The second stage, which usually begins abruptly, is characterized by true meningeal signs, such as nuchal rigidity, convulsions, increased deep tendon reflexes, hypertonia, vomiting, and cranial nerve palsies. The brain stem usually is the site of greatest involvement, with the third, sixth, and seventh cranial nerves being affected most often. Patients show varying degrees of symptoms compatible with encephalitis. The second stage correlates physiologically with the development of hydrocephalus, increased intracranial pressure, and meningeal irritation. The final stage is associated with coma, irregular pulse and respirations, high fever, and eventually death.

The CSF findings in tuberculous meningitis can be similar to those in aseptic meningitis. The WBC count is usually 100 to 1000 WBCs/mm^3, with a lymphocyte predominance. The protein concentration can be normal or markedly increased (more than 400 mg/dL) owing to hydrocephalus and static CSF. Although the glucose can be normal in 10 per cent of patients, the index of suspicion for tuberculous meningitis should be high when the blood glucose–to–CSF ratio is greater than 2:1. Other critical indicators for diagnosis include a history of exposure; a positive tuberculin skin test—although a negative PPD (purified protein derivative) is never exclusive—an abnormal chest radiograph; and a positive stain or culture of CSF, gastric aspirate, or urine. Polymerase chain reaction for *Mycobacterium tuberculosis* in the CSF is also available. Computed tomography scan with contrast enhancement may reveal basilar enhancement.

Fungal Infections

Cryptococcus neoformans, Blastomyces dermatitidis, Coccidioides immitis, Histoplasma capsulatum, and numerous other pathogens can cause infection in immunocompromised patients. The clinical findings in fungal infections are similar to those in tuberculous meningitis, and the CSF findings are very similar to those in viral meningitis. India ink stain or cryptococcal antigen quantitation can be helpful in diagnosing cryptococcal infection. Specific fungal stains may also be useful. Serum fungal titers can be helpful in infections due to *Coccidioides immitis* and *Cryptococcus neoformans* but are less helpful in infection due to *B. dermatitidis* or *H. capsulatum*. Positive cultures provide the definitive diagnosis. A chest film may reveal concurrent pulmonary infection. Skin lesions typical of blastomycosis or coccidioidomycosis or oral lesions characteristic of histoplasmosis can also provide clues to diagnosis. In patients with HIV infection and symptoms consistent with meningitis, the diagnosis of *C. neoformans* infection should be vigorously sought because it is common in this group of immunocompromised patients.

Mycoplasma Pneumoniae Infection

Involvement of the CNS can be seen in as many as 7 per cent of patients admitted to the hospital with *M. pneumoniae* infection. This statistic probably represents a skewed sample, and the percentage is probably an overestimation of the true incidence. However, this treatable infection can cause significant morbidity and mortality. This infection is unique in that it follows a respiratory illness by a few days to 3 weeks. Presumptive diagnosis can be made when tests for serum cold agglutinins and *Mycoplasma* antibodies are positive. Culture of *M. pneumoniae* from CSF requires a reference laboratory and is usually not done.

Vaccine and Drug Use

Although uncommon, aseptic meningitis resulting from the use of certain vaccines is well documented in children. The measles-mumps-rubella vaccine and mumps vaccine cause aseptic meningitis that is clinically similar to mumps meningitis in about 1 in 10,000 to 1 in 65,000 persons vaccinated. The onset of the inflammation occurs between 11 and 32 days after the administration of the vaccine. Mumps virus has been cultured from the CSF in these patients. Oral polio vaccine has been reported to cause aseptic meningitis in two children with ventriculoperitoneal shunts, with the infection being confirmed by positive CSF cultures for the vaccine strain of poliovirus. Aseptic meningitis can be caused by therapy with numerous drugs (Table 1).

Systemic Disease

Involvement of the CNS has been reported in conjunction with several systemic diseases. In one pediatric series, systemic lupus erythematosus produced neurologic signs and symptoms in 22 (44 per cent) of 50 patients. Sarcoidosis, Kawasaki disease, and Behçet's disease may cause a clinical picture consistent with aseptic meningitis. Migraine headaches can also cause a cellular reaction in the CSF.

Malignant Disease

Among children with acute leukemia, 5 per cent have CNS disease at presentation. Headache, nausea, vomiting, lethargy, irritability, nuchal rigidity, and aseptic meningitis

Table 1. Differential Diagnosis in Viral Meningitis

Bacterial Infections	**Systemic Diseases**
Partially treated bacterial meningitis	Kawasaki disease
Tuberculosis	Migraine headache
Lyme disease	Systemic lupus erythematosus
Leptospirosis	Sarcoidosis
Neurobrucellosis	Behçet's disease
Syphilis	**Use of Certain Vaccines**
Ehrlichia chaffeensis infection	Mumps-measles-rubella
Mycoplasma pneumoniae infection	Mumps
Rickettsia rickettsii infection	Polio
Fungal Infections	**Use of Certain Drugs**
Cryptococcus neoformans	Azathioprine
Coccidioides immitis	Ibuprofen
Histoplasma capsulatum	Intravenous immune globulin
Blastomyces dermatitidis	Isoniazid
Malignant Diseases	Muromonab-CD3
Leukemia	Sulfamethizole
Lymphoma	Trimethoprim-sulfamethoxazole
Parasitic Infections	Carbamazepine
Angiostrongylus cantonensis infection	Phenazopyridine
Cysticercosis	Cytarabine
Toxoplasmosis	Sulindac
	Tolmetin sodium
	Naproxen

may be part of the presentation of acute leukemia. The CSF specimens must be examined carefully for malignant cells with special Wright-stained smears of the sediment for blastocytes. Rarely, a primary CNS lymphoma can present in the same manner. The complete differential diagnosis of viral meningitis is presented in Table 1.

POLIOMYELITIS

By Stephen J. Ryan, M.D.,
and Kevin R. Nelson, M.D.
Lexington, Kentucky

Poliomyelitis is an acute infection of the anterior horns of the spinal cord, the medulla, and to a lesser extent the posterior horn, posterior ganglion, midbrain, cerebellum, basal ganglia, and cerebral cortex. The infectious agent is a single-stranded RNA enterovirus of the picornavirus group with three serotypes (polioviruses 1, 2, and 3).

PRESENTING SIGNS AND SYMPTOMS

Infection occurs by the fecal-oral route in wild-type infection, with symptoms appearing after a 1- to 5-day incubation period. Poliovirus is an extremely effective contagion, infecting nearly 100 per cent of susceptible (nonimmune) individuals who come in contact with an infected person. Ninety to 95 per cent of infections are asymptomatic, and 4 to 8 per cent of patients experience a nonspecific viral syndrome (referred to as the minor illness), which consists of malaise, myalgia, and low-grade fever lasting only a few days.

Only 1 to 2 per cent of patients experience the major illness—viral meningitis that sometimes ends with lower motor neuron (anterior horn cell) injury or paralytic polio (see further on).

The last case of indigenous wild-type poliomyelitis in the United States occurred in 1979. However, 30 cases of vaccine-associated paralytic polio (VAPP) occurred in recipients of the trivalent oral polio vaccine (TOPV) from 1980 to 1989. Thirty-two cases were found in household contacts of vaccine recipients, and four cases in community contacts. Immigrants accounted for five cases. Fourteen cases of VAPP occurred in immunocompromised individuals (most with hypogammaglobulinemia) who received TOPV. Intramuscular injections within 30 days of receiving TOPV increases the risk of VAPP, and such injections should be avoided during that time.

For all three doses of TOPV currently recommended, the risk of VAPP is approximately 1 in 2.5 million doses. However, 76 per cent of cases (in recipients or contacts) of VAPP are associated with the first dose, increasing the first-dose risk to 1 in 700,000 doses. In vaccine recipients, paralysis begins 4 to 30 days after inoculation. Community contacts experience VAPP 4 to 60 days after vaccination of recipients.

MENINGITIS AND PARALYTIC POLIOMYELITIS

Lower motor neuron (anterior horn cell) injury occurs in only 1 in 2000 susceptible individuals exposed to wild poliovirus. Infants rarely experience paralysis, but 1 in 1000 children suffer paralytic poliomyelitis (PP), as do 1 in 75 adults.

Seven to 14 days after the initial exposure, patients experience fever, headache, and stiff neck with backache as a consequence of viral meningitis. These symptoms resolve in a few days in about 50 per cent of patients. In the other half of patients, paralysis occurs in one or more limbs over hours to days, starting 2 to 5 days after the onset of meningismus. This is frequently accompanied by tingling, myalgias, and shooting pains. Weakness occurs more commonly in the legs than in the arms. Only 10 per cent of patients have clinically evident brain stem lower motor neuron involvement, with dysphagia, respiratory weakness (hypoventilation), or facial drooping. Neurons to the tongue and chewing muscles can occasionally be affected. Oculomotor involvement is rare but can lead to transient external ophthalmoplegia and nystagmus.

Dysautonomia (mainly from involvement of the brain stem reticular formation) occurs occasionally and can produce cardiovascular instability (arrhythmias, labile blood pressure and heart rate) as well as impaired bladder and bowel function.

Ten per cent of patients die in the acute phase of PP, with higher mortality in adolescents and adults. These deaths are most often from aspiration or respiratory compromise. Among survivors of PP, about half regain full function of the limbs, and the other half are left with residual weakness of varying degrees. Motor improvement occurs within weeks, and 80 per cent of recovery is complete by 6 months. Further improvement may take place over the next 2 to 3 years, with little or no improvement thereafter.

PHYSICAL EXAMINATION

In the early stage of the major illness, the patient appears ill and is often tremulous and agitated. Signs of meningismus may appear, including nuchal rigidity, Brudzinski's sign (flexion of the neck causing flexion of the hips), and Kernig's sign (pain on extension of the knee with a flexed hip).

In paralytic poliomyelitis, these signs are followed by flaccid weakness in one or more limbs, which is often asymmetrical. The weakness is frequently more proximal than distal. The muscles are tender and sometimes stiff. A muscle under strenuous use during the early stage of the illness is at risk for greater weakness. Hyporeflexia or areflexia is found in the affected limbs. There may be facial drooping or bulbar weakness, indicating brain stem involvement. Early hyperreflexia occurs in 20 per cent of patients with PP, with an extensor plantar sign in 6 per cent of these individuals. This hyperreflexia may persist throughout recovery. Atrophy of the affected muscles begins 1 to 2 weeks after paralysis and is accompanied by fasciculations.

When the diagnosis of PP is suspected, information on the vaccination history (including lot number if available) of patients and close contacts must be obtained. Suspected cases are reported to the state Board of Health and the Centers for Disease Control and Prevention. Vaccine-related cases are also reported to the Food and Drug Administration.

LABORATORY STUDIES

Routine blood counts and chemistry panels are unhelpful. Lumbar puncture reveals normal pressure (<200 mm

H_2O) in two thirds of patients with the major illness and is only slightly increased (200 to 300 mm H_2O) in the remaining one third of patients. Examination of spinal fluid in the meningeal period prior to paralysis typically reveals pleocytosis (10 to 300 cells/mm^3) with an average of 185 cells/mm^3. The average count falls to 50 cells/mm^3 1 week after the onset of paralysis and to 5 cells/mm^3 after 1 month. Neutrophils predominate during the first 5 days in 20 per cent of patients, but lymphocyte predominance is the rule in most cases. Protein concentrations are normal or slightly increased in the preparalytic stage and rise for 2 to 3 weeks after the onset of PP to an average peak of 164 mg/dL. By the second month, the protein concentration returns to normal in most patients. Red blood cells are not seen, and glucose concentrations are normal. Poliovirus is rarely cultured from cerebrospinal fluid. CSF is usually normal in the minor illness.

Poliovirus can be cultured from nasopharyngeal swabs and rectal swabs for the first week of the acute illness, and it can be cultured from the stool of 90 per cent of patients by 10 days. A rising antibody titer to poliovirus may be helpful in establishing the diagnosis. The titers should be obtained in the acute phase of illness and 3 to 4 weeks later (when titers peak). Nasopharyngeal swabs and rectal swabs can be cultured in contacts at risk. All positive viral isolates are submitted to a reference laboratory (e.g., Centers for Disease Control and Prevention or the state board of health) for serotyping and genotyping (especially in suspected vaccine-related cases).

Nerve conduction studies are usually normal in the first few days of paralysis and then show a gradual decrease of the compound motor action potential amplitude characteristic of motor axonal loss. Electromyography can show decreased motor units after the onset of PP, with spontaneous fibrillations appearing 2 to 3 weeks after the onset of paralysis. Reinnervation can be demonstrated in most cases after several weeks and remains evident throughout life. Sensory studies remain essentially unaffected.

DIFFERENTIAL DIAGNOSIS

Other entities that may cause or mimic acute lower motor neuron paralysis include acute inflammatory demyelinating polyradiculoneuropathy (Guillain-Barré syndrome), acute transverse myelitis, botulism, myasthenia gravis, arsenic poisoning, and tic paralysis. Coxsackievirus and echovirus have been reported rarely to cause a similar viral meningoencephalomyelitis with lower motor neuron injury.

COMPLICATIONS OF PARALYSIS

The paralyzed patient is susceptible to contractures, decubitus ulcers, stress ulcers, aspiration, constipation, urinary tract infections, and pneumonia. Respiratory involvement may require ventilator support temporarily (hours to months). Permanent respiratory compromise is exceptional.

POSTPOLIO SYNDROME

Postpolio syndrome (PPS; also known as delayed polio weakness or postpoliomyelitis progressive muscular atrophy) is now the most common late complication affecting survivors of previous poliomyelitis epidemics in the United States. PPS refers to the onset of new complaints of weakness in PP patients decades after the acute phase of the illness. The defining feature is new weakness in a previously recovered muscle, which typically presents as new *focal* weakness given the typical pattern of strength recovery in PP. The cause is unknown.

The new complaints usually occur two to four decades after the acute phase of illness (8 to 71 years, average 35 years). The rate of prevalence is difficult to determine because the diagnosis of PPS is based on the exclusion of other medical problems in an aging population. Various studies suggest that PPS affects 16 to 66 per cent of patients with PP. Risk factors for the development of PPS include (1) four-limb involvement in the acute phase of PP, (2) required hospitalization or ventilator support, and (3) age greater than 10 years at the time of onset of PP.

The new complaints consist of fatigability, weakness, myalgia, cramps, atrophy, joint pain, and back pain. The problems are generally limited to previously affected muscles, and the course is one of insidious onset and slow progression. The progressive weakness can lead to decreased mobility and ambulation as well as a decreased ability to climb stairs.

Although a neuromuscular mechanism is currently suspected, the problems may be exacerbated by arthritis in previously weakened and overtaxed limbs, progressive contractures, radiculopathy, compressive mononeuropathies (e.g., carpal tunnel syndrome), depression, and other general medical problems. In previously weakened limbs, joints have been at a mechanical disadvantage, and additional burdens have been placed on the unaffected limbs and the spine through compensatory overuse and abnormal postures.

Progressive respiratory problems may rarely lead to hypoventilation or sleep apnea. Patients with scoliosis, pulmonary disease, and cardiac disease are at increased risk for respiratory compromise, especially at night. In one uncontrolled series, 31 of 32 patients with PPS had swallowing abnormalities on video fluoroscopic evaluation. Only 14 patients complained of dysphagia and, interestingly, only 12 had dysphagia during the acute phase of PP.

No pathognomonic physical findings have been identified in PPS, but documented worsening muscular atrophy is strongly suggestive. The diagnosis is made by a history of new focal weakness and exclusion of other medical problems. The typical sequelae of long-standing PP (muscular atrophy, contractures, fasciculations, and rarely hyporeflexia and extensor plantar signs) are seen but constitute old findings. Serum creatine kinase activity can be mildly increased. Nerve conduction studies, electromyography, and muscle biopsy are not diagnostic but can be helpful if other illnesses, such as radiculopathy, are suspected. A sensitive measure of reinnervation is fiber density on single-fiber electromyography (SFEMG). This may be of value in establishing the diagnosis of PP in a patient with little residual weakness. PPS is a diagnosis of exclusion, and other diagnoses such as degenerative joint disease, depression, and compressive neuropathies should be considered.

RABIES

By Georgina Groleau, M.D.,
and Jeanne O'Connell, M.D.
Baltimore, Maryland

DEFINITION

Rabies is an acute encephalomyelitis caused by a neurotropic, bullet-shaped, enveloped, single-stranded RNA virus of the Rhabdoviridae family. The genome of this virus encodes five structural proteins—three associated with the genomic RNA and two associated with the bilayered envelope. It is the knoblike structures of the glycoprotein of the outer envelope that confer neurotropic properties by enabling the virus to bind to acetylcholine receptors.

The World Health Organization estimates that 50,000 people die of rabies every year. Most of these deaths occur in India and Asia. By contrast, the incidence of rabies in the United States remains low because of animal control and canine vaccination programs initiated during the 1950s and advances in human prophylaxis before and after exposure. To date, only three human survivors of rabies have been documented worldwide. With or without intensive medical support, the patient with rabies usually dies. Thus, emphasis is on prevention through immunization.

EPIDEMIOLOGY

Although rabies is rare in humans, exposure to the virus is a real threat because rabies is common in certain wild and domestic animals. The major reservoir worldwide is the dog. In countries with animal vaccination and control programs and modern postexposure prophylaxis, the reservoir has shifted from dogs to wild animals. In the United States, in 1993, there were 9498 cases of documented rabies reported by the Centers for Disease Control and Prevention. Only three were human infections. Racoons were the major wildlife reservoir (62 per cent), followed by skunks (17.3 per cent), bats (8 per cent), foxes (3.8 per cent), and other wild animals, rodents, and lagomorphs (2.3 per cent). Rabid skunks and bats can be found throughout the United States. In the south Atlantic, mid-Atlantic, and northeastern states, the racoon rabies epizootic has spread at alarming rates. From 1992 to 1993, the number of reported cases of rabies in racoons increased 37.1 per cent.

In the United States, infection of domestic animals usually results from exposure to rabid wild animals in areas where the disease is epizootic. In 1993, there were 606 cases of laboratory proven rabies in domestic animals, including dogs, cats, cattle, swine, sheep, and goats. Rabid cats outnumbered rabid dogs in the United States, continuing a 5-year trend. Human rabies tends to occur in areas where rabies is epizootic or enzootic in wild animals and the population of unimmunized domestic animals is high. Therefore, pet immunization of both dogs and cats against rabies can minimize the risk of exposure.

TRANSMISSION

Rabies is nearly always transmitted by animal bites or other actions that disrupt the integument, allowing introduction of infected secretions. Rabies will develop in 25 to 50 per cent of individuals who are not treated following a bite by a proven rabid animal. Head and neck insults and young age increase the risk of infection. For those in whom rabies does not develop, current hypotheses suggest that the infection is aborted by neutralizing antibodies, killer lymphocytes, and interferon.

Other forms of transmission are far less common. Aerosolized transmission has been reported in laboratory personnel and in spelunkers in bat-infested caves. There are also six reports worldwide of transmission from corneal transplants; these are the only known examples of human-to-human transmission of rabies. Transmission of virus to contacts of patients with rabies has not yet been documented.

The proportion of rabies patients lacking a history of definitive animal bite or other exposure has increased in the United States over the past 30 years. Therefore, rabies should be included in the differential diagnosis of any patient with a rapidly progressive encephalitis or myelitis.

PATHOPHYSIOLOGY

The rabies virus enters peripheral nerves and travels by retrograde axoplasmic transport to the central nervous system. Centrifugal neural spread is responsible for viral introduction into highly innervated extraneural sites. Thus the virus enters the retina, cornea, skin, adrenal medulla, kidney, lung, liver, skeletal muscle, intestine, olfactory epithelium and, most importantly, the salivary glands. This ensures the presence of infective virus in urine, feces, and saliva.

The incubation period varies from a few days to many years. The length of incubation depends on the site of inoculation, the size of the inoculum, the age of the patient, and the host defense mechanisms. Incubations associated with head and neck bites are often shorter in duration, especially in children. The average incubation for face bites is 5 weeks compared with 8 weeks for limb bites.

CLINICAL PRESENTATION

Two distinct clinical presentations of rabies exist. The classic furious form accounts for 80 per cent of cases, and the paralytic form accounts for 20 per cent of all patients with rabies.

The clinical course of classic rabies can be divided into three phases. The nonspecific prodromal phase lasts 2 to 10 days and probably represents the initial central nervous system infection. Typical nonspecific symptoms include malaise, myalgia, sore throat, anorexia, nausea, vomiting, and fever. Symptoms more specific for rabies include pain, paresthesias, and/or intense pruritus at the site of the inoculation, which is probably due to multiplication of the virus in the dorsal root ganglion of the sensory nerves at the site of inoculation. The acute neurologic phase, or encephalitic phase, is heralded by periods of anxiousness, agitation, excessive motor activity, and emotional lability. Episodes of dysphagia and hydrophobia occur. Lucid periods alternate with periods of extreme aggression. The final clinical phase of rabies, or the depressive phase, is complicated by dysrhythmias, autonomic motor system dysfunction, and coma. Autonomic dysfunction includes extremes of blood pressure, lacrimation, and salivation. Weakness, progressive paralysis, and hyporeflexia or areflexia indicate upper motor neuron dysfunction. The mechanism of death in most patients with rabies is attributed to respiratory center dysfunction and apnea.

The prominence of brain stem dysfunction distinguishes rabies from other viral encephalopathies. Hydrophobia, which is pathognomonic of rabies, involves painful, violent, involuntary spasms of the diaphragm and respiratory, pharyngeal, and laryngeal muscles initiated by swallowing of liquids. Opisthotonus, facial grimacing, and seizures may be seen. The patient experiences terror during these episodes. Hydrophobia occurs in approximately half of classic rabies cases. Episodes similar to hydrophobia can be triggered in some patients following sounds (phonophobia) or drafts of air across the face (aerophobia).

A patient with the paralytic form of rabies may present with a prodrome similar to that of classic rabies. Pain and paresthesias occur at the site of inoculation. The clinical course, however, differs. In paralytic rabies, the patient has an ascending paralysis that is symmetric or asymmetrical. The diagnosis of paralytic rabies is challenging because hydrophobia does not occur and many features of the illness resemble the Guillain-Barré syndrome.

DIAGNOSIS AND TREATMENT

The diagnosis of rabies is difficult because the initial manifestations are nonspecific. Furthermore, the patient may present with hallucinations and other features of psychosis. Fewer than 15 per cent of patients with rabies are diagnosed correctly on the first visit to a physician, and less than a third are correctly diagnosed at the time of hospital admission. A history of rabies exposure and/or the recognition of hydrophobia increases the likelihood of diagnosis before death. More than 20 per cent of rabies victims are first recognized after death. Isolation of virus or the detection of rabies antigen or antibody allows a definitive diagnosis. For diagnosis before death, the Centers for Disease Control and Prevention requires cerebrospinal fluid (CSF) and saliva for isolation of the virus, serum and CSF for rabies antibody titers, and skin biopsy of the highly innervated, hair-covered area of the neck for detection of rabies antigen using rabies fluorescent antibody (RFA). Although rabies virus may be isolated during the first 2 weeks of illness, most laboratories require 3 weeks for confirmation. If virologic test results are negative, the diagnosis of rabies is not excluded. The significance of serum antibodies to the virus depends on the status of rabies immunizations. Any detectable titer is significant in the unvaccinated patient. For patients with prior vaccination, the detection of rabies antibodies in the CSF indicates acute rabies infection. The results of RFA testing of neck skin are positive in approximately 50 per cent of patients with rabies. RFA testing of brain tissue, or mouse inoculation techniques, will confirm the diagnosis of rabies post mortem. Negri bodies are not detected post mortem in up to 20 per cent of proven cases of rabies.

After rabies has occurred, there is no cure. Despite intensive medical care, the patient usually dies. Therefore, early diagnosis benefits primarily the contacts of the victim by decreasing their exposure to the virus.

RABIES PROPHYLAXIS

In the absence of a cure for rabies, prevention must be emphasized. Pre-exposure immunization is indicated for those at high risk of exposure (e.g., rabies research laboratory personnel, veterinarians, spelunkers, animal control personnel in rabies epizootic areas, and travelers visiting rabies-endemic countries for more than 1 month). Three doses (1 mL) of human diploid cell vaccine (HDCV) are administered intramuscularly or intradermally on days 0, 7, and 28, with boosters every 6 months to 2 years. When intradermal vaccine is administered to travelers concurrently with chloroquine, the antibody response to rabies may be inhibited, leaving the patient unprotected.

For after exposure (Table 1), consider the type of exposure, the species of animal, the circumstances of the incident, and the immunization status of the patient. First, determine whether exposure involved a bite with actual penetration of the skin by animal teeth. Nonbite exposures include the contamination of abrasions, scratches, or mucosal surfaces with saliva containing the rabies virus and, rarely, exposure to aerosols in laboratories or bat-infested caves. If the exposure involves a wild animal, it should be regarded as rabid. Prophylaxis must be started immediately after exposure, with interruption of therapy only if laboratory testing indicates that the animal is not rabid. If the patient has been in contact with an apparently healthy domestic animal that is available for 10 days of observation, rabies prophylaxis is not indicated unless rabies develops in the animal. By contrast, if the domestic animal appears ill or rabid, initiate prophylaxis immediately. If the domestic animal is sacrificed and laboratory tests indicate the absence of infection, antirabies therapy can be discontinued. If exposure involves an unknown or escaped domestic animal or livestock animals, contact the local health department for information on rabies prevalence in the area. For all species of animals, an unprovoked attack is associated with a higher risk of rabies than is a provoked attack. When an apparently healthy animal bites during feeding or handling, most authorities view the event as a provoked attack.

Prophylaxis following exposure includes proper wound care, passive immunization with human rabies immune globulin (HRIG), and active immunization with the human diploid cell vaccine (HDCV). For the best outcome, begin prophylaxis within 72 hours of the exposure. Irrigate the wound with a soapy (viricidal) solution. Passively immunize with 20 IU/kg of HRIG. Whenever possible, administer one half of the dose intramuscularly and one half directly into the wound. Initiate the HDCV series on the first visit as well. Give 1 mL of HDCV intramuscularly, with subsequent doses on days 3, 7, 14, and 28. The recommended site for intramuscular injection of HDCV is the deltoid muscle in adults and the anterolateral upper thigh in children. HDCV should not be injected in the gluteal region. If the patient has received HDCV but not HRIG, and 8 days have passed, passive immunization is no longer indi-

Table 1. Rabies Prophylaxis Following Exposure

Proper wound care
Passive immunization
Human rabies immune globulin (HRIG)
Total 20 IU/kg
one-half intramuscularly
one-half into wound if possible
HRIG not needed if immunization has taken place before exposure
Active immunization
Human diploid cell vaccine (HDCV)
1 mL intramuscularly on days 0, 3, 7, 14, and 28
1 mL intramuscularly on days 0 and 3 if immunization before exposure has taken place

cated because active immunization should protect. For patients who have undergone immunization before exposure, administer two intramuscular doses (1 mL) of HDCV on day 0 and day 3. Rabies prophylaxis is not contraindicated or modified in pregnant or immunocompromised patients.

The side effects of rabies prophylaxis are typically mild. After HDCV therapy, pain, erythema, swelling, and pruritus at the injection site occur in approximately 25 per cent of patients. Fewer than 20 per cent of patients experience headache, dizziness, myalgias, and/or abdominal discomfort. Urticaria, arthritis, fever, vomiting, and/or anaphylaxis are rarely seen. Two cases of Guillian-Barré syndrome have been attributed to HDCV therapy. The side effects of HRIG are also mild; local pain and fever are most frequently noted. HRIG administration has been associated rarely with anaphylaxis. Rabies prophylaxis should not be discontinued for mild side effects.

PEARLS AND PITFALLS

Failure of rabies prophylaxis has not been reported in the United States when current recommendations for prophylaxis following exposure have been followed. Occasional cases of failure of rabies prophylaxis have been linked to the omission of passive immunization. Other cases have been associated with treatment administered more than 72 hours after exposure. Patients have developed rabies when the recommended dosing schedule of HDCV was not followed. Also, rabies may develop in immunized patients who are not given additional HDCV therapy after an exposure event.

If evaluating the patient presenting with rabies, remember that the diagnosis is often elusive initially during the prodrome. For any patient with rapidly progressing encephalomyelitis, consider rabies in the differential diagnosis (Table 2).

Table 2. Differential Diagnosis of Rabies

Classic Rabies
Other causes of viral encephalitis
Herpes simplex
St. Louis encephalitis
Eastern equine encephalitis
Venezuelan equine encephalitis
La Crosse viruses
Tetanus
Toxic encephalopathies
Psychiatric disorders
Paralytic Rabies
Guillian-Barré syndrome
Poliomyelitis
Neuroparalytic reactions following vaccination
Simian herpes virus encephalitis

TETANUS

By J. Brad Lichtenhan, M.D.
Paola, Kansas
and Rick Kellerman, M.D.
Salina, Kansas

Tetanus is a severe, acute poisoning caused by the potent neurotoxin tetanospasmin. Produced by the bacterium *Clostridium tetani,* tetanospasmin is considered one of the world's most toxic substances. This agent acts on the nervous system, blocking the release of inhibitory neurotransmitters. The result is unrestrained reflex excitability of the voluntary muscles and the autonomic nervous system.

ETIOLOGY

Clostridium tetani is a spore-forming, gram-positive obligate anaerobe. The sporulated form has a characteristic drumstick or tennis racket shape with a terminal spore. The spores are highly resistant to destruction and are found nearly everywhere, particularly in warm, cultivated soils that are rich in animal manure. The spores can also be recovered from house dust, operating rooms, clothing, splinters, thorns, rusty nails, and contaminated needles used by intravenous drug abusers.

Tetanus is a common and deadly disease in Third World countries, causing more than 500,000 deaths per year. Neonates are the most common victims, becoming infected because of unsanitary care of the umbilical cord after being born to unimmunized mothers. In the United States and other developed countries, there are few cases of neonatal tetanus; instead, tetanus has become a disease of the elderly (Fig. 1), occurring in unimmunized or inadequately immunized individuals.

Completion of a primary vaccination series is essentially 100 per cent protective. A previous history of adequate immunization practically eliminates tetanus from the differential diagnosis (Tables 1 and 2), and the adequate immunization of pregnant women prevents neonatal tetanus as well. Tetanus is not a self-immunizing disease; a person with a previous history of tetanus can get it again.

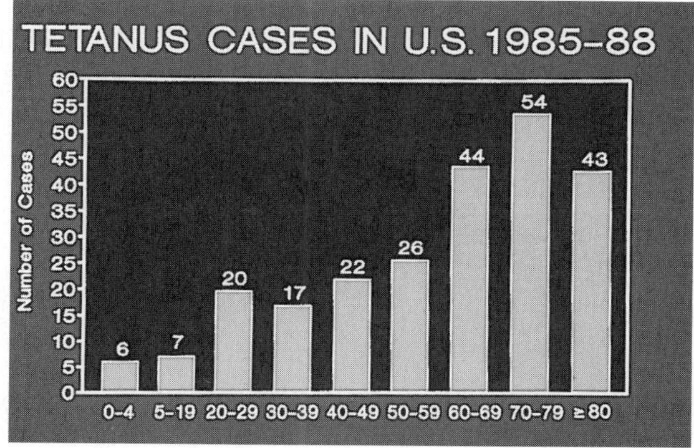

Figure 1. Age distribution of persons who contracted tetanus in the United States from 1985 to 1988. (Adapted from Centers for Disease Control and Prevention. Tetanus: United States, 1985–86. MMWR 36[29]:477–481, 1987; and Centers for Disease Control. Tetanus: United States, 1987–88. MMWR 39[3]:37–41, 1990.)

Table 1. Routine Diphtheria and Tetanus Vaccination Schedule for Persons Aged 7 Years and Older*

Dose	Interval
Primary 1	First dose
Primary 2	4–8 wk after first dose*
Primary 3	6–12 mo after second dose†
Booster	10 yr after third dose; then every 10 yr

*Diphtheria and tetanus toxoid, adult formulation (Td) is product used.
†Prolonging the interval does not require restarting series.
Adapted from Immunization Practices Advisory Committee (ACIP). Update on adult immunizations. MMWR 40(RR-12):16–19, 1991.

PATHOGENESIS

The tetanus spores are introduced into tissue through major trauma, chronic wounds, or mild inapparent skin injuries. Classic tetanus-prone wounds include deep punctures, crush injuries, burns, frostbite, and chronic decubitus. These wounds often contain devitalized tissue and contaminants, such as foreign bodies, animal feces, and soil. Also, any wound in an inadequately immunized person should be considered prone to tetanus. Approximately 20 per cent of individuals who contract tetanus have no obvious wound source by history or physical examination.

The time between wound occurrence and the first clinical manifestations of tetanus is called the incubation period. This varies from 0 to 60 days, but more severe disease is associated with incubation periods of less than 7 days. The period of onset is the length of time between the first symptoms and the first generalized muscle spasms and ranges from a few hours to several days. Again, the shorter this period, the more severe the illness. Longer incubation periods are usually associated with sites of injury rather distant from the spinal cord and brain stem, whereas central nervous system (CNS) and head wounds produce symptoms after a short interval.

Four types of tetanus are recognized. Local tetanus is a form of the illness most often related to an extremity wound, with muscle spasms restricted to that extremity. This is a rare, usually mild form of tetanus, but in its most severe form, very painful spasms occur in the muscle groups around the wound. These symptoms may persist for months and occasionally progress to generalized tetanus.

Cephalic tetanus is also uncommon. This form of local tetanus is associated with head injuries. In Third World countries, it is often associated with chronic otitis media. Manifestations include dysfunction of multiple cranial nerves and frequent progression to generalized tetanus. The prognosis for cephalic tetanus is usually poor.

Table 2. Centers for Disease Control Statistics 1985–1988

Reported Immunization Status (No. of Doses)	No.	Percentage
0	60	25
1	21	13
2	9	
3	6	5
≥4	8	
Unknown	135	57
TOTAL	239	100

Data from Centers for Disease Control and Prevention. Tetanus: United States, 1985–1986. MMWR 36(29):477–481, 1987; and Centers for Disease Control. Tetanus: United States, 1987–88. MMWR 39(3):37–41, 1990.

Neonatal tetanus is the most common form of the disease in Third World countries. It most often presents with poor sucking and excessive crying and rapidly progresses to varying degrees of trismus, dysphagia, and generalized tetanus. In the absence of aggressive medical intervention, death of the neonate usually occurs.

Generalized tetanus, which accounts for 80 per cent of all cases of tetanus, may be mild, moderate, or severe. Mild cases involve muscle rigidity without spasms. Moderate cases involve muscle rigidity with few spasms. Severe tetanus is characterized by muscle rigidity with multiple severe spasms.

The initial signs and symptoms of adult tetanus vary. A prodrome of restlessness, headaches, irritability, and vague discomfort in the jaws, neck, or lower back may be reported. Stiffness or cramping of the muscles around the wound is often present. Other symptoms include stiffness of the neck and jaw, facial pain, or dysphasia.

Early in the course of tetanus, the physical examination may reveal a wound and hyperreflexia of the involved extremity. As the disease progresses, trismus or lockjaw develops. The jaw muscles are so contracted that the patient is unable to voluntarily open the mouth, and the examiner may be unable to pry it open.

As the infection spreads to muscles of the face, the classic facial expression of risus sardonicus develops. Other muscles of the head, neck, and shoulders become tight and firm and then spasm occurs. The spread of rigidity to muscles of the chest, back, abdomen, and extremities causes the patient to "lie at attention" in bed, with all muscles hard to palpation. In severe tetanus, the rigidity progresses to severe muscle spasms.

Generalized muscle spasms reflect a sudden exacerbation of underlying rigidity. Although spasms may last only a few seconds, in severe tetanus they become alarming and dramatic events lasting several minutes. Spasms may be precipitated by minute stimuli (e.g., turning on a light or touching the patient), or they may occur spontaneously. Groups of muscles may suddenly and simultaneously contract, resulting in exaggerated posturing termed opisthotonus. The arms are held in flexion and adduction with the fist clenched tightly against the chest. The legs and feet are fully extended and the spine is hyperextended. Compression fractures of thoracic vertebrae may occur. The clavicles and long bones of the extremities may fracture as well.

The patient is unable to breathe during these generalized spasms owing to chest wall muscle contractions and laryngospasm. Severe hypoxia can occur. Excessive secretions accumulate in the mouth because the patient cannot swallow, and the risk of aspiration is clinically significant. If the patient's airway is not protected and appropriately ventilated, laryngeal and chest wall muscle spasms may rapidly cause death.

The victim of tetanus is mercilessly intact mentally, suffering pain and dread anticipation from the recurrent spasms. Sensory function remains intact, and multiple generalized spasms lead to profound exhaustion. Fortunately, survivors typically experience some degree of amnesia.

Severe tetanus also affects the autonomic nervous system. The patient may experience dramatic increases and decreases in blood pressure as well as tachycardia, bradycardia, profuse perspiration, high fever, tachypnea, apnea, flushing, urinary retention, constipation, arrhythmias, and cardiac arrest.

PROGNOSIS

The manifestations of successfully treated tetanus usually peak at 4 to 5 days, plateau for a few days, and then diminish gradually over several weeks, with respiratory assistance frequently required for 2 to 4 weeks. Hospitalization may exceed 2 months when complications occur. Sometimes patients suffer mild extended complications such as residual stiffness and sleeping difficulties. Despite modern medical care, the mortality rate of severe generalized tetanus approaches 50 per cent.

COMPLICATIONS

Respiratory compromise is the most common mechanism of death in patients treated conservatively. Respiration is impaired by spasm-induced respiratory muscle exhaustion, the aspiration of secretions, atelectasis, pneumonia, apnea, pulmonary embolus, and adult respiratory distress syndrome (ARDS). With intensive management via muscle blockade and mechanical ventilation, the mechanism of death is more commonly related to cardiac arrhythmias, septicemia, or the direct effects of the toxin on the brain stem.

Further complications in patients with tetanus include decubitus ulcers, urinary tract infection, rhabdomyolysis, renal failure, dehydration, malnutrition, fractures, traumatic glossitis, and myositis ossificans. However, if the patient recovers, serious long-term sequelae are rare.

LABORATORY AND DIAGNOSTIC TESTS

The diagnosis of tetanus is clinical. Definitive diagnostic laboratory tests for tetanus are not available. The leukocyte count may be slightly increased. With secondary infection, the leukocyte count may increase further. The serum concentration of creatine kinase (CK) reflects the degree of muscle spasms. Other routine blood tests are not altered. Gram-stained specimens from the infected wound rarely show organisms, and culture specimens may not grow *C. tetani.* A negative Gram stain or culture does not exclude tetanus. A positive result is helpful but is not diagnostic.

Although intracranial pressure may be increased, the cerebrospinal fluid is typically unremarkable. An electroencephalogram (EEG) shows a sleep pattern, and computed tomography (CT) or magnetic resonance imaging (MRI) should be unremarkable. Electromyography is of little diagnostic value. Anti–tetanus toxin antibody titers exceeding 0.01 IU/mL are considered protective, but some individuals with titers in the protective range have experienced signs and symptoms of tetanus.

DIFFERENTIAL DIAGNOSIS

The diagnosis is readily apparent once the disease has progressed to the severe form, but other disorders may simulate the early stages of tetanus toxicosis. Strychnine poisoning may closely resemble severe tetanus. However, the constant muscle rigidity of tetanus is not typically seen following strychnine exposure. Instead, periods of complete muscle relaxation occur between spasms, and the duration of strychnine poisoning is much shorter than that of tetanus toxicosis.

Drug and alcohol withdrawal may precipitate a dramatic event mimicking tetanus. However, the patient's history, laboratory test results, and altered mental status generally point to the correct diagnosis. Dystonic reactions to phenothiazines may resemble tetanus, but, again, the history is very helpful. The absence of trismus and a rapid response to intravenous diphenhydramine administration distinguish the phenothiazine reaction from tetanus.

The clinician should include meningitis, encephalitis, subarachnoid hemorrhage, and schizophrenia in the differential diagnosis. Hypocalcemia, alkalosis, and hepatic encephalopathy can be confirmed with laboratory tests. Rabies with drooling and apparent dysphagia may be confused with the early stages of tetanus. Hyperventilation with associated carpopedal spasms may also resemble tetanus, but hyperventilation quickly resolves with treatment.

A dislocated mandible, temporomandibular joint disease, peritonsillar abscess, dental infection, head and neck trauma, and tumor all can cause trismus or stiff muscles of the head and neck; the history and physical examination typically suffice to distinguish these disorders from tetanus.

Neonatal tetanus is difficult to diagnose in developed countries because it is rare. The differential diagnosis includes traumatic intracranial birth injury, drug withdrawal, hypoglycemia, metabolic alkalosis, hypomagnesemia, hypocalcemic tetani, meningitis, sepsis, and seizures from another cause. Usually the history of maternal immunizations and a description of the delivery and postdelivery care of the newborn provides the diagnosis.

SUMMARY

The key to the diagnosis of tetanus is the recognition of (1) inadequate tetanus immunization, (2) an injury or chronic wound, and (3) the early signs and symptoms of the illness, particularly in the elderly individual.

TRAUMA OF THE CENTRAL NERVOUS SYSTEM

By Kevin L. Boyer, M.D.,
and Roy A. E. Bakay, M.D.
Atlanta, Georgia

Trauma of the central nervous system encompasses injuries to the brain and spinal cord. In its broadest sense, the term head injury refers to all injuries of the scalp, face, skull, and intracranial contents—including the meninges, brain, and brain stem. Concerning injuries to the brain itself, the term traumatic brain injury is used. Similarly, spinal injury encompasses all injury to the paraspinal musculature, the bony spine, its ligaments, and the contents of the spinal canal, that is, the spinal cord and nerve roots.

More than 4 million incidents of total brain injury are estimated to occur annually, resulting in nearly 500,000 hospitalizations. The annual incidence of total brain injury requiring hospitalization is approximately 200 per 100,000 population. Extrapolating from estimates, an annual national expense of greater than $600 million may be conservative.

Most brain and spinal cord injuries result from transport-related events, with falls being the second most common cause. Other contributors include sporting and occupational accidents, interpersonal violence, and penetrating missile or knife wounds. Brain injury is the leading cause of death in most industrialized countries, accounting for 50 to 60 per cent of all motor vehicle trauma deaths.

APPROACH TO THE PATIENT WITH CENTRAL NERVOUS SYSTEM INJURY

The diagnosis of central nervous system injury begins with obtaining a thorough history of the incident, with emphasis on the mechanism of injury. Victims of motor vehicle accidents, those ejected from a vehicle, pedestrians struck by vehicles, those who have fallen or have been struck by a large or heavy object, and anyone with a reported loss or alteration of consciousness, seizure, or vomiting should be regarded as having a clinically significant head injury until it is proved otherwise.

The airway, breathing, and circulation are stabilized according to standard Advanced Trauma Life Support (ATLS) resuscitation protocols prior to addressing a head injury or determining the severity of brain or spinal cord injury in a trauma patient. Investigation for injuries to other systems are performed simultaneously. A rapid but thorough examination of the patient's head, neck, and back reliably discloses superficial evidence of head and spine injury and should be performed simultaneously with stabilization of the patient but should not delay evaluation of the patient's overall status. Specific injuries to the face, scalp, skull, or intracranial contents can be isolated, but often two or more injury-related problems appear concurrently. Disruptive injuries to the vascular scalp present with excessive bleeding around the head. Careful inspection, including shaving of the head, is necessary for confirming the presence of multiple scalp lacerations and for controlling bleeding, which may be lifesaving. Delicate finger palpation inside the wound can disclose underlying skull fractures but should be performed cautiously to avoid further brain injury. Scalp contusions, nonhemorrhagic abrasions, and subgaleal hematomas can also be diagnosed by palpation, but they are often small and can elude early diagnosis. Radiographic imaging is indicated to help define underlying bony injury. Fractures of the skull can be of the linear nondisplaced, linear displaced, basilar, or depressed type. If associated with scalp disruption, they are managed as open skull fractures. Plain films of the skull have been almost completely replaced by computed tomography (CT) for the evaluation of adult head injury because it is more sensitive for intracranial injury. Skull films are useful, however, in children and adults with depressed skull fractures and penetrating injuries. These injuries tend to occur in patients with more severe head trauma, and CT permits more accurate definition of the fracture. Linear fractures in the plane of the CT image may be missed, but they are usually clinically insignificant.

Basilar skull fractures are best diagnosed on the basis of clinical signs such as unexplained bleeding in the nasopharynx, oropharynx, or external auditory canal. Periorbital ecchymosis (raccoon eyes), hemotympanum, and retromastoid hematomas (Battle's sign) are other hemorrhagic signs of basilar skull fracture. Cerebrospinal fluid leak from the nose (rhinorrhea) or ear (otorrhea) is diagnostic.

Following resuscitation and stabilization of blood pressure and oxygenation, neurologic status is assessed as part of the initial evaluation. The level of consciousness and focal neurologic deficits help categorize the severity of brain injury and presence of spinal cord injury.

The Glasgow Coma Score (GCS) remains the most widely accepted grading scale for total brain injury classification (Table 1). It is based on the patient's best motor function, verbal response, and eye opening. Patients with a score of 13 to 15 are classified as mildly brain-injured, and those with scores of 9 to 12 as moderately brain-injured. Patients with a score of 8 or less are considered to have severe brain injury. This grade assignment assists subsequent clinical decisions concerning brain injury management. The GCS grade is not assessed until resuscitation measures have been completed because coexisting hypotension may skew the initial GCS score. The presence of toxic substances such as barbiturates, alcohol, and other central nervous system depressants must be considered. Metabolic causes of coma can usually be detected using routine laboratory tests.

Occasionally, patients may have severe injuries to the eyes or require intubation that precludes the GCS assignment in the categories of eye opening and verbal response. In this setting, assessment of motor function and assignment of a motor score is the best prognostic indicator of outcome and survival. Patients in whom an eye or a verbal score cannot be reliably determined and with a motor score of 5 or 6 should be categorized with the mild or moderate total brain injury patients. Only patients with a GCS score of 15, without reported loss of consciousness, nausea and vomiting, seizures, or retrograde amnesia, are released from care without further evaluation. All others undergo further diagnostic studies of the head or spine. Once a GCS score is assigned, focal neurologic changes can help localize specific parenchymal injuries to the central nervous system. Severe depression of mental status (GCS score of 8 or less) suggests diffuse injury to the brain and has a high likelihood of increased intracranial pressure (ICP).

Evaluation of the cervical spine is performed while the patient is in the emergency room. The coincidence of total brain injury and cervical spine injuries ranges from 2 to 19 per cent and is notably higher in persons involved in motor vehicle accidents and those suffering severe brain injury. Pupillary function is assessed for size, reactivity to light, and roundness. Asymmetry in size and unilateral loss of reactivity may be due to herniation of the temporal lobe over the tentorial edge causing third cranial nerve compression. This results from hemisphere edema or mass effect from a space-occupying lesion causing a shift of in-

Table 1. Glasgow Coma Scale (GCS)

Eye opening response (E)	
Spontaneous	4
To voice stimulation	3
To painful stimulation	2
Absent	1
Verbal response (V)	
Fully oriented	5
Confused	4
Inappropriate words	3
Incomprehensible sounds	2
Absent	1
Motor response (M)	
Follows commands	6
Localizes painful stimuli	5
Withdraws from pain	4
Flexion to pain	3
Extension to pain	2
Flaccid (absent)	1
Best possible score: 15	
Worst possible score: 3	

tracranial structures. Eye movements are also evaluated for spontaneity and gaze palsies or preferences. Corneal and gag reflexes and spontaneous respirations are also briefly assessed and can localize injury to the brain stem or suggest central herniation syndromes.

Motor skills are assessed as part of the assignment of a GCS score. Special reflexes can provide more information concerning spinal cord injury. An alert, cooperative patient can help localize the level of the spinal injury by allowing a detailed sensory examination. Perineal reflexes (bulbocavernosus and anal wink), as well as rectal tone (both resting and volitional) should be assessed.

RADIOGRAPHIC EVALUATION

In addition to plain film evaluations performed as part of the Advanced Trauma Life Support protocol, the lateral cervical spine films are obtained during the initial stabilization of the patient. This study includes the base of the skull, the first thoracic vertebra, and all vertebrae in between. It should adequately disclose the great majority of unstable fractures or dislocations of the cervical spine or cervicothoracic junction. Often, the lateral cervical spine film does not include C6, C7, or T1, and cervical spine immobilization must be maintained until further radiographic evaluation of this area can be performed.

The CT scan of the head provides precise anatomic diagnosis and guides further decisions regarding intervention. The value of the CT scan as a prognostic indicator for patients with mild brain injury is well established, and the incidence of neurologic deterioration is nil if the initial CT scan is normal. CT of the brain shows an abnormality in nearly 20 per cent of patients with mild head injuries accompanied by loss of consciousness or retrograde amnesia. This percentage is higher with more severe head injury. The CT scan of the head can include imaging of the cervical spine to assess areas inadequately visualized by the lateral cervical spine films.

The role of magnetic resonance imaging (MRI) in the management of brain-injured patients remains poorly defined. MRI has been shown to be superior to CT in the detection of many forms of intracranial pathology. Lack of availability, however, has prevented MRI from replacing CT in most centers. A small percentage of patients with unexplained neurologic deficits may benefit from an MRI scan.

Cerebral arteriography has been virtually replaced by the use of CT in the evaluation of a head-injured patient. In some patients with a normal CT scan and lateralizing neurologic signs suggesting specific cerebral injury, the cerebral angiogram may disclose vascular injury such as arterial disruption, dissection, or vascular thrombosis.

If the neurologic examination is suggestive of spinal cord injury, the CT scan should include the thoracic and/or lumbar spine. Newer CT equipment can be used to recreate sagittal images and three-dimensional images of the spine that can provide detailed information concerning the structural anatomy. Radiographic evaluation of patients who require immediate surgery for hemodynamic stabilization because of injuries to other systems may require other diagnostic procedures until a CT scan can be obtained. In these patients, diagnostic bur holes with placement of intracranial pressure monitors can be performed in the operating room. All patients must then undergo CT scanning immediately following surgery.

CRITERIA FOR HOSPITALIZATION

Only patients with a GCS score of 15 who have no history of loss of consciousness, seizures, or nausea and vomiting and do not present with retrograde amnesia are released from care. If a reliable relative is available to observe the patient for 24 hours subsequent to the injury, patients with loss of consciousness or retrograde amnesia may be observed at home with follow-up in the physician's office within 3 days. All patients with evidence of spinal cord injury are admitted for the administration of high-dose methylprednisolone (30 mg/kg per hour load followed by intravenous drip of 5.4 mg/kg per hour for 24 hours) and stabilization of spinal injury.

RECOGNITION OF SPINAL CORD INJURY

Recognition of a spinal cord injury can be difficult in a patient with a brain injury whose neurologic examination precludes an adequate peripheral neurologic examination. Even a motor examination can usually be performed on a comatose patient and remains the mainstay of evaluation in patients suspected of having spinal cord injury. Initial signs in a trauma patient with spinal cord injury include paraplegia, quadriplegia, bowel and bladder incontinence, lack of rectal tone, and autonomic dysregulation with profound hypotension unexplained by hemorrhage. Cerebral evaluation and physical examination in these patients helps localize a spinal cord lesion more accurately. In a quadriplegic patient, detailed attention is given to the cervical spine to delineate cervical spine injury. All patients should undergo plain film evaluation of the thoracic and lumbar spine. Once a spinal cord injury is apparent, a detailed sensory examination is the most sensitive indicator of the level of lesion. Sensation to pain and/or temperature based on dermatomal distribution accurately localizes the level of spinal cord injury to within two vertebral bodies. These patients should undergo CT to include the area of concern.

DIAGNOSIS AND CLASSIFICATION

Head Injury

Skull fractures can be divided into (1) linear fractures that may be displaced or nondisplaced and (2) depressed skull fractures. Unless associated with a marked deformity, skull fractures can be missed at the time of the initial evaluation of the trauma patient. Linear skull fractures are rarely of clinical significance, and further diagnostic evaluation is not necessary. Depressed skull fractures are often detected during examination of the head and scalp; however, specific characteristics of the fracture, such as its diameter, depth, and any associated bone fragments that may have been driven into the cerebral parenchyma, can be determined by CT.

Even when evidence of basilar skull fracture is found on physical examination, the lesion may not be seen on routine CT of the head. In this setting, coronal and axial CT images of the temporal bones may be necessary for defining the fracture. Associated cranial nerve deficits can also help localize basilar skull fractures.

Certain physical findings raise the suspicion of serious brain injury. A depressed GCS score without focal neurologic deficits is consistent with diffuse cerebral injury without a significant focal lesion. If a space-occupying lesion is not identified on the CT scan in these patients, intracranial pressure monitoring is instituted to diagnose increased ICP and help determine the required intensity of therapeutic intervention. If ICP cannot be maintained below 40 mm Hg, prognosis is poor. When pupils have become dilated and unreactive to light bilaterally, massive cerebral swelling with downward herniation of cranial contents toward and through the foramen magnum is likely. Focal neurologic deficits are more suggestive of specific parenchymal injuries and unilateral space-occupying lesions that can be difficult to define based on physical examination alone. In this setting, CT of the brain reliably provides the specific diagnosis (Table 2).

Cerebral contusions (Fig. 1) may be hemorrhagic or nonhemorrhagic, and they typically occur in areas of brain parenchyma adjacent to bony ridges at the base of the skull. The base of the frontal lobes, the tips of the temporal lobes, and the occipital poles are common locations. Even the smallest of cerebral contusions, if strategically placed, can result in profound neurologic deficits. Cerebral edema associated with contusion can cause a mass effect. Children, especially, can have markedly increased ICP associated with minimal parenchymal injury.

Epidural hematomas (Fig. 2) develop in the space between the skull and the dura mater. They tend to be associated with overlying skull fractures in the distribution of the middle meningeal artery. The classic description of a patient suffering from an epidural hematoma is a brief period of loss of consciousness followed by a lucid interval of several hours. The patient subsequently deteriorates rapidly as the epidural hematoma expands. A lenticular, hyperdense lesion intimately associated with the inner surface of the skull is seen on the CT scan. These lesions tend to occur in patients suffering a direct blow to the head.

Subdural hematomas (Fig. 3) occur in a space between the dura mater and the brain itself. These patients also suffer loss of consciousness at the time of injury but experience no lucid interval and in general present with marked neurologic compromise. CT scanning reveals a less regular hematoma that is often described as crescent-shaped be-

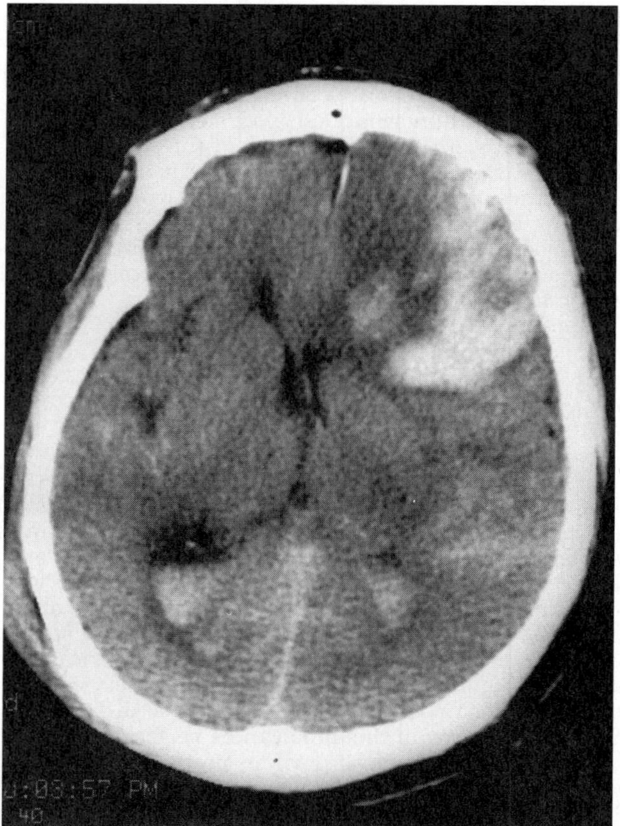

Figure 1. Hemorrhagic cerebral contusions in frontal lobe, with midline shift and intraparenchymal and layered interventricular blood.

Table 2. Classification of Head Injury Lesions

- Extracranial soft tissue injury
- Subgaleal hematoma
- Cranial fractures*
  - Linear
    - Displaced or nondisplaced
  - Depressed
  - Basilar skull fracture
- Intracranial pathology
  - Epidural hematoma
  - Dural laceration
  - Subdural hematoma
  - Subarachnoid hemorrhage
  - Intraparenchymal hematoma
  - Intraventricular hemorrhage
  - Parenchymal damage
    - Contusion
    - Cerebral edema
    - Diffuse axonal injury
- Missile (penetrating) injury
  - Bullet, spear, arrow, injuries
  - Knife injury
- Central nervous system vascular injury
  - Arterial disruption or dissection
  - Traumatic arterial aneurysms
  - Arteriovenous fistulas

*Head injuries are classified as open if there is disruption of the soft tissues overlying the bony skull.

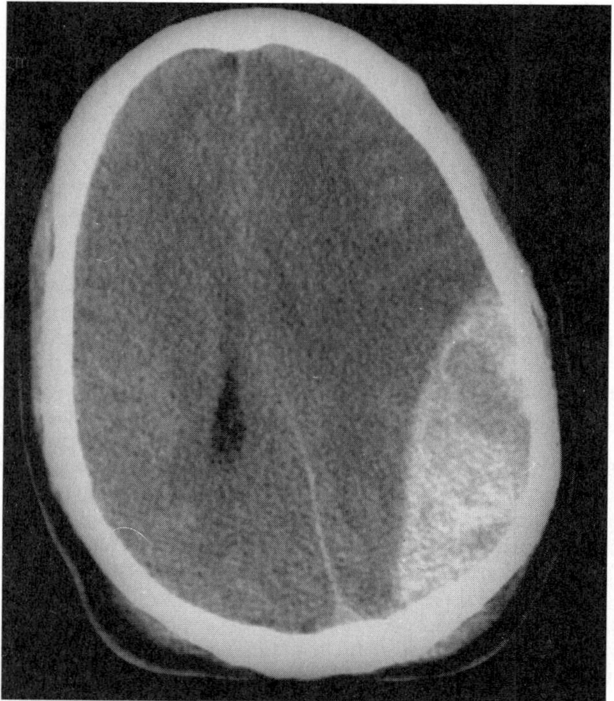

Figure 2. Epidural hematoma with edema in the ipsilateral hemisphere and midline shift. Note elliptic shape of hematoma.

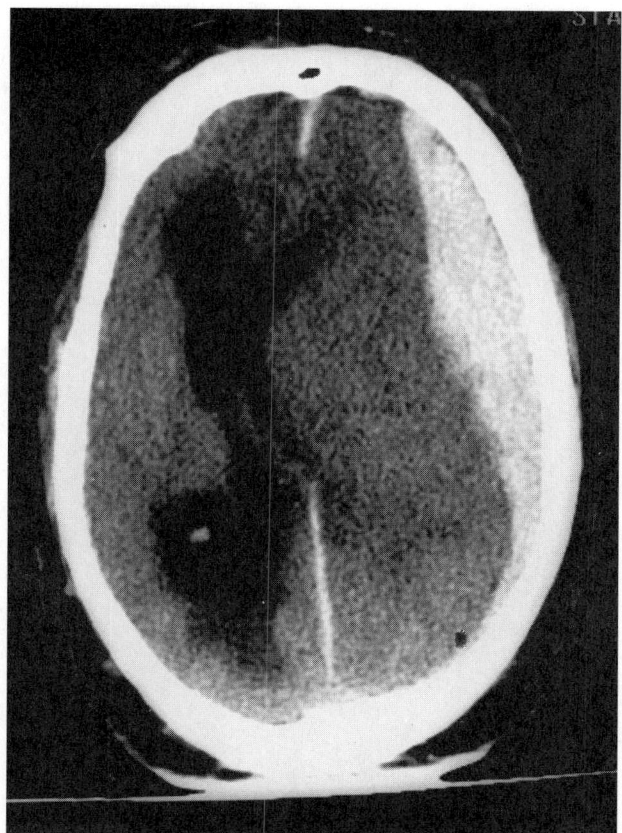

Figure 3. Acute subdural hematoma with midline shift and a dilated contralateral ventricle. Note crescent shape of hematoma.

cause it spreads over the surface of the brain (Fig. 4). As intracranial structures shift away from the hematoma, the uncus of the temporal lobe frequently herniates over the tentorial edge, causing third nerve compression and an ipsilateral oculomotor nerve palsy. In more extreme cases, the brain stem is thrust against the contralateral tentorial edge, causing compression of the cortical spinal fibers and resulting in ipsilateral hemiplegia. This false localizing sign can present a dilemma in diagnosis. Subdural hematomas typically occur in patients suffering rapid deceleration injuries to the head with resultant tearing of bridging cortical veins. Chronic subdural hematomas (Fig. 5) are more common in older patients, in whom they cause a higher mortality rate.

Subarachnoid hemorrhage is the result of bleeding into the space between the pia arachnoid and the brain parenchyma itself. Although this is of little consequence in trauma, it usually suggests a more severe head injury. On CT scanning, subarachnoid hemorrhage appears as a thin layer of hyperdense fluid that follows the intricate curvature of the surface of the brain. Hyperdensity often extends into the fine recesses of the sulci. Intraventricular hemorrhage is an even less common result of trauma. Patients with subarachnoid or intraventricular hemorrhage are at higher risk for the development of post-traumatic hydrocephalus. In patients with subarachnoid hemorrhage without overt signs of trauma, bleeding from a cerebral aneurysm or arteriovenous malformation must be considered.

Traumatic intraparenchymal hematoma is usually secondary to a hemorrhagic contusion and typically occurs in the areas defined earlier. These hematomas present on CT as irregular hyperdense lesions within the axis of the brain. They tend to track along white matter tracts causing neurologic deficits by mass effect, and not by direct cerebral injury.

The diagnoses of penetrating injuries to the brain are easily made on history and physical examination alone. Only a CT scan of the head can delineate the path of the penetrating trauma and ultimately locate foreign bodies and bony fragments (Fig 6). The CT scan can also disclose mass-occupying hematomas that may have been created by the penetrating injury.

Spinal Injury

Only in the alert, cooperative patient who complains of no pain or tenderness to the spinal axis can absence of injury to the spine be confirmed without further radiographic analysis. Spinal or spinal cord injury can be accurately localized in a patient who is able to cooperate with the physical examination. If a head injury results in an altered level of consciousness, neurologic evaluation of spinal cord function may not be possible.

Structural damage to the bony spine and its ligamentous structures varies in different regions of the spine. Most spinal injuries can be identified on plain film. This includes anteroposterior, lateral, two oblique, and open-mouth odontoid views of the cervical spine, as well as anteroposterior and lateral views of the thoracic and lumbar spine. Review of the films should include detailed attention to the paravertebral soft tissues and normal anatomic alignments. If no bony abnormality is found, flexion and extension films

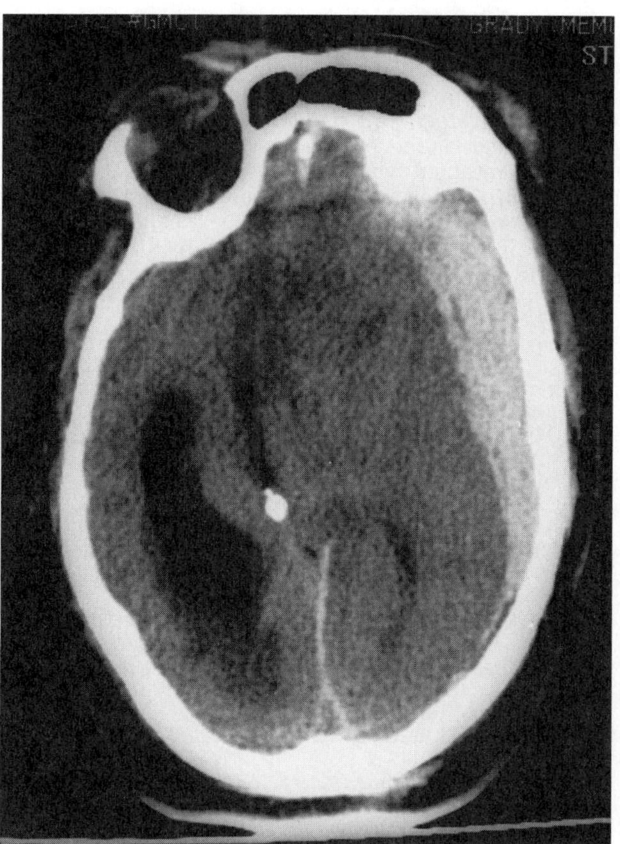

Figure 4. Acute subdural hematoma with herniation from mass effect.

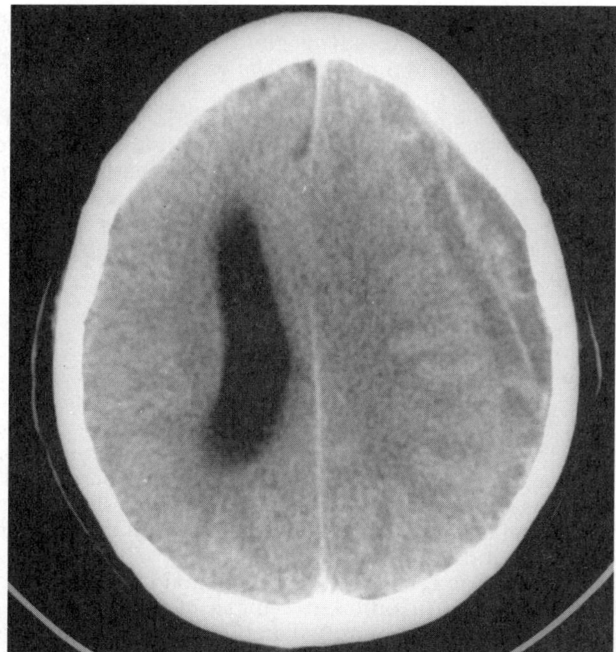

Figure 5. Chronic subdural hematoma with mass effect and hematoma membranes. Note hypodense appearance when compared with brain.

of the cervical spine complete the plain film evaluation and exclude ligamentous injury (Table 3).

Once an injury to the spine has been identified, further radiographic evaluation to characterize the lesion precisely is performed whether or not the patient suffers from a spinal cord injury. CT enhanced with subarachnoid injection of myelographic dye gives an image of the thecal sac and discloses the presence of foreign bodies or bone fragments retained within the spinal canal. This also allows identification of compression of the neural tissue within the spinal canal.

Spinal cord injuries can be divided into four basic categories (Table 4).

Table 3. Classification of Spinal Injury

Cervical injury	
C1	Craniocervical dislocation
	Jefferson fracture
	Transverse ligament avulsion
C2	Odontoid fractures (types I–III)
	Hangman's fracture
C3–C7	Ligamentous injury
	Fracture-dislocation
	Facet injury
	Unilateral dislocation-fracture
	Bilateral dislocation-fracture
	Acute herniated nucleus pulposus
	Spinous process fracture
Thoracic and lumbar injury	
Compression fracture	
Burst fracture	
Fracture-dislocation	
Chance fracture	
Acute herniated nucleus pulposus	
Ligamentous injury	
Spinous and transverse process fracture	

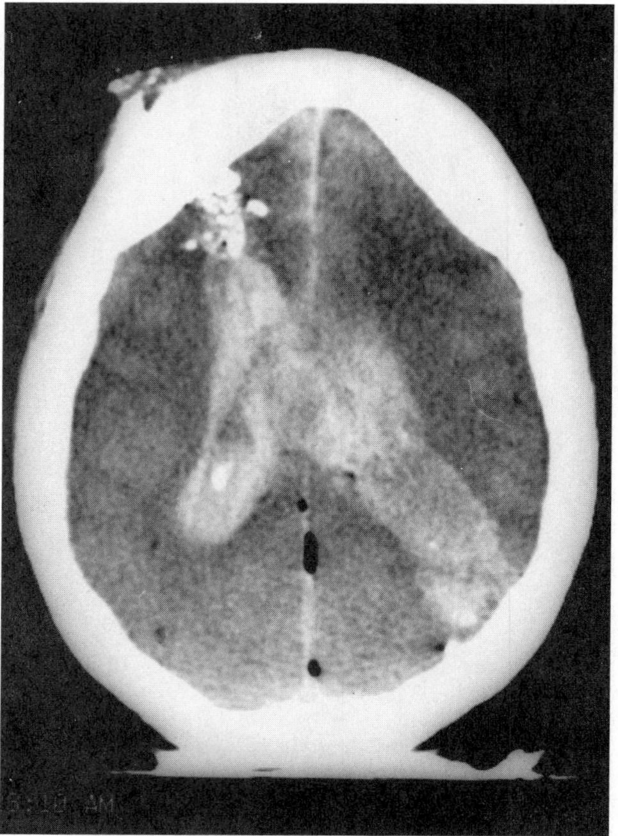

Figure 6. Interventricular and intraparenchymal hemorrhage resulting from gunshot wound to the head. Impaled bone fragments are seen near the entrance wound.

1. Diffuse spinal cord injury produces complete or nearly complete loss of function below the level of injury.
2. Injury to the anterior columns of the spinal cord results in paralysis and loss of pain and temperature sensation below the level of the lesion. Proprioceptive, vibratory, and some fine touch sensation is preserved.
3. Loss of motor function and dorsal column function ipsilateral to and below the level of lesion occurs as does

Table 4. Classification of Spinal Cord Injury

Complete	
	Total loss of neurologic function below the level of lesion
	Spinal shock common
Anterior cord syndrome	
	Complete motor loss below lesion
	Pain and loss of temperature sensation below lesion
	Dorsal column function intact
	Spinal shock common
Hemicord syndrome (Brown-Séquard syndrome)	
	Ipsilateral loss of motor and dorsal column function below level of lesion
	Contralateral loss of pain and temperature sense
	Spinal shock frequent
Central cord syndrome	
	Upper extremity weakness profound
	Lower extremity weakness mild if at all
	Severe upper extremity paresthesias
	Spinal shock unusual
	Suspended sensory loss

loss of pain and temperature sensation contralateral to and below the level of the lesion.

4. Central cord lesions result in asymmetrical loss of function that is worse in the upper extremities than in the lower extremities. Hypesthesias of the upper extremities is also common.

The specific level of spinal cord injury can be determined by finding the highest level of neurologic function. This portion of the neurologic examination is performed after the patient has been stabilized and is still in spinal immobilization. Thorough motor examination of the upper and lower extremities provides localization of a spinal cord injury in the cervical or lumbar spinal cord. Sensory examination based on dermatomal nerve root distribution then confirms and precisely localizes the level of spinal cord injury, recalling that the spinal cord terminates at the level of the second lumbar vertebra.

Myelographically enhanced CT is the study of choice in patients with spinal cord injury to fully define the spinal injury and to disclose any invasion of the spinal canal by bone fragments, foreign bodies, penetrating objects, or acutely herniated disk material. MRI has been shown to be particularly sensitive in detecting injuries to the spinal cord; however, the efficiency of obtaining an MRI scan in an emergency situation limits its use at this time.

Table 1. Listing of Tumors and Their Percentage of the Yearly Total of Newly Diagnosed, Histologically Verified, Primary Brain Tumors in the United States (Approximately 15,000 Cases)

Tumor	Percent of Total
Gliomas	
Glioblastoma multiforme	20
Astrocytoma	10
Ependymoma	6
Oligodendroglioma	5
Medulloblastoma	4
Meningioma	18
Pituitary adenoma	9
Schwannoma	7
Craniopharyngioma, epidermoid, dermoid, teratoma	4
Sarcomas	4
Angiomas	4
Miscellaneous (pineal tumors, chordoma, lymphoma)	4
Unclassified	5

From Newton, H.B.: Primary brain tumors: Review of etiology, diagnosis, and treatment. Am. Fam. Phys., 49:787–797, 1994, with permission of the American Academy of Family Physicians.

INTRACRANIAL NEOPLASMS

By Herbert B. Newton, M.D.
Columbus, Ohio

Intracranial neoplasms are a diverse group of tumors that can occur at any age and affect any region of the brain. They can be divided into two basic categories: primary brain tumors, which develop from cells of the brain, cerebral vasculature, and meninges, and metastatic brain tumors, which originate from systemic primary neoplasms. Intracranial neoplasms affect both adults and children but occur more frequently in the adult population. The peak age of incidence for primary brain tumors in adults is between 45 and 55 years; for children the incidence peaks between 4 and 9 years. Primary brain tumors represent 2 per cent of newly diagnosed malignancies each year in the United States, with an annual incidence across all age groups of 6 to 9 per 100,000 population. This corresponds to about 15,000 to 17,000 histologically verified new cases yearly (Table 1). The majority of these tumors are gliomas, meningiomas, and pituitary adenomas. In children, the age-specific annual incidence of primary brain tumor is only 2 to 3 per 100,000 population. However, brain tumors are still the most common solid neoplasm diagnosed in young patients; only leukemia is a more common cause of malignancy in children. The location and histologic features of primary brain tumor in children are distinctly different from those in adults (Table 2). In young patients, more than 60 per cent of tumors develop in the infratentorial cavity within the cerebellum, pons, and brain stem. In contrast, the majority of tumors affecting adults develop supratentorially within the cortical, subcortical, and basal ganglia regions of the brain.

Metastatic brain tumors occur in 20 to 40 per cent of cancer patients, accounting for another 18,000 to 20,000 new intracranial neoplasms each year. Metastases are the most common central nervous system complication of systemic cancer and may be the first manifestation of malignancy in more than one third of patients. Brain metastases are frequently documented in lung and breast cancer, melanoma, renal cell carcinoma, genitourinary tumors, and colorectal carcinoma.

The neurologic manifestations of primary and metastatic brain tumors are similar. Both can increase intracranial pressure (ICP), often causing generalized symptoms such as headache, nausea, and diplopia. Focal symptoms and signs can also develop, and tumors may compress, infiltrate, or invade areas of brain that mediate language, vision, or sensation. In benign tumors (e.g., meningioma),

Table 2. Distribution of Common Primary Brain Tumors by Age and Location

Tumor Type	Percent of Tumors (Age 1–20 years)	Percent of Tumors (Age >20 years)
Supratentorial		
Glioblastoma	<5	35–40
Astrocytoma	8–12	18–20
Craniopharyngioma	5–8	<2
Ependymoma	3–5	<1
Choroid plexus papilloma	2–3	<1
Pituitary tumors	<1	5
Pineal tumors	2	2
Meningioma	<1	17
Infratentorial		
Medulloblastoma	18–25	<1
Cerebellar astrocytoma	15–20	<1
Brain stem glioma	8–10	<1
Ependymoma	4–6	<1
Schwannoma	<1	3–5
Meningioma	<1	2–3

From Newton, H.B.: Primary brain tumors: Review of etiology, diagnosis, and treatment. Am. Fam. Phys., 49:787–797, 1994, with permission of the American Academy of Family Physicians.

the clinical course is slow and indolent, with symptoms developing over months to years. In more malignant tumors (e.g., glioblastoma multiforme, metastases), the onset of symptoms is more rapid, occurring over days, weeks, or a few months.

PRESENTING SIGNS AND SYMPTOMS

The most important feature of the clinical presentation of most patients with intracranial neoplasms is the *progressive nature* of the symptoms. The evolving presentation varies and depends on many factors, including the type of tumor and its method of growth (infiltrative versus expansile), the location of the tumor within the brain, the rapidity of growth, and the degree of associated edema and mass effect. Table 3 lists the common symptoms noted at presentation in a large series of adult patients with supratentorial gliomas. Individually, none of these symptoms is pathognomonic for an intracranial tumor. However, clinical suspicion should increase if several of these symptoms occur together in the context of a *progressive* neurologic illness. Generalized symptoms and signs of an intracranial neoplasm typically result from disturbed regulation of ICP, whereas focal signs and symptoms are produced by disruption of the function of specialized regions of the brain due to tissue destruction and/or compression.

Neurologic Symptoms

The most common symptoms of intracranial neoplasms are headache, generalized seizure activity, cognitive and personality changes, nausea and emesis, diplopia, and altered consciousness. These symptoms occur as the expanding tumor and associated edema raise ICP and compress specific structures within the nervous system. Compression of ventricular pathways by tumor and associated edema may cause hydrocephalus, which may further augment increased ICP.

Headache is the most common symptom produced by intracranial tumors; it is present in two thirds of patients with primary brain tumors and almost half of those with metastatic brain tumors. Headaches are probably caused by a combination of increased ICP and traction on blood vessels, dura mater, and other sensitive structures. The headache usually occurs in the frontal or vertex region but may be more diffuse. Headaches may be more severe in the morning because cerebrospinal fluid drainage is reduced in the recumbent position and because hypercarbia that develops during the hypoventilation of sleep increases cerebral blood volume and exacerbates peritumoral edema. However, morning headache is not specific for brain tumors. Patients with migraine can also demonstrate this pattern. Brain tumor–related headache pain is typically of moderate to severe intensity and often lasts for hours. The intensity of pain may be increased by coughing, sneezing, straining, or other maneuvers that increase intrathoracic (and consequently intracranial) pressure. In the majority of patients with intracranial neoplasms, the headaches become more frequent and more intense and are more resistant to analgesics than prior, non–tumor-related headaches. Nausea and emesis are present in one third of patients with intracranial tumors and are not always correlated with headaches. These conditions are caused by increased ICP and are also frequently most severe in the morning.

Table 3. Common Symptoms at Presentation of Patients With Gliomas

Symptom	All Gliomas (% Cases) (n = 653)
Headache	70
Seizure activity	54
Partial motor	23
Generalized tonic-clonic	20
Partial complex	9
Absence	2
Cognitive-personality change	52
Focal weakness	43
Nausea-vomiting	31
Speech disturbance	27
Alteration of consciousness	25
Sensory abnormalities	14
Visual disturbances	8

From Newton, H.B.: Primary brain tumors: Review of etiology, diagnosis, and treatment. Am. Fam. Phys., 49:787–797, 1994, with permission of the American Academy of Family Physicians.

Generalized convulsions occur in the form of tonic-clonic or absence seizures in one fifth of patients. Tumor growth leads to irritation and compression of neural tissues, producing epileptogenic activity that becomes generalized to the whole brain. Generalized seizures may be the first sign of an intracranial neoplasm, and brain tumors should always be included in the differential diagnosis of a first seizure, especially in patients older than 20 to 25 years of age.

Changes in cognition and personality may be caused by increased ICP, mass effect, and/or disruption of central pathways. Mild alterations of memory, concentration, and reasoning are commonly noticed by family members. Dulling of affect or loss of energy and initiative may also develop. Increased ICP can also disturb the patient's level of consciousness, producing lethargy, drowsiness, irritability, or coma. The most common alteration is excessive daytime sleepiness or lethargy that is typically noted by a spouse or parent.

Double vision and other visual disturbances may develop. Diplopia is caused by dysfunction of the sixth cranial nerve secondary to increased ICP. Diplopia is considered a false localizing sign because the dysfunction is not due to a direct effect of tumor on the nerve. Double vision is often apparent to the patient before dysconjugation is noted by the physician.

Focal symptoms that may localize a tumor are usually the result of destruction, compression, or irritation of specialized regions of the brain. Tumors near the cerebral cortex can induce focal motor or sensory seizures, most often affecting the contralateral face and arm. Todd's postictal paralysis (prolonged weakness of the limbs following seizures) is more common with intracranial tumors than with other conditions. Focal signs and symptoms, including personality or cognitive changes (e.g., apathy, dulling of affect, jocularity, forgetfulness), limb weakness, loss of sensation, speech disturbances, visual field changes, gait disturbances (e.g., ataxia, imbalance), and limb incoordination, occur frequently in patients with brain tumors and are commonly progressive.

Neurologic Signs

The neurologic examination is an important tool for analyzing the signs that develop in brain tumor patients. The common neurologic signs from a series of adults with supratentorial gliomas are listed in Table 4. Hemiparesis, cranial nerve palsies, and papilledema are noted in the

Table 4. Common Neurologic Signs in Patients With Gliomas

Neurologic Sign	All Gliomas (% Cases) (n = 1251)
Hemiparesis	57
Cranial nerve palsies	54
Papilledema	53
Cognitive changes—confusion	45
Depressed sensorium	37
Hemianesthesia	30
Hemianopsia	29
Dysphasia	25

From Newton, H.B.: Primary brain tumors: Review of etiology, diagnosis, and treatment. Am. Fam. Phys., 49:787–797, 1994, with permission of the American Academy of Family Physicians.

majority of patients. Hemiparetic weakness often involves the arm more than the leg and may be accompanied by an ipsilateral increase in tendon reflexes and Babinski's sign. Arm weakness is usually more severe in extensor than in flexor muscles. The most common cranial nerve palsies are lower facial weakness (ipsilateral to the hemiparesis), caused by seventh nerve dysfunction, and incomplete eye abduction, secondary to sixth nerve dysfunction. A detailed funduscopic examination is necessary when considering an intracranial neoplasm. Papilledema is seen as swelling of the optic nerve head with blurring of the disk margin and reduced venous pulsations; in more severe stages, retinal venous engorgement and hemorrhages may occur. Severe papilledema may produce central visual field defects because of enlargement of the blind spot. Hemianopic visual field defects are found on examination in almost one third of patients. If the defect develops slowly, the patient may remain unaware of the deficit. Speech disturbances can be manifested as difficulty with articulation (dysarthria), which is commonly seen in children with infratentorial tumors affecting the brain stem or cerebellum, or as a deficit in language (dysphasia), with an impaired ability to express or understand speech. Further characterization of the symptoms and signs of an intracranial neoplasm depends on the specific anatomic location of the tumor. The clinical manifestations of tumors located in different regions of the brain are discussed further on.

NEOPLASMS OF THE CEREBRAL HEMISPHERES

Tumors of the cerebral hemispheres typically occur in adults between 35 and 55 years of age. Metastatic tumors are diagnosed most commonly, followed by gliomas and extra-axial meningiomas. The degree of neurologic compromise depends on the size of the tumor, the specific lobe (or lobes) of the brain affected, and whether the tumor is on the dominant or nondominant side of the brain. In all right-handed patients and most left-handed patients, the left hemisphere is dominant for speech. Tumor growth within or near the pars opercularis of the dominant inferior frontal lobe (Broca's area) results in a nonfluent "expressive" language deficit (dysphasia), with an impaired ability to articulate speech. Patients are often frustrated and state that they can think of what they want to say but cannot get the words out. Comprehension remains intact, whereas repetition is disturbed in most patients. In addition to expressive language function, the frontal lobes also mediate many aspects of personality and executive activities. Symptoms are more severe in bifrontal lesions but can also occur with unilateral tumors. Orbitofrontal neoplasms (e.g., gliomas or metastases) often cause uninhibited behavior, irritability, jocularity, and lack of social awareness. Dorsal midline tumors may cause abulia, with profoundly slowed initiation of thought, speech, and motor behavior. Tumors affecting the dorsolateral convexity region usually cause apathy, depressed mentation, impaired planning, and lack of motivation. Bifrontal inferomedial lesions (e.g., olfactory groove meningioma, "butterfly" gliomas) may present as a dementia resembling Alzheimer's disease. Frontal lobe release signs, including the glabellar, snout, and palmomental reflexes, may appear with any of the frontal lobe tumors. Compression or destruction of the precentral gyrus (primary motor cortex) causes varying degrees of contralateral spastic hemiparesis. Parasagittal lesions (e.g., meningioma) can present in a manner similar to a myelopathy, with spastic paraparesis and impaired bowel and bladder function. Seizures are common with tumors of the frontal lobes. They can be generalized, focal, or partial complex. Focal seizures are usually manifested as clonic activity affecting the contralateral face and arm and less commonly the leg. They can also cause speech arrest and, if the frontal eye field (premotor cortex) is irritated, contralateral conjugate deviation of the eyes and head. Partial complex seizures may occur with tumors in the prefrontal region, as manifested by an altered level of consciousness and automatisms. In some patients with high-grade, infiltrative gliomas of the frontal lobes, the neurologic examination may be normal.

Tumors developing within the parietal lobes most often disturb the postcentral gyrus (primary sensory cortex), causing contralateral sensory loss, astereognosis, and agraphesthesia. Posteriorly placed tumors on the dominant side may disturb Wernicke's area, causing a fluent receptive language deficit with impaired repetition. These patients speak fluently, often with excessive "empty" speech yet lack comprehension of spoken or written words. Most patients with receptive aphasia are unaware of their deficit and do not appear frustrated. Dominant-side lesions near the angular gyrus may produce Gerstmann's syndrome, with agraphia, acalculia, right-left disorientation, and finger agnosia. Nondominant parietal lesions may result in a neglect syndrome, as manifested in mild cases by contralateral extinction to sensory stimuli. In more severe cases, parietal lobe neglect can cause severe spatial disorientation, with complete inattention to the contralateral side of the body and environment. Parietal lesions may also cause apraxia—the inability to formulate and execute complex motor behaviors such as dressing or constructions, despite intact strength and coordination. Tumors of either parietal lobe can cause apraxia, but this condition is more common with tumors of the nondominant side. Disturbance of the deep parietal white matter can affect the optic radiations, causing a contralateral lower homonymous quadrantanopsia. Generalized and focal seizures can also develop from tumors within the parietal lobes. Focal seizures usually present as intermittent sensory phenomena on the contralateral side of the body.

Temporal lobe tumors (e.g., glioma, meningioma) may be clinically silent if located anteriorly. Seizures are common with medial and posterior neoplasms. Although these seizures are most often partial complex and associated with altered consciousness and motor automatisms, generalized seizures can also occur. Large superomedial tumors may cause motor deficits by compressing the adjacent frontal lobe. Dominant-side, medially placed tumors may cause loss of verbal memory, whereas nondominant-side lesions may affect visuospatial memory. Disturbance of deep white matter can cause a contralateral superior homonymous quadrantanopsia. Tumors affecting the uncus or parahippocampal gyrus (e.g., sphenoid wing meningioma) may cause olfactory hallucinations (e.g., metallic or unpleasant odors) and impaired memory. If the posterior aspect of the dominant superior temporal gyrus is affected, a fluent receptive dysphasia may develop, similar to Wernicke's.

Lesions affecting the occipital lobes (e.g., meningioma, metastasis, glioma) usually cause a contralateral partial or complete homonymous hemianopsia. In association with damage to the posterior corpus callosum, dominant-side occipital lobe tumors may present with the syndrome of alexia without agraphia, in which the patient is unable to read but has intact spoken and written language skills. Seizures caused by tumors of the occipital region are usually manifested as intermittent flashing lights or unformed images.

NEOPLASMS OF THE POSTERIOR FOSSA

Neoplasms of the posterior fossa are found significantly more often in children than in adults (Table 2). Not surprisingly, poor appetite, a change in school performance, weight loss, ataxia, dizziness, posterior neck pain, dysphagia (difficulty swallowing), and head tilt (caused by vertical misalignment of the eyes) are more common in children than in adults. Similarly, truncal or limb ataxia, nystagmus, bulbar weakness (weakness of palatal and pharyngeal muscles), gaze palsy, and opisthotonos are more frequent in children.

All tumors of the posterior fossa can cause obstructive hydrocephalus by impeding the flow of spinal fluid through the aqueduct of Sylvius or out the fourth ventricle. Common symptoms include headache, urinary incontinence, gait disorder, and dementia. Infants with unfused sutures may not have typical signs of increased ICP from hydrocephalus but may have accelerated head growth, irritability, and episodes of opisthotonos or stiffening of the extremities.

Neoplasms of the midline cerebellum (medulloblastoma, ependymoma) usually cause hydrocephalus. In addition, they often present with morning headaches, nausea, emesis, truncal ataxia, limb incoordination, diplopia, nystagmus, and dysarthria. Hemispheric cerebellar tumors (e.g., pilocystic or low-grade astrocytomas) also cause hydrocephalus, headaches, papilledema, nausea, and ipsilateral limb dysmetria. Infiltration of cerebellar tumors into the brain stem may produce pyramidal tract signs, spasticity, and gaze palsies.

Brain stem gliomas (usually astrocytomas) typically develop in children. They usually originate from the pons and then spread by infiltration of adjacent regions of the brain stem. Gait ataxia is the most common presenting symptom, often appearing in combination with diplopia, dysphagia, dysarthria, and head tilt. Parents often notice behavioral changes as well, including apathy, withdrawal, poor school performance, and impaired memory. Nausea and emesis may occur from compression or irritation of posterior fossa structures. On neurologic examination, these patients demonstrate gait ataxia, pyramidal tract signs, dysarthria, dysmetria, nystagmus, and cranial neuropathies (fifth, sixth, seventh, ninth, and tenth cranial nerves). Gaze palsies are also possible when tumors infiltrate pontine gaze centers, abducens nuclei, and the medial longitudinal fasciculus. Lesions confined to the midbrain can present with cerebellar symptoms and signs or with upgaze abnormalities if the dorsal region is involved. Tumors of the lower brain stem (e.g., foramen magnum meningioma) cause downbeat nystagmus, dysphagia, dysphonia, and pyramidal tract signs.

Tumors of the cerebellopontine angle are usually acoustic schwannomas (derived from the eighth cranial nerve), meningiomas of the petrous bone, epidermoid and dermoid cysts, schwannomas of other cranial nerves, and rare ependymomas. The early symptoms include unilateral slow loss of hearing and tinnitus. As the tumor enlarges, the fifth and seventh cranial nerves can be compressed, causing ipsilateral facial numbness and weakness.

NEOPLASMS OF THE PITUITARY REGION

Tumors of the pituitary region develop within the pituitary gland itself (e.g., pituitary adenomas and carcinomas, metastases) or from suprasellar tissues (e.g., craniopharyngioma, meningioma, epidermoid). Patients with pituitary region tumors present clinically with endocrine abnormalities or symptoms of mass effect (e.g., headache and cranial nerve dysfunction), or both. Small tumors less than 1 cm in diameter (mostly pituitary microadenomas) may remain totally asymptomatic. The headaches are caused by disturbance of the diaphragma sellae and other dural structures, usually with retro-orbital or bifrontal pain. Visual loss occurs frequently as tumors enlarge and encroach on nearby optic nerves and the optic chiasm. The classic pattern of visual loss is bitemporal hemianopsia in which tumors compress the optic chiasm from below. Other patterns of visual loss, including unilateral or homonymous hemianopsia, can also be observed. Rarely, a pituitary tumor can hemorrhage, causing pituitary apoplexy. The apoplectic patient experiences acute severe headache, confusion, nausea, oculomotor palsies, and sudden visual loss. Pituitary apoplexy is a neurosurgical emergency that must be recognized and treated quickly. Lateral extension of a pituitary region tumor can affect the cavernous sinus, in which the third, fourth, fifth (V_1 and V_2) and sixth cranial nerves course. Compression of these nerves by tumor will cause diplopia, partial or complete ophthalmoplegia, and facial numbness. Large tumors (e.g., pituitary macroadenoma, craniopharyngioma) may compress the inferomedial frontal lobes and foramen of Monro, causing personality changes or dementia and hydrocephalus. Endocrine abnormalities are common with pituitary adenomas and include various hormonal deficiency states, as well as hormone overproduction when secretory tumors are present (e.g., prolactinoma, growth hormone, adenocorticotropic hormone [ACTH]). A complete endocrine evaluation is indicated in all patients with a neoplasm of the pituitary region.

NEOPLASMS OF THE PINEAL REGION

Various tumors can develop in the pineal region, especially germinomas and other germ cell tumors, pineocytomas and pineoblastomas, meningiomas, gliomas, and metastatic neoplasms. Headache is common and results from increased ICP with or without associated hydrocephalus. Pineal tumors often cause hydrocephalus by compressing the aqueduct of Sylvius during its course through the midbrain. Compression of the nearby dorsal midbrain by tumor often causes Parinaud's syndrome, which consists of paralysis of upgaze, retraction nystagmus, pupillary light-near dissociation, and impaired convergence. Further compression or infiltration of tumor into the brain stem or cerebellum results in pyramidal tract signs, cranial nerve palsies, dysmetria, and ataxia. Several tumors of the pineal region (e.g., germinoma, pineoblastoma, nongerminomatous germ cell tumors) have a predilection for spinal fluid dissemination and may present with back pain, radiculopathy, or cranial neuropathies. Rarely, endocrine abnormalities are noted with pineal tumors, including diabetes insipidus and the onset of precocious puberty in children.

OTHER PRESENTATIONS

In children, hypothalamic tumors (usually astrocytomas) can present with lethargy and progressive emaciation as part of the diencephalic syndrome. Colloid cysts of the third ventricle can cause intermittent or acute hydrocephalus, with signs of increased ICP. If the cyst ruptures, a severe chemical meningitis may develop. Thalamic tumors cause headache, contralateral sensory loss, and contralateral pyramidal tract signs if the mass compresses the internal capsule. On the dominant side, thalamic neoplasms may cause a nonfluent form of dysphasia as well as behavioral changes that may resemble dementia. Tumors of the skull base (e.g., metastases, meningiomas, chordomas, schwannomas) typically present with headaches and multiple cranial neuropathies.

RADIOLOGIC DIAGNOSIS

In a patient with a history and neurologic examination suspicious for an intracranial neoplasm, neuroimaging is an essential tool for diagnosis. Computed tomography (CT) and magnetic resonance imaging (MRI) are both excellent for an initial screening evaluation of a mass lesion. The advantages of CT are its availability, rapid scanning capability (helpful for agitated or severely ill patients), and relatively low cost. However, CT scans do expose patients to radiation and are not very sensitive for small supratentorial tumors or for tumors in the posterior fossa (because of bone artifact). MRI does not expose patients to radiation and delineates normal and pathologic brain anatomy far better than does CT. Because the quality of MRI scans is not affected by the presence of bone, posterior fossa masses are easily demonstrated. However, MRI scans are time-consuming and therefore difficult to perform in agitated, uncooperative, claustrophic, or severely ill patients. They are also considerably more expensive than CT scans. MRI scans are generally contraindicated in patients with surgically implanted ferromagnetic metals.

Despite these limitations, MRI, in combination with the paramagnetic contrast agent gadolinium–diethylenetriamine penta-acetic acid (DTPA) has become the modality of choice for diagnosing intracranial neoplasms. The tumor appears as a region of altered signal with surrounding edema and mass effect (Fig. 1). The majority of malignant tumors enhance with contrast medium because of an alteration of the blood-brain barrier within tumor vasculature. In addition, MRI clearly demonstrates low-grade tumors and small metastatic lesions and allows the differentiation of vascular masses from tumors. Because there is no bone artifact, MRI is more sensitive than CT for detecting tumors in the posterior fossa involving the brain stem and cerebellum (Fig. 2). Also, magnetic resonance images can be formatted as multiplanar axial, coronal, and sagittal sections, which can be useful for detection of tumors in certain regions of the brain, such as the pituitary gland, medial temporal lobes, and posterior fossa.

Despite the overall superiority of MRI for the diagnosis of intracranial tumors, CT remains an excellent diagnostic technique. After the addition of a contrast agent, CT can readily demonstrate the enhancing mass, surrounding edema, and mass effect of the majority of tumors, especially if they are supratentorial (Fig. 3). Injection of contrast material should always be ordered for CT or MRI scans in the investigation of a possible brain tumor. The presence of a brain neoplasm cannot be excluded on the basis of a nonenhanced scan (especially when using CT). Contrast enhancement increases the sensitivity for discovering the tumor and also helps distinguish it from other lesions that may have a similar appearance (Table 5).

In the modern neuroimaging era of MRI and CT, older

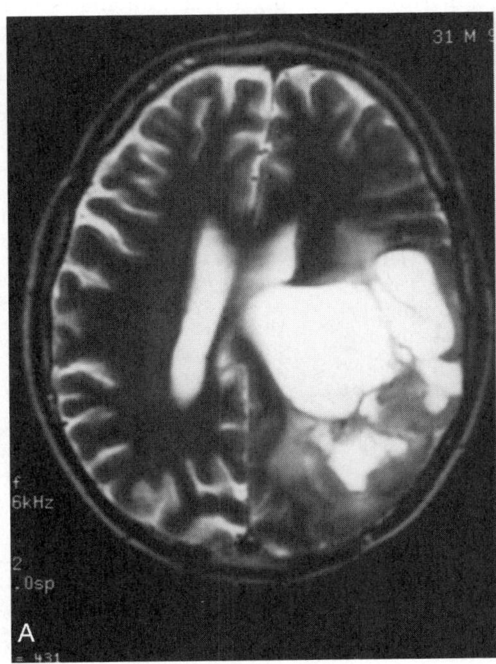

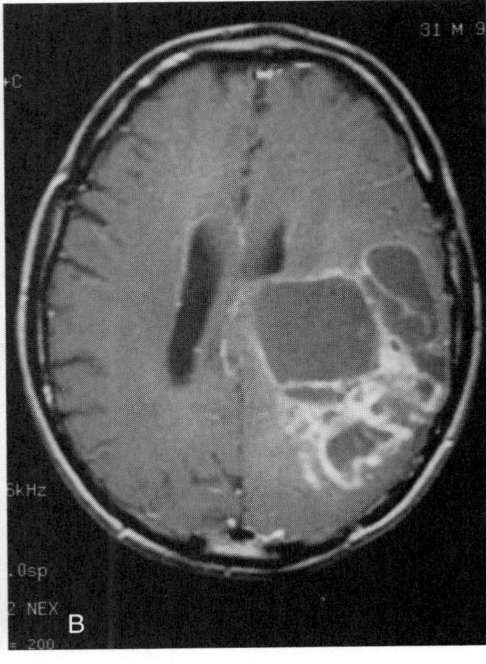

Figure 1. Magnetic resonance imaging (MRI) scan of a 28-year-old man with right arm focal seizures, mild dysphasia, and new headache. *A,* T2-weighted image demonstrating large, cystic lesion of mixed high signal within the left parietal lobe, with surrounding edema. *B,* T1-weighted image after contrast injection with gadolinium–diethylenetriamine penta-acetic acid (DTPA), demonstrating enhancment of the noncystic portions of the lesion. Resection and histopathologic examination revealed a glioblastoma multiforme. Note in both *A* and *B* the clear delineation of cystic and solid tumor from surrounding brain parenchyma and ventricles.

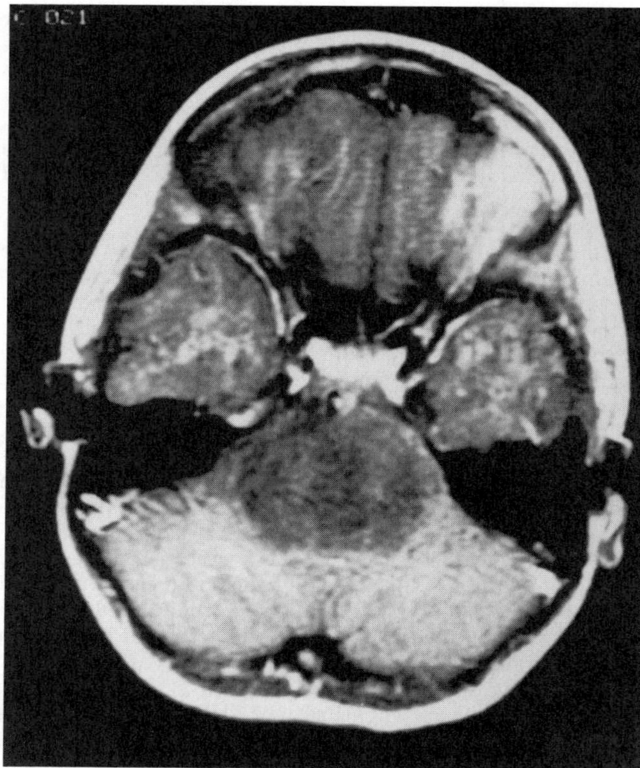

Figure 2. MRI scan of a 6-year-old boy with complaints of headache, slurring of speech, gait imbalance, leg stiffness, double vision, and weakness. This axial T1-weighted image shows a diffuse low-signal mass in the region of the pons. Histopathologic examination of the biopsy revealed a high-grade brain stem glioma.

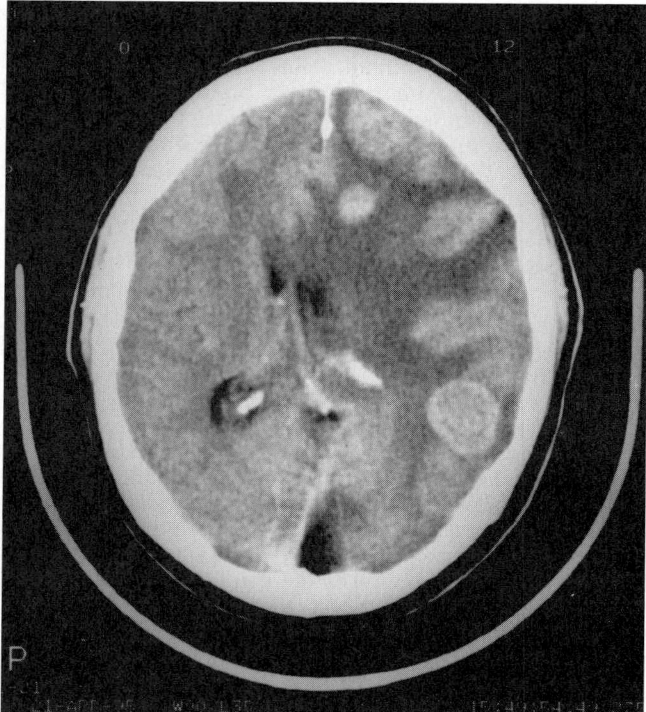

Figure 3. Computed tomographic scan of a 38-year-old man who complained of generalized seizures, headaches, expressive dysphasia, impaired memory, and gait instability. He was found to have a right lung mass that proved to be poorly differentiated adenocarcinoma at the time of resection. On the left side of the brain are two hyperdense metastatic lesions that enhance with contrast. The tumors are surrounded by hypodense peritumoral edema and cause a mass effect on the ipsilateral lateral ventricle.

techniques such as pneumoencephalography and radioisotopic brain scanning are no longer used to diagnose a suspected intracranial neoplasm. Cerebral angiography has also lost utility as an initial diagnostic modality for brain tumors. Before MRI, angiography was important for distinguishing a vascular malformation from a brain neoplasm. That distinction can now be made accurately with MRI in most patients. However, preoperative angiography may help the neurosurgeon evaluate the blood supply of a tumor or assess possible involvement of a tumor with major cerebral blood vessels.

All tumors that have a predilection for spread to the cerebrospinal fluid require further evaluation to determine the extent of disease. The evaluation frequently includes a myelogram or an enhanced MRI of the spine, as well as analysis of cerebrospinal fluid (see further on). Tumors that require this evaluation include medulloblastoma, germinoma, ependymoma, pineoblastoma, choroid plexus carcinoma, and nongerminomatous germ cell tumors. Evidence of tumor dissemination from the primary site to the spinal fluid or spinal neuraxis stratifies the patient into a high-risk group, thereby influencing subsequent treatment decisions.

OTHER DIAGNOSTIC TESTS

Because CT and MRI are so sensitive, ancillary tests such as electroencephalography and lumbar puncture are not required for routine diagnosis of intracranial neoplasms. Electroencephalography can be used to determine the presence of a seizure focus or to assist in seizure classification. However, the clinical presentation and history are generally more helpful than electroencephalographic testing for the diagnosis of a tumor-related seizure disorder. Lumbar puncture is not required for the diagnosis of the vast majority of brain tumors. In fact, a spinal tap is contraindicated in many patients owing to increased ICP and mass effect, which could induce herniation during the procedure. There are few indications for a lumbar puncture

Table 5. Differential Diagnoses of Primary Brain Tumors on Computed Tomography and Magnetic Resonance Imaging

Diagnosis	Comments
Abscess	Mature (capsule); bacterial, fungal
Multiple sclerosis	Large solitary demyelinated plaque
Hematoma	Distinguish from tumor with hemorrhage
Granulomatous lesions	Tuberculosis, sarcoidosis
Parasitic infections	Cysticercosis
Vascular malformations	Arteriovenous usually
Infarct	Enhancement and mass effect resolve with time
Progressive multifocal leukoencephalopathy	Uncommon

From Newton, H.B.: Primary brain tumors: Review of etiology, diagnosis, and treatment. Am. Fam. Phys., 49:787–797, 1994, with permission of the American Academy of Family Physicians.

in a brain tumor patient (if a myelogram is performed, spinal fluid can be obtained at that time). As mentioned earlier, an assessment is helpful in patients harboring tumors that often spread to the spinal fluid and neuraxis or for patients who have symptoms consistent with carcinomatous meningitis. Cerebrospinal fluid cytologic examination and tumor markers are useful for diagnosing meningeal tumor. The most helpful tumor markers are β-glucuronidase and β_2-microglobulin, unless the patient has a pineal region mass. Many of the germ cell tumors that arise from the pineal region (e.g., germinoma) are associated with increased cerebrospinal fluid concentrations of alpha-fetoprotein and human chorionic gonadotropin. These tumor markers can be used to assess the effectiveness of therapy and to monitor for possible recurrence. For patients with MRI scans that are consistent with a mass or large demyelinating plaque from multiple sclerosis, cerebrospinal fluid can be analyzed for IgG indices and the presence of oligoclonal bands.

Patients with tumors of the pituitary gland and surrounding region require a screening endocrine evaluation to assess for hormonal deficiency or hypersecretion. This information will be helpful for diagnosis and subsequent therapy. In patients with tumors that affect the visual pathways (including pituitary tumors), a neuro-ophthalmologic examination can document visual acuity, visual field deficits, and oculomotor function.

Tumors of the cerebellopontine angle (e.g., acoustic schwannoma) can be readily visualized by enhanced MRI. However, further assessment with audiologic, vestibular, and brain stem auditory evoked potential testing may add further information for a more precise diagnosis.

In many large academic and private hospital nuclear medicine departments, single photon emission computed tomography (SPECT) scans are available. Single photon emission tomography scans using thallium (which evaluates metabolic activity inside the target area) can be helpful when it is unclear whether a new or recurrent mass is viable tumor (which appears as a hot spot) or necrosis (e.g., following radiation, stroke, abscess; appears as a cold spot).

COMMON DIAGNOSTIC DILEMMAS

As mentioned earlier, many of the common neurologic signs and symptoms of patients with intracranial neoplasms (see Tables 3 and 4) are not specific to brain tumors. The progressive nature of these complaints will eventually distinguish them from their non-neoplastic counterparts. Headaches occur frequently in the general population. The vast majority of these headaches are not related to intracranial tumors. Acute and chronic tension headaches present with head and neck pain described as tight, pressing, squeezing, and bandlike. They are often precipitated by fatigue, family crises, work deadlines, or other stressful situations. Tension headaches respond well to mild analgesics and, after cessation of the causative stimulus, usually improve. Migraine headaches are typically described as pounding or throbbing and are often associated with nausea, emesis, and photophobia. Cluster headaches occur in periodic cycles and are extremely painful. The pain usually affects one eye and is associated with ipsilateral scleral injection, tearing, rhinorrhea, and sinus congestion. Distinguishing brain tumor–related headaches from other common headaches by history is difficult. Older patients who have previously been free from headaches and now experience them should be evaluated carefully. Patients with stable headache disorders that have a well-described pain pattern who then complain of a new type of headache, or of a progressive worsening of their headaches, need close observation and possibly neuroimaging. A normal neurologic examination and the absence of papilledema significantly decrease the likelihood of a brain neoplasm but do not exclude it. The possibility of glaucoma or temporal arteritis should be assessed with tonometry and measurement of the erythrocyte sedimentation rate. Other common conditions that may cause headaches, including hypertension, allergies, cervical degenerative joint disease, oral contraceptive use, and visual refractive errors, should be considered. Nausea and emesis are common symptoms of numerous gastrointestinal ailments. When these symptoms occur as part of the presentation of a brain tumor, the clinician may significantly delay proper diagnosis and treatment if a central nervous system cause is not considered. Extensive gastrointestinal evaluations are occasionally performed early in the course of brain neoplasms, when nausea and emesis may be prominent while other symptoms are more subtle (e.g., spasticity, gait difficulty, weakness, diplopia, and so on). This happens most often in children with posterior fossa tumors.

The clinical presentation of non-neoplastic disorders can occasionally suggest the presence of a brain tumor. Focal symptoms and signs can be seen with multiple sclerosis, stroke, abscess, enlarging aneurysm, encephalitis, infectious or neoplastic meningitis, and cerebral vasculitis. A detailed history and neurologic examination, enhanced MRI and, if necessary, cerebrospinal fluid analysis usually distinguish these diseases from an intracranial neoplasm. On occasion, the CT or MRI results are equivocal and the diagnosis remains unclear (see Table 5). Cerebral abscess is the only entity seen in Table 5 that typically has a progressive course and ring-enhancing appearance similar to that of a brain tumor on contrast-enhanced CT or MRI. Biopsy is often required to distinguish an intracranial tumor from an abscess or, less frequently, the other disorders listed in the table.

DELIRIUM AND DEMENTIA

By Michael H. Bross, M.D.,
and Nancy O. Tatum, M.D.
Jackson, Mississippi

Delirium and dementia are common conditions that impair cognitive function, especially in the elderly. Determining the cause of mental decline is often difficult, owing to the numerous medical and psychosocial factors that can adversely affect cognition. Delirium and dementia can coexist or can be complicated by underlying depression. The management and prognosis of delirium, dementia, and depression are very different. Delirium calls for quick diagnosis and correction, whereas dementia and depression are diagnosed and treated over a longer period of time. Correct diagnosis is essential for reducing the high morbidity and mortality of these disorders.

DELIRIUM

Synonyms include acute organic brain syndrome, toxic encephalopathy, acute confusional state, exogenous reaction, symptomatic psychosis, and toxic psychosis.

Definition and Presenting Signs and Symptoms

Delirium is defined by the *Diagnostic and Statistical Manual of Mental Disorders,* Fourth Edition (DSM-IV), of the American Psychiatric Association, as inattentiveness with a disturbance of consciousness. Delirium is acute or subacute and develops over hours or days. The diagnosis of delirium is based on observation, mental status testing, and reports from sources close to the patient. Treatment is determined by the specific cause identified.

Delirium is a very common condition in the hospitalized elderly. Thinking is disorganized, with the severity of the condition fluctuating during the day and often becoming worse at night. Incoherent or rambling speech may be the first evidence of delirium. Typically, the process is transient and characterized by clouded consciousness. Disorientation to time and place is common. Delusions, illusions, and hallucinations often occur. Short-term memory is impaired more often than remote memory.

Delirium is associated with three distinct presentations: hyperactive, hypoactive, and mixed. Restlessness, rapid speech, and irritability reflect increased psychomotor activity in the hyperactive delirious patient. The hypoactive delirious patient may be apathetic, with slowed speech and decreased alertness. The mixed patient tends to alternate between hypoactive and hyperactive characteristics.

Table 1. Common Causes of Delirium

Prescription drugs
- Sedative-hypnotics (intoxication and withdrawal)
- Anticonvulsants
- Antidepressants
- Antihistamines
- Antihypertensive drugs
- Antiparkinsonian drugs, including amantadine (Symmetrel)
- Corticosteroids
- Digitalis
- Histamine H_2 receptor antagonists
- Narcotics
- Phenothiazines

Drugs of abuse
- Alcohol
- Cocaine
- Lysergic acid diethylamide (LSD)
- Marijuana
- Amphetamines

Toxins
- Anticholinesterase substances
- Organophosphates
- Carbon monoxide
- Carbon dioxide

Volatile substances
- Fuel
- Paint
- Glue
- Solvents

Infections
- Meningitis
- Pneumonia
- Sepsis
- Pyelonephritis

Cardiac illness
- Arrhythmias
- Congestive heart failure
- Myocardial infarction

Metabolic disturbances
- Fluid and electrolyte disturbances
- Hypercalcemia
- Hypoglycemia and hyperglycemia
- Hypoxia
- Liver failure
- Renal failure

Central nervous system disorders
- Epilepsy
- Vascular injury

Neoplasms
- Metastases to brain
- Primary brain tumors

Urinary retention and/or fecal impaction

Trauma
- Anesthesia
- Burns
- Fractures (especially hips)
- Surgery

Location change
- Hospitalization (especially intensive care)

Course of the Process

The failure to recognize delirium or to identify its underlying cause in a timely manner can result in high morbidity and mortality. A high index of suspicion is therefore required in patients at risk if the complications associated with delirium are to be averted. The onset of delirium is usually abrupt, and its resolution may be equally abrupt. In many patients, delirium has several causes. The risk of delirium rises significantly as the number of potential coexisting causes increases.

The course of delirium as well as its classification is determined by its cause (Table 1). Delirium that accompanies a general medical condition must be a direct physiological consequence of the condition that causes the cognitive impairment. Through history taking, physical examination, or assessment of laboratory data, a temporal relationship is established that relates the onset, exacerbation, or remission of the delirium to the medical condition. Delirium may be induced by the side effects of medication, multiple toxins, drug intoxication, or withdrawal from various substances. The most frequently seen and best described delirium is the delirium tremens associated with alcohol withdrawal. Occasionally, delirium occurs in the absence of evidence of any of the causes listed in Table 1. In these patients, the disorder is classified as delirium not otherwise specified.

The outcome of delirium varies with the cause. Many patients fully recover to baseline status. Others progress to a more chronic condition that may be the result of previously unrecognized or irreversible processes. Death may also occur if the underlying causes of delirium are not determined and corrected.

Risk factors and How to Identify Them

A number of factors have been associated with the onset of delirium. The mnemonic SUNDOWNERS has been used to describe those risks:

*S*ick
*U*rinary retention/fecal impaction
*N*ew environment
*D*emented
*O*ld
*W*rithing in pain
*N*ot adequately evaluated
*E*yes and ears
*R*x—therapeutic drug intoxication
*S*leep deprived

One of the frequent precipitating causes of delirium, especially in the elderly, is hospitalization. Perhaps the changes in circadian hormones, superimposed on the reduced lighting of night, allow misinterpretation of auditory and visual stimuli. Delirium commonly occurs in the postoperative period and is frequently related to perioperative hypotension or hypoxemia, pain, and the use of anticholinergic or sedating drugs. Falls, especially in the elderly, are frequently associated with the agitation and disorientation of delirium. Fractures occur that may require surgery, increasing once again the risk of developing delirium.

Expected and Unusual Findings on Physical Examination

A diagnosis of delirium is based on the history and physical findings. Owing to the multitude of causes, there are no pathognomonic physical findings. Significant deviation from the patient's baseline mental status must be ascertained from family, friends, or healthcare personnel who have witnessed a decline in function. The clinician should determine the onset of confusion, alterations of sleep patterns, and any history of previous mental disturbance. Past medical history, current medications, social history, and a complete review of body systems may suggest one or more causes of the delirium.

The diagnosis of delirium requires an abnormal mental status examination. Screening tests, including the Mini-Mental State examination and Short Portable Mental Status Questionnaire, are useful and easy to administer. The Short Portable Mental Status Questionnaire (Fig. 1) tests for orientation, recent memory, remote memory, attention, and calculation. The test can be administered to patients with visual and motor impairments. The score is adjusted for age, race, and level of education. Three or more errors indicate intellectual impairment.

The Mini-Mental State examination (Fig. 2) tests for orientation, recent memory, registration, recall, attention, calculation, language, and praxis. The test has a maximum score of 30 points. A score of less than 24 points indicates cognitive impairment. Scores are artificially low in patients with less formal education, different cultural backgrounds, motor problems, and visual problems.

Further evidence of delirium includes rambling speech, misperceptions of stimuli, and poorly connected thoughts demonstrated by inconsistent responses to test questions. Inability to concentrate, distractibility, confabulation, and emotional lability are also characteristic of delirium.

A comprehensive physical examination may uncover the probable cause of delirium. Tachycardia and increased temperature suggest infection. Careful examination of the chest and abdomen may reveal a pulmonary, gastrointestinal, or genitourinary source of infection. Peripheral edema, basilar rales, tachycardia, and abnormal heart sounds suggest a cardiac cause. Focal neurologic deficits are consistent with head trauma or cerebrovascular accident. Restlessness or tremor may indicate alcohol withdrawal. Asterixis and myoclonus suggest metabolic encephalopathy. Urinary incontinence and anorexia occur in many types of delirium, especially in the elderly. Muscle wasting is also common in delirious elderly patients.

Useful Laboratory Procedures

The history and physical findings dictate the extent and direction of laboratory evaluation. Baseline evaluation

Short Portable Mental Status Questionnaire

Check Errors		
________	1.	What is the date today? (month, day, year)
________	2.	What day of the week is it?
________	3.	What is the name of this place?
________	4.	What is your telephone number?
________	4A.	What is your street address? (Ask only if patient does not have a telephone.)
________	5.	How old are you?
________	6.	When were you born?
________	7.	Who is the President of the United States?
________	8.	Who was the President just before him?
________	9.	What was your mother's maiden name?
________	10.	Subtract 3 from 20 and keep subtracting 3 from each new number, all the way down.
________		Total Number of Errors

Scoring the Short Portable Mental Status Questionnaire

Data suggest that education and race influence performance on the questionnaire, so they must be considered in evaluating an individual's score.

For scoring purposes, three educational levels have been established:

1. Grade school education only
2. Any high school education or high school graduation
3. Any education beyond high school: college, graduate school, or business school

For white subjects with at least some high school, but not more than high school education:

0–2 Errors	Intact intellectual functioning
3–4 Errors	Mild intellectual impairment
5–7 Errors	Moderate intellectual impairment
8–10 Errors	Severe intellectual impairment

Allow one more error if subject has had only a grade school education.
Allow one less error if subject has had education beyond high school.
Allow one more error for black subjects, using identical education criteria.

Figure 1. The Short Portable Mental Status Questionnaire. (Adapted from Pfeiffer, E.: A short portable mental status questionnaire for the assessment of organic brain deficits in elderly patients. J. Am. Geriatr. Soc. 22:433–443, 1975, with permission.)

MINI-MENTAL STATE

Maximum Score	Score	
		ORIENTATION
5	( )	What is the (year) (season) (date) (day) (month)?
5	( )	Where are we: (state) (county) (town) (hospital) (floor).
		REGISTRATION
3	( )	Name 3 objects: 1 second to say each. Then ask the patient all 3 after you have said them. Give 1 point for each correct answer. Then repeat them until he learns all 3. Count trials and record. Trials
		ATTENTION AND CALCULATION
5	( )	Serial 7's. 1 point for each correct. Stop after 5 answers. Alternatively spell "world" backwards.
		RECALL
3	( )	Ask for the 3 objects repeated above. Give 1 point for each correct.
		LANGUAGE
9	( )	Name a pencil, and watch (2 points) Repeat the following: "No ifs, ands, or buts." (1 point) Follow a 3-stage command: "Take a paper in your right hand, fold it in half, and put it on the floor" (3 points) Read and obey the following: CLOSE YOUR EYES (1 point) Write a sentence (1 point) Copy design (1 point)

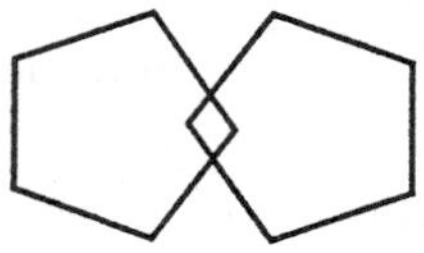

ASSESS level of consciousness along a continuum

Alert Drowsy Stupor Coma

30	
Maximum Score	Patient Total

*Score of 23 or less indicates cognitive disturbance.

Figure 2. Mini–Mental State examination. (Adapted from Folstein, M.F., Folstein, S.E, McHugh, P.R.: "Mini-mental state": A practical method for grading the cognitive state of patients for the clinician. J. Psychiatr. Res. 12:189–198, 1975, with permission.)

should include a complete blood count, chemistry profile, electrolytes, urinalysis, chest film, and electrocardiogram. Blood tests for syphilis, thyroid dysfunction, vitamin B_{12}, and folic acid may also be indicated. Low serum albumin, reflecting protein calorie malnutrition or major organ dysfunction, is commonly found. If poisoning or overdose is suspected, urine drug or heavy metal screens may be warranted. Any evidence of infection requires appropriate cultures, and suspicion of meningitis requires lumbar puncture. Abnormal cardiopulmonary findings necessitate an evaluation of cardiac enzymes and arterial blood gases. An abnormal electroencephalogram may help the clinician distinguish delirium from an acute psychotic state.

The radiographic studies used in the diagnosis of delirium are limited to those specifically needed to verify suspected underlying medical conditions. Chest films may provide evidence of pneumonia, tumor, or congestive heart failure. Computed tomography or magnetic resonance imaging of the brain may reveal signs of central nervous system trauma or vascular injury.

Pitfalls and Errors in Diagnosis

The differential diagnosis of delirium includes all other causes of confusion. Most commonly, the clinician must distinguish delirium from dementia, acute functional psychosis, and depression. However, delirium may also be superimposed on depression or dementia. In addition, the quiet, nondisruptive, hypoactive form of delirium may be seen more frequently in elderly patients and may be misdiagnosed as dementia.

The confusion associated with delirium has a sudden onset, whereas the confusion associated with dementia has an insidious onset. The course of dementia is stable, whereas the fluctuating pattern of delirium has nocturnal exacerbations. Both are associated with impaired cognition, but patients with dementia frequently have clear consciousness and can maintain attention. The hallucinations, fleeting delusions, illusions, and fluctuating psychomotor activity seen in delirium are frequently absent in dementia.

Like delirium, acute functional psychosis has a sudden onset. Consciousness is clear, whereas attention may be disordered. The course of the psychosis is typically stable, with auditory hallucinations predominating and delusions remaining sustained and systematic. The physical illness or drug toxicity associated with delirium is absent in acute functional psychosis.

A diagnosis of delirium requires a high index of suspicion in patients known to be at risk or in patients with the acute onset of confusion or altered mental status. The clinician should avoid the pitfall of merely ordering restraints, rather than carefully examining the patient, when a sudden change in behavior is reported. Rapid identification of the underlying organic cause can prevent the significant morbidity and mortality associated with this illness. By preventing permanent brain damage through rapid diagnosis and treatment, expensive institutional care can be avoided.

DEMENTIA

Synonyms include chronic organic brain syndrome and chronic encephalopathy.

Definition and Presenting Signs and Symptoms

Dementia is defined by the DSM-IV as a decline in the thought process that is severe enough to interfere with occupational or social functioning. Memory is always impaired, and at least one of the following disorders is present: aphasia, agnosia, apraxia, or a disturbance in executive functioning. Dementia is typically a chronic process with a duration of more than 1 month. Dementia cannot be diagnosed when an acute, fluctuating thought pattern is accompanied by altered consciousness. If significant disturbance of cognition persists after the sensorium clears, dementia becomes a likely diagnosis.

The memory impairment associated with dementia is more severe than mild day-to-day forgetfulness. Many people misplace their car keys or forget to feed the cat. This forgetfulness has little consequence. In contrast, a patient with dementia may get lost while walking around the neighborhood or forget where the bathroom is located. Forgetting to turn off the stove, forgetting appointments, and forgetting to stop the car before opening the door are other behaviors that often have serious consequences. Such memory problems can strain interpersonal relationships and may result in harm to the patient.

Aphasia is the disorder of language, with impairment of speaking and/or understanding speech. The patient may have difficulty in recalling a word and compensate by saying "small person" instead of child, for example. Substituting a word that sounds similar, such as "wild" for child, may also occur. When patients are unable to answer questions, they may compensate by responding with a vague answer such as, "Oh, you know." When a patient has trouble understanding speech, family members may interpret this as uncooperative behavior. A simple request, such as "please get ready for church," may not be followed by appropriate actions because the patient with dementia may not understand the meaning of "ready for church."

Agnosia is the inability to recognize or name objects despite the ability to see or feel them. A person with agnosia may not know the purpose or name of a toothbrush or fork. Progression of dementia can lead to failure to recognize family members and even oneself. Individuals with agnosia have mistaken mirror reflections of themselves for intruders.

Apraxia is indicated by a person's having problems with performing simple activities despite having the necessary sensation, motor function, and understanding. A person with apraxia may experience difficulty in brushing the teeth, tying shoes, cooking, going to the bathroom, bathing, and using eating utensils. Intense frustration may lead the person with apraxia to avoid simple tasks. When family members insist on certain behaviors, the individual with dementia may erupt in anger. Calm understanding, gentle assistance, and simplifying tasks are often effective interventions when dementia is the underlying problem.

Problems with executive function reflect the inability to think abstractly and to carry out complex activities. An elderly woman, formerly an outstanding cook, may develop problems with buying groceries and preparing meals. Financial mismanagement may occur, as in buying a second new car or failing to pay the mortgage despite many late notices. Problems with driving a car may result in traffic violations and accidents.

The prevalence of dementia rises sharply with advanced age. Dementia affects 5 to 10 per cent of persons older than 65 years of age. Nearly 50 per cent of the population older than 85 years of age is affected. Dementia is unusual in children and adolescents but, when it does occur, adversely affects development and school performance.

Atypical presentations of dementia make the diagnosis more difficult. Patients with early dementia may have insight into their loss of cognitive function and suffer from secondary depression, which directs attention away from the underlying dementia. A well-educated, organized person may compensate for the losses of early dementia with notes and reminders. Many social skills may remain, allowing for pleasant conversation. The activities of life that require higher function, such as driving a car and managing finances, may be severely affected and may go unnoticed until a crisis arises. Chronic diseases may also mask or mimic the signs of dementia. Decreased vision, poor hearing, incontinence, arthritis, and other common diseases often lead to social isolation. A supportive spouse or relative may compensate for physical problems without recognizing the mental decline. The slow progression of dementia may go unnoticed by family members and physicians as they concentrate on medical illnesses. When a severe medical illness occurs, the patient with dementia is placed in an unfamiliar hospital environment. Delirium often occurs and directs attention to the patient's mental status. With appropriate medical and supportive care, the delirium resolves, and the signs of early dementia become apparent.

Course of the Process

The course of dementia varies according to the underlying brain injury. If the dementia is secondary to a treatable systemic or neurologic disease, the dementia may remit. Occasionally, dementia is caused by a single brief episode of brain trauma or cerebral anoxia. The mental deterioration may stabilize and remain static for years. More often, the pathologic process continues and the patient experiences progressive intellectual deterioration over months to years. Close attention to the present and past medical history (Table 2) can alert the clinician to the correct cate-

Table 2. History and Physical Findings: Types of Dementia

Dementia Type	Common Findings
Alzheimer's dementia	Gradual onset in patients older than 65 years of age is typical; onset at younger age is associated with positive family history Frontal release signs may occur: root, snout, suck, grasp, and palm-chin reflexes
Vascular dementia	Prior cardiovascular disease and cerebrovascular accidents; abrupt steplike deterioration Hypertension, carotid bruits, decreased pulses, focal and lateralizing neurologic signs
Dementias Due to General Medical Conditions	
Pick's disease	Onset usually occurs after age 65 years Frontal release signs and temporal lobe signs
Creutzfeldt-Jakob disease	Rapidly progressive dementia; onset after age 50 years Myoclonic jerking, severe rigidity, asymmetrical reflexes
Huntington's disease	Onset in middle adult life; autosomal dominant inheritance Slowly progressive choreiform movements and dementia
Parkinson's disease	Onset after age 50 years Tremor at rest, cogwheel rigidity, bradykinesia, and shuffling gait Gradual onset of dementia in advanced Parkinson's disease
Normal-pressure hydrocephalus	History of prior head injury, meningitis, or subarachnoid hemorrhage Apractic gait, incontinence
Progressive supranuclear palsy	Onset after age 50 years; history of frequent falls Inability to gaze downward; dysarthria; and extrapyramidal signs Dementia is usually mild
Intracranial tumor	Severe headaches, seizures History of malignancy Focal neurologic signs, papilledema
Neurosyphilis	History of prior syphilis infection Progressive stroke symptoms may occur; Argyll Robertson pupils, optic atrophy, footslap, atactic gait
Multiple sclerosis	Onset usually in early adulthood; recurrent episodes of neurologic dysfunction and remission Gradual progression of disease; dementia may occur with extensive cerebral disease Optic disc pallor, brain stem signs, spinal cord signs, and cerebellar signs are common
Wilson's disease	Onset before age 40 years Personal and family history of hepatic and neurologic dysfunction Psychiatric disorders, extrapyramidal signs, corneal Kayser-Fleischer rings
Head trauma	Prior severe head injury or repeated trauma (as in boxing)
Subdural hematoma	History of falls
Other diffuse brain injuries	History of severe anoxia, hypoglycemia, encephalitis, exposure to radiation
Human immunodeficiency virus (HIV) disease	History of high-risk sexual behavior or intravenous drug use Weight loss, severe seborrheic dermatitis, Kaposi's sarcomas, and repeated infections
Renal dysfunction	Renal failure requiring dialysis Uremic symptoms
Hepatic dysfunction	Severe liver disease: asterixis, ascites, jaundice
Vitamin B_{12} deficiency	History of gastric surgery; loss of sense of vibration and position, hyperreflexia, spasticity
Hypothyroidism	History of thyroid surgery or replacement Delayed relaxation of deep tendon reflexes, dry skin, weight gain
Meningitis	Impaired immunity, as with HIV disease or chemotherapy Nuccal rigidity, headache
Substance-Induced Persisting Dementias	
Alcohol, inhalants	History of substance abuse; wide-based atactic gait and signs of liver disease
Medications	History of excessive sedative, hypnotic, or anxiolytic use Anticonvulsant medications and intrathecal methotrexate
Toxins	Toxic exposure to carbon monoxide, organophosphate insecticides, industrial solvents, lead, or mercury

gorization of the dementia. For the purposes of this article, the DSM-IV classification system has been applied.

Alzheimer's dementia characteristically begins after age 65 years but may occur between the ages of 40 and 90. Memory disturbances are gradually followed by aphasia, agnosia, and apraxia. In the later stages of the disease, abnormalities of gait and motor function occur. Patients are usually bedridden when death occurs from secondary complications such as pneumonia and sepsis.

Patients with vascular dementia have a history of vascular disease or associated risk factors (e.g., prior strokes, hypertension, diabetes, and cardiac disease). The course of vascular dementia is characterized by stepwise deterioration as additional cerebral infarcts occur.

Dementia can result from head trauma or a number of general medical conditions. Recent head trauma suggests subdural hematoma as the cause of the dementia. Remote head injury, subarachnoid hemorrhage, and meningitis all are risk factors for normal-pressure hydrocephalus. Frequently, the history does not indicate these risk factors, but a history of incontinence or gait disturbance is usually present with normal-pressure hydrocephalus. Prior gastric resection or thyroidectomy suggests vitamin B_{12} deficiency or hypothyroidism, respectively. A seizure history suggests a focal brain injury or a tumor. The onset of choreiform movements in early adulthood, coupled with a family history of early-onset dementia, suggests Huntington's disease. Human immunodeficiency virus (HIV) infection strongly suggests encephalopathy related to acquired immunodeficiency syndrome (AIDS), a more common type of dementia in young adults. The onset of hepatitis and extrapyramidal signs in adolescents and young adults suggests Wilson's disease. Myoclonus in a middle-aged patient, with rapid progression of dementia over several months, may indicate Creutzfeldt-Jakob disease. Extrapyramidal symptoms beginning in middle-aged and older adults are consistent with Parkinson's disease.

Substance-induced dementia can be diagnosed only when the symptoms of dementia persist long after the substance has been cleared from the body. A history of alcohol and drug abuse may be concealed or minimized, and additional family input may be required for diagnosis. Occupational and other exposures to lead, carbon monoxide, and other neurotoxic agents may also cause chronic dementia.

Physical Examination

The physical examination is essential in the diagnosis of dementia and greatly assists in determining the type of dementia. All findings must be interpreted with respect to the patient's social context and highest level of function. A man who had previously taught accounting at a university would not be expected to speak and dress the same as a man with a fourth-grade education who had worked as a day laborer.

Mental Status Examination

The mental status examination begins with the presentation and interview of the patient. Is the patient alert and medically stable? A decreased level of consciousness and acute illness suggest delirium, a condition that must be resolved before dementia can be reliably diagnosed. What is the patient's appearance and dress? A lack of attention to personal grooming may be a sign of significant cognitive decline. Does the patient speak for himself? The patient must be personally acknowledged and respected as the focus of the examination and given time to reply to questions. If visual and hearing problems are recognized, adjustments can be made to assist the patient. The clinician can sit close to the patient in a well-lit room, speak slowly in a clear voice, and have the patient use any available hearing aid. Can the patient answer written questions? Although hearing and visual impairments may suggest dementia, alternative methods of communication may verify intact cognitive function (as demonstrated so incredibly by Helen Keller). Is the patient's speech understandable and clear? Can the patient express complex thoughts? Limited use of specific words, with many vague descriptions, usually indicates expressive language problems. Are there signs of emotional distress, such as a flat affect, downcast eyes, and frequent sighing? Signs of depression must not be overlooked because depression may mimic dementia.

Many patients retain social skills and become adept at concealing day-to-day problems associated with dementia. Mental status screening tests can detect subtle cognitive decline and can provide a simple means of assessing changes in cognitive function over time. Two mental status screening tests are widely used in clinical practice: the Short Portable Mental Status Questionnaire and the Mini-Mental State examination (see Figs. 1 and 2).

Additional mental status examination techniques often prove valuable. Test agnosia by asking patients to name common objects, such as a pen, key, and watch. Test object identification by touch. Test apraxia by asking the patient to tie shoelaces or brush the teeth. Test reasoning and judgment by asking the patient: "What would you do if you found a wallet? What would you do if you were planning to go on vacation next week?" (Proverb interpretation is not recommended because many intellectually intact people experience difficulty with this test.) Test concentration by asking the patient to repeat a sequence of digits. The average mentally-intact individual can repeat at least five digits. Use clock drawing to test spatial ability and executive function.

Additional Physical Assessment

The clinician should perform a comprehensive physical examination to detect comorbid conditions that may contribute to cognitive dysfunction. Medical disorders are common in fragile elderly patients and are often overlooked. Physical signs of malnutrition, hypoxia from chronic lung disease, congestive heart failure, and drug toxicity must be recognized. Treatment of comorbid illness must precede any reliable diagnosis of dementia.

Thorough examination may also uncover specific signs associated with the different types of dementia. Common physical findings are summarized in Table 2. Cranial nerve evaluation must include an examination of visual fields. Homonymous hemianopia suggests infarction in the posterior cortex. Bitemporal hemianopia is a classic finding in patients with pituitary tumors. Unilateral central facial weakness suggests a lateralizing process, especially vascular dementia. Dysfunction of the glossopharyngeal and vagus nerves often produces dysphagia and dysarthria consistent with pseudobulbar palsy dementia and vascular dementia.

Motor examination should include tests of strength, evaluation of gait, and notation of any involuntary movements. Unilateral weakness and spastic gait are consistent with previous infarction. Bilateral lower extremity weakness may result from spinal cord impingement (possible tumor), neuropathic processes (e.g., alcoholic neuropathy), or normal-pressure hydrocephalus. Myoclonus, the random jerking of small muscle groups, suggests Creutzfeldt-Jakob disease. Chorea, the random movement of large muscle groups, is characteristic of Huntington's disease. Resting tremor, cogwheel rigidity, and a shuffling gait typify Parkinson's disease. A wide-based gait occurs in alcohol-induced dementia, neurosyphilis, and normal-pressure hydrocephalus.

Sensory, reflex, and cerebellar examinations are also indicated. Marked loss of position and vibratory sensation, with hyperreflexia and spasticity, suggests vitamin B_{12} deficiency. Peripheral neuropathy with hyporeflexia may indicate diabetic or toxin damage. Upper motor neuron disease often results in hyperreflexia, clonus, and Babinski's signs. The frontal release signs (see Table 2) may occur with normal aging and should be noted only if very prominent. The glabellar reflex, persistent blinking as the forehead is tapped, is present in dementia with Parkinson's disease. Cerebellar disease is indicated by prominent intention (action) tremor, dysarthria, and the inability to perform rapid alternating movements.

Useful Laboratory Procedures

Laboratory tests for suspected dementia are summarized in Table 3. Studies that have consistent value are listed

Table 3. Diagnostic Laboratory Tests for Suspected Dementia

Indicated Studies	Significance of Abnormalities
Complete blood count	Infection, anemia, possible vitamin B_{12} deficiency or alcoholism (with macrocytosis), blood disorders
Erythrocyte sedimentation rate	Inflammation (possible infection, malignancy, or collagen vascular disease)
Urinalysis	Infection, diabetes, liver disease, renal disease
Serum electrolytes	Hyponatremia suggests water intoxication, syndrome of inappropriate antidiuretic hormone (SIADH), excessive diuresis, or Addison's disease Hypernatremia suggests dehydration (consider immobility and neglect)
Calcium, phosphorus	Malignancy, hyperparathyroidism
Albumin	Severe chronic disease and/or malnutrition
Blood glucose	Diabetes, hypoglycemia
SUN/creatinine	Acute or chronic renal dysfunction
Liver function tests	Hepatocellular or obstructive liver disease; alcoholism, Wilson's disease
Thyroid function tests	Hypothyroidism, hyperthyroidism
Medication levels	Toxic levels
Serum vitamin B_{12}, folate	Pernicious anemia, malnutrition
VDRL; FTA-ABS or MHA-TP	Syphilis; obtain FTA-ABS or MHA-TP routinely, as VDRL often negative in late syphilis
Chest film	Pulmonary disease, cardiac disease, tumor
Electrocardiogram	Cardiac disease
Studies That May Be Indicated	
Computed tomography or magnetic resonance imaging scan	Cortical atrophy, ventricular enlargement, hematoma, hygroma, tumor, white and gray matter vascular lesions, infection
Neuropsychological testing	Objective measurement of cognitive dysfunction based on age, gender, and education Inconsistent performance and affective disturbance suggest depression
Electroencephalogram	Age-related changes with Alzheimer's disease Focal changes, seizures suggest mass Periodic sharp, triphasic synchronous discharges with Creutzfeldt-Jakob disease
Lumbar puncture	
Opening pressure	High intracranial pressure
Cell count and differential	Infection or inflammation
Protein, glucose	
Cultures	
Cryptococcal antigen, India ink stain	Cryptococcal meningitis (usually HIV related)
VDRL	Syphilis
Oligoclonal bands	Multiple sclerosis
HIV testing	Acquired immunodeficiency syndrome (AIDS)
Rheumatoid factor, ANA	Vasculitis, lupus
Serum, urinary copper excretion, liver biopsy, ceruloplasmin	Wilson's disease
Spot urine drug screen	Substance abuse
24-hour urine for heavy metals	Heavy metal intoxication
Arterial blood gases	Hypoxia, carbon dioxide narcosis
Holter monitoring	Cardiac arrhythmias
Echocardiogram	Cardiomyopathy, valvular heart disease, clots, vegetations
Carotid artery Doppler studies	Reduced cerebral blood flow
Cerebral angiography	Vascular lesions
Cisternogram	Normal-pressure hydrocephalus

ANA = antinuclear antibodies; FTA-ABS = fluorescent treponemal antibody absorption test; MHA-TP = microhemagglutination assay–*Treponema pallidum;* SUN = serum urea nitrogen; VDRL = Venereal Disease Research Laboratories test.

first. These tests assist in the diagnosis of concurrent diseases as well as diseases causing dementia. Fragile elderly patients are very prone to cognitive disturbances from many illnesses. Acute physiologic disturbances must be recognized and addressed, and the patient's condition optimized.

Additional studies should be guided by the history and physical examination. In patients younger than 40 years of age, clinicians should strongly consider HIV testing and determination of serum ceruloplasmin concentration. Signs of multiple sclerosis or meningitis warrant analysis of cerebrospinal fluid. Fever, heart murmur, and a history of drug abuse suggest bacterial endocarditis. Appropriate cultures and an echocardiogram are indicated.

African Americans and patients with diabetes or hypertensive vascular disease are very prone to vascular dementia. Carotid Doppler studies assist in diagnosing carotid artery stenosis and plaques. Holter monitoring and echocardiography identify patients prone to embolic strokes. Although not diagnostic, a computed tomography (CT) or magnetic resonance imaging (MRI) scan may also help support the diagnosis of vascular dementia. Magnetic resonance imaging is less affected by bony artifacts and is more sensitive in detecting infarctions of white and gray matter.

Any patient with focal neurologic signs or new-onset seizures warrants a CT or an MRI scan. Early tumors, subdural hematomas, and hygromas are readily diagnosed and often treatable. The classic signs of incontinence, gait disturbance, and dementia call for a scan or cisternogram to exclude normal-pressure hydrocephalus. Magnetic resonance imaging is especially helpful in detecting the plaques of multiple sclerosis.

The electroencephalogram (EEG) can assist with the diagnosis of dementia and its cause. Normal elderly patients, depressed patients, and patients with Alzheimer's disease have normal or nonspecific age-related changes. Focal intracranial pathology may be revealed by focal EEG changes. Creutzfeldt-Jakob dementia is characterized specifically by periodic sharp, triphasic synchronous discharges. In most patients with delirium, characteristic widespread slowing of the EEG pattern occurs, with fast wave changes in drug-withdrawal delirium.

The diagnosis of Alzheimer's disease can be supported—but not made—by laboratory tests. Serious systemic disturbances must be excluded as causes of the decline in cognitive function. In patients older than 65 years of age, a gradual onset of cognitive problems and the absence of neurologic abnormalities strongly suggest Alzheimer's disease. Both CT and MRI scanning have a low yield for diagnosing other pathology and are sometimes omitted. In patients younger than 65 years of age, other types of dementia are relatively more common than Alzheimer's disease, so CT and MRI scanning are more frequently helpful.

Other Useful Diagnostic Procedures

Neuropsychological assessment can often help diagnose dementia. When elderly patients experience hearing and/or visual problems, mental status testing is much more difficult. Patient performance on tests must be interpreted with regard to education attained, cultural background, and language. Affective disorders, especially depression, can impair performance. Neuropsychological assessment accounts for these variables and helps determine whether there has been a true cognitive decline. Such testing quantifies psychopathology and often helps diagnose specific types of dementia.

The Geriatric Depression Scale (Yesavage and Brink) or the Zung Self-Rating Depression Scale are easy-to-administer screening tests that can help the clinician differentiate dementia from depression.

Frequently Used Diagnostic Procedures That May Not Be Helpful

After the clinician has completed a thorough assessment, the diagnosis of dementia and its cause are usually clearly determined. Unfortunately, most dementias are irreversible, and the treatment options are limited. The families of patients with dementia are often devastated and may pressure physicians for more tests to "be sure." Further diagnostic tests have a very low yield and often lead to false-positive results, creating further anxiety. Patients with dementia and their families need physicians' compassion, support, and understanding to accept the diagnosis of dementia and to avoid unnecessary additional testing.

Therapeutic Tests

When depression cannot be readily separated from dementia, a brief trial of an antidepressant medication is warranted. It is best to use an antidepressant with low anticholinergic properties and to start with a low dose in elderly patients. If depression is the underlying disorder, dramatic improvement often occurs.

Pitfalls in Diagnosis

It is easy to miss early dementia because patients often hide their problems and seem to react in an appropriate way. For elderly patients at high risk, the routine use of mental status screening tests helps detect deficits. A thorough history and physical examination are essential for directing further testing. Acute and chronic medical problems must be appropriately addressed. If a CT or an MRI scan is obtained, clinical correlation is necessary to avoid an incorrect diagnosis. In difficult cases, consultation with a neurologist or a psychiatrist is often helpful.

EPILEPSY AND SEIZURE DISORDERS

By Allen R. Wyler, M.D.,
and David G. Vossler, M.D.
Seattle, Washington

The treatment of epilepsy, like that of most diseases, depends on an accurate diagnosis. However, unlike other disease entities resulting from a single cause, seizures are *symptomatic* of brain dysfunction that may be secondary to a wide variety of possible causes. Owing to this etiologic diversity, the natural history of the different epilepsies can be markedly different. Some epilepsies are relatively benign and self-limited and are easily treated. Other epilepsies may exist throughout the patient's lifetime and become refractory to control with even the best medical therapy. Therefore, to arrive at a diagnosis that carries with it a realistic prognosis, the physician must ascertain three determinants: (1) a seizure diagnosis, (2) an epilepsy diagnosis, and (3) a syndrome diagnosis. To achieve this goal, a clear understanding of critical diagnostic elements is necessary.

A *seizure* is a paroxysmal event by nature. It occurs only for a limited period of time, usually less than a minute, begins suddenly, and usually ceases quickly. During the seizure, normal nervous system function is disrupted. The manifestation of this disruption depends on the area and extent of nervous system involvement. For example, a seizure event involving only primary hand sensory cortex may manifest itself in the form of abnormal sensations, such as tingling, in the hand. In contrast, a seizure involving the basal ganglia and reticular areas may occur as a tonic-clonic convulsion with loss of consciousness. *Epilepsy* is diagnosed when a person experiences chronically recurring seizures.

A single lifetime seizure may result from various metabolic or physiologic stresses to the brain (e.g., electrolyte imbalances, high fever, central nervous system depressant drug withdrawal, infection, trauma, and many others). For example, if individuals are deprived of sleep for long enough, they are likely to have a seizure. The occurrence of a seizure does not mean, however, that they have epilepsy. On the other hand, a teenager who has had three unexplained convulsions over a period of a month has epilepsy.

OCCURRENCE OF SEIZURES AND EPILEPSY

The approximate incidence figures in the United States are 80 in 100,000 person-years for single and recurrent seizures and 40 in 100,000 person-years for epilepsy. Age and cause are included in the cumulative prevalence of seizures. Febrile seizures occur in 2 to 4 per cent of children before 5 years of age. About 4 per cent of white middle-class Americans experience a seizure by age 20 years, and about 10 per cent by age 80 years.

The highest incidence of epilepsy occurs in patients younger than 10 years of age. It drops to a minimum between ages 30 and 50 years, then steadily rises after age 50 years owing to acquired cerebral lesions or degenerative diseases. At most ages, the incidence of epilepsy is slightly higher in males. During childhood, the incidence of epilepsy characterized by generalized seizures is greater than epilepsy manifested by partial seizures, and the converse is true for adults. The prevalence of epilepsy in the population is slightly less than 1 per cent. By contrast, the cumulative prevalence of epilepsy is 1 per cent by age 29 years, 2 per cent by age 60, and 3.5 per cent by age 80 years. Thus, in an average lifetime the chance of developing epilepsy is about 3 per cent. Nevertheless, many cases remit, and the prevalence of epilepsy at age 80 years is just over 1 per cent. Higher prevalence is seen in lower socioeconomic classes.

CLASSIFICATION OF SEIZURES

As noted previously, the diagnosis requires three components: (1) a seizure diagnosis, (2) an epilepsy diagnosis, and (3) a syndrome diagnosis. Often, the epilepsy and syndrome diagnoses are the same. Initially, however, it is easiest to think of them separately.

A *seizure diagnosis* is made by considering what happens to the patient physically and neurologically from start to finish of the ictus. Achieving this goal requires careful consideration of the history from the patient and/or a careful observer or, in some cases, long-term electroencephalographic and video monitoring. For example, a seizure that begins with a blank stare and an arrest of motion and that several seconds later develops automatisms (automatic repetitive movements) is most likely a complex partial seizure (Table 1).

An *epilepsy diagnosis* is reached by considering the seizure type with its electroencephalographic correlates. For example, if the seizure described previously is accompanied by 1.5 to 2.5-Hz bilateral synchronous spike-and-wave discharges from the onset, the epilepsy diagnosis would most likely be atypical absence—rather than complex partial—and this is a form of symptomatic, generalized epilepsy. The distinction is important, because the treatments of these two forms of epilepsy are markedly different.

A *syndrome diagnosis* incorporates the seizure and epilepsy diagnoses in addition to genetic, historical, neurologic, and laboratory information. Frequently this pool of information includes data from structural studies, the most important of which is magnetic resonance imaging (MRI) of the brain. The syndrome diagnosis is most important for deriving a prognosis. A patient with atypical absence epilepsy, mental retardation, and a normal MRI scan probably has Lennox-Gastaut syndrome and has a markedly poorer prognosis than that of a person with normal intelligence and similar seizures due to a benign frontal lobe tumor.

Table 1. Simplified International Classification of Epileptic Seizures

I. Partial seizures (seizures beginning focally)
  A. Simple partial seizures (consciousness not impaired)
  B. Complex partial seizures (consciousness impaired)
  C. Partial seizures with secondary generalization
II. Generalized seizures (no focal onset)
  A. 1. Absence seizures
    2. Atypical absence seizures
  B. Clonic seizures
  C. Tonic seizures
  D. Tonic-clonic seizures
  E. Myoclonic seizures
  F. Atonic seizures
III. Unclassified seizures

CAUSES OF EPILEPSY

In general, partial seizures are most likely due to any one of a myriad of insults capable of causing focal damage to gray matter, or cortex. Seizures are seldom the result of white matter disease. Examples of common causes are trauma, infarction, and tumors. In contrast, generalized epilepsies are more clearly influenced by genetics. This relationship is exemplified by the balance of excitatory and inhibitory central nervous system neurotransmitters that are ultimately influenced by RNA synthesis and hence DNA. The etiologic distinction between partial and generalized seizures is a gross simplification and the two influences (genetic and symptomatic) are inextricably related. For example, 100 people may receive the same head injury, but some may go on to develop post-traumatic epilepsy whereas others do not. Those who develop epilepsy have a different genetic predisposition to epilepsy than those who do not.

DIFFERENTIAL DIAGNOSIS OF SEIZURES

Nonepileptic seizures (NES) are paroxysmal events that alter or appear to alter neurologic function and produce signs or symptoms that, at least superficially, resemble epileptic seizures. The term NES is preferred to the older term pseudoseizures, because the later implies that the patient is voluntarily feigning the episode (which sometimes occurs). An NES can be physiologic or psychological in origin, and the term psychogenic seizure refers to the latter.

Nonepileptic seizures are often misdiagnosed. Some psychiatric disorders that may be misdiagnosed as psychogenic seizures include panic attacks, hyperventilation, somatoform disorders (e.g., conversion disorder), dissociative disorders (e.g., fugue), Munchausen syndrome (either directly or by proxy), malingering, and learned habits. The manifestations of psychogenic seizures are highly variable and often difficult to diagnose by history alone. Reliable diagnostic signs of psychogenic seizures have not been identified. The duration of psychogenic seizures also varies widely, and they may last for periods of several minutes.

Other paroxysmal disorders capable of being confused with epilepsy are vasovagal syncope, cardiac arrhythmia, orthostatic hypotension (or decreased cardiac output for other reasons), transient ischemic attacks, transient global amnesia, migraine and migraine equivalents, narcolepsy, sleep apnea, parasomnias, myoclonus and other movement disorders, vertigo, hypoglycemia, drug intoxication, porphyria, and certain pediatric conditions (e.g., neonatal jitteriness or apnea, shuddering attacks, gastroesophageal reflux, breath-holding spells, and attention deficit disorder).

DIAGNOSIS OF STATUS EPILEPTICUS

Status epilepticus occurs when a seizure persists for more than 20 minutes or when seizures recur so frequently that they impair consciousness. The two forms of status epilepticus are convulsive and nonconvulsive. Both require immediate recognition and intervention, but convulsive status is a true emergency. When patients present to the physician, their motor activity may be less vigorous and may consist of only irregular, arrhythmic clonic jerks or twitching in limited muscle groups. Distinguishing this activity from myoclonus in coma can be aided by obtaining a history from those who witnessed the seizure onset, but the electroencephalogram (EEG) usually provides the most definitive diagnostic information. The response to intravenous benzodiazepines and phenytoin can also help. Common causes of convulsive status epilepticus include rapid changes or withdrawal of anticonvulsants, severe hypoglycemia, anoxic or ischemic encephalopathy, or central nervous system infection.

Nonconvulsive status epilepticus occurs in patients who suffer either complex partial or absence seizures. Patients may appear awake but confused and even drowsy; they may or may not be able to communicate. Often, unusual automatic behavior occurs and the EEG is crucial for establishing this diagnosis. The condition can be abruptly terminated by an intravenous injection of an appropriate benzodiazepine, and this result can be used as a diagnostic test if the EEG is unavailable.

DIAGNOSTIC EVALUATION

The diagnosis of epilepsy is based primarily on clinical information. The most important clue is a solid neurologic and physiologic history of seizures. Because seizures are paroxysmal and are seldom witnessed by the physician, the diagnosis depends far more on the history than on the physical examination.

History

The history is used to search for clues of illness or situations likely to result in cortical damage. Direct questioning for a history of infantile febrile seizures, head trauma, central nervous system infections, cerebral palsy, the chronic use of drugs that affect the central nervous system (alcohol), or other obvious factors, and a family history of seizures or central nervous system illness is important. A detailed history of the seizure itself provides the initial approach to diagnosis. An aura is nothing more than a simple partial seizure and, when described by a reliable patient, suggests that the seizures themselves are partial. If a parent or spouse has witnessed the seizures, the very first signs they recognize as the start of the seizure can provide clues as to seizure type. Most seizures are self-limited and last no more than 5 minutes; they are very stereotypical and often followed by postictal lethargy and/or confusion.

Electroencephalography

The diagnosis of seizures and epilepsy is the major indication for electroencephalography. In this test, electrodes are attached to multiple standardized points on the scalp. The small electrical potentials generated by the underlying brain are amplified and displayed. The EEG is usually recorded during both wakefulness and sleep. In some forms of epilepsy, interictal epileptiform abnormalities can be provoked by hyperventilation or stroboscopic stimulation.

Patients with seizures of any type must have at least one EEG. However, it is common for the initial EEGs not to be helpful in arriving at a diagnosis, and this test may need to be repeated. In some hard-to-diagnose cases, long-term electroencephalographic and video monitoring is required, with the use of specialized equipment. Although some neurologists advocate the use of portable (ambulatory) long-term recording systems, these devices have an unacceptable error rate, because visual confirmation of movement-induced artifacts (which can mimic epileptic activity) cannot be correlated with the tracings, and because the clinical signs of the seizures cannot be seen by the physician.

Neuroimaging Studies

As noted previously, partial seizures are commonly the result of focal cortical damage, and neuroimaging studies can often help identify this damage. The brain MRI scan is unquestionably the best study for this purpose. If complex partial seizures of temporal lobe origin are suspected, the MRI scan should include special thin-cut, magnified views perpendicular to the axis of the temporal horn. This study often demonstrates evidence of mesial temporal sclerosis, a common cause of complex partial seizures.

Routine computed tomography (CT) scans have been replaced by MRI, except in geographic regions where MRI is not readily available. For more complicated evaluations, computed tomography provides additional information, because, unlike MRI, it demonstrates intraparenchymal calcium deposits. This capability helps distinguish certain types of tumors and other central nervous system syndromes. The use of positron emission tomography (PET) or single-photon emission computed tomography (SPECT) scans adds little to the routine evaluation and diagnosis of epilepsy, and routine skull films are rarely of value.

Other Studies

Because epilepsy is a chronic problem in which the initial etiologic insult often occurs years before the symptomatic seizures begin, the use of acute diagnostic tests, such as lumbar puncture, is rarely indicated. However, new seizures thought to be symptomatic of an acute disease, such as meningitis or acquired immunodeficiency syndrome (AIDS), must be evaluated with whatever tests are medically appropriate.

TICS

By Sarah M. Roddy, M.D.
Loma Linda, California

DEFINITION

Tics are common movement disorders that are characterized by brief and intermittent movements or sounds. Motor and vocal tics can be classified as simple or complex. Simple motor tics are abrupt, recurrent, involuntary movements involving one group of muscles. Examples include eye blinking, shoulder shrugging, head jerking, and facial grimacing. Complex motor tics consist of distinct coordinated patterns of sequential movements such as touching, hitting, jumping, and kicking. Simple vocal tics are sounds produced by moving air through the mouth, nose, or throat that may be heard as throat clearing, sniffing, snorting, squeaking, or barking. Complex vocal tics involve more complicated sounds such as whistling or involuntary articulation of words, phrases, or sentences. Echolalia (repeating the words of another person) and palilalia (repeating one's own words) are complex vocal tics. Coprolalia (the involuntary utterance of obscenities) is one of the most disconcerting and socially unacceptable tics.

Tic disorders are classified along a spectrum based on severity. The American Psychiatric Association's Diagnostic and Statistical Manual of Mental Disorders, fourth edition (DSM-IV) outlines the clinical criteria for the diagnosis of tic disorders. The mildest and most common form is the transient tic. Patients have single or multiple motor and/or vocal tics that occur for at least 4 weeks, but no longer than 12 consecutive months. As many as 25 per cent of children have transient tic disorder. Next along the spectrum is chronic motor or vocal tic disorder, which is characterized by single or multiple motor or vocal tics but not both. Tics persist for a period of more than 1 year. Chronic tic disorder affects approximately 1.5 per cent of the population. The diagnosis of Tourette syndrome is made when patients have multiple motor and one or more vocal tics that have been present for more than 1 year. There is a spectrum of severity in Tourette syndrome, with some patients having mild symptoms and others more severe symptoms. The exact prevalence of Tourette syndrome is unknown. Estimates range from 2.9 to 49.5 per 100,000 children, but this may be an underestimate because many mild cases probably are not diagnosed.

PRESENTING SIGNS AND SYMPTOMS

Tics begin before 18 years of age, with a mean age of onset of 7 years. Males more commonly have tics than females. Tic disorders occur in all races, socioeconomic classes, and ethnic groups. Tics begin abruptly in many patients without any apparent precipitating factor. The most frequent initial tics are motor tics involving the head, especially the eyes, and include eye blinking, grimacing, and head jerks. Throat clearing and sniffing are often the first vocal tics to occur.

Tics vary in frequency, location, type, and severity. They may occur from many times a minute to a few per day. They wax and wane spontaneously, and there may be periods of days to months when all symptoms disappear. A particular tic may last weeks to years and then disappear, with another type of tic appearing. Although initial motor tics usually involve the head, over time the tics often involve the limbs and trunk. New tics may be triggered by environmental stimuli. A patient may hear a sound such as a siren or an animal sound and start imitating it. If the patient has an upper respiratory infection with sniffing, the sniffing may persist as a vocal tic long after the infection is gone.

Many patients with tics can voluntarily suppress them for varying periods. However, the suppression creates an inner tension, and eventually the tics must be released. Patients often suppress tics in public so that fewer are present in comparison with the number seen when they are at home. Stress and fatigue can exacerbate tics, whereas absorbed concentration may decrease them. Tics may also increase during times when patients are relaxing. Tics usually decrease or disappear during sleep, although family members may continue to observe some tics even when the patient is asleep.

Tourette syndrome has been associated with attention-deficit/hyperactivity disorder and obsessive-compulsive disorder. As many as 50 per cent of patients with Tourette syndrome have attention-deficit/hyperactivity disorder manifested by difficulty in sustaining attention and remaining seated, fidgeting, distractibility, and impulsivity. These symptoms often precede the onset of tics. Obsessive-compulsive behaviors are also present in approximately 50 per cent of patients with Tourette syndrome. Symptoms may begin in childhood or early adolescence and continue to progress into early adulthood. Behaviors include repetitive checking, arranging, counting, and making sure things are symmetric. Older patients may express concerns about contamination and may perform washing rituals.

Chronic tic disorders and Tourette syndrome are inherited and probably transmitted in an autosomal dominant pattern. Penetrance in females is 70 per cent and in males it is 99 per cent. Females may manifest symptoms of obsessive-compulsive disorder rather than tics.

Tic disorders may present atypically. Although motor tics are usually noted initially, some patients may have only vocal tics. The symptoms of throat clearing, sniffing, coughing, and noisy breathing often result in evaluation for allergies or upper respiratory infection before the diagnosis of a tic disorder is made. Occasionally, a patient may present with complex motor tics without simple motor tics. A thorough review of the history may reveal that the patient previously had simple motor tics that disappeared. Dystonic tics are also a less common presentation of a tic disorder. They are characterized by twisting, squeezing, and other abnormal postures and include sustained mouth opening, torticollis, ocular deviation, and blepharospasm.

COURSE

Although tics may be distressing to the child and parents, the course of transient tic disorder is relatively benign, with the tics disappearing within 1 year. By definition, patients with chronic tic disorder and Tourette syndrome have symptoms that persist for more than 1 year. There is considerable variability in the severity and course of Tourette syndrome. Many patients have tics that are mild and do not interfere with their social or academic functioning and therefore never need treatment. Others may have more significant symptoms and over time may develop more complex tics. These complex tics include complicated actions, such as squatting and touching the ground, twirling while walking, or doing deep knee bends. Dystonic tics such as bruxism, head tilting, and blepharospasm may occur. Coprolalia may develop 4 to 7 years after the onset of the initial symptoms but fortunately occurs in only a minority of patients. In some patients with Tourette syndrome, the symptoms associated with attention-deficit/hyperactivity disorder and obsessive-compulsive disorder may be more disabling than the tics and may require treatment.

From the time of the original description of Tourette syndrome more than a century ago until the late 1970s, this syndrome was considered to be a chronic, lifelong illness. However, it is now known that the long-term prognosis of Tourette syndrome is generally good. Approximately one third of patients have complete remission of their tics by late adolescence. An additional one third of patients report that their tics significantly lessen in frequency and severity by late adolescence. The remaining one third of patients continue to have symptoms into adulthood, although there is often continuing or gradual improvement throughout life. The severity of tics in childhood does not correlate with the degree of improvement in adolescence. Symptoms of attention-deficit/hyperactivity disorder also tend to improve during the adolescent years, although some patients continue to have difficulty into adulthood, with the symptoms affecting their ability to function in their occupation. Obsessive-compulsive behaviors, which tend to begin later than tics, may persist, and in some patients may have a negative impact on their lives.

COMMON COMPLICATIONS

Tic disorders are not degenerative and do not shorten the life span. They are not associated with any specific medical complications. In some patients, however, physical injury or pain may accompany tics or obsessive-compulsive behavior. Skin problems can result from picking at the skin. Orthopedic injuries may occur from repetitive movements, such as knee bending or head jerking.

Children with tic disorders may have significant impairment in social and academic functioning. Teachers may not understand the involuntary nature of the tics, and the child may be disciplined for symptoms over which he or she has no control. Because of embarrassment over the tics, children may experience increased anxiety, poor socialization skills, and low self-esteem. There is also an increased incidence of conduct disorder, aggressiveness, inappropriate sexual behaviors, and self-injurious behaviors. Because of the emotional energy expended in attempting to suppress tics, the child may have a low tolerance for frustration. Many children also have learning difficulties that lead to repeating grades in school. Intelligence is usually normal, but psychological testing of children with Tourette syndrome often reveals specific learning disabilities, including abnormal visual-perceptual performance and reduced visual-motor skills. Modifications in the school program may be required to accommodate the child's needs.

Adolescents tend to have a particularly difficult time coping with tics. Hormonal changes and stress relating to peer acceptance can increase the incidence and frequency of tics. There may be outbursts of anger or social withdrawal. The adolescent may even refuse to go to school when tics are severe.

The psychosocial complications associated with chronic tics may be accompanied or exacerbated by the side effects of neuroleptic agents, which are currently the most effective treatment for tics. Cognitive difficulties, impaired attention span, and decreased motivation may cause a decline in work performance or school marks. Acute dystonia and akathisia have been reported. Tardive dyskinesia rarely occurs in patients with tic disorders treated with neuroleptic agents, possibly because the dose of medication is rather low.

DIAGNOSTIC EVALUATION

Physical Examination

Tics are the main finding on physical examination. Tics can be suppressed, however, and patients may not exhibit motor or vocal tics while in the examining room. Sometimes, it is helpful to watch patients walk down the hall as they leave because suppressed tics may be released at that time. If no tics are seen and the description of sounds and movements is inconclusive, asking the family to make a video may be helpful. The examination is usually normal, although some children may have soft neurologic findings, such as awkwardness or mirror movements.

The history is often more helpful than the physical examination in making the diagnosis of a tic disorder. The history should include information about school performance, attention problems, learning difficulties, obsessive-compulsive tendencies, and drug and medication use. A detailed family history should also be obtained, including information about family members with any of the associated conditions such as obsessive-compulsive behaviors, attention-deficit disorder, learning problems, or conduct disorders. Tics often remit in adolescence and may be forgotten, so it is helpful to have the family contact extended family members and specifically ask about tics.

Laboratory Studies

There is no laboratory test that is diagnostic for tic disorders. The diagnosis is based on clinical criteria. Laboratory tests are almost always unremarkable in patients with tic disorders. Neuroimaging studies do not reveal structural abnormalities. In the future, positron emission tomography (PET) and single photon emission computed tomography (SPECT) may help define the pathophysiology of Tourette syndrome, but at this time, these tests are not used for diagnostic purposes. Electroencephalographic results are variable, nonspecific, and generally unhelpful in making the diagnosis.

Laboratory tests are not required for patients with tic disorders unless the history or physical examination suggests another possible diagnosis. Tics can usually be distinguished from chorea. If movements are choreiform, request streptococcal antibody titers and perform a cardiac evaluation to check for Sydenham's chorea. If Wilson's disease is suspected, measure serum copper and ceruloplasmin and perform a slit-lamp examination looking for Kayser-Fleischer rings. Seizures are rarely confused with tics, but if the diagnosis is not clear, an electroencephalogram (EEG) may be helpful.

Although biochemical and physiologic laboratory tests are not diagnostic for tic disorders, psychological tests may aid the diagnosis of learning disabilities, attention-deficit disorder, or obsessive-compulsive disorder.

POTENTIAL ERRORS AND PITFALLS

The best way of assuring accurate diagnosis of tic disorders is to obtain a detailed history and to perform a thorough physical examination. The history should be negative for cognitive decline or psychosis. The neurologic examination should be unremarkable except for tics and possible soft signs.

Tics should not be confused with other movement disorders (e.g., tremor, chorea, myoclonus, dystonia, or dyskinesias). Children with autism and developmental delay may have complex stereotyped movements that resemble tics, but complex stereotyped movements are usually intentional and more rhythmic than tics. The choreiform movements of Sydenham's chorea may be mistaken for tics. Choreiform movements are nonrepetitive and are usually more random than tics. Sydenham's chorea typically follows a streptococcal infection and may be associated with carditis, arthritis, or other manifestations of rheumatic fever. Often, many of these patients also display marked emotional lability and hypotonia. Huntington's chorea is not likely to be confused with tic disorders because dementia, rigidity, and/or ataxia are not seen in patients with tics.

Patients with Wilson's disease may have involuntary movements that could resemble tics. However, the additional findings of tremor, dystonia, dementia, and hepatic dysfunction distinguish Wilson's disease from tic disorders.

In most cases, seizure disorders are easily distinguished from tics. Myoclonic seizures typically consist of bilateral synchronous jerks of the body without the variability of tics. Patients with absence seizures may have eye blinking and, less often, mouth twitches or movements of the extremities. Absence seizures are characterized by a brief loss of consciousness, an event not seen in patients with tics.

The diagnostic criteria for tic disorders specify that the tics are not drug-induced. Approximately 1.5 per cent of patients who are taking methylphenidate, dextroamphetamine, or pemoline for attention-deficit disorder experience tics after starting the treatment. When the medication is stopped, the tics usually disappear. In some patients, however, the tics persist. These patients are probably genetically vulnerable and would experience tics later even if they had not been treated with stimulant medication. Stimulants may also exacerbate tics in up to one third of patients with tic disorders. Other medications that uncommonly exacerbate tics include antihistamines, antidepressants, and antiepileptic agents. The history of medication use and its temporal relationship to the onset of tics is essential in the evaluation of patients with tic disorders.

CONCLUSIONS

Tics are common movement disorders that are classified by severity. In transient tic disorders, the tics resolve in less than 1 year. If a patient has either motor or vocal tics that persist for more than 1 year, the diagnosis of chronic motor or vocal tic disorder is made. Tourette syndrome is diagnosed when both motor and vocal tics are present and the tics persist for more than 1 year. There are no diagnostic laboratory tests for tic disorders. The diagnosis is based on clinical criteria. The differential diagnosis of tic disorders is limited. A thorough history and physical examination usually eliminate other diagnostic possibilities. Tic disorders are not degenerative, and symptoms usually improve by late adolescence.

Table 1. Parkinsonism

I. Idiopathic Parkinson's disease
II. Secondary parkinsonism
  A. Pharmacologic agents
    1. Antipsychotics (e.g., phenothiazine)
    2. Antiemetics (e.g., metoclopramide)
    3. Antihypertensives (e.g., reserpine)
    4. Others (e.g., amiodarone, meperidine)
  B. Infectious and postinfectious disorders
  C. Toxins (e.g., manganese, carbon monoxide, MPTP)
  D. CNS structural disorders
    1. Normal-pressure hydrocephalus
    2. Stroke
    3. Tumor
    4. Trauma
    5. Subdural hematoma
    6. Syringomesencephalia
  E. Metabolic and/or heritable disorders
    1. Hypoparathyroidism and basal ganglia calcifications
    2. Chronic hepatocerebral degeneration
    3. Wilson's disease (hepatolenticular degeneration)
    4. Huntington's disease
    5. Hallervorden-Spatz disease
    6. Machado-Joseph disease (Azorean disease)
    7. Apathy, parkinsonism, and alveolar hypoventilation
III. Other neurodegenerative conditions with parkinsonian features
  A. Multiple system atrophies
    1. Progressive supranuclear palsy
    2. Shy-Drager syndrome
    3. Olivopontocerebellar degeneration
    4. Striatonigral degeneration
  B. Levodopa-responsive dystonia
  C. Cortical basal ganglionic degeneration
  D. Hemiatrophy-hemiparkinsonism
  E. Parkinsonism-ALS-dementia complex of Guam
  F. Alzheimer's and Pick's diseases
  G. Senile gait disorder
  H. Creutzfeldt-Jakob and Gerstmann-Sträussler-Scheinker diseases
  I. Rett's disease

MPTP = 1-methyl-4-phenyl-1,2,3,6-tetrahydropyridine; CNS = central nervous system; ALS = amyotrophic lateral sclerosis.

EXTRAPYRAMIDAL DISORDERS

By William C. Koller, M.D., Ph.D., Jean P. Hubble, M.D., Rajesh Pahwa, M.D., *and* Richard M. Dubinsky, M.D.
Kansas City, Kansas

PARKINSONISM

Parkinsonism is a symptom complex consisting of resting tremor, rigidity, bradykinesia, or slowed movement, and postural instability. The diagnosis of this condition is based on the presence of two or more of these clinical features. Parkinsonism may be caused by a variety of insults to the central nervous system (Table 1). Parkinson's disease, the most common type of parkinsonism, occurs in approximately 1 per cent of the United States population older than 60 years of age. The recognition of Parkinson's disease as a distinct nosologic entity is credited to James Parkinson, who meticulously detailed its unique clinical manifestations in his 1817 monograph, *The Shaking Palsy.* It was not until the mid-20th century that the pathologic and neurochemical basis of Parkinson's disease was established to be a loss of substantia nigra neurons with a concomitant reduction in striatal dopamine. The detection of this selective neurotransmitter loss led to the development of replacement therapy in Parkinson's disease (levodopa) and served as an impetus to neuropharmacologic investigation and treatment of other central nervous system disorders.

Diagnosis of Parkinson's Disease

Many conditions can mimic Parkinson's disease (see Table 1). Clues to the presence or absence of these disorders can frequently be gleaned from the history of the ailment (its onset and progression), a history of drug or toxin exposure, the family medical history, and the presence of other neurologic signs and symptoms. In some instances, diagnostic testing including bloodwork and brain imaging may be warranted. A trial of levodopa can be employed to attempt to clarify the diagnosis. The failure of levodopa to ameliorate the motor features of the ailment (particularly rigidity and bradykinesia) weighs strongly against the diagnosis of Parkinson's disease.

Although essential tremor is not a form of parkinsonism,

it is probably the most common condition misdiagnosed as Parkinson's disease. As its name implies, tremor is the single clinical feature of essential tremor; rigidity, bradykinesia, and postural disturbances are lacking. The hand tremor of essential tremor differs from that of Parkinson's disease in that it is usually accentuated by, or present only with, sustained posture of the limbs, that is, outstretched arms. Other features that distinguish Parkinson's disease from essential tremor are listed in Table 2.

No confirmatory diagnostic tests exist for Parkinson's disease; therefore, its accurate diagnosis ultimately depends on the clinician's ability to recognize its clinical manifestations and course. The onset of symptoms in Parkinson's disease usually occurs in the sixth decade of life or later. Early in the course of the disease, motor signs and symptoms occur exclusively or predominantly on one side of the body. Progression to involvement of the opposite side is typical. While resting tremor is frequently considered to be the most obvious feature of Parkinson's disease, its presence does not appear to be essential for diagnosis of the condition. Thus, stiffness and discomfort in a single limb ("frozen shoulder") may constitute the initial presentation of Parkinson's disease. Family members may note subtle changes in the patient's appearance and gait (the person stares, smiles less, loses arm swing, or drags a foot). Other early features of Parkinson's disease may include disturbed handwriting (micrographia), voice changes (loss of volume, stuttering), stooped posture, loss or lessening of the sense of smell, skin changes (seborrheic dermatitis), disturbances in salivation and swallowing, and constipation.

Psychological disturbances are common in Parkinson's disease and may include alteration in affect, personality, and cognition. Significant cognitive impairment (dementia) is usually seen in patients with Parkinson's disease who are aged or have advanced disease. The occurrence of dementia at the onset of illness or the progression of dementia when motor signs and symptoms remain mild should call into question the accuracy of the diagnosis. In such instances, complete diagnostic testing to identify a treatable cause of the dementia is appropriate.

Table 2. Comparison of Parkinson's Disease and Essential Tremor

	Parkinson's Disease	Essential Tremor
Characteristic		
Family history	Usually negative	Positive in 50%
Alcohol	No effect	Marked tremor reduction
Age at onset	Midadult	Childhood, adult, or elderly
Tremor type	Resting	Postural, kinetic
Body part affected	Hands, legs	Hands, head, voice
Medical attention sought	Early in course	Often late in course
Disease course	Progressive	Slowly progressive, static for long periods
Bradykinesia, rigidity, postural instability	May be present	Not present
Treatment		
Levodopa	Effective	No effect
Propranolol	May decrease tremor	Effective
Primidone	No effect	Effective

Parkinsonism Related to Infection

Parkinsonism can result from infectious and postinfectious causes. Encephalitis lethargica was an epidemic form of encephalitis in which parkinsonism (von Economo's disease) was a common complication. Encephalitis lethargica occurred in pandemics in Europe from 1915 to 1918 and in the United States from 1918 to 1919. Postencephalitic parkinsonism is mainly of historical interest at this time, since the encephalitis no longer occurs and new cases of this form of parkinsonism are not seen. The symptoms of encephalitis lethargica tended to vary. Acute manifestations frequently included fever, lethargy, somnolence, ocular nerve palsies, parkinsonism, chorea, myoclonus, restlessness, delirium, hypomania, and hallucinations. The diagnosis was based on the clinical signs and the presence of a known epidemic. Parkinsonism developed as a long-term sequela, months to years after the encephalitis, even when the acute stages did not manifest extrapyramidal symptoms. The rate of progression was either very slow or static. Dyskinetic movements, such as chorea and dystonia, could also be present in addition to parkinsonism. Other features common to the postencephalitic state were lateral curvature of the spine and oculogyric crisis, a fixation of the eyes in one position, usually upward. Oculogyric crisis is not seen in Parkinson's disease. Parkinsonism has been occasionally reported in temporal association with other encephalitides, including Japanese B encephalitis, western equine encephalitis, tick-borne encephalitis, influenza type A, and coxsackie virus type B infections. In these cases, parkinsonism has typically developed during the convalescent phase—and not after a latent period, as has been described in von Economo's postencephalitic parkinsonism. Cases of parkinsonism secondary to neurosyphilis have also been reported.

Toxin-Induced Parkinsonism

Various toxins can cause parkinsonism. Manganese intoxication is a serious occupational hazard and probably is responsible for more cases of parkinsonism than any other toxin. Miners, workers who grind manganese, and those who process the metal are at risk. Chronic exposure to a high concentration of manganese dust is apparently responsible for the production of this syndrome; however, only a minority of those who have been exposed develop symptoms. The reasons for individual susceptibility are unknown. Somnolence, apathy, bradykinesia, emotional lability, aggressiveness, and hallucinations (manganese madness) are frequent initial manifestations. A progressive parkinsonian syndrome eventually replaces these symptoms. Difficulty with gait, postural instability, and disturbed speech are prominent abnormalities. An action tremor, rather than a resting tremor, is usually present. Other neurologic signs that may occur include dementia, depression, cerebellar dysfunction, and impotency. Early recognition and withdrawal of the patient from further manganese exposure can result in total recovery. However, neurologic symptoms may progress even after removal.

Carbon monoxide (CO) is a colorless, odorless, nonirritating gas that produces damage to the central nervous system by anoxemic anoxia. Toxicity results from accidental exposure and from suicide attempts involving automobile exhaust. Carbon monoxide poisoning can occur acutely or chronically with repeated exposure, such as in workers in closed automobile garages. The most common manifestations of chronic CO intoxication are anorexia, apathy, weight loss, headache, dizziness, myoclonus, behavioral changes, and language difficulties. Acute CO poisoning occurs with inhalation of high concentrations and often results in coma. The severity of poisoning correlates with the degree of CO saturation in blood. Most cases of CO intoxication are either rapidly fatal or cause no residual effect. In one survey, 20 per cent of patients with acute poisoning died. While the incidence of permanent neurologic sequelae is low (2 to 10 per cent), diffuse nervous system dysfunction with some parkinsonian features can occur.

Cyanide, a potent, fast-acting toxin, inactivates cytochrome oxidase and other oxidative enzymes, resulting in cessation of cellular respiration and anoxia. The brain is particularly susceptible, and cyanide-produced damage results in failure of the medullary respiratory center. The mortality rate is approximately 95 per cent, and death usually occurs in less than 30 minutes. Major destructive changes may occur in the globus pallidus and putamen. A parkinsonian syndrome has been reported in several survivors. One case has been reported of a survivor of methanol poisoning who developed rigidity, bradykinesia, and tremor.

In 1982, several young adults (aged 22 to 44 years) in northern California presented with a profound parkinsonian syndrome after the intravenous use of what was purported to be a synthetic heroin. These individuals had been taking a "designer drug" produced by an illicit laboratory. The toxin (a byproduct of the drug synthesis) responsible for the parkinsonism was identified as 1-methyl-4-phenyl-1,2,3,6-tetrahydropyridine (MPTP). These patients displayed all the major motor features of Parkinson's disease, although clinical manifestations varied among individuals. Bradykinesia, rigidity, or tremor was the predominant symptom. A kyphotic posture was prominent in all patients. Improvement with sleep (sleep benefit) and worsening of symptoms with fatigue and stress occurred; these features are also common in Parkinson's disease. Thus, MPTP, unlike other toxins, appears to produce a pure parkinsonian syndrome. The hypothesis that MPTP selectively destroys nigrostriatal dopaminergic neurons has been confirmed in nonhuman primates and rodents. Thus, MPTP-induced parkinsonism has proved an excellent pathologic animal model of Parkinson's disease. However, the etiologic relationship of MPTP-induced parkinsonism to Parkinson's disease is unclear. Whether MPTP will provide key clues to the cause of Parkinson's disease remains to be determined.

Table 3. Neuroleptics and Related Agents

Brand Name	Generic Name
Phenothiazines	
Compazine	Prochlorperazine
Etrafon (Triavil)	Perphenazine and amitriptyline
Levoprome	Methotrimeprazine
Mellaril	Thioridazine
Phenergan	Promethazine
Prolixin	Fluphenazine
Norzine	Thiethylperazine
Serentil	Mesoridazine
Sparine	Promazine
Stelazine	Trifluoperazine
Thorazine	Chlorpromazine
Torecan	Thiethylperazine
Trilafon	Perphenazine
Butyrophenones	
Haldol	Haloperidol
Fentanyl	Droperidol
Thioxanthenes	
Navane	Thiothixene
Taractan	Chlorprothixene
Benzamides	
Reglan	Metoclopramide
Dihydroindolone	
Moban	Molindone
Dibenzoxazepine	
Loxitane	Loxapine
Dibenzodiazepine	
Clozaril	Clozapine

Drug-Induced Parkinsonism

Various drugs can induce a parkinsonian syndrome; for example, neuroleptics (antipsychotic drugs) produce parkinsonism as a side effect. Shortly after the introduction of these compounds, parkinsonism was described in patients treated with chlorpromazine and reserpine. Parkinsonism can result from the use of most of the drugs included in the class "neuroleptics" (Table 3). These drugs are used primarily as antipsychotic agents, but they also have nonpsychiatric uses, such as the control of nausea and vomiting. Metoclopramide, an atypical neuroleptic belonging to the benzamide class, is employed as an antiemetic and is used in the treatment of gastric stasis. The reported incidence of neuroleptic-induced parkinsonism is about 60 per cent, with clinically significant parkinsonism occurring in 10 to 15 per cent; however, this may be a gross underestimate.

Drug-induced parkinsonism probably occurs more commonly with the potent piperazine phenothiazines or with the butyrophenones. Thioridazine may have fewer extrapyramidal side effects, but controlled studies aimed at substantiating these speculations have not been performed. The occurrence of drug-induced parkinsonism does not appear to be directly related to length or dose of treatment. Epidemiologic studies suggest that increasing age increases the risk. After discontinuation of neuroleptics, the majority of patients are free from parkinsonian signs within a few weeks. However, the effects may last longer, in some cases up to several months. Neuroleptic-induced parkinsonism was once thought to resemble postencephalitic parkinsonism, rather than Parkinson's disease, but more recent observations suggest that the syndrome is clinically indistinguishable from Parkinson's disease. Bradykinesia, rigidity, postural abnormalities, and tremor may occur. Distinguishing drug-induced parkinsonism from idiopathic Parkinson's disease can be difficult. The characteristic parkinsonian unilateral "pill-rolling" tremor may be present, but bilateral postural hand tremor is more common in drug-induced parkinsonism. Drug-induced symptoms develop subacutely or acutely, are usually bilateral, and are often accompanied by orolingual movements (tardive dyskinesia). The drug-induced form improves with time, whereas Parkinson's disease progressively worsens.

The propensity to cause parkinsonism has been clearly demonstrated in virtually all antipsychotic medications, with the notable exception of clozapine. Parkinsonism and other extrapyramidal side effects are either rare or nonexistent with this drug. Clozapine use, however, has been somewhat restricted because of its association with agranulocytosis; weekly blood counts are required in all treated individuals. Other drugs that rarely have been implicated as causing or contributing to parkinsonism include alphamethyldopa, lithium, amiodarone, phenelzine, procaine, meperidine, amphotericin B, cephaloridine, and diltiazem.

Other Causes of Parkinsonism

Diseases with significant parkinsonism in association with other neurologic signs indicating degeneration of multiple neuroanatomic systems are referred to as the multiple-system atrophies or parkinsonism-plus syndromes. Early in their course, these and related disorders may be difficult to distinguish from Parkinson's disease; however, the fully developed syndromes have distinct clinical profiles.

In the past, parkinsonism was frequently classified into three major types: Parkinson's disease, postencephalitic parkinsonism, and arteriosclerotic parkinsonism. Whether a vascular form of parkinsonism exists is now questioned. Many cases formerly labeled as arteriosclerotic parkinsonism would now probably be classified as other known diseases. The incidence of clinical arteriosclerosis in parkinsonism is no different from that in age-matched control subjects. The term "arteriosclerotic" parkinsonism is probably best avoided except in instances when the onset of parkinsonism is temporally related to a well-defined stroke or when postmortem examination supports the diagnosis.

Elderly patients, even in the absence of a definable clinical entity, may have mild parkinsonian features, such as stooped posture, uncertainty and stiffness in turning, gait problems, and generalized slowness. Sometimes, the clinical picture in the very elderly may be difficult to distinguish from the akinetic-rigid form of Parkinson's disease. A therapeutic trial of levodopa may, at times, be necessary. Senile parkinsonism does not respond clinically to levodopa or other antiparkinsonism drugs.

Some other primary disorders of the central nervous system may occasionally present with parkinsonism. These include conditions such as normal-pressure hydrocephalus, head trauma sequelae, and structural lesions such as tumors and tuberculoma.

TREMOR DISORDERS

Shakiness or tremor is a common human experience, often occurring without adverse effects. However, tremor can occur in various neurologic conditions and is most commonly seen in disorders associated with advanced age. Appropriate treatment depends on accurate diagnosis.

Distinguishing Characteristics of Tremor

Tremor refers to rhythmic oscillations produced by involuntary contractions of reciprocally innervated antagonistic muscles. Tremor must be distinguished from other abnormal involuntary movement disorders to ensure proper diagnosis and treatment. The stereotyped and rhythmic nature of tremor usually allows it to be easily differentiated from other dyskinesias. In contrast, athetosis refers to slow, writhing movements of the fingers and hands. Chorea is characterized by irregular, purposeless movements of various body parts, giving the appearance of restlessness. Wild, forceful, flinging movements of proximal body parts characterize ballismus. Dystonia describes spasmodic and twisting movements with relatively sustained postural abnormalities. Tics are erratic, rapid, and repetitive stereotyped movements. Myoclonus consists of abrupt, involuntary single or repetitive jerks of muscle groups and is often arrhythmic.

Table 4. Causes of Pathologic Tremors

Essential tremor	Trauma
Parkinsonism	Infections
Demyelinating disease	Drugs
Vascular insult	Peripheral neuropathies
Tumors	Psychogenic causes

Table 5. Factors That May Enhance Physiologic Tremor

Emotions	Hypoglycemia
Anxiety	Thyrotoxicosis
Fright	Pheochromocytoma
Stress	Exercise
Fatigue	

Classification of Tremor

While tremor is an easily recognized clinical entity, specific characteristics of the tremor are associated with various disorders. Thus, it is useful to classify tremor according to the motor state in which it occurs. Currently, tremor is categorized as follows:

1. Resting tremor occurs at rest (e.g., hands lying in the lap)
2. Postural tremor becomes prominent during maintenance of sustained antigravity posture (e.g., holding the hands outstretched)
3. Kinetic tremor is produced by dynamic goal-directed performance of the hands (e.g., during finger-to-nose testing)

Etiology

Tremor can be due to a variety of conditions, both physiologic and pathologic (Table 4). For example, a slight tremor can be observed in most individuals when the hands are held outstretched. A variety of mechanisms have been proposed to explain this type of physiologic tremor, which appears to be the result of neural activity. The frequency of this tremor is 10 to 12 Hz until about the fifth decade of life, after which the frequency decreases with age. Physiologic tremor is not of clinical importance unless it is enhanced (Table 5).

Emotional stress, endocrine changes, and exercise can exacerbate physiologic tremor and result in symptomatic dysfunction. The mechanism of this enhancement is thought to be due to increased norepinephrine release. Also, drugs (i.e., amphetamines, certain anticonvulsants, antidepressants) and toxins can cause a symptomatic postural tremor (Table 6). Tremors also may be due to a variety of underlying pathologic conditions, some of which are reviewed later.

Table 6. Selected Pharmacologic Causes of Tremor

Beta-Adrenergic agonists	Psychiatric drugs
Theophylline	Lithium
Metaproterenol	Neuroleptics
Terbutaline	Tricyclic antidepressants
Amphetamines	Methylxanthines
Anticonvulsants	Coffee
Valproate	Tea
	Heavy metals

Essential Tremor

The most common tremor disorder, particularly in the elderly, essential tremor is a monosymptomatic illness that may affect as many as 3 to 4 million people in the United States. The pathologic lesion or mechanism of essential tremor is unknown. However, the prevalence of essential tremor increases with age, and the family history is positive for essential tremor in approximately 50 per cent of cases. Late-onset tremor, occurring in patients older than 65 years of age, has been referred to as senile tremor, although this tremor is no different from essential tremor or the inherited form of the disease.

Essential tremor commonly affects the hands, head, and voice. The legs and trunk are also sometimes involved. In essential tremor, the tremor of the hands occurs during a maintained posture and during kinetic movements, although no tremor is observed in the resting position. Accelerometric recording shows a tremor frequency of 5 to 9 Hz. The head tremor may be horizontal (no-no) or vertical (yes-yes). Some patients describe an intermittent head tremor that occurs during periods of stress. Voice tremor results in a characteristic quivering intonation that causes a fluctuating and rhythmic dysphonia.

The course of essential tremor is extremely variable, beginning insidiously and progressing slowly over many years with an increase in amplitude or a spreading of the abnormality to other body parts. A number of external factors can influence the severity of essential tremor. For example, emotions and stress can markedly worsen the tremor. Also, many patients relate that alcohol ingestion dramatically decreases the tremor, an effect that lasts for 30 minutes to 1 hour. This is an important historical feature of the disease, because alcohol has no effect on other tremor disorders. In one controlled study, the intravenous administration of alcohol reduced essential tremor by 70 per cent.

Although essential tremor has been referred to as benign, because it does not shorten life span, the quality of life may be dramatically affected. Patients with essential tremor are often functionally disabled, experiencing difficulty with handwriting, drinking liquids, fine manipulations, and eating. In fact, functional disability and social embarrassment frequently prompt the patient to seek medical attention.

Parkinsonism

Clinically, approximately 50 per cent of patients with Parkinson's disease present with tremor. However, 10 per cent never experience tremor during the course of their illness. When present, the classic tremor of Parkinson's disease is a resting tremor, although a tremor in the postural position is also frequently observed. The tremor, with a frequency of 4 to 6 Hz, is mainly distal, involves the hands, and causes a supination-pronation movement (pill-rolling tremor). Kinetic tremor (tremor when the hand is in motion) is absent. Tremor of the legs, jaw, or lower lip can also occur in some patients, but head tremor is uncommon. Mild to moderate tremor usually causes minimal functional disability, but embarrassment can be a major problem. Stress markedly enhances the tremor, and it disappears during sleep.

Cerebellar Disease

Patients with cerebellar disease may demonstrate both a postural and a characteristic kinetic tremor. The kinetic tremors, with a frequency of 3 to 5 Hz, are evident on finger-nose and heel-shin tests. The tremor appears on the initiation and during the course of a movement and is usually coarse with a side-to-side component. The amplitude of the tremor increases as the arm is extended or the limb approaches a target.

Cerebellar tremors are thought to be due to lesions of the lateral cerebellar nuclei (i.e., the dentate nucleus) or their projections. Lesions in the midbrain around the area of the red nucleus produce a wing-beating type of tremor (rubral or midbrain tremor). Midline cerebellar disease (lesion of the vermis) causes bilateral arm tremor or, more commonly, a rhythmic tremor of the head or trunk (titubation). Patients with cerebellar tremor also have other signs of cerebellar dysfunction, such as ataxia, nystagmus, and decomposition of movements. Common causes of cerebellar disease in the elderly include cerebrovascular disease and brain tumors. Neuroimaging of the brain using computed tomography or magnetic resonance imaging scans frequently demonstrates these lesions.

Alcohol Withdrawal Tremor

Tremor is a symptom of alcohol withdrawal precipitated by a period of absolute or relative abstinence of alcohol consumption. It may occur after a single night's sleep following one or more days of heavy alcohol usage. The tremulousness, when fully developed, consists of gross movements involving the entire body; this tremor has the characteristic of enhanced physiologic tremor. A more permanent tremor can sometimes develop in chronic alcoholics and may persist even after many years of total abstinence.

Psychogenic Tremor

Tremors can also occur on a psychogenic basis. The authors have seen many cases of hysterical tremors. The tremor in these patients has many unusual characteristics, such as occurring in all three positions, changing frequencies and amplitudes, and producing selective disabilities. Hysterical tremor is a difficult diagnosis, but a key feature is that the tremor dramatically diminishes or disappears when the patient's attention is distracted. A history of other somatizations and previous hysterical illnesses can often be elicited. In addition, psychiatric disease is frequently present. Treatment of the underlying disorder can result in disappearance of the tremor, but tremors often persist for long periods of time and remain refractory to all modes of therapy.

Neuropathies and Tremor

Tremor can occur as a rare complication of hereditary and acquired peripheral neuropathies. This tremor may be related to fatigue. In any event, a mild postural or kinetic tremor is often observed with neurologic disorders that cause weakness.

DYSTONIA

Dystonia is defined as "a syndrome of sustained muscle contractions, frequently causing twisting and repetitive movements, or abnormal postures" (Ad Hoc Committee of the Dystonia Medical Research Foundation, February 1984). The term was first coined by Oppenheim in 1911 to describe conditions in which the muscle was hypotonic on one occasion and in tonic spasm on another. Oppenheim also described several other characteristics of dystonia that are important in distinguishing dystonia from other disorders, including psychogenic disorders. These include the *lack of* atrophy, weakness, sensory abnormalities, sphincter disturbances, and psychological disturbances. Throughout the middle part of this century, many patients with focal or generalized dystonias were treated as if they had psychiatric disturbances. This confusion has caused inappropriate treatment of many patients with dystonia.

Classification of the Dystonias

Age at Onset

Dystonia can be subclassified by the age at onset. Onset in the first or second decade is associated with generalized dystonia. The first manifestation of generalized dystonia is unilateral foot inversion while the patient walks or stands. The dystonia progresses over the next few years to involve the other leg and then the entire body. No evidence of cognitive impairment has been found. Spasmodic dysphonia is uncommonly a component of generalized dystonia. Other childhood-onset dystonias include dopamine-responsive diurnal fluctuating dystonia (DRD) and tardive dystonic cerebral palsy. An inheritable disorder, DRD is reported with both autosomal dominant and autosomal recessive patterns. Within the course of a day, children as well as adults with DRD fluctuate from severe dystonic posturing to parkinsonian rigidity. Patients with DRD have a strong paroxysmal kinesis and can become almost manic while exercising. They respond well to small amounts of levodopa replacement. Tardive dystonic cerebral palsy presents in the first decade of life in children with a history of significant neonatal asphyxia. The disorder consists of progressive motor impairment, delay of motor milestones, and spasticity and dystonic movements.

Onset in the third decade and later is usually associated with a focal dystonia that is less likely to spread compared to those with onset under age 20 years. Occasionally, patients with a later onset of dystonia have the movements spread to involve the entire body. However, generalized dystonia is more commonly associated with other movement disorders, such as Huntington's disease, Wilson's disease, neuroacanthocytosis, and cortical basal ganglionic degenerations (CBG). Typical patients with CBG have a focal onset in one arm, with spread to the other arm within a few years accompanied by cognitive impairment.

Body Part Involvement

Another way of classifying dystonias is by the site that is involved (Table 7). Thus the dystonias can be subdivided into focal, segmental, multifocal, hemidystonia, and generalized dystonia.

Table 7. Classification of Dystonia

Type	Description
Focal dystonias	A single body part is affected (e.g., blepharospasm, torticollis, writer's cramp, oromandibular spasmodic dysphonia)
Segmental dystonias	Cranial: two or more parts of the cranial and neck musculature are involved Axial: neck and trunk are involved Brachial: one arm and axial, both arms ± neck ± trunk Crural: one leg and trunk; both legs ± trunk
Multifocal dystonia	Two or more noncontiguous parts are affected
Hemidystonia	Ipsilateral arm and leg are affected
Generalized dystonia	A combination of segmental crural dystonia and any other segment

The typical clinical manifestations of dystonia vary according to which body part is involved. Some features that are commonly seen in all dystonias include aggravation of the dystonia by the use of the involved limb (e.g., an upright posture worsens cervical dystonia), alleviation by sensory or proprioceptive tricks (the French term for this is *geste antagonique*), the presence of provocative factors (e.g., bright sunlight worsens the symptoms of blepharospasm), slight variations in severity throughout the day, and elimination of the movements during sleep.

The cranial dystonias consist of blepharospasm and Meige's syndrome. Blepharospasm can vary from a slight increase in the rate of blinking to functional blindness due to continuous contraction of the obicularis oculi muscles. Typically, blepharospasm is worsened by flickering lights, glare from the sun, and glare from car headlights at night. Two types of movements are seen; one is an increase in simple blinking and the other is frank blepharospastic contractions that force the eyelids shut for periods of several seconds. Many patients find that talking, coughing, or light pressure at the corner of the eye helps them keep their eyes open.

Meige's syndrome consists of blepharospasm in association with lower facial dyskinetic movements. The lower facial movements include wrinkling of the nose, puckering of the lips, dyskinetic tongue movements (e.g., roving of the tongue within the mouth and tongue protrusions), excessive jaw opening, and/or excessive jaw closing. Most of these movements are not present in the same patient. The mandibular movements can be so severe that they prevent the patient from eating, drinking, and talking.

Spasmodic dysphonia occurs when the vocal cords are involved. This condition can be an isolated dystonia or it can be associated with cranial and cervical dystonias. The two primary types are abductor dysphonia (in which the vocal cords are pulled apart, out of the air stream) and adductor dysphonia (in which the vocal cords are pulled together, stopping the air stream). Clinically, patients with abductor dysphonia have a whispering, quiet voice that fades toward the end of a phrase. Patients with adductor dysphonia have numerous glottal stops and a strangled quality to their speech.

Torticollis, or cervical dystonia, is the most widely recognized form of dystonia, possibly because many patients with less obvious dystonias (spasmodic dysphonia, limb dystonias) are not properly diagnosed. Most cases of cervical dystonia are idiopathic, but some patients can have secondary cervical dystonias induced by medications, trauma, meningiomas, and Arnold-Chiari type III malformation. Idiopathic cervical dystonias begin as a tendency to hold the head turned toward one side or to tilt the head and neck toward one side. Over a period of months to years, the movements become more common and more severe. Typically, at the onset, cervical dystonia is not a painful disorder. As the movement becomes more severe, patients often complain of pain and discomfort in muscles that are used to fight the abnormal movements. Limitation of the ability to turn the head and neck toward the opposite side develops. Many patients have a "honeymoon" period early in the morning when they are relatively free from abnormal movements. This period can last for a few seconds or as long as an hour. Whenever these patients rest the neck, by leaning back in a chair with neck support, leaning against a wall, or holding chin in hand, the movements are lessened if not eliminated. During a clinical examination, the movements become more severe when these patients are distracted by difficult motor tasks and are not allowed to use their "tricks." Occasionally, other movements are observed, such as shoulder elevation, retrocollis (pulling of the head backward), and/or anterocollis (pulling of the head forward).

Focal limb dystonias are primarily task-specific, but over time they can spread to involve other tasks as well. Focal limb dystonias are seen in patients who overuse the forearms and hands for diverse tasks such as typing, piano playing, writing, and the playing of other musical instruments. The pathophysiologic basis that causes one patient to develop a task-specific dystonia while the majority of typists and musicians perform without a problem is not known. Typical patterns seen with writer's cramp include excessive finger or wrist flexion, excessive finger or wrist extensions, and combinations of both. Analysis of a task-specific dystonia is best accomplished by observing the patient performing the task that causes the involuntary movement. The task-specific dystonias are most likely an overuse phenomenon in which excessive repetition of a well-learned movement leads to corruption of the original motor program in the motor cortex and basal ganglia or causes restructuring of the spinal cord inhibitory cells, resulting in diminished reciprocal inhibition.

Leg or crural dystonias are seen rarely outside the setting of generalized, juvenile-onset dystonia. Occasionally, crural dystonia can be induced by leg trauma or spinal cord trauma or as the result of a basal ganglia stroke. Regardless of the cause, these patients have excessive inversion of the foot at the ankle, causing them to walk on the outer aspect of their foot. Such gait is quite painful and frequently leads to falls. In cases induced by a stroke, there may be an additional component of tibialis anterior weakness, leading to footdrop.

The last group of dystonias are the paroxysmal types. Two types are well described; they are paroxysmal kinesogenic dystonia (PKD) and paroxysmal nonkinesogenic dystonia (PNKD). The PKDs, also known as reflex epilepsy, are triggered by specific actions by the involved limb, causing a painful involuntary movement that can last from seconds to minutes (though duration of less than 1 minute is typical) until the cramp is broken by the forceful extension of the involved limb. The PKD occurs every time the patient attempts to perform the triggering activity, often up to 100 times per day. Patients therefore avoid using the involved limb altogether for fear of triggering the pain. PKD responds well to the anticonvulsants phenytoin, carbamazepine, and clonazepam. The PNKDs occur less often throughout the day (three or four times per day) and last for minutes to hours. The attacks are triggered by exercise, caffeine, and alcohol, but they are not triggered by specific activities. Patients with PNKD do not avoid using the involved limb, and the disorder responds to clonazepam, oxazepam, and acetazolamide—but not to phenytoin or carbamazepine.

Clinical Evaluation of the Dystonias

The main goal of the clinical evaluation of the dystonias is to exclude other, secondary causes. These may be curable forms of dystonia (e.g., Wilson's disease) that warrant thorough evaluation. Conversely, if a patient has had the same movement disorder for decades, without a history of progression and a lack of cognitive changes, the search for a secondary cause is usually futile.

The onset of idiopathic dystonia usually occurs in the late first or the second decade. Onset within 1 to 4 years of birth is typical of athetotic (or dystonic) cerebral palsy. Occasionally, it presents at a later age and can be labeled tardive dystonic cerebral palsy. The first and second decades are the most common time for the onset of idiopathic dystonia. However, this is also the typical age at onset of the juvenile form of Parkinson's disease (Segawa's disease) and also a common age at onset of the parkinsonian form of Huntington's disease. A family history of hyperkinetic movements and mental changes should alert the clinician to the possibility of Huntington's disease, while atypical features such as bradykinesia and resting tremor are more typical of Segawa's disease. Idiopathic dystonia–parkinsonism with diurnal fluctuations, also known as dopamine-responsive dystonia with diurnal fluctuations, usually begins in the second decade and can affect several generations or several members of one generation.

Several neurodegenerative diseases can have dystonia as one of their features. Wilson's disease, characterized by hepatolenticular degeneration, can have both dystonic and athetotic features, while the primary manifestation is usually a severe tremor. Neuroacanthocytosis is characterized by hyperkinetic movements, usually choreiform, with oral self-mutilation, generalized seizures, and later progression to hypokinetic movements accompanied by motor neuron disease. This disease occurs in both an autosomal dominant and a recessive inheritance pattern. Ataxia-telangiectasia, Pelizaeus-Merzbacher disease, Machado-Joseph's disease, olivopontocerebellar atrophy, and the spinocerebellar atrophies all can have dystonic features; however, the primary manifestation is not dystonia.

Tourette's syndrome is an inherited disorder characterized by both motor and vocal tics, with a duration greater than 12 months and onset before age 21 years. Most of the motor tics in Tourette's are brief. However, dystonic tics are well described, as are complex stereotypes that can mimic dystonic posturing of a limb. The young age at onset, association with other motor or vocal tics, ability to voluntarily suppress the movements and alleviation of the abnormal movements when distracted by a difficult motor task help distinguish Tourette's syndrome from dystonia.

A variety of structural abnormalities can cause dystonia; these include perinatal trauma, direct central nervous system trauma, peripheral trauma, arteriovenous malformations, cerebrovascular accidents, and postencephalitic syndromes. Most of these can be detected by neuroimaging studies and a careful clinical history. Rarely, endocrine disorders, such as hyperthyroidism, can have dystonic or choreiform features. Dystonic features can also predominate in Sydenham's chorea.

Medications, both prescribed and illicit, can cause dystonia. Tardive dystonias, dyskinesias and akathisias, have been described in association with the use of neuroleptics, and a large number of antiemetics (specifically metoclopramide). Tardive dystonias are seen in three situations: breakthrough (appearance of the movements while the patient is on a steady dose of medication), dose reduction, and withdrawal emergent (appearance within 12 weeks of stopping a neuroleptic). If the movements have just started, often the patient undergoes a complete remission if the dopamine-blocking agent is discontinued. However, the longer the patient has been under dopamine blockade and the higher the dose of the causative agent, the more difficult it is to stop the movements after the causative agent is removed. Acute dystonic reactions are also described with these medications.

Some disorders can simulate focal dystonias. Orthopedic problems, such as atlantoaxial subluxation, perinatal trauma to the sternocleidomastoid muscle, and Klippel-

Feil syndrome, can cause a secondary torticollis. Trochlear nerve palsy is reported to cause a head tilt to compensate for the diplopia induced by external rotation of the involved eye. Ocular or corneal irritation can mimic blepharospasm. Stage III reflex sympathetic dystrophy is defined as dystonic posturing of the involved limb. This may represent either a true dystonia or a learned response in reaction to the pain provoked on movement of the involved limb. Last, dystonic movements can be manifestations of a psychogenic disorder, which can be difficult to prove and to treat. Clinical suspicion should be aroused in a patient who has obvious features that are not associated with dystonias, such as inconsistencies of abnormal movements, sphincter disturbances, gastrointestinal complaints, and dystonia that migrates to different parts of the body.

CHOREA

The term chorea is derived from the Greek for dance. It consists of brief, jerky involuntary movements that are irregular and unpredictable. These movements migrate from one part of the body to another in a continuous, random sequence. Chorea can be associated with a large number of disorders (Table 8).

Huntington's Disease

Symptoms usually appear between 35 and 40 years of age, although the disease may present in childhood or as late as the eighth or ninth decade. It usually begins insidiously with random fidgeting or purposeless movements that progress to chorea over a period of years. Chorea initially begins in the muscles of the face and arms but later becomes generalized. The early stages are typically associated with slight grimacing of the face, shrugging of the shoulders, and jerking movements of the limbs. As the disease progresses, the gait becomes stuttering and dancing in character owing to intermittent lordotic and flexion postures. Later, the choreiform movements can become incapacitating, and the patient may need assistance with the activities of daily living. Other hyperkinetic disorders, such as dystonia, athetosis, and myoclonus, may also occur. Parkinsonian features, such as bradykinesia and postural instability, emerge and worsen as the disease progresses. "Milkmaid grips" and inability to keep the tongue steadily protruded are typical and are due to motor impersistence or inhibitory pauses during voluntary contraction. Dysarthria and dysphagia are common findings in all stages of the disease.

The involuntary movements are associated with progressive changes in personality and dementia. Personality changes include inappropriate behavior, irritability, loss of social inhibitions, and low threshold of frustration. Emotional disturbances, such as depression and lack of motivation, are often present. Patients with early Huntington's disease have verbal and nonverbal memory deficits, dyscalculia, and problems with language usage. As the disease progresses, profound dementia can develop. On Mini-mental Status Examination testing, patients with Huntington's disease perform more poorly on serial sevens, registering three items, and writing a sentence compared with Alzheimer's patients.

Variations in the presentation of Huntington's disease include patients with only chorea or dementia. Some of these patients have subtle movements or mild cognitive impairment. Late-onset Huntington's disease is defined as the onset of motor impairment after the age of 50 years, and it may have a slower progression of symptoms. Motor impairment consisting primarily of rigidity and akinesia occurring before age 20 years is termed juvenile-onset Huntington's disease. Recurrent seizures and severe dementia are other features of this disorder. Rarely, patients with Huntington's disease have signs of cerebellar ataxia, amyotrophy, and autonomic abnormality.

The presence of chorea and dementia and a history of similar manifestation in family members make the diagnosis apparent. Few laboratory tests are helpful. The EEG may show nonspecific changes. Some neuropsychologic tests, such as Stroop Interference Test and the Trailmaking and Symbol Modalities subtests of the Wexler Adult Intelligence Scale-Revised, are sensitive indicators of early Huntington's disease. Computed tomography and MRI of the head may demonstrate caudate atrophy. Single-proton

Table 8. Common Causes of Chorea

Hereditary	**Infectious or Immunologic**
Huntington's disease	Sydenham's chorea
Benign familial chorea	Encephalitis
Wilson's disease	Systemic lupus erythematosus
Neuroacanthocytosis	Tuberculosis meningitis
Ataxia-telangiectasia	**Drug-Induced**
Inborn errors of metabolism	Neuroleptics, such as haloperidol, thiothixene, thioridazine
Hallervorden-Spatz disease	Antiparkinsonian drugs, such as levodopa, anticholinergics
Paroxysmal kinesogenic choreoathetosis	Anticonvulsants, such as phenytoin, carbamazepine
Metabolic and Endocrine	CNS stimulants, such as amphetamine, cocaine, pemoline
Hypernatremia	Birth control pills
Hyponatremia	**Cerebrovascular**
Hypocalcemia	Basal ganglia infarcts
Hyperglycemia	Subdural or epidural hematomas
Hypoglycemia	Arteriovenous malformations
Hypomagnesemia	CNS hemorrhage
Hyperthyroidism	**Other Causes**
Hypoparathyroidism	Chorea gravidarum
Hepatic encephalopathy	Senile chorea
Renal encephalopathy	Essential chorea

CNS = central nervous system.

emission computed tomography with labeled hexamethylpropyleneamineoxine may show decreased regional cerebral blood flow. Positron emission tomography scan with fluorodeoxyglucose typically reveals reduced metabolism in the caudate and putamen. MRI spectroscopy may demonstrate increased lactate concentrations in the basal ganglia and the cerebral cortex. With the discovery of the HD gene, genetic testing is the definitive diagnostic test. Counseling before genetic testing is essential for ethical and psychosocial reasons, and is especially important for presymptomatic diagnosis.

The disease has a progressive course but the rate of progression varies from patient to patient. The clinical picture can change from pure chorea to a combination of different movement disorders, including chorea, dystonia, and athetosis. Occasionally in the terminal stages of the disease, the severity of chorea can decrease and the patient may exhibit signs of terminal dementia. Huntington's disease is a fatal disorder, and the duration of the illness ranges from 13 to 15 years. Death typically occurs as the result of aspiration pneumonia, trauma due to falls, and sepsis.

Neuroacanthocytosis

Neuroacanthocytosis is the most common hereditary chorea after Huntington's disease. It is characterized by adult-onset chorea, seizures, dysarthria, and axonal neuropathy and may be associated with dementia and parkinsonism. Choreiform movements are particularly prominent in the face and mouth region. The presence of acanthocytosis in the peripheral blood smear helps make the diagnosis.

Benign Familial Chorea

Benign familial chorea (BFC) is a rare disorder with symmetrical and predominantly distal distribution. The disorder usually begins in early childhood, before the age of 5 years. The neurological examination is usually normal except for the presence of postural and kinetic tremor. Rarely, patients may have ataxia, dysarthria, or pyramidal tract signs. Intellectual impairment is a rare feature. The disorder is usually nonprogressive, although reports of initial worsening during adolescence are associated with a subsequent nonprogressive course. Distinguishing between benign familial chorea and Huntington's disease in an adult can be difficult, but the early age at onset, the nonprogressive course, and the absence of dementia provide essential clues.

Senile Chorea

Senile chorea typically presents after the age of 65 years as an isolated symptom. The movements are mild and may involve the limbs, face, mouth, and tongue. It is not associated with cognitive impairment, and no family history of a similar disorder can be elicited. Genetic testing for Huntington's disease may reveal that some of these patients have the disease even in the absence of a positive family history.

Paroxysmal Choreas

Paroxysmal kinesigenic choreoathetosis (PKC) and paroxysmal dystonic choreoathetosis are well-defined syndromes. The former is characterized by attacks of choreoathetosis precipitated by sudden movement. The age at onset ranges from 6 to 15 years. The attacks occur more than 100 times a day and last less than 1 minute. The neurologic examination between attacks is usually normal. There is often a family history of similar disorder. Paroxysmal kinesigenic choreoathetosis attacks decrease in frequency and severity in adulthood, and occasionally resolution may be complete. Rarely, metabolic abnormalities, such as hypoparathyroidism, hyperthyroidism, hypernatremia, hypoglycemia, and hyperglycemia, can present as PKC. Paroxysmal dystonic choreoathetosis is characterized by dystonic and choreoathetoid movements occurring less than once a day and lasting for several minutes. The age at onset is less than 5 years, and most cases are familial.

Sydenham's Chorea

Sydenham's chorea is associated with group A streptococcal infection and rheumatic fever. The age at onset is typically between 5 and 15 years. The initial symptom is usually irritability or behavior disturbance—rarely confusion. Chorea may have an abrupt or insidious onset and may be unilateral or bilateral, but it almost always involves the face. Other neurologic manifestations are uncommon but can include dysarthria, encephalopathy, and hyperreflexia. The chorea usually progresses during the first 2 to 4 weeks, persists for a variable amount of time, and then resolves completely over 3 to 6 months. Recurrent attacks may occur within 2 years in some patients, and antistreptolysin-O and antistreptokinase blood antibody titers may be elevated.

Chorea Gravidarum

Chorea gravidarum occurs most commonly during the first pregnancy in women who have a previous history of chorea. The choreiform movements typically begin in the first trimester and resolve spontaneously after a few months. Rarely, the chorea persists until delivery, and it may recur in subsequent pregnancies.

Systemic Lupus Erythematosus

Chorea is an uncommon manifestation of systemic lupus erythematosus (SLE). It usually occurs early in the course of the disease and may precede the diagnosis of SLE by years. Either focal or generalized chorea may occur. The erythrocyte sedimentation rate, antiphospholipid antibody titers, and antinuclear antibody (ANA) testing can suggest the diagnosis.

SPINOCEREBELLAR DEGENERATIVE DISORDERS

By Henry Paulson, M.D., Ph.D.,
and Howard Hurtig, M.D.
Philadelphia, Pennsylvania

The spinocerebellar degenerative disorders are a group of inherited neurologic conditions that are characterized clinically by progressive ataxia and pathologically by degeneration of the cerebellum and/or its afferent and efferent pathways. Despite similarities, the individual disorders usually can be distinguished from each other by the associated clinical features and precise pattern of neuropathologic degeneration seen in the cerebellum, brain stem, and spinal cord.

For years, a great deal of debate has surrounded the nomenclature and classification of these disorders, in part because the clinical features often vary widely and in part because until recently little was known about the underlying molecular mechanisms. In the past, classification was based on pathology, for example, olivopontocerebellar atrophy and cerebellar-cortical atrophy. Fortunately, genetic advances have begun to permit a rational biologic basis for classification. The identification of specific genes has led to the development of specific and sensitive genetic tests for several forms of spinocerebellar degeneration, and the molecular basis of others is likely to be discovered soon. Accordingly this article uses Harding's classification of hereditary ataxias in describing the most common forms of spinocerebellar degeneration.

The diagnosis of a particular spinocerebellar degenerative disorder is based on clinical assessment; a genetic test may or may not clinch the diagnosis. Attention to several characteristics certainly aids in the diagnosis. For example, the age at onset is critical because the list of candidate diseases differs for early- and late-onset ataxia. Especially in early-onset disease, evidence must be sought for a metabolic or nutritional deficiency. In the adult patient, the disease may be familial or sporadic. In addition, other neurologic signs may accompany the cerebellar dysfunction. In particular, ophthalmoparesis or peripheral neuropathy may be present. The major forms of spinocerebellar degeneration can often be distinguished based on the characteristics presented in Table 1. Describing every form of spinocerebellar degeneration is beyond the scope of this article because many metabolic and nutritional defects can lead to degeneration of the cerebellum and its afferent and efferent systems. Instead, the major forms of spinocerebellar degeneration are discussed, mentioning, when appropriate, less common diseases with similar neuropathologic features.

EARLY-ONSET FORMS OF SPINOCEREBELLAR DEGENERATION

Ataxia occurs in many inherited childhood disorders, most of them inherited in an autosomal recessive manner. *Intermittent ataxia* is seen in a number of metabolic disorders, including defects in urea cycle enzymes (the hyperammonemias), defects in pyruvate and lactate metabolism, and several aminoacidurias. *Progressive ataxia,* in contrast, characterizes the spinocerebellar degenerative disorders. Many of the rarer causes of spinocerebellar degeneration are also metabolic disorders and must be excluded in a child presenting with progressive ataxia (Table 2). However the most common and stereotyped form of early-onset spinocerebellar degeneration, Friedreich's ataxia, is a single-gene disorder without a known metabolic defect.

Friedreich's Ataxia

By far the most common form of hereditary ataxia, Friedreich's ataxia is an autosomal recessive disease characterized clinically by progressive gait and limb ataxia, lower limb areflexia, and onset in childhood. The distinctive neuropathologic feature of Friedreich's ataxia is degeneration of the dorsal columns, spinocerebellar and lateral corticospinal tracts, dorsal root ganglia, and large myelinated axons in peripheral nerves.

Patients usually present before puberty with gait ataxia,

Table 1. Major Forms of Spinocerebellar Degeneration

Disease	Inheritance	Associated Clinical Features	Site of Pathology	Specific Laboratory Tests
Early Onset				
Friedreich's ataxia	Recessive	Areflexia, cardiac and musculoskeletal defects	Dorsal columns, corticospinal and spinocerebellar tracts, myelinated nerves	Expanded trinucleotide repeat in FA gene (test pending)
Early-onset cerebellar ataxia with retained reflexes	Heterogeneous Most recessive	Pyramidal tract signs may be present	Cerebellum	None
Ataxia-telangiectasia	Recessive	Telangiectasias, immunodeficiency, infections, oculomotor dyspraxia, extrapyramidal, cognitive disturbance	Cerebellum	Increased alpha-fetoprotein, decreased IgA, translocations Mutations in *ATM* gene
Late Onset				
Type 1 autosomal dominant cerebellar ataxias (includes spinocerebellar ataxia, types 1 through 5)				
Spinocerebellar ataxia, type 1	Dominant	Ophthalmoparesis, pyramidal and extrapyramidal signs	Cerebellum, brain stem, spinocerebellar tracts	Expanded trinucleotide repeat in *SCA1* gene
Machado-Joseph disease (or spinocerebellar ataxia, type 3)	Dominant	As in SCA1; also peripheral and cranial nerve deficits, amyotrophy	Brain stem, sparing of cerebellar cortex and olives	Expanded trinucleotide repeat in *MJDI* gene
Late-onset pure cerebellar ataxia	Heterogeneous	Dysarthria	Cerebellum	None

Table 2. Progressive Ataxia Associated With Known Metabolic Disorders

Disease	Laboratory or Biopsy Abnormalities
Abetalipoproteinemia and hypobetalipoproteinemia	Abnormal serum protein electrophoresis Low vitamin E, high cholesterol
Isolated vitamin E deficiency	Low vitamin E
Ceroid lipofuscinosis	Lipopigment inclusions on skin and rectal biopsy specimens
Cholestanolosis	High serum cholestanol
GM_2 gangliosidosis	Hexosaminidase A or A and B deficiency
Leukodystrophies	
Adrenoleukodystrophy	Increased very long chain fatty acids
Late-onset globoid cell	Galactocerebrosidase deficiency
Metachromatic	Sulfatase A deficiency
Mitochondrial encephalomyopathies	Mitochondrial DNA mutations, red ragged fibers on skeletal muscle biopsy
Sialidosis	Neuraminidase deficiency
Sphingomyelin storage disorders	Increased lysosomal sphingomyelin
Niemann-Pick, type C disease	Sea-blue histiocytes in bone marrow, reduced cholesterol esterification
Defective DNA repair	
Ataxia-telangiectasia	Mutations in *ATM* gene Decreased IgA and IgG, increased alpha-fetoprotein
Cockayne's syndrome	Various defects in DNA repair enzymes
Xeroderma pigmentosum	Various defects in DNA repair enzymes

although in less than 5 per cent disease may begin in young adulthood. In infants, ataxia occurs as a delayed onset of walking and in the older child, it occurs as increased difficulty in walking. At or soon after the onset of ataxia, dysarthria, lower limb areflexia, and proprioceptive sensory loss become evident. Kyphoscoliosis or pes cavus may also be present at onset. In some patients, scoliosis and cardiac abnormalities may even precede neurologic signs of disease.

The rate at which neurologic disability progresses varies widely. Over several years, gait and lower limb ataxia worsens and spreads to the arms, leaving most patients unable to walk by age 25 to 30 years. Mobility is further compromised by distal weakness, hypotonia, and severe kyphoscoliosis, which often develop within a few years. Dysarthria, which is present in many patients at the onset of illness, becomes increasingly disabling, but intellect remains largely intact. Position and vibratory sensory loss, particularly in the legs, nearly always becomes evident as the disease progresses. Optic flutter and square wave jerks are frequently seen, but ophthalmoplegia does not occur. Disabling sensorineural hearing loss and optic atrophy occur in a substantial minority of patients.

As disabling as the neurologic symptoms are (most patients are unemployable as adults), the major threats to life are respiratory compromise, due to severe kyphoscoliosis and neuropathy, and cardiac abnormalities, which occur in up to 90 per cent of patients. Although the range of cardiac findings is wide, hypertrophic cardiomyopathy and arrhythmias are the most common life-threatening abnormalities. In addition, 10 to 15 per cent of patients have overt diabetes mellitus. Most patients live into their 30s, usually dying of cardiac failure or infection, but patients with minimal scoliosis or cardiac disease may live into their 50s. Early surgical repair of scoliosis may be of benefit, both in prolonging the patient's ability to walk and in making life more comfortable in the later stages of illness.

Onset after the age of 20 years is uncommon. The clinical picture of early- and late-onset disease is identical except that foot deformities, muscle wasting, and overt cardiomyopathy are seen less frequently if symptoms begin later in life.

Physical Examination

Neurologic signs vary depending on the stage of disease. Early on, the patient usually has gait ataxia, reduced or absent reflexes in the legs, and a positive Romberg's sign. Patients with more advanced disease also show dysarthria, dysmetria in heel-to-shin testing, and decreased position and vibratory sensation in the legs. Lower limb areflexia is a hallmark of disease; preservation of lower limb reflexes is distinctly unusual and should raise doubts about the diagnosis unless the patient is from a family known to be affected. The legs usually become hypotonic with distal wasting, although flexor spasms may also occur. As the disease progresses, the arms display distal weakness and areflexia. Plantar responses are extensor in most patients and neutral in the remainder. Optic flutter and fixation instability are the characteristic ocular findings, and nystagmus is seen in some patients. The vestibulo-ocular reflex is impaired, but optokinetic nystagmus is intact. Eye movements otherwise are largely unperturbed. Hearing loss and optic atrophy, which are present in a minority of patients, should be sought in advanced disease. A careful musculoskeletal and cardiac examination must be performed in all patients to document kyphoscoliosis, equinovarus deformities, and signs of heart failure.

Diagnostic Testing

The gene responsible for Friedreich's ataxia was recently identified on chromosome 9. The defect is an expansion of a trinucleotide repeat, and direct genetic testing for the expanded repeat should be available soon. The biochemical defect, however, remains unknown. The glucose tolerance test is abnormal in up to 30 to 40 per cent of patients, but other routine laboratory tests, including cerebrospinal fluid analysis, produce normal results. Abnormalities in pyruvate carboxylase, pyruvate dehydrogenase, and mitochondrial enzyme activity have been reported but are of uncertain significance. Testing for these abnormalities is probably unnecessary.

Magnetic resonance imaging (MRI) of the cervical cord usually demonstrates atrophy with occasional intramedullary signal abnormalities on T2-weighted images. MRI and computed tomography (CT) scans of the brain demonstrate mild cerebellar atrophy in up to two thirds of patients. It is of note that brain stem structures above the medulla are generally preserved, distinguishing Friedreich's ataxia from other spinocerebellar degenerations. Chest films reveal cardiomegaly in 30 per cent of patients. The severity of kyphoscoliosis can be documented with spinal films.

The electrocardiogram is useful in distinguishing Friedreich's ataxia from other childhood ataxias, because the most common abnormality, widespread T-wave inversion, is virtually diagnostic for this form of ataxia. An echocardiogram often shows symmetric ventricular hypertrophy or, less commonly, septal hypertrophy.

Electrophysiologic studies of the nervous system are useful in distinguishing Friedreich's ataxia from other diseases, including several hereditary motor and sensory neuropathies. Nerve conduction studies typically reveal absent or small sensory action potentials with normal or only slightly reduced motor conduction velocities. The electromyogram is usually normal. Somatosensory evoked potentials are severely abnormal, and brain stem auditory evoked potentials may be abnormal in up to half of patients. Nerve biopsy reveals loss of large myelinated fibers in peripheral nerve, but this test is rarely necessary.

In advanced disease, positron emission tomography (PET) may demonstrate decreased glucose metabolism in the cerebellum, brain stem, and thalamus, but early disease may show increased glucose metabolism in the same areas. In general, PET is not helpful in diagnosing Friedreich's ataxia.

Pitfalls in Diagnosis

In a patient from a family with documented disease, the diagnosis is straightforward. However, most patients do not have a positive family history because on average only 25 per cent of offspring are affected with this autosomal recessive disease. Still, its stereotyped features (the particular constellation of neurologic abnormalities with cardiac and musculoskeletal defects) usually make this a readily recognizable condition. Neurologic diseases that are mistaken for Friedreich's ataxia include several hereditary motor and sensory neuropathies and the myelopathy of vitamin E deficiency.

Friedreich's ataxia may be confused with the major demyelinating form of *hereditary motor and sensory neuropathy* (Charcot-Marie-Tooth disease) because patients with the latter can present in childhood with areflexia, clumsiness, and mild motor deficits (but without cerebellar ataxia). It is important to distinguish the two because hereditary motor and sensory neuropathy, type 1 is an autosomal dominant disorder with a better prognosis. The two can, in fact, be easily distinguished by nerve conduction studies. In hereditary motor and sensory neuropathy, type 1, nerve conduction velocities in the upper limbs will be less than 40 m per second (demyelinating range), whereas they are greater than 40 m per second in Friedreich's ataxia.

Hereditary motor and sensory neuropathy, type 4 (also known as *Refsum's disease*) is an autosomal recessive disorder characterized by ataxia, demyelinating polyneuropathy, and an increased serum concentration of phytanic acid. Signs of disease may first occur in children or adults and include progressive gait ataxia, polyneuropathy, pigmentary retinopathy, ichthyosis, and deafness. Clinically, it can be distinguished from Friedreich's ataxia by the ichthyosis, retinopathy, and prominent involvement of the arms. Diagnostic test results distinguishing it from Friedreich's ataxia include increased serum phytanic acid and lipid concentrations, decreased nerve conduction velocities, and denervation on electromyography (EMG).

Hereditary ataxia with muscular atrophy (also known as Roussy-Lévy syndrome) is another form of hereditary motor and sensory neuropathy characterized by mild cerebellar deficits and atrophy of leg muscles. Patients have mild gait ataxia accompanied by areflexia and wasting of the legs and kyphoscoliosis. They do not have the dysarthria and ocular findings of Friedreich's ataxia. Electrophysiologic studies show decreased nerve conduction and denervation, which are signs of a demyelinating neuropathy.

The group of conditions whose clinical and pathologic features most closely resemble Friedreich's ataxia are those due to abnormalities in vitamin E absorption or metabolism. The two most prominent causes of primary vitamin E deficiency are *abetalipoproteinemia* (Bassen-Kornzweig syndrome) and *familial isolated vitamin E deficiency* (in some cases due to mutations in the gene for the α-tocopherol transport protein). Secondary causes of vitamin E deficiency, however, are more common. Secondary deficiency can be caused by any disease leading to severe malabsorption, including cystic fibrosis, cholestatic liver disease, celiac disease, and short bowel syndrome. Patients with vitamin E deficiency experience gait and limb ataxia, areflexia, proprioceptive sensory loss, dysarthria, and pigmentary retinopathy. The presence of retinopathy helps distinguish abetalipoproteinemia from Friedreich's ataxia. Signs of malabsorption are not always overt, especially in abetalipoproteinemia, but a history consistent with fat malabsorption should always raise suspicion of vitamin E deficiency in the ataxic patient. A low serum concentration of vitamin E confirms the diagnosis. In abetalipoproteinemia, decreased serum cholesterol concentrations, acanthocytes in the peripheral blood smear, and a characteristic abnormal serum protein electrophoretic pattern are also seen.

The *progressive myoclonic ataxias* (formerly called the Ramsay-Hunt syndrome) are a group of childhood disorders characterized by action myoclonus and progressive cerebellar ataxia. Causes include mitochondrial disorders, in particular the Kearns-Sayre syndrome and myoclonus epilepsy with red ragged fibers; muscle biopsy reveals red ragged fibers, and analysis of mitochondrial DNA identifies a deletion in the Kearns-Sayre syndrome and a tRNA point mutation in myoclonus epilepsy with red ragged fibers. Other causes of progressive myoclonic ataxia include celiac disease and the juvenile onset form of dentatorubral-pallidoluysian atrophy. This latter condition is one of several neurodegenerative diseases now known to be caused by the expansion of a trinucleotide repeat within the disease-related gene (trinucleotide repeat diseases). Expanded trinucleotide repeats also cause at least two other forms of spinocerebellar degeneration, Machado-Joseph disease and spinocerebellar ataxia, type 1—both of which typically occur in adults and are discussed further on. Patients with progressive myoclonic ataxia have infrequent or no seizures and relatively little cognitive decline, which are features that distinguish this group of diseases from the closely related progressive myoclonic epilepsies. Because the progressive myoclonic ataxias and epilepsies overlap considerably, however, causes of the latter should also be sought in patients presenting with myoclonus and progressive ataxia. Causes of progressive myoclonic epilepsy include neuronal ceroid lipofuscinosis, Lafora's disease, the sialidoses, and Unverricht-Lundborg disease.

The list of metabolic disorders that cause progressive ataxia in children is extensive (see Table 2). The ataxic child who does *not* clearly have Friedreich's ataxia should undergo appropriate metabolic tests to exclude these individually rare but collectively significant causes of progressive ataxia. The evaluation should also include MRI of the brain to exclude a mass lesion in the posterior fossa.

Early-Onset Cerebellar Ataxia With Retained Tendon Reflexes

Early-onset cerebellar ataxia with retained tendon reflexes is one fourth as common as Friedreich's ataxia and is characterized by progressive ataxia beginning in childhood, dysarthria, and retained reflexes. It appears to be a genetically heterogeneous disorder, with most cases inherited in an autosomal recessive manner. The presentation is similar to Friedreich's ataxia, with patients usually displaying gait ataxia between 2 and 10 years of age. Pyramidal tracts signs are common: increased tone in the arms, mildly spastic gait, and brisk knee and arm reflexes (although ankle reflexes may be absent). Distal vibration and position sense may be decreased in some patients. Early-onset cerebellar ataxia is distinguished from Friedreich's ataxia by the retained reflexes and the absence of diabetes, cardiac defects, and musculoskeletal deformities. Prognosis is better than in Friedreich's ataxia, although life expectancy is slightly reduced when compared with that in unaffected individuals.

Diagnostic Tests

No specific laboratory test results are known to be abnormal in early-onset cerebellar ataxia with retained reflexes. MRI typically reveals cerebellar atrophy without the cervical cord atrophy seen in Friedreich's ataxia; although some scans show spinal atrophy. Results of electrophysiologic studies are highly variable, perhaps reflecting the heterogeneous nature of early-onset cerebellar ataxia. In approximately one third of patients, EMG reveals a sensorimotor axonal neuropathy. These same patients usually display abnormal somatosensory evoked potentials. In a small percentage of patients, the results of electrophysiologic studies do not permit clear distinction from Friedreich's ataxia.

Pitfalls in Diagnosis

Early-onset cerebellar ataxia with retained reflexes is a diagnosis of exclusion. Metabolic causes of progressive ataxia (see Table 2) must first be excluded. The combined results of physical examination, MRI, nerve conduction studies, and somatosensory evoked potentials typically distinguish early-onset cerebellar ataxia with retained reflexes from Friedreich's ataxia.

Early-onset cerebellar ataxia and Friedreich's ataxia are by far the most common causes of childhood ataxia without a known metabolic defect. However, rarer forms of early-onset ataxia without a known metabolic defect have also been reported, each occurring in association with one of the following clinical features: hypogonadism, congenital or childhood deafness, optic atrophy, pigmentary retinopathy, or cataract and mental retardation (Marinesco-Sjögren syndrome). Physical or clinical evidence to suggest any of these rare conditions must therefore be sought.

Ataxia-Telangiectasia

Ataxia telangiectasia or Louis-Bar syndrome is an autosomal recessive, multisystem disorder characterized by progressive ataxia, oculocutaneous telangiectasias, recurrent bronchopulmonary infections, immunodeficiency, and defective DNA repair. Truncal ataxia in infancy is usually the first sign of disease, manifesting as postural instability and difficulty learning to walk. Occasionally the ataxia begins later in childhood. Some patients may present with uncontrollable shaking of the head (titubation). Oculocutaneous telangiectasias usually do not appear until age 3 to 5 years, well after the onset of ataxia, but they are occasionally the first sign of disease.

Truncal ataxia typically worsens and spreads to all four limbs, leaving most patients wheelchair-bound by age 12 years. As the disease progresses, dysarthria, oculomotor dyspraxia, and coarse nystagmus become prominent features. Extrapyramidal signs also appear, most commonly dystonic posturing, athetoid movements, and myoclonic jerks. Most patients show either a decline in cognitive function or arrested intellectual development. Unusual temper tantrums may be prominent early on. Rarely, the disease follows a more protracted course and begins later, even in young adulthood.

Telangiectasias first appear in the bulbar conjunctivae at 3 to 5 years of age and subsequently develop over the face, ears, neck, and flexor creases. Both body growth and the development of secondary sexual characteristics are delayed. Signs of premature aging may also be present, including premature graying. Immunodeficiency leads to recurrent sinopulmonary infections, which begin in later childhood and result eventually in chronic bronchiectasis and pulmonary insufficiency. The frequency of neoplasms, particularly lymphoreticular cancers, is greatly increased. The mean age of death is approximately 20 years and usually is due to infection or neoplasm.

Physical Examination

Early in the disease, obvious difficulty in standing and learning to walk may be the only physical finding. Some children display titubation (postural tremor) of the head. The truncal and gait ataxia eventually spreads to the limbs and is accompanied by an intention tremor. The earliest ocular findings include slow saccades, obligatory blinking when redirecting gaze, and nystagmus; these later progress to ocular dyspraxia. Often within a few years of onset, involuntary movements arise, including dystonic hand posturing, choreoathetoid movements, and myoclonic jerks. In advanced disease, patients may experience a peripheral neuropathy with distal weakness and decreased position and vibratory sensation. Areflexia may occur, although it is not characteristic as it is for Friedreich's ataxia.

Telangiectasias can be found in the bulbar conjunctivae, face, mouth, skin creases, and exposed areas of skin. Other skin changes include freckling, café au lait spots, and progeric changes of hair and skin. Short stature and immature development are common. Auscultation of the lungs may reveal signs of bronchopulmonary infection. A thorough examination of all organ systems is necessary for detecting signs of cancer. Leukemias and lymphomas are most common, but solitary tumors can arise from almost any organ.

Diagnostic Testing

Mutations in the *ATM* (ataxia-telangiectasia mutated) gene are responsible for the disease. Genetic testing may soon be available commercially and currently is available through research institutes. Genetic testing is important for carriers as well as affected individuals, since heterozygous females have a significantly increased risk of breast cancer. Nearly all patients have increased alpha-fetoprotein concentrations and decreased or absent IgA. Other abnormalities of immune function are common, including decreased IgE and IgM, lymphocytopenia, low helper T-cell counts, and a failure to respond to common antigens on skin testing. Chromosomal translocations occur frequently, particularly between chromosomes 7 and 14. A glucose tolerance test result may be abnormal, and some patients have overt diabetes. Mild increases in liver enzyme activity may also be found. MRI usually reveals cerebellar atrophy and enlargement of the fourth ventricle. Calcification in the basal ganglia occurs in some patients and, rarely, diffuse white matter changes may be seen. The chest film may show signs of pulmonary infection. When the diagnosis is uncertain, fibroblasts can be screened for increased x-ray sensitivity and radioresistant DNA synthesis, two hallmarks of ataxia-telangiectasia. Although additional neurologic tests are rarely necessary, nerve conduction studies and EMG may corroborate the clinical impression of a peripheral neuropathy.

Pitfalls in Diagnosis

The diagnosis is straightforward in the ataxic patient with telangiectasias, increased alpha-fetoprotein concentrations, and decreased IgA. Many patients, however, have not yet developed telangiectasias when first seen by the clinician. The absence of skeletal deformities and the presence of reflexes helps distinguish ataxia-telangiectasia from Friedreich's ataxia. Unless the diagnosis is certain, metabolic causes of ataxia and a mass lesion of the posterior fossa must be ruled out.

Two other diseases of DNA repair—xeroderma pigmentosa and Cockayne's syndrome—can cause ataxia and progressive neurodegenerative disease. However, patients with these conditions differ from those with ataxia-telangiectasia in that they display extreme photosensitivity (both diseases) with skin cancers and facial erythema (xeroderma) or characteristic facies (Cockayne's syndrome). In Cockayne's syndrome, MRI reveals calcification of the basal ganglia and abnormal white matter signal intensity. Xeroderma pigmentosa and Cockayne's syndrome also fail to show the expected laboratory abnormalities of ataxia-telangiectasia.

LATE-ONSET FORMS OF SPINOCEREBELLAR DEGENERATION

Classification of the late-onset spinocerebellar degenerative disorders has been particularly difficult and contentious. This is in large part due to the markedly variable phenotype seen in these disorders. Even in members of the same family, age of onset and disease severity can vary widely. Some of these disorders also show anticipation, that is, the tendency for the disease to occur earlier in successive generations of a family. These unusual clinical features are now explained by the particular type of genetic defect underlying some (if not all) of these disorders—the expansion of a trinucleotide repeat within the disease gene. These "dynamic" mutations are unstable, tending to change size when passed from one generation to the next (Table 3). At least two of the dominantly inherited late-onset ataxias, spinocerebellar ataxia, type 1 and Machado-Joseph disease, are known to be caused by expanded repeats, and others are likely to have the same cause. Several other neurodegenerative diseases, including Huntington's disease, dentatorubral-pallidoluysian atrophy, and spinobulbar muscular atrophy (Kennedy's syndrome), are caused by similar expanded trinucleotide repeats.

The discovery of trinucleotide repeat mutations has direct relevance to the clinician. First, and most important, particular spinocerebellar degenerative disorders can now be diagnosed with certainty by a simple, sensitive, and specific genetic test. Second, because these are dominantly inherited disorders, a positive test result carries profound implications for other family members. The clinician must therefore make sure that families are provided with genetic and psychological counseling and that testing of presymptomatic individuals is performed only after appropriate counseling. Third, because trinucleotide repeats tend to expand in successive generations of a family, the clinician should ask about subtle signs of disease in a patient's ancestors. The sporadic case might, after all, prove to be inherited. Fourth, since some sporadic cases may represent newly expanded repeats arising from intermediate-sized alleles, it may be appropriate to test for particular expanded trinucleotide repeats in bona fide sporadic cases.

Table 3. Trinucleotide Repeat Diseases

General Features
Autosomal dominant recessive or X-linked inheritance
Variable phenotype
Unstable expanded repeats change size with transmission
Larger repeats correlate with more severe disease
Anticipation is common and is due to increased repeat length in successive generations
Sporadic cases may arise from intermediate-sized repeats
Direct test for expanded repeat is sensitive and specific
The Diseases
Type 1 (neurodegenerative disorders with CAG repeats encoding polyglutamine)
Huntington's disease
Spinocerebellar ataxia, type 1*
Machado-Joseph disease (spinocerebellar ataxia, type 3)*
Dentatorubral-pallidoluysian atrophy*
Spinal and bulbar muscular atrophy (or Kennedy's syndrome)
Type 2 (multisystem disorders with repeats outside of protein coding region)
Myotonic dystrophy
Fragile X syndrome
Friedreich's ataxia

*May present with progressive ataxia.

In the past, adult-onset forms were classified according to pathologic features, for example, olivopontocerebellar atrophy and cerebellar-cortical atrophy. This classification is being replaced because neuropathologic changes, as distinctive as they may be, permit only an oversimplified descriptive nomenclature. A pathologic classification does not take into account biochemical and molecular features associated with genetic disturbances. Harding's classification of autosomal dominant cerebellar ataxias (Table 4) is more rational in light of the molecular genetic discoveries of the last decade. Most cases previously labeled as familial olivopontocerebellar atrophy fall within the largest class of autosomal dominant cerebellar ataxias, the type 1 class. Spinocerebellar ataxia, type 1 and type 3 (Machado-Joseph disease), the two most common forms of type 1 autosomal dominant cerebellar ataxia are discussed further on. Also discussed is late-onset pure cerebellar ataxia, a clinical syndrome that is genetically heterogeneous. It includes but is not limited to autosomal dominant cerebellar ataxia, type 3. Many cases previously called cerebellar-cortical atrophy fall into this group.

Type 1 autosomal dominant cerebellar ataxia consists of at least five genetically distinct disorders—spinocerebellar ataxia types 1 through 5 (Table 5). They are characterized by progressive cerebellar ataxia with varying degrees of bulbar dysfunction, ophthalmoparesis, pyramidal and extrapyramidal signs, optic atrophy, and dementia. Neuropathologic studies show variable patterns of spinocerebellar degeneration. The precise genetic defect has been identified for only two of these conditions—spinocerebellar ataxia, type 1 and type 3 (Machado-Joseph disease). In both, the defect is an expanded trinucleotide repeat.

Table 4. Classification of Late-Onset Hereditary Ataxias

Class	Associated Features
Autosomal dominant cerebellar ataxia, type 1	Variable ophthalmoplegia, dementia, extrapyramidal features, optic atrophy and amyotrophy
Autosomal dominant cerebellar ataxia, type 2	Pigmentary retinopathy ± ophthalmoplegia and extrapyramidal features
Autosomal dominant cerebellar ataxia, type 3	Pure cerebellar ataxia
Periodic autosomal dominant cerebellar ataxia	Intermittent episodes of ataxia, dysarthria, and vertigo; may be normal between episodes

Spinocerebellar ataxia types 1 and 3 probably are the most common forms of autosomal dominant cerebellar ataxia, yet still account for slightly less than half of all affected families.

Spinocerebellar Ataxia Type 1

Spinocerebellar ataxia type 1 (SCA1) is an autosomal dominant disorder characterized by cerebellar ataxia, ophthalmoparesis, and variable pyramidal and extrapyramidal signs; it may be the most common hereditary ataxia in Europe. The defect responsible is an expanded trinucleotide repeat in the spinocerebellar ataxia, type 1 gene on chromosome 6. Like other neurodegenerative trinucleotide repeat diseases, SCA1 shows marked phenotypic variability and anticipation within families. Neuropathologic findings include neuronal loss in the cerebellum (principally Purkinje's cells) and brain stem, and degeneration of spinocerebellar tracts. Atrophy is most pronounced in the ventral pons and middle cerebellar peduncles and is variable in the cerebellum, inferior olives, cranial nerve nuclei, substantia nigra, and striatum. The cerebral cortex is usually spared.

Like other trinucleotide repeat disorders, SCA1 usually becomes symptomatic in the third to fifth decades and progresses over 10 to 20 years. It can also present in childhood or much later in life. Gait ataxia is a common early sign, followed by limb ataxia and dysarthria. Dysarthria and fatigue are the presenting complaints in some patients.

SCA1 is a progressive disorder, evolving to severe four-limb ataxia, titubation, dysmetria, dysdiadochokinesia, and dysarthria. Most patients are wheelchair-bound within 15 to 20 years of onset. Dysphagia is often present early and eventually becomes life-threatening. Weight loss, even before the onset of severe dysphagia, is common. In most patients, early nystagmus progresses to a disabling ophthalmoparesis. Variable degrees of amyotrophy, distal wasting, dystonia, and choreoathetosis may be seen, but parkinsonian features are uncommon. Intellect remains largely intact until the late stages of disease, when behavioral changes and a frontal lobe–like syndrome may become prominent. Life expectancy is shortened, and death often results from respiratory failure or infection. Juvenile-onset disease progresses more rapidly and is usually paternally transmitted, as in Huntington's disease, another trinucleotide repeat disorder.

Physical Examination

Depending on the stage of disease, signs of cerebellar dysfunction may be limited to gait and lower limb ataxia or include all the features listed previously. Oculomotor disturbances can include nystagmus, lid retraction, loss of optokinetic nystagmus, upward gaze palsy, or a nearly complete ophthalmoplegia. Hyperreflexia is present initially, but tendon reflexes usually become depressed as the disease progresses. Amyotrophy is common, and decreased position and vibratory sensation can occur. Dystonia and choreoathetosis, if they occur, appear late in the course. Testing for expanded repeats has shown that some presymptomatic individuals have subtle neurologic signs, including gaze-evoked upward-beating nystagmus, intermittent tremor, and occasional unsteadiness.

Diagnostic Testing

The only important laboratory test is detection of an expanded CAG repeat at the *SCA1* locus on chromosome 6. This simple, sensitive, and rapid test is performed with the polymerase chain reaction and is now available at most major academic centers. In unaffected individuals, the repeat is between 6 and 39 trinucleotides in length, and greater than 40 trinucleotides in affected individuals. Pa-

Table 5. Distinct Genetic Forms of Type 1 Autosomal Dominant Cerebellar Ataxia

Disease	Locus	Mutation	Distinctive Features
Spinocerebellar ataxia, type 1	Chromosome 6	CAG trinucleotide repeat	Ophthalmoparesis, pyramidal and extrapyramidal findings
Spinocerebellar ataxia, type 2	Chromosome 12	Unknown	Slow saccades, minimal extrapyramidal findings
Spinocerebellar ataxia, type 3 (Machado-Joseph disease)	Chromosome 14	CAG trinucleotide repeat	As in spinocerebellar ataxia, type 1; bulging eyes and facial fasciculations common
Spinocerebellar ataxia, type 4	Chromosome 16	Unknown	Early areflexia; prominent sensory axonal neuropathy
Spinocerebellar ataxia, type 5	Chromosome 11	Unknown	Milder disease than spinocerebellar atrophy, types 1 through 4

tients with juvenile-onset disease have repeat lengths of greater than 60 trinucleotides. Because the size difference between normal and expanded repeats is narrow, the physician should exercise caution in making the diagnosis of SCA1 in a patient with equivocal neurologic findings and an intermediate repeat length (approximately 38 to 42 trinucleotides).

CT and MRI show brain stem and cerebellar atrophy, particularly involving the ventral pons and middle cerebellar peduncle. Atrophy of the cerebellar cortex and medulla may help distinguish SCA1 from Machado-Joseph disease. Other tests are not necessary in the setting of a positive expanded repeat test. However, evoked responses and EMG and nerve conduction studies can document a peripheral neuropathy, nuclear magnetic resonance (NMR) spectroscopy may show increased lactate concentrations in advanced cases, and PET may demonstrate decreased glucose utilization in the cerebellum and brain stem.

Spinocerebellar Ataxia Type 3

Spinocerebellar ataxia type 3 (SCA3), or Machado-Joseph disease is characterized by progressive gait ataxia, supranuclear ophthalmoparesis, and variable degrees of pyramidal and extrapyramidal signs, peripheral and cranial nerve deficits, and amyotrophy. Originally described in inhabitants of the Portuguese islands of the Azores, it is now recognized to be widespread, occurring in patients of both Portuguese and non-Portuguese descent. It may be the most common form of type 1 autosomal dominant cerebellar ataxia in the United States. Neuropathologic findings include degeneration of most of the cerebellar afferent and efferent pathways, pontine and dentate nuclei, substantia nigra and subthalamic nucleus, cranial motor nerve nuclei, and anterior horn cells. The cerebral cortex, striatum, cerebellar cortex, corticospinal tracts, and olives tend to be spared.

As with other neurodegenerative diseases caused by trinucleotide repeats, signs of SCA3 appear most frequently when patients are in their 30s or 40s but may begin before age 20 years (juvenile onset) or as late as age 60 years. The first symptom is usually gait ataxia, often made worse by sudden turning of the head. Fewer than 10 per cent of patients may first present with ocular signs, including diplopia and a staring expression. Children may show signs of disease at an earlier age than their parents or grandparents, a phenomenon known as anticipation. Patients with early-onset disease are more likely to show rigidity and dystonia of limbs than are typical patients with adult onset of disease.

As with other trinucleotide repeat diseases, SCA3 progresses slowly, although the rate may vary even within a family. In most patients, the disease progresses over 15 to 20 years but can evolve more rapidly in juvenile-onset disease and more slowly in patients with the latest onset of disease. Gait ataxia worsens slowly and is later accompanied by lower limb ataxia and eventually upper limb ataxia. In more advanced stages, incoordination is severe enough that patients need help with feeding and other daily activities.

Within 3 years of onset, most patients show signs of progressive supranuclear ophthalmoplegia. Peripheral involvement tends to occur later, in some patients progressing to marked distal amyotrophy. Dysarthria usually begins after several years and is soon followed by bulbar signs such as dysphagia and dysphonia. Weight loss begins within 5 to 10 years, preceding the dysphagia in some patients. Eventually patients are terminally bedridden. Cognitive functions remain largely intact throughout the course of illness, but sleep disturbances occur in roughly half the patients.

Physical Examination

Depending on the stage of disease, ataxia may be limited to gait alone or may include incoordination of the legs and, less frequently, the arms. Hyperreflexia is usually present in early stages but disappears as the disease progresses. Early ocular findings include loss of upward gaze, slow saccades, mild ocular dysmetria, and nystagmus. Later, supranuclear ophthalmoplegia with sparing of downgaze is found. In one third of patients, lid retraction and decreased blinking lead to the characteristic appearance of bulging eyes. In addition to bulbar signs such as dysphagia and dysphonia, cranial motor nerve involvement can cause facial palsy, ptosis, and lingual atrophy in the patient with advanced disease. Facial fasciculations are more common in SCA3 than in other forms of type 1 autosomal dominant cerebellar ataxia. Dystonia appears in roughly one third of patients and may take the form of dystonic hand posturing, facial grimacing, or blepharospasm. Parkinsonian features such as rigidity and bradykinesia may occur, but are usually mild.

The most variable feature of SCA3 is the degree of peripheral involvement. Some patients show loss of ankle reflexes with hyperreflexia elsewhere, whereas marked distal amyotrophy with areflexia occurs in others. Limb fasciculations are common. Mild sensory disturbances occur frequently, but autonomic dysfunction is unusual.

Diagnostic Testing

The only critical laboratory test is a blood test to detect the expanded trinucleotide repeat at the *MJD* locus on chromosome 14. Unaffected individuals have a repeat length of 13 to 36 trinucleotides, whereas affected individuals have repeat lengths of greater than approximately 60 trinucleotides (lengths of 36 to 60 trinucleotides have not been reported). As in all the neurodegenerative triplet repeat diseases, the repeated trinucleotide in SCA3 is the sequence CAG.

MRI demonstrates variable atrophy of brain stem structures. The pons, midbrain, cerebellar peduncles, and vermis are commonly affected. Sparing of the cerebellar cortex and olives in SCA3 helps distinguish it from SCA1. The presence of a sensitive genetic test eliminates the need for other more expensive, less definitive tests. PET and single photon emission computed tomography (SPECT) may demonstrate decreased glucose metabolism and blood flow, respectively, in brain stem structures, but the pattern cannot distinguish SCA3 from other type 1 autosomal dominant cerebellar ataxias. EMG of limb muscles shows signs of denervation in many patients.

Pitfalls in Diagnosis of Type 1 Autosomal Dominant Cerebellar Ataxia

Distinguishing the various forms of type 1 autosomal dominant cerebellar ataxia is difficult on clinical grounds alone because considerable overlap exists between SCA1 and SCA3 and other type 1 autosomal dominant cerebellar ataxias. The patient with bulging eyes and staring expression, prominent peripheral signs, and radiographic evidence of sparing of the olives and cerebellar cortex is more likely to have SCA3 than spinocerebellar ataxia, type 1. The patient in whom MRI reveals prominent cerebellar atrophy is more likely to have SCA1. Still, the definitive answer lies in identifying the specific expanded repeat that underlies each disorder.

In the appropriate clinical context, a positive trinucleotide repeat test for SCA1 or SCA3 clinches the diagnosis. However, in most families with autosomal dominant cerebellar ataxia, type 1, a genetic diagnosis is still not possible. A negative test result for both repeats excludes SCA1 and SCA3 and raises the possibility of other forms of type 1 autosomal dominant cerebellar ataxia, for which only linkage analysis is currently available (Table 5). SCA2 initially described in a large Cuban family, is characterized by ataxia, slow saccades without nystagmus, peripheral neuropathy, and minimal or no corticospinal and extrapyramidal signs. Radiographic and pathologic studies usually show atrophy of the olives, distinguishing it from Machado-Joseph disease but not from SCA1. In patients with spinocerebellar ataxia, type 4, ataxia is accompanied by a prominent sensory axonal neuropathy, pyramidal tract signs, and normal eye movements. SCA5 usually causes a milder form of disease with a minimal shortening of life span.

The certainty of genetic diagnosis requires that patients and families have pretest psychological and genetic counseling. In spinocerebellar ataxia, types 1 and 3, the largest CAG trinucleotide repeats tend to cause more severe disease of earlier onset. However, repeat length should not be used to predict outcome because the correlation is imprecise for all but the largest repeats.

When an ataxic patient has a family history of similar neurologic disease, testing for the Machado-Joseph disease and SCA1 expanded repeats is clearly appropriate. It is not clear, however, whether testing should be performed in patients who have clinical and radiographic features suggestive of autosomal dominant cerebellar ataxia but lack a family history. As has been shown for sporadic Huntington's disease, some sporadic cases of spinocerebellar degeneration may represent newly expanded repeats that arose from intermediate-sized alleles. Therefore we currently favor testing for expanded repeats in sporadic cases, with strict adherence to guidelines for informed consent. The yield of such testing has yet to be fully determined, but results may be helpful in selected patients.

Another dominantly inherited trinucleotide repeat disease that may present as progressive ataxia is dentatorubral-pallidoluysian atrophy. This condition, like spinocerebellar ataxia, types 1 and 3, is characterized by phenotypic variability and anticipation. In addition to ataxia, affected individuals show varying degrees of choreoathetosis, dementia, myoclonus, and epilepsy. Testing for the expanded repeat in the *DRPLA* gene on chromosome 12 is available. Type 2 autosomal dominant cerebral ataxia is distinguished from type 1 solely by the presence of retinopathy. Therefore, a careful funduscopic examination is necessary in any patient presenting with progressive ataxia. One form of this disease has been localized to chromosome 3. *Periodic ataxia* is unlikely to be confused with the progressive ataxia of spinocerebellar degeneration. In some families, this autosomal disorder of episodic imbalance is due to mutations in the *KCN1A* potassium channel gene.

Sporadic Olivopontocerebellar Atrophy

Sporadic olivopontocerebellar atrophy is often the correct diagnosis in patients who have clinical features of type 1 autosomal dominant cerebellar ataxia yet lack a family history. Also called olivopontocerebellar degeneration, sporadic olivopontocerebellar atrophy is one of the three major phenotypic variants of the disease *multiple-system atrophy,* the other two being Shy-Drager syndrome and striatonigral degeneration. Multiple-system atrophy is a protean disease manifested by a wide spectrum of deficits in the extrapyramidal and pyramidal systems, the autonomic nervous system, and the cerebellum and its afferent and efferent pathways. All forms of multiple-system atrophy are characterized to some degree by parkinsonism, but the individual phenotypic variants of multiple-system atrophy are identified by predominant involvement of a specific neural system: the cerebellum in sporadic olivopontocerebellar atrophy, the autonomic nervous system in Shy-Drager syndrome, and the basal ganglia in striatonigral degeneration. Sporadic olivopontocerebellar atrophy may appear clinically identical to type 1 autosomal dominant cerebellar ataxia, except that patients also typically show parkinsonian features such as rigidity and bradykinesia and may have evidence of autonomic insufficiency, such as bowel or bladder symptoms, sexual dysfunction, or orthostatic hypotension. MRI usually demonstrates atrophy in the cerebellum and brain stem, much like type 1 autosomal dominant cerebellar ataxia. However, recent studies suggest that PET can distinguish the two. Both show reduced glucose metabolism in the cerebellum, but only sporadic olivopontocerebellar atrophy displays reduced glucose metabolism in the basal ganglia, thalamus, and cortex. Moreover, only sporadic olivopontocerebellar atrophy demonstrates reduced ^{18}F-fluorodopa in the striatum, a biologic marker of parkinsonism. Unfortunately no specific laboratory tests can be used to identify sporadic olivopontocerebellar atrophy. The diagnosis remains largely clinical, and it may be reached only after years of progression reveal the full array of signs and symptoms.

With sporadic cases, other causes of progressive ataxia must also be excluded, including a mass lesion of the posterior fossa, demyelinating disease, vitamin E deficiency, and several metabolic disorders that rarely first show signs of disease in adulthood (the leukodystrophies, hexosaminidase deficiency, mitochondrial disorders).

Late-Onset Pure Cerebellar Ataxia

Late-onset pure cerebellar ataxia is a heterogeneous group of disorders characterized by progressive cerebellar dysfunction without serious oculomotor disturbance, dementia, or extrapyramidal features. It is not a single gene disorder; rather it is a clinical spectrum syndrome that can be seen in both sporadic and familial disorders (for example, type 3 autosomal dominant cerebellar ataxia). Disorders within this group are characterized by later onset and milder neurologic deficits than are seen in type 1 autosomal dominant cerebellar ataxia. The neuropathologic hallmark is degeneration of the cerebellar cortex, with or without involvement of the dentate nuclei and inferior olivary nuclei.

Patients typically present with gait and lower limb ataxia after 50 years of age. Dysarthria and oculomotor disturbances usually are not present at the onset of ataxia. Given the heterogeneous nature of this group of disorders, the clinical course may vary. Compared with type 1 autosomal dominant cerebellar ataxia, neurologic dysfunction generally begins later, progresses more slowly, and remains confined to the cerebellum and its afferent and efferent pathways. Lower limb ataxia slowly progresses to the upper limbs. Dysarthria is common, and nystagmus and dysmetric saccades may be seen. Some patients have dorsal column loss. Pyramidal tract signs (hyperreflexia and extensor plantar responses) are found in some patients, but extrapyramidal features (parkinsonism, dystonia, choreoathetosis) do not occur. Dementia is not a feature of this group of diseases. Symptoms begin late and progress slowly, which usually allows patients to live a normal life span.

CT and MRI reveal cerebellar cortical atrophy, usually with prominent vermian atrophy and occasionally with olivary atrophy. No specific laboratory tests are known to produce abnormal results, and the underlying genetic defects have not been identified.

The clinical and radiographic features of this group of disorders closely mimic those seen in acquired or secondary cerebellar degeneration. In sporadic cases, the diagnosis of late-onset pure cerebellar ataxia cannot be made until underlying causes have been excluded. Chronic ethanol abuse (usually in combination with malnutrition) and chronic drug exposure (e.g., phenytoin) are the most common causes of acquired cerebellar atrophy. Paraneoplastic cerebellar degeneration is a rare but important cause that can be identified by finding anti-Purkinje cell (anti-*Yo* or, less commonly, anti-*Hu*) antibodies in patients with carcinomas of the ovary, lung, and breast in adults and neuroblastoma in children. Hodgkin's disease and tumors of the uterus, stomach, and colon have also been associated with a cerebellar syndrome. In most cases, the cerebellar dysfunction progresses over days to weeks, distinguishing it from the slower course seen in hereditary causes. A careful screening for occult neoplasm should include breast and pelvic examination, mammography, CT of the pelvis and/or abdomen, and measurement of CA-125 antigen concentration.

Additional causes of progressive ataxia in adults include Wilson's disease, chronic progressive multiple sclerosis, late-onset leukodystrophies, and mass lesions of the posterior fossa. In the absence of a family history of similar neurologic disease, any patient presenting with progressive ataxia should undergo MRI of the brain to exclude demyelinating disease, tumor, or vascular malformation.

MULTIPLE SCLEROSIS AND OTHER DEMYELINATING DISEASES

By Robert L. Knobler, M.D., Ph.D.
Philadelphia, Pennsylvania

Multiple sclerosis (MS) is a neurologic disorder characterized by immune-mediated destruction of the myelin sheaths insulating nerve fibers of the central nervous system (CNS). The consequence of the loss of myelin is interruption of nerve impulse transmission in the affected pathways, which can result in the production of neurologic symptoms. Clinical symptoms reflect involvement of the particular pathway involved (e.g., optic neuritis is the end result of demyelination in the optic nerve, and any myelinated CNS pathway may be affected). However, neurologic symptoms do not always correlate with the number or location of lesions observed in the brain by magnetic resonance imaging (MRI) because some lesions produce only subtle findings and may therefore be considered neurologically "silent" areas.

The cause of this autoimmune disease is unknown at present, but like other autoimmune diseases, it typically follows a relapsing-remitting course initially, which is later followed by a secondary progressive course. Less commonly, MS may follow a primary progressive course. A benign form of MS, in which lesions are present without associated clinical symptoms, has also been recognized.

CLINICAL SYMPTOMS

Symptoms in MS occur when a demyelinating lesion in a particular pathway has reached sufficient size to cause a recognizable disturbance of nerve impulse conduction. Because the demyelinating lesions are inflammatory, associated tissue edema also causes symptoms. In fact, it is the resolution of edema with treatment (e.g., with steroids), that can lead to rapid improvement in symptoms over a few days of treatment. The nature of symptoms in MS depends on which myelinated fiber pathways in the CNS are affected by demyelination and edema. Involvement of one or more neurologic pathways is typical, and many symptoms are possible (Table 1).

MS frequently affects memory, mood (euphoria and/or depression) and cognitive behavior, visual acuity and control of eye movements, sensation (numbness and tingling, pain), balance, coordination, and motor power as well as bowel, bladder, and sexual function (Table 2). Other clinical features can include increased muscle tone with spasticity, increased and pathologic reflexes (extensor plantar responses), spasms, and severe fatigue. Some of these clinical manifestations may not be recognized by family members and coworkers, which often leads to further problems such as reactive depression due to a severe loss of self-esteem and limitation of interpersonal interactions.

Clinical attacks (exacerbations), defined as the new onset or worsening of symptoms lasting longer than 24 hours, must be distinguished from transient worsening (pseudoexacerbation) that can occur when the core body temperature rises from any of several causes; increased temperature slows nerve conduction in demyelinated nerve fibers. Hot baths, ingestion of hot food or drinks, physical exertion or high ambient temperature and humidity that limit normal body cooling by perspiration can all cause transient worsening of symptoms. Subclinical lesions, as observed on MRI, may also provide the neuroanatomic basis for such phenomena. Several laboratory tests, including examination of the cerebrospinal fluid (CSF), electrophysiologic evaluations (evoked potential testing), and imaging studies (computed tomography [CT], MRI), can be used to corroborate the findings of MS (Table 3), but none is pathognomonic for MS.

Table 1. Clinical Features of Multiple Sclerosis: Symptom Development

Pathology
Demyelination and edema
Impaired nerve conduction
Symptoms Reflect Impaired Conduction
Loss of ability to sustain repetitive discharge (fatigue)
Negative Symptoms
Loss of function
Positive Symptoms
Aberrant discharges, seizures, myoclonic jerks, pain, itching, tingling

Table 2. Presenting Features of Multiple Sclerosis With Exacerbation

Cognitive

Decreased memory and altered mood (euphoria and/or depression)

Visual

Decreased acuity, often associated with eye pain on movement, and difficulty in control of eye movements, double vision, with or without nystagmus

Abnormal Sensation

Numbness and tingling, pain (trigeminal neuralgia), bandlike sensation around the waist or an extremity, an electriclike sensation on neck flexion (Lhermitte's sign), altered balance, with or without vertigo

Abnormal Motor Control

Decreased coordination and motor power in one or more limbs, or more rarely the face (Bell's palsy)

Bladder, Bowel, and Sexual Functions

Incontinence, impotence, lack of genital sensation (these symptoms must be sought specifically)

Other

Increased muscle tone with spasticity, increased and pathologic reflexes (extensor plantar responses), spasms, and severe fatigue

CEREBROSPINAL FLUID

The CSF is analyzed for cell count and protein and glucose concentrations. The CSF glucose concentration is usually in the reference range in MS; if decreased, it suggests an infectious or other process, such as tuberculous meningitis, fungal meningitis, meningeal carcinomatosis, lymphoma, or sarcoidosis. Increased CSF protein concentration can occur in MS, but it is rarely greater than 100 mg/dL. This is usually related to an increased IgG concentration in the CSF and is reflected in the IgG-to-albumin ratio or the CSF IgG index, which is typically greater than 15 per cent in MS. Discrete bands of IgG are found in MS on isoelectric focusing or high resolution electrophoresis of the CSF. These bands are referred to as oligoclonal bands, but they are not unique to this disease. Myelin basic protein (MBP) may be found in the CSF as well. However, detection of MBP or antibodies to MBP has no unique significance in the diagnosis of MS. A mild to moderate CSF pleocytosis may be found in MS, and it is often characterized by somewhat atypical "activated" cells, numbering in a range of 5 to 100 cells/mm^3. If the clinical setting warrants, and aseptic meningitis is suspected, lumbar puncture should be repeated within 1 week or sooner (see article on acute viral encephalitis and meningitis).

Table 3. Laboratory Tests in Multiple Sclerosis

Cerebrospinal Fluid Findings

Oligoclonal bands in the CSF
Increased IgG index in the CSF

Clinical Neurophysiologic Testing

Visual evoked potentials
Brain stem auditory evoked potentials
Somatosensory evoked potentials
Motor evoked potentials

Imaging Studies (MRI, CT)

New lesion activity
Total lesion burden

CSF = cerebrospinal fluid; MRI = magnetic resonance imaging; CT = computed tomography.

ELECTROPHYSIOLOGIC STUDIES

Evoked potential testing can be performed on the visual, brain stem auditory, and somatosensory and motor systems. These tests can be used to follow abnormalities over time. They do not show abnormalities that are specific for MS but simply demonstrate abnormalities of nerve conduction from any cause. These tests are most useful when a subclinical lesion is sought and found through the selected use of evoked potential testing. For example, detection of an abnormal visual evoked potential—for example, prolongation of the P100 latency—in the absence of clinical symptoms of visual involvement adds to the clinical data if MS is suspected.

MAGNETIC RESONANCE IMAGING IN MULTIPLE SCLEROSIS

MRI can help visualize the pathologic lesions of MS in the white matter pathways of the brain and spinal cord. However, care must be taken to distinguish between the demyelination, reactive gliosis, and edema characteristic of MS and white matter lesions with a similar location and appearance but due to other causes (e.g., hypertension, human immunodeficiency virus [HIV], Lyme disease, Alzheimer's disease). In this regard, the clinical history and associated laboratory findings are important for interpretation of the MRI findings to ensure that they are consistent with MS.

The use of gadolinium enhancement helps characterize new MS lesions (lesion activity) by identifying breakdown of the blood-brain barrier (BBB) and the presence of edema in the early stages of demyelinating lesion development. Gadolinium-enhanced lesions reflect new lesion activity. Frequent new lesion activity probably leads to the accumulation of an increased lesion burden over time, which is eventually reflected in more neurologic symptoms.

DIFFERENTIAL DIAGNOSIS

Other causes of demyelination that may mimic MS are listed in Table 4. They include vascular malformations and emboli, a variety of infectious and postinfectious causes, degenerative spinal diseases, other autoimmune disorders such as systemic lupus erythematosus and Behçet's disease, inherited metabolic disorders such as the leukodystrophies, a variety of acquired toxic-metabolic forms of demyelination, traumatic causes, misdiagnosis (e.g., spinocerebellar degeneration), and manifestations of neoplastic diseases.

PATHOGENESIS AND EPIDEMIOLOGY

The use of MRI as a research tool has also served to modify our current understanding of the pathogenesis of MS. Serial MRI studies have shown that subclinical lesions come and go on a continual basis, modifying the older notion that lesions form only when new clinical symptoms

Table 4. Differential Diagnosis of Multiple Sclerosis

Vascular

Arteriovenous malformation, multiple emboli, vasculitis

Infectious

Postinfectious encephalomyelitis, granulomatous disease, neurosyphilis, progressive multifocal leukoencephalopathy, progressive leukoencephalopathy of AIDS, HTLV-I (HTLV-I associated myelopathy), tropical spastic paraparesis, multiple abscesses, toxoplasmosis, Lyme disease, parameningeal infection with multiple cranial nerve involvement, recurrent or relapsing (Mollaret's) meningitis, tuberculoma

Trauma

Cervical spondylosis, craniovertebral junction lesions

Autoimmune

Systemic lupus erythematosus, Behçet's disease, Sjögren's syndrome, sarcoidosis

Metabolic

Hereditary metabolic demyelination, metachromatic leukodystrophy, Krabbe globoid cell leukodystrophy, adrenoleukodystrophy, Pelizaeus-Merzbacher disease, Alexander's disease, Canavan's disease, phenylketonuria, Refsum's disease, acquired toxic-metabolic demyelination (hexachlorophene, hypoxia, diphtheria toxin, chemotherapy [methotrexate]), nutritional demyelination (vitamin B_{12} deficiency, central pontine myelinolysis, Marchiafava-Bignami disease), traumatic demyelinating diseases (edema, barbotage), leukoaraiosis (periventricular leukomalacia)

Iatrogenic

Misdiagnosis (e.g., spinocerebellar degeneration)

Neoplastic

Carcinomatous meningitis, primary CNS lymphoma, multiple metastases, primary infiltrating neoplasm (glioma)

Degenerative

Arnold-Chiari malformation, syringomyelia

AIDS = acquired immunodeficiency syndrome; HTLV = human T-cell lymphotrophic virus; CNS = central nervous system.

appear (an exacerbation). In fact, some new lesions are observed to form at the time that older lesions are resolving. Therefore, not all new lesions detected by MRI are associated with clinical symptoms, and clinical silence does not assure that no new lesions have formed in the CNS.

This newer understanding of the pathogenesis of MS strongly justifies the use of ongoing treatments to alter the natural history of this demyelinating disease. The use of intravenous steroids (methylprednisolone) rapidly resolves the gadolinium-enhanced cerebral lesions detected by MRI and may delay the accumulation of these lesions. Furthermore, the use of recombinant human interferon beta (Betaseron) has dramatically limited new lesion formation as detected in noncontrast MRI studies, and it has reduced the frequency and severity of attacks of relapsing-remitting MS.

MS is most often diagnosed in individuals between the ages of 18 and 50 years and is almost twice as common in females as in males. Familial studies have shown that the disease has a higher incidence in identical twins, approaching 30 per cent compared with 4 per cent in fraternal twins and other siblings, suggesting that genetic factors do not act alone in the pathogenesis of MS. Epidemiologic studies provide further support for a role of a combination of genetic and environmental factors influencing the development of MS. Viral agents have long been suggested as the specific environmental trigger.

Although no consistent association between MS and a specific viral pathogen has emerged, MS patients have higher than normal CSF titers of antibodies to a number of common human viruses. The antibody concentrations generated in the CSF may reflect a capacity for increased antibody production as an inherited characteristic of this disease. These high titers of virus-specific antibody may provide survival value by protecting neuronal cells of the CNS from pathogens that would otherwise severely damage or destroy neuronal cells of the CNS. A consequence of this vigorous immune response in the CNS may be nonspecific damage to the myelin sheaths (demyelination).

Acute viral illnesses in patients with MS are frequently followed by a clinical exacerbation of MS symptoms. This may be due to the effects of fever causing slowing of nerve conduction in demyelinated nerve fibers (pseudoexacerbation) or activation of cells of the immune system, which then enter the CNS to produce demyelination. No evidence currently exists for entry of virus into the CNS during acute infections or for entry of virus-specific immune cells that react with CNS antigens or persistent viral antigens located in the CNS white matter.

A higher incidence of MS in northern climates has been attributed to geographic preferences for similar latitudes following population migrations. For example, northern Europeans, who have a higher incidence of MS, favor more northerly climates in North America. This geographic association more likely represents a genetic influence rather than an environmental one. Neither a specific gene nor a consistent environmental risk factor has yet been identified, although the HLA haplotypes A3, B7, and DR2 have frequently been associated with MS in whites of western European origin. Nevertheless, MS is probably an immunologically mediated demyelinating disease that requires an environmental trigger in genetically predisposed individuals.

PATHOPHYSIOLOGY

The major function of the myelin sheath is to enhance the speed of conduction of the nerve impulse efficiently. Loss of myelin (demyelination) leads to either slowed or blocked nerve impulse conduction along the nerve fiber. Conduction of nerve impulses can also be impaired along affected nerve fibers by inflammation and swelling (edema). Partially myelinated and remyelinated fibers can be transiently compromised by increased core body temperature.

Myelin in the CNS is synthesized and maintained by the oligodendrocyte, a cell that has been estimated to produce between 5 and 100 separate segments (internodes) of myelin. Histologically, myelin is easily recognized in cross section by its jelly roll form surrounding the nerve fiber. The spiral nature of this sheath accommodates the growth of axons of the developing nervous system by slippage and compaction of layers of the spiral. Axons that are demyelinated are already larger in diameter, and during remyelination, these axons are covered by only a thin myelin sheath, with compromise of conduction as temperature rises.

The normal function of the myelin sheath is to limit the energy required for nerve conduction to the sodium channel–rich regions of the nerve fiber, which are gaps between adjacent sheaths known as nodes of Ranvier. Normally, the nerve impulse jumps rapidly and efficiently from one node of Ranvier to the next in a process called saltatory conduction. Larger diameter axons have both thicker myelin sheaths and longer internodes, permitting greater speeds of nerve impulse transmission. Cytoplasmic channels of communication throughout the myelin sheath are most evident at the ends of the internode (i.e., the paranodal region). The axonal membrane underlying the paranodal region is rich in conduction-blocking potassium channels that help restrict nerve impulse conduction to the nodes of Ranvier. Following the loss of myelin internodes and their paranodal regions during demyelination, potassium channels spread into the nodal region, contributing to the block of nerve impulse conduction.

OTHER DEMYELINATING DISEASES

Postinfectious Encephalomyelitis

Demyelination may occur as a consequence of a prior viral infection in circumstances other than MS. This condition is known as postinfectious encephalitis, but it does not actually implicate late effects of viral replication on neural cells as the cause of neurologic damage. Instead, it represents indirect immunopathologic responses elicited by the virus and is characterized by a monophasic course and immune reactivity to MBP. A number of synonyms exist for this syndrome, including parainfectious encephalitis, acute disseminated encephalomyelitis, and allergic encephalomyelitis. This disorder may also occur following vaccination with brain-based preparations (e.g., rabies vaccinations) and has been termed postvaccination encephalomyelitis. The latter has been eliminated through the use of nonbrain inocula.

Postinfectious encephalomyelitis typically occurs within the 2-week period after recovery from an infection, such as a childhood exanthem or, more rarely, following a vaccination. The onset may be abrupt. The spinal cord, optic nerves, and peripheral nervous system are frequently involved. Patients often have headache, fever, nausea, vomiting, and focal neurologic signs. To a lesser extent, patients may experience seizures and altered levels of consciousness. Neuroimaging usually demonstrates multifocal white matter lesions that can be hemorrhagic in severe cases. Death may occur in as many as 20 per cent of affected individuals, specifically in association with measles. Other conditions associated with this disorder include chickenpox, rubella, mumps, Epstein-Barr–associated infectious mononucleosis, and *Mycoplasma pneumoniae* infection.

Acute Necrotizing Hemorrhagic Leukoencephalitis

Acute necrotizing hemorrhagic leukoencephalitis is a fulminant, often fatal form of demyelinating disease that can follow an upper respiratory infection. It often progresses to death over 48-hours and is associated with a heavy infiltration of polymorphonuclear leukocytes.

Transverse Myelitis

Transverse myelitis presents as either an acute or subacute onset of clinical symptoms, including lower extremity weakness, sensory abnormalities with a sensory level, and abnormalities of sphincter function that may or may not have associated back pain. Sometimes an associated prior history of infection can be elicited. Complete recovery occurs in about two thirds of affected individuals, but some are left with permanent deficits. Poor prognostic indicators include the severity of the deficit at onset and failure to respond to therapeutic intervention after about 3 months of effort.

Transverse myelitis may represent a spectrum of illnesses, including arteriovenous malformation (AVM), Lyme disease, lupus, MS, and cancer (particularly lymphoma and bronchogenic carcinoma). Some individuals have presented clinically with CNS demyelination, in the form of transverse myelitis, coupled with a radiculopathic Guillain-Barré pattern of peripheral demyelination.

PERIPHERAL NEUROPATHIES

By Michael E. Shy, M.D.
Detroit, Michigan

The peripheral nervous system (PNS) consists of motor, sensory, and autonomic neurons that extend outside the central nervous system (CNS) and are associated with Schwann cells or ganglionic satellite cells. The PNS includes the dorsal and ventral spinal roots, spinal and cranial nerves, sensory and motor terminals, and the bulk of the autonomic nervous system. Motor neurons extend from their cell body in the ventral horn of the spinal cord to the neuromuscular junctions at the muscle they innervate. The cell bodies of primary sensory neurons lie outside the spinal cord in the dorsal root ganglia (DRG), where they extend peripherally to specialized sensory end-organs, including nociceptors, thermoreceptors, and mechanoreceptors. Central projections from DRG enter the spinal cord through the dorsal roots. At each spinal segment, the ventral roots, carrying motor axons, and the dorsal roots, carrying sensory axons, join to form mixed sensorimotor nerves. In the cervical, brachial, and lumbosacral areas, the mixed spinal nerves form plexuses from which the major anatomically defined limb nerves emanate. Each mixed nerve is composed of large numbers of myelinated and nonmyelinated nerves of varying diameters. The large, myelinated axons include motor neurons and large-fiber sensory nerves, which subserve the position and vibration senses. Small, thinly myelinated or nonmyelinated axons subserve primarily nociception and autonomic modalities. Preganglionic sympathetic autonomic fibers begin in the intermediolateral column of the spinal cord and synapse in the sympathetic trunk with sympathetic ganglia. Preganglionic parasympathetic fibers travel long distances from their cell bodies in the brain stem or sacral spinal cord to reach terminal ganglia that are near the organs that the parasympathetic fibers innervate. The sympathetic and parasympathetic divisions work synergistically to mediate motivational and emotional states as well as to monitor the body's basic physiology. Peripheral neuropathy is a general term for disorders that affect peripheral nerves. These disorders can be genetic, toxic, immunologic, or metabolic. Some or all populations of peripheral nerves can be affected. Since in many cases mixed sensorimotor nerves are affected, the majority of peripheral neuropathies are sensorimotor, although isolated motor or sensory neuropathies do exist (see later).

The key in evaluating a patient with peripheral nerve disease is to take a systematic approach. A multitude of laboratory abnormalities, toxins, and hereditary and acquired disorders can cause peripheral neuropathy. A "shotgun" approach, in which every conceivable cause of neuropathy is excluded, is expensive and may not identify the cause of the neuropathy; therefore, it is not in the patient's best interests. The preferred approach is to use the history and physical examination to demonstrate peripheral nerve disease, utilize electroneuromyography (ENMG) to characterize the demyelinating or axonal nature of the process, and then to order the relevant tests for diagnosing the neuropathy (Fig. 1).

HISTORY AND PHYSICAL EXAMINATION

The first goal of the history and physical examination is to identify the problem as a peripheral neuropathy. This identification is based on characteristic motor, sensory, and autonomic features, which are discussed later. The next objective is to determine whether the onset is acute (less than 1 month), subacute (less than 6 months), or chronic (more than 6 months) and whether the disorder is symmetrical or asymmetrical.

In peripheral nerve disease, weakness is often distal and more severe in the legs than the arms. Extensor muscles tend to be more affected than are flexors. Therefore, the extensors of the great toe and of the foot in the lower extremity, and the wrist or finger extensors in the upper extremity, are particularly useful muscles for testing. When weakness is caused by axonal destruction, muscle wasting is more severe than when weakness is caused by CNS disease, such as that following a stroke. Wasting in the lower extremity is frequently detected on the anterior calf and in the upper extremity on the dorsal hand between the index finger and the thumb. Cramps, the painful knotting of a muscle, frequently occur in motor or sensorimotor neuropathies. Fasciculations appear as small twitches of the muscle. They represent the random firing of a motor unit, which consists of a motor neuron and all the muscle fibers that it innervates. When fasciculations are associated with weakness and wasting of muscle, they suggest the diagnosis of motor neuron disease or amyotrophic lateral sclerosis (ALS). However, fasciculations also occur in many normal people and are especially associated with fatigue and caffeine ingestion. Their presence in the absence of weakness and muscle wasting is not likely to be significant. Reflexes in motor neuropathies, as in sensorimotor or sensory neuropathies, are usually reduced. Although the vast majority of neuropathies are sensorimotor, a group of predominantly motor neuropathies has been identified (Table 1).

Sensory loss in peripheral nerve disease is also predominantly distal and can be separated into sensory modalities of large fibers (position and vibration) and small fibers (pain and temperature). Large fibers are usually ensheathed by myelin, while small fibers are only thinly myelinated or are not myelinated at all. Small-fiber neuropathies are often accompanied by burning or stabbing pain as well as by loss of sensation to pain and temperature. Numerous causes of predominantly sensory neuropathies have been reported (Table 2).

Autonomic symptoms frequently accompany neuropathies with small-fiber sensory predominance. These include orthostatic hypotension, urinary retention or incontinence, impotence, gastric motility dysfunction, pupillary dysfunction, heat intolerance, and diaphoresis. Causes of neuropathies with predominant autonomic features are listed in Table 3.

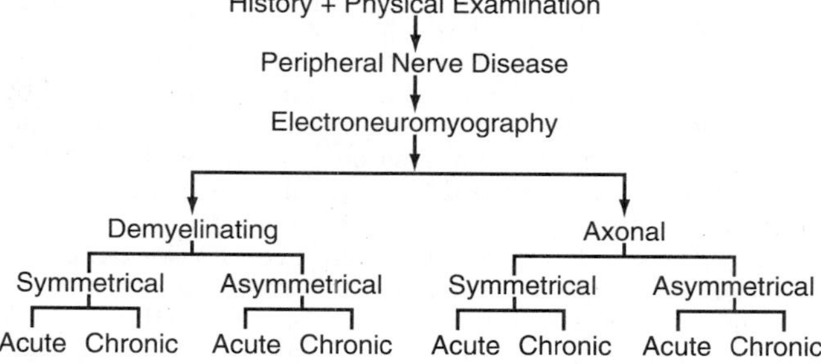

Figure 1. An approach to diagnosing peripheral neuropathies.

Table 1. Predominantly Motor Neuropathies

Immune Mediated
Guillain-Barré syndrome
Chronic inflammatory demyelinating polyneuropathy (CIDP)
Pure motor neuropathy (PMN), often with conduction block
Toxic
Lead
Dapsone
Paraneoplastic
Motor neuropathy associated with lymphoma
Hereditary
Porphyria
Hexosaminidase A deficiency

Table 2. Predominantly Sensory Neuropathies

Large-Fiber Neuropathies
Immune Mediated
Sensory neuropathy associated with Sjögren's syndrome
Toxic and Metabolic
Cisplatin
Paclitaxel
Vitamin E deficiency
Vitamin B_{12} deficiency
Paraneoplastic
Sensory neuropathy with "anti-Hu" antibodies
Hereditary
Hereditary sensory neuropathy
Abetalipoproteinemia
Small-Fiber Neuropathies
Associated With Systemic Disease
Diabetes mellitus
Amyloidosis
Human immunodeficiency virus (HIV)
Toxins
Metronidazole
Misonidazole
Vacor
Hereditary
Hereditary sensory neuropathy
Fabry disease
Tangier disease

ELECTRONEUROMYOGRAPHY (ENMG)

After the physical examination, ENMG is performed to determine whether a neuropathy is demyelinating or axo-

Table 3. Neuropathies With Autonomic Features

Associated With Systemic Disease
Diabetes mellitus
Amyloidosis
Toxins
Vacor
Hereditary
Riley-Day syndrome (familial dysautonomia)
Shy-Drager syndrome (chronic orthostatic hypotension)

nal. If the neuropathy is demyelinating, the ENMG helps distinguish between hereditary and acquired demyelinating neuropathy. If the neuropathy is axonal, the ENMG can help distinguish between uniform axonal neuropathies and the asymmetrical mononeuritis multiplex. Also, ENMG can help decide whether the neuropathy is chronic. These distinctions are important, because they identify potentially treatable neuropathies. Virtually all acquired demyelinating neuropathies respond to therapy directed at suppressing the immune response, as do many axonal forms of mononeuritis multiplex. Conversely, few effective treatments are available for the hereditary or chronic axonal neuropathies. After neuropathies have been classified by ENMG, appropriate decisions can be made about laboratory tests that may be useful to further characterize the neuropathy.

The ENMG study is typically divided into two sections: nerve conduction velocities and the needle electromyogram. Nerve conduction velocities measure conduction along the fastest conducting, myelinated motor and sensory nerves. Slowed conduction velocities (70 per cent of normal) suggest demyelinating neuropathy. For technical reasons, motor nerve conduction velocities measure conduction over the main body of nerves—but not their proximal or distal portion. Distal motor latencies and F-wave latencies measure velocities over the distal and proximal portions of the nerves. In inherited demyelinating neuropathies, such as Charcot-Marie-Tooth disease type 1, conduction velocities tend to be uniformly slowed. Conversely, in acquired demyelinating neuropathies, such as the Guillain-Barré syndrome, nerve conductions are likely to be slowed asymmetrically. In asymmetrical slowing, the conduction velocity of some nerves is slowed, but that of others is normal. Moreover, some regions of the same nerve may exhibit slow conduction, while other regions are normal. Nerve conduction velocities are also useful in diagnosing axonal neuropathies. In the case of motor conduction, the compound muscle action potential (CMAP) is the sum of action potentials of the individual muscle fibers that have been stimulated to fire by individual axons. The sensory nerve action potential (SNAP) is a summation of action potentials from individual sensory axons. In axonal neuropathies, axons are lost, so the sum of the action potentials is reduced in amplitude. Therefore, in axonal neuropathies, the magnitude of the CMAP, SNAP, or both is reduced.

The needle electromyogram also helps analyze axonal neuropathies. At rest, the muscle is electrically silent; however, when axons are acutely damaged, the muscle they innervate develops "spontaneous" activity characterized by fibrillations and positive sharp waves. If a nerve is transected (e.g., owing to trauma), portions of the axon distal to the lesion degenerate in a process called wallerian degeneration. In this setting, fibrillations and positive sharp waves develop within 2 to 3 weeks of the injury. In an axonal neuropathy, if the process is acute or subacute, fibrillations or positive waves are typically observed, although they may disappear in a chronic axonal neuropathy. Fasciculations, the random, spontaneous firing of motor units, also appear when the muscle is at rest. When healthy axons attempt to reinnervate denervated muscle fibers, the waveform of their motor units becomes more complex, or polyphasic. Thus, in chronic axonal neuropathies, a higher percentage of polyphasic potentials than normal is observed in early recruited motor units. Recruitment of motor units is also reduced in patients with axonal neuropathies because fewer axons and, therefore, fewer motor units are available for recruitment.

DEMYELINATING PERIPHERAL NEUROPATHIES

Evaluation of Demyelinating Neuropathies

When the history, physical examination, and ENMG suggest the presence of a demyelinating neuropathy, appropriate laboratory tests can further categorize and clarify the disorder. If the demyelination is uniform, particularly in the setting of a family history of neuropathy, the patient probably has a form of Charcot-Marie-Tooth disease (see later). These neuropathies are usually chronic and progress slowly over years. The appropriate test for these patients is genetic screening of DNA, from blood, for abnormalities in the genes encoding myelin proteins PMP-22 and PO or the myelin-related protein connexin 32.

When the history, physical examination, and electrophysiology suggest an asymmetrical process in the absence of a family history, the evaluation should include lumbar puncture. Spinal fluid examination helps characterize demyelinating neuropathies, many of which, such as the Guillain-Barré syndrome and chronic inflammatory demyelinating polyneuropathy (CIDP), have increased spinal fluid protein concentrations with only a few white blood cells. The evaluation for acquired demyelinating neuropathies also includes serum protein electrophoresis (SPEP) and an immunoelectrophoresis (IPEP) to detect monoclonal gammopathy.

The question of screening for the presence of specific autoantibodies in demyelinating (or axonal) neuropathies is controversial. Several commercial firms provide antibody testing for patients with neuropathy. Although detection of these antibodies—particularly anti–myelin-associated glycoprotein (MAG), anti-Hu, and anti-G_{M1} can be useful in specific circumstances (see later), they are expensive and, if ordered indiscriminately, can actually confuse the diagnosis and management. In fact, the antibodies may be associated with certain neuropathies, but may not be completely specific for them. Thus, treatment decisions based solely on the presence of autoantibodies lead to treatment of some patients who should not be treated. Additionally, many patients with treatable neuropathies do not have antibodies to MAG or G_{M1}. In these cases, appropriate treatment may be inappropriately withheld. Firm evidence of an acquired demyelinating neuropathy must be sought. If it is found, the patient is a likely candidate for immunosuppressive therapy. Then, a screen for antibodies to MAG or G_{M1} can be considered if the information is still deemed clinically useful.

Sural nerve biopsy is useful when it can answer a specific question about the neuropathy. It is rarely useful as part of a battery of tests ordered in the search for the cause of a neuropathy, when the clinician is simply hoping to find something helpful. Appropriate use of sural nerve biopsy

Table 4. Laboratory Evaluation of Acquired Demyelinating Neuropathies

Necessary Studies
ENMG
CSF evaluation (protein, cells, glucose)
SPEP, IPEP, UPEP
Useful Studies
Thyroid function studies
HIV screening
Sural nerve biopsy

HIV = human immunodeficiency virus; IPEP = immunoelectrophoresis; SPEP = serum protein electrophoresis; UPEP = urine protein electrophoresis.

in demyelinating neuropathies is to document CIDP (see later) or detect IgM deposits on nerve tissue suspected of being damaged by monoclonal IgM M-proteins. An outline for the evaluation of demyelinating neuropathies is given in Table 4.

Inherited Demyelinating Neuropathies

The diagnosis of many of the inherited neuropathies can now be made with certainty by DNA analysis (Table 5). The most frequently occurring is Charcot-Marie-Tooth disease type 1A (CMT1A), which is inherited as an autosomal dominant disorder. The incidence of CMT1A is about 1 in 2500, and the disease typically presents around 12 years of age with difficulties in running, climbing, or jumping. Calf muscles, in particular, may appear atrophied ("storklike legs"), and high arches or flat feet are frequent. Nerve conduction velocities are uniformly slowed, with rates as slow as 10 to 20 m per second (normal rates, 40 to 50 m per second). The disease is slowly progressive, and many patients need ambulatory aid as they grow older. However, the disease is variably expressed, and an affected family member may have only high arched feet, for example, making an accurate family history difficult to obtain. Sural nerve biopsies of patients with CMT1A show uniform demyelination, little if any inflammation, and many "onion bulb" formations, which are thought to represent concentric rings of Schwann cells trying to remyelinate axons. CMT1A is caused by a 1.5-megabase duplication on chromosome 17 in the region that contains the Schwann cell myelin-specific gene PMP-22. Point mutations in PMP-22 may also cause a phenotype that resembles CMT1A, suggesting that it is the abnormality of PMP-22 that causes CMT1A. Certain point mutations in PMP-22 lead to very severe, autosomal dominant demyelinating neuropathies that appear before the age of 5 years. Typically, severe demyelinating neuropathies presenting in young childhood are called Dejerine-Sottas disease. This disorder is often autosomal recessive; therefore, the relationship between PMP-22 mutations and all cases of Dejerine-Sottas disease is unknown.

When patients have a deletion of PMP-22, instead of a duplication or point mutation, they develop a distinct neuropathy termed hereditary neuropathy with liability to pressure palsies (HNPP). These patients have an increased tendency to develop entrapment syndromes, such as carpal tunnel or tarsal tunnel syndrome, but they typically do not develop clinical evidence of diffuse neuropathy.

Charcot-Marie-Tooth disease type 1B is much less frequent than CMT1A, with only rare cases reported. Type 1B is also an autosomal dominant neuropathy and is caused by various point mutations in the gene encoding the major PNS myelin protein, PO. Only a few families have been characterized, and no reliable method exists to distinguish CMT1B from CMT1A on clinical grounds alone. Some reports have noted that CMT1B may have larger numbers of onion bulbs on sural nerve biopsy and very thickened nerve roots that are apparent on magnetic resonance examination of the spinal cord. These associations are not certain, however, and neither sural nerve biopsy nor magnetic resonance imaging are required for routine evaluation of patients with Charcot-Marie-Tooth disease.

The X-linked form of Charcot-Marie-Tooth disease (CMTX) is more frequent than CMT1B but less frequent than CMT1A. Clinically, it is distinguished from CMT1A and CMT1B by the X-linked pattern (males get the neuropathy) of inheritance. CMTX is caused by point mutations in the Schwann cell gene connexin 32. The diagnosis of CMT1A, CMT1B, and CMTX can be made by analyzing DNA obtained from blood cells.

A small group of inherited disorders has been reported to have demyelinating neuropathies as a component of the disease, but not necessarily as the main feature. These conditions include Refsum's disease, phytanic acid accumulation with associated retinitis pigmentosa and cerebellar ataxia; metachromatic leukodystrophy, galactosyl-3-sulfate accumulation with associated CNS dysmyelination; adrenoleukodystrophy, long-chain fatty acid accumulation induced by mutations in the *ALD* gene on the X chromosome, with associated CNS dysmyelination and adrenal failure; Krabbe disease, galactocerebroside abnormalities associated with CNS dysmyelination; and Pelizaeus-Merzbacher disease, mutations in the myelin gene proteolipid protein (PLP) with associated CNS dysmyelination.

Table 5. Gene Defects in Inherited Demyelinating Neuropathies

Charcot-Marie-Tooth disease type 1A	Duplication on chromosome 17 (region containing PMP-22 gene)
Charcot-Marie-Tooth disease type 1B	Point mutations in P0 gene
Hereditary neuropathy with liability to pressure palsies (HNPP)	Deletion of PMP-22 allele
Charcot-Marie-Tooth disease type X	Point mutations in connexin 32

Acquired Demyelinating Neuropathies

Acquired demyelinating neuropathies are typically distinguished from inherited neuropathies by the lack of a family history and by their asymmetry. Moreover, in some types, the rapid onset is not consistent with the diagnosis of Charcot-Marie-Tooth disease (Table 6). Acquired demyelinating neuropathies must be correctly diagnosed, because virtually all of them are treatable.

Guillain-Barré Syndrome

The most frequent acquired demyelinating neuropathy is the Guillain-Barré syndrome. In two thirds of the cases, its onset occurs about 2 weeks following an upper respiratory infection or other viral illness. Patients develop the rapid onset of weakness, often in an ascending pattern from their legs to their arms and face. Breathing is often affected, and respiratory distress can be life-threatening. Approximately 50 per cent of patients reach their nadir within 2 weeks, 75 per cent within 3 weeks, and more than

Table 6. Acquired Demyelinating Neuropathies

Condition	Onset
Guillain-Barré syndrome	Rapid
CIDP	Subacute to chronic
Associated with plasma cell dyscrasia	
IgM anti-MAG	Subacute to chronic
IgG with POEMS	Subacute to chronic
MMN with conduction block	Subacute to chronic

CIDP = chronic inflammatory demyelinating polyneuropathy; MAG = myelin-associated glycoprotein; MMN = multifocal motor neuropathy; POEMS = polyneuropathy, organomegaly, endocrinopathy, monoclonal gammopathy, and skin changes.

90 per cent within 4 weeks of the onset of weakness. After a short period of stabilization, patients tend to spontaneously improve at about the same rate at which they became weak. More than two thirds of patients recover spontaneously. Sensation is also lost in Guillain-Barré syndrome, but usually to a lesser extent than strength. Plasmapheresis and intravenous immunoglobulin (IVIG) are effective in the treatment of Guillain-Barré syndrome, and they are often used to improve the rate and extent of recovery. The diagnosis of this condition is based on a triad: patchy demyelination on nerve conduction velocities, areflexia, and increased protein concentration in the absence of an increased cell count in the CSF. The amplitude of the CMAP on nerve conduction studies has been reported to be the best prognostic indicator for recovery; the more normal the CMAP, the better the chance for recovery. Typically less than 5 to 10 white blood cells/mm^3 are found in the CSF, and the protein may be above 100 mg/dL. In patients with human immunodeficiency virus (HIV) infection, a high CSF cell count is associated with Guillain-Barré syndrome. In this setting, the disease often occurs around the time of seroconversion and should raise suspicion of HIV infection. The cause of Guillain-Barré syndrome is not known, but some cases appear to be associated with prior infection by the enteropathogenic gram-negative rod *Campylobacter jejuni*. This bacteria contains the Galβ1-3GalNAc carbohydrate, which is also a part of the ganglioside G_{M1}. Some patients with Guillain-Barré syndrome have antibodies to G_{M1}, and an autoimmune process related to *Campylobacter* may play a role in the pathogenesis of some cases.

Two variants of Guillain-Barré syndrome deserve mention; the first, the Miller Fischer variant, consists of ophthalmoplegia, ataxia, and areflexia. The time course is similar to that of Guillain-Barré syndrome. The ataxia occurs in the absence of any obvious cerebellar lesion or extensive large-fiber sensory loss. The reason that typical patients with Guillain-Barré syndrome do not develop ophthalmoplegia and these patients *do* is unknown. Nerve conduction velocities are either normal or mildly slowed in the Miller Fischer variant. Recently, patients with the Miller Fischer variant have been found to have autoantibodies to the ganglioside G_{Q1b}, which may be involved in the pathogenesis of the disease. A second variant is an acute axonal form of Guillain-Barré syndrome, called acute motor axonal neuropathy (AMAN) syndrome, that has recently been discovered in northern China. Patients with AMAN are particularly likely to have had preceding *Campylobacter jejuni* infections and antibodies to G_{M1} implicating the organism and/or the infection in the cause of the disease. Cases of the AMAN syndrome are now being reported in North America.

The differential diagnosis of Guillain-Barré syndrome is usually straightforward, with the acute onset of a patchy demyelinating neuropathy; however, two rarer disorders can mimic the syndrome. The first is diphtheria, in which the toxin can induce an acute demyelinating neuropathy. The second is ingestion of buckthorn berries, which grow in the milder regions of the United States.

Chronic Inflammatory Demyelinating Polyneuropathy

Unlike Guillain-Barré syndrome, which is acute, CIDP, by definition, progresses more slowly over at least 4 months. Occasionally, the disease waxes and wanes (relapsing CIDP), but most patients become progressively weaker. Like Guillain-Barré syndrome, CIDP also is associated with asymmetrical slowing on nerve conduction velocities, increased protein concentration with few cells in the CSF, and areflexia. Unlike Guillain-Barré syndrome, a viral illness does not usually precede CIDP.

Neuropathies Associated With Plasma Cell Dyscrasia

Plasma cell dyscrasia (PCD) is associated with both axonal and acquired demyelinating neuropathies; the treatable forms are the demyelinating neuropathies. The others are discussed in the section on axonal neuropathies. In PCD, monoclonal antibodies are produced by individual clones of B lymphocytes and are detected by serum protein electrophoresis (SPEP), immunoelectrophoresis (IPEP), and urine protein electrophoresis (UPEP). In some cases the antibodies invade and damage tissue, causing multiple myeloma or Wäldenstrom's. Typically, however, the PCD is associated with no disease apart from the neuropathy and is termed monoclonal gammopathy of uncertain significance (MGUS). The presence of PCD with neuropathy, by itself, does not implicate the antibody in the disease. More than 1 per cent of the population older than 50 years have monoclonal gammopathy, frequently with no associated disorder.

Neuropathy and IgM Monoclonal Gammopathy

IgM monoclonal antibodies that bind to carbohydrate determinants shared by MAG, PO, PMP-22, and a glycolipid termed SGPG, are associated with an acquired sensorimotor, demyelinating neuropathy that has many features in common with CIDP. The neuropathies are chronic and usually evolve over years, beginning with the loss of large- and small-fiber sensory abnormalities. Weakness develops and eventually can become debilitating. The IgM antibody can be shown by Western blot or enzyme-linked immunosorbent assay (ELISA) to bind to the carbohydrate, and by immunohistochemistry to bind to peripheral nerve tissue. It has caused neuropathy when injected into cat nerve or when passively transferred to chickens.

Rarely, patients with IgM gammopathy have been described with a motor neuropathy that resembles a lower motor neuron form of ALS. These patients have weakness and wasting of muscle, occasional fasciculations, and decreased reflexes, rather than the increased reflexes associated with ALS. IgM antibodies from these patients bind to G_{M1} by ELISA or immuno thin-layer chromatography assays. Some of these patients have been shown to improve following immunotherapy. Other patients with this clinical syndrome have no monoclonal IgM but, instead, have polyclonal IgM antibodies that bind to G_{M1}. Many of these patients have also improved with immunotherapy. Careful, multisegment nerve-conduction analysis reveals that many, but not all, of the patients have conduction block, suggesting focal demyelination. These cases, usually known as multifocal motor neuropathy (MMN) associated with conduction block, may exist in the absence of antibodies to G_{M1} and are worth identifying because they represent a treatable disorder, unlike the ALS they resemble. Some IgM antibodies associated with demyelinating neuropathies do not bind to any known antigen in peripheral nerve. Nevertheless, these patients may improve when treated with immunotherapy.

Neuropathy and IgG Monoclonal Gammopathy

Most neuropathies with IgG monoclonal antibodies are axonal, but one important exception is osteosclerotic multiple myeloma and the related POEMS syndrome. About 3 per cent of myeloma patients have sclerotic lesions in bone, and more than 50 per cent of these patients have a demyelinating neuropathy that may respond to immunotherapy. When the peripheral neuropathy (P) and myeloma (M) are associated with organomegaly (O), endocrinopathy (E), and skin changes (S), the disorder is called the POEMS syndrome.

Table 7. Laboratory Evaluation of Axonal Neuropathies

Necessary Studies
ENMG
Knowledge of medications and drugs ingested
Routine fasting electrolytes (glucose, creatinine, SUN especially)
Urinalysis
Liver function tests
Erythrocyte sedimentation rate
Antinuclear antibodies
Rheumatoid factor
Useful Studies
Lyme disease titers
SPEP, IPEP, UPEP, cryoglobulins
Vitamin B_{12} assay (consider Schilling test)
Nerve biopsy (looking for specific abnormalities only)
Urine for porphyrias
Hair sample for arsenic

IPEP = immunoelectrophoresis; SPEP = serum protein electrophoresis; SUN = serum urea nitrogen; UPEP = urine protein electrophoresis.

AXONAL NEUROPATHIES

Symmetrical axonal neuropathies can also be divided into acute, subacute, and chronic forms. Acute axonal neuropathies are unusual. The axonal variant of Guillain-Barré syndrome, the AMAN syndrome, was discussed earlier. In addition, the acute ingestion of arsenic or thallium can lead to acute neuropathic pain, although the resultant neuropathy is more slowly progressive. Acute-onset axonal neuropathies can also occur with porphyria and tick bite paralysis. The vast majority of neuropathies associated with systemic disease, caused by metabolic abnormalities, medications, or toxins, are axonal neuropathies that occur over months to years. When an axonal neuropathy progresses for more than 5 years, it is more likely to be inherited, although some of the axonal neuropathies associated with systemic disease can progress over this period as well.

Evaluation of Axonal Neuropathies

When the axonal neuropathy is uniform, much of the initial screening is a natural outcome of the medical history, physical examination, and laboratory evaluation. For example, clinical awareness of neuropathy-causing disorders (e.g., diabetes mellitus and renal failure) or toxins (e.g., alcohol, drug abuse, chemotherapeutic agents) should emerge early in the evaluation. Protein electrophoresis is also helpful in diagnosing some cases of axonal neuropathy associated with monoclonal gammopathies (Table 7). Sural nerve biopsy can be useful in diagnosing amyloidosis, vasculitis, sarcoidosis, leprosy, or giant axonal neuropathy, but it should not be used indiscriminately.

Inherited Axonal Neuropathies

Charcot-Marie-Tooth disease type 2 is an axonal sensorimotor neuropathy that is inherited as an autosomal dominant disorder. Although not as frequent as CMT1A, it is not rare. The clinical presentation is similar to that of CMT1A, with the patient experiencing progressive difficulties in running, climbing, or jumping. However, CMT2 is likely to develop later in life and may be milder; indeed, patients may not even realize that a neuropathy may be the cause of foot and ankle problems in their middle years. The axonal nature of the process is illustrated by normal nerve conduction velocities with reduced CMAP and SNAP amplitudes. Sural nerve biopsy typically reveals axonal loss, but not demyelination. The genetic abnormality that causes CMT2 has not yet been identified, so the diagnosis remains clinical. Careful examination of family members may be necessary in demonstrating the autosomal dominant inheritance pattern.

Axonal neuropathies are typically associated with other inherited diseases that affect multiple organ systems. Predominantly sensory axonal neuropathies are a component of Friedreich's ataxia and Fabry disease. Certain rare hereditary sensory neuropathies can affect both large and small sensory fibers. Familial dysautonomia, known as Riley-Day syndrome, leads to a degeneration of unmyelinated autonomic and sensory fibers. Shy-Drager syndrome is a multisystem disorder in which autonomic dysfunction occurs secondary to the degeneration of autonomic neurons.

Acquired Axonal Neuropathies Associated With Systemic Disease

Diabetes Mellitus

Patients with type I (insulin-dependent) and type II (non–insulin-dependent) diabetes frequently develop neuropathies in middle age, although the neuropathy can occur earlier. The neuropathies are similar in both type I and type II. By far, the most frequent is the symmetrical predominantly sensory form that occurs as many as 50 per cent of diabetics. Typically, the neuropathy begins with paresthesias and loss of sensation in the feet. In some cases, the neuropathy progresses in an ascending fashion. When symptoms or signs reach the knees, problems begin to occur in the fingers. By this time, autonomic abnormalities, including orthostatic hypotension, diarrhea, impotence, incontinence, and anhidrosis, may appear. Although weakness is a minor component of the neuropathy, nerve conduction velocities show abnormalities of both sensory and motor nerves. Interpretation of the conduction velocities can be confusing, because evidence of both demyelinating and axonal damage is often present. Pathologically, however, the neuropathy appears axonal. The cause of the symmetrical sensory neuropathy is not known, but it probably involves a combination of vascular and metabolic abnormalities. Abnormalities of *myo*-inositol or sorbitol pathways may be involved, but this theory remains controversial. Usually, the more severe neuropathies are associated with poor glucose control.

Diabetic patients can also develop acute mononeuropathies, including mononeuritis multiplex (see later), although the incidence is much less than that for symmetrical sensory neuropathy. The basis of these mononeuropathies is probably nerve infarction. Typical clinical presentations of these focal neuropathies are ophthalmoplegia (third, fourth, or sixth nerve palsies), proximal leg weakness (femoral neuropathy or "diabetic amyotrophy"), and thoracic pseudoradiculopathy (intercostal neuropathies). The mononeuropathies usually present with pain followed by loss of function of the nerve involved; thus, symptoms may be either motor or sensory. Gradual recovery of function can occur over a period of months. Patients with diabetes also are more likely to develop compression neuropathies, such as carpal tunnel syndrome, tarsal tunnel syndrome, and ulnar neuropathy.

Malignancy

Sensorimotor axonal neuropathies occur in the presence of malignancy, but the association between the two is not always clear. In some cases, however, the neuropathy is clearly associated with the malignancy. The pure sensory neuropathy associated with "anti-Hu" antibodies is a paraneoplastic syndrome associated predominantly with small cell carcinoma of the lung. This neuropathy is predominantly large fiber, with severely decreased vibration and position sense, and can precede the malignancy by as long as 2 years. The osteolytic form of multiple myeloma is associated with neuropathy in more than 10 per cent of patients, and this neuropathy is usually axonal. As many as 25 per cent of patients with Waldenström's macroglobulinemia have neuropathy, and many of these conditions are also axonal. These neuropathies can be sensory or sensorimotor, involve large as well as small fibers, and respond poorly to treatment. Rarely, a lymphoma patient can have predominantly motor axonal neuropathies.

Several medications used to treat malignancy are associated with neuropathy. Vincristine (Oncovin) and vinblastine (Velban) cause a neuropathy that begins with paresthesias and then evolves into a predominantly motor axonal neuropathy. Cisplatin (Platinol) and paclitaxel (Taxol) cause predominantly large-fiber sensory neuropathy.

Collagen Vascular Disease

Collagen vascular diseases also cause mononeuritis multiplex (see later). However, as many as 50 per cent of patients with polyarteritis nodosa (PAN) have axonal neuropathy that can be the presenting symptom. Wegener's granulomatosis, Churg-Strauss vasculitis, and hypersensitivity vasculitis can be associated with axonal neuropathies. Approximately 10 per cent of patients with systemic lupus erythematosus have neuropathy. Rheumatoid arthritis is associated with an increased frequency of entrapment syndromes. Sjögren's syndrome may be accompanied by a large-fiber sensory neuropathy. Although not classically a collagen vascular disease, the inflammatory disorder sarcoidosis may be associated with a sensorimotor axonal neuropathy or polyradiculopathy.

Amyloidosis

Primary amyloidosis is caused by mutations in the transthyretin gene, and acquired amyloidosis is associated with deposits of monoclonal antibodies. Both forms are associated with small-fiber sensory and autonomic neuropathies. Predominant symptoms are painful dysesthesias accompanied by impotence.

Infection

Virtually all patients with HIV infection develop a peripheral neuropathy during the course of their disease. At the time of seroconversion, they may develop Guillain-Barré syndrome. However, after the CD4 count has dropped below 400, all patients eventually develop a predominantly small-fiber sensory axonal neuropathy associated with painful dysesthesias and decreased sensation to pain and temperature. The cause of the neuropathy is unknown. Some patients with acquired immunodeficiency syndrome (AIDS) develop a painful, lumbosacral polyradiculopathy caused by cytomegaloviral infection. The medications ddI (2′,3′-dideoxyinosine, didanosine), ddC (2′,3′-dideoxycytidine, zalcitabine), and d4T (2′,3′-didehydro-2′,3′-dideoxythymidine) used to treat AIDS all induce dose-dependent painful sensory neuropathies that mimic the small-fiber sensory neuropathy associated with the disease itself.

Lyme disease, caused by infection with the tick-borne spirochete *Borrelia burgdorferi,* can cause multiple cranial neuropathies and mononeuritis multiplex. Axonal sensorimotor neuropathies have occasionally been reported in patients.

Leprosy, the most common cause of neuropathy in the world, is increasingly present in the United States. The neuropathy is axonal, occurs in the lepromatous form of the disease, and is caused by direct infection of the nerve by *Mycobacterium leprae.* Since the bacteria grow best at 86°F, the neuropathy predominantly affects the cooler (distal) portion of the extremities.

Metabolic Diseases

The predominant metabolic disorders associated with neuropathy are renal, hepatic, and thyroid diseases. Patients with renal failure are likely to develop a painful axonal sensorimotor neuropathy that can progress and involve large-fiber sensory modalities and even cause weakness. The chances of neuropathy are increased if the renal failure progresses to the point at which dialysis or transplantation is needed. However, even patients with stable renal disease (creatinine >2 mg/dL) are susceptible to these neuropathies. The porphyrias (acute intermittent, variegate, and coproporphyric) are associated with predominantly motor axonal neuropathies that typically affect the arms more than the legs. Barbiturates, anesthetic agents, or other drugs can precipitate the neuropathy. Hypothyroidism can be associated with axonal neuropathy, and increased frequencies of entrapment syndromes are more probable sequelae.

Acquired Axonal Neuropathies Associated With Toxins

Alcoholic Neuropathy

Ethanol, the most common toxin that causes neuropathy, is associated with chronic alcohol abuse. Most patients with alcoholic neuropathy will have ingested at least 100 mL of ethanol daily for at least 3 years. The neuropathy is symmetrical and predominantly sensory during the early stages and affects both small and large fibers. Eventually, weakness also develops. Both sensory and motor loss depend on nerve length, with initial symptoms occurring in the feet. Painful paresthesias are a frequent early feature of the neuropathy. Whether the neuropathy is caused by the alcohol itself or by associated vitamin deficiencies remains unclear.

Vitamin Deficiencies

Sensorimotor axonal neuropathies occur with thiamine, pyridoxine, folate, and pantothenic acid deficiencies. These neuropathies frequently present with painful dysesthesias. They are rare in the United States except when they are associated with alcoholism, malabsorption, or fad diets. Vitamin B_{12} deficiency can occur when isoniazid therapy is given without supplementation of the vitamin. Vitamin B_{12} deficiency can induce a large-fiber sensory neuropathy as part of combined-system degeneration. Vitamin E deficiency, usually from malabsorption, results in a large-fiber sensory neuropathy associated with ataxia.

Heavy Metal Ingestion

Lead ingestion induces a motor neuropathy that appears axonal in adults, who are likely to present with bilateral wristdrops. In children and laboratory animals, lead appears to induce a demyelinating neuropathy. Patients who survive acute arsenic or thallium ingestion develop a painful predominantly sensory axonal neuropathy. Organic mercury poisoning may cause axonal sensorimotor neuropathy in addition to CNS damage. In all these situations, neuropathy rarely occurs without clinically significant exposure and involvement of other systems besides the PNS.

Drugs and Other Toxins

Axonal neuropathies are associated with medications used to treat HIV and malignancy (see above). Other drugs are also associated with axonal neuropathy; the antibiotics amphotericin, ethambutol, and chloroquine cause axonal neuropathies. Chronic metronidazole treatment for Crohn's disease can cause sensory neuropathy. Dapsone, used in the treatment of leprosy or skin diseases, is associated with a pure motor neuropathy. Sulfonamide or nitrofurantoin can cause axonal neuropathies. Phenytoin (Dilantin) leads to a sensorimotor axonal neuropathy after many years of use. Seafood (usually large tropical fish such as grouper) containing ciguatera toxin causes a painful sensory axonal neuropathy. Ingestion of the rat poison Vacor leads to a severe small-fiber sensory and autonomic neuropathy with orthostatic hypotension as a predominant feature.

Table 8. Axonal Causes of Mononeuritis Multiplex

Diabetes mellitus
Vasculitis
Polyarteritis nodosa (PAN)
Wegener's granulomatosis
Allergic granulomatous angiitis (Churg-Strauss syndrome)
Rheumatoid arthritis
Chronic inflammatory condition
Sarcoidosis
Infections
HIV (cytomegalovirus)
Leprosy
Cryoglobulinemia
Amphetamine abuse
Tumors (myeloma, neurofibromatosis)

Mononeuritis Multiplex

Asymmetrical neuropathies in which some peripheral nerves are spared and others damaged are called mononeuritis multiplex. Most of these are axonal, and the demyelinating forms, such as the Guillain-Barré syndrome or CIDP have been discussed above. The most frequent causes of axonal mononeuritis multiplex are diabetes mellitus and the collagen vascular diseases (see above). Other causes of mononeuritis multiplex include mixed cryoglobulinemia and inflammatory diseases, such as sarcoidosis and leprosy. The causes of mononeuritis multiplex are listed in Table 8.

MOTOR NEURON DISEASES

By Jeremy M. Shefner, M.D., Ph.D.
Boston, Massachusetts

The motor neuron diseases are a group of disorders that affect both adults and children. The genetic bases of some of these diseases are currently known, and other diseases are likely to have a genetic basis. For the adult neurologist, the most commonly encountered noninherited motor neuron disease is amyotrophic lateral sclerosis (ALS). The clinical definition of ALS is quite rigid, and many adult patients do not fulfill all the criteria at the time of initial presentation. These patients sometimes acquire other labels, such as progressive bulbar palsy, primary lateral sclerosis, and spinal muscular atrophy. However, many of these patients will ultimately exhibit enough clinical signs to support the diagnosis of ALS, and even in patients who do not, the pathology will usually be indistinguishable from that of ALS.

Although the majority of adults with motor neuron disease fall under the category of ALS or its related syndromes, other processes can produce similar clinical presentations. Among these are multifocal motor neuropathy with conduction block, and motor neuron disease associated with lead intoxication, hyperthyroidism, or infectious disease. Because treatment is available for a subset of patients with these secondary motor neuron diseases, their distinction is of critical importance.

Historically, the inherited motor neuron diseases were the province of the pediatric neurologist. However, adult-onset inherited motor neuron diseases are increasingly being identified. Classic ALS is familial in approximately 10 per cent of patients; of these, approximately 20 per cent have a defined mutation of the *SOD1* gene on chromosome 21. In addition, Kennedy's syndrome is an adult-onset spinal muscular atrophy with X-linked inheritance. Table 1 presents a classification of the more frequently encountered motor neuron diseases.

ADULT MOTOR NEURON DISEASE

The most common form of adult motor neuron disease is amyotrophic lateral sclerosis, defined as a disease involving progressive upper and lower motor neuron deterioration at multiple levels of the neuraxis. At presentation, patients may have signs and symptoms related only to

Table 1. Classification of Motor Neuron Diseases

Noninherited Adult Diseases
Amyotrophic Lateral Sclerosis
Primary lateral sclerosis
Progressive bulbar palsy
Spinal muscular atrophy
Motor Neuron Diseases Associated With Other Conditions
Multifocal motor neuropathy with conduction block
Motor neuron disease of hyperthyroidism
Postpolio syndrome
Lead neuropathy
Inherited Diseases
Adult Diseases
Familial amyotrophic lateral sclerosis
X-linked bulbospinal muscular atrophy
Pediatric Diseases
Werdnig-Hoffmann disease
Wohlfart-Kugelberg-Welander syndrome
Hexosaminidase deficiency

upper motor neuron or to lower motor neuron disease, but the diagnosis can be made with certainty only when both types of abnormalities are present. The World Federation of Neurology has established criteria for the diagnosis of ALS; on purely clinical grounds, the diagnosis of ALS requires the presence of both upper and lower motor neuron signs in the bulbar musculature as well as concurrent upper and lower motor neuron involvement in two of the three spinal regions (cervical, thoracic, and lumbosacral). Lower motor neuron signs include weakness, muscle wasting, and fasciculations, while upper motor neuron signs include increased deep tendon reflexes, spasticity, pseudobulbar features, extensor plantar responses, and other abnormal stretch reflexes.

When patients fulfill these criteria, the clinician is left with little in the way of differential diagnosis, even in the absence of confirmatory diagnostic tests. Most commonly, however, patients present with fragments of the above syndrome, and the clinician must make appropriate use of neurophysiologic and radiographic tests to eliminate other possible diseases. Common initial presentations are discussed below. With time, most patients who present with partial syndromes will show spread of abnormalities, and the diagnosis then becomes more obvious.

Occasionally, patients present with a purely spastic disorder, involving increased tone in bulbar and spinal musculature and slow, clumsy movements, but little muscle wasting or weakness. This syndrome, named primary lateral sclerosis, was described in the 1800s shortly after the original descriptions of ALS. In most cases, patients initially presenting with pure upper motor neuron signs will eventually develop classic ALS. However, a small subgroup of patients appear to have disease restricted to the descending cortical pathways. These patients have a relatively benign clinical course, with expected survival of more than 15 years.

Another group of patients present with signs limited to the bulbar musculature. At the initial evaluation, upper and lower motor neuron signs are seen together; most often, speech is spastic and fasciculations of the tongue are obvious. Historically, this presentation was called progressive bulbar palsy and was distinguished from classic ALS. The current view, however, is that these patients will develop classic disease and their clinical course is indistinguishable from that of other ALS patients.

Some patients present with purely lower motor neuron signs; in these patients, reflexes are usually absent or reduced. The presenting symptom is often limited to weakness in one limb; with time, the weakness spreads and involves multiple extremities. Some of these patients develop signs of upper motor neuron dysfunction and thus are classified as having classic ALS. Other patients remain with only lower motor neuron signs, showing increasing weakness and atrophy in multiple areas of the neuraxis. Such patients are often diagnosed as having progressive muscular atrophy and are distinguished from ALS patients by their lack of upper motor neuron signs and by the slow progression of the disease.

Rarely, a patient presents with slowly progressive weakness in one limb. Muscle atrophy may be dramatic, and deep tendon reflexes in the limb are usually absent. After root and peripheral nerve entrapments are excluded, motor neuron disease is usually considered; however, the process may remain localized indefinitely. This process has been named benign focal amyotrophy. It affects young males almost exclusively and is a reassuring though rare entity to be considered when dealing with such patients.

In some patients with clinical signs of motor neuron disease, an underlying or associated condition can be found. Recently, a subset of patients with pure lower motor neuron findings were discovered to have a motor neuropathy rather than an anterior horn cell disease. The diagnosis of this condition is made neurophysiologically; sensory nerve conduction studies are normal, but motor nerve conduction studies show multiple areas of conduction block. Clinically, arms are more often affected than legs, and deficits are usually asymmetrical. Although reflexes in very weak limbs are usually reduced, in less affected areas reflexes may be preserved or even relatively enhanced. However, no definite upper motor neuron signs are present. Disease progression is usually slower than that of other forms of motor neuron disease. This syndrome has been called multifocal motor neuropathy with conduction block (MMNCB). When first described, this disorder was causally linked to antibodies to the ganglioside GM_1; however, many patients with this syndrome do not have antiganglioside antibodies, and patients with classic ALS may have detectable anti-GM_1 antibodies. Correct diagnosis is essential, as many patients with MMNCB dramatically respond to immunosuppressive drugs or intravenous immunoglobulin.

Although MMNCB is not strongly associated with specific immunologic abnormalities, it is clear that as many as 10 per cent of patients with otherwise typical motor neuron disease have an associated paraproteinemia. The monoclonal spike may be IgA, IgG, or IgM, and treatment to reduce the concentration of antibody does not usually affect the course of the motor neuron disease other than MMNCB. Thus, the nature of the association is unclear.

Other medical disorders have also been associated with motor neuron disease. For example, although most hyperthyroid patients have muscle weakness due to myopathy, a few have developed motor neuron involvement. While acute polio is rare and does not present a significant diagnostic challenge for the neurologist, many patients who have recovered from childhood polio report new weakness decades after the infection. In this postpolio syndrome, the clinical and electrophysiologic findings may be indistinguishable from those of purely lower motor neuron disease; appropriate diagnosis depends on the history and lack of rapid disease progression. In most patients, progressive weakness occurs in the limbs that were originally affected. Many individuals report subjectively rapid deterioration, but objective assessment usually reveals a very slow decline that can be measured only over years. Finally, severe lead poisoning in adults may produce a lower motor neuron syndrome. Focal weakness of the wrist and finger extensors and bilateral footdrop have been described.

Presentation and Progression

Although patients with classic ALS present with characteristic signs and symptoms involving both the extremities and the bulbar musculature, most patients have focal signs and symptoms early in the course of their illness. In half of all patients with ALS, the most common initial symptom is arm weakness. Wristdrop is also a characteristic early sign, often noted with concurrent wasting of intrinsic hand muscles. By contrast, flexor compartment forearm muscles are usually affected later in the disease. This asymmetry of forearm involvement typically leads to a clawed posture of the hand. Classic ALS spreads from the distal to the proximal arm, where the biceps and deltoid muscles are usually affected before the triceps.

About one quarter of patients present with lower extremity symptoms, most commonly a unilateral footdrop. As in the upper extremity, weakness tends to spread regionally, first to more proximal muscles in the same leg and then to the opposite leg, before it ascends to involve the arms. Most of the remaining patients present with bulbar dysfunction or bulbar dysfunction combined with other symptoms. Altered clarity of speech is often the first sign of bulbar involvement; difficulty in swallowing is also noted early. Problems with liquids occur before problems with solids; carbonated and alcoholic beverages are not as well tolerated as thicker liquids.

Importantly, most of the signs and symptoms mentioned above are related to lower motor neuron dysfunction. By contrast, although upper motor neuron signs may be appreciated by the examining physician early in the course of ALS, they are rarely the cause of symptoms. It is the unusual ALS patient who initially reports limb stiffness and slowed movements. Even as the disease progresses and upper motor neuron signs become more flagrant, lower motor neuron loss continues to be the most important factor contributing to disability.

Other less common presentations of ALS include isolated respiratory failure and diffuse fasciculations. The latter are common in the general population and may precipitate a visit to a neurologist. However, in the absence of clear signs of motor neuron loss, fasciculations are almost never a harbinger of ALS. Electromyography can document the presence of fasciculations but cannot distinguish between those that are benign and those that are associated with ALS. Muscle cramps are commonly reported by patients with ALS, but the cramps are almost always associated with significant upper motor neuron disease. Cramps are not usually seen in otherwise normal limbs.

Some neurologic symptoms, when reported, should make the clinician doubt the diagnosis of ALS. Although end-position nystagmus and mild abnormalities of rapid eye movements can be seen, diplopia or vertigo is extremely uncommon. Reports of vague sensory symptoms are common, but objective sensory loss is rare and should prompt the clinician to consider alternative or concurrent disease processes. Patients often report dysesthetic sensations that could represent true sensory symptoms, but that could also be due to muscle soreness from overuse. Bowel or bladder incontinence is infrequent in ALS. By contrast, constipation is a common complaint, perhaps related to loss of abdominal muscle tone. Urinary urge incontinence is frequently reported, more by women than men. Urinary dysfunction is seen most often in two patient groups. Female patients who recall having temporary urge incontinence after childbirth are likely to have recurrence of such symptoms. In addition, women (and occasionally men) with significant upper motor neuron involvement may also report episodes of incontinence.

Laboratory Evaluation

Neurophysiologic tests are useful in the diagnosis of motor neuron disease. Sensory nerve conduction studies are typically unremarkable; motor nerve studies may be normal or may show reduced amplitude of motor potentials in the context of normal or mildly reduced conduction velocity. Electromyography typically shows widespread denervation of muscle, with fibrillation and fasciculation potentials, and changes in the shape of motor units consistent with reinnervation. Scans and radiographs should be used sparingly to exclude alternative diagnoses. For example, if a patient has diffuse upper motor neuron abnormalities and denervation in all limbs, facial muscles, and thoracic regions, there is no anatomic lesion that can produce such a syndrome, and scans or radiographs are unnecessary. However, in less clear cases, cranial, cervical, or lumbosacral magnetic resonance imaging may be useful. Serum thyroid-stimulating hormone and thyroxine (T_4), serum protein electrophoresis, and a urine screen for heavy metals should be considered; lumbar puncture and muscle biopsy are rarely useful.

HERITABLE MOTOR NEURON DISEASES

Adult Diseases

Approximately 10 per cent of patients with ALS have a family history of the disease. In most of these patients, the family tree suggests an autosomal dominant pattern of inheritance. A mutation in the *SOD1* gene on chromosome 21 has been identified in some patients with familial ALS (FALS); the association of this mutation with motor neuron disease has been strengthened by reports that transfection of the mutant human *SOD1* gene into mice produces an ALS-like syndrome. However, only 20 per cent of patients with FALS show mutations in the *SOD1* gene. Clinically, patients with FALS resemble those with sporadic disease. However, the age at onset of FALS is probably slightly earlier, and the rate of progression may be more rapid.

Another adult-onset inherited motor neuron disease is X-linked bulbospinal muscular atrophy, also known as Kennedy's disease. This disease affects only males and most commonly presents in the third decade of life with facial weakness, tongue fasciculations, and proximal leg weakness. Gynecomastia and mild testicular atrophy are seen, but affected patients are not necessarily infertile. The course of the disease is very slow, and patients are typically ambulatory until late in life.

Pediatric Diseases

The inherited spinal muscular atrophies are among the most devastating of the pediatric neurologic disorders. Different names have been given to the diseases on the basis of age at onset; Werdnig-Hoffmann disease has its onset from birth to 6 months of age, while Wohlfart-Kugelberg-Welander syndrome causes symptoms from 6 months to early adolescence. In Werdnig-Hoffmann disease, children have a flaccid quadriparesis, never sit, and usually die by 2 years of age. Most commonly, problems are evident at birth. Affected babies are floppy and lie with their legs externally rotated and knees flexed. Paradoxical respiration is a common sign. Deep tendon reflexes are absent. The electromyographic results are usually consistent with acute and chronic denervation.

Similarly, diffuse lower motor neuron signs are characteristic of Wohlfart-Kugelberg-Welander syndrome; however, the age at onset and the rate of progression are so variable that some patients remain ambulatory well into adulthood, and life span may be normal. Reflexes are depressed but not necessarily absent, and paradoxical respiration is uncommon.

The spinal muscular atrophies are usually autosomal recessive disorders. Most—if not all—patients have a genetic abnormality on chromosome 5. The location of the abnormality is probably identical in all variants of spinal muscular atrophy. Thus, different forms of the disease may be associated with different alleles of the same gene.

Although the spinal muscular atrophies are the most common forms of pediatric motor neuron disease, other inherited metabolic disorders may produce both upper and lower motor neuron abnormalities. Most of these diseases are associated with a wide spectrum of neurologic abnormalities; however, hexosaminidase deficiency can produce a relatively pure picture of motor neuron disease. The onset of symptoms in patients with hexosaminidase deficiency occurs at a later age than in patients with spinal muscular atrophy; either upper motor neuron or lower motor neuron signs may predominate. Although the disease may start with pure motor abnormalities, mental status changes, ataxia, and extrapyramidal abnormalities eventually appear in most patients.

MYASTHENIA GRAVIS

By K. Philip Lee, M.D.,
Woon-Chee Yee, M.D.,
and Alan Pestronk, M.D.
St. Louis, Missouri

Autoimmune myasthenia gravis (MG) is an acquired disorder of the neuromuscular junction associated with autoantibodies that bind to acetylcholine receptors in the postsynaptic membrane. This binding leads to an increased rate of degradation of acetylcholine receptors and damage to the postsynaptic membrane. The resulting failure of neuromuscular transmission produces the classic symptoms of myasthenia gravis—weakness and fatigability.

CLINICAL MANIFESTATIONS

The prevalence of myasthenia gravis is about 50 to 125 cases per million. The incidence is typically bimodal: one peak occurs in the second and third decades, with female predominance, while the other occurs in the sixth and seventh decades, affecting mostly men. The onset is generally insidious, with progression over weeks to months. Infections, emotional stress, or pregnancy may rapidly aggravate the symptoms of myasthenia gravis. Drugs that inhibit neuromuscular transmission, including anesthetics, antiarrhythmics, antibiotics, anticonvulsants, psychotropic drugs, cholinergic blocking agents, and muscle relaxants, can exacerbate myasthenia gravis. Penicillamine may induce myasthenia gravis de novo.

Weakness due to myasthenia gravis characteristically fluctuates, worsening through the day or with prolonged physical activity. Many patients with myasthenia gravis present initially with diplopia or ptosis due to the weakness of extraocular muscles or levator palpebrae. In some of these patients, the weakness remains limited to the extraocular and eyelid muscles during the entire course of the illness (ocular myasthenia). However, most patients develop weakness in other muscles. The bulbar and facial muscles are frequently affected, causing dysphagia, dysarthria, nasal speech, or weakness of mastication. When the systemic musculature is involved, the typical symptoms include proximal weakness, such as difficulty in arising from chairs or climbing stairs. In patients with severe myasthenia gravis, respiratory or bulbar muscle weakness can be life-threatening. Dysphagia caused by bulbar weakness may result in aspiration pneumonia. Diaphragmatic and intercostal muscle weakness may lead to respiratory failure. Respiratory insufficiency (documented by reductions in vital capacity or negative inspiratory force) and bulbar dysfunction constitute the two major causes of morbidity and mortality in myasthenia gravis. When a patient presents with these difficulties, a rapidly acting therapeutic intervention, such as plasma exchange, is usually required.

PHYSICAL EXAMINATION

Ocular, bulbar, and general motor examinations reveal the most prominent abnormalities. Ocular weakness is typically bilateral and often asymmetrical and may mimic isolated palsy of third or sixth cranial nerve or internuclear ophthalmoplegia. When unilateral disorders of eye movements are found, localized intracranial lesions should be excluded. Ptosis may be unilateral or symmetrical. Myasthenia gravis does not produce pupillary dysfunction. Bilateral facial muscle weakness is almost always present. Bulbar examination may reveal a poor gag reflex and palate elevation, dysphagia, dysarthria, or dysphonia. A weak tongue is very common when the bulbar musculature is involved. Weakness in the systemic musculature can be diffuse but is usually more prominent in proximal areas, including the neck, shoulder, and hip girdle muscles. The triceps muscles may be selectively weaker than others. Myasthenia gravis is one of the few diseases—along with amyotrophic lateral sclerosis and polymyositis—that can produce selective weakness of neck extensors, resulting in difficulty in holding the head erect (head ptosis).

The clinician may elicit weakness, even in initially strong muscles, by producing fatigue through repetitive muscle strength testing or prolonged tonic contraction. Timed upward gaze or forward arm abduction is useful in quantitating fatigue in patients with myasthenia gravis. Muscle wasting is uncommon, except when the disease is chronic and goes untreated. Deep tendon reflexes are usually preserved, and they may even be somewhat brisk, in clinically weak muscles. Objective sensory changes are not found.

ASSOCIATION WITH OTHER DISORDERS

Thymic tumors occur in about 10 to 15 per cent of patients with myasthenia gravis, especially those older than 30 years of age. A computed tomography scan of the thorax should be performed to search for a thymoma in myasthenia gravis patients 20 years of age and older. Magnetic resonance imaging of the chest is more expensive and is not clearly superior. Thymic hyperplasia may be present in as many as 80 per cent of myasthenia gravis patients, most prominently in patients from younger age groups. This association has therapeutic implications because thymectomy may promote long-term clinical improvement in patients younger than 50 years of age.

As many as 15 per cent of patients with myasthenia gravis also have thyroid disease. Hyperthyroidism is more common than hypothyroidism, but both can exacerbate the symptoms of myasthenia gravis. Laboratory studies to exclude thyroid disorders should always be performed during the evaluation for myasthenia gravis. The disease can be associated with various autoimmune disorders, including rheumatoid arthritis, lupus erythematosus, polymyositis, and pernicious anemia. Laboratory screening for other autoimmune syndromes is carried out as indicated by the symptoms and signs in each individual patient.

DIFFERENTIAL DIAGNOSIS

The differential diagnosis in patients with prominent ocular symptoms includes progressive external ophthalmoplegia (mitochondrial myopathy), oculopharyngeal muscular dystrophy, intracranial mass lesions, and senile ptosis. In patients with bulbar dysfunction, the differential diagnosis should encompass motor neuron syndromes, including amyotrophic lateral sclerosis (ALS) and X-linked bulbospinal muscular atrophy (Kennedy's disease); polymyositis; thyroid disorders; and oculopharyngeal dystrophy. In generalized myasthenia gravis, the clinician should consider Eaton-Lambert syndrome, an autoimmune disorder of presynaptic nerve terminals; botulism; congenital myasthenic syndromes; drug-induced myasthenia, especially penicillamine; and generalized myopathies or muscular dystrophies. Serum creatine kinase (CK) concentration, which is often increased in primary muscle disorders, is normal in myasthenia gravis. Inherited myasthenia gravis should be considered whenever persistent weakness begins in infancy or early childhood. However, because the inherited form of the disease is an uncommon and usually autosomal recessive disorder, positive family histories are the exception. Some forms of hereditary myasthenia gravis improve with anticholinesterase medications, but none respond to immunosuppression.

DIAGNOSTIC TESTING

The clinician must firmly establish the diagnosis of myasthenia gravis because thymectomy or long-term immunotherapy may be required. A firm diagnosis avoids inappropriate treatment and side effects in patients who do not have the disease. The primary approaches to diagnostic testing have traditionally been pharmacologic, serologic, and electrodiagnostic. In general, a firm diagnosis is based on a characteristic history and physical examination and two positive diagnostic tests (Table 1).

Edrophonium chloride (Tensilon) is a rapid-onset, short-acting medication that produces inhibition of acetylcholinesterase, thereby prolonging the presence of the neurotransmitter acetylcholine in the neuromuscular junction. Administration of edrophonium enhances muscle strength for a few minutes in patients with dysfunction of the neuromuscular junction. The Tensilon test is useful only in patients with objective, preferably measurable, findings on physical examination. The test should be performed with the patient free from all cholinesterase-inhibitor medications. A positive test result requires clear improvement in muscle strength. Subjective or minor responses, such as a reduction in the patient's sense of fatigue, should not be overinterpreted.

Table 1. Comparison of Diagnostic Tests in Myasthenia Gravis (MG)

Tests	Advantages	Limitations
Intravenous edrophonium	Can be done at bedside Inexpensive	Low sensitivity Subjective interpretation Potentially serious side effects Frequent false-positive results
Anti–acetylcholine receptor antibodies	Specific and sensitive in generalized MG Objective result	Less sensitive in childhood and ocular MG
Repetitive nerve stimulation	Sensitive in generalized MG Objective result	May be uncomfortable, especially with facial and proximal stimulation Less sensitive in ocular MG Occasional false-positive result
Single-fiber electromyography	Very sensitive	Technically demanding and time-consuming May be uncomfortable Not specific

Initially, a test dose (2 mg) of edrophonium is administered intravenously while the patient's heart is monitored for bradycardia or ventricular fibrillation. If no clear response develops within 2 minutes, as much as 8 additional mg of edrophonium can be injected. A double-blind protocol with saline injection as a placebo has been advocated. Most myasthenic muscles respond 30 to 45 seconds after injection with improved strength that may persist for as long as 5 minutes. The cholinergic side effects of edrophonium, including increased salivation and lacrimation, mild sweating, flushing, urgency, and perioral fasciculations, may occur. Injectable atropine should be readily available to reverse the effects of edrophonium should hemodynamic instability ensue. This extra precaution is especially important for elderly patients. The sensitivity of the Tensilon test is relatively low (60 per cent) compared with other diagnostic tests. False-positive results can occur in patients with Eaton-Lambert syndrome, ALS, or even localized, intracranial mass lesions. Tensilon testing is only rarely helpful in the diagnostic evaluation of equivocal presentations of myasthenia gravis. Also, a positive Tensilon test result does not necessarily predict that a patient will respond to a longer-acting cholinesterase inhibitor, such as pyridostigmine. Tensilon testing should not be used to adjust the dose of pyridostigmine.

Serum IgG antibodies that bind to acetylcholine receptors are measured by immunoprecipitation using human acetylcholine receptors labeled with ^{125}I-α-bungarotoxin. Measurement of serum anti–acetylcholine receptor antibodies is a relatively specific and sensitive test for myasthenia gravis. Although test results are positive in 85 to 90 per cent of adults with generalized myasthenia gravis, the test is less sensitive (50 to 70 per cent positive) in the childhood and ocular forms of the disease. Measuring serum antibodies that accelerate the degradation of acetylcholine receptors may be helpful in a few patients when the standard immunoprecipitation assay for antibodies that bind to the acetylcholine receptor is negative.

Repetitive nerve stimulation is the most frequently used electrodiagnostic test for myasthenia gravis. The nerve to be studied is electrically stimulated 6 to 10 times at 2 or 3 Hz. The compound muscle action potential (CMAP) is recorded with surface electrodes over the muscle. In normal muscle, no change in CMAP amplitude is seen. In myasthenic muscle, CMAP amplitudes progressively decline during the first four to five stimuli. The test result is positive when there is a decrement of more than 10 per cent in CMAP amplitude from the first to the fourth or fifth potential. Exercising the muscle briefly before testing may exacerbate the decremental response, an effect known as postexercise exhaustion.

Repetitive nerve stimulation is positive in about 75 per cent of patients with generalized myasthenia gravis when proximal and clinically involved muscles are tested. The sensitivity of repetitive nerve stimulation may be further enhanced by ensuring that the muscle is warm and by testing more than one muscle. The sensitivity of repetitive nerve stimulation is greatly reduced when distal muscles are tested. This testing is positive in only 50 per cent of patients with ocular myasthenia gravis. A decremental response to repetitive nerve stimulation is not specific for myasthenia gravis and may also be seen in presynaptic disorders, such as Eaton-Lambert syndrome, and in motor neuron diseases, including ALS.

Single-fiber electromyography (SFEMG) is a sensitive test for disorders of neuromuscular transmission. A physiologic effect of neuromuscular junction blockade in myasthenia gravis is increased variability of the latencies at which the muscle fibers innervated by an individual axon are activated. By simultaneously recording the potentials of two muscle fibers innervated by an individual axon, SFEMG is able to measure this variability, or "jitter." At times, the muscle fiber potential may even be "blocked" when transmission at its neuromuscular junction fails completely. This test is the most sensitive, with more than 95 per cent sensitivity in both generalized and ocular myasthenia gravis when the test site includes facial muscles. However, abnormal jitter may occur in other neuromuscular disorders, including ALS, polymyositis, and Eaton-Lambert syndrome.

In general, diagnostic investigations of myasthenia gravis should include repetitive nerve stimulation studies as well as testing for serum anti–acetylcholine receptor antibodies. Tensilon tests may be readily performed at the bedside but are not as sensitive as the serologic and electrophysiologic studies. SFEMG is reserved for selected patients in whom results of other tests have been negative or equivocal. Other diagnostic tests include motor-point muscle biopsies (to count acetylcholine receptors at neuromuscular junctions or to evaluate neuromuscular transmission by in vitro electrophysiologic methods), immunocytochemical staining of muscle end-plates for immunoglobulin and complement, tests of ocular movement, and genetic evaluation for defects in acetylcholine receptor subunits. However, these tests are generally not required or indicated in the great majority of patients with myasthenia gravis.

PARANEOPLASTIC SYNDROMES: DISORDERS OF THE PERIPHERAL MOTOR SENSORY UNIT

By H. Royden Jones, Jr., M.D.
Burlington, Massachusetts

OVERVIEW

Various well-recognized paraneoplastic syndromes can affect the peripheral motor sensory unit. Some of these unique processes represent remote autoimmune nonmetastatic complications of malignancy. Two illnesses, the Lambert-Eaton myasthenic syndrome and primary sensory neuropathy, occur predominantly in cigarette smokers who develop occult small cell lung cancer. The POEMS syndrome (*p*olyneuropathy, *o*rganomegaly, *e*ndocrinopathy, *M* protein, *s*kin changes) typically provides a clue to an otherwise unsuspected, frequently isolated, focal osteosclerotic myeloma. A small percentage of patients with myasthenia gravis harbor thymomas. Despite years of controversy, a significant epidemiologic link between dermatomyositis and cancer indicates that older individuals who develop dermatomyositis need careful evaluation for an occult neoplasm of the alimentary tract, female reproductive system, or lung. This chapter amplifies the clinical diagnostic approach to a number of paraneoplastic syndromes involving the peripheral nervous system.

MOTOR NEURON DISEASE

Amyotrophic Lateral Sclerosis (ALS)

Clinical Presentation

Disorders of the motor neuron are only rarely associated with occult malignancy. Occasionally, patients with Hodgkin's disease have developed motor neuron dysfunction within 1 year of their diagnosis and treatment with radiation. In contrast to patients who have rather more common, nonparaneoplastic disorders of motor neurons, these patients with Hodgkin's disease tend to have a self-limited illness.

Renal cell carcinoma has also been rarely associated with motor neuron dysfunction. In patients with hypernephroma, the motor neuron dysfunction has antedated the discovery of the tumor. Other malignancies associated with paraneoplastic motor neuron disease include small cell and large cell carcinoma and adenocarcinoma of the lung, thymoma, and Waldenström's macroglobulinemia.

Physical Findings

Patients with paraneoplastic motor neuron dysfunction typically experience the insidious onset of progressive weakness and atrophy of skeletal and bulbar muscles, most often accompanied by definite or probable upper motor neuron signs, as seen in amyotrophic lateral sclerosis (ALS). The first manifestation may be difficulty in using a hand, lifting an arm, or picking up a foot while walking. Some of these patients develop tongue fasciculations. Although weakness most often is variably distributed, the presentation in a few patients may be more symmetrical than that typically observed in the idiopathic forms of motor neuron disease.

Laboratory Studies

In patients with motor neuron disorders, abnormalities of various laboratory tests may indicate the presence and type of coincident neoplasm. An increased erythrocyte sedimentation rate (ESR), abnormal liver function studies, and slight anemia have been associated with renal cell carcinoma; paraproteinemia or increased anti G_{M1} or anti-asialo-G_{M1} antibody titers may suggest lymphoma. Some clinicians routinely request serum protein electrophoresis and anti-G_{M1} testing in all patients who develop ALS and other motor neuron disorders. Increased cerebrospinal fluid protein and the presence of oligoclonal bands may also be associated with occult lymphoma.

Electromyography (EMG) with nerve conduction studies may help the clinician distinguish primary motor neuron dysfunction from other abnormalities of the motor unit. In particular, potentially treatable axonal or multifocal demyelinating motor neuropathies should be excluded. In patients with primary motor neuron disease, the electromyogram should reveal widespread signs of active denervation-reinnervation manifested by long-duration high-amplitude motor units and well-defined fibrillation potentials and positive waves.

When the history and/or laboratory studies suggest the presence of occult malignancy in patients with ALS, selected imaging studies (e.g., chest films, computed tomography, abdominal ultrasound) may also be useful.

Finally, in patients known to have lymphoma, the possibility of leptomeningeal invasion by tumor must be considered. Cytologic analysis of spinal fluid, often necessitating multiple samplings, may be required for the exclusion of nonparaneoplastic nerve root invasion as a cause of apparent motor neuron dysfunction.

Course

The inexorable progression of classic ALS is not typically seen in patients with paraneoplastic motor neuron disorders. Some patients improve, especially if the primary malignancy is identified and treated. At least one patient has recovered muscle strength within 4 months of resection of a renal tumor identified with abdominal ultrasound and computed tomography. Other patients have reportedly stabilized for long periods of time. Autopsy in two patients with Hodgkin's disease complicated by paraneoplastic motor neuron dysfunction and central nervous system infection demonstrated anterior horn cell degeneration with patchy demyelination of lumbar and brachial nerve roots.

Summary

Paraneoplastic processes that primarily affect motor neurons are exceedingly rare. ALS-like syndromes have been identified in patients with lymphoma, renal carcinoma, lung carcinoma, and thymoma. Abnormal laboratory studies may suggest the presence of a paraneoplastic syndrome.

Clinicians caring for patients with presumed idiopathic ALS should routinely request chemistry screens, ESR, serum protein immunoelectrophoresis, anti-G_{M1} antibodies, nerve conduction studies, and possibly spinal fluid analysis. If any of these studies are abnormal, bone marrow biopsy and/or computed tomography of the chest and abdomen may be indicated. Paraneoplastic forms of ALS have a favorable prognosis. They should be considered in any patient who presents with evidence of primary motor neuron disease.

PARANEOPLASTIC NEUROPATHIES

Primary Sensory Neuropathy

Introduction

Denny-Brown provided the first description of a paraneoplastic neurologic syndrome in 1948. He reported a patient with primary sensory neuropathy associated with small cell lung cancer (SCLC). Dysfunction of the dorsal root ganglia in these patients has been attributed to autoimmune attack by antineuronal nuclear antibodies (ANNA-1), also known as anti-Hu. As with many of the paraneoplastic disorders, the symptoms of primary sensory neuropathy usually predate the recognition of the underlying malignancy (most often a SCLC).

Clinical Presentation

Patients with paraneoplastic primary sensory neuropathy (PPSN) typically present with the insidious onset of sensory symptoms reflecting the site of involvement at the dorsal root ganglion. The symptoms often include paresthesias or dysesthesias of the hands and/or feet; occasionally, the trunk or face is involved. Paresthesias may have a more proximal distribution in PPSN than in most other peripheral neuropathies. Sometimes the sensory symptoms are painful or asymmetrical or they may involve just one limb. Many patients with PPSN progress to total deafferentation and cannot locate their limbs in space. They cannot distinguish objects in their pockets or locate their feet in the dark, causing difficulty in accelerating or braking when driving. Sometimes, deafferentation leads to pseudoathetotic, involuntary movement of the fingers and hands.

The signs and symptoms of primary sensory neuropathy can broadly overlap with the Lambert-Eaton myasthenic syndrome or with paraneoplastic syndromes involving the limbic system, brain stem, or cerebellum. Thus, gait ataxia, changes in mental status, seizures, or proximal weakness may precede or accompany the sensory symptoms noted above.

Physical Findings

Patients with PPSN demonstrate severe deficits in all major sensory pathways. Loss of touch, temperature, pain, vibration, and position sense most often involves the distal limbs, but at times such loss can be demonstrated over the face or the trunk. Profound gait and appendicular ataxia, sometimes leading to pseudoathetosis, frequently develops. Damage to primarily large sensory fibers is the major cause of the patient's inability to perceive the location of limbs and digits in space. The deep tendon reflexes are universally suppressed, often asymmetrically. Muscle strength testing is nearly always normal.

Less common physical findings in PPSN include anisocoria, depressed pupillary light responses, nystagmus, extraocular muscle weakness, facial sensory loss, diminished hearing, and tongue weakness with an associated dysarthria. Dysfunction of every cranial nerve but the spinal accessory has been reported. Occasionally, patients with PPSN also have autonomic dysfunction, typically manifested by orthostatic hypotension.

Paraneoplastic intestinal pseudo-obstruction may accompany or, less commonly, precede the onset of PPSN related to SCLC. This rare syndrome is characterized by impaired motility with symptoms and signs appropriate to the site of involvement within the gastrointestinal tract.

Laboratory Results

The most important confirmatory blood test for the diagnosis of PPSN is the titer of type 1 antineuronal nuclear antibodies (ANNA-1), also known as anti-Hu antibodies. The ANNA-1, or anti-Hu, antibody test should also be positive in patients with occult SCLC who present with intestinal pseudo-obstruction. When the anti-Hu antibody cannot be detected, the clinician must fastidiously search for other known causes of primary sensory neuropathy. Exclude exposure to environmental agents (e.g., disulfiram, isoniazid, arsenic). Measure serum glucose, creatinine, vitamin B_{12}, protein immunoelectrophoresis, anti–SS-A/SS-B, and angiotensin converting enzyme (ACE). Collect a 24-hour urine specimen for heavy metal quantitation.

Cerebrospinal fluid analysis is also diagnostically useful. Most patients with PPSN have increased cerebrospinal fluid protein concentration; in one third, the concentration exceeds 100 mg/dL. Oligoclonal banding and anti-Hu antibodies are frequently detected while the cerebrospinal fluid glucose concentration is typically unremarkable.

In PPSN, electromyography is almost always characterized by a lack of detectable sensory nerve action potentials (SNAPs). However, there is an evolution of EMG findings. Early in the course of PPSN, both motor and sensory nerve conduction studies may be normal or show only the absence of the H-reflex. Later in the course of PPSN, the SNAPs gradually diminish in amplitude and eventually disappear, with preservation of motor nerve conduction. Needle EMG is typically unremarkable because the fundamental pathologic process is confined largely to the dorsal root ganglion.

Imaging Studies

Although chest films eventually demonstrate abnormalities in all patients with SCLC, these radiographs may be unremarkable during the early phases of PPSN. Occasionally, computed tomography or magnetic resonance imaging detects an occult tumor when the chest film is unrevealing.

Course

Patients with sensory manifestations often have a relatively rapid onset of signs and symptoms that may progress relentlessly over a few months.

In one study of patients with PPSN referred to a major cancer center, 78 per cent had a SCLC, 13 per cent had no detectable tumor, and the remainder had miscellaneous tumors, including adenocarcinoma of the lung, prostate, and adrenal, neuroblastoma, and chondromyxosarcoma. Importantly, even in major referral centers, patients presenting with primary sensory neuropathy most often do not harbor an underlying neoplasm. Rather, the sensory neuropathy is an idiopathic disabling process still awaiting precise pathophysiologic definition.

Summary

The syndrome of primary sensory neuropathy may at times be secondary to an occult neoplasm, most likely a SCLC. This is a very disabling clinical process that may evolve as rapidly as subacute demyelinating polyneuropathy. Electromyography is very useful for defining the primary sensory nature of the illness. Specific antibodies, known either as ANNA-1 or anti-Hu, may be found in either the serum or the cerebrospinal fluid. Identification of these antibodies should prompt imaging studies of the chest that may be unremarkable early in the course of the neuropathy but become abnormal with repeat study at a later date.

POEMS Syndrome

Introduction

The acronym POEMS was coined by Bardwick in 1978 to describe a rare but interesting paraneoplastic neuropathy. The P represents polyneuropathy, the O stands for organomegaly, the E relates to endocrine dysfunction, the M signifies the presence of a monoclonal gammopathy, and the S points to the skin changes that often provide an important clue to the diagnosis. This syndrome is related to myeloma that may be clinically occult when the patient first becomes ill. The typical patient with multiple myeloma is older than most patients with POEMS, who are typically diagnosed between the ages of 30 and 45 years.

Clinical Presentation

POEMS typically presents as a generalized sensorimotor neuropathy with distal paresthesias and weakness. The illness begins gradually but rapidly increases in severity. Some individuals do not progress beyond mild difficulties in walking, whereas others experience severe incapacitation, requiring hospitalization and occasionally intensive care monitoring.

Careful questioning may reveal symptoms of gonadal or thyroid hypofunction. Male patients, if asked, may describe diminishing sexual performance early in the course of the illness.

Physical Findings

Stocking-and-glove sensory loss is frequently accompanied by areflexia and distal weakness that may progress proximally. Some individuals eventually develop hearing loss, hoarseness, or other signs of cranial nerve involvement. Papilledema is occasionally noted, especially in patients with the IgA (Castleman) variant of the POEMS syndrome. Skin hyperpigmentation that varies from deep tan to erythematous purple may accompany the onset of neuropathy or may develop several years later. Organomegaly may be obvious (hepatosplenomegaly) or relatively subtle (a few enlarged lymph nodes).

Laboratory Results

In a patient with polyneuropathy, detection of an IgG lambda monoclonal gammopathy catalyzes the search for other components of the POEMS syndrome. More than 90 per cent of POEMS patients develop a gammopathy with lambda light chains. Patients who present with IgA lambda gammopathy may have a major variant of the POEMS syndrome known as Castleman's disease. This variant is characterized by the development of angiofollicular lymph node hyperplasia.

Concomitant serum abnormalities include increased thyroid stimulating hormone (TSH) and low testosterone. Some patients have unexplained thrombocytosis. The cerebrospinal fluid protein concentration is increased (100 to 200 mg/dL) without evidence of pleocytosis.

Electromyography demonstrates a diffuse demyelinating polyneuropathy characterized by prolonged distal latencies, dispersed compound muscle action potentials, absent sensory nerve action potentials, and marked slowing of conduction velocity, often to 20 to 35 m per second.

Imaging Studies

The clinician who finds the constellation of polyneuropathy (P), organomegaly (O), laboratory signs of endocrine (E) dysfunction, and a monoclonal (M) gammopathy in a patient with recent changes in skin (S) pigmentation must search for an occult myeloma. Typically, the lesion is focal and osteosclerotic and often involves one vertebra, or less commonly an osteolytic lesion is identified in a proximal bone, such as the pelvis. These lesions are best identified by performing a "metastatic" skeletal radiograph survey. Occasionally, physicians have suspected POEMS but have missed the correct diagnosis by erroneously requesting a radioisotopic bone scan that does not reveal these focal myelomatous lesions. Rarely, patients present with diffuse, rather than focal, myeloma. The diagnosis is confirmed by bone biopsy of the focal lesion or by bone marrow sampling when more diffuse changes are detected by imaging.

In the patient with IgA monoclonal lambda gammopathy, the bone survey is usually normal. Computed tomography of the chest or the abdomen may reveal subtle to marked lymphadenopathy, whereas biopsy shows the classic angiofollicular lymph node hyperplasia seen in the Castleman variant of POEMS.

Clinical Course

The course of POEMS varies. It may be relentlessly progressive in patients with multiple myeloma, fluctuating to moderately progressive in Castleman's disease, or dramatically reversible in patients with classic POEMS after the focal myeloma has been irradiated. Not all features of POEMS, including the monoclonal gammopathy, are apparent at the time of initial presentation. Endocrine and protein parameters must be re-evaluated in any patient with idiopathic progressive neuropathy, especially if the electromyogram defines a demyelinating polyneuropathy.

Summary

The POEMS syndrome is a rare but potentially treatable form of demyelinating polyneuropathy. The diagnosis primarily requires recognition of the constellation of systemic symptoms associated most commonly with an IgG lambda monoclonal gammopathy and the demonstration of an osteosclerotic or osteolytic focal myeloma.

DISORDERS OF NEUROMUSCULAR TRANSMISSION

Lambert-Eaton Myasthenic Syndrome

Introduction

The Lambert-Eaton myasthenic syndrome (LEMS) is the most prominent example of a presynaptic defect in neuromuscular transmission in adults. First defined as a paraneoplastic syndrome, LEMS typically is associated with SCLC in cigarette smokers but also occurs rarely with other malignancies. If a neoplasm is not identified within 4 years of the onset of symptoms, paraneoplastic LEMS is remote, especially in a nonsmoker. Instead, the syndrome may represent a primary autoimmune disorder unrelated to malignancy. The latter form of LEMS now occurs about as often as the paraneoplastic variety and is typically seen in younger individuals (age 20 to 40 years). Lambert-Eaton myasthenic syndrome occurs infrequently; the prevalence is estimated at 1 to 3 per cent of all new patients presenting with symptoms of myasthenia gravis.

Physiologic and immunologic investigations have identified voltage-gated calcium channels (VGCC) as the primary site of immunopathology. An IgG antibody adheres to the peripheral cholinergic nerve terminals and thus blocks the calcium influx that normally occurs with nerve depolarization. Inadequate calcium influx causes inadequate release of acetylcholine (ACh) from motor and autonomic cholinergic nerve terminals. The VGCCs present in the membrane of SCLC provide the presumed antigenic stimulus for antibody production in the paraneoplastic form of LEMS.

Clinical Presentation

The diagnosis of LEMS is often suspected clinically. Most LEMS patients are symptomatic for less than a year; however, recognition of LEMS has been delayed for as long as 8 to 25 years after the initial presentation of symptoms. Individuals with LEMS typically present with proximal weakness, vague numbness in the thighs, and various signs of autonomic dysfunction, including dry mouth and impotence. Conversely, LEMS has well-known protean clinical manifestations that may mimic myasthenia gravis, especially in patients with diplopia, ptosis, dysarthria, and other bulbar symptoms. The proximal weakness often suggests the diagnosis of polymyositis. Some LEMS patients present with gait ataxia and symptoms of cranial nerve involvement rarely mimicking multiple sclerosis. The vague sense of fatigue and the weight loss sometimes suggest the presence of an occult malignancy. Patients sometimes present with evanescent symptoms that may be mistaken for hysteria, stress, or a psychiatric disturbance.

The muscle weakness of LEMS is typically proximal and characterized by difficulties in arising, from a sitting position, walking, or climbing stairs. Although proximal arm and neck muscles are often weak on examination, it is uncommon for patients with these problems to have primary symptoms related to the arms. Fatigue is a prominent finding; it may be the initial manifestation of LEMS. At times, the initial neurologic examination may suggest inconsistent effort and a lack of true weakness. The facilitative component of this weakness is mistaken for the "give-way" weakness seen in patients with psychological disturbances. Muscle stiffness or tightness is occasionally prominent.

Bulbar symptoms are less prominent in LEMS than in classic myasthenia gravis. Their presence, however, should not exclude LEMS from diagnostic consideration. The most common bulbar symptoms are ptosis and facial weakness. With sustained upward gaze, a paradoxical lid elevation in LEMS may occur secondary to facilitation. This phenomenon contrasts with the situation in myasthenia gravis, where the same maneuver evokes increased ptosis. Paraspinal and proximal leg weakness may result in pseudoataxia. By contrast, some LEMS patients have true gait ataxia owing to concomitant paraneoplastic cerebellar degeneration. Primary paraneoplastic sensory neuropathy may precede the initial symptoms of LEMS. Ataxia or neuropathy in a patient with concomitant proximal limb weakness should suggest the diagnosis of LEMS.

Autonomic symptoms (e.g., dry mouth and sexual impotence) may provide important clues. The combination of vague weakness, dry mouth, and paresthesias may mimic hyperventilation and lead to an inappropriate psychiatric evaluation for anxiety or depression.

Physical Findings

Proximal limb and neck weakness is common in LEMS patients. Sometimes, the astute clinician can detect the ability of some of these patients to facilitate their strength. Initially, the patient appears to be weak; when asked to contract a muscle with greater force, the patient shows a few seconds of improved strength followed by deterioration in just another few seconds. The clinician should not misinterpret this event as the give-way weakness of conversion hysteria or malingering. When patients with suspected LEMS do not have detectable weakness on neurologic examination, subtle weakness may be discovered by watching the person arise from a chair or climb stairs. Deep tendon reflexes are typically absent or depressed in most LEMS patients. However, as many as 25 per cent of LEMS patients may have normally active deep tendon reflexes. Patients with areflexia or sluggish deep tendon reflexes characteristically have postexercise facilitation of strength and/or deep tendon reflexes. Sluggish pupillary light responses, a sign of autonomic dysfunction, may be observed in a minority of LEMS patients.

Laboratory Results and Diagnostic Testing

TENSILON (EDROPHONIUM) TESTING. Some patients require Tensilon testing because the clinical presentation of LEMS may suggest a diagnosis of myasthenia gravis. The Tensilon test may be "subjectively" or "objectively" positive in as many as two thirds of LEMS patients. This test should not be used as the sole means of distinguishing myasthenia gravis from LEMS.

Electromyography is the keystone of the diagnosis of LEMS. Motor nerve stimulation typically demonstrates diminished compound muscle action potentials (CMAPs) in LEMS. The amplitude of CMAPs may be less than 10 per cent of normal. Five per cent of patients with early LEMS have normal CMAPs. Sensory nerve action potentials (SNAPs) are normal in the absence of concomitant paraneoplastic sensory neuropathy.

Repetitive motor nerve stimulation (RMNS) at 2 to 3 Hz produces a decremental response in both LEMS and myasthenia gravis. The marked facilitation of the typical low-amplitude CMAPs following brief and maximal voluntary exercise is unique to patients with LEMS. These neurophysiologic characteristics in LEMS indicate a presynaptic lesion of the neuromuscular junction. This situation is a mirror image of myasthenia gravis, the more common postsynaptic disorder. Failure to recognize the significance of a low-amplitude CMAP at the time of routine motor conduction studies is the major reason the diagnosis of LEMS is missed by some electromyographers. If low-amplitude CMAPs are appreciated, it is a simple step to have the patient contract the relevant muscle and repeat the motor stimulation. The key maneuver is having the patient exercise no more than 10 to 15 seconds before checking for signs of post-tetanic facilitation. Patients with LEMS typically demonstrate at least 200 per cent facilitation. In selected patients, 600 to 1000 per cent increases in CMAP amplitude have been recorded.

ANTIBODY STUDIES. Antibodies to the VGCC are detected in 75 per cent of LEMS patients with SCLC and in 25 per cent of LEMS patients with other types of malignancy. Importantly, 43 per cent of LEMS patients with the autoimmune form of the illness (unrelated to an underlying malignancy) may also have significant titers of VGCC antibodies.

Acetylcholine receptor (AChR) antibodies are present in 13 per cent of LEMS patients. Rarely, the identification of VGCC and AChR antibodies in the same patient may confirm the simultaneous occurrence of LEMS and myasthenia gravis. However, patients who have bulbar symptoms and AChR antibodies should not be presumed to have myasthenia gravis. The electromyographer must perform careful EMG to distinguish presynaptic and postsynaptic defects. Early in the course of LEMS, CMAP amplitude may be relatively normal; and therefore a significant facilitation may not be observed with exercise or RMNS.

Imaging Studies

The diagnosis of LEMS frequently precedes an order for a chest film. If the patient is a smoker, the chest film most often shows a hilar mass that proves to be a SCLC. However, in some patients, the chest film is unremarkable; thus, computed tomography or magnetic resonance imaging of the chest is required for the detection of an occult neoplasm. Occasionally, all three imaging studies are normal, and bronchoscopy is required for diagnosis. If bronchoscopy is unremarkable, the clinician must search elsewhere for uncommon malignancies. In patients with LEMS, 4 years may pass before SCLC is observed on chest film, computed tomography, or magnetic resonance imaging. Other malignancies may also appear several years after the initial diagnosis of LEMS.

Clinical Course

The clinical course of patients with paraneoplastic forms of LEMS is exceedingly variable. Those with SCLC who respond to therapy may gradually experience resolution of their LEMS symptomatology. In others, the cancer is resistant to all forms of therapy, and, consequently, the LEMS is difficult to treat. Although some LEMS patients with SCLC may live for as long as 6 years, many die within 1 year of diagnosis of the malignancy. A few patients have remission of LEMS, with no detectable tumor for 3 to 4 years.

Summary

Lambert-Eaton myasthenic syndrome is a discrete paraneoplastic syndrome affecting presynaptic neuromuscular transmission. Most commonly, it is the presenting clinical feature of the malignancy. Occasionally, the typical symptoms do not manifest until after the tumor has been identified. Most patients present with symptoms of proximal weakness and autonomic dysfunction (e.g., dry mouth and erectile impotence). Bulbar symptoms may also occur and lead to confusion with the diagnosis of myasthenia gravis. The diagnosis of LEMS is best confirmed by EMG and VGCC antibody testing.

Paraneoplastic Myasthenia Gravis

Introduction

Myasthenia gravis is primarily an autoimmune disorder of postsynaptic neuromuscular transmission. Nearly 10 per cent of patients with myasthenia gravis have an associated thymoma. This subject is covered in greater detail elsewhere in this text; therefore, a relatively brief outline is included in this section on paraneoplastic disorders.

Clinical Presentation

The clinical presentation of the myasthenic patient who harbors a thymoma cannot be distinguished from the presentation of the patient with myasthenia gravis who does not have the tumor. Individuals with myasthenia gravis typically present with ptosis and diplopia; difficulties in chewing, swallowing, and speaking are observed less commonly. Some patients experience problems in climbing stairs or lifting the arms over the head. Severe myasthenia may result in respiratory embarrassment requiring intubation. Myasthenic symptoms may be accompanied by significant fatigue that is often most prominent in the late afternoon and early evening.

Physical Findings

The clinical findings in myasthenia gravis typically include ptosis, varying degrees of ophthalmoparesis, nasal speech, and weakness of the neck flexors. With more diffuse disease, weakness of the proximal muscles may exceed that of the distal muscles, especially in the extremities.

Laboratory Results

Electromyography shows a decremental response of at least 10 per cent in the amplitude of CMAPs following RMNS at 2 or 3 Hz, especially if three or more nerve-muscle groups are studied. Intravenous injection of edrophonium readily reverses the decrement. Other causes of postsynaptic defects in neuromuscular transmission must be excluded.

Antibody studies indicate an autoimmune process affecting the alpha subunit of the AChR of the postsynaptic membrane of the neuromuscular junction. These binding, modulating, and blocking antibodies are detected in 85 per cent of patients with myasthenia gravis.

Eighty per cent of patients with myasthenia gravis who have thymoma also have antibodies to striated muscle. The frequency of detection of this antibody increases with the age at onset of myasthenia gravis. Antistriated muscle antibodies are rarely present before age 20 years but are found in more than half of patients whose myasthenia gravis begins after age 60. These antibodies to striated muscle are found more often in myasthenia gravis patients with thymoma who are younger than 40 years of age. Although these antibodies rarely occur in patients who do not have myasthenia gravis, they have been detected in patients with LEMS and SCLC. Again, the clinician must consider LEMS even when much of the initial presentation and data may strongly point to the diagnosis of myasthenia gravis.

Imaging Studies

Routine chest films may occasionally reveal a thymoma, but computed tomography or magnetic resonance imaging is required for the identification of very small (1 cm) lesions.

Clinical Course

Although patients with myasthenia gravis and associated thymoma typically experience a clinical course similar to those who do not have thymoma, the prognosis may be poorer in patients who harbor especially malignant lesions.

Summary

Most patients with myasthenia gravis do not have an associated thymoma. However, the initial evaluation of any patient with suspected myasthenia gravis must include both antibody and radiographic studies in the search for an underlying thymoma.

MYOPATHIES

Paraneoplastic Dermatomyositis and Polymyositis

Introduction

The association between inflammatory myositis and malignancy has been debated for many years. Swedish epidemiologic studies support the concept of a paraneoplastic variant of dermatomyositis and polymyositis. The definitive diagnostic evaluation for inflammatory myopathy is covered elsewhere in this text; comments here relate primarily to the paraneoplastic forms of myositis.

Clinical Presentation

These patients typically present with proximal weakness; they have problems in climbing steps, arising from low positions, or performing activities that require the arms to be over the head. Less commonly, patients with myositis experience difficulty in chewing, swallowing, or holding up the head.

Physical Findings

Although proximal muscle weakness is easily demonstrated in most individuals with paraneoplastic myositis, a few patients may have to attempt squatting, standing, or stairclimbing to manifest their deficits. Three individual muscles are particularly useful for demonstrating subtle degrees of weakness—the neck flexors, triceps, and iliopsoas. Careful testing of these muscles may provide enough evidence of weakness to support a careful search for abnormalities of the peripheral motor unit. In some patients, careful inspection of the skin may reveal the heliotrope rash associated with dermatomyositis.

Laboratory Results

Serum creatine kinase (CK) is typically increased two- to fiftyfold. The ESR is not a reliable indicator of the presence of inflammatory myopathy.

Electromyography can help define the precise site of the abnormality in the peripheral motor unit, that is, the anterior horn cell, peripheral nerve, neuromuscular junction, or myocyte. When needle electromyography is characterized by numerous low-amplitude, short-duration, polyphasic motor unit potentials and markedly abnormal insertion activity, the site of the most profound electrical change should be the guide for selection of a biopsy site. The muscle tissue should be obtained from the contralateral homologue that was not sampled during the needle EMG.

Imaging Studies

Occult malignancy has been documented in patients with dermatomyositis; women are twice as likely as men to harbor a previously unexpected tumor. These individuals, especially the older patients, should be clinically evaluated for tumors of the stomach, pancreas, colon, breast, ovary, and lung. If the physical examination suggests a lesion of any of these organs, the appropriate imaging study must be undertaken. Routine imaging screens for cancer are not warranted, especially in patients with polymyositis.

Clinical Course

If an occult malignancy is found and successfully treated, some patients with dermatomyositis may improve remarkably, even in the absence of the immunosuppressive therapy typically advocated for the primary autoimmune forms of dermatomyositis.

Summary

Dermatomyositis and, even less commonly, polymyositis may rarely provide the clue to an occult underlying neoplasm. If an older individual develops an inflammatory myopathy, careful clinical evaluation may lead to diagnostic testing that uncovers an otherwise unsuspected cancer.

PARANEOPLASTIC CENTRAL NEURAL SYNDROMES

By José A. Gutrecht, M.D.
Burlington, Massachusetts

The paraneoplastic central neural syndromes (PCNS) are neurologic syndromes secondary to systemic cancer elsewhere in the body. They are not due to direct invasion by or metastasis of cancer and thus have also been known as "remote effects of cancer." In common neurologic practice, syndromes secondary to metabolic derangement, such as inappropriate secretion of antidiuretic hormone in lung cancer, and bleeding in the case of leukemia or infarcts secondary to a coagulopathy, are not considered paraneoplastic. Of course, the PCNS are not due to malnutrition, secondary infections, or cancer treatment.

The paraneoplastic central neural syndromes are rare but fairly clinically homogeneous constellations of symptoms and signs of subacute onset secondary to damage of central neural elements, such as the limbic system, cerebellum, and brain stem. Involvement may also include the peripheral nervous system, such as the dorsal root ganglion cells, peripheral nerve, and neuromuscular junction, or muscle. The pathogenesis of the PCNS is thought to be immunologically based, part of a reaction to the underlying cancer. It is postulated that serum antibodies directed against cancer antigens cross-react with organ-specific neural tissue, and this cross-reaction leads to degeneration and, eventually, cell death. In many cases, the early diagnosis of these syndromes is greatly aided by the presence of circulating antibodies. Prompt recognition is important, since early detection of the cancer may offer greater therapeutic choices, including cancer cures, and sometimes slow down or reverse the development of the neurologic disabilities. Unfortunately, in these patients, the cancer is often small and may escape detection initially. Close clinical monitoring is of paramount importance in this group of patients.

LIMBIC ENCEPHALITIS

Patients with this syndrome develop a marked amnestic syndrome reminiscent of Wernicke's encephalopathy but of subacute onset over a few days to weeks. Other manifestations include sleep disturbances, hallucinations, depression, anxiety, and personality changes. The latter symptoms are often quite dramatic and may lead to an incorrect psychiatric diagnosis. Seizures of focal onset with or without secondary generalization may occur. The syndrome usually develops in the sixth or seventh decade of life. The electroencephalogram is usually abnormal but nonspecific, with focal or generalized abnormalities. Computed tomography and magnetic resonance imaging scans may demonstrate contrast-enhancing abnormalities in one or both temporal lobes. Cerebrospinal fluid examination is generally abnormal, with increased mononuclear cell counts and modest increases in protein concentration. In many cases, cerebellar and brain stem symptoms or signs are present. Often, evidence of peripheral neuropathy exists as well.

The main histopathologic changes are located in the limbic structures, particularly the hippocampal gyrus, Ammon's horn, and the amygdala. These changes are characterized by neuronal loss, microglial proliferation, perivascular cuffing, and gliosis. The carcinoma most frequently associated with this syndrome is small cell carcinoma of the lung. Single cases of limbic encephalitis, malignant thymoma, and testicular or colon cancer have been reported.

Sometimes, features of limbic encephalitis are present to a lesser degree in combination with other, more prominent neurologic symptoms or signs, indicating a more widespread neurologic syndrome suggestive of brain stem encephalitis, cerebellar degeneration, and/or myelopathy. A peripheral, predominantly sensory neuropathy may be part of this picture.

PARANEOPLASTIC CEREBELLAR DEGENERATION

Paraneoplastic cerebellar degeneration is rare. It develops in a subacute manner in both sexes in the sixth and seventh decades of life. Most patients demonstrate severe, disabling pancerebellar deficits, such as gait and limb ataxia with ocular dysmetria, and nystagmus of variable degree, often downbeat, but rarely evidence of other symptoms or signs originating in the brain stem. Other symptoms or findings of cortical, pyramidal, or extrapyramidal origin or peripheral neuropathy are less frequent and generally mild. Cerebrospinal fluid examination usually reveals increased mononuclear cell counts with a mild increase in total protein concentration; increased IgG turnover and oligoclonal bands are often found. Computed tomography or magnetic resonance imaging scans are usually normal at first but may show cerebellar atrophy as the illness progresses. The pathologic findings in the cerebellum include cortical atrophy with degeneration and severe loss of Purkinje's cells, with some perivascular cuffing and gliosis.

Paraneoplastic cerebellar degeneration is seen most commonly in patients with small cell carcinoma of the lung, gynecologic cancer, breast cancer, and Hodgkin's disease. Some of the patients with this syndrome have antibodies in blood and cerebrospinal fluid that cross-react with Purkinje's cells. The best-known antibody found in this group is the so-called anti-Yo antibody (PCA-1). The presence of the anti-Yo antibody (PCA-1) in a woman almost invariably indicates an underlying gynecologic cancer, usually ovarian, and, less often, uterine or fallopian tube in origin. Unfortunately, cure of the underlying cancer does not translate into improvement of the neurologic deficits. In patients with paraneoplastic cerebellar degeneration and Lambert-Eaton myasthenic syndrome, small cell carcinoma of the lung is the usual cancer association. In the young population, particularly if male, Hodgkin's disease is the underlying cancer.

OPSOCLONUS-MYOCLONUS

This syndrome is the most common paraneoplastic syndrome in children. It is characterized by (1) involuntary conjugate continuous quick eye movements in any direction and occurring with irregular frequency made worse by visual fixation and persisting during eye closure (opsoclonus) and (2) lightning-quick muscle jerks with visible movements of the trunk or limbs (myoclonus). The latter may also involve the head, larynx, pharynx, or diaphragm. Opsoclonus may occur alone, but usually opsoclonus and myoclonus are present together. This syndrome is found in 50 per cent of children with neuroblastoma and sometimes is the presenting feature. In children with this syndrome, neuroblastoma tends to occur in the chest, the histology is more benign, and the condition has a better prognosis.

This syndrome may be encountered in adults, but it is very rare. It is often of acute onset and associated with other symptoms and signs, such as vertigo, ataxia, apathy, and confusion. Abnormally increased mononuclear cell counts or protein concentration has been noted in the cerebrospinal fluid. Computed tomography or magnetic resonance imaging scans are unremarkable. The electroencephalograms do not show epileptiform activity. This syndrome is usually associated with small cell carcinoma of the lung. It has also been reported in association with breast cancer, other types of bronchogenic cancer, and medullary cancer of the thyroid. Of interest, this syndrome often has a remitting and exacerbating course and may improve or stabilize after treatment of the underlying malignancy. The pathogenesis of this syndrome is not known. Adult patients with this syndrome and breast cancer may have the so-called anti-Ri antibody (ANNA-2) in serum and cerebrospinal fluid.

PARANEOPLASTIC RETINAL DEGENERATION

Paraneoplastic retinal degeneration is usually associated with small cell carcinoma of the lung. It is characterized by loss of visual acuity or scotomatous field defects that may develop suddenly or progress subacutely. Symptoms may start unilaterally, but eventually involve both eyes. These patients may have photosensitivity, dramatic light-induced glare, impaired visual acuity, diminished color vision, night blindness, and episodic visual obscurations. Funduscopic examination demonstrates narrowing of the central retinal arterioles and, often, some disc pallor. Visual evoked potentials are normal, but the electroretinogram is abnormal. The pathology in the retina is characterized by widespread loss of photoreceptor cells, loss of nuclei of the outer nuclear layer, and macrophage infiltration and eventual gliosis in these layers. Other retinal structures and the optic nerve appear preserved. Antibodies against retinal photoreceptors have been demonstrated in blood. Paraneoplastic retinal degeneration has also been described in conjunction with cutaneous melanomas.

PARANEOPLASTIC SUBACUTE MYELOPATHY

A subacute necrotic myelopathy has been described in association with lung cancer and lymphoproliferative malignancies. Single cases have also been described in several other types of cancer. The myelopathy tends to occur more frequently in males and involves the thoracic spinal cord in most cases.

FOOD-BORNE NEUROTOXINS

By Richard J. Hamilton, M.D.,
and Lewis R. Goldfrank, M.D.
New York, New York

In general, when groups of patients present with comparable signs and symptoms, it is helpful to consider their common sources of exposure—food, water, and air. If symptoms can be temporally related to a meal, a food-borne cause of illness must be strongly considered. Food-borne toxicity typically results in gastrointestinal manifestations. Food-borne neurotoxicity represents a small percentage of the reported cases of food-borne toxicity. When a single patient who denies gastrointestinal symptoms presents with neurologic symptoms dissociated from a meal by time and place, the diagnosis becomes more difficult. However, food-borne neurotoxins often produce illnesses that have characteristic symptom complexes, allowing the well-prepared clinician to recognize the etiology.

Classification of the biologic or chemical mediator of food-borne neurotoxicity can assist the clinician in searching for a diagnosis when characteristic symptom complexes are lacking, or when presenting symptoms are limited (Table 1).

FOODS INHERENTLY NEUROTOXIC

Neurotoxic Mushrooms

Eating improperly identified mushrooms may result in the ingestion of toxic substances. Most people who eat toxic mushrooms experience self-limited gastrointestinal disturbances. However, ingestion of neurotoxic mushrooms may produce a wide range of manifestations, from seizures to hallucinations. Some individuals seek mushrooms with hallucinatory properties for the purpose of substance abuse.

In the evaluation of a patient who has ingested potentially toxic mushrooms, it is often tempting to "solve the case" by first identifying the species of mushroom that has been ingested. Unfortunately, such identification is often extremely difficult, even for a mycologist! Some tests are available. Spore print analysis may take 12 to 24 hours and is usually only clinically useful in retrospect. The Melzer reaction, which involves chemical staining of microscopic spores, is most useful in identifying the hepatotoxic *Amanita virosa* or *Amanita phalloides.* Following the ingestion of a neurotoxic mushroom, the patient's clinical condition usually provides all the clues necessary for making the diagnosis.

Mushrooms in the *Gyromitra* genus contain gyromitrin. Humans can transform gyromitrin to monomethylhydrazine, a toxin that causes seizures and central nervous system excitation. *Gyromitra* species are usually found in the spring in northeastern North America. They have a characteristic cerebriform (brainlike) appearance and typically are mistaken by the mushroom hunter for the true morel (*Morchella esculenta*). *Gyromitra esculenta* (false morel) is the common species associated with human poisoning, which usually manifests within 6 to 10 hours of ingestion. Headache, nausea, and vomiting may progress to seizures and hepatorenal failure. The mortality rate ranges from 15 to 40 per cent.

Table 1. Food-Borne Neurotoxins

Food	Source	Toxin	Differential Characteristics
Foods Inherently Neurotoxic			
Mushrooms	*Gyromitra esculenta*	Gyromitrin	Status epilepticus, responds to vitamin B_6
	Clitocybe and *Inocybe* species	Muscarine	Peripheral cholinergic effects
	Amanita gemmata, Amanita muscaria, and *Amanita pantherina*	Ibotenic acid and muscimol	Somnolence, hallucinations, delirium
	Psilocybe and *Panaeolus* species	Psilocybin	Visual hallucinations, confusion
Herbal drinks, teas, and spices	*Datura stramonium* (jimsonweed)	Atropine Scopolamine	Dry skin, mydriasis, tachycardia, hyperthermia, seizures, anticholinergic toxidrome
	Myristica fragrans (nutmeg)	Myristin	Visual hallucinations, bizarre behavior, hypothermia
	Lobelia inflata (lobelia)	Lobeline, atropine	Nausea, vomiting, dry skin, mydriasis, tachycardia, hyperthermia, seizures
	Cola nitida (Kola nut, botu cola)	Caffeine	Nausea, vomiting, headache, anxiety
Plants	*Cicuta maculata*	Cicutoxin	Status epilepticus
	Conium maculatum	Conine	CNS depression, paralysis
Animals	Tetraodontiformes (puffer), blue ringed octopus, and newts	Tetrodotoxin	Rapidly ascending paralysis
	Ratfish, chimaeras, elephant fish	Unknown	Rapid CNS depression
	Red whelk	Tetramine	Curarelike effects
	Mullet, goatfish, rudderfish	Unknown	Hallucinogenic
Foods Contaminated With Biologic Neurotoxins			
Home-canned foods, foods preserved in oils, preserved seafood, vichyssoise (see table 2)	Contamination by *Clostridium botulinum* bacteria/spores and production of botulinum toxin in food	Exogenous botulinum toxin	Cranial nerve abnormalities, descending symmetrical motor paralysis, EMG shows brief, small, abundant motor unit action potentials

Mushrooms of the *Clitocybe* and *Inocybe* genus contain muscarine, a quaternary ammonium compound that typically causes peripheral cholinergic effects. Muscarinic effects on the autonomic nervous system (salivation, lacrimation, urination, defecation, bronchorrhea, and miosis) typically develop within one half to 2 hours of ingestion. Toxicity is otherwise limited, and fatalities have not been reported.

Mushrooms that contain ibotenic acid and muscimol include *Amanita gemmata, Amanita muscaria* (which contains little muscarine), and *Amanita pantherina.* Ingestion of these mushrooms produces somnolence, hallucinations, and delirium in adults. Children more often develop myoclonic movements and seizures. Mild nausea, vomiting, and diarrhea may occur in children as well as adults. Symptoms tend to resolve within 3 to 4 hours.

Mushrooms that contain psilocybin account for the great majority of neurotoxic mushroom exposures, and these intoxications are usually seen in patients seeking hallucinatory effects. The experience generated by the psilocybin and psilocin indoles in these mushrooms may be pleasant or unpleasant. The central nervous system effects include ataxia, hyperkinesis, and rarely seizures. Patients typically note visual hallucinations but retain a normal orientation to person, place, and time. Tachycardia and mydriasis may suggest anticholinergic poisoning. In contrast to the short-lived effect of intravenous benzodiazepines on the progression of anticholinergic syndromes, the dramatic response of psilocybin-intoxicated patients to benzodiazepines is typical and helps confirm the diagnosis. Importantly, the clinician must also consider the possibility of contamination of mushrooms with other drugs of abuse when the clinical picture is consistent with anticholinergic, opioid, or sympathomimetic toxicity.

Herbal Drinks, Teas, and Spices

Herbal preparations typically are not considered foods or drugs and are not regulated by the U.S. Food and Drug

Table 1. Food-Borne Neurotoxins *Continued*

Food	Source	Toxin	Differential Characteristics
Foods Contaminated With Biologic Neurotoxins Continued			
Commercial honey, corn syrup	*Clostridium botulinum* bacteria/spores	Proliferation in GI tract and endogenous production of botulinum toxin	Cranial nerve abnormalities, descending symmetrical motor paralysis, EMG shows brief, small, abundant motor unit action potentials
Honey	Bees utilizing *Rhododendron* species for nectar	Grayanotoxins	Salivation, paresthesias, hypotension, bradycardia
Fish	Red snapper, grouper, sea bass, amberjack, and other species of fish that have *Gambierdiscus toxicus* in their food chain	Ciguatoxin	Dysesthesias, temperature reversal, bradycardia
	Moray eel	Ciguatoxinlike neurotoxin	Dysesthesias, temperature reversal, bradycardia, cholinergic toxicity, seizures, respiratory paralysis
Mollusks	Shellfish that ingest *Ptychodiscus brevis*	Brevitoxin (neurotoxic shellfish poisoning)	Self-limited peripheral sensory symptoms
	Shellfish that ingest *Protogonyaulax catenella* and *Protogonyaulax tamarensis*	Saxitoxin (paralytic shellfish poisoning)	Paresthesias, facial paralysis, respiratory failure
	Mollusks of Prince Edward Island, Canada, that ingest *Nitzschia pungens*	Domoic acid (amnestic shellfish poisoning)	Bronchorrhea, hemiparesis, ophthalmoplegia, persistent disorders of memory
Restaurant and commercially prepared food	Flavor enhancers	Monosodium glutamate	Rapid onset of headache, facial pressure, and delayed bronchospasm
Fish, treated seed grain	Industrial waste, fungicides	Methylmercury	Abnormalities of sense organs (e.g., blindness, deafness, paresthesias), birth defects
Jamaican ginger extract, cooking oil	Adulterated oils	Triorthocresyl phosphate	Painful neuropathies, spasticity, extremity paralysis
Watermelons, hydroponic vegetables	Organophosphate or carbamate insecticides	Aldicarb, parathion	Salivation, lacrimation, bronchorrhea, miosis, respiratory paralysis

CNS = central nervous system; EMG = electromyography; GI = gastrointestinal.

Administration (FDA). As such, they are commonly ingested by naturalists or prescribed by herbalists for their "natural" pharmacologic activity. Table 1 lists several herbs that are potentially neurotoxic when consumed as teas or food. Natural products such as jimsonweed (*Datura stramonium*) and nutmeg (*Myristica fragrans*) deserve special attention owing to their periodic popularity as psychoactive substances.

Datura stramonium is also known as jimsonweed, Jamestown weed, locoweed, thorn apple, or sacred datura. Datura is a hardy plant that grows at roadsides and in cleared fields, has dark green, pointed leaves, and grows to 1 to 2 m. The white, tubular flowers bloom in late summer. Datura produces a spiny capsular fruit that contains 50 to 100 seeds. This collection of seeds contains as much as 6 mg of atropine as well as clinically significant quantities of scopolamine and hyoscyamine. Jimsonweed has been used as a source of a hallucinogen by teenagers, who eat the seeds, drink jimsonweed tea, or smoke preparations of this plant for psychogenic effects. *Datura stramonium* use causes an anticholinergic toxidrome. Patients present with agitation and bizarre behavior and may report dry mouth, feeling flushed or hot, and blurred vision. The pulse and temperature are typically increased. The pupils are markedly dilated and poorly reactive to light and accommodation. The skin is flushed and dry. The bladder is full, and bowel sounds are diminished or absent. Seizures may occur and are typically brief, but their presence indicates substantial poisoning. Severe untreated toxicity may persist for days, whereas milder symptoms resolve within 24 to 48 hours. Physostigmine (1 to 2 mg over 3 to 5 minutes, 0.5 to 1.0 mg in pediatric patients) is used to inhibit cholinesterase and to increase acetylcholine concentrations in synaptic clefts. Acetylcholine effectively competes with atropine or scopolamine to reverse toxicity. Physostigmine must be administered slowly and with caution because its use has led to seizures and arrhythmias. Physostigmine should be used only when the diagnosis is certain and the patient has not ingested tricyclic antidepressants; this drug should not be used to establish a diagnosis.

Nutmeg toxicity is encountered when this agent is abused as a euphoriant. Nutmeg contains essential oils with alkylbenzene derivatives and terpenes that are biotransformed to amphetaminelike compounds. Nausea, vomiting, headaches, chest pain, visual hallucinations, and bizarre behavior occur within several hours of the ingestion of 5 to 15 g of nutmeg. The physical examination shows tachycardia, hypertension, hypothermia, and mild diaphoresis.

Neurotoxic Plants

Eating plants that have not been properly identified may result in the ingestion of neurotoxic agents. *Daucus carota* ("wild carrot" or "Queen Anne's lace") has an edible root that tastes and smells like a carrot. Individuals who believe they are ingesting this member of the Umbilliferae (carrot) family may, instead, consume *Cicuta maculata* (water hemlock) or *Conium maculatum* (poison hemlock), two of the most poisonous plants in North America. An extract of the latter is almost certainly the poison that Socrates ingested. The alkaloids of poison hemlock have a nicotinelike effect that results in central nervous system depression and paralysis. By contrast, water hemlock contains cicutoxin, a potent proconvulsant. Refractory status epilepticus, which develops rapidly after ingestion, is responsible for the 30 per cent mortality rate associated with ingestion of water hemlock.

Tetrodotoxin Food Poisoning

Tetrodotoxin is present in nearly 100 fresh and saltwater fish of the order Tetraodontiformes. This toxin is also found in the blue-ringed octopus and certain newts. In Japan, the puffer fish, known as fugu, is considered a delicacy. The preparation and consumption of fugu involves a large industry and a loyal cadre of gourmets. The skin, ovaries, liver, intestines, and some muscles contain the toxin. Only licensed chefs may prepare fugu, as they have demonstrated the delicate art of removing the toxin-containing organs. In Japan, deaths commonly occur when fugu liver is ingested or when fugu is prepared at home. Methods for detoxifying the liver are not reliable, and chefs are not allowed to prepare it.

The symptoms of tetrodotoxin poisoning occur minutes after ingestion. Headache, a floating sensation, diaphoresis, and paresthesias of the lips, face, tongue, and hands occur rapidly. Nausea, salivation, vomiting, and abdominal pain are typical gastrointestinal symptoms. Weakness, ataxia, fasciculations, and malaise may ensue. The mental status is not significantly altered. Hypotension, bradycardia, and fixed dilated pupils indicate severe intoxication. An ascending paralysis may lead, within 4 to 24 hours, to respiratory arrest that is typically lethal if untreated.

Uncommon Seafood Poisonings

Red whelk poisoning, which produces curarelike symptoms, is frequently reported in Japan. Ingestion of mullet, goatfish, and rudderfish may cause hallucinations, while ratfish, elephant fish, or chimaeras may cause central nervous system depression.

FOODS CONTAMINATED WITH BIOLOGIC NEUROTOXINS

Food-Borne Botulism (Exogenous Toxin Formation)

Food-borne botulism results from the ingestion of foods containing exogenously formed botulinum toxin. When *Clostridium botulinum* spores proliferate in a favorable media, such as the anaerobic environment of canned foods or those preserved in oil, the toxin tends to form. Five important types of botulinum toxin (A, B, E, F, and G) have been associated with human poisoning.

Botulism typically presents with nausea, vomiting, abdominal pain, and a descending symmetrical paralysis. Patients who present early in their illness, prior to the onset of neurologic signs, are seldom correctly diagnosed because the initial symptoms resemble those of common gastrointestinal illnesses. The subtleties of this early presentation cannot be overemphasized. The patient may have nonspecific abdominal manifestations followed by constipation and sore throat. This symptom complex is commonly diagnosed as a viral syndrome, and observation is usually recommended.

Foods commonly associated with botulism vary (Table 2). The spores are ubiquitous in soil, air, and water and are heat resistant. In general, *C. botulinum* does not proliferate in food that is maintained at pH less than 4.5 or preserved with nitrites. Food contaminated with type A and B botulinum organisms often has a putrified appearance owing to proteolysis by bacterial enzymes. However, type E organisms lack these enzymes, and thus food contaminated with these organisms may appear and taste normal. Botulinum toxins have a relatively characteristic geographic distribution. Type A is found predominantly west of the Mississippi River, type B is found east of the Mississippi and in Europe (especially Portugal), and type E predominates in the Baltic states.

The initial gastrointestinal symptoms of botulism include nausea, vomiting, abdominal distention, and pain. In type E botulism, these symptoms are especially prominent. Additional symptoms typically follow a delay of several hours to several days. These delayed symptoms include constipation, symptoms related to the oropharynx, and cranial nerve disturbances. The oropharyngeal symptoms include dry mouth, odynophagia, and dysphagia; the cranial nerve manifestations are difficulty with visual accommodation, dysphonia, diplopia, ptosis, and mydriasis. Dilated and/or sluggishly reactive pupils are often noted early in the course of botulism.

Cranial nerve abnormalities or the progression of a descending symmetrical motor paralysis is usually present by the time the diagnosis of botulism is considered. The constellation of medial rectus palsy, ptosis, and mydriatic pupils that are sluggishly reactive correlates highly with subsequent respiratory paralysis.

Although mental status is normal, patients may express anxiety over their inexplicable symptoms. Often, the first

Table 2. Food Products That Cause Botulism Outbreaks

Toxin Type	Source
A	Vichyssoise, commercial potpies, fish (salmon), beaver, honey (infants), cheese spread, sautéed onions, chopped garlic in soy oil, home-canned foods (peppers, tomatoes, corn, mushrooms, beets, beans, potatoes, peas, carrots)
B	Home-canned figs, beets, tomatoes, mushrooms, pork and beans, applesauce, cabbage
E	Fish: fermented, frozen or air-dried fish eggs, seal, mussels
F	Liver pâté, venison jerky

Modified from Goldfrank, L.R., et al. (eds.): Botulism. *In Toxicologic Emergencies*, 5th ed. East Norwalk, CT, Appleton & Lange, 1994, p. 939, with permission.

signs of toxicity are cranial nerve abnormalities—usually abducens (CN IV) or occulomotor (CN III). The sensory examination is normal and remains so throughout the illness. Initially, the deep tendon reflexes are normal; however, if the paralysis descends, the respiratory muscles and those of the extremities are impaired.

Differential Diagnosis

Table 3 lists the various conditions that share many of the early clinical manifestations of botulism. In helping to distinguish these disorders from botulism, a handful of diagnostic maneuvers and tests have proved useful. The Tensilon (edrophonium) test is used to determine whether myasthenia gravis is the cause of muscular weakness. Edrophonium increases the amount of acetylcholine at motor end-plates by briefly inhibiting acetylcholinesterase, thereby improving motor function in many patients with myasthenia gravis. Edrophonium is commonly administered in a double-blind, placebo-controlled test to allow objective evaluation of effects. Edrophonium (10 mg) is placed in a coded syringe, and saline placebo is placed in a second syringe. The syringes are injected without the evaluating physician or the patient knowing which syringe contains the drug. The first 1 to 2 mg are given slowly to avoid nausea and vomiting, and the remainder is administered over 5 minutes. The patient is then examined thoroughly for improvement in motor function. Patients with myasthenia gravis demonstrate a dramatic improvement in strength that is noted 1 minute after administration and lasts for approximately 5 minutes. By contrast, patients with botulism manifest little or no increase in muscle strength following administration of edrophonium.

The electromyogram is a virtually diagnostic test for botulism. The electromyographic pattern is characterized by brief, small, abundant motor unit action potentials. Motor nerve conduction velocity is normal. In addition, an increment of small compound muscle action potential amplitude follows repetitive stimulation at 25 to 50 Hz. Stimulation at 2 Hz produces a decrement in the amplitude of muscle potential. Similar but more pronounced findings are seen in the Eaton-Lambert syndrome. When these changes in action potentials occur consistently in all muscle groups, the diagnosis of Eaton-Lambert syndrome is more probable. In patients with botulism, the action potentials vary substantially among muscle groups and the abnormalities progress from cephalad to caudad over time. Intrinsic or inflammatory diseases of muscle may show comparable electromyographic changes, but serum concentrations of muscle enzymes are also characteristically increased. The latter finding is not typically seen in botulism.

Table 3. Differential Diagnosis of Botulism

Amanita muscaria ingestion	Midbrain cerebrovascular accident
Anticholinergic ingestion	Myasthenia gravis
Carbon monoxide	Organophosphate poisoning
Chemical poisoning	Paralytic shellfish poisoning
Clostridium tetani	Poliomyelitis (bulbar)
Diphtheria	Porphyria, acute intermittent
Dystonic reaction	Postanesthetic paralysis
Eaton-Lambert syndrome	Primary muscle disorder
Encephalitis	Tick paralysis
Food poisoning (bacterial)	Trichinosis
Guillain-Barré, atypical	

Modified from Goldfrank, L.R., et al. (eds.): Botulism. *In Toxicologic Emergencies*, 5th ed. East Norwalk, CT, Appleton & Lange, 1994, p. 941, with permission.

A definitive test for botulism involves examination of potential food sources and the patient's serum, stool, vomitus, and gastric contents for *C. botulinum* bacteria and botulinum toxins. Botulinum toxin is potent even at picogram per kg (10^{-12} g/kg) concentrations; thus, small samples may contain enough toxin to perform an animal bioassay. In brief, mice are inoculated with material thought to contain botulinum toxin (e.g., food, serum, biologic fluids). The mice are observed for at least 24 hours for fatalities, even if adverse effects become obvious in a shorter period of time. If any mouse dies, the test is repeated on a second set of mice. During this second phase, one mouse acts as the control and is given placebo, while the remaining animals are administered specific botulinum antitoxins (types A, B, AB bivalent, E, ABE trivalent, and F). This last phase of testing establishes the toxin type and may guide antitoxin therapy, even if initial treatment is typically started prior to obtaining the results of the bioassay.

The prognosis is excellent when botulism is diagnosed early in the course and patients receive continuous observation, parenteral nutrition, and good respiratory support. Antitoxin has a modest effect on the course of the illness, which is often protracted. Full recovery takes several months to a year. Long-term sequelae include dry mouth, dysgeusia (parageusia), constipation, dyspepsia, arthralgias, exertional dyspnea, and easy fatigability.

The clinician who suspects botulism must contact the local health department or the Centers for Disease Control and Prevention (404–639–2206 days, or 404–639–2888 all other times) to assist in diagnosis, testing, and release of trivalent antitoxin.

Infant-Type Botulism (Endogenous Toxin Formation)

Infant botulism develops from the colonization of the gut by *C. botulinum* bacteria/spores. This illness is also associated with an extensive differential diagnosis (Table 4). The toxin is absorbed following enteric production, and the onset of symptoms is more gradual than in food-borne botulism. The use of honey and refined sugar syrups has been associated with botulism in infants. Breast-feeding is also frequently associated with infant-type botulism. The profile of the intestinal flora of the infant may be the most important determinant of disease acquisition. Breast-fed infants predominantly grow species of *Bifidobacterium,* an organism that does not inhibit the growth of *C. botulinum.* By contrast, bottle-fed infants are more likely to harbor coliforms, enterococci, and *Bacteroides* species that may inhibit the growth of *C. botulinum.* Most patients are 2 to 6 months of age, but infection has been reported in 7-day-old infants.

The signs and symptoms of infant botulism are remarkably constant. Initially, the infant demonstrates constipation. Subsequently, the vigor of the cry and/or sucking decreases. Progressive weakness descends symmetrically over hours to days. Muscles supplied by cranial nerves are impaired first; then descending motor paralysis impairs muscles of the trunk and extremities. The child displays little spontaneous movement or motor response to general stimulation. No abnormal sensory findings are noted. Autonomic dysfunction is manifested by variable heart rate and blood pressure, decreased salivation, and abdominal distention. The diagnostic electromyographic findings are similar to those seen in adult botulism. The diagnosis is confirmed in the mouse bioassay with the use of a filtrate of stool obtained spontaneously or through the use of enemas.

The CDC classifies adult-type infant botulism (endogenous toxin formation) as a separate entity. Patients older

Table 4. Differential Diagnosis of Infant Botulism

Initial Presentation	Subsequent Common Diagnoses	Subsequent Uncommon Diagnoses
Dehydration, failure to thrive, hypotonia of unknown etiology, sepsis, viral syndrome	Amino acid metabolism disorders, drug-or-toxin ingestion, metabolic encephalopathy, Guillain-Barré syndrome, lead or arsenic poisoning, Hirschsprung's disease, hypothyroidism, myasthenia gravis, poliomyelitis, viral polyneuropathy, Werdnig-Hoffmann disease	Bites or stings, carbon monoxide poisoning, atonic cerebral palsy, encephalitis, glycogen or lipid storage disease, hypotonia, mononucleosis, muscular dystrophy, myotonic dystrophy, organophosphate poisoning, polymyositis

Modified from Goldfrank, L.R., et al. (eds.): *Toxicologic Emergencies*, 5th ed. East Norwalk, CT, Appleton & Lange, 1994, p. 941; and modified from Johnson, R.O., Clay, S.A., and Arnon, S.S.: Diagnosis and management of infant botulism. Am. J. Dis. Child., 133:586–593, 1979, with permission.

than 1 year of age who develop botulism without an implicated food source are defined as having adult-type infant botulism. The mechanism of infection is similar to that of the infant type. Achlorhydria, antibiotic therapy, or prior intestinal surgery may increase susceptibility to colonization of the gut with spores of *C. botulinum.* The progression of adult-type infant botulism is similar to that of adult botulism; however, the nausea, vomiting, and diarrhea are much less prominent.

Toxic Honey

When beehives are located near large stands of *Rhododendron* species, the bees produce a large amount of honey tainted with grayanotoxins found in rhododendron nectar. Grayanotoxins produce salivation, emesis, circumoral and extremity paresthesias, profound hypotension, and bradycardia. Seizures have been reported. The symptoms resolve in 24 hours.

Seafood Neurotoxins

Ciguatera

Ciguatera poisoning is the most common type of seafood poisoning in the world. The term ciguatera is derived from the Spanish word for the snail (*cigua*) that was originally thought to be the cause of the poisoning. Ciguatoxin, the most common fish-borne neurotoxin, is actually a product of an algae dinoflagellate (*Gambierdiscus toxicus*) that grows abundantly between the north and the south 35th parallels. Small herbivorous fish feed on these algae, and the ciguatoxin accumulates in fish tissues. Larger carnivorous fish then feed on the smaller fish, and the toxin is further concentrated. Fish weighing 4 to 6 pounds are typically thought to carry sufficient quantities of ciguatoxin to cause human toxicity. Those who understand the risk of ciguatoxicity avoid the ingestion and sale of larger fish caught in the endemic areas. The ciguatoxin is heat stable, odorless, and tasteless and is most commonly found in red snapper, grouper, sea bass, and amberjack. The moray eel is the source of a particularly severe form of ciguatera poisoning (gymnothorax poisoning). No method of preparation diminishes the toxicity, and the meat itself does not display warning signs of the presence of toxin.

Most episodes of toxicity occur 2 to 6 hours following ingestion; rarely, a delay of more than 24 hours is noted. The patient usually notes the acute onset of gastrointestinal problems often associated with bizarre neurologic symptoms. Abdominal pain, nausea, vomiting, and profuse watery diarrhea may persist for 24 to 48 hours.

The characteristic neurologic manifestations of ciguatera poisoning include headache, the sensation of loose painful teeth, a strange metallic taste, circumoral numbness, and dysesthesias that may progress to involve the tongue and throat. Although the sensation of temperature reversal (cold objects feel hot or hot objects feel cold) is frequently reported, this symptom is also noted in neurotoxic shellfish poisoning (see later). Variations of this temperature reversal include the feeling of superficial skin warmth and deep cold. Arthralgias and myalgias are also commonly described.

Vertigo, ataxia, scotomata, transient blindness, and blurred vision have been reported; seizures and respiratory paralysis have led to fatalities. The physical examination reveals a diaphoretic patient with bradycardia, hypotension, orthostatic changes, dysesthesias, and paresthesias. Chronic weakness and sensory symptoms may persist for weeks but are not usually permanent. However, some patients report recurrence of symptoms during stress, illness, or after consumption of ethanol.

Although several assays can identify the presence of ciguatoxin, none is required for making the diagnosis. The latex solid-phase immunobead assay that employs monoclonal antibodies to ciguatoxin remains a research tool. The "dipstick" test for ciguatoxin has been used for rapid identification of contaminated fish in the field. Mice can be inoculated with a special extract from contaminated fish; the onset of tachypnea, cyanosis, ataxia, and death indicates the presence of ciguatoxin. None of the assays associated with ciguatera folklore have proved reliable or practical. Clinicians in endemic areas rely on the constellation of gastrointestinal, neurologic, and limited cardiovascular symptoms in making the diagnosis.

Shellfish Poisoning

Dinoflagellates are the source of several other neurotoxins. *Ptychodiscus brevis* contains brevitoxin, and *Protogonyaulax catenella* and *Protogonyaulax tamarensis* produce saxitoxin. Humans are exposed to these agents by consuming the mollusks that ingest and filter these dinoflagellates as food. These tiny organisms rapidly reproduce, or "bloom," from May through August and are responsible for the "red tides" or "brown tides" that may be seen along the eastern coastline of the United States, especially around Long Island and Cape Cod. The extreme dinoflagellate overgrowth and the excessive toxin production may be fatal to birds and fish. Toxins such as brevitoxin produce respiratory symptoms in humans who merely inhale the toxin aerosolized by the pounding surf. *Nitzschia pungens* produces domoic acid and has been identified only in Prince Edward Island, Canada.

Oysters, clams, mussels, and scallops are the common sources of shellfish poisoning. Brevitoxin causes neurotoxic shellfish poisoning, saxitoxin is responsible for paralytic shellfish poisoning, and domoic acid causes amnestic shellfish poisoning.

In some patients, neurotoxic shellfish poisoning may develop within minutes after seafood ingestion. Others, however, may experience a 24-hour delay following ingestion of a shellfish meal. The symptoms of gastrointestinal distress and peripheral sensory impairment are characteristic of this poisoning. Patients report nausea, vomiting, diarrhea, rectal burning, and abdominal pain. The neurologic symptoms consist of paresthesias, dysesthesias, and ataxia. This poisoning may also produce the sensation of temperature reversal, as described in ciguatera poisoning. Paralysis and respiratory failure do not occur, and no fatalities have been reported.

Paralytic shellfish poisoning is primarily a neurologic poisoning. The symptoms include paresthesias of the mouth and extremities, headache, ataxia, vertigo, and facial paralysis. Gastrointestinal symptoms are uncommon. Respiratory failure occurs within 12 hours and accounts for mortality. Affected muscles may remain weak for protracted periods of time.

Amnestic shellfish poisoning has been reported only in association with the consumption of mussels from Prince Edward Island, Canada (1987). These patients developed nausea, vomiting, diarrhea, and bronchorrhea. Hemodynamic instability, peripheral vasodilation, and hypotension were observed in the sickest patients. The neurologic symptoms included myoclonus, fasciculations, hyperreflexia, weakness, seizures, and coma. A novel syndrome of alternating hemiparesis and ophthalmoplegia also developed. Other patients demonstrated spastic hemiparesis, ophthalmoplegia, and diplopia. Electromyographic studies revealed an acute, nonprogressive neuronopathy involving anterior horn cells or a diffuse axonopathy predominantly affecting motor axons. Mortality was seen in older patients with the more severe neurologic symptoms. At postmortem examination, these individuals had necrosis of neurons in the amygdaloid nucleus and hippocampus. Severely poisoned patients who survived suffered persistent anterograde and retrograde amnesia, with preservation of other cognitive functions.

FOOD CONTAMINATED BY CHEMICAL NEUROTOXINS

Chinese Restaurant Syndrome

Monosodium glutamate (MSG) is used as a flavor enhancer in many foods. The syndrome of neurotoxicity typically occurs when foods containing monosodium glutamate are consumed on an empty stomach. Rapid absorption of this chemical results in headache, flushing, bronchospasm, burning, and facial pressure. Most patients report a sense of fear and distress. The burning symptoms are intense and frequently spread to the neck, torso, and abdomen. Gastrointestinal symptoms are minor. The syndrome usually resolves within 1 hour, but bronchospasm may be delayed and lead to respiratory compromise. In children, monosodium glutamate has been associated with seizurelike "shudder attacks."

Methylmercury

Methylmercury is a short-chain alkylmercury compound that has caused two large outbreaks of food-related neurotoxicity. During the 1940s, a vinyl chloride plant in Japan dumped hazardous waste into Minamata Bay. The methylmercury in the waste was bioaccumulated in the fish and poisoned the local community. Because methylmercury is lipophilic, it readily distributes into the central nervous system and placenta. The early signs and symptoms of this toxicity (also known as Minamata disease) develop over months and include headache, tremor, ataxia, paresthesias, fatigue, blurred vision, blindness, hearing disturbances, movement disorders, salivation, and dementia. The fetus is particularly at risk because maternal methylmercury ingestion that leads to minimal toxicity in the adult may produce severe fetal deficits. Decreased birth weight, developmental delay, spasticity, decreased muscle tone, seizures, deafness, and blindness are common neonatal manifestations of a maternal-fetal methylmercury exposure that may have resulted in limited symptoms for the mother. Breast-fed infants who were not exposed in utero can also develop this constellation of symptoms.

In Iraq in late 1971, 95,000 tons of seed grain treated with methylmercury fungicide were mistakenly baked into bread for human consumption. Within 6 months, 459 patients had died, and 6530 patients had been admitted to hospitals for methylmercury poisoning. The illness began with headaches, fatigue, tremor, and paresthesias of the lips, nose, and distal extremities and progressed to severe toxicity, comparable to the poisoning seen in the community surrounding Minamata Bay.

The Reinsch test and other classic metal screening tests are sensitive enough to detect low concentrations of mercury. Whole blood mercury concentrations are only useful in acute exposures. A 24-hour urine specimen is usually sufficient for the detection of chronic exposure to elemental mercury, mercury salts, or phenylmercury (which is rapidly metabolized to mercuric oxide). However, methylmercury is excreted through the biliary system and undergoes substantial enterohepatic recirculation that limits the utility of a urine assay. Urinary levels obtained in this manner do not accurately predict symptoms. Methylmercury accumulates in hair, and this substrate may serve as a biologic marker for exposure. Hair samples may be most useful when fetal birth defects prompt an evaluation for maternal fetal exposure. In this case, maternal hair samples reveal previous methylmercury exposure. The diagnosis is usually made in the presence of epidemiologic data, clinical evidence suggesting methylmercury intoxication, and the presence of slight increases in the concentration of mercury in the blood, urine, or hair. Recovery from the neurologic symptoms of methylmercury poisoning is limited.

Organophosphates and Carbamates

Organophosphates and carbamates inhibit acetylcholinesterase and cause an accumulation of acetylcholine at synapses. Thus, toxicity reflects the distribution of this neurotransmitter and can be divided into three categories: muscarinic, nicotinic, and central nervous system effects. The muscarinic receptors innervate the bronchial tree, gastrointestinal tract, heart, bladder, pupils, ciliary body, and sweat, lacrimal, and salivary glands. Muscarinic intoxication results in bronchorrhea, nausea, vomiting, diarrhea, diaphoresis, salivation, lacrimation, bradycardia, miosis, and blurred vision. The nicotinic receptors are located on striated muscle and sympathetic ganglia and, when poisoned, produce fasciculations, cramps, paralysis, hypertension, tachycardia, pallor, and mydriasis. The central nervous system manifestations range from emotional lability, restlessness, headache, and tremor to ataxia, seizures, and coma. Organophosphate intoxication is best characterized by miosis, fasciculations, bronchorrhea, increased gastrointestinal motility, and altered mental status.

In patients with insufficiently treated acute exposures and untreated chronic exposures, delayed neurotoxicity may develop. This condition usually occurs 1 to 3 weeks after exposure and is manifested as a distal axonopathy. Glove-and-stocking paresthesias, weakness, and ataxia may progress to bilateral flaccid paralysis. Recovery may occur, but spasticity results from insidious upper motor neuron damage.

Laboratory testing is useful as confirmation of acute toxicity or in the evaluation of chronic exposures, but such testing offers little assistance in making acute diagnoses. Red blood cell (RBC) cholinesterase activity reflects synaptic activity, but RBC cholinesterase measurements are not widely available. Plasma cholinesterase assays are more widely available and can serve as useful markers of toxicity. Plasma cholinesterase activity is a sensitive indicator of exposure but is not as reliable as RBC cholinesterase activity. Plasma cholinesterase may be depressed owing to genetic deficiency, medical illness, or chronic organophosphate exposure. Mild acute organophosphate poisoning is typically confirmed when plasma cholinesterase activity declines to 20 to 50 per cent of the values designated as the laboratory "reference range." In severe organophosphate poisoning, plasma cholinesterase activity typically falls to less than 10 per cent of the reference range values. Chronic exposures to organophosphates may result in gradual, asymptomatic depression of cholinesterase activity. The diagnosis is confirmed when activity returns to reference range values during subsequent analyses.

Organophosphates and carbamates may contaminate various food sources when they are improperly applied or persist in the environment from previous applications. The carbamate aldicarb is most frequently involved in food-borne exposures owing to its widespread use and low median lethal time (LD_{50}). Even food produced in soil that was sprayed with aldicarb during the previous year may be contaminated. The biologic persistence of this chemical is thought to be responsible for a large outbreak of toxicity associated with aldicarb-contaminated watermelons grown in Oregon. Aldicarb toxicity has also been associated with two smaller outbreaks attributed to hydroponically grown cucumbers.

Triorthocresyl Phosphate

In the 1930s, "Jamaican ginger paralysis" or "Jake leg" affected at least 50,000 people who purchased an ethanol extract of Jamaican ginger as an ethanol substitute during prohibition. Although this drink was originally safely adulterated with castor oil, it was later formulated with triorthocresyl phosphate (TOCP) when the price of castor oil increased. A second comparable epidemic of 10,000 cases of TOCP-induced paralysis occurred in Morocco when cooking oil was diluted with a turbojet lubricant containing TOCP. Many of the exposed patients had permanent painful neuropathies and spasticity.

CONCLUSION

Food-borne neurotoxicity can be a difficult clinical problem. Establishing the diagnosis is difficult because symptoms are similar and definitive tests for these toxins are not readily available. Once an appreciation is developed for the subtleties of presentation, as well as the manner in which food can be either inherently neurotoxic or function as a vehicle for biologic or chemical neurotoxins, the clinician can follow the analytical steps that will lead to the diagnosis.

Section Eleven

PSYCHIATRY

GERIATRIC PSYCHIATRY

By Gary J. Kennedy, M.D.,
and Pamela Silverman, M.D.
Bronx, New York

The diagnosis of mental disorders in old age is challenging. A single disorder is usually the sole cause of morbidity among younger persons, but most psychiatric disorders in late life coexist with physical illness. Simple diagnosis is insufficient to identify the range of interventions, from definitive to rehabilitative, that are necessary for restoring the person's well being. State-of-the art diagnosis in geriatrics seeks not only to reverse acute episodes of illness and prevent recurrence but to minimize the rate of decline and extent of disability in persistent or degenerative conditions. Thus, the diagnostic assessment needs to be both comprehensive and functionally oriented. When the illness is refractory or degenerative, maintenance of the patient's functional independence may become the principal goal of the diagnostic process, and diagnostic precision can lead to realistic goals for the patient, family, and physician.

GERIATRIC SYNDROMES

The concept of geriatric syndromes has evolved to characterize common late-life conditions that are not included in traditional diagnostic categories. The syndromes include incontinence, osteopenia (osteoporosis and falls), hearing and vision deficits, pressure sores, malnutrition, polypharmacy, immobility, and cognitive impairment. The terminology reflects the multifactorial causes of old-age health problems and the multidimensional interventions needed to maintain optimal function.

Implicit in the geriatric-syndrome approach is the concept of excess or avoidable disability. Excess disability is the disability that one condition adds to another and that may be lessened by some form of therapeutic intervention. One example of excess disability is the apathy, loss of hope, and increased confusion brought about by a depressive episode in a person with Alzheimer's disease. Treatment of the depression can restore the part of the person's functional capacities that has been impaired by the depression. Like dementia, depression in late life meets the criteria of a geriatric syndrome. Other mental disorders may not fit the geriatric-syndrome concept as well as depression and dementia, but emphasis on the optimization of functional outcome can be applied to all of them.

COMPREHENSIVE GERIATRIC ASSESSMENT OF MENTAL ILLNESS

The stigma of mental illness is more troubling for older than younger persons, and the fears and anxieties of the aged patient must be allayed for the psychiatric examination. A deferential, formal attitude is usually more effective than a familiar or casual approach. The history, review of systems, and the mental status and physical examinations of the older person take time. The sheer volume of detail can be burdensome for both the patient and the physician. Most older persons are brought to the physician by the family, and the older patient is usually more comfortable in the presence of a family member. The patient's permission for a conjoint or separate interview with the collateral informant can speed the history taking and lessen the burden on the patient.

The patient and/or the collateral informant should also be queried about the patient's personality, interests, activities of daily living, socially supportive relationships, and routines. Most older adults who are physically healthy and have a partner continue to make love into late life. The examiner should not hesitate to politely inquire about changes in sexual interest and activity. Prescribed and over-the-counter medications, the patient's nutritional habits, sleep and activity patterns, and exercise habits should also be assessed. In the social history, the developmental milestones of late life include the patient's management of retirement, the children's exit from the home, and previous episodes of illness or disability in the patient or the spouse. Because religious practice is prevalent among older persons, participation in the activities of personal devotion and attendance at services should also be elicited. The assessment need not be exhaustive to be comprehensive. Rather, it is designed to identify changes in behavior that clarify the diagnosis, that provide therapeutic leverage, and that establish realistic treatment goals.

Laboratory examinations for late-life mental illness include the electrocardiogram; complete blood count; glucose; electrolytes; urea nitrogen; creatinine; liver function tests; thyroid function, such as triiodothyronine (T_3), thyroxine (T_4), and thyroid-stimulating hormone (TSH); folate; and vitamin B_{12}. An assessment of VDRL should not be omitted owing to deference to age. Other tests are useful in clarifying treatment resistance or prognosis. These tests include the dexamethasone suppression test, electroencephalogram, computed tomography (CT) scan and magnetic resonance imaging (MRI) of the brain, neuropsychological examination, polysomnography, and examination of cerebrospinal fluid.

The mental status examination requires attention to cognitive function and a greater degree of deference and understanding for the patient. The Mini-Mental State Examination (normalized for age and education), the Short Portable Mental Questionnaire, or the Blessed Mental Status Test are commonly employed for quantifying cognitive performance. Serial instrumental assessments of cognition are particularly valuable when decline is questionable. The experienced examiner can administer each of these tests in a matter of minutes. When the testing becomes more time consuming, the examiner is often too forgiving toward patient errors. Subtle signs of cognitive impairment require a more sensitive test of cognitive function, such as the Mattis Dementia Rating Scale. Instruments for assessing cognitive impairment are measurement tools—not diagnostic interviews.

Some older persons will not tolerate or cannot participate in formal cognitive testing, and the examiner must infer cognitive impairment from the collateral informant's history and the clinical interview. Conversely, intellectually gifted or educationally advantaged seniors may give a history of substantial decline yet obtain perfect marks on the cognitive screening instrument. Again, the diagnosis is based on clinical judgment—not on the test score.

COGNITIVE DISORDERS

The modifier organic has been dropped from the diagnostic nomenclature to reflect contemporary awareness that the split between functional (e.g., schizophrenic) and organic disorders (e.g., dementia) has ceased to be meaningful. Indeed, efforts to exclude diagnoses rather than sort out the contributors to the patient's morbidity often frustrate the physician.

Delirium, a disturbance of awareness and attention, emerges following a precipitating event and has a fluctuating course. It may be acute or chronic depending on the cause. Heightened distractibility or inability to attend to the examiner should raise the suspicion of delirium. Memory, perception, and language may also be affected. Acute confusional states can be caused by sleep deprivation or overwhelming social stress, particularly in persons whose mental status is compromised by dementia. However, the most frequent cause of an acute change in mental status is delirium due to infection. The diagnosis is important to recognize not only because it signals an acute illness but also because the associated mortality due to agitation and inability to tolerate intravenous lines or life supports is considerable.

Unlike the reversible cognitive impairment of delirium, the dementias are characterized by progressive decline in at least two domains of intellectual function. These domains include recent and remote memory, learning, and other cognitive processes that, when damaged, lead to apraxia, aphasia, agnosia, and impaired capacity to regulate mood and aggression, to attain insight, to exercise good judgment, and to plan effectively. Pharmacologic interventions for cognitive impairment yield measurable but minimal benefits. However, a variety of agents can be used to treat the depression, sleep disturbance, delusions, and hallucinations that are frequent in dementia.

Alzheimer's disease, which accounts for a plurality of the dementias, is probable when vascular diseases are absent. The onset is insidious, and the course of decline is smooth rather than halting. Alzheimer's disease is definitively diagnosed at autopsy by the number of amyloid plaques and neuritic tangles in excess of that expected for age alone. Brain imaging typically reveals ventricular enlargement and cortical atrophy, particularly in the temporoparietal and hippocampal areas.

Second in prevalence is vascular or multi-infarct dementia, which is associated with focal neurologic signs, a history of cardiovascular and cerebrovascular disease, sudden onset, and stair-step decline. Periods of transient improvement and relative stability can occur. Subcortical lesions as well as atrophy and ventricular enlargement may be demonstrated with brain imaging. Multi-infarct and Alzheimer's pathology can co-exist and account for the largest minority of cases termed mixed dementias. Parkinson's disease is also frequently associated with dementia and depression.

The rare dementias are recognized by signature presentations. Normal-pressure hydrocephalus exhibits a triad of dementia, incontinence, and "magnetic" gait disturbance. Paraneoplastic dementia occurs with malignancies outside the central nervous system. In Pick's disease, the frontal lobes are atrophied, and changes in personality, feeding, and sexual behaviors are more marked than is the memory impairment. Jakob-Creutzfeldt disease, one of the rare transmissible dementias, is diagnosed by the presence of myoclonic twitching and periodic polyphasic sharp-wave electroencephalographic discharges superimposed on background slowing. Dementia caused by infection with human immunodeficiency virus (HIV), although uncommon in late life, may ultimately emerge as the most common infectious dementia, exceeding causes such as syphilis and tuberculosis. Dementia associated with alcoholism and chronic lung disease is far more frequent than are the rare forms of dementia. Korsakoff's amnestic syndrome, caused by alcohol abuse and nutritional deficiencies, is an example of disabling cognitive impairment that is potentially reversible and easily mistaken for dementia.

GERIATRIC MOOD DISORDERS

Diagnosis of depression in late life underwent a paradigm shift in the 1990s. The breadth and severity of symptoms and coexisting conditions that practitioners and clinical scientists considered significant have expanded. The introduction of selective serotoninergic reuptake inhibitors now permits treatment that is as effective as the tricyclic antidepressants, without life-threatening side effects. A uniform terminology for describing the dynamics of the illness has also emerged.

Depressed mood is not required for meeting the diagnostic criteria for mood disorder; apathy rather than sadness is sufficient in combination with other symptoms such as suicidal thought, delusional guilt or pessimism, irritability, and difficulty in concentrating or indecisiveness. Suicidal utterances and, particularly, suicidal intent are considered signs of depression until they are proved otherwise. Medically ill or bereaved persons may be sad—even pessimistic—but are usually free from suicidal thoughts or delusions of guilt or worthlessness. However, the medically ill, particularly those with cardiovascular and cerebrovascular disease, and the bereaved are at greater risk for a depressive episode. Their depressive symptoms may be "understandable" but, if persistent and disabling, should be considered diagnostic.

A major depressive episode is characterized by weeks, rather than months, of dysphoria and a symptom count of five or more. A minor depressive episode is similarly brief, but with fewer symptoms. Like minor depression, dysthymia is diagnosed by a low level of depressive symptoms but persistence over 2 years or more. Dysthymia may predispose the patient to a major depressive episode ("double depression") as well as prevent full recovery. Late-onset depression is most frequently associated with apathy, rather than sadness. Deep white matter MRI lesions (leukoaraiosis) in the basal ganglia, caudate, or thalamus are found in more than 50 per cent of these individuals.

Pseudodementia has come to mean the reversible cognitive impairment of mood disorder. However, whether the depression is late in onset or a recurrent disorder originating in early adulthood, the presence of cognitive impairment with depression in old age most often heralds dementia.

The emergence of a uniform terminology for describing the course of depression recognizes that depression is often a recurrent disorder. The term relapse is applied when symptoms reappear within the first few weeks following an initial remission before an extended period of recovery has occurred. The term recurrence is reserved for depression that re-emerges following the first months of recovery.

The diagnosis of psychosis and mania in depression is critical for effective choice of treatments. However, the psychotic or manic components may be subtle, expressed somatically, or mistaken for age-appropriate thoughts of mortality or simple irritability. Although bipolar illness is thought to abate with age, a small percentage of patients have a progressive course more typical of "bad-outcome" schizophrenia. The emergence of mania late in life without history of prior bipolar illness is most often associated with structural brain changes seen in stroke and subcortical dementia.

ANXIETY DISORDERS

The prevalence of anxiety disorders in late life is uncertain. Community surveys of physically healthy older adults indicate that anxiety disorders are more prevalent than is major depression, with agoraphobia (unreasoned fear of leaving the household) among women being the most frequent diagnosis. However, studies of primary care clinics and patients referred for psychiatric evaluations find that anxiety is actually more indicative of a depressive disorder. In any event the overlap between depression and anxiety seems not to be a sampling or measurement artifact. A careful search for the correct diagnosis has implications not so much for the choice of medications but for the choice of the psychotherapeutic techniques. Antidepressants are preferred to the benzodiazepines in elderly patients with an anxiety disorder. Cognitive behavioral and interpersonal psychotherapies are effective for depression, but cognitive behavioral techniques are preferred for panic attacks and agoraphobia.

The diagnosis of agoraphobia is complicated by the physical disability and transportation problems that the infirm elderly experience. However, finding that older homebound persons ceased to leave the house before the onset of a physical disability or that they now refuse to venture out for mail or fresh air even in the company of a family member or a home health aide suggests agoraphobia or some other mental disorder. Generalized anxiety disorder and panic attacks can be associated with cardiac illness or medications for pulmonary disease. However, these diagnoses are less often confounded by the physical disability so closely linked to depression.

The shared element of the anxiety disorders is fear without reasonable cause. Agoraphobic patients may experience a panic attack when events force them out of the house. The key components of panic are catastrophic thinking, autonomic discharge, and hyperventilation occurring spontaneously or from an encounter with the object of a phobia.

SLEEP DISTURBANCES AND DISORDERS

Sleep disturbances are less helpful for differential diagnosis because of age-related changes in sleep, and the frequency of sleep complaints in depression, dementia, and anxiety. Nonetheless, establishing the pretreatment pattern of disrupted sleep is helpful in evaluating the efficacy of therapy. Nearly a quarter of older adults report less-than-ideal sleep. Careful inquiry often uncovers unrealistic expectations, difficulties with scheduling, lack of exercise, or medications with stimulant or diuretic effects, all of which contribute to poor sleep hygiene and call for changes in behavior. Sleep disturbances brought about by physical conditions such as nocturnal dyspnea, arthralgia, diuretics, or stimulant medications are frequent. Analgesics and modifications in the medication regimen can be quite beneficial.

The insomnia of major mental illness is more often characterized by difficulty in falling asleep or early-morning awakening than by the frequent awakenings and shallow sleep typical of advanced age. Excessive daytime sleepiness, or hypersomnia, is less common and may be difficult to distinguish from lack of stimulation and exercise or boredom.

SUBSTANCE ABUSE AND DEPENDENCE

The prevalence of illicit substance use as well as alcoholism is thought to decline with age, but the phenomenon is poorly understood and probably represents a combination of factors. First, the current cohort of seniors had a low base rate of illicit substance use in early adulthood. Second, premature mortality is associated with heavy abuse of alcohol and drugs. Third, the criteria for abuse and dependence are poorly defined for older persons whose social responsibilities may have declined to the point where dysfunction is difficult to identify. Elders are more sensitive to the effects of alcohol but are less likely to exhibit the classic signs of dependence, namely tolerance, withdrawal, and escalating intake. Thus, the diagnosis of alcohol abuse or dependence should be considered even when the amount ingested and the resultant dysfunction is small. A history of falls, accidents, solitary drinking, or inability to reduce intake or to successfully care for others dependent on the patient suggests alcohol abuse. Overuse of nonprescription medications, such as analgesics and cathartics, and the misuse of prescribed medications, particularly sedative hypnotics, can be a greater problem than alcohol abuse. Alcohol and polypharmacy complicate the differential diagnosis and treatment of the aged, just as they do with younger patients.

PERSONALITY DISORDERS

Personality disorders must be distinguished from a change in personality that is often the result of stroke, major depressive disorder, or dementia. A life-long pattern of interpersonal distress and social dysfunction distinguishes the personality disorders from transient adjustment reactions. However, in either case, the patient, family, or staff typically seek assistance as a result of some precipitating event. Often, the need to negotiate with and rely on others to manage declining capacities causes severe emotional stress for the patient and can result in some of the most difficult behavioral management problems in nursing homes.

Personality disorders may be seen either as less disabling forms of major mental illnesses or as maladaptive exaggerations of normal personality traits. They are divided into three descriptive clusters that facilitate diagnosis. Cluster A, the odd eccentric disorders, includes paranoid, schizotypal (schizophrenialike) and schizoid (aloof). Cluster B comprises the overly dramatic, impulsive disorders, including antisocial, histrionic, borderline, and narcissistic. Cluster C encompasses the anxious personalities, including avoidant, dependent, and obsessive-compulsive disorders. The dramatic cluster disorders, especially antisocial, are less of a problem in late life because impulsiveness wanes with increasing age; however, the "ravages of old age" are not kind to histrionic narcissists. Obsessive-compulsive and schizotypal disorders seem to persist with little change. Individuals with personality disorders are vulnerable to episodes of major mental illness; specifically, anxiety and depressive disorders among clusters B and C and the psychoses in cluster A. Personality disorders also compromise the conduct and outcome of treatment (see the article on personality disorders).

SOMATOFORM DISORDERS

Somatic concerns are pervasive in late life; however, when symptoms that fail to reflect patterns of physical illness become a crippling preoccupation, the diagnosis of a somatoform disorder should be considered. Unlike the personality disorders, somatoform disorders are considered major mental illnesses with substantial disability. They include hypochondriasis, conversion, somatization, and pain disorders. These diagnoses should be approached with caution, because physical illness in late life often presents with atypical findings. However, family members or physicians who know the patient well can help identify signs and symptoms that diverge from the usual pattern of somatoform symptoms. The clinician must understand that the symptoms and disability are real, and that they are not imagined or feigned in a purposeful attempt at secondary gain.

Hypochondriasis is characterized by an unshakable conviction of serious physical illness despite findings to the contrary, the pursuit of procedures and examinations, and anger at physicians for failing to find a cause and a cure. This condition may emerge de novo in late life. *Conversion disorder* involves the disabling impairment of motor or sensory function, typically follows some overwhelming stress, protects the patient from intolerable responsibilities or expectations (e.g., living alone), and may be modeled on the illness of a friend or relative. It most often occurs in the context of another mental illness, such as depression and psychosis, or an episode of bereavement.

Somatization disorder begins early in adulthood and usually affects women. It is distinguished from other somatoform disorders by the breadth of organ systems involved and by the multitude of procedures, particularly gastrointestinal and gynecologic, which the patient has undergone. *Pain disorders* are usually associated with a physical condition but are disabling in excess of the anatomic findings. Untreated depression is frequently present in both younger and older patients. As with all somatoform disorders, recognition of the diagnosis protects patients from unnecessary procedures and physician-induced discomfort or disability.

PSYCHOSES

A substantial minority of schizophrenics experience a clinically significant lessening in symptom severity and associated disability with advancing age. Hallucinations and delusions become less prominent; however, negative symptoms, apathy, cognitive impairment, and intellectual and interpersonal impoverishment increase, particularly among institutionalized residents. Without an adequate history of neurodevelopmental and social decline early in adulthood, the diagnosis of *schizophrenia* with a preponderance of negative symptoms can be easily confused with dementia.

Late-onset schizophrenia is a psychotic disorder occurring after age 45 years and is associated with decline in self-care and social skills. Typically, the patient is an elderly woman with auditory hallucinations and persecutory delusions. A history of paranoid or schizoid personality is common, but frankly bizarre (implausible) behavior or thought content is observed less often.

Late-life delusional (paranoid) disorder is less disabling than late-onset schizophrenia, but it also occurs in persons with a paranoid or eccentric personality. Unwarranted accusations of a persecutory or jealous nature precipitated by trivial events are typical. Grandiose self-regard can be observed. Self-care and cognitive skills are preserved, but the capacity for trust and intimacy is severely impaired. Hallucinations are minimal or absent. Hearing impairment is frequent, and structural brain changes are often present.

ELDER ABUSE AND NEGLECT

Maltreatment of the older person, including misappropriation of funds and the failure to provide care despite the presence of entitlements from Medicare, Medicaid, or the Veterans Administration, is an increasing problem. Physical abuse is less frequent and more easily detected by signs of malnutrition, pattern bruises such as restraint marks, and pressure ulcers due to immobilization. A dubious history, provided most often by family caregivers, of frequent accidents with a pattern of visits to several hospitals or clinics is typical. Sadly, the older victim of abuse is often not the physician's best ally in detecting the problem. Fears of institutionalization or retribution from the perpetrator or the desire to protect an abusive family member can frustrate the diagnostic effort. The most valuable diagnostic evidence is provided by an unscheduled house call by the physician, visiting nurse, social worker, or a representative of the Adult Protective Services agency. Physically dependent women of advanced age with multiple health problems, including dementia and another mental disorder, make up the typical profile of the high-risk victim. The abuser, on the other hand, is more often a family member with mental illness or substance abuse problems as well as financial difficulties.

ASSESSMENT OF THE RISK OF SUICIDE

The assessment of suicide risk, a crucial element of psychiatric diagnosis, is even more crucial in the elderly, in whom suicide rates have increased by more than 20 per cent since the inception of Medicare. Suicide attempts in late life are more often planned than impulsive and are more likely to involve lethal means and preclude the chances of rescue. The highest-risk profile is characterized as patients with a previous attempt or family history of suicide, white males, divorced and socially isolated with physical health problems, financial distress, use of alcohol, and a firearm in the home. Suicide is most often committed in the context of a major depressive episode. However, the fact that most suicides in the aged occur within a month of the last visit to the physician suggests that the depression may be atypical and elusive. The assessment cannot be made without asking the question, and the clinician should not hesitate to inquire for fear of triggering the suicidal impulse.

ANXIETY DISORDERS

By Gene R. Corbman, M.D.
Elkins Park, Pennsylvania

Virtually everyone has experienced anxiety at some time in their lives, whether due to an examination in school, a date, or a meeting with a boss. Anxiety is often accompanied or even overshadowed by feelings of inadequacy or guilt. Although these feelings may or may not appear appropriate to the observer, the importance that the patient gives them must be recognized. This is significant because we all have our own idea of what it means to be anxious, and it helps to put into perspective the significance and severity of the anxiety that our patients describe to us. Anxiety is related to, but it is not the same as, an anxiety disorder. Both deserve our attention and treatment.

Anxiety is the perception of a danger by the individual, who may then feel paralyzed by that danger. Anxiety is related to fear and is an essential, built-in factor that warns us of danger and signals that something needs to be done. However, as can happen with the deer caught in the headlights of a car, fear can be incapacitating and dysfunctional. The threat or danger may be real, such as loss of job, of income, of a loved one, of prestige, and so on. This sense of helplessness and paralysis is a telltale sign of both anxiety and depression and shows how they are sometimes related.

Twenty-eight million Americans suffer from an anxiety disorder each year, which makes it the most prevalent form of mental disorder. Anxiety disorders are less related to external circumstances and more related to the individual's reaction to the internal environment, that is, the psyche and/or the body. However, because individuals tend to explain or rationalize why they feel anxious, it is often difficult to distinguish anxiety from an anxiety disorder. Both can have behavioral, cognitive, affective, and somatic symptoms (Table 1). No pathognomonic signs or symptoms of an anxiety disorder have been identified. The patient who enters the office complaining of anxiety may be surprisingly difficult to treat. An even greater challenge is posed by the anxious patient who does not complain of anxiety.

Table 1. Signs and Symptoms Associated With Anxiety Disorders

Motor and behavioral	Restlessness, trembling, pacing, shaking, hand wringing, rapid speech, hyperventilation
Cognitive	Fears of impending doom or something terrible happening, preoccupation with anxiety-provoking thoughts, inability to concentrate
Affective	Feeling anxious, tense, nervous, scared, breathless, distracted, "wired," "not part of things"
Somatic	Tightness in head, neck, chest, stomach, limbs; tingling, numbness, lightheadedness; difficulty breathing, swallowing; a lump in throat, choking sensation; palpitations; nausea, vomiting, diarrhea

PRESENTING SIGNS AND SYMPTOMS

Anxiety disorders are currently divided into 12 separate categories; common and distinguishing features are found in each.

Panic attacks occur in the context of several different anxiety disorders and are not by themselves an anxiety disorder, but they deserve separate attention. A panic attack is a discrete period characterized by a sudden onset of intense fearfulness or apprehension, which builds to a peak in 10 minutes or less and is often associated with feelings of impending doom and a need to escape. Typical symptoms include shortness of breath or a feeling of smothering, palpitations, chest pain or tightness, a feeling of choking, a fear of going crazy or of losing control, sweating, trembling or shaking, dizziness or lightheadedness, nausea or abdominal distress, a sense of derealization (feelings of unreality) or depersonalization (being detached from oneself), fear of dying, paresthesias and chills, or hot flushes. At least four of these symptoms must be present to diagnose a panic attack.

Panic attacks are classified into three characteristic types. The unexpected panic attack is not associated with a situational trigger and appears to occur "out of the blue." The occurrence of unexpected panic attacks is necessary for making a diagnosis of panic disorder. Situationally bound panic attacks occur almost invariably on exposure to, or in anticipation of, exposure to a specific situation; they are typically seen in social or specific phobias. Situationally predisposed panic attacks are likely to occur on exposure to a given situation, but they are not invariably associated with a situational trigger. As a result, they can cause considerable diagnostic confusion, which is compounded if the patient begins to anticipate the panic attacks.

ANXIETY DISORDERS

Agoraphobia

Agoraphobia has the essential feature of anxiety about and avoidance of places or situations from which the person feels an overwhelming need to escape. Patients typically fear that escape would be difficult and embarrassing or they fear that help may not be available. Usual situations include being in a crowd, standing in line, or traveling on public or commercial transportation. In other words, the patient may present with either inhibiting self-consciousness or dependency on others, or both. Agoraphobia may occur with or without panic attacks or in the context of panic disorder. The anxiety typically leads to avoidance of being outside the house, especially alone, or even of being alone at home. A careful history is necessary to distinguish agoraphobia from social phobia or specific phobia.

Panic disorder is characterized by and has the essential feature of recurrent, unexpected panic attacks. The frequency and severity of the attacks can vary considerably. However, within a short time, the person begins to always expect or anticipate an anxiety attack, which leads to anticipatory anxiety and a self-perpetuating condition. In fact, the criteria for making the diagnosis include at least a month of persistent concern about having another panic attack. A panic disorder may be seen with or without agoraphobia and vice versa. Additional criteria include worry about the implications of the attack, such as losing control, going crazy, or having a heart attack and a significant change in behavior related to the attacks. The change in behavior may be due to the panic attacks or the patient may be unable to confront some psychologic problem, and the panic attacks represent a "cry for help." The latter case, of course, warrants further psychiatric intervention.

Associated features include constant or intermittent feelings of generalized anxiety, excessive apprehension about the outcome of routine events, and a lowered tolerance for physical symptoms or for the side effects of medications. Major depression can develop in two thirds of these patients. Substance abuse should also raise the suspicion of an anxiety disorder. The course of this condition is variable, and the age of onset is typically between the teenage years and mid-30s. The usual course is chronic with periods of exacerbation and apparent remission, but some individuals have constant, severe symptoms. Evidence of familial patterns has been reported; however, up to 75 per cent of patients in the clinical setting have no family history.

Phobias

Specific phobia was formerly called simple phobia. The essential feature is excessive or unreasonable anxiety provoked by exposure to a specific feared object or situation. The diagnosis is made only if the avoidance is uncontrollable and incapacitating or the anxious anticipation of encountering the feared object or situation interferes significantly with some aspect of the patient's life. For example, children have many fears in the course of development that do not significantly impair their functioning and therefore do not warrant the diagnosis. In addition, for individuals younger than 18 years old, the duration must be at least 6 months. Associated features may include vasovagal fainting and avoidance of medical care. Predisposing factors also help in the diagnosis and include traumatic events and unexpected panic attacks that become associated with the circumstances that were in place at the time of the attack. The appearance of a specific phobia can occur at any age but it typically starts in childhood or early adulthood. Family patterns and traumatic events can be helpful diagnostically.

Social phobia is characterized by significant and persistent anxiety resulting from normal daily social contacts leading to avoidant behavior. Typically, the fear is of embarrassment or of "freezing." The embarrassment may be related to the fear that others will see the patient shaking, sweating, blushing, or stammering. A vicious cycle of anticipatory anxiety can result in impaired performance that reinforces the phobia. The diagnosis is made only if the avoidance or fear of the social situation significantly interferes with daily activities or if the patient is significantly distressed over having the phobia.

Associated features include extreme sensitivity to criticism or negative evaluation, difficulty being assertive, and low self-esteem. Persons with social phobia often have poor social and interpersonal skills and may make individuals around them uncomfortable. They often underachieve in school and at work. In younger children, crying, tantrums, extreme shyness, and clinging may be seen. The course is variable. Age of onset is often the midteens, but the disorder may develop in the previously withdrawn or shy child. Social phobia may develop spontaneously or following a humiliating experience. It is typically chronic, and a familial pattern is often evident.

The differential diagnosis between social phobia and agoraphobia may be difficult. A history of unexpected panic attacks leads one to diagnose agoraphobia. Similarly, avoidance of social situations for fear of having a panic attack is more properly diagnosed as a panic disorder. Children with separation anxiety disorder will avoid situations that require them to be separated from a parent or other caretaker. The avoidance personality disorder has many features in common with social phobia, and the patient typically avoids taking any responsibilities.

Obsessive-Compulsive Disorder

Obsessive-compulsive disorder is characterized by intrusive, repetitive, unwelcome thoughts; doubts; impulses; or images (obsessions) accompanied by involuntary actions or behaviors (compulsions) that are performed to counteract the obsessions. Compulsions are typically ritualistic and idiosyncratic and are often related to the obsessions in some magical, superstitious, or unrealistic manner. The symptoms are time-consuming (often taking more than 1 hour a day) and distressing, causing significant functional impairment. They are experienced as being unreasonable or ego-dystonic and as such they are different from ruminations or worries that are more related to real life events such as financial or health concerns. As alien or unwanted as the obsessions are, the individual recognizes them as self-generated rather than being imposed from the outside as in thought insertion, hallucinations, or delusions. The individual's insight into the unreasonableness of the compulsions, however, can be variable. The person may have an intellectual awareness of the unreasonableness but experiences growing tension and anxiety as he or she attempts to resist the behavior, ultimately rationalizing the need to perform the compulsive behavior. Typically, patients fear that they did not perform the compulsive act properly or that they may have actually caused the disaster they feared while trying to prevent it (referred to as undoing).

Associated features include avoidance of situations that tend to stimulate the individual's obsessions. Dermatologic stigmas are common. A pathologic sense of responsibility and sleep disturbances are also common and should suggest the diagnosis. A major depression or a paranoid psychosis may eventually develop. The age of onset of obsessive-compulsive disorder is usually in the teens but may begin in childhood or early adulthood. The natural course is chronic and can be aggravated by stress; evidence exists for a genetic component.

Stress Disorders

Post-traumatic stress disorder (PTSD) is characterized by the re-experiencing of an extremely traumatic event accompanied by symptoms of increased autonomic and sensory arousal and avoidance behavior. The traumatic event is usually of life-threatening proportions and can be either personal or witnessed. The person must experience intense fear, helplessness, or horror. Avoidance of situations associated with the trauma usually follows. Symptoms must last for at least 1 month with significant distress or impairment of functioning for PTSD to be diagnosed.

Symptoms include recurrent, intrusive recollections of the event, distressing dreams about the event, and brief periods of actually re-experiencing the event in a dissociative state. Intense startle reactions are common. A feeling of detachment and amnesia for some aspect of the event can occur. Sleep disturbances often develop. Although exposure to a traumatic event may well be apparent, development of PTSD may not be readily recognized. An associated feature is feelings of guilt for having survived, having caused the event, or having been unable to avoid it. Interpersonal relationships may deteriorate as self-esteem drops. Substance abuse and self-destructive behavior may follow. One of the other anxiety disorders may appear.

Acute stress disorder is similar in presentation to PTSD but occurs immediately following or within 1 month of a traumatic event. The essential cluster of symptoms includes a sense of emotional numbing or absence of emotional response, a sense of detachment, a reduction of awareness of one's surroundings, derealization, depersonalization, and dissociative amnesia. As in PTSD, the victim has persistent recollections of the event as thoughts, dreams, images, and flashbacks, with marked anxiety and increased autonomic arousal. Patients typically avoid anything that may consciously or unconsciously remind them of the event. To make the diagnosis, the symptoms must cause significant distress and interfere with or impair normal functioning. The disturbance persists for 2 days to 4 weeks and can include impaired concentration and anhedonia. If the symptoms last longer than 1 month and are of sufficient severity, the diagnosis of PTSD is made. If the symptoms do not meet the criteria of PTSD, the diagnosis of adjustment disorder may be appropriate. Individuals may feel guilty, usually rationalizing that "they should have done something (differently)" to have avoided the traumatic event. This can lead to the development of a major depressive disorder.

Generalized Anxiety Disorder

Generalized anxiety disorder is defined by a period of at least 6 months of persistent and excessive anxiety and worry about a variety of issues that occurs more days than not during the period under consideration. Strictly speaking, it is probably one of the more difficult diagnoses to make because the clinician must make value judgments that can easily be clouded by cultural bias. Patients may not consider their worries to be excessive, but they may describe feeling distress because of constant worry, which they are likely to blame on external circumstances. Associated symptoms must include at least three of the following to make the diagnosis: restlessness or feeling "keyed up," easy fatigability, impaired concentration, irritability, muscle tension, and sleep disturbance. The symptoms must be of sufficient severity to impair functioning.

None of these symptoms are specific, and they may be seen in a wide variety of conditions. An accurate and detailed psychiatric history must be elicited to exclude more specific anxiety disorders as well as to exclude medical conditions that cause anxiety. Familiarity with the patient's social history is helpful in recognizing a generalized anxiety disorder. In children, this disorder may present as unreasonable concern about performance or competence in school or other activities. These children often experience conforming and perfectionistic behavior that requires excessive reassurance. Most individuals with this disorder describe themselves as having been anxious most of their lives, but onset after the age of 20 years is not uncommon. The course tends to be chronic with exacerbation under stress; however, these individuals are more likely to feel stressed by everyday events. No consistent evidence exists that there is a family pattern for this condition.

Anxiety Disorder Due to a General Medical Condition

Anxiety disorder due to a general medical condition is characterized by prominent symptoms of anxiety that are a direct physiologic consequence of a general medical condition. This condition must be distinguished from a substance-induced anxiety disorder. Medical conditions giving rise to anxiety disorders are listed in Table 2. The symptoms of anxiety accompanying any of these conditions are indistinguishable from anxiety due to any other cause. A physiologic cause for a general medical condition must not be missed and attributed to simple anxiety. Somatic symptoms of palpitations, shakiness, shortness of breath, sweating, and stomach pains may be prominent but are not diagnostic of a general medical condition. The chronology of the symptoms may suggest a medical condition, but emotional events can interact with certain pathophysiologic events such as asthma and hypoglycemia and mitral valve prolapse to obscure the picture. A good medical and social history helps to make a judicious choice of laboratory tests (see further on).

Table 2. Common Medical Conditions to Consider in a Patient Presenting With Anxiety

Endocrine	Hypothyroidism and hyperthyroidism
	Hypoglycemia and hyperglycemia
	Hyperadrenocorticism
	Thyrotoxicosis
	Pheochromocytoma
Cardiovascular	Arrhythmias
	Mitral valve prolapse
	Congestive heart failure
	Pulmonary embolism
Respiratory	Chronic obstructive pulmonary disease (COPD)
	Emphysema
	Asthma
Metabolic	Vitamin B_{12} deficiency
	Porphyria
Neurologic	Traumatic brain injury
	Infection of the central nervous system

Substance-Induced Anxiety Disorder

Substance-induced anxiety disorder is characterized by symptoms of anxiety that are a direct physiologic or pharmacologic consequence of a drug or other exogenous toxin. This diagnosis is made instead of substance intoxication or substance withdrawal only when the symptoms of anxiety are in excess of those usually associated with the intoxication or withdrawal syndrome. An example is the person being treated with anxiolytic and/or sedative-hypnotic agents for sleep. As tolerance to the substance develops, the patient may experience a state of mixed intoxication and withdrawal that is often associated with increased anxiety and increased self-medication. A substance-induced anxiety disorder is then superimposed on the anxiety disorder being treated, but the former may be masked.

The differential diagnosis between a drug-induced anxiety and another anxiety disorder requires a careful history and close observation. In an older person, the appearance of anxiety should lead one to question the use of sedative-hypnotics or some form of barbiturate. In the younger person, illicit drugs should be suspected, especially if an attitude of evasiveness or hostility is encountered during the examination and interview. Signs of marked autonomic arousal are also suggestive but are not conclusive.

Anxiety Disorder Not Otherwise Specified

Anxiety disorder not otherwise specified includes conditions in which prominent features of anxiety or phobic avoidance are exhibited but do not meet the criteria for one of the specific anxiety disorders. Examples include mixed anxiety-depressive disorders or anxiety disorders that cannot be completely characterized. Also included are clinical situations in which significant anxiety and/or phobic symptoms are related to self-consciousness about some other medical or psychologic condition. Examples include Parkinson's disease, psoriasis, or stuttering.

OTHER PSYCHIATRIC DISORDERS ASSOCIATED WITH ANXIETY

Somatoform disorders, which include somatization disorder (formerly called hysteria or Briquet's syndrome), conversion disorder, pain disorder, hypochondriasis, and body dysmorphic disorder are all associated with significant anxiety. The common feature of this group of disorders is excessive concern or anxiety focused on physical symptoms in the absence of a causative medical or physical condition.

An adjustment disorder with anxiety or with mixed emotional features is a condition characterized by significant emotional or behavioral symptoms that develop in response to an identifiable psychosocial stressor. Typically the stress is not life-threatening, but it can result in excessive anxiety. The symptoms in this condition must appear within 3 months of the stressful event and last no longer than 6 months after the termination of the event.

Attention deficit disorder (ADD) is often missed in the adult. The person with ADD typically worries needlessly and may seem to be constantly looking for something to worry about. Patients may have a sense of impending doom and insecurity. Their difficulty focusing on a subject can suggest the diagnosis of an anxiety disorder. No diagnostic studies can identify an anxiety disorder, but this is one of the few conditions in which a therapeutic trial can help in the differential diagnosis. A psychostimulant such as methylphenidate permits patients with ADD to focus their attention, but it produces the opposite effect in those with an anxiety disorder. Conversely, the use of a minor tranquilizer in patients with ADD shows variable and inconsistent results.

Premenstrual syndrome (PMS) is often associated with a feeling of irritability, edginess, and anxiety. It is relatively easy to identify because of its cyclic nature. However, one must be careful not to attribute other sources of anxiety to this condition because increased sensitivity resulting from hormonal changes may be uncovering other sources of anxiety.

Whether one considers alcoholism a psychiatric disorder or a physiologic disorder, the relationship between alcoholism and anxiety is complex. Anxiety may be the causal risk factor leading to alcohol abuse. Alcoholism and anxiety may share a common underlying genetic disorder, or anxiety may be alcohol-induced. If after a 6-week alcohol-free period symptoms of anxiety persist, a diagnosis of an anxiety disorder can be made.

EVALUATION OF THE PATIENT

The most useful aspect of the evaluation of the patient with an anxiety disorder is general appearance and history. The physical examination may be entirely normal, or increased or labile blood pressure, tachycardia, and tachypnea may be observed. Other physical signs can include pupillary dilatation, diaphoresis, flushing or pallor, tremulousness, and restlessness. However, delusions, hallucinations, disorientation, and a fluctuating level of consciousness argue against anxiety disorder.

Many organic disorders can present with anxiety, but no specific tests can identify any of the anxiety disorders. Therefore, a detailed psychosocial medical history, together with a complete physical examination, is required to make a judicious choice of laboratory tests. Some of the more useful tests include a urine drug screen, liver function tests, and thyroid function tests. Electrocardiography should be considered if symptoms indicate; echocardiography can help diagnose or exclude mitral valve prolapse.

Patients with panic attacks or panic disorder tend to be more sensitive to certain substances such as caffeine, lactate, yohimbine, isoproterenol, and epinephrine. Indeed, panic attacks can be provoked by administering these substances, but provocative testing is not diagnostic and is not routinely used. Similarly, no therapeutic tests can confirm or exclude the diagnosis of anxiety disorder. Anxiolytic agents have at least a temporary beneficial effect on anxiety of any cause, but breakthrough anxiety while the patient is using an anxiolytic agent does not exclude the presence of an anxiety disorder.

MOOD DISORDERS

By Richard W. Hudgens, M.D.
St. Louis, Missouri

Depression and mania are called mood disorders, or affective disorders, because the moods and affect (outward manifestation of mood) of individuals with these conditions are conspicuously disturbed. However, much more than mood is disrupted in these illnesses. The ability to concentrate, as well as the quality of judgment, level of energy, physical functioning, sensory perception, general behavior, and the sufferer's very philosophy of life, may also be changed in one direction or another. To think of depression as extreme sadness, or mania as extreme happiness is to be naive about the essential quality of these syndromes. They are disorders of brain function that are different from normal mood states, and their occurrence is not dependent on the happiness- or sadness-producing events that influence mood changes in all of us.

The mood disorders are currently classifed into two major groups: depressive disorders and bipolar disorders. Depressive disorders include major depression, which is a severe and usually episodic illness, and dysthymic disorder, which is a milder chronic version of depression. Bipolar disorders consist of bipolar I disorder, in which mania has occurred at least once in the person's life with or without a history of depression, and bipolar II disorder, in which the person has not suffered full-blown mania but has experienced major depression and at least one episode of the milder version of mania called hypomania.

Other terms are still in common use to describe mood disorders. Manic-depressive disorder, or manic-depression, is the familiar synonym for bipolar disorder. Depressive disorders with no history of mania or hypomania are sometimes called unipolar. Melancholia, an ancient term, is used to describe a depressive illness (occurring in the course of either a unipolar or a bipolar illness) in which the person's mood is especially impervious to change by external events. Physical functions are prominently affected, and the capacity for rational thinking is disrupted. In secondary depression or mania, the mood disorder arises in the course of a medical illness (e.g., diabetes or coronary artery disease) or in the course of another psychiatric illness (e.g., alcohol dependence). The mood disorder is thus secondary in the temporal sense of the word. Causation of the mood disorder by the illness that came first is not implied, although this sometimes occurs. For example, hypothyroidism and some strokes can lead to depression.

MAJOR DEPRESSION

Presenting Symptoms

Epidemiologic studies have demonstrated that two thirds of depressions are not diagnosed. Often, this failure is because the professional to whom the patient presents fails to recognize the illness. Unless patients are acquainted with depression through prior experience or knowledge, they do not usually walk into a physician's office with the complaint, "I have depression." More commonly, individuals present with physical symptoms, especially fatigue, sleep disturbance, any of a variety of gastrointestinal symptoms, or headache. If the patient is told that he or she has depression, the reply is often, "Of course I'm depressed, but I'm depressed because I feel bad"; the patient makes the common mistake of confusing the mood of depression with the illness of depression, a different thing altogether.

Patients often report anxiety, irritability, lack of joy, or excessive worrying. They do not typically characterize their moods as simply sad. Usually, a patient with depression recognizes that something is wrong, but when the clinical picture is dominated by irritability and loss of insight, the problem may be erroneously characterized as external. Without real evidence to support his or her view, the patient may become convinced that a once-pleasant boss has become a tyrant or that a formerly loving spouse has become intolerable. Thus, depression can present as a marriage problem or a job problem. The problem may simply be that the individual with depression is unhappy and hard to get along with at this time. If depression is present, treating it should take precedence over marriage counseling and certainly over a precipitous change of job or divorce.

The ability to concentrate or to reason logically is often disturbed. Individuals whose jobs require a good deal of cognitive activity frequently complain most about the difficulty they have thinking. What depressed individuals think about may also be troublesome. The content of thought commonly runs on negative themes, sad memories, pessimistic expectations, past sins, and guilt. More severely ill individuals may have delusions, for example, an irrational belief that they are unforgivably evil or that they are persecuted by others, perhaps deservedly, or that they have a dreadful medical disease, usually acquired immunodeficiency syndrome (AIDS) or cancer.

Depressed patients and their physicians often mistakenly conclude that the things that individuals worry and obsess about when they are depressed are the cause of their depression. In this way, an undue amount of attention is paid to some instance of misbehavior occurring years before the depression; for example, some therapists now dredge up memories of childhood sexual abuse instead of sending the patient to a physician for effective treatment of the illness.

The potential for suicidal behavior in a depressed patient deserves the physician's special attention. As many as 15 per cent of those who suffer from major depression eventually die by suicide, a rate that is 15 times higher than that of the general population. Patients usually do not volunteer that they are suicidal. The physician must ask about it and should not worry about putting ideas into the patient's head; he or she is already thinking about it. Almost everyone with major depression considers suicide as a way of ending the misery or as a response to delusional beliefs, such as imagined disease or irredeemable sinfulness. These patients are embarrassed to mention suicidal ideas spontaneously. By doing so, they may fear that they are removing one of the options available to them for escaping the torments of depression. The physician must always ask whether the patient has thought of ending his or her own life. If this is the case, the physician should ask what suicidal plans have been made and whether the patient has the means to carry out the plan. Specific plans, coupled with a convincingly pessimistic view of the future or delusional distortions of reality, are ominous signs and often require immediate hospital admission.

Course of Major Depression

The risk of major depression begins in childhood, but the illness usually makes its appearance after puberty. Most individuals, regardless of when the illness first begins, are not treated for it until their 30s or 40s. Depression may begin suddenly, from a standing start to full-blown symptoms in a few weeks. However, it usually begins insidiously over several months. In the case of persons suffering from chronic dysthymia, it may arise in the course of long-standing milder symptoms. The typical patient presenting to a psychiatrist arrives in the office several months after the illness has begun. Even a first episode of depression may last for at least a year before remitting spontaneously. Individuals who have had multiple previous episodes need continuous treatment for 3 to 5 years. Up to one third of those treated by psychiatrists for major depression need treatment indefinitely, continuing even after they are asymptomatic. As individuals age, their depressions tend to last longer and are more resistant to treatment. Other illnesses, medical problems, and dementias complicate the diagnostic and treatment picture.

Diagnostic Tests

The diagnosis of major depression is made from the history, which is taken from both the patient and a reliable informant. No laboratory tests or imaging techniques can help diagnose major depression in an individual patient. Endocrine and electroencephalographic studies have been performed in depressed and manic patients since the middle of this century. Abnormalities of function in the hypothalamic-pituitary-adrenal axis have been uncovered, including a blunting in the normal suppression of serum cortisol levels after a dose of dexamethasone. This failure of suppression does not occur in everyone with major depression and does occur in other conditions at times, so it has no value as a diagnostic test. Similarly, in some depressed persons—but not all—blunting of the expected release of thyrotropin occurs after stimulation of the pituitary by thyrotropin-releasing hormone. By the 1960s, electroencephalographic studies had begun to show sleep abnormalities in some individuals with melancholic depression, especially a shortened time lag between the onset of sleep and the beginning of the rapid eye movement (REM), or dreaming, phase of sleep.

New imaging procedures, such as magnetic resonance imaging (MRI) and positron emission tomography (PET), have moved the study of mood disorders into an exciting phase. Changes in brain metabolism (and sometimes structure) in the frontal and temporal lobes and the basal ganglia are being reported as acute or chronic abnormalities in both depression and mania. Thus far, these findings have not been sufficiently consistent or correlated closely enough with specific symptoms to be of use as diagnostic tests. At present, detection of biologic correlates of major depression in an individual requires procedures that are too expensive except in supported research settings. Typically, the findings are nonspecific, and inexpensive laboratory tests for this illness do not yet exist. Clinicians must realize that diagnostic tests are unnecessary for identifying major depression. A good history and close attention to the patient's mental status are all that is needed.

Differential Diagnosis

The class of psychiatric disorder that most mimics major depression is substance abuse. Alcoholism and dependence on cocaine (and other central nervous system stimulants) or marijuana can present a clinical picture identical to that of major depression, including both mood symptoms and vegetative (physical) symptoms. Additional sources of history and urine or blood screening tests may be necessary for uncovering these often-concealed disorders. Until a patient's substance abuse is under control, the presence of major depression cannot be determined.

Schizophrenia is a disorder of brain function, and often of brain structure, which typically begins by the late teens and usually progresses to a disabling state of delusions, hallucinations, and severely impaired initiative over the next several years. Before all the symptoms develop, some patients present a distressed or apathetic picture that is identical to major depression. In the early stages of the illness, these patients may in fact be treated for depression, which at least does no harm.

Other disorders may present with the clinical picture of depression. Significant anemia from any cause, as well as either hyperthyroidism or hypothyroidism, may mimic major depression. These conditions can be excluded by laboratory tests, which should be obtained routinely in anyone presenting with symptoms of depression. Occult intra-abdominal cancers, especially of the pancreas, present on occasion with depressed mood and vague physical symptoms. Computed tomography and ultrasound studies are helpful in this clinical setting.

Medications given for nonpsychiatric disorders can affect mood significantly. Reserpine, still in use as an antihypertensive agent, can cause severe and persistent depression. Adrenal corticosteroids, naturally occurring or synthetic, can trigger depression or mania in susceptible individuals. Beta-adrenergic blocking agents are reported to cause depression, and estrogen and progesterone in birth control pills have a variable effect on mood. On rare occasions, benzodiazepines can cause a depressive picture, even when taken in recommended doses.

In the course of any chronic and debilitating medical illness, patients may have many physical symptoms of major depression, such as fatigue, loss of appetite, and apathy. In fact, some of these patients have a major depression in addition to their medical disorder, and it should be treated if there are no contraindications. Traumatic brain injury and strokes, often in the left hemisphere, may be followed by major depression. Parkinson's disease is also accompanied by depression with a greater frequency than would be expected by chance. The fact that a depression arises as an apparent consequence of structural brain damage is no contraindication to treating the patient vigorously, but in such cases the depression is likely to be less responsive to treatment.

BIPOLAR DISORDER

The depressive phases of bipolar disorder typically present the same clinical picture as major (unipolar) depression. The following sections deal with mania and its milder variety, hypomania.

Mania

Full-blown mania cannot be ignored and requires hospital treatment, which may be against the patient's wishes, since he or she usually lacks the insight that this is an illness.

Mania is marked by hyperactive behavior and talking; sleeplessness; an intense, contentious or inappropriately friendly manner; insensitivity to the feelings of others, coupled with extreme antagonism when faced with opposition or disagreement; plans that are often grandiose and impractical; excessive spending perhaps fueled by a belief in nonexistent riches; increased romantic attachments and sexual activity that may be inappropriate or promiscuous; and, at times, excessive alcohol and drug use, which complicates the clinical picture.

Concentration and attention are conspicuously impaired, with the occasional appearance of confusion, imprecision of memory, and even disorientation. When delusions are present, they seem to stem from this confusion, from grandiosity, or from antagonism to other individuals who are not cooperating with the patient's excessive plans or are trying to force the patient into treatment. In the hospital, for example, manic patients may misidentify other patients and staff as friends and relatives, or they may think that they are in the hospital to treat patients and that they are not sick themselves. Alternatively, they may believe that the members of the staff are devils and that their families have imprisoned and abandoned them; they may think that they are possessed with special powers and insight, with extrasensory perception and the solution to the world's problems. These patients may also believe themselves divine—that they are God, Jesus, or the Virgin Mary; female patients may have the delusion that they are pregnant in the absence of a recent sexual experience, or even of a uterus, in which case the conception may be through divine agency.

Hypomania and Cyclothymia (Bipolar II Disorder)

Bipolar disorder may be difficult to diagnose if full mania has never occurred in the patient's life. A careful history, however, usually elicits a tale of mood swings, with alternating highs and lows in the absence of significant drug abuse.

Occasionally, patients with bipolar II disorder do not have well-demarcated depressive and hypomanic phases distinct from each other. They may, instead, present with a history of stormy moods and contentious relationships with others that suggest a personality disorder. These features may have resulted in a chaotic life with multiple job changes, broken relationships and divorces, and repeated alienation from friends and associates. Woven into the picture and complicating the diagnosis may be a history of recurrent alcohol or drug abuse. Abstinence from intoxicating substances and a trial on a mood-stabilizing agent, such as lithium carbonate, carbamazepine, or valproic acid, may be necessary for establishing the diagnosis.

Course of Bipolar Disorder

Bipolar disorder begins early in life. As many as one third of individuals in whom the illness develops experience the first episode before the end of the teenage years, and up to two thirds of affected individuals have an episode by age 30 years. When a severe depression begins before puberty, especially in a child with a positive family history, bipolar disorder is the likely diagnosis, and a manic or hypomanic episode is likely to occur later. Clinicians must be cautious because evidence exists that giving such a child an antidepressant medication can precipitate a manic episode or frequent mood cycles.

Acute manic episodes may run a course of several weeks or months if untreated. Because of the urgency with which such an illness presents, it seldom goes untreated. At present, aggressive treatment should bring the disorder under control within 3 or 4 weeks, after which maintenance treatment can begin. Patients typically have several clearly demarcated manic and depressive episodes over the years, interspersed with months or years of being completely well. In such cases, the highs may be classically "speeded up" times and the lows "slowed down" times of inertia and melancholy. These patients are the easiest to treat. Just as often, however, the course of bipolar disorder is less well defined. In the rapid-cycling variety of the illness, four or more episodes occur per year. In many patients, whether or not they suffer from this type of illness, each episode may present a combined picture of chaotic hyperactivity and a mood of intense displeasure. This presentation is dysphoric mania or a mixed episode. These patients are more difficult to treat, are less likely to be blessed with long intervals of wellness, and are less likely to respond to monotherapy with a mood stabilizer. A minority of patients with bipolar disease never recover totally and are chronically disabled despite vigorous treatment. The wide variations in the severity of the course of bipolar disorder (as well as that of major depression) from one person to the next have never been explained by any theoretical model. Over the course of a person's lifetime, manic episodes typically become less frequent and depressive episodes more frequent and prolonged.

Diagnostic Tests

As with major depression, the diagnosis of bipolar disorder is made from the history and observation of the patient. Laboratory tests and imaging procedures are not helpful as yet, despite a growing number of correlations between mood disorders and brain metabolism, brain structure, and endocrine function.

Differential Diagnosis

Schizophrenia uncommonly presents with a stormy, confusional, affect-laden clinical picture that appears identical to mania. Actually, mania is more often erroneously diagnosed as schizophrenia. Still, from the cross-sectional appearance alone, distinction between the two illnesses can be difficult. A family history of bipolar disorder in the relative of a diagnostically confusing patient favors that illness. Schizophrenia usually proceeds to chronicity and prominent auditory hallucinations, bizarre delusions, and impairment of initiative even without symptoms of significantly depressed mood.

A picture resembling mania can be produced by intoxication with drugs, especially phencyclidine (PCP) and lysergic acid diethylamide (LSD), and more rarely by anabolic steroids (abused by some athletes), cocaine, methamphetamine, marijuana, and hashish. In some patients with bipolar disorder, an actual episode of mania or hypomania can be triggered by one of these drugs. Individuals with bipolar illness frequently abuse drugs or alcohol, and the disorder may coexist with substance dependence. The presence of bipolar disorder and its degree of severity can be determined with certainty only in the absence of drug and alcohol intoxication, unless there is a prior history of mania or hypomania.

The toxic effects of some prescribed medications may mimic mania and hypomania. Among these drugs are over-the-counter cold remedies, antihistamines, and pseudoephedrine if taken in excessive amounts as well as adrenal corticosteroids. The latter can precipitate an actual episode of mania or hypomania in someone who has bipolar disorder.

Either mania or depression can occur in Cushing's disease with its excess of adrenal corticosteroids. So-called secondary mania can also occur following brain injury or stroke and must be treated as primary mania. Some workers report that lesions of the right hemisphere are more likely to produce this picture. Finally a giddy, silly affect, resembling hypomania and often accompanied by confusion, can be produced by a variety of disorders in which brain metabolism is compromised, such as hypoglycemia, or hypoxia from any cause.

Faced with an apparent case of mania or hypomania in a patient who has never had bipolar disorder, the clinician must exclude other medical illnesses (see preceding discussion). This is almost always possible following a complete physical examination (including neurologic examination) and laboratory tests. These tests include thyroid studies, a complete blood count, and a general chemistry profile. The diagnosis of mood disorders is not one of exclusion; each has its own characteristic symptoms and historical course. Observation of the patient and a thorough history, taken separately from both the patient and a reliable informant, almost always makes the diagnosis clear.

SEASONAL AFFECTIVE DISORDER

By Brenda Byrne, Ph.D.,
and George C. Brainard, Ph.D.
Philadelphia, Pennsylvania

Studies published during the past 40 years unequivocally support the existence of seasonal physiology in many mammalian species. Similarly, considerable research and clinical intervention in the last 15 years indicates that alterations in human functioning may be linked in predictable ways to the cycle of the seasons. This recognition of the power of the natural environment to affect mood, energy, and cognition represents less of a discovery than a rediscovery; more than 2000 years ago Hippocrates noted that the change of seasons produced diseases, and in the second century AD Aretaeus recommended that lethargic individuals be placed in the sunlight to counteract their symptoms. More recent medical literature mentions at least an occasional case of seasonally linked emotional disorder, and a number of such case studies appeared in the 19th and early 20th centuries. By 1923, with the development of the electric light bulb, "artificial sunlight" had been recommended for its stimulating effect on persons depleted by a nervous or mental disorder.

Only since the late 1970s, however, has a seasonal disorder been named, noted in diagnostic manuals, systematically studied and treated, and made a major focus of study for a professional society (The Society for Light Treatment and Biological Rhythms). Although seasonal affective disorders (SADs) occur in the spring and summer as well as in the fall and winter months, SAD is virtually synonymous with fall-winter depression and has become the most widely recognized seasonal disorder. The onset of SAD is associated with decreases in environmental light, and treatment with bright light reverses many of its affective, cognitive, and vegetative symptoms. SAD in its spring-summer variant appears to be related to changes in temperature rather than changes in ambient light. More recently, some studies have identified seasonal variations in anxiety, panic, and eating disorders as well as in mood and menstrual disorders.

SAD is the name given to a cluster of depressive symptoms that tend to emerge as natural daylight decreases through the fall season and that remit as daylight increases in the spring. SAD is described in unipolar and bipolar forms; that is, alternation may be between depressed and euthymic states (unipolar) or between depressed and hypomanic or manic states (bipolar). The Diagnostic and Statistical Manual, Fourth Edition (DSM-IV) permits that, for mood disorders, the longitudinal course specifier "With seasonal pattern" be applied to major depressive episodes that occur in bipolar I disorder, bipolar II disorder, or major depressive disorder, recurrent. The DSM-IV notes, however, that a seasonal pattern may also describe recurrent depressive episodes that do not meet criteria for a major depressive episode (Table 1).

This set of criteria is similar to that proposed by Rosenthal (1984)* for the diagnosis of winter depression, except that his criteria specify that only one of the depressions occurring in 2 consecutive years must meet research diagnostic criteria for major depression, and that no other axis I pathologic condition must be found.

Recurrent spring-summer depression is the complement of fall-winter depression in its time of onset and symptom picture. Depressive symptoms in the spring-summer seasonal variant are more likely to display the "typical" pattern of reduced sleep and appetite and weight loss. This variant has not been well studied, and no specific treatments comparable to light treatment for fall-winter depression have emerged.

*Rosenthal, N.E., Sack, D.A., Gillin, J.C., et al.: Seasonal affective disorder: A description of the syndrome and preliminary findings with light therapy. Arch. Gen. Psychiatry 41:72–80, 1984.

Table 1. Criteria for Seasonal Pattern Specifier (DSM-IV)

A. There has been a regular temporal relationship between the onset of Major Depressive Episodes in Bipolar I or Bipolar II Disorder or Major Depressive Disorder, Recurrent, and a particular time of year (e.g., regular appearance of the Major Depressive Episode in the fall or winter).

Note: Do not include cases in which there is an obvious effect of seasonal-related psychosocial stressors (e.g., regularly being unemployed every winter).

B. Full remissions (or a change from depression to mania or hypomania) also occur at a characteristic time of the year (e.g., depression disappears in the spring).

C. In the last 2 years, two Major Depressive Episodes have occurred that demonstrate the temporal seasonal relationships defined in Criteria A and B, and no nonseasonal Major Depressive Episodes have occurred during that same period.

D. Seasonal Major Depressive Episodes (as described above) substantially outnumber the nonseasonal Major Depressive Episodes that may have occurred over the individual's lifetime.

PRESENTING SIGNS AND SYMPTOMS

SAD presents as a longitudinal course of recurrent episodes of depression with onset in the fall or early winter and remission in the spring or early summer. A typical cluster of complaints and symptoms include decreased activity, sadness, anxiety, social withdrawal, appetite disturbance (most often increased appetite and carbohydrate craving), weight gain, decreased libido, increased total sleep time, and daytime sleepiness. SAD patients sometimes report the more typical vegetative symptoms of appetite and weight loss and insomnia. Patients with SAD frequently report cold intolerance, stating that they never feel warm enough in winter, and women with SAD often report intensified premenstrual mood difficulties in the fall and winter.

The most common general complaints expressed by patients with SAD are an overwhelming lack of motivation or energy and a disinclination to "be bothered" by anyone. Typically, these individuals must push themselves through the fall and winter after onset of the syndrome and, despite the presumed causative element of light depletion, often acknowledge a preference for staying indoors and being left alone to eat and sleep. Periods of sleep may be longer and daytime sleepiness greater, but sleep itself is often described as being of poorer quality (i.e., lighter and less refreshing than sleep during asymptomatic periods). Persons predisposed to SAD commonly become symptomatic in response to prolonged dark or cloudy weather in any season. Symptoms may also increase when these individuals are exposed to dark indoor environments for prolonged periods.

Seasonal depressive symptoms may also be combined with other presentations of mood disorders. For example, persons with unipolar or bipolar depression or dysthymic disorders may be symptom-free only rarely and yet report that symptoms are regularly worse in the fall and winter. Recurrent brief depressions (episodes occurring at least once a month and lasting less than the 2 weeks necessary for diagnosis of major depression) may also follow a seasonal pattern.

Symptoms of SAD can also present in a milder subsyndromal form (termed S-SAD by researchers). Compared with symptoms of the full SAD syndrome, symptoms of S-SAD affect more persons but are less disruptive of mood, activity, and productivity.

Formal criteria for the diagnosis of SAD (Rosenthal, 1984) or of seasonal pattern (DSM-IV, 1994) should not dissuade the clinician from inquiring into seasonal changes that may present in less clear forms or fall into milder ranges of severity. Subsyndromal SAD has been shown to improve with light treatment, and light may also reduce the severity of winter symptoms in patients with combined seasonal and nonseasonal mood disturbances.

The assessment of SAD (Table 2) is based primarily on the patient's description of the longitudinal course of symptoms and so may be performed at any time of year. If treatment with light is foreseen, notice should be taken of a history of spring mania or hypomania; light treatment itself may trigger such responses in persons with seasonal bipolar mood fluctuations.

Table 2. Evaluation for Seasonal Affective Disorder

Presenting problem
Background-history of presenting problem (first symptoms of mood disorder, course of the difficulty, events leading to referral)
Symptoms associated with mood disorder (mood, affect, energy, motivation, cognitive functioning, self-esteem, sociability, libido, sleep, appetite, weight changes, suicidal behavior)
Evidence of hypomania or mania
Seasonal pattern (onset and cessation of symptoms, nadir, anticipatory anxiety, effects of travel to warm-sunny locales, evidence of "skipped" winters or year-round depression)
Treatment history (previous diagnosis of SAD, other psychiatric diagnoses and treatments, current medications, hospitalizations, suicide attempts)
Medical background (current medical problems-treatments, medications, significant past medical problems-treatment, ophthalmologic history, premenstrual syndrome, cold intolerance, substance use and abuse [alcohol, tobacco, drugs, caffeine])
Family and social history (family of origin, family history of SAD or other psychiatric disorders or substance abuse, education, job, military service-combat, current life circumstances and stressors, significant anniversaries, social system)
Mental status
Diagnoses
Recommendations and plan

SAD = seasonal affective disorder.

CLINICAL COURSE

Recurrent fall-winter depressions typically arise following puberty, with the age of onset usually occurring in the early to mid-20s. During their reproductive years, women outnumber men in their complaints of SAD, but in older populations rates of SAD in women and men are similar. The occurrence of fall-winter depression increases as latitude increases; for example, prevalence is estimated at about 1.4% in Florida and 9.7% in New Hampshire.

The typical course of SAD is defined by a characteristic cluster of symptoms recurring over a period of years and beginning during a 60-day window in the fall or early winter (although longer windows have been reported) and remitting in the spring. Patients with "pure" SAD report that since their first episode, they have had no winters that were free of depressive symptoms and no summers without remission of SAD. In bipolar presentations of SAD, springtime mania or hypomania may require active clinical management. Patients with seasonal symptoms combined with nonseasonal mood disorders present a more complex year-to-year course, although worsening in the winter and improvement in the summer typically persists.

Persons with SAD commonly experience remission of symptoms after a few days in a warm, bright climate, and they often seek out such places for winter vacations. Vacationing in cold or cloudy settings generally will not produce the same lift in mood and energy. Some patients with SAD who tolerate cold well report improvement when they are exposed to intense light from snowy conditions.

In some patients, the primary symptoms of SAD present as changes in energy and appetite along with sleepiness, with depression appearing to be a secondary manifestation. In these individuals, depressed mood may be a reaction to their difficulties in keeping up their ordinary levels of activity and meeting their own and others' expectations.

PHYSICAL EXAMINATION AND LABORATORY STUDIES

Routine physical examination in patients with SAD is unlikely to produce findings relevant to the seasonal diagnosis. If treatment with light is anticipated, the ophthalmologic and medication history is reviewed. Consultation is obtained for patients with a history of retinal disorders and for patients being treated with photosensitizing agents that expose the retina to a greater risk of damage by bright light.

No consensus currently exists for a single physiologically based theory that explains the mechanisms by which SAD develops or by which light treatment reverses winter symptoms. Patients with seasonal disorder may differ from other groups by a variety of physiologic parameters. Patients with SAD may have decreased central serotonergic activity, low serum prolactin concentrations, retinal abnormalities detected by electro-oculography, mild central hypothyroidism due to impaired secretion of thyroid-stimulating hormone (TSH) in response to thyroid-releasing hormone (TRH), and increased eye blink rate. Melatonin secretion, both entrained and suppressed by light, may be involved in the development of SAD, and patients with SAD may have abnormally delayed circadian rhythms. Pituitary release of corticotrophin in response to injections of corticotrophin-releasing hormone (CRH) has been shown to be abnormally low in patients with SAD, suggesting an impaired ability to handle stressors (and helping to explain symptoms of withdrawal and depression). Related animal studies suggest that in winter, patients with SAD also may have low concentrations of brain serotonin that are increased by exposure to bright light.

Given a lack of consensus about the underlying physiologic features of SAD, it is not surprising that to date no laboratory tests have been proposed to aid in the diagnosis of seasonal disorder. Even less is known or proposed about the physiologic mechanisms underlying spring-summer affective disorder. (These likely involve compromise of the body's thermoregulation relative to seasonal temperature change rather than, as in winter SAD, to seasonal light change.)

DIAGNOSTIC APPROACH

Diagnosis of seasonal mood disturbances is generally based on the clinical interview. Seasonal patterns may also be clarified by the use of self-report instruments developed for the diagnosis of SAD. The Seasonal Pattern Assessment Questionnaire (SPAQ)*, for instance, is a 2-page self-assessment tool that allows patients to identify seasonal symptoms and specify their pattern of occurrence. A numerical score for the severity of seasonal effect is derived from a single item of the SPAQ that assesses the degree of change for length of sleep, social activity, mood, weight, appetite, and energy level. The Seasonal Screening Questionnaire (Rosenthal, N.E., Hardin, T., and Wehr, T., unpublished) is a longer self-report instrument for eliciting information about the patterns and course of seasonal symptoms. Although not specific to SAD, the Beck Depression Inventory is frequently used to assess the severity of

*Rosenthal, N.E., Genhart, M., Sack, D., et al.: Seasonal affective disorder and its relevance to understanding and treatment of bulimia. *In* Hudson, J.L., and Pope, H.G. (eds.): *The Psychobiology of Bulimia.* Washington, D.C.: American Psychiatric Association Press, 1987, pp. 205–228.

depressed mood in SAD, and other self-report methods may help document other symptom clusters. For instance, treatment response in SAD shows clearly on the Visual Analogue Scale for Fatigue.*

Structured interview guides help the clinician assess both the depressed and hypomanic poles of SAD symptoms. The Structured Interview Guide for the Hamilton Depression Rating Scale—Seasonal Affective Disorder Version (SIGH-SAD)† and the Hypomania Interview Guide (current and retrospective versions) (HIGH-C and HIGH-R)† are widely used. These guides also are available in self-report forms.

THERAPEUTIC TREATMENT TRIALS

The most widely acknowledged confirmation of the diagnosis of SAD is the patient's response to treatment with bright light. Although light treatment may also be helpful in some nonseasonal depressive disorders, patients with SAD respond more quickly, often within 2 to 4 weeks and sometimes within a few days.

Positive response to light treatment is predicted, according to several studies, by the severity of atypical depressive symptoms (hypersomnia and hyperphagia). Positive response has also been associated with high intake of sweets in the second half of the day as well as by suicidal behavior, anxiety, and younger age.

Light treatment can be delivered by a variety of methods. Most of the research in the field has been done with light boxes containing fluorescent tubes. Some light treatment devices have been designed to illuminate work spaces so that treatment effects occur via light reflected from a work surface. Many patients obtain an active treatment effect from as little as 20 or 30 minutes of bright light exposure (10,000 lux) per day. Head-mounted light units have also been developed, as have "dawn simulators," or devices that provide gradually increasing levels of illumination, leading up to the time of morning rising.

PITFALLS IN DIAGNOSIS

Erroneous diagnoses of SAD can easily be made in the presence of seasonal stressors, "anniversary reactions," and exaggerated data on self-report instruments. The presence of seasonal stressors (e.g., regular unemployment) or of anniversary reactions (e.g., the death of a loved one in the winter) can lead to recurrent fall-winter depressions, which can be mistaken for SAD. Evidence of such life events elicited by careful inquiry can provide important information that leads to the correct diagnosis. The patient's positive response to a 2- to 4-week trial of light treatment strengthens the case for SAD as an active component of the disorder.

Patients occasionally exaggerate symptoms on self-report instruments for a variety of reasons, especially when they are aware of common SAD symptoms and fear being refused treatment if they do not present the "classic" picture. Diagnostic interviews must review all important features of the disorder to correct the bias that can emerge in self-report instruments.

*Lee, K.A., Hicks, G., and Nino-Murcia, G.: Validity and reliability of a scale to assess fatigue. Psychiatry Res., 36:291–298, 1991.

†By Janet B.W. Williams and Michael Terman. Available through Society for Light Treatment and Biological Rhythms, 10200 West 44th Avenue, No. 302, Wheat Ridge, CO 80033.

Missed diagnoses (failure to find SAD when it is present) may result if seasonal stressors, anniversary reactions, or the presence of other psychiatric disorders are taken to exclude seasonal effect as a possible factor. Failure to identify SAD can also occur when the patient minimizes the importance of symptoms or events that provide clues to the presence of the disorder. For example, reports of striking remission of symptoms during a winter visit to a warm, sunny place must not be overlooked, especially if vacations in cold, overcast places failed to result in improved mood or energy. A history of mania or hypomania suggests caution in the use of light therapy, which can trigger such responses in patients with bipolar SAD.

SOMATOFORM DISORDERS

By Timothy E. Stone, M.D.,
and Romaine Hain, M.D.
Birmingham, Alabama

The somatoform disorders are characterized by the presence of physical symptoms or deficits that cause significant distress and functional impairment. The symptoms or deficits cannot be explained by any recognized neurologic or medical disorder and are not produced consciously. An underlying psychological conflict is the cause of the physical symptoms. The somatoform disorders are often difficult to recognize and manage because patients typically seek treatment from several physicians and present with complex and dramatic histories. The patients and their caregivers become emotionally and financially drained by frequent visits to the physician. Major surgical procedures are occasionally performed in pursuit of a diagnosis, and the medical system can be taxed by the patient's overuse of services.

The American Psychiatric Association's *Diagnostic and Statistical Manual of Mental Disorders,* fourth edition (DSM-IV), recognizes five different somatoform disorders: (1) somatization disorder, (2) conversion disorder, (3) hypochondriasis, (4) body dysmorphic disorder, and (5) pain disorder. In addition, the DSM-IV lists two residual diagnostic categories: (1) undifferentiated somatoform disorder and (2) somatoform disorder not otherwise specified (Table 1).

SOMATIZATION DISORDER

Somatization disorder is characterized by reports of somatic symptoms arising from multiple organ systems. This disorder is distinguished from the other somatoform disorders by the numerous symptoms and organ systems affected. The disorder is chronic and usually begins before the age of 30 years (Table 2).

Presenting Signs and Symptoms

The most common symptoms on presentation are nausea, vomiting, shortness of breath, dizziness, and menstrual abnormalities. The DSM-IV requires the presence of four pain symptoms, two gastrointestinal symptoms, one sexual symptom, and one pseudoneurologic symptom to meet the criteria for this disorder (see Table 2).

Table 1. Somatoform Disorders

Diagnosis	Clinical Features	Epidemiology	Diagnostic Considerations
Somatization disorder	Multiple physical symptoms in multiple organ systems	Lifetime prevalence of 0.2 per cent Women outnumber men 5- to 20-fold Onset before age 30 years Commonly coexists with other mental disorders	Onset before age 30 years Functional impairment Somatic symptoms in multiple organ systems Medical illness is excluded
Conversion disorder	One or more symptoms or deficits suggesting neurologic or general medical condition	Conversion symptoms in up to one third of population Women outnumber men 2- to 5-fold Onset at any age Common in poorly educated, rural, lower socioeconomic populations	Symptom or deficit is symbolic of intrapsychic conflict Symptom or deficit is not intentionally produced Medical illness is excluded
Hypochondriasis	Preoccupation with fear of disease or illness	Prevalence of 5 per cent in clinic populations Men and women equally affected Onset in 20s	Preoccupation with disease exists despite evaluation and reassurance Preoccupation is not delusional in nature Duration of at least 6 months
Body dysmorphic disorder	Preoccupation with imagined defect in appearance	Poorly studied but likely rare Onset in late teens Commonly coexists with other mental disorders (major depression, anxiety disorder)	Concern with physical defect is excessive and associated with significant distress
Pain disorder	Pain in one or more anatomic sites severe enough to warrant clinical attention	Pain syndromes are common in clinical practice Women outnumber men 2-fold Onset in 50s to 60s Commonly coexists with other psychiatric disorders	Pain causes significant distress and impairment in functioning Closely associated with psychologic factors Symptom is not intentionally produced

Course

The course of somatization disorder is chronic, and the prognosis for resolution of the disorder is poor. Patients are subjected to the repeated evaluation of their symptoms and are at risk for complications secondary to unnecessary procedures and medications. Consistent follow-up with a single physician who has established a trusting relationship with the patient can minimize the number of unnecessary procedures and medications. The managing physician must remain alert for the appearance of true medical illness.

CONVERSION DISORDER

Conversion disorder is defined as the presence of one or more symptoms or deficits affecting motor or sensory function that cannot be explained by a recognized neurologic or general medical condition. Conversion symptoms symbolically represent psychological conflict, as in the case of a man whose arm becomes paralyzed when he is angry with his wife and wishes to strike her. The paralysis prevents him from striking his wife and diffuses his anger.

Presenting Signs and Symptoms

Paralysis, blindness, and mutism are the most common conversion symptoms. Pseudoseizure is another conversion symptom. Approximately one third of patients with pseudoseizure also have an epileptic seizure disorder, so differentiation of pseudoseizures and epileptic seizures can be difficult. Occasionally, patients with conversion symptoms exhibit *la belle indifference,* which is an unconcerned attitude regarding a serious physical symptom.

Course

Ninety per cent of patients with conversion disorder experience resolution of their symptoms within a month. Most never experience conversion symptoms again. Approximately 25 per cent of these patients will have recurrent conversion symptoms, and with longer duration the disorder is much more difficult to treat. Hypnosis and interviews using amobarbital (Amytal) are effectual tools in the diagnosis and treatment of this disorder.

HYPOCHONDRIASIS

Hypochondriasis is the persistent fear that one is suffering from a serious disease despite the fact that appropriate medical evaluation has revealed no abnormalities. The fear of disease leads to preoccupation with illness and significant impairment of personal, social, and occupational function.

Presenting Signs and Symptoms

As already stated, patients with hypochondriasis usually present with a preoccupation or obsession with the belief that they are suffering from a physical illness that is undetected. The conviction that they are afflicted with this illness can amplify vague somatic symptoms. When medical evaluation provides no evidence of organic illness, patients may seek evaluation from other physicians. They may become angry at the suggestion that nothing is physically wrong and accuse health care professionals of providing inadequate care or of being incompetent. Hypochondriasis is differentiated from somatization disorder by the

Table 2. Diagnostic Criteria for Somatization Disorder

A. A history of many physical complaints beginning before age 30 years that occur over a period of several years and result in treatment being sought or significant impairment in social, occupational, or other important areas of functioning.
B. Each of the following criteria must have been met, with individual symptoms occurring at any time during the course of the disturbance:
   (1) *four pain symptoms:* a history of pain related to at least four different sites or functions (e.g., head, abdomen, back, joints, extremities, chest, rectum, during menstruation, during sexual intercourse, or during urination)
   (2) *two gastrointestinal symptoms:* a history of at least two gastrointestinal symptoms other than pain (e.g., nausea, bloating, vomiting other than during pregnancy, diarrhea, or intolerance of several different foods)
   (3) *one sexual symptom:* a history of at least one sexual or reproductive symptom other than pain (e.g., sexual indifference, erectile or ejaculatory dysfunction, irregular menses, excessive menstrual bleeding, vomiting throughout pregnancy)
   (4) *one pseudoneurological symptom:* a history of at least one symptom or deficit suggesting a neurological condition not limited to pain (conversion symptoms such as impaired coordination or balance, paralysis or localized weakness, difficulty swallowing or lump in throat, aphonia, urinary retention, hallucinations, loss of touch or pain sensation, double vision, blindness, deafness, seizures; dissociative symptoms such as amnesia; or loss of consciousness other than fainting)
C. Either (1) or (2)
   (1) after appropriate investigation, each of the symptoms in Criterion B cannot be fully explained by a known general medical condition or the direct effects of a substance (e.g., a drug of abuse, a medication)
   (2) when there is a related general medical condition, the physical complaints or resulting social or occupational impairment are in excess of what would be expected from the history, physical examination, or laboratory findings
D. The symptoms are not intentionally produced or feigned (as in Factitious Disorder or Malingering).

From the American Psychiatric Association: Diagnostic and Statistical Manual of Mental Disorders, Fourth Edition. Washington, D.C., American Psychiatric AssocitION, 1994, pp. 449–450. Used with permission.

patient's emphasis on a specific disease rather than symptoms from multiple organ systems. Hypochondriasis is closely associated with major depression and anxiety disorder.

Course

The course of hypochondriasis is episodic. Generally, exacerbations of the illness occur in close association with increased psychosocial stressors. Bouts can last months or years. The belief that one is afflicted with the illness is not delusional in nature and may change during the course of the disorder. One third to one half of all patients with hypochondriasis improve significantly over time.

BODY DYSMORPHIC DISORDER

Body dysmorphic disorder is the preoccupation with an imagined defect in appearance. If a slight physical defect is present, distress regarding the defect is excessive.

Presenting Signs and Symptoms

The presenting complaint in body dysmorphic disorder typically involves an imagined flaw of the face. Other body areas may be involved. Commonly associated symptoms include concern that others notice the flaw, attempts to hide the deformity, excessive examination of the flaw in the mirror (or avoidance of mirrors), and social withdrawal for fear of ridicule. This disorder is commonly associated with major depression and anxiety disorder, and as many as one fifth of these patients may attempt suicide.

Course

Body dysmorphic disorder is a chronic illness. The onset is usually gradual, and concern with the perceived body defect may wax and wane with time. The patient may frequently seek medical or surgical help with the hope of treating the defect.

PAIN DISORDER

The hallmark of pain disorder is pain in one or more anatomic sites that causes significant impairment in social or occupational function and is associated through onset or exacerbation with psychological stressors. The presence of pain is not fully explained by a medical or neurologic condition.

Presenting Signs and Symptoms

Patients with pain disorder represent a heterogeneous group and may present with headache, low back pain, chronic pelvic pain, or pain from a multitude of other areas. The pain may be attributed to any number of causes, but in all cases a psychological stressor is associated with onset, exacerbation, or maintenance of the pain syndrome.

Course

Because of the heterogeneous nature of the population affected by this disorder, generalizations regarding course and prognosis are difficult to make. However, the disorder can be chronic and disabling. With clearly identifiable psychological stressors, the pain syndrome may be identified and treated quickly with standard therapy. Most cases of pain disorder are not straightforward, and a chronic course is the norm.

CONVERSION DISORDERS, MALINGERING, AND DISSOCIATIVE DISORDERS

By Robert M. Pascuzzi, M.D.,
and Mary C. Weber, M.D.
Indianapolis, Indiana

Nonphysiologic symptoms and signs are abundant in clinical medicine. A variety of terms and labels for nonphysiologic disorders can lead to confusion or misconceptions in the patients, their families, or their physicians. The term nonphysiologic is preferred to the terms functional or psychogenic. Nonphysiologic disorder is a clear-cut unambiguous term that is well understood by health care professionals and patients. Although the term functional is often acceptable to physicians and patients, its use can result in confusion, because many patients are assessed for "function" using "functional scales" that deal with the activities of daily living. The term psychogenic is considered pejorative by many patients, even though it accurately reflects the origin of the problem. The main subtypes of nonphysiologic disorders include conversion (hysteria), malingering, Munchausen syndrome, and dissociative disorders.

CONVERSION

Conversion disorder and hysteria are synonymous, but conversion is the preferred term. Hysteria is an imprecise term and is considered pejorative by many patients. Conversion symptoms represent a subconscious or unwilled mental mechanism for the relief of anxiety. They provide a primary gain that involves relief of anxiety. Secondary gains can include avoidance of duties or responsibilities and a sense of control over the responses of others. The symptoms and signs are unwilled, or unconscious, and are perceived as being valid or real by the patient (Table 1).

MALINGERING

In contrast with conversion, the malingerer is consciously or willfully feigning symptoms and/or signs to achieve an immediate goal or identifiable gain. The immediate goal is often to avoid duties or responsibilities, such as work or social commitments. In the legal system, some malingerers may attempt financial gain (disability benefits or compensation) through feigning injury.

The distinction between conversion disorder and malingering is difficult in most patients. Accusing a patient with conversion of faking an illness can precipitate more severe psychological difficulties and interfere with a developing doctor-patient relationship. When confronting a patient with a nonphysiologic disorder, the clinician can describe the various physiologic disturbances that have been considered and excluded, followed by an explanation that the patient's symptoms or examination findings are similar to those of other patients who were experiencing a form of "stress reaction." The terms conversion, hysteria, or malingering should usually be avoided when confronting the patient. The clinician should focus on the issue of a stress-related mechanism that should improve over time.

Table 1. Clinical Features of Conversion Disorder

A. Presence of symptoms that do not match a known pathophysiologic pattern of illness. Rather, the symptoms typically reflect the patient's own notion of body function and arrangement.
B. The absence of pathophysiologic or organic illness. Symptoms exist without objective signs of medical illness.
C. A history of stress or psychiatric illness.
D. Remission of the symptoms over time.
E. Conversion usually presents between the ages of 10 to 30 years, often preceded by a long history of emotional disturbance, personality disorders, or multiple stresses. Immediate mental or emotional stress frequently precipitates the conversion.
F. Some patients with conversion disorder display a bland indifference *(la belle indifference)* to their deficits or disability and seem inappropriately unconcerned about the disorder, its cause, or its prognosis. Many patients, however, appear overly concerned or overdramatic when they describe or react to their symptoms or signs.

PATTERNS OF NONPHYSIOLOGIC DISTURBANCE

Vision

Nonphysiologic visual disturbance usually consists of blindness, reduced vision, visual field defects, or monocular diplopia. The typical nonphysiologic visual field defect is a constriction of the visual fields in both eyes, producing tunnel vision or tubular vision. Patients with this disorder often demonstrate a "spiral visual field" in which the size of the visual field diminishes on repeated trials. A physiologic visual field disturbance produces a defect that increases in size with increasing distance to the target, but the size of a nonphysiologic defect does not change. Monocular diplopia suggests a nonphysiologic process. Some ocular disorders can produce monocular diplopia (e.g., retinal fold or detachment, dislocated lens, iris defect), but these can be detected by ophthalmologic examination.

Patients with nonphysiologic blindness often visually fix on moving objects in the room. The pupillary light reaction and fundus examination are normal. Optokinetic nystagmus is typically present, but some patients can willfully suppress this response. Patients with nonphysiologic blindness also show normal visual evoked potentials recorded over the occipital cortex. Occasionally, either acute optic neuritis or Anton's syndrome is confused with nonphysiologic blindness. The syndrome of acute retrobulbar neuritis or optic neuritis can cause complete monocular blindness of abrupt onset. These patients usually have an abnormal pupillary light reflex in the affected eye, but the early funduscopic examination may be normal. Anton's syndrome occurs with bilateral occipital lobe lesions (usually ischemic infarction), resulting in "cortical blindness." Patients typically deny blindness and describe seeing people and items that are not present. Pupillary light reflexes are normal.

Nonphysiologic Deafness

Nonphysiologic deafness can be detected when patients startle in response to a sudden loud noise or when they turn to a person who suddenly addresses them from the side. These responses indicate an intact auditory pathway, but absence of a response does not necessarily mean that the deafness is organic. Sleep electroencephalography and brain stem auditory evoked responses can also demonstrate the integrity of the auditory pathway.

Disorders of Somatic Sensation

Nonphysiologic sensory disorders include anesthesia, paresthesia, hyperesthesia, and pain. A region of anesthesia usually involves all sensory modalities (pain, temperature, light touch, position, and vibration). If only one sensory modality is lost, it is usually touch or pain sensation. Nonphysiologic sensory loss is almost never limited to vibration or position sense, and sensory deficits usually follow nonanatomic patterns of distribution. For example, nonphysiologic facial anesthesia typically extends up to the hairline and down to the angle of the jaw. In contrast, physiologic trigeminal nerve deficits extend to the vertex of the head and spare the angle of the jaw, which is supplied by the cervical nerve roots. In the limbs, nonphysiologic anesthesia usually involves the hand or foot, extends proximally, and stops abruptly at a joint line or skinfold.

A frequent nonphysiologic sensory disturbance is hemianesthesia. The patient loses all sensation on one half of the body. The border between the anesthetic and the normal side is usually distinct and exactly at the midline (although it may change or fluctuate with time). Patients with physiologic sensory loss on one side of the body usually have an indistinct midline loss or fading of sensation. Nonphysiologic hemisensory loss is typically associated with absent vibration sense when a tuning fork is applied to one side of the sternum or forehead. This phenomenon is nonphysiologic because vibration on the sternum or forehead is transmitted across the midline and is perceived on the nonanesthetic side.

Patients who report anesthesia for all sensory modalities without paralysis may use the affected limb in a completely normal manner. Such normal usage, along with normal muscle stretch reflexes, muscle tone, and coordination, indicates fairly normal sensory function. Physiologic complete sensory loss is associated with areflexia, hypotonia, and sensory ataxia.

Gait

In nonphysiologic inability to stand (astasia), or inability to walk (abasia), or a combination of both (astasia-abasia), patients gyrate wildly while standing or walking but rarely fall. If patients do fall, they fall into the examiner's arms or harmlessly in a chair without suffering injury. The very fact that these patients can gyrate or wobble wildly without falling suggests that their balance is actually quite good. Some may have no imbalance or wobbling while lying or sitting, but if asked to stand or walk they develop dramatic swaying.

While standing and closing the eyes to test for the Romberg sign (a test of position sense), patients with astasia-abasia often show increased swaying. When their attention is diverted (e.g., by performing a calculation or by testing finger-to-nose coordination), these patients can often maintain better balance with less swaying. In contrast, the patients who are truly ataxic become even more impaired if they try to perform other tasks simultaneously. A classic nonphysiologic gait is the "dragging leg." If the patient claims to have a weak leg and drags the foot from behind, it is nonphysiologic (real weakness results in circumduction of the leg or high steppage if footdrop is present).

Paralysis

Patients with nonphysiologic paralysis may appear dramatic in their efforts to move the limb, with grimacing, grunting, squirming, or straining. Nonphysiologic paresis (partial paralysis) is usually characterized by very slow movement of the part (the patient seems to be in slow motion). Weakness is inconsistent or variable, and patients typically "give way" abruptly with manual muscle testing; often, strong contractions of the supposedly weak muscles can be seen and felt by the examiner. Agonist and antagonist muscles are typically contracted simultaneously, and patients who report complete paralysis of the limb may be found to move the limb normally during sleep. For reasons that are not clear, the majority of patients with nonphysiologic hemimotor or hemisensory syndromes have symptoms affecting the left side of the body instead of the right. The patient with nonphysiologic paraplegia rarely has bladder or bowel involvement, in contrast with the patient with organic spinal cord or cauda equina disease.

Pseudoseizures

Nonphysiologic convulsive seizures have a variety of manifestations that often occur in the setting of strong emotional stimulus or unpleasant circumstance. These patients usually do not injure themselves, and they usually do not become incontinent. During pseudoseizures, blood pressure, heart rate, and pupillary size do not fluctuate. Patients with true convulsive seizures develop marked metabolic acidosis, which does not occur with pseudoseizures. In addition, serum prolactin concentration often increases following real seizures—but not pseudoseizures. Prolonged electroencephalogram (EEG) with video monitoring is useful for documenting and distinguishing real seizures from pseudoseizures with certainty.

Coma

Patients with nonphysiologic coma have no objective abnormalities on a neurologic examination. All show the fast phase of nystagmus with cold water caloric irrigation of the ear canals (the fast phase of nystagmus disappears in true coma). Nonphysiologic coma can be tested by lifting one of the patient's hands directly over the face and then dropping it while the examiner guards the patient's face. In physiologic coma, the hand drops straight onto the face. In nonphysiologic coma, the hand drops off to the side and thus misses the face.

MUNCHAUSEN SYNDROME

Munchausen syndrome is a subtype of factitious disorder characterized by multiple presentations for hospitalizations and various procedures, often invasive. The physical or psychological signs and symptoms of patients are intentionally produced or feigned, although there is typically not an identifiable secondary gain, as is found with malingering. Munchausen syndrome is somewhat overrepresented in groups of individuals with a background or knowledge of the health care system.

Symptoms begin in early adulthood and affect both men and women. These patients attempt to assume the role of a patient and often submit to a series of invasive and potentially dangerous tests or surgical procedures. Common presentations include abdominal pain, bleeding disorders, skin problems, and a variety of neurologic conditions, including recurrent severe headaches, recurrent comas, and pseudoseizures. The complaint of pain often leads to the use of narcotics. Because these patients often have a strong medical background, they may give a compelling history for organic disease and produce factitious abnormalities on tests, such as mixing blood with urine. Some of these patients purposely ingest anticoagulant medication to alter their physiologic bleeding time. Others inject various substances into the skin to produce skin lesions, rashes, fevers, and other objective abnormalities. During pseudoseizures, these patients are more likely to induce self-injury such as tongue biting, and they may demonstrate apparent incontinence. Patients with Munchausen syndrome often visit many physicians and institutions. The clinician must be alert to the patient with a long-standing history of recurrent surgical procedures and medical problems beginning at an early age in the absence of objective findings on physical examination or laboratory studies.

Munchausen syndrome by proxy involves children whose parents produce clinical histories and physical signs suggesting that the child needs hospitalization, a variety of tests, and/or treatment. These children often have real symptoms induced by inappropriate administration of medication that produces findings such as altered consciousness, coma, seizures, hypoglycemia, and diarrhea.

DISSOCIATIVE DISORDERS

When life experiences are traumatic, distortions in the formation of memory and/or identity sometimes occur. These distortions arise as a function of cognitive mechanisms that are designed to protect one's sense of self from the psychologically harmful effects of trauma. These defensive functions operate automatically outside of the individual's awareness. A list of briefly defined defense mechanisms appears in the *Diagnostic and Statistical Manual of Mental Disorders,* fourth edition (DSM-IV). In the DSM-IV glossary of terms, dissociation is defined as a "disruption in the usually integrated functions of consciousness, memory, identity, or perception of the environment."

When experiences are intensely painful, frightening, or threatening to one's life, they are difficult to assimilate sensibly and meaningfully into one's sense of self and others. Traumatic events that reduce individuals to objects of complete powerlessness in the face of human cruelty or natural disaster arouse an automatic cognitive response that strains to preserve sanity, yet in so doing distortions of memory and errors in the perception of reality may occur. The protective psychic response to horrifying or life-threatening events involves reconstruction of reality in a way that excludes memory of the event (or parts of it) or distorts sensory and perceptual awareness so that the trauma is rendered bearable.

The experience of trauma may be distorted so that when the event is recalled, no emotion is experienced, a process called psychic numbing. This emotional unresponsiveness can then extend to other aspects of the patient's life, including family and friends. Consequently, following the experience of severe trauma, victims may find that they can no longer feel close to significant people in their lives, such as spouses and children. Because they are unaware of the process that underlies this emotional numbing, they often feel unnecessarily guilty and worried about their ability to love those closest to them.

Sometimes, victims of trauma describe feeling as if they were watching the trauma happen rather than experiencing it directly. This distortion in perceptual awareness is an example of a process called depersonalization, which involves the splitting off of consciousness from the direct experience of the senses. In severe cases of chronic unrelenting trauma, such as that experienced early in life as childhood abuse, the patient's sense of personal identity may fail to develop in a well-integrated fashion, instead fragmenting into several separate and dissociated states of consciousness. This condition is called dissociative identity disorder (see below).

Dissociative Amnesia (Formerly Psychogenic Amnesia)

When exposed to a traumatic event that is severe enough to initiate psychic defenses, some people completely lose the ability to recall the event. Amnesia is typically restricted to the period of time surrounding the traumatic event. Memory of the event is usually recovered, sometimes spontaneously, often as the result of psychotherapeutic intervention. Recurrent amnesia for the traumatic event is rare after memory has fully recovered. Dissociative amnesia commonly occurs following wartime experiences, natural disasters, mass shootings, and other intense, brief traumatic episodes.

Occasionally, patients present knowing that they have survived a traumatic event but reporting a loss of memory for the event. Sometimes, they present with a complaint of general memory loss without knowledge of the trauma initiating the dissociation. In either case, organic causes for memory loss must first be excluded; some of these include postconcussive amnesia, substance-induced blackouts, and seizure disorders. In about 5 per cent of cases, the patient is found to be malingering. The diagnosis of this disorder and the determination of its cause require a complete medical history and physical and psychiatric examinations.

Dissociative Fugue (Formerly Psychogenic Fugue)

Patients with dissociative fugue travel away from home and leave behind all that is familiar, including memory of their own history and identity. The onset of the dissociative episode begins abruptly with the departure from home, and as with all the dissociative disorders, the activity is beyond the patient's control. The disorder is characterized by an absence of awareness of the psychodynamics that precipitate the event, and the onset is typically a result of traumatic stress.

In some cases, the patient spontaneously adopts a new persona or identity. However, the majority of cases are characterized only by the absence of identity without substitution of a new identity. The onset and cessation of the disorder are both discrete and sudden. After the event has resolved, the patient is typically amnestic for the period of time that passed during the fugue state.

Patients typically present with the chief symptom of memory loss, but they may occasionally report physical symptoms that are unrelated to the fugue state. Those that have physical symptoms are often poor historians who give vague responses to questions about their symptoms, or they may seem uncooperative and guarded. Organic causes of memory loss and confusion must be excluded. Patients with early dementing processes can also present as poor historians, confabulating to fill in the memory gaps. Dissociative fugue often coexists with alcoholism and personality disorders. When dissociative processes are suspected, psychiatric consultation may help distinguish between the various dissociative processes. The symptom presentation of dissociative fugue is similar to that of other dissociative disorders involving identity disturbance, a similarity that occasionally creates a diagnostic dilemma.

Depersonalization Disorder

In depersonalization disorder, perception and awareness are altered so that patients feel estranged or apart from themselves. Typically, either patients feel as if they are observers of, rather than participants in, their experience, or they become detached from affective components of experience, which causes their behavior to feel mechanical, automatic, and nonvolitional. Unlike the other dissociative disorders, depersonalization can be a normal variant in human experience. Severe distress and trauma, however, can lead to pathologic depersonalization. In either case, affected individuals sense that they are experiencing something strange or unusual, and this awareness is typically uncomfortable and disturbing.

Medical conditions that can lead to symptoms of depersonalization include drug-induced intoxication, withdrawal from psychoactive substances, and certain seizure disorders. Moreover, several serious psychiatric disorders, including schizophrenia, major depression, and panic disorder, are associated with depersonalized states.

Dissociative Identity Disorder (Formerly Multiple Personality Disorder)

With dissociative identity disorder, the patient's consciousness is split between two or more ego states. These states take on the character of separate personalities in the sense that they are each characterized by distinct histories, gender, and age and are often identified by different names. One dominant affective state often characterizes each separate alter state. For example, one alter may exclusively express angry affect, another may be depressive and suicidal, and yet another may be glib and effusive. Alter states are frequently encapsulated to the extent that they have no awareness of the others, and the core alter state is typically retiring and self-effacing. Almost invariably, these patients have suffered severe childhood abuse. The course of this disorder is chronic and unrelenting, but with competent long-term psychotherapeutic care, slow progress can be accomplished.

The diagnosis is extremely difficult to make. The typical patient presents on average 6.5 years before an accurate diagnosis is made. Presentational clues are usually subtle and involve little more than markedly different demeanors from one appointment to another. Close attention to detail sometimes reveals evidence of self-mutilating behavior, which is commonly associated with the disorder. Careful questioning sometimes reveals that patients are repeatedly unable to account for discrete periods of time, having no memory for intervals of hours or even days.

The patient may be perplexed to find clothing or other items in their homes and have no memory of how they got there. Unfortunately, prompt diagnosis is often delayed because the patient is too embarrassed to discuss the oddities of his or her experience. Once the dissociative identity disorder is suspected, psychiatric referral for diagnosis and treatment is essential.

SEXUAL AND GENDER IDENTITY DISORDERS

By John G. Halvorsen, M.D., M.S.
Peoria, Illinois

The American Psychiatric Association's *Diagnostic and Statistical Manual of Mental Disorders,* fourth edition (DSM-IV), recognizes the following sexual and gender disorder categories: sexual dysfunctions, paraphilias, and gender identity disorders. The sexual dysfunctions represent problems with sexual desire, disorders in the psychophysiologic processes of the sexual response cycle, and pain associated with sexual intercourse. All must be "persistent or recurrent," "cause marked distress or interpersonal difficulty," "not be better accounted for by another axis I disorder," or "due exclusively to the direct psychophysiologic effects of a substance (e.g., a drug of abuse or a medication) or a general medical condition." Paraphilias are recurring, "intense sexual urges, fantasies, or behaviors that involve unusual objects, activities, or situations." They must also cause "clinically significant distress or impairment in social, occupational, or other important areas of functioning." People with gender identity disorders experience strong, continuous identification with the opposite gender and often express a desire to become, or a strong belief that they are, the opposite sex. They must also demonstrate "persistent discomfort" with their assigned sex or show evidence that they cannot appropriately fulfill that gender's roles.

Clinicians must ascertain the level of diagnostic involvement they wish to pursue when patients present with sexual concerns. Any one of several levels may be appropriate; the first is limited to case finding. The initial sexual history is elicited to determine whether any problem exists, but affected patients are referred to another professional for further evaluation. The second level of involvement requires clinicians to fully evaluate the sexual concern as they would any other chief symptom. They collect the basic sexual history during routine visits and provide basic education about normal anatomy, physiology, and sexual functioning. When sexual problems are reported, they obtain a "history of the present problem," pursuing symptoms and performing a focused physical examination as appropriate. They then have the option to refer the patient to another professional for further diagnostic evaluation. Clinicians who practice at the third level conduct a comprehensive evaluation, obtaining a detailed sexual history, incorporating both the psychosocial and the medical histories. They also perform a comprehensive physical examination and coordinate any organic evaluation with appropriate laboratory tests and special diagnostic procedures.

Many clinicians infrequently ask patients about their sexual concerns, and patients, likewise, often hesitate to initiate the discussion. Most men and women, however, are grateful when their physicians ask, and they willingly discuss these issues. The physician-initiated discussion is therefore a critically important diagnostic step.

When both the patient and the physician identify a sexual problem, further inquiry may proceed in several stages. A brief history explores the problem as a "chief symptom" with questions about onset, chronicity, severity, exacerbations, and remissions; effects of any attempted management; presence of any associated symptoms in other body systems; what the patient believes is causing the problem; and whether the problem has been lifelong or is acquired, is generalized or situational, or is related to an existing general medical condition or substance use, including medication. In compiling the detailed sexual history, the clinician goes beyond the initial pursuit of symptoms to develop a thorough understanding of the problem by discussing the person's current sexual interactions, past sexual history, family history, marital history, current stressors, and complete medical history.

Inquiries about the person's current sexual interaction should determine the frequency of intercourse or sex play, frequency both partners would prefer, time of day for lovemaking, presence of fatigue during lovemaking, difficulties with privacy, verbal and nonverbal communication of desires, types and pleasurability of sex play that precedes intercourse, level of arousal during intercourse, orgasm frequency, cognitive activities that occur during sex (thoughts, visualizations, fantasies), pain during intercourse, type of contraception, and the presence of any paraphilias.

The sexual history explores the patient's early experiences, response to puberty, emotional reactions, attitudes toward sexuality, level of sexual knowledge, frequency and types of past sexual practices, acceptance of cultural myths, development of current sexual relationships, masturbation practices and fantasies, homosexual experiences, history of negative sexual experiences (e.g., multiple rejections, incest, sexual assault), body image, and physical sexual development.

Important family history data include information about family attitudes toward sexuality, parental modeling, religious influences, relationships with parents and siblings, family violence, and the level of family function in the couple's families of origin. The marital history describes the development and stability of the couple's relationship, changes in feelings toward each other, presence of unresolved conflict, loss of trust or fidelity, and problems with communication (e.g., failures to listen and understand, hidden agendas, use of sex for power in the relationship). The physician should also determine whether and to what extent any current stressors impact the family. These stressors include intrafamilial stresses (e.g., death, illness, problems with children), extrafamilial stresses (e.g., financial, occupational, legal), and stresses and strains that are normally associated with the stages and transitions of the family life cycle.

The complete medical history includes the details of acute or chronic illness, injuries, surgery, medications, habits, and drug or alcohol use and explores a complete review of systems. The comprehensive physical examination helps discover the general medical conditions that may contribute to a sexual disorder. It also can identify physical conditions that may affect sexual functioning or influence treatment for a diagnosed disorder.

SEXUAL DYSFUNCTIONS

The complete sexual response cycle progresses through four stages: desire, excitement, orgasm, and resolution. Sexual fantasies and an appetite for sexual activity characterize the desire phase. During excitement, men subjectively sense sexual pleasure and experience penile tumescence and erection along with secretions from the bulbourethral glands. Changes in women are more complex and include pelvic vasocongestion, vaginal lubrication, external genital swelling, narrowing of the outer third of the vagina from increased pubococcygeal muscle tension and vasocongestion, vasocongestion of the labia minora, breast tumescence, and lengthening and widening of the inner vagina.

Sexual pleasure peaks during orgasm and is accompanied by sexual tension release and rhythmic contractions in the perineal and pelvic reproductive organs. In men, a sensation that ejaculation is inevitable precedes the contractions in the prostate, seminal vesicles, and urethra that result in seminal emission. During orgasm in women, contractions occur in the distal third of the vaginal wall. Both men and women feel relaxed and free from muscular tension during resolution. Men are temporarily refractory to further erection and orgasm, but women can respond almost immediately to further stimulation. Inhibitions can occur at one or more phases of the sexual response cycle. Most clinically significant disorders, however, affect the first three phases.

Additional classification of the primary sexual disorders into subtypes further defines them according to onset, context, and etiologic factors. The onset can be characterized as lifelong (present since the onset of sexual functioning) or acquired (developing only after a period of normal functioning). The context is described as generalized (not limited to certain types of stimulation, situations, or partners) or situational (limited to certain types of stimulation, situations, or partners). Etiologic subtypes include disorders due to psychological factors, in which psychological variables play the primary role in the onset, severity, exacerbation, or maintenance of the dysfunction. Disorders due to combined factors typically involve psychological factors in the onset, severity, exacerbation, and maintenance of the dysfunction, but a general medical condition or substance use compounds the problem.

Hypoactive Sexual Desire Disorder

The essential diagnostic feature of hypoactive sexual desire disorder, also known as inhibited sexual desire, is insufficient, or even absent, sexual fantasy and appetite for sexual activity. The problem may affect all forms of sexual expression, or it may involve only specific partners or sexual activities. People with hypoactive desire disorder do not seek sexual stimuli or try to decrease sexual frustration when they are sexually deprived. They do not initiate sexual activity and only reluctantly participate when others initiate it. Their involvement in sexual activity is usually infrequent, although partner pressure may increase the level of activity more than the individual's desire would predict. The diagnosis rests on the clinician's judgment, taking into account multiple personal, cultural, and situational variables, since relatively little data exist to help define normative age- or gender-related frequency or degree of sexual desire.

The clinical history can also help determine whether the person's low interest level is primary or whether it is really secondary to another sexual problem. People often inhibit their desire when they experience problems with sexual arousal and orgasm as a way of protecting themselves from the consequences of sexual failure. Some individuals with low desire, however, can experience satisfactory sexual excitement and orgasm in response to adequate sexual stimulation. Puberty is usually the age at onset for individuals with primary hypoactive desire. Most, however, develop the disorder as adults after a period of normal sexual functioning. These cases are usually secondary to psychological distress, stressful life events, interpersonal difficulties, or relationship distress. For some, the lost interest is continuous, but for others it is episodic and related to varying degrees of relationship intimacy and commitment.

Hypoactive sexual desire disorder is the most difficult sexual dysfunction to treat. The outlook is better when the problem is secondary, the symptoms have been present a year or less, the couple's relationship is stable, both partners are emotionally calm, both partners view each other as physically attractive and loving, both find pleasure in sexual activity, and both comply with therapist recommendations during treatment.

No specific physical findings are unique to this disorder. The physical examination, however, helps identify general medical conditions that may cause a person to lose sexual desire. The clinician must search for physical signs associated with chronic systemic illness, the presence of disfiguring problems, neurologic disorders, and endocrine problems (e.g., diabetes mellitus or thyroid, adrenal, and pituitary disorders). The presence of secondary sex characteristics are noted in both sexes, including the presence or absence of pubic and axillary hair. Other important findings include the presence of testicular atrophy, castration, structural penile lesions, and gynecomastia in men, and galactorrhea and findings consistent with early pregnancy in women.

Further diagnostic evaluation in men usually begins with a serum testosterone concentration. If concentrations are low or borderline, or if the low-desire symptoms are associated with little or no masturbation history, follicle-stimulating hormone (FSH), luteinizing hormone (LH), and serum prolactin measurements can help distinguish between primary and secondary (pituitary-hypothalamic) testicular failure. When hypogonadotropic hypogonadism is found, computed tomography (CT) or magnetic resonance imaging (MRI) can evaluate the sella turcica for the presence of a pituitary tumor. Testosterone therapy has been recommended by some as a therapeutic trial, but no consistent evidence exists to document its effectiveness. Furthermore, its masculinizing side effects cause problems in most women.

The clinician must determine whether the person's hypoactive desire is due specifically to the physiologic effects of a specified general medical condition, in which case treatment also focuses on that condition, or whether it is directly related to the physiologic effects of a pharmacologic agent or drug of abuse, in which case substance elimination is required. One must also distinguish this disorder, where fantasy and desire are absent, from sexual aversion, where the person actively tries to avoid any genital contact or sexual activity with a partner.

Sexual Aversion Disorder

Those who suffer from sexual aversion disorder express an extreme dislike for sexual activity and actively avoid genital contact with a sexual partner. They experience anxiety, fear, or repugnance when confronted with sexual opportunities. Sometimes, the revulsion is generalized to all sexual stimuli, including kissing and touching. In others, the aversion is focused on specific parts of the sexual encounter (e.g., vaginal secretions or penetration). The reactions the individual displays also vary from moderate anxiety and displeasure to extreme anguish and panic attacks. Many display profoundly impaired interpersonal relationships with their partners. They may also design covert avoidance strategies, such as retiring early at night, traveling out-of-town, neglecting their personal appearance, substance use, and overcommitment to work, social, or family activities.

Sexual aversion may be lifelong or acquired, and it may be generalized or situational in context. Some consider hypoactive desire and aversion as different points on the same continuum, with aversion occurring less commonly. The clinical course of sexual aversion depends on its severity and the complexity of associated features (e.g., panic attacks, marital dissatisfaction, complex avoidance behaviors).

No physical findings are specific for sexual aversion. The same examination focus used for evaluating hypoactive desire is appropriate (see earlier). No specific laboratory, imaging, or special diagnostic procedures are indicated other than a laboratory screen to evaluate for underlying general medical conditions.

When evaluating a person's sexual aversion, the clinician determines whether another underlying sexual disorder is present. Occasionally, the aversion is actually an attempt to deal with dyspareunia, premature ejaculation, erectile dysfunction, or one of the paraphilias. The clinician must also determine whether the aversion is due to another axis I disorder, such as a major depressive disorder, obsessive-compulsive disorder, and post-traumatic stress disorder.

Female Sexual Arousal Disorder

Women with a sexual arousal disorder cannot reach or maintain an adequate lubrication-swelling response (pelvic vasocongestion, vaginal lubrication and lengthening, and labial swelling) until they complete sexual activity. They may also lack subjective pleasure during arousal.

The arousal disorder may be primary or secondary. Primary disorders are less common, and their onset coincides with the onset of sexual activity. Secondary disorders occur after a period of normal sexual functioning. Clinicians must determine whether a secondary disorder began after a medical condition was diagnosed, and whether it may be due exclusively to the physiologic effects of that condition. They must also ascertain whether the disorder is caused by the direct effects of a medication or an abused substance that may affect lubrication (e.g., antihypertensives or antihistamines) or vascular supply. An inadequate lubrication-swelling response may also result in painful intercourse, which can, in turn, cause sexual aversion and other disruptions in the couple's relationship.

The physical examination in a woman with an arousal disorder focuses on several areas. The clinician must carefully examine for signs of generalized cardiovascular and neurologic disease, as well as localized disease that affects only the genital system. The cardiovascular findings include bruits (especially femoral), decreased peripheral pulses, evidence of venous stasis or arterial insufficiency in the lower extremities, and a pulsatile abdominal mass. General neurologic findings include abnormalities in gait, coordination, motor strength, and deep tendon reflexes and the presence of pathologic reflexes. The examination must also include a search for findings associated with adrenal, thyroid, and pituitary disorders. Women need a complete pelvic examination evaluating general medical and gynecologic conditions (e.g., infectious vaginitis, atrophic vaginitis, diabetes mellitus, pelvic radiation) that may produce pain or inhibit the arousal response in other ways. In addition to a general laboratory screen for acute and chronic systemic disease, some authorities recommend measurements of testosterone, estrogen, and prolactin, because hormonal alterations are implicated in some arousal disorders. Techniques for measuring nocturnal vaginal blood flow have been used to demonstrate that vaginal engorgement cycles occur in women during rapid eye movement (REM) sleep with the same frequency that erectile cycles occur in men. This technique is still experimental, but validity and reliability for clinical use may emerge.

When considering the diagnosis of a sexual arousal disorder, the clinician must distinguish inadequate sexual excitement from hypoactive desire, even though limited evidence suggests that the two disorders often accompany each other. Women with arousal disorders alone desire sexual activity, but their sexual excitement is insufficient to maintain the necessary physiologic responses. If the arousal disorder relates to a primary axis I disorder, the clinician must determine whether the arousal disorder predates that disorder.

Male Erectile Disorder

Men with male erectile disorder (MED), also known as impotence or male arousal disorder, cannot attain or maintain an erection that allows them to complete sexual activity. Men report various dysfunctional patterns; some have been unable to achieve an erection since they became sexually active. Some obtain only partial tumescence. Others attain erection but lose it when they attempt vaginal penetration or when they begin penile thrusting. Still others report that erections occur only on awakening or with self-stimulation, but not with a partner.

The clinical course of MED varies considerably, depending on the underlying etiology. The few individuals with primary disorders who have never experienced adequate erections usually encounter chronic, lifelong problems. Those who acquire their disorder after a period of functioning normally experience spontaneous remissions in 15 to 30 per cent of cases when the cause relates to episodic organic or psychogenic factors. Some cases depend on the partner or the intensity and the quality of the relationship. These are also often episodic, but recurrent. Men whose erectile disorders are related to chronic, irreversible medical conditions require medical or surgical intervention to achieve adequate erections.

Whereas MED is often caused by other organic conditions, it can also create its own complications. Men with MED often experience performance anxiety, fears of failure, lost self-esteem, decreased desire for sexual activity, decreased sexual pleasure, and depression related to their real and perceived losses. In addition, MED can adversely affect the couple's relationship and may contribute to infertility.

The general physical examination in men is similar to that performed in women. In men, however, the physician must evaluate the genital system further for testicular size and consistency; penile size; penile structural abnormalities or lesions (e.g., plaques of Peyronie's disease); signs of infection in the urethra, prostate, or epididymis; and surgical scars that may indicate previous neurologic, vascular (e.g., aortic aneurysm, aortofemoral bypass), or genital (e.g., prostate, bladder) surgery. The neurologic examination should focus on the sacral dermatomes, and the integrity of the sacral reflex arc (S2 through S4) is assessed by evaluating perineal sensation, anal sphincter tone, cremasteric reflex, and the bulbocavernosus reflex.

The examiner obtains a penile blood pressure measurement during the physical examination by inflating a 3-cm pediatric blood pressure cuff around the base of the penis and auscultating the central artery of a corpus cavernosum with a 9.5-MHz Doppler stethoscope as the cuff is deflated. The pressure at which the arterial pulse is first heard is the penile systolic pressure. The ratio between the penile systolic pressure and the brachial systolic pressure (the penile-brachial index, or PBI) should be greater than .75. If it is less than .60, significant penile arterial insufficiency is probable.

In addition to the laboratory screen for associated systemic disease, a serum testosterone concentration is obtained to screen for hypogonadism. Low results are investigated further with the protocol described for hypoactive sexual desire (see earlier).

Nocturnal penile tumescence (NPT) measurements are also useful. Three or four erections typically occur each night during REM sleep. Sleep eliminates the psychological factors that can inhibit arousal, and erections should occur. Organic interference, however, persists during sleep, blunting or eliminating the erectile response. Methods for assessing NPT include the snap gauge, the Rigiscan, and NPT monitors.

The snap gauge is a ring of opposing Velcro straps that are connected by three plastic strips. Before sleep, men wrap the straps around the base of the penis. During sleep, a rigid erection will break all three plastic strips. By noting whether 0, 1, 2, or 3 bands break, one can estimate the maximal erectile response during sleep. This method is simple and inexpensive and can be done in the natural sleep setting. False-negative results occur when the band is not applied tightly enough. False-positive results occur when strips break while the patient turns during sleep. The gauge detects only the maximal erectile event during sleep and does not measure duration, number, or actual rigidity of erection. Erections cannot be correlated with REM sleep cycles by this technique.

The Rigiscan is a small computer with two cords leading to rings that fit around the base and tip of the penis. Inside each ring is a cable that the central unit can loosen or tighten during monitoring. The cables detect tumescence by passively expanding, and they determine rigidity by actively contracting and detecting resistance. This NPT method records all erectile events, measures duration, tumescence, and rigidity, and can be performed at home. It cannot correlate erections with REM sleep cycles, and the dynamic nature of the contracting bands may induce or augment erectile activity during testing.

Other NPT monitors use mercury strain gauges attached to the base and tip of the penis that are connected to a plethysmograph to record tumescence. Monitoring occurs in a sleep laboratory where electroencephalographic tracings can also detect sleep cycles. Rigidity is assessed visually or by applying a hand-held tonometer to the penis to detect the force required to "buckle" it. This NPT method records all erectile events, measures duration, tumescence, and rigidity (but not as well as the Rigiscan), and correlates erections with REM sleep. However,it is expensive and time and labor intensive and must be performed in an unnatural sleep environment.

Duplex ultrasound scanning provides high-resolution real-time ultrasound imaging and pulse Doppler analysis of the actual blood flow in the cavernous arteries before and after injection of a vasodilator (45 to 60 mg of papaverine or 40 μg of prostaglandin E_1 [PGE_1]). Normal vessels double in size with an initial peak systolic flow velocity greater than 30 cm per second, which decreases as the veno-occlusive mechanisms begin to operate. Low initial flows are associated with arterial insufficiency. Normal initial flows that persist may be associated with leaks in the venous system.

Intracavernous injections of papaverine or PGE_1 by themselves can also help screen for vascular causes of MED. An injection of 30 to 60 mg of papaverine or 40 μg PGE_1 typically produces within 10 minutes an erection that lasts at least 30 minutes. Delays greater than 15 to 20 minutes indicate arterial insufficiency, and a prompt rigid erection that dissipates quickly suggests a venous leak. When arterial lesions are suspected and the patient is a candidate for a surgical bypass, pudendal angiography can determine the site of a vascular block and help decide whether it could be corrected surgically. If the individual is not a candidate for vascular surgery, angiography is unnecessary.

Cavernosometry and cavernosography evaluate the veno-occlusive mechanisms of the corpora cavernosum. Initial pressure measurements are obtained from a corpus cavernosum through a butterfly needle, after which 20 μg of PGE_1 is injected. When pressures equilibrate (usually above 100 mm Hg in about 10 minutes), heparinized saline is infused at a rate sufficient to maintain the erection. Radiographic contrast material is then infused at the same rate, and films are taken to visualize leaks in specific veins and to evaluate leaks of the corpus spongiosum and glans penis.

Bulbocavernosus reflex latency tests measure the integrity of the sacral reflex arc. Electromyographic needles are inserted into the bulbocavernosus muscle to measure the length of time from glans stimulation by a pinch or squeeze to muscle contraction. Longer times suggest a neurologic cause of MED. Somatosensory evoked potentials can help localize neurologic lesions. The technique documents waveforms that are produced over the sacrum and the cerebral cortex in response to dorsal penile nerve stimulation and can localize neurologic lesions to peripheral, sacral, or suprasacral locations.

As is the case with other sexual disorders, the clinician must consider the possibility that MED represents an attempt to manage another sexual disorder. Men with premature ejaculation or those with paraphilic arousal patterns may consciously inhibit arousal in an effort to deal with a more severe sexual problem. One must also assess whether the MED is caused entirely by another axis I disorder, such as depression, post-traumatic stress, or an obsessive-compulsive disorder.

Female Orgasmic Disorder

Women with female orgasmic disorder, formerly known as inhibited female orgasm, experience normal sexual desire and excitement but encounter delayed or even absent orgasm. This diagnosis requires clinician judgment, since women differ in respect to the types and intensity of stimulation that arouses them to orgasm. One must determine whether a woman's orgasmic potential is greater than her experience, considering factors such as age, sexual experience, and the adequacy of sexual stimulation.

Primary orgasmic disorders are much more common in younger women; orgasmic capacity increases with age. Only about 50 per cent of women experience their first orgasm during adolescence, whereas 95 per cent of women older than 35 years of age have achieved orgasm. As women mature, they often become less psychologically inhibited. They also experience more types of sexual stimulation and begin to understand their own physiologic responses better. Secondary orgasmic disorders are therefore much more common. As many as 46 per cent of women encounter difficulty in reaching orgasm, and 15 per cent will become anorgasmic. The natural history of untreated orgasmic disorders in women is largely unknown. Women with a primary disorder respond rapidly, with high treatment success rates, to sexual therapy that is focused on a program of directed, progressive self-stimulation. Women with secondary disorders respond better when traditional marital therapy is added to the sexual therapy, and when partners are incorporated into treatment.

After a woman has learned how to reach orgasm, she retains that capacity unless some other factor intervenes. The intervening variables are usually psychological or relationship concerns that include sexual trauma, poor communication, unresolved relationship conflict, fear, guilt, hostility, and the inability to abandon oneself. No apparent association between orgasmic function and specific personality patterns or psychopathology exists. Likewise, orgasmic capacity is not related to pelvic muscle strength or vaginal size. Occasionally, a specific organic problem, such as a spinal cord lesion and major vaginal or vulvar surgery, may impair orgasm. Most often, however, general medical conditions, even problems such as diabetes and pelvic cancer, leave orgasm intact, but they may affect arousal. The physiologic effects of certain substances (e.g., antidepressants, benzodiazepines, neuroleptics, antihypertensives, opioids) may also interfere with orgasm. Complications caused by female orgasmic disorder are mainly psychosocial. Women may develop problems with their own self-esteem and body image. In addition to being caused by relationship problems, the disorder can also precipitate relationship dissatisfaction, conflict, distance, and communication difficulties.

The physical examination in these women should focus on identifying signs of localized genitourinary infection or inflammation, evidence of major pelvic surgery or irradiation, and signs of either generalized neurologic disease or localized sensory deficits. Other than baseline laboratory studies used to identify an underlying etiologically associated systemic disease, no specific laboratory tests or special procedures are indicated for evaluating women with orgasmic disorders.

When considering this diagnosis, the clinician must be certain that it is not part of the symptom complex for another axis I disorder, and that it is not exclusively due to another general medical condition or substance use. Both desire and arousal disorders frequently accompany female orgasmic disorders.

Male Orgasmic Disorder

Men with male orgasmic disorder, formerly known as inhibited male orgasm or retarded ejaculation, experience normal sexual desire and arousal but encounter either a delayed orgasm or none at all. The condition may be lifelong, in which case affected men have never experienced orgasm, or it may be acquired after a period of normal sexual functioning. In men, as in women, the clinician must use judgment when considering this diagnosis, taking into account the man's age and whether the stimulation he receives is sufficient in focus, intensity, and duration.

The disorder can present in various ways. Most commonly, men report that they cannot achieve orgasm during intercourse, but they can ejaculate in response to their partner's manual or oral stimulation. Some men reach coital orgasm only after prolonged, intense noncoital stimulation; others ejaculate only after self-stimulation. Many anorgasmic men describe feeling aroused initially during a sexual encounter with their partner, but that they then experience penile thrusting as burdensome rather than pleasurable.

Men can reach orgasm even when vascular or neurologic problems cause erectile dysfunction. Orgasmic sensations and the striated muscle contractions that occur during orgasm remain intact even in men whose prostate and seminal vesicles are removed during radical cancer surgery. Many substances, however, can adversely affect orgasm, including many anxiolytics, antihypertensives, antidepressants, antipsychotics, and sedative-hypnotic agents.

No reliable data exist to indicate the natural course of this disorder. Treatment using techniques similar to those used to treat women with female orgasmic disorder results in similar success rates. Male orgasmic disorder can complicate a couple's relationship by precipitating or augmenting relationship conflict and dissatisfaction. Some couples present with infertility because the husband has hidden his coital anorgasmy. Then, both fertility and communication issues must be addressed.

The physical examination in men with this disorder who experience normal desire and arousal should focus mainly on identifying suprasacral neurologic disorders. Other than the baseline laboratory studies that can help identify a systemic disease that could produce sexual problems as a complication, no specific laboratory tests are indicated for evaluating men with orgasmic disorders.

Male orgasmic disorder must be distinguished from retrograde ejaculation and anemission. In retrograde ejaculation, orgasm and emission occur normally, but the seminal fluid is directed retrogradely into the bladder because the bladder neck fails to close completely during emission. Men report a "dry" orgasm or only a very small fluid emission, and the cause is almost always organic. Men with anemission experience no seminal emission. This may result from anatomic problems, but it is almost always caused by a diagnosed neurologic disorder (e.g., spinal cord trauma, multiple sclerosis, severe autonomic neuropathy). In these men, orgasm may or may not occur, depending on the type and severity of the underlying condition.

Premature Ejaculation

Men with premature ejaculation reach orgasm and ejaculation quickly, in response to minimal stimulation. Ejaculation may occur before, during, or shortly after vaginal penetration and almost always before either partner wants it to happen. Premature ejaculation may be defined as the inability to delay ejaculation long enough to satisfy a sexual partner at least half of the time. Some men have had the problem since they became sexually active; in others, it arises after a period of normal functioning. A detailed sexual history coupled with astute clinical judgment is important for accurate diagnosis. Before making the diagnosis, the clinician must consider factors that affect the duration of sexual excitement. These include age, novelty of the sexual partner or situation, intensity of stimulation, and frequency of sexual activity. Men with this disorder can usually delay orgasm and ejaculation longer during self-stimulation than they can during coitus. In most cases, the cause of the disorder is psychogenic. In a few cases, surgical trauma to the sympathetic nervous system (e.g., during surgery for aortic aneurysm), local genital disease (e.g., prostatitis, urethritis), or drug withdrawal from narcotics or trifluoperazine may underlie the problem.

Long-standing cases of premature ejaculation can often be traced back to initial sexual experiences, which are frequently accompanied by anxiety and sexual inexperience. Ejaculation, therefore, comes quickly, and with repetition this pattern can become habitual. In addition, during early experiences men's sexual focus is often directed to their partner's body, rather than to their own. They therefore fail to learn the intricacies of their own sexual response, to recognize the erotic sensations that precede orgasm, and to control their own arousal and ejaculatory response. Most men learn to delay orgasm with age and sexual experience. Others learn to contain their sexual response in established relationships but lose control when exposed to a new partner or situation.

Several factors can cause men to lose the ability to control their ejaculatory response after functioning normally. These include decreased sexual activity, profound performance anxiety with a new partner, and problems with another sexual disorder. In some cases, men who are recovering alcoholics experience premature ejaculation if they had used alcohol previously to inhibit their orgasm. Premature ejaculation may create tension in a couple's relationship and cause a man's partner to become sexually frustrated. It may also precipitate problems with erectile failure. Recurring episodes of premature ejaculation can cause men to become so preoccupied with their condition that they consciously inhibit arousal and develop secondary erectile dysfunction. On the other hand, some men who can attain erections but lose them rapidly experience orgasm by training themselves to reach it quickly. In these men, the premature ejaculation masks an arousal disorder. No specific physical findings or laboratory procedures are indicated for evaluating premature ejaculation, other than the tests used to detect uncommon organic conditions (see later).

Dyspareunia

Genital pain that occurs during intercourse in either men or women is termed dyspareunia. Although pain usually occurs during coitus, it may appear either before or after the sexual act. Women may experience superficial pain during penile penetration, or deeper pelvic pain during thrusting. The intensity of the pain can vary from mild to severe discomfort.

In women, many medical conditions can cause dyspareunia, including multiple genitourinary disorders, estrogen deprivation states, gastrointestinal problems, connective tissue disorders, and dermatologic conditions. In addition, as many as 30 per cent of the surgical procedures performed on a woman's genital tract result in at least temporary dyspareunia, and 30 to 40 per cent of women seen in sex therapy clinics for dyspareunia have identified pelvic pathology. Men with dyspareunia frequently have structural abnormalities of the penis, such as Peyronie's disease, priapism, urethral strictures, genital infections, and a history of prior genitourinary surgery. Painful orgasm in both sexes has been reported in patients taking fluphenazine, thioridazine, and amoxapine. Most people with dyspareunia assume that their problem is organic in origin. Therefore, few seek their initial treatment from mental health clinicians but visit their primary physician instead.

The course of dyspareunia varies with the underlying etiology. Problems caused by surgical procedures are often remedied by time and natural healing processes. When dyspareunia relates to an underlying medical condition, managing the condition optimally often decreases the pain. When the cause is associated with underlying psychological factors, the course tends toward chronicity. Complications that originate from the disorder itself affect mainly the person's relationships. Experiencing recurrent pain with each coital episode can cause men or women to avoid sexual encounters and suppress their sexual desire to avoid subsequent pain. Avoidance may produce conflict and frustration in their current relationship or limit their ability to develop new relationships.

When examining men with dyspareunia, the clinician must search carefully for signs of genitourinary infections (e.g., urethritis, prostatitis, seminal vesiculitis, cystitis, tuberculosis, elephantiasis, orchitis), penile lesions (e.g., Peyronie's disease, condylomata, priapism, urethral stricture), and prior genitourinary trauma (e.g., pelvic fracture, urethral rupture, penile surgery).

Women need a careful pelvic examination. Examine the external genitalia for evidence of infection (e.g., herpetic lesions, condylomata, discharge), scars, vulvar inflammation, clitoral inflammation or adhesions, and dermatitis. Inspect the introitus for vaginal sphincter spasm, fourchette irritation, hymenal abnormalities, urethral carbuncle, and Bartholin's gland inflammation. On vaginal examination, look for atrophy, discharge, inflammation, stenosis, vaginal or cervical lesions, relaxation of supporting ligaments, tenderness along the vaginal urethra or posterior bladder wall, and inadequate lubrication. During the bimanual examination, feel for endometriosis, adnexal masses, and pelvic inflammatory disease. Also, note uterine position, size, mobility, and tenderness. Finally, examine the rectum for hemorrhoids, proctitis, constipation, and fissure.

The laboratory evaluation for dyspareunia is directed at confirming data collected during the clinical examination. Other tests used to evaluate specific concerns include examination of vaginal secretions to diagnose vaginitis; a urinalysis and urine culture to diagnose urinary tract infection; tests to identify chlamydial, herpes simplex, and gonococcal infections; colposcopy to detect human papillomavirus infections and other vaginal or cervical disease; ultrasonography to assess adnexal, uterine, or cul-de-sac abnormalities; laparoscopy to identify and, in some cases, treat adnexal or intraperitoneal conditions; and anoscopy or sigmoidoscopy to detect associated colorectal problems.

Dyspareunia is not the diagnosis if the sexual pain is better explained by another axis I disorder (e.g., when the reported pain is really part of a somatization disorder). Likewise, pain with intercourse that occurs only sporadically, but that does not persist or recur, is not considered dyspareunia.

Vaginismus

Women with vaginismus experience involuntary spasm in the perineal muscles that surround the distal third of the vagina during any attempt to insert an object (e.g., penis, finger, tampon, examination speculum) through the introitus into the vagina. Even the thought of penetration stimulates muscle spasm in some women. The spasm varies in degree from mild tightness and discomfort to contractions that are severe and impenetrable. Fortunately, the physiologic phases of the sexual response cycle are intact in most women and thus make this condition very treatable.

Vaginismus can be either lifelong or acquired. The onset of the lifelong subtype is usually acute and often occurs during initial attempts at sexual penetration or during the woman's initial pelvic examination. Acquired vaginismus may also appear acutely in response to sexual trauma or an underlying medical condition. Vaginismus usually occurs in younger women and often in those who have attained a higher education and from higher socioeconomic levels. Many women with the disorder have been sexually abused or traumatized, and many express negative attitudes toward sex. Most of the same organic factors that were previously discussed for dyspareunia can also produce vaginismus.

Because the muscle spasm associated with vaginismus usually prevents intercourse, newly forming sexual relationships can be seriously impeded. Vaginismus can also add stress, frustration, conflict, and dysphoria to existing relationships. Unconsummated marriages and infertility can also result from the disorder.

Physicians often discover the problem while performing a pelvic examination. Affected women typically adduct their thighs when the physician attempts the examination and contract the muscles surrounding the vaginal outlet. In addition to searching for these findings, the physician should complete a careful pelvic examination, as previously discussed for dyspareunia. Likewise, a laboratory evaluation similar to that described for dyspareunia is appropriate. When vaginismus is secondary to a medical condition or to major sexual trauma, such as rape, the physician must also diagnose and manage the accompanying medical and psychological problems.

Sexual Dysfunction Due to a General Medical Condition

When the evidence that the physician gathers from a comprehensive history, physical examination, appropriate laboratory studies, and diagnostic procedures identifies a medical condition whose physiologic effects directly explain any of the sexual dysfunctions that have been previously discussed, and when the problem is not accounted for by another axis I disorder, then this DSM-IV category is used. The predominant sexual dysfunction is stated first, followed by the implicated medical condition. For example, male erectile disorder due to . . . (indicate the general medical condition), or female hypoactive sexual desire disorder due to . . . (indicate the general medical condition).

Substance-Induced Sexual Dysfunction

This diagnostic category is used when the history, physical examination, or laboratory evaluation indicates that the person's sexual dysfunction is completely explained by substance use. When substance use is responsible for the sexual dysfunction, the symptoms develop during or within a month of intoxication with an abused substance, or they occur concurrently with medication use. Sexual dysfunctions that are not substance induced are usually characterized by the following criteria: the dysfunction predates the substance use; the symptoms last for more than a month after the substance is withdrawn; the symptoms are magnified beyond what one would expect, given the type, amount, or duration of substance use; or the history indicates that dysfunctions have occurred previously without substance use. When using this diagnostic category, the clinician should list the specific substance first, followed by the sexual dysfunction that relates to it; for example, (specific substance) use with impaired desire, or (specific substance) use with impaired arousal.

PARAPHILIAS

The term paraphilia originates from the Greek roots *para* (a prefix meaning beside, beyond, accessory to, apart from, against) and *philein* (to love). Paraphilias, then, represent sexual activity that is "apart from love." By DSM-IV definitions, paraphilias are recurring, intense, sexually arousing fantasies, sexual urges, or behaviors that involve nonhuman objects, the suffering or humiliation of oneself or one's partner, and children or other nonconsenting persons. To qualify as a disorder, the paraphilia must recur for at least 6 months. People incorporate paraphilias into their sexual activity differently. For some, the paraphilic fantasies or stimuli are required for sexual arousal and are always included in sexual activity. Others include them only episodically, perhaps during stressful life circumstances, and can otherwise function quite normally. To some extent, the diagnosis is culturally dependent: What is deviant in one culture may be acceptable in another. Almost all paraphilias occur in men. Sexual masochism also occurs in women, but even then the ratio is 20 men to each woman.

When a person acts out his or her paraphilic fantasies, particularly in cases of pedophilia or sexual sadism, he or she may injure a nonconsenting partner. Certain paraphilias often lead to legal apprehension and incarceration. Sexual offenses against children are among the most commonly reported criminal sex acts, and individuals with exhibitionism, pedophilia, and voyeurism are the sex offenders most commonly arrested.

People with paraphilic arousal patterns frequently cannot find a consenting adult to help them act out their fantasies. They may then either act them out with unwilling victims or use prostitutes. They may also seek certain hobbies or occupations that bring them into close contact with their desired sexual stimulus in more socially acceptable ways. They also frequently collect both written and visual material that depict their preferred paraphilic stimulus.

People respond to their paraphilias in various ways. Some report absolutely no personal distress and are bothered only by the reaction that their behavior causes in others. Others are bound by extreme guilt, shame, and depression when they participate in sexual activity that is socially unacceptable or morally reprehensible to them.

The paraphilias complicate social and sexual relationships when others object to the person's behavior or if partners refuse to cooperate in helping paraphiliacs act out their fantasies. Most individuals with paraphilias come to the attention of the medical profession when their behavior causes conflict with their partners or with society. These people are frequently unable to experience reciprocal, affectionate sexual activity, and sexual dysfunctions and personality disorders frequently coexist with the paraphilias.

Paraphilias are usually lifelong disorders. They often begin in childhood, become better defined and elaborated during adolescence, undergo further elaboration and revision during adulthood, and finally begin to diminish with advancing age. For many, the fantasies are always present, but the urges vary considerably in both frequency and intensity. They usually increase during periods of psychosocial stress, in relation to other mental disorders, and as more opportunities to act out the paraphilias present themselves. No general medical conditions underlie these disorders. They may, however, cause medical problems. Frequent unprotected sex with multiple unknown partners may cause or transmit a sexually transmitted disease. Engaging in sadistic or masochistic activity can cause significant, even life-threatening injury.

Exhibitionism

Exhibitionists are almost always men who expose their genitalia to strangers and then masturbate to orgasm during the exposure episode or later as they fantasize about it. Once they expose themselves, they usually do not attempt further sexual activity with the stranger. Some men who expose themselves want to surprise or shock the observer, but others fantasize that the observer will also become sexually aroused. Exhibitionism usually begins before age 18 and tends to become less severe after age 40.

Fetishism

Nonliving objects (the "fetish") provide the paraphilic focus in fetishism. Women's underpants, bras, stockings, shoes, boots, or other wearing apparel are common fetishes. People with fetishism often masturbate while holding, rubbing, or smelling the fetish. They may also ask their sexual partner to wear the object during sexual activity. The fetish is usually required for sexual arousal, and in its absence men may experience erectile disorders. Most fetishism begins in adolescence, although the particular object may have become imbued with special significance earlier in childhood. Once firmly incorporated into the person's sexual life, fetishism is usually lifelong. Fetishism is not the diagnosis when the objects are limited to female clothing that is used during cross-dressing, or when the person uses an object like a vibrator that is designed for genital stimulation.

Frottage

The sexually arousing fantasies, urges, and behaviors of frottage involve touching and rubbing against a nonconsenting person. The rubbing and touching often happens in crowded places from which the person can escape to avoid arrest (e.g., public transportation, sidewalks, elevators, or queue lines). The episode usually begins when the man rubs his genitals against the victim's thighs and buttocks or fondles her genitalia or breasts with his hands. During this phase he usually fantasizes that he has a caring, exclusive relationship with the person. After touching the victim, he usually recognizes the need to escape and flees to avoid arrest.

Frottage most often begins during adolescence, and most acts occur between the ages of 15 and 25, after which they gradually decline.

Pedophilia

Individuals with pedophilia experience intense sexual urges or arousal that is focused on children who are age 13 or younger. They must be at least 16 years of age themselves and 5 years older than the child victim. If the paraphiliac is younger than 16 years of age but in late adolescence, no precise age defines the disorder and the diagnosis depends on clinical judgment accounting for the maturity of the perpetrator and the victim. Most pedophiliacs are uniquely attracted to children of a specific age. The gender of the victims varies with the perpetrator, and some are equally attracted to both sexes. Sexual activity with girls is more frequently reported, and the most common victim age for girls is 8 to 10 years. Male victims tend to be slightly older. Some pedophiliacs are sexually attracted only to children, but others are also attracted to adults.

Pedophiliacs engage in sexual activity with children that varies in focus and intensity. Some only undress and look at the child. Others may expose themselves or masturbate in the child's presence. Still others involve the children by touching and fondling them, performing fellatio or cunnilingus, or using force to penetrate the child's vagina, mouth, or anus with their fingers, foreign objects, or penis. Genital fondling and oral sex are most frequent. Vaginal and anal penetration are rare, except in cases of incest. The pedophiliac often attempts to justify his behavior by arguing that the child enjoys it, needs to learn something from it, or was sexually provoking.

The children victimized may be the pedophiliac's own children, stepchildren, relatives, or children from other families. Some pedophiliacs threaten children to avoid disclosure. Others try to gain the child's affection and loyalty so that the child will not report the activity. Often, pedophiliacs create complicated schemes to gain access to their victims. For example, they may try to win the mother's trust or marry the mother of an attractive child. They may also trade children with other pedophiliacs, become foster parents, or abduct children from strangers.

The disorder usually begins in adolescence. Pedophiliacs rarely report that the paraphilia began in middle age. The acting out frequency depends on levels of psychosocial stress. The disorder tends to be lifelong. Among those who obtain treatment, recidivism is almost twice as frequent for those who prefer boys.

Sexual Masochism

The term masochism is derived from the name of a 19th century Austrian novelist, Leopold von Sacher-Masoch. His characters realized sexual pleasure from abuse and domination by women. In sexual masochism, the individual is humiliated, beaten, bound, or made to suffer in other ways. Masochism affects individuals in varying degrees. Some experience only masochistic fantasies of being raped or bound by others without possible escape. These often occur during sexual intercourse. Others perform masochistic acts on themselves in response to their urges (binding themselves, pricking themselves with pins, shocking themselves, or mutilating themselves). Still others engage a partner for physical restraint, blindfolding, paddling, spanking, whipping, beating, electrical shocks, cutting, infibulation, and subjection to acts of humiliation (e.g., forced cross-dressing, treatment as a helpless infant clothed in diapers, being forced to crawl and grovel like an animal, being urinated or defecated on).

One potentially lethal form of sexual masochism is termed hypoxyphilia—sexual arousal by oxygen deprivation. Hypoxia is produced by chest compression, noose, ligature, plastic bag, mask, or chemical (usually a volatile nitrate that temporarily decreases brain oxygenation by peripheral vasodilatation). Hypoxyphilic activities may occur alone or with a partner. Mistakes have caused accidental deaths.

Most masochistic fantasies originate in childhood but are not usually acted on until early adulthood. The disorder is usually lifelong and focuses on the same recurring masochistic acts. Many do not escalate the severity of their masochistic acts over time. Others, often in response to stress, escalate to the point that they can injure, or even kill, themselves.

Sexual Sadism

The term sadism also derives its origin from an author, the Marquis de Sade, an 18th century French writer who was infamous for committing violent sexual acts against women. The diagnostic category refers to individuals who become sexually excited when they commit actual acts against a victim that result in that person's psychological or physical suffering, including humiliation. The sadist's focus is on the victim's suffering. It is the suffering that stimulates sexual arousal.

As in masochism, sadism affects individuals in varying degrees. Some are bothered by sexual fantasies that focus on complete control over a victim who is frightened by the anticipated sadistic act. These fantasies usually occur during sexual activity and are not acted on. Others may act out their sadistic urges with a willing sexual partner (who may also be a sexual masochist) who submits to pain, suffering, and humiliation. Still other sadists act out their sexual urges with nonconsenting victims.

The fantasies and acts that the sadist uses vary in intensity and in the degree to which they include victims. Some focus on a need to dominate the victim (e.g., making the victim perform various humiliating acts or keeping the victim in a cage). They may also include restraint, blindfolding, paddling, spanking, whipping, pinching, beating, burning, electrical shocks, rape, cutting, stabbing, strangulation, torture, mutilation, or even murder.

Sadistic fantasies often begin during childhood, but sadistic acts usually begin in young adulthood. The disorder is usually lifelong, with the sadistic acts increasing in severity over time. When sadism involves nonconsenting victims it usually continues until the sadist is arrested. Those who seriously injure or even kill their victims most often also have an associated antisocial personality disorder.

Transvestic Fetishism

Transvestic fetishism is also known as cross-dressing or just transvestitism. Men with this disorder keep a wardrobe of women's clothing that they wear to stimulate sexual arousal. While wearing the clothing, they usually masturbate and imagine that they are both the male and the female partner in their sexual fantasy. To date, the disorder has been described only in heterosexual men. In fact, when not dressed in women's clothing, these men may appear hypermasculine and engage in stereotypically male-associated occupations. They tend to have few sexual partners and may have engaged in occasional homosexual acts.

Degrees of involvement with cross-dressing lie on a continuum from occasionally wearing female clothes in private to extensive involvement with a transvestic subculture. Some men wear only a single item of women's apparel hidden beneath their male clothing. Others try to appear entirely female, using make-up in addition to their women's apparel.

Cross-dressing usually begins in childhood or early adolescence, but it does not become public until early adulthood. It often begins with partial cross-dressing that progresses to complete cross-dressing. A particularly stimulating article of clothing may become erotic itself and be used in masturbation and coitus. Cross-dressing frequency may wax and wane. It is often used as a means of coping with anxiety or depression. A few individuals who cross-dress may become fixed on gender dysphoria and seek gender reassignment. This is the point at which people with transvestic fetishism often seek treatment.

Voyeurism

Individuals with voyeurism, also known as "peeping" or scopophilia, observe unsuspecting people, who are usually strangers, when they are naked, disrobing, or participating in sexual activity. They look to become sexually aroused, not to seek sexual activity with the person observed. They usually masturbate to orgasm while looking, or later as they recall the event. They may fantasize a sexual experience with the person they observed, but they rarely act out this fantasy. Voyeurism usually begins before age 15, and the course tends to be lifelong.

Paraphilia Not Otherwise Specified

This group of atypical paraphilias do not meet the criteria for any of the specific categories previously discussed. The following are some examples: zoophilia (incorporating animals into arousal fantasies or sexual activity), coprophilia (the desire to defecate on a partner, or to be defecated on, to achieve sexual pleasure), klismaphilia (using enemas as part of sexual stimulation), urophilia (sexual pleasure associated with the desire to urinate on a partner or to be urinated on), necrophilia (the act of obtaining sexual gratification from cadavers), partialism (focusing on one part of the body to the exclusion of all others), and telephone scatology (achieving sexual arousal through obscene phone calls).

GENDER IDENTITY DISORDERS

Four major factors must exist for the diagnosis of gender identity disorder. First, the individual must demonstrate a strong, persistent cross-gender identification—not merely a desire to be the opposite gender for cultural advantage. Second, the person must manifest persistent discomfort with his or her assigned gender or with the roles required of that gender. Third, no concurrent physical intersex condition can exist (e.g., androgen insensitivity syndrome or congenital adrenal hyperplasia). Fourth, the disorder must be clinically distressing and impair the person in social, occupational, and other important functional areas.

Children manifest cross-gender identification by (1) repeatedly telling people that they are or wish to become the opposite sex, (2) cross-dressing or simulating the attire of the other gender, (3) strongly and persistently preferring cross-sex roles in make-believe play or fantasizing about being the other sex, (4) intensely desiring to participate in stereotypical games and pastimes of the other gender, and (5) strongly preferring playmates of the opposite sex.

Adults and adolescents reveal their cross-gender identification by their stated desire to be the other sex, frequently passing or attempting to pass as the opposite sex, wanting to live and be treated as the other gender, or sincerely believing that they feel and react just like the other sex.

Children demonstrate their discomfort with their gender in many ways. Boys maintain that their penis or testes are revolting, that they will disappear, or that they would be better off without them. They also avoid rough-and-tumble play and refuse toys, games, and activities that are stereotypically male. Girls refuse to urinate while sitting, believe that they will grow a penis, do not want to grow breasts or menstruate, and actively avoid wearing feminine clothing.

Adolescents and adults manifest their distress by focusing intently, to the point of preoccupation, on obliterating their primary and secondary sex characteristics. To achieve this end, they frequently request hormones, surgery, or other procedures that will physically alter their sexual characteristics. They also firmly believe that they were born the wrong sex and that their real person is held captive in the wrong body.

The course of this disorder is variable. Parents of children who are referred for evaluation often report noticing the cross-gender behavior between 2 and 4 years. Most children are seen about the time they start school because the parents are concerned that this "phase" of their life does not seem to be passing. Over time, in response to peers, or with parental intervention, most of these children demonstrate less overt cross-gender behavior. By late adolescence or early adulthood, about 75 per cent of the boys report a homosexual or bisexual orientation. The remainder are heterosexual. Statistics for girls are currently unknown.

This disorder may follow one of two courses in adult men. The first course is to continue the gender identity disorder that began in childhood. These men usually present in late adolescence or in early adulthood. Men who follow this course and are sexually attracted to men usually present with a lifelong history of gender dysphoria. Men who follow the second course usually present in early to middle adulthood. Overt signs of the disorder develop more gradually in these men, and their cross-gender identification appears later. Sometimes it appears concurrent with transvestic fetishism. The degree of cross-gender identification in these men varies. They are more ambivalent toward sex-change surgery and less likely to be satisfied if they pursue it. They may also have a greater attraction for women. Gender dysphoria usually follows a chronic course, although spontaneous remission has occurred.

Problems with gender identity complicate many aspects of life. Children are unhappy and may become so preoccupied that the ordinary activities of living suffer. Older children often fail to develop age-appropriate same-sex peer relationships and skills and therefore become socially isolated. They may even avoid school to escape the teasing and pressure to appear and perform according to stereotypical gender expectations. Children are also at greater risk for anxiety disorders and depression. Adolescents may feel that they are unacceptable to their families because of their gender dysphoria. They are frequently teased and can become socially isolated and rejected by their peers. School and work performance is often impaired. Adolescents are also at greater risk for depression, suicidal ideation, and suicide attempts.

Adults can become totally preoccupied with activities that decrease their gender distress, especially when they are just beginning to live the opposite sex role. Some men attempt to treat themselves with female sex hormones, and a few have even attempted their own castration or penectomy. Some engage in sexual activity with prostitutes or other unknown partners, exposing themselves to greater risk of sexually transmitted disease. Depression, suicide attempts, and substance abuse are also commonly associated, and relationships with their families of origin are frequently destroyed.

Both men and women with gender identity disorders possess normal genitalia, although women with the disorder have a higher than anticipated incidence of polycystic ovarian disease. These men and women may, however, demonstrate physical findings that result from their attempts to manage the disorder. Breast enlargement in men may result from estrogen ingestion. Male hair patterns may be altered by epilation. Other cosmetic procedures such as rhinoplasty or surgical reduction in the thyroid cartilage may have been performed. Women may demonstrate breast rashes or breast distortion from breast binding. Women who have undergone sex-reassignment surgery may demonstrate prominent chest wall scars from breast excision. Men may experience vaginal strictures, rectovaginal fistulas, urethral stones, and misdirected urinary streams.

No specific diagnostic tests exist for gender identity disorder. If the physical examination is normal, karyotyping for sex chromosomes and sex hormone assays are unnecessary. Psychological testing may be pertinent if a concomitant psychiatric disorder is suspected.

Individuals with gender identity disorder frequently have associated psychiatric problems that must be diagnosed and managed. Common accompanying diagnoses include borderline, antisocial, or narcissistic personality disorders; substance abuse; depression and suicide; and other self-destructive behaviors. These individuals also frequently become demanding and manipulative, often resisting any management attempts that are not focused on their chosen method (usually sex-reassignment surgery).

SCHIZOPHRENIA

By John W. Goethe, M.D.
Hartford, Connecticut

Schizophrenia is a pathologic condition that affects mental functions and has traditionally been described and classified as a thought (cognitive) disorder that can cause psychosis. Patients with this illness have disturbed perception, behavior, communication, and affect, but not all cognitive functions are impaired. Dementia, for example, is not a feature of schizophrenia, even though deterioration in intellectual capacity has been described (e.g., "dementia praecox").

Although the modern concept of schizophrenia originated nearly 100 years ago, it remains to be determined whether schizophrenia is a single disease with a range of manifestations or a label for several distinct pathologic processes with shared clinical characteristics. The cause of schizophrenia is not known; diagnosis is based on clinical description. Historically, there have been inconsistencies and conceptual differences among the accounts that have provided benchmarks for the diagnosis of schizophrenia. Current diagnostic criteria are rather strict and emphasize the presumably observable manifestations of schizophrenia. This approach is particularly prominent in the *Diagnostic and Statistical Manual of Mental Disorders* (4th edition) (DSM-IV), published by the American Psychiatric Association (the official nomenclature for the classification of mental disorders in North America). The clinician should be aware, however, that clinical practice is also influenced by classic descriptions of schizophrenia (e.g., Bleuler's "4 A's") and other diagnostic systems (e.g., the International Classification of Diseases, published by the World Health Organization).

DIAGNOSTIC CRITERIA

The diagnosis of schizophrenia is based not only on (1) characteristic symptoms but also on the (2) historical data (duration and frequency of symptom episodes), (3) known consequences of the disorder (e.g., functional deficits or incapacities attributed to the illness), and (4) exclusion of other conditions. Some of these data are considered essential to the diagnosis, while others are viewed as "associated findings." What is essential in one diagnostic system, however, may not be in others. The symptoms of schizophrenia vary over time, with prodromal, active (acute), and residual phases. Therefore, information from all phases may be important to the diagnostic decision. DSM-IV defines the active phase rather narrowly compared with other diagnostic systems. Furthermore, DSM-IV limits the assignment of the diagnosis of schizophrenia by requiring at least one episode of illness in the active phase and by setting minimum criteria for the duration of both the active phase and the total episode of illness. Virtually all concepts of schizophrenia view it as a chronic disorder that typically impairs functioning. Evidence of such impairment, however, may not be required for the diagnosis under DSM-IV criteria. Finally, the need to exclude other causes of the patient's problems is common to all diagnostic approaches.

SYMPTOMS

In defining the active phase of schizophrenia, DMS-IV recognizes five symptom groups: (1) delusions, (2) hallucinations, (3) disorganized speech, (4) grossly disorganized or catatonic behavior, and (5) so-called "negative" symptoms. These symptoms are consistent with traditional descriptions of schizophrenia, but DSM-IV allows the diagnosis only if two or more of the five groups can be documented. Some symptoms are given more weight, and the active phase criteria can be satisfied simply by observing a particular type of delusion ("bizarre") or hallucination (voices conversing with one another or commenting about the patient). Other symptoms may contribute to the presentation, but in DSM-IV they have less diagnostic importance.

Delusions are strongly held but false beliefs pertaining to any theme and involving any life experience; patients typically cannot be persuaded that their beliefs are unfounded. Delusions may be widespread or narrowly focused, and their impact on overt behavior varies greatly. Common types of delusions are persecutory (probably the most common type in schizophrenia), grandiose, religious, and somatic. Some patients, in the absence of persecutory ideation, may believe that many aspects of their environment make reference to them (referential thoughts). Religious delusions may also be grandiose (e.g., believing that one is Jesus Christ). So-called "bizarre" delusions are given increased weight in DSM-IV because these false beliefs seem to be particularly characteristic of, if not truly unique to, schizophrenia. The distinction between what is and is not bizarre may be difficult. Common examples are beliefs that one's actions are being controlled or made to occur, that thoughts are inserted ("thought insertion") or taken away ("thought withdrawal"), or that one's thoughts are being broadcast ("thought broadcasting").

Hallucinations are false perceptions that occur when patients are fully awake and alert. Like delusional beliefs, they are "real" to the patient. By definition, hallucinations occur in the absence of an external stimulus, but patients may report associated events that they believe to be causal, perhaps in an attempt to explain the experience. Hallucinations may involve any sensory modality. Patients most commonly report hearing one or more voices; some individuals describe hearing their own thoughts "out loud." As with bizarre delusions, DSM-IV gives more diagnostic weight to hallucinations with a particular quality (e.g., a voice commenting on the patient or two or more voices conversing).

Disorganized thinking impairs the patient's ability to communicate. Although this group of symptoms is presumed to be a manifestation of "thought disorder," it is the patient's speech that is actually assessed. Patients may periodically "lose track" of what they are saying, in subtle or dramatic ways. The examiner may experience the patient's comment as generally vague or obscure, or there may be frank "breaks" in the conversation. The latter are referred to as "loose associations" or "derailments;" they may be obliquely related to the conversation ("tangentiality") or appear to be completely irrelevant. Speech may come to an abrupt halt ("thought blocking"), or there may be an abundance of apparently unconnected words ("word salad" or "incoherence") that sometimes resembles aphasia. Patients may also use words they have created ("neologisms").

Disorganized behavior, like disorganized thinking, can present in various ways. Patients may have stereotypic, repetitive movements, or they may refuse to follow instructions. General aimlessness and inability to perform the usual activities of daily living are frequently described. The most dramatic alterations in behavior are catatonic stupor and catatonic excitement.

So-called *negative symptoms* are those that reflect the partial or complete loss of normal mental or physical capabilities. Poverty of thought, diminished ideation, limited (or inappropriate) affective response, and slowness of movement are classically described negative symptoms. In DSM-IV, affective flattening, alogia, and avolition are recognized as part of the active phase of the illness. Anhedonia and apathy are also frequently observed in schizophrenic patients.

Affective flattening refers to a disturbance in the expression of feeling. The words "affect" and "mood" are sometimes used interchangeably, but the latter term technically refers to sustained states of feeling, rather than to moment-to-moment affective responses. If this distinction is applied, it is the alteration in affect that is characteristic of schizophrenia. In normal individuals, affective response shifts with changes in thought content. In schizophrenics, this capacity to modulate is deficient. Abrupt shifts in affect may occur in the absence of an observable stimulus.

The range and depth of feeling may be restricted. Affect may be blunted, with some preservation of responsiveness, or flat, with little or no expression in the face or in intonation. Even if a state of feeling is conveyed, it is often not congruent with the content of the conversation or with the immediate situation.

Alogia is poverty of speech. As noted earlier, disturbed speech probably results from the disordered thought characteristic of schizophrenia. In DSM-IV, disorganized speech (a "positive" symptom) is distinguished from alogia (a "negative" symptom) in which productivity and fluency are diminished. Similarly, disorganized behavior is distinguished from *avolition*, which represents a decreased ability to initiate and/or persist in goal-directed activities. This distinction between functions that are preserved but disorganized and those that are absent or deficient may be difficult.

In applying the DSM-IV diagnostic algorithm, the clinician must not count one finding as evidence of the presence of more than one of the five symptoms of the active phase. For example, a negative symptom cannot also be regarded as evidence of "disorganized behavior" or "disorganized thinking." It may also be difficult to distinguish between the negative symptoms of schizophrenia and some of the characteristic features of major depression. Depressed patients usually describe their feeling state as painful, and their appearance and speech content are typically consistent with affect and mood.

The symptoms of schizophrenia mentioned earlier are the most important in the DSM-IV diagnostic category. However, so-called associated symptoms also contribute to the overall clinical picture, and the presence of these symptoms may be critical for meeting the criteria of other (non–DSM-IV) diagnostic systems.

Anhedonia (the absence of pleasure) refers to what is believed to be a fundamental deficit in the ability to experience pleasure. Although anhedonia is conceptually different from the loss of pleasure that accompanies depressive disorders, this distinction may be difficult to make clinically.

Ambivalence refers to the "paralysis" of expression and action characteristic of schizophrenia. Ambivalence has been attributed to the fact that contradictory ideas exist simultaneously and carry equal weight for these patients, leaving them unable to resolve the conflict. Even minor decisions, such as whether to move from a chair, may be impossible because other issues, peripheral to the current situation and normally disregarded, are perceived as important. Although the word ambivalence sometimes refers to simultaneous conflicting feelings experienced by normal individuals (so-called "mixed feelings"), schizophrenic ambivalence is qualitatively and quantitatively different. Bleuler, among others, considered ambivalence to be a fundamental aspect of the disorder he described as schizophrenia.

Autism was also regarded by Bleuler as a fundamental feature of schizophrenia. Autism is not a single symptom. Rather, it describes a style of thinking or relating to the world. The clinical picture includes various distortions of reality and of self-perception. Patients may describe a "loss of boundaries" between themselves and the outside world or a disturbance in identity, with depersonalization or derealization. None of these experiences, however, is unique to schizophrenia. Moreover, the features of autism cannot be reliably assessed in many patients with schizophrenia.

Lack of insight is a common symptom of schizophrenia, as are *poor judgment* and *concrete thinking* (inability to abstract). Patients with schizophrenia may also exhibit or report depression, anxiety, anger, or other disturbances in mood. Sleep and eating patterns may be abnormal. Concentration, orientation, and memory may be impaired, and various abnormalities of psychomotor activity are common. Many of these symptoms are easily detected during routine mental status examination, but they have low diagnostic specificity.

Schizophrenic symptoms and associated features may aggregate in various ways. The recognized subtypes of schizophrenia represent some of the most frequently described clinical pictures. DSM-IV lists five subtypes: paranoid, disorganized, catatonic, undifferentiated, and residual. There are additional subtypes mentioned in other diagnostic systems, including previous editions of DSM. Some patients have symptoms characteristic of more than one category. Atypical is sometimes used as an alternative term for the undifferentiated subtype, but atypical more commonly refers to a condition that may be different from "typical schizophrenia" in its cause, course, or treatment response. Latent refers to symptoms and behaviors typical of the prodromal phase of schizophrenia. Subtypes similar to latent include prepsychotic, pseudoneurotic, pseudopsychopathic, and simple schizophrenia. Finally, despite its association with severely disturbed and even psychotic behavior, "borderline" properly refers to a personality disorder that should not be regarded as a form of schizophrenia.

HISTORY

The diagnosis of schizophrenia depends on the medical and psychiatric history (longitudinal data) as well as the present mental status examination (i.e., cross-sectional data). The characteristic symptoms of the active phase, while dramatic, may be relatively brief. The DSM-IV criteria require acute symptoms for at least 1 month (for a shorter period if the symptoms are interrupted by successful treatment), while other diagnostic systems, including earlier editions of DSM, do not specify a duration. The total episode of illness, including prodromal and residual phases, is emphasized in all diagnostic approaches; this period of illness typically must last for at least 6 months. Longitudinal data are critical for the diagnosis because many psychiatric and other illnesses can cause acute (active-phase) symptoms. A careful history may also reveal social and occupational dysfunctions typical of and, in DSM-IV, necessary for the diagnosis of schizophrenia.

CONSEQUENCES AND FUNCTIONAL IMPAIRMENT

In the absence of a definitive diagnostic test, the consequences of the mental disturbances associated with schizophrenia become important diagnostically. DSM-IV requires evidence of deterioration in at least one major area of performance (e.g., work or academic study, self-care, social and interpersonal activity).

DIFFERENTIAL DIAGNOSIS

DSM-IV emphasizes the need to exclude schizoaffective and mood disorders because both conditions share symptoms with schizophrenia and have features that may be difficult to distinguish from schizophrenia. DSM-IV also discourages the diagnosis of schizophrenia in patients with developmental disorders, unless prominent delusions or hallucinations have subsequently emerged and persisted.

Table 1. Diagnosis of Schizophrenia: Summary Table

Active-Phase Symptoms*	Subtype*,‡	Common Course Patterns	Differential Diagnosis§
Delusions Hallucinations Disorganized speech Disorganized or catatonic behavior	Paranoid Disorganized Catatonic Undifferentiated	Single episode, full remission Single episode, partial remission Episodic without residual symptoms Episodic with residual symptoms	Substance-induced disorder Mood disorders Schizophreniform disorder Brief psychotic disorder
Affective flattening† Alogia† Avolition†	Residual	Continuous Other Unspecified	Delusional disorder Pervasive developmental disorder Severe personality disorder

*Based on Diagnostic and Statistical Manual of Mental Disorders, 4th ed. (DSM-IV).
†"Negative symptoms."
‡Common presentations and/or dominant picture.
§Includes psychiatric disorders only.

Table 1 lists the most common psychiatric disorders in the differential diagnosis.

COURSE

The usual age at onset for schizophrenia is the late teens to middle 30s. Childhood- and late-onset forms have also been reported. Schizophrenia is defined as a chronic illness associated with functional impairments, but the course of schizophrenia is highly variable. Symptoms of the active phase (hallucinations, delusions, and/or gross disorganization) may be prominent and essentially continuous, or they may occur infrequently following the initial episode of illness. DSM-IV provides six "course specifiers" that describe common patterns: (1) single episode in full remission; (2) single episode in partial remission; (3) episodic with no residual symptoms between episodes; (4) episodic, with interepisode residual symptoms; (5) continuous; and (6) other, or unspecified. Recognizing this variability in course is important to the diagnosis because some clinicians continue to believe that deterioration is inevitable and that the more dramatic symptoms are always present. Knowledge of the variability in course also informs treatment decisions because some patients may not require continuous pharmacotherapy.

COMPLICATIONS

The principal complications of schizophrenia are social and behavioral. Inattention to self-care, however, places individuals with schizophrenia at increased risk for diseases related to malnutrition and untreated infections. The altered perceptions and odd behaviors may produce legal difficulties and interpersonal conflicts, sometimes resulting in injury or death to the patient or others. Approximately 10 per cent of schizophrenics commit suicide. Many of these patients do not meet developmental milestones or educational goals, and a myriad of occupational, interpersonal, and intrapsychic difficulties may ensue.

FINDINGS ON PHYSICAL EXAMINATION AND LABORATORY ASSESSMENT

There are no characteristic physical or laboratory findings in schizophrenia. However, neurologic, toxic, endocrine, and other conditions that can alter mental status and behavior should be excluded. Some imaging studies have demonstrated alterations in brain structure (e.g., increased ventricular size) and function (e.g., glucose metabolism), but none of these findings has clinical relevance at the present time. Neuropsychological assessment, while not diagnostic, may be useful in designing remedial learning and rehabilitation programs for these patients.

PITFALLS IN DIAGNOSIS

The diagnosis of schizophrenia and other mental disturbances is a complex task. The major obstacles to an accurate diagnosis are as follows: (1) absence of definitive diagnostic tests or pathognomonic signs and symptoms; (2) variability in the clinical presentation and course of the disorder; (3) subtlety, ambiguity, and low specificity of some of the "characteristic" signs and symptoms; and (4) difficulty in eliciting information (i.e., patients with schizophrenia may be unwilling to respond and/or may have difficulty in communicating). Diagnosis should be based on the cluster of symptoms and features, rather than on a single finding. In the setting of uncertain or incomplete data, a "provisional" diagnosis may be appropriate, especially if the degree of functional incapacity or symptom severity is great and there is no evidence of another disorder. The provisional diagnosis facilitates the initiation of treatment but also reminds the clinician that reassessment is required to confirm the diagnosis of schizophrenia.

PERSONALITY DISORDERS

By Robert Benjamin, M.D.
Dresher, Pennsylvania

Personality disorders have been defined as "an enduring pattern of inner experience and behavior that deviates markedly from the expectations of the individual's culture, is pervasive and inflexible, has an onset in adolescence or early adulthood, is stable over time and leads to distress or impairment."* While the foregoing is the precise definition, the more colloquial definition of personality disorder

**The Diagnostic and Statistical Manual of Mental Disorders, Fourth Edition (DSM-IV), p. 629.*

Table 1. General Diagnostic Criteria for a Personality Disorder

1. Personality disorders are enduring patterns of inner experience and behavior that deviate markedly from the expectations of the individual's culture and are manifested in at least two of the following areas:
   a. *Cognition* (ways of perceiving and interpreting self, other people, and events)
   b. *Affectivity* (emotional range, intensity, lability, and appropriateness of response)
   c. *Interpersonal Functioning*
   d. *Impulse Control*
2. This enduring pattern is inflexible and pervasive across a broad range of personal and social situations.
3. The pattern leads to clinically significant distress or impairment in social, occupational, or other important areas of functioning.
4. The pattern is stable and has long duration, and its onset can be traced back to at least adolescence or early adulthood.
5. This pattern is not better accounted for as a manifestation or consequence of another mental disorder.
6. The enduring pattern is not due to the direct physiologic effects of any substance (drugs of abuse, medications, etc.) or general medical condition (head trauma, and many others).

Adapted from the *Diagnostic and Statistical Manual of Mental Disorders*, Fourth edition. Washington, DC, American Psychiatric Press, Inc., 1994, p. 633, with permission.

is more impish: These are people who are not "crazy," but who drive everyone else crazy. That is, their symptoms are generally not annoying to the patient who possesses them but are profoundly disturbing to those around them. The clinician must take care not to use these diagnoses as sophisticated insults, but rather as tools for understanding the worldview of another. In this way, the chances for constructive interaction with the patient can be maximized despite an impairment in social relationships.

Personality disorders must be distinguished from personality traits, which are enduring patterns of perceiving, relating to, and thinking about the environment and oneself that are exhibited in a wide range of social and personal contexts. Only when these personality traits become inflexible, maladaptive, and the cause of significant functional impairment or subjective distress do they rise to the degree of a personality disorder (Table 1).

Personality disorders are divided into clusters A, B, and C (Table 2), as well as a fourth section called personality disorders not otherwise specified (NOS). This last category is reserved either for diagnoses of persons who fit criteria for more than one of the types of personality disorders or for diagnoses that fall into a category of personality disorders that have not yet been codified into the nomenclature but nevertheless are commonly used. The latter group includes passive-aggressive, sadistic, and self-defeating personality disorders. Table 1 describes each personality disorder in terms of the trigger phenomena that elicit the responses characteristic of that personality type. This table describes how the patient perceives the trigger and also how behavioral and emotional responses follow from these triggers.

CLUSTER A

The first group of personality disorders is known as the eccentric cluster. The common trigger for each of them is close interpersonal relations. In general, persons with these disorders appear emotionally cold and mistrustful. They may also have peculiarities of thinking that are noticeable to others but are not overtly disturbing to the person who displays them.

Paranoid Personality Disorder

This type of personality disorder is characterized by a pervasive distrust and suspiciousness of others. Motives of people with whom these patients associate are interpreted as malevolent and deceptive. Individuals with the paranoid personality suspect that others are trying to exploit, harm, or deceive them. They are preoccupied with unjustifiable doubts about the loyalty and trustworthiness of friends and associates. They are reluctant to confide in others as a result of unwarranted fear that this information will be used maliciously against them. They often find hidden meanings or threatening interpretations in benign remarks or events. They persistently bear grudges and are unforgiving of even inadvertent slights or insults. They perceive the actions of others as attacks on their character or reputation, and they are quick to react with anger or to counterattack against these imagined slights. Without justification, they have recurrent suspicions regarding the fidelity of a spouse or partner. As with all the personality disorders, these symptoms are not the consequences of other broader diagnoses (e.g., schizophrenia, mood disorders, anxiety disorders) and are not due to the direct physiologic effects of a general medical condition.

Schizoid Personality Disorder

These individuals demonstrate a pervasive pattern of detachment from social relationships. They also have a restricted range of expression of emotion in interpersonal settings. The pattern begins by early adulthood and exists in a variety of contexts. Patients neither desire nor enjoy close personal relationships, including those within a family. They almost always choose solitary activities and take pleasure in few, if any, social activities. They typically lack close friends or confidants other than their first-degree relatives and show little interest in being involved sexually with another person. They seem uninterested in either praise or criticism. In general, they display emotional coldness, detachment, and flattened affect. These symptoms must be distinguished from the premorbid characteristics of schizophrenia, a much more serious and pervasive chronic psychotic illness.

Schizotypal Personality Disorder

Individuals manifesting this personality disorder have a pervasive pattern of social and interpersonal deficits marked by discomfort with and reduced capacity for close relationships. They manifest cognitive and perceptual disturbances and eccentricities of behavior, including ideas of reference (but not rising to the degree of delusions); magical beliefs not consistent with cultural norms; unusual perceptual experiences, including illusions about their bodies; and odd speech patterns, including vague, circumstantial, metaphorical, overly elaborate, or stereotypic speech. They may also display paranoid ideation, inappropriate or constricted affect, and odd appearance or behaviors. They frequently lack close friends and show excessive social anxiety that tends not to diminish with familiarity.

Such behaviors need to be differentiated from the prodromal stages of a more serious disorder such as schizophrenia. In the past, such individuals have sometimes been labeled as "latent schizophrenics." Although these patients share some characteristics with the schizoidal individuals

Table 2. Personality Disorders as Maladjusted Response to Triggers

Personality Disorder	Trigger	Perception of Trigger	Behavioral Response	Emotional Response
Cluster A				
Paranoid	Close interpersonal relations	"People sneak up on me and harm me."	Guarded distance, secretive, devious, scheming, counterattacking	Suspicious, jealous, angry, hypervigilant
Schizoid	Close interpersonal relations	"People are meaningless to me."	Avoids social involvement	Cold, stiff, distant, aloof
Schizotypal	Close interpersonal relations	"Others have special magic intentions."	Imagines love or rejection without evidence	Inappropriate excitement, hostile aloofness
Cluster B				
Antisocial	Social standards and rules	"Rules limit me from fulfilling my needs."	Violation of social rules, standards, and law	Impulsively angry, hostile, cunning
Borderline	Personal goals, close relations	"Goals are good; no, they are not; people are great; no, they are not."	Changing goals, ambivalent relations	Labile mood and affect
Histrionic	Heterosexual relations	"I have to show intense emotions to impress."	Flirts, shows exaggerated, nongenuine emotions	Excited by positive, dysphoric by negative response
Narcissistic	Evaluation of self	"I'm the only person that counts."	Self-centeredness, expects recognition without contributions	Labile, grandiose, inflated feelings
Cluster C				
Avoidant	Close interpersonal relations, public appearance	"People reject and criticize me."	Escapes and avoids social appearances	Anxious, withdrawn
Dependent	Self-reliance, being alone	"I had to be alone."	Giving up own goals to cling to others (e.g., parents)	Anxious, panicky
Obsessive-compulsive	Close relationships, unstructured situations, authority	"My rules must prevail; uncertainty is frightening; feelings interfere with thinking."	Emotional restriction, rigid, angry if his rules are broken; defiance of authority	Anxious, angry, resentful
Personality Disorders Not Otherwise Specified (NOS)				
Passive-aggressive	Deadlines, demands to perform	"They impose on my freedom, but it is dangerous to resist openly."	Procrastination, broken commitments	Anxious, angry, resentful
Sadistic	Weak, dependent persons	"I have to show them who is boss; I can make them eat crap."	Cruel, restrictive acts against defenseless people	Pleasure derived from the suffering of others
Self-defeating	Situations and relationships difficult to master	"I have to endure hardship to prove myself worthwhile."	Enters or creates situations that promise hardship	Indulges in suffering

Adapted from Othmer, E., and Othmer, S.C.: *The Clinical Interview Using DSM-IV, vol. 1, Fundamentals.* American Psychiatric Press, Inc., 1994, pp. 235–236.

described earlier, they are more bizarre and eccentric in their presentation.

The three preceding personality disorders present significant challenges for the practicing physician. Owing to their difficulty in interpersonal relations and their frequently distorted sense of reality, these individuals are apt to misinterpret comments made to them during discussion of their physical ailments. Special effort must be made to communicate with them carefully. The clinician must converse precisely with paranoid patients and then meticulously document what was said in order to correct later misinterpretations if they occur. These patients typically challenge conversational statements and interpret them in a personalized and idiosyncratic way as being "unfair to them."

Schizoid patients often neglect their medical care owing to their social withdrawal. Their tendency to withdraw defensively is intensified during times of physical illness or stress. Misinterpretation of physical ailments can occur owing to the patients' superstitions and unusual beliefs. When possible, the clinician should involve family members and other caregivers to ensure cooperation with treatment.

Patients' reasons for noncompliance with medical regimens should be explored. Lack of cooperation may be related to their idiosyncratic interpretations of the course of events, side effects of medications, and the meanings of symptoms.

CLUSTER B

Individuals with this group of disorders appear dramatically and emotionally labile. Their interpersonal relationships are frequently unstable, intense, and superficial. They are perceived by others as being manipulative, but they do not appear to be eccentric or odd, as do those in Cluster A. As their difficulties with interpersonal relations gradually become clearer, interactions with them can be extremely vexing to the clinician.

Antisocial Personality

This category is particularly controversial, and serious concerns have been raised about its misuse. The essential feature of antisocial personality disorder is a pervasive pattern of disregard and violation of the rights of others that begins in childhood or early adolescence and continues into adulthood. By definition, it cannot be diagnosed before 18 years of age and then only if a history of conduct disorder symptoms begins before age 15. For individuals older than 18, the diagnosis of conduct disorder is used only if the criteria for antisocial personality disorder are not met. Synonyms for antisocial personality have included psychopathy, sociopathy, or dissocial personality disorder. Because deceit and manipulation are essential features of this diagnostic category, information obtained from collateral sources must be integrated with the information gathered from the individual patient.

Some have expressed concern that this disorder is overly diagnosed in lower socioeconomic groups, and that it is underdiagnosed in women, particularly owing to the emphasis on aggressive features in the definition. The clinician must take care that this diagnosis is not inappropriately applied to individuals of lower socioeconomic strata whose apparent antisocial behavior is, in fact, part of a protective survival strategy in dysfunctional situations. Individuals with this disorder frequently appear to lack empathy and functional parenting skills.

The diagnostic criteria for antisocial personality disorder include failure to conform to social norms, especially with respect to lawful behaviors; deceitfulness, including lying and conning others for personal profit or pleasure; irritability and aggressiveness with reckless disregard for the safety of self or others; impulsivity, with failure to plan ahead; and irresponsibility in work habits and financial affairs. Persons with this disorder begin to manifest during the early teenage years dysfunctional behaviors such as lying, stealing, fighting, truancy, substance abuse, and precocious sexuality. During adulthood, these symptoms may continue as vagrancy, promiscuity, and criminal behavior. Although the hallmark of antisocial personality disorder is the inability to live within or abide by societal norms, the most pathognomonic feature is the incapacity to feel guilt or remorse. Physicians who deal with such individuals need to be on guard for malingering, drug-seeking behavior, attempts at manipulation, and real illness underlying the annoying behavior.

Borderline Personality

Often used imprecisely and incorrectly to categorize any generally difficult patient, borderline personality disorder has strict criteria for its diagnosis. Careful, as opposed to casual and pejorative, use of this term is essential, because completed suicide is reported to occur in 8 to 10 per cent of these patients, and suicide threats and attempts are very common. Other self-destructive acts, including self-mutilation, are common, and they are usually precipitated by threats of separation or rejection by important others. Self-harm, typically by burning or cutting, may bring transient relief from emotional anguish by reaffirming the ability to feel bodily sensations or by allowing the person to punish the self for being "bad." Self-mutilation often occurs during dissociative episodes, and dissociative disorders may overlap with borderline personality diagnoses. Borderline personality disorder also commonly coexists with mood disorders, and the depressions can be severe.

Impairment from the disorder and the risk of suicide are greatest in the young adult years and gradually decrease with advancing age. The majority of individuals with this disorder attain greater stability in their thirties and forties in their relationships and in their vocational functioning. Borderline personality disorder is diagnosed about three times more commonly in females than in males, and it must be distinguished from more transient identity problems occurring in adolescents and young adults, particularly when such problems are accompanied by substance abuse.

The formal diagnostic criteria for borderline personality disorder include a pervasive pattern of instability of interpersonal relationships, self-image, and affects. Other characteristics include desperate efforts to avoid real or imagined abandonment, chronically unstable but intense interpersonal relationships with alternations between extremes of ideation and devaluation, and identity disturbances with inconsistent self-image and sense of self. Patients often exhibit marked impulsivity in activities such as spending money, sex, substance abuse, reckless driving, and binge eating. Chronic feelings of emptiness and inappropriately intense feelings of anger are typical, and patients have difficulty in controlling their temper, as marked by physical and sometimes violent outbreaks. This marked reactivity of mood also extends to depression and anxiety, with intense episodes of dysphoria punctuating a baseline generalized sense of unhappiness. More transient stress may be related to paranoid ideation or significant dissociative symptoms.

Borderline personality patients invoke strong reactions in the individuals who attempt to treat them. They often lull practitioners into a false sense of security during the initial overidealization phase, only to turn on them later with sudden extreme ferocity when disappointed by the lack of fulfillment of unrealistic expectations. These patients can become vindictive and severely paranoid, greatly overpersonalizing the nature of the interaction with the health care professional. They may allege inappropriate sexual behavior on the part of the practitioner when, in fact, their own behavior may be flirtatious and seemingly inviting. They may elicit inappropriate boundary-crossing relationships with the physician and staff, thereby causing anger and confusion among the caregivers. The caregivers must establish firm professional boundaries at the outset when dealing with these patients to avoid overreaction to their provocations.

Histrionic Personality Disorder

Persons with this disorder display excessive emotionality and attention-seeking behaviors. They appear uncomfortable in groups in which they are not the center of attention, and their interactions with others are characterized by inappropriate, sexually seductive, or provocative behaviors. They use their physical appearance to draw attention to themselves and display rapidly shifting and shallow emotions. Their speech is typically excessively impressionistic and lacking in detail, with frequent overdramatization and exaggerated expressions of emotion. Patients with this disorder are easily influenced by others, and they often attempt inappropriate intimacy in professional or social relationships. They also have difficulty in achieving and maintaining genuine emotional intimacy in romantic or sexual relationships, often assuming the role of "victim" or "princess" in their relationships with others.

They may seek to control their partners through emotional manipulation or seductiveness on one level while displaying a marked dependency on them at another level. They often have impaired relationships with same-sex friends because they are sexually provocative in a way that may be threatening to others. They also alienate friends because of their excessive demands for constant attention, and when they are not the center of attention, they become depressed and upset. They crave novelty, stimulation, and excitement and typically become easily bored with their usual routine. These individuals are often intolerant of and frustrated by situations that involve delay of satisfaction, and their actions are often directed at obtaining immediate gratification. Although they may initiate a job or a project with great enthusiasm, their interest lags quickly. Long-term relationships may be neglected to make way for the excitement of new relationships.

Individuals with histrionic personality disorder often exaggerate their symptoms and display low tolerance for discomfort or pain. Stress, such as that induced by physical illness, may increase their anxiety and demanding behavior. They require repeated reassurance from the clinician as they seek increased contact and attention. Reassurance must be combined with limit-setting in the clinical setting.

Narcissistic Personality Disorder

The essential features of narcissistic personality disorder are a pervasive pattern of grandiosity, a need for admiration, and lack of empathy. These individuals have a grandiose sense of self-importance, and expect to be acknowledged as having exceptional attributes without commensurate achievements. They are preoccupied with fantasies of boundless power, success, brilliance, beauty, or idealized romantic love. They harbor the belief that they are "special" and unique and thus can be understood only by or should associate only with other equally special or high-status persons. This sense of entitlement leads to unreasonable expectations of especially favorable treatment. Others perceive them as exploitative and preoccupied with achieving their own ends while disregarding the needs or feelings of others. They are frequently arrogant and envious of people around them.

Many highly successful individuals display personality traits that can be considered narcissistic. Only when these traits become inflexible, maladaptive, and persistent and cause significant functional impairment or subjective distress do they constitute a personality disorder. Narcissistic patients may have special difficulties in adjusting to the onset of the physical and occupational limitations that are part of the normal aging process. Illness or disability is typically perceived as a personal humiliation, leading to denial of physical problems and assumption of invulnerability. Because their own self-esteem mirrors the idealized value that they assign to those with whom they associate, they are quite likely to insist on being affiliated with only the "best institutions," and they wish to have only the "top person" help them. In turn, they may devalue the credentials of anyone whose performance disappoints them, however unrealistic their expectations were.

CLUSTER C

Individuals in the groups included in cluster C are characterized by anxiety, fearfulness, and rigidity in their approach to life circumstances. Although they are not manipulative, their behaviors under stress become inappropriate and dysfunctional.

Avoidant Personality

Individuals with this disorder have a pervasive pattern of social inhibition, feelings of inadequacy, and hypersensitivity to negative evaluation. They avoid occupational activities that involve significant interpersonal contact because of fears of criticism, disapproval, or rejection. They typically consider themselves to be socially inept, personally unappealing, or inferior to others. They are unwilling to become involved with other people unless they are certain of being liked and appreciated. Fear of shame and ridicule causes restraint within intimate relationships, and preoccupation with criticism or rejection in social situations inhibits formation of new interpersonal relationships.

Avoidant behavior may begin early in life with shyness, isolation, and fear of strangers in new situations. Although some degree of shyness in children is common, it tends to gradually decrease with age. In contrast, individuals who develop avoidant personality disorder become increasingly shy and avoidant during adolescence and early adulthood when social relationships are becoming especially important. They react strongly to even the most subtle cues that suggest disapproval by others, and they exaggerate the potential dangers of ordinary situations while living a restricted lifestyle that satisfies their need for certainty and security.

Cooperative behavior with physicians may be difficult for these patients, and the clinician must remain consistently supportive and noncritical. Such an attitude helps avoid embarrassment and withdrawal behaviors that may cause noncompliance with the medical regimen.

Dependent Personality Disorder

This disorder is characterized by a pervasive and excessive need to be cared for and leads to submissive and clinging behaviors with fears of separation. Patients with dependent personality disorder have difficulty in making everyday decisions without excessive advice, assistance, and reassurance from others, and often require others to assume responsibility for most areas of their lives. They have difficulty in expressing disagreement because they unrealistically fear the loss of support or approval from others. They dread initiating projects or accomplishing tasks on their own because they lack self-confidence in their judgment or abilities. They go to excessive lengths to obtain support and nurture from others, even to the point of volunteering to perform unpleasant tasks. They feel helpless or uncomfortable when alone owing to exaggerated fears of being unable to care for themselves.

Individuals with dependent personality disorder are typically passive and allow others to take the initiative and assume responsibility for them. They often believe that others can do things better than they can and are convinced that they are incapable of functioning independently. When a close relationship with a partner or caregiver ends (e.g., because of separation or death), these patients become obsessed with the need to find someone to replace the loss. They are typically preoccupied with fears of being left to fend for themselves. In some situations, such a fear is realistic, but persons with dependent personality disorder carry their concerns to unjustifiable lengths.

These individuals can become inappropriately and excessively attached to the clinician, and the patient's dependency needs can become an onerous burden. One useful strategy is to assure them that they are being closely supervised by their doctor, accompanied by signs of approval that doctor's orders are being precisely followed. In this way, rather than fearing that they will be abandoned because they are incompetent, they are assured that they will continue to receive support and guidance from the professional whose approval and advice they crave.

Obsessive-Compulsive Personality Disorder

Obsessive-compulsive personality disorder is a well-known pattern of behavior in which individuals are preoccupied with orderliness, perfectionism, and control. This extreme need for perfection comes at the expense of flexibility, openness, and efficiency. It is characterized by a preoccupation with details, rules, lists, order, organization, or schedules to the extent that the major point of the activity is lost. These patients show perfectionism that interferes even with task completion owing to overly strict adherence to unreasonable personal standards. Excessive devotion to work often leads to the exclusion of leisure activities and friendships. Patients with this disorder are overly conscientious, scrupulous, and stubborn about matters of morality, ethics, or values. They are reluctant to delegate tasks or to work with others unless they can dictate exactly the way things will be done. They adopt a miserly spending style toward both themselves and others, and they are often unable to discard worn-out or worthless objects. Overall, their style is one of rigidity, recalcitrance, and preoccupation with perfection to the extent that it interferes with daily functioning. They are uncomfortable in the presence of others who are emotionally expressive, because they restrict their emotions in a tightly controlled or stilted fashion.

Obsessive-compulsive personality disorder must be distinguished from the similarly named condition, obsessive-compulsive disorder (OCD), which is a more serious psychiatric problem. Classified as a subtype of anxiety disorders, OCD is increasingly recognized as a medication-responsive condition. It can be differentiated from the personality disorder when behaviors such as extreme hoarding are escalated to the point of dangerousness, day-to-day functioning is impaired to a marked extent, or most especially importantly when true obsessions and compulsions present as symptoms.

Some degree of obsessive-compulsive behavior is actually adaptive in certain occupations that require great precision. Accountants, engineers, and some physicians are caricatured as behaving in these ways. The clinician must delineate when such behaviors are useful and when they are carried to excessive and unreasonable extremes. Obsessive-compulsive personality traits in moderation may be desirable, particularly in situations that reward high performance. However, when these traits are carried to an inflexible, maladaptive degree, causing significant functional impairment or subjective distress, they then constitute a personality disorder.

Patients with obsessive-compulsive personality disorder are overly devoted to exactitude in instructions, particularly concerning medication and rules of behavior, and they become easily frustrated when they perceive that the clinician's instructions regarding treatment or medication are insufficiently precise. When these patients are ill, the loss of self-control may be so overwhelming and frightening to them that it further rigidifies their inflexible behavior, leading to struggles with the health care providers caring for them. However, when they are given adequate information so that they can apply their skills at orderliness and exactitude, they are extraordinarily cooperative and obedient to the treatment plan.

PERSONALITY DISORDERS NOT OTHERWISE SPECIFIED (NOS)

This mixed category includes individuals who fulfill the criteria for more than one of the personality disorders described previously. It is also used as a miscellaneous category for several other well-known conditions that do not meet sufficiently rigorous criteria to be delineated as specific disorders.

Passive-Aggressive Personality Disorder

Individuals with passive-aggressive personality disorder mask their hostility with an overt display of cooperation. They have a pervasive pattern of passive resistance to reasonable demands for adequate social and occupational performance. Although superficially cooperating with what is demanded of them, they covertly resist by procrastinating, being irritable, having low productivity, or poor performance, protestation, forgetfulness, and unwarranted resistance to reasonable demands of authority. Chronic interpersonal difficulties develop when behavior patterns are recognized by their superiors. Their self-image is marked by a sense of victimization associated with a smoldering defense of anger and pessimism.

Because they are often unaware of the impact of their passive resistance, direct confrontation about the self-defeating nature of their behaviors is usually fruitless and can lead to destructive power struggles. The preferred strategy is to encourage them to acknowledge their frustrations and to encourage them to channel their anger into more reasonable and socially acceptable ways of behaving. These patients can be challenging for the clinician, because they voice no open opposition to a treatment plan. Instead, they subtly undermine it, complain about it, or seek to prove it worthless.

Sadistic Personality Disorder

This pervasive pattern of behavior is marked by cruel, demeaning, and aggressive behavior toward others. These individuals derive pleasure from causing suffering in others. In both social and sexual spheres, they are preoccupied with control and domination. Their repetitive patterns of cruel and restrictive actions toward those who depend on them may be a transparent defense against their own underlying feelings of weakness and dependency. These behaviors can become exaggerated when a patient loses control owing to infirmity or illness. Conversely, this pattern of behavior can emerge in caretakers of the aged or ill, particularly when a reversal of roles occurs, such as a formerly domineering parent being cared for by a previously oppressed child. The grown offspring can now seek revenge for years of past abuse by exhibiting sadism toward the ill and helpless patient. These situations may require that the authorities be alerted to elder abuse. A more common manifestation, however, is extreme impatience and intolerance of the infirmity of an elderly patient.

Self-Defeating Personality Disorder

Individuals with this disorder put themselves in situations that chronically victimize them. They have pervasive ways of interacting with others that lead to suffering and humiliation. They fail to care for themselves appropriately in many activities of daily life and may avoid seeking and complying with timely medical care, putting themselves at risk by delaying necessary treatment. They endure suffering, such as excessive pain, without complaining and deny themselves adequate opportunities for healing. They usually rationalize their maladaptive self-defeating behaviors by denying that they are putting themselves at risk by their noncompliance. Attempts to manage underlying medical illness are typically met with frustration for the clinician. Gentle confrontation and reassurance that they require and deserve good medical care can often facilitate cooperation with the care plan.

CLINICAL IMPLICATIONS

The personality disorders, as a group, present significant challenges for the clinician. Their hallmark is that they evoke extraordinary distress for those around them. The clinician's own emotional reaction to these patients is often the first clue that a personality disorder is present. Collateral information from caretakers, relatives, and others is often necessary for confirming the diagnosis when adequate evidence is not available from the patients themselves. Because the maladaptive behaviors of personality disorders are accentuated by stress, the clinicians who see these patients when they are ill are often seeing them at their worst. People whose personality disorders are merely annoying in other aspects of their lives can become vexing and frustrating for the clinician who attempts to care for them when they are sick and vulnerable. In such circumstances, these patients rely on tried and true mechanisms that have allowed them to have some sense of control over their lives.

Many medical conditions and a long list of psychiatric disorders may be initially manifested by personality changes. The differential diagnosis includes substance abuse, varieties of affective disorders (depression and its various subtypes), anxiety disorders, impulse control disorders, post-traumatic stress disorder, dissociative disorders, attention deficit disorders, late luteal phase dysphoric disorder (premenstrual syndrome [PMS]), and factitious disorders. A host of medical conditions, including neurologic problems such as postconcussion syndrome or infection with human immunodeficiency virus (HIV), can also present as changes in personality. Besides the direct effects of medical illness, personality disorders can also present as stress reactions to physical illness or fatigue in otherwise well-adapted individuals.

In the medical setting, the treatment of personality disorders is often subsumed under "good bedside manner." The experienced clinician develops a repertoire of ways of reacting to "difficult patients." Occasionally, judicious use of psychiatric consultation may confirm a diagnosis, suggest better ways of interacting with the patient, or result in referral for various types of psychotherapy. Psychotherapeutic approaches may involve individual, group, or family therapies as well as pharmacologic interventions. Useful medications include the use of antidepressants and antianxiety agents to lessen the stress and tension so that symptomatic behavior is reduced.

Hospitalization is rarely helpful or effective in the treatment of patients with personality disorders, except when their behavior escalates to life-threatening or possibly self-harmful behaviors such as suicide attempts, gestures, and self-mutilation. For the less severe types of personality disorders, self-help groups can be beneficial. These groups include "12-step groups" such as Alcoholics Anonymous (AA) and Narcotics Anonymous (NA) when coexistent abuse of alcohol or drugs is diagnosed. In other cases, involvement in supportive social organizations, such as religiously affiliated, fraternal, or civic groups, can be helpful.

Personality disorders, by definition, are pervasive and lifelong, and the prognosis usually depends on the patient's capacity for insight and willingness to cooperate with treatment. The main goal for the nonpsychiatric physician is to recognize these patterns and adjust his or her interactional style with the patient accordingly to improve patient cooperation with needed medical or surgical treatment.

SUBSTANCE USE DISORDERS

By John R. Steinberg, M.D.,
and Joel L. Sereboff, Ph.D.
Baltimore, Maryland

Substance abuse disorders, including both alcohol and drug-related dependencies, have become very prevalent and prominent national health care problems. Most individuals with these problems present at some time to a primary care health provider. Clinicians must be conversant with the signs, symptoms, and relevant diagnostic features of these disorders, which have been variously described as substance use disorders, dependencies, and addictions or given specific names such as alcoholism or cocaine addiction. All of them have certain common features.

As in any disease state, damage is minimized by early diagnosis, but a confounding issue complicates substance use disorders. The earlier in the course of disease the individual presents, the more ambiguous are the findings and historical information obtained. It is impossible to state on what given day or at what given moment a substance use disorder developed. Therefore, emphasis is placed on the core features of all addictive disorders that fall within the comprehensive generic category of chemical dependency.

At the core of the diagnosis are three concepts: loss of control, compulsive pattern of use, and adverse consequences related to use. Patients may present a rebuttal argument for these various criteria. For example, they typically claim that they are perfectly able to control their drug use or their drinking in most instances. The appropriate response is that while loss of control may not be absolute and may also be intermittent, it remains absolutely unpredictable. The individual who has a substance use disorder cannot reliably predict when control over use or drinking will be lost.

The compulsive pattern of use does not mean that all users or drinkers follow a maintenance or daily-use pattern. The compulsive pattern of use refers rather to an inappropriate emotional investment in the substance of choice. The patients often respond, "I can stop anytime I want." The health practitioner may respond by reminding patients that they certainly can stop, but that they cannot stop indefinitely and, more importantly, even when they have stopped, they cannot stop thinking about the substance.

The third core item of diagnosis is the adverse consequences that are directly related to the substance use pattern and that do not impede a return to further use. Obviously, these adverse consequences can be experienced in many different areas of life. Familial disruption and dysfunction often occur early in chemical dependency. Familial disruption may include impairment of parenting skills and disruption of marital and other intimate or significant-other relationships. Social relationships are also disrupted early in the course of disease. Individuals typically withdraw from community activity and from circles of friends not directly related to patterns of use of the substance. Financial problems may occur owing to loss of employment related to problems in the work area, a common occurrence among cocaine users. Common legal problems include arrests related to driving while intoxicated, or associated with drug possession or related criminal charges. The individual's health can be adversely affected, with changes in sexual function, appetite, and sleep patterns as well as specific organ system–related health consequences.*

PRESENTING SIGNS AND SYMPTOMS

No specific findings are absolutely diagnostic of substance use disorder, but certain general aspects of the presentation are characteristic. The presenting affect can cover a wide range of mood states, including depression, anhedonia, and emotions inappropriate to the situation in which the patient is seen. Evasiveness in response to specific questions is typical. Stimulant users may present with rapid speech or an almost hypomanic press of speech. The patient's general appearance and hygiene, or lack thereof, provides helpful clues, but the clinician should not conclude that "this patient does not look like an addict or alcoholic." Absolutely stereotypical substance use disorder patients do not exist.

COURSE OF DISEASE AND COMPLICATIONS

The course of chemical dependency disorders or substance use disorders has been described as progressive. These diseases are more aptly thought of as processes rather than events. The progression may be rapid or slow with worsening of the illness occurring in either a continuous or an intermittent fashion interspersed with periods of relative stability. Often, an increasing number of drugs are used; many individuals start with so-called gateway drugs (marijuana, nicotine, alcohol) and then proceed to use other drugs. Alcoholism typically involves increasing alcohol consumption due to both tolerance and progression of disease. Complications related to substance use disorders include trauma, infections, and exacerbations of underlying primary illnesses, such as diabetes and hypertension.

*Diagnostic and Statistical Manual of Mental Disorders, fourth edition, published in 1994 by the American Psychiatric Association, Washington, D.C.

PHYSICAL EXAMINATION

Any organ system may be involved in substance use disorders, and a comprehensive physical examination is crucial in screening for and diagnosing substance use disorders. The examination of the head, eyes, ears, and nose should focus especially on trauma resulting from falls during periods of diminished levels of consciousness. Erythematous mucosa may be seen in the nasal passages in conjunction with the insufflation of cocaine or other substances. Conjunctival injection (redness of the eyes) is a relatively nonspecific finding that may occur in conjunction with any recent drug or alcohol use. Nystagmus has also been noted in users of marijuana or phencyclidine (PCP). Pupillary dilatation or constriction can suggest drug use. Dilation of the pupils often indicates hallucinogenic or stimulant abuse, whereas constriction may indicate opiate use.

Dermatologic findings can include a number of excoriations or scabbed-over sores related to the efforts of cocaine or amphetamine users to alleviate symptoms of an imaginary infestation of parasites. Other dermatologic findings more specific to drug use include sclerosed veins or punctate sites of previous drug injections, known as "tracks."

Rapid pulse rates can be associated with volume depletion or stimulant use, and heart murmurs can result from valvular infections secondary to intravenous substance use. Refractory hypertension—in particular systolic hyperten sion—often occurs secondary to alcoholism or stimulant use.

Dry inspiratory crackles in the lungs of individuals who smoke cocaine, marijuana, or PCP may be due to fibrotic changes in the alveoli. Edema associated with pulmonary hypertension or congestive heart failure can develop after years of intravenous drug use, owing to obstruction of the pulmonary capillary bed by insoluble material used as a "cutting" agent in the preparation of street drugs.

Early in the course of alcoholism, fatty infiltration produces an enlarged, nontender liver, that can evolve into alcoholic hepatitis with tenderness to palpation in addition to enlargement. In late-stage alcoholism, the liver is often shrunken, nodular, sclerosed, and hard, indicating cirrhotic liver damage. Alcoholic pancreatitis may present with pain radiating to the back or diffuse abdominal pain.

The genitourinary system must be examined for evidence of sexually transmitted diseases. Individuals who are habitually intoxicated often engage in risky sexual behaviors. Testing for human immunodeficiency virus (HIV) infection must be considered and discussed with the patient. Individuals involved in illicit drug use on the streets may also engage in prostitution to secure drugs or money. Diffuse generalized lymphadenopathy may be an early indication of HIV infection, and specific areas of tender, swollen adenopathy suggest infection secondary to intravenous or subcutaneous drug administration.

Tremulousness or abnormal deep tendon reflexes, including hyperactive patellar reflexes, suggest alcohol-related damage. Peripheral neuropathy related to chronic alcohol use is often found in the form of a footdrop or a painful mononeuritis in peripheral nerve distributions. Use of illicit synthetic opiates has produced a parkinsonianlike syndrome due to destruction of neurons in the substantia nigra that is probably irreversible.

LABORATORY STUDIES

Laboratory data related to diagnosis of substance use disorders are obtained from toxicologic screening and other laboratory tests. Toxicologic screening procedures are designed to identify the presence of drugs or their metabolites. Other laboratory findings may reflect organ damage or abnormalities associated with illnesses induced by the substance use disorder.

Ethyl alcohol can be measured in either blood or breath. A direct relationship between the concentration of alcohol in the blood and the concentration of alcohol in the breath validates alcohol measurement by breath analysis. For clinical purposes, a blood alcohol concentration of 100 mg/dL during a routine office visit, a concentration of 200 mg/dL without impairment, or a concentration of 300 mg/dL at any time strongly suggests a diagnosis of alcoholism. For many patients, a blood alcohol concentration of 100 mg/dL implies the recent ingestion of approximately three oz of 80 proof (40 per cent) beverage alcohol and is inappropriate during a routine office visit. This information can be used to initiate the investigation of an ethyl alcohol–related disorder. Any individual who can maintain a blood alcohol concentration of 200 mg per cent without demonstrating impairment has developed tolerance, which implies regular consumption of large amounts of alcohol. A blood alcohol concentration of 300 mg/dL in a nontolerant subject typically produces stupor, sedation, ataxia, and/or slurred speech.

Other laboratory tests are also useful in diagnosing substance use disorders. Hypomagnesemia and hypophosphatemia and B vitamin deficiencies are attributed to malnutrition in alcoholics. Hypersegmented neutrophils and macrocytic anemia suggest vitamin B_{12} deficiency. Occasionally, nutritional anemia in alcoholics is reported as normocytic and normochromic because microcytic as well as macrocytic erythrocytes are present in the peripheral blood.

Increased serum γ-glutamyltransferase (GGT) activity has been touted as a sensitive indicator of significant alcohol consumption. Increased serum transaminases often reflect alcoholic liver damage. In alcoholic hepatitis, the serum concentration of aspartate aminotransferase (AST) activity is typically more than twice the concentration of alanine aminotransferase (ALT). Increased serum amylase activity suggests alcoholic pancreatitis.

Leukocytosis should be evaluated in patients with substance use disorders. Immune suppression, metabolic abnormalities, and parenteral injection of microorganisms may contribute to an increased incidence of infection in these patients.

Proteinuria has been reported in patients with heroin-induced nephropathy. Pulmonary infections may be present in individuals who smoke or inhale illicit substances. Fungal contamination of marijuana has been associated with an increased incidence of *Aspergillus* infection in cannabis users.

DIAGNOSTIC PROCEDURES AND TESTS

For many years, clinicians have used the CAGE and MAST tests to facilitate the diagnosis of alcoholism. The CAGE test asks the patient four basic questions. "C" relates to the question, "Have you ever cut down on your drinking? "A" refers to the question, "Do you get angry when people discuss your drinking with you?" "G" refers to the question, "Do you ever feel guilty about your drinking?" "E" refers to the question, "Do you ever take an eye opener in the morning?" The CAGE test is quite sensitive, but it lacks specificity. Clinicians who receive a "yes" answer to any one of the four questions should obtain a more detailed history.

The MAST test, or Michigan Alcoholism Screening Test, consists of 26 questions. Positive and negative responses are assigned various values. MAST discrepancy has become a useful diagnostic tool. First, the patient takes the MAST and self-scores it. Zero to three is negative, four to nine is suspicious, and 10 or more points is considered diagnostic of alcoholism. With the patient's permission, a "significant other" answers the same set of questions on behalf of the patient. A discrepancy of more than five points suggests excessive alcohol consumption. For example, the alcoholic spouse may score himself or herself at 6 (nondiagnostic), while the nonalcoholic spouse taking the test for the alcoholic spouse may produce a score of 20. Discrepancies in this area are more often large than small.

With the permission of the patient, the family may provide valuable corroborative information related to the patient's substance use disorder. Family members often ask the physician to raise the issue of drug or alcohol use with the patient. Psychogenic or functional illness in a family member who does not use drugs may provide a clue to a patient's substance use disorder. For example, the diagnosis of alcoholism in a female patient was made when her adolescent son presented with diffuse abdominal pain but no objective physical signs or laboratory abnormalities. Further inquiries prompted the son to say, "It's the way my mother drinks."

The clinician seeking to diagnose substance use disorder should focus on patterns, not incidents. A single incident is never diagnostic of a substance use disorder, but an overall pattern of problems related to the use of alcohol or other substances should produce a high degree of clinical suspicion.

Drug-seeking behavior (for controlled or psychoactive substances) is common in individuals whose principal substance use disorder is alcoholism or the use of illicit street drugs. Examples of drug-seeking behavior include the request for a controlled substance at the initial visit, the genuine or feigned history of allergy to nonsteroidal anti-inflammatory drugs that may compel the physician to prescribe an opiate, and the patient's air of sophisticated knowledge of drugs or false and disingenuous sense of naiveté concerning drugs. The patient who presents late at night, as the office is closing, asking for a controlled substance, may also suffer from a substance use disorder.

The clinician should focus more on the emotional tone of the patient's speech, and less on the specific content. When drug or alcohol issues are discussed, a strong emotional response most often indicates a strong emotional involvement with these substances. This emotionality can be related to the compulsive pattern of use of drugs.

PITFALLS IN DIAGNOSIS

There are several common diagnostic pitfalls and errors. The most common error is the failure to diagnose the disorder. As stated previously, no individual is exempt from this prevalent disorder. Some clinicians assign inappropriate value to laboratory data. Hematologic and metabolic tests are not very sensitive, and toxicologic tests are seldom diagnostic. No single physical finding, with the possible exception of needle injection scars, is pathognomonic of chemical dependency. Therefore, the physician should avoid excessive reliance on specific findings and rather should focus on global patterns that result from a synthesis of laboratory, historical, and physical findings.

CONCLUSION

The clinician should recall several basic principles when suggesting the diagnosis of substance use disorder to the patient. Importantly, the patient must accept the diagnosis, because individuals will not accept or comply with treatment for illnesses they do not believe they have. Physicians who diagnose and treat substance use disorders must be objective, nonjudgmental, and supportive. The diagnosis as presented to the patient should be based on objective historical, physical, and laboratory data. The physician must avoid the tiniest hint of condescension or pejorative judgment when presenting the diagnosis of a substance use disorder. Furthermore, clinicians should reassure the patient that these disorders have excellent prognoses when properly treated.

When the physician creates an atmosphere of comfortable acceptance and reassurance, the patient is more likely to accept the diagnosis of substance use disorder. This disease is common and eminently treatable, but to obtain a good outcome, the clinician must first obtain an accurate diagnosis.

ATTENTION-DEFICIT/ HYPERACTIVITY DISORDER

By Rachel E. Fargason, M.D.,
Crayton A. Fargason, Jr., M.D., M.M.,
and Lee I. Ascherman, M.D.
Birmingham, Alabama

Attention-deficit/hyperactivity disorder (ADHD) is the current term used to describe a syndrome characterized by attention difficulties and problems with impulse control and hyperactivity. The previous names used to describe this constellation of symptoms include minimal brain dysfunction; childhood hyperactivity syndrome; hyperkinetic disorder of childhood; and attention deficit disorder. ADHD is a descriptively defined syndrome that exhibits great variability in symptom clusters and symptom severity between individuals.

Historically, ADHD was believed to be a disorder of childhood that was outgrown through the process of neurologic and psychological maturation. This notion was challenged in the 1980s, when long-term follow-up studies of children with ADHD demonstrated that the syndrome persists into early adulthood in approximately one third of cases. Current estimates of the prevalence of ADHD suggest that 3 to 5 per cent of children have the disorder. Consequently, the number of adults with ADHD symptoms is probably substantial. However, the prevalence has not been reliably estimated in the general adult population. ADHD is more common in males. Females may be diagnosed later in life than males because they display less of the disruptive and aggressive behaviors that often lead to treatment in childhood.

PRESENTING SIGNS AND SYMPTOMS

The diagnosis of ADHD is based on specific criteria developed for the *Diagnostic and Statistical Manual of Mental Disorders* (DSM-IV), Fourth Edition, published by the American Psychiatric Association. These are the criteria that are most widely available. Clinicians who care for large numbers of adults with ADHD should also familiarize themselves with the Utah Criteria.* According to DSM-IV, a patient can be diagnosed with ADHD by meeting criteria for inattention ("ADHD, Predominantly Inattentive Type") or hyperactivity-impulsivity ("ADHD, Predominantly Hyperactive-Impulsive Type"). This classification is based on recent evidence that there are at least two distinct subtypes of ADHD. A patient is diagnosed "ADHD, Combined Type" when criteria for both of these subtypes are met.

To meet the DSM-IV hyperactivity-impulsivity criteria for ADHD, the patient must suffer from a dysfunctional level of hyperactivity or impulsivity as evidenced by six or more of the following symptoms:

SYMPTOMS OF HYPERACTIVITY

1. fidgets or squirms when seated
2. has difficulty in remaining seated when it is appropriate to do so
3. displays excessive motor activity when inappropriate or experiences subjective feelings of restlessness
4. has difficulty in engaging in leisure activities quietly
5. often appears "on the go" or driven
6. talks excessively

SYMPTOMS OF IMPULSIVITY

1. blurts out answers before questions are completed
2. has difficulty in waiting
3. interrupts or intrudes on others' conversations or activities

Patients with predominant symptoms of hyperactivity and impulsivity are often intrusive and lacking in social skills. They tend to be easily overaroused, hyperesthetic, and sometimes aggressive. These patients have difficulty in effectively regulating their responses to external stimuli and to internal stimuli (e.g., their own thoughts and impulses).

To meet DSM-IV criteria for ADHD, predominantly inattentive type, the patient must suffer from a dysfunctional level of inattention as reflected by at least six of the following symptoms:

1. fails to pay attention to details; has a tendency to make careless mistakes
2. has difficulty in sustaining attention
3. fails to listen when directly addressed
4. has difficulty in following through on instructions and completing tasks
5. shows disorganization in tasks and activities
6. avoids tasks requiring sustained mental effort
7. frequently loses things
8. becomes easily distracted by extraneous stimuli
9. tends to be forgetful

Patients with ADHD, inattentive type are often described as "daydreamers" or "absentminded." They often appear underactive, mentally sluggish, socially withdrawn, and clumsy. Associated learning disabilities and anxiety problems are common. Females are more likely to be diagnosed with this subtype of the disorder. Symptoms must

---

*Wender, P. H.: Pharmacological treatment of attention deficit disorder, residual type in adults. Psychopharmacol. Bull., 21:222–231, 1985.

appear before age 7, but patients may not present for treatment until much later. Adults who continue to suffer impairing symptoms without meeting full criteria are coded in DSM-IV as "ADHD, in partial remission." Patients with partial manifestations of the syndrome also benefit from diagnosis and treatment.

ADHD is a pervasive disorder, and patients are significantly impaired in at least two settings (i.e., school, work, or home or social environment). In school, they are unable to sustain attention in lectures, while reading, or when performing classroom assignments. They often procrastinate when faced with difficult assignments and then rapidly perform tasks in an impulsive manner. They misplace learning materials, books, and assignments. During examinations, they are easily distracted, and academic failure or underachievement is common.

In the workplace, patients with ADHD frequently change jobs or are fired. Impatient behavior and inappropriate comments generate conflict with superiors and customers. Careless errors, incomplete work, failure to meet deadlines, and inadequate planning of projects lead to poor performance evaluations. As a result, patients with ADHD often do not advance as expected.

Individuals with ADHD have difficulty in sustaining interpersonal relationships. Temper outbursts, craving for novelty, and impulsive behaviors can disrupt relationships. Partners are often irritated by the patient's failure to follow through on household tasks, and their inability to listen attentively. Multiple failures at school and work lead to a lack of stability, which strains spousal support.

Satisfactory school or work performance does not necessarily protect a patient from interpersonal distress. Successful ADHD patients often expend inordinate amounts of time and energy compensating for their ADHD symptoms. For example, a businessman with ADHD may work long hours in order to sustain an average performance. Success, therefore, often comes at high personal cost.

Although symptoms affect multiple aspects of a patient's life, the severity of symptoms may vary substantially in relation to the task at hand. A patient who is excited about a project may focus quite well for a period of time, sometimes even becoming hyperfocused. Performance often deteriorates, however, when the patient must address tedious details of the project or when the patient becomes fatigued or stressed. The variability in performance is often confusing to patients, family members, and clinicians because it suggests that patients can voluntarily control their behavior. As a result, performance failures are often incorrectly ascribed to poor effort.

Patients with ADHD may not recognize that they are inattentive, impulsive, or hyperactive. Instead, they often have a sense that vague personal problems explain their failure to live up to their potential. Therefore, patients often present to physicians with nonspecific complaints such as depression, insomnia, or stress-related physical symptoms. Some patients may request an evaluation for "yeast," "thyroid," or other "fad" disorders that they hope will explain their problems. Other patients present in crises from disruptions in employment and personal relationships. Because many physicians are not aware of adult ADHD, and many patients present with vague symptoms, ADHD is underdiagnosed in adults.

COURSE

No longitudinal studies have followed ADHD patients from childhood through adult life. Clinical experience suggests several possible courses for the disorder, as displayed in Figure 1.

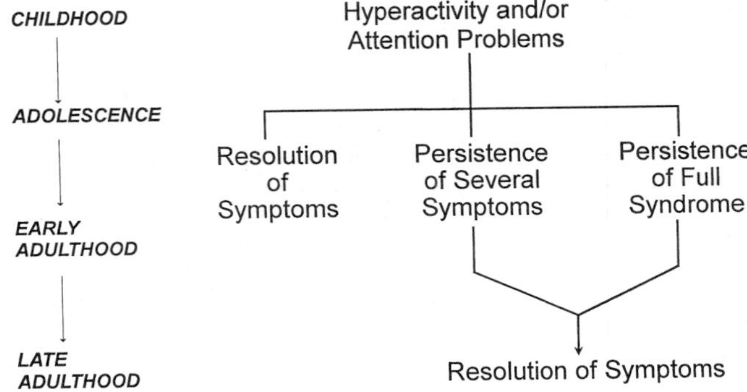

Figure 1. Course of ADHD.

ADHD begins in childhood. Hyperactivity typically peaks in early childhood; however, attention problems may not be appreciated until school age. During adolescence, most patients have noticeable improvement in their symptoms. Some experience complete remission, while others continue to experience one or two residual impairing symptoms. Hyperactivity and impulsivity resolve more frequently with maturation than do attention problems. Approximately one third of children with ADHD continue to meet DSM-IV criteria for ADHD as they enter adulthood. Individuals whose symptoms persist beyond adolescence experience a chronic course characterized by a very gradual improvement in symptoms. After adolescence, an acute exacerbation or a remission of symptoms independent of changes in medical therapy should lead the clinician to reconsider the diagnosis. By age 60, minimal symptoms remain.

COMPLICATIONS

During childhood, ADHD patients are often labeled as lazy, defiant, or dull by parents and teachers. Because of their poor social skills, patients are often spurned by peers. Such global rejection can have a negative impact on patient self-esteem. As the patient matures, the cumulative experience of failure in multiple settings results in demoralization, despair, frustration, and even suicidal thoughts. To protect themselves emotionally, ADHD patients can develop maladaptive character defenses, such as obsessional, controlling, or avoidant traits. Antisocial personality disorder frequently complicates ADHD, particularly in patients with the hyperactive-impulsive symptom complex. Adolescents with ADHD may feel that they have little to lose. They may engage in delinquent behaviors to obtain approval, even if it comes from disturbed individuals. Disturbances in personality structure create long-term functional difficulties that persist even after the ADHD symptoms have been controlled.

Substance abuse problems frequently complicate ADHD, particularly in patients with antisocial personality traits. Use of alcohol or illicit substances can begin at an early age. Such behaviors may persist, in part, as an effort to self-medicate mental or motor restlessness. Stimulant medications used in the pharmacologic management of ADHD are rarely abused by this population.

ADHD patients are at high risk for accidental injury. Impulsivity, impatience, and inattention, combined with clumsiness, can lead to frequent automobile accidents, occupational injuries, and injuries in the home. Poor regulation of temper can result in frequent physical disputes and personal injury.

DIAGNOSTIC ASSESSMENT

History and Physical Examination

The diagnosis of ADHD is established by the clinical interview. First, the clinician documents the presence of one or both of the DSM-IV symptom clusters listed earlier; a history of symptoms in childhood; and the impact of symptoms on the patient's functioning at school, work, and home. Progression of symptoms from childhood to the present is documented. Second, the clinician excludes other significant pathology. Specifically, inquiry should be made about birth trauma, congenital abnormalities, lead or other toxic exposure, central nervous system trauma, seizure disorders, and hearing or vision problems. A substance use and psychiatric history is also obtained. A legal and accident history may objectively corroborate the impact of symptoms on the patient's life.

Family members are encouraged to attend the initial interview. Spouses can provide useful information about the patient's current behavior. An older relative who remembers the patient as a child can provide a history of childhood symptoms. Old report cards reveal teachers' past perceptions of the patient in the classroom. Care should be taken to review previous diagnostic evaluations and therapeutic interventions. A previous response to psychostimulant medications, such as methylphenidate (Ritalin), does not, in isolation, establish the diagnosis. Psychostimulants have nonspecific performance-enhancing properties, even in normal individuals. A family history often reveals that other family members suffer from ADHD, substance abuse, antisocial personality disorder, and/or learning disabilities.

Minor physical anomalies are sometimes found on the physical examination. On neurologic examination, soft neurologic signs such as motor overflow movements, sequential errors in successive finger-tapping, problems with right-left discrimination, and motor clumsiness may be noted. The presence of motor or vocal tics should be assessed, as ADHD symptoms may be the earliest manifestation of Tourette's disorder. On mental status examination, the patient may show excessive motor activity, inattentiveness, distractibility, poor ability to follow long explanations or sequential instructions, and a disorganized style of answering open-ended questions. Gross disorientation, pervasive memory problems, or focal neurologic findings always suggest other neurologic conditions. While the abnormalities on mental status and physical examination, described earlier, support the diagnosis of ADHD, many patients with ADHD have no objective findings. Both children and adults with ADHD display fewer clinical signs in one-on-one interactions, such as the clinical interview, than in less structured settings.

Rating Scales

No empirically validated scales exist for diagnosing ADHD in adults. Wender designed the Parents Rating Scale* to help the clinician establish a childhood history of ADHD when evaluating an adult for the disorder. The checklist in Figure 2 can be used as a tool in establishing the diagnosis. This scale is based on the DSM-IV symptom criteria, modified to better reflect adult manifestations of the syndrome.

*Wender, P.H.: Attention-deficit/hyperactivity disorder in adults. Arch. Gen. Psychiatry, 38:449–456, 1981.

Psychological Tests

When diagnostic uncertainty persists, psychological testing can be helpful. Tests that screen for attention difficulties and impulsive tendencies are available (Table 1). Formal testing environments also allow the clinician to observe the patient while he or she works on a defined task for a prolonged period of time. A complete assessment of cognitive strengths and weaknesses is helpful to patients who face important academic or career choices. Psychological testing can also document learning disabilities or exclude other neuropsychiatric disorders. Specially trained clinicians should administer and interpret tests.

Clinicians can selectively use tests to answer specific diagnostic concerns. In addition to tests that evaluate different aspects of attention, intelligence tests, educational achievement tests, and psychiatric screening tests can be helpful. Intelligence (IQ) testing enhances the interpretation of scores on attention tasks. Educational achievement tests establish the presence of learning disorders. The Minnesota Multiphasic Personality Inventory (MMPI) and projective testing facilitate diagnosis of other psychiatric disorders. Although psychological tests are useful adjuncts to diagnosis, they are costly. When the clinical diagnosis is certain, formal testing is unnecessary.

Laboratory Evaluation

Routine laboratory tests are not indicated in the evaluation of a patient for ADHD. Laboratory studies may be performed selectively, based on the results of the history, physical examination, and psychological testing. For example, thyroid function tests are ordered in patients with clinical evidence of thyrotoxicosis or when resistance to thyroid hormone (a condition that often includes ADHD) is suspected. Toxicology screens are appropriate in patients with suspected substance abuse problems, and magnetic

Table 1. Complete Psychological Testing Battery

I. Measures of focused attention/executive function
   A. Trail Making test
   B. Wechsler Adult Intelligence Scale–Revised, Digit Symbol subtest
   C. Wisconsin Card Sorting test
   D. Verbal and Nonverbal Selective Reminding tests
II. Measures of ability to encode/manipulate information
   A. Wechsler Adult Intelligence Scale–Revised, Digit Span and Arithmetic subtests
III. Measures of sustained attention
   A. Continuous Performance test
   B. Paced Auditory Serial Addition test
IV. IQ measures
   A. Wechsler Adult Intelligence Scale–Revised
V. Achievement tests
   A. Wide Range Achievement test–Revised
   B. Woodcock Johnson Psychoeducational Battery
VI. Personality tests
   A. Minnesota Multiphasic Personality Inventory
   B. Project Personality tests
      1. Rorschach test
      2. Thematic Appreciation test

Adapted from Barkley, R. A.: *Attention Deficit Hyperactivity Disorder: A Handbook for Diagnosis and Treatment.* New York, Guildford Press, 1990; and Denckla, M. B.: Attention-deficit/hyperactivity disorder, residual type. J. Child Neurol., 6:S44–S50, 1991, with permission.

Please rate the degree to which the symptoms listed below have been a lifelong problem for you:

SYMPTOMS	Absent	Mild	Moderate	Severe
Poor attention to details; frequent mistakes				
Short attention span				
Failure to listen to others				
Avoidance of tasks requiring sustained mental effort				
Losing things				
Being easily distracted				
Forgetfulness				
Failure to follow through on duties				
Disorganization in tasks and activities				
Fidgeting or squirming when seated				
Difficulty remaining seated or feeling uncomfortable when sedentary				
Mental restlessness or moving excessively in inappropriate situations				
Difficulty engaging in quiet activities; loudness				
Being often "on the go"; "driven"				
Talking excessively				
Acting or speaking without thinking; speaking out of turn				
Interrupting or intruding on others				
Impatience, difficulty waiting				

Additional comments: ______________________________

____

____

Figure 2. Checklist of adult ADHD symptoms. (Data from American Psychiatric Association: *Diagnostic and Statistical Manual of Mental Disorders,* Fourth Edition. Washington, DC, American Psychiatric Association, 1994.)

resonance imaging and computed tomography are performed only when clinically indicated to help exclude other neurologic disorders.

POTENTIAL ERRORS AND PITFALLS IN DIAGNOSIS

A common error in the assessment of patients for ADHD is the failure to allot adequate time for the clinical interview of the patient. To compensate for an inadequate clinical assessment, some clinicians rely too heavily on the results of screening checklists or psychological tests. Psychological tests cannot replace a careful patient history. Attention problems in ADHD patients are often muted in structured and novel settings, such as a testing environment. Thus, results in the normal range on neuropsychological tests do not exclude ADHD. Conversely, severe organic or psychiatric pathology may present solely as nonspecific attention problems on some psychological tests. Correctly diagnosing ADHD requires integrating the history provided by the patient and family members with observations made during the clinical interview and testing.

Attention problems, impulsivity, and hyperactivity are nonspecific symptoms that can suggest a variety of psychiatric, medical, and neurologic conditions. ADHD should be diagnosed only after these conditions are excluded. Medical conditions that cause attention problems and hence mimic ADHD include metabolic disorders (e.g., hypoglycemia and hyponatremia); hypoxia; renal or hepatic disease; vitamin deficiency states; traumatic brain injury; sleep disorders (e.g., narcolepsy and sleep apnea); absence or complex-partial seizures; or chronic delirium of any etiology. Dementia, mental retardation, significant learning disabilities, and sensory deficits (e.g., partial deafness) may mimic ADHD. Medical syndromes that can produce symptoms of motor restlessness include hyperthyroidism, amphetamine or cocaine intoxication, alcohol or sedative withdrawal, medication toxicity (e.g., theophylline, caffeine), akathisia due to medications such as fluoxetine or antipsychotics, or agitated delirium. A history of the characteristic clustering of problems with hyperactivity, impulsivity, or attention that begin in childhood and follow a chronic, unremitting course usually distinguishes ADHD from other medical problems. Adults with acute or progressive symptoms do not have ADHD.

Psychiatric conditions often affect concentration and activity level and must also be considered in the differential diagnosis. Psychiatric problems that can be confused with ADHD include agitated major depression, thought disorders, bipolar disorder, cyclothymia (characterized by more subtle manic and depressive symptoms), or generalized anxiety disorder. Unlike ADHD, these disorders typically have a later onset, with fluctuating courses that often include periods of normalcy. Unlike the apathetic depressed patient, individuals with ADHD are enthusiastic and productive when engaged in projects that interest them. ADHD patients are excitable but do not develop the euphoria or grandiosity characteristic of mania. While symptoms of ADHD and other psychiatric disorders can be aggravated by environmental stressors, only ADHD patients characteristically become more symptomatic when bored.

Patients with personality disorders, such as antisocial or borderline personality disorders, have impulsivity and temper problems that resemble ADHD. However, these patients do not have persistent, pervasive attention problems or motor restlessness. Unlike the antisocial patient, the ADHD patient generally feels remorse following impulsive acts. While ADHD patients can be reckless, they do not demonstrate the overt self-destructive behaviors displayed by patients with borderline personality disorder.

Many psychiatric conditions coexist with ADHD. More than half of adults with ADHD suffer from generalized anxiety disorder; as many as one fourth suffer from comorbid dysthymia and cyclothymia. A significant minority of patients also have major depression, personality disorders, or obsessive-compulsive disorder. The reasons that these disorders coexist with ADHD are not clear. Patients with such psychiatric conditions may not respond to standard treatments for ADHD unless comorbid psychiatric conditions are recognized and treated. Psychiatric consultation may be helpful when psychiatric disorders are considered as the primary diagnosis, or when such conditions complicate ADHD.

While the establishment of a retrospective childhood history of ADHD is an important part of the diagnosis, a reliable childhood history may be impossible to obtain. Many individuals' memories of how they behaved as children are selective or distorted. Brighter patients with inattentive symptoms may not have experienced academic or occupational difficulties until later in life, when the intellectual complexity or time demands of their work exceeded their compensatory mechanisms. In addition, parents may minimize their child's past difficulties or may simply be unaware of them when they provide a history. Finally, parents or others who could provide information may be unavailable.

SLEEP DISORDERS

By Philip M. Becker, M.D.
Dallas, Texas

Sleep is a basic biologic function that restores mind and body. When the ability to sleep is disturbed or sleep intrudes into normal daytime activities, the cause must be investigated. With more than 70 possible sleep disorders, the clinician must employ some organizing principles to diagnose the patient's sleep disturbance. Although sleep medicine specialists have altered their nosology of sleep disorders to reflect physiology, the nonspecialist usually prefers the clinically oriented organizing principles of the disorders of insomnia, hypersomnia, biologic rhythms, and parasomnia.

Insomnia is a multifactorial disturbance of sleep that is remarkably common. Disturbances related to the initiation and/or maintenance of sleep are experienced by approximately 35 per cent of adults in industrialized countries during any year. In the United States, irregularities of sleep onset, sleep maintenance, or the restorative capacity of sleep impair the daytime function of 9 per cent of adults for months at a time. The chronic disturbance of sleep has an impact on the performance of cognitive tasks, such as complex problem solving, and on memory and lessens the patient's ability to manage shifting emotional states.

Hypersomnia is a more specific state than being tired, fatigued, or depressed. Patients may initially report these more socially acceptable symptoms. Patients with hypersomnia report that on becoming still they doze off to sleep. About 6 per cent of adults experience hypersomnia or excessive daytime sleepiness. Unlike the situation with the unwanted wakefulness of insomnia, patients who suffer from the disorders of hypersomnia may have only a vague awareness that their sleepiness intrudes into their conscious functioning. For this reason, they are involved in industrial and motor vehicle accidents two to three times more frequently than the general public.

Biologic rhythms are features of single-cell organisms and human beings alike. The rhythms of greatest importance to sleep approximate the solar day and are termed circadian rhythms (L. *circa,* about; *dies,* day). The sleep-wake cycle itself is an example. When subjects are confined in isolation from light and social cues, the hormonal processes and core body temperature, electrolyte balance, and other bodily processes demonstrate a consistent pattern of higher and lower values. Disturbances of the circadian rhythm include common problems such as shift work, jet lag, and the sleep-timing disorders of delayed sleep phase syndrome and advanced sleep phase syndrome, which are discussed later.

Parasomnias, or disorders of arousal, represent abnormal behaviors that present out of sleep. Somnambulism (sleepwalking) and sleep terrors are common in children between 3 and 8 years of age. If abnormal behaviors become dangerous, continue after age 14, or arise in adults, investigation becomes necessary. Parasomnias also encompass sleep-related seizures, enuresis, rhythmic movement disorder (head or body rocking), sleep-related bruxism, dream anxiety attacks (nightmares), and others, to be described.

Sleep disorders hide in the darkness of the night. The unconsciousness of sleep leaves the patient often unaware of the source of the problem. As soon as the patient shifts from sleep into wakefulness, the symptom disappears. It is often the bedpartner who brings the symptoms or problem to the attention of the patient and the physician. Such information is invaluable for correct diagnosis. The symptom of insomnia may herald an important emotional or lifestyle change for the patient. In the months before a clinical diagnosis of major depressive disorder can be made, patients report problems of sleep onset and maintenance. Loss, grief, and threat, whether real or imagined, are sufficient reasons in susceptible individuals to produce wakefulness in the patient who yearns to sleep.

APPROACH TO DIAGNOSIS OF SLEEP DISORDERS

The evaluation of a sleep-related symptom combines elements of both medical and psychiatric histories. Physical examination is usually of limited value. Basic information, such as age and sex, provide clues. Older patients are more likely to experience insomnia and hypersomnia from a variety of causes. Sleep apnea, periodic limb movements disorder (sleep-related myoclonus), and depression increase in incidence in patients older than 50 years of age. Older women are more likely to report insomnia, while older men experience more snoring and sleep apnea. Narcolepsy presents most commonly in young adulthood, with both sexes affected equally.

Symptom development guides the evaluation. Again, the bedpartner can offer invaluable information. For example, the physician evaluating snoring in older men often finds that the spouse can identify a worsening of the volume and quality of snoring during a period of significant weight gain in the husband. Later, excessive daytime sleepiness and the observed pauses in breathing are manifested. Specifying the onset of symptoms becomes essential in diagnosing the causes of insomnia. It is the rare insomnia patient who can state exactly when the poor sleep began. It is often helpful to ask the question, "When was the last time you were a good sleeper?" The patient who reports "never" or before age 12 years may have many complicating factors. The abrupt onset of a period of insomnia is often due to crises of anxiety—feelings of acute threat to security or ego. Far more common is the patient who had occasional bouts of insomnia that progressed into increasing difficulties of sleep onset, numerous or extended awakenings, and worsening daytime fatigue. Often, the events that precipitated the initial bouts of insomnia are of less importance in perpetuating the insomnia; factors of negative expectancy, increasing performance anxiety, and poor sleep habits often interact to maintain poorly restorative sleep.

Sleep logs help both the patient and the physician begin to specify the frequency of, severity of, and potential factors contributing to the symptom of disordered sleep. Figure 1 shows a typical sleep log. Information is best gathered for at least 7 days and nights, since weekend sleep can vary greatly from sleep during the rest of the week. The pattern and frequency of napping may point to an important factor in the symptom of insomnia. Patients with hypersomnia often report that short naps of 10 to 20 minutes prove quite refreshing and help them function during the day. Medication, both prescribed and over-the-counter, and alcohol use in the 5 hours before bedtime needs to be specified.

SLEEP DIARY

Name: ______________________ Sleep Medicine Associates of Texas

INSTRUCTIONS: Please complete each time upon awakening in the morning by rating from 1 to 5 (worst to best score).

Day & Date	Day Fatigue Level	? Minutes in Naps	Medication	Lights Out	Minutes to Fall Asleep	Times Up	Final Waking Time	Hours Slept	Type of Sleep	Rest Score
Example 5·27·91	2	2 pm for 30 min.	Aspirin 1 Beer	11:15 p.m.	75 min.	2 for 40 min.	5:15 a.m.	4 hours, 5 mins.	3	1
1										
2										
3										
4										
5										
6										
7										
8										
9										
10										

DAY FATIGUE LEVEL: use the numbers 1 (extremely tired) - 5 (rested & full of energy) to show how you felt during the past day
MINUTES IN NAPS: estimate as accurately as possible the total number of minutes you napped
MEDICATION: any over-the-counter medications, prescription drugs or alcohol taken within five (5) hours of bed
LIGHTS OUT: time when you first tried to fall asleep
MINUTES TO FALL ASLEEP: estimate as accurately as you can
TIMES UP: how often you woke up and total minutes of awake time after falling asleep
FINAL WAKING TIME: when you awake and do not fall asleep again
HOURS SLEPT: approximate time, including brief periods when you temporarily awoke after first falling asleep
TYPE OF SLEEP: use the numbers 1 (very restless) - 5 (very sound) to best show how your sleep was
REST SCORE: use the numbers 1 (exhausted) - 5 (very refreshed) to show how you feel upon awakening

Figure 1. Sleep diary.

At times patients use a medication, for example, decongestants, without realizing its disruptive effects on sleep. Alcohol is a short-lived sedative that is converted to an aldehyde, which results in sleep disruption. Many patients with insomnia develop a very irregular pattern of bedtime. They vary their times of turning out the lights or trying to fall asleep and then vary their time of final awakening. The subjective ratings of the type of sleep and its degree of refreshment help the physician determine whether the hours of reported sleep coincide with the subjective assessment of sleep quality. Individuals with sleep disorders report that no matter how many hours of sleep are obtained, refreshment of normal energy and alertness during the day does not occur.

Some sleep medicine specialists prefer to utilize a circadian sleep diary (Fig. 2). It provides a visual representation of how sleep and wakefulness occur during the 24-hour day. Circadian sleep diaries prove valuable to the clinician in assessing circadian disorders such as shift work, irregular sleep-wake schedules, delayed or advanced sleep phase syndromes, and patients who take frequent naps that may have an impact on the sleep-wake schedule.

Psychological testing proves of greatest value in assessing the symptom of insomnia. Many patients focus on the biologic disturbance in their sleep, appetite, or physical comfort. The somatic symptoms are an expression of the underlying disturbance in mood or cognitive functioning arising from psychological distress or psychiatric disorder. Standardized instruments of assessment such as the Minnesota Multiphasic Personality Inventory (MMPI), the Beck Depression Inventory, and the Zung Depression Scale can assist the physician in characterizing the nature and degree of psychological disturbance. The Millon clinical multiaxial inventory (MCMI) is particularly helpful in characterizing personality function and outlining therapeutic strategies. For disorders other than insomnia, psychological testing is best reserved for the complex or confusing case. Sleep disorders can also be an expression of an early dementing process. If memory disturbance is present on mental status examination, referral for neuropsychological assessment is indicated.

A new self-rating scale for sleepiness can also assist physicians. Dr. Murray Johns of the Epworth Hospital in Australia has developed an eight-item self-report form that correlates well with objective findings of daytime sleepiness. The patients rate themselves on a scale from 0 to 3 regarding their "chance of dozing off" in eight different situations. Figure 3 provides an example of the Epworth Sleepiness Scale. The scores range from 0 to 24. A normal score is 6 or less. Mild sleepiness yields scores between 7 and 10. A score of 11 to 15 indicates moderate sleepiness. Scores of 16 or above represent severe daytime sleepiness requiring active intervention.

Polysomnography is an overnight diagnostic study that evaluates multiple physiologic parameters simultaneously during sleep. Traditionally, such monitoring required the constant attention of a trained technologist in a sleep laboratory. Portable, in-home recording of specified physiologic channels is seeing increased use, particularly for sleep disordered breathing. The advantages of in-laboratory polysomnography come primarily with the observation and response capabilities of the trained technologist who monitors the recording of the electroencephalogram (EEG), eye movements, various electromyograms (EMGs), nasal-oral airflow, respiratory effort, electrocardiographic rhythm strip, pulse oximetry, and so forth. Specialized methods of assessment are employed for each of the disorders.

The multiple sleep latency test (MSLT) and its variants provide an objective measurement of the degree of daytime sleepiness. The MSLT is based on the principle that the speed with which a person enters sleep during a series of planned daytime naps under controlled conditions provides a measurement of the degree of daytime sleepiness. This test is often used to characterize hypersomnia and to determine whether patients enter rapid eye movement (REM) sleep during monitored (10-minute) sleeping at 2-hour intervals. The pathologic sleepiness that is found in narcolepsy and severe obstructive sleep apnea results in a mean sleep latency of 5 minutes or less from the four- or five-nap opportunities. When a patient enters REM sleep two or more times, the diagnosis of narcolepsy is made, if the patient was not sleep-deprived or had not just discontinued REM-suppressing medications. Variations of the MSLT, such as the maintenance of wakefulness test and modified assessment of sleepiness test, study the propensity of sleep onset when subjects are asked to passively resist sleepiness.

Portable or ambulatory technology continues to be devel-

2-Week Sleep Diary

1. Answer the questions in the shaded portion.
2. Draw a line through the times you were asleep.
3. Put down arrows (↓) at the times you went to bed and up arrows (↑) at the times you got up.

(1=Poor, 2=Fair, 3=Good)

	Date	Night	I took a sleeping pill: Yes	No	Each tick mark represents 1 hour (9:00 PM – Midnight – 9:00 AM)	Rate the quality of your sleep (1-3)	Rate your level of daytime alertness (1-3)	Rate your mood (1-3)
Example	1/27	Example		✓	↓ ——— ↑	2	2	1
		Night 1						
		Night 2						
		Night 3						
		Night 4						
		Night 5						
		Night 6						
		Night 7						
		Night 8						
		Night 9						
		Night 10						
		Night 11						
		Night 12						
		Night 13						
		Night 14						

Figure 2. Circadian 2-week sleep diary. (From Searle, Chicago, IL, with permission. © 1994.)

EPWORTH SLEEPINESS SCALE

Name____________________ Date____________

In contrast to just feeling tired, how likely are you to doze off or fall asleep in the following situations? (Even if you have not done some of these things recently, try to work out how they would have affected you.) Use the following scale to choose the most appropriate number for each situation:

0 = *Would never* doze
1 = *Slight chance* of dozing
2 = *Moderate chance* of dozing
3 = *High chance* of dozing

Situation	**Chance of Dozing**
Sitting & Reading	______
Watching TV	______
Sitting inactive in a public place (i.e. theatre)	______
As a car passenger for an hour without a break	______
Lying down to rest in the afternoon	______
Sitting & talking to someone	______
Sitting quietly after lunch without alcohol	______
In a car, while stopping for a few minutes in traffic	______
TOTAL SCORE	______

Figure 3. Epworth sleepiness scale: a self-report of daytime sleepiness. (From Johns, M.W.: A method for measuring daytime sleepiness: The Epworth Sleepiness Scale. Sleep 14:540–545, 1991, with permission.)

oped and refined. The experience with portable testing is limited, but promising. Actimeters, small, wristwatchlike microprocessors, record movement and assess the sleep-wake pattern by analyzing the presence or absence of limb movements. Actimeters show promise in the assessment of insomnia and disorders of circadian rhythm. In the clinical research setting, portable polysomnography has been successful in assessing various forms of insomnia, sleep apnea, sleep-related seizures, and narcolepsy. Specialized physiologic channel recorders, developed for assessing obstructive sleep apnea syndrome, range from pulse oximeters to 16-channel home polysomnography.

ASSESSING PRIMARY SLEEP DISORDERS

The history and physical examination constitute the cornerstone of proper diagnosis. In-laboratory polysomnography provides the most comprehensive assessment—but at significant cost. When sleep must be accurately evaluated, a central EEG site referenced to an opposite ear provides the standard for defining wakefulness (beta: >16 Hz). Other defined stages include relaxed wakefulness (alpha: 8 to 12 Hz), stage 1 sleep (theta: 4 to 7 Hz), stage 2 sleep (sleep spindles: 12- to 14-Hz bursts), and stage 3 and 4 sleep (delta: 0.5 to 3 Hz). Stage REM demonstrates a theta EEG plus rapid eye movements on electro-oculography and a loss of muscle tone on submental EMG. REM sleep occurs in a regular, periodic pattern at 90- to 120-minute intervals that total 18 to 25 per cent of all sleep. The percentages of the other sleep stages change with age. After age 50 years, the quantities of stage wakefulness, stage 1, and stage 2 sleep increase, whereas stages 3 and 4 constitute 0 to 5 per cent of all sleep. Sleep disorders produce even more pronounced disruptions of sleep-stage distribution.

Sleep Apnea Syndromes

Obstructive and central sleep apnea syndromes are described in detail in the respiratory section. Obstructive sleep apnea syndrome and its variants generally present as hypersomnia associated with loud, disruptive snoring. Central sleep apnea syndrome can cause hypersomnia or insomnia and is frequently associated with central nervous system pathology or heart failure.

Narcolepsy

Narcolepsy is a lifelong disorder that affects about 250,000 persons in the United States and is equally distributed between the sexes. Daytime sleepiness is usually severe and intrudes into any sedentary activity no matter how much sleep the patient has had. Persistent sleepiness typically presents between ages 12 and 25 (although younger children have been identified) with the ancillary symptoms of cataplexy, sleep paralysis, and hypnagogic hallucinations presenting 2 to 5 years later. The symptoms of narcolepsy represent the abnormal expressions of REM sleep during wakefulness. Cataplexy, reported by 50 to 70 per cent of patients, is often the most disabling symptom. Highly charged, emotional situations that involve surprise, anger, or stress often cause the embarrassing presentation of partial to complete muscular paralysis. Commonly, patients report that a funny joke or tense confrontation causes them to slur their speech, to lose head or eyelid control, and sometimes to collapse to the floor. Sleep paralysis, reported by 30 to 50 per cent of patients, represents the early onset or continuation of the normal paralysis of REM sleep while the patient is shifting from wakefulness to sleep or from sleep to wakefulness. Sleep paralysis can be frightening, as many patients struggle to breathe. Hypnagogic hallucinations, reported by 20 to 40 per cent of patients, are waking dreams that occur before drifting into sleep. Hypnopompic hallucinations occur when the patient passes from sleep into wakefulness and can be seen occasionally in normal individuals. Commonly, the patient reports sleep paralysis associated with the seemingly real appearance of a person, voices, or other sounds in the room. Only after the experience does the patient recognize it as a hallucination. Owing to the bizarre nature of cataplexy, sleep paralysis, and hypnagogic hallucinations, some patients are reluctant to share this information with their physician.

Bedpartners are often both aware of and frustrated with the symptoms of narcolepsy in their partner. The severe sleepiness can disrupt social and occupational function and the normal confrontations of a relationship can lead to the onset of cataplexy. Often, the bedpartner intervenes during the moaning of sleep paralysis or the fear of a hypnagogic or hypnopompic hallucination. In older patients with narcolepsy, bedpartners often observe snoring, pauses in breathing, and periodic limb movements of sleep, because mild to moderate obstructive sleep apnea and sleep-related myoclonus occur frequently in this group.

Sleep logs reveal normal or increased total sleep time with frequent, planned naps, but increased sleep only minimally improves daytime alertness. To diagnose a disorder of excessive sleepiness, patients are encouraged to sleep for 8 hours or more per night for 7 or more days. If daytime sleepiness continues to intrude even after adequate sleep in a patient who is not using sedating medication, narcolepsy or another cause of hypersomnia should be considered. Some narcoleptics show the paradoxical ability to maintain later bedtimes. These patients typically report that they discover themselves to be most alert in the evening.

Laboratory studies are valuable for excluding metabolic disturbances, such as hypoglycemia, hypothyroidism, and various muscle disorders. The routine EEG typically reveals a drowsy alpha pattern with no epileptiform discharges. HLA typing is most helpful in excluding narcolepsy. In white and Asian patients, nearly 100 per cent demonstrate DR2 and DQw1 positivity; both African American and white patients show positivity for DQB1*0602 and DQA1*0102. Even with this high association between DR2 and narcolepsy, narcoleptics represent only 0.3 to 1 per cent of all DR2-positive individuals in the general population, whereas 10 to 35 per cent DR2 positivity is found.

Polysomnography and MSLT must be completed after 2 weeks of abstinence from medications that affect the central nervous system or alcohol. Sleep onset at night occurs rapidly, and in nearly half of patients a sleep-onset REM period follows in about 20 minutes. REM sleep should occupy 15 to 25 per cent of total sleep. As patients with narcolepsy age, they show a reduction in sleep quality. The older patient should show only mild obstructive sleep apnea and/or periodic limb movements of sleep. In questionable cases, the apnea and movements need to be effectively treated before the MSLT is completed. On MSLT, patients with narcolepsy average a mean sleep latency of 5 minutes or less during the four- or five-nap trials. Two or more of the naps should result in the onset of REM sleep during the 10 minutes of sleep. After the initiation of treatment, the maintenance of wakefulness test provides a better means of assessing response to treatment. Portable monitoring techniques are currently being studied but are not in regular clinical use.

Idiopathic Hypersomnia (Non-REM Narcolepsy)

The excessive daytime sleepiness of idiopathic hypersomnia presents in a manner very similar to narcolepsy. Both sexes are affected equally between ages 15 and 25, frequently during times of stress. The prevalence is unknown in the general population. Sleep attacks similar to narcolepsy can occur, although many patients report a pervasive feeling of sleepiness that slows mental function. Often, long periods of sleep or naps offer no gain in alertness. Patients deny cataplexy, sleep paralysis, or hypnagogic hallucinations. Patients must have no history of central nervous system infection or trauma, since post-traumatic hypersomnia generally progresses over the 12 to 18 months after central nervous system insults. A significant minority of patients may also have associated migraines, syncope, orthostatic hypotension, and peripheral vascular changes in the hands and feet similar to Raynaud's phenomenon. Bedpartner reports should be free from snoring, apnea, myoclonus, or other abnormal behaviors in sleep.

Sleep logs reveal long sleep periods of 9 to 12 hours when the patient is allowed to sleep. The lack of refreshment results in long daytime naps as well. Epworth sleepiness scales range between 10 and 20. Laboratory testing reveals no thyroid, adrenal, or other endocrinologic abnormalities. Chemistry tests and blood counts are normal. HLA typing is not helpful; the DR2 haplotype occurs at the same frequency as that of the distribution in the general population, while the frequency of Cw2 is slightly increased. Polysomnography and MSLT reveal patterns of extended, normal nocturnal sleep with continued daytime sleepiness that commonly average a mean of 5 to 10 minutes for the four- or five-nap trials. Latency to the first period of nocturnal REM sleep is a normal 70 minutes or longer, and there are no REM onset naps. Any apnea or myoclonus that is found must be insufficient to account for the sleepiness. A trial of a central nervous system psychostimulant, such as methylphenidate or dextroamphetamine, offers little improvement in the sleepiness and frequently produces the side effects of headache and dysphoria. Actimeters can document the long sleep periods with minimal movements.

Restless Legs Syndrome

The disagreeable leg sensations that intensify in the hours before bedtime significantly affect 2 to 5 per cent of adults, with both sexes equally represented. Some investigators estimate the frequency of restless legs syndrome (RLS) to be as high as 18 per cent of individuals who are middle-aged or older. Patients typically describe the sensation as variable, bilateral restlessness deep in the calves that increasingly compels them to move. Movement relieves the sensation, which is variously reported as "creepy," "crawly," "like worms," "heebie-jeebies," "pulling," or "aching." In its most severe presentations, RLS can progress to affect the thighs, the feet, and, rarely, the arms. The increased activity of RLS in the evening often impedes sleep onset. Other times of extended rest, such as when the patient is a passenger in a car or plane, can also cause RLS to appear during the day. Patients often report that they obtain their best sleep after 4:00 AM, when RLS lessens in intensity. Although sleep-onset insomnia represents the most common symptom, periodic limb movement disorder (PLMD), or sleep-related myoclonus, to be described later, often creates sleep-maintenance insomnia and/or hypersomnia during the day. Unless a coexistent neuropathy is present, the patient with RLS should show no deficits in sensory or motor testing. RLS is commonly noted during pregnancy, anemia, nephritis, and rheumatoid arthritis.

Bedpartner reports reveal the presence of restlessness and tossing and turning at sleep onset. Some report that their partner rubs or stretches the legs. When the RLS patient finally falls asleep, the observant bedpartner may note regular flexion, jerks, or periodic leg movements of sleep in the feet and legs. In its most severe form, the bedpartner may be kicked awake. Sleep logs show sleep onsets of 20 to 120 minutes in length. At times, patients are so tired that they fall asleep rapidly but then awaken 15 to 60 minutes later and pace for 1 to 2 hours before returning to bed. Awakenings due to leg restlessness can occur, as well as extended awakenings from unrecognized PLMD. In more severe cases, patients show total sleep times of 3 or 4 hours, with the best sleep obtained just before arising. Daytime naps are frequent if they can be taken.

Psychological testing often reveals higher levels of anxiety and depression, which at times can be severe and debilitating. Treatment of depression can be more difficult because antidepressants are known to exacerbate RLS. To exclude metabolic or neurologic disorders, laboratory testing includes a complete blood count (CBC), iron, folate, vitamin B_{12}, liver profile, thyroid function tests, and creatinine. Neuropathies may require electromyographic or nerve conduction studies. Myelopathies are generally not confused with RLS. Polysomnography reveals extended periods of wakefulness punctuated by both voluntary and involuntary movements. At times, the restriction of the monitoring environment becomes stressful for the patient. When sleep arrives, myoclonic movements often result in arousals and sometimes full awakenings (see section on PLMD later). The movements typically decrease, and sleep quality improves in the last half of the sleep period. MSLT reveals moderately excessive daytime sleepiness, with the mean sleep latencies falling between 5 and 10 minutes. Portable monitoring is being tested. Actimeters placed on the legs show increased activity in the evening and while the patient sleeps. Some recorders measure electromyographic activity, acceleration or movement by piezoelectric strain gauge often in association with EEG monitoring. These techniques will see greater use in the future.

Periodic Limb Movement Disorder (Sleep-Related Myoclonus)

Periodic limb movement disorder (PLMD) most commonly presents as a brief Babinski-like extension of the great toe with partial flexion of the ankle and knee, and sometimes the hip. Patients are usually unaware of the 1- to 2-second flexion of the lower limb but may report poorly restorative sleep and awakening for uncertain reasons during the night. Daytime sleepiness, reflected in Epworth Sleepiness scores above 10, is often present. The frequency of PLMD can vary greatly from one night to the next. PLMD is less common in the upper extremities. As noted previously, periodic movements of sleep are seen in more than 80 per cent of patients who have RLS. In the most severe forms, daytime movements can occur. PLMD is an expression of an underlying neuromuscular process that appears more commonly during metabolic dysfunction, such as uremia, and during ingestion of or withdrawal from agents that affect the central nervous system, such as caffeine, antidepressants, barbiturates, anticonvulsants, and anticholinergic agents. The prevalence remains unknown, although estimates range from 1 per cent of young adults to 30 per cent or more of patients older than 60 years of age who report sleep-maintenance insomnia.

Bedpartners may or may not be aware of the movements. Observation must occur over a period of 10 minutes or more to recognize the periodic flexion and relaxation of the leg movements. The more severe disorder that produces vigorous flexion and frequent movement is the one that bedpartners usually recognize, particularly if they have been kicked. Sleep logs do not help the physician arrive at the diagnosis of PLMD. Typically, the log reveals increased awakenings, poorly restorative sleep, and daytime sleepiness that seems more severe than would be expected by reported sleep loss alone. Patients with PLMD often nap when they are able.

Psychological testing may show mild or moderate anxiety and depression that can confuse the diagnostic impressions. Polysomnography is often the method of discovery of PLMD. The stereotypical, repetitive movements are most commonly recorded from bilateral anterior tibialis EMG during non-REM sleep. The EMG contractions last from 0.5 to 5 seconds in either one or both of the legs, followed by 5 to 90 seconds of normal EMG activity. At fixed intervals that are often 20 to 40 seconds in length, the EMG bursts occur. Recording from the central EEG reveals an associated brief arousal of 3 to 15 seconds. Sometimes, a fully conscious awakening occurs. The diagnosis of PLMD can be made if the patient reports insomnia and/or hypersomnia in association with an hourly rate of five or more of the stereotypical, repetitive movements that lead to arousals or awakening. Most patients with significant PLMD show 25 or more movement-related arousals per sleep hour. MSLT is usually not needed unless the symptom of daytime sleepiness produces significant occupational dysfunction. As described for RLS, portable testing is under investigation with equipment that can characterize the frequency and intensity of movements and also the EEG arousals and awakenings.

ASSESSING INSOMNIA

The evaluation of insomnia can be approached with a variety of methods. Transient insomnia is easily identified, as it is common and occurs in good sleepers who find themselves under acute stress or time zone changes. Short-term insomnia lasts for up to 3 weeks and represents a shift in lifestyle, a real or potential threat or loss, or bereavement. In the predisposed individual, the changes in sleep may develop into chronic insomnia. The patient with insomnia typically experiences reduced daytime cognitive function, diminished emotional control, or sleepiness and tiredness. Short sleepers who require less than 6 hours of sleep per night may be falsely characterized as insomniacs.

Clinical Evaluation

Insomnia is a symptomatic complaint that can arise from over 20 different disorders. When the symptom of lengthened sleep onset, frequent or extended awakenings, early-morning awakening, or poorly restorative sleep has gone on for months, more than one disorder is usually responsible for the perpetuation of the complaint. Chronic insomnia affects 9 per cent of adults, and older individuals, particularly women, are more significantly represented. Psychiatric disorders, particularly depression and anxiety, may be the primary factors in approximately 50 per cent of chronic insomnia sufferers. RLS and PLMD are the most common primary sleep disorders, causing chronic insomnia in about 15 per cent of patients. The majority of patients also develop maladaptive behaviors in relation to their increasingly frustrating attempts to sleep. When maladaptive behaviors become conditioned negative responses that produce activation as the patient retires to the bedroom, the disorder is called psychophysiologic insomnia. With any chronic insomnia, the patient must learn to follow a routine that promotes good sleep hygiene and enhances sleep-compatible behaviors. Substances such as caffeine, alcohol, and some sleeping pills can also interfere with sleep and should be avoided.

A 3-minute interview for the evaluation of insomnia can direct the further exploration and treatment of patients with chronic insomnia. When the symptoms of sleep disturbance and daytime dysfunction have lasted for 3 weeks or more, six lines of symptomatic exploration are warranted. Line 1 requires the physician to establish whether any neurologic, metabolic, endocrinologic, or cardiopulmonary disorder accounts for the problem. For the vast majority of patients, an occult disease is very unlikely without other symptomatic presentations of an illness. Line 2 of investigation is helpful when the insomnia has developed during the last year. The physician inquires about any correlated changes in substance use (e.g., caffeine, alcohol, decongestant pills or spray), prescribed or over-the-counter medication, stressful experiences at work or in the home (even when the patient dismisses their significance), or chronic medical problems that result in pain or a threat to normal function.

Line 3 investigates psychiatric causes by asking a general question such as, "Are you feeling sad, blue, down, or depressed?" or "How nervous, tense, worried, or stressed do you feel?" Some may prefer a symptomatic report on a scale "1 to 10": "How depressed (or anxious/stressed) do you feel this week, with 1 being the most depressed (anxious) you've ever felt and with 10 being the best?" Higher levels of agitation, irritability, guilt, hopelessness, or changes in appetite or libido increase suspicions about mood disorders, such as major depression or mania-hypomania, and anxiety disorders such as generalized anxiety disorder or panic disorder. Anxiety disorders usually persist through both night and day, and worry, apprehension, and dread concern the anxious patient more as bedtime approaches. Many patients, some with psychiatric disorders, report that they have "no problems."

When the physician is reasonably certain that the patient's moods are stable, line 4 of investigation seeks conditioned factors that have become linked to attempts to sleep. A helpful question is "Do you sometimes sleep better out of your own bedroom, such as on the couch or in another bed at home or on a trip?" Patients with psychophysiologic insomnia report improved sleep in unexpected places, since these locations are not linked to the activation of trying to sleep. Such patients tend to practice sleep-incompatible behaviors, such as napping, using caffeine to improve daytime alertness, using alcohol to assist sleep onset, varying bedtimes, and then sleeping late whenever possible. They often remain in bed for hours at a time in the hope of capturing any minute of sleep. The practice of lying in bed while awake often results in light sleep and wakefulness during sleep, defeating the expected result.

Line 5 of questioning explores misalignment of the circadian sleepy phase with society's sleep schedule of 11:00 PM to 7:00 AM. Delayed and advanced sleep phase syndromes are described later. When patients are free from responsibilities, they often sleep when their bodies want to sleep. When the history offers few clues to the diagnosis, line 6 of inquiry pursues the primary sleep disorders of obstructive and central sleep apnea, RLS, and PLMD, as described previously. Polysomnography can be helpful in further documenting and elucidating possible causes. Polysomnography becomes essential when pharmacologic and behavioral interventions have failed or have lost effectiveness.

Sleep logs of 7 to 14 days of data represent a helpful tool in the diagnosis of insomnia. Both patients and physicians make unexpected discoveries from the data. Patterns of better sleep on weekends and poor sleep on Sunday night point to irregularity in the sleep-wake cycle or work-related stresses. Patients should keep track of one or two possible factors that worsen sleep, for example, conflicts with spouse or coworkers, late-night work, and evening conversations. The sleep log can reveal whether the presence or absence of the factors influences sleep either positively or negatively. The sleep log also helps during therapy because patients tend to remember the bad nights, but not the good nights. Exploring better nights helps patients realize that they can successfully sleep.

Psychological testing with the MMPI, Beck or Zung Depressive Inventory, or MCMI may reveal psychological issues and personality styles that worsen sleep. When psychopathology is significant, referral to a psychiatrist or psychologist is indicated. Polysomnography is reserved for the diagnostic dilemma, therapeutic failures, or patients who present with possible sleep apnea or myoclonus. In as many as 60 per cent of cases, polysomnography can focus treatment, but it only occasionally results in the discovery of totally unexpected findings. Often, a patient's response to the monitoring environment reveals important issues of perception, control, anxiety, and expectancy that were not as prominent during daytime sessions or even in psychological testing. The MSLT is usually of little to no clinical value in diagnosing insomnia. Portable testing remains an area of serious study in insomnia. Studying patients in their natural environment is helpful. The most widely used instrument is the actimeter, which records the time of movement over 7 to 30 days. Portable polysomnographic systems have also been successfully utilized.

CIRCADIAN DISORDERS

The biologic rhythm of sleep remains closely linked to the nighttime hours for more than 90 per cent of the population. When the sleep-wake rhythm strays from the nighttime hours by design, habit, or internal abnormality, a circadian disorder arises. The most common disorders involving misalignment of biologic time with solar time include time zone change (jet lag) syndrome, shift work sleep disorder, delayed sleep phase syndrome, and advanced sleep phase syndrome.

Time Zone Change (Jet Lag) Syndrome

On rapid time zone change of 2 hours or more, most people experience symptoms of insomnia, hypersomnia, and daytime problems of reduced alertness, decreased mood, diminished performance, and physical discomfort. Eastward jet flight, e.g., such as from the United States to Europe, typically results in the most significant problem of adjustment. An 11:00 PM bedtime in Paris would be a 5:00 PM alert phase in Chicago or Dallas. The circadian rhythm asynchrony of the midwestern visitor to Paris results in sleep-onset insomnia, frequent awakenings, and then sleepiness during the Parisian morning that continues for 2 or 3 days. Adjustment of physiologic processes may take 8 days or more. Westward flights tend to be easier on travelers in their adjustment to the new sleep-wake rhythm. Older individuals report more symptoms of jet lag, including insomnia, malaise, daytime sleepiness, reduced concentration, inattentiveness, and gastrointestinal upset. Evaluation beyond symptom reports or sleep logs is not needed. When symptoms last for 2 weeks or longer, other sleep disorders must be investigated. Prophylactic treatment has been proposed. Experimental methods of evaluation have included polysomnography, MSLT, actimeters, core body thermometry, and hormonal rhythms.

Shift Work Disorder

Night work and rotating shifts are required of as many as 8 per cent of the adult population in industrialized countries. On completion of the night shift, between 40 and 50 per cent of workers report sleep-onset insomnia and early awakening from sleep before they feel rested. Total daytime sleep averages 3 to 6 hours, and return to work on the next night increases the chances of falling asleep on the job. Patients report fatigue, malaise, reduced alertness on the job, irritability, and gastrointestinal upset. Again, older subjects tend to be affected more severely. Some research suggests chronic night work increases the risks of cardiovascular disease, family conflict, and abuse of alcohol and sedative or stimulating drugs.

Evaluation is most appropriate for the severe case or when symptoms of other sleep disorders are elicited and require further assessment. Circadian sleep logs aid the clinician in evaluating the pattern over 2 weeks or longer of normal and abnormal sleep. Portable testing with the actimeter can be unobtrusively offered to document the pattern of sleep, wakefulness, and lapses into sleep while the patient is on the job. Polysomnography is used infrequently, because it must be repeated during both work and nonwork periods.

Delayed Sleep Phase Syndrome

Delayed sleep phase syndrome results in sleep-onset insomnia and major difficulties in arising at the usual times of the morning. When patients with delayed sleep phase syndrome are allowed to sleep for a week or longer on their own schedule, they typically fall asleep at about the same hour sometime after 2:00 AM and then sleep well with few awakenings until 11:00 AM or later. These patients are the ultimate "night owls," who struggle with sleepiness when awake in the morning. This syndrome appears to be a disorder of young adults; as many as 7 per cent of adolescents have academic and social impairment due to their delayed sleepy phase. The parent often brings an adolescent or young adult child to the physician. Oppositional behavior and conflicts are often apparent. If a sedative-hypnotic agent has been tried, it usually loses effectiveness within a week or two.

Evaluation includes a review of other potential sources of insomnia, including depression, psychophysiologic insomnia, and RLS. Psychological testing can be helpful in assessing mood and personality issues. Some patients may have anxiety disorders or avoidant personality disorder. A circadian sleep diary kept for a period of 2 weeks or more reveals delayed sleep onsets during the school or work week, with arising times on weekends in the midafternoon. Experimental testing includes portable testing with actimeters, rectal temperature recording, and the dim-light melatonin onset test. Polysomnography reveals normal sleep without primary sleep disorders after the delayed onset of sleep. Polysomnography and MSLT are usually not needed unless other sleep disorders, particularly narcolepsy, are suspected. The patient with delayed sleep phase syndrome infrequently experiences sleepiness past 3:00 PM, but the patient with narcolepsy experiences sleepiness through most of the day.

Advanced Sleep Phase Syndrome

Advanced sleep phase syndrome is the reverse of the delayed form. The patient, usually older than 50 years of age, reports awakening too early, after only 3 or 4 hours of sleep. Questioning reveals that the patient must resist sleepiness in the later evening. Older patients often choose to retire at 8:00 or 9:00 PM and then awake in the middle of the night, complaining about their inability to return to sleep. Patients often avoid evening social gatherings because of their difficulties with drowsiness.

Evaluation must consider major depression as a potential factor. If the clinical history and psychological testing show normal mood, a circadian sleep diary should be kept for 2 weeks. Polysomnography may have a role in excluding the sleep apnea and myoclonus that occur at a greater frequency in the over-50 age group. Portable testing, similar to that for delayed sleep phase syndrome, can offer documentation of the advanced sleepy phase.

PARASOMNIAS

Nearly 30 disorders result from a physical disturbance that arises during sleep-related arousal, partial arousal, or sleep stage transition. Parasomnias are subclassified into the arousal disorders, the sleep-wake transition disorders, REM-related disorders, and other parasomnias.

The arousal disorders are the most common and best described parasomnias. Sleepwalking (somnambulism) and sleep terrors (pavor nocturnus in children or incubus in adults) are seen most frequently in younger children who have an abrupt presentation of sitting up, walking, or confused screaming during the first 1 to 3 hours of sleep. In its most severe presentation, the person may engage in dangerous behavior, such as running into walls or windows or exiting the home. Attempts at awakening can result in striking out or fighting. Sleepwalking and sleep terrors occur out of stage 3 and 4 sleep, which accounts for the high prevalence of all arousal disorders throughout childhood as well as the typical complete or partial amnesia for the event. Confusional arousals (sleep drunkenness, excessive sleep inertia) also present out of stage 3 and 4 sleep with disorientation, slowed cognition, and memory disturbance lasting from minutes to, rarely, hours. Evaluation with polysomnography is helpful when the clinical diagnosis alone is uncertain, the behavior presents *de novo* in adults, or partial complex seizures with automatisms are suspected.

Sleep-wake transition disorders—rhythmic movement disorder (jactatio capitis nocturna, head or body rocking or rolling), sleep starts (hypnic jerks, predormital myoclonus), sleeptalking (somniloquism), and nocturnal leg cramps (charley horse)—occur as a normal physiologic response to drifting into or out of sleep.

Rhythmic movement disorders, with the head being the most common site of movement, appear to be a normal self-rocking motion of young childhood that assists sleep onset. Movements in older children are more commonly associated with mental retardation, autism, psychopathology and, rarely, epilepsy. Sleep starts, sleeptalking, and nocturnal leg cramps are normal behavioral responses, particularly during times of increased fatigue and stress. The history alone is usually adequate for diagnosis unless the presentation is obscured by other factors; in this case, polysomnography or an EEG should be considered.

Parasomnias are usually associated with REM sleep owing to the unique cognitive and physiologic characteristics of REM sleep. In nightmares patients are able to describe in detail the frightening or anxious dream. Nightmares are common in children and are also seen more frequently in adults with personality disorders or in family members of patients with psychiatric disorder. Medications can also induce nightmares in adults. REM behavior disorder exhibits not only nightmares but also the physical acting out of their content. Bedpartners report yelling, kicking, running, or fighting, while the patient can describe in detail the dream content. Patients with REM behavior disorder have lost the ability to maintain the paralysis of REM sleep. In sleep paralysis, patients enter or awaken from sleep with the recognition of the paralysis. The disorder represents a state of dissociation between REM sleep and wakefulness that can prove frightening, as the motor control of arms, legs, and accessory respiratory muscles is temporarily interrupted. Sleep paralysis is a common feature of narcolepsy; therefore, other symptoms of narcolepsy—daytime sleepiness, cataplexy, hypnagogic hallucination, automatic behavior—should be reviewed. Polysomnography for these disorders can prove helpful in documenting their behavioral presentation during REM sleep, although the variability in their presentation may make confirmation on a single night difficult.

PSYCHIATRIC EMERGENCIES

By Michelle Biros, M.S., M.D.
Minneapolis, Minnesota

An acute psychiatric emergency is any condition that causes impairment of thought, behavior, mood, or social interactions and requires immediate intervention to prevent patient injury or further deterioration. In the emergent setting, this diagnosis is usually initiated by individuals who know the patient and who are not health care providers. These concerned individuals can usually describe the specifics of the presentation much better than the patient, who may not have adequate insight into his or her present condition.

As many as 30 per cent of all patients evaluated in urban emergency departments (EDs) are seen for symptoms related to a change in mental status or behavior. As many as 40 per cent of all urban ED patients also carry a previous diagnosis of a psychiatric disease. One goal of the ED evaluation of these patients is to distinguish medical causes from psychiatric causes of the acute change in mental status.

In patients with known psychiatric illnesses, ED visits are often prompted by a worsening of the mental disorder, suicidal or homicidal behavior, indiscriminate assaultive actions or violence toward social contacts, or unacceptable side effects of medications used for treatment. In patients with no known psychiatric diagnosis, the acute presentation may be the first indication of an undiagnosed mental disorder or a medical condition presenting with behavioral or thought abnormalities. As many as 40 per cent of patients with acute changes in mental status may have a mixture of both. A previous history of a psychiatric disorder should not bias the clinician in evaluating the current problem. Various medical causes of acute changes in mental status are potentially life-threatening; thus, all patients presenting with altered mental status should be thoroughly evaluated for medical conditions before the clinician assumes that the current presentation can be attributed to a previously diagnosed psychiatric disorder.

ACUTE PSYCHOSIS

Psychosis is generally defined as dysfunction of thought process from any cause. Psychosis attributed to medical causes can be related to definable pathophysiologic abnormalities. When psychosis occurs secondary to psychiatric disease, the neuropathologic basis of the psychosis may not yet be defined or may not be apparent on initial or routine testing. Distinguishing medical causes from psychiatric causes of psychoses can be extremely important because the medical disorders underlying an acute psychotic episode can involve rapidly progressing, life-threatening pathophysiologic processes.

Medical psychoses can present as either dementia or delirium. Dementia reflects chronic, gradually progressive brain dysfunction. Many demented patients come to medical attention as a result of recent changes in behavior. However, a careful history obtained from family members often reveals a long-standing chronic decline in mental functioning. By contrast, delirium reflects acute brain dysfunction. Delirious patients often deteriorate rapidly due to progression of their underlying disorder.

In urban areas, most acute psychoses have medical causes. Abuse, intoxication, and withdrawal from alcohol and other drugs are among the most frequent causes of acute psychoses. Other frequent causes of acute psychosis include infection, metabolic disturbances, central nervous system disorders, hypoxia, and any cardiac dysfunction that interrupts cerebral blood flow. Acute psychoses associated with psychiatric diseases can be classified as disorders of thought content (the schizophrenic disorders) or disorders of mood (affective disorders).

Table 1. Diagnostic Precepts for Acutely Psychotic Patients

Assume that all patients have a medical cause of acute psychosis until proved otherwise
The current episode may not have the same etiology as previous ones
Demented patients may lie to cover up memory deterioration
Medical and psychiatric dysfunction can occur in the same patient
Mental status changes in the extremes of age are usually due to medical diseases
Immediate diagnosis may not be possible; exclude life-threatening conditions
Never leave a suicidal or violent patient unmonitored

Table 3. Pertinent Medical History in Acute Psychosis

Recent trauma, surgery, illness
Recent medications and changes
Past medical problems and medications
Recent symptoms
Onset and duration of symptoms
Acute changes in symptoms
Prior similar episodes
Substance use and/or abuse
Exposure to toxins
Current medications

Initial Stabilization

Even before distinguishing whether the acute psychosis is due to a medical or psychiatric cause, the physician must make decisions regarding the emergency management of these critically ill patients (Tables 1 to 3). When an acutely psychotic patient presents to the ED, health care providers should have a realistic expectation of what can be done for him or her. These patients are psychotic and therefore are irrational in their behavior. For the benefit of the patient, as well as for the protection of those around them, it is important to ensure that the environment is safe. Steps must be taken to control and limit potential physical aggression so as to reduce the number of individuals exposed to a potentially harmful situation. If possible, the patient should be isolated so that the noise and confusion of the ED does not aggravate the patient's condition. Extremely agitated patients who are isolated require frequent monitoring. In some institutions, video cameras are available that allow this monitoring to occur from a distance. When patients are not in the direct line of vision of health care providers, it is essential that the video monitor be checked at regular intervals to ensure the patient's level of consciousness and level of activity.

As with any acutely ill patient, the psychotic patient should be evaluated immediately. It is not appropriate to delay the initial medical assessment of the acutely psychotic patient until he or she becomes cooperative. At the very least, the airway, breathing, and circulatory status (ABC) of the patient should be assessed, and any identified compromise should be addressed immediately. Vital signs should be obtained as soon as it is feasible to do so. The finer points of the examination can be pursued later. Abnormal neurologic findings sometimes identify potentially lethal causes of acute psychoses. Therefore, the neurologic examination needs to be performed as soon as possible. In patients who are acutely psychotic, a basic neurologic examination should be considered part of the primary survey. This examination should include pupillary findings, mental status, and motor movement.

Agitated psychotic patients typically do not respond to verbal attempts to control behavior, but unless the patient's agitation or threatening behavior is controlled, an adequate assessment is impossible. Physical restraints provide one means of reducing physical threat to caretakers as well as reducing the potential for self-injury to the patient. Often, a show of force defuses potential violence, and a team approach to physical restraint is advocated by most authorities. Caretakers must remember that overly enthusiastic physical restraint may result in physical injury. Restraining a patient is an attempt to control and subdue the patient so that subsequent evaluation and management can occur. During physical restraint, the patient must be frequently and carefully monitored. Restrained patients can writhe around, struggle against the restraint, and do themselves harm. These patients lose many survival skills and are prone to complications from this loss. For example, restrained patients who vomit can aspirate the vomitus if they are not positioned properly or have, through struggling, moved themselves into an unsafe position.

Table 2. Emergency Management of Acutely Psychotic Patients

Assess vital functions and vital signs
Establish a safe, controlled treatment environment
Recognize and reverse life-threatening conditions
Assess mental and neurologic status
Determine whether psychosis is organic or functional
Prevent progression or complications of the causative disorder
Initiate definitive therapy based on the cause
Determine appropriate disposition as a patient advocate

In some patients, agitation or violent behavior prevents any reasonable examination. This situation has the potential to delay the diagnosis of a serious medical problem. Under these circumstances, antipsychotic medication may be required in addition to physical restraints. Since these drugs can often cause sedation, the patient must be frequently reassessed for respiratory and hemodynamic status. Antipsychotic drugs are very effective in reducing agitation or aggressive behavior from any cause. Haloperidol and droperidol are most frequently administered. Doses are determined by the presence of target symptoms such as acute agitation and hallucinations. If the psychosis is due to a psychiatric cause, these drugs are the first step in definitive treatment.

Blood glucose should be measured, and hypoglycemia treated. Cardiac dysrhythmias with concurrent blood pressure alterations should be treated as indicated, because decreased cerebral blood flow may be the basis of the abnormal mental status. Hypoxia, from any cause, can also alter mental status, and supplemental oxygen should be initiated. Most ambulance services do not carry antipsychotic drugs, such as haloperidol and droperidol, but most carry diazepam for use in seizure control. In circumstances where an extremely agitated patient is being brought to the ED by ambulance, sedation should be considered for reducing agitation and anxiety. A pertinent medical history may need to be elicited from a friend or relative who is well acquainted with the patient prior to the onset of the acute episode (see Table 3).

Emergency Evaluation

After the patient has been stabilized and agitated behavior has been controlled, continued evaluation in the ED can occur. Patients with acute psychoses typically have poor insight into their own needs. Patients who are disheveled and have apparently neglected their self-care are at risk for harboring other injuries or illnesses in addition to their acute psychoses. Therefore, in all psychotic patients, a complete physical examination is required for detecting occult injury or signs of systemic illness.

On completion of the physical examination, attention is given to the mental status examination to help distinguish between medical and psychiatric causes of acute psychosis. Often, much information can be obtained from simple observation of the patient. The patient's general appearance and behavior provide insight into the current level of functioning. It is often easy to determine whether a patient is acutely hallucinating by watching them when they believe they are not being observed.

A formal mental status examination may not always be possible if the acutely psychotic patient is unable to cooperate with the examination. Some key elements to be assessed include the following:

PATIENT MOOD. Patient mood assessment examines the patient's current affect. A good way of gauging patient mood is to see what kind of emotional response your interaction with the patient elicits in you. If you feel unsafe or threatened by a psychotic patient after completion of the medical interview, you probably are.

PATIENT ORIENTATION. Determining the patient's orientation is important, since it assists in the differentiation between medical and psychiatric causes of acute psychoses. In most cases of medical delirium, orientation to person is the last point of orientation to be lost. Some patients with dementia confabulate to avoid detection of their condition. They understand that their thinking is not clear and are embarrassed by this, so they attempt to delude interviewers into believing that their thinking is actually normal. In this circumstance, it is important to avoid asking orientation questions in a manner that allows the patient to evade the question. This can sidetrack the inexperienced clinician.

TRAIN AND CONTENT OF THOUGHTS. This assessment determines whether the thought process that the patient is undergoing is logical and whether the ideas expressed are consistent with reality. The easiest way of assessing for these qualities is to determine if what the patient says makes sense or if it confuses the interviewer.

PERCEPTION. Hallucinations are false perceptions of reality that occur when the patient is fully awake and conscious. In psychoses from psychiatric disorders, patients usually reveal their hallucinations if directly asked. They have poor insight into their condition and therefore do not believe that their hallucinations are abnormal. In psychiatric disorders, most hallucinations are auditory. If the patient states that auditory hallucinations consist of more than one voice or that there are several voices arguing or partaking in an ongoing conversation, the diagnosis of schizophrenia should be entertained. The hallucinations from medical causes of psychosis may be visual or auditory and can often be assessed by direct observation of the behavior of the patient. Delusions are fixed false perceptions of reality that are not changeable by argument or fact and are not held by other individuals with the same cultural background as the patient. Delusions may take many forms, but delusions of grandeur or persecution are most common. The examination should attempt to determine whether delusions are consistent or are changing, since this quality is a distinguishing point between medical and psychiatric psychosis.

COGNITIVE FUNCTION. This assessment is aimed at determining whether the patient can think something through and whether the thought process is logical.

JUDGMENT AND INSIGHT. Most patients who have psychosis from a medical cause understand that their thought processes are abnormal and they freely acknowledge this when asked. Most patients whose psychosis is from a psychiatric disorder do not recognize abnormality in their behavior. The goal of assessing judgment and insight is to determine whether the patient knows that there is something wrong with his or her thinking.

MEMORY TESTING. The function of both short-term and remote memory should be assessed, since the type of memory affected distinguishes medical causes from psychiatric causes of psychosis.

ATTENTION. Assessment of attention determines whether the patient can attend to questions asked, can remember what is being asked of him, and can perform as directed. A three-part command allows the investigator to determine the patient's attention to the request, the ability of the patient to think through a process and consequently to perform the task in three parts. Therefore, this test assesses attention, memory, and cognition.

RECOGNITION. This test assesses the ability of patients to recognize objects, people, places, and other common factors in their environment.

LEVEL OF CONSCIOUSNESS. The patient's level of consciousness should be described in detail. Terms such as stupor, lethargy, and obtundation may have different meanings for different examiners. To ensure that the presentation of the patient is accurately described, the clinician should supply more detail than what is provided by these standard terms.

Laboratory and Imaging Studies

Potentially useful screening laboratory studies for the patient with acute psychosis are listed in Table 4. The choice of studies should be guided by the history and physical examination. It is often easy to determine laboratory needs when a patient appears to have a medical cause of acute psychoses. A pitfall in assessment is failure to perform laboratory studies in psychotic patients who are suspected of having psychoses from psychiatric causes. However, mixed disorders (medical and psychiatric) exist in almost 40 percent of patients with altered mental status, and a stable psychiatric patient can be thrown into acute decompensation under conditions of physical stress, such as an acute infection. In several retrospective studies, acutely psychotic ED patients medically cleared for psychiatric admission were eventually found to have a medical cause of their acute presentation.

Imaging studies may be useful in distinguishing between

Table 4. Laboratory Studies in Acute Psychosis

CBC, electrolytes, blood sugar
Creatinine, SUN
Urine toxicology screen
Blood alcohol concentration
Arterial blood gases
Urine analysis
Thyroid and liver function studies
ECG
Chest radiograph
Lumbar puncture
CT scan

CBC = complete blood count; CT = computed tomography; ECG = electrocardiogram; SUN = serum urea nitrogen.

Table 5. Selected Potentially Life-Threatening Causes of Acute Psychosis

Medical Psychoses	Psychiatric Psychoses
Infections	Major depression and its complications
Pulmonary infections	
CNS infections	
Sepsis from any cause	Suicide
Metabolic	
Diabetes, uncontrolled	Substance abuse
Encephalopathies	
Acute endocrine dysfunction	Violence to self, others
Chemical	
Drug and/or ethanol withdrawal	
Acute drug overdose	Personal neglect
Accidental toxic exposure	
Medication reaction	Autonomic overactivity
Hypertension, hypotension	
Metabolic abnormalities	
End-organ failure	
Decreased cerebral perfusion	
CNS disease, trauma	
Mass lesions, cerebral edema	
Infection	
Trauma	
Spontaneous intracranial bleeds	
Seizures, postictal state	
Cardiac dysfunction	
Any reason for reduced cardiac output	
Postresuscitation "confusion"	
Pulmonary	
Hypoxia from any cause	
Infection	
Pulmonary embolism	
Hypothermia, hyperthermia	

CNS = central nervous system.

medical and psychiatric problems. In patients with hypoxia, a chest film is particularly useful for excluding pneumonia or other pulmonary disorders. A CT scan of the head without contrast enhancement is a useful emergent study in patients whose altered mental status may be due to recent head trauma.

DISTINGUISHING ACUTE PSYCHOTIC ILLNESS FROM MEDICAL ILLNESS

Because medical disorders can rapidly become life-threatening, all psychoses should be considered secondary to a medical problem until proved otherwise (Table 5). A list of several features that can be used to distinguish acute psychoses caused by medical or psychiatric disease is presented in Table 6. Schizophrenic patients have extremely bizarre complex delusions and hallucinations that do not change over time. They are able to think things through, but they have no insight into their problem. Their perceptions are often based on familiar items in their reality, but somehow these familiar things have taken on an unfamiliar aspect. Interviewing the manic patient is often very unrewarding, simply because he or she cannot attend to questions or follow a thought through to completion. It is difficult to assess the manic patient's orientation because they often do not attend to the examiner's questions. Their delusions change as rapidly as their focus of attention, but in general, they are grandiose. Manic patients are so hyperactive that it may be fatiguing to watch them. Depressed patients look normal in many ways, but like the manic, they are difficult to question because they cannot attend. Their attention wanders, and interviewing them can be frustrating and tiring.

Speech patterns and context help distinguish acute psychoses. Patients with acute psychoses due to thought disorders frequently demonstrate disorganized speech with decreased content or production. They may also present with perseverations or other abnormalities of speech. Depressed patients often respond slowly to questions, and manic individuals demonstrate a pressured speech with flight of ideas or clanging, which is the use of words for their sound instead of their meaning. Patients with medical problems that present as acute psychoses often exhibit a paucity of speech or an extremely slow rate of production.

Table 6. Distinctions Between Medical and Psychiatric Psychoses

	Psychiatric Disorders			Medical Disorders	
Feature	***Schizophrenic***	***Affective (Mania)***	***"Pseudodementia" (Depression)***	***Delirium***	***Dementia***
Onset	Variable	Variable, often acute	Relatively rapid	Acute (hours–days)	Gradual (months–years)
Age	<40 yr	30–40 yr	Any age	Any age	>60 yr
Course	Progressive (acute exacerbations)	Fluctuating	Progressive	Fluctuating	Progressive
Vital signs	Usually normal	Often abnormal	Normal	Often abnormal	Usually normal
Symptoms	Consistent	Fluctuating	Consistent	Often fluctuating (worse at night)	Consistent
Wakefulness	Normal (agitated, anxious)	Increased	Normal	Fluctuating (usually hyperalert)	Usually normal
Attentiveness	Fluctuating	Impaired	Fluctuating	Fluctuating	Impaired
Disorientation	Rare	Intermittent	Intermittent	Intermittent	Constant
Hallucinations	Usually auditory (fixed, bizarre, grandiose)	Usually auditory (changing, grandiose)	None	Usually visual (disorganized)	Usually none
Delusions	Familiar-unfamiliar (complex, fixed)	Grandiose (fluctuating)	Rare (pessimistic)	Unfamiliar-familiar (simple, inconsistent)	Variable
Sleep-wake dysfunction	Rare	Frequent	Frequent	Frequent	Frequent
Cognition	Intact (lack of insight)	Abnormal (cannot attend)	Abnormal (cannot attend)	Abnormal (fluctuating)	Abnormal
Recent memory	Intact	Variable (cannot attend)	Decreased	Decreased	Decreased (recent and distant)
Motor movements	Normal or repetitive, posturing, rocking	Hyperactive	Normal, slow	Hyperactive, hypoactive, tremor, ataxia	Normal or hypoactive
Neurologic signs	None	None	None	Occasional deficit	No acute changes
Most common cause of acute psychosis	Nonmedical compliance	Nonmedical compliance	Major depression	Intoxicants, withdrawal	Alzheimer's disease, ethanol dementia

The recognition of medical delirium is a key goal in the ED evaluation of acutely psychotic patients. Medical delirium is an acute brain dysfunction that may be life-threatening but is often reversible. These patients are disoriented and usually have problems with recent memory. It is sometimes difficult to obtain or interpret their former mental status examination. Often, patients with medical delirium have abnormal vital signs that may be due to a toxin or an acute infection. The only other group of acutely psychotic patients with abnormal vital signs are the acutely manic patients. Symptoms of medical delirium become worse at night, and the mental status examination fluctuates. The hallucinations during acute medical delirium are usually not auditory, and they tend to change. Perceptions of reality are very simple, and what is unknown is considered familiar.

An important factor that distinguishes medical psychoses from psychoses due to psychiatric disease is the patient's age. The first presentation of a psychiatric disorder usually occurs in patients in their late teens or 20s. Psychoses from psychiatric illness rarely develop in patients after 40 years of age. Therefore, a first-time psychotic episode in a patient younger than 20 or older than 40 year of age should be considered a medical delirium until proved otherwise.

Memory of recent events is also a distinguishing factor. In patients with psychiatric psychoses, intact recent memory is present. Therefore, an impairment of memory of recent events suggests a medical problem. The patient's level of consciousness also assists in distinguishing the cause of the psychoses. In psychiatric disorders, the level of consciousness is typically normal, but it may be altered in patients with medical disease.

PATIENT DISPOSITION

When patients present to the ED with psychosis of medical origin, hospitalization is warranted if serious medical illness is identified with persistently abnormal vital signs and metabolic abnormalities that require gradual reversal. With psychosis from acute psychiatric illness, the indications for hospitalization include the first episode of acute psychosis, psychosis in an established psychiatric patient that fails to respond to ED neuroleptic therapy, suicidal, homicidal, or violent behavior or ideation, acute anxiety unrelieved by medications, and uncontrollable mania.

Because many psychotic patients are unable to care for themselves or their families are unable or unwilling to care for them, it is important to ensure that these patients have adequate support systems prior to any discharge planning. Patients with previously diagnosed psychiatric illness, whose acute psychotic episode has been effectively treated with neuroleptic medications in the past, can be safely discharged from the ED after resolution of the acute episode. However, a strong support system must be in place, and these patients must be considered likely to return for follow-up. If these patients have no place to go or appear to have been noncompliant with previous medications, hospital admission may be warranted. Social Service contact and consultation may provide other options, such as a sheltered environment, a home health aide, or a visiting nurse.

Drug or alcohol intoxicated patients can be discharged from the ED after they have been medically cleared and their mental status has returned to normal. Discharge is also possible in patients with easily reversible organic dysfunctions, such as the diabetic who has become hypoglycemic or whose symptoms abate after the administration of intravenous glucose. A summary of appropriate ED dispositions of acutely psychotic patients is presented in Table 7.

Table 7. Disposition of Acutely Psychotic Patients From the Emergency Department

Admission, Psychiatric Psychosis	Admission, Other Considerations
Initial episode of acute psychiatric psychosis	Demented patient unable to care for self
Acute psychosis not responsive to neuroleptics in the emergency department	No strong support systems
Suicidal, homicidal, violent patients	Psychosis with unclear, indeterminate, or mixed etiology
Acute anxiety unrelieved with medications	**Discharge**
Uncontrollable mania	Previously diagnosed psychiatric psychosis, controlled in the emergency department with neuroleptics
Admission, Medical Psychosis	Drug and/or alcohol ingestion, observed and now cleared
Serious identifiable medical illness	Reversible medical psychoses (i.e., hypoglycemia)
Persistent abnormal vital signs	
Metabolic abnormalities requiring slow reversal	

Section Twelve

MUSCLE, BONE, AND JOINT DISORDERS

MUSCULAR DYSTROPHIES

By Kathryn N. North, M.D.
Camperdown, Sydney, Australia
and Geoffrey Miller, M.D.
Houston, Texas

The muscular dystrophies (MDs) are genetically determined disorders of muscle. They are characterized by primary myopathic change that leads to degeneration and wasting of muscle fibers. Skeletal muscle is always affected, although some of the MDs also involve smooth and cardiac muscle. The degree of muscle weakness is very variable within some genotypes as well as between phenotypes, and in some allelic variations weakness is minimal or absent. The different genotypes include dystrophinopathies (Duchenne and Becker MD), myotonic dystrophy, congenital MD, facioscapulohumeral MD, Emery-Dreifuss MD, limb-girdle MD, oculopharyngeal MD, and distal myopathy. The diagnosis is based on (1) clinical findings, which include involvement of other systems apart from muscle; (2) family history; (3) serum creatine kinase (CK) activity; (4) electromyography; (5) muscle histopathology; and (6) molecular genetic analysis.

X-LINKED DYSTROPHINOPATHIES (DUCHENNE AND BECKER MUSCULAR DYSTROPHY)

Duchenne muscular dystrophy (DMD) and the milder phenotype Becker muscular dystrophy (BMD) are allelic disorders caused by mutations in the dystrophin gene on the X chromosome. Heterozygous female DMD carriers occasionally show mild symptoms, and rarely their condition may be severe owing to failure of X-inactivation, monosomy X, or X autosome translocation. These manifesting carriers or affected females have increased CK activity in their sera. The tissue-specific expression of dystrophin, in muscle and brain, correlates with the phenotypic expression of the disease—progressive muscular weakness, cardiomyopathy, and static encephalopathy. The different phenotypes of DMD and BMD are due to the differing effects of gene mutations on the translational reading frame. The severe DMD phenotype is caused by mutations that disrupt the translational reading frame and result in severe truncation of the 427-kd dystrophin isoform. Mutations that cause BMD allow production of internally deleted or duplicated proteins owing to conservation of the translational reading frame and a milder and more variable phenotype. However, occasional exceptions to this rule are observed.

DMD occurs in 1 in 3500 live male births and typically presents with proximal limb-girdle weakness between 3 and 5 years of age. Early gross motor milestones may be delayed, and a delay in walking until 18 months or more is common. Language delay is frequently present. Apart from the late appearance of lower facial weakness, the extraocular and facial muscles are not clinically affected. Patients are usually never able to run or jump and develop progressive difficulty in climbing stairs or arising from the floor. A lumbar lordosis develops with toe walking, a waddling gait, and frequent falls. On examination, a Gowers sign is observed, and pseudohypertrophy of the calves or other muscle groups is variably present. The Achilles tendons are short. Tendon reflexes are initially present but are later lost as weakness inexorably progresses. Loss of independent ambulation usually occurs by 10 to 12 years, followed by a decline in pulmonary function. Without active intervention, contractures and scoliosis ensue. Death due to respiratory insufficiency or, less commonly, cardiac failure or arrhythmia occurs in the second or third decade. The mean full-scale IQ score of boys with DMD is approximately 1 standard deviation below the mean for the population, and consequently a greater proportion are retarded. Delay in acquisition of language may precede development of muscle weakness. Cardiomyopathy often presents as sinus tachycardia in young patients, and a minority of patients develop significant dysrhythmias or congestive heart failure. Gastric hypomotility can also occur.

With an incidence of 1 in 30,000 live male births, BMD is a more heterogeneous disorder, having variable age at onset and rate of progression. Proximal muscle weakness, the most frequent presenting feature, is found in the same distribution as that in DMD. Calf hypertrophy and muscle cramps with exercise are common. Patients generally remain ambulatory into their 20s and may continue walking into their 50s and 60s. Cardiomyopathy and static encephalopathy are more variable. The atypical variants of BMD include cardiomyopathy alone, myalgia without significant weakness, and increases in serum CK activity in the absence of muscle weakness. Patients with BMD may also present with mental retardation or neurobehavioral disturbance in the absence of muscle weakness. The latter includes attention-deficit/hyperactivity disorder and specific learning disability. Other presentations are listed in Table 1. Both DMD and BMD are susceptible to malignant hyperthermia.

Laboratory Diagnosis

Beginning in infancy, CK activity is markedly increased in serum, usually 100 to 700 times the upper limit of the reference range. The electromyogram is abnormal and myopathic, but this test is rarely necessary in the evaluation of suspected cases, unless the diagnosis is in doubt after completion of other testing. Muscle biopsy demonstrates dystrophic changes, with marked variation in fiber size, small clusters of degenerating and regenerating fibers, prominent large hypercontracted fibers, and a

Table 1. List of Possible Clinical Presentations of Dystrophinopathy

Duchenne Muscular Dystrophy

Presentation at birth or during early infancy
Psychomotor delay, language disorder, or neurobehavioral difficulty of early onset
Typical DMD: loss of unassisted ambulation by age 13 years
Duchenne "outlier": loss of unassisted ambulation by age 16 years

Becker Muscular Dystrophy

Severe BMD: loss of unassisted ambulation by age 20 years
Moderate BMD: loss of independent ambulation by age 30 years
Mild BMD: independent ambulation beyond age 30 years

Other Male Phenotypes

Cardiomyopathy with or without mild skeletal muscle weakness
Mild limb-girdle weakness or quadriceps myopathy
Myalgia or cramps on exercise with minimal or no weakness
Asymptomatic increase in CK activity in serum
Mental retardation
Neurobehavioral disorders, such as attention-deficit/hyperactivity disorder or specific learning disability

Manifesting Female Carrier

Asymptomatic increase in CK activity in serum
Myalgia or cramps on exercise
Isolated calf hypertrophy
Varying degrees of muscle weakness

Affected Female (Monosomy X or X-Autosome Translocation)

DMD
Severe BMD

BMD = Becker muscular dystrophy; DMD = Duchenne muscular dystrophy.

marked increase in endomysial connective and adipose tissues.

With DNA testing of peripheral blood, 65 per cent of patients with DMD or BMD have deletions in their dystrophin gene and 7 per cent have duplications. The remainder probably have point mutations. Polymerase chain reaction (PCR)–based assays that screen mutational "hot spots" in the gene can identify as many as 98 per cent of detectable deletions. Southern blot analysis is required for detecting duplications. Furthermore, if the reading frame of the mutation is determined (by PCR alone, or in conjunction with Southern blot), the severity of the phenotype, that is, DMD versus BMD, can be established with 92 per cent accuracy. If a deletion or duplication is identified, carrier status, or presymptomatic testing in relatives, can also be performed with these techniques. Males suspected of having DMD or BMD should have DNA testing included as part of the initial evaluation. If unequivocal results are obtained, invasive procedures such as electromyography and muscle biopsy are not necessary to establish the diagnosis.

For patients without a demonstrable mutation on DNA analysis, and for patients in whom the reading frame is not determined or the severity of the phenotype is in doubt (i.e., early in the course of disease), muscle biopsy is essential for establishing the diagnosis and predicting disease severity. Indirect immunofluorescence on frozen sections of muscles with antibodies directed against dystrophin can be used to distinguish between the absence of dystrophin staining (DMD) and the presence of altered dystrophin (BMD) in vitro. In BMD, the staining may range from almost normal to patchy and significantly lighter. Although this method can detect a subset of DMD female carriers (who often have patches of negative fibers among positive fibers owing to X-chromosome inactivation), it is not completely reliable. Immunofluorescence does not typically detect BMD carriers.

Western blot analysis, using antibodies against both the amino-terminal and carboxyl-terminal regions of dystrophin, establishes the laboratory diagnosis of DMD versus BMD versus other MDs. However, as noted earlier, it may be restricted to cases in which the diagnosis and phenotype (DMD or BMD) is found to be equivocal with the use of other methods. The quantity and quality (size) of dystrophin can be accurately assessed. In general, the complete absence of dystrophin is predictive of DMD with an accuracy of more than 99 per cent. The presence of a variably sized dystrophin protein, or one of reduced abundance, establishes the diagnosis of BMD with an accuracy of more than 95 per cent. Patients with molecularly defined BMD, but with levels of dystrophin less than 20 per cent of normal, often exhibit an intermediate phenotype, becoming wheelchair bound in their middle to late teens. In the absence of a detectable deletion, immunoblotting is also the most accurate way of detecting carriers of DMD and BMD.

As with any diagnostic approach, exceptions to the rules exist. Occasionally, patients with predicted out-of-frame deletions following molecular analysis have presented with a BMD phenotype, and the reverse (i.e., a DMD patient with an in-frame mutation) can also occur—albeit infrequently. Usually, dystrophin analysis using immunologic techniques resolves the discrepancy. However, if Western blot is performed using only antibodies raised toward a region of dystrophin that is deleted, no dystrophin is detected. Usually, this problem is overcome with the use of antibodies to two or three nonoverlapping regions of the protein.

Differential Diagnosis

While dystrophin testing now provides accurate diagnosis of the dystrophinopathies, other disorders may be considered during the initial evaluation. Markedly increased serum CK activity in a child with muscle weakness raises the possibility of inflammatory disorders such as dermatomyositis, which are important to exclude because of their implications for therapy. DMD and BMD must also be distinguished from limb-girdle MD, congenital MD, various congenital myopathies, metabolic myopathies, and spinal muscular atrophy. The diagnosis should be considered in young males who present with developmental delay or neurobehavioral difficulties and in male patients with unexplained cardiomyopathy or muscle cramps on exercise.

MYOTONIC DYSTROPHY (DYSTROPHIA MYOTONIA, STEINERT'S DISEASE)

Myotonic dystrophy (DM) is an autosomal dominant disorder characterized by the presence of myotonia, that is, sustained contraction of skeletal muscle in response to electrical or physical stimulus. Myotonia and weakness usually present in adulthood, but marked clinical variability occurs both within and between families. A multisystem disorder, DM involves the heart, smooth muscle, central nervous system, eyes, and endocrine glands. Patients may be asymptomatic, or the predominant symptoms may be non-neurologic. The recent identification of the DM gene has revolutionized diagnosis, prenatal diagnosis, and presymptomatic testing as well as an understanding of the phenotypic heterogeneity of the disorder.

In the classic, adult-onset form of the disorder, muscle weakness is the most frequent presenting symptom and tends to be progressive in nature. Preferential involvement of the face, jaw, and anterior neck muscles gives rise to a characteristic facial appearance—with ptosis, a flat smile, and slight forward carriage of the head. Hollowed cheeks and temples reflect temporalis and masseter muscle wasting. Extraocular muscle weakness rarely, if ever, occurs. Dysphagia and respiratory muscle weakness can occur and may be life-threatening. The distal limb muscles are preferentially affected, in contrast with other MDs. Tendon reflexes are lost early. Myotonia tends to appear before the dystrophic process, usually in the second or third decade. Many patients are unaware of it or complain only of "stiffness." Myotonia may be elicited by direct percussion of muscles (e.g., thenar eminence) or by testing for rapid relaxation after sustained contraction (handgrip, eye closure).

Systemic features of DM may occur in the absence of significant muscular weakness and are of special importance with respect to prognosis and management (Table 2). Cardiac involvement can result in potentially lethal conduction defects, in particular heart block and atrial arrhythmias. Cataracts are usually not present until the second or third decade and then become more prominent at older ages. Systems review, including electrocardiography and slit-lamp examination, should be performed in any patient in whom a diagnosis of DM is suspected. More than 80 per cent of gene carriers never present to a physician with problems related to DM, and thus a family history may not be elicited from the patient.

Laboratory Diagnosis

Biochemical tests are usually not informative. Creatine kinase activity in serum is normal or only slightly increased. Electromyography demonstrates typical myotonic discharges, with or without myopathic features, even in asymptomatic patients. On muscle biopsy, type I fiber atrophy and a high prevalence of centrally placed nuclei are the most characteristic changes. Dystrophic changes, including variation in fiber size and fibrosis, are also observed.

Table 2. Systemic Manifestations of Myotonic Dystrophy

Heart
80% of patients
Conduction abnormalities; bradycardia, heart block
Cardiomyopathy
Sudden death
Smooth Muscle
Dilatation and hypomotility of esophagus or bowel
Dysphagia, aspiration, constipation, colic, diarrhea
Gallstones
Uncoordinated contraction of the uterus during labor
Eyes
Subcapsular, multichromatic cataracts
Pigmentary retinal degeneration
Ptosis
Endocrine Glands
Testicular and ovarian atrophy
Hyperinsulinemia in response to glucose load
Premature balding
Central Nervous System
Mild mental retardation or low-normal intelligence
Socialization difficulties: hostile, suspicious, uncooperative
Hypersomnia

Differential Diagnosis

The distribution of muscle weakness, with predominantly facial and distal limb involvement, distinguishes DM from the X-linked dystrophinopathies and many of the other autosomal dystrophies. The pattern of weakness may cause diagnostic uncertainty because of its similarity to facioscapulohumeral dystrophy, myasthenia gravis, or primary neuropathic conditions, such as hereditary motor and sensory neuropathy type I (HMSN I). A combination of neuromuscular and systemic symptoms can also occur in mitochondrial myopathies. Recognition of myotonia, clinically or on electromyography, provides ready distinction from these disorders. DM also must be distinguished from the nonprogressive inherited myotonic disorders, such as myotonia and paramyotonia congenita and chondrodystrophic myotonia (Schwartz-Jampel syndrome). In these disorders, myotonia is usually the predominant symptom, without systemic involvement or significant muscle weakness or atrophy.

Congenital Myotonic Dystrophy

Twenty per cent of the affected offspring of mothers with DM present with congenital myotonic dystrophy. The mothers themselves may be mildly affected, or they may be unaware that they have the disorder. Much more severe than the adult form, congenital DM is frequently fatal. A history of reduced fetal movements and polyhydramnios (hydramnios) is often elicited. Infants are usually extremely weak and hypotonic, with a high incidence of respiratory insufficiency, feeding difficulties, and joint contractures. Bilateral facial weakness, marked jaw weakness, and a tented upper lip produce a characteristic appearance. Myotonia is not present clinically or on electromyography during the newborn period but may become apparent in the first decade. If children survive the neonatal period, they often show moderate to severe mental retardation that is nonprogressive.

The clinical presentation in these infants may be difficult to distinguish from severe myotubular or nemaline myopathy, neonatal myasthenia, spinal muscular atrophy, or severe hypomyelinating polyneuropathies. Furthermore, birth asphyxia with basal ganglia hemorrhage may mimic the condition. The mainstay of diagnosis is a high index of clinical suspicion, coupled with clinical and electromyographic evaluations for myotonia in the mother.

Molecular Testing

With the identification of the DM gene on chromosome 19q13.3, a clinical diagnosis of DM or congenital DM can now be confirmed with DNA analysis by Southern blotting or PCR. In patients with DM, an expansion of an unstable DNA sequence (trinucleotide repeat CTG) occurs within the 3′ untranslated region of the gene. In the normal population, the number of CTG repeats varies between 5 and 30. In patients with DM, mutations result in a variable increase in the number of trinucleotide repeats. The mutation is "dynamic"—that is, the insert does not remain a constant size in individuals within a pedigree, and a correlation between repeat number and age at onset is observed. Minimally affected individuals have 50 to 80 repeats. More typically affected adult-onset patients have a wide and variable repeat number, in the range of 100 to 500 copies, and the number of copies does not closely correlate with disease severity. The size of the CTG repeat varies between tissues in the same individual and may be the basis of variable expressivity. Therefore, blood DNA analysis cannot always predict the severity of disease in an individual. The length of the trinucleotide repeat tends to increase in subsequent generations, which accounts for the anticipation (increased severity in subsequent generations) that has been observed in families with DM. Patients with congenital onset show the largest expansions (usually 500 to 1500 repeats), and unlike the adult form, the congenital form exhibits repeat length in tissues that corresponds to repeat length in blood DNA. The size of the dynamic mutation locus probably explains the severe, early, uniform clinical manifestations in congenital DM.

CONGENITAL MUSCULAR DYSTROPHY

The congenital MDs are a heterogeneous group of muscle diseases characterized by early onset of weakness (at birth or during the first year of life), hypotonia, delayed achievement of motor milestones, and a high incidence of severe and early contractures. The weakness is generalized and usually involves the face. Bulbar and respiratory muscle involvement is variable but may be severe. The primary muscle pathology includes a striking variation in muscle fiber diameter, depletion of muscle fibers and replacement by fat, and a conspicuous increase in endomysial and perimysial collagenous connective tissue in the absence of specific ultrastructural changes. Creatine kinase activity in serum may be normal or increased. Electromyography is abnormal and reveals brief, small-amplitude, polyphasic potentials. Inheritance is thought to be autosomal recessive or sporadic. The congenital MDs must be distinguished from the congenital myopathies, spinal muscular atrophy, storage disorders, DMD and myotonic dystrophy, all of which can present in the first months of life.

Within the group of diseases classified as congenital MDs, several distinct autosomal recessive subtypes have been identified on the basis of their differing degrees of central nervous system involvement. Fukuyama congenital MD, prevalent in Japan, is associated with neuronal migration defects and mental retardation. Affected babies present with generalized weakness, hypotonia, and varying degrees of arthrogryposis. Facial and bulbar involvement is usually present, and seizures are sometimes frequent. Only a small percentage of children can stand by 4 years of age, weakness and contractures tend to worsen, and the majority of children die by adolescence. The gene has been localized to chromosomes 9q31-q33. Abnormalities that distinguish the condition from Walker-Warburg syndrome include macrogyria (pachygyria) and polymicrogyria, rather than agyria (lissencephaly), and areas of more normal gyral patterns. The cortex also has a more widespread "cobblestone" appearance. Other distinguishing features are white matter changes that improve with age and only mild ventriculomegaly and cerebellar polymicrogyria. In addition, eye anomalies are only minor. Both Walker-Warburg congenital MD and Santavuori congenital MD (muscle-eye-brain disease) are associated with developmental defects of the eye and brain and are distinguished clinically on the basis of age at onset and severity of disease. In Walker-Warburg congenital MD, structural defects of the eye (e.g., retinal dysplasia) and brain (agyria) are obvious at birth. The head can be abnormally large in conjunction with progressive hydrocephalus, or microcephaly and an occipital encephalocele may be observed. The brain is markedly abnormal, with agyria, white matter dysmyelinization or cystic changes, ventriculomegaly, and brain stem and cerebellar hypoplasia. The findings on neuroimaging are striking. Axial views show the classic smooth surface and figure-8 configuration of agyria. In contrast with other forms of agyria, the white matter is poorly myelinated and appears dark on computed tomography and abnormally bright on T2-weighted magnetic resonance imaging. The corpus callosum may be absent, or only the genu and a small portion of the anterior body is seen. The vermis is dysplastic, and the cerebellar hemispheres are small. Dandy-Walker malformations are common, and an occipital encephalocele may be present. The prognosis in Walker-Warburg syndrome is poor. Profound mental retardation is typical, seizures occur as the baby ages, and few survive more than a few months, although prolonged survival is possible with gastrostomy feeding, avoidance of aspiration, and vigorous management of respiratory tract infection. In congenital MD of the Santavuori type, there may be frontal macrogyria and polymicrogyria posteriorly, in addition to retinal hypoplasia with reduced or absent responses on electroretinogram. Other findings can include white matter changes that are similar to those found in Walker-Warburg syndrome, progressive hydrocephalus, absent septum pellucidum, and an absent or a dysgenetic corpus callosum. Other possible eye findings include myopia, choroidal hypoplasia, optic nerve pallor, glaucoma, iris hypoplasia, cataracts, and colobomas. Neonates present with hypotonia, weakness, feeding difficulties, poor vision, and apathy. Distal contractures may be present. All develop mental retardation, and seizures are common. In contrast with Walker-Warburg syndrome, most have a prolonged survival; however, independent ambulation is unusual. The development of high-amplitude visual evoked potentials by 2 years of age is a particular feature, and the electroencephalogram becomes abnormal by 1 year of age. Serum CK activity may be normal within the first year, but it is always increased later. Milder forms may exist.

Classic congenital MD is a relatively nonprogressive disease that is distinguished from the aforementioned subtypes by the lack of clinical involvement of the central nervous system. The considerable clinical variability that exists within the classic phenotype suggests that it may be etiologically heterogeneous. Arthrogryposis multiplex congenita may or may not be present, CK activity may be normal or increased, and white matter changes on magnetic resonance imaging have been detected in a subset of cases.

Recently immunohistochemical studies have demonstrated a complete absence of merosin, a component of the extracellular matrix protein laminin, in a subset of patients with the classic non-Japanese form of congenital MD. Significant linkage of merosin-negative congenital MD to the merosin locus on 6q2 has subsequently been demonstrated. These findings suggest that a proportion of patients with the classic congenital MD phenotype can now be distinguished on the basis of immunohistochemistry for merosin.

Merosin-negative congenital MD patients have a number of clinical features that distinguish them from the merosin-positive group. In merosin-negative patients, CK activity is more likely to be increased above 2000 U/L, weakness is more pronounced, ambulation may not be achieved, and respiratory problems such as hypoventilation are more common. White matter changes on magnetic resonance imaging are evident in all merosin-negative patients, but these changes do not affect intellectual development. Peripheral neuropathies and unspecified ocular abnormalities have also been observed in this subgroup.

LIMB-GIRDLE MUSCULAR DYSTROPHY

Limb-girdle MDs make up a heterogeneous group of disorders characterized by muscle weakness that predominantly affects proximal limb and girdle muscle and spares the face and extraocular muscles. The dystrophic muscle biopsy picture is not due to an abnormality of the X-linked dystrophin gene, which distinguishes the condition from BMD or manifesting carriers of a dystrophinopathy. Inheritance is autosomal recessive or dominant, and the former is more common. The initial symptoms are due to proximal muscle weakness, and onset usually ranges from early childhood into the 20s. Autosomal dominant forms may present later, although early childhood presentation of this form has been described. Calf hypertrophy and ankle contractures are common. Serum CK activity is significantly increased in the autosomal recessive forms. In the autosomal dominant form, the increase is variable, except with clinical presentation in early childhood, when the enzyme activity is very high. Electromyography produces myopathic findings.

The clinical course is variable. In the majority of cases, the disorder is incompletely defined, but three syndromes have been recognized. The severe childhood autosomal recessive MD (SCARMD) presents in early childhood and behaves like an intermediate or severe dystrophinopathy. Laboratory diagnosis is made by detection of a deficiency of the 50-kd component of the dystrophin-associated protein complex linked to chromosome 13q or 17q (adhalin-deficient). The autosomal recessive type of limb-girdle MD linked to chromosome 15q usually presents in middle childhood, with progression to loss of ambulation around 30 years. An autosomal dominant form linked to chromosome 5q that presents in early adult life is slowly progressive and is sometimes associated with dysarthria. Respiratory muscle involvement is frequent, and in some patients, early severe weakness of the diaphragm occurs. Cardiomyopathy also occurs but is less common.

The diagnosis of limb-girdle MD is one of exclusion. The differential diagnosis includes a dystrophinopathy, and in female patients, a chromosome analysis is required for excluding monosomy X or X-autosomal translocation. Other considerations include chronic spinal muscular atrophy; endocrine myopathies; some congenital, mitochondrial, and metabolic myopathies; and polymyositis.

FACIOSCAPULOHUMERAL MUSCULAR DYSTROPHY

Facioscapulohumeral muscular dystrophy (FSHD) affects the facial and shoulder-girdle muscles and, to a variable extent, the anterior compartment muscles of the lower leg. Later involvement of the pelvic-girdle muscles can occur. The clinical age at onset is variable but is most often during the teens with weakness of eye closure and the perioral muscles. The muscles of mastication, extraocular muscles, and lingual and pharyngeal muscles are spared. Weakness and wasting of the muscles that fix the scapula give rise to scapula winging, prominence of the upper border of the scapula, and a sloped appearance of the shoulders. Early asymmetrical involvement may occur. Although this disorder is usually relatively benign, intrafamilial and interfamilial variability occurs, and the disease can present during early infancy. Progression is usually slow, with long periods of clinical arrest, although exceptions have been noted. In many cases, bilateral sensorineural hearing loss is present. Retinal vascular abnormalities may also be found, and these telangiectasias sometimes progress to exudation and detachment.

The disorder is autosomal dominant or sporadic, although on careful inspection one of the parents may have minimal or subclinical involvement. The gene for FSHD is located on chromosome 4q35, and presymptomatic diagnosis may be available in the near future. Creatine kinase activity rarely exceeds five times normal and may not be increased at all. Muscle biopsy of an affected muscle may show only mild myopathic change. Other findings include small angular fibers, "moth-eaten fibers," and cellular infiltrates that may be extensive and may appear inflammatory although a family history is often present and steroids are not beneficial. Electromyography typically shows a myopathic pattern, and occasionally some neurogenic features are present.

EMERY-DREIFUSS MUSCULAR DYSTROPHY

Apart from potentially life-threatening cardiac involvement, Emery-Dreifuss MD (EMD) is relatively benign. It presents in childhood with early contractures at the elbows and ankles that result in the characteristic semiflexed position of the arms and toe walking. Limited neck movement also occurs early from contractures in the posterior cervical muscles and may be followed by paraspinal muscle involvement and a rigid spine. Mild, slowly progressive humeroperoneal muscle weakness and wasting occur. Later in the course of the disease, limb-girdle muscles become affected. Calf hypertrophy is not a feature. Cardiac conduction defects, manifested by bradycardia, appear as muscle weakness progresses, but may occur before this. The potential for sudden cardiac death should always be anticipated.

EMD is X-linked and mapped to Xq28. Possible rarer autosomal dominant forms have been described. Creatine kinase activity may be only moderately increased and decreases with age. The muscle biopsy reveals myopathic or dystrophic change. Angular fibers may be present in addition to type I fiber atrophy. Electromyography yields myopathic findings.

OCULOPHARYNGEAL MUSCULAR DYSTROPHY

Oculopharyngeal MD is an autosomal dominant disorder that usually presents in middle life with progressive ptosis and dysphagia. The progressive ptosis, which can be asymmetrical, leads to the typical facial appearance of raised eyebrows and wrinkled forehead. Eye movements are unaffected until late in the disease, and even then complete ophthalmoplegia is unlikely. Dysphagia initially occurs with ingestion of solids but later includes liquids. Aspiration may result from palatal weakness, and laryngeal muscle involvement causes dysphonia. As the disease slowly progresses, weakness and wasting of other muscles become apparent. Included are the lingual, temporalis, and masseter muscles, and later the girdle muscles. Distal involvement may also occur.

Creatine kinase activity in serum is normal or only mildly increased, and electromyography produces myopathic findings. Muscle biopsy reveals a myopathic picture, with loss of muscle fibers and interstitial fat and fibrosis. Necrosis and myophagocytosis are rare. Histochemical stains may show "rimmed vacuoles." The rims stain red with Gomori's trichrome stain. On electron microscopy, characteristic tubulofilamentous inclusions are found.

Family history, typical presentation, and histopathologic

and electron microscopy findings distinguish oculopharyngeal MD from other neuromuscular disorders. Ptosis and dysphagia can be found in myotonic dystrophy, myotubular myopathy, and polymyositis, but clear clinical and pathologic differences from oculopharyngeal MD are observed. Dysphagia also occurs in inclusion body myositis, in which "rimmed vacuoles" and ultrastructural filaments can be seen. In inclusion body myositis, inflammatory change is found and accompanied by early limb weakness. Prominent ptosis is not a feature. Muscle biopsy and electromyography distinguish oculopharyngeal MD from mitochondrial disorders, such as the Kearns-Sayre syndrome, and from myasthenia.

MYOPATHIES

By Lawrence J. Kagen, M.D.
New York, New York

The voluntary or skeletal muscles account for one of the largest tissue or organ systems in the body. They are responsible for our movements, our expressions, and, in large measure, our body shape. Even so, on many occasions, dysfunction of this system (myopathy) can be difficult to recognize and diagnose. Many different conditions may affect muscle function, and myopathies may be secondary to abnormalities of other organ systems. Therefore, attention may not focus initially on the musculature in many patients. Several factors in addition to the complexity of muscle-viscera relationships can delay recognition of myopathies. Myopathic disorders may begin insidiously, and the patient may not be able to define an abnormality to which he or she has slowly adapted. Moreover, the language used to describe muscular abnormalities is often imprecise or vague. For example, weakness can be viewed as a general state of fatigue or lack of energy. The patient or physician may also believe that symptoms of weakness, muscle aches, or soreness reflect the effects of aging rather than those of a specific muscle disorder. Therefore, despite the fact that muscles and their actions are, in general, observable and easily perceived, the suspicion of myopathy may be delayed or clouded by the presence of various interrelated factors or by the imprecision of terms used to characterize muscle function. (Table 1 lists four important symptoms that can provide early clues to the presence of myopathy.) In some patients, however, the first suspicion of muscle disease occurs when routine laboratory evaluation shows an increased concentration of serum creatine kinase (CK) in an otherwise normal individual.

SYMPTOMS AND SIGNS

The dominant finding in patients with myopathy is weakness. The clinician should ask the patient to specify the muscle groups that are involved. Upper extremity proximal weakness is characterized by a decreased ability to lift objects, especially overhead. Using a hairbrush, hanging up clothing, reaching for objects in cabinets, and lifting food or liquids from the upper shelves of a refrigerator can be difficult for patients in this group. By contrast, distal upper extremity weakness is uncommon in most myopathies, unless the condition has progressed to an advanced stage. Proximal muscle weakness of the lower extremities may be suggested by difficulty in arising from a chair or toilet seat or trouble in climbing stairs or getting in and out of an automobile. Stepping onto the sidewalk from the street may also be difficult. Distal or foot weakness may occur, but it is unusual in myopathic disorders. An abnormal gait with a high step, or tripping on curbs, uneven ground, or pavement may be the consequence of weakness of foot dorsiflexion.

Weakness of the musculature of the trunk can be hard to recognize, but patients so affected have difficulty in arising from bed. A characteristic maneuver involving rolling to the side and swinging the legs downward while using the arms to press against the bed is employed to raise the upper body from the supine position. Weakness of the muscles of the face (e.g., ptosis of the eyelids or facial droop) is not common in most myopathies. Tongue weakness is also uncommon. Palatal weakness with swallowing difficulties and altered speech patterns has been reported and may increase the risk of aspiration.

As much as possible, functional abnormalities should be quantified. For example, how far can the patient walk? How much can he or she lift? The clinician can then perform muscle testing to confirm the nature and degree of muscle dysfunction suggested by the history. Measuring muscle weakness during the physical examination requires experience and skill. Importantly, the patient must be able to cooperate fully. Pain or fatigue may interfere with maximal effort and preclude objective assessment of muscle strength. The most commonly used technique employs a numerical grading system (Table 2). The distinction between good (4) strength and normal (5) strength in such a system depends on the relationship of the examiner's force to the patient's strength. Subjective variability in the perception of clinicians who test muscle strength is well documented. Therefore, these tests should be performed in precisely the same manner with the patient assuming standard joint positions. For example, the quadriceps femoris produces more force when tested isometrically at 60 degrees rather than at 30 degrees of knee extension. If some examiners test at 30 degrees, whereas others test at 60 degrees, scoring will not be uniform.

The clinician should also assess gait, including toe-and-heel walking as well as the ability to step up onto a low platform. The patient's ability to rise from a chair, as well as from the supine position, should also be tested. Muscle tenderness, muscle volume, spontaneous movements, deep tendon reflexes, and sensory findings should be recorded.

Table 1. Clues to the Presence of Muscle Disease

Muscle pain
Muscle weakness
Fatigue
Exercise intolerance

Table 2. Scoring Muscle Strength

Grade	Characteristics
0	No voluntary contraction evident
1 trace	Trace of contraction—no limb motion
2 poor	Limb can be moved but cannot overcome gravity
3 fair	Muscle can overcome gravity
4 good	Muscle can overcome moderate applied resistance
5 normal	Muscle can overcome considerable resistance

Table 3. Myopathy Versus Lower Motor Neuron Disease

Finding	Myopathy	Lower Motor Neuron Disease
Muscle volume	Initially preserved	Atrophic
Deep tendon reflexes	Preserved	Lost
Spontaneous twitching	Absent	Present
Cramping	Absent	Present
Weakness	Present	Present

Table 3 compares these findings in patients with myopathy with the findings in patients with lower motor neuron disease. If the history and physical examination raise the possibility of myopathy, laboratory analyses, electromyography, ultrasound, magnetic resonance imaging (MRI), and muscle biopsy can be used to identify the basis for clinically significant muscle dysfunction more precisely.

LABORATORY ASSAYS

The most useful laboratory tests are those that measure the release of myoplasmic components into the circulation and the urine.

Enzymes

Serum enzyme activity is increased in many patients with myopathy. However, proper interpretation of these enzyme assay results requires knowledge of preanalytic variables that may influence the values reported by various laboratories. Most assays reflect enzyme activity, rather than amount, so that artifacts induced by inhibitors, specimen handling, or dilution may affect the values reported by the laboratory. In addition, hemolysis may produce spurious increases of lactate dehydrogenase (LD) and aspartate aminotransferase (AST) that reflect release of enzyme from erythrocytes, not myocytes. Despite these potential pitfalls, serum enzyme values continue to be the most useful laboratory indicators of muscle disease (Table 4).

Creatine kinase (CK) is present in highest concentration in muscle and in appreciable amounts in the nervous system. CK controls the flow of energy within cells by catalyzing the interconversion of adenosine triphosphate (ATP) and creatine phosphate. More than 90 per cent of the CK in skeletal muscle consists of dimers composed of two M subunits. Skeletal muscle also contains traces of the MB isoform composed of one M subunit and one B subunit. Cardiac muscle also contains primarily MM, but the MB isoform comprises 20 to 30 per cent of the total. CK is also present in smooth muscle and in the nervous system, but in smaller amounts than in skeletal or cardiac muscle. In the central nervous system (CNS) and smooth muscle, BB dimers compose 95 to 100 per cent of the total CK. Therefore, skeletal muscle damage causes the release of CK-MM, whereas cardiac muscle injury causes the release of CK-MM and CK-MB. Increased amounts of CK-MB in the circulation can provide a useful marker of cardiac disease in many individuals. In patients with chronic myopathy, however, increased amounts of CK-MB may be present both in skeletal muscle and in the circulation. Indeed, CK-MB concentrations of up to 20 and 30 per cent have been noted in various skeletal muscle disorders, including muscular dystrophy and inflammatory muscle disease. Increased concentrations of CK-MB have even been observed in the skeletal muscle and circulation of long distance runners. Therefore, increased CK-MB in serum may indicate cardiac damage, but in patients with diseases of skeletal muscle, reliance on total CK-MB or on the ratio of CK-MB to total CK cannot be used alone for the diagnosis of myocardial injury. Large molecular weight complexes of mitochondrial CK, or macro-CK, have been observed in patients with severe tissue damage or certain neoplasms. Macro-CK of another type may be the result of a complex between the enzyme and immunoglobulin. The clinical significance of this latter form of CK is uncertain.

Table 4. Enzymes

Creatine kinase
MB form in higher concentrations in myopathic skeletal muscle
Macroforms rarely present in serum
Aspartate aminotransferase
Found in many tissues
Lactate dehydrogenase
Found in many tissues
Aldolase
Found in many tissues
Carbonic anhydrase III
Not found in cardiac muscle

Although release of CK is most dramatic and rapid in the course of myopathy, other enzymes are also released into the serum of patients with skeletal muscle disease. AST is found in many tissues including heart, liver, skeletal muscle, and kidney. Its values rise less rapidly and to a lesser degree than those of CK during the course of muscle disease. Smaller amounts of ALT may also be present in muscle, and increases of this enzyme to a lesser extent may also occur.

LD, a tetrameric protein that catalyzes the interconversion of pyruvate and lactate, is found in many tissues. During acute myopathy, the rise in serum LD is less dramatic, generally occurs later, and is more prolonged than that of CK. In patients with inflammatory myopathy who are responding to treatment, serum LD concentrations may remain increased for hours to days following normalization of serum CK. There are five LD isoenzymes, and different muscles may contain different proportions of all forms. Thus, electrophoresis and isoenzyme identification and/or quantitation has not been useful in the management of myopathies. In general, patients with skeletal muscle disease release many if not all LD isoenzymes into the circulation, with a relative disproportionate increase in the cathodal forms. The precise degree and pattern of release varies with age, extent of disease, and site of muscle involvement. Markedly increased serum LD is observed in liver disease and hemolysis and, like AST, LD has less specificity than does CK for the diagnosis of myopathy. Aldolase is another widely distributed enzyme with various protein forms. Increased serum aldolase concentrations are not specific for skeletal myopathy.

Most patients with active myopathy demonstrate increased serum activity of all the enzymes mentioned. Occasionally, however, patients with muscle disease do not release significant amounts of enzyme into the circulation. For example, during the course of the eosinophilia-myalgia syndrome (an epidemic illness that occurred in patients who ingested certain commercial lots of tryptophan) serum CK concentrations were normal despite clear evidence of inflammatory muscle disease in biopsy specimens.

Carbonic anhydrase III is found in many tissues, including skeletal muscle. Importantly, it has not been found in cardiac muscle. Although it is possible that serum concentrations of carbonic anhydrase may be helpful in distinguishing skeletal from cardiac myopathy, clinical utility has thus far been limited to recent studies.

Myoglobin

Myoglobin is the respiratory protein of both skeletal and cardiac muscle. It may leak from the cell and appear in the circulation during the course of muscle disease (Table 5). In the laboratory, myoglobinuria may be detected if the amount of myoglobin released is substantial. Following trauma, drug-related rhabdomyolysis, or exercise-induced rhabdomyolysis in genetically susceptible individuals, large amounts of myoglobin are released rapidly, and visible myoglobinuria occurs. Myoglobinemia regularly accompanies myopathic states even in the absence of visible pigmentation of serum or urine. Therefore, assay of serum myoglobin is another useful laboratory indicator of myopathy or cardiac disease. Clinicians must remember that patients with muscle disease and persistent large increases of myoglobin in the circulation are at increased risk for the development of renal failure resulting from myoglobinuria.

Creatine

The urinary excretion of creatine may provide a measure of the severity and activity of myopathy, even in patients with normal serum concentrations of enzymes and myoglobin.

Creatine is synthesized in the liver and transported to muscle where, as creatine phosphate, it plays a key role in energy metabolism. It is cleared at the glomerulus on its release from the myocyte as creatinine. The total excretion of creatinine depends on muscle mass. In myopathic states, the urinary concentration of creatine increases because myocytes do not take it up efficiently from the circulation and because its retention and storage within muscle cells is impaired. The measurement and assessment of creatinuria, however, has some difficulties. Collection may be logistically difficult, and daily excretion rates may vary. Creatinuria occurs normally in children and is also seen in patients with hyperthyroidism.

Ischemic Lactate Testing

An interesting and rare subset of patients with metabolic myopathy has striking exercise intolerance manifested by pain, cramping and, in severe cases, rhabdomyolysis. Defects in a number of muscle enzymes that metabolize glycogen and glucose to produce adenosine triphosphate and lactate have been identified in some of these patients. When abnormalities of this type are suspected, ischemic lactate testing can provide further diagnostic support. This outpatient procedure begins with venous sampling for lactate without a tourniquet. The clinician then produces forearm muscle ischemia by inflating a blood pressure cuff to greater than systolic pressure for 60 seconds. During this time, the patient rapidly opens and clenches the fist to its maximal extent. The cuff is then released and postischemic exercise samples are obtained from the vein of that forearm after 1, 2, 3, and 5 minutes. Normal individuals show a striking, rapid rise in lactate concentrations (usually three times the initial control value), whereas patients with enzyme defects in the lactate-generating pathway fail to show increases in blood lactate concentrations under these conditions. The diagnosis of metabolic myopathy can then be confirmed by biopsy and specific biochemical assay. Ammonia production is normally increased during ischemic exercise as a consequence of purine metabolism. If the ammonia concentration does not increase in venous samples obtained during the ischemic test, abnormalities of myoadenylate deaminase must be considered.

Table 5. Myoglobin

Respiratory heme protein of skeletal muscle
Myoglobinemia common in myopathic states
Myoglobinuria carries risk of renal failure

ELECTROMYOGRAPHY

Electromyographic studies are designed to evaluate the patterns of activity of several muscles and their response to stimulation. The pattern of response may suggest abnormalites of neural stimulation, abnormalities of the motor end-plate, or abnormalities of the muscle cell. The experience and patience of the electromyographer are critical contributors to the sensitivity of this technique.

Lower motor neuron lesions are accompanied by fibrillation potentials and the loss of activity of motor units, precluding the normal interference pattern seen with voluntary contraction. Synchronization of motor unit activity following reinnervation of previously denervated myofibers produces larger than normal amplitudes of response with prolonged duration.

In disorders of the muscle cell, loss of myofibers decreases the duration of the motor unit potential and increases the number of polyphasic responses. In some muscle disorders, especially the inflammatory myopathies, irritative phenomena with fibrillation potentials may be observed.

The response of muscle to repetitive stimulation can provide evidence for the presence of motor end-plate disorders (e.g., myasthenia gravis). Measurements of the speed of impulse conduction in peripheral nerves can provide evidence of neuropathy. Taken together, the electromyogram plus nerve conduction studies can provide specific evidence of myopathy, neuropathy, or motor end-plate disease. The patterns of abnormalities can also be used to localize lesions anatomically.

MUSCLE BIOPSY

At present, muscle biopsy continues to provide the most specific and precise approach to the diagnosis of muscle disorders. Importantly, careful technique produces the most diagnostically useful information. First, the investigator must decide which muscle to sample for analysis. In general, the muscle selected should be involved but not severely atrophic or at the end stage of disease. Second, the proper techniques required for analysis should be available. Light microscopy with conventional staining is generally always useful. Enzyme assay staining techniques can be employed to distinguish fiber types and to evaluate neuropathies as well as metabolic disorders. Electron microscopy can be particularly helpful in the diagnosis of mitochondrial myopathies and inclusion body myositis. Biochemial assay of muscle enzyme content may be appropriate in metabolic and mitochondrial myopathies; for example when McArdle's disease or other disorders of glycogen breakdown are suspected. The response of muscle to exogenous agents can be tested, as has been performed in the malignant hyperthermia syndrome. Communication and cooperation among clinicians, pathologists, and relevant laboratory personnel prior to muscle biopsy will ensure the best results. Open surgical or closed needle biopsy techniques may be employed.

NEWER TESTS

Newer approaches to the evaluation of the patient with myopathy include MRI, computed tomography, and ultrasound (Table 6). MRI may be helpful in localizing abnormal muscles and in guiding the biopsy of inflamed muscles in patients with patchy involvement. Spectroscopic analysis of the nuclear magnetic resonance of phosphorus has also been used to study energy metabolism of muscles and to follow the clinical progress of patients with myopathies.

DIFFERENTIAL DIAGNOSIS

To construct a reasonable differential diagnosis of a muscle disorder, the clinician should focus the initial inquiry on pain and weakness. First, what signs and symptoms can be directly ascribed to the musculoskeletal system? If pain is present, is it localized, suggesting an injury or tendinitis? Remember that shoulder impingement and osteoarthritis of the spine may produce localized pain of contiguous musculature. By contrast, generalized muscle pain is commonly reported in systemic disorders, including viral infections, hypothyroidism, and toxicity associated with the use of lipid-lowering agents. Patients with fibromyalgia and polymyalgia rheumatica can also present with marked muscle pain. Polymyalgia frequently leads to pain in muscles of the shoulder and pelvic girdle, which is often accompanied by severe morning stiffness and disability.

If weakness is present, what is the pattern? Asymmetric weakness may be caused by focal lesions in the nervous system. Distal symmetric weakness is consistent with neuropathy or lower motor neuron disease. Spinal stenosis or vascular disease of the lower extremities may produce exertional pain and weakness. Inclusion body myositis may also present with distal weakness that accompanies proximal muscle dysfunction. Weakness of cranial muscles occurs in central nervous system disorders, myasthenia gravis, myotonic dystrophy, and facioscapulohumeral dystrophy. Symmetric proximal weakness is a classic presentation for skeletal myopathy. Cramps, fasciculations, abnormal sensation, and abnormal deep tendon reflexes point to disease of the nervous system. Deep tendon reflexes may be difficult to elicit when the responding muscle is at the end stage of disease or is severely atrophic.

When the history and physical examination suggest myopathy, at least nine basic causes of muscle disease should be considered (Table 7). In the United States, viruses are the most common infectious causes of myopathy. Influenza, human immunodeficiency virus (HIV), and coxsackievirus are most commonly implicated. Bacterial pyomyositis is unusual in temperate climates in otherwise normal hosts. Lyme disease with myopathy is thus far unusual. *Toxoplasma* may produce a flulike illness with myopathy.

Table 6. Newer Tests for Evaluating Myopathy

- Magnetic resonance imaging
- Magnetic resonance phosphorus spectroscopy to evaluate biochemical function
- Computed tomography
- Ultrasound

Table 7. Causes of Myopathy

- Trauma
  - Localized
  - Generalized with risk of myoglobinuria
- Infections
  - Viral (influenza, coxsackievirus, human immunodeficiency virus)
  - Bacterial (pyomyositis, Lyme disease)
  - Toxoplasmosis
  - Parasitic (*Trichinella*)
- Vascular
  - Ischemic myopathy
- Pharmacologic agents
  - Lipid-lowering agents, diuretics, illicit drugs
- Electrolyte disorders
  - Sodium, potassium, phosphorus, calcium, magnesium
- Endocrine and metabolic disorders
  - Thyroid, adrenal, parathyroid
  - Alcohol exposure
- Hereditary dystrophies and myopathies
  - In adults (e.g., facioscapulohumeral, limb-girdle, distal dystrophies)
  - Carbohydrate pathway disorders (e.g., McCardle's disease)
  - Lipid pathway disorders (e.g., carnitine palmitoyl transferase deficiency, carnitine deficiencies)
  - Mitochondrial myopathies
- Neoplasms
  - Paraneoplastic states
    - Myasthenic syndromes
    - Paraneoplastic myopathy
    - Dermatomyositis
  - Direct involvement of muscle uncommon
- Inflammatory disorders
  - Connective tissue diseases
    - Scleroderma
    - Sarcoid
    - Rheumatoid arthritis
    - Sjögren's syndrome
    - Systemic lupus erythematosus
  - Primary myositis
    - Dermatomyositis
    - Polymyositis
    - Inclusion body myositis

Vascular (ischemic) disorders, electrolyte imbalance, and drugs are also well-established causes of myopathy. Although electrolyte disturbances are unusual in outpatients who are not receiving parenteral fluids, measurement of serum sodium, phosphorus, potassium, calcium, chloride, and magnesium concentrations may be useful in selected patients. Chronic diuretic use with electrolyte depletion occasionally causes muscle weakness, and the recent focus on correcting hypercholesterolemia has led to widespread use of lipid-lowering agents that may produce a painful myopathy. Alcohol consumption can produce acute or chronic myopathy, with or without increased serum enzyme activity. Intravenous drug use (e.g., heroin, cocaine) has also been associated with severe myopathy. Thyroid function must be evaluated in any patient with persistent systemic muscle dysfunction. Hypothyroid individuals frequently experience muscle pain and stiffness and markedly increased serum CK activity. In hypothyroidism, generalized weakness may develop insidiously. Myopathy frequently develops in patients with excess glucocorticoid concentrations due to endocrinopathy or steroid administration. Adrenal insufficiency and pituitary disorders may also cause muscle dysfunction. Parathyroid conditions associated with hypercalcemia or hypocalcemia may present with neuromyopathic symptoms. Exhaustive endocrine evaluation is not required in all patients with myopathy. Rather, the possibilities should be considered and specific testing employed when appropriate.

Although hereditary myopathy typically appears in childhood, facioscapulohumeral dystrophy and some forms of limb-girdle and distal dystrophy may appear in early adulthood. McArdle's disease and other disorders of carbohydrate metabolism may also first appear in young adults. Family history can be especially valuable in the diagnosis of hereditary myopathy, but it may be difficult to obtain.

Chronic generalized myopathy, dermatomyositis, and a myasthenic syndrome of progressive weakness with exertion have all been associated with underlying or occult neoplasm. Thus, in selected patients, a search for cancer may be appropriate. Electromyography can help the clinician seeking to distinguish myasthenia gravis from the paraneoplastic myasthenic syndrome most frequently associated with cancer of the lung. Patients with scleroderma, systemic lupus erythematosus, sarcoidosis, and rheumatoid arthritis may present with myopathy. Weakness, increased serum enzyme activity, and histologic evidence of muscle inflammation can be detected in some patients with connective tissue disorders. The presence of Raynaud's phenomenon, dysphagia, nodules, or joint pain and swelling may be helpful in suggesting the presence of other connective tissue disorders in certain patients with inflammatory muscle disease.

Finally, primary idiopathic inflammation of muscle (e.g., polymyositis, dermatomyositis, and inclusion body myositis) presents with weakness, increased serum enzyme activity, and characteristic biopsy findings. A characteristic rash may be noted on the face, neck, chest, upper arms, and thighs and over bony prominences, especially in the hands, in patients with dermatomyositis. Periungual telangiectasia may also be a significant finding.

PERIODIC PARALYSES

By Louis S. Binder, M.D.
Chicago, Illinois
and Albert C. Cuetter, M.D.
El Paso, Texas

Acute presentation of periodic generalized muscular weakness is an uncommon yet important and challenging medical emergency. There are many causes of acute periodic muscular weakness. Table 1 shows a convenient grouping of the periodic paralyses into two major groups: the familial, primary periodic paralyses and the secondary periodic paralyses.

Table 1. Classification of Periodic Paralyses

Familial Primary Periodic Paralyses

- Hypokalemic
- Hyperkalemic without myotonia, or with myotonia (paramyotonia congenita, von Eulenberg-Gamstorp disease)
- Andersen's syndrome

Secondary (Acquired) Periodic Paralyses

- Due to urinary potassium loss
  - Primary hyperaldosteronism
  - Thiazide therapy
  - Ureterocolostomy
  - Renal tubular acidosis
- Due to gastrointestinal potassium loss
  - Sprue
  - Severe diarrhea
  - Repeated vomiting
  - Draining gastrointestinal fistula
- Due to intracellular shift of potassium
  - Thyrotoxic periodic paralysis
  - Barium poisoning

FAMILIAL PRIMARY PERIODIC PARALYSES

The familial primary periodic paralyses are a group of conditions with several common features. They are inherited as autosomal dominant disorders, and a positive family history is a crucial clinical factor in establishing the diagnosis. Localized or generalized episodic muscular weakness is associated with changes in serum potassium during the attacks of paralysis. Weakness usually begins in the proximal muscles and then spreads to the distal musculature. The patient may experience the weakness on arising in the morning, and the muscular weakness is generally limited to the limbs and limb girdles. Respiratory and cranial nerve muscles tend to be spared in early attacks, but they may be involved during subsequent attacks.

The incidence of attacks increases in cold weather. Exposure to cold may produce the weakness, while continuous mild exercise may abort the attacks. The patient may be able to "walk off" an attack of paralysis, and complete recovery typically occurs after the attack. Rest following a period of exercise tends to provoke weakness of the muscles exercised. Muscle fibers become unresponsive to electrical stimulation during the attacks of paralysis. The frequency of attacks tends to diminish with age, but permanent weakness and irreversible vacuolar myopathy can develop after repeated attacks.

New genetic information indicates that the simple classification of familial primary periodic paralyses into *hypokalemic periodic paralysis* and *hyperkalemic periodic paralysis* is still valid. Both hypokalemic periodic paralysis and hyperkalemic periodic paralysis can have normal serum potassium values during the attacks of weakness. It is the response to factors that raise or lower serum potassium that characterizes these disorders.

SECONDARY PERIODIC PARALYSES

Secondary periodic paralyses are usually associated with urinary potassium loss, gastrointestinal potassium loss, or intracellular potassium shifts. Periodic paralysis secondary to primary hyperaldosteronism, thiazide therapy, ureterocolostomy, or renal tubular acidosis is typically associated with loss of potassium in the urine. Periodic paralysis secondary to sprue, severe diarrhea, repeated vomiting, or draining gastrointestinal fistula is typically associated with loss of potassium from the gastrointestinal tract. Periodic paralysis secondary to thyrotoxicosis or barium poisoning is most often associated with intracellular shifts of potassium.

PRESENTING SYMPTOMS AND SIGNS

Familial Primary Hypokalemic Periodic Paralysis

Familial primary hypokalemic periodic paralysis (FPHypoKPP) is inherited as an autosomal dominant disorder.

The attacks of paralysis typically begin in adolescence but may start as late as the third decade. A male predominance of 3:1 reflects reduced penetrance and expression of the disease in females. FPHypoKPP is more common in whites than other races. Episodes of paralysis are most common at night, with patients typically awakening unable to walk. The weakness may last up to 36 hours. Attacks occur as infrequently as once a year, but in severe cases can appear daily. Initially, attacks are infrequent, but eventually they may recur daily. The muscular weakness is limited to the limbs. Cranial and respiratory muscles are rarely involved. During the attacks, the muscle stretch reflexes are diminished.

Factors that may precipitate an attack of weakness include large meals rich in carbohydrates, metabolic alkalosis, surgery, hypothermia, excitement, or the administration of epinephrine, hydrocortisone, insulin, or sodium chloride. Attacks are alleviated by the administration of potassium.

The paralysis is related to hypokalemia in patients with adequate total body potassium stores. Potassium moves from extracellular spaces into the cell. This shift causes resting membrane depolarization, making the muscle fibers electrically unexcitable. No muscle contractions occur, and paralysis ensues. The exact method of potassium translocation is unknown, but it is increased by rest, a diet rich in carbohydrates, and infusion of glucose and insulin. The serum potassium concentration is usually decreased during the attacks, but it may be normal.

Familial Primary Hyperkalemic Periodic Paralysis

The clinical spectrum of familial primary hyperkalemic periodic paralyses (FPHyperKPP; von Eulenberg-Gamstorp disease, paramyotonia congenita) includes episodes of periodic weakness with or without myotonia, and attacks of myotonia with or without weakness. The episodic weakness induced or worsened by potassium is called FPHyperKPP; the episodic myotonia and weakness induced or worsened by muscle cooling is called paramyotonia congenita. Thus, FPHyperKPP and paramyotonia congenita are genetic muscle disorders sharing the common features of episodic myotonia and weakness. Some patients present with features of both disorders.

FPHyperKPP and paramyotonia congenita are transmitted as autosomal dominant allelic disorders. Both conditions are associated with mutations in genes (on chromosome 17q) that code for the alpha subunit of adult skeletal muscle voltage–dependent sodium channels. Molecular alterations of the alpha subunits lead to abnormal sodium currents, which, in turn, cause muscle paralysis.

The attacks in FPHyperKPP typically begin in childhood. Weakness and/or myotonia is first noted between 4 and 18 years of age. Most patients have mild and brief attacks, especially in the daytime. A few patients with FPHyperKPP have brief attacks several times per day. Nocturnal attacks are typically more prolonged than daytime episodes. Most patients with FPHyperKPP have clinical or electromyographic myotonia. Attacks begin with a stiff feeling in the legs after prolonged sitting; weakness becomes apparent when the patient tries to walk. Weakness may remain confined to the legs, but stiffness and weakness may spread to the back, arms, and neck, typically within 30 minutes. In some patients, attacks of weakness subside after adolescence; in others, proximal weakness gradually develops after many years of repeated attacks. Muscle wasting is not generally observed in FPHyperKPP. Attacks of weakness can be elicited by sleep, fasting, cold weather, emotional stimulation, menstruation, pregnancy, intercurrent infections, anesthesia, rest after exercise, and by oral loading with potassium salts. Warming of the muscles diminishes the weakness.

Cold exposure precipitates myotonia and weakness in patients whose clinical picture includes myotonia. The myotonic phenomenon may affect the cranial, thenar, and finger extensor muscles. The patient may complain of stiff eye muscles, tightness of the face and throat, dysphagia, dysarthria, and the inability to relax the hand and forearm muscles after a contraction. The alert clinician may observe lid-lag myotonia when the patient is asked to look down after looking up. Percussion myotonia has been reported in the thenar muscles. Some patients with other typical features of FPHyperKPP do not have clinical myotonia, but needle electrode examination may show myotonic discharges. These repetitive discharges of 50 to 70 Hz may produce a characteristic musical sound in the audio display of the electromyograph that has been likened to the sound of a "dive bomber."

Although serum potassium concentration is often normal in FPHyperKPP, it tends to be high when attacks reach maximal severity. Attacks may occur with serum potassium concentrations of 6 to 7.5 mEq/L, and the critical concentration tends to be relatively constant for a given patient. An increased serum potassium concentration between attacks suggests secondary periodic paralysis, rather than primary familial periodic paralysis.

Andersen Syndrome

Andersen syndrome is a potassium-sensitive periodic paralysis associated with cardiac arrhythmias and dysmorphic features. Spontaneous attacks of weakness are associated with hyperkalemia, but myotonia is not a prominent feature. The dysmorphic features of Andersen syndrome include microcephaly, low-set ears, hypoplastic mandibles, hypertelorism, clinodactyly, and short stature. The inheritance is autosomal dominant in some patients. The defect in Andersen syndrome is not genetically linked to other forms of potassium-sensitive periodic paralyses.

Hyperaldosteronism

Hyperaldosteronism frequently accompanies hyperplasia or tumor of the adrenal cortex. The combination of sodium retention, potassium loss, and metabolic alkalosis produces recurrent muscular weakness and hypertension. The Conn syndrome (primary aldosteronism) is most commonly seen in Asian patients.

"Pseudohyperaldosteronism" has been reported as a complication of chronic licorice ingestion. Licorice is prepared from the *Glycyrrhiza glabra* plant, which contains glycyrrhizic acid. This agent has mineralocorticoid activity that suppresses the renin-angiotensin-aldosterone axis and thus produces sodium retention, hypokalemia, and paralysis. This effect can be seen with a single dose or repeated doses as small as 100 to 200 g (two to four confectionery twists) of licorice per day. Carbenoxolone, a derivative of glycyrrhizic acid, has also been associated with hypokalemic paralysis.

Renal Tubular Acidosis

Renal tubular acidosis (RTA) refers to a group of syndromes characterized by the impaired ability to secrete hydrogen ions in the distal nephron (type I RTA) or to resorb bicarbonate ions in the proximal tubules (type II RTA). Chronic metabolic acidosis occurs in both forms of

RTA, but potassium depletion and hypokalemic paralysis are more common in the distal form. Distal RTA (type I) usually is a sporadic disorder, but familial cases occur as autosomal dominant disorders or in association with other genetic diseases. Sporadic, spontaneous distal RTA occurs as a primary disease that is more common in women than men. However, sporadic, spontaneous distal RTA also develops as a secondary disorder in patients with Sjögren's syndrome, renal medullary cystic disease, nephrocalcinosis, renal transplanation, chronic obstruction, and chronic toluene exposure, and in patients treated with lithium or amphotericin B. By contrast, proximal RTA (type II) accompanies several inherited diseases, including Fanconi's syndrome, Wilson's disease, Lowe (oculocerebrorenal) syndrome, and hereditary fructose intolerance as well as multiple myeloma, vitamin D deficiency, hypocalcemia with secondary hyperparathyroidism, renal transplantation, and treatment with acetazolamide, sulfonamides, streptozocin, and outdated tetracycline.

Other disorders associated with urinary potassium loss and possible hypokalemic paralysis include nephrotic syndrome, the diuretic phase of acute tubular necrosis, the treatment phase of diabetic ketoacidosis, chlorothiazide-associated hypokalemia, and hypokalemia following ureterocolostomy.

Patients with severe diarrhea may lose as much as 100 mEq/L of potassium per day. Hypokalemic paralysis has been associated with gluten-induced enteropathy (celiac disease), tropical sprue, Salmonella enteritis, Strongyloides enteritis, Yersinia enterocolitis, and malabsorption due to short bowel syndrome.

Thyrotoxic Periodic Paralysis

Thyrotoxic periodic paralysis (TPP) resembles the familial primary periodic paralyses. Onset of the paralytic attacks coincides with onset of hyperthyroidism, but overt signs of thyrotoxicosis are rarely present during the initial paralytic attack. Although hyperthyroidism is generally more common in females, TPP occurs with a male-to-female ratio of 20 to 1. More than 90 per cent of all cases of TPP have been reported in Asian patients, and the disease affects as many as 25 per cent of thyrotoxic Asian males. The onset of TPP is in the second to fourth decades. As with familial primary periodic paralysis, there is a translocation of potassium into the muscle cells. Acetazolamide administration may exacerbate the attacks of paralysis in TPP, and attacks can be blocked with propranolol.

Barium Toxicity

Oral ingestion of 0.8 to 15 g of absorbable barium chloride or barium carbonate (used for glazing pottery) has been reported to cause hypokalemic paralysis and death. Epidemics of poisoning have occurred after barium carbonate contamination of flour or salt. Industrial accidents and suicide attempts have also been reported.

COMPLICATIONS

In FPHypoKPP, cardiac symptoms, especially bradycardia, may occur during an attack of weakness. Electrocardiographic changes, including T-wave alterations and prolongation of PR, QRS, and QT intervals, are typically seen when the serum potassium concentration drops below 3.3 mEq/L.

Cardiac arrhythmias between attacks are not a feature of FPHypoKPP, but fixed electrocardiographic abnormalities occur infrequently after many years of disease. These electrocardiographic changes include ectopy, most commonly bigeminy, and ventricular tachycardia. Some patients with both types of familial primary periodic paralyses develop a chronic vacuolar myopathy after many years of repeated attacks. The permanent weakness in FPHypoKPP may be disabling. Thyrotoxicosis is associated with arrhythmias, and a slightly greater risk of arrhythmias may exist in thyrotoxic periodic paralysis. Respiratory paralysis and/or failure is rare in all forms of periodic paralyses.

DIAGNOSTIC EVALUATION

History and Physical Examination

A positive family history and adequate documentation of an attack of weakness are crucial factors in the diagnosis of familial periodic paralyses. However, secondary causes of periodic paralysis must be excluded (see Table 1). Patients who present beyond age 30 with episodic paralysis most likely have a secondary, rather than a primary, form of periodic paralysis.

Between attacks, the physical examination typically shows normal strength. During the attacks of weakness in FPHypoKPP, the muscle stretch reflexes are diminished. Patients with FPHyperKPP may have clinical percussion myotonia in the tongue and thenar muscles. They cannot relax the hand muscles after making a grip, and lid-lag myotonia may be seen on downward gaze after they have looked up.

Useful Laboratory Procedures

Blood count, urinalysis, blood chemistry, chest radiograph, electrocardiogram, and thyroid function studies should be performed; serum potassium concentration should be measured every 30 minutes during attacks. Although the serum potassium concentration is usually low or low-to-normal during attacks of FPHypoKPP, it may be normal late in the attacks. Potassium concentrations are often normal in FPHyperKPP; hyperkalemia may be noted as attacks begin to subside.

Provocative tests are necessary for confirming the diagnosis unless the attacks can be precipitated with changes in diet and/or physical activity. Provocative tests should not be performed in patients with cardiac disease, renal insufficiency, or unequivocally abnormal concentrations of serum potassium. During provocative testing, the muscle strength, electrocardiogram, and serum potassium concentration should be monitored. The best known provocative test in FPHypoKPP involves the oral administration of 2 g/kg of glucose plus 20 U of crystalline insulin. Weakness typically develops within 3 hours. If weakness does not develop, the test can be repeated after exercise and after salt loading (2 g of sodium chloride dissolved in water and administered orally every hour for 4 doses). The results of these tests may help the clinician predict the response to treatment with potassium.

The potassium exercise test can also be useful in confirming the diagnosis of FPHypoKPP. Normal individuals usually reveal increased serum potassium concentrations after 30 minutes of vigorous exercise. By contrast, patients with FPHypoKPP have little or no increase in serum potassium concentrations after exercise.

To precipitate or exacerbate weakness and myotonia in FPHyperKPP, 2 to 10 g of potassium chloride is administered orally in an unsweetened solution immediately following exercise in the fasting state. Patients should be monitored closely because potassium loading may produce respiratory paralysis or cardiac conduction disturbances. Immersion of the hand in water at 10°C for 5 minutes may elicit localized weakness or exacerbate weakness in patients with myotonia.

Other Useful Diagnostic Procedures

In both forms of familial primary periodic paralysis, serum creatine kinase activity may be increased following an attack of weakness. Between attacks of primary familial periodic paralyses, the electrocardiogram is usually unremarkable. During the attacks, electrocardiographic changes reflect the variation of serum potassium concentrations.

Nerve conduction studies show normal compound muscle action potentials (CMAPs) during supramaximal stimulation. In patients at rest, repetitive nerve stimulation at 2 Hz produces little or no decrement in the amplitude of CMAPs. By contrast, if stimulation at 2 Hz is performed 20 minutes after prolonged exercise lasting 5 minutes, a 40 per cent reduction in the amplitude of CMAPs is frequently observed. This finding correlates with the clinical occurrence of weakness while the patient is at rest after a period of prolonged exercise. Needle electrode examination during attacks shows a full interference pattern with motor unit action potentials of reduced amplitude and duration.

During needle electrode examination, myotonic discharges are seen only in patients with FPHyperKPP. Their presence can help the clinician distinguish FPHyperKPP from FPHypoKPP. In addition, the electromyographic myotonia of FPHyperKPP differs from other myotonias in two ways. First, the myotonia of FPHyperKPP worsens with repetitive muscular contraction; second, that myotonia disappears electrographically with cooling. The latter feature is the electrical expression of the cold-induced weakness seen clinically in FPHyperKPP with myotonia.

The various forms of familial primary periodic paralysis cannot be distinguished by light microscopic or electron microscopic evaluation of muscle biopsy tissue. However, the observation of distended sarcoplasmic reticulum, multiple intracellular vacuoles, and increased intrafibrillary glycogen supports the diagnosis of periodic paralysis in patients who report episodic weakness.

A response to treatment during attacks of weakness or a response to prophylaxis in patients with documented familial primary periodic paralyses may have diagnostic significance. Attacks of FPHypoKPP are diminished by potassium and are prevented by small feedings, a low-carbohydrate diet, spironolactone, and acetazolamide. Attacks of FPHyperKPP are diminished by foods rich in carbohydrates and by inhalations of salbutamol; attacks can be prevented by administration of kaliuretic agents.

In Andersen syndrome, the oral potassium challenge induces significant proximal weakness. Hypokalemia aggravates cardiac abnormalities. The electrocardiogram shows premature ventricular contractions, ventricular bigeminy, and unsustained ventricular tachycardia. The QT interval is prolonged.

In RTA, the principal clinical features are a hyperchloremic metabolic acidosis, hypokalemia, nephrolithiasis, and nephrocalcinosis. The associated hypokalemia may present with paralysis. Distal RTA can be confirmed with an acid loading test. The oral administration of ammonium chloride, 100 mg/kg, normally reduces urine pH below 5.2 within 3 to 6 hours. In patients with distal RTA, urine pH remains above 6.0. Proximal RTA can be identified with a bicarbonate titration test. Sodium bicarbonate is slowly infused to raise the serum bicarbonate concentration. In proximal RTA, bicarbonate classically appears in the urine before serum bicarbonate reaches the reference range.

Genetic Testing

Patients with Von Eulenberg-Gamstorp disease have single base pair mutations in the gene that codes for the alpha subunit of the voltage-dependent sodium channel. This genetic defect can be identified by DNA testing performed in specialized centers.

PITFALLS IN DIAGNOSIS

Many patients who complain of episodic weakness do not have true weakness at all. Furthermore, true recurrent weakness is more likely an acquired or a secondary condition than a familial or inherited primary disorder. The fluctuating weakness and fatigability of myasthenia gravis that is aggravated by continuous or repetitive activity and improved by rest should not be confused with periodic paralyses. Ocular, facial, and bulbar muscles are more commonly impaired in myasthenia gravis, and other clinical and laboratory features of myasthenia (e.g., response to edrophonium and presence of antibodies to acetylcholine receptors) are not seen in the periodic paralyses.

Serum potassium values are low or low-to-normal early in the attack of HypoKPP but may be normal late in the attack. Potassium values are often normal in HyperKPP but may increase when attacks reach their nadir. When the serum potassium concentration is normal in patients with periodic paralyses, provocative testing can secure the diagnosis.

RHABDOMYOLYSIS AND MYOGLOBINURIA

By Jen-Tse Cheng, M.D.
New York, New York

and Donald A. Feinfeld, M.D.
East Meadow, New York

Rhabdomyolysis is a clinical syndrome resulting from injury to skeletal muscle that breaks down the cell membranes, with consequent liberation of intracellular constituents (e.g., enzymes, potassium, phosphate, creatinine, and myoglobin) into the circulation. The most serious complication of rhabdomyolysis is myoglobinuria. Myoglobinuria refers to the excretion of increasing amounts of myoglobin in the urine and is often associated with the hypermyoglobinemia of rhabdomyolysis. However, not all rhabdomyolysis results in clinical myoglobinuria, and not all myoglobinuria is caused by rhabdomyolysis. In its most serious form, myoglobinuria can lead to myoglobinuric acute renal failure. The reported causes of rhabdomyolysis are many (Table 1). They can be classified into factors that (1) decrease oxygen delivery to the muscle, as in ischemic rhabdomyolysis; (2) directly injure skeletal muscle, as in traumatic rhabdomyolysis, or toxic and drug-induced rhabdomyolysis; (3) decrease energy storage or utilization of the

Table 1. Causes of Rhabdomyolysis

I. Decreased oxygen delivery to the skeletal muscles
  A. Arterial occlusion
  B. Severe vasoconstriction in cocaine or "crack" users
  C. Prolonged pressure compression of the muscles
    1. Crush injury
    2. Prolonged coma with pressure ischemia
  D. Hypokalemia with severe potassium depletion
    1. Diuretics, chronic diarrhea, vomiting
    2. Massive black licorice ingestion, carbenoxolone
    3. Amphotericin B
  E. Carbon monoxide poisoning
II. Direct injury to skeletal muscles
  A. Trauma
  B. Burns
  C. Toxins
    1. Ethanol, heroin, isopropyl alcohol, ethylene glycol, quail ingestion, snake bite, hornet stings, brown recluse spider bite, Haff disease, mercuric chloride, toluene
  D. Infections
    1. Viral: influenza, coxsackievirus, infectious hepatitis
    2. Bacterial: tetanus, Legionnaire's disease
  E. Primary muscle diseases
    1. Polymyositis and dermatomyositis
    2. Muscular dystrophies
III. Decreased energy storage or utilization
  A. Hypophosphatemia with severe phosphate depletion
  B. Disorders in carbohydrate metabolism
    1. Diabetic ketoacidosis
    2. Nonketotic hyperosmolar coma
    3. McArdle's disease
  C. Disorders of lipid metabolism
    1. Carnitine deficiency
    2. Carnitine palmityltransferase deficiency
    3. Lovastatin or gemfibrozil with concomitant renal failure or administration of cyclosporine, niacin, or erythromycin
  D. Myxedema
  E. Hypothermia
  F. Zidovudine (AZT)
IV. Increased energy consumption
  A. Seizures
  B. Delirium tremens
  C. High-voltage shock
  D. Tetanus
  E. Malignant hyperthermia
  F. Heat stroke
  G. Drugs
    1. Cocaine
    2. Amphetamine
    3. Phencyclidine (PCP, "angel dust")
    4. Malignant neuroleptic syndrome
    5. Succinylcholine

muscle, as in metabolic rhabdomyolysis; and (4) increase energy consumption, as in exertional rhabdomyolysis.

PRESENTING SYMPTOMS AND SIGNS

The presenting symptoms and signs of rhabdomyolysis (Table 2) depend largely on the underlying cause of the syndrome. The common manifestations include muscle pain, cramps, swelling, and weakness and, sometimes, loss of sensation in the overlying skin. Excretion of reddish-brown urine is observed in some patients with massive rhabdomyolysis, signaling the presence of severe myoglobinuria.

Patients with traumatic rhabdomyolysis typically present with a history of crush injury to the limb suffered during an automobile accident, a seismic disaster, or a bomb explosion. The affected limb appears swollen, discolored, and indurated, with decreased or absent muscle power. The presence of tachycardia, hypotension, and shock in the absence of external blood loss are signs of severe muscle damage, with osmotic influx of extracellular fluid into the injured muscle and consequent contraction of intravascular volume with hemoconcentration.

Patients with ischemic rhabdomyolysis usually present with symptoms of severe muscle pain with pallor, cyanosis, or coldness of the affected extremity. The arterial pulse of the affected limbs may be absent. However, in patients with cocaine-associated rhabdomyolysis, signs of severe vasoconstriction with muscle damage can be masked by the agitated, aggressive, and combative behavior, only to be recognized later by the passage of dark urine associated with early development of hyperkalemia and renal failure.

Patients with alcohol-induced rhabdomyolysis can present with muscle pain and weakness following heavy consumption of alcohol. Affected muscles are painful, swollen, and tender. Patients with heroin-induced rhabdomyolysis may be brought in to the emergency room in deep coma, with muscle swelling, and weakness and discoloration of the affected limb that has sustained prolonged compression.

Patients with metabolic rhabdomyolysis can present with severe proximal muscle weakness associated with severe hypophosphatemia or diabetic coma, severe hypokalemia secondary to gastrointestinal fluid loss or use of diuretics or amphotericin B, and severe magnesium depletion. Patients with genetic disorders of carbohydrate metabolism (e.g., myophosphorylase deficiency in McArdle's disease) can present with a history of recurrent muscle cramps and muscle weakness following exercise. Patients with genetic disorders of lipid metabolism, such as carnitine palmityltransferase deficiency, may develop muscle

Table 2. Symptoms and Signs of Rhabdomyolysis and Myoglobinuria

Rhabdomyolysis

General findings in rhabdomyolysis
  Muscle pain, cramps
  Muscle swelling
  Weakness and loss of sensation
Traumatic rhabdomyolysis
  History of crush injury
  Discoloration of injured area
  Signs of volume depletion (hypotension, tachycardia)
Ischemic rhabdomyolysis
  Severe muscle pain
  Pallor, cyanosis, or coldness in affected extremity
  Agitation, combative behavior in cocaine toxicity
Alcoholic rhabdomyolysis
  Muscle pain, weakness
  Muscle swelling and tenderness
Metabolic rhabdomyolysis
  Proximal muscle weakness
  Hypokalemia or hypophosphatemia
  History of recurrent cramps
  History of taking high-dose lovastatin with cyclosporine
Exertional rhabdomyolysis
  Seizures of delirium tremens
  Use of stimulants
  Hyperthermia

Myoglobinuria

Reddish-brown or smoky urine
Oliguria if renal failure is present

weakness and pass pigmented urine following prolonged fasting. Rhabdomyolysis with muscle pain and weakness occurs in a minority of patients receiving high doses of lipid-lowering agents, such as lovastatin and gemfibrozil, in the presence of renal failure or when combined with the use of cyclosporine or niacin.

Exertional rhabdomyolysis can occur in patients with a history of seizures, delirium tremens, use of stimulant drugs, or vigorous exertion. These events are then followed by the development of muscle pain, swelling, tenderness, and weakness and the excretion of dark urine. Hyperthermia can complicate severe muscle exertion, as seen in exercise-induced heat stroke. Many patients with rhabdomyolysis not due to trauma may not present with the typical clinical symptoms and signs of muscle injury. The clues to the presence of rhabdomyolysis can be found later in a routine urinalysis and serum chemistries.

Myoglobinuria can be totally asymptomatic, especially in its early phase. If the urinary myoglobin concentration is very high, the patient may note brown, reddish-brown, or smoky urine ("like tea or cola"). No specific physical findings are typically observed. Decreased urine volume can occur as the result of volume depletion from sequestration of fluid or from true myoglobinuric acute renal failure.

LABORATORY FINDINGS (Table 3)

A complete blood count typically reveals hemoconcentration (increased hemoglobin concentration and hematocrit) in patients with severe and extensive muscle injury, owing to sequestration of extracellular fluid in the damaged muscles. Thrombocytopenia may be seen in patients who develop disseminated intravascular coagulation. Since myoglobin does not bind strongly to plasma protein and is rapidly cleared from the plasma by the kidneys while they are functioning, inspection of the plasma from centrifuged blood in patients with rhabdomyolysis and myoglobinuria does not reveal the pink color characteristic of hemolysis.

Table 3. Laboratory Findings in Rhabdomyolysis and Myoglobinuria

Complete Blood Count

- Hemoconcentration (high hematocrit and hemoglobin)
- Thrombocytopenia (with disseminated intravascular coagulation)

Examination of Serum or Plasma

- Clear serum, indicating absence of hemoglobinemia

Blood Chemistries

- Creatinine concentration rising faster than urea nitrogen
- Early hyperkalemia
- Metabolic acidosis with high anion gap
- Hyperphosphatemia
- Hypocalcemia
- Hyperuricemia
- Increased muscle enzyme activity in serum
  - Creatine kinase (CK)-MM isotype
  - Aspartate aminotransferase (AST)
  - Lactate dehydrogenase (LD)
  - Aldolase

Coagulation Tests (In Disseminated Intravascular Coagulation)

- Increased prothrombin time, partial thromboplastin time, and fibrin degradation products
- Decreased plasma fibrinogen

Urinalysis

- Appearance: reddish-brown or "cola-colored"
- Acid urine (pH <5.5)
- Protein positive
- Positive dipstick orthotolidine test for "blood"
- Few, if any, red blood cells in urine sediment
- Pigmented granular casts
- Renal epithelial cells
- Uric acid crystals

Routine blood chemistry tests invariably show a marked increase in serum creatine kinase (CK), aldolase, lactate dehydrogenase (LD), and aspartate aminotransferase (AST) activities due to the release of these intramuscular enzymes into the circulation following rhabdomyolysis. Examination of the CK isoenzymes reveals the predominance of CK-MM isozyme, indicating the origin of the CK from skeletal muscle and excluding the heart and brain as the source of CK. A disproportionate increase in serum creatinine and serum potassium concentrations early in the course of the illness is consistent with the liberation of intracellular muscle constituents into the circulation. Decreased serum bicarbonate and increased anion gap is a frequent finding in rhabdomyolysis and signifies the development of metabolic acidosis from renal failure and/or excessive release of organic or inorganic anions into the circulation. This finding should be confirmed by arterial blood gases. Severe but asymptomatic hypocalcemia and hyperphosphatemia are common in rhabdomyolysis, resulting from the release of intracellular phosphate into the blood with subsequent sequestration of circulating plasma calcium as calcium phosphate in the damaged muscles. Marked hyperuricemia can occur as a result of increased catabolism of cellular nucleic acids. Increased prothrombin time, partial thromboplastin time, and fibrin degradation products with decreased fibrinogen activity indicate disseminated intravascular coagulation secondary to release of thromboplastin into the circulation.

In myoglobinuria, a disproportionate increase in the concentration of creatinine in the serum compared with that of urea nitrogen indicates increased creatinine release secondary to rhabdomyolysis. However, a subsequent progressive daily increase in both urea nitrogen and serum creatinine concentrations denotes the development of acute renal insufficiency.

On examination, the urine may appear cola-colored or reddish-brown. Inspection of a centrifuged specimen reveals pigmented supernatant and brownish sediment. A reagent strip chemistry test of the supernatant urine shows acid urine (pH less than 5.5), the presence of protein, and a large amount (3+ to 4+) of blood. This test for blood actually detects the peroxidase activity of heme, which is observed in either hemoglobinuria or myoglobinuria. The absence of pink color in the plasma excludes hemoglobinuria. The absence of red blood cells in the urine sediment then confirms that the positive reagent strip test for blood is due to soluble myoglobin. The urine sediment of a patient with uncomplicated rhabdomyolysis usually contains fewer than 10 red blood cells per high power field. Microscopic examination of the urine sediment reveals many pigmented granular casts and increased numbers of renal epithelial cells in the absence of significant microhematuria. Myoglobinuria can be distinguished from hemoglobinuria by spectrophotometric scan, electrophoresis, differential solubility, or differential ultrafiltration. Radioimmunoassay is, by far, the most sensitive and specific test for myoglobin.

As in acute myocardial infarction with release of myoglobin into the circulation, serum myoglobin is markedly increased in patients with rhabdomyolysis, especially in the presence of renal failure. The presence of increased quantities of myoglobin in serum can be detected by the very sensitive radioimmunoassay or by nonisotopic immunoassays.

DIAGNOSIS OF RHABDOMYOLYSIS AND MYOGLOBINURIA

The key to the diagnosis of rhabdomyolysis and myoglobinuria is a high index of suspicion in patients with risk factors for this syndrome (e.g., trauma, prolonged coma, ischemia, alcohol and drug abuse, electrolyte disorders, and seizures). They may present with typical or atypical symptoms of muscle injury. The history should be followed by a careful physical examination and a thorough search for muscle swelling, induration, tenderness, or weakness. The most sensitive laboratory test for rhabdomyolysis is a greatly increased serum CK-MM fraction that is usually more than 10 times the basal concentration in serum. The possibilities in the differential diagnosis of increased serum CK activity include myocardial infarction, primary muscle disease, acute cerebral disease, and thyroid disease, which can be distinguished clinically in most circumstances. The concomitant increase in serum activity of other muscle enzymes, such as AST and LD, also suggests rhabdomyolysis, but other disorders that may cause liver disease or hemolysis should be excluded clinically. Increased serum aldolase activity, an enzyme found in skeletal muscle, can confirm the diagnosis of muscle breakdown. The magnitude of the increase of these muscle enzymes in serum is not as pronounced as that of CK.

Measurement of serum myoglobin concentration by radioimmunoassay is a very sensitive and specific method for detection of the muscle damage caused by either acute myocardial infarction or rhabdomyolysis. Measurement of urine myoglobin by immunoassay is both sensitive and specific for diagnosing myoglobinuria. Patients with renal failure from any cause can excrete small quantities of myoglobin in their urine (see later), but only the presence of a high concentration of myoglobin in urine (more than 1000 ng/mL according to one study) is associated with the subsequent development of acute renal failure. Other methods for detecting myoglobinuria are not sensitive or specific enough to be recommended for routine use in the diagnosis of myoglobinuria.

Imaging Procedures

No specific imaging procedures are helpful in rhabdomyolysis or myoglobinuria. If the metastatic calcification resulting from the hyperphosphatemia is severe, a plain film of an injured area may reveal flecks of extraosseous calcium. Occasionally, in cases of compartment compression syndrome the soft tissue swelling can be seen on computed tomography (CT) or magnetic resonance imaging (MRI).

Definitive Diagnosis

Rhabdomyolysis is certain when unequivocal evidence of skeletal muscle injury is present. This evidence usually includes increased serum CK, perhaps confirmed by increased serum aldolase, in a setting where muscle injury would be an expected complication, such as crush injury, trauma, seizures, and drug overdose. Myoglobinuria is certain whenever an increased concentration of myoglobin is measured in urine. However, in the presence of renal failure, myoglobinuria can be diagnosed as the cause of the renal failure only when there has been rhabdomyolysis (see next section).

It is not helpful to rely solely on the measurement of urinary myoglobin to make the diagnosis of myoglobinuric acute renal failure. The mere presence of myoglobin in the urine of an azotemic patient is not sufficient to establish this diagnosis. Pre-existing renal failure of any cause can increase urinary myoglobin excretion to the point where the reagent strip test for blood becomes positive. In these cases, however, the serum CK is usually not markedly increased, as would be expected in primary rhabdomyolysis. This increase in urine myoglobin is not sufficient to cause further renal injury. Myoglobinuric acute renal failure invariably occurs only in the setting of rhabdomyolysis, when the amount of myoglobin that reaches the renal tubules is sufficient to cause tubular obstruction and breakdown.

Another test that is of no value in the diagnosis of rhabdomyolysis and myoglobinuria is the use of urinary sodium excretion to distinguish acute tubular necrosis from acute prerenal azotemia. The fractional excretion of sodium (FE_{Na}), and the renal failure index, which usually serve as reliable indicators of tubular function, are typically normal in myoglobinuric acute renal failure and cannot differentiate this condition from pure volume contraction.

COURSE AND COMPLICATIONS OF RHABDOMYOLYSIS

The clinical course of rhabdomyolysis and myoglobinuria is widely varied and depends on the underlying cause, the extent and severity of muscle damage, the presence or absence of complications, and the preventive management at the scene of muscle injury. For example, an exercise-induced rhabdomyolysis and myoglobinuria may remain asymptomatic and unnoticed until a serum CK or a urinalysis is performed. On the other hand, in a patient suffering the crush syndrome following the collapse of a building, aggressive fluid replacement early in the course of injury can be successful in preventing the development of acute renal failure and lead to a relatively uncomplicated course of rhabdomyolysis. A patient with drug (especially cocaine)-induced rhabdomyolysis may present with coma, extensive rhabdomyolysis, hyperthermia, hypotension, acute oliguric renal failure, hepatic failure, disseminated intravascular coagulation, and respiratory failure. The course is usually fulminant, and the outcome is usually fatal.

The most serious complication of rhabdomyolysis is acute myoglobinuric renal failure. This condition is caused by both a prerenal component of decreased renal blood flow secondary to loss of circulating blood volume into the damaged skeletal muscle and a renal component of acute tubular necrosis secondary to the tubular toxicity of myoglobin and tubular obstruction by myoglobin casts. The clinical picture of acute renal failure in rhabdomyolysis is characterized by a rapid and progressive increase in urea and creatinine concentrations in the serum shortly after muscle injury. Furthermore, it is usually characterized by an initial ratio of serum urea nitrogen (SUN) to serum creatinine that is frequently less than 5, compared with the usual ratio of 10. The presenting serum creatinine may also have predictive value: in one large study, only 20 per cent of patients presenting with serum creatinine less than 3 mg/dL developed acute intrinsic renal failure, compared with 73 per cent of those presenting with a creatinine of 3 mg/dL or more. Signs of intravascular volume depletion (secondary to third spacing), such as tachycardia and postural hypotension, are common, yet patients may not show weight loss or decrease in skin turgor. Oliguria is common, and examination of the urine shows small amounts of reddish-brown urine containing large numbers of pigmented granular casts. The urine sodium concentration is usually low, and the fractional excretion of sodium is typically less than 1 per cent. If the patient does not respond to initial aggressive fluid therapy and if oliguria persists despite adequate volume repletion, the clinical course parallels that of hypercatabolic acute renal failure. These patients are likely to require aggressive and prolonged dialysis (hemodialysis, continuous hemoperfusion, peritoneal dialysis, or some combination of these treatments until life-sustaining renal function is recovered) for as long as 3 months. However, if the clinical course is not further complicated by bleeding, multiorgan failure, or sepsis, complete recovery of life-sustaining renal function can be anticipated in most patients.

Severe, life-threatening hyperkalemia can develop very early in the course of acute renal failure and is due to the leakage of large quantities of cellular potassium from skeletal muscle into the circulation, combined with the failure of the kidneys to excrete potassium. Metabolic acidosis can further exacerbate the hyperkalemia. Severe hyperkalemia may develop before acute renal failure is evident but is more likely to develop in patients with oliguric renal failure than in those with nonoliguric renal failure.

Severe hypocalcemia is another complication of rhabdomyolysis. Hypocalcemia results from the release of large amounts of intracellular phosphate to the circulation, with consequent formation of calcium phosphate and the sequestration of circulating calcium in the damaged skeletal muscle. However, this severe hypocalcemia is usually asymptomatic and seldom causes neuromuscular irritability, seizure, or tetany. Hypocalcemia can, however, potentiate hyperkalemic cardiac toxicity.

Hypercalcemia sometimes occurs as a late complication during the recovery phase of myoglobinuric acute renal failure. Most patients who develop hypercalcemia are those who had hypocalcemia during the early stage of rhabdomyolysis. Hypercalcemia appears to be due to the reabsorption of trapped calcium from the injured muscle and is associated with inappropriately normal or high concentrations of serum parathyroid hormone and 1,25-dihydroxycholecalciferol during the repairing process.

Severe hyperuricemia, with serum uric acid concentrations sometimes exceeding 35 mg/dL, resulting from the metabolism of purines released from the injured muscle, is a distinctive complication of rhabdomyolysis. While profound hyperuricemia is often associated with renal failure, marked hyperuricemia in rhabdomyolysis can occur in the absence of renal failure.

Disseminated intravascular coagulation secondary to the release of thromboplastin from the damaged muscle is a serious complication of severe rhabdomyolysis and is associated with a high mortality, as reported in cocaine-induced rhabdomyolysis.

Acute compartment syndrome is also a serious complication of rhabdomyolysis. Because muscle groups in the extremities are surrounded and bounded by tough, unyielding fascial envelopes called compartments, swelling of the injured muscle in the extremities can cause a rapid rise in the intracompartmental pressure, causing ischemic damages to the muscles and nerves within the compartment. Patients with the acute compartment syndrome typically report severe muscle pain out of proportion to the injury and loss of sensation or motor function of the involved muscle. On examination, the involved area appears pale and cold, with diminished pulses and pain on passive stretching. Emergency measurement of intracompartmental pressure provides definitive diagnosis, and the patient may require emergency fasciotomy for relief of muscle tamponade.

ERRORS AND PITFALLS IN DIAGNOSIS

The most important diagnostic error in dealing with rhabdomyolysis is underestimating the severity of the muscle injury, which can, in turn, lead to less-than-aggressive intravenous fluid treatment of the high blood and urine myoglobin, thus making renal injury more likely. Therefore, a history of crush injury, ischemia to a limb, seizures, envenomations, drug or alcohol overdose, or heat stroke should result in a high index of suspicion for rhabdomyolysis. Subtle signs of volume depletion must be sought.

It is also important to distinguish between substantial myoglobinuria that may lead to acute tubular necrosis and secondary myoglobinuria from pre-existing renal failure or myocardial infarction, in which urinary myoglobin is present but not in sufficient quantity to damage renal tubules. The latter occurs exclusively after rhabdomyolysis; therefore, evidence of severe muscle injury must be sought. A history of pre-existing renal disease or an acute myocardial injury can help make this distinction.

TUMORS OF MUSCLE AND SOFT TISSUE

By Howard G. Rosenthal, M.D.
Kansas City, Missouri

Tumors involving the musculoskeletal system constitute a heterogeneous group of neoplastic processes that are commonly grouped together as soft tissue sarcomas. More than 50 types of soft tissue sarcomas originate from mesenchymal tissues located anywhere in the body. The rarity of these tumors has resulted in few clinicians having extensive experience in their diagnosis and treatment, and pathologic classification is often incomplete or inaccurate. Even when the correct diagnosis is made, physicians skilled in cancer management may lack the knowledge necessary for the treatment of soft tissue sarcomas.

Soft tissue sarcomas arise from the mesenchymal elements of the extraskeletal system. Soft tissue tumors can be defined as masses that arise from or within the nonepithelial extraskeletal tissues of the body. Tumors that arise within the reticuloendothelial system, glial tissues, and supportive tissues of various parenchymal organs are not classified as soft tissue tumors. Conversely, tumors that arise from the peripheral nervous system (neuroectodermal origin) are included. Soft tissue tumors are described histologically based on the mature tissue that they resemble (Table 1). For example, the microscopic appearance of liposarcomas resembles that of adult fatty tissue, with mature lipocytes appearing adjacent to malignant-appearing lipoblasts. Rhabdomyosarcoma, or striated muscle sarcoma, exhibits malignant-appearing striated muscle cells.

The incidence of soft tissue tumors is difficult to ascertain. Approximately 100 benign soft tissue tumors are diagnosed for every malignant soft tissue sarcoma. A significant number of soft tissue benign tumors probably do not

Table 1. Histologic Diagnoses Based on Tissue Type

Benign	Malignant
Fibrous Tumors	
Nodular fasciitis Fibroma Elastofibroma Aggressive fibromatosis Myofibromatosis Desmoid tumor	Fibrosarcoma Inflammatory fibrosarcoma Desmoid tumor
Fibrohistiocytic Tumors	
Benign fibrous histiocytoma Xanthogranuloma Reticulohistiocytoma Xanthoma Fibroxanthoma Dermatofibroma protuberans	Malignant fibrous histiocytoma Dermatofibroma protuberans Myxoid malignant fibrous histiocytoma Malignant giant cell tumor Inflammatory malignant fibrous histiocytoma
Lipomatous Tumors	
Lipoma Atypical lipoma Angiolipoma Spindle cell lipoma Hibernoma Lipoblastoma	Liposarcoma Myxoid liposarcoma Round cell liposarcoma Pleomorphic liposarcoma Dedifferentiated liposarcoma
Smooth Muscle Tumors	
Leiomyoma Angioleiomyoma Epithelioid leiomyoma	Leiomyosarcoma Epithelioid leiomyosarcoma
Skeletal Muscle Tumors	
Adult rhabdomyoma Genital rhabdomyoma Fetal rhabdomyoma	Rhabdomyosarcoma (embryonal rhabdomyosarcoma, alveolar, etc.) Mesenchymoma
Blood Vessel and Lymph Tumors	
Hemangioma Lymphangioma Lymphangiomatosis Angiomatosis	Hemangioendothelioma Angiosarcoma Lymphangiosarcoma Kaposi's sarcoma
Perivascular Tumors	
Glomus tumor Hemangiopericytoma	Malignant glomus tumor Malignant hemangiopericytoma
Synovial or Synovial-Like Tumors	
Tenosynovial giant cell tumor Extra-articular pigmented villonodular synovitis	Synovial sarcoma Maligant giant cell tumor of tendon sheath
Neural Tumors	
Neuroma Neuromuscular hamartoma Nerve sheath ganglion Schwannoma Neurothekeoma Neurofibroma	Malignant peripheral nerve-sheath tumor (malignant schwannoma) Clear cell sarcoma (melanoma of soft parts) Primitive neuroectodermal tumor
Extraskeletal Soft Tissue Tumors	
Myositis ossificans Extraskeletal chondroma Extraskeletal osteoma	Extraskeletal chondrosarcoma Extraskeletal osteosarcoma
Miscellaneous Tumors	
Tumoral calcinosis Myxoma Angiomyxoma Amyloid tumor (nodular amyloidosis) Parachordoma	Alveolar soft part sarcoma Epithelioid sarcoma Desmoplastic small cell tumor

come to the physician's attention. For example, many patients with lipomas never seek the attention of a physician. Therefore, the annual incidence of benign soft tissue tumors probably exceeds 300 in 100,000 people in the United States. At some point, malignant soft tissue tumors nearly always come to the physician's attention.

The National Cancer Institute's Surveillance, Epidemiology, and End Results Program, which measures the incidence of various tumors, estimates that approximately 5700 new soft tissue sarcomas are diagnosed each year in the United States. An estimate of the overall annual incidence is approximately 1.4 in 100,000 patients. Soft tissue sarcomas therefore represent fewer than 1 per cent of all cancers seen in the United States. More than half of these sarcomas affect patients older than 50, whereas 15 per cent affect patients younger than 15 years. No significant racial or social predominance has been observed, and while there is a very slight male predominance, this varies among histologic types.

Soft tissue sarcomas arise in any location within the body. Two thirds of all soft tissue sarcomas occur in the extremities, with two thirds of those in the lower extremity. The trunk, including the abdominal and chest walls and the retroperitoneum, accounts for 30 per cent, while the remainder are typically located within the head and neck region. Any soft tissue mass that develops in a child must be considered a soft tissue sarcoma until proven otherwise. In the adult, soft tissue sarcoma must be considered in the differential diagnosis of any soft tissue mass that is greater than 5 cm in diameter or that lies deep to the limiting fascia of the extremity. While most of these tumors are benign, the clinician must evaluate them appropriately with radiographic studies, clinical examination, and biopsy before excluding the possibility of sarcoma. Poor prognostic factors include a higher grade, increased size, deep-seated tumors, and proximity to the axial part of the body. The larger the tumor, the greater risk of metastatic spread at the time of diagnosis. The size of the tumor usually has a significant impact on the feasibility of performing limb-salvage surgery. With regard to selection of treatment, the most important determining factor is the histologic grade of the tumor. Two staging systems are utilized. The American Joint Committee on Cancer Staging (AJCCS) System, which is based on the TMMG System, uses tumor size and histologic grade as the major determinants of tumor stage. Nodal and distant metastases are also determining factors in this system. By contrast, the Musculoskeletal Tumor Society (MTS) Staging System, a surgical staging system, is concerned with the histologic grade as well as anatomy of the tumor itself. Tumors are described as high or low grade as well as intracompartmental or extracompartmental. An intracompartmental tumor lies within one muscle compartment group. An extracompartmental tumor extends beyond fascial boundaries into another compartment. For example, a primary bone tumor with erosion through the cortex of the bone and development of a soft tissue mass is classified as extracompartmental. Most high-grade sarcomas are MTS stage IIb. Therefore, the appropriate studies for determining a specific diagnosis for large, deep-seated soft tissue masses must include clinical examination, radiographic studies, and biopsy for staging purposes.

CLINICAL APPROACH

The clinical examination determines the size of the tumor, the location, and whether the lesion is attached or fixed to nearby structures, including bone and neurovascular structures. Lymph node involvement, while unusual for soft tissue sarcomas, must be addressed, as should the neurovascular status of the limb involved. Evaluation of the functional status of the involved limb includes range of motion of the joints surrounding the lesion. Range of motion of the joints above and below the lesion assesses whether contractures have developed. This evaluation assists in determining whether the tumor is fixed to specific tendons or muscles.

When the biopsy is performed, the pathologist must be told the age of the patient, the location of the tumor, and its size and growth characteristics. The results of radiographic studies and, most importantly, the magnetic resonance imaging (MRI) findings must become an integral part of the pathologist's clinical information. The age of the patient can help separate the histologically similar tumors. Pleomorphic types of malignant fibrous histiocytoma are extraordinarily rare in young children; conversely, neuroblastoma and angiomatoid malignant fibrous histiocytoma rarely occur in adulthood.

The location of the tumor also aids in the differential diagnosis. Most malignant fibrous histiocytomas are located deep to the limiting fascia of the extremity; however, lesions such as dermatofibroma protuberans and epithelioid sarcoma frequently present in superficial locations. Dermatofibroma protuberans and certain forms of malignant fibrous histiocytoma are histologically similar, and location or depth of the tumor can be very helpful in the diagnosis.

The size and location of the tumor influence the approach to limb-sparing surgery. The relationship of the tumor to adjacent structures such as bone and neurovascular bundles is determined radiographically and by MRI scan. The radiologist must be apprised of all pertinent clinical information so that optimal diagnostic studies can be performed. Plain films obtained in patients with soft tissue sarcomas can frequently identify the soft tissue matrix. As many as one third of synovial sarcomas show calcifications within the tumor on plain film, while lipomas and low-grade liposarcomas are visualized as fatty densities. Gallium scan, bone scan, and other scintigraphic methods are no longer necessary, and computed tomography (CT) is rarely required for evaluating the primary tumor. Angiography has been replaced by MRI for evaluation of the proximity of the tumor to the vessels. Angiography can help monitor chemotherapeutic response and assist in visualization of vascular compression by an overlying tumor.

Radiographic studies are used to fully stage the tumor. Most soft tissue sarcomas spread hematogenously, and metastases to the lung must be evaluated by CT scan, with and without contrast enhancement, of the pulmonary parenchyma. Only about 5 per cent of soft tissue sarcomas spread via the lymphatic route. Each soft tissue mass must be evaluated individually, and the biology of the tumor itself must be considered. For example, malignant fibrous histiocytoma, the most common soft tissue sarcoma of the extremities, typically invades and erodes through bone. For this reason, plain films are diagnostically more helpful than MRI in the evaluation of bony involvement. Magnetic resonance imaging cannot demonstrate cortical erosion as clearly as plain films or CT of the extremity.

The biopsy is an integral part of the diagnostic evaluation for the patient with soft tissue sarcoma, and it is crucial to the selection of appropriate therapy. The goal of the biopsy is to obtain a specimen large enough to permit complete histopathologic examination of the tumor. Additional specimens for cytology, cytogenetic analysis, electron microscopy, and special stains are often required, and for this reason at least 1 cm^3 of tissue must be obtained. An open, or incisional, biopsy is most commonly used and typically requires a longitudinal incision over the tumor mass with the patient receiving regional anesthesia. Infiltration of the region with a local anesthetic increases the risk of metastasis and is to be avoided.

The incisional biopsy provides a sample of tumor and pseudocapsule, permitting orientation of the architecture of the tumor by the pathologist. Excessive manipulation and crushing must be avoided, and hemostasis must be maintained during the procedure. Additional immunohistochemical stains and cytogenetic studies are often needed for complete diagnosis. For example, extraskeletal Ewing's sarcoma can appear histologically indistinguishable from many other small, round, blue cell tumors. Extraskeletal Ewing's sarcoma can be evaluated with the use of cytogenetic analysis, which typically demonstrates a distinct and specific alteration in karyotype, that is, translocation of chromosomes 11 and 22. Plans must be made *before* the biopsy is performed to obtain fresh tissue for this study, because it may be the only way of distinguishing Ewing's sarcoma from other tumors. The diagnosis and treatment of these tumors is a highly specialized area of medical practice. Patients with suspected soft tissue tumors should be promptly referred to clinicians who are skilled and experienced in their management. Both the initial studies, such as MRI, and the definitive biopsy procedure must be performed in close consultation with all the physicians who will be involved with the patient's care.

PAGET'S DISEASE OF BONE

By Henry G. Bone, M.D.
Detroit, Michigan

Paget's disease of bone is a focal or multifocal bone disorder that may cause pain, deformity, functional disturbance, and rarely malignancy. The primary lesion is characterized by greatly accelerated, dysfunctional bone resorption by oversized, hypernucleated osteoclasts. Secondary accelerated bone formation by osteoblasts may occur at affected sites, but the bone so formed is qualitatively abnormal and structurally deficient. Small haphazard "mosaic" patches of lamellar bone may be formed from the disorderly pattern of resorption and formation, as may patches of loosely constructed "woven" bone. In the evolution of pagetic lesions, either the lytic effects of osteoclasts or the radiographically sclerotic effects of osteoblasts may predominate. However, pagetic bone is generally weakened regardless of the balance between lytic and sclerotic lesions. Although pagetic bone may actually expand in volume, the architectural changes compromise its strength, resulting in a tendency toward deformity and fracture. The more frequent complications include degenerative disease in weight-bearing joints adjacent to pagetic bone, deafness associated with damage to the cochlear capsule by Paget's disease of the temporal bone, and neurologic deficits, perhaps due to vascular "steal" as a result of the greatly increased blood flow to pagetic bone.

After osteoporosis, Paget's disease is the second most

common bone disease. However, its prevalence in the United States is not known with certainty. While perhaps 1 per cent of adults older than 50 years of age have the disorder, far fewer have disease requiring treatment. The prevalence is highly variable. For example, in parts of Britain the prevalence reaches 5 per cent or more of adults older than 50 years, whereas in Scandinavia and Africa, Paget's disease is quite rare. In African Americans, however, the prevalence is comparable to that in whites. Paget's disease is rare among Asians who live in Asia, Australia, or the United States.

One hypothesis suggests that Paget's disease may begin in childhood or adolescence, perhaps as a consequence of a paramyxovirus infection. However, the disorder is rarely diagnosed before middle age, and overt clinical manifestations are usually seen in elderly patients whose disease has progressed over many years.

PRESENTATION

Paget's disease is often detected during the investigation of specific signs and symptoms, but the disorder may also be discovered incidentally in patients with abnormal radiographs or increased serum alkaline phosphatase activity.

Symptomatic Paget's disease may have many forms and presentations. When the skull is involved, the clinician may observe bony thickening of the frontal or maxillary region or mandibular enlargement producing prognathism. Deafness is fairly common when the petrous temporal bone is involved. Fortunately, basilar invagination, hydrocephalus, and cranial nerve syndromes are rare. Spinal involvement may not be clinically apparent in the absence of vertebral compression fracture or spinal cord dysfunction due to impingement and vascular steal. Involvement of the pelvis is often associated with pain and degenerative changes in the hip. When the femur is involved, pain, bowing, and degenerative hip joint changes may occur, as may fracture. Bowing is typical in the tibias. The humerus and scapula may be affected, predisposing to degenerative changes in the shoulder. The radius and ulna are occasionally abnormal, leading to deformity and ulnar neuropathy. Pagetic changes of the hands and feet are uncommon.

Symptomatic patients typically report localized or multifocal skeletal pain. Some patients think that they have "arthritis"; they may have consumed nonspecific analgesic and anti-inflammatory preparations for months to years. Radiographs may be taken, revealing pagetic changes, often in the pelvis or the femur. A bone scan may disclose additional sites of the disease, and plain films characterize the structural status of each site. Biochemical tests, particularly the serum alkaline phosphatase test and one of the urine markers of bone resorption described later, are employed to characterize disease activity and to measure the response to treatment.

Asymptomatic patients are often discovered incidentally when radiographs are taken for unrelated reasons (e.g., excretory urogram) or when the serum alkaline phosphatase activity exceeds the reference range. Once the increased alkaline phosphatase is shown to be of skeletal origin, a bone scan is commonly obtained. Plain films of the areas of excess uptake may help confirm the diagnosis of Paget's disease.

CLINICAL ASSESSMENT

The primary goals of treatment of Paget's disease are to relieve symptoms, to prevent complications, and, if possible, to achieve remission. The clinician should carry out the evaluation of patients with these goals in mind. The effect of the disease on the patient's functional and symptomatic status, its potential for causing complications, and its degree of activity all are important considerations. The anatomic and functional status of affected areas and their proximity to vulnerable structures should be thoroughly evaluated at baseline.

When a patient with Paget's disease is identified, radiologic evaluation can define the anatomy of the disease and provide a baseline for assessment of its structural progression. Biochemical testing is used to characterize the activity of the disease and its response to treatment.

IMAGING METHODS

Radionuclide scanning with a bone-seeking agent (e.g., bisphosphonate) linked to a radionuclide (e.g., technetium [^{99m}Tc]) is generally considered the most useful test for determining the extent and location of pagetic lesions. A few hours after injection, the scanner can highlight the sites where scanning agent has been concentrated owing to its affinity for exposed bone mineral. These are sites of excessively rapid, pathologic bone remodeling, characteristic of Paget's disease as well as other disorders. Although the distribution of the radionuclide may be typical of Paget's disease and provide strong clues to the diagnosis, definitive diagnosis generally requires plain films or computed tomography (CT) images of the sites detected by the bone scan. Bone scans are mainly useful for the initial detection of the disease and its distribution. Since the distribution does not change, serial bone scans are of limited use unless quantitative scintigraphy is performed to measure the response to treatment. Ordinarily, biochemical tests are adequate for this purpose, but quantitative scintigraphy can be particularly helpful when a very small volume of bone is involved.

Plain films are usually adequate for the specific diagnosis of Paget's disease. At the sites of lytic lesions, plain films may also provide good evidence of the structural response to treatment. This is particularly true of lytic lesions in long bones and osteoporosis circumscripta in the skull. When plain films are used for assessing the progress of the disease or its response to treatment, the greatest possible care must be taken with respect to positioning of the patient for serial studies. Even small degrees of rotation can make comparisons extremely difficult or impossible. In patients with small lesions or an extensive mixture of lytic and sclerotic changes, plain films may not provide clear evidence of treatment effect, and CT may be more helpful.

Typical radiographic changes of Paget's disease include a mixture of lysis and sclerosis with thickened cortices and trabeculae and sometimes increased diameter of the affected bone. In the skull, areas of lysis without sclerosis are referred to as osteoporosis circumscripta, while thickening and sclerosis are described as "cotton-wool" changes. In long bones, a progressive wedge of osteolysis produces the characteristic "flame" or "blade-of-grass" lesion. Subtle Paget's disease in the pelvis may be signaled by thickening of the iliopectineal line. Bowing of the femur or tibia may be particularly apparent deformities, as may an increased angle of the femoral neck, or protrusio acetabuli.

Computed tomograms demonstrate that most of the lytic changes seen on plain films occur in the cortices. Also well seen on CT are thickened trabecular structures. Computed tomography provides much better information about the cross-sectional structure of bone than does plain radiography. Thus, CT can be very helpful in diagnosis when plain films are not conclusive. Computed tomography is also extremely helpful in assessing the response to treatment in small lesions or complex regions of involvement. Small variations in positioning may decrease the clinician's ability to interpret or compare serial CT studies. However, methodology under development can now transform three-dimensional CT data sets so that positioning discrepancies are eliminated in the postprocessing of the images.

In general, magnetic resonance imaging (MRI) is less useful than CT in the evaluation of Paget's disease. However, MRI can be highly useful in evaluating the spinal cord or brain when Paget's disease is associated with neurologic deficits.

BIOCHEMICAL TESTS

The magnitude of biochemical abnormalities is related to *both* the intensity and the extent of disease. This fact has several implications. First, the clinician should not assume that relatively modest abnormalities of biochemical markers reflect mild disease. Importantly, disease activity may be quite intense at very limited sites. Second, when the activity and extent of disease are considered, the clinician has some basis for determining an initial dose of pamidronate. Third, reductions in the serum concentrations of biochemical markers mainly indicate decreased intensity, because the anatomic extent of disease changes relatively little. Occasionally, an imbalance between resorption and formation markers is observed, especially in lytic disease, or in recently treated patients. In the latter, markers of bone formation will often remain increased for several months after resorption is suppressed. Thus, resorption markers generally provide a better early indication of efficacy of treatment.

The serum alkaline phosphatase concentration has been the preferred biochemical measurement for assessment of disease activity and response to treatment. The recent development of bone-specific alkaline phosphatase assays has greatly enhanced the clinical utility of this test. When an increased serum alkaline phosphatase concentration is detected and the etiology is unknown, a bone specific alkaline phosphatase measurement should be requested. If this value is abnormal, skeletal scintigraphy and radiography should be pursued in the asymptomatic patient.

Osteocalcin is a protein constituent of bone matrix, produced by osteoblasts. The serum osteocalcin concentration is increased in Paget's disease and may decrease following treatment. This measurement, however, has not proved to be as useful as that of serum alkaline phosphatase in evaluating patients with Paget's disease.

Among the tests that measure the rate of appearance of collagen degradation products in urine, the measurement of hydroxyproline has been used most extensively. This test is particularly useful when the results are expressed as a ratio of hydroxyproline to creatinine excretion in a fasting, second-voided urine specimen. Obtaining the specimen in this way minimizes the influence of dietary collagen on urinary hydroxyproline excretion. Measurement by high-performance liquid chromatography is preferred; many of the other hydroxyproline assays are less specific, owing to confounding interfering substances. The quest for more convenient and specific tests has led to attempts to measure deoxypyridinoline, pyridinolines, and N- or C-telopeptides of type I collagen. These tests can produce results qualitatively similar to those of hydroxyproline testing, but with more convenience and greater specificity for bone collagen. Although it is not yet clear which of these assays will be adopted as standard clinical tests, it does seem likely that faster, more convenient methods will replace the measurement of hydroxyproline within the next several years.

EVALUATION OF HEARING LOSS

In patients with hearing loss and Paget's disease, careful evaluation is required to determine the cause of the deafness. Many patients with Paget's disease have alternative or additional causes of impaired hearing, including cumulative noise exposure or presbycusis. Conductive hearing loss due to otosclerosis should be considered because specific intervention is available. Audiograms of patients with pagetic deafness typically demonstrate sensorineural hearing loss characterized by high-frequency threshold increases and air-bone gaps. When the clinical picture suggests hearing loss due to Paget's disease, CT examination of the petrous temporal bone is informative. Pagetic hearing loss is generally *not* the result of ossicular changes or impingement on the eighth cranial nerve. The degree of pagetic involvement of the cochlear capsule strongly correlates with alteration of hearing thresholds.

AGGRAVATING CONDITIONS

Calcium and/or vitamin D deficiency due to insufficient intake or impaired absorption may aggravate Paget's disease. Increased parathyroid hormone may indirectly stimulate pagetic osteoclasts, while insufficient vitamin D and calcium intake may impair mineralization of newly repaired bone. Measurement of 24-hour urine calcium as well as serum calcium, parathyroid hormone, and vitamin D metabolites may help identify these aggravating conditions.

Systematic evaluation of the patient with Paget's disease, with respect to the extent, anatomy, and activity of the disease provides the basis for well-founded management. Omission of the baseline bone scan and radiographs or insufficient biochemical follow-up data may greatly handicap the long-term management of the disease.

OSTEOARTHRITIS

By David T. Felson, M.D.
Boston, Massachusetts

Osteoarthritis, also called osteoarthrosis or degenerative joint disease, is by far the most prevalent rheumatic disease. Microscopic evidence of osteoarthritis exists in almost 90 per cent of persons older than 70 years of age. Osteoarthritis has highly characteristic pathologic, biochemical, clinical, and radiographic features. The clinical and radiographic features that the clinician uses to establish the diagnosis develop after disease has already begun in the cartilage.

Osteoarthritis is characterized by progressive loss of articular cartilage and by sclerosis in the bone underneath the cartilage. Also seen are osteophytes, outgrowths of cartilage and bone at the joint margin. Osteoarthritis progresses and ultimately involves the entire articular structure. The joint capsule is thickened, the synovium is inflamed, and the muscles that bridge the joint become atrophic.

The causes of osteoarthritis are multifactorial. The incipient lesion is cartilage damage caused by blunt trauma or other identifiable injury (e.g., a football injury) or by wear and tear due to increased loads across normal joints or abnormal misshapen joints. Muscles, tendons, and subchondral bone are designed to protect joints from injury. When muscles or tendons fail, owing to poor conditioning or impaired somesthetic input, the increased load is transmitted to the joint cartilage, which begins to deteriorate. Muscle and tendon failure occurs when neuropathy alters the sense of position, when muscles are poorly conditioned, or when impact loads are applied to joints so rapidly that muscles and tendons fail to serve as adequate shock absorbers. Repeated damage to cartilage must occur for osteoarthritis to develop.

The prevalence of osteoarthritis increases with age, and osteoarthritis occurs more frequently in women than in men, especially after age 50 years. The modifiable risk factors for osteoarthritis include excessive weight; major joint injuries, including those leading to meniscectomies; and work-related cumulative trauma. By contrast, genetic predisposition to osteoarthritis and concomitant arthritic conditions (e.g., rheumatoid arthritis) are risk factors that cannot be modified.

The risk factors for osteoarthritis may not be the same for all joints. Heredity and age may influence all joints similarly, but specific injuries and excessive weight may influence some joints more than others. Importantly, some cases of hip osteoarthritis are caused by developmental abnormalities (e.g., congenital dysplasias, Legg-Calvé-Perthes disease).

The natural history of osteoarthritis varies, but many patients can be clinically stable for long periods of time. The natural history of clinical osteoarthritis is different from radiographic osteoarthritis. In clinical osteoarthritis, with good clinical care, one third of patients may experience substantial improvement in symptoms, one third deteriorate, and one third remain stable over several years. By contrast, radiographic osteoarthritis rarely improves, but stability or very slow progression is more likely than rapid deterioration. Indeed, the films of some patients with hip osteoarthritis may actually improve with time.

SYMPTOMS AND SIGNS

The primary symptoms of osteoarthritis are pain on motion, relief of pain with rest, and localized stiffness lasting a short time after joint motion. In the later stages of osteoarthritis, night pain is common. The symptoms of osteoarthritis may be episodic, but acute inflammatory flares with hot swollen joints should raise concern about coexistent crystal-induced synovitis.

Evidence of osteoarthritis on physical examination includes joint line tenderness and crepitation on motion. Bony enlargement of the hands and knees can be seen in advanced osteoarthritis.

PRIMARY SITES OF INVOLVEMENT

Hands

Osteoarthritis of the hands is often remarkably symmetrical. Bony enlargements of the distal interphalangeal (DIP) joints of the hands are called Heberden's nodes. Swelling is typically observed over the dorsolateral aspects of these joints. Similarly enlarged Bouchard's nodes can be found over the lateral aspects of the proximal interphalangeal (PIP) joints. Both Heberden's and Bouchard's nodes are more common in women than in men and may be inherited. The symptoms associated with osteoarthritis of the DIP and PIP joints are variable and often minor and are frequently noted incidentally, without associated pain or functional disability. However, some patients present with acute pain, redness, swelling, and tenderness. The swollen DIP or PIP joint may be soft and fluctuant. Occasionally, patients present with cysts that are thought to communicate with the joint space. If punctured, these cysts may release viscous material rich in hyaluronic acid. When compared with the interphalangeal joints, the metacarpophalangeal (MCP) joints are involved less frequently and later in the course of osteoarthritis.

The first carpometacarpal (CMC) joint commonly deteriorates in osteoarthritis, especially in elderly women. Pain and swelling of the CMC joint are frequent, and physical examination reveals a squared-off appearance at the base of the thumb. The adjoining trapezioscaphoid joint may also be involved. Patients present with pain at the base of the thumb, and examination discloses tenderness over the joint line. The clinician can often elicit pain by grasping the patient's first MCP joint and rotating it up and down, applying pressure proximally.

Knees

Symptomatic osteoarthritis of the knee afflicts 3 to 9 per cent of adults and frequently causes significant pain and disability. Patients with osteoarthritis of the medial or lateral compartment report pain while walking on level ground, whereas those with patellofemoral involvement have knee symptoms when they go up and down stairs or sit with the knees bent. Patients with patellofemoral involvement may also experience knee buckling and even falling. Examination reveals tenderness over the joint line of the involved compartment, and passive range-of-motion movement may cause crepitation. Quadriceps atrophy may develop, especially in the presence of substantial joint effusion. Severe loss of medial compartment joint space frequently leads to a genu varum deformity.

Hip

Although osteoarthritis of the hip is half as common as osteoarthritis of the knee, it is often a source of considerable pain and disability. Patients with hip osteoarthritis often have pain localized to the groin or the inner aspect of the thigh, but they can also have buttock pain, sciatic pain, or even pain over the lateral hip. Sometimes, hip osteoarthritis can manifest as pain in the distal thigh or even the knee.

Spine

Osteoarthritis of the spine is a heterogeneous disorder. Disease can occur in the apophyseal articulation (the facet joints), the vertebral bodies, or the intervertebral disks. The association of common, episodic low back pain with osteoarthritis is tenuous and poorly understood, and patients should not be regarded as having spinal osteoarthritis if they have episodic low back pain associated with radiographic evidence of osteoarthritis. The two conditions may be unrelated. The most common site of spinal osteoarthritis discovered by radiograph is the lumbar spine, followed by the cervical and thoracic spines. Osteoarthritis should be suspected as a cause of back or neck pain when symptoms persist and correlate anatomically with the radiographic location of joint space and bony lesions.

RADIOGRAPHIC FINDINGS

Early in the course of osteoarthritis, radiographs are unremarkable. Cartilage loss and bony changes can evolve with few or no visible abnormalities on plain films. Magnetic resonance imaging (MRI) is more sensitive for detecting the early changes of osteoarthritis. Later in the disease, the characteristic changes of osteoarthritis that can be seen in radiographs include loss of joint space, often in a nonuniform distribution throughout the joint; subchondral bony sclerosis, known as eburnation; subchondral cyst formation, especially in the hips; and osteophytes at the margin of the joint. Gross deformity of the joint space, loose bodies, and bony attrition can develop when osteoarthritis is severe.

The radiographic changes that characterize hand osteoarthritis are similar to those for osteoarthritis in other joints. A posteroanterior view of the hand is usually sufficient to make the diagnosis.

The radiographic changes of osteoarthritis in the knee include joint space narrowing, osteophytes, and subchondral sclerosis. These changes are most often seen in the medial and patellofemoral compartments. To make a radiographic diagnosis of knee osteoarthritis, weight-bearing knee films in the anteroposterior view must be obtained. However, anteroposterior views do not reveal abnormalities in the patellofemoral joint. Therefore, a skyline view for the patellofemoral joint or a lateral view for both the patellofemoral and the femorotibial joints may be indicated. Finally, a tunnel view may provide the best evidence of abnormalities of the femoral condyle.

In the spine, each type of osteoarthritis has characteristic radiographic features. Disk narrowing and linear collections of gas within the disk (vacuum phenomenon) are frequently seen. Apophyseal joint osteoarthritis is best detected with multiple views of the spine, including oblique views that may reveal bony encroachments on the foraminal exits of nerves.

Magnetic resonance imaging has been used to diagnose joint disease. The current cost, however, makes MRI less desirable as a primary imaging tool for osteoarthritis.

SYNOVIAL FLUID FINDINGS

Synovial fluid analysis can be helpful, but the results are not diagnostic of osteoarthritis. Synovial fluid in the osteoarthritic joint usually has good viscosity and a normal or slightly increased cell count, usually fewer than 1000 cells/mm^3. The synovial fluid glucose concentration in osteoarthritis is typically unremarkable.

EROSIVE OR INFLAMMATORY OSTEOARTHRITIS

Erosive or inflammatory osteoarthritis has a predilection for the DIP and PIP joints. Inflammation and joint destruction can occur rapidly over several months. This disease affects primarily women within 10 to 20 years of the onset of menopause. In addition to the usual radiographic changes of osteoarthritis, erosions at the joint margin can be seen. The synovium may reveal a proliferative synovitis that suggests a diagnosis of rheumatoid arthritis.

DIFFUSE IDIOPATHIC SKELETAL HYPEROSTOSIS (DISH)

DISH is characterized by extensive hyperostosis and large joint spurs in the appendicular skeleton. The lower thoracic spine is typically involved, primarily on the right side. The anterior longitudinal ligament of the spine is ossified, with bridging of multiple vertebral bodies on radiograph. The symptoms include spinal stiffness and various peripheral joint complaints. DISH has its highest prevalence in middle-aged and elderly men.

CHARCOT'S JOINTS

Patients with disorders of vibration and position sense, such as luetic (syphilitic) neuropathy and diabetic neuropathy, can develop severe, rapidly progressive osteoarthritis in a denervated joint. The feet, ankles, and knees are most commonly affected. Charcot's osteoarthritis is a rather severe and impressively destructive condition, with fragmentation of bone as well as cartilage. The diagnosis is made by observing the characteristic radiographic findings of osteoarthritis in a patient with the appropriate neuropathy.

OSTEOPOROSIS

By Clifford J. Rosen, M.D.
Bangor, Maine

DEFINITION

Osteoporosis is a systemic disorder characterized by decreased bone mass, microarchitectural deterioration of bone tissue, increased bone fragility, and susceptibility to fracture. The osteoporotic "syndrome" refers to the triad of decreased bone density, vertebral fractures, and back pain. It has been called idiopathic osteoporosis, senile osteoporosis, involutional osteoporosis, age-related osteoporosis, primary or secondary osteoporosis, and postmenopausal osteoporosis. This syndrome is associated with functional disability and impaired quality of life. Osteopenia has been defined as the appearance of decreased bone mineral content on radiography, but the term more appropriately refers to a phase in the continuum from decreased bone mass to fractures and infirmity. By the time the diagnosis of osteopenia is made radiographically, significant and irreversible bone loss has already occurred.

PRESENTATION

The earliest stages of bone loss are asymptomatic. Once skeletal mass is reduced, fragility increases and the risk of fracture is heightened. The presentation of osteoporosis varies from acute fracture to chronic recurrent pain from previous fractures. The typical presentation of a new osteoporotic fracture features the acute onset of back pain following trauma (Fig. 1). The first fracture is often localized

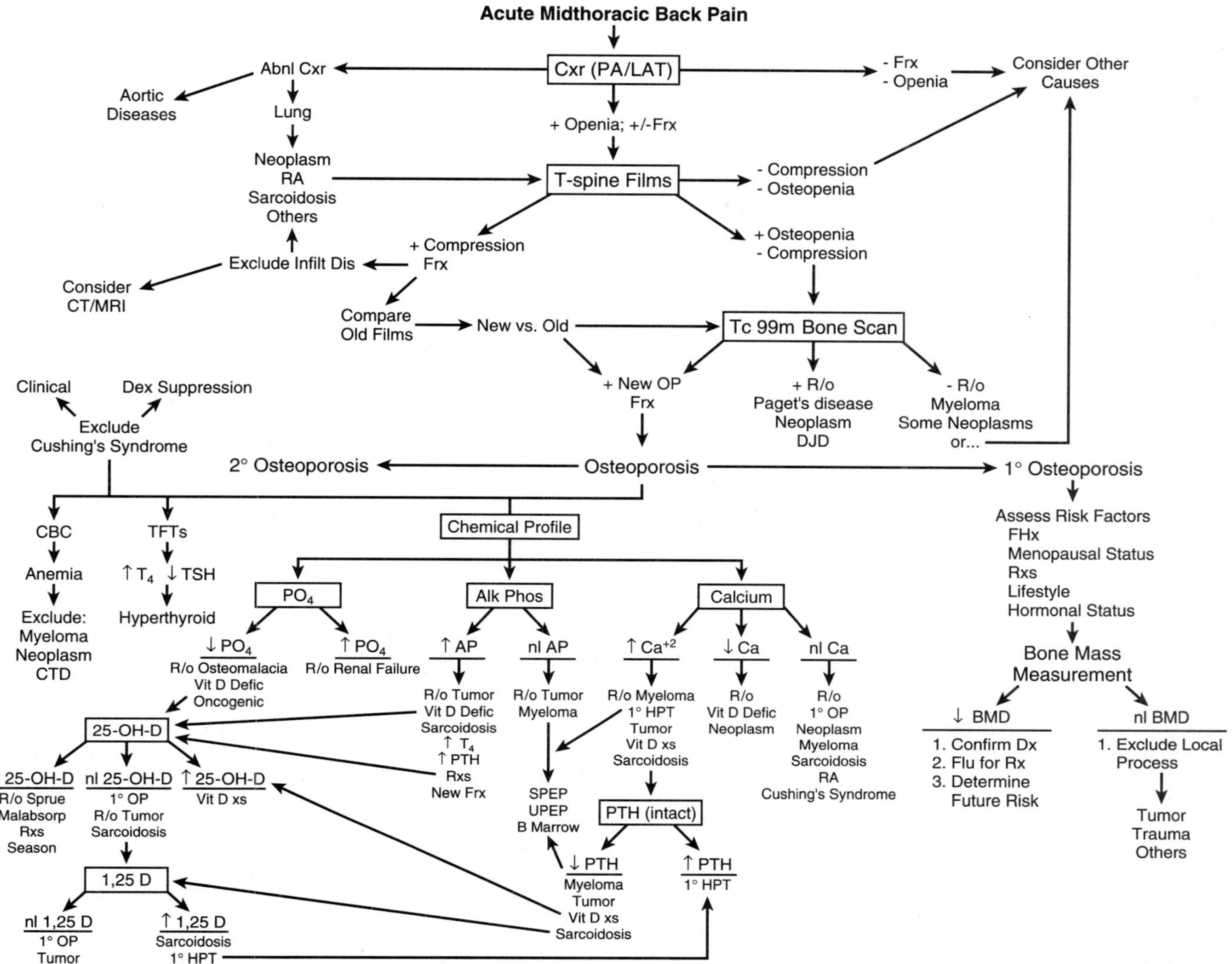

Figure 1. This algorithm presents the case of a 54-year-old woman with the acute onset of midthoracic back pain. Although the diagnosis of osteoporosis can be made from radiographs and bone density in an asymptomatic individual (see text), new back pain is often the presenting symptom of the disease. The following abbreviations are part of the algorithm: T-spine = thoracic spine films; Frx = no evidence of fracture; Infilt = infiltrative diseases of bone (sarcoid, neoplasm, other granulomatous disorders); CTD = connective tissue diseases; BMD = bone mineral density; 25-OH-D = 25(OH) vitamin D_3; Dex suppression = the overnight 1-mg dexamethasone suppression test; Rxs = drugs; RA = rheumatoid arthritis.

to the L2–L3 region or the midthoracic area (T8–T10). Low back pain, which is excruciating and knifelike, often awakens the patient during the night. Pain results from irritation of the periosteum, stretching of back ligaments, pressure from edema and hemorrhage, and spasm of the deep paraspinous muscles. Lumbar fractures cause discomfort that may radiate to the lower abdomen and mimic appendicitis, diverticulitis, or incarcerated hernia. Referred pain to the buttocks and inguinal region has also been described. Dermatomal pain radiating to the lower extremities is much less common. Thoracic compression fractures are also associated with severe discomfort that occasionally radiates to the anterior chest, simulating pleural, myocardial, or pericardial pain. Anterior rib pain may be the first manifestation of a thoracic compression fracture.

Atypical presentations of compression fracture include (1) pain radiating to the shoulder or scapula (simulating acute bursitis), (2) severe sacroiliac or perineal pain, (3) flank pain that mimics renal colic in location and intensity, and (4) right upper quadrant pain, simulating acute cholecystitis. Rarely, the first manifestation of osteoporosis is a hip fracture with acute pain in the groin, hip, or buttocks. Nausea and vomiting can result from bone pain and/or medications prescribed to treat pain.

Infrequently, fractures of the appendicular skeleton are the first sign of systemic bone loss and osteoporosis. Stress fractures of the fourth metatarsal bone result in acute foot pain. Tibial plateau fractures cause knee pain, hemarthrosis, and swelling after trauma. Distal tibial pain can occur from stress fractures in the lower leg resulting from repetitive trauma and decreased bone mass. Painful extremities can cause incapacitation and limit ambulation. Rarely, chronic limb pain and sympathetic dystrophy can result from small bone fractures of the foot.

The precipitating traumatic event in a compression fracture (e.g., lifting an object, carrying a child, vacuuming, taking a roast out of the oven) is usually recalled after careful questioning. However, patients with decreased bone mass can sustain a fracture with minimal trauma (e.g., coughing, sneezing, rolling over in bed), which may not be specifically remembered. In addition, the onset of pain after injury may be delayed from several hours to days.

Chronic back pain results from multiple fractures of the thoracic and/or lumbar spine. Although the source of pain may not be clear, the patient often presents with intense paraspinous muscle spasm. Movement is difficult, especially in the supine position. The pain is dull and gnawing and typically does not radiate. After several thoracic compressions, a dermatomal pattern of referred pain, much like a neuropathic process, may be reported. The pain is often accompanied by a "tired" feeling in the back. The patient frequently describes a sense of back "weakness" and intense fear of further pain with specific movements. For older women, daily activities such as vacuuming or cooking are tedious and painful. Sometimes the patient specifically complains of loss of height and exhibits dorsal thoracic kyphosis; other patients with thoracic compression fractures relate absolutely no symptoms. The first indication of osteoporosis may be found in a chest film obtained for other reasons. Asymptomatic compression fractures of the lumbar spine are uncommon.

COURSE OF THE DISEASE

Osteoporosis is a progressive and unrelenting disease. At first, bone loss is asymptomatic. After an indeterminate latency period, a spinal compression or appendicular fracture is reported. Further fractures (especially in the spine) are almost certain to occur if therapy is not begun. Loss of height, pain, and infirmity often progress over 5 to 10 years. To predict future fractures, measurement of bone mass has been advocated. Decreased bone mineral density (BMD; measured by densitometry [see further on]) is the best predictor of risk for future fracture. A patient with a BMD 1 SD below the mean has a relative risk of two to two and one-half times for a future spinal fracture when compared with a height- and weight-matched 35-year-old individual. The presence of a previous spinal fracture represents an independent risk factor for another fracture. Decreased bone density plus previous spinal fractures increases the relative risk of new fracture exponentially. Two spinal fractures plus a bone density 1 SD below the mean presents an eightfold greater risk for a future fracture.

The time course of symptoms from a single vertebral fracture varies. Acute bone pain can last from 1 week to 3 months. Back discomfort can wax and wane but typically persists and is not relieved by conventional non-narcotic medications. In 3 to 6 months, the pain subsides and the patient is well until the next fracture. In patients with multiple fractures, chronic pain can persist, and each new fracture causes intense muscle spasm and pain. The onset of severe back pain in a patient with known osteoporosis usually means a new compression injury or a microfracture. The repeating cycle of fracture, pain, and relief is characteristic of the chronic osteoporosis syndrome. Disability is common in such patients, and activities of daily living may be completely curtailed.

Hip fractures are a late but devastating presentation of osteoporosis in older individuals. Long-standing bone loss accompanied by multiple asymptomatic fractures may leave the patient unaware of osteoporosis. In that situation, a hip fracture may be the first manifestation of the disease. Elders are more susceptible to complications resulting from hip fractures. Mortality as high as 20 per cent may be due to infections, septicemia, venous thrombosis, pulmonary embolus, or the sequelae of accelerated catabolism and malnutrition. Those who survive face a difficult rehabilitation process. One third to one half of all patients with hip fracture leave their previous living situation and enter a long-term health care facility. The degree of chronic pain associated with hip fracture varies with the type of device inserted and the extent of complications. Problems with balance and ambulation frequently accompany femoral neck fracture. Fear of falling is a significant complaint among elders with osteoporosis and a history of previous fractures.

COMPLICATIONS

Single or recurrent spinal fractures cause pain and disability. Although thoracic and lumbar fractures result in loss of height, they are rarely associated with life-threatening complications. Patients with chronic lung disease and a new thoracic spinal fracture have extreme difficulty breathing and impaired respiratory excursions. Rib, spinal, or thoracic fractures also increase the risk of atelectasis and/or pneumonia. Administration of narcotics may cause carbon dioxide retention and worsening acidosis. Severe thoracic kyphosis can aggravate already compromised pulmonary function, making aggressive management more difficult. The use of glucocorticoids for chronic obstructive pulmonary disease (COPD) increases the risk of additional fractures and their sequelae. In susceptible individuals (diabetics, patients taking glucocorticoids), a rib fracture from osteoporosis can puncture the lung, causing pneumothorax, empyema, abscess, or other complications.

Lumbar compression fractures from osteoporosis occasionally produce neurologic complications. In elders with mild spinal stenosis, changes in vertebral alignment may further compromise the spinal canal and the cauda equina. In progressive spinal stenosis, pain and symptoms of leg or buttocks claudication typically increase. In general, however, osteoporotic spinal fractures do not cause neurologic impairment because posterior fragmentation into the spinal canal is rare. As detected by magnetic resonance imaging (MRI), retropulsion of small fragments from a fracture of the lumbar spine can occasionally occur, but these fragments rarely produce spinal cord compromise or compression. When the spinal canal is threatened, bowel and bladder functions typically are preserved despite the onset of dermatomal pain due to nerve root irritation.

Appendicular fractures generally follow a benign course. Colles' fracture of the wrist may be the first sign of osteoporosis but is generally uncomplicated unless nonunion results. Colles' fracture with nonunion is more prevalent in patients with type I diabetes or in patients taking high-dose glucocorticoids or immunosuppressive agents. In diabetics, recurrent fractures of the feet may produce Charcot's joint deformities. Finally, tibial plateau fractures may be complicated by hemarthrosis, pain, and immobility.

PHYSICAL EXAMINATION

The physical examination of the patient with osteoporosis may or may not be helpful. The patient who has suffered a new fracture is usually in significant distress and unable to move quickly or lie down. Extreme spasm of the deep paraspinous muscles is often present. Sometimes pinpoint tenderness over the affected thoracic or lumbar vertebrae can be elicited.

In the chronic osteoporotic syndrome, kyphosis (lumbar or thoracic) is obvious. In the standing position, the abdomen often protrudes and the lower rib cage can be palpated near the pelvic brim. Significant downward angulation of the ribs occurs and the head often appears to be bent and fixed. In severe cases, pelvic tilt, hamstring contractures, stiff ankles, and pronated feet are seen. A shuffling, unsteady gait and a fixed downward gaze may suggest Parkinson's disease.

Paraspinous muscle spasm is often noted adjacent to the thoracic and lumbar spine. However, deep tendon reflexes are intact (except in diabetes mellitus), and muscle strength is usually normal. Evaluation of the patient in the supine position can accentuate the pain. A straight, upright posture may be nearly impossible, and the horizontal distance from a wall to the base of the neck can be useful in determining the severity of the kyphosis. Straight leg raising is usually unremarkable even after new lumbar fractures. However, with a Valsalva maneuver, back pain may be accentuated. Costovertebral angle tenderness typically is not present, but movement worsens the back pain. Sphincter tone remains intact.

In patients with osteoporosis and vitamin D deficiency (osteomalacia), muscle weakness may be profound and leg or bone pain may be intense. These patients often respond to vitamin D with increased motor strength, but relief of pain may take 12 to 18 months. Examination of other organs and tissues to exclude metastatic disease is especially important. This includes careful evaluation of the lungs, breasts, thyroid gland, prostate gland, and lymph tissues.

Unusual findings on examination that might suggest a secondary cause of osteoporosis include (1) exophthalmos and/or goiter (thyrotoxicosis); (2) blue sclerae, triangular facies, hearing and/or tooth loss, joint laxity, skin hyperelasticity (osteogenesis imperfecta or a forme fruste); (3) ectopic or scleral calcification (primary hyperparathyroidism); (4) tetany (due to severe osteomalacia in patients with nontropical sprue or malabsorption); (5) supraclavicular fullness, easy bruisability, thin skin, and facial puffiness (Cushing's syndrome); (6) episodic macular patches and erythema (mastocytosis); (7) increased height with a span-to-height ratio of less than a factor of 1 (Klinefelter's syndrome with osteopenia); (8) a marfanoid appearance (Marfan's syndrome or homocystinuria); (9) kyphosis with mucosal neuromas (multiple endocrine neoplasia [MEN] type IIb); (10) acromegalic facies (acromegaly); or (11) short stature and a webbed neck (Turner's syndrome).

LABORATORY PROCEDURES

The diagnosis of osteoporosis often rests on the radiographic features of a fracture, usually a compression fracture of the dorsal or lumbar spine. Other radiographic appearances of the spine, however, can also support the diagnosis of osteoporosis. Demineralization causes loss of the normal trabecular pattern and false accentuation of the superior and inferior cortical edges. With further progression of the disease, there is biconcave compression of the end-plates, resulting in a "codfish" type of appearance. Progressive demineralization leads to wedge fractures that are almost always anterior and often noted in the thoracic spine. The combination of anterior wedge fractures and biconcavity of the vertebral body is common.

Compression fractures of the T7–T8 or T12–L3 region are routinely associated with evidence of osteopenia elsewhere. However, not every compression fracture is due to osteoporosis. For example, fractures above the fourth thoracic vertebra are atypical for osteoporosis and may point to another disorder. Posterior wedging of the vertebrae strongly suggests an underlying disorder such as Paget's disease, trauma, or malignancy. Thinning of the superior or inferior cortical edges is seldom seen in primary osteoporosis; its presence should prompt the clinician to exclude neoplasms, disk disease, osteomyelitis, and other causes of inflammation.

Demineralization and cortical thinning in long bones may provide an early clue to the diagnosis of osteoporosis. Loss of trabecular components in the radius and distal humerus suggests diffuse osteoporosis. Spotty demineralization is consistent with osteoporosis but could also reflect multiple myeloma or other lymphoproliferative diseases.

Hip fractures are easily recognized on plain films. Impaction of the femoral head or fractures of the femoral neck can also be seen in patients with a history of trauma or of a fall. Stress fractures of the femur are more difficult to detect radiographically; tomography or bone scanning (see further on) may be required. Occasionally, "pseudofractures" or "loose zones" are seen in the femur or other sites. These insufficiency zones are characteristic of osteomalacia. The coexistence of osteoporosis and osteopenia is common in elders with vitamin D deficiency.

Analysis of body fluids may support the diagnosis of osteoporosis or exclude secondary causes. In primary osteoporosis, the serum concentrations of calcium, alkaline phosphatase, phosphate, total protein, and creatinine should be normal. By contrast, after a new fracture serum alkaline phosphatase activity is often increased for up to 6 months. Similarly, the total serum alkaline phosphatase may be increased in patients with metastatic tumor or Paget's disease. Chronic phenytoin administration and thyrotoxicosis (treated or untreated) may also be associated with increased alkaline phosphatase activity. Plain films and/or tomography provide the best means for distinguishing new osteoporotic fractures from Paget's disease.

Hypocalcemia is consistent with osteomalacia, whereas hypercalcemia suggests primary hyperparathyroidism, sarcoidosis, or neoplasm. Hyperproteinemia can be seen in multiple myeloma, whereas hypophosphatemia may uncover osteomalacia due to vitamin D deficiency, X-linked hypophosphatemia, or tumor-related osteomalacia.

The complete blood count is typically normal in patients with primary osteoporosis. By contrast, anemia is often found in patients with secondary causes of osteoporosis (e.g., metastatic disease to bone, multiple myeloma, chronic infections, underlying connective tissue disorders, or renal insufficiency). Most cases of multiple myeloma can be detected with serum and urine protein electrophoresis. However, bone marrow aspiration and biopsy are needed to confirm the diagnosis because nonsecretory variants occur in 1 to 5 per cent of patients with myeloma. Although both myeloma and hyperparathyroidism may cause anemia, hypercalcemia, fractures, and bone pain, the serum parathyroid hormone concentration is increased in primary hyperparathyroidism and suppressed in multiple myeloma.

OTHER IMAGING PROCEDURES OR LABORATORY STUDIES THAT ASSIST IN THE DIAGNOSIS

Radiographic diagnosis of fracture resulting from osteoporosis is often obscured by previous fractures or artifacts unrelated to osteoporosis (e.g., degenerative changes). Sometimes the patient complains of severe back or hip pain, but the plain films do not show a fracture. Technetium Tc 99m (^{99m}Tc) bone scanning may be particularly useful in detecting a new fracture in the spine or a stress fracture in the hip. Bone scans may remain positive for up to 6 months after the initial fracture. However, increased uptake of ^{99m}Tc is not pathognomonic for osteoporotic fracture and can be seen with degenerative arthritis, overlying soft tissue or bony infections, granulomas, Paget's disease, inflammatory disk disease, and metastatic or primary neoplasm of bone. Conversely, negative bone scans are observed in some metastatic processes and in multiple myeloma.

"Insufficiency" fractures have been reported with increasing frequency in elders with osteopenia. Typical sites of involvement include the sacrum, the iliac bones, and the pubis. Presenting complaints include low back pain, sacroiliac discomfort, perineal or inguinal pain, and difficulty walking. Radiographs of the lumbosacral spine and pelvis are usually normal, but ^{99m}Tc scanning reveals intense uptake in the affected area.

CONFIRMATION OF THE DIAGNOSIS

Measurements of bone mass (BMD, densitometry) can detect the extent of bone loss from the spine, hip, wrist, or total body with tremendous accuracy and precision. Various techniques (dual energy x-ray absorptiometry [DEXA], computed tomography [CT] scanning, single energy x-ray absorptiometry [SXA], dual photon absorptiometry [DPA], radiogrammetry) can be employed to measure bone density. BMD measurements can confirm the diffuse nature of osteoporosis, thereby providing critical information about the risk of future fractures. In addition, the precision error of most of these techniques is low enough that the tests can provide a reference point for clinicians to assess treatment outcomes or rates of bone loss. Bone loss by densitometry may predict osteoporotic fracture better than hypercholesterolemia predicts heart disease or excessive blood pressure predicts stroke.

Magnetic resonance imaging may provide additional information about the relationship of a compression fracture to the spinal canal and specific nerve roots. Magnetic resonance imaging is the most sensitive means of measuring the degree of spinal stenosis and the extent of retropulsion from a fracture.

Pyridinoline molecules cross-link the three peptide chains that compose type I collagen within the bony matrix. During bone resorption, these cross-links are broken. Clearance of the cross-linking molecules (deoxypyridinoline and pyridinoline) can be measured in 2-hour or 24-hour collections of urine. These assays have not found widespread clinical use, but they may become important tools for gauging response to therapy or for detecting bone loss in asymptomatic individuals.

Serum concentrations of vitamin D_3 are decreased in the elderly, especially those living in northern latitudes and in nursing homes. Twenty to 40 per cent of elders with new hip fractures have borderline or low serum 25-hydroxycholecalciferol (25(OH)D) concentrations that typically reflect poor diet and inadequate sun exposure (especially in winter months). Decreased serum 25(OH) vitamin D_3 also occurs in patients with tropical sprue, malabsorption, primary biliary cirrhosis, or chronic anticonvulsant therapy. In most of these conditions, oral administration of ergocalciferol or cholecalciferol normalizes the serum 25(OH)D concentration. Vitamin D therapy can eliminate deficiency of this vitamin as a contributing factor to the progression of osteoporosis. Appropriate vitamin D treatment may also decrease the incidence of fracture in some high-risk patients.

Bone biopsy following tetracycline labeling may help distinguish osteoporosis from osteomalacia. Biopsy may also reveal Paget's disease or neoplastic invasion of bone. However, bone biopsy is costly and is not required for the diagnosis of osteoporosis. In many patients, the histomorphometric appearance of the bone does not correlate with the clinical course.

PITFALLS IN THE DIAGNOSIS OF OSTEOPOROSIS

In patients with decreased BMD and radiographic evidence of a compression or appendicular fracture, the diagnosis of osteoporosis can be made relatively easily. In the absence of bone density measurement, the diagnosis can be established by radiographic features, especially if there are multiple spinal fractures. Distal stress fractures are part of the osteoporosis syndrome, but without previous fractures or evidence of decreased BMD, the definitive diagnosis is more elusive. The clinical phenotype of osteoporosis, which includes kyphosis, frailty, and back pain, is easily recognized in older patients. Loss of height and back pain, however, are not sufficient for diagnosing osteoporosis because degenerative arthritis can also lead to disk degeneration, loss of height, and pain. Decreased bone mass without fracture is the earliest phase of the osteoporotic process; at this stage, and in the absence of fracture, the diagnosis requires bone density measurements. In the future, markers of bone resorption (collagen cross-links) may be sufficient to diagnose the earliest stages of osteoporosis.

DIAGNOSTIC PROCESS

Diagnosing osteoporosis is not difficult when an elderly patient suffers a hip fracture. At that stage, however, most preventive and therapeutic measures are ineffective. Osteoporosis remains clinically silent for many years as bone loss progresses. Eventually fractures occur. The goal for every patient with osteoporosis is to prevent fracture. Hence, early diagnosis is critical for the institution of appropriate therapy. The clinician must search for important risk factors (e.g., early gonadal steroid deprivation, family history, use of certain medications, and so forth) in men and women of all ages. Early identification of asymptomatic premenopausal women with decreased bone mass increases the likelihood that early treatment will prevent bone loss and reduce the number of fractures from osteoporosis.

The clinician's greatest challenge in the diagnosis of osteoporosis lies in excluding secondary causes of an osteoporotic fracture. The diagnosis of multiple myeloma may be straightforward in a patient with new back pain, osteopenia, increased serum creatinine concentrations, hypercalcemia, anemia, and a markedly increased sedimentation rate. Older patients, however, may have mild anemia, an increased sedimentation rate, and back pain that suggests multiple myeloma but is also consistent with age-related osteoporosis. When serum and urine protein studies are inconclusive and the bone marrow does not contain significantly increased numbers of plasma cells, a bone biopsy may be helpful. Is an older patient's first compression fracture a delayed manifestation of osteoporosis or is it metastatic disease to bone? Serum studies are often indeterminate. Decreased bone density, especially in the elderly, does not exclude malignancy. ^{99m}Tc bone scanning may provide important information but can be positive in many conditions, including neoplasm, trauma, inflammation, granulomatous processes, and Paget's disease. Computed tomography may be useful because it can reveal soft tissue as well as bony changes due to primary or secondary tumors. In managing patients with significant pain and persistent symptoms, imaging is better than following the clinical course or repeating certain blood tests.

Subtle radiographic changes often are not detected or reported, especially at the first reading. Thus, review of earlier films is useful. Serial spinal films may show relative changes in the size, shape, or position of the vertebrae, suggesting either a new fracture or an infiltrative process. Thinning of the superior or inferior cortical margins suggests tumor or infection. Posterior wedging or loss of a distinct posterior vertebral cortical margin may also indicate infiltration by tumor or infection.

Paget's disease of the appendicular skeleton is easily recognized. However, pagetic involvement of the spine may be confused with idiopathic osteoporosis. Early in the disease, the vertebrae may appear osteoporotic, whereas the ^{99m}Tc scan is strongly positive. Vertebral collapse may occur. Later, the vertebrae appear expanded, suggesting an infiltrative process. Radiographic evidence of coarse vertical striations and thickened margins is consistent with invasion by tumor. However, markedly increased alkaline phosphatase concentrations and a positive bone scan narrow the diagnostic possibilities. In addition, neurologic impairment is more often seen in pagetic than in osteoporotic vertebral collapse. Spastic paraparesis, numbness, paresthesias, and bowel and bladder dysfunction have been reported. In some patients, CT and MRI can further narrow the differential diagnosis and help define the extent of neurologic impairment.

In summary, the diagnosis of osteoporosis can be easy or elusive. To increase the benefits of treatment, early diagnosis is essential. Secondary causes of osteoporosis must be excluded. Clinically useful measurements of bone mass are now available to aid in early diagnosis.

RICKETS AND OSTEOMALACIA

By Florence N. Hutchison, M.D.,
and Norman H. Bell, M.D.
Charleston, South Carolina

Rickets and osteomalacia represent a spectrum of diseases that are characterized by defective mineralization of bone matrix. Rickets is a disease of children in which impaired mineralization of the epiphyseal growth plates is the most prominent feature. If unrecognized, the defective mineralization leads to disorganization of bone growth with resultant growth retardation and skeletal deformities. In the adult skeleton, in which growth has ceased, mineralization of newly formed osteoid matrix occurs in the process of bone remodeling, and a defect in mineralization of bone is referred to as osteomalacia. Failure of osteoid to mineralize normally results in loss of bone strength and rigidity so that the bones, particularly in the axial skeleton, are deformed by weight bearing and muscle tension.

REGULATION OF BONE FORMATION

Bone mineralization is a complex process that is not completely understood. During skeletal growth and remodeling, an organic matrix, osteoid, is produced by osteoblasts and must undergo a period of maturation prior to mineralization. Calcium is taken up by osteoblasts and concentrated in matrix vesicles along with alkaline phosphatase. Phosphorus is made available for reaction with calcium by the action of alkaline phosphatase, and the resulting amorphous calcium phosphate is deposited in the osteoid matrix. Amorphous calcium phosphate must then be converted to mature hydroxyapatite to complete the process of mineralization. This process is dependent on the normal production of osteoid by osteoblasts, the availability of calcium and phosphorus, and the presence of substances, both local and systemic, that regulate the activity of osteoblasts and the serum concentrations of calcium and phosphorus.

Vitamin D and parathyroid hormone (PTH) are the primary regulators of calcium and phosphorus metabolism. Figure 1 illustrates the metabolism of vitamin D and the relationship of defects in its metabolism to diseases that result in rickets or osteomalacia. Vitamin D_3 (cholecalciferol) is derived from ultraviolet conversion of epidermal 7-dehydrocholesterol. The plant-derived ergocalciferol (vitamin D_2) and cholecalciferol are ingested in fortified foods and multivitamins. Since ergocalciferol and cholecalciferol are fat soluble, uptake is dependent on normal intestinal fat absorption. Uptake may be impaired in the presence of pancreatic or biliary disease. Both forms of vitamin D undergo a similar metabolic activation and have equivalent metabolic activity. Vitamin D is sequentially hydroxylated to 25-hydroxycholecalciferol (25(OH)D) in the liver and to 1,25-dihydroxycholecalciferol ($1,25(OH)_2D$) in the kidney. $1,25(OH)_2D$ is the most potent metabolite and stimulates intestinal calcium and phosphorus absorption, stimulates bone resorption, and suppresses PTH synthesis and secretion. Renal hydroxylation is inhibited by calcium and phosphorus and is stimulated by PTH.

PTH is critical to the maintenance of a normal serum calcium concentration. This peptide hormone induces release of calcium from bone stores by stimulating osteoclast activity. It also increases renal tubular calcium reabsorption and phosphorus excretion. PTH also indirectly stimulates intestinal calcium absorption by increasing renal 1α-hydroxylase activity for synthesis of $1,25(OH)_2D$. The interaction of $1,25(OH)_2D$ and PTH produces a closed negative feedback loop in which increased PTH stimulates $1,25(OH)_2D$ synthesis, and the increased serum $1,25(OH)_2D$ then suppresses PTH synthesis. Primary or secondary abnormalities in the production or action of these hormones and hypophosphatemia account for most cases of osteomalacia and rickets.

CLINICAL FEATURES

Although rickets and osteomalacia may be caused by a diverse group of nutritional, genetic, or metabolic abnormalities, or may be associated with other chronic systemic diseases, the clinical signs and symptoms are remarkably similar (Table 1). Unfortunately, many of the symptoms are nonspecific so that early diagnosis is difficult. Additionally, it is not possible to distinguish which of the many pathophysiologic causes of rickets or osteomalacia is operative based on the clinical evaluation alone. Nevertheless, recognition of the clinical features is of paramount importance so that the diagnosis can be confirmed, the specific

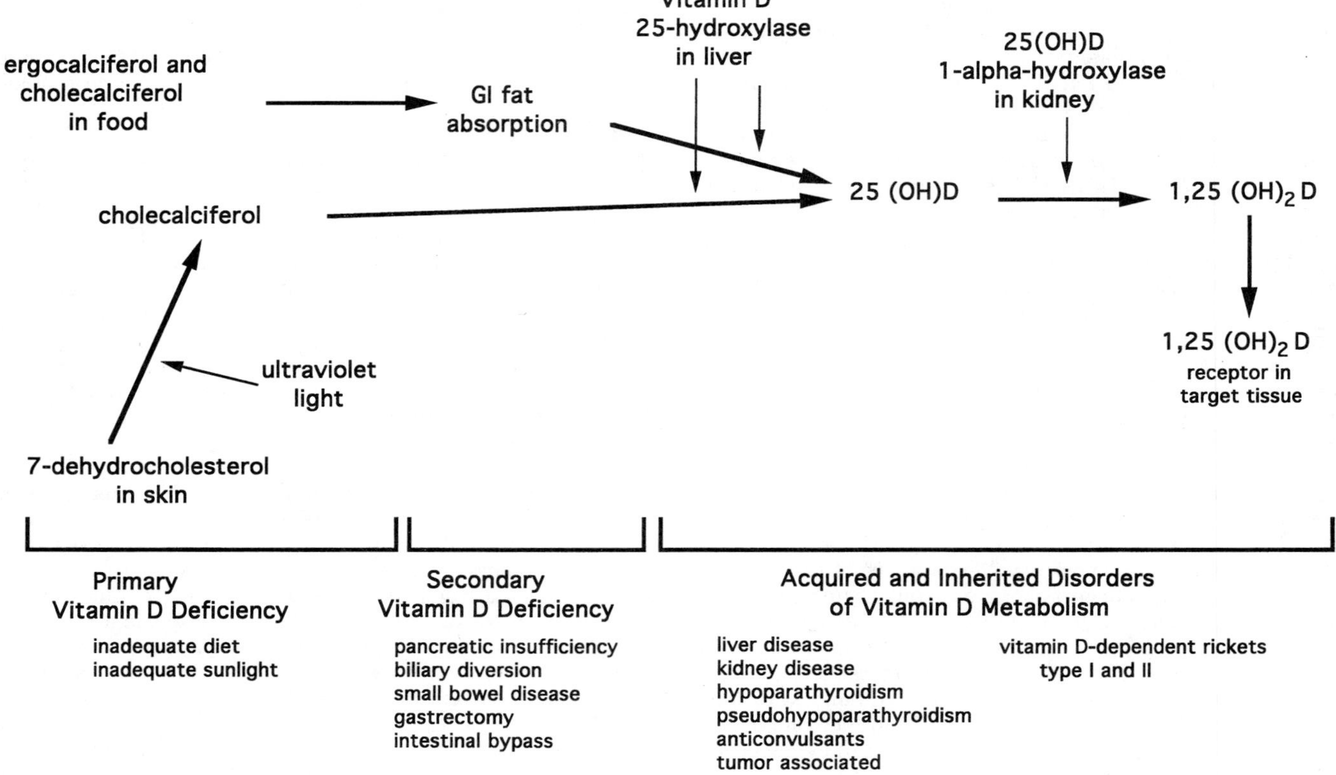

Figure 1. Vitamin D metabolism and osteomalacia. The availability of substrate for, and the synthesis of, $1,25(OH)_2D$ is crucial to the process of bone mineralization. Abnormalities at any of the steps of vitamin D metabolism may produce rickets or osteomalacia. Ergocalciferol is vitamin D_2, and cholecalciferol is vitamin D_3.

cause of the disease identified, and appropriate management initiated.

An early feature of rickets is growth retardation, and the diagnosis of rickets should be considered in any child below the 5th percentile in height. Generally, wasting is not a feature of rickets, and body weight is appropriate to height. More subtle symptoms include irritability, depression, or loss of interest in activities and withdrawal from physical activities. Skeletal deformities occur in bones that undergo rapid growth. Since the growth rate of different bones varies with age, the particular bones most affected are dependent on age at the time of onset of the disease. Frontal bossing, widened cranial sutures, and the softening and deformity of the cranial bones referred to as craniotabes are characteristic of neonatal rickets and are not present when the onset of rickets occurs late in childhood. Chest wall abnormalities such as the funnel chest deformity caused by abnormal rib growth and the rachitic rosary caused by nodular thickening of the costochondral joints are more typical of early childhood rickets. The classic bowing deformities of the extremities in advanced rickets, either bowleg (genu varum) or knock-knee (genu valgum), result from weight bearing and are rarely present in very young children. Tooth formation also may be affected by rickets, with enamel hypoplasia and carious disease being prominent features. Fractures are a common feature, and the diagnosis of rickets should be considered in children presenting with frequent fractures, fractures at unusual sites, or fractures not associated with significant physical trauma.

Table 1. Clinical and Radiographic Features of Rickets and Osteomalacia

Symptoms and Signs	Radiographic Findings
Growth retardation	Decreased bone density
Irritability, depression	Craniotabes
Malaise	Frontal bossing
Muscle weakness	Rachitic rosary
Premature tooth loss	Harrison's groove
Pain with physical activity	Pseudofractures
Bone pain	Looser's zones
Bone deformity	Concave "codfish" vertebrae
Fractures	Biconvex vertebral disks
	Bowing of long bones

Osteomalacia is frequently asymptomatic. It is estimated that as many as 25 per cent of hip fractures in the geriatric population are due to previously asymptomatic and unrecognized osteomalacia. The most common complaints are nonspecific symptoms of malaise, fatigue, generalized weakness, and diffuse bone pain. The bone pain is described as a dull, aching pain in the lower back and hips or at sites where fractures have occurred; the pain is worsened by physical activity. Fractures are observed most commonly in ribs, vertebrae, and long bones, and repeated fractures may lead to significant skeletal deformity. Muscle weakness also may be a prominent feature on clinical examination and most frequently affects proximal muscle groups. Severe involvement of the hip girdle muscles results in a peculiar waddling gait (abductor lurch). Muscle wasting and tenderness and hyperreflexia also have been described in patients with osteomalacia.

LABORATORY DIAGNOSIS OF OSTEOMALACIA AND RICKETS

Blood chemistry panels may provide supportive evidence for osteomalacia or rickets but cannot be considered diagnostic. Serum alkaline phosphatase activity, specifically that of the skeletal isoenzyme, is elevated in 80 to 90 per cent of patients. Hypocalcemia and hypophosphatemia may be present. Urinary calcium excretion may be increased and urinary phosphorus excretion decreased. Serum 25(OH)D concentrations may be decreased, and serum PTH concentrations are frequently increased because of hypocalcemia or vitamin D deficiency. A list of laboratory investigations recommended for the evaluation of patients with rickets or osteomalacia is provided in Table 2. Given the heterogeneous pathophysiologic disorders that produce osteomalacia, these tests are more helpful in characterizing the specific metabolic or nutritional disorder once the diagnosis of osteomalacia or rickets has been confirmed radiologically or histologically.

RADIOGRAPHIC FEATURES

The common radiographic findings in rickets and osteomalacia are listed in Table 1. Reduced bone density is the most common radiographic finding in osteomalacia, but it is nonspecific and provides little useful diagnostic information. More helpful, if present, are Looser's zones or pseudofractures. Looser's zones are linear radiolucencies that transect and lie perpendicular to the cortical bone margin. Looser's zones are commonly found at the axillary margins of the scapulae, the lower ribs, the superior and inferior pubic rami, the femoral neck, and the proximal ulnae. Multiple pseudofractures with a bilateral, symmetrical distribution are referred to as Milkman's syndrome. The pathogenesis of Looser's zones is not known. These lesions may represent a pseudofracture that has healed by deposition of inadequately mineralized osteoid or, alternatively, a site of mechanical erosion from overlying arterioles. In advanced disease, the vertebral bodies soften and become concave, producing the typical "codfish" vertebrae. In contrast, the vertebral disks appear large and biconvex. Vertebral compression fractures may be observed but are less frequent than in osteoporosis.

Because of the high incidence of secondary hyperparathyroidism in patients with long-standing rickets or osteomalacia, bone changes typical of osteitis fibrosa cystica are common. In particular, subperiosteal resorption of the phalanges, clavicles, and humeri may be apparent on radiographic examination and may confound the diagnosis of osteomalacia.

Bone mass is reduced both radiographically and as measured by single-photon and dual-photon or dual-energy absorptiometry but, as noted previously, is a nonspecific finding common to a variety of other bone disorders. A technetium Tc 99m pyrophosphate bone scan typically shows increased uptake by the long bones, wrists, skull, and mandible. Uptake of isotope at the costochondral junctions may highlight the rachitic rosary, or more diffuse uptake by the sternum may produce the so-called tie sternum. Pseudofractures appear as hot spots (areas of increased uptake of isotope) and may be confused with metastatic bone lesions.

Table 2. Recommended Laboratory Investigations

Serum phosphorus and calcium concentrations
Serum creatinine, urea, potassium, bicarbonate concentrations
Serum alkaline phosphatase activity
Serum 25-hydroxyvitamin D concentration
Serum 1,25-dihydroxyvitamin D concentration
Serum intact parathyroid hormone concentration
Urinary calcium and phosphorus excretion
Fecal fat (if malabsorption is suspected)

HISTOLOGIC FEATURES OF BONE IN RICKETS AND OSTEOMALACIA

The underlying pathophysiologic process common to rickets and osteomalacia, defective bone mineralization, results in characteristic histologic abnormalities of bone. In rickets, impaired mineralization of the epiphyseal growth plate results in a hypertrophic cartilaginous zone with disorganized bone formation and increased uncalcified osteoid. In osteomalacia, newly synthesized osteoid laid down in areas of bone remodeling fails to mineralize and accumulates in wide bands of uncalcified osteoid along bony trabeculae.

Wide osteoid seams resulting from increased osteoid synthesis are also present in hyperthyroidism, Paget's disease, and primary hyperparathyroidism but are not associated with the defective mineralization characteristic of osteomalacia. Thus, it is imperative to assess the degree of mineralization to distingush among these diseases. This can be accomplished by double tetracycline labeling. Tetracycline antibiotics bind to the amorphous calcium phosphate that is deposited as the initial step in bone mineralization and can be visualized as a fluorescent band along the zone in which mineralization is actively occurring. By administering two courses of tetracycline 10 days apart, it is possible not only to visualize the mineralization front but also to measure the rate of mineralization by determining the distance between the two labels. Tetracycline hydrochloride fluoresces green and demeclocycline fluoresces yellow, allowing accurate measurement of the mineralization rate even under conditions of impaired bone formation. In normal adults, mineralization occurs at a rate of 1 μm per day; this rate is markedly reduced in bone affected by osteomalacia. In severe osteomalacia, the rate of mineralization may be so reduced that only a single, poorly defined band of fluorescent label is visible.

In the absence of specific radiographic findings, the definitive procedure for the diagnosis of rickets or osteomalacia consists of dynamic bone histomorphometry with double tetracycline labeling to demonstrate wide osteoid seams and impaired mineralization. Bone biopsy, although invasive, has low morbidity and can provide the diagnostic information that is crucial to appropriate management of osteomalacia. However, the cause of osteomalacia or rickets cannot be determined on the basis of bone biopsy alone.

DIFFERENTIAL DIAGNOSIS OF RICKETS AND OSTEOMALACIA

The conditions that result in rickets or osteomalacia can be broadly grouped into three categories: abnormalities of vitamin D metabolism, phosphate deficiency, and primary defects in mineralization.

Primary Vitamin D Deficiency

Nutritional deficiency of vitamin D is rare in the United States because dairy products are fortified with vitamin D and sunlight exposure is adequate in most parts of the country. Only 2.5 μg of dietary vitamin D per day in adults and 10 μg per day in children, or 10 to 15 minutes of sunlight exposure per day, is required to prevent osteomalacia. Black infants are prone to the development of rickets, particularly those who are breast-fed. Elderly individuals and those who are institutionalized may be at increased risk for vitamin D deficiency because of limited sun exposure and consumption of diets containing insufficient quantities of fortified foods. Recently vitamin D deficiency has been recognized as a problem in Asian immigrants in the United Kingdom because of the combination of greater skin pigmentation, reduced sun exposure, and a vegetarian diet. Chupatti flour, a traditional dietary staple in the Indian and Pakistani populations, chelates dietary calcium and impairs fat absorption, which is necessary for absorption of dietary vitamin D.

Secondary Vitamin D Deficiency

Conditions that impair or prevent vitamin D absorption also result in vitamin D deficiency and osteomalacia and are the most common causes of vitamin D deficiency osteomalacia in the United States. These conditions include pancreatic insufficiency, chronic biliary diversion, and small bowel diseases such as regional enteritis, scleroderma, celiac disease, and sprue. Osteomalacia resulting from vitamin D deficiency may also occur as a complication of partial or total gastrectomy or intestinal bypass procedures performed for the treatment of morbid obesity. A detailed medical and dietary history is useful to evaluate the possibility of either primary or secondary vitamin D deficiency; this diagnosis can be confirmed by measuring serum 25(OH)D. The normal range for 25(OH)D is 10 to 60 ng/mL, and values less than 6 ng/mL should be considered diagnostic of vitamin D deficiency.

Acquired Disorders of Vitamin D Metabolism

Vitamin D must be hydroxylated in the liver and the kidney to be converted to active metabolites. As a result, any defects in these processes result in a secondary vitamin D deficiency. Impaired 25-hydroxylation in the liver may be associated with hepatocellular disease, primary biliary cirrhosis, or biliary atresia, but it is unusual. In these conditions, both absorption and biosynthesis may be impaired. Serum 25(OH)D concentrations are decreased and may not increase significantly after supplementation with vitamin D, necessitating the supplemental use of $25(OH)D_3$ or $1,25(OH)_2D_3$.

Since PTH exerts a stimulatory effect on renal 1α-hydroxylase, hypoparathyroidism or pseudohypoparathyroidism (target organ resistance to the action of PTH) limits conversion of 25(OH)D to $1,25(OH)_2D$. Typically, serum 25(OH)D concentrations are normal and $1,25(OH)_2D$ concentrations are decreased. Hypocalcemia is commonly present in these diseases and also contributes to the development of osteomalacia or rickets.

Renal failure produces complex disturbances in calcium and phosphorus metabolism, including impaired synthesis of $1,25(OH)_2D$, metabolic acidosis, retention of inhibitors of bone calcification, and abnormal collagen synthesis. Osteomalacia or rickets may be a component of the renal osteodystrophy that commonly occurs in patients with advanced renal failure. Synthesis of $1,25(OH)_2D$ from 25(OH)D is reduced in patients with renal failure because of the loss of functional renal mass and retention of phosphorus. Serum $1,25(OH)_2D$ increases only modestly in response to treatment with vitamin D or 25(OH)D. Serum calcium concentrations are typically decreased and serum phosphorus concentrations are increased in untreated patients. Serum PTH concentrations increase when serum $1,25(OH)_2D$ and calcium values are low so that osteitis fibrosa cystica due to secondary hyperparathyroidism is frequently observed and may occur along with osteomalacia. Accumulation of aluminum may also contribute to impaired mineralization, and aluminum-induced osteomalacia may be worsened by parathyroidectomy or treatment with $1,25(OH)_2D$. The diagnosis of aluminum-induced osteomalacia is discussed further in the discussion of inhibition of mineralization. A tetracycline-labeled bone biopsy is recommended in patients with renal failure and symptomatic bone disease because this population frequently has mixed bone disease with components of vitamin D–dependent osteomalacia, secondary hyperparathyroidism, and/or aluminum intoxication.

Osteomalacia and rickets are well recognized complications of anticonvulsant drugs, particularly phenytoin and phenobarbital. Although symptomatic bone disease due to anticonvulsant therapy is uncommon in patients who are not institutionalized, hypocalcemia and increased serum alkaline phosphatase activity is not uncommon. It is likely that immobilization, inadequate diet, and lack of exposure to sunlight also contribute to osteomalacia and rickets in the institutionalized population. Phenytoin and phenobarbital increase the hepatic synthesis of 25(OH)D from vitamin D and increase the subsequent conversion of 25(OH)D to biologically inactive metabolites. Although serum concentrations of 25(OH)D are reduced, serum concentrations of $1,25(OH)_2D$, the more biologically active metabolite, are usually normal, suggesting that factors other than vitamin D deficiency contribute to the development of bone disease. These drugs may also inhibit intestinal absorption of calcium and mobilization of calcium from bone, suggesting an acquired defect in target organ response to $1,25(OH)_2D$.

Osteomalacia has been reported in association with a variety of neoplasms, both benign and malignant, including sarcomas, hemangiomas, giant cell tumors of bone, and breast and prostate carcinoma. Patients with oncogenous osteomalacia present with the typical features of osteomalacia—bone pain and muscle weakness—and improve with removal or effective treatment of the tumor. Tumor-associated osteomalacia is characterized by decreased renal synthesis of $1,25(OH)_2D$ and renal phosphate wasting. It is probable that substances produced by the tumors interfere with $1,25(OH)_2D$ synthesis and impair renal tubular phosphorus reabsorption. Serum phosphate concentrations are decreased, serum calcium concentrations are normal or slightly reduced, serum alkaline phosphatase activity is elevated, and serum $1,25(OH)_2D$ concentrations are reduced. Urinary calcium and phosphorus concentrations are increased.

Inherited Disorders of Vitamin D Metabolism

Several inborn errors of vitamin D metabolism have been identified as causes of osteomalacia. Vitamin D–dependent rickets, type I is transmitted as an autosomal recessive trait and has been attributed to an abnormality of renal 25(OH)D-1α-hydroxylase. As a result, serum 25(OH)D concentrations are normal and serum $1,25(OH)_2D$ concentrations are low or undetectable. Hypocalcemia and hypophosphatemia are invariably present, and serum PTH concentrations and alkaline phosphatase activity are increased. Children affected by vitamin D–dependent rickets appear normal at birth, but the clinical features of rickets develop in the first year of life. Symptoms and biochemical abnormalities can be readily corrected by administration of $1,25(OH)_2D_3$ in physiologic doses.

Vitamin D–dependent rickets, type II is characterized by target organ resistance to $1,25(OH)_2D$ because of abnormal vitamin D receptor function. This disorder is transmitted as an autosomal recessive trait but may occur sporadically. Familial studies have identified mutations at several sites in the vitamin D receptor gene, and this genetic heterogeneity accounts for the disparity in disease severity among families. Clinical symptoms may present at any time from birth to adolescence. Hypocalcemia is common, and alopecia occurs in patients with severe forms of this genetic disorder. A predisposition to pulmonary infections has been attributed to immune dysfunction and respiratory muscle weakness. Serum $1,25(OH)_2D$ concentrations are usually high; values in excess of 700 pg/mL have been reported. Secondary hyperparathyroidism is common, and skeletal changes resulting from excess PTH are not unusual. Unlike type I vitamin D–dependent rickets, the response to $1,25(OH)_2D_3$ supplementation is variable, depending on the mutation. Chronic calcium infusions may be helpful in patients refractory to $1,25(OH)_2D_3$.

Mineralization Defects

The availability of calcium and phosphorus is critical to bone mineralization, so sustained hypocalcemia or hypophosphatemia of any cause can produce the clinical features of rickets or osteomalacia. The serum calcium concentration is tightly regulated by PTH and $1,25(OH)_2D$, and hypocalcemia usually occurs in the setting of hypoparathyroidism or impaired vitamin D metabolism, as previously discussed. In adults, dietary calcium deficiency sufficient to produce hypocalcemia usually results in secondary hyperparathyroidism with the bone disease characteristic of this disorder. Diet-induced hypocalcemia in children has been reported to produce rickets, perhaps because of the greater amount of calcium required to support skeletal growth. Hypophosphatemia may be inherited or acquired as a primary disorder or may occur secondary to another disease process. Hypophosphatemia due to inadequate dietary phosphorus is usually associated with severe protein malnutrition and alcoholism because phosphorus is found ubiquitously in protein-rich foods and dairy products. Hypophosphatemia can also be induced by chronic ingestion of antacids that bind dietary phosphorus and prevent its intestinal absorption. Nutritional hypophosphatemia is associated with decreased urinary excretion of phosphorus and hypercalciuria and may be complicated by nephrolithiasis.

Rickets resulting from hypophosphatemia is an X-linked dominant disorder that is characterized by hypophosphatemia and renal phosphate wasting. The latter results from defective PTH-dependent tubular phosphate reabsorption, but phosphate reabsorption in the intestinal mucosa is also impaired, indicating that the defect is not limited to the renal tubular epithelium. Clinical symptoms, if present, usually appear at 12 to 18 months of age. Delayed or abnormal dentition is a common presenting feature. The severity of disease is variable, ranging from asymptomatic hypophosphatemia (usually in females) to severe rickets. Fasting hypophosphatemia appears to be the most common clinical finding. Serum calcium and PTH concentrations are normal. Serum $1,25(OH)_2D$ concentrations are low relative to the degree of hypophosphatemia and do not increase appropriately in response to exogenous PTH. Supplementation with $1,25(OH)_2D_3$ does not reverse the tubular defect in phosphorus reabsorption, and correction of hypophosphatemia does not normalize $1,25(OH)_2D$ synthesis.

Osteomalacia and rickets are common complications of untreated renal tubular acidosis and other forms of chronic acidosis. Chronic acidemia produces renal phosphorus wasting, which indirectly limits deposition of amorphous calcium phosphate, and acidosis directly impairs conversion of amorphous calcium phosphate to hydroxyapatite. Acidemia also enhances PTH action on bone and may contribute to loss of calcium from bone. Acidosis is frequently accompanied by hypercalciuria, which further depletes body calcium stores. Renal tubular acidosis is not associated with defective synthesis of $1,25(OH)_2D$ unless there is associated renal failure. Serum calcium concentrations are usually normal, whereas serum phosphorus concentrations may be normal or decreased, reflecting secondary hyperparathyroidism. Serum alkaline phosphatase activity is increased. Most patients with renal tubular acidosis also have hypokalemia, which may serve as a clue to the diagnosis.

Hypophosphatasia is transmitted as an autosomal recessive trait and is classified as infantile, childhood, or adult depending on the age at onset of symptoms. The disease results from defects in the structure and function of alkaline phosphatase. The diagnosis is confirmed by the findings of decreased alkaline phosphatase activity and increased serum and urinary phosphoethanolamine and pyrophosphate concentrations in patients with skeletal abnormalities due to rickets.

Infantile hypophosphatasia is the most common form of this rare disease and is usually apparent within 6 months of birth. Skeletal disease is prominent and is accompanied by increased intracranial pressure, hypercalciuria, and nephrocalcinosis. Mortality is greater than 50 per cent in patients with infantile hypophosphatasia. Childhood phosphatasia presents with premature loss of deciduous teeth, retarded growth, and increased susceptibility to infection. Bowing deformities of the skeleton, fractures, and craniosynostosis are common features. Adult hypophosphatasia is less common than the infantile or childhood variants. Poorly healing fractures are a common presenting symptom. The medical history may reveal early loss of deciduous teeth in childhood and signs and symptoms of rickets.

A variety of substances may act as inhibitors of mineralization, usually by forming a complex with skeletal calcium and phosphorus. Since the rate of mineralization is decreased, serum alkaline phosphatase activity usually is not increased. The diphosphonates, etidronate and pamidronate, are analogues of pyrophosphate that are used to pharmacologically inhibit bone mineralization in high turnover bone diseases such as Paget's disease. Bone changes due to osteomalacia have been reported after administration of high doses of diphosphonates, but they can usually be avoided by using lower doses.

Osteomalacia due to aluminum intoxication is common in patients with renal failure resulting from the use of aluminum-containing antacids as dietary phosphate binders. Aluminum accumulation causes defective bone mineralization and may cause or worsen pre-existing osteomalacia and obscure coexistant hyperparathyroid bone disease. Unlike osteomalacia caused by vitamin D deficiency, aluminum-induced osteomalacia is associated with normal or minimally increased serum PTH concentrations, and treatment with $1,25(OH)_2D_3$ may produce hypercalcemia but does not improve the bone disease. Aluminum-induced osteomalacia has also been reported to result from contaminated amino acid solutions used for parenteral nutrition and contaminated dialysate water supplies but is an unusual source of aluminum intoxication today. This disease is common in the population of hemodialysis patients but is rare in the absence of advanced renal failure. Aluminum intoxication can be demonstrated by the finding of a large increase in plasma aluminum concentrations after administration of the chelator deferoxamine, and treatment requires long-term chelation therapy for removal of aluminum in bone.

Chronic fluoride intoxication can impair normal bone mineralization and produce the signs and symptoms of osteomalacia. In children, a brown mottling of the teeth may occur during the period of tooth development. Fluoride intoxication may develop when fluoride is administered chronically as a dental prophylaxis or for treatment of osteoporosis; it may also occur from fluoride ingested in untreated water supplies. Municipal water supplies are tested regularly for fluoride content, and residents should use treated water if fluoride levels are excessive. Fluoride content of water from untreated sources such as ground wells can be tested commercially.

OSTEOMYELITIS

By Jon T. Mader, M.D.,
Roxanne Halencak, P.A.-C,
Billy R. Ledbetter, M.D.,
and Jason H. Calhoun, M.D.
Galveston, Texas

Osteomyelitis refers to an infection of the bone, generally of the cortical and/or medullary portions. Many different types of microorganisms can cause osteomyelitis. The most commonly isolated organisms are bacterial, but fungal and mycobacterial infections are also seen. Osteomyelitis can be described by duration (acute, chronic), etiology (trauma, hematogeneous, surgery, true contiguous spread), site (spine, hip, tibia, foot), extent (size of defect), and type of patient (infant, child, adult, compromised host).

Based on the Waldvogel system, bone infections are currently classified as either hematogeneous osteomyelitis or osteomyelitis secondary to a contiguous focus of infection. Contiguous-focus osteomyelitis has been subdivided further into osteomyelitis in patients with relatively normal vascularity and osteomyelitis in patients with generalized vascular insufficiency.

An alternative classification system has been developed by Cierny and Mader.* This classification takes into consideration the quality of host, the anatomic nature of the disease, treatment, and prognostic factors (Table 1). The Cierny and Mader staging system combines four anatomic disease types and three physiologic host categories to define 12 discrete clinical stages of osteomyelitis. Stage 1, or medullary osteomyelitis, equates with early hematogeneous osteomyelitis in which the primary lesion is endosteal. An infected intramedullary rod in a stable bone is another example of stage 1 osteomyelitis. In stage 2, or superficial osteomyelitis, the bone infection results from an adjacent soft tissue infection and represents a true contiguous-focus lesion. The outer surface of bone at the base of a soft tissue wound is exposed, infected, and necrotic. Stage 3, or localized osteomyelitis, is characterized by full-thickness

Table 1. Anatomic Classification of Osteomyelitis, Etiology, and Host Factors

Anatomic Stage and Etiology

Stage 1 Medullary Osteomyelitis

Necrosis limited to medullary contents and endosteal surfaces.
Etiology: Hematogeneous

Stage 2 Superficial Osteomyelitis

Necrosis limited to exposed surface.
Etiology: Contiguous soft tissue infection

Stage 3 Localized Osteomyelitis

Well marginated and stable before and after debridement
Etiology: Trauma, evolving stages 1 and 2, iatrogenic

Stage 4 Diffuse Osteomyelitis

Circumferential and/or permeative
Unstable prior to or after debridement
Etiology: Trauma, evolving stages 1, 2, and 3, iatrogenic

Host Factors

A Host—normal host
B Host—systemic compromise (Bs)
local compromise (Bl)

Systemic (Bs)	*Local (Bl)*
Malnutrition	Chronic lymphedema
Kidney, liver failure	Major vessel compromise
Chronic hypoxia	Arteritis
Immune disease	Extensive scarring
Malignancy	Radiation fibrosis
Extremes of age	Small vessel disease
Immunosuppression or immune deficiency	Complete loss of local sensation
Tobacco abuse	

C Host—treatment worse than the disease

cortical sequestration that can be surgically removed without compromising the stability of the infected bone. Stage 4, or diffuse osteomyelitis, represents a through-and-through section of the bone and usually requires segmental resection of the bone. The patient with stage 4 disease may also have bone infection on both sides of a nonunion or major joint. Diffuse osteomyelitis includes infections with a loss of bony stability either before or after debridement surgery. In this system, patients are classified as A, B, or C hosts. A hosts are patients with normal physiologic, metabolic, and immunologic capabilities. B hosts (see Table 1) are patients who are either locally compromised or systemically compromised, or both. It is important to improve the factors and diseases that make the patient a B host. The goal of host modification is to make a B host as much like an A host as possible. The final category, or C host, represents the patient in whom treatment of the bone infection is worse than the osteomyelitis itself. This staging system has been used to determine optimal treatment protocols and prognosis and to compare therapy results among institutions. The stages are dynamic and may be altered by therapeutic outcome or a change in host status.

NATURAL HISTORY

Osteomyelitis may be acute or chronic. Acute osteomyelitis may be characterized by suppurative infection accompanied by edema, vascular congestion, and small vessel thrombosis. The vascular supply to the bone is compromised as the infection extends to the surrounding soft

*Cierny, G., Mader, J.T., Penninck, J.J.: A clinical staging system of adult osteomyelitis. Contemp. Orthop., 10:17–37, 1985.

tissues. Large areas of dead bone (sequestra) may be formed when both the medullary and the periosteal blood supplies are compromised. Despite appropriate therapy (surgery, antibiotics) and a host response, viable colonies of bacteria may be harbored within the necrotic and ischemic tissues. On the discontinuation of antibiotics and a decline in host response, the organisms may proliferate, leading to recurrence of the infection. This is termed chronic osteomyelitis. This condition is composed of a nidus of infected bone or scar tissue and an ischemic soft tissue envelope. Often, this leads to a refractory clinical course.

CLINICAL MANIFESTATIONS

The clinical features of osteomyelitis are dependent on the age of the patient and the pathogen or pathogens. Infants and children are at greater risk for hematogeneous osteomyelitis. The terminal vessels of the growth plates form large sinusoids that are easy targets for infection. Infants and children with hematogeneous osteomyelitis usually present one of two ways. The most common presentation is an abrupt onset of fever, irritability, lethargy, and local signs of infection, which include redness, swelling, tenderness, and dysfunction of 3 weeks' or less duration. Also, a joint effusion adjacent to the bone is present in 60 to 70 per cent of infants. The second group of patients present with vague symptoms, including pain in the involved limb of 1 to 3 months' duration and minimal, if any, temperature elevation. The metaphyses of the long bones (femur, tibia) are the most frequently involved. The clinical signs of soft tissue extension may dominate the clinical picture, which may lead to inappropriate diagnostic and/or therapeutic measures unless the clinician has an index of suspicion for osteomyelitis.

A single pathologic organism is almost always recovered from bone in hematogeneous osteomyelitis. Polymicrobic infection is rare. In the infant, *Staphylococcus aureus*, *Streptococcus agalactiae*, and *Escherichia coli* are the most frequently recovered bone isolates. In children older than 1 year of age, *S. aureus*, *Streptococcus pyogenes*, and *Haemophilus influenzae* are the most common organisms isolated. However, after the age of 4 years, the incidence of *H. influenzae* decreases. With the recent licensing and use of the *Haemophilus* sp. vaccine, the incidence of *H. influenzae* will decrease even further.

Hematogeneous osteomyelitis also occurs in adults. The most common site is in the vertebrae. The infection is usually monomicrobic, with *S. aureus* and aerobic gram-negative rods having the highest incidence. *Pseudomonas aeruginosa* and *Serratia marcescens* have a high incidence among intravenous drug abusers. The lumbar vertebral bodies are most often involved, followed by the thoracic and cervical vertebrae. Spread of the infection to adjacent vertebral bodies may occur rapidly via the rich venous networks in the spine. The patient commonly presents with vague signs and symptoms: dull, constant back pain; spasms of the paravertebral muscles; point tenderness over the involved vertebrae; and no or low-grade fever.

When bacteria are introduced into the bone by direct trauma or by extension of adjacent soft tissue infections, contiguous-focus osteomyelitis results. Common predisposing conditions include open fractures, surgical reduction and internal fixation of fractures, chronic soft tissue infections, and radiation therapy. Multiple bacterial organisms are usually isolated from the bone. The bacteriologic features are diverse, but the most common organism isolated is *S. aureus*. In addition, aerobic gram-negative bacilli and anaerobic organisms are frequently isolated. Bone necrosis, soft tissue damage, and loss of bone stability occur, often making this form of osteomyelitis difficult to manage. The signs and symptoms include local pain, draining sinuses, tenderness, and erythema over the involved bone.

Another form of osteomyelitis occurs in individuals with vascular insufficiency. The small bones of the feet are most commonly involved. Decreased tissue perfusion to the lower extremities predisposes the patient to infection by blunting the local inflammatory response. The infection usually occurs after minor trauma to the feet, infected nail beds, cellulitis, or trophic skin ulcerations. This form of osteomyelitis may develop insidiously owing to the absence of fever and pain and the development of peripheral neuropathy. Multiple bacteria are usually isolated from the infected bone. The most common organisms are *S. aureus*, *Streptococcus epidermidis*, *Enterococcus* spp., gram-negative rods, and anaerobes. The desirable outcome for these patients is a cure, but a more realistic goal of therapy is to suppress the infection and maintain the functional integrity of the affected limb. Even after presumed successful treatment, the majority of patients have a recurrence of infection with eventual resection of the infected areas.

LABORATORY STUDIES

Although hematologic studies do not confirm the diagnosis of osteomyelitis, they do indicate a response to treatment. The leukocyte count may be increased in acute osteomyelitis but normal in more chronic cases. The sedimentation rate is usually increased in both acute and chronic osteomyelitis. Sedimentation rates and leukocyte counts may decrease with appropriate therapy, but both may increase acutely following debridement surgery. A sedimentation rate that decreases during the course of therapy is a favorable prognostic sign. This laboratory determination, however, is not reliable in the compromised host, as these patients are constantly challenged by minor illnesses and peripheral lesions that may increase this index. Laboratory studies are necessary to monitor the nutritional status of the patient and any toxic effects from antibiotic treatment regimens. Blood and any drainage should be cultured prior to the start of antibiotic therapy. Historically, 50 to 75 per cent of blood cultures are positive in patients with acute hematogeneous osteomyelitis.

The definitive diagnosis of osteomyelitis requires isolation of the causative bacteria from bone or blood. In hematogeneous osteomyelitis, positive blood cultures can often obviate the need for a bone biopsy when there is associated evidence of osteomyelitis by radiography or radionuclide scanning. Chronic osteomyelitis is rarely associated with bacteremia unless there is acute extension of the infection into the soft tissues. Cultures from the sinus tract are not reliable for predicting which organisms will be isolated from the bone. Antibiotic treatment of osteomyelitis should be based on deep bone biopsy cultures and specific antimicrobial susceptibilities. Tube dilution sensitivities are preferred to disk diffusion assays.

IMAGING STUDIES

Changes on routine radiographs in acute hematogeneous osteomyelitis accurately reflect the destructive process but lag at least 2 weeks behind the evolution of the infection. The earliest changes on plain films are soft tissue swelling, periosteal thickening and/or elevation, and focal osteopenia. These findings may be subtle and are frequently missed. The more diagnostic lytic changes are delayed and may take several weeks to months to appear. Later, when the patient is receiving appropriate antimicrobial therapy, radiographic improvement may lag behind clinical recovery. In contiguous-focus and chronic osteomyelitis, the radiographic changes are even more subtle, are often found in association with other nonspecific radiographic findings, and require careful clinical correlation to achieve diagnostic significance.

Earlier diagnosis of osteomyelitis may be achieved with radionuclide imaging. The three-phase technetium (^{99m}Tc) scan demonstrates increased isotope accumulation in areas of increased blood flow and reactive new bone formation. False-negative ^{99m}Tc scans can occur, presumably from impairment of the blood supply to the bone by the infection. A second class of radiopharmaceuticals used for the diagnosis of osteomyelitis includes the gallium and indium scans. Gallium and indium attach to transferrin, which leaks from the bloodstream into areas of inflammation. They also show increased isotope uptake in areas concentrating polymorphonuclear leukocytes. In contrast to gallium, indium is more heavily concentrated by hematopoietic tissue and is not found to accumulate in areas of reactive bone. Indium-labeled leukocyte scans are used in the evaluation of osteomyelitis. Indium leukocyte scans are positive in approximately 40 per cent of patients with acute osteomyelitis and in 60 per cent of patients with septic arthritis. Indium-labeled leukocyte scans are not useful in chronic osteomyelitis. Since gallium-labeled and indium-labeled leukocyte scans do not show bone detail well, it is often difficult to distinguish between bone and soft tissue inflammation. Comparison of these scans with a ^{99m}Tc scan helps resolve this problem.

Computed tomography (CT) may play a role in the diagnosis of osteomyelitis. Increased marrow density occurs early in the infection. Computed tomography can also help identify areas of necrotic bone and assess the involvement of the surrounding soft tissue. One disadvantage of this study is the scatter phenomenon, which occurs when metal is present in or near the area of bone infection. This scatter results in a significant loss of image resolution.

Magnetic resonance imaging (MRI) has been recognized as a useful modality for diagnosing the presence and extent of musculoskeletal sepsis. The spatial resolution of MRI makes it useful in differentiating among cellulitis, soft tissue abscess formation, and bone infection, which is often a problem with radionuclide studies. Magnetic metallic implants in the region of interest may produce focal artifacts, thereby decreasing the utility of the image. Initial MRI screening usually consists of a T1-weighted and a T2-weighted spin-echo pulse sequence. In a T1-weighted study, edema is dark and fat is bright. In a T2-weighted study, the reverse is true. The typical appearance of osteomyelitis is a localized area of abnormal marrow with decreased signal intensity on T1-weighted images and increased signal intensity on T2-weighted images. Post-traumatic or surgical scarring of the marrow is seen as a region of decreased signal intensity on T1-weighted images, with no change seen on the T2-weighted image. Sinus tracts are seen as areas of high signal intensity on the T2-weighted image extending from the marrow and bone through the soft tissues and out of the skin. Cellulitis is seen as diffuse areas of intermediate signal in the T1-weighted images of the soft tissues, with increased signal on the T2-weighted images of the same area. Distinguishing infection from neoplasm on the basis of MRI may be difficult. Clinical and radiographic confirmation is therefore necessary.

SEPTIC ARTHRITIS

By Ratanavadee Nanagara, M.D.,
Daniel G. Baker, M.D.,
and H. Ralph Schumacher, Jr., M.D.
Philadelphia, Pennsylvania

Septic arthritis is defined as the invasion of joint tissues by viable microorganisms. It is also called infectious arthritis, pyogenic arthritis, bacterial arthritis, and suppurative arthritis.

PRESENTING SYMPTOMS AND SIGNS

The classic clinical picture of septic arthritis is acute inflammation of a single weight-bearing peripheral joint. Typically, pain is felt with active or passive motion of the joint. Most patients have fever, but it may be low grade. Shaking chills can occur and are found most frequently in patients with positive blood cultures. Patients with septic arthritis usually recognize the gradual onset of these symptoms over a few days to 1 to 2 weeks. This is of some help in distinguishing infection from crystal-induced arthritis or traumatic arthritis in which symptoms more often peak within 24 hours.

A significant number of patients have a predisposing factor such as recent injury of the joint, coexisting infection elsewhere, underlying rheumatic disease, previous needle aspirations of the joint or corticosteroid injections into the joint, intravenous (IV) drug abuse, and immunosuppressed conditions, including human immunodeficiency virus (HIV) infection. The presence of risk factors favors consideration of septic arthritis and can be helpful in determining the probable causative microorganisms. *Staphylococcus aureus* is the most common cause of nongonococcal septic arthritis. The other causative pathogens, determined by age and risk factors, are shown in Tables 1 and 2.

Polyarticular septic arthritis can occur in up to 20 per cent of adults with septic arthritis. Patients with polyarticular infection often have serious underlying chronic illnesses or chronic arthritis, especially rheumatoid arthritis. Septic arthritis may be the initial presentation of various systemic diseases, including bacterial endocarditis, HIV infection, hypogammaglobulinemia, and multiple myeloma. Diagnosis of the underlying disease is important, because treatment of both the infection and associated disease may be critical to a desirable outcome.

Atypical presentations of septic arthritis can be found in individuals at the extreme ends of age, IV drug abusers, patients with prosthetic joints, patients with rheumatoid arthritis, and immunocompromised patients. Diagnosis depends on a high index of suspicion of joint infection when such patients present with joint pain with or without fever.

Neonates and Infants

Most septic arthritis in neonates and infants is hospital-acquired and usually associated with umbilical catheters or septicemia. Multiple joint infection is frequent and usually involves the hips, knees, and shoulders. Patients are

Table 1. Predilection for Causative Agents in Septic Arthritis by Age Group

Age Group	Causative Agents
Neonates	
Community acquired	Group B streptococci
Hospital acquired	*S. aureus,* MRSA (during outbreaks) Gram-negative bacilli *Candida*
Children	
2 mo–2 yr	*H. influenzae* *S. aureus* *Streptococcus* spp.
Older than 2 yr	*S. aureus* *Streptococcus* spp. *N. meningitides*
Adults	
15–40 yr	*N. gonorrhoeae* *S. aureus* *Streptococcus* spp.
Older than 40 yr	*S. aureus* *N. gonorrhoeae* *Streptococcus* spp. Gram-negative bacilli
Menstruating women and elderly individuals	*N. gonorrhoeae* *S. aureus* *Streptococcus* spp. Gram-negative bacilli

MRSA = methacillin-resistant *Staphylococcus aureus.*

often afebrile and present with pseudoparesis of the involved extremity and cry on passive or active movement of the joint. If the hip joint is infected, the infant may lie in a frog-legged position, with the thigh flexed, abducted, and externally rotated.

Children

Acute febrile illness with leg or knee pain is characteristic of septic arthritis in children. In children younger than 2 years of age, ankle and hip joints are the common sites of infection, which is preceded by upper respiratory tract infection in 50 per cent of patients. In children older than 2 years of age, hip and knee joints are more frequently affected, usually in association with cutaneous infection. In hip joint infection, pain is often referred to the thigh and knee. The child usually refuses to move the leg and holds it in external rotation and abduction. There may be hip or leg edema and pain over the groin. Septic arthritis should be distinguished from transient synovitis of the hip, which occurs commonly in children.

Elderly Individuals

Many elderly patients are afebrile. More than half of these individuals also have underlying articular disease. Septic arthritis of the shoulder in the elderly is often misdiagnosed as tendinitis or "frozen" shoulder. Septic arthritis should always be suspected in elderly patients who present with acute or subacute shoulder complaints.

Gonococcal Arthritis

The characteristic patient with gonococcal arthritis is a young woman presenting with acute migratory oligopolyarthralgia with low-grade fever, especially during pregnancy or menstruation. Associated skin lesions, often found over the dorsum of the hands or feet, and tenosynovitis are important clues for diagnosis. Since the organisms are infrequently detected by Gram staining of joint fluid, the initial diagnosis usually depends on recognition of the clinical characteristics. Occasionally, the diagnosis can be made only after a dramatic response to antibiotic treatment, because the organisms fail to grow even with appropriate culture technique.

Intravenous Drug Abusers

Infection in IV drug abusers may involve unusual joints, such as vertebral joints and fibrocartilaginous articulations, that is, sternoclavicular joints, sacroiliac joints, the manubriosternal joint, and the pubic symphysis. In drug addicts, infection of the axial skeleton is usually caused by gram-negative bacilli. Axial infections usually have more insidious clinical presentations, with less toxicity and a longer duration of symptoms than do acute infections of peripheral joints, which are more commonly caused by *S. aureus.*

Prosthetic Joints

The clinical presentation of prosthetic joint infection varies with the interval that has elapsed since surgery. Early prosthetic joint infection, mostly occurring within the first month after surgery, presents with swelling, drainage, and sometimes fever. The major diagnostic challenge is to determine whether the infection is confined to the superficial

Table 2. Predilection for Causative Agents in Septic Arthritis Determined by Risk Factors

Risk Factors	Causative Agents
IV drug abusers	*S. aureus,* MRSA *Streptococcus* spp. Gram-negative bacilli (*Pseudomonas, Serratia, Escherichia coli*) *Candida*
Prosthetic joint	Coagulase-negative staphylococci *S. aureus* Gram-negative bacilli Anaerobes *Candida*
Rheumatoid arthritis	*S. aureus* *Streptococcus pneumoniae* (Felty's syndrome after splenectomy)
Intra-articular steroid injection	*S. aureus* Gram-negative bacilli
Joint trauma or surgery	*S. aureus* *Streptococcus* spp. Gram-negative bacilli Anaerobes
Sickle cell anemia	*Salmonella* spp. *Streptococcus pneumoniae*
SLE	*Salmonella* spp. Non-group A *Streptococcus* spp.
HIV infection	*S. aureus* Non-group A *Streptococcus* spp. *Streptococcus pneumoniae* *H. influenzae* *Salmonella* spp. Gram-negative bacilli
Immunocompromised patients	Gram-negative bacilli
Gastrointestinal cancer	Gram-negative bacilli Anaerobes
Rattlesnake ingestion	*Salmonella arizoni*
Cat or dog bite	*Pasteurella multocida*

IV = intravenous; SLE = systemic lupus erythematosus; HIV = human immunodeficiency virus.

tissues (i.e., infected hematoma) or has involved the joint. Disproportionate pain after insertion of a prosthesis, failure of pain to abate with time, and exacerbation of pain are suggestive of infection. If present, risk factors for early prosthetic joint infections (e.g., prolonged duration of surgery, the number of operating room personnel, an inexperienced primary surgeon, advanced age of the patient, rheumatoid arthritis or other systemic illness, and perioperative nonarticular infections) may be helpful in the recognition of early prosthetic joint infection.

Late prosthetic joint infections, occurring between 6 and 24 months after surgery, are difficult to diagnose. The most common feature is a prolonged, indolent course of increasing joint pain aggravated by joint activity. Fever is usually absent, and the patient may have no features suggesting local inflammation. Diagnosis may be delayed by confusion with aseptic loosening of the prosthesis.

Rheumatoid Arthritis

Distinguishing disease exacerbation from complicating infection is the diagnostic problem in patients with rheumatoid arthritis. A clinical history of long-standing severe seropositive rheumatoid arthritis and administration of oral or intra-articular corticosteroids within 2 weeks prior to the onset of symptoms may be helpful in the clinical diagnosis. Approximately one third of patients present with poly-articular arthritis. The indolent course of symptoms and the vague local signs of inflammation, sometimes without fever, lead to a delayed diagnosis. A high suspicion of joint infection should exist when one or more joints become inflamed out of phase with other joints or when the affected joints do not respond well to the usual means of treatment of rheumatoid arthritis.

Immunocompromised Patients

In immunocompromised patients, infection of the joints may present with an unusual clinical picture, such as insidious onset of bacterial arthritis or acute onset of fungal arthritis in acquired immunodeficiency syndrome (AIDS), acute or chronic *Salmonella* polyarthritis in systemic lupus erythematosus (SLE) and sickle cell anemia, ureaplasma in hypogammaglobulinemia, or complicated bacterial arthritis in hemophilic arthritis associated with HIV infection.

Unusual Risk Factors of Septic Arthritis

Septic arthritis associated with unusual situations has been reported increasingly. Examples include septic arthritis of the shoulder following mastectomy and radiotherapy for breast carcinoma, septic arthritis occurring during neurosurgical convalescence, septic hip following gunshot wounds of the abdomen, psoas abscess, postpartum sepsis, or severe burns.

Infections of Specific Joints

Patients with pyogenic sacroiliitis complain of pain in the lower back, buttock, hip, upper thigh, or lower abdomen. The clinical picture may mimic a protruded disk or hip joint infection. In women, the misdiagnosis of pelvic infection is possible. Septic arthritis of the symphysis pubis is also difficult to diagnose due to the poorly localized pain and the potentially misleading physical findings suggestive of hip disease. Patients with sternoclavicular joint infection usually complain of anterior chest discomfort, fever, and restricted range of motion of the homolateral shoulder. Substernal chest pain may be the initial presentation of sternomandibular septic arthritis. Patients with temporomandibular joint (TMJ) infection typically present with acute joint pain associated with swelling and erythema. Malaise, nausea, and vomiting may also present. Risk factors for temporomandibular joint infection are head and neck infection, underlying articular disease, and trauma.

CLINICAL COURSE AND COMMON COMPLICATIONS

Staphylococcus aureus, the most common cause of septic arthritis, can destroy cartilage in as little as 1 to 2 days. Articular cartilage and adjacent bone may be destroyed, followed by articular subluxation or dislocation. Occasionally, spontaneous fibrous ankylosis may occur. Bacteremia or septic shock can contribute to a mortality rate of up to 30 per cent, particularly in rheumatoid arthritis patients with polyarticular infection. Bacterial infection may extend into the neighboring soft tissues with abscess formation or may form sinus tracts. Spinal cord compression with a neurologic deficit may be associated with infection of the spine. Infection of the hip joint in both children and adults can result in avascular necrosis of the femoral head.

The most common sequela of septic arthritis is osteoarthritis. The determining factors are a delay between the onset of symptoms and treatment, virulence of the organism, and host characteristics. Osteomyelitis of the adjacent bone is commonly associated with septic arthritis in neonates and infants, delayed and/or inadequate treatment, and certain types of pathogens such as mycobacteria or fungi. Septicemia and distant infection to other target organs can be found.

PHYSICAL EXAMINATION

When a joint has been infected, the patient usually holds it in mild flexion and resists either active or passive movement. Joint swelling or effusions are present in 90 per cent of patients. Tenderness is invariably present, but erythema and warmth may be imperceptible, particularly in deep-seated joint infection.

Little evidence of local inflammation may be present in immunosuppressed patients, IV drug abusers, or patients with septic arthritis caused by less virulent organisms (e.g., *Streptococcus epidermidis, Mycobacterium* sp., or fungus). Physical findings of joint infection may be masked or difficult to distinguish from inflammation caused by underlying articular disease. This is particularly true in rheumatoid arthritis. Findings in early prosthetic joint infection may mimic a postoperative infected hematoma, and findings in late prosthetic joint infection may mimic mechanical aseptic hip loosening. Patients who cannot complain (e.g., neonates or elderly, severely ill, or comatose patients) may present with fever of unknown origin only. Physical examination, looking for warmth or swelling of the joints that may be the primary source of infection, should be performed carefully.

USEFUL LABORATORY PROCEDURES

The most valuable laboratory test for the diagnosis of septic arthritis is synovial fluid (SF) analysis with Gram stain and culture. Direct joint aspiration should be performed in virtually every case of joint disease in which infection is suspected. Large volumes of lidocaine should not contact the SF because lidocaine may interfere with bacterial growth. Needle irrigation with sterile normal saline may be performed if joint fluid samples are not obtained from difficult to aspirate joints such as the sternoclavicular joints, the manubriosternal joint, or the sacroiliac joints. Orthopedic or rheumatologic consultation should be sought if there is difficulty in obtaining fluid or in cases of presumed prosthetic joint infection that may require aspiration.

If only a few drops of SF are obtained, at least Gram staining, culture, and examination of a wet drop should be performed. These will provide definitive diagnosis of septic arthritis and crystal-induced arthritis, which may have a similar clinical picture.

Gram staining of SF is especially helpful if the patient has received antibiotics before evaluation. It is not unusual for the Gram stain to be the only documentation of joint infection; these results may guide the choice of antibiotics and duration of treatment. If SF is not purulent, positive yields are increased if Gram staining is performed on a centrifuged or cytocentrifuged pellet.

For optimal culture yield, the SF should be sent to the laboratory promptly in the sealed syringe. Routine aerobic and anaerobic cultures should be performed. Special culture requests must be carefully considered according to the organism suspected (e.g., *Neisseria gonorrhoeae, Haemophilus influenzae, Mycobacterium spp.,* fungus, *Borrelia burgdorferi,* and *Chlamydia trachomatis*).

Bacteriologic studies of specimens from primary sources of infection and blood may be helpful in the diagnostic evaluation. In the sexually active young adult, careful culturing for gonococci must be performed (obtaining specimens from the cervix, urethra, pharynx, and rectum as appropriate).

Synovial tissue biopsy, with cultures and histologic examination, may be indicated in ill-defined or chronic processes in which routine joint fluid study has been unrewarding. This is particularly true when gonococcal, chlamydial, or granulomatous disease or Lyme disease is suspected. Such studies occasionally may be helpful in cases of pyogenic arthritis, but they are not usually necessary.

A SF leukocyte count and differential cell counts may support a diagnosis of septic arthritis, especially when the SF cell count is greater than 100,000 cells/mm^3, with greater than 90 per cent polymorphonuclear cells. However, an SF leukocyte count greater than 100,000 cells/mm^3 may be observed in settings other than infection, and many infections produce less than 100,000 cells/mm^3.

Although the lowest concentrations of glucose in SF are generally observed in septic arthritis, a normal concentration should not greatly reduce the suspicion of this diagnosis.

In patients who have had prior antibiotic treatment, apart from SF Gram stain, SF counterimmunoelectrophoresis (CIE) may be helpful if septic arthritis caused by *H. influenzae* or *Streptococcus pneumoniae* is suspected. Polymerase chain reaction (PCR) for bacterial DNA or RNA is available for some organisms.

In classic septic arthritis, erythrocyte sedimentation rate (ESR) and C-reactive protein (CRP) determinations are not necessary. However, an increased ESR and CRP favors an infectious process in the differential diagnosis between septic arthritis and transient synovitis of the hip joint in children and between late prosthetic joint infection and aseptic loosening of hip joint in adults.

Peripheral blood leukocytosis is relatively common (60 to 75 per cent of patients) but may be absent in the immunosuppressed patient or in the individual with a prosthetic joint infection. A peripheral blood smear may aid in the diagnosis of underlying diseases such as sickle cell anemia, systemic lupus erythematosus, or hematologic malignancy.

USEFUL IMAGING PROCEDURES

Neither radiographs nor radioisotope scans are specific for infection. In the early phase, radiographic findings are nondiagnostic. Abnormal radiographic findings typically do not appear until 10 to 14 days after the onset of infection. However, initial plain radiographs should be obtained to provide a baseline assessment of the infected joint and evaluation of underlying joint disease and possible contiguous osteomyelitis. They are particularly helpful in slowly developing infectious arthritis (e.g., tuberculous or fungal arthritis).

Unusual radiologic features of bacterial arthritis can be diagnostically useful. Gas formation within the joint suggests infection, especially that due to anaerobic organisms. Dystrophic calcification may follow rupture of an infected joint with soft tissue extension. The radiologic findings in prosthetic joints with suspected infection are difficult to distinguish from mechanical loosening of the prosthesis because both may cause zones of radiolucency at the bone-cement interface.

Further imaging studies are seldom necessary for septic arthritis except in cases of hip, sacroiliac joint, and other deep-seated joint infections or when the diagnosis is uncertain because of a vague clinical presentation. Abnormal findings on bone scanning are not specific for the diagnosis of septic arthritis, but normal bone scans are strong evidence against septic arthritis. Magnetic resonance imaging (MRI) and computed tomography (CT) have comparable sensitivity and remarkably improved anatomic resolution when compared with bone scans.

In general, serodiagnosis is not particularly helpful, except when Lyme arthritis is suspected. Both false-positive and false-negative results may occur. Test results should be carefully correlated with clinical characteristics.

THERAPEUTIC DIAGNOSIS

When the clinical setting is highly suggestive of septic arthritis, but the causative microorganism cannot be revealed by Gram stain, therapeutic diagnosis may be needed. This is commonly used in gonococcal arthritis in which SF Gram stain results are frequently negative. Dramatic response to penicillin treatment within 2 days is characteristic. A Herxheimer reaction may support successful killing of infecting spirochetes.

PITFALLS IN DIAGNOSIS

Both overdiagnosis and underdiagnosis can occur. Several rheumatic diseases may mimic septic arthritis, for example, crystal-induced arthritis, traumatic arthritis, viral arthropathy, acute rheumatic fever, transient synovitis of the hip joint in children, or Still's disease. In such patients, severe joint pain with fever may be misleading. A careful history, physical examination, and synovial fluid examination are important clinical tools to avoid unnecessary antibiotic administration and prolonged hospitalization.

In most cases of severe soft tissue infection around a

joint, a small, sterile sympathetic effusion develops. An uninfected joint will maintain a good degree of mobility with less pain than seen in an infected joint. If arthrocentesis is necessary, the needle should not transgress an area of cellulitis to avoid inoculating bacteria into the joint.

Septic arthritis can coexist with other types of arthritis. The presence of crystals in SF does not exclude septic arthritis. A "positive" crystal identification in the inflammatory SF of a young, sexually active woman is most likely an error (e.g., resulting from talc from a surgical glove or a corticosteroid crystal from prior injection) because crystal-induced arthritis in a young woman is rare. Notably, the crystals found in such situations are usually not associated with SF leukocytes.

A negative SF culture does not absolutely exclude septic arthritis, but it provides stong evidence against nongonococcal bacterial infection, especially if the patient has not received antibiotics prior to joint aspiration. However, cultures may be negative because of mishandling of the SF, inappropriate culture media, or fastidious organisms. The absence of fluid leukocytosis and polymorphonuclear predominance does not exclude septic arthritis; this situation may be seen most commonly in a compromised host. Hemorrhagic SF may also need to be sent for culture, particularly when conventional treatment for primary articular disease is unsuccessful because coexisting infection in hemophiliac arthritis, Charcot's joint disease, and traumatic arthritis are possible. SF aspirated from patients with rheumatoid arthritis should be sent for culture, especially if the patient is febrile, there is an unexplained exacerbation, and intra-articular corticosteroid therapy is being considered.

If Gram staining of the SF is not helpful, empirical antibiotic therapy according to the host's characteristics should be started after acquisition of culture specimens from the joint and other possible sources of infection. Clinical observation and reaspiration should be performed within 24 hours to evaluate the antibiotic response. During this period, nonsteroidal anti-inflammatory drug (NSAID) administration should be avoided. The use of these medications may cause confusion in patients in whom a firm bacteriologic diagnosis has not been reached. Improvement secondary to nonsteroidal anti-inflammatory drug use may delay realization of inadequate antibiotic coverage.

SKELETAL NEOPLASMS

By Richard D. Lackman, M.D.
Philadelphia, Pennsylvania

A large variety of lesions can present as a mass within bone or in supporting soft tissues. These lesions can be neoplastic, reactive, developmental, infectious, or traumatic. The more common entities are addressed below.

BENIGN BONE TUMORS

Osteochondroma

Osteochondroma is synonymous with the term exostosis and refers to lesions that grow on the surface of a bone during childhood and adolescence. They are composed of a cartilaginous cap and the underlying bone that it produces. The cartilaginous cap functions as epiphyseal cartilage and causes growth of bone in an abnormal direction. As the individual reaches puberty, the cartilaginous cap thins to usually no more than a few millimeters, and further growth ceases. The tumors may be pedunculated (stalklike) or sessile (moundlike). They may occur as multiple lesions but most commonly are singular. Osteochondromas usually come to medical attention during adolescence. They can present clinically with pain, as a mass, or both. The pedunculated lesions are frequently painful as they press into adjacent soft tissue, creating a bursitislike condition locally.

The most feared complication related to the presence of an exostosis, malignant transformation, typically occurs in the fifth decade or beyond. Osteochondromas as a whole share a 1 per cent risk of this occurrence. Malignant transformation is signaled by the onset of growth of the remaining cartilaginous cap in individuals beyond puberty. Patients who experience this problem present with a history of increase in the size of a previously stable lesion with or without associated pain. Low-grade chondrosarcoma is the most frequent histologic diagnosis, although high-grade sarcomas of various types can occasionally occur. Any growth of a previously stable lesion or the onset of pain in exostosis in an adult should be considered evidence of malignant transformation until proved otherwise.

Plain films, bone scans, CT, and MRI are useful in distinguishing a painful benign exostosis from one with malignant change. Benign osteochondromas have a smooth margin on their surface, and the cartilaginous cap in adults is usually just a few millimeters thick. The thickness of the cartilaginous cap can be assessed with CT or MRI as long as associated overlying bursae are not confused with additional thickness of cartilage. Malignant transformation is defined as the presence of a cartilaginous cap thicker than 2 cm in a mature individual. Technetium Tc-99m bone scans in adults show signals from exostosis that are similar to those from normal bone, but in transformed lesions they show markedly increased uptake. The most useful and reliable means of diagnosing malignant change is by histologic examination that measures the thickness of the cartilaginous cap directly and searches for the usual histologic features of malignant cartilage.

Exostosis can be distinguished from other lesions growing on the surface of a bone, because the cortex of the exostosis is always confluent with the cortex of the bone itself. As a result, the exostosis draws normal medullary bone up into its base and is the only lesion on the surface of a bone to contain normal medullary bone and marrow. Any lesion immediately adjacent to an intact cortex, by definition, cannot be an osteochondroma.

Enchondroma

Enchondroma, a benign cartilage tumor that occurs in bone, typically appears in the long bones, especially the proximal humerus, the femur, or the tibia near the knee. Enchondromas are also common in the small bones of the hands and feet. These lesions usually develop in early adulthood and are rarely found in children. They are typically encountered as incidental findings on plain films obtained for other reasons. The major diagnostic problem with any central cartilage tumor is to distinguish benign enchondroma from chondrosarcoma.

The first hallmark of an enchondroma is that the lesion is painless. The physician must carefully distinguish true lesional bone pain from the frequent symptoms associated with inflammatory and traumatic conditions of adjacent joints, such as bursitis, tendonitis, and contusions. Radiographically, enchondromas appear as areas of stippled calcification within the medullary canal and show no evidence of destruction of the medullary or cortical bone. Chondrosarcomas, conversely, are typically painful and the pain tends to be worse at night. The x-ray findings of chondrosarcoma include lysis within the lesion, scalloping of the adjacent endosteal surface, and frequently cortical thickening as the bone responds to the expanding lesion. Computed tomography and MRI are very useful in assessing central cartilage lesions, and these studies readily show areas of malignant progression per the criteria noted previously. Bone scans usually show increased uptake in all enchondromas, and this study is not a reliable indication of benign versus malignant behavior.

One major pitfall for physicians lies in the diagnosis of low-grade malignant cartilage tumors. Distinguishing clearly benign cartilage tumors from those that are clearly malignant is usually straightforward. Between these two extremes, however, lies a continuum that includes atypical benign lesions as well as borderline low-grade malignant chondrosarcomas. Given this subtle distinction, appropriate imaging studies as well as representative pathology slides and a thorough patient history all must be evaluated by a skeletal pathologist and a skeletal radiologist so that histologic, radiographic, and clinical data can be combined to allow the best possible assessment. Even so, periodic follow-up studies are often necessary for accurately determining the biologic potential of a tumor. The usual follow-up for benign enchondroma is a yearly plain film and an understanding by patients that they must alert their physician to any onset of pain or progressive enlargement.

Chondroblastoma

Chondroblastoma is a benign tumor that usually occurs as a lytic lesion in the epiphysis of a growing child. It causes pain and is treated with curettage and bone grafting. The major differential diagnosis is infection, which is usually associated with systemic signs and symptoms, such as fevers, chills, and an increased white blood cell count. The histologic picture of chondroblastoma shows the presence of large, polygonal, well-delineated cells in association with some chondroid matrix. Also noted frequently is the presence of "chicken-wire" calcification that is seen as black lines running between the stromal cells of the tumor.

Giant Cell Tumor

Giant cell tumors are aggressive but typically benign lesions that begin to appear following closure of growth plates in late adolescence and can occur into the seventh decade. The most common age range for patients with this tumor is 20 to 50 years. The lesions have a typical radiographic appearance. They are always juxta-articular within the bone and appear very lytic, with moth-eaten margins. Giant cell tumors frequently cause cortical thinning and erosion but show little periosteal reaction. The tumors are usually not painful when small and often reach a very large size prior to coming to medical attention. As a result, resection of the end of the bone is often necessary for establishing local control. Pathologic fracture is common in the large lesions and may be the presenting symptom.

Physical examination usually shows localized tenderness with painful motion of the adjacent joint and often the presence of a palpable mass. Imaging studies, such as radiography, CT, and MRI easily show the lesion. Computed tomography is most useful in assessing the adequacy of adjacent cortical and subchondral bone, while MRI can best assess extraosseous extension of the lesion into the surrounding soft tissues. The radiographic differential diagnosis of giant cell tumors includes osteosarcoma and aneurysmal bone cyst in young adults and metastasis, chondrosarcoma, and plasmacytoma in older adults.

Ultimately, the diagnosis of giant cell tumor depends on histologic examination of tumor tissue. Histology shows a spindle cell tumor with plump stromal cells and giant cells, and the nuclei of the stromal cells appear identical to the nuclei of the giant cells. The presence of fibroblastic elements within the lesion or the presence of neoplastic osteoid suggests the potential diagnosis of giant cell–rich sarcoma, which may occasionally masquerade as a giant cell tumor.

While giant cell tumors are typically benign, 2 per cent of these lesions eventually show evidence of systemic metastasis, usually to the lung. This metastasis is most common in tumors that have multiple local recurrences, with extensive soft tissue invasion, or in large lesions with soft tissue extension at initial diagnosis. Pathologic examination in these cases frequently shows intravascular invasion by the tumor leading to shedding of cells into the circulation and the phenomenon of metastasis in an otherwise benign lesion. These metastases can take two distinctly different clinical courses; some patients do well with excision of the metastatic lesions, while others follow an aggressive course and die from a clinical picture similar to that of a metastatic high-grade sarcoma. The usual follow-up procedure for giant cell tumors is a yearly chest film to evaluate for pulmonary nodules.

Bone Cysts

The two common forms of bone cysts include simple (or unicameral) bone cysts and aneurysmal bone cysts. Simple bone cysts are lytic lesions occurring in the metaphysis or diaphysis of a bone in the first or second decade of life. These lesions are frequently large and always occupy the full width of the bone but usually are not expansile. A pathologic fracture is often the first sign of the lesion, although many patients also present with mechanical pain. Simple bone cysts vary in terms of local aggressiveness; the younger the child and the closer the cyst lies to the adjacent growth plate, the more aggressive the lesion is and the more aggressive its treatment must be. Simple bone cysts typically fill in and heal spontaneously by the age of 18 to 20 years, and the diagnosis of a benign cyst after the age of 20 years is rare.

Physical examination typically reveals tenderness in symptomatic cysts, but the examination may be normal in asymptomatic cysts, which are frequently found incidentally on plain films obtained for unrelated reasons. The aspiration of a unicameral or benign bone cyst yields at least a few milliliters of clear fluid, followed by grossly bloody fluid as more is aspirated. This finding is in contrast with aneurysmal bone cysts, where the aspirate is always grossly bloody.

The common diagnostic studies that are useful for unicameral bone cysts include plain films, CT, and MRI. They typically show a well-demarcated lesion with no surrounding edema and no periosteal reaction. As cysts heal, bone begins to fill in the void, and multiple septations can be observed with various imaging techniques. The differential diagnosis of unicameral bone cyst on imaging studies includes aneurysmal bone cyst and fibrous dysplasia. The histology of unicameral bone cyst shows large, fluid-filled spaces with thin epithelial lining. Very little solid material is contained within a unicameral bone cyst, and most of its volume is clear fluid.

Aneurysmal bone cysts, unlike unicameral cysts, tend to be eccentric within the metaphysis of the bone, and they typically erode one side of the cortex to involve the surrounding soft tissues. As the name suggests, they cause aneurysmal dilatation of the bone and usually have a fine rim of cortex surrounding the expanded area with no significant periosteal reaction. They are very aggressive lesions clinically and may erode through adjacent growth plates.

Aneurysmal cysts usually occur during the first three decades of life and rarely present after the age of 30 years. Occasionally, they are self-limited and may resolve spontaneously over the course of many months. Most, however, are very destructive and require treatment to prevent local damage to the involved bone and adjacent joint. Unlike simple bone cysts, aneurysmal cysts can occur in the spine, where they are typically seen as expansile lytic lesions in the posterior elements. Patients typically present with painful scoliosis. Physical examination of aneurysmal bone cysts in the limbs usually shows localized swelling and tenderness with decreased and painful motion of the involved joint.

Imaging studies such as plain films, CT, and MRI help narrow the differential diagnosis, which includes osteosarcoma in children and giant cell tumor and round cell tumors in young adults. One frequent finding on MRI scans of aneurysmal cysts is the "fluid-fluid level." This is a phenomenon in which a distinct line is observed through the cyst due to sedimentation of its contents. While this finding is typical of aneurysmal bone cyst, it is not diagnostic and can be observed in malignant lesions, such as osteosarcoma.

The cause of aneurysmal bone cysts is poorly understood. Most authorities theorize that aneurysmal bone cysts arise de novo from various primary disorders, including abnormalities in the local bone circulation. Others speculate that aneurysmal bone cysts develop following disruption of the circulation by another primary tumor, such as giant cell tumor and chondroblastoma. Documented secondary aneurysmal bone cysts are observed in association with a variety of primary bone lesions, and the primary lesion itself usually remains clearly visible on imaging studies and pathologic examination. The histologic diagnosis of aneurysmal bone cyst requires the presence of large blood-filled spaces aligned with bland-appearing epithelial cells. Giant cells and mononuclear inflammatory cells can also be seen in these fibrous septa.

MALIGNANT BONE TUMORS

Osteosarcoma

Osteosarcoma (osteogenic sarcoma) is a primary malignant tumor of bone that occurs most commonly in adolescence but also shows a smaller increase in incidence associated with Paget's disease in the elderly. These lesions are aggressive, destructive tumors that typically present with both pain and a palpable mass. About 20 per cent of patients have evidence of pulmonary metastases at the time of presentation, and the prognosis for these patients remains dismal. The development of effective chemotherapy, however, has improved the overall survival of individuals with localized osteosarcoma to approximately 70 per cent at 5 years. Five-year disease-free survival equates to a cure of this disease in most patients.

The usual imaging studies are useful in the evaluation of patients with suspected osteosarcoma. Radiographically, these lesions typically show neoplastic osteoid production and an associated characteristic "hair-on-end" or "sunburst" periosteal reaction. Not all osteosarcomas show radiographically visible bone formation; therefore, this lesion must be considered in the differential diagnosis of every permeative bone lesion in all age groups.

Magnetic resonance imaging provides the best demonstration of the extension of osteosarcoma into bone and soft tissue. Computed tomography can be used to estimate the degree of cortical involvement, but MRI is the preferred study. The bone scan is part of the usual evaluation of patients with osteosarcoma, but metastatic lesions to other areas in the same bone or to other bones are rare. The histologic diagnosis of osteosarcoma requires the presence of tumor osteoid in association with malignant spindle cell stroma. While malignant osteoid can be difficult to find, the presence of even small amounts of osteoid justifies the diagnosis of osteosarcoma.

When seen in association with Paget's disease, osteosarcomas present with a distinct change in the underlying symptoms, most commonly with a significant increase in pain and/or the development of a mass. Any patient with Paget's disease and a change in symptoms must be evaluated for the possibility of malignant transformation.

Chondrosarcoma

Chondrosarcomas are primary malignant bone tumors that produce malignant cartilage and occur more commonly as histologically low-grade lesions. These tumors occasionally present during the third decade of life, but they occur more commonly in elderly patients. The typical presenting symptom of chondrosarcoma is pain that is independent of activity and associated with a palpable mass. Physical examination often shows tenderness, swelling, and limited range of motion if the lesion abuts a joint. Because most chondrosarcomas are low grade, the symptoms can be insidious and take months or years to fully develop. The clinician must suspect the diagnosis when speed of recovery does not coincide with the initial diagnosis.

In these instances, appropriate imaging studies are essential for avoiding prolonged delay in diagnosis. As with other bone tumors, plain films, CT, and MRI usually provide a clear image of the location and extent of these lesions. The clinical hallmarks of chondrosarcoma include a painful lesion in bone showing stippled calcification, intralesional lysis, endosteal scalloping, and cortical thickening or expansion.

Typical benign enchondromas that show none of the aforementioned changes should not be biopsied routinely, but must be followed with annual plain films. Clinicians must realize that the diagnosis of borderline low-grade malignant cartilage tumor is extremely difficult and suspected cases must be referred to pathologists with considerable experience in the evaluation of cartilage tumors. Pathology and radiology consultation must be sought prior to any definitive treatment in patients with suspected low-grade tumors so that diagnosis and management can be optimized.

The pathology of chondrosarcoma includes a spectrum of changes from subtle in very low-grade lesions to bizarre and exaggerated in the rare high-grade chondrosarcoma. The histologic hallmarks of low-grade chondrosarcoma include plumping of chondrocyte nuclei, increased cellularity, binucleate cells, the presence of more than one cell in some lacunae, cells outside of lacunae, and degradation of the quality of the chondroid matrix.

Malignant Round Cell Tumors

The malignant round cell tumors comprise Ewing's sarcoma in children and plasmacytoma and lymphoma in adults. These are typically diaphyseal lesions, although they can occasionally occur in metaphyseal locations. They are permeative, destructive tumors that often reach large size prior to diagnosis. The presenting symptoms include pain and localized swelling, especially when soft tissue extension is present. A total of 20 per cent of patients with Ewing's sarcoma present with an acute illness that includes fever, chills, and increased sedimentation rate, all of which can mislead the treating physician to a presumptive diagnosis of infection. The location of systemic metastases from these lesions varies greatly. Ewing's sarcoma often spreads via the hematogenous route to the lung, while lymphomas tend to appear in adjacent lymph nodes. Plasmacytomas usually spread to diffuse marrow sites.

No screening laboratory tests exist for most sarcomas, but multiple myeloma can be discovered by abnormalities in the serum or urine protein electrophoresis. Occasionally, solitary plasmacytoma can be nonsecretory and, therefore, show no paraprotein on electrophoresis. Imaging studies for these lesions are essential for proper staging. Ewing's sarcoma typically appears radiographically as a permeative lesion with "onionskin" periosteal reaction in a large soft tissue mass. The soft tissue extension is frequently greater than the amount of bone involvement. Lymphomas, however, tend to fill the marrow cavity, and only after extensive marrow replacement do they break into the surrounding soft tissues. Both of these lesions are best imaged with MRI, which readily shows marrow replacement processes and the soft tissue extension of primary bone tumors. Plasmacytomas are typically lytic "soap-bubble"–appearing lesions that are better localized than either Ewing's sarcoma or lymphoma. On occasion, plasmacytoma can simulate osteoporosis, with diffuse demineralization not associated with specific lytic lesions. In all patients with radiographically visible osteoporosis and bone pain, laboratory evaluation for myeloma should be performed.

The histologic diagnosis of round cell tumors can be very difficult. Plasmacytoma is recognized on light microscopy by the plasma cells, which have a typical appearance with eccentric plump nuclei, a cartwheel nucleolar pattern, and pink cytoplasm. Lymphomas are readily diagnosed via immunohistochemistry with markers such as leukocyte common antigen (LCA) and specific T- and B-cell markers. The diagnosis of Ewing's sarcoma is suggested by a uniform population of small round cells that stain with periodic acid–Schiff stain (PAS). Specific immunohistochemical markers for Ewing's sarcoma are also available. Another useful tool in the diagnosis of Ewing's sarcoma is the recognition of the 11-22 translocation.

SOFT TISSUE NEOPLASMS

Benign Lipoma

Lipomas are benign fat tumors that occur commonly in subcutaneous locations, where they are easily palpable and visible. They are a common cause of concern to patients, who bring them to the attention of their physicians. Lipomas are usually painless and have a typical soft, doughy feel. They do not cause local erythema or soft tissue edema.

Small lesions (less than 3 cm) in the subcutaneous fat that fit the clinical description of lipoma and that do not grow or cause symptoms can usually be followed without surgical excision or biopsy. Any soft tissue mass, however, that feels firm, enlarges, or causes pain should be biopsied to confirm the histologic diagnosis. Malignant soft tissue tumors occasionally grow slowly, are frequently painless, and, when small, are quite inconspicuous. The clinician must maintain a high index of suspicion and refer for appropriate evaluation any lesion that does not appear clinically to be a benign lipoma.

Occasionally, lipomas occur as large, deep-seated soft tissue masses in the extremities. They are most common in the thigh and can attain very large dimensions, occasionally reaching 20 to 25 cm in diameter. Both MRI and CT are useful in evaluating these tumors and can establish the diagnosis of benign lipoma. They typically show uniform fat density with occasional strands through the lesion, but with no other interstitial markings.

On CT, a benign lipoma appears as a uniform black mass that is identical to subcutaneous fat, and on MRI benign lipomas mimic subcutaneous fat on all pulse sequences. Histologically, lipomas show a picture of uniform mature fat.

Soft Tissue Sarcomas

Soft tissue sarcomas are primary malignant tumors of the supporting soft tissues in the body and may be found in muscle or fat or adjacent to neurovascular bundles. They are rare lesions, and only about 5000 new cases are seen in the United States each year. Many different types of soft tissue sarcoma exist, and they are typically not named for the cell of origin, but for their direction of differentiation. Liposarcomas, for example, are not necessarily tumors that arise in fat, but they are tumors in the soft tissue that differentiate toward the production of fat cells. The most common forms of soft tissue sarcomas are malignant fibrinous histiocytoma, liposarcoma, and synoviosarcoma. Other less common examples include fibrosarcoma, epithelioid sarcoma, leiomyosarcoma, and malignant schwannoma.

Typically, these tumors grow quietly in the soft tissues, and pain is usually not a prominent feature. They often come to the attention of the patient as palpable masses that may be remarkably large when first noted, especially if they develop in the thigh or groin, where deep-seated masses are not palpable until they have attained a fairly large size. Any deep-seated soft tissue mass must be evaluated with either MRI or CT. Magnetic resonance imaging is superior to CT for assessing these lesions within the soft tissue.

Histologic conformation of cell type and tumor grade are essential prerequisites to the institution of appropriate treatment. The major delay in the diagnosis of soft tissue tumors is that patients commonly attribute the onset of soft tissue masses to localized trauma. The clinician must carefully evaluate the history and physical findings while maintaining a high index of suspicion to avoid further delay in diagnosis. The prognosis for patients with soft tissue sarcoma is optimistic, especially in patients whose tumor is histologically low grade and less than 5 cm in diameter.

BURSITIS AND TENDINITIS

By John Waterman, M.D.
Farmington, Connecticut
and Aitezaz Ahmed, M.D.
Hartford, Connecticut

Although the human body has more than 150 bursae, only a few are commonly inflamed, with resulting discomfort. Likewise, most tendons perform their functions silently and without producing pain. When inflammation of tendons or bursae does occur, it may reflect a localized or a systemic process.

Bursae are categorized as subcutaneous and deep. The subcutaneous bursae (e.g., the olecranon bursa), develop after birth in response to external friction. Deep bursae, such as the iliopsoas bursa, are present before birth and develop in response to fetal movement. A third type of bursa, the so-called adventitious bursa, forms in response to abnormal shearing forces. The most common adventitious bursa forms over the head of the first metatarsal bone. Histologically, bursae are relatively unremarkable. They have a thin lining of sparse synovial cells. Normal bursal fluid exists as a thin film. Tendon sheaths are very similar in their structure. They usually facilitate movement over areas of stress rather inconspicuously.

The biologic function of a tendon is to transmit muscle power. Tendon function can be impaired by numerous processes: trauma, inflammation, vascular compromise, and atrophy. While most of the body's tendons are short and do not have sheaths, tendon sheaths form where extensive tendon movement occurs or in areas where tendons bridge joints. Tendon sheaths are lined by fibroblasts and synovial cells. Despite the fact that tendon ruptures are frequent, the rupture rarely occurs in the tendon itself due to its great tensile strength; rather, it occurs at the muscle-tendon boundary or at the insertion of the tendon into the bone. Direct trauma accounts for only 25 per cent of tendon ruptures.

Inflammation in a tendon sheath or bursa usually causes pain and swelling. Impaired musculoskeletal function results. The keys to the diagnosis of bursitis and tendinitis are (1) a high index of suspicion; (2) a knowledge of anatomy; (3) the recovery of bursal or tendon sheath fluid (although this is rarely accomplished), and (4) the effects of a local injection of lidocaine. The pain seen with bursitis and tendinitis is usually aggravated by motion and relieved by rest. However, nocturnal pain is common, and so is radiated pain. Bursitis and tendinitis that occur in the setting of constitutional symptoms, such as weight loss, fever, and malaise, are probably associated with a systemic rheumatic disease.

Inflamed bursae or tendon sheaths may become infected. Septic bursitis may be acute, with all the classic signs of inflammation, or it may be insidious. Usually, the subcutaneous bursae are affected, primarily the prepatellar bursa or the olecranon bursa. The source of the infection is local in the vast majority of cases. Alcoholics, diabetics, and immunocompromised patients are more commonly affected. Eighty-five per cent of patients with either septic olecranon or prepatellar bursitis are men. Tendinitis associated with infection includes the migratory tenosynovitis associated with disseminated gonococcal disease. Rarely, tuberculosis, including the atypical mycobacterial, can cause tenosynovitis. Fungal infections can also cause bursitis and tendinitis, especially in the immunocompromised host.

Aspiration of bursal fluid, when possible, is an important part of the initial evaluation. The fluid should be examined for the presence of bacteria with Gram stain and for crystals with polarized light microscopy. In addition, the fluid should be sent for a white blood cell count and differential count as well as a culture. White blood cell counts vary widely in inflamed bursal fluid, with mononuclear cells usually predominating. In traumatic bursitis, the fluid is often hemorrhagic. Tendon sheath effusions are difficult to aspirate; however, when infection or microcrystalline disease are suspected, an attempt should be made to obtain fluid.

Inflammatory diseases associated with bursitis and tendinitis are varied in their etiologies. For example, tendinitis may occur early in the course of rheumatoid arthritis. Tendon nodules causing snapping or "trigger" fingers have been noted in 32 per cent of rheumatoid arthritis patients. With dorsal wrist tenosynovitis in rheumatoid arthritis, tendon rupture frequently occurs. Other inflammatory conditions associated with bursitis and/or tendinitis include sarcoidosis, systemic lupus erythematosus, the spondyloarthropathies (e.g., Reiter syndrome), and the microcrystalline diseases (gout and pseudogout). Granulomatous tendinitis can be seen with beryllium poisoning and injury due to thorns.

Many types of bursitis are related to occupation. These are summarized in Table 1.

ROTATOR CUFF TENDINITIS

Also known as impingement syndrome, rotator cuff tendinitis is the most common cause of shoulder pain. In some cases, the subacromial bursa may be secondarily involved. The onset may be acute or insidious. A history of forceful abduction or strain may be present in acute cases but is usually lacking in the insidious-onset cases. In the subacute type of onset, the symptoms consist of a dull ache in the shoulder that is increased with abduction of the arm between 60 and 120 degrees as well as when the arm is lowered. Internal rotation of the shoulder, for example, reaching behind the back, is also painful. Patients may experience pain at night and may report difficulty in finding a comfortable position while lying on the affected side. In younger patients, the onset is often acute with excruciating pain, even at rest. Such cases may be associated with calcific tendinitis on radiographs. The degree of pain in rotator cuff tendinitis is less with passive range-of-motion

Table 1. Occupational Bursitides

Miner's elbow Student's elbow	Olecranon bursitis
Housemaid's knee Wrestler's knee	Prepatellar bursitis
Weaver's bottom	Ischial bursitis
Cavalryman's knee	Anserine bursitis
Haglund's disease (pump bumps)	Retrocalcaneal bursitis
Policeman's heel	Postcalcaneal bursitis

movements, a point that distinguishes it from subacromial bursitis. A useful clue is the impingement sign: the patient's arm is raised forward against resistance while the examiner prevents scapular motion with the other hand (Fig. 1). Pain occurring before 180 degrees of forward flexion indicates a positive test.

A therapeutic injection of lidocaine often provides significant improvement in pain and range of motion, helping confirm the diagnosis. Radiographs should be performed in patients with post-traumatic pain to exclude bony injury, in cases of acute onset to exclude calcifications, and in unresponsive cases to assess mechanical factors, such as osteophytes. Arthrograms may be performed to detect tears of the supraspinous tendon. Magnetic resonance imaging is noninvasive but much more expensive.

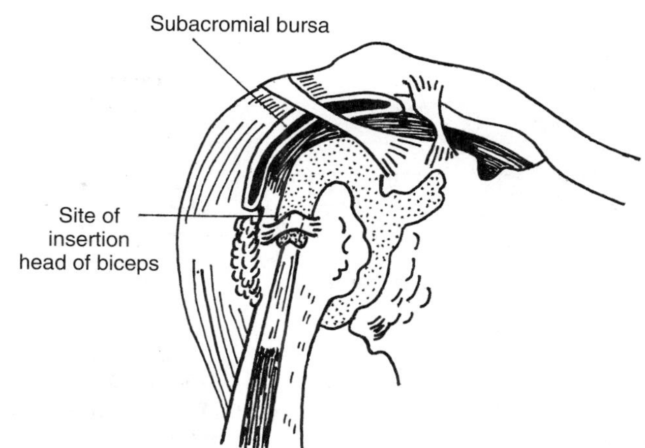

Figure 2. Biceps tendinitis.

BICEPS TENDINITIS

The tendons of the biceps muscle may become inflamed and painful at both its upper and lower ends. Tendinitis of the long head of the biceps is felt as pain and discomfort over the anterior aspect of the shoulder (Fig. 2). Tenderness is elicited by palpation over the greater tuberosity of the humerus, medial to the coracoid process of the scapula. Pain may be also elicited by supination of the forearm against resistance (Yergason's sign) or shoulder flexion against resistance (Speed's sign). Extension of the shoulder backward can also reproduce the pain. The antecubital syndrome, a burning pain over the lateral aspect of the antecubital fossa, is caused by inflammation at the insertion of the biceps tendon at the elbow. Resisted flexion of the elbow and forearm supination accentuate this pain.

Rupture of the long head of the biceps tendon and subluxation of the biceps tendon are two conditions seen with biceps tendinitis. Rupture of the long head of the biceps tendon occurs with prolonged irritation, is usually painless, and produces no functional impairment. Flexion of the arm causes a characteristic bulge in the midarm region. Subluxation of the biceps tendon is characterized by a popping sensation and pain in the shoulder with forward flexion. A snap over the anterior aspect of the shoulder may be noted as the arm is moved back and forth in a horizontal position. Biceps tendinitis is self-limited unless there is repetitive strain or underlying mechanical or inflammatory arthritis.

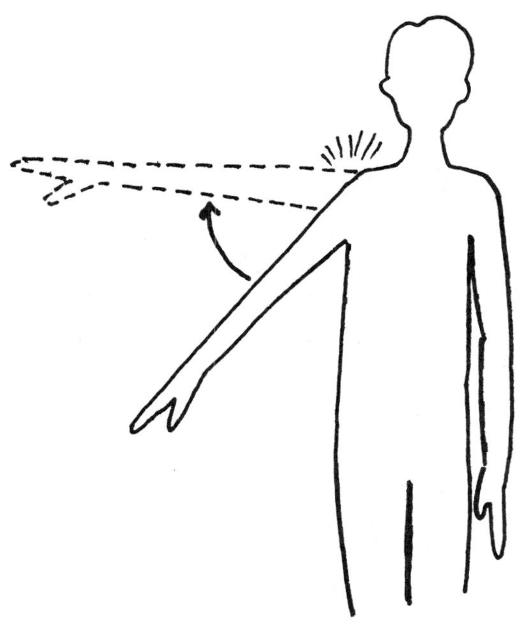

Figure 1. Positive impingement test.

ADHESIVE CAPSULITIS

Adhesive capsulitis is a chronic, painful condition of the shoulder with various synonyms, including pericapsulitis, frozen shoulder, periarthritis, and obliterative bursitis, which point to its poorly understood pathogenesis. Any chronic, painful, or inflammatory condition of the shoulder may lead to fibrosis and adhesions; however, adhesive capsulitis is usually seen without such associations. Nevertheless, a well-known association does exist with diabetes and, less commonly, with other conditions, such as myocardial infarction, thoracic surgery, and cervical herpes zoster. The condition consists of three phases: the "freezing" phase, characterized by a persistent, dull, aching pain lasting 3 to 6 months; the "frozen" phase, distinguished by a severe restriction of motion as well as pain on motion; and, finally, the "unfreezing" phase, during which gradual improvement in pain and motion occurs. Arthrography confirms the diagnosis by showing severe loss of joint volume. The prognosis is usually good.

LATERAL EPICONDYLITIS (TENNIS ELBOW)

This condition is characterized by pain noted over the lateral elbow region. In spite of its eponym, only about 10 per cent of cases are associated with the game of tennis. Any minor repetitive motion involving wrist extension and forearm supination can cause it. Handshakes, gardening, and briefcase carrying all can exacerbate the symptoms. The pain is dull and may radiate to the dorsal aspect of the forearm. Palpation of the lateral epicondyle usually elicits sharp pain (Fig. 3). Additional maneuvers include forced dorsiflexion of the wrist with the forearm in midsupination.

MEDIAL EPICONDYLITIS (GOLFER'S ELBOW)

Similar to lateral epicondylitis, this condition is characterized by pain at the insertion of the wrist and finger

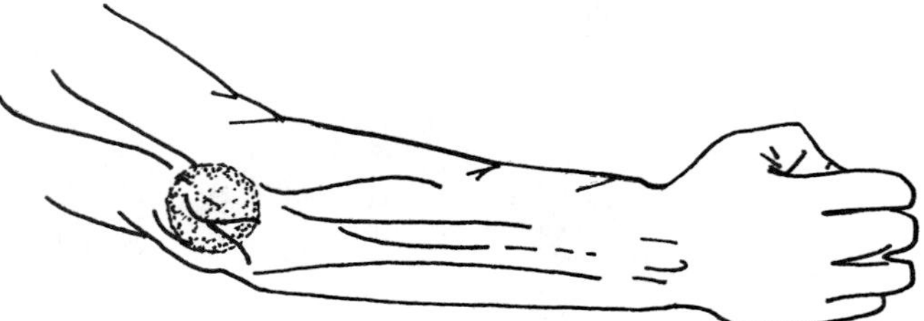

Figure 3. Lateral epicondylitis: site of tenderness over lateral epicondyle.

flexor muscles into the medial humeral epicondyle. Medial epicondylitis is usually less painful and disabling than lateral epicondylitis. Examination reveals local tenderness over the medial epicondyle that is exacerbated with forced flexion of the wrist.

OLECRANON BURSITIS (STUDENT'S ELBOW, MINER'S ELBOW)

The olecranon bursa, a subcutaneous bursa overlying the olecranon process of the humerus, is one of the bursae that are commonly involved in inflammatory processes (Fig. 4). Chronic trauma is a frequent cause of bursitis at this site. Infection and inflammatory conditions, such as gout and rheumatoid arthritis, are often the etiology of olecranon bursitis. Pain is minimal, although a sizable effusion may be present. Range of motion movement of the elbow is usually painless. Erythema and warmth may give a hint of infection; however, a culture of aspirated fluid is essential, since subacute infection is often present. In addition to culture, polarized light microscopy should be performed on all fluid to look for microcrystalline disease. Palpation of the bursa may detect nodules and suggest rheumatoid arthritis, gout, sarcoidosis, or other granulomatous conditions.

DEQUERVAIN'S TENOSYNOVITIS

This is the name given to tenosynovitis of the extensor pollicis brevis and abductor pollicis longus tendons. The condition is seen with repetitive movements involving pinching with the thumb while moving the wrist, for example, using heavy shears in the clothing industry. It is also seen frequently in young mothers. Pain is noted along the radial styloid, which may be increased with pinching movements such as using a key, unscrewing a jar lid, or opening a car door. Tenderness may be present along the course of the tendons over the radial styloid and the posterior boundary of the anatomic snuffbox, and swelling may be seen in some cases. The Finkelstein test is often positive: adduction of the patient's wrist by the examiner toward the ulnar side, while the thumb is folded across the palm with the fingers flexed over it, elicits pain over the affected tendon sheaths. The list of possibilities in the differential diagnosis of this condition includes two other painful conditions affecting the same area, including ununited fracture of the scaphoid, where a history of trauma may be available, and osteoarthritis of the first carpometacarpal joint, in which the Finkelstein test is negative. Sometimes, radiographs are needed for distinguishing between these two conditions in cases where the physical examination is not helpful.

FLEXOR TENOSYNOVITIS (TRIGGER FINGER)

Flexor tenosynovitis is usually a minimally painful condition that affects the flexor tendon sheaths of the fingers. Repetitive friction causes the tendon fibers to shear off and form a small nodule, which becomes detached from the tendon. The nodule slips with difficulty through the tendon sheath and hangs up under the A-1 pulley (Fig. 5). As a result, patients report a "snapping" sensation when the finger is flexed or extended. Often, the finger may become stuck in a flexed position, and active force is then required to release it. The third digit is most commonly affected. Examination often reveals a palpable nodule at the level of the metacarpophalangeal joint. Localized tenderness may also be noted at this location. The majority of patients have no obvious etiology; however, patients with both rheumatoid arthritis and diabetes mellitus have an increased incidence of this flexor tenosynovitis.

TROCHANTERIC BURSITIS

The trochanteric bursa is a superficial bursa that separates the gluteus medius tendon from the lateral aspect of

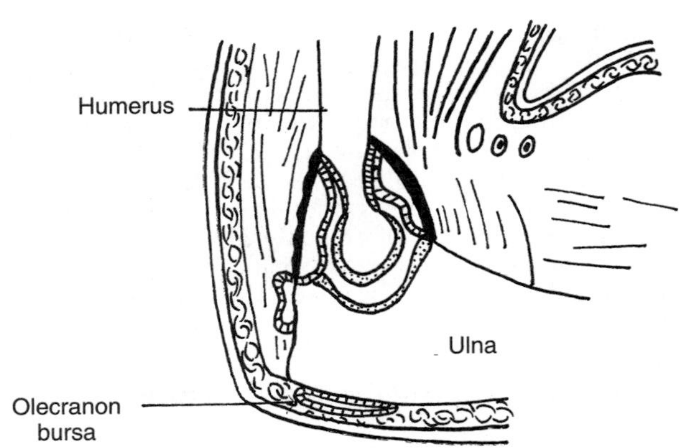

Figure 4. Olecranon bursitis.

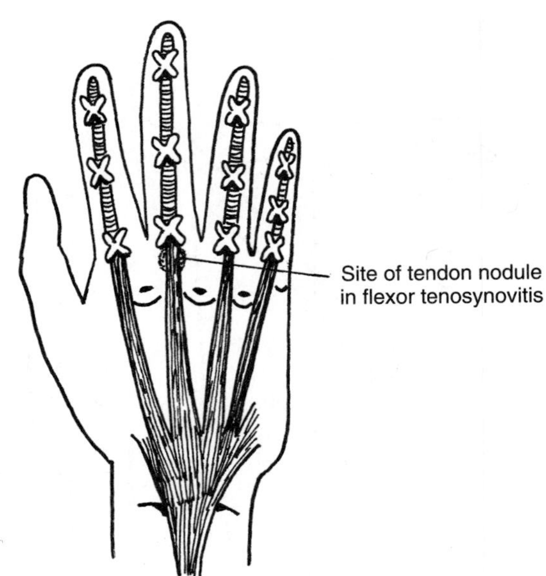

Figure 5. Flexor tenosynovitis.

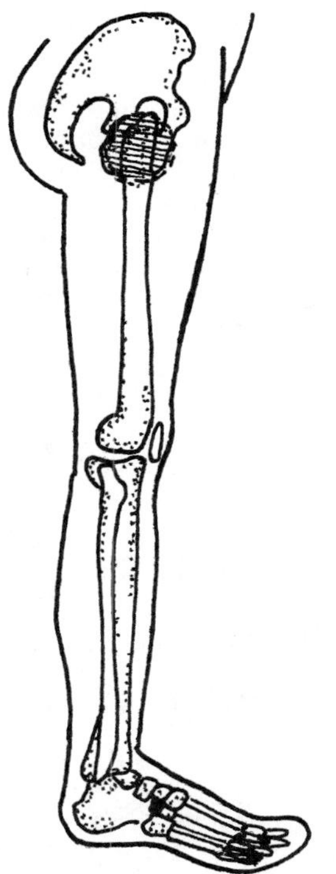

Figure 6. Site of tenderness in trochanteric bursitis.

the greater trochanter (Fig. 6). The trochanteric bursa is the most commonly involved bursa around the hip joint, and trochanteric bursitis is most commonly misdiagnosed. Patients often report "hip" pain and point to the lateral aspect of the greater trochanter, whereas true hip pain is referred to the groin or buttock areas. The pain is often increased by walking or by lying on the affected side. Exiting an automobile may be painful. The most useful physical finding is localized tenderness over the area of the greater trochanter with relatively painless motion of the hip joint. However, the pain may be increased with external rotation and forced abduction of the hip. The cause is usually idiopathic; however, a recent increase in activity may be a clue.

PREPATELLAR BURSITIS (HOUSEMAID'S KNEE)

Located between the skin and the lower half of the patella and the upper half of the patellar tendon (Fig. 7), this bursa is subject to trauma. Friction due to prolonged kneeling may lead to swelling. Pain is minimal, and a fluctuance over the lower half of the patella is commonly seen. Warmth, redness, and tenderness suggest septic bursitis. This bursa does not communicate with the knee joint.

INFRAPATELLAR BURSITIS (CLERGYMAN'S KNEE)

The two infrapatellar bursae are a deep bursa that lies between the tibia and the back of the patellar tendon and a superficial bursa between the skin and the insertion of the patellar tendon. Both nuns and priests often acquire this type of bursitis, rather than prepatellar bursitis, as they kneel in an upright position (see Fig. 7). Inflammation or infection of the deep infrapatellar bursa causes swelling

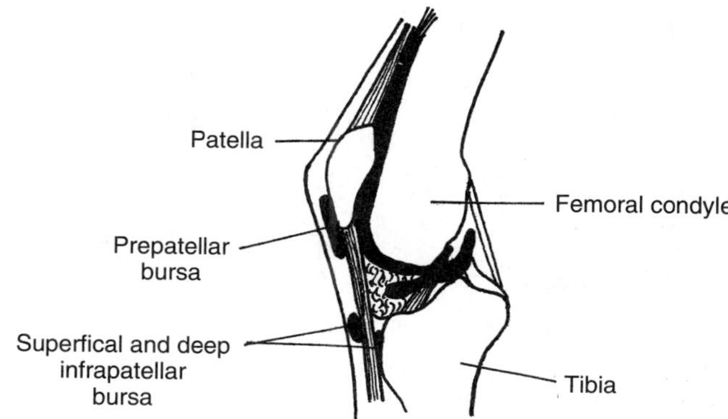

Figure 7. Sites of prepatellar and infrapatellar bursitis.

and fluctuance on either side of the patellar ligament with tenderness to palpation as well as pain on knee flexion.

ANSERINE BURSITIS (CAVALRYMAN'S KNEE)

Anserine bursitis is a common, often overlooked cause of pain in the knee area. The anserine bursa lies between the insertion of the conjoint tendon of the semitendinosus, sartorius, and gracilis and the medial collateral ligament of the knee. Inflammation of this bursa occurs owing to chronic knee instability and strain on the surrounding tendons. Most patients are obese, middle-aged, and female. While most report "knee pain," the true area of tenderness is approximately 2 to 3 cm below the joint line on the medial side (Fig. 8). The pain may keep the patient awake at night. Physical examination reveals discrete tenderness below the true knee joint on the medial aspect. Range-of-motion movement of the knee is usually painless.

PATELLAR TENDINITIS (JUMPER'S KNEE)

Pain is felt in the anterior aspect of the knee over the patellar tendon in athletes who sustain repetitive strain of

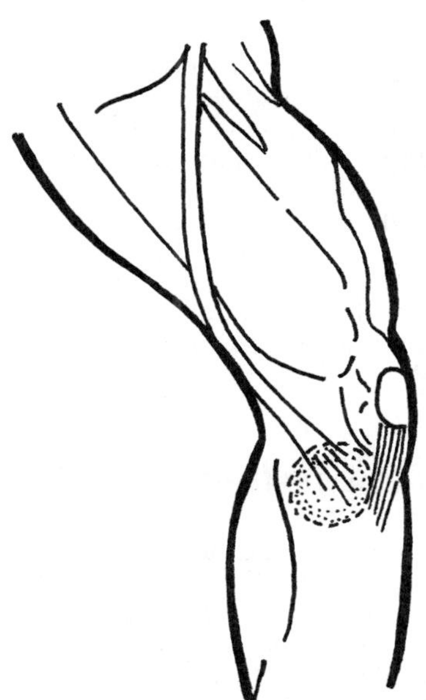

Figure 8. Site of tenderness in anserine bursitis.

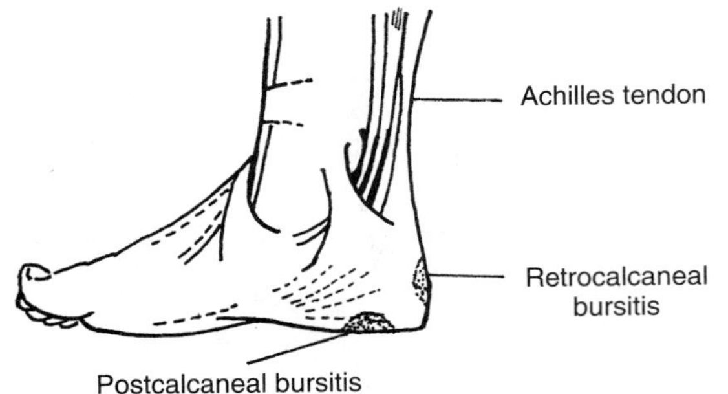

Figure 9. Sites of Achilles tendinitis, retrocalcaneal bursitis, and postcalcaneal bursitis.

the tendon (pole-vaulters and high jumpers). The pain is exacerbated by forced knee extension.

ACHILLES TENDINITIS

Chronic strain of the Achilles tendon and ill-fitting shoes as well as systemic conditions, especially the spondyloarthropathies, may cause pain and tenderness over the Achilles tendon. The pain is felt at the insertion of the tendon into the heel and along the posterior ankle as well as occasionally along the calf (Fig. 9). The pain is worse with dorsiflexion, and localized tenderness over the tendon itself may be seen, thus distinguishing it from retrocalcaneal bursitis. Prolonged friction or inflammation may lead to partial or complete rupture of the tendon, indicated by compression of the calf with the patient kneeling over a chair that does not cause dorsiflexion of the foot (Thompson test). Both heterotrophic calcification and osseous metaplasia have been described in Achilles tendinitis, although it is not clear whether these conditions cause, or are a result of, the tendinitis.

RETROCALCANEAL AND POSTCALCANEAL BURSITIS ("PUMP BUMPS")

The retrocalcaneal bursa is interposed between the posterior surface of the calcaneus and the anterior aspect of the Achilles tendon. Inflammation of this bursa causes heel pain and swelling, which may be difficult to distinguish from Achilles tendinitis. Fluctuation may be seen near the heel on either side of the calcaneus anterior to the Achilles tendon. The postcalcaneal bursa is an adventitious bursa lying between the insertion of the Achilles tendon and the skin (see Fig. 9). Pump pumps is the name given to the inflammation of this bursa in association with bony exostoses on the heel.

POSTERIOR TIBIAL TENDINITIS

The patient reports pain behind the medial malleolus. The pain is exacerbated by forced inversion or passive eversion. This condition is seen with chronic overuse or with systemic inflammatory disease. Associated tenderness or swelling may be seen on examination. Other movements of the ankle are painless, distinguishing it from true ankle involvement.

PLANTAR FASCIITIS AND CALCANEAL BURSITIS

These two conditions cause similar symptoms and, consequently, are often used interchangeably. However, calcaneal bursitis occurs in older individuals and is usually due to local factors, whereas plantar fasciitis may often be associated with systemic diseases, such as the spondyloarthropathies or microcrystalline disease. Both conditions are aggravated by obesity. Heel pain with localized tenderness on examination is the major feature (see Fig. 9). The significance of heel spurs seen on radiographs is unclear. However, they probably play an etiologic role in isolated calcaneal bursitis that occurs in the absence of systemic disease.

CARPAL TUNNEL SYNDROME

By Richard T. Katz, M.D.
St. Louis, Missouri

Carpal tunnel syndrome (CTS) as a complication of trauma was first noted by Sir James Paget in 1854. The more common idiopathic (and often bilateral) CTS was described by Lord Brain, a pre-eminent neurologist, in 1947. Since that time, CTS has been recognized as an extremely common entrapment syndrome. Today, CTS is a diagnosis for any primary practitioner.

The carpal tunnel is bordered posteriorly by the carpal bones of the wrist and anteriorly by the inelastic flexor retinaculum, also known as the transverse carpal ligament (Fig. 1). Because of its anatomic restrictions, the carpal tunnel is the site of the most common of all entrapment neuropathies. Ten structures traverse the carpal tunnel: four tendons of the flexor digitorum superficialis and four of the flexor digitorum profundus, the tendon of the flexor pollicis longus, and the median nerve. The ulnar nerve, artery, and palmar cutaneous nerve (which innervates part of the skin of the palm) do not traverse the carpal tunnel. In most persons, the median nerve innervates all but one of

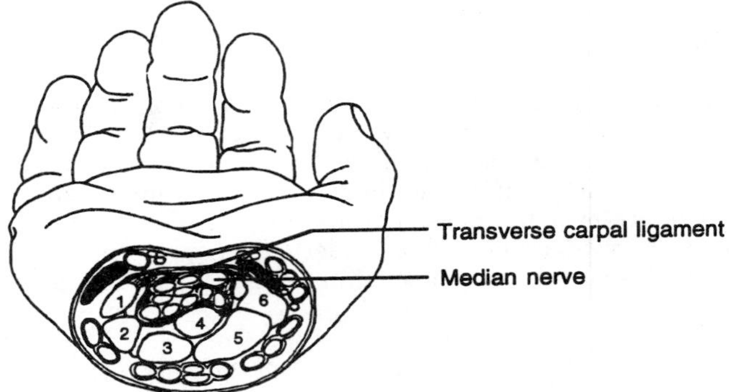

Figure 1. The carpal tunnel is bounded on the volar aspect by the inelastic transverse carpal ligament, and dorsally by the carpal bones. These are the pisiform (1), the triquetral bone (2), the lunate (3), the capitate (4), the scaphoid (5), and the trapezium (6). The 10 structures that traverse the carpal tunnel include the four tendons of the flexor digitorum superficialis, the four tendons of the flexor digitorum profundus, the flexor pollicis longus, and the median nerve.

Table 1. Physical Examination for Carpal Tunnel Syndrome

1. Examine thenar eminence for wasting.
2. Observe for *Tinel's sign* (for CTS)—pain, numbness, and dysesthesias in a median distribution on tapping over the carpal tunnel.
3. Look for *Phalen's sign*—flexing the wrist 90 degrees for 1 min causes numbness and dysesthesias in a median distribution.
4. Test for *Reverse Phalen's sign*—extending the wrists 90 degrees for 1 min (as if in a prayer position).
5. *Carpal compression test*—the examiner presses the thumbs over the patient's carpal tunnel for 30 sec to elicit symptoms.
6. *Flick test*—the patient is asked "What do you actually do with your hand or hands when symptoms are at their worst?" The patient exhibits movement similar to shaking down a thermometer.

CTS = carpal tunnel syndrome.

the thenar muscles, including the abductor pollicis brevis, opponens pollicis, and the superficial head of the flexor pollicis brevis. The deep head of the flexor pollicis brevis is innervated by the ulnar nerve.

CLINICAL SYNDROME

CTS most commonly affects women in midlife. Patients frequently complain of pain in the distal arm or wrist. The pain classically radiates into the thumb and index and middle fingers and is exacerbated by motion of the wrist. The pain may also radiate proximally into the arm, shoulder, or even the neck. Thus, a careful differential diagnosis must be made to exclude other causes of neck, shoulder, or upper extremity pain or dysesthesias, as described further on.

A hallmark of CTS is nocturnal pain. Up to 95 per cent of patients relate a history of awakening in the middle of the night with painful numbness. Patients commonly describe electrical sensations and dyesthesias in the distribution of the median nerve. Patients may also indicate that symptoms begin when they hold the steering wheel of a car.

The clinician should ask the patient to draw his or her numbness on a diagram of a hand. Numbness outlined in a median nerve distribution is highly predictive of carpal tunnel syndrome. There may be concomitant loss of grip strength in patients with more severe CTS. In almost 50 per cent of patients, CTS is bilateral. Therefore, both upper extremities should be carefully examined. Ask the patient to complete a standardized questionnaire, such as the Carpal Tunnel Severity Scale (Fig. 2).

Useful clinical signs of CTS are summarized in Table 1. The thenar eminence should be examined carefully for evidence of atrophy. The presence of swelling, redness, or warmth should suggest other diagnoses. Tinel's sign is positive in 60 to 70 per cent of patients with classic CTS. Phalen's sign is positive in up to 80 per cent of patients, and the carpal compression test is positive in up to 90 per cent of patients with classic CTS. Most recently, the Flick test has been shown to be highly sensitive (93 per cent) and specific. By contrast, the tourniquet test is performed by placing a blood pressure cuff on the upper arm and inflating it to greater than systolic blood pressure. Paresthesias and numbness in the median nerve distribution after inflation for less than 1 minute is considered a positive test result. Unfortunately, the tourniquet test is neither sensitive nor specific.

CONDITIONS ASSOCIATED WITH CARPAL TUNNEL SYNDROME

Although most cases of CTS are idiopathic, several conditions (Table 2) predispose a person to its development. Nonspecific synovial proliferation within the carpal tunnel is the most common predisposing factor. Pregnant patients commonly experience symptoms of CTS that resolve post partum. Hypothyroid and acromegalic patients are also at increased risk for the development of CTS. The diagnosis is commonly overlooked in patients with fractures of the distal radius or ulna. The possibility that reduced carpal tunnel cross-sectional area predisposes to CTS remains to be established.

The concept of the "double crush" suggests that patients with nerve compression in one site are more vulnerable to compression at a second site. Specifically, it has been suggested that patients with cervical radiculopathy may be more susceptible to the development of carpal tunnel syndrome. The validity of this "sick" nerve concept has not been confirmed.

Repetitive flexion or extension of the wrist may predispose a person to CTS. Flexion of the wrist displaces the finger flexor tendons against the palmar side of the carpal tunnel, producing pressure on the tendons and the median nerve. Extension of the wrist displaces the tendons against the dorsal side of the tunnel and radial head, again produc-

Table 2. Causes of Carpal Tunnel Syndrome

Increased Canal Volume

Nonspecific synovial proliferation*
Rheumatoid tenosynovitis
Edema
- Pregnancy*
- Following injury
- Thyroid disease*
- Congestive heart failure
- Renal failure
- Acromegaly

Aberrant anatomy
- Proximal lumbrical insertion
- Distal extension of the flexor superficialis muscle
- Persistent or thrombosed median artery
- Abnormal palmaris longus

Mass lesion
- Benign tumor (lipoma, ganglion)
- Hematoma
- Gouty tophus
- Calcium
- Amyloid
- Malignant tumors
- Multiple myeloma

Decreased Canal Volume

Acute fracture or callus from healing fracture
Arthritis or wrist malalignment
Congenitally small canal
"Sick" nerve with minimal compression (double crush)
- Cervical radiculopathy
- Thoracic outlet syndrome
- Proximal median neuropathy
- Diabetes mellitus*

*One of the most common causes.
Modified from Stevens, J.C., Beard, C.M. O'Fallon, W.M., and Kurland, L.T.: Conditions associated with CTS. Mayo Clin Proc 67:541–548, 1992.

The following **eleven** questions refer to your symptoms for a typical twenty-four hour period during the past two weeks (check one answer for each question).

1) How severe is the hand or wrist pain that you have at night? ☐ 1 I do not have hand or wrist pain at night ☐ 2 Mild pain ☐ 3 Moderate pain ☐ 4 Severe pain ☐ 5 Very severe pain	2) How often did hand or wrist pain wake you up during a typical night in the past two weeks? ☐ 1 Never ☐ 2 Once ☐ 3 Two or three times ☐ 4 Four or five times ☐ 5 More than five times
3) Do you typically have pain in your hand or wrist during the daytime? ☐ 1 I never have pain during the day ☐ 2 I have mild pain during the day ☐ 3 I have moderate pain during the day ☐ 4 I have severe pain during the day ☐ 5 I have very severe pain during the day	4) How often do you have hand or wrist pain during the daytime? ☐ 1 Never ☐ 2 Once or twice a day ☐ 3 Three to five times a day ☐ 4 More than five times a day ☐ 5 The pain is constant
5) How long, on average, does an episode of pain last during the daytime? ☐ 1 I never get pain during the day ☐ 2 Less than 10 minutes ☐ 3 10 to 60 minutes ☐ 4 Greater than 60 minutes ☐ 5 The pain is constant throughout the day	6) Do you have numbness (loss of sensation) in your hand? ☐ 1 No ☐ 2 I have mild numbness ☐ 3 I have moderate numbness ☐ 4 I have severe numbness ☐ 5 I have very severe numbness

Figure 2. Carpal tunnel syndrome symptom severity scale. (From Levine, D.W., Simmons, B.P., Koris, M.J., et al.: Self-administered questionnaire for the assessment of severity of symptoms and functional status in carpal tunnel syndrome. J Bone Joint Surg Am 75A[11]:1585–1592, 1993, with permission.) *Figure continued*

7) Do you have weakness in your hand or wrist?		8) Do you have tingling sensations in your hand?	
☐ 1	No weakness	☐ 1	No tingling
☐ 2	Mild weakness	☐ 2	Mild tingling
☐ 3	Moderate weakness	☐ 3	Moderate tingling
☐ 4	Severe weakness	☐ 4	Severe tingling
☐ 5	Very severe weakness	☐ 5	Very severe tingling
9) How severe is numbness (loss of sensation) or tingling at night?		10) How often did hand numbness or tingling wake you up during a typical night during the past two weeks?	
☐ 1	I have no numbness or tingling at night	☐ 1	Never
☐ 2	Mild	☐ 2	Once
☐ 3	Moderate	☐ 3	two or tree times
☐ 4	Severe	☐ 4	Four or five times
☐ 5	Very severe	☐ 5	More than five times
11) Do you have difficulty with the grasping and use of small objects such as keys or pens?			
☐ 1	No difficulty		
☐ 2	Mild difficulty		
☐ 3	Moderate difficulty		
☐ 4	Severe difficulty		
☐ 5	Very severe difficulty	Total	_______

Figure 2 *Continued*

Table 3. Electrodiagnostic Confirmation of Carpal Tunnel Syndrome

1. CTS usually involves both large sensory and motor fibers, but occasionally only one type of nerve fiber is involved; therefore the clinical neurophysiologist must study sensory *and* motor fibers.
2. Other nerve conduction studies must be performed to exclude peripheral neuropathy.
3. Sensitivity of the test can be increased by comparing the median conduction study with that of an adjacent nerve—ulnar or superficial radial—or the corresponding nerve in the contralateral limb.
4. Measuring short segments of the median nerve (by stimulating the palm and recording over the wrist) increases diagnostic accuracy.
5. It is sometimes useful to obtain an electromyogram of the entire upper extremity and corresponding paraspinal muscles in addition to one of the thenar eminence to exclude double-crush syndrome.
6. Nerve conduction studies do not correlate well with the severity of the patient's symptoms.

CTS = carpal tunnel syndrome.

ing increased pressure. Carpal tunnel pressures have been measured by transducers placed within the canal. Pressures are often much higher in symptomatic patients when compared with control subjects, and pressures increase significantly during flexion or extension.

CONFIRMATORY TESTS

Nerve conduction studies and electromyography can aid the clinician who seeks to confirm or refute the diagnosis of CTS. Essentially all patients should be referred for nerve conduction studies if the diagnosis is suspected. Although some hand surgeons have argued that nerve conduction studies are superfluous, several countervailing arguments exist. Nerve conduction studies are critical to (1) confirming the diagnosis, (2) facilitating appropriate early treatment, (3) verifying the diagnosis prior to surgery, and (4) excluding other conditions. For example, the differential diagnosis of CTS includes motor neuron disease, cervical canal (intraspinal) lesions, neurogenic thoracic outlet syndrome, multiple sclerosis, plexopathy, polyneuropathy, and hysteria. The clinician must balance the patient's mild to moderate discomfort during electrodiagnostic studies against the alternative of unnecessary surgery. Some clinicians have argued that a favorable response to surgery provides sufficient proof of the diagnosis of CTS, even when electrodiagnostic studies are normal. However, the powerful placebo effect of a surgical procedure strongly undermines this argument. Also, patients whose electrodiagnostic studies are normal or nearly normal often benefit from conservative treatment, whereas severe CTS should, as a rule, be surgically treated. Nerve conduction studies are also important as a baseline for comparison with the postoperative result. Sensory and motor latencies often improve after surgery, but they seldom completely return to normal.

Electrodiagnostic studies can generate both false-positive and false-negative results. There is no "ideal" way of performing nerve conduction studies in the diagnosis of CTS, but some useful guidelines for the interpretation of reports are provided in Table 3.

As employed in clinical practice, nerve conduction studies primarily evaluate large myelinated motor and sensory nerve fibers. Thus, if the patient's discomfort results from changes in small myelinated or unmyelinated fibers, standard nerve conduction studies may not detect significant abnormalities.

Although portable, hand-held nerve-stimulating units have been offered as alternatives to sophisticated electrodiagnostic equipment, the clinical utility of these portable devices has not been established. Portable testing has many pitfalls, and clinicians should understand that most hand-held devices are used by individuals with little or no formal training in electrodiagnosis.

Two-point discrimination (which can be simply performed with an electrocardiogram [ECG] caliper and a ruler graduated in millimeters) has been used in the diagnosis of CTS. Normal individuals can distinguish two points 5 mm or more apart; many CTS patients cannot. Two-point discrimination, however, is normal in more than 50 per cent of CTS patients. Vibration testing with a 256-Hz tuning fork is more sensitive than two-point discrimination, but the rate of false-positive and false-negative results remains unacceptably high.

The sensory threshold associated with pressure on the fingertips can be measured with a series of Semmes-Weinstein monofilaments. Perception of light touch is as-

Table 4. Classification of Median Neuropathies at the Carpal Tunnel

Class 0	Asymptomatic	No signs or symptoms; electrodiagnostic evidence of definite dysfunction of median nerve myelinated fibers
Class 1	Intermittently symptomatic	Intermittent paresthesias with normal examination; paresthesias may be reproduced with provocative tests
Class 1A	Subclinical median nerve irritability	Excessive neuronal firing occurs only with provocative tests; hands intermittently go to sleep
Class 1B	Mild CTS	Transient symptoms of CTS (e.g., with pregnancy), then become asymptomatic; electrodiagnostic abnormalities may resolve; some require no treatment, others respond to ergonomic-conservative treatment
Class 1C	Moderate intermittent CTS	Symptoms many times per week; neurologic examination usually normal; electrodiagnostic studies usually positive; some benefit from conservative therapy, others require surgery
Class 2	Persistently symptomatic CTS	More commonly have neurologic findings; usually have abnormal median nerve conduction; usually require surgery
Class 3	Severe CTS	Clinical evidence of median axonal interruption; thenar atrophy, needle examination findings; most patients improve after surgery but some incompletely

CTS = carpal tunnel syndrome.
Modified from Rosenbaum, R.B., and Ochoa, J.L.: Carpal Tunnel Syndrome. Boston, Butterworth-Heinemann, 1993, pp. 51–53, with permission.

sessed by applying a series of standardized monofilaments to the digital surfaces, and recording the thinnest detectable filament. Each probe is marked with the number that represents the log of 10 times the force (in milligrams) required to bend the monofilament. A threshold value greater than 2.83 has been considered abnormal.

Despite the attractiveness and simplicity of techniques such as monofilament testing, electrodiagnostic studies remain the focal point of the evaluation for carpal tunnel syndrome. Although probably not a gold standard, nerve conduction studies continue to provide the most reliable technique for determining the presence and severity of CTS. On the basis of the history, physical examination, and electrodiagnostic studies, patients can be classified (Table 4) in ways that can help the clinician steer the patient toward proper management.

SPORTS MEDICINE

By G. Klaud Miller, M.D.
Evanston, Illinois

Since almost any disease or injury can occur in an athlete or affect an athlete's performance, in the strictest sense, "sports medicine" covers an extremely broad area of medical knowledge. Almost any fracture or dislocation can occur in sports such as football, lacrosse, or Rugby. To delineate all variations of trauma, tendinitis, or bursitis simply duplicates conventional orthopedic textbooks. This author has attempted to select problems that either are common in popular sports or are a common diagnostic dilemma. No attempt was made to enumerate all the possible injuries in each individual sport. Representative sports have been used to help the physician understand the mechanisms of injury and disease involved.

Several organizational schemes are possible. Discussion according to a strict enumeration by anatomic area would require significant repetition of diagnoses such as tendinitis and bursitis. Therefore, this author has chosen first to classify problems by broad etiologic groups and then to subclassify them by anatomic areas. This classification also helps the treating physician find information more quickly.

Even the definition of injury or disease may be problematic at times. Is muscle soreness from running too far an injury? Is the bony hypertrophy seen in a tennis player's dominant arm a disease? Can arthritis be attributed to earlier participation in sports? For purposes of discussion in this article, an injury is defined as any medical problem, from whatever cause, that can limit participation in a sporting endeavor (practice or a game) for at least 1 day. It is acknowledged that an "injury" in one sport, according to this definition, may not limit participation in another sport and therefore may not fulfill the strict definition of injury under all circumstances. As an example, a fractured left wrist would certainly limit a wrestler but would have much less effect on a right-handed tennis player. Clearly, the athlete has suffered an injury in each case even though the performance implications are vastly different.

TRAUMA

Macrotrauma is defined as a single episode or, at most, a few distinctly identifiable episodes of trauma that are sufficient to result in functional limitation of participation in the athlete's chosen sport. Microtrauma is the repetitive application of forces that are not great enough to cause injury when applied only a few times. Typical overuse injuries are tendinitis, bursitis, stress fractures, and a chronic compartmental syndrome. The common etiology is relative overuse of an anatomic structure. It is critical to remember that overuse is a relative term. Overuse injuries in an untrained runner obviously require much less mileage than those in the marathon runner who may be used to training 100 miles or more per week. Overuse injuries tend to occur in certain sensitive areas of the body and are predictable in specific sports.

Sprains

Ligaments are bands of tough connective tissue that allow motion of a joint in some direction (e.g., up or down) but limit or constrain displacement in another (e.g., side to side). A sprain of a joint is a stretching injury of one or more ligaments. All sprained joints are swollen and tender, and all but the mildest manifest restricted motion in the planes of normal motion. Often, little quantitative difference exists between the signs and symptoms of sprains of different degrees of severity. This ambiguity makes predictions of time to return to sports participation difficult. Total recovery time depends primarily on the severity of the injury and the total tissue damage. A grade 1 injury stretches the ligament within its elastic limits so that no physical lengthening of the ligament occurs. The joint, by definition, is still totally stable even though painful and swollen. The ligament functions like a spring. If the energy is great enough, a grade 2 sprain results as the ligament is stretched beyond its point of plastic deformation and is permanently lengthened. The spring is permanently stretched out. In grade 3 sprains, the stress is great enough to completely tear the ligament, and all resistance to applied forces in that direction is lost. If the forces are great enough or enough ligaments are torn, joint instability can result. Subluxation of a joint is defined as a partial loss of joint surface contact as a result of one or more ligament sprains. A dislocation occurs when the total ligament damage or applied forces are great enough to cause total loss of contact between the two joint surfaces so that the bones separate. Subluxations and dislocations may be acute, chronic, or recurrent and may spontaneously reduce. A "chip sprain" is a variation of a grade 3 injury in which the ligament is still intact, but instability results because the normal attachment of the ligament from one side of the joint is pulled off, with a small chip of bone. The net effect is ligamentous instability even though, anatomically, the ligament itself may be completely intact. Although such an injury is technically a fracture, it is really a sprain.

Strains

Strains are stretching injuries of a muscle-and-tendon unit. Think "T" for tendon to remember the difference between sprains and strains. Because of the much greater elasticity of the musculotendinous system, complete structural failures (tendon rupture or muscle tear) are much less common than sprains. Children usually avulse apophyses or fracture through epiphyseal plates because the tendons and ligaments are stronger than the cartilage plates. The tendon attachments pull bone off, rather than the tendon tearing. These injuries are usually classified as Salter-type fractures even though technically they also are chip sprains (see the section on pediatric injuries later in this article).

Tendinitis

Tendinitis is inflammation of the long, thin collagen bundles that connect muscles to bone. In sports, the inflammation is almost always the result of overuse. The tendon is painful and swollen. Radiographs are rarely helpful.

Bursitis

Bursae are synovium-lined sacs that minimize friction and allow one anatomic structure (i.e., skin or tendon) to slide over another deeper structure (i.e., bone). Bursae can become inflamed and swollen. Pain and tenderness are common, but not universal. Swelling is sometimes dramatic. A direct blow can rupture the capillaries in the bursal wall, and the resultant blood-filled sac is known as traumatic bursitis. If there is an associated abrasion, the blood can become contaminated, and a septic bursitis results. Aspiration of fluid for culture is reasonable if pain and erythema are present.

MACROTRAUMA

Neurologic Trauma

Concussion

Concussion is a word derived from the Latin word *concutere* (to shake violently). A concussion, by definition, is a post-traumatic, transient, self-improving disturbance of neural function. The only difference is the severity of the alterations and the duration. This category includes states ranging from minor alterations of consciousness, such as a "ding" (minor dizziness, a temporary loss of memory, either antegrade or retrograde), to severe alterations, such as loss of consciousness for a period of time. Football is the sport in which concussions occur most commonly, but concussions do occur in lacrosse, boxing, and horseback riding and when an athlete falls off a piece of gymnastics equipment.

GRADE 1 CONCUSSION (MILD). Grade 1 concussion is characterized by retrograde amnesia for less than 30 minutes, headache, dizziness, fatigue, nausea or vomiting, or difficulties with concentration. By definition, there is no loss of consciousness.

GRADE 2 CONCUSSION (MODERATE). This category includes any of the features of a grade 1 concussion plus loss of consciousness for less than 5 minutes or amnesia for more than 30 minutes.

GRADE 3 CONCUSSION (SEVERE). This grouping includes any of the features of a grade 2 concussion plus loss of consciousness for more than 5 minutes or amnesia for more than 24 hours. There may be asymmetrical motor, reflex, or cranial nerve changes, and seizures are possible.

One must not forget the more severe problems that can occur in these individuals with concussions. Cerebral edema, skull fractures, and intracranial bleeding all can lead to severe neurologic residuals, and are covered elsewhere in this text. The physician must not assume that only the head is injured. Cervical spine and facial fractures or ear, nose, and throat (ENT) injuries must also be sought, especially in the unconscious athlete. Patients with cerebrospinal fluid or blood draining from the nares or an ear or a palpably depressed skull fracture, and all patients with grade 2 or 3 concussions should be transported immediately for neurosurgical evaluation.

Postconcussion syndrome consists of neurologic signs and/or symptoms that persist after the patient is otherwise alert and oriented. These findings can include headaches, dizziness, blurred vision, double vision, nausea, vomiting, and, occasionally, paresthesias. The patient may also have difficulty in concentrating and with memory. With postconcussion syndrome, by definition, there are no objective neurologic findings, such as muscle weakness and objective sensory or reflex changes. These deficits usually spontaneously improve, and no specific treatment other than reassurance and observation is required. Amnesia can result from either a concussion or any of the other problems mentioned earlier. Most commonly, amnesia is antegrade, which means that the memory loss is from the time of the injury forward for a variable period. However, sometimes the amnesia is retrograde, in that the loss of memory includes a variable period of time before the neurologic insult. This type of amnesia indicates a more severe injury.

Ear, Nose, and Throat Trauma

Cauliflower Ear

Because of the unique requirements of wrestling, there is frequent rubbing of body parts across each other. In the past, wrestlers did not wear protective headgear and the ears were subject to trauma as the wrestlers performed the various wrestling maneuvers. The ear is primarily cartilage with a superficial blood supply. With trauma to the ears, superficial blood vessels can be broken, creating a hematoma between the skin and isolating the auricular cartilage from its vascular supply. The hematoma may undergo necrosis and eventually calcify. The swelling may be severe if left untreated and can expand to give the appearance of a cauliflower, hence the name. A cauliflower ear usually does not compromise function, but it can swell so badly that the external auditory canal becomes blocked. It is a significant cosmetic problem. No true ecchymosis formation occurs. The problem tends to occur in practice, when the individuals for vanity or other purposes do not wear their headgear. Most reputable competitions require the use of headgear for protective purposes. Treatment should consist of early recognition, cool packs, and a referral to an ENT specialist for immediate evacuation of the hematoma and application of a cast.

Laryngeal Trauma

Laryngeal injuries are unusual but potentially devastating. A "clothesline tackle" in football, a lacrosse or hockey stick to the throat, or any other form of direct trauma to the laryngeal area can fracture either the hyoid bone or the larynx. Several variations are possible. The hyoid bone is the most cephalic of the laryngeal structures. Pain, localized tenderness, and crepitus should make the clinician suspicious. Subcutaneous emphysema is common. The larynx itself can also be traumatized, with mucosal swelling and obstruction of the airway. Severe dyspnea can result from epiglottis edema but is rare. Sometimes, the thyroid or cricoid cartilage can be cracked. Supraglottic injuries tend to cause less rapid development of dyspnea and stridor than do more distal injuries. The common denominator is mucosal swelling and restriction of the airway. The airway can become rapidly compromised, with catastrophic results. One or both recurrent laryngeal nerves may be injured, with resultant hoarseness or paralysis of the vocal cords and dyspnea. Any individual with anterior neck trauma of any kind who reports shortness of breath should be closely monitored.

Soft tissue swelling and subcutaneous emphysema in the anterior aspect of the neck can make the differential diagnosis difficult. Differentiation between hyoid, cricoid, and thyroid cartilage fractures is important because with a tracheal or cricoid fracture an adequate airway may not be established with the standard cricothyroidotomy taught for emergency ventilation purposes. A true tracheostomy must be performed on an emergent basis to provide an adequate airway for these injuries. The team physician's responsibility is early recognition and immediate transfer to a hospital at the slightest evidence of these injuries.

Spine Trauma

Cervical Fractures

The variety of cervical spine fractures is too great to allow a detailed discussion of the specific types of fractures. Moreover, field identification of individual fractures is not possible. Detailed x-ray studies, including computed tomography (CT), tomograms, and magnetic resonance imaging (MRI), are usually necessary for complete identification of all components of fractures. However, several diagnostic signs and symptoms are consistent with a fracture, and the team physician should assume that these findings are the result of a fracture until proved otherwise and treat appropriately. Any individual with a neck or head injury and paresthesias, hypoesthesias, or weakness in any of the extremities should be assumed to have a fracture until proved otherwise. Reflex loss and muscle strength asymmetry are additional indications. Tenderness over the spinous processes or obvious gaps between the spinous processes are suggestive. Paraspinal muscle spasm is common in fractures but is also commonly seen in contusions and sprains. True muscle paralysis or severe apprehension if the neck is moved that persists for even a short period of time is an indication for spine immobilization, removal of the athlete from the game, and x-ray examination. The details of helmet removal, immobilization, and transfer of cervical spine injuries are also beyond this article, but every team physician should be aware of these procedures.

While cervical spine injuries can occur as the result of falls from horses, bicycles, or pieces of gymnastic equipment, they probably occur most commonly in football. It is well known that a technique called spearing predisposes to cervical spine injuries. Spearing is a technique in which a tackler strikes the runner with the top of his head (known as the crown). This type of impact causes axial compression, which fractures the vertebral bodies. This injury often leads to severe neurologic impairment, such as tetraparesis (quadriparesis) and nerve root injuries. In recent years, spearing has been banned, and coaches have been instructed to teach the proper tackling technique, in which the forehead strikes the opposing player first. This change in technique has significantly decreased the incidence of cervical spine injuries.

Burners (Brachial Plexus Neurapraxia)

"Burner" is a descriptive term for a stretch injury of the brachial plexus, most commonly seen in football players. As the tackler strikes the body of the running back, the shoulder is depressed and the head and neck are forced to the opposite side, stretching the brachial plexus. The net effect is a nerve dysfunction involving the shoulder and/or hand, depending on the particular nerve roots involved. These injuries may be simply sensory (hypoesthesia or burning dysesthesias) in nature or may be severe enough to cause temporary or even prolonged weakness. A positive Tinel sign may be present at the site of the injury. Because the C5 roots are the most proximal and, therefore, the most exposed, it is common to see normal sensory motor examinations in the hand but an inability to abduct the shoulder. The clinician must specifically look for weakness of abduction of the shoulder because the player may hide this finding and move his hands and elbows in an attempt to convince the coach or team physician that he can return to play. A hyperabduction injury can injure the lower roots. Lesions involving the more proximal roots (to the rhomboids and serratus anterior), multiple root involvement, and lesions with an associated sympathetic dysfunction (Horner's syndrome) tend to have a worse prognosis. Return to play cannot be sanctioned until full motor and sensory recovery has occurred. Repeated or frequent burners are grounds for removal of the athlete from participation for the season.

Shoulder Trauma

It is conceptually useful to classify shoulder problems into several areas: extra-articular, intra-articular, capsular, and rotator cuff problems. The extra-articular problems consist of acromioclavicular and sternoclavicular dislocations as well as biceps tendon subluxations and ruptures. Intra-articular problems consist of conditions such as arthritis, loose bodies, superior labrum anterior posterior (SLAP) lesions, and a torn labrum. Capsular problems include shoulder instability.

Acromioclavicular Joint Injuries

Acromioclavicular joint injuries usually result from a fall on the shoulder with the arm at the side. The acromion is driven down and underneath the clavicle, rupturing the coracoclavicular ligaments and the acromioclavicular ligaments. The standard three grades of ligamentous injury are utilized. A grade 2 injury is defined as a separation between the acromion and the clavicle of less than the thickness of the clavicle. A grade 3 injury is actually a true dislocation, in which the acromion and clavicle are separated by a distance greater than the width of the clavicle. The diagnosis is made by noting the characteristic tenderness at the acromioclavicular joint and the limited range of motion of the shoulder. Stress radiographs taken with weights held in the hands may be necessary for accurate demonstration of the full extent of the instability. In the more severe grades, tenderness associated with a palpable step-off is seen. Unusual variations occur, in which the clavicle goes either posteriorly or, extremely rarely, distal to the acromion and coracoid. Occasionally, the clavicle is impaled in the trapezius. Appropriate treatment is early referral to an orthopedic surgeon for discussion of the options.

Sternoclavicular Injuries

Sternoclavicular injuries usually result from a crushing-type injury, such as being caught in a football or Rugby pile-up and, occasionally, falling off a piece of gymnastic equipment. Tenderness at the sternoclavicular joint is the hallmark. A grade 2 or 3 injury results in a palpable step-off. However, the displacements, even when significant on radiograph, are clinically not dramatic. The medial clavicle is displaced anteriorly more than 90 per cent of the time. In rare conditions, the unstable medial clavicle is displaced posteriorly. The great vessels and trachea pass directly behind the sternum. The potential for injuries to these structures is present. Tenderness with a palpable step-off and shortness of breath should make the physician suspicious of this diagnosis. Computed tomography scans are recommended for definitive diagnosis.

In the young adult, an unusual injury may occur. The medial epiphysis of the clavicle is one of the last in the body to ossify and close. It closes between ages 22 and 25 years and, in some individuals, as late as age 30. Therefore, in the otherwise physiologically mature individual, which includes most college football players, an injury to this area usually results in an epiphyseal fracture, rather than a sternoclavicular dislocation. This difference must be appreciated and included in the diagnostic and treatment decisions. The clinical examination is identical to a true dislocation.

Biceps Tendon Dislocation

The biceps tendon runs in a groove on the anterior aspect of the proximal humerus between the greater and the lesser tuberosities and is covered by the transverse humeral ligament. This ligament keeps the biceps tendon in the groove throughout rotation of the shoulder. If the transverse humeral ligament is disrupted, the tendon can sublux out of the groove, creating a characteristic snapping and anterior tenderness. This displacement usually occurs with external rotation, as the tendon subluxes and reduces with internal rotation. This snapping can usually be felt. Localizable tenderness in the area of the bicipital groove is almost always present. Exercises help, but treatment is usually surgical. Computed tomography arthrograms may document the tendon displacement from the bicipital groove.

Bicipital Tendon Rupture

Bicipital tendon rupture is distinctly unusual in individuals younger than age 40. The individual is characteristically lifting a weight, which is not always extremely heavy. There is usually a snap, and the muscle "rolls up" like a window shade. Ninety-five per cent or more of the ruptures occur proximally and involve only the long head of the biceps. The muscle is found to be contracted distally in an irregular lump, proximal to the antecubital fossa. Distal ruptures, which do rarely occur, are sometimes missed because the only pain is in the elbow itself. The muscle has rolled up proximally and can be nearly normal in appearance. The major symptom in each is usually weakness of supination. The brachial muscle allows elbow flexion, and elbow flexion weakness is usually not significant. There is usually ecchymosis from distal ruptures. Ecchymosis can occur from proximal ruptures, but this finding is less common. Some argument exists about whether proximal bicipital tendon ruptures ever occur without rotator cuff pathology, but cuff pathology should always be sought.

Torn Labrum and SLAP Lesion

The biceps muscle is a diarthrodial muscle. It crosses two joints. The proximal attachment of the biceps tendon is to the anterosuperior glenoid of the scapula, at approximately a one o'clock position in the right shoulder. The biceps muscle attaches distally to the bicipital tuberosity of the radius. A common injury is a fall in which the individual attempts to save himself or herself by grabbing something. The force brings the arm into an extended and abducted position. The biceps muscle contracts and literally pulls off its proximal attachment (the SLAP lesion). This injury can occur in gymnastics or, sometimes, in football during a tackle. The net effect is a painful shoulder. Pain is usually felt during the follow-through phase of throwing. Tenderness is felt frequently, but not invariably, along the proximal anterior glenohumeral joint line. A click may be heard with rotation. The "hands-on-hips test" has been advocated by some as a specific test, but it has low sensitivity. No definitive diagnostic test exists that can be performed, except for arthroscopy. Treatment consists of arthroscopic repair of the detachment.

Shoulder Instability

Instability of the shoulder takes several forms. A subluxation is an incomplete loss of normal congruity of the joint. By definition, the two joint surfaces are always at least partially in contact. A dislocation is loss of joint congruity in which all contact between the two bones is lost. Actually, four joints make up the shoulder girdle: the sternoclavicular, acromioclavicular, glenohumeral, and scapulothoracic joints. By far the most common joint instability seen is that of the glenohumeral joint. Ninety-seven per cent of all glenohumeral joint dislocations occur anteriorly, with the humeral head moving anteriorly relative to the scapular glenoid. Approximately 2 per cent are posterior and 1 per cent are multidirectional, inferior, or involuntary. A very small percentage of dislocations have an associated greater tuberosity fracture of the humerus.

In the typical anterior glenohumeral dislocation, the arm is held slightly abducted and externally rotated as the external rotator muscles are stretched and become taut as the head is "stuck" on the anterior aspect of the glenoid. An area of hypoesthesia may be found at the insertion of the deltoid muscle. This finding is due to a stretch injury of the recurrent axillary nerve. Vascular injuries are possible but rare. After reduction, the integrity of the deltoid muscle strength must also be tested, as the axillary nerve may have suffered a stretch neurapraxia. All these findings must be carefully documented both before and after the reduction.

Examination after a dislocation may show excessive anterior laxity (anterior drawer test). The shoulder may be distracted with longitudinal pressure, this distraction creating a hollow inferior to the acromion (the "sulcus sign"). External rotation at 90 degrees of abduction causes pain and withdrawal ("apprehension test"). If posterior pressure applied to the anterior shoulder relieves the pain of the apprehension test, the "relocation test" is considered positive. A posterior dislocation theoretically has the reverse deformity; that is, the arm is fixed in internal rotation and abduction. However, frequently the deformity is more appropriately described as a loss of full external rotation, rather than the arm truly being held in internal rotation. The arm is usually not abducted but has limited abduction. A characteristic hollow may be found anteriorly, and a prominence posteriorly, but these findings are clinically very subtle. A posterior drawer test may be missed. The clinician may even be able to push the head posteriorly out of the glenoid (a positive "push-pull test"). More than 50 per cent of posterior shoulder dislocations are missed initially. The surgeon should be suspicious of a posterior dislocation in anyone who has fallen forward on the outstretched hand or has suffered a direct blow to the anterior shoulder and has less than a completely normal range of motion. Inferior dislocations are classically manifested as luxatio erecta with the arm fixed in an abducted position and an inability to adduct the arm because the humeral head is buttonholed through the inferior capsule. This latter finding results from the humeral head being locked distal to the glenoid labrum. This instability is the rarest type. Multidirectional instability can result from repetitive dislocations or diffuse soft tissue laxity, and in this injury, by definition, the shoulder can dislocate in at least two of the three directions. Such a problem is very disabling and must be carefully sought on questioning. Involuntary subluxation is instability of the shoulder that cannot be controlled or prevented by the individual. Some people, especially those with multidirectional instability, can voluntarily dislocate their shoulders and perform the dislocation as a "party trick." Involuntary dislocators are individuals who literally cannot control the instability. They frequently started out as voluntary dislocators; however, through repetitive insults and dislocations, the joint is now totally unstable with minimal provocation and is functionally incompetent.

Any dislocation can suffer a concomitant fracture of the greater tuberosity; thus, prereduction radiographs are important. While the diagnosis of a greater tuberosity fracture is important for reduction, its most significant value is its effect on the prognosis for recurrence. In addition to routine views of the shoulder, an axillary, or "Y," view shows the dislocation. The radiograph may show a notch in the posterior humeral head (the Hill-Sachs lesion) from the humeral head impacting on the anterior glenoid rim. Fractures of the anterior glenoid rim can occur and are more common in recurrent dislocations.

Statistically speaking, the chance of recurrence is dependent primarily on age. Individuals younger than 20 years of age at the time of initial dislocation may have a redislocation rate as high as 90 per cent. An individual older than age 40 at the time of initial dislocation has at most a 10 to 15 per cent chance of a second dislocation. A fracture of the greater tuberosity, even in a young individual, seems to be highly protective against recurrent dislocations. The incidence of redislocation drops dramatically to, at most, a few percentage points. Males have a higher recurrence rate than females.

Rotator Cuff Tendinitis

The rotator cuff tendons consist of the four "SITS muscles": the supraspinatus, infraspinatus, teres minor, and subscapularis. The common denominator in rotator cuff tendinitis is inflammation of the cuff tendons. Frequently, the biceps tendon is secondarily involved as it passes through the inflamed rotator cuff, and biceps tendinitis results. Classic rotator cuff tendinitis occurs in the 40- to 60-year-old active person. It is primarily degenerative in nature and occurs in persons such as painters and wallpaperers, who use their arms repetitively. Of course, rotator cuff tendinitis can also occur in the younger athlete who participates in activities that involve throwing, such as baseball, tennis, handball, and racquetball. Classic rotator cuff tendinitis has a so-called painful arc syndrome. The arm is not painful for 0 to 90 degrees of abduction, and at approximately 90 to 110 degrees of abduction the shoulder becomes painful. Classically, the pain decreases or is eliminated at 160 to 180 degrees of motion. Thus, there is approximately a 60-degree arc that is painful. Crepitation may occur with rotation of the shoulder. The shoulder is tender to palpation in the lateral subacromial area. Tenderness may be felt over the anterior subacromial area also. Patients commonly report that the pain is at the insertion of the deltoid muscle, and they may not report pain more proximally. The patient's pain is relieved and the tendinitis treated by a subacromial injection of cortisone and local anesthetic.

The differential diagnosis must include subacromial bursitis or cervical radiculitis, which may also cause radiation of pain to the deltoid area. Commonly, an associated acromioclavicular joint degeneration or arthritis may be found, especially in the older individual. Usually, point tenderness is felt over the acromioclavicular joint, and palpable spurs may even be noted. If simple tendinitis exists, the cuff muscles may be weak secondary to pain. Subacromial bursitis can occur without rotator cuff tendinitis, but both are usually involved eventually. Clinical differentiation is difficult.

A variation of rotator cuff tendinitis found in a much younger age group is the impingement syndrome. This condition involves primarily the anterior rotator cuff as a result of repetitive activity in the forward plane. Three stages exist. Stage 1 is tendon edema; stage 2 is tendon fibrosis; and stage 3 is a true rotator cuff tear. Stage 1 occurs in the 20- to 30-year-old person who is active in a throwing sport or in swimming. The symptoms are very similar to those of standard rotator cuff tendinitis except that there is tenderness in the anterior, but not the lateral, subacromial area. The patient may have some weakness with isolated supraspinatus testing, but rarely a true-positive "drop arm test" (see later). When the arm is brought up to 90 degrees and then maintained at that level as the arm is brought across the chest to the opposite shoulder, pain frequently results. This maneuver is called the impingement test and results from pressing the anterior portion of the rotator cuff under the anterior aspect of the acromion and the coracoclavicular ligament. The impingement syndrome or subacromial bursitis can be confirmed by injection of local anesthetic into the anterior subacromial area. Elimination of the pain confirms the diagnosis and is considered a confirmatory test for the impingement sign. Care must be taken to eliminate biceps tendinitis or acromioclavicular degenerative changes as either an independent diagnosis or an associated problem. Radiographs may be completely normal or may show anterior acromion and acromioclavicular spurs.

Rotator Cuff Tears

The rotator cuff tear classically presents with a sudden onset of pain while the person attempts to lift something. However, the pain can occur spontaneously without any significant repetitive traction on the cuff. Rarely does a true tear of the rotator cuff occur in a person younger than 40 to 45 years of age. An exception to this is the elite throwing athlete who may have articular-surface partial-thickness tears of the rotator cuff due to trauma. If the symptoms are ignored, an elite-level performer with long-standing rotator cuff tendinitis can progress through the three stages of the impingement syndrome to a true tear as early as age 35 years. The symptoms are similar to those of rotator cuff tendinitis. The physical examination is also similar to that of rotator cuff tendinitis. The supraspinatus muscle is tested by abducting the arm 90 degrees, bringing it 30 degrees forward, and internally rotating the thumb to point toward the floor. Elevation of the arm from this position has been shown to be almost exclusively done by the supraspinatus muscle. Classically, in this position the arm drops when a true tear of the rotator cuff exists (the so-called drop arm test).

Radiographic findings are variable but can include all the findings of rotator cuff tendinitis as well as greater tuberosity irregularity and cysts. Late findings in chronic rotator cuff tears show proximal migration of the humeral head (narrowing of the acromiohumeral space) and may progress to overt osteoarthritis (rotator cuff arthropathy). A positive arthrogram is the standard for the diagnosis of a rotator cuff tear. Magnetic resonance imaging is accurate for complete tears but less helpful for distinguishing between partial tears and true rotator cuff tendinitis. Only diagnostic arthroscopy allows complete evaluation of the whole joint.

A symptom complex also exists in which an unstable shoulder allows the humerus to sublux anteriorly and cause a true impingement syndrome. The subluxed humeral head rides forward and causes impingement of the rotator cuff underneath the curved acromion. Therefore, before a true impingement syndrome can be diagnosed, instability of the glenohumeral joint must be excluded.

Elbow Trauma

Dislocation can occur in any direction, but the most common is a posterolateral dislocation, in which the ulna and radius are dislocated posteriorly and laterally relative to the humerus. Dislocation can also occur with fractures of the radius or the olecranon. As the bones go laterally and posteriorly, the ulnar nerve may be injured. In severe injuries, the brachial artery can be traumatized. Care must be taken to differentiate between a true dislocation of the elbow and a fracture through the distal humerus, which externally appear very similar. Compartmental syndrome is an unusual but well-described complication of elbow dislocations. Serial circulation, motor, and sensation examinations must be performed for diagnosis.

Olecranon Fracture and Triceps Tendon Rupture

A fall on the "point" of the elbow can fracture the olecranon. This injury usually manifests as swelling and a palpable step-off in the olecranon. Triceps rupture without fracture can occur in activities such as weightlifting and, occasionally, in gymnastics. A cortisone injection for triceps tendinitis predisposes to tendon rupture and therefore should be avoided. The bony architecture is intact, and a defect can be palpated proximal to the olecranon. Of course, findings include antecubital pain, tenderness, and loss of active elbow extension. The biceps tendon can rupture distally from the bicipital tuberosity. Elbow flexion may be weakened. What is consistently weak, however, is supination of the forearm because the biceps is a significant forearm supinator. The individual may be able to flex the elbow but cannot drive in a screw. Frequently, the reason that patients present is an inability to open a doorknob or drive in a screw.

Wrist and Hand Injuries

As stated earlier, almost any fracture can occur in sporting activities. However, a complete discussion of all possibilities is beyond the scope of this article. Several fractures, however, are commonly associated with sports injuries. The hamate is one of the bones on the ulnar side of the wrist, in the proximal row. It can be injured under two circumstances. The classic situation is in a golf swing in which the club strikes the ground. The sudden deceleration is transmitted through the shaft, into the palm of the hand, and the hook of the hamate is fractured. This injury can also occur during the swing of a baseball bat in which the butt end of the bat strikes the hand or, even more rarely, a tennis racket. Examination shows grip weakness and tenderness directly over the hamate. Diagnosis is by a carpal tunnel–view radiograph or even a CT scan. Diagnosis requires a high index of suspicion, and treatment is surgical excision.

A mallet finger is an injury of the distal interphalangeal joint that results from a forced flexion injury. This injury typically occurs when a ball strikes the end of the finger and flexes the distal phalanx. The strength of the finger extension is exceeded, and the extensor tendon is either torn or detached from the distal phalanx, with a variably sized chip of bone. The net effect is a loss of the active extensor movement, and the distal phalanx droops but maintains full passive range of motion. The treatment is splinting, unless overt instability exists. Surgical treatment is rarely necessary.

A jersey finger results from the exact opposite mechanism and classically involves the fourth finger or, less commonly, the third. The mechanism is grasping for a jersey as the finger is pulled away from the flexed grasp into forced extension. An avulsion of the flexor digitorum profundus tendon, from the distal phalanx, results. The distal interphalangeal joint is held in full extension and cannot be actively flexed. A chip of bone may be avulsed. This chip can be seen on a radiograph at the decussation of the flexor digitorum sublimis tendon, at the level of the proximal phalanx. This particular combination of a flake, at this level, with the inability to actively flex the finger is classic. Treatment is early referral for surgical repair.

Gamekeeper's thumb is an acute avulsion or chronic stretching of the ulnar collateral ligament of the metacarpophalangeal joint of the thumb. The acute injury commonly occurs from a fall on a ski pole. The pole abducts the thumb and avulses the distal end of the collateral ligament. Diagnosis is confirmed by valgus stress, showing an unstable collateral ligament. Pinch is painful and weak. Stability should be tested at 30 degrees of flexion, as a false stability can be obtained if the thumb is tested in full extension. Sometimes, there are no radiologic findings. In a significant number of cases, however, the ligament is avulsed with a chip of bone from the distal side of the joint (from the proximal phalanx). This piece, visible on radiograph, is the so-called Stener lesion. The injury requires surgical repair because the collateral ligament is displaced superficial to the adductor aponeurosis and prevents the ligament from returning to its original attachment site whether or not there is a bone chip.

Dislocations of the proximal interphalangeal and distal interphalangeal joints are, of course, common and, unless there is an associated fracture, merely require closed reduction. Rarely are there neurologic difficulties. Closed reduction is usually successful. A special variation is a complex metacarpophalangeal dislocation. This injury most commonly involves the second metacarpophalangeal joint and is anatomically unique because the volar plate of the metacarpophalangeal joint is caught on the dorsum of the second metacarpal. The flexor tendons cross the volar aspect of the metacarpal neck and lock the dislocation. The proximal phalanx is almost parallel to the metacarpal in a "bayonet"-type position on the dorsum of the metacarpal. A characteristic "dimple" is noted on the volar aspect. A single attempt at reduction is reasonable. When a dimple exists and a single attempt at reduction is not successful, further attempts will probably be fruitless and referral to an orthopedic surgeon for surgical reduction is indicated.

Boxer's fracture is a fracture of the metacarpal neck, usually the fourth or fifth metacarpal. It results from striking a firm object with the fist. The metacarpal head is flexed and occasionally shortened, resulting in a decreased prominence of the knuckle involved. Treatment is almost always nonsurgical. If the metacarpophalangeal joint cannot be actively fully extended, surgical referral is appropriate.

Boutonnière deformity can occur as a complication of a simple dislocation of a proximal interphalangeal joint. The deformity results from avulsion of the central slip of the extensor tendon from the middle phalanx. The characteristic position is flexion of the proximal interphalangeal joint and hyperextension of the distal interphalangeal joints. This injury can be treated nonsurgically with splinting before contracture develops. A late deformity requires surgical treatment.

Subungual hematoma is a collection of blood that occurs underneath the fingernail. These hematomas appear as dark-blue or reddish spots and are usually exquisitely painful. Subungual hematoma sometimes occurs from a crush injury, but more commonly it is the result of a partial lifting of the nail. Sometimes, this injury accompanies underlying fractures of the distal phalanx. Pain results from the pressure. Release of the hematoma relieves the pressure and the pain.

Hip Injuries

A hip pointer is a subperiosteal hematoma along the iliac crest. This extremely painful injury occurs in football or hockey, when the hip pads displace and expose the crest to direct trauma. A palpable mass may or may not be present directly over the anterior crest, depending on the size. Side bending is painful. All hip pointers are locally tender and require only conservative treatment and padding for protection against repeated injury.

While unusual in sports, hip dislocation is one of the few true orthopedic emergencies. The femoral head dislocates posteriorly from a fall, such as in football, from a piece of gymnastic equipment, or from a horse. The hip is flexed, slightly internally rotated, and adducted. As the hip dislocates, the sciatic nerve may be stretched. Dislocation of the hip is a true orthopedic emergency. The hip must be reduced within 8 hours, or the chances of avascular necrosis, because of disruption of the vascular supply of the femoral head, are great. Immediate transfer of the patient to an orthopedic surgeon for reduction is imperative.

Myositis ossificans, a problem seen primarily in the thigh, occurs when a hematoma in the quadriceps muscle calcifies. A similar process can occur around the elbow, after an elbow dislocation. In the thigh, the classic mechanism is a direct blow to the thigh from a helmet, when a thigh pad shifts during football or hockey. The direct blow causes bleeding within the quadriceps muscle that initially is painful and swollen and ultimately calcifies. At first, radiographs are always negative; only after several weeks or months do they show calcium deposits. Initially, the diagnosis is based primarily on the history. Sometimes, the diagnosis is not obvious in long-standing cases and can even be confused with a neoplastic condition. Radiographs and MRI scans show a calcific density within the quadriceps muscle, usually anteriorly. Characteristically, the mass is detached from the shaft. However, such a finding is not universal. In some viewing planes, it is difficult to distinguish the mass from the femur. Sometimes, the margins are ill defined, especially in a relatively recent injury. This finding may make a differential diagnosis with sarcoma very difficult. Classically, the most histologically immature portion of the osseous metaplasia is in the center of the myositis ossificans, whereas the most immature osseous metaplasia is at the periphery of the sarcoma. Because the vascular invasion, and therefore the calcium, must come from the periphery of the hematoma toward the avascular center, the most mature osseous tissue is at the periphery of the myositis. Therefore, if biopsy is undertaken, proper labeling of the biopsy specimen with regard to site is critical.

Knee Injuries

Entire books have been written about the knee and knee injuries. Only the more common diagnostic tests and injuries can be discussed here. Knee injuries can be subclassified into ligament injuries, meniscal injuries, articular cartilage injuries, and synovial injuries. Meniscus tears are certainly numerically the most common. The menisci perform several functions, including contributing to the stability of the knee; increasing the contact area between the femur and the tibia, and therefore distributing the body weight over a larger area; and providing nutrition to the articular cartilage. The menisci can be injured in association with other structures, but most commonly meniscal injury occurs in an isolated pattern. One or both menisci can be torn from a twisting-type injury, usually on the flexed weight-bearing leg. While there is no single test or even a combination of tests whose results are consistently associated with a torn cartilage, several symptoms commonly occur. Effusions, buckling, locking, a sense of impending buckling, pain with prolonged standing, and the feeling of something moving inside of the knee are commonly reported. A torn meniscus is classically painful going down stairs and with squatting. Frequently, joint line tenderness occurs over the torn cartilage and an effusion is present. A twisting maneuver of the loaded knee can elicit a click or pain—a positive McMurray test. The patient may experience a loss of full extension, a "locked knee." An intra-articular injection of local anesthetic eliminates the pain. Differential diagnosis is difficult because many of these same signs and symptoms occur in other pathologic conditions, and these conditions respond to local anesthetic in the same way.

The most common ligament injury is a torn anterior cruciate ligament. The two cruciate ligaments crisscross within the intercondylar notch of the knee. The anterior cruciate ligament limits anterior translation of the tibia on the femur and restricts excessive tibial internal rotation. A common history is a twisting-type injury followed by a pop and effusion within 12 hours. An effusion that develops this rapidly is almost always secondary to intra-articular bleeding—a hemarthrosis. Only four structures can bleed in the knee: the bone, the meniscus, a cruciate ligament, and the synovium. It has been well shown that a knee with this three-symptom complex has a 95 per cent chance of surgical pathology, a 75 per cent chance of an anterior cruciate ligament tear, a 50 per cent chance of meniscus tear, and a 10 to 15 per cent chance of an osteochondral fracture or loose body. The 5 per cent of injuries that are not surgically significant are due to synovial injury and bleeding. Diagnosis of a torn anterior cruciate ligament is made by excessive anterior translation of the tibia, relative to the femur. The classic test is the anterior drawer test, in which the knee is flexed to 90 degrees and an anteriorly directed force is applied with the hands. The Lachman test is the same action performed at 30 degrees of flexion. All ligamentous instabilities are graded on a 3+ scale. Grade 1 laxity is common physiologically. Grade 2 is not even necessarily pathologic. Therefore, while the Lachman test is considered the more sensitive of the two, even a grade 2 finding on the Lachman test is not necessarily diagnostic of pathology. Any laxity must be compared to the opposite "normal" knee.

In the pivot-shift test, the lateral side of the joint is impacted, with stress applied laterally at the knee and medially at the ankle. The knee is extended, with the tibia internally rotated from approximately 45 degrees of flexion toward full extension. At approximately 30 degrees, the anterolateral tibia suddenly subluxes anteriorly relative to the femur, this subluxation causing what is described as a pivot-shift phenomenon. This test, which also has different degrees of severity, is considered the sine qua non of anterior cruciate ligament laxity. A physiologic pivot shift does exist in individuals with extremely lax ligaments, but such patients are exceedingly rare. The anterior cruciate ligament tear can exist as an isolated injury but commonly is associated with a torn meniscus. A Segond fracture (a chip from the anterolateral tibia) may be seen, but radiographs are otherwise useful only in excluding tibial plateau fractures or loose bodies.

The medial collateral ligament protects the knee from valgus forces. Valgus forces stretch the inner aspect and classically occur during a football tackle from the side. The diagnosis is confirmed by showing valgus laxity with the knee flexed at 30 degrees. If the forces are great enough, the medial collateral ligament is torn, the medial meniscus is torn, and finally the anterior cruciate ligament is torn. This combination of injuries is known as the "Terrible Triad of O'Donoghue."

The lateral collateral ligament tear is a rare isolated injury; however, it is devastating. It requires a varus stress. Force is applied to the inside of the knee, stretching the outside. The leg collapses to the outside and the opposite leg cannot protect the individual from falling. Diagnosis is confirmed by showing lateral laxity with the knee flexed at 30 degrees. This injury commonly occurs in association with a posterior cruciate ligament injury—posterolateral instability (see later).

The posterior cruciate ligament can be injured in several ways. Classically, the mechanism is a direct blow to the anterior aspect of the tibia, driving it posteriorly, relative to the femur. A direct blow to the anterior aspect of the knee or hyperextension of the knee can also cause a tear of the posterior cruciate ligament. Injury of the posterior cruciate ligament is diagnosed by a posterior drawer sign, which is the exact opposite of the anterior drawer sign. With the knee flexed at 90 degrees, the tibia can be pushed posteriorly. A combination of both cruciate injuries sometimes makes it very difficult to determine whether anteroposterior laxity represents an anterior drawer sign, a posterior drawer sign, or a combination of the two, because the neutral position cannot be well defined. Posterior cruciate and lateral collateral ligament injuries are commonly found in association. Posterolateral instability is characterized by an increase in varus stress and the so-called reverse-pivot shift, in which the lateral aspect of the tibia shifts posteriorly with the pivot-shift maneuver while it maintains external tibial rotation.

Knee dislocation usually results from severe trauma. Typically, both cruciates and the medial collateral ligament are torn. The presumptive diagnosis must sometimes be made based on the presence of severe medial collateral ligament instability, along with severe anteroposterior instability. Examination shows the tenderness and laxity consistent with the individual ligament injuries. Rarely does a hemarthrosis occur, because the capsule is torn and allows the blood to extravasate into the soft tissues. Radiographs show tibiofemoral displacement, which is an important diagnosis to make because there is commonly an associated posterior tibial artery injury. This injury must be diagnosed quickly, as complete obstruction can occur suddenly. The patient should be immediately referred to both an orthopedic and a vascular surgeon after any diagnosis of a true tibiofemoral knee dislocation is made.

Patella Injuries

Patellar instability has a very wide degree of variability in severity. The mildest form, the patellar malalignment syndrome, is not a true injury. A patellar subluxation can occur, usually from a twisting-type injury. This mechanism is the same as the one that may cause a torn meniscus. The tenderness is felt along the medial aspect of the patella—not along the joint line, as in a meniscus tear—and usually does not present with an effusion. If the patellar instability is great enough, a true dislocation results and the limb is physically incapable of support; the leg collapses. An acute hemarthrosis is common. Sometimes, the patella can be physically seen in its dislocated position. More commonly, the dislocation reduces spontaneously, this reduction making the diagnosis difficult. Pushing the patella laterally re-creates the instability. The patient feels this instability and involuntarily tightens the quadriceps mechanism to prevent movement. This maneuver is the so-called apprehension test.

Radiographs can help confirm the diagnosis by showing residual asymmetrical subluxation. Loose bodies can result and may be visible on radiograph if bone is involved. The incongruity caused by lateral displacement of the patella can cause sheer forces that knock off a piece of articular cartilage, with or without bone attached, and create the osteochondral or chondral fracture. The clinical manifestations of these loose bodies are pain, effusions, and true locking. In true locking, the knee is physically stuck and cannot be either flexed or extended. Locking must be differentiated from catching, which is a momentary "hang-up." Catching is like going over a speed bump with a car, whereas locking is like hitting a brick wall. Locking is a mechanical sign, as something is being caught within the joint and disrupting the normal kinematics. This disruption requires either a large torn meniscus or a large loose body. Free cartilage pieces can be knocked off and grow large enough in the synovial fluid to cause true locking. Long-standing loose bodies can become calcified and show up on radiograph, even though they began as pure cartilaginous loose bodies. Normally, loose bodies are not visible with simple radiography.

Patellar tendon rupture, an unusual injury, commonly is the end result of a chronic jumper's knee (see section on microtrauma that follows). The diagnosis is obvious from an inability to actively extend the knee, a palpable defect in the patellar tendon, and point tenderness at the distal pole of the patella. The patella is proximally displaced on the lateral radiograph. Sometimes, the quadriceps tendon ruptures from the proximal pole of the patella, but this finding is unusual. The signs and symptoms are identical to patellar tendon rupture except that the tenderness and defect are at the proximal pole of the patella and the position of the patella is normal on the lateral radiograph.

The medial synovial shelf (medial patellar plica) is a normal structure that stretches from midpatella along the medial and inferomedial aspect of the patella. A normal synovial fold, it is usually injured by a direct blow, becomes bruised, and thickens. Injury to this plica can cause all the symptoms of a torn meniscus, including swelling, buckling, locking, and snapping. Occasionally, the plica can be palpated, but this finding is not consistent. The diagnosis results purely from a high index of suspicion or diagnostic arthroscopy.

The fat pad syndrome is a somewhat controversial diagnosis. The fat pad, located directly behind the patellar tendon, is a normal structure. Just as in a medial synovial shelf, the fat pad can become contused from direct trauma to the anterior knee, swell, and create a physical impediment within the knee. No unique findings exist, and fat pad syndrome can present with all the common symptoms of buckling, locking, and, especially, pain with full knee extension. The diagnosis is made only when there is clinical suspicion or after diagnostic arthroscopy.

Chondral Fracture

Chondral fractures result from a fall on "hands and knees" or from a direct blow to the knee, such as with a blunt instrument. Under these circumstances, the articular cartilage does not tear as does a meniscus, but rather cracks like a windshield. The symptoms include any of those seen in a torn meniscus. Clinical diagnosis is by suspicion only. There may be tenderness of the articular cartilage of the medial or lateral femoral condyles. Magnetic resonance imaging, arthrograms, and CT scans are notoriously useless. Chondral fracture is a diagnosis made only with diagnostic arthroscopy.

Baker Cyst

A Baker cyst is the normal popliteal bursa filled with fluid. The bursa is normally empty. Whenever there is a source of fluid, be it torn meniscus, arthritis, or fracture, the popliteal bursa fills. This filled sack is known as the Baker cyst. It must be emphasized that the fluid is the result of some other problem. Aspiration of the cyst does *not* help unless the underlying pathology is also treated. The Baker cyst is slightly medial to the midline, larger at the end of the day, and less symptomatic and smaller in the morning. The patient frequently reports feeling a fist in the back of the knee at the end of the day. This symptom is, of course, associated with symptoms of the primary problem (e.g., a torn meniscus). A distended Baker cyst can stretch the tibial nerve and cause sciatialike pain radiating from the knee, down the posterior calf.

A unique problem exists when a Baker cyst ruptures. Synovial fluid in the soft tissue creates tremendous inflammation. The patient may present with a very swollen and tender calf. The classic description is "woody hard." This presentation creates significant difficulty with the differential diagnosis of thrombophlebitis. However, it has been the author's experience that if someone has a clinical diagnosis of thrombophlebitis and has any pre-existing knee problems, the more likely scenario is a ruptured Baker cyst. This diagnosis can be confirmed with negative studies for Doppler flow, or, more specifically, by injecting radioactive material into the knee and watching it extravasate down the posterior aspect of the calf. Arthrograms can also be performed, and the dye extravasation can be observed proceeding down the calf. The radiopaque dye tends to be even more irritating than the radionuclide and is not generally recommended.

A ganglion can be confused with a Baker cyst. A ganglion is rarely larger than 3 to 4 cm and occurs more anteriorly, and while it may vary in size, the size does not vary with the degree of knee effusion. A meniscus cyst, resulting from degeneration of the meniscus, is more commonly medial and usually does not vary in size. An MRI scan is useful for showing underlying degenerative changes in the meniscus. A ganglion should have no direct connection with the joint.

Tibia Trauma

Compartmental Syndrome

Fractures of the tibia are, of course, common in impact sports, such as football and lacrosse, but are beyond the scope of this article. A compartment syndrome begins when the tissue pressure is elevated above end capillary closing pressure. This process can be initiated by a tibia or fibula shaft fracture with postinjury swelling from trauma or, as discussed later, in a chronic overuse situation. With the capillary flow obstructed, the tissue pressure builds and causes edema from the anoxic muscle. Large-vessel venous outflow is obstructed, pressure ultimately builds further, and the muscle eventually undergoes necrosis. If the problem causing the elevated pressure persists, ultimately arterial inflow may cease and overt necrosis results. The "six P's" are the classic six signs: pain, pallor, paresthesia, poikilothermy, pulselessness, and paralysis. The pain, which is always present and usually the earliest sign, is characteristically unrelieved, even with narcotic analgesics. Pallor, a relatively late finding, usually is not seen except in advanced cases. Paresthesias are common but are not always present, and the clinician cannot rely on them in making the diagnosis. Theoretically, the sensory nerves are the earliest affected as the tiny arteriolar circulation is obstructed. However, clinically, paresthesia is a relatively late finding. Poikilothermy, a decrease in temperature due to obstructed blood flow, is a relatively late finding. The clinician certainly should not rely on it in formulating a diagnosis. Paralysis and pulselessness are extremely late findings and may never occur.

The diagnosis of compartmental syndrome depends on a high degree of suspicion and measuring compartment pressures early and frequently. Recommendations for surgical intervention vary, but most recommendations are for surgical decompression if there is a compartment pressure of 60 mm Hg or 30 mm Hg less than the diastolic blood pressure (whichever is lower). Great care in diagnosis must be taken in the hypotensive individual, as a true compartmental syndrome can develop at tissue pressures that would be unremarkable in the normotensive individual.

Plantaris Tendon Rupture

The plantaris is a very small muscle in the calf that in humans provides no significant function. Because it has a very long tendon, it is routinely used in hand surgery as a source of tendon grafts without loss of function. However, clinically plantaris tendon rupture presents a problem in differentiating between a gastrocnemius and an Achilles tendon rupture. The classic plantaris tendon rupture occurs in the fourth and fifth decades in an active person. The classic description is the tennis player who makes a sudden move and hears a pop or snap. Sometimes, the description is that of a gunshot, and the individual feels as if he or she has been shot in the leg. Severe pain occurs, frequently with difficulty in ambulation and swelling. In a few days, ecchymoses develop at the ankle. However, the tenderness is proximal in the muscle belly of the gastrocnemius, and the Achilles tendon itself is not tender and is clinically intact. Although painful, active plantar flexion is possible. The differential diagnosis is important, as a plantaris tendon rupture requires only supportive treatment.

Ankle Trauma

Sprains

A discussion of all the variations of fractures of the ankle is beyond the scope of this article. Sprains are, obviously, a very common problem within the sporting community. By far the most common is the lateral ankle sprain, in which the lateral ligaments are stretched. The typical grade 1 or 2 sprain requires only ice, support, and a graded exercise program. Recurrent sprains, however, are much more problematic. Several theories exist as to why an individual progresses to recurrent sprain. One theory is that normal proprioception is disrupted. The individual is unable to sense where the foot is in space, lands in a nonplantigrade position, and repetitively sprains the ankle. Another explanation is that the initial injury was, in fact, a grade 3 ligament sprain that healed in an elongated position.

Grade 3 sprains are diagnosed with the anterior drawer test, analogous to the same test in the knee. Lateral tenderness is always noted. Frequently, medial-sided tenderness results from mild injury to the deltoid ligaments as the talus tilts in the mortise. Rarely, medial tenderness is noted in grade 1 or 2 sprains. The normal anterior displacement of the talus on the tibia is less than 5 mm. The diagnosis of a third-degree sprain is also made by measuring the angle between the dorsal talar surface and the distal tibial surface on the anteroposterior radiograph. Normally, a difference of 6 degrees or less exists between the two sides. An absolute measurement of talar tilt of greater than 10 degrees on the injured side is also consistent with a grade 3 sprain. Several arguments exist in the orthopedic literature regarding primary surgical versus nonsurgical treatment. Referral to an orthopedic surgeon is the recommendation.

Peroneal Tendon

In an inversion sprain, the peroneal tendons can be stretched and either disrupted or completely torn. The diagnosis is made by noting tenderness along the peroneal tendons, usually as they pass directly behind the lateral malleolus. The findings include persistent pain, tenderness, and, occasionally, catching or even true locking. Diagnostic confirmation of peroneal tendon involvement is achieved with a local anesthetic injection into the tendon sheath. The peroneal tendons are held in their groove behind the lateral malleolus by the peroneal retinaculum. If this structure is disrupted, the tendons may sublux out of their normal track and sometimes can cause confusion with an ankle sprain diagnosis. Radiographs may show a flake of the distal fibula from the avulsed retinaculum. The tendons usually can be shown to sublux by asking the patient to actively evert and dorsiflex the foot against resistance. Under these circumstances, the tendons are felt to sublux around the lateral malleolus.

Achilles Tendon

Achilles tendon rupture classically involves the athlete in the fourth or fifth decade who is usually intermittent in pursuit of sporting activities. The typical history is a sudden movement, such as in basketball or tennis. The patient feels an acute rip or snap at the heel. The tendon is swollen and tender and usually has a palpable defect or thinned area. Sometimes, the tendon ruptures more proximally at the muscle-tendon junction. Such ruptures may not have a palpable defect.

The individual with an Achilles tendon rupture usually demonstrates that the injured side is dorsiflexed slightly relative to the resting position of the normal foot and ankle. The classic Thompson test is performed by having the patient lie on the stomach and examining the foot. The test is performed by squeezing the calf and noting whether the foot plantar-flexes. A positive test occurs when the calf is squeezed and the foot does not plantar-flex owing to disruption of the gastrocnemius-soleus mechanism. Orthopedic opinion differs on surgical versus nonsurgical treatment, but the individual should be referred for orthopedic evaluation.

Osteochondral Fractures and Osteochondritis Dissecans

Osteochondral fractures and osteochondritis dissecans also occur in the ankle, just as in the knee. Multiple arguments are found in the orthopedic literature about whether these conditions are separate entities. Trauma is clearly not a requirement. If they occur as a flake fracture off the dorsal lateral aspect of the talus, they are usually considered osteochondral fractures. Lateral ligament laxity and talar tilt allow the dorsolateral talus to impinge on the fibula. This impingement occurs after ankle fractures. It usually presents with pain and swelling, often with clicking. If the piece is completely displaced, true locking or buckling may occur. The medial-sided lesions are often called osteochondritis dissecans, although a significant percentage of these too are probably true osteochondral fractures from medial impaction at the time of talar tilt. They tend to be slightly more posterior. The best diagnostic confirmation is an MRI scan, which shows great detail and whether the piece is still attached, or whether the articular cartilage has been completely disrupted and the fragments are free. True loose bodies in the ankle do occur from purely cartilaginous chips but are relatively unusual.

Foot Trauma

Sesamoid Injuries

The sesamoid bone underneath the first metatarsophalangeal head can be fractured during a fall from a height, or with repetitive trauma, and create great pain in running. Treatment is usually conservative, although surgical excision is occasionally necessary in the intractable case. Fractures of the base of the fifth metatarsal are very commonly caused by avulsion fracture of the peroneus brevis from the base of the fifth metatarsal during an inversion injury. These fractures usually require only supportive therapy. A much more difficult fracture is the Jones fracture. This fracture, which is found at the junction of the diaphysis and metaphysis of the fifth metatarsal, can occur as either a true stress fracture or an acute traumatic fracture. In either case, healing is often prolonged and incomplete and presents great treatment problems. The clinical examination shows that the maximal point of tenderness is approximately 3 cm distal to the base of the fifth metatarsal. Standard cast treatment frequently fails. Treatment often includes electrostimulation and, sometimes, surgical intervention and bone grafting. Sesamoid injuries pose difficult treatment problems, and it is important to make an early diagnosis.

Turf toe (runner's toe) occurs from either a single episode or repetitive episodes of banging the toe on the playing field or from ill-fitting shoes. This injury can cause the same painful subungual hematoma as occurs in the hand. Eventually, the nail turns black and frequently sloughs. The individual may have to wear protective-toed shoes to avoid a recurrent problem.

MICROTRAUMA

Tendinitis

Tennis elbow and bowler's elbow are essentially identical problems occurring on opposite sides of the elbow. They are overuse injuries that result in tendinitis of the attachment of the common extensor origin (tennis elbow) on the lateral epicondyle of the humerus or the common flexor origin (bowler's elbow) on the medial epicondyle. The symptoms of tennis elbow are localized tenderness over the lateral epicondyle and pain with resisted wrist extension or supination. Tennis elbow occurs because the improperly trained tennis player attempts to use the wrist during the backhand stroke, instead of maintaining a rigid wrist and using the power of the shoulder for the stroke. The repetitive wrist motion, analogous to a badminton stroke, exceeds the muscular capabilities, and a tendinitis develops. In reality, the most common cause of tennis elbow is keyboard typing with the wrist extended.

Bowler's elbow presents with tenderness over the medial epicondyle and pain on resisted wrist flexion or pronation. Bowler's elbow derives its name from the inappropriate pronation seen when some bowlers try to incorrectly develop a large hook. By pronating the arm at the moment the ball is released, the bowler causes the ball to rotate in a counterclockwise direction. This maneuver is not the most efficient method of achieving this rotation, however. The repetitive motion causes a flexor overuse. This syndrome also results from repetitive weightlifting while the weightlifter is trying to develop either forearm or upper arm musculature. Bowler's elbow develops when a high-performance tennis player attempts to get that extra little bit of speed on his or her serve by snapping the wrist. Proverbially, the good tennis player gets bowler's elbow, whereas the poor tennis player gets tennis elbow.

Triceps tendinitis occurs from a repetitive throwing-type activity—either pitching or using a racquet. The tendon is tender just proximal to its insertion on the olecranon. Treatment is with anti-inflammatory medicine. Occasionally, the inflammation involves the cubital tunnel sympathetically, and ulnar nerve paresthesia results.

DeQuervain's disease is tendinitis of the short extensor and long abductor tendons of the thumb (the first extensor compartment) as they run through a fibrous tunnel on the subcutaneous border of the radius. Ulnar deviation of the wrist with the thumb held inside a clenched fist is very painful (Finkelstein's test). This injury is not associated with any specific sporting injury. In DeQuervain's disease, swelling occurs approximately 2 to 3 cm proximal and 1 cm dorsal to the point of maximal tenderness. At this point, the abductor pollicis brevis and extensor pollicis longus cross over the deeper long wrist extensors. The intersection syndrome is a tendinitis on the dorsum of the hand in the second extensor compartment.

The iliotibial band is a fascial band extending from the iliac crest to the tibia that can be involved at the hip but is actually more commonly involved at the knee. The iliotibial band syndrome is caused as the band rubs over the lateral femoral epicondyle with knee motion. The typical individual is a runner who runs the same path around the track day after day. Especially on a banked track, the involved limb will be the inside (downhill) leg. With the downhill limb weighted, a slight extra varus component is applied to the knee and the iliotibial band becomes stretched and irritated as the knee is repetitively flexed and extended. A localizable tenderness is noted over the lateral femoral epicondyle. The area of tenderness characteristically moves posteriorly relative to the condyle as the iliotibial band moves posteriorly with knee flexion. Extra-articular injection of local anesthetic at the tender point eliminates the pain and confirms the diagnosis.

Quadriceps tendinitis can occur from an increase in activity level in a relatively short period of time or even over a single particularly severe activity session. Examination shows tenderness only at the proximal pole of the patella. Patellar tendinitis (jumper's knee) is more commonly an overuse-type injury from running or repetitive jumping. Volleyball players, basketball players, and high and broad jumpers commonly suffer from it. This injury can also occur in the runner who runs up hills or stairs. The pathologic finding is point tenderness at the extreme distal pole of the patella. In its mildest form, patellar tendinitis may be painful only during running or jumping. As the symptoms progress in severity and duration, the individual may have pain with simple walking and, finally, even at rest. Catastrophic failure is possible. A patellar tendon rupture can occur with minimal trauma. A patellar tendon rupture in a young athletic individual almost always is the result of an untreated jumper's knee, rather than some sort of connective tissue disorder.

Popliteal tendinitis causes symptoms of pain on the posterolateral aspect of the knee. Posterolateral joint line tenderness may occur. More commonly, tenderness is found along the posteromedial and proximal tibia at the origin of the popliteal muscle. No effusion, buckling, or locking is seen, in contrast with a meniscus tear. Popliteal tendinitis commonly results from a sudden increase in running, especially downhill or on the "uphill" leg of a runner who habitually runs on a banked track. Both of these mechanisms cause increased internal rotation of the tibia and stress the popliteal tendon.

Pes anserinus tendinitis involves the three hamstring tendons (sartorius, gracilis, and semitendinous) along the anterior proximal medial tibial plateau. Examination shows local tenderness that is clearly distal to the joint line and sometimes with resisted knee flexion. Pes anserinus bursitis occurs in the bursa that lies under the pes anserinus tendons. Pes anserinus tendinitis and bursitis are eliminated by an injection of local anesthetic—but not by an intra-articular injection. The two cannot be distinguished on clinical grounds, but such distinction is unimportant because treatment is the same for both. Stress fractures almost never occur in such a proximal location.

Achilles tendinitis or paratenonitis results from repetitive jumping or running. The tendon is swollen and tender at its insertion to the calcaneus or for some 1 to 2 inches proximally. Crepitation may be present. A common clinical variation involves tendinitis at the musculotendinous junction. Such an injury is probably more aptly called a strain, rather than a true tendinitis. Peritenonitis, or tenosynovitis, also occurs. In this condition, the peritenon tissue is inflamed, but the tendon itself is not. Differentiation on clinical grounds alone is impossible, and an MRI scan must be obtained. With prolonged symptoms, the Achilles tendon may undergo central degeneration with necrosis, which ultimately calcifies, and a calcific tendinitis results. When calcification has occurred, the first radiographic changes are usually seen. An MRI scan can occasionally find subclinical deposits of calcium, not visualized on the standard radiograph. MRI scans are useful for determining the diagnosis of chronic, versus acute, Achilles tendinitis.

Most tendinitis of the foot results from running. However, these problems are certainly not limited to runners. A pes planus foot is a foot with a decreased arch. A pes cavus foot has an increased arch. A pes planus foot is hyperflexible and tends to have exaggerated motion. This foot "rolls over" more with repetitive weight bearing, as in running, and tends to cause increased stress on the posterior tibial tendons. The posterior tibial tendon's job is to support the longitudinal arch and control the normal pronation of the foot. Without intrinsic ligamentous support, the posterior tibial tendon may be overstressed, and a tendinitis results.

The anterior tibial tendon inserts slightly medially on the dorsum of the foot and controls the normal deceleration of the foot at foot strike. It can be overstressed in running and develop a tendinitis. Anterior tibial tendinitis exhibits local tenderness and swelling. Active dorsiflexion of the foot is painful.

Peroneal tendinitis has been discussed as part of ankle sprains. A pes cavus foot has a high arch that decreases foot shock absorption and tends to concentrate the forces in the metatarsals. This type of foot also tends to have an increased incidence of plantar fasciitis. Tendinitis can occur in the common toe extensors in swimmers. Repetitive plantar flexion during the flutter kick may cause irritation under the extensor retinaculum. Flexor hallucis longus tendinitis is a problem limited largely to professional and elite ballet dancers. This problem, due to repetitive en pointe work and jumps, is very disabling for a dancer. The tenderness is usually directly behind the medial malleolus. It may progress to triggering.

Bursitis

Subscapular bursitis involves a bursa occurring between the chest wall and the scapula. This injury presents with pain along the medial border of the scapula and, frequently, crepitation. Pain is sometimes elicited with a deep breath. Subscapular bursitis occurs primarily in throwing sports. The differential diagnosis must include pain radiating from the neck and a primary pulmonary problem. However, the pain is usually only with shoulder motion—not with a deep breath. Crepitation can sometimes be appreciated with scapular movement.

Olecranon bursitis can occur either traumatically, such as after a fall on the ground that causes bleeding into the bursa, or occasionally from repetitive weightlifting that produces pressure on the point of the elbow, as in doing arm curls. This bursitis is somewhat atypical in that it may be very large and yet produce very little pain. Wrestling or football can cause an abrasion over the olecranon bursa that can become infected, with a resultant septic bursitis.

Trochanteric bursitis can occur in runners from overuse as well as traumatically from falls on the ground, such as in football. The greater trochanter is tender, and sleeping on that side may be painful. The pain can radiate distally down the thigh and may be confused with lumbosacral radiculitis. Local anesthetic injections into the trochanteric bursa confirm and treat the diagnosis. The iliotibial band can also cause a painful snapping over the underlying greater trochanter. While bony abnormalities are sometimes the cause, significant irregularity is usually not present.

Ischial bursitis can result either from localized trauma from a fall or, more commonly, chronically from prolonged sitting, as in bicycling and rowing. The diagnosis is made by finding point tenderness over the ischial spines.

Prepatellar bursitis (housemaid's knee) usually results from a fall on the knee, such as in football and basketball. The bursal wall is traumatized, and the bursa fills with blood. Examination shows the fluid-filled bursa anterior to the patella. No effusion is present. If the skin is abraded, the blood can become infected and cause a septic bursitis.

A pump bump is a bony prominence of the posterior aspect of the calcaneus. The counter of the shoe pushes in on the posterior aspect of the Achilles tendon and presses the tendon against the underlying bony prominence. This pressure creates a painful tendinitis and/or bursitis at the Achilles insertion. The inflammation frequently aggravates the problem. Treatment consists primarily of protection and anti-inflammatory drugs or, in severe cases, surgical excision of the underlying prominence. The pre-Achilles bursa can be involved in bursitis, independent of the Achilles tendinitis, and such involvement is characterized by tenderness a fingerbreadth anterior to the Achilles tendon. The Achilles tendon itself is neither tender nor swollen.

Spine Trauma

While weightlifters and, especially, basketball players may have problems in the low back with degenerative and acute slipped disks, there is nothing unusual about their presentation. However, two spine problems are more specific to sports. Spondylolysis is a defect in the pars interarticularis (the portion of the vertebra between the facet joints). This injury is commonly seen in football linemen, gymnasts, and weightlifters as a result of high stresses on the lumbar spine. Spondylolysis represents a true stress fracture of this area. Diagnosis is by radiographs with oblique views or a bone scan. The bone scan is most accurate and can be supplemented with CT or MRI to determine the exact position of the defect and to exclude any associated disk problems. Acute treatment is usually bracing and activity modification.

Segmental spinal fragmentation arises from participation in elite-level gymnastics. Participation in high-intensity training by athletes younger than 8 years causes vertebral body end-plate failure from multiple small fractures. This injury is primarily a problem of elite-level gymnasts who started training before age 6 and who practice more than 4 to 6 hours per day; it usually does not present in the "club gymnast." The injuries result from repetitive dismounts and lumbosacral flexion-extension, causing repetitive axial loads. The thoracolumbar spine is most commonly involved. Because of the biologic plasticity of the juvenile skeleton, this condition can progress to end-plate failure, vertebral body deformity, spinal stenosis, and low back pain in the adolescent years.

Shoulder Trauma

Shoulder problems were discussed in the macrotrauma section. Sometimes, the distinction between macrotrauma and microtrauma blurs in the shoulder. As alluded to previously, a rotator cuff tear may be an acute injury or the result of a degenerative process. Refer to the earlier section for discussion of subacromial bursitis and impingement syndromes.

A peculiar disorder is seen primarily in weightlifters: the disappearing clavicle syndrome or traumatic osteolysis of the clavicle. In this condition, radiographs show an osteolysis and tapering of the distal inch of the clavicle. The syndrome is almost always unilateral. The weakness of abduction and tenderness are relatively mild, and the diagnosis can be made only with radiographs. Long thoracic nerve palsy is not well understood but may be a stretch neurapraxia of the long thoracic nerve to the serratus anterior muscle. Diagnosis is made by one-sided scapular winging. Scapular winging is best visualized with the person doing a "push-up" while leaning against the wall. The scapula is abnormally prominent in this position, as the primary purpose of the serratus anterior is to maintain the scapula against the chest wall.

Tennis Shoulder

Tennis shoulder is a drooping of the dominant shoulder without any other neurologic findings. This condition results from many years of aggressive playing and stretching out of the shoulder musculature (especially the trapezius). With tennis shoulder, the shoulder is stable, as the capsule itself is intact. However, the repetitive ball striking stretches the muscles around the shoulder. The shoulder droops as a result. The musculature is actually hypertrophied from use and is not atrophic.

Elbow Trauma

Cubital tunnel syndrome results from stenosis of the ulnar nerve as it passes through the cubital tunnel just posterior and distal to the medial humeral epicondyle. This condition can result from fibrosis secondary to acute or repetitive trauma, such as that seen in throwing athletes. A significant number occur idiopathically. Tenderness in this area can sometimes be confused with bowler's elbow. The characteristic findings do not include the tenderness, but rather the paresthesias and neurologic symptoms referred to the ulnar nerve distribution. Sensation is decreased in the fifth finger and the ulnar half of the fourth. Weakness may be noted in the ulnarly innervated musculature of the hand, and the patient may report dropping things or decreased coordination. Flexion of the elbow frequently aggravates the symptoms. Tinel's sign may be present. Electromyography confirms the diagnosis.

The pronator teres syndrome is secondary to median nerve impingement by the pronator teres muscle in the proximal forearm. The symptoms are differentiated from those of the more distally impinged carpal tunnel syndrome by the involvement of the median nerve branches to the long and short flexors of the hand and thumb, causing weakness and painful grip. Pain is felt in the proximal forearm or elbow area with activities. Phalen's test is negative. Tinel's test is negative at the wrist. Resisted pronation is painful. Therefore, the sensory disruption of the median nerve distribution with motor involvement of the long finger and thumb flexors suggests a proximal median nerve involvement. Electromyography confirms the diagnosis.

Wrist and Hand Trauma

Carpal tunnel syndrome is an impingement of the median nerve at the wrist. Impingement of the median nerve can rarely result after wrist fractures. This injury has not been associated with sports such as handball, in which obvious direct trauma occurs to the palm of the hand. Paresthesias and pain occur in the thumb, the second finger, the third finger, and the radial half of the fourth finger. The person commonly wakes up at 2 AM with pain. Pain is felt with prolonged wrist flexion (Phalen's test) and with percussion of the nerve (Tinel's test). Electromyography confirms the diagnosis. An electromyogram is negative approximately 10 to 15 per cent of the time.

Trigger finger is a problem in which a nodular thickening of the tendon gets caught within the tendon sheath tunnels, causing a partial restriction of motion and a snapping. The flexor muscles are stronger and can pull the tendon nodule into the pulleys of the tendon sheath, and the extensor muscles may or may not be strong enough to pull it out. Sometimes, manual extraction with the opposite hand is necessary. The nodule is palpable at the distal palmar flexion crease or into the case of the thumb in the metacarpophalangeal flexion crease. The diagnosis is made by the palpable snapping, local tenderness, and the palpation of a nodule that moves with excursion of the tendon.

The ulnar nerve lies just to the ulnar side of the hook of the hamate. Therefore, a fracture of the hook of the hamate, as outlined earlier, can also cause an ulnar nerve neurapraxia. Usually, this neurapraxia is not permanent and resolves with time. Pressure on the hand for prolonged periods, such as in bicycling on the "drops" of the handlebars, can cause ulnar nerve neurapraxia. The manifestations of this injury depend on the exact site of pressure—a sensory and/or a motor disruption is seen. Both can result if the common digital nerve is pinched prior to its decussation into two separate motor and sensory branches just proximal to Guyon's canal. The characteristic numbness of the fourth and fifth fingers results from sensory branch compression. If the motor branch is involved, the intrinsic muscles and the first dorsal interosseous muscle are also weakened. The individual is unable to actively abduct the second finger.

Hip Trauma

The piriformis muscle is the most superior of the small external rotator muscles applied to the posterior aspect of the proximal femur. The sciatic nerve exits the pelvis and goes underneath this muscle on its way down the leg. A tight piriformis muscle can pinch and irritate the sciatic nerve and cause true sciatica. The pain is poorly localized in the area of the buttocks, groin, coccyx, and/or ischium. Differential diagnosis between the back and the *piriformis syndrome* consists of a localized tenderness over the posterior aspect of the proximal femur, along with a totally normal low back examination. Hip internal rotation may aggravate the symptoms as the piriformis muscle is tightened over the sciatic nerve.

A stress fracture of the femoral neck occurs most commonly in runners who have dramatically increased their training mileage. Initially, the pain is deep in the groin and occurs only after a period of running. As the severity progresses, the pain may occur with any sort of weight bearing and, even, with walking. In its most severe form, just prior to total failure, walking without crutches may even be impossible. This injury has the potential to be extremely severe. Progression to true fracture is a medical emergency in these individuals. The femoral neck has a tenuous blood supply, and fracture can result in avascular necrosis of the femoral head even when the fracture is surgically repaired immediately. Radiographs should always be performed but are frequently initially negative. A bone scan and/or MRI is the definitive diagnostic test.

Osteitis pubis is a poorly understood problem resulting from an inflammation of the symphysis pubis secondary to repetitive shearing forces. Occurring more commonly in females, osteitis pubis is diagnosed by noting persistent pain in the midline over the symphysis pubis and, possibly, with radiation into the groin. Localized tenderness is felt directly over the symphysis pubis. The symptoms can usually be reproduced with hip abduction or adduction. Radiographs are frequently normal but may show at most a mild sclerotic pattern. Running and bicycling are the two most common sports that produce this injury. A bone scan will be positive.

Knee Trauma

Patellar "tracking" disorders are not technically injuries but are commonly aggravated by sports. As alluded to in the patellar dislocation section, the milder forms of patellar malalignment syndrome consist of the patella staying within the trochlear groove but being either abnormally tilted or partially subluxed through a portion of the range of motion. The net effect is a concentration of forces on the lateral facet of the patella that causes pain. Typical symptoms consist of pain with bent-knee sitting, squatting, kneeling, and going up stairs. It must be emphasized that the patellar tracking disorders are the great imitators of orthopedics and can present with almost any symptom.

Pseudolocking, pseudobuckling, crepitation, catching, locking, and effusions can also be manifestations of this syndrome. Several factors predispose to the problem. The female-to-male ratio is 9:1. In the so-called "miserable malalignment syndrome," anteverted femurs, externally rotated tibias, and pes planus all exaggerate the tendencies for lateral tracking. The "Q angle," the angle formed by the lines from the anterosuperior iliac spine, to the center of the patella, to the tibial tubercle, is normally 10 to 12 degrees in females and 7 to 8 degrees in males. This angle is commonly increased, creating a greater lateral vector force when the quadriceps muscle is tightened. Nonsurgical treatment is successful in more than 90 per cent of patients. Alterations of the normal anatomy of the patellar configurations and of the length of the patellar tendon can also predispose to these problems. Patella alta, in which the patellar tendon is more than 120 per cent of the length of the patella on lateral radiograph, predisposes to patellar instability and problems. Patella baja, in which the patellar tendon is less than 80 per cent of the length of the patella as seen on the lateral view, predisposes to abnormal compression syndromes and patellar tendinitis.

Breaststroker's knee is a problem found primarily in swimmers who do the breaststroke, in which the medial collateral ligament is stretched and irritated on a chronic basis. This problem is painful but otherwise is not serious.

Tibia Trauma

A stress fracture is a microscopic failure of bone. Stress fractures most commonly result from repetitive overuse at such a level that the body cannot repair itself in between workouts. The normal physiologic reserve is progressively compromised. Eventually, the site of the stress fracture becomes painful. Initially, the fracture is painful only with high-intensity activities. With time and progression, greater and greater amounts of bone are left unrepaired and the pain becomes prominent with simple activities. Rest will still diminish the pain. Ultimately, the injury can progress to such a point that the bone may even catastrophically fail and a "standard" fracture develops. Stress fractures are primarily a problem of runners but can occur in any repetitive impact sport. The tibia is most commonly involved and usually presents with tenderness over the medial subcutaneous border. The tenderness is very localized and may be associated with swelling in severe cases. The sites of tenderness should be distinguished from pes anserinus bursitis and hamstring tendinitis. The area of tenderness in a stress fracture is commonly in the middle third or at the junction of the middle and distal thirds of the tibial shaft. The fibula can also be involved, although much less commonly. Characteristic tenderness is usually found in the middle of the shaft. Radiographs are always negative initially; the periosteal reaction that is characteristic of the healing response frequently takes several weeks to develop. A bone scan is necessary for early diagnosis.

Shin splints, a "wastebasket" term no longer appropriate, was used to describe any pain in the calf or anterior tibia. It included things such as posteromedial stress syndrome, stress fractures, and tendinitis. This term has no place in current medical diagnosis.

The posteromedial stress syndrome is an inflammatory reaction, or periosteitis, due to repetitive overuse at the origin of the soleus muscles. This condition is distinct from a stress fracture, as there is never any compromise of the structural integrity of the tibia. However, the symptoms are somewhat similar. Localized tenderness is felt at the junction of the middle and proximal thirds, but it is on the posterior margin of the tibia, as opposed to the more typical anterior margin for a true tibial stress fracture. Bone scans show different characteristic patterns. The posteromedial stress syndrome has a longitudinal orientation to the increased uptake on the posterior aspect of the tibia. Stress fractures show a transverse orientation on the anterior aspect.

Chronic compartmental syndromes should be differentiated from acute compartmental syndrome. Chronic compartmental syndromes result primarily from high-mileage running, but they can occur in any sport. The patient reports an aching-type pain, which increases with activity. The pain can become so severe that it prevents activity. The pain is felt in the anterior tibia, is poorly localized, and usually resolves within 30 minutes after discontinuing the activity. In between episodes, there may not be any objective findings whatsoever. Baseline compartment pressures may or may not be elevated. However, they are dramatically elevated with exercise. A chronic compartmental syndrome is defined as baseline compartment pressures greater than 15 mm Hg or pressures remaining elevated above 30 mm Hg for more than 20 minutes after activity is discontinued. Chronic compartmental syndromes respond very well to surgical release.

Ankle Trauma

Anterior synovial impingement develops in individuals who are runners or football linemen or sometimes as the result of an ankle sprain. This injury can occur from repetitive foot dorsiflexion, from a synovial contusion, or as a result of the ankle sprain itself. The only findings are synovial impingement and swelling. In chronic cases, one may see an anterior spur off the distal tibia. Pain results from either the spur or the synovitis. However, pain is not a consistent finding. Occasionally, MRI is performed to exclude other associated problems. Intra-articular injection of local anesthetic confirms the location of the pathology. However, the only reliable diagnostic tool for anterior synovial impingement is arthroscopy.

Superficial nerve palsies can occur over the anterior ankle area from ill-fitting ski boots. The pressure results from the forward lean during skiing. Paresthesias extend from the ankle to the dorsal aspect of the toes. These can last for several days.

Foot Trauma

If the arch of the foot is the bow, the bowstring is the plantar fascia. Plantar fasciitis results from repetitive weight bearing, especially in the cavus foot. As the bow tries to flatten with weight bearing, the bowstring is stretched. One end is repetitively pulled and irritated. Theoretically, either end can be involved, but for practical purposes, only the end at the calcaneus insertion is involved. Plantar fasciitis is characterized by tenderness at the origin of the plantar fascia at the proximal end of the longitudinal arch. Tenderness is felt on toe walking, because this gait stresses the plantar fascia. Radiographs may or may not show a calcaneal spur. The spur is the result of the inflammation and is not the cause.

A difficult differential diagnosis is the fat pad syndrome. An inflammation of the fat pad of the heel, this syndrome occurs approximately 1 inch posterior to the origin of the plantar fascia. The fat pad performs a shock-absorbing function at heel strike. Repetitive running, or sometimes even a single trauma to the area, can induce swelling. A fat pad syndrome is painful with heel walking, but not with toe walking. Both of these syndromes have variable degrees of severity and may be painful only with running or after activity.

Tarsal tunnel syndrome can occur in a pes planus or hypermobile foot as the plantar branch of the posterior tibial nerve is repetitively stretched. Shoes can cause inflammation, resulting in scarring as the inflammation runs underneath the arch formed by the first abductor muscle. The diagnosis is confirmed by noting localized tenderness on the medial aspect of the talus and, frequently, burning dysesthesias on the plantar aspect of the heel. Tinel's sign may be positive. Electromyography can be positive, but it is not necessary for making the diagnosis. Injections of local anesthetic and cortisone eliminate the pain, confirm the diagnosis, and also treat the condition.

Like any other stress fracture, a calcaneus stress fracture results from repetitive running. The diagnosis is made by finding tenderness along the medial and/or lateral aspect of the calcaneus. The intensity of the symptoms varies, and the injury may be symptomatic only with running or, if it is severe, at rest. Definitive diagnosis frequently requires a bone scan. The medial tenderness from a stress fracture must be differentiated from that of tarsal tunnel syndrome. In tarsal tunnel syndrome, no comparable tenderness is felt on the lateral aspect of the calcaneus.

Navicula stress fractures have been, unfortunately, only relatively recently recognized. Professional basketball players such as Bill Walton and Michael Jordan have made this diagnosis famous. These injuries act like typical stress fractures and exhibit pain and local tenderness. They are notoriously difficult, if not impossible, to see on plain films and usually require a CT scan or bone scan for diagnosis.

Sinus tarsi syndrome is a chronic irritation, inflammation, and fibrosis of the area on the lateral side of the foot, approximately 1 cm anterior and 1 cm distal to the tip of the fibula. Sinus tarsi syndrome can occur after an ankle sprain. Fractures of the anterior process of the calcaneus are also found here and after a "simple" sprain. Fracture of the anterior process of the calcaneus is a diagnosis that can be made with simple radiography. The anterior process of the calcaneus is approximately 1 cm distal and 5 mm plantar to the point of tenderness on the sinus tarsi fracture.

Metatarsal stress fractures occur commonly in running with the pronated foot and are characteristically found in the middle of the shaft. The most commonly involved metatarsal is the second, followed by the third metatarsal. These fractures occur as a result of a large increase in mileage over a short period of time.

Sesamoiditis is inflammation involving the sesamoid bones on the plantar aspect of the first metatarsophalangeal joint. The sesamoids can even become fragmented and fracture from repetitive stress. Examination shows local tenderness and an inability to walk on tiptoes secondary to pain.

Hallux rigidus limitus is an idiopathic problem that frequently presents as unremitting pain and limited motion in the first metatarsophalangeal joint (hallux limitus). Eventually, large spurs form as the range of motion diminishes, and the metatarsophalangeal joint may be functionally fused (hallux rigidus). This problem can become significant in runners, as the toe cannot dorsiflex sufficiently to allow normal running. Radiographs taken early in the course may show squaring of the first metatarsal head before the spurs develop.

Köhler's disease is avascular necrosis of the tarsal navicula. This idiopathic process causes pain and must be differentiated from a stress fracture. Freiberg's infraction is osteochondrosis of the head of the second metatarsal bone, usually resulting from overuse. This injury causes localized pain and usually presents with tenderness localized to the second metatarsophalangeal joint, but relatively normal motion. The characteristic radiologic change is flattening and squaring of the metatarsal head.

Hallux valgus, a bunion, or tailor's bunion can cause running difficulties owing to difficulty in shoe fit. Hallux valgus, a deformity of the first toe deviating toward the second toe, tends to run in families. With shoe wear, the toe deviates further. Ultimately, an exostosis of the first metatarsal head results, and a formal bunion develops. An overlying factitious bursa may aggravate the apparent deformity. A bunion may result from an overly long second toe (Morton's foot). As the second toe is forced by shoe wear to the level of the first toe, the second toe flexes, resulting in a mallet toe or clawtoe. The gap formed by the deformity of the second toe allows the first toe to be pushed into this space, aggravating the natural tendency to hallux valgus. Tailor's bunion is a prominence of the lateral aspect of the fifth metatarsal, from persistent pressure. This name is derived from the bunion that resulted from the ancient tailor's habit of sitting cross-legged. Tailor's bunion is usually seen in skiers and skaters with a very wide foot, which makes the fitting of boots difficult.

Metatarsalgia, a nonspecific term somewhat analogous to shin splints, describes any source of pain on the plantar aspect of the foot and the metatarsal heads. The most common cause is a plantar-flexed second metatarsal, causing excessive pressure on the second, relative to the other metatarsals. Sprinters who use starting blocks (frequent hyperextension of the toes) and run on their toes are at increased risk. This type of running frequently results in a plantar callus and pain. Metatarsalgia must be differentiated from metatarsal stress fractures and Morton's neuroma.

Morton's neuroma is a thickening of the common digital nerve, between the metatarsal heads. The most common area is between the third and fourth toes, but any web space can be involved. The patient reports pain with shoe wear, which is relieved by removing the shoes. The pain is also aggravated by mediolateral compression of the foot and local pressure in the web space. The diagnosis is confirmed when local anesthetic injection eliminates the pain.

Posterior tibial tendon rupture usually results from a chronic tendinitis that has been ignored. The tendon may fail insidiously or catastrophically. Onset of unilateral pes planus is usually sudden. The foot also tends to be pronated and externally rotated slightly. When the foot is viewed from behind, more toes are seen on the injured side than on the uninjured side (the "too many toes sign"). The patient also has great difficulty in rising onto tiptoes because of the loss of medial support.

Fat pad atrophy is one of the conditions that should be considered in the differential diagnosis of metatarsalgia. The normal pads of fat over the plantar aspect of the metatarsal head simply seem to atrophy. This resultant reduced shock absorption results in pain. Fat pad atrophy is usually seen in the older runner.

PEDIATRICS

There are relatively few unique pediatric sports medicine injuries. However, several problems require special treatment because of the immature skeleton. Scheuermann's disease is apophysitis of the thoracic spine. An idiopathic phenomenon, this condition does not appear to be traumatic (as opposed to segmental spinal fragmentation) but is painful. Scheuermann's disease must be included in the differential diagnosis of adolescent back pain, especially in the elite gymnast, as discussed earlier.

Scoliosis is a side-to-side curvature of the spine. This condition does not produce tenderness and should not be used as an explanation for pain. A herniated nucleus pulposus is, of course, possible in the pediatric age group but is rarely the cause of back pain.

Spondylolysis (discussed earlier) can certainly occur in the adolescent age group. After simple muscular strain of the spine, spondylolysis is probably the most common cause of low back pain.

Shoulder Trauma

The author has already alluded to the extremely late closure of the medial epiphysis of the clavicle. The acromion has an epiphysis that is also very late in closing. This structure can remain as an unfused epiphysis, called a mesoacromion. This condition must be distinguished from fractures on radiographs taken for other purposes. It is not pathologic. True dislocations of the humeral joint can certainly occur in the adolescent age group. However, they must be differentiated from a Salter fracture of the proximal humerus. Clinically, the fractured humerus does not show the empty subacromial space of the dislocated shoulder. Usually, no tenderness is felt along the anterior glenohumeral joint line. The fracture has maximal tenderness approximately 2 to 3 inches distal to the acromion, an area that is not tender in a dislocation. Simple radiographs easily differentiate between the two problems.

Little league shoulder is a painful condition found in the throwing athlete with an open epiphysis of the proximal humerus. Repetitive stress causes a stress fracture of the epiphysis. Radiographs show widening of the epiphyseal plate, demineralization, accelerated growth, and even apparent fragmentation of the epiphysis itself.

When a true shoulder dislocation does occur in an adolescent, an extremely high chance of redislocation exists. Redislocation rates are dependent largely on the age at the initial dislocation. The chance of repeated dislocation in a first-time dislocation in a person older than 40 is, at most, 5 to 10 per cent. The chance of repeat dislocation in a person with a primary dislocation who is younger than 20 is 90 per cent or more. The treatment does not change, but the prognosis is much worse.

Little league elbow, or Panner's disease, occurs from repetitive stress on the immature skeleton. Medial overload, medial stretch, and valgus compression occur. A chronic inflammatory response may exist, owing to stretch on the medial aspect, and impaction forces on the lateral aspect of the elbow can result in cartilaginous damage. This inflammation can also progress to osteochondrosis of the capitellum (Panner's disease). Radiographs show a fragmentation of the capitellum (lateral aspect), the distal humerus, and sometimes even loose bodies in the elbow. Dislocations in the elbow are very unusual in the adolescent population, as Salter fractures usually predominate.

True hip dislocations are rare in the adolescent population, but they do occur. Because of the persistent growth left in the proximal femur, emergency reduction is even more important than in the adult. Despite immediate reduction, avascular necrosis still occurs in 10 per cent of cases. The longer the delay in reduction, the higher the chance of necrosis. The incidence of avascular necrosis climbs rapidly if the hip is left dislocated for more than 8 hours. Therefore, emergency transfer of the patient for orthopedic treatment is imperative.

Slipped capital femoral epiphysis (SCFE) is an unusual problem and usually is not related to sports, but it must be differentiated from a true dislocation. The femoral epiphysis slips posteriorly with little or no trauma. The child presents with the limb slightly flexed and externally rotated and resists internal rotation. The SCFE typically occurs in the 12- to 14-year-old male who may be somewhat developmentally delayed and is characteristically overweight. Unfortunately, an SCFE commonly presents only with limp and knee pain and no symptoms referable to the hip itself. Any adolescent presenting with knee pain should have a hip examination. An SCFE must be differentiated from a true femoral neck fracture, which although rare does occur. This fracture usually results from significant trauma, such as a motor vehicle accident, or occasionally from a football injury. Radiography distinguishes the two conditions.

Legg-Calvé-Perthe's disease (Perthe's disease) is not a sports-related injury, but an osteochondrosis of the proximal femur. This condition tends to occur in males younger than age 10 but can be found in the adolescent population. It can present as only knee pain. Legg-Calvé-Perthes disease is beyond the scope of this discussion, but it is mentioned to reiterate the importance of a good hip examination in any adolescent presenting with knee pain.

Many apophyses can be avulsed in the adolescent. These avulsions are apophyseal injuries—not epiphyseal injuries. The apophyses do not contribute to longitudinal growth and usually merely require supportive treatment. X-ray examination usually makes the diagnosis. The ischial apophysis can be avulsed in a fall, such as in football. The patient is tender over the weight-bearing ischial spines. Avulsion of the lesser trochanter is caused by the pull of the iliopsoas muscle during a football or soccer kick. Sudden deceleration while cutting or twisting or a football tackle may also cause it. The sartorius muscle may avulse the anterior superior iliac spine in young runners. The rectus femoris muscle may avulse the anterior inferior iliac spine.

Osgood-Schlatter disease, apophysitis of the tibial tubercle, is not truly an athletic injury but occurs in athletic individuals. This condition presents with localized pain, tenderness, and swelling of the tibial tubercle. It is aggravated by activities, such as sports. Radiographs may show fragmentation of the tubercle. Occasionally, a calcified nidus is seen in the tendon of older athletes. Sinding-Larsen disease, the pediatric equivalent of jumper's knee, has all the characteristics of the adult problem.

At one time, knee ligament injuries were thought to be exceedingly rare, as it was believed that the epiphyseal plate failed first and effectively protected the ligaments from injuries. This theory has now been disproved. True middle substance anterior cruciate ligament tears can occur in the adolescent. The medial collateral ligament attaches distal to the femoral epiphyseal plate and distal to the epiphyseal plate of the tibia. Therefore, the most common injury is a Salter fracture of the distal femur, rather than a ligament injury. True medial collateral ligament injuries have been reported, however. The diagnosis of fracture is made with stress radiographs, which show separation of the epiphyseal plate. One fracture that is commonly confused with anterior cruciate ligament injury is avulsion of the tibial apophysis. This fracture usually does not involve the attachment of the anterior cruciate ligament. Only severely displaced, large fractures involve the anterior cruciate ligament.

Sever's disease, osteochondrosis of the posterior aspect of the calcaneus, is similar to Osgood-Schlatter disease or

Sinding-Larsen disease. The individual is tender over the extreme posterior aspect of the heel. Sever's disease typically occurs in the athletic male 8 to 12 years of age. Radiographs may or may not show sclerosis and fragmentation of the apophysis. The syndrome is usually self-limited.

TRAUMA IN WOMEN

Female athletes are subject to all the problems found in male athletes. Although controversial, some evidence seems to support the theory that women may actually have a higher incidence of anterior cruciate ligament tears than do men who participate in the same sports. Much discussion has occurred about whether increased ligamentous laxity predisposes to injury, but no line of reasoning is universally accepted.

Breast contusions can result from sports such as field hockey or fast-pitch baseball. Nipple abrasions occur from jersey friction, especially in long-distance runners.

MISCELLANEOUS TRAUMA

Runner's diarrhea is a poorly understood problem that results in loose or frequent bowel movements after prolonged running. This condition normally responds to simple training alterations, with the athlete eating more than 2 hours before the time of exercise. The etiology is felt to be either increased parasympathetic tone or, more likely, relative bowel ischemia due to shunting of blood during heavy exercise.

Leg length discrepancy is not an injury resulting from sports. However, leg length discrepancies have been blamed for much back pain. It has been well shown that some three fourths of the population have a leg length discrepancy between 5 and 7 mm when critically measured. Moreover, a study has been done in which marathon runners who had never had a history of back pain were noted to have up to 1 inch of leg length discrepancy. They never realized that they had such a severe discrepancy. Therefore, back pain is rarely due to leg length discrepancies.

Heat disorders are due to impairment of the body's ability to control its core temperature. Most commonly, these conditions result from dehydration and poor conditioning with a compromise of the normal cooling mechanisms. This compromise is usually aggravated by the environmental factors of heat and high humidity. Sporting equipment, such as full football pads, may limit cooling by evaporation. Heat cramps present with muscle cramps, heavy sweating, and fatigue. The athlete's temperature is normal. Heat exhaustion is characterized by the patient's still maintaining a normal rectal core temperature of less than 40°C. The patient reports burning in the legs, extreme weakness, headaches, dizziness, rapid pulse, and profuse sweating with cool skin. A large orthostatic drop in blood pressure occurs, with a narrow pulse pressure. Heat stroke occurs when the body can no longer control its temperature. The body's core temperature rises, often to extreme levels, and rectal core temperature is greater than 41°C. The gait is staggering. The patient is often incoherent and can even lose consciousness. The body may actually stop sweating because of the severity of dehydration. The skin is hot and dry. A wide pulse pressure is noted, with a very low diastolic pressure. Heat exhaustion is a serious problem. Heat stroke is a potentially fatal problem if not aggressively treated.

Section Thirteen

CONNECTIVE TISSUE AND AUTOIMMUNE DISORDERS

RHEUMATOID ARTHRITIS

By John Baum, M.D.
Rochester, New York

DIAGNOSIS

Rheumatoid arthritis (RA) as a specific syndrome has become well established, if not always well defined. Over the years, various criteria for the diagnosis of RA have been used in different countries by different investigators or committees. Among the best were those devised by committees of the American Rheumatism Association (now the American College of Rheumatology [ACR]). The most clinically significant were the criteria of 1958 and the revised criteria of 1987 (Table 1). The latter criteria are simplified by omitting laboratory tests (other than analysis for rheumatoid factor) and by omitting microscopic evaluation of the synovial membrane and rheumatoid nodule.

The examining physician should always remember that criteria are helpful, but not absolute. If it looks like RA, feels like RA, and sounds like RA, it probably is, even if the criteria are not strictly met. The experienced clinician who encounters a patient with a 5-week history of arthritis at only two sites should never categorically reject the diagnosis of RA simply because the American College of Rheumatology criteria require arthritic signs and symptoms for more than 6 weeks at three or more sites.

Accurate diagnosis of RA requires recognition and documentation of the objective manifestations of the disorder. Joint pain is a subjectively reported symptom, whereas tenderness following pressure is a more objective sign because the examiner can assess the responses of multiple joints to varying degrees of pressure. Although not commonly observed in RA, erythema (redness) is also an objective sign of inflammation. Increased temperature (warmth) is another objective feature of inflammation that can be assessed in multiple joints. Joint swelling per se may or may not reflect inflammation. Effusions are frequently detected by palpation. The "patellar click" (felt by snapping the patella down through the fluid in which it is floating) is typically associated with the presence of at least 15 mL of synovial fluid. Larger effusions may fill the available space and prevent movement of the patella. Early in the course of RA, the range of motion of affected joints is restricted because of pain and swelling; later in the course, decreased range of motion is attributed to structural changes in the joints. Range of motion during the early stages may improve following treatment with nonsteroidal anti-inflammatory drugs.

Only 10 per cent of patients with RA who are seen by rheumatologists go into remission. At least 20 per cent of RA patients experience progressively erosive, deforming, and eventually crippling disease. Most patients with RA show progressive radiographic changes and declines in functional capacity. Ten years after diagnosis, more than half of all patients with RA will have measurable impairment that may result in a determination of partial or total disability.

Rheumatoid nodules are easily detected and virtually diagnostic of RA. These nodules typically appear 2 inches below the elbow on the extensor surface of the forearm, but can also be seen as "pump bumps" over the Achilles tendons. Although the rheumatoid nodule is a vasculitic lesion, it is not considered a marker of systemic vasculitis. Some clinicians perform a biopsy on these nodules to exclude gouty tophi, amyloid deposition, or keloid formation.

Rheumatoid nodules may appear early but are not typically seen until the disease process is well established. Thus, in most patients, the initial diagnosis is based on the history and physical examination of the joints. In RA, morning stiffness usually lasts for more than an hour. By contrast, in osteoarthritis, morning stiffness rarely exceeds 30 minutes. Patients with fibromyalgia typically emphasize back and neck stiffness rather than joint stiffness.

NONSPECIFIC FEATURES

Nonspecific features of chronic disease should be recorded early because their evolution can help the clinician gauge the progression of RA over time. Weight loss is seen in many chronic inflammatory and infectious disorders. In the patient with RA, persistent or increasing weight loss indicates poor control of the inflammatory process. By contrast, weight gain may indicate control or remission of disease.

Fatigue can be seen in RA patients with minimal or active joint disease. Scales are available for measuring the intensity and duration of fatigue, but for initial diagnosis it is sufficient to recognize its presence. Reduced fatigue is a sign of improvement. Increased duration and/or intensity of fatigue indicates that the inflammatory process has not been well controlled or suppressed.

EXTRA-ARTICULAR MANIFESTATIONS

Ischemic ulcers and peripheral neuropathy (mononeuritis multiplex), especially of the lower extremities, are well-known extra-articular manifestations of vasculitis in patients with RA. Mesenteric ischemia has also been described. Necrotizing vasculitis in RA is associated with male sex, erosive joint disease, rheumatoid nodules, decreased serum complement, circulating immune complexes, and high titers of rheumatoid factor.

Rheumatoid pulmonary disease is characterized by pleural effusions, fibrosing alveolitis, and nodules. In the heart, mitral valve lesions, conduction defects, and pericarditis have been documented, whereas in the skin, pyoderma gangrenosum, vasculitis, and palmar erythema have been reported. The patient with RA who complains of dry or

Table 1. The American Rheumatism Association 1987 Revised Criteria for the Classification of Rheumatoid Arthritis*

Criterion	Definition
1. Morning stiffness	Morning stiffness in and around the joints, lasting at least 1 hr before maximal improvement
2. Arthritis of three or more joint areas	At least three joint areas simultaneously have had soft tissue swelling or fluid (not bony overgrowth alone) observed by a physician. The 14 possible areas are right or left PIP, MCP, wrist, elbow, knee, ankle, and MTP joints.
3. Arthritis of hand joints	At least one area swollen (as defined above) in a wrist, MCP, or PIP joint
4. Symmetric arthritis	Simultaneous involvement of the same joint areas (as defined in criterion 2) on both sides of the body (bilateral involvement of PIPs, MCPs, or MTP joints is acceptable without absolute symmetry)
5. Rheumatoid nodules	Subcutaneous nodules, over bony prominences, or extensor surfaces, or in juxta-articular regions, observed by a physician
6. Serum rheumatoid factor	Demonstration of abnormal amounts of serum rheumatoid factor by a method for which the result has been positive in <5 per cent of normal control subjects
7. Radiographic changes	Radiographic changes typical of rheumatoid arthritis on posteroanterior hand and wrist radiographs, which must include erosions or unequivocal bony decalcification localized in or most marked adjacent to the involved joints (osteoarthritis changes alone do not qualify)

*For classification purposes, a patient shall be said to have rheumatoid arthritis if he or she has satisfied at least four of these seven criteria. Criteria 1 through 4 must have been present for a least 6 weeks. Patients with two clinical diagnoses are not excluded. Designation as classic, definite, or probable rheumatoid arthritis is *not* to be made.

PIP = proximal interphalangeal; MCP = metacarpophalangeal; MTP = metatarsophalangeal.

Modified from Arnett, F.C., Edworthy, S.M., Bloch, D.A., et al.: American College of Rheumatology 1987 Revised criteria for the classification of rheumatoid arthritis. Arthritis Rheum., 31:315, 1988, with permission.

gritty eyes may have Sjögren's (or sicca) syndrome, which is seen mostly in females late in the course of RA. Painful scleritis in RA may be accompanied by thinning and perforation of the sclera. Finally, the incidence of osteoporosis, depression, and infections is increased in patients with RA.

LABORATORY TESTS

Although the presence of rheumatoid factor in the serum can be used to confirm the diagnosis of RA, the clinician must understand the significant pitfalls and limitations of this test. For example, rheumatoid factor is detected in only 15 to 20 per cent of children (typically older girls) with polyarticular juvenile arthritis. Conversely, many older individuals with gout, septic arthritis, osteoarthritis, and other chronic illnesses have detectable rheumatoid factor and antinuclear antibody. However, when the titer of rheumatoid factor is 1:1280 or higher, RA is the most likely diagnosis, especially if clinical criteria are met. Importantly, titers do not predictably vary with the course of the disease or treatment. Some clinicians believe that high titers of rheumatoid factor correlate with the onset or intensity of vasculitis, but there is no consensus that titers can be used to assess the benefit of immunosuppressive therapy.

In 35 to 60 per cent of patients with RA, antinuclear antibody (ANA) can be detected in the serum. The titers do not correlate with the onset, intensity, or course of the disease. Moreover, titers of antinuclear antibody cannot be used to assess the impact of treatment.

Normocytic, normochromic anemia is common in patients with RA. If microcytosis is observed, iron deficiency should be excluded, especially in patients treated with nonsteroidal anti-inflammatory drugs that may cause gastric bleeding. Neutropenia is occasionally detected in RA; when neutropenia is accompanied by splenomegaly, the diagnosis of Felty's syndrome can be made. Thrombocytosis, increased serum alkaline phosphatase activity, and mild polyclonal hypergammaglobulinemia are also seen in RA.

The erythrocyte sedimentation rate (ESR) is increased in 90 per cent of RA patients. Early in the disease process, however, measurement of C-reactive protein may be an even more sensitive indicator of inflammation than is the erythrocyte sedimentation rate. Serum C-reactive protein concentrations may correlate with radiographic progression of RA; moreover, C-reactive protein concentrations may decrease in patients treated with immunosuppressive agents.

RADIOGRAPHIC STUDIES

Standard radiographs are not helpful in the first 6 months of the disease. Soft tissue swelling and mild periarticular osteoporosis may be the only abnormalities seen. With disease progression, other features become apparent. Narrowing of the joint space and marginal erosions are seen. Although most of these changes appear within 3 years of the onset of RA, the rate of radiologic deterioration, like the rate of clinical deterioration, is highly variable. Radiographs of the feet may be more sensitive than hand films in detecting changes secondary to RA. Magnetic resonance imaging (MRI) provides an even more sensitive method of identifying joint inflammation and cartilage destruction because soft tissue changes appear earlier than the bony abnormalities seen in standard radiographs. Some of the changes seen on MRI may be nonspecific. Current research is designed to improve the capacity of imaging techniques to distinguish synovial hypertrophy, capsular thickening, and fluid. Unfortunately, the cost of MRI currently prohibits its use for the routine evaluation of patients with RA. Joint scans can also provide evidence of inflammation, but the findings are too nonspecific for routine clinical use.

MEDICAL RECORDS

A drawing or stamp of the skeleton emphasizing the joints should be used to record each of the features of joint inflammation. Using a scale of 1 to 4, warmth, swelling, effusion, redness, and tenderness can be described at appropriate intervals. This record-keeping process can provide an overall estimate of joint activity and a basis for comparison with subsequent examinations. A visual analogue scale provides a rather more objective method of recording joint pain. A 10-cm line is anchored at one end by the word "none" and at the other end by the words "severest pain." After the patient marks the point on the line representing the degree of pain at the time of examination, the mark is overlaid with a 10-cm ruler and a numerical value is assigned. If used at each examination, this analogue scale can help the clinician monitor disease activity and assess response to treatment. Finally, the physician should define the total duration of morning stiffness by reviewing the patient's morning routine in excruciating detail.

DIFFERENTIAL DIAGNOSIS

Most other disorders that cause arthritis must be excluded. Acute rheumatic fever, Lyme disease, gonococcal arthritis, psoriatic arthritis, ankylosing spondylitis, gout, osteoarthritis, chondrocalcinosis, amyloidosis, and Whipple's disease can involve joints, and infection can be superimposed on a rheumatoid joint. During active joint inflammation in RA, the synovial fluid is cloudy and sterile and has reduced viscosity. The RA joint fluid typically has 3000 to 50,000 leukocytes/mm^3. Most of the cells are usually neutrophils, but occasionally lymphocytes and other mononuclear cells predominate. Crystals are not typically seen in RA joint fluids.

EPIDEMIOLOGY

In Europe and North America, the prevalence of RA ranges from 0.5 to 0.9 per cent. A 3:1 female-to-male ratio is frequently cited, but this gender distribution seems more characteristic of younger patients. In older patients, there is a tendency toward equal prevalence between the sexes. Women tend to be 5 years younger than men at the time of onset of RA.

PROGNOSIS

Some features of RA are associated with a poor prognosis (Table 2), whereas others correlate with a high risk of early mortality (Table 3).

CORRECT DIAGNOSIS

The presence of an inflamed joint and the detection of serum rheumatoid factor are not enough to support the diagnosis of RA. Several disorders can produce joint inflammation and circulating antibodies to altered gamma globulin. However, as the duration of active joint inflammation increases, and the number of involved joints increases, the certainty of the diagnosis of RA also increases. Although a correct diagnosis of RA can be made at the onset of disease, it is more likely to be correct after 6 weeks to 6 months of persistent signs and symptoms.

Table 2. Poor Prognostic Features in Rheumatoid Arthritis

Persistently increased erythrocyte sedimentation rate (or C-reactive protein concentrations)
Persistent high titers of rheumatoid factor
Reduced functional capacity after 1 yr of disease activity
Persistent anemia
Appearance of subcutaneous nodules

Table 3. High Risk of Early Mortality in Rheumatoid Arthritis

Many involved joints
Presence of cardiovascular disease
Poor functional status (can be seen after first year of disease)

FIBROMYALGIA

By George F. Duna, M.D.
Cleveland, Ohio

To effectively manage fibromyalgia, one must first establish the correct diagnosis. Confusing terminology (e.g., fibrositis, fibromyositis, diffuse myofascial pain syndrome, generalized soft tissue rheumatism) and the lack of uniform criteria for diagnosis have interfered with our understanding of fibromyalgia in the past. In 1990, the American College of Rheumatology (ACR) published criteria for the classification of fibromyalgia. This stimulated further research interest and resulted in enhanced recognition of the syndrome. Fibromyalgia now accounts for as many as 6 per cent of new patients seen in general medical clinics and 20 per cent of those evaluated in rheumatology centers. Its prevalence in the general population is about 2 per cent, with a female predominance (female-to-male ratio of 7:1).

DEFINITION

Fibromyalgia is a disorder of widespread pain characterized by the presence of typical tender points by digital palpation. Symptoms must have been present for at least 3 months. Widespread pain is defined as pain on both sides of the body, above and below the waist, including the axial skeleton. Pain on digital palpation (using $\approx$4 kg of pressure) defines the presence of a tender point. For the diagnosis of fibromyalgia, the ACR criteria require the presence of at least 11 tender points from a list of 18 suggested sites (9 on each side of the body) (Fig. 1). Finally, the presence of a second clinical disorder does not exclude the diagnosis of fibromyalgia.

PRESENTING SYMPTOMS

Pain Characteristics

Widespread pain is the most characteristic symptom of fibromyalgia. It is usually described as continuous, deep, and aching, with diffuse radiation. It is typically worse when patients assume a stationary position for a significant length of time (e.g., driving or performing desk duties). Although symptoms are less pronounced during physical activity, postexertional pain and fatigue are common.

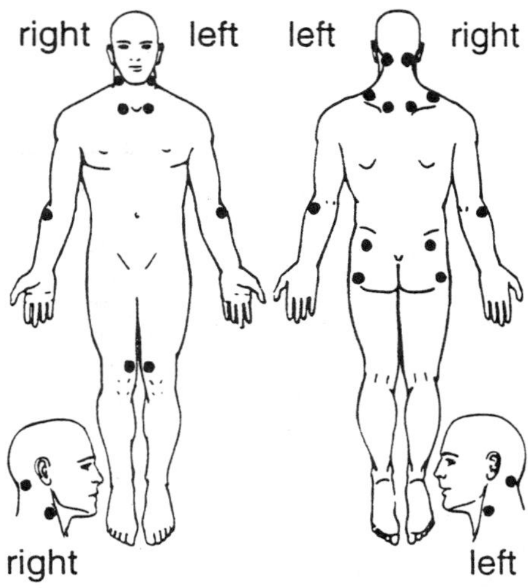

1. Occiput
2. Low cervical
3. Trapezius
4. Supraspinatus
5. Second rib
6. Lateral epicondyle
7. Gluteal
8. Greater trochanter
9. Knees

Figure 1. The sites of the 18 tender points of the 1990 ACR criteria for the classification of fibromyalgia.

Heat (e.g., a warm shower) provides temporary relief, whereas cold usually aggravates the condition. Other negative modulating factors may include humidity, noise, poor sleep, fatigue, stress, and anxiety (discussed further on). A reduction in pain thresholds results in an amplification process—that is, extensive and severe pain is perceived following relatively mild nocioceptive stimuli.

Associated Symptoms

Fatigue, stiffness, and sleep disturbances are reported by the majority (≥75 per cent) of patients with fibromyalgia. Fatigue is typically prominent after physical exertion and may further limit the patient's functional capacity. However, it is a nonspecific symptom and may be related to the presence of alternative or concurrent diagnoses. Moreover, fibromyalgia may be present in patients with chronic fatigue syndrome.

Morning stiffness (or stiffness following periods of inactivity) is often present and may be prolonged. This symptom may indeed suggest the presence of a systemic inflammatory condition (e.g., rheumatoid arthritis or polymyalgia rheumatica). However, making the distinction should be relatively easy because patients with fibromyalgia alone lack other specific features of inflammatory diseases (see discussion of differential diagnosis).

Sleep disturbances may include difficulty in falling asleep and frequent and/or early morning awakening. As a result, patients feel "unrefreshed" in the morning. More subtle abnormalities have also been detected during sleep studies, for example, "alpha-delta intrusion." When present, sleep disturbances may lead to further reduction in pain thresholds and pain amplification.

Other commonly reported symptoms include headaches (migraine or tension headaches), paresthesias, gastrointestinal complaints suggestive of irritable bowel syndrome, dysmenorrhea, urinary urgency, and sicca symptoms (e.g., dry eyes, dry mouth). Because of such symptoms, many patients may undergo extensive diagnostic evaluation prior to the recognition of fibromyalgia (e.g., brain scans, electromyography and nerve conduction studies, upper and lower gastrointestinal studies, repeated gynecologic examinations, pelvic ultrasound, and others).

PHYSICAL FINDINGS

Except for the presence of multiple tender points, the physical examination is usually unremarkable. Nonetheless, the clinician should always look for physical signs that may suggest associated conditions or alert one to the presence of alternative diagnoses (discussed further on). Although ACR criteria require the presence of at least 11 tender points, the diagnosis of fibromyalgia may still be made in individual patients with characteristic symptoms and fewer tender points.

LABORATORY FINDINGS

Fibromyalgia is a clinical diagnosis. There are no laboratory markers for the disease. In the absence of concurrent medical conditions, laboratory test results (e.g., complete blood counts, serum chemistry panels, muscle enzyme activity, thyroid function tests, urinalysis, and sedimentation rate, rheumatoid factor, and antinuclear antibody determinations) are expected to be normal. The extent of diagnostic testing in patients with suspected fibromyalgia should be guided by clues gathered during history taking and physical examination. Subjecting all patients to a random battery of tests is unlikely to be cost-effective. In the absence of specific symptoms or signs, ordering an "autoimmune panel" (e.g., rheumatoid factor, antinuclear antibody [ANA] profile, immunoglobulin concentrations, complement, and others) is particularly inappropriate. False-positive results are commonly encountered and may lead to further unnecessary tests and diagnostic confusion.

USEFUL TOOLS FOR EVALUATING PATIENTS WITH FIBROMYALGIA

The functional evaluation of patients with fibromyalgia is more useful than any form of laboratory testing. Self-assessment tools are preferred. Examples include sensory diagrams (Fig. 2), visual analogue scales for pain and general function (Fig. 3), and a self-administered Health Assessment Questionnaire (e.g., modified Health Assessment Questionnaire). Such functional measurements may be repeated at regular intervals and are invaluable in assessing response to therapy.

MEDICAL CONDITIONS ASSOCIATED WITH FIBROMYALGIA

Most patients with fibromyalgia have no other medical problems. Conversely, studies have suggested the associa-

Mark in the areas of your body where you now feel your typical pain. Include all affected areas. Use the appropriate symbols indicated below:

ACHE	>>>>	NUMBNESS	-----	PINS &	oooo	BURNING	xxxx	STABBING	////
	>>>>		-----	NEEDLES	oooo		xxxx		////
	>>>>		-----		oooo		xxxx		////

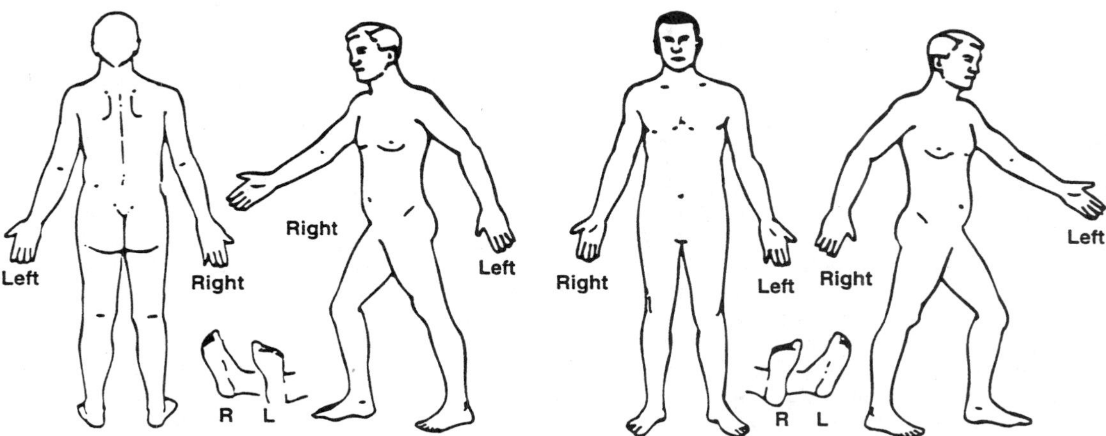

Figure 2. Sensory diagrams used in evaluating patients with fibromyalgia.

tion of fibromyalgia with a wide variety of conditions, including physical trauma, infections (e.g., human immunodeficiency virus [HIV], Lyme disease), connective tissue diseases (e.g., systemic lupus erythematosus, Sjögren's syndrome, rheumatoid arthritis), endocrine disorders (e.g., hypothyroidism), and others. The observed associations do not necessarily imply a causal relationship. Furthermore, the presence of fibromyalgia should not be equated with active associated disease. For example, patients with systemic lupus erythematosus may have fibromyalgia at a time when their lupus is clinically inactive. Escalating immunotherapy in such patients may be detrimental. Similarly, patients with Lyme disease may continue to have symptoms of fibromyalgia even in the absence of active infection. Further antibiotics therapy is unlikely to be effective.

Psychological factors have been extensively studied in patients with fibromyalgia. With the use of different instruments, various studies have documented an increased prevalence of active or past psychological abnormalities, including depression, anxiety, somatization, and a history of physical and/or sexual abuse. Nonetheless, most patients with fibromyalgia have a normal psychological status.

PITFALLS IN DIAGNOSIS

All that hurts is not fibromyalgia. When present, certain symptoms and signs should alert the clinician to the presence of alternative diagnoses. In patients older than 50 years of age, the presence of widespread pain should lead one to consider polymyalgia rheumatica (PMR) as a potential diagnosis. Pain and stiffness in the shoulder and hip girdles is characteristic of PMR. Pain may increase with movement of the affected joints owing to synovitis. Synovial swelling and tenderness may occasionally be present in peripheral joints as well (e.g., hands and wrists). PMR may be associated with temporal or giant cell arteritis (GCA) in as many as one third of patients. The following symptoms or signs may then be elicited: headaches, fever, visual disturbances, scalp tenderness, jaw or extremity claudication, neurologic deficits, and a tender or pulseless temporal artery. Suspicion of PMR or GCA should be promptly followed by diagnostic testing and therapeutic decisions to prevent the occurrence of ischemic events (e.g., stroke or blindness in GCA). Anemia, thrombocytosis, and an increased Westergren sedimentation rate and C-reactive protein concentration are the most commonly encountered laboratory abnormalities. Temporal artery biopsy may be considered.

Patients with fibromyalgia may complain of generalized "weakness" (i.e., fatigue). However, pain itself remains the dominant complaint. When weakness is prominent, a thorough neuromuscular examination is necessary for detecting neurologic deficits suggestive of other diagnoses. Proximal muscle weakness may indicate the presence of inflammatory muscle disease (e.g., polymyositis, dermato-

Please place an "X" on the line below indicating the level of your pain over the past two weeks:

None |——————————————————————| Severe

Considering all the ways that your illness affects you, rate how you are doing by placing an "X" on the line below:

Very well |——————————————————————| Very poor

Figure 3. Visual analogue scales for patients with fibromyalgia.

myositis). In such instances, muscle enzyme (creatine kinase, aldolase) activity should be determined, followed by electrophysiologic studies and/or muscle biopsy. Progressive weakness with exertion (fatigability) may suggest the presence of myasthenia gravis. Focal neurologic deficits should lead to the consideration of alternative diagnoses, for example, cerebrovascular disease, demyelinating conditions, peripheral neuropathy or neuritis, or somatization disorders. In the absence of neurologic symptoms or signs, specific laboratory testing and neuroimaging procedures are of extremely low yield.

COURSE OF DISEASE

Studies from tertiary referral centers have suggested that fibromyalgia is a chronic and unremitting disease: the majority of patients have persistent symptoms and continue to fulfill diagnostic criteria a few years after their initial evaluation. In contrast, a recent community-based study reported close to 25 per cent remission rates within 2 years. In addition, almost half the patients no longer fulfilled the diagnostic criteria. These observed differences are probably due to referral bias—that is, patients with refractory fibromyalgia of long-standing duration are likely to be referred to tertiary centers, whereas patients with less severe disease may not even seek medical care.

Although fibromyalgia does not lead to a progressive pathologic muscle condition, the chronic pain itself may be disabling. Work disability figures vary tremendously, depending on the country and social system. The impact of litigation and compensation (e.g., post-traumatic fibromyalgia) and coexistent psychological disorders on the ultimate prognosis of fibromyalgia remains unclear. Comprehensive pain management may improve the functional status of patients with fibromyalgia by encouraging physical activity rather than avoidance and work modification rather than unemployment.

ANKYLOSING SPONDYLITIS AND RELATED ARTHROPATHIES

By Robert M. Bennett, M.D.
Portland, Oregon

Ankylosing spondylitis (AS) is the prototype for a group of interrelated disorders collectively known as the spondyloarthropathies (SAs) (Table 1). These disorders are characterized by an inflammatory synovitis, persistently negative test results for rheumatoid factor, sacroiliac (SI) joint involvement, and several other commonalities (Table 2).

Table 1. The Spondyloarthropathies

Ankylosing spondylitis
Reactive arthritis (Reiter syndrome)
Psoriatic arthritis
Arthropathy of Crohn's disease
Arthropathy of ulcerative colitis

Table 2. Common Clinical Features of the Spondyloarthropathies

Asymmetrical arthritis in lower limbs	Skin and nail lesions*
Negative rheumatoid factor test results	Balanitis circinata
Sacroiliitis	Mucosal ulcers (gut, mouth, genitals)
Enthesopathy	Variable presence of HLA B27
Eye inflammation	Familial aggregation

*Skin lesions include psoriasis, keratoderma blennorrhagicum, pyoderma gangrenosum, erythema nodosum. Nail lesions include pitting, onycholysis, and thickening.

ANKYLOSING SPONDYLITIS

Ankylosing spondylitis predominantly afflicts young men. The essential two elements in diagnosis are (1) a history of inflammatory lower back pain and (2) the radiographic imaging of the SI joints. The only blood test result that may be of use is the finding of a moderately increased Westergren sedimentation rate. HLA B27 is present in 99 per cent of patients with AS, but it is also found in about 10 per cent of the normal white population and thus lacks specificity in the setting of exquisite sensitivity. The odds *against* an HLA B27–positive individual having AS are about 20 to 1. Uncritical use of HLA B27 testing accounts for many false diagnoses of AS in patients who have a mechanical cause for their lower back pain. A carefully taken history is essential for distinguishing inflammatory back pain from mechanical back pain. Inflammatory back pain is characterized by prominent stiffness on arising and after inactivity and improvement of pain with activity. In contradistinction, mechanical back pain is improved by rest and aggravated by activity. If the history suggests inflammatory back pain, a plain film of the pelvis should be obtained. The features of early sacroiliitis are pseudowidening of the SI joints (grade 2), blurring of the cortical margin on the iliac side, and erosions of the SI joints (grade 3). In advanced disease, the SI joints become progressively narrowed with marginal sclerosis (grade 4) and eventually fuse (grade 5). In patients with classic AS, these radiographic changes are symmetrically bilateral within the first year, whereas in some of the other related SAs, the changes are more likely to be asymmetrical. Problems commonly arise in the interpretation of SI joint changes in three situations: (1) in young individuals before the joints have fused (usually by age 20 years in 90 per cent of individuals); (2) in osteitis condensans ilii—sclerosis of the lower portion of the iliac side of the SI joints, which is sometimes associated with nonprogressive lower back pain (predominantly in women and often occurring post partum), and (3) in elderly persons with sclerosis of the joint margins and joint narrowing, which is a result of degenerative joint disease. This latter diagnosis is suggested by the finding of osteophytes projecting into the pelvis at the lower end of the SI joints. When interpretation of plain films is questionable, requesting a computed tomography (CT) scan of the SI joints is the most cost-effective way of resolving the issue.

The advanced stages of AS are usually self-evident. As the axial skeleton becomes progressively involved, a loss of mobility occurs first in the lumbar spine (in both the coronal and the sagittal planes) and later in the neck. Eventually, the patient may develop a distinctive stooped appearance with a forward thrust of the pelvis. A unilateral uveitis is the most common extra-articular manifestation of AS; rare problems include aortitis with aortic incompetence, conduction defects, apical lung fibrosis, and a cauda equina syndrome (sphincter dysfunction and sensory-motor findings in the lower limbs). The radiographic manifestations of spinal involvement are (in chronologic order) increased sclerosis at the inferior and superior margins of the vertebral bodies, squaring of the vertebral bodies, and syndesmophyte formation. Syndesmophytes are bony bridges that arise from the margins of the vertebrae and project upward or downward parallel to the axis of the spine. In contradistinction, the osteophytes of degenerative disease project almost at right angles to the spinal axis. Syndesmophyte formation is part of the specific inflammatory process that is a common denominator in the SAs, so-called enthesopathy. This term refers to an inflammation of attachments of ligaments to bone. Enthesopathy causes pain at ligamentous insertions; characteristic sites of such involvement are plantar fascia (heel pain), Achilles tendon (posterior heel pain), and hamstring origins from the pelvis (buttock pain). In the earliest stages, enthesopathies are radiologically transparent, but with chronicity they show up as "whiskery" new bone formation at the ligament-bone junction. In the most advanced stages of AS, the spinal ligaments become ossified, giving rise to the classic radiologic finding of a "bamboo spine." Several diagnostic sets have been proposed for standardizing the diagnosis of AS, the most commonly used criteria are the revised New York criteria (Table 3).

REACTIVE ARTHRITIS

The term reactive arthritis refers to an SA that is triggered by an antecedent infection. This term embraces the older concept of Reiter syndrome, which is somewhat restrictive because of the inclusion of conjunctivitis in the diagnostic criteria—conjunctivitis is a transient feature that is usually gone by the time the patient is first seen. Classic Reiter syndrome is more common in males (15:1 male-to-female predominance), but postdysenteric arthritis often has an equal sex ratio. The clinical syndrome commonly follows the infection after a lag of 1 to 4 weeks. The associated infections involve either the urogenital tract or the gut (Table 4).

The clinical clues to this diagnosis are a subacute asymmetrical oligoarthritis that predominantly involves the lower limbs and an enthesopathy; this usually causes heel pain (resulting from enthesitis of the Achilles or plantar fascia) or a sausage digit. Other useful diagnostic features are buccal ulcers (often painless), balanitis circinata (about 25 per cent of patients), keratoderma blennorrhagicum on the soles (about 15 per cent of patients); the latter resembles pustular psoriasis. In the early stages, there may be conjunctivitis; later there may be iridocyclitis. In a minority of patients, prominent systemic features occur, with high fevers and weight loss, raising concerns about septicemia and lymphoma. Other extra-articular problems are the same as in AS, except for erythema nodosum, which is a unique feature of *Yersinia*-associated disease. Lower back pain due to sacroiliitis is rarely an early complaint but becomes a problem later on in about 25 per cent of cases. Reactive arthritis is more common in human immunodeficiency virus (HIV)–positive individuals, who may have a particularly severe disease with prominent keratoderma blennorrhagicum. Approximately 85 per cent of patients with reactive arthritis are HLA B27–positive. The same caveats cited in regard to AS apply to using HLA B27 as a diagnostic test. The most useful finding is the demonstration of a recent infection with one of the known inciting organisms. The erythrocyte sedimentation rate (ESR) and white cell count are increased as expected in any subacute inflammatory state. Synovial fluid usually contains more than 10,000 cells/mm^3 (mainly neutrophils) and should be examined with Gram stain and culture to exclude infection. A common concern in patients with a history of urethritis is a gonococcal infection; in such patients, appropriate urethral, cervical, rectal, and pharyngeal cultures should be obtained. Occasionally, a dual infection occurs, and a reactive arthritis follows a treated case of disseminated gonococcal disease. Periostitis of the phalanges may be seen in severe cases of reactive arthritis. When sacroiliitis develops, it is often unilateral. Later, if the spine becomes involved, the distribution of syndesmophytes is asymmetrical, and they are more "bulky" than in classic AS. A chronic disease course with intermittent episodes of subacute attacks occurs in half of all patients; about 15 per cent of patients with classic Reiter syndrome develop a destructive arthritis.

Table 3. Revised New York Criteria for Ankylosis Spondylitis

Radiographic evidence of sacroiliitis
Either Bilateral involvement with grade 2 or greater *or*
Unilateral involvement with grade 3 or greater

plus
one of the following three features

History of inflammatory lower back pain for 3 mo or more
Reduced lumbar spine motion in sagittal and frontal planes
Reduced chest expansion for age and sex

Table 4. Infectious Agents Associated With Reactive Arthritis

Usual Pathogens	Less Common Pathogens
Chlamydia trachomatis	*Shigella sonnei*
Shigella flexneri	*Salmonella enteritidis* serotype *paratyphi B*
Shigella dysenteriae	*Salmonella enteritidis* serotype *paratyphi C*
Salmonella typhimurium	*Salmonella enteritidis* serotype *heidelberg*
Salmonella enteritidis	*Salmonella choleraesuis*
Yersinia enterocolitica 03	*Yersinia enterocolitica* 08
Yersinia enterocolitica 09	*Clostridium difficile*
Yersinia pseudotuberculosis	*Borrelia burgdorferi*
Campylobacter jejuni	

PSORIATIC ARTHRITIS

The association of arthritis with psoriasis is usually self-evident. The sex ratio is equal. As in reactive arthritis, infection with human immunodeficiency virus is an aggravating cofactor. There are two situations in which diagnostic problems may arise. First, the arthritis may antedate the skin disease; this occurs in about 15 per cent of cases. Second, the patient may have "subtle" psoriasis that is easily missed unless a thorough search is made. Locations where so-called hidden psoriasis occur are the scalp, natal cleft, and umbilicus. The nails are involved in about 70 per cent of patients with psoriatic arthritis with pitting, onycholysis, and thickening. Both the mild skin lesions and the nail changes can be confused with fungal infections, which should be excluded with scrapings. The arthritis associated with psoriasis is characteristically asymmetrical and oligoarticular; however, a polyarticular distribution is the most common presentation. In this respect psoriatic arthritis differs from the other SAs and may be mistaken for rheumatoid arthritis. One clinical feature, the sausage digit (resulting from a combination of arthritis and tenosynovitis of the adjacent flexor tendon) is a useful clue to the diagnosis of psoriatic arthritis. The persistence of negative test results for rheumatoid factor is another feature that should suggest a diagnosis of psoriatic arthritis in a patient with inflammatory polyarthritis. In patients with advanced disease, there are several radiographic features that distinguish psoriatic arthritis from rheumatoid arthritis, namely, preservation of bone density, pencil-and-cup deformities of interphalangeal joints, periarticular osteolysis, periostitis, and bony ankylosis. The SI joints are involved in about 20 per cent of patients with psoriatic arthritis. These patients are usually HLA B27–positive, whereas there is no distinct HLA association with the peripheral arthritis of PSA. The comments regarding the radiographic features of SI and spinal changes in reactive arthritis also apply to psoriatic arthritis.

ARTHRITIS OF INFLAMMATORY BOWEL DISEASE

Joint involvement in patients with inflammatory bowel disease (IBD) predominantly involves the knees, ankles, elbows, shoulders, and digits. The incidence of IBD sex is equal in both sexes. Peripheral arthritis occurs in about 10 per cent of patients with ulcerative colitis and 20 per cent of patients with Crohn's disease. It is usually oligoarticular (typically two to eight joints), asymmetrical, and intermittent. The arthritis is often subacute and may last a few weeks to several years. In general, attacks are related to the severity of the bowel disease and are more common in patients with extraintestinal complications. However, axial disease is unrelated to the activity of the IBD. Sacroiliitis develops in about 15 per cents of patients with IBD. In about 10 per cent of patients, the joint involvement antedates the symptomatic phase of the bowel disorder. Careful questioning of these patients usually elicits a history of mild intermittent diarrhea, which was considered irrelevant by the patient. A persistently increased erythrocyte sedimentation rate and/or a hypochromic anemia, even when the bowel disease is quiescent, is often a clue to subclinical IBD. In the setting of an unexplained seronegative arthritis, these features dictate the need for ileocolonoscopy and biopsy. The presence of HLA B27 is less common in IBD-related arthropathy (about 50 per cent). Unlike the other SAs, the radiographic changes in the SI joints and spine most resemble classic AS. Extra-articular complications include pyoderma gangrenosum, erythema nodosum, uveitis, stomatitis and, rarely, clubbing.

POLYMYALGIA RHEUMATICA AND GIANT CELL ARTERITIS

By Jo Ann Allen, M.D.,
and James E. Brick, M.D.
Morgantown, West Virginia

Polymyalgia rheumatica (PMR) and giant cell arteritis (GCA) are idiopathic disorders typically affecting persons older than 50 years of age. These conditions are usually discussed together because they are thought to be closely related, occurring in the same population of patients, having overlapping clinical features, and, in some cases, occurring in the same patient. Both have a mean age at onset of about 70 years, occur twice as often in women as in men, and are extremely rare in African Americans.

POLYMYALGIA RHEUMATICA

Polymyalgia rheumatica manifests as a clinical syndrome of aching pain in the neck and pelvic and shoulder girdles. It is classically associated with pronounced stiffness and an increased Westergren erythrocyte sedimentation rate (WESR). The onset of the arthralgias and myalgias may be insidious or abrupt. The shoulder girdle is the first to be involved in most patients. Occasionally, symptoms are unilateral at onset, involving one shoulder or hip, with gradual progression over several weeks to become bilateral. The pain is often severe enough to significantly interfere with the patient's ability to complete the activities of daily living. Constitutional symptoms, including anorexia, weight loss, low-grade fever, malaise, and fatigue, are common and may be the presenting symptoms. High fevers are not typical. Adhesive capsulitis of the shoulders and muscle atrophy from disuse may develop late in untreated disease. The weight loss and fever may raise suspicion of a malignant process. Depression may be present, clouding the clinical picture and leading to diagnostic delays.

The physical examination is remarkable for a paucity of abnormal findings. True muscle weakness is not present, but the muscle pain and tenderness may make resistive testing difficult to interpret. Range of motion may be limited by pain but is often normal.

The most characteristic and consistent laboratory abnormality is an increased WESR. Only a small number of patients have a WESR less than 40 mm per hour, and values greater than 100 mm per hour are frequently seen. Increased serum concentrations of other acute-phase reactants (C-reactive protein, α_2-globulins, and ferritin) are also seen. A mild to moderate normochromic anemia is common. Leukocyte and platelet counts are generally normal, although thrombocytosis may be seen. Serum alkaline phosphatase activity may be increased. Liver biopsy results are unremarkable. Serum creatine kinase concentrations are normal. Electromyography (EMG) and muscle biopsies, if performed, usually produce normal results. Synovial fluid analysis may reveal mild inflammation. Rheumatoid factor and antinuclear antibody test usually produce negative results. The diagnosis of PMR can be confirmed by a trial of low-dose prednisone (10 to 15 mg a day). Clinical improvement is often reported within 24 to 72 hours.

The WESR usually declines with decreasing symptoms. Efforts should be made to slowly taper the prednisone over months after a response occurs. Most patients with PMR must be treated for 18 to 24 months, although a sizable minority may require treatment longer or indefinitely. Patients should be monitored for the development of arteritic symptoms, such as headache, jaw claudication, and visual problems, because GCA may occur concomitantly with or subsequent to the development of PMR.

Some patients with classic symptoms of PMR go on to develop typical rheumatoid arthritis, with prominent peripheral joint swelling, nodules, erosive changes, and or a positive result on rheumatoid factor testing. Polymyositis can be distinguished from PMR by the presence of increased serum creatine kinase activity, proximal muscle weakness, and an abnormal electromyogram. Fibromyalgia is distinguished from PMR by a normal WESR and the classic tender points of that disorder. Chronic infections, including subacute bacterial endocarditis, can mimic PMR.

GIANT CELL ARTERITIS

Giant cell arteritis, also called temporal arteritis and cranial arteritis, is a vasculitis that most often involves the branches of the aortic arch. The inflammation is usually segmental. Forty to 60 per cent of patients with PMR develop GCA.

PMR may begin before, coincident with, or following the diagnosis of GCA. Presenting symptoms vary widely, but headache is most common, occurring in at least two thirds of patients. The characteristic headache is severe and located over the temporal areas. Scalp tenderness may be identified over the temporal or occipital arteries. Weight loss, anorexia, arthralgias, myalgias, and fever are frequent, as in PMR, and may be the presenting symptoms. Jaw claudication, or pain in the masseter muscle with chewing that resolves with rest, is produced by facial artery disease leading to ischemia.

Visual changes, which may be unilateral or bilateral, include blurred vision, partial field cuts, diplopia, amaurosis fugax, or complete and permanent blindness. These changes are usually caused by arteritis of branches of the ophthalmic or posterior ciliary arteries. Visual loss, once present, typically is not reversible. The most common neurologic manifestations are neuropathies (mononeuropathies and peripheral polyneuropathies), transient ischemic attacks, and strokes. Gangrene of an extremity, the scalp, or the tongue may occur if marked vascular narrowing occurs. Myocardial infarction, angina pectoris, congestive heart failure, sore throat, cough, and hoarseness may also occur.

Physical examination may reveal tenderness over one or both temporal arteries, erythematous or nodular scalp arteries, and/or decreased temporal artery pulses. In patients without visual symptoms, the ophthalmoscopic examination is usually normal. The early funduscopic changes in patients with loss of vision reflect ischemic optic neuritis with pallor of the disk, cotton-wool patches, and small hemorrhages. Optic atrophy follows with time. Bruits may be heard over the arteries of the head, neck, upper torso or arms, but are not specific to GCA in this age group.

As in PMR, laboratory studies reveal a characteristically increased WESR. Normochromic anemia and mild abnormalities of liver function tests are also seen. Tests for antinuclear antibody and rheumatoid factor typically produce negative results. Angiography, which is not usually recommended for diagnosis, reveals a segmental tapering stenosis without plaque of the medium-sized to large arteries, often involving the subclavian, axillary, or brachial arteries.

If the diagnosis of GCA is seriously considered, the patient should receive high-dose corticosteroid therapy (40 to 60 mg of prednisone daily). A temporal artery biopsy should be performed promptly. Temporal artery biopsy is not generally indicated in patients with signs of PMR alone. However, patients with PMR who experience temporal headache, visual change, jaw claudication, or tender temporal arteries should undergo temporal artery biopsy. A clinically abnormal or symptomatic portion of the artery should be selected for biopsy because of the patchy nature of the arterial involvement. If the temporal artery is clearly abnormal, only a small portion need be removed. In the absence of clinically apparent lesions, a longer segment (2 to 5 cm) should be obtained and examined. The entire surgical specimen should be sectioned serially. Biopsy of the contralateral side is recommended when there is a high index of suspicion and the first arterial biopsy does not show inflammation. As in PMR, the response to steroids should be dramatic, with prompt relief of the headache, fever, and other symptoms. As in PMR, steroids should be tapered slowly over many months; the patient should be monitored for recurrent symptoms and a rise in the WESR.

GCA may be more difficult to diagnose when temporal artery symptoms are absent. Fever, weight loss, and an increased WESR often suggests an underlying malignancy. GCA in the setting of a normal WESR or in persons 50 years of age or older requires a high index of suspicion based on clinical symptoms. Other forms of arteritis can generally be distinguished by the distribution of lesions, pathologic findings, patient population, and affected organs.

POLYMYOSITIS AND DERMATOMYOSITIS

By Ira N. Targoff, M.D.
Oklahoma City, Oklahoma

Polymyositis (PM) and dermatomyositis (DM) are types of idiopathic inflammatory myopathy (IIM) (Table 1). The predominant clinical manifestation of these conditions is muscle weakness, and the pathologic hallmark is muscle inflammation. The cause of IIMs is unknown. The three major types of IIM are PM, DM, and inclusion body myositis (IBM). Both PM and DM are described by the criteria of Bohan and Peter (Table 2). By definition, DM has an associated characteristic rash, but typical DM can be distinguished by important microscopic features as well. Neither PM nor IBM is associated with a rash, but IBM is clinically and histologically distinct from PM. Other forms of IIM occur rarely (see Table 1). Often, PM and DM are separated clinically into five classes: adult PM, adult DM, juvenile DM, PM or DM associated with malignancy, and PM or DM associated with other connective tissue diseases. Other IIMs are considered separately.

PRESENTATION

Polymyositis is more common than DM in adults in most studies (PM:DM, 1 to 2:1), while DM is much more common

Table 1. Clinical Classification of Idiopathic Inflammatory Myopathies

I. Polymyositis and Dermatomyositis (see Bohan, A., and Peter, J.B. N. Engl. J. Med., 292:344–447, 1975)
  A. Adult polymyositis
    Adults with no rash, malignancy, or diagnosed second CTD
  B. Adult dermatomyositis
    1. Adults with Gottron's papules, heliotrope, and/or erythematous-poikilodermatous lesions, but no malignancy or diagnosed second CTD
      a. Subclass: amyopathic dermatomyositis (Patients with cutaneous DM without myositis)
  C. Polymyositis or dermatomyositis with malignancy
    Adults with PM or DM who also have a malignancy, usually diagnosed within 2 years of each other
  D. Juvenile dermatomyositis (or polymyositis)
    Children (usually younger than 16 years) with PM or DM; usually DM
  E. Overlap syndrome of polymyositis or dermatomyositis with another connective tissue disease
    Patients with PM or DM who also satisfy criteria for a second CTD; usually lupus, scleroderma, rheumatoid arthritis, or Sjögren's syndrome; Raynaud's syndrome, arthritis, or interstitial lung disease alone would not qualify
II. Inclusion Body Myositis
  Patients who satisfy the criteria of Calabrese and Chou (Rheum. Dis. Clin. North Am., 20:955–972, 1994)
III. Rare Forms
  A. Granulomatous myositis
  B. Eosinophilic myositis
  C. Focal myositis
  D. Orbital myositis

CTD = connective tissue disease; DM = dermatomyositis; PM = polymyositis.

(20:1) in children. The peak incidence of PM and DM occurs in the 40 to 60 age group, with a smaller peak in childhood. In adults, the female-to-male ratio is approximately 2:1 overall, higher in childbearing years, and higher with connective tissue disease (CTD) features or overlap. Although PM and DM occur in only 5 to 10 per million population per year, the IIMs are the most common idiopathic acquired myopathies and thus should be considered in any patient with new-onset muscle weakness. Early recognition of PM or DM is vital because those patients who experience prolonged delay from the onset of symptoms to the start of treatment have a decreased likelihood of full recovery.

Myositis

Symptoms

The typical clinical problem in PM and DM is symmetrical proximal muscle weakness. Lower extremity weakness may lead to difficulty in walking up stairs, standing up from a chair without pushing up with the arms, or disturbance of gait. Upper extremity involvement can cause difficulty in reaching or working with the arms over the head. Neck weakness may cause difficulty in raising the head from the bed, and paraspinal and trunk weakness may impair the ability to sit up or turn in bed. The pharyngeal and upper esophageal muscles may be involved, with resultant dysphagia, nasal regurgitation, and risk of aspiration. Some patients may have respiratory muscle weakness, with respiratory compromise in severe cases. Facial weakness and extraocular muscle dysfunction are rare and should suggest myasthenia gravis. Muscle aches and pains may occur in as many as 50 per cent of these patients; pain is occasionally severe and predominant, but weakness is usually the main problem. A family history of myopathy may be important; it suggests dystrophy or other muscle disease because familial PM and DM are quite rare.

Course

Most patients with PM and DM have a subacute onset, over weeks to months. Dermatomyositis tends to develop more rapidly than PM. Acute onset over days is unusual. A chronic, slow onset with gradual progression over years is also unusual, and IBM should be considered in such cases. Lower extremity weakness often occurs first, but usually weakness also involves the upper extremity.

Examination

Muscle strength is assessed by manual testing and by observing activities. The patient should be observed while walking, standing up from a chair without using the arms, stepping up, sitting up from supine, and raising the head or raising the legs off the examining table. More subtle weakness may be revealed by having the patient squat or stand up from the floor or walk up a flight of stairs. Timing by the clinician of the patient repeatedly standing up from a chair or holding the head or legs off the table can provide quantitation. The patient exerting strength against the examiner's manual resistance should also be assessed in extremity muscle groups; in PM and DM, the hip, shoulder, thigh, and upper arm muscles are typically more affected than the grip, or lower arm and leg muscles. Mechanical devices have been used to measure muscle strength and to

Table 2. Diagnosis of Polymyositis and Dermatomyositis

I. Criteria: 3 criteria = probable PM or DM; 4 criteria = definite PM or DM. (Bohan, A., and Peter, J.B. N. Engl. J. Med. 292:344–447, 1975)
  1. Thyroid disease, HIV and HTLV-1 infection, and drug-induced myopathy should be excluded, and Table 4 considered. Excluding other conditions is most important in PM without MSA.
  2. Symmetrical proximal muscle weakness
  3. Increased activity of serum muscle enzymes
  4. Electromyographic findings typical of polymyositis or dermatomyositis
     Myopathic potentials with increased spontaneous activity (fibrillations, positive sharp waves, and/or complex repetitive discharges). Myopathic recruitment pattern and increased insertional activity also seen.
  5. Muscle biopsy findings typical of polymyositis or dermatomyositis
     Inflammation with necrosis, phagocytosis, and regeneration. Perifascicular atrophy is characteristic of dermatomyositis but not required for diagnosis.
  6. Dermatologic features of dermatomyositis
     Gottron's papules or sign and/or heliotrope sign. Erythematous and/or poikilodermatous rash, nail fold capillary changes, and calcinosis would support diagnosis but do not qualify as criteria.
II. Additional Suggestions
  1. Myositis-specific autoantibodies (see Table 3) could serve as an additional criterion in the same framework.
  2. If the above studies fail to establish PM or DM, but these conditions are still suspected, magnetic resonance imaging (MRI) may be helpful. Areas of increased intensity on T2-weighted images would suggest inflammatory myopathy and can be used to direct a biopsy.
  3. Positive ANA or positive MRI can support the diagnosis but cannot establish it.

follow individual patients over time. Atrophy may be present, typically later in the course. Weakness of the muscles of a region is seen, rather than isolated involvement of individual muscles. PM and DM are not associated with sensory or neuropathic changes.

Skin Lesions

The identifying cutaneous features of DM are Gottron's papules or sign, the heliotrope sign, and the erythematous-poikilodermatous rash. Gottron's papules are raised, erythematous or violaceous, often scaly lesions that typically occur over the metacarpophalangeal and interphalangeal joints. The term Gottron's sign refers to similar lesions that are macular and may include lesions over the knees, elbows, and other extensor surfaces. Gottron's lesions are among the most common (70 to 80 per cent of DM) and most specific manifestations of DM. The heliotrope, a violaceous suffusion around the eyes, is often accompanied by periorbital edema. A similar change is occasionally seen in patients with trichinosis or allergies, but the presence of heliotrope strongly suggests DM, especially in association with Gottron's lesions. Although erythematous or violaceous rash may involve almost any area in DM, the upper back, shoulders, base of the neck ("shawl" pattern), "V" of the neck, extremities, hands, and scalp are most frequently affected. Alopecia may be noted with scalp involvement. Photosensitive induction or exacerbation of the rash is common. Poikiloderma, a pattern of varying hypopigmentation and hyperpigmentation with atrophy and telangiectasia, also commonly develops.

Other findings are supportive, but not specific. Nailfold capillary changes are common, including dilatation, telangiectasia, and capillary loss similar to that seen in scleroderma. Children, and rarely adults, may develop cutaneous ulcers. Cuticular overgrowth may cause a thick, rough appearance. Calcinosis may occur, usually later in the course, more commonly in children, but occasionally in adults. Calcinosis appears as plaques or as nodules in the skin or subcutaneous tissue (calcinosis circumscripta). Calcinosis may also extend along fascial planes or extensive subcutaneous deposits (calcinosis universalis). Deposits may become inflamed, and may ulcerate and drain. A skin lesion termed "mechanic's hands" has also been associated with myositis, with or without DM features, more often with certain autoantibodies. "Mechanic's hands" refers to hyperkeratosis, scaling, and fissuring along the edges of the fingers, giving the appearance of "dirty" lines resembling changes from heavy work with the hands. Signs of overlapping connective tissue disorders (CTDs) may also be observed.

Course

The rash and muscle disease usually occur within weeks or a few months of each other, but the rash more commonly occurs first. Occasionally, the delay in onset of weakness is more prolonged. When the delay is more than 2 years, the condition is considered amyopathic DM (or DM sine myositis).

Other Clinical Manifestations and Complications

Fever can occur during exacerbations of myositis, and this fever must be distinguished from that caused by infection. Fatigue, malaise, and weight loss are common. Features of CTD may occur, including Raynaud's phenomenon, puffy edematous fingers, and arthritis. Overt overlap with lupus, scleroderma, rheumatoid arthritis, and Sjögren's syndrome has been reported.

Interstitial lung disease due to PM and DM is similar to that seen with other CTDs and is found in 10 to 30 per cent of PM/DM patients overall. Pulmonary fibrosis may be seen on chest film or high-resolution computed tomography (CT), but in early stages, it may be detected only as pulmonary function abnormalities, with a restrictive defect, decreased lung diffusing capacity for carbon monoxide, and hypoxemia with exercise. Pulmonary fibrosis may be asymptomatic but can be progressive or fulminant, and may contribute to mortality. The severity of the interstitial lung disease is independent of the myositis and can precede it. Interstitial lung disease must be distinguished from opportunistic infections due to immunosuppressive treatments and from hypersensitivity pneumonitis caused by methotrexate.

Respiratory compromise may be caused by respiratory muscle weakness (e.g., diaphragm, intercostals) in a small proportion of patients and may require mechanical ventilation. Measurement of peak flow or inspiratory pressure may be used to assess respiratory muscle strength. Respiratory weakness is potentially fatal but usually responds to treatment of the myositis. Muscle weakness, with impaired cough, dysphagia, and difficulty in turning in bed, may also predispose to aspiration.

Cardiac abnormalities can be demonstrated in one half to three quarters of PM and DM patients. Most common are conduction disturbances (fascicular block, bundle branch block, and, occasionally, advanced heart block), arrhythmias (extrasystoles, tachyarrhythmias), and, less often, myocarditis with congestive heart failure. Patients with palpitations or abnormal electrocardiograms should have Holter monitoring. Pericarditis should raise the suspicion of an overlap syndrome with another connective tissue disease.

Dysphagia is the most common gastrointestinal manifestation and, occasionally, is the presenting symptom. It usually results from pharyngeal muscle weakness and usually responds to treatment of the myositis. Sometimes, fibrosis of the cricopharyngeus causes dysphagia, requiring myotomy. Vascular disease in the intestine may lead to perforation in children, but this complication is quite rare in adults.

Association With Malignancy

Malignant tumors are detected in approximately 15 per cent and 10 per cent of DM and PM patients, respectively. The cancer may precede, be concurrent with, or follow the DM. The nature of the association is not established, but 20 per cent of DM patients with malignancy show a "paraneoplastic" course, in which the conditions appear linked. For example, DM may worsen with recurrence of malignancy or may resist treatment until the malignancy is resected. The risk of malignancy in amyopathic DM seems to be at least as high as that in the usual form of DM. The most common tumors are those of the lung and breast, but there is an increase in the proportion of ovarian cancer. Many ovarian cancers in DM patients have been occult and difficult to treat.

USEFUL LABORATORY PROCEDURES

Muscle Markers

Most patients with active PM or DM have increased serum activity of muscle-associated enzymes. Creatinine kinase (CK) is the most useful enzyme because of its high sensitivity (increased in 70 to 90 per cent on presentation), its relative muscle specificity, its degree of increase (often 50- to 100-fold normal), and the correlation with disease activity over time. Increases in CK activity can predict a disease flare, with increases occurring 6 weeks or more before muscle weakness. Normalization with treatment usually indicates a response. Increases in CK activity may occur in various conditions associated with muscle necrosis, including trauma, strenuous physical activity, intramuscular injections, certain drugs, viral infections, and hypothyroidism. The reference range for CK activity is higher in blacks than in whites and in men than in women. This may be associated with occasional, false-positive increases in serum CK. Most of the CK is the MM isoenzyme, but some patients have increases in the MB fraction. This finding does not necessarily correlate with cardiac involvement, and is probably due to regenerating skeletal muscle.

Normal CK activity despite active myositis can occur, more often in DM than PM, and more with recurrence than presentation. Most patients, however, have increased activity of some enzyme at some point in their course. Creatine kinase activity may be increased above the patient's baseline, but it may remain within the reference range for the laboratory. It may then decrease with treatment. Persistent or recurrent increases above baseline within the reference range may also reflect disease activity.

In addition to CK, other serum enzymes, including aldolase, lactate dehydrogenase (LD), and transaminases, are usually increased in PM and DM and other muscle injury. These enzymes are less specific for muscle than CK, and thus their diagnostic value is less. However, they correlate with muscle inflammation and are sometimes increased when CK is not, so they may be useful for monitoring disease activity. Serum myoglobin has also been used to monitor disease activity in PM and DM and appears to be as effective as CK for this purpose, but its analysis is less readily available.

Autoantibodies

Most patients with PM and DM produce autoantibodies. The antinuclear antibody (ANA) test is positive in 50 to 80 per cent. Nuclear patterns are most common, but nucleolar or cytoplasmic patterns are also seen. Autoantibodies in response to defined cellular antigens have been associated with myositis; some autoantibodies are considered "myositis-specific" (MSA) (Table 3). Each is present in a small proportion of patients, with individual patients having only one. The presence of autoantibodies is useful for diagnosis because almost all patients with the antibody have myositis. Specific autoantibodies also can aid classification because each antibody is associated with characteristic clinical features. The MSA (when present) may be a better predictor of course, prognosis, or associated features than the clinical classification. Anti–Jo-1 is the most common and most clinically available antibody associated with PM and DM. The antigen, histidyl-tRNA synthetase, is one of a family of enzymes (aminoacyl-tRNA synthetases), and autoantibodies to other enzymes in the family are also associated with PM and DM. Patients with any "antisynthetase" have a similar clinical syndrome: myositis with a high frequency of interstitial lung disease, arthritis (potentially deforming but not erosive), and other features (see Table 3). Some investigators have found a high frequency of sclerodermatous or sicca features as well. Antisynthetase patients are more likely to have recurrence of myositis as treatment is tapered, and survival is reduced compared with that of antibody-negative patients. These antibodies are rare in children and unusual in myositis with malignancy. Other MSAs of importance and their clinical associations are described in Table 3. Although often not included among patients with MSAs, most patients with anti–PM-Scl have myositis, and this antibody defines a clinical subgroup with PM/DM, scleroderma, or, most commonly, an overlap syndrome with features of both condi-

Table 3. Myositis Autoantibodies

Autoantibody	Percentage of PM and DM	Associated Syndrome
Myositis-Specific Autoantibodies (MSAs)		
I. Anti–Jo-1 and other "antisynthetases" (60–80% of antisynthetases are anti–Jo-1, [anti-histidyl-tRNA synthetase]; others are anti–PL-7, PL-12, OJ, and EJ)	25–30	"Antisynthetase syndrome" (Myositis, ≈95%; arthritis-arthralgia, ≈90%; interstitial lung disease, ≈80%; Raynaud's phenomenon, ≈60%; fever during flare, ≈80%; flares during taper, 60%; mechanic's hands, 70%); PM:DM = 60:40, mortality = 20%
II. Anti-SRP (anti–Signal recognition particle)	4–5	Almost all PM (rash is rare); often severe, acute in onset, relatively resistant to treatment, increase in cardiac involvement (up to 40%)
III. Anti–Mi-2 (antibody to unidentified nuclear protein)	5–10 (10–20% of adult DM)	Almost all DM (≈95% have DM rash), adult or juvenile; rash often prominent; no increase in antisynthetase syndrome features
Autoantibodies in Myositis That Are Not "MSAs"		
IV. Anti-PM-Scl (antibody to a nuclear-nucleolar protein complex)	5–10	Myositis-scleroderma overlap syndrome, or syndrome with features of both conditions ("scleromyositis") or myositis or scleroderma alone
V. Anti-RNP (antibody to U1 small nuclear ribonucleoprotein; rarely other RNPs)	10–15	In myositis, often associated with overlap with systemic lupus erythematosus and/or scleroderma or syndrome with features of these conditions ("mixed connective tissue disease")
VI. Anti-Ro/SSA	10	In myositis, often associated with connective tissue disease overlap syndromes (especially Sjögren's syndrome or systemic lupus erythematosus) or with antisynthetases

Reviewed in Miller, JAMA, 270:1846–1849, 1993.

tions, often with milder myositis. Other antibodies, such as anti-U1RNP and anti-Ku, have an association with myositis overlap syndromes but are not myositis-specific.

Electromyography and Nerve Conduction Studies

Electromyography and NCS nerve conduction studies are useful for distinguishing myopathic from neuropathic processes. They can also detect muscle involvement in patients who present with other features (rash, CTD features, interstitial lung disease, MSAs), but no detectable weakness. The normal nerve conduction and repetitive stimulation studies in PM and DM can help exclude other conditions. Some electromyographic abnormality is found in approximately 90 per cent of patients with PM/DM. The electromyogram (EMG) typically shows myopathic motor unit action potentials (low amplitude, short duration, polyphasic), a myopathic recruitment pattern (early recruitment and full interference), increased insertional activity, and spontaneous activity, including fibrillations, positive sharp waves, and complex repetitive discharges, but not fasciculations. Spontaneous activity suggests active inflammation.

Biopsy

Muscle biopsy is important both for demonstrating the typical features of PM and DM and for excluding other conditions. Although an open biopsy is traditional, often has less artifact, and provides more tissue to decrease sampling error, its accuracy for diagnosis of PM and DM is only marginally better than needle biopsy with multiple sampling. Furthermore, open biopsy causes a larger scar and more morbidity and cannot be repeated as easily. An involved but not severely atrophic muscle is chosen (usually quadriceps or deltoid). If not clear on clinical grounds, the best muscle may be inferred by EMG evidence of involvement on the contralateral side. However, a muscle recently subjected to electromyography should not be used, since the needle injury can cause changes. Magnetic resonance imaging (MRI) can also be used to identify involved muscles and areas of focal activity within them.

Mononuclear cells, predominantly lymphocytic inflammatory infiltrates, are seen in about 75 per cent of patients. Fiber necrosis, degeneration, and phagocytosis may be seen as well as regeneration. Atrophy, fibrosis, and fat replacement are later findings. In typical PM, the infiltrates are predominantly endomysial. CD8+ T cells have been shown to surround and invade non-necrotic fibers, and antigen-directed T-cell cytotoxicity is thought to be the primary pathogenetic mechanism of muscle injury. In juvenile and typical adult DM cases, the infiltrates are predominantly perimysial. Deposition of membrane attack complex of complement in the muscle microvasculature and capillary loss are very early findings; the primary mechanism of DM is believed to be complement-mediated vascular injury. This injury often leads to perifascicular atrophy, a characteristic finding of DM. Other evidence of vascular injury may also be seen, such as endothelial cell tubuloreticular inclusions and circumscribed areas of myofibrillar loss. The muscle biopsy should not contain evidence of IBM (no rimmed vacuoles or cytoplasmic or nuclear filamentous inclusions), metabolic myopathies (no glycogen or lipid accumulation and normal enzymes by histochemistry), mitochondrial myopathies (no abundant ragged red fibers or mitochondrial abnormality by electron microscopy), or other conditions.

In DM, skin biopsy is usually not definitive and often is not necessary, but it may be helpful when there are other diagnostic considerations. The pathology resembles lupus, with vacuolar degeneration at the basal layer. In DM, however, the mononuclear infiltrate at the dermal-epidermal junction is usually milder, there tends to be more mucin in the dermis, and, most importantly, little if any immunoglobulin deposition is seen at the dermal-epidermal junction.

USEFUL IMAGING PROCEDURES

Magnetic resonance images of the thighs are usually obtained for screening, and these studies can sensitively detect inflammation in muscles as increased intensity on T2-weighted images. Fat-suppression techniques further enhance the images, but gadolinium is not needed. Involvement noted with MRI is often focal and varies with disease activity, normalizing with disease suppression. Magnetic resonance imaging is useful for initial diagnosis, for detecting activity when EMG, biopsy, and/or enzymes are normal, and for following disease activity. Phosphorus-31 magnetic resonance spectroscopy can measure muscle metabolic products and is highly sensitive for PM and DM, even showing subtle changes in amyopathic DM. The findings in PM and DM are similar to those in other myopathies, but they can vary with disease activity.

OTHER USEFUL DIAGNOSTIC PROCEDURES

Evaluation for Malignancy

The extent of testing to uncover occult malignancy in patients with DM (or PM) is controversial. Some physicians believe that a thorough general evaluation, with pursuit of any abnormalities, is sufficient; this evaluation should include a history, a physical examination, routine laboratory tests, a chest film, and studies tailored to the individual (mammography, gynecologic examination, rectal examination with occult blood testing, prostate examination and PSA, testicular examination, and so forth, as appropriate). Others do more extensive testing, including computed tomography (CT) of the chest and abdomen and gastrointestinal studies. The latter course may be considered in those at highest risk: those with DM, older than 45 years of age, without connective tissue disease features or specific antibodies, those with resistant disease, weight loss, and possibly, those with vasculitis. Particular attention should be given to excluding ovarian cancer; patients at risk should at least have a physical examination, transvaginal ultrasound, and CA-125 determination.

Other Tests

The erythrocyte sedimentation rate and C-reactive protein (CRP) may be increased in about 50 per cent but are not reliable indicators of disease activity and can be normal in active disease. Rheumatoid factor can be positive, more so in overlap syndromes, but there is no specific association. Gamma globulin can be increased but severe hypogammaglobulinemia or agammaglobulinemia should suggest echovirus-induced myositis. Complement is usually normal. The clinician should obtain a chest film to look for pulmonary fibrosis, and an electrocardiogram (ECG) should be performed. Other testing for nonmuscular features (e.g., pulmonary function testing, esophageal manometry, echocardiogram) or overlapping CTDs should be performed when suggested by symptoms and signs.

DIFFERENTIAL DIAGNOSIS

The criteria proposed by Bohan and Peter, shown in Table 2, can be very useful in approaching the diagnosis. An inflammatory myopathy is demonstrated by the presence of weakness, increased activity of muscle enzymes in serum, and compatible findings on EMG and biopsy.

Usually, DM is easier to diagnose because of the characteristic rash. When the rash is seen in association with muscle weakness, the diagnosis of DM should be suspected. Increased CK activity supports the diagnosis, and an EMG and nerve conduction studies can confirm the presence of a compatible myopathy. Thyroid function should be checked, the possibility of medication effect reviewed, and testing for human immunodeficiency virus (HIV) or human T-cell lymphotropic virus type I (HTLV-I) considered. A typical rash, along with a compatible myopathy and these exclusions, can be enough to consider the diagnosis established. The more typical the rash, the greater the diagnostic confidence. The combination of Gottron's papules and heliotrope is particularly strong diagnostic evidence, and nail fold capillary changes and the erythematous, poikilodermatous rash are supportive. Adult patients should be evaluated, as detailed above, for the presence of malignancy. If a question remains, or the rash is incomplete or atypical, a muscle biopsy should be performed.

The diagnosis of PM usually requires more extensive testing to confirm the diagnosis and exclude other conditions. Proximal muscle weakness with increased CK activity should suggest PM. Electromyography and nerve conduction studies can help confirm a myopathy, but unless clear evidence of a neuropathy (e.g., amyotrophic lateral sclerosis [ALS]) is seen, a muscle biopsy should be performed. However, the association of an antisynthetase, anti–Mi-2, anti–PM-Scl, or anti-SRP with clinical evidence of myopathy provided by weakness, enzymes, and EMG, can be sufficient (assuming that MSA testing is accurate). In distinguishing PM from other myopathies, evidence of systemic inflammatory or autoimmune disease suggests PM. Such evidence includes unexplained fever, increased erythrocyte sedimentation rate, positive ANA in significant titer (especially a defined autoantibody such as an MSA or anti-U1RNP), another connective tissue disease, or new-onset Raynaud's phenomenon. However, PM patients may not show these features, and their absence should not preclude further evaluation for PM and DM. Although the association with malignancy is not certain for PM, a thorough general evaluation is still advisable.

Numerous conditions can be confused with PM (Table 4). For all patients, it is important to exclude thyroid disease; hypothyroidism commonly causes increased CK activity and weakness. The clinician must consider HIV infection because it can be associated with a typical inflammatory myositis (which may be the first manifestation), and treatment for PM would be immunosuppressive. HTLV-1 has been found in a significant proportion of PM patients in endemic areas, and the clinician should check for "this pathogen" where appropriate. Acute, self-limited viral myopathy may occur and can lead to increased CK activity and rhabdomyolysis; this condition can be confused with PM. A myositis that resembles PM may occur in toxoplasmosis; the significance of the increased frequency of positive toxoplasma serology in idiopathic PM and DM is unclear. Metabolic myopathies can be excluded with enzyme histochemistry, and such testing should be considered when the history is suggestive or a forearm ischemic exercise test demonstrates abnormalities in serum lactate and ammonia. Finally, drug-induced myopathy is a common and important consideration. A myositis similar to PM or DM can be caused by D-penicillamine; even occasional production of anti–Jo-1 has been reported. Therapeutic doses of colchicine have caused neuromyopathy that resembles PM in patients with renal insufficiency. Most cholesterol-lowering agents have been reported to cause myopathy. Lovastatin myopathy occurs more frequently when this drug is used in combination with cyclosporine or gemfibrozil. Zidovudine (AZT) can cause a mitochondrial myopathy that may cause problems by itself or in combination with HIV-associated myositis. Corticosteroids can cause proximal muscle weakness, which can be confused with exacerbation of disease in treated patients, but serum CK activity is usually normal.

Pitfalls

A delay in diagnosis may occur if muscle weakness is not recognized and pursued or is attributed to generalized weakness or fatigue. However, patients have been unnecessarily treated with corticosteroids and/or immunosuppressive agents when noninflammatory conditions such as colchicine-induced myopathy, myophosphorylase deficiency, and hypothyroidism were not properly excluded.

The diagnosis is sometimes not pursued because of normal results on important tests. The CK activity may be normal in 10 per cent of patients with PM and in more with DM; evaluation for PM and DM should proceed despite a normal CK test if unexplained proximal muscle weakness is present. A normal EMG is found in approximately 10 per cent and should not prevent muscle biopsy if the clinical picture is suggestive. Muscle biopsy may be normal in roughly 10 per cent of patients with PM and DM and is equivocal or fails to show the typical picture in at least another 10 to 20 per cent. In this situation, muscle MRI can be particularly helpful; a normal study should lead the clinician to seriously question the diagnosis. On the other hand, if areas of increased intensity are found, biopsy can be directed to the muscle and the area of involvement. Autoantibody testing should also be performed in such patients, since the presence of MSA can help establish the diagnosis. However, MSA testing has low sensitivity, and the absence of MSAs should not be considered evidence against a diagnosis of PM or DM. If PM cannot be established confidently with biopsy (or MSA), the diagnosis remains provisional.

The rash of DM commonly precedes the myositis, sometimes for prolonged periods (amyopathic DM), and such DM patients cannot satisfy the diagnostic criteria, which depend on the presence of myositis. The diagnosis must be based, in such patients, on dermatologic criteria. It is important not to dismiss the diagnosis under these circumstances; associated malignancy must be considered, and these patients should be followed to avoid delay in treatment if myositis appears.

INCLUSION BODY MYOSITIS

Inclusion body myositis represents 15 to 30 per cent of IIM but is often misdiagnosed as PM. The onset is usually after age 50 years, and it is two to three times more common in men. Proximal muscle weakness is usually present, but distal weakness is much more common than in PM (50 to 90 per cent), as is asymmetrical involvement (60 per cent). Problems in the lower extremities are usually detected first, with severe quadriceps involvement, loss of the knee reflex, and frequent falling. Dysphagia is common

Table 4. Differential Diagnosis of PM and DM

Other Forms of Myositis

Myositis in Infection

- Viruses
  - HIV: Associated with a PM-like myositis; also, increased frequency of other infections of muscle
  - HTLV-I: associated with a PM-like myositis, usually in endemic areas
  - Enteroviruses: (1) acute self-limited myopathy; (2) chronic infection in agammaglobulinemia (usually echovirus) that can cause myositis with encephalitis, and other problems
  - Influenza: acute self-limited myositis
  - Hepatitis B, EB-virus, cytomegalovirus, and others associated with myositis
- Bacteria
  - Pyomyositis: one or more spontaneous muscle abscesses; classic form affects males in tropical areas, usually due to *Staphylococcus;* found increasingly in nontropical areas in predisposed individuals (AIDS, older patients with diabetes or other medical illnesses), often due to other organisms
  - Lyme myositis: usually focal, probably from direct infection
  - Other (tuberculosis, mycoplasmosis, leprosy, streptococcal infection, etc.)
- Protozoa
  - Toxoplasmosis: Direct infection appears capable of producing myopathy that can be confused with PM clinically; must be distinguished from reactivated toxoplasmosis due to immunosuppression; increase in positive serologies in PM and DM of unknown significance
  - Chagas' disease (American trypanosomiasis, *Trypanosoma cruzi* infection)
- Parasites
  - Trichinosis: can infect muscle and cause periorbital edema that can be confused with heliotrope
  - Cysticerosis
- Fungi
  - *Candida*

Idiopathic

- Inclusion body myositis (see text)
- Connective tissue diseases: scleroderma, systemic lupus erythematosus, Sjögren's syndrome, rheumatoid arthritis
- Vasculitis: polyarteritis nodosa, Wegener's granulomatosis, rheumatoid arthritis
- Polymyalgia rheumatica: pain and stiffness predominate, but occasional PM patients may have prominent pain
- Granulomatous myositis: may be seen in sarcoidosis, etc.
- Eosinophilic myositis: alone or as part of hypereosinophilic syndrome
- Focal myositis

Noninflammatory Myopathies

Dystrophies

- Suspect if a family history exists; sporadic dystrophies in adults are most likely to be confused with PM, especially limb-girdle or facioscapulohumeral muscular dystrophy

Congenital Myopathies

- Mitochondrial myopathies: ragged red fibers seen on biopsy
- Nemaline rod, central core, etc.

Metabolic

- Myophosphorylase deficiency (McArdles's disease) and phosphofructokinase deficiency
  - MP and PFK deficiencies can be identified by specific testing for enzyme by histochemistry, and forearm ischemic exercise test with impaired increase of lactate, but not ammonia
- Myoadenylate deaminase deficiency: impaired increase of ammonia, but not lactate
- Acid maltase deficiency
- Lipid storage diseases
  - Carnitine deficiency
  - Carnitine palmitoyltransferase deficiency

Neuropathic Disorders

- Motor neuron diseases: amyotrophic lateral sclerosis may cause increases in CK activity
- Myasthenia gravis or Eaton-Lambert syndrome
- Guillain-Barré syndrome

Endocrine and Metabolic Disorders

- Thyroid disease: increased CK activity with hypothyroidism; muscle effects with hypothyroidism or hyperthyroidism
- Hypercortisolism
- Hyperparathyroidism or hypoparathyroidism, or hypocalcemia
- Hypokalemia, including periodic paralyses
- Diabetes and neurologic complications
- Malnutrition

Drugs

- D-Penicillamine: can induce PM and DM indistinguishable from idiopathic
- Cimetidine: rare
- L-Tryptophan: contaminated L-tryptophan caused epidemic eosinophilia-myalgia syndrome
- Zidovudine: leads to myopathy through mitochondrial toxicity
- Colchicine: neuromyopathy, usually seen in renal insufficiency
- Chloroquine or hydroxychloroquine: vacuolar myopathy; may have cardiac involvement
- Lipid-lowering agents
  - HMG-CoA reductase inhibitors: appears most common with lovastatin; increased frequency when used with cyclosporine, fibrates, or niacin
  - Fibrates: clofibrate, gemfibrozil
- Cyclosporine
- Ipecac, emetine
- Aminocaproic acid
- Carbimazole, propylthiouracil
- Alcohol and drugs of abuse (cocaine, amphetamines, heroin, phencyclidine, barbiturates): alcohol, cocaine, and some others have direct drug effects on muscle; trauma and crush can also increase CK activity
- Anesthetics: can cause malignant hyperthermia
- Psychotropics: can cause neuroleptic-malignant syndrome
- Corticosteroids: steroid myopathy; worse with long-acting fluorinated; CK activity usually normal
- Others

(40 per cent). Evidence of neuropathy may help distinguish IBM from PM. Most patients have no family history, although a rare, usually noninflammatory familial condition can resemble IBM.

Course

Inclusion body myositis has an insidious onset and slow progression that may lead to prolonged delay (3 to 6 years) in proper diagnosis. IBM is relatively resistant to treatment, and weakness typically slowly progresses over ten to fifteen years.

Laboratory Procedures

Creatine kinase activity is increased, but seldom markedly. Antinuclear antibodies are uncommon, and MSAs are uniformly negative. The EMG and nerve conduction studies resemble those of PM except for the neuropathic features, when present. Magnetic resonance imaging can show increased intensity on T2-weighted imaging, with predominantly anterior thigh involvement.

Biopsy is required to establish the diagnosis. The inflammatory infiltrate may range from intense to absent. As in PM, typically endomysial infiltration is present, with T cells surrounding and invading non-necrotic fibers. Necrosis and regeneration are also seen. There is no capillary dropout or complement deposition in vessels. The characteristic features are rimmed vacuoles and filamentous inclusions. The cytoplasmic inclusions are 15- to 21-nm helical filaments (with smaller inclusions in the nucleus) that are paired and resemble those of Alzheimer's disease. Electron microscopy is necessary for definitive identification of the inclusions and confirmation of the diagnosis. Inflammatory features may predominate early, and the diagnosis may be missed. If patients with apparent PM are not responding to treatment and the clinical picture is suspicious for IBM, rebiopsy should be considered. However, the diagnosis, which may affect treatment decisions, requires histologic confirmation. Criteria have been proposed (Calabrese and Chou, Rheum. Dis. Clin. North Amer. 20:955–972, 1994), based on combining the vacuoles and filaments with clinical evidence of myopathy.

SCLERODERMA

By Walter G. Barr, M.D.,
and Mary C. Massa, M.D.
Maywood, Illinois

Scleroderma, or systemic sclerosis, is a multisystem disease of the connective tissues characterized by fibrosis, vascular obliterative disease, and variable expressions of disordered immunity. Fibroblasts, T lymphocytes, endothelial cells, and mast cells interact in complex ways to produce local as well as systemic abnormalities. Until the pathogenesis of this disorder is more completely understood, diagnostic and therapeutic interventions will remain imperfect. The disease is uncommon, but not rare. Ten to 15 new cases per million population are documented each year. Scleroderma is found across racial and geographic lines and is three to four times more common in women. The peak age at onset is 30 to 50 years of age.

CLASSIFICATION AND ITS SIGNIFICANCE

The term scleroderma ("hard skin") is often used interchangeably with systemic sclerosis. The latter terminology is preferred to the older term progressive systemic sclerosis because not all patients follow a progressive course. Scleroderma may be classified in various ways (Table 1). Most schemes broadly contrast localized with generalized disease (systemic sclerosis). Localized disease is limited to the skin and includes entities such as morphea and linear scleroderma. Recent reports of serologic and other laboratory abnormalities suggest that localized scleroderma may not be completely confined to the skin. Nonetheless, these abnormal test results typically do not carry major implications for systemic involvement, and transition to generalized disease is rare.

Generalized disease can be divided into two major categories based largely on the extent of cutaneous involvement. Patients with diffuse scleroderma or diffuse cutaneous systemic sclerosis have widespread cutaneous thickening. Patients with limited skin involvement are classified as having limited scleroderma, limited cutaneous systemic sclerosis, or CREST syndrome. The acronym CREST (*c*alcinosis, *R*aynaud's phenomenon, *e*sophageal disease, *s*clerodactyly, *t*elangiectasias) has fallen into disfavor because this constellation of features is not always found in patients with limited scleroderma, nor are these features restricted to patients with limited cutaneous disease. Clearly, sclerodactyly too narrowly defines the extent of cutaneous disease in limited scleroderma.

Occasional patients present with characteristic internal organ involvement of scleroderma without skin disease. The term scleroderma sine scleroderma has been used to describe scleroderma without hard skin. Some patients have features of scleroderma coexisting with those of other connective tissue diseases. These conditions are known as overlap syndromes. By contrast, undifferentiated connective tissue disease is a useful term for patients having Raynaud's phenomenon with serologic and/or capillary microscopic abnormalities of scleroderma but lacking definite skin thickening or evidence of internal organ involvement of systemic sclerosis.

The classification of scleroderma has implications for management because the natural history of diffuse disease and that of limited disease are distinctly different. Patients with diffuse disease have skin involvement proximal to the elbows and knees and can be absolutely distinguished from patients with limited cutaneous disease by the presence of chest or abdominal skin involvement. These patients are most likely to have heart, lung, gut, and kidney involvement. Disease progression is most evident in the first 5 years of disease, and mortality at that point may be as

Table 1. Classification of Scleroderma

Localized Scleroderma
Linear scleroderma
Morphea
Generalized Scleroderma (Systemic Sclerosis)
Diffuse scleroderma
Limited scleroderma (CREST)
Scleroderma sine scleroderma
Scleroderma in overlap syndromes
Undifferentiated connective tissue disease

CREST = calcinosis, Raynaud's phenomenon, esophageal disease, sclerodactyly, telangiectasias.

Table 2. Early Generalized Scleroderma (Less Than 5 Years After Onset)

	Diffuse Scleroderma	Limited Scleroderma
Skin thickening	Proximal to elbows and knees, face, trunk; may progress rapidly	Absent or limited to fingers and hands
Raynaud's phenomenon	May be absent at outset	Present for long periods prior to skin thickening
Organ involvement	Gastrointestinal, pulmonary interstitial fibrosis, renal, myocardial	Heartburn, dysphagia
Constitutional	Fatigue	None
Serum autoantibodies	Anti-Scl 70	Anticentromere
Musculoskeletal involvement	Arthritis, tendon, friction rubs, early contractures	None or puffy fingers

high as 30 to 40 per cent. Therefore, patients with diffuse scleroderma warrant early consideration for potentially disease-modifying therapy.

Patients with diffuse scleroderma may often be distinguished from patients with limited scleroderma by the presence of Scl-70 antibody (antitopoisomerase I). However, 10 to 15 per cent of patients with limited scleroderma are also Scl-70–positive. In the early stages of cutaneous disease, tendon friction rubs may provide another clue to the diagnosis of diffuse scleroderma.

Patients with limited scleroderma may experience Raynaud's phenomenon for many years prior to the onset of demonstrable cutaneous disease. Skin changes are often limited to the fingers and hands, although some patients have involvement of the forearms. Early clinical problems for this subset of patients include heartburn and recurrent digital ulcerations, whereas late manifestations include severe pulmonary hypertension, malabsorption, and biliary cirrhosis. Patients with limited scleroderma rarely have major renal involvement. Most of these patients are identified serologically by detecting anticentromere antibodies rarely found in patients with diffuse scleroderma. Survival in the limited form is most often measured in decades, and patients generally are not considered candidates for potentially hazardous disease-modifying therapy. Furthermore, the prolonged survival and slow evolution of limited disease (Table 2) makes it difficult to assess the efficacy of long-term, potentially toxic treatments.

EARLY DIAGNOSIS

Few diseases are misdiagnosed with greater frequency than scleroderma in its earliest stages. A typical scleroderma patient has multiple encounters with physicians prior to appropriate diagnosis. Too often, early complaints of puffiness, fatigue, and tingling sensations in the extremities are considered "functional." Only the development of frank skin tightening may resolve otherwise puzzling symptoms. The current emphasis on accurate early diagnosis will become even more important as more effective treatment becomes available. Success with agents currently under study presumes intervention in the early prefibrotic phase of the illness.

Raynaud's phenomenon is seen in most patients with scleroderma. However, most patients with Raynaud's phenomenon do not acquire diffuse connective tissue disease. Such a benign clinical course is most often seen in younger women with an onset of Raynaud's phenomenon as teenagers or in the early 20s. The onset of Raynaud's phenomenon after age 40 years should prompt a careful search for an underlying cause. Among the connective tissue diseases, scleroderma accounts for many of these cases. Patients with limited scleroderma usually have Raynaud's phenomenon as their first clinical symptom. Patients with diffuse disease may experience edema prior to the onset of Raynaud's phenomenon. This early edematous phase can progress without Raynaud's phenomenon ever developing. Patients often have a greater appreciation of the hand swelling than the physician does. The edematous phase of this illness may be mistaken for postoperative edema or reflex sympathetic dystrophy. Other clinical presentations include carpal tunnel syndrome, ischemic digits, arthritis, and esophageal symptoms (Table 3).

Autoantibodies detected in serum have not been as useful in the diagnosis and treatment of scleroderma as they have been in systemic lupus erythematosus. Current use of human cells in culture as substrates for antinuclear antibody (ANA) reveals a much higher prevalence of detectable ANA than formerly appreciated. As many as 95 to 98 per cent of patients with scleroderma have ANA when their serum is tested with the human oral carcinoma cell line HEp-2. The anticentromere pattern of autoantibodies seen in limited scleroderma is not typically observed in mouse organ substrates.

Raynaud's phenomenon and anticentromere antibody may be the only findings in early limited cutaneous disease. Antinucleolar antibodies, which are typically expressed in the later stages of scleroderma, are not as specific for this disorder as the anticentromere pattern is. Detection of ANA in a nucleolar pattern in the absence of characteristic clinical features should not prompt an exhaustive search for scleroderma.

The only other widely available serologic marker for scleroderma is Scl-70 (antitopoisomerase I). This antibody is found in a subset of patients with diffuse scleroderma and is often associated with pulmonary interstitial fibrosis. PM-Scl antibody identifies an overlap syndrome with features of polymyositis and scleroderma. Mixed connective tissue disease is associated with antibody to nuclear ribonucleoprotein (anti-nRNP), high-titer ANA in a speckled pattern, and overlapping features of multiple connective tissue disorders. Mixed connective tissue disease may evolve to classic scleroderma.

The role of skin biopsy in the early identification of scleroderma requires further investigation. Epidermal at-

Table 3. Presenting Manifestations of Scleroderma

Raynaud's phenomenon
Puffy hands
Polyarthritis
Carpal tunnel syndrome
Digital ischemia
Esophageal or gastrointestinal symptoms

rophy and dermal fibrosis are generally found in areas of skin with clinically detectable abnormalities. Early microscopic changes include diffuse or perivascular infiltration with T lymphocytes and monocytes. Direct skin immunofluorescence is not observed, but an increased number of mast cells may be seen. The skin biopsy can also provide evidence of diseases that mimic scleroderma (e.g., scleredema and eosinophilic fasciitis).

The characteristic microvascular changes of scleroderma can be detected in vivo with nailfold capillary microscopy. Capillary loops in the nailfold normally appear as hairpins on end. By contrast, in scleroderma these loops become distorted, dilate, and disappear. Abnormal capillaries may be seen early in scleroderma, even in the absence of classic skin changes. Therefore, all patients with Raynaud's phenomenon should be evaluated with nailfold capillary microscopy.

In the limited as well as the diffuse forms of scleroderma, the disease process commonly involves the esophagus. Altered motility of the lower two-thirds of the esophagus and diminished lower esophageal sphincter pressure often occur early in the illness in the absence of symptoms involving other internal organs.

Restrictive airway changes and reduced diffusion capacity may be seen in early scleroderma, but the findings are nonspecific. The early diagnosis and classification of scleroderma is a challenging problem for even the most experienced rheumatologist. However, with appropriate use of multiple diagnostic tools, the clinician can increase the chances of success.

EVALUATION OF SKIN THICKENING

The extent and progression of skin thickening determines the disease classification, provides a surrogate marker for internal organ involvement (more skin disease equals more internal organ disease), and can be used to monitor therapy. Clinical research trials typically rely on a semiquantitative evaluation of skin thickening that generates a total skin score. Skin scoring methods vary, but they all provide a number based on the severity of palpable thickening (e.g., 0 = normal skin, 1 = mild thickening, 2 = moderate thickening, and 3 = severe thickening) at a specified number of sites. Thus, in a system based on 17 sites and a scale of 0 to 3, the maximal total skin score is 51. This methodology is reliable and reproducible when used by properly trained clinicians.

OTHER LABORATORY AND IMAGING PROCEDURES

Anemia may be associated with rapid deterioration of renal function and the onset of sclerodermatous renal crisis. Such patients may also experience severe hypertension and other features of microangiopathy, including thrombocytopenia, increased serum lactate dehydrogenase (LD) activity, and red cell fragmentation in the peripheral smear.

Polyclonal hypergammaglobulinemia can be documented in one third of patients with scleroderma. Serum complement concentrations are typically normal but may increase as acute-phase reactants. The erythrocyte sedimentation rate (ESR) ranges from normal to moderately increased, but the erythrocyte sedimentation rate has not proved useful in monitoring the course of patients with scleroderma. The presence of rheumatoid factor may create diagnostic confusion in patients with significant arthralgia and arthritis. Serum concentrations of interleukin 2, interleukin 4, and soluble interleukin 2 receptor may be increased, but these measurements have yet to find a routine role in the diagnosis and management of scleroderma.

After Raynaud's phenomenon and skin changes, gastrointestinal involvement is the third most common clinical feature of scleroderma. Esophageal dysmotility is seen in 80 to 90 per cent of these patients. Esophageal dysfunction can be documented by manometric, barium, or radionuclide transit studies. Barium swallow is generally well tolerated and often sufficient for diagnosis. Endoscopy may confirm the presence of stricture as a cause of dysphagia.

The presence of more than 10 g of fat in a 72-hour collection of stool may indicate malabsorption. Decreased urinary excretion of D-xylose suggests malassimilation rather than maldigestion as the cause of malabsorption. Stasis and bacterial overgrowth of small bowel contents may lead to diarrhea and bloating that responds to treatment with rotating oral antibiotic therapy. Small bowel hypomotility is characterized by dilatation of the lumen and by delayed transit of contrast in small bowel radiographs. Decreased peristalsis of the colon resulting in constipation or pseudo-obstruction may be confused with mechanical obstruction. Barium enema occasionally reveals wide-mouthed diverticula on the antimesenteric border of the transverse and descending colon. These lesions are nearly pathognomonic of scleroderma.

The chest film is an insensitive tool for detecting interstitial fibrosis (seen in 70 per cent of patients with diffuse scleroderma and 35 per cent of patients with limited scleroderma) but should be part of the baseline assessment. Pulmonary function testing remains the cornerstone for detection and serial monitoring of lung involvement and should likewise be part of the baseline evaluation. Reduced lung volumes and diffusing capacity are frequently observed; diffusing capacities measuring less than 40 per cent of the reference values are associated with a poor prognosis. High-resolution computed tomography (HRCT) is more sensitive than the chest film in detecting early interstitial disease, but it does not enable the clinician to distinguish inflammation from fibrosis. Bronchoalveolar lavage (BAL) may provide a useful guide to disease activity in the hands of experienced investigators. Bronchoalveolar lavage in patients with sclerodermatous lung disease typically reveals increased neutrophils, lymphocytes, and eosinophils. Gallium scanning currently has no role in the assessment of established sclerodermatous lung disease. Lung biopsy is rarely indicated for early sclerodermatous lung disease. The incidence of lung cancer may be increased in scleroderma patients with long-standing pulmonary fibrosis. In scleroderma patients with unexplained dyspnea, ECHO doppler may suggest pulmonary hypertension that should be confirmed by right-heart catheterization.

Echocardiographic evidence of pericardial disease (thickening and/or fluid) can be seen in up to 50 per cent of patients. The large extramural coronary arteries are typically normal, and myocardial infarction is rare. However, both radionuclide studies and autopsy data have documented small vessel occlusive disease. Holter monitoring is appropriate for selected patients, because atrial and ventricular tachyarrhythmias occur in scleroderma and are associated with increased mortality and sudden death.

Two types of muscle disease in scleroderma can be distinguished by electromyography (EMG) and muscle biopsy. Some patients have inflammatory myopathy that is indistinguishable from polymyositis. More commonly, a bland myopathy with normal or slightly increased concentrations creatine kinase (CK) is seen. The latter is characterized by electromyographs showing few polyphasic potentials and little or no insertional activity. Muscle biopsy reveals interstitial fibrosis and nonspecific fiber changes. The course is typically indolent and most often does not require treatment.

The vascular lesion in scleroderma is characterized by bland intimal hyperplasia rather than the necrotizing vasculitis seen in other collagen-vascular diseases. Rarely, microscopic changes in the digital artery at the time of amputation provide the basis for a diagnosis of scleroderma. Angiography of an extremity seldom aids diagnosis but may indicate a surgically correctable large vessel occlusion. Increased serum concentrations β-thromboglobulin (reflecting platelet activation) and factor VIII (von Willebrand factor; suggesting endothelial cell disruption) have been reported, but the clinical utility of these measurements has not been demonstrated.

In patients with early diffuse disease, urine should be collected for 24 hours to determine the protein concentration and the creatinine clearance. Although plasma renin concentrations are uniformly increased in patients with sclerodermatous renal crisis, routine measurement of renin does not help predict sclerodermatous renal disease.

Renal biopsies may reveal vascular abnormalities even in the absence of clinically demonstrable renal disease; however, renal biopsy is uncommonly performed in scleroderma. The main role of biopsy is to establish an alternative cause of renal disease. For example, the presence of red cell casts or large amounts of protein in the sediment should prompt a biopsy because these findings are rarely found in scleroderma.

Hand radiographs may show resorption of the digital tufts (acro-osteolysis) or soft tissue calcifications (calcinosis cutis). Resorption of the mandibular condyles may also be seen. Erosive arthritis is uncommon and at times represents an overlap with rheumatoid arthritis. Synovial fluid in scleroderma primarily contains mononuclear cells. Calcification of the synovium is occasionally associated with chalky fluid laden with calcium phosphate crystals. Hypothyroidism is common and insidious in scleroderma. Thyroid function should be measured annually.

CLINICAL COURSE

Most patients with scleroderma have either diffuse or limited disease. Patients with diffuse disease typically have a uniphasic illness with maximal expression 2 to 3 years after onset. A subset of these patients may progress from first symptom to death within 18 months. Others experience an illness that unfolds over longer periods in stepwise fashion, but scleroderma (unlike lupus) is not a disease of remissions and exacerbations. It is uncommon for patients with diffuse disease to develop new internal organ involvement or skin progression after 5 years, and late morbidity is typically related to early disease events.

Limited scleroderma (CREST) evolves slowly and usually begins with Raynaud's phenomenon. Clinically detectable skin tightening may follow months to years later. Internal organ involvement likewise unfolds slowly. Major morbidity and mortality in limited disease is often related to severe pulmonary hypertension or malabsorption that may not develop until the second decade of the illness. Most patients with scleroderma follow one of the paths described, but individual variability precludes assigning a definite prognosis to any specific patient. Even patients with diffuse scleroderma may experience an indolent and relatively benign course.

DISEASES THAT MIMIC SCLERODERMA

The differential diagnosis for scleroderma is extensive and includes all disorders associated with Raynaud's phenomenon, skin thickening, and similar visceral features (e.g., esophageal dysfunction, primary pulmonary hypertension, and idiopathic pulmonary fibrosis). Some of the more commonly considered disorders (e.g., eosinophilic fasciitis and eosinophilia-myalgia syndrome) can be distinguished by the absence of Raynaud's phenomenon and sparing of the fingers. Patients that may have scleroderma should be evaluated by a rheumatologist or a dermatologist. Long-term management should include periodic consultation or primary care by the rheumatologist.

COMMON ERRORS AND PITFALLS IN DIAGNOSIS

Most young women with Raynaud's phenomenon do not have nor will they ever acquire scleroderma or other connective tissue disorder. Detection of ANA plus Raynaud's phenomenon increases the index of suspicion for collagen-vascular disease, but these two findings are not enough to make the diagnosis of scleroderma. An 18-year-old woman with nothing more than Raynaud's phenomenon and a weakly positive ANA test result should not be burdened with a premature and most likely inaccurate diagnosis of scleroderma. Conversely, a small subset of patients with scleroderma will never manifest Raynaud's phenomenon or will acquire Raynaud's phenomenon only after the onset of hand edema.

Serologic testing can be both helpful and misleading. A nucleolar pattern of ANA suggests scleroderma but is not diagnostic. Anti-Scl antibody can be detected in limited as well as in diffuse variants of scleroderma. Most, but not all, patients with limited disease can be identified by the presence of anticentromere antibody. A small subset of patients with scleroderma may not reveal any of the commonly available serologic markers. The diagnosis of scleroderma is ultimately based on clinical assessment and judgment. The accuracy of diagnosis is enhanced by clinical experience with the variable expressions of this enigmatic disorder.

SJÖGREN'S SYNDROME

By Robert I. Fox, M.D., Ph.D.
La Jolla, California

Sjögren's syndrome (SS) refers to the combination of a particular form of dry eyes (keratoconjunctivitis sicca [KCS]) and dry mouth due to characteristic lymphocytic infiltration of the salivary gland. Considerable controversy has surrounded the criteria used to classify SS, leading to uncertainty in clinical practice and in publications. While the ocular findings (namely, KCS) in SS have been well defined, the oral component (i.e., xerostomia) has not found similar consensus.

At one end of the spectrum of proposed classification criteria, the "San Diego" criteria for definite SS require objective clinical evidence of decreased lacrimal or salivary

Table 1. San Diego Criteria for Diagnosis of Primary and Secondary Sjögren's Syndrome

I. Primary Sjögren's syndrome (SS)
  A. Symptoms and objective signs of ocular dryness
    1. Schirmer's test result less than 8 mm of wetting per 5 minutes *and*
    2. Positive rose bengal test or staining of cornea *or* conjunctiva to demonstrate keratoconjunctivitis sicca
  B. Symptoms and objective signs of dry mouth
    1. Decreased parotid flow rate using Lashley cups or other methods *and*
    2. Abnormal biopsy of minor salivary gland (focus score of 2 or higher based on an average of four evaluable lobules)
  C. Evidence of a systemic autoimmune disorder
    1. Increased rheumatoid factor ≥1:320 *or*
    2. Increased antinuclear antibody ≥1:320 *or*
    3. Presence of anti–SS-A (Ro) or anti–SS-B (La) antibodies

II. Secondary Sjögren's syndrome
  Characteristic signs and symptoms of SS (described above) plus clinical features sufficient to allow a diagnosis of rheumatoid arthritis, systemic lupus erythematosus, polymyositis, scleroderma, or biliary cirrhosis

III. Exclusions
  Sarcoidosis, pre-existent lymphoma, acquired immunodeficiency syndrome, and other known causes of keratitis sicca or salivary gland enlargement

*Definite Sjögren's syndrome requires objective evidence of dryness of the eyes or mouth and a systemic autoimmune process, including a characteristic minor salivary gland biopsy.

†Probable Sjögren's syndrome does not require a minor salivary gland biopsy but can be diagnosed with demonstration of decreased salivary function (I.B.1).

gland function and laboratory evidence of a systemic autoimmune process characterized by increased titers of autoantibodies and microscopic abnormalities of minor salivary glands (Table 1). These rigorous criteria are designed for patients participating in research protocols, where the aims are to identify underlying pathogenetic mechanisms, establish prognosis, and evaluate specific therapies. At the other end of the spectrum of classification criteria, the recently proposed preliminary European criteria do not have an absolute requirement for either autoantibodies or minor salivary gland histopathology (Table 2). As a result, more people fulfill the European classification criteria than fulfill the San Diego criteria for definite SS. Dryness of the eyes or mouth and swelling of lacrimal or salivary glands can accompany many different illnesses (discussed later). However, the diagnosis of SS should not be made when human immunodeficiency virus (HIV) infection, sarcoidosis, lymphoma (pre-existent), hepatitis C viral infection, or other known causes of dry eyes and dry mouth are present (see Table 1).

Sjögren's syndrome may exist as a primary disorder (primary SS, 1° SS) or as a secondary condition (2° SS) associated with rheumatoid arthritis (RA), systemic lupus erythematosus (SLE), or progressive systemic sclerosis (PSS). Even when "rigorous" criteria for 1° SS are chosen, this group of patients remain heterogeneous with regard to laboratory and clinical features, including extraglandular involvement of the kidneys, liver, lungs, and nervous system. To expedite the clinician's evaluation of relevant symptoms, the current International Classification of Diseases-9-CM code assignments are provided in Table 3.

PRESENTING SYMPTOMS AND SIGNS

Patients with SS frequently describe a "foreign" body sensation in their eyes. Complaints of "itching," however, are ubiquitous and not helpful in the diagnosis of SS. Decreased basal tear flow, especially at night, is often the initial complaint. Symptoms of eye discomfort develop despite the patient's ability to generate tears during crying or exposure to onions or other stimuli. The clinician can measure tear volume by inserting paper strips under the lower eyelid for 5 minutes in the absence of topical anesthesia (Schirmer's test I). Maximally stimulated tear flow (Schirmer's test II) can be rapidly measured by gently inserting a Q-tip into the nose to stimulate the nasolacrimal reflex. However, tear volume and flow correlate poorly with signs and symptoms of KCS. Moreover, a wide range of tear volumes and flows can be seen in normal individuals. The volume of saliva produced as basal secretion or after stimulation also correlates poorly with symptoms of dry mouth and signs of periodontal disease.

The clinician who evaluates a complaint of dry eyes should determine whether objective signs of dry eyes are commensurate with the patient's symptoms. The integrity of the corneal surface and tear film can be easily measured with the rose bengal test, fluorescein staining, or the tear break-up time (see Table 1). If the results of one or more of these tests are not clearly abnormal, the clinician should look for other causes of the patient's ocular symptoms. These causes may include eye strain (poor refraction), blepharitis (irritation of the lids), blepharospasm (uncontrolled blinking due to an increased local reflex), uveitis, retinitis, or symptoms due to anxiety or depression.

The principal oral symptom of SS is dryness of the mouth with a broad range of severity. One of the most significant initial symptoms is difficulty in swallowing food without taking sips of water. Interruption of sleep to take sips of water strongly suggests a significant sicca syndrome. Not all patients specifically complain of dryness; many describe difficulty in wearing dentures, changes in their sense of taste, increased incidence of dental caries, chronic burning symptoms, intolerance to acidic or spicy foods, and the inability to eat dry food or speak continuously for more than a few minutes. Nutrition may be compromised, and patterns of sleep disturbed.

The SS patient lacks the normal salivary pooling under

Table 2. Preliminary Classification Criteria Developed by the European Economic Community

I. Primary SS (if at least 4 items present)
  A. Ocular symptoms (at least 1 present)
    1. Daily, persistent, troublesome dry eyes for more than 3 months
    2. Recurrent sensation of sand or gravel in the eyes
    3. Use of a tear substitute more than 3 times a day
  B. Oral symptoms (at least 1 present)
    1. Daily feeling of dry mouth for at least 3 months
    2. Recurrent feeling of swollen salivary glands as an adult
    3. Drinking of liquids to aid in washing down dry foods
  C. Objective evidence of dry eyes (at least 1 present)
    1. Schirmer's test I
    2. Rose bengal test
    3. Lacrimal gland biopsy with focus score ≥1
  D. Objective evidence of salivary gland involvement (at least 1 present)
    1. Salivary gland scintigraphy
    2. Parotid sialography
    3. Unstimulated whole sialometry (≤1.5 mL per 15 minutes)
  E. Laboratory abnormality (at least 1 present)
    1. Anti–SS-A or anti–SS-B antibody
    2. Antinuclear antibody (ANA)
    3. IgM rheumatoid factor (anti-IgG Fc)

Table 3. Current International Classification of Diseases-9-CM Code Assignments for Sjögren's Syndrome Manifestations, Related Symptoms, and Related Disorders

710.2	Sicca syndrome (Sjögren's syndrome)
375.15	Tear-film insufficiency (dry eye without Sjögren's syndrome)
370.33	Keratoconjunctivitis sicca (without Sjögren's syndrome)
521.1	Hypertrophy of the salivary glands (without Sjögren's syndrome)
527.7	Disturbance of salivary gland function (without Sjögren's syndrome)
714.0	Rheumatoid arthritis
710.0	Systemic lupus erythematosus
710.1	Progressive systemic sclerosis (scleroderma)
710.3	Dermatomyositis
710.4	Polymyositis
112.0	Candidiasis of mouth
125.8	Dyspareunia
245.2	Autoimmune thyroiditis
273.0	Polyclonal hypergammaglobulinemia
285.9	Anemia (unspecified)
202.8	Lymphoma
357.5	Polyneuropathy (coded secondary to Sjögren's syndrome)
359.6	Symptomatic myopathy (coded secondary to Sjögren's syndrome)
517.8	Symptomatic lung involvement (coded secondary to Sjögren's syndrome)
373.0	Blepharitis
443.0	Raynaud's syndrome
447.6	Arteritis
521.0	Dental caries
530.81	Esophageal reflux
571.5	Cirrhosis of liver without alcohol
571.6	Biliary cirrhosis
595.1	Interstitial cystitis
704.0	Alopecia
729.1	Myalgia and myositis
730.7	Myalgia and fatigue
787.2	Dysphagia
790.1	Elevated erythrocyte sedimentation rate
785.5	Enlarged lymph nodes
780.1	Rash (nonspecific)

the tongue and may have rapidly progressive caries. Examination may reveal caries at the base of the tooth, petechial lesions on the hard palate, and lichen planus–like lesions (fine, white, lacy strands) on the buccal mucosa. Chronic oral candidiasis is common in the SS patient, but it is unusual to see the plaquelike appearance (thrush) found in severely immunocompromised patients. SS patients also develop angular cheilitis, a condition that must be treated at the same time as the buccal mucosal candidiasis.

CLINICAL COURSE

The manifestations of SS are nonvisceral (fatigue, arthralgias, myalgias, skin lesions) and visceral (lung, heart, kidney, and nervous system abnormalities) (Table 4). These features may be present at the time of initial clinical diagnosis or develop during subsequent years.

Skin

Vasculitis in SS patients takes multiple forms. The characteristic vasculitis among SS patients is hypergammaglobulinemic purpura, with multiple nonpalpable 2- to 3-mm lesions distributed symmetrically over the lower extremities. These lesions are often seen in SS patients who develop a type II mixed cryoglobulinemia (i.e., a monoclonal rheumatoid factor plus a polyclonal IgG). As these acute lesions fade, they are replaced by hyperpigmentation that may persist from months to years. In addition, SS patients may develop palpable purpura owing to leukocytoclastic vasculitis, urticarial vasculitis, erythema nodosum, erythema multiforme, and photosensitive maculopapular skin lesions. Periungual telangiectasias may be detected in some SS patients; their presence in large numbers has been associated with an increased risk of later development of scleroderma.

Dryness of the skin may be related to decreased secretory capacity of sebaceous glands. Oral candidiasis and angular cheilitis frequently cause mouth pain and decreased sensation of taste. Oral candidal infection is particularly common in SS patients treated with glucocorticoids.

Respiratory

Patients with SS often develop tenacious secretions in the nasopharynx and upper airways. An apparently minor case of bronchitis can be complicated by mucus plugs that obstruct the bronchial tree. SS patients may also develop

Table 4. Extraglandular Manifestations in Patients With Primary SS

Respiratory

- Chronic bronchitis secondary to dryness of the upper and lower airway with mucus plugging
- Lymphocytic interstitial pneumonitis
- Pseudolymphoma with nodular infiltrates
- Lymphoma
- Pleural effusions
- Pulmonary hypertension, especially with associated scleroderma

Gastrointestinal

- Dysphagia associated with xerostomia
- Atrophic gastritis
- Liver disease, including biliary cirrhosis and sclerosing cholangitis

Skin

- Candidiasis, oral and vaginal
- Vaginal dryness
- Hyperglobulinemic purpura, nonthrombocytopenic
- Raynaud's phenomenon
- Vasculitis

Endocrine, Neurologic, and Muscular

- Thyroiditis
- Peripheral neuropathy, symmetrical involvement of hands and/or feet
- Mononeuritis multiplex
- Myalgias

Hematologic

- Neutropenia, anemia, thrombocytopenia
- Pseudolymphoma
- Angioimmunoblastic lymphadenopathy
- Lymphoma and myeloma

Renal

- Tubulointerstititai nephritis (TIN)
- Glomerulonephritis, in the absence of antibodies to DNA
- Mixed cryoglobulinemia
- Amyloidosis
- Obstructive nephropathy due to enlarged periaortic lymph nodes
- Lymphoma
- Renal artery vasculitis

polyserositis, with pleuritic chest pain and pleural effusion. Persistent infiltrates in chest films may reflect lymphocytic interstitial pneumonitis or lymphoma.

SS patients with unexplained dyspnea should be carefully examined for pulmonary hypertension. SS patients may produce anticardiolipin antibodies that predispose to deep vein thrombophlebitis and occult pulmonary emboli. Interstitial fibrosis on chest film or high-resolution chest CT is consistent with scleroderma as a cause of SS. Patients with sarcoidosis can present with sicca symptoms, parotid swelling, fever, and increased ANAs (Heerfordt's syndrome).

Gastrointestinal

Decreased saliva production in patients with primary SS causes difficulty in swallowing and deglutition. This problem is particularly common in patients with dentures who cannot chew their food adequately. Abnormal motility in the upper third of the esophagus can also be demonstrated in some SS patients. Heartburn due to gastroesophageal reflux may require the use of agents that block hydrogen ion production.

Significant abnormalities of liver function are unusual and should prompt a search for drug effect, viral hepatitis (especially hepatitis C), primary biliary cirrhosis (PBC), or fatty change in patients chronically treated with steroids. Although PBC may coexist with SS, antimitochondrial antibodies (AMAs) are closely correlated with histologic evidence of PBC, and anti–SS-A and anti–SS-B antibodies are not commonly found in PBC patients with sicca symptoms.

Renal

Renal dysfunction in SS patients is typically subclinical and may be detected during laboratory screening or studies of renal tubular function. Decreased serum bicarbonate, hypokalemia, or increased serum creatinine concentration may result from interstitial lymphoid infiltrate or from medication that exacerbates a previously mild interstitial nephritis. Hypokalemic periodic paralysis and decreased renal function in some SS patients have been attributed to the use of herbal agents.

Proteinuria is uncommon in patients with SS; however, those with associated disorders (e.g., SLE, amyloidosis, or mixed cryoglobulinemia) may develop glomerulonephritis. Decreasing renal function may also signal renal vasculitis, uncontrolled hypertension, or obstruction by abdominal lymphoma.

Hematologic

Leukopenia is relatively common in SS patients but rarely reaches a point of clinical significance. Bone marrow aspirates indicate that this neutropenia results from increased peripheral immune destruction as well as margination of leukocytes in the spleen and other mesenteric vessels.

SS patients experience a 40-fold increased incidence of lymphomas when compared with age-matched control subjects. These are typically IgM-kappa B-cell lymphomas. Lymphadenopathy and recurrent swelling of the parotid and submandibular glands usually precede the development of frank lymphoma. With persistently enlarged nodes or glands, biopsy is often required for excluding neoplasia. DNA analysis of biopsy material is not diagnostic, because oligoclonal DNA rearrangements may be seen in myoepithelial sialadenitis as well as in lymphoma. SS patients who are infected with HIV may also develop a pseudolymphomatous condition.

Neurologic, Psychiatric, and Endocrine Manifestations

Various types of neurologic and psychiatric dysfunction may occur in SS patients. The most common symptoms include fatigue, memory deficit, and depression. Although SS may be associated with subtle alterations in neurochemistry and sleep patterns, it is not clear that changes in affect are caused by autoimmune dysfunction.

SS patients may develop both central and peripheral nervous system manifestations of vasculitis and demyelination. The reported frequency of these complications varies. By contrast, patients with multiple sclerosis have an increased frequency of sicca symptoms, but their dryness results from central nervous system autonomic neuropathy, rather than autoimmune dysfunction of the salivary and lacrimal glands.

Patients with Sjögren's syndrome can present with hypothyroidism or develop this problem later in their course. Thyroid function should be evaluated annually. Adrenal insufficiency may occur, but it usually results from iatrogenic suppression by therapeutic corticosteroids. Adrenal insufficiency can be life-threatening during surgical intervention or other systemic stresses such as septicemia. The association of Sjögren's syndrome with other endocrine disorders is much less common. Nutritional deficits may be encountered as a result of sicca complaints (difficulty in swallowing certain foods), particularly in the edentulous patient who cannot chew meats or other solid foods. Zinc is a critical co-factor for several metalloproteins required in gustatory response; zinc is lacking in many diets and most vitamin supplements, and zinc deficiency may contribute to decreased sense of taste in some patients. Fluoride is important in the maintenance of dental enamel; the absence of fluoride in the water supply in some parts of the country may predispose to progressive dental erosion.

COMMON COMPLICATIONS

Nasal Dryness and Sinusitis

Many SS patients report nasal dryness and postnasal drip. Upper respiratory tract or sinus inflammation may linger for months because decreased secretions and inadequate drainage predispose SS patients to bacterial infection. A change of secretions from clear to yellow or green often indicates bacterial infection, which may require treatment with antibiotics.

Gynecologic

Vaginal dryness often leads to painful intercourse (dyspareunia). Vaginal problems, however, do not occur in all SS patients, even those with severe mouth and eye dryness. When dryness does occur as part of SS, the spouse must be reassured that this problem is not due to failure of sexual arousal. Vaginal dryness in perimenopausal or postmenopausal women is often related to vaginal atrophy that may respond to vaginal estrogen creams.

Fatigue and Depression

Fatigue is a common complaint with many causes that may or may not be related to SS. Two types of fatigue should be considered. The first type is late-morning or early-afternoon fatigue, where the patient arises with adequate energy but "runs out of gas" in the early afternoon. Patients compare this type of fatigue to "having the flu." Fatigue due to active inflammation is often associated with increased erythrocyte sedimentation rate, increased C-reactive protein, and polyclonal hypergammaglobulinemia. The incidence of hypothyroidism is increased in patients with SS; periodic thyroid hormone analysis can exclude this cause of fatigue.

A second type of fatigue is "morning fatigue," where the patient arises with feelings of inadequate sleep. This type of fatigue is also quite common in SS and may accompany "inflammatory" fatigue. For example, patients may have inadequate sleep owing to joint or muscle pain. Increased fluid intake to relieve dry mouth and throat may cause nocturia that disrupts sleep and leads to morning fatigue. Saliva substitutes in place of fluid ingestion may help to reduce nocturia.

SS patients who are depressed experience difficulty in concentrating, poor appetite, or sleep disturbances. The precise contribution of inflammation and hormone imbalances to depression in SS patients remains unclear. Stress, poor sleep, and chronic illness can also contribute to depression.

Anesthesiology and Surgery

SS patients have particular problems during the preoperative, perioperative, and postoperative periods. The normal preoperative instruction is "no fluids by mouth" after dinner or midnight on the day prior to surgery. In the absence of normal saliva flow, these patients have great discomfort that can be reduced by the use of artificial salivas.

Operating rooms and postoperative recovery areas tend to be dry, and patients are further exposed to nonhumidified oxygen via face masks. Therefore, SS patients have increased risk of developing corneal abrasions during surgery and postoperatively. A decreased blink reflex during anesthesia also contributes to the risk of abrasions. The administration of ocular lubricants prior to surgery and in the postoperative recovery suite can reduce the chance of this complication.

Upper airway dryness may lead to mucus plug inspissation and obstructive pneumonias postoperatively. The use of humidified oxygen, avoidance of medications that excessively dry the upper airways, adequate hydration, and appropriate respiratory care can prevent this problem. Poor dentition in SS patients increases the risk of damage to and aspiration of teeth during intubation.

In RA patients with secondary SS, the anesthesiologist must be alerted to arthritic involvement of the neck (especially C1–C2 level). Attempts to hyperextend the neck during intubation may cause transection of the cervical spinal cord and paraplegia. Fitting the patient with a soft cervical collar prior to intubation may avoid this problem.

Finally, assessment of the "fluid status" of the SS patient during the postoperative period may be relatively difficult. Evaluation of the moisture in the ocular and oral membranes may be quite misleading. Also, some SS patients have interstitial nephritis that prevents adequate urine concentration and maintenance of fluid balance. Renal insufficiency may be exacerbated by aminoglycosides and other antibiotics.

DIAGNOSTIC PROCEDURES

Salivary Gland Biopsy and Sialography

Biopsy of the minor salivary gland is perhaps the most specific procedure for the diagnosis of SS. The San Francisco criteria define a focus score, with each "focus" representing a cluster of at least 50 mononuclear cells. The average focus score is based on at least 4 evaluable glands. "Focal sialadenitis" in labial biopsies should be distinguished from "chronic nonspecific sialadenitis." The latter biopsies contain scattered mononuclear cell infiltrates (rather than focal clusters of lymphocytes), and the salivary ducts are often distended and/or obstructed by mucinous material. In some cases of chronic sialadenitis, neutrophils migrate to periductal tissues in response to leakage of inspissated mucus. This "chronic" sialadenitis is commonly found in older patients and can be distinguished from the focal sialadenitis found in SS patients. In other patients with dryness, salivary glands may reveal fibrosis, amyloid, or fat; these types of biopsies must also be distinguished from focal sialadenitis.

Minor salivary gland biopsies should be obtained from clinically normal mucosa because biopsies taken from an area of mucositis may give false-positive results. At least 4 evaluable salivary glands should be obtained. An average "focus score" (a focus is defined as a cluster of at least 50 lymphocytes) per mm^2 should be reported, based on evaluation of at least 4 glands. A focus score from a single lobule is not acceptable for diagnosis. Moreover, focus scoring should not include evaluation of lobules where "nonspecific" inflammatory infiltrate is produced by obstruction of salivary duct tubules by inspissated mucus.

Sialography, parotid scanning, and magnetic resonance imaging (MRI) have been used to examine the function and size of the major salivary glands. Avoidance of oil-base contrast media for sialography eliminates the risk of chronic "granulomatous" reactions due to dye extravasation. However, the use of water-base sialographic materials may exacerbate an acute flare of parotitis. When sialography is employed to evaluate the ducts, specific criteria for head positioning and the timing of postinfusion imaging must be carefully met.

Scanning of the parotids with technetium Tc-99m provides a noninvasive method for evaluation of secretory function. However, it is difficult to determine whether delayed excretion is specifically related to focal sialadenitis or is the result of any process associated with sicca symptoms. If salivary glands are palpably enlarged, soft tissue MRI of the neck and glands can identify some lesions prior to biopsy.

Autoantibody Analysis

The frequency of ANAs in SS patients varies with the criteria used to make the diagnosis. With the use of immunofluorescence and Hep-2 cells, a homogeneous or fine speckled pattern is most commonly observed. SS sera contain antibodies directed against SS-A (Ro) antigen and SS-B (La) antigen. However, the production of anti–SS-A and anti–SS-B antibodies is more closely associated with specific HLA class II antigens than with specific clinical manifestations of autoimmune disease.

Antibodies against SS-A and SS-B are predominantly IgG (typically IgG1). Although these antibodies may cross the placenta and contribute to neonatal SLE and congenital heart block, their role in the pathogenesis of SS is unclear because the target antigens are found in all nucleated cells. Immunoblotting and immunoprecipitation studies indicate that anti–SS-A binds to proteins weighing 60 and 52 kd, respectively; these proteins are associated with small RNA molecules termed hYRNAs. The pattern of SS-A reactivity in SS patients does not closely correlate with clinical features. Anti–SS-B antibodies react with a 48-kd phosphoprotein that complexes with products of RNA polymerase III activity.

Other autoantibodies are found in some SS patients. The identification of antibodies against nucleolar and centromere antigens suggests overlap with scleroderma. Antibodies against Golgi-associated and cytoplasmic antigens have not been correlated with clinical features or prognosis.

DIFFERENTIAL DIAGNOSIS

Other causes of keratitis include pemphigoid, sarcoidosis, trauma, infection, vitamin deficiency, neuropathy, and allergy (Table 5). Some SS patients have recurrent swelling of the parotid and submandibular glands. The swelling of these glands and cervical lymph nodes may suggest the presence of lymphoma, particularly in patients with low-grade fever and night sweats. In these SS patients, biopsy of major salivary gland or lymph node may be indicated because the risk of lymphoma is 50-fold greater than that in age-matched control subjects. The lymphomas are generally IgM-kappa B-cell malignancies. In some SS patients, lymph node or salivary gland biopsy reveals "reactive" lymphoid hyperplasia (pseudolymphoma). The majority of infiltrating lymphocytes are CD4-positive T cells. One or more oligoclonal rearrangements of the immunoglobulin or T-cell antigen receptor genes may be identified, and these patients have an increased risk of developing non-Hodgkin's lymphoma.

Other causes of salivary gland enlargement (see Table 5) include sarcoidosis, infection, drug hypersensitivity, tumors, and HIV infection. Any history of intravenous drug abuse, multiple sexual encounters, or blood transfusions should prompt a request for HIV screening. Importantly, anti–SS-A and anti–SS-B are rarely found in HIV-positive individuals with lymphadenopathy and hyperglobulinemia. While HLA-DR5 is more common in HIV-positive patients, HLA-DR3 is more common in whites with SS.

Table 5. Causes of Keratitis and Salivary Gland Enlargement Other Than SS

Keratitis

- Mucous membrane pemphigoid
- Sarcoidosis
- Infections: viral (adenovirus, herpes virus, vaccinia), bacterial, or chlamydial (i.e., trachoma)
- Trauma (i.e., from contact lenses) and environmental irritants, including chemical burns, exposure to ultraviolet lights, or radiographs
- Neuropathy, including neurotrophic keratitis (i.e., damage to fifth cranial nerve and familial dysautonomia [Riley-Day syndrome])
- Hypovitaminosis A
- Erythema multiforme (Stevens-Johnson syndrome)

Salivary Gland Enlargement

- Sarcoidosis, amyloidosis
- Bacterial infections, including gonorrhea and syphilis, and viral infections (i.e., infectious mononucleosis, mumps)
- Tuberculosis, actinomycosis, histoplasmosis, trachoma, leprosy
- Iodide, lead, or copper hypersensitivity
- Hyperlipidemic states, especially types IV and V
- Tumors (usually unilateral), including cysts (Warthin's tumor), epithelial (adenoma, adenocarcinoma), lymphoma, and mixed salivary gland tumors
- Excessive alcohol consumption
- Human immunodeficiency virus (HIV) infection

POTENTIAL PITFALLS IN DIAGNOSIS

The clinical terms used to describe SS patients are relatively vague. For example, patients are said to have xerostomia. Late in the 19th century, this term was used to identify patients with a truly dry mouth (i.e., no clinical evidence of saliva and nothing expressible from the ducts). At the close of the 20th century, a wide range of salivary flow rates have been reported in clinically normal individuals. Investigators have therefore questioned the validity of arbitrarily defined cutoff rates for normal salivary flow. Indeed, maintenance of the integrity of oral tissues may depend not only on the quantity of saliva but also on its protein and mucin composition.

Some clinicians rely more heavily than others on serologic evidence to support a diagnosis of SS. However, all physicians who care for SS patients should be aware of artifacts leading to both false-positive and false-negative autoantibody profiles.

For example, a laboratory report may state that the ANA is negative but antibody to SS-A is positive. Since all dividing human cells require the SS-A antigen for a critical step in post-translational modification of RNA, any serum that reacts with SS-A antigens should also react with a human cell line that is dividing. Thus, the absence of ANA reactivity in an SS-A antibody–positive serum sample must represent a technical artifact in the detection of either ANA or anti–SS-A antibody. Possible explanations for this discrepancy include the following:

1. The ANA result could be artifactually negative. Cultured human cells (e.g., Hep-2 cells) are frequently used as substrate for indirect immunofluorescent detection of ANA in patient's serum. However, the use of alcohol, acetone, or formaldehyde to preserve cells on slides may solubilize or denature the SS-A antigen, leading to a false-negative result. The method of preservation differs significantly among vendors of kits for detection of ANA and, occasionally, among lots of substrate provided by the same vendor. Further, the methods of preservation are often "proprietary" secrets not available for review by the rheumatologist or the clinical laboratory. The problem of variability in ANA substrates is more frequently encountered in SS patients than in SLE patients because the SS-A antigen is less stable than the Sm or DNA antigens detected in SLE sera. Although sera from SLE patients are generally analyzed as positive controls for ANA tests, sera from SS patients are typically not included as positive controls. Further, no "standard human sera for SS" are available for use as uniform positive controls.
2. The antibody to SS-A could be artifactually positive. In some laboratories, antigens are prepared from human cell lines or extracts of calf thymus. In other laboratories, recombinant antigens are utilized. Cell extracts may be contaminated with other proteins, while recombinant antigens may not have the correct post-translational modifications required for antigenicity or may have partial aggregation that causes artifactual reactivity. The frequency of these problems has increased with the detection of anti–SS-A antibody by ultrasensitive enzyme-linked immunosorbent assay (ELISA) techniques. In general, little debate exists about sera that strongly react with SS-A antigen in ELISA because these antibodies can be confirmed by Ouchterlony diffusion and Western blotting. However, the significance of weakly reacting anti–SS-A antibodies by ELISA remains unclear. The method used to "validate" such weak

ELISAs may be their reactivity with sera from a panel of SS patients. However, since the criteria for SS remain controversial, the validation of weak ELISA tests by this method may be misleading. The interpretation of anti–SS-A activity is also challenging because some SS patients react with either the 60-kd or the 52-kd molecules, but not with both. Also, a variety of epitopes on each protein are present in some, but not in other, SS sera. Although murine monoclonal antibodies have been prepared against human SS antigens, they cannot be used as standard positive controls because they react with a pattern of epitopes that differs from those of human SS sera. Finally, fresh mouse kidney (a substrate used in some ANA tests) contains one or more SS-A proteins that are antigenically distinct from human SS-A protein.

3. The antibody to SS-B antigen is artifactually positive. SS-B protein is more stable during fixation and cross-reacts with antibodies to mouse SS-B antigen. Thus, fewer standardization problems have been encountered in the detection of SS-B proteins with the use of Ouchterlony methods. In general, antibodies against SS-B are found only in sera that also contain antibodies against SS-A. However, ultrasensitive ELISA testing has demonstrated an increased frequency of anti–SS-B reactivity in sera lacking anti–SS-A activity. Although a false-positive ELISA for SS-B seems most likely, further studies are required.

Finally, it deserves emphasis that every patient with an enlarged salivary or lacrimal gland and a positive ANA does not necessarily have SS. Low titers of ANAs are occasionally present in patients with sarcoidosis, and the presence of a noncaseating granuloma on biopsy confirms this diagnosis. Other patients with dryness and enlarged salivary glands have amyloidosis or hemochromatosis in association with chronic arthritis. Other causes of enlarged glands include fatty infiltrates associated with diabetes mellitus, hepatic cirrhosis, hyperlipoproteinemia, and chronic pancreatitis.

The author wishes to thank his coworkers at the Scripps Clinic for their suggestions, including Drs. M. Friedlaender (Ophthalmology), R. Simon (Allergy), F. Izuno (Dermatology), S. Poceta (Neurology), J. Willems (Gynecology), R. Stewart (Oral Medicine), and the members of the Rheumatology Department.

SYSTEMIC LUPUS ERYTHEMATOSUS

By H. Michael Belmont, M.D.
New York, New York

Systemic lupus erythematosus (SLE) is an autoimmune disease characterized by immune dysregulation, production of antinuclear antibody (ANA), generation of circulating immune complexes, and activation of the complement system. SLE is notable for unpredictable exacerbations and remissions and a predilection for clinical involvement of the joints, skin, kidney, brain, serosa, lung, heart, and gastrointestinal tract. The pathologic hallmark of SLE is recurrent, widespread, and diverse vascular lesions.

SLE is not a rare disorder. Although reported at both extremes of life (e.g., diagnosed in infants and in the 10th decade of life), SLE chiefly affects women of child-bearing age. In children, SLE occurs three times more commonly in females than in males. In the 60 per cent of patients with SLE who experience the onset of disease between puberty and the fourth decade of life, the female-to-male ratio is 9:1. Thereafter, the female preponderance again falls to that observed in prepubescents.

The disorder is three times more common in African Americans than in white Americans. SLE is also more common in Asians than in whites. In China, SLE may be more common than rheumatoid arthritis; African Caribbean blacks are at greatest risk for SLE. The worldwide annual incidence of SLE ranges from 6 to 35 new cases per 100,000 population. The prevalence of SLE in the United States is debated. Traditional prevalence estimates of 250,000 to 500,000 cases are contradicted by a recent nationwide telephone poll suggesting a prevalence of 1 to 2 million cases.

The clinical features of SLE are protean and may mimic infectious mononucleosis, lymphoma, or other systemic disease. Therefore, the American College of Rheumatology has developed criteria to include patients with SLE and exclude those with other disorders (Table 1). These criteria are best used for inclusion of appropriate patients in epidemiologic or other research studies. Many patients do not fulfill the rigid criteria at first encounter. However, many will eventually meet the criteria if followed for a sufficient time.

The cause of SLE remains unknown. A genetic predisposition, sex hormones, and an environmental trigger or triggers most likely contribute to the disordered immune response that underlies the disease. A role for heredity is suggested by the disproportionate presence of two histocompatibility antigens (HLA-DR2 and HLA-DR3) in patients with SLE. The extended haplotype HLA-A1, B8, DR3 is also found more frequently in patients with SLE. The role for heredity is further supported by the concordance for SLE among monozygotic twins. However, the polygenic nature of this genetic predisposition and the significant role of environmental factors are suggested by the relatively moderate concordance rate of 25 to 60 per cent.

The origin of autoantibody production in SLE is unclear, but antigen-driven processes, spontaneous B-cell hyperresponsiveness, and/or impaired immune regulation could play a role. Regardless of the cause of autoantibody production, SLE is associated with impaired clearance of circulating immune complexes due to decreased CR1 expression, deficient C4A, or defective Fc receptors.

The cellular and molecular aspects of the vascular changes are better understood than the origins of autoimmunity in SLE. Manifestations of disease are related to recurrent vascular injury due to immune complex deposition, leukothrombosis, or thrombosis (Table 2). In addition, cytotoxic antibodies mediate autoimmune hemolytic anemia and thrombocytopenia, whereas antibodies to specific antigens disrupt cellular function. For example, the production of antineuronal antibodies has been correlated with the neuropsychiatric manifestations of SLE.

The functional status of a patient with SLE is related not only to the baseline disease activity but also to the damage that results from recurrent episodes of disease flare and the adverse effects of treatment. Recurrent flares of SLE are associated with deforming arthropathy, shrinking lung, end-stage renal disease, and organic mental syndromes. Well-known adverse effects of treatment of SLE include avascular necrosis of bone, infections, and premature atherosclerosis.

Table 1. The 1982 Revised Criteria for Classification of Systemic Lupus Erythematosus*

Criterion	Definition
Butterfly rash	Fixed erythema, flat or raised, over the malar eminences, tending to spare the nasolabial folds
Discoid lupus	Erythematous raised patches with adherent keratotic scaling and follicular plugging; atrophic scarring may occur in older lesions
Photosensitivity	Skin rash as a result of unusual reaction to sunlight, diagnosed by patient history or physician observation
Oral ulcers	Painless oral or nasopharyngeal ulceration observed by a physician
Arthritis	Nonerosive arthritis involving two or more peripheral joints, characterized by tenderness, swelling, or effusion
Serositis	Pleuritis—convincing history of pleuritic pain or rub heard by a physician or evidence of pleural effusion *or* Pericarditis—documented by ECG or rub or evidence of pericardial effusion
Renal disorder	Persistent proteinuria greater than 0.5 g/d or greater than 3+ if quantitation not performed *or* Cellular casts—may be red cell, hemoglobin, granular, tubular, or mixed
Neurologic disorder	Seizures—in the absence of offending drugs or known metabolic derangements (e.g., uremia, ketoacidosis, or electrolyte imbalance) *or* Coma—in the absence of offending drugs or known metabolic derangements (e.g., uremia, ketoacidosis, or electrolyte imbalance)
Hematologic disorder	Hemolytic anemia with reticulocytosis *or* Leukopenia—less than 4000/mm^3 total on two or more occasions *or* Thrombocytopenia—less than 100,000/mm^3 in the absence of offending drugs
Immunologic disorder	Positive LE cell preparation *or* Antibody to native DNA (n-DNA) in abnormal titer *or* antibody to Sm nuclear antigen *or* False-positive STS for patients known to be positive for at least 6 months and confirmed by TPI or FTA tests
Antinuclear antibody	An abnormal titer of ANA by immunofluorescence or an equivalent assay at any point in time and in the absence of drugs known to be associated with drug-induced lupus erythematosus syndrome

*For the purpose of identifying patients in clinical studies, a person shall be said to have systemic lupus erythematosus if any 4 or more of the 11 criteria are present, serially or simultaneously, during any interval of observation.

TPI = *Treponema pallidum* immobilization; FTA = fluorescent treponema antibody; ECG = electrocardiogram; LE = lupus erythematosus; STS = serologic test for syphilis; ANA = antinuclear antibody.

Modified from Tan, E.M., Cohen, A.S., Fries, J.F., et al.: The 1982 revised criteria for the classification of systemic lupus erythematosus. Arthritis Rheum., 25:1271–1276, 1982.

PRESENTING SIGNS AND SYMPTOMS

Eighty per cent of patients with SLE present with skin or joint problems. For example, photosensitive rash, with or without alopecia, is a common presenting complaint. Alternatively, patients may present with arthralgia or frank arthritis. However, patients may also present with fever and single organ involvement. Typical examples of the latter presentation include serositis, glomerulonephritis, neuropsychiatric disturbance, autoimmune hemolytic anemia, or thrombocytopenia. Rarely, patients present with severe, acute lupus crisis involving multiple organs and systems.

Constitutional Symptoms

Ninety per cent of patients with SLE experience fatigue. Arthralgia and myalgia often accompany complaints of malaise. A less common but more serious constitutional feature of SLE is persistent fever and weight loss.

Musculoskeletal Symptoms

Approximately 90 per cent of patients with SLE have musculoskeletal symptoms. The typical clinical manifesta-

Table 2. Pathologic and Clinical Spectrum of Vascular Injury in Systemic Lupus Erythematosus

Pathologic Features	Pathogenesis	Clinical Phenomenon
Capillaritis* Vasculitis*	Immune complex deposition Activation of complement, neutrophils, and endothelium Modeled by Arthus lesion	Glomerulonephritis, pulmonary alveolar hemorrhage Cutaneous purpura, polyarteritis nodosa–like systemic and cerebral vasculitis
Leukothrombosis	Intravascular activation of complement, neutrophils, and vascular endothelium Absence of local immune complex deposition Modeled by Shwartzman lesion	Widespread vascular injury, hypoxia, cerebral dysfunction, systemic inflammatory response syndrome (SIRS)
Thrombosis	Antibodies to anionic phospholipid-protein complexes interact with endothelial cells, platelets, or coagulation factors Modeled by antiphospholipid antibody syndrome Disseminated intravascular platelet aggregation	Arterial and venous thrombosis, fetal wastage, thrombocytopenia, pulmonary hypertension Thrombotic thrombocytopenia purpura (TTP)

*Capillaritis or microvascular angiitis and lupus vasculitis share a similar pathogenesis but are associated with different clinical phenomena.

tion is arthralgia. The joints most commonly involved are the proximal interphalangeal, metacarpophalangeal, wrist, and knee joints. In contrast to rheumatoid arthritis, lupus is rarely accompanied by frank articular erosions. When arthritis does occur in SLE, it typically follows periarticular inflammation with involvement of tendons. This can lead to Jaccoud's arthropathy with characteristic reducible deformities. Myalgias are another common feature of SLE. Less common is frank inflammatory myositis, which may be confused with steroid-induced myopathy. However, with inflammatory muscle disease, serum concentrations of creatine phosphokinase, lactate dehydrogenase, and aldolase are typically increased.

Mucocutaneous Symptoms

Mucosal ulcers are documented in 30 per cent of patients with lupus. Ulcers most often occur on the hard or soft palate but also may be found on the nasal septum. The lesions are usually painless and undetected by the patient but may be painful when oral candidiasis or other secondary infection develops. In some patients, the cause of the ulcers may be simple inflammatory mucositis. In others, the cause may be frank vasculitis of the mucous membranes.

Approximately 80 per cent of patients with SLE have dermatologic manifestations during the course of their illness. The classic acute skin eruption is described as a photosensitive rash with a butterfly appearance because the lesion involves the bridge of the nose and malar areas of the face. This "butterfly" rash characteristically spares the nasolabial folds. Photosensitivity is less common in patients of color but nevertheless occurs in 50 per cent of all patients with SLE. The rash of subacute cutaneous lupus is observed in patients with circulating anti-Ro antibodies. This eruption is moderately photosensitive and may have a papulosquamous, pityriasiform, psoriasiform, or annular polycyclic appearance. Twenty-five per cent of patients with SLE have nonphotosensitive discoid skin lesions, most frequently seen on the face and the inner pinna of the ear. Discoid lesions are characterized clinically by follicular plugging, skin atrophy, scaling, telangiectasia, and skin erythema.

Alopecia occurs in 50 per cent of patients with SLE and is typically described as reversible hair thinning during periods of exacerbation of the disease. Hair can be plucked easily from the scalp, and short strands of "lupus hairs" develop at the scalp line. In the wake of an acute, usually febrile, exacerbation of SLE, patients may experience precipitous generalized hair loss as part of a telogen effluvium following an arrest of hair growth. Discoid lesions of the scalp typically lead to scarring alopecia.

Unusual skin manifestations of lupus include urticaria, angioedema, bullae, and panniculitis known as lupus profundus. Raynaud's phenomenon is observed in 30 per cent of patients with SLE. Livedo reticularis is also more frequently seen in patients with SLE. The presence of livedo may identify patients with SLE and the secondary antiphospholipid antibody syndrome. Digital and palpable purpura most likely reflect the intensity of leukocytoclastic vasculitis in patients with SLE.

Serosal Symptoms

Inflammation (serositis) of the pleura, pericardium, and peritoneum occurs in 50 per cent of patients with SLE. Pleuritis, pericarditis, and medical peritonitis in SLE may be accompanied by large effusions or no effusion at all. Effusions in SLE are typically inflammatory and exudative. Frank cardiac tamponade is rare.

Hematologic Symptoms

Anemia of chronic inflammation is a common feature of exacerbated SLE. Coombs' test–positive hemolysis occurs in 10 per cent of patients. Some patients with SLE present with thrombocytopenic purpura, whereas others acquire this condition later in the course of illness. Thrombocytopenia as a consequence of the antiphospholipid antibody syndrome has also been described in SLE. Leukopenia with lymphopenia is a characteristic feature of SLE that may not be associated with a significantly increased risk of infection in the absence of exposure to cytotoxic drugs.

Renal Symptoms

Although most SLE patients have microscopic evidence of glomerulopathy, only 50 per cent manifest clinically significant renal disease. SLE glomerulopathy is typically associated with deposition of immune complexes containing anti-DNA. Serum anti-DNA antibodies provide a clinically useful marker for the onset of renal disease. Hypocomplementemia is also a harbinger of active renal disease. Mesangial lupus nephropathy is generally associated with an excellent prognosis, whereas proliferative lupus nephropathy, especially the diffuse variant, is often characterized by hypertension, red cell casts, and significant deterioration of renal function. Nephrotic syndrome in the absence of hypertension, active urine sediment, or significant hypocomplementemia suggests the membranous variant of lupus nephropathy.

Central Nervous System Symptoms

Neuropsychiatric complications occur in 50 per cent of SLE patients. Acute and chronic as well as focal and diffuse manifestations have been described. Cerebrovascular accidents are the consequence of either inflammatory or noninflammatory thrombotic vasculopathy in the central nervous system. Seizures complicate the course in 25 per cent of patients with lupus. Diffuse cerebral dysfunction may present as personality disorder, psychosis, affective disorder, or coma. Vascular or migraine headaches occur in 10 per cent of lupus patients. Recurrent complications in the central nervous system may lead to organic brain syndrome and dementia.

Secondary Antiphospholipid Antibody Syndrome

Patients with SLE acquire autoantibodies against negatively charged phospholipids. The antiphospholipid antibody syndrome occurs most frequently in SLE patients with high-titer IgG anticardiolipin antibodies or lupus anticoagulant. Patients with this disorder are at increased risk for recurrent arterial and venous thrombosis, thrombocytopenia, and fetal wastage. The mechanisms of this prothrombotic diathesis (hypercoagulable state) are uncertain, but these autoantibodies, perhaps interacting with co-factors, bind to target antigens on endothelial cells, platelets, and coagulation factors.

Ocular Symptoms

Patients with lupus may experience anterior uveitis or iridocyclitis. Frank retinal vasculitis, central retinal artery occlusion, central retinal vein occlusion, and ischemic optic neuropathy have been described. Xerostomia with keratoconjunctivitis sicca is seen in 10 per cent of patients with lupus.

Pulmonary Symptoms

The most common disorder of the lung in lupus is inflammatory serositis producing pleuritis. However, patients with lupus also experience transient hypoxia due to pulmonary leukosequestration, inflammatory pneumonitis, interstitial pulmonary fibrosis, pulmonary hypertension, diaphragmatic dysfunction, and phrenic nerve palsy.

Cardiac Symptoms

Although the most common cardiac complication is pericarditis with or without effusion, lupus patients can also experience myocarditis. In addition, nonbacterial verrucous endocarditis or Libman-Sacks endocarditis produces millimeter vegetations on the mitral and aortic valves. These vegetations are usually asymptomatic and found incidentally at autopsy. Rarely, they may cause cerebral or coronary artery embolization. Thrombotic valvulitis and thrombosis of cardiac chambers have been described in patients with the antiphospholipid antibody syndrome. Coronary artery vasculitis has been documented in active lupus, but this condition rarely produces myocardial infarction.

The incidence of atherosclerotic heart disease is increased in patients with lupus. Premature atherosclerosis may be initiated by immune complex deposition in coronary arteries and aggravated by chronic steroid treatment that produces hyperlipidemia and hyperglycemia. In addition, the hyperlipidemia that accompanies lupus nephritis promotes atherosclerosis. When SLE patients with antiphospholipid antibody syndrome experience myocardial infarction, the most common cause is bland coronary artery thrombosis.

Gastrointestinal Symptoms

Medical peritonitis with or without ascites is a well-documented manifestation of lupus serositis. Less common gastrointestinal complications include mesenteric ischemic vasculitis and pancreatitis. The latter can be a manifestation of lupus or, less commonly, a consequence of treatment with steroids. Although nonspecific hepatic inflammation has been described in lupus, abnormalities of liver function most commonly result from idiosyncratic reactions to aspirin, anti-inflammatory drugs, hydroxychloroquine, or azathioprine. Progression of inflammatory liver disease to cirrhosis is rare in SLE.

SUBSETS OF SYSTEMIC LUPUS ERYTHEMATOSUS

Discoid, drug-induced, neonatal, and Ro (ANA-negative) lupus are related to SLE and warrant a brief description.

Discoid lupus is a chronic, nonphotosensitive, potentially scarring skin disorder. ANA and other autoantibodies are not usually detected. Perhaps 10 per cent of patients with discoid lupus acquire the systemic disorder.

Procainamide, hydralazine, and other drugs can induce the formation of ANA, especially antihistone antibodies. Drug-induced lupus is usually characterized by fever, autoimmune hemolytic anemia, autoimmune thrombocytopenia, and/or serositis. Skin, renal, and neurologic manifestations are uncommon.

Neonatal or congenital lupus occurs when the transplacental acquisition of anti-Ro (SS-A) autoantibodies produces a transient photosensitive rash, congenital complete heart block, thrombocytopenia or, rarely, hepatobiliary dysfunction.

ANA-negative or Ro lupus is defined by the absence of ANA and the presence of a lupuslike illness. Ro lupus is most often characterized by a partially photosensitive skin rash referred to as subacute cutaneous lupus erythematosus. These patients often demonstrate anti-Ro antibodies in the serum.

LABORATORY PROCEDURES

In patients with suspected SLE, appropriate laboratory studies include a complete blood count, erythrocyte sedimentation rate, urinalysis, biochemical profile, and ANA testing. SLE is associated with the anemia of chronic inflammation, acute hemolytic anemia, leukopenia, lymphopenia, and thrombocytopenia. Increased sedimentation rates are typical of exacerbation episodes. Lupus glomerulonephritis is accompanied by hypoalbuminemia, hyperlipidemia, and azotemia. The urinalysis in nephrotic lupus patients may show increased protein only. By contrast, patients with proliferative nephritis show hematuria, red cell casts, and white cell casts. The occasional patient with SLE myositis may have increased aspartate aminotransferase (AST), lactate dehydrogenase (LD), creatine kinase (CK), and aldolase in the serum. Ninety to 95 per cent of patients with SLE have speckled, diffuse, or peripheral patterns of serum ANA in titers exceeding 1:40.

When the ANA is not detected but the diagnosis of SLE is strongly suspected, testing for anti-Ro (SS-A) and anti-La (SS-B) can be used to identify the rare patient with ANA-negative, Ro lupus. Moreover, a serum CH_{50} value of zero can identify the unusual ANA-negative patient with homozygous complement deficiency (e.g., C1q, C2, C4) who is at risk for the development of an SLE-like illness.

Additional testing may confirm the diagnosis of SLE in selected patients. Thirty to 70 per cent of patients with SLE have anti-DNA antibodies in the serum, whereas 30 per cent have anti-Sm antibodies. The presence of anti–double-stranded DNA antibodies and decreased complement in the serum strongly suggests the diagnosis of lupus and identifies the patient at increased risk for glomerulonephritis.

In patients with a history of recurrent thrombosis or recurrent fetal wastage, the diagnosis of antiphospholipid antibody syndrome can be confirmed by detecting anticardiolipin antibodies and by demonstrating an abnormal VDRL, partial thromboplastin time (PTT), and/or dilute Russell's viper venom time.

DIAGNOSTIC PROCEDURES

Plain radiographs are not routinely useful in the diagnosis or management of SLE. Magnetic resonance imaging (MRI) is now recognized as the most sensitive technique for identifying avascular necrosis of bone in lupus patients treated with steroids. Chest films and chest computed tomography (CT) scans may help the clinician distinguish infectious from inflammatory lung disease. Thoracentesis, pericardiocentesis, and paracentesis may be necessary for evaluating patients with effusive serositis, especially if fever is present. Electrocardiography (ECG) may show changes consistent with pericarditis. Electrocardiography may also provide evidence of myocardial infarction in SLE patients with chest pain. Echocardiograms may show pericardial effusions or valvulitis. Electroencephalograms are nonspecifically abnormal in 75 per cent of SLE patients with acute diffuse cerebral dysfunction. Quantitative electroencephalography may provide more specific information but is not routinely available. Computed tomography of the brain is also nonspecific and has proved less sensitive than MRI in evaluating the central nervous system. MRI, in turn, is more useful in patients with focal rather than diffuse cerebral dysfunction. Finally, positron emission tomography (PET) and single photon emission computed tomography (SPECT) scans of the nervous system may prove diagnostically helpful in the future.

Biopsies are required infrequently for the diagnosis of SLE. Occasionally, biopsies of the skin can distinguish cutaneous manifestations of lupus from coincidental skin disorders. Lymphadenopathy occurs in 40 per cent of patients with SLE, and biopsies typically show reactive or immunoblastic hyperplasia. Lymphomas, however, are more frequent in patients with SLE, and lymph node biopsy may be necessary for excluding the possibility of malignancy. Renal biopsies are often required in the management of SLE. The timing of the biopsy remains controversial because many rheumatologists recommend empirical treatment of initial episodes of nephritis with corticosteroids. However, a biopsy is useful for refractory, recently relapsed, or frequently relapsed renal disease, especially for the identification of candidates for cytotoxic therapy. Importantly, the nature and extent of renal microscopic abnormalities correlate with prognosis. Renal histopathologic characteristics can be categorized using a World Health Organization (WHO) or a National Institutes of Health (NIH) classification system. In the WHO classification, mesangial and membranous lupus nephropathy have a better prognosis than proliferative lupus nephritis. Membranous disease with persistent nephrotic syndrome can lead to progressive renal dysfunction, but patients with focal or diffuse proliferative glomerulonephritis clearly have the worst prognosis. Renal biopsies are most useful when evaluated by light microscopy, immunofluorescence, and electron microscopy, using the WHO classification and NIH activity and chronicity indices.

COMMON PITFALLS AND ERRORS

Misinterpretation of ANA results is common. Abnormal ANA titers are not diagnostic of SLE. Importantly, 25 to 40 per cent of normal, healthy women are ANA-positive but never acquire lupus or other connective tissue disease. The ANA determination may be transiently positive in response to commonplace viral infections, in the presence of chronic infections, or as a consequence of prescription drug use. The ANA determination may also be positive in patients with lymphoproliferative disorders or chronic liver disease. Titers in patients with false-positive ANA determinations are usually low, tend to fluctuate (reverting at times to negative), and are not accompanied by cardinal signs and symptoms of SLE. The more specific autoantibodies seen in SLE, including anti-DNA, anti-Sm, and anti-Ro, are also not detected. Therefore, patients with myalgia and arthralgia who may, in fact, have fibromyalgia or nonrheumatic causes for their complaints should not be diagnosed with SLE simply because ANA has been detected.

The clinician must be able to recognize a benign systemic variant of SLE. Patients with benign or incomplete SLE are ANA-positive, but the manifestations of their disorder are limited to mild constitutional, articular, cutaneous, and serosal changes. These patients do not experience the more serious renal, neurologic, hematologic, and visceral manifestations of classic SLE. Avoidance of sun as well as the administration of topical steroids, nonsteroidal anti-inflammatory agents, and/or hydroxychloroquine are the typically adequate measures for managing patients with benign or incomplete SLE.

At the other extreme, a potential pitfall is to consider the diagnosis of SLE but to fail to perform an adequate history, physical examination, and evaluation of laboratory studies to identify a patient with severe lupus. Subtle signs, symptoms, or laboratory abnormalities (e.g., shortness of breath, forgetfulness, agitation, proteinuria, hematuria, hypocomplementemia, and so on) may be a harbinger of serious organ injury that warrants aggressive medical therapy. Failure to recognize the significance of these findings and failure to initiate appropriate treatment may cause unnecessary morbidity, if not mortality.

POLYARTERITIS NODOSA

By Lee D. Kaufman, M.D.,
and Ranjan Roy, M.D.
Stony Brook, New York

The vasculitides are a heterogeneous group of disorders characterized by inflammation of blood vessels. The spectrum of vasculitic disease has been traditionally classified on the basis of vessel size, the pathologic lesion (presence or absence of granuloma), and the organ system or systems involved (Table 1). Most patients with a clinical syndrome consistent with vasculitis fall into one of the following categories: (1) small-vessel or leukocytoclastic vasculitis (associated with specific drugs, infections, neoplasms, or connective tissue diseases), (2) polyarteritis nodosa (which classically affects small and medium-sized muscular arteries), (3) Wegener's granulomatosis (WG; a necrotizing granulomatous vasculitis of small to medium-sized vessels of the upper airways and kidney), and (4) the large-vessel diseases of temporal (cranial) arteritis and Takayasu's arteritis. In patient populations served by primary care physicians, leukocytoclastic vasculitis and temporal arteritis followed by polyarteritis are likely to be the most common forms of vasculitis encountered.

The multisystem disease associated with classic polyarteritis nodosa (PAN; also referred to as systemic necrotizing vasculitis [SNV]) is the focus of this discussion, and the terms PAN and SNV should be considered interchangeable. PAN is a rare condition with an annual incidence of 4.6 to 9 cases per 1 million population. There is no racial predilection, and men are affected twice as often as women. The peak age at onset is between 40 and 60 years. An aggressive and thoughtful diagnostic strategy is necessary for this potentially lethal disease, which has an estimated 5-year survival of 58 per cent.

CLINICAL MANIFESTATIONS

The clinical spectrum of SNV is characterized by local or systemic disease. As indicated in Table 1, isolated forms of PAN occur predominantly in the gastrointestinal and genitourinary tracts. These localized forms of disease are rare, are generally not suspected clinically, and are often diagnosed following careful histopathologic review of surgical or biopsy specimens.

The onset of SNV may be protean or organ-specific. Fever, fatigue, weight loss, arthralgia (with or without arthritis), and myalgia occur in one half to two thirds of patients.

Table 1. Classification of Vasculitis

Small-Vessel (or Leukocytoclastic or Hypersensitivity) Vasculitis

- Serum sickness
  - Drugs
    - Penicillin
    - Sulfonamide
    - Phenytoin
    - Allopurinol
    - Nonsteroidal anti-inflammatory agents
    - Propylthiouracil
  - Infection
    - Hepatitis B>C>A
    - Cytomegalovirus
    - Parvovirus
    - Human immunodeficiency virus type 1
  - Foreign protein (heterologous antiserum)
- Cryoglobulinemia
- Henoch-Schönlein purpura
- Vasculitis of connective tissue diseases
  - Systemic lupus erythematosus
  - Rheumatoid arthritis
  - Sjögren's syndrome
- Behçet's disease
- Buerger's disease (thromboangiitis obliterans)
- Tumor-associated
  - Hairy cell leukemia
  - Lymphoma
  - Myeloma

Medium-Sized Vessel Vasculitis (Polyarteritis Nodosa Group)

- Classic polyarteritis nodosa
- Churg-Strauss allergic granulomatosis
- Overlap systemic necrotizing vasculitis
- Microscopic polyarteritis
- Kawasaki disease (childhood polyarteritis)
- Localized arteritis
  - Appendix
  - Gallbladder
  - Kidney
  - Epididymis
  - Uterus

Wegener's Granulomatosis

Large-Vessel Vasculitis

- Temporal arteritis
- Takayasu's arteritis

In a patient with constitutional symptoms in whom infection and neoplasm have been excluded, weight loss (which may be profound) can be an important indicator of SNV. The systemic features are usually the consequence of renal, neurologic, pulmonary, cutaneous, gastrointestinal, and/or musculoskeletal disease. The diagnostic categorization of a patient with SNV depends on the target organs involved. The Churg-Strauss variant of SNV usually occurs in atopic patients, always involves the lungs, and is associated with peripheral eosinophilia. Microscopic polyarteritis is a less commonly recognized subset that is frequently associated with necrotizing glomerulitis. The relative differences among the polyarteritis variants are outlined in Table 2.

Organ-Specific Disease

Renal involvement occurs in 70 to 100 per cent of patients with SNV. Renal failure due to vasculitis, glomerulonephritis, or hypertensive vascular disease occurs in as many as one half of patients with classic polyarteritis. Nephrotic-range proteinuria suggests renal vein thrombosis. Spontaneous rupture of a microaneurysm within the renal circulation can produce flank pain and hypotension.

Peripheral neuropathy develops in 60 to 76 per cent of patients with polyarteritis. The most common presentation is a polyneuropathy with diffuse paresthesia. In some patients with SNV, a mononeuritis multiplex presents with severe pain in the affected limb or limbs, which evolves over the course of hours to days and is usually associated with motor and sensory dysfunction that may be transient or persist for months. The peroneal, sural, radial, ulnar, and median nerves are the most commonly affected peripheral nerves. Cranial neuropathies also occur, typically involving cranial nerves I, VII, and VIII.

Central nervous system (CNS) disease is seen in 40 per cent of individuals with SNV. Typical presentations include seizures, encephalopathy, and focal abnormalities. The latter may be caused by a cerebrovascular accident. Ocular abnormalities in patients with SNV may be related to hypertension, episcleritis, and central retinal artery or choroidal vasculitis. Retinovascular abnormalities often lead to amaurosis fugax, monocular blindness, or retinal detachment.

Pulmonary involvement has not been a feature of classic PAN. However, pulmonary infiltrates are an integral component of the Churg-Strauss syndrome (allergic granulomatosis) and a frequent finding in patients with microscopic polyarteritis. Pleural disease is an uncommon manifestation of SNV and should suggest an infectious process.

Skin lesions in SNV are easily recognized by the experienced clinician and can be important clues for the diagnosis of SNV. Morphologically, skin lesions resemble those seen in the smaller vessel vasculitic syndromes and include palpable nonthrombocytopenic purpura, urticaria, vesicles, livedo reticularis, extremity ulcers, and, occasionally, painful subcutaneous nodules.

Gastrointestinal manifestations are generally the result of a ruptured aneurysm or a small bowel and/or liver infarction secondary to celiac or superior mesenteric artery occlusion. These events occur in 31 to 50 per cent of patients and manifest with severe, usually acute, abdominal pain associated with fever, diarrhea, and often upper or lower gastrointestinal bleeding. Signs of peritonitis may develop as a complication of intra-abdominal bleeding or, less often, of pancreatitis, cholecystitis, or appendicitis directly related to the vasculitic syndrome.

Cardiac involvement is more common in the juvenile form of polyarteritis (Kawasaki disease or the mucocutaneous lymph node syndrome) than in adults. This is principally due to coronary arteritis and the development of congestive heart failure, frequently complicated by coexisting hypertension. Nevertheless, in adults, coronary involvement is well recognized as causing myocardial ischemia, angina, or infarction. Pericarditis (unrelated to

Table 2. Contrasting Features of the Polyarteritis Group of Systemic Vasculitis

Organ System or Manifestation	Polyarteritis Nodosa (%)	Microscopic Polyarteritis (%)	Churg-Strauss Syndrome (%)
Renal	70	100	38
Neurologic	80	30	63
Pulmonary	Absent	50	100
Gastrointestinal	50	50	42
Cardiac	40	Absent	40
Arthralgia-arthritis	50	75	20
Skin	40	50	70
Oral ulcers	Absent	20	Absent

uremia or ischemic heart disease) and conduction disturbances are additional features of cardiac disease in SNV.

PATHOLOGIC FEATURES

Although PAN affects primarily the medium-sized and small arteries, arterioles and venules may also be involved. The histopathologic abnormalities are primarily focal and segmental; that is, only a portion of a vessel or only a part of the circumference of a vessel wall may be affected. The inflammatory lesion is typically transmural (panarteritis), and the vascular infiltrate usually contains mononuclear cells and variable numbers of neutrophils and eosinophils. Fibrinoid necrosis is often considered one of the hallmarks of acute necrotizing PAN. However, this lesion is not specific for vasculitis and is frequently found in patients with malignant hypertension. The site of vascular damage in PAN may be complicated by superimposed thrombosis with luminal occlusion and regional ischemia or weakening of the vessel wall with microaneurysm formation. The chronic lesion is associated with fibrotic healing. It is important to recognize that both acute and chronic changes may be observed in a single biopsy sample.

DIFFERENTIAL DIAGNOSIS OF SUSPECTED POLYARTERITIS NODOSA OR SYSTEMIC NECROTIZING VASCULITIS

In 1990, the Diagnostic and Therapeutic Criteria Committee of the American College of Rheumatology established diagnostic criteria for the classification of polyarteritis. The committee reported that when at least 3 of the 10 criteria listed in Table 3 are present, the sensitivity and specificity for a diagnosis of PAN are 82.2 per cent and 86.6 per cent, respectively. Nevertheless, several other diseases that mimic SNV must be considered in the differential diagnosis (Table 4). The most significant disorders to be excluded in the diagnosis of SNV are those associated with thromboembolic phenomena (e.g., bacterial endocarditis, cholesterol emboli [atheroemboli] and atrial myxomas). Each of these entities often presents with digital ischemic lesions, renal disease, and, in the case of atheroemboli, eosinophilia. Thrombotic thrombocytopenic purpura, which manifests with fever, renal insufficiency, CNS dysfunction, microangiopathic hemolytic anemia, purpura, and, occasionally, angiographic microaneurysms, also reveals many of the features of SNV. The vasculopathy associated with the antiphospholipid syndrome may also present with occlusive vascular lesions of the skin and viscera that can be clinically confused with (or rarely overlap) the features of PAN.

Table 3. American College of Rheumatology 1990 Criteria for the Diagnosis of Polyarteritis Nodosa*

1. Weight loss of ≥4 kg
2. Livedo reticularis
3. Testicular pain or tenderness (excluding infection and trauma)
4. Myalgia (excluding proximal thoracic and pelvic girdles), weakness, or leg tenderness
5. Mononeuropathy or polyneuropathy
6. Diastolic blood pressure >90 mm Hg
7. Increased serum urea nitrogen (>40 mg%) or creatinine (>1.5 mg%)
8. Hepatitis B surface antigen or antibody
9. Arteriographic demonstration of an aneurysm or occlusion of a visceral artery not related to atherosclerosis or fibromuscular dysplasia
10. Histologic evidence of a polymorphonuclear or mononuclear infiltrate in the wall of a small- or medium-sized artery

*When three criteria are present, the sensitivity and specificity for a diagnosis of polyarteritis are 82.2 per cent and 86.6 per cent, respectively.

Table 4. Disorders That Mimic Vasculitis

- Coagulopathies
  - Disseminated intravascular coagulation
  - Thrombotic thrombocytopenic purpura
- Infection
  - Endocarditis
  - *Neisseria* bacteremia
  - Echovirus infection
  - Coxsackievirus infection
  - *Rickettsia* infection
- Cholesterol emboli
- Atrial myxoma
- Antiphospholipid antibody syndrome
- Vasoconstriction due to recreational drug use
  - Cocaine
  - Methamphetamine
- Scurvy
- Amyloidosis
- Schamberg's disease (benign capillaritis)
- Intravascular lymphomatosis (malignant angioendotheliomatosis)

DIAGNOSTIC APPROACH

The principal goals of the clinician in the evaluation of suspected SNV are (1) to exclude the disorders with which they may be confused (see Table 4), thereby avoiding catastrophic errors in therapy, and (2) to follow a logical progression of studies that will provide a definitive diagnosis using the procedures that have the least risk and greatest yield for an individual patient.

Although a diagnostic algorithm can be created for SNV, the clinician should recognize that evaluation must be individualized and tailored to the needs of each patient. In the majority of patients, diagnosis depends on a constellation of clinical and laboratory findings. In SNV, routine laboratory studies reveal a nonspecific acute-phase response that includes an increased erythrocyte sedimentation rate, leukocytosis, and thrombocytosis. A prominent eosinophilia suggests the Churg-Strauss form of SNV. Rheumatoid factor, antinuclear antibody, and decreased serum complement are generally found in no more than 25 to 50 per cent of patients with SNV. Furthermore, a low-titer rheumatoid factor or antinuclear antibody test often serves to confuse rather than clarify the diagnosis, especially when coexisting arthralgia, arthritis, serositis, and constitutional symptoms suggest the presence of rheumatoid arthritis or systemic lupus erythematosus.

Antineutrophil cytoplasmic antibodies (ANCA) are highly sensitive and specific for the diagnosis of WG. ANCA was the first serologic test to be helpful in the diagnosis of an idiopathic vasculitis and is now universally available through many commercial laboratories. These antibodies are of two types that are determined by the pattern of indirect immunofluorescence on ethanol-fixed neutrophils. The more specific ANCA is characterized by a cytoplasmic pattern (c-ANCA) and is due to antibodies directed against a serine protease known as proteinase 3. The c-ANCA strongly suggests a diagnosis of WG in a

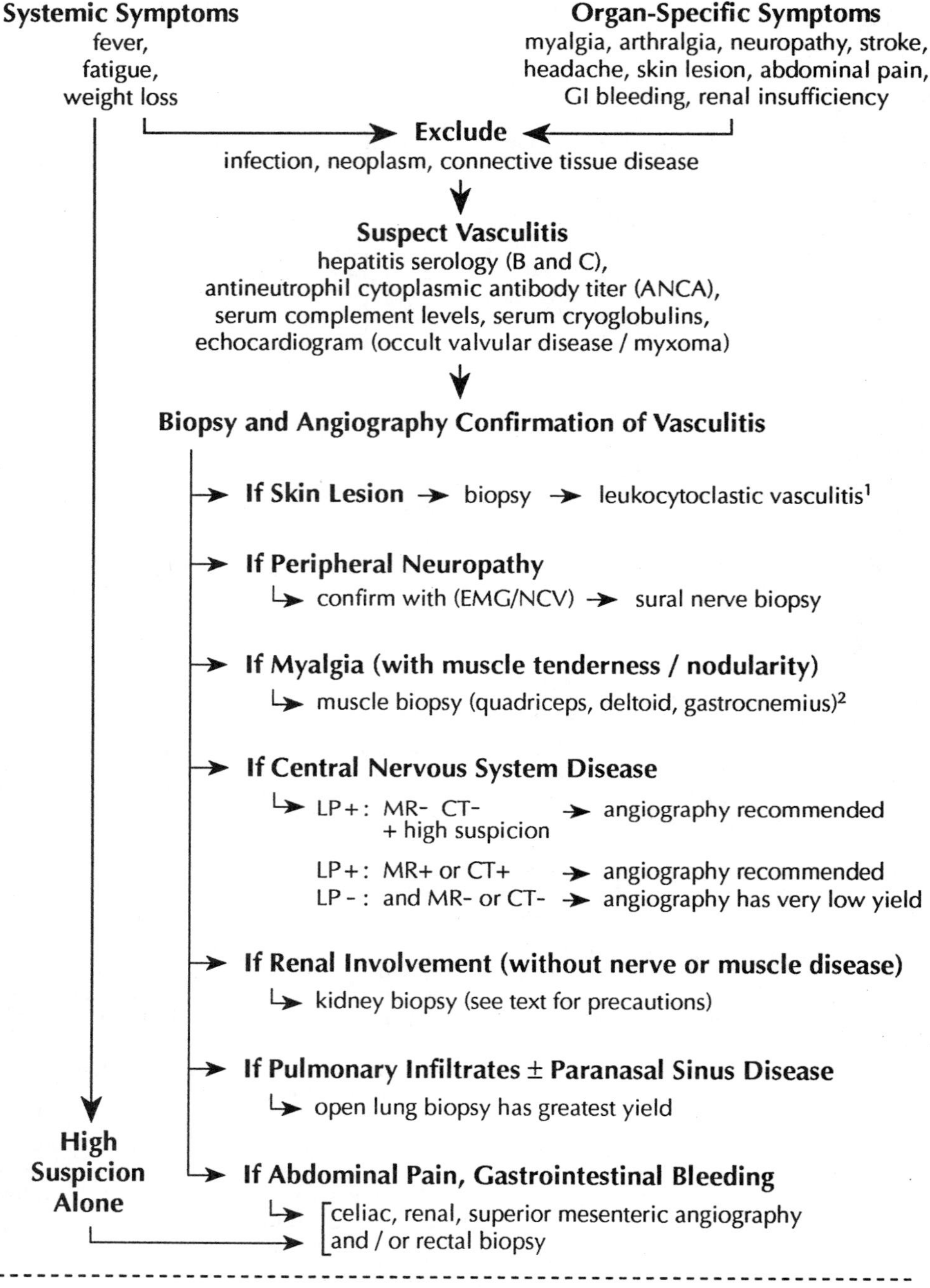

[1] If etiology is apparent (drug, infection, lymphoproliferative disease, connective tissue disease) or there are no other symptoms to suggest systemic involvement, additional work-up is not necessary.

[2] Yield of muscle biopsy may also be increased in the presence of abnormalities by EMG and elevated creatine kinase.

Figure 1. Diagnostic evaluation for suspected vasculitis.

patient with otherwise typical paranasal sinus and pulmonary abnormalities. The second ANCA is distinguished by a peripheral pattern (p-ANCA) with indirect immunofluorescence and is usually produced by antibodies against neutrophil myeloperoxidase or elastase. The p-ANCA is less specific and has been described in PAN, Churg-Strauss syndrome, microscopic polyarteritis, Henoch-Schönlein purpura, Kawasaki disease, rheumatoid arthritis, inflammatory bowel disease, human immunodeficiency virus type 1 infection, and idiopathic necrotizing glomerulonephritis. There have also been recent reports of drug-associated p-ANCA positivity (e.g., hydralazine and propylthiouracil). Therefore, the interpretation of positive ANCA reports should be made with caution and never out of clinical context. Ultimately, the diagnosis of SNV requires definitive histopathologic or angiographic confirmation prior to initiating therapy.

The most helpful clinical signs of SNV consist of cutaneous, neurologic, and renal abnormalities. The biopsy of skin lesions is easily accomplished and accompanied by low morbidity. Some clinicians believe that biopsy is critical in all patients with cutaneous vasculitic lesions because the clinical morphologic features are not always distinctive, and microscopic evaluation may reveal nonvasculitic lesions that would require different therapy. The most important clinical issue in a patient with cutaneous vasculitis is whether the skin involvement is a manifestation of systemic illness with visceral disease. In some patients, the clinical findings may help distinguish SNV from other diseases associated with cutaneous vasculitis. For example, a distinctive serpiginous eruption along the borders of the palms and soles has been described in human serum sickness, but not in PAN, Henoch-Schönlein purpura, or vasculitis associated with connective tissue disorders. Furthermore, purpuric, nodular, bullous, and ulcerative lesions are more likely to be seen in systemic disease than are petechiae, maculopapular, or urticarial eruptions. In addition, large plaques with multifocal areas of hemorrhage in a livedoid pattern are closely associated with the deposition of IgA and may be predictive of Henoch-Schönlein purpura.

A rational approach to tissue biopsy should be pursued from the least to the most invasive site. In view of the high prevalence of neuromuscular symptoms in SNV, biopsy of nerve and muscle is common. The presence of peripheral neuropathy confirmed by abnormal electrophysiologic studies increases the yield of a sural nerve biopsy from 19 per cent (random yield based on autopsy data) to 71 per cent for the diagnosis of SNV. Skeletal muscle is an alternative low-morbidity site for biopsy. The yield from muscle is greater when sampling (1) areas demonstrated to be abnormal by electromyography, (2) tender or painful muscles (often distal groups), and (3) palpable nodules, as well as (4) disease of less than 6 months' duration and (5) prior to corticosteroid therapy. When these guidelines are used, the reported diagnostic yield is from 29 per cent (autopsy data) to 80 per cent (highly abnormal examination). Although blind muscle biopsies may occasionally be helpful, they are associated with a significant degree of sampling error and are therefore not recommended. Sites previously examined by electromyography should not be blindly biopsied because the risk of histopathologic artifact is high. In some institutions, biopsy of rectal mucosa provides a suitable alternative. In patients with pulmonary infiltrates, an open lung biopsy is the procedure with the greatest yield. Lung biopsy can define the size of the vessel involved and determine the presence or absence of granuloma (present in Churg-Strauss syndrome and WG, but absent in classic PAN). A renal biopsy remains the last option for histopathologic confirmation and should be pursued if the cause of a systemic illness associated with renal disease remains otherwise unclear. Percutaneous renal biopsy is generally not considered a first choice for tissue sampling by most physicians evaluating suspected SNV because it is invasive, carries a small but identifiable risk of microaneurysm perforation, and most often demonstrates focal nonspecific segmental glomerulonephritis. Therefore, in pulmonary-renal syndromes in which systemic vasculitis is suspected, a lung biopsy would be the procedure of choice.

In the absence of histologic confirmation of SNV, angiography should be pursued in an individual with multisystem disease in whom SNV is considered. To increase the probability of detecting microaneurysms, both renal arteries, the celiac axis, and the superior mesenteric artery must be evaluated. If CNS manifestations are present, cerebral angiography may be helpful. In patients with CNS vasculitis, detection of abnormalities with the use of a combination of lumbar puncture and either computed tomography or magnetic resonance imaging correlates well with detection of abnormalities by angiography. This observation suggests that the yield by CNS angiography is low when both an imaging study and a lumbar puncture are normal. Importantly, CNS angiography in patients with possible CNS vasculitis is considered a low-risk procedure (<1 per cent prevalence of persistent neurologic deficits). However, caution should be observed in patients with renal impairment because contrast-associated renal failure has occurred following angiography in patients with PAN. Angiographic findings that support a diagnosis of SNV include multiple aneurysms, stenotic segments, or ectasia. The results of angiography must also be interpreted cautiously because they are not pathognomonic of polyarteritis. For example, microaneurysms, considered to be a classic finding in PAN, may also be observed in systemic lupus erythematosus, Kawasaki disease, WG, thrombotic thrombocytopenic purpura, endocarditis, atrial myxoma, drug abuse, fibromuscular dysplasia, and pseudoxanthoma elasticum. These "false-positive" angiographic findings during the evaluation of multisystem disease serve to emphasize the extensive differential diagnosis for SNV.

A recommended strategy for the diagnosis of SNV based on currently available literature is displayed in Figure 1. Judicious use of the laboratory, tissue biopsy selection, and angiography provides the most expeditious path to establishing a diagnosis of polyarteritis.

WEGENER'S GRANULOMATOSIS

By Rex M. McCallum, M.D.,
and Nancy B. Allen, M.D.
Durham, North Carolina

Wegener's granulomatosis (WG) is a distinct clinicopathologic entity of unknown etiology. Almost all patients have upper and/or lower respiratory tract involvement that is associated with clinically evident renal disease in 70 to 80 per cent of patients. Joints, ears, eyes, and skin are also affected in more than 45 per cent of cases. Involvement of every organ system has been described. The pathologic hallmark is necrotizing granulomatous inflammation of small arteries and veins. Generalized and limited forms of

WG have been described. Generalized disease involves at least two of the following three areas: upper airways, lungs, and kidneys. Limited disease occurs in only the upper or lower respiratory tract. Limited renal disease, while it may occur, cannot be recognized as WG until either upper or lower respiratory disease has developed. A definitive diagnosis requires appropriate clinical findings combined with appropriate pathologic findings on a biopsy of one or more sites of disease activity. The presence of antineutrophil cytoplasmic antibodies (ANCA) may be helpful in the diagnosis.

PRESENTING FEATURES

Although patients have been described in the second through the ninth decades, WG typically presents in the fourth or fifth decade of life. Males and females are affected in equal numbers. The exact incidence and prevalence are unknown. The majority of patients present with upper respiratory tract symptoms, such as sinusitis, rhinitis, nasal obstruction, otitis media, ear pain, and decreased hearing. Less frequently, other head and neck problems occur at presentation; these findings include gingival inflammation, epistaxis, sore throat, laryngitis, ocular inflammation, proptosis, and saddle-nose deformity. Lower respiratory tract symptoms are noted in one third of patients and include cough, sputum production, hemoptysis, and pleuritis. At presentation, 45 per cent of patients have pulmonary nodules, infiltrates, or both. These findings may be asymptomatic and fleeting. Ocular symptoms are noted in 15 per cent of patients initially and can include ocular pain, loss of vision, red eyes, and diplopia. At presentation, 15 per cent of all patients have fever, weight loss, and cutaneous disease. Even less frequently, presenting symptoms are nonspecific and include anorexia, malaise, myalgias, and arthralgias. Rarely, patients present with oral ulcers, headache, cutaneous disease, polyarthritis, orchitis, mastoiditis, cranial nerve dysfunction, parotid mass and pain, breast mass, thyroiditis, peripheral neuropathy, anosmia, pericarditis, diabetes insipidus, asthma, and Raynaud's phenomenon. Notable is the lack of symptoms related to the gastrointestinal and urinary tracts; only 11 per cent of patients have renal impairment at presentation. Patients have been reported who present with renal disease consistent with WG 4 to 78 months before the development of diagnostic respiratory tract disease. Other disease manifestations may precede diagnostic clinical and pathologic findings by weeks to years.

CLINICAL FEATURES

The course without treatment is progressive, and the majority of patients develop renal disease. From historical data, the disease is rapidly fatal if untreated. The mean survival from diagnosis is approximately 5 months, with 82 per cent of patients dying within the first year. Early recognition and treatment improve the prognosis significantly, with 75 per cent complete remission rates and 91 per cent marked improvement or partial remission reported with the use of the conventional therapy of prednisone and cyclophosphamide. Unfortunately, 50 per cent of remissions are followed by relapses, which may occur months to years after therapy is completed. Therefore, a high degree of suspicion and careful monitoring of all patients with a history of WG is essential. Organ involvement during the course of WG is summarized in Table 1.

Table 1. Clinical Manifestations of Wegener's Granulomatosis

Organ System	Percentage of Patients (%)
Ear, nose, and throat	90
Lung	85
Kidney	75
Joints	70
Eye	50
Skin	45
Neurologic	
Peripheral	15
Central	10
Heart	5–15
Muscle	4

Upper Airway Disease

The pattern and degree of involvement with WG vary widely. Sinus disease occurs in 85 per cent of patients. The most frequently affected sinuses are the maxillary, sphenoid, and ethmoids, with approximately 70, 30, and 15 per cent involvement, respectively. Superimposed infections, with *Staphylococcus aureus* the predominant organism, are common. Antibiotic therapy, aggressive sinus care, daily sinus irrigation, and occasional drainage procedures are frequently required.

Inflammatory and/or vasculitic lesions can occur at any site in the upper airways. Cartilage destruction in the nasal septum may result in saddle-nose deformity in as many as 25 to 30 per cent of patients. Nasal obstruction by inflammatory tissue is common. Severe and persistent sore throat can be a major symptom. Oral and nasal lesions are generally shallow ulcers with sharp margins. Gingivitis, gingival bleeding, tooth loss, and alveolar bone resorption occur less frequently. Unlike the upper airway midline neoplastic and destructive diseases, such as midline malignant reticulosis and midline granuloma, WG does not erode through the subcutaneous tissues of the face, skin of the face, or hard palate. Wegener's granulomatosis can involve the bony walls of the sinuses and frequently erodes the lamina papyracea (thin, bony plate covering the middle and posterior ethmoidal cells forming a large part of the medial wall of the orbit) in patients with ethmoidal disease. Otitis media is usually secondary to blockage of the eustachian tube and is seen in 40 per cent of patients. Hearing loss occurs in 40 per cent of patients. Less frequently noted are suppurative otitis, primary auricular granulomatous inflammation, otorrhea, cholesteatoma, ear pain, auricular chondritis, and temporal bone granuloma.

Granulomatous vasculitis is not often found on biopsies from upper airway sites. The majority of biopsies show nonspecific changes of acute and chronic inflammation with necrosis. Vasculitis and granulomatous inflammation are seen in 20 per cent of upper airway biopsies, and only 15 per cent of such biopsies reveal vasculitis, necrosis, and granulomatous inflammation all present at the same time. This finding may be related to the relatively small biopsy size and the extensive necrosis that often occurs.

Pulmonary Disease

The best site to biopsy and find the classic pathologic findings of WG is the lung. Granulomatous changes and vasculitis are found in 90 per cent of open lung biopsies. Open lung biopsy is the best method for obtaining diagnostic pathologic material. In addition, this allows infection and neoplasm to be definitively excluded as diagnostic possibilities. An endobronchial biopsy may be diagnostic in the 15 per cent of patients who have endobronchial involvement; however, some patients develop this problem later in the course of disease. Endobronchial involvement may lead to subglottic and/or bronchial stenosis with stridor or atelectasis. Endobronchial disease is also associated with obstructive findings, and subglottic stenosis is suggested by flattening or squaring of the flow-volume loops on pulmonary function testing.

Radiographic findings are typically multiple, bilateral nodular infiltrates with cavitation; they typically occur more frequently in the upper lobes than the lower ones. Single lesions and unilateral abnormalities with or without cavitation have been noted. While discrete nodular lesions occur in 25 per cent of patients, infiltrates can be associated with adjacent atelectasis and may lack sharply defined margins. Pleural effusions are seen in 10 per cent but are rarely massive. The unusual findings include mediastinal mass, peritracheal mass, hilar adenopathy, diffuse pulmonary hemorrhage, large cavitary lesion, calcified nodule, miliary pattern, and lower lobe interstitial disease.

Renal Disease

Renal involvement is usually asymptomatic at presentation, with urinary sediment or functional abnormalities occurring in 75 per cent of patients during the course of the disease. Glomerulonephritis and/or renal insufficiency can progress rapidly over hours to days in the absence of appropriate therapeutic interventions. Rarely, perinephric hematoma or ureteral vasculitis with obstruction is noted; hypertension is unusual. In clinical protocol situations, 50 per cent of patients with WG who manifest no clinical renal disease show evidence of disease activity on renal biopsy, although renal biopsy is not routinely recommended under these circumstances.

Histopathologically, granulomas and true vasculitis are rarely found on renal biospy. The broad range of pathologic findings runs from mild focal and segmental glomerulonephritis to fulminant diffuse necrotizing glomerulonephritis with proliferative and crescentic changes. Immune complex deposition is uncommon. For these reasons, a renal biopsy is rarely diagnostic of WG, but it can exclude differential considerations, such as Goodpasture's syndrome or systemic lupus erythematosus, and thus provide support for aggressive treatment in the patient in whom a diagnostic biopsy is not forthcoming.

Joint Disease

A total of 70 per cent of patients report joint symptoms during the course of their disease. Most manifest arthralgias that are polyarticular and symmetrical and involve large and small joints. True arthritis occurs in 30 per cent, generally with large lower-extremity joint synovitis that is nondeforming. Joint effusions have rarely been analyzed, and reported patients' studies have revealed nonspecific findings. Infrequently, symmetrical, small-joint arthritis suggestive of rheumatoid arthritis is seen.

Eye Disease

Ocular involvement, which occurs in 50 per cent of patients, may result from direct involvement of ocular structures or from the spillover of sinus disease into the orbital space. The heterogeneous manifestations include conjunctivitis, scleritis, episcleritis, corneoscleral ulcer, uveitis, retinal vasculitis, optic nerve vasculitis, proptosis, and nasolacrimal duct obstruction. Proptosis occurs in 15 per cent of patients and is generally secondary to a retroocular mass lesion. Biopsies of ocular tissues reveal acute and chronic inflammation with or without granulomatous vasculitis. Proptosis is generally slow to respond to therapy for the underlying disease. Occasionally, it is refractory to medical therapy and thus requires surgical orbital decompression. Rapid functional impairment can occur from ocular involvement with WG. Ophthalmologic assistance and follow-up with computed tomography and/or magnetic resonance imaging are essential in the evaluation and treatment of patients with ocular problems related to WG.

Skin Disease

Cutaneous disease occurs in 45 per cent of patients; more than one type of lesion can develop in the same patient. Palpable purpura are frequently noted, but ulcers, papules, vesicles, subcutaneous nodules, and petechiae are also seen. Rarely, nonhealing of surgical wounds, digital ischemic necrosis, and necrosis of the penis have been noted. The histopathologic findings range from nonspecific acute and chronic inflammation to leukocytoclastic vasculitis and characteristic necrotizing granulomatous vascular inflammation. Cutaneous difficulties rarely dominate the clinical situation.

Nervous System Disease

Overall, neurologic involvement occurs in 20 to 30 per cent of patients with WG. Peripheral disease is noted in 15 per cent of patients with typical patterns of mononeuritis multiplex, carpal tunnel syndrome, polyneuropathy, or polyneuritis that can be confirmed by electromyographic and nerve conduction velocity studies. Central nervous system disease is found in 10 per cent of patients with WG and may represent primary involvement with WG or secondary spread of the inflammatory process from the nasal or paranasal sinuses. Cranial neuropathies, central nervous system vasculitis with or without subarachnoid or intracerebral hemorrhage, cerebritis, unexplained syncope, and diabetes insipidus have been observed. Cranial neuropathies particularly involve the first, second, sixth, seventh, and eighth cranial nerves. A sural nerve biopsy may reveal necrotizing granulomatous vasculitis. Computed tomography, magnetic resonance imaging, arteriography, and lumbar puncture are helpful in evaluating central nervous system difficulties.

Heart Disease

Cardiac disease occurs in 5 to 15 per cent of patients clinically and as many as 50 per cent of patients in autopsy series. While pericarditis is most common, any cardiac structure may be involved in WG. Pancarditis with or without congestive cardiomyopathy, valvulitis, endomyocardial inflammation, coronary arteritis, and intractable arrhythmias have been observed.

Skeletal Muscle

Symptomatic myopathy may be seen in as many as 5 per cent of patients and may manifest in a manner similar to polymyositis. A biopsy may reveal nonspecific inflammation with or without small-vessel arteritis and, occasionally, typical necrotizing granulomatous vasculitis.

Miscellaneous

As many as one third of patients have increased activity of alkaline phosphatase and/or transaminases; the liver biopsy may reveal triaditis with or without granuloma. Symptomatic giant cell arteritis has been described in patients with WG. Unusual sites of involvement with WG are seen in acute thyroiditis, unexplained ascites, recurrent pancreatitis, and granulomatous masses of the vocal cord, tympanic membrane, cervical vertebral body, parotid gland, breast, prostate, gastrointestinal tract, esophagus, and posterior larynx. These signs may precede, occur simultaneously with, or follow the more typical manifestations of WG.

LABORATORY FEATURES

Often, characteristic but nonspecific abnormalities are noted in early untreated WG. The erythrocyte sedimentation rate is almost invariably increased, ranging from 50 to 140 mm/hour. Increased C-reactive protein is frequent, and in European studies this test is used more often than the erythrocyte sedimentation rate. Leukocyte counts are increased in the majority of patients and are normal in the others. Increased numbers of band forms may be seen. Anemia is present in the majority of patients and is typically normocytic, normochromic, and compatible with anemia of chronic disease. Thrombocytosis is noted in one third of patients. Leukopenia and thrombocytopenia are not seen before therapy.

Rheumatoid factor is found in 60 per cent of patients, usually of moderate titer, but this may lead to the inappropriate diagnosis of rheumatoid arthritis in patients with WG who present with musculoskeletal symptoms. Increased concentrations of immunoglobulins (IgA, IgG, and IgM) occur in the majority of patients. An increase in IgE concentration is rarely noted. Circulating immune complexes are found in almost one half of patients. Cryoglobulins are noted in a few patients. Antinuclear antibodies, hepatitis B surface antigen, hepatitis C antibody, and anti-DNA antibody determinations are uniformly negative. Whole hemolytic complement activity may be decreased, normal, or increased in patients with WG. Skin test anergy is unusual.

Urinary sediment abnormalities are seen in 70 to 80 per cent of patients; the most common findings are microscopic hematuria, with or without red blood cell casts, and proteinuria. Proteinuria may be in the nephrotic range. Renal function abnormalities are noted in 11 per cent at presentation and can progress rapidly, to oliguria or frank anuria. Careful and close monitoring of the urinalysis and creatinine is important, particularly early in the course of the illness.

The best available single laboratory test is ANCA, which is detected in 34 to 92 per cent of patients with WG. In a recent literature review and meta-analysis, the pooled sensitivity of cytoplasmic ANCA (cANCA) was 66 per cent, and the pooled specificity was 98 per cent. The antigen responsible for cANCA is thought to be proteinase 3, a serine protease in the cytoplasm of neutrophils. Tests for proteinase 3 have been developed and are available in some centers. Perinuclear ANCA (pANCA), another pattern, is found in approximately 10 per cent of patients with WG.

Table 2. Summary of Typical Biopsy Findings

Site	Typical Pathologic Findings	Probability of Diagnostic Biopsy
Lung		
Transbronchial	Acute or chronic inflammation with or without giant cells	+
Open	Necrotizing granulomatous vasculitis	+ + + +
Upper airways	Acute or chronic inflammation with or without giant cells or vasculitis, but rarely both	+ +
Kidney	Focal or proliferative glomerulonephritis with or without crescents; nonspecific immunofluorescence	+
Eye	Acute or chronic inflammation with or without granuloma or vasculitis, but rarely both	+ +
Skin	Leukocytoclastic vasculitis	+
Sural nerve	Acute axonopathy	+

Differential Diagnosis

The differential diagnostic possibilities are broad and depend on the presenting manifestations of WG. Pulmonary-renal syndrome presentations are common; differential diagnostic possibilities include other systemic necrotizing vasculitis syndromes (e.g., Churg-Strauss syndrome), systemic lupus erythematosus, systemic sclerosis, lymphomatoid granulomatosis, Goodpasture's syndrome, pneumonia complicated by glomerulonephritis, bacterial endocarditis, uremic pneumonitis, paraneoplastic syndrome, sarcoidosis, and acute inflammatory myopathy with myoglobin-related renal failure. Open lung biopsies are more helpful and provide more specific information than do renal biopsies in pulmonary-renal syndrome patients who require a biopsy for diagnosis. Renal biopsies can provide the diagnosis in systemic lupus erythematosus and Goodpasture's syndrome, which can also be diagnosed by clinical and laboratory features. Most other differential diagnostic considerations, including Goodpasture's syndrome, can be clarified by lung biopsy. In addition, biopsy allows the definite exclusion of infection and neoplastic disorders in the lungs. Other differential diagnostic considerations include berylliosis, tuberculosis, histoplasmosis, blastomycosis, mucormycosis, coccidioidomycosis, syphilis, relapsing polychondritis, and primary or secondary neoplasms of the lung or upper respiratory tract.

Therefore, the diagnosis of WG requires the identification of an appropriate clinical setting with subsequent biopsy revealing *both* granulomatous inflammation and necrotizing vasculitis. Pathologic specimens manifesting only granuloma or vasculitis are compatible with WG but are not pathologically diagnostic. Pathologically diagnostic material must be found before a definite diagnosis can be made. If pulmonary disease is present, the lung is clearly the best site to biopsy. Biopsies of sites other than the lung less frequently reveal pathologically diagnostic material. Several different biopsies may be required before a definite diagnosis can be made. The ANCA test is often helpful, but awareness of the existence of false-negative and false-positive tests still leads to the recommendation of biopsy confirmation of WG. Paraneoplastic and infection-related vasculitic syndromes may also mimic WG. Unlike the situation with other vasculitic syndromes, angiography is rarely helpful in the diagnosis of WG.

The presence of renal disease should raise a sense of urgency in the clinician who is considering the diagnosis of WG. Rapid progression to frank renal failure can occur, therefore, establishing a diagnosis quickly and instituting appropriate therapy with proven benefit is very important. For this and the aforementioned reasons, open lung biopsy should be rapidly undertaken in patients with active renal disease who also manifest pulmonary disease and in whom WG is a major differential consideration. Attempts to perform diagnostic biopsies in other more readily available sites may do the patient a great disservice by delaying the institution of appropriate therapy. A summary of typical biopsy findings appears in Table 2. While some biopsy sites are more commonly diagnostic, biopsies of virtually any involved site can be diagnostic. Meticulous consideration of the differential possibilities, judicious use of cultures and laboratory studies, appropriate biopsies, and careful interpretation of pathologic specimens permit the correct diagnosis to be established and the proper therapy instituted in patients with WG.

Section Fourteen

GENITOURINARY SYSTEM

INFECTIONS OF THE URINARY TRACT

By Gayle J. Weaver, M.D.,
and Byungse Suh, M.D., Ph.D.
Philadelphia, Pennsylvania

Urinary tract infection (UTI) is one of the most common human infections and affects women far more often than men. In the United States, UTI is the reason for more than 5 million visits to physicians' offices per year. Also the leading cause of nosocomial infection, UTI contributes significantly to inpatient morbidity and mortality as well as hospital costs. Although UTI may initially involve any anatomic site from the urethral meatus to the kidney, the entire system is at risk for invasion by the causative organism after a part of the urinary tract has been infected.

Urinary tract infection can be divided into two broad categories on the basis of host factors: uncomplicated, or simple, infections, which occur in the absence of structural or functional abnormalities of the urinary tract, and complicated infections, which occur in the setting of anatomic or functional abnormalities of the urinary tract (e.g., obstruction, stones, and neurologic dysfunction). In addition, UTI can be classified on the basis of the location of the infection; lower tract infection refers to infection of the bladder (cystitis), while upper tract infection refers to infection involving the kidney (e.g., pyelonephritis).

A clinical diagnosis of simple UTI can often be made on the basis of the history and physical examination alone, with few laboratory tests. The usual presentation of acute bacterial cystitis is that of a young female with no prior history of urinary tract pathology presenting with a sudden onset of urgency, frequency, dysuria, low back pain, and possibly nocturia of several days' duration. In this clinical setting, the only common positive physical finding is suprapubic tenderness. Conversely, the patient with acute pyelonephritis typically appears acutely ill at presentation and may have fever, flank pain, and rigors. Gastrointestinal symptoms such as vomiting, abdominal pain, and diarrhea may also be present. Patients with acute pyelonephritis often have costovertebral angle tenderness and abdominal tenderness on palpation. These clinical manifestations are variable, and localization of the infection to the upper or lower urinary tract based solely on the presenting signs and symptoms may be less than 60 per cent accurate. Correct diagnosis and localization of UTI requires carefully planned microbiologic studies and, occasionally, may require diagnostic imaging procedures.

DETECTION OF BACTERIURIA

Urine represents a sterile filtrate of the blood, and normal urine remains sterile when obtained by aseptic means, such as suprapubic aspiration of the bladder and aspiration from an aseptically placed catheter. Voided urine specimens, however, are usually contaminated with bacteria and they typically contain at least 10^2 colony-forming units (CFU) per milliliter. Bacteriuria (the presence of bacteria in the urine) is the hallmark of UTI, and a reliable documentation of "significant bacteriuria" is useful in the diagnosis of UTI.

Two broad categorical methods, microbiologic and chemical, are currently available for quantitating the presence of bacteria in the urine. Bacteriuria is clinically significant when colony counts reveal at least 10^5 CFU/mL. The majority (95 per cent) of UTIs are characterized by the presence of at least 10^5 CFU/mL except those caused by *Staphylococcus saprophyticus* or *Candida* species, in which smaller numbers of the organisms have been associated with UTIs.

Specimen collection is the most important step in the diagnosis of UTI, because falsely high colony counts due to contamination or falsely low counts due to the introduction of an antibacterial substance during the specimen collection can lead to a misdiagnosis followed by mismanagement. Early-morning midstream clean-catch urine is the best specimen for urinalysis and culture. Each patient must receive clear and easily understandable instructions on how to obtain a proper urine specimen. Specimens for culture must be processed as soon as possible because the multiplication of bacteria at room temperature leads to falsely increased counts and a falsely positive diagnosis. If immediate processing is not possible, the specimen is refrigerated or transferred to transport media containing an appropriate preservative. Some examples of the preservatives are boric acid (1.8 per cent), boric acid–glycerol sodium formate or sodium chloride–polyvinyl pyrrolidone. A sufficient amount of specimen (a minimum of 3 mL) needs to be added to dilute the preservative, since it can inhibit or kill bacteria.

Direct microscopic examination is an easy, readily available technique for evaluating bacteriuria. A freshly voided unspun urine specimen can be gram-stained and examined in the office. The presence of one or more organisms per high-power (oil) field suggests UTI. A centrifuged wet mount preparation suggests UTI if it contains 20 or more organisms per high-power field.

Cultures of the urine enable the clinician to identify and obtain antimicrobial sensitivities of infecting organisms as well as to quantitate the organisms present. Two major standardized culture techniques are used: the pour plate method and the streak plate method.

With the pour plate method, 0.1 mL of urine is diluted in 10 mL of broth (1:100) and mixed, and 0.1 mL is placed in a Petri dish. Approximately 10 mL of liquid agar (45°C) is added and gently mixed, and the plate is incubated at 37°C overnight. This method permits quantitation of the number of CFUs in the urine. On the plate, one colony represents approximately 1000 living organisms per milliliter of the original specimen. Addition of 0.1 mL of the diluted urine (1:100) into an additional 10 mL of diluent (1:10,000), which is then processed similarly, provides more accurate counts when bacterial counts are higher. One colony on this plate represents 100,000 living organisms per milliliter of the original urine specimen.

The streak plate method uses a fixed amount of urine (0.001 mL) streaked onto an agar plate with a standardized sterile loop. This method also permits quantitation and antibiotic sensitivity testing of the infecting organism. On this plate, 100 colonies is equivalent to 100,000 colonies per milliliter of urine. The streak plate method is used more frequently than is the pour plate method because it is simple and inexpensive, but it may still not be convenient for use on a routine basis in the office setting.

A number of commercially available kits can be used for urine culture in the office. All the methods require delivery of a constant, standardized aliquot of urine onto a prepared culture medium with overnight incubation. In the dip-slide method, a glass slide or plastic template coated with an agar medium on each side is dipped into the urine specimen and incubated overnight. The results correlate well with those obtained with the quantitative methods described earlier.

Using the filter paper method, a trypticase soy agar plate is inoculated with a standardized filter paper strip that has been dipped into the urine and incubated at 37°C overnight. The same amount of urine is transferred each time, and 25 colonies are equivalent to 100,000 living organisms per milliliter of the original urine. Fewer than 5 per cent of results are false positive or false negative. Neither the dip-slide nor the filter paper method provides identification of the causative organisms, and both require subculture onto appropriate media.

The nitrite method represents the chemical test with the greatest potential for mass screening and for following treated patients. This test is based on the ability of most organisms that cause UTI to reduce urinary nitrate to nitrite. Detection of this bacterial metabolite indirectly demonstrates the presence of bacteria in the urine. This test is most accurate when performed on a first voided morning specimen, because the organism in the urine has had an ample opportunity overnight to convert nitrate to nitrite. A positive test strongly suggests and is specific for "significant bacteriuria," but a negative test does not exclude infection because gram-positive organisms do not reduce nitrate. The immediate appearance of a pink color as the test strip is immersed into a freshly passed first-morning urine specimen indicates a positive test result. A positive nitrite test result in the presence of significant bacteriuria confirmed by urine culture is considered diagnostic.

DETECTION OF PYURIA

Pyuria refers to the presence of white blood cells (WBCs) or pus in the urine. The most frequent cause of pyuria is UTI. The noninfectious causes of pyuria include interstitial nephritis, glomerulonephritis, renal stones, neoplasms, appendicitis, and rejection of a transplanted kidney. "Sterile" pyuria can also result from infection of the urinary tract caused by slow-growing and/or fastidious organisms, such as mycobacteria, fungi, and chlamydia.

Several clinically useful methods have been developed for determining significant pyuria. Microscopic examination of a fresh, uncentrifuged urine specimen is a simple, commonly used method of establishing the presence of pyuria. One to two WBCs per high-power field (30 per low-power field) correlates well with the presence of a UTI. The finding of WBC casts on microscopy strongly suggests pyelonephritis. Examination of an unspun urine specimen in a cell-counting chamber is also a reliable method. By this method, at least 10 WBCs/mm^3 is considered to be significant pyuria. Microscopic evaluation of a centrifuged urine specimen typically provides less reliable results owing to the introduction of more variables, including changes in pH, osmolality, temperature, and reconstitution volume.

The leukocyte esterase test detects the presence of esterases of leukocyte origin (not derived from serum, urine, or renal tissue) and is available as a reagent strip test. Leukocyte esterase hydrolyzes indoxylcarboxylic acid ester impregnated in the filter-paper pad to indoxyl, which subsequently oxidizes at room temperature and produces an indigo color. The enzyme activity is proportional to the intensity of the blue color, and a 90 per cent correlation between the positive leukocyte esterase test and the chamber count method has been reported. Although both pyuria and bacteriuria are present in the majority of UTIs, pyuria is not synonymous with bacteriuria.

Pyuria with low colony counts or no growth is a dissociation phenomenon, also known as pyuria-dysuria syndrome or acute urethral syndrome. It is common and accounts for about half the female patients with dysuria. The exact cause of this problem has not been well defined, and several different agents, such as *Chlamydia trachomatis,* herpesvirus, and, less frequently, *Neisseria gonorrhoeae,* have been implicated. Vaginitis can also mimic this syndrome, and a careful pelvic examination should be part of the evaluation process. A therapeutic trial of doxycycline has been performed, with varying success rates.

Asymptomatic female patients with a single culture revealing significant bacteriuria (10^5 CFU/mL) have an 80 per cent probability of UTI, and this value rises to 95 per cent when a second culture reveals bacteriuria with the same organism. Therefore, at least two, preferably three, separate cultures should be performed in this clinical setting before therapy is instituted. If the colony counts are lower (e.g., 50,000 CFU/mL), the organisms obtained from three consecutive specimens must be identical to the level of species or the phage type before a certain diagnosis of UTI is made. Similar principles apply to males with asymptomatic bacteriuria. The morbidity due to UTI is high in certain patient populations. Thus, the threshold for initiation of therapy is considerably lower in these populations, which include patients with poorly controlled diabetes mellitus, pregnant women, and renal transplant recipients.

LOCALIZATION OF INFECTION

When one anatomic site of the urinary tract is infected, infection can spread to other parts of the system and eventually involve the whole urinary system. Fortunately, exact localization of the infection in the management of UTI is less important than distinguishing a complicated UTI from an uncomplicated one. Several different methods have been proposed, but the most reliable approach is the cystoscopic differential culture method. A cystoscope is introduced into the bladder, with proper preparation, and the urine specimen representing the bladder urine is obtained. The bladder is then thoroughly washed with irrigating solution, followed by cannulation of the ureters. The serial urine specimens obtained from the ureters represent renal urine. Microscopic and microbiologic studies are then performed to determine the origin of infection. Again, exact localization of the infection is rarely necessary and is used primarily as a research tool.

Another approach is based on the principle that the host

mounts a significant local antibody response when tissue invasion is present and the presence of antibody-coated bacteria (ACB) represents an upper tract infection. Although this test carries an acceptable correlation with pyelonephritis (62 per cent), other local infections, including acute hemorrhagic cystitis (67 per cent) and prostatitis (67 per cent), are also associated with a positive ACB test. The ACB test appears to be a good predictor of the patients who require prolonged antimicrobial therapy. The ACB-negative patients respond favorably to single-dose or short-course therapy, but prolonged therapy is needed for patients with positive ACB test results.

LOWER URINARY TRACT INFECTION IN MEN

In men, UTI is rare unless the urinary tract has undergone instrumentation or trauma. However, the incidence of UTI in males sharply increases with prostatic hypertrophy. The prostate gland is a common site of bacterial infection, mostly by the ascending route, and often becomes the source of recurrent UTIs. For the determination of the anatomic site of infection, the three-cup test is still used.* This approach should be reserved for patients who experience recurrent UTIs when the source of infection cannot be determined. The three-cup test is not a routine laboratory procedure and should be performed by an experienced physician in a facility equipped with reliable microscopy and microbiologic handling of the specimens.

The subject must be well hydrated, with a full bladder, for the procedure to be carried out successfully. The utmost care is observed throughout the procedure to avoid contamination of the specimens. All test tubes and other specimen containers must be sterile. The patient is asked to fully retract the foreskin and hold it in place until the last urine specimen (third voided bladder urine [VB_3]) is obtained. The glans is cleansed with a detergent soap, followed by a wet sponge, and then dried with a sterile sponge. The patient is then asked to void into a test tube, and the specimen (10 mL) is labeled as the first voided bladder urine (VB_1). The patient continues to void another 200 mL, at which point another 5- to 10-mL urine specimen (VB_2) is obtained, to be used as the midstream urine specimen. The patient is then asked to stop voiding, and the clinician performs a prostatic massage as the patient holds a cup to catch the drops of prostatic secretion (EPS, expressed prostatic secretions). Immediately following the massage, the patient is asked to void into another test tube, and a urine specimen (VB_3) of approximately 5 to 10 mL is collected. The patient is then allowed to empty the bladder. All the specimens, including VB_1, VB_2, EPS, and VB_3, are sent for microscopy and quantitative colony counts. In urethritis, VB_1 shows the highest colony counts, but in cystitis, the counts in VB_1, VB_2, and VB_3 are the same. Higher counts in EPS or VB_3 than those in VB_1 and VB_2 (by at least 10-fold) strongly suggest prostatitis.

DIAGNOSTIC IMAGING STUDIES IN URINARY TRACT INFECTION

A number of different diagnostic imaging studies are employed in the evaluation of patients with UTIs, especially with complicated UTIs. They are particularly useful in the investigation of the structural integrity of the urinary tract and when surgical intervention may lead to eradication of the infection and/or prevention of future UTIs. Intravenous pyelography is the gold standard with which all other diagnostic imaging studies are compared. Accurate evaluation of the renal parenchyma, the collecting system, and excretory function can be accomplished with this procedure. Its use, however, is restricted to well-hydrated patients who have no contraindications.

Renal ultrasonography is a safe and useful procedure in patients who present with impaired renal function or other relative contraindications for intravenous pyelography. When combined with a plain abdominal film (kidney, ureter, bladder [KUB]), this procedure provides results similar to those of intravenous pyelography in assessing renal pelvicaliceal distention, renal masses (abscesses), and renal calculi. Ultrasonography does not provide functional information about the kidney. This study can be normal in as many as 50 per cent of patients with documented pyelonephritis. When patients with UTI fail to respond favorably to a standard course of antimicrobial therapy, these diagnostic studies can be used to investigate the presence of mechanical or structural abnormalities, as listed earlier.

Computed tomography (CT) is rapidly becoming the diagnostic imaging procedure of choice in the assessment of infections of the urinary tract, including pyelonephritis, renal or perinephric abscesses, and emphysematous pyelonephritis and/or cystitis. Computed tomography studies are superior to ultrasonography in defining the extent of mass lesions, such as abscesses. With the availability of these newer methods, the reliance on intravenous pyelography for the assessment of UTIs is diminishing.

*Meares, E.M., Stamey, T.A.: Bacteriologic localization patterns in bacterial prostatitis and urethritis. Invest. Urol. 5:492–518, 1968.

ACUTE RENAL FAILURE

By Murray L. Levin, M.D.
Chicago, Illinois

COMPLICATIONS OF ACUTE RENAL FAILURE

Acute renal failure is a severe, relatively common clinical affliction. Approximately 5 per cent of all hospitalized patients develop acute renal failure as a complication of their hospitalization. Of those patients who develop acute renal failure in the hospital, 30 to 60 per cent will survive (average about 50 per cent). This terrible human cost is compounded by a large financial cost, since the length of stay is increased by 2 to 3 weeks in patients who develop the syndrome. Thus, an understanding of the clinical pathogenesis of acute renal failure and attempts to prevent it from occurring are of extreme importance. Acute renal failure is defined as a sudden interruption in normal renal function that results in a decrease in the filtration of plasma. As a consequence, this decrease in renal function is manifested as rising serum urea nitrogen (SUN) and creatinine concentrations and/or a decrease in urine output. If the decrease in filtration is nearly complete, the average increase in the serum creatinine concentration each day is 0.5 to 1.5 mg/dL, depending on the muscle mass of the patient, the age of the patient, and whether acute muscle injury is part of the overall disease state that induced the acute renal failure. The usual increase in SUN is 10 to 20 mg/dL per day. The rate of increase in SUN can be accelerated by a hypercatabolic state, the use of corticosteroids, and sepsis. Also, gastrointestinal bleeding can cause a more rapid increase in SUN. The rate of increase in SUN and creatinine will be less in patients whose renal functional decrease is incomplete.

In acute renal failure, urine volume is typically less than necessary for maintaining fluid homeostasis and less than that necessary for excreting the nitrogenous load of metabolites. Thus, most cases of acute renal failure are called oliguric. The 24-hour urine volume is less than 400 mL per day. However, many patients may have so-called nonoliguric renal failure, especially those with renal failure caused by aminoglycoside toxicity or intravenous radiocontrast materials. The urine volumes of these patients typically range between 400 and 1200 mL per day but may be even higher. Anuria is usually defined as a total 24-hour urine volume of less than 100 mL. Total anuria, zero output, is caused either by total obstruction to urine flow or by a vascular or glomerular lesion that results in zero filtration. Occasionally, total anuria can be seen in acute tubular necrosis. Severe hypotension can also cause anuria.

Patients may present with acute renal failure in the outpatient or the inpatient setting. Patients who present with acute renal failure as outpatients most likely have drug toxicity (nonsteroidal anti-inflammatory drugs [NSAIDs], angiotensin converting enzyme [ACE] inhibitors, toxin ingestion) or severe volume depletion from hemorrhage, vomiting, diarrhea, or overdiuresis. Outpatients may also present with acute renal failure secondary to sepsis, glomerulonephritis, vasculitis, or obstructive uropathy.

Inpatients present with acute renal failure syndromes that are frequently secondary to volume depletion from mechanisms as described earlier, drug toxicity (antibiotics, NSAIDs, ACE inhibitors), or toxicity from exposure to radiocontrast material. In addition, many patients develop acute renal failure postoperatively, from intraoperative hypotension. Aortic catheterization may cause acute renal failure by inducing atheroembolic renal disease.

The major clinical complications of acute renal failure are loss of the excretory and regulatory functions of the kidney. The excretory function of the kidney is designed to rid the organism of potential toxins. If these toxins are not excreted, patients can become lethargic, nauseated with vomiting, confused, semicomatose, and then fully comatose. Ultimately, seizures and death ensue. Loss of the regulatory functions of the kidney causes a failure to excrete a volume load of salt and water, with resultant vascular congestion, pulmonary edema, and hypoxia. Hyperkalemia may become life-threatening. Severe acidosis may ensue, compromising cardiac function and increasing the hyperkalemia. Serum phosphorus concentration rises with time, causing a reduction in serum calcium as calcium phosphate solubility product is exceeded. Anemia may be attributed not only to the underlying disorder that led to acute renal failure but also to reduced serum erythropoietin.

CAUSES OF ACUTE LOSS OF RENAL FUNCTION

The most common cause of acute loss of renal function is underperfusion of the kidneys (Table 1). The clinician must recognize states in which the kidneys are underperfused because quick reversal of the condition may prevent the onset of true acute renal failure with all its complications.

Table 1. Causes of Acute Renal Failure

Prerenal Causes (Renal Underperfusion)
Hypovolemia: GI or urinary loss, inadequate replacement; hemorrhage; third spacing; congestive heart failure (inadequate cardiac output)
Hypotension: Sepsis; drug-induced hypotension; hypotension controlled below patient's autoregulatory levels; anesthesia-induced hypotension
Pharmacologic: NSAIDs, ACE inhibitors
Arterial obstruction
Intrarenal Causes
Acute tubular necrosis: Sepsis; hypovolemia and hypotension; contrast nephropathy; aminoglycosides
Atheroembolic disease
Interstitial disease: Acute allergic interstitial nephritis, drug-induced; necrotizing papillitis (bilateral)
Glomerular: Acute glomerulonephritis, especially rapidly progressive; Wegener's granulomatosis; acute and chronic vasculitis; scleroderma kidney; light chain and cryoglobulin disease
Infiltrative: Lymphoma, sarcoidosis
Intratubular obstruction: Tumor lysis syndrome, acyclovir, light chain disease
Postrenal Causes
Bladder neck and urethral obstruction, including obstructed indwelling catheters
Intrabladder: tumors
Ureteral: One calculus or tumor on side of single functioning kidney; retroperitoneal tumors; bilateral stones
Intrarenal: Infiltrative diseases

ACE = angiotensin converting enzymes; GI = gastrointestinal; NSAIDs = nonsteroidal anti-inflammatory drugs.

Prerenal Causes

Volume depletion is an important cause of decreased renal perfusion. Loss of fluid volume to the external environment is typically associated with vomiting, nasogastric suction, diarrhea, overdiuresis, and hemorrhage. In addition, intravascular volume depletion and inadequate cardiac output with resultant underperfusion of the kidneys can occur with sequestration of fluid in an operative wound, in retroperitoneal hemorrhage, in severe pancreatitis, or in severe compartment syndromes, especially of the lower extremities. In some patients, renal hypoperfusion may be exacerbated by inadequate fluid replacement for normal volume losses.

Hypotension is a common cause of renal underperfusion, especially in hospitalized patients whose blood pressures are maintained at levels below those ordinarily experienced. Thus, an elderly patient with a typical blood pressure of 150 to 160/80 to 90 mm Hg may experience severe renal hypoperfusion following vasodilator treatment for angina pectoris. Maintaining a patient's blood pressure at 100 to 110/60 mm Hg may reduce the perfusion pressure below the autoregulatory range for that individual, and renal perfusion will fall, with resultant oliguria and an increase in SUN and creatinine concentrations. Similarly, maintenance of low blood pressures in the cardiac-surgical intensive care unit after coronary artery bypass may induce the same phenomenon. Reducing the dosage of nitroglycerin, beta-blockers, or other vasodilators or restoring vascular volume in the postoperative patient may assist considerably in returning renal function to normal. Sepsis with accompanying vasodilatation, hypotension, and renal underperfusion is another major cause of renal failure. It should be considered whenever a patient becomes hypotensive or oliguric or experiences a change in mental status.

Hypotension during surgery is a cause of renal failure that can be discovered by review of intraoperative anesthesia records. The patient's renal pressure may fall below autoregulatory levels, with resultant oliguria and acute tubular necrosis. Intraoperative hypotension is a common cause of an increasing SUN and creatinine on the first postoperative day. Intravascular volume deficits should be replaced with isotonic saline—not half-normal saline. Twice as much of the isotonic solution remains within the blood vessels.

Congestive heart failure and cirrhosis of the liver may also contribute to renal hypoperfusion. Similarly, obstruction of renal blood flow (with renal hypoperfusion) can occur with thrombus in the aorta, embolus to a single functioning kidney, bilateral renal arterial thrombi or emboli, atherosclerotic emboli to both kidneys following spontaneous embolization from intra-aortic atherothrombus or the introduction of a catheter into the aorta for angiography. Such atheroembolic events can be catastrophic for renal function.

Intrarenal Causes

The four major targets of intrarenal causes of acute renal failure are the tubules, the interstitium, the glomeruli, and the blood vessels. The most frequent target is the tubular cell, and the most important syndrome is acute tubular necrosis (ATN). Patients typically develop ATN when the duration or severity of hypoperfusion leads to irreversible tubular cell injury prior to correction or repair of the original insult. Thus, prolonged hypotension for any reason, prolonged intravascular volume depletion, prolonged sepsis, and severe hemorrhage with prolonged hypotension all lead to ATN. In addition, ATN may be caused by exposure to various renal toxins and renally active drugs, especially contrast material, aminoglycosides, NSAIDs, and ACE inhibitors. Patients who are volume-depleted are especially prone to the development of ATN if they are also consuming NSAIDs or ACE inhibitors. By preventing the normal prostaglandin-stimulated afferent arteriolar vasodilation in the face of volume depletion or decreased cardiac output, NSAIDs can increase the duration and/or severity of the renal effects due to the underlying state of hypoperfusion. Similarly, because ACE inhibitors prevent the well-known efferent arteriolar vasoconstriction necessary for compensatory maintenance of glomerular filtration pressure in underperfused states, they may also cause ATN and acute renal failure.

Ingestion of methanol or ethylene glycol may lead to ATN. Exposure to ethanol and/or cocaine can also cause ATN, primarily by initiating rhabdomyolysis. Methotrexate and platinum-containing compounds can cause ATN and/or vascular disease, leading to slowly progressive loss of renal function. In addition, rapid lysis of tumor cells (e.g., lymphomas, leukemias) may precipitate urates and phosphates, causing irreversible tubular obstruction. If this syndrome is suspected, dialysis should be initiated as soon as possible to lower serum urate and phosphate concentrations. Acyclovir can also precipitate in renal tubules, whereas cryoglobulins precipitate in glomeruli and light chains precipitate in glomeruli and/or tubules in light chain disease or in multiple myeloma.

Other intrarenal causes of acute renal failure include acute glomerulonephritis, vasculitis, and allergic interstitial nephritis. Classic causes of the latter condition include thiazides, cimetidine, sulfa drugs, penicillin derivatives, and NSAIDs. Some medications can increase the serum creatinine concentration without changing the glomerular filtration rate. For example, cephalosporins may falsely increase serum creatinine by interfering with the chemical determination of creatinine. Trimethoprim, cimetidine, and ranitidine may increase the serum creatinine concentration by interfering with its secretion. Ordinarily, about 10 per cent of urinary creatinine is the product of secretion. Therefore, if a patient has normal renal function, an increase in the serum creatinine concentration from 1.0 to 1.1 mg/dL may be anticipated with the use of one of these agents. Most clinicians would not consider this to be a clinically significant increase. However, with increasing degrees of renal failure, secretion of creatinine represents an increased percentage of the amount of excreted creatinine. Thus, at a serum creatinine of 3 to 4, creatinine secretion may represent 20 to 25 per cent of excreted creatinine. With trimethoprim, cimetidine, or ranitidine use, a serum creatinine of 4 may increase to a serum creatinine of 5 simply because secretion is not occurring. This increase in serum creatinine concentration may unnecessarily alarm many clinicians. To distinguish a true decrement in renal function from a drug-induced increase in serum creatinine concentration, the responsible agent should be stopped and the serum creatinine monitored.

Postrenal Causes

Postrenal causes of acute renal failure are associated with obstruction that can occur anywhere from the urethral orifice to the renal parenchyma. A single renal calculus or a renal or ureteral tumor on the side of a single functioning kidney can cause enough obstruction to induce acute renal failure. Retroperitoneal fibrosis and retroperitoneal adenopathy can cause obstructive acute renal failure, as can obstruction of urine flow at the bladder trigone by infiltrating bladder or prostate carcinoma. Infiltration by cervical, uterine, or rectal carcinoma can also occlude urine flow in both ureters. The most common cause of obstruction to urine flow is disease of the prostate, benign or malignant. Finally, infiltrative diseases of the renal parenchyma, bilateral renal calculi, urethral strictures, and obstructed indwelling bladder catheters all have been associated with acute reductions in renal function.

EVALUATION OF THE PATIENT WITH ACUTE RENAL FAILURE

History and Physical Examination

Optimal evaluation of the patient with acute renal failure requires an appropriate history from the patient and a review of the patient's record. In particular, a detailed and compulsive chart review must be performed whenever a patient develops acute renal failure in the hospital. Any history of volume loss from diarrhea, vomiting, nasogastric suction, diuresis, or excessive diaphoresis should be documented. Fluid intakes, urine output, diarrhea, and stool losses should be determined and recorded. Stool output should include any ostomy drainage that occurs. Blood pressure readings and anesthesia records should be reviewed for evidence of hypotension. The patient's typical blood pressure during the preceding 2 to 3 days should be compared to the blood pressure recorded at the onset of acute renal failure. As mentioned earlier, renal hypoperfusion caused by controlled, drug-induced hypotension may lead to acute renal failure. The patient should be asked if he or she has had any angiograms, cardiac catheterizations, or contrast-enhanced tomographic studies. Medication use should be reviewed, especially use of antibiotics,

NSAIDs, and ACE inhibitors. A history consistent with obstruction (e.g., dribbling, decreased urinary stream and/or frequency, and nocturia) should be sought. Any patient with an increasing SUN and serum creatinine should have intake and output recorded to determine the degree of oliguria so that appropriate reduction in fluid intake can be ordered after the patient has been judged not to be volume depleted. Finally, a history of bloody or dark urine, pharyngitis, rash, bloody diarrhea, joint pains, hemoptysis, sinusitis, and sinus pain and drainage should be sought as evidence of glomerulonephritis or vasculitis that may have caused or contributed to the acute renal failure.

During the physical examination, check for orthostasis by measuring blood pressure and pulse first with the patient lying flat and then with the patient sitting with legs dangling. If the patient begins to get dizzy or looks as if he or she is about to have syncope, the diagnosis of orthostasis is made immediately and the patient should be placed back in the reclining position. The patient should never be brought from reclining to standing without sitting for a while with the legs dangling. If the patient does not become symptomatic, take the pulse and blood pressure. If the diastolic blood pressure falls more than 4 to 6 mm Hg, the systolic falls more than 10 mm Hg, and the pulse rises more than 8 beats per minute, orthostasis is present. If such phenomena do not occur, ask the patient to stand for 3 minutes. Measure the pulse and blood pressure again. If there is no orthostasis and skin turgor is adequate, significant volume depletion probably does not exist, but a fluid challenge can still be given. Check skin turgor on the chest and upper extremities, then observe skin turgor of the forehead by rotating the thumb on the forehead and determining the rapidity with which the skin returns to its usual configuration. This maneuver can be especially helpful in elderly patients whose chest wall skin elasticity may be considerably decreased, especially if they are quite thin. The skin should also be examined for rash, petechiae, and changes in color. A cool lower extremity with mottling may be the result of underperfusion or atheroembolic disease. Petechiae and hemorrhage may suggest hemolytic-uremic syndrome or thrombotic thrombocytopenic purpura (TTP). Finally, check for evidence of congestive heart failure by searching for distended neck veins, hepatojugular reflux, an S_3, rales, pleural effusions, hepatic congestion, and peripheral edema.

Laboratory Tests

With regard to laboratory tests, the most important examination is the urinalysis (Table 2). A bland urine, without many cells or casts, usually reflects obstructive uropathy or an underperfused state without true ATN. Once ATN ensues, brownish, broad casts can be seen, along with epithelial cells, in the urinary sediment. If a glomerulonephritic or vasculitic syndrome is present, red blood cells and red blood cell casts may appear. Proteinuria, especially greater than 100 mg/dL, is rarely seen in ATN or in obstructive uropathy. If proteinuria greater than 100 mg/dL is documented, consider a vasculitic or nephritic syndrome.

Measure the SUN and creatinine concentrations and determine their ratio. If the ratio is greater than 15:1, underperfusion of the kidneys has most likely occurred. However, underperfusion may occur in protein deficiency states or in cirrhosis of the liver. These conditions are associated with decreased urea formation. Therefore, in patients with these conditions, an SUN-creatinine ratio of only 10 to 12:1 may still be high for those particular patients. In addition, steroids always increase the SUN-to-creatinine ratio because steroid-induced gluconeogenesis requires amino acid catabolism to synthesize glucose. Tetracycline and its derivatives may also increase the SUN. Urinary osmolality should be obtained. A urine osmolality greater than 400 mOsm/kg is frequently associated with volume depletion or nephritis. A urine–to–plasma osmolality ratio greater than 1.3 to 1, a urinary sodium concentration of less than 20 mEq/L, a urinary fractional excretion of sodium of less than 1 per cent, and a renal failure index of less than 1 typically indicate prerenal azotemia, volume depletion, and renal underperfusion, rather than ATN (Table 3).

Complete blood count (CBC) and platelet count are occasionally helpful in the diagnosis and management of acute renal failure. The clinician who observes microangiopathic hemolysis and thrombocytopenia should consider sepsis, vasculitis, hemolytic-uremic syndrome, or TTP. During pregnancy or immediately post partum, the clinician must consider postpartum renal failure or the HELLP syndrome (*h*emolysis, *e*levated *l*iver enzymes, *l*ow *p*latelet count) occurring in association with pre-eclampsia. The percentage or number of eosinophils should be determined in blood as well as urine. Eighty-five per cent of patients with acute allergic interstitial nephritis have peripheral eosinophilia (>500 eosinophils/μL). To detect eosinophiluria, evaluate the first morning urine with Hansel's stain. Alternatively, Wright's stain can be used, but the urine pH should be adjusted to 7 so that eosinophils will show the bright-red staining. Eosinophilia is also present in patients with atheroembolic renal disease, but only 15 per cent of cases of NSAID-induced interstitial nephritis are associated with increased numbers of eosinophils in blood or urine.

If the patient's urine chemistries suggest glomerulonephritis (see Table 3), request antistreptolysin O (ASO) and antihyaluronidase titers if there is a history of sore throat or previous skin infections. Streptococcal infection of the skin typically does not cause an increase in ASO but does cause an increase in antihyaluronidase titers. If a sinus-pulmonary-renal syndrome is suspected, request serologic testing for the presence of antineutrophil cytoplasmic antibodies (ANCA) and anti-glomerular basement membrane antibodies. If systemic lupus erythematosus is suspected, request antinuclear antibody and anti–double-stranded DNA antibody testing. Search for cryoglobulins when a

Table 2. Urinalysis in Acute Renal Failure

	Hypovolemia	Acute Tubular Necrosis	Acute Interstitial Nephritis	Glomerulonephritis	Obstructive Uropathy
Sediment	Bland	Broad, brownish casts Epithelial cells	White cells, eosinophils, cellular casts	Red cells, RBC casts	Bland or bloody
Protein	Negative or low	Negative or low	May be increased with NSAIDs	Increased (>100 mg/dL)	Low

RBC = red blood cell.

Table 3. Renal Tubular Function in Acute Renal Failure

	Hypovolemia	Acute Tubular Necrosis	Interstitial Nephritis	Glomerulo-nephritis	Obstructive Uropathy
Urine sodium concentration (mEq/L)	<20*	>40	>30	<20	<20†
Urinary osmolality (mOsm/kg)	>400	<350	<350	>400	<350
U/P creatinine	<40	<20	<40	>40	<30
RFi $\frac{\text{U Na}}{\text{(U/P) Cr}}$	<1	>1	?	<1	<1
FENa $\frac{\text{(U/P) Na}}{\text{(U/P) Cr}} \times 100$	<1%	>1%	?	<1%	<1%

*Hypovolemia in presence of continued vomiting or nasogastric suction causes Na > 30, low U Cl.
†Values given are for acute obstructive uropathy. Values for chronic obstruction (more than a few days) approach those for chronic renal failure: high sodium concentration, urinary osmolality same as plasma, RFi and FENa > 1.
FENa = excreted fraction of filtered sodium; RFi = renal failure index; U Cl = urine chloride concentration; U Na = urine sodium concentration; Cr = urine creatinine concentration; U/P = urine-to-plasma ratio.

patient has a purpuric rash and ulcerating lesions on the legs. Finally, look for immunoglobulin light chains in the urine and blood because light chain nephropathy can occur even in the absence of myeloma and clinically significant anemia.

If acute glomerulonephritis or rapidly progressive nephritis is considered the most probable diagnosis, proceed to renal biopsy while awaiting the results of serologic testing. Histopathologic features of the biopsy may provide sufficient basis for appropriate initial treatment.

THERAPEUTIC TRIALS

When a patient has all the historical and physical signs of volume depletion, request urine chemistries and cautiously begin a therapeutic trial of saline. Keep in mind, however, that patients who are oligo- or anuric and only slightly dry may be tipped into circulatory overload and pulmonary congestion when large amounts of saline are administered. Partial correction of volume depletion with saline may increase urinary sodium concentration and the fractional excretion of sodium. Diuretics may increase urinary sodium concentration, decrease urinary osmolality, increase the renal failure index, and increase the fractional excretion of sodium. Thus, high values for these indices, when obtained after saline or diuretic use, may not be meaningful, whereas low values would suggest continued volume depletion. Many physicians attempt to increase urine flow by administering loop-acting diuretics and/or mannitol. While there is no consensus that the use of these agents reduces the incidence of acute renal failure, the conversion of oliguric to nonoliguric renal failure may provide the physician with more freedom in managing fluid balance in patients with acute renal failure. In addition, nonoliguric renal failure may run a shorter course than that of oliguric renal failure. Therefore, it is reasonable to attempt to convert an oliguric patient to a state of nonoliguria even though the glomerular filtration rate continues to be quite low.

OTHER DIAGNOSTIC STUDIES

When obstructive uropathy is a likely diagnosis, the clinician should obtain ultrasound images of the bladder and kidney if the patient has not yet been catheterized. Ultrasound can also help the physician distinguish acute renal failure from chronic renal failure. Small kidneys and/or increased cortical echogenicity usually indicate chronic disease but do not distinguish pure chronic disease from chronic disease with superimposed acute renal failure. Ultrasound may reveal sites of obstruction to urine flow at various levels of the genitourinary tract, but computed tomography (CT) scans, cystoscopy with retrograde pyelography, and antegrade pyelography with nephrostomy drainage may be necessary for determining intrarenal obstruction. In addition, CT scans can be very helpful in evaluating unilateral or bilateral ureteral obstruction by tumors, or retroperitoneal granulomas or fibrosis. Cystoscopy and retrograde urography are useful in assessing intrabladder obstruction, bilateral obstruction, and bilateral papillary necrosis. Doppler flow studies may suggest arterial obstruction that can be confirmed by angiography.

The physician must do everything possible to prevent acute renal failure because this disorder is still associated with a 40 to 70 per cent mortality rate. Rapid correction or prevention of volume depletion, judicious use of antibiotics, and avoidance of NSAIDs in the volume-depleted patient are critical to this effort. When aminoglycosides are administered, the dosage should be adjusted on the basis of the true creatinine clearance. The preferred formula for estimating creatinine clearance in a patient with stable renal function is as follows:

$$\text{Ccr} = \frac{[140 - \text{age (years)}] \times \text{ideal body weight (kg)}}{72 \times \text{serum creatinine (mg/dL)}}$$

(for women, substitute 85 for 72).

SUMMARY

The clinician must not forget that acute renal failure is largely a preventable disorder. When this condition is not preventable, the cause should be investigated and all pathophysiologic disturbances reversed whenever possible. The physician's highest priority is adequate renal perfusion. Hemodialysis may be life-saving when the patient's SUN is greater than 100 mg/dL, when severe hyperkalemia or acidosis is difficult to control, and when hypervolemia causes pulmonary congestion in an oliguric patient who cannot excrete excessive fluid volume. Dialysis is also required when the patient becomes symptomatically uremic with nausea, vomiting, lethargy, coma, and/or seizures. Timely intervention, however, emphasizing fluid management, decreased potassium intake, correction of hypovolemia, and prevention of hypervolemia, can decrease the number of patients who eventually require hemodialysis.

CHRONIC RENAL FAILURE

By Nicolaos Athienites, M.D.,
and Ronald D. Perrone, M.D.
Boston, Massachusetts

A decrease in the glomerular filtration rate (GFR) that allows the accumulation of nitrogenous waste products produces a state of renal insufficiency or renal failure. Renal insufficiency indicates any decrement in renal function, whereas renal failure refers to a severe and life-threatening loss of renal function. The level of renal function (GFR in milliliters per minute) is used to roughly categorize whether renal insufficiency is mild (50 to 80 mL/min), moderate (25 to 50 mL/min), or severe (10 to 25 mL/min). Acute renal failure occurs over a few days to several weeks, whereas chronic renal failure occurs over months to years. Acute renal failure is frequently reversible, whereas chronic renal failure is not. Azotemia refers to the accumulation of nitrogenous waste products of metabolism (i.e., urea) owing to decreased renal excretion. Uremia refers to the constellation of symptoms and signs induced by the accumulation of large amounts of uremic toxins, most of which are poorly defined. The term end-stage renal disease (ESRD) refers to a level of kidney function for which renal replacement therapy (dialysis or transplantation) is necessary. The GFR at this stage is less than 10 mL/min, and uremic signs or symptoms are present. According to the United States Renal Data System 1994 report, on December 31, 1991, there were 188,591 patients with ESRD in the United States.

UREMIC SYMPTOMS AND SIGNS

Patients with mild to moderate decrements in renal function are usually asymptomatic. Abnormalities of renal function may be found during routine laboratory evaluation or urinalysis. A typical-case scenario is the presentation of an elderly patient with minimal or nonspecific symptoms, such as fatigue and weight loss, where routine laboratory work reveals azotemia. In some cases, kidney disease is diagnosed during the initial evaluation for newly diagnosed hypertension. Foamy urine indicates heavy proteinuria, found in glomerulonephritis. Impaired urine concentrating ability present in chronic renal insufficiency leads to urinary frequency and nocturia. Renal failure due to systemic disease is usually associated with other features of the systemic disorder. For example, lupus erythematosus often presents with arthralgia or photosensitivity rash. Polycystic kidney disease may present with flank pain or hematuria. Diabetic nephropathy, a common cause of ESRD, is often accompanied by other diabetic complications, including retinopathy and neuropathy.

Advanced renal failure may present with multiple symptoms. In the absence of treatment with dialysis, anorexia, weight loss, cachexia, fatigue, and decreased exercise tolerance are common in the advanced stages of renal failure. Symptoms and signs of fluid overload or congestive heart failure appear early in the course of renal failure in patients with coexisting cardiomyopathy, but they appear later in the absence of heart disease. Uremic pericarditis may develop with or without pericardial effusion; pleuritis and pleural effusion may produce dyspnea and chest pain. Nausea, vomiting, dysgeusia, (parageusia), and ammoniacal breath odors are common. The tongue may have a brown discoloration. The skin may be dry, pruritic, and pale or yellow; scratching may have caused excoriation and lichenification. Reversible alopecia and body hair loss occur frequently. Nail changes associated with renal failure and other chronic conditions include wide transverse parallel bands (Muercke's lines) and a single transverse white line (Mees' line). Central nervous system manifestations of advanced renal failure include mood changes, euphoria, hallucinations, memory deficits, delirium, and seizures or coma in the terminal stages. Sleep disturbances include the inability to fall asleep at night, daytime lethargy, altered sleep patterns, and the sleep apnea syndrome. Asterixis, or flapping of the hands when arms are extended and hands are in dorsiflexion, is a well-documented sign of uremia. Manifestations of peripheral neuropathy in chronic renal failure include numbness and paresthesias, muscle twitching, hyperreflexia, myoclonus, loss of vibratory sensation and restless legs syndrome (inability to keep legs still while at rest).

LABORATORY FINDINGS

Symptoms and signs of renal failure appear late in the natural history. Therefore, the diagnosis of renal failure is most commonly made by laboratory testing. The traditional measures of renal function include the serum urea nitrogen (SUN) or blood urea nitrogen (BUN), serum creatinine, and 24-hour urine collections for determination of urea and creatinine clearance. Urinalysis and measurement of protein excretion in the 24-hour urine or in a random-voided "spot" urine (protein-to-creatinine ratio) remain important tools for the diagnosis of chronic renal disease.

Serum Urea Nitrogen (SUN)

The normal range of the SUN is 11 to 23 mg/dL. Urea is an end product of protein metabolism. Increased SUN concentrations reflect increased production or decreased excretion of urea. Increased production of urea is associated with corticosteroid therapy, sepsis and other hypercatabolic states, and protein loading during hyperalimentation or major upper gastrointestinal bleeding. When protein intake is very low, urea production is decreased, and SUN can be normal even in the presence of severe renal insufficiency. Decreased excretion of urea occurs when the GFR is reduced or when tubular reabsorption of urea increases owing to volume depletion or decreased cardiac output. When renal function is normal, 40 to 60 per cent of the filtered urea is reabsorbed. Thus, the SUN concentration is affected by a number of variables, including the GFR, protein intake, renal blood flow, and volume status. As such, SUN is not an accurate indicator of the level of renal function and must be interpreted in the light of these other factors. Increased SUN in a patient with normal serum creatinine suggests a prerenal and therefore potentially reversible condition.

Serum Creatinine

The normal range is 0.6 to 1.2 mg/dL. Creatinine is an end product of creatine catabolism. The main source of creatinine is endogenous creatine found in muscle. However, the ingestion of meat also contributes to the total creatine pool and ultimately to serum creatinine concentrations. Ingestion of a meal rich in red meat increases serum creatinine without decreasing renal function. Rhabdomyolysis also increases serum creatinine (regardless of renal function) and may produce acute renal failure. Daily creatinine production is related to muscle mass, that ultimately depends on age, weight, and gender. Thus, serum creatinine typically underestimates the degree of renal insufficiency in the elderly and in patients with muscle wasting, cirrhosis, and other chronic wasting illnesses. A normal serum creatinine may be found in these conditions even with significant reduction in renal function. On the other hand, large muscular men may have normal renal function despite mildly increased serum creatinine. Assessment of muscle mass is important in every patient with increased serum creatinine because cachectic patients with serum creatinine concentrations in the range of 3 to 4 mg/dL could have ESRD. Ketoacids and certain cephalosporins falsely increase serum creatinine concentration measured by the Jaffe reaction, whereas 5-flucytosine falsely increases serum creatinine measured by enzymatic methods.

Creatinine Clearance

The normal GFR in young adults is approximately 130 mL/min for males and roughly 120 mL/min for females (adjusted for 1.73 m^2 body surface area). GFR decreases by approximately 10 mL/min per decade after age 40. The ideal marker for measurement of GFR is a substance that is freely filtered by the glomerulus and is neither absorbed nor excreted by the renal tubules. Creatinine is an endogenous substance that fulfills the above criteria with the limitation that it is secreted by the proximal tubule; the endogenous creatinine clearance overestimates the true GFR by 10 to 40 per cent in normal individuals and to a greater degree in moderate to severe renal insufficiency. Medications that inhibit the tubular secretion of creatinine, such as trimethoprim and cimetidine, increase serum creatinine without affecting GFR. Some authors administer cimetidine to utilize the creatinine clearance as a more accurate measure of GFR. The use of endogenous creatinine clearance as a reflection of GFR is based on the assumptions that the patient is in a steady state with regard to the level of renal function and creatinine production. Cockcroft and Gault have derived the following equation for estimating creatinine clearance:

$$\text{Ccr} = \frac{[140 - \text{age (years)}] \times \text{ideal body weight (kg)}}{[72 \times \text{serum creatinine (mg/dL)}]}$$

(for women, substitute 85 for 72)

For routine clinical purposes, creatinine clearance is typically calculated using the 24-hour urine creatinine and serum creatinine drawn at the midpoint or end of the collection. Typical errors are undercollection or overcollection of urine and the use of a serum creatinine value that was obtained long before or long after the collection. To avoid collection errors, patients should be given specific instructions: on the day of the scheduled collection, the first morning urine void will be discarded and the time noted; for the next 24 hours, all urine will be collected in a given container, including the first morning void obtained the next day.

The formula for calculating creatinine clearance based on a timed urine collection is as follows:

$$\text{Ccr} = \frac{\text{urine creatinine (mg/dL)} \times \text{urine volume (mL)}}{\text{serum creatinine (mg/dL)} \times \text{time of collection (min)}}$$

Assessment of Proteinuria

Protein excretion that exceeds 150 mg/day is abnormal. Increased urinary excretion of protein usually indicates the presence of renal disease but provides no information about the level of renal function. Abnormal proteinuria of less than 1 g/day may be found in benign orthostatic proteinuria and in physiologic conditions not associated with kidney disease (e.g., heavy exercise or a febrile illness). By contrast, most cases of chronic renal insufficiency due to diseases affecting the glomerulus are associated with proteinuria exceeding 1 g/day. In diseases that affect primarily the renal interstitium, protein excretion is typically less than 1 g/day, and it is not unusual for patients with severe renal insufficiency due to renal artery disease to have little or no proteinuria. Urinary protein associated with light chain disease or multiple myeloma is most often detected by urine protein electrophoresis and may be missed by urine dipsticks. Although the level of proteinuria does not correlate with the severity of renal insufficiency, heavy proteinuria is associated with a faster rate of progression to ESRD. Measuring the excretion of small amounts of albumin (20 to 250 mg/day) in the urine requires a specific radioimmunoassay or other sensitive test. Microalbuminuria correlates with the development of diabetic nephropathy and progression to ESRD. Proteinuria may be assessed in a 24-hour urine collection or in a single voided specimen. Measurement of the 24-hour urine creatinine excretion is also necessary for determining the adequacy of the collection. Undercollection shows falsely decreased and overcollection falsely increased amounts of proteinuria. A spot urine protein-to-creatinine ratio correlates well with the results of timed collections. A ratio greater than 1 indicates significant proteinuria, and a ratio exceeding 3.5 indicates nephrotic-range proteinuria.

DIFFERENTIAL DIAGNOSIS

The initial evaluation for chronic renal failure should include assessment of the level and stability of renal function. Serum creatinine and SUN, serum electrolytes, calcium and phosphorus, complete blood count, and urinalysis should be obtained. These values should be compared to previous measurements because documentation of abnormal renal function tests over months is essential in distinguishing chronic renal failure from acute renal failure. Three major categories of renal disease can be defined, as follows:

1. Proteinuria (greater than 1.5 g/day) and hematuria with or without red blood cell casts typically indicates glomerulonephritis. Measurement of serum complement proteins, antinuclear antibodies (ANA), anti-DNA antibodies, antineutrophil cytoplasmic antibodies (ANCA), cryoglobulins, and hepatitis B and C antibodies may help the clinician identify a specific cause of glomerulonephritis.
2. Proteinuria greater than 1.5 g/day without hematuria generally indicates a noninflammatory glomerular disorder most often associated with diabetes, amyloidosis, membranous nephritis, focal and segmental glomerulosclerosis, and heroin or human immunodeficiency virus (HIV) nephropathy.

3. A benign urine sediment (proteinuria < 1.5 mg/day and absence of hematuria) is typically seen in atherosclerotic renal artery disease, analgesic nephropathy, myeloma kidney, and chronic obstructive uropathy.

Imaging Studies

Ultrasonography is the most common imaging study performed in the evaluation of renal disease. Ultrasound has largely replaced the intravenous pyelogram (IVP) because it is simple to perform and patients are not exposed to the risk of anaphylaxis or acute renal failure following administration of contrast material. Renal ultrasound can detect obstruction and reveal kidney size, symmetry, location, and the thickness of the renal cortex. The finding of small kidneys with thin cortex and increased echogenicity confirms the presence of advanced, irreversible disease. Enlarged kidneys are seen in patients with diabetes and amyloidosis while multiple bilateral cysts are observed in polycystic kidney disease. Renal asymmetry in a patient with hypertension and generalized atherosclerosis suggests renal artery disease.

Diagnostic Reasoning

In the differential diagnosis of renal failure, the clinician must first distinguish acute disease from chronic and reversible disease from irreversible. Readily reversible conditions (e.g., volume depletion or obstruction) must be considered early and treated if present. Plotting serial measurements of serum creatinine or creatinine clearance may show both the chronicity and the rate of progression of renal disease. Acute renal failure, by definition, evolves within days to weeks, whereas chronic renal failure evolves over months to years. If prior measurements of serum creatinine are unavailable, the detection of small atrophic kidneys by any imaging modality almost always confirms the presence of chronic disease. The clinician must then distinguish glomerular processes from interstitial ones. Finally, the clinician must identify treatable systemic causes of renal disease, such as the nephritis of systemic lupus erythematosus, ANCA-associated nephritis, membranous nephritis, or light chain disease. The absence of nonrenal symptoms, signs, or laboratory abnormalities increases the likelihood of primary kidney disease rather than secondary. The principal causes of ESRD in the United States are shown in Table 1.

Table 1. Causes of Renal Failure in New Patients With End-Stage Renal Disease

	Percentage
Diabetes	33.8
Hypertension	28.3
Glomerulonephritis	12.6
Cystic kidney disease	3.0
Interstitial nephritis	3.0
Obstructive nephropathy	2.0
Collagen vascular diseases	2.1
Malignancies	1.2
Metabolic diseases	0.4
Congenital and other hereditary disease	0.7
Sickle cell disease	<0.1
AIDS-related	0.3
Other causes	1.0
Cause labeled unknown	5.7
Missing information	5.1

AIDS = acquired immunodeficiency syndrome.
Causes of renal failure in 1989–1991, from the United States Renal Data System. The National Institutes of Health, 1994 Annual Data Report, July, 1994. Bethesda, Maryland.

COURSE OF RENAL FAILURE

Chronic renal failure usually progresses to ESRD. The rate of progression depends on the nature of the kidney disease, the level of renal function, the amount of proteinuria, and the age and gender of the patient. Hypertension is present in 80 per cent of ESRD patients. Patients with hypertension and proteinuria greater than 1 g/day reach ESRD earlier than patients who do not have hypertension or proteinuria. Patients with diabetic nephropathy and moderate renal insufficiency progress rapidly to ESRD, while patients with polycystic kidney disease usually progress to ESRD over several decades.

COMPLICATIONS

The complications of renal failure are usually evident when the GFR falls below 20 mL/min. Metabolic complications classically result in hyperkalemia, metabolic acidosis, hypocalcemia, hyperphosphatemia, and hyperuricemia. Abnormal calcium-phosphorus metabolism leads to hyperparathyroidism relatively early in the course of renal insufficiency. Radiologic evidence of hyperparathyroidism (renal osteodystrophy) appears later. Anemia of chronic renal disease due to decreased production of erythropoietin occurs close to ESRD. The anemia of ESRD is normocytic and normochromic and responds to the administration of erythropoietin. Patients with abnormal bleeding time due to platelet dysfunction may develop epistaxis, gastrointestinal bleeding (in combination with uremic gastritis or colitis), or rarely, hemorrhagic pericardial effusion.

POTENTIAL ERRORS AND PITFALLS IN DIAGNOSIS

Renal insufficiency and renal failure are easily diagnosed with laboratory measurements of serum urea nitrogen and serum creatinine concentrations. The most common error is underestimating the severity of renal insufficiency, particularly in elderly patients whose SUN and creatinine may be only moderately increased due to reduced muscle mass and decreased protein intake. Overestimation of the GFR often leads to toxicity due to errors in dose adjustment for medications excreted by the kidneys. In patients with cirrhosis or other chronic wasting diseases, a severely decreased GFR is not necessarily accompanied by substantially increased values of SUN and serum creatinine.

Lack of review of previous measurements of serum creatinine may lead to misdiagnosis of acute renal failure as chronic, and vice versa. As the population ages, the incidence of obstructive uropathy, multiple myeloma, and atherosclerotic renal artery disease as the cause of renal failure increases. Renal ultrasound, which conveys the most useful information regarding renal size, texture, and presence or absence of obstruction, should be obtained in every new case of renal insufficiency and failure. Two problems deserve special emphasis: myeloma kidney and atherosclerotic renovascular disease. Both disorders usually present with a bland urinary sediment. Focused investigation, including serum or urine protein electrophoresis for myeloma and renal arteriography for renovascular disease, is required for accurate diagnosis.

NEPHROTIC SYNDROME

By Jean Lee, M.D.,
and Ziauddin Ahmed, M.D.
Philadelphia, Pennsylvania

Many glomerular diseases cause massive proteinuria. The various complications that accompany massive proteinuria are collectively known as the nephrotic syndrome. This clinical entity was originally defined by its four most striking features: proteinuria, hypoalbuminemia, hyperlipidemia, and edema. The clinician must recall, however, that other, less obvious complications of proteinuria can also have serious sequelae.

ETIOLOGY

The cause of nephrotic syndrome may be localized or systemic. By themselves, the light microscopic features of a renal biopsy rarely, if ever, permit the clinician to distinguish primary causes of nephrosis from secondary ones. For example, membranous glomerular lesions may be idiopathic and primary to the kidney or secondary to lupus, syphilis, drugs, or solid tumors. Table 1 provides a list of secondary causes of nephrotic syndrome. Etiology, incidence, and prognosis varies with age. Table 2 highlights important differences between adult and childhood nephrotic syndrome. The prognosis is usually better in children.

SPECIFIC SECONDARY DISEASES

Diabetic nephropathy is probably the most common cause of nephrotic syndrome and renal failure in adults. Nephropathy can occur in both type I (40 per cent) and type II (60 per cent) diabetics. Clinical evidence of renal disease is initially masked by an early increase in the glomerular filtration rate and by the relative insensitivity of the urinary dipstick for protein. In early diabetic nephropathy, albumin excretion is increased above the reference range, but the total protein excretion is normal. Early detection is now possible by screening for microalbuminuria (more than 20 mg/day), which is highly predictive of the subsequent development of clinically evident disease. The presence of diabetic nephropathy is usually suggested by a long history of diabetes, increasing proteinuria, progressive renal failure (end-stage renal failure in 3 to 7 years), and concurrent evidence of retinal involvement. Recent evidence suggests that tight control of blood sugar early in the course of disease may prevent the development of nephropathy and may retard its progression.

Table 1. Secondary Causes of Nephrotic Syndrome

Malignancies	Multiple myeloma, solid tumors, lymphomas
Drugs and Nephrotoxins	Nonsteroidal anti-inflammatory drugs, gold, pencillamine, heavy metals, street heroin
Infections	HIV, syphilis, hepatitis B, hepatitis C, subacute bacterial endocarditis, shunt nephritis, poststreptococcal glomerulonephritis, malaria, parasitic diseases, leprosy
Collagen Vascular Diseases	Lupus, Henoch-Schönlein purpura, mixed cryoglobulinemia
Systemic Illnesses	Diabetes, sarcoidosis, amyloidosis
Hereditary Disorders	Alport's syndrome, sickle cell disease, Fabry disease, congenital nephrotic syndrome, nail-patella syndrome
Allergens	Bee stings, snake venom, poison ivy, and poison oak
Other	Congestive heart failure, pregnancy, preeclampsia, hypothyroidism, renal transplant, obstructive uropathy, renal vein thrombosis

HIV = human immunodeficiency virus.

Lupus can present with nephrotic syndrome alone or in combination with other symptoms. The renal biopsy can show any of five different histologies. Diffuse proliferative disease more often results in renal failure and is treated more aggressively with cytotoxic agents. Low complements, C3 and C4, may also be markers for more severe disease.

Dysproteinemias should be sought in middle-aged to elderly people presenting with nephrotic syndrome. Abnormal plasma cells secrete parts of immunoglobulin chains, which then deposit in the kidney. The renal lesion depends on the type of chain being excreted by the abnormal plasma cell. Both glomerular and tubular lesions may be present. The glomerular lesions may appear as amyloid. In amyloid disease, the urine protein consists mainly of albumin, which can be detected by urine dipstick. In light-chain disease, urine protein is composed of various light chains (Bence Jones proteins). These light-chain proteins are not detected by the dipstick, which is sensitive only to albumin, but they can be detected with the use of protein precipitation tests, such as the sulfosalicylic acid test. The diagnosis can be made with serum and urine electrophoresis.

Patients infected with human immunodeficiency virus (HIV) can develop nephrotic syndrome and rapidly progressive renal failure. The kidneys have a characteristic large echogenic appearance on ultrasonography. The glomeruli are sclerotic, with a large amount of tubular damage as well.

Many primary glomerulopathies present with nephrotic syndrome (Table 3). The classification is made according to the histologic appearance on renal biopsy. Again, it must be emphasized that the many secondary glomerular lesions mimic primary glomerular diseases. Thus, the renal biopsy alone cannot exclude a systemic cause of renal disease.

SPECIFIC PRIMARY DISEASES

Membranous glomerulonephritis is the most common primary lesion found on renal biopsy in adults with nephrotic syndrome. The capillary loops look diffusely thickened on light microscopy, and subepithelial immune deposits are found on electron microscopy. Membranous glomerulonephritis can be idiopathic or secondary. It has a variable prognosis. Some patients remit, others stay nephrotic for years but maintain good renal function, while a third group unfortunately develops renal failure. Some response to steroid and other cytotoxic agents may occur, but it may not be complete. Membranous glomerulonephritis commonly recurs in transplanted kidneys.

Minimal change, or nil disease, is by far the most common lesion in childhood. The incidence of minimal change disease is so great and the response to steroids so good, that many pediatric nephrologists first give a trial of corticosteroids before proceeding to renal biopsy. The glomeruli

Table 2. Some Differences Between Adult and Childhood Nephrotic Syndrome

	Childhood	Middle and Old Age
Incidence	20–25 new cases/10^6/yr	10–11/10^6/yr
Causes	*In order of frequency* Minimal change disease (>70%) Focal segmental GN Membranoproliferative GN Others ***Young Adult*** *Almost equal in frequency* Minimal change disease Focal segmental GN Membranoproliferative GN Lupus Others	*In order of frequency* Diabetes Membranous GN Amyloid disease Minimal change disease Others
Complications		
Thrombosis	Less common, but arterial and venous thrombosis are equally frequent Renal vein thrombosis is rare in children with membranous GN	Thromboses of deep vein in legs are common Arterial thrombosis is rare Renal vein thrombosis is common, occurring in 30–50% of adults with membranous GN
Hypovolemia	Common	Rare
Infection with *Streptococcus pneumoniae*	Common in all types of childhood nephrotic syndrome	Never seen in patients older than 20 yr
Response to treatment	Minimal change disease responds promptly (8 wk) to steroids and cyclophosphamide Relapses are common Membranoproliferative GN type I responds to steroids	Minimal change disease responds less promptly (16 wk) to treatment Relapses less common Membranoproliferative GN type I is resistant to all forms of treatment

look normal on light microscopy and show only foot-process fusion on electron microscopy. The response to steroids is excellent, although some patients relapse when the steroids are withdrawn. The disease generally remits over time. Renal function remains well preserved.

Focal sclerosis can be difficult to diagnose because not all glomeruli are involved in early stages. Due to this partial involvement, focal sclerosis is frequently confused with minimal change disease, especially when only a few glomeruli are obtained on renal biopsy. Focal sclerosis produces focal and segmental sclerosis of parts of glomeruli. If the nephrotic syndrome remits with corticosteroids, the prognosis is good. Patients who continue to be proteinuric usually develop renal failure in a few years.

PRESENTATION AND COMMON COMPLICATIONS

Edema, the most dramatic manifestation of the nephrotic syndrome, can occur suddenly or with a more gradual onset. The amount of edema present in nephrotic patients depends on the level of hypoalbuminemia, the salt and water intake, and the degree of renal dysfunction. Findings can range from trace ankle edema to anasarca. Some patients have significant proteinuria but only slight decreases in serum albumin concentrations. These patients typically have little or no edema. At the other extreme are patients who have massive swelling as well as ascites and pleural effusions. Quite frequently in adults, these signs of fluid overload are confused with right-sided congestive heart failure. Children typically present with periorbital edema, while adults often develop lower-extremity edema with pretibial pitting. Since edema is dependent, it is important to look for edema over the lumbosacral area in bedbound patients.

Table 3. Primary Glomerulopathies With Nephrotic Syndrome

Minimal change disease
Focal sclerosis
Membranous glomerulonephritis
Membranoproliferative glomerulonephritis
IgM nephropathy
IgA nephropathy (rare)

Hypercoaguability is a troublesome feature of the nephrotic syndrome. Increased thrombosis occurs because of the loss of various anticoagulant factors, such as antithrombin III, in urine, increased platelet aggregation, and, most importantly, hyperfibrinogenemia. Venous stasis, poor mobility, and dehydration may further predispose to thrombus formation. Venous thrombosis is a frequent complication in adult nephrotics. Venous thrombosis with nephrotic syndrome has been reported in virtually every organ system, although deep venous and renal vein thrombosis are the most common. Often these venous thromboses migrate to the lungs and cause pulmonary emboli. Renal venous thrombosis can cause flank pain, hematuria, and loss of renal function. Arterial thrombosis, a much-feared complication, occurs mainly in children. The incidence of subclinical thromboembolic complications can be as high as 60 per cent in adults and 28 per cent in children.

Infection is a major cause of morbidity in nephrotic patients. Opsonization of encapsulated bacteria is impaired owing to defects in the complement pathway. White blood cell function is impaired, and IgG concentrations are decreased. Many of the medications used to treat various forms of nephrotic syndrome are themselves immunosuppressive. In children, pneumococcal peritonitis is a serious complication. Peritonitis can also be caused by other organisms, such as *Haemophilus influenzae* and *Escherichia coli*. Cellulitis can occur in both children and adults, especially when patients are very edematous. Skin flora, such as beta-hemolytic streptococci, are the most common offending organisms.

Malnutrition can result from heavy ongoing urinary protein losses of albumin and other proteins. These losses result in abnormalities in calcium and vitamin D metabolism, which in turn, can cause osteomalacia in adults and a failure to grow in children. In addition, concentrations of some trace metals, that is, iron, copper, and zinc, fall owing to urinary loss of their binding proteins.

Renal function in the nephrotic syndrome depends on several factors: those caused by the underlying disease and those caused by the nephrotic syndrome. The nephrotic syndrome itself may change renal hemodynamics. It can cause decreased effective circulating volume and/or intrarenal swelling. These changes lead to decreased renal blood flow and an acute fall in the glomerular filtration rate. The situation improves with treatment of the underlying factors and with remission of the nephrotic syndrome. The nature of the underlying disease also determines renal function. Renal function remains excellent in many diseases, most notably minimal change disease. In other diseases, the kidney is progressively damaged, and steady declines in renal function occur over months to years.

LABORATORY FINDINGS

Urinalysis is the single most helpful test in the detection of nephrotic syndrome. The urine dipstick measures urine albumin and is very sensitive in detecting nephrotic-range proteinuria. However, dipstick readings for protein can be artificially increased if the urine is concentrated, or falsely decreased if the urine is very dilute. Blood in the urine and a urine pH greater than 8 can falsely increase dipstick readings. Protein precipitation methods, such as adding sulfosalicylic acid to a urine sample, can also be used to detect urine protein. These methods precipitate out all proteins, not just albumin. False-positive reactions can occur when radiocontrast material, cephalosporins, or penicillin analogues are present in the urine.

The urine sediment may contain lipid droplets, which appear as Maltese crosses when examined under polarized light microscopy. These lipids may be found as free droplets, trapped in lipid-laden casts, or in epithelial cells known as oval fat bodies. Waxy casts and, rarely, a few red blood cells may be found.

Protein excretion varies throughout the day, depending on whether the patient is ambulatory or at rest. Generally, protein excretions are higher if the patient has been upright for some period of time. Therefore, the amount of protein in the urine should be quantitated through a 24-hour urine collection. Classically, nephrotic-range proteinuria was defined by a urine protein excretion equal to or greater than 3.5 g in 24 hours. However, a decline in the glomerular filtration rate and marked hypoalbuminemia can lead to a reduction in protein excretion below that expected in nephrotic syndrome. Since 24-hour urine collections can be difficult to perform correctly, a urine protein-to-creatinine ratio obtained on a random daytime urine specimen can be substituted in some cases. A ratio greater than 3.5 is compatible with nephrotic-range proteinuria; one less than 2 is probably normal. The urine sample should be collected during the day, since protein excretion diminishes after the patient has been supine for some time.

Measurements of serum albumin are generally less than 3.5 g/dL. Concentrations of serum cholesterol and triglycerides are increased and are at times extremely high. Concentrations of very low density lipoprotein (VLDL), intermediate-density lipoprotein (IDL), and low-density lipoprotein (LDL) tend to be increased. HDL may be decreased owing to urinary loss. These laboratory values return to normal after the nephrotic syndrome has resolved. The role of hyperlipidemia in cardiovascular complications is still being debated.

DIAGNOSIS

A careful history and physical examination are important, as is careful questioning about specific risk factors, infections, and medications. The funduscopic examination is particularly important in diabetics. Nephrotic syndrome can be a manifestation of malignancy; thus, patients should also be examined carefully, with special attention given to the lymph node, breast, rectal, and gynecologic examinations. Age-appropriate cancer screening should be performed. A chest film should be obtained. Laboratory screening should be performed for specific infectious etiologies, including HIV, Venereal Disease Research Laboratories (VDRL), and hepatitis B and C testing. In the older age group, serum protein electrophoresis (SPEP) and urine protein electrophoresis (UPEP) may be helpful in detecting dysproteinemias. Antinuclear antibody and complement testing may reveal lupus. Patients who have resided in endemic areas should have the appropriate screening for malaria and schistosomiasis because they are important worldwide causes of nephrotic syndrome.

If no systemic cause can be found, a renal biopsy is often necessary. This procedure can be performed percutaneously with the use of ultrasonography or computed tomography guidance. Prothrombin time (PT), partial thromboplastin time (PTT), platelet count, and bleeding time should be checked prior to biopsy. In rare cases when a closed biopsy cannot be done, an open biopsy may be attempted. Renal biopsy is usually a safe procedure. The major complication is bleeding.

GLOMERULONEPHRITIS

By Mary H. Foster, M.D.
Philadelphia, Pennsylvania

Glomerulonephritis (GN) is defined pathologically by characteristic morphologic changes in the glomerulus. It is usually recognized clinically by the presence of hematuria, proteinuria, and red blood cell (RBC) casts, that is, the functional manifestations of the structural abnormalities. The hematuria may be gross or microscopic, and the quantity of proteinuria may vary considerably. The association of hematuria with heavy proteinuria (>2 g per 24 hours) strongly suggests the diagnosis. The presence of RBC casts is diagnostic of GN; however, they may not be visible on microscopic examination of the urine sediment in all patients. Glomerulonephritis is a manifestation of several systemic and primary renal diseases (Table 1), and the diagnosis of a specific disease depends on correlation of clinical, serologic, and/or pathologic evaluation.

Table 1. Major Causes of Acute Nephritis Categorized by Serum Complement Concentration

	Decreased Serum Complement*	Normal Serum Complement
Systemic diseases	Systemic lupus erythematosus (focal, 75%; diffuse, 90%)	Polyarteritis nodosa group
	Subacute bacterial endocarditis (focal, 60%; diffuse, 90%)	Hypersensitivity vasculitis
		Wegener's granulomatosis
	Acute bacterial endocarditis (diffuse, 68%)	Henoch-Schönlein purpura
	"Shunt" nephritis (90%)	Goodpasture's syndrome
	Cryoglobulinemia (85%)	Visceral abscess
Renal diseases	Acute poststreptococcal GN (90%)	IgA nephropathy
	Membranoproliferative GN	Idiopathic RPGN
	Type I (50–80%)	Anti-GBM disease
	Type II (80–90%)	ANCA-positive pauci-immune GN

ANCA = antineutrophil cytoplasmic autoantibody; CH_{50} = total serum hemolytic complement; GBM = glomerular basement membrane; RPGN = rapidly progressive glomerulonephritis.

*Percentages indicate the approximate frequencies of depressed C3 or CH_{50}.

Data from Madaio, M. P., and Harrington, J. T.: The diagnosis of acute glomerulonephritis. The New England Journal of Medicine, 309:1299–1302, 1983.

CLINICAL PRESENTATION

The initial signs and symptoms of GN are diverse, ranging from asymptomatic hematuria to edema and severe uremia. However, several syndromes dominate the clinical presentation (Table 2). Acute GN refers to the abrupt onset of disease. The most common symptom is edema. In children and young adults, the edema is usually dependent and involves the face after recumbency and the lower extremities after ambulation. In the elderly and in patients with pre-existing heart disease, congestive heart failure may be the initial manifestation. Microscopic hematuria is almost universal. Gross hematuria, apparent at presentation in more than one third of patients, is often accompanied by proteinuria and hypertension. Other disorders to be considered in the differential diagnosis of this presentation include allergic interstitial nephritis, atheroembolism, and hemolytic-uremic syndrome or thrombotic thrombocytopenia purpura.

Rapidly progressive glomerulonephritis (RPGN) is the term used to describe GN associated with acute renal failure (increase in serum creatinine of more than 1.0 mg/dL per week). This subset of patients with acute GN initially presents with uremia, oliguria, and/or a progressive decrease in GFR over days to weeks, in addition to the signs and symptoms described earlier.

Chronic GN refers to an irreversible reduction in the glomerular filtration rate (GFR) secondary to GN. The kidneys are reduced in size as a result of chronic inflammation and/or fibrosis. This reduction may be either the sequela of an episode of acute GN or the initial presentation of previously asymptomatic or unrecognized disease. The initial presentation includes signs and symptoms of end-stage renal disease (uremia). In the absence of a pathologic diagnosis (biopsy is typically precluded by the small kidney size), the diagnosis is inferred from patient or family history, hematuria and/or proteinuria on urinalysis, and/or evidence of an associated systemic disease.

Occasionally, individuals with GN present with asymptomatic urinary abnormalities (hematuria, proteinuria, and/or RBC casts), discovered on routine urinalysis. Hematuria, in the absence of proteinuria, dysmorphic RBCs (detection requires phase-contrast microscopy), or RBC casts, can originate from any site in the urinary tract. Detection of isolated hematuria requires a thorough investigation of the entire urinary tract to exclude structural abnormalities (i.e., bladder carcinoma, stones). Patients with glomerulonephritis (i.e., IgA nephropathy) occasionally present with a nephrotic, rather than nephritic, clinical syndrome. Conversely, the diseases typically associated with the nephrotic syndrome occasionally present with the urinary sediment abnormalities typical of GN (see the article on the nephrotic syndrome).

In individuals with GN associated with systemic disease, the clinical signs and symptoms are due to multiorgan involvement. Frequently, those due to nonrenal involvement dominate the clinical presentation (i.e., massive hemoptysis in Goodpasture's syndrome; fever and cardiac manifestations in bacterial endocarditis; purpura and abdominal pain in Henoch-Schönlein purpura). The initial approach to patients with GN must always include consideration of selected systemic diseases.

Table 2. Major Clinical Presentations of Glomerulonephritis

Acute glomerulonephritis
Rapidly progressive glomerulonephritis (RPGN)
Chronic renal failure
Asymptomatic urinary abnormalities (proteinuria or hematuria)
Nephrotic syndrome
Symptoms related to underlying systemic disease

DIFFERENTIAL DIAGNOSIS

The initial approach to the evaluation of patients with suspected GN is to estimate the GFR with serial serum creatinine measurements and to quantitate the total protein excretion in a 24-hour urine specimen. If renal failure is present or is rapidly progressive, the patient should be hospitalized for further evaluation and consideration of an immediate renal biopsy (see below). In a stable patient with a normal serum creatinine measurement, evaluation can proceed in the outpatient setting.

Measurements of serum complement have proved particularly useful in the differential diagnosis of acute GN. During the initial evaluation C3, C4, and total serum hemolytic complement (CH_{50}) should be measured on at least two occasions, because the results may fluctuate. Because CH_{50} assesses components C1 through C8 (C9 is not necessary), low CH_{50} activity can identify patients with systemic diseases similar to systemic lupus erythematosus (SLE) and GN associated with deficiencies of components of the early classic complement pathway. The clinical presentation and serum complement measurements allow provisional narrowing of the differential diagnosis to one of two major groups of disorders that cause acute GN: those associated with a normal serum complement and those usually accompanied by hypocomplementemia (see Table 1). Clinical and laboratory evaluations also readily distinguish patients with renal-limited disease (primary GN) from those with systemic disease. Additional serologic and laboratory tests frequently permit definitive diagnosis, as outlined later for SLE, endocarditis, cryoglobulinemia, vasculitis, and Goodpasture's syndrome or anti–glomerular basement membrane (GBM) disease. Serum C4 or serial complement measurements can be particularly useful in distinguishing membranoproliferative GN (MPGN) from acute poststreptococcal GN (APSGN; see later). Hypocomplementemia, however, can also result from numerous nonimmunologic conditions, including those that cause renal disease and/or mimic vasculitis (i.e., atheroembolism, hemolytic-uremic syndrome or thrombotic thrombocytopenic purpura, severe sepsis, and acute pancreatitis).

GLOMERULONEPHRITIS DUE TO SYSTEMIC DISEASES WITH HYPOCOMPLEMENTEMIA

Decreased serum complement activity indicates that consumption of complement exceeds its production. Settings in which this decreased activity occurs include activation and depletion of the complement system by immune complexes within the kidney and other organs (most common); stabilization of the C3 or C4 convertase enzyme by autoantibodies (termed nephritic factors) directed against components of the complement cascade, thus leading to continuous complement breakdown; decreased production of complement; and genetic deficiency of an individual complement component (disorders associated with an increased incidence of GN). The initial clinical approach to patients with GN and hypocomplementemia is to distinguish systemic diseases from primary glomerular diseases. This distinction is usually obvious from the clinical presentation and laboratory evaluation.

Systemic Lupus Erythematosus

An autoimmune disease involving multiple organs, SLE primarily affects women (9:1 female-to-male ratio) between the ages of 15 and 40 years. The clinical presentation is variable; common signs and symptoms include arthralgias, malar rash, fever, alopecia, and malaise. Clinical renal involvement is present in 50 per cent of patients at onset and 70 to 75 per cent of patients during the course of the disease. Autoantibodies to a variety of intracellular and extracellular antigens may be present. The indirect immunofluorescence assay (antinuclear antibody [ANA]), positive in 95 to 99 per cent of patients with untreated SLE, is a sensitive (although not very specific) screening assay. A negative ANA is present in 1 to 5 per cent of patients with typical SLE, particularly if the assay employs rodent tissue substrate; antibodies against SSA/Ro, SSB/La/Ha, or single-stranded (ss) DNA are usually detected in these patients. If a positive ANA is identified, assays for detecting specific autoantibodies should be performed. The majority of patients with untreated SLE have high titers of antibodies to one or more of the following antigens: double-stranded (ds) DNA (40 to 70 per cent of patients), Smith antigen (Sm; 17 to 30 per cent), ribonucleoprotein (RNP; 32 per cent), SSA/Ro (35 per cent), and histone (70 per cent). Anti-dsDNA and anti-Sm are highly specific for SLE. Anti-SSA/Ro or antihistone is also found in 60 per cent of patients with Sjögren's syndrome and 70 per cent of patients with drug-induced lupus, respectively. Low titers of ANA and antibodies to ssDNA are frequently observed in a variety of other clinical conditions with acute or chronic inflammation, and they increase in frequency in the normal population with age.

Serum C3 and C4 concentrations are also usually decreased during active GN. Notably, neither complement nor anti-dsDNA concentrations consistently correlate with disease severity, renal histopathology, clinical relapses, or response to therapy. Complement activity may remain low and anti-dsDNA concentration may remain increased in some patients despite adequate therapy and clinical remission; conversely, exacerbations of disease activity have occurred in the setting of normal laboratory values. Although typically serum C3 and C4 concentrations fluctuate predictably with disease activity in SLE, C3 should be measured to serially monitor complement status. The high incidence of C4 null genes in SLE and the wider range of normal for serum C4 concentration reduce its diagnostic utility in SLE.

Kidney biopsy is used to define the severity of disease and to guide therapy. Lupus GN is classified into four pathologic types: mesangial (mesGN), focal proliferative (FPGN), diffuse proliferative (DPGN), and membranous (MGN). The terms describe the appearance of glomeruli on light microscopy. The quantity and location of glomerular immune deposits on immunofluorescence microscopy generally correlate with the histologic abnormalities: DPGN is associated with subendothelial, mesangial, and subepithelial immune deposits; mesGN is associated with mesangial deposits only; and FPGN is an intermediate class. In MGN, subepithelial immune deposits predominate. The most common and severe form, DPGN occurs in approximately 40 to 60 per cent of patients, whereas each of the other types occurs in approximately 10 to 20 per cent of patients. Clinically, patients with DPGN usually have the most severe disease, including an active urine sediment, nephrotic-range proteinuria, and an increased serum creatinine. These patients are easily distinguished, and biopsy is not necessary for determining the diagnosis. In patients with less severe clinical disease, the histologic abnormalities cannot always be predicted from the clinical and laboratory presentation, and a biopsy is usually necessary for determining the need for immunosuppressive therapy. Additionally, in patients with more severe disease (DPGN), the kidney biopsy is often used to determine the need for additional treatment (i.e., prolonged course of steroids and/or cyclophosphamide).

Development of new urinary sediment abnormalities (for example, RBC casts), nephrotic syndrome, or acute renal failure in patients with a previous history of mild disease suggests a transformation to a more severe form. A kidney biopsy is usually necessary for defining the histology. Furthermore, in patients with slowly progressive renal failure, in the absence of extrarenal or serologic disease activity, the biopsy is used to distinguish active renal disease from progressive renal scarring. In the former case, more immunosuppressive treatment is administered; in the latter, therapy should be discontinued.

Bacterial Endocarditis and "Shunt" Nephritis

The changing epidemiology of endocarditis, including antibiotic prophylaxis in valvular heart disease, the increased frequency of *Staphylococcus aureus* etiology, and the high incidence of parenteral drug abuse, has similarly altered the epidemiology of the associated GN. An incidence range in endocarditis patients from 2 to 60 per cent has been reported in the postantibiotic era. Several studies report a

20 to 25 per cent incidence of focal or diffuse proliferative immune-complex GN at autopsy in fatal endocarditis. Patients with parenteral drug abuse and/or *S. aureus* acute endocarditis have a particularly high incidence of clinical renal involvement in some series. Most patients present with the signs and symptoms of endocarditis, including weakness, fever, arthralgias, rash, congestive heart failure, heart murmur, and hepatosplenomegaly. Hypertension is rare. The renal abnormalities range from asymptomatic urinary abnormalities to RPGN; however, the nephrotic syndrome is unusual. Acute GN is particularly common in intravenous drug abusers and may occur at presentation or shortly after the initiation of therapy. Blood cultures are usually positive in patients with endocarditis, but some organisms may be fastidious. Of note, renal infarction, often associated with hematuria and/or flank or abdominal pain, is reported in 30 to 60 per cent of fatal cases of bacterial endocarditis. Children with infected ventriculoatrial shunts may develop GN ("shunt nephritis"). Hematuria is the most common abnormality, and nephrotic syndrome is present in more than 30 per cent of these patients. Positive culture of the shunt fluid provides the diagnosis.

Serum complement concentrations are often depressed at presentation but return to normal with adequate antibiotic therapy and, in the case of patients with shunt nephritis, removal of the infected shunt. Hypocomplementemia is more common in subacute endocarditis and diffuse GN (see Table 1). In these settings, persistent hypocomplementemia indicates active nephritis and ineffective therapy. Hypocomplementemia can also occur in the absence of histologic evidence of GN. Initial improvement followed by recurrent fever or rash suggests an allergic process (e.g., secondary to penicillin). Other laboratory abnormalities due to endocarditis include leukocytosis, increased erythrocyte sedimentation rate, circulating rheumatoid factors, and cryoglobulinemia. An antinuclear antibody may be present at a low titer. The presence of the latter findings may suggest either SLE or essential mixed cryoglobulinemia, but blood cultures usually confirm the diagnosis. Renal pathology is variable, but most often FPGN with subendothelial and mesangial immune deposits is detected with electron microscopy. Eradication of the infection with antibiotics and removal of the source, if necessary, usually results in resolution of the GN. Occasionally, patients develop chronic renal failure.

"Essential" Mixed Cryoglobulinemia ("Idiopathic" Cryoglobulinemia)

Cryoglobulins are immunoglobulins that form a precipitate in the cold and redissolve on warming. Their detection requires special attention to the method of blood specimen collection, because some cryoglobulins precipitate between 22°C (room temperature) and 37°C. The needle and syringe should be warmed to 37°C prior to venipuncture. Cryoglobulins are classified into three major groups based on their immunoglobulin composition (Table 3). The amount and type of cryoprecipitable immunoglobulin are usually determined by immunoelectrophoresis. The cryocrit, which measures all cryoprecipitable protein (i.e., not limited to immunoglobulins) and can range from 1 to 70 per cent, is not recommended. Type II and III cryoglobulins contain rheumatoid factor (RF), usually in high titer; however, RF activity may not be detected in standard assays if a cryoprecipitate forms and removes it from solution during processing of the serum. Low concentrations of cryoglobulins (<80 ng/mL) are present in as many as 38 per cent of normal individuals; mildly to moderately increased concentrations are present in the sera of patients with a wide variety of disorders (see Table 3). In the past, 30 per cent of mixed cryoglobulins were found not to be associated with an underlying disease and were termed idiopathic or "essential." However, recent reports of a very high prevalence of hepatitis C virus (HCV) infection (HCV RNA positivity) or exposure (anti-HCV antibody positivity) in most of these patients implicate an HCV etiology. Thus, most patients with the syndrome known as "essential" mixed cryoglobulinemia (EMC) probably have secondary cryoglobulinemia due to HCV.

Glomerulonephritis may occur in any type of cryoglobulinemia but is most common in type II EMC. Essential mixed cryoglobulinemia refers to a clinical syndrome due to a small-vessel vasculitis that typically presents in middle-aged females with recurrent episodes of palpable purpura involving the lower extremities, accompanied by arthritis or arthralgias, Raynaud's phenomenon, livedo reticularis, skin ulceration or necrosis, lymphadenopathy, peripheral neuropathy, and liver abnormalities. More than 50 per cent of patients with EMC have evidence of GN. The initial clinical presentation is variable and ranges from asymptomatic urinary abnormalities (50 per cent) to nephrotic syndrome (20 to 25 per cent) and/or acute nephritic syndrome (20 to 25 per cent). Cryoglobulins, usually type II, are typically present in the serum in concentrations in the range of 0.2 to 1.0 g/L or higher; however, the concentrations are extremely variable (between different patients and in the same patient at different times) and may not correlate with disease activity. A high mixed IgM-IgG cryoglobulin titer (>100 mg/dL, or >1 g/L) with a monoclonal IgM component in the appropriate clinical setting is considered diagnostic of EMC, but lower concentrations are more common and often require a skin or kidney biopsy to support or confirm the diagnosis (see later).

Testing for HCV must be performed in any patient with suspected EMC. Hepatitis C virus RNA has been detected in the sera of more than 80 per cent of patients with EMC and in almost 100 per cent of those with GN. Notably, evidence of active HCV infection detected by the HCV RNA polymerase chain reaction (PCR) occurs in the sera of patients who test negative for anti-HCV antibody by the enzyme-linked immunosorbent assay (ELISA) and recombinant immunoblot assay (RIBA), respectively, which demonstrates a significant incidence of false-negative serologic test results in patients with EMC. The latter may be due to precipitation of the anti-HCV antibody in the cryoprecipitate, as described earlier for RF. Thus, PCR testing for HCV genome (RNA) is recommended. Because HCV virus coprecipitates with the antibody, the serum can test negative for HCV even by the sensitive PCR method in low viral carriage states, despite persistent viremia. Precautions to maintain the blood specimen at 37°C (as outlined earlier) may avert this problem. Finally, as many as one third of patients with HCV liver disease test positive for the presence of mixed cryoglobulins, but few of these cryoglobulin-positive patients have overt disease manifestations of cryoglobulinemia, such as nephropathy and vasculitis. Notably, interferon-α therapy has been effective in patients with symptomatic HCV-associated mixed cryoglobulinemia.

Early components of the classic pathway of the complement system, particularly C2 and C4, are often profoundly depressed in EMC. In contrast, C3 levels may be only slightly decreased or within the normal range. The concentrations may not correlate with the severity of nephritis, and they can remain decreased despite clinical remission.

Table 3. Three Major Groups of Cryoglobulins

Type	Composition	Disease Associations
I	Single cryoprecipitable monoclonal Ig, IgG, IgM, or IgA class, or light chain (Bence Jones protein)	Multiple myeloma MGUS Waldenström's macroglobulinemia
II	Mixed cryoglobulins consisting of monoclonal rheumatoid factor, usually IgM, directed against polyclonal IgG	Lymphoproliferative disorders EMC*
III	Mixed cryoglobulins consisting of polyclonal rheumatoid factor, directed against polyclonal IgG	Autoimmune and infectious diseases†

EMC = essential mixed cryoglobulinemia; MGUS = monoclonal gammopathy of undetermined significance.

*Historically, approximately 30% of mixed cryoglobulinemias had no underlying or associated disease. Recent studies indicate that most of these patients probably have secondary cryoglobulinemia due to hepatitis C infection (see text).

†Disorders include, but are not limited to, vasculitis, endocarditis, systemic lupus erythematosus, acute poststreptococcal glomerulonephritis, chronic inflammatory liver disease, and collagen vascular diseases.

Bilirubin concentration and liver enzyme activities are frequently increased in serum; however, normal transaminase activities do not preclude the presence of HCV infection. Skin biopsy of affected areas reveals the pathologic changes of hypersensitivity vasculitis, and immunoglobulins deposited within vessel walls are of the same isotype as those present in the serum cryoprecipitate. Renal biopsy can be helpful in patients with an ambiguous clinical presentation. The typical findings are mesangial and endothelial cell proliferation, monocyte exudation, and basement membrane thickening due to interposition and subendothelial and mesangial deposits of IgM, IgG, and complement; MPGN is common. Intraluminal thrombi of precipitated cryoglobulins have a diagnostic fibrillar or crystalloid structure on electron microscopy.

PRIMARY GLOMERULONEPHRITIDES ASSOCIATED WITH HYPOCOMPLEMENTEMIA

Acute Poststreptococcal Glomerulonephritis

Acute poststreptococcal glomerulonephritis (APSGN) is a disease primarily of children older than 2 years of age. It occurs in epidemic and sporadic forms following skin or throat infections; however, the epidemic form is most often associated with impetigo. Only certain strains of group A beta-hemolytic streptococci are associated with GN (i.e., type 49 in impetigo, type 12 in pharyngitis). Symptoms usually occur suddenly and include edema (85 per cent), gross hematuria (30 per cent), and back pain (5 to 10 per cent). In the elderly, congestive heart failure may be the initial manifestation. Hypertension due to volume expansion is common. In children, lethargy, vomiting, and confusion alert the clinician to the possibility of hypertensive encephalopathy. Presentation as RPGN is rare in children (<1 per cent) but is more common in adults (5 to 10 per cent).

The diagnosis of APSGN should be suspected from a history of recent skin or throat infection. Owing to the relatively long latency period (10 days from the onset of pharyngitis, or more than 21 days from the appearance of skin infection) and the frequent use of antibiotic therapy, cultures are often negative at the time of diagnosis. Serologic tests may provide confirmatory evidence of a recent streptococcal infection if the patient has not received antibiotics. Antibodies to five (see later) of a large number of extracellular group A streptococcal antigens are commonly sought. Because the immune response to streptococcal antigens varies considerably, depending on the site of infection, antibody titers must be measured individually. Anti-DNase B and antihyaluronidase titers are increased in more than 80 to 90 per cent of untreated patients with pyoderma, whereas antistreptolysin O (ASO) and anti-NADase responses are often absent or weak in these patients. In contrast, the ASO and anti-NADase titers are increased in more than 90 per cent of untreated patients with previous pharyngitis. The Streptozyme test is a rapid, passive hemagglutination test that assesses antibody responses to five extracellular antigens (the four listed earlier and streptokinase) present in a crude preparation derived from streptococcal culture broth. Studies comparing the Streptozyme test with individual antibody tests are not yet conclusive.

Titers become increased 1 to 5 weeks after infection and may remain so for 3 to 6 months or longer. Serial measurements may reveal a titer rise consistent with a recent infection. However, the antibody response is abolished by early antibiotic therapy. In patients with GN, titers do not correlate with the severity of clinical disease. Notably, the incidence of streptococcal infection in children is relatively high, so that antistreptococcal antibodies are often present in children with unrelated GN. Conversely, anti–group A streptococcal antibodies are absent in the occasional outbreak of APSGN due to group C streptococci.

More than 90 per cent of patients have a decreased C3 concentration in the first week, which returns to normal in most patients within 2 to 6 weeks. Occasionally, normalization of C3 may take as long as 3 months. C4 levels are normal or minimally depressed. Persistent hypocomplementemia or profound depression of C4 concentrations at presentation suggest MPGN (see later). A normal serum complement at the time of the initial clinical presentation suggests an alternative diagnosis (i.e., IgA nephropathy).

Many pediatricians rely on the clinical presentation and lack of evidence of another cause of GN to make a presumptive diagnosis of APSGN. Renal biopsy is usually unnecessary in children and is reserved for patients with persistent renal failure or persistently low complement concentrations. In adults, especially those with atypical presentations, early biopsy establishes the diagnosis. Proliferative GN with polymorphonuclear leukocyte and monocytic infiltration, immune deposits of IgG and C3, and electron-dense deposits in subepithelial, mesangial, and subendothelial locations is typical; dome-shaped subepithelial deposits may be present, but they are not diagnostic.

With supportive care, nearly all children recover, including the occasional patient with RPGN. Serum creatinine concentration typically returns to normal within 1 month, although non–nephrotic range proteinuria may persist for more than 10 years. The long-term prognosis is good, but decreased GFR can persist in as many as 5 per cent of patients. Progressive renal failure accompanied by severe hypertension is somewhat more common in adults.

Membranoproliferative Glomerulonephritis

The initial clinical presentation of MPGN usually occurs in adolescents and young adults. It varies from asymptomatic urinary abnormalities to acute GN. Recurrent episodes of gross hematuria associated with respiratory or gastrointestinal infections are common. IgA nephropathy, Henoch-Schönlein purpura (HSP), and APSGN are usually considered in the differential diagnosis. More than 50 per cent of patients develop nephrotic-range proteinuria during the course of the disease. Approximately 50 per cent of patients develop chronic renal failure within 10 years. Poor prognostic indicators include male sex, older age, hypertension, nephrotic syndrome, and increased serum creatinine at onset. An association of MPGN with partial lipodystrophy and a strong association with viral hepatitis (HBV and, particularly, HVC), with or without concurrent cryoglobulinemia, has been observed. Evidence of viral hepatitis infection, liver damage, and cryoglobulinemia (see earlier) must be sought in patients with histologic evidence of MPGN.

Serum C3 concentration is reduced at initial presentation in more than 70 per cent of patients, and it decreases during the course of disease in an additional 15 per cent. In contrast with APSGN, low C3 concentration tends to persist. MPGN is divided into two types based on histologic criteria (see later). MPGN type I, the more common form, is associated with decreased serum C4 concentrations. In MPGN type II, like APSGN, the serum C3 can be profoundly decreased, but the C4 concentration is usually normal. C3 and C4 nephritic factor may be present in the sera of patients with either type of MPGN and in occasional patients with other forms of nephritis (APSGN, SLE).

The histologic findings are diagnostic, and a biopsy is usually performed to confirm the diagnosis. Mesangial hypercellularity and increased mesangial matrix are characteristic, and crescents may be observed. MPGN type I is associated with C3 and immunoglobulin deposits on immunofluorescence microscopy, along with subendothelial and mesangial electron-dense deposits. MPGN type II is characterized by heavy C3 deposits without immunoglobulins and with pathognomonic electron-dense deposits within the basement membrane (termed dense deposit disease). Interposition of mesangial matrix between basement membrane and endothelial cells is commonly found in both types. Current therapy, consisting of daily aspirin and dipyridamole (Persantine), delays the development of renal failure. In patients with associated HCV infection, proteinuria and/or viremia may resolve with interferon-α therapy.

GLOMERULONEPHRITIS DUE TO SYSTEMIC DISEASES WITH NORMAL SERUM COMPLEMENT CONCENTRATIONS

Normal serum complement activity indicates that complement production is keeping pace with complement consumption. Normocomplementemia does not exclude a role for complement in the pathogenesis of GN. Proteinuria due to experimental membranous nephropathy (Heymann's nephritis) is clearly complement dependent, but the serum complement concentration is normal. Additionally, prominent glomerular complement deposition is a common finding on kidney biopsy in patients with GN and either decreased or normal complement concentrations (see Table 1). Immunoreactive complement (C3 and C4) must be measured on at least two occasions because the concentrations may fluctuate (see earlier). Finally, the initial clinical approach to patients with GN and normal serum complement is the same as that described earlier for patients with hypocomplementemia; that is, systemic diseases must be distinguished from primary glomerular disorders on the basis of the clinical presentation and laboratory evaluation.

Polyarteritis Nodosa

Classic polyarteritis nodosa (PAN), a necrotizing vasculitis of small to medium-sized muscular arteries, can occur at any age but typically presents in middle-aged men. The clinical manifestations are highly variable and depend on the organ systems involved; frequently affected vessels include the coronary arteries, mesenteric arteries, kidneys, muscles, and vasa nervorum. General malaise, fever, weakness, weight loss, arthralgias, and myalgias are common presenting symptoms. Nervous system involvement, typically manifested as an asymmetrical polyneuropathy (mononeuritis multiplex), occurs in more than 40 per cent of patients. Involvement of the central nervous system can lead to focal (seizures, stroke) or global (headache, confusion, lethargy, psychosis) disturbances. Vasculitis of coronary vessels can cause congestive heart failure, angina, or myocardial infarction. Intestinal ischemia or infarction can result in severe abdominal pain or may present as an acute abdomen. Less common findings in classic polyarteritis nodosa are pulmonary infiltrates and cutaneous involvement, including subcutaneous nodules, livedo reticularis, palpable purpura, and necrosis. Disorders associated with this disease include hepatitis B or C infection, intravenous drug abuse, and hairy cell leukemia. The incidence of HBV surface antigen carrier state in PAN varies by location; in the United States, the incidence of HBV-related PAN ranges from 6 to 40 per cent.

Renal vasculitis is common and causes ischemia and necrosis. The clinical presentation depends on the type of vessels affected. Hypertension, due to large and/or medium-sized vessel vasculitis, is present in more than 50 per cent of patients and may be malignant. With isolated large-vessel vasculitis, asymptomatic nonspecific urinary abnormalities predominate. Small-vessel vasculitis often leads to glomerular inflammation and necrosis, with either acute GN or RPGN. Nephrotic-range proteinuria is present in 25 per cent of patients. Both large and small vessels are involved in some patients, and this can lead to overlap of symptoms and clinical findings (see later in section on microscopic polyarteritis).

In the presence of a multisystem disorder, the diagnosis of vasculitis must be considered. Evaluation must be rapid, because effective early therapy limits inflammation and minimizes irreversible scarring. A definitive diagnosis of PAN requires angiographic or histologic demonstration of the vascular lesions in the appropriate clinical setting. Angiography of the celiac and renal arteries is abnormal in 80 per cent of patients with classic PAN. Microaneurysms at vessel bifurcations and abrupt cutoff of small arteries is diagnostic in the appropriate clinical setting. Similar angiographic findings may also be observed in vasculitis associated with SLE, fibromuscular dysplasia, and atrial myxoma with embolization; all these conditions should be considered in the differential diagnosis. Histologic demonstration of vasculitis in a symptomatic organ is an alternative approach. Biopsy of involved nerve (i.e., sural nerve) or muscle, preferably guided by electrophysiologic testing, can be positive in as many as 87 and 50 per cent of patients, respectively. However, blind muscle biopsy can also provide the diagnosis in some patients. If pulmonary disease is prominent, open lung biopsy is preferable to percutaneous renal biopsy, because the focal vascular lesions are usually not observed in renal biopsy specimens. Biopsy of skin lesions may show leukocytoclastic vasculitis, supporting the diagnosis, although this nonspecific finding is common to other vasculitides, connective tissue diseases, and malignancy. The clinical presentation in patients with atheroembolic disease, in which the skin lesions, renal failure, hypertension, hypocomplementemia, and eosinophilia may closely resemble vasculitis, can be distinguished by the demonstration of cholesterol emboli on biopsy of the kidney or another organ. Only 50 per cent of patients with untreated classic polyarteritis nodosa survive for more than 3 months, and the 6-month survival is 35 per cent. Treatment with steroids and cytotoxic agents markedly improves the prognosis, and definitive diagnostic procedures should not be delayed.

The finding of necrotizing GN without immune deposits on renal biopsy should always alert the clinician to the possibility of vasculitis, either systemic or limited to the kidney. Determination of serum autoantibodies to neutrophil cytoplasmic antigens (ANCAs; see later) may help to further narrow the differential diagnosis. The limited data available suggest that ANCAs, usually antimyeloperoxidase, are present in approximately 25 per cent of cases of "classic" PAN, but the incidence is lower in PAN associated with HBV markers. Antiproteinase 3 (cANCA) and antimyeloperoxidase (pANCA) are typically observed in patients with untreated Wegener's granulomatosis and microscopic polyarteritis; they are also occasionally seen in patients with SLE and other disorders (see later).

Hypersensitivity Vasculitis

Small vessels are predominantly affected in hypersensitivity vasculitis. The disorder can occur at any age, and it is often associated with exposure to a new drug or foreign antigen (viral, tumor). Palpable purpura, the most prominent feature, is usually present over the lower extremities and buttocks. Demonstration of leukocytoclastic vasculitis on skin biopsy is diagnostic, and the kidney and gastrointestinal tract are also frequently involved. Similar findings may be found in myeloproliferative or autoimmune disorders. Kidney biopsy is usually not required for diagnosis, but vasculitis and GN are typical features. Any drug suspected of causing the disease should be discontinued. The drugs most commonly implicated include penicillins, sulfonamides, thiazides, and allopurinol. Some patients with severe disease (i.e., Stevens-Johnson syndrome) require a short course of high-dose steroids.

Glomerulonephritis Associated With Antineutrophil Cytoplasmic Autoantibody (ANCA)

The characterization of serum ANCA has revolutionized the diagnosis and classification of systemic and renal-limited vasculitis. The two ANCA subtypes, cANCA and pANCA, have distinct disease associations (Table 4), although both can be found across the spectrum of ANCA-associated disease. A positive cANCA, or antiproteinase 3 by solid-phase assay, is specific (up to 96 per cent) for classic Wegener's granulomatosis (WG), Wegener's vasculitis (a category recognized by some investigators and including patients with disease typical of WG but without histologic demonstration of necrotizing granulomas), microscopic polyarteritis (MPA), and a subset of patients with pauci-immune crescentic and necrotizing GN with no evidence of extrarenal disease (see Table 4). Positive cANCAs are rarely observed in other systemic diseases considered in the differential diagnosis of pulmonary-renal syndrome (e.g., SLE, Goodpasture's syndrome, and classic PAN). Positive cANCAs are occasionally observed in other disorders, including rare patients with a clinical syndrome initially suggesting vasculitis (systemic mycobacterioses, myeloproliferative disorder).

The antigen specificities and disease associations with pANCA are more heterogeneous (see Table 4). Most patients with ANCA-positive crescentic and necrotizing GN, with or without systemic disease manifestations, have antimyeloperoxidase pANCA. Most assays detect only IgG ANCA, but a group of patients with an MPA-like illness and predominant IgM ANCA have been described. Given the low prevalence of ANCA-associated disease in the general population and the lack of 100 per cent specificity of ANCA for vasculitis, ANCA testing is useful primarily in patients with pulmonary-renal syndrome or RPGN; that is, those clinically suspected of having a small-vessel vasculitis.

Wegener's Granulomatosis

Wegener's granulomatosis is a granulomatous vasculitis found in middle-aged adults. Patients typically present with vasculitis of the upper (nasopharynx, paranasal sinuses) and lower respiratory tracts and with necrotizing GN. Early in the disease, urinalysis and renal function may be normal, but eventually most patients develop GN (see the article on Wegener's granulomatosis).

Microscopic Polyarteritis (Polyangiitis)

Microscopic polyarteritis (MPA) is a small-vessel (capillary, venule, arteriole) necrotizing vasculitis that shares many clinical and pathologic similarities with WG but lacks the prominent upper respiratory tract involvement and granulomas. Renal involvement is almost invariably present, and pulmonary hemorrhage due to alveolar capillaritis is common. Although most patients with MPA are positive for cANCA, as many as 20 per cent are positive for antimyeloperoxidase pANCA (see Table 4). Microscopic polyarteritis is clinically, pathologically, and serologically distinct from the medium-sized to large vessel vasculitis of classic PAN. However, precise classification of patients is sometimes not clinically possible owing to overlapping features.

Churg-Strauss Syndrome (Allergic Granulomatosis)

Young adults with this syndrome typically have a history of allergy, asthma, and peripheral eosinophilia preceding symptoms of systemic vasculitis. As in polyarteritis nodosa, multiple organs are involved, including peripheral nerves, gut, and lung. Cardiac involvement is less common but is a major cause of mortality. Renal involvement is usually mild, but severe focal necrotizing GN can develop. Clues to the diagnosis include eosinophilia, increased plasma IgE concentrations, and patchy or nodular pulmonary infiltrates on chest film examination. The limited available data suggest that ANCAs, usually antimyeloperoxidase, are present in approximately 60 per cent of patients. Biopsy of involved tissue, including kidney, typically demonstrates eosinophilic infiltrates and granulomas.

Table 4. Characteristics of ANCA Subtypes and Major Disease Associations

	cANCA	pANCA
Staining pattern on ethanol-fixed neutrophils	Diffuse cytoplasmic	Perinuclear
Major antigen specificity	Serine proteinase 3 (>95%)	Myeloperoxidase* Elastase Lactoferrin Cathepsin G Additional unidentified antigens
Major disease associations	Systemic vasculitis: WG/WV/MPA Renal-limited vasculitis (pauci-immune necrotizing GN) 40% of all ANCA+ RPGN† 20% of ANCA+ RPGN with renal-limited disease	Systemic vasculitis: WG/WV/MPA* (5–20% of ANCA+ cases) Renal-limited vasculitis* (pauci-immune necrotizing GN) Spontaneous SLE Hydralazine-induced lupus Inflammatory bowel disease Autoimmune liver disease 60% of all ANCA+ RPGN† 80% of ANCA+ RPGN with renal-limited disease

MPA = microscopic polyarteritis; RPGN = rapidly progressive glomerulonephritis; WG = Wegener's granulomatosis; WV = Wegener's vasculitis.
*Greater than 95% of pANCA in the setting of WG, WV, MPA, or renal-limited vasculitis is specific for myeloperoxidase.
†Patients with RPGN constitute a subset of all patients listed above with either systemic or renal-limited vasculitis. Among all ANCA-positive patients with RPGN, approximately 75% have evidence of extrarenal (systemic) disease (see text).
Adapted from Foster, M.H.: Serologic evaluation of the renal patient. *In* Jacobson, H., Klahr, S., and Striker, G. (eds.): Principles and Practice of Nephrology, 2nd ed. St. Louis, Mosby-Year Book, 1995.

Henoch-Schönlein Purpura

Henoch-Schönlein purpura is a small-vessel vasculitis that typically affects children in late winter or early spring, but it can also occur sporadically in adults. It is frequently preceded by an upper respiratory tract infection. The classic clinical presentation is palpable purpura, arthritis, or arthralgias of large joints, gross hematuria, and abdominal pain. The renal presentation varies considerably, but acute GN and/or nephrotic syndrome are the most common presenting manifestations. Biopsy of a skin lesion demonstrating IgA deposits in the dermal vessels is diagnostic, but IgA may not be demonstrable in older lesions. Renal biopsy is usually not necessary, but in the absence of skin lesions it can be diagnostic. Histologic findings include mesangial proliferation with prominent mesangial IgA deposits.

PRIMARY GLOMERULONEPHRITIDES ASSOCIATED WITH NORMAL SERUM COMPLEMENT CONCENTRATIONS

IgA Nephropathy (Berger's Disease)

IgA nephropathy is the most common cause of primary GN worldwide. It occurs at all ages but most commonly presents in adolescents and young adults. Typical clinical presentations include macroscopic hematuria (40 to 45 per cent of patients) and asymptomatic microscopic hematuria and proteinuria (35 to 40 per cent). Macroscopic hematuria may be recurrent, following upper respiratory tract or gastrointestinal infections. The latency period between infection and hematuria is 1 to 3 days, distinguishing it from APSGN. A variety of systemic disorders have been associated with IgA nephropathy, including cirrhosis, dermatitis herpetiformis, gluten enteropathy, and ankylosing spondylitis. Their presence should alert the clinician to the possibility of the diagnosis. Less frequently, patients present with acute GN, RPGN, or the nephrotic syndrome.

IgA concentration is increased in as many as 50 per cent of patients, but this finding is nonspecific and of limited diagnostic value. An increased concentration of IgA-fibronectin aggregates unaccompanied by IgG-fibronectin aggregates has demonstrated specificity for idiopathic nephropathy in some laboratories. Complement concentrations are usually normal, but hypocomplementemia may occasionally be observed in patients with liver disease. Thus, the diagnosis of IgA nephropathy depends primarily on histopathologic examination of the kidney. Renal biopsy typically reveals predominant IgA mesangial deposits; IgG, IgM, and C3 are variably observed. On light microscopy, the abnormalities vary with clinical activity from mild mesangial abnormalities to crescentic GN. During an episode of clinical activity, mesangial proliferation is usually observed. Mesangial IgA deposition is also prominent in HSP and SLE, but these disorders usually can be distinguished from IgA nephropathy by clinical and serologic criteria.

Despite recurrent episodes of acute GN, the majority of patients maintain normal renal function for many years. However, 40 to 50 per cent of patients have a gradual increase in serum creatinine, and 20 to 30 per cent of patients develop chronic renal failure after 20 years. Poor prognostic signs include heavy proteinuria, hypertension, and renal insufficiency. In a recent prospective controlled trial, dietary fish oil therapy proved effective in slowing the progression of IgA nephropathy.

Goodpasture's Syndrome and Anti-GBM Disease

Goodpasture's syndrome is defined as acute GN with pulmonary hemorrhage mediated by autoantibodies that react with the glomerular and alveolar basement membranes. When pulmonary hemorrhage is absent, the term anti-GBM disease is used to define the disorder. These rare disorders typically present in young males (reported male-to-female ratio ranges from 2:1 to 9:1) between the ages of 20 to 30 years, but the disease can present at virtually any age. Symptoms due to pulmonary hemorrhage (hemoptysis, cough, and/or dyspnea), acute GN, and RPGN are the most common clinical presentations. More than 50 per cent of patients with anti-GBM antibody–mediated disease have Goodpasture's syndrome at initial presentation, and 82 to 94 per cent of these present with hemoptysis. Although hemoptysis typically precedes overt GN in GS by months, laboratory evidence of GN (microscopic hematuria and proteinuria and/or RBC casts) is almost always present (83 to 100 per cent) at presentation. Pallor and anemia are also common at presentation with Goodpasture's syndrome. The syndrome is occasionally preceded by an upper respiratory tract infection or a flulike illness (20 to 61 per cent of patients with Goodpasture's syndrome). A history of smoke inhalation is common, and pulmonary hemorrhage is more likely in cigarette smokers. Exposure to hydrocarbon solvents or chemicals is documented in fewer than 5 per cent of cases. In the absence of symptoms, chest film can reveal bilateral pulmonary infiltrates due to hemorrhage. Heme-positive stools can be a sign of unrecognized hemoptysis. Other clinical conditions that can present with pulmonary hemorrhage and GN include the ANCA-associated vasculitides, systemic lupus erythematosus, necrotizing vasculitis, and Henoch-Schönlein purpura. Clinical evidence of other organ involvement (e.g., skin rash or purpura, synovitis, arthritis, pleuritis, mononeuritis multiplex, abdominal pain) and laboratory studies (ANA, ANCA, complement concentrations) usually distinguish these disorders. In some series ANCA-associated disease is a more common cause of hemoptysis in patients with crescentic and necrotizing GN than is Goodpasture's syndrome.

Definitive diagnosis is based on demonstration of circulating anti-GBM antibodies in serum and/or characteristic linear immunostaining for Ig on kidney biopsy. The pathogenic anti-GBM antibodies bind to an epitope of the noncollagenous domain (NC1) of the α3 chain of type IV collagen. Testing for anti-GBM is indicated in the clinical setting of RPGN, pulmonary-renal syndrome, or unexplained hemoptysis. The assays in current use employ a variety of substrates as target antigen, so that they vary in their specificity and sensitivity for disease (Table 5). Conventional assays detect only IgG, although an occasional patient with isolated IgA or IgM anti-GBM antibodies has been reported. Anti-GBM titers do not predictably correlate with disease severity, but serial anti-GBM antibody titers are useful in monitoring disease activity during therapy and follow-up. Late recurrences are infrequent; however, the disease may recur in transplanted kidneys.

Some anti-GBM assays (see Table 5) also detect nonpathogenic antibodies restricted to other collagen subunits, including other chains (α1 or α4) of type IV collagen. Occasionally, these antibodies appear in the serum of either patients with Goodpasture's syndrome or anti-GBM disease (at low titer in 15 per cent of patients, in addition to the pathogenic antibodies that react with the NC1 domain of the α3 chain of type IV collagen), or patients with pulmonary signs and symptoms due to other diseases (i.e., carcinoma, vasculitis). A clinicopathologic syndrome characterized by clinical features and serologies that suggest an anti-GBM–ANCA overlap syndrome has been described. The syndrome remains poorly defined but includes patients with multisystem disease suggesting systemic vasculitis and variably characterized by pulmonary-renal syndrome, skin rash, arthritis, polyneuropathy, and/or uveitis. Renal biopsy typically demonstrates crescentic GN, with variable amounts of necrosis, diffuse linear deposition of IgG along the GBM, and, in some patients, evidence of renal vasculitis (arteriolitis, granulomas). Diagnostic confusion arises because both anti-GBM antibodies and ANCAs are detected in the sera. As many as 10 to 30 per cent of sera positive for anti-GBM antibodies have also been reported positive for ANCA and/or anti-MPO. Conversely, fewer than 10 per cent of ANCA-positive sera are positive for anti-GBM antibodies. In one center, the majority of the sera positive for anti-GBM antibodies from patients with ANCA showed no specific reactivity with the true Goodpasture antigen (NC1 domain of type IV collagen). In contrast, true-positive cANCAs (antiproteinase 3) have been reported in patients with Goodpasture's syndrome who were demonstrated to have developed either concurrent or sequential Wegener's granulomatosis.

The characteristic histopathologic feature is linear deposition of IgG along the GBM demonstrable by direct immunofluorescence microscopy. Crescentic GN is usually present with no deposits observed on electron microscopy. False-positive results with kidney biopsy (i.e., linear staining for immunoglobulin) have been reported in diabetic nephropathy and, rarely, in focal segmental glomerulosclerosis, polyarteritis nodosa, and APSGN. False-negative results occasionally occur in aggressive GN in which the typical linear immunofluorescence pattern is disrupted. Lung biopsy findings are often nonspecific; immunoglobulin along the alveolar basement membrane is variably demonstrable and can confirm, but not exclude, the diagnosis. However, open lung biopsy is indicated when the clinical suspicion of vasculitis is strong.

Rapid evaluation is essential for institution of immediate therapy (plasmapheresis, prednisone, and cyclophosphamide) to prevent both life-threatening pulmonary hemorrhage and irreversible loss of renal function. Recovery of renal function is uncommon if the serum creatinine concentration exceeds 6.0 mg/dL prior to initiation of therapy.

Rapidly Progressive Glomerulonephritis

A clinicopathologic syndrome of diverse etiology, RPGN is characterized by acute crescentic GN and rapidly progressive renal failure. It may be secondary to any cause of acute GN (see Table 1), or it may have no identifiable underlying disorder (idiopathic RPGN). Rapid evaluation

Table 5. Assays for Detecting Anti-GBM Autoantibodies

Assay	Substrate	Sensitivity (%)*	Specificity (%)
Indirect immunofluorescence	Human kidney tissue sections	60–87†	>99‡
Solid-phase assays (RIA, ELISA, immunoblotting)	Purified intact type IV collagen Purified NC1 domain Purified M2 subunit of NC1 domain Collagenase-digested human GBM§	90–100	95–99

ELISA = enzyme-linked immunosorbent assay; GBM = glomerular basement membrane; RIA = radioimmunoassay.
*Sensitivity is for acute untreated biopsy-proven Goodpasture's syndrome or anti-GBM disease.
†The indirect immunofluorescent antibody assay is least sensitive in patients with GN without pulmonary hemorrhage.
‡Specificity of indirect immunofluorescence in the laboratory of C.B. Wilson et al. Kidney International 6:114a, 1974.
§The assays employing collagenase-digested GBM are less specific than those employing purified antigen.

is essential so that immediate therapy can be instituted to avoid irreversible renal failure.

The first step is consideration of the causes of acute GN. This process includes (1) a thorough history and physical examination and (2) performance of the laboratory tests described earlier for the individual systemic diseases (i.e., serum C3 and other appropriate serologic and histologic tests). A kidney biopsy early in the course is recommended by some authorities, because once the serum creatinine concentration exceeds 6 mg/dL, the probability of response to therapy is poor regardless of etiology.

The pathologic diagnosis of RPGN is usually confirmed by renal biopsy, which demonstrates more than 50 to 60 per cent of glomeruli with cellular or fibrous crescents. The findings on immunofluorescence microscopy divide RPGN into three major pathologic categories that are broadly associated with pathogenetic mechanisms and clinical syndromes. These categories include linear deposits of IgG (anti-GBM disease) in 5 to 20 per cent, no immune deposits (pauci-immune) in 34 to 65 per cent, and granular immunoglobulin deposits in 25 to 45 per cent of patients. The presence of granular deposits of immunoglobulin may provide clues to an underlying disease process. For example, subepithelial "humps" on electron microscopy suggest APSGN; and the presence of IgG, IgM, and IgA in subendothelial, mesangial, and subepithelial locations suggests SLE. The absence of immune deposits on biopsy may be due either to an underlying vasculitis (especially with associated necrotizing GN) or to idiopathic RPGN.

Serologic tests are particularly useful in the differential diagnosis when biopsy is contraindicated or delayed or fails to provide the correct diagnosis. The presence of anti-GBM indicates Goodpasture's syndrome or anti-GBM disease. In the setting of RPGN, ANCAs are highly specific and sensitive for crescentic necrotizing pauci-immune GN. These antibodies are present in 80 per cent at presentation, and an additional 10 per cent develop them during the course of disease. Approximately 75 per cent of these patients have evidence of extrarenal disease suggesting systemic vasculitis (Wegener's granulomatosis, Wegener's vasculitis, microscopic polyarteritis, see earlier), and the remaining 25 per cent have renal-limited vasculitis with no evidence of systemic disease. Of these latter patients, 80 per cent have pANCA (antimyeloperoxidase specificity), and 20 per cent have cANCA (see Table 4).

The prognosis of untreated RPGN is poor regardless of the etiology. As many as 80 per cent of untreated patients develop end-stage renal disease or die within weeks to months. Poor prognostic signs include a serum creatinine concentration greater than 6 to 8 mg/dL, anuria, and more than 80 per cent crescents or abundant fibrous crescents on kidney biopsy. An important exception is RPGN due to APSGN; in this disorder, recovery of renal function is common even in patients with acute oliguric renal failure.

Hereditary Nephritis (Alport's Syndrome)

Hereditary nephritis is a familial disorder characterized by glomerulonephritis, sensorineural deafness, and anterior lenticonus due to the production of abnormal basement membrane type IV collagen. It typically presents with symptomatic urinary abnormalities or recurrent gross hematuria. Blood pressure and renal function are usually normal at the time of diagnosis. Other signs and symptoms depend on the age and sex of the patient and the particular abnormalities present in the kindred. The most common extrarenal findings are sensorineural hearing loss and eye abnormalities such as anterior lenticonus and cataracts. Owing to the various modes of inheritance (X-linked, autosomal dominance segregating with the X chromosome, and autosomal recessive), males are affected more severely and earlier than females. Almost 50 per cent of affected boys have hematuria by age 5 years. Both the renal disease and the hearing loss are typically slowly progressive, although they are generally less common and less severe in females. End-stage renal disease typically occurs between the ages of 16 and 35 years, varying between families but remaining relatively constant within a kindred.

The diagnosis is suggested by the family history and the extrarenal involvement, and it can be confirmed by renal biopsy. In some patients with no family history and isolated renal disease, hereditary nephritis is diagnosed by the typical laminated appearance and thickening and thinning of the GBM demonstrated by electron microscopy.

Approximately 5 to 10 per cent of patients with Alport's syndrome who undergo renal transplantation develop anti-GBM nephritis in their allograft. These patients lack the reactive epitope (NC1 domain) in Goodpasture's syndrome owing to the inherited defects in the different alpha chains (α3, 4, or 5) of type IV collagen. The role for routine measurement of anti-GBM levels in Alport's syndrome patients who have undergone renal transplantation is unclear. The clinical course is benign in some patients, and others have linear IgG staining of the GBM on biopsy without evidence of nephritis. Moreover, circulating anti-GBM antibodies that react with the Goodpasture epitope have not been invariably detected in patients with nephritis.

OBSTRUCTIVE NEPHROPATHY

By M. David Schwalb, M.D.
Bronx, New York
and Barry Lifson, M.D.
Valhalla, New York

Obstructive nephropathy, also referred to as obstructive uropathy, is the term given to diseases of the urinary tract caused by obstruction. When obstruction occurs, the increased pressure exerted proximal to the obstruction may result in a deleterious effect on the involved renal parenchyma. Outflow obstruction can occur at any point from the renal papilla to the urethral meatus. If an obstruction exists distal to the bladder, it may result in bilateral obstructive changes of the upper urinary tract. Ureteral or intrarenal obstruction may be unilateral or bilateral. Descriptive terms for ectasia of the upper urinary tract due to increased pressure proximal to an obstruction include pyelocaliectasis and hydrocalyx. Dilatation of the entire upper (supravesical) urinary tract is called hydroureteronephrosis.

The degree of damage to the renal parenchyma following obstruction depends on several factors. Is the obstruction unilateral or bilateral? Is it complete or partial? Has it been present for hours or weeks or years? Has the obstruction been complicated by infection? Increased ureteral and intrarenal pressure reduces renal blood flow and usually causes distal tubular atrophy followed by proximal tubular atrophy. With time, all phases of renal function except diluting capacity are adversely affected. Concentrating ability is typically altered first.

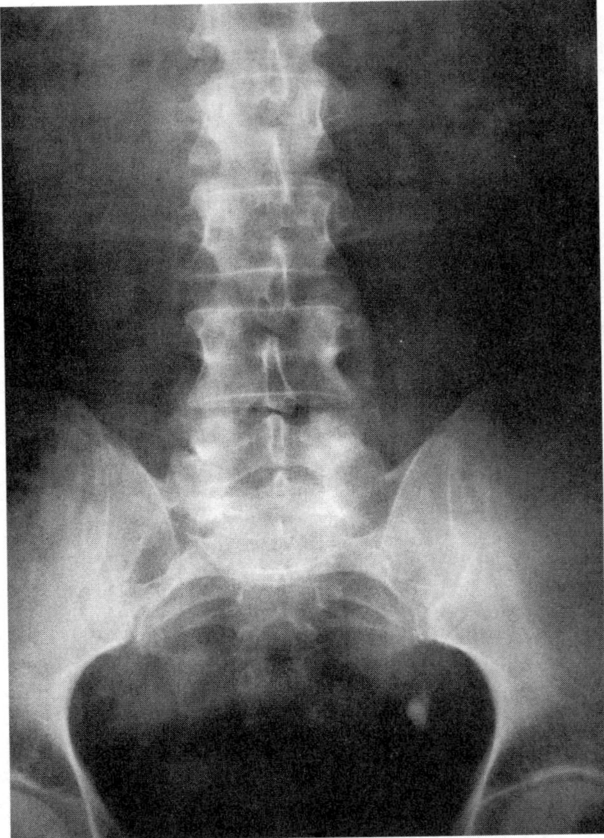

Figure 1. Kidney, ureter, bladder (KUB) film in a patient with a large left lower ureteral stone.

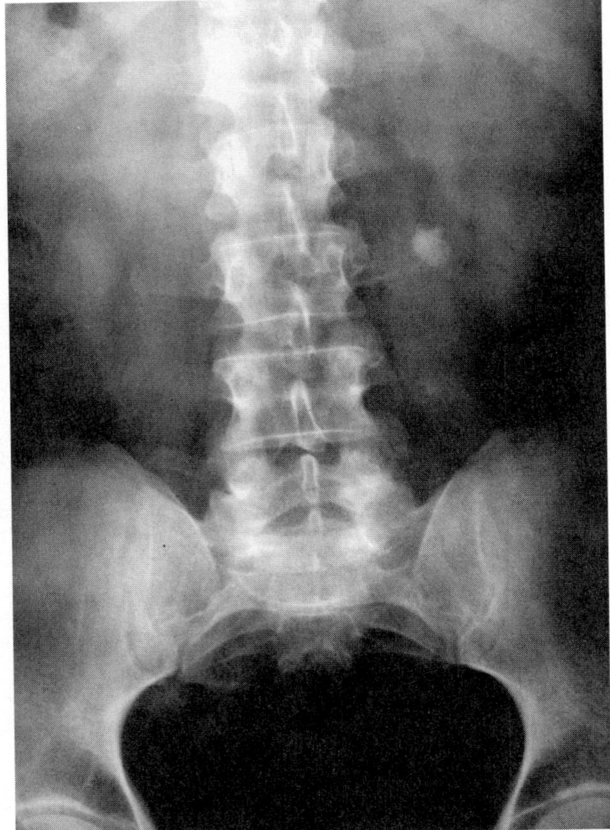

Figure 2. A KUB film performed 2 years earlier revealed a stone in the region of the left ureteropelvic junction (UPJ); however, this patient was lost to follow-up at that time.

PRESENTING SIGNS AND SYMPTOMS

Flank pain, or renal colic, is commonly associated with acute unilateral ureteral obstruction. Intramural obstruction is typically caused by stone, blood clot, or tumor. Extrinsic ureteral obstruction due to retroperitoneal disorders tends to occur gradually and is frequently asymptomatic. Chronic bilateral ureteral obstruction may present with oliguria or anuria, or it may cause silent deterioration of renal function. Although chronic unilateral ureteral obstruction may present with intermittent vague flank pain, gastrointestinal symptoms, or a flank mass (palpable kidney), this condition may also be clinically silent, with detection occurring incidentally (Figs. 1 to 5) or during an evaluation for hypertension. Often, these nonfunctioning kidneys are unsalvageable (Figs. 6 and 7). Obstruction of the lower urinary tract usually produces irritative or obstructive voiding signs, such as hesitancy (slow start), decreased force of stream, pushing to void, daytime or nighttime frequency, and postvoid dribbling. Occasionally, lower urinary tract obstruction may be asymptomatic in chronic cases and eventually produce a decompensated (atonic) bladder.

Pain

Acute ureteral obstruction frequently presents as colicky flank pain that radiates anteromedially. The pain is attributed to overdistention of the upper urinary tract and renal capsule. The pain is acute and severe and is unrelieved by changes in position. Pain may also present as vague upper abdominal discomfort with upper tract obstruction or as vague lower abdominal pain with bladder distention.

Fever

The fever that accompanies urinary tract obstruction is usually not related to the obstruction itself but results

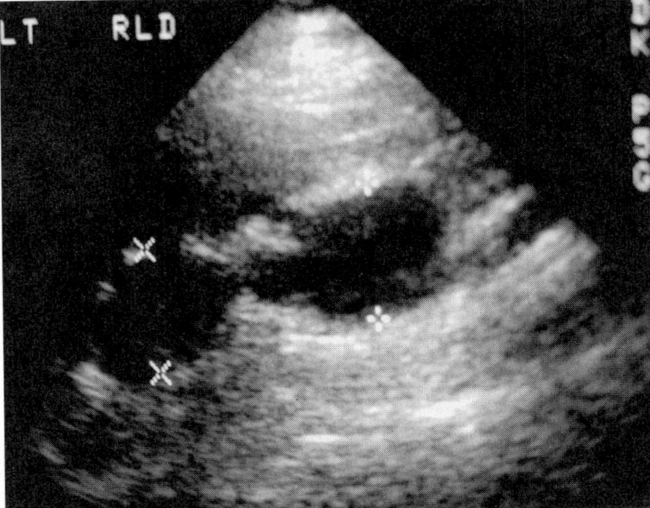

Figure 3. Renal ultrasound scan demonstrating massive hydronephrosis with apparent cortical loss. Symbols indicate boundaries of dilated collecting system.

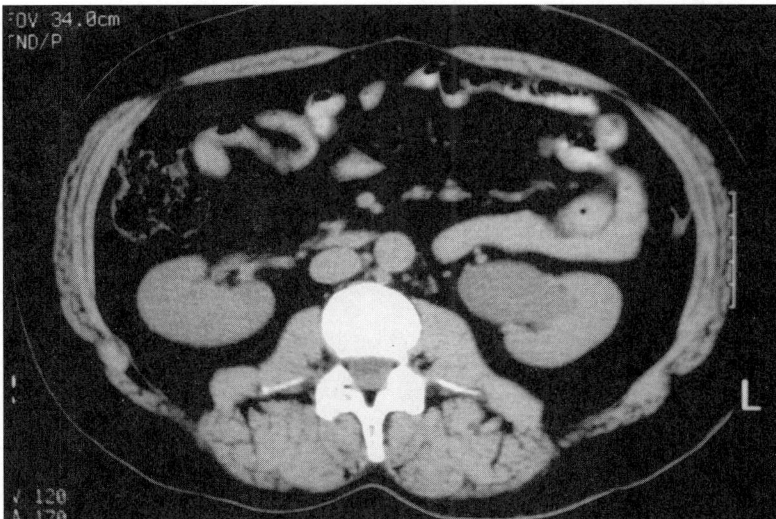

Figure 4. Computed tomography (CT) scan showing massive hydronephrosis with good renal parenchyma despite long-standing obstruction.

from infection that may complicate the clinical picture. When irritative voiding symptoms are accompanied by fever, an obstruction of the lower urinary tract should be suspected. When acute pyelonephritis is accompanied by fever that persists despite appropriate antibiotic therapy, obstruction of the upper tract, renal abscess, or perinephric abscess should be considered.

Gastrointestinal Symptoms

Nausea, vomiting, and recurrent diarrhea in patients with obstructive nephropathy are most likely related to overlapping autonomic innervation in the gastrointestinal and genitourinary tracts.

Voiding Symptoms

The inability to empty the bladder effectively may be caused by prostatic obstruction, urethral stricture, or posterior urethral valves. Although urethral stricture is uncommon in women, failure of the urinary sphincter to relax frequently causes infravesical obstruction (non-neurogenic neurogenic bladder). True neuropathic voiding dysfunction occurs in both sexes and produces symptoms that mimic infravesical obstruction. The classic symptoms of obstruction include frequency and urgency of urination, decreased force of urinary stream, pushing to void, and, in severe cases, inability to urinate (retention).

Hematuria

Gross or microscopic hematuria must be investigated to exclude a mass or other obstructing lesion in the upper urinary tract. An enlarged or a carcinomatous prostate and even a urethral stricture may occasionally present with hematuria.

Abdominal Mass

A palpable flank mass may occur secondary to long-standing hydronephrosis. In patients with urinary retention, a distended bladder may be felt as a lower abdominal mass.

DIAGNOSIS

The investigation of urinary obstruction should proceed from the history and physical examination to laboratory

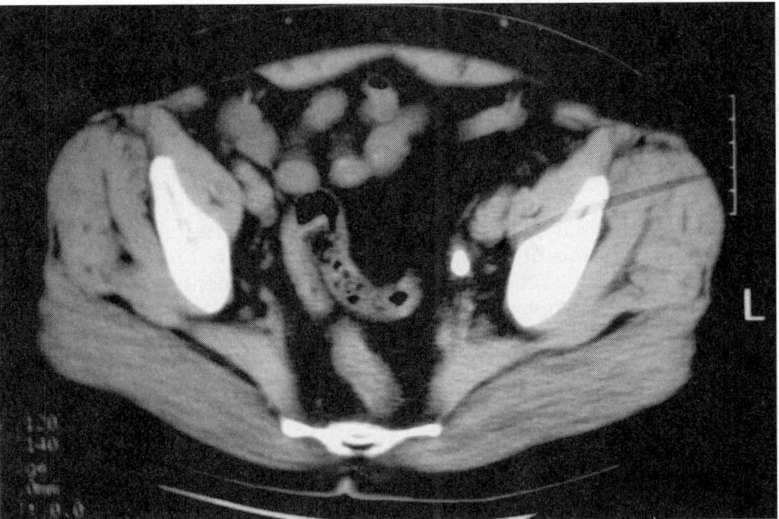

Figure 5. Pelvic CT section demonstrating ureteral dilatation to the level of the stone.

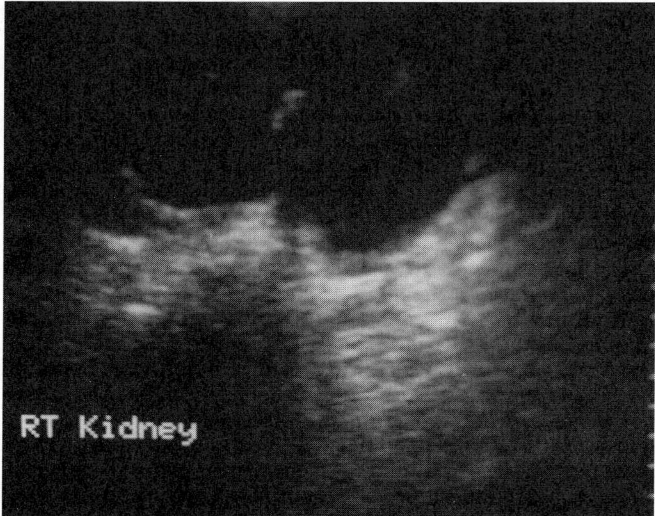

Figure 6. Renal ultrasound scan in a patient with a nonfunctioning hydronephrotic kidney who presented with long-standing recurrent bouts of urinary tract infections and vague right flank pain.

and imaging studies. Renal colic is immediately evident in some patients, whereas others present with vague abdominal pain, fever, obstruction, irritative voiding symptoms, hematuria, or anuria. Gastrointestinal symptoms may occasionally be related to urinary tract obstruction.

The classic physical findings include a flank mass, flank tenderness, or a distended bladder. Pelvic and bimanual examination can identify urethral or bladder induration, uterine enlargement, colon disease, or adnexal disorders that may cause bladder outlet or ureteral obstruction. Rectal examination may identify benign prostatic hyperplasia or carcinoma as a cause of obstruction. Although the male urethral meatus should be inspected for obstruction, many patients with visually apparent stenosis have normal results on uroflowmetry.

Measurements of serum creatinine and serum urea nitrogen concentrations and urinalysis are useful in the investigation of obstructive nephropathy. The urinary sediment should be examined for the presence of cells, casts, crystals, and bacteria. The creatinine clearance should be calculated from analysis of a 24-hour urine collection. Prostate-specific antigen should be measured in the serum of patients suspected of having carcinoma of the prostate.

Imaging studies are used to determine the presence of obstruction and its location. Ultrasound is noninvasive, avoids radiation, often identifies the presence of obstruction, and may pinpoint its location. However, ultrasonography must be interpreted with caution because a dilated collecting system is not always obstructed and an obstructed system is not always dilated. Real-time ultrasonography of the kidneys can be used to assess intrarenal collecting system dilatation, upper ureteral dilatation, and the presence of renal calculi. Although decreased thickness of the renal parenchyma may reflect the chronicity of an obstructive process as well as the reduced functional reserve of the renal unit, ultrasound images do not always correlate with biochemical function (see Figs. 3 and 4). Ultrasound of the bladder examines its ability to empty completely. The normal postvoid residual amount should not exceed 50 mL. Occasionally, a dilated distal ureter or a distal ureteral stone is visualized during ultrasound of the bladder.

Excretory urography (intravenous pyelography [IVP]) is the most useful test for determining the anatomic location and extent of an obstruction. Renal parenchymal thickness can be measured, and filling defects of the collecting system can be delineated. IVP can be particularly useful in the evaluation of septic patients with unilateral flank pain and normal serum urea nitrogen and serum creatinine concentrations. Delayed images may be necessary for identifying the exact site of obstruction in the setting of reduced blood flow and excretion of contrast medium by the involved renal unit. The disadvantages of excretory urography include the potential for allergic and anaphylactic reactions, exposure to ionizing radiation, and adverse cardiovascular and renal effects of iodinated contrast administration, particularly in patients with compromised renal function. These complications have led many to advocate renal ultrasound and abdominal plain films (kidney, ureter, bladder [KUB]) as the frontline imaging procedures in patients with hematuria or renal colic.

When a mass is suspected, an abdominopelvic computed tomography (CT) scan can delineate the extent of the lesion and its relationship to the urinary tract. If intravenous contrast material is used, a plain abdominal film taken immediately after the CT scan may add important information concerning the site of an obstructing lesion ("poor man's IVP").

The radionuclide renal scan can help the clinician distinguish true obstructive dilatation from simple nonobstructive dilatation (megacalycosis). If renal obstruction is suggested by failure of the involved unit to clear the isotope in a timely fashion, furosemide is administered when peak counts have been recorded (typically by 30 minutes). In the absence of anatomic obstruction, the isotope rapidly leaves the collecting system and the renogram curve shows a sharp decline in the counts. The diuretic typically has little effect on a truly obstructed kidney. If vesicoureteral reflux is suspected or bladder outlet obstruction is present, a bladder catheter should be maintained during the study to prevent artifacts.

Other, more invasive studies for the delineation of uri-

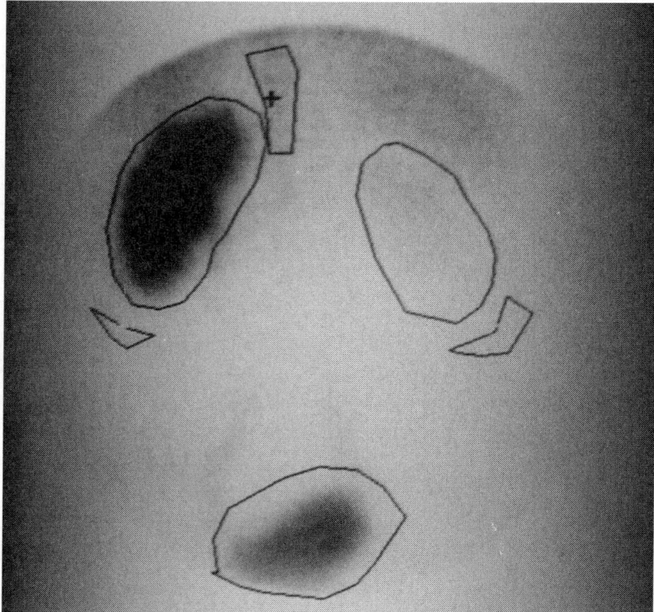

Figure 7. Renal scan confirming the absence of function in the involved kidney.

nary tract obstruction include cystourethroscopy, retrograde ureteropyelography, and antegrade ureteropyelography. If the obstruction is located, site-specific treatment can be started after the patient is stabilized.

POTENTIAL ERRORS AND PITFALLS

Whenever possible, the investigation of obstructive nephropathy should proceed from the least invasive to the more invasive procedures. Renal sonography is usually the first test employed, followed by other imaging procedures as needed. Invasive procedures are rarely required for diagnosis of obstruction. Inappropriate instrumentation of the urinary tract may cause infection or other adverse sequelae.

Occasionally, an obstruction develops without dilatation of the intrarenal collecting system, especially in dehydrated patients. If the index of suspicion is high, renal scanning should be performed or renal ultrasonography should be repeated after hydration.

Increased serum urea nitrogen and serum creatinine concentrations and hypertension frequently occur in patients with chronic bilateral obstructive hydronephrosis. In many patients, release of the obstruction promotes physiologic diuresis and natriuresis, with concomitant reductions in serum urea nitrogen and creatinine concentrations and normalization of blood pressure. To prevent cardiovascular collapse and fatal arrhythmias from postobstrutive diuresis, blood pressure and serum electrolyte concentrations should be monitored and hydration initiated when appropriate.

The clinician must have a high index of suspicion for silent obstruction, especially in elderly and debilitated patients. Chronic obstruction often produces few symptoms and may lead to progressive and irreversible loss of renal function.

CYSTIC DISORDERS OF THE KIDNEY

By Gregory A. Anderson, M.D.
Marshfield, Wisconsin

Renal cystic disease is hereditary, congenital, or acquired (Table 1). Within these broad categories, a specific diagnosis can be incidental, such as an unexpected radiographic finding, or it can be made by evaluation of findings on the initial history and physical examination. The diagnosis of syndromic renal cystic disease (e.g., von Hippel-Lindau disease, tuberous sclerosis) cannot be made solely by studying the kidneys; instead, it requires identification of renal cysts in conjunction with other extrarenal hallmarks of the syndrome.

Table 1. Classification of Renal Cystic Disease

Hereditary
- Autosomal recessive polycystic kidney disease
- Autosomal dominant polycystic kidney disease
- Syndromic cystic disease
  - von Hippel-Lindau disease
  - Tuberous sclerosis
  - Cerebrohepatorenal syndrome
  - Jeune's syndrome (asphyxiating thoracic dystrophy)
  - Orofaciodigital syndrome, type I
  - Others
- Hereditary cystic nephrosis
- Medullary tubulointerstitial disease
  - Juvenile nephronophthisis
  - Renal-retinal dysplasia
  - Renal medullary cystic disease
  - Alström's syndrome

Congenital
- Multicystic dysplastic kidney
- Multilocular cyst
- Pyelogenic renal cyst (caliceal diverticula)
- Infantile glomerulocystic disease
- Sponge kidney

Acquired
- Simple cysts
  - Solitary or multiple
  - Unilateral or bilateral
- Cysts in end-stage renal disease or in patients on dialysis

HEREDITARY CYSTIC DISEASE

Autosomal Recessive Polycystic Kidney Disease

Autosomal recessive polycystic kidney disease (ARPKD) presents as a syndrome of cystic dilatation of renal urine-collecting ducts and urine-collecting tubules and congenital hepatic fibrosis (CHF). Cystic changes in the liver and pancreas, as well as cerebral berry aneurysms, have been reported, although much less commonly than in autosomal dominant polycystic kidney disease (ADPKD). The disease can present in adulthood but is typically more common and severe in infancy; hence, its earlier designation, infantile polycystic kidney disease. In the severe renal form, kidneys are markedly enlarged bilaterally and manifest as palpable abdominal masses that may interfere with delivery. Oligohydramnios can occur antenatally, and infants are often stillborn with characteristic Potter facies, or they die in the early postpartum period of respiratory failure secondary to pulmonary hypoplasia. Pneumothorax and pneumomediastinum also suggest the diagnosis.

Radiographically, the kidneys are symmetrically enlarged but retain their reniform shape. Ultrasonography typically shows increased echogenicity from innumerable small, uniform cortical cysts that are not seen individually. Intravenous urogram (IVU) exhibits a characteristic "sunburst," or irregularly mottled, nephrogram.

Less severe renal disease is typical in patients with CHF, who present at an older age with hepatosplenomegaly, systemic and portal hypertension, and varying degrees of renal insufficiency and growth retardation. In these patients, the IVU usually shows medullary ductal ectasia identical to that seen in sponge kidney. Distinguishing between ARPKD and sponge kidney involves finding CHF and renal cortical cystic changes as well as medullary ductal ectasia and a positive family history in the former condition. Severe ARPKD of infancy is usually fatal; however, survival in the less severe renal forms may be quite prolonged, and such patients are candidates for renal transplantation when renal failure ensues.

Autosomal Dominant Polycystic Kidney Disease

Autosomal dominant polycystic kidney disease (ADPKD) occurs in 1 in 1000 live births, affects approximately 500,000 people in the United States, accounts for approximately 10 per cent of all cases of end-stage renal disease, and is the most common hereditary disease. A total of 93 per cent of ADPKD cases have been linked to one or more mutations on chromosome 16, and a screening test has been developed to identify these patients.

The disease may present in childhood but is typically seen in adult patients; thus, its earlier designation, adult polycystic kidney disease. The presenting clinical manifestations are age-related. Patients in the fourth decade exhibit flank pain, hematuria, kidney stones, and recurrent urinary tract infections. Those in the fifth decade demonstrate progressive cystic renal failure and hypertension. The cystic changes in other organs (liver, pancreas, spleen, lungs) can be dramatic. Cerebral aneurysms occur in as many as 22 per cent of autopsied patients and account for 9 per cent of adult deaths from ADPKD.

Cysts can occur anywhere along the nephron, are disparate in size, and may distort the renal outline and collecting system on IVU. Ultrasonography and computed tomography also demonstrate these renal cystic changes as well as the solid renal neoplasms that can develop and cystic processes in other organs. The mean survival is about 50 years, and death is usually caused by cardiac disease, renal failure, and cerebral hemorrhage. Radiographic screening for ADPKD may require serial studies in younger subjects to detect evolving cystic disease. Evaluation for chromosome 16 abnormalities may provide an earlier answer in these patients.

Medullary Tubulointerstitial Disease

Several related conditions are included under this heading: juvenile nephronophthisis (JN), renal-retinal dysplasia (RRD), and renal medullary cystic disease (RMC). The importance of these conditions lies in their often subtle presentation, and JN, in particular, is a common cause of childhood renal failure. Both JN and RRD are autosomal recessive disorders and occur in younger patients (younger than age 20). RMC disease is probably autosomal dominant and is seen predominantly in older patients (older than age 20).

Patients with RRD can present with progressive blindness, usually secondary to retinitis pigmentosa. All three conditions can cause renal salt wasting and decreased urine-concentrating ability with secondary polyuria and polydipsia as well as anemia and advanced renal failure. Hypertension is uncommon, even in advanced disease. Urinalysis typically is unremarkable, and proteinuria seldom exceeds 2+. All patients suspected of JN or RMC disease should have an ophthalmologic evaluation, and patients with retinitis pigmentosa should be assessed for renal disease. Ultrasonography and computed tomography show shrunken kidneys and may demonstrate small cortical cysts clustered around the cortical medullary junction, although cysts are present in only 75 per cent of cases. Intravenous urography is not helpful. A definitive diagnosis relies on family history, demonstration of progressive renal failure with normal or nearly normal urinalysis, and a lack of radiographic or extrarenal findings that point to other causes of chronic renal failure. Renal biopsy is often needed to support the clinical suspicion.

Multicystic Dysplastic Kidney

Multicystic dysplastic kidneys (MCDKs) of clinical significance present in infancy, are unilateral (bilateral disease occurs but is incompatible with life), and range in size from nonpalpable to massive enough to impair respiration. Indeed, in newborns most palpable abdominal masses are due to either hydronephrosis or MCDK. Flank or abdominal pain, as well as urinary tract infection, and decreased renal function are related to commonly associated contralateral renal disease (ureteropelvic junction obstruction, vesicoureteral reflux) and may also lead to the diagnosis. Ultrasonography can confirm the diagnosis antenatally as well as after birth by demonstrating (1) noncommunicating, simple cysts; (2) no large central cysts suggestive of a renal pelvis; (3) the lack of a renal sinus. These criteria help distinguish between MCDK and hydronephrosis, which exhibits a dilated central renal pelvis communicating with smaller peripheral calices.

An IVU or a renal isotope scan showing absence of function on the affected side supports the diagnosis and helps distinguish between MCDK and hydronephrosis as well as multilocular cysts (MLCs), both of which typically exhibit function on the studies (Table 2). Patients with MCDK should have a thorough evaluation of the contralateral renal unit (IVU, voiding cystourethrogram) and should probably be followed serially for hypertension, although the risk of hypertension and renal tumors in these patients does not appear to be significantly different from that of the general population.

Multilocular Cysts

Multilocular cysts (MLCs) can present as abdominal masses with or without pain at any age. Table 2 outlines important features of this condition, which cannot be reliably distinguished from cystic Wilms' tumor. Exploration is therefore mandatory when this entity is identified.

Pyelogenic Renal Cysts

Pyelogenic cysts, also known as caliceal diverticula, are dilated outpouchings of the renal collecting system

Table 2. Comparison of Multicystic Dysplastic Kidney (MCDK), Multilocular Cysts (MLC), and Hydronephrosis

	MCDK	MLC	Hydronephrosis
Age	Infancy	Any	Any
Ultrasound findings	Noncommunicating cysts No large central cyst No normal kidney	Cysts within cysts Usually some normal kidney present	Large central renal pelvis communicating with peripheral dilated calices Usually, identifiable renal cortex present
Renal scan/IVU findings	Nonfunction	Function	Function
Pathology	Dysplasia	No dysplasia	Occasional dysplasia
Ipsilateral ureteral defect	Yes	No	Yes
Contralateral renal disease	Common, 20–70%	No	Relatively uncommon

Table 3. Cyst Classification

	Ultrasound	Computed Tomography	Clinical Impression
I	Thin, smooth wall No septations No internal echogenicity	Thin, smooth wall No septations Nonenhancing	Nonsuspicious No follow-up needed
II	Scanty calcification in smooth cyst wall Few, thin septations	Scanty calcification in smooth cyst wall Few, thin septations Hyperdense without contrast enhancement; nonenhancing with contrast	Nonsuspicious Possible follow-up for hyperdense cysts
III	Thick, irregular wall Many septations Nodular calcification	Thick, irregular wall Many septations Nodular calcification Thin, enhancing septa Nonenhancing wall	Suspicious for neoplasm Exploration indicated
IV	Same as type III	Same as type III except wall enhances with contrast, or thick enhancing septa present	Overt neoplasm Exploration indicated

branching from caliceal fornices. Most caliceal diverticula are asymptomatic and are discovered incidentally on ultrasonography (which shows simple cortical cysts but does not usually provide the diagnosis) or on IVU, which clearly demonstrates the pathologic anatomy and confirms the diagnosis. The diverticula contain no renal papillae and must fill retrogradely with contrast material from the rest of the collecting system; therefore, delayed films may be needed to visualize narrow-necked lesions. Calculi and milk of calcium are commonly noted on plain films and ultrasonography. Flank pain, urinary tract infection, and hematuria are typical presenting symptoms associated with calculi.

Sponge Kidney

Sponge kidney (medullary sponge kidney) is a congenital dilatation of medullary urine-collecting ducts that can present as flank pain, urinary tract infection, or hematuria; however, many cases are discovered incidentally during intravenous urography. Despite its congenital nature, the diagnosis is most commonly made after age 20. The IVU is diagnostic, showing prominent papillary striations (papillary brush) or cystic dilatations (bouquet of flowers). Presentation is often bilateral (75 per cent) and diffuse, although only one papilla may be affected in some cases. Calculi are frequently present, and sponge kidney must be considered in patients with medullary nephrocalcinosis. An association between distal renotubular acidosis and sponge kidney has been observed, and evaluation of the former condition is performed with appropriate blood and urine tests.

The coarse papillary striations of sponge kidney must be distinguished from the more diffuse papillary "blush," which does not reveal individual striations and which is a normal variant. Decreased renal function and hypertension are uncommon unless chronic pyelonephritis from calculus disease or urinary tract infection has supervened.

ACQUIRED RENAL CYSTIC DISEASE

Simple Cysts

Simple cysts can be single or multiple and unilateral or bilateral. They are usually silent and are identified only during ultrasonography or computed tomography for other reasons. The IVU may suggest the presence of a cyst but is not diagnostic; the cyst is usually confirmed via ultrasonography. Ultrasonographic and computed tomography criteria for cyst classification are listed in Table 3. Diagnostic cyst puncture and cystography are rarely necessary, with the newer imaging techniques available. An estimated 50 per cent of individuals older than 50 years of age have one or more simple renal cysts, typically without impaired renal function or hypertension. The clinical manifestations (flank pain, hematuria, urinary tract infection) stem from complicating events, such as cyst trauma, hemorrhage, or secondary infection. Multiple bilateral simple acquired renal cysts must be distinguished from ADPKD by family history, evaluation of serial renal function studies, and the presence or absence of extrarenal cystic disease. Patients with acquired cystic disease lack a family history and extrarenal manifestations and typically exhibit stable renal function. Renal biopsy and screening for chromosome 16 abnormalities can be helpful in difficult cases.

Cysts Associated With Renal Failure

Progressive cystic degeneration is a recognized outcome of long-term dialysis, occurring in as many as 90 per cent of patients after 5 to 10 years. Dialysis itself does not appear to be responsible, however, because cystic changes are observed to a lesser degree in milder cases of renal insufficiency that do not require dialysis. Cysts are usually silent but may present as flank pain or hematuria due to cyst hemorrhage or infection. Renin-mediated hypertension in proportion to the degree of cystic change can also occur. Ultrasonography and computed tomography demonstrate atrophic kidneys with multiple simple cysts of varying sizes, some having wall calcifications.

Controversy surrounds the frequency of renal cell carcinoma in cystic end-stage kidneys and the need to serially evaluate for tumor development. Large autopsy series have recently shown the incidence of local and metastatic renal cell carcinoma to be similar in patients with end-stage renal disease and the general population, this similarity making the need for screening patients with end-stage renal disease consequently less compelling. If screening is undertaken, computed tomography is superior for the overall detection of solid neoplasms in the cystic end-stage kidney. Ultrasonography may be superior for the detection of small lesions (less than 1 cm in diameter) and is less expensive.

CARCINOMA OF THE KIDNEY

By Susan K. Stevens, M.D.,
and Jeffrey H. Reese, M.D.
San Jose, California

Renal cell carcinoma, also known as renal adenocarcinoma and formerly as hypernephroma, accounts for more than 90 per cent of the solid renal malignancies found in adults. Approximately 27,000 new cases of renal cell carcinoma are diagnosed each year, and about 10,000 deaths are attributed to this disease. The male-to-female ratio is approximately 6:4, and the tumor occurs most commonly in the fifth to seventh decades of life. Renal cell carcinoma may occur sporadically or as part of a familial cluster. In particular, patients with von Hippel-Lindau syndrome often present with multiple and recurrent tumors.

Although renal cell carcinoma is by far the most common adult solid renal mass, other tumors, including angiomyolipoma, sarcoma, renal transitional cell carcinoma, and metastatic lesions such as lymphoma must be considered in the differential diagnosis. Most of these other lesions cannot be distinguished preoperatively, and the diagnosis is made after the kidney has been removed. In children, the most common renal neoplasm is Wilms' tumor.

SIGNS AND SYMPTOMS

Signs and symptoms of renal cell carcinoma often are not observed until late in the course of the disease because the kidney occupies a well-protected locale within the body. The classic triad of hematuria, flank pain, and an abdominal mass occurs in only 10 per cent of patients with this tumor. Flank pain and/or hematuria are the most common presenting complaints in as many as 40 per cent of patients with renal cell carcinoma. Hematuria may be either gross or microscopic. Other signs include weight loss, fever, night sweats, and bone pain.

As many as 50 per cent of patients presenting with renal cell carcinoma have metastatic disease at the time of diagnosis. The most common sites of metastases are regional lymph nodes, lung, bone, liver, skin, and brain. In recent years, many renal cell tumors have been detected incidentally during abdominal ultrasound, computed tomography (CT), or magnetic resonance imaging (MRI) for other disease processes. Unlike tumors that cause symptoms, many of the incidental renal cell tumors are localized at the time of discovery.

Renal cell carcinoma is sometimes called the "internist's tumor" because it has been associated with numerous paraneoplastic syndromes. The tumors themselves may produce renin, erythropoietin, prostaglandins, parathormonelike substances, glucagon, and insulin. An increased erythrocyte sedimentation rate occurs in 50 to 60 per cent of patients with renal cell carcinoma. Serum ferritin concentrations are increased, especially in patients with larger tumors. Various syndromes are also associated with renal cell carcinoma. For example, hypertension due to increased renin can be documented in as many as 40 per cent of patients with renal cell carcinoma. The clinician should recall, however, that polycythemia, hypercalcemia, arteriovenous fistulas within the tumor, or occlusion of segmental renal arteries may also contribute to an increased blood pressure.

Liver function abnormalities can occur in as many as 40 per cent of patients with renal cell carcinoma. Liver metastases may cause some hepatic dysfunction. Patients may also develop abnormal liver function tests, fever, fatigue, weight loss, and anemia (Stauffer's syndrome) that are not associated with metastases. Resolution of liver dysfunction following nephrectomy increases the likelihood of surviving 1 year, whereas persistence of abnormalities portends a dismal prognosis.

Anemia develops in 30 to 40 per cent of patients with renal cell carcinoma, while polycythemia occurs in 3 to 5 per cent. Patients with polycythemia are more likely to experience cerebrovascular accidents. Neuropathy and amyloidosis have been reported in as many as 5 per cent of patients with renal cell carcinoma.

Physical Examination

Palpation of a renal abdominal mass is unusual because the kidneys are located deep within the body cavity. In advanced disease, however, adenopathy or cutaneous nodules may be palpable. In males, the sudden development of a varicocele, particularly on the left side, may be the first sign of renal cell carcinoma.

LABORATORY TESTS

The evaluation of a patient for renal cell carcinoma should include a complete blood count (CBC) and chemistry panel (Fig. 1). Unfortunately, valid and reliable serum or cytogenetic markers are not yet available for the diagnosis and prognosis of renal cell carcinoma. In the future, analysis of DNA ploidy and evaluation of nuclear antigens may provide information that helps the clinician predict the biologic behavior of a specific tumor in a specific patient.

CLINICAL COURSE

Clinical staging currently provides the most reliable indication of prognosis in patients with renal cell carcinoma. Patients with tumors confined to the kidney can expect a 5-year survival rate approaching 90 per cent. By contrast, fewer than 30 per cent of patients with lymph node metastases and less than 10 per cent of patients with organ metastases survive 5 years. Factors associated with decreased rates of survival include metastases to lymph nodes, metastases to multiple organs, decreased Karnofsky status, and high histologic grade of tumor. The presence of tumor thrombus in the renal vein or vena cava is not, by itself, associated with decreased rate or decreased time of survival. Patients with a single surgically resectable metastasis, especially in the lung, have a 5-year survival rate as high as 35 per cent.

Patients with surgically resectable tumor in solitary kidneys can expect a survival with parenchyma-sparing surgery similar to that of radical nephrectomy. The prognosis in these patients depends on the stage of the tumor at the time of surgery.

IMAGING OF RENAL CELL CARCINOMA

Investigation of patients suspected of having renal cell carcinoma usually begins with excretory urography. In some patients, however, the evaluation begins when a renal lesion is found during abdominal ultrasonography or

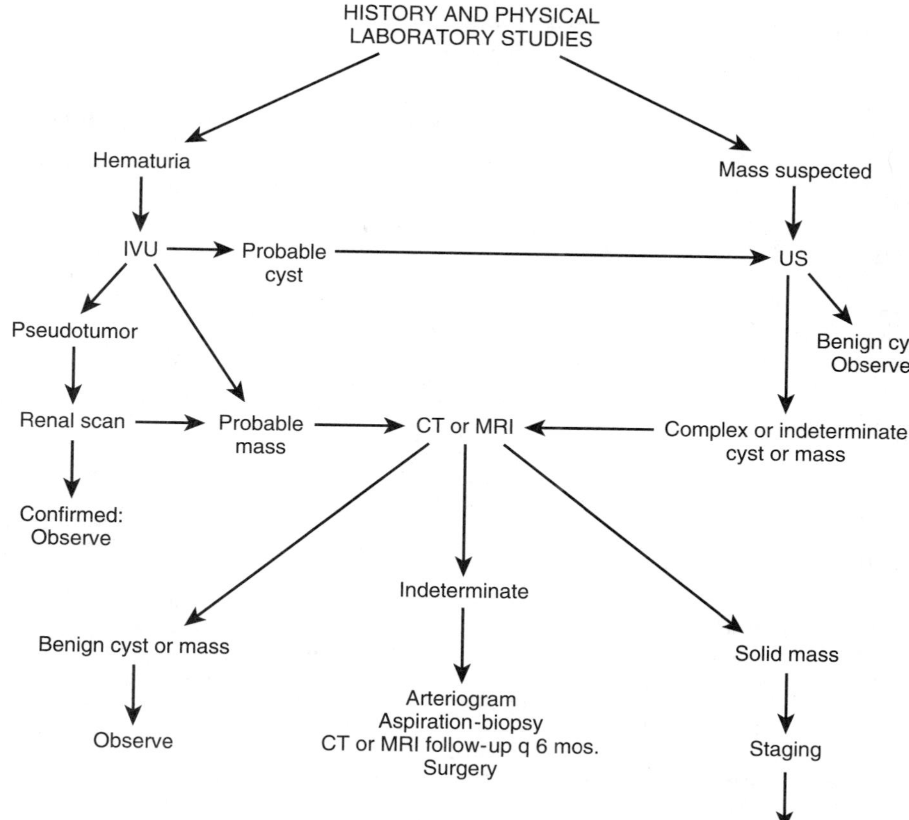

Figure 1. Algorithm for diagnosis of carcinoma of the kidney. CT = computed tomography; IVU = intravenous urography; MRI = magnetic resonance imaging; US = ultrasound.

CT performed for other reasons. The introduction of power Doppler ultrasound, spiral CT, and ultrafast gradient echo MRI has clearly improved the rate of detection and the preoperative precision of diagnosis of some kidney disorders. Although the intravenous urogram (IVU) remains the preferred initial study in the search for renal masses, this technique has significant limitations. For example, in patients with renal masses confirmed by CT, the IVU detects only 10 per cent of lesions less than 1 cm in diameter, 21 per cent of lesions between 1 and 2 cm, 52 per cent of lesions between 2 and 3 cm, and 85 per cent of lesions exceeding 3 cm. Thus, a normal IVU does not exclude the presence of a renal mass. When a mass is detected by IVU, it is often impossible to distinguish a cystic lesion from a solid one. Further studies with ultrasound, CT, or MRI may be required for determining the character of the mass. If the IVU reveals a cystic mass (5 to 15 per cent of renal cell carcinomas are cystic), ultrasound is indicated. By contrast, if a solid lesion is suspected, either CT or MRI should be requested.

Intravenous Urography (Excretory Urography)

Despite its limitations, IVU can provide several radiographic signs that support the diagnosis of renal cell carcinoma. Calcification, for example, is seen in 8 to 18 per cent of renal cell carcinomas but in only 1 per cent of simple renal cysts. As many as 87 per cent of lesions with central calcification are malignant. Segmental enlargement, focal bulging, renal contour deformities, and tilting of the renal axis are frequently seen in kidneys harboring tumors. Irregularity of the urothelial surface or complete occlusion of a calix or infundibulum suggests involvement of the collecting system.

Filling defects that represent blood clot or tumor invasion may be identified within the collecting system. Highly vascular or cystic tumors may be difficult to distinguish from cysts on the IVU, but if the wall of a cystic mass can be detected on the IVU, the lesion is not a simple cyst. Further evaluation with either CT or MRI is warranted. Intravenous urography with tomography cannot definitively distinguish benign lesions from malignant ones. Therefore, the masses that are most likely benign cysts are best confirmed sonographically, while lesions that are most likely complex cystic or solid masses are best evaluated with CT or MRI.

Ultrasound

Ultrasound can distinguish solid renal masses from cystic renal masses. The ultrasound criteria for the diagnosis of a simple renal cyst include absence of internal echoes, sharply marginated smooth walls, and increased transmission of sound. Simple benign renal cysts are usually readily distinguished from complicated renal cysts or solid renal masses. Lesions that do not meet the criteria for a simple cyst require CT or MRI evaluation. Specifically, lesions characterized by septal or mural thickening, calcification, nodularity, and/or irregularity require further evaluation. Magnetic resonance imaging, angiography, cyst puncture, local excision, and/or complete nephrectomy may be indicated.

The ultrasound appearance of renal cell carcinoma varies considerably. Approximately 86 per cent of tumors are isoechoic, 4 per cent are hyperechoic, and the remainder are hypoechoic. Highly echogenic carcinomas may mimic the increased echogenicity of fat-containing tumors, such as angiomyolipoma. Observation of an anechoic rim surrounding the lesion and/or intratumoral cysts within a hyperechoic mass suggests renal cell carcinoma rather than angiomyolipoma. Of the 5 to 15 per cent of renal cell carcinomas that are cystic, at least half are unilocular and 30 per cent are multilocular on ultrasound examination. Multilocular tumors consist of multiple noncommunicating cystic spaces often containing blood. Isoechoic or solid tumors can be difficult to detect with ultrasound, especially if they are small and do not displace the collecting system or produce a contour deformity. Less echogenic masses may simulate more homogeneous tumors, such as lymphoma. Although useful in characterizing renal masses, ultrasound is not considered adequate for staging renal cell carcinoma. However, the renal veins and inferior vena cava are typically well visualized on ultrasound, and the use of Doppler often provides an excellent means of assessing the presence of tumor thrombus within either of these structures.

Computed Tomography

Computed tomography can detect cystic or solid renal lesions with 89 to 99 per cent sensitivity. The accuracy of contrast CT in distinguishing solid from cystic masses exceeds 95 per cent. The CT appearance of renal cell carcinoma varies with tumor size and vascularity. Both nonenhanced and contrast-enhanced scans are required for correct diagnosis. Assessment of the degree of enhancement following contrast administration requires comparison with non–contrast-enhanced images. In addition, the observation of fat on an unenhanced CT scan suggests that angiomyolipoma is more likely present than renal cell carcinoma.

Some of the CT features of renal cell carcinoma include irregular parenchymal interface or margin, contour deformity, mass effect, calcification, and heterogeneous enhancement following contrast administration. Renal cell carcinomas typically enhance somewhat less than the surrounding tissue. Cystic renal cell carcinomas typically reveal tumor nodules and thick irregular walls. Computed tomography may also show lymph node enlargement, invasion of adjacent organs, metastases, and invasion or hemorrhage into the perinephric space. Invasion of the renal vein or inferior vena cava is usually seen as enlargement of the renal vein or inferior vena cava with or without filling defects.

Computed tomography can help the clinician distinguish renal cell carcinoma from some benign renal masses. For example, the observation of a central, stellate, nonenhancing scar suggests oncocytoma, while the presence of low attenuation fat (Hounsfield unit <0) suggests angiomyolipoma. Renal abscesses containing gas are readily distinguished from renal cell carcinoma by CT, whereas xanthogranulomatous pyelonephritis is not easily distinguished from renal cell carcinoma preoperatively.

Magnetic Resonance Imaging

The role of MRI in imaging renal masses continues to expand. Magnetic resonance imaging has a unique role in evaluating patients with renal failure or contrast allergy in whom iodinated contrast media should be avoided. Non–contrast-enhanced MRI (conventional spin echo T1- and T2-weighted images) detects solid renal lesions less than 3 cm in diameter with a sensitivity as low as 63 per cent, whereas contrast-enhanced MRI (using gadolinium-containing agents) detects both cystic and solid lesions with a sensitivity equal to that of CT (94 to 97 per cent).

Magnetic resonance imaging has been shown to be superior to conventional CT in depicting lymph node necrosis, tumor invasion of adjacent organs, and the presence and extent of tumor thrombus in the renal vein or inferior vena cava. Spiral CT, however, due to its multiplanar reconstruction and three-dimensional imaging, has been shown to have a sensitivity equal to that of MRI in delineating the presence and extent of tumor thrombus in the renal vein. It is also a useful surgical aid when planning partial nephrectomy. The limitations of MRI include inconsistent detection of calcification and poor delineation of gastrointestinal or mesenteric disease. Fortunately, the latter is uncommon in patients with renal cell carcinoma.

Angiography

Angiography is no longer part of the initial imaging and staging evaluation of patients with renal cell carcinoma. Angiography is not required for diagnosis, but it may be helpful when renal-sparing surgery is contemplated for patients with solitary kidneys or when the renal parenchyma is abnormal or distorted as in patients with polycystic kidneys or von Hippel-Lindau disease. Delineation of tumor vascularity and the number and location of renal arteries may contribute to a safer, more precise surgical resection. Arteriography may also aid the evaluation of renal cell carcinomas that are indeterminate on CT or MRI. Intra-arterial epinephrine, which causes normal renal vessels to constrict but leaves tumor vessels unaffected, may help characterize these tumors. Finally, arteriography may be a necessary prelude to angioembolization of larger tumors prior to surgical resection.

Radionuclide Studies

Technetium-99m glucoheptonate and dimercaptosuccinic acid (DMSA) are the preferred agents for evaluating the columns of Bertin detected by intravenous urography, ultrasound, or CT. Pseudotumors demonstrate normally functioning parenchyma, whereas all other masses are nonfunctioning. In screening patients for possible skeletal metastases, technetium-99m hydroxymethylene diphosphonate (HDP) is the radiopharmaceutical of choice. Metastases present as areas of increased radionuclide uptake.

Venacavography

Inferior venacavography was used widely in the past to detect the extension of tumor into the inferior vena cava. Venacavography has largely been replaced by Doppler ultrasound, MRI, and other less invasive techniques.

INVASIVE DIAGNOSTIC TECHNIQUES

Cyst Aspiration

The role of cyst aspiration in the evaluation of renal cell carcinoma is limited. Aspiration is usually reserved for poor surgical risks who have cystic lesions that do not meet the strict criteria for benign cysts. Patients with hemorrhagic cysts may also undergo cyst puncture because malignancy has been reported in as many as 30 per cent of hemorrhagic cysts. Unfortunately, the false-negative rate (for detection of tumor cells) is even higher in hemorrhagic cysts.

Fine-Needle Aspiration Biopsy

Currently, there is little role for percutaneous needle biopsy in the evaluation of renal masses. Occasionally, needle biopsy provides a nonsurgical means of confirming the presence of a primary renal tumor in a patient presenting initially with distant metastases or of identifying a nonrenal primary tumor that has metastasized to the kidney. In addition, the diagnosis of benign or inflammatory lesions by needle biopsy allows the clinician to begin definitive treatment. The major drawback to this technique remains sampling error; specifically, lack of evidence of malignancy in a needle aspirate cannot be taken as proof that malignancy is not present in some other part of the mass. Complications of needle aspiration biopsy include pneumothorax, hematoma, and hematuria. Tumor seeding along the needle biopsy tract is rarely seen.

Cystoscopy

Cystoscopy should be performed in any patient with gross hematuria to exclude the presence of bladder lesions. As many as 85 per cent of patients with upper tract transitional cell tumors develop bladder lesions.

CONCLUSION

Patients with early-stage renal cell carcinoma have an excellent survival following surgical resection of the tumor. Once the lesion has spread beyond the confines of the kidney, however, renal cell carcinoma remains remarkably resistant to nonsurgical treatment. Thus, to identify these tumors as early in their course as possible, the clinician must be familiar with the wide variety of signs and symptoms that herald the presence of renal cell carcinoma.

Early detection, characterization, and staging of renal cell carcinoma are critical in identifying the patients who will benefit from surgical management. Although the IVU remains the most widely used screening test, studies with ultrasound and CT have shown that small renal tumors are often overlooked at excretory urography. Ultrasound and CT have generally replaced intravenous urography in the characterization of renal masses. High-resolution conventional and spiral CT scanning with dynamic contrast enhancement have become the preferred methods for evaluating and staging suspected renal cell carcinoma. Magnetic resonance imaging is reserved for patients with inconclusive staging by CT, especially with respect to vascular extension. In addition, MRI is indicated in patients with renal failure or allergy to iodinated contrast media and in selected cases of cystic renal masses considered indeterminate by ultrasound and CT.

BLADDER AND URETERAL CANCERS

By Mary E. Watson, M.D.,
and G. Daniel Rath, M.D.
Canton, South Dakota

Malignant tumors of the ureter and bladder are the fifth most common malignancies, accounting for 4.5 per cent of newly diagnosed malignant neoplasms each year and 1.9 per cent of cancer deaths each year in the United States. Approximately 50,500 new cases of bladder cancer were diagnosed in the United States in 1995. Nearly 11,200 deaths in the United States in 1995 were caused by bladder cancer, which is the most common form of urinary tract cancer. Transitional cell carcinoma accounts for more than 90 per cent of bladder tumors, followed by squamous cell carcinoma (5 per cent), adenocarcinoma (fewer than 2 per cent), and rhabdomyoscarcoma (fewer than 1 per cent). Primary tumors of the upper part of the urinary tract, that is, the ureters, are rare (fewer than 10 per cent of transitional cell carcinoma).

BLADDER CANCER

Carcinoma of the bladder, most prevalent in the 50- to 70-year-old age group, peaks in the sixth decade and affects men more frequently than women, by a 3:1 ratio. Bladder cancer before the age of 40 is relatively rare, and younger patients tend to have low-grade, papillary, noninvasive transitional cell carcinomas, which also have less of a chance of recurrence than the same tumor in an older patient. However, bladder cancers can occur in people younger than 40, and even in children; therefore, a high index of suspicion must still be maintained in the evaluation of individuals in this age group who have unexplained hematuria. Most bladder cancers (70 to 80 per cent) are early-stage superficial papillary lesions at the time of diagnosis; 20 per cent are initially diagnosed as invasive disease. Superficial tumors have a greater propensity for recurrence, and 10 to 20% progress to invasion of the bladder wall. Patients with invasive tumors are at high risk for disease progression despite therapy, and the overall 5-year mortality rate is almost 50 per cent.

Epidemiology

Bladder cancer was one of the first malignancies shown to result from exposure to chemical carcinogens. Rehn's 1895 report established the relationship of bladder cancer to exposure to specific chemicals in the "aniline dye industry" in Germany. Exposure to 2-naphthylamine, a potent carcinogen, accounted for the development of tumors in exposed workers in the dye and rubber industry. Owing to this association, the chemical has been removed from the modern workplace. However, epidemiologic studies show a continued increased risk in occupations with exposure to gasoline, paints, oils, chromium, and zinc. Bladder cancer typically appears 15 to 40 years after the initial exposure to the chemicals, even if the time of exposure was relatively short. Although industrial carcinogens are important, the number of individuals exposed to these potent carcinogens is small compared with the numbers exposed to the less potent carcinogen, tobacco.

More than 50 per cent of the cases of bladder cancer in men and 25 to 33 per cent of the cases in women are due to cigarette smoking. Therefore, cigarette smoking is clearly the most important single cause of bladder cancer. The highest risk is associated with the use of dark tobacco (cigarettes), whereas the risk associated with the use of cigars or smokeless tobacco appears to be small. The mechanism by which cigarette smoking produces bladder cancer is not totally understood but is most probably related to the numerous chemicals in cigarette smoke, such as aromatic amines. Nicotine and its metabolites as well as tobacco-specific nitrosoamines do not appear to be related to the development of bladder cancer.

Additional risks for bladder cancer include chronic infection and inflammation, abuse of phenacetin-containing analgesics, cyclophosphamide, and pelvic irradiation. Studies have also been done to determine whether caffeine plays a role in bladder cancer. The results vary from no effect to a slight increase in the relative risk. Epidemiologic studies have not verified a relationship between exposure to sodium saccharin and cyclamate (artificial sweeteners) or tryptophan and bladder cancer. A viral cause of bladder cancer may possibly play a role in patients who are immunosuppressed owing to genetic immunodeficiencies, prevention of allograft rejection, or acquired immunodeficiency syndrome.

Dietary factors are poorly defined, but individuals who consume greater quantities of vitamin A or carotene may have a lower rate of bladder cancer than individuals who do not consume these substances. High doses of vitamin C may suppress the development of bladder cancer, although this theory has not been supported by experimental evidence.

Pathology

Ninety per cent of bladder cancers are transitional cell carcinoma, 5 per cent are squamous cell carcinoma, fewer than 2 per cent are adenocarcinoma, and fewer than 1 per cent are rhabdomyosarcoma. Squamous cell carcinomas probably arise in transitional epithelium via the process of squamous metaplasia. Metaplastic changes can be associated with the chronic inflammatory changes seen with foreign bodies, such as indwelling catheters, and parasitic infections, such as schistosomiasis. Adenocarcinomas of the bladder are thought to arise from embryonic hindgut remnants, such as a persistent urachus in the dome of the bladder. Rhabdomyosarcomas arise from the muscular wall of the bladder and are very rare.

Signs and Symptoms

The most common presenting feature of all urologic malignancies is the presence of gross or microscopic hematuria that can be intermittent and painless (Table 1). More than 85 per cent of patients with urothelial cancers develop hematuria, but as many as 13 per cent of all adults can have microscopic hematuria at some time. A total of 68 to 97 per cent of individuals with bladder cancer actually present with asymptomatic microscopic hematuria. Malignant disease can be found in as many as 10 per cent of asymptomatic patients with microscopic hematuria, but 33 per cent of patients with bladder cancer report symptoms related to bladder irritability, such as frequency, urgency, and dysuria, mimicking the more common diseases, such as cystitis and prostatism. High-grade tumors, including carcinoma in situ (CIS), are more likely to produce these symptoms than are low-grade papillomas.

Typically, primary care providers diagnose only one new bladder cancer every few years. To avoid missing that one patient, the physician must maintain a high index of suspicion and evaluate any high-risk male or female with painless hematuria, any female with a urinary tract infection that fails to respond to appropriate antibiotics or has persistent unexplained bladder symptoms, or any male with frequency, urgency, and dysuria.

Table 1. Causes of Hematuria

Renal (Nonglomerular)

Perirenal hematoma (infants)
Cortical necrosis
Papillary necrosis
Trauma
Vascular malformation
Tumors
Interstitial nephritis (drug allergy, infection)
Sponge kidney
Polycystic kidney
Pyelonephritis
Tuberculosis
Renal vein thrombosis
Renal infarct
Nephrosclerosis secondary to hypertension

Renal (Glomerular)

Acute proliferative glomerulonephritis (poststreptococcal GN)
Primary mesangiopathic GN (Berger's disease)
Focal proliferative GN associated with systemic disease (Schönlein-Henoch purpura, vasculitis)
Rapidly progressive GN
Lupus nephritis
Membranoproliferative GN
Alport's syndrome
Benign familial hematuria
Any other glomerular lesion

Postrenal

Stones
Periureteritis secondary to extraurinary pathology
Tumors of the lower urinary tract
Cystitis (idiopathic, radiation, drug-induced, viral, bacterial, schistosomal)
Prostatitis
Epididymitis
Meatal ulceration (circumcised boys)
Urethral stenosis
Foreign bodies of bladder or urethra (including Foley catheter)
Strenuous exercise
Urethritis
Phimosis
Benign prostatic hypertrophy
Obstruction
Vascular malformations
Endometriosis
Vesicoureteral reflux

Hematologic

Coagulopathy
Anticoagulation
Sickle cell anemia, trait, thalassemia; hemoglobin C–thalassemia disease
"False" hematuria
Red diaper syndrome
Vaginal bleeding
Bleeding circumcision
Factitious
Pigmenturia: porphyria, hemoglobinuria, myoglobinuria, food (beets, blackberries, rhubarb), drugs

Diagnostic Evaluation

Physical Examination

Physical examination plays a limited role in the diagnosis of most cases of bladder cancer, but as with any disease a thorough history and physical examination must be completed. A history of trauma, past urinary tract infection, renal stones, previous tumors, and local and constitutional symptoms must be elicited. Special attention during the physical examination is given to the abdomen, flank, prostate, and external and internal genitalia. A thorough abdominal examination is performed with the patient under general anesthesia at the time of cystoscopy.

Laboratory Studies

The presence of more than three to eight red blood cells per high-power field on any urine specimen is considered abnormal, and these urine specimens should be cultured to exclude infection. A normal repeat urinalysis *should not* reassure the clinician that the initial results were spurious, because bleeding from a bladder tumor can be intermittent. Under phase-contrast microscopy, red blood cells from bladder cancer appear normal in size and shape, but red blood cells of glomerular origin appear crenated and small. Pyuria, proteinuria, and bacteriuria aid in the diagnosis. Unexplained microhematuria merits further testing. Routine screening for bladder cancers in the general population with reagent strip urinalysis for hematuria is not cost-effective. Exceptions include those individuals at high risk (i.e., cigarette smokers) and those exposed to other bladder carcinogens, such as 1- and 2-naphthylamines, benzidine-4-aminobiphenyl, and 4,4-methylenebis(2-chloroaniline).

Voided urine cytology is diagnostic when positive, but it has a high rate of false-negative results. The test result is most often positive in those individuals with higher grade tumors and carcinoma in situ, and it has also been found to be positive when cystoscopic examination has failed to disclose a lesion. Cytologic specimens obtained by vigorous bladder barbotage during cystoscopy are considered to be the most reliable. These specimens are expected to be positive in 10 per cent of patients with grade I tumors, 50 per cent of those with grade II tumors, 90 per cent of those with grade III tumors, and 80 per cent of those with carcinoma in situ.

Automated flow cytometry, which uses lasers to count the chromatin content of urothelial cells, is one of the newest techniques to be developed. Normal cells are diploid, and therefore aneuploidy may be an early marker of malignancy. The sensitivity of flow cytometry, like that of urine cytology, is higher in the high-grade lesions, but low-grade lesions can be missed. Flow cytometry is useful in following recurrent bladder carcinoma and defining the presence of carcinoma in situ.

Developments of monoclonal antibodies that bind to the Lewis X (Le) blood group antigen, a determinant expressed on 90 per cent of superficial bladder tumors, and several other monoclonal antibodies to antigens associated with bladder tumors have shown promise as new treatment and prognostic markers. Compared with standard cytologic methods, immunocytologic detection of Le on exfoliated cells in urine increases the discovery of superficial bladder tumors. The antigen detected by antibodies M344 and 19A211 on tissue specimens is expressed on 70 per cent of superficial bladder tumors but is rarely expressed in invasive lesions. When immunocytologic tests with these markers are used, along with tests for DNA ploidy and cytologic examinations, the ability to detect bladder cancer cells in urine specimens is improved. The antigen detected by antibody T138 is associated with decreased survival. These tissue antigens may also be helpful in the treatment of bladder tumors. Chromosomal abnormalities involving the long arm of chromosome 9 and the short arm of chromosome 17 have also been associated with bladder cancer. Many of these tests are beginning to move from research facilities into the diagnostic laboratory.

Imaging Studies

Intravenous urography remains the mainstay of radiographic evaluation for urologic malignancies, because it provides efficient visualization of both the upper and the lower urinary tract. Close attention is paid to abnormalities observed in the bladder, including hydronephrosis, nonfunction of a kidney, lack of bladder distensibility, and filling defects. However, only 60 per cent of *known* bladder cancers are seen on intravenous urograms, and therefore a negative examination should not be viewed as the end of the evaluation. Obstruction of the ureteral orifice on intravenous urography with hydronephrosis or a nonfunctioning kidney is usually caused by an invasive bladder tumor. Filling defects in the upper tracts require further evaluation with retrograde urography and selective urinary cytology. However, if a bladder tumor is present, ureteroscopy is contraindicated because upper tract seeding can occur. Intravenous urography is also useful in the subsequent management of patients with bladder cancers, because 2 to 3 per cent progress to develop upper tract tumors, and more will develop carcinoma in situ.

Ultrasonography, computed tomography, and magnetic resonance imaging all are better suited for local staging than the diagnosis of bladder cancer and are therefore neither useful nor cost-effective in the initial diagnostic evaluation.

RENAL PELVIS AND URETER

Fewer than ten per cent of tumors involving urothelium arise in the upper portion of the urinary tract (ureters and renal pelvis). When tumors are found in the ureters, the majority are found in the distal third of the ureter. The tumors may arise spontaneously or by seeding from the renal pelvis, bladder, or contralateral ureter. Very rarely, the ureter is the site of symptomatic metastatic disease. These cancers typically arise in the breast, colon, rectum, cervix, prostate, or bladder or are retroperitoneal lymphomas. Most become symptomatic when the patient is preterminal or they are observed at autopsy. Occasionally, tumors of the colon or cervix or retroperitoneal lymphomas grow onto the ureter. This encroachment usually results in compression rather than invasion.

Signs and Symptoms

Ureteral cancer should be considered in the older patient with gross or microscopic hematuria, previous urothelial tumors, ureteral obstruction, or hydronephrosis. Renal colic is rare because the obstruction is insidious. A total of 50 per cent of ureteral cancers seed to the bladder, and 80 per cent bleed. Bleeding can be intermittent; hence, rechecking a urinalysis to see whether the hematuria has cleared is not appropriate in the high-risk individual.

Diagnostic Studies

Excretory urography, in combination with cystoscopy and ureteroscopy, constitutes the initial evaluation. Retrograde pyelography is helpful when excretory urography is nondiagnostic or contraindicated. The differential diagnosis of a filling defect in the ureter includes ureteral tumors, radiolucent stones, clots, sloughed renal papilla, and fungus balls. Urine cytology is often negative, does not give location, grade, or depth, and is laboratory dependent (i.e., an experienced cytology laboratory is required). Flow cytometry has similar pitfalls. If positive, urine cytology and flow cytometry are diagnostic, but cystoscopy is still required. Cytology and flow cytometry can be useful in management, but the more cost-effective approach is to proceed to cystoscopy and uretoscopy after initial excretory urography.

PITFALLS IN DIAGNOSIS

The most common diagnostic pitfall is delay in diagnosis. This frequently occurs because signs and symptoms are attributed to benign diseases, such as cystitis, prostatism, benign prostatic hypertrophy, and vaginal prolapse. Benign diseases improve with treatment; therefore, the clinician must maintain a high index of suspicion when the patient's symptoms fail to improve. Care must also be taken not to disregard hematuria and irritative voiding symptoms in the high-risk patient. Intravenous urograms can miss lesions in the bladder; therefore, the clinician must guard against false reassurance by a negative examination. Flow cytometry and urine cytology can easily miss low-grade lesions and are best performed on fresh washings from the bladder, not voided urine specimens. The most important point to remember is to maintain a high index of suspicion when dealing with the patient who has either hematuria or irritative voiding symptoms.

URETHRITIS AND PROSTATITIS

By E. James Seidmon, M.D.
Philadelphia, Pennsylvania

NONGONOCOCCAL URETHRITIS

Inflammation of the urethra can occur in both sexes and may be caused by a sexually transmitted disease or an infection. Nongonococcal urethritis (NGU) is also called nonspecific urethritis (NSU) and is diagnosed when *Neisseria gonorrhoeae* cannot be specifically detected by either bacterial culture or staining.

Nongonococcal urethritis is more often observed in the sexually active adult, is more likely to be observed and reported by men rather than women, and occurs mostly in the 15- to 35-year-old age group. In addition, NGU is encountered following diagnosis and treatment of gonorrhea and as a postgonococcal urethritis. *Chlamydia trachomatis* and *Ureaplasma urealyticum* are the most common organisms diagnosed and are isolated in 70 to 80 per cent of cases. Less found but still associated with NGU are *Trichomonas vaginalis*, herpes simplex virus, *Candida albicans*, and *Bacteroides* species. In approximately 20 per cent of cases, the cause cannot be determined. In university clinics as well as outlying patient clinic centers, NGU occurs in more than 50 per cent of cases of urethritis and is more frequent in heterosexual men.

The clinical manifestations present after an incubation period of 7 to 21 days and include dysuria with a mucoid, opalescent, or clear urethral discharge that is often scant but can be thick and purulent. Urethral itching, meatal stickiness, and crusting or concomitant staining of the patient's underwear are typical. Discharge from the male urethra is best observed in the morning prior to urination. The examination should include close observation of the genital field, including the inguinal region, for any cutaneous lesions or lymphadenopathy. The scrotal contents are assessed, and in the female the labia are carefully examined. The perianal region is examined for discharge or lesions, and anoscopy is performed if indicated. The urethra is carefully palpated for tenderness and induration. If exudate can be obtained by urethral massage or endourethral swab, it can be cultured and gram-stained. Alternatively, the patient can void the first 10 to 15 mL of urine for culture and Gram stain. If fewer than 4 polymorphonuclear leukocytes (PMNs) per oil immersion field are observed, urethritis is unlikely. However, more than 4 PMNs noted in the absence of intracellular diplococci is diagnostic for NGU. Alternatively, if the microscopic examination of the spun urine sediment sample reveals 15 or more PMNs in 5 random high-power fields (400×), clinical urethritis exists. Monoclonal antibody tests and rapid immunoassays (enzyme-linked immunosorbent assay [ELISA]) are available for detecting *C. trachomatis*. These tests can be very helpful in early diagnosis and treatment.

Complications occur more often in men with epididymitis or Reiter syndrome (urethritis, conjunctivitis, arthritis, and mucocutaneous lesions). *Chlamydia trachomatis* is the most common cause of epididymitis in men younger than 35 years of age, whereas coliform infections secondary to a history of urologic disease or urologic instrumentation are more common in men older then 35.

Table 1. Prevalence of Bacteriuria in Males

Age	Percentage (%)
Infants	2
Young boys	0.1–5
Young adults	<0.03
30–60 years	0.1
>60 years	5–15

PROSTATITIS (ACUTE AND CHRONIC)

An acute bacterial infection of the prostate is most commonly associated with bacteriuria (Table 1). In infants, urinary tract infection is more common in males than females, probably owing to the increased incidence of congenital genitourinary disorders in the male. After infancy, bacteriuria is rare in men until they reach the seventh decade, and then the prevalence is similar to that of women.

As men age, the prostate enlarges, and many men experience changes in their voiding pattern (frequency, nocturia, urgency, dysuria, hesitancy, double voiding, dribbling). Age, however, does not necessarily make the male more susceptible to an acute or chronic bacterial infection of the prostate. The routes of infection include the ascent through the urethra, reflux of infected urine into the prostatic ducts, hematogenous or lymphatic spread, and direct extension of bacteria from the rectum. Acute bacterial prostatitis is typically associated with a urinary tract infection (e.g., cystitis), and the clinical presentation usually defines the infected site (Table 2). Acute cystitis does not necessar-

Table 2. Incidence of Causative Organisms in Acute Prostatitis

Organism	Percentage (%)
Escherichia coli	80
Klebsiella	10–15
Streptococcus faecalis	5
Pseudomonas	1–2

Table 3. Symptoms of Prostatitis or Prostatodynia

Frequency	"Ball" in perineum
Urgency	Decreased stream
Nocturia	Postejaculatory pain

ily lead to an acute bacterial infection of the prostate, whereas the converse is much more likely.

Clinical Findings

Acute prostatitis is associated most commonly with low back (sacral) and/or perineal pain, urinary frequency and urgency, dysuria, nocturia, fever, chills, generalized malaise, and some form of bladder outlet obstruction (Table 3). The voiding dysfunction can vary from difficulty in micturition and/or dribbling to actual urinary retention. Occasionally, hematuria or painful erections can be a part of this acute condition, and pain on ejaculation or at the tip of the penis has also been reported.

The abnormal signs are typically confined to the prostate. In the acute stage of the disease, the gland is tense, swollen, and exquisitely tender. Rectal pain and difficulty with defecation are often reported. On gentle rectal examination, the prostate feels nodular and indurated. Early in the acute infection, the prostate may be very tender but may feel normal to palpation. *Prostate massage should not be performed.* Typically, an acute urinary tract infection from the bladder accompanies the prostatitis, and hazy urine is noted on visual inspection. Microscopic examination shows red blood cells, white blood cells, and bacteria. Culture of the specimen identifies the pathogen, and the sensitivities guide the treatment. During the acute stage of the infection, transurethral instrumentation must be avoided, and if the patient develops urinary retention, suprapubic drainage is performed. Once antibiotic therapy has been initiated, the patient is observed and periodic rectal examinations are performed over the next several weeks to monitor resolution of the prostatitis. If the prostate becomes boggy and fluctuant, an abscess may be developing. Spontaneous rupture of an abscess can occur, with pus draining into the urethra, bladder, or rectum. Alternatively, if fever and pain persist along with physical findings consistent with an abscess, surgical intervention becomes necessary, and transurethral or perineal drainage of the abscess is performed.

The histologic findings of prostatitis include leukocytes in the prostatic stroma. These PMNs partially destroy the glandular epithelium and lumen as well as the adjacent stroma. The density of the intraluminal infiltrate of PMNs is histologically documented, and the increase of stromal involvement is noted. With more severe infection, abscess or microabscess formation may be observed. Acute infection causes focal or multifocal—but not diffuse—disease.

Chronic infection of the prostate can present with a variety of symptoms (see Table 3) or with no real symptoms at all. The physical examination can be completely normal even with a history of recurrent urinary tract infections caused by the same organism. This finding means that while the bladder infection has been treated, the nidus (i.e., the prostate) has been ineffectively treated. To make the diagnosis of bacterial prostatitis, examination of the prostatic fluid must be performed by the three-glass technique. Voided bladder one (VB_1) is the first 10 to 15 mL of the patient's urine. This collection is followed by a midstream urine voided bladder two (VB_2). Following this, a vigorous prostatic digital massage is performed, with the resultant discharge of several drops of fluid that are collected in a wide-mouth container for bacterial culture. This collection is called the expressed prostatic secretion (EPS). Finally, another small voided specimen is collected immediately following the EPS and is labeled as the voided bladder three (VB_3). Leukocytosis of 10 or more white blood cells per high-power field in the EPS and a positive bacterial culture of VB_3 is diagnostic for prostatic infection.

Those patients who suffer from acute urinary retention or who have unusual risk factors, such as diabetes mellitus, immunosuppression, or fever higher than 102°F, need to be hospitalized for intensive intravenous antimicrobial therapy, hydration, and pain medication. Treatment of chronic prostatitis is typically more difficult due to the poor concentration of the antibiotic in the tissue of the prostate, whereas in acute prostatitis the drug rapidly diffuses from the plasma into the prostatic tissue and its secretions, initiating rapid improvement.

Chronic prostatitis can lead to destruction of the gland as well as scarring of the bladder neck and stricture formation. Additional concerns include acute epididymitis or pyelonephritis and the development of bacteremia with overwhelming sepsis. Cystourethroscopy can help diagnose a bladder neck contracture or a urethral stricture and voiding cystourethrogram can demonstrate prostatic calculi or diverticuli. Prostatic ultrasound is useful in detecting smaller prostatic calculi missed by radiograph, and biopsies may be necessary for distinguishing prostatitis from prostatic carcinoma. Sometimes, radical transurethral resection of the prostate or open prostatectomy is required for removing the local nidus (i.e., the infected prostatic calculi and chronically infected prostate tissue).

Nonbacterial Prostatitis

Nonbacterial prostatitis (Table 4) is characterized by irritative or obstructive voiding symptoms, and pain is localized to the low back region, pelvis, or perineum. These patients may also report voiding dysfunction or ejaculatory pain. The complaints are almost always the same as those offered by patients diagnosed with chronic prostatitis. While the leukocyte count is similar in the EPS, these patients lack documented bacterial infection of VB_3. Studies attempting to link *Ureaplasma urealyticum* and *C. trachomatis* to the disorder have been inconclusive. Because the cause is unknown, treatment is not always successful, but a therapeutic trial with tetracycline, erythromycin, or doxycycline is reasonable. Concomitant use of nonsteroidal

Table 4. Classification of Benign Painful Prostate

Prostatitis/Prostatodynia	Systemic Signs	Purulent Fluid	Bacteria	Pain	Flow Decrease
Acute bacterial	Yes	Yes	Yes	Yes	Yes
Chronic bacterial	No	Yes	Yes	Yes	Yes
Nonbacterial	No	Yes	No	Yes	Yes
Prostatodynia	No	No	No	Yes	Yes

anti-inflammatory drugs and hot baths can provide some symptomatic relief.

Prostatodynia

These patients often have symptoms that mimic prostatitis, but the EPS is normal and the VB_3 is culture negative. Perineal pain and musculoskeletal abnormalities are often responsible for this symptom complex. Because the cause is unknown, treatment is often empiric, and the patient should be so informed. Pelvic floor dysfunction with pelviperineal pain can be treated with selective alpha-adrenergic blocking agents (terazosin or doxazosin) in low doses at bedtime. Diazepam and hot baths may relieve muscle spasm. Antibiotic therapy in this situation is not beneficial and is not recommended.

BENIGN PROSTATIC HYPERPLASIA

By William J. Ellis, M.D.
Seattle, Washington

Benign prostatic hyperplasia (BPH) is a benign neoplasm of the prostate that arises in the periurethral transition zone. The progressive growth of this periurethral tissue leads to obstruction of normal bladder outflow. Most men experience symptoms of bladder outlet obstruction during their lifetime; approximately one fourth are treated for these symptoms. In the future, two factors are expected to increase the number of men receiving treatment for bladder outlet obstruction. First, medical treatments and less invasive procedures are being introduced to treat BPH. Second, the number of men suffering from this disorder will increase as the population ages.

Although the etiology of BPH is unknown, androgens may contribute to the development of the disease. Men who have been castrated prior to puberty do not develop prostatic hyperplasia. In normal men, histologic evidence of the disease can be detected as early as the third or fourth decade of life; microscopic changes are ubiquitous by the eighth decade of life. Growth factors are thought to be involved in the disease process, but no clear links have been established. Although a familial predisposition to BPH has been reported, specific genetic alterations have not been identified. Benign prostatic hyperplasia is not associated with the subsequent development of prostatic carcinoma.

The histopathology of BPH is characterized by stromal hyperplasia with interspersed epithelial and glandular elements. The stromal component contains both smooth muscle and connective tissue. Hyperplasia often begins as a small stromal nodule in the transition zone. Progressive growth of these stromal nodules leads to the formation of multinodular adenomas as large as 100 to 200 g. Normal prostatic parenchyma is stretched around the adenoma, forming a pseudocapsule known as the surgical capsule.

Obstruction due to BPH may be produced in two ways. The static component of bladder outlet obstruction is due to urethral occlusion by the bulk of the prostatic adenoma. The dynamic component of obstruction is due to constricting forces applied by the prostatic and bladder neck smooth muscle. The relative contribution of each of these elements varies among men. The correlation between prostate size and bladder outlet obstruction is poor and unreliable.

SYMPTOMS

The symptoms associated with BPH may be classified as obstructive or irritative. The obstructive symptoms include a slow stream, often with hesitancy or a delay in initiation of the stream; an intermittent stream that starts and stops; and a sensation of incomplete emptying that may be associated with double voiding. Eventually, the patient develops urinary retention. Often, patients in urinary retention void small amounts with great frequency but are unable to adequately empty the bladder. Only a small percentage of men with BPH progress to urinary retention, but this possibility must always be considered in the male with bladder outlet obstructive symptoms.

The irritative symptoms are generally the most bothersome to patients with BPH. They frequently develop progressive urinary frequency, nocturia, and dysuria. Increasing voiding pressures lead to increasing urgency, occasionally accompanied by incontinence. Severe urgency can be socially crippling because many men with BPH are reluctant to venture far beyond the known safety of a restroom. Irritative symptoms appear to be due to changes in bladder structure and innervation related to chronic outflow obstruction.

DISEASE COURSE

The course of symptomatic BPH varies. In some patients, symptoms tend to wax and wane, with periodic exacerbations that may or may not progress. The majority of men, however, note a gradual increase in symptoms over time. Initially, a slow stream and occasional nocturia may be the only symptoms present. At this point, the detrusor muscle can adapt to the mild degree of obstruction, and residual volumes of urine are small. As voiding pressures increase, bladder irritability and the sense of urgency increase. Eventually, the obstruction leads to decompensation of the detrusor muscle. The bladder begins to dilate, and postvoid residual urine volumes increase. Ultimately, complete bladder decompensation occurs, and chronic urinary retention develops. Intervention to restore normal voiding at this point is generally fruitless. To enhance recovery in patients with BPH, the clinician should remember that interventions are best undertaken before the detrusor decompensates.

DIAGNOSIS

The diagnosis of symptomatic BPH is based primarily on the history. Most men report a gradual onset of symptoms that evolve over several years. By contrast, the sudden onset of voiding symptoms often suggests another problem. Voiding symptoms in men younger than 50 years are rarely due to BPH because little macroscopic enlargement of the prostate occurs prior to this age. Therefore, other diagnoses should be entertained. The American Urological Association has developed a questionnaire designed to quantitate symptoms. The symptom score runs from 0 to 35, with 0 to 7 classified as mild, 8 to 19 as moderate, and 20 or more as severe symptoms. The past medical history should be thoroughly probed regarding urinary tract infections, sexually transmitted diseases, diabetes, congestive heart failure, neurologic disorders, back injuries, pelvic surgery, diuretic use, alcohol use, and decongestant use.

Several caveats in the interpretation of symptoms are important. Daytime frequency alone may indicate habitual voiding. Frequency associated with a good stream may indicate polydipsia. A daily diary listing the time and volume of all ingested fluids and urine output may help clarify the patient's urinary pattern.

The physical examination should include a careful evaluation of the lower abdomen to assess the degree of bladder emptying. Suprapubic dullness to percussion generally correlates with a distended urinary bladder. Inguinal hernias may be associated with straining to initiate urination. The phallus should be inspected for signs of meatal stenosis and chronic urinary leakage. Careful digital rectal examination of patients with BPH reveals a symmetrical, firm, rubbery enlarged prostate gland. The absolute size of the prostate correlates poorly with the degree of urinary symptoms. Any nodularity, induration, or asymmetry of the prostate should be further evaluated to exclude carcinoma. An extremely tender prostate suggests prostatitis. If prostatitis is suspected, prostatic massage for evaluation of expressed prostatic secretions should be performed. In febrile patients, however, a tender prostate may represent an acute bacterial prostatitis where vigorous rectal examination or prostatic massage can produce bacteremia. A tender asymmetrical or focally fluctuant prostate suggests a prostatic abscess. Transrectal ultrasound should be performed with aspiration of any visible fluid collection.

Uroflowmetry can be used to evaluate the urinary stream. Both the peak urinary flow rate and the flow pattern can be useful in determining the cause of voiding dysfunction. Postvoid residual urine volumes provide an objective measure of bladder emptying. The residual urine volume may be determined by catheterization or by use of ultrasound units designed for this purpose. Young men generally have residual urine volumes of less than 10 mL. With bladder outlet obstruction, the residual urine volume increases. Men with postvoid residual urine volumes of more than 100 mL should undergo thorough urologic evaluation.

When a neurologic cause of bladder dysfunction is suspected, urodynamic evaluation of voiding may be indicated. This evaluation may range from a simple filling cystometrogram to video urodynamics.

The decision to treat BPH is based primarily on symptoms. Where the diagnosis remains uncertain after the history, physical examination, and uroflowmetry, endoscopy (cystourethroscopy) may be useful. Mucosal trabeculation is the hallmark of a chronically obstructed bladder. However, the cystoscopic appearance of the prostate is a poor indicator of the degree of prostatic obstruction. For most patients, cystoscopy is not necessary prior to surgery.

Laboratory tests are rarely useful in the diagnosis of BPH. However, serum concentrations of prostate-specific antigen (PSA) should be obtained in all patients with prostate symptoms who have a life expectancy of more than 10 years. Increased serum PSA is not diagnostic of prostatic carcinoma, but abnormal PSA concentrations can identify the men at increased risk for occult prostatic malignancy. Importantly, prostatic enlargement alone can produce modest increases in serum PSA. Serum creatinine should be measured in men with moderate to severe symptomatic BPH to exclude renal dysfunction due to urinary retention.

Routine imaging of the upper urinary tract with intravenous pyelography or ultrasound is not cost-effective. Imaging should be reserved for patients with hematuria, abnormal renal function, or persistent urinary tract infection.

DIFFERENTIAL DIAGNOSIS

A number of disorders produce symptoms that may be confused with BPH. Prostatic carcinoma is the most common malignancy in the aging male. Most prostate carcinoma develops in the periphery of the gland and produces few voiding symptoms in its early stages. Yet approximately one fourth of prostatic carcinomas develop in the transition zone, where they are more likely to produce obstructive symptoms. If a man has a normal digital rectal examination and a normal serum PSA, his symptoms are probably not related to unsuspected carcinoma of the prostate.

The predominant symptom of urethral stricture is a slow stream. Frequency and urgency are seen less commonly than in BPH. Iatrogenic injury following urethral catheterization is now the most common cause of urethral strictures. A history of gonococcal urethritis should also raise the suspicion of urethral stricture, which classically produces a "flat-topped" pattern on uroflowmetry, as the peak flow rate is fixed by the smallest diameter of the urethra. Strictures can be identified by retrograde urethrograms or cystoscopy.

Lower urinary tract infection can produce many of the irritative symptoms described in BPH, including a sensation of incomplete emptying. In addition, because patients with urinary tract infections often void small volumes, they may have weak streams. Acute or chronic prostatitis may also contribute to irritative voiding symptoms, and prostatic edema may increase prostatic urethral obstruction. Urinalysis is useful in patients with voiding symptoms, and microscopic examination of expressed prostatic secretions can exclude prostatic inflammation.

Bladder tumors, particularly carcinoma in situ, can produce bladder irritation, and large, pedunculated tumors may prolapse into the bladder outlet, producing obstruction. Most bladder tumors, however, cause hematuria or pyuria detectable by urinalysis.

Both upper and lower neurologic disorders can produce voiding symptoms. The peripheral motor and sensory neuropathy of diabetes mellitus produces a hypocontractile bladder with poor sensation. Often, diabetic patients carry large residual urine volumes and feel the urge to void infrequently. A timed voiding program is ideal for such patients. Surgical procedures in the pelvis, particularly colorectal surgery, can acutely produce a denervated bladder. Strokes and spinal cord injuries alter the ability to inhibit the voiding reflex. In these patients, the primary urinary symptom is urgency, often accompanied by urge incontinence. Congestive heart failure is frequently associated with nocturia that follows mobilization of fluid sequestered in the lower extremities. Heart failure patients also take diuretics that may produce transient urinary frequency.

A few medications may exacerbate the symptoms of BPH. Most systemic decongestants contain alpha-adrenergic agonists that contract the smooth muscle of the prostatic urethra and increase bladder outflow resistance. Psychoactive and other medications with anticholinergic effects can decrease the strength of detrusor contractions. Alcohol intoxication transiently decreases bladder awareness, and the associated diuresis may lead to acute overdistention of the bladder.

SUMMARY

Benign prostatic hyperplasia is a common disorder in aging males. Therefore, a thorough understanding of the pathogenesis and the other conditions considered in the differential diagnosis is important to all physicians. The diagnosis of BPH is based primarily on symptoms. A careful history and urinalysis can exclude many of the possibilities in the differential diagnosis. Serum PSA, residual urine determinations, and uroflowmetry may be needed to complete the initial evaluation. Treatment of the obstruction should be initiated before bladder decompensation occurs, as many of the bladder changes are irreversible.

CARCINOMA OF THE PROSTATE

By Joseph D. Schmidt, M.D.
San Diego, California

Because of a growing and aging United States male population, carcinoma of the prostate now is its most common malignancy. In 1996, 317,000 men will be diagnosed with, and 41,400 will die from, the disease. In 1994, the distribution of prostate cancer was 36 per cent among all male cancer patients (lung cancer was 14 per cent), and it was responsible for approximately 14 per cent of the cancer deaths reported. The true incidence is unknown because of confusion between clinical and latent disease but increases with age. African American men tend to have a higher incidence and a decreased 5-year survival, reflecting both higher stage and grade of cancer at diagnosis.

The great majority of these tumors are adenocarcinomas arising from prostatic acini. Ductal adenocarcinoma, mucinous adenocarcinoma, squamous cell carcinoma, transitional cell carcinoma, and sarcoma are responsible for approximately 5 per cent of the tumors arising in the prostate. Cancer metastatic to the prostate from a distant primary, although reported occasionally, does not generally present a clinical problem. Primary rectal cancer rarely invades the prostate.

SIGNS AND SYMPTOMS

Localized prostate cancer is usually asymptomatic. By contrast, men with symptoms of outlet obstruction (hesitancy, dribbling, straining to void, decreased stream) have coincidental benign enlargement or diffuse prostatic malignancy. A total of 20 to 30 per cent of patients with prostatic cancer present with local extension of the tumor or with distant metastases. These men often have symptoms of outlet obstruction. Those who present with metastases frequently report back pain secondary to bone involvement. Pathologic fractures are seen occasionally. Cord compression presents as abrupt onset of weakness or paraplegia and is considered a neurosurgical emergency. Weight loss, anemia, and renal failure may occur in advanced disease. Ureteral obstruction and hydronephrosis may present with flank pain, fever, and chills, the latter from secondary urinary infection.

At autopsy, rectal involvement is found in 0.6 to 11 per cent of all males; it presents in one of four ways: anterior mass with compression, annular rectal stricture (most common), mucosal ulceration with an anterior rectal mass (most closely resembling primary rectal carcinoma), and metastasis to the proximal rectosigmoid.

PHYSICAL EXAMINATION

Digital rectal examination should be performed yearly on every male 50 years of age or older up to the age of 75 to 80. African American patients and patients with a family history of prostate cancer should undergo annual rectal examination starting at age 40. Glandular size and consistency, and the presence of a firm nodule, should be noted. Any abnormality, even minimal induration, should be further evaluated. The seminal vesicles generally are not palpable. The examination is often performed with the patient bent over at the waist. If this position is unsatisfactory (a frequent occurrence in obese patients), ask the patient to kneel on the table with his head down to facilitate complete examination.

DIAGNOSIS

Diagnosis is made by histologic examination of a core needle biopsy or cytologic examination of a fine-needle aspiration. Needle biopsy specimens can be obtained through the transrectal or the transperineal approach. The transrectal approach is more accurate but is associated with a higher incidence of complications, mainly infection and hemorrhage.

In the past, needle biopsy was carried out with either the Franklin modification of the Vim-Silverman needle or the disposable Tru-Cut needle. Recently, spring-loaded biopsy guns with disposable 18-gauge needles have become available. This system, used with transrectal ultrasound guidance, fires rapidly with little patient discomfort and minimal displacement of the gland and provides more uniform core samples.

Fine-needle aspiration has been used extensively in Europe and has gained some acceptance in the United States, only to be displaced by the biopsy guns. The major advantages of fine-needle aspiration are patient comfort and very low complication rates. Open biopsy is the most accurate method of biopsy but is infrequently used today. Transurethral biopsy generally is not performed because most lesions are located in the periphery of the gland. Cytologic examination of expressed prostatic secretions may provide the correct diagnosis but is considered unreliable.

Use of transrectal ultrasonography (TRUS) in the detection of prostate cancer remains controversial. Routine screening is neither practical nor cost-effective. Furthermore, small lesions may be identified that may not be clinically significant. Ultrasound may be helpful in staging in patients who are believed clinically to have prostate cancer but in whom finger-guided biopsy findings are normal. Biopsy under ultrasound guidance can increase the likelihood that the lesion in question has been sampled adequately.

Only 50 per cent of patients with a palpable nodule or abnormality are found to have cancer of the prostate. The remainder have nodular benign prostatic hypertrophy (BPH), chronic prostatitis, prostatic calculi, tuberculosis, or granulomatous prostatitis.

STAGING

Treatment of prostate cancer is based on the extent of disease at the time of presentation as well as the age and general health of the patient. In the United States, urologists still prefer the Whitmore-Jewett staging system to the TNM (tumor, node, metastasis) classification, but the latter is gaining in popularity.

STAGE A (T1). Stage A tumors are those that are discovered following a TUR-P (transurethral resection of the prostate) or open prostatectomy for clinical benign disease. The preoperative rectal examination is not suspicious for malignancy. Cancer is found in approximately 10 per cent of these patients. Stage A_1 (T1a) is defined as either three or fewer positive chips or involvement of less than 5 per cent of the total volume, and a well-differentiated tumor. Once thought to be clinically insignificant, as many as 16 per cent of stage A_1 tumors have been found to progress by 8 years. Stage A_2 (T1b) involves more than 5 per cent of the tissue. Any tumor grade other than well-differentiated places the patient in stage A_2. Stage A_2 tumors tend to behave more like stage B_2 and C tumors and are associated with lymph node metastases in 23 per cent of patients. Stage T1c implies that the cancer is not recognized clinically but has been detected via an abnormal PSA (prostate-specific antigen) blood test and biopsy.

STAGE B (T2). Stage B tumors are clinically detectable by digital rectal examination. By definition, stage B tumors are confined within the capsule. Tumors in stage B_1 (T2a) are less than 1.5 to 2 cm in diameter, whereas stage B_2 (T2b) denotes a larger volume of tumor confined to one lobe. Bilateral involvement is considered stage T2c.

STAGE C (T3). Stage C tumors represent tumor extension outside the capsule of the prostate gland, but with no evidence of distant metastases. These tumors may be subdivided into C_1 (T3a) (minimal extension) or C_2 (T3b, T3c) (more extension, fixation, or involvement of the seminal vesicles).

STAGE D (N+, M+). Stage D tumors are those associated with distant metastases. As in the other stages, there are subdivisions within this category. Stage D_0 tumors are clinically localized, and the bone scan is normal; however, serum acid phosphatase activity is increased. Stage D_1 (N1–3) tumors represent involvement of regional pelvic lymph nodes. Stage D_2 (M1) denotes distant nodal (outside the pelvis), bone, or visceral metastases. Stage D_3 represents progression of metastatic disease after appropriate endocrine therapy.

Radiologic Studies Used in Staging

A bone scan (technetium 99m) is obtained in most patients, as is a chest film. Bone scans are more sensitive than skeletal surveys. It is often necessary to obtain a plain film of an area that is positive on bone scan to exclude benign disease, such as Paget's disease, arthritis, fractures, and osteomyelitis. Radionuclide bone scanning is rarely positive in patients with a serum PSA less than 10 ng/mL.

Computed tomography (CT) scans are not used routinely because they are insensitive for demonstrating pelvic lymph nodes. These scans may be useful in evaluating patients with high-grade tumors and a high risk of nodal metastases. Fine-needle aspiration plus CT scanning obviates the need for surgical staging, with an obvious decrease in associated morbidity in many of these patients.

Lymphangiography is rarely used. Lymph nodes less than 5 mm in diameter are generally not seen. The hypogastric nodes in general may not be well visualized. In addition, lymphangiography is invasive and often difficult to perform.

Transrectal ultrasonography is of limited use in staging patients with prostate cancer, for example, identifying extracapsular extension and/or seminal vesicle involvement. Occasionally, a patient who appears to have stage C disease clinically is downstaged based on transrectal ultrasound examination; that patient becomes a candidate for surgical cure.

Magnetic resonance imaging (MRI) with an endorectal coil can distinguish normal or benign prostatic tissue from abnormal tissue. Although expensive, MRI can also distinguish pelvic lymph node and bone metastases. The role of MRI in detecting extraprostatic disease is still evolving.

Laboratory Studies

Numerous laboratory studies are obtained in the evaluation of the patient with prostate cancer. Serum prostatic acid phosphatase (PAP) activity is increased in roughly 80 per cent of patients with metastases. However, prostate massage, needle biopsy, and TUR-P also increase the serum PAP (as well as PSA). Patients with increased PAP and a negative bone scan often have pelvic nodal metastases. PAP is not useful for screening.

PSA is a more sensitive and specific test than PAP. PSA is also useful in evaluating response to therapy and falls to zero or near zero, depending on the assay used, after successful radical prostatectomy. Persistent increases indicate residual tumor. PSA is also useful as an indicator of early recurrence. In one study, only 35 per cent of patients treated with radiation had serum PSA below 2.5 ng/mL, and only 13 per cent had undetectable PSA. The reference range for serum PSA is 0 to 4.0 ng/mL.

A complete blood count and a chemistry profile can help the clinician identify anemia, urinary tract obstruction, and liver or bone metastases.

Staging by Surgical Lymphadenectomy

Prostate cancer is understaged clinically in about 50 per cent of men. Therefore, a staging lymphadenectomy is often performed prior to radical prostatectomy. If evidence of more than minimal microscopic lymph node involvement is found, radical prostatectomy is not performed because the chance for cure is nil. A modified or limited node dissection is now performed; less morbidity is encountered, with little difference in detection of metastases. The percentage of patients with positive lymph nodes increases with the grade of tumor. Staging lymphadenectomy is not routinely required in patients who have opted for radiation therapy; however, if laparoscopic node dissection has shown the patient to be free from metastases, limited-field prostatic irradiation can be delivered. Laparoscopic node dissection may also be indicated for patients with a higher risk of metastases (e.g., higher grade, PSA exceeding 20 ng/mL).

CONCLUSION

Digital rectal examination *plus* PSA blood testing is now preferred for identifying patients at risk for prostate cancer. Approximately 10 per cent of patients undergoing a TUR-P for BPH are found to have cancer of the prostate. Treatment is based on the stage of the tumor at the time of presentation. Transrectal ultrasound is useful mainly for directed biopsy; however, neither TRUS nor any radiologic study is recommended for screening. Proper staging allows the selection of the most appropriate treatment, with minimal associated morbidity.

INTRASCROTAL MASSES AND TUMORS

By Joel C. Hutcheson, M.D.,
and Jerome P. Richie, M.D.
Boston, Massachussetts

The majority of intrascrotal masses are associated with benign conditions. More than 70 per cent of intrascrotal masses are caused by infection, hydrocele, and other inflammatory conditions. However, the potential for testicular malignancy, torsion of the spermatic cord, and other serious disorders makes prompt evaluation and management essential. Although accurate diagnosis frequently can be established with only the history and presenting signs and symptoms, some patients require additional laboratory and radiologic testing to distinguish among various disorders, especially those that present with acute onset of scrotal pain. In this article, intrascrotal lesions are discussed in the context in which they typically occur, either associated with acute scrotal pain or as a nontender mass. Note that this schema presents an oversimplification for purposes of organization.

NONACUTE SCROTUM

A nontender, palpable mass, often of long-standing duration, may reflect a benign or malignant process. This section addresses tumors of the testis and adnexae, as well as hernias, hydroceles, varicoceles, sarcoidosis, and spermatoceles.

Testicular Tumors

Presentation

Testicular cancer is the most common malignancy in men between the ages of 15 and 35. A total of 90 to 95 per cent of testicular tumors are of germ cell origin; the remainder are germ cell tumors and metastatic lesions. In men older than 50, lymphoma is the most frequent neoplasm.

The risk factors for testis cancer include cryptorchidism and hormone exposure. Patients with cryptorchidism have a risk of testicular malignancy 20 to 48 times greater than that of the general population. The risk of testicular cancer in patients whose mothers were exposed to diethylstilbestrol is 2.8 to 5.3 per cent higher. Testicular neoplasia may be detected following trauma, but a cause-and-effect relationship has not been demonstrated.

Patients with testicular tumors typically present with a nodule or painless swelling in one gonad. As many as 10 per cent of patients present with pain. A total of 30 to 40 per cent of patients report a dull ache or heavy sensation in the lower abdomen, anal region, or scrotum. Ten per cent of patients present with symptoms attributable to metastases, including dyspnea secondary to pulmonary metastases, bone pain due to skeletal metastases, and lower extremity swelling due to retroperitoneal and iliac adenopathy.

Physical Examination

A testicular mass may be palpable as a discrete nodule or as diffuse enlargement producing asymmetry. Synchronous bilateral tumors are noted in 2 to 3 per cent of patients with testicular lesions; therefore, the contralateral testis should be examined carefully. Acute onset of a hydrocele may occur in conjunction with the tumor and may compromise the physical examination. Hemorrhage within highly vascular lesions may cause acute enlargement. Gynecomastia is noted in five per cent of patients with testicular tumors.

Laboratory Studies

A complete blood count (CBC), urinalysis, and serum chemistries are usually normal, but serum lactate dehydrogenase (LD) activity is commonly increased when bulky metastatic disease is present. Serum alpha-fetoprotein (AFP) and serum beta-human chorionic gonadotropin (β-hCG) are useful as tumor markers but are not specific for testicular malignancy. Serum concentrations of AFP and β-hCG should be measured prior to orchiectomy.

Other Diagnostic Tests

Scrotal ultrasonography is a rapid, reliable, and highly accurate test that should be requested if the clinician has any doubt about the presence of an intratesticular lesion. Clinical staging, routinely performed subsequent to orchiectomy and final pathologic classification, consists of chest films and abdominal-pelvic computed tomography (CT) scans. Bipedal lymphangiography and supraclavicular node biopsy are no longer performed routinely.

Pitfalls in Diagnosis

Testicular malignancies sometimes occur in patients with epididymitis, trauma, and torsion. The clinician should suspect malignancy in any lesion that fails to resolve after an appropriate course of therapy. In any patient with a solid intratesticular mass, cancer must be the working diagnosis until proof of another lesion is obtained.

Non–Germ Cell Tumors

Non–germ cell neoplasms constitute about five to ten per cent of tumors arising in the testis. Most non–germ cell tumors arise from the Leydig or Sertoli cells; only ten per cent are malignant. The presentation of non–germ cell neoplasms is similar to that of germ cell tumors; thus, these lesions are typically diagnosed after orchiectomy.

The epidermoid cyst is a benign tumor arising within the testis; this lesion probably represents a monolayer of teratoma. Most are asymptomatic and present as a painless mass. Epidermoid cysts are typically diagnosed after orchiectomy; frozen-section diagnosis is difficult because these lesions can resemble teratoma. However, surgery that spares the testis and appropriate follow-up surveillance may provide a viable treatment option when the diagnosis is suspected preoperatively.

Paratesticular Tumors

A wide range of benign and malignant tumors arise from the epididymis, tunics, and spermatic cord. Most of these tumors are of mesenchymal origin; approximately 3 per cent are malignant. A majority of paratesticular lesions arise from the spermatic cord—most are lipomas. In most patients, the final diagnosis is established after exploration and histologic evaluation of the surgical specimen.

Epididymis

Most epididymal tumors are benign. Adenomatoid tumors are the most common, followed by leiomyomas and cystadenomas. Most of the malignant tumors are sarcomas; cystadenocarcinomas of the epididymis are rare.

The benign tumors usually present as a painless mass posterior to the testis. Adenomatoid tumors classically occur in the lower pole. Leiomyomas and cystadenomas occur bilaterally in 15 per cent of cases, and cystadenomas are often multiple. An associated hydrocele is present in 20 to 50 per cent of patients. Von Hippel-Lindau disease is noted in 30 to 50 per cent of patients with cystadenomas.

Most of the malignant epididymal tumors are sarcomas; rhabdomyosarcoma is the most common and most aggressive lesion. Both sarcomas and carcinomas typically present as a painful tender mass. Metastases from the stomach, prostate, kidney, colon, and other organs may also manifest as an epididymal mass. Although treatment generally entails orchiectomy, local excision is possible in patients with obviously benign lesions. Adjunctive treatment for sarcomas includes radiotherapy and chemotherapy.

Spermatic Cord

Lipomas, fibromas, dermoid cysts, and remnants of the wolffian duct (mesonephros) all may present as a benign cord mass. Lipomas are by far the most common growths arising in the spermatic cord. Lipomas and cysts are soft and mobile on physical examination and may mimic a hernia or hydrocele. Fibromas are usually hard, nontender masses and may be suspected of being malignancies.

Sarcomas, the most common malignancies of the spermatic cord, usually arise from the scrotal cord. Sarcomas are rarely diagnosed preoperatively; they often mimic hernias or hydroceles. When the diagnosis is suspected, ultrasonography and CT may help characterize these lesions. Benign lesions are usually diagnosed at the time of surgery. The highest survival rates in patients with sarcomas are achieved with extirpative surgery, followed by radiation or chemotherapy.

Scrotal Tunic Tumors

Fibromas of the tunics present as a painless mass or masses and may be located anywhere in the scrotum. Fibromas can usually be distinguished from the testicle. Rhabdomyosarcoma, the most common malignancy of the tunics, usually presents as a painless, hard mass.

Mesotheliomas of the tunic are extremely rare and present as a painless, firm mass. Fifteen per cent are malignant. As in mesotheliomas arising elsewhere, asbestos exposure and trauma may be risk factors. Mesotheliomas often occur in association with a hydrocele. Treatment has not been standardized, but surgical excision and close follow-up are essential.

Other Painless Masses

Sarcoidosis

Sarcoidosis is a multisystem granulomatous disease of uncertain etiology that rarely affects the genitourinary tract. Nevertheless, sarcoidosis may occur as a testicular and/or epididymal mass that may be the only detectable manifestation of the disease. Granulomatous inflammation leads to irreversible fibrosis and a hard, nontender mass. Preoperative diagnosis is often difficult but may be suspected in a patient with a scrotal mass and evidence of sarcoidosis elsewhere. Patients are usually explored for final tissue diagnosis because testicular tumors have been reported in patients with genitourinary sarcoidosis.

Hernias

Inguinal hernias can usually be diagnosed by the history and physical examination. A reducible mass and abdominal wall defect are usually palpated in the scrotum and/or groin. A more detailed discussion is found elsewhere in this text.

Spermatocele and Epididymal Cyst

Spermatoceles and epididymal cysts are benign cystic lesions that have been detected in as many as forty per cent of asymptomatic individuals presenting for ultrasonography. These two lesions can be distinguished only by the presence or absence of sperm in aspirated fluid. Spermatoceles and epididymal cysts are often subclinical and are frequently diagnosed at ultrasonography requested for other reasons. These lesions typically measure less than one cm but may grow as large as 3 cm and are located at the head of the epididymis. Treatment is not indicated in the absence of discomfort.

Hydroceles

The parietal and visceral layers of the tunica vaginalis form a potential space in which serous fluid may collect and form a hydrocele. Hydroceles may be congenital, idiopathic, secondary to tumors or inflammation, or related to renal transplantation. Congenital hydroceles occur in neonates with a patent processus vaginalis. These hydroceles often resolve during the first year of life as the processus closes. Adult patients typically present with a painless scrotal mass; discomfort may be noted in some larger hydroceles. Lymphatic obstruction due to filariasis is a common cause of hydroceles in areas where the parasitic infection is endemic.

On physical examination, the hydrocele may surround the ipsilateral testis or may be entirely separate from it and occur higher on the cord. Transillumination enables the examiner to distinguish the hydrocele from solid lesions. However, if the testis and cord structures cannot be thoroughly examined, or if a solid mass is suspected, scrotal ultrasonography should be requested.

Treatment is usually conservative for asymptomatic hydroceles. In the symptomatic patient, aspiration and sclerosis has a high recurrence rate; surgical treatment is quite effective for most patients.

Varicocele

Dilatation and tortuous elongation of the veins that constitute the pampiniform plexus can result in a clinically detectable varicocele. Although present in as many as twenty per cent of normal males, varicoceles have been noted in 39 per cent of males presenting to infertility clinics. Patients may report a nontender, soft mass or infertility. Sudden development of a varicocele in an older man is an ominous sign and may indicate possible renal vein invasion by a renal tumor.

Diagnosis is usually based on palpation of a plexus of distended veins. Most varicoceles arise on the left side. The patient should be examined in the standing position to maximize distention of the veins. Asking the patient to initiate a Valsalva maneuver may cause the veins to engorge. Ultrasonography may reveal subclinical varicoceles in infertile patients with abnormal semen parameters and an equivocal physical examination.

Treatment of infertile men with varicoceles is safe and effective and thus is commonly undertaken. By contrast, treatment of varicoceles in adolescents is controversial.

Some urologists favor treatment only of those patients who develop clinically detectable atrophy after months to years.

ACUTE SCROTUM

The patient presenting with acute scrotal pain represents a *clinical emergency.* The decision to undertake surgery is challenging because the presentation of some nonsurgical and surgical conditions may be quite similar. Conditions known to produce pain in the scrotum include inflammation, infection, trauma, and vascular lesions, especially torsion of the spermatic cord. These diseases, as discussed here, should form the framework for a differential diagnosis of the acute scrotum.

Epididymo-orchitis

Epididymitis, orchitis, and epididymo-orchitis represent inflammatory conditions of the epidiymis and/or testis that may occur unilaterally or bilaterally. An infectious etiology is most common, and orchitis typically develops from ascending infection due to epididymitis. Trauma and exposure to amiodarone have also been associated with epididymitis. Tuberculous epididymo-orchitis is relatively uncommon. Most patients with epididymo-orchitis experience the gradual onset of scrotal pain over hours to days. Urethritis or cystitis may also develop, with characteristic symptoms of dysuria, frequency, and urgency. In men younger than 35 years of age, the most common pathogens are *Chlamydia* and *Neisseria gonorrhoeae*. In men older than 35, enteric gram-negative organisms are the most common pathogens. Infection in older men is usually related to urethral instrumentation or obstruction of the urinary tract.

On physical examination, most patients with epididymo-orchitis are febrile. The scrotum may be hyperemic, with edema and loss of rugae as the illness progresses. A reactive hydrocele may be observed. The epididymis is indurated and tender to palpation; abscess formation may be detected as fluctuation. The inflamed testis is swollen, tense, and tender. Relief of pain with elevation of the affected side (Prehn's sign) is unreliable and may give false-positive results when one attempts to distinguish epididymitis from torsion. The urethral meatus should be inspected for urethral discharge.

Diagnostic Tests

The white blood cell count is often increased in acute epididymitis and may help distinguish this lesion from acute torsion, in which the count is usually normal. Urinalysis often reveals leukocytes and bacteria. Culture of the abnormal urine may guide therapy, and culture of urethral swabs is appropriate if a discharge is observed.

To exclude the presence of torsion, Doppler ultrasonography and radionuclide scintigraphy are sometimes requested. A pattern of increased flow or marker accumulation may be related to the hyperemia of infection or inflammation. However, the clinician should not place absolute faith in these tests because false-negative results are noted. Ultrasonography may also demonstrate the presence of an abscess.

Treatment with the appropriate antibiotic is based on clinical presentation, suspected pathogens, and culture results. Oral antibiotics are usually sufficient, but if the patient shows signs of urosepsis or is otherwise debilitated (e.g., by persistent nausea and vomiting), admission for intravenous antibiotics and closer monitoring should be considered. Surgical intervention is routinely required when an abscess is present.

Mumps orchitis occurs without antecedent epididymitis. One third of adult males with paramyxoviral infection develop orchitis; the infection is bilateral in 16 to 65 per cent of cases. Most patients experience testicular pain and swelling, along with malaise, fever, and bilateral parotitis. Early treatment with interferon alpha-2b may reduce the risk of testicular atrophy and subsequent infertility.

Trauma

Blunt and penetrating trauma may cause serious injury to the scrotum and its contents. Virtually all penetrating scrotal injuries should be explored for potential injury to the testes and cord structures. Rupture of the testis should be suspected in any patient who has sustained blunt trauma to the inguinoscrotal region. Disruption of the tunica albuginea may cause protrusion of the seminiferous tubules and is usually associated with hematocele or a collection of blood between the layers of the tunica vaginalis. Blunt trauma may also cause scrotal hematoma, hematocele, or intratesticular hematoma without associated rupture.

Patients with trauma usually present in severe distress. The pain is often accompanied by nausea and vomiting. Physical examination typically reveals an ecchymotic scrotum. The hematocele, if present, is palpable as a soft mass around the testis. The scrotum is often exquisitely tender, and appropriate examination can be difficult.

Testicular rupture is a surgical emergency and early exploration may reduce the risk of testicular loss due to necrosis or secondary infection. Clinical symptoms alone do not enable the clinician to distinguish testicular rupture from conditions that may be treated conservatively (e.g., scrotal hematoma). Ultrasonography may help the clinician distinguish hematoma from hematocele and may also demonstrate disruption of the tunica albuginea. Some clinicians advocate treating patients with blunt testicular trauma and no hematocele with observation, bedrest, and scrotal elevation. However, the presence of a hematocele is related to rupture, and thus these patients should be explored. Unequivocal findings on ultrasonography mandate immediate surgical intervention.

Torsion of the Spermatic Cord

Torsion of the spermatic cord requires prompt diagnosis and surgical intervention if the testis is to be saved. Irreversible damage to the testis can occur within four to six hours if the torsion is left untreated. The presentation of torsion may be mistaken for that of epididymitis, causing a delay in diagnosis and treatment. The diagnosis of torsion often must be made on clinical grounds alone.

Torsion typically occurs in postpubertal adolescents but can occur in any age group. As opposed to the gradual onset of pain in acute epididymitis, the classic presentation is one of acute onset of pain, often awakening the patient from sleep. There may be a history of recent similar attacks that resolved spontaneously. The patient may even note that twisting the testis relieved the symptoms. The pain is usually severe. Nausea, vomiting, and anorexia are frequently reported. Most patients with torsion typically lie motionless because movement intensifies their discomfort.

On physical examination, the affected testis is often tense and swollen. A reactive hydrocele may be present. Usually no fever is present. As discussed earlier, elevation of the scrotum classically does not relieve the pain, but this is an unreliable sign. The cremasteric reflex is usually absent on the affected side. The testis may have a "horizontal lie," with the poles oriented in the transverse plane.

The leukocyte count is usually normal, as is the urinalysis. Imaging studies can be helpful in the decision-making process but should not be obtained if they will cause an unnecessary delay in treatment. In fact, when there is little doubt of the diagnosis, imaging studies should not be obtained. In patients in whom the diagnosis is questionable, radionuclide scintigraphy and scrotal ultrasonography with Doppler flow have reasonable sensitivity and specificity, exceeding ninety per cent. Ultrasonography is considered less reliable by some because of its dependence on the experience of the examiner. The main pitfall in both modalities is that in very early torsion, arterial blood flow to the testis can often be detected. At scrotal exploration, the affected side is detorsed and then fixed to the scrotal tunics. Orchiopexy is then performed on the contralateral side owing to the risk of torsion on that side.

The presentation of patients with torsion of the appendix testis may be similar to that of patients with torsion of the spermatic cord. If the pain is localized to the upper pole of the testis and the classic "blue dot" sign (the necrosed appendage visible through the scrotal skin) is observed, conservative treatment is indicated. In these patients, a radionuclide scan or Doppler ultrasonography can demonstrate normal blood flow to the testis.

INTERSTITIAL NEPHRITIS

By Andre A. Kaplan, M.D.,
and Orly F. Kohn, M.D.
Farmington, Connecticut

The term interstitial nephritis describes a major group of kidney diseases in which pathologic renal features are most prominent in the interstitial compartment, with relative sparing of the glomeruli. Most forms of interstitial nephritis present with a reduction in creatinine clearance, often accompanied by modest proteinuria (<2 g per day). Tubular disorders (e.g., renal tubular acidosis, urinary concentrating defects, hyper- or hypokalemia, and magnesium wasting) may dominate the clinical picture. The interstitial nephritides are usefully classified as acute or chronic because the clinical presentations are often distinctly different. There are, however, well-known types of interstitial nephritis that are associated with acute and chronic forms (e.g., oxalate deposition and autoimmune disorders) (Table 1).

Table 1. Interstitial Nephritides

Acute Interstitial Nephritis	Chronic Interstitial Nephritis	Immune Complex–Mediated Nephritis
Drug-induced (see Table 3)	Analgesic abuse	Lupus erythematosus
Infectious	Lithium nephropathy	Sjögren's syndrome
Oxalate nephropathy	Cyclosporine nephropathy	
	Urate nephropathy	
	Oxalate nephropathy	
	Hypercalcemic nephropathy	
	Sarcoidosis	
	Radiation nephritis	
	Metal intoxication: lead, cadmium, and so on	

Table 2. Clinical Setting of Acute Interstitial Nephritis

Recent increase in creatinine (days to weeks)
No evidence of volume contraction or hydronephrosis
Occasionally with flank pain
Occasionally with oliguria and dark-colored urine
Normal or enlarged kidneys
Often with hyperkalemia and hyperphosphatemia
Urinalysis
  Hematuria, pyuria, white cell casts, modest proteinuria (<2 g per day)

Acute interstitial nephritis (AIN) is suspected when a rapid increase in serum creatinine concentration is associated with drug hypersensitivity or infection (Table 2). Renal inflammation and acute distention of the renal capsule frequently produce flank pain. Results of urine chemistry panels are not well characterized, but a fractional excretion of sodium greater than 1 per cent in the setting of oliguric renal failure (<500 mL per day) is a sign of tubular dysfunction similar to that observed with acute tubular necrosis. Hypertension is not as common in AIN as it is in glomerular disorders. Fever, rash, and eosinophilia suggest drug hypersensitivity. Perhaps most characteristic of AIN are pyuria and white cell casts. If AIN is related to drug allergy or viral infection, the standard urine culture will not produce microorganisms.

Chronic interstitial nephritis is far more difficult to identify because the presentation is insidious and urinary findings may be unimpressive. Suspicion of chronic interstitial nephritis is most often raised when slowly increasing serum creatinine concentrations and modest proteinuria (<2 g per day) cannot be attributed to diabetic nephropathy, hypertensive nephrosclerosis, or polycystic kidney disease. Support for the diagnosis of chronic interstitial nephritis is often provided by a history of chronic analgesic abuse, prolonged cyclosporine therapy, or occupational exposure to lead or cadmium. The diagnosis of interstitial nephritis requires confirmation by renal biopsy. However, the histopathologic changes seldom reflect a specific cause, and the background history remains the major factor in determining the etiology.

ACUTE INTERSTITIAL NEPHRITIS

Allergic Interstitial Nephritis

Allergic interstitial nephritis has been described as acute renal failure in patients with fever, rash, and eosinophilia. Importantly, however, only 30 per cent of patients exhibit the complete triad. The incidence of presenting signs and symptoms is listed in Table 3. The drugs most commonly implicated include antibiotics, diuretics, and nonsteroidal anti-inflammatory drugs (NSAIDs) (Table 4). Following

Table 3. Incidence of Presenting Signs and Symptoms of Drug-Induced Allergic Interstitial Nephritis

Proteinuria	80%	Rash	40%
Hematuria	90%	Fever	75%
Pyuria	80%	Eosinophilia	80%
Eosinophiluria	80%	Fever, rash, eosinophilia	30%

Table 4. Drug-Induced Interstitial Nephritis

Antibiotics
Penicillins, cephalosporins, sulfonamides, rifampin, para-aminosalicylic acid, nitrofurantoin
NSAIDs
All—can present with proteinuria in the nephrotic range
Diuretics
Thiazides, furosemide, chlorthalidone, ethacrynic acid
ACE inhibitors
Captopril, enalapril
Anticonvulsants
Phenobarbital, phenytoin
Miscellaneous
Allopurinol, cimetidine, omeprazole

NSAIDs = nonsteroidal anti-inflammatory drugs; ACE = angiotensin-converting enzyme.

primary exposure, symptoms may not be manifested for several weeks. By contrast, in patients with prior exposure, symptoms may develop within a few days. Allergic interstitial nephritis should be suspected when there is a history of recent drug exposure and urinalysis indicates sterile pyuria with or without leukocyte casts. Proteinuria is usually modest but may be in the nephrotic range (>3 g per day) if there is an associated minimal-change glomerulopathy, described most often with NSAIDs. Eosinophilia and eosinophiluria support the diagnosis, but their absence is common, particularly in NSAID-induced interstitial nephritis. Eosinophiluria is most commonly sought with Wright's staining of the urinary sediment and has been defined as a ratio of urine eosinophil count to urine total leukocyte count of at least 30 per cent. By contrast, with Hansel's stain of the urine, eosinophiluria is diagnosed if eosinophils compose more than 1 per cent of the urinary leukocytes. Although Hansel's stain is considered more sensitive than Wright's stain, it appears to be less specific because it identifies eosinophiluria in a substantial percentage of patients with rapidly progressive glomerulonephritis, prostatitis, and cholesterol emboli. Renal ultrasound demonstrates normal to enlarged kidneys. Gallium scanning often shows prolonged (>72 hours), intense, bilateral renal uptake, but this finding can also be seen in acute glomerulonephritis, bilateral pyelonephritis, and nephrotic syndromes. Unilateral uptake of gallium strongly suggests infectious pyelonephritis. The fractional excretion of sodium often exceeds 1 per cent, rendering prerenal azotemia unlikely. Although the diagnosis is best supported by a renal biopsy showing intense interstitial inflammation, the diagnosis is typically made presumptively; the offending drug is then discontinued and the patient is observed for recovery. Most patients with drug-induced interstitial nephritis recover in a few weeks. A short trial of steroids may shorten the course of the disease if renal dysfunction is severe and recovery is not manifested within 1 to 2 weeks of discontinuance of the suspected offending agent.

Infections and Interstitial Nephritis

As a primary infection localized in the interstitium of the kidney, pyelonephritis can be considered an interstitial nephritis. In addition, some systemic infections tend to cause interstitial nephritis, especially infections associated with streptococci, diphtheria, leprosy, syphilis, leptospirosis, and several viruses. Most infectious causes of interstitial nephritis can be identified with routine bacterial culture of the urine. Viral infections of the interstitium often present with systemic manifestations that may dominate the clinical picture. Adenovirus infection is most often suspected in immunocompromised hosts with massive urinary tract hemorrhage, but adenovirus may also cause acute renal failure. The diagnosis of adenovirus-induced interstitial nephritis is supported by culturing adenovirus from the urine, but a positive viral culture does not distinguish renal involvement from a purely lower urinary tract infection. Renal biopsy is rarely performed because these patients are typically thrombocytopenic.

A unique form of bacterial interstitial nephritis that can lead to renal failure is malacoplakia. Patients typically present with symptoms of pyelonephritis, urinalysis showing full-field pyuria, a culture positive for coliform bacteria, and a gallium scan that is intensely positive. The response to antibiotic therapy is slow because the patients have a defect in bacterial clearance by macrophages. The renal biopsy is diagnostic when von Hansemman bodies are observed.

A disease of recent interest in the United States is the hemorrhagic fever and renal syndrome caused by the Hantaan virus. This virus is spread by inhalation of rodent feces, and it typically causes endothelial damage that leads to widespread microvascular hemorrhage and shock. The disorder was originally recognized by American physicians during the Korean war and was labeled Korean hemorrhagic fever. A recent outbreak in the southwestern United States was dominated by pulmonary manifestations. Hantaan virus has a broad distribution and is a major cause of renal failure in Eurasia and Scandinavia. The disease is recognized by the progression of symptoms from fever to shock, renal failure, and convalescence. Renal biopsy reveals interstitial hemorrhage rather than inflammation. The diagnosis can be confirmed with appropriate antibody tests available from the Centers for Disease Control and Prevention and a few commercial laboratories.

CHRONIC INTERSTITIAL NEPHRITIS

Analgesic Nephropathy

Renal damage is associated with the chronic, massive ingestion of mixed analgesics containing aspirin, phenacetin, and acetaminophen. Analgesic nephropathy has been considered to be the cause of end-stage renal disease in 30 per cent of all dialysis patients in Australia but is diagnosed less often in the United States. The typical patient is a middle-aged woman with chronic discomfort who has consumed several kilograms of analgesics over a period of years. Renal damage may be accompanied by gastritis or peptic ulcer disease due to chronic ingestion of NSAIDs. Renal insufficiency is slowly progressive, and the urinary sediment varies from bland to sterile pyuria. Renal biopsy in the early stages reveals patchy necrosis of the interstitium of the inner medulla. Papillary necrosis may be the first indication of the disease and can present with ureteral obstruction, flank pain, and hematuria. Papillary necrosis can be detected by intravenous or retrograde pyelography or, less accurately, by renal ultrasound. This lesion is not specific to analgesic nephropathy and may be seen in other conditions (diabetes, sickle cell disease and trait, urinary tract obstruction). With advanced disease, the kidneys shrink and become more echogenic. The calyces are often blunted. Analgesic abusers may also have increased risk of urologic tumors; a full evaluation is appropriate if hematuria develops.

Lithium-Induced Nephropathy

Long-term (10 to 15 years) use of lithium has been associated with a microcystic form of chronic interstitial nephritis. It is uncommon, however, for the renal damage to progress to substantial renal failure. Occasionally, acute lithium intoxication causes tubular injury and acute renal failure. The most common renal abnormality associated with lithium use is nephrogenic diabetes insipidus resulting in polyuria and nocturia.

Uric Acid Nephropathy

Excessive uric acid may cause three patterns of renal disease known as (1) uric acid lithiasis, which is the formation of uric acid stones; (2) acute urate nephropathy, characterized by massive tubular deposition of uric acid following chemotherapy-induced tumor lysis; and (3) urate nephropathy, which is a chronic nephritis characterized by sodium urate deposition in the interstitium.

Postmortem studies indicate that most patients with gout have some renal damage associated with urate deposition in the interstitium. However, a direct correlation between increased serum uric acid concentrations and decreased renal function has not been shown. Several authors believe that urate nephropathy does not occur unless there is comorbidity with hypertension, obesity, or diabetes. One study suggests that all patients with renal dysfunction secondary to uric acid actually have lead nephropathy. At present, treatment of chronic hyperuricemia is not recommended in the absence of gouty arthritis or uric acid lithiasis.

Oxalate Nephropathy

Calcium oxalate is a highly insoluble salt that will precipitate in various tissues as a result of increased oxalate production or absorption. Oxalate deposits in the kidney can result from inherited enzyme deficiencies (primary hyperoxalosis) or acquired increases in oxalate absorption or production. Primary hyperoxalosis usually presents early in life with recurrent kidney stones, pain, hematuria, and pyuria, leading to end-stage renal disease before the age of 20 years. Acquired hyperoxaluria due to increased absorption of oxalate may accompany small bowel resection, malabsorption syndromes, chronic pancreatitis, and Wilson's disease. Increased production of oxalate may follow the ingestion of ethylene glycol (antifreeze) or large doses of ascorbic acid or the administration of methoxyflurane anesthetic. Pyridoxine deficiency can decrease the conversion of glyoxylic acid to glycine, facilitating glyoxylate metabolism to oxalate.

Renal biopsy in chronic oxalate nephropathy reveals oxalate deposits within the interstitium sometimes surrounded by a fibrotic reaction that may include giant cells. The deposits are strongly birefringent with polarized light. In patients with recurrent urinary stones, the diagnosis can be made by demonstrating hyperoxaluria in a 24-hour urine collection. Normal patients produce 15 to 30 mg per day/1.73 m^2, whereas patients with hyperoxaluria produce 50 to 250 mg per day/1.73 m^2.

Acute oxalate nephropathy can result from ingestion of ethylene glycol (antifreeze) or the administration of methoxyflurane. Under these conditions, deposition of calcium oxalate crystals within the tubules can cause a clinical picture of acute tubular necrosis. The diagnosis can be supported by the observation of birefringent, square, envelope-shaped crystals in the urine sediment. Unfortunately, this finding is not diagnostic because the poorly soluble calcium oxalate can precipitate even in normal urine, especially if the sample is allowed to cool.

Hypercalcemic Nephropathy

Acute renal manifestations of hypercalcemia include nephrogenic diabetes insipidus, renal tubular acidosis, and hypertension. These abnormalities can be reversed with correction of the serum calcium concentration. Prolonged hypercalcemia associated with primary hyperparathyroidism, bone metastases, multiple myeloma, vitamin D intoxication, or sarcoidosis can lead to nephrocalcinosis with interstitial and intraluminal deposition of calcium, interstitial fibrosis, and tubular atrophy. The diagnosis of hypercalcemic nephropathy is further supported by radiographic demonstration of scattered flecks of intrarenal calcification. Definitive diagnosis, however, requires renal biopsy.

Cyclosporine Nephropathy

Cyclosporine is a potent immunosuppressive agent that has been used to prevent organ transplant rejection and to treat uveitis, early insulin-dependent diabetes mellitus, rheumatoid arthritis, inflammatory bowel disease, severe psoriasis, and other autoimmune conditions. During high-dose intravenous administration, cyclosporine predictably causes renal vasoconstriction, decreased renal perfusion, and low fractional excretion of sodium and urea. Oligoanuria may ensue but is rapidly reversible when serum drug concentrations decline. Prolonged use of cyclosporine has been associated with progressive, irreversible renal failure due to chronic, fibrosing, interstitial nephritis. In some patients, the renal failure can progress to end-stage renal disease, especially in heart transplant recipients. The serum creatinine concentration, which is not a sensitive marker of cyclosporine-induced renal failure, rises over the course of months to years. The onset of hyperkalemia, hypomagnesemia, and hyperuricemia may reflect defects in tubular transport. The urinalysis is usually bland. Renal biopsy reveals ischemic collapse and scarring of glomeruli accompanied by "striped" interstitial fibrosis and tubular atrophy. Stripes of interstitial fibrosis and atrophic tubules may alternate with normal-appearing interstitium. The diagnosis is usually suspected on clinical grounds, most commonly in an organ transplant recipient receiving high-dose, maintenance cyclosporine therapy. The diagnosis can be confirmed only by renal biopsy. In the kidney transplant recipient, other causes of renal dysfunction (e.g., transplant rejection) must be excluded.

Sarcoidosis

Although interstitial nephritis with granuloma formation is histologically common in patients with sarcoidosis, it rarely leads to renal failure. By contrast, nephrocalcinosis, which can be seen on renal tomograms, may lead to impaired renal function in patients with sarcoidosis. Systemic signs of sarcoidosis usually precede or present concomitantly with the renal dysfunction. Hypercalcemia and hypercalciuria secondary to increased production of 1,25-dihydroxyvitamin D may respond favorably to treatment with corticosteroids.

Radiation Nephritis

With improvement in radiation therapy methods, attention to cumulative dose, and precise localization of delivery ports, radiation nephritis has become a rare disease. Nevertheless, clinicians must be familiar with the presentation of this disorder because total body irradiation and intense chemotherapy are still provided in many bone marrow transplantation protocols. Patients receiving more than 20

Gy to the kidney may present within 6 months to a year with renal insufficiency often associated with severe hypertension and disproportionate anemia. Urinalysis typically shows modest proteinuria and microscopic hematuria. Renal insufficiency progresses to end-stage renal disease. Patients who have received less than 20 Gy may present years after radiation therapy with a decline in renal function, hypertension, and a reduction in kidney size. Renal biopsy reveals interstitial fibrosis, glomerular sclerosis, and scarcity of inflammatory infiltrates.

Lead Nephropathy

Chronic lead exposure (e.g., from moonshine alcohol or occupational exposure in welders and battery workers) can result in chronic interstitial nephritis associated with hyperuricemia, gout, and hypertension. A normal blood lead concentration is not uncommon and does not exclude the diagnosis of lead nephropathy. X-ray fluorescence or an ethylenediamine tetraacetic acid (EDTA) infusion test may provide evidence of an excessive body burden of lead.

IMMUNE COMPLEX–MEDIATED INTERSTITIAL NEPHRITIS

Peritubular granular deposits of immunoglobulins and complement are found in up to two thirds of patients with lupus nephritis, especially those with glomerular lesions. Pure interstitial nephritis without glomerular involvement is rare in patients with systemic lupus erythematosus. Interstitial involvement may be suspected in the presence of renal glucosuria, renal tubular acidosis, or hyperkalemia secondary to defective tubular function.

Interstitial nephritis with lymphocytic infiltration can be seen in Sjögren's syndrome. This may progress to interstitial fibrosis and tubular atrophy. Urinalysis often produces benign results, but proximal and distal renal tubular acidosis, nephrogenic diabetes insipidus, and severe hypokalemia due to renal potassium wasting may be prominent.

Section Fifteen

GYNECOLOGIC MEDICINE

BREAST CANCER

By Susan Rosenthal, M.D.,
and Deborah Rubens, M.D.
Rochester, New York

EPIDEMIOLOGY AND ETIOLOGY

Breast cancer is the most common malignant disease of women and the second leading cause of cancer deaths after lung cancer among women in the United States. It currently accounts for 32 per cent of new cancers in American women and 18 per cent of cancer deaths in this group. In 1996, 185,700 new cases of breast cancer and 44,560 deaths from this disease occurred in the United States. About one in every eight American women will acquire breast cancer at some time during her life—a risk that was 1 in every 14 in 1960.

Breast cancer incidence becomes appreciable at about age 30 years, and the incidence rate increases with each succeeding decade. About 6 per cent of breast cancers occur in women younger than 40 years of age. No American woman is at "low risk" for this malignancy, but epidemiologic studies have identified women who are at higher than average risk. Those who have a first-degree relative with breast cancer have a risk two to three times that of the general population, and this risk increases further if the relative had breast cancer at an early age or had bilateral disease. Women with fibrocystic changes in the breasts are not at increased risk unless atypical hyperplasia is recognized in a biopsy specimen.

The recent identification of *BRCA1,* a susceptibility gene for inherited breast and ovarian cancer, suggests that genetic screening for families with inherited breast cancer may become a reality in the foreseeable future. Women who carry a germline mutation in the *BRCA1* gene have an 85 per cent lifetime risk of breast cancer (50 per cent before age 50 years). Two to 4 per cent of all cases of breast cancer may result from mutations in the *BRCA1* gene on chromosome 17. The role of the *BRCA1* gene in sporadic breast cancers, which account for the vast majority of cases of the disease, remains uncertain.

SCREENING

The goal of cancer screening is the detection of early, potentially curable cancers in asymptomatic individuals in the general population and in high-risk groups. Screening for breast cancer using the combination of physical examination of the breasts and mammography has clearly proved effective. Screening detects smaller and lower stage breast cancers, with consequent improvement in survival. The effects of physician examination, self-examination by the patient, and mammography are hard to separate, but all contribute to the early detection of breast cancer. The American Cancer Society currently recommends that

- Women older than age 20 years should perform breast self-examination every month
- Women between the ages of 20 and 40 years should have a breast examination by a physician every 3 years; women aged 40 years and older should have a yearly breast examination
- Women between the ages of 40 and 50 years should undergo mammography every 1 to 2 years, and women age 50 years and older should undergo annual mammography

Women at high risk (family history of breast cancer in a first-degree relative, previous breast cancer, previous breast biopsy showing atypical hyperplasia) require more intensive screening, beginning at an earlier age.

Tremendous controversy surrounds the issue of screening mammography in women between the ages of 40 and 50 years. A number of studies have failed to demonstrate a survival benefit in this group, but screening proponents point to flaws in these trials and to their failure to study sufficiently large groups of women to permit detection of a beneficial effect (beta error). Most oncologists, radiologists, and surgeons strongly support the American Cancer Society recommendations for screening mammography in this age group, and many urge annual screening (rather than biannual) for these women.

Mammography in Asymptomatic Women

Positive findings detected with screening mammography include abnormal microcalcifications, soft tissue mass, soft tissue asymmetry, and distortion of the normal breast architecture. An ultrasound examination of a focal nonpalpable mass may demonstrate a simple cyst; such a diagnosis under these circumstances is highly reliable, and no further intervention is required. Other nonpalpable mammographic abnormalities may be subjected to close follow-up at 3- to 6-month intervals or, if suspicious for malignancy, biopsied immediately by fine-needle aspiration (FNA) or core-needle biopsy (often under ultrasound guidance), stereotactic biopsy, or excisional biopsy with needle localization.

The overall sensitivity of screening mammography is 75 to 80 per cent. Mammography is more likely to miss breast cancers in young women with dense breasts and in women with lobular carcinomas. Approximately 45 per cent of cancers are detected by mammography alone. About 25 to 35 per cent of biopsies recommended for nonpalpable lesions seen on mammography reveal cancer.

Needle Localization Biopsy

Biopsy of a mammographically detected, nonpalpable lesion poses a problem for the surgeon. In this situation, the radiologist and the surgeon collaborate to perform a biopsy with needle localization technique. The radiologist localizes the lesion and passes a very fine needle into it under mammographic guidance; methylene blue dye is injected, and the localization wire is left in place to guide the surgeon to the lesion. Most localizations do not require anesthesia or sedation; they are performed as outpatient procedures in the mammography suite immediately prior to surgery. The patient is then taken to the operating room for an excisional biopsy, usually performed under local anesthesia.

PALPABLE BREAST MASSES

Clinical Presentation

Breast cancer usually presents as a painless mass detected by the patient herself or by the physician during the course of a routine physical examination. All palpable breast masses must be evaluated, but certain characteristics—hardness, immobility, fixation to skin, satellite lesions, peau d'orange skin changes, and axillary adenopathy—strongly suggest malignancy. Bloody discharge from the nipple may be an initial symptom; an underlying mass is usually present. A swollen, tender, inflamed breast is usually caused by acute mastitis but may be due to inflammatory breast cancer. Neglected breast cancers can present as large, malodorous masses with ulceration of the skin and, sometimes, with destruction of the entire breast.

Patients themselves and inexperienced examiners often express concern over lumpy breasts or fibrocystic disease (a nondisease). Both of these terms refer to a normal physiologic condition: increased nodularity in the breast as a result of hormonal stimulation, either in premenopausal women or in postmenopausal women who are taking replacement hormones. Premenopausal women should optimally be examined 5 to 7 days after the onset of menses, a time when hormonal effects on the breast are minimal. If the examiner is uncertain about the significance of a palpable abnormality, the patient should be re-examined in 1 to 3 months to ascertain whether the suspected lesion really is present. Once the examiner convinces himself or herself that a dominant mass is present, biopsy is indicated (see further on). All patients with palpable breast masses should undergo bilateral mammography, primarily to detect other, clinically occult lesions. (Patients younger than 30 to 35 years of age should undergo ultrasonography rather than mammography. If the ultrasound reveals anything other than a simple cyst, these patients should also have mammograms.)

The role of ultrasonography in the evaluation of palpable breast masses is controversial. Some authorities, particularly radiologists, recommend ultrasonography for all palpable masses. If the ultrasound examination shows a cyst, these authorities advise observation only. Solid masses, however, require biopsy by either fine-needle aspiration or surgical excision. Other authorities, particularly surgeons, believe that ultrasonography is unnecessary in the evaluation of palpable breast masses and that every such mass should be biopsied. If the mass is a cyst that can be evacuated, the patient is spared the expense of an ultrasound examination, and no further intervention is required. Any solid mass, regardless of findings on imaging studies, requires FNA and cytologic evaluation.

Fine-Needle Aspiration

Fine-needle aspiration permits the distinction of cystic from solid masses. If fluid is aspirated and the cyst disappears, no further evaluation is necessary unless the fluid is bloody. If the lesion is solid, the FNA may yield sufficient cellular material for a cytologic diagnosis of malignancy. In this case, the next step is discussion of treatment options with the patient (lumpectomy plus breast irradiation versus modified radical mastectomy). However, confirmation by frozen-section evaluation during the surgical procedure is strongly recommended to detect the very rare instance of a false-positive cytologic diagnosis.

If the FNA yields normal or suspicious material, or if a mass persists after aspiration of a cyst, excisional biopsy is required. Biopsy may reveal cancer or various benign conditions, including fat necrosis, scar tissue, sclerosing adenosis, fibroadenoma, intraductal papilloma, hematoma, and cyst.

STAGING OF BREAST CANCER

Clinical Staging

After a diagnosis of breast cancer has been made following FNA, needle biopsy, or excisional biopsy, clinical staging should be undertaken before local therapy is considered. In most cases, a thorough history and physical examination with attention to common sites of metastases (regional lymph nodes, lungs, pleura, bones, liver), and a routine complete blood count, chest film, and screening blood chemistries are sufficient. If signs or symptoms or abnormal test results suggest the possibility of metastases, further diagnostic evaluation should precede surgical intervention. For example, in a patient who reports severe back pain, a bone scan is indicated to evaluate for possible bone metastases. If serum chemistries reveal unexplained abnormalities of liver function tests, computed tomography (CT) of the upper abdomen should be performed to assess the liver. An unexplained increase of serum alkaline phosphatase justifies a bone scan. In the absence of signs or symptoms or of abnormalities in blood work or the chest film, screening imaging studies for metastases are unnecessary.

Certain clinical findings in patients with locally advanced breast cancer denote inoperability, at least with curative intent, and suggest the need for local irradiation and/or systemic therapy as the initial treatment. These findings include supraclavicular adenopathy; edema of the arm; large, fixed axillary lymph nodes; ulceration of the tumor; fixation of the tumor to the chest wall; satellite skin nodules; and inflammatory carcinoma.

Surgical Staging

Surgical staging consisting of operative and histopathologic evaluation results in the assignment of a TNM (tumor, nodes, metastases) stage, which then indicates the need for further local and/or systemic therapy and provides prognostic information. TNM staging of breast cancer is universal, and physicians dealing with this disease must be conversant with the TNM definitions for breast cancer.

Pathologic Evaluation

Full evaluation of a lumpectomy or mastectomy specimen should include tumor size, histologic type, nuclear grade, determination of the presence or absence of lymphatic and/or blood vessel invasion, determination of involvement of surgical margins, and report of positive axillary lymph nodes (if any). Each of these factors has prognostic significance and, in combination with receptor concentrations and oncogene and other assays (see further on), may indicate the need for systemic adjuvant therapy.

Breast cancer specimens can also be analyzed for S phase and ploidy (flow cytometry) and for various oncogenes, proteins, growth factors, and growth factor receptors. These parameters may help determine the likelihood of subsequent systemic dissemination.

Hormone Receptor Analysis

Hormone receptors are proteins that are present in the cytosol of many breast cancer cells. These receptors (estrogen receptor [ER], progesterone receptor [PR]) mediate the effects of estrogen and progesterone within the cell. If the receptors are decreased or lacking, tumor growth is less hormonally dependent. Biochemical assays measure receptor concentrations in fresh tumor tissue; immunohistochemical techniques allow semiquantitative determination of hormone receptor status in fixed, embedded material. Hormone receptor positivity predicts responsiveness to all forms of endocrine therapy, but the assay is most reliable in identifying patients unlikely to respond.

SURVEILLANCE FOR RECURRENT BREAST CANCER

In the past, surgeons and medical oncologists followed breast cancer patients several times yearly with physical examinations, blood work, chest radiographs, and annual or even semiannual bone scans and other imaging procedures. Recent prospective studies demonstrate that this type of intensive follow-up confers no advantage. Most systemic recurrences of breast cancer occur between visits and are heralded by symptoms. Early diagnosis of metastatic breast cancer (even if achievable) provides no improvement in survival because no curative therapy is available.

Patients who have been treated with lumpectomy and breast irradiation should undergo annual mammography and breast examination by a physician at least twice yearly for the first 5 years after diagnosis. Early detection of in-breast recurrence is valuable; mastectomy at the time of recurrence may be curative. All patients with previous breast cancer should have annual mammograms for life. Whether these patients benefit from routine blood work and general physical examinations more often than would otherwise be recommended is not currently known. Many oncologists and surgeons, however, are comfortable returning these patients to the care of their primary physicians.

ADVANCED BREAST CANCER

The course of breast cancer varies. Most patients with stage I and stage II disease are cured with local treatment plus systemic adjuvant therapy, if appropriate. In other individuals, the disease may progress rapidly with widespread dissemination to vital organs, or it may follow an indolent course with slowly progressive local growth. In elderly women with bone metastases, progression may be slow, and the duration of survival may be relatively long.

Occasionally, patients with breast cancer present with metastases before the primary tumor in the breast is detected. Careful physical examination of the breasts and mammography should be the first steps in the evaluation of any woman presenting with metastatic adenocarcinoma of unknown origin.

Regional Lymph Node Metastases

In a woman with a persistent suspicious axillary mass, biopsy is indicated. If the biopsy reveals adenocarcinoma and the patient has no previous history of malignancy and no evidence of a primary tumor elsewhere, the diagnosis should be metastatic breast cancer, even if the breast examination and mammograms are normal. Such patients often present with breast masses at a later date, and the natural history and pattern of metastatic spread resemble those of typical breast cancer. These cancers also respond to the usual modalities used to treat advanced breast cancer. Supraclavicular and cervical adenopathy is uncommon in patients with breast cancer unless the ipsilateral axillary nodes are involved as well.

Bone Metastases

All too often the initial symptom of a woman with breast cancer is back pain or pain in another bony site. In some cases, the patient has ignored a large, often ulcerated breast mass, but on occasion the breast mass is inapparent and the manifestations of metastases precede those of the local tumor. In patients with a previous diagnosis of breast cancer, bone metastases represent one of the most common sites of initial systemic dissemination. Any woman with a history of breast cancer who subsequently experiences back pain, "arthritis," "sciatica," or similar symptoms should undergo a bone scan and plain films of the painful area before a diagnosis of a benign condition is accepted. Bone scans usually identify bone metastases before the abnormality can be detected on plain films. In rare patients, especially those with purely lytic metastases, plain films may reveal lesions not evident on bone scan. In patients who have persistent pain despite normal bone scans and plain films, computed tomography (CT), and even magnetic resonance imaging (MRI) of the painful area should be performed to exclude metastatic disease.

Hypercalcemia

Patients with lytic bone metastases from breast cancer (or other malignancies) may experience hypercalcemia. The symptoms may be subtle and consist only of fatigue, malaise, nausea, constipation, anorexia, and thirst—symptoms that may arise from numerous other causes in cancer patients. In some patients, however, hypercalcemia may present more dramatically with vomiting, dehydration, obtundation, or even coma. A serum calcium concentration should always be checked in a patient with known bone metastases and acute onset of any of these symptoms. Early recognition of hypercalcemia is important because it can be treated easily and usually successfully.

Bone Marrow Involvement

Patients with extensive and long-standing skeletal metastases (from breast cancer and other malignancies) often experience bone marrow failure owing to replacement of the marrow by metastatic tumor. This process is termed myelophthisic anemia. The diagnosis is suggested by anemia, often accompanied by granulocytopenia and/or thrombocytopenia, in excess of that expected as a consequence of the chemotherapy and radiotherapy the patient may have received. The peripheral blood smear reveals nucleated red blood cells and immature myeloid forms (leukoerythroblastosis) and teardrop-shaped poikilocytes. Bone marrow aspiration frequently yields a dry tap, but biopsy demonstrates tumor in the marrow in most patients. Normal bone marrow biopsy results do not exclude the diagnosis; a second biopsy should be performed. Magnetic resonance imaging (MRI) can reveal marrow abnormalities that suggest bone marrow involvement by tumor.

Spinal Cord Compression

Spinal cord compression is a true oncologic emergency. Any patient with vertebral metastases is at risk for this devastating complication. Virtually all cases of spinal cord compression in patients with breast cancer represent epidural tumor extending from vertebral disease (rather than intramedullary metastasis). Therefore, nearly every patient presents with back pain as well as with some combination of weakness, numbness, paresis, or paralysis. The extremities are affected equally, and a sensory level is usually detectable. In advanced cases, paralysis of bowel and bladder function may also occur. A high index of suspicion and early diagnosis are critical; patients who can still walk when the diagnosis is made have a much greater chance of retaining the ability to ambulate after treatment; those unable to walk at diagnosis rarely if ever ambulate again. Diagnosis depends on the clinical picture and plain films of the spine; a magnetic resonance scan provides clinical certainty in most cases. Myelography is rarely indicated unless MRI is unavailable.

Lung and Pleural Metastases

Dyspnea due to unilateral pleural effusion is occasionally the first symptom of breast cancer. More commonly, a unilateral pleural effusion represents the first manifestation of metastases in a patient with a past history of breast cancer. Pleural fluid cytologic findings usually reveal malignant cells consistent with breast cancer, but multiple pleural fluid samples may be required before a cytologic diagnosis can be made. Pleural fluid cell counts, chemistry panels, and special enzyme concentrations have little or no value in making the diagnosis of metastatic breast cancer, and pleural biopsy is rarely indicated.

Parenchymal pulmonary involvement in metastatic breast cancer is rarely present at the time of diagnosis but is not uncommon in patients with advanced disease. The lungs may contain multiple pulmonary nodules or an interstitial pattern of involvement unilaterally or bilaterally (which may mimic congestive heart failure radiographically). Hilar and mediastinal adenopathy is often detected as well. Rarely, multiple tumor emboli may produce pulmonary hypertension. Physical examination of the chest may be completely normal, even in patients with extensive parenchymal disease. A chest film should be obtained in any patient with a history of breast cancer and respiratory symptoms.

Liver Metastases

Liver metastases are commonly found in patients with advanced disease but only rarely found at initial diagnosis. Patients with liver metastases often complain of right upper quadrant pain, nausea, vomiting, anorexia, and early satiety. Fever, jaundice, and ascites may be present. An enlarged, often tender liver with palpable nodules is readily detected on palpation of the abdomen, and ultrasound or CT scanning confirms the diagnosis. Tissue diagnosis is rarely required, but easily obtained (when indicated) with FNA biopsy under CT or ultrasound guidance. Cutting needle liver biopsy should be avoided.

Gastrointestinal Metastases

Breast cancer, especially the lobular type, has a predilection for the gastric mucosa. About 5 per cent of patients with breast cancer have clinically evident metastases to the stomach. These patients may present with ulcer symptoms or with upper abdominal distention and early satiety. A CT scan may show thickening of the gastric wall suggesting gastric metastases. Upper gastrointestinal series or gastroscopy confirms the diagnosis.

Patients with mediastinal adenopathy from metastatic breast cancer may experience dysphagia due to extrinsic compression of the midesophagus. Barium swallow and/or esophagoscopy reveals extrinsic compression without an intrinsic abnormality. The chest film usually reveals the mediastinal tumor, but chest CT is required in some patients.

Rarely, patients with metastatic breast cancer acquire ascites. Cytologic evaluation of the peritoneal fluid reveals adenocarcinoma (except in patients in whom very advanced liver metastases produce ascites due to portal hypertension). In a patient with extensive metastases from breast cancer, the ascites is presumed to result from peritoneal carcinomatosis due to breast cancer. However, in a patient with minimal or no metastases from breast cancer, the possibility of primary ovarian cancer arises. There is no sure way to make this distinction; an ovarian mass may be present with either disease, and the serum CA-125 concentration (an ovarian tumor marker) may be increased in peritoneal carcinomatosis from any cause. An experienced oncologist should be consulted under these circumstances.

Brain Metastases

About 6 to 20 per cent of patients with breast cancer have clinical evidence of brain metastases at some point in their course. Brain involvement usually occurs in patients with extensive extracranial metastases. Presenting symptoms include subtle changes in mental function, cranial nerve disturbances, motor deficits, or seizures. Careful neurologic examination usually detects focal abnormalities, and CT scanning with contrast or MRI confirms the clinical suspicion. Lumbar puncture and electroencephalography (EEG) are rarely indicated. On occasion, however, patients present with cranial nerve abnormalities and normal head CT scans. Such patients may have meningeal involvement, and their cerebrospinal fluid (CSF) often contains tumor cells. MRI with contrast may reveal subtle enhancement and nodularity of the meninges.

MALE BREAST CANCER

Carcinoma of the male breast is rare, accounting for 1000 new cases and 300 deaths annually in the United States. The median age of men at the time of initial diagnosis of breast cancer is almost 10 years older than the median age in women. The cause is unknown, but the incidence is clearly increased in patients with Klinefelter's syndrome and may be increased in patients with endogenous and exogenous hyperestrogenism.

Breast cancer in males presents as it does in females—with a painless, firm to hard mass in the breast. It can be confused with unilateral gynecomastia that may cause a tender discoid subareolar mass. Mammography is sometimes helpful in making this distinction, but biopsy is required for definitive diagnosis. Unlike breast masses in women, most masses (other than gynecomastia) in the male breast are malignant; benign tumors (such as fibroadenomas) of the male breast are extremely rare.

Male breast cancer often presents in a more advanced stage than does female breast cancer, and because of the limited amount of breast tissue, it frequently involves the pectoral muscles. Stage for stage, however, the prognosis is similar to that of female breast cancer. The natural history and pattern of metastases are also similar. In males as in females, axillary node involvement at the time of diagnosis is the most important prognostic factor.

PITFALLS IN DIAGNOSIS

- Failure to biopsy a palpable breast mass because of a negative mammogram
- Failure to fully evaluate a palpable breast mass because of young age and/or negative family history
- Failure to excise a palpable breast mass because of normal or nondiagnostic FNA
- Attribution of back pain or other musculoskeletal complaint in a patient with breast cancer to a benign cause without obtaining a bone scan and/or plain films
- Failure to recognize the symptoms of hypercalcemia in a patient with metastatic breast cancer involving bone
- Failure to recognize the early symptoms of spinal cord compression in a patient with metastatic breast cancer involving the spine

URETHRITIS AND STRESS INCONTINENCE

By James N. Kvale, M.D.,
and Janice K. Kvale, Ph.D., C.N.M.
Austin, Texas

Urinary incontinence is defined as the involuntary loss of urine or an increase in the frequency of voiding that the patient perceives as a problem. The prevalence of incontinence increases with advancing age. Because urinary incontinence is a factor that commonly precipitates the decision to enter a nursing home, the prevalence in nursing homes is high. Community-based studies report the prevalence of urinary incontinence in adults to be between 14 and 51 per cent.

Four types of urinary incontinence have been identified to facilitate recognition and to enable the clinician to accurately diagnose the type of incontinence. Each type of incontinence is characterized by the pathophysiologic mechanism that causes the symptom. First, stress incontinence is the involuntary leakage of urine when intra-abdominal pressure is increased. Coughing, laughing, standing, sitting, or a Valsalva maneuver results in a leakage of urine from the urethra. The mechanism is the loss of effective sphincter function as well as structural changes in the tissues that surround the urethra. Second, urge incontinence is the sensation of a need to void with an inability to retain control for a sufficient time to reach the toilet. This response is caused by an erratic and unstable response of the detrusor muscle. Third, overflow incontinence occurs when the urethra becomes partially blocked. In women, overflow incontinence is commonly due to neurologic changes resulting from diabetes or other progressive neurologic disease that impair normal flow of urine from the bladder. In overflow incontinence, the bladder remains full and distended, and subsequently the person experiences continuous dribbling. Fourth, the incontinence that occurs when people are cognitively, psychologically, or physically unable or unwilling to use the toilet is called functional incontinence. Very commonly, patients present with a mixture of mechanisms of incontinence. An understanding of the pathophysiology is central to management.

An accurate history of voiding patterns is crucial for establishing the type of incontinence. Because incontinence does not become a significant problem for most women until sometime after the child-bearing period, it is important to recognize the structural and endocrine changes that occur in the perimenopausal and postmenopausal periods.

NORMAL CHANGES OF AGING

After menopause, the ratio between estradiol and estrone changes; estrone becomes the dominant estrogen. This change is the result of increased peripheral conversion of androstenedione to estrone and, to a lesser degree, the conversion of estrone to estradione. This process is normal and does not necessarily represent an indication for estrogen replacement therapy.

The condition of the entire female genital tract is dependent on estrogen, and the hormonal changes have obvious structural and physiologic effects. The ovaries and uterus atrophy after menopause and are typically not palpable in women older than the age of 75. Moreover, the vagina shortens, and the barrel of the vagina constricts in sexually inactive women. In sexually active females, the vaginal mucosa lubricates slowly, if at all. The urethra and sphincters atrophy, resulting in less effective control of urination. The pelvic muscles relax, stretch, and fail to maintain structural integrity. And finally, the vulva atrophies and is predisposed to dysplastic and neoplastic changes.

Several normal aging processes contribute to stress incontinence. Sphincter dysfunction and detrusor instability result in part from the normal slowing of the complex neuromuscular functions that attend aging. Sphincters and periurethral structures are estrogen dependent and become less efficient as estrogen concentrations change. The pelvic relaxation that results from childbirth trauma predisposes to cystocele, cystourethrocele, rectocele, and enterocele.

DIAGNOSIS

An accurate understanding of the history of patient symptoms and patterns is the key to an accurate diagnosis of the type of urinary incontinence. In addition, the clinician must be aware of other clinical issues that can affect control of urination. A disability caused by any chronic degenerative disease (e.g., lung disease, congestive heart failure, and degenerative arthritis) hinders efficient mobility and thus the ability of the patient to respond to the urge to urinate.

Medications that are used to manage chronic diseases may aggravate the symptoms of incontinence. For example, the use of a diuretic may increase the frequency of urination and decrease a patient's willingness to venture far from a toilet. Any medication that impedes mental clarity (e.g., sedatives, hypnotics, neuroleptics, and benzodiazepines) can worsen stress incontinence.

When obtaining the medical history, the clinician should inquire about the patient's living environment. A good assessment of the living environment yields important clues to potential interventions that may help the patient improve his or her control of urination.

The goal of the physical examination is to understand

what structural changes have occurred and how these changes affect urinary control. The clinician can obtain an appreciation of the vigor of muscle tone by watching how the patient walks or moves the body. Therefore, the examination for incontinence begins the moment the patient is seen.

The use of cystometry can provide an understanding of the pathophysiologic mechanisms of incontinence. Cystometry is a diagnostic technique that determines whether the incontinence is caused by detrusor instability, sphincter dysfunction, or both. The test enables the clinician to distinguish between the different types of incontinence and to plan effective interventions. Some cystometric techniques are complex and sophisticated and are typically performed by a urologist. Alternatively, a simplified office version, which yields equally accurate information in most cases, can be performed. The necessary supplies are available in most office settings.

Office Cystometry for Stress Incontinence

Office evaluation for stress incontinence is easily done and requires no special equipment.

Materials and Supplies

1. Toweling or incontinence pads, for placement under the patient
2. Graduated container (mL) for measuring urine
3. Sterile catheterization tray with a straight 14 Fr. to 16 Fr. rubber catheter
4. Sterile irrigation syringe (50 to 60 cc) that fits the catheter
5. Sterile saline solution (1 L)

Procedure

Ask the patient to empty her bladder and then lie on her back on the examination table. Insert the catheter into the urethra and empty the bladder into the container. Fill the syringe with saline solution. Attach the barrel of the irrigation syringe to the catheter and hold it 15 cm (6 inches) above the symphysis pubis. Gradually fill the bladder with sterile saline using less than 600 mL, because a greater quantity may injure the bladder. If bladder contractions begin to force the saline back into the syringe barrel or cause leaks around the catheter, record the volume of saline instilled at the time of the initial contraction. Most bladders can comfortably tolerate 300 to 400 mL. Remove the catheter with a comfortable quantity (about 300 mL) of saline remaining in the bladder. Ask the patient to cough, or perform a Valsalva maneuver. Observe the urethra for leakage. Ask the patient to stand, and repeat the same maneuver. Once again, observe for leakage.

Interpretation of Results

More than 100 mL of residual urine in the bladder indicates a dystonic bladder that is not emptying adequately. It also indicates detrusor dysfunction, resulting in ineffectual contraction and emptying. During filling of the bladder, spontaneous contractions with a strong urge to void are interpreted according to the volume of saline in the bladder when the contractions begin. When contractions occur with less than 300 mL of saline in the bladder, the detrusor is unstable and contracting uncontrollably. When contractions occur with 400 to 600 mL of saline in the bladder, the sphincters are not effective in controlling the egress of urine. Leakage around the catheter may be caused by sphincter dysfunction. After the catheter has been removed with 300 mL of saline remaining in the bladder, leakage occurring when the patient is supine or upright indicates detrusor instability.

PELVIC RELAXATION AND UTERINE PROLAPSE

Loss of tone in the musculature of the pelvic sling and stretching of ligaments may lead to protrusion of pelvic structures through the vaginal introitus. When the anterior wall of the vagina and the bladder or urethra are involved, the protrusion is a cystocele or a cystourethrocele. When the posterior wall of the vagina and the rectum or small bowel are affected, the condition is known as a rectocele or enterocele.

Loss of support for the uterus results in protrusion of the uterine corpus into the vaginal barrel. Protrusion that extends into the upper portions of the vagina is described as a first-degree prolapse. Protrusion that extends to the vaginal introitus is a second-degree prolapse. When prolapse is complete, with protrusion of the cervix beyond the introitus, the condition is described as procidentia, or third-degree prolapse.

Nonsurgical treatment of these conditions involves placing an object known as a pessary into the vagina to support surrounding structures. Pessaries have existed since the beginning of recorded history. The advent of surgical plastics and inventive designs have led to an array of devices that are effective in a high percentage of women.

Women usually present with stress incontinence to gynecologists, and the typical treatment recommendation is some form of surgical intervention. However, no large-scale, long-term outcome studies of reconstructive surgery have been reported. Therefore, a nonsurgical modality provides the best initial approach to the management of urinary incontinence, and surgical methods can be reserved for refractory situations.

Recently urologists have been performing periurethral injections with processed bovine dermal collagen (Contigen). The rationale is that the collagen enhances sphincter efficiency by improving urethral function. Multisite studies, with two years of follow-up, indicate that the procedure seems to benefit "carefully selected" patients, and women apparently derive greater benefit than men. Information about long-term benefits or complications from this intervention requires further study.

DYSFUNCTIONAL UTERINE BLEEDING

By David Frankfurter, M.D.
Boston, Massachusetts

and Joseph T. Chambers, M.D., Ph.D.
New Haven, Connecticut

INTRODUCTION

At some point in life, almost all women experience vaginal bleeding that is perceived as abnormal. In fact, approximately 20 per cent of all general gynecologic office visits are prompted by irregular or abnormal vaginal bleeding.

The medical lexicon is filled with a broad spectrum of terms that aim to characterize atypical vaginal bleeding. These terms include dysfunctional uterine bleeding, anovulatory bleeding, perimenopausal bleeding, postmenopausal bleeding, and breakthrough bleeding. Unfortunately, these terms are often used interchangeably and incorrectly to describe a wide array of histopathologic or clinical conditions that present with similar signs and symptoms. Dysfunctional uterine bleeding is defined as abnormal uterine bleeding in the absence of pelvic organ or systemic disease. It is a diagnosis of exclusion that is frequently associated with anovulation. An appropriate clinical approach to pathologic uterine bleeding requires an understanding of the physiology of the normal menstrual cycle.

MENSTRUAL CYCLE

Regular menstrual cycles are the product of precise and coordinated communications among the hypothalamus, anterior pituitary gland, and ovary. The end result of this orderly process is a cyclic alteration of the histologic architecture of the endometrial lining of the uterus. The purpose of this cyclic coordination is to produce a mature oocyte that is receptive to fertilization and an endometrium that is hospitable for implantation. If fertilization does not occur, the endometrial lining is sloughed in a synchronous, controlled manner. Central to this cyclicity is the pulsatile release of gonadotropin-releasing hormone (Gn-RH) from the hypothalamus and the concomitant increased release of follicle-stimulating hormone (FSH) by the anterior pituitary during the follicular phase of the menstrual cycle.

Ovarian follicles continuously progress through phases of gonadotropin-dependent growth and atresia. During the early follicular phase of the menstrual cycle, FSH stimulation of the ovary leads to the recruitment of a cohort of follicles that have developed the capacity to respond to gonadotropins. From this point on, follicular growth is gonadotropin dependent. The rate of mitosis increases within these follicles, and under the influence of FSH, granulosa cells convert androgens produced by theca cells into estradiol. Granulosa cells also secrete a glycoprotein, inhibin, that feeds back to the pituitary and hypothalamus to decrease synthesis and release of FSH as the follicular phase progresses. Thus, as this phase continues, follicular development and estradiol production must be accomplished despite the diminishing levels of FSH. Normally, this level of development is achieved only by the follicle whose granulosa cells have a critical concentration of FSH receptors and can remain responsive despite a decreasing FSH concentration. Toward the end of the follicular phase, serum estradiol concentrations increase significantly. A sustained increase in estradiol concentrations exerts a positive feedback on the pituitary, causing a precipitous and marked release of luteinizing hormone (LH). The LH surge causes changes within the follicle leading to maturation, rupture, and ovulation. The ruptured follicle now attains a characteristic yellow appearance and becomes increasingly vascular. Within this corpus luteum, granulosa cells begin to produce large amounts of progesterone as well as estradiol. These processes herald the onset of the luteal phase.

FSH is suppressed by continued production of inhibin. LH alone cannot indefinitely support the corpus luteum, and in the absence of embryonic production of human chorionic gonadotropin (hCG), luteolysis begins approximately 10 to 12 days after ovulation. As the corpus luteum begins to involute, serum estradiol, progesterone, and inhibin concentrations fall. This in turn frees the hypothalamic-pituitary axis of its negative feedback. FSH starts to rise, and another cycle begins.

The ovarian steroids produced throughout the menstrual cycle in response to pituitary gonadotropins act in a phasic manner to promote conception and to prepare the endometrium for implantation. The proliferative phase of endometrial development is associated with the follicular phase of the ovarian follicle and increased estradiol concentrations. Re-epithelialization of the endometrium and proliferation of the stromal and glandular components are most prominent. After ovulation, the endometrium is under the influence of both estrogen and progesterone. Proliferation ends and maturation begins. The glands begin to secrete glycoproteins and peptides in anticipation of blastocyst implantation. If fertilization does not occur, luteolysis ensues and estradiol and progesterone concentrations begin to fall. Lysosomes within endometrial cells are stabilized under the influence of progesterone. As progesterone falls, these cells undergo autolysis. Spasmodic contraction of spiral arteries within the endometrium causes tissue ischemia, necrosis, and eventual desquamation of the endometrial lining. Hemostasis is preserved as vessels constrict, platelets and fibrin are deposited, and estrogen increases in the early follicular phase. This rhythmical progression leads to a coordinated, synchronous, controlled, and self-limiting sloughing of the entire endometrium.

MENSES

Menstrual bleeding is considered abnormal if it causes anemia or lasts for less than 3 days or longer than 7 days, or the quantity is greater than 80 mL per menses. Menstrual periods that occur more frequently than every 23 days or less frequently than every 35 days are also considered aberrant. Normally, menses lasts 4 to 6 days and results in the loss of approximately 30 mL of blood. The various terms used to describe these aberrations include oligomenorrhea, polymenorrhea, menorrhagia (hypermenorrhea), hypomenorrhea, metrorrhagia, menometrorrhagia, and amenorrhea.

The normal menses follows progesterone withdrawal at the end of the luteal phase of the menstrual cycle. Uterine bleeding is considered dysfunctional when it is irregular and no overt abnormalities are present. Dysfunctional uterine bleeding is usually the result of estrogen breakthrough, estrogen withdrawal, or progesterone breakthrough—and not usually of progesterone withdrawal. This diagnosis is one of exclusion, as the clinician must be certain that there are no other pathologic explanations for the bleeding.

DIFFERENTIAL DIAGNOSIS

The differential diagnosis is vast, but a handful of clinically useful disease categories are often suggested by age and hormonal status. For women in the child-bearing years, pregnancy must be excluded. Spontaneous abortion, retained products of conception, ectopic pregnancy, molar pregnancy, and even a "normal" gestation may present with vaginal bleeding. During the first 20 weeks of gestation, between 20 and 40 per cent of pregnancies are complicated by bleeding. Of these, approximately one half end in miscarriage. Fifty to eighty per cent of patients with an ectopic pregnancy have vaginal bleeding, and almost all have significant abdominal or pelvic pain. In the absence of intrauterine pregnancy (IUP), plateauing hCG titers in patients with abdominal or pelvic pain strongly suggest ectopic pregnancy, while markedly increased hCG titers and a fundal height exceeding that predicted by dates is consistent with molar pregnancy.

Bleeding dyscrasias may initially present as abnormal vaginal bleeding. Twenty per cent of adolescents who present with increased menstrual bleeding have a coagulation disorder, most frequently von Willebrand's disease. Platelet dysfunction associated with idiopathic thrombocytopenic purpura and thrombotic thrombocytopenic purpura may result in vaginal bleeding. Severe liver disease causes decreased clotting factor production that can lead to bleeding irregularities. Medications can impair platelet function or the clotting cascade, leading to menstrual irregularities. Among the best-documented culprits are antiviral medications, salicylates, furosemide, heparin, warfarin, and ginseng.

Severe systemic or medical disorders may cause menstrual irregularities. Both hyperthyroid and hypothyroid conditions produce menstrual irregularities. Liver and kidney disease impair estrogen metabolism and clearance; administration of glucocorticoids and opiates may cause anovulation. The clinician must also be alert for genital tract infection as a possible cause of vaginal bleeding. Endometritis, vaginitis, and cervicitis often produce friable epithelium that can bleed.

Thirty per cent of women with uterine leiomyomas experience abnormal bleeding that may be minimal or profuse. Irregular vaginal bleeding has also been reported in patients with adenomyosis, uterine polyps, or cervical polyps. Tumors arising in the vagina, cervix, uterus, or ovary may present with bleeding. Vaginal and cervical cancers are typically associated with postcoital bleeding, while endometrial hyperplasia and carcinoma can present with irregular vaginal bleeding. Estrogen- or progesterone-secreting tumors of the ovary may induce endometrial hyperplasia or atrophy that produces irregular uterine bleeding.

Atypically, patients with perineal or genital trauma may describe acute or abnormal vaginal bleeding. Lacerations of the vulva, cervix, and vagina produced by falls, accidents, coitus, or forced penetration can bleed profusely. Rarely, surgical trauma secondary to electrocoagulation of the fallopian tubes has been linked to irregular bleeding patterns. Other causes of abnormal genital tract bleeding include intrauterine devices granulation tissue, or retained suture material.

ANOVULATORY BLEEDING

Anovulation is physiologic at the beginning and end of the reproductive years. Prior to menarche, the positive feedback mechanism that is responsible for the LH surge has not yet matured. As menopause ensues, the remaining follicles do not produce sufficient estrogen to stimulate the LH surge.

Anovulatory bleeding is usually a manifestation of estrogen breakthrough or withdrawal bleeding. This bleeding is excessive and is due to prolonged endometrial exposure to high estrogen concentrations. The bleeding is asynchronous and irregular and occurs in focal areas of the fragile endometrium.

Anovulation may be secondary to hypothalamic, pituitary, or ovarian dysfunction. Ovulation depends on hypothalamic pulsatile secretion of Gn-RH; if an appropriate pulse frequency is not achieved, ovulation cannot occur. Profound weight loss through exercise or dieting or as the result of an eating disorder can disturb this hypothalamic function.

Hyperprolactinemia leads to hypothalamic dysfunction and anovulation. Increased prolactin may be secondary to pituitary tumors, central nervous system tumors, or aberrations in the dopaminergic pathways of the hypothalamus. Despite a functioning hypothalamus, persistently increased estrogen concentrations produce chronic FSH inhibition, especially during pregnancy, stress, thyroid disturbance, adrenal or ovarian tumors, or increased extraglandular production of estrogen.

An imbalance of autocrine and paracrine factors within the ovary may produce ovulatory dysfunction resulting in androgen excess. This produces an ovarian microenvironment that impairs follicular maturation and ovulation. This polycystic ovary syndrome is associated with increased estradiol and androgen concentrations as well as android obesity and insulin resistance. These patients are at significant risk for the comorbidity of diabetes mellitus, atherosclerotic cardiovascular disease, and endometrial cancer. Thus, disruption of menses can be produced by aberrations at any point along the hypothalamic-pituitary-ovarian axis.

EVALUATION

Irregular vaginal bleeding is a common manifestation of many disorders. Therefore, taking an appropriate history is important for ensuring focused and effective use of subsequent diagnostic measures. From the patient's menstrual history, the clinician can obtain a sense of the pattern of bleeding. Is the bleeding acute or chronic? Have menses ever been regular? Are blood clots present? Does the patient feel pregnant? Has she noticed any changes in hair growth or distribution? Has she noted an increase in acne? Has she been a victim of sexual abuse or domestic violence? Has she experienced recent weight loss? Does she feel that her level of psychosocial stress has increased? Is she experiencing midcycle spotting? From the patient's history, the clinician can eliminate systemic or pharmacologic causes of abnormal bleeding and may establish that the bleeding is not from the genital tract, but rather from a urinary or gastrointestinal source.

The physical examination is the essential next step. Look for general signs of virilization, trauma, bleeding disorder, or systemic disease. After the general examination, inspect the external genitalia, beginning with the vulva, the vagina, and the cervix. If signs of infection are present, obtain cultures and prepare a wet mount. In the absence of a visible lesion, obtain a Papanicolaou (PAP) smear of the cervix. If a lesion is visible, biopsy is required. Check for clitoral enlargement and signs of vulvar or vaginal atrophy. On bimanual examination, the uterus may feel enlarged, soft, nodular or firm. An enlarged uterus is consistent with pregnancy, adenomyosis, or endometrial cancer; nodularity suggests uterine leiomyomas or an adnexal mass. The adnexa should be evaluated during the rectovaginal examination. Adnexal masses include pedunculated uterine leiomyomas, benign or malignant disease of the ovary, metastases to the ovary, or even an ectopic pregnancy. Evaluation of the stool for occult bleeding can be performed at this time or by the patient at home.

Laboratory evaluation should include a pregnancy test in women of reproductive age, a coagulation profile in adolescents, and a complete blood count (CBC). The presence of iron deficiency anemia indicates that bleeding is quantitatively significant. If the patient's history does not indicate ovulation (no cyclic breast tenderness, menstrual cramping, or water weight gain), assess the ovulatory status with basal body temperatures, urine LH, or luteal-phase serum progesterone. Tissue samples that reveal secretory-phase endometrium are also consistent with ovulation.

Measure serum thyroid-stimulating hormone (TSH), prolactin, FSH, and LH in all patients with anovulatory bleeding. The FSH concentration may help determine whether a patient is menopausal or has ovarian failure. Serum LH concentrations that are twice the FSH concentrations suggest anovulation. In patients with signs of virilization, cancer and endocrinopathies must be excluded. Androgen-secreting tumors are associated with rapid onset of virilizing characteristics, and androgen profiles can help determine whether the source is adrenal or ovarian. Patients who are anovulatory, hirsute, and obese must be monitored for diabetes mellitus, cardiovascular disease, and endometrial cancer.

Although endometrial cancer generally occurs in postmenopausal women, nearly 25 per cent of patients with this tumor are premenopausal, and 5 per cent are younger than 40 years. If the patient is older than 35 years of age and presents with irregular menstrual bleeding, perform endometrial sampling and endocervical curettage. If the patient has been anovulatory for more than 1 year, sample the endometrium. Most women younger than 35 who present with endometrial cancer experience chronic anovulation. These women have a high incidence of endometrial hyperplasia and a threefold increased risk of developing endometrial cancer.

The Papanicolaou smear alone is not effective in making the diagnosis of endometrial cancer. One half to two thirds of patients with endometrial carcinoma have normal PAP smears. However, if cytology reveals endometrial cells with atypia, further evaluation of the endometrium is mandatory.

Various instruments can be used to obtain a specimen for histopathologic evaluation. Formerly, a D&C (dilatation and curettage) would have been performed; however, this procedure is costly and requires an operating room. Furthermore, D&C is associated with a 1 per cent incidence of uterine perforation and a one tenth of 1 per cent incidence of hysterectomy. Also, tumors are missed in as many as 10 per cent of patients undergoing blind D&C. Today, most clinicians use a flexible plastic endometrial sampler in the office; anesthetics and cervical dilatation are not required, and patient discomfort is minimal. Endometrial sampling devices are disposable, inexpensive, and easy to use. Sampling of the endometrium with these plastic cannulas can lead to detection of neoplasia with a sensitivity as high as 97.5 per cent.

The clinician should pursue hysteroscopy-directed biopsy if endometrial sampling does not provide sufficient information. Office hysteroscopy provides direct visualization of the endometrial cavity and does not add significantly to the time and cost of the office visit. Importantly, hysteroscopy enables the clinician to diagnose and treat at the same time. Diagnostic hysteroscopy with the patient under anesthesia may be appropriate if the cervix is stenotic or an examination under anesthesia is indicated. Hysteroscopy has been particularly useful for obtaining directed biopsies and for diagnosing and treating submucosal uterine leiomyomas, intrauterine adhesions, and endometrial polyps. Hysteroscopy plus endometrial sampling provides reliable evaluation of the endometrium in 98 per cent of patients.

Transvaginal ultrasonography can be utilized for assessing uterine size, fluid within the endometrial cavity, uterine leiomyomas, endometrial thickness, and the consistency of the adnexa. For postmenopausal women with irregular vaginal bleeding, an endometrial stripe greater than 6 mm is associated with an increased incidence of endometrial hyperplasia, polyps, and cancer. If ultrasound reveals an endometrial stripe less than 5 mm, the clinician can safely exclude endometrial carcinoma as a cause of abnormal bleeding. This may obviate the need for hysteroscopy. Ultrasonography is also useful in diagnosing endometrial polyps and uterine leiomyomas. Magnetic resonance imaging provides a sensitive means for diagnosing adenomyosis and very accurately detects uterine leiomyomas.

TREATMENT

Treatment is designed to control acute bleeding, prevent future bleeding, and prevent any comorbidity related to anovulation. When bleeding is profuse and the patient is hemodynamically unstable, then, after appropriate resuscitation, the patient should undergo endometrial sampling or a definitive operative procedure. If bleeding is less severe, the patient can be managed medically. The evaluation helps direct treatment.

When a diagnosis of dysfunctional uterine bleeding is made, the clinician has various treatment options. Primary therapy utilizes a progestational agent. These agents work to stabilize the endometrium by reversing estrogenic effects and, on withdrawal, lead to synchronous and universal desquamation of the endometrium. Choice of agent and duration of treatment vary considerably. For adolescents with anovulatory cycles secondary to immaturity of positive feedback on the pituitary, a short course of oral contraceptives usually normalizes bleeding episodes. Cessation of medication usually results in regular menses as the feedback system matures.

Women frequently experience midcycle spotting secondary to the postovulatory drop in estrogen. This type of vaginal bleeding is easily controlled with oral contraceptive pills (OCPs). In patients with chronic anovulation who desire contraception, OCPs can be used as well. If contraception is not an issue, a synthetic progesterone can be administered for the first 12 days of the month, with vaginal bleeding expected thereafter.

If endometrial sampling reveals adenomatous hyperplasia, therapy consists of continuous progesterone therapy for 2 to 3 months followed by repeat sampling. For perimenopausal patients with no evidence of hyperplasia or neoplasia on endometrial sampling, synthetic progesterone can be given for the first 12 days of the month. These women should be advised that they may still ovulate and require contraception. U.S. Food and Drug Administration (FDA) has approved the use of low-dose OCPs up to the age of menopause in women who do not have a history of hypertension, hyperlipidemia, or smoking as well as any other condition that would contraindicate their use. Once withdrawal bleeding has ceased, hormone replacement treatment should be encouraged.

If the patient cannot comply with medical management and reproductive capacity is not desired, the clinician should consider a definitive operative treatment. Surgical options include hysterectomy or endometrial ablation. The advantages of the latter include decreased short-term morbidity, lower cost, and decreased recovery time. Hysterectomy has been associated with premature ovarian failure as well as psychosexual dysfunction. These complications can be avoided with endometrial ablation. Unfortunately,

25 per cent of patients who have undergone endometrial ablation continue to have menstrual flow.

HORMONE REPLACEMENT THERAPY AND TAMOXIFEN

By the year 2000, more than 700 million women worldwide will be older than 45 years of age. As the number of postmenopausal women increases, more patients will be maintained on hormone replacement therapy (HRT). Estrogen replacement has been shown to decrease low-density lipoprotein (LDL) cholesterol, increase high-density lipoprotein (HDL) cholesterol, retard atherosclerosis, improve peripheral glucose metabolism, reduce the risk of bone fracture from osteoporosis, and improve cognitive function. Although it is not necessary to routinely screen all women on HRT for endometrial cancer, women on hormone replacement with irregular bleeding or breakthrough bleeding or those who start bleeding after a long period of amenorrhea require evaluation of the endometrium.

Patients who take tamoxifen have a higher incidence of developing endometrial carcinoma than control subjects, especially if they have been receiving this medication for 2 years or more. The routine evaluation of these patients remains undecided, but the practitioner must be alert for any signs of endometrial abnormalities, especially if patients on tamoxifen present with vaginal bleeding.

LEIOMYOMA UTERI

By Robert J. Kiltz, M.D.
Skaneateles, New York

Leiomyoma uteri (uterine myomas or fibroids) are among the most common tumors of the female reproductive tract. Fibroids are found in 20 to 30 per cent of women of reproductive age. The incidence at autopsy has been reported as high as 50 per cent.

Myomas arise from smooth muscle cells that proliferate to form well-circumscribed solid tumors primarily composed of whorls of smooth muscle cells interlaced with varying amounts of fibrous tissue. Myomas may be single but are most often multiple. Two thirds of myomas show some degree of degeneration. Hyaline degeneration (65 per cent) is most commonly observed, followed by myxomatous degeneration (15 per cent), and calcific degeneration (10 per cent). Estrogen facilitates the growth of leiomyomas, but the actual cause of tumor formation remains a mystery. In hypoestrogenic states (e.g., menopause or treatment with gonadotropin-releasing hormone [GnRH] agonists), myomas regress in size. The greater prominence of fibroids in African American women than in white women suggests a genetic predisposition. Fibroids are benign in most patients. Malignant changes are seen in 0.3 to 0.7 per cent of myomas. Fibroids are classified by their anatomic relationship to the layers of the uterus. The most common types of myomas are submucous (beneath the endometrium), intramural (within the myometrium but distorting neither the endometrium nor the serosa), and subserosal (beneath the uterine serosa). Fibroids that involve all layers are referred to as transmural. Myomas may also be found in the broad ligament and cervix and as pedunculated lesions on narrow stalks. Myomas may be microscopic or they may fill the entire abdomen. The center of the lesion is relatively avascular, whereas one or two blood vessels surround the pseudocapsule.

PRESENTING SYMPTOMS AND SIGNS

Twenty to 50 per cent of women with uterine myomas are asymptomatic. The severity of symptoms is directly related to the size, number, and location of the myomas. Up to 30 per cent of women with myomas present with menorrhagia or abnormal uterine bleeding. Mechanical distortion of the uterine cavity or distortion of the vascular drainage may explain the abnormal bleeding associated with leiomyomas. Five to 10 per cent of myomas are submucous, and many of these lesions produce abnormal uterine bleeding. As a myoma outgrows its blood supply, degeneration and central necrosis may be associated with episodes of pelvic pain. A large pedunculated myoma may twist on its narrow stalk, leading to necrosis and pain. Direct pressure on the bladder from a lower anterior uterine or cervical myoma may cause frequent urination.

Although infertility and complications of pregnancy are believed to be rare in women with fibroids, large submucous myomas may interrupt the implantation site, causing failure of implantation or early abortion. A cornual myoma may cause infertility by obstructing the fallopian tube.

DIAGNOSIS

The identification of uterine myomas begins with a careful history of presenting symptoms. Many patients present without complaints and their fibroids are detected during routine annual examinations. When myomas are suspected on physical examination, further documentation of their size, number, and location is often necessary. Tools for accomplishing this task include pelvic or abdominal ultrasound, plain abdominal radiographs, intravenous pyelograms, hysteroscopy, hysterosalpingography, magnetic resonance imaging (MRI), computed tomography (CT), laparoscopy, and/or laparotomy.

The selective use of these diagnostic tests depends on the patient's anatomy and willingness to cooperate during examination. The need for further studies may be guided by the patient's age or desire to become pregnant. In addition, accurate preoperative definition of the number, location, and size of myomas can decrease the required number of uterine incisions. Also, third-party payors may request that evidence of uterine myomas identified by physical examination be confirmed by other diagnostic modalities prior to surgical intervention.

PHYSICAL EXAMINATION

A bimanual examination often detects an irregular and/or enlarged, firm uterus. The clinician may also palpate individual myomas. An eccentrically located leiomyoma may be mistaken for an ovarian or adnexal mass, pregnancy, or adenomyosis. Inspection and palpation of the abdomen may detect myomas exceeding 15 weeks in gestational size.

Although the experienced clinician may have little difficulty identifying uterine myomas on physical examination, this method does not permit accurate definition of the number, size, and location of these lesions.

PLAIN RADIOGRAPHS

Plain films of the abdomen and pelvis may reveal the calcifications present in 5 per cent of leiomyomas. Plain films may also provide evidence of cholelithiasis, ascites, renal calculi, bowel obstruction, perforation, or other abdominal disorders, but they are not useful for defining the size, number, or location of uterine fibroids.

INTRAVENOUS PYELOGRAPHY

Intravenous pyelography (IVP) can be used to identify ureteral obstruction, renal pelvic dilatation, and displacement of the ureters secondary to leiomyomas. IVP does not identify myomas directly. Although IVP has been used preoperatively to identify ureteral location, this may be unnecessary because the ureters must also be located during the pelvic dissection. If surgical removal is not yet indicated, or if the patient is otherwise being managed conservatively, IVP may be performed in selected patients to exclude hydronephrosis secondary to ureteral dilatation.

ULTRASOUND

Abdominal or pelvic ultrasound is considered the procedure of choice for evaluating the suspected pelvic mass or fibroid uterus. Ultrasound is accurate and readily available at a reasonable cost. Ultrasound uses transducers with frequencies between 1 and 10 MHz. Higher frequencies produce greater detail, but tissue penetration by the beam is reduced. Transabdominal scans use frequencies between 3 and 5 MHz and generally require a full bladder for optimal visualization of pelvic organs. The typical focal length of transabdominal probes is between 5 and 10 cm. Transvaginal probes provide more detailed views of the pelvis and reduce patient discomfort by eliminating the need for a full bladder, thereby placing the probe closer to the structures of interest. Transvaginal probes use frequencies between 5 and 7.5 MHz.

Typical myomas may appear isoechoic or hypoechoic when compared with adjacent myometrium. Myomas with central hypolucency may have developed central necrosis and degeneration. Ultrasound does not allow the clinician to distinguish benign from malignant myomas. An enlarged, diffusely irregular uterus may contain foci of adenomyosis rather than leiomyomas.

The vaginal probe also has limitations in patients with large pelvic myomas or masses outside the pelvic field of view. In these patients, abdominal scans are preferred. Abdominal ultrasound also permits evaluation of ureteral or renal pelvic dilatation. Ultrasound seldom detects myomas less than 2 cm in greatest dimension.

HYSTEROSONOGRAPHY

A relatively new diagnostic aid, hysterosonography, coupled with pelvic ultrasound can significantly enhance the visualization of uterine filling defects, including submucous or pedunculated myomas. Hysterosonography can be performed using the Soules intrauterine insemination catheter (Cook OB/GYN, Indianapolis, Indiana), which is 25 cm in length and 1.88 mm in diameter. The catheter is inserted through the cervical os into the fundus. Sterile saline is flushed through the catheter prior to its insertion. The vaginal probe (transducer) is then inserted into the vagina and the uterus is scanned. Approximately 10 to 20 ml of sterile saline flows into the uterine cavity during the scanning procedure.

In the office, hysterosonography is an excellent adjunct to ultrasound because it is inexpensive and well tolerated and may provide documentation of tubal patency.

HYSTEROSALPINGOGRAPHY

Hysterosalpingography uses radiopaque contrast to fill the uterine cavity, which can identify uterine filling defects from submucous or transmural myomas. Hysterosalpingography is performed prior to ovulation but after menstruation has stopped. A balloon-tipped catheter is placed in the cervical canal and oil- or water-soluble contrast material is injected slowly under fluoroscopic guidance. Early films are taken with small amounts of contrast to improve detail and the identification of filling defects or tubal patency. If the balloon is placed in the uterine cavity, it should not be mistaken for a myoma. The administration of doxycycline or other antibiotics may reduce the incidence of infection following hysterosalpingography.

HYSTEROSCOPY

Hysteroscopy allows direct visualization of the uterine cavity. Carbon dioxide, sorbitol, or high-viscosity dextran is instilled into the cavity following paracervical anesthesia and intravenous sedation. A narrow endoscope (3 to 5 mm in diameter) permits identification of myomas impinging on the uterine cavity. Video recording facilitates the hysteroscopy and enhances patient education. Outpatient hysteroscopy is performed early in the follicular phase after menses have ceased. Operative hysteroscopy may facilitate the resection of myomas and the ablation of endometrium in patients with abnormal uterine bleeding. Laparoscopy is often combined with operative hysteroscopy to avoid uterine perforation during a resection.

MAGNETIC RESONANCE IMAGING

MRI uses radiofrequency waves in varying magnetic fields to produce cross-sectional images with high soft tissue contrast discrimination. T2-weighted images provide excellent views of the uterus that frequently enable the clinician to distinguish fibroids from the normal myometrium.

MRI is considered the most accurate and precise imaging technique for the detection and location of leiomyomas. Unlike many of the previously mentioned techniques, MRI is not limited by mass size or myoma location. Unfortunately, the high cost, long scanning times, and claustrophobic atmosphere for some patients may limit the routine use of MRI.

Table 1 compares the previously discussed techniques.

COMPUTED TOMOGRAPHY

The identification of uterine myomas by CT is poor because CT does not adequately discriminate the tissue density of the uterus. MRI is superior to CT because MRI avoids ionizing radiation, provides better soft tissue contrast, and has the capacity to scan in coronal as well as

Table 1. Comparison of Magnetic Resonance Imaging, Sonography, and Hysterosalpingography in Detection of Leiomyomas and Approximate Cost of Each Modality

Modality	Sensitivity (%)	Specificity (%)	Accuracy (%)	Cost ($)
MRI	86	100	97	1300
Sonography	60	99	87	250
HSG	9	97	76	500

MRI = magnetic resonance imaging; HSG = hysterosalpingography.
Adapted from Dudiak, C.M., Turner, D.A., Patel, S.K., et al.: Uterine leiomyomas in the infertile patient: Preoperative localization with MR imaging versus US and hysterosalpingography. Radiology 167:627, 1988, with permission.

sagittal planes. Both CT and MRI are relatively expensive and may not be as readily available as ultrasound.

LAPAROSCOPY AND LAPAROTOMY

Persistent diagnostic uncertainty occasionally justifies an exploratory laparoscopy or laparotomy. Uterine or pelvic masses larger than 15 weeks' gestational size may necessitate open laparoscopy or laparotomy. If indicated, clinicians with appropriate training and experience may perform myomectomy during the "diagnostic" surgical procedure. With the recent development of a 2-mm high-resolution endoscope, office diagnostic laparoscopy may become more common.

With the use of many of these diagnostic modalities, the routine removal of the myomatous uterus that is larger than 12 to 14 gestational weeks in size should be questioned. Since malignant changes are rare, observation and conservative therapy may become more common in the case of an asymptomatic patient and a uterus larger than 12 to 14 weeks' gestational size.

Malignant changes of leiomyomas fortunately are rare, occurring in fewer than 1 per cent of hysterectomies (for myomas). Currently, there are no noninvasive modalities capable of distinguishing benign from malignant leiomyomas. Although some have attempted to utilize MRI, it is not accurate enough for clinical use. Uterine curettage remains the most commonly used method of evaluating for uterine malignancy and can identify malignant leiomyomas invading the endometrium. An alternative method utilizing ultrasound-directed transabdominal or transvaginal needle biopsy of a leiomyoma might be used in rare circumstances where surgery is relatively contraindicated and significant concerns regarding the possibility of malignancy exist.

OTHER STUDIES

Assay of serum tumor markers (e.g., CA-125) is not helpful in the diagnosis of leiomyomas or in defining their malignant potential. Urine or serum pregnancy testing, complete blood counts, and coagulation studies are useful in evaluating the patient with abnormal uterine bleeding or a pelvic mass, but the results of these tests are not diagnostic of leiomyomas.

DIAGNOSTIC PITFALLS

A bimanual examination may fail to detect an adnexal mass or may erroneously identify an eccentric myoma. If uncertainty exists at the time of the pelvic or abdominal examination, the clinician should request abdominal ultrasound. If ultrasound fails to confirm the diagnosis of leiomyomas, further studies are indicated.

Use of GnRH agonists prior to myomectomy may cause small myomas to be undetectable at the time of surgery. Thus, follow-up diagnostic studies may be helpful prior to surgery to document the presence of leiomyomas in patients pretreated with GnRH agonists.

CONCLUSION

A careful history and physical examination will identify most leiomyomata uteri. Pelvic ultrasound provides the most cost-effective method for identifying the origin of a pelvic mass and the location of the ovaries. The diagnosis of malignant degeneration of a uterine fibroid requires examination of relevant tissue under the microscope.

DIAGNOSIS AND SELECTED MEDICAL PROBLEMS IN PREGNANCY

By Joanne Armstrong, M.D., MPH,
and Richard Depp, M.D.
Philadelphia, Pennsylvania

DIAGNOSIS OF PREGNANCY

The diagnosis of pregnancy relies largely on a combination of symptoms and physical signs that may be confirmed by biochemical and/or ultrasonographic testing.

HISTORY AND PHYSICAL EXAMINATION

Amenorrhea is one of the first presumptive signs of pregnancy. Cessation of menses is most reliable in women with previously regular menstrual cycles. It is an unreliable sign in women with a history of irregular menstrual bleeding or in women who have taken or are currently taking oral contraceptives. Irregular bleeding is never normal in pregnancy but may represent benign implantation bleeding that occurs approximately 6 days after fertilization or 20 days after the first day of the last menstrual period (LMP). Approximately 20 per cent of pregnancies are associated with first-trimester bleeding. Nearly 80 per cent of those with bleeding maintain a viable pregnancy. Irregular first-trimester bleeding may also suggest a nonviable intrauterine pregnancy or an ectopic pregnancy. These conditions require further evaluation.

Nausea and vomiting occur in as many as 70 per cent of all pregnancies, usually between 2 and 12 weeks of gestation. Although most commonly reported in the morning, nausea and vomiting may occur at any time of the day. Treatment includes emotional support, dietary changes, and antiemetics. Approximately 2 per cent of patients develop severe, protracted nausea and vomiting (hyperemesis gravidarum) that requires rehydration and, occasionally, parenteral nutrition. Ptyalism, or excess production of saliva, is an unusual manifestation of pregnancy that may result from excess production of saliva or from a decreased ability of the nauseated patient to swallow normal amounts of saliva.

Breast tenderness (mastodynia) and breast enlargement occur as early as 4 weeks after the LMP. Breast enlargement in the first 8 weeks of gestation is the product of vascular engorgement. Thereafter, it is due to estrogen-driven ductal growth and progesterone-driven alveolar hypertrophy. Nipple enlargement and areolar hyperpigmentation are also noted. Supernumerary breasts (polymastia) and nipples (polythelia), which may be found along the "milk line" extending from the axilla to the vulva, may become more prominent during pregnancy. Accessory nipples may undergo hyperpigmentation. Precolostrum (plasma exudate rich in immunoglobulins, lactoferrin, and serum albumin) may be secreted as early as 16 weeks of gestation.

Pelvic pressure is often reported in early pregnancy and represents progressive enlargement of the uterus. The uterus is palpable at the pubic symphysis at 12 weeks and at the umbilicus at 20 weeks of gestation. The uterus increases approximately 1 cm in vertical length per week when measured by the McDonald technique (from the pubic symphysis to the top of the uterine mass) from the first trimester through the early part of the third trimester. When fundal height measurements are consistent with estimated gestational age, the clinician can be reasonably assured that fetal growth is appropriate. When fundal height measurements are discordant with calculations of gestational age (within 3 cm), further evaluation is warranted to confirm gestational age or to exclude intrauterine growth restriction (IUGR), macrosomia, or polyhydramnios (hydramnios). Discordant fundal height measurements, however, are poorly predictive of IUGR, and when IUGR is known to exist, it is rarely detected by size-date discrepancies.

Quickening, the first perception of fetal movement by the mother, may be helpful in gestational dating but is experience dependent. Nulliparous women first appreciate fetal movement at about 19 weeks; multiparous women can first perceive fetal movement at 17 weeks.

The pelvis undergoes characteristic changes in response to the increased vascularity of early pregnancy. Chadwick's sign refers to the bluish discoloration of the vagina and cervix. Goodell's sign, or softening of the cervix, may be noted at 4 weeks of gestation. Hegar's sign, or softening of the uterine isthmus, can be detected at 6 to 8 weeks.

Irregular hyperpigmentation of the forehead, upper lip, nasal bridge, and cheeks is known as the "mask of pregnancy," or melasma. Hyperpigmentation in the midline of the lower abdomen is described as the linea nigra. Hyperpigmentation is also seen in the umbilicus, axillae, and perineum. This hyperpigmentation is a response to increased concentrations of estrogen, progesterone, and melanocyte-stimulating hormone. Excess estrogen production also leads to the development of spider angiomas and palmar erythema. Pigmented nevi darken during pregnancy and should be evaluated to exclude malignancy.

Confirmatory diagnostic tests of pregnancy include the auscultation of fetal heart tones, the palpation of a fetus, ultrasound identification of a pregnancy, or the identification of human chorionic gonadotropin (hCG) in urine or blood. Electronic Doppler devices usually detect fetal heart activity between 8 and 12 weeks of gestation, while fetal heart tones are typically first heard with obstetric stethoscopes at 19 weeks of pregnancy. Inaccurate gestational dating, maternal obesity, and nonviable fetal status should be considered when fetal heart tones are not audible at appropriate gestational ages.

Palpation of the fetus is a positive, albeit late, diagnostic sign of pregnancy. Palpation can be accomplished at 22 weeks. Fewer than 40 per cent of twin gestations can be diagnosed by palpation. By contrast, more than 95 per cent of multiple gestations delivered as twins can be diagnosed prenatally by ultrasonography.

Ultrasound can be useful in diagnosing pregnancy or in determining or confirming gestational age. A gestational sac can be identified by transvaginal ultrasound at 5 weeks of gestation, and fetal heart activity can be identified during the sixth week of pregnancy. The accuracy of vaginal probe ultrasound in determining gestational age during the first trimester is excellent. First-trimester measurements of fetal crown-rump length can confirm gestational dating to within 5 days in 95 per cent of patients. Routine ultrasound is not, however, an efficient way of diagnosing pregnancy or establishing gestational age in women whose menstrual histories are accurate and available.

PREGNANCY TESTS

Historically, biologic tests using mice, rabbits, rats, and frogs were used to diagnose pregnancy. Urine from pregnant women was injected into the test animal, and changes in corpora lutea or the extrusion of eggs was evaluated. These biologic endpoints were observed more frequently as the number of weeks beyond the missed period increased. Biologic tests of pregnancy were eventually replaced by qualitative and quantitative immunoassays of hCG.

Human chorionic gonadotropin, luteinizing hormone (LH), follicle-stimulating hormone (FSH), and thyrotropin-stimulating hormone (TSH) are glycoproteins composed of identical alpha-subunits and varying beta-subunits. The beta-subunits of hCG and LH have similar, but not identical, amino acid sequences. Secreted by placental syncytiotrophoblasts, hCG can be detected in maternal serum as early as 6 to 8 days after fertilization. Most currently available pregnancy assays permit the detection of hCG in urine 3 to 4 days after implantation (day 25 of a 28-day menstrual cycle).

Qualitative urine pregnancy tests are based on antibody agglutination inhibition assays (Fig. 1). In direct agglutination inhibition assays, test reagents of red blood cells or latex particles coated with hCG and antibodies directed against hCG are added to urine from the patient. If that urine contains hCG, it will selectively bind the test antibodies and no agglutination of the latex particles will occur. If the urine does not contain hCG, the test antibodies will bind the hCG-coated latex particles and agglutination will occur. A positive test result is indicated by deposition of a ring at the bottom of the test tube. The most recent generation of these tests has a detection limit of 200 mIU/mL and is positive 4 to 7 days after the first missed period. Although these agglutination tests are well known and inexpensive, they are not specific for pregnancy because the assay uses antibodies raised against the intact (entire) hCG molecule. False-positive results may be seen in patients with hypothyroidism, immunologic disorders, renal failure, or conditions associated with increased concentrations of LH.

The use of antibodies raised against the purified beta-subunit of hCG has increased the sensitivity and specificity of urine pregnancy tests (Fig. 2). In the technique known as enzyme-linked immunosorbent assay (ELISA), a solid-

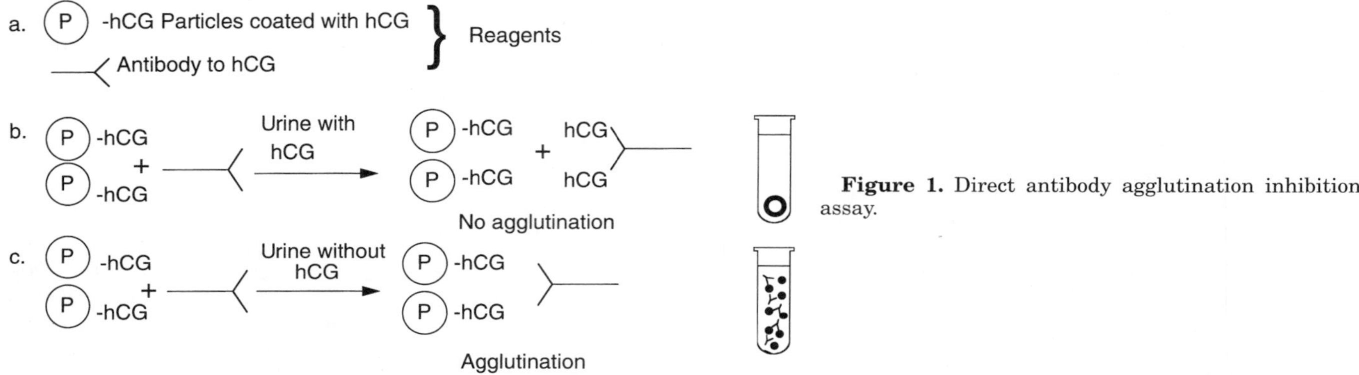

Figure 1. Direct antibody agglutination inhibition assay.

phase anti–alpha-subunit antibody is mixed with patient serum or urine. An enzyme-labeled anti–beta-subunit antibody is then added. If the patient's urine contains hCG, the resultant antibody sandwich will cause a reagent to change colors. The use of two antibodies increases the sensitivity of the test because the capture antibody concentrates hCG on the surface of the solid phase. Antibody sandwich assays also improve specificity because the two antibodies are directed against two different sites found only on the hCG molecule. The detection limit of ELISA-based pregnancy tests is 25 to 50 mIU/mL of urine. The predictive value of both a negative and a positive qualitative pregnancy test with a detection limit of 25 to 50 mIU/mL is excellent. A negative test result obtained more than 1 week after the expected time of the missed period almost always excludes pregnancy. False-negative results can occur when conception takes place later than would be expected by LMP dating. Retesting in 1 week eliminates residual false-negative results. False-positive results usually reflect low circulating concentrations of hCG in nonpregnant women, but may also be produced by hCG-secreting tumors or therapeutic injections of hCG administered in ovulation induction programs. The rate of false-positive results in ELISA test kits varies from 1 to 2 per cent. False-positive values are typically in the range of 5 to 25 mIU/mL; concentrations exceeding 25 mIU/mL usually reflect pregnancy. In general, values less than 5 mIU/mL are considered true-negative results, while values greater than 25 mIU/mL are considered true-positive results. If the first urine hCG concentration is greater than 5 mIU/mL but less than 25 mIU/mL, the test should be repeated in 48 hours.

Quantitative serum pregnancy tests utilize radiolabeled antibodies (iodine-125) directed against hCG. Using scintillation counting techniques, laboratories can detect serum concentrations as low as 2 to 4 mIU/mL. Quantitative analysis allows calculation of hCG "doubling times" that may confirm appropriate progression of the pregnancy. In early viable pregnancies, hCG titers increase rapidly with doubling times of 1.3 to 3.5 days. Typically, hCG concentrations peak around 100,000 mIU/mL at 7 to 10 weeks of pregnancy. When hCG concentrations are measured every 48 hours, 85 per cent of normal intrauterine pregnancies demonstrate appropriate doubling times. Although beta-hCG concentrations do not predict exact gestational age, titers higher than expected for gestational age should increase the index of suspicion for inaccurate gestational dating, the presence of multiple gestations, or gestational trophoblastic neoplasia. By contrast, titers lower than expected at a particular gestational age may reflect inaccurate dating or nonviable status of the pregnancy. Human chorionic gonadotropin doubling times probably should not be used to assess the normalcy of pregnancies known to have progressed beyond 8 to 10 weeks.

Early diagnosis of abnormal pregnancies, including ectopic pregnancy, is crucial. Ectopic pregnancy is the leading cause of first-trimester maternal death in the United States. A fivefold increase in the incidence of ectopic pregnancy over the past 2 decades has been attributed to an increased incidence of pelvic inflammatory disease, increased use of assisted reproductive technologies, and increased use of progestational contraceptives that alter tubal motility. Earlier identification of ectopic pregnancies that would otherwise have remained subclinical has also contributed to the apparent increase in the incidence of this disease. The history and clinical examination, alone, do not reliably identify the women who have ectopic pregnancies. The symptoms of an ectopic pregnancy include adnexal-pelvic pain, amenorrhea, abnormal bleeding, nausea, syncope, and passage of tissue. The classic triad of pain, bleeding, and adnexal mass is observed in only 14 to 33 per cent of patients with ectopic pregnancies. In classic studies of women who died from ectopic pregnancy during the period 1979 to 1980, 47 per cent of cases were misdiagnosed as gastrointestinal disorders (25 per cent), intrauterine pregnancy (18 per cent), pelvic inflammatory disease (14 per cent), psychiatric disorders (9 per cent), spontaneous abortions (9 per cent), and other conditions (25 per

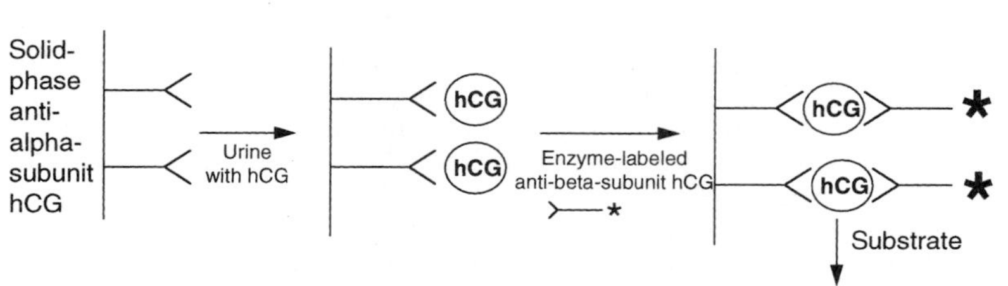

Figure 2. Enzyme-linked immunosorbent assay used in pregnancy testing.

cent). A retrospective review of women who were medically evaluated prior to death from ectopic pregnancy revealed pain, abnormal bleeding, and adnexal mass in 100 per cent, 63 per cent, and 17 per cent of patients, respectively. The knowledge that ectopic pregnancies are associated with impaired hCG secretion has improved diagnostic accuracy and has been an important determinant of the decrease in the case fatality rate for this condition. Approximately 85 per cent of ectopic pregnancies have less than a 66 per cent increase in hCG secretion over 48 hours of monitoring. Unfortunately, this also means that 15 per cent of ectopic pregnancies have normal doubling times. Moreover, approximately 10 to 15 per cent of viable intrauterine pregnancies have abnormal doubling times and must be distinguished from nonviable pregnancies.

Knowledge of the free beta-subunit hCG value can help the clinician select other testing modalities. The "discriminatory zone," or minimal concentration of beta-subunit hCG below which a gestational sac cannot be visualized by transvaginal ultrasound, is 1000 mIU/mL. Most ultrasonography units require 1500 to 2000 mIU/mL for visualization. The discriminatory zone for transabdominal ultrasound is about 6500 mIU/mL, which means that transvaginal ultrasound can detect a viable intrauterine pregnancy about 5 to 7 days earlier than transabdominal ultrasound. Ultrasound evaluation of early pregnancy in a patient with serum hCG below the discriminatory zone for transvaginal ultrasound is expected to be unrevealing. In a stable patient, the clinician should allow the appropriate number of doubling times to pass so that the beta-subunit hCG exceeds the discriminatory zone for the available ultrasound unit. Conversely, the inability to identify an intrauterine pregnancy by ultrasound when the beta-subunit hCG exceeds the relevant discriminatory zone suggests an ectopic pregnancy and warrants immediate attention. Although hCG testing is superior to ultrasound for diagnosis of early pregnancy, it is inferior to ultrasound for dating the pregnancy.

The clinician should be aware of the particular reference units employed by the laboratory to report beta-subunit hCG because serial quantitative hCG measurements can be compared only if they are reported in the same units. The most commonly used standard is the first international reference preparation (IRP), which is obtained from highly purified hCG.

Measurement of serum progesterone has been suggested as an adjunct to serum hCG for the diagnosis of ectopic pregnancy. Unlike the case with hCG, serum concentrations of progesterone, which reflect corpus luteum function, vary little through the first 8 to 10 weeks of pregnancy. Although serum progesterone may be helpful in distinguishing a viable pregnancy from a nonviable one, it is not helpful in distinguishing a nonviable intrauterine pregnancy from an extrauterine pregnancy. When progesterone concentrations are 5 ng/mL or less, a nonviable pregnancy is almost always found. When progesterone is 25 ng/mL or more, a viable intrauterine pregnancy is identified in 98 per cent of patients. Only 2 per cent of ectopic pregnancies have associated progesterone concentrations of 25 ng/mL or more. Progesterone values are less helpful in the range of 5 to 25 ng/mL (the range associated with most ectopic pregnancies). Thus, serum progesterone measurement has limited value in the diagnosis of ectopic pregnancy.

SELECTED MEDICAL PROBLEMS IN PREGNANCY

Diabetes and Pregnancy

Approximately 2 to 3 per cent of all pregnancies are complicated by diabetes mellitus. Among those whose pregnancies are accompanied by diabetes, 10 per cent have pregestational diabetes and 90 per cent have gestational diabetes (GDM). Pregestational diabetics who experience poor glycemic control during embryogenesis have an increased incidence of spontaneous abortions and a fourfold increase in the incidence of major congenital anomalies, including caudal regression syndrome, neural tube defects, cardiac anomalies, and renal anomalies. Women with underlying vascular disease have an increased prevalence of preeclampsia and IUGR. Moreover, pregnancy may worsen the progression of diabetic retinopathy in women with active retinopathy at the time of conception. Optimal glycemic control achieved before and during pregnancy reduces perinatal mortality rates to those of nondiabetic women. The Priscilla White classification of diabetes mellitus categorizes patients according to age at onset, duration of diabetes, and presence of associated vasculopathy (Table 1). This classification has been used historically to predict and explain pregnancy risks to the mother and fetus. A newer classification system, based on the presence or absence of good maternal metabolic control and the presence or absence of vasculopathy, appears to be a more reliable predictor of maternal and fetal outcomes.

Assessment of maternal and fetal risks should begin prior to conception and should focus on ophthalmologic, cardiac, and renal status. An ophthalmologic evaluation should be completed as early as possible in pregnancy, and women with proliferative retinopathy should be monitored closely. Chronic hypertension, pregnancy-induced hypertension, and poor glycemic control are risk factors for progression of proliferative retinopathy. Baseline electrocardiographic and thyroid function studies should be considered in pregestational diabetics. A 24-hour urine collection for measurement of creatinine clearance and total protein excretion should be obtained. Although proteinuria tends to worsen during pregnancy, permanent worsening of diabetic renal disease has not been demonstrated.

The goal of glycemic control during pregnancy is to prevent hyperglycemia and ketoacidosis. Plasma glucose values should be monitored several times throughout the day with portable reflectance meters and recorded in the permanent memory of the instrument for review. Recommended values for plasma glucose are listed in Table 2.

The percentage of glycosylated hemoglobin (hemoglobin A_{1C}) reflects glycemic control over the previous 4 to 8 weeks. Although the ideal value for hemoglobin A_{1C} has not been established for pregnant women, the rate of major congenital malformations among diabetic women with hemoglobin A_{1C} values less than 8.5 per cent (normal) is

Table 1. Modified White's Classification of Diabetes Mellitus

Gestational diabetes: discovered for the first time during pregnancy	
Class A:	Diagnosed before pregnancy—any age at onset or duration; managed by diet alone
Class B:	Insulin treatment necessary before pregnancy; Onset: ≥20 years of age, *or* Duration: <10 years
Class C:	Onset: 10–19 years of age, *or* Duration: 10–19 years
Class D:	Onset: before age 10; *or* Duration: ≥20 years; *or* Chronic hypertension; or background retinopathy
Class F:	Renal disease
Class H:	Coronary artery disease
Class R:	Proliferative retinopathy
Class T:	Renal transplant

Table 2. Recommended Values for Plasma Glucose

Time of Testing	Range of Plasma Glucose (mg/dL)
Fasting	60–90
Before lunch, dinner, bedtime snack	60–105
After meals	1-hour postprandial <130–140 2-hour postprandial <120
Early morning 2 AM to 6 AM	60–90

equal to that of the nondiabetic population. By contrast, hemoglobin A_{1C} values greater than 11 per cent are associated with a major congenital malformation rate of 26 per cent. Hemoglobin A_{1C} should be measured at the first prenatal visit and regularly thereafter in cases of poor metabolic control.

Gestational diabetes describes carbohydrate intolerance with onset or first recognition during pregnancy. Poorly controlled gestational diabetes is associated with an increased risk of several adverse perinatal outcomes, including excessive fetal growth and associated birth trauma, fetal death, neonatal hypoglycemia, and hyperbilirubinemia. Although the maternal risks are usually less severe than those with pregestational diabetes, women diagnosed with gestational diabetes have as much as a 50 per cent chance of developing overt diabetes mellitus within 20 years. Screening for gestational diabetes is recommended between 24 and 28 weeks of pregnancy or earlier if the patient has a previous history of gestational diabetes. Although universal screening is not currently recommended, selective screening of women at high risk (family history of diabetes, prior unexplained stillbirth, prior infant with birth weight of more than 4000 g, macrosomia by ultrasound, hydramnios, maternal obesity, hypertension, glycosuria, age older than 30 years) identifies only 50 per cent of gestational diabetics.

Screening for GDM begins with administration of 50 g of glucose by mouth. Plasma glucose is measured 1 hour later. If plasma glucose exceeds 130 to 140 mg/dL, a 3-hour glucose tolerance test should be performed. Although fasting improves the sensitivity, the initial 1-hour test can be done at any time of day and in the nonfasting state. The sensitivity of the test is also influenced by the cutoff value for a normal screen. An abnormal value defined as more than 130 mg/dL identifies almost all gestational diabetics with a false-positive rate of 25 per cent. A higher threshold of 140 mg/dL reduces the number of false-positive screens to 15 per cent but misses approximately 10 per cent of cases of GDM. Women with 1-hour screen values that exceed 185 mg/dL have GDM and do not require 3-hour glucose tolerance testing (GTT). Women who had unremarkable 1-hour screening prior to 24 weeks of gestation should have repeat testing between 24 and 28 weeks. Glycosylated hemoglobin determinations do not provide the degree of sensitivity and specificity required for effective primary screening for GDM.

Formal 3-hour GTT should be offered to all women with abnormal 1-hour values. A total of 100 grams of glucose is administered by mouth following an overnight fast of at least 8 hours (and not longer than 14 hours). Fasting, 1-, 2-, and 3-hour venous plasma glucose concentrations are measured. Normal values are listed in Table 3. O'Sullivan and Mahan originally established normal values based on whole blood glucose determinations. These investigators employed the Somogyi-Nelson method, which measures other saccharides as well as glucose. Their criteria are the most widely used in the United States. By contrast, the National Diabetes Data Group (NDDG) developed criteria based on plasma glucose analysis. Plasma glucose concentrations are 15 per cent higher than whole blood concentrations. Carpenter and Coustan modified the gestational diabetes criteria even further to account for specimen and methodologic differences. Using any of these three sets of glucose tolerance criteria, the clinician can establish the diagnosis of GDM when any two values are met or exceeded. Approximately 15 per cent of women with abnormal 1-hour screens have two abnormal values on 3-hour testing. Women with a single abnormal value on 3-hour testing should be considered for repeat 3-hour testing because 34 per cent will ultimately meet the formal criteria of GDM on retesting. Women with a single abnormal value on retesting (25 per cent) are at risk for the development of fetal macrosomia and should be carefully monitored. The treatment of women with one abnormal value on 3-hour GTT may decrease the incidence of macrosomia, large-for-gestational-age infants, preeclampsia, and cesarean sections.

Fetal screening efforts are designed to prevent and identify major congenital anomalies, to ensure timely initiation of antenatal fetal surveillance, and to reduce fetal morbidity using appropriately timed delivery. Screening tools for major congenital anomalies include measurement of maternal serum alpha-fetoprotein and hemoglobin A_{1C} and ultrasound evaluation of fetal anatomy. Maternal serum alpha-fetoprotein (MSAFP) screening between 16 and 20 weeks of pregnancy may increase the detection rate for neural tube defects but not for other major congenital anomalies. In diabetic women, the sensitivity of MSAFP for detecting major anomalies ranges from 17 to 34 per cent, and the predictive value of a positive test is 7 to 17 per cent. The specificity is 75 to 86 per cent, and the negative predictive value is 89 to 94 per cent. The clinician who interprets MSAFP values in diabetic patients must keep in mind that the median value for diabetic women is lower than that for nondiabetic women. A screening test more useful than MSAFP for the identification of anomalies is targeted ultrasonography performed between 18 and 20 weeks of pregnancy. Ultrasound in this context has a sensitivity and specificity of 59 per cent and nearly 100 per cent, respectively. The positive predictive value ap-

Table 3. Detection of Gestational Diabetes

Test	Plasma Glucose Level* (mg/dL)		
Screening			
50-g, 1-h screen	130–140		
Diagnostic		***O'Sullivan Criteria (1964)***	
100-g oral glucose tolerance test†		NDDG Conversion (1979)	Carpenter Conversion (1982)
Fasting		105	95
1 h		190	180
2 h		165	155
3 h		145	140

*Result is upper limit of normal.

†Diagnosis of gestational diabetes is made when any two values are met or exceeded.

From American College of Obstetricians and Gynecologists. Diabetes and Pregnancy. ACOG Technical Bulletin No. 200, December 1994, p. 5, with permission from American College of Obstetricians and Gynecologists, Washington, D.C.

proaches 100 per cent, and the negative predictive value is 97 per cent. Fetal echocardiography performed between 20 and 22 weeks is useful when cardiac anomalies are suspected.

The timing and frequency of outpatient fetal testing, including the nonstress test, contraction stress test, and biophysical profile, depend on the degree of underlying maternal vascular disease and the level of glycemic control during the pregnancy. In a pregnancy complicated by nephropathy, vascular disease, or other risk factors, weekly nonstress testing may begin at 28 weeks. Antenatal testing may begin later in gestation in the absence of high risk factors. Assessment of fetal well-being should also include periodic ultrasound evaluation of fetal growth. Women with poor glycemic control in the third trimester experience a threefold greater rate of macrosomia and large-for-gestational-age infants than do women with euglycemia.

The timing of delivery is determined by maternal and fetal risk factors. Patients with poor or undocumented glycemic control are at risk for delayed biochemical maturation of the fetal lung; thus, documentation of fetal pulmonary maturity should be considered before elective delivery. Fetal pulmonary maturity is confirmed by an amniotic fluid lecithin–to–sphingomyelin ratio of 2.0 or more, or phosphatidylglycerol of 2 to 5 per cent or more.

Postpartum management of women diagnosed with GDM should include 2-hour oral GTT using a 75-g glucose load within the first few months following delivery, and yearly thereafter (Table 4). Approximately 2 per cent of women diagnosed with GDM have abnormal 2-hour screens in the immediate postpartum period. Of the remaining population of former gestational diabetics, those who required insulin have a 50 per cent risk of developing diabetes within 5 years. Women who required only dietary modification have a 60 per cent likelihood of developing diabetes within 10 to 15 years. Breast-feeding may decrease the incidence of nongestational diabetes mellitus in former gestational diabetics.

Thyroid Disorders

Abnormalities of thyroid function are commonly encountered in pregnancy. The symptoms of hyperthyroidism may mimic the normal hypermetabolic state of pregnancy. Physical diagnosis is challenging because benign enlargement of the thyroid gland is observed in normal pregnancy as a result of glandular hyperplasia and increased vascularity. The laboratory evaluation of thyroid disorders may also be confusing because commonly used thyroid function tests are altered in normal pregnant women owing to increases in total and free estrogen concentrations in the first trimester (Table 5). Estrogen stimulates hepatic biosynthesis of thyroxine-binding globulin (TBG), a major carrier of thyroxine (T_4). The total amount of circulating thyroxine and triidothyronine (T_3) is increased, but the amounts of biologically active free T_4 and free T_3 are unchanged. Direct measurements of TBG, free T_4, and T_3 are difficult, so indirect measurements using competitive binding assays are employed. The T_3 resin uptake (T_3RU) is an indirect measure of TBG concentration. Radiolabeled T_3 is incubated with a serum sample (containing TBG) and an artificial resin column. Radiolabeled T_3 selectively binds to available TBG molecules before binding to the artificial resin. Thus, binding of radiolabeled T_3 to the resin decreases in proportion to increases in TBG. Conditions that increase TBG (e.g., pregnancy) cause a reciprocal decrease in T_3RU. Many laboratories find it impractical to measure serum TBG and the metabolically active free T_4. Instead, they provide an indirect measure of free hormone concentration that adjusts for pregnancy-associated increases in TBG by calculating the free thyroxine index (FTI, or T_7). This index is a multiple of the total T_4 times the ratio of the patient's T_3RU to the normal T_3RU value. The FTI remains unchanged during normal pregnancy and is a reliable test of thyroid function. An increased FTI suggests hyperthyroidism; a low FTI suggests hypothyroidism.

Table 4. Postpartum Evaluation for Carbohydrate Intolerance

	Plasma Glucose Level* (mg/dL)		
Time Tested	***No Diabetes***	***Impaired Glucose Tolerance***	***Diabetes Mellitus***
Fasting	<115	<140	≥140†
½, 1, 1½ h	All <200	1 value ≥200	1 value ≥200
2 h	<140	140–199	≥200

*Values are based on a 2-h, 75-g oral glucose tolerance test.

†Fasting plasma glucose determinations of ≥140 on two occasions establish the diagnosis.

From American College of Obstetricians and Gynecologists. Diabetes and Pregnancy. ACOG Technical Bulletin No. 200, December 1994, p. 1, with permission from American College of Obstetricians and Gynecologists, Washington, D.C.

Table 5. Influence of Pregnancy on Thyroid Function Tests

Test	Normal Pregnancy	Hyperthyroidism
TBG	Increased	No change
Total T_4	Increased	Increased
Free T_4	No change	Increased
Total T_3	Increased	Increased
Free T_3	No change	Increased
T_3RU	Decreased	Increased
TSH	No change	Decreased

T_3 = triiodothyronine; T_4 = thyroxine; T_3RU = triiodothyronine resin uptake; TSH = thyroid-stimulating hormone.

Hyperthyroidism that develops during pregnancy is most commonly caused by Graves' disease, but acute and subacute thyroiditis, toxic nodular goiter, and toxic adenoma have also been reported. Graves' disease is an autoimmune disorder characterized by production of thyroid-stimulating immunoglobulins (TSI) that stimulate thyroid function or cause glandular disruption and release of stored thyroid hormone. The clinical symptoms of thyrotoxicosis include nervousness, fatigue, excessive sweating, weight loss, resting maternal tachycardia, diffuse thyroid enlargement, exophthalmos, tremors, and onycholysis. Thyroid storm results from undiagnosed or untreated hyperthyroidism and is marked by hyperpyrexia (>103°F), tachycardia, and agitation. Cardiovascular collapse may occur without appropriate treatment. Serum T_4 concentrations exceed those normally seen in pregnancy, while the expected decrease of T_3RU is not observed. Therefore, FTI is increased.

Women who remain clinically hyperthyroid throughout pregnancy are at increased risk for preeclampsia, congestive heart failure, and adverse perinatal outcomes, including preterm labor, preterm delivery, and stillbirth. In about 1 per cent of infants born to mothers with Graves' disease, thyroid-stimulating immunoglobulins cross the placenta and bind to the fetal thyroid gland, causing fetal thyrotoxicosis. Fetal death may occur in 15 to 25 per cent of affected pregnancies. Propylthiouracil (PTU), the drug of choice for treating maternal thyrotoxicosis during pregnancy, also crosses the placenta, increasing the risk of neonatal hypothyroidism and goiter. PTU is cleared from the neonatal circulation more rapidly than is TSI. Therefore, neonates who are euthyroid (or hypothyroid) at birth may become hyperthyroid within the first days of life. Approximately 2 per cent of women with hydatidiform mole develop clinical signs of hyperthyroidism. Increased serum T_4 concentrations have been attributed to stimulation of thyroid hormone production by estrogens.

The development or enlargement of thyroid nodules does not normally occur in pregnancy and should be further investigated. True toxic adenomas function independent of TSH stimulation. The patient may or may not have classic signs of frank thyrotoxicosis. Ultrasound can detect nodules smaller than 0.5 cm and may enable the clinician to distinguish solid lesions from cystic ones. Solid masses are more likely to harbor malignancy, but there are no specific sonographic criteria for distinguishing benign lesions from malignant ones. Fine-needle aspiration biopsy provides the most sensitive and specific means for distinguishing malignant disease from benign. Radionuclide imaging with ^{131}I is contraindicated in pregnancy.

Overt hypothyroidism is uncommon in pregnancy. Decreased thyroid hormone production is associated with increased rates of infertility, intrauterine fetal demise, and low birth weight. Common causes of hypothyroidism include Hashimoto's thyroiditis, iatrogenic destruction of the gland, antithyroid medications, and iodine deficiency. Hashimoto's thyroiditis is the most common cause of hypothyroidism and is believed to be an autoimmune disorder.

The signs and symptoms of hypothyroidism that may be indistinguishable from symptoms of pregnancy include fatigue, weakness, sleep disturbances, constipation, skin dryness, cold intolerance, hair loss, and myxedema. Classically, hypothyroid patients have a palpable goiter and delayed deep tendon reflexes. Patients with subclinical hypothyroidism may be asymptomatic. Laboratory analysis typically reveals increased TSH and decreased T_4 concentrations in the serum. Ultrasensitive TSH assays are now preferred for the diagnosis of primary hypothyroidism. Serum TSH should be normal during pregnancy, but increased in primary hypothyroid states. TSH determinations can also be used to monitor the adequacy of thyroid hormone replacement.

Anemia in Pregnancy

Anemia is one of the most common hematologic problems in pregnancy. In the United States, about 60 per cent of women of reproductive age show evidence of iron deficiency and 5 per cent are anemic. About 40 to 80 per cent of pregnant women not receiving iron supplements develop iron deficiency anemia during pregnancy. Pregnancy, itself, induces a "physiologic anemia" because maternal plasma volume increases by 40 to 50 per cent, while total erythrocyte mass increases by 25 per cent. A decreased hematocrit may be noted as early as 8 weeks of gestation and typically reaches a nadir in the second trimester. In the absence of significant hemorrhage at delivery, hematocrit values return to normal by 6 weeks after delivery. Most anemias are due to iron deficiency, but other acquired anemias (folic acid and vitamin B_{12} deficiency, chronic disease, parasite infestation, autoimmune disease, blood loss, hemolytic processes) and inherited anemias (thalassemias, hemoglobinopathies) should be considered.

The signs and symptoms of anemia vary with the rapidity of onset as well as the underlying cardiovascular status of the patient. Slowly developing nutritional anemias permit gradual volume expansion and cardiovascular compensation. Thus, symptoms are subtle and nonspecific. Fatigue, pallor of the skin and mucous membranes, cheilosis (fissuring of the angles of the mouth), koilonychia (spoon nails), and a smooth, beefy tongue are classically reported in advanced nutritional anemias. By contrast, a history of rapid blood loss is associated with tachycardia, postural hypotension, vasoconstriction in the extremities, and dyspnea.

The laboratory evaluation of anemia begins with a complete blood count (including the hemoglobin, hematocrit, platelet count, and red cell indices) and a peripheral blood smear. A significant anemia in pregnancy is defined by a hemoglobin of less than 11 g/dL or a hematocrit of less than 33 per cent. The mean corpuscular volume (MCV) can be useful in the differential diagnosis of anemia. Microcytic anemia (MCV <80 μm³) is more common than normocytic (MCV 80 to 100 μm³) or macrocytic (MCV >100 μm³) anemia. Microcytosis occurs in iron deficiency, thalassemia trait, and chronic disease; normocytosis occurs in acute blood loss; and macrocytosis is characteristic of folic acid and vitamin B_{12} deficiencies. The peripheral blood smear may reveal sickle cells, target cells, schistocytes, nucleated red blood cells, or erythrocytes harboring parasites. In addition, the peripheral smear can be used to identify the neutrophil abnormalities characteristic of megaloblastic anemia and to distinguish platelet clumping from true thrombocytopenia.

About 95 per cent of nutritional anemia in pregnancy is caused by iron deficiency. Pregnant women need 1 g of elemental iron to meet the demands of increased maternal red blood cell production (450 mg), fetal erythropoiesis (350 mg), and anticipated blood loss at delivery (200 mg). Lactation requires 1 mg per day of elemental iron. In the United States, the usual diet supplies 15 mg of elemental iron daily, but only 10 per cent is absorbed. The average daily requirement for iron during pregnancy is 4 mg in the second trimester and 6 to 8 mg in the third trimester. Women with malabsorption syndromes or who ingest nonnutritive substances (pica) such as starch or clay are at increased risk for the development of iron deficiency anemia.

The first change to occur in iron deficiency anemia is a depletion of iron stores (in the form of ferritin and its derivative, hemosiderin) in the bone marrow, liver, and spleen. Following this, total iron-binding capacity (TIBC) increases, plasma iron concentration falls, and the percentage saturation of transferrin decreases. Reduced hemoglobin and hematocrit are then observed. Initially, erythrocytes remain normocytic and normochromic while the hematocrit falls, but eventually, microcytic, hypochromic red blood cells are released into the peripheral circulation. Serum ferritin concentrations below 10 ng/dL may be the most useful corroborating test of iron deficiency anemia despite an expected decline of serum ferritin as plasma volume increases during pregnancy (Table 6). Bone marrow aspiration is rarely required for making the diagnosis of iron deficiency anemia.

Table 6. Changes in Iron Studies With Progressing Anemia

Hemoglobin (g/dL)	MCV (μm³)	Serum Ferritin (μg/mL)	Serum Iron (μg/dL)	Bone Marrow Biopsy
≥13	≥100	14–150	50–150	Fe present
10–12	≥100	<10	↓(<60)	Fe absent
8–10	80–100	<10	↓↓	Fe absent
≤8	≤80	<10	↓↓↓	Fe absent

To correct iron deficiency anemia, prescribe the ingestion of 60 mg of elemental iron two to three times a day. The reticulocyte count should increase within 2 weeks of initiating treatment. Hemoglobin values rise about 0.5 g/dL per week.

Folic acid deficiency is the major cause of megaloblastic anemia during pregnancy. Vitamin B_{12} deficiency (pernicious anemia) is exceedingly rare in women of childbearing age. Pregnancies complicated by multiple gestation, malabsorption syndromes, sickle cell anemia, alcoholism, and prior use of phenytoin may be at increased risk for folic acid deficiency. Diagnosis is made by review of the peripheral smear in combination with serum and red blood cell folate measurements. A decreased serum folate (≤4 ng/mL) may be the first indication of deficiency, but folate analyses may be unreliable because serum folate falls as plasma volume increases in normal pregnancy. Hypersegmentation of neutrophils (usually more than 5 per cent of cells demonstrating five or more lobes) then occurs, followed by depletion of red blood cell folate. Megaloblasts observed in bone marrow aspirates are a late sign. If the aforementioned criteria cannot be satisfied and folate deficiency is still suspected, a therapeutic trial of folic acid may be indicated. The response to folic acid replacement is immediate. Reticulocytosis is observed within a few days, and the hematocrit rises by 1 per cent daily after 1 week of replacement. Approximately 70 per cent of patients with folic acid deficiency are also iron deficient and should be treated with iron.

INFERTILITY

By Dale W. Stovall, M.D.
Iowa City, Iowa

Infertility is a common condition with important psychological, economic, demographic, and medical implications. Evaluation of the infertile couple is a clinical challenge that requires a broad perspective. Infertility is defined as the inability to conceive after 1 year of intercourse without contraception. Patients who have previously conceived and subsequently become infertile are said to have secondary infertility. The average monthly probability of pregnancy (fecundity) for normally fertile couples is approximately 20 per cent. Assuming a 20 per cent monthly fecundity, the cumulative probability of pregnancy after 12 months is 93 per cent (Table 1). That is, after 12 months, the likelihood of being normally fertile and not pregnant is only 7 per cent. Thus, in couples who have not been able to conceive despite 12 months of unprotected intercourse, a standard infertility evaluation is warranted.

Table 1. Cumulative Conception Rate in Normally Fertile Couples

Month	Monthly Fecundity	Cumulative Conception Rate
1	0.2	0.20
3	0.2	0.49
6	0.2	0.74
9	0.2	0.87
12	0.2	0.93

Table 2. Incidence of Infertility With Respect to Age

Age (yr)	Per Cent Infertile
25–29	9
30–34	14
35–39	25
40–44	27

Population studies that have attempted to estimate the prevalence of infertility can be difficult to interpret, as both the number of infertile couples (the numerator) and the number of women "at risk" for pregnancy (the denominator) depend on the definition used for infertility and the questions being asked. In the United States, recent changes in the population have had an impact on the prevalence of infertility in this country. Because of the "baby boom" that occurred from 1947 through 1961, the percentage of the population in their middle to late 30s and early 40s has increased. Age has a negative influence on fertility. The incidence of infertility rises as age increases (Table 2). Thus, the percentage of the U.S. population of a "subfertile" reproductive age has increased. In response to a changing social and economic environment, couples are delaying childbearing; the U.S. birth rate for women younger than 30 years of age is decreasing, while the birth rate in women older than 30 years of age is increasing. In addition, those who have been unsuccessful in starting a family have become aware of the highly publicized advances in infertility therapy. Thus, the number of physician visits for infertility has significantly risen over the past decade.

The relative frequency of factors associated with infertility has been evaluated in numerous studies. Short of an absolute infertility factor, such as azoospermia and bilateral tubal occlusion, it cannot be said with certainty that any abnormality found during infertility testing is "the" cause of infertility in a particular patient. Thus, any effort to specify the relative frequency of "causes" of infertility is necessarily imprecise. Nonetheless, it is instructive to estimate the frequency with which various factors are found in association with infertility as a rough approximation of their relative importance. For this purpose, some estimated rates of various factors associated with infertility are listed in Table 3. The clinician must keep in mind that a significant percentage of couples who are infertile will have a completely normal infertility evaluation.

INITIAL VISIT

The Couple

The infertility evaluation should be recorded on an easy-to-read flow sheet. Information obtained during the initial

Table 3. Distribution of Factors Associated With Infertility

Cause	Percentage of Infertile Couples
Unexplained	28
Abnormal semen analysis	23
Ovulatory dysfunction	18
Tubal disease	14
Endometriosis	6
Coital problems	5
Cervical factor	3

visit, infertility testing, and subsequent visits can be quickly reviewed and updated on this sheet. Initially, the infertile couple should be evaluated together. Obtain a detailed history, as described later, and instruct the couple regarding the conditions that are required for fertility. Explain that the male must produce a sufficient number of spermatozoa to ensure penetration of the cervical mucus and migration to the fallopian tubes. Indicate that normal cervical mucus and uterine secretions must be present to support sperm transport. Describe the timely release of a mature oocyte, the uptake and transport of the oocyte, and the normal hormonal production by the ovary to support endometrial development and implantation. Instruct the couple regarding the most likely time for conception (within 24 to 48 hours of ovulation), and urge them to avoid coital lubricants that may be spermicidal. Determine the duration of the couple's current infertility, and discuss any previous infertility evaluation or therapy. Record the frequency of intercourse.

The Female Partner

Record the female's obstetric history, including gravidity and parity. Assess ovarian function by recording the patient's menstrual history. Regular cyclic menses of 28 ± 4 days are consistent with ovulation. Evaluate women with irregular menstrual cycles for hirsutism, weight gain, galactorrhea, and hot flashes. Galactorrhea is associated with hyperprolactinemia, while hot flashes can signal a decreased ovarian reserve. A history of dysmenorrhea or intermenstrual pelvic pain suggests endometriosis. Record the previous method of contraception. In particular, women who have previously used intrauterine devices (IUDs) for contraception are at increased risk for pelvic infection and tubal occlusion. Pelvic inflammatory disease and appendicitis may also produce pelvic abnormalities and associated infertility. A history of abdominopelvic surgery for appendicitis, ovarian cysts, pelvic pain, endometriosis, or uterine leiomyomas suggests the possibility of pelvic adhesions with distortion of pelvic anatomy. Smoking has been linked to infertility, and couples who smoke should be encouraged to stop.

The Male Partner

Obtain a thorough history from the male partner. Explore the history to assess the development of the external genitalia, androgen production, spermatogenesis, potency, and ejaculatory function. Assess the onset and development of secondary sexual characteristics as indicators of the appropriate onset of testosterone production. A history of undescended testes (cryptorchidism) is occasionally found. If this condition is not treated before puberty, azoospermia or oligospermia and infertility commonly occur. Testicular trauma, especially straddle injuries, may impair spermatogenesis. Any testicular trauma, including vasectomy, that breaks the blood-testes barrier may lead to the formation of sperm antibodies, which can impair sperm motility. Ask the male partner about exposure to toxic chemicals, radiation, illicit drugs, and tobacco. A medical history of diabetes mellitus, hypertension, or other vascular diseases is also associated with infertility. Finally, assess male sexual function, with special attention to potency, erection, and ejaculation.

Physical Examination

The Female Partner

Record the vital signs and weight of the female partner, and examine the skin. Patients with irregular menses often have hirsutism, which is defined as an increase in the distribution of secondary sexual hair on the face, chest, lower abdomen, lower back, and extremities. Hirsutism is the clinical manifestation of hyperandrogenemia. The triad of obesity, hirsutism, and irregular menstrual cycles is consistent with chronic anovulation and the polycystic ovarian syndrome. Some patients with this syndrome have insulin resistance and hyperinsulinemia. A common observation in patients with insulin resistance is acanthosis nigricans, a pigmentation of the skin commonly found on the neck and axilla and in skinfolds.

Examine the breasts, looking for expressible breast milk. During the pelvic examination, look for an enlarged clitoris and/or male pubic hair patterns that suggest hyperandrogenemia. Highly rugate vaginal mucosa indicates normal estrogen production. When the examination is performed 3 to 4 days before ovulation, the cervical mucus should be clear and abundant, providing further evidence of normal estrogen production. Perform a bimanual examination to determine the size and contour of the uterus and ovaries. An enlarged or irregularly shaped uterus may harbor leiomyomas. Pelvic discomfort during a bimanual examination is a nonspecific finding. Patients with pelvic tenderness may suffer from pelvic inflammatory disease, pelvic adhesions, leiomyomas, ovarian cysts, and/or endometriosis. Definitive diagnosis of pelvic adhesions and/or endometriosis requires direct visualization of the pelvis via laparoscopy or laparotomy. Endometriosis should always be considered if the pelvic examination reveals nodularity beneath the cervix (along the uterosacral ligaments), especially in a patient with pelvic tenderness and infertility. Office ultrasonography is not routinely performed during the initial visit, but it may be helpful in the assessment of adnexal masses and uterine abnormalities.

The Male Partner

The male partner is not routinely examined during the first visit. Rather, a detailed history is obtained and semen is analyzed. If the semen is abnormal or the history reveals a specific abnormality, physical examination is warranted. As in the female, the male body habitus may provide clues to the status of gonadal function. In particular, gynecomastia and reduced sexual hair distribution suggest hypoandrogenemia. Men with Klinefelter's syndrome (47, XXY), the most common disorder causing male hypogonadism, have a eunuchoid body habitus. Their arm span is usually more than 2 cm longer than their height, and their upper-to-lower body ratios are less than 1. In these patients and others with abnormalities in spermatogenesis, the testes are often small and firm.

Inspect the urethral meatus for evidence of hypospadias. Severe hypospadias may result in ejaculation of spermatozoa outside the vagina or at great distances from the cervix. Use an orchidometer to assess testicular volume. The normal, postpubertal testicular volume is approximately 25 cm^3. Palpate the vas deferens and epididymis. Examine the scrotal sac for the presence of a varicocele or hydrocele. A varicocele is a varicose enlargement of the veins of the spermatic cord. Varicoceles are most easily detected in standing patients during Valsalva maneuvers. These venous enlargements may impair spermatogenesis by increasing the temperature within the testes. In contrast, hydroceles are collections of serous fluid. Although hydroceles may cause discomfort, they are less likely to impair spermatogenesis. Finally, perform a rectal examination to exclude prostatic enlargement, tenderness, and/or irregularity.

INFERTILITY TESTING

When the initial history and physical examination have been completed, the clinician should schedule infertility testing. The standard infertility tests include a semen analysis; serum progesterone or endometrial biopsy to assess ovulation; postcoital testing to assess the cervical factor; hysterosalpingogram to assess uterine contour and tubal patency; and laparoscopy to identify pelvic adhesions or endometriosis. With efficient scheduling, all but the laparoscopy can be completed in a single menstrual cycle. The remainder of this article reviews the purpose, technique, and timing of these procedures. As the infertility evaluation proceeds, each abnormal test must be interpreted with respect to its degree of departure from "normality."

Semen Analysis

Spermatogenesis occurs in the seminiferous tubules. Spermatozoa move from the seminiferous tubules into the epididymis, where they continue to mature and attain their motility. The seminiferous tubules contain a "wave" of spermatozoa at different stages of development. This wave ensures a continuous supply of spermatozoa. However, no two ejaculates contain the same number or concentration of spermatozoa. Thus, one semen analysis may not provide an adequate assessment of the overall process of spermatogenesis. Furthermore, the production of mature spermatozoa, beginning with the division of a spermatogonia and progressing through spermatogenesis, spermiogenesis, and sperm maturation, takes approximately 94 days. Therefore, any testicular injury or insult that impairs spermatogenesis may not affect the results of a semen analysis for several months.

After a thorough history has been obtained from the male partner, he is instructed to collect a semen sample. Semen is typically collected by masturbation without the use of lubricants. Before collection, instruct the patient to abstain from intercourse for 2 to 7 days. Ask the patient to deliver the sample to the andrology laboratory within 45 minutes of collection. If possible, collect the semen in the same building as the andrology laboratory. Clearly label each container. Clearly mark the collection time on the container. Do not allow the seminal fluid to be exposed to extremes in temperature. Special condoms are available for men who cannot or will not collect semen by masturbation. Condoms used for contraception should not be used to collect semen for analysis.

The normal semen analysis parameters are listed in Table 4. Distinguishing normal from abnormal sperm parameters is difficult. At one extreme, azoospermia represents an absolute barrier to pregnancy; at the other, men producing large numbers of motile spermatozoa with normal morphology will probably be fertile. Importantly, men who have one or more abnormal semen analysis parameters may still be fertile, while men with no abnormal parameters may nevertheless be subfertile. Infertility treatment outcome studies indicate that sperm motility and morphology are the most sensitive predictors of pregnancy. However, most laboratories that perform semen analysis do not use standardized objective criteria in defining abnormal motility or morphology. Thus, different laboratories evaluating the same specimen may reach different conclusions.

Table 4. Reference Values for Semen Analysis Parameters

Semen Parameters	Reference Value
Semen volume (mL)	2–5
Sperm density ($\times$ 10^6/mL)	20–250
Sperm motility (%)	>50
Normal sperm morphology (%)	>50

Men with azoospermia require further investigation. If one or more semen analyses reveal an absence of spermatozoa, the seminal fluid should be evaluated for the presence of fructose. The seminal vesicles produce fructose; its presence in the ejaculate makes obstruction of the male reproductive tract unlikely. If the seminal plasma does not contain fructose, the patient may have congenital absence of the seminal vesicles or obstruction of the vas deferens. Patients with decreased sperm density (oligospermia), decreased sperm motility (asthenospermia), or decreased percentage of normally shaped spermatozoa (teratospermia), on two occasions, require further assessment. These patients should have a physical examination and measurement of serum follicle-stimulating hormone (FSH) and testosterone. In the patient with severe oligospermia or azoospermia, normal serum concentrations of FSH and testosterone are consistent with obstruction of the epididymis or vas deferens, arrest of sperm maturation, and the Sertoli-cell–only syndrome. Testicular biopsy is required for identifying the latter two disorders. Of these abnormalities, only an obstruction can be repaired. Increased serum FSH concentrations, coupled with decreased serum testosterone, indicates gonadal failure that is difficult, if not impossible, to treat. By contrast, a patient with decreased FSH and decreased testosterone most likely has hypothalamic or pituitary dysfunction that usually responds to the administration of gonadotropins.

Postcoital Test

After deposition in the upper vagina, spermatozoa enter the uterine cavity at varying rates of speed. For most of the menstrual cycle, the cervical os contains thick, sparse mucus that serves as a barrier to the penetration of sperm. In the periovulatory period, under the influence of estrogen, the cervical mucus becomes thin and abundant, allowing easy passage of spermatozoa into the uterine cavity. To assess the interaction between spermatozoa and cervical mucus, the postcoital test (PCT) is performed 1 to 3 days prior to ovulation. Approximately 2 to 12 hours after coitus, obtain two cervical mucus samples with a Randall Stone forceps or a plastic angiocatheter attached to a syringe. Take the first sample from the cervical os, and the second from the vaginal pool. Place the latter sample on a microscope slide, and cover with a coverslip. Identification of spermatozoa in this vaginal pool specimen is consistent with adequate coitus. Assess one half of the mucus obtained from the cervical os for the presence of ferning as the sample dries. Examine the other half with a microscope. Record the number of leukocytes and motile spermatozoa per 1 high-power field. The cervical mucus is usually thin, abundant, and elastic and demonstrates ferning when allowed to dry. It contains few inflammatory cells, and at least five forwardly motile sperm per 1 high-power field. Cervicitis, if present, may interfere with sperm motility. In the absence of inflammation, when the spermatozoa move in place, "shake," or do not move at all, the probability of finding sperm antibodies in the cervical mucus or seminal fluid is increased.

The validity and clinical utility of postcoital testing are not established. Universal criteria that distinguish normal findings from abnormal ones have not been adopted, and there is no indication that PCT results distinguish fertile populations from infertile ones.

Assessment of Ovulation

Fertility requires the timely release of a mature oocyte and normal production of the ovarian hormones that support endometrial development and implantation. Cyclic, predictable menses implies consistent ovulation; amenorrhea signifies the absence of ovulation; and oligomenorrhea, or irregular menses, implies erratic ovulation. Although oligo-ovulation does not represent an absolute barrier to pregnancy, the likelihood of pregnancy in a given time interval is reduced.

To confirm a clinical impression of ovulation, the clinician can instruct the patient to perform basal body temperature (BBT) charting. During an ovulatory cycle, the BBT curve is "biphasic," with temperature increases of 0.5 to 1.0°F in the luteal phase owing to progesterone production by the corpus luteum. BBT charting is inexpensive, but it is also subjective and often difficult to interpret. By contrast, a serum progesterone exceeding 10 nmol/L, or a biopsy showing secretory endometrium, provides more objective confirmation of ovulation. After ovulation, the serum progesterone concentration rises slowly and reaches a plateau in approximately 7 days. Thus, the serum progesterone concentration should be measured 7 to 10 days after ovulation, and endometrial biopsies should be obtained 10 to 12 days after ovulation. Luteinizing hormone (LH) surge kits can be used to time the serum progesterone measurements and endometrial sampling. When an LH surge is detected, ovulation ensues in the next 36 hours. The sensitivity and reliability of urine LH assays are clinically acceptable if the patient closely follows the instructions in the kit. Also, LH surge kits are useful in helping couples time intercourse.

If the menstrual history typically provides reliable information about the presence or absence of ovulation, why are serum progesterone measurements and endometrial biopsies so important? The primary concern is the luteal phase defect (LPD) that may cause infertility by impairing nidation, or implantation. Luteal phase deficiency is defined as a defect in corpus luteal production of progesterone or in the endometrial response to progesterone stimulation. The gold standard for assessment of LPD is the endometrial biopsy. Histologic changes in the glands and stroma of the endometrium during the secretory phase of the menstrual cycle are used to "date" the endometrium. Luteal phase defects typically delay endometrial maturation by more than 2 days. The endometrial biopsy should be obtained 10 to 12 days after ovulation, and the date of the next menses should be recorded to determine luteal phase length. Luteal phase defects are more prevalent in infertile women, and they may provide at least a partial explanation for a specific patient's inability to complete a pregnancy.

If menses are cyclic and predictable, the infertility evaluation does not require measurement of prolactin, thyrotropin, gonadotropins, or androgens. By contrast, the concentration of these hormones should be measured in the serum of infertile patients with amenorrhea or irregular menses. Prolactin surges normally occur several times per day and may also accompany food intake or physical exertion. Therefore, serum for prolactin measurement should be obtained in the fasting state, between 8 and 10 AM. Patients with serum prolactin concentrations exceeding 50 ng/mL should undergo imaging studies to exclude a pituitary adenoma. Patients with a history of amenorrhea or advanced reproductive age (40 years old or more) should have serum for FSH measurement drawn on the third day of menses. An increased "day 3 FSH" concentration indicates reduced ovarian reserve and a decreased probability of induction of ovulation or conception. In a patient younger than 30 years of age with secondary amenorrhea, an increased serum FSH concentration is consistent with gonadal dysgenesis, as found in Turner's syndrome (45, X, or XO). Karyotype analysis is required for confirming this diagnosis.

Uterine Factors

Many uterine abnormalities have been linked to infertility and/or spontaneous abortion, including congenital uterine anomalies, particularly uterine septa; abnormalities associated with in utero exposure to diethylstilbestrol (DES; e.g., T-shaped uterus); leiomyomas, especially if submucous or cornual; endometrial polyps; and intrauterine adhesions or synechiae from prior intrauterine manipulation. Although each of these conditions may be related to infertility, each can also occur in association with pregnancy. Therefore, a causal link between infertility and these conditions has yet to be established. Importantly, there are no large-scale studies comparing the incidence or prevalence of the aforementioned uterine conditions in infertile women and properly matched fertile control subjects. Nevertheless, many infertility evaluations include a hysterosalpingogram to evaluate both uterine and tubal factors. Performing a hysterosalpingogram involves the instillation of radiopaque dye through the cervical os under fluoroscopic observation. The dye fills the uterine cavity, revealing its shape and the presence of intrauterine filling defects. If the fallopian tubes are patent, the dye fills the fallopian tubes and eventually spills into the peritoneal cavity. During the procedure, several radiographs are obtained. The first is a scout film. The second is taken when the uterine cavity has been filled, and a third is taken to document tubal patency. Occasionally, air bubbles enter the uterine cavity; they can be mistaken for an intrauterine filling defect. When air bubbles are detected, turn the patient to the lateral recumbent position. This position may improve the visualization of the uterine cavity. If tubal abnormalities are present, the hysterosalpingogram can be quite painful. Patients should be given a nonsteroidal anti-inflammatory drug or other analgesic prior to the procedure.

Hysteroscopy is used to further evaluate and treat intrauterine synechiae, submucous leiomyomas, endometrial polyps, uterine septa, and other abnormalities detected by hysterosalpingography. Office hysteroscopy using carbon dioxide as a distending media can be performed without cervical dilation and is best suited for evaluating the patient with dysfunctional uterine bleeding. Conversely, outpatient hysteroscopy using an operative, hysteroscopic sheath and liquid distending media is preferred for the diagnosis and treatment of infertile patients with intrauterine lesions. Distention of the uterine cavity during hysteroscopy gives the surgeon a panoramic view of the endometrial cavity. This panoramic view affords clear visualization of both intrauterine lesions and the tubal ostia. Endometrial polyps, synechiae, and submucous leiomyomas can be removed via operative hysteroscopy, and metroplasty can be performed in patients with uterine septa.

Tubal and Peritoneal Factors

The most common cause of tubal infertility is pelvic inflammatory disease. Severe endometriosis and pelvic adhesions secondary to nonpelvic, intra-abdominal infections or pelvic surgery may also interfere with egg pick-up by the fallopian tube. Both hysterosalpingography and laparoscopy can detect tubal abnormalities. Using laparoscopy as the gold standard for correct diagnosis of tubal occlusion, the sensitivity and specificity of a hysterosalpingogram for correct diagnosis of tubal obstruction exceeds 90 per cent. By contrast, the hysterosalpingogram is less effective than laparoscopy for diagnosis of damaged tubal epithelia, partial tubal obstruction, or peritubal adhesions. Hysterosalpingography may miss 20 to 30 per cent of these tubal abnormalities that would otherwise be identified by laparoscopy.

In addition to missing a substantial portion of tubal abnormalities in infertile women, a hysterosalpingogram does not detect cases of endometriosis in which peritoneal and/or ovarian implants coexist with mobile and patent fallopian tubes that are unaffected by the disorder. Endometriosis occurs with high frequency among infertile women, often without symptoms. The rate of endometriosis in infertile women is about 10 times that in fertile control subjects. The substantial difference in the incidence of endometriosis between fertile and infertile women suggests an association between endometriosis and infertility. Such an association may seem sufficient to prompt laparoscopy in asymptomatic, infertile women with a normal hysterosalpingogram. However, the efficacy of endometriosis treatment for infertility in early-stage disease has not been confirmed.

The hysterosalpingogram should be a standard component of the initial infertility evaluation. In some patients, the hysterosalpingogram may eliminate the need for laparoscopy. A woman in her late 30s who is found to have severe bilateral hydrosalpinges may be counseled to proceed with in vitro fertilization, thus bypassing the discomfort and risks of laparoscopy and general anesthesia. Moreover, a woman who is found to have a normal hysterosalpingogram and who is otherwise a candidate for donor insemination because of azoospermia, or for ovulation induction because of chronic anovulation, may reasonably undergo such treatment without first having laparoscopy. If no conception occurs after a specific number of cycles (e.g., six), laparoscopy may be warranted for evaluating a potential false-negative hysterosalpingogram. The technique of selective tubal cannulation under fluoroscopic guidance can be employed to reduce the rate of false-positive hysterosalpingographic diagnoses of proximal obstruction, and to probe beyond an apparent proximal obstruction to evaluate the distal tube. Laparoscopy is warranted in the initial infertility evaluation when symptoms suggest endometriosis or when a history of appendicitis, previous pelvic surgery, pelvic inflammatory disease, or other conditions suggest pelvic abnormalities. Diagnostic laparoscopy is also indicated in unexplained infertility when the standard evaluation fails to identify a recognized cause.

CONCLUSION

Prior to initiating an infertility evaluation, the clinician should counsel the couple about the risks, potential benefits, and alternatives to each test. The evaluation should proceed with an appreciation of the limitations of each diagnostic test. The medical history and initial test results can help the clinician design an appropriate and efficient diagnostic pathway that meets the needs of a specific couple. The essential components of the standard infertility evaluation are outlined in Table 5. Once the initial evaluation is performed, couples who do not have an absolute barrier to pregnancy should be informed that they may eventually conceive on their own, without medical intervention. Treatments that attempt to correct specific abnormalities should continue only as long as the likelihood of pregnancy warrants the cost, both financial and emotional.

Table 5. Components of the Standard Infertility Evaluation

Test	Day Performed
Semen analysis	Any day of cycle
Hysterosalpingogram	May be performed from cessation of bleeding until ovulation
Ovulation prediction kit (urine)	Testing should begin 1–5 days before the anticipated day of ovulation
Postcoital test	Performed 1–3 days before the anticipated day of ovulation
Endometrial biopsy	Performed 10–12 days after ovulation
Laparoscopy	May be performed during a subsequent cycle, depending on the findings of the above tests

ENDOMETRIOSIS

By David L. Olive, M.D.
New Haven, Connecticut

DEFINITION

Endometriosis, a disease that has been recognized since the late 1800s, has been defined in various ways over time. The traditional histologic criteria require the presence of both endometrial glandular tissue and stroma in an ectopic location. The basis for the inflexible requirement of both components of normal endometrium arose not from a well-studied linkage to the adverse effects of the disease but rather as an arbitrary ploy to maintain uniformity of diagnosis among pathologists. Thus, it is unclear whether one or both endometrial components should be required for making the diagnosis.

Location, too, has varied over time in the definition of endometriosis. Originally, any endometrium outside the uterine cavity was considered to be endometriosis. If identified within the myometrium, it was termed endometriosis interna; if identified elsewhere, it was called endometriosis externa. Subsequent investigation, however, demonstrated that the symptoms, risk factors, and the affected populations for endometriosis interna differed from those for endometriosis externa. Thus, given a different pathophysiologic process, endometriosis interna was renamed adenomyosis, whereas the moniker endometriosis persisted for remaining sites.

PATHOGENESIS AND EPIDEMIOLOGY

Endometriosis is a disease found almost exclusively in women of reproductive age. The disease has been observed in a handful of girls younger than 10 years. Most postmenopausal women with symptomatic endometriosis are taking female hormones. Menstrual characteristics currently viewed as significant risk factors for endometriosis include early menarche, late menopause, and heavy or lengthy menses. Women with lower parity are also at increased risk, with nulliparity being a strong risk factor. Reproductive disorders predisposing to the disease include müllerian anomalies with outflow obstruction, infertility, and structural abnormalities (e.g., leiomyomas) producing a greater menstrual flow or abnormal uterine bleeding. Conversely, the disease is seen less frequently among women with high parity or an early first pregnancy, prolonged amenorrhea, or blocked fallopian tubes.

Such risk factors suggest an important role for the quantity of menstrual debris in the pathogenesis of endometriosis. This is consistent with the transplantation theory that endometriosis derives from endometrium translocated to ectopic sites. Although such a process may occur via lymphatic dissemination, hematogenous spread, direct extension, or even iatrogenically during surgery, the most likely route is via retrograde menstruation. Such a mechanism is consistent with the previously mentioned risk factors and the anatomic distribution of the disease, which is most commonly seen in gravity-dependent areas of the pelvis and abdomen.

Although the quantity of retrograde menstruation may be a vital factor in the pathogenesis of endometriosis, quality may also be an issue. A genetic predisposition to the disease has been illustrated by several studies; the mode of inheritance may be polygenic and multifactorial or autosomal dominant with variable penetrance. Thus far, however, there is no clear evidence of a racial predisposition to endometriosis; instead, racial and ethnic differences in disease prevalence can be explained by confounding factors, including reproductive and breast-feeding patterns and access to health care.

Endometriosis is most commonly diagnosed in the second and third decades of life. This may reflect hesitation by clinicians to pursue the diagnosis aggressively in the teenage years. Studies investigating the prevalence of endometriosis among symptomatic teenagers demonstrate that it is not rare. Symptoms of endometriosis, however, are infrequent in the first few years after menarche; most symptomatic women are diagnosed in their late teenage years.

SYMPTOMS

There are two chief symptoms associated with endometriosis: pain and infertility. Pain is by far the most frequent symptom; it is reported by as many as 75 per cent of women with endometriosis. Although pain can be experienced wherever endometriosis occurs, pelvic and lower abdominal pain are the most frequent manifestations because the pelvis and lower abdomen are the most common sites of implantation. Dysmenorrhea, dyspareunia, and noncyclic lower abdominal and pelvic pain are frequent complaints, whereas dysuria and dyschezia are less commonly reported.

Infertility is commonly associated with endometriosis. Infertility may be a risk factor for development of the disease, but it may also be a direct result of the disease process. For example, fibrosis and scarring induced by endometrial implants destroy the normal relationship between fallopian tubes and ovaries and may even cause tubal obstruction.

Implantation of endometrium in unusual locations produces unusual complaints. Thus, renal endometriosis may cause hematuria, pulmonary implants may cause hemoptysis, and brain implants may produce neurologic dysfunction. Finally, an unknown proportion of women with endometriosis remain totally asymptomatic.

PHYSICAL FINDINGS

Although many findings on pelvic examination are consistent with endometriosis, no such signs are unequivocally diagnostic. Cul-de-sac tenderness, particularly with nodularity, adnexal tenderness or masses, and decreased mobility of the pelvic viscera strongly suggests the diagnosis. Many patients, however, have an unremarkable pelvic examination.

Endometriosis of the bowel, colon, bladder, or other pelvic viscera is rarely identified on physical examination. Even rectal palpation of a nodule is unreliable as a predictor of true bowel wall invasion. When the disease results from iatrogenic spread following uterine surgery, it is frequently manifested as incisional endometriosis. This often presents as a mass in a surgical scar that is more tender at the time of menses. Other uncommon sites of endometriosis that may be visualized on physical examination are the umbilicus and the vagina.

LABORATORY TESTING

Laboratory analysis of body fluids is not useful for the diagnosis of endometriosis. The serum concentration of the CA-125 antigen is increased in any inflammatory process involving the peritoneal epithelium. Thus, the sensitivity and specificity of the CA-125 assay for the diagnosis of endometriosis are too low: most studies place them at 60 to 80 per cent at best. Moreover, the CA-125 assay has not proved useful in combination with other diagnostic methods. Whether CA-125 concentrations in the serum will prove valuable in following response to therapy is currently under study.

IMAGING STUDIES

Computed tomography (CT) scanning is not helpful in the diagnosis or localization of peritoneal or ovarian endometriosis. By contrast, ultrasonography can be useful for detecting ovarian endometriomas. When combined with Doppler flow technology, the overall efficiency (sensitivity and specificity) of this technique may exceed 70 per cent. However, ultrasound has not been useful in detecting peritoneal endometriosis.

The best available imaging technique for detecting endometriosis is magnetic resonance imaging (MRI). In experienced hands, ovarian endometriomas are detected by MRI with greater than 90 per cent accuracy. MRI can also detect endometriomas in unusual soft tissue sites, including the pelvic side wall, thigh, or lung. Unfortunately, MRI does not consistently detect peritoneal lesions.

Specialized imaging studies may be employed to diagnose endometriosis in unusual locations. For example, if ureteral involvement is suspected, an intravenous pyelogram may reveal the site and extent of the lesion and the degree of ureteral compromise. Similarly, upper and lower gastrointestinal fluoroscopic studies may confirm the diagnosis of bowel endometriosis.

SURGICAL PROCEDURES FOR DIAGNOSIS

Direct visualization of the pelvic and abdominal contents by laparoscopy is currently the gold standard approach to the diagnosis of pelvic and abdominal endometriosis. Implants may appear as red, white, clear, or hemosiderin-stained lesions or as bluish black "powder burns." Implants may be polypoid or plaquelike in appearance. The same lesion may have multiple appearances. The rule of thumb is that any visibly abnormal peritoneum may harbor endometriosis and should be assumed to do so until proved otherwise.

A biopsy of suspicious lesions for histologic confirmation of endometriosis is highly desirable. The purpose of such a biopsy is not to make the diagnosis, for the absence of endometrial glands and stroma in a biopsy specimen does not prove the absence of disease. Rather, the biopsy of suspicious lesions is used to exclude other disorders of similar appearance and to confirm the physician's visual impression.

Pelvic and abdominal adhesions are frequent manifestations of endometriosis. One third of such adhesions contain endometrial tissue within them. The external surface of the capsule of an ovarian endometrial cyst (endometriosis) may appear unremarkable, but entry into the cyst often reveals thick, chocolate-colored fluid consistent with chronic hemorrhage. This fluid is presumptively, but not necessarily, diagnostic of endometriosis.

As mentioned previously, endometriotic lesions are most commonly observed in gravity-dependent areas of the abdomen and pelvis. Thus, frequent sites of implantation include the anterior and posterior cul-de-sacs, the ovaries, the rectum, and the pararectal gutters. Importantly, endometriosis can be found in the abdominal paracolic gutters in more than 90 per cent of women with endometriosis-associated pain.

Invasive endometriotic lesions of the bladder are most often diagnosed with the aid of cystoscopy in conjunction with laparoscopy. Similarly, invasive bowel lesions may require colonoscopy for complete evaluation. Finally, soft tissue disease may necessitate dissection (and eventual excision) of the involved area.

DIFFERENTIAL DIAGNOSIS

Pain associated with endometriosis is typically chronic. Dysmenorrhea, dyspareunia, adenomyosis, irritable bowel syndrome, other chronic bowel disorders, and the chronic effects of acute disorders (e.g., appendicitis, pelvic inflammatory disease) all may produce similar discomfort.

Occasionally, the patient with endometriosis may experience acute abdominal pain from ovarian torsion or rupture of an endometrioma. Of course, acute pelvic inflammatory disease, appendicitis, diverticulitis, Crohn's disease, and even ectopic pregnancy may also present with acute abdominal pain.

Any ovarian or paraovarian mass can be initially confused with an endometrioma, but imaging studies should help distinguish these disorders. Nodularity of the cul-de-sac can be secondary to prior infection, inflammation, or tumor and may occasionally be confused with endometriosis. Laparoscopic visualization and excisional biopsy facilitate appropriate diagnosis.

PELVIC INFLAMMATORY DISEASE

By Martin A. Quan, M.D.
Los Angeles, California

Acute pelvic inflammatory disease (PID) is defined as an ascending infection of the upper genital tract in the female involving the uterus (endometritis), fallopian tubes (salpingitis), ovaries (oophoritis), and adjacent pelvic structures (parametritis, pelvic peritonitis). It is a community-acquired disorder that has reached epidemic proportions in the United States and is responsible for more than 250,000 hospital admissions and 2.5 million outpatient visits each year. Direct and indirect costs of PID were estimated at more than $3.5 billion in 1990.

In addition to its short-term impact, acute PID is responsible for a number of important sequelae as well. Tubo-ovarian abscesses are present in 3 to 16 per cent of patients hospitalized with PID, and recurrent PID is a complication seen in 4 to 23 per cent of cases. A single episode of acute PID increases the risk for the development of an ectopic pregnancy 7- to 10-fold; nearly 50 per cent of patients with ectopic pregnancies manifest evidence of prior PID on laparoscopy. Acute PID is also an important cause of infertility, rendering 21 per cent of those afflicted infertile. This risk of infertility increases with each succeeding infection, with an incidence of 13 per cent after the first episode, 35 per cent after the second episode, and 75 per cent following the third episode. Finally, an estimated 17 per cent of patients experience chronic pelvic pain syndromes following an episode of acute PID, including dyspareunia and painful pelvic adhesions.

EPIDEMIOLOGY

A number of epidemiologic risk factors have been linked to the development of acute PID. Awareness of these factors can facilitate early recognition and treatment of this condition. Historical factors that would identify a patient at higher risk for having acute PID include an age less than 25 years, sexual activity prior to age 16 years, single marital status, multiple sex partners, a past history of PID or other sexually transmitted diseases, the presence of bacterial vaginosis, and vaginal douching three or more times a month.

The patient's method of contraception also has an impact on the risk of PID. Although some data suggest that patients using combined oral contraceptives may be at higher risk for cervicitis due to *Chlamydia trachomatis,* other data suggest that combined oral contraceptives reduce the risk of PID by 50 per cent. Similarly, the regular use of barrier methods of contraception (i.e., condoms, diaphragm) may also reduce the likelihood of PID. Finally, in women using the intrauterine device (IUD), the increased risk of PID related to the device is confined primarily to the first 3 to 4 months following insertion.

CLINICAL FINDINGS

Acute PID causes a broad spectrum of illness ranging from mild subclinical changes to severe symptoms with signs of peritonitis (i.e., rebound and rigidity). The most common complaint of patients with PID is lower abdominal pain; many investigators require that it be present for the diagnosis of PID to be considered. Importantly, however, lower abdominal pain may be absent in up to 6 per cent of cases. The duration of pain is less than 14 days in 80 per cent of patients and typically is aggravated by coitus, movement, and the Valsalva maneuver. Other common complaints include abnormal vaginal discharge in 38 to 73 per cent of patients, vaginal bleeding in 16 to 50 per cent of patients, urinary symptoms in 19 to 37 per cent of patients, and gastrointestinal symptoms in 25 per cent of patients.

Cervical motion tenderness and adnexal tenderness are the physical findings most frequently elicited in patients with acute PID. The adnexal tenderness is unilateral in 10 to 20 per cent of patients. An adnexal mass or fullness can be found in 16 to 49 per cent of patients and an abnormal vaginal discharge can be noted in 38 to 73 per cent of patients. Other findings include fever in 24 to 60 per cent of patients and right upper quadrant tenderness (Fitz-Hugh–Curtis syndrome) in 5 to 10 per cent of patients.

DIFFERENTIAL DIAGNOSIS

Although the history and physical examination may suggest the diagnosis of PID, several laparoscopic studies have demonstrated that a diagnosis of acute PID made on clinical grounds can be confirmed in only two thirds of cases. Surprisingly, a normal pelvis has been a common laparoscopic finding in these studies, being reported in more than 20 per cent of cases. Other entities that should be considered in the differential diagnosis of acute PID can be conveniently divided into three major categories:

- Pregnancy-related causes—ectopic pregnancy, septic abortion, and intrauterine pregnancy with corpus luteal bleeding
- Gynecologic causes—torsion of the adnexa, ruptured ovarian cyst, endometriosis, corpus luteal cyst bleeding, hemorrhagic follicular cyst, septic abortion, ovarian tumor, uterine leiomyoma, and pelvic adhesions
- Nongynecologic causes—acute appendicitis, mesenteric lymphadenitis, inflammatory bowel disease, and urinary tract infection

LABORATORY EVALUATION

Hematologic Studies

Nonspecific indicators of inflammation that are of diagnostic value in the patient with suspected PID include the leukocyte count, the erythrocyte sedimentation rate (ESR), and the serum C-reactive protein (CRP) concentration. Although these laboratory values are typically increased in patients with PID (i.e., leukocyte count exceeding 10,500 cells/mm^3, ESR exceeding 15 mm per hour, CRP exceeding 20 mg/L), it is important to recognize that the leukocyte count can be normal in up to 50 per cent of patients and that the ESR and CRP can be normal in one fourth of patients with PID.

Cervical Gram Stain

For patients with acute pelvic pain, a Gram stain of cervical scrapings can provide useful diagnostic information. For example, the finding of 10 or more white cells per oil immersion field is diagnostic for mucopurulent cervicitis and is generally considered to substantiate the clinical diagnosis of acute PID. Similarly, in the patient with suspected PID, the finding of gram-negative intracellular diplococci on cervical Gram staining is highly specific for gonococcal cervicitis and supports the diagnosis of gonococcal PID.

Examination of the Male Partner

If available for examination, the male partner of the patient should be evaluated for the presence of urethritis, a finding that would corroborate the diagnosis of acute PID in the female patient. Examination of the male partner can provide confirmatory evidence for the diagnosis of PID in as many as 50 per cent of patients.

Pregnancy Testing

The clinical presentations of acute PID and ectopic pregnancy can be remarkably similar. Therefore, all patients of reproductive age presenting with acute pelvic pain or abnormal vaginal bleeding should routinely undergo pregnancy testing. The urine monoclonal antibody pregnancy test becomes positive at human chorionic gonadotropin (hCG) concentrations as low as 50 IU/L and detects 90 to 96 per cent of ectopic pregnancies. The qualitative serum tests, which rely on monoclonal antibody or radioimmunoassay techniques, can detect serum hCG concentrations as low as 25 IU/L. These serum hCG tests are positive in 97 per cent of tubal pregnancies. Quantitative serum pregnancy tests can detect hCG concentrations as low as 5 IU/L with a sensitivity for ectopic pregnancy of 98.8 to 100 per cent; thus, a negative result effectively excludes the diagnosis of ectopic pregnancy.

Cervical Studies

Laboratory confirmation of an endocervical infection with *Neisseria gonorrhoeae* or *Chlamydia trachomatis* is regarded as strong evidence for the diagnosis of acute PID. Although cultures remain the "gold standard" for diagnosis, rapid nonculture methods have become widely available. For example, gonorrhea can be detected with enzyme immunoassay or DNA probes, whereas *C. trachomatis* can be detected with enzyme immunoassay, DNA probes, or immunofluorescent antibody tests.

Culdocentesis

Culdocentesis is a rapid and relatively simple technique for detecting and sampling fluid in the cul-de-sac. Purulent fluid obtained by culdocentesis corroborates a diagnosis of acute PID, but purulent fluid can also be aspirated from the cul-de-sac in patients with acute appendicitis, a ruptured diverticular abscess, or other causes of peritonitis. To ensure proper handling of specimens for gonococcal, aerobic, and anaerobic cultures, the clinician should communicate with the microbiology laboratory prior to aspiration of the cul-de-sac. Contraindications to culdocentesis include a mass in the cul-de-sac (absolute) and a markedly retroflexed uterus (relative).

Pelvic Ultrasonography

Pelvic sonography is occasionally useful in the diagnosis of acute PID. Sonographic findings consistent with PID include distention and dilatation of the fallopian tubes; enlargement of the ovaries, tubes, and ligaments; fluid in the cul-de-sac; and the appearance of a complex, multiloculated mass with cystic and solid elements incorporating the uterus. Although image resolution has improved with the introduction of endovaginal sonography, careful clinical correlation is required because the sonographic abnormalities associated with PID can be mimicked by other intrapelvic disorders. Nevertheless, ultrasound can be helpful when pain, obesity, or uncooperativeness precludes an adequate pelvic examination. Moreover, pelvic ultrasound can be used to detect pelvic abscesses and to monitor their response to treatment.

Endometrial Biopsy

Transcervical endometrial biopsy (in the office) has been proposed as an alternative to laparoscopy for the diagnosis of acute PID. The histopathologic diagnosis of endometritis is based on the finding of plasma cells in the endometrial stroma, with the severity of disease proportionate to the degree of stromal infiltration. Unfortunately, in some facilities the results of endometrial biopsy may not be available for several days.

Diagnostic Laparoscopy

Diagnostic laparoscopy is an invaluable technique that permits direct visualization of structures within the peritoneal cavity. Laparoscopic features of PID include erythema, edema, spontaneous or expressible inflammatory exudate, tubo-ovarian abscess, and/or pyosalpinx of the fallopian tube. Although some authorities have recommended routine performance of laparoscopy in all patients with suspected PID, such an approach is not logistically or economically feasible. Diagnostic laparoscopy is considered a safe procedure when performed by an experienced laparoscopist, but it is not without risk; there are an estimated five deaths for every 100,000 laparoscopies performed and five major morbid events for every 1000 laparoscopies performed. Nevertheless, diagnostic laparoscopy should be strongly considered for (1) patients with suspected PID that is unresponsive to medical therapy, (2) patients in whom the diagnosis remains unclear despite a comprehensive evaluation, and (3) patients who may have a life-threatening disorder such as ectopic pregnancy or acute appendicitis.

ESTABLISHING THE DIAGNOSIS

In all sexually active patients with acute pelvic pain (or any other clinical finding consistent with PID), the clinician must first distinguish pregnancy-related disorders from non–pregnancy-related disorders. This determination requires a serum pregnancy test or, at a minimum, a sensitive urine monoclonal antibody pregnancy test.

For patients with acute pelvic pain unrelated to pregnancy, acute PID becomes a leading diagnostic consideration. However, the clinical diagnosis of PID cannot be made with confidence and reliability until specific criteria derived from laparoscopic studies are fulfilled. Therefore, aggressive efforts to corroborate the diagnosis by fulfilling such criteria seem particularly prudent in patients presenting with moderate to severe symptoms. Current criteria for the diagnosis of PID include lower abdominal, cervical motion, and adnexal tenderness plus at least one of the following:

- Temperature exceeding 38°C
- Leukocytosis exceeding 10,500 cells/mm^3
- Purulent material aspirated on culdocentesis
- Inflammatory mass on pelvic ultrasonography
- ESR exceeding 15 mm per hour
- Culture or nonculture evidence of gonococcal or chlamydial infection of the endocervix
- Mucopurulent cervicitis associated with more than 5 to 10 leukocytes per oil immersion field on Gram staining of the endocervical discharge

Recognizing that insistence on a rigid set of diagnostic criteria would result in many cases of mild PID going undiagnosed and untreated, the Centers for Disease Control (CDC) published guidelines in 1991 that lowered the clinical threshold for making a presumptive diagnosis of PID in patients with mild disease. The CDC now recommends that a tentative diagnosis of PID be made in any patient who manifests lower abdominal, bilateral adnexal, and cervical motion tenderness on examination provided that competing diagnoses have been adequately excluded. For many of these patients, the clinician may recommend a trial of antibiotic therapy. The CDC has offered guidelines for hospitalization (Table 1) as well as options for inpatient and outpatient antibiotic regimens (Tables 2 and 3).

Regardless of how the diagnosis of PID is made, the importance of close clinical follow-up cannot be overstated. Patients treated for PID require frequent evaluations. If no clinical improvement is seen in 2 to 3 days, other diag-

Table 1. Criteria for Hospitalization of Patients With Acute Pelvic Inflammatory Disease

The diagnosis is uncertain and surgical emergencies such as appendicitis and ectopic pregnancy cannot be excluded
Pelvic abscess is suspected
The patient is pregnant
The patient is an adolescent
The patient has HIV infection
Severe illness or nausea preclude outpatient management
The patient is unable to follow or tolerate an outpatient regimen
The patient has failed to respond clinically to outpatient therapy
Clinical follow-up within 72 hours of starting antibiotic treatment cannot be arranged

HIV = human immunodeficiency virus.
Adapted from Centers for Disease Control: MMWR 42(RR-14):75–81, 1993.

Table 2. 1993 Centers for Disease Control and Prevention Recommended Inpatient Treatment Options for Acute Pelvic Inflammatory Disease

Regimen A
Cefoxitin, 2 g IV every 6 hr, or cefotetan, 2 g IV every 12 hr, plus doxycycline, 100 mg IV or orally every 12 hr
Continue for at least 48 hr after the patient demonstrates substantial clinical improvement, after which doxycycline, 100 mg orally two times a day, should be continued for a total of 14 days
Regimen B
Clindamycin, 900 mg IV every 8 hr, plus gentamicin loading dose IV or IM (2 mg/kg) followed by a maintenance dose (1.5 mg/kg) every 8 hr
Continue for at least 48 hr after the patient demonstrates substantial clinical improvement, then follow with doxycycline, 100 mg orally two times a day, or clindamycin, 450 mg four times a day, to complete 14 days of therapy

IV = intravenously; IM = intramuscularly.
Adapted from Centers for Disease Control: MMWR 42(RR-14):75–81, 1993.

Table 3. 1993 Centers for Disease Control and Prevention Recommended Outpatient Treatment Options for Acute Pelvic Inflammatory Disease

Regimen A
Cefoxitin, 2 g IM, plus probenecid, 1 g orally in a single dose concurrently, or ceftriaxone, 250 mg IM, or other parenteral third-generation cephalosporin (e.g, ceftizoxime or cefotaxime), plus doxycycline 100 mg orally two times a day for 14 days
Regimen B
Ofloxacin, 400 mg orally two times a day for 14 days, plus either clindamycin, 450 mg orally four times a day, or metronidazole, 500 mg orally two times a day for 14 days

IM = intramuscularly.
Adapted from Centers for Disease Control: MMWR 42(RR-14):75–81, 1993.

noses (e.g., appendicitis, endometriosis, ruptured ovarian cyst, or adnexal torsion) must be seriously reconsidered. Diagnostic laparoscopy (or possibly endometrial biopsy) may be necessary for these patients as well as for patients whose clinical symptoms are severe enough to require rapid, definitive diagnosis.

THE MENOPAUSE

By Gloria A. Bachman, M.D.,
and George Tweddel, M.D.
New Brunswick, New Jersey

Many terms are used to describe the time of life when a woman ceases to menstruate. The three processes that are important to define are the menopause, the perimenopause, and the climacteric. The menopause is defined as that point in time when permanent cessation of menstruation occurs following the loss of ovarian activity. A generally accepted clinical definition of menopause is a period of six months of amenorrhea in a women older than 45 years of age. The perimenopause is the period immediately before the menopause when changes in menstrual pattern and flow, vasomotor symptoms, and declining fertility may become obvious. The climacteric is a more encompassing word, indicating the period of time when a woman passes through a transition from the reproductive stage to the postmenopausal years, a period of waning ovarian function.

Designating average ages for these conditions has been difficult. In the Massachusetts Women's Health Study, women who reported the onset of menstrual irregularity were considered perimenopausal. The median age at onset of the perimenopause was 47.5 years. For most women, this transitional period was approximately 4 years. The median age for menopause was 51.3 years, and the range was 48 to 55 years. Menopause before age 40 occurs in approximately 1 per cent of women and should be considered premature ovarian failure.

The age at which menopause occurs is probably genetically predetermined. Oral contraceptives, socioeconomic status, marital status, race, parity, height, weight, and age at which menarche occurred appear to have no effect on the age at which menopause occurs. By contrast, smoking, malnutrition, and living at high altitudes have been associated with younger age at menopause.

Since 1960, the number of older people in the United States has been growing faster than the number of younger people. By the year 2050, more than one of five people will be elderly, and by 2000 the number of women older than 45 will exceed 700 million worldwide. Postmenopausal patients are requiring increased attention from primary care providers because women can now expect to live nearly one third of their lives after menopause. The clinician should focus on efforts to decrease the risk of complications of osteoporosis and cardiovascular disease. The menopause marks the end of a woman's reproductive life and a confrontation with the process of aging. Clinicians should therefore provide support, encouragement, and attention to emotional and sexual issues. Comprehensive counseling and medical care can help menopausal women remain physically and mentally fit for many years.

HORMONAL CHANGES

After age 40, the frequency of both long and short menstrual cycles increases. A progressive decline in estradiol production by the ovary leads to increased circulating concentrations of follicle-stimulating hormone (FSH) and luteinizing hormone (LH), a shortened follicular phase, an inadequate luteal phase, and resultant irregular bleeding. Menopause is typically confirmed when serum estradiol falls below 20 pg/mL and serum FSH exceeds 40 mIU/mL. Low concentrations of estrogen are maintained in the postmenopausal years by peripheral synthesis from androgens secreted by the adrenals and the stromal cells of the ovary. Overall, the concentrations of testosterone and androstenedione produced by the ovary decrease, although less dramatically than do estradiol concentrations. This decrease in androgens may be associated with the adverse changes in sexual function many menopausal women report, including a decrease in libido, less frequent and less intense orgasms, and a loss of sexual daydreaming. Decreased androgens also lead to a decreased estrogen-to-testosterone ratio, which can result in male-pattern hair thinning as well as hirsutism. In obese patients who are menopausal and are not ovulating, the peripheral conversion of androgens to estrogens can be exaggerated, this increase resulting in unopposed estrogen concentrations. The free estrogen concentration can also be increased owing to decreased concentrations of sex hormone binding globulin. These patients are at increased risk for endometrial hyperplasia and endometrial cancer.

In addition, the decreased estrogen production can lead to shifts in total cholesterol, triglyceride, high-density lipoprotein (HDL) and low-density lipoprotein (LDL) cholesterol concentrations, contributing to an increased risk of cardiovascular disease in the menopausal patient.

SIGNS AND SYMPTOMS

Abnormal bleeding patterns are most commonly reported by patients approaching menopause. Oligomenorrhea or amenorrhea is usually the first clinical sign of menopause, but anovulatory bleeding can be varied. The abnormal bleeding pattern must be evaluated during this period because endometrial disease and malignancy can present in this fashion.

The differential diagnosis of abnormal bleeding includes pregnancy; malignancies of the cervix, vagina, and uterus; retained intrauterine devices (IUDs) or foreign bodies; fibroids; polyps; and infection. Endocrine causes, including hypothyroidism, hyperthyroidism, and prolactinomas, and diseases such as idiopathic thrombocytopenic purpura (ITP) and cirrhosis of the liver should be considered. Patient evaluation should be individualized and may include a pregnancy test, Papanicolaou (PAP) smear, pelvic sonogram, thyroid-stimulating hormone (TSH), prolactin, complete blood count (CBC), and liver function tests. The evaluation of abnormal vaginal bleeding in the perimenopausal and menopausal patient should include office endometrial sampling or office hysteroscopy to exclude hyperplasia, cancer, polyps, or submucous fibroids. If patients are unable to tolerate office sampling, outpatient dilation and curettage should be performed.

Vasomotor instability or hot flashes are a classic sign of menopause and a predominant symptom in the perimenopause. A hot flash is the sudden, transient sensation of intense heat that spreads over the body, particularly on the chest, face, and head. Hot flashes are typically accompanied by flushing, tachycardia, and perspiration and are often followed by a chill. The magnitude and duration of these components can vary. The prevalence of hot flashes is highest during the first two postmenopausal years, ranging from 58 to 93 per cent, and lessens with time. In perimenopausal women, reports of hot flashes range from 28 to 65 per cent. An individual hot-flash episode typically lasts 3 to 6 minutes, although it can be of shorter duration. On occasion, a hot flash can last for 30 minutes. The period of time over which hot flashes are most often experienced is 6 months to 2 years; however, women can have hot flashes for 10, 20, or even 40 years. The mechanism for the hot flash is unknown, but a sudden lowering of the thermoregulatory set-point in the hypothalamus may occur. Estrogens influence thermoregulatory centers as well as vascular tissue. A complex interaction of sex steroids, opioid peptides, and gonadotropin-releasing hormone (Gn-RH) and LH is likely involved in the physiology of the hot flash.

During menopause, atrophic changes occur in all tissues with estrogen receptors. The decrease in genital epithelium can lead to atrophic vaginitis, with symptoms of burning, itching, bleeding, and dyspareunia, and urethritis with symptoms of dysuria, frequency, urgency, and incontinence. Additional symptoms, including fatigue, anxiety, headaches, depression, palpitations, insomnia, myalgias, and irritability often, are collectively referred to as the menopausal syndrome. Controversy exists as to which of these symptoms are directly related to estrogen.

HEALTH CONSEQUENCES

Osteoporosis

Osteoporosis, a consequence of declining estrogen concentrations, is characterized by a decreased density of bone. Two types of osteoporosis attributed to the aging process have been identified. Type 1 is associated with accelerated bone loss in women during the menopausal years. This loss is primarily from trabecular bone and leads to an increased incidence of vertebral and wrist fractures in the decade following menopause. Type 2 is associated with slow, progressive bone loss in men and women and leads to fractures predominantly in the hip and vertebrae of women older than 70. Type 1 osteoporosis can be treated and is usually the focus of physician efforts at prevention via education and early identification of perimenopausal and menopausal patients who are at risk. Small-framed, white and Asian hypoestrogenic women with lifestyles or medical conditions associated with impaired calcium metabolism have the greatest risk of developing osteoporosis. Smoking, alcohol consumption, and sedentary lifestyle are risk factors. Cushing's syndrome, hyperthyroidism, hyperparathyroidism, neoplastic diseases, chronic renal failure, intestinal malabsorption, and malnutrition are other possible causes that may require evaluation.

Approximately 1.2 million fractures related to osteoporosis occur in the United States each year. Vertebral fractures occur in one third of women older than 65. By age 90, 33 per cent of women have sustained hip fractures, with a 5 to 20 per cent mortality rate within the first six months after the fracture. A total of 15,000 women die of osteoporosis or its complications annually, with a health cost of more than 9 billion dollars per year. Early detection of the patients at risk and early institution of therapy are the clinician's main goals.

Cardiovascular Disease

Cardiovascular disease is the leading cause of morbidity and mortality in women, significantly outweighing other causes, including cancer, cerebrovascular disease, lung disease, infectious disease, diabetes, suicide, and renal disease. In women, 46 per cent of deaths are due to cardiovascular disease, and 50 per cent of these are due to coronary artery heart disease. These statistics indicate that in the United States, a woman has a 23 per cent lifetime chance of dying of ischemic heart disease.

Premenopausal women uncommonly develop coronary heart disease, whereas postmenopausal women have rates similar to those of men. This observation has led many to speculate that estrogen is a protective factor in premenopausal women. A plausible biologic mechanism for the protective effect of estrogen is its impact on the lipid profile. Multiple studies have demonstrated a relationship between increased cholesterol concentrations and death from cardiovascular disease. Subsequent clinical trials have shown that decreasing cholesterol concentrations decreases the risk of first heart attack. The process of atherosclerosis is related to increased LDL cholesterol concentrations and decreased HDL cholesterol concentrations. In women, the strongest predictor of coronary heart disease is low HDL cholesterol. On the other hand, women who have HDL concentrations greater than 55 to 60 mg/mL have essentially no increased risk of heart disease. Estrogen deficiency correlates with a moderate increase in total and LDL cholesterol, and a lowering of HDL cholesterol. Thus, it is not surprising that menopause is associated with an increased risk of cardiovascular disease.

MANAGEMENT

Menopause has multiple health consequences. These range from the discomfort of a hot flash or vaginal irritation to osteoporosis and increased risk of adverse cardiovascular events. An aggressive approach to prevention and treatment of these conditions improves the transition to the postmenopausal years and increases the quality and length of life.

Estrogen administration is currently the most effective treatment for hot flashes, which are associated with a decline in ovarian function. The effect of estrogen is not typically immediate. Full benefit may require several months of therapy. In the United States, the most commonly used regimen for treating hot flashes is oral conjugated equine estrogen (Premarin), 0.625 mg or 1.25 mg PO every day. Transdermal estradiol (Estraderm), 0.05

to 0.10 mg/day, and other oral and transdermal estrogen preparations are also available. Estrogen is also prescribed as subcutaneous implants, injectables, and vaginal creams. Most are effective in treating hot flashes. Other symptoms that may be improved following estrogen therapy include insomnia, vaginal dryness, memory lapses, lower urinary tract problems, and mood.

Alternatives to estrogen treatment exist for patients who cannot take estrogen or who find the side effects unacceptable. Medroxyprogesterone acetate and megestrol acetate are nonestrogen steroids that can decrease the number of hot flashes. Clonidine, an alpha-adrenergic receptor agonist that influences vascular responses, has been used with some success. Propranolol, a beta-adrenergic receptor antagonist, has been used with mixed results. Bellergal, which is a combination of belladonna alkaloids, ergotamine acetate, and phenobarbital, appears to be more effective than placebo in reducing the frequency of hot flashes. The specific mechanism is unknown. Nonpharmacologic treatments, including acupuncture, exercise, vitamin E, diet, and changes in ambient air temperature, have also been advocated.

Management of osteoporosis begins in the premenopausal years. Clinicians can identify patients at risk and educate them as to the proper exercise, diet, and lifestyle changes necessary for keeping bones healthy. In adult women before the onset of menopause, the rates of bone formation and bone resorption are approximately equal; calcium balance is maintained, and no loss of bone mass occurs. After menopause, although both bone formation and bone resorption rates increase, the rate of bone resorption increases more rapidly, resulting in calcium imbalance and a net loss of bone. Therefore, the first goal of therapy for osteoporosis should be the restoration of bone resorption and bone formation to premenopausal levels. Optimally, bone formation should be maintained at a slightly higher rate than that of bone resorption, producing a positive calcium balance and preventing bone loss.

It is clear that hormone replacement therapy (HRT) helps prevent bone loss. Although the benefit of HRT is greatest when HRT is begun early in a patient's postmenopausal years, there is evidence that HRT prevents bone loss at all stages of postmenopausal life. Oral estrogen doses of 0.625 mg and transdermal doses of 0.05 mg are effective for prevention of bone loss. Estradiol gel also can prevent bone loss.

The role of calcium intake in the development of decreased bone mass and susceptibility to fractures remains the subject of intense debate. The current daily requirement of calcium is 1000 mg for premenopausal women and 1500 mg for postmenopausal women. However, calcium alone is not as effective as HRT in preventing bone loss. When given with low-dose estrogen, calcium may enhance the maintenance of bone mass in some patients.

Other regimens for established osteoporosis include calcitonin, anabolic steroids, parathyroid hormone, coherence therapy, and alendronate sodium tablets. The latter drug, which acts as an inhibitor of osteoclast-mediated bone resorption, has been shown to increase bone mineral density of the lumbar spine, femoral neck, and trochanter when given at a dose of 10 mg per day.

Hormone replacement therapy appears to lower cardiovascular risk in postmenopausal women. The concentrations of plasma LDL-cholesterol and HDL-cholesterol are modulated by the effect of estrogen on hepatic lipid metabolism. Estrogens may also directly influence cardiac and coronary artery cells, modulating atherogenesis and endothelial cell hyperplasia and even causing direct coronary vasodilatation.

Hormone Replacement Therapy Regimens

The biggest problem with HRT is patient compliance. Approximately 15 to 25 per cent of postmenopausal women are currently taking HRT. As many as 35 per cent of women on HRT stop the treatment after one year. The biggest complaint is either renewed or irregular vaginal bleeding. Some patients also report symptoms typically associated with premenstrual syndrome (PMS), breast-swelling, fluid retention, and depression. Formulations that augment benefits and minimize risk and side effects are obviously preferred. Currently, popular methods include sequential and continuous oral HRT. With both regimens, estrogens are administered daily throughout the month. Synthetic progesterone, such as medroxyprogesterone acetate, 10 mg, is given for 10 to 14 days monthly with sequential therapy and 2.5 mg daily with continuous therapy. Sequential therapy is the most thoroughly studied. Its advantages include predictable withdrawal bleeding and easy implementation during the perimenopausal years. Continuous therapy is gaining popularity because of ease of administration (no cycling) and eventual scant or absent bleeding. The disadvantages include irregular bleeding during the first 6 months of use. The addition of androgens should be considered for women who do not have adequate symptomatic relief with estrogens alone or who report decreased libido and sexual desire. For women who have mainly genital symptoms from estrogen deficiency, locally applied estrogen should be considered. Low-dose estrogen can be delivered to the vaginal tissue as a vaginal cream or as a vaginal ring that remains active for 3 months.

Patients receiving HRT may be more compliant if they are reevaluated in 4 to 6 months. Once a patient is stable on a particular HRT regimen, she should be evaluated annually. During these evaluations, breast and pelvic examinations should be performed, a Papanicolaou smear obtained, and attention directed to cholesterol, blood pressure, and the effectiveness of treatment. In women taking adequate progestins, endometrial biopsy should be reserved for women with excessive or prolonged bleeding or other clinical problems (see later).

RISKS AND CONTRAINDICATIONS

A causal relationship between high blood pressure and the doses of estrogen used for HRT has not been established. In addition, an increased risk of myocardial infarction and stroke has not been demonstrated. In fact, as noted previously, estrogen therapy provides a protective effect. Finally, thromboembolic phenomena have not been associated with HRT.

In postmenopausal women, the incidence of endometrial cancer is 1 in 1000 per year. Unopposed estrogen stimulation is associated with the development of atypical hyperplasia and endometrial cancer. Estrogen replacement therapy alone increases the risk of adenocarcinoma of the endometrium two- to ten-fold. This risk is eliminated when estrogen is combined with a progestational agent. Although estrogens promote endometrial growth, progestational agents oppose it. Therefore, postmenopausal estrogen should always be accompanied by progestin therapy in patients who have not undergone hysterectomy. The number of days and the dose required for adequate progestin exposure are controversial. Studies indicate, however, that at least 10 days of progestin therapy at a dose equivalent to 10 mg of medroxyprogesterone acetate per cycle will prevent hyperplasia. Fortunately, the antiestrogen effect of progestin does not reverse the positive effect of estrogen on osteoporosis. In fact, progestin seems to complement estrogen by further reducing bone loss. Decreases in HDL cholesterol also have been demonstrated with several progestational agents, but a dose-response relationship exists and progestins have a minimal impact, if any.

Approximately 10 per cent of women in the United States will develop breast cancer in their lifetimes. Evidence supporting an association between ERT and breast cancer is inconsistent. In one meta-analysis, the combined estimate of the relative risk from 23 studies was 1.1. Most studies suggest that low-dose and/or short-term use of estrogen replacement does not substantially increase the risk of breast cancer.

Absolute contraindications to HRT include the presence of an embolus or thrombophlebitis. By contrast, well-controlled hypertension, fibroids, varicose veins, or gallstones should not preclude HRT. Estrogen-sensitive tumors should not be considered an absolute contraindication to HRT. In patients previously treated for stage 1 adenocarcinoma of the endometrium, estrogen therapy has not been shown to increase the risk of recurrence. Similar data are being collected regarding HRT in breast cancer patients. Clinicians must weigh the severity of menopausal symptoms versus the unknown risk of recurrence in each patient.

CONCLUSION

The menopause is one phase in the life cycle of women that provides an opportunity for enhancing the physician-patient relationship. This physiologic event brings clinicians and patients together and provides an opportunity for counseling, medical intervention, and enrollment of patients in preventive health care programs. Contrary to popular opinion, the menopause is not a signal of impending decline, but rather a phenomenon that can signal the start of a good health program and something positive in a woman's life cycle.

VULVAR AND VAGINAL DISEASE

By David C. Foster, M.D., M.P.H.
Rochester, New York

For the purposes of organizing vulvar complaints according to predominant symptoms and signs, this article groups vulvar problems into four major categories: (1) pain and inflammation, (2) ulcers and blisters, (3) nodules, cysts, and masses, and (4) pigmented lesions.

PAIN AND INFLAMMATION

Inflammatory conditions of the vulva present a dermatologic challenge to the clinician. In addition to infections specific to the vulva or vagina, other dermatologic conditions produce vulvovaginal itching or burning and are classified as "dermatoses." These conditions include lichen sclerosus, squamous cell hyperplasia, and "other dermatoses." The category of "other dermatoses" includes psoriasis, allergic or irritant dermatitis, lichen simplex chronicus, lichen planus, and other vesiculobullous diseases. With any type of dermatologic process on the vulva, the gross appearance may differ from the classic lesions found elsewhere on the body owing to the moist environment of the perineum. Consequently, careful evaluation of the entire patient and a complete history are essential for making an accurate diagnosis.

Acute Dermatitis

Acute dermatitis is a common affliction of the vulva and can arise from a myriad of sources. The clinician may distinguish "contact," or irritant, dermatitis from "allergic" dermatitis through visible characteristics of each form of inflammation. In the acute phase of contact dermatitis, the vulva becomes erythematous and often excoriated through scratching. Such reactive lesions are caused by various locally active agents, including hygiene sprays and lotions; soaps or detergents used for washing the patient or her clothes; colored or perfumed toilet paper; tight-fitting, poorly absorbent underwear and slacks; and local anesthetics. By contrast, allergic dermatitis develops more slowly, with skin reactions that resemble those seen following exposure to poison ivy.

Monilial Vulvovaginitis

Vaginal discharge varies considerably in candidiasis. The classic "cottage cheese" discharge is seen primarily in florid cases. Monilial vulvovaginitis can result from infection by various types of *Candida* fungi. Asymptomatic carriers have been detected in as many as 25 per cent of women. The false-negative rate of vaginal potassium hydroxide smears is high, and therefore culture of the discharge in Sabouraud or Nickerson's medium improves diagnostic accuracy, especially in patients with "recurrent yeast." In patients with recurrent vaginal candidiasis, treatment of intestinal candidiasis does not appear to significantly reduce the recurrence rate. It is thought that a majority of relapses occur from oral-genital contact and that treatment of the sexual partner significantly reduces the recurrence rate compared with topical treatment alone.

Bacterial Vaginosis

On examination, this infection is associated with a thin, white, odoriferous, and often copious vaginal discharge. Burning or itching symptoms can be quite variable. Bacterial vaginosis is thought to be due to an overgrowth of anaerobic bacteria with a concomitant decrease in peroxide-producing lactobacilli. This situation results in the diagnostic triad: (1) a characteristic fishy odor that is magnified by the addition of 10 per cent potassium hydroxide ("positive whiff test"); (2) an increase in the vaginal pH to more than 4.5; and (3) the presence of "clue cells" by wet-mount microscopy.

Trichomonas Vulvovaginitis

The vaginal discharge of a *Trichomonas* infection commonly has a white or green and foamy appearance. Confirmation of the diagnosis commonly depends on the identification of the flagellated organism found, microscopically, with an admixture of saline and vaginal secretions. Occasionally, spermatozoa may be mistaken for *T. vaginalis* by the less experienced microscopist. *Trichomonas*, like *Candida*, may have a high false-negative rate by saline smear; therefore, culture with a commercial liquid medium (modified Diamond) may be preferable for confirming the diagnosis. A poor response to therapy is due primarily to reinfection or failure of the patient to complete the treatment regimen.

Atrophic Vulvovaginitis

Atrophic change grossly results in loss of vaginal rugae, narrowing of the introitus, development of urethral carunculae, reduction of external vulvar hair, and vaginal inflammation. Atrophy can be confirmed by evidence of parabasal cells in a cytologic maturation index (MI). The symptoms of atrophic vulvovaginitis generally occur later than the onset of hot flashes in the postmenopausal state. Nevertheless, atrophic problems are not restricted only to the postmenopausal patient. Because of the significantly higher mean percentage of parabasal cells in postpartum women with symptomatic vaginitis, it is thought that vaginal atrophy is a common cause of postpartum vaginitis, particularly in the patient who breast-feeds. Another disorder associated with an "atrophic" MI is the phenomenon of "erosive vaginitis." This disorder presents with vulvovaginal pain and burning without evidence of the common vaginal infections noted previously. Two proposed sources of erosive vaginitis include a form of lichen planus or an overgrowth of vaginal streptococci. The latter theory is difficult to prove, since streptococcal species can be normal vaginal flora.

Vestibular Pain and Inflammation

With "vulvar vestibulitis," the patient relates a history of painless coitus for 1 year or more prior to the development of long-standing dyspareunia. The patient has commonly been diagnosed as having chronic vaginitis, and a multitude of therapies have been instituted, without improvement. Other agents have been employed on the supposition that this problem may be related to herpes or human papillomavirus (HPV) infection. The diagnosis is confirmed by the presence of pain (allodynia) or hypersensitivity (hyperalgesia) to the light pressure of a cotton-tip applicator. The pain should be well demarcated between the point of loss of vulvar keratinization (Hart's line) and the caruncula hymenalis. It is important that the clinician exclude other vulvovaginal infections and atrophy before making this diagnosis.

Hidradenitis Suppurativa

This inflammatory condition of the apocrine gland can involve the vulva (sparing the labia minora) and extend up the "milk line," which runs from labia majora over the breasts and into the axillae. In these cutaneous regions, apocrine sweat glands can become inflamed and develop recurrent abscesses and chronic drainage. In severe cases, fistulous tracts form between one area of apocrine gland infection and another, and can be demonstrated by passage of a silver wire probe within the tract. The clinician can distinguish this condition from the common furuncle by examining the breasts and axillae for similar inflammatory lesions. Obesity may increase the risk of developing hidradenitis.

Other Causes of Pain and Inflammation

A number of other causes of vulvar and vestibular pain have been highlighted. One group of patients with vulvar burning and pain demonstrated allodynia, hyperesthesia, and hyperalgesia in a pudendal nerve distribution. The suggested cause of the pain was trauma to the perineum and resultant injury to the pudendal nerve from a variety of sources (e.g., a bicycle seat). In addition to trauma, a suggested source of pudendal neuralgia has been herpetic infection (possible herpes zoster or simplex). This proposal has been difficult to prove because of the high prevalence of herpes antibodies combined with the low prevalence of pudendal neuralgia in the general population. Recently, vulvar pain has been associated with sacral-meningeal (Tarlov) cysts, which may result in sacral nerve root compression. Tarlov cysts are best confirmed with lumbosacral magnetic resonance imaging (MRI). A less common inflammatory lesion known as vulvitis circumscripta plasmacellularis (VCP) or Zoon's disease has been described. Grossly, the striking feature is an orange hue surrounding the erythematous lesion. The histology includes dermal thinning, edema, small horizontally disposed keratinocytes, dermal inflammation, and the splitting of the dermoepidermal junction. Some authors consider "VCP" a useful term for the idiopathic form of erosive vulvitis with specific clinicopathologic findings.

ULCERS AND BLISTERS

Owing to the difficulty in the gross distinction of vulvovaginal ulcers, the diagnostic approach should be systematic and should generally include examination of oral mucosa, darkfield evaluation, syphilis serology, herpes culture, chlamydial culture, Giemsa stain of material from the ulcer base, biopsy of the leading ulcer edge, and photography (Table 1).

Herpes Vulvovaginitis

Herpetic infections may occur via oral or genital contact from another individual who is actively shedding virus. Although active virus has been isolated via fomites, such as a warm moist cloth with infected semen, this route of transmission is rare, if it occurs at all. The incubation period is approximately 3 to 7 days; thus, the source of infection is commonly identifiable. The primary symptom during the vesicular stage is burning or tingling. Subsequently, with rupture of the vesicle and superimposed bacterial infection, increasing pain results. During the primary viremic phase, signs and symptoms can include significant regional lymphadenitis, fever, malaise, and, rarely, central nervous system involvement. Once the shallow, painful ulcers are present on the vulva, they are also commonly located in the vagina, cervix, urethra, and bladder. Primary infection is commonly very painful, with swelling, urinary retention, and pain on defecation. Viral shedding lasts for 1 to 2 weeks. Labial adhesions are a rare complication of genital herpes infection, presumably owing to contact of contiguous ulcerated surfaces and the formation of fibrotic scar. Clinical recurrence develops in approximately 50 per cent of cases, and the symptoms are usually less severe than those associated with the primary infection. Viral shedding can occur in both men and women without the presence of symptoms.

Syphilis

Between 1981 and 1989, the incidence of primary and secondary syphilis increased from 13.7 to 18.4 cases per 100,000 persons in the United States. This incidence is higher than that at any time since 1949. The greatest

Table 1. Diagnostic Modalities for Vulvovaginal Disorders

Modality	Technique and Comments
Inspection with photography	Photography with "macro" (close-up) lens very helpful in documenting the response to therapy
Colposcopy with 5% acetic acid	Acetic acid opacifies areas of acanthosis and hyperkeratosis and helps identify potential areas for biopsy
2% Toluidine blue with 5% acetic acid rinse	Helps identify parakeratosis, but caution is needed because of "false-positive" staining of excoriated areas as well
Cystoscopy (air or water)	May be helpful in examining prepubertal girls for possible foreign bodies in vagina
Vaginal pH	In postmenarchal women, important for determining normal acidic milieu (pH < 4.5)
Papanicolaou smear and maturation index	May be combined with DNA probe for HPV: maturation index useful in determining hormonal milieu
Cultures: herpes simplex, *Mycoplasma* / *Ureaplasma,* fungal, gonococcal/*Chlamydia*	May contribute to vulvar pathology; fungal culture important because of false-negative rate of potassium hydroxide (KOH) wet-mount
Wood's lamp	Helpful in specific skin mycoses
Vaginal wet-mount (saline and KOH)	Helpful in screening for *Trichomonas,* moniliasis, and *Gardnerella vaginalis*
Darkfield microscope	Confirms diagnosis of *Treponema pallidum* in primary chancre or condylomata lata
Special stains: Giemsa/ Wright's	Confirms diagnosis of granuloma inguinale (Donovan bodies)
Vulvar biopsy	Of primary importance in the diagnosis of many dermatologic disorders; review of previous biopsy slides as well as written pathology reports also very important

increases in the decade of the 1980s occurred in heterosexual blacks and Latinos in urban areas. Coexisting human immunodeficiency virus (HIV) infection can influence both the diagnosis and the progression of syphilis and result in more frequent and earlier neurosyphilis. An additional concern is the possibility that genital ulcers of any sort, such as syphilis, herpes, and chancroid, may be a route of transmission of HIV infection.

Syphilis is usually transmitted through sexual intercourse or other forms of intimate contact. Congenital syphilis is usually transmitted via spirochetemia but may also be transmitted during birth. The primary stage of syphilis is manifested by the painless chancre (ulcer) at the site of inoculation. This lesion develops, on the average, 3 weeks after exposure and heals spontaneously even without treatment in 4 to 6 weeks. Secondary syphilis occurs 2 to 8 weeks after the primary stage, with generalized systemic symptoms similar to those of a viral infection. Macular and condylomatous lesions, occasionally meningitis, hepatitis, and nephrotic syndrome, can develop. Tertiary syphilis results in gummatous lesions in skin, bone, and the central nervous system.

Two nontreponemal tests, the VDRL (Venereal Disease Research Laboratories) and RPR (rapid plasma reagin) tests, can be used as a screening tool and for measurement of treatment efficacy. An automated reagin test and VDRL-ELISA (enzyme-linked immunosorbent assay) are two additional nonspecific tests. If a nonreactive treponemal test, such as the fluorescent treponemal antibody absorption test (FTA-AbS), follows a reactive nontreponemal test, the result of the nontreponemal test is considered a biologic false-positive. A number of illnesses can produce such results, including collagen vascular diseases, cirrhosis, infectious mononucleosis, genital herpes, and lepromatous leprosy. False-negative results can occur in early infection, immunodeficiency, and HIV infection.

Recommendations offered by an expert panel convened by the Centers for Disease Control and Prevention (CDC) in 1988 included the following:

1. Patients infected with HIV via the sexual or intravenous drug abuse route should be tested for syphilis.
2. If clinical findings suggest syphilis and serologic tests are negative, alternative tests including darkfield evaluation and fluorescent antibody test should be used.
3. Laboratories should titrate nontreponemal antibody tests to final endpoint, which can be used as a baseline for following the response to therapy.
4. Neurosyphilis should be in the differential diagnosis in HIV-infected individuals with neurologic manifestations.
5. Consultation with specialists is recommended in the evaluation and follow-up of individuals with unusual test results.

Other Ulcerogenic Sexually Transmitted Diseases

Other venereal diseases that are less common in the United States but are still seen in some tropical countries, particularly in the islands of the Caribbean, include granuloma inguinale, lymphogranuloma venereum (LGV), and chancroid. Granuloma inguinale and LGV are minimally symptomatic during the initial phase of the disease, presenting with a papule, shallow ulcer, erosion, or urethritis. Lymphogranuloma venereum, a chronic infection of *Chlamydia trachomatis*, develops a rather dramatic enlargement in the inguinal region after an incubation period of 10 to 30 days. These enlargements are usually diagnosed as masses of lymph nodes; however, they also include subcutaneous buboes. The pus obtained from the incision of these enlargements was used in the original Frei test. This test, and the complement fixation test, have been supplanted by the McCoy cell culture, immunofluorescence and ELISA as the primary modes of diagnosis. Late manifestations of this infection include perirectal abscess, ischiorectal fistulas, anal fistulas, and rectal stricture.

In contrast to LGV, the multiple small, superficial ulcers of granuloma inguinale often coalesce into larger, slightly elevated painless granulomas. Granuloma inguinale is associated with an encapsulated gram-negative bacillus. Diagnosis is made by biopsy or smears from these granulomatous masses. The Donovan body is identified microscopically as a "closed safety pin" structure either in the large mononuclear cells or in an extracellular position. The primary ulcerations may respond adequately to treatment; however, in the chronic stages of both granuloma inguinale and LGV, surgery may be necessary for removing the chronically infected distorted vulvar tissue. These granulomatous lesions in the chronic phase may be associated with the development of vulvar cancer.

Behçet's Disease

This ulcerative lesion is relatively nonspecific in its initial appearance. Nevertheless, the diagnosis is established when the clinician notes the presence of vulvar ulceration, similar ulcerations on the buccal mucous membrane, and two of the following: iridocyclitis, synovitis, cutaneous vasculitis, or meningoencephalitis. The ulcerative lesions of the vulva are rather sharply marginated, with a grayish-white necrotic center. The disease is characterized by spontaneous remissions and recurrences. Patients often give the history that they have had the ulcerations intermittently for many years. They are usually asymptomatic. Nevertheless, the ophthalmologic involvement is most serious and has been associated with patients carrying the HLA-B5 histocompatibility antigen. The ophthalmic pathology may lead to blindness and progression to meningoencephalitis and death. Patients with milder manifestations often develop recurrent arthritis with the accompanying disability. Biopsy of the lesion often reveals rather dramatic vasculitis and suggests that the disease is of the autoimmune variety. A characteristic response to cutaneous trauma with the development of a sterile pustule is termed "pathergy." This finding is considered pathognomonic of the disease.

Vulvar Cancer

The gross appearance of vulvar cancer may be ulcerative or proliferative. The labium majus is the most common site of origin, but any area of the vulva may be involved, including the clitoris and fourchette. Invasive carcinoma of the vulva constitutes about 4 to 5 per cent of all primary malignancies in the female genital canal, and more than 90 per cent of all invasive vulvar malignancies are found in the postmenopausal woman. Associated symptoms are similar to most vulvar diseases, namely, pruritus, pain, and bleeding. Other symptoms depend on extension of the lesion into the urethra, rectum, vagina, or deeper tissues. The diagnosis is made by biopsy, which should be taken of any suspicious lesion, particularly of the chronic irritative variety. Histopathologically, 75 per cent of the lesions are of the mature variety, and 25 per cent are less well differentiated. It is common, however, to find both histopathologic alterations immediately adjacent to one another.

Blistering Vulvovaginal Disease

Blistering diseases can involve the vulva and lead to misdiagnosis of a vulvar ulcer or a more common vulvar dermatitis. The diseases include bullous pemphigoid, cicatricial pemphigoid, epidermolysis bullosa acquisita, linear IgA disease, and pemphigus. In these diseases, autoantibodies are directed toward normal components of the epidermis and are diagnosed by direct immunofluorescence with a fresh biopsy. Common misdiagnosis includes herpes simplex and sexual abuse. Vulvar involvement in pediatric patients most commonly includes lichen sclerosus, linear IgA disease, and bullous impetigo. Each of these problems is relatively characteristic on inspection. However, vulvar biopsy may be necessary for confirmation.

Other Vulvar Ulcers

In addition to herpes vulvitis, many painful lesions of the vulva appear initially as ulcers, for example, the granulomatous diseases, Crohn's disease, and traumatic lesions. These ulcers do not fall into one of the preceding categories but must be identified so that appropriate therapy can be started.

NODULES, CYSTS, AND MASSES

Size, shape, and location are important parameters in distinguishing the etiology of vulvar nodules, cysts, and masses. A common cystic nodule seen on the vulva is the epidermal inclusion cyst, which has a smooth surface and commonly carries a yellow hue. This nodule can be located from the external surface of the labia minora outward, generally is symptom free, and has no malignant potential. Another common nodule is the small umbilicated lesion of molluscum contagiosum, which is very characteristic in appearance and commonly involves the labia majora and perineum. A larger, umbilicated lesion, the hidradenoma is commonly found in the interlabial sulcus. The exophytic cauliflowerlike lesions of condyloma acuminatum are also very characteristic. Conversely, smaller, papillomatous lesions, particularly of the vestibule, have probably been overdiagnosed as condyloma. It is now thought that these lesions are frequently normal variations. Care must also be taken to distinguish condylomata lata from condylomata acuminata. Condyloma latum generally has a smoother, flatter surface; however, errors in distinguishing the two are common, and testing via darkfield evaluation and serology should be done for any lesion in question.

Bartholin's Abscess or Cyst

Bartholin's gland, which enters the introitus just above the fourchette at the vaginal outlet, may be dilated as a result of chronic infection or cyst formation. It was previously suggested that the majority of Bartholin gland abscesses and residual chronic infection are of gonorrheal origin; however, this is not the case. Cultures of infected material reveal the presence of the gonococci in 25 to 30 per cent of cases, and culture usually reveals a mixed bacterial flora. Cysts usually arise from occlusion of the duct by surgery or scarring. The clinician should have a high level of suspicion when examining a Bartholin mass in the postmenopausal patient, since carcinoma of Bartholin's gland may be overlooked if such a solid mass is small and nontender. Biopsy or surgical excision should be considered.

Hydrocele, Hernia, and Cysts of the Canal of Nuck

Cystic lesions appearing in the labium majus either near the external inguinal ring or in the middle of the vulva commonly represent fluid accumulations (hydrocele) along the extension of the peritoneal sac through the inguinal ligament into the vulva. Swelling in the labium majus near the point of insertion of the round ligament may indicate the presence of bowel because the peritoneal investment of the round ligament is continuous with the peritoneum of the abdominal cavity. Such lesions should be evaluated accurately by careful palpation with the patient standing and coughing before any surgery is contemplated. Usually, the sac contains only fluid, or a "cystic tumor." However, bowel in the sac may be injured if the possibility of its presence is not taken into account. Furthermore, incision and drainage of a hydrocele misdiagnosed as a Bartholin duct cyst leads only to recurrence of the condition. Accurate diagnosis is imperative.

Verrucous Lesions

Verrucous lesions of the vulva occur in one of two forms: as papilloma or as condyloma acuminatum. The true papilloma appears as a warty growth, usually arising from the labia majora in the perimenopausal or postmenopausal patient and having a treelike microscopic structure. A micropapillomatous growth can also be observed within the vestibule on the inner aspects of the labia majora in younger women. These structures, best visualized by colposcopy, are probably present congenitally and become more prominent during inflammatory processes. Both warty structures especially need to be distinguished from condylomata acuminata. As noted earlier, this lesion originates from infection with HPV, a sexually transmitted disease.

Acuminate warts are currently the most prevalent sexually transmitted disease. The common wart virus (HPV) has been studied extensively, and although HPV-associated acuminate warts appear, on gross examination, similar to the common skin wart (verruca vulgaris), they are antigenically different. Currently, at least 60 varieties of HPV have been described. Types 6, 11, 16, 18, 31, 33, 35, and 41 are sexually transmitted and involve primarily the genitalia and laryngeal area. These lesions are almost epidemic in our culture. With no means of preventing recurrences, the patient is faced with the necessity of repeated local ablative treatments to eliminate the external evidence of infection, although she may be infectious for an indeterminate period of time in the absence of gross lesions.

As noted, the incubation period from contact to the appearance of the lesion is a long one, approximately 3 to 6 months; consequently the initial lesion, if there is one, is not recognized. The development of antibodies undoubtedly occurs; however, in contrast to herpetic infection, titers for such antibodies cannot be evaluated at present. Certainly, the immunosuppressed patient, for example the patient with acquired immunodeficiency syndrome (AIDS), is prone to developing extensive lesions and to recurrences regardless of therapy. The pregnant patient demonstrates similar problems, although following termination of the pregnancy the lesions may disappear spontaneously. If the lower genital tract is markedly involved with condylomata, cesarean section should be considered as the method of delivery, to reduce the possibility of massive hemorrhage secondary to massive lacerations. Furthermore, some instances of laryngeal papillomata and genital infections in the infant are thought to be secondary to maternal-infant transmission at birth. In a recent case control study, condylomata acuminata were found to increase the risk of vulvar malignancy more than 15-fold, and if a history of cigarette smoking was also present, this risk increased to 35-fold.

Hidradenoma

This nodule is rarely more than 1 to 1.5 cm in diameter and commonly appears in the interlabial sulcus between labia majora and minora. These nodules are easily removed by simple excision and often “pop out” with an apparently well-defined capsule. Despite their “benign” gross appearance, the histopathology may be confusing, characterized by a complex papillary-adenomatous pattern. Despite their intricate pattern, these lesions are benign and need no postoperative therapy. Hidradenomas are routinely solitary lesions, although multiple nodules have been recognized on occasion, particularly near the anal orifice.

Other Masses

Other benign masses seen on the vulva with characteristic pathologic findings on biopsy include seborrheic keratosis, acrochordon, fibroma, neurofibromatosis, accessory breast tissue, granular cell myoblastoma, and sebaceous adenoma.

PIGMENTED LESIONS

The junction of the vestibule with the remaining vulva manifests a normal color change known as Hart’s line. This color change corresponds, histologically, to an area of reduced keratinization. The vulva can present other color changes varying from black, to brown, red, or white. The extent to which such color changes mark a significant pathologic problem is also variable. A safe “rule of thumb” is to perform skin biopsies of any questionable pigmented lesion.

Squamous Cell Hyperplasia

Patients describe a long-standing problem of vulvar irritation, itching, or burning. Often, an inciting agent is obvious, such as chronic moniliasis in the patient with diabetes mellitus. Although the number of inciting problems are numerous, the final common presentation is a hyperpigmented, irritated, often excoriated vulva with squamous cell hyperplasia. Histologically, this condition is characterized by hyperkeratosis, elongation of the rete pegs (acanthosis), and essentially normal maturation of the epithelium with associated underlying inflammatory infiltrate. Thus, the classic picture is one of chronic dermatitis with hyperkeratosis (previously called leukoplakia). All keratotic lesions are white or gray—white owing to the absorption of fluid into the overlying keratin. Conversely, parakeratosis (incomplete keratinization) produces a red or reddish-brown appearance. Given the diverse array of conditions associated with hyperkeratosis, the term leukoplakia should be eliminated from the nomenclature of vulvar disease.

Lichen Sclerosus

Lichen sclerosus, previously designated lichen sclerosus et atrophicus, may be seen in any age group, although it is most common in postmenopausal patients. Grossly, the lesions are characterized by a thin, white surface (“cigarette paper” or “parchment” skin) and loss of normal architecture often associated with disappearance of the labia minora, constriction of the vaginal outlet (kraurosis), and superficial ecchymoses. In the early stages of development, particularly during the menstrual years, the lesions may be asymptomatic. Nevertheless, in the postmenopausal patient, itching and irritation are prevalent, and superficial excoriations often develop. Biopsy should be performed in such cases. Histologically, lichen sclerosus is characterized by a mild to moderate degree of hyperkeratosis, thinning of the epithelium with loss of the rete pegs, “homogenization” of the subepithelial layer (a generally acellular zone often with dilated vascular channels), and inflammatory infiltrate of the subepithelial layer. Keratin frequently plugs the superficial invaginations, such as hair follicles and sebaceous glands. It is important to confirm the diagnosis by biopsy, often at multiple foci, specifically those with marked keratin (whitish) deposits or ulcerations.

Vulvar Intraepithelial Neoplasia

On inspection of the vulva, vulvar intraepithelial neoplasia (VIN) can present as a dark lesion, a red lesion, a white lesion, or an ulcer. Older terminology has confused the pathologic diagnosis of vulvar carcinoma in situ because of a myriad of designations, such as Bowen's disease, erythroplasia of Queyrat, bowenoid papulosis, and atypical pigmentation. Currently, all these lesions are incorporated under the heading VIN, as multiple histopathologic patterns are commonly found within the same lesion. Particularly in the young patient, they pursue a proliferative recurrent pattern but rarely, if ever, invade, metastasize, or result in death. The incidence is increasing, and currently the average age at occurrence is in the late third and early fourth decades of life. However, patients in the seventh, eighth, and ninth decades are not exempt, nor are teenagers.

It may be difficult to distinguish the gross appearance of the benign lesion from the malignant lesion. Thus, biopsy is necessary for recurrent lesions or those that change color, particularly the hyperpigmented wart. A major diagnostic problem today is overinterpretation of the condylomata as an "in situ" or, even, an invasive cancer. The proliferation of the basal and parabasal zones with associated multinucleate cells gives the impression of hyperactivity, although both alterations are classic findings in viral disease. Tangential cutting of the specimen offers an additional challenge to the pathologist. These common "warty" changes must be taken into consideration in the evaluation of both the tissue specimen and the vaginal cytopathologic preparation.

Malignant Melanoma

After squamous cell carcinoma, malignant melanoma is the second most common malignancy that occurs on the vulva. Malignant melanoma makes up approximately 2 to 3 per cent of all melanomas in the human body and is no more common on the vulva than elsewhere. It is two to four times more common in white women than in black women, and the mean age at diagnosis is 60 years. Melanomas may be of the spreading or nodular variety and usually arise on the labia minora. Visible signs that should raise suspicion of melanoma include (1) lesion size greater than 6 mm (larger in diameter than a standard pencil eraser), (2) irregular lesion border, (3) variable color (especially red, white, or blue), and (4) irregular lesion surface. Biopsy of all suspicious lesions is mandatory, and obviously follow-up therapy must be instituted promptly if there is any question as to the interpretation of the pathology. The prognosis is based largely on the level of involvement, commonly referred to Clark's levels. For example, Clark's levels I and II are "intraepithelial" and "invasion in the interpapillary ridges," respectively.

Paget's Disease of the Vulva

Paget's disease of the vulva is commonly seen in the fifth and sixth decades of life with primary symptoms of burning and pruritus. Grossly, the lesions are fiery-red with white patches involving multifocal areas of the vulva. Swelling occasionally occurs, although it is usually seen in the later stages of the disease. Thorough inspection of the perianal area and the breasts is important in the recognition of multifocal disease. The breast is the most common site of Paget's disease. Histopathologically, the Paget cell is seen initially just above the basal layer, which suggests that it originates from the undifferentiated "embryonal stratum germinativa." The large, pale cells are occasionally arranged in a glandlike pattern. Commonly, the entire surface epithelium is involved, with individual or small groups of the classic large, pale cell. These cells are periodic acid–Schiff (PAS)– and mucicarmine-positive, which clearly distinguishes them from the cells of the amelanotic melanoma. The appendages are also involved in approximately 75 to 80 per cent of cases. The condition is then termed Paget's disease with gland involvement, but the prognosis remains the same. Lesions on the vulva remain largely intraepithelial, although recurrences are frequent. Progression from intraepithelial to invasive Paget's disease appears to be rare. Nevertheless, patients should be followed carefully, and biopsies taken of new areas of involvement. On rare occasions, an underlying adenocarcinoma in the apocrine system has been recognized in the removed tissue. However, for the most part, the histopathologic signs of malignancy have been those noted with many in situ cancers: the "breaking through" of the so-called basement membrane with extension into the underlying tissue by the Paget's disease, and undifferentiated epithelial cells in the basal layer.

Other Pigmented Conditions

A number of benign pigmented conditions of the vulva can often be mistaken for melanoma, vulvar cancer, or lichen sclerosus. These conditions include seborrheic keratosis and lentigo (dark lesions), leukoderma and vitiligo (white lesions), and inflammatory conditions (red lesions). It should be reiterated that the clinician should not hesitate to biopsy and photograph questionable pigmented lesions, given the importance of excluding potentially life-threatening conditions.

INTRAEPITHELIAL AND INVASIVE CERVICAL CANCER

By James M. Davison, D.O.,
and Verda Hunter, M.D.
Kansas City, Missouri

Death from cervical cancer represents the endpoint of a disease continuum that begins with mild atypical cellular changes. The transition from preinvasive to frankly malignant disease is the point on that continuum at which a quantum change in biologic behavior, clinical presentation, and patient prognosis occurs. In the premalignant stages, there is no direct threat to the patient's life or health and no overt signs or symptoms of disease; at this point, cure is easily effected. Once the change to invasive cancer has occurred, the patient has a disease that, unless adequate and timely treatment is undertaken, will prove fatal. It would, therefore, seem logical to divide the discussion of cervical neoplasia into preinvasive or intraepithelial and invasive disease.

Cancer of the cervix may arise from either the squamous epithelium of the ectocervix or the glandular tissue of the endocervix. Although adenocarcinoma of the cervix appears to be increasing in incidence, squamous cell carcinoma is by far the more common type. The natural history of squamous cell carcinoma of the cervix is well understood, and most screening programs are directed at the detection of precursor lesions of this disease. Because adenocarcinoma of the endocervix is rarely diagnosed prior to the development of invasive disease, it will be discussed under the heading of invasive cancer.

About 600,000 new cases of cervical intraepithelial neoplasia (CIN) are diagnosed in the United States each year. They result in about 13,000 new cases of cervical cancer and 4500 deaths. In the past, cancer of the cervix was the leading cause of cancer death among women. With the establishment of screening programs, cervical cancer has dropped to seventh among all cancers and to third among gynecologic cancers. Indeed, the incidence of cervical cancer has decreased by 50 per cent in the last half-century. The decreased incidence of cervical cancer has been attributed, in part, to the increased number of women undergoing screening and has occurred despite a marked increase in the incidence of preinvasive disease. Screening with the Papanicolaou smear may reduce the risk of death from cervical cancer by as much as 90 per cent. Even adequately screened patients in whom cancer develops are likely to have earlier, more curable lesions at the time of diagnosis.

The American College of Obstetricians and Gynecologists has stated that "All women who are or have been sexually active should undergo an annual Pap test and pelvic examination. After a woman has had three consecutive, satisfactory annual examinations with normal findings, the Pap smear may be performed less frequently at the discretion of her physician." Importantly, only women at low risk (those who have always been in a strictly monogamous relationship or who have never been sexually active) are candidates for less than yearly screening. If all women followed this recommendation, the number of deaths from cervical cancer would be further reduced.

NATURAL HISTORY

The development of cervical neoplasia most likely requires exposure of susceptible cervical epithelium to carcinogens and a loss of host capacity to recognize and eliminate abnormal or transformed cells. Under the influence of an acidic vaginal environment caused by high estrogen states, glandular cells that normally line the upper vagina, cervix and endocervical canal during fetal life are converted to stratified squamous epithelium in a process called metaplasia. Cells undergoing metaplasia seem to be particularly susceptible to the effects of carcinogenic agents, which are believed to be (although this has not been proved) certain subtypes of the human papillomavirus (HPV). When metaplasia is complete, the resulting mature squamous epithelium is relatively resistant to malignant transformation. Epidemiologic data indicate that the carcinogen must be sexually transmitted. Women who have not experienced sexual intercourse are at low risk for the development of cervical cancer. Most cancers arise at the interface of the columnar epithelium and the squamous epithelium (the squamocolumnar junction) because the most active metaplasia occurs in this area. This squamocolumnar junction may be found on the ectocervix, within the cervical canal or, rarely, in the upper vagina. As previously noted, estrogen increases metaplastic activity by lowering the pH of the vagina and everting the cervix, exposing more columnar epithelium to both the low pH and the carcinogen, if it is present. When a metaplastic cell is exposed to the carcinogenic agent, and possibly certain cofactors, it may undergo changes that cause it to appear somewhat atypical. These changes may evolve to a premalignant lesion and eventually to invasive cancer. Progression to malignancy does not necessarily occur in an orderly, stepwise manner. Some cancers progress rapidly over a period of months, whereas others arise de novo without passing through a preinvasive stage. On rare occasions, squamous cell carcinoma may arise outside the transformation zone.

RISK FACTORS

Sexual activity is the major risk factor for the development of cervical cancer. Multiple partners and an early age at first intercourse place the patient at greatest risk. The rate of metaplastic activity is highest in young girls and the likelihood of exposure to sexually transmitted carcinogens increases with the number of sexual partners. Intercourse with a high-risk male (one with a previous partner with cervical cancer) also substantially increases a woman's risk of acquiring cancer.

Additional, independent risk factors for cervical cancer have been described. The immune compromised woman is more likely to get cancer, and tumors are more likely to behave aggressively in this type of patient. The use of oral contraceptives increases the risk of cervical cancer independent of sexual history, presumably by causing a state of excess estrogen. Barrier contraceptives decrease the risk by reducing exposure to sexually transmitted carcinogens. Women who smoke are more likely to acquire cervical cancer. There is an ethnic bias in the incidence of cervical cancer: Hispanics are at greatest risk, followed by African Americans and whites who are at a somewhat lower risk. The increased risk of cervical cancer in women of lower socioeconomic status has been attributed to poor access to health services, lack of preventive care, and excessive risk-taking behavior.

Although many clinicians believe that HPV infection is a cause of cervical cancer, not all cervical tumors contain HPV. Moreover, the HPV subtypes most frequently associated with malignancy are found in as many as 80 per cent of normal women. Despite the strength of the association between HPV and cervical malignancy, the vast majority of women infected with HPV do not acquire either preinvasive disease or cancer.

PREINVASIVE DISEASE

Signs and Symptoms

Premalignant disease of the cervix is usually asymptomatic, and inspection of the cervix rarely reveals diagnostic abnormalities. If visible abnormalities are present, they are likely to be cauliflowerlike condylomatous lesions or flat, white plaques. Either of these abnormalities should be biopsied, as should any visible abnormality, regardless of the results of the Papanicolaou smear. Occasionally, endocervical polyps or nabothian cysts may be sources of confusion for the inexperienced observer.

The nomenclature of preinvasive disease is confusing because of frequent changes in terminology over the last several years. The relationships among the various systems of classification are presented in Table 1. Currently, the Bethesda classification is the most commonly used in the United States. Under this system, squamous cell changes are divided into atypical changes of uncertain significance, premalignant changes, and changes that typify invasive cancer. Premalignant changes are further divided into low-grade and high-grade intraepithelial lesions. Low-grade lesions encompass those changes consistent with infection by HPV and changes formerly termed mild dysplasia or CIN I. These changes are felt to pose a low risk of progression to invasive disease. High-grade lesions are those formerly termed moderate dysplasia (CIN II),

Table 1. Classification of Preinvasive Cervical Disease

Papanicolaou Classes	Dysplasia	Cervical Intraepithelial Neoplasia	Bethesda
I	Normal	Normal	Normal
II	Atypia	Atypia	Atypical squamous cells of uncertain significance
II or III	Mild dysplasia	CIN I	Low-grade squamous intraepithelial lesion
III	Moderate dysplasia	CIN II	High-grade squamous intraepithelial lesion
	Severe dysplasia	CIN III	
III or IV	Carcinoma in situ		
V	Cancer	Cancer	Cancer

CIN = cervical intraepithelial neoplasia.

severe dysplasia, and carcinoma in situ (CIN III). Fifty per cent of CIN III lesions progress to invasion over 10 years, whereas less than 1 per cent of women with low-grade lesions go on to get cervical cancer.

Diagnosis

Premalignant lesions of the cervix are usually discovered with routine screening tests. As already mentioned, the most commonly used screening tool is the Papanicolaou smear in which cells exfoliated from the cervix are stained and examined microscopically. The Papanicolaou smear is fast, inexpensive, easy to perform, and suitable for mass screening programs. The clinician should recall, however, that as many as 27 per cent of women with stage I cancers have had normal results within 1 year of the diagnosis of their malignancy. Furthermore, the majority of intraepithelial lesions diagnosed with screening colposcopy or cervicography are associated with normal smear results at the time of examination. The sensitivity of the Papanicolaou smear probably does not exceed 50 per cent. The success of the Papanicolaou smear in reducing the incidence of cervical cancer rests on repetitive screening, thereby decreasing the number of slowly progressing premalignant lesions that are missed. The low sensitivity of the Papanicolaou smear requires the clinician to pursue with diagnostic testing any result suggesting an intraepithelial lesion. Attempts to confirm initial Papanicolaou smear results with repeat smears are not recommended. Any finding of atypical cells of undetermined significance should also trigger further diagnostic testing.

The Papanicolaou smear is generally performed in two steps. After removal of discharge from the cervix, a sample is obtained from the endocervical canal with one of several devices. Classically, cotton-tipped applicators moistened with saline have been used. Modern endocervical brushes increase the number of endocervical cells obtained at the time of screening. It is not yet clear that brushing decreases the number of falsely normal smear results. Nevertheless, most authorities now advocate the use of a brush rather than the cotton-tipped applicator to obtain the endocervical specimen because it may help in the early diagnosis of endocervical cancers. Various other devices also can be used to obtain endocervical specimens, but their use is unsupported by clinical data.

Once the specimen is obtained, the swab or brush is *rolled* across the surface of a clean glass slide, producing a thin, smooth layer of cells for examination. The slide must be rapidly fixed with commercial fixative or 95 per cent ethanol; otherwise drying artifact will render the specimen difficult to interpret. A second specimen is obtained from the vaginal portion of the cervix by scraping it with a specially shaped (Ayer's) wooden spatula. This specimen is also smeared onto a glass slide and fixed. The clinician must ensure that a reputable laboratory interprets the slides. Some commercial laboratories have been cited for the use of substandard techniques and procedures that may contribute to the problem of falsely normal test results.

Other tests for the detection of cervical cancer include screening colposcopy and cervicography. Screening colposcopy, like diagnostic colposcopy, should be performed by clinicians specifically trained in this technique. Cervicography employs a specially designed camera to photograph the cervix after it has been treated with acetic acid. An office nurse can obtain the photographs with minimal training, but the pictures should be interpreted by specially trained physicians. The use of parallel testing protocols, in which one of these ancillary tests is used in conjunction with cytologic testing, can drastically reduce the number of lesions that are missed by cytologic studies alone. This type of parallel testing scheme may be particularly appropriate for use in high-risk populations or in populations in which frequent repeat testing cannot reasonably be performed.

Work-Up of the Abnormal Papanicolaou Test

Most clinicians use series rather than parallel testing. An abnormal Papanicolaou smear is typically followed by one or more diagnostic tests, which are, in turn, followed by definitive therapy if appropriate. The most commonly used diagnostic test is colposcopy, which involves examination of the cervix with a low-power, stereo-optic binocular microscope. The cervix is painted with 5 per cent acetic acid (vinegar) after it has been cleansed of any discharge. The acetic acid causes whitening of abnormal squamous epithelium and renders visible various vascular changes associated with cervical neoplasia. Punch biopsies are performed on abnormal areas, and scrapings are obtained from the endocervical canal. The colposcope should also be used to evaluate lesions of the vagina and vulva because up to 20 per cent of patients with CIN have associated vulvar or vaginal intraepithelial neoplasia. Colposcopy with directed biopsy offers a safe, rapid, and relatively painless diagnosis.

The goal of diagnostic testing is to exclude the presence of invasive disease. When colposcopy is not readily available or when the entire potentially abnormal area (the transformation zone) cannot be visualized, a cone biopsy of the cervix must be performed. Cone biopsy is also indicated if the Papanicolaou smear suggests a higher grade lesion than is found on colposcopy-directed biopsy or if the punch biopsy demonstrates microinvasive cancer. This procedure involves a circumferential excision of an area of the cervix that includes a portion of the endocervical canal. If the disease process is completely excised, the cone procedure may provide cure as well as definitive diagnosis. Complications of cone biopsy include hemorrhage, which can be severe, and infertility because of removal of important mucus-secreting glands of the endocervical canal. In addition, pregnancy loss may result if the cervix is weakened by removal of significant amounts of supporting tissue. The

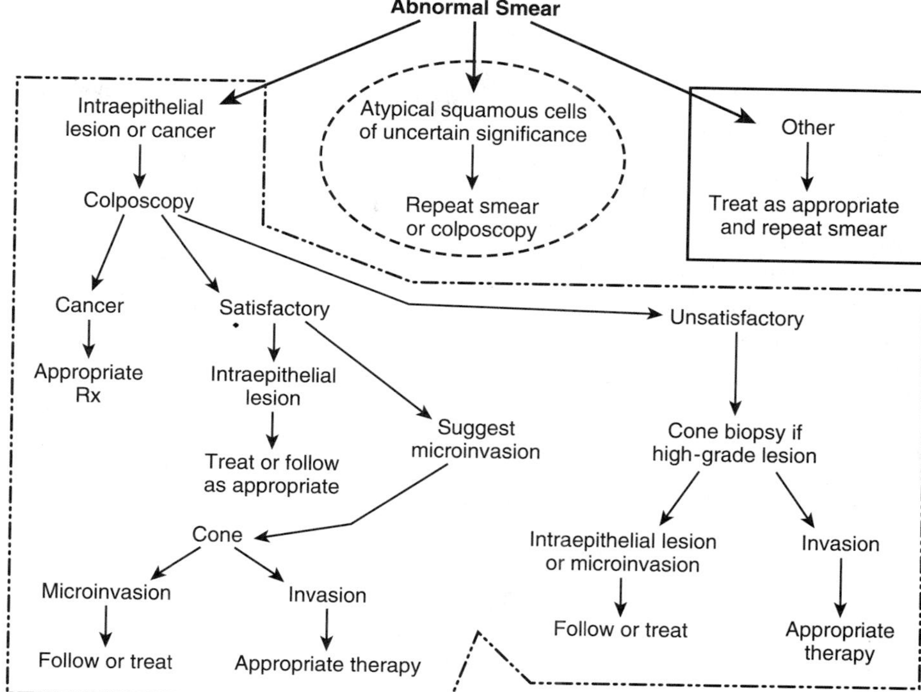

Figure 1. Algorithm for evaluation of abnormal Papanicolaou smear.

disadvantage of cervical cone biopsy without colposcopic examination is the lack of optimal evaluation of other potentially abnormal areas of the reproductive tract. Whenever possible, the clinican should insist on colposcopic examination for the patient with an abnormal Papanicolaou smear. Cone biopsy should be used only when absolutely indicated or when colposcopy is unavailable (Fig. 1). Causes of abnormal Papanicolaou smear are presented in Table 2.

INVASIVE DISEASE

Signs and Symptoms

Although early cancer of the cervix is typically asymptomatic, some patients report an increased vaginal discharge that may be misinterpreted as infection. By contrast, frankly invasive cervical cancer frequently presents with a history of postcoital and intermenstrual bleeding that may be associated with increased vaginal discharge. Pain may be present in the advanced stages of cervical cancer with extension of tumor into the parametrium. With further extension of tumor to the pelvic side wall, lymphedema of the extremity and ureteral obstruction with ipsilateral renal failure may occur. Concurrent occlusion of the pelvic veins may result in deep venous thrombosis. Bladder or rectal extension of tumor may present with dysuria and hematuria or tenesmus and rectal bleeding. Rarely, more advanced cases may present with obstruction of the small or large intestine, jaundice from hepatic metastasis, cough from pulmonary metastasis, or lymphadenopathy.

Table 2. Causes of Abnormal Papanicolaou Smears

Cancer	Infection
Vulva	Viral
Vagina	Bacterial
Cervix	Parasitic
Endocervix	Fungal
Uterus	Estrogen deficiency
Tube	Healing (repair)
Ovary	Pelvic irradiation
Intraepithelial disease	
Vulva	
Vagina	
Cervix	

In some patients, physical examination may reveal no overt signs of cancer. In others, however, carcinoma of the cervix may present as a small, friable ulceration or as a large, necrotic, exophytic lesion. Cervical cancer tends to spread by direct extension through the cervix and into surrounding tissues. Thus, endophytic tumors often present as an enlarged, hardened, barrel-shaped but otherwise normal-appearing cervix. If extension beyond the cervix has occurred, both the cervix and uterus may be immobile and fixed, with induration palpable in the surrounding tissues.

Diagnosis

In patients with invasive cervical tumors, an abnormal Papanicolaou smear typically leads to colposcopy and biopsy of detectable lesions. If microinvasion (to a depth less than 3 mm below the basement membrane) is observed in the cervical punch biopsy specimen, conization must be performed to exclude more extensive invasion. Definitive invasion exceeding 3 mm on punch biopsy does not require conization for confirmation.

Staging

Once a definitive histopathologic diagnosis is obtained, the tumor must be staged. The staging for cervical cancer is clinical rather than surgical. The staging of early cervical cancer is currently debated. The standard staging is presented in Table 3. By convention, staging includes a medical history, physical examination, laboratory studies

Table 3. Staging of Cervical Cancer

Stage I	Limited to the cervix
IA	Microinvasive (various definitions)
IB	Frankly invasive
Stage II	Spread beyond cervix
IIA	To upper vagina
IIB	To parametrium but not onto side wall
Stage III	
IIIA	Spread to lower third of vagina
IIIB	Parametrial involvement to side wall
	Ureteral dilatation is presumptive evidence of spread to side wall
Stage IV	Spread beyond reproductive tract
IVA	Involvement of rectal or bladder mucosa
IVB	Distant metastasis

(including assessment of liver and kidney function), chest film, and intravenous pyelography. In some patients, a barium enema may be indicated. Under anesthesia, cystoscopy and proctoscopy can also be performed. Lymphangiography, computed tomography (CT), magnetic resonance imaging (MRI), and ultrasound are frequently used by gynecologic oncologists or radiation therapists in planning treatment, but these procedures are not part of traditional staging protocols for cervical cancer.

Adenocarcinoma

Adenocarcinoma of the cervix arises from the glandular epithelium of the endocervix. The incidence appears to be rising worldwide, especially in women younger than 35 years of age. Women with cervical adenocarcinoma tend to be nulliparous, single, and of a higher socioeconomic class when compared with women in whom squamous carcinoma of the cervix develops.

Before the introduction of the endocervical brush for obtaining the endocervical portion of the Papanicolaou smear specimen, screening for adenocarcinoma was rarely discussed in the medical literature. Although the natural history of this tumor is not as well understood as that of squamous cell cancer, atypical glandular cells, endocervical glandular dysplasia, and adenocarcinoma in situ can be identified by cytologic findings and are felt to represent precursor lesions in the development of endocervical adenocarcinoma.

Signs and symptoms of adenocarcinoma of the cervix are similar to those described for invasive squamous cell cancer of the cervix. Bleeding is the most common presenting complaint. The bleeding may be intermenstrual or may be associated with intercourse. Adenocarcinoma may also present with a mucoid or watery cervical-vaginal discharge. This discharge, which may contain many leukocytes and may be confused with the discharge of cervicitis, typically fails to respond to antibiotic therapy.

Cervical adenocarcinomas classically present as barrel-shaped lesions that expand the cervix prior to causing visible surface changes. As with squamous cell cancer, the diagnosis is established using colposcopy and cone biopsy. The staging process for adenocarcinoma is the same as the staging process for squamous cell cancer of the cervix.

HYPERPLASIA AND CARCINOMA OF THE ENDOMETRIUM

By Barbara S. Apgar, M.D., M.S.
Ann Arbor, Michigan

and Gregory Brotzman, M.D.
Milwaukee, Wisconsin

The endometrium comprises a morphologic spectrum that ranges from normal secretory glands, through various degrees of hyperplasia, to carcinoma. Endometrial hyperplasia is a benign proliferation of the endometrium that frequently involves both glands and stroma. Although atypical endometrial hyperplasia is considered a precursor to endometrial adenocarcinoma, the exact relationship remains controversial. Pathologists have used various terms, including proliferative, cystic, glandular, complex, adenomatous, and carcinoma in situ, to describe the various endometrial proliferations. While most of the simple and complex architectural patterns regress spontaneously, atypical hyperplasia has a much greater tendency to persist or progress if it is not specifically treated.

For many years, there has been uncertainty over the diagnostic criteria for distinguishing the various types of hyperplasia. Interpretation of these lesions varies among pathologists. At times, it may be difficult to distinguish atypical hyperplasia from well-differentiated carcinoma. The interpretation of what is actually an atypical hyperplasia as invasive disease can be fraught with the potential for overdiagnosis and inappropriate treatment. A recent attempt to achieve a definitive histopathologic diagnosis for each precursor lesion has led to the classification of noninvasive and invasive terms according to the presence of stromal invasion. The presence of stromal invasion, in and of itself, is the best criterion for determining whether cancer is present. The deeper the stromal invasion, the worse the prognosis.

The goal of the pathologist is to identify those lesions that have the minimal potential for invasion versus those that will readily metastasize. The classification system proposed by the International Society of Gynecological Pathologists recognizes that regardless of which diagnostic technique is used, there are a certain number of malignant cells that will defy all attempts to categorize them until invasive disease occurs.

NORMAL ENDOMETRIAL FINDINGS

An understanding of the histologic events in the menstrual cycle is required for an effective comprehension of the evolution of endometrial hyperplasia. The proliferative or preovulatory endometrium is characterized by a proliferation of gland cells, stromal fibroblasts, and endothelial cells. As a result of the increased mitotic activity during this phase, the glands become progressively more abundant and tortuous as ovulation is approached. Estradiol concentrations peak by day 10 of the menstrual cycle, producing a thick and voluminous endometrium. The secretory or postovulatory phase undergoes rapid differentiation under the influence of progesterone. By the middle of the secretory phase, small vacuoles appear in the base of the gland cells. These vacuoles are the first reliable histologic indication that ovulation has occurred. These glycogen vacuoles in the lining cells of the gland and the presence of the gland cell nuclei arranged in a palisade definitely establish the secretory phase.

As the supranuclear cytoplasmic secretions are dispatched into the glandular lumen, the apical portions of the cells are detached. The active mitoses that were so abundant in the proliferative phase are now inhibited by progesterone and cease by day 19. The edematous stroma actively begins to change in response to the coiling of the spiral arteries and the predecidualization process. These changes are under the influence of prostaglandin F_2, which encourages capillary permeability. By day 26, coinciding with the decrease of estradiol and progesterone concentrations, the glands exhibit coiling. The action of lysosomal enzymes digests the cytoplasmic elements, the intracellular desmosomes, and results in the entire collapse of the cellular system.

CLASSIFICATION OF THE ENDOMETRIAL PRECURSOR LESIONS

The various architectural abnormalities of the endometrial cancer precursors are divided into two different types of hyperplasia: the simple or cystic and the complex or adenomatous. These two groups are further subdivided into groups defined by the presence or absence of cytologic atypia. Approximately 2 per cent of hyperplasia without atypia and 25 per cent with atypia progress to endometrial cancer. Because atypia may be associated with either simple or complex hyperplasia, most pathologists use the term atypical hyperplasia (also called endometrial intraepithelial neoplasia) as a separate category without attaching the terms simple or complex to it. There are no distinguishing features of these various types of hyperplasia that can be clinically visualized, so the clinician must rely on the histopathologic diagnosis. Additionally, the diagnosis of hyperplasia does not rely on the volume of tissue obtained by sampling devices.

A common method of identifying the various endometrial precursor abnormalities involves classifying the architectural abnormalities by identifying the relationship of the glands and the stroma. The extent of the "crowding" of the glands and the resulting degree of stromal obliteration determine the severity of the preinvasive changes. When back-to-back crowding is absent, and the glands are evenly distributed throughout the stroma, the hyperplasia is referred to as simple or cystic. If the glands are overly developed or hypertrophied and obliterate the stromal space, the hyperplasia is classified as complex or adenomatous. The presence of these closely packed glands along with the additional features of cytologic atypia are the most difficult for the pathologist to interpret.

The morphologic abnormalities are further classified by the presence of cytologic or nuclear atypia. The normal epithelial cells lining the endometrial glands are oval shaped, with basal-oriented oval nuclei. The cells are interpreted as atypical when the nuclei become round and enlarged (so there is less cytoplasmic space) and hyperchromatic and lose polarity near the surface. The roundness of the nuclei results in a cleared appearance secondary to the margination of the chromatin. The presence of cytologic atypia is the single most important histologic finding because only atypical hyperplasia has a significant risk of developing into endometrial carcinoma.

The corpus of the endometrium can be divided into two histologic areas: the basalis and the functionalis. The basalis area is the zone between the myometrium and the functionalis area. Cells in the basalis layer respond to estrogen by undergoing proliferation but do not respond to progesterone. The basalis layer plays a critical role by serving as a zone of reserve cells for the rest of the endometrium. Glands of the basalis layer appear slightly proliferative during the entire menstrual cycle. The functionalis layer consists of an epithelial and a stromal component. The epithelial component can contain proliferative or basalis-type cells, secretory cells and ciliated cells. The stromal component of the endometrium contains two cell types: the endometrial stromal cell and stromal granulocytes. The stromal cells are the cells that undergo predecidualization. Both epithelial and stromal cells of the endometrium can possess estrogen and progesterone receptors. Estrogen receptors tend to be present throughout the menstrual cycle, whereas progesterone receptors are present only under the influence of estrogen.

Morphologic interpretation is determined by the status of the functionalis layer of the endometrium. If an endometrial sample does not contain the functionalis layer and diagnosis is made on the basis of the basalis layer alone, an erroneous diagnosis may be obtained. The earliest histologic features indicating that ovulation has occurred appear on day 16. The best time to obtain an endometrial sample to confirm ovulation is on days 22 to 23. Secretory endometrium may be somewhat more difficult to date than menstrual endometrium. Secretory endometrium may demonstrate subtle changes and combinations of histologic patterns that result in errors of several days. The dates of the endometrial samples should be based on the endometrial findings that represent the most advanced phase of the menstrual cycle.

SIGNIFICANCE OF A HYPERPLASTIC ENDOMETRIUM

Progestins control the estrogen-primed endometrial glands by decreasing the numbers of estrogen receptors in epithelial cells. Progestins are effective in stopping the cell-mediated events related to growth and proliferation in the endometrium caused by estrogen stimulation. The incidence of endometrial cancer in postmenopausal women treated with both estrogen and progestin is lower than that observed in the general population. The regulation of mitoses in fully differentiated epithelial cells can be accomplished by progesterone, but the effect of progesterone on halting the mitoses and subsequent proliferation of atypical cells is less clear. In high doses, progestins cause pseudodecidualization of the stroma with atrophy of the glandular component.

Atypical complex hyperplasia has the greatest risk of progressing to invasive endometrial cancer. If this type of hyperplasia is not treated, the risk of malignant progression within 5 years is approximately 30 per cent. For this reason, it should be considered a true cancer precursor. In contrast, 8 per cent of atypical simple hyperplasia, 3 per cent of complex hyperplasia, and 1 per cent of simple hyperplasia will progress to cancer within 10 years. Although the risk of malignant transformation is low with these types of hyperplasia, a small risk does exist. The majority of these lesions are hormonally derived, and if the hormonal status is not altered, the risk continues.

ENDOMETRIAL CARCINOMA

Endometrial carcinoma accounts for about 90 per cent of malignant tumors of the uterus and is the fourth most common malignancy in women but the most frequent invasive gynecologic malignancy. Its frequency increases with the age of the population, and most cases occur after the age of 50. The incidence rises steeply between the ages of 45 and 55 and peaks in the late 60s, with a modest decline thereafter. The incidence of endometrial cancer in Asian and African women is lower than that in North American and European populations. The lifetime risk of a North American woman developing endometrial cancer is about 3 per cent. Endometrial cancer now exceeds cervical cancer by a factor of more than 2.

The endometrial carcinomas range from well differentiated to poorly differentiated. More than 70 per cent of endometrial cancers are stage I at the time of presentation. The majority of women with endometrial carcinoma are obese or have a history of unopposed estrogen. Since it has become common practice to add a progestin to estrogen replacement therapy in women with an intact uterus, the rate of endometrial carcinoma has decreased. Data from the steroid and hormone study from the Centers for Disease Control and Prevention demonstrated that the use of oral contraceptive pills (OCPs) for 12 months or longer reduces the risk of endometrial cancer by about 50 per cent. This protection increases with the duration of use and may persist for up to 15 years after OCPs are discontinued. This protection may offer a dramatic way of lowering the endometrial carcinoma rate in future years.

Risk Factors for Endometrial Cancer

Unopposed Estrogen

Although nonhormonal factors are associated with endometrial cancer, the majority of these tumors are etiologically related to unopposed estrogen, either endogenous or exogenous. Unopposed estrogen administration may accelerate the progression from simple to atypical hyperplasia and, ultimately, to carcinoma. Simple, or atypical, hyperplasia will regress if the unopposed estrogen is discontinued. The regression of the hyperplasia may occur because spontaneous ovulation occurs and production of progesterone increases, or because the production of estradiol decreases after weight loss or menopause.

Women who use unopposed estrogens for at least two years develop endometrial cancer 2 to 20 times more frequently than nonusers. The risk increases with higher doses and longer use. After 10 years of use, the risk of developing endometrial cancer approaches 10 per 1000 postmenopausal women. Even after therapy with the unopposed estrogen is discontinued, a residual risk may persist for up to 15 years. Endometrial cancer associated with estrogen use is associated with a significantly higher risk of extrauterine dissemination than that in women who have not taken estrogen. Endometrial cancer related to unopposed estrogen use has a slightly lower mortality rate than the same cancer diagnosed in women who do not take estrogen. This variance may be due to the fact that endometrial cancer in estrogen users may be detected earlier because of more frequent examinations or may be pursued by more aggressive therapy. Therefore, when correction is made for grade, stage, and depth of invasion, survival among estrogen users is no better than that among the general population. Endometrial cancer that is not diagnosed in early stages has a greater probability of metastasis at the time of eventual diagnosis.

The endometrial cancers in estrogen users are frequently better differentiated than the tumors in those who have not taken estrogen. Only a small percentage of estrogen users have well-differentiated endometrial cancer; thus, the presence of highly differentiated adenocarcinoma of the endometrium may be unrelated to hormonal factors. The presence of endometrial hyperplasia is the most important risk factor correlating with a favorable prognosis. A low tumor grade and the lack of myometrial invasion are characteristically associated with the presence of hyperplasia. High-grade tumors are more often associated with an atrophic endometrium. These high-grade cancers, such as serous carcinoma and clear cell carcinoma, tend to occur at a later age than estrogen-related endometrial cancers. The frequency of the high-grade carcinomas is higher in African American women than in white American women.

Prolonged Endogenous Estrogen Exposure

Prolonged exposure to endogenous estrogens due to chronic anovulation can be seen in women who are obese, have hyperandrogenic chronic anovulation (formally polycystic ovarian syndrome), are infertile, or reach menopause at a later age. One mechanism may be the greater conversion of androstenedione to estrone in adipose tissue. There is a ninefold increased risk of endometrial cancer in women who are more than 50 pounds overweight. This mechanism helps explain the decreased probability of developing endometrial cancer in women who smoke. Smokers are known to experience a shorter perimenopause and an earlier menopause owing to decreased estrogenic stimulation and increased estrogen clearance following induction of hepatic microsomal enzymes.

Other Risk Factors

A hereditary link has been postulated for endometrial cancer, especially in women with first-degree relatives who have breast cancer. Hypertension is common in women with endometrial cancer but does not appear to act as an independent risk factor. Diabetes mellitus has a relative risk for endometrial cancer of 2.8, after controlling for age, weight, and socioeconomic status. Increased risks have also been found in nulliparous patients. The protective effect of pregnancy seems to reflect the influence of delivering a term birth. Spontaneous and induced abortions seem to be unrelated to risk. Early age at menarche and longer days of menstrual flow increase the risk of developing endometrial cancer. After adjustment for other reproductive characteristics, age at first birth and duration of breast-feeding do not seem to be related to increased risk. Hirsutism developing at an older age is also associated with increased risk.

Long-term tamoxifen use has an estrogenic effect on the postmenopausal endometrium. Compared with control subjects, tamoxifen-treated patients have a thicker endometrium and a larger uterine volume. Hysteroscopy performed on patients receiving tamoxifen reveals an atrophic endometrium in a significantly lower percentage than in control subjects.

Findings of Endometrial Carcinoma

The various endometrial cancers cannot be distinguished by gross clinical appearance. The endometrial surface is shaggy, glistening, and focally hemorrhagic. The gross and microscopic hemorrhage accounts for the vaginal bleeding, which is the most common presenting symptom of endometrial cancer.

A variety of histologic types exist. They include endometrial, mucinous, clear cell, papillary serous, mixed adenosquamous, and pure squamous cell carcinomas. The most common types are endometrial and mucinous. The most important prognostic factors include the degree of histologic differentiation and the depth of stromal invasion. The grade of histologic differentiation is determined by the percentage of solid areas.

Methods of Detection

Cervical Cytologic Screening

The Papanicolaou smear should not be used to "screen" for endometrial cancer. Some patients with endometrial carcinoma, however, have endometrial cells detected by previous cervical cytology. Patients with malignant cervical cytology are at increased risk for having a high-grade tumor. Of the patients with malignant endometrial cells on cervical cytology, almost 70 per cent have deep myometrial invasion. This finding would suggest the utility of the Papanicolaou smear in preoperative assessment of the risk of myometrial invasion, but the smear should not be the only method of assessment. Surgical staging and intraoperative evaluation are still needed.

Endometrial Aspiration

Several office endometrial sampling devices have demonstrated a diagnostic accuracy similar to Vabra aspiration, the Novak biopsy curet, and dilatation and curettage (D & C). They are highly sensitive for the detection of endometrial cancer, but endometrial polyps and submucous myomas are frequently missed. One of the primary advantages of the endometrial sampling devices is that a histologic diagnosis can be made at the time the patient presents to the office with vaginal bleeding. Common aspiration devices include the Pipelle, the Endosampler, and the Explora. Although the Pipelle may obtain an adequate specimen for histologic assessment, the specimen has been shown to represent only a small focus of the endometrial cavity, usually only a fraction of the anterior or posterior surface. The office sampling devices are inexpensive, cause minimal discomfort to the patient, and do not require anesthesia in most cases. Perforation has not been reported with their use. The sensitivity for endometrial carcinoma may be 97.5 per cent or higher. The poor sensitivity of the endometrial aspirator in detecting disease other than endometrial cancer is due mainly to its failure to detect polyps and submucous myomas.

A disadvantage of the endometrial aspiration device is the lack of adequate sampling of atrophic endometria because the device works by shearing rather than by curettage. The insufficiency rate or method failure of the various sampling devices is approximately 15 per cent.

Ultrasonography

The thicker the endometrial lining of postmenopausal women, as seen on vaginal ultrasonography, the greater the risk of endometrial disease. Most endometrial cancers are represented sonographically by a thickened endometrial lining, called a "stripe." The negative predictive value for the diagnosis of cancer or hyperplasia is 100 per cent when a postmenopausal endometrium measures less than 5 mm in thickness. The different cutoff points of endometrial thickness above which endometrial lesions are suspected range from 4 to 8 mm. In women with endometrial thicknesses less than 5 mm, D & C commonly yields atrophic tissue or none at all. Most clinicians adhere to the less than 5 mm cutoff point. If endometrial sampling has recently been performed, this sonographic abnormality is not valid. For this examination to be accurate, the endometrium must be identified in a sagittal view of the uterus, perpendicular to the long axis of the probe. There is no currently proven method of sonographically distinguishing a superficial endometrial cancer from hyperplasia that measures more than 5 mm.

Even in the presence of fluid in the lumen of the uterus, endometrial polyps, or myomas, the thickened lining is more predictive of endometrial disease than the other features. Because the sonographic picture of the endometrial lining cannot identify the histologic pattern, it has recently been recommended that ultrasonography and endometrial sampling be combined in women not receiving exogenous estrogen who present with symptoms of endometrial disease. If a thin lining of 4 mm or less is present on ultrasonography, no further investigation is necessary. Women who have a lining greater than 4 mm should proceed to endometrial sampling. If endometrial sampling fails to confirm disease in the presence of a thickened endometrium on ultrasonography, hysteroscopy should be performed. If office sampling is precluded by the patient's weight or mental state, cervical stenosis, or other reasons, the sonographic findings can assist the clinician in determining the need for examination of the patient under general anesthesia. The endometrium of tamoxifen-treated patients reveals a well-defined lining that is typically consistent with various forms of endometrial hyperplasia.

Hysteroscopy

The combination of hysteroscopy and endometrial biopsy can provide nearly 100 per cent accuracy in the diagnosis of endometrial carcinoma and its precursors. Furthermore, hysteroscopy is a useful tool for excluding further investigations in patients who have no disease. Hysteroscopy can be used in the selection of the patients who are at risk for endometrial carcinoma or its precursors as well as to help direct the endometrial biopsy to establish an accurate diagnosis. Hysteroscopic visualization has no place in the evaluation of patients with endometrial hyperplasia with or without nuclear atypia.

With endometrial hyperplasia, the mucosa is thickened, and it is possible to estimate the thickness by indenting the mucosa with the hysteroscope. On hysteroscopic examination, endometrial hyperplasia demonstrates an irregular arrangement and concentration of glandular orifices and cystic dilatation. It is possible to follow the conversion of hyperplastic glands to those demonstrating a secretory effect after progestin therapy has been initiated. If the patient has prolonged bleeding after a progestational agent has been administered, hysteroscopy may help distinguish atrophy from persistent hyperplasia.

Mencaglia* classified the hysteroscopic diagnosis of endometrial hyperplasia into low-risk and high-risk categories according to the pathologic classification of potential risk. A total of 618 women older than 45 years of age who had abnormal uterine bleeding were examined. The following hysteroscopic diagnoses were demonstrated: functional endometrium (42 per cent), atrophic endometrium (0.2 per cent), dysfunctional endometrium (1.8 per cent), endometritis (0.2 per cent), fibroids (9.6 per cent), polyps (9.8 per cent), low-risk hyperplasia (12.6 per cent), high-risk hyperplasia (1.3 per cent), and adenocarcinoma (10.6 per cent). Immediately following the hysteroscopy, endometrial sampling was performed. This study demonstrated that hysteroscopy has considerable diagnostic accuracy, directly proportional to the severity of the lesion. In

*Mencaglia, L., and Perino, A.: Hysteroscopy and microcolpohysteroscopy in gynecologic oncology. *In* Baggish, M.S., Barbot, J., and Valle, R.F. (eds.): *Diagnostic and Operative Hysteroscopy: A Text and Atlas.* St. Louis, Mosby-Year Book, 1989, pp. 114–120.

Table 1. Grading of Endometrial Carcinoma

Grade 1	5% or less of a solid growth pattern (does not include squamous patterns)
Grade 2	6–50% of the tumor has a solid growth pattern
Grade 3	More than 50% solid growth

adenocarcinoma, the agreement between hysteroscopy and histologic diagnosis was 95 per cent, in high-risk endometrial hyperplasia it was 87.5 per cent, and in low-risk endometrial hyperplasia it was 65.2 per cent. In the low-risk category, there were 34.8 per cent false-positive results and no false-negative results.

The appearance of endometrial carcinoma by hysteroscopy is extremely characteristic. The adenocarcinoma reveals cerebroid projections that are necrotic and friable. Vascularization is irregular and bizarre. A distinct delineation between normal and abnormal epithelia may be seen. Small carcinomas deep within the cornu or behind a submucosal myoma missed at D & C can be found at hysteroscopy. Staging the tumor is an important part of the hysteroscopic examination to determine whether the carcinoma is confined to the uterus corpus (stage I) or whether there is cervical involvement (stage II). Treatment and prognosis are significantly different between the two stages. Errors in staging can occur 10 to 15 per cent of the time with D & C alone. It remains to be determined whether the information obtained at hysteroscopy has any long-term impact on survival.

Method of Staging Endometrial Carcinoma

The International Federation of Gynecology and Obstetrics (FIGO) revised its system for staging endometrial carcinoma. The new system utilizes a combination of surgical and pathologic criteria. The new system considers the natural history of endometrial cancer and defines certain prognostic factors, such as myometrial invasion, presence of metastasis, status of pelvic lymph nodes, and peritoneal cytology. This system abolishes the old practice of performing a D & C for staging purposes. Table 1 lists the grading criteria, and Table 2 lists the criteria for tumor invasion. Tumor grade and depth of myometrial invasion correlate well with nodal metastases.

Table 2. FIGO Staging of Endometrial Carcinoma

Stage IA	Tumor limited to endometrium
Stage IB	Invasion to less than 50% of the myometrium
Stage IC	Invasion to more than 50% of the myometrium
Stage IIA	Endocervical gland involvement only
Stage IIB	Cervical stromal invasion
Stage IIIA	Tumor invades serosa and/or adnexae, and/or positive peritoneal cytology
Stage IIIB	Vaginal metastases
Stage IIIC	Metastases to pelvic and/or para-aortic lymph nodes
Stage IVA	Invasion of bladder and/or bowel mucosa
Stage IVB	Distant metastases, including intra-abdominal and/or inguinal lymph nodes

BENIGN AND MALIGNANT OVARIAN TUMORS

By Thomas J. Rutherford M.D.,
and Peter E. Schwartz, M.D.
New Haven, Connecticut

Ovarian neoplasms are a common clinical problem affecting women of all ages. Although the majority of these neoplasms are benign, the goal in evaluating the patient is to identify those that are malignant. The incidence of malignancy in patients with ovarian neoplasm increases with age, and a patient in whom a malignant lesion develops often has decreased survival. Treatment of a neoplasm in a premenopausal patient may disrupt hormonal function, resulting in the loss of reproductive capacity. Methods for preoperative evaluation and diagnosis of an ovarian neoplasm have evolved with advances in diagnostic imaging and monoclonal antibody technology. However, these techniques have had little impact on the definitive management procedure, namely, surgical extirpation. It is estimated that 5 to 10 per cent of women will have a surgical procedure in their lifetime for a suspected ovarian neoplasm.

PREMENARCHAL CYSTS

At the time of birth, infants occasionally exhibit ovarian cysts. These abdominal masses are usually follicular cysts caused by maternal hormonal stimulation of the fetal ovaries. The masses tend to regress with hormonal withdrawal during the first few months of life. Thereafter, neoplasms of the ovaries in infants and young children are rare. Generally, nongynecologic abdominal masses that present in the pediatric population are most often neuroblastomas or Wilms' tumors. Ovarian neoplasms are rare in this age group but when present tend to be germ cell malignancies (Table 1). Solid or solid and cystic neoplasms in this age group are most often dysgerminomas or immature teratomas.

MENARCHAL CYSTS

In adolescents, most ovarian masses are functional cysts. These cysts reflect ovarian physiologic variation and include the follicular cyst, corpus luteum cyst, and theca-lutein cyst.

Follicular cysts are the most common cystic structure

Table 1. Serum Tumor Markers in Malignant Germ Cell Tumors of the Ovary

Histologic Features	Alpha-Fetoprotein	Human Chorionic Gonadotropin
Dysgerminoma	−	±
Endodermal sinus tumor	+	−
Embryonal	±	+
Polyembryoma	+	+
Choriocarcinoma	−	+
Immature teratoma	±	−

found in the normal ovary. They range in size from 1 mm to 8 cm and are commonly found in menstruating females. These cysts arise in the ovarian cortex when the dominant follicle fails to rupture or the incomplete follicle does not involute. When follicular cysts fill with blood, they are called follicular hematomas. Management of a presumed follicular cyst is conservative because these lesions usually reabsorb over one or two menstrual cycles. Some clinicians advocate the use of oral contraceptives to suppress the growth of these cysts. A persistent cyst requires further evaluation and conservative operative intervention.

A corpus luteum cyst develops from a mature graafian follicle. Spontaneous but limited bleeding often fills the cystic cavity with blood. These cysts can rupture and bleed into the peritoneal cavity. If the cystic central cavity persists, blood is reabsorbed and the cavity fills with clear fluid resulting in a corpus albicans cyst. Management is conservative.

The least common of the physiologic ovarian cysts is the theca lutein cyst. This lesion is caused by overstimulation of the ovaries by exogenous or endogenous gonadotropins. Theca lutein cysts are typically associated with pregnancy, hydatidiform mole, choriocarcinoma, or gonadotropin excess. Theca lutein cysts usually regress as the concentrations of the stimulant, human chorionic gonadotropin (hCG), decline. However, an occasional theca lutein cyst may rupture spontaneously, causing signs and symptoms of peritoneal irritation.

The most common ovarian neoplasm is a benign cystic teratoma. These tumors have thickened capsules and may contain bone or teeth that can be detected by a sonogram or plain film of the abdomen. Complexed (solid and cystic) or solid ovarian masses are more likely to harbor germ cell malignancies, especially dysgerminomas or immature teratomas (see Table 1).

During the reproductive years, ovarian functional cysts are the most common mass identified and mature cystic teratomas are the most common benign neoplasm. Endometriosis and ovarian endometrial cysts are also common benign processes detected in these years. Up to 40 per cent of malignant ovarian neoplasms are borderline serous or mucinous adenocarcinomas. Sex cord–stromal neoplasms (Table 2) may cause hormonal effects that may be recognized in the premenarchal, reproductive, or postmenopausal years. Diagnosis and therapy are primarily designed to preserve ovarian function during the reproductive years.

POSTMENOPAUSAL TUMORS

Ovarian neoplasms arising after menopause may be benign, but the risk of malignancy increases with age. Epithelial ovarian neoplasms (Table 3), which are infrequent in women younger than 40 years, account for 60 per cent of all ovarian tumors (benign and malignant) in postmenopausal women. The development of bilateral, complex masses with ascites suggests malignancy. The most common epithelial ovarian malignancy is the serous cystadenocarcinoma.

Table 2. World Health Organization Classification of Sex Cord–Stromal Tumors

Granulosa-stromal cell tumors
- Juvenile
- Adult

Thecoma-fibroma group
- Thecoma
- Fibroma
- Fibrosarcoma

Sertoli-stromal cell tumors
- Sertoli cell tumor
- Sertoli-Leydig cell tumor

Gynandroblastoma

Steroid (lipid) cell tumors
- Stromal luteoma

Leydig cell tumor

Table 3. Histologic Classification of Epithelial Tumors of the Ovary

- Serous tumor
- Mucinous tumor
- Endometrioid tumor
- Clear cell tumor
- Brenner tumor
- Mixed epithelial tumor

PRESENTATION AND EVALUATION

Clinically useful screening tests for the detection of early-stage ovarian cancer are not yet available. Unfortunately, most patients with ovarian cancer present with advanced disease because early-stage ovarian tumors are asymptomatic. The most common presenting symptoms in women with ovarian neoplasms are abdominal discomfort or pain and distention or fullness caused by ascites or enlargement of the pelvic tumor. Nonspecific gastrointestinal symptoms include dyspepsia, nausea, early satiety, and altered bowel movements. Genitourinary symptoms include pressure, frequency, or urinary retention. Acute abdominal pain due to torsion of the ovarian mass is common in patients with germ cell neoplasms, especially benign cystic teratomas. Functional granulosa cell tumors can present with premenarchal precocious puberty, postmenopausal vaginal bleeding, or menorrhagia-amenorrhea in the menstruating patient. Sertoli-Leydig cell tumors occur most often in the reproductive years and may cause defeminization or masculinization. Women with advanced ovarian cancer often present with weight loss and cachexia.

In evaluating a woman with a pelvic mass, the clinician must obtain a careful and thorough personal history and family history and perform a careful physical examination. Note the patient's age, reproductive history, and family history of relatives with cancer. Examine the lymph nodes, chest, and breasts. Inspect the abdomen and palpate for masses, ascites, and tenderness. During the bimanual examination, attempt to characterize any pelvic mass as cystic or solid, unilateral or bilateral, fixed or mobile, and smooth or irregular. Remember that large neoplasms can fill the entire cul-de-sac of Douglas, but the size of the mass does not predict or guarantee malignancy.

TUMOR MARKERS

Tumor markers have a limited role in the diagnosis and management of ovarian malignancies. The serum concentration of the CA-125 protein is increased in 80 per cent of patients with epithelial ovarian malignancies. However, serum CA-125 is also increased during menses and the first trimester of pregnancy and in patients with endometriosis, pelvic inflammatory disease, and nonepithelial ovarian tumors. Nongynecologic conditions associated with increased serum CA-125 concentrations include diverticulosis, pancreatitis, cirrhosis, peritonitis, and carcinomas of the pancreas, breast, colon, and lung. For premenopausal women with adnexal masses, if the concentration of CA-125 is less than 35 U/mL, the mass is statistically likely to be benign. If the concentration of CA-125 is greater than 200 U/mL, the mass is statistically likely to be malignant. If the CA-125 concentration is between 35 and 200 U/mL, the mass is most likely benign, but the patient must be instructed that the risk of malignancy is clinically significant. When a pelvic mass has been detected and the serum CA-125 concentration is increased, the premenopausal patient should be placed on a preoperative bowel preparation. Prior to surgery, the patient should be informed that if a malignant tumor is discovered, chemotherapy or radiation therapy may be recommended in addition to removal of the lesion. Any postmenopausal woman with a pelvic mass and a serum CA-125 concentration exceeding 35 U/mL should be evaluated for an ovarian neoplasm.

Germ cell tumors express alpha-fetoprotein (AFP) and hCG (see Table 1). Endodermal sinus tumors and choriocarcinomas, for example, produce AFP and hCG, respectively. Dysgerminomas are associated with increased serum lactate dehydrogenase (LD), especially when the primary ovarian tumor exceeds 10 cm in diameter. Mixed germ cell tumors may contain elements of any germ cell neoplasm and may be associated with increased serum hCG and AFP concentrations.

DIAGNOSTIC RADIOGRAPHIC EVALUATION

Ultrasonography is less expensive than other imaging modalities and is commonly used in an attempt to distinguish benign masses from malignant ovarian tumors. Ascites can be detected and benign tumors can be identified with a morphologic scoring system that emphasizes septations, echogenicity, wall structure, and shadowing. Color Doppler flow imaging uses blood flow indices to distinguish benign from malignant neoplasms. Doppler imaging is based on evidence that malignant tumors have neovascularized vessels with decreased resistance to blood flow. The pulsatility index (PI) and resistive index (RI) tend to be lower in neovascularized (malignant) tissue ($RI < 0.4$, $PI < 1.0$). In turn, the peak systolic velocity tends to be increased in malignancies. A peak systolic velocity exceeding 25 cm per second has been measured in some ovarian tumors. The reliability of this technique depends on the expertise of the operator and the ability to obtain flow data. The routine use of ultrasound to screen postmenopausal patients for ovarian or other pelvic cancer is not cost-effective.

Computed tomography (CT) is superior to ultrasound for evaluation of the liver, pelvic and para-aortic nodes, omentum, and mesentery. Unfortunately, CT does not consistently detect lesions less than 2 cm in diameter. Preoperative CT may help distinguish gynecologic disease from gastrointestinal or pancreatic disease in patients with intra-abdominal carcinomatosis who do not have an ovarian mass. CT may also identify those patients who may benefit from neoadjuvant chemotherapy because their ovarian or pelvic masses are not surgically debulkable initially. In women who present with gross ascites, increased serum CA-125 concentrations, and no palpable ovarian masses, CT can detect hepatic cirrhosis as the cause of ascites.

Magnetic resonance imaging (MRI) provides no advantage over CT for the assessment of ovarian masses. Ascites, retroperitoneal adenopathy, omental metastases, and peritoneal implants larger than 1 cm can be detected by MRI. The major disadvantages of MRI are expense and the inability to visualize the bowel and urinary tract with contrast.

LABORATORY EVALUATION

For patients with suspected ovarian malignancies, the clinician should obtain a chest film and electrocardiogram preoperatively. Pleural effusions should be tapped to improve pulmonary function prior to surgery. Pulmonary function testing should be undertaken in patients with a history of lung disease. A complete blood count (CBC), hepatic profile, serum urea nitrogen, creatinine, and electrolyte concentrations should be ordered. Hemodynamically capable patients should be allowed to autodonate blood prior to nonemergent surgery.

SURGICAL EXPLORATION

Definitive diagnosis of an ovarian mass requires surgical exploration by laparoscopy or laparotomy. In the premenarchal and reproductive age groups, the aim of surgery is to preserve the ovary and remove the tumor. A persistent ovarian tumor greater than 6 cm in diameter should be removed. If microscopic evaluation indicates a malignant growth, the standard of care includes surgical staging and optimal tumor debulking.

Section Sixteen

IMMUNE SYSTEM

IMMUNODEFICIENCY

By Arthur Kavanaugh, M.D.
Dallas, Texas

Immunodeficiency diseases are a diverse group of disorders that result from various quantitative or qualitative defects in the immune system. The primary purpose of the immune system is immunosurveillance, that is, the differentiation of self from nonself. Among the most relevant functions of the immune response is the identification and elimination of foreign microbial pathogens. Therefore, the most important clinical characteristic of immunodeficiency diseases is an increased susceptibility to infection. However, patients with immunodeficiencies may also have characteristic clinical presentations that depend on the specific component of the immune response that is affected.

PRIMARY VERSUS SECONDARY IMMUNODEFICIENCY

Immunodeficiency diseases may be categorized as primary or secondary. Primary immunodeficiencies are relatively uncommon. They often represent focal defects in a particular component of the immune response (Table 1). Analysis of the cellular and molecular defects underlying the various primary immunodeficiencies has provided substantial insight into the complex interactions and function of the normal immune system. Significant primary immunodeficiency diseases occur with an incidence of 1 in 10,000 to 1 in 100,000, a frequency comparable to that of leukemias plus lymphomas in children.

Secondary immunodeficiencies represent impairments of the immune response that accompany severe systemic disease, infection, the use of immunosuppressive medications, and several other conditions (Table 2). Some secondary immunodeficiencies are characterized by defects in a specific arm of the immune system, while others reflect a compromise of the integrity of multiple distinct immune functions. Corticosteroids, for example, are potent immu-

Table 1. Selected Primary Immunodeficiencies

B-Lymphocyte (Antibody) Defects
X-linked (Bruton's) agammaglobulinemia
Common variable immunodeficiency (CVID)
IgA deficiency
IgG subclass deficiency (IgG1, IgG2, IgG3, IgG4)
Immunoglobulin deficiency with increased IgM
Combined B-Lymphocyte / T-Lymphocyte Defects
Severe combined immunodeficiency (SCID)
Wiskott-Aldrich syndrome
Ataxia-telangiectasia
T-Lymphocyte Defects
DiGeorge syndrome
Adenosine deaminase (ADA) deficiency
Purine-nucleoside phosphorylase (PNP) deficiency
Phagocytic Cell Defects
Chronic granulomatous disease
Leukocyte adhesion deficiency (CD11/CD18 deficiency)
Chediak-Higashi syndrome
Complement Component Deficiency

Table 2. Causes of Secondary Immunodeficiency

Pharmacologic Agents
Corticosteroids
Chemotherapeutic drugs (e.g., cyclophosphamide, chlorambucil, cisplatin, etoposide)
Medications that may be associated with myelosuppression as an adverse effect (e.g., phenothiazines, semisynthetic penicillins, nonsteroidal anti-inflammatory drugs, antithyroid drugs, gold salts, D-penicillamine, captopril)
Nonpharmacologic Therapeutic Interventions
X-irradiation
Plasmapheresis
Leukopheresis
Lymphoproliferative Diseases
Hodgkin's disease
Non-Hodgkin's lymphoma
Leukemia
Multiple myeloma
Infectious Diseases
HIV-1 and HIV-2 infection
Rubella
Cytomegalovirus infection
Influenza
Varicella
Systemic Inflammatory Diseases
Rheumatoid arthritis
Systemic lupus erythematosus
Sarcoidosis
Vasculitis
Loss of Anatomical Integrity
Instrumentation (e.g., catheters)
Mucosal inflammation (e.g., related to atopic disease, irritants such as cigarette smoke)
Mucociliary elevator dysfunction (e.g., related to cystic fibrosis or the immotile cilia syndrome)
Impaired dermatologic barrier function (e.g., related to burns, psoriasis, atopic dermatitis)
Protein Loss
Protein-losing enteropathy
Nephrotic syndrome
Miscellaneous
Diabetes mellitus
Renal failure
Postsplenectomy
Sickle cell disease
Solid organ malignancy
Severe liver disease
Nutritional deficiency (e.g., protein-calorie malnutrition, zinc deficiency)
Presence of foreign-bodies (e.g., prosthetic joints, cardiac valves)

HIV = human immunodeficiency virus.

nosuppressive agents that influence several aspects of the immune response. Importantly, secondary immunodeficiencies occur more frequently than primary immunodeficiencies and are thus more likely to come to the clinician's attention.

APPROACH TO THE EVALUATION OF THE PATIENT

The most important contributor to the accurate diagnosis of an immunodeficiency state is a high index of suspicion. Increased susceptibility to infection may be manifested in various ways (Table 3). For example, immunodeficient patients may experience an increased frequency or recurrence of infections, when compared with age-matched control subjects with comparable exposure. Importantly, the frequency of infection must be properly related to exposure and the clinical situation. Thus, when a 37-year-old executive suffers eight episodes of pharyngitis in 1 year, an impaired immune response should certainly be considered. However, the same number of infections in 1 year may not be unexpected in a 3 year old repeatedly exposed to other ill children at a day-care center. Immunodeficiency may also be seen in patients whose infections with common pathogens seem more severe than anticipated. For example, a typically minor upper respiratory infection due to *Haemophilus influenzae* may progress to pneumonitis, osteomyelitis, meningitis, or sepsis. For most patients, repeated episodes of progressive infection should heighten the clinical suspicion of immunodeficiency. Another clue in infected patients may arise from suboptimal responses to appropriate antibiotics or surgical drainage. Finally, infections with normally nonpathogenic organisms and complicated infections with usual pathogens should suggest the possibility of immunodeficiency. Opportunistic infections such as cryptosporidiosis or *Pneumocystis carinii* pneumonia are infrequently seen in normal hosts and more frequently seen in patients with immunodeficiency.

Although the clinical hallmark of immunodeficiency is an increased susceptibility to infection, other symptoms can also be attributed to impairment of the immune system. For example, a normal immune system efficiently distinguishes self from nonself, but an impaired immune system may not. Failure to recognize self may lead to the development of autoimmune disease. Indeed, the incidence of idiopathic thrombocytopenic purpura (ITP), autoimmune hemolytic anemia, systemic lupus erythematosus (SLE), rheumatoid arthritis, and systemic vasculitis is increased in patients with primary immunodeficiency. Another potential outcome of defective recognition of self versus nonself is impaired immunosurveillance. As a result, patients with primary immunodeficiencies may have an increased risk of developing malignancy. As many primary immunodeficiencies represent abnormalities of bone marrow progenitor cells, it should perhaps not be surprising that anemia, leukopenia, and thrombocytopenia can accompany these syndromes. In some cases, these accompanying abnormalities may provide important clues to the diagnosis. For example, thrombocytopenia is characteristic of the Wiskott-Aldrich syndrome. Finally, additional symptoms that may be associated with primary immunodeficiency, particularly in infants and young children, include suboptimal growth and development, and gastrointestinal symptoms such as diarrhea. Sometimes, the diarrhea can be attributed to infection; in other patients, inflammatory bowel disorders may be responsible.

Table 3. Clues to the Presence of an Immunodeficiency

Infections that are
- of increased frequency (when compared with age-adjusted patients with comparable exposure)
- of excessive severity (e.g., requiring aggressive antibiotic therapy, surgical drainage)
- of prolonged duration (e.g., requiring prolonged antibiotic therapy)
- complicated (e.g., by spread of the infection to other organ systems)
- caused by unusual organisms (organisms that are not usually pathogenic, that is, opportunistic infections)

In evaluating the patient with suspected immunodeficiency, other features of these conditions should be kept in mind. Most patients whose clinical course is consistent with immunodeficiency do not have a primary immunodeficiency disease. Typically, one of the secondary causes of immunodeficiency (see Table 2) is responsible for the increased susceptibility to infection.

Most of the primary immunodeficiencies present in youth. Two thirds of the patients with primary immunodeficiency are diagnosed before the age of 15, and 80 per cent before the age of 20. Many of these children have symptoms for months or even years before the diagnosis is established. The age at presentation of an immunodeficiency may depend on the nature and severity of the disorder. Severe T-cell or phagocytic immunodeficiencies become evident soon after birth, and failure to thrive is commonly observed. By contrast, antibody deficiencies may develop at any age. Infants tend not to develop problems before maternal antibody has waned, at approximately 6 months of age. Premature infants, however, may not receive normal amounts of placentally transmitted maternal immunoglobulin due to early delivery. Thus, they may have an antibody deficiency unless and until their own immune systems mature.

Many primary immunodeficiencies are genetically determined. Thus, a careful family history, with particular attention to recurrent infections, problems with vaccinations, unexplained early deaths, and malignancies may provide meaningful information. Owing to the X-chromosome involvement in many of these disorders, three quarters of the patients with primary immunodeficiency are male.

EVALUATION OF THE PATIENT

Documentation is very important in the evaluation of a patient with suspected immunodeficiency. A detailed record of all episodes of infection should include the causative agent, the treatments required, and the complications, if any. Such documentation provides a basis for the clinical suspicion of immunodeficiency and therefore determines the necessity of immunologic evaluation. Moreover, documentation of the sites of infection and the infecting organisms may provide critical clues to the nature of the immunodeficiency. Thus, defects in the different arms of the immune response are characteristically associated with infections by specific pathogens (Table 4). The immune response is mediated by four functional components: (1) B cells (antibody), (2) T cells, (3) phagocytes, and (4) complement proteins. Defects in antibody function most commonly present with recurrent upper and lower respiratory tract infections. The pathogens often are organisms enclosed by polysaccharide capsules that resist cell-mediated destruction and require antibody responses for their removal. On the other hand, T-cell deficiencies leave the

Table 4. Organisms Associated With Specific Immunodeficiencies

B-cell/antibody deficiency	Polysaccharide-encapsulated pyogenic organisms *(Streptococcus pneumoniae, Haemophilus influenzae* type b, *Streptococcus pyogenes, Moraxella catarrhalis)*; also *Staphylococcus aureus, Giardia lamblia, Campylobacter jejuni*
T-cell deficiency	Fungi (e.g., *Candida albicans*), viruses (e.g., cytomegalovirus, varicella-zoster, herpes simplex virus), bacteria *(Listeria monocytogenes)*, protozoa *(Pneumocystic carinii)*, mycobacteria (e.g., *Mycobacterium tuberculosis, M. avium-intracellulare*)
Phagocytic deficiency	*Staphylococcus aureus,* gram-negative enteric bacteria (*Escherichia coli, Proteus mirabilis, Serratia marcescens, Pseudomonas cepacia* and *aeruginosa*), fungi
Complement deficiency	*Neisseria meningitidis* and *gonorrhoeae;* gram-negative and pyogenic infections

patient susceptible to intracellular pathogens (e.g., viruses and mycobacteria, fungi, and protozoa). Infections with these organisms are often systemic and severe. Phagocytic defects most often present with recurrent infections, especially of the skin and mucosal surfaces. Characteristic organisms include *Staphylococcus aureus* and enteric, gram-negative bacteria. Complement deficiencies, although classically associated with neisserial infections, may also be associated with pyogenic and gram-negative infections.

Every patient suspected of having immunodeficiency should have a thorough history and physical examination. The clinician should note the use of potentially immunosuppressive medications or the previous diagnosis of a severe systemic disorder. Recurrent sinusitis every fall and spring in a patient with antecedent sneezing and nasal pruritus suggests atopic diathesis to aeroallergen rather than primary immunodeficiency. Patients with recurrent infections related to lymphoproliferative disease typically have historical and physical evidence of that disease (e.g., night sweats and lymphadenopathy).

Laboratory evaluation of patients with suspected immunodeficiency has two goals: (1) to establish the presence of a secondary cause of immunodeficiency, and (2) to qualitatively and quantitatively assess the different arms of the immune system. A complete blood count with differential demonstrates immunodeficiencies associated with neutropenia (e.g., cyclic neutropenia, chemotherapy-induced myelosuppression); abnormal neutrophil forms (e.g., Chédiak-Higashi syndrome); abnormal red cell forms (e.g., Howell-Jolly bodies associated with functional asplenia); lymphopenia, which is suggestive of T-cell deficiency (e.g., DiGeorge syndrome, acquired immunodeficiency syndrome [AIDS]); and thrombocytopenia (which is seen in the Wiskott-Aldrich syndrome). Secondary causes of immunodeficiency may be suggested by the results of routine serum chemistries, urinalysis, and radiographic studies. For example, the presence of uremia or diabetes can be readily established by serum chemistries, and nephrosis can be revealed by urinalysis. In addition, if a particular secondary immunodeficiency is suggested by the history, further specialized testing may be appropriate. For example, in a child with recurrent respiratory infections, failure to thrive, and gastrointestinal symptoms, referral for sweat chloride determination is appropriate to exclude cystic fibrosis. If such a concomitant condition is found and is sufficient to explain the difficulty with infections, further immunologic testing may not be necessary. Following these initial screening procedures, analysis of the various components of the immune response should reveal most immunodeficiency diseases.

COMPONENTS OF THE IMMUNE RESPONSE

The normal components of the immune response can be divided into nonspecific and specific mediators. The nonspecific factors, which constitute the so-called innate part of the immune response, are not specific in their relationship to a particular antigen and thus are not influenced by previous antigenic exposure. Nonspecific elements include the various cells that phagocytose and serum components capable of damaging pathogens (e.g., the proteins of the complement cascade). The specific or adaptive immune response consists of B cell (antibody-mediated) and T cell (cell-mediated) immune responses. These components of the immune system have both antigen specificity and immunologic memory and are enhanced with subsequent antigen encounter. Primary immunodeficiency disorders can be viewed as qualitative or quantitative defects in discrete parts of the immune response. An organized approach to the evaluation of a patient with suspected immunodeficiency, which includes the determination of the integrity of the different arms of the immune response, can help delineate the defect and guide therapy.

Deficiencies of the B-cell/antibody component of the immune response are the most common causes of primary immunodeficiency. Specific syndromes are shown in Table 1. Isolated B-cell/antibody deficiencies account for 50 per cent of all primary immunodeficiencies, and combined B-cell plus T-cell deficiencies account for an additional 20 to 30 per cent. Therefore, evaluation of B-cell function is of paramount importance in the diagnosis of primary immunodeficiency. Isolated T-cell deficiencies cause 10 to 15 per cent of immunodeficiencies. Phagocytic defects are uncommon, accounting for less than 10 per cent of all primary immunodeficiencies. Deficiencies of the various complement components are even more uncommon.

EVALUATION OF B-CELL/ANTIBODY FUNCTION

The contribution of B cells to host defense derives from their ability to secrete large quantities of high-affinity antibody. B-cell immunodeficiencies are therefore characterized by infections with organisms that are most efficiently eliminated by antibody (see Table 4). Often, patients with B-cell immunodeficiencies present with recurrent respiratory infections, sometimes in association with gastrointestinal symptoms. Some of these syndromes (see Table 1) have characteristic physical findings (e.g., the paucity of lymphoid tissue in patients with X-linked agammaglobulinemia).

IgG antibodies migrate in the gamma region on serum protein electrophoresis (SPEP), and therefore deficiencies of IgG may be suggested by a decreased gamma fraction on SPEP. However, SPEP is not very sensitive, and the diagnosis of serum antibody deficiency is more definitively established by measuring serum immunoglobulins (IgG,

IgA, IgM) by nephelometry. These tests uncover not only primary B cell/antibody immunodeficiencies but also conditions accompanied by hypogammaglobulinemia (e.g., nephrotic syndrome). Importantly, approximately 1 in 700 persons have serum concentrations of IgA that fall below the reference range. Only a small minority of these patients, however, are symptomatic. This fact is not surprising, because the serum concentration of IgA does not necessarily provide information about the integrity of the more functionally relevant IgA that is synthesized and secreted in various mucosal surfaces. Thus, the results of quantitative serum immunoglobulin analysis must be interpreted in the appropriate clinical context.

Normal total serum concentrations of the various immunoglobulins do not preclude the presence of a significant deficiency of the antibody-mediated immune response. If such a condition is strongly suspected on clinical grounds, two additional tests may be done. The first is a quantitative determination of the serum IgG subclasses. Patients with deficiencies of the IgG subclasses (IgG1, IgG2, IgG3, IgG4) may present with symptoms identical to those of patients with hypogammaglobulinemia, yet the total serum IgG concentration may be within the age-adjusted reference range. The second type of testing involves the determination of specific antibody responses. Because the function of the B cell/antibody–mediated arm of the immune response is to bind and eliminate specific antigens, the "gold standard" test of this component of the immune response is the determination of antigen-specific antibody responses. As in IgG subclass deficiencies, normal total serum immunoglobulin concentrations may mask functionally impaired antibody response. This response may be evaluated in several ways. Patients older than 1 year of age who are not of the AB blood group (i.e., patients of blood group O, A, or B) can be tested for the presence of naturally occurring isohemagglutinin antibodies (i.e., anti-A and/or anti-B). Alternatively, the ability to mount an antibody response to vaccination with various antigens can be assessed. Ideally, this test would include protein (e.g., diphtheria, tetanus) as well as carbohydrate (e.g., pneumococcus) antigens, with the development of antibodies assessed 2 to 4 weeks after immunization. These tests typically must be sent to a reference laboratory. Importantly, if antibody deficiency is strongly suspected, immunization with live viral vaccines should be avoided. Finally, additional tests of the B-cell component of the immune response include enumeration of the numbers of circulating B cells and analysis of the proliferative response of B cells in vitro to various stimuli. These tests are not part of the routine laboratory evaluation and are best performed by specialized research laboratories.

EVALUATION OF T-CELL FUNCTION

The T-cell or cell-mediated component of the immune response is critical for the host defense against intracellular pathogens, including viruses, mycobacteria, fungi, and protozoa. Severe primary T-cell immunodeficiencies (see Table 1) are often life-threatening immediately after birth. Recent attention to AIDS, the manifestations of which result from profound depletion of CD4+ T cells by human immunodeficiency virus (HIV), has brought heightened recognition of the importance of the T-cell component of the immune response.

The T-cell arm of the immune response is most easily assessed by delayed-type hypersensitivity testing (DTH). More than 5 mm of cutaneous induration 48 to 72 hours after the intradermal administration of antigen indicates intact cell-mediated immunity. With the use of a panel of at least three common recall antigens (e.g., mumps, *Candida* and *Trichophyton*), the majority of adults are noted to be responsive. Multiple antigen devices are now commercially available. DTH testing may be negative, yet many patients may not have impaired T-cell function, especially those with acute viral illness or young children who have not had sufficient exposure to the test antigens.

T-cell function may be assessed in other ways. The white blood cell count and the percentage of lymphocytes in the differential count provide a good estimate of circulating T-cell numbers. Enumeration of specific subsets of circulating T cells using flow cytometry is widely available. The number of T cells that stain positive with antibodies to CD4 (a marker of the T-cell population responsible for providing help to B cells and other T cells) and CD8 (a marker for the suppressor and cytotoxic T-cell populations) can now be readily determined. Various primary and secondary immunodeficiencies are characterized by alterations in the numbers of circulating T cells or subsets of T cells. Finally, the clinician can request analysis of the ability of T lymphocytes to proliferate in vitro when exposed to plant lectins. However, this test is expensive and requires an experienced laboratory.

EVALUATION OF PHAGOCYTE FUNCTION

Primary immunodeficiencies characterized by impaired phagocyte function are uncommon. Appropriate evaluation includes assessment of both quantitative and qualitative aspects of phagocyte function. The numbers of circulating neutrophils can be determined from the white blood cell count and the differential count. Morphologic analysis of neutrophils may reveal abnormal forms characteristic of a primary immunodeficiency (Chédiak-Higashi syndrome) or indicative of systemic infection (e.g., toxic granulations of neutrophils, as seen in sepsis). Cell surface expression of CD11/CD18, which is absent in the leukocyte adhesion deficiency syndrome, can be readily determined by flow cytometry.

The assessment of qualitative phagocytic defects is more complex because different tests are required for demonstrating various phagocytic abnormalities. One example is the nitroblue tetrazolium dye reduction test, which assesses the ability of neutrophils to generate oxygen radicals and form hydrogen peroxide. This important microbial killing mechanism is abnormal in chronic granulomatous disease. Neutrophil function can also be assessed by analyzing chemotaxis, either in vivo or in vitro. These complex tests, however, are probably best performed in a research laboratory.

EVALUATION OF COMPLEMENT FUNCTION

To screen for deficiencies of complement proteins, the CH_{50} test (total serum hemolytic complement) is appropriate. The CH_{50} provides a functional estimate of the ability of the entire complement cascade to lyse a target. Alternatively, the serum concentrations of individual complement components can be measured. However, because complement protein deficiencies are quite rare, the predictive value of any given laboratory result is minimal. Aside from measurements of serum C3 and C4, other complement analyses are performed infrequently, and results should be interpreted with caution.

CONCLUSION

Stepwise evaluation of patients with suspected immunodeficiency should be initiated when clinical evidence suggests an impaired ability to respond to infections. Initially, the more common secondary immunodeficiency states should be excluded. If necessary, the clinician can investigate the function of the various arms of the immune system, guided by the clinical presentation.

RHINITIS

By Hueston C. King, M.D.
Venice, Florida
and Richard L. Mabry, M.D.
Dallas, Texas

Rhinitis is a broad term used to describe a variety of nasal conditions that are frequently dissimilar and unrelated. The primary structure affected is the nasal mucosa, which may be inflamed and irritated, resulting in an altered mucus production, congestion with vascular engorgement, and edema. The symptoms and physical findings vary widely, depending on the underlying cause, and the general term rhinitis is truly appropriate only as a localizing designation, not as a diagnosis or disease entity. For a diagnostic evaluation to be of value, the specific type of rhinitis must be identified.

ALLERGIC RHINITIS

Allergic rhinitis is the most common cause of persistent or recurrent nasal discomfort. The condition may be classified as seasonal or perennial.

Seasonal Allergic Rhinitis

More commonly known as hay fever, seasonal allergic rhinitis is the condition usually associated by the public with allergy. Repeated episodes of sneezing, clear rhinorrhea, itching of the eyes, and occasional urticaria make the condition apparent to anyone near the victim. The condition is most commonly produced by pollen and is therefore seasonal in nature, although different blooming times for different plants make any season a potential offender. The onset of symptoms occurs over a few days, without fever or malaise, but with much discomfort. Nasal mucosal pain is minimal until repeated sneezing and blowing of the nose produce secondary trauma. Severe itching of the eyes and itching of the nose and skin are common accompanying symptoms. The symptoms usually resolve rapidly when the exposure ceases, as when the person enters a room with air conditioning. The symptoms generally increase throughout the duration of a blooming season and resolve within a week or so after the blooming season is completed. A history of allergy in the family is common, and the condition usually presents in youth, although the severity of attacks can increase into early adulthood, recurring with each seasonal exposure.

Physical Findings

The typical nasal findings of allergy include edematous nasal mucosa, usually bluish in color, with profuse clear watery discharge and no pharyngeal erythema. The conjunctiva is usually edematous and pale, although injection can occur from rubbing the eyes. Tearing is typical.

Common Complications

The most common complications of seasonal allergic rhinitis are eustachian tube or sinus obstruction from mucosal edema. These obstructions may result in a barometric partial vacuum, with pain or secondary serous effusion. They may be distinguished from an infectious condition by the absence of fever or altered polymorphonuclear neutrophil (PMN) leukocyte count.

Laboratory Tests

While the diagnosis of allergic rhinitis is traditionally made by the history and physical examination, confirmation is available from laboratory tests. The presence of an increased eosinophil count is suggestive but not diagnostic, because other conditions can also increase the eosinophil count. An increased total IgE concentration (PRIST) is suggestive but may also be misleading, as other conditions can raise IgE concentrations, and a low IgE concentration does not eliminate the possibility of atopy.

Nasal smears are sometimes performed to diagnose allergic rhinitis. In preparing a nasal smear, the clinician passes a fine swab over the inferior or medial surface of the inferior or middle turbinate, carefully rolls it on a slide, and stains it with Wright-Giemsa stain. A heavy concentration of eosinophils suggests allergy, but this finding is not always the case (see N.A.R.E.S. in the section on nonallergic rhinitis that follows). The complexity and degree of specificity of testing necessary is dictated by the patient's motivation for a specific type of therapy.

Testing for specific allergens, chosen by a careful history of exposure, is of much greater value. This may be done with skin testing, but such testing requires equipment usually only available to the practicing allergist. More convenient is in vitro testing, which can be performed by sending serum to an allergy reference laboratory for radioallergosorbent test (RAST) or enzyme-linked immunosorbent assay (ELISA) screening of regional allergenic offenders. Such screens usually include local pollens, molds, and some epidermals. Usually 8 to 10 tests are enough to establish the diagnosis. Some laboratories offer single-test screening, with each test containing a variety of regional allergens. Such tests are not quantitative but can confirm the diagnosis.

Alternatively, office in vitro tests for regional offenders are available. These tests consist of kits that allow reagent strips containing bands impregnated with regional allergens to be passed through the patient's serum. A series of washes produce color changes that indicate the degree of sensitivity present. The tests are semiquantitative and inexpensive. Radiographs are of little value in allergic rhinitis except in eliminating complications such as sinusitis or mucoceles.

Perennial Allergic Rhinitis

The allergens that produce perennial allergic rhinitis are those present throughout the year; they typically include molds, dust, and animal danders to which the patient is exposed. Basically, the symptoms are those of seasonal allergic rhinitis except that the violent sneezing and conjunctivitis tend to be less pronounced. The congestion and drainage are the same as that found in seasonal allergic rhinitis. The condition is an ongoing one, fluctuating somewhat from time to time but present all year. It may improve with a major change of environment, but many perennial allergens are present worldwide, especially those found primarily indoors.

The physical findings are similar to those found in seasonal allergic rhinitis. The bluish mucosa may at times be replaced with a drier, thickened mucosa from prolonged edema, but this finding is inconstant. At times, especially in the presence of a purely dust allergy, the mucosa may be dry and inflamed and resemble a viral infection. In such a case, the diagnosis is made by the perennial nature of the condition and laboratory findings typical of allergy. The laboratory findings in perennial allergic rhinitis are the same as those found in seasonal allergic rhinitis, except that the allergens are predominantly those that are constantly present. Complications are also similar to those that occur in seasonal allergic rhinitis.

Pitfalls in Diagnosis

Few pitfalls are likely in the basic diagnosis of seasonal allergic rhinitis. One potential error of omission is the failure to identify a complication, such as sinusitis, that can follow osteomeatal obstruction from allergic congestion. In the allergic patient, this complication can perpetuate the symptoms from a reaction to the entrapped bacteria and should be considered when the normal symptom pattern fails to change with the season. Another pitfall is failing to recognize the tendency of allergens to be carried in the victim's hair and clothing, making the offender more difficult to identify, because the symptoms can persist in the absence of immediate exposure. The prolonged nature of perennial allergic rhinitis predisposes the patient to chronic sinus obstruction and to mucosal polyp formation. Careful rhinoscopy with an endoscope after the use of nasal vasoconstrictors can help clarify the situation. Sinus films or a limited computed tomography (CT) scan (see later) can also be useful.

NONALLERGIC RHINITIS

Nonallergic, or hypersensitivity, rhinitis is nearly as common as allergic rhinitis if all of its forms are included. The conditions grouped under this heading are perennial nonallergic rhinitis, nonallergic rhinitis with eosinophilia (N.A.R.E.S.), vasomotor rhinitis, rhinitis of pregnancy, rhinitis medicamentosa, geriatric rhinitis, and pediatric rhinitis. By definition, all specific tests for allergy are negative in these conditions.

Perennial Nonallergic Rhinitis

The symptoms of perennial nonallergic rhinitis are essentially identical with those of perennial allergic rhinitis, making identification by the history alone both difficult and unreliable. Little or no variation in symptoms occurs with seasonal change, geographic location, or specific allergen exposure. As in perennial allergic rhinitis, conjunctivitis, itching, and violent sneezing tend to be less pronounced than in seasonal allergic rhinitis, but these are variable factors. The consistent feature is chronic nasal congestion, with or without a viscous nasal discharge.

The physical findings are identical with those of perennial allergic rhinitis. The only reliable means of separating allergic from nonallergic rhinitis is by testing for immunoglobulin E with the use of either serum or skin testing. All laboratory studies directed toward the identification of specific IgE are negative if the diagnosis is perennial nonallergic rhinitis. Nasal smears may produce uncertainty if the N.A.R.E.S. variant is present (see later).

Skin responses are affected by a variety of factors, including antihistamines, tranquilizers, and other related drugs. The failure to recognize this may lead to an incorrect diagnosis of nonallergic rhinitis based on skin test responses. In vitro assays are not so affected and provide a reliable diagnostic tool. Nasal smears for eosinophils can be positive if the N.A.R.E.S. form is present, or negative in the case of perennial nonallergic rhinitis. Therefore, they are of no value.

N.A.R.E.S.

Nonallergic rhinitis with eosinophilia (N.A.R.E.S.) is a variant of perennial nonallergic rhinitis in which all laboratory and skin tests for allergy are negative, but a nasal smear may be heavily loaded with eosinophils. The cause of this anomaly is unknown, and the presence of the eosinophils in the smear is inconstant. Fortunately, the diagnosis in this disorder does not affect the therapy. The physical findings are identical to those found in perennial nonallergic rhinitis, and laboratory studies fail to detect any allergen-specific IgE. The use of a nasal smear for eosinophils alone is misleading, and when the diagnosis of N.A.R.E.S. is considered it should always be confirmed by in vitro laboratory testing.

Vasomotor Rhinitis

The existence of vasomotor rhinitis as a separate entity is still questioned by some, but most investigators now recognize it as a unique condition. Under stable conditions, the patient with vasomotor rhinitis is relatively asymptomatic. When exposed to any of a variety of stimuli, however, the nose abruptly becomes congested, sneezing may be spasmodic, and a clear, watery drainage appears and may become profuse. Stimuli include an abrupt change of temperature, such as entering an air-conditioned building from summer heat, or going outside from a heated building. Placing warm food in the mouth may also precipitate an episode. Other stimuli include turbulent air, fumes, and irritants such as nonorganic dust. The onset of symptoms is quite prompt, and remission occurs rapidly when the stimulus is removed. There is no fever, generally no surface discomfort in the nasal mucosa, and no conjunctivitis or itching of the skin. All laboratory tests including nasal smears are normal. No complications should be expected except the high degree of discomfort and embarrassment experienced by the patient.

Rhinitis of Pregnancy

In both animals and humans, the increase of estrogen in early pregnancy as well as puberty and other conditions is capable of inducing nasal mucosal edema. Pregnancy reliably produces progressive nasal congestion that can become a symptomatic problem. However, surveys of pregnant women show that about one third report nasal congestion, one third feel no change, and one third feel better while pregnant. Rhinitis of pregnancy, therefore, is not a predictable condition. It must be considered in the differential diagnosis when appropriate, but it must not be expected to occur in all pregnancies. Studies have shown that rhinitis of pregnancy is more properly termed "rhinitis during pregnancy," and it may have elements of vasomotor rhinitis, rhinitis medicamentosa, infection, and allergy.

Nasal congestion alone is both the primary complaint

and the primary physical finding in rhinitis of pregnancy. The nasal mucosa is typically boggy and red, rather than pale. All tests for allergy or infection are normal, except when intercurrent disease complicates the clinical picture. The only complication to be expected is rhinitis medicamentosa, because the patient becomes so uncomfortable that she overuses topical nasal decongestants.

Rhinitis Medicamentosa

Rhinitis medicamentosa may be the direct result of misuse of medication, usually topical drugs applied to the nasal mucosa (rebound rhinitis), or a side effect of systemic drugs administered for therapeutic reasons. The most common cause is overuse of vasoconstrictors in the form of nose drops or nasal sprays. The nasal mucosa appears dry, erythematous, and irritated, with the airways either wide open or tightly closed. Discharge is minimal. Mucosal response to vasoconstrictors is significantly reduced. Similar findings in the nose appear with the use of cocaine and with excess smoking.

Several drug families are capable of inducing nasal congestion. The most common of these is the antihypertensive group, including many beta-blockers. Estrogens may also produce nasal congestion, if given in high enough doses. The findings are nonspecific; mucosal congestion is present without significant change in discharge. Laboratory findings are unremarkable.

Because rhinitis medicamentosa resembles none of the other forms of allergic or nonallergic rhinitis (other than a superficial resemblance to dust allergy), the only problem to be expected is that of a mistaken diagnosis of infectious rhinitis. Rhinitis medicamentosa takes some time to develop; therefore a reliable history should suffice to separate the two. Drug abusers are often reluctant to admit their habit; however, a sympathetic approach to the patient can help elicit this problem. The side effects of systemic drugs are often overlooked, and the failure to recognize this factor may cause the patient to overuse topical decongestants, compounding rather than relieving the problem.

Geriatric Rhinitis

Only recently has geriatric rhinitis been recognized as a unique entity, although the elderly have complained about the symptoms for decades. The condition is a normal development of aging, as the nasal mucosa thins and the mucosal glands atrophy. The chief complaint is usually congestion, accompanied by a thick postnasal drip with frequent clearing of the throat. These symptoms are frequently accompanied by the symptoms of vasomotor rhinitis. On examination, the nasal airways are dry and wide open, with little discharge. The sensation of congestion is apparently a paradoxical one, engendered by the dryness and mucosal sensitivity. What mucus is present is thick and adherent, frequently visible in the pharynx, but with little or no pharyngeal irritation or erythema. Frequently, a pooling of mucus in the hypopharynx is present, sometimes obscuring the vocal cords. All laboratory studies are normal.

Pediatric Rhinitis

Rhinitis in the very young is a frequently seen and commonly misdiagnosed entity, primarily owing to its clinical insignificance. The infant is born with all the nasal mucosal glands that will be present throughout life, and the nasal airway is at its smallest. Moderate clear nasal discharge is to be expected at this age. Only if other evidence of infection appears does the child need to be treated. The nasal mucosa shows normal coloration, and moderate to increased clear, somewhat tenacious mucus, and no fever or pharyngeal erythema is present. All laboratory findings, including cultures, are normal.

INFECTIOUS RHINITIS

The nose is a common target for infection in anyone who interacts with the public. Most nasal infections are viral, despite the frequent tendency to treat them with antibiotics. The most common form of infectious rhinitis is the common cold, which usually resolves in about a week. An ever-increasing variety of respiratory viruses, however, are producing symptoms that may continue for several weeks. More important diagnostically is the nature of onset of the nasal infection.

While frequently prolonged, nasal respiratory infections are not continual. The condition starts rather abruptly and is usually accompanied by malaise and a feeling of nasal irritation and, often, by a low-grade fever. The early stage of inflammation is accompanied by scant, usually clear drainage. During this time, even gentle blowing of the nose is painful, and the patient often describes a nasal burning. Over a variable period, usually only a few days, the inflammatory stage gives way to an exudative stage, during which much of the sensitivity subsides, and thick mucoid or mucopurulent discharge appears. This stage may be prolonged, but it marks the beginning of resolution. It is followed by progressive improvement unless some unrelated problem ensues, such as a secondary bacterial infection. This pattern is not typical of other forms of rhinitis and is characteristic of respiratory virus infection.

Physical Findings

In infectious rhinitis, the mucosa is congested and red, with clear to mucopurulent exudate as the condition progresses. Frequently pharyngeal erythema and tenacious exudate are visible below the soft palate. Cervical adenopathy may be present. Much of the erythema resolves after the inflammatory stage clears.

Complications

The most common complications are secondary bacterial infections, sometimes leading to sinusitis or otitis media. Sinusitis usually develops secondary to obstruction of the osteomeatal complex, trapping purulent secretions in the ethmoid and maxillary sinuses. These sinus infections rarely progress to orbital cellulitis and even intracranial extension. Middle ear infections occur more commonly in children owing to direct extension via the eustachian tube or as a result of an effusion in the middle ear cleft.

Diagnostic Tests

A white blood cell count often shows leukopenia and relatively few immature forms with a viral infection, or a leukocytosis and increased numbers of immature forms with a bacterial infection. Nasal cultures are of value if secondary bacterial infection has occurred, but in the early viral stages cultures may show only normal flora. A nasal smear stained with Wright-Giemsa can show PMN leukocytes, bacteria, and sloughing of damaged basement membrane cells if the infection is viral. This study is no more difficult to perform than a peripheral blood smear and, in prolonged cases, can be of considerable value. Sinus films can be helpful if sinusitis is suspected owing to localizing symptoms or a severe or prolonged course. Computed tomography is especially useful for detecting ethmoid sinusitis.

HEREDITARY ANGIOEDEMA

By D. Michael Elnicki, M.D., *and* Paris T. Mansmann, M.D.
Morgantown, West Virginia

Although urticaria and angioedema are common problems affecting nearly 20 per cent of the population, hereditary angioedema (HAE) is a rare disorder. It accounts for about 2 per cent of clinical angioedema and has an incidence of about 1 in 150,000 persons. Hereditary angioedema is caused by a genetic insufficiency of C1 esterase inhibitor (C1-INH). Defects in this protein allow unchecked activation of the classic complement pathway and other biochemical systems. Patients can present with any combination of cutaneous angioedema, abdominal pain, or acute airway obstruction. Prior to the development of effective therapy, the mortality rate was reported at 20 to 30 per cent. Although preventable and treatable, the complications of this disease do not respond well to the usual therapies for angioedema, and thus the establishment of the diagnosis is critical.

HISTORY

Patients who have HAE typically report episodic attacks that begin during adolescence, although some may present as children. Attacks are often preceded by a prodrome associated with anxiety, which led to the inappropriate term angioneurotic edema. Trauma precipitates about half the attacks, and coexisting illnesses, such as infections, may trigger others. However, many attacks have no clear inciting event. The frequency of attacks varies greatly between affected individuals, with some experiencing weekly episodes while others have attacks less frequently than once a year.

The most common and most noticeable symptom is cutaneous edema. Patients first notice a tightness or tingling of the skin, followed by the appearance of a nonpruritic, nonpainful rash that evolves over several hours. The initial site of the edema is often that of relatively minor trauma, such as athletic contact. The cutaneous lesions typically resolve over 1 to 3 days.

Often, patients with HAE first seek medical attention because of abdominal pain, which they may or may not associate with the skin lesions. Attacks are frequently preceded by feelings of bloating, anorexia, and nausea. Constipation and vomiting are common early in the attack, followed often by diarrhea as the pain resolves. The abdominal pain of HAE is described as colicky and poorly localized. Some patients are able to distinguish their HAE pain from that of other disorders, such as dyspepsia and biliary pain.

The most feared complication of HAE is laryngeal edema, which can cause an immediate, life-threatening emergency. Dental work and surgery involving the head and neck are common precipitants, but laryngeal edema can be spontaneous. Patients describe a choking sensation, as if something were caught in their throat. They may rapidly progress to stridor and airway obstruction and require emergency intubation or tracheostomies to ensure adequate airways.

Less common presentations reflect edema at other sites. Some patients report cough and pleuritic pain due to pleural involvement, and pleural effusions may develop. Others can develop swelling in the genitalia following intercourse. Rarely, patients develop headaches, seizures, or focal neurologic defects from intracranial edema.

Hormonal fluctuations play a role in HAE, and the surges that occur during adolescence are associated with the disease's usual presentation at that age. Women often have attacks during menses, but attacks are less frequent during pregnancy. The frequency and intensity of attacks often lessen after menopause. Both estrogen and antiandrogen therapy have been described as precipitating HAE attacks.

PHYSICAL EXAMINATION

When patients present with acute attacks of HAE, they may appear severely ill. The first priority in evaluating them is to ensure an adequate airway. With severe attacks, patients can develop hypotension owing to sequestration of fluid in the extravascular space. They should not be febrile if HAE is their only active problem.

The angioedema of HAE most often involves the upper extremities and oropharynx. The trunk and lower extremities are less commonly involved. Not associated with urticaria, the lesions are nonpitting and mildly erythematous, tend to remain in a single lymphatic area, and typically do not extend beyond a major joint (Fig. 1). They resolve without scarring. Histologically, the angioedema of HAE is indistinguishable from that of other types.

The abdominal pain of HAE is caused by edema of the gastrointestinal tract and can mimic peptic disease, biliary colic, appendicitis, or a perforated viscus. The intensity can approximate that of an acute abdomen, often resulting in unnecessary surgery in these patients. Decreased gastrointestinal motility, to the point of mechanical bowel obstructions, can develop. The gastrointestinal edema generally

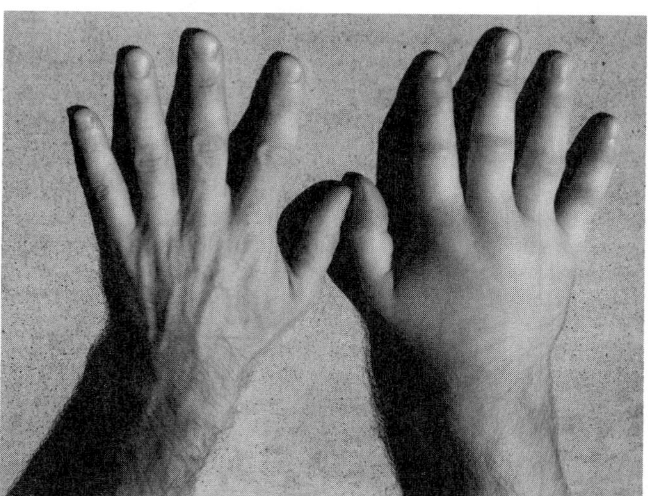

Figure 1. Cutaneous edema involving the right hand of a patient with hereditary angioedema.

follows the same time course to resolution as that of the cutaneous attacks.

Laryngeal edema is the major source of HAE-related mortality, and case series indicate that more than half of HAE patients develop involvement in this area. The patient's clinical condition may deteriorate rapidly following the inciting event, progressing through mild discomfort to complete airway obstruction. The soft tissue edema can be readily seen when it involves the throat and uvula.

GENETICS

Abnormal C1-INH production is the most common genetic defect in the complement system, and the genetics of HAE have recently become well characterized. The C1-INH gene is located on chromosome 11 in the p11-q13 region. Restriction endonuclease techniques have demonstrated that multiple mutations can result in the affected phenotype. The inheritance is autosomal dominant with incomplete penetrance. Those inheriting the abnormal gene can be anywhere on a clinical spectrum from asymptomatic to severely affected.

Two genetic types of HAE result in essentially the same phenotypic expression (Table 1). In the most common form (type I), which accounts for about 85 per cent of cases, synthesis of C1-INH is blocked at the site of the faulty gene but occurs at the normal gene. The result is transcription of the normal protein, yielding serum concentrations of C1-INH that are about 10 to 30 per cent of normal. In type II HAE, about 15 per cent of cases, ample amounts of a nonfunctional C1-INH are synthesized by the abnormal gene. The presence of the mutated C1-INH decreases the synthesis of the normal protein, and both are rapidly catabolized. Whereas type I patients have normal concentrations of cleaved, inactive C1-INH, some type II patients have markedly increased concentrations of the catabolized protein. Recently, a third type of HAE has been described in which the abnormal C1-INH protein binds to albumin. Both antigenic and functional C1-INH concentrations are reported to be decreased in these patients.

LABORATORY TESTING

Most routine laboratory tests performed on HAE patients are normal. Patients with HAE typically do not have increased erythrocyte sedimentation rates (ESR) or eosinophilia; if either of these are present, the clinician should consider another or a coexisting diagnosis. During attacks, patients can demonstrate hemoconcentration or prerenal azotemia, both of which reflect intravascular volume loss. The white blood cell count can become increased during attacks. Imaging studies are usually unrevealing, but occasionally mechanical bowel obstructions are observed during attacks of gastrointestinal edema. Ultrasonographic examination of the abdomen of a patient with gastrointestinal edema shows edema inside and outside the intestinal lumen and within the intestinal wall.

The screening test for HAE is the C4 concentration, as it is always decreased during attacks. Between attacks, the C4 concentration may be equivocal. The concentrations of C3 and C1q should be normal in HAE patients, regardless of the clinical status of their disease. During attacks, the total serum hemolytic complement (CH_{50}) is typically decreased, but it returns to normal with recovery.

The diagnosis of HAE is confirmed by obtaining both functional and quantitative concentrations of C1-INH. Obtaining both demonstrates the presence of HAE and the type, something relevant in choosing therapy. Concentrations of C1-INH correlate poorly with clinical disease severity and do not need to be regularly monitored after the diagnosis has been made.

When sending a specimen for C1-INH analysis, those handling it must do so with care. The components of complement degrade after 24 to 48 hours at room temperature. Although stable if refrigerated, C1-INH degrades when heated, and it is completely inactivated at temperatures higher than 60°C.

Other types of urticaria without angioedema, referred to as acquired angioedema (AAE), can complicate the process of diagnostic evaluation. Like patients with HAE, those with AAE suffer from decreased C1-INH concentrations and experience the same spectrum of clinical disease. The two conditions differ in several respects, however. Patients with AAE do not have affected family members and typically present later in life than those with HAE. Acquired angioedema is not a genetic disorder, and normal or even supranormal concentrations of C1-INH are synthesized. The problem is that the protein is being rapidly consumed by massive activation of C1. Type I AAE is typically seen in patients with lymphoproliferative disorders, but it has also been described in association with a variety of malignancies and chronic inflammatory conditions. Patients with type II AAE have an autoantibody that binds to C1-INH at the active site, thereby inactivating the enzyme. This antibody can occur as an isolated defect or as part of a more widespread autoimmune problem, such as rheumatoid arthritis or systemic lupus erythematosus. On laboratory testing, AAE patients demonstrate decreased C1q concentrations in addition to decreased C4 and C1-INH concentrations (see Table 1).

Table 1. Laboratory Values Characterizing the Forms of C1-INH Deficiency

	Hereditary Angioedema			Acquired Angioedema	
	Type I	*Type II*	*Type III*	*Type I*	*Type II*
C4 concentration	↓	↓	↓	↓	↓
C1-INH quantitative	↓	N	↓	↓	↑
C1-INH functional	↓	↓	↓	↓	↓
C1-INH cleaved	N	↑ ↑	N	N	↑
C1q protein concentration	N	N	N	↓	↓

↓ = decreased; ↑ = increased; N = normal.

BIOCHEMISTRY

C1-INH is a member of the serpin family of proteases, along with $alpha_1$-antitrypsin, antithrombin III, and angiotensinogen. These proteins stoichiometrically inactivate their target proteases, forming stable, one-to-one complexes. Synthesized primarily by hepatocytes, C1-INH is also synthesized by monocytes. The regulation of the protein's production is not completely understood, but androgens stimulate C1-INH synthesis.

Although named for its action on activated first component of complement (C1 esterase), C1-INH also inhibits components of the fibrinolytic, clotting, and kinin pathways. Specifically, C1-INH inactivates plasmin, Hageman factor (factor XII), and kallikrein. Within the complement system, C1-INH blocks the activation of C1 and the rest of the classic complement pathway. Without C1-INH, unchecked activation of C1, C2, and C4 occur before other inhibitors (C4 binding protein and factor I) can halt the cascade.

The actual factor or factors responsible for the edema formation in HAE remain somewhat controversial. Some researchers have demonstrated activation of the kinin system and increased bradykinin concentration associated with clinical flares. Bradykinin is an important inflammatory mediator that causes neutrophil chemotaxis, capillary dilatation, and smooth muscle relaxation, and it has been linked to other forms of angioedema. Others have implicated C2 kinin, a metabolite of C2b, as the active agent in the presence of plasmin.

C1-INH is not needed for intact immune function, and HAE patients have no increase in the incidence or severity of infections. Other biochemical pathways where C1-INH is active, such as fibrinolysis and clotting, also function normally without it. Unlike other forms of angioedema, histamine is not involved in the pathogenesis of HAE.

SUMMARY

Although rare, HAE is a disease with potentially catastrophic consequences for those affected. These effects include acute respiratory compromise and unnecessary abdominal surgery, both of which can be prevented by and treated after recognition of the disease.

The clinician should be alerted by a history of intermittent attacks, usually beginning in young adulthood and involving cutaneous edema, unexplained abdominal pain, or laryngeal edema. Attacks evolve over 4 to 8 hours, last 1 to 3 days, and are often precipitated by trauma. A history of affected family members and the lack of an association with atopic features should heighten suspicions. During an attack, patients have erythematous, nonpitting edema of the face, trunk, or extremities—often at the site of recent trauma. The abdominal pain is colicky and can reach the intensity of an acute abdomen. Laryngeal edema often presents as choking and can rapidly evolve to airway obstruction.

When clinical suspicion exists, the presence of HAE can be confirmed or excluded with a few laboratory tests. Serum C4 concentration is always decreased during an attack and is typically decreased between attacks. While a low C4 concentration is a good screening test, the presence of the disease is confirmed by finding decreased serum C1-INH concentration (type I) or decreased functional activity (type II). Other tests are usually helpful only in the negative sense. After the diagnosis has been established, patients can be treated chronically or can reach prophylaxis for stressful events, such as surgery, dental work, or athletic competition, so that disruption of their lives is minimized.

URTICARIA

By Joe Venzor, M.D.,
and David P. Huston, M.D.
Houston, Texas

Urticaria, commonly known as "hives," manifests as pruritic, palpable, erythematous skin lesions that are well demarcated, blanch with pressure, and often exhibit central clearing. Urticarial lesions range from millimeters to centimeters in diameter and may exist singly but are usually numerous. Urticaria is often classified as acute or chronic. In acute urticaria, individual lesions resolve within hours of appearance and are histologically characterized by dermal edema, dilatation of blood vessels, and a paucity of inflammatory cells (Fig. 1*A* and *B*). In chronic urticaria, individual lesions resolve more slowly, sometimes persisting for more than 24 hours, and are characterized histologically by perivascular cuffing with mononuclear cells (Fig. 2*A* and *B*), which implicates a more complex pathophysiology. Although the term chronic urticaria is sometimes used to describe patients who have clinical symptoms that persist or recur for longer than 6 weeks, this definition does not always correlate with the histopathologic definition.

Angioedema is clinically characterized by cutaneous

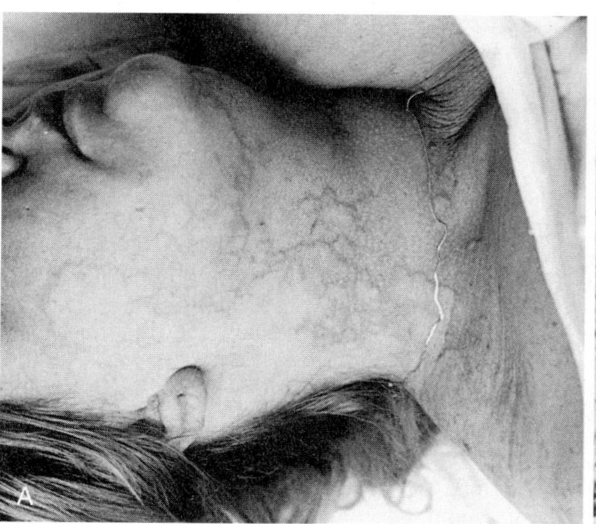

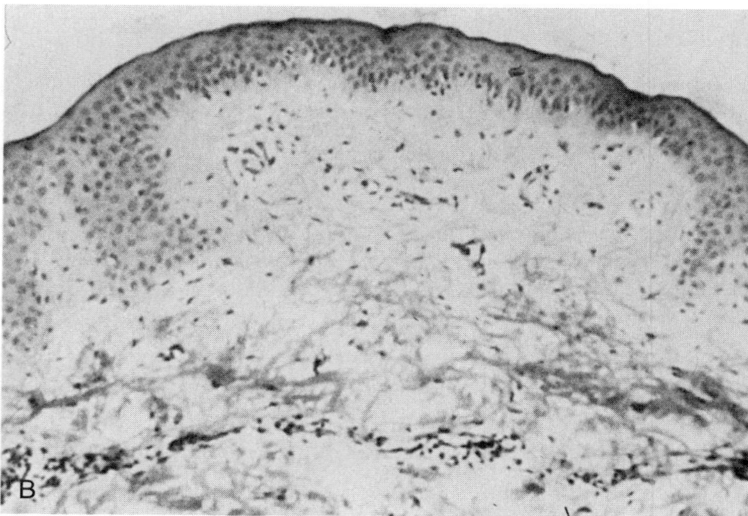

Figure 1. Acute urticaria. *A,* Clinical appearance of cutaneous lesions, which have a characteristic well-demarcated erythematous border and pale center. *B,* Histopathology demonstrating dermal edema and minimal cellular infiltrates. (From Huston, D.P., and Bressler, R.B.: Urticaria and angioedema. Med. Clin. North Am., 76:809, 1992, with permission.)

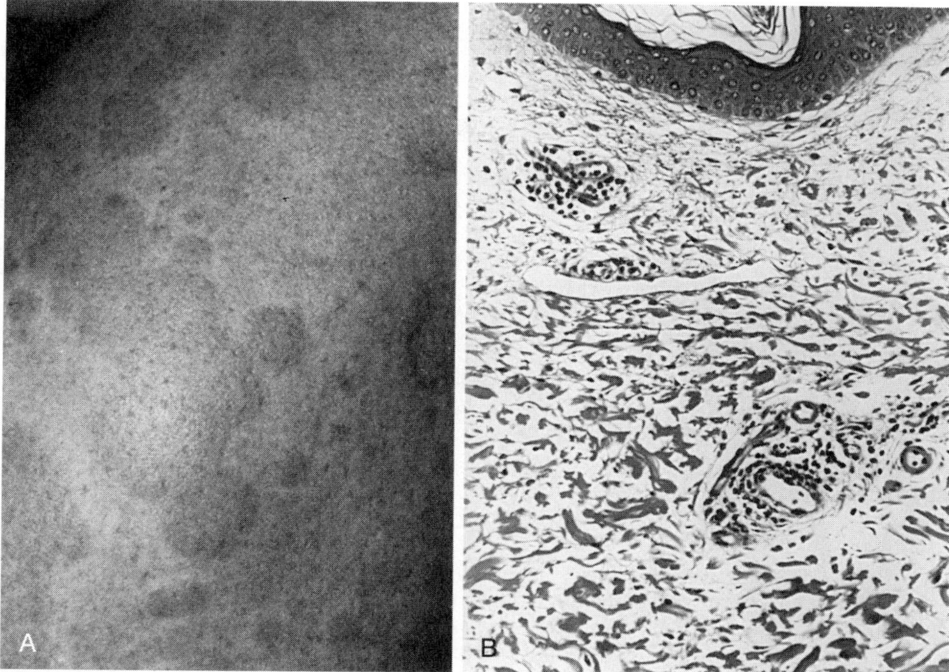

Figure 2. Chronic urticaria. *A,* Clinical appearance of cutaneous lesions, which are more indurated than those with acute urticaria. *B,* Histopathology demonstrating perivascular mononuclear cell infiltrate. (From Huston, D.P., and Bressler, R.B.: Urticaria and angioedema. Med. Clin. North Am., 76:809, 1992, with permission.)

edema without the well-demarcated erythema of urticaria (Fig. 3*A*), and it is usually associated with a burning or tingling sensation, rather than pruritus. The lesions may involve the mucosal tissues, and involvement of the oropharynx can cause asphyxiation (see Fig. 3*B*). Angioedema is histologically similar to acute or chronic urticaria except that the edema extends into the deeper dermis and subcutaneous tissues. This more extensive edema often requires a longer time for resolution. Approximately 20 per cent of the population have at least one episode of urticaria or angioedema during their lifetime. Urticaria and angioedema coexist in 50 per cent of affected individuals, and angioedema occurs alone in 10 per cent.

Urticaria is also the hallmark of a subset of patients with leukocytoclastic vasculitis. These urticarial vasculitis lesions can be clinically indistinguishable from acute or chronic urticaria and may appear as angioedema. However, clinical characteristics that should raise suspicion of urticarial vasculitis include persistence of individual lesions for several days, the sensation of pain or burning in addition to pruritus, coexistent purpura, and hyperpigmentation after lesion resolution (Fig. 4*A*). The classic histopathologic features of urticarial vasculitis include a predominantly neutrophilic perivascular infiltrate and neutrophils within the walls of the blood vessels (see Fig. 4*B*). Extravasation of erythrocytes and leukocytoclasis with fragmentation of neutrophils into scattered nuclear debris are characteristic of the infiltrate. Lesional skin biopsies reveal deposition of immunoglobulins, complement, and fibrinogen within the vessel walls of more than 50 per cent of patients.

Central to the pathogenesis of urticaria is mast cell activation, with the release of preformed and newly synthesized mediators. However, the mechanism by which the mast cells are activated and the intensity and cellular composition of the subsequent inflammatory cascade are

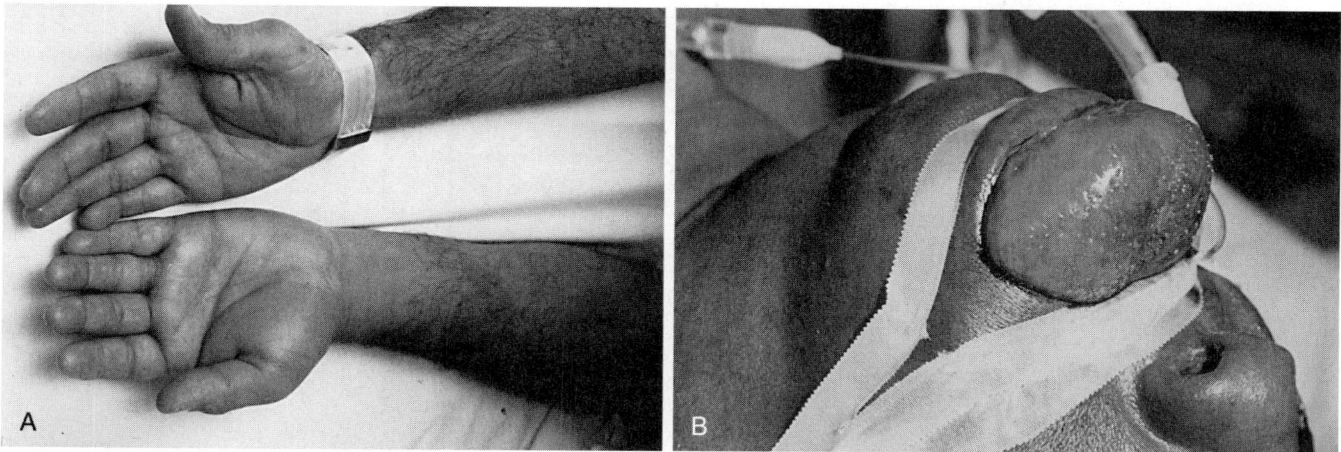

Figure 3. Angioedema. *A,* Acute angioedema. *B,* Oropharyngeal angioedema requiring intubation. (From Huston, D.P., and Bressler, R.B.: Urticaria and angioedema. Med. Clin. North Am., 76:809, 1992, with permission.)

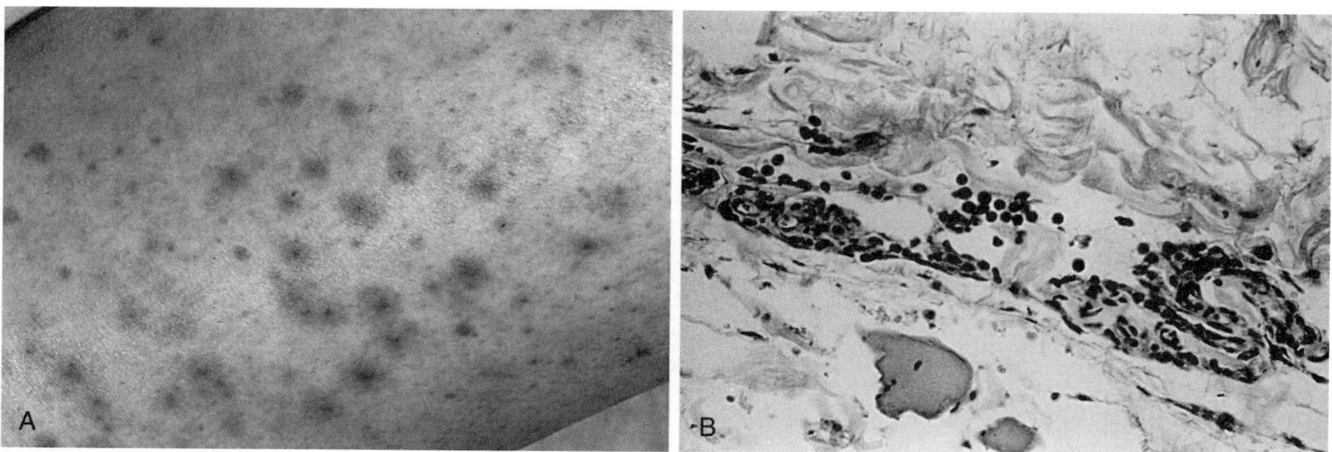

Figure 4. Urticarial vasculitis. *A,* Indurated lesions of urticarial vasculitis, which may be difficult to clinically distinguish from those of chronic urticaria. *B,* Histopathology demonstrating leukocytoclastic vasculitis.

important for selecting the most appropriate diagnostic evaluation and therapy. Angioedema is also due to mast cell activation in the vast majority of patients. Rarely, angioedema is the manifestation of a deficiency of C1 esterase inhibitor (C1-INH). Because the management of angioedema due to C1-INH deficiency is different from the treatment of mast cell-dependent angioedema, diagnostic distinction of these conditions is imperative.

PATHOPHYSIOLOGIC MECHANISMS

Mast cell activation and degranulation can be a consequence of antigen cross-linking of mast cell membrane–bound IgE (anaphylactic) or of non–IgE-mediated (anaphylactoid) mechanisms, including direct activation of the mast cell by drugs, chemicals and physical stimuli, complement activation, or alterations in the mast cell arachidonic acid pathway, such as those caused by nonsteroidal anti-inflammatory drugs (Fig. 5). Inflammatory mediators (e.g., histamine, tryptase, and leukotrienes) produced and released during mast cell degranulation are important acute effectors of urticaria and angioedema. The late-phase reaction, which appears 6 to 12 hours after mast cell activation, is characterized by mononuclear, neutrophil, and eosinophil cellular infiltrates induced by chemokines and cytokines generated during the inflammatory process.

DIFFERENTIAL DIAGNOSIS (Table 1)

Aeroallergens, Contactants, and Insect Allergy

Aeroallergen-induced urticaria is uncommon and usually exists concurrently with symptoms of asthma or allergic rhinitis. Both seasonal and perennial aeroallergens have been pathogenically implicated. Direct contact of an antigen with the skin can also induce urticaria. These antigens can be as diverse as feline salivary proteins or latex.

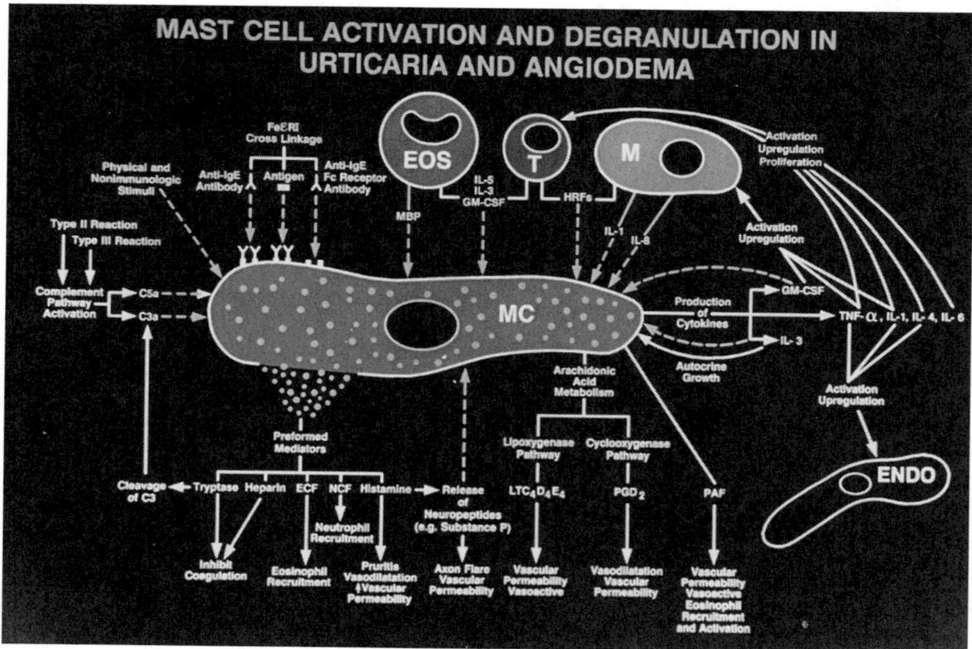

Figure 5. Mast cell activation and degranulation in urticaria and angioedema. MC = mast cell; T = T cell; M = monocyte; EOS = eosinophil; ENDO = endothelial cell; MBP = major basic protein; HRF = histamine-releasing factor; GM-CSF = granulocyte-macrophage colony-stimulating factor; ECF = eosinophil chemotactic factor; → = degranulation stimulus. (*A* from Huston, D.P., and Bressler, R.B.: Urticaria and angioedema. Med. Clin. North Am., 76:814, 1992, with permission.)

Table 1. Potential Causes of Urticaria and Angioedema

- Idiopathic causes
- Food allergy
- Food additives and preservatives: benzoic acid derivatives, dyes (especially tartrazine), flavorings (aspartame)
- Drug reactions
  - Antibiotics: penicillin, cephalosporins, sulfa derivatives, vancomycin
  - Over-the-counter medications: vitamins, cold formulas
  - Antihypertensive medications: diuretics
  - Psychotropics: sedatives, tranquilizers
  - Opiates: morphine sulfate, codeine
  - Muscle relaxants: D-tubocurarine
  - Hyperosmolar radiocontrast media
  - Cyclooxygenase inhibitors: aspirin, nonsteroidal anti-inflammatory drugs (NSAIDs)
  - Hormonal: birth control pills, thyroid replacement, adrenocorticotropic hormone (ACTH), insulin
  - Chemotherapeutic medications: doxorubicin (Adriamycin)
  - Intravenous gamma globulin
  - Protamine
  - Enzymes: papain
  - Vaccines
  - Antiserum
  - Immunotherapy injections
- Insect bites and stings
  - Hymenoptera: wasp, honeybee, yellow jacket, hornet, fire ant
  - Biting insects: kissing bug (conenose), mosquitoes, horseflies and deerflies
- Physical causes
  - Dermatographism
  - Cholinergic
  - Localized heat
  - Cold
  - Delayed pressure
  - Exercise-induced anaphylaxis
  - Solar
  - Vibratory
  - Aquagenic
- Collagen vascular diseases
  - Systemic lupus erythematosus
  - Rheumatoid arthritis
  - Sjögren's syndrome
- Infection
  - Viral: hepatitis, infectious mononucleosis
  - Bacterial
  - Parasitic: invasive helminths, giardiasis
  - Fungal
- Malignancy: lymphoma, solid tumors, myeloproliferative disorders
- Vasculitis
  - Hypocomplementemic urticarial vasculitis
  - Normocomplementemic urticarial vasculitis
  - Associated with systemic diseases
  - Serum sickness: heterologous protein administration, drugs
  - Schnitzler's syndrome: chronic urticaria, vasculitis, high levels of monoclonal IgM
- C1 esterase inhibitor deficiency syndromes (angioedema only)
  - Hereditary angioedema
  - Acquired angioedema
- Contactants: latex, animals, food, plants, sea nettles
- Aeroallergens
- Transfusion reaction
- Rare miscellaneous causes
  - Familial cold urticaria
  - Amyloidosis with nerve deafness and limb pain
  - Episodic angioedema with eosinophilia
  - Carboxypeptidase N deficiency

Adapted from Huston, D. P., and Bressler, R.B.: Urticaria and angioedema. Med. Clin. North Am., 76:810, 1992, with permission.

Stinging and biting insects also cause acute urticaria. The stinging insects belong to the order Hymenoptera and include bees, wasps, hornets, yellow jackets, and fire ants. Retention of the stinger in the skin is characteristic of a bee sting because only bees have a barbed stinger. In the absence of visual identification of the responsible hymenopteran, immediate hypersensitivity skin testing with venom extracts can be used to identify the offending antigen. The biting insects that commonly induce urticaria are the kissing bug (conenose), mosquitoes, horseflies, and deerflies. Usually, the reaction to an insect bite is localized and is referred to as papular urticaria.

Drug Reactions

Virtually all medications have been reported to cause urticaria. Most of these reactions occur via IgE-mediated mechanisms. The most frequent offenders include antibiotics such as the penicillins, sulfa drugs, quinolones, and cephalosporins in addition to certain narcotics, antihypertensives, vaccines, and diuretics. Vaccine-induced urticaria is usually the result of egg sensitivity. Direct mast cell degranulation is produced by morphine, codeine, vancomycin (red man syndrome), intravenous radiocontrast media, doxorubicin, and the muscle relaxant D-tubocurarine. Aspirin, nonsteroidal anti-inflammatory drugs, and food additives such as benzoate and dyes produce urticaria by an unknown mechanism possibly related to an imbalance between prostaglandin and leukotriene production. Blood products, intravenous gamma globulin, and antisera produce urticaria as result of immune complex formation that activates complement anaphylatoxins (C3a and C5a), which, in turn, induce mast cell degranulation.

Food Allergy

Food allergy is a common cause of acute urticaria, but it is rarely a cause of chronic urticaria. The foods most likely to be implicated are fish, nuts, legumes, shellfish, eggs, and milk. However, certain food additives, such as benzoate and sulfites, dyes such as tartrazine, and flavorings such as aspartame may cause urticaria by direct activation of mast cells. Many times, a diagnosis of food allergy can be made on the basis of the history alone. Immediate hypersensitivity skin testing with selected food extracts can be useful if the diagnosis is unclear. Positive skin tests that occur in the absence of clinical food allergy must be interpreted in the context of a patient's history. Conversely, negative skin tests almost completely exclude allergy to that food. Although food-elimination diets may support a diagnosis, double-blind, placebo-controlled challenge is required for a definitive diagnosis. Owing to the risk of anaphylaxis during skin testing or ingestion challenge, these procedures should be performed only under the supervision of a qualified physician. Most foods cause urticaria through IgE-mediated mechanisms.

Physical Urticarias

Physical urticarias are induced by physical stimulation and present as recurrent acute urticaria. Dermatographism, cholinergic urticaria, and cold urticaria, the most common physical urticarias, account for approximately 15 per

Table 2. Tests Useful for the Diagnosis of the Physical Urticarias

Type of Urticaria	Test	Positive Result
Dermatographism	Application of pressure to the skin with a narrow object	Linear wheal and flare (2–5 min)
Delayed dermatographism	Same	Linear wheal and flare (3–8 hr)
Cholinergic	1. Methacholine skin test 2. Increase core body temperature 0.7 to 1.0°C by immersion in warm water or exercise	Characteristic satellite lesions or urticaria
Exercise-induced anaphylaxis	Exercise challenge	Urticaria
Cold urticarias		
Primary	Localized cold challenge (i.e., ice cube test)	Pruritus and urticaria or angioedema within 5 min of rewarming
Secondary (associated with systemic disease)	Not indicated or recommended	None
Exercise cold-induced	Exercise in cold temperature	Urticaria
Systemic	1. Generalized cold exposure 2. Local cold challenge	1. Generalized urticaria 2. Negative
Cold-induced dermatographism	Chilling lightly scratched skin	Linear wheal and flare
Delayed pressure	Application of a 15-lb weighted sling to shoulder for 15 min	Painful swelling 4–12 hr later
Solar	1. Monochrometer testing with specific wavelengths of light 2. Testing for porphyrins of type 6	Hives over light-exposed area Elevated erythrocyte protoporphyrin
Vibratory	Vibration to forearm for 5 min	Localized urticaria
Aquagenic	Room-temperature water compress to upper back for 30 min	Localized urticaria

Adapted from Huston, D.P., and Bressler, R.B.: Uriticaria and angioedema. Med. Clin. North Am., 76:820, 1992, with permission.

cent of all urticarias. Younger adults are more commonly affected. Tests useful in the diagnosis of physical urticarias are shown in Table 2.

Dermatographism

Dermatographism, or "writing on the skin," is the most common of the physical urticarias, but it carries a low morbidity in most patients. Unfortunately, some patients experience severe pruritus and swelling in areas of friction from clothing, scratching, or minor trauma (Fig. 6). Hot baths, exercise, and emotional stress are often exacerbating factors. Simple stroking of the skin with a tongue blade or a pen results in urticaria formation within a few minutes and is diagnostic. The use of a spring-loaded dermographometer set at 3600 g/cm^2 of pressure may allow for more accurate reproduction of dermatographism. Two rare forms of dermatographism exist. One form occurs with only simultaneous cold exposure. The other is a delayed form of dermatographism that presents 36 hours after the initial stimulation.

Cholinergic Urticaria

Cholinergic urticaria is characterized by wheals 2 to 4 mm in diameter surrounded by a large area of macular

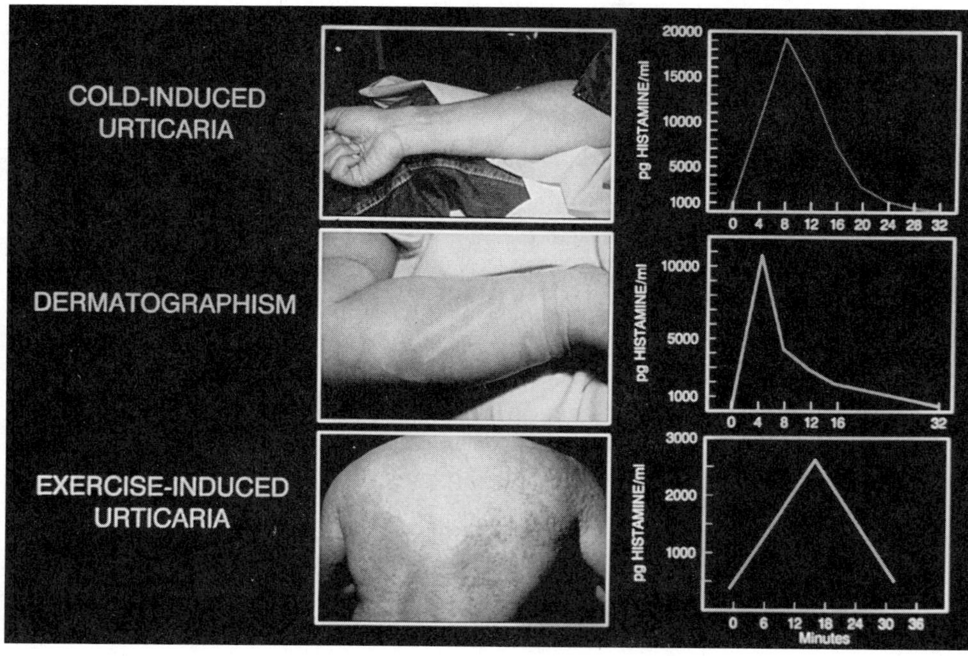

Figure 6. Evidence of mast cell degranulation in physical urticarias. Increase in plasma histamine concentrations in draining venous blood following cold challenge *(top),* stroking of the skin *(middle),* and exercise *(bottom).* (From Huston, D.P., and Bressler, R.B.: Urticaria and angioedema. Med. Clin. North Am., 76:821, 1992, with permission.)

erythema (see Fig. 6). These wheals are distinctive in appearance from other types of urticaria. Cholinergic urticaria is produced when the core body temperature is increased by approximately 1°C, as with a hot bath or exercise. Angioedema, hypotension, shortness of breath, wheezing, headaches, abdominal pain, and other systemic symptoms can occur simultaneously. A positive methacholine skin test, with both a central wheal and satellite wheals, occurs in about one third of patients. Inducing the characteristic urticarial lesions in a hot room or with exercise until the patient begins to sweat confirms the diagnosis. The plasma histamine concentration is transiently increased at the onset of the urticarial lesions.

Cold Urticaria

Several forms of cold-induced urticaria have been described. The most common subgroup is primary cold urticaria that occurs within a few minutes after rewarming of an area that has been exposed to cold (see Fig. 6). Lesions occur only at the site of cold exposure and often have the appearance of angioedema. Systemic symptoms are related to the extent of mast cell mediator release and may include life-threatening hypotension. The diagnosis is confirmed by either immersion of the hand in water at 10°C for 10 minutes or the application of an ice pack to the forearm for 5 minutes.

Secondary cold urticaria is acquired as the result of systemic disorders such as cryoglobulinemia, collagen vascular diseases, syphilis, and hematologic malignancies. Cold challenge testing is *not recommended* because tissue ischemia can result.

Familial cold urticaria is a rare autosomal dominant disorder in which urticaria develops a half hour to 3 hours after generalized cold exposure, along with systemic symptoms of headache, fever, chills, and arthralgias. Skin biopsies reveal leukocytoclastic vasculitis. The local cold challenge test is negative in familial cold urticaria.

Delayed Pressure Urticaria

Delayed pressure urticaria appears 4 to 6 hours after sustained pressure is applied to the skin. Urticaria is precipitated by the use of tight clothes or elastic straps, prolonged standing or sitting, clapping, or pressure applied to an extremity. The lesions are characteristically more tender and diffuse than other urticarias and are accompanied by angioedema. Flulike symptoms and leukocytosis may occur. The application of a 15-pound weighted sling across the shoulder for 15 minutes is diagnostic.

Exercise-Induced Anaphylactic Syndrome

Patients with the exercise-induced anaphylactic syndrome present with urticaria in addition to the classic clinical signs of anaphylaxis, including hypotension, shortness of breath, gastrointestinal symptoms, and angioedema. Exercise—and not the resultant increase in core body temperature, as in cholinergic urticaria—is required for producing the syndrome. A subset of patients have symptoms during exercise only after the ingestion of certain foods, including celery, shellfish, and wheat.

Solar Urticaria

Solar urticaria occurs within a few minutes after exposure to light. Most patients react to specific wavelengths of light, which may change with time. Erythropoietic porphyria should be excluded in patients with reactivity between 400 and 500 nm. Therapeutic tolerance can be induced in some patients with repetitive sunlight exposure, such as that which occurs on the exposed extremities of many patients.

Vibratory Angioedema

Local angioedema presents within 1 to 5 minutes after exposure to a vibratory stimulus, such as a lawnmower, motorcycle, or massage. Autosomal dominant and idiopathic cases have been described. Urticaria is uncommon in this disorder. The diagnosis is confirmed with the application of a vibratory stimulus to the forearm for 5 minutes, producing an increase in arm circumference.

Aquagenic Urticaria

Aquagenic and localized heat urticaria are extremely uncommon disorders, with fewer than 25 cases of each reported in the literature. Aquagenic urticaria occurs within 30 minutes after water exposure. The lesions are similar in appearance to those of cholinergic urticaria. However, no relationship to core body temperature or reaction to methacholine skin testing is observed.

Localized Heat Urticaria

The application of a heated object to the skin for 5 minutes results in urticaria formation. Systemic symptoms can occur with excessive skin exposure. The ingestion of hot liquids can induce oropharyngeal lesions.

Urticaria Associated With Systemic Disorders

Collagen Vascular Diseases

Patients with systemic lupus erythematosus, Sjögren's syndrome, and rheumatoid arthritis may have urticaria as part of the spectrum of disease, presumably through immune complex formation. An increased incidence of urticarial vasculitis exists in these disorders.

Infection

Urticaria has been associated with a wide variety of infectious agents. Common viral causes include hepatitis, infectious mononucleosis, and coxsackievirus infections. Rarely, bacterial infections such as sinusitis and dental or abdominal abscesses are associated with the development of urticaria. In patients with coexisting gastrointestinal symptoms, screening for parasitic organisms is indicated.

Malignancies

Urticaria or urticarial vasculitis can occur in the context of malignancies, such as myeloproliferative disorders, lymphoma, and other solid tumors. The occurrence of angioedema with these underlying diseases requires diagnostic assessment for acquired C1-INH deficiency.

Urticaria Pigmentosa and Mast Cell Dyscrasias

The characteristic lesions of urticaria pigmentosa are light brown to red, persist for years, and form urticaria with light trauma (Darier's sign), as seen in Figure 7. Urticaria pigmentosa is the most common form of cutaneous mastocytosis in children and adults. A lesional skin biopsy demonstrates increased numbers of mast cells. Systemic mastocytosis or mastocytosis with an associated hematologic disorder is present in a minority of cases. Systemic mastocytosis is confirmed by the presence of increased numbers of mast cells in a bone marrow biopsy.

Urticarial Vasculitis

Urticarial vasculitis is a subtype of leukocytoclastic vasculitis that manifests as urticaria. Cutaneous characteristics of urticarial vasculitis include a painful or burning sensation in addition to pruritus, the persistence of individual lesions for longer than 24 hours, and residual pigmentation following resolution. The disorder may be idiopathic, associated with systemic diseases such as systemic lupus erythematosus, or triggered by antigens present in medications or foods. Patients are classified according to serum complement levels, with normocomplementemia associated with a good prognosis and mild systemic involvement. Hypocomplementemic patients are more likely to have multiorgan involvement, including the kidneys, lungs, gastrointestinal tract, and musculoskeletal system. Urticarial vasculitis associated with increased concentrations of monoclonal IgM, bone pain, fever, and weight loss is known as Schnitzler's syndrome.

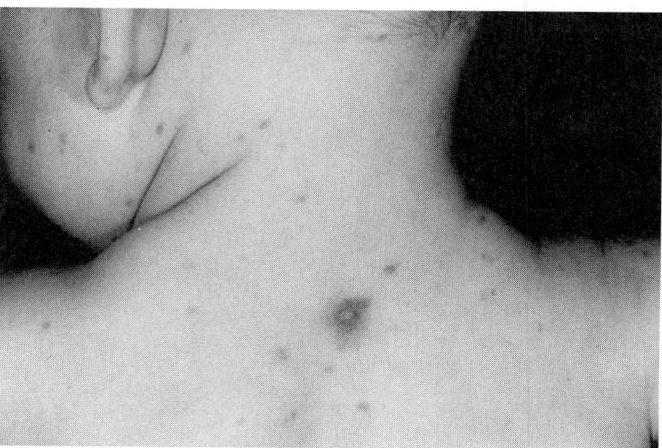

Figure 7. Young child with urticaria pigmentosa. Darier's sign, which is urticaria formation after an individual lesion is scratched, is demonstrated.

Idiopathic Urticaria

More than 80 per cent of chronic urticaria patients fall into this category after extensive evaluations for primary causes. Episodes of idiopathic chronic urticaria can recur for a prolonged period and then resolve suddenly. Repeated episodes can occur years later. Anti-IgE and anti-IgE Fc receptor autoantibodies have been reported in the sera of a few patients with chronic idiopathic urticaria.

PITFALLS IN DIAGNOSIS

Well-performed history taking and physical examination are usually sufficient for making the diagnosis of urticaria. Most forms of acute urticaria are temporally associated with a causative factor that is easily discerned. On the other hand, chronic urticaria is usually idiopathic, and extensive testing often yields negative results. Therefore, unless relevant clinical findings are evident from the history and physical examination, laboratory testing is not indicated. Despite the occasional diagnosis of systemic disorders during the diagnostic evaluation, urticaria is rarely the sole manifestation of a systemic disease. If any clinical characteristics of urticarial vasculitis are present, a skin biopsy is required, because a positive diagnosis changes the prognosis and therapeutic regimen. The differential diagnosis is most important in the patient who presents with angioedema but lacks urticaria. C1-INH deficiency must be considered in these patients. A normal serum C4 concentration excludes C1-INH deficiency, but a decreased serum C4 concentration requires further assessment of antigenic and functional C1-INH concentrations in the serum.

Section Seventeen

SKIN

APPROACH TO SKIN DISORDERS

By Tracy F. Gannon
Minneapolis, Minnesota

Dermatology, unlike other areas of medicine where practitioners have had some exposure to commonly encountered diseases, is a specialty unto itself, with unfamiliar nomenclature and unique diagnostic tools. The skin is the most accessible organ, and clinicians can easily develop a reliable method of approaching and diagnosing the myriad of skin diseases encountered during routine office visits. Although the classic approach to diagnosis begins with the history, the dermatologic assessment first emphasizes the physical examination. This, together with a brief history, often provides adequate information for diagnosing distinctive lesions. The clinician can then decide whether additional information from a general medical examination, a follow-up history, or the use of special diagnostic aids is necessary for generating a differential diagnosis and, ultimately, for selecting the correct diagnosis.

PHYSICAL EXAMINATION

For the skin to be adequately inspected, the patient must be placed on an examination table in a gown with illumination from either natural or overhead fluorescent light. By encouraging this routine, the clinician may find additional lesions to help confirm the diagnosis, and he or she will not miss important incidental lesions. Special areas, such as the scalp, mouth, nails, and plantar surfaces, may need to be examined. The physician must then be ready to look for, not at, the skin changes presented.

Three major characteristics of cutaneous findings are important—distribution, arrangement, and morphology—with the latter by far the most critical. An easy way of organizing these terms is to imagine inspection starting at some distance from the patient, taking in the picture as a whole (distribution), and concluding close up, with the focus on one individual lesion (morphology). The arrangement of lesions is appreciated at an intermediate distance.

Distribution

The distribution of skin lesions is characterized by their extent and location. Regarding extent, are lesions localized, regional, or generalized? Regarding location, are lesions random, symmetrical or asymmetrical, on flexor or extensor surfaces, on exposed or intertriginous areas, or at sites of pressure?

Arrangement

The arrangement is observed by the pattern or relationship of nearby, but not confluent lesions. Examples include scattered discrete, grouped, linear, annular, arcuate, polycyclic, herpetiform, zosteriform, gyrate, and reticulate lesions (Fig. 1).

Morphology

Most importantly, proper classification of the morphology or appearance of an individual lesion is critical to arriving at a correct diagnosis. This process can be viewed as choosing a noun while constructing a descriptive dermatologic sentence. Three classes of lesions (nouns) as well as several additional descriptive terms are listed in Table 1.

Primary Lesion

The primary lesion is the earliest, basic lesion that has not been changed by time or outside forces (see Table 1, part A). This lesion provides the key to accurate interpretation, description, initial orientation, and formulation of a differential diagnosis. The names of primary lesions are based on size.

Secondary Lesion

A secondary lesion is one that has evolved sequentially over the natural course of a disease or was created by scratching or infection (see Table 1, part B). If a secondary lesion is the only type present, the primary disease process must be inferred.

Table 1. Morphologic Terminology of Skin Lesions

A. Primary Lesions	
Less than 1 cm	*Greater than 1 cm*
Macule	Patch
Papule	Plaque
Nodule	Tumor
Wheal	Wheal
Vesicle	Bulla
Pustule	Abscess
Purpura	Ecchymosis
B. Secondary Lesions	
Scale	
Crust	
Erosion	
Ulcer	
Fissure	
Scar	
C. Special Lesions	
Comedo	
Cyst	
Burrow	
Telangiectasia	
D. Descriptive Terms	
Lichenification	
Atrophy	
Sclerosis	
Pigmentation	
Poikiloderma	

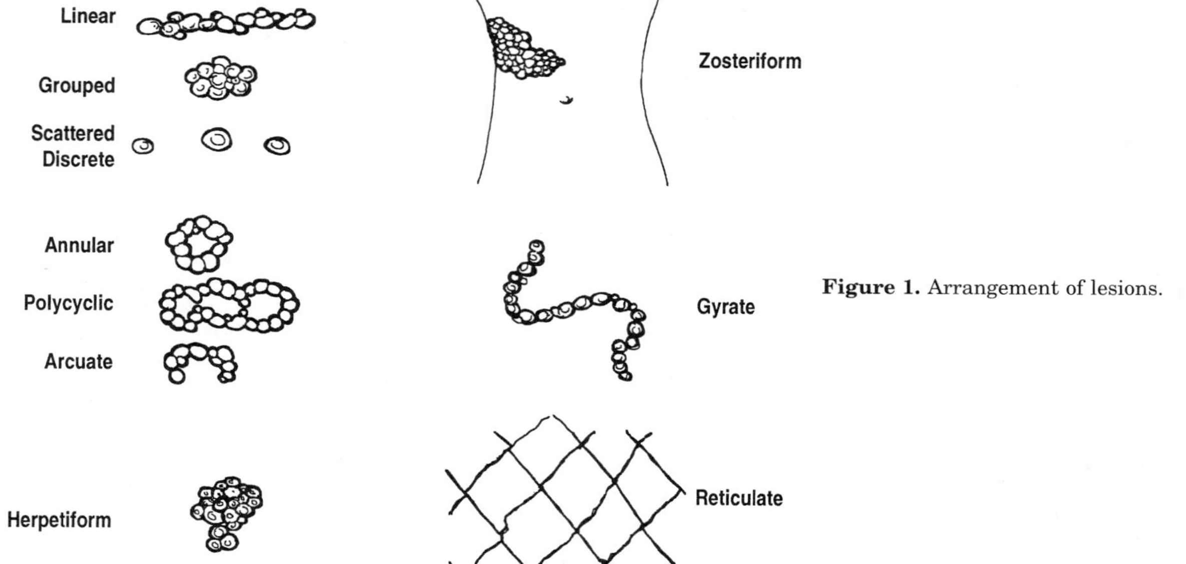

Figure 1. Arrangement of lesions.

Special Lesion

Special lesions have additional structure unique to dermatology (see Table 1, part C).

Descriptive Terms

Descriptive terms denote unusual changes that may accompany or may be superimposed on a primary lesion (see Table 1, part D).

Characteristics

For a description to be complete, several aspects of the primary lesion must be included. These are size, color, configuration, margination, and surface characteristics.

Size

Some estimate of the size of a lesion is implied in the noun chosen for the primary lesion (e.g., macule versus patch, papule versus plaque). The point of demarcation is approximately 1 cm in diameter. An actual measurement of the diameter should be recorded. (Ulcer margins can be traced with a permanent marker onto the top side of a plastic bag, after which the underside touching the ulcer can be discarded, and the drawing added to the chart for later size comparison.)

Color

The basic colors encountered in the skin include red, white, blue, brown, black, and "flesh-colored" or "skin-colored." Additional shades of red or brown plus yellow, orange, violet, and gray may also be observed. The true color is more accurately found at the periphery of a lesion, where secondary changes such as scale or crust are less prominent. "Flesh-colored" lesions must be considered in terms of the patient's own skin color; that is, tan to white in a light-skinned individual versus brown in a dark-skinned individual. Erythema is often hard to appreciate in a dark-skinned individual and may appear violaceous.

Configuration

The outline of a lesion as viewed from above is its configuration. Most lesions are circular. Others are oval or irregularly shaped. All the shapes in Figure 1, depicting the arrangement of multiple, nonconfluent lesions, apply here as well. The difference is that here they represent the shape of one lesion (which may be large due to overlap with adjacent lesions).

Margination

The shape of a lesion as viewed in cross-section, or from the side, is its margination. This term describes the transition zone between lesional and normal skin and is usually referred to as well defined or ill defined. Margination can distinguish papulosquamous from eczematous disease, with the former being well defined, and the latter ill defined. Margination also provides information about the surface contour (Fig. 2). This information can help further

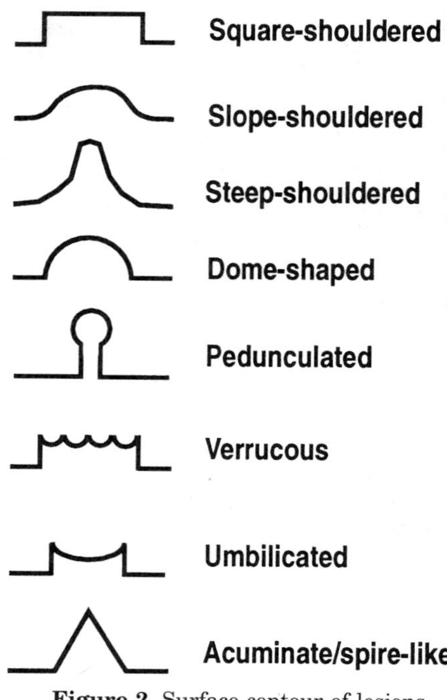

Figure 2. Surface contour of lesions.

delineate the transition zone and may reflect the depth of pathologic change because superficial lesions tend to be "square-shouldered" and deeper lesions tend to be "slope-shouldered."

Surface Characteristics

By palpating the surface of a lesion, the clinician can discern either smooth or rough texture. Roughness occurs from scale or crust. Crust is always visible, whereas scale may or may not be visible. Therefore, roughness without visible change is always due to scale. This distinction is important because scale occurs with hypertrophic disorders (e.g., psoriasis), whereas crust occurs with disruptive disorders (e.g., eczema). A few additional comments about the primary lesion can be added to complete the assessment. These include consistency (soft, firm), temperature (warm, cool), mobility (mobile, fixed), and odor (malodorous).

HISTORY

As noted above, the physical examination often takes precedence over the history in a dermatologic assessment. This prioritization does *not* mean that the history is unimportant. In fact, many clinicians obtain much of the history *during* the physical examination. This preliminary history is comparable to the information that would be obtained from the chief complaint and the history of the present illness. To elicit the chief complaint, an opening inquiry such as, "What can I do for your skin today?" can be asked at the beginning of each examination. Additional questions then follow to fill in the details of the history of the present illness.

These questions should reveal points about the chronology, evolution, symptoms, and treatment of each problem presented. (a) *Chronology*: "When did it start?" "How long has it lasted?" "Has it occurred before?" The chronology concerns the order of events and includes the date of first onset, duration of the present episode, and occurrence of past episodes. (b) *Evolution*: "Where did it start?" "How has it changed?" "What makes it better or worse?" The evolution covers information about the site of onset, the character of the earliest lesion, the pattern of spread, and provocative factors that make the problem better or worse. (c) *Symptoms*: "Is it bothersome?" The most important subjective symptom is the presence or absence of pruritus. Other sensations include pain, burning, tingling, crawling sensation (formication), and dysesthesia. (d) *Treatment*: "What has been used for treatment?" Treatment includes both past and present therapies, and both topical and systemic, as well as prescription and nonprescription medications. Medications not only may cause skin diseases but also can aggravate many others (e.g., perpetuation of an allergic contact dermatitis secondary to treatment with a topical sensitizer, such as bacitracin). This information may also prevent repetitive use of an ineffective medication.

A standard history and physical examination may be sufficient for diagnosis. When the diagnosis remains elusive, however, a follow-up history may be necessary to explore other areas of the traditional medical history, such as past medical history, family history, social history, and review of systems.

Past Medical History

ILLNESSES, OPERATIONS, AND HOSPITALIZATIONS. Concentrate on previous skin disorders and systemic conditions likely to involve the skin (e.g., thyroid, connective tissue, and inflammatory bowel diseases; diabetes; malignancies). The possible role of psychological factors (i.e., depression, anxiety) should also be considered, since they may initiate, exacerbate, or perpetuate many dermatoses.

MEDICATIONS. A complete list of medications must be compiled, including those unrelated to the present skin problem and those recently discontinued.

ALLERGIES. Especially important are drug sensitivities and the recognition of atopy and the atopic triad (asthma, respiratory and/or food allergies, and atopic dermatitis).

HABITS. Include dietary habits, tobacco and alcohol usage, and daily toiletry routine with products used for skin, hair, nails, and so forth.

Family History

Inquire about skin diseases, atopic disorders, and other pertinent medical illnesses in family members.

Social History

The clinician should ask about occupational and recreational exposures and contactants; travel history, including short trips; sexual practices, with attention to risk factors for sexually transmitted diseases; and ethnic traditions, especially attitudes toward disease and treatment.

Review of Systems

Inquire about constitutional symptoms that may indicate acute illness (i.e., fever, headache, nausea) or chronic illness (e.g., fatigue, anorexia, weight loss). Indications of systemic disease, whether or not they are related to the skin lesions, require a complete medical examination, which must precede any special studies.

SPECIAL APPROACHES TO DERMATOLOGIC DISEASE

Many special diagnostic procedures are used in dermatology to confirm a clinical diagnosis or to provide additional information when a diagnosis cannot be made on clinical grounds alone. These approaches may involve the use of clinical tests, laboratory studies, or special instrumentation unique to dermatology.

Clinical Tests

Special Signs

The *Asboe-Hansen sign* refers to the lateral extension of a blister produced after pressure is applied directly over an intact bulla in patients with blistering diseases (e.g., pemphigus vulgaris). *Nikolsky's sign* refers to the extension produced after lateral pressure is applied to a bulla or to normal-appearing adjacent skin in some blistering diseases (e.g., pemphigus vulgaris and toxic epidermal necrolysis). *Auspitz's sign* refers to the appearance of pinpoint hemorrhages from ruptured capillaries when scale is removed from a plaque (e.g., psoriasis). *Darier's sign* refers to the development of a palpable wheal after firm stroking of a macule or papule (e.g., urticaria pigmentosa). The wheal may not appear for 5 to 10 minutes. *Dermatographism*, one of the physical urticarias, refers to the wheal that forms after firm stroking of apparently normal skin. *Fitzpatrick's sign* refers to lateral compression of a papule between the thumb and the index finger causing it to become depressed, or "dimpled" (e.g., dermatofibroma).

Magnification

Magnification of lesions can be accomplished with a simple hand-held magnifying lens (5× to 10×), a hand-held lens to which built-in lighting has been added (10× to 30×), or a binocular microscope (5× to 40×). The latter two improve the visualization of details when used with a drop of oil, which makes the skin more transparent and permits inspection of deeper layers. This technique, called *epiluminescence microscopy*, is especially useful for visualization of telangiectasias in connective tissue diseases, Wickham's striae in lichen planus, and color changes in malignant melanoma and other pigmented skin lesions.

Lighting

Oblique lighting refers to side lighting done in a darkened room to visualize the surface contour of a lesion. By observing the subsequent shadow that is cast, the clinician can appreciate slight degrees of elevation or depression. With *subdued lighting*, low illumination enhances the contrast between hyperpigmented or hypopigmented lesions and the surrounding normal skin.

Wood's Lamp

The Wood's lamp emits ultraviolet light at a wavelength of 360 nm. To see skin contrasts clearly, this lamp should be used in a darkened room. The Wood's lamp is useful to characterize pigmentation and conditions that have characteristic fluorescent patterns. The site of melanin deposition (epidermal versus dermal) can be localized in hyperpigmented lesions. Epidermal lesions become more accentuated (e.g., lentigo, melasma), whereas dermal lesions do not accentuate (e.g., mongolian spot). This distinction is not observed in dark-skinned individuals.

The variation in the lightness of lesions compared with the normal skin color can also be estimated. Hypopigmented lesions are off-white or cream colored (e.g., pityriasis alba), while depigmented lesions are stark white (e.g., vitiligo). This finding applies to all skin types. Detection of fluorescence is useful in certain dermatophytoses, erythrasma, and porphyria. The zoophilic dermatophytes fluoresce a *green to yellow* color on hair shafts. The corynebacteria that cause erythrasma produce a porphyrin that fluoresces a *coral-red* color. The uroporphyrins in the urine of porphyria fluoresce a *pinkish-red* color. Multiple exogenous substances, including lint, dyes, and lipsticks, can also fluoresce in various colors on the skin. The Wood's lamp examination can reveal more widespread involvement than initially appreciated on routine skin examination.

Diascopy

Diascopy refers to the process of compressing a skin lesion (usually with a microscope slide) and observing the changes. All red-to-blue and yellow-brown lesions should be tested. Lesions due to vascular dilatation blanch or disappear with compression and then gradually refill after pressure has been removed. Lesions due to extravasation of blood are nonblanchable (some may blanch slightly), and nonblanchable palpable purpura indicates *vasculitis* until proved otherwise. Many granulomatous diseases have an "apple-jelly" color, which becomes more prominent with diascopy (e.g., sarcoidosis, tuberculosis).

Acetowhitening

Acetowhitening is a test that can enhance the detection of subclinical condylomata acuminata (penile warts). Gauze is soaked with 5 per cent acetic acid (white vinegar) and wrapped around the penis or over the vulva for 5 to 10 minutes. The area is then examined with a magnifying lens for the small, white papules that indicate condylomata. False-positive results can be seen if lesions have been treated in the preceding 3 to 4 weeks with conventional therapies (e.g., cryotherapy, chemical therapy). Under these circumstances, normal components of the skin, altered by treatment, can also appear white.

Patch Testing

Patch tests are used to identify contact allergy (e.g., allergic contact dermatitis). The test involves application of suspect allergens to the skin for 2 days. The patches must be kept dry and undisturbed during that time. The test sites are then inspected for erythema, induration, or vesiculation, (signs of a positive reaction). Standard patch test kits contain a large variety of commonly encountered contact antigens. Direct patch testing with suspect contactants (e.g., clothing, cosmetics, occupational products), known as a *"use test,"* can also be helpful. Use tests are inappropriate for the evaluation of strong industrial or laboratory chemicals, because severe reactions (allergic or irritant) can occur. When patch test results are interpreted, false-positive results may occur if reactions to any tape used for occlusion are read as positive. A positive patch test reaction does not automatically confirm the diagnosis of allergic contact dermatitis. In addition, patients must show improvement in their condition when the suspect allergen is removed from their environment.

Phototesting

In some photosensitivity diseases, phototesting is performed to assess a patient's reaction to various wavelengths of ultraviolet radiation. In general, longer wavelength ultraviolet A (UVA) is more important in these conditions than shorter wavelength ultraviolet B (UVB). Keep in mind that UVA passes through window glass, whereas UVB does not.

A special variant of phototesting involves the use of photopatches *(photopatch testing)*. This test combines the use of the patch test, described earlier, with ultraviolet light. Photopatch testing is helpful in identifying photoallergic contact dermatitis, in which an antigen forms only in the presence of ultraviolet light.

Laboratory Studies

Direct Microscopy

Potassium Hydroxide Preparation

The potassium hydroxide (KOH) preparation is a sensitive and specific test for identifying dermatophytes or hyphae responsible for superficial fungal diseases, pityriasis (tinea) versicolor, and candidiasis. The KOH preparation is the most commonly used microscopic test in dermatology. Scale, pustules, blister roofs, and clippings from hair or nails may be examined, and a rapid diagnosis established. A No. 15 scalpel blade (or the edge of a glass microscope slide) can be used to scrape the edge of a scaling lesion. If the scale has been moistened with either water or an alcohol swab, it sticks to the edge of the blade and can easily be transferred to a microscope slide. One to two drops of 10 per cent KOH is added to the slide, followed by a coverslip. Gentle pressure is applied to the coverslip to disperse air bubbles.

Scale can usually be examined immediately, especially if dimethyl sulfoxide (DMSO) has been added to the KOH. The DMSO helps dissolve the cell walls and thus makes the hyphae more visible. If a blister roof, hair, or nails are being examined, let the preparation sit for 15 to 20 minutes, or heat it gently over an alcohol flame (avoid boiling) to accelerate the clearing process. The specimen is scanned initially under low or medium power with low illumination (turn the condenser down and dim the light source). Bright light obscures the hyphae. The high-power objective is used to confirm the presence of suspected hyphae, which often appear slightly refractile. Both dermatophyte hyphae and candidal pseudohyphae are long, thin, and branching. Therefore, distinguishing between the two can be difficult and may require clinical impression, along with subsequent cultures. Pityriasis versicolor hyphae are short and "stubby," surrounded by clusters of small round spores, termed "spaghetti and meatballs" or "grapes on a branch." Artifacts are often encountered and can be mistaken for hyphae. Cell walls have an irregular linearity; threads are thicker, uniform, and lack branching; and hairs lack branching. Manual compression of the coverslip may break up false lines produced by cell walls.

Tzanck Preparation

The Tzanck preparation (or smear) provides rapid diagnosis of herpesvirus infections, including herpes simplex, herpes zoster, and varicella. The test cannot, however, distinguish between the three. Tzanck preps are also useful in pemphigus vulgaris and in distinguishing between staphylococcal scalded skin syndrome (SSSS) and toxic epidermal necrolysis (TEN). In herpesvirus infections, the roof of a fresh, often umbilicated, vesicle is opened with a No. 15 scalpel blade. The base is gently scraped, and the fluid is smeared onto a microscope slide, air-dried, alcohol-fixed, and then stained, according to standard methods, with Giemsa or Wright's stain. Examination under low or medium power demonstrates multinucleated giant cells with deep purple-blue cytoplasm. In pemphigus vulgaris, rounded acantholytic cells are seen, with cytoplasmic contents concentrated at the periphery. In staphylococcal SSS, broad epithelial cells without accompanying inflammation are observed, while TEN produces inflammation plus cuboidal cells with a higher nuclear-to-cytoplasmic ratios.

Mineral Oil Preparation

The mineral oil preparation can facilitate the immediate diagnosis of scabies. The preferred lesion for clinical study is the linear burrow, but an unexcoriated papule or vesicle will suffice. The adult female scabies mite *(Sarcoptes scabeii)* is found in a subcorneal location on finger webs or anterior wrists and in intertriginous areas, such as the male genitalia. A No. 15 scalpel blade is coated with mineral oil (so the skin adheres to the blade) and scraped vigorously over a suspicious lesion. Anesthesia is not necessary. Fine bleeding demonstrates that the proper depth has been reached. The specimen is then transferred to a microscope slide, covered, and examined under low power for mites, eggs, or feces. Potassium hydroxide, if used instead of mineral oil, dissolves the feces.

Gram Stain

Both bacteria and candida can be identified with the Gram stain, which is prepared according to standard methods outlined in microbiology texts. Gram stain is most useful in the setting of a blistering or pustular dermatosis (e.g., *Staphylococcus aureus* in bullous impetigo or *Candida albicans* in candidiasis). Intact lesions must be examined, because a previously ruptured vesicle or pustule may be contaminated with surface bacteria. For similar reasons, superficial crusts and medications should first be removed from erosive or ulcerative lesions.

Darkfield Examination

Darkfield examination is useful for early diagnosis of syphilis; this test may be positive even when sensitive serologic tests are not. Most physicians are not equipped to perform this microscopic examination in the office. However, if a specimen is collected for evaluation, an adequate amount of serous fluid must be obtained from the lesion (usually a genital ulcer). The clinician may need to perform an initial curetting, followed by compression of the lesion between gloved fingers. The serous fluid is touched to a coverslip, which is diluted with a drop of saline on a microscope slide. The specimen must be examined immediately; if left to dry, it cannot be interpreted. Specimens from the oral cavity must be read with caution, because spirochetes resembling *Treponema pallidum* are present in the normal oral flora.

Cultures

Many organisms that are initially identified with direct microscopy can be confirmed and further characterized by culture. Although cultures for bacteria and fungi are most commonly requested, the availability of cultures for viruses (e.g., herpesviruses) has increased in recent years.

Bacterial and Atypical Mycobacterial Cultures

Material for bacterial culture is best obtained from intact vesicles, bullae, or pustules. Lesions are opened with sterile technique and swabbed or aspirated with a needle. If crusts are present, they should be lifted first so that the underlying exudate is sampled. Skin biopsy specimens can be cultured after mincing the tissue in a sterile mortar; this procedure is especially useful for mycobacteria, which are difficult to grow from a swab of exudate. Some atypical mycobacteria grow only at room temperature, and the laboratory must be informed if these organisms are included in the differential diagnosis. Cellulitis cannot be easily cultured. Injection and then aspiration of the lesion with nonbacteriostatic saline generally produces a low yield. Needle punctures through diseased skin are easily contaminated, and cultures obtained in such a manner must be interpreted with caution.

Fungal Cultures

Both superficial (dermatophyte) and deep (systemic) fungi can be cultured. For dermatophytes, samples of scale, nails, or plucked hairs are collected and implanted in Sabouraud's and Mycosel media. Cultures often require 3 to 4 weeks of incubation for positive identification. They are most useful for confirming an equivocal KOH examination or for diagnosing tinea capitis (where the KOH preparation is difficult to interpret), or when systemic antifungal medication is required (e.g., onychomycosis). For systemic fungal infections, minced tissue from a skin biopsy is preferred. *Candida* species can be cultured from a swab sample (i.e., exudate from a pustule) and identified in a few days, but *Pityrosporum* species cannot be easily cultured in the microbiology laboratory.

Viral Cultures

Cultures for the herpesviruses are easily obtained by swabbing the base of a suspected vesicle or erosion. Herpes simplex grows out in 2 to 3 days, while herpes zoster takes as long as 14 days.

Other Studies

Many other available studies can assist in the diagnosis, ranging from routine laboratory tests to the more sophisticated imaging studies. Each should be considered and ordered as indicated.

Skin Biopsy

Correlation of the clinical findings with histopathologic changes is often necessary for reaching a dermatologic diagnosis. The skin is easily accessible for three types of biopsy: shave, punch, and ellipse. All are performed after cleansing the site with alcohol and infiltrating with a local anesthetic. Most routine office procedures are done in a clean, rather than sterile, setting. Timing and site are critical factors for a successful biopsy. Early lesions (less than 24 hours old) are usually preferred for diseases involving immune complex deposition, while older lesions (2 to 6 weeks old) are better for granulomatous processes. Biopsies are typically obtained from the center of a lesion, except for blistering disorders, annular eruptions, or ulcers, where a sample from the border or advancing edge is indicated.

The shave biopsy is usually reserved for elevated lesions confined to superficial portions of the skin where little bleeding or scarring occurs. It is often performed with a thin razor blade bent into an arc, and the lesion is shaved off with a back-and-forth "sawing" motion. This method leaves a base that is more "flush" with the surrounding skin than that left by a No. 15 scalpel blade. Hemostasis is obtained with a chemical cauterant (e.g., Monsel's solution or aluminum chloride) or with light electrocautery. This method should *never* be used if melanoma is suspected, because the depth of the lesion is essential for prognosis.

The punch biopsy is used for lesions extending into the deep dermis or subcutaneous tissues. A small, cylindrical knife, usually 3 or 4 mm in diameter (but available in sizes from 2 to 8 mm), is rotated between the thumb and the index finger over taut skin. The specimen is then held gently with forceps while the base is cut with a scissors at the level of the fat. Crushing of the specimen must be avoided to prevent tissue disruption. Hemostasis is achieved with a chemical cauterant, by packing the defect with absorbable gelatin (Gelfoam), or by suturing. Sutures are used for any defect 4 mm or more in diameter to reduce scarring.

The elliptical biopsy is excisional and is used whenever the lesion involves the deep dermis or fat, where a punch biopsy is unlikely to provide a specimen sufficient for diagnosis. Using a No. 15 scalpel blade held perpendicular to the skin (to avoid beveling the edges), the clinician cuts a fusiform or "football-shaped" incision around the lesion, with a length-to-width ratio of 3 to 1. Undermining may be necessary for reducing skin tension. Sutures are used for closure, producing a fine, linear scar.

After the biopsy has been obtained, the appropriate diagnostic tests must be ordered. Part of the tissue may be used for cultures, but most often it will be sent for light microscopy, immunofluorescence, electron microscopy, or special staining. For routine histologic processing and most special stains, the specimen is placed in 10 per cent formalin. For immunofluorescence, the sample must be immediately snap-frozen or placed in a special buffered transport medium. If electron microscopy is required, the specimen is placed in buffered glutaraldehyde. Immunofluorescence testing is especially useful in the diagnosis of blistering diseases and lupus erythematosus. Both direct tests and indirect tests are available for detecting autoantibodies associated with these conditions. Electron microscopy is indicated less often, but is helpful in several uncommon disorders, such as histiocytosis X and epidermolysis bullosa.

DERMATITIS

By Elizabeth F. Sherertz, M.D.,
and Christine J. Hashem, M.D.
Winston-Salem, North Carolina

Dermatitis refers to inflamed skin. The term is overused as a diagnostic label because "dermatitis" says little about the underlying process or about the signs and symptoms an individual patient may have. The term eczema is also confusing because it is sometimes used interchangeably with dermatitis to refer to any skin inflammation and is sometimes used to specify atopic dermatitis. It is important to try to determine the nature and contributing factor or factors of the dermatitis in any one patient to provide optimal patient management as well as effective education about the prevention of recurrence and prognosis. By far, the history and physical examination are the key factors in the correct diagnosis of the common types of dermatitis.

SEBORRHEIC DERMATITIS

Seborrheic dermatitis is a common erythematous scaling condition that occurs in infants and adults. Typically, the scalp and areas around the ears are involved, and there is often extension to the central portion of the face. In patients with human immunodeficiency virus (HIV) infection, seborrheic dermatitis may be severe and can be an early clinical finding.

Clinical Symptoms and Signs

Infantile seborrheic dermatitis generally presents between 2 weeks and 6 months of age. Patches of greasy, yellow-brown, adherent scale are often seen in the scalp, and there may be erythema extending to the face around the ears. Erythema without much scale may occur in flexural folds of the neck, axillae, and groin, and thus seborrheic dermatitis is in the differential diagnosis of diaper dermatitis. The absence of pruritus helps distinguish seborrheic dermatitis from atopic dermatitis in this age group.

Adult seborrheic dermatitis may develop indolently, initially being considered "bad dandruff," or may have an abrupt, florid onset of bright erythema and greasy fine scale of the eyebrows, central face, beard area, and scalp. In the more acute form, involvement of the presternal area and flexural areas may occur. Patients usually complain of itching scalp and the appearance of scaling and/or redness. In African American patients, hypopigmentation may develop at the inflamed sites on the face.

Course

Infantile seborrhea usually clears by the age of 2 years. Adult seborrheic dermatitis has a variable course with a tendency toward chronicity and recurrence. Some patients note improvement in the warmer months and exacerbation in the winter. Other patients report flares temporally related to psychological or physical stress. Effective topical therapy can significantly improve the pruritus and clinical signs in most patients.

Variants and Complications

Patchy involvement of only the scalp or facial areas is a common variant of seborrheic dermatitis in both children and adults. An acute onset can mimic contact dermatitis or a photodermatitis, but history and distribution are helpful. Involvement of the eyelids (seborrheic blepharitis) and copresentation with acne rosacea in adults may occur. There is some clinical overlap between seborrheic dermatitis and psoriasis. A family history should be taken, and a skin examination for signs of psoriasis should be performed. In seborrheic dermatitis, there are no associated nail changes, and lesions are typically not found on the extremities. If scratching or attempting to remove scale is vigorous, secondary bacterial infection, especially with *Staphylococcus aureus* or group A streptococci, may occur. Likewise, removal of adherent scalp scale may cause a reversible, nonscarring alopecia. Ear involvement with secondary infection may trigger otitis externa.

Infantile seborrheic dermatitis that is not responsive to therapy should be distinguished from atopic dermatitis, Leiner's disease or Letterer-Siwe disease. In an adult with severe seborrheic dermatitis, risk factors for infection with HIV should be assessed. Diagnosis of seborrheic dermatitis is based almost wholly on the clinical constellation of signs and symptoms. Skin biopsy may be supportive of the diagnosis but is not specific. Laboratory studies are not routinely necessary.

ATOPIC DERMATITIS

Atopic dermatitis is one of the most common skin disorders in infants and children, affecting 10 to 15 per cent of the childhood population. It is a chronic, relapsing disease that begins at a young age and is characterized by a number of different morphologic lesions. It is frequently associated with a personal and/or family history of atopic dermatitis, childhood-onset asthma, or environmental allergies with resulting allergic rhinitis (this constellation is sometimes referred to as the atopic history).

Clinical Symptoms and Signs

The primary complaint of patients who have atopic dermatitis is itching, and subsequent scratching leads to the typical appearance and distribution of skin lesions. The results of repeated scratching and rubbing include ill-defined thickened patches and plaques, with exaggerated skin markings (lichenification). Excoriations and areas of weeping and crusting may occur. The exact morphologic features vary, depending on the age of the patient and the stage of presentation.

The infantile form of atopic dermatitis begins between 2 and 6 months of age. It is characterized by intense itching, erythema, scattered papules and scaling plus or minus crusting. At this age, it often begins at the sites most accessible to scratching: the face, scalp, and extensor surfaces of the extremities. Characteristic flexural involvement of the antecubital and popliteal fossae begins to appear at about 18 months of age.

Signs of atopic dermatitis may first be brought to medical attention in children between the ages of 4 and 10 years. These patients tend to have more chronic, lichenified lesions. Dry, circumscribed, thick, scaling patches are often seen on the wrists, the ankles, flexural surfaces, the posterior aspect of the thighs, and the buttocks. The soles of the feet may be involved, with peeling that may mimic a fungal infection. Superficial excoriations and discrete, thickened hyperkeratotic nodules (prurigo nodules) may develop as the result of significant pruritus. Vesicular finger and foot dermatitis may occur. Areas where there has been active inflammation may become hypo- or hyperpigmented, which is particularly noticeable in darker skin.

In addition to the skin findings already outlined, several associated clinical features support a diagnosis of atopic dermatitis. An extra infraorbital eyelid fold, termed Dennie-Morgan fold, suggests atopy. Dry skin, hyperlinear palms, keratosis pilaris (sandpaper-like dry follicular papules typically on the upper arms or thighs), and ichthyosis vulgaris (fishscale-like dry skin, especially on the lower extremities) can also be associated with atopic dermatitis. Atopic patients may have a lower threshold to pruritic stimuli, such as rough clothing fibers (e.g., wool).

Course

As patients become educated about their skin, and control scratching and avoid external trigger factors, the skin findings associated with atopic dermatitis often improve or resolve. However, these individuals persist in having atopy and sensitive, reactive skin. A small percentage of individuals may not experience an initial outbreak of atopic dermatitis until after age 30 years. Eczematous lesions may develop where the skin becomes dry or irritated by materials coming into contact with the skin. In adults, atopic dermatitis is often exacerbated by irritant contact exposures, such as frequent exposure to water or detergent, chemicals, or solvents, or low environmental humidity. Topical skin care products and cosmetics may irritate the skin. Thus, in adults, lesions of atopic dermatitis develop most often on the hands and arms with contact exposures or on the face with cosmetic exposures. It is important to recognize occupational aggravation of atopic dermatitis so that accommodation in the workplace can take place.

Variants and Complications

The major clinical variable that affects the management of atopic dermatitis is recognition and treatment of secondary bacterial infection. Such infection (usually *S. aureus* plus or minus group A beta-hemolytic streptococci) triggers acute flares of lesions, and bright erythema, vesicles, pustules, crusting, and occasionally cellulitis may develop. Strong evidence exists for the use of antibiotics in treating flares of atopic dermatitis. Herpes simplex infections can spread cutaneously in patients with atopic dermatitis, leading to eczema herpeticum, with characteristic grouped, umbilicated vesicles and punched-out erosions. Varicella tends to be severe and can become secondarily infected with *S. aureus,* which may lead to extensive bullous lesions. The diagnosis of these viral infections is supported by the clinical examination and the finding of multinucleated giant epithelial cells on a Tzanck smear of an intact vesicle. Viral culture can confirm the diagnosis.

Contact dermatitis from topical medications, repeated wet-dry-wet exposures, skin care products, or other irritants is another common complication of atopic dermatitis. External contactants must be considered, particularly if an adult patient with a history of atopy experiences worsening or persistent dermatitis, especially involving the hands.

Immediate contact urticaria from latex (e.g., rubber gloves) is recognized as a possible life-threatening complication in atopic patients and must be considered if a patient has a history of urticaria, angioedema, or anaphylaxis after a medical or dental procedure involving latex gloves or devices. In its most extreme form, atopic dermatitis may evolve into a generalized exfoliative erythroderma.

Diagnostic Procedures

The diagnosis of atopic dermatitis is made primarily on the basis of the aggregate of the history and clinical signs and symptoms. Laboratory tests usually are not needed except in the case of an atypical presentation or a confounding disorder. An increased serum IgE concentration may occur but is not a major diagnostic finding. The routine use of skin testing is not advocated for atopic dermatitis. In some situations, an oral double-blind, placebo-controlled food challenge may be useful to investigate dietary exacerbations of atopic dermatitis. Allergic contact dermatitis due to specific allergens can be confirmed by skin patch tests. Contact urticaria from latex can be confirmed by careful interpretation of skin prick tests or radioallergosorbent (RAST) tests. Skin biopsy results of atopic dermatitis lesions are often nonspecific.

CONTACT DERMATITIS

Contact dermatitis is the term used for inflamed skin resulting from external contactants. The two broad categories of contact dermatitis are *irritant* contact dermatitis, in which a substance or exposure causes direct damage to the skin without prior immunologic sensitization, and *allergic* contact dermatitis, in which an external contactant triggers immunologic events that lead to inflammation at the sites of skin contact.

Clinical Symptoms and Signs

Failure to consider a contact exposure as the cause of dermatitis is the most important obstacle to making the correct diagnosis. The history of contact exposure may be obvious in some cases, but other presentations may require a high index of suspicion. For example, a history of poison ivy or poison oak exposure on a weekend followed several days later by an acute, streaky, erythematous and vesicular eruption at exposed sites is straightforward. However, recurrent vesicular hand dermatitis when a patient claims there is "nothing new" or that he or she "has changed everything" can make clinical diagnosis of a specific contactant difficult. Irritant or allergic contact dermatitis should be included in the differential diagnosis for any patient with dermatitis, and any topical agent should be "suspect." The most common skin irritants and allergens are listed in Table 1. Often, a patient gives a history of more than one topical exposure and at certain sites (especially eyelids, face, and hands), mixed irritant and allergic contact factors may contribute to the dermatitis. Because there is such overlap, it may be difficult to distinguish irritant from allergic contact dermatitis on clinical grounds alone.

Table 1. Common Irritants and Allergens That May Cause Contact Dermatitis

Irritants	Comments
Water Soap and detergents Housecleaning products Solvents Chemicals Mechanical friction Cutting oils Plant and animal products	Especially with frequent or recurrent contact
Allergens	**Comments**
Poison ivy, poison oak	Even minimal contact could trigger dermatitis
Nickel	Jewelry, metal in skin contact >3 minutes
Fragrance	Cosmetics, skin care products, airborne particles
Preservatives	
Quaternium 15 Imidazolidinyl urea Methylchloroisothiazolinone Methylisothiazolinone	Cosmetics and skin care products/biocides
Rubber ingredients	Gloves, shoe insoles, make-up sponges
Formaldehyde	Multiple industrial uses
Paraphenylenediamine	Hair dyes
Epoxy	Adhesives, glues
Neomycin, bacitracin	Topical antibiotic creams or drops

Irritant Contact Dermatitis

Individual susceptibility to irritants varies; however, irritants affect everyone. It is known that atopic individuals with dermatitis, for example, are more susceptible to irritant reactions. The clinical presentation of irritant reactions varies from patient to patient, based on the chemical involved, any underlying inflammation or sensitivity of a patient's skin, the site of exposure, and the length of exposure time. Irritant contact dermatitis may result from acute exposure to irritating agents, such as acids and alkalis, or may result from cumulative damage from less toxic agents.

Affected sites are those in contact with the suspected chemical irritant, but objective findings of severity vary, based on the factors mentioned previously. Frequently affected sites include the face and dorsum of the hands. Palms and soles are relatively less affected because of the thick protective stratum corneum. An irritant reaction usually occurs minutes to hours after initial exposure. Acute contact can result in erythema, edema, and vesiculation resembling a chemical burn. A "dripping" effect where the dermatitis follows the path of gravitational forces of poured liquid may be seen. Burning or stinging sensations are often felt acutely.

Cumulative exposure to a less caustic irritant typically produces a more chronic picture of hyperkeratosis, fissuring, and lichenification. These chronic lesions can be indistinguishable from chronic allergic contact dermatitis. Patch testing is warranted to determine if there is an allergic component, especially when the hands and feet are chronically affected. Acute cases of irritant contact dermatitis are usually diagnosed by history and physical findings. Crusting and purulent drainage may signify secondary infection and should be treated accordingly. The differential diagnosis includes allergic contact dermatitis and atopic dermatitis.

Allergic Contact Dermatitis

Only certain individuals experience allergic contact dermatitis. It is a specific, immunologically mediated response. Allergy can develop to products that the patient has been using for years. Therefore, a thorough history must be sought, including the use of over-the-counter creams, make-up products, fragrances, fabrics, topical medications such as neomycin or benzocaine as well as work exposure, including chemicals and rubber.

The clinical appearance of allergic contact dermatitis may vary, depending on the site of involvement and the duration of the problem. The initial reaction is often delayed until several days after exposure, unlike irritant contact dermatitis, which may arise within minutes to hours of the inciting event. Pruritus is a common complaint. Erythema, edema, and vesiculation are often prominent in the acute phase. On sites such as the eyelids and genitals, vesiculation may be less prominent than edema. Conversely, chronic allergic contact dermatitis is marked by lichenification, scaling, and overlying fissuring with or without small papulovesicles. When a patient first seeks medical attention at the chronic stage, clinical diagnosis alone is more difficult.

The intensity of the allergic response may be different bilaterally despite a similar exposure history; thus, lesions may not be symmetric (e.g., glove or shoe contact dermatitis). However, the most important clue to the diagnosis of allergic contact dermatitis is often the distribution of lesions. The most severe reaction tends to be where exposure to the allergen is greatest. There are notable exceptions to this, however, because body sites differ in their responsiveness to allergens. A classic example is eyelid dermatitis resulting from nail cosmetics. The fingertips themselves are relatively nonreactive to the nail polish, but when it is transferred to the eyelids by rubbing the eyes, for example, it may cause an allergic contact dermatitis. Allergens can also be transferred via air currents, leading to dermatitis on exposed sites such as the face and arms (e.g., fragrance, epoxy).

Course

The course of contact dermatitis depends on the nature and type of exposure, the accurate recognition of the contactants, and the ability to prevent future skin contact through avoidance and protective clothing, when applicable.

Variants and Complications

Once a dermatitis develops, particularly if it is chronic, the inflamed skin is prone to further damage from otherwise "harmless" contactants such as water or certain topical ingredients. This can complicate and frustrate attempts at specific diagnosis and management. Secondary bacterial infection, most often due to *S. aureus* plus or minus group A beta-hemolytic streptococci, can develop in cracked, fissured sites, leading to impetigo or cellulitis. Certain contactants cause a reaction only in combination with ultraviolet light, causing a photocontact dermatitis. There can be variable penetration of allergens depending on heat, sweat, and body site; thus, the clinical lesions may be seasonal or patchy.

Diagnostic Procedures

A high index of suspicion is necessary to make the diagnosis of contact dermatitis. Skin biopsy is not useful to differentiate irritant from allergic contact dermatitis and usually cannot distinguish contact dermatitis from other types of dermatitis. The diagnosis of irritant contact dermatitis is made strictly on clinical grounds with a compatible history and physical examination. When allergic contact dermatitis is suspected clinically, patch testing to look for delayed-type hypersensitivity reactions to specific standardized cutaneous allergens is a useful confirmatory tool. Patch testing is performed primarily by dermatologists, since proper patient selection, test application, and interpretation of results for relevance to the active dermatitis are key points in the value of this test. Patch testing should not be used to test unknown substances, or in nonstandardized concentrations, because false-positive or false-negative results can occur. Radioallergosorbent, scratch, and prick tests are not useful for the diagnosis of allergic contact dermatitis. Diagnostic trials of avoidance of suspected contactants are occasionally useful in clearing a dermatitis without concomitant therapy, but failure of a dermatitis to clear does not confirm that the avoided product is harmless. Repeated open application tests or "use" tests, in which a suspected substance is applied to normal skin in a manner similar to usual skin exposure (e.g., lotion applied twice daily to the skin of the upper arm) is sometimes useful to reproduce an allergic dermatitis. Use tests should be carried out only with products known to be nonirritating when left on the skin (e.g., lotions, topical medications, *not* soaps or solvents). Because this method only "narrows down" the culprit without identifying a specific allergen, it is not a substitute for patch tests.

OCCUPATIONAL DERMATITIS

A working definition of occupational dermatitis is "any skin disorder that would not have been present had the affected person not been involved in the current work environment." As indicated in the section on atopic dermatitis, some dermatoses can be aggravated by the workplace, such as situations in which pre-existing dermatitis develops at new sites compatible with workplace exposure or significantly worsens at those sites.

Clinical Signs and Symptoms

The majority of occupational dermatitis is contact dermatitis. The clinical diagnostic features of contact dermatitis were summarized previously. Determining the link between the occupation and the dermatitis requires insight into the workplace tasks and exposures as well as experience in the evaluation of contact dermatitis. Table 2 summarizes points in the history and examination that support an occupational cause for a dermatitis. As with other contact dermatitis, changes in types of exposures or "new" exposures are not necessary for dermatitis to develop, even in a long-standing employee. Frequent, repeated, or cumulative exposure to low-grade irritants may lead to the eventual development of dermatitis. Documentation of more

Table 2. Clues to an Occupational Cause of a Dermatitis

Clinical appearance of a contact dermatitis
Workplace exposures to potential skin irritants or allergens
Body sites involved with dermatitis are consistent with exposure during job
Temporal relationship between exposure and onset of dermatitis
Improvement of dermatitis away from work exposure to the suspected irritant or allergen
In patients with pre-existing dermatitis, occurrence of dermatitis at new body sites that would be exposed during work or worsening of dermatitis at those sites coincident with work exposures

than one employee having a similar dermatitis is suggestive of an irritant contact dermatitis or, less likely, a strong cutaneous allergen. Common environmental exposures should not be overlooked as sources of occupational dermatitis, especially poison ivy and poison oak or sunburn dermatitis in outdoor workers.

Course

The recognition of contributing factors and modification of workplace exposures are important in determining the course of occupational dermatitis. Certain irritant allergens (e.g., epoxy) and occupations (e.g., hairdressers, machinists) are associated more often with chronic dermatitis, even with avoidance measures.

PHOTODERMATITIS

The term photodermatitis can generally be defined as an abnormal response to ultraviolet radiation in which skin inflammation develops or as a pre-existing dermatitis that worsens. Photodermatoses can be divided broadly into four categories: acquired idiopathic photodermatoses, phototoxicity or photosensitization by exogenous drugs or chemicals, genetic-metabolic photodermatoses, and pre-existing dermatoses exacerbated by ultraviolet radiation.

Clinical Symptoms and Signs

Patients with suspected photodermatitis are evaluated by a careful history determining current medication, topical plants and products that may have been in contact with the skin, the time course of the eruption in relation to sun exposure, affected sites, and family history. The classic distribution of a photodermatitis involves the face—sparing the upper eyelids and the shaded areas of nasolabial creases—the area under the nose, and beneath the chin. Exposed areas of the neck, especially the "V" area of the sternoclavicular notch, are often involved. Depending on clothing, the outer surfaces of the arms, backs of hands, and tops of the feet may be involved. Some photoeruptions can extend to sites that had been covered by clothing.

Diagnostic Procedures

The findings from the clinical history and physical examination of a photodermatitis can narrow the alternative diagnostic possibilities without the need for further confirmatory studies. However, laboratory tests, including an antinuclear antibody (ANA) screen, anti-SSA (Ro), and anti-SSB (La), can help exclude subacute cutaneous lupus. Urinary, stool, and/or blood porphyrin concentrations are useful to exclude porphyria cutanea tarda, variegate porphyria, and erythematosus, phototoxic reactions, or other photodermatoses. Photopatch tests, photosensitivity (minimal erythema dose) testing, and tests for solar urticaria are reserved for use in specific circumstances in which screening diagnostic studies have been unrevealing.

Acquired Idiopathic Photodermatoses

Polymorphous light eruption is the most common photodermatosis. It is characterized by nonscarring, pruritic, erythematous papules-vesicles that appear on light-exposed skin within hours of ultraviolet exposure. In any one patient, the lesions are morphologically similar and in similar locations. Lesions develop over a period of hours to days and usually resolve within a week if further sun exposure is avoided. The process may be intermittent, typically occuring in the spring or with an initial period of sun exposure to a site, such as the chest, after a period of little exposure. Polymorphous light eruption occurs more often in females, with onset before the age of 30 years, and a familial incidence can occur.

The diagnosis of polymorphous light eruption is based primarily on the history and the morphologic features and distribution of the lesions. However, other light-sensitive conditions must be excluded.

Photodermatitis Caused by Topical Agents

As with contact dermatitis, certain materials react with ultraviolet light to cause a direct irritant or toxic effect on the skin. Most commonly this occurs with plants containing furocoumarins or natural psoralens, such as figs or juice or peel from limes. The resulting phototoxic dermatitis is usually a mildly symptomatic, streaky, irregular burn at the sites of plant contact, occurring within hours; the lesions may gradually become hyperpigmented. The extremities are involved most often. A history of being outdoors among such plants or squeezing fresh limes in the sunshine is helpful. Some perfume ingredients can cause a similar eruption if the sites to which the perfume is applied are subsequently exposed to the sun, but this is not commonly seen today. Coal tar derivatives that come into contact with skin can also cause a toxic burn reaction with ultraviolet exposure, termed tar smarts.

The second type of photocontact dermatitis is a photoallergic type, in which a substance becomes allergenic when placed on the skin and then exposed to light. Photoallergic dermatitis is usually intensely pruritic, with an eczematous papulovesicular, weeping, edematous appearance in a photodistribution pattern. It may develop rather indolently or abruptly. Among the more common culprits for photoallergic contact dermatitis are fragrance or aftershave containing musk ambrette, airborne material from the chrysanthemum family of plants and, ironically, sunscreen ingredients such as benzophenones and methoxycinnamates. The history of exposure, physical examination, and a modified form of patch testing with allergen-skin exposure to ultraviolet light (photopatch testing) can be performed to confirm the diagnosis.

Photodermatitis Caused by Systemic Agents

A review of oral medications should also be carried out with any patient suspected of having a photodermatitis. The morphologic features and distribution of a drug-induced photodermatitis are similar to the phototoxic and photoallergic contact reactions described earlier. The duration of medication use prior to the onset of a photodermatitis can vary from days to years, depending on ultraviolet exposure to other factors, so, once again, the culprit may not be a "new" drug.

Drugs causing phototoxic (exaggerated sunburn) reactions include tetracycline, doxycycline, phenothiazines, amiodarone, oral contraceptives, oral psoralens, and some nonsteroidal anti-inflammatory drugs. Examples of photosensitizing (immunologic reaction) medications include thiazides, sulfonamides, nonsteroidal agents (e.g., piroxicam), and tricyclic antidepressants. Certain drugs cause specific clinical eruptions. For example, some nonsteroidal agents have triggered lesions similar to porphyria, and hydralazine and procainamide are known to induce lupus erythematosus (usually with minimal skin involvement). Most photodrug eruptions clear in several days to weeks after the triggering agent is discontinued. The history, clinical course, and physical examination help distinguish drug eruptions secondary to ultraviolet radiation from other primary photodermatoses.

Genetic-Metabolic Photodermatoses

The diverse group of metabolic or heritable disorders associated with photodistribution of skin eruption includes porphyrias, disorders of DNA repair (e.g., xeroderma pigmentosum), and Hartnup disease. The signs and symptoms referable to the skin can occur from early childhood to adulthood. The important clinical history includes familial incidence, exacerbating factors, time course and morphologic features of skin eruptions, and medication use. The porphyrias, as an example of metabolic photodermatoses, are disorders due to either inherited or acquired enzymatic deficiencies of heme synthesis. The most common porphyria associated with skin findings is porphyria cutanea tarda. Cutaneous lesions are primarily noninflamed vesicles and bullae on light-exposed areas, especially on the dorsal aspect of the hands and forearms and on the cheeks. Skin fragility, erosions, and milia with scarring of the bullae are also prominent features. The scarring may resemble scleroderma, and hypertrichosis at involved sites can also develop. Adult onset is most typical and may be triggered by estrogen, iron, or ethanol intake in susceptible individuals. The clinical course consists of intermittent skin eruptions that are often exacerbated by sunlight or ingested drugs.

Pre-existing Dermatoses Exacerbated by Ultraviolet Light

Atopic dermatitis, some types of contact dermatitis, and occasionally psoriasis are among the dermatoses that may worsen with sun exposure. Other skin conditions, such as vitiligo, may be prone to sunburn because of the lack of functional melanocytes. In other situations, such as any inflammatory dermatoses in a dark-skinned individual, sun exposure during the healing phase may exacerbate the appearance of postinflammatory hyperpigmentation. Because protection from the sun is regularly stressed to many patients with skin diseases, patients with photodermatitis must be questioned about sunscreen use. Sunscreen ingredients in addition to para-aminobenzoic acid (PABA) have been implicated in sunscreen photodermatitis.

EXFOLIATIVE DERMATITIS

Exfoliative dermatitis is a descriptive term for a generalized eruption characterized by erythema and overlying scale. The onset can be abrupt, over days to weeks, as from a drug eruption, or can be a progression of some chronic papulosquamous disorders, such as psoriasis and atopic dermatitis. Rarely, a nonspecific exfoliative dermatitis may herald an internal malignancy.

When an exfoliative dermatitis becomes generalized, the nonspecific appearance may make precise clinical diagnosis difficult. The history of the site of initial involvement and subsequent spread may be useful. For example, psoriasis may begin on the scalp, and contact dermatitis may have a specific pattern early on that becomes obscured as the process extends. Predominance of involvement at some sites, such as a thick "candle-dipped" appearance of hyperkeratosis on palms and soles accompanied by skipped areas of normal skin, can help a dermatologist diagnose pityriasis rubra pilaris. A history of medication use is important. Anticonvulsants, allopurinol, trimethoprim-sulfamethoxazole, diuretics, calcium channel blockers (e.g., diltiazem), and angiotensin-converting enzyme (ACE) inhibitors (e.g., captopril) are examples of medicines that can cause exfoliative erythroderma. An atopic history (eczema, hay fever, asthma) and use of topical products can provide insight about contributing factors. With extensive exfoliative dermatitis, the clinical involvement can include secondary nonscarring hair loss, nail dystrophy, and palm-sole desquamation. Mucous membranes are usually spared. Patients with exfoliative erythroderma may have difficulty with temperature regulation (e.g., they may not mount a febrile response and are easily chilled). Resting tachycardia, dependent edema, and generalized lymphadenopathy can occur.

The course and prognosis of exfoliative dermatitis depend largely on the underlying process. Identifying a drug reaction and changing therapy usually lead to gradual (over weeks to months) improvement. Primary skin diseases, such as psoriasis or atopic dermatitis, that become erythrodermic can be managed but usually do not clear totally. In about one third of cases, a specific underlying cause may not be identifiable. These patients tend to have a prolonged course.

Breakdown of the skin barrier and fissuring may provide entry for organisms, and secondary bacterial impetigo or cellulitis may occur. Lack of fever and the camouflage effect of the baseline erythema may hinder clinical diagnosis of cellulitis or even sepsis. Hemodynamic instability with high-output cardiac failure and heat and fluid loss may also occur. An "exfoliative enteropathy" of diarrhea and malabsorption rarely occurs. Skin biopsy of exfoliative dermatitis is often nonspecific, but it may be helpful in revealing the primary pathologic process, especially if the biopsy is performed early in the course or at a previously untreated site. Otherwise, screening laboratory studies are not routinely performed for diagnosis.

COMMON BACTERIAL AND FUNGAL INFECTIONS OF THE INTEGUMENT

By Steven M. Hacker, M.D.
Boca Raton, Florida

The skin has many natural mechanisms enabling it to protect itself from the bacterial and fungal environment to which it is so often exposed. Particularly, an intact stratum corneum, rapid epidermal turnover, skin surface lipids, and skin surface pH all contribute to natural resistance and consequently aid in protection against potential pathogens. Additionally, the resident and transient flora that harmlessly colonize skin can in some instances protect it. Normal skin flora, for example, may release protein-complex antibiotics (bacteriocins) that act antagonistically toward potential pathogens.

INFECTIONS DUE TO BACTERIA

Furunculosis

A furuncle, or boil, is an acute perifollicular staphylococcal abscess of the skin and subcutaneous tissue. Carbuncles represent interconnected furuncles that drain through a number of points in the skin surface. The exact pathogenesis is unknown. Typically, a furuncle forms around a hair follicle or sebaceous gland. The most common cause of furuncles is either an ingrown hair or an obstructed sebaceous gland resulting in the growth of coagulase-positive *Staphylococcus aureus.*

Typically, the patient presents with complaints of a tender, inflamed "sore," "boil," or "pimple." A furuncle is an indurated, dull red nodule with a central purulent core that may be fluctuant. A carbuncle appears similar, although it is typically larger, more painful, and has multiple drainage sites overlying it. Furuncles occur most commonly on the nape, face, buttocks, thighs, perineum, breast, and axillae. Carbuncles favor these sites but tend to occur in thicker skin, allowing for lateral extension of the abscess. The diagnosis is based on clinical appearance and history. Purulent material should be cultured from all lesions. The differential diagnosis may include acne conglobata and folliculitis, but separating these diagnoses is in general fairly straightforward.

Typically, a furuncle ruptures spontaneously, discharges pus, and slowly decreases in redness and edema over 1 to 2 weeks. However, the more persistent lesions typically are seen by the physician. They often require treatment for relief of symptoms and prevention of uncommon complications. A furuncle is a focus of bacterial infection; therefore, bacteremic spread at any time is a possibility, resulting in sepsis, endocarditis, or osteomyelitis. Probably the most bothersome complication is recurrent furunculosis. With this disorder, painful red lesions can recur for years.

Factors that predispose an individual to furunculosis include poor hygiene, occupational exposure to grease or oil, infection of pre-existing dermatoses, malnutrition, alcoholism, and underlying immunosuppression. Recurrent furunculosis is a common problem that is often difficult to treat. The mainstay of prevention includes avoidance of irritants and diligent hygiene with the use of strong antibacterial soaps such as chlorhexidine gluconate. In patients carrying *S. aureus,* treatment of the carriage site (nasal vestibule in most cases) has been reported to be effective. Treatment includes the use of topically applied mupirocin (Bactroban) several times daily to the carriage site.

Impetigo

Impetigo occurs in a nonbullous form, with thick golden crusts, as well as a bullous form. The nonbullous form is also referred to as impetigo contagiosa. Impetigo is seen in all age groups, although it represents one of the most common pediatric infections of the skin. The nonbullous form of impetigo can be caused by either *S. aureus* or group A beta-hemolytic streptococci. The bullous form, however, appears to be caused primarily by *S. aureus.* Specifically, in this disorder, the bullae may be toxin-induced lesions resulting from the group II phage 71 strain of *S. aureus.* This strain has also been associated with neonatal bullous impetigo, staphylococcal scalded skin syndrome, and staphylococcal scarlet fever.

In nonbullous impetigo, lesions begin as small superficial vesicles that either fill with pus or develop a crusting with a golden honey color. On removal of the crust, the undersurface appears smooth, red, and slightly exudative. Occasionally, a halo of erythema surrounds these lesions. Common sites of involvement include the exposed surface where minor trauma, insect bites, abrasions, and contact dermatitis can occur. Pain is usually absent and pruritus is mild. In bullous impetigo, lesions start as small vesicles and enlarge to form bullae. The bullae typically rupture in 1 to 2 days, leaving a thin, varnishlike crust. These lesions can occur anywhere on the body.

The diagnosis of impetigo is based on clinical presentation with laboratory confirmation. Laboratory evaluation includes a Gram stain and culture of an early lesion or undersurface of crust. Impetigo can resolve spontaneously without antibiotics but the course is typically prolonged. A serious complication of nonbullous impetigo is acute glomerulonephritis (AGN). This may be seen when streptococci are implicated as a pathogen in this disorder. The incidence of AGN varies from 2 to 15 per cent, depending on the strain of *Streptococcus.* Acute glomerulonephritis is a complication most commonly seen in children younger than 6 years of age, and treatment of impetigo does not alter the risk for the development of AGN. Bullous impetigo is not associated with AGN. Other disorders associated with streptococcal skin infections include scarlet fever, lymphangitis, erysipelas, and cellulitis. Rheumatic fever has not been reported following nonbullous impetigo. The most serious complications of bullous impetigo occur in neonates in whom bacteremia, pneumonia, and meningitis have been reported.

Cellulitis

Cellulitis is a diffuse suppurative inflammatory process involving the subcutaneous tissue. The most common causes of cellulitis are beta-hemolytic streptococci and *S. aureus.* However, in patients with underlying immunosuppression or diabetes, atypical organisms such as gram-negative bacilli and cryptococci have been implicated as causative agents. The most common scenario is that of a preceding wound, trauma, or stasis dermatitis that is followed by erythema and warmth over the course of the following 1 to 2 days.

The affected area is characterized by red, hot, tender, and edematous skin. The redness can be distinguished from normal-appearing skin and is often used to judge clinical response. The causative organism has been recovered by skin biopsy, blood culture, or aspiration of the leading edge. However, these diagnostic maneuvers tend to be inconsistent and unreliable.

Cellulitis is typically responsive to systemic antibiotic therapy. As the disease responds to therapy, the redness, swelling, and pain diminish. Also, the systemic symptoms of malaise, fever, and chills dissipate with appropriate treatment. Uncommon complications include gangrene, metastatic abscess, and sepsis. These complications are seen more frequently in immunocompromised patients or very young children. In older patients, involvement of the lower extremity can be complicated by thrombophlebitis.

Folliculitis

Folliculitis refers to inflammation and infection that involves the hair follicle. Most commonly, it is bacterial in origin. However, fungal and dermatophytic infection can also involve the hair follicle. Typically, folliculitis is classified according to the depth of hair follicle involvement and the causative organism.

Superficial folliculitis is caused by coagulase-positive *S. aureus.* As the name suggests, it involves the superficial aspects of the hair follicle. The clinical diagnosis is confirmed on culturing and Gram staining of a pustule. Clinically, this disorder presents as fine, small, superficial pustules centered around the orifice of a hair follicle. A terminal hair may project through the dome-shaped pustule. The disease may resolve spontaneously; however, patients often complain of "itchy" recurrent "pimples" on hair-bearing areas. This group of patients benefits most from therapy, and empirical topical antibiotics can be effective at accelerating the clearing process.

Gram-negative folliculitis is a form of folliculitis that may be either deep or superficial. The superficial form typically presents with pustules in the paranasal area. The deep form presents with nodulocystic lesions. Gram-negative folliculitis most often occurs as a superinfection in a patient who has received long-term antibiotics for acne vulgaris. Cultures of lesions often reveal *Klebsiella* or *Enterobacter* in the superficial variant and *Proteus* in the deeper variant. Only topical antibiotics may be required in the superficial variant, whereas systemic antibiotics such as ampicillin-clavulanate, trimethoprim-sulfamethoxazole, or ciprofloxacin may be necessary in the deeper variant. In severe recalcitrant cases, the treatment of choice is isotretinoin.

Paronychia

Paronychia refers to inflammation of the nail folds, and pyonychia refers to pyoderma involving the paronychium. The presence of a potential space surrounding the nail fold provides an excellent setting for infection. Minor trauma that results in a break of the skin is often sufficient to allow infection to occur. The most common bacteria causing acute paronychia include staphylococci, beta-hemolytic streptococci, and gram-negative enteric bacteria. Chronic paronychia is a separate entity that is usually caused by *Candida* species. It is frequently seen in hands that are repeatedly exposed to or submersed in water.

The diagnosis is apparent and therefore based on clinical grounds. The paronychium is typically inflamed, red, tender, and sore. Pus may be seen either through the nail or at the paronychial fold. Often, gentle pressure on the tender paronychium expresses pus from the affected area. The distal edge of the finger pad and paronychium is usually spared. The disorder tends to occur over the course of a few days. Resolution may proceed spontaneously within a few days. However, if the inflammation persists and progresses to involve the nail matrix, permanent nail dystrophy can result.

INFECTIONS DUE TO DERMATOPHYTES (SUPERFICIAL FUNGI)

Dermatophytes are superficial fungi that appear to have a "keratinophilic" capacity and consequently colonize the stratum corneum of the epidermis, nails, and hair. Taxonomically, three genera are recognized: *Microsporum, Trichophyton,* and *Epidermophyton.* Ecologically, these species are further classified based on their preferred location: geophilia (found in the soil), zoophilia (found in association with domestic and wild animals), and anthrophilia (found in association with human beings).

Tinea Versicolor

Tinea versicolor is a chronic, recurrent, scaly dermatophytic infection characterized by scaly, hypo-, and hyperpigmented macules usually located on the upper torso and proximal extremities. It is caused by *Pityrosporum orbiculare* (formerly known as *Malassezia furfur*), a dimorphic, lipophilic dermatophyte that is often found as a nonpathogen on normal skin. Under appropriate conditions, it becomes a pathogenic yeast responsible for the signs and symptoms of the disorder. It therefore represents an opportunistic infection when favorable factors such as a warm, humid environment; Cushing's disease; immunosuppression; malnourishment; and inherited predisposition are present.

Clinical infection most commonly presents with papulosquamous lesions. Less common presentations include folliculitis and inverse tinea versicolor. The papulosquamous lesions are often fawn-colored or hypo- or hyperpigmented. They are oval to guttate in shape and often have a dustlike superficial scale adherent to them. The scale can be produced by light scraping of the fingernail over the involved area. This diagnostic maneuver has been referred to as "the fingernail sign" or coup d'angle. The term versicolor is derived from the color variation seen among the lesions, particularly the white to reddish brown to fawn-colored. The variation in color is accentuated by the presence or absence of tan. Pruritus is mild or absent.

The diagnosis is established by scraping a lesion and examining it with a KOH preparation. Easily identifiable, short, stubby hyphae and clusters of round spores are seen yielding the so-called franks and beans or spaghetti and meatball appearance. Typically, tinea versicolor is recurrent and chronic despite treatment. No serious complications occur except the cosmetic debilitation that some patients endure with severe outbreaks.

Tinea and Onychomycosis

Tinea corporis represents dermatophytic infections involving glabrous skin, with the exception of the palms, soles, and the groin. The three most common causative organisms are *Trichophyton rubrum, Microsporum canis,* and *Trichophyton mentagrophytes.* Tinea manum is a dermatophytic infection of the palmar and interdigital areas of the hand. *T. rubrum* produces a dry, hyperkeratotic pattern on the hands. *T. mentagrophytes* may produce a vesicular pattern. Tinea pedis is a dermatophytic infection of the feet. *T. rubrum, T. mentagrophytes,* and *Epidermophyton floccosum* are the most common causes. The chronic intertriginous type is seen most frequently and is characterized by fissuring, scaling, and maceration often involving the lateral toe webs.

Tinea cruris is a dermatophytosis involving the groin area and includes infection of the genitals, pubic area, and perineal and perianal skin. This infection occurs more commonly in the summer months. The most common organisms are *E. floccosum, T. rubrum,* and *T. mentagrophytes.* The disease occurs almost exclusively as a male dermatophytosis, whereas candidiasis, a yeast infection, affects both sexes. In men, candidiasis is distinguished by a greater incidence of obvious scrotal involvement with the presence of satellite pustules. Tinea cruris has more extensive involvement of the medial thigh.

Onychomycosis includes all infections of the nail caused by any fungus, including nondermatophytes and yeast. Four main clinical types are recognized: (1) distal subungual onychomycosis, (2) proximal subungual onychomycosis, (3) white superficial onychomycosis, and (4) candidal onychomycosis.

Tinea infection can be transmitted by direct contact with other infected individuals or by infected animals or fomites. Typically, the initial pathogenic sequence is invasion of the stratum corneum in the presence of moist, humid, occlusive conditions. The host epidermis attempts to shed the organism by increasing the epidermal turnover rate. This defense mechanism probably accounts for the clearing of the center of the annular lesion. The most common presentation is the typical annular lesion with an active, erythematous, vesicular border. The patient often complains of scaly, itchy lesions. Typically, tinea infection gradually progresses to involve a greater surface area. Without treatment, the disorder becomes chronic. Serious complications from this infection are rare, but recurrences are common.

The diagnosis is confirmed by obtaining a scraping of the leading edge of the scaly plaque. The scraped scale is placed on a slide with KOH. This preparation reveals septate, branching hyphae in the stratum corneum. A fungal culture can also be performed. Commonly used media include Sabouraud's dermatophyte test medium (DTM). The latter is simple to interpret because the phenol indicator turns the agar red in the presence of dermatophytes.

Tinea capitis is a dermatophyte that involves the scalp, typically occurring in children. In the 1950s and 1960s, the most common cause was the fluorescent *Microsporum audouinii.* The most common cause today is the nonfluorescent, endothrix variety produced by *Trichophyton tonsurans.* The infection is spread easily among family members, classmates, and infants. Arthroconidia have been isolated from couches, pillows, sheets, combs and brushes. These fomites have been implicated in person-to-person transmission. Scalp colonization has led to the persistence of this infection as 30 per cent of asymptomatic adults and 25 per cent of asymptomatic children may harbor this fungus.

The appearance of tinea capitis may be either inflammatory or noninflammatory. The noninflammatory type can present without scale and minimal hair loss. The inflammatory type is more typical and can present with pustules, abscesses, hair loss, and scaling. A boggy, intense, suppurative mass is often found, representing a severe inflammatory reaction referred to as kerion. Additionally, autoeczematization (id) reactions may occur. They typically present as pinhead papules on the neck or upper torso. Cervical lymphadenopathy is often palpable.

The diagnosis is made by scraping the affected area, particularly that under a dried yellow crust (scutulum). The KOH preparation typically reveals endothrix arthroconidia within dystrophic hair shafts. Culture of the hair and scrapings should be performed to confirm the diagnosis. Typically, the disease is responsive to oral antifungal therapy. Recurrences may occur. Complications are rare.

FLIES, LICE, MITES, AND BITES

By Larry E. Millikan, M.D.
New Orleans, Louisiana

Within the broad category of arthropod bites and infestations are a number of signs and symptoms reflecting the multifold causes of such a condition. Organisms included in this group include flying, crawling, and biting arachnids and insects, as well as other mites and lice that live in close contact with their human hosts. The signs and symptoms are variable in presentation. Involvement of exposed areas of the skin is related largely to flying insects, environmental arachnids, and other insects. The pattern is confined primarily to the exposed areas. In contrast, other smaller organisms that are in a more intimate relationship with the host include various types of mites and lice. This category includes tropical rat mites, bird mites, and sarcoptic mites (including *Cheyletiella*) that are acquired from their animal hosts after close contact with the host. Under these circumstances, the bites may appear on both the exposed and the covered areas of the skin. Several categories of lice (including body lice, crab lice, and head lice) cause pathologic conditions of the skin. With careful examination, the lice or their eggs may be seen on or in the skin, on hair (nits), or in clothing seams (body lice). Mites can occur in the home (e.g., bird mites and rat mites) and result in a more chronic exposure. Scabies infestation is also a chronic condition that is related to hygiene, crowding, and transfer from one person to another.

The single most common presenting sign in this vast array of arthropod-caused disease is pruritus. The amount of pruritus can be variable and is related to the host's immune status. With human scabies, for example, the initial exposure may be subtle and asymptomatic, but subsequent exposures after host immunity has become apparent causes severe pruritus, resulting in the scabies mite being called the itch mite. Subsequent exposures to Hymenoptera, Diptera, and *Solenopsis* after the patient has become sensitized result in pruritic urticarial or burning reactions around the site of the bite. In very sensitive patients, urticaria and angioedema can occur as complications, and invariably pruritus is an important presenting sign. The source of the disorder can often be elucidated by a careful history and a careful examination to determine the distribution (exposed versus nonexposed skin); association of outdoor, indoor, or intimate exposure; and a history of symptoms or lack thereof in persons having intimate contact with the patient. Patients who present acutely after a single exposure reveal much to the careful observer regarding bite sites (i.e., whether they are single or multiple) and the distribution of the findings (i.e., whether they are limited to the site of the bite or are present with peripheral signs and symptoms). After a single exposure, spontaneous resolution is typical, and in a patient with subsequent reactions, appropriate questioning helps patients recall previous exposures, allowing the physician to pinpoint probable causes.

In contrast to an acute first reaction, subsequent episodes usually result in increasing urticaria around the site of the bite (as a manifestation of IgE reactions to the venom) or expanding skin involvement from secondary infection, autoeczematization, or other mechanisms. Common, easily diagnosed examples of acute cases include *Solenopsis* (fire ant) in which grouped pustular lesions are the sequelae of exposure to mounds or hills of these ants. Diagnosis is usually not a problem; the patient rapidly becomes aware of the bites and after the initial sting, the pustular reactions are characteristic. The bite of certain deer flies (Tabanidae) causes obvious urticarial reactions around the site of the bite and can cause severe angioedema in bites around the face. Also included in this group of arthropod-related reactions are the characteristic but uncommon reactions to various caterpillars resulting from contact with the stinging hairs. Typically, an immediate intense urticarial reaction occurs with burning and stinging sensations. Acute reactions may be prolonged in the hypersensitive host, but those in the naive host usually resolve spontaneously and promptly.

Chronic, recurring lesions are sometimes confused with various types of urticaria. Several arthropod agents have been implicated in these situations, but perhaps the most common are mites and various types of lice (see earlier). The reactions observed in chronic syndromes are largely eczematous, but sometimes the hypersensitive patient experiences urticaria and edema.

COMMON COMPLICATIONS

Perhaps the most significant dermatologic complication with widespread pruritic disorders from various arthropods is secondary infection. Scabies has been reported to cause secondary infection and recurrent outbreaks of *Streptococcus*-associated disease such as glomerulonephritis. With more virulent and antibiotic-resistant organisms, the additional risk of severe life-threatening bacterial infections must now be anticipated. In various infestations, especially those presenting with pruritus and eczematization, autoeczematization is a significant risk and mandates early treatment to prevent widespread extension of the disease beyond the areas of infestation with possible systemic complications. This again requires early and expectant therapy.

Of particular interest are the complications due to various arachnid bites (spiders, ticks, and certain mites). Perhaps the best known of the arachnid bites is the syndrome associated with envenomation from *Loxosceles reclusa.* This spider, also known as the brown recluse spider, has become a familiar problem, especially in the Mississippi, Missouri, and Ohio River valleys of the United States. Complications from these bites include tissue necrosis and bulla formation, followed by signs of systemic involvement that include a coagulopathy (sometimes with disseminated intravascular coagulation), hemolysis, and myolysis. If a large amount of venom is injected, renal damage requiring dialysis can ensue. The venom of the black widow spider (*Latrodectus mactans*) is associated with autonomic changes, and those at greatest risk are the very young and the hypertensive elderly in whom a hypertensive crisis or severe hypotension can be precipitated by the bite. Complications from tick bites are mostly infectious, and include Lyme borreliosis and the rickettsiae (see articles on Lyme disease and the Rickettsia). In patients at risk, anticipation of these infections is important and testing and early therapy are crucial.

PHYSICAL EXAMINATION

The pattern of the signs and symptoms is the key to the evaluation, and primary distribution of skin lesions relates to whether the offending agent is a flying insect, an arachnid, or a mite. The clinical picture may well relate to the sensitivity of the host; for example, patients with Diptera bites or Hymenoptera stings and hypersensitivity can present with impressive urticarial reactions. Fire ant bites begin as painful erythematous, edematous papules that subsequently develop into pustules. The exposure is usually obvious to the patient, and diagnosis is not difficult.

On the covered areas of the body where the migration is stopped by elastic clothing, mites such as *Eutrombicula* (chiggers) show a characteristic pattern. The distribution of scabies on the hands can also be an important clue in addition to the typical periareolar and periumbilical distributions. The presence of burrows can also be observed by the discerning examiner. Patients with compromised immunity (especially acquired immunodeficiency syndrome [AIDS] patients or the elderly) can acquire Norwegian scabies, characterized by widespread disease with heavy infestation of mites and an atypical distribution. The more typical distribution of cutaneous lesions from mites and lice involves primarily the covered areas of the body.

USEFUL DIAGNOSTIC STUDIES

Few laboratory tests are useful in these cutaneous disorders. An exception is the hematologic tests used to evaluate possible coagulopathy in patients with *Loxosceles* envenomation, including prothrombin time, partial thromboplastin time, and fibrin split products. The patient should also be evaluated for proteinuria, hemoglobinuria, myoglobinuria, and signs and symptoms of deep tissue necrosis and underlying myolysis. Increased IgE concentrations can be observed in the serum of patients with exaggerated urticarial responses to various arthropod bites and stings. No imaging procedures are diagnostically useful in these disorders.

SKIN TUMORS

By Scott W. Fosko, M.D.,
and Neal S. Penneys, M.D., Ph.D.
St. Louis, Missouri

Cancer of the skin is categorized as nonmelanoma and melanoma. The former consists primarily of basal cell carcinoma (BCC) and squamous cell carcinoma (SCC). Although nonmelanoma skin cancer (NMSC) is usually locally confined, it may result in extensive local morbidity and infrequent metastases. Nearly 1 million new cases of skin cancer will be diagnosed in 1996. Most of these lesions will be categorized as basal cell and squamous cell carcinomas. This volume exceeds the incidence of cancers of the lung, breast, colon, rectum, prostate, bladder and all lymphomas combined. The incidence of NMSC is similar in magnitude to that of the total incidence of all noncutaneous malignancies.

The incidence of melanoma is also increasing significantly. It was projected that in 1995, 34,000 cases would be diagnosed. Unlike nonmelanoma, melanoma has a significant mortality rate, and it is projected that nearly 7300 deaths will occur primarily in men. This accounts for 1.3 per cent of all deaths due to cancer. Melanoma accounts for 5 per cent of all skin cancers but 75 per cent of deaths from skin cancer. Melanoma is the most common cancer in people aged 25 to 29 years and is second to breast cancer in women aged 30 to 34 years. In 1935, 1 of 1500 individuals was diagnosed with melanoma. In the year 2000, it is estimated that 1 of every 75 individuals will be diagnosed with melanoma.

ETIOLOGY

The cause of skin cancer is strongly linked to ultraviolet radiation exposure. Ultraviolet B (290 to 320 nm) plays a role in cutaneous carcinogenesis, and recent data support a role for longer wavelength ultraviolet radiation, ultraviolet A (320 to 400 nm), as well. The role of ultraviolet radiation in cutaneous carcinogenesis is supported by both the anatomic distribution of these carcinomas and the increased incidence seen in populations closer to the equator.

Genetic influences also play a role, as seen in individuals with xeroderma pigmentosum and the nevoid basal cell nevus syndrome. In xeroderma pigmentosum, individuals acquire both NMSC and melanoma at an early age. In xeroderma pigmentosum, patients are unable to repair ultraviolet-induced thymidine dimers in DNA. Nevoid basal cell nevus syndrome often presents with multiple BCCs in sun-exposed areas in young individuals and is also associated with other organ involvement, especially bone.

Exogenous factors also play a role, especially with SCC. It is known that NMSC can develop in scars, chronically draining ulcers and sinuses, and radiation-damaged skin. Exposure to arsenic in medicaments; well water; pesticides; and the mining, sheep dipping, and smelting industries has also been reported to play a role in SCC. Human papillomavirus has been associated with cutaneous SCCs, primarily of the genital region but also of the periungual area. With the increasing incidence of organ transplantation and the use of immunosuppressive agents, these individuals often present with numerous wartlike lesions that can progress to SCC. These individuals have a much greater incidence of nonmelanoma and melanoma skin cancers and may die at an early age from metastatic disease.

BASAL CELL CARCINOMA

Clinical Diagnosis

BCC is the most common skin cancer and the most common cancer of all types. It occurs most often in individuals older than 60 years of age, but there is an increasing incidence in younger individuals. BCC occurs most frequently on the head and neck, with the nose being the most common site on the face. Several clinical and histologic variants of BCC exist. Nodular BCC, previously called "rodent ulcer," is the most common subtype of BCC. Usually, the lesion is translucent and pink to pearly and often has overlying telangiectasias. At times the lesions may be pigmented and brownish. These lesions often grow slowly but with time may ulcerate, bleed, or become secondarily infected. Superficial multicentric BCC is seen more commonly on the trunk and extremities. This lesion is often red to brown, flat, and slightly scaly, and at times has an expanding, rolled border. These lesions can mimic dermatitis or dermatophyte infection. One of the more difficult BCCs to recognize is the morpheaform or sclerosing BCC. This tumor has a distinctive histologic appearance but can be subtle clinically. At times, there is minimal skin change, only a subtle, scarredlike, porcelain-to-white change. Textural changes and firmness may be present. Often, the patient presents with a history of an "enlarging scar," without a history of trauma or prior surgery to the area. A less common variant of BCC is cystic BCC. Clinically, these lesions mimic a nodular BCC, but on close examination a cystic component is noted. The color may vary from white to pink. Micronodular BCC represents another unique histopathologic variant and can present clinically as a flat, firm, translucent, ill-defined plaque. Finally, fibroepithelioma of Pinkus is an infrequently seen BCC that also has striking histologic features. Most commonly, it presents as flat, pink to fleshy-colored thin plaques on the lower back. At times, they may be slightly raised and pedunculated.

Several reports have described BCCs with aggressive growth characteristics. The histologic extent of these tumors is much greater than the apparent clinical involvement. Often, they contain morpheaform and micronodular histopathologic patterns. Young individuals may be more predisposed to these aggressive BCCs, with the upper lip a frequent site in women. These tumors must be managed aggressively because they are often extensive and have a high propensity for recurrence with conventional modes of treatment.

Evaluation

Basal cell carcinoma rarely metastasizes. Despite this, BCC may be locally extensive and result in significant morbidity because of local invasion and destruction of underlying and adjacent tissue structures. This is especially true of BCCs of the central face, which includes the perinasal, periocular, periauricular, and perioral regions. A clear understanding of why tumors in this location extend is lacking; however, histopathologic evaluation has documented their aggressive nature.

Less than 1 per cent of BCCs metastasize. Metastasis most commonly occurs in the context of recurrent BCCs. Although the majority of metastatic BCCs are from large, grossly obvious lesions, small lesions have also been reported to metastasize. The most common metastatic sites are the primary draining regional lymph node basins, followed by the lung. Physical examination should focus on defining the local extent of the tumor clinically, with a thorough lymph node examination for higher risk lesions.

Procedural Diagnosis

Cutaneous carcinomas are easily accessible to rapid diagnosis through skin biopsies. For superficial and nodular-type BCCs, shave biopsies may provide adequate tissue for diagnosis. For micronodular and morpheaform BCCs, the pathology may be deeper, and a punch biopsy may be more appropriate. This procedure is easily performed in an outpatient setting with the patient under local anesthesia and has minimal morbidity. The clinician must understand the nature of the cutaneous lesion and provide the appropriate biopsy of that lesion.

SQUAMOUS CELL CARCINOMA

SCC is the second most common NMSC. Unlike BCC, SCC has a much greater propensity to metastasize, with 4 per cent on average (reported range, 0.5 to 16 per cent) of cutaneous SCCs having evidence of metastasis at the time of initial presentation. The metastatic rate is influenced by causative factors; lesion size, location, and duration; histopathologic depth of invasion; degree of differentiation; and the presence of perineural invasion.

Diagnosis

SCC also presents with a variety of clinical and histopathologic subtypes. Unlike BCC, a precursor lesion exists for SCC, which is called actinic keratosis. These lesions are most commonly seen in fair-complexioned individuals of Celtic descent, occur in sun-exposed areas, and are characterized by a gritty, scaly papule. At times they may be inflamed and slightly red or may even have a variable amount of brownish pigmentary change. The rate of malignant transformation is widely debated and previously was reported in the range of 5 to 20 per cent. More recent studies estimate the risk to be much less at 1 per 1000 cases per year. For an individual with a single lesion, the risk of SCC would be low. However, in a person with numerous actinic keratoses, the risk of malignant degeneration is greater, and these patients need to be managed aggressively and with close regular follow-up.

SCC may be confined to the epidermal layer. This is called SCC in situ or Bowen's disease. SCC in situ is clinically similar to actinic keratosis but may have greater scale and thickness and more erythema. Squamous cell carcinoma in situ involving the glans penis is also called erythroplasia of Queyrat. It can have less scale and can be a smooth, red-brown, thin plaque. It is important to recognize that SCC in situ can also extend deeply into the appendage structures, especially hair follicles, which may extend into the subcutis (fat). This must be kept in mind when managing the patient. In addition, when serial sections are performed in SCC in situ, a focus of invasive carcinoma may be seen in the dermis.

SCC most commonly presents as erythematous to pink nodules and plaques. The pearly, translucent, and superficial telangiectasias often seen with BCC are usually lacking. Ulceration may occur. SCC can also develop in chronic ulcers and prior sites of trauma, such as burns and osteomyelitis, as well as in areas of radiation dermatitis. Clinically, SCC may have a more rapid growth pattern than that of BCC.

One subset of SCC is verrucous carcinoma. This carcinoma is a well-differentiated SCC and goes by one of three names, depending on the tumor's location. Lesions of the oral cavity are called oral-florid papillomatosis; anogenital lesions are giant condyloma of Buschke-Löwenstein; and those of the lower extremity, especially the foot, are epithelioma cuniculatum. Histopathologically, these can be difficult to diagnose because the SCC is well differentiated. Despite an indolent clinical appearance, they also have an ability to metastasize.

A clinical and histopathologic challenge distinguishes SCC from pseudoepitheliomatous hyperplasia. The latter is a reactive proliferation of the epidermis that is secondary to either inflammatory processes or infections. Separating these two entities can be difficult.

Less frequently seen variants of SCC include spindle cell SCC (reported to have an increased incidence of perineural invasion and more aggressive clinical behavior), clear cell carcinoma, adenosquamous cell carcinoma, and signet ring SCC.

Keratoacanthoma is considered by some to be a well-differentiated SCC, and by others to be a benign, self-limited lesion. It has the striking clinical presentation of rapid onset over several days to weeks, forming a large, crater-filled papule or nodule. The lesion may become large and can be locally destructive, especially in the central face. After rapid evolution, there is a period of stable growth followed by resolution in some cases. Certain histopathologic features assist in making the diagnosis of a keratoacanthoma, but differentiation from SCC is not always possible. An incisional or excisional biopsy is required to demonstrate the entire architecture of the lesion, a feature that is important in making this diagnosis. Several reports of keratoacanthoma metastasizing suggest that some of these lesions were indeed SCC initially. We consider keratoacanthoma to be a well-differentiated SCC, and it should be treated as such.

Evaluation

Patients with SCC need a thorough clinical evaluation. This includes examination of the draining regional lymph nodes. After lymph node involvement, the second most common site of involvement is the lung. Risk factors for SCCs with a greater likelihood of metastases include a tumor located on the lip, ear, dorsum of the hand, or genitals. Other risk factors include recurrent lesions, known perineural involvement, immunosuppression, depth of invasion of the SCC (Breslow's depth), and degree of differentiation, with poorly differentiated lesions having a higher propensity to metastasize. Individuals who have features of high-risk SCCs should be considered for diagnostic imaging because clinical examination is not as sensitive, especially for lymph nodes of the head and neck region. In addition, a chest film should be considered.

Procedural Diagnosis

A proper biopsy for SCC is imperative for accurate diagnosis. For suspected invasion, tissue samples to the level of the subcutis must be provided. Incisional, excisional, or deep-punch biopsies are employed. In clinical situations in which the clinician is considering keratoacanthoma, pseudoepitheliomatous hyperplasia, or SCC of the verrucous carcinoma subtype, adequate representative sampling is required because the histopathologic diagnosis is dependent on the amount of tissue examined. Incisional or excisional biopsies should be employed.

MELANOMA

Melanoma is a malignant proliferation of melanocytes and may be in situ or invasive. It is most commonly seen in adults with a mean age at presentation of 50 years, but children can also be affected. Risk factors for the development of melanoma include a fair complexion (blond to red hair, blue eyes), a history of childhood blistering sunburns, the inability to tan, atypical nevocellular nevi, a congenital nevocellular nevus, or a first-degree relative with melanoma. A higher socioeconomic status is also a risk factor, probably as a result of outdoor vacations with intense sun exposure. An individual with a history of melanoma has an approximately 5 per cent risk of acquiring a second primary melanoma. Darkly pigmented individuals are at less risk for melanoma overall but are more likely to acquire melanoma in an acral location. A genetic link in the development of melanoma has recently been identified at chromosome 9. Individuals and family members with this mutation are at increased risk for the development of melanoma. The mortality rate from melanoma is increasing faster than that from any other cancer. Women have a lower mortality rate, which may be related to more frequent self-examination.

Diagnosis

The most common forms of melanoma are superficial spreading melanoma (including melanoma in situ), nodular melanoma, lentigo maligna melanoma, and acral-lentiginous melanoma. Superficial spreading melanoma accounts for 70 per cent of all melanomas and most commonly occurs on the upper trunk in men and on the legs of women. Lentigo maligna melanoma makes up 4 to 10 per cent of melanomas and occurs on chronically sun-exposed skin of elderly patients, arising from a lentigo maligna (a form of melanoma in situ). Clinically, lentigo maligna grows and progresses slowly. Lentigo maligna melanoma represents the development of an invasive component within a lentigo maligna. Once an invasive component develops in lentigo maligna, its prognosis is similar to that of other melanomas based on the depth of invasion (Breslow's depth). Acral-lentiginous melanoma accounts for 2 to 8 per cent of melanomas and is usually found on the palms, soles, and nail beds. It occurs more commonly in darkly pigmented individuals such as African Americans and Asians than in white individuals. Nodular melanoma grows rapidly and accounts for 15 to 30 per cent of melanomas. This melanoma accounts for a large percentage of melanomas in childhood.

The early recognition of melanoma has been greatly assisted by the American Cancer Society's program of "ABCDs." This algorithm was developed by the melanoma group at New York University and highlights features often seen in melanoma. *A*symmetry, *b*order irregularity, *c*olor variegation, and *d*iameter greater than 6 mm are the criteria; however, they are not absolute. Melanomas often have pigmentary variegation ranging from dark tannish brown to black but may also have areas of red, blue, and white, the latter color representing clinical regression. At times melanoma will be amelanotic. Nodular melanoma often does not fit the algorithm, as it has rapid growth, symmetric borders, and is often amelanotic. Lentigo maligna melanoma should be suspected when an individual presents with a long-standing, previously uniformly pigmented tannish brown patch in a sun-exposed area that has developed a focus of pigment irregularity and elevated growth within the lesion (this focus often fails the ABCD criteria). Acral-lentiginous melanoma should be suspected in darkly pigmented individuals who present with an atypical lesion of the palms or soles, and especially in individuals who have an isolated pigmented streak of the nail bed. All melanomas may ulcerate and form a nonhealing sore. Melanoma should be suspected in any pigmented lesion that meets the ABCD criteria or presents with unusual continued growth, especially in the elderly. In Australia, which has the highest incidence of melanoma worldwide, the criteria for suspicion of melanoma are broader. In addition to the ABCDs, it is also emphasized that *any* change in the clinical characteristics of a suspected nevocellular or melanocytic lesion warrants further evaluation for melanoma.

Evaluation

Breslow's depth is the single most important prognostic indicator for melanoma. The depth of invasion of the tumor is measured in millimeters from the granular layer of the epidermis to the deepest part of the tumor. Breslow's depth is the most significant prognostic indicator regarding risk of metastasis, local recurrence, and overall survival.

The evaluation of individuals is also guided by Breslow's depth but more importantly is dictated by a thorough history, review of symptoms, and physical examination. Some melanoma centers recommend a baseline chest film for lesions greater than 1 mm. Extensive evaluation with laboratory blood tests and diagnostic imaging has not proved to be of significant benefit in the absence of clinical signs. Once regional lymph node or distant disease is suspected, more thorough evaluation is warranted to assist with proper staging. Survival rates have consistently correlated with the depth of melanoma invasion (Breslow's depth). Reported 5-year survival rates for clinical stage I (localized disease, no lymph node involvement) are shown in (Table 1).

Table 1. Survival Rates and Breslow's Depth in Stage I Melanoma

Breslow's Depth (mm)	5-Year Survival Rate (%)
<0.85	99
0.86–1.69	94
1.70–3.64	78
>3.65	42

Proper evaluation and treatment is based on the Breslow's depth of melanoma. To determine this depth, adequate tissue must be obtained, primarily by excisional biopsies whenever possible and incisional or punch biopsy only in special situations. In not sending the entire thickness of the lesion to the pathologist, a sampling error may occur and the true depth of invasion may not be observed.

Precursor Lesions

Melanoma may occur de novo or in a pre-existing melanocytic nevocellular nevus. Individuals may have nevocellular nevi or common "moles," such as junctional or intradermal nevi, that have clinical features such as border irregularity or color variegation but show no melanoma histopathologically. These nevi have been designated by the National Institutes of Health Consensus Development Conference Statement on the Diagnosis and Treatment of Early Melanoma as *atypical moles.* It is estimated that 5 to 10 per cent of the general population has an atypical mole. Former nomenclature referred to these as *dysplastic nevi.* This conference also described certain histopathologic features that assist in making the diagnosis of an atypical mole. The rate of melanoma development in an atypical mole is widely debated. However, it has been documented in large population-based studies that individuals with atypical moles have an increased incidence of melanoma. Melanoma has been shown to arise histopathologically in an atypical mole. At times, persons will have numerous atypical moles (greater than 100). These individuals have the atypical mole syndrome and should be evaluated thoroughly. Other family members should be examined as well. Individuals with atypical mole syndrome and a family history of melanoma in first-degree relatives have been designated as having familial atypical mole and melanoma syndrome. These individuals have a greater risk of developing melanoma.

Another precursor lesion is the congenital nevocellular nevus. Approximately 1 per cent of newborns have a congenital nevus. The rate of malignant change with this clinical lesion is also debated and ranges from 4.6 to 6.3 per cent. The size of the congenital nevocellular nevus appears to play a role, with small lesions (<1.5 cm), having a lower rate of malignant degeneration, when compared with large lesions (>1.5 to 20 cm) or giant lesions (>20 cm). These congenital nevocellular nevi should be monitored closely and biopsied if any atypical features develop. The risks and benefits of elective excision, which sometimes involves serial procedures if the lesion is large, versus close follow-up must be reviewed.

Evaluation of Precursor Lesions

As with melanoma lesions, adequate tissue of atypical moles must be obtained at the time of biopsy. The overall architecture of the lesion, as well as cytologic features, assist in distinguishing between an atypical mole and melanoma. Accurate histopathologic interpretation by a dermatopathologist or a surgical pathologist with experience with melanocytic lesions is the cornerstone to management of melanoma and atypical nevi.

SUMMARY

The incidence of melanoma and nonmelanoma skin cancer continues to increase. Both forms of cancer are curable at an early stage. Patient education and patient self-examination can assist in early diagnosis. Accurate clinical diagnosis in conjunction with accurate histopathologic evaluation is critical.

PARANEOPLASTIC SYNDROMES OF THE SKIN

By Philip R. Cohen, M.D., *and* Razelle Kurzrock, M.D.
Houston, Texas

The clinical features of a paraneoplastic syndrome of the skin may be the initial presentation of a previously asymptomatic cancer in an otherwise healthy individual or the first sign of a recurrence of neoplasm in an oncology patient. Paraneoplastic syndromes of the skin (which have also been referred to as cutaneous paraneoplastic syndromes) are a group of disorders in which the mucocutaneous lesions precede, occur concurrently, or follow the detection of an associated internal malignancy. For some of these disorders, an underlying neoplasm is virtually always present, and a diligent evaluation for cancer is warranted. However, several of these conditions can also occur without the coexistence or subsequent discovery of an associated malignancy. Therefore, once a "potential" paraneoplastic syndrome of the skin has been discovered, an appropriately focused search for a possible related neoplastic process should be performed.

DIAGNOSTIC CRITERIA FOR PARANEOPLASTIC SYNDROMES OF THE SKIN

The diagnostic criteria for a paraneoplastic syndrome of the skin appeared originally in 1976 in a chapter by Helen Ollendorff Curth entitled Skin Lesions and Internal Malignancy in the book *Cancer of the Skin: Biology-Diagnosis-Management*. These criteria follow:

1. Both conditions start at about the same time (i.e., dermatomyositis).
2. Both conditions follow a parallel course (e.g., malignant acanthosis nigricans).
3. In certain syndromes, neither the course nor the onset of one of the two manifestations is dependent on those of the other manifestation, because the two conditions are part of a genetic syndrome and are therefore coordinated with each other (e.g., Gardner's syndrome).
4. It is a specific tumor (i.e., adenocarcinoma in malignant acanthosis nigricans) that occurs in connection with a certain dermatosis.
5. The dermatosis is usually not common (e.g., erythema gyratum repens).
6. A high percentage of the association of the two conditions is noted (e.g., reticulohistiocytoma).

Currently, criteria 4, 5, and 6 are not essential for a dermatosis to be considered a paraneoplastic syndrome of the skin. Also, conditions that fulfill criterion 3 have more appropriately been reclassified as genodermatoses with malignant potential: hereditary conditions with mucosal and cutaneous manifestations in which the individuals are susceptible to the development of disease-associated malignancies. Therefore, only the first and second of Curth's criteria are important in establishing a relationship between a dermatosis and an internal malignancy.

CANCER-RELATED MUCOCUTANEOUS DISORDERS

Two groups of cancer-related mucocutaneous disorders are recognized: genodermatoses with malignant potential and paraneoplastic syndromes of the skin (Table 1). For persons with the former group of dermatoses, chromosomal abnormalities or defective DNA repair, or both, result in an inherent susceptibility for the affected individual not only to manifest disease-related mucocutaneous lesions but also to develop malignancies subsequently. In patients with paraneoplastic syndromes of the skin, three, not necessarily mutually exclusive, mechanisms for the pathogenesis of the malignancy-associated dermatosis are postulated: (1) production (or release or induction) by the tumor of a substance or substances (such as cytokines) that directly or indirectly cause the dermatosis, (2) depletion by the tumor of a specific substance or substances that, in turn, can result in the paraneoplastic manifestations, and (3) a normal or aberrant host response to the cancer to which the dermatosis is etiologically related.

Because disease-associated internal malignancies occur in patients with either genodermatoses with malignant potential or paraneoplastic syndromes of the skin, evaluation for cancer is essential in individuals with either of these conditions. However, it is important to distinguish between these dermatoses. In contrast to genodermatoses with malignant potential, neither screening of the patient's family nor genetic counseling is necessary for individuals in whom the diagnosis of a paraneoplastic syndrome of the skin is established (Table 2).

ACANTHOSIS NIGRIGANS AND TRIPE PALMS

Acanthosis Nigricans

Acanthosis nigricans is a dermatosis with a predilection for the posterior neck, axillae, and other intertriginous areas such as the groin and submammary region. The confluent, small, hyperkeratotic papules have a hyperpigmented, mosslike appearance and a velvety texture. The diagnosis of acanthosis nigricans is usually based solely on the clinical presentation of the lesions. Microscopic examination shows hyperkeratosis (thickening of the uppermost layer of the epidermis—the stratum corneum) and papillomatosis (irregular undulation of the surface of the epidermis). Hence, acanthosis nigricans is a histologic misnomer because neither acanthosis (thickening of the entire epidermis) nor nigricans (basal layer hyperpigmentation) are typically noted on histologic examination; the clinically observed hyperpigmentation results from the hyperkeratosis.

Acanthosis nigricans can occur in a benign, often familial, form in children. It can also be associated with endocrinopathies. The new onset of acanthosis nigricans in an adult—especially when the lesions appear on mucosal membranes such as the lips, periocular areas, and anus—may be indicative of an underlying tumor. Adenocarcinoma of the abdomen is the most common malignancy—most often cancer of the stomach. Therefore, in addition to a thorough history and physical examination, a complete blood count with differential and platelet counts, serum chemistry panels, a chest film, and imaging studies of the stomach (radiographic or endoscopic) should be obtained. Additional investigation for an intra-abdomi-

Table 1. Characteristics of Genodermatoses With Malignant Potential and Paraneoplastic Syndromes of the Skin

Characteristics	Genodermatoses With Malignant Potential*	Paraneoplastic Syndromes of the Skin
Occurrence of disease-associated internal malignancies	Yes	Yes
Appearance of cutaneous and/or mucosal lesions in relation to the time of diagnosis of the associated malignancy	Always precedes	Precedes, occurs concurrently, or follows†
Periodic examination of patient for new or recurrent internal malignancies	Yes	Yes
Genetic predisposition of the patient for the development of malignancy	Yes	No
Increased risk of family members developing cancer	Yes	No
Necessity of screening family members for mucocutaneous disorder	Yes	No
Genetic counseling for the patient and the patient's family	Recommended	Not necessary

*These conditions include ataxia-telangiectasia, Beckwith-Wiedemann syndrome, Birt-Hogg-Dube syndrome, Bloom's syndrome, Carney complex, Chédiak-Higashi syndrome, common variable immunodeficiency, Cowden's syndrome, dyskeratosis congenita, epidermal nevus syndrome, familial atypical multiple mole melanoma syndrome, Fanconi's anemia, Gardner's syndrome, hemochromatosis, hereditary tylosis, ichthyosis, incontinentia pigmenti, Maffucci's syndrome, Muir-Torre syndrome, multiple endocrine neoplasia type 2 or 2A, multiple endocrine neoplasia type 2B or 3, neurofibromatosis, nevoid basal cell carcinoma syndrome, Peutz-Jeghers syndrome, porphyria cutanea tarda, Rothmund-Thomson syndrome, supernumerary nipples, tuberous sclerosis, Werner's syndrome, Wiscott-Aldrich syndrome, xeroderma pigmentosum, X-linked agammaglobulinemia, and X-linked lymphoproliferative disorder. Some of the listed conditions include genodermatoses in which malignancies have developed in some patients, but the link is not yet considered clear-cut.

†By definition, in order for a dermatosis to be considered a paraneoplastic syndrome of the skin, the malignancy must be present first in order to promote the development of the paraneoplastic condition; yet, in the clinical setting, the mucocutaneous lesions may present first because the associated tumor is not of sufficient mass to permit detection.

Data from Cohen, P.R., Kurzrock, R.: Preface (genodermatoses with malignant potential). Dermatol Clin 13:79–89, 1995, with permission.

nal neoplasm should be based on the results of these primary studies.

Tripe Palms

Tripe palms is considered a distinct paraneoplastic syndrome of the skin. It has also been referred to as acanthosis palmaris and may merely represent the palmar manifestations of acanthosis nigricans. However, tripe palms have been observed both in patients with acanthosis nigricans and in those without. Tripe palms are thickened palms in which there is exaggeration of the normal ridges and furrows of the skin. Hence, the ventral hand and fingers are mosslike and velvety in texture or cobbled and/or honeycombed in appearance (Fig. 1). Tripe palms are found most commonly in patients with either pulmonary or gastric carcinoma. An associated malignancy has been detected in more than 90 per cent of individuals in whom these palmar changes develop. Therefore, once the diagnosis of tripe palms has been established, a thorough evaluation for malignancy is mandatory. Specifically, in addition to routine screening laboratory tests, a chest film and an endoscopic examination of the stomach should be performed.

ACQUIRED ICHTHYOSIS

Ichthyoses are a group of inherited dermatoses that typically appear either at birth or within the first few months of life. The onset of ichthyosis later in life can be secondary to systemic diseases (acquired immunodeficiency syndrome, endocrinopathies, connective tissue diseases, and sarcoidosis), medications (primarily cholesterol-lowering drugs), or visceral malignancies (most commonly Hodgkin's lymphoma). Clinically and microscopically, the lesions of

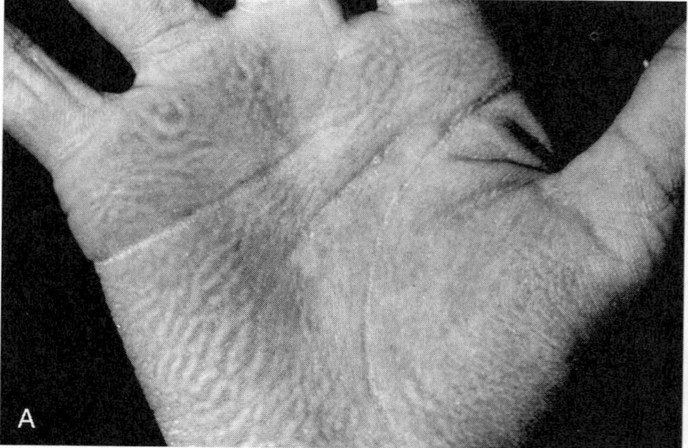

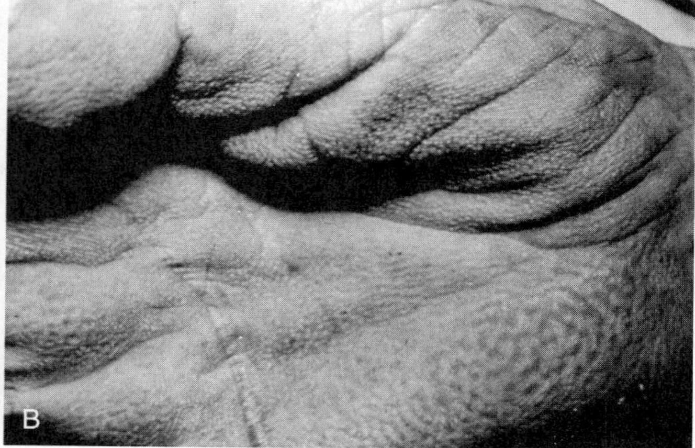

Figure 1. Tripe palms in a man with pulmonary adenocarcinoma, demonstrating exaggerated ridges and furrows with a mosslike velvety texture *(A)* and in a woman with squamous cell carcinoma of the lung showing a honeycombed, cobbled pattern *(B)*. (With permission from Cohen, P.R., Grossman, M.E., Almeida, Kurzrock, R.: Tripe palms and malignancy. J. Clin. Oncol. 7:669–678, 1989. Copyright 1989, Harcourt Brace, Orlando, FL.)

Table 2. Malignancies Commonly Associated With Paraneoplastic Syndromes of the Skin

Paraneoplastic Syndromes of the Skin	Clinical Characteristics	Site or Type of Associated Malignancies
Acanthosis nigricans	Flexural (axillae and posterior neck) verrucous, velvety-textured, hyperpigmented epidermal hyperplasia	Intra-abdominal (stomach)
Acquired ichthyosis	Diffuse rhomboid scales with free edges	Hodgkin's lymphoma
Acquired tylosis	Palmar and plantar keratoderma	Lung cancer (most common); also esophageal and gastric cancer
Amyloidosis	Purpura, macroglossia and/or tongue papules, periocular purpura and/or waxy papules	Myeloma, Hodgkin's lymphoma, kidney
Bazex's syndrome (acrokeratosis paraneoplastica)	Erythematous, scaling papulosquamous lesions on the fingers, toes, ears, and nose; nail dystrophy; palmoplantar keratoderma	Squamous cell carcinomas of the upper aerorespiratory tract or a neoplasm with cervical lymph node metastases in white men over the age of 40 years
Bowen's disease	Erythematous plaque on a photodistributed or non–sun-exposed site	Controversial (age-associated neoplasms)
Bullous pemphigoid	Erythematous-based, subepidermal tense bullae on flexor thighs and forearms	Controversial (lung, larynx, breast, gallbladder, kidney, bladder, ovary, uterus, rectum, prostate, cervix, thyroid, stomach)
Dermatitis herpetiformis	Pruritic, papulovesicles on the elbows and knees, upper back, and buttocks	Lymphoma (gastrointestinal and nongastrointestinal), lung, small intestine, bladder
Dermatomyositis	Periocular heliotrope rash, Gottron's papules, periungual telangiectasias, poikiloderma	Age-associated neoplasms
Epidermolysis bullosa acquisita	Adult-onset, subepidermal blisters at trauma sites	Controversial (myeloma, lung, lymphoma, chronic lymphocytic leukemia)
Erythema annulare centrifugum	Expanding, annular erythema with a raised edge, peripheral scale, and central clearing	Lung, lymphoma (Hodgkin's and non-Hodgkin's), histiocytosis, prostate
Erythema gyratum repens	Advancing erythematous rings with "wood grain" or striped appearance	Lung, esophagus, uterus, cervix, breast, stomach
Erythroderma and exfoliative dermatitis	Generalized erythema with or without scaling	Lymphoma (cutaneous T-cell and Hodgkin's), chronic lymphocytic leukemia, acute and chronic myelogenous leukemia, uterus, lung, stomach, prostate, thyroid, liver, larynx
Erythromelalgia	Severe burning pain, erythema, and warmth of the distal extremities relieved by cold exposure and/or elevation of the extremity	Polycythemia vera, essential thrombocythemia, agnogenic myeloid metaplasia, chronic myelogenous leukemia
Extramammary Paget's disease	Erythematous, exudative plaque located on the vulva, perianal area, penis, scrotum, and/or groin	Cutaneous adnexal carcinoma; internal malignancies: breast, uterus, rectum, bladder, vagina, prostate
Florid cutaneous papillomatosis	Verrucous papillomas on the trunk and the extremities	Intra-abdominal (stomach, bladder, bile ducts, ovary, uterus)
Glucagonoma syndrome	Necrolytic migratory erythematous patch, glossitis, angular stomatitis	Alpha-cell pancreatic carcinoma (glucagonoma)
Hypertrichosis lanuginosa acquisita	Generalized, pale, fine-textured hair growth	Lung, colorectal, breast, uterus, bladder, lymphoma
Hypertrophic pulmonary osteoarthropathy and clubbing	Clubbing of fingers and toes with tender swelling of the distal arms, legs, and adjacent joints	Lung, mediastinal tumors, sarcomas
Multicentric reticulohistiocytosis	Papules, nodules, and rapidly progressive, debilitating polyarthritis	Breast, lymphoma, cervix, stomach, ovary, colon, lung, pleura, acute myelogenous leukemia
Palmar fasciitis–arthritis syndrome	Flexion contracture of all fingers and nodular thickening of the palmar fascia	Ovarian carcinoma and lung cancer
Paraneoplastic pemphigus	Polymorphous pruritic papules and blisters; cutaneous and painful mucosal erosions	Lymphoma, chronic lymphocytic leukemia, sarcoma, lung, thymoma
Pemphigus vulgaris	Intraepidermal bullae of the skin; oral blisters and erosions	Lymphoreticular (Kaposi's sarcoma), thymus, breast, skin
Pityriasis rotunda	Noninflammatory, geometrically perfect, circular patches of scales	Liver

Table continued on following page

Table 2. Malignancies Commonly Associated With Paraneoplastic Syndromes of the Skin *Continued*

Paraneoplastic Syndromes of the Skin	Clinical Characteristics	Site or Type of Associated Malignancies
Porphyria cutanea tarda	*Early:* photodistributed subepidermal vesicles, skin fragility, facial hypertrichosis and hyperpigmentation *Late:* scarring, milia, sclerodermoid changes, calcinosis cutis, alopecia	Controversial (liver)
Pruritus	Excoriations, prurigo nodularis, lichen simplex chronicus	Lymphoma (Hodgkin's and cutaneous T-cell), polycythemia vera
Pyoderma gangrenosum	Papulopustule that develops into a nodule that ulcerates with an irregular, violaceous, undermined border	Hematologic malignancies
Raynaud's phenomenon	Triphasal reaction: pallor, cyanosis, and hyperemia of digits	Genitourinary (testicular) and gastrointestinal
Sign of Leser-Trélat	Seborrheic keratoses (may be pruritic)	Stomach, lymphoma, breast, lung
Sweet's syndrome (acute febrile neutrophilic dermatosis)	Tender, erythematous pseudovesicular plaques on the arms, head, and neck	Acute myelogenous leukemia
Tripe palms	Thickened, velvet or moss textured, honeycombed or cobbled palms with pronounced dermatoglyphics	Lung, stomach
Trousseau's syndrome	Thrombophlebitis (often superficial and migratory)	Pancreas, lung, stomach
Vasculitis	Palpable, nonblanchable purpura; erythematous nodules	Leukemia (hairy cell and chronic myelogenous), myeloma, lymphoma, myelodysplastic syndrome

Modified from Cohen, P.R.: Cutaneous paraneoplastic syndromes. Am Fam Physician 60:1273–1282, 1994, with permission. Copyright 1994, American Academy of Family Physicians, Kansas City, MO.

acquired ichthyosis are identical to those of the autosomal dominant ichthyosis vulgaris. Morphologically, they appear as small, white to brown scales with a free edge and are most often located on the trunk and the limbs.

The lesions of acquired ichthyosis can be mimicked by those of asteototic dermatitis (eczema); however, the distribution of acquired ichthyosis is usually restricted to the extensor surfaces of the extremities, whereas asteotFotic dermatitis typically involves the entire surface of the limbs. If acquired ichthyosis cannot be distinguished from asteototic dermatitis clinically, a skin biopsy readily differentiates these conditions: An absence of the normally present granular layer of the epidermis is pathognomonic for acquired ichthyosis.

Once the diagnosis of acquired ichthyosis has been established, dermatosis-associated causes, including malignancy, should be considered. After a detailed history is taken (looking particularly for ichthyosis-inducing medications and symptoms of ichthyosis-related systemic diseases) and a physical examination is performed, a complete blood count with differential and platelet counts, a human immunodeficiency virus serologic assay, and a chest film (with specific attention to lymphadenopathy) completes the initial evaluation. In addition, if these preliminary studies are normal, computed tomography of the abdomen to exclude Hodgkin's lymphoma should be considered.

CLUBBING AND HYPERTROPHIC PULMONARY OSTEOARTHROPATHY

Clubbing of the digits is characterized by an increased convexity of the nail plate and a thickening of the distal phalanges. Clinically, there is a loss of the 15- to 20-degree angle between the downward curve of the proximal nail plate and the adjacent proximal nail fold. Unfortunately, this can sometimes be difficult to evaluate visually. However, there is a simple and rapid screening test that is useful for determining the presence of clubbing. After the distal dorsal phalanges of similar fingers are placed against each other, a small diamond-shaped "window" is formed by the proximal nail folds and the proximal nail plates in an individual without clubbing (Fig. 2*A*). In contrast, in patients with clubbing, the window is obliterated and the opposing distal nail plates form a wide angle (see Fig. 2*B*).

Clubbing can be primary (hereditary or idiopathic) or secondary to systemic diseases such as chronic lung disorders, cyanotic heart disease, endocarditis, gastrointestinal disorders, hyperthyroidism, or tumors (most commonly bronchogenic carcinoma and mesothelioma). Hypertrophic pulmonary osteoarthropathy is a paraneoplastic syndrome of the skin that includes not only digital clubbing but also painful swelling and tenderness of the distal third of the arms, legs, and adjacent joints, joint effusions, and periosteal new bone formation along the shafts of the tubular bones of the extremities. Because hypertrophic pulmonary osteoarthropathy can present with polyarthritis or joint pain, this disorder can be confused with rheumatoid arthritis. The gold standard for diagnosing hypertrophic pulmonary osteoarthropathy is the changes observed on bone radiographs. Yet, radionuclide bone scanning is more sensitive for detecting the skeletal changes of hypertrophic pulmonary osteoarthropathy.

All patients with hypertrophic pulmonary osteoarthropathy should have a thorough evaluation for cancer—especially lung tumor. An associated malignancy—most frequently a peripherally located non–small cell pulmonary carcinoma—is eventually detected in as many as 90 per cent of patients in whom hypertrophic pulmonary osteoarthropathy develops. Hypertrophic pulmonary osteoarthropathy has also been noted in patients with other intrathoracic tumors and, less often, in association with extrathoracic neoplasms that have pulmonary metastases (most commonly sarcoma).

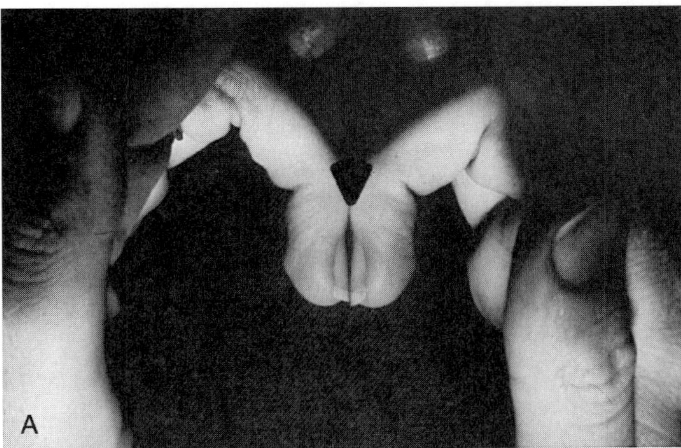

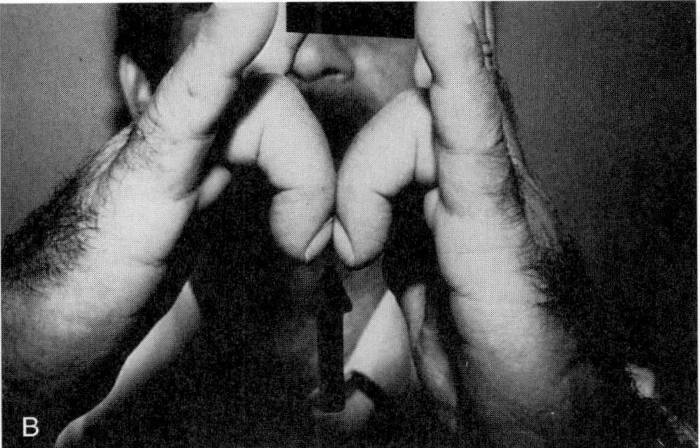

Figure 2. A small diamond-shaped "window" *(arrow)* is formed by the proximal nail folds and the proximal nail plates when the distal dorsal phalanges of similar fingers are placed against each other in an individual without clubbing *(A)*. The window is obliterated and the opposing distal nail plates form a wide angle *(arrow)* in a patient with clubbing *(B)*. (With permission from Cohen, P.R.: Cutaneous paraneoplastic syndromes. Am Fam Physician 60:1273–1282, 1994. Copyright 1994, American Academy of Family Physicians, Kansas City, MO.)

EXTRAMAMMARY PAGET'S DISEASE

Extramammary Paget's disease typically occurs in apocrine gland–bearing regions of the body. Common sites include the groin, perineum, and perianal area. Establishing the diagnosis of extramammary Paget's disease is often delayed because the lesions present as erythematous eczematous plaques mimicking either dermatitis or candidiasis (Fig. 3). Therefore, the possibility of extramammary Paget's disease should be considered in patients with either a chronic eczema that does not resolve with topical corticosteroid therapy or a monilial intertrigo that does not improve with topical antifungal therapy. A biopsy of the lesion is necessary to confirm the diagnosis of extramammary Paget's disease: Microscopic examination reveals round cells with abundant pale cytoplasm and a large reticulated nucleus (Paget's cells) within the epidermis.

Extramammary Paget's disease represents a cutaneous adenocarcinoma. Therefore, appropriate local therapy (complete excision and/or radiotherapy) is warranted. In addition, an internal malignancy is also discovered in nearly half the patients with extramammary Paget's disease. The tumor site is usually related to the location of the dermatosis—adenocarcinoma of the digestive tract for perianal extramammary Paget's disease and malignancy of the genitourinary tract for penile-scrotal-groin extramammary Paget's disease. Therefore, the cancer evaluation for a patient with extramammary Paget's disease should include imaging studies and/or endoscopic evaluation of the gastrointestinal and genitourinary tracts.

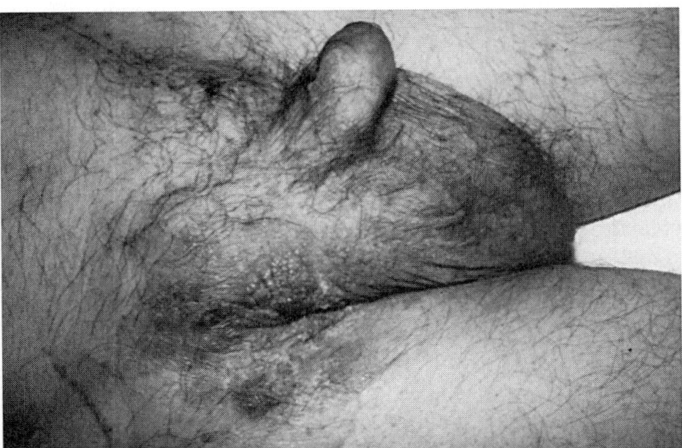

Figure 3. Extramammary Paget's disease presenting as a pruritic erythematous plaque involving the groin and scrotum. (With permission from Cohen P.R.: Cutaneous paraneoplastic syndromes. Am Fam Physician 60:1273–1282, 1994. Copyright 1994, American Academy of Family Physicians, Kansas City, MO.)

NEUTROPHILIC DERMATOSES: PYODERMA GANGRENOSUM AND SWEET'S SYNDROME

Two paraneoplastic syndromes of the skin are neutrophilic dermatoses—pyoderma gangrenosum and Sweet's syndrome. Microscopically, both dermatoses show a dense infiltrate of mature polymorphonuclear leukocytes in the dermis. Pyoderma gangrenosum begins as a small pustule that rapidly enlarges into a boggy, necrotic-based ulcer whose undermined borders are violaceous. No associated cause for pyoderma gangrenosum is discovered in more than one third of the individuals with this disorder; other dermatosis-related conditions include Behçet's syndrome, chronic active hepatitis, inflammatory bowel disease, and rheumatoid arthritis. A bullous or atypical form of pyoderma gangrenosum may occur in association with hematologic malignancies—particularly acute myelogenous leukemia and multiple myeloma.

Sweet's syndrome, also known as acute febrile neutrophilic dermatosis, is characterized by pyrexia, neutrophilia, and tender erythematous pseudovesicular plaques (Fig. 4). This syndrome occurs most frequently as an idiopathic condition following a streptococcal throat infection in middle-aged women; the signs and symptoms promptly respond to systemic corticosteroids and may recur episodically. However, in up to one fifth of individuals with Sweet's syndrome, the dermatosis is associated with malignancy. Acute myelogenous leukemia is the most common malignancy. Less commonly, Sweet's syndrome can also appear in patients with solid tumors—specifically carcinomas of the genitourinary organs, breast, and gastrointestinal organs. The absence of pyrexia or an increased neutrophil count does not eliminate the possibility of Sweet's syn-

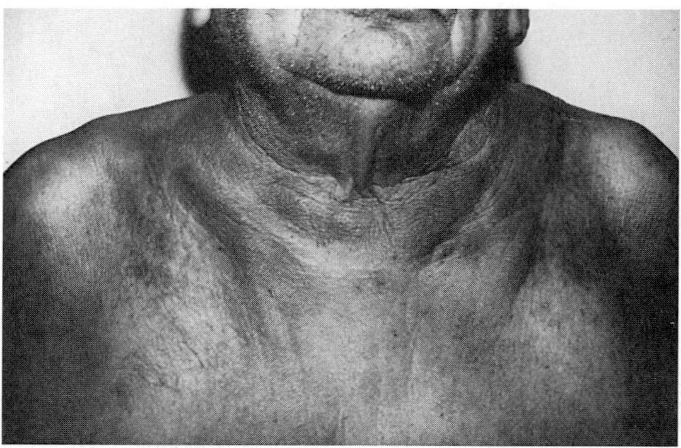

Figure 4. Tender erythematous pseudovesicular plaques of Sweet's syndrome on the shoulder of a man with acute myelogenous leukemia. (With permission from Cohen, P.R., and Kurzrock, R.: Paraneoplastic Sweet's syndrome. Emerg Med 26(2):37–38, 1994. Copyright 1994, Excerpta Medica, New York, NY.)

drome in an oncology patient because, in contrast to patients with idiopathic Sweet's syndrome, fever and/or neutrophilia may not be present in cancer patients with biopsy-confirmed Sweet's syndrome.

A biopsy of a suspected neutrophilic dermatosis lesion should be performed. The specimen should be bisected—half to be sent for routine hematoxylin and eosin staining and half for bacterial, fungal, and mycobacterial cultures. Once the diagnosis of either pyoderma gangrenosum or Sweet's syndrome is established, the evaluation begins with a history and physical examination. Laboratory studies should include a complete blood count with differential and platelet counts. If any blood count abnormality (other than isolated neutrophilia) is present, a bone marrow biopsy should be performed.

PARANEOPLASTIC PEMPHIGUS

Paraneoplastic pemphigus is a recently described paraneoplastic syndrome of the skin. The cutaneous lesions may be widely distributed and polymorphous: erythematous patches, vesicles and bullae, papules and plaques, and erosions. Individuals with this condition also have severe erythema multiforme–like mucosal lesions that present as painful blisters or erosions of the oral cavity and conjunctivitis. The variable clinical morphologic features can be misinterpreted as a bullous drug eruption or as a viral infection (such as a herpesvirus infection) or as a primary bullous disorder. The findings on microscopic examination are also variable, corresponding to the clinical lesions: The combination of suprabasal acantholysis (pemphigus-like lesions) and dyskeratotic keratinocytes (erythema multiforme–like lesions) is suggested to be diagnostic of paraneoplastic pemphigus. In order to confirm the diagnosis of paraneoplastic pemphigus, tissue for direct immunofluorescence studies and serum for indirect immunofluorescence studies (on both stratified squamous epithelia such as monkey esophagus and simple, columnar, and transitional epithelia such as rat bladder) should be collected. Serum should also be evaluated (using immunoprecipitation techniques with carbon 14–labeled human keratinocyte extracts) for the presence of polypeptide proteins of specific molecular weights characteristic for this condition: (1) 250 kd (desmoplakin I), (2) 230 kd (bullous pemphigoid antigen I), (3) 210 kd (desmoplakin II), (4) 190 kd (currently unidentified antigen), and (5) 170 kd (currently unidentified antigen).

An associated benign (thymoma or Castelman's pseudotumor) or malignant neoplastic process has been discovered in nearly all patients with paraneoplastic pemphigus. The most common malignancies are chronic lymphocytic leukemia and non-Hodgkin's lymphoma; others include acute myelogenous leukemia, pulmonary squamous cell carcinoma, sarcoma, and Waldenström's macroglobulinemia. Hence, a thorough evaluation for a hematologic or lymphoproliferative malignancy is warranted in all patients in whom paraneoplastic pemphigus is diagnosed.

PRURITUS

Pruritus refers to itching; it is attributed to an unknown origin when the cause cannot be determined. Cutaneous stigmata of pruritus are variable and include excoriations, itchy papules and nodules (nodular prurigo), normal-appearing skin, and pruritic plaques (lichen simplex chronicus). An associated systemic disease may be found in about 30 per cent of patients with pruritus, and an associated malignancy may be the inducing cause in up to 11 per cent of patients with pruritus.

Primary dermatologic disorders can cause pruritus, including dermatoses such as cutaneous infestations (pediculosis and scabies), dermatitis (e.g., asteototic, chronic, contact, eczematous, and irritant dermatitis), drug reactions, lichen planus, psoriasis vulgaris, urticaria, and vesiculobullous diseases (e.g., dermatitis herpetiformis). In addition, pruritus of unknown origin can be the result of a generalized condition such as hepatic, renal, or thyroid disease. Therefore, in the patient who presents with generalized itching without an attributable primary dermatosis, biochemical tests to exclude dysfunction of the liver, kidneys, and thyroid should be performed.

Lymphoma (most commonly Hodgkin's and less often non-Hodgkin's, e.g., premycotic stage of cutaneous T-cell lymphoma and the Sézary syndrome) is the most frequently associated malignancy in patients with paraneoplastic pruritus. Pruritus can also, albeit less commonly, occur in patients with leukemia and a variety of solid tumors. A marker for polycythemia rubra vera is pruritus following a warm bath or shower as the patient begins to cool off. Interestingly, in some patients with advanced brain tumors, chronic and persistent pruritus localized to the nostrils has been described.

The evaluation for a person presenting with pruritus should be directed toward determining the cause. In patients who have pruritus and a rash, the examination should focus on the possibility of establishing a diagnosis of a primary dermatologic condition. However, in patients having either pruritus without a rash or pruritus with excoriations and/or secondary cutaneous lesions, the initial investigation for an underlying cause should include a thorough history (particularly to exclude an allergic disorder) and physical examination. Additional laboratory studies should include a chest film and blood tests to assess hepatic, renal, and thyroid function. If a cause for the pruritus is not apparent, computed tomography of the abdomen should be considered.

REACTIVE ERYTHEMAS

Reactive erythemas are flat, red skin lesions that appear in a circinate, arcinate, or polycyclic pattern. Conceptually, they can be considered secondary dermatoses; they represent a nonspecific cutaneous response to a primary systemic cause that can either be identified or remain undiscovered (idiopathic). Erythema gyratum repens and necrolytic migratory erythema are two paraneoplastic syndromes of the skin that present as reactive erythema.

Erythema Gyratum Repens

Erythema gyratum repens is a reactive erythema with a distinctive clinical appearance: erythematous, migratory, scaly, concentric annular rings that have a "wood grain" or striped appearance (Fig. 5). The trunk and proximal extremities are typical sites for lesions to appear. The diagnosis of this dermatosis is primarily based on the dramatic, yet characteristic, morphologic features of the clinical lesions. However, extensive tinea corporis secondary to dermatophyte infection could mimic erythema gyratum repens. The pathologic changes of a lesion seen on biopsy are nonspecific and show a moderate perivascular lymphohistiocytic infiltrate in the dermis with mild patchy spongiosis and parakeratosis of the overlying epidermis; the absence of hyphae after staining with periodic acid–Schiff or Gomori–methenamine silver stain excludes the possibility of fungus.

More than 80 per cent of patients with erythema gyratum repens have an associated internal malignancy—most often lung cancer. Other common neoplasms in these patients include tumors of the genitourinary organs, upper gastrointestinal tract, and breast. CREST (calcinosis, Raynaud's phenomenon, esophageal dysmotility, sclerodactyly, and telangiectasia) syndrome, tuberculosis, and virginal breast hypertrophy, are some of the non-neoplastic conditions that have been present in patients with non–malignancy-associated erythema gyratum repens; in at least two individuals, no detectable underlying problem was discovered.

Erythema gyratum repens appears from 1 month to 6 years prior to the detection of an associated malignancy. Therefore, once the diagnosis of erythema gyratum repens has been established, a complete history and physical evaluation (including pelvic examination with Papanicolaou's smear) should be followed by a thorough investigation for an asymptomatic visceral tumor. In addition to routine laboratory studies (a complete blood cell count with differential and platelet counts and serum chemistry panels), a chest film, mammogram, and endoscopy of the upper gastrointestinal tract should be performed. An initial evaluation that is negative for malignancy does not exclude the possibility of a dermatosis-related cancer that is currently undetectable. Hence, complete re-evaluation of individuals with persistent erythema gyratum repens should be carried out periodically—annually or more often if new signs and/or symptoms of a possible neoplasm appear.

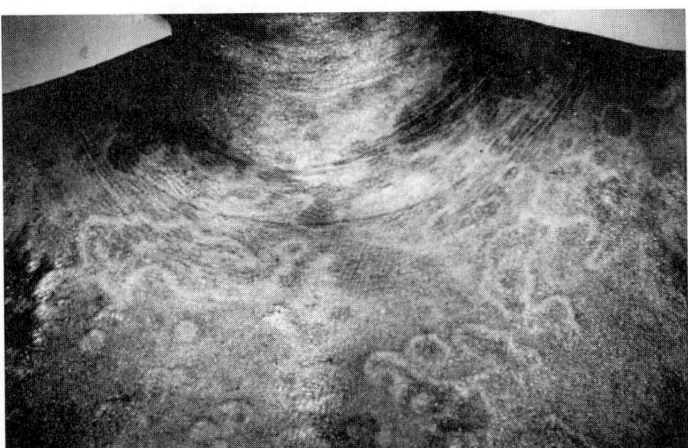

Figure 5. Erythema gyratum repens appearing as serpiginous, concentric, erythematous bands of erythema in a woman with breast carcinoma. (With permission from Kurzrock, R., Cohen, P.R.: Erythema gyratum repens. [photo/essay] JAMA 273:594, 1995. Copyright 1995, American Medical Association, Chicago, IL.)

Necrolytic Migratory Erythema

Necrolytic migratory erythema is often associated with a glucagon-secreting alpha–islet cell tumor of the pancreas; less often, it has been described in patients without pancreatic neoplasms. It is a cyclic (7 to 14 days) eruption that appears initially as erythematous patches that progress to plaques with central blisters. As the blisters rupture, the "new" lesions expand peripherally in an annular fashion, and the old lesions heal with postinflammatory hyperpigmentation. The clinical lesions can mimic either zinc deficiency or candidiasis; in addition, superimposed monilial intertrigo—especially in perineal lesions of necrolytic migratory erythema—may also be present. Therefore, the diagnosis of necrolytic migratory erythema should be considered in a patient with presumptive candidiasis of the perineum that is not appropriately responding to either topical or systemic antimonilial therapy.

Biopsy of the lesion is helpful to confirm a suspected diagnosis of necrolytic migratory erythema. The pale, eosinophilic upper epidermis reflects sudden death (necrolysis) of the epithelium. Additional pathologic changes include confluent parakeratosis, absence of the granular layer, vacuolated keratinocytes with pyknotic nuclei and intracellular edema, neutrophilic infiltration of the epidermis, and possible intraepidermal cleft formation. Acquired zinc deficiency, acrodermatitis enteropathica, Hartnup disease, pellagra, and pemphigus foliaceus are other clinical conditions that have microscopic features similar to those observed in necrolytic migratory erythema.

Necrolytic migratory erythema is one of the mucocutaneous manifestations observed in patients with the glucagonoma syndrome; others include glossitis and a painful angular stomatitis. In addition to weight loss, laboratory features of glucagonoma syndrome include anemia, decreased serum amino acid levels, and increased serum glucagon and glucose levels. Therefore, the detection of glucagonemia should prompt a diligent evaluation for pancreatic carcinoma.

SIGN OF LESER-TRÉLAT

The sudden appearance, or sudden increase in number and size, of pruritic (or asymptomatic) seborrheic keratoses in association with the detection of an internal malignancy is known as the sign of Leser-Trélat. Although Hollander is likely to have been the first author to have associated seborrheic keratoses with internal malignancies in 1900, this paraneoplastic syndrome of the skin is named after Edmund Leser and Ulysse Trélat—two European surgeons who actually described patients in whom eruptive cutaneous senile angiomas were a presenting sign of either mammary carcinoma or visceral malignancy in the 1890s.

Seborrheic keratoses are common lesions, especially in the elderly. Hence, most individuals with multiple seborrheic keratoses do not have a related tumor. The diagnosis of a seborrheic keratosis can often be made based on the clinical appearance—the lesions typically appear as "stuck-on" plaques. Microscopically, there are several histologic variants. Common pathologic changes include hyperkeratosis, acanthosis, papillomatosis, horned pseudocysts, and hyperpigmentation.

Gastrointestinal adenocarcinoma and lymphoma are the more commonly associated malignancies in patients who exhibit the sign of Leser-Trélat. Following a history and physical examination, a complete blood count with differential and platelet counts should be evaluated. To exclude gastric cancer, upper endoscopy with visualization of the stomach should be considered.

TROUSSEAU'S SYNDROME

The association of migratory thrombophlebitis with cancer was initially described by Trousseau in 1860. He subsequently diagnosed his own cancer of the pancreas. In acknowledgment of this French physician, malignancy-associated superficial thrombophlebitis is also referred to as Trousseau's syndrome.

Superficial migratory thrombophlebitis presents as a tender linear erythema that follows the distribution of an underlying large vein. It may be recurrent or occur as a single episode. A bleeding diathesis, arterial emboli, and thrombotic endocarditis are other features that may be present in patients with malignancy-associated superficial migratory thrombophlebitis. Pancreatic carcinoma (nearly always involving the body and tail) is the most common visceral tumor in these individuals; next in frequency are carcinomas of the lung and stomach. Although superficial migratory thrombophlebitis occurs prior to the detection of an asymptomatic malignancy in more than half of patients with this condition, the tumor has already metastasized in more than 90 per cent of individuals by the time the diagnosis of cancer is established. Therefore, in addition to a chest film, a computed tomography scan of the abdomen (with emphasis on the pancreas and stomach) should be performed in patients with superficial migratory thrombophlebitis.

VASCULITIS

Inflammation and necrosis of blood vessels defines vasculitis. The classification of vasculitis has previously been based on vessel size (small and large) and type of infiltrate (neutrophilic, lymphocytic, and granulomatous). A classification scheme based on multiple criteria was proposed by the American College of Rheumatology in 1990. The cutaneous lesions of vasculitis are polymorphous and may appear as erythematous papules and nodules, livido reticularis (with a netlike pattern of erythema), palpable purpura, subcutaneous nodules, ulcers, and urticarial plaques. Therefore, when the diagnosis of vasculitis is suspected, a biopsy of the lesion is necessary for confirmation.

Leukocytoclastic Vasculitis

Leukocytoclastic vasculitis is characterized pathologically by (1) leukocytoclasia (fragmented neutrophil nuclei), (2) neutrophils in the vessel walls, (3) fibrinoid necrosis of the vessels, and (4) extravasation of erythrocytes into the surrounding dermis. Leukocytoclastic vasculitis typically involves small vessels in the upper dermis. Clinically, palpable purpura is one of the most common presentations.

Since most individuals with biopsy-confirmed leukocytoclastic vasculitis do not have a related underlying malignancy, a complete evaluation for other causes of vasculitis should be performed initially. After a careful history and physical examination, a complete blood cell count with differential and platelet counts and a chest film should be performed. Indeed, tumor-associated vasculitis may be considered a diagnosis of exclusion after other conditions (such as drug reaction, hepatitis, lupus erythematosus, rheumatoid arthritis, sepsis, and Sjögren's syndrome) have been appropriately excluded. An associated neoplastic process is present in approximately 5 per cent of patients with vasculitis; in individuals with leukocytoclastic vasculitis, these processes include both hematologic malignancies (leukemias, lymphomas, and multiple myeloma) and solid tumors (most commonly non–small cell carcinoma of the lung). Evaluation for a previously undiagnosed or relapsing hematologic malignancy should be performed in all patients with vasculitis who also have abnormal blood counts, lymphadenopathy, or splenomegaly.

Polyarteritis Nodosa

Vasculitis involves the small arteries in polyarteritis nodosa; an associated septal panniculitis may also be present. The condition is characterized microscopically by minimal perivascular inflammation surrounding thrombotic vessels whose necrotic walls contain inflammatory cells. Polyarteritis nodosa often presents as linear subcutanous nodules (Fig. 6); it can also appear as erythematous papules, livido reticularis, or ulcerations. Hairy-cell leukemia is the most commonly associated malignancy in patients with polyarteritis nodosa.

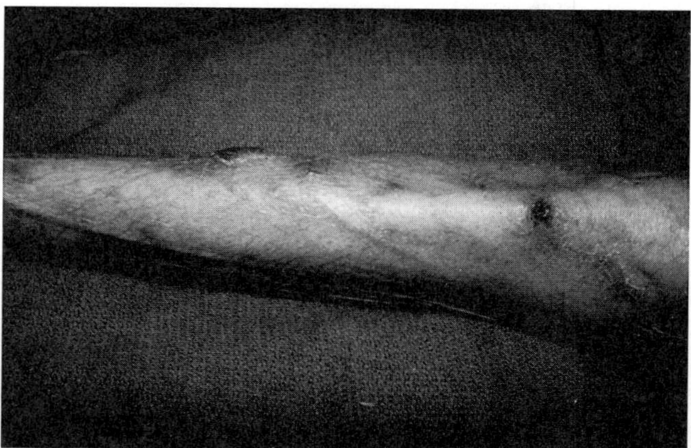

Figure 6. Erythematous nodules of polyarteritis nodosa on the leg of a woman with hairy-cell leukemia. (With permission from Kurzrock, R., Cohen, P.R.: Vasculitis and cancer. Clin Dermatol 11:175–187, 1993. Copyright 1993, Elsevier Science Publishing Co., Inc., New York, NY.)

Section Eighteen

NUTRITION

NUTRITIONAL ASSESSMENT

By Adil A. Abbasi, M.D.,
and Marla M. Buth, R.D.
Milwaukee, Wisconsin

Nutritional problems frequently complicate the course of a medical illness. Both obesity and undernutrition are associated with adverse clinical outcomes. Undernutrition in hospitalized and institutionalized patients has been linked to increased morbidity, mortality, and medical care expenditures. Undernutrition is frequently treatable, but physicians often fail to recognize and optimally treat this problem. This article briefly addresses the basic principles of clinical nutrition and nutritional assessment in adults.

PRINCIPLES OF CLINICAL NUTRITION

A review of basic principles of clinical nutrition provides a useful starting point. Our food, composed of recently living plant and animal tissue, has all the chemical complexity of living organisms. Many food components are physiologically indispensable, but only a few are nutritionally indispensable (i.e., must be supplied by the diet). The identification of members of the second group has been the goal of several generations of nutrition scientists. The problem is practical as well as theoretical; it sometimes becomes necessary to nourish patients with a simplified, even synthetic, diet either enterally or parenterally. The correct formulation of such elemental diets depends on a basic understanding of essential nutrients.

Identification of essential nutrients became feasible when nutrition investigators developed purified diets. An animal or a person under study was fed a mixture consisting only of known purified nutrients. If the transition from mixed foods to the restricted diet caused a failure of growth or other indication of illness, it was concluded that one or more essential nutrients must have been withdrawn. Indicators that are sensitive to the withdrawal of an essential nutrient in healthy growing subjects (animal or human) are body weight gain and nitrogen retention and, in healthy adult subjects, maintenance of zero nitrogen balance and constant body weight. Furthermore, the purified restricted diet often caused lesions specific for the withdrawal of a particular essential nutrient. Classic examples include rachitic bone (vitamin D), scorbutic skin (vitamin C), beriberi opisthotonos (vitamin B_1), and canine black tongue (niacin). Thus, it was recognized early in the 20th century that crude lipid and water-soluble extracts of liver were required for the growth and integrity of rats fed highly purified diets. Two or more essential factors (fat-soluble and water-soluble vitamins, among others) were subsequently demonstrated in each of these extracts. Each factor corrected a different component of the disorder induced by the purified diet. For most (but not all) nutrients, signs of nutritional deficiency are more likely caused by protracted, rather than short-term, consumption of the restricted diet. For example, only by prolonged feeding of purified diets was the essentialness of polyunsaturated fatty acids and the trace elements revealed.

The essential nutrients that have been identified in this fashion can be divided into macronutrients (more than 100 mg per day required in humans) and micronutrients (less than 100 mg per day required in humans). They can also be divided into organic factors (protein, essential fatty acids, vitamins) and inorganic factors (water, minerals, trace elements). The catalog of the 40 essential nutrients includes 23 organic compounds (9 essential amino acids, 13 vitamins, 1 fatty acid), 15 elements, water, and an energy source (Table 1).

For each essential nutrient, there are three dosage thresholds: minimum daily requirement (MDR), recommended daily allowance (RDA), and maximal daily tolerance. The MDR is determined in a group of healthy subjects of a specified age, sex, and physiologic status (e.g., level of physical activity; whether pregnant or lactating) and represents the mean value, in the subjects tested, of the lowest amount of nutrient that will prevent clinical or chemical manifestations of a deficiency illness. The RDA—the amount estimated to prevent deficiency in at least 97 per cent of the population—takes into account the interindividual variation in the MDR and is usually 30 to 100 per cent higher than the MDR. The maximal daily tolerance reflects the fact that every dietary component, essential or nonessential, will cause illness if sufficient excess is taken for a sufficient time.

RDAs that specifically address the needs of patients older than 65 years do not exist. Current RDAs are the same for everyone 50 years and older. Surveys of older adults (aged 60 to 80 years) living independently indicate that caloric intake is less than the RDA in about one third and the consumption of minerals and vitamins is less than the RDA in up to one half of this group of healthy older adults. The blood concentrations of vitamins and minerals are also subnormal in 10 to 30 per cent of this group. The quality and quantity of the nutritional intake of institutionalized older adults is not as good as that of their independently living counterparts and tends to vary from institution to institution. Low calorie, protein, vitamin, and mineral intake is more prevalent in institutionalized older adults. Calorie requirements decline progressively beyond age 60 years. Two thirds of this decline is due to a decline in energy expenditure (decreased activity level) and one third of the decline is attributed to a decreased metabolic rate associated with decreased lean body mass. Although the RDA for calcium is 800 to 1200 mg per day, most experts recommend that the elemental calcium intake for women older than 50 years and for men older than 65 years should exceed 1000 to 1500 mg per day. More work is needed, however, to define the nutritional requirements of independently living healthy older adults and those living in institutions. Importantly, older adults with a reduced caloric intake are at increased risk for various nutritional deficiencies.

Table 1. Catalog of the 40 Known Essential Nutrients

Essential Amino and Fatty Acids	Vitamins	Elements	Other
Amino acids	Thiamine	Sodium	Water
L-Threonine	Niacin	Potassium	Energy sources
L-Valine	Riboflavin	Calcium	
L-Isoleucine	Pyridoxine	Magnesium	
L-Leucine	Folic acid	Chloride	
L-Lysine	Vitamin B_{12}	Phosphorus	
L-Tryptophan	Ascorbic acid	Iron	
L-Methionine-cyst(e)ine	Biotin	Copper	
L-Phenylalanine-tyrosine	Pantothenic acid	Zinc	
L-Histidine	Vitamin A	Chromiun	
	Vitamin D	Manganese	
Fatty acids	Vitamin E	Selenium	
Linoleic acid	Vitamin K	Molybdenum	
		Iodine	
		Fluoride	

NUTRITIONAL ASSESSMENT

Nutritional assessment involves anthropometric and biochemical measurements, clinical observations during physical examination, evaluation of a patient's diet, and recognition of possible drug-nutrient interactions.

ANTHROPOMETRIC MEASUREMENTS

Anthropometry specifically refers to the measurement of height, weight, body mass index, triceps skinfold, midarm muscle circumference, and subscapular skinfold thickness.

Body Weight

Weight loss is common in hospitalized patients and is associated with adverse clinical outcomes. A weight loss exceeding 5 per cent in 1 month, 7.5 per cent in 3 months, and 10 per cent over 6 months is considered a significant weight loss, and an investigation to find its cause is warranted. Body weight less than 80 per cent of ideal is frequently associated with adverse clinical outcomes. Hamwi's method provides a quick and commonly used way of estimating ideal body weight (IBW). However, Hamwi's formula (shown below) tends to underestimate the IBW for people older than 60 years of age.

For men: IBW = 106 lb + 6 lb for every inch greater than 5 ft

For women: IBW = 100 lb + 5 lb for every inch greater than 5 ft

The Metropolitan Life tables can be used to estimate IBW, but these tables do not take into account the change in weight that occurs with age. The Gerontology Research Center age-specific weight-for-height table includes body weight for each decade of life from age 25 years to age 65 years. The National Institute on Aging included a copy of the Metropolitan Life 1983 weight table for ages 25 to 59 years alongside a copy of the Gerontology Research Center weight table, showing a progressive increase in body weight from 1 decade to the next (Table 2).

Body Mass Index

Body mass index (BMI) is a ratio of body weight (kg) to height² (m²). A BMI of 23 or less and 30 or more has been shown to be associated with increased mortality in the 60-year and older age group. The formula to calculate BMI is

$$\text{BMI} = \frac{\text{body weight (in kgs)}}{\text{height}^2\text{ (in m}^2\text{)}} \text{ or } \left(\frac{\text{kg}}{\text{m}^2}\right)$$

Skinfold and Muscle Mass Measurements

The triceps skinfold and subscapular skinfold thickness are used to estimate subcutaneous fat reserves, whereas midarm muscle circumference is used to estimate skeletal muscle mass. These measurements are less reliable in older adults (>60 years) because of age-related decline in lean body mass and an increase in body fat.

Alternative Methods of Measuring Height in Nonambulatory Patients and Patients With Disabilities and Deformities

Total arm length is a useful method of estimating height in nonambulatory patients and in older individuals with abnormal posture (e.g., kyphosis). Total arm length is measured from the tip of the acromial process of the scapula to the end of the arm at the styloid process of the ulna. The results are compared with height equivalent standards. Arm span is another acceptable alternative to height, especially in nonambulatory older individuals. Arm span is measured from fingertip to fingertip (middle finger), passing in front of the clavicles.

Knee height can be used to estimate total height in a nonambulatory patient. The knee and ankle are bent at 90 degrees with the patient in a supine position. A caliper is used to measure the knee height from under the heel of the left foot and top of the knee cap. The formula for estimating height from knee height is

Height (women) = [(1.83 × knee height) − (0.24 × age)] + 84.88

Height (men) = [(2.02 × knee height) − (0.04 × age)] + 64.19

BIOCHEMICAL INDICATORS OF NUTRITIONAL STATUS

Several biochemical measures can be used to assess nutritional status, including serum albumin, cholesterol, insulin-like growth factor-I (IGF-I), prealbumin, retinol-binding protein, and transferrin.

Table 2. Body Weight for Height Comparing Metropolitan Life Table and Gerontology Research Center Weight Range for Men and Women*

	Metropolitan 1983 Weights for Ages 25–59 Yr†		Gerontology Research Center Weight Range for Men and Women by Age (Yr)‡				
Height (ft-inches)	*Men*	*Women*	*25*	*35*	*45*	*55*	*65*
4'10"	—	100–131	84–111	92–119	99–127	107–135	115–142
4'11"	—	101–134	87–115	95–123	103–131	111–139	119–147
5'0"	—	103–137	90–119	98–127	106–135	114–143	123–152
5'1"	123–145	105–140	93–123	101–131	110–140	118–148	127–157
5'2"	125–148	108–144	96–127	105–136	113–144	122–153	131–163
5'3"	127–151	111–148	99–131	108–140	117–149	126–158	135–168
5'4"	129–155	114–152	102–135	112–145	121–154	130–163	140–173
5'5"	131–159	117–156	106–140	115–149	125–159	134–168	144–179
5'6"	133–163	120–160	109–144	119–154	129–164	138–174	148–184
5'7"	135–167	123–164	112–148	122–159	133–169	143–179	153–190
5'8"	137–171	126–167	116–153	126–163	137–174	147–184	158–196
5'9"	139–175	129–170	119–157	130–168	141–179	151–190	162–201
5'10"	141–179	132–173	122–162	134–173	145–184	156–195	167–207
5'11"	144–183	135–176	126–167	137–178	149–190	160–201	172–213
6'0"	147–187	—	129–171	141–183	153–195	165–207	177–219
6'1"	150–192	—	133–176	145–188	157–200	169–213	182–225
6'2"	153–197	—	137–181	149–194	162–206	174–219	187–232
6'3"	157–202	—	141–186	153–199	166–212	179–225	192–238
6'4"	—	—	144–191	157–205	171–218	184–231	197–244

*Values in this table are for height without shoes and weight in pounds without clothes.
†The weight range is the lower weight for small frame and the upper weight for large frame.
‡Data from Andres.
Modified from Reporter, National Institute on Aging information programs. National Institute on Aging. 301, 496, 1986. Courtesy of the National Institute on Aging 1992.

Serum albumin is a good predictor of morbidity and mortality, but its value as an indicator of nutritional status is limited. Albumin in serum has a half-life of 2 to 3 weeks; thus, hypoalbuminemia (serum albumin <3.5 g/dL), reflects chronic rather than acute protein depletion. Serum prealbumin, which has a short half-life (2 to 3 days), is a sensitive indicator of visceral protein status and can be used to monitor nutritional status. Prealbumin concentrations of 10 to 15 mg/dL, 5 to 10 mg/dL, and less than 5 mg/dL are correlated with mild, moderate, and severe visceral protein depletion, respectively.

CLINICAL INDICATORS OF NUTRITIONAL STATUS

Several clinical indicators of specific nutritional deficiencies have been described (Table 3). Dry, flaky skin with poor elasticity is commonly observed in moderate to severe protein-calorie undernutrition (PCU). Hair loss is associated with deficiency of several essential nutrients, including protein and zinc. Perifollicular petechiae and ecchymoses have been reported with vitamin C and vitamin K deficiency. Wound healing may be delayed in patients with protein, vitamin C, or zinc deficiency. Dry eyes and night blindness may accompany vitamin A deficiency. Cheilosis and angular fissures are seen in niacin and riboflavin deficiency. A painful red tongue (glossitis) may indicate deficiency of various B vitamins and folic acid. Loss of or distorted taste has been associated with zinc deficiency. Spooning of nails (koilonychia) suggests iron deficiency, whereas a decrease in vibratory and position sense suggests vitamin B_{12} deficiency.

DRUG-NUTRIENT INTERACTIONS

Drug-induced nutritional deficiencies are caused by drug-induced malabsorption, drug-induced renal loss, or inhibition of nutrient biosynthesis. These deficiencies are more common in patients with poor oral intake and compromised nutritional status and in those with prolonged or chronic illnesses. Older adults are at increased risk for drug-induced deficiencies because they often take several medications and because protein-calorie undernutrition is common among the elderly, especially those who reside in institutions.

Many drugs can cause anorexia, thereby increasing the risk of protein-calorie undernutrition. The anticholinergic effects of antihistamines, antipsychotics, cyclic antidepressants, and other drugs can cause dry mouth and impaired oral intake. Both loop and thiazide diuretics can cause dehydration and sodium, potassium, and magnesium deficiencies. Concurrent use of a laxative and a diuretic can

Table 3. Clinical Indicators of Nutritional Status

Clinical Indicators	Deficiency
Dry, lax skin	Protein, calorie
Hair loss	Protein, biotin, zinc, essential fatty acids
Ecchymosis and perifollicular petechiae	Vitamins C and K
Delayed wound healing	Protein, vitamin C, and zinc
Dryness of eyes and night blindness	Vitamin A
Cheilosis and angular fissures	Niacin and riboflavin
Glossitis	Vitamins B_6 and B_{12}, riboflavin, niacin, and folic acid
Dysgeusia (parageusia)	Zinc
Koilonychia	Iron
Absence of vibratory and position sense	Vitamin B_{12}

Table 4. Drug-Nutrient Interaction

Nutrient Deficiency	Medications
Calcium (osteoporosis)	Loop diuretics, corticosteroids, thyroxine, heparin, alcohol abuse, anticonvulsants
Magnesium	Loop diuretics, thiazides, alcohol abuse
Potassium	Loop diuretics, thiazides, lithium, levodopa, corticosteroids, laxatives
Sodium	Loop diuretics, thiazides, spironolactone, ACE inhibitors
Zinc	Alcohol abuse, corticosteroids, penicillamine
Folate	Phenytoin, phenobarbital, sulfasalazine, triamterene, trimethoprim, alcohol abuse
Riboflavin	Amitriptyline
Niacin	Isoniazid
Thiamin	Alcohol abuse
Vitamin B_6	Isoniazid, alcohol abuse
Vitamin B_{12}	Colchicine, cimetidine
Vitamin A	Alcohol abuse
Vitamin D	Phenytoin, phenobarbital, isoniazid, aluminum-containing antacids
Vitamin K	Coumadin (warfarin sodium), cholestyramine, tetracycline
Caloric intake	Digoxin, antihistamines, antipsychotics, tricyclic antidepressants, anticholinergic agents

ACE = angiotensin-converting enzyme.

worsen the electrolyte deficiency (especially potassium) and dehydration (drug-drug interaction). Several drugs can adversely influence calcium and vitamin D metabolism. Drugs such as anticonvulsants, corticosteroids, heparin, thyroxine, and loop diuretics can negatively influence bone mineral density (osteoporosis). Drugs such as phenytoin, phenobarbital, aluminum-containing antacids, and isoniazid can adversely influence vitamin D metabolism (osteomalacia). Table 4 summarizes some of the commonly encountered drug-nutrient interactions.

NUTRITIONAL ASSESSMENT OF HOSPITALIZED PATIENTS

Several studies have demonstrated a relationship between nutritional status and adverse clinical outcomes in hospitalized patients. An unintentional weight loss of >10 per cent, a depressed serum albumin concentration, depressed grip strength, and an anergic skin response to common antigens often predict increased morbidity during hospitalization. Protein-calorie undernutrition is common is hospitalized patients. In patients with body weight less than 90 per cent of ideal, a serum albumin concentration less than 3.5 g/dL or a serum prealbumin concentration less than 10 mg/dL, a diagnosis of moderate protein-calorie undernutrition should be considered.

The nutritional status of hospitalized patients can be assessed by various methods. The traditional methods of nutritional assessment rely heavily on objective anthropometric and laboratory test results. Nutritional assessment can also be based on the findings of history and physical examination. Subjective global assessment (SGA) was developed by Detsky and associates to identify hospitalized patients at nutritional risk. This subjective tool of nutritional assessment is based on the findings of history and physical examination. The assessment is made by obtaining the following six features of the patient's condition (Table 5): (1) weight change, (2) dietary intake, (3) gastrointestinal symptoms, (4) functional capacity, and (5) physical signs. Based on this assessment, a score of A is given if there is no evidence or minimal evidence of nutritional compromise, a score of B is given if there is clear evidence of food restriction with functional changes but little evidence of any changes in body mass, or a score of C is given if there is overwhelming evidence of nutritional compromise. This is a subjective screening tool, and various categories can be interpreted as follows:

- *Class A* indicates less than 5 per cent weight loss or more than 5 per cent total weight loss but recent evidence of weight gain and improvement in appetite (well nourished).
- *Class B* indicates 5 to 10 per cent weight loss without recent weight gain, poor dietary intake, and mild (1+) loss of subcutaneous fat (moderately malnourished).
- *Class C* indicates weight loss of more than 10 per cent with severe loss of subcutaneous fat and muscle wasting, often with edema (severely malnourished).

NUTRITIONAL ASSESSMENT OF OLDER ADULTS

The proportion of older Americans continues to grow in our society. This segment of our population is at increased nutritional risk for a variety of reasons. The caloric intake declines after age 60 years, and this may also cause a reduced intake of essential nutrients. An older person is more likely to have a functional disability, undesirable psychosocial environment, and one or more medical problems, and is more likely to consume one or more medications. All these factors put an older person at increased nutritional risk. Since a compromised nutritional status has been shown to be associated with adverse clinical outcomes, early recognition and treatment of an older person at nutritional risk is recommended.

The Nutrition Screening Initiative was developed by the American Academy of Family Physicians, the American Dietetic Association, and the National Council on the Aging, Inc., to screen older Americans for nutritional risk. This is a tiered approach to screening. The first level of screening is a checklist to be completed by the older person or the caregiver, which is followed by a two-level approach accomplished in a professional setting. The Nutrition Screening Initiative is designed for early recognition and treatment of nutritional deficiencies in older Americans.

SCALES (Sadness, Cholesterol, Albumin, Loss of weight, Eat, Shopping) is a simple nutritional risk screening tool

Table 5. Subjective Global Assessment of Nutritional Status

(Select appropriate category with a checkmark or enter numerical value where indicated by "#")

A. History

1. Weight change

   Overall loss in past 6 months: amount = # ______ kg; % loss = # ______

   Change in past 2 weeks: ______ increase

   ______ no change

   ______ decrease

2. Dietary intake change (relative to normal)

   ______ No change

   ______ Change ______ duration = # ______ weeks

   ______ type: ______ suboptimal solid diet, ______ full liquid diet ______

   ______ hypocaloric liquids, ______ starvation

3. Gastrointestinal symptoms (persisting for >2 weeks)

   ______ none, ______ nausea, ______ vomiting, ______ diarrhea, ______ anorexia

4. Functional capacity

   ______ No dysfunction (e.g., full capacity)

   ______ Dysfunction ______ duration = # ______ weeks

   ______ type: ______ working suboptimally,

   ______ ambulatory,

   ______ bedridden

B. Physical (for each trait specify: 0 = normal, 1 + = mild, 2+ = moderate, 3+ = severe)

______ loss of subcutaneous fat (triceps, chest)

______ muscle wasting (quadriceps, deltoids)

______ ankle edema

______ sacral edema

______ ascites

C. SGA rating (select one)

______ A = well nourished

______ B = moderately (or suspected of being) malnourished

______ C = severely malnourished

SGA = subjective global assessment.

Adapted from Detsky, A. S., McLaughlin, J. R., Baker, J. P., et al.: What is subjective global assessment of nutritional status? J. Parenter. Enter. Nutr. 11:8–13, 1987, with permission.

developed by Morley (Table 6). This tool highlights the importance of depression, weight loss, feeding dependence, psychosocial factors, low serum cholesterol, and low serum albumin as indicators of nutritional risk in older persons.

Institutionalized older adults are at the greatest risk for protein-calorie undernutrition in the United States. Frequently, one or more treatable causes of protein-calorie undernutrition can be identified in this population. Table 7 lists some of the commonly observed causes of protein-calorie undernutrition in institutionalized older adults. Failure to recognize and treat depression, lack of feeding assistance, medications, oral diseases, and inappropriate use of a restricted diet are some of the commonly observed treatable causes of protein-calorie undernutrition in institutionalized older adults.

Table 6. The Nutritional Risk Screening for Older Adults (Scales)

*S*adness	Yesavage Geriatric Depression Scale of 15 or greater out of 30
*C*holesterol	Less than 160 mg/dL
*A*lbumin	Less than 4 g/dL
*L*oss of weight	2 lb in 1 mo or 5 lb in 6 mo
*E*at	The individual has problems feeding self because of either physical (e.g., tremor) or cognitive problems
*S*hopping	Insufficient money to buy food and the inability to obtain and prepare it

Adapted from Morley, J. E.: Why do physicians fail to recognize and treat malnutrition in older persons? J. Am. Geriatr. Soc. 39:1139–1140, 1991; with permission.

CONCLUSION

Nutritional assessment should be an essential part of every patient's clinical database. Most of the information

Table 7. Modifiable Causes of Undernutrition in the Institutionalized Elderly Population

Inappropriate use of restricted or modified diet
Drugs that cause anorexia (e.g., digoxin) or affect ability to eat (drugs with anticholinergic action causing dryness of mouth, e.g., antihistamines, antipsychotics, tricyclic antidepressants)
Lack of feeding assistance
Inadequate caloric intake and prescription
Depression
Inadequate nutritional support during intercurrent illness
Unmet need for modified diet
Poor dental status

needed to assess nutritional status can be obtained from a history and physical examination. Physicians often underestimate the significance of nutritional status in disease outcome and the well-being of patients. Patients with compromised nutritional status have increased morbidity and mortality.

ANOREXIA AND BULIMIA

By Steven J. Romano, M.D.,
and Katherine A. Halmi, M.D.
White Plains, New York

Eating disorders have gained clinical and research attention, paralleling an increase in their prevalence over the last few decades. They are best viewed as clinical syndromes rather than specific diseases because they do not have a single cause or course. As such, eating disorders are defined largely by a constellation of behaviors and attitudes that persist over time, producing characteristic complications that contribute to physical sequelae and psychosocial dysfunction. Knowledge of the behavioral characteristics of eating disorders can lead to improved recognition and implementation of effective treatment strategies. Eating disorders involve a complicated interplay of psychiatric, psychosocial, and medical consequences; therefore, treatment beyond initial medical stabilization generally requires referral to specialists.

MULTIDIMENSIONAL MODEL

A multidimensional model can illustrate the role of various factors in the genesis of clinically significant eating disturbances and may help the clinician who confronts such complicated syndromes. In this multidimensional "stress diathesis" model, psychological, biologic, and sociocultural stressors contribute to the expression of symptoms.

Psychological contributors include personality features (e.g., the anorectic patient's obsessive-compulsive qualities, constrained affect, and sense of ineffectiveness, or the bulimic's impulsivity) as well as developmental stressors and family dynamics. Biologic factors include the adverse effects of starvation and the physiologic imbalances caused by malnutrition and purging behaviors (e.g., vomiting and the misuse of laxatives and diuretics). Caloric restriction and malnourishment not only contribute to the development of anxiety and depression but also intensify the distinctive psychological features of the eating disorders. The possibility of pre-existing biologic vulnerability has been suggested by preliminary reports of dysfunctional neuromodulation and the development of amenorrhea in some anorectic patients prior to significant weight loss. Sociocultural factors, including the idealization of thinness, contribute to dieting behavior that often begins in early adolescence. Importantly, dieting almost always precedes the development of an eating disorder. Also, periods of illness may lead to weight loss that, in vulnerable individuals, may be followed by willful dieting.

The multidimensional model aids conceptualization and improves recognition of the eating disorders. In anorexia nervosa, multiple factors including biologic vulnerability, may initiate illness. Weight loss and malnourishment may cause physiologic changes that intensify dieting behavior and a psychological mindset. In bulimia nervosa, disordered intake and purging may generate neurochemical alterations that sustain abnormal ingestion behaviors.

ANOREXIA NERVOSA

Description

Anorexia nervosa is a relatively rare disorder that afflicts less than 1 per cent of young women. The most striking behavior of patients with anorexia nervosa is the willful restriction of intake that may cause death in 5 to 7 per cent of patients within 10 years of the disorder's onset. These patients harbor irrational fears of becoming overweight, and they view themselves as overweight even in the presence of severe emaciation. Anorectic individuals often display a phobic response to food, especially fatty and other calorically dense items. These women are obsessively preoccupied with food, eating, dieting, weight, and body shape. They often exhibit ritualistic behavior in the course of choosing, preparing, and ingesting meals. For example, many anorectic patients cut food into very small pieces or chew each bite a specific number of times.

Early in the course of anorexia nervosa, women begin to avoid many types of food. As the disorder progresses, the anorectic individual's menu becomes excessively and rigidly constricted. Minor variations in meal content may produce tremendous anxiety. Unlike the average dieter, the anorectic individual pursues thinness to an extreme and becomes psychologically dependent on the daily registration of weight loss. Reduction of weight spurs further restrictions of caloric intake. Exercise is often compulsive, and hyperactivity is frequently noted. Weakness, myalgias, sleep disturbances, constipation, postprandial bloating, and amenorrhea are common complaints.

Some anorectic individuals adopt bulimic behavior, including binging and purging. Self-induced vomiting and the misuse of laxatives and diuretics are frequently seen in the absence of binging. The combination of purging and self-starvation increases the risk of medical complications in anorexia nervosa.

Anorectic patients typically minimize their symptoms and the negative consequences of the disorder. Thus, they are rarely motivated to undergo treatment. Both the manifestations of illness and the lack of desire for treatment are intensified with weight loss. Family and friends become increasingly anxious, even angry, as their loved one regresses and their efforts are thwarted by mounting opposition. Superficial compliance, as is sometimes seen, belies a profound resistance. Treatment of anorectic individuals becomes increasingly complex as they cling tenaciously to their beliefs and behaviors.

Psychosocial dysfunction is common in patients with anorexia. Although educational milestones may be attained by adolescent patients, their social relationships diminish and deteriorate, and sexual interest is reduced or absent.

Differential Diagnosis

The classic features of anorexia nervosa, especially the intense fear of becoming overweight and the relentless pursuit of thinness, are absent in medical and psychiatric conditions that may confound the diagnosis. The term anorexia, which denotes an absence of appetite, is a misnomer as used in anorexia nervosa. True anorexia accompanies a host of medical conditions, especially cancer and gastrointestinal disorders.

Decreased appetite or food intake, with or without subsequent weight loss, is also encountered in depression, psychosomatic disorders, schizophrenia, and some delusional disorders. Patients with anorexia nervosa typically do not manifest the persistent mood disturbance and associated depressive ideation seen in major depression, the fear of choking seen in patients with globus hystericus, or the fear of poisoning predicated on false belief or delusional ideation seen in patients with paranoid delusions. Patients with obsessive-compulsive disorder (OCD) may exhibit bizarre behavior regarding food, eating, or meal preparation, but their actions are often a response to obsessional ideation (e.g., the fear of contamination). In contrast to patients with anorexia nervosa, individuals with obsessive-compulsive disorder typically acknowledge their discomfort with the need to perform such compelling and often excessive or senseless acts. In summary, although comorbid psychopathologic conditions may be encountered in patients with anorexia nervosa, the hallmark of the disorder (i.e., the morbid fear of becoming fat and the relentless pursuit of thinness) is absent in other psychiatric syndromes. The goal of weight loss does not drive the behavior in any of those disorders.

Medical Complications

Most of the medical consequences of anorexia nervosa occur in starvation states or as a direct result of purging behaviors. Medical complications can be reversed, however, with nutritional rehabilitation and the discontinuation of purging behaviors. For example, with nutritional rehabilitation, decreased leukocyte counts normalize and do not require further evaluation.

Metabolic alkalosis, hypokalemia, hypochloremia, and increased serum bicarbonate concentrations are frequently seen in patients who induce vomiting. By contrast, some patients who abuse stimulant-type laxatives acquire metabolic acidosis. Dehydration and volume depletion in those who fast or purge may increase aldosterone production and potassium excretion. Thus, indirect renal loss of potassium may compound its direct loss from the gastrointestinal tract.

Emaciation and electrolyte disturbances may cause other problems, especially in anorectic individuals who purge. The electrocardiogram may show flat or inverted T waves, ST-segment depression, and a prolonged QT interval. Severe hypokalemia increases the risk of serious arrhythmias and cardiac arrest. Excessively rapid refeeding of emaciated anorectic patients may cause heart failure.

Parotid gland enlargement and increased amylase concentrations are often seen in anorectic patients who binge and practice self-induced vomiting. Acute gastric dilatation is a rare medical emergency in patients who binge. Delay in gastric emptying may cause postprandial discomfort and early satiety.

BULIMIA NERVOSA

Description

Bulimia nervosa has been described in 2 to 3 per cent of young women; bulimic behavior, however, may be encountered in many more women, especially during periods of restrictive dieting. Bulimic individuals engage in regular episodes of binge eating, followed by compensatory behavior that attempts to counteract the weight gain resulting from ingested calories. Binge eating is characterized by rapid consumption of large amounts of food over a distinct period, usually 1 to 2 hours. Binging is accompanied by a sense of loss of control and is often followed by feelings of guilt or shame. Frequently, other dysphoric affective states (e.g., depression or anxiety), follow the binging and purging. Some patients report a brief alleviation of dysphoria during or immediately following the binge-purge episode. During a binge, the patient may consume several thousand calories. Some women describe trigger foods (e.g., chocolate) that can precipitate a binge. Macroanalysis of nutrient content indicates that the sources and nutrients of the food consumed vary significantly. The bulimic individual binges almost exclusively in private because the act of excessive food consumption is humiliating. Embarrassment in bulimic individuals can lead to varying degrees of social avoidance or isolation.

The need to compensate for consumption further contributes to avoidance behavior. Most bulimic individuals induce vomiting during or after a binge; some also use laxatives or diuretics. A few patients employ laxatives or diuretics alone. Two subtypes of compensatory behavior are encountered in bulimia nervosa, namely, purging and nonpurging. Nonpurging compensatory behavior involves compulsive exercising and restrictive dieting or fasting between binges.

Bulimic individuals are not satisfied with their body shape or weight, and they may become obsessively preoccupied with their dissatisfaction. In turn, the bulimic woman's self-evaluation is excessively influenced by her perception of her physical characteristics. The profound effect of body image on self-esteem is suggested by the comorbid depression seen in bulimic individuals. Significant impulsiveness is encountered in many patients with bulimia nervosa; in some bulimic individuals, associated behaviors include substance abuse, sexual promiscuity, and stealing or shoplifting.

Differential Diagnosis

Bulimia nervosa is seldom confused with other medical or psychiatric disorders. Frequently, the observation of specific physical signs or symptoms in a young woman who does not admit to binging or purging behaviors may lead the clinician to search for another primary medical diagnosis. Usually the complaints are a direct result or consequence of self-induced vomiting and diuretic or laxative use. Signs and symptoms associated with gastritis, esophagitis, dehydration, or electrolyte disturbances lead to consultation with primary care physicians or to emergency room visits, postponing psychiatric consultation and evading more primary interventions. If the patient is underweight and amenorrheic and is binging and purging, she has anorexia nervosa, binge-purge subtype.

Medical Complications

The majority of medical complications due to bulimia nervosa are consequences of purging behaviors. Self-induced vomiting can lead to gastritis, esophagitis, periodontal disease, and dental carries, the latter caused by the corrosive effect of acidic stomach contents on the dental enamel. Gastric dilatation and gastric or esophageal rupture are rare medical emergencies that may lead to shock. Metabolic alkalosis and clinically significant hypokalemia in patients who vomit is not unusual. Electrocardiographic changes in this setting carry significant import because arrhythmias can lead to cardiac arrest if hypokalemia and related disturbances are not corrected effectively. The use of diuretics cause similar disturbances. Metabolic acidosis can be encountered in individuals who use a significant amount of stimulant-type laxatives. Dehydration that may require intravenous fluid administration may accompany various purging behaviors. General physical complaints, such as fatigue and muscle aches, are more often associated with bulimic behaviors. Although it is becoming seen less frequently in clinical practice, the long-term use of the emetic, ipecac, can lead to myopathies, including (most seriously) cardiomyopathy. The latter is not an infrequent cause of death in patients abusing this toxic substance.

CONCLUSION

Eating disorders represent a broad spectrum of psychopathologic behaviors, not limited to disturbances in appetite, and are best understood in terms of multiple causative factors influencing the development of clinical syndromes. Recognition of the complexity of these disorders, including the array of comorbid psychiatric features, and understanding the more specific eating-disordered behaviors and attitudes aids in the recognition of clinically significant cases.

OBESITY

By C. Laird Birmingham, M.D.,
Elliot M. Goldner, M.D.,
and Iain G.M. Cleator, M.B., Ch.B.
Vancouver, British Columbia, Canada

Obesity, which is defined as an excess of total body fat, presents with the complaint of overweight, as a functional impairment such as hypertension, in the context of an eating disorder, or as an observation at the time of assessment for another complaint.

In defining obesity, two difficulties are encountered: how to measure body fat accurately and how to determine what constitutes an excess. In most clinical situations, simple inspection of the body habitus and pinching an area of skin to determine the depth of subcutaneous fat ("pinch an inch") is adequate to demonstrate excess. Changes in body fat in obese individuals are then documented routinely by weighing the patient. Although weight does not provide an independent estimate of body fat, changes in weight while dieting are easily and accurately measured and over time reflect changes in body fat. Short-term changes in weight are often confounded by fluid shifts, however. Thus, on a very low calorie diet, most of the initial weight loss is loss of fluid, but long-term weight loss without loss of significant amounts of edema results mostly from loss of fat.

Based on studies and consensus panels, most authors and tables arbitrarily define obesity as a body weight 20 per cent greater than ideal or a body mass index (BMI) (see further on) greater than the 85th percentile. A normal weight for gender can be simplistically estimated by defining normal weight for a female as 100 lb for the first 5 ft and an additional 5 lb for every inch thereafter and for a male as 106 lb for the first 5 ft and an additional 6 lb for each additional inch. Correction for gender, height, and body frame can be achieved by using tables such as the Metropolitan Life tables; however, these tables were based on actuarial data obtained from a life insurance reference population, and using them in other patient populations may not be valid.

Sometimes the diagnosis is more difficult if the obesity is less marked or if other tissues (e.g., muscle mass) or fluids (e.g., edema) may be contributing to the increased weight. Methods that attempt to estimate body fat separately include dual-energy x-ray absorptiometry (DEXA). Unfortunately, these tests are time-consuming and expensive, and some involve a dose of radiation. In addition, the tests have inherent errors, (often >2 per cent), and in edematous states and very obese individuals they can have a much higher error.

"Synonyms" for obesity are often used clinically because overweight, excess body fat, and high BMI are more acceptable terms to the patient than obesity. Conversely, morbid obesity is sometimes used inappropriately to convince the patient of the seriousness of the disease. Discussing the limitations of these synonyms raises some important issues about obesity.

Adiposity means excess subcutaneous fat. Therefore, obese patients do have excess adiposity. Some, however, may have localized adiposity, as in the common familial distribution of excess body fat to the hips. The term adiposity does not mean the patient has excess total body fat and therefore does not always imply obesity. Importantly, however, even modest central adiposity is a strong risk factor for the metabolic complications of obesity such as diabetes, hypertension, and hyperlipidemia. Although overweight, or weight in excess of that found in standard tables, is often used as a synonym for obesity, it does not specifically identify fat as the tissue in excess. Although the excess weight is usually fat, it may be due to muscularity, as in weight lifters; to fluid, as in states of severe edema, lymphedema, or ascites; or rarely to another tissue, as in the case of massive intra-abdominal tumors. The BMI is weight corrected to height by dividing the weight in kilograms by the square of the height in meters. Many misinterpret this correction of weight for height as a more accurate measurement of obesity. It is not, but because it produces a single number with abstruse dimensions, it is often given greater importance than weight and height interpreted in the context of standard weight tables. Adolescents are often aware of their BMI and strive to be a certain "number" without considering the important variables of frame size or muscularity. So, although BMI is useful in normalizing the results of research relating to weight in groups of individuals by height, it must be used with caution in individual patient care.

Morbid obesity means body fat 100 per cent greater than normal (100 lb in the case of men or women less than 5 ft in height). This term is commonly used as one criterion for assessing a candidate for obesity surgery, because the mortality rate in this group of patients is known to be high. For example, a female 100 per cent above her ideal weight and between 25 and 35 years of age has a 12-fold increase in the risk of death over a matched control subject of normal weight. Nonetheless, the term morbid obesity is misleading to some because its use is not dependent on the presence of morbidity.

Obesity usually presents with the patient complaining of being overweight. In the case of children, parents may bring the child to the physician with the complaint of weight gain. Obesity can also be defined according to functional impairment. Thus, a middle-aged man who has gained 20 lb over his previous weight and has acquired hypertension, non–insulin-dependent diabetes, and hypertriglyceridemia, all of which disappear with weight loss, clearly has a functional excess of total body fat. Obesity may present in this way as non–insulin-dependent diabetes mellitus, hypertension, gout, hyperlipidemia, osteoarthritis or exacerbation of pre-existent arthritic syndromes, sleep apnea, the pickwickian syndrome, or with other complications of functional status. Lastly, obesity can present as part of an eating disorder. Obese patients who present with physical complaints frequently encounter a tendency among clinicians to reflexly ascribe them to the obesity. This is simplistic and only decreases trust and rapport between patient and physician.

CLINICAL COURSE

Obesity can begin at any time in life from infancy to old age. Obesity due to genetic or familial factors often has a similar time of onset among family members. Obesity secondary to medications, such as psychotropic agents, or diseases, such as hypothyroidism, is often temporally related to the use of the medication or onset of the disease. An increase in body fat resulting in a weight gain of more than 20 lb lasting more than a few months usually results in persistence and often a gradual increase in obesity even if a preventable cause is found and treated. Common clinical presentations are childhood obesity, obesity in females occurring in the setting of recurrent pregnancies, central obesity occurring most frequently in middle-aged men, perimenopausal obesity in females, and obesity associated with depression.

The onset of obesity usually occurs during childhood, adolescence, in relation to pregnancies, or in middle life. In childhood, when genetic or food-related obesity typically begins, isolation and depression caused by the condition can cause the child to be less active, to avoid exercise such as swimming, and to eat in response to negative feelings. Childhood obesity usually causes a hyperplasia of fat cells (adipocytes), and these increased numbers of fat cells remain throughout life. During puberty, females experience an increase and redistribution of total body fat; with pregnancy, a physiologic increase in body fat occurs. Following pregnancy, women are often instructed not to restrict caloric intake during breast-feeding. If the new mother then becomes pregnant before much weight has been lost, a cycle of weight gain, along with feelings of hopelessness, isolation, and depression leading to further eating, often begins.

Later in life, in the sixth and seventh decades, most individuals experience a gradual decrease in lean body mass and an increase in fatty mass, the significance of which is unclear. Central adiposity in middle-aged men is common. Often referred to as a "beer belly," this fat often results in a 15- to 40-lb weight gain and is associated with hypertension, hypertriglyceridemia, hyperuricemia, and a gradual impairment of glucose tolerance. It usually results from a sedentary lifestyle in the face of significant caloric intake. Early intervention (perhaps because weight loss usually rapidly normalizes the biochemical derangements) often is at least moderately successful in achieving initial weight loss and long-term stabilization in this group. Perimenopausal women can experience significant increases in weight and body fat over a few years. This weight gain is variable and does not respond to exogenous estrogens.

Obesity secondary to other diseases or processes bears a temporal relationship to that disease or process and may be just one part of a cluster of signs and symptoms. Thus, with hypothyroidism, other signs and symptoms of hypothyroidism are typically present. Adiposity in Cushing's syndrome is primarily deposited centrally, with prominent supraclavicular fat pads; buttock wasting is common, in contrast with primary obesity in which the buttocks usually increase in size. Insulinoma is a rare cause of obesity that can cause an initial weight gain resulting from the anabolic effect of excess circulating insulin. Initiation of insulin in insulin-dependent diabetes does not usually cause obesity unless there is dietary excess or concomitant bulimia nervosa. Tumors such as craniopharyngiomas or other processes such as cerebrovascular accidents that involve the hypothalamus rarely cause obesity. A rapid onset of weight gain is often caused by medications such as estrogens, tricyclic antidepressants, lithium, and centrally acting antihistamines.

Obesity is an excess of total body fat and is not to be confused with localized adiposity, such as lipomas. A protuberant abdomen is commonly misdiagnosed as obesity when it may be due to another cause, such as ascites, feces or flatus retention, pregnancy, or an intra-abdominal mass. The distribution of the adiposity in genetic obesity is usually similar to that in other family members, especially those of the same sex. Women in certain families have a hip and thigh distribution of fat. Rarely, genetic syndromes include obesity as well as other unique abnormalities. These syndromes include Laurence-Moon-Biedl syndrome, which is characterized by retinitis pigmentosa, mental retardation, skull deformities, polydactyly, and syndactyly; Prader-Willi syndrome, with hypotonia, mental retardation, and diabetes mellitus; Fröhlich's syndrome in boys, characterized by hypogonadism and a variable incidence of diabetes insipidus, visual impairment, and mental retardation; Alström syndrome, with retinitis pigmentosa, nerve deafness, diabetes mellitus, and primary gonadal failure; and Biemond syndrome, with diabetes mellitus, hypogonadism, polydactyly, and iris colobomas. These syndromes are typically associated with onset of obesity at an early age.

COMMON COMPLICATIONS

Non–Insulin-Dependent Diabetes Mellitus

Ninety per cent of non–insulin-dependent diabetes is accompanied by obesity and is at least partially controlled by weight loss. The onset of hyperglycemia is usually gradual, with few or no symptoms. Hyperglycemia can significantly antedate symptoms; therefore fasting serum glucose and hemoglobin A_{1c} determinations are performed on the initial evaluation of the obese patient. With continued weight gain or even with weight maintenance, the insulin resistance increases and symptomatic diabetes eventually emerges. Asymptomatic hyperglycemia carries the same risk for vascular and metabolic complications as does symptomatic hyperglycemia; it must therefore be detected, monitored, and treated.

Hypertension

All obese patients should have their blood pressure checked at regular intervals with an appropriately sized blood pressure cuff. The blood pressure cuff must have a wide diameter with a bladder 20 per cent wider than the diameter of the arm. A blood pressure cuff that is too small results in a falsely increased blood pressure measurement. Hypertension in obese patients is associated with insulin resistance and may appear over time, even when a steady weight is maintained. Conversely, even minimal weight loss with maintenance on a low-calorie diet is often associated with significant lowering of blood pressure. If patients fail to maintain dietary control and to lose weight, other treatments must be used as necessary.

Hyperuricemia and Gout

Hyperuricemia and gout are more common in obese individuals, particularly in those on diets that result in the formation of ketone bodies in the liver from the metabolism of triglycerides, which, in turn, compete with the excretory pathway for uric acid and result in hyperuricemia. Serum uric acid concentrations should be measured on initial assessment of the obese patient, especially in those with tophi or a history of renal dysfunction or gout.

Hyperlipidemia

Hyperinsulinemia caused by insulin resistance (see previous discussion) results in increased release of very low density lipoprotein (VLDL) from the liver. This is assessed by measuring fasting triglycerides and cholesterol. The high serum VLDL results primarily in hypertriglyceridemia but also in some degree of hypercholesterolemia with a relative decrease in high-density lipoproteins (HDLs). Screening is indicated at initial presentation and at regular intervals during treatment. The hyperlipidemia due to VLDL excess is often responsive to weight loss or even compliance with a low-calorie diet with maintenance of modest weight loss. Obesity also appears to increase the risk of atherosclerosis independent of diabetes, hypertension, and hyperlipidemia.

Musculoskeletal Complications

Obese individuals suffer more commonly from significant osteoarthritis and varicose veins. Neither of these disorders is reversed by weight loss, but symptoms and progression may be lessened. Hernias, intertrigo, and deep venous thrombosis are also more common in obese persons.

Respiratory Complications

Sleep apnea (see article on sleep disorders) is associated with an increased neck diameter and obesity in about two thirds of patients. Closure of the upper airway causes recurrent attempts at respiration before full inspiration is possible. This results in oxygen desaturation and is associated with nocturnal snoring, choking, apnea, restless sleeping, morning headaches, and daytime somnolence. A history of these symptoms must be elicited, often from the bed partner, because most patients do not volunteer a history of nocturnal snoring, choking, or apnea. Unrecognized sleep apnea in the preoperative patient presents a significant risk of postoperative apnea.

The pickwickian syndrome is associated with massive obesity. In this rare disorder, the energy required to maintain normal breathing is so great relative to the body's need for oxygen that respiration is subnormal, resulting in hypercapnia, hypoxemia, polycythemia, and pulmonary hypertension. The patient with pickwickian syndrome is somnolent, extremely obese, and often cyanotic. Most patients with this syndrome also suffer from sleep apnea.

Malignancy

The incidence of breast and uterine cancer is increased in obese patients, and screening for these disorders is important for proper management. The obese female often has large breasts that must be carefully examined by palpation and mammography. Detection of uterine cancer is complicated because the gynecologic examination is difficult in obese women. Patience and vigilance in obtaining a Papanicolaou smear, and investigating abnormal menstrual bleeding is crucial. Moderate to severe obesity is usually associated with oligomenorrhea.

Hepatobiliary Disease

Obese patients usually have fat deposition in the liver that presents a characteristic picture on ultrasound or computed tomography. Fatty liver is usually asymptomatic and does not alter liver function or liver function tests. However, mild increases in liver enzyme activity can occur secondary to hepatic steatosis, which, when severe, can increase portal pressure. Cholelithiasis is also more common in obese patients, particularly with recurrent weight loss.

PHYSICAL FINDINGS

Obese patients typically have a generalized distribution of fat; however, some patients with primary obesity have a "buffalo hump," silvery striae on the abdomen, and some degree of excess central adiposity. Large buttocks and hirsutism are also more common in obese individuals. Breath sounds are audible but may be distant. The cardiac apex usually is not displaced, but heart sounds may be faint. Blood pressure is frequently increased, and some dependent edema may be present. The abdominal and gynecologic examinations are usually difficult. Mild to moderate hepatomegaly is common because of hepatic steatosis, and it does not regress even with significant long-term weight loss. Intertrigo beneath the breasts and abdominal pannus occurs often, particularly in diabetic patients if personal hygiene is not maintained.

Unusual findings on physical examination should prompt a consideration of other primary disorders. Papilledema due to empty sella syndrome is more common in obese persons, although it is still rare. Signs of Cushing's syndrome include supraclavicular fat pads, buttock wasting, and purplish striae of the abdomen. Pituitary disease can cause bitemporal hemianopsia. An enlarged thyroid gland, dry skin, and a delayed relaxation phase of the deep tendon reflexes suggest hypothyroidism. Most obese patients present with moist skin, sparse clothing, and perspiration with minimal exertion. The obese patient who appears cold, is dressed normally, and does not perspire may have hypothyroidism. Breasts must be examined for the presence of masses.

LABORATORY AND OTHER DIAGNOSTIC TESTS

Obese patients are best assessed by weight and height. As stated previously, the BMI, which corrects weight for height, must not be overemphasized. Patients with a lean body mass have a higher weight than normal for sex, age, and build, and therefore a high BMI. Simply raising a fold of fat between the thumb and the index finger provides a useful estimate of excess body fat. This can be measured using skinfold calipers to document an increased thickness of subcutaneous fat. Specific measures of body fat are less reliable as obesity becomes more severe, but distinguishing normal body fat from a significant excess is simplified by using skinfold calipers. Other less useful methods of documenting fat thickness and total body fat include densitometry by underwater weighing, bioelectrical impedance analysis (BIA), dual-energy x-ray absorptiometry, tritium and deuterium dilution methods of total body water, total body computed tomography, and subcutaneous ultrasonography. None of these tests is without error, cost, and inconvenience, and therefore they are not employed routinely.

Biochemical tests have similar reference ranges in both obese and nonobese populations. Commonly, however, hepatic steatosis causes a mild increase in lactate dehydrogenase and alkaline phosphatase activity, whereas aspartate aminotransferase activity remains normal. Sex hormone–binding globulin can be decreased in association with the hepatic steatosis. With the onset of glucose intolerance, the fasting and postprandial glucose and hemoglobin A_{1c} concentrations gradually increase. Serum insulin concentrations are supranormal even in obese nondiabetic patients. As glucose intolerance progresses, VLDL becomes increased, with a concomitant increase in triglycerides and a lesser increase in cholesterol. Renal function is normal in obese patients, but pulmonary function tests typically show a reduction in the functional residual capacity.

DISORDERS OF VITAMIN AND SUPPLEMENT EXCESS

By Jack W. Snyder, M.D., J.D., Ph.D.
Philadelphia, Pennsylvania

In developed countries where food is abundant, many people supplement their diet by ingesting vitamins, minerals, hormones, amino acids, plant extracts, pharmaceuticals, and other over-the-counter agents. Billions of dollars are spent on hundreds of products whose consumption is believed to enhance muscle growth, decrease appetite, increase libido and sexual potency, decrease the effects of aging, and prevent acne, psoriasis, osteoporosis, atherosclerosis, and cancer. There is, however, no evidence that the most common diseases in developed nations are caused by nutritional deficiency or that daily supplementation of the diet with vitamins and minerals is required for optimal functioning. It is therefore not surprising that convincing evidence of the specific efficacy of these supplements is difficult to obtain or is nonexistent. Nevertheless, their use continues unabated in the 1990s, and clinicians must understand that the consumption of megadoses and other excessive or inappropriate uses of supplements have been associated with significant adverse health effects.

Counterbalancing this documented risk of harm are three proposed bases for the rational use of high-dose vitamins. First, a patient may have a vitamin-dependent genetic disease. Second, a patient may have a disorder characterized by defective transport of vitamins across cell membranes. Third, a patient may require the use of vitamins as antidotes for the toxicity of methotrexate, antifolates, or other agents that interfere with vitamin production or function. When confronted with a patient who consumes or would like to consume large doses of vitamins or other supplements, the clinician should consider whether any of these rationales may legitimize megadoses. If not, the physician should advise the patient of the potential health risks associated with megadoses.

VITAMIN A (RETINOL) (RECOMMENDED DAILY ALLOWANCE = 5000 IU, 1 mg = 3333 IU)

Vitamin A, or retinol, serves as a cofactor in several biochemical pathways. This fat-soluble vitamin is required for growth, bone development, proper ovarian and testicular function, and visual adaptation to darkness. Vitamin A derivatives have been used to treat Darier's disease, ichthyosis, malabsorption syndromes, acne, sun-damaged and aging skin, and psoriasis. Vitamin A has also been promoted as an antioxidant, anticancer agent, and cure for attention deficit disorder. In the diet, preformed vitamin A comes from animals, vitamin A precursors (β-carotene and other carotenoids) come from vegetables, and high concentrations (100,000 IU/g) of vitamin A can be obtained from fish-liver oils. Vitamin A is also available in capsular, liquid, tablet, and injectable products. Vitamin A derivatives available by prescription include isotretinoin (oral retinoic acid, Accutane), tretinoin (topical retinoic acid, Retin-A), and etretinate (oral retinoic acid, Tegison).

Vitamin A toxicity is an uncommon but well-known problem that correlates with dose and duration of exposure and the total body vitamin A content. Acute hypervitaminosis A typically requires ingestions exceeding 25,000 IU/kg body weight, whereas chronic toxicity is associated with consumption of at least 4000 IU per day/kg body weight. Acute toxicity is more common in children than in adults, whereas chronic hypervitaminosis A occurs in food faddists, consumers of beef and polar bear livers, and patients treated for dermatologic conditions.

Acute vitamin A toxicity is characterized initially by headache from increased intracranial pressure, dizziness, fatigue, irritability, nausea, vomiting, anorexia, and abdominal pain. Within 24 to 72 hours, petechiae, erythema, and peeling of the skin as well as perioral fissures, hair loss, hypercalcemia, and abnormal liver function test results ensue.

By contrast, chronic hypervitaminosis A is characterized by protean abnormalities involving the eyes, brain, bones, joints, skin, mucous membranes, liver, and gastrointestinal tract. Pseudotumor cerebri (benign intracranial hypertension) with papilledema, diplopia, blurred vision, and headaches is probably the most well-known and feared complication because persistent visual impairment due to optic atrophy is the only major long-term effect of vitamin A toxicity. By contrast, most of the other abnormalities resolve within weeks to months after cessation of vitamin A intake.

In addition to pseudotumor cerebri, the signs and symptoms most helpful in the diagnosis of chronic vitamin A toxicity include teratogenesis, spontaneous abortions, mucocutaneous changes (especially loss of hair, brittle nails, rough scaly skin, and peripheral edema), bone and joint discomfort, gastrointestinal disturbances, and hepatomegaly with or without cirrhosis. Radiographic changes include bone demineralization, new bone formation, and abnormal calcification. Diagnostically significant laboratory abnormalities include hypercalcemia, hyperuricemia, hypertriglyceridemia, hypercholesterolemia, anemia, leukopenia, and increased serum bilirubin concentrations and alkaline phosphatase and transaminase activity. Chronic vitamin A toxicity is associated with serum concentrations of retinol exceeding 100 μg/dL.

VITAMIN B_2 (RIBOFLAVIN) (RECOMMENDED DAILY ALLOWANCE = 2 mg)

Excessive doses of riboflavin have not been reported to cause adverse human health effects. Moreover, no specific benefit has been observed in nondeficient persons who consume large amounts of riboflavin. Megadoses of B vitamins may intensify the yellow color of urine, and riboflavin may produce yellow perspiration.

VITAMIN B_3 (NIACIN) (RECOMMENDED DAILY ALLOWANCE = 20 mg)

Niacin is an essential vitamin that consists of two isomers—nicotinic acid and nicotinamide. The terms niacin and nicotinic acid are typically used interchangeably, as are the terms niacinamide and nicotinamide. Niacin is required for glycogenolysis, lipid metabolism, and tissue respiration. Depending on the dose, niacin is partially converted to niacinamide, which, in turn, undergoes hepatic metabolism. Reports dating back to 1955 suggest that ingestion of niacin, but not niacinamide, may lower serum cholesterol concentrations by decreasing the synthesis of low-density lipoproteins (LDLs) and apoprotein B. Nicotinic acid consumption at doses 10 to 100 times the Recommended Daily Allowance (RDA) may also reduce serum triglyceride and increase serum high-density lipoprotein (HDL) cholesterol concentrations. Niacin is inexpensive, widely available over the counter, and generally well tolerated. Its extensive use, however, especially in high doses, has been linked to clinically significant adverse effects. Initial use often causes nausea, vomiting, gastric irritation, diarrhea, pruritus, skin rash, vasodilation and cutaneous flushing, headache, blurred vision, dizziness, hypotension, tachycardia, vasovagal reactions, and syncope that may result, at least in part, from the release of prostaglandins. Extended use of niacin may cause or aggravate asthma, hyperglycemia, hyperuricemia, myopathy, coagulopathy, amblyopia, and hyperpigmentation. Dose-related, sometimes chronic hepatotoxicity has been reported, especially in individuals who consume sustained-release preparations.

If niacin is indicated, begin treatment at 150 to 300 mg per day. Gradually increase the dose (at 1- to 2-month intervals), but do not exceed 1 to 3 g per day. To determine efficacy and to decrease the risk of clinically significant toxicity, measure serum transaminase activity and cholesterol and bilirubin concentrations 1 month after each major change of dose.

VITAMIN B_6 (PYRIDOXINE) (RECOMMENDED DAILY ALLOWANCE = 2 mg)

The phosphate ester of pyridoxine (pyridoxal phosphate) is an important cofactor for many enzyme reactions. Widely available in 50- to 500-mg tablets, pyridoxine is consumed by some body builders and has been used to treat premenstrual syndrome, attention deficit disorders, autism, and schizophrenia. Pyridoxine is commonly employed as an antidote for poisoning by isoniazid (INH) and monomethylhydrazine (MMH), an agent found in rocket propellant and also produced following ingestion and metabolism of mushrooms known as the false morels.

Although the minimum daily requirement (MDR) is 2 to 4 mg, pyridoxine is occasionally consumed in gram quantities per day. Daily doses of 2 to 6 g for 2 to 40 months have caused progressive (but often reversible) sensory ataxia, loss of position and vibration sense, perioral dysesthesias, peripheral neuropathy, altered reflexes, and impaired sense of pain, temperature, and touch. Doses as low as 200 to 500 mg of pyridoxine per day have also been associated with neurotoxicity. Low-dose pyridoxine may also antagonize the action of various drugs, including phenytoin, barbiturates, and levodopa.

Volunteers given 1 to 3 g of pyridoxine per day simultaneously experienced dose-dependent, abnormal (increased) quantitative sensory thresholds and altered sensation on physical examination. Nerve biopsies from symptomatic patients consuming megadoses of pyridoxine have shown widespread, nonspecific axonal degeneration, which may be reversible with early diagnosis and cessation of supplementation.

VITAMIN B_{12} (CYANOCOBALAMIN) (RECOMMENDED DAILY ALLOWANCE = 6 μg)

Cyanocobalamin serves as a cofactor in protein synthesis, fat and carbohydrate metabolism, and hematopoiesis. Excessive doses of cyanocobalamin rarely, if ever, cause adverse human health effects. Urticaria, pruritus, diarrhea, thrombosis, and hypokalemia may rarely occur with parenteral use. Ingestion of large amounts is typically innocuous because the gut will not generally absorb more than 2 to 3 μg from any single dose. No specific benefit has been observed in nondeficient persons who consume large amounts of vitamin B_{12}.

VITAMIN C (ASCORBIC ACID) (RECOMMENDED DAILY ALLOWANCE = 60 mg)

Ascorbic acid, or vitamin C, is required for collagen formation and tissue repair. Despite the lack of documented efficacy, megadosing (>500 mg per day) with vitamin C (ascorbic acid) remains popular for the treatment or prevention of viral syndromes, heart disease, cancer, aging, and stress and for the treatment of burns or other wounds. Ascorbic acid is converted to oxalate, and chronic ingestions exceeding 1 to 2 g per day may cause nausea, vomiting, flushing, heartburn, diarrhea, dental erosion or decalcification, decreased uric acid clearance, hyperoxaluria, and kidney stones containing cystine or oxalate. Ascorbic acid has induced hemolysis in patients with glucose-6-phosphate dehydrogenase deficiency. Vitamin C also increases the absorption of iron, so consumption of megadoses should be discouraged in patients with thalassemia, hemochromatosis, or sideroblastic anemia.

VITAMIN D (CHOLECALCIFEROL) (RECOMMENDED DAILY ALLOWANCE = 400 IU = 10 μg)

Vitamin D stimulates calcium and phosphate absorption from the small intestine and promotes the release of calcium from bone into blood. Most humans meet the daily requirement for vitamin D through exposure to sunlight for 5 to 10 minutes, four to five times per week. Vitamin D is available in capsule, liquid, tablet, topical, and injectable forms and has been used to treat rickets, hypoparathyroidism, hypophosphatemia, vitamin D–deficient states, psoriasis, and osteoporosis. Topical use of vitamin D (calcipotriene) commonly causes skin irritation, but hypercalcemia is extremely rare. Chronic ingestion of 1600 to 2000 IU per day causes hypervitaminosis D, which is characterized by anorexia, weakness, stiffness, bone pain, weight loss, nausea, vomiting, constipation, polyuria, hypertension, hypercalcemia, hyperphosphatemia, nephrocalcinosis, soft tissue or ectopic calcification, anemia, acidosis, proteinuria, irreversible renal failure, and falsely increased serum cholesterol concentrations. Rarely, excessive milk intake may cause hypervitaminosis D.

VITAMIN E (α-TOCOPHEROL) (RECOMMENDED DAILY ALLOWANCE = 30 IU)

At least eight naturally occurring forms of tocopherol possess vitamin E activity. In animal tissues, the most quantitatively significant form of vitamin E is α-tocopherol, which serves as the primary lipid antioxidant in biologic membranes. Parenteral vitamin E has been administered to infants to prevent intraventricular hemorrhage and retinopathy of prematurity and to reduce oxygen-mediated eye and lung injury in retrolental fibroplasia and bronchopulmonary dysplasia. Adults seeking to reduce their risk of atherosclerosis ingest large doses (>200 IU per day) of vitamin E to decrease the oxidation of low-density lipoproteins. Some individuals use vitamin E topically as well as orally in the belief that it will prevent cancer. However, the efficacy of α-tocopherol as an antiatherogenic and anticancer agent remains to be established.

Widespread adverse health effects have not been reported following long-term ingestion of vitamin E at doses of 100 to 1000 IU per day. However, patients taking large doses may occasionally describe headache, blurred vision, dizziness, fatigue, weakness, nausea, flatulence, and/or diarrhea. Ingestion of high doses of vitamin E may also interfere with the absorption, storage, and function of vitamins A and K. A prolonged prothrombin time and clotting time have been noted rarely. Skin rashes, contact dermatitis, and erythema multiforme may result from topical use. The potential long-term hazards of chronic high-dose vitamin E consumption remain unknown.

PSEUDOVITAMINS

Pseudovitamins are not really vitamins at all. A vitamin is typically defined as an organic substance required in relatively small amounts in the diet for the proper functioning of an organism. Thus, carnitine (so-called vitamin B_7), pangamic acid (so-called vitamin B_{15}), laetrile (so-called vitamin B_{17}), and bioflavinoids (so-called vitamin P) are not recognized as true vitamins because there is no evidence that these substances are required in the diet for proper functioning of human tissues.

MINERALS AND TRACE ELEMENTS

Zinc is an essential trace metal that serves as a cofactor for enzymes such as alcohol dehydrogenase, carbonic anhydrase, and carboxypeptidase. Zinc has become a popular dietary supplement. When consumed daily in gram quantities, zinc salts may interfere with copper absorption, impair leukocyte function, reduce serum HDL:LDL ratios, and cause reversible sideroblastic microcytic anemia. Zinc chloride and zinc phosphide are corrosive to the gastrointestinal tract and can cause vomiting and gastrointestinal distress that may significantly limit toxicity.

Selenium is an essential trace element required for the action of glutathione peroxidase, an enzyme that catalyzes the synthesis of oxidized glutathione. Selenium-deficient animals are more sensitive to oxygen radical or free radical cell injury. The antioxidant and proposed anticarcinogenic properties of selenium have increased its use as a diet supplement and as a controversial treatment for cystic fibrosis. The ingestion of microgram amounts of elemental selenium or selenium salts does not cause problems, but chronic consumption of milligram quantities may cause nausea, vomiting, cramps, diarrhea, garlic breath odor, fatigue, irritability, hair loss, nail changes or loss, paresthesias, and polyneuropathy.

AMINO ACIDS

Among the amino acids, L-arginine, L-lysine, and L-ornithine can be obtained over the counter for ingestion as dietary supplements. There are no recognized indications for their consumption, but there are also no reports of clinically significant human toxicity. By contrast, L-tryptophan is a nutritional supplement that was promoted for the treatment of insomnia, dysmenorrhea, anxiety, and lower back pain. In the early 1990s, hundreds of reports of adverse effects (including death) were associated with ingestion of 150 to 8400 mg per day of L-tryptophan for 2 weeks to 8 years. Symptoms and signs included intense myalgias, weakness, weight loss, dyspnea, paresthesias, and thickening of the skin with edema. Laboratory data revealed eosinophil counts greater than 1000 cells/mm^3 and occasional pulmonary infiltrates. Muscle biopsy confirmed the presence of inflammation. The disorder was named eosinophilia-myalgia syndrome (EMS). It deserves emphasis that high-dose L-tryptophan was probably not the cause of the eosinophilia-myalgia syndrome. Rather, the presence of one or more specified contaminants is believed to have triggered the inflammation. The Food and Drug Administration has now recalled all products containing L-tryptophan.

γ-HYDROXYBUTYRATE

γ-Hydroxybutyric acid (GHB) ($CH_2OH—CH_2—CH_2—COOH$) is a metabolite of γ-aminobutyric acid (GABA). GHB is a central nervous system (CNS) depressant that has been used in obstetric anesthesia and to treat narcolepsy. Although recalled by the Food and Drug Administration in 1990, GHB has been sold over the counter as an agent that can produce a "high," control weight, and increase muscle mass. Although hypotonia and amnesia start at doses as low as 10 to 30 mg/kg, most life-threatening events have followed ingestions exceeding 50 to 70 mg/kg. Reported dose-related effects include anesthesia, dizziness, confusion, ataxia, nystagmus, tremors, bradycardia, hypotension, seizures, coma, and respiratory depression.

GINSENG

Ginseng is one of the most commonly used herbal remedies in the world. Available in cigarettes, capsules, teas, extracts, and the roots of *Panax ginseng* or *Panax quinquefolium*, this dietary supplement has been advocated for centuries as a treatment for dyspepsia, fatigue, stress, neurosis, anemia, leukopenia, cancer, motion sickness, and disorders of the heart, thyroid, and adrenal glands. In the 1990s, ginseng has been heavily promoted as a tonic, stimulant, aphrodisiac, and mood enhancer. Twentieth-century peer-reviewed Western biomedical literature does not provide evidence of therapeutic or preventive efficacy, but it does document clinically significant adverse effects attributed to steroidal saponin glycosides in products containing ginseng. Chronic, excessive use (in doses up to 50 g) has been associated with a syndrome characterized by excitation, arousal, hypertension, insomnia, nervousness, skin eruptions, morning diarrhea, and possibly postmenopausal bleeding.

ANABOLIC-ANDROGENIC STEROIDS

Anabolic steroids are synthetic derivatives of testosterone that have been used in the treatment of bone marrow failure, anemia of renal disease, hereditary angioneurotic edema, and metastatic breast cancer. As dietary supplements, these compounds are consumed to stimulate protein synthesis, antagonize glucocorticoid catabolic effects, increase red blood cell production, decrease fatigue, increase motivation, enhance performance, increase lean body mass and strength, and reduce recovery time between workouts. The biomedical literature does not provide convincing evidence that anabolic steroids actually improve performance, but it does document clinically significant adverse effects.

Anabolic steroids typically are administered parenterally and orally in 12- to 18-week cycles interrupted by drug-free intervals of 4 to 6 weeks. "Stacking" refers to the simultaneous administration of more than one steroid, "plateauing" refers to overlap dosing designed to prevent tolerance on discontinuation of one agent, and "pyramiding" refers to intervals of abstinence alternating with intervals of consumption. To avoid rapid degradation of testosterone in plasma or the liver, most steroids are sold in alkylated or esterified forms that undergo biotransformation more slowly. However, the concentration of steroids in many products is often not known, and a growing "black market" provides materials whose purity, strength, and consistency are largely unregulated. With passage of the Anabolic Steroids Control Act of 1990 (which classifies anabolic steroids as Schedule III controlled substances and criminalizes physician prescription of anabolic steroids for any use other than treatment of disease), this black market and self-administration of these agents will most likely continue to flourish.

Controlled, long-term longitudinal studies of the adverse effects of steroids in athletes and others who use these supplements are not yet available. However, patients taking steroids for hematologic or neoplastic disorders may experience behavioral, hepatic, and endocrine abnormalities, including aggression, irritability, paranoia, anxiety, mania, and violent mood swings (so-called roid rage); cholestatic hepatitis, liver tumors, and liver cysts (peliosis hepatis); decreased sperm counts, altered sperm morphologic characteristics, and testicular atrophy in men; and virilization in women. The doses of anabolic-androgenic steroids at which these effects occur vary considerably among patients.

PITFALLS IN DIAGNOSIS

The most likely pitfall in the diagnosis of the disorders discussed in this chapter is failure to consider the possibility that vitamin and/or supplement excess could explain a particular patient's problem. When asked about their use of medications or over-the-counter products, patients may not mention diet aids because they do not view them as medications or drugs. Thus, the clinician must make specific inquiry regarding the use of large doses of vitamins and other supplements. As long as persons in the United States and other developed nations continue to use and promote these widely available products, clinicians must increase their vigilance and index of suspicion for new as well as previously described adverse effects.

NUTRIENT DEFICIENCY DISORDERS

By Jane V. White, Ph.D., R.D.
Knoxville, Tennessee
and Richard J. Ham, M.D.
Syracuse, New York

NAME OF THE DISEASE OR CONDITION

Nutrient deficiency disorders encompass a wide range of diseases and conditions that have as their cause an inadequate supply of nutrients to the body. This inadequacy may result from

- Inadequate nutrient intake
- Increased nutrient requirement
- Altered nutrient utilization

In developing nations, nutrient deficiency disorders are common and are associated with considerable morbidity and mortality. The lack of a safe and adequate water supply, with resultant high infection rates, is a significant contributor to nutrient deficits in many countries. In these areas, access to food is often limited because of poverty, political upheaval, and/or difficulties in food distribution and storage. Individuals in many of these countries rely exclusively on plant sources for nutrients. Protein-energy malnutrition in such settings is common, particularly in more rural or isolated sections of these countries and in the urban poor. In developing areas of the world where the soil in which crops are grown is deficient in minerals and transportation of food is difficult, deficiency states such as goiter (iodine), Keshan disease (selenium), and other mineral deficit disorders may be common. A leading cause of blindness in developing nations is vitamin A deficiency. The nutritional anemias, particularly those related to iron, vitamin B_{12}, and folate deficiency; riboflavin deficiency; and zinc deficiency are also common. Population subgroups at particularly high nutritional risk in developing nations are children and women from poor families.

In the United States and other Western societies, and in the affluent segments of developing nations, malnutrition is often associated with excessive consumption of nutrients rather than with the nutrient deficiency disorders. Older individuals in the United States and other Western societies do, however, have a much higher prevalence of macronutrient deficiency than most clinicians expect. Inadequate calorie and protein intakes contribute to the syndrome of protein-energy malnutrition frequently seen in these patients. In the United States, the nutrient deficiency disorders are most often seen in association with one or more of the following:

- Inadequate economic resources (general, medical, or food assistance programs)
- Dependence on others to meet basic needs (the frail elderly, institutionalized individuals)
- Impediments to eating (physical, i.e., poor oral health, severe arthritis; cognitive, i.e., mental retardation, dementia; emotional, i.e., depression, eating disorders)
- Recent severe trauma
- Recovery from major surgery
- Immunodeficiency disorders
- Disease-induced digestive, absorptive, or metabolic changes

- Excessive physical activity or immobility
- Substance abuse, cigarette smoking
- Chronic medication use, adverse drug reactions
- Restrictive dietary behaviors (self-imposed or prescribed)

SYNONYMS

Malnutrition is the synonym most often used when referring to a nutrient deficiency state. However, depending on the nutrient or nutrients that are lacking, nutrient deficiency disorders may be described as protein-energy malnutrition—marasmus or kwashiorkor (protein), wet or dry beriberi (thiamine), pellagra (niacin), scurvy (ascorbic acid), rickets-osteomalacia (vitamin D), goiter (iodine), and so forth. The principal nutrients and a description of the clinical presentation of deficiency states associated with a lack of them are provided in Table 1.

PRESENTING SIGNS AND SYMPTOMS

Evidence of poor nutritional status frequently exists long before the classic signs and symptoms of overt nutrient deficiency occur. Malnutrition is seldom diagnosed by a single physical sign or symptom. The nutrient deficiency disorders are complex and are often multifactorial. Many of the physical signs and symptoms of nutrient deficiency disorders may include non-nutritional as well as nutrition-related causes in the differential diagnosis. For example, oral candidiasis, a lack of teeth, or ill-fitting dentures that cause the oral cavity to collapse can produce the cheilosis or angular scars seen with riboflavin or vitamin B complex deficiency. Thus, the diagnosis of a nutrient deficiency disorder should be based on the *constellation* of signs and symptoms that appear in an individual (see Table 1) combined with a dietary evaluation, nutritional assessment, physical examination, and other appropriate anthropometric, laboratory, or diagnostic information.

When a patient presents with one or more signs or symptoms suggestive of a nutrient deficit disorder, Tables 1 and 2 may be cross-referenced to facilitate further evaluation and diagnosis. For example, if a patient presents with one or two physical signs or symptoms common to more than one nutrient deficiency (Table 2), a comprehensive listing of the deficiency symptoms associated with a specific nutrient (see Table 1) can be compared with the patient's presenting complaints, thus facilitating diagnosis.

COURSE OF THE PROCESS

Nutrient deficiency disorders follow a fairly steady progression. Tissue depletion occurs initially and may evolve over a considerable period, especially for the macronutrients (protein, fat, energy), the minerals, and the stored vitamins (A, D, E, K). Biochemical changes then result, followed by reductions in blood or urinary concentrations of the nutrient. Functional changes, histologic changes, and the appearance of the classic signs and symptoms of the nutritional deficiency disorders are relatively late occurrences. Thus, an awareness of vulnerable population groups in the United States (the frail old, those recovering from severe trauma or infection, and so forth) and lifestyle factors associated with an inability to obtain, prepare, or consume an adequate diet (poverty, poor oral health, depression, and so on) is essential to the prevention and early detection of these disorders.

HISTORY

Dietary evaluation is an essential component of the history taken to evaluate nutritional status. The frequency of food intake and the quantity and quality of food eaten are critical determinants of nutritional status. A consistent absence of food intake; lack of a habitual pattern of eating; the inability to obtain, prepare, or consume an adequate diet; or lack of sufficient food that is acceptable to eat are significant potential contributors to nutrient deficiency states.

The assessment of customary food intake can be accomplished in a number of ways:

- Ask the person to describe what they have actually eaten in the last 24 hours.
- Request that the person record actual food intake over a period of 1, 3, or 7 days.
- Use a food frequency questionnaire to ascertain how frequently foods are consumed over a defined time span (3, 6, or 12 months).

The information obtained can then be compared with known food sources of nutrients and to established dietary recommendations for health. Table 3 lists food sources of nutrients and Table 4 provides a listing of the recommended servings of foods from each food group whose consumption is consistent with good health in adults.

Individuals who habitually fail to consume the minimal number of recommended servings from one or more food groups or whose diets lack variety or are extremely restrictive are at increased risk for deficient intakes of one or more vitamins and minerals and possibly calories and macronutrients. In the United States, only 13 per cent of adults consume the minimal number of servings of fruit and vegetables daily. Intakes of dairy products are often inadequate, particularly in females and blacks.

In addition to the assessment of food intake, assessment of the following physical and psychosocial parameters are useful in determining increased nutritional risk and in making the decision to provide a supplement:

- Body weight (change of >10 per cent over a period of 6 months)
- Access to economic resources (fixed income, reliance on economic assistance programs)
- Oral health status (poor dentition, poorly fitting dentures, chronic mouth pain, difficulty chewing or swallowing)
- Functional status (physical, cognitive, emotional)
- Social history (isolation, inability to cook, limited transportation)
- Food preparation and storage facilities (availability, adequacy)
- Appetite or sense of taste or smell (chronic alterations)
- Gastrointestinal complaints (chronic nausea, vomiting, diarrhea, early satiety)
- Presence of chronic or severe acute diseases or conditions
- Food intolerance; allergy; restrictive religious, cultural, or health-related food practices
- Alcohol, cigarette, or illicit substance use
- Prescribed or over-the-counter medication use
- Dietary supplement use

A registered dietitian or other qualified nutrition professional can provide assistance in obtaining and assessing this type of information.

LABORATORY PROCEDURES

The laboratory assessment of micronutrient status can be difficult and expensive and may be of indeterminate

Table 1. Deficiency States Associated with Lack of Nutrients

Nutrient	Signs and Symptoms	Synonyms and Comments
Macronutrients		
Protein	Soft, pitting, painless edema of the feet and legs extending to the perineum, upper extremities, and face in severe cases; *skin:* erythematous, hyperpigmented, hyperkeratotic; *hair:* dry, brittle, easily plucked, dull brown, red, or yellowish white, alternating bands of color (flag sign); subcutaneous fat is present; muscle wasting; apathy; irritability; anorexia; postprandial vomiting; diarrhea; hepatomegaly with severe fatty infiltration; abdominal distention; tachycardia; hypothermia	Kwashiorkor
Protein-energy	Generalized muscle wasting and absence of subcutaneous fat; edema; *hair:* sparse, thin, dull brown or reddish, easily plucked; *skin:* dry, thin, little elasticity, wrinkled; apathy; postprandial vomiting; constipation and/or diarrhea; low heart rate and blood pressure; hypothermia, abdominal distention	Marasmus
Essential fatty acid(s)	Dry, flaky skin, scaling, eczematoid dermatosis of face and neck; poor wound healing, anemia; enlarged fatty liver	Usually found in prolonged, lipid-free enteral or parenteral formula feeding
Water	Weight loss, thirst, oliguria, tachycardia, postural hypotension, hemoconcentration	Dehydration
Fat-Soluble Vitamins		
A (retinoids)	*Eyes:* night blindness, xerosis, Bitot's spots, xerophthalmia, punctate keratopathy, keratomalacia; *skin:* perifollicular hyperkeratosis, phrynoderma; impaired taste; anorexia	
D (calciferol)	Bone pain and tenderness; skeletal deformity; weakness of proximal muscles; frequent fractures; waddling gait; difficulty getting up and down stairs	Osteomalacia: simulates paraplegia in elderly, muscular dystrophy in younger adults
E (tocopherol)	Nervous system disorders, muscle wasting	Uncommon
K (quinones)	Hypoprothrombinemia, abnormal blood clotting, bleeding	Usually the result of chronic liver disease, obstructive jaundice, or anticoagulant therapy in combination with prolonged antibiotic therapy or certain cephalosporins
Water-Soluble Vitamins		
Thiamine (B_1)	*Cardiovascular:* chronic high-output right- and left-sided heart failure, tachycardia, rapid circulation time, elevated peripheral venous pressure, sodium retention, edema	Beriberi (wet)
	Neurologic: mental confusion, ophthalmoplegia, coma, loss of memory for distant events, inability to form new memory, loss of insight and initiative	Wernicke's encephalopathy Korsakoff's psychosis
	Peripheral neuropathy: symmetric foot drop; tenderness of calf muscles; disturbance in sensation over outer aspects of legs and thighs and in patches over abdomen, chest, forearms; ataxia with loss of position and vibratory sense; burning paresthesias in feet; amblyopia	
Riboflavin (B_2)	Reddened, scaly, greasy, painful, and pruritic skin in the nasolabial folds, alae nasi, external ears, eyelids, scrotum in males and labia majora in females; dyssebacia (sharkskin); angular stomatitis; cheilosis; sore, magenta-colored tongue; photophobia; lacrimation; conjunctival injection	Symptoms common to many nutrient deficiencies
Niacin (B_3)	Symmetric dermatosis and desequamation of sun-exposed areas of the skin, erythema, keratosis, scaling with pigmentation; reddened, scaly, greasy, painful, pruritic skin in areas containing many sebaceous glands; bright red, swollen, painful tongue; gastritis; diarrhea; malabsorption; depression; insomnia; headaches; dizziness; tremulous movement or rigidity of the limbs with loss of tendon reflexes, numbness, and paresis of extremities; encephalopathy	Pellagra
Pyridoxine (B_6)	Irritability; depression; seborrheic dermatitis affecting nasolabial folds, cheeks, neck, and perineum; glossitis; cheilosis; angular stomatitis; blepharitis; peripheral neuropathy	Seen in volunteers fed a pyridoxine-deficient diet; rarely seen in clinical practice

Table 1. Deficiency States Associated with Lack of Nutrients *Continued*

Nutrient	Signs and Symptoms	Synonyms and Comments
Biotin	Dry, shining, scaly skin on face and hands; swelling of oral mucosa and tongue; painful, magenta-colored tongue, severe loss of body hair	Infrequently seen in patients consuming large amounts of raw egg white or in those receiving enteral or parenteral formulas lacking biotin
Cobalamin (B_{12})	Megaloblastic anemia; *neurologic changes* (often precede anemia): sensory neuropathy with "glove-and-stocking" distribution, paresthesias, areflexia, subacute combined degeneration of the spinal cord; red, smooth, shining, painful tongue; hyperpigmentation of skin; anorexia; weight loss; indigestion; episodic diarrhea; optic atrophy	*Pernicious anemia:* neurologic changes precede anemia *Dietary deficiency:* megaloblastic anemia is prominent feature
Folic acid	Megaloblastic anemia; peripheral neuropathy; red, painful tongue progressing to atrophy of papillae (shiny, smooth surface); hyperpigmentation of skin; gingival hyperplasia; *pregnancy:* increased incidence of neural tube defects	
Ascorbic acid (C)	Weakness; fatigue; listlessness; shortness of breath; aching bones, joints, muscles; perifollicular hemorrhages and perifollicular hyperkeratosis; acne; broken, coiled body hairs and loss of body hair; spongy, swollen, and bleeding gums; poor wound healing; hemorrhage	Scurvy
Minerals		
Calcium	*Tetany:* paresthesias (lips, tongue, fingers, feet), carpopedal spasm (Trousseau's sign), generalized muscle aches, spasm of facial muscles (Chvostek's sign); depression; psychosis; dementia; encephalopathy; cataracts	Rarely due to dietary deficiency
	Osteoporosis: bone deformity; localized bone pain; loss of height; fracture of neck of femur; Colles' fracture	Seen more often in women, associated with poor calcium intake and estrogen deficiency
Potassium	Muscle weakness leading to respiratory failure, paralytic ileus, hypotension tetany; *electrocardiographic changes:* ST-segment depression greater than U-wave amplitude, T-wave amplitude less than U-wave amplitude in same lead, polymorphous atrial and ventricular contractions, ventricular and atrial tachycardias; polyuria; polydypsia	Sometimes seen in starvation, absence of potassium in intravenous solutions, or as the result of diuretic therapy; cardiac effects more often seen in patients taking digitalis
Magnesium	*Neuromuscular:* Trousseau's and Chvostek's signs, muscle fasciculations, tremor, muscle spasm; personality changes; anorexia; nausea; vomiting	Frequently accompanied by hypocalcemia and hypokalemia
Phosphorus	Circumoral and extremity paresthesias; red cell fragility, hemolysis	Restricted phosphate diets may cause deficiency in renal patients receiving phosphate binders
Iodine	Thyroid enlargement, hypothyroidism, impaired mental function	Goiter; iodine added to salt and salt substitutes has virtually eliminated this problem in the United States
Iron	Pallor; fatigue; hypochromic anemia; koilonychia; nonspecific glossitis with loss of filliform papillae; angular stomatitis; *cardiorespiratory:* exertional dyspnea, tachycardia, palpitations, angina, claudication, night cramps, cardiac enlargement, cardiac failure, basal crepitations, peripheral edema, ascites; *neuromuscular:* headache, tinnitus, vertigo, cramps, faintness, increased cold sensitivity, retinal hemorrhage; *gastrointestinal:* anorexia, nausea, constipation, diarrhea, pica; low-grade fever; menstrual irregularity; urinary frequency; loss of libido	
	Anemia, glossitis, dysphagia, achlorhydria, postcricoid web, malignancy	Patterson-Kelly (Plummer-Vinson) syndrome
Copper	Hypochromic anemia unresponsive to iron, neutropenia, osteoporosis	Seen occasionally with excessive zinc supplementation
Fluoride	Tooth decay, osteoporosis(?)	
Selenium	Cardiomyopathy, muscle pain and tenderness, dyschromotrichia, white nail beds, macrocytosis	Keshan disease; occasionally seen in patients receiving unsupplemented parenteral nutrition formulations
Zinc	Growth retardation, delayed sexual maturation, impotence, hypogonadism, hypospermia, alopecia, acro-orificial skin lesions, glossitis, nail dystrophy, immune deficiencies, behavioral disturbances, night blindness, impaired taste, delayed wound healing, anorexia, photophobia, poor dark adaptation, bilateral xerosis, keratomalacia	Seen in adults chronically fed enteral or parenteral formulations lacking zinc

Table 2. Nutrient Deficiencies

Signs and Symptoms	Possible Deficiency
General	
Generalized muscle wasting, absence of subcutaneous fat	Protein, protein-energy
Bilateral edema	Protein, thiamine
Skin	
Slow wound healing	Vitamin C, zinc, essential fatty acids
Psoriaform rash, eczematous scaling	Zinc
Perifollicular hyperkeratosis, dryness, thickening	Vitamin A, essential fatty acids, B-complex vitamins
Bruising	Vitamin C, K
Dryness, mosaic, sandpaper feel, flakiness	Vitamin A
Erythema, keratosis, pigmentation, desquamation of sun-exposed areas	Niacin
Red, scaly, greasy, painful, pruritic	Riboflavin, biotin
Petechiae, purpura, perifollicular hemorrhage	Vitamin C
Pallor	Iron, copper, folate, vitamin B_{12}
Scrotal or vulvar dermatosis	Riboflavin
Seborrheic dermatitis of nasolabial folds, cheeks, neck, perineum	Pyridoxine, riboflavin, biotin, essential fatty acid
Head	
Temporal muscle wasting	Protein-energy
Increased intracranial pressure	Vitamin A
Hair	
Dull, dry, lack of natural shine	Protein-energy
Thin, broken, sparse, absent	Vitamin C
Color changes, depigmentation, easily plucked	Protein, copper
Abnormal spiral twisting	Copper
Eyes	
Pale membranes	Iron, folate, vitamin B_{12}
Night blindness, dry membranes, dull or soft cornea, impaired visual recovery after glare	Vitamin A, zinc
Bitot's spots, conjunctival xerosis, corneal xerosis, keratomalacia	Vitamin A, zinc
Photophobia, lacrimation, conjunctival injection	Riboflavin
Redness and fissures of corners of eyelids	Niacin
Optic atrophy with visual loss	Vitamin B_{12}
Lips	
Redness and swelling, angular fissures, scars at corner of mouth	Niacin, riboflavin, pyridoxine, iron
Gums	
Spongy, swollen, bleeding	Vitamin C
Gingivitis	Vitamin A, niacin, riboflavin, folate
Gingival hyperplasia	Folate, vitamin C
Mouth	
Cheilosis, angular scars	Riboflavin, folate, pyridoxine
Tongue	
Sores, swollen, scarlet, raw	Folate, niacin
Smooth, atrophic filiform papillae	B-complex vitamins
Glossitis	Iron, B-complex vitamins
Purplish or magenta	Riboflavin
Taste	
Diminished sensation	Zinc
Geophagia	Iron, zinc
Pica	Iron

Table 2. Nutrient Deficiencies *Continued*

Signs and Symptoms	Possible Deficiency
Teeth	
Caries	Fluoride
Missing or erupting abnormally	Generally poor nutrition
Face	
Depigmentation, dark cheeks and eyes, enlarged parotid glands, nasolabial seborrhea	Protein-energy, niacin, riboflavin, pyridoxine
Heart	
Electrocardiographic changes, polyventricular contractions; tachyarrhythmias	Potassium
Small, decreased output	Protein
Cardiomegaly, tachycardia, rapid circulation time, increased peripheral venous pressure	Thiamine
Neck	
Thyroid enlargement, signs of hypothyroidism	Iodine
Nails	
Fragility, banding	Protein
Koilonychia (spoon-shaped)	Iron
Gastrointestinal System	
Anorexia	Vitamin A, zinc
Anorexia, flatulence, indigestion, episodic diarrhea	Vitamin B_{12}
Gastritis, diarrhea	Niacin
Hepatomegaly	Protein
Muscular System	
Weakness, wasting	Protein-energy, vitamin D, selenium, phosphorus, potassium
Bilateral calf tenderness, hyporeflexia, bilateral wrist-foot drop	Thiamine
Aching muscles, bones, joints	Vitamin C
Muscle twitching, tremor, spasm, cramps	Magnesium, potassium, calcium
Skeletal System	
Dwarfism, growth retardation	Zinc
Demineralization of bone	Calcium, vitamin D, phosphorus
Bowed legs, epiphyseal enlargement, pain/fracture, stunted growth	Vitamin D, calcium
Osteoporosis	Calcium, copper
Rickets, osteomalacia	Vitamin D
Nervous System	
Confusion, loss of distant memory, psychosis	Thiamine
Listlessness	Protein-energy
Ataxia, loss of position and vibratory sense, hyporeflexia	Thiamine, vitamin B_{12}
Dementia	Niacin, vitamin B_{12}
Seizures, impaired memory, behavioral disturbances	Magnesium, zinc
Peripheral neuropathy, dementia	Pyridoxine, vitamin B_{12}, thiamine
Depression, psychosis	Thiamine, calcium
Vestibular disturbance	Vitamin A, phosphorus
Hematologic System	
Anemia, hypochromic	Copper
Anemia, macrocytic	Folate, vitamin B_{12}
Anemia, microcytic	Iron
Red cell fragility, hemolysis	Phosphorus

Table 3. Food Sources of Nutrients

Nutrient	Sources
Macronutrients	
Protein	Eggs, milk, yogurt, cheese, lean meat, poultry, fish, soy beans, tofu, dried beans and peas, nuts, seeds, peanut butter
Complex carbohydrate–fiber	Breads, rolls, muffins, cereals, rice, pasta, crackers, dried beans and peas, vegetables, fruit
Fat	Oils, margarines, dairy fats, shortening, mayonnaise, salad dressings, nuts, seeds, olives, avocado, peanut butter, bacon, lard, fatty meats, poultry skin
Fat-Soluble Vitamins	
A (retinoids)	*Preformed:* fish liver oils, liver, organ meats, whole eggs, dairy products, whole small fish *Carotenoids:* carrots, dark green leafy vegetables, spinach, tomatoes, yellow maize, papayas, ripe mangos, oranges, peaches, apricots, cantaloupe
D (calciferol)	Sunlight, fortified milk, egg yolks, eel, herring, salmon, liver
E (tocopherol)	Vegetable and seed oils, seeds, nuts, wheat germ, margarine, mayonnaise and salad dressings made with oils
K (quinones)	Broccoli, cabbage, kale, lettuce, spinach, turnip greens, green tea, liver, cigarettes (tobacco)
Water-Soluble Vitamins	
Thiamine (B_1)	Yeast, lean pork, legumes, rice bran, enriched or fortified breads, rolls, crackers, and cereals
Riboflavin (B_2)	Milk, eggs, lean meats, broccoli, enriched or fortified breads and cereals
Niacin (B_3)	Liver, meats, fish, legumes, peanuts, enriched or fortified breads and cereals, coffee, tea
Pyridoxine (B_6)	Wheat bran, avocado, sunflower seeds, cashews, walnuts, peanuts, poultry, dried beans, soybeans, potatoes, bananas
Biotin	Liver, egg yolk, soybeans, yeast, cereals, legumes, nuts, cauliflower, mushrooms
Cobalamin (B_{12})	Meats, dairy products, liver, eggs, clams, oysters, salmon, sardines
Folic acid	Yeast, liver, organ meats, asparagus, green beans, beats, broccoli, cauliflower, corn, peas, tomatoes, oranges, bananas
Ascorbic acid (C)	Citrus fruit and juices, melon, berries, kiwi, cabbage, broccoli, tomatoes, potatoes
Minerals	
Calcium	Yogurt, milk, cheese, broccoli, nuts, tofu precipitated with calcium, soft bones of fish, calcium fortified fruit juice
Potassium	Milk, bran cereals, oatmeal, meats, asparagus, broccoli, carrots, tomatoes, potatoes, bananas, oranges
Magnesium	Milk, bran cereals, oatmeal, wheat cereals, fish, beets, corn, potatoes, bananas, cocoa, green vegetables
Phosphorus	Poultry, fish, meats, milk, eggs, cereals, nuts, legumes, soft drinks
Iodine	Iodized salt, seafood, kelp, breads made by continuous batch process
Copper	Shellfish, nuts, seeds, legumes, bran and germ portions of grains, liver, organ meats
Iron	Meat, poultry, fish, soybeans, potatoes with skins, broccoli, tomatoes, cauliflower, cabbage
Selenium	Organ meats, seafood, meats, cereals and grain products
Zinc	Seafood, meat, liver, eggs, milk

significance. Table 5 lists laboratory procedures that are sometimes used to evaluate micronutrient status. Comments are included when relevant. Radiologic findings suggestive of nutrient deficiency disorders may be present in deficiencies of vitamins D and C (particularly in children) and in certain malabsorption syndromes (i.e., sprue, scleroderma), parasitic diseases, and protein-losing enteropathies. Neoplastic diseases, which often result in significant nutrient deficits, may also be observed radiologically. (Refer to the article on nutritional assessment for a discussion of nutritional anthropometry and biochemical indices diagnostic of protein-energy malnutrition. A discussion of drug-nutrient interactions is also provided in that article.)

PROTEIN-ENERGY MALNUTRITION

Although the prevalence of protein-energy malnutrition is uncommon in healthy, independently living adults in the United States, in long-term care facilities its prevalence is estimated to range from 19 to 27 per cent, whereas in acute care settings prevalence estimates from general medical and surgical services range from 33 to 58 per cent. The elderly, hospitalized individuals, and those who reside in institutions are at increased risk of protein-energy malnutrition in the United States. In developing countries, it is more often children and poor women who are vulnerable to this condition. As the percentage of older persons in developing countries rises, the frail elderly are more frequently recognized as a group at increased risk of protein-energy malnutrition.

Protein-energy malnutrition incorporates two syndromes of macronutrient deficiency: *kwashiorkor* (protein deficiency or hypoalbuminemic malnutrition) and *marasmus* (deficiency of calories and to a lesser extent, protein). Protein-energy malnutrition is often accompanied by a number of concurrent micronutrient deficiencies and secondary infections. Depending on the part of the world in which this deficiency is seen as well as the age of the patient, the presence of concurrent diseases or conditions, and the associated medical and psychosocial parameters mentioned previously, the constellation of accompanying physical signs, symptoms, and functional outcomes will differ.

The early symptoms of protein-energy malnutrition tend to be nonspecific: anorexia, fatigue, lassitude, irritability, anxiety, and confusion. Signs seen on physical examination

Table 4. Recommended Daily Food Consumption Pattern for American Adults

Food Group	Servings Per Day	Equivalent* Serving Sizes
Grain products†	6–11+	1 slice whole grain or enriched bread 1/2 bun, bagel, English muffin, pita 1/2 cup rice, pasta, cooked cereal 1 oz cold cereal 3–6 crackers
Fruit	2–4+	Citrus or other vitamin C source 1 medium piece 1/2 cup juice or canned fruit
Vegetables	3–5+	Dark green or deep yellow 1 cup raw 1/2 cup cooked
Dairy Products†	2–4+	1 cup fluid milk, yogurt, custard, pudding, soft serve ice cream or frozen yogurt 1½ oz cheese 1½ cup soup made with milk 2 cups cottage cheese, ice cream or ice milk
Meat, meat alternates†	2–3+	2–3 oz meat, fish, poultry 2 eggs 1 chicken breast or leg and thigh 1/3 cup tofu 2 Tbsp peanut butter 1/2–1 cup dried beans or peas
Fats and sweets	As needed for calories	
Fluid	4–8+	1 cup water or other liquid

*Calcium equivalent milk group, protein equivalent meat group.
†Lower fat, lower calorie items may be recommended depending on health status.
Adapted from United States Department of Agriculture, United States Department of Health and Human Services: Nutrition and your health: Dietary guidelines for Americans, 3rd ed. Home and Garden Bulletin No. 232, U.S. Government Printing Office, Washington, DC, 1990.

include fat and/or muscle wasting, muscular weakness, thin and sparse hair with a flaking dermatitis, peripheral edema and/or abdominal distention in some individuals, and occasionally hepatomegaly, parotid gland enlargement, and changes in skin pigmentation (see Tables 1 and 2). Weight loss is often significant in marasmus but may be less obvious in kwashiorkor. A variety of anthropometric, clinical, and biochemical parameters can be used to diagnose protein-energy malnutrition and to distinguish between the two types. (See article on nutritional assessment for a more complete review of these issues.)

Protein-energy malnutrition should be considered as an explanation for any involuntary weight loss in an older person constituting more than 5 per cent in the prior month or 10 per cent in the prior 6 months. A diagnosis of protein-energy malnutrition should also be considered in adults with pressure sores, poor wound healing, frequent or nosocomial infections, or apparent failure to thrive, especially if they are frail, homebound, institutionalized, or poor. Any individual with a long-term chronic condition (particularly dementia and especially if physically dependent or poor), persons recently discharged from the hospital (especially if the hospitalization was prolonged or if a hip or long-bone fracture is present), and any person with impaired physical or emotional status is at increased risk of protein-energy malnutrition and other nutrient deficiency disorders.

ISOLATED NUTRIENT DEFICIENCIES

Isolated nutrient deficiencies occur infrequently in the United States. When they occur, they are generally the result of overly restrictive dietary behaviors that result in the elimination of specific foods or food groups that contain the nutrient in question; an adverse drug-nutrient interaction; cigarette, alcohol, or drug abuse; or a disease-induced digestive, absorptive, or metabolic change. Examples of diseases or conditions associated with nutrient deficiency diseases are found in Table 6. These types of deficiency syndromes may respond well to single-nutrient supplementation.

MIXED NUTRIENT DEFICIENCIES

When the more common protein-energy, multiple vitamin-mineral deficiency syndromes do occur, they are usually the result of the presence of one or more chronic or severe acute diseases or conditions combined with an inadequate food intake or an inappropriate or inadequate enteral or parenteral formula. In such instances, the provision of an adequate diet, or an appropriate type and amount of nutritionally complete enteral or parenteral formula, will reverse the generalized symptoms of malnutrition.

SUMMARY

Malnutrition, secondary to a combination of poor intake and poor individual and public health, particularly when secondary to poverty, is a widely recognized world problem. Even in Western society, the classically described syndromes of nutritional deficiency are surprisingly prevalent, especially among the chronically ill and the old and frail. Many specific illnesses are associated with specific nutrient deficiencies, which can therefore be anticipated. However, the most important clinical issue is that all who care for those at special risk maintain constant vigilance for under-

Table 5. Laboratory Assessment of Selected Micronutrient Parameters in Adults

Nutrient, Test	Reference Value	Comments
Fat-Soluble Vitamins		
Vitamin A		
Serum (retinol)	360–1200 μg/L	
Plasma	20–200 μg/dL	Reference range (higher concentrations in men)
	<10 μg/dL	Significantly decreased (increased carotenoid concentration may cause falsely low value)
Carotene		
Blood	40–180 μg/dL	
Vitamin D		
25-hydroxycalciferol (serum)	14–42 ng/mL	Winter reference range
	15–80 ng/mL	Summer reference range
	<15 ng/mL	Deficiency
1,25-dihydroxycalciferol (serum)	15–60 pg/mL	
Vitamin E		
α-Tocopherol (blood)	0.7–2 mg/dL	
	<0.5 mg/dL	Deficiency
	0.3 mg/dL	Sprue
	0.4 mg/dL	Chronic pancreatitis
	0.2 mg/dL	Cystic fibrosis
	<0.1 mg/dL	Biliary obstruction
Water-Soluble Vitamins		
Thiamine (B_1)		
Blood	5.3–7.9 μg/dL	Increased pyruvic acid concentrations seen in deficiency states
Red blood cell transketolase	<8 IU	Thiamine deficiency; adding thiamine causes >20 per cent increase
Riboflavin (B_2)		
Red blood cell	20–28 μg/dL	
	<10 μg/dL	Deficiency
Niacin (B_3)		
Whole blood	30 μg/mL	
	<24 μmol/L	Deficiency, decreased excretion of niacin metabolites in urine, plasma tryptophan decreased
Red blood cell	90 μg/mL	
Serum	0.5 μg/mL	
White blood cell	70 μg/mL	
Pyridoxine (B_6)		
Plasma	37–68 pmol/mL	Higher in males and pregnant women
Folic acid		
Serum	3–18 ng/mL	
	<3.0 ng/mL	Deficiency
Red blood cell	<140 ng/mL	Deficiency
Vitamin B_{12} (cobalamin)		
Serum	180–960 pg/mL	
	100–200 pg/mL	Indeterminate
	<100 pg/mL	Deficient
Vitamin C (ascorbic acid)		
Plasma	0.5–1.5 mg/dL	
	Absent	Frank scurvy
White blood cell (buffy coat)	30 mg/dL	
	Absent	Frank scurvy

Table 5. Laboratory Assessment of Selected Micronutrient Parameters in Adults *(Continued)*

Nutrient, Test	Reference Value	Comments
Minerals		
Calcium		
Total serum	8.4–10.6 mg/dL	
	<6 mg/dL	Critically low
Serum ionized	4.25–5.25 mg/dL	
Potassium		
Serum	3.5–5.0 mEq/L	
	<2.5 mEq/L	Critically low
Magnesium		
Serum	1.3–2.1 mg/dL	
Phosphorus		
Serum	3.0–4.5 mg/dL	
	<1 mg/dL	Critically low
Copper		
Plasma	70–155 μg/dL	Influenced by gender, females have higher mean copper concentrations than males; pregnancy and oral contraceptives increase concentrations
Ceruloplasmin	23–44 mg/dL	Higher in smokers
Iron		
Blood ferritin	20–250 ng/mL	Males
	10–120 ng/mL	Females
	10–20 ng/mL	Indeterminate, males or females
	<25 ng/mL	Deficiency, inflammation
	<50 ng/mL	Deficiency, hemodialysis
	<100 ng/mL	Deficiency, liver disease (most sensitive test to detect iron deficiency, may be increased in coexisting liver disease, inflammation)
Serum iron	75–175 μg/dL	Males
	65–165 μg/dL	Females
	<40 μg/dl	Deficiency
Total iron binding capacity	250–450 μg/dL	
	350–460 μg/dL	Increase suggestive of deficiency
Per cent saturation	20–50%	
	<15%	Suggestive of deficiency
Hemoglobin	12–16 g/dL	Females
	14–18 g/dL	Males
	<5 g/dL	Critical deficiency
Hematocrit	37–47 vol %	Females
	42–52 vol %	Males
	<15 vol %	Critical deficiency
Selenium		
Serum	95–165 ng/mL	
Urine (24 hr)	<35 μg per day	
Zinc		
Plasma	70–130 μg/dL	

*Values vary, depending on individual laboratories and methods used. Each clinician should assess the applicability of these data to their

Table 6. Selected Diseases or Conditions Associated wih Nutrient Deficiency

Disease, Condition	Potential Nutrient Deficit
Gastrointestinal	
Achlorhydria, pernicious anemia	Vitamin B_{12}
Blind loop syndrome	Vitamins B_{12} and D; calcium
Cholestatic disorders	Vitamins D and B_{12}
Gastrectomy	Vitamins A, D, E, K, and B_{12} and folic acid; iron and calcium
Inflammatory bowel disease (Crohn's disease, regional enteritis, ulcerative colitis, others)	Protein; calories; vitamins B_{12} and D and folate; calcium, iron, magnesium, and zinc; other fat- and water-soluble vitamins, depending on site and severity of inflammation
Liver disease, alcohol abuse	Vitamins A, D, C, and B_6, thiamine, riboflavin, niacin, and folic acid; magnesium, calcium, and zinc
Obstructive jaundice	Vitamins A and K
Pancreatic insufficiency	Vitamins A, D, E, K, and B_{12}
Peptic ulcer disease (chronic)	Iron
Pica	Iron and zinc
Short bowel syndrome, ileal resection	Vitamins A, D, K, and B_{12}, folic acid, and other B-complex vitamins; calcium, magnesium, and iron
Sprue (gluten enteropathy)	Vitamins A and D and folic acid; iron
Endocrine	
Hypothyroidism	Iodine
Thyrotoxicosis	Vitamins A, B_6, B_{12}, and C, thiamine, and folic acid
Hematopoietic	
\nemia	Iron and copper; vitamins B_{12}, B_6, and E, folic acid, and thiamine
ectious	
AIDS	Protein; calories; multiple vitamins and minerals
ions, fever (chronic)	Vitamins A and C, thiamine, riboflavin, and folic acid; calories
psychiatric	
disorders (anorexia nervosa)	Calories and protein; multiple vitamins and minerals
romatosis	Vitamin D
ure (chronic)	Magnesium and calcium; vitamin D; calories
	Calories; vitamins A and C and niacin; copper
ctive pulmonary disease	Calories; vitamins A, D, E, and K
tarians)	Vitamin B_{12} (possibly protein; riboflavin; calcium, iron, and zinc)
	Vitamin D

virus; AIDS = acquired immunodeficiency syndrome.

nutrition as a contributing factor in, and potential cause for, a variety of symptoms.

Undernutrition contributes to the prevalent dwindling and failure to thrive that occurs in many chronically ill, dependent individuals, especially during and after the stress of acute illness and hospitalization. Undernutrition is often underrecognized and inadequately considered and addressed as the frequent contributing factor that it is in situations producing dependency and ultimately mortality. The clinician must recognize that the presence of one nutrient deficiency is likely to be associated with others. All health care providers must adopt a proactive, preventive approach to ensure that individuals reach old age and dependency in as good nutritional condition as possible and therefore are best prepared for the extra stresses and strains that intercurrent illness will ultimately produce.

Section Nineteen

LABORATORY VALUES OF CLINICAL IMPORTANCE

REFERENCE INTERVALS FOR THE INTERPRETATION OF LABORATORY TESTS

By William Z. Borer, M.D.
Philadelphia, Pennsylvania

Most of the tests performed in a clinical laboratory are quantitative in nature—that is, the amount of a substance present in blood or serum is measured and reported in terms of concentration, activity (e.g., enzyme activity), or counts (e.g., blood cell counts). The laboratory must provide reference values to assist the clinician in the interpretation of laboratory results. These reference ranges specify the physiologic quantities of substance (concentrations, activities, or counts) to be expected in healthy individuals. Deviation above or below the reference range may be associated with a disease process, and the severity of the disease process may be associated with the magnitude of the deviation. Unfortunately, a sharp demarcation between physiologic and pathologic values rarely exists, and the transition between these two is often gradual as the disease process progresses.

The terms normal and abnormal have been used to describe the laboratory values that fall inside or outside the reference range, respectively. Use of these terms is now discouraged because it is virtually impossible to define normality and because "normal" may be confused with the statistical term gaussian. Reference ranges are established from statistical studies in groups of healthy volunteers. Although these study subjects must be free from disease, they may have lifestyles or habits that result in subtle variations in their laboratory values. Examples of these variables include diet, body mass, exercise, and geographic location. Age and gender may also affect reference values. When the data from a large cohort of healthy subjects fit a gaussian distribution, the usual statistical approach is to define the reference limits as two standard deviations above and below the mean. By definition, the reference range excludes the highest and the lowest 2.5 per cent of the population. Nongaussian distributions are handled by different statistical methods, but the result is similar in that the reference range is defined by the central 95 per cent of the population. In other words, the odds are 1 in 20 that a healthy individual will have a laboratory result that falls outside the reference range. If 12 laboratory tests are performed, the odds increase to about 1 in 2 that at least one of the results is outside the reference range. This means that all healthy individuals are likely to have a few laboratory results that are unexpected. The clinician must then integrate these data with other clinical information, such as the history and physical examination, to arrive at the appropriate clinical decision. The reference range for many tests (especially enzyme and immunochemical measurements) varies with the method used. It is important that each laboratory establish reference ranges appropriate for the methods it employs.

SI UNITS

During the 1980s, a concerted effort was made to introduce SI units (le Système International d'Unités). The rationale for conversion to SI units is sound. Laboratory data are scientifically more informative when the units are based on molar concentration rather than mass concentration. For example, the conversion of glucose to lactate and pyruvate or the binding of a drug to albumin is more easily understood in units of molar concentration. Another example is illustrated as follows:

CONVENTIONAL UNITS
1.0 gram of hemoglobin
Combines with 1.37 mL of oxygen
Contains 3.4 mg of iron
Forms 34.9 mg of bilirubin

SI UNITS
4.0 mmol of hemoglobin
Combines with 4.0 mmol of oxygen
Contains 4.0 mmol of iron
Forms 4.0 mmol of bilirubin

The international use of SI units would also enhance the standardization of nomenclature to facilitate global communication of medical and scientific information. The units, symbols, and prefixes employed in the International System are shown in Tables 1, 2, and 3.

Unfortunately, problems have arisen with the implementation of SI units in the United States. Their introduction in 1987 prompted many medical journals to report laboratory values in both SI and conventional units in anticipation of complete conversion to SI units in the early 1990s. The lack of a coordinated effort toward this goal has forced

Table 1. Base SI Units

Property	Base Unit	Symbol
Length	Meter	m
Mass	Kilogram	kg
Amount of substance	Mole	mol
Time	Second	s
Thermodynamic temperature	Kelvin	K
Electric current	Ampere	A
Luminous intensity	Candela	cd
Catalytic amount	Katal	kat

Table 2. Derived SI Units and Non-SI Units Retained for Use with the SI

Property	Unit	Symbol
Area	Square meter	m^2
Volume	Cubic meter	m^3
	Liter	L
Mass concentration	Kilogram/cubic meter	kg/m^3
	Gram/liter	g/L
Substance concentration	Mole/cubic meter	mol/m^3
	Mole/liter	mol/L
Temperature	Degree Celsius	°C = °K − 273.15

a retrenchment on the issue. Physicians continue to think and practice using laboratory results expressed in conventional units and few, if any, American hospitals or clinical laboratories exclusively use SI units. It is not likely that complete conversion to SI units will occur in the foreseeable future, yet most medical journals will probably continue to publish both sets of units. For this reason the tables of reference ranges in this Appendix are given in both conventional units and SI units.

Table 3. Standard Prefixes

Prefix	Multiplication Factor	Symbol
yocto	10^{-24}	y
zepto	10^{-21}	z
atto	10^{-18}	a
femto	10^{-15}	f
pico	10^{-12}	p
nano	10^{-9}	n
micro	10^{-6}	μ
milli	10^{-3}	m
centi	10^{-2}	c
deci	10^{-1}	d
deca	10^{1}	da
hecto	10^{2}	h
kilo	10^{3}	k
mega	10^{6}	M
giga	10^{9}	G
tera	10^{12}	T

TABLES OF REFERENCE VALUES

Some of the values included in the tables have been established by the Clinical Laboratories at Thomas Jefferson University Hospital, Philadelphia, PA, and have not been published elsewhere. Other values have been compiled from the sources cited herein. These tables are provided for information and educational purposes only. They are intended to complement data derived from other sources, including the medical history and physical examination. Users must exercise individual judgment when employing the information provided in this appendix.

References

AMA Drug Evaluations, Annual. Chicago, American Medical Association, 1994.

Bick, R.L. (ed.): *Hematology—Clinical and Laboratory* Practice. St. Louis, Mosby–Year Book, 1993.

Borer, W.Z.: Selection and use of laboratory tests. *In* Tietz, N.W., Conn, R.B., and Pruden, E.L. (eds.): *Applied Laboratory Medicine.* Philadelphia, W.B. Saunders Co., 1992, pp. 1–5.

Campion, E.W.: A retreat from SI units. *N. Engl. J. Med.* 327:49, 1992.

Friedman, R.B., and Young, D.S.: *Effects of Disease on Clinical Laboratory Tests,* 2nd ed. Washington, D.C., AACC Press, 1989.

Henry, J.B.: *Clinical Diagnosis and Management by Laboratory Methods,* 18th ed. Philadelphia, W.B. Saunders Co., 1991.

Hicks, J.M., and Young, D.S.: *DORA 1992–1993: Directory of Rare Analyses.* Washington, D.C., AACC Press, 1992.

Jacobs, D.S., Kasten, B.L., Demott, W.R., et al.: *Laboratory Test Handbook,* 2nd ed. Baltimore, Williams & Wilkins Co., 1990.

Kaplan, L.A., and Pesce, A.J.: *Clinical Chemistry—Theory, Analysis, and Correlation,* 2nd ed. St. Louis, C.V. Mosby, 1989.

Kjeldsberg, C.R., and Knight, J.A.: *Body Fluids—Laboratory Examination of Amniotic, Cerebrospinal, Seminal, Serous, and Synovial Fluids,* 3rd ed. Chicago, ASCP Press, 1993.

Laposata, M.: *SI Unit Conversion Guide.* Boston, New England Journal of Medicine Books, 1992.

Scully, R.E., McNeely, W.F., Mark, E.J., et al.: Normal reference laboratory values. *N. Engl. J. Med.,* 327:718, 1992.

Speicher, C.E.: *The Right Test—A Physician's Guide to Laboratory Medicine,* 2nd ed. Philadelphia, W.B. Saunders Co., 1993.

Tietz, N.W. (ed.): *Clinical Guide to Laboratory Tests,* 2nd ed. Philadelphia, W.B. Saunders Co., 1990.

Wallach, J.: *Interpretation of Diagnostic Tests—A Synopsis of Laboratory Medicine,* 5th ed. Boston, Little, Brown, 1992.

Young, D.S.: Determination and validation of reference intervals. *Arch. Pathol. Lab. Med.,* 116:704, 1992.

Young, D.S.: *Effects of Drugs on Clinical Laboratory Tests,* 3rd ed. Washington, DC, AACC Press, 1990.

Young, D.S.: Implementation of SI units for clinical laboratory data. *Ann. Intern. Med.,* 106:114, 1987.

Reference Values for Hematology

	Conventional Units	SI Units
Acid hemolysis (Ham test)	No hemolysis	No hemolysis
Alkaline phosphatase, leukocyte	Total score 14–100	Total score 14–100
Cell counts		
Erythrocytes		
Males	4.6–6.2 million/mm³	4.6–6.2 × 10^{12}/L
Females	4.2–5.4 million/mm³	4.2–5.4 × 10^{12}/L
Children (varies with age)	4.5–5.1 million/mm³	4.5–5.1 × 10^{12}/L
Leukocytes, total	4500–11,000/mm³	4.5–11.0 × 10^{9}/L
Leukocytes, differential counts*		
Myelocytes	0%	0/L
Band neutrophils	3–5%	150–400 × 10^{6}/L
Segmented neutrophils	54–62%	3000–5800 × 10^{6}/L
Lymphocytes	25–33%	1500–3000 × 10^{6}/L
Monocytes	3–7%	300–500 × 10^{6}/L
Eosinophils	1–3%	50–250 × 10^{6}/L
Basophils	0–1%	15–50 × 10^{6}/L
Platelets	150,000–400,000/mm³	150–400 × 10^{9}/L
Reticulocytes	25,000–75,000/mm³ (0.5–1.5% of erythrocytes)	25–75 × 10^{9}/L
Coagulation tests		
Bleeding time (template)	2.75–8.0 min	2.75–8.0 min
Coagulation time (glass tube)	5–15 min	5–15 min
D-Dimer	<0.5 μg/mL	<0.5 mg/L
Factor VIII and other coagulation factors	50–150% of normal	0.5–1.5 of normal
Fibrin split products (Thrombo-Welco test)	<10 μg/mL	<10 mg/L
Fibrinogen	200–400 mg/dL	2.0–4.0 g/L
Partial thromboplastin time (PTT)	20–35 s	20–35 s
Prothrombin time (PT)	12.0–14.0 s	12.0–14.0 s
Coombs' test		
Direct	Negative	Negative
Indirect	Negative	Negative
Corpuscular values of erythrocytes		
Mean corpuscular hemoglobin (MCH)	26–34 pg/cell	26–34 pg/cell
Mean corpuscular volume (MCV)	80–96 μm³	80–96 fL
Mean corpuscular hemoglobin concentration (MCHC)	32–36 g/dL	320–360 g/L
Haptoglobin	20–165 mg/dL	0.20–1.65 g/L
Hematocrit		
Males	40–54 mL/dL	0.40–0.54
Females	37–47 mL/dL	0.37–0.47
Newborns	49–54 mL/dL	0.49–0.54
Children (varies with age)	35–49 mL/dL	0.35–0.49
Hemoglobin		
Males	13.0–18.0 g/dL	8.1–11.2 mmol/L
Females	12.0–16.0 g/dL	7.4–9.9 mmol/L
Newborns	16.5–19.5 g/dL	10.2–12.1 mmol/L
Children (varies with age)	11.2–16.5 g/dL	7.0–10.2 mmol/L
Hemoglobin, fetal	<1.0% of total	<0.01 of total
Hemoglobin A_{1C}	3–5% of total	0.03–0.05 of total
Hemoglobin A_2	1.5–3.0% of total	0.015–0.03 of total
Hemoglobin, plasma	0.0–5.0 mg/dL	0.0–3.2 μmol/L
Methemoglobin	30–130 mg/dL	19–80 μmol/L
Erythrocyte sedimentation rate (ESR)		
Wintrobe		
Males	0–5 mm/h	0–5 mm/h
Females	0–15 mm/h	0–15 mm/h
Westergren		
Males	0–15 mm/h	0–15 mm/h
Females	0–20 mm/h	0–20 mm/h

*Conventional units are percentages; SI units are absolute counts.

Reference Values* for Clinical Chemistry (Blood, Serum, and Plasma)

	Conventional Units	SI Units
Acetoacetate plus acetone		
Qualitative	Negative	Negative
Quantitative	0.3–2.0 mg/dL	30–200 μmol/L
Acid phosphatase, serum (thymolphthalein monophosphate substrate)	0.1–0.6 U/L	0.1–0.6 U/L

Table continued on following page

Reference Values* for Clinical Chemistry (Blood, Serum, and Plasma) *Continued*

	Conventional Units	SI Units
ACTH (see corticotropin)		
Alanine aminotransferase (ALT, SGPT), serum	1–45 U/L	1–45 U/L
Albumin, serum	3.3–5.2 g/dL	33–52 g/L
Aldolase, serum	0.0–7.0 U/L	0.0–7.0 U/L
Aldosterone, plasma		
Standing	5–30 ng/dL	140–830 pmol/L
Recumbent	3–10 ng/dL	80–275 pmol/L
Alkaline phosphatase (ALP), serum		
Adult	35–150 U/L	35–150 U/L
Adolescent	100–500 U/L	100–500 U/L
Child	100–350 U/L	100–350 U/L
Ammonia nitrogen, plasma	10–50 μmol/L	10–50 μmol/L
Amylase, serum	25–125 U/L	25–125 U/L
Anion gap, serum, calculated	8–16 mEq/L	8–16 mmol/L
Ascorbic acid, blood	0.4–1.5 mg/dL	23–85 μmol/L
Aspartate aminotransferase (AST, SGOT), serum	1–36 U/L	1–36 U/L
Base excess, arterial blood, calculated	0 ± 2 mEq/L	0 ± 2 mmol/L
β-Carotene, serum	60–260 μg/dL	1.1–8.6 μmol/L
Bicarbonate		
Venous plasma	23–29 mEq/L	23–29 mmol/L
Arterial blood	21–27 mEq/L	21–27 mmol/L
Bile acids, serum	0.3–3.0 mg/dL	0.8–7.6 μmol/L
Bilirubin, serum		
Conjugated	0.1–0.4 mg/dL	1.7–6.8 μmol/L
Total	0.3–1.1 mg/dL	5.1–19.0 μmol/L
Calcium, serum	8.4–10.6 mg/dL	2.10–2.65 mmol/L
Calcium, ionized, serum	4.25–5.25 mg/dL	1.05–1.30 mmol/L
Carbon dioxide, total, serum or plasma	24–31 mEq/L	24–31 mmol/L
Carbon dioxide tension (P_{CO_2}), blood	35–45 mmHg	35–45 mmHg
Ceruloplasmin, serum	23–44 mg/dL	230–440 mg/L
Chloride, serum or plasma	96–106 mEq/L	96–106 mmol/L
Cholesterol, serum or EDTA plasma		
Desirable range	<200 mg/dL	<5.20 mmol/L
LDL cholesterol	60–180 mg/dL	1.55–4.65 mmol/L
HDL cholesterol	30–80 mg/dL	0.80–2.05 mmol/L
Copper	70–140 μg/dL	11–22 μmol/L
Corticotropin (ACTH), plasma, 8 AM	10–80 pg/mL	2–18 pmol/L
Cortisol, plasma		
8:00 AM	6–23 μg/dL	170–630 nmol/L
4:00 PM	3–15 μg/dL	80–410 nmol/L
10:00 PM	<50% of 8:00 AM value	<50% of 8:00 AM value
Creatine, serum		
Males	0.2–0.5 mg/dL	15–40 μmol/L
Females	0.3–0.9 mg/dL	25–70 μmol/L
Creatine kinase (CK), serum		
Males	55–170 U/L	55–170 U/L
Females	30–135 U/L	30–135 U/L
Creatine kinase MB isoenzyme, serum	<5% of total CK activity <5% ng/mL by immunoassay	<5% of total CK activity <5% ng/mL by immunoassay
Creatinine, serum	0.6–1.2 mg/dL	50–110 μmol/L
Estradiol-17β, adult		
Males	10–65 pg/mL	35–240 pmol/L
Females		
Follicular phase	30–100 pg/mL	110–370 pmol/L
Ovulatory phase	200–400 pg/mL	730–1470 pmol/L
Luteal phase	50–140 pg/mL	180–510 pmol/L
Ferritin, serum	20–200 ng/mL	20–200 μg/L
Fibrinogen, plasma	200–400 mg/dL	2.0–4.0 g/L
Folate, serum	3.0–18.0 ng/mL	6.8–41.0 nmol/L
erythrocytes	145–540 ng/mL	330–1220 nmol/L
Follicle-stimulating hormone (FSH), plasma		
Males	4–25 mU/mL	4–25 U/L
Females, premenopausal	4–30 mU/mL	4–30 U/L
Females, postmenopausal	40–250 mU/mL	40–250 U/L
γ-Glutamyltransferase (GGT), serum	5–40 U/L	5–40 U/L
Gastrin, fasting, serum	0–110 pg/mL	0–110 mg/L
Glucose, fasting, plasma or serum	70–115 mg/dL	3.9–6.4 nmol/L
Growth hormone (hGH), plasma, adult, fasting	0–6 ng/mL	0–6 μg/L
Haptoglobin, serum	20–165 mg/dL	0.20–1.65 g/L
Immunoglobulins, serum (see Reference Values for Immunologic Procedures)		
Insulin, fasting, plasma	5–25 μU/mL	36–179 pmol/L

Reference Values* for Clinical Chemistry (Blood, Serum, and Plasma) *Continued*

	Conventional Units	SI Units
Iron, serum	75–175 μg/dL	13–31 μmol/L
Iron binding capacity, serum		
Total	250–410 μg/dL	45–73 μmol/L
Saturation	20–55%	0.20–0.55
Lactate		
Venous whole blood	5.0–20.0 mg/dL	0.6–2.2 mmol/L
Arterial whole blood	5.0–15.0 mg/dL	0.6–1.7 mmol/L
Lactate dehydrogenase (LD), serum	110–220 U/L	110–220 U/L
Lipase, serum	10–140 U/L	10–140 U/L
Lutropin (LH), serum		
Males	1–9 U/L	1–9 U/L
Females		
Follicular phase	2–10 U/L	2–10 U/L
Midcycle peak	15–65 U/L	15–65 U/L
Luteal phase	1–12 U/L	1–12 U/L
Postmenopausal	12–65 U/L	12–65 U/L
Magnesium, serum	1.3–2.1 mg/dL	0.65–1.05 mmol/L
Osmolality	275–295 mOsm/kg water	275–295 mOsm/kg water
Oxygen, blood, arterial, room air		
Partial pressure (PaO_2)	80–100 mm Hg	80–100 mm Hg
Saturation (SaO_2)	95–98%	95–98%
pH, arterial blood	7.35–7.45	7.35–7.45
Phosphate, inorganic, serum		
Adult	3.0–4.5 mg/dL	1.0–1.5 mmol/L
Child	4.0–7.0 mg/dL	1.3–2.3 mmol/L
Potassium		
Serum	3.5–5.0 mEq/L	3.5–5.0 mmol/L
Plasma	3.5–4.5 mEq/L	3.5–4.5 mmol/L
Progesterone, serum, adult		
Males	0.0–0.4 ng/mL	0.0–1.3 mmol/L
Females		
Follicular phase	0.1–1.5 ng/mL	0.3–4.8 mmol/L
Luteal phase	2.5–28.0 ng/mL	8.0–89.0 mmol/L
Prolactin, serum		
Males	1.0–15.0 ng/mL	1.0–15.0 μg/L
Females	1.0–20.0 ng/mL	1.0–20.0 μg/L
Protein, serum, electrophoresis		
Total	6.0–8.0 g/dL	60–80 g/L
Albumin	3.5–5.5 g/dL	35–55 g/L
Globulins		
$Alpha_1$	0.2–0.4 g/dL	2.0–4.0 g/L
$Alpha_2$	0.5–0.9 g/dL	5.0–9.0 g/L
Beta	0.6–1.1 g/dL	6.0–11.0 g/L
Gamma	0.7–1.7 g/dL	7.0–17.0 g/L
Pyruvate, blood	0.3–0.9 mg/dL	0.03–0.10 mmol/L
Rheumatoid factor	0.0–30.0 IU/mL	0.0–30.0 kIU/L
Sodium, serum or plasma	135–145 mEq/L	135–145 mmol/L
Testosterone, plasma		
Males, adult	300–1200 ng/dL	10.4–41.6 nmol/L
Females, adult	20–75 ng/dL	0.7–2.6 nmol/L
Pregnant females	40–200 ng/dL	1.4–6.9 nmol/L
Thyroglobulin	3–42 ng/mL	3–42 μg/L
Thyrotropin (hTSH), serum	0.4–4.8 μIU/mL	0.4–4.8 mIU/L
Thyrotropin-releasing hormone (TRH)	5–60 pg/mL	5–60 ng/L
Thyroxine (FT_4), free, serum	0.9–2.1 ng/dL	12–27 pmol/L
Thyroxine (T_4), serum	4.5–12.0 μg/dL	58–154 nmol/L
Thyroxine-binding globulin (TBG)	15.0–34.0 μg/mL	15.0–34.0 mg/L
Transferrin	250–430 mg/dL	2.5–4.3 g/L
Triglycerides, serum, after 12-hr fast	40–150 mg/dL	0.4–1.5 g/L
Triiodothyronine (T_3), serum	70–190 ng/dL	1.1–2.9 nmol/L
Triiodothyronine uptake, resin (T_3RU)	25–38%	0.25–0.38
Urate		
Males	2.5–8.0 mg/dL	150–480 μmol/L
Females	2.2–7.0 mg/dL	130–420 μmol/L
Urea, serum or plasma	24–49 mg/dL	4.0–8.2 nmol/L
Urea nitrogen, serum or plasma	11–23 mg/dL	8.0–16.4 nmol/L
Viscosity, serum	1.4–1.8 × water	1.4–1.8 × water
Vitamin A, serum	20–80 μg/dL	0.70–2.80 μmol/L
Vitamin B_{12}, serum	180–900 pg/mL	133–664 pmol/L

*Reference values may vary, depending on the method and sample source used.

Reference Values for Therapeutic Drug Monitoring (Serum)

	Therapeutic Range	Toxic Concentrations	Proprietary Names
Analgesics			
Acetaminophen	10–20 μg/mL	>250 μg/mL	Tylenol Datril
Salicylate	100–250 μg/mL	>300 μg/mL	Aspirin Bufferin
Antibiotics			
Amikacin	25–30 μg/mL	Peak >35 μg/mL Trough >10 μg/mL	Amikin
Chloramphenicol	10–20 μg/mL	>25 μg/mL	Chloromycetin
Gentamicin	5–10 μg/mL	Peak >10 μg/mL Trough >2 μg/mL	Garamycin
Tobramycin	5–10 μg/mL	Peak >10 μg/mL Trough >2 μg/mL	Nebcin
Vancomycin	5–10 μg/mL	Peak >40 μg/mL Trough >10 μg/mL	Vancocin
Anticonvulsants			
Carbamazepine	5–12 μg/mL	>15 μg/mL	Tegretol
Ethosuximide	40–100 μg/mL	>150 μg/mL	Zarontin
Phenobarbital	15–40 μg/mL	40–100 ng/mL (varies widely)	Luminal
Phenytoin	10–20 μg/mL	>20 μg/mL	Dilantin
Primidone	5–12 μg/mL	>15 μg/mL	Mysoline
Valproic acid	50–100 μg/mL	>100 μg/mL	Depakene
Antineoplastics and Immunosuppressives			
Cyclosporin A	50–400 ng/mL	>400 ng/mL	Sandimmune
Methotrexate, high dose, 48 hr	Variable	>1 μmol/L 48 hr after dose	Mexate Folex
Tacrolimus (FK-506), whole blood	3–10 μg/L	>15 μg/L	Prograf
Bronchodilators and Respiratory Stimulants			
Caffeine	3–15 ng/mL	>30 ng/mL	
Theophylline (aminophylline)	10–20 μg/mL	>20 μg/mL	Elixophyllin Quibron
Cardiovascular Drugs			
Amiodarone (obtain specimen more than 8 hours after last dose)	1.0–2.0 μg/mL	>2.0 μg/mL	Cordarone
Digitoxin (obtain specimen 12–24 hours after last dose)	15–25 ng/mL	>35 ng/mL	Crystodigin
Digoxin (obtain specimen more than 6 hours after last dose)	0.8–2.0 ng/mL	>2.4 ng/mL	Lanoxin
Disopyramide	2–5 μg/mL	>7 μg/mL	Norpace
Flecainide	0.2–1.0 ng/mL	>1 ng/mL	Tambocor
Lidocaine	1.5–5.0 μg/mL	>6 μg/mL	Xylocaine
Mexiletine	0.7–2.0 ng/mL	>2 ng/mL	Mexitil
Procainamide	4–10 μg/mL	>12 μg/mL	Pronestyl
Procainamide plus NAPA	8–30 μg/mL	>30 μg/mL	
Propranolol	50–100 ng/mL	Variable	Inderal
Quinidine	2–5 μg/mL	>6 μg/mL	Cardioquin Quinaglute
Tocainide	4–10 ng/mL	>10 ng/mL	Tonocard
Psychopharmacologic Drugs			
Amitriptyline	120–150 ng/mL	>500 ng/mL	Elavil Triavil
Bupropion	25–100 ng/mL	Not applicable	Wellbutrin
Desipramine	150–300 ng/mL	>500 ng/mL	Norpramin Pertofrane
Imipramine	125–250 ng/mL	>400 ng/mL	Tofranil Janimine
Lithium (obtain specimen 12 hours after last dose)	0.6–1.5 mEq/L	>1.5 mEq/L	Lithobid
Nortriptyline	50–150 ng/mL	>500 ng/mL	Aventyl Pamelor

Reference Values for Clinical Chemistry (Urine)

	Conventional Units	SI Units
Acetone and acetoacetate, qualitative	Negative	Negative
Albumin		
Qualitative	Negative	Negative
Quantitative	10–100 mg/24 hr	0.15–1.5 μmol/day
Aldosterone	3–20 μg/24 hr	8.3–55 nmol/day
δ-Aminolevulinic acid (δ-ALA)	1.3–7.0 mg/24 hr	10–53 μmol/day
Amylase	<17 U/hr	<17 U/hr
Amylase/creatinine clearance ratio	0.01–0.04	0.01–0.04
Bilirubin, qualitative	Negative	Negative
Calcium (regular diet)	<250 mg/24 hr	<6.3 nmol/day
Catecholamines		
Epinephrine	<10 μg/24 hr	<55 nmol/day
Norepinephrine	<100 μg/24 hr	<590 nmol/day
Total free catecholamines	4–126 μg/24 hr	24–745 nmol/day
Total metanephrines	0.1–1.6 mg/24 hr	0.5–8.1 μmol/day
Chloride (varies with intake)	110–250 mEq/24 hr	110–250 mmol/day
Copper	0–50 μg/24 hr	0.0–0.80 μmol/day
Cortisol, free	10–100 μg/24 hr	27.6–276 nmol/day
Creatine		
Males	0–40 mg/24 hr	0.0–0.30 mmol/day
Females	0–80 mg/24 hr	0.0–0.60 mmol/day
Creatinine	15–25 mg/kg/24 hr	0.13–0.22 mmol/kg/day
Creatinine clearance (endogenous)		
Males	110–150 mL/min/1.73 m^2	110–150 mL/min/1.73 m^2
Females	105–132 mL/min/1.73 m^2	105–132 mL/min/1.73 m^2
Cystine or cysteine	Negative	Negative
Dehydroepiandrosterone		
Males	0.2–2.0 mg/24 hr	0.7–6.9 μmol/day
Females	0.2–1.8 mg/24 hr	0.7–6.2 μmol/day
Estrogens, total		
Males	4–25 μg/24 hr	14–90 nmol/day
Females	5–100 μg/24 hr	18–360 nmol/day
Glucose (as reducing substance)	<250 mg/24 hr	<250 mg/day
Hemoglobin and myoglobin, qualitative	Negative	Negative
Homogentisic acid, qualitative	Negative	Negative
17–Hydroxycorticosteroids		
Males	3–9 mg/24 hr	8.3–25 μmol/day
Females	2–8 mg/24 hr	5.5–22 μmol/day
5–Hydroxyindoleacetic acid		
Qualitative	Negative	Negative
Quantitative	2–6 mg/24 hr	10–31 μmol/day
17–Ketogenic steroids		
Males	5–23 mg/24 hr	17–80 μmol/day
Females	3–15 mg/24 hr	10–52 μmol/day
17–Ketosteroids		
Males	8–22 mg/24 hr	28–76 μmol/day
Females	6–15 mg/24 hr	21–52 μmol/day
Magnesium	6–10 mEq/24 hr	3–5 mmol/day
Metanephrines	0.05–1.2 ng/mg creatinine	0.03–0.70 mmol/mmol creatinine
Osmolality	38–1400 mOsm/kg water	38–1400 mOsm/kg water
pH	4.6–8.0	4.6–8.0
Phenylpyruvic acid, qualitative	Negative	Negative
Phosphate	0.4–1.3 g/24 hr	13–42 mmol/day
Porphobilinogen		
Qualitative	Negative	Negative
Quantitative	<2 mg/24 hr	<9 μmol/day
Porphyrins		
Coproporphyrin	50–250 μg/24 hr	77–380 nmol/day
Uroporphyrin	10–30 μg/24 hr	12–36 nmol/day
Potassium	25–125 mEq/24 hr	25–125 mmol/day
Pregnanediol		
Males	0.0–1.9 mg/24 hr	0.0–6.0 μmol/day
Females		
Proliferative phase	0.0–2.6 mg/24 hr	0.0–8.0 μmol/day
Luteal phase	2.6–10.6 mg/24 hr	8–33 μmol/day
Postmenopausal	0.2–1.0 mg/24 hr	0.6–3.1 μmol/day
Pregnanetriol	0.0–2.5 mg/24 hr	0.0–7.4 μmol/day

Table continued on following page

Reference Values for Clinical Chemistry (Urine) *Continued*

	Conventional Units	SI Units
Protein, total		
Qualitative	Negative	Negative
Quantitative	10–150 mg/24 hr	10–150 mg/day
Protein/creatinine ratio	<0.2	<0.2
Sodium (regular diet)	60–260 mEq/24 hr	60–260 mmol/day
Specific gravity		
Random specimen	1.003–1.030	1.003–1.030
24-Hour collection	1.015–1.025	1.015–1.025
Urate (regular diet)	250–750 mg/24 hr	1.5–4.4 mmol/day
Urobilinogen	0.5–4.0 mg/24 hr	0.6–6.8 μmol/day
Vanillylmandelic acid (VMA)	1.0–8.0 mg/24 hr	5–40 μmol/day

Reference Values for Toxic Substances

	Conventional Units	SI Units
Arsenic, urine	<130 μg/24 hr	<1.7 μmol/day
Bromides, serum, inorganic	<100 mg/dL	<10 mmol/L
Toxic symptoms	140–1000 mg/dL	14–100 mmol/L
Carboxyhemoglobin, blood	*% Saturation*	*Saturation*
Urban environment	<5%	<0.05
Smokers	<12%	<0.12
Symptoms		
Headache	>15%	>0.15
Nausea and vomiting	>25%	>0.25
Potentially lethal	>50%	>0.50
Ethanol, blood	<0.05 mg/dL <0.005%	<1.0 mmol/L
Intoxication	>100 mg/dL >0.1%	>22 mmol/L
Marked intoxication	300–400 mg/dL 0.3–0.4%	65–87 mmol/L
Alcoholic stupor	400–500 mg/dL 0.4–0.5%	87–109 mmol/L
Coma	>500 mg/dL >0.5%	>109 mmol/L
Lead, blood		
Adults	<25 μg/dL	<1.2 μmol/L
Children	<15 μg/dL	<0.7 μmol/L
Lead, urine	<80 μg/24 hr	<0.4 μmol/day
Mercury, urine	<30 μg/24 hr	<150 nmol/day

Reference Values for Cerebrospinal Fluid

	Conventional Units	SI Units
Cells	<5/mm^3; all mononuclear	<5 × 10^6/L, all mononuclear
Protein electrophoresis	Albumin predominant	Albumin predominant
Glucose	50–75 mg/dL (20 mg/dL less than in serum)	2.8–4.2 mmol/L (1.1 mmol less than in serum)
IgG		
Children under 14	<8% of total protein	<0.08% of total protein
Adults	<14% of total protein	<0.14% of total protein
IgG index $\left(\frac{\text{CSF/serum IgG ratio}}{\text{CSF/ serum albumin ratio}}\right)$	0.3–0.6	0.3–0.6
Oligoclonal banding on electrophoresis	Absent	Absent
Pressure, opening	70–180 mmH_2O	70–180 mmH_2O
Protein, total	15–45 mg/dL	150–450 mg/L

Reference Values for Tests of Gastrointestinal Function

Test Name	Conventional Units
Bentiromide	6-hr urinary arylamine excretion greater than 57% excludes pancreatic insufficiency
β-Carotene, serum	60–250 ng/dL
Fecal fat estimation	
Qualitative	No fat globules seen by high-power microscope
Quantitative	<6 g/24 hr (>95% coefficient of fat absorption)
Gastric acid output	
Basal	
Males	0.0–10.5 mmol/hr
Females	0.0–5.6 mmol/hr
Gastric acid output *(continued)*	
Maximum (after histamine or pentagastrin)	
Males	9.0–48.0 mmol/hr
Females	6.0–31.0 mmol/hr
Ratio: basal/maximum	
Males	0.0–0.31
Females	0.0–0.29
Secretin test, pancreatic fluid	
Volume	>1.8 mL/kg/hr
Bicarbonate	>80 mEq/L
D-Xylose absorption test, urine	>20% of ingested dose excreted in 5 hr

Reference Values for Immunologic Procedures

	Conventional Units	SI Units
Complement, serum		
C3	85–175 mg/dL	0.85–1.75 g/L
C4	15–45 mg/dL	150–450 mg/L
Total hemolytic (CH_{50})	150–250 U/mL	150–250 U/mL
Immunoglobulins, serum, adult		
IgG	640–1350 mg/dL	6.4–13.5 g/L
IgA	70–310 mg/dL	0.70–3.1 g/L
IgM	90–350 mg/dL	0.90–3.5 g/L
IgD	0.0–6.0 mg/dL	0.0–60 mg/L
IgE	0.0–430 ng/dL	0.0–430 μg/L

Lymphocyte Subsets, Whole Blood, Heparinized

Antigen	*Cell Type*	*Percentage*	*Absolute*
CD3	Total T cells	56–77	860–1880
CD19	Total B cells	7–17	140–370
CD3 and CD4	Helper-inducer cells	32–54	550–1190
CD3 and CD8	Suppressor-cytotoxic cells	24–37	430–1060
CD3 and DR	Activated T cells	5–14	70–310
CD2	E rosette T cells	73–87	1040–2160
CD16 and CD56	Natural killer (NK) cells	8–22	130–500

Helper/suppressor ratio: 0.8–1.8.

Reference Values for Semen Analysis

	Conventional Units	SI Units
Volume	2–5 mL	2–5 mL
Liquefaction	Complete in 15 min	Complete in 15 min
pH	7.2–8.0	7.2–8.0
Leukocytes	Occasional or absent	Occasional or absent
Spermatozoa		
Count	60–150 × 10^6/mL	60–150 × 10^6/mL
Motility	>80% motile	>0.80 motile
Morphology	80–90% normal forms	>0.80–0.90 normal forms
Fructose	>150 mg/dL	>8.33 mmol/L

Index

Page numbers in *italics* refer to illustrations; numbers followed by t indicate tables.